Textbook of Clinical Neuropsychology

"Simply superb! Kudos to the Editors for producing a sequel that outshines the original and continues to set the standard for textbooks in clinical neuropsychology in its scope and scholarship. Morgan and Ricker have amassed an all-star cast of contributors who present a well curated coverage of the essential aspects of contemporary evidence-based neuropsychological practice with the expertise and depth that will satisfy the ardent graduate student as well as the seasoned academic and clinician. Every neuropsychologist should have the *Textbook of Clinical Neuropsychology* on his or her bookshelf."

– Gordon J. Chelune, University of Utah School of Medicine

The first edition of the *Textbook of Clinical Neuropsychology* set a new standard in the field in its scope, breadth, and scholarship. This second edition comprises 50 authoritative chapters that will both enlighten and challenge readers from across allied fields of neuroscience, whether novice, mid-level, or senior level professionals. It will familiarize the young trainee through to the accomplished professional with fundamentals of the science of neuropsychology and its vast body of research, considering the field's historical underpinnings, its evolving practice and research methods, the application of science to informed practice, and recent developments and relevant cutting-edge work. Its precise commentary recognizes obstacles that remain in our clinical and research endeavors and emphasizes the prolific innovations in interventional techniques that serve the field's ultimate aim: to better understand brain-behavior relationships and facilitate adaptive functional competence in patients.

The second edition contains 50 new and completely revised chapters, written by some of the profession's most recognized and prominent scholar-clinicians, broadening the scope of coverage of the ever-expanding field of neuropsychology and its relationship to related neuroscience and psychological practice domains. It is a natural evolution of what has become a comprehensive reference textbook for neuropsychology practitioners.

Textbook of Clinical Neuropsychology

2nd Edition

Edited by

Joel E. Morgan and Joseph H. Ricker

Routledge
Taylor & Francis Group
NEW YORK AND LONDON

Second edition published 2018
by Routledge
711 Third Avenue, New York, NY 10017

and by Routledge
2 Park Square, Milton Park, Abingdon, Oxon, OX14 4RN

Routledge is an imprint of the Taylor & Francis Group, an informa business

First edition published by Routledge 2008

Library of Congress Cataloging-in-Publication Data
Names: Morgan, Joel E., editor. | Ricker, Joseph H., editor.
Title: Textbook of clinical neuropsychology / [edited by] Joel E. Morgan, Joseph H. Ricker.
Description: 2nd edition. | New York, NY : Routledge, 2018. | Includes bibliographical references and index.
Identifiers: LCCN 2017034746 | ISBN 9781848726956 (hb : alk. paper) | ISBN 9781315271743 (eb)
Subjects: MESH: Central Nervous System Diseases—diagnosis | Central Nervous System Diseases—therapy | Neurocognitive Disorders | Neuropsychology—methods
Classification: LCC RC346 | NLM WL 301 | DDC 616.8—dc23
LC record available at https://lccn.loc.gov/2017034746

ISBN: 978-1-84872-695-6 (hbk)
ISBN: 978-1-315-27174-3 (ebk)

Typeset in Times
by Apex CoVantage, LLC

MIX
Paper from responsible sources
FSC® C014174

Printed and bound in the United States of America by Sheridan

Dedicated to the memory of
Manfred F. Greiffenstein, PhD, ABPP (CN, FP),
scientist, scholar, clinician, devoted husband and
father, and generous friend. His wit, intellectual
integrity, and fearless pursuit of truth are indelibly
etched in our minds and hearts.

Contents

About the editors x
List of contributors xi
Preface xiv
JOEL E. MORGAN AND JOSEPH H. RICKER
Foreword xv
IDA SUE BARON
Acknowledgments xvii

Part I
Foundations of Clinical Neuropsychology 1

1 **Historical Trends in Neuropsychological Assessment** 3
WILLIAM B. BARR

2 **Specialty Training in Clinical Neuropsychology: History and Update on Current Issues** 14
LINAS A. BIELIAUSKAS AND ERIN MARK

3 **Psychometric Foundations of Neuropsychological Assessment** 22
GLENN J. LARRABEE

4 **Assessment of Neurocognitive Performance Validity** 39
KYLE BRAUER BOONE

5 **Differential Diagnosis in Neuropsychology: A Strategic Approach** 51
DAVID E. HARTMAN

6 **Neuroanatomy for the Neuropsychologist** 62
CHRISTOPHER M. FILLEY AND ERIN D. BIGLER

7 **The Central Nervous System and Cognitive Development** 91
KATHRYN C. RUSSELL

8 **Genomics and Phenomics** 102
ROBERT M. BILDER

9 **Functional and Molecular Neuroimaging** 111
JOSEPH H. RICKER AND PATRICIA M. ARENTH

Part II
Disorders in Children and Adults 125

10 **Genetic and Neurodevelopmental Disorders** 127
E. MARK MAHONE, BETH S. SLOMINE, AND T. ANDREW ZABEL

11 **Traumatic Brain Injury in Children and Adolescents** 141
KEITH OWEN YEATES AND BRIAN L. BROOKS

12 **Pediatric Cancer** 158
CELIANE REY-CASSERLY AND BRENDA J. SPIEGLER

13 **Autism Spectrum Disorder** 184
GERRY A. STEFANATOS AND DEBORAH FEIN

14 **Neurodevelopmental Disorders of Attention and Learning: ADHD and LD Across the Life Span** 281
JEANETTE WASSERSTEIN, GERRY A. STEFANATOS, ROBERT L. MAPOU, YITZCHAK FRANK, AND JOSEPHINE ELIA

15 **Consciousness: Disorders, Assessment, and Intervention** 332
KATHLEEN T. BECHTOLD AND MEGAN M. HOSEY

16 **Cerebrovascular Disease** 350
C. MUNRO CULLUM, HEIDI C. ROSSETTI, HUNT BATJER, JOANNE R. FESTA, KATHLEEN Y. HAALAND, AND LAURA H. LACRITZ

17 **Moderate and Severe Traumatic Brain Injury** 387
TRESA ROEBUCK-SPENCER AND MARK SHERER

18 **Concussion and Mild Traumatic Brain Injury** 411
HEATHER G. BELANGER, DAVID F. TATE, AND RODNEY D. VANDERPLOEG

19 **Neurocognitive Assessment in Epilepsy: Advances and Challenges** 449
JOSEPH I. TRACY AND JENNIFER R. TINKER

20 **Neurotropic Infections: Herpes Simplex Virus, Human Immunodeficiency Virus, and Lyme Disease** 477
RICHARD F. KAPLAN AND RONALD A. COHEN

21 **Hypoxia of the Central Nervous System** 494
RAMONA O. HOPKINS

22 **Parkinson's Disease and Other Movement Disorders** 507
ALEXANDER I. TRÖSTER AND ROBIN GARRETT

23 **Cognitive Functions in Adults With Central Nervous System and Non–Central Nervous System Cancers** 560
DENISE D. CORREA AND JAMES C. ROOT

24 **Toxins in the Central Nervous System** 587
MARC W. HAUT, JENNIFER WIENER HARTZELL, AND MARIA T. MORAN

25 **Multiple Sclerosis and Related Disorders** 603
PETER A. ARNETT, JESSICA E. MEYER, VICTORIA C. MERRITT, AND LAUREN B. STROBER

26 **Neuropsychological Functioning in Autoimmune Disorders** 618
ELIZABETH KOZORA, ANDREW BURLESON, AND CHRISTOPHER M. FILLEY

27 **Sports-Related Concussion** 659
WILLIAM B. BARR, LINDSAY D. NELSON, AND MICHAEL A. MCCREA

28 **The Three Amnesias** 678
RUSSELL M. BAUER AND BRETON ASKEN

29 **Neuropsychological Functioning in Affective and Anxiety-Spectrum Disorders in Adults and Children** 701
BERNICE A. MARCOPULOS

30 **Dementia** 717
GLENN SMITH AND ALISSA BUTTS

31 **Complexities of Metabolic Disorders** 742
MARC A. NORMAN, OLIVIA BJORKQUIST HARNER, AND S. JOSHUA KENTON

32 **Clinical Assessment of Posttraumatic Stress Disorder** 757
JIM ANDRIKOPOULOS

33 **Military Service–Related Traumatic Brain Injury** 792
LOUIS M. FRENCH, ALISON N. CERNICH, AND LAURA L. HOWE

34 **Pain and Pain-Related Disability** 823
KEVIN W. GREVE, KEVIN J. BIANCHINI, AND STEVEN T. BREWER

35 **Neuropsychological and Psychological Assessment of Somatic Symptom Disorders** 846
GREG J. LAMBERTY AND IVY N. MILLER

Part III

Forensic, Ethical, and Practice Issues 855

36 **Forensic Neuropsychology: An Overview of Issues, Admissibility, and Directions** 857
JERRY J. SWEET, PAUL M. KAUFMANN, ERIC ECKLUND-JOHNSON, AND AARON C. MALINA

37 **Basics of Forensic Neuropsychology** 887
MANFRED F. GREIFFENSTEIN AND PAUL M. KAUFMANN

38 **Assessment of Incomplete Effort and Malingering in the Neuropsychological Examination** 927
SCOTT R. MILLIS AND PAUL M. KAUFMANN

39 **Pediatric Forensic Neuropsychology** 942
JACOBUS DONDERS, BRIAN L. BROOKS, ELISABETH M. S. SHERMAN, AND MICHAEL W. KIRKWOOD

40 **Clinical Neuropsychology in Criminal Forensics** 960
ROBERT L. DENNEY, RACHEL L. FAZIO, AND MANFRED F. GREIFFENSTEIN

41 **Disability** 980
MICHAEL CHAFETZ

42 **Ethical Practice of Clinical Neuropsychology** 1000
SHANE S. BUSH

43 Evidence-Based Practice in Clinical Neuropsychology **1007**
JERRY J. SWEET, DANIEL J. GOLDMAN, AND LESLIE M. GUIDOTTI BRETING

44 Medical and Psychological Iatrogenesis in Neuropsychological Assessment **1018**
DOMINIC A. CARONE

45 Complementary and Alternative Medicine for Children With Developmental Disabilities **1032**
KAREN E. WILLS

Part IV
Interventions **1043**

46 Psychotherapy and the Practice of Clinical Neuropsychology **1045**
GEORGE P. PRIGATANO

47 Mindfulness-Based Interventions in Neuropsychology **1054**
PATRICIA M. ARENTH

48 Collaborative Therapeutic Neuropsychological Assessment **1068**
TAD T. GORSKE

49 Empirically Based Rehabilitation of Neurocognitive Disorder **1078**
ANTHONY Y. STRINGER

50 Clinical Psychopharmacology **1089**
SAMUEL ALPERIN AND LENARD A. ADLER

Author index 1099
Subject index 1110

About the editors

Joel E. Morgan, PhD, ABPP, was Director of Training at the Veterans Administration New Jersey Healthcare System and Clinical Associate Professor of Neurosciences at Rutgers New Jersey Medical School prior to entering full-time private practice in 2001. Dr. Morgan maintains a life span private practice in clinical and forensic neuropsychology. He is licensed as a psychologist in New Jersey and is board certified by the American Board of Professional Psychology in both Clinical Neuropsychology and the subspecialty of Pediatric Neuropsychology. Dr. Morgan has served as a member of the editorial boards of four peer-reviewed journals and was an Oral Examiner for the American Board of Clinical Neuropsychology for ten years. He has more than 50 scholarly publications as book editor and chapter author, and has presented more than 25 invited addresses at national conferences.

Joseph H. Ricker, PhD, ABPP (CN, RP) is the Director of Psychology for Rusk Rehabilitation at New York University Medical Center and is a Professor in the departments of Rehabilitation Medicine, Psychiatry, and Radiology at New York University School of Medicine. He has been licensed as a psychologist in five states and is board certified by the American Board of Professional Psychology in both Clinical Neuropsychology and Rehabilitation Psychology. He has served as a member of the editorial boards of five peer-reviewed journals (*Journal of Clinical & Experimental Neuropsychology, Journal of Head Trauma Rehabilitation, The Clinical Neuropsychologist, Rehabilitation Psychology, and Archives of Clinical Neuropsychology*). Dr. Ricker has a long record of federally funded research examining cognitive impairment, recovery, and rehabilitation following traumatic brain injury. His current research interests include the examination of altered cerebral blood flow and functional connectivity as they relate to cognitive impairment after brain injury, using modalities such as functional MRI, positron emission tomography, and diffusion tensor imaging.

Contributors

Lenard A. Adler, MD, Professor of Psychiatry and Child and Adolescent Psychiatry, Director, Adult ADHD Program, New York University (NYU) School of Medicine, New York

Samuel Alperin, MD, Hofstra Northwell School of Medicine, Hempstead, New York

Jim Andrikopoulos, PhD, ABPP (CN), Northwestern Medicine Regional Medical Group /Neurosciences, Winfield, Illinois

Patricia M. Arenth, PhD, Department of Physical Medicine and Rehabilitation, University of Pittsburgh School of Medicine, Pittsburgh, Pennsylvania

Peter A. Arnett, PhD, Professor and Director, Neuropsychology of Sports Concussion and MS Programs, Pennsylvania State University, Psychology Department, University Park

Breton Asken, ATC, MS, Department of Clinical and Health Psychology, University of Florida, Gainesville

Ida Sue Baron, PhD, ABPP (CN), Independent Private Practice Professor, Departments of Pediatrics and Neurology, University of Virginia School of Medicine, Charlottesville, VA & Clinical Professor, Department of Pediatrics, The George Washington School of Medicine, Washington, DC.

William B. Barr, PhD, ABPP (CN), NYU School of Medicine, New York

Hunt Batjer, MD, FACS, ABNS, Professor and Chairman of Neurological Surgery, University of Texas Southwestern Medical Center, Dallas

Russell M. Bauer, PhD, ABPP (CN), Department of Clinical and Health Psychology, University of Florida, Gainesville

Kathleen T. Bechtold, PhD, ABPP (CN, RP), Associate Professor, Department of Physical Medicine and Rehabilitation, The Johns Hopkins University School of Medicine, Baltimore, Maryland

Heather G. Belanger, PhD, ABPP (CN), James A. Haley Veterans Hospital and University of South Florida, Tampa

Kevin J. Bianchini, PhD, ABN, Independent Practice, Jefferson Neurobehavioral Group, Metairie, Louisiana

Linas A. Bieliauskas, PhD, ABPP (CP, CN), Professor, University of Michigan Health System and Staff Psychologist, Ann Arbor Veterans Administration Healthcare System, Ann Arbor

Erin D. Bigler, PhD, ABPP (CN), Professor of Psychology and Neuroscience, Brigham Young University, Provo, Utah; Adjunct Professor of Psychiatry, University of Utah, Salt Lake City

Robert M. Bilder, PhD, ABPP (CN), Michael E. Tennenbaum Family Professor of Psychiatry and Biobehavioral Sciences and Psychology, University of California, Los Angeles

Olivia Bjorkquist Harner, PhD, Northwestern University, Feinberg School of Medicine, Chicago, Illinois

Kyle Brauer Boone, PhD, ABPP (CN), California School of Forensic Studies, Alliant International University, Los Angeles, California

Steven T. Brewer, PhD, Angelo State University, San Angelo, Texas

Brian L. Brooks, PhD, Neurosciences program, Alberta Children's Hospital; Departments of Pediatrics, Clinical Neurosciences, and Psychology, University of Calgary; and Alberta Children's Hospital Research Institute, Calgary, Alberta, Canada

Andrew Burleson, MS, National Jewish Health, Denver, Colorado

Shane S. Bush, PhD, ABPP (CN, CP, RP, GP), Independent Practice, Long Island Neuropsychology, PC, Lake Ronkonkoma, New York

Alissa Butts, PhD, Department of Psychiatry and Psychology, Mayo Clinic, Rochester, Minnesota

Dominic A. Carone, PhD, ABPP (CN), State University of New York (SUNY) Upstate Medical University, Syracuse

Alison N. Cernich, PhD, ABPP (CN), Department of Veterans Affairs, Defense Centers of Excellence for Psychological Health and Traumatic Brain Injury, Washington, DC

Michael Chafetz, PhD, ABPP (CN), Independent Practice, Algiers Neurobehavioral Resource, LLC, New Orleans, Louisiana

Ronald A. Cohen, PhD, ABPP (CN), Evelyn McKnight Chair for Cognitive Aging and Memory; Professor, Departments of Neurology, Psychiatry and Aging; Director, Center for Cognitive Aging and Memory, University of Florida, Gainesville, Florida

Denise D. Correa, PhD, ABPP (CN), Department of Neurology, Memorial Sloan Kettering Cancer Center, New York, New York

C. Munro Cullum, PhD, ABPP (CN), Professor of Psychiatry, Neurology, and Neurological Surgery, University of Texas Southwestern Medical Center, Dallas, Texas

Robert L. Denney, PsyD, ABPP (CN, FP), Neuropsychological Associates of Southwest Missouri, Springfield

Jacobus Donders, PhD, ABPP (CN, RP), Chief Psychologist, Mary Free Bed Rehabilitation Hospital, Grand Rapids, Michigan

Eric Ecklund-Johnson, PhD, ABPP (CN), Department of Neuropsychology, University of Kansas Hospital, Fairway, Kansas; Departments of Neurology and Psychiatry, University of Kansas Medical Center, Kansas City, Kansas

Josephine Elia, MD, Department of Psychiatry, University of Pennsylvania, Philadelphia, Pennsylvania; Nemours Neuroscience Center, Wilmington, Delaware; Department of Pediatrics and Psychiatry, Sidney Kimmel Medical College, Thomas Jefferson University; A.I. DuPont Hospital for Children, Wilmington, Delaware

Rachel L. Fazio, PsyD, Private Practice, Bradenton, Florida

Deborah Fein, PhD, ABPP (CN), University of Connecticut (UConn) Board of Trustees Distinguished Professor, Department of Psychology, Department of Pediatrics, University of Connecticut, Mansfield

Joanne R. Festa, PhD, Department of Neurology, Icahn School of Medicine at Mt. Sinai, New York, New York

Christopher M. Filley, MD, Director, Behavioral Neurology Section, Professor of Neurology and Psychiatry, University of Colorado School of Medicine, Senior Scientific Advisor, Marcus Institute for Brain Health

Yitzchak Frank, MD, Pediatric Neurologist and Clinical Professor in Pediatrics, Neurology and Psychiatry at the Icahn School of Medicine, Mount Sinai in New York

Louis M. French, PsyD, Walter Reed National Military Medical Center, Bethesda, Maryland

Robin Garrett, PsyD, Movement Disorders Center of Arizona, Scottsdale, Arizona

Daniel J. Goldman, PhD, Independent Practice, Edina, Minnesota

Tad T. Gorske, PhD, Assistant Professor, Director of Outpatient Clinical Neuropsychology, Division of Neuropsychology and Rehabilitation Psychology, University of Pittsburgh School of Medicine, Pittsburgh, Pennsylvania

Manfred F. Greiffenstein, PhD, ABPP (CN, FP), Psychological Systems Inc., Royal Oak, Michigan

Kevin W. Greve, PhD, ABPP (CN), Independent Practice, Jefferson Neurobehavioral Group, Metairie, Louisiana

Leslie M. Guidotti Breting, PhD, ABPP (CN), Department of Psychiatry and Behavioral Neuroscience, University of Chicago, Pritzker School of Medicine, Chicago; Department of Psychiatry and Behavioral Sciences, North Shore University Health System, Evanston, Illinois

Kathleen Y. Haaland, PhD, ABPP (CN), Professor, Departments of Psychiatry and Behavioral Sciences and Neurology, University of New Mexico, Albuquerque

Marc W. Haut, PhD, ABPP (CN), Departments of Behavioral Medicine and Psychiatry, Neurology, and Radiology, West Virginia University School of Medicine, Morgantown

David E. Hartman, PhD, MS, ABN, ABPP, (CP), Medical and Forensic Neuropsychology, Chicago, Illinois

Jennifer Wiener Hartzell, PsyD, ABPP (CN), Departments of Supportive Oncology and Neuropsychology, Levine Cancer Institute, Carolinas HealthCare System, Charlotte, North Carolina

Ramona O. Hopkins, PhD, Professor of Psychology and Neuroscience, Psychology Department, Brigham Young University, Provo, Utah; Department of Medicine, Pulmonary and Critical Care Medicine, Intermountain Medical Center, Murray, Utah

Megan M. Hosey, PhD, Assistant Professor, Division of Rehabilitation Psychology and Neuropsychology, Department of Physical Medicine and Rehabilitation, The Johns Hopkins University School of Medicine, Baltimore, Maryland

Laura L. Howe, JD, PhD, Veterans Administration Palo Alto Health Care System, Palo Alto, California

Richard F. Kaplan, PhD, ABPP (CN), Professor of Psychiatry and Neurology, Department of Psychiatry, University of Connecticut Health Center, Farmington

Paul M. Kaufmann, JD, PhD, ABPP (CN), University Compliance Officer, University of Arizona, Tucson

S. Joshua Kenton, PsyD, Commander, U.S. Navy; Neuropsychologist, Naval Hospital, Camp Pendleton, Oceanside, California

Michael W. Kirkwood, PhD, ABPP (CN), Department of Physical Medicine and Rehabilitation, Children's Hospital, Colorado and University of Colorado School of Medicine, Aurora

Elizabeth Kozora, PhD, ABPP (CN), Professor, Department of Medicine, National Jewish Health Professor, Departments of Psychiatry and Neurology, University of Colorado School of Medicine, Denver

Laura H. Lacritz, PhD, ABPP (CN), Professor of Psychiatry and Neurology and Neurotherapeutics, Associate Director, Neuropsychology, University of Texas Southwestern Medical Center, Dallas

Greg J. Lamberty, PhD, ABPP (CN), Minneapolis Veterans Administration Health Care System, Minneapolis, Minnesota

Glenn J. Larrabee, PhD, ABPP (CN), Independent Practice, Sarasota, Florida

E. Mark Mahone, PhD, ABPP (CN), Director, Department of Neuropsychology, Kennedy Krieger Institute, Professor of Psychiatry & Behavioral Sciences, Johns Hopkins University School of Medicine, Baltimore, MD

Bernice A. Marcopulos, PhD, ABPP (CN), Professor, Department of Graduate Psychology, James Madison University, VA and Associate Professor, Department of Psychiatry and Neurobehavioral Sciences, University of Virginia School of Medicine, Charlottesville, VA

Aaron C. Malina, PhD, ABPP (CN), Private Practice, Lake Barrington, Illinois

Robert L. Mapou, PhD, ABPP (CN), Independent Practice, Silver Spring, Maryland and Rehoboth Beach, Delaware

Erin Mark, PhD, Independent Practice, Complete Neuropsychology Services, Ann Arbor, Michigan

Michael A. McCrea, PhD, ABPP (CN), Medical College of Wisconsin, Milwaukee

Victoria C. Merritt, MS, Psychology Department, Pennsylvania State University, University Park

Jessica E. Meyer, MS, Psychology Department, Pennsylvania State University, University Park

Ivy N. Miller, PhD, Minneapolis Veterans Administration Health Care System, Minneapolis, Minnesota

Scott R. Millis, PhD, ABPP (CN, CP, RP), CStat, PStat; Professor, Wayne State University School of Medicine, Detroit, Michigan

Maria T. Moran, PhD, Department of Physical Medicine and Rehabilitation, Pennsylvania State, Milton S. Hershey Medical Center, Hershey

Joel E. Morgan, PhD, ABPP (CN), Independent Practice, Morristown, New Jersey

Lindsay D. Nelson, PhD, Medical College of Wisconsin, Milwaukee

Marc A. Norman, PhD, ABPP (CN), University of California, San Diego

George P. Prigatano, PhD, ABPP (CN), Emeritus Chairman of Clinical Neuropsychology and the Newsome Chair of Neuropsychology, Barrow Neurological Institute, Phoenix, Arizona

Celiane Rey-Casserly, PhD, ABPP (CN), Director, Center for Neuropsychology, Boston Children's Hospital, Harvard Medical School, Boston, Massachusetts

Joseph H. Ricker, PhD, ABPP (CN, RP), Professor of Rehabilitation Medicine, Psychiatry and Radiology, NYU School of Medicine, New York

Tresa Roebuck-Spencer, PhD, ABPP (CN), Independent Practice, Jefferson Neurobehavioral Group, New Orleans, Louisiana

James C. Root, PhD, Department of Psychiatry and Behavioral Sciences, Memorial Sloan Kettering Cancer Center, New York, New York

Heidi C. Rossetti, PhD, Assistant Professor of Psychiatry, University of Texas Southwestern Medical Center

Kathryn C. Russell, PhD, Seattle, Washington

Mark Sherer, PhD, ABPP (CN), FACRM, Associate Vice President for Research, TIRR Memorial Hermann, Houston, Texas

Elisabeth M. S. Sherman, PhD, Director, Brain Health and Psychological Health, Copeman Healthcare Centre, Adjunct Associate Professor, Departments of Paediatrics and Clinical Neurosciences, University of Calgary, Alberta, Canada

Beth S. Slomine, PhD, ABPP (CN), Director of Training, Department of Neuropsychology, Kennedy Krieger Institute, Associate Professor of Psychiatry & Behavioral Sciences, Johns Hopkins University School of Medicine, Baltimore, Maryland

Glenn Smith, PhD, ABPP (CN), University of Florida Department of Clinical and Health Psychology, Gainesville

Brenda J. Spiegler, PhD, ABPP (CN), Hospital for Sick Children, Toronto, Ontario, Associate Professor, Department of Pediatrics, University of Toronto, Canada

Gerry A. Stefanatos, DPhil, Associate Professor, Director, Cognitive Neurophysiology Laboratory, Department of Communication Sciences and Disorders, Temple University, Philadelphia, Pennsylvania; Department of Psychiatry, Drexel University School of Medicine, Philadelphia, Pennsylvania

Anthony Y. Stringer, PhD, ABPP (CN), Professor, Department of Rehabilitation Medicine, Emory University, Atlanta, Georgia

Lauren B. Strober, PhD, Senior Research Scientist, Neuropsychology and Neuroscience Laboratory, Kessler Foundation, Assistant Professor, Rutgers, New Jersey Medical School, West Orange

Jerry J. Sweet, PhD, ABPP, (CN, CP), Department of Psychiatry and Behavioral Neuroscience, University of Chicago, Pritzker School of Medicine, Chicago, Illinois; Department of Psychiatry and Behavioral Sciences, North Shore University Health System, Evanston, Illinois

David F. Tate, PhD, Associate Professor–Research, Missouri Institute of Mental Health, University of Missouri–St. Louis

Jennifer R. Tinker, PhD, Assistant Professor, Neurology Department, Thomas Jefferson University/Sidney Kimmel Medical College, Philadelphia, Pennsylvania

Joseph I. Tracy, PhD, ABPP (CN), Professor, Neurology and Radiology Departments, Director, Neuropsychology Division, Thomas Jefferson University/Sidney Kimmel Medical College, Philadelphia, Pennsylvania

Alexander I. Tröster, PhD, ABPP (CN), Professor and Chair, Department of Clinical Neuropsychology and Center for Neuromodulation, Barrow Neurological Institute, Phoenix, Arizona

Rodney D. Vanderploeg, PhD, ABPP (CN), James A. Haley Veterans Hospital and University of South Florida, Tampa

Jeanette Wasserstein, PhD, ABPP (CN), Independent Practice and Faculty at Mt. Sinai Medical School, New York, New York

Karen E. Wills, PhD, ABPP (CN), Neuropsychologist, Children's Hospitals and Clinics of Minnesota, Minneapolis

Keith Owen Yeates, PhD, ABPP (CN), Ronald and Irene Ward Chair in Pediatric Brain Injury, Professor of Psychology, Pediatrics, and Clinical Neurosciences, University of Calgary, Alberta, Canada

T. Andrew Zabel, PhD, ABPP (CN), Clinical Director, Department of Neuropsychology, Kennedy Krieger Institute, Associate Professor of Psychiatry & Behavioral Sciences, Johns Hopkins University School of Medicine, Baltimore, Maryland

Preface

The second edition of the *Textbook of Clinical Neuropsychology* brings changes in the form of updated and new chapters and eliminates any that are no longer considered contemporary. As in the first edition, we strove to provide readers with the fundamentals of the science of neuropsychology, its historical underpinnings, the application of science to informed practice, and a look at recent developments and relevant cutting-edge work. Readers will take note that some chapters from the first edition have been combined into larger, integrated discussions of related concepts and domains, providing more depth. The addition of new chapters broadens the scope of coverage of the ever-expanding field of neuropsychology and its relationship to related neuroscience and psychological practice domains. This second edition is a natural evolution of what has become a comprehensive reference textbook for neuropsychology practitioners.

Joel E. Morgan and Joseph H. Ricker

November 2017

Foreword

There can be no more meaningful a volume in neuropsychology today than one that has embraced the essential importance of a life span focus while providing essential and contemporary knowledge about both classic and nascent segments of the broadening profession of neuropsychology. Editors Joel Morgan and Joseph Ricker made a significant contribution to the scientific literature with publication of the *Textbook of Clinical Neuropsychology* (2008). With the newest edition they entrusted their vision for this volume to extraordinarily gifted contributors, each of whom has produced authoritative chapters that will both enlighten and challenge readers from across allied fields of neuroscience, whether novice, mid-level, or senior-level professionals.

While one can selectively read a chapter in one's particular area of interest, the reader who considers the merits of all 50 chapters will come to realize that this volume is superlative in both the quality and breadth of its coverage. Further, there is a unifying message about the practice of neuropsychology and the populations served by members of the profession. Most notably is the extensive range of topics covered outside the constraints of the sometimes inflexible and artificial lines dividing pediatric from adult neuropsychology. Blurring these lines allows the reader to truly understand an individual's developmental course over his or her lifetime. This analytical posture can and should make a meaningful difference for the individual, the family, and, more broadly, society. This exemplary textbook should be mandatory reading.

One is struck in reading this second edition that there is a richness associated with the numerous and rapid gains made in the accumulation of neuropsychological knowledge over decades that is foundational. The efforts of many, well cited in this volume, served to move forward intentions to advance rigorous research protocols, extend clinical diagnostic methods, introduce effective interventions, and sharpen practitioners' clinical acuity for the effects of central nervous system and systemic disease and disorder, or lack thereof. This volume is a testament to the vital contributions of colleagues past and present to whom are owed an enormous debt of gratitude, and to those in the profession who pursue study cognizant of these achievements.

The advances documented throughout this volume highlight vividly the contrast between a less well-understood profession that endorsed early the scientist-practitioner model of neuropsychology but had yet to define many of its fundamental tenets and neuropsychology's current expanded position and range of accomplishments. Each chapter author engages the reader with an intellectual depth for the content in his or her respective area of expertise but also highlights the more global and pragmatic strengths that are inherent to our field. This combination of established knowledge and pursuit of knowledge has sustained rapid and remarkable growth, passion, and collegiality among neuropsychologists who have diverse but compatible interests, experiences, and openness to the teachings of their colleagues. The second edition goes far to support these objectives.

The second edition will familiarize the young trainee through to the accomplished professional with a now vast and at times overwhelming database that places neuropsychology within its correct context of historical growth, evolving practice and research methods, and therapeutic gains. Yet, it contains precise commentary that recognizes obstacles that remain in our clinical and research endeavors along with a hopeful emphasis on the prolific innovations in interventional techniques that fully serve an ultimate aim, to better understand brain-behavior relationships and facilitate adaptive functional competence in patients. An objective to provide ethical, evidence-based, and compassionate care for our patients who entrust us to be knowledgeable in order to improve their health and well-being is truly supported by this volume's content, which considers the past yet sets standards for how the field might advance critical future directions for the whole person across their life span, and that will further support magnificent growth and accomplishment by those who pursue their career in the specialty of neuropsychology.

Ida Sue Baron, PhD, ABPP (CN)
Professor of Pediatrics and Neurology
University of Virginia School of Medicine
Charlottesville
and
Clinical Professor of Pediatrics
The George Washington University
Washington, DC
Independent Private Practice
Potomac, Maryland

Acknowledgments

No project of this size and scope is possible without considerable collaboration and assistance. We are indebted to our many contributors for their generous work on this volume and are grateful for their scholarship. They truly embody the 'scientist-practitioner.' We would like to thank our editors, Georgette Enriquez and Paul Dukes, for their guidance and publication acumen, and Renata Corbani, our production editor, for her extraordinary organizational skills and for actually producing this book. Finally, we wish to thank our editorial assistant, Denise Krouslis, for her tireless devotion to seeing this project through and coordinating our large cadre of contributors. We could not have done this without all of you!

Joel Morgan and Joseph Ricker

Part I

Foundations of Clinical Neuropsychology

1 Historical Trends in Neuropsychological Assessment

William B. Barr

Clinical neuropsychology continues to be one of the most popular and fastest growing fields of psychological practice. At last look, the Society of Clinical Neuropsychology (Division 40) has vaulted over the past several years into the role as the largest division of the American Psychological Association (APA) (Barr, 2011). The number of clinical neuropsychologists who have gone on to receive board certification through the American Board of Clinical Neuropsychology (ABCN) has recently exceeded the landmark number of 1,000, making it the fastest growing specialty of the American Board of Professional Psychology (Stringer & Postal, 2015). The number of published studies using neuropsychological methods continues to grow exponentially.

To accompany its growth, clinical neuropsychology also faces a growing number of obstacles as a profession. In the age of health care reform, there are increasing pressures for clinical neuropsychologists to increase clinical productivity and to streamline the methodology they use for patient assessment (Puente, 2011). Based on developments with computers and the Internet, there is a call to adapt assessment technology in a rapid manner with the goal of meeting growing technological and marketing demands. There is also a demand to extend the reach of neuropsychological testing to reach all individuals in our communities, including those who do not speak English as a native language (Rivera-Mindt, Byrd, Saez, & Manly, 2010). However, before moving on to developing any "new" or "advanced" approaches to neuropsychological assessment, it is important to come to a full understanding of how our field arrived at this point in its development, by examining its history.

There are numerous clichés on the need to study history, such as the avoidance of being doomed to repeat it. Some argue that studying the history of one's profession can be a fascinating and rewarding experience in its own right (Henle, 1976). The goal of this chapter is to focus on the development of various approaches to neuropsychological assessment as they developed from the middle part of the 20th century. There exist a number of excellent summaries of the origins of specific tests and accounts of neuropsychology's pioneers (Boake, 2002; Goldstein, 2009; Meier, 1992; Reitan, 1994; Stringer, Cooley, & Christensen, 2002). This chapter will differ from those contributions by emphasizing the development of neuropsychological assessment and some of the major approaches developed in North America that are used today in modern-day practice.

Development of Assessment Methods in Clinical Neuropsychology

Neuropsychological assessment developed as a methodology from extending the use of clinical test batteries that had been developed for the purpose of experimentation or the evaluation and characterization of a more broadly defined category of psychopathology. The professional field of clinical neuropsychology has held debates over the years on a variety of issues that are not unlike those that were mounted for years in the field of clinical psychology, regarding "statistical" versus "clinical" approaches to assessment (Meehl, 1954). Ongoing debate between practitioners of these two approaches has continued for a half-century (Grove, Zald, Lebow, Snits, & Nelson, 2000) and similar debates continue in neuropsychology to the present day (Bigler, 2007).

On the one hand, there is one view of neuropsychological assessment that emphasizes quantification. It is characterized by the use of a fixed battery of tests and the application of empirically based cutoff scores to aid in decision making. There are other approaches typified by a more flexible battery with a selection of tests resulting from clinical hypotheses, the referral question at hand, or by characteristics of the patient's behavior during the interview or in the solution of various tasks. Some might consider this second approach to be more "qualitative" in nature. When viewing these two approaches together, they appear to be so different as to possibly representing separate schools or systems of neuropsychology. The goal in the following pages is to summarize the historical origins of these different approaches to neuropsychological assessment and discuss how the issues of quantification versus characterization continue in the contemporary practice of neuropsychology.

Quantitative Approaches to Neuropsychological Assessment

The interest of psychology as a science to the study of brain disorders in human beings dates back to the mid-19th century (Boring, 1950). **Wilhelm Wundt's** (1832–1920) laboratory in Germany provided the first experimental approach to psychology, characterized by rigorous quantification and analysis of consciousness. This methodology was taken outside of the psychology laboratory by Wundt's student, the famous psychiatrist **Emil Kraepelin** (1856–1926), who is known to have used some of the first applications of experimental psychological methods to study basic traits such as memory, fatigue, and learning ability associated with psychopathology.

The American **James McKeen Cattell** (1860–1944) imported **Wilhelm Wundt's** methods from Germany, but with less interest in laboratory studies and more of an emphasis on using psychological instrumentation for the study of individual differences. Cattell is credited for having first used the term *mental tests* and for being the first proponent for developing a standardized psychological test battery that could be used to compare results obtained in experiments performed by different investigators (Cattell, 1890). His student **Shepard Ivory Franz** (1874–1933) is credited for being the first to take an extended battery of psychological tests for use in a clinical setting. Franz developed what is likely to be the first neuropsychological test battery (see Table 1.1) given to patients in the United States (Franz, 1919). The battery was developed when he worked at McLean Hospital of Boston and followed him with use at St. Elizabeth's Hospital in Washington, DC. Many consider Franz to have been the first clinical and experimental neuropsychologist in the United States (Colotla & Bach-y-Rita, 2002). His work is known to have also included early studies of neuropsychological rehabilitation in addition to defining the psychologist's to clinical interviewing.

Table 1.1 Battery of mental tests used by Shepard Ivory Franz (1919)

1 ***Tests of Sensation***
2 ***Tests of Movement***
3 ***Speech and Aphasia***
- **a** Voluntary Speech
- **b** Reading Aloud
- **c** Writing
- **d** Repeating
- **e** Reading Comprehension
- **f** Simple Commands
- **g** Recognition of Objects and Their Uses
- **h** Figures on Skin
- **i** Speech Errors

4 Attention, Apprehension, and Perception
- **a** Qualitative Observation
- **b** Fluctuations of Attention
- **c** Apprehension Test
- **d** Ebbinghaus Test
- **e** Heilbronner Test

5 ***Memory***
- **a** Qualitative Tests of Memory
- **b** Span of Memory
- **c** Memory for Connected Words
- **d** Memory for Complex Events
- **e** Number of Repetitions for Memory
- **f** Memory for Connected Trains of Thought
- **g** Memory for School Subjects

6 ***Association***
- **a** Ideas
- **b** Words

7 Calculation
8 General Intelligence
- **a** Knowledge of Common Things
- **b** Ziehen Test
- **c** Collective Terms
- **d** Masselon Test
- **e** Word Completion
- **f** Reading Backwards and Upside Down
- **g** Proverbs
- **h** Logical Tests
- **i** Absurdities
- **j** Word Building
- **k** Vocabulary
- **l** Maze Test

Origins of the Halstead–Reitan Neuropsychological Test Battery

The development of neuropsychological methodology was influenced subsequently by academic and research activities at the University of Chicago, beginning with studies on the physiological basis of behavior that extended well into the middle portion of the 20th century. **Karl Lashley** (1890–1958) was a member of that faculty from 1929 to 1935, where he was joined by a group of students that would go on to have a significant impact on the early development of psychology (Dewsbury, 2002). With more specific regard to neuropsychology, the students at that time included **Donald O. Hebb** (1904–1985), who was the author of the classic book *Organization of Behavior: A Neuropsychological Theory* (Hebb, 1949) and is now regarded as the founder of cognitive neuroscience.

In Chicago, members of the university's medical faculty were also becoming interested in the study of psychological phenomena in the patients they were treating. Interactions between the university's medical and psychology faculty led to the collaboration of **Heinrich Kluver** (1897–1979) and **Paul Bucy** (1904–1993) and their famous observations on the psychological effects of bilateral medial temporal resection in monkeys (Kluver & Bucy, 1937).

Ward Halstead (1908–1969) joined the medical faculty at Chicago in 1935 after completing his graduate study in the psychology department at nearby Northwestern University. Halstead is now regarded as one of the major pioneers, if not the "founding father" of the field of neuropsychology as practiced by many in the United States (Goldstein, Weinstein, Reed, Hamsher, & Goodglass, 1985; Reitan, 1994). His name is associated with the creation of the first laboratory devoted to the study of brain and behavior relationships in human beings. He is also known for providing the origins of the Halstead–Reitan battery (HRB; see Reitan & Wolfson, 1985), which was one of the most influential approaches of clinical neuropsychological assessment to have evolved in the 20th century.

Many of Halstead's aims are outlined in the introductory chapters of his classic work, *Brain and Intelligence: A Quantitative Study of the Frontal Lobes* (Halstead, 1947). In the book's introductory chapters, he clearly states that his goal was to study a form of biological intelligence that differed from the type intelligence that was measured by standard IQ tests. He sought to determine whether this form of intelligence contributed to man's survival as an organism. He wanted to know if it was similar or different to the mental functions possessed by other organisms. Attempts to study this form of intelligence through a battery of psychological tests was the result of his desire to know whether biological intelligence could, in fact, be measured quantitatively and whether it was composed of unitary or multiple factors. He was also interested in knowing whether quantitative indices developed as a measure of biological intelligence would be helpful in furthering our understanding of normal and pathological ranges of human behavior.

Halstead assembled a combination of 27 indices, taken from 21 separate tests, in an effort to develop a battery used to provide a quantitative measure of biological intelligence. The test battery (listed in Table 1.2) included a number of measures created by Halstead as well as those developed by others. The selection of tests was based on their ability to distinguish between "brain-injured" and "normal" individuals or through their capacity to measure various aspects of psychometric intelligence, personality, or basic sensory abilities. He acquired test data from 237 individuals, with each of them examined in his laboratory over a period of two days.

Table 1.2 Halstead's quantitative indicators (Halstead, 1947)

1	Carl-Hollow Squares Test
2	Halstead Category Test
3	Halstead Flicker-Fusion Test
4	Halstead Performance Test (TPT)
5	Multiple Choice Inkblots
6	Minnesota Multiphasic Personality Inventory
7	Henmon-Nelson Tests of Mental Ability
8	Hunt Minnesota Test for Organic Brain Damage
9	Halstead Schematic Face Test
10	Seashore Measures of Musical Talent
11	Speech-Sounds Perception Test
12	Halstead Finger Oscillation Test
13	Halstead Time Sense Test
14	Halstead Dynamic Visual Field Test
15	Manual Steadiness Test
16	Halstead-Brill Audiometer
17	Halstead Aphasia Test
18	Shlaer-Hecht Anomaloscope
19	Halstead Weight Discrimination Test
20	Halstead Color Gestalt Test
21	Halstead Closure Test

The experimental sample for Halstead's test battery included neurosurgical patients who had undergone cerebral lobectomies, head-injured patients, and some control subjects (Loring, 2010). The test scores were subjected to a factor analysis, which was a new statistical method that had been developed by Chicago colleague **L. L. Thurstone** (1887–1955). Halstead's analysis is, in fact, one of the first applications of this new analytic technique. The resulting solution was composed of four factors, with the first characterized as a central integrative factor, which Halstead labeled as Factor C. This was accompanied by separate factors for abstraction (Factor A), power (Factor P), and differentiated abilities (Factor D). Halstead's book concludes with chapters reviewing how these four factors coincide with what was known in the existing literature (Halstead, 1947).

It must be emphasized that Halstead assembled his battery of tests in an effort to conduct an experimental analysis of biological intelligence. He did not originally intend its clinical use in a medical or psychiatric setting. He left the development of these clinical applications in the capable hands of his students, with **Ralph Reitan** (1922–2014) as the most successful among them. In his initial work, Reitan used Halstead's test battery to examine brain functioning in brain-injured soldiers from World War II and continued with the study in various forms of medical and psychiatric illness (Reitan, 1989; Russell, 2015). After moving to the University of Indiana in 1951, Reitan continued to modify the test battery for more extended use in diagnosing the presence of brain damage as well as etiology and location of various brain lesions (Reed & Reed, 2015). This was accomplished by reducing the number of tests to those most sensitive for identifying the presence of brain disorders as well as including other tests that were proven useful for clinical analysis (Reitan, 1974). The final selection of tests used in the HRB is provided in Table 1.3.

Reitan and his followers argued that a fixed battery of tests has the clinical advantage of employing a central "impairment index" that can be used in a quantitative manner to

Table 1.3 Halstead-Reitan battery (Halstead, 1947; Reitan & Wolfson, 1985)

1	Category Test
2	Tactual Performance Test
3	Trail Making Test
4	Seashore Rhythm Test
5	Speech Sounds Perception Test
6	Finger Oscillation Test
7	Grip Strength
8	Sensory Perceptual Examination
9	Aphasia Screening Test
10	Wechsler Adult Intelligence Scale
11	Minnesota Multiphasic Personality Inventory

identify the presence or absence of brain damage (Goldstein, 1984; Reitan & Wolfson, 1985; Russell, Neuringer, & Goldstein, 1970). Validating and co-norming a set of procedures together also enables the clinician to determine how interrelations among various tests can be used to identify more specific patterns of brain dysfunction. Reitan's followers, using variants of the HRB and other fixed clinical batteries (see Table 1.4), have continued with successful ventures into the study of epilepsy, traumatic brain injury, and stroke. The HRB was one of the first neuropsychological tests to have been used in conjunction with a computerized scoring system (Russell et al., 1970) and one of the largest normative databases in the field has been conducted on a modified version of the HRB in conjunction with other tests (Heaton, Grant, & Matthews, 1991). While other quantitative test batteries have come and gone (Golden, Purisch, & Hammeke, 1979), Halstead and Reitan's battery continues currently as the most successful example of using a fixed battery of neuropsychological tests.

Table 1.4 Description of psychological tests and experimental procedures (Reitan & Davidson, 1974)

1 Wechsler Scales
2 Halstead's Neuropsychological Test Battery for Adults
- **a** Category Test
- **b** Tactual Performance Test
- **c** Rhythm Test
- **d** Speech-Sounds Perception Test
- **e** Finger Oscillation Test
- **f** Time Sense Test
- **g** Critical Flicker Frequency

3 The Halstead Neuropsychological Test Battery for Adults Category Test
4 Reitan-Indiana Neuropsychological Test Battery for Children
5 Specialized Neuropsychological Test Batteries
- **a** Reitan-Klove Sensory Perceptual Examination
- **b** Klove-Matthews Motor Steadiness Battery
- **c** Reitan-Klove Lateral Dominance Examination

6 Additional Test Batteries
- **a** Wide Range Achievement Test
- **b** Minnesota Multiphasic Personality Inventory

7 Individual Tests and Experimental Procedures
- **a** Aphasia Screening Test
- **b** Ballistic Arm Tapping
- **c** Benton Right-Left Orientation Test
- **d** Benton Sound Recognition Test
- **e** Boston University Speech Sounds Discrimination Test
- **f** Dynamometer
- **g** Index Finger Tapping
- **h** Klove-Matthews Sandpaper Test
- **i** Modified Tactual Formboard Test
- **j** Peabody Picture Vocabulary Test
- **k** Porteus Maze Test
- **l** Reitan-Klove Tactual Performance Test
- **m** Trail Making Test
- **n** Visual Space Rotation Test

Qualitative Approaches to Neuropsychological Assessment

The roots of a more qualitative approaches to neuropsychological assessment, characterized by the use of flexible test batteries, can be traced back to a more descriptive European approach to clinical assessment, as exemplified by **Jean-Martin Charcot's** (1825–1893) method of eliciting and describing complex psychological phenomena in asylum patients. The major difference is that, as opposed to relying solely on clinical impression, psychologists extended the use of these methods by submitting them to empirical analysis through the use of standardized tests.

Among the first systematic clinical applications of a more qualitatively oriented test battery can be seen in the work of **Kurt Goldstein** (1878–1965) in collaboration with psychologist **Adhemar Gelb** (1887–1936). Goldstein obtained a medical degree and developed an interest in brain disorders, especially aphasia, after an introduction to the topic by **Karl Wernicke** (1848–1904) (Eling, 2015; Goldstein, 1967; Goldstein, 2009; Simmel, 1968). In contrast, Gelb was a psychologist colleague of Wertheimer's who performed a number of influential experimental studies on the perception of color constancy. These investigators together provided a number of detailed descriptions of the effects of focal brain lesions on behavior in German soldiers injured during World War I (Goldstein & Gelb, 1918). Their view was that neurological syndromes such as aphasia and agnosia were based on a basic impairment in "abstract behavior," a characteristic that could be elicited reliably through administration of standardized assessment techniques.

Like many others, Goldstein fled Europe in the 1930s and continued his work in the United States. He was known in this country as a proponent of a holistic view of brain functioning that was consistent with findings reported in laboratory studies by Karl Lashley and through clinical descriptions by the English neurologist **Henry Head** (1861–1940). He was also recognized for an approach emphasizing the effects of psychopathology on the organism as a whole including not only cognition, but also various aspects of personality.

Goldstein's collaboration with psychologist **Martin Scheerer** (1900–1961) led to further refinement of the psychological test methods that he had initially developed in Germany (Eling, 2015; Goldstein, 2009). The monograph describing the use of the test battery listed in Table 1.5 provides one of the first systematic descriptions of how to

Table 1.5 Goldstein–Scheerer battery (Goldstein & Scheerer, 1941)

1 Cube Test
2 Color Sorting Test
3 Object Sorting Test
4 Color Form Sorting Test
5 Stick Test

examine patients for psychological signs of brain dysfunction (Goldstein & Scheerer, 1941). Included in this methodology is the view that the effects of brain dysfunction cannot be captured adequately through analysis of test scores as found in standard approaches to quantitative testing. Their view was that "test results can be evaluated only by analyzing the *procedure* by which the patient has arrived at his results" (Goldstein & Scheerer, 1941).

During the 1930s **Molly Harrower** (1906–1999), one of the lesser-known pioneers in the field of clinical neuropsychology, began to explore the use of psychological tests with neurosurgical patients in **Wilder Penfield's** (1891–1976) neurosurgical unit in Montreal (Harrower, 1939). Harrower was influenced greatly by Gestalt psychology, having studied with **Kurt Koffka** (1886–1941), one of its founders, for her doctoral degree at Smith College. She also spent an influential three-month period with Kurt Goldstein before joining Penfield's group. Harrower is known for adapting Rubin's reversible figures for clinical purposes as a means to study the disruption of perceptual organization processes in patients with brain disorders and other forms of psychopathology (Harrower, 1939). Her formal work in neuropsychology terminated for the most part upon leaving Penfield's unit in 1941. Harrower went on in her career to become a major influence on clinical psychology and an expert on use of psychological tests in appraising both normal and pathological personality (Dewsbury, 1999).

The influence of training in clinical psychology on the development of neuropsychology during that period is also seen in **Arthur Benton's** (1909–2006) early work, with the test battery used in his first publication in the field of neuropsychology (Benton & Howell, 1941). Benton went on to have a profound influence on the development and maturation of the field of neuropsychology. He had obtained his first clinical experience working with patients at the New York State Psychiatric Institute while a graduate student at Columbia University in the late 1930s (Goldstein, 2009; Levin, Sivan, & Hannay, 2007). Exposure to neuropsychology was obtained through his attendance at Kurt Goldstein's weekly Saturday lectures at Montefiore Hospital (Goldstein, 2009; Meier, 1992). His interest in the brain and behavior was solidified in World War II when he began to conduct evaluations on brain-injured soldiers at the Naval Hospital in San Diego with **Morris Bender** (1905–1983) a neurologist who was known for an interest in the study of higher-order cerebral functions (Hamsher, 1985; Meier, 1992). Bender had exposed Benton to the classic literature in neurology, forming a long-standing interest in an historical approach to the study of well-known neurological syndromes.

Benton originated some of the neuropsychological tests bearing his name to meet the demands of clinical practice. For example, he developed what eventually became the Benton Visual Retention Test as a set of designs drawn informally out of the immediate need for a reliable measure of nonverbal memory. The designs were eventually redrawn by a graphic artist and later published by The Psychological Corporation (Benton, 1997). Benton moved to the University of Iowa in 1948, after spending a brief period of time at the University of Louisville. His initial role at Iowa was the Director of the Graduate Training Program in Clinical Psychology. He established a clinical assessment service for the Department of Neurology in 1950. His research efforts during that period focused on the study of somatosensory processes associated with Gerstmann's syndrome. His research program expanded significantly in 1957 when research funding enabled him to establish a full-time neuropsychological laboratory.

Benton criticized the classic neurological literature for its lack of standardized methodology. His research goals consisted of the study of well-known neurological syndromes such as aphasia, apraxia, and agnosia through the use of well-validated test procedures that enabled him to factor out the influence of unspecified variables such as age and education. A list of the procedures developed in Benton's laboratory for use in experimental studies is provided in Table 1.6 (Benton & Hamsher, 1989; Benton, Hamsher, Varney, & Spreen, 1983). Many of these measures are now standard components of neuropsychological test batteries used by those employing a hypothesis-testing approach to clinical assessment.

A similar approach to neuropsychological assessment is seen in the work of Benton's contemporary **Hans Lukas Teuber** (1916–1977). Teuber was born in Germany and came to

Table 1.6 Benton's neuropsychological tests

1 Tests of Orientation and Learning (Benton et al., 1983)
- **a** Temporal Orientation
- **b** Right-Left Orientation
- **c** Serial Digit Learning
- **d** Visual Retention Test*

2 Perceptual and Motor Tests
- **a** Facial Recognition
- **b** Judgment of Line Orientation
- **c** Pantomime Recognition
- **d** Tactile Form Perception
- **e** Finger Localization
- **f** Phoneme Discrimination
- **g** Three-Dimensional Block Construction
- **h** Motor Impersistence

3 Multilingual Aphasia Examination (Benton & Hamsher, 1978)
- **a** Visual Naming
- **b** Oral Spelling
- **c** Token Test
- **d** Reading Comprehension of Words and Phrases
- **e** Sentence Repetition
- **f** Written Spelling
- **g** Aural Comprehension of Words and Phrases
- **h** Controlled Word Association
- **i** Block Spelling
- **j** Rating of Articulation
- **k** Rating of Praxic Features of Writing

the United States in 1941 (Hurvich, Jameson, & Rosenblith, 1987). He received his PhD in psychology from Harvard University in 1947. He had an indirect link to Gestalt psychology: his father was Director of the scientific station for the study of primates on the island of Tenerife when the Gestalt psychologist **Wolfgang Köhler** (1887–1967) arrived there in 1913 to conduct his famous studies of problem-solving abilities in apes (Köhler, 1925). Teuber's initial exposure to neuropsychology was at Harvard, where he interacted with Karl Lashley and attended lectures given by Kurt Goldstein, who was a visiting professor there in 1941 (Goldstein, 2009). In an interesting coincidence, Teuber also worked at the San Diego Naval Hospital in 1944 with Morris Bender, where he was exposed to working with patients with brain damage and to the classical literature in neurology. Following the war, Bender helped him develop a laboratory for the study of brain disorders at New York University (NYU). It was there that he went on to conduct a number of classic studies on perceptual disturbances of visual and somatosensory regions in brain-injured subjects in collaboration with Bender and a host of psychologist colleagues (Semmes, Teuber, Weinstein, & Ghent, 1960; Teuber, Battersby, & Bender, 1960).

Teuber, much like Benton, advocated the use of standardized procedures developed for conducting a reanalysis of many of the classical neurobehavioral syndromes described by 19th century investigators (Teuber, 1950). However, Teuber also demonstrated an interest in using the knowledge obtained from these investigations for understanding the basis of "normal" brain functioning. He is known for developing the concept of "double dissociation," which has become a standard method for verifying the relationship between a given deficit and a specific lesion site (Teuber, 1955). He also advocated using a battery of tests "to analyze numerous specific performances in an individual patient" rather than devising "omnibus instruments purporting to detect 'the' brain injured patient as such" (Teuber, 1950 p. 31. An example of the battery used in his laboratory is provided in Table 1.7. For Teuber, neuropsychological tests provided a valid means of assessing brain–behavior relationships. His interests extended from the study of perceptual processes to include a means to solve the "riddle" of frontal lobe functioning (Teuber, 1964). He moved from NYU to the Massachusetts Institute of Technology in 1961 where he was responsible for establishing the foundation for the institute's strong reputation as a center for the study of cognitive neuroscience.

Our discussion of flexible test batteries extends above the U.S. border, into Canada, to the Montreal Neurological Institute (MNI). Neuropsychological studies have continued to flourish at the center as a result of **Wilder Penfield's** interests in behavior and his early collaborations with **Molly Harrower** and **Donald Hebb** on the surgical treatment of epilepsy (Loring, 2010). **Brenda Milner** arrived at MNI following World War II as a graduate student at McGill after having studied with **Oliver Zangwill** (1913–1987) in Cambridge, England (Meier, 1992). She conducted her doctoral thesis on the neuropsychological effects of temporal lobectomy (Milner, 1954). She is best known for a series of studies on the behavioral effects of left versus right temporal lobe ablation on memory and other psychological functions (Milner, 1967). She also made important observations on the differences between patients with temporal and frontal lobe dysfunction, particularly as it applies to the effects of surgery (Milner, 1964).

While the focus of the work was on experimentation, Milner and her colleagues at MNI have developed and utilized a number of neuropsychological methods that have been

Table 1.7 Teuber's battery of neuropsychological tests (Teuber, 1950)

- **1** Occipital Lobes
  - **a** Flicker Fusion: Perimetry
  - **b** Tests of Perception and Apparent Movement
  - **c** Double Simultaneous Stimulation
  - **d** "Mixed Figures" Tests
    - **i** Werner and Strauss Figures
    - **ii** Poppelreuter Figures
  - **e** Reversible Figures
    - **i** Harrower Figures
    - **ii** Necker Cube
- **2** Temporal Lobes
  - **a** Melodic Patterns
  - **b** Reversible Melodies
- **3** Parietal Lobes
  - **a** Somato-Sensory Functions
    - **i** Simultaneous Tactile Stimulation
    - **ii** Tactile Thresholds
    - **iii** Prolonged After-Sensations
  - **b** Spatial Orientation
    - **i** Finger Gnosis
    - **ii** Human Figure Drawing
    - **iii** Clock Test
    - **iv** Bisection Tests
    - **v** Three-String Experiment
    - **vi** Field of Search Test
- **4** Frontal Lobes
  - **a** Rylander's Battery
    - **i** Figure Matching Test
    - **ii** Abstract Words
    - **iii** Kraepelin's Test of Continued Addition
    - **iv** Goldstein's Object Sorting Test
    - **v** Stanford-Binet IQ
  - **b** Halstead's Battery
    - **i** Formboard Recall
    - **ii** Flicker Fusion: Frequency
    - **iii** Category Test
    - **iv** Finger Oscillation
    - **v** Flicker Fusion: Thresholds
  - **c** Sorting Tests
    - **i** Weigl Figures
    - **ii** Wisconsin Card-Sorting Test

Table 1.8 Neuropsychological test procedures used and developed at the Montreal Neurological Institute

A Clinical Battery (Kolb & Whishaw, 1990)
- **1** Wechsler Intelligence Scale
- **2** Wechsler Memory Scale
- **3** Mooney Faces Test
- **4** Rey Osterrieth Complex Figure
- **5** Kimura Recurring Figures
- **6** Semmes Figures
- **7** Right-Left Orientation
- **8** Newcombe Fluency Tests
- **9** Wisconsin Card Sorting Test
- **10** Chicago Fluency

B Testing Hippocampal Function (Jones-Gotman, 1987)
- **1** Recognition of Unfamiliar Face, Tonal Melodies, and Nonsense Figures
- **2** Recall of 18 Simple Designs
- **3** Repeating Supraspan Digit and Block Sequences
- **4** Delayed Recall of Words Generated as Synonyms or Rhymes
- **5** Recall of Consonant Trigrams
- **6** Subject-Ordered Pointing to Abstract Words or Designs
- **7** Recall of a Spot on a Line
- **8** Tactual and Visual Maze Learning
- **9** Recall of Spatial Location of Objects

incorporated for use by other psychologists. An example of the clinical and experimental test battery developed and used at MNI is provided in Table 1.8 (Jones-Gotman, 1987; Kolb & Whishaw, 1989). The popularity of measures such as the Design Fluency Test (Jones-Gotman & Milner, 1977) and the Recurring Figures Test (Kimura, 1963), which were developed for neurosurgical studies, provides an excellent example of how experimentally derived measures can be incorporated into a flexibly defined battery of clinical tests.

Origins of the Boston Process Approach

Many associate the type of flexible battery used today with the work of neuropsychologists at the Boston Veterans Administration (VA) Medical during the 1960s through the 1980s and the development of what now called the *Boston Process Approach* to neuropsychological assessment (Kaplan, 1988). The theoretical origins of the Boston Process Approach, with its emphasis on qualitative analysis of test behavior, are commonly attributed to the writings of **Heinz Werner** (1890–1964). In a classic paper published in 1937, Werner argued that the analysis of test scores or achievements is useful only when it is "supplemented by an analysis of the mental processes which underlie the achievements themselves" (Werner, 1937). Werner was raised in Vienna and developed interests in philosophy and science early in his life. After receiving his degree at the University of Vienna, he moved to Hamburg where he worked under the direction of **William Stern** (1871–1938). Stern is known for his work in child development and is regarded as the originator of the concept of the IQ. It is interesting to note that Goldstein's collaborator, **Martin Scheerer**, was a junior collaborator of Stern's at Hamburg during the same time period.

Werner immigrated to the United States in the 1930s and held initial positions at the University of Michigan and Harvard before moving on to Brooklyn College and Clark University. He gained a reputation for a series of studies on "feeble-minded" children at a state institution located outside of Detroit, Michigan. His view was that normal and pathological development proceeded in terms of a qualitative change in patterns of functions rather than quantitative increases in accomplishments, as measured by the IQ (Werner, 1948). Werner drew parallels between his work and the work of Soviet psychologists **Alexander Romanovich Luria** (1902–1977) and **Lev Vygotsky** (1896–1934). While Luria is known for his structured approach to using qualitative methods for analyzing brain disorders (Luria, 1962), Vygotsky is known for his approach to analyzing mental growth by studying an individual's *zone of proximal development,* which is the precursor to the method that is currently called *testing the limits* (Vygotsky, 1978).

The group at the Boston VA Hospital was comprised of a number of talented physicians, psychologists, and linguists who would challenge the holistic orientation to brain functioning and its disruption that was prominent in the field of neurology for much of the century. The group was led by neurologist **Fred Quadfasel** (1902–1974), who had been exposed to the 19th-century European literature in neurology while receiving his medical training in Germany. Quadfasel made an effort to expose his younger colleagues to this classic literature. **Norman Geschwind** (1976–1984) was the most prominent of these individuals. Geschwind is known in the field of neurology for reviving study of the neuroanatomic basis of language and other higher-order processes. He also exposed a new generation to detailed clinical investigative methods of observation and analysis, as popularized by Charcot and his colleagues in Europe before the turn of the century.

Geschwind was joined at the Boston VA by a rather large and talented group of clinical and research psychologists. The list included **Harold Goodglass** (1926–1984), who had an ongoing interest in studying the psychological and linguistic basis of aphasias as well as **Edith Kaplan** (1924–2009) who had an interest in the analysis of development through interactions with her undergraduate and graduate school mentor, Heinz Werner (Delis, 2010). **Sheila Blumstein**, **Edgar Zurif**, and others conducted a number of neurolinguistic studies of language and aphasia. **Nelson Butters** (1937–1995) was another student of Werner's who made a transition from the study of primates to humans. Butters, in collaboration with his colleague, **Laird Cermak** (1942–1999), conducted a number of influential studies on the psychological processes disrupted in memory disorders, combining the use of neuropsychological methods and those developed in the cognitive psychology laboratory (Butters & Cermak, 1980). Butters later moved to the University of California, San Diego, where he formed a group that performed studies on dementia and other neuropsychological conditions in a manner that was consistent with the Boston tradition. Cermak remained at the Boston VA to establish the Memory Disorders Research Center.

Goodglass and Kaplan worked together to develop what was a rather unique approach to neuropsychological assessment characterized by a combination of neurological investigative methods combined with Werner's emphasis on the study of process over achievement (Goodglass & Kaplan, 1979). This culminated in the introduction of the Boston Diagnostic Aphasia Examination (BDAE), which provided a systematic means of measuring and classifying aphasic disorders in a manner that was consistent with the clinical investigative model (Goodglass & Kaplan, 1972). An emphasis on performing a systematic analysis of behavior during testing led the group to develop specifications and materials for adapting commonly used tests such as the Wechsler Adult Intelligence Scale (WAIS) and Wechsler Memory Scale (WMS) and other tests, such as the Rey-Osterrieth Complex Figure and Clock Drawing Test, to enable clinicians to elicit and observe behaviors that are not easily captured through standard test administration guidelines. An example of the clinical test battery used at the Boston VA is provided in Table 1.9. Some of the methods developed at Boston for "testing the limits" during administration of routine tests have been incorporated for standardized use by publishers of tests including the WAIS-III and WAIS-IV (Wechsler, 1997; 2008).

Kaplan went on to coin the term *process approach* based on her use of qualitative observations (Kaplan, 1988). Although similar to what provided in observations of her predecessors, Goldstein and Scheerer (1941), the methods recommended by Kaplan are more systematic in nature. It would not be accurate to characterize the process approach as "solely qualitative" or with the goal of simply noting a patient's behavior when administering tests. The process approach, in its true form, calls for developing standardized methods for observing, scoring, and analyzing qualitative features of behavior in addition to interpreting traditional test scores (Kaplan, 1988). The approach is seen most clearly in a number of tests developed by Kaplan and her colleagues, including the California Verbal Learning Test (CVLT; see Delis, Kaplan, Kramer, & Ober, 1987) and the Delis-Kaplan Executive Function System (DKEFS; see Delis, Kaplan, & Kramer, 2001). The process approach, in its intended form, provides a means of observing the behavior of clinical subjects systematically in a manner that qualifies it as a qualitative analysis using quantitative methods.

Table 1.9 Neuropsychological test battery used at the Boston VA (Goodglass & Kaplan, 1979)

1	Wechsler Adult Intelligence Scale
2	Wechsler Memory Scale
3	Boston Diagnostic Aphasia Examination
4	Boston Diagnostic Parietal Lobe Battery
5	Paper-and-Pencil Drawings
6	Modified Bender-Gestalt Designs
7	Rey-Osterrieth Complex Figure
8	Word Lists (Category, FAS)
9	Stroop Test
10	Wisconsin Card Sorting Test
11	Interleaved Series (Competing Programs, Luria Three-Step)
12	Porteus Mazes
13	Money Roadmap Test
14	Hooper Visual Organization Test
15	Benton Test of Visual Recognition

Update on Today's Trends

Proponents of the quantitative methods used in neuropsychology continue to argue that fixed test batteries, such as the HRB, are the only ones that have been fully validated for clinical decision making and diagnosis (Hom, 2003; Russell, Russell, & Hill, 2005). They also issue the criticism that the flexible nature of other test batteries, with their focus on qualitative aspects of behavior, is "unscientific." Some have gone as far as to argue that the methodology used in flexible test batteries does not meet *Daubert* standards (*Daubert v. Merrell Dow,* 1993) to be admissible in court for scientific testimony (Reed, 1996).

Opponents of fixed test batteries argue that those batteries take too long to administer and contain a number of redundant measures that offer little to address the clinical question at hand. They also argue that the validation studies performed on fixed batteries are outdated. Using today's standards for identifying the presence of brain damage through modern imaging techniques, combined with development of tests enhancing our ability to rule out the presence of motivational factors, the accuracy of the diagnoses used in those original validation studies and their relevance to modern-day practice becomes unclear. There are ample data from clinical and research studies indicating that, properly administered and interpreted, flexible test batteries do meet legal standards for neuropsychologists involved in forensic work (Bigler, 2007; Larrabee, Millis, & Meyers, 2008).

Lessons from social psychology inform us that it is normal to perceptually widen the gap between our personal views and those of our opponents. It is unlikely that those emphasizing a quantitative approach to assessment have no interest in observations of test behavior. In fact, Halstead himself is known to have regarded discrepancies between test scores and abilities in brain-damaged subjects to be a "patent absurdity" (Halstead, 1947). This chapter has also pointed out that followers of the process approach to assessment are not disinterested in the analysis of test scores and are, in fact, more interested in developing new ones, emphasizing a careful analysis of test behavior. A continuation of competing approaches to neuropsychology perpetuates a negative "us" and "them" mentality that has been carried into our professional organizations and boards. A failure to understand and address divisions in neuropsychology not only hinders scientific progress but also delays development of the field at large.

There is now ample evidence indicating that neuropsychologists are moving away from polarized positions to one that combines features from both quantitative and qualitative approaches to clinical assessment. In the most recent survey conducted by the AACN, it was found that the majority of neuropsychologists are now using a "fixed flexible battery" approach to assessment, consisting of a relatively standard set of tests in evaluations of diagnostically related groups, combined with some flexibility to add or subtract tests from the battery to meet individual needs of the patient (Sweet, Meyer, Nelson, & Moberg, 2011).

The results of recent survey data also indicate that neuropsychologists have remained rather stagnant in their development and utilization of new test methodology over the past ten years (Rabin, Paolillo, & Barr, 2016). Based on these results, it appears that most neuropsychologists are particularly reluctant to utilize computer technology for existing tests or to develop new tests based on more novel conceptions of brain and behavior (Bilder, 2011; Rabin et al., 2014). There are also indications that much of the methodology currently in use fails to meet society's needs based on ongoing changes in culture and demographics, particularly with regard to our country's Spanish-speaking population (Elbulok-Charcade et al., 2014; Rivera-Mindt et al., 2010). It is clear that the field needs to initiate efforts to update its assessment methodology. However, returning to the aim of this chapter, it is important for those individuals tasked with developing "new and better" assessment methodology to gain some knowledge of the rich and interesting history of neuropsychology and the lessons it teaches us to ensure clinical neuropsychology's successful move into the future.

References

Barr, W. B. (2011). American Psychological Association (APA), Division 40. In J. S. Kreutzer, J. Deluca, & B. Caplan (Eds.), *Encyclopedia of Clinical Neuropsychology* (pp. 135–138). New York: Springer.

Benton, A. (1997). On the history of neuropsychology: An interview with Arthur Benton. *Newsletter 40*, *15*(2), 1–14.

Benton, A., & Hamsher, K. D. (1989). *Multilingual Aphasia Examination*. Iowa City, IA: AJA Associates.

Benton, A. L., Hamsher, K. D., Varney, N. R., & Spreen, O. (1983). *Contributions to Neuropsychological Assessment: A Clinical Manual*. New York: Oxford University Press.

Benton, A. L., & Howell, I. I. (1941). The use of psychological tests in the evaluation of intellectual function following head injury: Report of a case of post-traumatic personality disorder. *Psychosomatic Medicine*, *III*, 138–152.

Bigler, E. (2007). A motion to exclude and the 'fixed' versus 'flexible' battery in 'forensic' neuropsychology: Challenges to the practice of clinical neuropsychology. *Archives of Clinical Neuropsychology*, *22*, 45–51.

Bilder, R. M. (2011). Neuropsychology 3.0: Evidence-based science and practice. *Journal of the International Neuropsychological Society*, *17*, 7–13.

Boake, C. (2002). From the Binet-Simon to the Wechsler-Bellevue: Tracing the history of intelligence testing. *Journal of Clinical & Experimental Neuropsychology*, *24*(3), 383–405.

Boring, E. G. (1950). *A History of Experimental Psychology* (2nd ed.). New York: Appleton-Century-Crofts.

Butters, N., & Cermak, L. S. (1980). *Alcoholic Korsakoff's Syndrome: An Information-Processing Appproach*. New York: Academic Press.

Cattell, J. M. (1890). Mental tests and measurement. *Mind*, *15*, 373–381.

Colotla, V. A., & Bach-y-Rita, P. (2002). Shepherd Ivory Franz: His contributions to neuropsychology and rehabilitation. *Cognitive, Affective, & Behavioral Neuroscience*, *2*(2), 141–148.

Daubert V. Merrell Dow, 509 (United States 1993).

Delis, D. C. (2010). Edith Kaplan (1924–2009). *American Psychologist*, *65*, 127–128.

Delis, D. C., Kaplan, E., & Kramer, J. H. (2001). *Delis-Kaplan Executive Function System*. San Antonio, TX: The Psychological Corporation.

Delis, D. C., Kaplan, E., Kramer, J. H., & Ober, B. A. (1987). *The California Verbal Learning Test*. San Antonio, TX: The Psychological Corporation.

Dewsbury, D. A. (1999). Molly Harrower (1906–1999). Lover of life. *The Feminist Psychologist*, *26*, 1–2.

Dewsbury, D. A. (2002). The Chicago five: A family group of integrative psychobiologists. *History of Psychology*, *5*, 16–37.

Elbulok-Charcade, M. M., Rabin, L. A., Spadaccini, A. T., & Barr, W. B. (2014). Trends in the neuropsychological assessment of ethnic/racial minorities: A survey of clinical neuropsychologists in the U.S. and Canada. *Cultural Diversity and Ethnic Minority Psychology*, *20*, 353–361.

Eling, P. (2015). Kurt Goldstein's test battery. *Cortex*, *63*, 16–26.

Franz, S. I. (1919). *Handbook of Mental Examination Methods* (2nd ed.). New York: MacMillan.

Golden, C. J., Purisch, A. D., & Hammeke, T. A. (1979). *The Luria-Nebraska Neuropsychological Battery*. Lincoln: University of Nebraska Press.

Goldstein, G. (1984). Comprehensive neuropsychological assessment batteries. In G. Goldstein & M. Hersen (Eds.), *Handbook of Psychological Assessment* (pp. 231–262). New York: Pergamon Press.

Goldstein, G. (2009). Neuropsychology in New York City. *Archives of Clinical Neuropsychology*, *24*, 137–143.

Goldstein, G., Weinstein, S., Reed, J., Hamsher, K. D., & Goodglass, H. (1985). The history of clinical neuropsychology: The role of some American pioneers. *International Journal of Neuroscience*, *25*(3–4), 273–275.

Goldstein, K. (1967). Kurt Goldstein. In E. G. Boring & G. L. Lindzey (Eds.), *A History of Psychology in Autobiography* (Vol. 5, pp. 147–166). New York: Appleton-Century-Crofts.

Goldstein, K., & Gelb, A. (1918). Psychologische Analysen hirnpathologischer Falle auf Grund von Untersuchungen Hirnverletzer. *Zeitschrift fur die gesamte Neurologie und Psychiatrie*, *41*, 1–142.

Goldstein, K., & Scheerer, M. (1941). Abstract and concrete behavior: An experimental study with special tests. *Psychological Monographs*, *53*(2), 1–151.

Goodglass, H., & Kaplan, E. (1972). *The Assessment of Aphasia and Related Disorders*. Philadelphia, PA: Lea & Febiger.

Goodglass, H., & Kaplan, E. (1979). Assessment of cognitive deficit in the brain-injured patient. In M. S. Gazzaniga (Ed.), *Handbook of Behavioral Neurology* (Vol. 2, pp. 3–22). New York: Plenum Publishing Corporation.

Grove, W. M., Zald, D. H., Lebow, B. S., Snits, B. E., & Nelson, C. E. (2000). Clinical vs. mechanical prediction: A meta-analysis. *Psychological Assessment*, *12*, 19–30.

Halstead, W. C. (1947). *Brain and Intelligence: A Quantitative Study of the Frontal Lobes*. Chicago: The University of Chicago Press.

Hamsher, K. D. (1985). The Iowa group. *International Journal of Neuroscience*, *25*(3–4), 295–305.

Harrower, M. (1939). Changes in figure-ground perception in patients with cortical lesions. *British Journal of Psychology*, *30*, 47–51.

Heaton, R. K., Grant, I., & Matthews, C. G. (1991). *Comprehensive Norms for an Expanded Halstead-Reitan Battery: Demographic Corrections, Research Findings, and Clinical Applications*. Odessa, FL: Psychological Assessment Resources.

Hebb, D. O. (1949). *The Organization of Behavior: A Neuropsychological Theory*. New York: Wiley.

Henle, M. (1976). Why study the history of psychology? *Annals of the New York Academy of Sciences*, *270*, 14–20.

Hom, J. (2003). Forensic' neuropsychology: Are we there yet? *Archives of Clinical Neuropsychology*, *18*, 827–845.

Hurvich, L. M., Jameson, D., & Rosenblith, W. (1987). Hans-Lukas Teuber, 1916–1977. *Biographical Memoirs*, *57*, 461–490.

Jones-Gotman, M. (1987). Commentary: Psychological evaluation: Testing hippocampal function. In J. Engel (Ed.), *Surgical Treatment of the Epilepsies* (pp. 203–211). New York: Raven Press.

Jones-Gotman, M., & Milner, B. (1977). Design fluency: The invention of nonsense drawings after focal cortical lesions. *Neuropsychologia*, *15*, 653–674.

Kaplan, E. (1988). A process approach to neuropsychological assessment. In T. Boll & B. K. Bryant (Eds.), *Clinical Neuropsychology and Brain Function: Research, Measurement, and Practice* (pp. 125–167). Washington, DC: American Psychological Association.

Kimura, D. (1963). Right temporal lobe damage. *Archives of Neurology*, *8*, 264–271.

Kluver, H., & Bucy, P. C. (1937). "Psychic blindness" and other symptoms following bilateral temporal lobectomy in rhesus monkeys. *American Journal of Physiology*, *119*, 352–353.

Köhler, W. (1925). *The Mentality of Apes*. London: Routledge & Kegan Paul.

Kolb, B., & Whishaw, I. Q. (1989). *Fundamentals of Human Neuropsychology*. New York: W. H. Freeman and Company.

Larrabee, G. J., Millis, S. R., & Meyers, J. E. (2008). Sensitivity to brain dysfunction of the Halstead-Reitan vs an ability-focused neuropsychological battery. *The Clinical Neuropsychologist*, *22*, 813–825.

Levin, H., Sivan, A. B., & Hannay, H. J. (2007). A tribute to Arthur Benton. *Cortex*, *43*, 572–574.

Loring, D. W. (2010). History of neuropsychology through epilepsy eyes. *Archives of Clinical Neuropsychology*, *25*, 259–273.

Luria, A. R. (1962). *Higher Cortical Functions in Man*. New York: Basic Books.

Meehl, P. E. (1954). *Clinical vs. Statistical Prediction: A Theoretical Analysis and Review of the Evidence*. Minneapolis, MN: University of Minnesota Press.

Meier, M. J. (1992). Modern clinical neuropsychology in historical perspective. *American Psychologist*, *46*, 550–558.

Milner, B. (1954). Intellectual function of the temporal lobes. *Psychological Bulletin*, *51*, 42–62.

Milner, B. (1964). Some effects of frontal lobectomy in man. In J. M. Warren & K. Akert (Eds.), *The Frontal Granular Cortex and Behavior* (pp. 313–334). New York: McGraw-Hill.

Milner, B. (1967). Brain mechanisms suggested by studies of the temporal lobes. In C. H. Millikan & F. L. Darley (Eds.), *Brain Mechanisms Underlying Speech and Language* (pp. 122–132). New York: Grune & Stratton.

Puente, A. E. (2011). Psychology as a health care profession. *American Psychologist*, *66*, 781–792.

Rabin, L. A., Paolillo, E., & Barr, W. B. (2016). Stability in test-usage practices of clinical neuropsychologists in the United States and Canada over a 10-year period: A follow-up survey of INS and NAN members. *Archives of Clinical Neuropsychology*, *31*, 206–230.

Rabin, L. A., Spadaccini, A. T., Brodale, D. L., Grant, K. S., Charcape, M. M., & Barr, W. B. (2014). Utilization rates of computerized tests and test batteries among clinical neuropsychologists in the U.S. and Canada. *Professional Psychology: Research & Practice*, *45*, 368–377.

Reed, J. E. (1996). Fixed versus flexible neuropsychological test batteries under the Daubert standard for the admissibility of scientific evidence. *Behavioral Sciences and the Law*, *14*, 315–322.

Reed, J. C., & Reed, H.B.C. (2015). Contributions to neuropsychology of Reitan and associates: Neuropsychology Laboratory, Indiana University Medical Center, 1960s. *Archives of Clinical Neuropsychology*, *30*, 770–773.

Reitan, R. M. (1974). Methodological problems in clinical neuropsychology. In R. M. Reitan & L. A. Davison (Eds.), *Clinical Neuropsychology: Current Status and Applications* (pp. 19–46). New York: John Wiley & Sons.

Reitan, R. M. (1989). A note regarding some aspects of the history of clinical neuropsychology. *Archives of Clinical Neuropsychology*, *4*(4), 385–391.

Reitan, R. M. (1994). Ward Halstead's contributions to neuropsychology and the Halstead-Reitan Neuropsychological Test Battery. *Journal of Clinical Psychology*, *50*(1), 47–70.

Reitan, R. M., & Davison, L. A. (Eds.). (1974). *Clinical Neuropsychology: Current Status and Applications.* Washington, DC: Winston.

Reitan, R. M., & Wolfson, D. (1985). *The Halstead-Reitan Neuropsychological Test Battery: Theory and Clinical Interpretation.* Tucson: Neuropsychology Press.

Rivera-Mindt, M., Byrd, D., Saez, P., & Manly, J. (2010). Increasing culturally competent neuropsychological services for ethnic minority populations: A call to action. *The Clinical Neuropsychologist*, *24*, 429–453.

Russell, E. W. (2015). Ralph Reitan: A scientist in neuropsychology. *Archives of Clinical Neuropsychology*, *30*, 770–773.

Russell, E. W., Neuringer, C., & Goldstein, G. (Eds.). (1970). *Assessment of Brain Damage: A Neuropsychological Key Approach*. New York: Wiley-Interscience.

Russell, E. W., Russell, S. L., & Hill, B. D. (2005). The fundamental psychometric status of neuropsychological batteries. *Archives of Clinical Neuropsychology*, *20*, 785–794.

Semmes, J., Teuber, H. L., Weinstein, S., & Ghent, L. (1960). *Somatosensory Changes After Penetrating Missile Wounds in Man*. Cambridge, MA: Harvard University Press.

Simmel, M. L. (1968). Kurt Goldstein: 1878–1965. In M. L. Simmel (Ed.), *The Reach of Mind: Essays in Memory of Kurt Goldstein* (pp. 3–12). New York: Springer Publishing Company, Inc.

Stringer, A. Y., Cooley, E. L., & Christensen, A. L. (Eds.). (2002). *Pathways to Prominence in Neuropsychology: Reflections of Twentieth Century Pioneers*. New York: Psychology Press.

Stringer, A. Y., & Postal, K. (2015). Representing the underrepresented: American Board of Clinical Neuropsychology (ABCN) and American Academy of Clinical Neuropsychology (AACN) Diversity Initiatives. *The Specialist*, *35*, 31–32.

Sweet, J. J., Meyer, D. G., Nelson, N., & Moberg, P. (2011). The TCN/AACN 2010 "Salary Survey": Professional practices, beliefs, and incomes of U.S. neuropsychologists. *The Clinical Neuropsychologist*, *25*, 12–61.

Teuber, H. L. (1950). Neuropsychology. In M. R. Harrower (Ed.), *Recent Advances in Diagnostic Psychological Testing: A Critical Summary* (pp. 30–52). Springfield, IL: Charles C. Thomas Publisher.

Teuber, H. L. (1955). Physiological psychology. *Annual Review of Psychology*, *6*, 267–296.

Teuber, H. L. (1964). The riddle of frontal lobe function in man. In J. M. Warren & K. Akert (Eds.), *The Frontal Granular Cortex and Behavior* (pp. 410–444). New York: McGraw-Hill.

Teuber, H. L., Battersby, W. S., & Bender, M. B. (1960). *Visual Fields Defects After Penetrating Missile Wounds of the Brain*. Cambridge, MA: Harvard University Press.

Vygotsky, L. S. (1978). *Mind in Society: The Development of Higher Psychological Processes*. Cambridge, MA: Harvard University Press.

Wechsler, D. (1997). *Wechsler Adult Intelligence Scale: Third Edition (WAIS-III)*. San Antonio, TX: The Psychological Corporation.

Wechsler, D. (2008). *Wechsler Adult Intelligence Scale: Fourth Edition (WAIS-IV)*. San Antonio, TX: Pearson.

Werner, H. (1937). Process and achievement: A basic problem of education and developmental psychology. *Harvard Educational Review*, *7*, 353–368.

Werner, H. (1948). *Comparative Psychology of Mental Development*. New York: Science Editions, Inc.

2 Specialty Training in Clinical Neuropsychology

History and Update on Current Issues

Linas A. Bieliauskas and Erin Mark

Since its nascence in the experimental work of Lashley, Hebb, and Halstead, and early development of clinical applications by Reitan, Goldstein, and Benton (Meier, 1992), clinical neuropsychology can be justifiably proud of having become one of the most developed and formalized fields of practice within psychology. This is most apparent in the evolution of a training model that gives the profession a recognizable roadmap providing a rational basis for the construction and composition of education and training programs.

As described by Meier (1992), "the organizational structure for clinical Neuropsychology originated as much with the formation of the International Neuropsychological Society (INS) as any other single development" (p. 556). INS was formed in 1966 and held its first formal meeting in New Orleans in 1973. As Meier indicated, at the time, there was not sufficient support for clinical neuropsychology to form a division within the American Psychological Association (APA). Interest in clinical neuropsychology continued to grow, however, and in 1980, the Division of Clinical Neuropsychology (Division 40) was formed and is now one of the largest divisions within the APA. In 2013, the division changed its name to the *Society of Clinical Neuropsychology*.

Education and training in clinical neuropsychology were undergoing continued development during this period, though not all of it was systematic and much of it came from different points of view. It was not at all uncommon for individuals to enter the practice of clinical neuropsychology coming from a primary training background in animal Neuropsychology, education, or human development. More extensive reviews of the evolution of training in clinical neuropsychology during this time can be found in Meier (1981) and Bieliauskas and Steinberg (2003). Milestones in the development of a formalized training model in clinical neuropsychology, as well as more recent advances in the maturation of the field, and contemporary issues and challenges are summarized below.

A large number of acronyms for training bodies and other organizations with ties to clinical neuropsychology have developed and reference to these will be made throughout this chapter. For ease of use by the reader, a glossary of these acronyms is appended to the conclusion of this chapter.

Developments in the 1980s

In 1977, INS formed a task force on education, accreditation, and credentialing that began a systematic exploration of current training practices in clinical neuropsychology with the goal of establishing guidelines. This effort was joined by Division 40 in 1980, and in 1984, the Joint APA Division 40/INS Task Force on Education, Accreditation, and Credentialing in Clinical Neuropsychology issued a report describing current training practices in clinical neuropsychology (INS/APA, 1984). That report concluded that "training in clinical neuropsychology was far from standardized and that there was an increasing number of individuals who claimed competency in this area without indication of effective background or training" (p. 21, Bieliauskas & Matthews, 1987). One outcome of the existence of multiple routes toward obtaining competence in clinical neuropsychology was the establishment of the American Board of Clinical Neuropsychology (ABCN) board certification procedures so that the public and other professionals would have a recognizable standard by which to judge the capabilities of those calling themselves clinical neuropsychologists.

The task force then issued a series of reports in order to further identify the essential components of training programs at various levels and to provide guidelines for the further development of such training programs. These reports were consolidated in the INS/APA Guidelines report (1987), and included guidelines for clinical neuropsychology training programs at the doctoral, internship, and postdoctoral levels. Consideration was given to clinical and experimental psychology core knowledge areas, training in the neurosciences, desirable didactic and experiential training, and exit criteria from each of the levels of training. These guidelines were eventually adopted as official documents by Division 40 of APA and were employed as a guide to create a list of those programs at each level (i.e., doctoral, internship, and postdoctoral) that purported to be in compliance with these guidelines. It was the goal of Division 40 to provide a central listing of programs in response to increasing demand from students who wished to explore such training, as well as to provide some guidance to programs wanting to develop training programs in clinical neuropsychology. A listing of graduate, internship, and postdoctoral programs that report they are in compliance with the Division 40 guidelines can be found online at www.Div40.org and is regularly updated. As of the writing of this chapter, Division 40 listed 40 doctoral programs, 50 internships, and 96 postdoctoral programs claiming adherence to Division 40 training guidelines. It should be noted, however, that like other program listings, a program's adherence to the Division 40 guidelines is purely by self-report.

In 1988, Division 40 adopted a "Definition of a Clinical Neuropsychologist" that broadly outlined training expectations for those wishing to identify themselves as specialists in the field. Basically, it indicated that clinical neuropsychologists need to have acquired systematic didactic and experiential training in neuropsychology and neuroscience and that his or her competencies had been reviewed by their peers and found acceptable, with board certification through the American Boards of Professional Psychology (ABPP) showing the clearest evidence of such. In 2006, the Division 40 Executive Committee decided to reevaluate and update a definition of neuropsychology that had been adopted by the Division some years earlier. To that end, the Executive Committee published a survey seeking the views of Division 40 members on this topic and also appointed a group to review the responses, formulate a proposed course of action, and report back to the Executive Committee. At its August 2007 meeting, the Executive Committee reviewed the work of that group, including a proposed revised definition of neuropsychology. After conferring with APA staff, the Executive Committee decided to proceed with a broader approach to provide guidance both to the public and the profession regarding the specialty of neuropsychology, through promulgation of guidelines for neuropsychology. These proposed guidelines for neuropsychology will be drafted in accordance with governing policy regarding both practice and education guidelines.

As training became more organized, another significant development was the establishment of training organizations for each of the different levels of training in clinical neuropsychology. This permitted the various training programs to come together to discuss areas of mutual interest and concern and lead to increased standardization of training experiences across the United States and Canada. The first of these organizations to form was the Midwest Consortium of Postdoctoral Programs in Clinical Neuropsychology in 1988, which eventually developed into the Association of Postdoctoral Programs in Clinical Neuropsychology (APPCN) in 1994. The Midwest Consortium, and then APPCN, developed formal bylaws, criteria for postdoctoral program membership, and devised self-study forms to better identify a uniform training standard. APPCN has also been active in developing accreditation standards for specialty postdoctoral training while working closely with APA, a process that is discussed in more detail on p. 18. At the time of this writing, APPCN listed 67 member programs on its website (www.appcn.org/member-programs), of which many are also listed by Division 40.

As indicated earlier, the ABCN was established in 1981 and was subsequently incorporated into the parent board of the ABPP in 1983. ABCN has always employed the generally accepted guidelines adopted by Division 40 as its basic credentialing requirements for taking the board specialty examination, a practice that is becoming increasingly common, especially among clinical neuropsychologists who have recently completed their training. As of April 2016, 1,141 individuals have become board certified clinical neuropsychologists (i.e., ABPP-CN) from across the United States and Canada. APPCN requires that the director of postdoctoral training of its member programs be board certified through ABCN. Initial descriptions of the formation of the history of the board can be found in Bieliauskas and Matthews (1987), with an update of ABCN policies and procedures in Yeates and Bieliauskas (2004), and in Lucas, Mahone, Westerveld, Bieliauskas, and Barron (2014). Further information about ABCN can be found online at www.theabcn.org.

The membership organization associated with ABCN is the American Academy of Clinical Neuropsychology (AACN). Full AACN membership is restricted to individuals who have been board certified by ABCN, though anyone with an interest in clinical neuropsychology who is not board certified may join AACN as an affiliate member. Whereas ABCN is strictly an examining body for board certification, AACN offers a continuing education program, develops position statements related to the field of clinical neuropsychology, and advocates for the maintenance of quality standards of practice. AACN hosts an annual meeting and sponsors regional neuropsychology educational presentations. More information about AACN can be found online at www.theaacn.org.

Developments in the 1990s

In the 1990s, doctoral and internship programs that provided specialty training in clinical neuropsychology also began to organize in response to the Houston Conference guidelines. The Association for Doctoral Education in Clinical Neuropsychology (ADECN; www.adecnonline.org) and the Association of Internship Training in Clinical Neuropsychology (AITCN; www.aitcn.org) were in place by 1995. Fifty internship programs identifying clinical neuropsychology as a special emphasis are listed on the Division 40 website, with approximately half of these also belonging to AITCN (listed online at www.aitcn.org/member_programs). Those programs that are APA-accredited are designated as internships in clinical *psychology*, even though they offer significant specialty training in clinical neuropsychology. According to the Division 40 guidelines (INS/APA, 1987), 50% of an intern's training should include supervised experiences in clinical neuropsychology in order for an internship program to be viewed as a specialty training program.

In 1995, the Clinical Neuropsychology Synarchy (CNS) was formed to provide a unified forum for all major organizations in clinical neuropsychology to discuss training and professional issues and the CNS continues to meet for this purpose on a regular basis. The members of CNS include APPCN, ADECN, and AITCN, as well as the ABCN, AACN, Division 40, the National Academy of Neuropsychology (NAN), and the Association of Neuropsychology Students in Training (ANST). The impetus for development of the CNS was, in part, based on the recognition of clinical neuropsychology as a specialty by the APA and, in part, a decree of the Interorganizational Council for Accreditation of Postdoctoral Programs in Psychology (IOC)—an organization composed of all the regulatory bodies in professional psychology in North America and representatives of the specialties. Both of these organizations recognized that as new psychology specialties developed and were recognized, a consensus voice of the specialty would be needed to foster standards of education and credentialing. Thus, development of a *synarchy*, which means "governance through joint sovereignty," was encouraged for each specialty. While CNS has served this purpose for clinical neuropsychology, similar synarchies/specialty councils exist for 13 other specialties in professional psychology. The INS sends an observer to CNS meetings, but does not consider itself a participating member of CNS since it is a scientific rather than professional organization and it is not discipline-specific in its membership (i.e., its membership is multidisciplinary). Typically CNS summit meetings of the organizational representatives are held two or three times annually. To date, CNS has opted not to develop bylaws and instead, decision making is by consensus. More information about CNS can be found on the organization's website (www.appcn.org/clinical-neuropsychology-synarchy).

In 1996, after an approximately ten-year application process, clinical neuropsychology was the first psychology specialty to be formally recognized as such by the APA. The 14 psychology specialties currently recognized by the APA with their respective year of initial recognition are listed in Table 2.1. Division 40 has since led the necessary periodic reapplication process for clinical neuropsychology specialty status, which is currently approved until 2017. A listing of APA-recognized psychological specialties and proficiencies can be found online at the organization's website (www.apa.org/ed/graduate/specialize/recognized.aspx).

Table 2.1 APA-recognized specialties in professional psychology

Specialty Name	*Year Initially Recognized*
Clinical Neuropsychology	1996
Industrial-Organizational Psychology	1996
Clinical Health Psychology	1997
Clinical Psychology	1998
Clinical Child Psychology	1998
Counseling Psychology	1998
Psychoanalysis in Psychology	1998
School Psychology	1998
Behavioral and Cognitive Psychology	2000
Forensic Psychology	2001
Family Psychology	2002
Geropsychology	2010
Police and Public Safety Psychology	2013
Sleep Psychology	2013

Information from APA's web page listing specialties in psychology (APA, n.d.)

The Houston Conference

With the recognition of specialty status in 1996, there came the realization that clinical neuropsychology had now matured as a profession and that the model of training should be specified. Julia Hannay proposed a consensus conference and, with the support of the University of Houston, the conference was organized in the fall of 1997. A planning committee was formed by the CNS and the Houston Conference was organized with the co-sponsorship of the University of Houston, the board of Educational affairs of APA, AACN, ABCN, Division 40, APPCN, and NAN. All members of Division 40 and NAN and all training programs in the Division 40 listing were invited to submit applications to attend the conference. From these submissions, 40 delegates were chosen by the planning committee, bringing the total number of conference participants to 46 (including the planning committee). Delegates to the conference were chosen to be broadly representative of the field based on such parameters as geographic region, practice setting, level of training, gender, cultural diversity, subspecialization within the field, and seniority. Delegate selection and the format of the conference were modeled on earlier successful training conferences in psychology such as the Conference on Postdoctoral Training (Belar et al., 1993) and the Conference on Internship Training (Belar et al., 1989). The Houston Conference produced a policy statement formally recognizing training appropriate to the development of specialization in clinical neuropsychology. The statement can be accessed at the Division 40 or AACN website (www.theaacn.org/position_papers/Houston_Conference.pdf), though the reader is encouraged to read the proceedings of the conference to achieve a full appreciation of the development of the document (Hannay et al., 1998). While there was considerable discussion and debate at the Houston Conference regarding training models, a consensual training model was eventually developed that acknowledged the need for both specialized and generalized clinical training throughout a systematic program of doctoral studies, internship, and postdoctoral residency. For example, education and training were to be completed at accredited training programs, a provision that will be further discussed later in this chapter. Clinical neuropsychology was acknowledged as a postdoctoral specialty, with residency training viewed as an integral part of the training background, leading to eligibility for specialty board certification through the ABPP, the parent board of ABCN. There was clear consensus that while *continuing education*, such as that provided by workshops, lectures, online learning, etc., was an expected activity for all specialists, continuing education was *not* seen as sufficient for establishing core knowledge or skills or for primary career changes. Concern was raised at the time about whom the recommended training should affect and it was agreed that the policy would apply to future training in clinical neuropsychology (i.e., to those *entering* training after the document was to be implemented) and was not intended to be retroactive. CNS and all its member organizations, endorsed the Houston Conference document within one year, such that the Houston Conference model of training became the recommended route to becoming a clinical neuropsychologist for those *beginning* their training in 1999 or later.

The Houston Conference Guidelines for Training in Clinical Neuropsychology

The Houston Conference guidelines laid out a recommended sequence of training, starting at the undergraduate level, for students wishing to eventually specialize in clinical neuropsychology. At the undergraduate level, student typically complete an undergraduate degree in psychology, with emphases on the biological bases of behavior, cognition, and basic neuroscience (although a psychology major continues *not* to be an absolute requirement to enter graduate training). Students then enter a graduate program in applied psychology, most often clinical psychology, which provides either specialty *track* training in clinical neuropsychology or substantial training opportunities in subject areas germane to clinical neuropsychology. Next, the graduate student typically completes an internship offering at least some specialty training in clinical neuropsychology. Finally, the student attends a two-year postdoctoral residency specializing in clinical neuropsychology. The completion of a postdoctoral residency, though a relatively new aspect of specialty training, is now a credentialing *requirement* for candidates seeking board certification by ABCN who completed their training as of January 1, 2005 or later. While the residency requirement may seem unnecessary to some, it places specialists in clinical neuropsychology at the same level of training as their counterparts in the medical specialties of neurology or psychiatry and further eliminates distinctions that can be perceived as markers of second-class professional status.

In addition to specifying the recommended training sequence for specialization in clinical neuropsychology, the Houston Conference also specified a *knowledge base* and *skill base* thought to be necessary for specialization in clinical neuropsychology. The knowledge base includes training in core general psychology topics (e.g., statistics, learning theory, biological bases of behavior), core clinical psychology topics (e.g., psychopathology, psychometrics, interview and assessment techniques, intervention, ethics), foundations of brain-behavior relationships (e.g., functional neuroanatomy, neurological and related disorders, neuroimaging techniques, neuropsychology of behavior), and foundations for the practice of clinical neuropsychology (e.g., specialized neuropsychological assessment and intervention, research design and analysis, practical implications). The skill base is comprised of the following areas: assessment; treatment and intervention; consultation to patients, families, and institutions; research; and teaching and supervision. It is worth noting here that the Houston Conference guidelines permitted some degree of flexibility with respect to when in the training sequence students could acquire their knowledge and skill base. Thus, for example, students may acquire their knowledge base in brain-behavior relationships during their graduate, internship, or postdoctoral training. The Conference also placed importance on research activities and recommended that students' research skills go beyond basic skills (i.e., research design, literature review) and include the ability to execute research, monitor its progress, and evaluate its outcome. Thus, per the Houston Conference Guidelines, clinical neuropsychologists were expected to be not just consumers of research but also to be capable of producing research. From start to finish (including undergraduate education), the typical time to completion of specialty training in clinical neuropsychology is approximately 11 years, which is similar to the training period in medical specialties.

Effectively, the Houston Conference produced a formal model for training in clinical neuropsychology that is essentially equivalent to models developed for specialties in medicine. The model specified general and specific training at the doctoral, internship, and postdoctoral level. Board certification in clinical neuropsychology, through the parent body of ABPP, was identified as the desirable exit goal—again, making the specialty similar to medical specialties. In actuality, the model stipulated by the Conference guidelines did not *create* novel training requirements for neuropsychologists, but rather codified the kind of training that most clinical neuropsychologists had already undergone. Nevertheless, with the Houston Conference guidelines, clinical neuropsychology became the first of psychology's specialties to forward such a detailed training model.

Later Developments: APA Accreditation and Postdoctoral Residency

The Houston Conference, which identified clinical neuropsychology as a postdoctoral specialty, also specified that training should occur in *accredited* programs. APA has long accredited doctoral and internship training programs in professional psychology (APA, 2013a; APA, 2013b), the current listing of which can be found online at www.apa.org/ed/accreditation/programs. Accreditation of postdoctoral programs, however, has started to occur relatively recently. APA has moved to accrediting postdoctoral residency programs by two designations. First, programs can be accredited as providing training in professional psychology. This designation covers programs that offer training in multiple areas of concentration, though without having being accredited as offering "substantive" training in a designated specialty area. Such programs may offer training in clinical neuropsychology as part of their curriculum, but their graduates may not designate themselves as having completed an accredited postdoctoral residency in clinical neuropsychology. Their designation reflects completion of an accredited postdoctoral residency in professional psychology.

Second, APA offers accreditation of postdoctoral residencies in substantive specialty areas, including clinical neuropsychology. These programs must meet specialty-specific criteria as well as more general criteria for training in professional psychology. APA is steadily moving forward with formal accreditation under both designations, but the development has been recent, and its accreditation criteria for clinical neuropsychology largely derive from the Houston Conference (Hannay et al., 1998). Since the publication of the first edition of this volume, the number of accredited postdoctoral residency programs has increased dramatically, almost quadrupling. At the time of this writing, APA listed 22 formally accredited postdoctoral programs offering specialty training in clinical neuropsychology (APA, 2013b).

The recommendation by the Houston Conference, that training occur at accredited programs, was not intended to restrict training opportunities. Indeed, the Houston Conference document simply indicates that postdoctoral programs will *pursue* accreditation according to specific criteria. As such, ABCN currently requires that training in clinical neuropsychology be in conformity with the Houston Conference document and does not currently require that the postdoctoral residency be accredited by APA.

Although the number of APA-accredited postdoctoral programs offering specialty training in clinical neuropsychology has increased significantly in the last decade, the previously slow pace of formal accreditation necessitated alternative means of specialty designation. The earliest was a general designation for postdoctoral programs instituted by the Association of Psychology Postdoctoral and Internship Centers (APPIC) in 1968. APPIC criteria for membership as a postdoctoral training center includes general requirements (including organized training experiences), supervision requirements, and a minimum of 25% time in providing professional services (APPIC Directory, 2013). APPIC criteria was most recently revised in May 2006, with later clarification of the criteria occurring in June 2011. As June 2014, APPIC listed 163 agencies as offering postdoctoral training, 100 of which described themselves as offering "supervised experiences" in adult or child clinical neuropsychology (https://membership.appic.org/directory/search).

Designation of postdoctoral programs as offering specialty training in clinical neuropsychology has been offered by APPCN since 1994. While APPCN initially considered the development of an accreditation process, it chose not to pursue this when it became clear that APA was ready to formally accredit specialty postdoctoral training in clinical neuropsychology. APPCN has always required, and continues to require, that each member program complete a self-study covering specific training criteria. APPCN has cooperated with APA in developing accreditation criteria and APPCN's self-study guide has been largely incorporated by APA into its accreditation procedures. As mentioned earlier, there are currently 67 postdoctoral training programs listed by APPCN. Both their listing of programs and the self-study guide can be found at the AAPCN's website (www.appcn.org).

In addition to providing a list of designated training programs, APPCN also organizes an annual postdoctoral match (i.e., "the match") that matches candidates to programs. Prior to the advent of the match, neuropsychology postdoctoral programs relied on advertising, word-of-mouth, organizational listing, and other informal methods for recruitment of postdoctoral candidates. Candidates generally completed multiple program applications, traveled for invited interviews, and then received offers when the candidate and the program agreed that there would be a good match. It was becoming clear in the 1990s that the growing number of candidates and programs made this informal process unwieldy and inefficient. In 2001, APPCN established a match system for candidates seeking specialty postdoctoral training. This system approximated the match system employed for specialty training in medical residencies and psychology internships and established a central listing of available postdoctoral programs, a uniform application form, a uniform application date, and a uniform match date, which occurs in February. Once candidates and programs commit to the match, they are bound by its results, avoiding the older method of scrambling phone calls, offers and counter-offers, and anxiety-inducing delays. A standard interview time and space has been provided at the annual North American meeting of the INS, which takes place in February at an annual meeting (meeting information for INS can be obtained at its website: www.the-ins.org/), affording programs and candidates an opportunity to meet without being limited by time, expense, and the inconvenience of traveling to multiple long-distance on-site interviews. It should be noted, however, that not all programs participate in the match, which may complicate the application process for program directors bound by match-imposed timelines, and candidates who are receiving competitive offers from programs not participating in the match.

Acknowledging the possibility that not all programs and candidates would find suitable matches during the initial match process, the APPCN created a secondary "clearinghouse." This clearinghouse service provides a listing of both candidates and programs that did not find a suitable match on match day. A description of these match-related services can also be found on the APPCN website.

Another service offered through APPCN is the residency examination, an objective examination for postdoctoral students-in-training. The examination is designed to identify whether the student is progressing effectively in the different areas of clinical neuropsychology and moving toward success on the board certification examination. The residency examination provides effective feedback for postdoctoral training programs and can be used to assess overall effectiveness of APPCN programs when test results are aggregated.

Recent Developments and Continuing Controversies

The movement toward board certification has steadily gained momentum in the last decade, and among early career neuropsychologists board certification is becoming increasing more commonplace. In an effort to increase rates of board certification among newly trained neuropsychologists, ABPP provides students with an opportunity to start the board certification process before completion of their training by allowing students to submit and maintain their credentials for a one-time fee of $25.00.

Multiple support resources exist for neuropsychologists interested in pursuing board certification in clinical neuropsychology. As mentioned earlier, neuropsychologists interested in pursuing board certification should go to ABPP.org for more information about starting the certification process. Additional resources can be found on the AACN website Study Materials page, which has links to useful resources, including information about the AACN membership program. The AACN membership program offers candidates (i.e., individuals who have had their credentials accepted by ABPP/ABCN) the opportunity to request a mentor to assist them through the various stages of the process. Individuals interested in textbooks on the subject of board certification in clinical neuropsychology will surely find the following two volumes helpful: *Board Certification in Clinical Neuropsychology: A Guide to Becoming ABPP/ABCN Certified Without Sacrificing Your Sanity* (2008) by Kira Armstrong, Dean Beebe, Robin Hilsabeck, and Michael Kirkwood; and *Clinical Neuropsychology Study Guide and Board Review* edited by Kirk Stucky, Michael Kirkwood, and Jacobus Donders (2013). Finally, an excellent resource that acts both as a study group and as a source for free neuropsychology-related study materials is the BRAIN group (i.e., Be Ready for ABPP in Neuropsychology). BRAIN is a peer-based support and study group that was started in 2002, has grown over time, and is now partnered with AACN. See BRAIN's Wikipedia page for more information (www.brain.aacnwiki.org).

The most recent development to effect board certification opportunities came early in 2014 when the ABCN announced the creation of its first subspecialty board: Pediatric Clinical Neuropsychology. The creation of this subspecialty board is the result of many years of effort on the part of many committed pediatric neuropsychology professionals. At the time of this writing, application for ABCN subspecialty certification in pediatric clinical neuropsychology is available only to those *currently* board certified in clinical neuropsychology through ABPP/ABCN. Further details concerning subspecialty certification can be obtained from the ABCN website.

Another important aspect of training that continues to evolve is the role of technologies, such as functional imaging techniques and computerized testing batteries. Some practitioners are apprehensive about the potential negative impact of such technological advances on the practice of clinical neuropsychology. Innovation in this context, however, is not something to fear. On the contrary, neuropsychologists, with their strong background in the neurosciences, and continually updated training programs, are well poised to take advantage of continuing developments in the field of health care.

As with any efforts at formalization and establishment of standards, some controversies have arisen. Some have objected to the establishment of the training model specified by the Houston Conference. In particular, there remains some questioning of the need for formal postdoctoral training and the specification that specialty training cannot be established through continuing education (CE) activities. As described earlier (Bieliauskas, 1999), the rightful aspiration of the professional specialty of clinical neuropsychology to command respect and be equally regarded by other professional specialties, such as those in medicine, requires that it behave in a similar way. A profession without a model will command no respect. Just as a patient has the right to expect that his or her medical specialist has completed recognized residency training and does not profess to have developed her or his diagnostic and treatment capability online, or in weekend workshops, so does a patient have the same right to expect residency training when he or she seeks specialist services from a clinical neuropsychologist. Just as a patient has the right to expect his or her medical specialist to have demonstrated the competence established during her or his training by undergoing examination for recognized board certification, the patient has the right to expect no less of his or her specialist in clinical neuropsychology. Again, the establishment of the two-year postdoctoral residency requirement for the field puts clinical neuropsychology on par with fellow medical specialties.

There are numerous opportunities to obtain CE in clinical neuropsychology and related areas of interest. Extensive workshop programs are sponsored by AACN during its annual meeting and in regional presentations (www.theaacn.org). The National Academy of Neuropsychology also provides an extensive workshop program at its annual meeting and provides online opportunities for CE (http://nanonline.org/). The American Academy of Neurology (AAN) offers many behaviorally related neurology educational offerings at its annual meeting as well (www.aan.com/professionals/). APA and many other organizations also offer multiple CE opportunities. The perspective developed at the Houston Conference is that CE is a valuable and necessary method of keeping updated in one's specialty and keeping abreast of current developments. It is *not*, however, an appropriate means for establishing the basis for specialization.

The argument has also been raised that formalization of training in clinical neuropsychology unnecessarily restricts the number of training opportunities for students and short-changes public needs for clinical neuropsychology services. Hopefully, from the review in this chapter, it is apparent that the field has grown considerably, most notably with respect to the number of designated postdoctoral programs in the last decade, and that numerous training opportunities are available. To repeat, the Division 40 website lists 40 doctoral programs, 50 internship programs, and 96 postdoctoral training programs. Along with the other listings described in this chapter, this does not appear to represent a shortage.

Finally, some have said that the establishment of a training model such as that represented by the Houston Conference is premature. That argument is obviated by the formal recognition by APA of clinical neuropsychology as a specialty. Once a specialty is thus formally established, it is important that it can reliably and validly describe the training and experience required to attain it. Any model for training to standards is, by nature, a living entity and, thus, a work in progress, and there is no doubt that further refinements and modifications in training will take place in the future. This is true for all the specialties in psychology, including, for example, clinical psychology, which has had major training conferences and emerging policies dating from the Boulder Conference in 1949 (Kelly, 1950) to the Conference on Postdoctoral Training in Professional Psychology in 1992 (Larsen et al., 1993). If one were to call the Houston Conference policy a "work in progress," it should be noted that the same can be said for the government of the United States, which continually amends its constitution, the latest amendment (27th) being ratified in 1992 after being initially proposed in 1789.

The evolution of training for the specialty of clinical neuropsychology has been remarkable in terms of its exciting beginnings, gradual coalescence, and systematic development toward a formal model. Students benefit by having a clear roadmap to becoming a clinical neuropsychologist, training programs benefit by having guidance on establishing curricula and training experiences that meet consensual standards, and the profession benefits by having a degree of confidence that its members have undergone a specific program of didactic and experiential training. There is a need to respect this systematic development (Bieliauskas, 1999) and the aspirations it represents for the good of our patients and the health of our profession. clinical neuropsychology can certainly be proud of its current professional status, which is due, in large part, to the development of its training model. Ongoing evolution is the mark of the health of the profession and exciting developments in this regard await all of us.

Glossary

AACN American Academy of Clinical Neuropsychology
AAN American Academy of Neurology
ABCN American Board of Clinical Neuropsychology
ABPP American Board of Professional Psychology
ADECN Association for Doctoral Education in Clinical Neuropsychology
AITCN Association of Internship Training in Clinical Neuropsychology
APA American Psychological Association
APPCN Association of Postdoctoral Programs in Clinical Neuropsychology
APPIC Association of Psychology Postdoctoral and Internship Centers
ANST Association of Neuropsychology Students in Training
CNS Clinical Neuropsychology Synarchy
INS International Neuropsychological Society
IOC Inter-organizational Council for Accreditation of Postdoctoral Programs in Psychology
NAN National Academy of Neuropsychology

References

American Association of Clinical Neuropsychology (AACN). (2014, June 26). *Study Materials webpage*. Retrieved from https://www.theaacn.org/studymaterial.aspx

American Board of Clinical Neuropsychology (ABCN). (2014, June 26). *FAQs webpage*. Retrieved from http://www.abpp.org/i4a/pages/index.cfm?pageid=3405

American Psychological Association (APA). (2013a). Accredited doctoral programs in professional psychology. *American Psychologist*, *68*(9), 861–876. http://dx.doi.org/10.1037/a0035066

American Psychological Association (APA). (2013b). Accredited internship and postdoctoral programs for training in psychology. *American Psychologist*, *68*(9), 833–860. http://dx.doi.org/10.1037/a0035064

American Psychological Association (APA). (n.d.) *APA's Recognized Specialties and Proficiencies webpage*. Retrieved June 26, 2014 from http://www.apa.org/ed/graduate/specialize/recognized.aspx

Armstrong, K., Beebe, D., Hilsabeck, R., & Kirkwood, M. (2008). *Board Certification in Clinical Neuropsychology: A Guide to Becoming ABPP/ABCN Certified Without Sacrificing Your Sanity*. New York: Oxford University Press.

Association of Psychology Postdoctoral and Internship Centers (APPIC). (2013). *APPIC Directory OnLine*. http://www.appic.org/Directory

Belar, C. D., Bieliauskas, L. A., Klepac, R. K., Larsen, K. G., Stigall, T. T., & Zimet, C. N. (1993). National Conference on Postdoctoral Training in Professional Psychology. *American Psychologist*, *48*(12), 1284–1289. doi: 10.1037/0003-066X.48.12.1284

Belar, C. D., Bieliauskas, L. A., Larsen, K. G., Mensh, I. N., Poey, K., & Roelke, H. J. (1989). The National Conference on Internship Training in Psychology. *American Psychologist*, *44*(1), 60–65. doi: 10.1037/0003-066X.44.1.60

Bieliauskas, L. A. (1999). Mediocrity is no standard: Searching for self-respect in Clinical Neuropsychology. *The Clinical Neuropsychologist*, *13*, 1–11.

Bieliauskas, L. A., & Matthews, C. G. (1987). American Board of Clinical Neuropsychology: Policies and procedures. *The Clinical Neuropsychologist*, *1*, 21–28.

Bieliauskas, L. A., & Steinberg, B. A. (2003). The evolution of training in clinical neuropsychology: From hodgepodge to Houston. In G. J. Lamberty, J. C. Courtney, & R. L. Heilbronner (Eds.). *The Practice of Clinical Neuropsychology* (pp. 17–30). Lisse, the Netherlands: Swets & Zeitlinger.

Definition of a Clinical Neuropsychologist. (1989). *The Clinical Neuropsychologist*, *3*, 22.

Division 40 of the APA, Society for Clinical Neuropsychology. (2014, June 26). *List of training programs*. Retrieved from http://www.div40.org/training/index.html

Hannay, H. J., Bieliauskas, L., Crosson, B. A., Hammeke, T. A., Hamsher, K., & Koffler, S. (1998). Proceedings of The Houston Conference on Specialty Education and Training in Clinical Neuropsychology. *Archives of Clinical Neuropsychology*, *13*, 157–250.

INS/APA. (1984). Report of the Task Force on Education, Accreditation and Credentialing in Clinical Neuropsychology. *The INS Bulletin*, 5–10. *Newsletter 40*, 1984, *2*, 3–8.

INS/APA. (1987). Reports of the INS-Division 40 Task Force on Education, Accreditation, and Credentialing. *The Clinical Neuropsychologist*, *1*, 29–34.

Kelly, E. L. (1950). *Training in Clinical Psychology*. New York: Prentice-Hall.

Larsen, K. G., Belar, C. D., Bieliauskas, L. A., Klepac, R. K., Stigall, T. T., & Zimet, C. N. (1993). *Proceedings of the National Conference on Postdoctoral Training in Professional Psychology*. Washington, D.C.: Association of Psychology Postdoctoral and Internship Centers.

Lucas, J.A., Mahone, M., Westerveld, M., Bieliauskas, L., & Baron, I.S. (2014). The American Board of Clinical Neuropsychology: Updated milestones past and present. *The Clinical Neuropsychologist*, *28*, 889–906.

Meier, M. J. (1981). Education for competency assurance in human neuropsychology: Antecedents, models, and directions. In S. B. Filskov & T. J. Boll (Eds.), *Handbook of Clinical Neuropsychology* (pp. 754–781). New York: Wiley.

Meier, M. J. (1992). Modern clinical neuropsychology in historical perspective. *American Psychologist*, *47*, 550–558.

Stucky, K., Kirkwood, M., & Donders, J. (Eds)., (2013). *Clinical Neuropsychology Study Guide and Board Review*. New York: Oxford University Press.

Yeates, K. O., & Bieliauskas, L. A. (2004). The American Board of Clinical Neuropsychology and American Academy of Clinical Neuropsychology: Milestones past and present. *The Clinical Neuropsychologist*, *18*, 489–493.

3 Psychometric Foundations of Neuropsychological Assessment

Glenn J. Larrabee

Plan of Chapter

The present chapter reviews the psychometric foundations of neuropsychological assessment. The reader is referred to Chapter 1 by William Barr for a review of the historical underpinnings of modern neuropsychological assessment. The current chapter begins with an overview of basic definitions of what a test is, and what psychometrics entails. This is followed by discussion of reliability, validity, normative issues, and data on test score variability pertinent to the interpretation of neuropsychological test results.

What Is Psychometric Testing?

Cronbach (1990) defines a *test* as a systematic procedure for observing and describing behavior with the aid of numerical scales or fixed categories. In other words, observations are quantified, then assigned some meaningful values that can be ranked as representing more or less of some trait, ability, or behavior. In neuropsychological assessment, tests comprise measures of abilities, such as language, perception, motor skills, working memory, processing speed, and learning and memory, as well as questionnaires completed either by the examinee (MMPI-2-RF, Tellegen & Ben-Porath, 2008/2011; Postconcussion Checklist, Gardizi, Millis, Hanks, & Axelrod, 2012) or by someone who knows the examinee, rating them on various traits or behaviors (Behavior Rating Inventory of Executive Function–Adult Version, Roth, Isquith & Gioia, 2005; note that self-report ratings are also available with this scale). Irrespective of whether the test is a measure of ability or a symptom questionnaire, the quantification and scaling of behaviors and responses captured by the test allows a meaningful ranking of a person's behavioral characteristics that are being assessed. Cronbach (1990) describes psychometric testing as summing up performance in numbers, and follows what he refers to as "two famous old pronouncements: If a thing exists, it exists in some amount; if it exists in some amount, it can be measured" (p. 34).

Nunnally and Bernstein (1994) discuss the role of measurement in science as consisting of rules for assigning symbols (e.g., numbers) to objects (in the case of psychology, attributes) so as to (a) represent quantities of attributes numerically (scaling) or (b) define whether the objects fall in the same or different categories regarding a given attribute. They note that much of what is historically called *measurement* involves scaling, and therefore properties of numbers, but classification can be of equal importance. Of course, neuropsychological examples exist wherein a collection of scaled attributes can be subjected to cluster analysis to yield different categories as defined by differential patterns of strengths and weaknesses on those attributes; for example, profiles of scaled attributes that characterize subtypes of learning disabilities (Fletcher & Satz, 1985).

Both Cronbach (1990) and Nunnally and Bernstein (1994) emphasize the importance of standardization. Measures are standardized to the extent that the rules for use are clear, practical to apply, do not demand great skill of administration beyond the initial learning period, are not dependent upon the specific test administrator, and include some form of norms that describe the numerical scores obtained in a population of interest, by quantifying how much of the attribute is present. The fundamental purpose of standardization is that users of a particular test should obtain similar results; in other words, absent practice effects, the same intelligence test administered to the same patient, but by different examiners should yield the same overall IQ score.

Nunnally and Bernstein (1994) review four different levels of measurement, originally proposed by Stevens (1951).

1. Nominal (equal vs. not equal): Permissible statistics include numbers of cases and mode, e.g., handedness.
2. Ordinal (> versus <): Permissible statistics include median, percentiles, order statistics, e.g., class rank.
3. Interval (equality of intervals or differences): Permissible statistics include arithmetic mean, variance, Pearson correlation, e.g., Wechsler Adult Intelligence Scale–IV (Wechsler, 2008) Index scores or Halstead-Reitan Battery (HRB) T scores (Heaton, Miller, Taylor, & Grant, 2004).
4. Ratio (equality of ratios), permissible statistics include geometric mean, e.g., temperature (Kelvin).

The level of measurement that best characterizes most neuropsychological test scores is the interval level, which allows general linear transformations of the type $x' = bx + a$.

Test procedures are typically designed to yield scores that follow the standard normal distribution with mean of 0 and standard deviation of 1. Through linear transformation one can obtain different descriptive mean scores and standard deviation units such as scores that follow an IQ metric, with a mean of 100 and standard deviation of 15, or IQ subtests with mean of 10 and standard deviation of 3. Other familiar transformations of mean and standard deviation values include the use of T scores with mean of 50 and standard deviation of 10 (Heaton et al., 2004). For test scores that do not approximate the standard normal distribution but rather yield a skewed distribution, performance is ranked following ordinal scaling using percentiles based on the frequency distribution of scores (e.g., many measures from the Benton Neuropsychology Laboratory are scored in this fashion; Benton, Sivan, Hamsher, Varney, & Spreen, 1994).

Reliability, Measurement Error, and Reliable Change Scores

Reliability refers to the consistency or stability of a test score; it is the degree to which an experiment, test, or any other measurement procedure yields the same results on repeated trials (Carmines & Zeller, 1979). In classical test theory, an observed test score is considered to be comprised of a true score component (i.e., the actual amount of the attribute being measured) as well as a component that is due to error (i.e., any component condition that is irrelevant to the purpose of the test; Anastasi & Urbina, 1997). Over several observations, the variance in observed scores is comprised of both true score and error variance. Reliability can then be considered as the ratio of true score variance to the observed score (total) variance (true score variance + error variance), or r_{tt} = True-score variance/Observed score variance (Cronbach, 1990).

There are four main ways of computing reliability (Anastasi & Urbina, 1997; Cronbach, 1990): (a) test-retest reliability, in which the same test is repeated following a temporal delay with scores at Time 1 correlated with scores at Time 2; (b) alternate or parallel form reliability, in which two (or more) equivalent test forms are administered, following a temporal delay, with correlations computed between scores obtained on the alternate forms (note, there is usually counterbalancing of alternate form order to control for practice effects, something that cannot be controlled in the test-retest paradigm); (c) split-half reliability, computed by correlating the score on both halves of the test (e.g., odd–even; obviously inappropriate for a speeded test such as Digit Symbol or Trail Making); and (d) internal consistency based on the consistency of responses to all items in the test.

Calamia, Markon, and Tranel (2013) have published a meta-analysis of the test-retest reliabilities of several commonly used neuropsychological tests, including the Wechsler Adult Intelligence Scale (WAIS), Auditory Verbal Learning Test (AVLT), California Verbal Learning Test (CVLT), Complex Figure Test (CFT), Trail Making Test (TMT), Benton Visual Retention Test (BVRT, Administration A), Boston Naming Test (BNT), Controlled Oral Word Association Test (COWA), and the Wisconsin Card Sorting Test (WCST) perseverative error count. The magnitude of these retest correlations was adequate to high, with several exceeding .70. Retest correlations were robust and related to the effects of age (estimated reliability increases slightly with increase in age), use of alternate forms (decreasing test-retest correlations based on alternate forms), and duration of retest interval (decreasing test-retest correlations in association with longer retest intervals). For the tests studied, retest correlations ranged from .706 for Matrix Reasoning to .915 for Information for the WAIS, .284 (recognition) to .881 (long delay) for the AVLT, .505 (Trial 1) to .749 (trials 1–5 total) for the CVLT, .500 (copy) to .741 (immediate recall) for the CFT, .658 (Trail A) to .769 (Trail B) for the TMT, .797 for BNT; .632 for BVRT, .794 for COWA, and .616 for WCST.

The correlation computed between split halves must be corrected for being based on only one-half of the total test items; all other things being equal, the longer a test the more reliable it will be (Anastasi & Urbina, 1997). The effect that lengthening or shortening a test can have on the reliability coefficient can be estimated by the Spearman-Brown formula, wherein $r_{nn} = nr_{tt} / 1 + (n - 1)\, r_{tt,}$ in which r_{nn} is the estimated coefficient, r_{tt} is the obtained coefficient, and n is the number of times the test is lengthened or shortened; e.g., if the number of test items is increased from 25 to 100, $n = 4$ (Anastasi & Urbina, 1997). When applied to a split-half computation, the formula simplifies to $r_{tt} = 2r_{hh} / 1 + r_{hh}$ where r_{hh} is the correlation of the half-tests (Anastasi & Urbina, 1997).

The interitem consistency upon which internal consistency reliability applies, is influenced by two sources of error variance: (a) content sampling (which also influences alternate form and split half reliability), and (b) the heterogeneity of the behavior domain being sampled (Anastasi & Urbina, 1997). Domains in which the content is homogeneous will have higher interitem consistency and greater internal consistency reliability coefficients. Anastasi and Urbina (1997) note that the most common procedure for finding interitem consistency was developed by Kuder and Richardson (1937) and is known as *Kuder-Richardson Formula 20.* The formula for Kuder-Richardson 20, provided by Anastasi and Urbina (1997) is:

$$r_{tt} = (n / n - 1)\,(SD_t^2 - \textstyle\sum pq) / SD_t^2$$

where r_{tt} is the reliability of the whole test, n is the number of items in the test, and SD_t is the standard deviation of total scores on the test. The value, $\sum pq$, is found by multiplying the number of persons who pass each item (p) multiplied by the number who fail each item (q) summing these item products over all items to give $\sum pq$. Anastasi and Urbina (1997) note that since p for each item is often recorded during test development to find the difficulty level of each item, the Kuder-Richardson Formula 20 involves little additional computation. They also report that Cronbach (1951) demonstrated mathematically that the Kuder-Richardson reliability coefficient is actually the mean of all split-half coefficients resulting from different splittings of a test.

Dick and Haggerty (1971) discuss an alternate to Kuder-Richardson Formula 20: *Kuder-Richardson 21,* which can substitute for Formula 20 when individual item statistics are unavailable. This formula is:

$$r_{tt} = (n / n - 1) / (SD_t^2 - np_{av}q_{av}) / SD_t^2$$

where p_{av} is the mean difficulty level (ratio of total test mean to the total number of test items) and q_{av} is $1 - p_{av}$. Dick and Haggerty note that Kuder-Richardson 21 yields a lower-bound estimate of internal consistency, i.e., a conservative or low estimate of test reliability.

A more general internal consistency formula is coefficient alpha (α; Cronbach, 1951). This is presented in Anastasi and Urbina (1997) as $\alpha = (n / n - 1) (SD_t^2 - \sum (SD_i^2) / SD_t^2$, where SD_i^2 is the sum of the variances of item scores, replacing $\sum pq$. Cronbach (1990) notes that what testers call α statisticians refer to as an *intraclass correlation*.

Although internal consistency reliabilities are not typically thought of as providing evidence of validity, there are times when validity is also addressed by demonstration of internal consistency, particularly when the test contains an apparently heterogeneous set of items. An example of this is the investigation by Butcher, Arbisi, Atlis, and McNulty (2003) of the MMPI-2 Symptom Validity Scale (FBS; Lees-Haley, English, & Glenn, 1991). These authors noted the original heterogeneous nature of the scale, designed to capture both faking good and faking bad self-report characteristics of personal injury malingerers (cf. Lees-Haley et al., 1991). Butcher et al. computed Cronbach's α for the FBS for a variety of subject groups, including psychiatric patients, medical patients, chronic pain, and forensic samples of personal injury litigants and correctional facility inmates. Excluding the personal injury sample, Cronbach's α ranged from a low of .47 for chronic pain patients to a high of .64 for psychiatric inpatients, reflecting the heterogeneous nature of the items comprising FBS. By contrast, Cronbach's α for the personal injury sample was substantially higher, .85, providing supporting evidence for the original test development strategy of Lees-Haley et al. (1991) that emphasized a hybrid pattern of personal injury exaggeration, mixing fake good and fake bad self-report.

Reliability is an important property of psychometric tests, for it places an upper limit on the validity of a test that cannot exceed the square root of the reliability of the test (Dick & Haggerty, 1971). Thus, for a test with a reliability of .81, the validity coefficient cannot exceed .90. Reliability is also directly related to the measurement error of a test.

The standard error of measurement (SEM) is equal to $SD_t\sqrt{1 - r_{tt}}$, where r_{tt} is the reliability of the test, and SD_t is the standard deviation of the test. The SEM is informative for interpretation of test scores, since tests are always less than perfectly reliable. Consequently, several different examinations of the same person would yield a normal distribution of performance, with the mean of this distribution likely representing an individual's true score. Like any other standard deviation, the SEM can be interpreted relative to the standard normal distribution, such that +/− 1 SEM would encompass approximately 68% of the distribution. For example, using Trail Making B, the Heaton et al. (2004) T score normative data (mean = 50, SD = 10), and the .769 reliability for Trail Making B reported by Calamia et al. (2013), for an individual who obtains a T score of exactly 50 on Trail Making B, representing her or his true score, actual obtained scores will fluctuate +/− 1 SEM, $10\sqrt{1 - .769}$, or +/− 4.81, 68% of the time.

Measurement error also impacts comparisons of score differences between two different tests. The standard error of the difference between two scores is $SE_{diff} = \sqrt{(SEM_1)^2 + (SEM_2)^2}$. Since $SEM_1^2 = SD\sqrt{1 - r_{11}}$, and $SEM_2^2 = SD\sqrt{1 - r_{22}}$, the formula can be rewritten to: $SE_{diff} = SD\sqrt{2 - r_{11} - r_{22}}$ (see Anastasi & Urbina, 1997). So, if the SE_{diff} for a comparison of two scores equals five T score points, for a score difference to be significant, $p = .05$ two-tail (nondirectionally), it must exceed (5)(1.96) or +/− 9.8 T score points.

Most modern test manuals contain not only data on test reliability, but also data on the SEMs of tests such as the WAIS-IV (Wechsler, 2008), and Wechsler Memory Scale IV (Wechsler, 2009). These manuals also contain data on the frequency of normative subjects who obtain various differences between test scores from different domains of performance, for example, Table B-11 of the Wechsler Memory Scale–IV (WMS-IV) manual shows the percentage of the theoretically normal distribution (base rates) of varying magnitudes of difference scores between the WAIS-IV General Ability Index (GAI) and various WMS-IV Indexes. It is noteworthy to compare the values in Table B-11, representing the actual frequency distribution of difference scores, to the data presented in Table B-10, which displays the values needed to obtain a significant difference between the WAIS-IV GAI and the WMS-IV Indexes. Take the comparison of the WMS-IV Auditory Memory Index, for example, which in Table B-10 shows a difference of 10.95 is needed to reach the .01 level of significance using the formula for the SEM for comparison of two difference scores. By contrast, Table B-11 shows that a WAIS-IV GAI minus WMS-IVAMI difference of 10 points occurs in 19% of theoretically normal subjects, and that a person must achieve a WAIS-IVGAI minus WMS-IVAMI difference of 34 points for this to occur in the bottom 1% of the normal population.

This apparent discrepancy is best understood by returning to classic test theory, which considers test scores as being comprised of both true score variance and error. The data in B-10 reflect the effects of measurement error alone, whereas the base rate data in Table B-11 reflect both true score variance (variability of the abilities of individual subjects) and error effects, for the difference scores reported. It is this author's opinion that the more informative data are those presented in tables reflecting the actual base rate of test score differences, such as contrasts between the GAI and AMI, rather than relying upon the statistical significance of this contrast as related to the combined measurement error of the two tests.

Since a common use of neuropsychological testing is to evaluate change over time, either in someone who is recovering from a cerebral insult, such as severe traumatic brain injury (TBI), or to monitor the deterioration over time that can occur with a dementing condition, it is important to understand the statistical and measurement issues attendant to evaluating change scores. Jacobson and Truax (1991) have proposed a reliable change index (RC) for determination of change in performance from Time 1 (x_1, baseline) to Time 2 (x_2, follow-up), which is divided by the standard error of the difference (SE_{diff}). SE_{diff} is defined as $\surd 2(SEM)^2$. SEM is defined as $SD\surd 1 - r_{xx,}$ with r_{xx} representing the reliability of the test used as the baseline and follow-up measure; so, RC = $x_2 - x_1 / \surd 2(SEM)^2$. If this value exceeds a z value of 1.98, it represents a reliable (significant) change (note that this formula is a variation of the formula for determining whether differing scores on two *different* tests, such as WAIS-IV GAI and WMS-IV AMI represent a reliable difference; in the case of RC, the change being compared is based on a second administration of the *same* test).

Chelune, Naugle, Luders, Sedlak, and Awad (1993) proposed a modification to the RC index of Jacobson and Truax (1991), taking into account the average practice effect that occurs on neuropsychological tests that are repeated. Chelune et al. determined practice effect size by repeat assessment of seizure disorder patients undergoing medical management of their seizures, with both the WAIS-R and WMS-R. They then used this practice effect information and the RC index for determination of significant change in seizure patients undergoing either left or right temporal lobectomy, finding better detection of change when the average practice effect was included in the RC formula. In Chelune et al.'s modification, the average practice effect is subtracted from the score difference in the numerator of the Jacobson and Truax formula, so that RC = $x_2 - x_1 - pe_{avg} / \surd 2\,(SEM)^2$, where pe_{avg} is the mean practice effect.

McSweeney, Naugle, Chelune, and Luders (1993) have taken an alternative approach for detection of change on repeat assessments. Using expanded samples of the seizure patients studied by Chelune et al., they determined T scores for change based on regression equations that utilized baseline performance on the WAIS-R or WMS-R, to predict follow-up performance on these measures, using the medically treated but nonoperated seizure patients for determination of the T scores. Simply, the equation becomes $y_p = \beta x + c$, where y_p is the predicted score on follow-up, β is the slope of the regression equation, x is the baseline score, and c is the regression constant. Predicted scores are then converted to T scores for change, with $T = 50 + [10\,(y_o - y_p) / SE_{est}]$. In this equation, y_o is the observed score on retest, y_p is the predicted score, and SE_{est} is the standard error of estimate. Better characterization of change over time was obtained using the regression estimated T scores for change, than using the unadjusted WAIS-R and WMS-R scores alone. In this regression procedure, SE_{est} replaces SEM and SE_{diff}, but returning to classical test theory, the scores entered into the regression equation include both true score and error score variance, so these factors are implicitly present in the model. Moreover, the regression approach also takes into account regression to the mean, an important factor in considering change scores for persons whose baseline performance is extreme relative to the mean score; scores at the extreme have greater regression effects than those closer to the mean.

Duff (2012) provides a comprehensive review of the evaluation of change scores in neuropsychological assessment, including RCI, RCI adjusted for practice effect, and both simple and complex regression equations for estimation of change. RCI proved inferior to both RCI adjusted for practice effect and regression-based approaches, which did not differ substantially from one another.

Validity, or Does the Test Measure What It Is Intended to Measure?

Generally defined, *validity* characterizes the scientific utility of a measuring instrument, in terms of how well it measures what it purports to measure (Nunnally & Bernstein, 1994). There are three main types of validity: content validity, criterion or predictive validity, and construct validity (Anastasi & Urbina, 1997; Cronbach, 1990; Nunnally & Bernstein, 1994). Content validity refers to how well the test that has been constructed was sampled from the items relevant to performance on that test; for example, did the Wide Range Achievement Test-IV (WRAT-IV) Arithmetic subtest adequately sample the domain of basic calculational ability? Criterion validity refers to how well the test predicts some external criterion, either at or near the same time the test is administered (concurrent validity, e.g., how well does the test predict ability to drive a car) or at some point in the future (predictive validity, e.g., how well does this test predict future development of dementia).

Construct validity is a more abstract concept. Cronbach and Meehl (1955) define a *construct* as some postulated attribute of people, assumed to be reflected in test performance. Anastasi and Urbina (1997) define the construct validity of a test as the extent to which the test may be said to measure a theoretical construct or trait. Neuropsychologically relevant examples of constructs include working memory, processing speed, verbal learning and memory, etc. Construct validity can be tested various ways: for example, comparison of groups that are expected to show low levels of a particular attribute in the context of evidence for preserved ability on unrelated attributes, such as persons behaviorally identified as amnestic scoring poorly on a verbal memory test, but normally on measures of intelligence and working memory. Correlational methods are also appropriate for the investigation of construct validity. Campbell and Fiske (1959) argued that construct validity is established not only by showing the relationship of measures of a construct to other measures of the same construct, but also by showing no relationship with measures not related to the construct—in other words, showing both convergent and discriminant validity. They proposed a method for analysis of construct validity by use of a multitrait–multimethod matrix of correlations. Another common way to evaluate the construct validity of a test is to factor analyze a data set containing the test and other tests that define the purported construct the test is hypothesized to measure, as well as tests unrelated to the purported construct, again, addressing both convergent and discriminant validity. (e.g., memory tests should load on a memory factor, but not on a factor defined by measures of intelligence and problem solving).

The remaining discussion of neuropsychological test validity draws heavily from a recent paper that presents a framework for developing a core neuropsychological test battery (Larrabee, 2014). This framework recommends reviewing previously conducted factor analyses to identify a core set of neuropsychological domains of performance, thereby determining the construct validity of test procedures. The patient groups recommended for investigating criterion validity include moderate and severe TBI, Alzheimer-type dementia, and unilateral left and right hemisphere stroke. Analysis of test performance in the TBI and Alzheimer groups can be used to address different criteria including sensitivity to the presence of neurological trauma or disease, identification of those tests most sensitive to the severity of cerebral injury or disease, and identification of those tests that are the best predictors of activities of daily living, including financial competency, ability to drive a motor vehicle, and ability to work. The unilateral left and right hemisphere groups can be used to evaluate the best procedures for identification of lateralized neuropsychological impairment, as well as for evaluation of the moderating effects of language comprehension impairment in left hemisphere stroke and neglect in right hemisphere stroke on specific neuropsychological abilities. Finally, as part of the validity section of this chapter, I will describe a hypothetical core neuropsychological battery based on these various aspects of test validity that I have proposed (Larrabee, 2014), which also incorporates embedded/derived measures of performance validity (a topic discussed in detail in Dr. Boone's chapter in the current volume).

Factor Analyses of Neuropsychological Tests

Factor analysis is frequently used to determine the construct validity of neuropsychological test procedures (Delis, Jacobson, Bondi, Hamilton, & Salmon, 2003; Floyd & Widaman, 1995; Larrabee, 2003a). Factor analysis can be used to summarize patterns of correlations among observed variables, reduce a larger number of observed variables into a smaller number of factors, provide an operational definition for an underlying process (e.g., memory) by using observed variables (i.e., memory test scores), and test a theory about the nature of underlying processes (Floyd & Widaman, 1995; Tabachnick & Fidell, 2005). A basic assumption is that tests loading on a particular factor (i.e., correlated with that factor) are explained by the underlying factor. For example, if a test is truly a measure of the construct of verbal memory, then it should load primarily on a factor defined by other tests known to be measures of verbal memory; conversely, the test should not show primary loadings on either a verbal symbolic factor or working memory factor, otherwise the purported verbal memory test is nothing more than another way of measuring verbal symbolic abilities or working memory.

As I have described in another paper (Larrabee, 2014), factor analyses of neuropsychological test batteries (Holdnack, Zhou, Larrabee, Millis, & Salthouse, 2011; Larrabee, 2000; Larrabee & Curtiss, 1992, 1995; Leonberger, Nicks, Larrabee, & Goldfader, 1992; Tulsky & Price, 2003) generally define six domains of function:

1. *Verbal symbolic abilities* including measures of word definition, word knowledge, and general facts such as measured by the WAIS-IV Vocabulary subtest, Similarities and Information subtests (Wechsler, 2008), and measures of word-finding ability such as Controlled Oral Word Association (COWA), and the Benton Visual Naming test (Benton, Hamsher, & Sivan, 1994). Also loading on this factor are measures of academic achievement such as the Wide Range Achievement Test–Revised (Jastak & Wilkinson, 1984) Arithmetic, Spelling and Reading, subtests (Greenaway, Smith, Tangalos, Geda, & Ivnik, 2009; Larrabee, 2000; Larrabee & Curtiss, 1992).
2. *Visuoperceptual and visuospatial judgment and problem solving abilities* including measures such as Visual Form Discrimination, Facial Recognition, and Line Orientation, (Benton et al., 1994; Greenaway et al., 2009; Larrabee, 2000; Larrabee & Curtiss, 1992). This factor also includes the subtests defining the Perceptual Reasoning Index of the WAIS-IV, including Visual Puzzles, Block Design, and Matrix Reasoning (Wechsler, 2008).
3. *Sensorimotor function* includes procedures such as Finger Tapping, Grip Strength, Purdue Pegboard, Grooved Pegboard, and Benton Finger Localization and Tactile Form Perception. There are very few factor analyses of these tests in the context of a larger set of nonsensorimotor neuropsychological procedures. Curtiss and I have reported loadings of Grooved Pegboard and Purdue Pegboard on a

visuoperceptual visuospatial factor, along with Benton Tactile Form Perception and WAIS-R Performance IQ subtests such as Block Design and Object Assembly, with a separate motor factor on which Finger Tapping and Grip Strength loaded (Larrabee & Curtiss, 1992; see Larrabee, 2000). In another investigation, Finger Tapping loaded with processing speed measures such as Trail Making B and Digit Symbol (Leonberger et al., 1992; also see Larrabee, 2000). Carroll (1993) has also reported loadings of sensorimotor variables on a psychomotor ability factor.

4 *Attention/working memory* includes the subtests comprising the Working Memory Index for the WAIS-IV (Wechsler, 2008) and WMS-IV (Wechsler, 2009) including Digit Span, Arithmetic, Letter-Number Sequencing, and Symbol Span (Holdnack et al., 2011). This dimension also includes measures such as the Paced Auditory Serial Addition Test (PASAT), which measures both processing speed and working memory (Larrabee & Curtiss, 1992; 1995; also see Larrabee, 2000). WAIS-IV Arithmetic, which loads primarily on a working memory factor, has a secondary loading on the *verbal symbolic* factor (Holdnack et al., 2011).

5 *Processing speed* includes measures such as Coding and Symbol Search, which comprise the WAIS-IV Processing Speed Index (Holdnack et al., 2011). Also included in this domain is the TMT (Reitan & Wolfson, 1993; Larrabee & Curtiss, 1992, see Larrabee, 2000; and Leonberger et al., 1992) and the PASAT. The Stroop Test is also considered by Carroll (1993) as a measure of cognitive speed. Controlled Oral Word Association measures word-finding skills under time constraints and loaded equivalently on a *verbal symbolic* factor and on a *processing speed* factor in one investigation (Larrabee & Curtiss, 1992; Larrabee, 2000).

6 *Learning and memory* tests can actually be divided into separate domains of *verbal learning and memory*, and *visual learning and memory. Verbal learning and memory* tests include three basic paradigms: text recall, paired associate learning, and supraspan list learning tasks. Exemplars of the text recall and paired associate paradigms include WMS-IV Logical Memory and Verbal Paired Associates. Tests of supraspan list learning include the CVLT-II (Delis et al. 2000), the Rey AVLT (Rey, 1964; Schmidt, 1996), and the Verbal Selective Reminding Test (VSRT, Buschke, 1973; Larrabee, Trahan, Curtiss, & Levin, 1988). *Visual learning and memory* tests usually include measures of design reproduction from memory such as the BVRT (Sivan, 1992), WMS-IV Visual Reproduction, or the CFT (Meyers & Meyers, 1995; Rey, 1941). Visual learning and memory tests also include recognition memory measures such as the Continuous Visual Memory Test (CVMT; Trahan & Larrabee, 1988), and the Faces subtest of the Recognition Memory Test (Warrington, 1984). On the one hand, factor analysis has shown that immediate design reproduction from memory is more closely associated with visuospatial/constructional tasks such as Block Design and Object Assembly, but that the delayed reproduction task causes a shift in loadings so that the stronger association is with memory, with a secondary association with visuospatial/constructional skills (Larrabee & Curtiss, 1995; Larrabee, Kane, Schuck & Francis, 1985). On the other hand, recognition memory tests such as the Continuous Recognition Memory test (CRM) for detection of recurring familiar figures such as insects and seashells (Hannay, Levin, & Grossman, 1979) show primary loadings with a memory factor for both the learning trials as well as for the delayed recognition trial (Larrabee & Curtiss, 1995). These data suggest that use of delayed reproduction attenuates the spatial/constructional confound inherent in assessing visual memory by having someone draw designs from memory. Visual recognition memory tasks appear to be purer measures of visual memory, from a factor analytic perspective.

Exceptions to the above six factors have been reported. A combined general memory factor, rather than separate verbal and visual learning and memory factors, has been reported using confirmatory factor analysis of WAIS-IV and WMS-IV subtests, including a hierarchical general ability factor in the model (Holdnack et. al., 2011). Confirmatory factor analysis also provides evidence supporting separate verbal and visual memory factors, rather than a combined factor, when a hierarchical model is not specified and the factors are allowed to correlate with one another (Holdnack et al., 2011). In one investigation, academic achievement measures such as the Wide Range Achievement Test–Revised (Jastak & Wilkinson, 1984) demonstrated primary loadings for Reading, Spelling, and Arithmetic on a *verbal symbolic* factor, with secondary loadings on a factor defined by measures of processing speed, attention and working memory including Wechsler Memory Scale Mental Control, TMT–B, and the PASAT (Larrabee & Curtiss, 1992; see Larrabee, 2000). Tests described as measures of *executive function* (Lezak, Howieson, Bigler, & Tranel, 2012) typically show loadings on factors of *processing speed* (TMT–B; COWA), *working memory* (Letter-Number Sequencing), or *visuoperceptual and visuospatial judgment and problem solving ability* (Category Test; WCST; see Larrabee, 2000; Leonberger et al., 1992), rather than on an *executive function* factor. Others have also found relationships between tests of executive function and tests of problem solving, general intelligence, and processing speed (Barbey, Colom, & Grafman, 2013; Keifer & Tranel, 2013; Salthouse, 2005). Last, the factor structure of collections of neuropsychological tests appears to be relatively invariant of age over the adult years (Crook & Larrabee, 1988; Larrabee & Curtiss, 1995; Wechsler, 2008), demonstrating that the same constructs are identified over the adult age range.

Criterion Validity

The original primary criterion for neuropsychological tests was sensitivity to the presence of brain damage or dysfunction, which was generally characterized by composing a sample of patients with a variety of different neurological disorders. In other words, "brain damage" was considered to be a *unitary* (present vs. absent) or *unidimensional* (more of or less of) construct. Early test batteries reinforced this assumed criterion by utilizing global impairment scores such as the Halstead Impairment Index, which used a cutting score to define presence or absence of brain damage (Reitan & Wolfson, 1993). Of course, this did not restrict further analysis of test data—for example, the analyses recommended by Reitan (1974) to include consideration of level of impairment, evaluation for pathognomonic signs, analysis of differential scores or patterns of ability, and comparisons of the functional efficiency of both sides of the body. Early investigations also compared the neuropsychological test performance of groups of subjects with diffuse, or left or right hemisphere damage (Russell, Neuringer, & Goldstein, 1970; Spreen & Benton, 1965). These groups, however, were comprised of subjects who had varying etiologies for their diffuse or lateralized brain damage with some cases likely including subjects who had both diffuse and lateralized damage, e.g., lateralized contusion or hematoma superimposed upon diffuse damage following severe TBI.

To better evaluate these original criteria for validity, as well as criteria that have evolved over time, it is helpful to use effect size analysis. The *standardized mean effect size,* generally defined, refers to the difference, in standard deviation units, between the mean performance of two groups on some dependent measure (Cohen, 1988). Typically, the standard deviation for this contrast is the pooled standard deviation of the control group and comparison group (Borenstein, Hedges, Higgins, & Rothstein, 2009), and the letter d is typically used to represent this effect size. The larger the effect size, the greater the separation of the test performance of the two comparison groups. Cohen (Table 2.2.1, p. 22, 1988) has provided percent nonoverlap for various magnitudes of d. Zakzanis, Leach, and Kaplan (Table 2.1, p. 13, 1999) have reported the percent of overlap as a function of the magnitude of d. For example, for a d of 1.0, the overlap percent is 44.6%, dropping to 18.9% for a d of 2.0, and 7.2% for a d of 3.0. As can be seen, the larger the value of d, the smaller the overlap percent, and the smaller the diagnostic error for both false positives and false negatives, resulting in an increase in both sensitivity (true positives) and specificity (true negatives).

The effect size is also related to the area under the receiver operating characteristic (ROC) curve. The ROC is derived by plotting the false positive error rate (1.0 − specificity) on the x-axis and the true positive rate (sensitivity) on the y-axis for each potential cutting score comparing two groups on a diagnostic test (Hsaio, Bartko, & Potter, 1989; Swets, 1973). In ROC analysis, perfect discrimination is achieved at an area under curve (AUC) of 1.00, with chance discrimination falling at an AUC of .50, represented as the diagonal line traversing from zero false positive rate, and zero sensitivity, to perfect sensitivity and 100% false positives. AUC represents the probability of correctly classifying a randomly selected individual with the condition of interest as well as correctly classifying a randomly selected individual without the condition of interest. AUC of 0.7 to 0.8 have been characterized as acceptable, 0.8 to 0.9 as excellent, and 0.9 or more as outstanding (Hosmer & Lemeshow, 2000). When the distributions for the false positive errors and sensitivity each are normally distributed, there is a 1:1 correspondence between ROC AUC and the effect size, d (Rice & Harris, 2005). Thus, in studies where the effect size alone is either reported or calculable from the data presented, the effect size can serve as a proxy for the ROC AUC. In investigations where ROC AUC and the effect size are both reported, ROC AUC provides a more accurate quantification of diagnostic accuracy, as it encompasses the entire range of test scores for the two groups being compared (i.e., those with and those without the condition of interest).

ROC AUC can be used to compare the diagnostic accuracy of single tests, as well as of multiple measures utilizing the logit obtained from logistic regression analysis. Greve, Ord, Curtis, Bianchini, and Brennan (2008) demonstrated equal ROC AUCs for the Portland Digit Recognition Test, Test of Memory Malingering, and Word Memory Test, for discriminating nonmalingering patients with either TBI or chronic pain, from litigants characterized as malingering cognitive impairment of TBI or chronic pain. Loring et al. (2008) found a Cohen's d of .47 for the Rey AVLT (Rey, 1964) scores of right vs. left temporal lobe epilepsy, which was substantially higher than the d of 0.29 for the same comparison employing the CVLT (Delis, Kramer, Kaplan, & Ober, 1987). Comparing the performance of right versus left temporal lobe epilepsy groups on the BNT (Kaplan, Goodglass, & Weintraub, 1983) yielded a Cohen's d of 0.56, compared to a Cohen's d of 0.36 for the Benton Visual Naming Test (Benton, Hamsher, & Sivan, 1994). Colleagues and I reported a slightly greater ROC AUC derived from logistic regression for an ability-focused neuropsychological battery than for the primary HRB subtests in discriminating brain-injured patients from a pseudoneurologic control sample (Larrabee, Millis, & Meyers, 2008).

Loring and I (Loring & Larrabee, 2006) used Reitan's original validation data to derive effect sizes for contrasts of brain-impaired and nonimpaired subjects for subtests of the Wechsler–Bellevue. In some cases these effect sizes surpassed those of subtests comprising the HRB, although the HRB did show the largest effect sizes overall. In the same paper, we reviewed subsequent publications that used the WAIS (Vega & Parsons, 1967; Kane, Parsons, & Goldstein, 1985) or WAIS-R (Sherer, Scott, Parsons, & Adams, 1994) that showed equal or superior effect sizes for the Wechsler scales in comparison to the HRB. For example, Sherer et al. found that the Full Scale IQ effect size, d = .92, was more than double that of the HRB Impairment Index, d = .43. Data analyzed from Kane et al. showed a WAIS Performance IQ (PIQ) effect size, d = 1.74, essentially equal to an HRB average T score, d = 1.63, and HRB Average Impairment Rating, d = 1.88. In a subsequent paper (Loring & Larrabee, 2008), we reported that the Verbal IQ (VIQ) effect size for the Kane et al. data, d = 2.40, was greater than any HRB effect size, as well as greater than the PIQ effect size.

As we emphasized (Loring & Larrabee, 2008), WAIS and HRB data that we reviewed show two interesting results. First, the similar and in some cases, greater effect sizes for the Wechsler scales versus the HRB in discriminating neurologically impaired from nonneurologically impaired subjects argues against the older notion that the HRB measures "biologic" intelligence whereas the Wechsler scales measure "psychometric" intelligence. These findings are best understood by the factor analyses of the WAIS-R, WMS-R, and HRB conducted by Leonberger et al. (1992), which showed that the HRB subtests loaded on the same factors as the subtests comprising the WAIS-R. The TPT and Category Test loaded on the same factor as the Picture Completion, Picture Arrangement, Block Design, and Object Assembly subtests. The Seashore Rhythm and Speech Sounds Perception tests loaded on the same factor as WAIS-R Arithmetic and WMS-R Digit Span and Mental Control. TMT–B split loadings between a perceptual organization factor and a processing speed factor, with Digit Symbol showing the same split in loadings, and Finger Tapping loading on the processing speed factor alone. Second, these data underscore that brain damage or dysfunction is not a unitary or unidimensional construct, otherwise why would WAIS VIQ show the largest effect size in the Kane et al. (1985) investigation, in comparison to PIQ and the HRB average impairment rating, and why would Sherer et al. (1994) find a PIQ effect size one-half of that reported by Kane et al., but double that found for the HRB Impairment Index in their own study?

Over the years, it has become obvious that "brain damage" is not a unitary or unidimensional construct, and in modern neuropsychology, the criterion is typically presence or absence of a particular *type* of brain dysfunction, and its differential impact on key neuropsychological abilities. For example, Zakzanis, Leach, and Kaplan (1999), reported larger effect sizes for measures of delayed recall for Alzheimer's and depression, relative to other neuropsychological abilities. For subjects with Alzheimer's disease, the delayed recall effect of 3.23 was nearly four times the effect of manual dexterity, 0.85, but in subjects who had Parkinson's disease with dementia, the delayed recall effect size of 1.82 was less than the manual dexterity effect of 2.42, consistent with the primary effects of this disease on motor functions. These data show how different disorders differentially impact performance in the major domains of neuropsychological abilities.

The most commonly seen disorders include those resulting from TBI, stroke, and dementia (Lezak et al., 2012). TBI and dementia allow for analysis of the effects of diffuse brain dysfunction on neuropsychological domains of ability. TBI and dementia also allow for analysis of change in neuropsychological abilities over time, that is, recovery over time in moderate or severe TBI, and deterioration over time in dementia. Stroke allows for analysis of the effects of unilateral hemispheric dysfunction on both lateralized cognitive abilities, as well as on sensorimotor skills.

Certain modifiers of criterion validity are also important to consider, such as disease severity, and presence/absence of language comprehension impairment in left hemisphere stroke, and presence/absence of neglect in right hemisphere stroke. Tests that are sensitive to presence/absence of disease may not be the same tests that are sensitive to severity of disease in either TBI or dementia, nor may such tests show sensitivity to the everyday functional consequences of a particular disorder such as Alzheimer's disease. On the one hand, failure of a task such as WAIS-III Block Design may represent a visuospatial problem solving deficit in a person with a right hemisphere stroke. On the other hand, patients with left hemisphere stroke may perform poorly on Block Design due to the effects of language comprehension impairment and disrupted verbal symbolic processes (employed by these subjects for problem solution, even on "nonverbal" tasks), rather than represent a purely visuospatial impairment.

In TBI, persisting impairments at one-year postinjury are not typically found, until the initial time to follow commands is between 1 to 24 hours (one hour to 24 hours of coma, Dikmen, Machamer, Winn, & Temkin, 1995). The only measures in a comprehensive neuropsychological battery that were sensitive to persistent deficit in this injury severity group were Verbal Selective Reminding (Buschke, 1973; Larrabee et al., 1988), a sensitive measure of verbal supraspan learning, and TMT–B (Reitan & Wolfson, 1993), a measure of psychomotor speed and set shifting. Additionally, the effect size for Verbal Selective Reminding, .46, was three times the effect size for TMT–B, 0.15, reflecting greater sensitivity of verbal memory than processing speed (Dikmen et al., 1995). Neuropsychological effects are clearly related to severity of TBI, as defined by time to follow commands, and using an overall test battery mean represented as an average z score (Dikmen et al., 1995; Rohling, Meyers, & Millis, 2003). In TBI, effect size for neuropsychological performance at one year posttrauma was $d = -0.02$ for time to follow commands (TFC) of < one hour contrasted with the performance of an orthopedic trauma control group, increasing linearly to $d = -0.22$ for 1–23 hours TFC, $d = -0.45$ for 1–6 days TFC, $d = -0.68$ for 7–13 days TFC,

$d = -1.33$ for 14–28 days TFC, and $d = -2.31$ for > 28 days TFC (Rohling et al., 2003). The most severely injured group, which took more than one month to follow commands, produced an effect size of $d = -2.31$, more than two standard deviations worse than the least severely injured group, whose performance was basically identical to that of orthopedic trauma controls, with $d = -0.02$.

Similar results showing sensitivity of processing speed and memory to acquired deficits related to moderate and severe TBI have been reported for the WAIS-IV and WMS-IV (Wechsler, 2009). The WAIS-IV and WMS-IV index scores most sensitive to discriminating moderate to severe TBI subjects from demographically matched controls were Processing Speed ($d = 1.32$) and all three WMS-IV primary indices (Auditory Memory Index, $d = 1.25$; Visual Memory Index, $d = 1.07$, and Visual Working Memory Index, $d = 1.26$).

Complimentary results have been reported by Miller, Fichtenberg, and Millis (2010), who evaluated the diagnostic discrimination of a group of subjects with mild, moderate, and severe TBI, as well as other neurologic disorders, from subjects who had cognitive complaints but no evidence for acquired neurological dysfunction (a "pseudoneurologic" control group). Miller et al. used an ability-focused battery covering five domains: language/verbal reasoning, visual-spatial reasoning, attention, processing speed and memory, using WAIS-III domain scores and select measures of neuropsychological function such as the CVLT-2, and TMT. ROC AUC was .89 based on the five domains, and .88 based on an average of the five domain scores. Based on processing speed and memory alone, the ROC AUC was .90.

In a neurological group that was comprised primarily of TBI and seizure disorder patients, performance on the AVLT Trial V (Rey, 1964; Lezak et al., 2012) was more sensitive to discriminating the neurologic group from a normal control group, than any other measure of performance, including tasks of verbal cognitive function, visual cognitive function, processing speed, attention/working memory, and visual memory function (Powell, Cripe, & Dodrill, 1991).

These data demonstrate that measures of verbal supraspan learning and processing speed are the most sensitive neuropsychological tests for detection of residual cognitive impairment following TBI. Effects of Alzheimer-type dementia also impact memory functioning and processing speed.

In Alzheimer's disease (AD), the tests that are typically most sensitive to discriminating patients with AD from normal elderly are those measuring learning and memory, particularly tests involving a delayed recall trial (Larrabee, Largen, & Levin, 1985; Welsh et al., 1994; Zakzanis et al., 1999). On the WMS-IV (Wechsler, 2009), effect sizes for Auditory Memory ($d = 2.24$) and Visual Memory ($d = 2.00$) are substantial, with greater differences for delayed recall ($d = 2.39$) than immediate recall ($d = 2.16$), accompanied by effect sizes of similar magnitude for processing speed ($d = 2.25$). Colleagues and I found a large effect size for WAIS Digit Symbol, $d = 1.57$, which was eclipsed by the effect size for Verbal Selective Reminding of $d = 2.53$ for words in consistent long-term retrieval, and $d = 3.41$ for total words recalled (Larrabee et al., 1985).

Despite the sensitivity of memory tests to detection of cognitive impairment associated with AD in Larrabee et al. (1985), memory tests were not sensitive to severity of the disorder. In particular, we found that Verbal Selective Reminding, the most sensitive measure discriminating AD from normal elderly, did not correlate at all with severity of AD. By contrast, WAIS Information and Digit Symbol reflected significant correlation with disease severity, as measured by the Clinical Dementia Rating Scale (CDR; Hughes, Berg, Danziger, Coben, & Martin. 1982), or functional impairment, as measured by the Blessed, Tomlinson, and Roth (1968) dementia rating scale. Similarly, Griffith et al. (2006) found that subjects with Mild Cognitive Impairment (MCI), many of whom are likely in the beginning stages of AD, were discriminated from normal controls by the Hopkins Verbal Learning Test (HVLT; Brandt, 1991; $d = 1.50$), but the HVLT did not discriminate MCI from AD ($d = 0.06$); rather, it was semantic fluency that discriminated AD and MCI ($d = 0.71$).

Studies of patients experiencing unilateral stroke allow not only for comparisons of the effects of lateralized brain insult on the six domains of function previously reviewed, but also allow for analysis of the moderating effects of conditions common to lateralized stroke. This includes analysis of the effects of auditory comprehension impairment consequent to aphasia following left-hemisphere stroke, and hemispatial neglect, which is common following right-hemisphere stroke.

Benton et al. (1994) have analyzed performance on a variety of visuoperceptual and visuospatial tasks in relation to language comprehension impairment, and visual field defect. Performance on Facial Recognition, a task requiring the subject to match a black-and-white photograph of an unfamiliar person to photographs of the same person presented in different shading contrasts, is performed more poorly by patients with posterior right-hemisphere lesions (53% failure rate) than anterior right hemisphere lesions (26% failure rate). By contrast, Facial Recognition is passed by 100% of left-hemisphere stroke patients without aphasia (anterior and posterior), and 100% of left-hemisphere stroke patients with aphasia (anterior and posterior), but who have normal auditory comprehension. Before concluding that Facial Recognition performance can contribute to discrimination of lateralized brain dysfunction, however, it is important to note that 29% of anterior left-hemisphere stroke patients, and 44% of left-posterior stroke patients who have auditory comprehension impairment fail the Facial Recognition Test.

In an investigation of the effects of unilateral hemisphere damage on WAIS Verbal and Performance IQ, I found (Larrabee, 1986) that overall severity of language dysfunction in the group with left-hemisphere damage (LHD) was significantly correlated, at equal levels of magnitude, with WAIS Verbal IQ (−.77) and Performance IQ (−.74). Additionally, aphasia severity in the LHD group correlated significantly with a number of so-called nonverbal subtests, including Block Design (−.44) and Object Assembly (−.72).

These data demonstrate that aphasia, in particular when accompanied by auditory comprehension impairment, is a moderating variable for performance on visual cognitive tasks, and must be considered in interpretation of what has traditionally been thought of as "nonverbal" performance in aphasic patients (e.g., WAIS-IV Block Design, Visual Puzzles). Benton, Sivan, et al. (1994) provide data showing that performance on Judgment of Line Orientation does not seem to be affected by presence/absence of auditory comprehension impairment, making this task important for the differential diagnosis of cognitive impairment secondary to one versus multiple infarctions. Hamsher (1991) also reported that performance on measures of global stereopsis was not disrupted by auditory comprehension impairment.

Hemispatial neglect, or inattention to the left hemispace in a right-handed individual, modifies the neuropsychological effects of right-hemisphere disease. Hemispatial neglect is a cognitive rather than a purely sensory phenomenon in that the lesions producing this condition need not involve sensory projection systems or primary sensory cortex (Heilman, Watson, & Valenstein, 2012). Neglect represents a failure of directed attention. Patients with a visual field cut without neglect will move the to-be-perceived object so that it will fall in the preserved visual field, whereas patients with neglect do not compensate for the field cut. On the Facial Recognition Test, patients with posterior right hemisphere stroke and field cut had a 58% failure rate, whereas those without field cut had a 40% failure rate (Benton, Sivan et al., 1994; note this difference was not statistically significant, and the authors did not differentiate the field cut group as to which subjects had or did not have neglect). Indeed, Trahan (1997) found that in particular, patients with left visual neglect showed impaired performance on the Facial Recognition Test. On the Line Orientation Test there was a nonsignificant trend toward a higher frequency of failure in patients with field defects (Benton, Sivan, et al., 1994). Although Benton, Sivan, et al. (1994) did not analyze the effects of neglect on the Visual Form Discrimination test, they do point out that the use of peripheral figures in both the right and left hemispace allows for analysis of neglect in the individual case.

The presence of neglect in association with right-hemisphere injury may reflect a more generalized attentional impairment following right-hemisphere stroke. Trahan, Larrabee, Quintana, Goethe, and Willingham (1989) reported a 56% rate of impairment for acquisition, and 48% rate of impairment for delayed recall on the Expanded Paired Associate Test (EPAT; Trahan et al., 1989) for left-hemisphere stroke patients, which was approximately double the failure rate of patients who had right-hemisphere stroke (25% for acquisition, and 23% for delayed recall). Performance on WAIS-R Digit Span, a measure of attention and working memory, was related to EPAT performance for the right- but not the left-hemisphere stroke patients. This suggested that reduced attention may have contributed to poor EPAT test performance in the right hemisphere stroke group. Data were unavailable, however, to determine whether there was a higher rate of neglect in those right CVA patients with attentional impairment, who also performed poorly on the EPAT.

Criterion validity also is evaluated by correlation of neuropsychological performance with important activities of daily living such as working, driving a car, and making financial decisions. This has also been referred to as *ecologic validity*. Measures of working memory, processing speed, verbal fluency, visuospatial ability, and calculational skills appear to be particularly significant predictors of these activities of daily living.

Williams, Rapport, Hanks, Millis and Greene (2013) found that neuropsychological tests predicted outcome on the Disability Rating Scale, and return to work, independent of and in addition to predictions based on admission Glasgow Coma Scale, and presence of CT scan abnormalities. Particularly significant predictors were Trail Making A and B, Grooved Pegboard, the Symbol Digit Modalities test, and measures of visuospatial ability. Interestingly, verbal learning and memory skills measured by tests such as the AVLT or CVLT, were *not* sensitive predictors of important activities of daily living.

Driving ability has been correlated with performance on Trail Making B in patients who have suffered severe TBI (Novack et al., 2006), and in patients with questionable dementia (Whelihan, Dicarlo, & Paul, 2005). Rizzo and Kellison (2010) recommend that predictions of driving ability be made based on performance on raw scores that have not been demographically corrected for age and education, since what matters on the road is pure ability regardless of demographic characteristics.

Financial capacity in Alzheimer's disease was related to performance on a variety of neuropsychological tests measuring working memory and oral calculational abilities (Earnst et al., 2001). Digits Forward was related to understanding a bank statement, whereas Digits Reversed related to all four aspects of basic monetary skills. WAIS-III Letter-Number Sequencing related to several domains of monetary capacity. The Arithmetic subtest related to basic monetary skills, and checkbook and bank statement management (Earnst et al., 2001). Sherod et al. (2009) found that written arithmetic skill (WRAT-3, Wilkinson, 1993) predicted financial capacity for control subjects, those with mild Alzheimer-type dementia, and those with amnestic MCI.

Marson, Ingram, Cody, and Harrell (1995) found that capacity to make medical decisions was related to word fluency (Controlled Oral Word Association), but not to memory performance or overall severity of cognitive impairment, in patients with AD. This was despite significant differences in global cognitive function, and memory function, between patients with AD and normal controls. This result is strikingly similar to the findings of Larrabee et al. (1985); Griffith et al. (2006); and Earnst et al. (2001), showing that although memory tests are the most sensitive discriminators of AD and normal elderly, nonmemory cognitive skills, specifically, verbal symbolic abilities, are more sensitive to severity of dementia, and to accompanying impairments in activities of daily living.

A Hypothetical Ability-Focused Neuropsychological Battery

In Larrabee (2014) I proposed a hypothetical ability-focused neuropsychological battery based upon (a) factor analytic support for each test as measuring one of the six primary neuropsychological factors with (b) evidence showing sensitivity to presence of neuropsychological deficits, and/or (c) showing evidence of sensitivity to the severity of effects of a neurobehavioral disorder such as what occurs with moderate and severe TBI or AD, and/or (d) showing significant correlations with activities of daily living, and/or (e) containing an embedded/derived measure of performance validity. Choice of a particular test for inclusion in this battery would depend largely upon how many of these five criteria were met by the measure. Primary criterion groups would include moderate and severe TBI, probable AD, and left- and right-hemisphere stroke for analysis of lateralized neuropsychological deficits as well as for evaluation of moderating effects of language comprehension impairment in left-hemisphere stroke, and left unilateral neglect in right-hemisphere stroke.

With the exception of discussing tests of performance validity, I have reviewed much of the same validity literature in this chapter as I did in Larrabee (2014). The reader is referred to Boone (Chapter 4 in this volume) for in-depth discussion of embedded/derived measures of performance validity, and to Larrabee (2014) for more in-depth discussion of the framework for development of an ability-focused neuropsychological battery. I have previously made the distinction between performance validity tests (PVTs), which assess whether the examinee is providing an accurate measure of his or her actual ability, and symptom validity tests (SVTs), which assess whether an examinee is giving an accurate report of his or her actual symptom experience, as would be captured on omnibus personality inventory validity scales, pain scales, and scales assessing self-reported cognitive functions (Larrabee, 2012a). Embedded and derived PVTs typically capture extremely poor performance on simple motor skills, unrealistically low basic visual perceptual discrimination skills, extremely poor working memory, poor recognition compared to recall on memory testing procedures, and atypical errors on recognition memory scores and on problem solving tasks. In other words, performance is either atypically low/poor, or falls in a pattern that is atypical for what is seen in patients who have bona fide neuropsychological impairments from significant neurologic, developmental, or psychiatric disorders.

The hypothetical battery I proposed (Larrabee, 2014) included the following.

- *Verbal symbolic ability*: COWA, Animal Naming, WAIS-IV Information and Similarities, WRAT-IV Reading and Arithmetic
- *Visuoperceptual visuospatial judgment and problem solving ability*: Benton Visual Form Discrimination, WAIS-IV Block Design, Visual Puzzles, WCST
- *Sensorimotor skills*: Grip Strength, Finger Tapping, Grooved Pegboard
- *Attention/working memory*: WAIS-IV Digit Span, Arithmetic, Letter-Number Sequencing, WMS-IV Symbol Span
- P*rocessing speed*: TMT, WAIS-IV Symbol Search, Coding, and the Stroop
- *Learning and memory* (*verbal*): the AVLT, WMS-IV Logical Memory and Verbal Paired Associates
- *Learning and memory* (*visual*): WMS-IV Visual Reproduction, CVMT, CRM (Hannay et al., 1979)

This hypothetical ability-focused battery contains 27 measures (11 of which require 5 minutes or less to administer, with a total estimated time of administration of 4.5 hours). Additionally, this hypothetical core battery includes ten embedded and derived measures of performance validity based on the following tests: Visual Form Discrimination (Larrabee, 2003b), Finger Tapping (Arnold et al., 2005; Larrabee, 2003b), Logical Memory Recognition and Verbal Paired Associates Recognition (Pearson, 2009), AVLT (Barrash, Suhr, & Manzel, 2004; Boone, Lu, & Wen, 2005; Davis, Millis, & Axelrod, 2012), Visual Reproduction Recognition (Pearson, 2009), CVMT (Larrabee, 2009), CRMT (Hannay et al., 1979; Larrabee, 2009), WAIS-IV Digit Span (Jasinski, Berry, Shandera, and Clark, 2011), and the WCST (Greve, Heinly, Bianchini, & Love, 2009; Larrabee, 2003b).

This compares to 34 measures if one were to administer all of the tests comprising the Heaton et al. (2004) normative data (23), plus all of the WAIS-R subtests (11) in this database, and 36 tests if the entire Neuropsychological Assessment Battery (NAB; Stern & White, 2003) is administered. The Meyers Neuropsychological Battery (MNB; Meyers & Rohling, 2004) contains 22 measures, with 11 embedded and derived PVTs, but uses single tests to represent motor and tactile ability, verbal and visual memory. Additionally, tests were selected for the MNB based upon their discrimination of various neurological groups; i.e., sensitivity to presence of disorder. Test selection was not also based on sensitivity to severity of impairment, or prediction of activities of daily living.

Psychometric Issues Related to Interpretation of Test Scores

Neuropsychological test scores for test procedures falling in each of the domains of ability including *verbal symbolic, visuoperceptual visuospatial judgment and problem solving, sensorimotor, working memory, processing speed*, and *learning and memory*, are measures of human capabilities and vary as a function of several factors that are independent of brain dysfunction, psychiatric, or developmental disorders, including age, education, sex, and ethnicity (Heaton et al., 2004; Holdnack & Weiss, 2013). Consequently, these factors that are independent of disease or clinical disorders must be taken into consideration in demographic adjustments to raw test scores. Otherwise, one runs the risk of overidentifying impairment (elevated false positive rate) in persons with low premorbid ability, and underindentifying impairment (elevated false negative rate) in persons with high premorbid ability. Key demographic factors include age, which shows greatest impact (cross-sectionally) on measures of *verbal* and *visual learning and memory*, *processing speed*, and novel *visuoperceptual visuospatial problem-solving* skills such as the Category Test (Heaton et al., 2004; Larrabee, 2014); educational and occupational attainment, which are most-strongly associated with *verbal symbolic* and *attention/working memory* abilities (Heaton et al., 2004; Holdnack & Weiss, 2013; Larrabee, 2014); and sex, which is correlated with performance on *verbal learning and memory* measures such as the VSRT (Larrabee et al., 1988), and CVLT (Delis et al., 1987), as well as related to performance on measures of *sensorimotor* skills such as Finger Tapping and Grip Strength (Heaton et al., 2004). Holdnack and Weiss (2013) present case examples of how appropriate adjustment for demographic factors can alter findings in two clinical cases.

Demographic adjustments are typically done in one of two ways. The first is to simply aggregate normative (i.e., nonclinical) subjects into groups with similar demographics (e.g., adult males with less than high school education, in ten-year increments of age, with age groups repeated for males with high school education, etc., with the same done separately for females). Numerous examples of this type of normative process are reported in Strauss, Sherman, and Spreen (2006). A second major approach uses multiple regression to predict test scores by the relevant demographic characteristics, with norms based on the residuals that remain after adjustment for the demographic factors (e.g., Heaton et al., 2004; also see Mitrushina, Boone, Razani, & D'Elia, 2005, for a regression approach based on meta-analytically derived normative data).

A third way, at least for WAIS-IV scores, is to administer a measure of accuracy of sight reading, the Wechsler Test of Premorbid Function (TOPF; Pearson, 2009), which is used in conjunction with demographic factors to estimate premorbid level of function for the four WAIS-IV Index scores, and compare the examinee's current level of function to his or her premorbid estimates. This is based on the long-supported evidence that sight reading—in particular, sight reading of irregularly spelled words such as *corps*—is relatively preserved even in patients with disorders such as early stage Alzheimer-type dementia (Holdnack, Schoenberg, Lange, & Iverson, 2013; Pearson, 2009). Of course, one must compare current reading ability to demographically estimated level, to ensure that reading ability itself is not affected by suspected acquired impairment; if this is the case, prediction is recommended based on demographics alone (Pearson, 2009). This approach is best reserved for the WAIS-IV, as the premorbid estimates for the WMS-IV have relatively large errors of estimate, and there is only a predictive relationship when demographic factors are included with the TOPF; demographic factors alone (e.g., educational and occupational attainment) do not predict WMS-IV performance (Holdnack et al., 2013), with the obvious exception of age. Holdnack et al. (2013) also discuss use of the Oklahoma Premorbid Intelligence Estimate (OPIE), which includes current performance on WAIS-IV subtests, as well as demographic factors to predict premorbid level of function. Of course, this approach results in a contamination of predictor with criterion, in which subtests comprising Full Scale IQ are also used to predict IQ, referred to by Holdnack et al. as inflation of prediction due to auto-correlation of the test with itself.

Thus, someone using demographically corrected index scores for the WAIS-IV is already adjusting for premorbid level of function, in contrast to using unadjusted (with the exception of age) scores, in comparison to estimated premorbid level of function. An interesting comparison, which I do not think has been conducted, would be to see whether demographically corrected WAIS-IV index scores are comparable in sensitivity to mild Alzheimer-type dementia, contrasted with an approach using demographically uncorrected (with the exception of age-correction) scores which themselves are compared to TOPF-estimated premorbid level of function.

Some have recommended comparing current level of performance for all neuropsychological tests to estimated premorbid level of intellectual function (i.e., premorbid IQ; Tremont, Hoffman, Scott, & Adams, 1998; Miller & Rohling, 2001). This approach would be expected to work better, that is, be more accurate, for those abilities more closely associated with IQ, including *verbal symbolic ability* and *visuoperceptual visuospatial judgment and problem solving ability*, *working memory*, and *processing speed*. Such an approach would work less well with abilities such as memory, which are less strongly related to traditional IQ scores (Holdnack et al., 2013; Larrabee, 2000), but show their strongest associations with age (Larrabee, 2014).

Scores on individual tests that have been scored using the appropriate normative base are typically interpreted, on a test-by-test basis, in reference to their standing in comparison to the normative group, either relying upon z or T scores relative to the standard normal curve, or by percentile rank for test scores that do not follow a normal distribution. This interpretive approach is somewhat akin to that in clinical medicine in which ranges of performance for normal and abnormal results are described for various laboratory values (e.g., white blood cell count, hematocrit, etc.). In the case of neuropsychological test score interpretation, the focus is a deficit-based approach. Different authors have recommended different interpretive schemes. For example, Heaton et al. (2004) use a T score based approach (mean = 50, SD = 10) to define 55+ as *above average*, 45–54 as *average*, 40–44 as *below average*, 35–39 as *mild impairment*, 30–34 as *mild to moderate impairment*, 25–29 as *moderate impairment*, 20–24 *as moderate to severe impairment*, and 0–19 as *severe impairment*. Using a global composite score, the Average Impairment Rating, Heaton et al. (2004) reported that defining impairment as a cutting score of T < 40 correctly classified 85.6% of 1,212 normal subjects as nonimpaired (85.6% specificity), and 77.1% of 436 brain-damaged patients as impaired (77.1% sensitivity). Benton, Sivan, et al. (1994) define *defective* as the bottom 5%, with scores in the bottom 1% as *severely defective*, and scores in the range of the sixth to 16th percentile considered to be *borderline*. On the WAIS-IV (Wechsler, 2008), scores in the range of 70–79 (third to 10th percentile) are considered to be *borderline*, with scores of 69 and below (second percentile) considered to be *extremely low*.

Heaton et al. (2004) caution against overinterpreting performance on the HRB as impaired, based solely on tabulating the number of scores falling in the impaired range. They report that in a large sample of 1,189 neurologically normal individuals, only 13.2% had no T score in the impaired range, and the group median was three abnormal scores out of 25. Binder, Iverson, and Brooks (2009) review the extensive literature on this topic, noting that it is common not only to find multiple impaired scores consequent to administering batteries of individual tests, but also to find large discrepancies between separate neuropsychological skills such as *verbal symbolic* functions and *verbal learning and memory*. Binder et al. (2009) conclude that abnormal performance on some proportion of tests in a battery is psychometrically normal, thus several abnormal scores in a large test battery do not necessarily imply the presence of acquired brain dysfunction. They also conclude that although people with higher IQ scores tend to have fewer low scores than people with lower IQ scores, normal persons of high intelligence often have some low test scores, large variability between highest and lowest scores is psychometrically normal, and the degree of normal variability is greater in those people with higher IQ scores.

In order to minimize the error of misinterpreting low scores or large variability between scores as showing impairment when such patterns are normal, Binder et al. (2009) recommend looking for consistencies across the data, and checking to see if the data match with the clinical history, neurodiagnostic data, and other clinical information. For example, consider two cases that each show three poor performances. The first is a 70-year-old man with a two-year history of memory decline, who produces poor performance on WMS-IV Logical Memory, Verbal Paired Associates, and the AVLT. The second case is a 25-year-old man who has vague cognitive complaints leading to referral, and produces poor performance on Finger Tapping, WAIS-IV Arithmetic, and Animal Naming, with normal Grooved Pegboard, Trail Making B, and AVLT performance. The history and context for evaluating these two sets of poor scores lead to different conclusion regarding the consequences of the three poor performances in each of these two cases. I have offered a four-part model for analysis of consistency of test performance (Larrabee, 1990; Larrabee, 2012b):

1. Are the data consistent within and between domains?
2. Is the neuropsychological profile consistent with the suspected etiology?
3. Are the neuropsychological data consistent with the documented severity of the injury (or illness)?
4. Are the neuropsychological data consistent with the subject's behavioral presentation?

Crawford, Garthwaite, and Gault (2007) provide a statistical approach based on the Monte Carlo simulation, which allows determination of the number of "impaired" scores occurring by chance, as a function of the number of tests administered, and the average intercorrelation between those tests. The Crawford et al. (2007) procedure also allows determination of the significance of large discrepancies occurring in a battery of tests as a function of the number of tests administered. While this provides very helpful statistical guidance, one must still analyze the clinical history and other contextual information to arrive at the most appropriate interpretation of the data.

Co-normed batteries such as the comprehensive norms for an expanded HRB (Heaton et al., 2004), the NAB (Stern & White, 2003), and the WAIS-IV/WMS-IV (Wechsler, 2009) allow for direct comparisons using different subtests with a common normative basis. Rohling and colleagues have developed an approach for aggregating individually normed tests: the Rohling Interpretive Method (RIM; Miller & Rohling, 2001; Rohling, Miller, & Langhinrichsen-Rohling, 2004), which is derived from effect size methodology with creation of linear composite scores including an Overall Test Battery Mean, and domain means for *verbal comprehension*, *perceptual organization*, *executive functions*, *memory*, *attention concentration*, and *processing speed*, with separate measurement of *symptom validity*, *personality factors*, *premorbid level of function*, *language comprehension*, and *sensory perceptual skills* (Miller & Rohling, 2001; Rohling et al., 2004). This procedure has been incorporated into the MNB, to aggregate norms developed independently for separate tests such as the AVLT and the TMT. The MNB norms, based on aggregated norms across different samples, are smoothed for demographic effects of age, gender, and education, based on a large sample of neurological, pain, and psychiatric patients (i.e., the norms are based on nonclinical subjects, with further smoothing of the norms using multiple regression to account for any additional effects of age, gender, and education, as based on clinical patient performance, essentially creating a normative "hybrid"). In a recent comparison of normative databases for tests common to the MNB, expanded HRB (Heaton et al., 2004), and the normative data presented by Mitrushina et al. (2005), there were essentially identical results for the performances scored using the co-norms of Heaton et al. (2004), meta-analytic (composite) norms of Mitrushina et al. (2005), and the hybrid (composite and regression smoothed) norms of the MNB (Rohling et al., 2015). Similarly, the hybrid normative database yielded essentially identical overall effect size and correlation with severity of TBI comparing an independent sample of TBI patients to the TBI sample investigated by Dikmen et al. (1995) using an expanded HRB, that included additional measures of memory and intellectual function (Rohling et al., 2003). This direct comparison of the aggregated norm approach characteristic of flexible battery approaches to the co-normed approach characteristic of fixed batteries supports the comparability of aggregated norm approaches, particularly when employing a statistically based approach such as the RIM (Miller & Rohling, 2001; Rohling et al., 2004).

In contrast to the earlier discussion regarding the importance of using demographically corrected scores in assessment and diagnosis of brain dysfunction, there is evidence suggesting that for prediction of functional outcome in activities of daily living, uncorrected or "absolute" scores can provide information above and beyond that provided by the corrected scores. As already noted, Rizzo and Kellison (2010) found that raw scores may be better predictors of driving ability than are scores corrected for age and education. Silverberg and Millis (2009) reported that absolute scores (Heaton et al., 2004)—norms for a general healthy adult population—predicted selected measures of functional outcome and functional status better than demographically adjusted scores (adjusted for age, gender, education, and race) for patients with TBI (median Glasgow Coma Scale [GCS] of 9).

Summary

This chapter reviewed the psychometric foundations of neuropsychological assessment, starting with the definition of what a test entails. This was followed by discussion of reliability and validity. The discussion of validity followed a recent paper (Larrabee, 2014) that provided a framework for comprising an ability-focused neuropsychological battery that is based on factor-analytically derived domains of performance, populated by procedures showing sensitivity to presence of impairment, sensitivity to severity of impairment, and prediction of instrumental activities of daily living, and containing embedded/derived measures of performance validity. In the final section of the chapter, psychometric issues related to normal test score variability were considered, as well as issue related to utilization of co-normed versus individually normed tests.

References

Anastasi, A., & Urbina, S. (1997). *Psychological Testing* (7th ed.). Upper Saddle River: Prentice Hall.

Arnold, G., Boone, K. B., Lu, P., Dean, A., Wen, J., Nitch, S., et al. (2005). Sensitivity and specificity of finger tapping test scores for the detection of suspect effort. *The Clinical Neuropsychologist*, *19*(1), 105–120.

Barbey, A. K., Colom, R., & Grafman, J. (2013). Dorsolateral prefrontal contributions to human intelligence. *Neuropsychologia*, *51*, 1361–1369.

Barrash, J., Suhr, J., & Manzel, K. (2004). Detecting poor effort and malingering with an expanded version of the Auditory Verbal Learning Test (AVLTX): Validation with clinical samples. *Journal of the International Neuropsychological Society*, *26*, 125–140.

Benton, A. L., Hamsher, K. de S., & Sivan, A. B. (1994). *Multilingual Aphasia Examination* (3rd ed.). Iowa City: AJA.

Benton, A. L., Sivan, A. B., Hamsher, K. de S., Varney, N. R., & Spreen, O. (1994). *Contributions to Neuropsychological Assessment: A Clinical Manual* (2nd ed.). New York: Oxford University Press.

Binder, L. M., Iverson, G. L., & Brooks, B. L. (2009). To err is human: "Abnormal" neuropsychological scores and variability are common in healthy adults. *Archives of Clinical Neuropsychology*, *24*, 31–46.

Blessed, G., Tomlinson, B. F., & Roth, M. (1968). The association between quantitative measures of dementia and of senile change in the cerebral gray matter of elderly subjects. *British Journal of Psychiatry*, *114*, 797–811.

Boone, K. B., Lu, P., & Wen, J. (2005). Comparisons of various RAVLT scores in the detection of noncredible memory performance. *Archives of Clinical Neuropsychology*, *20*, 301–319.

Borenstein, M., Hedges, L. V., Higgins, J.P.T., & Rothstein, H. R. (2009). *Introduction to Meta-Analysis*. Chichester, West Sussex: U. K.

Brandt, J. (1991). The Hopkins Verbal Learning Test: Development of a new verbal memory test with six equivalent forms. *The Clinical Neuropsychologist*, *5*, 124–142.

Buschke, H. (1973). Selective reminding for analysis of memory and learning. *Journal of Verbal Learning and Verbal Behavior*, *12*, 543–550.

Butcher, J. N., Arbisi, P. A., Atlis, M. M., & McNulty, J. L. (2003). The construct validity of the Lees-Haley Fake Bad Scale. Does this scale measure somatic malingering and feigned emotional distress? *Archives of Clinical Neuropsychology*, *18*, 473–485.

Calamia, M., Markon, K., & Tranel, D. (2013). The robust reliability of neuropsychological measures: Meta-analyses of test-retest correlations. *The Clinical Neuropsychologist*, *27*, 1077–1105.

Campbell, D. T., & Fiske, D. W. (1959). Convergent and discriminant validation by use of the multitrait-multimethod matrix. *Psychological Bulletin*, *56*, 81–105.

Carmines, E. G., & Zeller, R. A. (1979). *Reliability and Validity Assessment*. Newbury Park: Sage Publications.

Carroll, J. B. (1993). *Human Cognitive Abilities: A Survey of Factor Analytic Studies*. New York, NY: Cambridge University Press.

Chelune, G. J., Naugle, R. I., Luders, H., Sedlak, J., & Awad, I. A. (1993). Individual change following epilepsy surgery: Practice effects and baserate information. *Neuropsychology*, *1*, 41–52.

Cohen, J. (1988). *Statistical Power Analysis for the Behavioral Sciences* (2nd ed.). Mahwah, NJ: Lawrence Erlbaum Associates.

Crawford, J. R., Garthwaite, P. H., & Gault, C. B. (2007). Estimating the percentage of the population with abnormally low scores (or abnormally large score differences) on standardized neuropsychological test batteries: A generic method with applications. *Neuropsychology*, *21*, 419–430. Test Software www.abdn.ac.uk/~psy086/dept/PercentAbnormKtests.htm.

Cronbach, L. J. (1951). Coefficient alpha and the internal structure of tests. *Psychometrica*, *16*, 297–334.

Cronbach, L. J. (1990). *Essentials of Psychological Testing* (5th ed.). NY: Harper Collins.

Cronbach, L. J., & Meehl, P. E. (1955). Construct validity in psychological tests. *Psychological Bulletin*, *52*, 281–302.

Crook, T. H., & Larrabee, G. J. (1988). Interrelationships among everyday memory tests: Stability of factor structure with age. *Neuropsychology*, *2*, 1–12.

Davis, J. J., Millis, S. R., & Axelrod, B. N. (2012). Derivation of an embedded Rey Auditory Verbal Learning Test performance validity indicator. *The Clinical Neuropsychologist*, *26*, 1397–1408.

Delis, D. C., Jacobson, M., Bondi, M. W., Hamilton, J. M., & Salmon, D. P. (2003). The myth of testing construct validity using factor analysis or correlations with normal or mixed clinical populations: Lessons from memory assessment. *Journal of the International Neuropsychological Society*, *9*, 936–946.

Delis, D. C., Kramer, J. H., Kaplan, E., & Ober, B. A. (1987). *California Verbal Learning Test (CVLT): Adult Version* (Research ed.). San Antonio, TX: Psychological Corporation.

Delis, D. C., Kramer, J. H., Kaplan, E., & Ober, B. A. (2000). *California Verbal Learning Test, II*. San Antonio, TX: Psychological Corporation.

Dick, W., & Haggerty, N. (1971). *Topics in Measurement: Reliability and Validity*. New York: McGraw-Hill.

Dikmen, S. S., Machamer, J. E., Winn, H. R., & Temkin, N. R. (1995). Neuropsychological outcome at 1-year post head injury. *Neuropsychology*, *9*, 80–90.

Duff, K. (2012). Current topics in science and practice. Evidence-based indicators of neuropsychological change in the individual patient: Relevant concepts and methods. *Archives of Clinical Neuropsychology*, *27*, 248–250.

Earnst, K. S., Wadley, V. G., Aldridge, T. M., Steenwyk, A. B., Hammond, A. E., Harrell, L. E., & Marson, D. C. (2001). Loss of financial capacity in Alzheimer's Disease: The role of working memory. *Aging, Neuropsychology, and Cognition*, *8*, 109–111.

Fletcher, J. M., & Satz, P. (1985). Cluster analysis and the search for learning disability subtypes. In B. P. Rourke (Ed.), *Neuropsychology of Learning Disabilities: Essentials of Subtype Analysis* (pp. 40–64). New York: Guilford.

Floyd, F. J., & Widaman, K. F. (1995). Factor analysis in the development and refinement of clinical assessment instruments. *Psychological Assessment*, *7*, 286–299.

Gardizi, E., Millis, S. R., Hanks, R., & Axelrod, B. (2012). Rasch analysis of the postconcussion symptom questionnaire: Measuring the core construct of brain injury symptomatology. *The Clinical Neuropsychologist*, *26*, 869–878.

Greenaway, M. C., Smith, G. E., Tangalos, E. G., Geda, Y. E., & Ivnik, R. J. (2009). Mayo older Americans normative studies: Factor analysis of an expanded neuropsychological battery. *The Clinical Neuropsychologist*, *23*, 7–10.

Greve, K. W., Heinly, M. T., Bianchini, K. J., & Love, J. M. (2009). Malingering detection with the Wisconsin Card Sorting Test in mild traumatic brain injury. *The Clinical Neuropsychologist*, *23*, 343–362.

Greve, K. W., Ord, J., Curtis, K. L., Bianchini, K. J., & Brennan, A. (2008). Detection of malingering in traumatic brain injury and chronic pain: A comparison of three forced choice symptom validity tests. *The Clinical Neuropsychologist*, *22*, 896–918.

Griffith, H. R., Netson, K. L., Harrell, L. E., Zamrini, E. Y., Brockington, J. C., & Marson, D. C. (2006). Amnestic mild cognitive impairment: Diagnostic outcomes and clinical prediction over a two-year time period. *Journal of the International Neuropsychological Society*, *12*, 166–175.

Hamsher, K. de S. (1991). Intelligence and aphasia. In M. T. Sarno (Ed.), *Acquired Aphasia* (2nd ed., pp. 339–372). San Diego: Academic Press.

Hannay, H. J., Levin, H. S., & Grossman, R. G. (1979). Impaired recognition memory after head injury. *Cortex*, *15*, 269–283.

Heaton, R. K., Miller, S. W., Taylor, M. J., & Grant, I. (2004). *Revised Comprehensive Norms for an Expanded Halstead-Reitan Battery: Demographically Adjusted Norms for African American and Caucasian Adults (HRB)*. Lutz, FL: Psychological Assessment Resources.

Heilman, K. M., Watson, R. T., & Valenstein, E. (2012). Neglect and related disorders. In K. M. Heilman & E. Valenstein (Eds.), *Clinical Neuropsychology* (5th ed., pp. 296–348). New York: Oxford University Press.

Holdnack, J. A., Schoenberg, M. R., Lange, R. T., & Iverson, G. L. (2013). Predicting premorbid ability for WAIS-IV, WMS-IV, and WASI-II. In J. A. Holdnack, L. W. Drozdik, L. G. Weiss, & G. L. Inverson (Eds.), *WAIS-IV, WMS-IV, and ACS: Advanced Clinical Interpretation* (pp. 217–278). San Diego: Elsevier.

Holdnack, J. A., & Weiss, L. G. (2013). Demographic adjustments to WAIS-IV/WMS-IV norms. In J. A. Holdnack, L. W. Drozdik, L. G. Weiss, & G. L. Inverson (Eds.), *WAIS-IV, WMS-IV, and ACS: Advanced Clinical Interpretation* (pp. 171–216). San Diego: Elsevier.

Holdnack, J. A., Zhou, X., Larrabee, G. J., Millis, S. R., & Salthouse, T. A. (2011). Confirmatory factor analysis of the WAIS-IV/WMS-IV. *Assessment*, *18*, 178–191.

Hosmer, D. W., & Lemeshow, S. (2000). *Applied Logistic Regression*. New York: Wiley InterScience.

Hsaio, J. K., Bartko, J. J., & Potter, W. Z. (1989). Diagnosing diagnoses: Receiver operating characteristics methods and psychiatry. *Archives of General Psychiatry*, *46*, 664–667.

Hughes, C. P., Berg, L., Danziger, W. L., Coben, L. A., & Martin, R. L. (1982). A new clinical scale for the staging of dementia. *British Journal of Psychiatry*, *140*, 566–572.

Jacobson, N. S., & Truax, P. (1991). Clinical significance: A statistical approach to defining meaningful change in psychotherapy research. *Journal of Consulting and Clinical Psychology*, *59*, 12–19.

Jasinski, L. J., Berry, D.T.R., Shandera, A. L., & Clark, J. A. (2011). Use of the Wechsler Adult Intelligence Scale Digit Span subtest for malingering detection: A meta-analytic review. *Journal of Clinical and Experimental Neuropsychology*, *33*, 300–314.

Jastak, J., & Wilkinson, G. S. (1984). *The Wide Range Achievement Test-Revised*. Wilmington, DE: Jastak Associates.

Kane, R. L., Parsons, O. A., & Goldstein, G. (1985). Statistical relationships and discriminative accuracy of the Halstead: Reitan,

Luria-Nebraska, and Wechsler IQ scores in the identification of brain damage. *Journal of Clinical and Experimental Neuropsychology*, *7*, 211–233.

Kaplan, E. F., Goodglass, H., & Weintraub, S. (1983). *The Boston Naming Test* (2nd ed.). Philadelphia, PA: Lea & Febiger.

Keifer, E., & Tranel, D. (2013). A neuropsychological investigation of the Delis-Kaplan Executive Function System. *Journal of Clinical and Experimental Neuropsychology*, *35*, 1048–1059.

Kuder, G. F., & Richardson, M. W. (1937). The theory of estimation of test reliability. *Psychometrika*, *2*, 151–160.

Larrabee, G. J. (1986). Another look at VIQ-PIQ scores and unilateral brain damage. *International Journal of Neuroscience*, *29*, 141–148.

Larrabee, G. J. (1990). Cautions in the use of neuropsychological evaluation in legal settings. *Neuropsychology*, *4*, 239–247.

Larrabee, G. J. (2000). Association between IQ and neuropsychological test performance: Commentary on Tremont, Hoffman, Scott, and Adams (1998). *The Clinical Neuropsychologist*, *14*, 139–145.

Larrabee, G. J. (2003a). Lessons on measuring construct validity: A commentary on Delis, Jacobson, Bondi, Hamilton, and Salmon. *Journal of the International Neuropsychological Society*, *9*, 947–953.

Larrabee, G. J. (2003b). Detection of malingering using atypical performance patterns on standard neuropsychological tests. *The Clinical Neuropsychologist*, *17*, 410–425.

Larrabee, G. J. (2009). Malingering scales for the Continuous Recognition Memory Test and the Continuous Visual Memory Test. *The Clinical Neuropsychologist*, *23*, 167–180.

Larrabee, G. J. (2012a). Performance validity and symptom validity in neuropsychological assessment. *Journal of the International Neuropsychological Society*, *18*, 625–630.

Larrabee, G. J. (2012b). A scientific approach to forensic neuropsychology. In G. J. Larrabee (Ed.), *Forensic Neuropsychology: A Scientific Approach* (pp. 3–22). New York: Oxford.

Larrabee, G. J. (2014). Test validity and performance validity: Considerations in providing a framework for development of an ability focused neuropsychological test battery. *Archives of Clinical Neuropsychology*, *29*, 695–714.

Larrabee, G. J., & Curtiss, G. (1992). Factor structure of an ability-focused neuropsychological battery (abstract). *Journal of Clinical and Experimental Neuropsychology*, *14*, 65.

Larrabee, G. J., & Curtiss, G. (1995). Construct validity of various verbal and visual memory tests. *Journal of Clinical and Experimental Neuropsychology*, *17*, 536–547.

Larrabee, G. J., Kane, R. L., Schuck, J. R., & Francis, D. J. (1985). The construct validity of various memory testing procedures. *Journal of Clinical and Experimental Neuropsychology*, *7*, 239–250.

Larrabee, G. J., Largen, J. W., & Levin, H. S. (1985). Sensitivity of age-decline reistant ("Hold") WAIS subtests to Alzheimer's disease. *Journal of Clinical and Experimental Neuropsychology*, *7*, 497–504.

Larrabee, G. J., Millis, S. R., & Meyers, J. E. (2008). Sensitivity to brain dysfunction of the Halstead Reitan vs. an ability-focused neuropsychological battery. *The Clinical Neuropsychologist*, *22*, 813–825.

Larrabee, G. J., Trahan, D. E., Curtiss, G., & Levin, H. S. (1988). Normative data for the Verbal Selective Reminding Test. *Neuropsychology*, *2*, 173–182.

Lees-Haley, P. R., English, L. T., & Glenn, W. J. (1991). A fake bad scale on the MMPI-2 for personal injury claimants. *Psychological Reports*, *68*, 203–210.

Leonberger, F. T., Nicks, S. D., Larrabee, G. J., & Goldfader, P. R. (1992). Factor structure and construct validity of a comprehensive neuropsychological battery. *Neuropsychology*, *6*, 239–249.

Lezak, M. D., Howieson, D. E., Bigler, E. D., & Tranel, D. (2012). *Neuropsychological Assessment* (5th ed.). New York: Oxford University Press.

Loring, D. W., & Larrabee, G. J. (2006). Sensitivity of the Halstead and Wechsler test batteries to brain damage: Evidence from Reitan's original validation sample. *The Clinical Neuropsychologist*, *20*, 221–229.

Loring, D. W., & Larrabee, G. J. (2008). "Psychometric Intelligence" is not equivalent to "Crystallized Intelligence," nor is it insensitive to brain damage: A reply to Russell. *The Clinical Neuropsychologist*, *22*, 524–528.

Loring, D. W., Strauss, E., Hermann, B. P., Barr, W. B., Perrine, K., Trenerry, M. R., Chelune, G. . . .Bowden, S. C. (2008). Differential neuropsychological test sensitivity to left temporal lobe epilepsy. *Journal of the International Neuropsychological Society*, *14*, 394–400.

Marson, D. C., Ingram, K. K., Cody, H. A., & Harrell, L. E. (1995). Assessing the competency of patients with Alzheimer's disease under different legal standards: A prototype instrument. *Archives of Neurology*, *52*, 949–954.

McSweeney, A. J., Naugle, R. I., Chelune, G. J., & Luders, H. (1993). "T scores for change": An illustration of a regression approach to depicting change in clinical neuropsychology. *The Clinical Neuropsychologist*, *7*, 300–312.

Meyers, J. E., & Meyers, K. (1995). *The Meyers Scoring System for the Rey Complex Figure and the Recognition Trial: Professional Manual*. Odessa, FL: Psychological Assessment Resources.

Meyers, J. E., & Rohling, M. L. (2004). Validation of the Meyers Short Battery on mild TBI patients. *Archives of Clinical Neuropsychology*, *19*, 637–651.

Miller, J. B., Fichtenberg, N. L., & Millis, S. R. (2010). Diagnostic efficiency of an ability focused battery. *The Clinical Neuropsychologist*, *24*, 678–688.

Miller, L. S., & Rohling, M. L. (2001). A statistical interpretive method for neuropsychological test data. *Neuropsychology Review*, *11*, 143–169.

Mitrushina, M., Boone, K. B., Razani, J., & D'Elia, L. F. (2005). *Handbook of Normative Data for Neuropsychological Assessment* (2nd ed.). New York: Oxford.

Novack, T. A., Banos, J. H., Alderson, A. L., Schneider, J. J., Weed, W., Blankenship, J., & Salisbury, D. (2006).UFOV performance and driving ability following traumatic brain injury. *Brain Injury*, *20*, 455–461.

Nunnally, J. C., & Bernstein, I. H. (1994). *Psychometric Theory* (3rd ed.). New York: McGraw Hill.

Pearson (2009). *Advanced Clinical Solutions for Use With WAIS-IV and WMS-IV*. San Antonio, TX: Pearson Education.

Powell, J. B., Cripe, L. I., & Dodrill, C. B. (1991). Assessment of brain impairment with the Rey Auditory Verbal Learning Test: A comparison with other neuropsychological measures. *Archives of Clinical Neuropsychology*, *6*, 241–249.

Reitan, R. M. (1974). Methodological problems in clinical neuropsychology. In R. M. Reitan & L. A. Davison (Eds.), *Clinical Neuropsychology: Current Status and Applications* (pp. 19–46). New York: John Wiley and Sons.

Reitan, R. M., & Wolfson, D. (1993). *The Halstead-Reitan Neuropsychological Test Battery: Theory and Clinical Interpretation* (3rd ed.). Tucson, AZ: Neuropsychology Press.

Rey, A. (1941). L'examen psychologique dans les cas d'encephalopathie traumatique. *Archives de Psychologie*, *28*, 286–340.

Rey, A. (1964). *L'examen Clinique en Psychologie*. Paris: Presses Univeritaires de France.

Rice, M. E., & Harris, G. T. (2005). Comparing effect sizes in follow-up studies: ROC Area, Cohen's *d*, and *r*. *Law and Human Behavior*, *29*, 615–620.

Rizzo, M., & Kellison, I. L. (2010). The brain on the road. In T. Marcotte & I. Grant (Eds.), *Neuropsychology of Everyday Functioning* (pp. 168–208). New York: Guilford.

Rohling, M. L., Meyers, J. E., & Millis, S. R. (2003). Neuropsychological impairment following traumatic brain injury: A dose-response analysis. *The Clinical Neuropsychologist*, *17*, 289–302.

Rohling, M. L., Miller, R., Axelrod, B. N., Wall, J. R., Lee, A.J.H., & Kinikini, D. T. (2015). *Is Co-norming Required? Archives of Clinical Neuropsychology*, *30*, 611–633.

Rohling, M. L., Miller, L. S., & Langhinrichsen-Rohling, J. (2004). Rohling's interpretive method for neuropsychological data analysis: A response to critics. *Neuropsychology Review*, *14*(3), 155–169.

Roth, R. M., Isquith, P. K., & Gioia, G. A. (2005). *Behavior Rating Inventory of Executive Functions-Adult Version*. Lutz, FL: Psychological Assessment Resources, Inc.

Russell, E. W., Neuringer, C., & Goldstein, G. (1970). *Assessment of Brain Damage: A Neuropsychological Key Approach*. New York: Wiley-Interscience.

Salthouse, T. A. (2005). Relations between cognitive abilities and measures of executive function. *Neuropsychology*, *19*, 532–545.

Schmidt, M. (1996). *Rey Auditory and Verbal Learning Test*. Los Angeles: Western Psychological Services.

Sherer, M., Scott, J. G., Parsons, O. A., & Adams, R. L. (1994). Relative sensitivity of the WAIS-R subtests and selected HRNB measures to the effects of brain damage. *Archives of Clinical Neuropsychology*, *9*, 427–436.

Sherod, M. G., Griffith, H. R., Copeland, J., Belue, K., Kryzwanski, S., Zamrini, E. Y., . . . Marson, D. C. (2009). Neurocogntiive predictors of financial capacity across the dementia spectrum: Normal aging, MCI, and Alzheimer's disease. *Journal of the International Neuropsychological Society*, *15*, 258–267.

Silverberg, N. D., & Millis, S. R. (2009). Impairment *versus* deficiency in neuropsychological assessment: Implications for ecological validity. *Journal of the International Neuropsychological Society*, *15*, 94–102.

Sivan, A. B. (1992). *Benton Visual Retention Test* (5th ed.). San Antonio, TX: The Psychological Corporation.

Spreen, O., & Benton, A. L. (1965). Comparative studies of some psychological tests for cerebral damage. *Journal of Nervous and Mental Disease*, *140*, 323–333.

Stern, R., & White, T. R. (2003). *Neuropsychological Assessment Battery: Manual*. Lutz, FL: Psychological Assessment Resources.

Stevens, S. S. (1951). Mathematics, measurement, and psychophysics. In S. S. Stevens (Ed.), *Handbook of Experimental Psychology* (pp. 1–49). New York: Wiley.

Strauss, E., Sherman, E.M.S., & Spreen, O. (2006). *A Compendium of Neuropsychological Tests: Administration, Norms, and Commentary* (3rd ed.). New York: Oxford.

Swets, J. J. (1973). The relative operating characteristic in psychology. *Science*, *182*, 990–1000.

Tabachnick, B. G., & Fidell, L. (2005). *Using Multivariate Statistics* (5th ed.). Boston, MA: Allyn & Bacon.

Tellegen, A., & Ben-Porath, Y. S. (2008/2011). *MMPI-2-RF (Minnesota Multiphasic Personality Inventory-2 Restructured Form technical manual)*. Minneapolis, MN: University of Minnesota Press.

Trahan, D. E. (1997). Relationship between facial discrimination and visual neglect in patients with unilateral vascular lesions. *Archives of Clinical Neuropsychology*, *12*, 57–62.

Trahan, D. E., & Larrabee, G. J. (1988). *The Continuous Visual Memory Test*. Lutz, FL: Psychological Assessment Resources.

Trahan, D. E., Larrabee, G. J., Quintana, J. W., Goethe, K. E., & Willingham, A. C. (1989). Development and clinical validation of an expanded paired associates test with delayed recall. *The Clinical Neuropsychologist*, *3*, 169–183.

Tremont, G., Hoffman, R. G., Scott, J. G., & Adams, R. L. (1998). Effect of intellectual level on neuropsychological test performance: A response to Dodrill. *The Clinical Neuropsychologist*, *12*, 560–567.

Tulsky, D. S., & Price, L. R. (2003). The joint WAIS-III and WMS-III factor structure: Development and cross-validation of a six factor model of cognitive functioning. *Psychological Assessment*, *15*, 149–162.

Vega, A., Jr., & Parsons, O. A. (1967). Cross-validation of the Halstead: Reitan tests for brain damage. *Journal of Consulting Psychology*, *31*, 619–625.

Warrington, E. K. (1984). *Recognition Memory Test*. Los Angeles: Western Psychological Services.

Wechsler, D. (2008). *WAIS-IV: Technical and Interpretive Manual*. San Antonio, TX: Pearson.

Wechsler, D. (2009). *WMS-IV: Technical and Interpretive Manual*. San Antonio, TX: Pearson.

Welsh, K. A., Butters, N., Mohs, R. C., Beekly, D., Edland, S., Fillenbaum, G., & Heyman, A. (1994). The Consortium to Establish a Registry for Alzheimer's Disease (CERAD): Part V. A normative study of the neuropsychological battery. *Neurology*, *44*, 609–614.

Whelihan, W. M., DiCarlo, M. A., & Paul, R. H. (2005). The relationship of neuropsychological functioning to driving competence in older persons with early cognitive decline. *Archives of Clinical Neuropsychology*, *20*, 217–228.

Wilkinson, G. S. (1993). *WRAT-3: The Wide Range Achievement Test Administration Manual* (3rd ed.). Wilmington, DE: Wide Range.

Williams, M. W., Rapport, L. J., Hanks, R. A., Millis, S. R., & Greene, H. A. (2013). Incremental validity of neuropsychological evaluations to computed tomography in predicting long-term outcomes after traumatic brain injury. *The Clinical Neuropsychologist*, *27*, 356–375.

Zakzanis, K. K., Leach, L., & Kaplan, E. F. (1999). *Neuropsychological Differential Diagnosis*. New York: Taylor & Francis.

4 Assessment of Neurocognitive Performance Validity

Kyle Brauer Boone

Prior to the 1990s, little literature existed on psychometric methods to document noncredible performance during neurocognitive testing, but in the intervening decades there has been an explosion in the development and validation of techniques to objectively identify failure to perform to true ability (see Boone, 2007, 2013; Larrabee, 2007; Victor, Kulick, & Boone, 2013a,b), termed *performance validity tests* (PVTs; Larrabee, 2012). Practice recommendations indicate that PVTs are to be interspersed "throughout the evaluation" (National Academy of Neuropsychology, Bush et al., 2005), and that both "embedded" and "freestanding" PVTs should be utilized (American Academy of Clinical Neuropsychology; Heilbronner et al., 2009).

Freestanding PVTs serve a single purpose in assessing for negative response bias, while embedded indicators are derived from standard neurocognitive tests, and thus serve "double duty" both as measures of performance validity but also as techniques to evaluate neurocognitive function. The field of clinical neuropsychology will likely move to primary, if not exclusive, use of embedded PVTs because they do not require extra test administration time, and are more shielded from attempts at coaching and education because of their main purpose as measures of neuropsychological function. Further, they allow for evaluation of performance validity in "real time" rather than requiring that results from PVTs administered at one point in the exam be used to determine validity of neurocognitive test performance at a different point in the testing. Unfortunately, embedded indicators have developed a reputation as "second-rate" PVTs because it has been widely believed that they are less sensitive in identifying noncredible performance than "dedicated" PVTs. However, this is not entirely accurate: While overall sensitivity rates are probably lower for embedded PVTs as a group, as shown in tables in Boone (2013), dedicated and embedded PVTs both have sensitivity rates within the range of >20% to 80%. For example, at cutoffs recommended by the test developer, sensitivity of the Test of Memory Malingering (TOMM; Tombaugh, 1996) to noncredible performance in traumatic brain injury is only 48% to 56% (Greve, Ord, Curtin, Bianchini, & Brennan, 2008). While many embedded indicators also have sensitivity rates that approximate 50% (Digit Span variables, Babikian, Boone, Lu, & Arnold, 2006; Finger Tapping, Arnold et al., 2005; CVLT-II; Donders & Strong, 2011, Wolfe et al., 2010; Stroop A and B, Arentsen et al., 2013), others equal or exceed 65% (Picture Completion Most Discrepancy Index, Solomon et al., 2010; RAVLT effort equation, Boone, Lu, & Wen, 2005), while still others achieve at least an 80% detection rate (Digit Symbol recognition; Kim, N., et al., 2010; RO effort equation, Reedy et al., 2013).

Negative response used to be viewed as a unitary and static characteristic of the test taker, but available data indicate that that only a minority of noncredible patients engage in negative response bias on every measure administered during a neuropsychological exam. Rather, the large majority (>80%; Boone, 2009) "pick and choose" tests on which to demonstrate impairments, under the apparent belief that poor performances on all tasks will not be credible. Test takers may elect to underperform at particular times during the exam (e.g., at the end when "fatigued," at the beginning to illustrate that they do not function early in the day, etc.). Alternatively, they may decide to display deficits on particular types of tasks that they believe are consistent with their claimed condition. For example, research suggests that test takers performing in a noncredible manner in the context of claimed mild traumatic brain injury (mTBI) overselect verbal memory tests on which to underperform, whereas individuals feigning cognitive impairment in the setting of claimed psychiatric disorder appear to target timed, continuous performance test (CPT)–type tasks on which to perform poorly (Nitch, Boone, Wen, Arnold, & Warner-Chacon, 2006; Roberson et al., 2013). Further, even within the same claimed condition, test takers may adopt differing approaches to underperformance. The following two cases illustrate examples of differing strategies of feigning in the context of claimed mTBI.

Case #1: Feigned Verbal Memory and Math Impairment

This 41-year-old female litigant worked in public relations and had completed an AA degree. She was tested five years after a motor vehicle accident in which she, at most, sustained a mTBI; any loss of consciousness was equivocal, there was no retrograde or anterograde amnesia, and she was alert and oriented in the hospital and released the same day. She continued to work, and handled all activities of daily living (ADLs) independently. At the time of the exam she was reporting headaches, back pain, numbness/tingling in her right arm, cognitive difficulties including "struggles" with memory, and anxiety/depression.

She failed PVTs confined to verbal memory: Warrington Words: (total = 32; time = 201"; failed cut-offs for women; Kim, M., et al., 2010) and RAVLT (recognition false positives = 5 [failed]; effort equation = 13 [passed]; Boone et al., 2005). However, she passed indicators from nine other tests mostly tapping other cognitive domains: b Test (E-score = 42; Roberson et al., 2013), Rey Word Recognition (12; Bell-Sprinkel et al., 2013), Digit Symbol recognition (178; Kim, N., et al., 2010), Picture Completion Most Discrepant Index (5; Solomon et al., 2010), Digit Span variables (Age-Corrected Scale Score [ACSS] = 11; Reliable Digit Span [RDS] = 10; three-digit time = 1.5"; Babikian et al., 2006), Rey-Osterrieth (RO) Effort equation (61; Reedy et al., 2013), Logical Memory equation (64.5; Bortnik et al., 2010), and Trails A (18"; Iverson, Lange, Green, & Franzen, 2002), and Stroop A and B (A = 39"; B = 56"; Arentsen et al., 2013).

Across the neuropsychological battery, all scores were within the average range or higher with the exception of a borderline score in math calculation ability and a low average score in delayed verbal recall (verbal memory scores ranged from low average to average). On previous testing six months after the injury, math calculation ability was average, and verbal memory was average to high average. Thus, the weaknesses observed on current testing were not corroborated on testing completed closer in time to the injury. Minnesota Multiphasic Personality Inventory – 2 – Restructured Form (MMPI-2-RF) scales were unelevated with the exception of sanitizing of negative personal characteristics (L-r = 66T). The patient attributed her headaches to the mTBI, but chronic headache is not found post-mTBI in countries without a tort system (Mickeviciene et al., 2004), and the patient in fact had well-documented headaches, as well as an extensive history of chronic pain and vague medical symptoms, prior to the accident.

Case #2: Feigned Impairment in Visual Memory, Vigilance/Processing Speed, and Sensory Function

This 59-year-old female litigant worked as a mid-level executive and had completed an MBA. She was tested four years after a motor vehicle accident in which she sustained equivocal loss of consciousness. She called emergency personnel to the scene but did not seek medical attention except for chiropractic care. She continued to be active in her profession and church, and to handle all ADLs independently. When asked as to symptoms related to the accident, the patient reported multiple cognitive difficulties including lack of focus, mental slowness, difficulty processing information, "dyslexia," problems in multitasking, and becoming "visually lost," as well as orthopedic pain, difficulty hearing, development of sleep apnea, and emotional dyscontrol.

She failed PVTs involving processing speed/vigilance, such as b Test time (805"; E-score = 58 [passed]; Roberson et al., 2013), Dot Counting Test E-score (23; Boone, Lu, & Herzberg, 2002), Stroop (A = 98"; B = 123"; Arentsen et al., 2013), and Digit Symbol (ACSS = 4 [failed]; recognition equation = 80 [passed]; Kim, N., et al., 2010), as well as PVTs involving visual perception/spatial skill/memory (Picture Completion Most Discrepant Index = 2, Solomon et al., 2010; RO effort equation = 49, Reedy et al., 2013), basic attention (Digit Span: mean time per digit =1.05" [failed], ACSS = 7 [passed], and RDS = 8 [passed]; Babikian et al., 2006), and finger speed and sensation (Tapping dominant = 26, Arnold et al., 2005; Finger Agnosia errors = 4, Trueblood & Schmidt, 1993). In contrast, she passed all verbal memory PVTs (Warrington Words =50, 82," Kim, et al., 2010; Rey Word Recognition = 9, Bell-Sprinkel et al., 2013; RAVLT effort equation = 18, Boone et al., 2005), as well as Trails A (45"; Iverson et al., 2002) and Rey 15-item plus recognition (30; Boone, Salazar, Lu, Warner-Chacon, & Razani, 2002).

Across the neuropsychological exam, impaired scores were observed in motor dexterity, while impaired to low average scores were documented in processing speed and visual perceptual/constructional skill, and basic attention was low average; all other scores were average or higher. The failed PVT performances predicted which standard cognitive scores were lowered. The abnormal neurocognitive scores, if accurate, would be inconsistent with the patient's functionality in all activities of daily living. Further, on testing completed two years after the injury, all scores on measures of attention, processing speed, and motor dexterity were average; thus, low scores on current exam were not corroborated on the exam closer in time to the injury. On the MMPI-2-RF, the only elevated validity scale was FBS-r (80T), suggestive of noncredible overreport of physical and cognitive symptoms, and substantive scales involving physical symptom report were also elevated. In addition, multiple scales were elevated reflecting anxiety, depression, cycling mood disorder, and anger-related disorder. Such psychiatric symptoms are not empirically verified sequelae of remote mTBI (Panayiotou, Jackson, & Crowe, 2010), nor are the patient's complaints of chronic headache, loss of hearing, and development of sleep apnea.

In these cases, if PVTs had not been administered that covered a wide range of cognitive domains, the nature and extent of the negative response bias would not have been documented. Fortunately, numerous PVTs have now been validated within each of the cognitive domains (i.e., attention, processing speed, verbal and visual memory, executive, motor dexterity, sensory, visual perceptual/spatial, and language), and are listed and described in tables found in Boone (2013) and Victor et al. (2013a, 2013b).

Interpretation of Data From Multiple PVTs

Given that the recommendation is now to check for performance validity repeatedly during neuropsychological exams and within each cognitive domain (with the eventual goal of performance validity indicators for every task to check for performance veracity in real time), it is imperative to develop sound methods for interpreting the data from the various measures in combination. PVT cutoffs are traditionally set to allow a false positive rate of <10%. If a single PVT is administered, credible patients are not adequately protected (i.e., if they perform abnormally, they could be within the 10% of credible patients who fail the measure, yet they will be determined to be noncredible). The best method to protect credible patients is to administer multiple PVTs because while a single failure is not particularly unusual across several PVTs administered (i.e., 41% of credible neuropsychology clinic outpatients with various neurologic and psychiatric diagnoses fail a single PVT; Victor, Boone, Serpa, Beuhler, & Ziegler, 2009; see also Schroeder & Marshall: 19% of psychotic and 17% of nonpsychotic psychiatric patients failed a single PVT), failure on multiple PVTs is relatively rare. For example, Victor et al. (2009) found that only 5% of their credible sample failed two PVTs (out of four), Schroeder and Marshall (2011) reported that 5%–7% of psychiatric patients failed two PVTs (out of seven), and Larrabee (2003) observed that 6% of his credible moderate to severe traumatic brain injury sample failed two validity measures (out of four PVTs and one SVT), a remarkably consistent pattern of findings. Victor et al. (2009) further reported that only 1.5% of their sample failed three PVTs, and zero failed four, while Larrabee (2014) reported that 4% of his sample failed three measures (out of six PVTs and one SVT), with no false positive identifications after three failures. Other researchers have documented that two to three PVT failures are associated with 100% specificity (Chafetz, 2011; Davis & Millis, 2014; Meyers & Volbrecht, 2003; Meyers et al., 2014; Schroeder & Marshall, 2011; Sollman, Ranseen, & Berry, 2010; Vickery et al., 2004). Larrabee (2008) demonstrated that, using posterior probabilities, the probability that a test taker who fails three PVT cutoffs is in fact noncredible is essentially 99%, a finding recently confirmed by Meyers et al. (2014).

Berthelson, Mulchan, Odland, Miller, and Mittenberg (2013), citing results from a Monte Carlo simulation, argued that if PVTs are correlated at approximately .3 (as documented by Davis & Millis, 2014; Nelson et al., 2003), the false positive rate for two PVT failures (with cutoffs set to 90% specificity) in a credible population is 11.5%. They further assert that if PVT cutoffs are adjusted to result in 85% specificity, two failures occur in nearly 20% of credible patients. However, cutoffs typically are selected to achieve a false positive rate of <10%, precisely so that credible patients are adequately protected. To check the accuracy of Berthelson et al.'s (2013) simulation, Davis and Millis (2004) subsequently examined PVT false positive rates in a neurologic population with no motive to feign impairment, and observed that when six to eight PVTs are administered (with cutoffs set to 90% specificity), the actual occurrence of one or two failures was lower than predicted by Berthelson et al. (2013), and there was no significant relationship between number of PVTs administered and number failed (r = .10). Similarly, Larrabee (2014) also found that the Monte Carlo simulation overestimated that rate of multiple PVT failures in credible populations, likely because PVT data do not have normal score distributions required for use of the simulation model.

The question arises as to whether "passed" PVTs "cancel out" any failures. However, there is an inverse relationship between test sensitivity and specificity, such that when test cutoffs are selected to enhance specificity (i.e., allowing only a 10% failure rate), sensitivity will be lowered, thereby rendering failed performances more informative than passing scores. That is, if specificity of individual PVTs is >90%, and sensitivity rates range from <50% to 80%, scores on individuals PVTs will be more effective in ruling in than ruling out noncredible performance. Further, as discussed earlier, noncredible test takers are likely selecting specific tasks, and particular times, during the exam on which to underperform, rather than electing to fail to perform to true ability on all tests administered. As such, it is expected that they will pass some PVTs during the portions of the exam that they are choosing not to perform poorly.

To summarize, the current recommendation in the field of clinical neuropsychology, particularly in the context of a forensic exam in which there is compensation seeking or other external motive to present oneself as more impaired than is actually the case, is that multiple PVTs are to be administered, interspersed throughout the exam, to cover multiple cognitive domains (if not for every task administered), so that performance validity is repeatedly sampled.

In addition to failing scores on PVTs, additional confirming evidence of a noncredible presentation is typically present, including: (a) nonsensical change in scores on sequential neuropsychological examinations, particularly dramatic declines in scores remote from the injury; (b) mismatch between performance on PVTs and evidence as to how the test taker actually functions in activities of daily living; (c) report of nonplausible symptoms (inability to recall birth date and other overlearned personal and family information; chronic headache, loss of hearing, development of sleep apnea, etc., in the context of mTBI); and (d) evidence from personality inventories, such as the MMPI-2-RF, of noncredible cognitive symptom overreport (e.g., MMPI-2-RF RBS and FBS-r), often in conjunction with denial of antisocial and exploitive behaviors (Cottingham et al., in press). In most cases, observations gleaned from these sources of information and PVT data render conclusions straightforward.

However, there are two noteworthy exceptions: individuals with dementia and individuals with very low intellectual scores (Full Scale IQ [FSIQ] <70). As discussed earlier, multiple failures on PVTs virtually never occur in credible populations, but patients with dementia and low IQ have been documented to fail PVTs at a high rate despite performing to true ability (Dean, Victor, Boone, & Arnold, 2008; Dean, Victor, Boone, Philpott, & Hess, 2009; Meyers & Volbrecht, 2003; Rudman, Oyebode, Jones, & Bentham, 2011; Victor & Boone, 2007). For example, Dean et al. (2009) reported that in individuals with diagnosed dementia, 36% of PVTs were failed in those patients with Mini-Mental State Exam (MMSE) >20, 47% were failed when MMSE scores were 15 to 20, and 83% of PVTs were failed with MMSE <15. Similarly, in neuropsychology clinic patients with an IQ range of 60–69, 44% of administered PVTs were failed, while the failure rate was 60% in those with IQ of 50–59 (Dean et al., 2008). Performance validity indicators are based on the premise that simple tasks that appear relatively difficult will be passed by actual patients with brain injury, but failed by noncredible test takers. However, in patients with dementia or low IQ, most "simple" tasks are in fact difficult. The question then arises as to how to arrive at an accurate differential diagnosis of actual versus feigned dementia or intellectual disability.

The remainder of this chapter will address determination of performance validity in the context of possible dementia. The following case illustrates some of the techniques available in this endeavor.

Differential Diagnosis of Actual Versus Feigned Dementia

This 69-year-old patient with eight years of education and subsequent attainment of a GED sustained at most a mTBI in a motor vehicle accident five years prior to evaluation. Medical records indicate that he self-extricated at the scene and was standing at the accident site upon arrival of emergency medical personnel. The patient was described as alert and oriented with no loss of consciousness (Glasgow Coma Scale [GCS] was 15), although subsequently he displayed some mild confusion and was amnestic for the event. He required suturing of a laceration on his head, and was found to have a left hand fracture. Brain CT was normal, but brain MRI obtained two days later showed an area of acute infarction/ischemia in the left basal ganglia and left cerebral peduncle region, as well as mild atrophy with mild nonspecific periventricular and deep white matter changes judged likely related to chronic ischemic white matter disease. He was discharged to home after three days. He filed a lawsuit alleging reduced cognitive function secondary to direct effects of traumatic brain injury, as well as the effect of stroke, which was claimed as caused by the traumatic brain injury, and that precluded him from returning to work as a taxi driver. Symptoms reported at the time of evaluation included decline in memory, reduced balance, back and right leg pain, pain at the fracture site, periodic headaches, insomnia, and depression and anxiety.

The patient's medical history was rather extensive, including chronic hypertension (with associated borderline hypertrophy on echocardiogram and calcification of the aorta), high cholesterol, elevated blood sugar levels, low testosterone, possible sleep apnea, lengthy smoking history, treatment for gastrointestinal (GI) cancer in the year prior to the accident including six months of chemotherapy, chronic depression, thyroid and parathyroid dysfunction, and possible excessive alcohol use (current use of two glasses of wine three to four nights per week). Additionally, the patient had performed poorly in school due to difficulty "concentrating," but he stated that he did not know whether he had an actual learning disability or attention deficit disorder. Family history was noteworthy for a disabling psychiatric condition in his only child (a daughter), and apparent substance abuse in at least one parent. He resided with his wife and adult daughter, and no concerns were expressed regarding his ability to function within the community. He had an active driver's license.

Scores from the neurocognitive exam are reproduced in the Table 4.1.

The patient in fact failed 100% of PVTs administered (15 of 15 separate tests); the graphs in Figures 4.1, 4.2, and 4.3 contrast the patient's PVT scores against mean scores for credible and noncredible groups.

Results of neurocognitive testing revealed impaired scores in finger dexterity, visual perceptual/spatial skills, visual memory, and word retrieval; impaired to borderline scores in processing speed; impaired to low average scores in verbal memory; and low average performance in basic attention. In a test taker in the patient's age range who has documented evidence of small strokes and multiple medical illnesses, the question arises as to whether he has developed cognitive deterioration to the level of a dementia, and if this accounts for the widespread PVT failures.

The determination as to whether a patient's performance validity failures reflect noncredible performance versus the effects of an actual dementia is made by examining (a) the patient's functionality in ADLs to see if it is consistent with dementia; (b) the patient's test scores and spontaneously displayed skills for evidence of consistency of impairment; (c) whether performance on PVTs matches that expected for dementia, and (d) whether the patient still fails PVTs when cutoffs are selected that adequately protect against false positive identifications of malingering in credible dementia patients. Additionally, when a patient has been repeatedly tested, consistency of test scores across exams can be analyzed.

As outlined below, the evidence in the current case indicated that the patient did not in fact have a dementia and that his neuropsychological test performance was noncredible.

Evidence From PVT Performance

- The patient obtained a MMSE score of 19 (out of 29 possible points), which would suggest a mild/moderate dementia. Yet, he failed 100% of PVTs administered, which is markedly higher than that expected for this MMSE score. Specifically, Dean et al. (2009) found that with a MMSE score of 15 to 20, an average of 47% of PVTs are failed (in contrast to 36% with MMSE score of >20, and 83% with MMSE scores <15).
- The only PVT employed in the Dean et al. (2009) study that maintained 90% specificity in dementia at published cutoffs was mean time to recite four digits on forward Digit Span (cutoff >4"); the patient's score markedly exceeds this cutoff.

Table 4.1 Neuropsychological test scores in noncredible test taker

Gross Cognitive Function				
Mini-Mental State Exam	19 (out of 29 possible)			
Information Processing Speed			***PVT***	
b Test				Roberson et al. (2013)
E-score	102		***failed***	
Omissions	55		***failed***	
Commissions	0		passed	
Time	11'47"		***failed***	
Dot Counting Test				Boone et al. (2002)
E-score	31		***failed***	
Grouped dot time	12.5"		***failed***	
Ungrouped dot time	13.0"			
Errors	5		***failed***	
Trails A	79"	<1st %	***failed***	Iverson et al. (2002)
Stroop A (Word Reading)	2'29"	<1st %	***failed***	Arentsen et al. (2013)
Digit Symbol				Kim, N., et al. (2010)
ACSS	5	5th %	passed	
Recognition equation	8		***failed***	
Recognition total	4		***failed***	
Attention				
Digit Span				Babikian et al. (2006)
ACSS	6	9th %	passed	
Reliable Digit Span	7		passed	
Mean three-digit time	4"		***failed***	
Mean four-digit time	16.5"		***failed***	
Language				
Boston Naming Test	32	impaired	***failed***	Whiteside et al. (2015)
Visual Perceptual/Spatial Skills				
WAIS-III Picture Completion				Solomon et al. (2010)
ACSS	3	1st %	***failed***	
Most Discrepant Index	0		***failed***	
Rey Complex Figure				Reedy et al. (2013)
Copy	12.5	<1st %	***failed***	
Memory—Verbal				
WMS-III Logical Memory				Bortnik et al. (2010)
I	19	2nd %	***failed***	
II	9	9th %	***failed***	
Recognition	18	chance	***failed***	
Effort equation	36		***failed***	
Rey Auditory Verbal Learning Test				Boone et al. (2005)
Total	17		***failed***	
Trial 1	2	1st %		
Trial 2	4	2nd %		
Trial 3	3	1st %		
Trial 4	4	5th %		
Trial 5	4	1st %	***failed***	
List B	3	12th %		
Short delay	3	7th %	***failed***	
Long delay	3	22nd %	passed	
Recognition	3 (0 FP)<1st %		***failed***	
Effort equation	4		***failed***	
Rey Word Recognition	2		***failed***	Bell-Sprinkel et al. (2013)
Warrington Recognition Words				Kim, M., et al. (2010)
Total correct	19		***failed***	
Recognition time	399"		***failed***	

(*Continued*)

Table 4.1—continued

Memory—Visual				
Rey Complex Figure				Reedy et al. (2013)
Three-minute delay	4.0	<1st %	***failed***	
Recognition correct	3.0	<1st %	***failed***	
Effort equation	21.5		***failed***	
Rey 15-item				Boone, et al. (2002)
Recall	6.0		***failed***	
Recognition correct	6.0		***failed***	
Combination score	12.0		***failed***	
Test of Memory Malingering				
Trial 1	21		***failed***	Denning (2012)
Motor Dexterity				
Tapping				Arnold et al. (2005)
Dominant	19.0	<1st %	***failed***	
Nondominant	16.3	<1st %	***failed***	
Personality Function				
MMPI-2-RF				
Validity Scale				
VRIN-r	39T		low	
TRIN-r	73F		Within normal limits	
F-r	65T		Within normal limits	
Fp-r	59T		Within normal limits	
Fs	66T		Within normal limits	
FBS-r	67T		Within normal limits	
RBS	67T		Within normal limits	
L-r	62T		Within normal limits	
K-r	48T		Within normal limits	
Elevated Scales				
RC1	77T			
RC2	95T			
MLS	81T			
HPC	72T			
NUC	86T			
HLP	79T			
STW	65T			
MSF	65T			
IPP	68T			
SAV	75T			
INTR-r	93T			

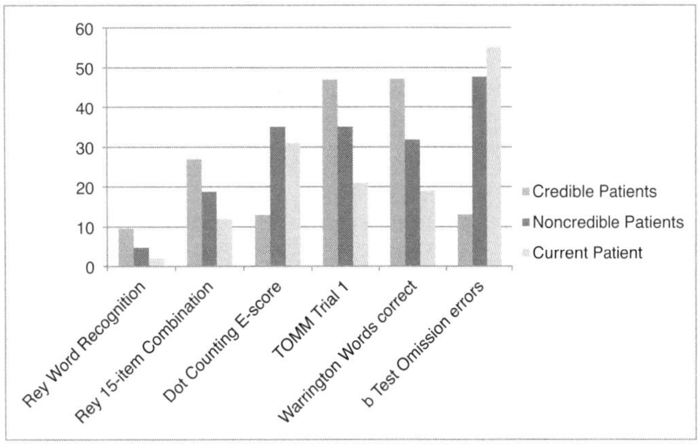

Figure 4.1 Scores on dedicated PVTs

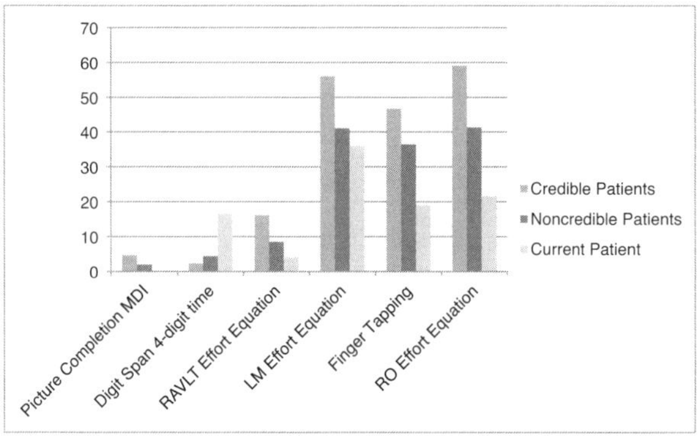

Figure 4.2 Scores on embedded PVTs involving attention, visual perception/spatial skills, motor dexterity, and verbal and visual memory

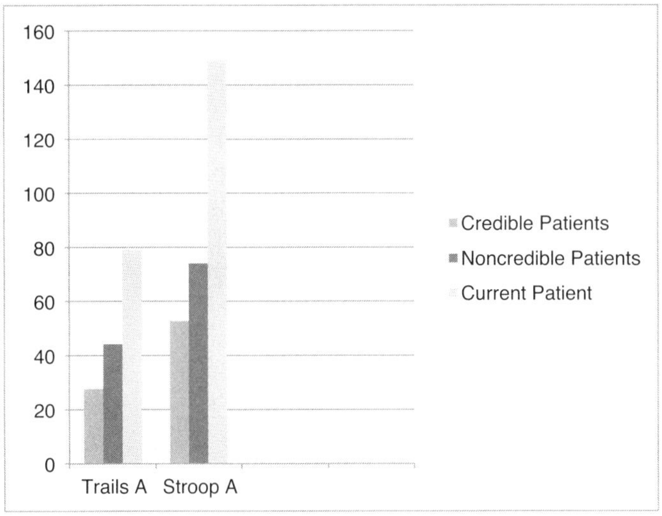

Figure 4.3 Scores on embedded PVTs involving processing speed

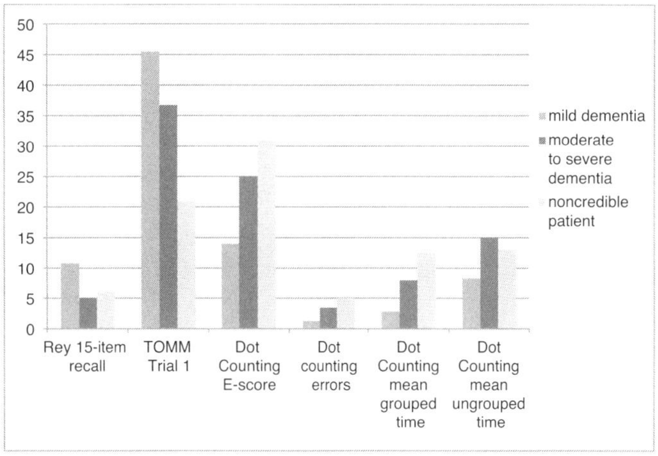

Figure 4.4 PVT Performance as compared to patients with mild and moderate/severe dementia

data for rey 15-item, TOMM Trial 1, and Dot Counting errors, mean grouped time, and mean ungrouped time from Rudman et al. (2011); data for Dot Counting E-score from Boone et al. (2002)

- When cutoffs were adjusted per the Dean et al. (2009) study to maintain a <10% false positive rate in dementia patients, the patient still failed the Warrington Words (cutoff <26), finger tapping dominant hand (cutoff <21), and Rey Word Recognition (cutoff <5).
- As shown in Figure 4.4, the patient's scores on the Dot Counting Test, Rey 15-item total recall, and TOMM Trial 1 were worse than mean scores obtained by patients with mild dementia, and most scores (with the exception of Rey 15-item recall and mean ungrouped dot counting time) were worse than mean scores obtained by patients with moderate to severe dementia who were residing in a locked residential facility.
- On a forced choice measure (Warrington–Words), the patient obtained a score significantly below chance (19/50). This performance would suggest that the patient knew correct answers that he did not provide, in contrast to patients with significant dementia (i.e., who have little to no ability to learn new information), and who would be expected to perform at worst at chance levels on the test.

Mismatch Between Test Scores and Demonstrated Functionality

- The patient was able to provide detailed information regarding the accident and his symptoms/treatment in his deposition and on interview, and showed no memory lapses in his interactions with the examiner (e.g., did not re-ask questions already asked, did not require test instructions be repeated, etc.), behaviors that would be inconsistent with his dementia-level word recall scores on the RAVLT. He scored below chance levels on one forced choice recognition memory test, arguably performing worse than a blind person (who would be predicted to perform at chance levels).
- His very low scores on measures of visual perceptual/constructional skills, visual memory, and processing speed would likely preclude ability to drive, yet he was driving at the time of the exam.
- His low confrontation naming score would be indicative of a significant word-retrieval difficulty, yet no such expressive language difficulties were observed in spontaneous speech.
- He obtained very low finger tapping scores yet used his fingers normally during the exam (to turn booklet pages, hold and use a pen, etc.), and did not report dysfunction of his fingers when asked regarding physical symptoms.
- He made excessive errors in counting (on the Dot Counting Test), a preschool level skill, but in his deposition he was able to provide detailed information regarding the amount and source of his income.
- He scored within the markedly impaired range in rapid word reading, yet he was able to complete the 338-item MMPI-2-RF in less than an hour. No significant overreport was documented on validity scales; however, of note, he obtained a below average score on VRIN-r (39T), which measures consistency in answering similar sets of items. His low score, reflecting more carefulness and consistency in responses than the typical test taker, would not be likely in an individual with actual dementia.

Marked Inconsistency in Test Scores Across Cognitive Exams

- Three years prior to current testing (but after the accident at issue in the lawsuit), the patient scored in the high average range on a visual spatial reasoning task, in contrast to the impaired scores obtained on current testing.

- Two years prior to current exam, the patient scored in the average range in processing speed, in contrast to the borderline to impaired scores obtained on current exam.
- Six months prior to current exam, the patient scored in the average range on visual memory testing, in contrast to the impaired visual memory scores observed on current testing.
- MMSE scores were widely discrepant across evaluations by different neurologists: One to two years after the accident the patient was described as displaying intact memory and concentration, but in the following year MMSE scores ranged from 15 to 18, and rose to 25 the year after that.
- Particularly poor finger tapping performance was documented on current exam and two years previously, but no neurologist or other physician had reported dysfunction of the patient's fingers.

Literature on PVTs in Dementia

The review of PVT performance in dementia provided by Dean et al. (2009), and the empirical data reported by Dean et al. (2009), Duff et al. (2011), Rudman et al. (2011), and Bortnik, Horner, and Bachman (2013), show that most PVTs (e.g., TOMM, Digit Span indices, Warrington, Digit Memory Test, Victoria Symptom Validity Test, Word Memory Test [WMT], Medical Symptom Validity Test [MSVT], Nonverbal Medical Symptom Validity Test [NVMSVT], Rey 15-item, Dot Counting, Amsterdam Short Term Memory Test, b Test, Rey Word Recognition, RAVLT effort equation, RO effort equation, RAVLT/RO discriminant function, RBANS Effort Index, Trailmaking Test Ratio) are found to have high false positive identification rates in dementia samples. For example, Rudman et al. (2011) reported specificity rates of 64% for TOMM (Trial 2 and retention <45), 54.8% for Rey 15 total (<8), 45.2% for MSVT, and 33.3% for NV-MSVT. Attempts have been made to identify a unique performance pattern on the WMT ("general memory impairment profile" [GMIP]) and MSVT ("severe impairment profile") that can be used to flag patients with actual severe cognitive dysfunction and thereby reduce the test false positive rate in these patients (Green, Montijo, & Brockhaus, 2011). However, Chafetz and Biondolillo (2013) showed that noncredible patients can easily produce the severe impairment profile, and others have argued that the requirement that the severe impairment profile only be considered if there is a probability that the patient has true impairment is circular (Axelrod & Schutte, 2010). Further, when impairment profiles are employed, specificity does increase, but sensitivity declines; for example, Fazio, Sanders, and Denney (2015) documented 95.1% sensitivity and 68.4% specificity for the WMT in a criminal forensic population, and with use of the GMIP, specificity was increased to 94.7%, but sensitivity declined to 56.1%. However, as discussed later, sensitivity rates of approximately 50% or less may be typical for techniques used to differentiate actual versus feigned dementia.

Perhaps the most research on performance validity in dementia populations has involved the RBANS. Silverberg, Wertheimer, and Fichtenberg (2007) developed an Effort Index (EI) using weighted scores from the Digit Span and List Recognition subtests of the RBANS. Using a cut-off of >3, specificity in a mixed clinical sample was 94%, while sensitivity in a noncredible mTBI sample was 53.3%. Similar sensitivity rates have been reported in geriatric suspect effort groups (51.1% to 64.4%; Barker, Horner, & Bachman, 2010). However, research has demonstrated excessive false positive rates for the EI in geriatric samples that included patients with mild cognitive impairment and Alzheimer's disease (e.g., 69% specificity; Hook, Marquine, & Hoezle, 2009). The EI appears to have good specificity in geriatric patients who are cognitively intact or have only mild impairment (97%), but specificity declines to unacceptable levels in nursing home residents and in patients with Alzheimer's disease (63% to 66%; Duff et al., 2011). Further, older age and less education negatively impacts EI scores in cognitively intact geriatric patients (Duff et al., 2011).

Because of the elevated false positive rates for the EI in dementia samples, Novitski, Steele, Karantzoulis, and Randolph (2012) developed the RBANS Effort Scale (ES) for use in an amnestic population. The ES involves calculation of the discrepancy between performance on list recognition and recall subtests, to which is then added the digit span subtest score. The authors cautioned that while this equation would result in lowered false positive identifications in truly amnestic patients, false positive identifications would be elevated in patients with normal memory. Several subsequent publications have confirmed lowered false positive rates for an ES cut-off of <12 as compared to the EI in dementia patients. For example, Dunham, Shadi, Sofko, Denney, and Calloway (2014) observed that EI specificity in a genuine memory impairment group was 41% as compared to specificity of 81% for the ES. However, in line with the cautions provided by Novitski et al. (2012), further analyses revealed that specificity was moderated by level of impairment; specificity was higher for the EI (75%) when the RBANS total score was average to mildly impaired, while ES specificity was 96% when RBANS total score was severely impaired, leading the authors to conclude that selection of which RBANS performance validity score to use depends on level of impairment. Burton, Enright, O'Connell, Lanting, and Morgan also reported higher specificity for ES (86%) as compared to EI (52%) in a mixed dementia sample, but noted that specificity rates depended on dementia type; ES specificity was 96% in patients with Alzheimer's disease, but only 69% in non-Alzheimer's dementia. In this vein, examination of performance validity RBANS scores in patients with Parkinson disease revealed an 8% false positive rate for the EI, but a 62.6% false positive rate for the ES (Carter, Scott, Adams, & Linck, 2016). Thus, the ES scale appears to be most appropriate for use in patients with prominent amnesia, but false positive rates are problematic in other types of dementia.

In the Dean et al. (2009) study, mean time to recite four digits in forward order on Digit Span maintained 90% specificity at established cutoffs in 48 dementia patients, although sensitivity has been reported as low (28% to 37%; Babikian et al., 2006). In the Dean et al. (2009) study, specificity for finger tapping cutoffs was low in the overall sample of 55 dementia patients with finger tapping scores, but was 100% in subgroups of patients with Alzheimer's disease and fronto-temporal dementia (but only 43% in vascular dementia), although subgroup sample sizes were small. Sensitivity levels for dominant finger tapping cutoffs are at least moderate (50% to 61%; Arnold et al., 2005). Finally, a recent study showed that use of Digit Span RDS <7 and RAVLT recognition <10 in combination only misclassified 5% of 178 early Alzheimer's dementia patients (Loring et al., 2016), although sensitivity of these cut-offs is unknown.

Additionally, other measures appear to have promise in distinguishing actual versus feigned dementia. Schindler, Kissler, Kuhl, Hellweg, and Bengner (2013) described performance on a yes/no recognition task (presentation of 20 unfamiliar faces, followed by a recognition trial in which the 20 faces are interspersed with 20 new faces, with the test taker instructed to report whether each face was previously seen) in a small sample of dementia patients (n = 13) and suspected malingerers (n = 11) as well as other groups. The dementia patients exhibited an inflated "yes" response bias, while the suspected malingerers displayed an increased "no" response bias. At a cutoff of nine false negative responses, sensitivity was 54% and specificity was 100%. Schroeder, Peck, Buddin, Heinrichs, and Baade (2012) reported data on the forced choice Coin-in-the-Hand Test in 45 hospitalized patients with moderate to severe cognitive deficits (mean RBANS Global score = first percentile; mean MMSE score = 21.47). More than one error (out of ten possible) occurred in 11% of the sample, and a cutoff of >2 errors resulted in 96% specificity, while specificity was 100% at a cutoff of >4 errors. Dementia subtype was not related to test performance. Rudman et al. (2011) had reported somewhat lower specificity for this measure in 42 patients of varying types of dementia; using a cutoff of <7, specificity was 88.1%, although it achieved the second highest specificity rate among various PVTs examined. The highest hit rate (100%) was observed for the discrepancy between grouped and ungrouped dot counting times on the Dot Counting Test (failure was defined as total ungrouped dot counting time < total grouped dot counting time).

These measures appear to warrant further study in the differential of actual versus feigned dementia, although, for the latter two indicators, while specificity may be relatively high, information as to whether they are in fact effective (i.e., have adequate sensitivity rates in real world settings) is lacking. As a caution, Vocabulary minus Digit Span was initially reported to be a useful PVT (Miller, Ross, & Ricker, 1998), and was documented to have a specificity rate of 97% in 38 patients with probable Alzheimer's disease (Dean et al., 2009). However, other research has demonstrated that this index does not discriminate credible and noncredible groups (Curtis, Greve, & Bianchini, 2009) and has low sensitivity (Harrison, Rosenblum, & Currie, 2010), thereby indicating that it has virtually no clinical utility. Thus, without real world sensitivity data for the Coin in Hand Test and the Dot Counting discrepancy score, it is unknown whether they are in fact effective PVTs in dementia evaluations.

Other avenues that might warrant exploration in distinguishing actual versus feigned dementia are development of PVTs that rely on old, overlearned information and implicit memory, which are relatively intact in patients with dementia. For example, Cuddy and Duffin (2005) reported spared recognition for music in a woman with advanced dementia (MMSE = 8) as measured by recognition of familiar from unfamiliar melodies, and detection of "wrong" notes in known melodies as well as distinguishing distorted versus correctly played melodies. Horton, Smith, Barghout, and Connolly (1992) observed that normal individuals and amnestic patients both showed typical priming effects on word or fragment completion tasks, in contrast to an amnesia simulation condition in which word completion rates were substantially below baseline performances. Hilsabeck, LeCompte, Marks, and Grafman (2001) subsequently reported data for a PVT involving priming, the Word Completion Memory Test, that requires test takers to complete word stems with previously studied words (Inclusion subtest), and then after exposure to a new list of words, test takers are asked to complete word stems *without* using these latter words (Exclusion subtest). Normal controls and a small group of memory disordered patients (n = 14), including two patients with dementia, used more list words on the first task than on the second, while simulators showed the opposite pattern, obtaining a mean difference score that was negative.

Considered as a whole, the available literature suggests that recognition memory tasks,, time scores for simple tasks (number repetition and counting), finger speed (except in vascular dementia patients), and implicit memory measures and those involving overlearned information, appear to show the most potential as PVTs in dementia populations, in that these tasks are performed relatively normally by these patients. Additionally, recognition techniques that capitalize on the "yes" response bias found in dementia patients and the "no" response bias that appears to characterize noncredible subjects may also be a fruitful avenue of investigation. Severity of dementia requires consideration in that patients with mild dementia are consistently found to outperform patients with more severe dementia on virtually all PVTs (see Dean et al., 2009). Use of multiple PVTs with cut-offs set to achieve at least 90% specificity for dementia will likely be shown to be adequately protective of dementia patients; as a model, Smith et al. (2014) demonstrated that when PVT cut-offs are selected to result in 90% specificity in a credible population with low intellectual level (FSIQ <75), ≥ 2 failures (across seven PVTs most sensitive in detecting likely feigning of intellectual disability) was associated with 85.4% specificity and 85.7% sensitivity, while a cut-off of ≥ 3 failures resulted in 95.1% specificity and 66.0% sensitivity.

In conclusion, the field of neuropsychology has made considerable strides in developing methods to accurately identify noncredible neurocognitive test performance, and a next important step will be to refine and perfect techniques to assist in distinguishing actual versus feigned dementia.

References

Arentsen, T., Boone, K., Lo, T., Goldberg, H., Cottingham, M., Victor, T., . . . Zeller, M. (2013). Effectiveness of the Comalli Stroop Test as a measure of negative response bias. *The Clinical Neuropsychologist*, *27*, 1060–1076.

Arnold, G., Boone, K. B., Lu, P., Dean, A., Wen, J., Nitch, S., & McPherson, S. (2005). Sensitivity and specificity of Finger Tapping test scores for the detection of suspect effort. *The Clinical Neuropsychologist*, *19*, 105–120.

Axelrod, B. N., & Schutte, C. (2010). Analysis of the dementia profile on the Medical Symptom Validity Test. *The Clinical Neuropsychologist*, *24*, 873–881.

Babikian, T., Boone, K. B., Lu, P., & Arnold, G. (2006). Sensitivity and specificity of various digit span scores in the detection of suspect effort. *The Clinical Neuropsychologist*, *20*, 145–159.

Barker, M. D., Horner, M. D., & Bachman, D. L. (2010). Embedded indices of effort in the repeatable battery for the assessment of neuropsychological status (RBANS) in a geriatric sample. *The Clinical Neuropsychologist*, *24*, 1064–1077.

Bell-Sprinkel, T., Boone, K. B., Miora, D., Cottingham, M., Victor, T., Ziegler, E., Zeller, M., & Wright, M. (2013). Cross-validation of the Rey Word Recognition symptom validity test. *The Clinical Neuropsychologist*, *27*, 516–527.

Berthelson, L., Mulchan, S. S., Odland, A. P., Miller, L. J., & Mittenberg, W. (2013). False positive diagnosis of malingering due to the use of multiple effort tests. *Brain Injury*, *27*, 909–916.

Boone, K. B. (Ed.). (2007). *Assessment of Feigned Cognitive Impairment: A Neuropsychological Perspective*. New York: Guilford Press.

Boone, K. B. (2009). The need for continuous and comprehensive sampling of effort/response bias during neuropsychological examinations. *The Clinical Neuropsychologist*, *23*, 729–741.

Boone, K. B. (2013). *Clinical Practice of Forensic Neuropsychology: An Evidence-Based Approach*. New York: Guilford.

Boone, K. B., Lu, P., & Herzberg, D. (2002). *The Dot Counting Test*. Los Angeles: Western Psychological Services.

Boone, K. B., Lu, P., & Wen, J. (2005). Comparison of various RAVLT scores in the detection of noncredible memory performance. *Archives of Clinical Neuropsychology*, *20*, 310–319.

Boone, K. B., Salazar, X., Lu, P., Warner-Chacon, K., & Razani, J. (2002). The Rey 15—item recognition trial: A technique to enhance sensitivity of the Rey 15-item memorization test. *Journal of Clinical and Experimental Neuropsychology*, *24*, 561–573.

Bortnik, K. E., Boone, K. B., Marion, S. D., Amano, S., Cottingham, M., Ziegler, E., Victor, T., & Zeller, M. (2010). Examination of various WMS-III logical memory scores in the assessment of response bias. *The Clinical Neuropsychologist*, *24*, 344–357.

Bortnik, K. E., Horner, M. D., & Bachman, D. L. (2013). Performance on standard indexes of effort among patients with dementia. *Applied Neuropsychology*, *20*, 233–242.

Burton, R. L., Enright, J., O'Connell, M. E., Lanting, S., & Morgan, D. (2014). RBANS embedded measures of suboptimal effort in dementia: Effort Scale has a lower failure rate than the Effort Index. *Archives of Clinical Neuropsychology*, *30*, 1–6.

Bush, S. S., Ruff, R. M., Troster, A. I., Barth, J. T., Koffler, S. P., Pliskin, N. H., . . . Silver, C. H. (2005). Symptom validity assessment: Practice issues and medical necessity: NAN Policy & Planning Committee. *Archives of Clinical Neuropsychology*, *20*, 419–426.

Carter, K. R., Scott, J. G., Adams, R. L., & Linck, J. (2016). Base rate comparison of suboptimal scores on the RBANS effort scale and effort index in Parkinson's disease. *The Clinical Neuropsychologist*, *30*, 1118–1125.

Chafetz, M. (2011). Reducing the probability of false positives in malingering detection of social security disability claimants. *The Clinical Neuropsychologist*, *25*, 1239–1252.

Chafetz, M., & Biondolillo, A. M. (2013). Feigning a severe impairment profile. *Archives of Clinical Neuropsychology*, *28*, 205–212.

Cottingham, M. E., Boone, K. B., Goldberg, H. E., Victor, T. L., Zeller, M. A., Baumgart, M., Ziegler, E., Wright, M. (in press). Use of MMPI-2-RF over- and under-report data in a noncredible neuropsychology sample. In Boone, K. B. (Ed.), *Assessment of Feigned Cognitive Impairment: A Neuropsychological Perspective* (2nd Ed). New York: Guilford Press.

Cuddy, L. L., & Duffin, J. (2005). Music, memory, and Alzheimer's disease: Is music recognition spared in dementia, and how can it be assessed? *Medical Hypotheses*, *64*, 229–235.

Curtis, K. L., Greve, K. W., & Bianchini, K. J. (2009). The Wechsler Adult Intelligence Scale—III and malingering in traumatic brain injury. *Assessment*, *16*, 401–414.

Davis, J. J., & Millis, S. R. (2014). Examination of performance validity test failure in relation to number of tests administered. *The Clinical Neuropsychologist*, *28*, 199–214.

Dean, A. C., Victor, T. L., Boone, K. B., & Arnold, G. (2008). The relationship of IQ to effort test performance. *The Clinical Neuropsychologist*, *22*, 705–722.

Dean, A. C., Victor, T., Boone, K. B., Philpott, L., & Hess, R. (2009). Dementia and effort test performance. *The Clinical Neuropsychologist*, *23*, 133–152.

Denning, J. H. (2012). The efficiency and accuracy of the test of memory malingering trial 1, errors on the first 10 items of the test of memory malingering, and five embedded measures in predicting invalid test performance. *Archives of Clinical Neuropsychology*, *27*, 417–432.

Donders, J., & Strong, C.A.H. (2011). Embedded effort indicators on the California Verbal Learning Test—II (CVLT-II): An attempted cross-validation. *The Clinical Neuropsychologist*, *25*, 173–184.

Duff, K., Spering, C. C., O'Bryant, S. E., Beglinger, L. J., Mose, D. J., Bayless, J. D., Culp, K. R., Mold, J. W., Adams, R. L., & Scott, J. G. (2011). The RBANS Effort Index: Base rates in geriatric samples. *Applied Neuropsychology*, *18*, 11–17.

Dunham, K. J., Shadi, S., Sofko, C. A., Denney, R. L., & Calloway, J. (2014). Comparison of the repeatable battery for the assessment of neuropsychological status Effort Scale and Effort Index in a dementia sample. *Archives of Clinical Neuropsychology*, *29*, 633–641.

Fazio, R. L., Sanders, J. F., & Denney, R. L. (2015). Comparison of performance of the Test of Memory Malingering and Word Memory Test in a criminal forensic sample. *Archives of Clinical Neuropsychology*, *30*, 293–301.

Green, P., Montijo, J., & Brockhaus, R. (2011). High specificity of the Word Memory Test and Medical Symptom Validity Test in groups with severe verbal memory impairment. *Applied Neuropsychology*, *18*, 86–94.

Greve, K. W., Ord, J. S., Curtin, K. L., Bianchini, K. J., & Brennan, A. (2008). Detecting malingering in traumatic brain injury and chronic pain: A comparison of three forced choice symptom validity tests. *The Clinical Neuropsychologist*, *22*, 896–918.

Harrison, A. G., Rosenblum, Y., & Currie, S. (2010). Examining unusual digit span performance in a population of postsecondary students assessed for academic difficulties. *Assessment*, *17*, 283–293.

Heilbronner, R. L., Sweet, J. J., Morgan, J. E., Larrabee, G., Millis, S., & conference participants. (2009). American Academy of Clinical Neuropsychology Consensus Conference Statement on the neuropsychological assessment of effort, response bias, and malingering. *The Clinical Neuropsychologist*, *23*, 1093–129.

Hilsabeck, R. C., LeCompte, D. C., Marks, A. R., & Grafman, J. (2001). The Word Completion Memory Test (WCMT): A new test to detect malingered memory deficits. *Archives of Clinical Neuropsychology*, *16*, 669–677.

Hook, J. N., Marquine, M. J., & Hoelzle, J. B. (2009). Repeatable battery for the assessment of neuropsychological status effort index performance in a medically ill geriatric sample. *Archives of Clinical Neuropsychology*, *24*, 231–235.

Horton, K. D., Smith, S. A., Barghout, N. K., & Connolly, D. A. (1992). The use of indirect memory tests to assess malingered amnesia: A study of metamemory. *Journal of Experimental Psychology: General*, *121*, 326–351.

Iverson, G. L., Lange, R. T., Green, P., & Franzen, M. D. (2002). Detecting exaggeration and malingering with the Trail Making Test. *The Clinical Neuropsychologist*, *16*, 398–406.

Kim, M. S., Boone, K. B., Victor, T. L., Marion, S. D., Amano, S., Cottingham, . . . Zeller, M. (2010). The Warrington Recognition Memory Test for words as a measure of response bias: Total score and response time cutoffs developed on "real world" and noncredible subjects. *Archives of Clinical Neuropsychology*, *25*, 60–70.

Kim, N., Boone, K. B., Victor, T., Lu, P., Keatinge, C., & Mitchell, C. (2010). Sensitivity and specificity of a digit symbol recognition trial in the identification of response bias. *Archives of Clinical Neuropsychology*, *25*, 420–428.

Larrabee, G. J. (2003). Detection of malingering using atypical performance patterns on standard neuropsychological tests. *The Clinical Neuropsychologist*, *17*, 410–425.

Larrabee, G. J. (2007). *Assessment of Malingered Neuropsychological Deficits*. New York: Oxford University Press.

Larrabee, G. J. (2008). Aggregation across multiple indicators improves the detection of malingering: Relationship to likelihood ratios. *The Clinical Neuropsychologist*, *22*, 666–679.

Larrabee, G. J. (2012). Performance validity and symptom validity in neuropsychological assessment. *Journal of the International Neuropsychological Society*, *18*, 625–631.

Larrabee, G. J. (2014). False positive rates associated with the use of multiple performance and symptom validity tests. *Archives of Clinical Neuropsychology*, *29*, 364–373.

Loring, D. W., Goldstein, F. C., Chen, C., Drane, D. L., Lah, J. J., Zhao, L., & Larrabee, G. J. (2016). False-positive error rates for reliable digit span and auditory verbal learning test performance validity measures in amnestic mild cognitive impairment and early Alzheimer disease. *Archives of Clinical Neuropsychology*, *31*, 313–331.

Meyers, J. E., Miller, R. M., Thompson, L. M., Scalese, A. M., Allred, B. C., Rupp, Z. W., Dupaix, Z.P., & Lee, A. J. (2014). Using likelihood ratios to detect invalid performance with performance validity measures. *Archives of Clinical Neuropsychology*, *29*, 224–235.

Meyers, J. E., & Volbrecht, M. E. (2003). A validation of multiple malingering detection methods in a large clinical sample. *Archives of Clinical Neuropsychology*, *18*, 261–276.

Mickeviciene, C. H., Schrader, B., Obelienienec, D., Surkiene, D., Kunickas, R., Stovner, L. J., & Sand, T. (2004). A controlled prospective inception cohort study on the post-concussion syndrome outside the medicolegal context. *European Journal of Neurology*, *11*, 411–419.

Miller, S. R., Ross, S. R., & Ricker, J. H. (1998). Detection of Incomplete Effort on the Wechsler Adult Intelligence Scale-Revised: A cross-validation. *Journal of Clinical and Experimental Neuropsychology*, *20*, 167–173.

Nelson, N. W., Boone, K., Dueck, A., Wagener, L., Lu, P., & Grills, C. (2003). Relationships between eight measures of suspect effort. *The Clinical Neuropsychologist*, *17*, 263–272.

Nitch, S., Boone, K. B., Wen, J., Arnold, G., & Warner-Chacon, K. (2006). The utility of the Rey Word Recognition Test in the detection of suspect effort. *The Clinical Neuropsychologist*, *20*, 873–887.

Novitski, J., Steele, S., Karantzoulis, S., & Randolph, C. (2012). The repeatable battery for the assessment of neuropsychological status effort scale. *Archives of Clinical Neuropsychology*, *27*, 190–195.

Panayiotou, A., Jackson, M., & Crowe, S. F. (2010). A meta-analytic review of the emotional symptoms associated with mild traumatic brain injury. *Journal of Clinical and Experimental Neuropsychology*, *32*, 463–473.

Reedy, S., Boone, K., Cottingham, M., Glaser, D., Lu, P., Victor, T., . . . Wright, M. (2013). Cross-validation of the Lu et al. (2003) Rey-Osterrieth Complex Figure effort equation in a large known groups sample. *Archives of Clinical Neuropsychology*, *28*, 30–37.

Roberson, C. J., Boone, K. B., Goldberg, H., Miora, D., Cottingham, M. E., Victor, T. L., . . . Wright, M. (2013). Cross-validation of the b Test in a large known groups sample. *The Clinical Neuropsychologist*, *27*, 495–508.

Rudman, N., Oyebode, J. R., Jones, C. A., & Bentham, P. (2011). An investigation into the validity of effort tests in a working age dementia population. *Aging and Mental Health*, *15*, 47–57.

Schindler, S., Kissler, J., Kuhl, K.-P., Hellweg, R., & Bengner, T. (2013). Using the yes/no recognition response pattern to detect memory malingering. *BMC Psychology*, *1*, 12.

Schroeder, R. W., & Marshall, P. S. (2011). Evaluation of the appropriateness of multiple symptom validity indices in psychotic and non-psychotic psychiatric populations. *The Clinical Neuropsychologist*, *25*, 437–453.

Schroeder, R. W., Peck, C. P., Buddin, W. H., Heinrichs, R. J., & Baade, L. E. (2012). The Coin-in-the-Hand Test and dementia: More evidence for a screening test for neurocognitive symptom exaggeration. *Cognitive and Behavioral Neurology*, *25*, 139–143.

Silverberg, N. D., Wertheimer, J. C., & Fichtenberg, N. L. (2007). An effort index for the Repeatable Battery for the Assessment of Neuropsychological Status (RBANS). *The Clinical Neuropsychologist*, *21*, 841–854.

Smith, K., Boone, K., Victor, T., Miora, D., Cottingham, M., Ziegler, E., Zeller, M., Wright, M. (2014). Comparison of credible patients of very low intelligence and non-credible patients on neurocognitive performance validity indicators. *The Clinical Neuropsychologist*, *28*, 1048–1070.

Sollman, M. J., Ranseen, J. D., & Berry, D.T.R. (2010). Detection of feigned ADHD in college students. *Psychological Assessment*, *22*, 325–335.

Solomon, R. E., Boone, K. B., Miora, D., Skidmore, S., Cottingham, M., Victor, T., Ziegler, E., Zeller, M. (2010). Use of the WAIS-III picture completion subtest as an embedded measure of response bias. *The Clinical Neuropsychologist*, *24*, 1243–1256.

Tombaugh, T. (1996). *Test of Memory Malingering (TOMM)*. North Tonawanda, NY: MultiHealth Systems.

Trueblood, W., & Schmidt, M. (1993). Malingering and other validity considerations in the neuropsychological evaluation of mild head injury. *Journal of Clinical and Experimental Neuropsychology*, *15*, 578–590.

Vickery, C. D., Berry, D.T.R., Dearth, C. S., Vagnini, V. L., Baser, R. E., Cragar, D. E., et al. (2004). Head injury and the ability to feign neuropsychological deficits. *Archives of Clinical Neuropsychology*, *19*, 37–48.

Victor, T. L., & Boone, K. B. (2007). Identification of feigned mental retardation. In K. B. Boone (Ed.), *Assessment of Feigned Cognitive Impairment: A Neuropsychological Perspective* (pp. 310–345). New York: Guilford Press.

Victor, T. L., Boone, K. B., Serpa, G., Beuhler, J., & Ziegler, E. A. (2009). Interpreting the meaning of multiple effort test failure. *The Clinical Neuropsychologist*, *23*, 297–313.

Victor, T. L., Kulick, A. D., & Boone, K. B. (2013a). Assessing noncredible attention, processing speed, language and visuospatial/perceptual function in mild TBI cases. In D. A. Carone & S. S. Bush (Eds.), *Mild Traumatic Brain Injury: Symptom Validity Assessment and Malingering* (pp. 231–267). New York: Springer Publishing Company.

Victor, T. L., Kulick, A. D., & Boone, K. B. (2013b). Assessing noncredible sensory-motor function, executive function, and test batteries in mild TBI cases. In D. A. Carone & S. S. Bush (Eds.), *Mild Traumatic Brain Injury: Symptom Validity Assessment and Malingering* (pp. 269–301). New York: Springer Publishing Company.

Whiteside, D. M., Kogan, J., Wardin, L., Phillips, D., Franzwa, M. G., Rice, L., Basso, M., & Roper, B. (2015). Language-based embedded performance validity measures in traumatic brain injury. *Journal of Clinical and Experimental Neuropsychology*, *37*, 220–227.

Wolfe, P. L., Millis, S. R., Hanks, R., Fichtenberg, N., Larrabee, G. J., & Sweet, J. J. (2010). Effort indicators within the California Verbal Learning Test—II (CVLT-II). *The Clinical Neuropsychologist*, *24*, 153–168.

5 Differential Diagnosis in Neuropsychology

A Strategic Approach

David E. Hartman

The word *diagnosis* dates from the late 1600s, a latinate derivation of the Greek διάγνωσις from the root word διαγιγνώσκειν (*diagignoskein*) generally translated as to "discern" or "distinguish." The *practice* of medical diagnosis was performed from ancient times, with differential diagnostic formulations filtered through prevailing theories of disease causation. Hippocrates, for example, understood that different imbalances among various bodily fluids or "humors" caused the spectrum of diseases, and in order to obtain the clearest picture of disease patterns, he proposed a diagnostic protocol that included tasting the urine, listening to the lungs, and noting skin color and other appearance changes (Berger, 1999). While neuropsychology has its own history of measurement and classification, aphasia insights and phrenological dead-ends, the focus of this chapter is an attempt to deconstruct the process of diagnosis as it is used in present-day clinical neuropsychology.

In contrast with the medical profession, it is not clear that neuropsychological "diagnosis" has consistent meaning or methodology within the profession. In medicine, there is a reasonably well established approach to diagnosis, where symptom complaints are mapped on to medical disorders; it has been proposed that 36 symptoms account for more than 80% of patient complaints and "the physician who has mastered the differential diagnosis of these symptoms will be able to diagnose accurately almost all the problems seen in a typical medical practice" (Seller & Symons, 2007, p. v).

No such agreement is found for *diagnosis* as it is practiced within neuropsychology. A PUBMED search of the phrase *neuropsychological diagnosis* elicited 55 results: 28 investigated brain abnormality, ten examined medical or substance-caused patterns of test abnormality, two described neuropsychological correlates of a psychiatric disorder, three discussed learning and educational issues, three reviewed aspects of neuropsychological rehabilitation, and nine described test development or test pattern research. Only one of these, "Syndrome Analysis" (MacFarland, 1983) suggested the need to identify symptom clusters in neuropsychology, but restricted symptoms to behavioral evidence of brain syndromes, e.g., aphasia, apraxia, perseveration.

The ambiguity of the term *neuropsychological diagnosis* suggests that the term is used differently according to both job characteristic and perhaps the orientation of the practitioner. Examining the ways that neuropsychologists use the term *diagnosis* suggest that the word describes a clinical methodology of varying complexity, level of information integration, and even accuracy.

The purpose of this chapter is an attempt to deconstruct the meanings of *diagnosis* in a neuropsychological context, to guide the student and practitioner into a general clinical approach to patient examination, and to recognize the multiple meanings of the word *diagnosis* and learn to distinguish the appropriate clinical strategy and pitfalls of each approach.

Perhaps the most basic meaning of the word *diagnosis* in neuropsychology is what might be termed *descriptive diagnosis*. Descriptive diagnosis involves the use of neuropsychological procedures to detect the existence or measure the severity of a single, known/assumed brain syndrome. The neuropsychologist who examines individuals for entry into a dementia treatment program is performing descriptive diagnosis; the patient's a priori diagnosis of dementia is required to merit entry into the program. It is the task of the neuropsychologist to measure the degree of dementia—either to provide additional justification for program entry, gauge the need for services, or shape the pattern of services to be provided.

Descriptive Diagnosis is synonymous with *measurement*. "Diagnosis" in this sense of the word does not require consideration of alternatives, but measurement of an agreed upon construct. Neuropsychologists asked to measure the severity of Parkinsonism, for example, might choose tests that explicate the Parkinsonian fronto-striatal axis of dysfunction with tests of fronto-executive ability, bradyphrenia, memory impairment, and motor signs. Basal ganglia damage would produce impairments of procedural memory, perceptual learning, and skill acquisition (Robbins & Cools, 2014); the neuropsychologist chooses tests appropriate to measuring the range of expected dysfunction.

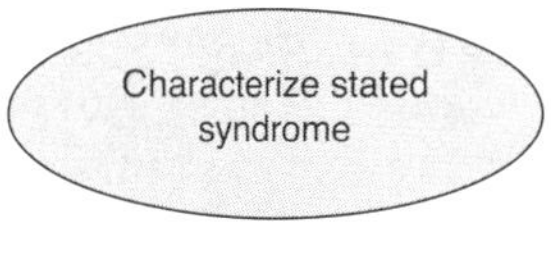

Figure 5.1 Descriptive diagnosis

This is typically a noncontroversial, common and necessary neuropsychological diagnostic task. However, clinicians asked to provide neuropsychological syndrome measurement are expected to familiarize themselves with available research and to determine expectable diagnostic patterns, range of severity, and even the viability of the construct. Neuropsychologists employed by a brain injury facility and requested to examine *postconcussion syndrome* should be familiar with expected acute symptomatology, neuropsychological severity levels, and recovery time. Finding severe test impairment and chronic or worsening neuropsychological dysfunction should prompt the neuropsychologist, not simply to conclude that tests reflect "severe, worsening postconcussion syndrome" but to consider that postconcussion complaints overlap with non–head-injury-based symptom complaints (Lees-Haley & Brown, 1993) including preexisting psychopathology or malingered impairment (Gunstad & Suhr, 2002; Satz et al., 1999) that the World Health Organization has criticized the diagnosis for its nonspecificity (Carroll et al., 2004) and that *severe worsening postconcussion syndrome* is almost certainly something *other* than postconcussion syndrome. Similarly, neuropsychologists examining athletes for *chronic traumatic encephalopathy* should understand that their neuropsychological tests may actually be measuring a multifactorial (Solomon & Zuckerman, 2014), or even an inappropriately diagnosed, condition (Andrikopoulos, 2014). Neuropsychologists asked to measure a single syndrome should investigate the origin of the referral. Is the referral source a clinician who advocates for the existence of a particular disorder? One physician's website likened her own personal reaction to toxic exposures as that of "canary in a coal mine," alluding to caged birds that miners took into their tunnels, to provide early warning of carbon monoxide exposure. The website of this physician stated that

> We 'human canaries' are here to warn the rest of you that, unless you become informed and start making changes to avoid as many toxic chemicals as possible, you too may become very ill, or even die, from the consequences.
>
> (Gilbere, 2000)

It is often useful to ask patients how they "discovered" their diagnosis, including asking about whether they have researched literature or particular Internet sites that support the diagnosis. Neuropsychologists should be wary when asked to validate what have been termed *fashionable illnesses*, typically characterized by vague fluctuating, multisystem psychosomatic complaints, buttressed by pseudoscientific explanations (Ford, 1997).

The greatest risk for neuropsychologists who perform descriptive diagnosis is *confirmatory bias*— assuming both the validity of the working diagnosis and the imprimatur to "measure" it. In fact, for many cases the diagnostic question may be incorrect, poorly worded, or completely irrelevant, given the patient's actual difficulties (Lezak, 1995, p. 110). Neuropsychologists would do well to recall Rosenhan's classic experiments during the 1970s, where healthy volunteers were asked to feign mental illness symptoms in order to gain admission to a psychiatric hospital. Once admitted, they were told to act completely normally. All were diagnosed with a psychiatric disorder, all told they required antipsychotic drugs, and all but one were diagnosed with schizophrenia "in remission" prior to their release (Rosenhan, 1973).

A simple rule to lessen confirmatory bias is to always view the referral question as a *hypothesis*, rather than the *presumptive diagnosis*. Referral sources may have limited access to information or propose their diagnosis from a circumscribed professional skill set. The fact that a diagnosis has been written in a chart does not necessarily make it correct. This author recalls a referral where the only question of concern was "degree of depression." The patient's chart repeatedly referenced the patient's "depressive demeanor." In my office, the patient proved to be a very pleasant older woman with no signs of depression. Her masked facies, lack of initiation, flat affect, and loss of executive function had been charted as "withdrawal" and "reactive depression," rather than, as proved to be the case, early signs of dementia and advancing parkinsonism.

In another case, the referral question was a single question to be measured, and was not neuropsychological but personality-related. A surgeon was referred by his hospital practice for loud and aggressive arguments with colleagues. He appeared to show insight on clinical interview that his behaviors had been truculent and argumentative, but attributed staff reactions to their unfamiliarity with his "urban" interpersonal style.

He did not appear immediately abrasive or unusual during the initial interview, but created a disturbing scenario on the elevator up to the testing laboratory. Here the doctor began to speak with a young child riding in the elevator with mother. He told the girl how "pretty" her coat was, and then bent over to feel the fabric on the coat's lapel. He was oblivious to her mother's surprised and horrified reaction.

This physician produced unremarkable results on personality tests, but failed several tests of executive function. My report to the referral source concluded that his "interpersonal pathology" better resembled frontal lobe abnormality and a neurological evaluation was strongly recommended. The doctor's brain MRI was found to demonstrate a lemon-size slow-growing tumor immediately posterior to the frontal lobe, which had the effect of degrading frontal lobe function without obvious sensory-motor or posterior impairment; in effect, inducing a very slow "frontal lobotomy." Surgery was reportedly performed immediately.

Another risk for neuropsychologists in a practice that is that while they are "often well practiced in the integration of findings from multiple test within multiple cognitive domains in an ongoing hypothesis-testing model" this approach may be "abandoned in favor of a unitary analysis of a single data source when psychological findings are addressed in the evaluation"(Allen, 2004, p. 17).

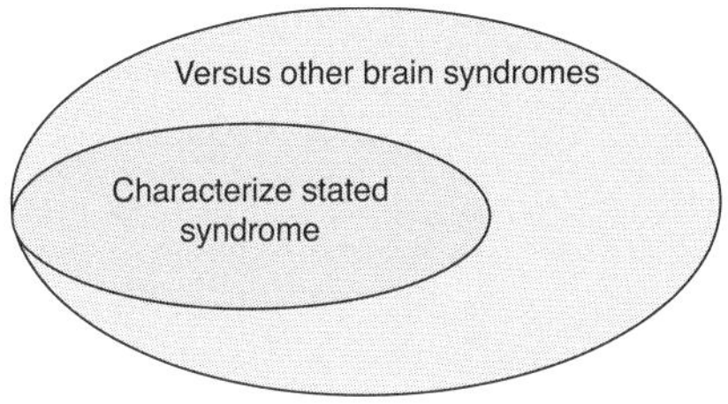

Figure 5.2 Domain-specific differential diagnosis

A more complex layer of diagnostic inference could be termed *domain-specific differential diagnosis*. Here the diagnostic task is to differentiate between patterns of at least two brain-based disorders: e.g., Alzheimer's disease versus vascular dementia, or traumatic brain injury versus stroke. The preparatory task is similar to that of descriptive diagnosis, with required understanding as to whether test patterns resemble one or more diagnostic entities; this level of diagnosis now includes *syndrome analysis.* While there is always processing overlap and interdependence of cognitive functions at the behavioral level of neuropsychological tests, syndrome analysis is frequently possible. Neurodegenerative dementias differ in their neuropsychological profiles. Compared to Alzheimer's disease, a vascular dementia profile "is characterized by better verbal memory performance worse quantitative executive functioning and prominent depressed mood" (Levy & Chelune, 2007). Compared to Alzheimer's, both dementia with Lewy bodies and Parkinson's disease can produce impaired visual information processing, degraded executive function, and mood-congruent hallucinations (Levy & Chelune, 2007).

Neuropsychological reports that require domain-specific differential diagnosis should outline the factual basis for concluding that a particular pattern of test results and history can be differentially diagnosed. Including research citations as scientific support is appropriate.

A third layer of diagnostic consideration includes differential functional localization-specific diagnoses while also considering the influence of medical disorders and their medications. This three-layered approach to diagnostic decision-making might be labeled *multidomain neuropsychological diagnosis*, where diagnostic considerations transcend focal central nervous system phenomena to include areas of non–central nervous system "medical" illness, along with the medications that are used to treat those same conditions.

Multidomain neuropsychological diagnosis requires the perspective that "many diseases affect behavior and cognitive without directly involving brain substance" (Lezak, 2012, p. vii) and more clearly mandates neuropsychological expertise at the level of medical neuropsychology. Interaction of organ system disease, metabolic disorder, genetic aberration, infection, autoimmune condition, or toxicant exposure with neuropsychological function make this level of diagnosis far more complex and challenging, but absolutely essential for neuropsychologists who diagnose as health care providers. While neuropsychologists may take the position that their

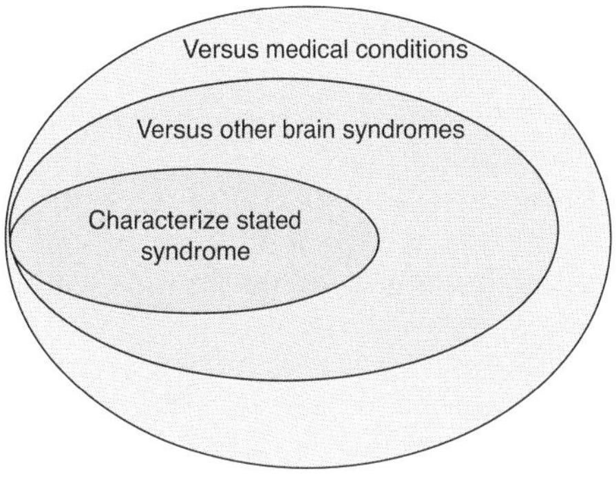

Figure 5.3 Multidomain neuromedical diagnosis

referral questions address brain–behavior phenomena, the fact is that patients sent for diagnosis are: (a) rarely perfectly healthy, and (b) rarely exhibit pathological patterns of behavior that are uniquely caused by central nervous system dysfunction. More typically, the patient's "neuropsychological" condition is influenced by layers of pathology and patients entering the neuropsychologist's office have diseases that "are actually relatively common, yet their neuropsychological symptoms and mechanisms are not often examined closely"(Armstrong, 2012, p. xii). Not only the type, but also the number of medical disorders may affect neuropsychological function. Patients with an aggregation of medical pathologies show cumulative deterioration that predicts cognitive deficits over and above age, mood, neuropathology, or psychiatric status (Patrick, Gaskovski, & Rexroth, 2002).

Neuropsychological pathology at a multidomain level of differential diagnosis requires appreciating that, referral question to the contrary, the influence of medical disorders may be additive or even primarily explanatory vis-à-vis test results, and also that these disorders are extremely common among patients who are referred for something more "neuropsychological." For example, the National Health and Nutrition Examination Survey (NHANES) data from 2005–2008 suggest age-standardized hypertension prevalence of 29.8 but rate of hypertension control at only 45.8% (Crim et al., 2012). Subpopulations (i.e., Mexican Americans) have higher rates and lower treatment levels (Burt et al., 1995). and prevalence of hypertension among African Americans at is considered to be "among the highest in the world and increasing" (Hall, Duprez, Barac, & Rich, 2012, p. 302). Hypertension contributes to progressive cognitive impairment (Birns, Morris, Jarosz, Markus, & Kalra, 2009) and elevates risk for stroke and myocardial infarction. Long-standing hypertension causes reductions in cerebral blood flow, metabolism, and cognitive function (Fujishima, Ibayashi, Fujii, & Mori, 1995). Hypertension is associated with greater degrees of cortical atrophy in older adults and is a risk factor for cognitive decline (Meyer, Rauch, Rauch, & Haque, 2000). Neurochemical disturbances are found among hypertensives, particularly in central nervous system catecholamines that mediate attention and memory (Waldstein,

Manuck, Ryan, & Muldoon, 1991). Hypertensives perform consistently more poorly than individuals with normal blood pressure on neuropsychological tests of memory, attention, and abstract reasoning.

Migraine headache history, in the absence of brain lesions or trauma, and typically seen as a "nuisance" symptom, reduces both cerebral blood flow and metabolism, producing transient cognitive impairments lasting for about an hour (Meyer, 2012) but chronic migraine sufferers may suffer orbitofrontal cognitive impairments from medication overuse, with a neuropsychological profile similar to substance abusers (Biagianti et al., 2012). Chronic cluster headache sufferers can be impaired on executive tasks, (e.g., Trails, Stroop), consistent with proposed prefrontal involvement in this headache syndrome (Dresler et al., 2012). It is almost impossible to obtain a complete medical history from clinical interview. Use of a checklist (see Table 5.1) prior to the evaluation, may allow additional inquiry and alert the neuropsychologist to possible diagnostic rule-outs.

Table 5.1 Disease/health history

Please check if you have a history of, have been told you have, or have been diagnosed with any of the following:

- Abuse: Physical, Sexual, or Verbal
- Addiction (Any)
- Attention deficit/hyperactivity disorder (ADHD)
- Adverse Childhood Experiences (Describe on Back Page)
- AIDS (Acquired Immune Deficiency Syndrome)
- Alcohol Abuse/Dependence
- ALS (Amyotrophic Lateral Sclerosis)
- Alzheimer's Disease
- American Trypanosomiasis/Chagas Disease
- Anemia
- Anthrax
- Anxiety or Panic
- Aortic Aneurysm
- Aortic Dissection
- Arthritis
- Childhood Arthritis
- Lupus (SLE) (Systemic Lupus Erythematosus)
- Osteoarthritis (OA)
- Rheumatoid Arthritis (RA)
- Aspergillus Infection (Aspergillosis)
- Asthma
- Autism Spectrum Disorder
- Bacterial Meningitis
- Balance Problems
- Bioterrorism Agents/Diseases
- Bipolar disorder
- Birth Defects
- Black Lung (Coal Workers' Pneumoconioses)
- Blast Injuries
- Blood disorders
- Botulism (Clostridium Botulinim)
- Bovine Spongiform Encephalopathy (BSE)
- BSE (Mad Cow Disease)
- Carpal Tunnel Syndrome
- Cerebral Palsy
- Cancer (Any) ________________
- CFS (Chronic Fatigue Syndrome)
- Chagas Disease (Trypanosoma Cruzi Infection)
- Chikungunya Fever (CHIKV)
- Childhood Injuries (Describe on Back Page)
- Child Abuse
- Childhood Overweight and Obesity
- Chlamydia (Chlamydia Trachomatis Disease)
- Chronic Fatigue Syndrome (CFS)
- Chronic Kidney Disease (CKD)
- Chronic Obstructive Pulmonary Dis. (COPD)
- Ciguatera Fish Poisoning
- Classic Creutzfeldt-Jakob Disease (CJD, Classic)
- Clostridium Botulinim
- Clotting disorders
- Coal Workers' Pneumoconioses Black Lung
- Complex Regional Pain Syndrome (CRPS)
- Concussion or Postconcussion Syndrome
- Congenital Hearing Loss
- Crohns Disease
- Decompression Sickness
- Deep Vein Thrombosis (DVT)
- Delirium (Any)
- Depression
- DES [Diethylstilbestrol] Exposure prenatally
- Dementia, any ________________
- Developmental Disabilities
- Diabetes
- Dizziness
- Domestic Violence
- Down Syndrome (Trisomy 21)
- Drug Abuse (Any) ________________
- Drycleaning Work-Related Solvent Exposure
- DVT (Deep Vein Thrombosis)
- Ear Infection (Otitis Media)
- Ebola Virus Disease (EVD)
- EBV Infection (Epstein-Barr Virus Infection)
- Electric and Magnetic Fields (EMF) Chronic Exposure
- Electrical Injury
- Elephantiasis
- Epilepsy/Seizure Disorder
- Epstein-Barr Virus Infection (EBV Infection)
- Ergonomic and Musculoskeletal Disorders
- Ethylene Glycol Poisoning
- Ethylene Oxide Poisoning
- Fungal Diseases (Mycotic diseases)
- Extreme Cold (Hypothermia)
- Extreme Heat (Hyperthermia)
- Fasciitis, Necrotizing (Strep)
- Fetal Alcohol Syndrome
- Fibromyalgia
- Fifth Disease (Parvovirus B19 Infection)
- Fireworks Injuries
- Flavorings-Related Lung Disease
- Food Poisoning

- Food-Related Diseases
- Formaldehyde in the Workplace
- Fragile X Syndrome (FXS)
- Fungal Meningitis
- FXS (Fragile X Syndrome)
- GA (Tabun) Poisoning
- Gambling Problems
- GB (Sarin) Poisoning
- Gout
- Guillain-Barre Syndrome
- H, HD, and HT (Mustard Gas)
- Hallucinations
- Hansen's Disease
- Hantavirus Pulmonary Syndrome (HPS)
- Headache Disorder (any)
- Hearing Loss, Occupational
- Heart Disease
- Heat Stress
- Hemochromatosis
- Hemoglobinopathies
- Herbicide Exposure
- Hereditary Bleeding Disorders
- Herpes, any
- Hexavalent Chromium Exposure
- High Blood Pressure
- High Cholesterol
- Hydrogen cyanide
- Hydrogen Sulfide
- Infertility
- Inflammatory Bowel Disease (IBD)
- Intimate Partner Violence
- Invasive Candidiasis
- Iron Overload (Hemochromatosis)
- Iron Storage Disease
- Isocyanates
- Japanese Encephalitis (JE)
- Kawasaki Syndrome (KS)
- KFD (Kyasanur Forest Disease)
- Kidney Disease (CKD)
- KS (Kawasaki Syndrome)
- La Crosse Encephalitis (LAC)
- Lead Poisoning
- Learning Disability
- Legionnaires' Disease (Legionellosis)
- Liver Disease and Hepatitis
- Lockjaw/ Tetanus Disease
- Lupus (SLE) (Systemic lupus erythematosus)
- Lyme Disease (Borrelia burgdorferi Infection)
- Malaria
- Manganese
- Marburg Hemorrhagic Fever
- Marine Toxins Exposure
- Menopause-Related Problems
- MD (Muscular Dystrophy)
- Meningitis
- Meningococcal Disease
- Mental Retardation
- Mercury Exposure
- MERS-CoV (Middle East Respiratory Synd. Coronavirus)
- Metalworking Fluids Exposure
- Methyl Alcohol Exposure
- Methyl Ethyl Ketone Exposure
- MRSA (Methicillin Resistant Staphylococcus aureus)
- Multiple Sclerosis (MS)
- Muscular Dystrophy (MD)
- Mustard Gas (H, HD, and HT) (Sulfur Mustard)
- Mycoplasma Pneumoniae Infection
- Myelomeningocele/Spina Bifida
- Myiasis
- Naegleria Infection (Primary Amebic Meningoencephalitis (PAM))
- Narcotic/Opioid Abuse/Dependence
- Necrotizing Fasciitis
- Ni (Nickel)
- Nitrous Oxide Overdose
- Nodding Syndrome
- Norovirus Infection
- OA (Osteoarthritis)
- Obesity and Overweight
- Obsessive-Compulsive Problems
- OD (Drug Overdose)
- Organic Solvents
- Osteoarthritis (OA)
- Osteoporosis or Osteopenia
- Overweight and Obesity
- Ozone exposure
- PAD (Peripheral Arterial Disease)
- Pain, Chronic
- Painkiller Dependence or Overdose
- Paraquat Exposure
- Parasitic Diseases
- PE (Pulmonary Embolism)
- Pelvic Inflammatory Disease (PID)
- Peripheral Arterial Disease (PAD)
- Pertussis (Whooping Cough)
- Phosgene (CG) Exposure
- Phosphine Exposure
- Phosphorus Burn
- PID (Pelvic Inflammatory Disease)
- Piercing Infections
- Plague (Yersinia Pestis Infection)
- Pneumoconioses (Black Lung)
- Poisoning (Any)
- Polio Infection (Poliomyelitis Infection)
- Polycystic Ovary Disease
- Postpartum Depression
- Posttraumatic Stress Disorder (PTSD)
- Potassium Cyanide Exposure
- Premature Birth
- Prion Disease
- Psychiatric Hospitalization
- Psoriasis
- Rabies
- Reflex Sympathetic Dystrophy (RSD)
- Rheumatoid Arthritis (RA)
- Ricin Exposure
- Rickettsial Diseases

- Riot Control Agent Exposure
- Scarlet Fever
- Schizophrenic Disorder
- Sepsis (Septicemia)
- Syphilis (Treponema Pallidum Infection)
- Shingles (Varicella Zoster Virus (VZV))
- Sick Building Syndrome
- Sickle Cell Disease
- Sinus Infection (Sinusitus)
- SLE (Lupus)
- Sleep Apnea
- Sleep Disorder (Any)
- SLEV (St. Louis Encephalitis)
- Smallpox (Variola Major and Variola Minor)
- Small Vessel Disease
- Smokeless (Oral) Tobacco use
- Smoking and Tobacco Use
- Snoring
- Stress, Occupational
- Stroke
- Strychnine Exposure
- Styrene Exposure
- Substance Abuse/Dependence
- Suicide Attempt
- Syncope (Fainting for Any Reason)
- Syphilis (Treponema Pallidum Infection)
- Tabun (GA) Poisoning
- TB (Tuberculosis)
- TBI (Traumatic Brain Injury)
- Tear Gas Exposure
- Tetanus (Lockjaw) Infection
- Tetrachloroethylene Exposure
- Thallium Poisoning
- Thyroid Disease (Over or Underactive)
- Lyme Disease (Borrelia burgdorferi Infection)
- Toluene Exposure
- Tourette Syndrome (TS)
- Transient Ischemic Attack (TIA)
- Traumatic Incident Stress
- Trichinellosis (Trichinosis)
- Trichloroethylene
- Ulcers
- Venomous Snakes/Spiders
- Vibration, Nervous System Iinjury
- Visual Impairment (Any)
- Wilson's Disease
- Xylene Exposure

Neuropsychological diagnosis which includes these four layers of information is enhanced by reviewing and ordering laboratory blood and urine tests. Lab tests can provide useful clues to neuropsychological diagnosis at the medical symptom level, and are important to identify pathognomonic signs, monitor medication levels, detect drug or alcohol abuse, and consider the possible influence of lab result abnormality upon neuropsychological diagnosis (McConnell, 2014). While most lab testing is performed by hospital or medical personnel, psychologists licensed to prescribe medications, depending upon state law, may order such tests directly. In either case, neuropsychologists practicing at this level of differential diagnostic expertise have the responsibility to collaborate with medical providers by reviewing and even requesting such tests.

Just as medical diagnosis influences neuropsychological diagnosis, prescription medications can significantly alter neuropsychological presentation and require the influence effects of medications prescribed to treat a medical diagnosis requires consideration in neuropsychological diagnosis. The influence of medication on neuropsychological diagnosis is as ubiquitous as are patients taking medication, and increases with age. Ninety percent of persons aged 65 and older take at least one prescription medication, and almost half are given five drugs or more (Tannenbaum, Paquette, Hilmer, Holroyd-Leduc, & Carnahan, 2012). Consideration of medication effects and their interactions by neuropsychologists is still relatively rare, even though "consumption of medication that can negatively affect cognition is an alternate explanation that may be under-recognized" (Tannenbaum et al., 2012, p. 640). Neuropsychologists are responsible for understanding the individual and interactive effects of medications in terms of dose, frequency of occurrence, and severity with respect to the patient's overall cognitive and emotional status. Some medication effects are fairly common, e.g., the effects of acute benzodiazepine ingestion upon memory. Alternatively, a neuropsychologist who routinely "finds" statin-related cognitive impairment is likely overdiagnosing a rare occurrence (Rojas-Fernandez & Cameron, 2012). Diagnostic conclusions should include possible neuropsychological medication effects and drug interactions; websites such as epocrates (www.epocrates.com) offer free drug interaction checks to professionals. Arguably, neuropsychologists should be aware of potentially dangerous or even lethal effects of medications, doses, and interactions, since prescriptions may be obtained from multiple physicians who are not in communication with one another and are unable to observe the patient outside the office. Patients themselves may fail to appreciate drug-related dangers that develop over time.

The next layer of neuropsychological diagnostic inference, *multidomain neuromedical diagnosis*, includes the influence of psychiatric disorder, both active and historical. Patients who are being evaluated for neuropsychological impairment may or may not have discussed their psychiatric history with the same health care practitioners who are treating them for neurologic or general medical concerns. As is the case with medical conditions, a comprehensive interview and/or history questionnaire concerning personal and familial psychiatric morbidity may suggest additional testing, neuropsychological inquiry, and psychiatric/psychological referral. Due to the high genetic loading of many psychiatric disorders (e.g., bipolar disorder), obtaining a family history of psychiatric presentation may guide questions addressed to the current patient. Psychiatric history is directly germane to

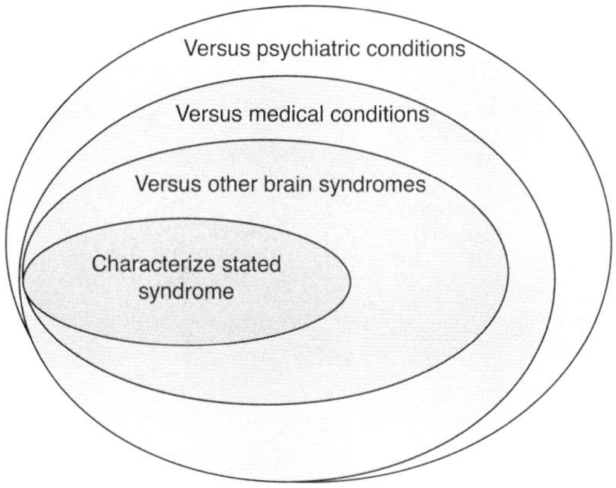

Figure 5.4 Neuromedical psychiatric diagnosis

neuropsychological conclusions since cognitive impairment profiles are common among individuals with certain psychiatric disorders, and may differ according to diagnosis. Patients with certain schizophrenic disorders, for example, may be neuropsychologically impaired, but stable, over the first ten years of illness (Bozikas & Andreou, 2011). In contrast, premorbid neuropsychological function in patients diagnosed with bipolar disorder is relatively normal, but deteriorates over time until chronic bipolar disorder patients "may be virtually indistinguishable" from patients with schizophrenic disorder (Woodward, 2016). Patients with bipolar disorder continue to display neuropsychological impairments that persist even during euthymic (normal mood) intervals.

> Cognitive deficits involving attention, executive function, and verbal memory are evident across all phases of bipolar disorder. . . . differentiating medication- from illness-induced cognitive dysfunction requires comprehensive assessment with an appreciation for the cognitive domains most affected by specific medications. No current pharmacotherapies substantially improve cognition in bipolar disorder.
>
> (Goldberg & Chengappa, 2009, p. 123)

Diagnostic history, family history of psychopathology, and use of objective psychological assessment instruments (e.g., Minnesota Multiphasic Personality Inventory-2 Restructured Form; Personality Assessment Inventory, Millon Clinical Multiaxial Inventory IV) provide valuable normative comparisons and symptom validity measurement as well.

The fifth layer of diagnostic consideration includes objective assessment of effort and motivation. Perhaps more than any other layer of influence, this may be a unique neuropsychological contribution to the understanding of patient symptoms. Clinicians listening to self-report may do little more than reify that self-report in the medical record. This does not advance accurate diagnosis unless the pattern of self-report provides reliable clinical data. Psychologists and neuropsychologists have the best and most widely researched procedures to provide objective assessment of response pattern credibility.

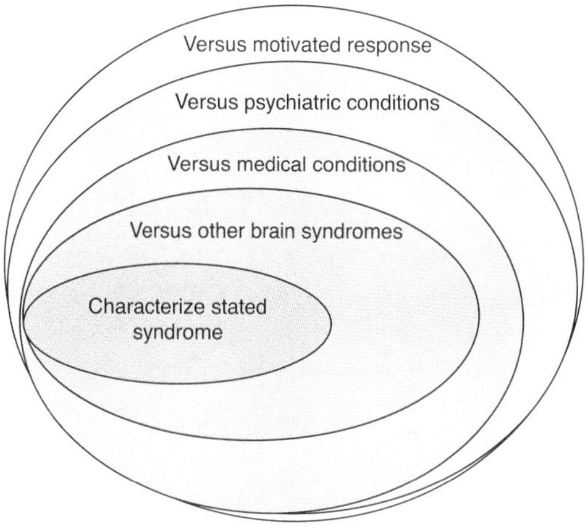

Figure 5.5 Forensic neuromedicopsychiatric diagnosis

The fifth layer of diagnostic inference, gradual and growing acceptance by the neuropsychological community that: "malingering or deficit exaggeration must be specifically addressed to support either a conclusion of faking bad or putting forth good effort at task performance" (Loring, 1995). Most neuropsychologists now agree that any neuropsychological evaluation is incomplete without the careful consideration of patient motivation (Iverson, 2003), and the specialized methodology employed to measure motivation has proven demonstrably superior to clinical judgment. Subjective clinical judgment in the absence of tests that determine motivation and effort do

> not make optimal or near-optimal use of information bearing on malingering when evaluating cases, for it that were so, clinicians [not making use of such tests] would at least be matching, if not outperforming, formal decision rules and success, which they are not doing.
>
> (Faust & Ackley, 1998, p. 2)

In one study, three-quarters of neuropsychologists who did not have access to formal tests of exaggeration indicated moderate or greater confidence in their *wrong* conclusions and "not a single neuropsychologist identified malingering in those patients who were instructed to fake brain injury" (Binder, 1997, p. 226).

There is no reasonable rationale to remove consideration of motivation distortion just because there is no active lawsuit. Poor effort and exaggeration occur for nonlitigious reasons: The patient may wish to be taken care of, avoid adult responsibility, or obtain family support; these may not require litigation, just formal validation of clinical disability.

The *National Academy of Neuropsychology*, representing the neuropsychological community, concluded that symptom validity testing was necessary in both medical and forensic contexts.

> Symptom exaggeration or fabrication occurs in a sizeable minority of neuropsychological examinees, with greater

> prevalence in forensic contexts. Adequate assessment of response validity is essential in order to maximize confidence in the results of neurocognitive and personality measures and in the diagnoses and recommendations that are based on the results. . . .Assessment of response validity, as a component of a medically necessary evaluation, is medically necessary. When determined by the neuropsychologist to be necessary for the assessment of response validity, administration of specific symptom validity tests is also medically necessary.
>
> (Bush et al., 2005, p. 419)

Specific test measures of effort and symptom distortion are not simply an adjunct to clinical impression, but must be *part* of that clinical impression. There is no corpus of data to suggest that motivation effects disappear if patients are not engaged in lawsuits. Apparently nonlitigating patients may be intending to litigate *after* testing; others may deny active litigation and attempt to route their referral through a treating physician, in order to have the evaluation covered as a clinical procedure. They may intend to have the neuropsychologist testify as a *fact* witness, unwittingly colluding with their search for disability. Some patients may not reveal litigation participation because their evaluation would be covered by insurance if it was a clinical procedure but *not* as part of a legal claim. Others who have no intention to sue shape their behavior for nonlitigation-related reinforcers, e.g., avoiding adult responsibilities. One frequently sees reports and studies where individuals are concluded to be well-motivated if *they have already obtained disability benefits,* as though the reason to feign impairment disappears when benefits are granted. More likely, because such patients undergo periodic disability review, they are well aware that the disability pretense must continue to ensure the continuation of benefits.

Others patients deliberately self-injure to *become* medically disabled. Some are obsessed with obtaining mutilating surgeries, which may actually occur unless they are correctly diagnosed with a *factitious* disorder. I asked one such patient, who had recurring episodes of lymphedema, infection, and sepsis in a leg, what he understood as a plan for treatment. He replied, with a fascinated expression,

> well, the doctor says that if my infection and lymphedema continues, they may have to amputate the leg at the knee . . . but that may not be enough, so they may have to amputate the leg at the thigh . . . but *that* may not be enough and they may have to amputate the leg above the thigh, all the way above the hip!

He described these morbid possibilities like that of a child being offered ever more desirable toys. The patient's medical record contained numerous exploratory operations, some of which found objects, such as broken-off pencil points, in muscle or joint tissue. Surgeons blithely recorded the patient's explanations, e.g., "He thanked us for removing the object, which had been embedded in his leg since childhood."

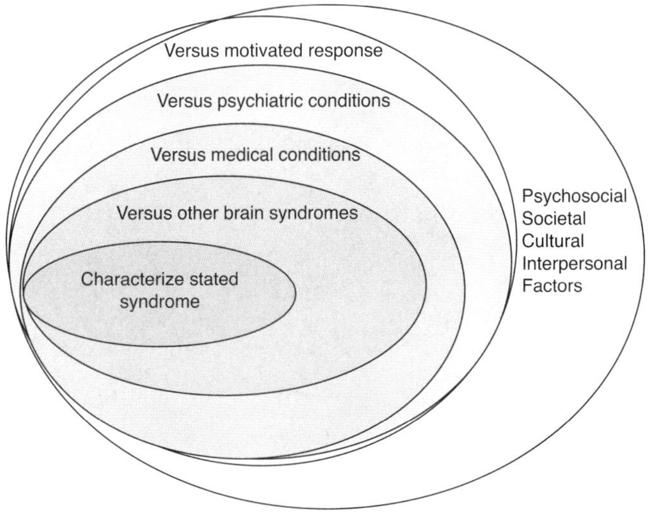

Figure 5.6 Differential forensic biopsychosocial diagnosis

The final layer of diagnostic consideration *differential forensic biopsychosocial diagnosis* includes a culture-fair biopsychosocial assessment as to how a particular diagnosis may be shaped by the patient's culture, language facility, societal differences, and attitude toward the examination. It is tempting for neuropsychologists to assume that their tests measure concrete, invariant aspects of brain function but of course, they do not. This author recalls the rather horrifying conclusion of one self-identified neuropsychologist who pronounced that a low IQ score per the Bell Curve was evidence, *ab aeterno*, of defective brain function; he indicated that it did not matter whether the patient given the IQ test was English- or Spanish-speaking, poorly or well-educated. Contrary to this egregiously incorrect understanding of what tests measure across languages and cultures, the *Ethical Principles of Psychologists and Code of Conduct* (American Psychological Association, 2010) requires psychological practitioners to respect the rights and welfare of all populations, and attempt to eliminate biases related to age, cultural, ethnicity, race, religion, sexual orientation, disability, language, and socioeconomic status (*Ethical Principles—Preamble: General Principle E*, 2010). For neuropsychological diagnosis, such respect comes with the understanding that neuropsychological differences are not indicia of immutable brain function, but may be related to health disparities, cultural approach to authority and testing, and many other factors. Even tasks as simple and universally administered as Digit Span are affected by linguistic and cultural differences (Ostrosky-Solis & Lozano, 2006).

The reasons behind cultural differences in neuropsychological test responses may be linguistic or cultural. Other authors have suggested that such differences reflect evidence of a "different" brain. Chee, Zheng, Goh, Park, and Sutton (2011) found young predominantly White American adults had higher cortical thickness in frontal, parietal, and medial-temporal polymodal association areas in both hemispheres, compared with Chinese residents of Singapore. They proposed that varying gray matter patterns could be the result of ethnic-cultural cognitive differences, genetics, or environmental factors. Regardless of whether neuropsychological differences are structural or psychosocially derived, neuropsychological diagnosis, in the largest sense, requires consideration of whether these influences shape or even change the diagnosis.

In conclusion, neuropsychological diagnosis requires a strategic approach with layered consideration of causal influences upon neuropsychological behavior. Detailed test measurement is only the most basic layer of that diagnostic inference. Depending upon the referral question and the complexity of the case, neuropsychological diagnosis can require detailed understanding, not only of brain-behavior relationships, but also brain-behavior-medical and medication-relationships. Neuropsychological diagnosis additionally requires the appreciation of mental health history, motivation, and psychosocial influences upon the final interpretation of what our tests measure, and what the patient actually "has." Neuropsychological test selection and numerical result interpretation is just the beginning.

If I have any final advice about *how to diagnose*, it is to explicitly justify one's diagnostic conclusions in the body of the report. Be clear about sources of data and how those data were integrated into final conclusions. The reader of a neuropsychological report should be clear as to each link in the chain of diagnostic inference. Footnotes to research and decision-making strategy included in the report allow the reviewer to trace or dispute your reasoning. A well crafted report should be clear, in and of itself. There should be no question in the mind of the reader why you made a particular diagnosis.

The following brief ABCDE of neuropsychological diagnosis could be considered an initial checklist when determining the influence of neuropsychological test results on behavior.

A(scertain) which level of diagnostic inference is required. Does "diagnosis" require measurement of an agreed-upon construct, or differential diagnosis at a more complex level of consideration? Is the construct generally agreed upon, e.g., Degree of Alzheimer's Dementia, or is the diagnostic request itself controversial or implausible, e.g., chronic postconcussion syndrome, multiple chemical sensitivity, chronic lime disease, toxic mold encephalopathy, etc.

B(ase) rate consideration of diagnostic influences and whether they are supported by peer-reviewed research. The effect of Benzodiazepines on neuropsychological function is generally agreed upon; statin effects upon neuropsychological function are probably rare. Ascribing Autism to vaccination is junk science.

C(onsideration) of reasonable alternatives and aggregate influences upon diagnosis. There should be an explicit set of considerations leading to your diagnosis.

D(e-bias) conclusions and reports. Sweet and Moulthrop (1999) remind the diagnostician that reports should be written to a standard that a panel of neuropsychological peers would find acceptable. The report should be reviewed for emotional or scientific bias and even if the report has no likelihood of being professionally critiqued, the diagnosing neuropsychologist should be prepared to dispassionately explain how diagnosis flows from data, rather than clinical lore or personal belief system.

E(ffort) examination is critical to understanding whether results are actual clinical neurobehavioral patterns or whether those same results are overridden by motivational

Table 5.2 Sample biopsychosocial questions. Each of these questions has potential import for understanding test results and diagnostic considerations

Is anyone in your family currently disabled, or has been disabled in the past? If so, who?
Have you or any members of your family been physically, sexually or chronically verbally abused?
Are you a member of any group with a diagnosis like yours?
Have you read any books that influence the way you understand your condition?
Are there any Internet sites that you particularly recommend in understanding your condition?
If you have limitations in your daily activities, who helps you?
How much coffee, tea or other caffeinated beverage do you drink each day?
How many alcohol drinks will you typically drink each week?
Do you take supplements, health foods, herbs or other nonprescribed treatments for your condition(s)?
What are you current favorite activities?
Have there been any major changes in your life or family in the past several years? (e.g., death, marriage, divorce, financial problems, addiction, violence) Please list ______________________________
Were you ever in the military or National Guard? Were you honorably discharged? At what rank? Do you have a military disability?
What is your primary language spoken at home? What languages do you speak?
Does anyone in your family have a history of depression, bipolar disorder, thyroid disorder, schizophrenic disorder, attention deficit, alcohol or drug abuse, attempted or completed suicide, tics, problems with the law, anxiety or panic, posttraumatic stress disorder, heart attack, high blood pressure, stroke, dementia, learning disability. Please explain.
Have you been sued or have you sued anyone? If yes, please describe each lawsuit and date.
If you are in a current lawsuit, how much stress does this cause you? 0(none)______ 10(extreme) ______

distortion. While poor effort is not the same as malingering, neither describes an accurate pattern of brain-behavior relationships. Given the preponderance of research and professional statements regarding this issue, examination of effort and motivation should be considered standard procedure for almost every diagnostic evaluation. It is arguably unethical to perform evaluations (e.g., Social Security Disability evaluations) that actually forbid the use of effort measures.

To conclude, neuropsychological diagnosis requires a *strategy*; specifically a multilayered series of considerations which lie between the initial referral question and the final diagnosis. Utilizing this methodology does not ensure perfect diagnosis, but using a multi-layered strategic approach increases the likelihood that appropriate incluences diagnosis are weighed before conclusions are drawn. We strive for understanding of our complex selves, and if we cannot yet understand a grand design, we can at least, be clear about the path we have taken.

Declaration of Conflicting Interests

The author declared no potential conflicts of interest with respect to authorship and/or publication of this chapter.

Funding

The author received no financial support for the research and/or authorship of this chapter.

References

Allen, J. B. (2004). Psychosocial factors in differential diagnosis. In J. H. Ricker (Ed.), *Differential Diagnosis in Adult Neuropsychological Assessment* (p. 1–26). New York: Springer Publishing Company.

American Psychological Association (2010). Ethical Principles of Psychologists and Code of Conduct. https://www.apa.org/ethics/code/principles.pdf

Andrikopoulos, J. (2014). Clinical presentation of chronic traumatic encephalopathy. *Neurology*, *83*, 1991–1993.

Armstrong, C. L. (2012). Preface. In C. L. Armstrong & L. Morrow (Eds.), *Handbook of Medical Neuropsychology* (p. xi). New York. Springer.

Berger, D. (1999). A brief history of medical diagnosis and the birth of the clinical laboratory, Part 1: Ancient times through the 19th *Medical* century. *Laboratory Observer*, *31*, 28–30, 32, 34–40.

Biagianti, B., Grazzi, L., Gambini, O., et al. (2012). Decision-making deficit in chronic migraine patients with medication overuse. *Neurological Science*, *33*, S151–S155.

Binder, L. (1997). Malingering on intellectual and neuropsychological measures. In R. Rogers (Ed.), *Clinical Assessment of Malingering and Deception* (p. 226). New York, Guildford Press.

Birns, J., Morris, R., Jarosz, J., Markus, H. S., & Kalra, L. (2009). Hypertension-related cognitive decline: Is the right time for intervention studies? *Minerva Cardioangiologica*, *57*, 813–830.

Bozikas, V. P., & Andreou, C. (2011). Longitudinal studies of cognition in first episode psychosis: A systematic review of the literature. *Australia and New Zealand Journal of Psychiatry*, *45*, 93–108.

Burt, V. L., Whelton, P., Roccella, E. J., et al. (1995). Prevalence of hypertension in the US Adult population. *Hypertension*, *25*, 305–313.

Bush, S. S., Ruff, R. M., Troster, A. I., Barth, J, T., Koffler, S. P., Pliskin, N. H., . . . Silver, C. H. (2005). NAN position paper: Symptom validity assessment: Practice issues and medical necessity. *Archives of Clinical Neuropsychology*, *20*, 419–426.

Carroll, L. J., Cassidy, D., Peloso, P. M., Borg, J., Hoist, H., Holm, L., . . . Pepin, M. (2004). Prognosis for mild traumatic brain injury: Results of the WHO collaborating centre task force on mild traumatic brain injury. *Journal of Rehabilitation Medicine, Supplement*, *43*, 84–105.

Chee, M.W.L., Zheng, H., Goh, J.O.S., Park, D., & Sutton, B. P. (2011). Brain structure in young and old East Asians and Westerners: Comparisons of structural volume and cortical thickness. *Journal of Cognitive Neuroscience*, *23*, 1065–1079.

Crim, M. T., Yoon, S. S., Ortiz, E. W., et al. (2012). National surveillance definitions for hypertension prevalence and control among adults. *Circulation, Cardiovascular Quality and Outcomes*, *5*, 343–351.

Dresler, T., Lurding, R., Paelecke-Habermann, Y., et al. (2012). Cluster headache and neuropsychological functioning. *Cephalalgia*, *32*, 813–821.

Faust, D., & Ackley, M. A. (1998). Did you think it was going to be easy? Some methodological suggestions for the investigation and development of malingering detection strategies. In C. Reynolds (Ed.), *Detection of Malingering During Head Injury Litigation* (p. 1–54). New York: Plenum Press.

Ford, C. V. (1997). Somatization and fashionable diagnoses: Illness as a way of life. *Scandinavian Journal of Work Environment and Health*, *23*(Suppl 3), 7–16.

Fujishima, M., Ibayashi, S., Fujii, K., & Mori, S. (1995). Cerebral blood flow and brain function in hypertension. *Hypertension Research*, *18*, 111–117.

Gilbere, G. (2000). Allergic reactions and chemical sensitivity. Retrieved from www.ourlittleplace.com/article1.html

Goldberg, J. F., & Chengappa, K. N. (2009). Identifying and treating cognitive impairment in bipolar disorder. *Bipolar Disorders*, *11*(Suppl 2), 123–137.

Gunstad, J., & Suhr, J. A. (2002). Perception of illness: Nonspecificity of postconcussion syndrome symptom expectation. *Journal of the International Neuropsychological Society*, *8*, 37–47.

Hall, J. L., Duprez, D. A., Barac, A., & Rich, S. S. (2012). A review of genetics, arterial stiffness and blood pressure in African Americans. *Journal of Cardiovascular Transplant Research*, *5*, 302–308.

Iverson, G. (2003). Detecting malingering in civil evaluations. In. A. M. Horton & L. C. Hartlage (Eds.), *Handbook of Forensic Neuropsychology* (p. 138). New York: Springer Publishing Company.

Lees-Haley, P. R., & Brown, R. S. (1993). Neuropsychological complaint base rates of 170 personal injury claimants. *Archives of Clinical Neuropsychology*, *8*, 203–209.

Levy, J. A., & Chelune, G. J. (2007). Cognitive-behavioral profiles of neurodegenerative dementias: Beyond Alzheimer's disease. *Journal of Geriatric Psychiatry and Neurology*, *20*, 227–238.

Lezak, M. D. (1995). Chapter 5: The neuropsychological examination process. In *Neuropsychological Assessment* (3rd ed.). New York: Oxford University Press.

Lezak, M. D. (2012). Forward. In C. L. Armstrong & L. Morrow (Eds.), *Handbook of Medical Neuropsychology* (p. VII–X). New York: Springer.

Loring, D. W. (1995, February 9). *Ethical issues in medicolegal consultations*. Paper presented at the Annual North American Meeting of the International Neuropsychological Society, Seattle, Washington.

MacFarland, K. (1983). Syndrome analysis in clinical neuropsychology. *British Journal of Clinical Psychology*, *22*, 61–74.

McConnell, H. W. (2014). Chapter 3: Laboratory testing in neuropsychology. In M. W. Persons & T. A. Hammerke (Eds.), *Clinical Neuropsychology: A Pocket Handbook for Assessment* (pp. 53–89). Washington, DC: American Psychological Association.

Meyer, J. S. (2012). Cognitive declines during migraine and cluster headaches are caused by cerebral 5HT neurotransmitter dysfunction. In C. L. Armstrong & L. Morrow (Eds.), *Handbook of Medical Neuropsychology* (pp. 123–128). New York: Springer.

Meyer, J. S., Rauch, G., Rauch, R. A., & Haque, A. (2000). Risk factors for cerebral hypoperfusion, mild cognitive impairment, and dementia. *Neurobiology of Aging. Mar–Apr*, *21*, 161–169.

Ostrosky-Solis, F., & Lozano, A. (2006). Digit span: Effects of education and culture. *International Journal of Psychology*, *41*, 333–341.

Patrick, L., Gaskovski, P., & Rexroth, D. (2002). Cumulative illness and neuropsychological decline in hospitalized geriatric patients. *Clinical Neuropsychology*, *16*, 145–156.

Robbins, T. W., & Cools, R. (2014). Cognitive deficits in Parkinson's Disease: A cognitive neuroscience perspective. *Movement Disorders*, *29*, 597–607.

Rojas-Fernandez, C. H., & Cameron, J. C. (2012). Is statin-associated cognitive impairment clinically relevant? A narrative review and clinical recommendations. *Annals of Pharmacotherapeutics*, *46*, 549–557.

Rosenhan, D. (1973). On being sane in insane places. *Science*, *179*, 250–258.

Satz, P., Alfano, M., Light, R., Morgenstern, H., Zaucha, K., Asarnow, R., & Newton, S. (1999). Persistent post-concussive syndrome: A proposed methodology and literature review to determine the effects, if any, of mild head and other bodily injury. *Journal of Clinical & Experimental Neuropsychology*, *21*, 620–628.

Seller, R. H., & Symons, A. B. (2007). *Differential Diagnosis of Common Complaints* (6th ed.). Philadelphia, PA: Elsevier/Saunders.

Solomon, G. S., & Zuckerman, S. L. (2014). Chronic traumatic encephalopathy in professional sports: Retrospective and prospective views. *Brain Injury*, *29*, 1–7.

Sweet, J. J., & Moulthrop, M. A. (1999). Examination questions as a means of identifying bias in adversarial assessments. *Journal of Forensic Neuropsychology*, *1*, 73–88.

Tannenbaum, C., Paquette, A., Hilmer, S., Holroyd-Leduc, J., & Carnahan, R. (2012). A systematic review of amnestic and non-amnestic mild cognitive impairment induced by anticholinergic, antihistamine, GABAergic and opioid drugs. *Drugs and Aging*, *39*, 639–658.

Waldstein, S. R., Manuck, S. B., Ryan, C. M., & Muldoon, M. F. (1991). Neuropsychological correlates of hypertension: Review and methodologic considerations. *Psychological Bulletin*, *110*, 451–468.

Woodward, N. D. (2016). The course of neuropsychological impairment and brain structure abnormalities in psychotic disorder. *Neuroscience Research*, *102*, 39–46.

6 Neuroanatomy for the Neuropsychologist

Christopher M. Filley and Erin D. Bigler

Introduction

The details of human neuroanatomy are vast, intricate, and continually expanding. As a result, the study of neuroanatomy may seem forbidding to clinicians and researchers whose focus is on clinical behavioral assessment. Nevertheless, a working knowledge of neuroanatomy is fundamental for neuropsychologists. This chapter will endeavor to develop such an understanding, presenting an overview of human neuroanatomy while emphasizing the most relevant aspects for those engaged in the neuropsychological study of higher functions.

Historical Background

The origins of human behavior and consciousness are an enduring source of fascination. Few have not had occasion to ponder the sources of thought and feeling, and the personal immediacy of daily conscious experience is an inescapable aspect of human existence. Whereas richly descriptive literary and artistic accounts of mental life have been offered by the humanities for generations, the biomedical sciences have also advanced our understanding of these phenomena through formal investigation of the nervous system. From ancient times, physicians have been intrigued by the role of the brain in human behavior. In the fifth century B.C., Hippocrates held that the brain was the seat of all mental faculties, and that afflictions of the brain led to a wide range of mental and emotional disorders. Galen, in the second century A.D., believed that the brain was the primary modulator of mental capacities, although he and many medieval physicians asserted that these capacities were to be found within the ventricles. With the appearance of detailed studies of the brain by the Renaissance anatomist Vesalius in the 16th century, the identification of the brain as the site of cognition and emotion steadily gained credence. The rise of neurology and its allied basic neuroscience disciplines in the last two centuries buttressed this association with descriptive data on the clinical phenomenology of normal and abnormal brain functions. Even the psychoanalytic thinking of Sigmund Freud in the early 20th century acknowledged that the ultimate goal of psychological research was to establish a scientific basis for human behavior. Today, with the advent of sophisticated methods in neuroscience including modern neuroimaging, no doubt exists in the scientific community that the brain is the organ of the mind (Filley, 2011; Mesulam, 2001; Cummings & Mega, 2003).

Philosophy and the Brain

Despite the identity of brain and mind that is widely accepted among neuroscientists, considerable debate on this question remains in society as a whole. Many people are reluctant to attribute the extraordinary phenomena of human behavior to the activity of such physical entities as nerve cells and chemicals in the brain. This uncertainty stems from a long and persisting controversy in Western philosophy known as the mind-brain problem (Filley, 2011). Most closely linked with the work of the 16th century French philosopher Rene Descartes, this debate centers on the relationship of the mental and physical worlds. Descartes, sometimes called the father of modern philosophy, acknowledged that both mental and physical realities exist (*res cogitans* and *res extensa*, respectively), but maintained that they are strictly separated (Searle, 2000). For Descartes, the mental world is represented by the soul, an inherently subjective entity, whereas the physical world is an objective reality to which the soul cannot be reduced. This view, known as *dualism,* has dominated much of philosophical thinking for hundreds of years, and finds many adherents today. The soul, however, does not lend itself to scientific scrutiny, and postulation of its existence is not helpful to those wishing to study a physical phenomenon. Whereas proof that a soul does not exist is most difficult to acquire, there is also no evidence to support that it does. On the contrary, much information favors the idea that the brain makes an essential contribution to all aspects of mental existence. As modern neuroscientific data on the brain accumulate, it is increasingly apparent that both cognition and emotion—thinking and feeling, respectively—may be completely explained by brain science. Even consciousness, a formidable concept that until recently intimidated neuroscientists, appears to be nothing more—or less—than a product of the brain at work (Searle, 2000).

The Neuroanatomy of Higher Function

Neuroanatomy is the study of the structure of the nervous system, the major integrative organ system in the human body. The nervous system is an exceedingly complex assembly of excitable cells and their supporting structures, and is most usefully considered in terms of its major divisions (Table 6.1). As a first step, the major division in neuroanatomy is between the central nervous system (CNS), which is made up of the brain and the spinal cord, and the peripheral nervous system (PNS), consisting of numerous spinal and cranial nerves (CNs) with branches that reach virtually the entire body and transmit information to and from the CNS. The autonomic nervous system, organized to regulate many aspects of visceral function, is made up of selected components of both the CNS and the PNS. For clinicians primarily engaged in the assessment and care of individuals with disorders of the brain, the anatomy of the brain is the most critical portion of neuroanatomy. In this chapter, therefore, a clinically relevant depiction of brain anatomy will be provided. Special attention will be devoted to the representation of the singular mental capacities of *homo sapiens*, often referred to as the higher cerebral or *cognitive functions*, or simply the *higher functions*.

The first task will be to develop a thorough understanding of the structure of the brain. This foundation is a necessary basis for a basic task of clinical neuroscience: the localization of normal and disturbed brain function. For this process, not only do brain areas devoted to higher functions deserve attention, but also those anatomically related regions that enable identification of behaviorally relevant areas by virtue of their "neighborhood" proximity. With this background, a brief discussion will follow on major unifying themes in brain-behavior relationships, including the phylogenetic organization of the brain; the functions of cortical, subcortical, and white matter regions; and cerebral lateralization. These considerations will lead directly to the concept of neural networks, a notion that offers a comprehensive organizing principle for understanding all the domains of cognition and emotion. Finally, a synopsis of the major functional affiliations of the four cerebral lobes will be presented.

Table 6.1 Major neuroanatomic divisions

Nervous System
Central
Peripheral
Autonomic
Central Nervous System
Brain
Spinal Cord
Brain
Brain Stem
Midbrain
Pons
Medulla
Cerebellum
Cerebrum
Diencephalon
Thalamus
Hypothalamus
Cerebral hemispheres
Gray Matter
Cortex
Basal Ganglia
White Matter
Cerebral Cortex
Frontal Lobe
Temporal Lobe-Limbic System
Parietal Lobe
Occipital Lobe

Neuroanatomy Through Neuroimaging

Since the introduction of computed tomography (CT) in the early 1970s, the fidelity of brain imaging to visualize gross brain anatomy has improved at a rapid pace hastened by the development of magnetic resonance (MR) imaging (MRI). Today much of neuroanatomy is now taught via neuroimaging methods (Leichnetz, 2006; Nowinski & Chua, 2013). This chapter will use the basic information from the first edition of this book, as the fundamentals of neuroanatomy have not changed, and fuse this traditional approach with MR methods of imaging that highlight neuroanatomical detail. For example, the middle and right-hand images in Figure 6.1 are from an axial MRI section of the brain, which has the appearance of an actual gross postmortem neuroanatomical specimen as shown on the left. The distinct boundaries between white and gray matter are readily visualized with this type of MRI sequence as well as key major structures, which are identified in the scan on the right. The

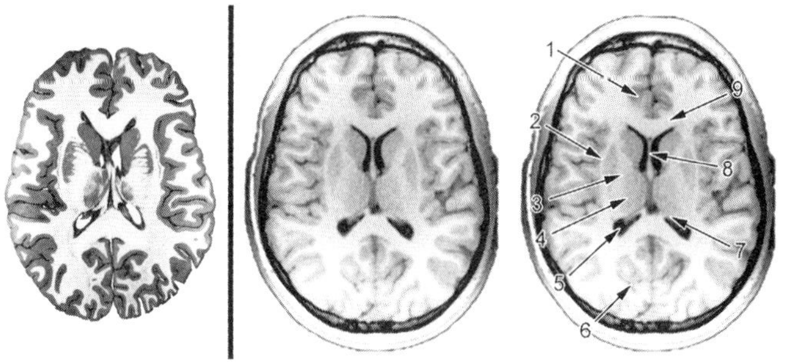

Figure 6.1 The postmortem stained horizontal (also referred to as axial) section on the left appears very similar to the living, in vivo T1-weighted axial MRI next to it (middle image). Used with permission from (Roberts & Hanaway, 1970). The similarities between the postmortem brain and MRI clearly demonstrates how MRI approximates gross anatomy. A duplicate of the middle image on the far right identifies common brain regions at this level: (1) cingulate gyrus, (2) corpus callosum (forceps minor), (3) internal capsule, (4) thalamus, (5) atria of the lateral ventricle, (6) visual cortex, (7) posterior fornix (crus forni), (8) septum pellucidum.

cortical ribbon of gray matter is clearly demarcated from white matter as are the ventricles, filled with cerebrospinal fluid (CSF) in both the histologically stained postmortem brain as well as the very much alive, in vivo brain image in the middle and right. Throughout this chapter various MR imaging techniques will be used to highlight neuroanatomy. An appendix to this chapter overviews CT and MRI methods for neuroanatomic identification.

The Structure of the Human Brain

Neuroanatomy is an enormous and growing area of neuroscience, and a complete description of the human brain alone is far beyond the scope of this chapter. However, the goal in this section is to provide a focused consideration of the brain that is useful for the purposes of clinical and research neuropsychologists. Additional details to amplify the account of general neuroanatomy can be found elsewhere (Blumenfeld, 2011; Brodal, 1981; Catani & Thiebaut de Schotten, 2012; DeArmond, Fusco, & Dewey, 1989; Kandel, Schwartz, & Jessell, 2000; Nolte, 2002; Paxinos, 1990).

Gross Anatomy

The human brain is a roughly spherical organ situated within the cranium and weighing about 1,400 grams (three pounds) in the adult. It has a soft, gelatinous consistency, and its visibly obvious delicacy immediately explains the protective role of the rugged skull in which it is encased. The surface of the brain is folded into many rounded ridges called *gyri,* between which are grooves known as *sulci* or *fissures.* At its base, the brain is continuous with the spinal cord, as the medulla oblongata of the brain stem merges into the cord as it exits the skull through an opening called the *foramen magnum.* A prominent external feature of the brain is its trio of three covering layers: the thick, fibrous *dura mater* just below the inner table of the skull, the weblike *arachnoid* that attaches itself to the inner surface of the dura, and the thin *pia mater* that directly invests the brain surface.

The brain is ordinarily divided into three gross anatomic segments: the cerebrum, cerebellum, and the brain stem (Figure 6.2). The cerebrum is made up of the paired cerebral hemispheres, joined by a large white matter tract called the *corpus*

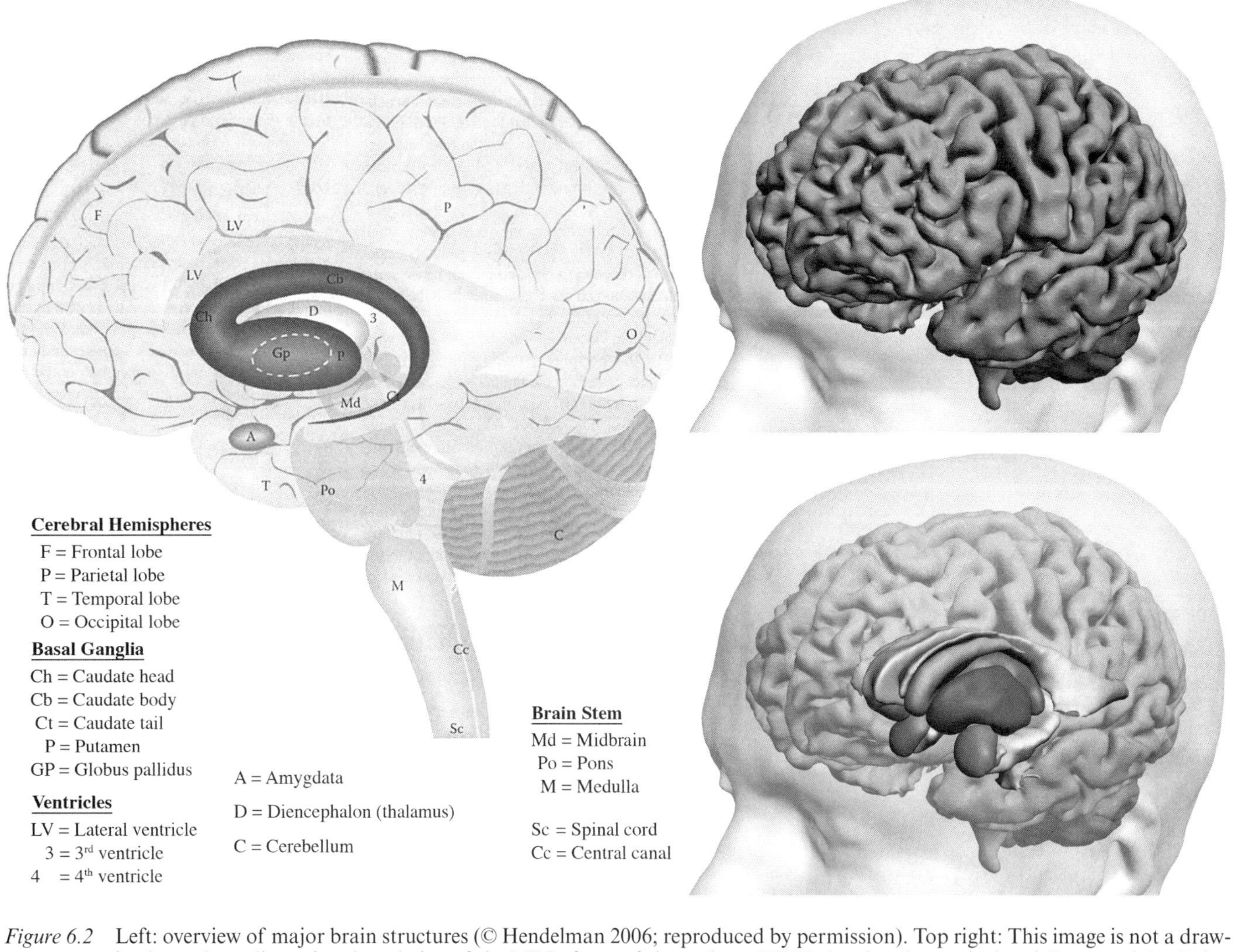

Figure 6.2 Left: overview of major brain structures (© Hendelman 2006; reproduced by permission). Top right: This image is not a drawing but a three-dimensional rendering of the MRI of one of the authors (EDB) showing the cortical gyri. Bottom right: Using see-through technology, each major region of interest can be isolated and classified. *A color version of this figure can be found in Plate section 1*

callosum, and the *diencephalon,* which includes the *thalamus* and *hypothalamus*. The cerebellum is a relatively large and discrete structure situated posterior to the brain stem. The brain stem itself consists of the *midbrain, pons,* and *medulla* (commonly used as a synonym for the *medulla oblongata*). Within the brain are four cavities known as *ventricles*—the two lateral ventricles in the cerebral hemispheres, the third ventricle lying between the two thalami, and the fourth ventricle between the brain stem and cerebellum—each filled with CSF. Numerous blood vessels are also visible grossly. Four major arteries in the neck provide a rich and constant flow of oxygenated blood to meet the high oxygen demand of the brain. These are the two carotid arteries and the two vertebral arteries, which link at the base of the cerebrum in a complex anastomotic structure, called the *circle of Willis,* where major arteries irrigating specific cerebral regions originate. On the venous side of the circulation, a widespread network of venous sinuses returns deoxygenated blood to the paired internal jugular veins in the neck.

Despite its relatively small size (about 2% of the total body weight in adults), the brain houses an extraordinary number of cells. The cellular composition of the brain includes neurons (nerve cells), the basic functional units of the nervous system, and glial cells (glia), that perform a variety of supporting roles. Although estimates differ, it is possible that the brain contains 100 billion neurons and as many as ten times as many glial cells. Even more impressive is the fact that neurons are believed to connect with at least 1,000 others via contacts known as *synapses*. Neurons are excitable cells that function to integrate signals they receive and transmit impulses to other cells, and the brain can thus be considered a densely interconnected electrical organ. The computational power conferred by the enormous number of neurons and synapses is thought to account in large measure for the singular capacities of the human brain.

Another important anatomic distinction in the brain can be drawn between the gray matter and white matter. These two components can be clearly discerned in the freshly cut brain because of the glistening white appearance of the latter that is imparted by its major constituent, myelin. Whereas the gray matter largely consists of the cell bodies of neurons and their synaptic connections, the white matter is the collective mass of myelin-coated axons that travel within and between the hemispheres to link cortical and subcortical gray matter areas. The white matter in the brain, which constitutes roughly half its volume and weight, thus enables connectivity between all brain areas, and is a crucial component of the many neural networks that are believed to subserve neurobehavioral functions.

Microscopic Anatomy

At a microscopic level, the brain can be regarded as a collection of neurons, glial cells, and blood vessels. The essential elements for neurobehavioral function are the neurons, but the glia and vasculature also perform important supportive roles.

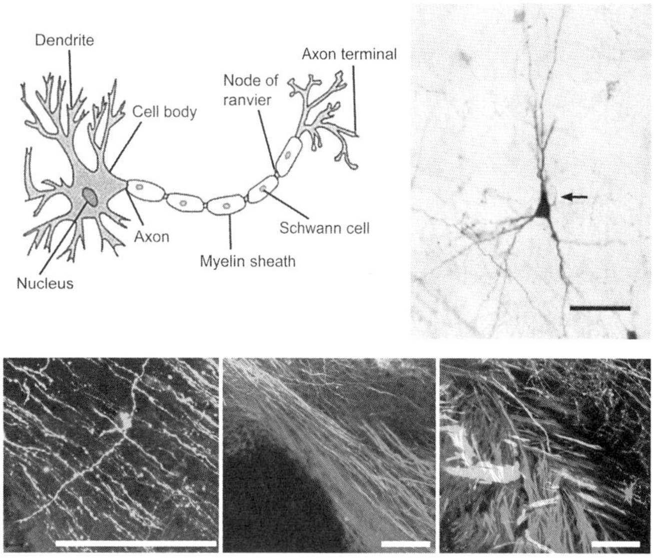

Figure 6.3 Upper left: drawing of a typical neuron, showing its characteristic cell body, dendrites, and axon. Upper right: The simplicity of the diagram to the left belies the true complexity of neurons, axonal projections, and dendritic fields. This is an actual photomicrograph of a hippocampal pyramidal cell in the pigeon. The arrow points at the axon with all of the other appendages being dendrites. The horizontal unit bar is 50μ. (Used with permission from Atoji, Wild, & Wiley, 1956). *A color version of this figure can be found in Plate section 1.*

Neurons are the fundamental units of the nervous system (Figure 6.3). These are cells that are anatomically and physiologically specialized to transmit or process information. Neurons are thus responsible for transmitting sensory stimuli to the brain from the periphery, for sending motor signals from the brain destined to produce movement in a muscle, and for the intermediary processing of information between stimulus and response. In the brain, the great majority of neurons are called *interneurons* because they are structurally interposed between sensory input and motor output; these cells mediate all the cognitive and emotional operations traditionally subsumed under the headings of mentation, higher function, and behavior. To accomplish these objectives, neurons have a typical arrangement that includes a cell body, a variable number of dendrites, and an axon as schematically shown in Figure 6.3. The cell body, also known as the *soma* or *perikaryon,* houses the cell's nucleus and other organelles that maintain the metabolic status of the neuron and synthesize its essential macromolecules. Dendrites are relatively short neuronal processes that extend from the cell body and receive input from other neurons via synaptic contacts. The axon, in contrast, is a long, cylindrical process that provides for the output of the neuron, again by means of synaptic contact with adjacent neurons.

Information transfer within the nervous system is both electrical and chemical in nature. In an individual neuron, the signal is electrical and takes the form of an action potential.

This electrical impulse, often referred to as a *spike* because of its characteristic appearance when recorded experimentally, is propagated along the axon by virtue of a sudden influx of sodium ions that transiently reverses the polarity of the axonal membrane. After the action potential passes, a short refractory period occurs and then another spike can be propagated. An important feature of the action potential is that it is an "all or none" phenomenon, so that its generation depends on the balance between the excitatory and inhibitory inputs received by neuronal dendrites. At the synapse, however, neuronal information transfer is chemical. The synapse is a specialized region of the neuron where a chemical messenger known as a *neurotransmitter* diffuses from one neuron (presynaptic) across a narrow synaptic cleft to activate another neuron (postsynaptic). When the neurotransmitter binds with its receptor on the postsynaptic membrane of the adjacent neuron, it may produce either a depolarization (excitatory stimulus) or a hyperpolarization (inhibitory stimulus), and the summation of these competing influences determines whether an action potential is generated in the postsynaptic neuron. Neurotransmitters are typically small amines, amino acids, and neuropeptides, the pharmacology of which promises many avenues for the successful manipulation of abnormal physical and mental states.

Returning to Figure 6.3, it must be emphasized that this schematic figure merely represents a characterization of a neuron. Actual neurons are far more complex, delicate, and intertwined with adjacent neurons and glia cells than what may be appreciated in the schematic. The diameter of axons is but a few microns, with axon membranes and synaptic gaps measured in nanometers. As will be shown in later illustrations, axon projections may be very short, some under a millimeter in length. However, some axons are very long and aggregate together to form distinct and identifiable tracts. The longest projecting axons within a distinct, well-identified tract are found within the corticospinal tract. In a tall basketball player, some axons from cortex to spine may be more than a meter in length! Axons within complex neural systems, such as those involved in working memory that connect parietal attentional networks with frontal areas involved in executive control and interhemispheric integration, vary in length from a few to several centimeters. Except for the shortest projections, axons course within the brain parenchyma in circuitous nonlinear pathways through densely compacted cellular arrays. Appreciating the microscopic size of the individual neuron, and the complex environment of billions of cells within which each neuron must navigate from origin to terminus, underscores the intricacy of these fundamental units of the brain. The histological staining techniques in Figure 6.3 show how projecting axons interlace one with another. As demonstrated in this figure, the interlacing of projecting axons only a few microns in length constitutes the basis of an extremely complex neuronal network (note that the horizontal bar in the upper right of Figure 6.3 indicates a micron scale—a millionth of a meter).

Glial cells are far more abundant in the CNS than neurons. Glia are classified into four types: *astrocytes, oligodendrocytes, microglia,* and *ependymal cells*. Each type of glial cell has special functions in the brain. Astrocytes are star-shaped cells found in both gray and white matter that participate in the mechanical support of neurons, the metabolic regulation of the microenvironment, and the response of the brain to injury. Oligodendrocytes are located mainly in white matter, where they are responsible for the myelination of central axons, just as Schwann cells carry out this function in the PNS. Microglia are small cells found in gray and white matter that serve as phagocytes, migrating as needed to damaged areas where they dispose of pathogens and neuronal debris. Ependymal cells line the ventricular system, and at a specialized structure known as the *choroid plexus,* one of which is located in each ventricle, ependymal cells form a secretory epithelium that produces CSF; this fluid fills the ventricles and also bathes the entire CNS.

The major vessels that transport blood to and from the brain are the arterial and venous structures discussed in the next section. At the microscopic level, numerous cerebral capillaries serve as the bridging vessels between the arterial and venous systems. These capillaries consist of tightly packed endothelial cells where blood containing oxygen and glucose is delivered to the brain, and then recirculated after these nutrients are extracted. An important feature of the capillaries is that they make up a major part of the blood-brain barrier, which protects the brain from the entry of many pathogens that may circulate in the bloodstream.

Blood Supply

The steady delivery of well-oxygenated blood to the brain is vital. Brain ischemia or anoxia causes neurologic symptoms within seconds, and irreversible neuronal damage and ultimately death will occur if either condition lasts for minutes. A complex system of arteries and veins transports blood to and from the brain, and a working knowledge of this vasculature is necessary for understanding the neurobehavioral effects of many neurologic disorders, including the common and often devastating stroke.

The arterial supply of the brain comes entirely from four large arteries, sometimes called *great vessels of the neck,* all of which ultimately derive from the aorta. The right and left common carotid arteries arise from the right subclavian artery and the ascending aorta, respectively, and within a few centimeters of its origin, each bifurcates into an external branch that supplies extracranial structures, and an internal carotid artery (ICA) that irrigates a substantial portion of the brain (Figure 6.4). The paired vertebral arteries, somewhat smaller than the common carotids, arise from the subclavian arteries and ascend in parallel to a level just below the pons, where they merge to form the single basilar artery. The four great vessels then combine to form the circle of Willis, a vascular loop at the base of the brain from which arise all the arteries supplying the cerebrum. As shown in Figure 6.4a, the

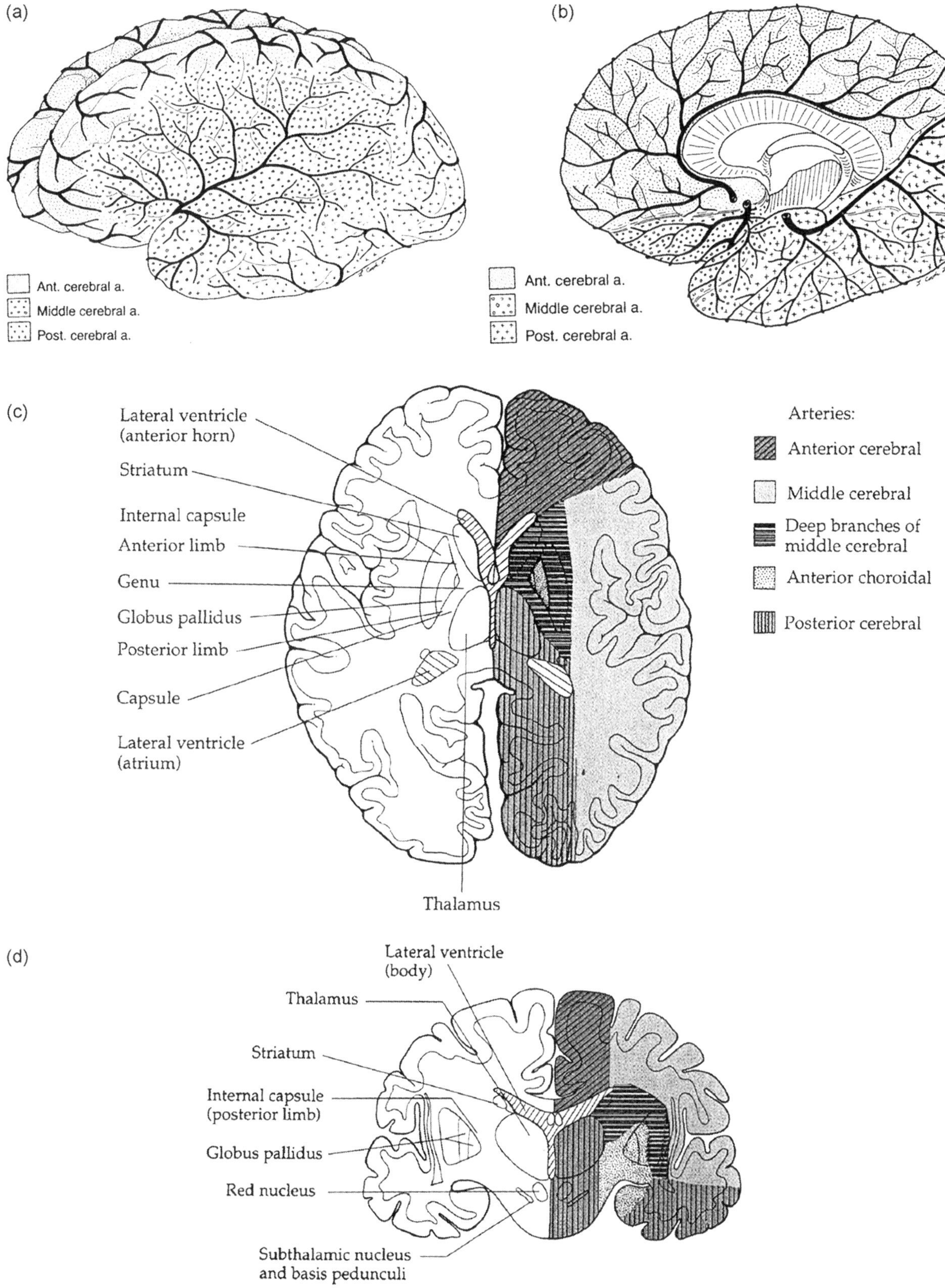

Figure 6.4a Left: the blood supply of the brain, showing the major arteries of the neck and their relationship to the circle of Willis. Right: (A) lateral, somewhat oblique, view of the convexal surface of the left cerebral hemisphere and the paramedian portion of the right cerebral hemisphere showing the anterior, middle, and posterior cerebral arteries and their territories (reprinted with the permission of Cambridge University Press); (B) sagittal section of the right cerebral hemisphere showing the anterior, middle, and posterior cerebral arteries and their territories (reprinted with the permission of Cambridge University Press); (C and D) arterial circulation of deep cerebral structures illustrated in this schematic horizontal (c) and coronal (d) section. (The figure on the left is from Martin 1996, while the figure on the right is adapted from Lim & Alexander, 2009.)

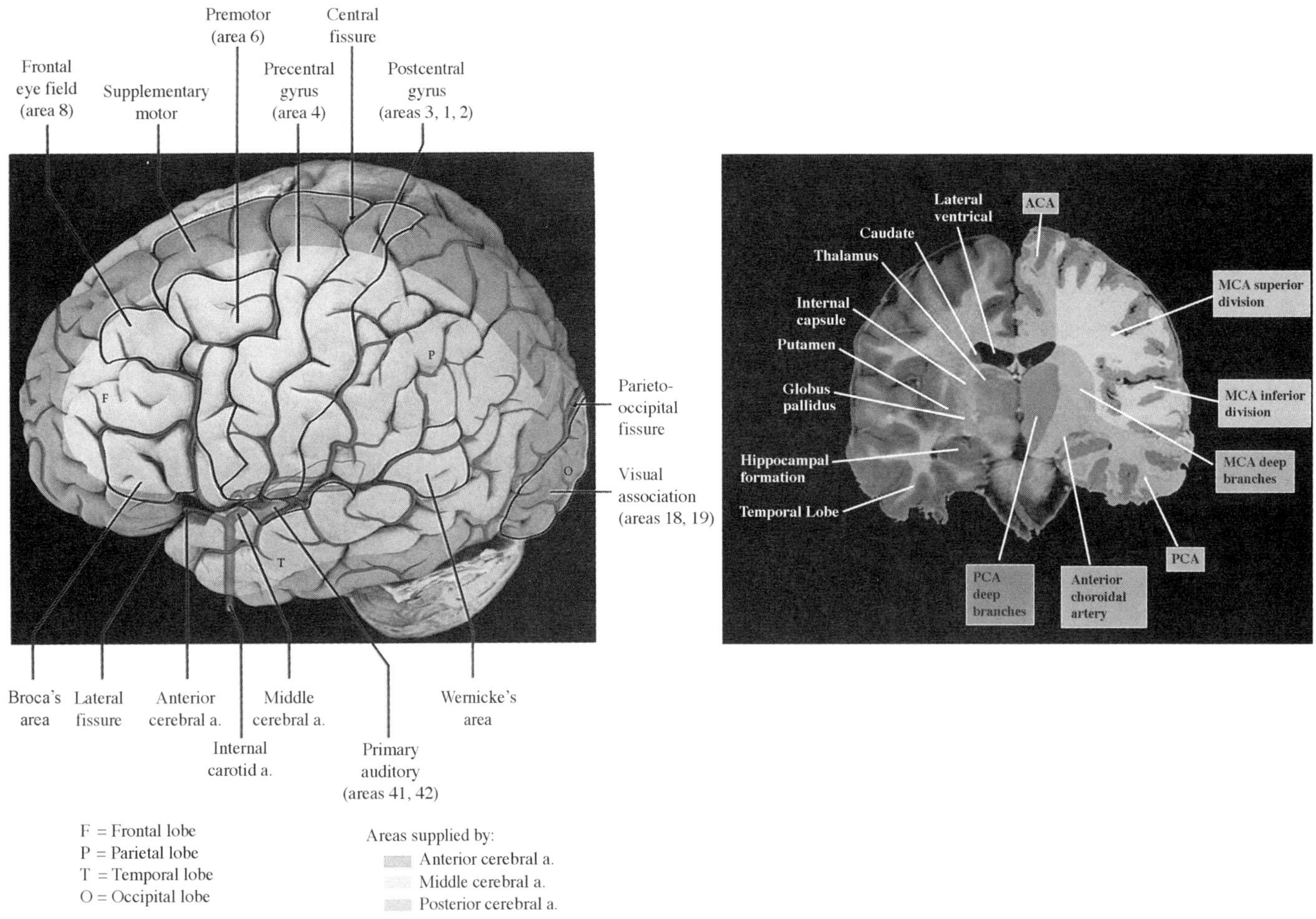

Figure 6.4b Left: coronal MRI section at the level of the thalamus depicting the differences in vascular distribution. Right: the distributions of the anterior, middle, and posterior cerebral arteries as depicted on the dorsolateral surface of the cerebral hemisphere. (© Hendelman 2006; reproduced with permission.) *A color version of this figure can be found in Plate section 1.*

circular appearance of the paired posterior cerebral arteries (PCAs) that bifurcate from the top of the basilar artery and proceed to supply posterior cerebral regions, the paired posterior communicating arteries (PCoAs) that connect the PCAs with the ICAs, the paired anterior cerebral arteries (ACAs) that arise from the ICAs and go on to irrigate anterior regions of the cerebrum, and a single anterior communicating artery (ACoA) that joins the two ACAs form what is referred to as the 'Circle of Willis', as depicted in Figure 6.4. Another important artery that arises from the circle of Willis is the middle cerebral artery (MCA): One MCA is found on each side, and each one ascends to the ipsilateral hemisphere to nourish the lateral aspect of the cerebrum. Whereas vascular disease of many kinds can affect any of these vessels and dramatically disrupt neurologic function, the MCA, ACA, and the PCA are most important arteries in terms of neurobehavioral function because these are the arteries that supply the cerebral hemispheres (see Figures 6.4b and 4c).

The venous drainage of the brain is accomplished by a richly anastomosed system of cerebral veins, conventionally divided into superficial and deep groups, both of which empty into a network of dural sinuses. Superficial veins near the brain surface typically drain into the superior sagittal sinus, a long, tubular structure that runs in the interhemispheric fissure at the top of the brain. Deep veins drain into the paired straight sinuses that are found superior to the cerebellum. The major dural venous sinuses merge at the confluence of sinuses, and then the straight sinuses drain into the internal jugular veins to return blood to the heart. Vascular disorders involving the cerebral venous system are far less common than those of the arterial system, but the outcome can be similarly catastrophic.

Ventricles and Cerebrospinal Fluid

Within the brain, there are four internal cavities called *ventricles* (Figure 6.5). These cavities are filled with CSF, a watery fluid produced within the ventricles that surrounds the entire CNS. The ventricular system is important in governing the pressure and fluid dynamics of the brain. The CSF plays a

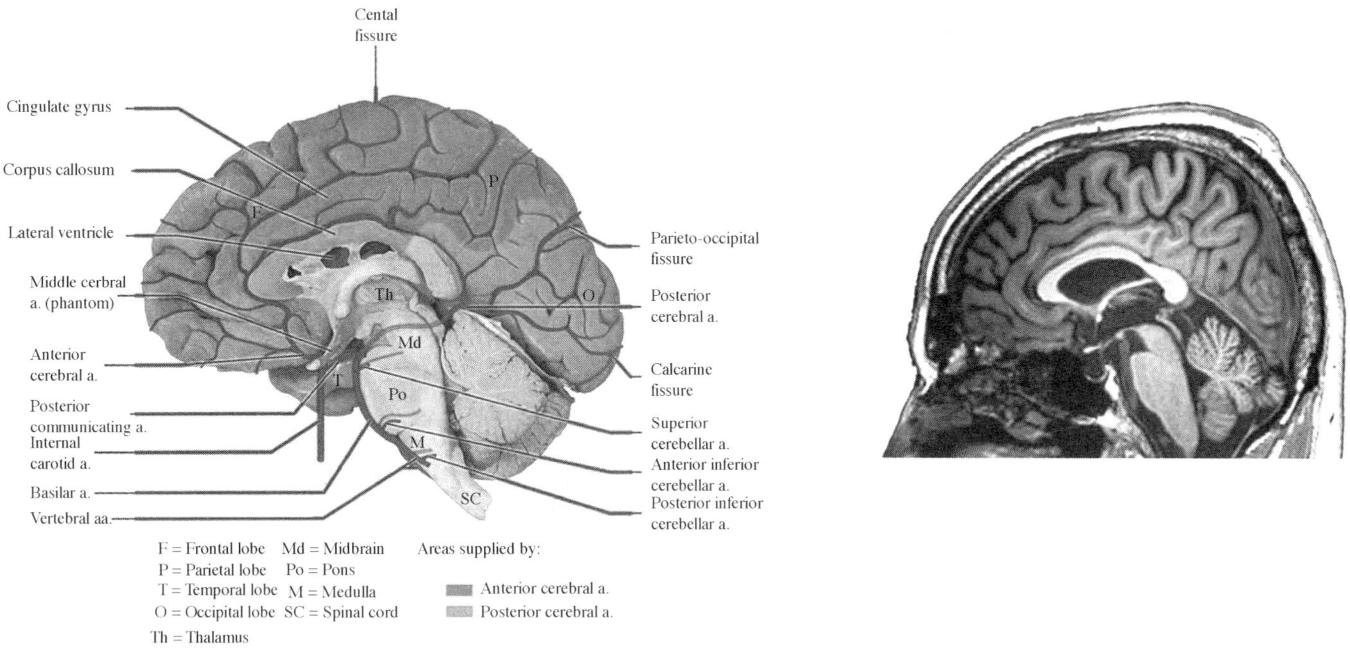

Figure 6.4c Left: the distributions of the anterior and posterior cerebral arteries on the medial surface of the cerebral hemisphere (copyright © Hendelman 2006; reproduced with permission). Right: MRI of one of the authors (EDB) at approximately the same level of the colorized postmortem sagittal section with the vasculature colored in on the left. The cut through the cerebral hemisphere is slightly off center so that the cortical gyri may be observed; these gyri are covered in part by the falx cerebri, an extension of the dura mater that is situated between the two cerebral hemispheres. *A color version of this figure can be found in Plate section 1.*

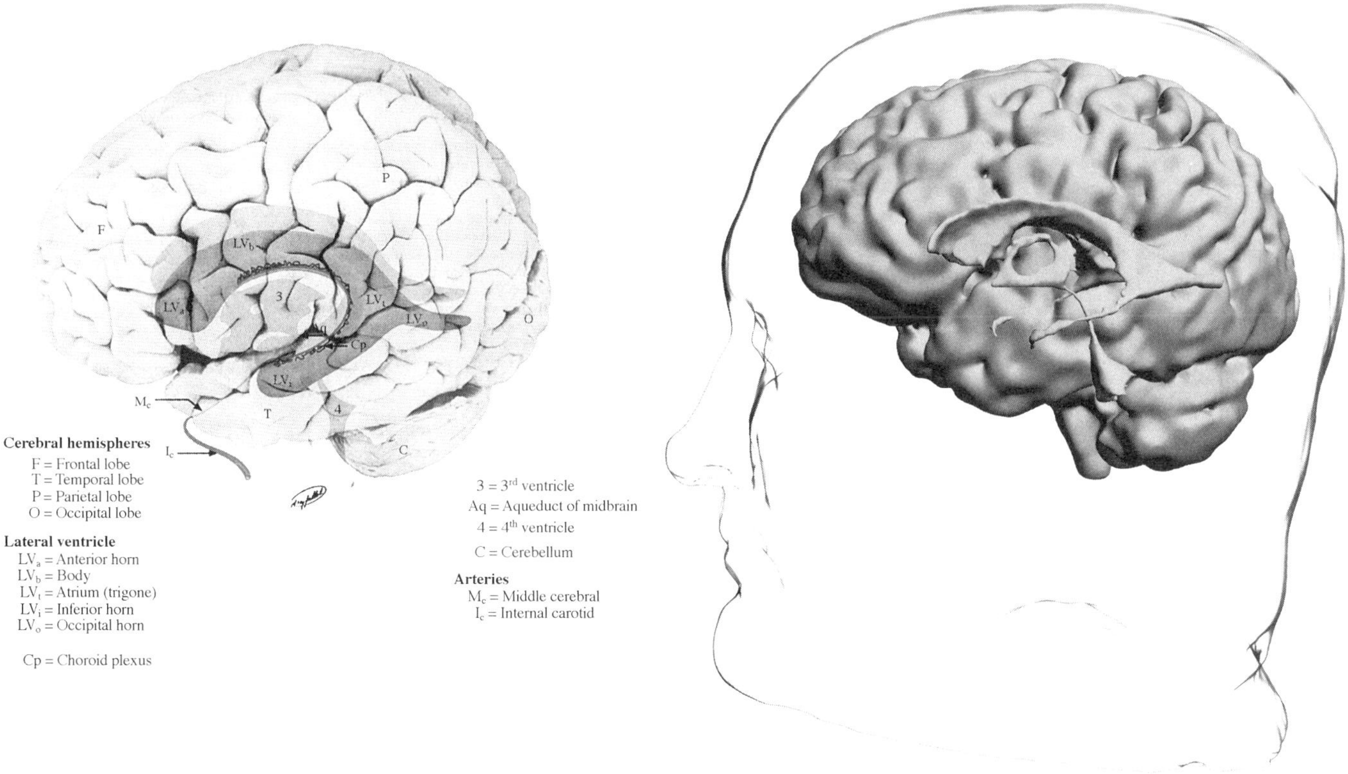

Figure 6.5 Left: the position of the four ventricles within the brain. (copyright © Hendelman 2006; reproduced with permission.) Right: three-dimensional MRI rendering of the ventricular system of one of the authors (EDB). To highlight the ventricular system, the surface of the brain has been smoothed to some extent. *A color version of this figure can be found in Plate section 1.*

supportive role in normal CNS function, and abnormalities of the CSF are critical in the diagnosis of many neurologic disorders.

The two largest ventricles are the lateral ventricles, one in each hemisphere, which are situated deep to the frontal, temporal, parietal, and occipital lobes. These communicate with a single third ventricle, which is narrow and located between the two thalami, via an opening in each lateral ventricle called the *foramen of Monro.* The tent-shaped fourth ventricle lies just dorsal to the brain stem and is connected to the third ventricle by a small conduit in the midbrain known as the *cerebral aqueduct.* In turn, the fourth ventricle empties into a region of the subarachnoid space called the *cisterna magna* through three apertures, the midline *foramen of Magendie* and the two lateral *foramina of Luschka*. The CSF then circulates caudally to the lower end of the spinal canal and then rostrally to the convexities of the brain, where it is eventually absorbed into the cerebral venous sinuses through structures called the *arachnoid villi.*

CSF is steadily produced by the choroid plexus in all four ventricles. The total volume of CSF in and around the CNS is approximately 140 ml, whereas the volume of CSF within the ventricles is a small fraction of this, about 25 ml. As the CSF is produced at a rate of about 450 ml per day, the CSF volume turns over about three times daily. The neuroanatomical importance of the CSF is twofold: In structural terms, it serves a supportive role in providing a buoyancy that prevents the brain from settling down upon the rigid bony protuberances of the skull, and functionally, the CSF takes part in regulating the chemical environment of brain neurons.

Clinically, the ventricular system and the CSF have many important implications. Enlargement of the ventricular system from an excess of CSF, as occurs with hydrocephalus and certain mass lesions, can have major neurologic consequences. Analysis of the constituents of the CSF after lumbar puncture is crucial for diagnosis of many neurologic disorders, such as meningitis and encephalitis. In disorders associated with parenchymal volume loss, such as many neurodegenerative diseases or moderate to severe traumatic brain injury, reduction of brain volume is accompanied by a compensatory increase in ventricular size, often readily identifiable on MRI or CT imaging.

Cranial Nerves

The 12 CNs provide for motor and sensory innervation of the head and neck, and their anatomy is inextricably associated with that of the brain. All of the CNs are regarded as components of the PNS, with one exception: The second CN, the optic nerve, is actually a tract of the brain. The CNs each exist in pairs, and their crossed and uncrossed connections with central structures are important in understanding the anatomy of the brain.

The first CN is the olfactory nerve, which subserves the sense of smell. Olfaction is far more highly developed in lower animals, but this chemical sense exists in humans as a reminder of the evolutionary background of *homo sapiens.* The olfactory system originates as a collection of olfactory receptor cells called the *olfactory epithelium* in the roof of the nasal cavity. The olfactory nerve consists of the collected axons of these cells. Ascending through the cribriform plate of the ethmoid bone, the olfactory nerve terminates in the olfactory bulb at the base of the frontal lobe. From there, the olfactory tract projects to the olfactory cortex in the medial temporal lobe.

The sense of vision is of central importance in human life, as signified by the large number of CNS neurons devoted to it. Incoming visual stimuli are initially processed in the eye, where photoreceptor cells in the retina—known as *rods* and *cones*—transduce patterns of light into electrical signals that are sent to the brain. The optic nerve can be seen by physicians at the back of the eye, where examination with an ophthalmoscope permits visualization of the optic disc. The optic disc contains the axons of neurons that transmit visual information to the lateral geniculate nucleus of the thalamus. From there, additional relays through the temporal and parietal lobes project to the primary visual cortex in the occipital lobes (Figure 6.6). On its way to the thalamus, the optic nerve divides into two components, one remaining on the same side as the eye from which it came and the other passing over to the other side of the brain. This neuroanatomical feature is important because it results in each hemisphere receiving input from the contralateral visual field. Thus the left hemisphere receives input from the right visual field and vice versa. Crossed function such as this is typical of a number of systems in the brain and has many clinical and neurobehavioral implications. In Figure 6.6 the neuroanatomical dissection next to the schematic shows the visual projections emanating from the lateral geniculate nuclei and how they fan through the temporal and parietal lobes to their destination in the visual cortices. The gross projections from the optic nerves to the visual cortices may now be identified in vivo using structural MRI along with the newer technique of diffusion tensor imaging (DTI).

CNs three, four, and six are typically considered as group because of their exclusive role in eye movements. These three nerves—the oculomotor (CN III), the trochlear (CN IV), and the abducens (CN VI)—arise from the brain stem and allow for normal conjugate gaze by linking the movement of the two eyes so that a single visual image is presented to the brain. CN III also provides the afferent limb of the important pupillary light reflex, which has much localizing value in neurologic diagnosis.

CN V, the trigeminal nerve, has both motor and sensory functions. It is the general sensory nerve of the face, mediating ipsilateral somatic sensation via three divisions: ophthalmic (V1), maxillary (V2), and mandibular (V3).

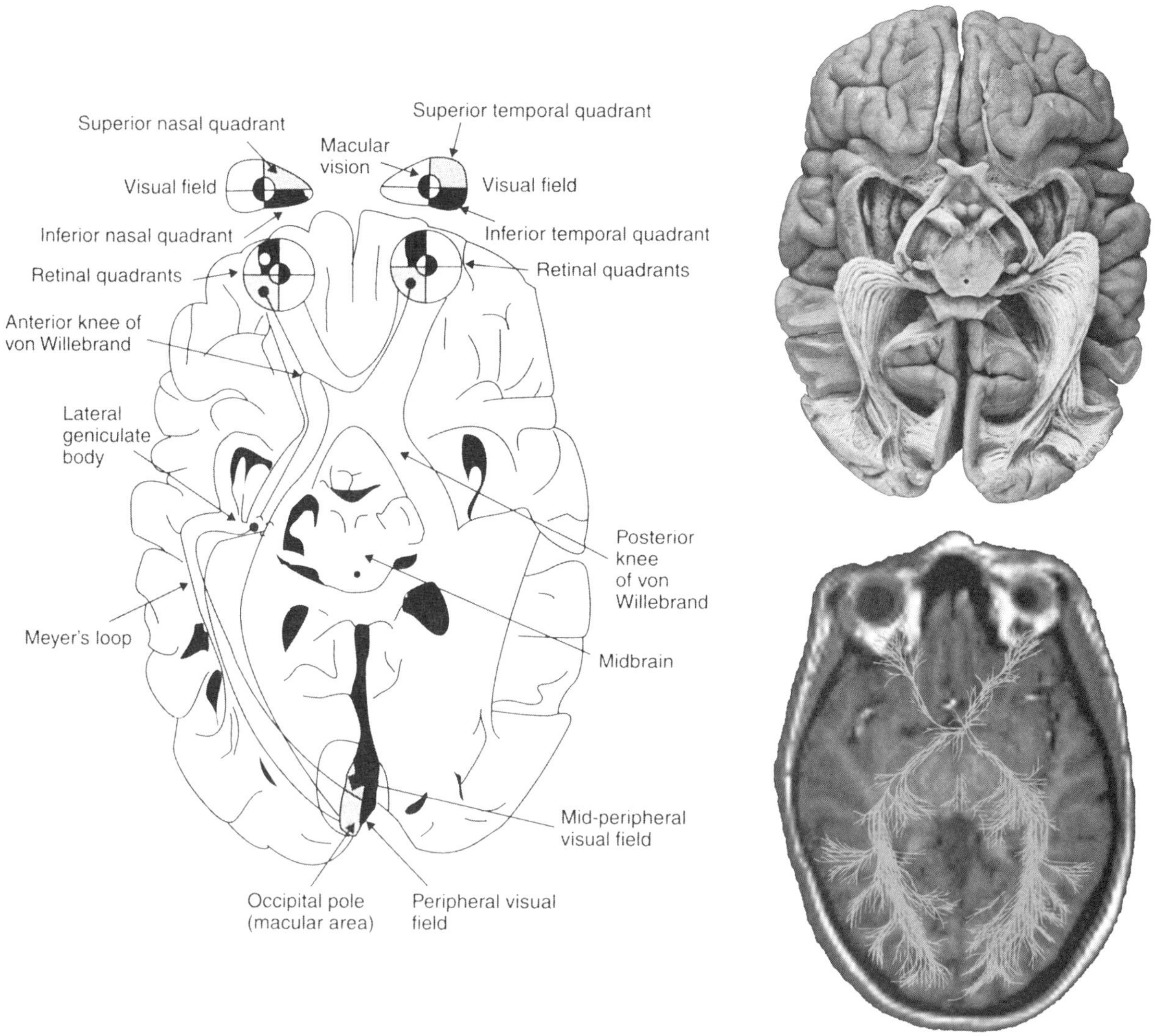

Figure 6.6 The course of the visual image is shown from the retina through the optic nerve, optic tract, lateral geniculate body, and optic radiation, to the visual cortex (reproduced with permission from Arslan, 2001). Top right: meticulous dissection of the visual projections from the optic chiasm to the visual cortex (reproduced with permission from Glubegovic & Williams, 1980). Bottom right: DTI of aggregate tracts from the visual projection system, plotted on a T1-weighted image (from Staempfli et al., 2007, and reproduced with permission from Wiley). *A color version of this figure can be found in Plate section 1.*

These divisions join in the trigeminal ganglion outside the brain stem, and then enter the pons as a single nerve. A secondary relay then sends this facial somatosensory information to the ventral posterior medial (VPM) nucleus of the thalamus, where it undergoes further processing. The motor function of CN V is to supply the muscles of mastication (chewing).

The facial nerve (CN VII) is primarily motor in its function. This nerve originates from the facial nucleus in the pons and innervates the ipsilateral muscles of facial expression. Facial weakness related to dysfunction of this nerve or its connections is frequently seen in clinical neurology. CN VII also has one notable sensory function, which is to convey taste from the anterior two-thirds of the tongue via a branch called the *chorda tympani* to the solitary tract in the pons and medulla.

The eighth CN is known as the *vestibulocochlear nerve* because it has two special sensory components called the *vestibular* and *cochlear* divisions. These two divisions mediate the vestibular (balance) system and the sense of audition (hearing), respectively. Each division of CN VIII makes use of mechanoreceptors found in the inner ear: Cells of the vestibular division are sensitive to positional head movements, and those of the cochlear division respond to sound stimuli. Complex mechanisms of transduction then permit the transmission of positional and auditory stimuli to the vestibular and cochlear nuclei in the pons. From there, vestibular input is extensively processed in the brain stem and cerebellum, and auditory input is relayed rostrally up the brain stem to the medial geniculate nucleus of the thalamus and finally to the primary auditory cortex of the temporal lobe (Heschl's gyrus). Among the central functions of hearing in humans is that it serves as a necessary precursor to language.

The ninth CN, the glossopharyngeal nerve, participates in motor, sensory, and autonomic functions of the face. Motor fibers of CN IX innervate the pharynx; sensory fibers mediate somatic sensation of the tongue, nasopharynx, and middle and outer ear as well as taste from the posterior one-third of the tongue; and autonomic fibers supply parasympathetic input to the parotid gland. The tenth CN, the vagus nerve, is the most widely distributed of the CNs, providing parasympathetic input to many thoracic and abdominal organs, and contributing to the motor and sensory innervation of the larynx, pharynx, and outer ear. CN XI, the accessory nerve, is a pure motor nerve that arises from the lower medulla and upper spinal cord. CN XI supplies ipsilateral sternocleidomastoid and trapezius muscles. The 12th CN, the hypoglossal, is also purely motor in function. It arises from the medulla and enters the tongue ipsilaterally to supply its musculature.

Brain Stem

The brain stem is the most caudal portion of the brain, serving structurally as a bridge between the spinal cord and the cerebrum and as an anchor for the cerebellum posterior to it. Its three divisions are the midbrain, lying just below the diencephalon and continuous with the thalamus; the pons, immediately caudal to the midbrain and anterior to the fourth ventricle; and the medulla, below the pons and continuous with the spinal cord. In addition to many CN nuclei, several ascending and descending tracts to and from higher structures are found within the brain stem, and also within this region is the important integrative structure known as the *reticular formation.*

An important point is that CNs III–XII have their central termini in the brain stem. This arrangement indicates that the brain stem serves as a general relay station conveying sensory, motor, and autonomic information between the CNS and the tissues and organs of the face and body. Damage to the brain stem can therefore have a major impact on CN function, and the diagnosis of many neurologic disorders is based on the localization of lesions causing CN deficits.

The long tracts in the brain stem are all continuations of fiber systems that originate at higher or lower levels of the nervous system. Four major tracts are most relevant clinically. First is the *corticospinal tract*, which begins in the precentral gyrus of the frontal lobe, descends to the spinal cord, and provides supraspinal input to motor neurons that directly innervate voluntary muscles. Within the brain stem, this tract occupies the ventral portion of the midbrain, pons, and medulla, and as it nears the most caudal portion of the medulla it crosses (decussates) so that most corticospinal fibers travel to the opposite side of the spinal cord. As in the visual system, therefore, there is a crossing of motor fibers that renders one side of the cerebrum responsible for nervous activity on the other side of the body. The second major tract is the *corticobulbar tract,* which has a similar origin and role as the corticospinal tract, but which terminates on various brain stem motor nuclei. The remaining two brain stem tracts of note are sensory. The *medial lemniscus,* a continuation of the dorsal column system in the spinal cord, conveys information regarding vibratory and position sensation to the contralateral ventral posterior lateral (VPL) nucleus of the thalamus and then to the somatosensory cortex of the parietal lobe. The *spinothalamic tract* is a similar sensory tract that transmits pain and temperature sensation from the periphery to the contralateral VPL thalamic nucleus and then the parietal lobe.

The *reticular formation* is a diffusely organized collection of nuclei and tracts within the core of the brain stem that serves a vital integrative function. This area, defined more by its physiologic characteristics than by discrete anatomic boundaries, harbors the nuclei of several neurotransmitters that supply more rostral brain regions, among them norepinephrine from the locus ceruleus and serotonin from the dorsal raphe nuclei. Although the reticular formation participates in sensation, movement, and autonomic function, perhaps its most important role is in consciousness. In the upper pons and midbrain lies a portion of the reticular formation called the *ascending reticular activating system* (ARAS). The ARAS serves as a general activating system for the brain, sending fibers to the intralaminar nuclei of the thalamus, which in turn project to the entire cerebrum (Figure 6.7). The ARAS has a major role in wakefulness and sleep and is largely responsible for the normal circadian rhythm of humans, a schematic of which is also shown in Figure 6.7. Damage to the ARAS, as from a brain stem stroke or traumatic brain injury, may result in a loss of normal arousal and produce the dramatic state of coma. The ARAS therefore contributes to human consciousness in a fundamental way. By virtue of its capacity to enable the general arousal system of the brain, the ARAS underlies all the operations of higher function. Neurologists have long employed a useful distinction that brings some order to the neurobiology of consciousness: In this formulation, the ARAS can be regarded as responsible for the *level* of consciousness, in contrast to the *content* of consciousness that is elaborated by more rostral regions of the brain (Plum & Posner, 1982). These distinctions are further elaborated in Figure 6.7.

Cerebellum

The cerebellum is a prominent structure of the brain lying posterior to the brain stem, to which it is extensively attached. Although it receives considerable sensory input, the cerebellum is considered part of the motor system because of its primary involvement with coordination, postural control,

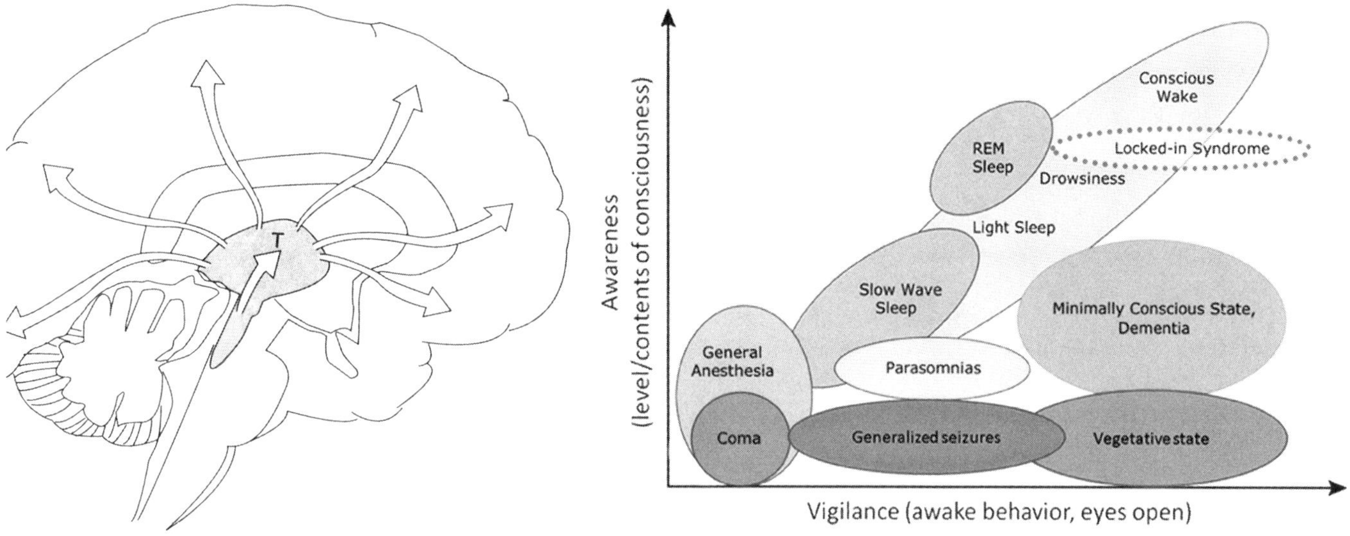

Figure 6.7 Left: midsagittal view of the brain showing structures responsible for arousal, including the ascending reticular activating system (ARAS) depicted as the upward projecting arrows and the thalamus (T). Right: The level of consciousness can be dissociated from behaviors that are traditionally regarded as signs of arousal (such as eye opening.). Higher levels of consciousness are associated with an increased range of conscious contents (with permission from Boly et al., 2013).

equilibrium, and motor control. Recent information has suggested that the cerebellum also participates in neurobehavioral function.

Grossly, the cerebellum can be divided into the body of the cerebellum (*corpus cerebelli*) and the smaller *flocculonodular lobe*. In functional terms, however, a more useful distinction can be drawn between the two lateral cerebellar hemispheres and the centrally located *vermis* (Figure 6.8a). This division is important because the cerebellar hemispheres are devoted to coordination of the limbs whereas the vermis is involved with postural adjustment. Damage to these areas of the cerebellum thus causes, respectively, limb ataxia and postural instability (also known as *truncal ataxia*).

Like the cerebrum, the cerebellum contains both gray and white matter. The gray matter is found in the cerebellar cortex, where neuronal cell bodies are arranged in three layers—the superficial molecular cell layer, the intermediate Purkinje cell layer, and the deeper granular cell layer—and in four collections of cell bodies within the cerebellum called the *dentate, globose, fastigial,* and *emboliform* nuclei. The white matter consists of myelinated axons coursing to and from the cerebellar cortex, and three cerebellar peduncles—inferior, middle, and superior—that connect the cerebellum with the medulla, pons, and midbrain, respectively (Figure 6.8b).

The importance of the cerebellum in the motor system stems from its intermediate position between multiple sensory inputs and its connections with motor regions of the cerebral hemispheres. A variety of vestibular, spinal, and cerebral cortical inputs are received by the cerebellum through the inferior and middle cerebellar peduncles. After extensive processing occurs, cerebellar output is sent via relays from the four deep nuclei through the superior cerebellar peduncle to the midbrain, and then to the contralateral ventral anterior (VA) and ventral lateral (VL) nuclei of the thalamus. These thalamic connections allow the cerebellum to influence the motor cortex, providing for the fine-tuning of limb and truncal movements. An important point for clinicians is that ataxia on one side of the body reflects damage on the same side as the cerebellar lesion: Unlike lesions of the cerebral hemispheres, cerebellar deficits are ipsilateral to the lesion because the cerebellar motor output crosses to the opposite thalamus, and then the corticospinal tract subserving voluntary movement crosses again to the side of the lesion.

Ataxia is the most characteristic feature of cerebellar damage, and may be most apparent in the limbs, the trunk, or in speech (as in a type of dysarthria called *scanning speech*). A wide-based gait and muscle hypotonia are also commonly encountered with cerebellar lesions. A contribution of the cerebellum to neurobehavioral function is being increasingly recognized. The acquisition of a skill such as playing a musical instrument (an example of procedural learning) appears to depend in part on the cerebellum, and mounting clinical evidence supports the notion the cognitive and emotional deficits can develop in individuals who have sustained cerebellar damage (Schmahmann & Sherman, 1998).

Figure 6.8b shows a sagittal MRI view off the midline showing the superior cerebellar peduncle and its attachment to the brain stem, with a coronal section cut somewhat obliquely that shows both cerebellar hemispheres (green lines

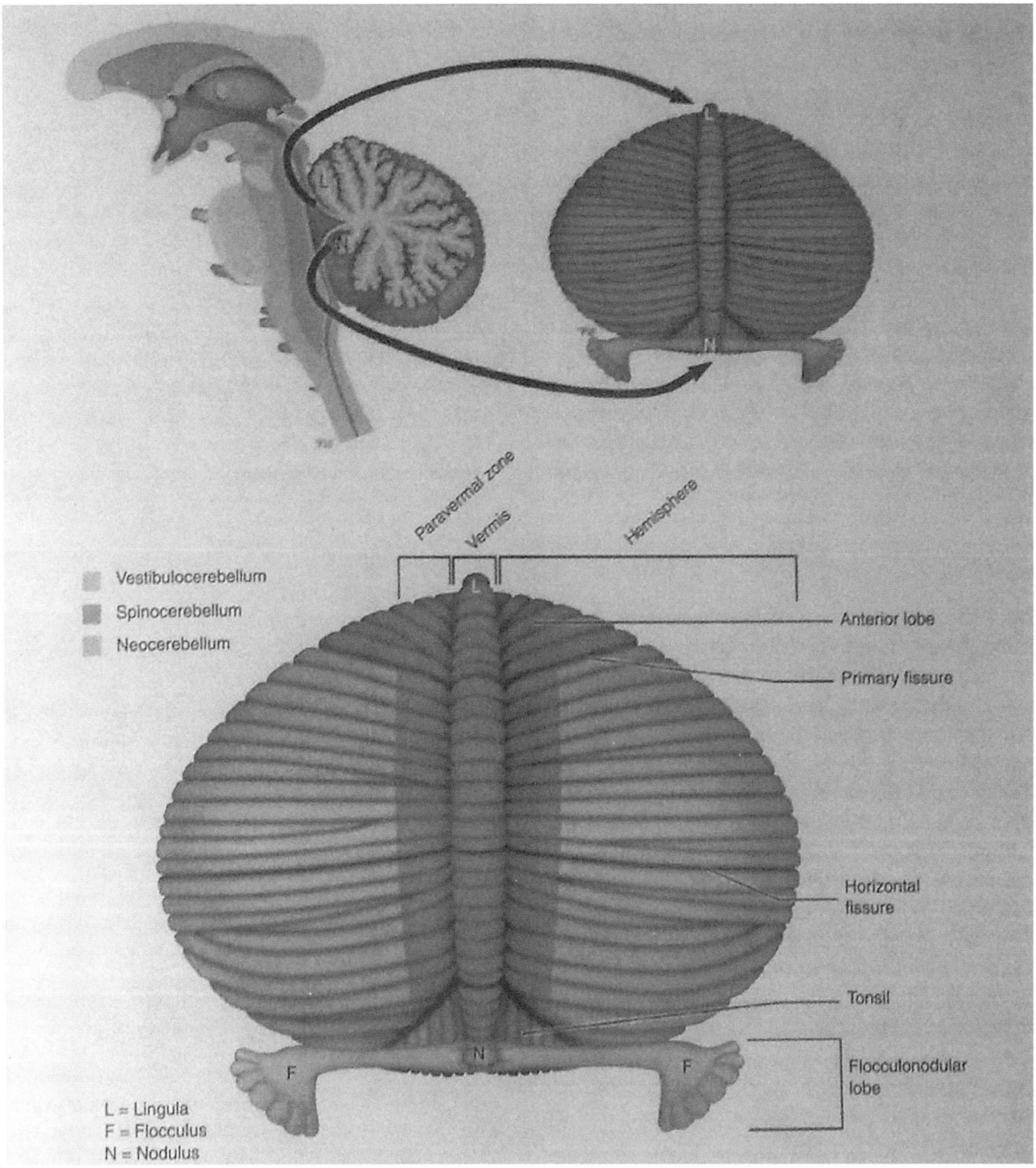

Figure 6.8a The cerebellum and functional lobes (© Hendelman 2006; reproduced with permission).

indicate the orientation and plane of each MR image). A close up of the cerebellar vermis is also shown with a midline MRI slice through the aqueduct of Sylvius and the fourth ventricle (upper right-hand image) depicting the ten lobules of the cerebellum. Lastly, sagittal DTI tractography shown in different colors depicts different trajectories of white matter pathways connecting the cerebellum and brain stem.

Diencephalon

The diencephalon is a collection of four structures located deep in the cerebral hemispheres immediately rostral to the midbrain and surrounding the third ventricle: the thalamus, hypothalamus, subthalamus, and epithalamus. Although small in size, the diencephalon has many important roles in

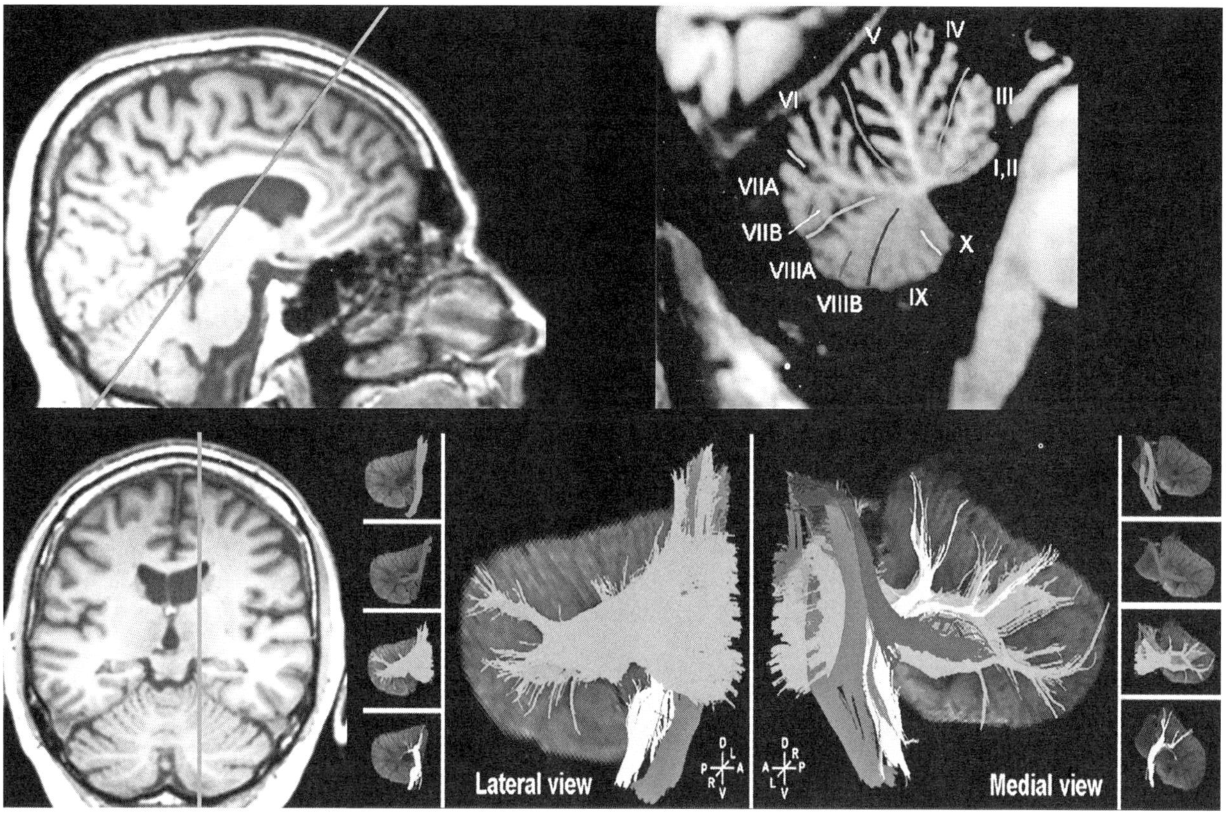

Figure 6.8b Upper left: a sagittal MR image cut off midline showing a section through the bulk of the cerebellum, with the coronal MRI demonstrating the appearance of the cerebellum in this plane. Lower left: a coronal image showing the level of cut (the vertical line) for the section shown in the upper image. Upper right: the traditional ten lobes of the cerebellar vermis as identified in the mid-sagittal cut. Bottom right: DTI tractography of the cerebellum and brain stem depicting the various major projections in this region. The left panel larger view of the cerebellum shows a lateral view, and the right larger panel shows a medial view where the smaller outside images depict the orientation of the superior (b), middle (c), inferior (d) cerebellar peduncles, and the corticospinal tract (a). Small insets show each pathway separately. The letters on each panel indicate the following: (A) anterior, (P) posterior, (D) dorsal, (V) ventral, (L) left, (R) right. (From Takahashi, Song, Folkerth, Grant, & Schmahmann, 2012; used with permission from Elsevier.) *A color version of this figure can be found in Plate section 1.*

nervous system function, particularly through the activities of the thalamus and hypothalamus.

The thalamus is an egg-shaped collection of nuclei that comprises about 80% of the diencephalon (Figure 6.9). Although primarily involved with sensation, the thalamic nuclei also participate in movement, arousal, cognition, and emotion. The most familiar thalamic function is to serve as a sensory relay station for stimuli that will eventually reach the cerebral cortex. All sensory systems with the exception of olfaction traverse the thalamus en route to their respective cortical areas. Accordingly, somatosensory information from the contralateral body and face reach the VPL and VPM nuclei, respectively, and taste fibers also project to the VPM nucleus. Similarly, visual projections from the optic nerve synapse in the lateral geniculate nucleus and auditory fibers in the medial geniculate nucleus. The VA and VL nuclei receive fibers from the cerebellum, and they also send fibers to the basal ganglia to enable their participation in the motor system. The intralaminar nuclei—the two largest of which are the centromedian and parafascicular nuclei—subserve the arousal system by receiving input from the brain stem ARAS and then relaying this input rostrally to activate the cerebrum. The dorsal medial nucleus and the pulvinar are the major thalamic nuclei for association regions of the cerebral cortex, and they contribute to cognition by connecting with the frontal and parietal-temporal-occipital cortices, respectively. The anterior nucleus plays a role in emotion by virtue of its position within the limbic system. Contemporary neuroimaging methods permit the identification and parcellation of thalamic regions and their cortical projections, as shown in Figure 6.9.

The hypothalamus is much smaller than the thalamus but exerts a powerful influence on autonomic, endocrine, and emotional function. Situated inferior to the thalamus and superior to the pituitary gland, the hypothalamus contains many tiny nuclei that in general help maintain bodily homeostasis. As the control center of the autonomic nervous system, the hypothalamus regulates aspects of body temperature, digestion, circulation, water balance, and sexual function. The autonomic nervous system is divided into a parasympathetic branch, which is generally associated with anterior regions,

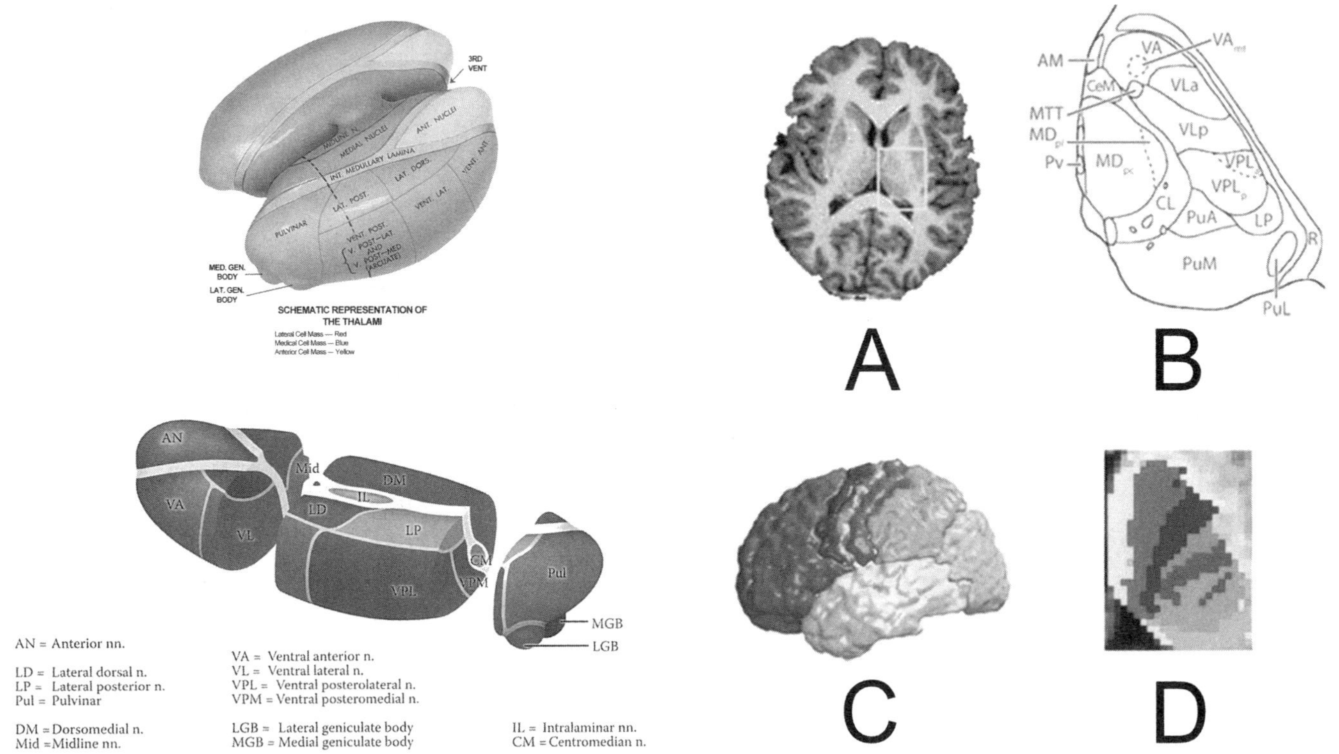

Figure 6.9 Left: the thalamus and its many constituent nuclei. These nuclei function as relay stations for information traveling to and from the cerebral cortex. (© Hendelman 2006; reproduced with permission). Right: (A) standard T1-weighted axial MR image with the yellow box highlighting and outlining one half of the thalamus; (B) thalamic nuclei (this will be coordinated with the Handelman diagram), which provides seed regions to examine cortical projections from thalamic nuclei; (C) cortical projections; (D) the aforementioned seed regions. Note how thalamic regions have specialized areas of cortical projection. *A color version of this figure can be found in Plate section 1.*

and a sympathetic branch that is affiliated with posterior sites. Endocrine function is also governed by the hypothalamus via its extensive neural and vascular connections with the two lobes of the pituitary gland. Lastly, the hypothalamus is a key component of the limbic system, and thus contributes to emotional function. The "flight or fight" response to threat, for example, is an illustration of the dramatic emotional display that requires the activity of the hypothalamus.

The remaining diencephalic regions have more limited significance. The subthalamus is a small area inferior to the thalamus that contains the subthalamic nucleus and the zona incerta; these areas have connections to the basal ganglia and cerebral cortex, but their functions are largely obscure. The epithalamus lies superior and caudal to the thalamus, and consists of the pineal gland and the habenular nuclei. The pineal gland is an unpaired brain structure that was once considered by Rene Descartes to be the seat of the soul; today it is known to secrete a hormone called *melatonin* that is thought to contribute to sleep and gonadal function.

Basal Ganglia

The basal ganglia include a number of gray matter structures located deep in the cerebral hemispheres. Their importance derives from their major role in motor function, and because increasing evidence from clinical populations also relates these regions to cognitive and emotional functions.

No uniformity of opinion exists about which structures should be included within the basal ganglia. However, most authorities would agree that the caudate nucleus, globus pallidus, and putamen should be listed under this heading, and many also include the midbrain substantia nigra and the subthalamic nucleus of the thalamus. For purposes of this chapter, the caudate, putamen, globus pallidus, and substantia nigra will serve to focus the discussion (see Figures 6.1, 6.2, and 6.4b), as these nuclei are most frequently implicated in clinical disorders. Other terminology of these structures is also worth reviewing: the caudate and putamen are often called the *striatum,* and the putamen and globus pallidus are alternatively referred to as the *lenticular nucleus.*

The principal function of the basal ganglia is to serve as an integrated unit in the modulation of the cerebral cortical control of voluntary movement. In performing this role, the basal ganglia make use of a series of parallel loops that mediate their involvement in cortical motor output. The most prominent of these loops involves the following: a number of cortical inputs reach the striatum by means of white matter tracts called the *internal* and *external capsules;* from this point, connections proceed first to the globus pallidus and then to the VA and VL thalamic nuclei; the final link involves connections returning from these nuclei back to the motor cortex, again via the internal capsule. The basal ganglia thus join the cerebellum as regions strongly connected to the voluntary motor system via specific thalamic relays. Whereas the cerebellum has a prominent role in coordination, the basal ganglia can be thought of as contributing to the initiation and timing of movements.

A final aspect of basal ganglia anatomy deserving attention is its neurochemical input, which arises from the midbrain substantia nigra (the general location of the midbrain is shown in Figures 6.4c and 6.6). Pigmented cells of the substantia nigra send axons rostrally to deliver the neurotransmitter dopamine to the striatum. Among the many functions of this important neurotransmitter, dopamine serves to activate the basal ganglia and the motor system in general, and its deficiency or absence within this system results in dramatic alterations in motor function. Parkinson's disease is the well-known neurologic disorder in which dopamine depletion in the substantia nigra causes classic clinical features of bradykinesia (slowness of movement), rigidity, and resting tremor. This is the most significant movement disorder because of its high prevalence, progressive course, and favorable response to dopaminergic drugs. Parkinson's disease has also served as a prototype disorder for the syndrome of subcortical dementia, an important concept in behavioral neurology and neuropsychology (Cummings, 1990).

Limbic System

The limbic system has long been a confusing but crucial concept in neuroanatomy and clinical neuroscience. The term *limbic* derives from the Latin *limbus*, meaning "border." The limbic system was identified by the French neurologist Paul Broca in 1878 as a collection of structures at the junction of the diencephalon and the cerebral hemispheres. Whereas some authors consider the limbic system to be a discrete lobe of the brain, its extensive thalamic, hypothalamic, and cortical connections justify its consideration as a transitional zone between the diencephalon and the hemispheres. Although opinions differ about what regions should be designated as the limbic system, there is little disagreement that the hippocampus, amygdala, cingulate gyrus, and parahippocampal gyrus deserve inclusion (Figure 6.10); other structures are variably listed in neuroanatomic accounts, but these details are less crucial than understanding the notion of the limbic system as a functional unit. It is now clear that the human limbic system, at one time thought to have a central role in olfaction, is actually much more devoted to memory and emotion. The two most important limbic components—the

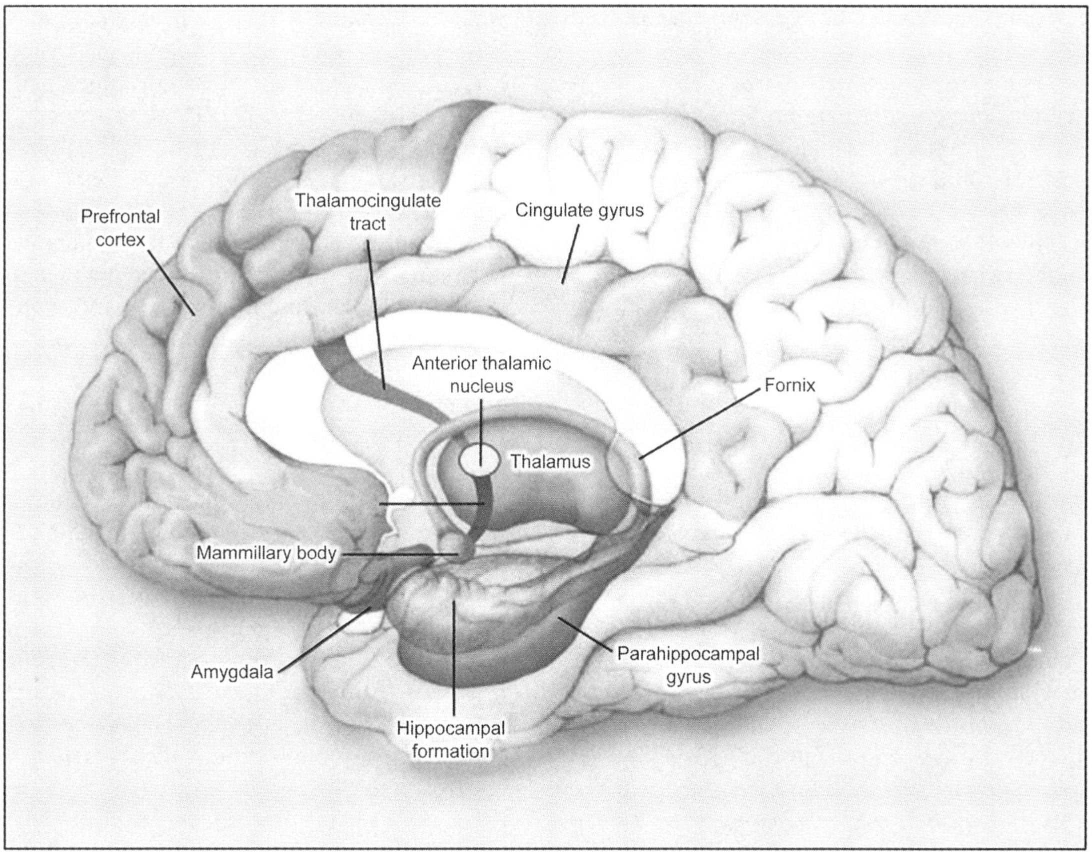

Figure 6.10 Medial view of the brain showing key components of the limbic system. Used with permission from Budson & Price (2005) and the *New England Journal of Medicine*.

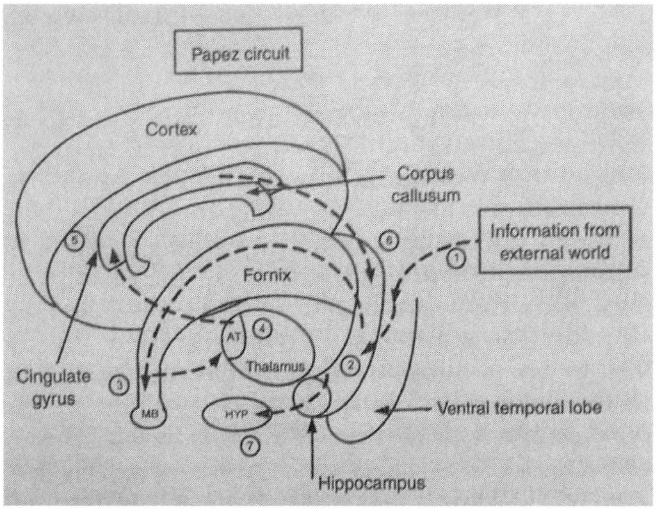

Figure 6.11 The Papez circuit (reproduced and adapted with permission from Pliszka, 2005).

hippocampus and amygdala—serve as nodal points for these two critical limbic circuits. The location of these structures within the temporal lobe suggests a strong linkage of limbic and temporal systems, and the terms *temporal lobe-limbic* and *temporolimbic* are often used to signify their extensive neuroanatomic and functional overlap.

The role of the limbic system in emotion is firmly established. In 1937, James Papez published an influential paper proposing that an interconnected network of structures including the cingulate gyrus, the parahippocampal gyrus, the hippocampus, the fornix, the mammillary bodies, the mammillothalamic tract, and the anterior nucleus of the thalamus comprised the cerebral basis of emotion (Papez, 1937). After decades of study and debate, this network, known as the *Papez circuit* (Figures 6.10 and 6.11) endures as a central concept in the still poorly understood area of emotion. Studies in recent years have identified the amygdala, a dense collection of nuclei in the anterior temporal lobe, as centrally involved in emotional learning and response, and the amygdala has now assumed major status in the neuroanatomy of emotion (LeDoux, 1996). Sensory input to the brain is extensively funneled to the amygdala, where it undergoes processing that produces an assessment of emotional valence: This processing may involve powerful emotional experiences such as intense fear and influence an equally impressive response such as the "flight or fight" reaction that is mediated through autonomic and endocrine systems of the hypothalamus.

In parallel with this expanding knowledge of the representation of emotions in the brain, the prominence of the hippocampus in memory has become more apparent (Squire & Zola, 1996). *Hippocampus* serves as a shorthand term for a trio of regions called the *dentate gyrus, hippocampus proper,* and the *subiculum.* This curved sheet of three-layered (archi-)cortex is tucked into the medial temporal lobe (Figure 6.12a). Figure 12b shows a ventral schematic view of the base of the brain depicting the relative position of the hippocampus in relation to other temporal lobe strucutres. To the right of the schematic is an actual post-mortem view of an intact ventral surface of the right temporal lobe compared to a dissected right temporal lobe revealing the different structures of the temporal lobe. The acquisition of declarative memory, which refers to the learning of facts and events as opposed to skills, is dependent in large part on the hippocampus, as it is well known that bilateral destruction of the hippocampus leads to severe and disabling dysfunction of recent declarative memory. Memory loss of this type may also follow damage to the dorsal medial nucleus of the thalamus and the basal forebrain (Figures 6.9 and 12a, b), implying that a network of interconnected structures subserves this domain. However, the centrality of the amygdala and hippocampus in the dual and tightly interconnected networks of emotion and memory is an intriguing neuroanatomic feature. The close proximity of these structures, and the systems they represent, likely accounts for the common experience that events with the greatest emotional significance are those most likely to be encoded in declarative memory.

White Matter

White matter occupies nearly one half the volume of the brain, and it serves in general to link cortical and gray matter regions with each other. The white matter consists of collections of CNS axons ensheathed with myelin that are most commonly called *tracts,* but that may also be termed *fasciculi, bundles, lemnisci, funiculi,* and *peduncles*. In the brain, these tracts travel between often widely dispersed gray matter areas to integrate cortical and subcortical areas into functionally unified neural networks (Figure 6.13). These networks in turn subserve the many unique functions of the brain, from basic sensation and motor function to cognition and emotion. The dramatic increase in conduction velocity that is conferred by the myelin of white matter axons allows for the rapid transfer of information along white matter tracts, a feature that permits not only efficient communication in sensory and motor systems, but also the integration of higher functions mediated by networks involving neocortical systems. White matter is thus essential for the normal operations of all neural networks (Filley, 2012).

White matter tracts in the brain are generally classified into three major categories: projection fibers, commissural fibers, and association fibers. Projection fibers are solely involved with elemental sensory and motor function; thus they either ascend to the cerebral cortex from lower structures corticopetally, or descend from the cortex to lower regions corticofugally. Major corticopetal (afferent) tracts are the thalamic radiations, relaying somatosensory information from the thalamus to the parietal cortex, and the optic radiations, projecting from the lateral geniculate body to the occipital cortex. The most important corticofugal (efferent) tract is the corticospinal tract, which projects from the motor cortex to lower motor neurons in the spinal cord. The corticobulbar tract occupies a similar position but descends to lower motor neurons in the brain stem. Knowledge of the course of these motor tracts is regularly exploited in neurologic diagnosis. Both of these tracts first travel through the internal capsule, and then cross at different levels; corticospinal fibers decussate

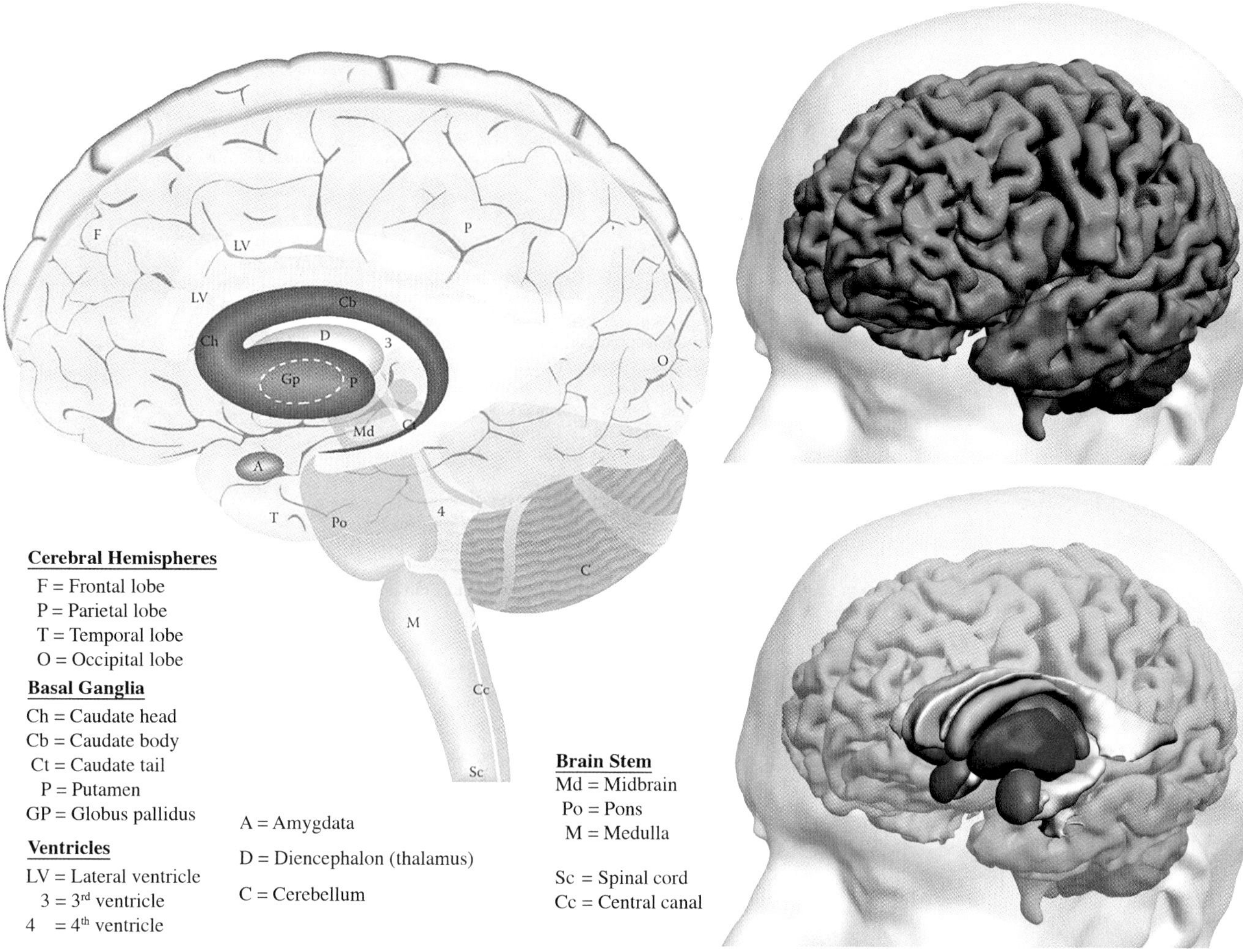
F
LV
P
LV
Cb
D
3
Ch
Gp
P
O
Md
Ct
A
T
Po
4
C
M
Cc
Sc
Cerebral Hemispheres
F = Frontal lobe
P = Parietal lobe
T = Temporal lobe
O = Occipital lobe
Basal Ganglia
Ch = Caudate head
Cb = Caudate body
Ct = Caudate tail
P = Putamen
GP = Globus pallidus
Ventricles
LV = Lateral ventricle
3 = 3rd ventricle
4 = 4th ventricle
A = Amygdata
D = Diencephalon (thalamus)
C = Cerebellum
Brain Stem
Md = Midbrain
Po = Pons
M = Medulla
Sc = Spinal cord
Cc = Central canal

Figure 6.2

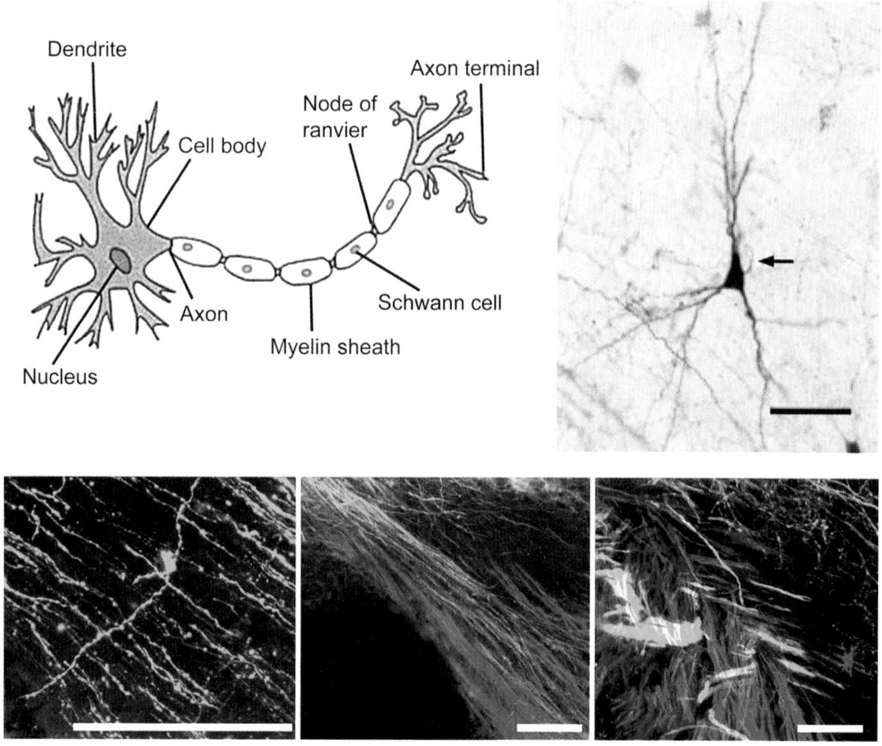
Dendrite
Cell body
Node of ranvier
Axon terminal
Axon
Schwann cell
Myelin sheath
Nucleus

Figure 6.3

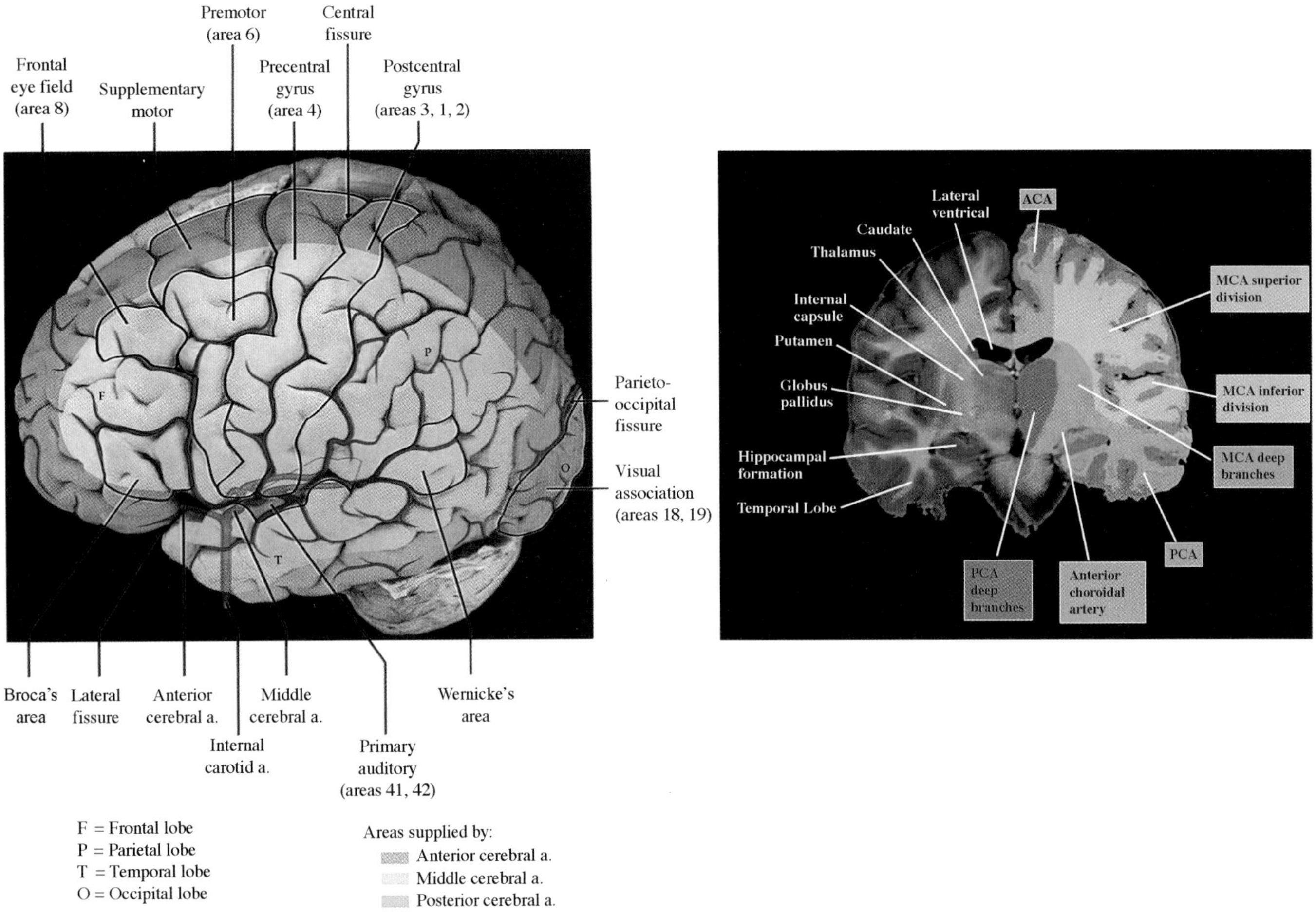
Premotor (area 6)
Central fissure
Frontal eye field (area 8)
Supplementary motor
Precentral gyrus (area 4)
Postcentral gyrus (areas 3, 1, 2)
F
P
T
O
Parieto-occipital fissure
Visual association (areas 18, 19)
Broca's area
Lateral fissure
Anterior cerebral a.
Middle cerebral a.
Internal carotid a.
Primary auditory (areas 41, 42)
Wernicke's area
F = Frontal lobe
P = Parietal lobe
T = Temporal lobe
O = Occipital lobe
Areas supplied by:
Anterior cerebral a.
Middle cerebral a.
Posterior cerebral a.
Lateral ventrical
ACA
Caudate
Thalamus
Internal capsule
Putamen
Globus pallidus
Hippocampal formation
Temporal Lobe
MCA superior division
MCA inferior division
MCA deep branches
PCA
PCA deep branches
Anterior choroidal artery

Figure 6.4b

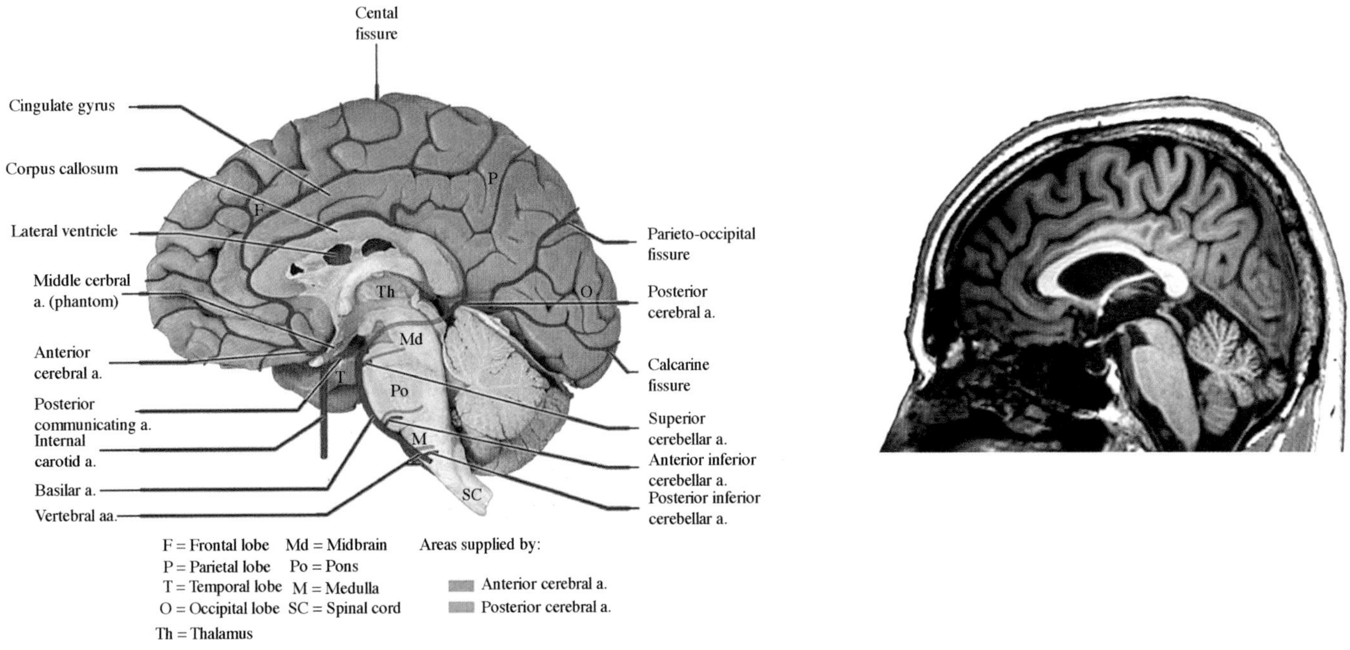
Cental fissure
Cingulate gyrus
Corpus callosum
Lateral ventricle
Middle cerbral a. (phantom)
Anterior cerebral a.
Posterior communicating a.
Internal carotid a.
Basilar a.
Vertebral aa.
F
P
O
T
Th
Md
Po
M
SC
Parieto-occipital fissure
Posterior cerebral a.
Calcarine fissure
Superior cerebellar a.
Anterior inferior cerebellar a.
Posterior inferior cerebellar a.
F = Frontal lobe
P = Parietal lobe
T = Temporal lobe
O = Occipital lobe
Th = Thalamus
Md = Midbrain
Po = Pons
M = Medulla
SC = Spinal cord
Areas supplied by:
Anterior cerebral a.
Posterior cerebral a.

Figure 6.4c

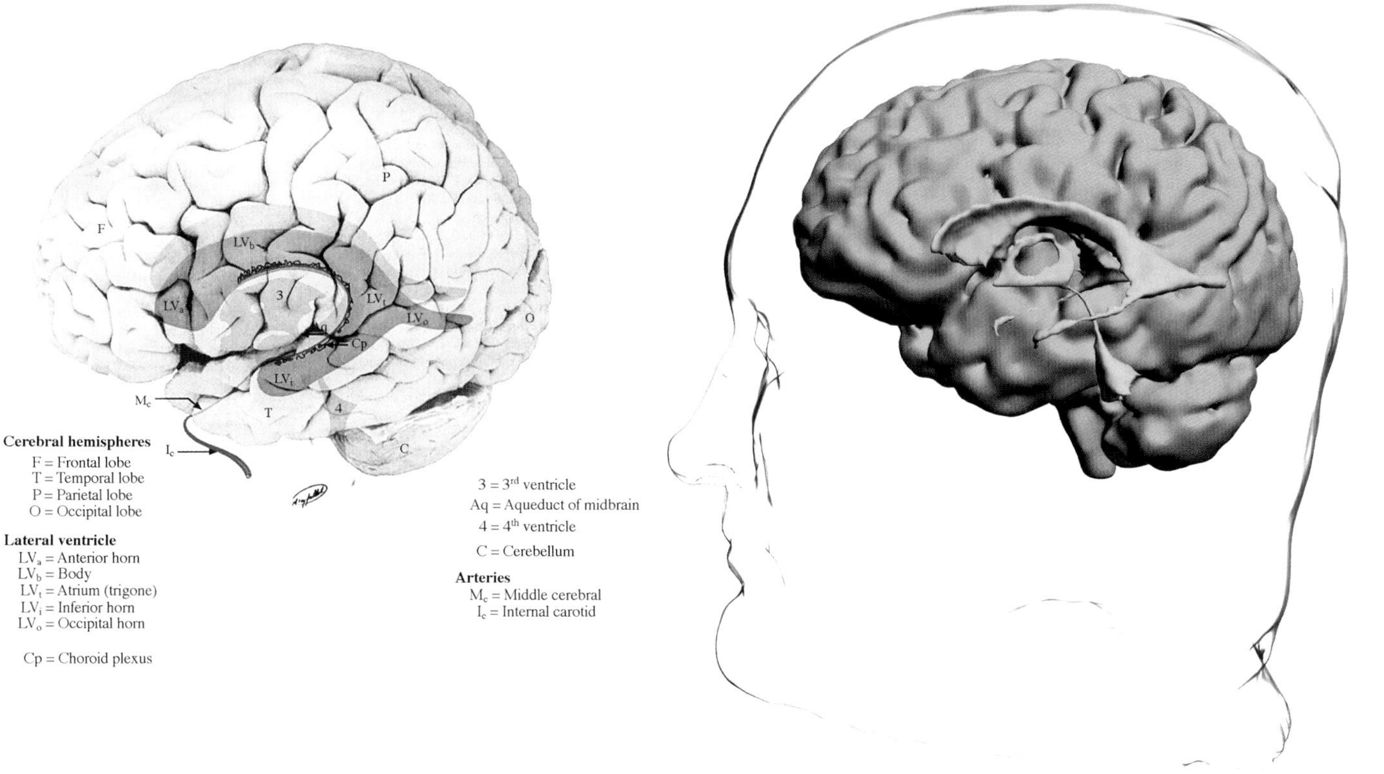
F
P
LVb
LVa
3
LVt
LVo
O
Cp
LVi
Mc
T
4
Ic
C
Cerebral hemispheres
F = Frontal lobe
T = Temporal lobe
P = Parietal lobe
O = Occipital lobe
Lateral ventricle
LVa = Anterior horn
LVb = Body
LVt = Atrium (trigone)
LVi = Inferior horn
LVo = Occipital horn
Cp = Choroid plexus
3 = 3rd ventricle
Aq = Aqueduct of midbrain
4 = 4th ventricle
C = Cerebellum
Arteries
Mc = Middle cerebral
Ic = Internal carotid

Figure 6.5

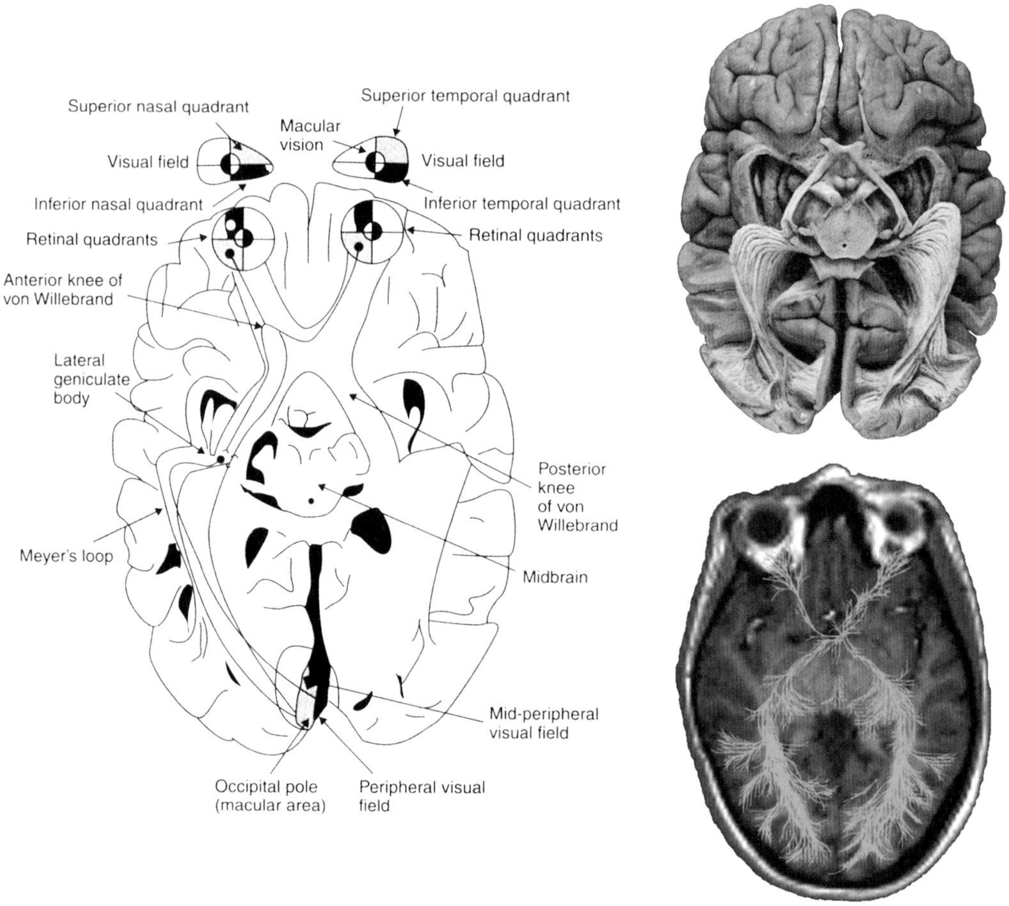
Superior nasal quadrant
Superior temporal quadrant
Macular vision
Visual field
Visual field
Inferior nasal quadrant
Inferior temporal quadrant
Retinal quadrants
Retinal quadrants
Anterior knee of von Willebrand
Lateral geniculate body
Posterior knee of von Willebrand
Meyer's loop
Midbrain
Mid-peripheral visual field
Occipital pole (macular area)
Peripheral visual field

Figure 6.6

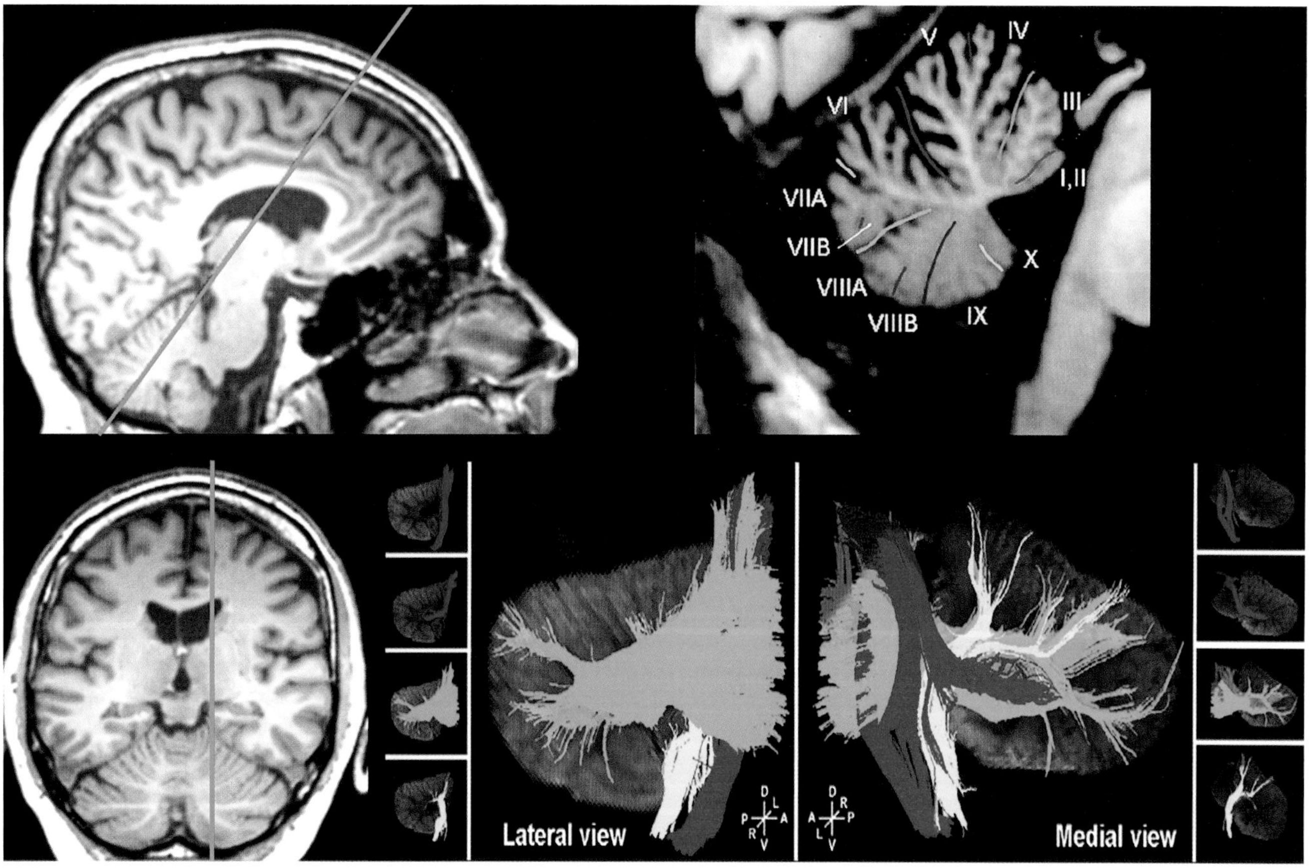
V
IV
VI
III
I,II
VIIA
VIIB
X
VIIIA
VIIIB
IX
Lateral view
Medial view
D
L
P
A
R
V
D
R
A
P
L
V

Figure 6.8b

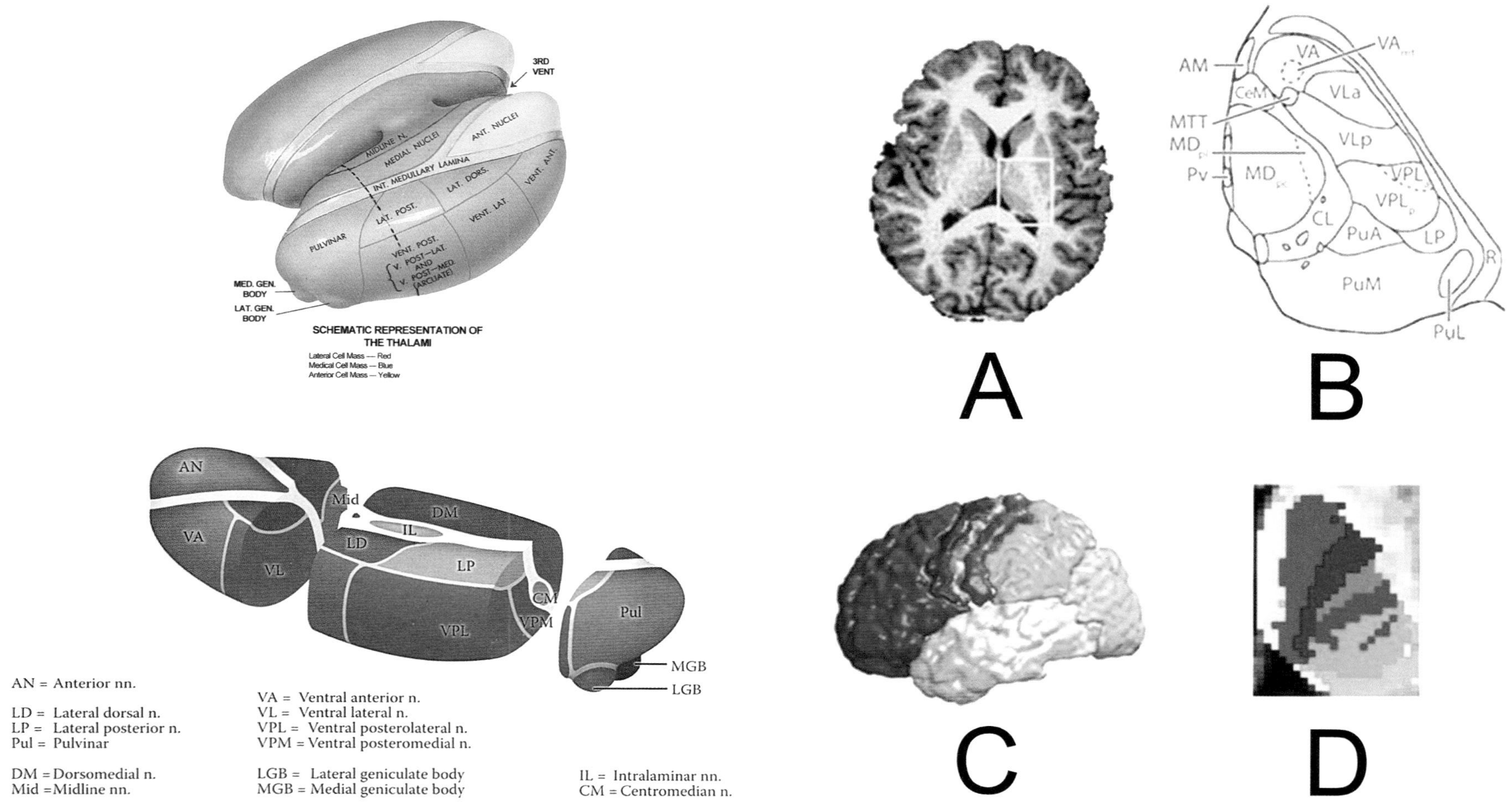
3RD VENT
MIDLINE N.
MEDIAL NUCLEI
ANT. NUCLEI
INT. MEDULLARY LAMINA
LAT. DORS.
VENT. ANT.
LAT. POST.
VENT. LAT.
PULVINAR
VENT. POST.
V. POST-LAT. AND V. POST-MED. (ARCUATE)
MED. GEN. BODY
LAT. GEN. BODY
SCHEMATIC REPRESENTATION OF THE THALAMI
Lateral Cell Mass — Red
Medical Cell Mass — Blue
Anterior Cell Mass — Yellow
AN
VA
VL
Mid
DM
IL
LD
LP
VPL
CM
VPM
Pul
MGB
LGB
AN = Anterior nn.
LD = Lateral dorsal n.
LP = Lateral posterior n.
Pul = Pulvinar
DM = Dorsomedial n.
Mid = Midline nn.
VA = Ventral anterior n.
VL = Ventral lateral n.
VPL = Ventral posterolateral n.
VPM = Ventral posteromedial n.
LGB = Lateral geniculate body
MGB = Medial geniculate body
IL = Intralaminar nn.
CM = Centromedian n.
A
AM
VA
CeM
VLa
MTT
VLp
Pv
CL
PuA
LP
R
PuM
PuL
B
C
D

Figure 6.9

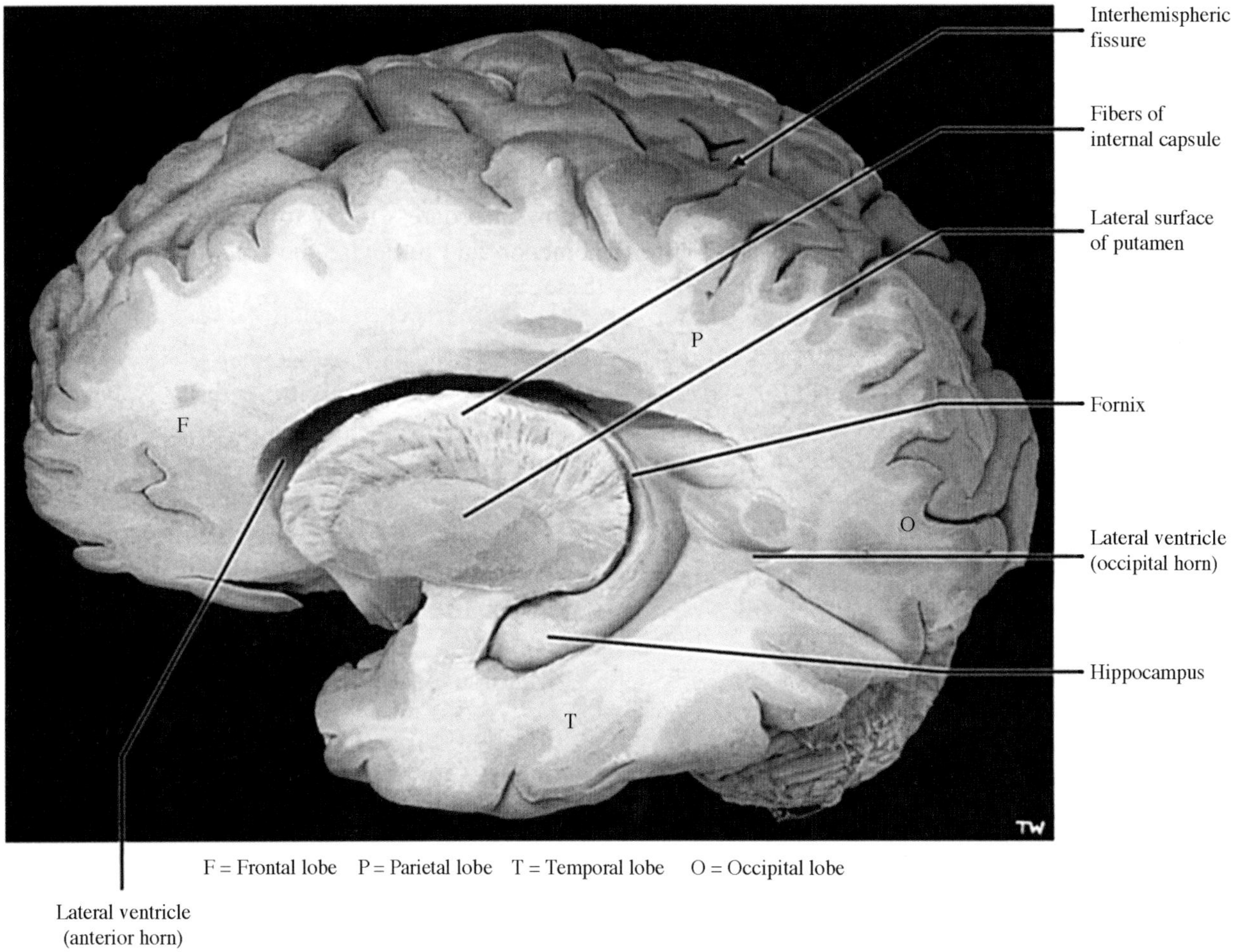
Interhemispheric fissure
Fibers of internal capsule
Lateral surface of putamen
P
F
Fornix
O
Lateral ventricle (occipital horn)
Hippocampus
T
TW
F = Frontal lobe P = Parietal lobe T = Temporal lobe O = Occipital lobe
Lateral ventricle (anterior horn)

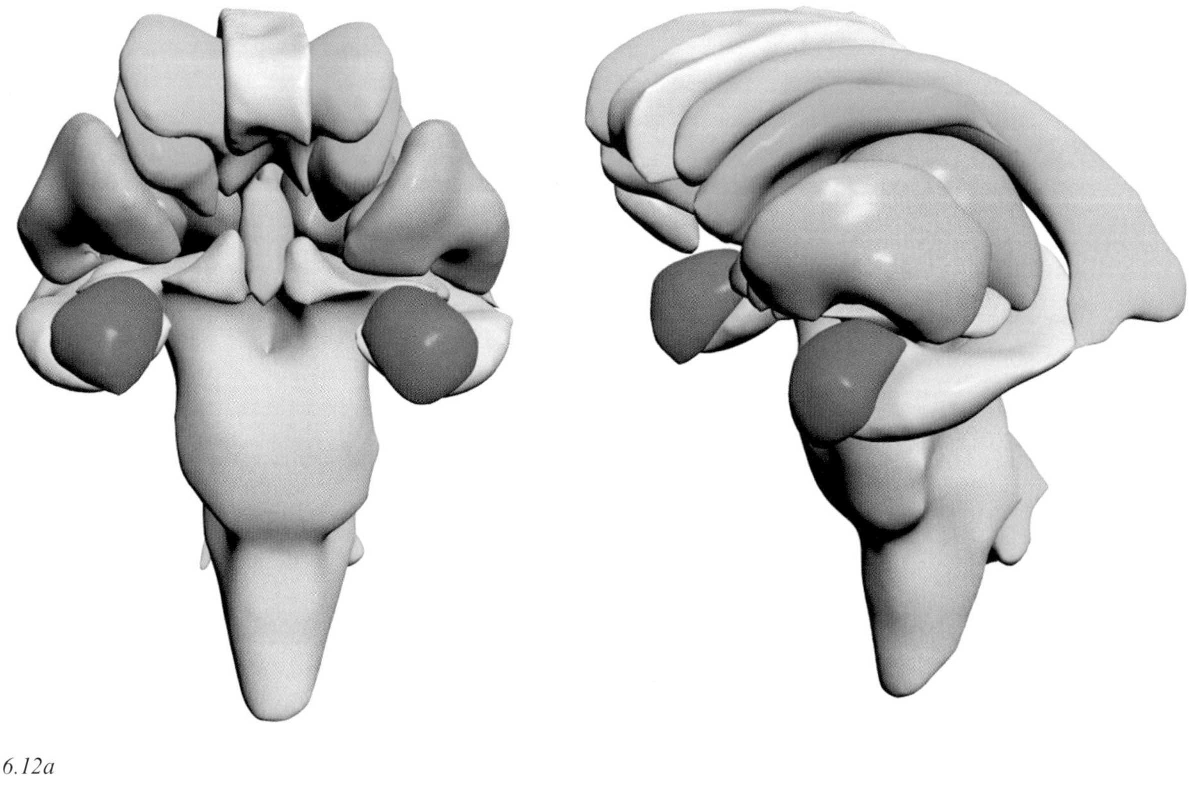

Figure 6.12a

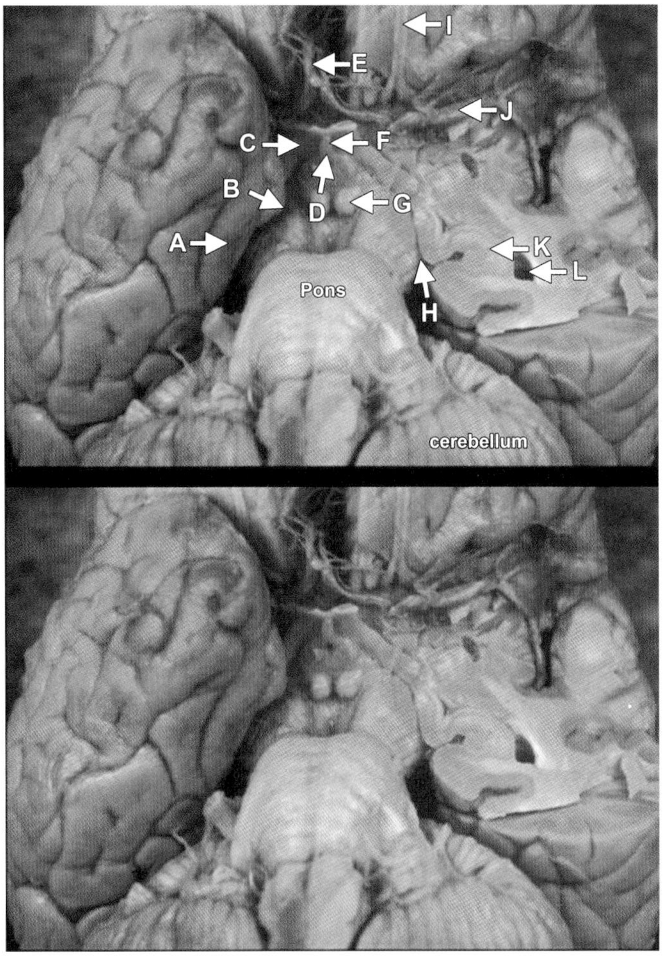

Figure 6.12b

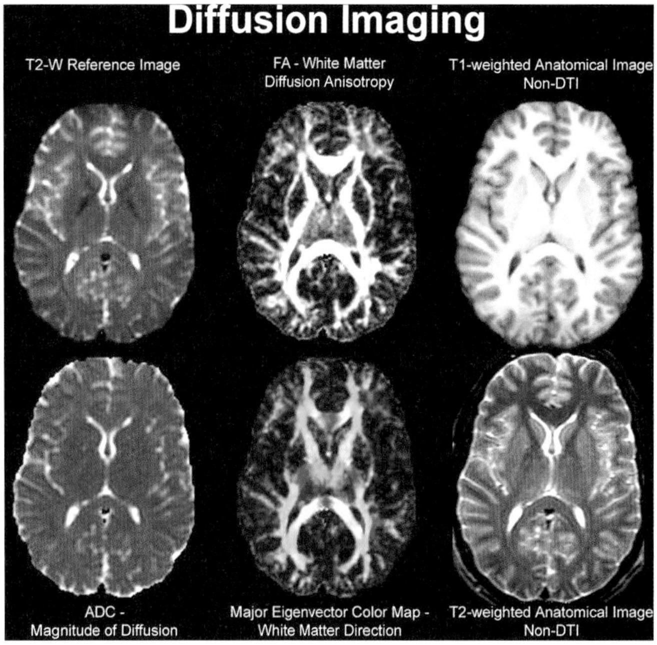

Figure 6.16

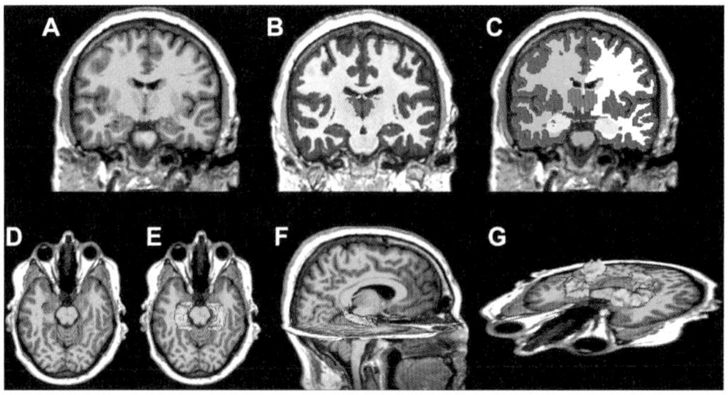

Figure 6.17

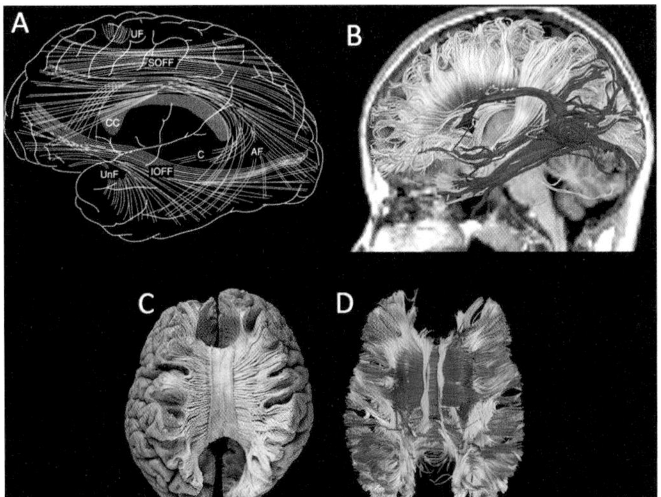

Figure 6.13

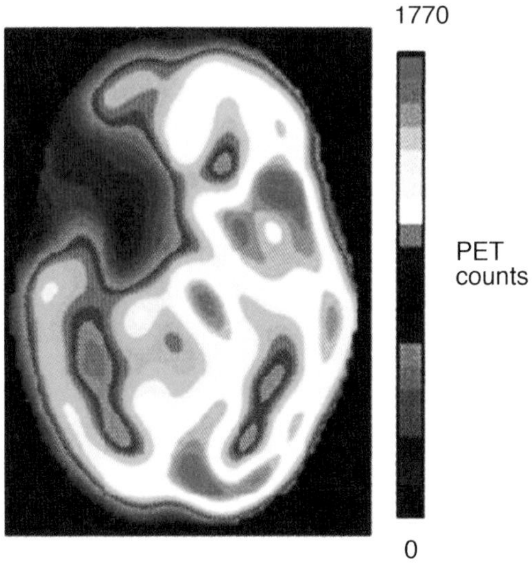

Figure 9.1

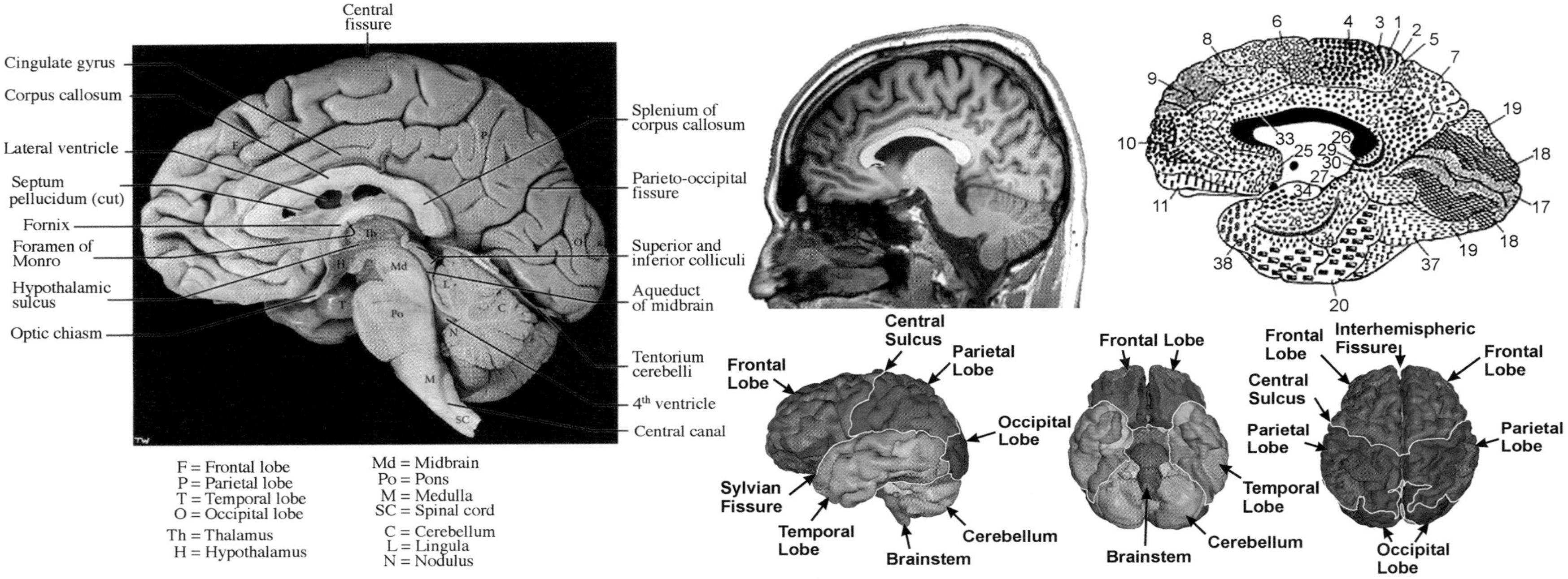

Figure 6.14

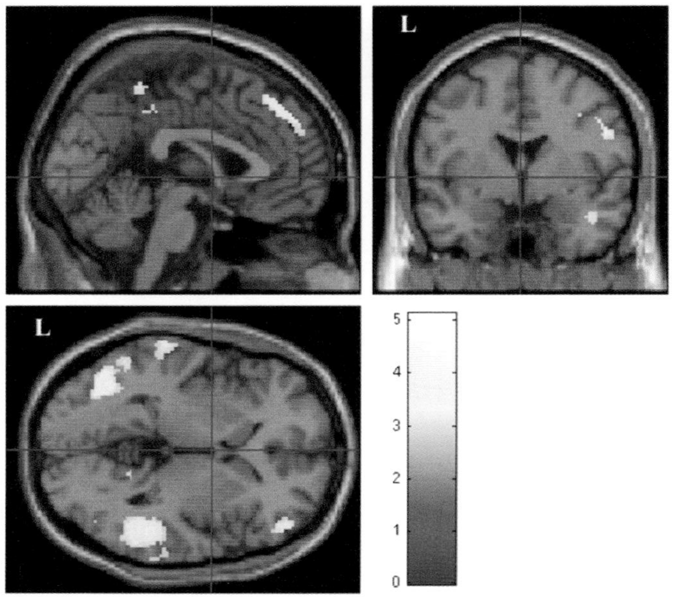

Figure 9.2

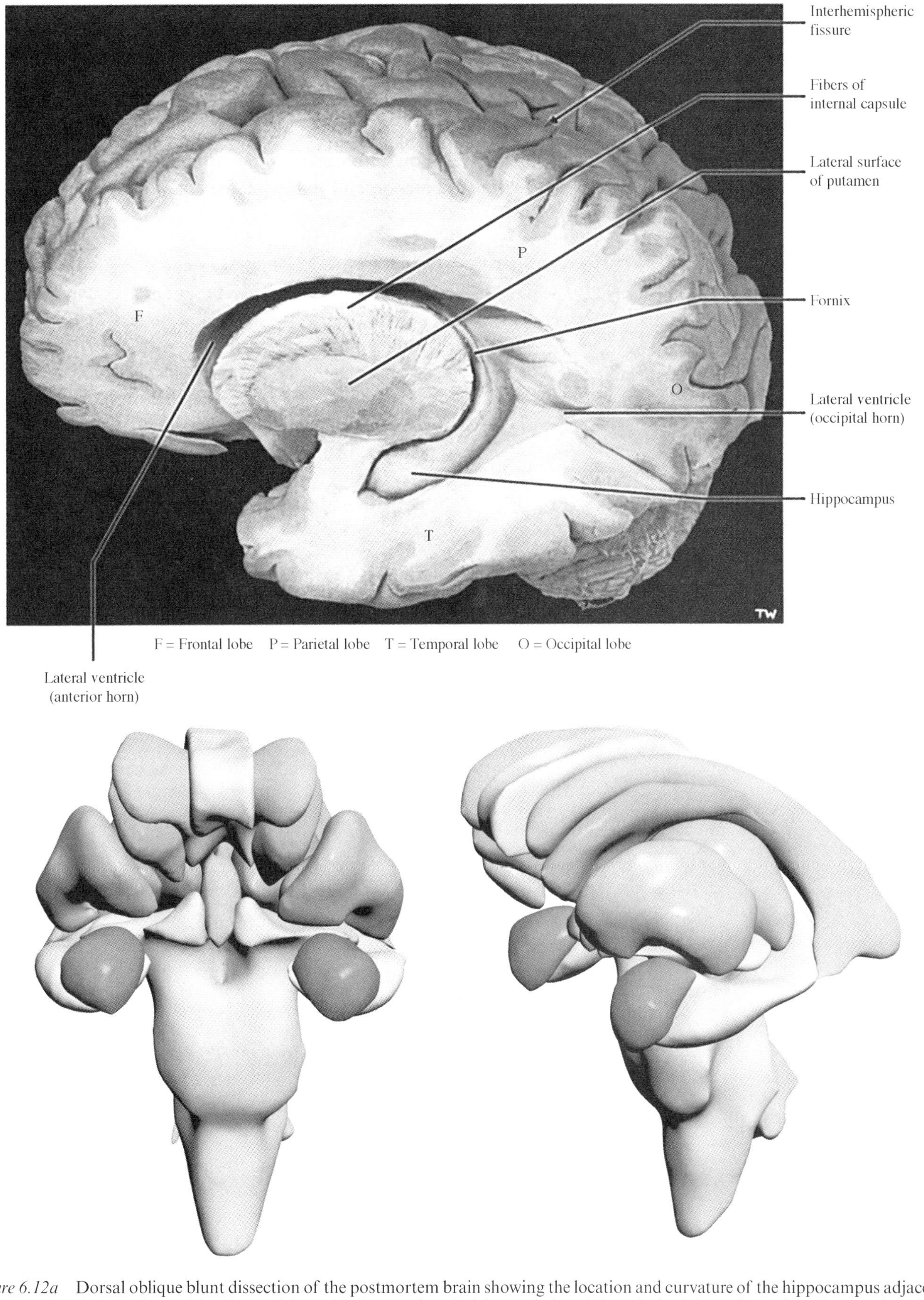

Figure 6.12a Dorsal oblique blunt dissection of the postmortem brain showing the location and curvature of the hippocampus adjacent to the lateral ventricle. (© Hendelman 2006, reproduced with permission). The colorized three-dimensional images (left, frontal view; right, left lateral oblique) are derived from the MRI first shown in Figure 6.2. (see Figure 6.2 for color legend). *A color version of this figure can be found in Plate section 1.*

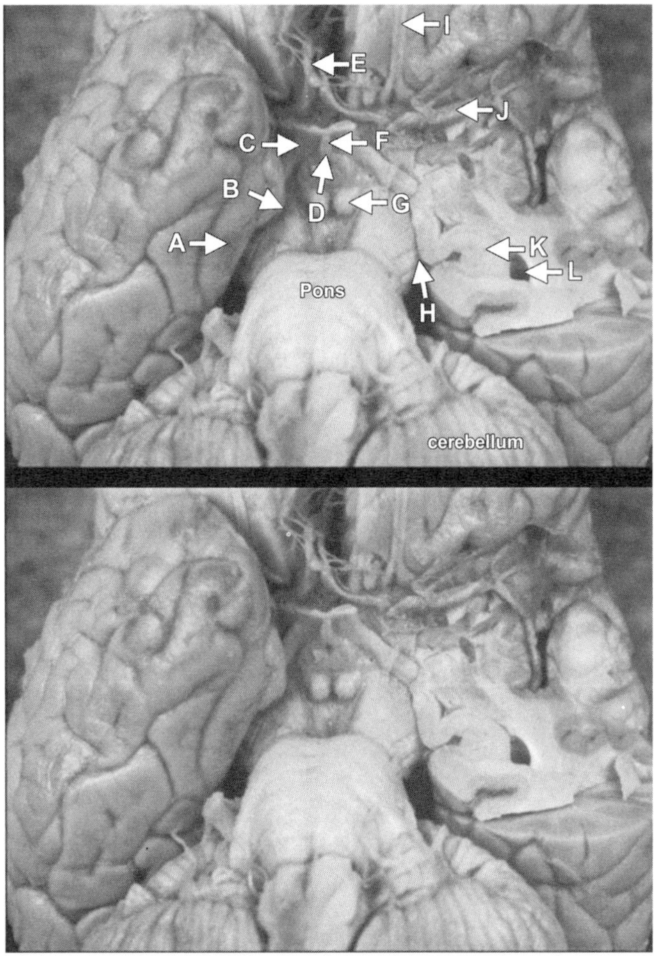

Figure 6.12b Left: diagrammatic representation of the hippocampal formation and its various constituents (reproduced with permission from Arslan, 2001). Right: ventral view of the postmortem brain showing the anatomical location of medial temporal lobe and other structures: (A) parahippocampal gyrus, (B) uncus, (C) optic tract, (D) region of the chiasmatic cistern and infundibulum, (E) anterior cerebral artery, (F) optic chiasm at the top of the arrow, (G) mammillary body, (H) note the proximity of the medial temporal lobe with the cerebral peduncle of the midbrain, (I) olfactory bulb, (J) middle cerebral artery. *A color version of this figure can be found in Plate section 1.*

in the lower medulla to reach the contralateral spinal cord, whereas corticobulbar fibers cross in the brain stem before synapsing on the motor neurons to which they project.

More critical in the mediation of higher functions are the commissural and association fibers (Figure 6.13). Commissural fibers are those that course between the hemispheres via the cerebral commissures. By far the largest of these commissures is the *corpus callosum,* a massive tract that connects the four lobes of the brain with homologous regions on the contralateral side; the anterior and hippocampal commissures are much smaller commissural fiber systems. The association tracts, in contrast, join gray matter regions within each hemisphere. Among these, neuroanatomists have distinguished two types: short and long association fibers. Short association fibers, also called *arcuate* or *U fibers,* connect adjacent cortical gyri throughout the cerebrum. Long association fiber systems are longer and link ipsilateral cerebral lobes; these are the *superior occipitofrontal fasciculus,* the *inferior occipitofrontal fasciculus,* the *arcuate fasciculus,* the *uncinate fasciculus,* and the *cingulum.* An interesting neuroanatomic feature of these tracts is that they all have one terminus in frontal lobe, while the other terminus is variably in more posterior regions.

Many other white matter tracts can be identified, but two deserve special mention. The *fornix* is a prominent arched tract of the limbic system that connects the hippocampus and the mammillary bodies within the Papez circuit. The *medial forebrain bundle* joins the hypothalamus with both caudal and rostral brain regions and participates in the hypothalamic control of the autonomic nervous system.

Contemporary neuroimaging techniques, most impressively DTI, provide methods to extract aggregate images of white matter pathways from the brain, as shown in Figure 6.13. Beyond the capacity of DTI to show dramatic images of the brain and its major pathways, anisotropic measurements can also be made that actually reflect the microscopic integrity of the tissue. Thus not only can an image of a white matter pathway be generated in the living individual, but also quantification is possible regarding the condition of the pathway and its viability.

Cerebral Cortex

The surface of the brain is grossly visible as the *cortex*, meaning "bark" in Latin. The cerebral cortex is the outermost layer of the cerebrum, and it consists of a thin sheet of neurons averaging 3 mm in thickness. The number of cerebral cortical neurons is estimated at 25 billion, and the number of synapses between these neurons may be an extraordinary 300 trillion. The computational power made possible by this remarkable number of contacts renders the cerebral cortex as the locus of the most advanced functions of the human brain. An understanding of cortical structure and function is a prerequisite for the neuroscientific study of the mind and all that this pursuit entails.

Microscopically, the cerebral cortex has a horizontally laminated structure. More than 90% of the cortex is classified as *neocortex,* a term that signifies the relatively recent arrival of this structure in the course of evolution. The neocortex consists of six layers: the outermost molecular layer, the external granular cell layer, the external pyramidal cell layer, the internal granular cell layer, the internal pyramidal cell layer, and the innermost multiform layer. A vertical organization to the neocortex can also be defined physiologically. Columns of cells, arranged perpendicular to the cortical surface, respond as a unit to a given stimulus. Hundreds of millions of these columns exist, connected with each other and many more caudal areas by the axons of pyramidal cells.

The remaining cortical regions are classified as *allocortex,* which is in turn made up of *paleocortex* and *archicortex,* ancient cortical types that are more prominent in lower animals than humans. The olfactory system is largely allocortical in composition, and one of the most important allocortical

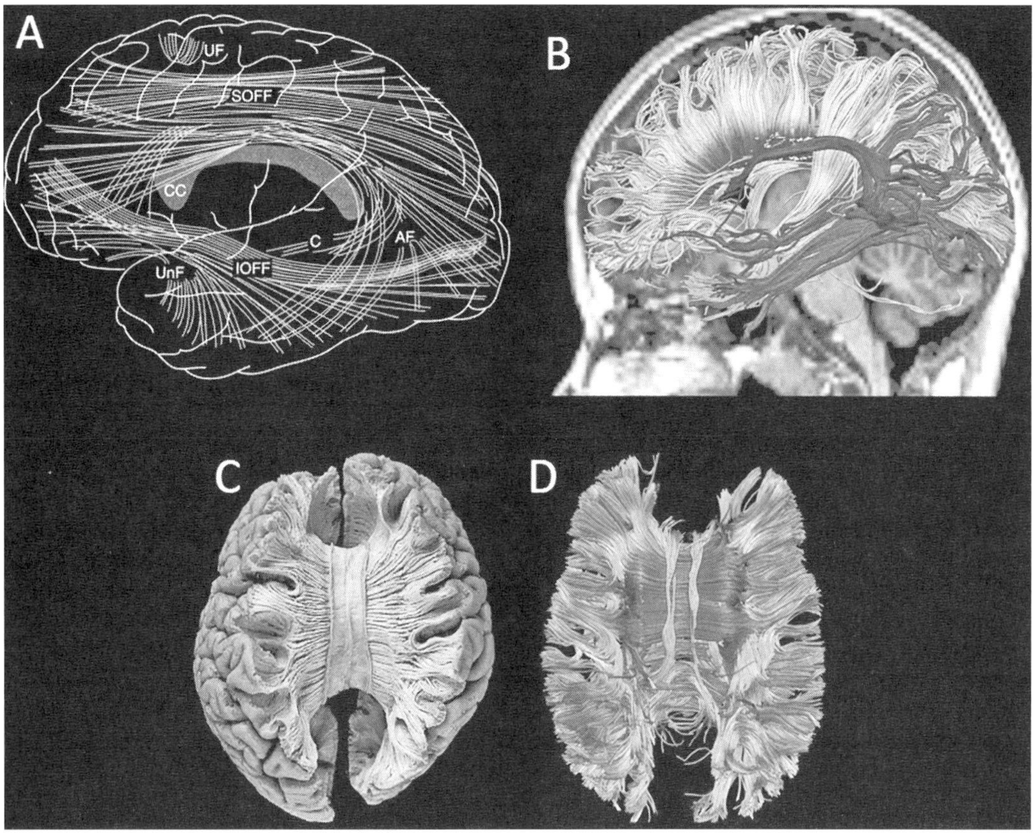

Figure 6.13 (A) Drawing of the commissural and association white matter tracts of the cerebrum. Abbreviations: CC, corpus callosum; UF, U fibers; SOFF, superior occipitofrontal fasciculus; IOFF, inferior occipitofrontal fasciculus; AF, arcuate fasciculus; UnF, uncinate fasciculus; C, cingulum. Reprinted with permission from Filley (2012). (B) Side view of some of the major tracts as derived from DTI. (C) Dorsal view of a meticulous blunt dissection showing the back-and-forth projections of the callosal fibers and how they may be imaged using DTI tractography methods as shown on the bottom right. *A color version of this figure can be found in Plate section 1.*

zones is the hippocampus. As reviewed earlier, the hippocampus is a cortical area of the limbic system that is involved with the memory and emotional systems of the brain. The hippocampus has three layers: the outer molecular layer, the pyramidal cell layer, and the inner polymorphic layer.

Neuroanatomists have often attempted to divide the cerebral cortex into discrete zones in an effort to understand its functional affiliations. The best known of these cortical parcellations is that of Korbinian Brodmann (Brodmann, 1994), who described about 50 areas of the cortex, based on distinct histological characteristics he found in each (Figure 6.14). Although some of these areas have been found to have clear functional roles, the significance of many still remains undetermined. Nevertheless, the cortical map of Brodmann has endured for almost a century, and reference to his carefully numbered zones is commonplace in accounts of neocortical anatomy and function.

The cortical surface serves as the basis for the definition of the four lobes of the cerebrum: the frontal, temporal, parietal, and occipital lobes (Figures 6.2, 6.4b, 6.9, and 6.14). These lobes are widely employed as convenient divisions of the cerebral hemispheres that facilitate conceptualizations of neurobehavioral functions in the brain. The frontal lobe is the most rostral of the four, positioned anterior to the Rolandic fissure and superior to the Sylvian fissure. The temporal lobe lies inferior to the Sylvian fissure, and its posterior boundary is determined by the junction of two lines: one from the parietooccipital sulcus to the preoccipital notch and the other running posteriorly from the end of the Sylvian fissure (Figure 6.4b). The parietal lobe is found posterior to the Rolandic fissure, and its inferior margin is also defined by the two lines that form the posterior extent of the temporal lobe. The occipital lobe is located posterior to both the temporal and parietal lobes. Another small neocortical region, not visible on the brain surface, is the *insula,* or *island of Reil,* concealed under the Sylvian fissure by portions of the frontal, temporal, and parietal lobes.

The Relationship of Brain and Behavior

The foregoing synopsis of neuroanatomy, however truncated, may appear overwhelming in its complexity. Moreover, the relevance of much neuroanatomic detail to neuropsychology may seem uncertain. In this section, an attempt will be made to develop a series of conceptual themes in neuroanatomy

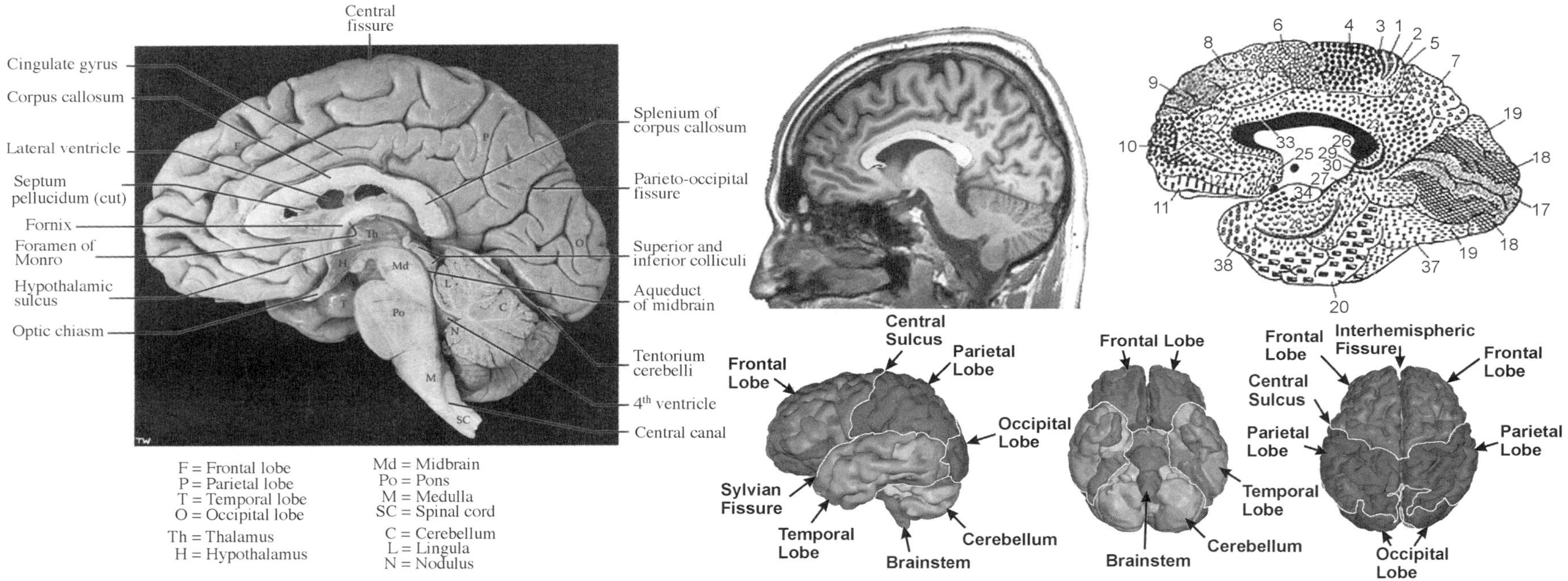

Figure 6.14 Left: medial illustration of the brain showing the position of the four lobes of the cerebral hemispheres (© Hendelman, 2006; reproduced with permission). Middle: MR image at a similar level (slightly off the midline, so as to reveal the gyral pattern of the medial surface unobscured by the falx cerebri, as it will most typically appear on a mid-sagittal cut with conventional MRI). Right: The original line drawing from Brodmann depicting the mid-sagittal view of designated Brodmann regions. Note that the general Brodmann areas can be identified when viewing MRI. *A color version of this figure can be found in Plate section 1.*

that are particularly useful to the clinical practice and research goals of neuropsychology. A working knowledge of neurobehavioral anatomy is clearly an essential prerequisite for the study of brain-behavior relationships (Cummings, 2003; Filley, 2012; Mesulam, 2001).

General Principles

An initial grasp of the brain as the organ of human behavior can be gained by considering some general organizational principles. As a first step, brain function can be broadly considered by reference to a series of distinctions based on the vertical, longitudinal, and horizontal dimensions of the cerebral hemispheres.

Vertical organization. Seen in the context of its evolutionary development or phylogeny, the vertical organization of the brain becomes apparent (Cummings, 2003). The course of evolution has endowed human beings with a highly developed brain that enables unique behaviors permitting unprecedented mastery of the environment. This development mainly entails the progressive expansion of the cortical mantle seen in mammalian evolution, particularly the frontal lobes. However, many features of the human brain are shared in common with other animals, such as those concerned with basic needs such as feeding, defensive aggression, and reproduction. Humans have neuroanatomic residua of ancient neural systems common to many animals, but also harbor more recently evolved brain systems that confer a set of unique adaptive abilities. In this sense, the human brain can be seen as the most highly developed nervous structure in nature.

The hierarchical structure of the brain has been described by MacLean as the "triune" brain (MacLean, 1970). In his formulation, three levels of neural development can be identified: reptilian, paleomammalian, and neomammalian. The reptilian brain—including the brain stem, cerebellum, and thalamus—is a primitive inner core concerned with arousal, autonomic, cardiovascular, respiratory, and visceral functions. The paleomammalian brain, consisting of the limbic system, reflects early mammalian development and the advent of drives, child rearing, communal bonding, and territoriality. The neomammalian brain, essentially the cerebral cortex, harbors the most recent mammalian capacities that are generally referred to as cognition and emotional behavior.

Whereas the triune brain of MacLean has had considerable theoretical impact, a distinction based on the levels of neuroanatomic organization in the human cerebrum may have more direct applicability to clinicians and researchers in neuropsychology. In recent decades, much work has been devoted to contrasting the neuropsychological affiliations of the cerebral cortex with those of the subcortical gray matter (Cummings, 1990), and, more recently, the cerebral white matter (Filley, 2012). Although the disorders affecting these three broad regions are necessarily diffuse in their distribution, and thus these lines of inquiry do not assist in establishing specific brain-behavior relationships based on the study of focal lesions, the distinction between cortical, subcortical, and white matter dysfunction is relevant to the majority of patients seen by neuropsychologists who have diffuse cognitive dysfunction from dementia or traumatic brain injury. Consideration of these categories therefore extends the classic lesion method of behavioral neurology to the study of diffuse brain disorders that are so common and challenging to medicine and society.

Longitudinal organization. Along its longitudinal axis, the brain can immediately be seen to have a clear division of functional specialization. In brief, this separation divides the anterior cerebrum, devoted to motor function, from the posterior cerebrum, dedicated to sensory function.

The frontal lobe is the most anterior lobe of the brain, and it harbors the neocortical basis of motor activity. The corticospinal and corticobulbar tracts originate in the precentral gyrus of the frontal lobe, enabling the cortical control of voluntary movement. In addition, the frontal lobes mediate motor aspects of language and emotional prosody by the operations of Broca's area on the left and its analogous region on the right. The medial frontal regions also have a role in motor function in that they are thought to subserve the motivation to engage in voluntary action; damage to these regions may result in apathy or abulia, and, in extreme cases, akinetic mutism.

The posterior lobes of the cerebrum—temporal, parietal, and occipital—are primarily devoted to sensation. Audition and the comprehension of language and other sounds are functions of the temporal lobes. The parietal lobes are directly involved with the mediation of somatic sensation, and the right parietal lobe is selectively dedicated to the interpretation of visuospatial information. The occipital lobes are primarily dedicated to the sense of vision, which has assumed much greater importance in humans as the sense of olfaction has diminished in value with higher levels of adaptation.

Horizontal organization. A final dimensional distinction in the brain can be seen in the functional differences between the two sides of the cerebrum (Springer & Deutsch, 1989). Since the time of Broca, one of the best-recognized features of the human brain is its asymmetry with respect to function, an observation that led to the concept of *cerebral lateralization*. The most obvious of these functional asymmetries is the dominance of the left hemisphere for language in most individuals. The right hemisphere has also been recognized to possess dominant functions of its own. The reason for this arrangement is not known, as there appears to be no such lateralization of function in paired organs elsewhere in the body, such as the lungs and kidneys. Nevertheless, the neurobehavioral specializations of the cerebral hemispheres are increasingly well understood, and should always be considered in the assessment and care of neurologic patients.

The left hemisphere is dominant for language in most people. The great majority of right-handers and even most left-handers have their language skills primarily organized in the left hemisphere. It is commonly asserted that 99% of right-handers are left-dominant for language, and that 67% of left-handers are also left-dominant for this domain (Filley, 2012). While this generalization is adequate for routine clinical purposes, a more refined view is that 70% of the population is dextral and strongly left-dominant for language, 10% is sinistral and right-dominant for language, and 20%

is ambidextrous with anomalous (bilateral) language representation. These statistics find support in the asymmetry of the *planum temporale,* a structure of the superior temporal lobe concerned with language processing, in that about 70% of brains have a larger left side, 10% a larger right side, and 20% roughly equal sizes (Filley, 2012).

The right hemisphere, long considered the "nondominant" or "silent" hemisphere because of its relative inability to process linguistic information, has an impressive range of functions for which it can be regarded as dominant. The most uncontroversial domains that can be regarded as right-hemisphere dominant are constructional ability, spatial attention, and language prosody (Filley, 2012). Also attributed by many to the right hemisphere is music, although contributions from the left hemisphere also contribute to this highly complex capacity (Filley, 2012). In any case, the broad range of higher functions organized by both hemispheres, separately or in combination, clearly indicates that neither side is dominant in any absolute sense, that brain areas work together to produce optimal performance, and that, in neurobehavioral terms, there are no silent areas of the cerebrum.

Neural Networks

As the preceding discussion suggests, the localization of higher function in the brain is a central goal of neuroscience. Whereas generalizations regarding the functional organization of the brain are useful, more specific localization of higher functions within the hemispheres remains an imperative of neuroscience research. The representation of cognitive and especially emotional function in the brain has long been vigorously debated because the precise determination of the locus of these skills has often proven elusive. It should be recalled that much of the history of neuropsychology and behavioral neurology took place during an era when the only means of determining brain-behavior relationships was through postmortem study, but even in the age of modern neuroimaging, uncertainty remains about the consistency with which a given function can be said to be represented in a specific brain region.

Traditionally, the debate about cerebral representation of higher function has had two major factions: *localizationists* and *equipotential theorists.* The former group begins with the time-honored practice of neurologists that emphasizes detailed understanding of nervous system structure and the localization of functions within it. This process permits the application of the lesion method to the study of higher functions, theoretically producing a secure map of brain-behavior relationships. Whereas this approach is highly effective in localizing elemental neurologic deficits such as CN deficits and hemiparesis, it has not proven as reliable in identifying the sites of higher functions. There is no simple correspondence, for example, between a given gyrus and a discrete cognitive domain, and this kind of localization of higher function has proven to be inadequate for capturing the complexity of brain-behavior relationships. In this regard, strict localization has been justifiably criticized for too closely resembling its intellectual predecessor, the phrenology of Franz Joseph Gall (Filley, 2012).

Equipotential theorists have contended that any specific localization of higher functions in the brain is impossible. Most closely associated with the early 20th century Karl Lashley, the equipotential theory held that all cerebral cortical areas are capable of supporting the operations of higher functions (Filley, 2012). The cortex was considered to be essentially undifferentiated with respect to mentation, and thus a lesion in any cortical zone could be expected to diminish neurobehavioral capacity in proportion to the amount of tissue damaged. Much clinical and experimental evidence—most obviously that supporting the lateralization of language function discussed earlier—contradicts this claim, and it is clear from numerous clinical and neuroimaging studies that considerable specialization of cerebral areas exists with regard to the higher functions. Thus, like strict localization, pure equipotentiality is insupportable in light of current knowledge.

The resolution of this debate appears to come from the concept of distributed neural networks (Mesulam, 2001). As a compromise position, the notion of neural networks postulates that integrated ensembles of interconnected cerebral structures subserve specific neurobehavioral domains. Thus there is no singular and exclusive relationship between a brain structure and a mental function, but neither is there a diffuse representation of functions in which no cerebral specialization exists. Rather, a given domain is represented within a neuroanatomically linked network that operates as a functional unit. Familiar examples of these networks include the left perisylvian language zone and the medial temporal lobe memory system. Other neural networks, such as those subserving executive function and visual perception, are being elucidated with the assistance of modern structural and functional neuroimaging. Increasingly supported by the emergence of new information, the notion of neural networks represents a satisfying resolution of an old debate, and points the way toward many research opportunities designed to explicate the workings of the human brain.

Functional Affiliations of the Cerebrum

The clinical method used for the assessment of neurobehavioral disorders is based on the localization of higher functions in the brain (Filley, 2012; Mesulam, 2001; Cummings, 2003). Although the concept of neural networks increasingly influences thinking about brain-behavior relationships, an understanding of the basic functional affiliations of major brain regions is essential for clinical practice and research in neuropsychology. Individuals are typically referred for neuropsychological evaluation of a specific syndrome—a constellation of symptoms and signs that indicates the origin of clinical dysfunction. The neuropsychologist plays a crucial role in characterizing the nature and severity of the syndrome, defining the likely localization of the problem, helping to guide further diagnostic testing, assisting with providing the best possible medical care, and contributing to neuroscientific research on cerebral localization. Later chapters present detailed discussions of individual conditions that produce these syndromes; what follows here is a brief consideration

Table 6.2 Functional affiliations of the cerebrum

Frontal Lobe	
	Voluntary Movement
	Language fluency (left)
	Motor prosody (right)
	Working memory
	Executive function
	Comportment
	Motivation
Temporal Lobe	
	Audition
	Language comprehension (left)
	Sensory prosody (right)
	Memory
	Emotion
Parietal Lobe	
	Tactile sensation
	Visuospatial function (right)
	Attention (right)
	Reading (left)
	Calculation (left)
Occipital Lobe	
	Vision
	Visual perception

of the neurobehavioral functions of the four cerebral lobes, those brain areas most relevant to the neuropsychologist (see Table 6.2; Cummings, 2003; Filley, 2012; Mesulam, 2001).

The frontal lobe is the largest lobe of the human brain, occupying more than a third of the cortical surface, and it houses a variety of motor, cognitive, and emotional functions. However, because it has appeared most recently in phylogeny and its development seems to parallel that of human behavior, the frontal lobe is regarded as being particularly associated with the highest of human functions. Indeed, the lasting preoccupation of neuroscientists with this part of the brain stems from the enticing likelihood that singularly human capacities are most likely to be explained by reference to this lobe. Yet the essential role of the frontal lobe in human behavior remains elusive, even though much progress has been made in exploring its many contributions.

The most obvious role of the frontal lobe is in voluntary movement, which is based on the origin of corticospinal and corticobulbar tracts in the precentral gyrus (Brodmann area 4). Also important in movement is the supplementary motor area (area 6), which seems to have a special role in the initiation of voluntary movement and speech. In neurobehavioral terms, many other domains are securely associated with the frontal lobes, in particular those areas not concerned with motor function that are known as prefrontal cortex. Language fluency is clearly related to the function of Broca's area (areas 44 and 45) on the left side, and its counterpart in the right hemisphere is thought to subserve motor prosody. Working memory, a recently described domain that is related to both attention and memory, is likely affiliated with the dorsolateral prefrontal cortex (areas 9 and 46). The important concept of executive function, among the most critical domains for effective human performance, is thought to be mediated by a larger area of prefrontal cortex that includes areas 8, 9, 10, 46, and 47. Comportment, the ability to inhibit limbic impulses and maintain an appropriate behavioral repertoire, largely depends on the integrity of orbitofrontal regions (areas 11, 12, and 25). Lastly, motivation is most closely associated with medial frontal structures including the anterior cingulate gyrus (areas 24, 32, and 33).

The temporal lobe has a primary role in audition, receiving sound stimuli in the primary auditory cortex (Heschl's gyrus, areas 41 and 42) that arise from the ear and ascend through CN VIII, the brain stem, and the thalamus. Further processing of these stimuli then occurs in the temporal lobe as well. On the left, speech sounds are decoded in Wernicke's area (the posterior part of area 22), allowing for the comprehension of language, while in a homologous region on the right, other aspects of sound are interpreted to permit the perception of prosody and related areas such as melody. In addition, the strong associations of the temporal lobe with the limbic system, reviewed earlier, provide the neuroanatomic substrate for the involvement of this lobe in the mediation of memory and emotion.

The parietal lobe has a primary somatosensory affiliation, and interpretation of tactile information occurs in the postcentral gyrus (areas 3, 1, and 2) of each hemisphere. Higher order sensory cortex in the parietal lobe (areas 5 and 7) subserves the perception of tactile stimuli to permit the appreciation of stereognosis and graphesthesia. On the right side, the parietal lobe in general is specialized for visuospatial function, without which the ability to negotiate three-dimensional space is compromised. The right parietal lobe is also specialized for the domain of spatial attention, a feature that explains the curious and often devastating phenomenon of left hemineglect in patients with right parietal damage. These specializations are among those that make the right hemisphere primarily responsible for a wealth of nonverbal skills that significantly enhance human existence. On the left side, in contrast, the predominantly verbal domains of reading and calculation are primarily organized in the angular gyrus (area 39) and the supramarginal gyrus (area 40).

The occipital lobe has the most unified functional affiliation of all the cerebral lobes. Located at the rear of the brain and dominated by the medially located calcarine cortex (area 17), the occipital lobe is devoted to vision. Of all the senses, vision requires the greatest amount of neural tissue, and the occipital cortices represent the neocortical destination of the visual information processed by the eyes. After the first order visual neurons from the retinae synapse in the lateral geniculate body of the thalamus, second order visual neurons project to the calcarine cortex and enable primary visual function at the cortical level. From there, further processing occurs in the visual association cortex (areas 18 and 19) adjacent to the primary occipital cortex, permitting the perception of visual stimuli. Still further visual processing occurs in temporal and parietal regions that are involved in visual recognition. Recent data have supported the existence of two parallel visual systems of visual processing, termed the "what" and "where" systems, involving ventral and dorsal streams, respectively, of the visual association cortices. These streams begin in the visual association regions subserving visual perception, and then proceed anteriorly to inferior temporal cortices for the "what" system, and parietal cortices for the "where" system.

The affiliations of the four lobes of the brain serve as a useful introduction to the behavioral geography of the brain. In the succinct words of the influential behavioral neurologist Norman Geschwind: "Every behavior has an anatomy" (Geschwind, 1975). The anatomy of higher function is an amalgam of traditional neuroanatomic inquiry, the clinical study of neurologic patients, and the methods of modern neuroscience, all of which are expanding our insights into brain-behavior relationships as never before. Based on this knowledge, the neurobiologic basis of normal cognition, emotion, and consciousness becomes ever more clear. For those concerned with clinical assessment and treatment, this knowledge is a necessary precursor to the care of patients with disorders of the brain.

References

Arslan, O. (2001). *Neuroanatomical Basis of Clinical Neurology*. Boca Raton, FL: CRC Press.

Atoji, Y., & Wild, J. M. (2004). Fiber connections of the hippocampal formation and septum and subdivisions of the hippocampal formation in the pigeon as revealed by tract tracing and kainic acid lesions. *Journal of Comparative Neurology*, *475*(3), 426–461.

Bigler, E. D. (2015). Structural image analysis of the brain in neuropsychology using magnetic resonance imaging (MRI) techniques. *Neuropsychology Review*, 25(3), 224–249. doi: 10.1007/s11065-015-9290-0.

Blumenfeld, H. (2011). *Neuroanatomy Through Clinical Cases* (2nd ed.). Sunderland, MA: Sinauer Associates.

Boly, M., Seth, A. K., Wilke, M., Ingmundson, P., Baars, B., Laureys, S., . . . Tsuchiya, N. (2013, October 31). Consciousness in humans and non-human animals: Recent advances and future directions. *Frontiers in Psychology*, *4*, 625.

Brodal, P. (1981). *Neurological Anatomy* (3rd ed.). New York: Oxford University Press.

Brodmann, K. (1994). *Localisation in the Cerebral Cortex*. London: Smith-Gordon.

Budson, A. E., & Price, B. H. (2005, February 17). Memory dysfunction. *New England Journal of Medicine*, *352*(7), 692–699.

Catani, M., & Thiebaut de Schotten, M. (2012). *Atlas of Human Brain Connections*. New York: Oxford University Press.

Cummings, J. L. (Ed.). (1990). *Subcortical Dementia*. New York: Oxford University Press.

Cummings, J. L., & Mega, M. S. (2003). *Neuropsychiatry and Behavioral Neuroscience*. Oxford: Oxford University Press.

DeArmond, S. J., Fusco, M. M., & Dewey, M. M. (1989). *Structure of the Human Brain: A Photographic Atlas* (3rd ed.). New York: Oxford University Press.

Filley, C. M. (2011). *Neurobehavioral Anatomy* (3rd ed.). Boulder, CO: University Press of Colorado.

Filley, C. M. (2012). *The Behavioral Neurology of White Matter* (2nd ed.). New York: Oxford University Press.

Geschwind, N. (1975). The borderland of neurology and psychiatry: Some common misconceptions. In D. Blumer & D. F. Benson (Eds.), *Psychiatric Aspects of Neurologic Disease* (Vol. 1, pp. 1–8). New York: Grune and Stratton.

Glubegovic, & Williams (1980). *The Human Brain, a Photographic Guide*. New York: Harper & Row, figure 5–24, page 147.

Hendelman, W. J., (2006). *Atlas of Functional Neuroanatomy* (2nd ed.). London: Routledge/Taylor & Francis Group, LLC.

Jensen-Smith, H., Gray, B., Muirhead, K., Ohlsson-Wilhelm, B., & Fritzsch, B. (2007). Long-distance three-color neuronal tracing in fixed tissue using NeuroVue dyes. *Immunol Invest*, *36*(5–6), 763–789.

Kandel, E. R., Schwartz, J. H., & Jessell, T. M. (Eds.). (2000). *Principles of Neural Science* (4th ed.). New York: McGraw-Hill.

LeDoux, J. (1996). *The Emotional Brain*. New York: Simon and Schuster.

Leichnetz, G. R. (2006). *Digital Neuroanatomy*. New York: John Wiley & Sons. doi: 10.1002/047004554X

Lim, C., & Alexander, M. P. (2009, December). *Neuropsychologia*, *47*(14), 3045–3058. doi: 10.1016/j.neuropsychologia.2009.08.002. Epub 2009, August 8. Stroke and episodic memory disorders.

MacLean, P. D. (1970). The triune brain, emotion and scientific bias. In F. O. Schmitt (Ed.), *The Neurosciences: Second Study Program* (pp. 336–349). New York: Rockefeller University Press.

Martin, J. H. (1966). *Neuroanatomy: Text and Atlas, 1996*. Stamford: Appleton & Lange.

Mesulam, M.-M. (2001). *Principles of Behavioral and Cognitive Neurology* (2nd ed.). New York: Oxford University Press.

Nolte, J. (2002). *The Human Brain: An Introduction to Its Functional Anatomy* (5th ed.). St. Louis: Mosby.

Nowinski, W. L., & Chua, B. C. (2013, January). Bridging neuroanatomy, neuroradiology and neurology: Three-dimensional interactive atlas of neurological disorders. *The Neuroradiology Journal*, *26*(3), 252–262.

Papez, J. W. (1937). A proposed mechanism of emotion. *Arch Neurol Psychiatry*, *38*, 725–743.

Paxinos, G. (Ed.). (1990). *The Human Nervous System* (3rd ed.). San Diego: Academic Press.

Pliszka, S. R. (2005). *Neuroscience for the Mental Health Clinician*. New York: Guilford Press.

Plum, F., & Posner, J. B. (1982). *The Diagnosis of Stupor and Coma* (3rd ed.). Philadelphia, PA: F. A. Davis.

Roberts, M., & Hanaway, J. (1970). *Atlas of the Human Brain in Section*. Philadelphia, PA: Lea & Febiger. Copyright © 2006 from Atlas of Functional Neuroanatomy (2nd ed.) by W. J. Hendelman.

Schmahmann, J. D., & Sherman, J. C. (1998). The cerebellar cognitive affective syndrome. *Brain*, *121*, 561–579.

Searle, J. R. (2000). Consciousness. *Annual Review of Neuroscience*, *23*, 557–578.

Springer, S. P., & Deutsch, G. (1989). *Left Brain, Right Brain* (3rd ed.). New York: W. H. Freeman.

Squire, L. R., & Zola, S. M. (1996). Structure and function of declarative and nondeclarative memory systems. *Proceedings of the National Academy of Sciences*, *93*, 13515–13522.

Staempfli, P., Rienmueller, A., Reischauer, C., Valavanis, A., Boesiger, P., & Kollias, S. (2007 October 26). Reconstruction of the human visual system based on DTI fiber tracking. *Journal of Magnetic Resonance Imaging*, *26*(4), 886–893.

Takahashi, E., Song, J. W., Folkerth, R. D., Grant, P. E., & Schmahmann, J. D. (2013, March). Detection of postmortem human cerebellar cortex and white matter pathways using high angular resolution diffusion tractography: A feasibility study. *Neuroimage*, *68*, 105–111. doi: 10.1016/j.neuroimage.2012.11.042. Epub 2012 December 11.

Appendix: Structural Neuroimaging Basics for Understanding Neuroanatomy

Viewing neuroanatomy from brain imaging typically involves either CT or MRI, with MRI clearly superior for anatomical detail. In the same subject, Figure 6.15 compares CT with various MR pulse sequences that have different sensitivities to tissue type. In the mid-1990s MR DTI came on the scene, with the discovery that aggregate white matter tracts could be identified and extracted from the image because healthy axonal membranes constrain the direction of water diffusion perpendicular with the orientation of the fiber tract. By assessing directionality of water diffusion, fiber tract projections may be inferred. As shown in Figure 6.16, the diffusion scan from which DTI is derived has a rather fuzzy appearance in native space, but the actual diffusion color maps are rich in information about the directionality of water diffusion where green reflects anterior-to-posterior projecting

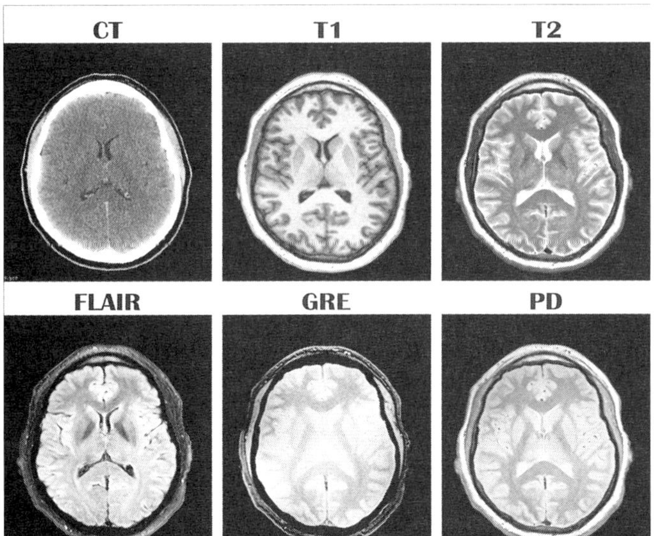

Figure 6.15 Comparison of CT imaging in the axial plane with other standard MRI pulse sequences all from the same indiviudal and all at approximately the same level and imaging plane. Note how each imaging sequence highlights differences in tissue type (see Table 6.3 for tissue characterization). FLAIR: fluid attenuated inversion recovery sequence. GRE: gradient recalled echo sequence. PD: proton density–weighted sequence.

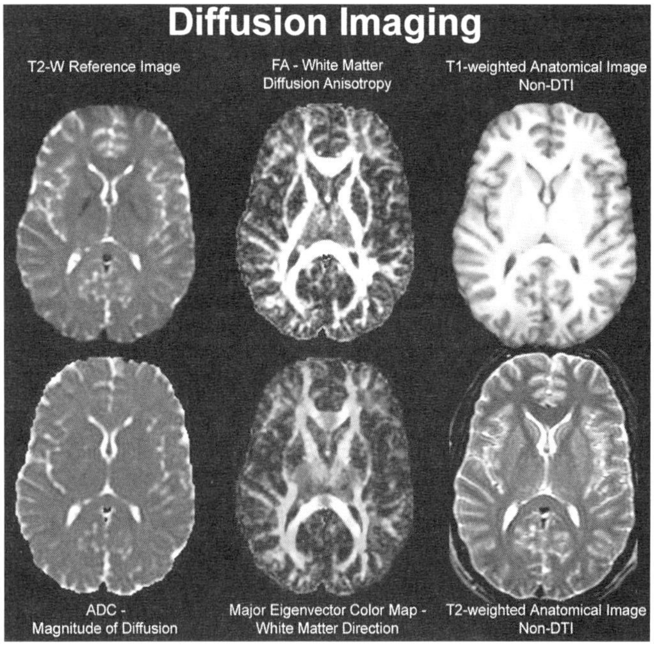

Figure 6.16 Diffusion imaging showing the diffusion scan in native space in the top center, compared to the T2- and T1-weighted images on either side, with the actual color map centered in the bottom row bordered by the apparent diffusion coefficient (ADC) map on the bottom left and the T2 weighted antomical image. *A color version of this figure can be found in Plate section 1.*

tracts, warm colors (orange to red) side-to-side projections, and cool colors (blues) vertically oriented tracts. Figures 6.6, 6.8b and 6.12a and b all present white matter fiber tracts derived from DTI.

Understanding neuroanatomy from neuroimaging is facilitated by the sensitivity of both CT and MRI in detecting differences in white matter and gray matter. Because specific white matter and gray matter boundaries may be distinctly differentiated with high-field MRI, the actual gray matter cortical ribbon and subcortical nuclei can be readily identified, as shown in Figure 6.17. Also, CSF has very different signal intensity from brain parenchyma, meaning it too can be segmented as shown in Figure 6.17. Segmenting tissue also provides the basis for identifying classic brain regions, like the hippocampus as presented in Figure 6.17. By defining

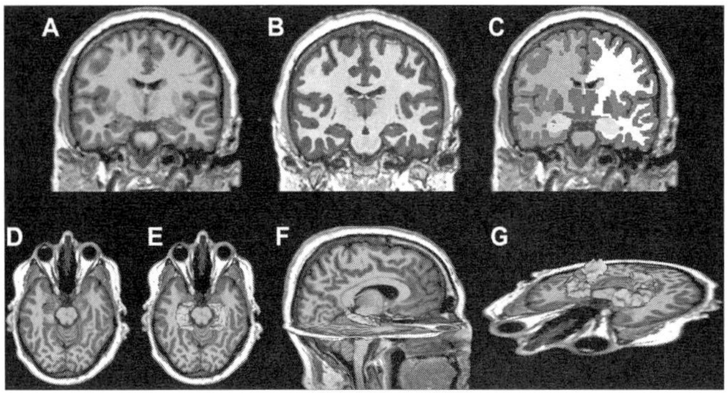

Figure 6.17 Standard T1-weighted coronal image that has been segmented to differentiate gray matter from white matter and CSF. The image is then classified into identifiable regions of interest or actual anatomical structures. *A color version of this figure can be found in Plate section 1.*

the boundaries of the hippocampus, that region of interest (ROI) may be extracted from the image and depicted in three-dimensional space, also demonstrated in Figure 6.17. Using similar techniques, any neuroanatomical ROI may be extracted from an image showing its anatomical position in relation to other structures as well as quantified in terms of volume, surface area, and shape, to name the most common quantitative measurements.

Figure 6.18 shows the same sagittal view of Figures 6.4c and 6.14 but this time with a vertical line showing the approximately level of a cut through the frontal and anterior temporal lobes (although at the mid sagittal level the anterior temporal lobe cannot be visualized in the mid-sagittal cut), with the resulting coronal image below (on the left). Adjacent to the coronal image from the MRI is a formalin-fixed coronal cut of a postmortem brain in approximately the same plane. Note the similarity of the MR image with that of the postmortem image, proof of the anatomical approximation of MRI findings to identify gross anatomy. From this image, the beautiful symmetry of the typical developed human brain also becomes apparent. Notice how the structures in one hemisphere mirror the other. This symmetry principle applies throughout the brain as depicted in a different coronal section more posterior to the position previously shown in Figure 6.19 or in the axial plane in Figure 6.20. Starting with

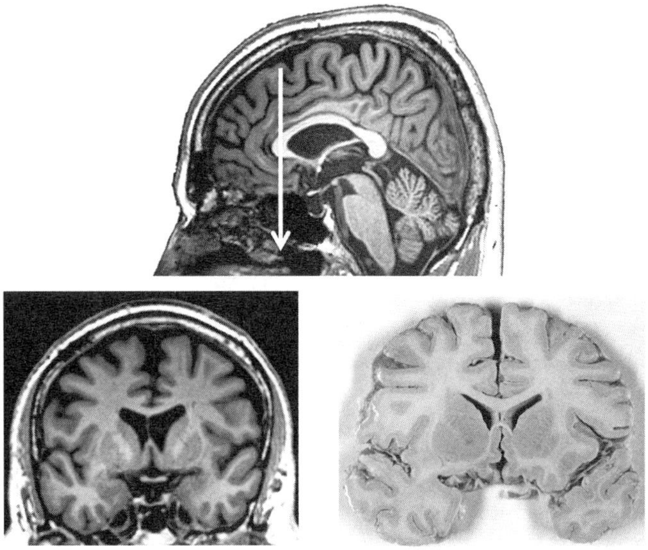

Figure 6.18 The mid-sagital view shown at the top of this figure is the same as in Figures 6.4c and 6.14, with the downward arrow showing the coronal plane where the approximate cut occurred to generate the image in the lower left panel. The lower right panel shows a similar location in a formalin-fixed postmortem brain sectioned at approximately the same level. Note the similarity of the postmortem section to the MRI-derived coronal image as well as the general symmetry of the brain.

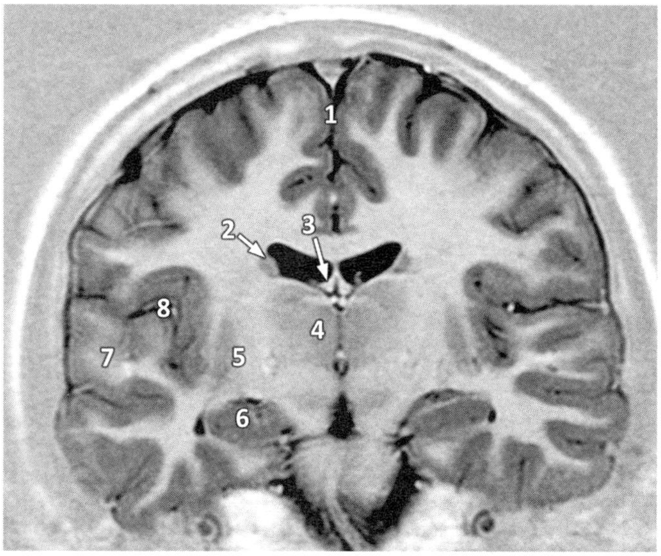

Figure 6.19 This is a coronal image using a true inversion recovery sequence that provides exquisite anatomical detail. Note how each hemisphere is the mirror of the other in terms of the distribution and organization of major brain areas and ROIs: (1) interhemispheric fissue; (2) the number sits in the central white matter of the frontal lobe, with the arrow pointing to the caudate (gray matter) and lateral ventricle (dark space); (3) the lower part of the number sits in the corpus callosum, with the top of the number in the cingulum bundle within the cingulate gyrus, and the arrow points to the body of the fornix; (4) thalamus; (5) the number sits in the lenticular nucleus, which is formed by the lighter (meaning more white matter) globus pallidus (to the right of the number) and the putamen (darker gray, to the left of the number); (6) hippocampus; (7) superior temporal gyrus of the temporal lobe, which forms the top of the temporal lobe, with in descending order followed by the middle temporal gyrus, inferior temporal gyrus, fusiform, and parahippocampal gyrus; (8) Sylvian fissure to the left of the number, frontal lobe above, temporal lobe below and to the right of the number, insular cortex.

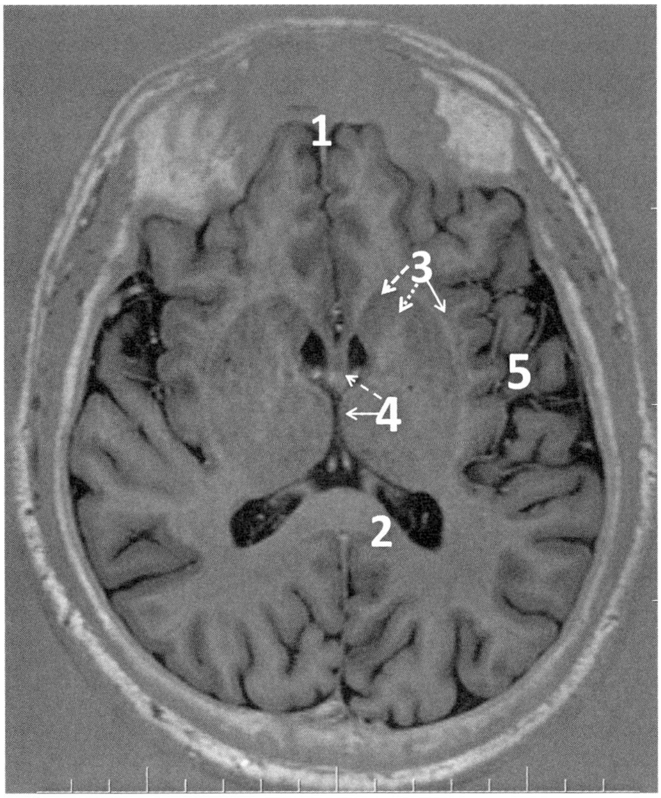

Figure 6.20 This is also a true inversion recovery sequence but in the axial plane, showing the same symmetry than can be visualized in the coronal plane: (1) interhemispheric fissure; (2) the number sits within the posterior corpus callosum, with the bottom of the number within the posterior cingulum bundle within the cingulate gyrus and the right top of the number adjacent to the posterior aspect (atria) of the lateral ventricle; (3) dashed arrow points to the caudate, dotted arrow points to the internal capsul and the straight arrow to the claustrum, where to the left of the claustrum the external capsule may be visualized and to the right, the extreme capsule; (4) the number is within the thalamus, with the left arrow pointing to the third ventricle and the dashed arrow to the column of the fornix; (5) the insular cortex within the Sylvian fissure.

the interhemispheric fissure (see label Number 1, in either the coronal image of Figure 6.19 or the axial image of Figure 6.20), essentially one hemisphere duplicates the other. So as to not clutter the image, labelling numbers are given only in one hemisphere in these two figures, but it is readily apparent that the brain structures numbered in one hemisphere appear nearly identical to that of the other hemisphere.

For normal anatomical appearance the above description represents the symmetry principle of a typical, healthy brain (Bigler 2015). Typical brain development is dynamic, so understanding normal brain anatomy also means understanding changes that may be relevant to the age of the individual being scanned. However, in the "normal" aging process, purely age effects will be registered within this normal symmetry, so that for a particular age ROIs appear symmetric across both hemispheres as reflected in Figures 6.18 to 6.20.

Combined with the principle of symmetry, also reflected throughout this chapter is the anatomical principle of normal "similarity" across healthy brains. In other words, in a very general sense, one brain appears similar to another. Returning to Figure 6.18, even though one image is based on an in vivo MRI section in a very much alive human adult and the other is postmortem, both are recognizable for their similar appearance at about the same point in the frontal and temporal regions of the brain in the coronal plane. Likewise the coronal image in Figure 6.17A is from a different pulse sequence than in Figure 6.19, yet there are obvious similarities. By applying the similarity and symmetry principles to understanding age-typical brain anatomy, in most cases a scan image may be straightforwardly identified as normal in appearance or not.

That last piece of a general overview to understand anatomy from imaging is understanding how the underlying physics of CT and MRI provide the basis for generating the resulting image. CT is based on x-ray beam technology where the physical density of tissue influences the speed of the x-ray beam as it passes through skin, the skull, and brain parenchyma. Reconstructing this information in two- or three-dimensional space provides an image as shown in the top left of Figure 6.15. By convention, on CT, bone is white, reflecting the greatest density encountered by the x-ray beam, whereas CSF and air pockets (as in a sinus area) provide the least density and are categorized as dark in a CT image. Because white matter is largely comprised of myelinated axons, it has a different density and water content compared to gray matter comprised of cell bodies. Accordingly, in viewing CT, white matter is darker gray, gray matter is lighter gray, CSF is dark gray to black, air is black, and bone bright white.

The MR signal is the result of a resonance interaction between hydrogen nuclei and externally applied magnetic fields spatially encoded to provide a mapping of the image area in two or three dimensions. The signal intensity depends on the density and the magnetic environment of the hydrogen nuclei (i.e., protons). Since white matter and gray matter differ in water content and have characteristically different MR signal properties, MR images of the brain with visible and distinguishable differences in gray and white matter may be shown as depicted in the various illustrations within this chapter, especially Figures 6.15 and 6.16. How distinct white and gray matter may be differentiated depends on the pulse sequence used, which will yield different findings as outlined in Table 6.3.

The use of innovative methods for varying the magnetic field strength, the delays between the sending and receiving of the radio waves, and the acquisition and display of the signal intensity allow a wide range of images to be produced.

Table 6.3 Neuroanatomy MRI appearance of commonly scanned tissues

Tissue	*T1-Weighted*	*T2-Weighted*	*Proton Density–Weighted*
Gray Matter	Gray	Light Gray	Light Gray
White Matter	White	Dark Gray	Gray
CSF or Water	Black	White	Dark Gray
Fat	White	Black	Black
Air	Black	Black	Black
Bone or Calcification	Black	Black	Black
Edema	Gray	White	White
Demyelination or Gliosis	Gray	White	White
Ferritin Deposits (e.g., in Basal Ganglia)	Dark Gray	Black	Black

Note: On fast spin echo (FSE) sequences (a faster variant of the SE sequence), fat appears bright in T2-weighted and proton density–weighted images.

For example, the behavior of the protons is characterized by two time constants, called Tl and T2. Tl reflects the rapidity with which protons become realigned with the magnetic field after a radio frequency (RF) pulse. Scans that are Tl-weighted tend to show greater detail but less contrast between structures; these images are therefore optimum for showing anatomy. T2 reflects the decay of in-phase precession (desynchronization or "dephasing") of protons after the pulse. Scans that are T2-weighted generally show normal structures as having an intermediate (gray) intensity, while fluid and many pathologic abnormalities appear with high intensity (white). These images provide excellent contrast between normal and abnormal structures and are, therefore, used for identifying both anatomy and pathology. Sequences that provide an average of Tl and T2 weighting are called *proton density sequences.* The appearance (brightness) on the various sequences can be used to characterize the tissue.

The true inversion recovery sequence shown in Figures 6.19 and 6.20 depicts the exquisite detail that can be achieved with MRI for portraying anatomy. For example, in Figure 6.19 the very thin band of gray matter that forms the claustrum may be visualized. Another sequence that uses subtle changes in magnetic field strength, called *gradient echo* (GRE), allows excellent image detail in short imaging times and has the added advantage of being sensitive to the presence of blood as well as blood breakdown products (hemosiderin) as a result of hemorrhage. A *susceptibility-weighted imaging* sequence (SWI) that uses a GRE pulse sequence is particularly sensitive in detecting venous blood as shown in Figure 6.21 and in pathological conditions, is sensitive in demonstrating presence of microhemorrhages. SWI impressively demonstrates the complex architecture of venous blood in a healthy individual as seen in Figure 6.21 (same as shown in Figures 6.18 and 20). The fluid attenuated inversion recovery (FLAIR) sequence is particularly sensitive to white matter pathology, but within a normal brain, as shown in Figure 6.15, signal in the parenchyma offers little distinction between white and gray matter.

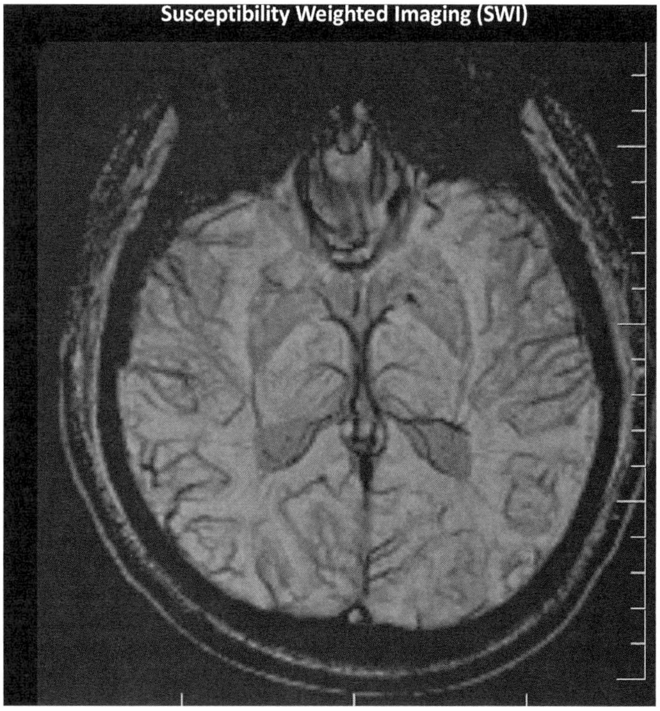

Figure 6.21 Susceptibility weighted image at a level just below what was shown in Figure 6.20, from the same individual, showing venous distribution to the thalamus, posterior lateral ventricle, and basal ganglia as well as cortical surface–draining veins.

7 The Central Nervous System and Cognitive Development

Kathryn C. Russell

Introduction

Anyone who has met a child knows that children's abilities change over time—sometimes faster than seems natural. They make great gains in the major skills of cognition, from the most basic kinds of perceptual and learning skills to memory, attention, executive functions, and language. These changes over time are the essence of development. With cognitive development specifically, it may be useful to consider brain structural changes along with function, though the interplay between these two is only beginning to be addressed in the literature. You might imagine that a change in brain structure can bring about or facilitate a change in cognitive ability; but alternatively improvements in cognition might incite brain changes. To complicate matters, other factors such as experience and motivation are likely to influence this relationship (see Bates, Thal, Finlay, & Clancy, 2003). Finally, the changes that the brain undergoes, at least as we understand them now, tend to develop on a longer time scale than cognitive changes. If the state of affairs is truly that complex, what is to be done? There are certain periods of time when things are happening to the structure of the brain and there are contemporaneous enhancements in cognition. At this point, what we can do is describe these, which will be the focus of this chapter. While we often talk about "development" as shorthand for child development, both the brain and one's cognitive abilities continue to develop over the course of one's lifetime, with periods of greater and lesser noticeable change. Our discussion will thus extend through adulthood. Finally, when neurotypical development is prevented, interrupted, or somehow altered, there are consequences to cognitive ability; an example will also be briefly reviewed here.

Prenatal Central Nervous System Development and Basic Principles

For a point of reference, the cortex of the brain is commonly divided into lobes, including the frontal, parietal, temporal, occipital, and limbic. They have a rough correspondence to functions, with somatosensory areas in the parietal lobe; visual processing falling largely under the occipital lobe's domain; auditory processing under the purview of the temporal lobe; and motor and many aspects of language, planning, behavioral control, etc., being subsumed by the frontal lobe. Some cognitive processes, such as language, often draw on resources from multiple lobes. Smaller subdivisions are made possible by a pattern of ridges and grooves known as *gyri* and *sulci*. On the whole, our brains are largely like those of other mammals—what seems to be unique is the expansion and resulting convolution of the cortex that humans exhibit, which leads to the pattern of gyri and sulci we see, and allows greater connectivity between regions (Nolte, 1999, p. 50). The cortex itself is a folded sheet with a thickness of only a few millimeters and is composed of six layers of cells. Regional differences between areas of cortex are a topic of great interest to researchers, and these regions can show differences in their developmental timelines. For instance, changes are still being made to the prefrontal cortex (PFC; part of the frontal lobe) well into adolescence and early adulthood. Cortical regions are often thought to have default specialties/typical representation patterns, but it is well-established that there are circumstances under which some area of cortex can take on a function it is not known for—for example, in congenitally blind participants, the visual cortex can assume some tactile and auditory processing. One recent example reported increased brain activity in an area of visual cortex known for higher-level processing of visual motion (V5/MT+) in response to pure auditory tone presentation in blind participants (Watkins et al., 2013).

Formation of the basic structures of the brain happens in the prenatal period; however, once these are formed, the brain undergoes more fine-grained tuning processes, and it is these that are likely correspondent with the changes we see in cognition during postnatal development. These processes include both additive and subtractive events (Elman et al., 1996). The former, on the one hand, add new structure on the small scale, such as the birth and proliferation of neurons, the migration of neurons to their final destinations, production or extension of both long-range connections (axonal) and local (dendritic) branching, and additive synaptic changes (Elman et al., 1996), as well as increased myelination of existing neurons. (In myelination, a fatty coating is introduced around axons that speeds message transmission.) Subtractive events, on the other hand, change neural organization by way of reduction or elimination of existing structures through cell death, axonal retraction, and synaptic pruning (Elman et al., 1996). These processes are also likely reflected in changes in brain metabolism over time. The general pattern that these processes follow is overproduction (of neurons, of synapses, etc.) followed by pruning, or selective reduction, with the former more rapid and the latter slower (Goldman-Rakic, 1987).

Additive processes: The birth of new neurons was originally thought to take place exclusively in the prenatal phase, though there is now evidence that there are exceptions to this limitation, including the olfactory bulb and the dentate gyrus of the hippocampus, in which new neurons have been found to be generated throughout the lifespan (see Lledo, Alonso, & Grubb, 2006, for a review). Most neurons, however, are generally thought to be born during the prenatal period and most are in place by the seventh month of gestation (Hoffelder & Hoffelder, 2007). Cell migration is the method by which neurons come to be "in place." Brain cells are generally born in special zones known as *proliferative zones.* They migrate to their new destinations either passively (having been pushed out by newly emerging neurons) or actively, in most areas along a scaffold of glial cells (Nicholls, Martin, Wallace, & Fuchs, 2001 includes a good description). The former state of affairs is more common and produces an organization in which the older cells are nearer to the surface of the brain. When young cells move actively past the older cells, the gradient is reversed (Nowakowski, 1987). Sprouting and growth of new connections (*synaptogenesis*) takes place after the migration has occurred. There is evidence that these processes occur throughout life, and they have been observed even in aging animals as a result of experience in brain areas that were otherwise undergoing degradation (Greenough, Black, & Wallace, 1987). While the previous two additive methods seem to be more predetermined, the formation of new branches is likely highly experience-dependent, and related to learning (Elman et al., 1996). It also has been suggested that it is necessary for there to be a critical mass of synapses before a behavior will emerge, with fully mature levels of the behavior then being dependent on elimination of excess synapses (Goldman-Rakic, 1987). In studies with monkeys, Goldman-Rakic determined that the timing and rate of increase of synapses seems to be similar between cortical areas; beginning before birth, and continuing to increase until a peak at around 2–4 months, after which time is a longer elimination period of excess synapses (see Goldman-Rakic, 1987, for a review). Interestingly, it is around the time of synaptogenic peak in the dorsolateral prefrontal cortex (DLPFC) where monkeys started to be able to perform tasks dependent on DLPFC functions at longer delays (Goldman-Rakic, 1987). In humans, cortical areas are not thought to reach peak cortical thickness at the same rate, with areas such as DLPFC reaching peak thickness later than, for example, primary sensory areas (Shaw et al., 2008). As will be seen throughout the rest of this chapter, the differential time course of these events has bearing on the course of cognitive development as well.

Subtractive processes: It may seem counterproductive that we should have neurons that were born only to die. While some cells that die have failed to make synapses or have innervated incorrect targets, it is thought that cell death is a way for the size of neuronal input to be matched to the size of the target (Nicholls et al., 2001). This feature is more easily illustrated in the motor realm: When looking at death in motor neurons innervating a limb, removal of the limb bud leads to more cell death than normal while adding a second limb bud yields less death (Hollyday & Hamburger, 1976). As compared to cell death, synaptic pruning is more of a refinement mechanism, and refers to a loss of some terminal branches and synapses through competition. It has been thought to play a role in helping functional organization and correcting mistakes, among other things (e.g., Nakamura & O'Leary, 1989). Activity can be involved in the rate and outcome of the competition that results in pruning (Nicholls et al., 2001), providing the possibility for learning to have influence on this process. Both axon degeneration as well as axon retraction help increase the precision of relationships between neuronal processions and target areas (see Luo & O'Leary, 2005, for a review).

Plasticity: Plasticity refers to changes that take place in the brain as a result of experience—it is part of the normal workings of the brain. It is not only called upon in response to some kind of insult, but also happens in response to learning. One commonly cited example involves reorganization of brain function in persons who are blind, such that cortex which generally contains visual representation can take on other functions (Kupers & Ptito, 2014), but can be as simple as the changes at a single synapse. The adult brain seems to be less plastic, which raises arguments about "sensitive" or "critical" periods during which some learning milestones must be reached if they are to be (fully) achieved. In humans, this argument often gets discussed in terms of language learning. There are a number of cases of children who were discovered late in life and who had not been exposed to typical language input (e.g., "Genie," Fromkin, Krashen, Curtiss, Rigler, & Rigler, 1974, and see Curtiss, 1989 for a review). These cases are not without controversy, but it is generally reported that if the children are discovered after puberty, their speech tends to lack common features. In the second-language-learning realm, learners who begin later seem to show more difficulty in achieving fluency, and show differential representation for the language in neuroimaging studies (see Newport, 2002 for a brief review). Other researchers believe these outcomes arise because experience has shaped both the brain and what it can learn, producing effects that look like sensitive periods (see Bates et al., 2003). Numerous examples have also shown us that the adult brain does, in fact, retain some plastic abilities. For instance, persons taught to juggle were shown to have brain changes postlearning on MRI that receded to baseline levels with subsequent loss of the skill (Draganski et al., 2004). Similar changes were also observed in elderly participants (Boyke, Driemeyer, Gaser, Büchel, & May, 2008). Overall, it seems that plasticity is an enduring feature of the brain, though there may be changes in the amount, location, or type of plasticity available over the life span.

Time Periods

With the basic mechanisms reviewed, we now turn to the time periods with what may be the clearest examples of structural and functional concurrent change. In the developmental literature, a range is almost always given. This convention reflects the fact that not every person develops at the same rate, but also that a lot of our understanding of central nervous system (CNS) development relies upon animal models from species with slightly different trajectories, but similar patterns of development. The time periods we will be considering, which should not be considered an exhaustive set of examples, include: at birth, 2–3 months, 8–12 months, 16–24 months, 4 years through adolescence, and adulthood and normal aging, as these are periods where known changes are taking place in the brain that may be relevant to cognition (Elman et al., 1996; though see Bates et al., 2003 for reexamination of this evidence).

Birth

Much of the general structure of the CNS is developed before birth, but many more studies of observed behavior have been done after birth, so this is the first time period to be discussed. By the time of birth, the neurons of the brain should have all been formed (save for the examples given on p. 92), and they should have finished migrating to their final positions. The brain as we know it is basically ready to learn, and although neonates have been described as experiencing the world as "a blooming, buzzing confusion" (James, 1890, p. 488), we now know that they actually come into the world with a set of tools to help them come to understand their surroundings, including basic reflexes and learning mechanisms. Predominant among those are reflexes that allow classical conditioning, the ability to learn by operant conditioning, and a preference for novelty. Imitation and statistical learning also play a role.

Examples of classical conditioning are easy to find in the newborn's life—any parent who has kept a strict feeding schedule can tell you that a baby can learn to anticipate the timing of that schedule. The ability of newborns to learn by way of operant conditioning has also been demonstrated: for instance, newborns will suck faster to hear auditory stimuli (Floccia, Christophe, & Bertoncini, 1997). Babies are further born with a preference for novelty that helps guide their attention. Habituation is the process of becoming used to something—in the baby's case, it means ceasing to prefer a given stimulus when it becomes familiar. When there is a change in the stimulus, it again becomes attractive, with this process being known as *dishabituation*. Together, these processes exert a rudimentary kind of control on the infant's attention without which it would be difficult for him or her to select a stimulus on which to focus. Researchers can use habituation and dishabituation to study basic perceptual, memory, and attentional processing in young babies. Newborns are also able to imitate observed behavior such as facial expressions like mouth opening and tongue protruding (see Meltzoff & Moore, 1983, for a review). Imitation, too, can be a powerful mechanism for learning. Statistical learning (the ability to extract and use patterns found in sensory input), was originally investigated in older babies as a method of learning how to segment a constant stream of speech (Saffran, Aslin, & Newport, 1996), but has recently been demonstrated in newborns in both language (Teinonen, Fellman, Näätänen, Alku, & Huotilainen, 2009) and visual (Bulf, Johnson, & Valenza, 2011) paradigms, suggesting this is a domain-general mechanism that is active from birth. Altogether, these findings would suggest that the newborn has a sophisticated bag of tricks for making sense of the environment, to the extent that his or her perceptual abilities are ready.

As far as perception is concerned, vision is the most discussed sense. It is quite poor at birth, as much as 20/600. Focus improves within the first couple of months, and acuity has progressed to 20/100 by 6–8 months (Courage & Adams, 1990). Newborns do show the ability to discriminate visual stimuli, as evidenced by habituation/dishabituation paradigms. As compared to vision, the sense of touch is more developed, and plays a role in many of the brain stem reflexes present at birth. Newborns can hear a variety of sounds, as discussed in more detail in the section on language at birth. What, then, about more common markers of "cognition" in the newborn? Glucose utilization as measured by positron emission tomography (PET) suggests the greatest functional activity is in primary sensory and motor cortex, as well as brain stem areas (Chugani, 1998). Cognitive activities, including memory, attention or executive functioning, and language tend to be heavily dependent upon these areas, and will now be considered in turn.

Memory: Most of us cannot recall instances from our very early life, thanks to a phenomenon known as *infantile amnesia,* which typically lasts until a child is between 3 to 5 years of age (Mullally & Maguire, 2014). The causes of this phenomenon are still under debate (see Rovee-Collier, 1999, for review). The use of the word "amnesia" does not mean that a newborn acts exactly as an adult with amnesia would, however; for instance by 3–4 days of age the newborn can recognize his or her mother's face (Bushnell, Sai, & Mullin, 1989), suggesting that some retention of information is taking place.

Attention and executive function: During the newborn period, there are but short periods of alertness during the day. Ruff and Rothbart (1996) describe this initial state of attention as being about orienting and investigating and driven by novelty. These periods are characterized by organized and selective looking—suggesting that rudimentary attention exists. Visual looking preferences have been noted for patterns with large features and high contrast (Fantz, 1963). Higher-level control is lacking, however, as newborns have been shown to have difficulty disengaging attention from a stimulus, even to the point of distress (see Ruff & Rothbart, 1996).

Language: It may be strange to talk about "language" in any real sense in the neonate, yet there are some communicative abilities and pre-language skills even at birth, such as the ability to imitate facial expressions. On the receptive side, newborns prefer "complex" sounds like noises and voices to pure tones (Bench, Collyer, Mentz, & Wilson, 1976), within a few days show sensitivity to word stress (Sansavini, Bertoncini, & Giovanelli, 1997), and by at least 1 month of age can make basic discriminations between speech sounds (categorical perception; Eimas, Siqueland, Jusczyk, & Vigorito, 1971). These abilities set the stage for language learning. Social abilities such as gazing at the face of a caregiver and making smiling-type motions, which tend to be reinforced by the caregiver early on, are also developing and will bolster language learning.

2–3 Months

During this time period, increases in glucose utilization in parietal, temporal, and primary visual areas are seen (Chugani, 1998), suggesting that these areas are increasingly functionally active. Experience-dependent changes are focused in these areas as well (Casey, Tottenham, Liston, & Durston, 2005), and synaptic density in visual and auditory cortices are nearing peak values (Huttenlocher & Dabholkar, 1997). The ratio of symmetric to asymmetric synapses increases, suggesting a move from predominantly excitatory to more balanced activation, and more synapses are also seen on dendritic spines, which is thought to allow more specificity of information transfer (see Bates et al. 2003). Long connective pathways are forming, and myelination is of course continuing. Again, in this time period there are changes in memory, attention and executive functioning, and language.

Memory: Memory abilities are increasing during this time, though there is debate about the nature of memory processing being used. One interesting method of examining memory has been used by Rovee-Collier (reviewed in Rovee-Collier, 1999). Infants had ribbons tied to their legs that moved an interesting mobile when they kicked. (A version wherein an infant manipulates a train can be used for older infants.) She found that 2-month-olds could remember the information for a day or two, and 3-month-olds for about a week (Rovee-Collier, 1999). Memory ability was found to increase over time, such that older babies could retain information about the task for longer periods of time. Interestingly, changing the training parameters or adding priming could make even younger babies show better performance (Rovee-Collier, 1999).

Attention and executive function: While executive functions are not evident at this time in development, there is reason to believe that attentional processes are developing. These gains in attention are bolstered by the infant's tendency to spend longer periods of time awake and looking around, as well as increases in visual ability and maturation of pathways associated with vision (Lewis, Maurer, & Brent, 1989). During this period, the infant selects a pattern for attention on design features, not just salience; objects are more readily followed visually; and there is a greater ability to disengage attention (see Ruff & Rothbart, 1996, for a review). All of these features suggest that attention is becoming somewhat more mature and under at least rudimentary control of the infant.

Language: While it is still early for language to emerge, it is clear that the foundations are being laid as during this time babbling can begin. Between 2 and 6 months vowel sounds are produced in cooing or play-type activities (Bates et al., 2003), suggesting development in both the intentional production of speech sounds as well as interest in communication.

8–12 Months

During this period of time, long-range connections between major regions of cortex are being established (Elman et al., 1996), and prefrontal and association cortexes are starting to see more of the experience-dependent changes than is the sensorimotor cortex (Casey et al., 2005). The distribution of metabolic activity between regions becomes more adult-like, with an increase in glucose utilization in frontal areas (Chugani, 1998). Synaptogenesis has been taking place since before birth, and cortical areas are beginning to reach high points, with peaks happening some time between now and 2 years of age, differing by location (Huttenlocher, 1979). Myelination of these connections is continuing. Along with these processes there is a corresponding significant jump in various cognitive abilities. At this point, important brain networks are coming online and there is a watershed in cognitive abilities associated with this time period. Examples can again be seen in the areas of memory, attention and executive function, and language.

Memory: One of the most touted enhancements in cognition during this time is in the area of memory, even though some forms of memory can be difficult to measure in prelinguistic children. There are many accounts of younger babies learning associations, and even using them flexibly, but around 9 months seems to be the time that babies begin to exhibit hippocampal-dependent memory processing (see Mullally & Maguire, 2014, for a review). This claim has evidence in that 9-month-olds who can complete a memory task show a different pattern of event-related potentials (ERPs) than do age-matched babies who cannot do the task

(Carver, Bauer, & Nelson, 2000). Interestingly, this pattern of results may represent a replacement of old, associative-heavy memory patterns, in that 12-month-old participants fail to perform on a memory task that younger babies can do and that relied upon an associative strategy (see Rovee-Collier & Giles, 2010). One focus of laboratory testing of memory in infants is how long events can be remembered. While 6-month-olds are rarely tested past 24 hours due to low success even at that time span, 9-month-olds show memory for testing events up to 1 month after presentation, and 10-month-olds for at least 3 months after presentation (Carver & Bauer, 2001).

Attention and executive function: Attention is another area of cognition that shows improvement around this time. In support of visual attention, acuity and binocular vision have been enhanced by this point (Aslin & Smith, 1988) and the infant is now able to manipulate objects. There is evidence that the posterior orienting network commonly believed to contribute to attentional processing is active by 6 months (e.g., Hood, 1993). Behavioral developments include longer durations of looking (e.g., at a toy during free play, see Ruff & Saltarelli, 1993), as well as an increase in shared attention (Bakeman & Adamson, 1984).

Working memory span also shows improvement during this period; Ross-Sheehy and colleagues (Ross-Sheehy, Oakes, & Luck, 2003) found that 10- and 13-month-olds showed signs of increased visual short-term memory spans as compared to 6.5-month-old infants. There is also an increase in the amount of delay after which an infant will still be able to succeed at the A$\bar{B}$ Object Permanence task (Diamond, 1985), where a learned response must be inhibited. Animal models of this task show that use of the PFC is necessary for success (see discussion in Goldman-Rakic, 1987). An increase in working memory is also beneficial for gains in language, as both comprehension and production require keeping sequences of information (perceived sounds and vocal gestures, respectively) in mind.

Language: As such, language and communicative abilities are growing in leaps and bounds during this time as well. At the beginning of this period, the infant goes from babbling nonselectively to preferring sounds in his or her native language. Work by Werker and Tees (1984) has shown that while 6-month-olds show categorical perception for speech sounds in their own native language as well as an unfamiliar one (Hindi and Salish for English learners), fewer babies can do this by 8 months, with the ability to perceive the nonnative contrast dropping out for most babies by 10–12 months. These results hold whether a longitudinal or a cross-sectional design is employed. Also around this time period, utterances may begin to have language-like intonation. The learning of first words often occurs during this time period as well (Bloom & Markson, 1998), with the comprehension of words surging beyond production abilities (Benedict, 1979).

16–24 Months

This period is characterized by change at the level of the synapse such that there is a fast acceleration in the number of synapses within regions of cortex as well as between them. (Elman et al., 1996). At this point, these changes tend to be in association cortex areas as well as PFC (Casey et al., 2005). Myelination is continuing, and around 18 months, the corpus callosum reaches about 50% of full myelination (Rodier, 1994). Synaptic density in frontal areas is nearing peak levels at this point (Huttenlocher & Dabholkar, 1997). During the latter part of this period, the PFC and the dentate gyrus (part of the hippocampus) gain functional maturity and begin to take over their functions in memory (Bauer, 2007). While most of these changes are not unique to this period, there is cognitive growth in the areas we have been considering throughout.

Memory: Along with the changes in the hippocampus and frontal lobes, there is an increase in the length of time that events can be remembered during this period, going from around 1 month in duration of recall at 9 months of age up to one year in duration at 20 months of age (Bauer, 2007). Diamond, Towle, and Boyer (1994; Experiment 2) tested 1- to 2.5-year-olds on a delayed nonmatch-to-sample task, where reaching for a new object (and ignoring a remembered one) is rewarded. They found a major improvement on this task by 21 months of age.

Attention and executive function: Attention during this time is characterized by longer periods of sustained attention (Ruff & Lawson, 1990) and fully developed joint (shared) attention capabilities (Morales et al., 2000), including now following glances and points by others, as well as attempting to direct the gaze of another person. Eighteen-month-olds have been described as having greater executive abilities than younger children (see Posner, Rothbart, Thomas-Thrapp, & Gerardi, 1998). Indeed, as additional frontal cortex tracts develop, control of attention becomes the major attentional gain during this time period. In Diamond et al.'s 1994 study using the delayed nonmatch-to-sample task, it seems to be not only improvements in memory that allow better performance at 21 months, but also a complex relationship between the delay and the kind of reward used. These latter factors are suggestive that attentional control may be part of what generates the improvement.

Language: At this point, children are "proficient" at word learning, and there is the beginning of a rapid acceleration in vocabulary acquisition (Bloom & Markson, 1998). While the set of first words learned tends to include few verbs, there is now an increase in verbs and adjectives (Bates et al., 2003). With this increased vocabulary and increased knowledge of predicates, grammar begins in the form of two-word combinations around 18–20 months (Bates et al., 2003). The exact syntactic status of these combinations continues to be under debate, but these utterances seem to follow patterns. Also related to language is the skill of categorization. While certain, largely perceptually based, categorization tasks can be completed before this time period, at around 18 months more active categorization becomes possible and seems to be related to vocabulary gains (Gopnik & Meltzoff, 1987). Overall, at this point language learning is beginning to rapidly increase.

4 Years Through Adolescence

While this is not a focused time period, there are long-developing processes that begin around 4 years of age and continue up to or through adolescence. Around this time there is a peak in the overall level of brain metabolism. Patterns of glucose metabolism have become qualitatively more adult-like, and overall rates of glucose utilization have been rising from birth until age 4. At this point they are twice the level of an adult (Chugani, 1998). They are maintained at this level between ages 4 and 10, and gradually decline to adult levels at around 16–18 years of age (Chugani, 1998). During this period, synaptic density is on the decline, starting with somatosensory areas and continuing with association areas and finally the PFC (Casey et al., 2005), a process that continues into adolescence. Experience-based growth in dendrites and synapses also continues throughout this period, as does myelination of the frontal lobes and connecting tracts. In one MRI study examining this myelination of tracts that connect to the frontal lobes, Paus et al. (1999) reported linear increases of left and right internal capsule and left arcuate fasciculus between ages 4 and 17. All of these processes contribute to the brain's efficiency in carrying out neural tasks. Processing time, as measured by various tasks, does decrease during this period (e.g., Kail, 1988). While we think of efficiency as purely a time- or energy-saving perk, there may also be cases where a certain amount of efficiency is necessary to perform a cognitive task. Neural efficiency also can help one to perform a task well, and given the coarse grain of most behavioral tasks, it may mean the difference between recording a success or a failure. Consequently, increases in cognitive abilities are seen during this time period even though there are not rapid changes in brain structure. This growth, however, is seen mainly in functions that rely on the brain areas undergoing the most tuning—i.e., attention and executive function, as well as the cognitive skills they support, like memory and language.

Memory: By age 4, recognition memory is often thought to be at adult-like levels (Brown & Campione, 1972; though see Sophian & Stigler, 1981), but there are improvements in other areas of episodic memory processing during middle childhood. While these gains partially rely upon the developments in the PFC and connecting white matter tracts (see Ghetti & Bunge, 2012, for a review), there are also other developments that are likely playing a role. During the period between age 4 and 25, the anterior hippocampus has been shown to lose mass while the posterior hippocampus gains mass (Gogtay et al., 2006). As the anterior hippocampus has been associated with more flexibly bound memory representations, which in turn are associated with better performance, it has been hypothesized that the pruning of this area leads to specialization (see Ghetti & Bunge, 2012). In one study examining whether participants were able to use an episodic representation of an item versus simple recognition, 8-year-olds showed activation patterns consistent with the latter, 14-year olds and adults preferred an activation pattern more consistent with the former, and 10–11-year-olds seemed to be in transition between these, supporting the authors' hypothesis of increased selectivity over this time period (Ghetti, DeMaster, Yonelinas, & Bunge, 2010). Memory increases during this period also come about due to use of beneficial strategy: for example, Yim, Dennis, & Sloutsky (2013) show that the use of one type of complex memory structure emerged between 4 and 7 years of age and developed further between age 7 and adulthood, and Shing & Lindenberger (2011) review studies suggesting that strategy instruction and practice could boost memory performance in children up to adult levels.

Attention and executive function: An improvement in attention around this time period has been noted in the literature, though the timing of the change is still under debate, and seems to be task dependent. Some place it between ages 5 and 7 (see Bartgis, Thomas, Lefler, & Hartung, 2008, for a review), though others have found improvements past the age of 7 as well (Klimkeit, Mattingley, Sheppard, Farrow, & Bradshaw, 2004). Still others place it earlier, or show multiple stages of improvement (see Ruff & Rothbart, 1996, for a review). These studies all indicate a "spurt" of development that does not correspond to anything sudden we know about brain development happening at this point, although attention would be expected to improve gradually over time with the previously discussed ongoing brain changes. There are a few reasons why this might be the case. For example, many of the studies addressing this issue include children of only a couple of ages, while any gradual change would require a continuum of ages to be included. The effect of strategy development can also not be factored out; during this period strategies for focusing attention could be learned, especially since many of these children are attending school.

Multiple studies (see Tsujimoto, 2008, for a brief review) have pinpointed 4 years of age as a time after which more adult-like processing in PFC-reliant cognition—such as inhibition, executive control, and working memory—begins to emerge. For example, between ages 3 and 4, children become able to better perform a card-sorting task that involves inhibition (Carlson, 2005). This finding does seem to be tempered by complexity, however: When another sorting dimension is added in the previous study, older children can no longer complete the task (Carlson, 2005), but when the dimensions are separated, they can succeed at the task 6 months earlier (Diamond, Carlson, & Beck, 2005). Similar findings are reported in working memory and shifting executive processing as well, both for the initial emergence of the ability, as well as the continued improvements that are often revealed through increasingly complex tasks (see Best & Miller, 2010, for a review). Short-term memory span, regardless of modality, shows linear increases throughout childhood and adolescence (Gathercole, 1999). Often, improvements in executive functions have been found even until early adulthood (Huizinga, Dolan, & van der Molen, 2006). These boosts in executive functions are also associated with differences in neuroimaging studies. In the original work on the topic, Casey and colleagues found that, while children and adults showed brain activation in the same areas using fMRI, children had larger volumes of activation in both working memory (Casey et al., 1995) and inhibition (Casey et al., 1997) tasks, again suggesting that the development of these skills is due to some tuning process or gains in efficiency. Further studies on the topic have found similar results (see Casey et al., 2005, for a review).

Overall, this literature is difficult to draw clear age-range conclusions from, due largely to difficulties in scaling a task to allow persons of a large range of ages to participate. What does seem fairly clear, however, is that during early childhood, the ability to use these processes emerges, and it shows improvement throughout childhood into adolescence, and in the cases of some tasks, up into adulthood—a trajectory that mirrors the changes taking place in the PFC.

Language: By 4 years of age, language is largely mature. Major syntactic features have been acquired (Bates et al., 2003; Bickerton, 1992). Communicative levels of vocabulary are in place, and improvements during this period seem more gradual. Vocabulary is still being acquired very rapidly, however—estimates place a 6-year-old's vocabulary at around 10,000 words and a high school graduate's at 60,000 (see Bloom & Markson, 1998). Grammatical development continues at least until the age of 9 (Bickerton, 1992) and some sentence constructions may not be fully ingrained until later. Discourse cohesion abilities are also continuing to develop.

Adulthood and Normal Aging

When talking about developmental issues, a touchstone period is needed to compare performance—this is typically adulthood. During this time people have achieved what are generally considered to be mature cognitive abilities. Behaviorally, there appears to be a steady state for many years. Brain-based changes are continuing, however, with the previously discussed pruning continuing to the third decade of life (Petanjek et al., 2011), and eventually these changes lead to noticeable decrements in various cognitive skills. Other brain modifications begin as soon as one's mid-20s (such as the decline in gray matter volumes as noted by Good et al., 2001). Eventually these changes include a loss of white matter, the extent of which varies between studies (see Peters, 2007, for discussion), but that does seem to affect certain areas differently. It has been suggested that areas that myelinate last are first to be affected (Peters, 2007), with particular losses noted in the frontal lobes and tracts that connect these to other brain areas (Hedden, 2007; Peters, 2007). There is further a reduction in microvascular plasticity in the aging brain that is often associated with changes in synaptic plasticity, though the relationship between these is still debated (see Sonntag, Eckman, Ingraham, & Riddle, 2007, for a review).

Cognitive changes are also noticed in the aging adult. Not surprisingly, these are most commonly seen in the areas of attention and various kinds of memory (Glisky, 2007), which are also the last to finish developing as frontal areas complete myelination. Working memory and episodic memory seem to be most affected while performance on semantic memory can be better than that of younger adults (Glisky, 2007). This time period is also characterized by much variability: Some older adults seem to retain complete control of cognition, while others noticeably suffer with everyday tasks. These patterns are also reflected in results from neuroimaging studies, where older adults often show a different pattern of brain activation to a task than do younger adults. For example, one study examining dual-tasking found older adults to activate areas not active in the younger adult group as a whole (Smith et al., 2001). Bilateral brain activation is also commonly seen wherein younger adults display unilateral activation. In one study examining verbal and spatial memory, younger adults show frontal activation in the left hemisphere for the former and the right for the latter, while older adults have bilateral activation for both types of stimuli (Reuter-Lorenz et al., 2000). Similar bilateral activation has been observed in posterior areas as well (Huang, Polk, Goh, & Park, 2012). In some studies (e.g., Huang et al., 2012; Rosen et al., 2002), persons in the group of older adults who show this kind of activation pattern have better performance than those who do not, perhaps pointing to a compensatory strategy.

Overall, this brief review suggests that the brain changes with aging are associated with cognitive declines, especially in memory and attention, but that there is variability within these, and that they may be ameliorated in some cases by the use of compensatory strategies.

Challenges to Development

The course of events described in the previous section can be understood as being fairly typical. While the exact timing of events can differ from person to person, the general course tends to be accurate for most people, most of the time. What happens, then, when there are cases that do not follow this timeline? There are numerous things that can affect development; both congenital and acquired events can alter the course, and the outcome of such events is dependent upon the period of development during which they occur. An exhaustive categorization of such events is unfortunately beyond the scope of this chapter, but a brief example may help illustrate this point.

Spina bifida occurs very early during prenatal development, and subsequently affects much of cognitive development to come. It comes about when a portion of the neural tube fails to close properly at the level of the spine (Juranek & Salman, 2010). In the most common type of spina bifida, brain development is subsequently affected: Studies have noted incomplete generation of the corpus callosum, and some other white matter tracts also appear less well-organized or complete (see Juranek & Salman, 2010, for a review). Although there are many physical sequelae associated with this condition, and they are sometimes thought of as comprising most of this disorder, cognitive complications are also quite common. Attention has been found to be affected from infancy (Dennis & Barnes, 2010), and skills like executive functioning do not seem to improve with age (Tarazi, Zabel, & Mahone, 2008). Deficits have been noted in areas such as timing, attention, movement, and perception (reviewed by Dennis & Barnes, 2010), and there is a high incidence of learning disabilities in this population, with one study reporting that 60% of their sample showed reading, math, or writing issues (Mayes & Calhoun, 2006). Without doubt, the early timing of the original insult plays a significant role in the widespread effects on cognition.

Discussion

In this chapter, contemporaneous gains in cognitive functioning and changes in brain structure have been described. While it may seem as if brain structure and cognitive functions are the only things influencing each other, it should be reiterated that this is not the complete picture. Let us consider the role of experience. During the 8–12 month cognitive watershed period, there are often motoric leaps as well. This period is exactly when crawling tends to either emerge or become a highly practiced skill. With the ability to move around, babies gain new perceptual perspectives, and these perspectives undoubtedly influence the brain structure/function relationship. Take for example a study by Bell and Fox (1996) that examined the influence of crawling on intrahemispheric EEG coherence in 8-month-olds. They found that novice crawlers (1–4 weeks experience) had greater coherence than either prelocomotor infants or more experienced crawlers, a pattern they interpreted as showing that the onset of crawling was associated with changes in cortical organization (Bell & Fox, 1996). In the work by Rovee-Collier (1999) discussed on p. 94, memory in 2–6-month-old infants was effectively cued only by the original mobile they experienced, while 9–12-month-old infants could be cued by a novel item for shorter delays, suggesting that context is more flexible in the older infants who have some mobility and more experience with different contexts.

Another caveat to note is that, although the examples given in this chapter tended to relate changes in brain structure to *gains* in cognitive functioning, this is not always the case. In some cases, a change in brain structure can disrupt previous improvements in functioning. For example, babies become faster to dishabituate to previously viewed stimuli up until 2 months or so, when there is growth in visual processing and dishabituation slows down dramatically (Hood et al., 1996). A similar disruption is seen in the strength of handedness preference during intense periods of language (Ramsay, 1985) and locomotor (Corbetta, Williams, & Snapp-Childs, 2006) learning. In these cases, gains are still being made in other areas, however.

Finally, learning and cognitive change is not static during the time periods that were not discussed here. While some highlights were chosen, it should not be believed that these are the only periods of interesting development. There are also smaller spurts and plateaus within some of the larger time periods. On the whole, there are many problems with the granularity of our knowledge of both brain changes as well as cognitive abilities. While a fascinating and worthwhile topic, the relationship between brain development and cognitive development is still only beginning to be investigated, and the variables are numerous—the interplay between them is likely to keep researchers busy for many decades to come.

References

Aslin, R. N., & Smith, L. B. (1988). Perceptual development. *Annual Reviews of Psychology*, *39*, 435–473. doi: 10.1146/annurev.psych.39.1.435

Bakeman, R., & Adamson, L. B. (1984). Coordinating attention to people and objects in mother-infant and peer-infant interaction. *Child Development*, *55*, 1278–1289. doi: 10.2307/1129997

Bartgis, J., Thomas, D. G., Lefler, E. K., & Hartung, C. M. (2008). The development of attention and response inhibition in early childhood. *Infant and Child Development*, *17*, 491–502. doi: 10.1002/icd.563

Bates, E., Thal, D., Finlay, B. L., & Clancy, B. (2003). Early language development and its neural correlates. In F. Boller & J. Grafman (Series Eds.) & S. J. Segalowitz & I. Rapin (Vol. Eds.), *Handbook of Neuropsychology, Vol. 8, Part II: Child Neuropsychology* (2nd ed., pp. 525–592). Amsterdam: Elsevier Science B. V.

Bauer, P. J. (2007). Recall in infancy: A neurodevelopmental account. *Current Directions in Psychological Science*, *16*, 142–146. doi: 10.1111/j.1467-8721.2007.00492.x

Bell, M. A., & Fox, N. A. (1996). Crawling experience is related to changes in cortical organization during infancy: Evidence from EEG coherence. *Developmental Psychobiology*, *29*, 551–561. doi: 10.1002/(SICI)1098-2302(199611)29:7<551::AID-DEV1>3.0.CO;2-T

Bench, J., Collyer, Y., Mentz, L., & Wilson, I. (1976). Studies in infant behavioral audiometry: I. Neonates. *International Journal of Audiology*, *15*, 85–105. doi: 10.3109/00206097609071766

Benedict, H. (1979). Early lexical development: Comprehension and production. *Journal of Child Language*, *6*, 183–200. doi: 10.1017/s0305000900002245

Best, J. R., & Miller, P. H. (2010). A developmental perspective on executive function. *Child Development*, *81*, 1641–1660. doi: 10.1111/j.1467-8624.2010.01499.x

Bickerton, D. (1992). The pace of syntactic acquisition. In L. A. Sutton, C. Johnson, & R. Shields (Eds.), *Proceedings of the 17th Annual Meeting of the Berkeley Linguistics Society: General*

Session and Parasession on the Grammar of Event Structure (pp. 41–52). Berkeley, CA: Berkeley Linguistics Society

Bloom, P., & Markson, L. (1998). Capacities underlying word learning. *Trends in Cognitive Sciences*, *2*, 67–73. doi: 10.1016/s1364-6613(98)01121-8

Boyke, J., Driemeyer, J., Gaser, C., Büchel, C., & May, A. (2008). Training-induced brain structure changes in the elderly. *The Journal of Neuroscience*, *28*, 7031–7035. doi: 10.1523/jneurosci.0742-08.2008

Brown, A. L., & Campione, J. C. (1972). Recognition memory for perceptually similar pictures in preschool children. *Journal of Experimental Psychology*, *95*, 55–62. doi: 10.1037/h0033276

Bulf, H., Johnson, S. P., & Valenza, E. (2011). Visual statistical learning in the newborn infant. *Cognition*, *121*, 127–132. doi: 10.1016/j.cognition.2011.06.010

Bushnell, I.W.R., Sai, F., & Mullin, J. T. (1989). Neonatal recognition of the mother's face. *British Journal of Developmental Psychology*, *7*, 3–15. doi: 10.1111/j.2044-835X.1989.tb00784.x

Carlson, S. M. (2005). Developmentally sensitive measures of executive function in preschool children. *Developmental Neuropsychology*, *28*, 595–616. doi: 10.1207/s15326942dn2802_3

Carver, L. J., & Bauer, P. J. (2001). The dawning of a past: The emergence of long-term explicit memory in infancy. *Journal of Experimental Psychology: General*, *130*, 726–745. doi: 10.1037/0096-3445.130.4.726

Carver, L. J., Bauer, P. J., & Nelson, C. A. (2000). Associations between infant brain activity and recall memory. *Developmental Science*, *3*, 234–246. doi: 10.1111/1467-7687.00116

Casey, B. J., Cohen, J. D., Jezzard, P., Turner, R., Noll, D. C., Trainor, R. J., . . . Rapoport, J. L. (1995). Activation of prefrontal cortex in children during a nonspatial working memory task with functional MRI. *Neuroimage*, *2*, 221–229. doi: 10.1006/nimg.1995.1029

Casey, B. J., Tottenham, N., Liston, C., & Durston, S. (2005). Imaging the developing brain: What have we learned about cognitive development? *Trends in Cognitive Sciences*, *9*, 104–110. doi: 10.1016/j.tics.2005.01.011

Casey, B. J., Trainor, R. J., Orendi, J. L., Schubert, A. B., Nystrom, L. E., Giedd, J. N., . . . Rapoport, J. L. (1997). A developmental functional MRI study of prefrontal activation during performance of a go-no-go task. *Journal of Cognitive Neuroscience*, *9*, 835–847. doi: 10.1162/jocn.1997.9.6.835

Chugani, H. T. (1998). A critical period of brain development: Studies of cerebral glucose utilization with PET. *Preventative Medicine*, *27*, 184–188. doi: 10.1006/pmed.1998.0274

Corbetta, D., Williams, J., & Snapp-Childs, W. (2006). Plasticity in development of handedness: Evidence from normal development and early asymmetric brain injury. *Developmental Psychobiology*, *48*, 460–471. doi: 10.1002/dev.20164

Courage, M. L., & Adams, R. J. (1990). Visual acuity assessment from birth to three years using the acuity card procedure: Cross-sectional and longitudinal samples. *Optometry and Vision Science*, *67*, 713–718. doi: 10.1097/00006324-199009000-00011

Curtiss, S. (1989). The independence and task-specificity of language. In A. Bornstein & J. Bruner (Eds.), *Interaction in Human Development* (pp. 105–138). Hillsdale, NJ: Erlbaum

Dennis, M., & Barnes, M. A. (2010). The cognitive phenotype of spina bifida meningomyelocele. *Developmental Disabilities Research Reviews*, *16*, 31–39. doi: 10.1002/ddrr.89

Diamond, A. (1985). Development of the ability to use recall to guide action, as indicated by infants' performance on A$\bar{B}$. *Child Development*, *56*, 868–883

Diamond, A., Carlson, S. M., & Beck, D. M. (2005). Preschool children's performance in task switching on the dimensional change card sort task: Separating the dimensions aids the ability to switch. *Developmental Neuropsychology*, *28*, 689–729. doi: 10.1207/s15326942dn2802_7

Diamond, A., Towle, C., & Boyer, K. (1994). Young children's performance on a task sensitive to the memory functions of the medial temporal lobe in adults—the delayed nonmatching-to-sample task—reveals problems that are due to non-memory-related task demands. *Behavioral Neuroscience*, *108*, 659–680. doi: 10.1037//0735-7044.108.4.659

Draganski, B., Gaser, C., Busch, V., Schuierer, G., Bogdahn, U., & May, A. (2004). Neuroplasticity: Changes in grey matter induced by training. *Nature*, *427*, 311–312. doi: 10.1038/427311a

Eimas, P. D., Siqueland, E. R., Jusczyk, P., & Vigorito, J. (1971). Speech perception in infants. *Science*, *171*, 303–306. doi: 10.1126/science.171.3968.303

Elman, J. L., Bates, E. A., Johnson, M. H., Karmiloff-Smith, A., Parisi, D., & Plunkett, K. (1996). Brain development. In *Rethinking Innateness: A Connectionist Perspective on Development* (pp. 239–317). Cambridge, MA: The MIT Press. doi: 10.1017/s0272263198333070

Fantz, R. L. (1963). Pattern vision in newborn infants. *Science*, *140*, 296–297. doi: 10.1126/science.140.3564.296

Floccia, C., Christophe, A., & Bertoncini, J. (1997). High amplitude sucking and newborns: The quest for underlying mechanisms. *Journal of Experimental Child Psychology*, *64*, 175–198. doi: 10.1006/jecp.1996.2349

Fromkin, V., Krashen, S., Curtiss, S., Rigler, D., & Rigler, M. (1974). The development of language in Genie: A case of language acquisition beyond the "critical period." *Brain and Language*, *1*, 81–107. doi: 10.1016/0093-934x(74)90027-3

Gathercole, S. E. (1999). Cognitive approaches to the development of short-term memory. *Trends in Cognitive Sciences*, *3*, 410–418. doi: 10.1016/s1364-6613(99)01388-1

Ghetti, S., & Bunge, S. A. (2012). Neural changes underlying the development of episodic memory during middle childhood. *Developmental Cognitive Neuroscience*, *2*, 381–395. doi: 10.1016/j.dcn.2012.05.002

Ghetti, S., DeMaster, D. M., Yonelinas, A. P., & Bunge, S. A. (2010). Developmental differences in medial temporal lobe function during memory encoding. *Journal of Neuroscience*, *30*, 9548–9556. doi: 10.1523/jneurosci.3500-09.2010

Glisky, E. L. (2007). Changes in cognitive function in human aging. In D. R. Riddle (Ed.), *Brain Aging: Models, Methods, and Mechanisms* (pp. 3–20). Boca Raton, FL: CRC Press. doi: 10.1201/9781420005523.sec1

Gogtay, N., Nugent, T. F., III, Herman, D. H., Ordonez, A., Greenstein, D., Hayashi, K. M., & Thompson, P. M. (2006). Dynamic mapping of normal human hippocampal development. *Hippocampus*, *16*, 664–672. doi: 10.1002/hipo.20193

Goldman-Rakic, P. S. (1987). Development of cortical circuitry and cognitive function. *Child Development*, *58*, 601–622. doi: 10.1111/j.1467-8624.1987.tb01404.x

Good, C. D., Johnsrude, I. S., Ashburner, J., Henson, R.N.A., Friston, K. J., & Frackowiak, R.S.J. (2001). A voxel-based morphometric study of ageing in 465 normal adult human brains. *NeuroImage*, *14*, 21–36. doi: 10.1006/nimg.2001.0786

Gopnik, A., & Meltzoff, A. (1987). The development of categorization in the second year and its relation to other cognitive and linguistic developments. *Child Development*, *58*, 1523–1531. doi: 10.1111/j.1467-8624.1987.tb03863.x

Greenough, W. T., Black, J. E., & Wallace, C. S. (1987). Experience and brain development. *Child Development*, *58*, 539–559. doi: 10.1111/j.1467-8624.1987.tb01400.x

Hedden, T. (2007). Imaging cognition in the aging human brain. In D. R. Riddle (Ed.), *Brain Aging: Models, Methods, and Mechanisms* (pp. 251–278). Boca Raton, FL: CRC Press. doi: 10.1201/9781420005523.ch11

Hoffelder, A. M., & Hoffelder, R. L. (2007). *How the Brain Grows*. New York: Infobase Publishing

Hollyday, M., & Hamburger, V. (1976). Reduction of the naturally occurring motor neuron loss by enlargement of the periphery. *The Journal of Comparative Neurology*, *170*, 311–320. doi: 10.1002/cne.901700304

Hood, B. M. (1993). Inhibition of return produced by covert shifts of visual attention in 6-month-old infants. *Infant Behavior and Development*, *16*, 245–254. doi: 10.1016/0163-6383(93)80020-9

Hood, B. M., Murray, L., King, F., Hooper, R., Atkinson, J., & Braddick, O. (1996). Habituation changes in early infancy: Longitudinal measures from birth to 6 months. *Journal of Reproductive & Infant Psychology*, *14*, 177–185. doi: 10.1080/02646839608404515

Huang, C.-M., Polk, T. A., Goh, J. O., & Park, D. C. (2012). Both left and right posterior parietal activations contribute to compensatory processes in normal aging. *Neuropsychologia*, *50*, 55–66. doi: 10.1016/j.neuropsychologia.2011.10.022

Huizinga, M., Dolan, C. V., & van der Molen, M. W. (2006). Age-related change in executive function: Developmental trends and a latent variable analysis. *Neuropsychologia*, *44*, 2017–2036. doi: 10.1016/j.neuropsychologia.2006.01.010

Huttenlocher, P. R. (1979). Synaptic density in human frontal cortex: Developmental changes and effects of aging. *Brain Research*, *163*, 195–205. doi: 10.1016/0006-8993(79)90349-4

Huttenlocher, P. R., & Dabholkar, A. S. (1997). Regional differences in synaptogensis in human cerebral cortex. *The Journal of Comparative Neurology*, *387*, 167–178. doi: 10.1002/(SICI)1096-9861(19971020)387:2<167::AID-CNE1>3.0.CO;2-Z

James, W. (1890). *The Principles of Psychology* (Vol. 1). New York: Henry Holt & Company

Juranek, J., & Salman, M. S. (2010). Anomalous development of brain structure and function in spina bifida myelomeningocele. *Developmental Disabilities Research Reviews*, *16*, 23–30. doi: 10.1002/ddrr.88

Kail, R. (1988). Developmental functions for speeds of cognitive processes. *Journal of Experimental Child Psychology*, *45*, 339–364. doi: 10.1016/0022-0965(88)90036-7

Klimkeit, E. I., Mattingley, J. B., Sheppard, D. M., Farrow, M., & Bradshaw, J. L. (2004). Examining the development of attention and executive functions in children with a novel paradigm. *Child Neuropsychology*, *10*, 201–211. doi: 10.1080/09297040409609811

Kupers, R., & Ptito, M. (2014). Compensatory plasticity and cross-modal reorganization following early visual deprivation. *Neuroscience and Biobehavioral Reviews*, *41*, 36–52. doi: 10.1016/j.neubiorev.2013.08.001

Lewis, T. L., Maurer, D., & Brent, H. P. (1989). Optokinetic nystagmus in normal and visually deprived children: Implications for cortical development. *Canadian Journal of Psychology*, *43*, 121–140. doi: 10.1037/h0084225

Lledo, P.-M., Alonso, M., & Grubb, M. S. (2006). Adult neurogenesis and functional plasticity in neuronal circuits. *Nature Reviews Neuroscience*, *7*, 179–193. doi: 10.1038/nrn1867

Luo, L., & O'Leary, D.D.M. (2005). Axon retraction and degeneration in development and disease. *Annual Review of Neuroscience*, *28*, 127–156. doi: 10.1146/annurev.neuro.28.061604.135632

Mayes, S. D., & Calhoun, S. L. (2006). Frequency of reading, math, and writing disabilities in children with clinical disorders. *Learning and Individual Differences*, *16*, 145–157. doi: 10.1016/j.lindif.2005.07.004

Meltzoff, A. N., & Moore, M. K. (1983). Newborn infants imitate adult facial gestures. *Child Development*, *54*, 702–709. doi: 10.2307/1130058

Morales, M., Mundy, P., Delgado, C.E.F., Yale, M., Messinger, D., Neal, R., & Schwartz, H. K. (2000). Responding to joint attention across the 6- through 24-month age period and early language acquisition. *Journal of Applied Developmental Psychology*, *21*, 283–298. doi: 10.1016/s0193-3973(99)00040-4

Mullally, S. L., & Maguire, E. A. (2014). Learning to remember: The early ontogeny of episodic memory. *Developmental Cognitive Neuroscience*, *9*, 12–29. doi: 10.1016/j.dcn.2013.12.006

Nakamura, H., & O'Leary, D.D.M. (1989). Inaccuracies in initial growth and arborization of chick retinotectal axons followed by course corrections and axon remodeling to develop topographic order. *The Journal of Neuroscience*, *9*, 3776–3795

Newport, E. L. (2002). Critical periods in language development. In L. Nadel (Ed.), *Encyclopedia of Cognitive Science* (pp. 737–740). London: Macmillan Publishers Limited./Nature Publishing Group

Nicholls, J. G., Martin, A. R., Wallace, B. G., & Fuchs, P. A. (2001). *From Neuron to Brain* (4th ed.). Sunderland, MA: Sinauer Associates, Inc.

Nolte, J. (1999). *The Human Brain: An Introduction to its Functional Anatomy* (4th ed.). St. Louis, MO: Mosby-Year Book, Inc.

Nowakowski, R. S. (1987). Basic concepts of CNS development. *Child Development*, *58*, 568–595. doi: 10.2307/1130199

Paus, T., Zijdenbos, A., Worsley, K., Collins, D. L., Blumenthal, J., Giedd, J. N., . . . Evans, A. C. (1999). Structural maturation of neural pathways in children and adolescents: In vivo study. *Science*, *283*, 1908–1911. doi: 10.1126/science.283.5409.1908

Petanjek, Z., Judaš, M., Šimić, G., Rašin, M. R., Uylings, H.B.M., Rakic, P., & Kostović, I. (2011). Extraordinary neoteny of synaptic spines in the human prefrontal cortex. *Proceedings of the National Academy of Sciences*, *108*, 13281–13286. doi: 10.1073/pnas.1105108108

Peters, A. (2007). The effects of normal aging on nerve fibers and neuroglia in the central nervous system. In D. R. Riddle (Ed.), *Brain Aging: Models, Methods, and Mechanisms* (pp. 97–126). Boca Raton, FL: CRC Press. doi: 10.1201/9781420005523.ch5

Posner, M. I., Rothbart, M. K., Thomas-Thrapp, L., & Gerardi, G. (1998). The development of orienting to locations and objects. In R. D. Wright (Ed.), *Visual Attention: Vancouver Studies in Cognitive Science* (Vol. 8, pp. 269–288). New York: Oxford University Press. doi: 10.1037/1196-1961.48.2.301

Ramsay, D. S. (1985). Fluctuations in unimanual hand preference in infants following the onset of duplicated syllable babbling. *Developmental Psychology*, *21*, 318–324. doi: 10.1037/0012-1649.21.2.318

Reuter-Lorenz, P. A., Jonides, J., Smith, E. E., Hartley, A., Miller, A., Marshuetz, C., & Koeppe, R. A. (2000). Age differences in the frontal lateralization of verbal and spatial working memory revealed by PET. *Journal of Cognitive Neuroscience*, *12*, 174–187. doi: 10.1162/089892900561814

Rodier, P. M. (1994). Vulnerable periods and processes during central nervous system development. *Environmental Health Perspectives*, *102*, 121–124. doi: 10.1289/ehp.94102121

Rosen, A. C., Prull, M. W., O'Hara, R., Race, E. A., Desmond, J. E., Glover, G. H., . . . Gabrieli, J.D.E. (2002). Variable effects of aging on frontal lobe contributions to memory. *NeuroReport*, *13*, 2425–2428. doi: 10.1097/00001756-200212200-00010

Ross-Sheehy, S., Oakes, L. M., & Luck, S. J. (2003). The development of visual short-term memory capacity in infants. *Child Development*, *74*, 1807–1822. doi: 10.1046/j.1467-8624.2003.00639.x

Rovee-Collier, C. (1999). The development of infant memory. *Current Directions in Psychological Science*, *8*, 80–85. doi: 10.1111/1467-8721.00019

Rovee-Collier, C., & Giles, A. (2010). Why a neuromaturational model of memory fails: Exuberant learning in early infancy. *Behavioural Processes*, *83*, 197–206. doi: 10.1016/j.beproc.2009.11.013

Ruff, H. A., & Lawson, K. R. (1990). Development of sustained, focused attention in young children during free play. *Developmental Psychology*, *26*, 85–93. doi: 10.1037/0012-1649.26.1.85

Ruff, H. A., & Rothbart, M. K. (1996). *Attention in Early Development: Themes and Variations*. New York: Oxford University Press. doi: 10.1017/s0021963097211327

Ruff, H. A., & Saltarelli, L. M. (1993). Exploratory play with objects: Basic cognitive processes and individual differences. *New Directions for Child and Adolescent Development*, *59*, 5–16. doi: 10.1002/cd.23219935903

Saffran, J. R., Aslin, R. N., & Newport, E. L. (1996). Statistical learning by 8-month-old infants. *Science*, *274*, 1926–1928. doi: 10.1126/science.274.5294.1926

Sansavini, A., Bertoncini, J., & Giovanelli, G. (1997). Newborns discriminate the rhythm of multisyllabic stressed words. *Developmental Psychology*, *1*, 3–11. doi: 10.1037/0012-1649.33.1.3

Shaw, P., Kabani, N. J., Lerch, J. P., Eckstrand, K., Lenroot, R., Gogtay, N., . . . Wise, S. P. (2008). Neurodevelopmental trajectories of the human cerebral cortex. *The Journal of Neuroscience*, *28*, 3586–3594. doi: 10.1523/jneurosci.5309-07.2008

Shing, Y. L., & Lindenberger, U. (2011). The development of episodic memory: Lifespan lessons. *Child Development Perspectives*, *5*, 148–155. doi: 10.1111/j.1750-8606.2011.00170.x

Smith, E. E., Geva, A., Jonides, J., Miller, A., Reuter-Lorenz, P., & Koeppe, R. A. (2001). The neural basis of task-switching in working memory: Effects of performance and aging. *Proceedings of the National Academy of Sciences of the United States of America*, *98*, 2095–2100. doi: 10.1073/pnas.98.4.2095

Sonntag, W. E., Eckman, D. M., Ingraham, J., & Riddle, D. R. (2007). Regulation of cerebrovascular aging. In D. R. Riddle (Ed.), *Brain Aging: Models, Methods, and Mechanisms* (pp. 279–304). Boca Raton, FL: CRC Press

Sophian, C., & Stigler, J. W. (1981). Does recognition memory improve with age? *Journal of Experimental Child Psychology*, *32*, 343–353. doi: 10.1016/0022-0965(81)90085-0

Tarazi, R. A., Zabel, T. A., & Mahone, E. M. (2008). Age-related differences in executive function among children with Spina Bifida/Hydrocephalus based on parent report. *The Clinical Neuropsychologist*, *22*, 585–602. doi: 10.1080/13854040701425940

Teinonen, T., Fellman, V., Näätänen, R., Alku, P., & Huotilainen, M. (2009). Statistical learning in neonates revealed by event-related brain potentials. *BMC Neuroscience*, *10*, 21–28. doi: 10.1186/1471-2202-10-21

Tsujimoto, S. (2008). The prefrontal cortex: Functional neural development during early childhood. *Neuroscientist*, *14*, 345–358. doi: 10.1177/1073858408316002

Watkins, K. E., Shakespeare, T. J., O'Donoghue, M. C., Alexander, I., Ragge, N., Cowey, A., & Bridge, H. (2013). Early auditory processing in area V5/MT+ of the congenitally blind brain. *The Journal of Neuroscience*, *33*, 18242–18246. doi: 10.1523/jneurosci.2546-13.2013

Werker, J. F., & Tees, R. C. (1984). Cross-language speech perception: Evidence for perceptual reorganization during the first year of life. *Infant Behavior and Development*, *7*, 49–63. doi: 10.1016/s0163-6383(84)80022-3

Yim, H., Dennis, S. J., & Sloutsky, V. M. (2013). The development of episodic memory: Items, contexts, and relations. *Psychological Science*, *24*, 2163–2172. doi: 10.1177/0956797613487385

8 Genomics and Phenomics

Robert M. Bilder

Overview

This chapter aims to provide the clinical neuropsychologist with information about the genetic bases of cognitive functioning and disorders of cognition. The chapter begins by introducing basic principles of modern genomic research and review of some key genetic concepts. The next section surveys existing findings about genetic associations with cognitive phenotypes, including both normal function and dysfunction. The final section provides an overview of the complexities involved in formulating and testing hypotheses that span multiple levels of analysis from genome to neuropsychiatric syndrome.

Basic Principles

The Central Dogma of Biology

Before moving on to consider more complex associations between genotype and phenotype, it is important to review the central dogma of molecular biology. In brief, the central dogma of biology states that DNA is used to create RNA, which in turn is used to create proteins. The process through which DNA is "read out" to form messenger RNA (mRNA) is referred to as *transcription*. The process through which RNA is used for protein synthesis is referred to as *translation*. Additional features of central dogma that are important to understand are that DNA undergoes self-replication. The transcription of DNA to RNA relies on RNA polymerase. The translation of RNA and proteins relies on ribosomes, and tRNA is involved in assembly of amino acids into protein chains. These principles are reviewed in most elementary textbooks of molecular biology, and have been the subject of several videos (see for example, *Animation: The Central Dogma* at http://youtu.be/J3HVVi2k2No).

A few additional basics are important to appreciate much of what you will read in papers describing genetic studies. First, it should be recognized that the entire human DNA sequence of approximately 3 billion base pairs is the basis for coding approximately 20,000 genes. We may recall that these base pairs are formed from nucleotides: for DNA, adenine, guanine, cytosine, and thymine (A, G, C, T); for RNA, thymine is replaced by uracil). The "coding" in DNA is accomplished by triplets of these four nucleotides, with each triplet coding for one of the 20 standard amino acids that are the basic structural units of proteins.

The classic use of the term *gene* in this context refers to the "chunk" of DNA (in more formal definitions, a *locatable region*) that is used to code for a single specific protein (or again, because there are now many exceptions to this "rule," the region that is associated with functional outputs as manifest through regulation or transcription). If we were to divide the total number of base pairs by the total number of genes, we would estimate that each gene contains approximately 150,000 base pairs. But most human genes contain only about 1,000 to 30,000 base pairs (albeit certain genes are exceptionally large; e.g., dystrophin is 2.4 million base pairs). Thus large segments of the human genome sequence are not used specifically for encoding proteins. These sections of noncoding DNA were once thought to be "junk" DNA, but subsequently have been found to serve other functions. Among these functions, some noncoding DNA has been found to produce transfer RNA, regulatory RNA, and ribosomal RNA; other noncoding DNA sections may serve regulatory purposes by determining how the process of transcription unfolds.

Certain regions of the DNA sequence are known to have special purposes. For example, the "promoter" region of DNA is the location adjacent to where transcription starts. This is where RNA polymerase and other transcription factors bind to initiate transcription of mRNA. Other specialized regions of DNA include *enhancers* (which activates transcription when they bind *activator* proteins), and *silencers* (which antagonize enhancers by binding proteins that are referred to as *repressors*). The parts of the DNA in parenthesis and RNA) sequences that code for proteins are referred to as *exons*. In contrast, *introns* do not code for proteins and are "spliced" out of the pre-mRNA sequence to yield the final mRNA that is used for translation into proteins.

It should be recognized that the process of transcription from DNA to mRNA and translation of mRNA into a sequence of amino acids is only the first step to creation of a functioning protein. In brief, the sequence of amino acids comprising the protein undergoes a complex process of folding, which is under the influence of the local chemical environment, in order to form the ultimate three-dimensional protein structure.

Classical Genetics Research Strategies

Before considering modern genetic research strategies, it is important to review some of the "classical" approaches that have provided the foundation of genetics research findings for biomedicine. In general, the idea of these studies has been to identify the "gene for" a specific phenotype: the set of observable characteristics of an individual resulting from the interaction of its genotype with the environment. In the case of biomedical research, the phenotype of interest is usually a disease state. The analytic process involves identifying a group of people with a specific phenotype or disease ("cases") and then comparing them to a group of healthy people ("controls"). This is the basis of the *case–control* design. Before researchers had access to genotyping methods that now enable us to directly examine DNA differences between individuals, the structure of genes was often determined by inference from patterns of inheritance. Thus, we may recall the classical experiments of Gregor Mendel, who found through selective breeding of peas that certain characteristics would be passed down from one generation to the next (for example, that some genes coded for a round shape, while others coded for a wrinkled shape). Documenting these patterns led to the definition of *alleles,* which are alternative forms of a gene that may lead to different expressed phenotypes (e.g., round = R, and wrinkled = r; thus a single plant might have the RR, Rr or rr, and in this case given that "R" is dominant and "r" is recessive, both RR and Rr lead to the same round phenotype, while the rr genotype leads to the wrinkled phenotype).

Decades of genetic research have revealed that organisms may possess many alleles at a particular genetic region or locus, and that most phenotypes are the product of multiple allelic effects and their interactions. Indeed, these allelic effects may span multiple genes. For example, eye color reflects the interaction of allelic variation across multiple genes. Complex traits such as neuropsychiatric syndromes or cognitive functions are associated with variation across many genes. For example, recent studies suggest that the genetic risk for a disorder like schizophrenia (which is about 80% heritable), is accounted for by approximately 8,000 genes, or more than one-third of the entire human genome.

In most early genetic mapping studies, variation in the genome was identified using genetic "markers," or identifiable sequences of DNA, and their proximity to each other was documented based on the likelihood that the markers would be inherited together (since closer segments of DNA are more likely to end up together during reproduction). With advances in the mapping of the human genome and high-throughput methods for testing DNA sequences, it is now routine to examine millions of locations across the entire human genome to conduct genome-wide association studies (GWAS), and it is becoming increasingly common to measure all 3 billion bases in the genome (whole genome sequencing). This has been technically feasible for almost two decades, but in 2014 the cost fell below $1,000, considered by some to be the "magic number" that will enable more widespread application.[1]

In brief, the methods for GWAS and whole genome sequencing involve examining specific genomic locations to determine exactly which nucleotides are present within a sequence of DNA. At some locations, there is not much variation across individuals, but some genetic loci are highly variable. These regions may have different forms or *polymorphisms.* If the difference occurs at a single nucleotide, that is referred to as a *single nucleotide polymorphism* (SNP). Most studies in the literature report on the frequencies of either specific "candidate" SNPs, or in the case of GWAS, enough SNPs that a picture of variation across the entire genome is possible (as provided by collecting hundreds of thousands to millions of SNPs). The primary reason for collecting a panel of SNPs rather than the entire genome, however, is cost. Now that the price for whole genome sequencing is dropping we can expect whole genome sequencing to become much more common, first in research reports, and ultimately in clinical databases.

Evaluating the Quality of Genetic Association Results

It may be very confusing for anyone not familiar with genetic association studies to appreciate the results of these studies and distinguish those that are high quality from those that are not. It is useful for readers to familiarize themselves with recent guidelines. Following the development of standards for reporting results of epidemiology studies called "Strengthening the Reporting of Observational Studies in Epidemiology" (STROBE; see Gallo et al., 2011), a new statement was developed specifically for genetic studies: STrengthening the REporting of Genetic Association studies (STREGA; see Little et al., 2009). Many of these guidelines may seem obvious to neuropsychologists. For example, the guidelines indicate that authors should clearly report the study design, sample characteristics, all key variables to be analyzed, and the statistical analysis plan. There are two particularly important characteristics, however, that deserve some further explanation because these so frequently impact study quality and the conclusions that are reasonable to draw from a genetic association study: (a) control for false positive findings and (b) control for population stratification.

The greatest single challenge for genetic association studies is claiming that a statistically significant finding has emerged that adequately corrects for the number of statistical tests performed, when there may be hundreds of thousands or millions of tests. To help *control for reported false-positive findings,* one guideline in wide use is to claim "genome-wide significance" only for individual associations with probability values of less than 5×10^{-8} or 1×10^{-8} (to reflect approximate alpha levels of .05 and .01 respectively). This standard is derived from a Bonferroni correction, with the assumption that there may be approximately 1 million independent variants in the human genome. There is a reasonable concern that the Bonferroni correction may be overly conservative, but even modified approaches that attempt to explicitly model the degree to which different genetic variants are not truly independent but instead correlated (in large part due to linkage disequilibrium, or the tendency of DNA segments to be inherited together), require P values of approximately 1×10^{-7}. It may seem somewhat alien to demand such stringent thresholds for claiming statistical significance, but there is now ample evidence that claims based on less rigorous thresholds have often turned out to be false positives.

The literature contains many reports of "candidate gene" associations, where usually a small number of SNPs is tested for association with one or more phenotypes. Authors sometimes claim that these studies do not require adjustments for multiple comparisons because they have only examined one SNP. But this strategy is unfortunately likely to yield an unacceptably high false positive rate, because there may be many SNPs in the genome that are associated with a complex trait (in some well-done studies, about one-third of the entire genome!), and if we consider the number of SNPs that may be in linkage disequilibrium with the selected SNP, it is clear why more stringent thresholds are needed to establish statistical significance. There are some methods that employ alternative methods for controlling false discovery rates (FDR) using "stepup," "adaptive," and "dependent" procedures; these may better control for Type I error without as much sacrifice of statistical power (van den Oord, 2005). But the thresholds remain far more stringent than we are accustomed to in neuropsychology research, usually by five or six orders of magnitude!

Regardless of the threshold selected for declaring a particular finding to be "significant," readers should remain skeptical. Ioannidis (2005) has crafted criteria to grade the "credibility" of molecular evidence. This framework suggests that the following factors be evaluated.

1. Effect size: Large effects are more likely to be true than small effects.
2. Replication: Multiple, independent replications increase credibility.
3. Bias: Studies with bias are less credible; those with protection against bias are more credible.
4. Biological plausibility: The more functional/biological data, the more credible.
5. Relevance: The stronger the potential application in clinical practice or public health, the more credible.

One sobering message from this work is that many findings of interest to neuropsychologists that have very small effects (for example, most of the putative associations between cognitive function and genetic variants have relative risk less than 1.2) are unlikely to be credible. Ioannidis and colleagues estimate that even the extensively replicated effects of this magnitude have credibility in the range of only 2% to 30% (Ioannidis, 2009).

Among the different kinds of bias (which also include bias in phenotype definition, bias in genotyping [lack of quality control], and selective reporting biases), the problem of *population stratification* deserves special attention. In brief, population stratification refers to the presence of differences in allele frequency associated with a particular subpopulation. If the subpopulation also differs in some phenotype of interest, then it is possible to observe a spurious association between genotype and phenotype due to this confound rather than a true association. There are several ways to handle this problem, including sampling within a specific subpopulation, using certain family based designs, and/or developing statistical representations of the population substructure (for example, using principal components analysis, or a "genomic control" strategy, which basically examines the hypothesis of association in subgroups defined specifically based on their genetic background (Devlin, Roeder, & Bacanu, 2001; Enoch, Shen, Xu, Hodgkinson, & Goldman, 2006; Kang et al., 2010).

It should be recognized that even when genetic studies reveal compelling associations that are considered significant at genome-wide levels and replicated, the identified variants may still account for only a small amount of the known heritability. Human height is a good example phenotype: Despite a heritability near 80%, only about 5% of phenotypic variance is explained by more than 40 known loci (Visscher, 2008). This has been referred to as the problem of "missing heritability" or the "dark matter" of heritability, and may be due to many reasons, including: (1) variants that the GWAS arrays are missing (i.e., the SNPs that have yielded association findings may not be the causative SNPs, and the true causative SNPs might have larger effects); (2) gene-gene interactions (epistasis) and/or gene-environment interaction effects too complicated to assess given current sample sizes and analytic strategies; (3) epigenetic effects; (4) much larger numbers of genetic variants with even smaller effects remaining to be found; and (5) inadequate accounting for shared environmental variance among relatives (Manolio et al., 2009).

Overall, those interested in surveying genetic associations with cognitive phenotypes of interest will be best served by large-scale meta-analyses that consider carefully the quality of studies based on all the factors noted in this section. Unfortunately, we still lack such evidence for the vast majority of cognitive or neuropsychological phenotypes. But given the increasing attention to harmonizing phenotype assessment, along with the increase in number of repositories for collecting genetic and phenotype data, the availability of high-quality association data should grow rapidly.

Genetics of Cognitive Function and Dysfunction

A challenge faces those interested in understanding the genetic bases of cognitive impairment. Specifically, most studies have focused on understanding the genetic bases of "disease" rather than the genetic bases of cognitive function or dysfunction, per se. Therefore, most of what is known about the genetics of cognition derives from studies about the genetic bases of cognitive syndromes.

Indeed, some of the most successful approaches have led to identification of very specific genetic associations with complex syndromes such as intellectual disabilities (formerly known as "mental retardation") that are primarily characterized by cognitive deficits. Intellectual disabilities, while hardly representing a uniform or homogeneous set of cognitive dysfunction phenotypes, have been linked to more than 300 distinctive monogenic causes, albeit each of these specific conditions is relatively rare, so even this large number of genetic "causes" of cognitive deficit account for only about .01% of all cases (Butcher, Kennedy, & Plomin, 2006).

Despite the low frequency of these conditions, they may be informative about mechanisms important to brain development and cognition. For example, the study of Fragile X syndrome has led to multiple insights about the genetics of trinucleotide repeats, X-linked genetic disorders, and the enormous pleiotropy of single-gene deficits on neural and other systems (Heulens & Kooy, 2011). Similarly the study of neurofibromatosis, and the NF1 gene, has yielded major insights into the molecular basis of these syndromes, yielded novel transgenic rodent models in which mutants have superior abilities, and may stimulate novel treatment development (Lee & Silva, 2009; Silva, Zhou, Rogerson, Shobe, & Balaji, 2009).

Studies of dementia risk offer further clues to the genetic bases of cognitive deficit. Perhaps the most robust identified genetic associations for any neuropsychiatric syndrome is the association of apolipoprotein E, epsilon 4 allele (APOE*E4) genotype with risk for dementia of the Alzheimer's type or Alzheimer's disease (AD; Corder et al., 1993; Saunders et al., 1993), with increased risk of clinical AD being large (with odds ratios ranging from twofold up to tenfold, depending on the population studied; see Online Mendelian Inheritance in Man or OMIM for reviews; Hamosh et al., 2005). While initial hypotheses centered on the possible role of this genotype in directly altering the formation of neurofibrillary plaques or tangles, subsequent hypotheses have focused attention on other cerebrovascular mechanisms or response to oxidative stress (Horsburgh, McCarron, White, & Nicoll, 2000; Wagle et al., 2009). Despite these efforts, the genetic basis of cognitive dysfunction associated with the APOE4 effect remains unknown.

A range of other associations between genetic variations and cognitive functions have been reported but, other than the association with APOE4 noted, none of these would satisfy the criteria for credibility of genetic findings as stipulated by Ioannidis and colleagues (see p. 104). Sabb and colleagues reviewed prior work on candidate genes for which investigators reported associations with cognitive phenotypes comprising "memory" (51 effects) and "intelligence" (42 effects) (Sabb et al., 2009). They found generally modest associations of candidate genes with varying cognitive phenotypes, with most effect sizes (Cohen's *d* for the effect distinguishing alleles) ranging from .09 to .23. An interesting result of this survey was that among genes investigated, two had relations specifically with intelligence (CHRM2 and DRD2), two had relations specifically with memory phenotypes (5-HTT and KIBRA), and four had reported links to both intelligence and memory phenotypes (DTNB1, COMT, BDNF, and APOE). Other researchers have highlighted the replication of selected findings related to rare variants in key genetic regions (such as PDE10A, CYSIP1, KCNE1/KCNE2, CHRNA7) and their possible connection to both schizophrenia and cognitive impairment phenotypes (Tam et al., 2010). Finally, recent intriguing findings suggest that a variant of the KLOTHO gene (which increases klotho protein in serum) is associated with a beneficial effect on cognition in both humans and rodents, along with increasing longevity, possibly mediated by enhancement of long-term potentiation, via an NMDAR mechanism (Dubal et al., 2014). Notably, the effect size for KLOTHO on cognitive function was .34 (Cohen's *d*), which is larger than the effect of the APOE genotype, and larger than the effects of any FDA-approved treatments for Alzheimer's disease (Dubal et al., 2014).

I and my colleagues have made an effort to catalog genetic association studies pertinent to cognitive phenotypes in the development of a Web-based resource (CogGene) and enable automated meta-analysis (Bilder, Howe, Novak, Sabb, & Parker, 2011), in a way similar to the tools available for examining other phenotypes such as the diagnosis of Alzheimer's disease (AlzGene) and schizophrenia (SczGene). Our analysis revealed only 12 associations that were nominally significant as reported in the original studies (that is, the 95% confidence intervals around the average effect size did not include zero). The "hits" included: APOE, CHRM2, DTNBP1, DRD2 (two SNPs), CHRM2/CHRNA4, IL1B, KIBRA, SNAP25 (two SNPs), IL1RAPL1, and CACNA1C. The only one of these putative candidates that has high credibility as a risk factor for cognitive impairment is the APOE*E4 genotype.

Chabris and colleagues (Chabris et al., 2012) attempted to replicate published associations between 12 genetic variants and estimates of general intelligence (*g*) in three independent, relatively large samples (totaling nearly 10,000 individuals). They demonstrated that about half of the variance in *g* is accounted for by common genetic variation, but could not replicate any of the associations as being statistically significant. There was adequate power to detect even small effects. For example, in the first analysis they had 99% power to detect a joint effect of 12 variants of .52% (about half of 1% variance explained in phenotype by all 12 variants). Similarly, Lencz and colleagues in the Cognitive Genomics consorTium (COGENT) (Lencz et al., 2014), looked for genetic associations to cognitive phenotypes in more than 5,000 people, and while they demonstrated shared polygenic risk between schizophrenia and cognitive impairment, they could find no genome-wide significant loci for cognitive function.

It should further be noted that in the analysis of Chabris and colleagues (Chabris et al., 2012), APOE*E4 was not significantly associated with *g*. This makes it clear that the effects of APOE*E4 may be expressed primarily through pathological processes later in life. Indeed, the APOE effect may be seen as a special case of the general finding that the heritability of intelligence increases with age. Recent summaries suggest that H^2 for IQ may increase from about .2 during infancy up to .80 in late adulthood (Haworth et al., 2010; Plomin & Deary, 2015). These authors highlight an alternate interpretation of this temporally increasing heritability or genetic amplification. They suggest that this may occur as "small genetic differences are magnified as children select, modify and create environments correlated with their genetic propensities" (Plomin & Deary, 2015; p. 100).

Research on the heritability of intelligence, other cognitive abilities, and academic skills and disabilities, further illustrates that so far we have not found more specific effects, and that we may be unlikely to find more specific genes for more specific neuropsychological domains. Meta-analysis suggests an average intercorrelation of about 0.3 among tests of different cognitive abilities, but the *genetic correlations* (that is, the amount of shared variance between tests due to shared genetic causes) tend to be greater than 0.6 (Plomin & Deary, 2015). These observations led to the formulation of the *Generalist Gene* hypothesis (Calvin et al., 2012; Plomin & Kovas, 2005), which suggests that common genetic factors are responsible for most cognitive abilities and skills, as well as for inherited dysfunctions affecting those abilities and skills.

It would be logical to reason that we could seek more specific associations between genetic variation and specific abilities by covarying for general abilities, and examining the residual variance in special abilities that may be associated with unique circuits or neural system-level functions. Unfortunately, given that traits like *g* are currently thought to reflect the operation of a very large number of very small genetic effects, extremely large samples may be needed to detect more subtle genetic effects that may only be apparent after "controlling for" the genetic backgrounds that govern general ability.

The perspective afforded by genetic studies may be very valuable to clinical neuropsychology, however, especially in helping to overcome "domain-specific" hypotheses that may not clearly reflect the true pathological processes suffered by our patients. For example, we frequently see neuropsychological reports organized in special sections with "domain" headings for "Language," "Executive Functions," and "Learning/Memory Functions" (to name only a few). But these "classic" domain headings were derived largely from the study of individuals with focal brain lesions following relatively normal development. In contrast, most genetic disorders are by definition "developmental," regardless of whether the genetic impacts are revealed early in life (as in Fragile X disorders) or later in life (as in those with APOE*E4 genotype).

If we consider the ultimate mechanistic paths through which these genetic variants exert their effects, then it becomes clearer why specific gene effects do not usually translate into neuropsychologically specific variation. For example, even without detecting any of the specific genetic variants associated with cognitive function at a level that provides high credibility, it is possible to examine groups of genes and determine if there is statistical support for the involvement of one or more *gene networks* (i.e., a group of genes that may be clustered by the involvement of their gene products in a specific metabolic pathway or other biological process). Several studies using this approach have suggested that cognitive function/dysfunction may be linked to glutamatergic signaling and more specifically the NMDA receptor complex (Hill et al., 2014; Ohi, Kimura, & Haji, 2015); immunologic function (e.g., major histocompatibility complex class 1)(McAllister, 2014; Ohi et al., 2015); glial cell function, inflammatory response, and neurotransmission (Levine, Horvath, et al., 2013; Levine, Miller, et al., 2013); or other general processes including mitochondrial function, oxidative stress, posttranslational modifications, protein folding, and protein trafficking (Bhattacharya & Klann, 2012).

There is further promise that research on molecular and cellular processes in animal models will yield dramatic progress in understanding not only healthy cognitive function, but also disorders of cognitive function and possibly trigger development of new treatments. An excellent review of mechanisms that may *enhance* synaptic plasticity, long-term potentiation, and learning-memory functions in transgenic rodent models points to multiple potentially valuable molecular targets (Lee & Silva, 2009; Silva et al., 2009). Examples include multiple approaches to enhance NMDA receptor function, methods to regulate cyclic-AMP response-element-binding protein (CREB) function, manipulation of proto-oncogenes such as H-ras, and possibly enhancement of glial cell function. Through integration of these basic neuroscientific findings with emerging studies of molecular biomarkers in humans, which are enabling the assessment of genome-wide expression patterns and metabolic functions, there is hope that we will one day possess reliable roadmaps capable of explicating the final common paths for both disruption of systems that lead to cognitive impairment, and specifying the molecular targets that may correct deficits or even enhance healthy functions.

*Omics Strategies for Understanding Brain Systems

Following the advent of *genomics* to represent the systematic study of the entire genome (rather than selected genes), the last 15 years has seen a burgeoning list of "*omics" strategies, including proteomics, metabolomics, and connectomics.

Early in these developments, Freimer and Sabatti (2003) argued that the ever-decreasing costs of genotyping would lead to the situation where the limiting step in discovery of molecular mechanisms would be found in characterizing the multitude of phenotypes, not genotypes. After all, the human genome contains only about 3 billion base pairs, comprising only four relatively simple nucleotides, in a linear sequence. In contrast, the collection of phenotypes is virtually infinite. Thus Freimer and Sabatti used the term *phenomics* to refer to the systematic investigation of phenotypes on a genome-wide scale. Implicit in this definition is the necessity to characterize multiple phenotypes simultaneously, thereby increasing the specificity of composite phenotype definition and presumably increasing the power to detect genetic association.

A fundamental distinction between the phenomics strategy and the more traditional strategy for GWAS is that the latter most often focuses on a "univariate" approach to seeking associations of an individual phenotype with a genome-wide assessment of variation. This is basically the equivalent of conducting a large number of statistical tests (as many as there are genetic variants in the assay, usually a million or more with current chips) and then correcting for multiplicity of testing to constrain the false-positive error rate. In contrast, the phenomics strategy implies assessment of multiple phenotypes both within a specific level of analysis (for example, multiple protein products) along with multiple phenotypes *across* levels of analysis (for example, not only proteins, but also cellular, neural system, and cognitive or behavioral phenotypes; see Bilder et al., 2009). Considering the complexity of establishing links across levels of analysis, and the number of levels that are interposed in any causal model linking structural genetic variation to a high-level behavioral phenotype, it can be demonstrated with simple calculations that most complex phenotypes would be likely to share only 0.01% up to 1.6% of variance with any specific genetic variant. A corollary of this calculation is that about 5,000 common variants may be necessary to explain the 50% heritability statistics reported for many cognitive traits such as *g* (Bilder & Howe, 2013; Plomin & Deary, 2015).

There is no consensus yet about how to navigate this vast search space, identify the most important variables, and prioritize the selection of paths that connect variables to each other most meaningfully. Development of novel informatics approaches holds promise. I and my colleagues have described an approach to visualization of variance (ViVA) and introduced graphical tools for visualization of the analysis of variance (VISOVA), to help navigate large data sets and detect patterns across large numbers of variables, and explore hypotheses about the correlates of neuropsychiatric phenotypes (Parker, Congdon, & Bilder, 2014). We have developed other approaches to represent specific multilevel hypotheses using graphical models (Bilder & Howe, 2013). For example, we assembled graphical representations of a few hypotheses about the cognitive construct *working memory* to include multiple levels of analysis including genes, gene expression, proteomics, cellular systems and signaling pathways, neural systems/circuits, cognitive phenotypes, symptom phenotypes, and syndromal or diagnostic phenotypes (Bilder & Howe, 2013). At the more basic levels of analysis, there exist already good knowledge bases that can be queried (for example: Entrez Gene; Gene Ontologies; Gene Expression Omnibus; Entrez Protein, UniProt/SwissProt; NextProt; Ingenuity Pathways Analysis; KEGG Pathway). At the "highest" level of syndromes (as manifest for example in the *Diagnostic and Statistical Manual of Mental Disorders*) there is clear definition of each diagnostic class in terms of its constituent symptoms; this is straightforward to make explicit in graphical models. Similarly, formal definitions of cognitive or neuropsychological constructs can be articulated using structural equation models that make clear exactly what objective measurements are used to define each latent construct. The biggest gap exists at the level of neural systems, and while we have some outstanding frameworks for representing neural networks and neuroanatomic structure, there remains no widely accepted map of human neural circuits to serve as a scaffold for hypotheses about circuit functions. I and my colleagues established a neural circuit description framework in order to specify selected hypotheses about neural circuit functions (Bilder & Howe, 2013), but this was conceptual and lacked links to an explicit spatial map of the brain. We hope that future implementations of this approach to modeling may include direct mapping onto atlases of human connectional anatomy that are emerging from the Human Connectome Project (Kocher et al., 2015).

If we can develop formal models about genetic hypotheses about cognitive phenotypes, this may enable fundamental advances. Much as drug discovery is now benefiting from *in silica* modeling of molecular species that can be designed to impact selected receptor targets, we hope that multilevel modeling may one day enable prediction of high-level cognitive consequences of genetic, proteomic, or metabolomic manipulations. These developments may have a profound impact on our understanding of the true dimensions of cognitive and other brain functions. For example, the current taxonomy of mental disorders specifies many classes of illness (diagnostic categories) for which there is sparse evidence of validity. For example, the current distinction between schizophrenia and bipolar disorder rests mostly on historical precedent—dating back to the time of Kraepelin—but more recent neurocognitive, neuroimaging, and neurogenetic data fail to support a clear distinction between these variants of psychotic illness, and may be better understand as reflecting a severity dimension (Bilder, 2015).

This effort to better carve nature "at its joints" is the desideratum of the National Institute of Mental Health (NIMH) Research Domains Criteria (RDoC) initiative, which also specifies the examination of key domains of function at multiple levels (or units) of analysis from genome to syndrome (see the NIMH's RDoC web page at www.nimh.nih.gov/research-priorities/rdoc/index.shtml). The goal of the RDoC is to create new diagnostic systems that will use biologically based dimensions and categories to replace the current taxonomy, which is both atheoretical and based almost exclusively on clinical interviews and observation of symptoms. Within each of the research domains in the master RDoC "matrix," there is a level to represent "genes"—albeit that level of the matrix remains lightly populated, given that we possess few well-validated candidate genes for these domains. We may note, however, that the domain of cognitive systems is relatively rich territory for neuropsychology, encompassing the following constructs and subconstructs (and associated genes where these were proposed):

- Attention (dopamine receptor genes (e.g., D4, D5); DAT1; serotonin receptor gene)
- Perception
  - Visual perception (Dysbindin/NRG1/Neuroligin/Neurexin)
  - Auditory perception (BDNF)
  - Olfactory, somatosensory, and multimodal perception
- Declarative memory (BDNF, KIBRA [hippocampal circuit]; FOXP2 [cortical, based on songbird model])
- Language behavior (FOXP2)
- Cognitive (effortful) control (COMT, BDNF, DISC1, 5HT2A, DRD4, DRD2, 5-HTTLPR, CHRM4, DAT1, MAO-A, 5-HTT)
  - Goal selection, updating, representation and maintenance
  - Response selection, inhibition or suppression
  - Performance monitoring
- Working memory (NRG1/Neuregulin, DISC1, DTNBP1/Dysbindin, BDNF, COMT, DRD2, DAT1)
  - Active maintenance
  - Flexible updating
  - Limited capacity
  - Interference control

It should be recognized, however, that most of the suggested candidate genes do not pass the threshold for credibility based on genome-wide significance, replication, and understanding of biological function. As data accumulate in RDoC projects, however, it is likely that more of the relevant evidence will be assembled, and new genetic targets and their biological correlates will be identified, ushering in a new era of *precision medicine* for neuropsychiatric disorders (Insel & Cuthbert, 2015). Insel and Cuthbert (2015) cite as an example recent work subtyping attention deficit/hyperactivity disorder (ADHD) into *mild*, *surgent*, and *irritable* subtypes, based on a combination of observations about temperamental characteristics, physiology, and neuroimaging measures (Karalunas et al., 2014). Whether these syndromal groups will prove to possess clearer genetic bases remains an open question, but at least by defining categories that have some biological validation, it seems more likely that the links to underlying genetic differences will be found.

The ultimate promise of these strategies is to provide more complete pathophysiological explanations of neuropsychiatric syndromes that can serve as the basis for the design of rational interventions. In theory, complete knowledge of the genetic architecture for syndromal risk can lead to both highly specific preventative interventions, along with early detection and treatment of emergent dysfunction. The better we understand the mechanisms at a genetic level, along with the manifold expressions of gene action at proteomic, metabolomic, cellular and systems levels, the more clearly we can determine what is the optimal level to intervene in order to maximize benefits and minimize adverse effects. Paralleling this increase in understanding of biological processes and treatments, there is also a burgeoning knowledge of the biology, including *molecular* biology, nonsomatic treatments. Thus, for example, we are learning more about the patterns of gene induction accompanying cognitive training (Klingberg, 2010), epigenetic modification following meditation practice (Kaliman et al., 2014), and the possible mediating roles that certain genetic backgrounds may have for the efficacy of cognitive therapy (Bakker et al., 2014). Insel and Cuthbert (2015) noted the paradox that this new focus on basic biological processes may lead to a renaissance in the appreciation of psychotherapy as an intervention strategy capable of remodeling neural circuits, and leveraging the brain's inherent neuroplastic capacities, in a highly personalized way.

Acknowledgement

This work was supported by a grant from the National Institute of Mental Health (R01MH101478).

Note

1 "Illumina Sequencer Enables $1,000 Genome." News: Genomics & Proteomics. *Gen. Eng. Biotechnol. News*, 34(4). February, 15, 2014. p. 18.

References

Bakker, J. M., Lieverse, R., Menne-Lothmann, C., Viechtbauer, W., Pishva, E., Kenis, G., . . . Wichers, M. (2014). Therapygenetics in mindfulness-based cognitive therapy: Do genes have an impact on therapy-induced change in real-life positive affective experiences? *Translational Psychiatry*, *4*, e384. doi: 10.1038/tp.2014.23

Bhattacharya, A., & Klann, E. (2012). The molecular basis of cognitive deficits in pervasive developmental disorders. *Learning & Memory*, *19*(9), 434–443.

Bilder, R. M. (2015). Dimensional and categorical approaches to mental illness: Let biology decide. In L. J. Kirmayer, R. Lemelson, & C. A. Cummings (Eds.), *Re-Visioning Psychiatry: Cultural Phenomenology, Critical Neuroscience, and Global Mental Health* (pp. 179–205). New York: Cambridge University Press.

Bilder, R. M., & Howe, A. G. (2013). Multilevel models from biology to psychology: Mission impossible? *Journal of Abnormal Psychology*, *122*(3), 917.

Bilder, R. M., Howe, A., Novak, N., Sabb, F. W., & Parker, D. S. (2011). The genetics of cognitive impairment in schizophrenia: A phenomic perspective. *Trends in Cognitive Sciences*, *15*(9), 428–435. doi: 10.1016/j.tics.2011.07.002

Bilder, R. M., Sabb, F. W., Cannon, T. D., London, E. D., Jentsch, J. D., Parker, D. S., . . . Freimer, N. B. (2009). Phenomics: The systematic study of phenotypes on a genome-wide scale. *Neuroscience*, *164*(1), 30–42. doi: 10.1016/j.neuroscience.2009.01.027

Butcher, L. M., Kennedy, J. K., & Plomin, R. (2006). Generalist genes and cognitive neuroscience. *Current Opinions in Neurobiology*, *16*(2), 145–151. doi: S0959-4388(06)00029-8 [pii] 10.1016/j.conb.2006.03.004

Calvin, C. M., Deary, I. J., Webbink, D., Smith, P., Fernandes, C., Lee, S. H., . . . Visscher, P. M. (2012). Multivariate genetic analyses of cognition and academic achievement from two population samples of 174,000 and 166,000 school children. *Behavioral Genetics*, *42*(5), 699–710. doi: 10.1007/s10519-012-9549-7

Chabris, C. F., Hebert, B. M., Benjamin, D. J., Beauchamp, J., Cesarini, D., van der Loos, M., . . . Laibson, D. (2012). Most reported genetic associations with general intelligence are probably false positives. *Psychological Science*, *23*(11), 1314–1323. doi: 10.1177/0956797611435528

Corder, E. H., Saunders, A. M., Strittmatter, W. J., Schmechel, D. E., Gaskell, P. C., Small, G. W., . . . Pericak-Vance, M. A. (1993). Gene dose of apolipoprotein E type 4 allele and the risk of Alzheimer's disease in late onset families. *Science*, *261*(5123), 921–923.

Devlin, B., Roeder, K., & Bacanu, S. A. (2001). Unbiased methods for population-based association studies. *Genetic Epidemiology*, *21*(4), 273–284.

Dubal, D. B., Yokoyama, J. S., Zhu, L., Broestl, L., Worden, K., Wang, D., . . . Mucke, L. (2014). Life extension factor klotho enhances cognition. *Cell Reports*, *7*(4), 1065–1076. doi: 10.1016/j.celrep.2014.03.076

Enoch, M. A., Shen, P. H., Xu, K., Hodgkinson, C., & Goldman, D. (2006). Using ancestry-informative markers to define populations and detect population stratification. *Journal of Psychopharmacology*, *20*(Suppl 4), 19–26.

Freimer, N., & Sabatti, C. (2003). The human phenome project. *Nature Genetics*, *34*(1), 15–21. doi: 10.1038/ng0503-15

Gallo, V., Egger, M., McCormack, V., Farmer, P. B., Ioannidis, J. P., Kirsch-Volders, M., . . . Statement, S. (2011). STrengthening the Reporting of OBservational studies in Epidemiology—Molecular Epidemiology (STROBE-ME): An extension of the STROBE statement. *Public Library of Science, Medicine*, *8*(10), e1001117. doi: 10.1371/journal.pmed.1001117

Hamosh, A., Scott, A. F., Amberger, J. S., Bocchini, C. A., & McKusick, V. A. (2005). Online Mendelian Inheritance in Man (OMIM), a knowledgebase of human genes and genetic disorders. *Nucleic Acids Research*, *33*(suppl_1), D514–D517.

Haworth, C. M., Wright, M. J., Luciano, M., Martin, N. G., de Geus, E. J., van Beijsterveldt, C. E., . . . Plomin, R. (2010). The heritability of general cognitive ability increases linearly from childhood to young adulthood. *MolecularPsychiatry*, *15*(11), 1112–1120. doi: 10.1038/mp.2009.55

Heulens, I., & Kooy, F. (2011). Fragile X syndrome: From gene discovery to therapy. *Frontiers in Bioscience: A Journal and Virtual Library*, *16*, 1211.

Hill, W. D., Davies, G., van de Lagemaat, L. N., Christoforou, A., Marioni, R. E., Fernandes, C. P., . . . Deary, I. J. (2014). Human cognitive ability is influenced by genetic variation in components of postsynaptic signalling complexes assembled by NMDA receptors and MAGUK proteins. *Translational Psychiatry*, *4*, e341. doi: 10.1038/tp.2013.114

Horsburgh, K., McCarron, M. O., White, F., & Nicoll, J. A. (2000). The role of apolipoprotein E in Alzheimer's disease, acute brain injury and cerebrovascular disease: Evidence of common mechanisms and utility of animal models. *Neurobiology of Aging*, *21*(2), 245–255.

Insel, T. R., & Cuthbert, B. N. (2015). Medicine: Brain disorders? Precisely. *Science*, *348*(6234), 499–500. doi: 10.1126/science.aab2358

Ioannidis, J. P. (2005). Molecular bias. *European Journal of Epidemiology*, *20*(9), 739–745. doi: 10.1007/s10654-005-2028-1

Ioannidis, J. P. (2009). Population-wide generalizability of genome-wide discovered associations. *Journal of the National Cancer Institute*, *101*(19), 1297–1299. doi: djp298 [pii] 10.1093/jnci/djp298

Kaliman, P., Alvarez-Lopez, M. J., Cosin-Tomas, M., Rosenkranz, M. A., Lutz, A., & Davidson, R. J. (2014). Rapid changes in histone deacetylases and inflammatory gene expression in expert meditators. *Psychoneuroendocrinology*, *40*, 96–107. doi: 10.1016/j.psyneuen.2013.11.004

Kang, H. M., Sul, J. H., Service, S. K., Zaitlen, N. A., Kong, S. Y., Freimer, N. B., . . . Eskin, E. (2010). Variance component model to account for sample structure in genome-wide association studies. *Nature Genetics*, *42*(4), 348–354. doi: ng.548 [pii] 10.1038/ng.548

Karalunas, S. L., Fair, D., Musser, E. D., Aykes, K., Iyer, S. P., & Nigg, J. T. (2014). Subtyping attention-deficit/hyperactivity disorder using temperament dimensions: Toward biologically based nosologic criteria. *JAMA Psychiatry*, *71*(9), 1015–1024. doi: 10.1001/jamapsychiatry.2014.763

Klingberg, T. (2010). Training and plasticity of working memory. *Trends in Cognitive Sciences*, *14*(7), 317–324. doi: 10.1016/j.tics.2010.05.002

Kocher, M., Gleichgerrcht, E., Nesland, T., Rorden, C., Fridriksson, J., Spampinato, M. V., & Bonilha, L. (2015). Individual variability in the anatomical distribution of nodes participating in rich club structural networks. *Frontiers in Neural Circuits*, *9*, 16. doi: 10.3389/fncir.2015.00016

Lee, Y. S., & Silva, A. J. (2009). The molecular and cellular biology of enhanced cognition. *Nature Reviews Neuroscience*, *10*(2), 126–140. doi: nrn2572 [pii] 10.1038/nrn2572

Lencz, T., Knowles, E., Davies, G., Guha, S., Liewald, D. C., Starr, J. M., . . . Malhotra, A. K. (2014). Molecular genetic evidence for overlap between general cognitive ability and risk for schizophrenia: A report from the Cognitive Genomics Consortium (COGENT). *Molecular Psychiatry*, *19*(2), 168–174. doi: 10.1038/mp.2013.166

Levine, A. J., Horvath, S., Miller, E. N., Singer, E. J., Shapshak, P., Baldwin, G. C., . . . Langfelder, P. (2013). Transcriptome analysis of HIV-infected peripheral blood monocytes: Gene transcripts and networks associated with neurocognitive functioning. *Journal of Neuroimmunology*, *265*(1–2), 96–105. doi: 10.1016/j.jneuroim.2013.09.016

Levine, A. J., Miller, J. A., Shapshak, P., Gelman, B., Singer, E. J., Hinkin, C. H., . . . Horvath, S. (2013). Systems analysis of human brain gene expression: Mechanisms for HIV-associated neurocognitive impairment and common pathways with Alzheimer's disease. *Biomed Central Medical Genomics*, *6*, 4. doi: 10.1186/1755-8794-6-4

Little, J., Higgins, J. P., Ioannidis, J. P., Moher, D., Gagnon, F., von Elm, E., . . . Birkett, N. (2009). STrengthening the REporting of Genetic Association Studies (STREGA)--an extension of the STROBE statement. *Genetic Epidemiology*, *33*(7), 581–598. doi: 10.1002/gepi.20410

Manolio, T. A., Collins, F. S., Cox, N. J., Goldstein, D. B., Hindorff, L. A., Hunter, D. J., . . . Chakravarti, A. (2009). Finding the missing heritability of complex diseases. *Nature*, *461*(7265), 747–753.

McAllister, A. K. (2014). Major histocompatibility complex I in brain development and schizophrenia. *Biological Psychiatry*, *75*(4), 262–268. doi: 10.1016/j.biopsych.2013.10.003

Ohi, Y., Kimura, S., & Haji, A. (2015). Modulation of glutamatergic transmission by presynaptic N-methyl-D-aspartate mechanisms in second-order neurons of the rat nucleus tractus solitarius. *Neuroscience Letters*, *587*, 62–67. doi: 10.1016/j.neulet.2014.12.031

Parker, D. S., Congdon, E., & Bilder, R. M. (2014). Hypothesis exploration with visualization of variance. *BioData Mining*, *7*, 11. doi: 10.1186/1756-0381-7-11

Plomin, R., & Deary, I. J. (2015). Genetics and intelligence differences: Five special findings. *Molecular Psychiatry*, *20*(1), 98–108. doi: 10.1038/mp.2014.105

Plomin, R., & Kovas, Y. (2005). Generalist genes and learning disabilities. *Psychological Bulletin*, *131*(4), 592–617. doi: 2005-08334-006 [pii] 10.1037/0033-2909.131.4.592

Sabb, F. W., Burggren, A. C., Higier, R. G., Fox, J., He, J., Parker, D. S., . . . Bilder, R. M. (2009). Challenges in phenotype definition in the whole-genome era: Multivariate models of memory and intelligence. *Neuroscience*, *164*(1), 88–107. doi: S0306-4522(09)00795-7 [pii] 10.1016/j.neuroscience.2009.05.013

Saunders, A. M., Strittmatter, W. J., Schmechel, D., George-Hyslop, P. H., Pericak-Vance, M. A., Joo, S. H., . . . Roses, A. D. (1993). Association of apolipoprotein E allele epsilon 4 with late-onset familial and sporadic Alzheimer's disease. *Neurology*, *43*(8), 1467–1472.

Silva, A. J., Zhou, Y., Rogerson, T., Shobe, J., & Balaji, J. (2009). Molecular and cellular approaches to memory allocation in neural circuits. *Science*, *326*(5951), 391–395. doi: 326/5951/391 [pii] 10.1126/science.1174519

Tam, G. W., van de Lagemaat, L. N., Redon, R., Strathdee, K. E., Croning, M. D., Malloy, M. P., . . . Grant, S. G. (2010). Confirmed rare copy number variants implicate novel genes in schizophrenia. *Biochemical Society Transactions*, *38*(2), 445–451. doi: 10.1042/BST0380445

van den Oord, E. J. (2005). Controlling false discoveries in candidate gene studies. *Molecular Psychiatry*, *10*(3), 230–231. doi: 10.1038/sj.mp.4001581

Visscher, P. M. (2008). Sizing up human height variation. *Nature Genetics*, *40*(5), 489–490. doi: 10.1038/ng0508-489

Wagle, J., Farner, L., Flekkoy, K., Wyller, T. B., Sandvik, L., Eiklid, K. L., . . . Engedal, K. (2009). Association between ApoE epsilon4 and cognitive impairment after stroke. *Dementia and Geriatric Cognitive Disorders*, *27*(6), 525–533. doi: 10.1159/000223230

9 Functional and Molecular Neuroimaging

Joseph H. Ricker and Patricia M. Arenth

Introduction

In conjunction with traditional physical examination and, in the case of neuropsychology, formal psychometric evaluation, functional brain imaging continues to advance the literature on the neural substrates of human cognition. This has resulted in exponential growth of the neuroimaging literature, and for increasing enthusiasm in the pursuit of clinical applications of these technologies. As with any technology or test (including psychometric tests), it important to always be mindful of what dependent variable is actually being measured, how reliably the dependent variable is being measured, and how valid any finding in an individual case might actually be in terms of clinical symptoms and functional outcome. This chapter will provide an overview of the major categories and types of functional imaging technologies that are likely to be encountered by clinical neuropsychologists in research and, to a more limited degree, clinical practice.

While the present authors recognize and acknowledge that virtually all of the imaging modalities to be discussed in this chapter are, rightly, classified as investigational for most clinical circumstances, it is also believed that having an appreciation of these technologies makes clinical neuropsychologists more informed consumers of research and the myriad (and, at times, speculative or even dubious) claims that are made for what various techniques add to clinical diagnosis and treatment.

Resting Versus Activated Functional Imaging Paradigms

Historically, functional imaging procedures could be grossly divided into two types of studies: "resting" studies and "activated" studies (Ricker, 2014). Resting neuroimaging paradigms acquire functional images during periods of no overt activity, such as might occur in a baseline condition, or when acquiring images while participants are quietly in the scanner with their eyes closed. There is no explicit or experimental requirement or consideration beyond what may be technically necessary to acquire a reliable set of images (Kilts & Ely, 2012). While participants in a resting condition have been explicitly instructed to not engage in any overt or covert activity, this represents more of an ideal scenario rather than what may be actually achieved. Indeed, it has been established through functional connectivity studies that the "resting" brain is actually quite "restless" (Raichle, 2015), in the sense that there are multiple brain networks that are active even when the brain is not task-engaged. There are numerous types of dependent variables that are examined in resting studies, such as cerebral blood flow (through single photon emission computed tomography, or SPECT; positron emission tomography, or PET; and certain magnetic resonance imaging, or MRI, applications); glucose uptake (using PET); or the detection of certain biomarkers, i.e., "molecular neuroimaging" (Price, 2012) using SPECT, PET or MRI-based techniques.

Activated imaging studies make use of explicit stimuli and/or activity in order to functionally "probe" regional brain activity during the processing of information or performance of a motor or cognitive task during a specified time period (Baribeau & Anagnostou, 2013). In a true experimental design, stimuli or tasks would be administered following a predetermined protocol. Such protocols will typically require some type of overt or objective response from the participant (Wilde, Hunter, & Bigler, 2012), although functional connectivity studies could be considered somewhat of an exception as these types of studies are evaluating networks of activation rather than specific focused areas of activation in response to overt stumli.

In view of the biophysical properties of the dependent variables investigated (e.g., briefer half-lives of radioisotopes, or transient changes in hemodynamic response), activation studies have much briefer windows for time sampling than resting studies. Certain imaging technologies can delineate changes in a continuous manner (e.g., event related functional magnetic resonance imaging, or fMRI, and magnetoencephalography). With this degree of experimental control, investigators are in a better position to infer the specific cerebral regions subserving the cognitive process under examination (Hutzler, 2014).

Radioisotope-Based Imaging

Single Photon Emission Computed Emission Tomography (SPECT)

SPECT is a functional imaging technology that derives from the concept that regional changes in cerebral activity or brain chemistry may be indirectly measured through the use of external gamma radiation detectors ("cameras") that identify localized accumulation of tracer flow or receptor-binding isotopes (Hutton, 2014). While most of the application of SPECT technology has been used to study regional cerebral blood flow (rCBF), characterization of some neuroreceptors or neurotransmitter systems can be accomplished with certain SPECT tracers (Palumbo et al., 2014).

rCBF has historically been studied as a primary dependent variable given the fact that, in most circumstances, increased regional cerebral activity is correlated with an increase in blood flow. In other words, when the relative activity of the brain increases, related energy utilization is also increased (Ingvar & Risberg, 1965). Thus, while blood flow is being reflected, actual neural activity is not directly measured. Radioisotopes employed in SPECT (and, for that matter, PET) are actually incorporated into the glia that are proximal to the active neurons. The absorbed radioisotopes are not immediately excreted from glia, thus allowing the isotopes to remain in greater concentration in the more active regions of the brain (Kim & Mountz, 2011). There are two main blood flow tracers that are used in SPECT: Tc-99m Hexamethylpropylene Amine Oxime (HMPAO) and Tc-99m Ethyl Cysteinate Dimer (ECD), which is better for high flow rates, such as seen in ictal states (Heiss, 2014). As the isotopes undergo normal radioactive decay, they emit annihilated radioactive particles (i.e., photons) that are then detected by external gamma cameras. Computerized reconstruction allows for characterization of isotope concentration within a spatial array (Takaki et al., 2009). This reconstruction may then be depicted graphically, often in the depiction of a brain map.

SPECT has some practical advantages over other neuroimaging technologies (Palumbo et al., 2014). For example, because the technology and technical requirements are not as extensive as those of PET or fMRI, it is generally more widely available. In addition, most of the radiotracers used for SPECT are sufficiently stable enough to be shipped rather than needing to be made per use using a cyclotron and thus necessitating the involvement of a radiochemist. In fact, the radioisotopes most commonly used in SPECT may be taken into by the brain within two minutes, but might have half-lives of several hours to days, giving SPECT an additional advantage over PET (Rahmim & Zaidi, 2008; Lin et al., 2012).

While brain SPECT is used primarily to examine resting cerebral blood flow or static biomarkers, the technology has some limited use in evaluating temporally linked changes in brain physiology. For example, SPECT is routinely used in the examination of pre-ictal, and ictal states (Kim & Mountz, 2011). SPECT may, in some highly controlled circumstances, be used to characterize physiological changes associated with circumscribed behavioral engagement and related inferred cognitive events (Ludwig, Chicherio, Terraneo, Magistretti, de Ribaupierre, & Slosman, 2008). That stated, the previously mentioned long half-lives of SPECT ligands have functional significance for imaging, such that once the tracer has been administered, the resulting images that are acquired will remain relatively static over the next several hours. As a result, SPECT would not be a good choice for the measurement of fluctuating changes such as those encountered in cognitive processes, where fMRI may be more advantageous (Ricker, Arenth, & Wagner 2013).

As is the case for any test (psychometric, physiological, or otherwise), measurement error is always present and must be seriously considered; SPECT is no different in this regard. In contrast to other technologies (for instance, PET), SPECT requires that regional counts be normalized to an anatomic area that is assumed to be free from injury and/or physiologic abnormality (Lin et al., 2012). While SPECT's resolution does not yet approach that of PET imaging, this concern has been attenuated somewhat with the increased availability of combined SPECT and computed tomography (CT) technology (Maebatake et al., 2014). Color SPECT image reconstruction can produce striking images, particularly when spatially rendered into three-dimensional "maps," but reliable and valid interpretation is best accomplished through quantitative approaches given the subjectivity and lack of standardization associated with interpreting three-dimensional images (Habert et al., 2011). It must be emphasized, however, that although SPECT can be used quantitatively, this is not the case in most settings. Visual inspection of SPECT maps is a qualitative process, and selection of regions of interest and interpretation may vary across clinicians or others viewing these images (Christen et al., 2013; Eo et al., 2014). In addition, image reconstruction is typically based on presumptions about which brain regions are "normal." Relative flow values in SPECT are often based upon a region such as the thalamus or cerebellum. While such assumptions might be valid for some populations with focal lesions (e.g., stroke), they might not be valid for populations whose involvement is more diffuse (Hagerstrom et al., 2012). SPECT is quite sensitive to detecting regional differences in resting blood flow, but there is little specificity to the patterns that are obtained and the results depicted in series of SPECT images can be affected by many factors, including acute or chronic emotional disturbances, medications, or current substance use (Granacher, 2008; Ricker, 2012).

SPECT is also objectively less sensitive than PET, with PET being considered to be two to three times more sensitive (Rahmim & Zaidi, 2008). SPECT radioligands emit single photons, rather than two diametrically opposed photons as in PET. In addition, only photons that are essentially parallel to the holes in the lead collimators used in SPECT will reach the detectors, thus filtering out much of the potential source of data (Dougherty, Rauch, & Rosenbaum, 2004; Ogawa & Ichimura, 2014). SPECT image quality may also be impacted by many factors beyond its inherent biophysical limitations (Sohlberg, Watabe, & Iida, 2008). Obviously, patient motion can affect image acquisition (Kyme, Hutton, Hatton, Skerrett, & Barnden, 2003), but motion effects are by no means restricted to the head, as movement of the extremities may result in changes in cerebral blood flow during SPECT scanning (Takekawa, Kakuda, Uchiyama, Ikegaya, & Abo, 2014). The patient's own biochemical status may also be a source of error. For example, caffeine and alcohol may impact cerebral blood flow, and sedating medications are known to impact SPECT tracer distribution (Juni et al., 2009).

Positron Emission Tomography

PET is another imaging technology that utilizes radioisotopes. The dependent variable of interest is usually glucose utilization (indexed by fluorodeoxyglucose uptake), although blood flow may also be assessed, particularly for activated imaging studies (Kudomi et al., 2013). Nitrogen (^{13}Nitrogen) and carbon (^{11}Carbon) are additional radionuclides that are used in PET. Various tracers that are specific to certain transmitter systems are also available (Billard, Le Bars, & Zimmer, 2014; Fuchigami, Nakayama, & Yoshida, 2015), as well as for specific cell types or cellular components (e.g., glia and myelin (Matthews & Datta, 2015). In resting PET studies, a radioisotope is injected peripherally into the bloodstream via a vehicle of intravenous saline. Brain regions of greater activity will take up proportionally greater amounts of glucose relative to less active brain regions, which leads to a greater concentration of protons relative to electrons (Nasrallah & Dubroff, 2013). This is depicted in Figure 9.1.

Unlike SPECT, the physics that underlie PET capitalize on the fact that the radioactive process involves results in the release of two diametrically opposed particles, known

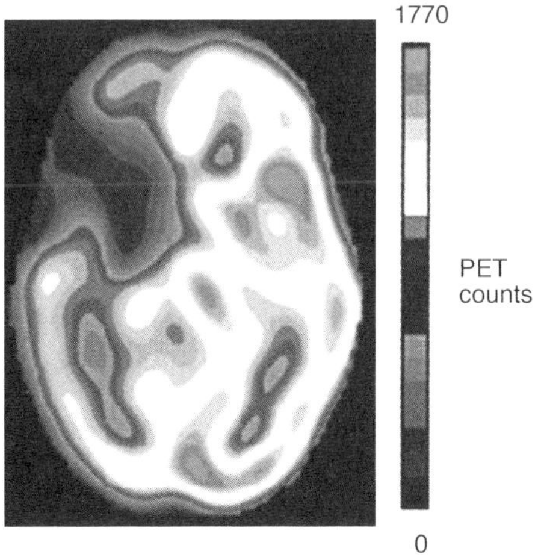

Figure 9.1 Oxygen-15 PET blood flow image of a patient with a left frontal stroke. Note decreased blood flow in the compromised region (depicted in blue). Adapted with permission from M. Corbetta and L. T. Connor (2006). Neurological recovery after stroke (p. 140). In M. D'Esposito (Ed.), Functional MRI: Applications in clinical neurology and psychiatry. Abingdon: Informa Healthcare. *A color version of this figure can be found in Plate section 1.*

as *photons* (Sossi, 2007). In PET, highly unstable radionuclides are injected into the participant. As the positrons from these radionuclides collide with electrons they annihilate each another, thus releasing radiation in the form of emitted photons, which are detected by a crystalline ring external to the head (Heiss, 2014). Both the location and level of photon release are subsequently calculated geometrically. Because there is a much larger array of crystalline detectors surrounding the head in PET (as contrasted with the holes within SPECT collimators), many more data points may be realized. Thus, PET provides a much richer data set for analysis and superior resolution than SPECT (Palumbo et al., 2014).

The half-life of the radioisotope used dictates the type of inferences that can be hypothesized regarding physiological activity during the scan. For example, the half-life of 18-FDG is several minutes, thus only very gross inferences can be made regarding an 18-FDG PET image and the underlying cognitive or motor activity. With oxygen-15, however, the half-life is two minutes, which permits briefer imaging periods and shorter wash-out periods between scans (Chugani, 2012). Thus, more reliable and valid inferences about cognitive or motor activity can be made, once, of course, one has introduced appropriate control conditions to account for general brain activation associated with task execution, such as button pressing, passive listening, ambient noise, and other factors that are controlled through cognitive subtraction analysis (Herrmann, Obleser, Kalberlah, Haynes, & Friederici, 2012).

A primary limitation of PET is that it remains a procedure with relatively limited availability, often only at academic medical centers or larger community hospitals. This is primarily because PET is a very expensive procedure, requiring an on-site chemist and, depending on the tracers needed, an on-site cyclotron (Wey, Desai, & Duong, 2013). Combined PET and CT systems (PET/CT) and magnetic resonance imaging (PET/MR) are now commercially available and are seeing use in nonacademic centers, but their use is typically more limited to very specific diagnostic questions, e.g., tumor characterization (Disselhorst, Bezrukov, Kolb, Parl, & Pichler, 2014; Shah et al., 2013).

Molecular Imaging With SPECT and PET

Receptor-specific binding agents can be radioactively labeled or "tagged," allowing for the characterization of regional concentrations of particular biochemicals—such as neuroreceptors, transporters, hormones, or enzymes—through the detection of the gamma particles that they emit (Kim & Mountz, 2011; Palumbo et al., 2014). Labeling neuroreceptors with radionuclides is by no means novel. The first approaches to molecular imaging actually developed in animal research through the process of receptor autoradiography, a process by which pharmacologic agents were radioactively tagged and introduced to the brains of animal subjects either in vivo through intravenous or direct intracerebral injection, or in vitro through direct application to brain specimens (Cherry, 2004). The brains were then sectioned and exposed directly to photographic emulsions, and the emitted radiation from specific receptor sites or other relevant brain regions resulted in photographic exposure and highly accurate depictions of localized concentrations of ligands. Obviously, such an approach cannot be applied to the living human brain, but by using external gamma-detecting cameras, as well as computerized spatial reconstruction, areas in which radiopharmaceuticals bound to high-affinity receptors can be accurately depicted using SPECT (although still not with a precision afforded by autoradiography or PET). Molecular imaging using PET is similar to that for SPECT, but with a larger variety of potential ligands available (Hutton, 2014), and, of course, greater anatomic and temporal resolution (Heiss, 2014; Price, 2012). There are many markers available that are specific to receptors and neurotransmitters (e.g., dopamine, serotonin) and drug classes (e.g., benzodiazepines, opioids). PET and SPECT markers have been developed for specific types of neuropathology, such as beta amyloid and tau, which have been subjected to much research in Alzheimer's dementia and are now receiving attention in the context of traumatic brain injury (Cohen & Klunk, 2014; Watanabe, Ono, & Saji, 2015).

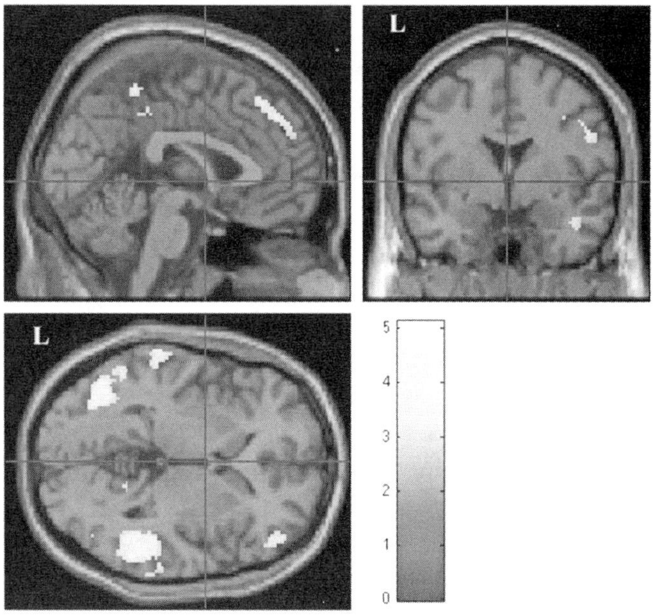

Figure 9.2 fMRI demonstrating regions of increased blood flow during a verbal list-learning task in persons with TBI. Adapted from Arenth, Russell, Scanlon, Kessler, and Ricker (2012). *A color version of this figure can be found in Plate section 1.*

Magnetic Resonance–Based Imaging

Overview and Biophysics

All MRI techniques capitalize on the presence of hydrogen in all of the body's tissues. When hydrogen atoms are placed in a strong magnetic field, their nuclei align in parallel to the field's direction. In MRI, radio frequency (RF) pulses are presented at a 90° angle relative to the magnetic field. When this occurs, the hydrogen nuclei realign and begin spinning in a different direction (a phenomenon referred to as *excitation*). When the RF pulse is then stopped, these nuclei return to their original alignment and direction of spin. The physical process of resuming previous nuclei states results in the emission of a minute electrical signal that can be detected by the scanner (Plewes & Kucharczyk, 2012). Although only approximately 1% of the hydrogen atoms in the magnetic field emit a response, this results in enough signal change to permit the acquisition of images. Given that most of the atoms that are excited in this process are found within water molecules, water content (and thus tissue density) dictate the signal intensity that is detectable by the scanner and ultimately digitally reconstructed into an image (Kim & Ogawa, 2012).

Functional Magnetic Resonance Imaging

In structural brain MRI, the primary goal is to generate high-resolution anatomic images of brain structure, but fMRI additionally allows the investigator to make inferences about regional changes in brain activity and to depict regions of activation or deactivation within the context of brain anatomy (see Figure 9.2).

As with other blood-flow related techniques, in fMRI specific tasks or stimuli are introduced to the individual while in the scanner in order to provoke a change in cerebral activity (Gaillard & Berl, 2012). When neural activity increases in a brain region, there is a related increase in blood flow to that region. While at rest, there is a tight correlation among rCBF) regional cerebral metabolic rate for glucose (rCMRglc) and regional cerebral metabolic rate for oxygen ($rCMRO^2$). When a brain region becomes active, however, rCBF may increase by more than 50%, which greatly exceeds metabolic demands. The physiologic basis for this is not clear, however (Nagaoka et al., 2006). With an excess of blood flow to the region and only a minimal increase in oxygen extraction, there results a localized abundance of oxyhemoglobin relative to deoxyhemoglobin in the venous and capillary beds that perfuse active regions of cortex. Oxyhemoglobin is naturally diamagnetic, while deoxyhemoglobin is paramagnetic (i.e., becomes readily magnetized within a magnetic field). This results in an increase in signal intensity that can be detected externally, and is represented as higher signal intensity on T2* ("T2-star") weighted scans. This change in signal intensity referred to as the blood oxygen level dependent (BOLD) effect (Kim & Ogawa, 2012). The signal changes obtained are very small, on the order of 1% to 6%, and occur over approximately a 2 to 6 second time frame, depending on brain region, tasks being performed, and the participant's age, among other factors (Simon & Buxton, 2015).

An additional technique known as arterial spin labeling (ASL) may be used in conjunction with fMRI. ASL is a noninvasive approach to characterizing cerebral blood flow by using biophysical "labeling" to provide an endogenous "contrast agent." Through ASL, a secondary pulse sequence is applied distal from the brain (e.g., at the level of the neck). This alters that area's blood's molecular spin and effectively "labels" that blood so that, upon reaching the brain, the difference in spin can be detected by the head coil and compared to the brain's own magnetic signal both before and after labeling, thus permitting direct inferences about brain perfusion (Aguirre & Detre, 2012).

Because fMRI utilizes the body's natural physical responses to high-strength magnetism, no exogenous tracers, radioisotopes, or contrast agents are necessary, and the anatomic resolution of fMRI is superior to that of SPECT or PET (Disselhorst et al., 2014). There are numerous activation paradigms that can be carried out in fMRI, and it allows for greater flexibility in paradigm with reference to repeatability and brevity of overall session (Kilts & Ely, 2012). In fMRI scanners of typical magnet strength (e.g., 1.5 Tesla), the signal changes that appear emanate from veins and large venules. In high-field magnets (e.g., 3 or 4 Tesla or higher), signal change in nonclinical populations is more likely obtained from microvessels, small venules, and capillaries (Buxton, 2013).

There are many technical considerations with regard to fMRI data acquisition and interpretation. Overt responses to tasks must be minimal at most. Movements of the jaw required for conversational speech are considered too excessive during fMRI, although some paradigms do allow for some degree of overt verbal responding (Gracco, Tremblay, & Pike, 2005), and the use of silent intervals within block designs allows for the use of fMRI to study the brain substrates of speech production (Berken et al., 2015). The normal high-frequency noise emitted by the scanner must be considered. The technician must also monitor the participant for idiosyncratic responses such as claustrophobia (Munn & Jordan, 2013). Most clinicians will know that any MRI-based technology presents safety issues in terms of obvious ferromagnetic objects and devices such as pacemakers, surgical clips, and other implanted devices, but image reconstruction artifacts and even misinterpretation may result from less obvious factors such as makeup, tattoos, or certain types of clothing (Krupa & Bekiesinska-Figatowska, 2015). Although virtually any contemporary MRI scanner can be adapted to functional imaging, fMRI is still investigational in most clinical populations with whom clinical neuropsychologists are likely to work (American College of Radiology, 2015), and is thus primarily a research tool at this time, mostly, though not exclusively, limited to academic medical centers, universities, and biomedical research centers.

A single fMRI session does not automatically generate clinically useable brain maps, although semi-automated techniques have been developed (Karmonik et al., 2010). The resulting images must be carefully and skillfully reconstructed, and this reconstruction process could still be considered to be as much art as science. As with all imaging technologies, the approach that one takes (and the hypotheses that one holds) in reconstructing and displaying the data in the form of brain images data will impact the portrayal and interpretation of the end product.

fMRI has been used as a research tool in humans for well over 20 years, with the first studies appearing in 1992. Yet, there have been essentially no routine clinical applications of fMRI outside of its use in presurgical mapping for epilepsy surgeries and tumor resections (Greicius, 2008; Ricker, 2014). There are many technical limitations that contribute to this poor clinical representation (e.g., poor signal-to-noise ratio of fMRI, and difficulties when applying findings derived from group data to individual cases), but another major contributor is also the necessary engagement and reliable execution of the experimental cognitive or motor task being administered. This may prove to be challenging for some patient populations and essentially limits most clinical generalizations to higher functioning patients.

Functional Connectivity Magnetic Resonance Imaging

While fMRI studies require an active administration of a stimulus or cognitive paradigm, with varying degrees of participant response or input, resting-state connectivity studies offer an opportunity to study the brain's functional connectivity without participants having to engage in prolonged, repetitive tasks during the scanning procedure. First, during "traditional" fMRI, the participant must be fully engaged in putting forth a good effort. As is the case with traditional psychometric testing, full effort during cognitive tasks in the scanner is imperative. Second, there is a relationship between task difficulty and cognitive activation. Greater levels of task difficulty usually result in more neural activation during cognitive task blocks, but if the task is too difficult a participant may become overwhelmed or simply disengage from the task, thus causing activation levels to return to a resting baseline level. These limitations can be partially mitigated through the use of fMRI during the resting state (Ricker, 2013).

Huettel and colleagues (Huettel, Song, & McCarthy, 2014) define functional connectivity as a "pattern of functional relationships among regions, inferred from common changes in activation over time, that may reflect direct or indirect links between those regions" (p. 293). The analyses used in functional connectivity studies are comprised of cross-correlations among activity concourses within separate brain regions, for which one assumes a priori functional relationships.

Resting-state studies are presently the most commonly used in functional connectivity MRI (fcMRI), but functional connectivity analyses may also be accomplished during cognitive tasks. There are two broad methodological approaches for examining resting-state fMRI data (Peterson, Thome, Frewen, & Lanius, 2014). The first approach is to examine how resting-state configurations may affect functional connectivity. This involves comparing long periods of rest (rest blocks) with rest blocks that alternate with cognitive tasks. Event-related designs may also be applied in which activity is elicited through short but continuous events rather than in blocks. The second major fcMRI approach is voxel-based and emphasizes comparisons among the regions of interest. This requires a greater degree of a priori selection of brain regions to be studied during resting the fMRI periods. The first studies of functional connectivity often examined only functional interrelations, and did not really concern themselves with structural connectivity or anatomic explanations for the functional relationships (Medaglia, Lynall, & Bassett, 2015). At present, however, several reliable functionally connected cerebral networks have been identified through fcMRI, three of which are likely to be of greatest interest and relevance to clinical neuropsychologists.

The first, and most frequently studied to date, is the default mode network (DMN). The DMN represents a broad network of cerebral areas thought to result in an interrelated system of self-referential cognitive activities, such as self-monitoring, autobiographical processing, and social functions (Whitfield-Gabrieli & Ford, 2012). The DMN is comprised of the medial prefrontal cortex, retrosplenial neocortex (i.e., posterior cingulate and precuneus), and the inferior parietal lobes, bilaterally (Peeters et al., 2015). The DMN demonstrates its most prominent activity during passive rest (Hsu, Broyd, Helps, Benikos, & Sonuga-Barke, 2013), but it is active during some higher-level reflective tests that tap prospective thinking, accessing of autobiographical memory, and activities associated with making inferences about the mental states of others, in others words, the "theory of mind" (Dunbar, 2012).

Second, a specific central executive network has been characterized through use of functional connectivity investigations. The central executive network spans dorsolateral prefrontal cortex and the posterior parietal lobes (Chen et al., 2013). In general, it underlies externally driven and cognitive demanding mental activities, and its associated cognitive operations include executive control and working memory (Shaw, Schultz, Sperling, & Hedden, 2015).

Third, the salience network, comprised of the anterior insula and anterior cingulate, mediates dynamic switching between the DMN and the central executive network and thus functions to mediate attention between endogenous and exogenous events (Kiverstein & Miller, 2015).

While seemingly more straightforward and to a large degree, less demanding in terms of study design (i.e., investigators do not need to develop reliable cognitive paradigms that work within the constraints imposed by conventional fMRI, fcMRI is not without its own challenges and limitations. For example, even subtle motion during fcMRI may result in spurious signal perturbations that might be erroneously interpreted as having significance relative to the construct being studied (Power, Schlaggar, & Petersen, 2015).

Molecular Imaging With MRI

Magnetic resonance spectroscopy (MRS) is an MR-based technique that offers the capacity to localize and characterize brain-based biomarkers. As an MR-based technology, it is based on the same biophysics as MRI, fMRI, and fcMRI. It differs, however, in that it derives its signal not only from water-bound or lipid-bound hydrogen, but is also capable of localizing other endogenous biomaterials based on their own unique signal waveform properties (Cecil, 2013).

MRS is capable of differentiating the unique magnetic profiles of biomarkers markers such as glutamate (Glu), creatine or phosphocreatine (Cre), n-acetyl aspartate (NAA), and choline (Cho) related compounds (Bertholdo, Watcharakorn, & Castillo, 2013). Each biomarker possesses different numbers of electrons in its nuclei, and the greater the number of electrons, the greater the local reduction within the magnetic field, resulting in a reduced spectral peak (Dale, Brown & Semelka, 2015). This allows for the localization and quantification of biomarkers in space, although MRS data are usually represented as spectral waveforms rather than topographic brain maps commonly depicted in other neuroimaging modalities.

Sodium MR imaging is an MRI-based molecular imaging technique that reflects sodium homeostasis, and is therefore considered to be an index of cellular viability (Price, 2012). Sodium ion homeostasis is lost when cells die in the brain (Boada et al., 2005). Sodium MRI is similar to MR spectroscopy in the sense that it yields metabolic information, but because it focuses solely on the resonance of one biomarker (i.e., sodium), pulse sequences may be acquired at much higher resolution (Ouwerkerk, 2011). Several critical processes at the cellular level depend on a balance of high extracellular and low intracellular sodium content, but many conditions (e.g., ischemia, injury, neoplasm) may lead to an increase in intracellular sodium, thus making sodium a potential biomarker for pathology or response to treatment (Madelin, Kline, Walvick, & Regatte, 2014).

Electrophysiological Brain Mapping Techniques

Quantitative Electroencephalography

Electroencephalography (EEG) is electrophysiologically based technology that is used to monitor gross brain electrical activity, such as normal neuronal firing and seizure activity. Traditional EEG output does not, however, permit characterization of the wave frequency continua that occur in a human brain. But, when Fourier transformation analyses are applied to EEG, continuous monitoring and quantification across cerebral wave frequencies may be achieved. This approach to data transformation is referred to as *quantitative EEG* (QEEG; see Haneef, Levin, Frost, & Mizrahi, 2013).

QEEG is an general term applied to a group of interrelated technologies that derive from a mathematical approach referred to as spectral analysis (Billeci et al., 2013). Basically, the EEG signal is digitally processed and the relative contributions of each frequency are identified and quantified. When digitized, the individual component frequencies of a complex waveform (i.e., the amounts of alpha, beta, delta, and theta activity contained within the signal) may be discerned in a manner superior to that of traditional visual analysis of EEG printed output (Trambaiolli et al., 2011).

There are various approaches for portraying spectral data from QEEG. In a compressed spectral array format, frequencies within specified time blocks (e.g., 30 seconds) are quantified. The output is then represented sequentially either in print or graphically, permitting interpretation of changes in the EEG signal over time (Williamson, Wahlster, Shafi, & Westover, 2014).

A common approach is to display QEEG spectra in the form of topographical maps. In this format, each electrode in the EEG montage is assigned a color or gray value representing each frequency range, with the shading or color intensity representing the frequency level that underlies the corresponding electrode. The shading or color gradient is subsequently superimposed on a head-shaped or brain-shaped oval. The resulting brain map thus resembles (somewhat) the topographical maps generated by a resting SPECT or PET scan. It needs to be understood, however, that a QEEG topographic map is really derived from a rather minimal number of solely cortical data points, and has numerous interpolated color values—specifically, all of the shades or colors between electrodes are actually interpolated (Kamarajan & Porjesz, 2015).

Another approach to depicting QEEG data is through probability mapping. This approach utilizes a topographic map as its basis, but then maps to a normative database (the "composite map"). An individual's map may then be statistically compared to the normative map, and inferences are made based on deviation from the normal distribution (Trimble & George, 2010).

Magnetoencephalography (MEG)

Neuronal activity generates minute magnetic fields, which may be detected through a technology referred to as *magnetoencephalography* (MEG). The physiological basis of MEG derives from normal neuronal membrane signal conduction. When a neuronal synapse becomes active, there is a current flow across the neural membrane. This current diffuses intracellularly, and subsequently emerges extracellularly at a consistent distance from where it began, i.e., from dendrite to synapse. This yields extracellular *sources* and *sinks*. In a neuron that is oriented asymmetrically in space, the sources and sinks create dipolar electromagnetic fields that cancel out one another and signals may be localized (Slater, Khan, Li, & Castillo, 2012). The intracellular current between the area of synapse activity and the area at where the current returns to extracellular space does not cancel out, which results in a change in the magnetic field that may can be externally recorded (Owen, Sekihara, & Nagarajan, 2012).

MEG uses an array of electromagnetic conducting coils placed around a person's head to detect changes in neuronal activity. Each coil is cooled by liquid helium to a temperature of almost absolute zero. Such super-cooling greatly dampens the electrical resistance of the conductor, which allows very small magnetic field changes to be detected The field changes are, however, still quite minute, and must be amplified through the use of what are known as superconducting quantum-interference devices (SQUIDs; see Schneiderman, 2014). A MEG scanner differs somewhat in configuration from other scanning devices such as those for SPECT and PET, allowing participants to be seated upright during scanned (as shown in Figure 9.3).

Although intuitively similar to EEG, MEG has several advantages. MEG frequencies are actually simpler to record than those from EEG, given that the detectors are placed in a helmet adjacent to the scalp and do not have to be individually applied and interconnected. Magnetic fields are also not affected by the variability in skull thickness over different regions of cortex. That said, however, there are some disadvantages to MEG. For example, it is not widely available and the physical facilities that must be specially constructed to support it are very expensive. In addition, MEG, similar to EEG, lacks the anatomic precision of other neuroimaging techniques and does not localize subcortical activity sources (Wilde et al., 2015).

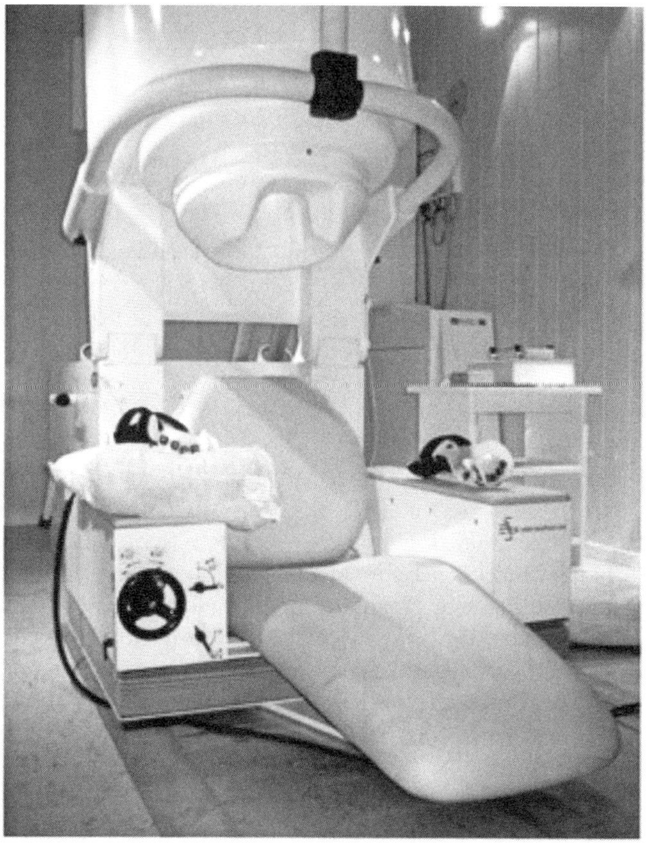

Figure 9.3 A MEG scanner. Note that the configuration allows for upright seating of the person being scanned. Reproduced with permission, from J. Ward (2015). *The student's guide to cognitive neuroscience,* 3rd edition (p. 46). East Sussex: Taylor & Francis.

Other Technologies

Optical (Near-Infrared) Imaging

The category of optical imaging techniques includes those that derive from the biophysical principles of light absorption and reflectance. Of interest for human brain imaging is the application of near-infrared spectroscopy. The near-infrared light spectrum includes the range of nonionizing (and, thus, not harmful to living tissue) electromagnetic radiation with wavelengths between 700 and 1,000 nm. Similarly to fMRI, functional near-infrared spectroscopy (fNIRS) characterizes changes in the ratio of oxyhemoglobin to deoxyhemoglobin, which, in addition to having differing magnetic properties, also have differing light-absorption properties (Arenth, Ricker, & Schultheis, 2007)

When used as a neuroimaging modality, fNIRS requires the placement of light emitting diodes (LEDs) and detectors directly against a person's scalp. FNIRS measures many of the same physiological parameters as fMRI and O-15 PET, but also has possesses some unique advantages over these techniques (Amyot et al., 2015). FNIRS is noninvasive, has no ionizing radiation, and does not require the use of high-field magnetization, thus making it essentially risk-free. FNIRS has the unique advantage of being quite portable and mostly unaffected by subject movement.

Functional Transcranial Doppler Ultrasonography

Transcranial Doppler (TCD) is used to depict blood flow within intracerebral arteries through the application of Doppler ultrasound technology. Ultrasound is capable of reflecting changes in blood flow through the placement of a sound source and receiver at the same location. The ultrasound beam that is projected into the skull is reflected back by blood cells that flow through the vessel that intersects the sound wave (Naqvi, Yap, Ahmad, & Ghosh, 2013).

Because sound does not travel well through bone, the ultrasound source must be placed against a thin or accessible skull region, referred to as an acoustic "window." The most common window for cognitive studies is the temporal window, which is located in the squamous region of the temporal bone. Additional windows include the transorbital, submandibular, and suboccipital windows (Kristiansson et al., 2013).

The data are initially represented as waveforms that reflect blood flow velocity, but are often subsequently portrayed using spectral analysis methods similar to those described above for QEEG. TCD has many positive features as an imaging modality. As is the case with near-infrared spectroscopy, TCD is noninvasive, emits no ionizing radiation, does not require a high-field magnet, is inexpensive, and is highly portable. Notably, however, TCD's spatial resolution is quite limited given that it is able to cover a very small number of cerebral regions (Purkayastha & Sorond, 2012).

Methodological Considerations in Clinical Interpretation

For the most part, most functional imaging technologies remain tools of research as this volume goes to press. But, there is increasing clinical use of some of these technologies in limited forms of differential diagnosis (e.g., vascular cognitive impairment vs. a primary progressive dementia), and functional imaging appears as evidence in forensic cases with increasing frequency (often in the absence of any scientific support for its application in the injury, illness, or defense in question). It is therefore important that clinical neuropsychologists consider several general methodological issues that are relevant to essentially all functional neuroimaging modalities and clinical syndromes.

Injury and Illness Characteristics

The impact of changes to brain morphology on image reconstruction must be considered. Functional imaging data from a brain that has been altered anatomically by surgery (e.g., resection of a tumor or lobe), injury (e.g., massive contusion), or disease process (e.g., progressive atrophy or an infarction) must be normalized, analyzed, and depicted carefully in order for regions of activation and deactivation to be represented in a reliable and valid manner (Ashburner & Friston, 2005).

Different image acquisition platforms (e.g., General Electric, Philips, Siemens) and image analysis and reconstruction software (e.g., AFNI, Brain Voyager, Statistical Parametric Mapping, or one of the numerous lab-specific specialized programs), may yield somewhat different findings across anatomic localization or activation intensity (Poldrack, Mumford, & Nichols, 2011).

Comorbid conditions, peripheral injuries, and pain can alter brain activation patterns independently of any relationship to actual brain status cognition, thus it is important to take into account a person's entire medical and physical status (which includes past and current medication and substance use) before making inferences and drawing conclusions from functional neuroimaging data. As just one example, sleep disorders—which are frequently encountered comorbidly (and premorbidly) in neuropsychological populations—are associated with differences in functional (De Havas, Parimal, Soon, & Chee, 2012) and even structural (Castronovo et al., 2014) neuroimaging findings, even in the absence of a primary neurological condition or injury.

There has been much debate in the functional imaging literature as to test-retest reliability and the nature of change (Aron, Gluck, & Poldrack, 2006) (Freyer et al., 2009), and functional imaging findings are often cited to support hypotheses about change in cognitive or brain status (e.g., as evidence of "decline," "improvement," "reorganization," etc.). Such inferences have no logical or empirical basis unless there have been are two or more sessions of imaging data acquired, thus making the way one operationalizes "change" as critical if one is using functional imaging to support such hypotheses. Furthermore, signal changes that are observed in the population of interest in a single study may actually represent a more general response to neurological disruption rather than a change that is specific to one clinical population (Hillary et al., 2015).

Conclusions and Future Directions

Functional neuroimaging has seen increased use in the study of cognitive and emotional functioning, and has changed many ways that brain-behavior relationships are conceptualized. While these technologies are intuitively appealing, it should be noted that virtually all of the types discussed in this chapter are classified as investigational for most clinical uses. Until much more benchmarking research is conducted, and numerous technical, methodological, and biophysical issues have been addressed, most functional neuroimaging technologies remain primarily research tools.

Interpretation of functional imaging examination results should vary in a reliable and predictable manner in relation to severity or degree of functional impairment. For example, it is counterintuitive—and scientifically unsupported—for imaging findings in a person, or sample of persons, with mild TBI to be interpreted as demonstrating greater pathology or dysfunction than would be expected using the same imaging procedure in a more severely injured person or sample. And, as scientifically trained psychologists first and foremost, clinical neuropsychologists should be able to readily appreciate that a "difference" or "change" cannot be not reflexively equated with pathology, dysfunction, or disability. The clinical utility of a given functional imaging tool may appear "self-evident" to some, but the evidence base has yet to be adequately established for the vast majority of populations likely to be evaluated and treated by clinical neuropsychologists (American College of Radiology Appropriateness Criteria, 2015; Ryan et al., 2014; Shetty et al., 2016). While often visually striking, functional imaging reconstructions must not be seen as literal "pictures" of brain status (Ward, 2015).

None of this should be misconstrued as taking a negative position; rather, it is a scientific and ultimately optimistic one. As existing approaches are deployed increasingly in clinical populations, and as even newer approaches such as optogenetic (Lu et al., 2015) and photoacoustic (Yao et al., 2015) imaging are eventually translated into humans, functional neuroimaging will eventually likely be a common adjunct to traditional assessment and intervention. For example, as reviewed recently (Ricker, DeLuca, & Frey, 2014), contemporary functional neuroimaging technologies have several potential applications to neurological populations. First, functional imaging could be used to evaluate the efficacy of behavioral or pharmacological interventions by potentially providing objective demonstration of long-term changes at the cerebral level. Second, functional imaging might eventually be used as a primary assessment tool in and of itself. For example, once neurofunctional correlates (i.e., "markers") of specific cognitive impairments have been established, it may be possible to compare an individual's performance to that of large samples with a known disease or impairment. Finally, functional imaging may eventually be used as an additional clinical prognostic tool, either in isolation, or preferably, in conjunction with other biomarkers and objective neuropsychological data. For example, if after an intervention patients do not show any impact at the cerebral level, and this is corroborated by lack of change at a behavioral level, future strategies and planning might be directed toward compensating for permanent deficits. Ultimately, it appears likely that the future holds promise for the integration of functional neuroimaging as a complement to the practice of clinical neuropsychology.

Acknowledgements

This work was supported, in part, by NIH grants K23-HD049626–01 (Arenth), R01-NS048178–01 (Ricker), and R01-NS049142–01 (Ricker).

References

Aguirre, G. K., & Detre, J. A. (2012). The development and future of perfusion fMRI for dynamic imaging of human brain activity. *Neuroimage*, *62*(2), 1279–1285. doi: 10.1016/j.neuroimage.2012.04.039

American College of Radiology Appropriateness Criteria. (2015). Retrieved from American College of Radiology website https://acsearch.acr.org/list

Amyot, F., Arciniegas, D. B., Brazaitis, M. P., Curley, K. C., Diaz-Arrastia, R., Gandjbakhche, A., . . . Stocker, D. (2015). A review of the effectiveness of neuroimaging modalities for the detection of traumatic brain injury. *Journal ofNeurotrauma*, *32*(22), 1693–1721. doi: 10.1089/neu.2013.3306

Arenth, P. M., Ricker, J. H., & Schultheis, M. T. (2007). Applications of functional near-infrared spectroscopy (fNIRS) to Neurorehabilitation of cognitive disabilities. *Clinical Neuropsychologist*, *21*(1), 38–57. doi: 10.1080/13854040600878785

Arenth, P. M., Russell, K. C., Scanlon, J. M., Kessler, L. J., & Ricker, J. H. (2012). Encoding and recognition after traumatic brain injury: Neuropsychological and functional magnetic resonance imaging findings. *Journal of Clinical & Experimental Neuropsychology*, *34*(4), 333–344.

Aron, A. R., Gluck, M. A., & Poldrack, R. A. (2006). Long-term test-retest reliability of functional MRI in a classification learning task. *Neuroimage*, *29*(3), 1000–1006. doi: 10.1016/j.neuroimage.2005.08.010

Ashburner, J., & Friston, K. J. (2005). Unified segmentation. *Neuroimage*, *26*(3), 839–851. doi: 10.1016/j.neuroimage.2005.02.018

Baribeau, D. A., & Anagnostou, E. (2013). A comparison of neuroimaging findings in childhood onset schizophrenia and autism spectrum disorder: A review of the literature. *Front Psychiatry*, *4*, 175. doi: 10.3389/fpsyt.2013.00175

Berken, J. A., Gracco, V. L., Chen, J. K., Watkins, K. E., Baum, S., Callahan, M., & Klein, D. (2015). Neural activation in speech production and reading aloud in native and non-native languages. *Neuroimage*, *112*, 208–217. doi: 10.1016/j.neuroimage.2015.03.016

Bertholdo, D., Watcharakorn, A., & Castillo, M. (2013). Brain proton magnetic resonance spectroscopy: Introduction and overview. *Neuroimaging Clinics of North America*, *23*(3), 359–380. doi: 10.1016/j.nic.2012.10.002

Billard, T., Le Bars, D., & Zimmer, L. (2014). PET radiotracers for molecular imaging of serotonin 5-HT1A receptors. *Current Medicinal Chemistry*, *21*(1), 70–81.

Billeci, L., Sicca, F., Maharatna, K., Apicella, F., Narzisi, A., Campatelli, G., . . . Muratori, F. (2013). On the application of quantitative EEG for characterizing autistic brain: A systematic review. *Frontiers in Human Neuroscience*, *7*, 442. doi: 10.3389/fnhum.2013.00442

Boada, F. E., LaVerde, G., Jungreis, C., Nemoto, E., Tanase, C., & Hancu, I. (2005). Loss of cell ion homeostasis and cell viability in the brain: What sodium MRI can tell us. *Current Topics in Developmental Biology*, *70*, 77–101. doi: 10.1016/S0070-2153(05)70004-1

Buxton, R. B. (2013). The physics of functional magnetic resonance imaging (fMRI). *Reports on Progress in Physics: Physical Chemistry*, *76*(9), 096601. doi: 10.1088/0034-4885/76/9/096601

Castronovo, V., Scifo, P., Castellano, A., Aloia, M. S., Iadanza, A., Marelli, S., . . . Falini, A. (2014). White matter integrity in obstructive sleep apnea before and after treatment. *Sleep*, *37*(9), 1465–1475. doi: 10.5665/sleep.3994

Cecil, K. M. (2013). Proton magnetic resonance spectroscopy: Technique for the neuroradiologist. *Neuroimaging Clinics of North America*, *23*(3), 381–392. doi: 10.1016/j.nic.2012.10.003

Chen, A. C., Oathes, D. J., Chang, C., Bradley, T., Zhou, Z. W., Williams, L. M., . . . Etkin, A. (2013). Causal interactions between fronto-parietal central executive and default-mode networks in humans. *Proceedings of the National Academy of Sciences U S A*, *110*(49), 19944–19949. doi: 10.1073/pnas.1311772110

Cherry, S. R. (2004). In vivo molecular and genomic imaging: New challenges for imaging physics. *Physics in Medicine and Biology*, *49*(3), R13–R48.

Christen, M., Vitacco, D. A., Huber, L., Harboe, J., Fabrikant, S. I., & Brugger, P. (2013). Colorful brains: 14 years of display practice in functional neuroimaging. *Neuroimage*, *73*, 30–39. doi: 10.1016/j.neuroimage.2013.01.068

Chugani, D. C. (2012). Neuroimaging and neurochemistry of autism. *Pediatric Clinics of North America*, *59*(1), 63–73, x. doi: 10.1016/j.pcl.2011.10.002

Cohen, A. D., & Klunk, W. E. (2014). Early detection of Alzheimer's disease using PiB and FDG PET. *Neurobiology of Disease*, *72*(Part A), 117–122. doi: 10.1016/j.nbd.2014.05.001

Dale, B. M., Brown, M. A., & Semelka, R. (2015). *MRI: Basic Principles and Applications* (5th ed.). New York: Wiley-Blackwell.

De Havas, J. A., Parimal, S., Soon, C. S., & Chee, M. W. (2012). Sleep deprivation reduces default mode network connectivity and anti-correlation during rest and task performance. *Neuroimage*, *59*(2), 1745–1751. doi: 10.1016/j.neuroimage.2011.08.026

Disselhorst, J. A., Bezrukov, I., Kolb, A., Parl, C., & Pichler, B. J. (2014). Principles of PET/MR imaging. *Journal of Nuclear Medicine*, *55*(Suppl 2), 2S–10S. doi: 10.2967/jnumed.113.129098

Dougherty, D. D., Rauch, S. L., & Rosenbaum, J. F. (2004). *Essentials of Neuroimaging for Clinical Practice*. Washington, DC: American Psychiatric Publishing.

Dunbar, R. I. (2012). The social brain meets neuroimaging. *Trends in Cognitive Sciences*, *16*(2), 101–102. doi: 10.1016/j.tics.2011.11.013

Eo, J. S., Lee, H. Y., Lee, J. S., Kim, Y. K., Jeon, B. S., & Lee, D. S. (2014). Automated analysis of (123)I-beta-CIT SPECT images with statistical probabilistic anatomical mapping. *Nuclear Medicine & Molecular Imaging*, *48*(1), 47–54. doi: 10.1007/s13139-013-0241-5

Freyer, T., Valerius, G., Kuelz, A. K., Speck, O., Glauche, V., Hull, M., & Voderholzer, U. (2009). Test-retest reliability of event-related functional MRI in a probabilistic reversal learning task. *Psychiatry Research*, *174*(1), 40–46. doi: 10.1016/j.pscychresns.2009.03.003

Fuchigami, T., Nakayama, M., & Yoshida, S. (2015). Development of PET and SPECT probes for glutamate receptors. *Scientific World Journal*, *2015*, 716514. doi: 10.1155/2015/716514

Gaillard, W. D., & Berl, M. M. (2012). Functional magnetic resonance imaging: Functional mapping. *Handbook of Clinical Neurology*, *107*, 387–398. doi: 10.1016/B978-0-444-52898-8.00024-0

Gracco, V. L., Tremblay, P., & Pike, B. (2005). Imaging speech production using fMRI. *Neuroimage*, *26*(1), 294–301. doi: 10.1016/j.neuroimage.2005.01.033

Granacher, R. P., Jr. (2008). Commentary: Applications of functional neuroimaging to civil litigation of mild traumatic brain injury. *Journal of the American Academy of Psychiatry and Law*, *36*(3), 323–328.

Greicius, M. (2008). Resting-state functional connectivity in neuropsychiatric disorders. *Current Opinion in Neurology*, *21*(4), 424–430. doi: 10.1097/WCO.0b013e328306f2c5

Habert, M. O., Horn, J. F., Sarazin, M., Lotterie, J. A., Puel, M., Onen, F., . . . Dubois, B. (2011). Brain perfusion SPECT with an automated quantitative tool can identify prodromal Alzheimer's disease among patients with mild cognitive impairment. *Neurobiology of Aging*, *32*(1), 15–23. doi: 10.1016/j.neurobiolaging.2009.01.013

Hagerstrom, D., Jakobsson, D., Stomrud, E., Andersson, A. M., Ryding, E., Londos, E., . . . Edenbrandt, L. (2012). A new automated method for analysis of rCBF-SPECT images based on the active-shape algorithm: Normal values. *Clinical Physiology and Functional Imaging*, *32*(2), 114–119. doi: 10.1111/j.1475-097X.2011.01063.x

Haneef, Z., Levin, H. S., Frost, J. D., Jr., & Mizrahi, E. M. (2013). Electroencephalography and quantitative electroencephalography in mild traumatic brain injury. *Journal of Neurotrauma*, *30*(8), 653–656. doi: 10.1089/neu.2012.2585

Heiss, W. D. (2014). Radionuclide imaging in ischemic stroke. *Journal of Nuclear Medicine*, *55*(11), 1831–1841. doi: 10.2967/jnumed.114.145003

Herrmann, B., Obleser, J., Kalberlah, C., Haynes, J. D., & Friederici, A. D. (2012). Dissociable neural imprints of perception and grammar in auditory functional imaging. *Human Brain Mapping*, *33*(3), 584–595. doi: 10.1002/hbm.21235

Hillary, F. G., Roman, C. A., Venkatesan, U., Rajtmajer, S. M., Bajo, R., & Castellanos, N. D. (2015). Hyperconnectivity is a fundamental response to neurological disruption. *Neuropsychology*, *29*(1), 59–75. doi: 10.1037/neu0000110

Hsu, C. F., Broyd, S. J., Helps, S. K., Benikos, N., & Sonuga-Barke, E. J. (2013). "Can waiting awaken the resting brain?" A comparison of waiting- and cognitive task-induced attenuation of very low frequency neural oscillations. *Brain Research, 1524*, 34–43. doi: 10.1016/j.brainres.2013.05.043

Huettel, S. A., Song, A. W., & McCarthy, G. (2014). *Functional Magnetic Resonance Imaging* (3rd ed.). Sunderland, MA: Sinauer Associates.

Hutton, B. F. (2014). The origins of SPECT and SPECT/CT. *European Journal of Nuclear Medicine and Molecular Imaging, 41*(Suppl 1), S3–S16. doi: 10.1007/s00259-013-2606-5

Hutzler, F. (2014). Reverse inference is not a fallacy per se: Cognitive processes can be inferred from functional imaging data. *Neuroimage, 84*, 1061–1069. doi: 10.1016/j.neuroimage.2012.12.075

Ingvar, D. H., & Risberg, J. (1965). Influence of mental activity upon regional cerebral blood flow in man: A preliminary study. *Acta Neurologica Scandinavica, 14*, 183–186.

Juni, J. E., Waxman, A. D., Devous, M. D., Sr., Tikofsky, R. S., Ichise, M., Van Heertum, R. L., . . . Society for Nuclear, M. (2009). Procedure guideline for brain perfusion SPECT using (99m)Tc radiopharmaceuticals 3.0. *Journal of Nuclear Medicine Technology, 37*(3), 191–195. doi: 10.2967/jnmt.109.067850

Kamarajan, C., & Porjesz, B. (2015). Advances in electrophysiological research. *Alcohol Research, 37*(1), 53–87.

Karmonik, C., York, M., Grossman, R., Kakkar, E., Patel, K., Haykal, H., & King, D. (2010). An image analysis pipeline for the semi-automated analysis of clinical fMRI images based on freely available software. *Computers in Biology and Medicine, 40*(3), 279–287. doi: 10.1016/j.compbiomed.2009.12.003

Kilts, C., & Ely, T. D. (2012). Human functional neuroimaging. *Handbook of Clinical Neurology, 106*, 97–105. doi: 10.1016/B978-0-444-52002-9.00007-3

Kim, S., & Mountz, J. M. (2011). SPECT imaging of epilepsy: An overview and comparison with F-18 FDG PET. *International Journal of Molecular Imaging, 2011*, 813028. doi: 10.1155/2011/813028

Kim, S. G., & Ogawa, S. (2012). Biophysical and physiological origins of blood oxygenation level-dependent fMRI signals. *Journal of Cerebral Blood Flow and Metabolism, 32*(7), 1188–1206. doi: 10.1038/jcbfm.2012.23

Kiverstein, J., & Miller, M. (2015). The embodied brain: Towards a radical embodied cognitive neuroscience. *Frontiers in Human Neuroscience, 9*, 237. doi: 10.3389/fnhum.2015.00237

Kristiansson, H., Nissborg, E., Bartek, J., Jr., Andresen, M., Reinstrup, P., & Romner, B. (2013). Measuring elevated intracranial pressure through noninvasive methods: A review of the literature. *Journal of Neurosurgical Anesthesiology, 25*(4), 372–385. doi: 10.1097/ANA.0b013e31829795ce

Krupa, K., & Bekiesinska-Figatowska, M. (2015). Artifacts in magnetic resonance imaging. *Polish Journal of Radiology, 80*, 93–106. doi: 10.12659/PJR.892628

Kudomi, N., Maeda, Y., Sasakawa, Y., Monden, T., Yamamoto, Y., Kawai, N., . . . Nishiyama, Y. (2013). Imaging of the appearance time of cerebral blood using [15O]H2O PET for the computation of correct CBF. *European Journal of Nuclear Medicine and Molecular Imaging, 3*(1), 41. doi: 10.1186/2191-219X-3-41

Kyme, A. Z., Hutton, B. F., Hatton, R. L., Skerrett, D. W., & Barnden, L. R. (2003). Practical aspects of a data-driven motion correction approach for brain SPECT. *IEEE Transactions on Medical Imaging, 22*(6), 722–729. doi: 10.1109/TMI.2003.814790

Lin, A. P., Liao, H. J., Merugumala, S. K., Prabhu, S. P., Meehan, W. P., 3rd, & Ross, B. D. (2012). Metabolic imaging of mild traumatic brain injury. *Brain Imaging and Behavior, 6*(2), 208–223. doi: 10.1007/s11682-012-9181-4

Lu, Y., Truccolo, W., Wagner, F. B., Vargas-Irwin, C. E., Ozden, I., Zimmermann, J. B., . . . Nurmikko, A. V. (2015). Optogenetically induced spatiotemporal gamma oscillations and neuronal spiking activity in primate motor cortex. *Journal of Neurophysiology, 113*(10), 3574–3587. doi: 10.1152/jn.00792.2014

Ludwig, C., Chicherio, C., Terraneo, L., Magistretti, P., de Ribaupierre, A., & Slosman, D. (2008). Functional imaging studies of cognition using 99mTc-HMPAO SPECT: empirical validation using the n-back working memory paradigm. *European Journal of Nuclear Medicine and Molecular Imaging, 35*(4), 695–703. doi: 10.1007/s00259-007-0635-7

Madelin, G., Kline, R., Walvick, R., & Regatte, R. R. (2014). A method for estimating intracellular sodium concentration and extracellular volume fraction in brain in vivo using sodium magnetic resonance imaging. *Scientific Reports, 4*, 4763. doi: 10.1038/srep04763

Maebatake, A., Sato, M., Kagami, R., Yamashita, Y., Komiya, I., Himuro, K., . . . Sasaki, M. (2014). An anthropomorphic phantom study of brain dopamine transporter SPECT images obtained using different SPECT/CT devices and collimators. *Journal of Nuclear Medicine Technology*. doi: 10.2967/jnmt.114.149401

Matthews, P. M., & Datta, G. (2015). Positron-emission tomography molecular imaging of glia and myelin in drug discovery for multiple sclerosis. *Expert Opinion on Drug Discovery, 10*(5), 557–570. doi: 10.1517/17460441.2015.1032240

Medaglia, J. D., Lynall, M. E., & Bassett, D. S. (2015). Cognitive network neuroscience. *Journal of Cognitive Neuroscience*, 1–21. doi: 10.1162/jocn_a_00810

Munn, Z., & Jordan, Z. (2013). Interventions to reduce anxiety, distress and the need for sedation in adult patients undergoing magnetic resonance imaging: A systematic review. *International Journal of Evidence Based Healthcare, 11*(4), 265–274. doi: 10.1111/1744-1609.12045

Nagaoka, T., Zhao, F., Wang, P., Harel, N., Kennan, R. P., Ogawa, S., & Kim, S. G. (2006). Increases in oxygen consumption without cerebral blood volume change during visual stimulation under hypotension condition. *Journal of Cerebral Blood Flow and Metabolism, 26*(8), 1043–1051. doi: 10.1038/sj.jcbfm.9600251

Naqvi, J., Yap, K. H., Ahmad, G., & Ghosh, J. (2013). Transcranial Doppler ultrasound: A review of the physical principles and major applications in critical care. *International Journal of Vascular Medicine, 2013*, 629378. doi: 10.1155/2013/629378

Nasrallah, I., & Dubroff, J. (2013). An overview of PET neuroimaging. *Seminars in Nuclear Medicine, 43*(6), 449–461. doi: 10.1053/j.semnuclmed.2013.06.003

Ogawa, K., & Ichimura, Y. (2014). Simulation study on a stationary data acquisition SPECT system with multi-pinhole collimators attached to a triple-head gamma camera system. *Annals of Nuclear Medicine, 28*(8), 716–724. doi: 10.1007/s12149-014-0865-2

Ouwerkerk, R. (2011). Sodium MRI. *Methods in Molecular Biology, 711*, 175–201. doi: 10.1007/978-1-61737-992-5_8

Owen, J. P., Sekihara, K., & Nagarajan, S. S. (2012). Non-parametric statistical thresholding for sparse magnetoencephalography source reconstructions. *Frontiers in Neuroscience, 6*, 186. doi: 10.3389/fnins.2012.00186

Palumbo, B., Buresta, T., Nuvoli, S., Spanu, A., Schillaci, O., Fravolini, M. L., & Palumbo, I. (2014). SPECT and PET serve as molecular imaging techniques and in vivo biomarkers for brain metastases. *International Journal of Molecular Science*, *15*(6), 9878–9893. doi: 10.3390/ijms15069878

Peeters, S. C., van de Ven, V., Gronenschild, E. H., Patel, A. X., Habets, P., Goebel, R., . . . Outcome of, P. (2015). Default mode network connectivity as a function of familial and environmental risk for psychotic disorder. *PLoS One*, *10*(3), e0120030. doi: 10.1371/journal.pone.0120030

Peterson, A., Thome, J., Frewen, P., & Lanius, R. A. (2014). Resting-state neuroimaging studies: A new way of identifying differences and similarities among the anxiety disorders? *Canadian Journal of Psychiatry*, *59*(6), 294–300.

Plewes, D. B., & Kucharczyk, W. (2012). Physics of MRI: A primer. *Journal of Magnetic Resonance Imaging*, *35*(5), 1038–1054. doi: 10.1002/jmri.23642

Poldrack, R. A., Mumford, J. A, & Nichols, T. E. (2011). *Handbook of Functional MRI Data Analysis*. Cambridge: Cambridge University Press.

Power, J. D., Schlaggar, B. L., & Petersen, S. E. (2015). Recent progress and outstanding issues in motion correction in resting state fMRI. *Neuroimage*, *105*, 536–551. doi: 10.1016/j.neuroimage.2014.10.044

Price, J. C. (2012). Molecular brain imaging in the multimodality era. *Journal of Cerebral Blood Flow and Metabolism*, *32*(7), 1377–1392. doi: 10.1038/jcbfm.2012.29

Purkayastha, S., & Sorond, F. (2012). Transcranial Doppler ultrasound: Technique and application. *Seminars in Neurology*, *32*(4), 411–420. doi: 10.1055/s-0032-1331812

Rahmim, A., & Zaidi, H. (2008). PET versus SPECT: Strengths, limitations and challenges. *Nuclear Medicine Communications*, *29*(3), 193–207. doi: 10.1097/MNM.0b013e3282f3a515

Raichle, M. E. (2015). The restless brain: How intrinsic activity organizes brain function. *Philosophical Transactions of the Royal Society of London – B: Biological Sciences*, *370*(1668). doi: 10.1098/rstb.2014.0172

Ricker, J. H. (2012). Functional neuroimaging in forensic neuropsychology. In G. Larrabee (Ed.), *Forensic Neuropsychology: A Scientific Approach* (2nd ed., pp. 160–178). New York: Oxford University Press.

Ricker, J. H. (2013). Connectivity studies in neuropsychology. In J.E.M.S. Koffler, I. S. Baron, & M. F. Greiffenstein (Eds.), *Neuropsychology Science and Practice* (pp. 208–221). New York: Oxford University Press.

Ricker, J. H. (2014). The neurological examination, radiologic, and other diagnostic testing: A review for neuropsychologists. In J.D.K.J. Stucky & M. Kirkwood (Eds.), *American Academy of Clinical Neuropsychology Study Guide and Board Review* (pp. 139–153). New York: Oxford University Press.

Ricker, J. H., Arenth, P. M., & Wagner, A. K. (2013). Functional neuroimaging of traumatic brain injury. In D.I.K.N.D. Zasler & R. D. Zafonte (Eds.), *Brain Injury Medicine: Principles and Practice* (2nd ed., pp. 218–229). New York: Demos Publishing.

Ricker, J. H., DeLuca, J., & Frey, S. H. (2014). On the changing roles of neuroimaging in rehabilitation science. *Brain Imaging and Behavior*, *8*(3), 333–334. doi: 10.1007/s11682-014-9315-y

Ryan, M. E., Palasis, S., Saigal, G., Singer, A. D., Karmazyn, B., Dempsey, M. E.,. . . Coley, B. D. (2014). Appropriateness criteria for head trauma–child. *Journal of the American College of Radiology*, *11*(10), 939–947. doi: 10.1016/j.jacr.2014.07.017

Schneiderman, J. F. (2014). Information content with low- vs. high-T(c) SQUID arrays in MEG recordings: The case for high-T(c) SQUID-based MEG. *Journal of Neuroscience Methods*, *222*, 42–46. doi: 10.1016/j.jneumeth.2013.10.007

Shah, N. J., Oros-Peusquens, A. M., Arrubla, J., Zhang, K., Warbrick, T., Mauler, J., . . . Neuner, I. (2013). Advances in multimodal neuroimaging: Hybrid MR-PET and MR-PET-EEG at 3 T and 9.4 T. *Journal of Magnetic Resonance*, *229*, 101–115. doi: 10.1016/j.jmr.2012.11.027

Shaw, E. E., Schultz, A. P., Sperling, R., & Hedden, T. (2015). Functional connectivity in multiple cortical networks is associated with performance across cognitive domains in older adults. *Brain Connectivity*. doi: 10.1089/brain.2014.0327

Shetty, V. S., Reis, M. N., Aulino, J. M., Berger, K. L., Broder, J., Choudhri, A. F. . . . Bykowski J. (2016). *Journal of the American College of Radiology*, *13*(6), 668–679. doi: 10.1016/j.jacr.2016.02.023

Simon, A. B., & Buxton, R. B. (2015). Understanding the dynamic relationship between cerebral blood flow and the BOLD signal: Implications for quantitative functional MRI. *Neuroimage*, *116*, 158–167. doi: 10.1016/j.neuroimage.2015.03.080

Slater, J. D., Khan, S., Li, Z., & Castillo, E. (2012). Characterization of interictal epileptiform discharges with time-resolved cortical current maps using the helmholtz-hodge decomposition. *Frontiers in Neurology*, *3*, 138. doi: 10.3389/fneur.2012.00138

Sohlberg, A., Watabe, H., & Iida, H. (2008). Three-dimensional SPECT reconstruction with transmission-dependent scatter correction. *Annals of Nuclear Medicine*, *22*(7), 549–556. doi: 10.1007/s12149-008-0170-z

Sossi, V. (2007). Cutting-edge brain imaging with positron emission tomography. *Neuroimaging Clinics of North America*, *17*(4), 427–440, viii. doi: 10.1016/j.nic.2007.07.006

Takaki, A., Soma, T., Kojima, A., Asao, K., Kamada, S., Matsumoto, M., & Murase, K. (2009). Improvement of image quality using interpolated projection data estimation method in SPECT. *Annals of Nuclear Medicine*, *23*(7), 617–626. doi: 10.1007/s12149-009-0281-1

Takekawa, T., Kakuda, W., Uchiyama, M., Ikegaya, M., & Abo, M. (2014). Brain perfusion and upper limb motor function: A pilot study on the correlation between evolution of asymmetry in cerebral blood flow and improvement in Fugl-Meyer Assessment score after rTMS in chronic post-stroke patients. *Journal of Neuroradiology*, *41*(3), 177–183. doi: 10.1016/j.neurad.2013.06.006

Trambaiolli, L. R., Lorena, A. C., Fraga, F. J., Kanda, P. A., Nitrini, R., & Anghinah, R. (2011). Does EEG montage influence Alzheimer's disease electroclinic diagnosis? *International Journal of Alzheimers Dissease*, *2011*, 761891. doi: 10.4061/2011/761891

Trimble, M. R., & George, M. S. (2010). *Biological Psychiatry* (3rd ed.). Oxford, UK; Hoboken, NJ: Wiley-Blackwell.

Ward, J. (2015). *The Student's Guide to Cognitive Neuroscience* (3rd ed.). East Sussex: Taylor & Francis.

Watanabe, H., Ono, M., & Saji, H. (2015). Novel PET/SPECT probes for imaging of Tau in Alzheimer's disease. *Scientific World Journal*, *2015*, 124192. doi: 10.1155/2015/124192

Wey, H. Y., Desai, V. R., & Duong, T. Q. (2013). A review of current imaging methods used in stroke research. *Neurological Research*, *35*(10), 1092–1102. doi: 10.1179/1743132813Y.0000000250

Whitfield-Gabrieli, S., & Ford, J. M. (2012). Default mode network activity and connectivity in psychopathology. *Annual Review of*

Clinical Psychology, *8*, 49–76. doi: 10.1146/annurev-clinpsy-032511-143049

Wilde, E. A., Bouix, S., Tate, D. F., Lin, A. P., Newsome, M. R., Taylor, B. A., . . . York, G. (2015). Advanced neuroimaging applied to veterans and service personnel with traumatic brain injury: State of the art and potential benefits. *Brain Imaging and Behavior*, *9*(3), 367–402. doi: 10.1007/s11682-015-9444-y

Wilde, E. A., Hunter, J. V., & Bigler, E. D. (2012). A primer of neuroimaging analysis in neurorehabilitation outcome research. *NeuroRehabilitation*, *31*(3), 227–242. doi: 10.3233/NRE-2012-0793

Williamson, C. A., Wahlster, S., Shafi, M. M., & Westover, M. B. (2014). Sensitivity of compressed spectral arrays for detecting seizures in acutely ill adults. *Neurocritical Care*, *20*(1), 32–39. doi: 10.1007/s12028-013-9912-4

Yao, J., Wang, L., Yang, J. M., Maslov, K. I., Wong, T. T., Li, L., . . . Wang, L. V. (2015). High-speed label-free functional photoacoustic microscopy of mouse brain in action. *Nature Methods*, *12*(5), 407–410. doi: 10.1038/nmeth.3336

Part II

Disorders in Children and Adults

10 Genetic and Neurodevelopmental Disorders

E. Mark Mahone, Beth S. Slomine, and T. Andrew Zabel

Introduction

Neurodevelopmental disorders are conditions that involve early insult or abnormality in the developing brain or central nervous system and are associated with a wide spectrum of abilities and deficits in children. The behavioral and cognitive dysfunction associated with early neural damage can range from subtle (or absent) to diffuse and profound. Importantly, the functional disability observed in children with neurodevelopmental disorders is variable, and is rarely predicted by a child's IQ (or developmental quotient) scores alone.

In children with neurodevelopmental disorders, it can be assumed that there has been early interference to the developing nervous system, which can take place during prenatal, perinatal, or postnatal development. For the purposes of this chapter, we define "early" as occurring within the first three years of life. These early occurring insults set the stage for what is often a chronic course, beginning in early childhood, in which the "normal" development of the central nervous system has been altered. The result of this alteration is *reorganization* within the nervous system in an unexpected manner, and ultimately, *competition* among available brain structures to support the development of cognitive and behavioral function. In other words, early insults stimulate alternate neural pathways; subsequently, the functional effect occurs not only on the damaged brain region, but also the regions that support the new functions.

The timing of the reorganization is critical, and outcome is a function of *when* the change occurs relative to critical periods in brain development. Functional reorganization that affects a particular brain region during a critical period of growth may result in "crowding," in which outcome (i.e., performance of critical life skills) is often less efficient. This inefficiency in performance of life functioning is the hallmark trait of children with neurodevelomental disorders. Performance on routine skills is often slower and more effortful than would be expected for the child's age, with new learning and skill development requiring more trials to master than in children without neurodevelopmental disorders.

Sensitive periods in development involve rapid periods of neural and functional growth and occur when specific regions and cells are also susceptible to insult at specific periods of brain development (i.e., selective vulnerability; Johnston, 2004). Given the importance of a sequential unfolding of multiple processes during these times, these sensitive periods represent great periods of vulnerability. The developmental neuropsychological framework necessarily considers how *timing* of central nervous system disruption can lead to different outcomes. For example, disruption in the first trimester can lead to major structural anomalies and often diffuse and pervasive neuropsychological deficits. Disruption in the second trimester affects neuronal migration. Disruption in the late second and early third trimester and postnatal is associated with more focal white and gray matter damage (Hoon & Melhem, 2000).

In neurodevelopmental disorders, the concept of the *time-referenced symptom* is critical. As a result of reorganization, functional impairments can be observed immediately; however, more often, the full range of functional deficits may not manifest until later in life, even though the neurobiological basis of the condition is present earlier (Rudel, 1981). The relationship between the biological vulnerability and psychological test performance may reside in the "take-a-test" demands with which assessment presents to the child, and the extent to which psychometric tests relate to functioning in the real-life (e.g., classroom) settings (Holmes-Bernstein & Waber, 1990).

Understanding brain-behavior relationships in children is challenging to the neuropsychologist for a variety of reasons. Frequently, no imaging studies will have been performed. Moreover, often there is no focal lesion as is the case in adults, and even when one is present, the neuropsychological deficits that manifest throughout the child's development are typically not consistent with a focal deficit.

In many instances, the early neural disruption occurs in multiple brain systems, leading to several types of functional reorganization. In typical development, functional skills develop along the same developmental timelines as nervous system development. In children with neurodevelopmental disorders, the development is often "off developmental track" behaviorally, and maturational timelines based on normal development become less applicable. Outcomes in children with neurodevelopmental disorders depend on the age of the child at the time of insult, the type of insult, whether the insult is chronic or acute, functional development prior to insult, and development that is not yet complete at the time of the insult. Each of these factors should be considered when assessing children with neurodevelopmental disorders.

Functional outcomes in children with neurodevelopmental disorders are also considered in the context of the child's changing educational demands. As children mature, they are expected to work more independently. As a result of this expectation, classrooms progressively minimize and eventually withdraw the structures and supports that enable young students to accomplish their goals. For example, in first grade, a student's primary task is to learn how to be a student, i.e., to learn *how* to learn. First graders learn how to read and write, how to pay attention, and how to follow the rules. Teachers provide extensive structure and support developing executive control functions. By fourth grade, however, students are expected to have learned how to read and are required to use reading as the primary means of mastering other subjects. If reading capability is not in place at this time, new difficulties will emerge. By middle school, students are expected to organize themselves and, increasingly, to learn on their own. By high school, students are expected to be well organized and self-motivating.

Transition Into Adulthood

Medical advances have sharply changed the life course of a number of genetic and developmentally involved conditions, making some conditions more survivable/compatible with life (e.g., very low birth weight preterm infants, hydrocephalus) and extending the expected life span for others (e.g., cystic fibrosis, sickle cell disease, and spina bifida). Due to higher survival rates and life spans extending into adulthood, increased attention has been given to the development of self-management and independence skills, and the transition into older adolescence and young adulthood. This transition is considerably different than transitions that have occurred earlier in development. For example, the academically based transitions of childhood (e.g., fourth grade, middle school, high school) have in many instances been scaffolded by parents, teachers, and entitlement-based accommodations and interventions. In contrast, the transition of youth with genetic and developmental conditions into young adulthood is often complicated by increased expectations of independence, a withdrawal of supports in general, and a transition into "eligibility"-based supports that may not be adequately available or funded.

During the period of "early adulthood," between the ages of 18 and 34 (Furstenberg, Rumbaut, & Settersten, 2005), individuals with genetic and developmental conditions are typically presented with a variety of opportunities and challenges, including employment, financial management, intimate relationships, parenting, etc. While early research suggests a more favorable adult outcome for some medically involved populations (e.g., prematurity; Saigal et al., 2006), adults with developmental disabilities in general still fall well behind age-matched peers in the attainment and performance of these early adult milestones. For instance, the rate of employment of individuals diagnosed with intellectual disability is less than half that of nondisabled peers during late adolescence (Butterworth, Leach, McManus, & Stansfeld, 2013), and this gap widens in early adulthood (Sulewski, Zalewska, Butterworth, & Migliore, 2013). In addition to the more typical adult level expectations, the transition into adulthood for individuals with genetic and developmental conditions can be further complicated by the challenge of assuming responsibility from parents for the reliable completion of medical self-management tasks, ranging from less-complicated daily medication administration (e.g., sickle cell disease) to more-complicated bowel and bladder management procedures (i.e., spina bifida) and respiratory therapies (i.e., cystic fibrosis). Finally, many of these conditions are further complicated by cognitive changes experienced during adulthood, ranging from "early aging" processes (e.g., spina bifida; Dennis, Nelson, Jewell, & Fletcher, 2010) to more overt declines in memory, language, and cognitive functioning (Down syndrome; Zigman, 2013).

Classification of Neurodevelopmental Disorders

There are two primary approaches to classification of neurodevelopmental disorders—one emphasizing *behavior*, and the other emphasizing *neurology* (see Table 10.1). Functional

Table 10.1 Examples of behavioral and neurological diagnoses in neurodevelopmental disorders

Behavioral Diagnoses
Intellectual disability
Communication disorders
Autism spectrum disorder
Attention deficit/hyperactivity disorder
Specific learning disorder
Motor disorders
Neurological Diagnoses
Known genetic cause
Down syndrome
Rett syndrome
Fragile X syndrome
22q deletion syndromes
Storage disorders
Neurocutaneous disorders
Known environmental cause
Fetal alcohol spectrum disorder
Traumas
Infections
Teratogens—lead, mercury
Multifactoral cause
Spina bifida
Cerebral palsy
Prematurity

independence, as well as disability in children with neurodevelopmental disorders, should be considered through these frameworks. In general terms, a *disability* involves personal limitations that produce a disadvantage when attempting to function in one's society. The disability is necessarily considered within the context of the environment, personal factors, and individualized supports (Wehmeyer et al., 2008). Function is thus understood as the interaction between one's own biology and the environmental demands/supports. Disability occurs when there is a discrepancy between biological attributes and environmental demands. Given the ever-changing environment experienced by the child, the discrepancy (and thus the functional disability) can change over time.

Behaviorally Defined Neurodevelopmental Disorders in DSM-5

Four of the *behaviorally* defined neurodevelopmental disorders outlined in the *Diagnostic and Statistical Manual for Mental Disorders,* fifth edition (DSM-5; American Psychiatric Association, 2013) that are most commonly encountered by neuropsychologists are described next. These include intellectual developmental disorder, specific learning disorders, attention deficit/hyperactivity disorder, and autism spectrum disorder.

Intellectual Disability (Intellectual Developmental Disorder)

The prevalence of intellectual disability is estimated to be 1% of the population (Maulik, Mascarenhas, Mathers, Dua, & Saxena, 2011) with approximately 3 million people diagnosed with intellectual disability in the United States (Larson et al., 2011). Multiple etiologies occurring during various sensitive periods of development have been associated with intellectual disability, including a variety of genetic conditions, teratogen exposures, prenatal/perinatal traumatic events, and postnatal injuries and infections.

Although the name of the condition was changed from *mental retardation* to *intellectual disability* (coupled with the term *intellectual developmental disorder*) in the DSM-5, the general diagnostic criteria for intellectual disability that were previously contained in the DSM-IV-TR (American Psychiatric Association, 2000) were retained, including the requirement for deficits in both adaptive functioning and intellectual functioning (American Psychiatric Association, 2013). Intellectual deficits are defined as impairment in "general mental abilities such as reasoning, problem solving, planning, abstract thinking, judgment, academic learning, and learning from experience," with a guideline of an IQ score of ≤ 70 (± 5 standard score points for error; American Psychiatric Association, 2013, p. 37). Adaptive deficits in at least one broad domain (i.e., conceptual, social, or practical) are determined by "both clinic evaluation and individualized, culturally appropriate, psychometrically sound measures" (American Psychiatric Association, 2013, p. 37), and the DSM-5 provides a descriptive table to help determine the severity of adaptive impairment. In the DSM-5, deficits in adaptive functioning have become central in the determination of intellectual disability severity (compared to the DSM-IV-TR practice of setting intellectual disability severity based upon IQ score), as extent of adaptive dysfunction is considered more relevant than IQ score for the determination of level of support required. The quantification of adaptive deficits remains an area of ongoing discussion in the field of assessment, with criticism over current practices of assessing adaptive "skills" (e.g., activities of daily living) rather than "real-world" problem solving, gullibility, and vulnerability to exploitation (Greenspan, 2006).

The diagnostic formulation of intellectual disability is contingent upon a causal relationship between the intellectual and adaptive deficits, in that "the deficits in adaptive functioning must be directly related to the intellectual impairments described" (American Psychiatric Association, 2013, p. 37). This is an important clinical consideration of diagnosis, as adaptive dysfunction is commonly reported in individuals with a variety of developmental disorders, and may be attributable to physical limitations or cognitive variables other than intelligence (e.g., executive functioning; Culhane-Shelburne, Chapieski, Hiscock, & Glaze, 2002; Papazoglou, Jacobson, & Zabel, 2013).

Learning Disorders

Learning disorders are neurodevelopmental disorders that affect the brain's ability to receive, process, store, and respond to information (Mahone & Mapou, 2013). Learning disorders typically have onset in early childhood, persist into adulthood, and are associated with academic underachievement problems that are otherwise unexpected, presumably related to underlying cognitive impairment. In this context, poor academic achievement is considered "unexpected" when it is not associated with low intelligence, sensory impairments, emotional disturbances, or limited opportunities to learn. Like most neurodevelopmental disorders, developmental learning disorders occur along a continuum, with significant variability in severity and characteristic features.

The diagnostic criteria in the American Psychiatric Association's DSM-5 for specific learning disorder reflect a hybrid model, in which diagnosis is made using synthesis of the individual's history (development, medical, family, education), psychoeducational reports of test scores and observations, and response to intervention. With learning disorders, there is a recognition that individuals may "grow into" their deficits (i.e., time-referenced symptoms), thus the full range of problems may not be fully manifest until a later age.

Attention Deficit/Hyperactivity Disorder

Attention deficit/hyperactivity disorder (ADHD) is the second most common behaviorally defined neurodevelopmental disorder (behind learning disorders). Affecting as many as 9%–11% of school age children, the onset of behaviors occurs most often in the preschool years and can persist into adulthood (Akinbami, Liu, Pastor, & Reuben, 2011). The primary symptom complex (inattention, hyperactivity, impulsivity) emerges and changes over time, and is associated with a wide range of comorbid behavioral conditions (Larson et al., 2011). Despite often having "normal" intelligence, children with ADHD manifest considerable functional difficulties, including higher rates of learning problems, missed school, troublesome relationships, and mental and physical conditions that result in 33% reduced earning as adults (Fletcher, 2013).

The DSM-5 retained most of the diagnostic criteria for ADHD that were previously contained in the DSM-IV-TR (American Psychiatric Association, 2000). Several important changes were introduced and may ultimately lead to an increase in the rates of diagnosis. First, the DSM-5 age of onset criterion was changed to require that symptoms are present prior to age 12, compared to the DSM-IV criterion of before age 7. Second, in DSM-5, the symptoms of inattention and/or hyperactivity-impulsivity are only required to be present, whereas in DSM-IV, the symptoms were required to cause impairment. Third, unlike the DSM-IV, the DSM-5 includes a provision for adult diagnosis (ages 17 and older), for which the symptom criterion is met with five (rather than six) symptoms of inattention and/or hyperactivity-impulsivity.

As a group, childen with ADHD demonstrate widespread reductions in cortical volume, as well as disruption to the development of subcortical structures, including basal ganglia and cerebellum (Mahone et al., 2011). Moreover, recent research has suggested that these ADHD-related anomalies can be detected in preschool children as young as age 4 years (Mahone et al., 2011). Nevertheless, at the individual level, MRI scans of children with ADHD are routinely read as normal, without individually identifiable lesions. The scan of a 4-year old boy with ADHD, which was read as entirely normal, is shown in Figure 10.1.

Autism Spectrum Disorder

Autism spectrum disorder also represents a behaviorally defined phenotype. The Centers for Disease Control and Prevention estimates that in the United States, one in 68 8-year-old children have been diagnosed with autism spectrum disorder (Centers for Disease Control and Prevention, 2014). According to the DSM-5, autism spectrum disorder represents a continuum of impairment from mild to severe and includes all four diagnoses that were previously separated in the DSM-IV, including autism, Asperger's disorder, childhood disintegrative disorder, and pervasive developmental disorder–not otherwise specified. Autism spectrum disorder is characterized by a selective impairment in social interaction as well as restricted and repetitive patterns of behavior (American Psychiatric Association, 2013). Within the DSM-5, difficulties with language and communication were deemphasized as a core feature of autism spectrum disorder because communication ability can vary greatly in individuals with autism spectrum disorder. While the risk factors are heterogeneous and complex (Willsey & State, 2015), over the last two decades several diagnosable genetic conditions commonly seen by neuropsychologists have been associated with this autism spectrum disorder, including Fragile X (Budimirovic & Kaufmann, 2011), tuberous sclerosis (Muzykewic, Newberry, Danforth, Halpern, E. F., & Thiele, 2007), and 22q13.3 deletion (Cusmano-Ozog, Manning, & Hoyme, 2007).

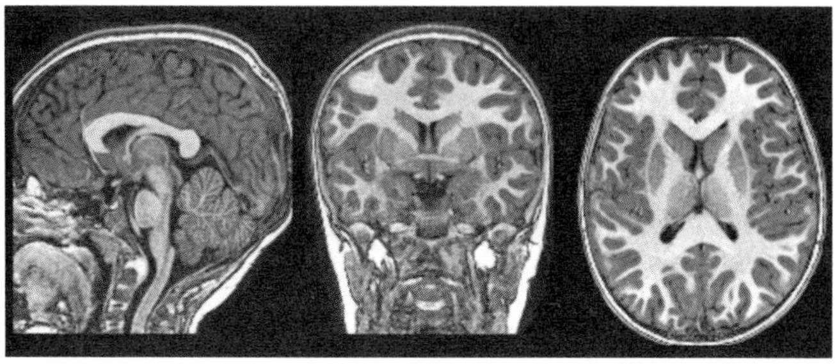

Figure 10.1 MRI scan of a 4-year old boy with ADHD

Neurodevelopmental Disorders Associated With Neurological Conditions

The *neurological* approach to classification of neurodevelopmental disorders provides for an understanding of the neurological development as well as the associated physical abnormalities. Children with neurological diagnoses can display many of the behaviorally defined disorders outlined in DSM-5. The behavioral diagnosis, however, provides little insight into the etiology of the condition, and the DSM framework is often agnostic with regard to etiology. More likely, childen with known medical or neurological conditions manifest symptoms of several behaviorally defined conditions, including ADHD, intellectual disability, learning disorders, communication disorders, motor disorders, and/or autism spectrum disorder. This observation highlights the limitations of relying only on the behavioral definitions outlined in DSM-5 when working with children with neurodevelopmental disorders.

Professionally, neuropsychologists work within these two schema in two ways. They search for neurological correlates of behaviorally defined conditions (ADHD, dyslexia, autism). At the same time, they search for behavioral phenotypes of genetic or neurologically defined disorders (e.g, Williams syndrome, Neurofibromatosis Type 1, Down syndrome). In clinical care, understanding the evidence-based research is needed when interpreting data, formulating clinical impressions, and providing recommendations.

Common Neurodevelopmental and Genetic Disorders

Down Syndrome

Down syndrome, also called *trisomy 21*, is a chromosomal disorder that typically results in an extra chromosome 21 (i.e., instead of 23 pairs of chromosomes, children are born with 22 pairs and one set of three chromosomes). Down syndrome is the most common known *genetic* cause of intellectual disability. It occurs in one out of every 732 live-births in the United States with advance maternal age as the most significant risk factor (Sherman, Allen, Bean, & Freeman, 2007). Down syndrome has a high prevalence of many medical conditions including cardiac, neurological, gastrointestinal, immunological, respiratory, sensory, and orthopedic abnormalities, although medical advances have resulted in increased longevity (Bittles, Bower, Hussain, & Glasson, 2006).

Cognitive deficits are also prominent among individuals with Down syndrome. While cognitive assessment can be challenging due to associated difficulties with communication, vision, and hearing, Down syndrome is commonly associated with intellectual disability, ranging from mild to profound intellectual disability (Lott & Dierssen, 2010). Additionally, while the pattern of impairment is variable, the behavioral phenotype of Down syndrome is usually associated with impairments in verbal short-term memory and long-term memory, with relative strengths in visuospatial short-term memory, associative learning, and implicit long-term memory functions (Lott & Dierssen, 2010). A variety of age-related changes occur earlier in individuals with Down syndrome (Bittles et al., 2006). Several physical, neurological, and psychiatric conditions develop early in individual with Down syndrome (Trotter Ross & Olsen, 2014). With age, individuals with Down syndrome often develop neuropathology and declines in memory, language, and cognitive functioning consistent with dementia of the Alzheimer's type (Zigman, 2013).

Fragile X Syndrome

Fragile X syndrome is the most common known *inherited genetic* cause of intellectual disability. Fragile X is a genetic condition resulting from mutations to the Fragile X mental retardation 1 (FMR1) gene on the X chromosome. The full mutation of the gene, defined as having > 200 CGG repeats, occurs in 1 in 4,000–7,000 ; however, permutation carriers are more common, and are estimated to include one in 130–250 females and one in 250–810 males ((Lozano, Rosero, & Hagerman, 2014). Given the significant overlap between the mutation and premutations, the term *Fragile X spectrum disorder* has been proposed to include the range of FMR1 mutations (Lozano et al., 2014).

Since the full mutation of FMR1 leads to absence or severe deficiency of FMR1 protein, a critical protein for synaptic plasticity, the lack of protein often leads to intellectual disability in males with Fragile X. In females with the full mutation, due to their other normal X chromosome, some FMR1 protein is produced, which results in IQ scores ranging from intellectual disability to normal. Deficits in executive functions, including response inhibition and working memory as well as visuospatial processing and visuomotor skills, are also associated with Fragile X (Fung, Quintin, Haas, & Reiss, 2012). Additionally, Fragile X is the most common known cause of autism spectrum disorder and accounts for 5% of cases (Budimirovic & Kaufmann, 2011). Premutations in both males and females are also associated with developmental problems including learning disabilities, autism spectrum disorder, ADHD, and prominent anxiety, although these difficulties are more pronounced in males (Lozano et al., 2014).

Cerebral Palsy

Cerebral palsy affects approximately two in 1,000 children, and is the most common motor disorder of early childhood (Menkes & Sarnat, 2000). While most commonly diagnosed in the early developmental period (i.e., by age 3 years), in less-severe cases, it can also be diagnosed later in the childhood years. Cerebral palsy refers to a group of motor impairment syndromes in which a static and nonprogressive cerebral lesion produces abnormal motor control—resulting in problems with muscle tone, strength, and fluidity of movement—as well as a variety of cognitive and behavioral deficits (Johnston & Hoon, 2006). The term *cerebral palsy* describes a syndrome, not an etiology, and diagnosis is made based upon a pattern of motor symptoms.

There are numerous genetic and acquired etiologies of cerebral palsy, including prematurity, neonatal encephalopathy, and various postnatal insults (Fennell & Dikel, 2001; Korzeniewski, Birbeck, DeLano, Potchen, & Paneth., 2008). The concept of selective vulnerability (Johnston, 2004) is particularly important when considering etiology, as the varieties of etiology in cerebral palsy are associated with susceptibility to injury of specific cells and brain regions at different sensitive periods of prenatal and neonatal development. Disruptions of neuron migration during the first trimester can result in brain malformations (i.e., lissencephaly, heterotopia, schizencephaly, etc.; Barkovich, Kuzniecky, Jackson, Guerrini, & Dobyns, 2001) and subsequent cerebral palsy. During the late second and early third trimesters of pregnancy, immature oligodendroglia are particularly vulnerable to injury secondary to hypoxia-ischemia or infection, which can in turn lead to another etiology of cerebral palsy, i.e., periventricular white matter injury (Johnston, Hoon, & Kaufmann, 2008). Finally, developing neuronal circuits are sensitive to injury in the weeks leading up to and following a term pregnancy, and are vulnerable to various disruptions that underline cerebral palsy, such as perinatal stroke (Johnston & Hoon, 2006). Given the different mechanisms of injury presenting at different sensitive periods of development, it is not surprising that the concept of cerebral palsy includes a broad range of phenotypic and neurologic presentations, with broad divisions (i.e., spastic vs. extrapyramidal), topigraphical distinctions (e.g., limb involvement), and specific motor subtypes (e.g., dystonia, dyskinesia, ataxia, hypotonia, etc.).

The diversity of etiologies of cerebral palsy has slowed the development of a cognitive phenotype. In general, severity of motor impairment is associated with intellectual functioning in individuals with cerebral palsy, and co-occurring seizure disorder increases the likelihood of intellectual disability (Fennell & Dikel, 2001). A variety of other neuropsychological findings have been reported, including nonverbal reasoning deficits (Pirila et al., 2004; Sigurdardottir et al., 2008), attention problems (Christ, White, Brunstrom, & Abrams, 2003), and visuospatial/visuoperceptual deficits (Kozeis et al., 2007). Of note, significant motor impairments (e.g., fine motor, oromotor, etc.) associated with cerebral palsy can complicate neuropsychological assessment. To help manage these threats to validity, a combination of targeted assessment with accommodations, process observations, and informal assessment techniques are suggested for the neuropsychological assessment of individuals with cerebral palsy (Zabel & Schmidt, 2011).

Prematurity

Prematurity is a broad term used for neonates born less than 37 weeks gestation. Due to advances in obstetric and neonatal care, there has been decreased mortality rates as well as increased age of viability among preterm infants since the 1970s. With these advances, there has been increased morbidity among preterm children, especially at the lower limits of viability (Allen, 2008). The literature in the area is complicated by the multitude of terms used to describe premature gestational age and low birth weight as well as the decreasing threshold of viability. At this time, the American College of Obstetricians and Gynecologists uses the term "threshold of viability" for preterm newborns born less than 25 weeks gestation or who weigh less than 1,000 grams, although extremely low birth weight has been commonly used to describe children less than 1,000 grams (American College of Obstetricians and Gynecologists, 2002, reaffirmed 2010).

Children with higher gestational age and more recent year of birth have lower rates of neurodevelopmental impairment; however, outcome studies with adolescents and young adults are needed to better understand the long-term outcome of extremely preterm birth (Vohr, 2014). Extremely preterm and extremely low birth weight children are at greatest risk for severe neurodevelopmental disabilities. At the threshold of viability, children have a high rate of cerebral palsy, intellectual disability, blindness, and sensorimotor hearing loss (Jarjour, 2014). In school-aged children and adolescents who were born very preterm (<32 weeks of gestation), neuropsychological deficits have been identified in many areas, including processing speed, attention, visuoperceptual and motor skills, memory, executive functioning, and language (Anderson, 2014). Importantly, until recently late preterm births (34–36 weeks gestation) were thought to be associated with low risk for neuropsychological impairment; however, recent research suggests that while these children function better than very preterm children, they display significantly more subtle neuropsychological deficits relative to full term children (Baron, Litman, Ahronovich, & Baker, 2012). Figure 10.2 shows the MRI of a 2-year-old former preterm infant with a history of posthemorrhagic hydrocephalus. Axial T2–weighted images of the brain (A and B) show loss of white matter volume predominantly in the bilateral parietal and occipital lobes (arrows) with moderate dilatation of the lateral ventricles and third ventricle, consistent with periventricular leukomalacia.

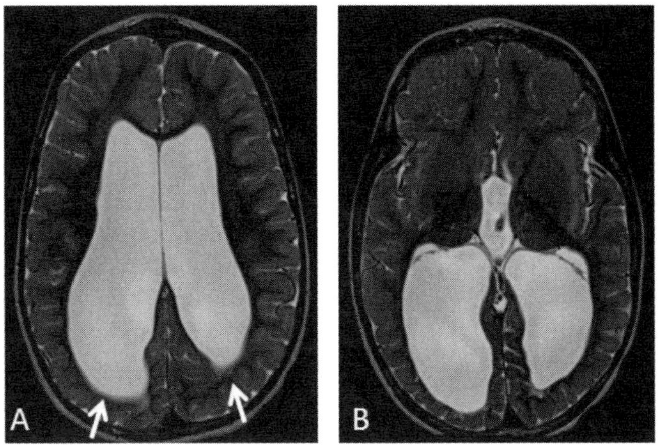

Figure 10.2 MRI scan of former preterm infant (courtesy of Thangamadhan Bosemani, Andrea Poretti, and Thierry A.G.M. Huisman)

Spina Bifida

Spina bifida is the second most common birth defect after cerebral palsy, and had an overall prevalence of 3.39 cases per 10,000 live births in 2003–2004 (Boulet et al., 2008). This represents a decline in cases relative to the prevalence of spina bifida prior to 1998, at which time the U.S. Food and Drug Administration began requiring folic acid fortification of cereal grain products (Centers for Disease Control and Prevention, 2004). Folate deficiency has been established as a risk factor for spina bifida, as have maternal factors such as diabetes mellitus, obesity, exposure to high heat during pregnancy, and certain anti-convulsant medications. A gene-environment interaction is suspected as a cause, but has not yet been specifically identified.

Spina bifida is a neural tube defect occurring in the sensitive period of the third and fourth weeks of pregnancy. It is caused by an incomplete closure of the spinal canal, and can include protrusion of the meninges (menigocele) or spinal cord (myelomeningocele) outside of the spinal column. While typically corrected surgically shortly after birth, emerging evidence suggests that prenatal surgical repair of spina bifida results in improved neurologic functioning (Adzick et al., 2011). Associated neurological complications frequently include Chiari II malformation (Treble-Barna, Kulesz, Dennis, & Fletcher, 2014), partial agenesis of the corpus callosum (Hannay, Kramer, Blaser, & Fletcher, 2009), increased (abnormal) cortical thickness of the frontal lobes (Juranek et al., 2008), and neurogenic bowel and bladder (Charney, 1992). Obstructive hydrocephalus is also a commonly associated condition with spina bifida, and shunt placement has been the conventional treatment for hydrocephalus since the 1960s. Approximately 50% of shunts in children fail within the first two years of placement, and alternative treatment approaches are being explored, including a "wait and see" monitoring of infants with hydrocephalus as well as consideration of minimally invasive procedures such as endoscopic third ventriculostomy (Warf & Campbell, 2008).

Intellectual functioning of individuals with spina bifida is typically grossly intact. Neuropsychological functioning was originally described within a nonverbal learning disability model, but has more recently been conceptualized within the "cognitive phenotype of spina bifida" model (Dennis & Barnes, 2010). This model proposes core deficits in motor, timing, and attentional processes. Within this context, persons with spina bifida frequently have strengths in associative processing (e.g., in the case of language, associating words with word meanings) and weaknesses in assembled processing (e.g., constructing text understanding). Time-referenced symptom presentation is noteworthy, as youngsters with spina bifida frequently experience functional academic issues when the demands for assembled processing increase (i.e., in fourth grade). Learning disability in math is particularly problematic for individuals with spina bifida, extended well into young adulthood (Hetherington, Dennis, Barnes, Drake, & Gentili, 2006). Executive dysfunction is also commonly reported by parents and teachers (Tarazi, Zabel, & Mahone, 2008; Zabel et al., 2011).

Fetal Alcohol Syndrome

While genetic factors may be responsible for many neurodevelopmental conditions, other common neurodevelopmental conditions may be due to external factors, such as fetal exposure to neurotoxins. Fetal alcohol syndrome (FAS) is the most common and significant condition resulting from exposure to an external agent. *Fetal alcohol spectrum disorder* is an umbrella term used to describe the entire continuum of clinical deficits related to prenatal alcohol exposure. In addition to a likely history of prenatal alcohol exposure, at the one end of the continuum, fetal alcohol spectrum disorder is characterized by a specific pattern of minor facial dysmorphic features (flattened philtrum, think upper lip, short palpebral fissures), growth deficiency at any point in the child's life (height and weight <10th percentile), and structural and/or functional central nervous system features (microcephaly, intellectual disability, psychiatric conditions; Hoyme et al., 2005), although specific diagnostic criteria are still debated (Dorrie, Focker, Freunscht, & Hebebrand, 2014). Additionally, this narrow set of criteria is most commonly used to identify children with FAS. Children with other types of fetal alcohol spectrum disorder—including those with partial fetal alcohol syndrome, alcohol-related neurodevelopmental disorder, and alcohol-related birth defects—do not exhibit all criteria. Prevalence estimates vary, but when all disorders falling under the umbrella of fetal alcohol spectrum disorder are included in population-based studies, prevalence rates may be as high as 2%–5% in elementary school–aged children (May et al., 2009). While not included in the DSM-IV, the DSM-5 mentions fetal alcohol spectrum disorder as an example of a condition that may be used for the code Other Specified Neurodevelopmental Disorder. In addition, "Neurobehavioral Disorder associated with Prenatal Alcohol Exposure" has been included in the conditions for further study section (American Psychiatric Association, 2013).

Fetal alcohol spectrum disorder has been associated with a range of neurobehavioral abnormalities. While intellectual functioning ranges from intellectual disability to high average functioning, many individuals with fetal alcohol spectrum disorder have significant deficits with attention, executive functioning, and adaptive skill development (Dorrie et al., 2014). Population based studies of school-aged children, however, suggest that many children with fetal alcohol spectrum disorder do not display significant neurobehavioral deficits (May et al., 2009).

22q11.2 Deletion Syndrome

22q11.2 deletion is in most cases a sporadic, de novo mutation occurring in parental sperm or ovum, with an estimated minimal prevalance of one in 4,417 to one in 8,224 births (Botto et al., 2003). Originally named after constellations of symptoms (i.e., velocardiofacial syndrome) and/or the researchers who first described them (Kirkpatrick & DiGeorge, 1968; Shprintzen et al., 1978), the syndrome was eventually linked to a microdeletion in the long arm of chromosome 22 in the 1990s (Carey et al., 1992; Driscoll, Budarf, & Emanuel, 1992) and was later unified under the term *22q11.2 deletion syndrome.* For diagnosis, identification of small interstitial 22q11.2 deletions is verified by fluorescence in situ hybridization (FISH). The physical phenotype is highly heterogeneous, with various combinations of "midline abnormalities" arising from impaired migration of neural crest cells, including cardiac abnormalities (e.g., interrupted aortic arch, Tetralogy of Fallot, ventricular septal defect, persistent truncus arteriousus), abnormal facies (e.g., small cup-shaped ears, narrow eye opening, long narrow face/flat cheeks), and palatal insufficiency (Gothelf, 2007).

Within the context of presentation heterogeneity, the possibility of a cognitive/neuropsychological phenotype has been explored. Moss and colleagues identified relative and significant deficits in areas such as nonverbal reasoning, attention, visual memory, and arithmetic performance (Wang, Woodin, Kreps-Falk, & Moss, 2000; Woodin et al., 2001). ADHD is the most common behavioral diagnosis made in individuals with 22q11.2 deletion syndrome (35% to 46%; Arnold, Siegel-Bartelt, Cytrynbaum, Teshima, & Schachar, 2001; Feinstein, Eliez, Blasey, & Reiss, 2002), but anxiety and mood disorders are also commonly identified during childhood (Baker & Skuse, 2005). Perhaps of most concern, however, is a prolonged and gradual evolution of subthreshold psychotic and neuropsychiatric features occurring in approximately one-third of individuals with 22q11.2 syndrome (Gothelf, 2007). The combination of psychiatric concerns and cognitive deficits is particularly problematic for the transition of youth with 22q11.2 into adulthood, as many of these symptoms manifest during adolescence and contribute to a decline in adaptive functioning and autonomy.

Framework for Conceptualization of Neurodevelopmental Disorders

The primary role for the neuropsychologist when working with children with genetic and/or neurodevelopmental disorders is to help better understand the current fit between the child's unique biology and the ever-changing demands (and supports) in the environment. Developmental neuropsychologists focus not only on understanding the child's current needs, but also—and just as importantly—on helping to predict and plan for future needs.

A *family practice* model of developmental neuropsychology is most effective when working with children with neurodevelopmental disorders and their families. In this model, the neuropsychologist frequently works with the child and family over multiple years—often from preschool through young adulthood. Assessments are completed within a framework of changing developmental needs and supports. The goal of the neuropsychologist is not to simply provide diagnosis and recommendations on a one-time basis, but rather to assess the developing child–environment interaction in developmental context, not only uncovering current needs, but also helping the family plan for changing needs throughout the child's lifetime. Psychological care is often comprehensive and continuing, and emphasizes the critical role of the child's family, schools, friends, and leisure activities. Importantly, the goal of neuropsychologial interventions with children with neurodevelopmental disorders is prevention, reduction, and amelioration of disability, and promotion of healthy and adaptive neuropsychological functioning throughout childhood and into adulthood. Multiple types of assessments are used over the lifetime within this model, and are described in the next section. In this family practice model, the neuropsychologist is an active treating provider for the child, rather than simply a consultant, and commonly works collaboratively with the child's school to provide translation of how medical and neurological dysfunction affects behavior and learning in the classroom.

Assessment of Neurodevelopmental Disorders

Our approach to assessment draws information from three primary sources—history, observations, and formal testing (Bernstein & Waber, 1990)—but takes into account the unique life circumstances and the chronicity of illness seen in children with neurodevelopmental disorders. Additionally, neuropsychologists are now called upon to draw information from a fourth source—the relevant research literature—in order to increase the evidence-based validity to their conclusions, and to apply assessment principles in light of research findings applicable to their patient's unique characteristics.

In applying these methods, review of the child's neurologic history is crucial to determine whether the "lesion" is *static* or *unstable*. The neuropsychologist also needs to consider current testing needs or adaptations, based on known deficits in communication skills and stamina, as well as motor or sensory needs. It is also critical to carefully review prior assessments, not only from psychologists, but also from other service providers (occupational therapists, speech/language pathologists, physical therapists, teachers). The *interdisciplinary model* is frequently used in hospitals or large centers working with children with neurodevelopmental disorders. In this model, the neuropsychologist's role may be more circumscribed and can defer to other members for focused assessment of other domains (e.g., language, motor skills).

Before assessing a child with a genetic or neurodevelopmental disorder, it is critical to determine what type of neuropsychological assessment is most appropriate. There are at least four common types of neuropsychological assessments used in children with neurodevelopmental disorders, and the clinician's approach should be different for each:

1. *Baseline assessment*, which is typically completed early in a child's life, is necessarily broad-based and comprehensive. Baseline evaluations have the purpose of setting the stage for planned, future follow-up, and are most effective when initially completed in the preschool years. Often, baseline assessments can help medical teams by mapping out the phenotype in order to assist with genetic diagnosis. As part of the baseline assessment, the neuropsychologist works with the family to understand and predict future life transitions and stress points for the child, based on the biological risk and early identified needs, with the goal of preparing the family for the changing (and often increasing) challenges the child faces as he or she "grows into" additional deficits.
2. *Planned follow-up assessments* may be broad-based or focused, and allow the clinician to compare both raw score data (to assess for loss or development of skills) as well as standard score data (to assess rate

of progress relative to peers). Among young children with neurodevelopmental disorders, planned follow-up assessments are most effective when implemented just before known transition points in the child's life (Mahone & Slomine, 2008)—for example, just before the child enters first grade, fourth grade, middle school, and high school.

3 *Neuropsychological screening* is used to determine if there is a need for a more comprehensive neuropsychological assessment (i.e., either a baseline or follow-up assessment). By definition, a screening should rapidly (e.g., 15–20 minutes) assess several neurobehavioral domains in order to answer the questions: "Is this skill generally intact? Are the child's needs being met in the current setting? Is more diagnostic information needed?" In certain contexts, this screening can take the form of a brief, focused "check in," which is not as comprehensive as a planned follow-up, but more extensive than the screening done in busy clinic settings. These check-in sessions are often completed between regular full assessments. The information collected in a brief check-in can be used to tailor recommendations in the moment. One recommendation may be to return for a full evaluation, but other recommendations may be related to more subtle changes in the child's treatment plan.
4 *Problem-focused assessment* typically involves focused follow-up to assess decline or improvement in a specific problem area following some treatment (e.g., reassessing attention skills following introduction of stimulant medication; reassessment of memory following an introduction or change in anticonvulsant medication). This type of assessment is also crucial to assess for pre-post treatment change among children who require surgery. For example, children with congenital hydrocephalus who require shunt revision may have planned neuropsychological assessment pre- and post-surgery to document change.

Developmental Neuropsychological Formulation for Neurodevelopmental Disorders

When working with children with genetic and/or neurodevelopmental disorders, the neuropsychologist is challenged to consider results in the context of child's condition, life situation, and current interventions. Often brain imaging or mapping has not been completed, and the clinician is required to make interpretations based on the clinical presentation. Developmental formulation is based on the timing of follow-up, relative to the onset of the brain anomaly. In formulating the developmental neuropsychological diagnosis, the child's full history should be clearly reviewed, with reference to the known or expected sequelae of the particular type of disorder. Assessment (considering history, observations, and testing) is synthesized in light of the available research. Optimally, the neuropsychologist is able to tell the family what the literature says about difficulties and outcomes with their child's disorder, and how what is known (generally) fits with their particular child's own neuropsychological profile.

Neuropsychological evaluation of individuals with genetic and developmental conditions should take into consideration the extent of typical and atypical demands placed upon the individual. Tarazi, Mahone, and Zabel (2007) describe a model that differentiates typical and atypical adaptive demands placed upon individuals with developmental and medical conditions, and the extent to which atypical demands may increase the burden of executive functioning. Most typically developing individuals are faced with the challenge of meeting typical adaptive demands over their developmental course. Individuals with developmental and genetic conditions are faced with these same challenges, but are often presented with additional atypical self-care requirements associated with their conditions. For example, an individual with spina bifida is expected to master typical adaptive skills such as personal hygiene, housekeeping, food preparation, etc., but may also be presented with atypical adaptive demands such as clean intermittent self-catheterization, bowel management programs, skin inspection, and other self-management requirements. These atypical self-management requirements may increase the demands placed upon the individual's prospective memory, initiation, organization, planning, and other executive functions. Tarazi et al. (2007) contend that the context of these atypical adaptive requirements may make the individual appear "more dysexecutive," and/or legitimately increase the need for executive functioning accommodations/supports. In this model, it is those individuals with both atypical adaptive skill requirements *and* impaired executive functioning who are considered the most vulnerable, and require the greatest degree of intervention/accommodation.

Challenges to Conceptualization and Service Provision for Children With Neurodevelopmental Disorders

There are a variety of challenges to understanding brain-behavior relationships in children with genetic and/or neurodevelopmental disorders. For example, many theories employed in child neuropsychology were developed on adults. Children, in contrast, have developing brains, which represent moving targets when attempting to understand function in relation to an early neurological insult. In children, these early insults change the child's course of learning and behavior, and disrupt the availability of brain systems to perform the developmental tasks intended. The result can be a disability in which the child's own neurology leads to interfering behaviors, which ultimately impede new learning opportunities, which serve to further impact the child's overall functional outcomes. In other words, children have a wide range of variability with respect to timetables of development. Children with neurological compromise are more vulnerable to problems with regulation of behavior, attention, and stamina—affecting integrity of test data (Mahone & Zabel, 2001).

Terminology

Some of the challenge to conceptualization involves clarity in *terminology*. For example, the term *delay* is often confusing to families. Use of the term *delay* simply implies that the child has slower than expected development in one or more domains of learning or behavior. When hearing this term, parents often assume that their child will catch up to peers following a period of intervention, remediation, or extra practice. In some situations (especially when opportunities to learn skills have been limited) this expectation may be realistic. In other cases, however (as in a child with intellectual disability), the use of the term *developmental delay* interchangeably with the more specific diagnosis can be misleading.

The term *deficit* can also be troublesome to families because it is not time-referenced (Mahone, 2007). In this context, the term *deficit* simply suggests absence of a behavior or skill; however, it is also used to indicate significantly impaired performance. Without clear reference to expected levels of functioning for a child's age, the term *deficit* can also be misleading. For example, a behavioral or cognitive deficit (i.e., absence of a skill) at one age may be abnormal, whereas while at another age it may represent age-appropriate functioning.

In children with neurodevelopmental disabilities, parents and clinicians often express concerns regarding behavioral or cognitive *regression*. The challenge for the neuropsychologist in these instances is to determine (often with objective performance-based tests) whether there is a true loss of skill in an absolute sense, or (as is more commonly the case), decline in *relative standing* to peers. Using objective, performance-based assessment, the psychologist can often clarify the nature of the regression by comparing a child's raw score performance on one or more standardized tests to his or her raw score performance on the same tests at a later point in time. True regression occurs when a child manifests an actual loss of skill from one time to the next. Conversely, *failure to keep pace* in skill acquisition may be present in children with neurodevelopmental disabilities when the environmental demands increase at a faster rate than skill development, and the child's rate of improvement is more protracted than that of peers (resulting in decreases in standard scores over time).

High-Stakes Educational Testing

An additional challenge to service provision comes in the form of the politics of high-stakes testing. Developmental neuropsychologists often assess children who have been simultaneously assessed within the school system. This scenario leads to three specific areas of difficulty. First, the focus of assessments within schools is to determine whether the child meets criteria for one or more of the 14 federally defined educational disabilities, and if so, what functional needs are present that would need to be addressed within an individual education plan (IEP). Unfortunately, the 14 federal educational disability definitions do not map directly onto the DSM-5 behavioral criteria. The result is that the school assessment is focused on the educational requirements of the school district. In contrast, the neuropsychologist functioning outside a school is more interested in identifying all potential areas of dysfunction, and recommending evidence-based interventions that can ameliorate the functional deficits. While the goals of the school and the neuropsychologist are often in harmony, at times (often as a result of limited resources), school systems feel pressure to provide only "appropriate" interventions, while outside neuropsychologists seek to implement "optimal" levels of service.

Second, the fact that most children with neurodevelopmental disorders receive some type of psychological assessment within the school system leads third-party insurers to be more reluctant to pay for assessment of diagnostic conditions that are considered "educational." Examples of the diagnostic categories typically rejected by third-party payers include autism spectrum disorders, communication disorders, learning disorders, intellectual disabilities, and (increasingly) ADHD. Given that these conditions are present in the vast majority of children with neurodevelopmental disorders, it becomes a challenge to the neuropsychologist working outside the school setting to receive third-party payment for neuropsychological assessment services, unless the child otherwise has a qualifying medical condition that can serve as the primary billing diagnosis.

Third, given the increasingly limited resources within educational systems, frontline school psychologists are often instructed by their administrators not to make certain diagnoses (e.g., intellectual disability), despite having the training, expertise, and evidence to do so. At the same time, neuropsychologists find themselves having to provide diagnostic formulations for these types of conditions later in life, when the evidence within the school records indicates that the diagnosis could have been made earlier.

Multiple Assessments

Because children with neurodevelopmental disabilities often require multiple neuropsychological assessments it is imperative to understand the challenges involved in interpreting repeat assessments. There are several ways in which to compare age-corrected standard scores across multiple assessments, including regression-based approaches and reliable change indices (RCI) (Duff, 2012; Heilbronner et al., 2010).

These types of statistical procedures account for the reliability of the test measures used, and are helpful in determining if a statistically rare change in a test score has occurred. If a statistically rare decline in a score has occurred, additional raw score analysis is necessary. Because standardized scores are typically corrected for age, a child with a declining standardized score over time may appear as if he or she is losing skills when he or she is actually gaining skills, but not acquiring skills at the same rate as same-aged peers. In these situations, it is helpful to examine changes in raw scores as a way to assess ongoing development or identify a true decline in skills. Making these raw comparisons, however, is possible only if the same exact measure is used on each occasion.

Flynn Effect

While using the same measure on multiple occasions can be helpful in the individual level, when comparing the individual to him- or herself, it may be problematic when comparing the child to same-aged peers. Flynn and others have documented an upward drift in normative performances on intelligence tests (Carlton & Sapp, 1997; Flynn, 1984, 1985, 1987; Truscott & Frank, 2001). Known as the *Flynn effect,* these score increases in the United States amount to approximately three IQ points per decade. Correspondingly, as time passes, normative samples used to develop new measures of intelligence can represent a higher-functioning group than their cohorts who acted as the normative sample for previous versions of the same test. As a result, when an IQ test is renormed, which occurs every 15–20 years, the mean is reset to 100, and children may have to become "smarter" or otherwise show improvement in performance in order to maintain a constant performance level (Kanaya, Scullin, & Ceci, 2003).

Practice Effects

In addition to thinking about comparing raw score changes using the same test, and considering the Flynn effect in interpretation, it is important to consider practice effects. While practice effects are typically considered when testing occurs close in time (a few months apart), repeat assessment for longer intervals can result in practice effects especially if the same test is given several times. Unfortunately, there is little literature to guide our interpretation in these situations.

Conclusions

Neuropsychologists who practice in a developmental and/or life span context will undoubtedly encounter individuals with neurodevelopmental and/or genetic conditions. These individuals represent a diverse population, requiring an understanding of both neuropsychological principles and child development. The neuropsychologist should be fluent in both the behavioral and neurological approaches to classification, and should be prepared to work alongside colleagues in the school system. It is, in fact, necessary for the neuropsychologist to access school observations, records, and assessments when considering the "history" of a child with a neurodevelopmental condition. The DSM-5 even references this requirement in the revised diagnostic criteria for ADHD, by noting, "confirmation of substantial symptoms across settings typically cannot be done accurately without consulting informants who have seen the individual in those settings" (American Psychiatric Association, 2013: 61). Given these considerations, ecologically valid neuropsychological assessment of children with neurodevelopmental disorders is necessarily a collaborative effort between the referred patient, parents, schools, and (often) multiple treating clinicians.

The developmental course of genetic and neurodevelopmental disorders is often chronic, necessitating a "family practice" approach to neuropsychological assessment and consultation, in which the clinician provides care in different contexts and in different formats throughout the life of the individual with the condition. This approach requires flexibility in assessment methodology and a willingness to understanding diagnostic formulations as dynamic, rather than static, regardless of the level of stability of the neurological condition itself. In this context, it is essential for the clinician to recognize how changing environmental demands interact with the individual's neurobiology, and how these interactions may change over the child's lifetime.

Despite the complex and often diffuse nature of the neurological conditions in children with neurodevelopmental and genetic disorders, thoughtful neuropsychological assessment can be extremely helpful in elucidating strengths and weaknesses and planning appropriate interventions, especially considering the many challenging life transitions. When considering these transitions, clinicians working with children with neurodevelopmental disorders and their families are challenged to understand the unique way that services are provided in the community, and the difficulties associated with accessing such services upon transition into adulthood. As such, the developmental framework is essential, and the neuropsychologist is often in the unique position to provide the life span approach to assessment and intervention, throughout childhood, and (often) well into adulthood.

References

Adzick, N. S., Thom, E. A., Spong, C. Y., Brock, J. W., III., Burrows, P. K., Johnson, M. P., . . . MOMS Investigators. (2011). A randomized trial of prenatal versus postnatal repair of myelomeningocele. *The New England Journal of Medicine*, *364*(11), 993–1004. doi: 10.1056/NEJMoa1014379

Akinbami, L. J., Liu, X., Pastor, P. N., & Reuben, C. A. (2011). Attention deficit hyperactivity disorder among children aged 5–17 years in the United States, 1998–2009. *NCHS Data Brief*, *70*. Hyattsville, MD: National Center for Health Statistics.

Allen, M. C. (2008). Neurodevelopmental outcomes of preterm infants. *Current Opinion in Neurology*, *21*, 123–128. doi: 10.1097/WCO.0b013e3282f88bb4

American College of Obstetricians and Gynecologists. (2002). Perinatal care at the threshold of viability. *ACOG Practice Bulletin no. 38.* Washington, DC: Author.

American Psychiatric Association. (2000). *Diagnostic and Statistical Manual for Mental Disorders* (4th ed., Text Revision). Washington, DC: Author.

American Psychiatric Association. (2013). *Diagnostic and Statistical Manual for Mental Disorders* (5th ed.). Washington, DC: Author.

Anderson, P. J. (2014). Neuropsychological outcomes of children born very preterm. *Seminars in Fetal & Neonatal Medicine*, *19*, 90–96. doi: 10.1016/j.siny.2013.11.012

Arnold, P. D., Siegel-Bartelt, J., Cytrynbaum, C., Teshima, I., & Schachar, R. (2001). Velo-cardio-facial syndrome: Implications of microdeletion 22q11 for schizophrenia and mood disorders. *American Journal of Medical Genetics*, *105*(4), 354–362. doi: 10.1002/ajmg.1359

Baker, K. D., & Skuse, D. H. (2005). Adolescents and young adults with 22q11 deletion syndrome: Psychopathology in an at-risk group. *The British Journal of Psychiatry*, *189*, 115–120. doi: 10.1192/bjp.186.2.115

Barkovich, A. J., Kuzniecky, R. I., Jackson, G. D., Guerrini, R., & Dobyns, W. B. (2001). Classification system for malformations of cortical development. *Neurology*, *57*(12), 2168–2178. doi: 10.1212/WNL.57.12.2168

Baron, I. S., Litman, F. R., Ahronovich, M. D., & Baker, R. (2012). Late preterm birth: A review of medical and neuropsychological childhood outcomes. *Neuropsychology Review*, *22*(4), 438–458. doi: 10.1007/s11065-012-9210-5

Bernstein, J.H., & Waber, D.P. (1990). Developmental neuropsychological assessment: The systemic approach. In A.A. Boulton, G.B. Baker, & M. Hiscock (Eds.). *Neuromethods: Neuropsychology* (pp. 311–371). Clifton, NJ: Humana Press.

Bittles, A. H., Bower, C., Hussain, R., & Glasson, E. J. (2006). The four ages of Down syndrome. *European Journal of Public Health*, *17*(2), 221–225. doi: 10.1093/eurpub/ckl103

Botto, L. D., May, K., Fernhoff, P. M., Correa, A., Coleman, K., Rasmussen, S. A., . . . Campbell, R. M. (2003). A population-based study of the 22q11.2 deletion: Phenotype, incidence, and contribution to major birth defects in the population. *Pediatrics*, *112*(1), 101–107.

Boulet, S. L., Yang, Q., Mai, C., Kirby, R. S., Collins, J. S., Robbins, J. M., . . . Mulinare, J. (2008). Trends in the postfortification prevalence of spina bifida and anencephaly in the United States. *Birth Defects Research Part A: Clinical and Molecular Teratology*, *82*(7), 527–532. doi: 10.1002/bdra.20468

Budimirovic, D. B., & Kaufmann, W. E. (2011). What can we learn about autism from studying FFragile X syndrome? *Developmental Neuroscience*, *33*, 379–394. doi: 10.1159/000330213

Butterworth, P., Leach, L. S., McManus, S., & Stansfeld, S. A. (2013). Common mental disorders, unemployment and psychosocial job quality: Is a poor job better than no job at all? *Psychological Medicine*, *43*(8), 1763–1772. doi: 10.1017/S0033291712002577

Carey, A. H., Kelly, D., Halford, S., Wadey, R., Wilson, D., Goodship, J., . . . Scambler, P. J. (1992). Molecular genetic study of the frequency of monosomy 22q11 in DiGeorge syndrome. *The American Journal of Human Genetics*, *51*(5), 964–970.

Carlton, M., & Sapp, G. L. (1997). Comparison of WISC-R and WISC-III scores of urban exceptional students. *Psychological Reports*, *80*(3), 755–760. doi: 10.2466/pr0.1997.80.3.755

Centers for Disease Control and Prevention (CDC). (2004). Spina bifida and anencephaly before and after folic acid mandate—United States, 1995–1996 and 1999–2000. *Morbidity and Mortality Weekly Report*, *53*(17), 362–365.

Centers for Disease Control and Prevention (CDC). (2014). Prevalence of autism spectrum disorder among children aged 8 years: Autism and developmental disabilities monitoring network, 11 sites, United States, 2010: Morbidity and mortality weekly report, March 28, 2014. *Surveillance Summaries*, *63*(2), 1–24.

Charney, E. B. (1992). Neural tube defects: Spina bifida and myelomeningocele. In M. Batshaw & Y. Perret (Eds.), *Children with Disabilities: A Medical Primer* (pp. 471–488). Baltimore, MD: Paul H. Brookes.

Christ, S. E., White, D. A., Brunstrom, J. E., & Abrams, R. A. (2003). Inhibitory control following perinatal brain injury. *Neuropsychology*, *17*(1), 171–178. doi: 10.1037/0894-4105.17.1.171

Culhane-Shelburne, K., Chapieski, L., Hiscock, M., & Glaze, D. (2002). Executive functions in children with frontal and temporal lobe epilepsy. *Journal of the International Neuropsychological Society*, *8*(5), 623-632.

Cusmano-Ozog, K., Manning, M. A., & Hoyme, H. E. (2007). 22q13.3 deletion syndrome: A recognizable malformation syndrome associated with marked speech and language delay. *American Journal of Medical Genetics Part C (Seminars in Medical Genetics)*, *145C*, 393–398. doi: 10.1002/ajmg.c.30155

Dennis, M., & Barnes, M. A. (2010). The cognitive phenotype of spina bifida meningomyelocele. *Developmental Disabilities Research Reviews*, *16*(1), 31–39. doi: 10.1002/ddrr.89

Dennis, M., Nelson, R., Jewell, D., & Fletcher, J. M. (2010). Prospective memory in adults with spina bifida. *Child's Nervous System*, *26*(12), 1749–1755. doi: 10.1007/s00381-010-1140-z

Dorrie, N., Focker, M., Freunscht, I., & Hebebrand, J. (2014). Fetal alcohol spectrum disorders. *European Child & Adolescent Psychiatry*, *23*, 863–875. doi: 10.1007/s00787-014-0571-6

Driscoll, D. A., Budarf, M. L., & Emanuel, B. S. (1992). A genetic etiology for DiGeorge syndrome: Consistent deletions and microdeletions of 22q11. *The American Journal of Human Genetics*, *50*(5), 924–933.

Duff, K. (2012). Evidence-based indicators of neuropsychological change in the individual patient: Relevant concepts and methods. *Archives of Clinical Neuropsychology*, *27*(3), 248–261. doi: 10.1093/arclin/acr120

Feinstein, C., Eliez, S., Blasey, C., & Reiss, A. L. (2002). Psychiatric disorders and behavioral problems in children with velocardiofacial syndrome: Usefulness as phenotypic indicators of schizophrenia risk. *Biological Psychiatry*, *51*(4), 312–318. doi: 10.1016/S0006-3223(01)01231-8

Fennell, E. B., & Dikel, T. N. (2001). Cognitive and neuropsychological functioning in children with cerebral palsy. *Journal of Child Neurology*, *16*(1), 58–63. doi: 10.1177/088307380101600110

Fletcher, J. M. (2014). The effects of childhood ADHD on adult labor market outcomes. *Health Economics*, *23*, 159–181.

Flynn, J. R. (1984). The mean IQ of Americans: Massive gains 1932 to 1978. *Psychological Bulletin*, *95*(1), 29–51. doi: 10.1037/0033-2909.95.1.29

Flynn, J. R. (1985). Wechsler intelligence tests: Do we really have a criterion of mental retardation? *American Journal of Mental Deficiency*, *90*(3), 236–244.

Flynn, J. R. (1987). Massive IQ gains in 14 nations: What IQ tests really measure. *Psychological Bulletin*, *101*(2), 171–191.doi: 10.1037/0033-2909.101.2.171

Fung, L. K., Quintin, E., Haas, B. W., & Reiss, A. L. (2012). Conceptualizing neurodevelopmental disorders through a mechanistic understanding of Fragile X syndrome and Williams syndrome. *Current Opinion in Neurology*, *25*(2), 112–124. doi: 10.1097/WCO.0b013e328351823c

Furstenberg, F. F., Jr., Rumbaut, R. G., & Settersten, R. A. Jr. (2005). On the frontier of adulthood: Emerging themes and new directions. In R. A. Settersten, Jr., F. F. Furstenberg, & R. G. Rumbaut (Eds.), *On the Frontier of Adulthood: Theory, Research, and Public Policy* (pp. 3–25). Chicago, IL: University of Chicago Press.

Gothelf, D. (2007). Velocardiofacial syndrome. *Child and Adolescent Psychiatric Clinics of North America*, *16*(3), 677–693. doi: 10.1016/j.chc.2007.03.005

Greenspan, S. (2006). Mental retardation in the real world: Why the AAMR definition is not there yet. In H. N. Switzky & S. Greenspan (Eds.), *What Is Mental Retardation? Ideas for an Evolving Disability in the 21st Century* (pp. 167–185). Washington, DC: American Association on Intellectual and Developmental Disabilities.

Hannay, H.J., Dennis, M., Kramer, L., Blaser, S., & Fletcher, J.M. (2009). Partial agenesis of the corpus callosum in spina bifida meningomyelocele and potentially compensatory mechanisms. *Journal of Clinical and Experimental Neuropsychology*, *31*, 180–194. doi: 10.1080/13803390802209954

Heilbronner, R. L., Sweet, J. J., Attix, D. K., Krull, K. R., Henry, G. K., & Hart, R. P. (2010). Official position of the American Academy of Clinical Neuropsychology on serial neuropsychological assessments: The utility and challenges of repeat test administrations in clinical and forensic contexts. *The Clinical Neuropsychologist*, *24*(8), 1267–1278. doi: 10.1080/13854046.2010.526785

Hetherington, R., Dennis, M., Barnes, M., Drake, J., & Gentili, F. (2006). Functional outcome in young adults with spina bifida and hydrocephalus. *Child's Nervous System*, *22*(2), 117–124. doi: 10.1007/s00381-005-1231-4

Holmes-Bernstein, J., & Waber, D. P. (1990). Developmental neuropsychological assessment: The systemic approach. *Neuropsychology*, 311–371. doi: 10.1385/0-89603-133-0:311

Hoon, A.H., & Melhem, E.R. (2000). Neuroimaging: Applications in disorders of early brain development. *Journal of Developmental and Behavioral Pediatics*, *21*, 291–302.

Hoyme, H. E., May, P. A., Kalberg, W. O., Kadituwakku, P., Gossage, J. P., Trujillo, P. M., . . . Robinson, L. K. (2005). A practical clinical approach to diagnosis of fetal alcohol spectrum disorders: Clarification of the 1996 Institute of Medicine criteria. *Pediatrics*, *115*(1), 39–47. doi: 10.1542/peds.2004-0259

Jarjour, I. T. (2014). Neurodevelopmental outcome after extreme prematurity: A review of the literature. *Pediatric Neurology*. Advance online publication. doi: 10.1016/j.pediatrneurol.2014.10.027

Johnston, M. V. (2004). Selective vulnerability in the neonatal brain. *Annals of Neurology*, *44*(2), 155–156. doi: 10.1002/ana.410440202

Johnston, M. V., & Hoon, A. H. Jr. (2006). Cerebral palsy. *NeuroMolecular Medicine*, *8*(4), 435–450. doi: 10.1385/NMM:8:4:435

Johnston, M. V., Hoon, H. A., & Kaufmann, W. E. (2008). Neurobiology, diagnosis, and management of cerebral palsy. In P. J. Accardo (Ed.), *Capute & Accardo's Neurodevelopmental Disabilities in Infancy and Childhood, Vol. 2: The Spectrum of Neurodevelopmental Disabilities* (pp. 61–81). Baltimore, MD: Paul H. Brookes Pub.

Juranek, J., Fletcher, J. M., Hasan, K. M., Breier, J. I., Cirino, P. T., Pazo-Alvarez, P., . . . Papanicolaou, A. C. (2008). Neocortical reorganization in spina bifida. *Neuroimage*, *40*(4), 1516–1522. doi: 10.1016/j.neuroimage.2008.01.043

Kanaya, T., Scullin, M. H., & Ceci, S. J. (2003). The Flynn effect and US policies: the impact of rising IQ scores on American society via mental retardation diagnoses. *American Psychologist*, *58*(10), 778. doi: 10.1037/0003-066X.58.10.778

Kirkpatrick, J. A., & DiGeorge, A. M. (1968). Congenital absence of the thymus. *The American Journal of Roentgenology, Radium Therapy, and Nuclear Medicine*, *103*(1), 32–37.

Korzeniewski, S.J., Birbeck, G., DeLano, M.C., Potchen, M.J., & Paneth, N. (2008). A systematic review of neuroimaging for cerebral palsy. *Journal of Child Neurology*, *23*, 216–227. doi: 10.1177/0883073807307983

Kozeis, N., Anogeianaki, A., Tosheva Mitova, D., Anogianakis, G., Mitov, T., & Klisarova, A. (2007). Visual function and visual perception in cerebral palsied children. *Ophthalmic & Physiological Optics*, *27*(1), 44–53. doi: 10.1111/j.1475-1313.2006.00413.x

Larson, S. A., Lakin, K. C., Anderson, L., Kwak, N., Lee, J. H., & Anderson, D. (2011). Prevalence of mental retardation and developmental disabilities: Estimates from 1994/1995 National Health Survey Disability Supplement. *American Journal of Mental Retardation*, *106*(3), 231–252.

Lott, I. T., & Dierssen, M. (2010). Cognitive deficits and associated neurological complication in individuals with Down's syndrome. *Lancet Neurology*, *9*(6), 623–633. doi: 10.1016/S1474-4422(10)70112-5

Lozano, R., Rosero, C. A., & Hagerman, R. J. (2014). Fragile X spectrum disorders. *Intractable & Rare Diseases Research*, *3*(4), 134–146. doi: 10.5582/irdr.2014.01022

Mahone, E. M. (2007). Psychological assessment. In A. Capute & P. Accardo (Eds.), *Neurodevelopmental Disabilities* (3rd ed., vol. 2, pp. 261–281). Baltimore, MD: Brookes Publishing Company.

Mahone, E. M., Crocetti, D., Ranta, M. E., Gaddis, A., Cataldo, M., Slifer, K. J., Denckla, M. B., & Mostofsky, S. H. (2011). A preliminary neuroimaging study of preschool children with ADHD. *The Clinical Neuropsychologist*, *25*(6), 1009–1028.

Mahone, E. M., & Mapou, R. (2014). Learning disabilities. In K. Stucky, M. Kirkwood, J. Donders, & C. Liff (Eds.). *Clinical Neuropsychology Study Guide and Board Review* (pp. 184–201). New York: Oxford University Press.

Mahone, E. M., & Slomine, B. S. (2008). Neurodevelopmental disorders. In J. Morgan & J. Ricker (Eds.), *Textbook of Clinical Neuropsychology* (pp. 105–127). New York: Taylor and Francis.

Mahone, E. M., & Zabel, T. A. (2001). Challenges to executive function. *Insights Into Spina Bifida*, *7*(5), 1A–8A.

Maulik, P. K., Mascarenhas, M. N., Mathers, C. D., Dua, T., & Saxena, S. (2011). Prevalence of intellectual disability: A meta-analysis of population-based studies. *Research in Developmental Disabilities*, *32*(2), 419–436. doi: 10.1016/j.ridd.2010.12.018

May, P. A., Gossage, J. P., Kalberg, W. O., Robinson, L. K., Buckley, D., Manning, M., & Hoyme, H. E. (2009). Prevalence and epidemiologic characteristics of FASD from various research methods with an emphasis on recent in-school studies. *Developmental Disabilities Research Reviews*, *15*(3), 176–192. doi: 10.1002/ddrr.68

Menkes, J. H., & Sarnat, H. B. (2000). Periuatal asphyxia and trauma. In J. H. Menkes & H. B. Sarnat (Eds.), *Child Neurology* (pp. 427–436). Philadelphia, PA: Lippincott Williams and Wilkins.

Muzykewicz, D.A., Newberry, P., Danforth, N., Halpern, E.F., & Thiele, E.A. (2007). Psychiatric comorbid conditions in a clinic population of 241 patients with tuberous sclerosis complex. *Epilepsy and Behavior*, *11*, 506–513.

Papazoglou, A., Jacobson, L. A., & Zabel, T. A. (2013). More than intelligence: Distinct cognitive/behavioral clusters linked to adaptive dysfunction in children. *Journal of the International Neuropsychological Society*, *19*(2), 189–197. doi: 10.1017/S1355617712001191

Pirila, S., van der Meere, J., Korhonen, P., Ruusu-Niemi, P., Kyntaja, M., Nieminen, P., & Korpela, R. (2004). A retrospective neurocognitive study in children with spastic diplegia. *Developmental Neuropsychology*, *26*(3), 679–690. doi: 10.1207/s15326942dn2603_2

Rudel, R.G. (1981). Residual effects of childhood reading disabilities. *Annals of Dyslexia*, *31*(1), 89–102.

Saigal, S., Stoskopf, B., Streiner, D., Boyle, M., Pinelli, J., Paneth, N., & Goddeeris, J. (2006). Transition of extremely low-birth-weight infants from adolescence to young adulthood. *Journal of the American Medical Association*, *295*(6), 667–675. doi: 10.1001/jama.295.6.667

Sherman, S. L., Allen, E. G., Bean, L. H., & Freeman, S. B. (2007). Epidemiology of Down syndrome. *Mental Retardation and Developmental Disabilities Research Reviews*, *13*, 221–227. doi: 10.1002/mrdd.20157

Shprintzen, R. J., Goldberg, R. B., Lewin, M. L., Sidoti, E. J., Berkman, M. D., Argamaso, R. V., & Young, D. (1978). A new syndrome involving cleft palate, cardiac anomalies, typical facies, and learning disabilities: Velo-cardio-facial syndrome. *The Cleft Palate Journal*, *15*(1), 56–62.

Sigurdardottir, S., Eiriksdottir, A., Gunnarsdottir, E., Meintema, M., Arnadottir, U., & Vik, T. (2008). Cognitive profile in young Icelandic children with cerebral palsy. *Developmental Medicine & Child Neurology*, *50*(5), 357–362. doi: 10.1111/j.1469-8749.2008.02046.x

Sulewski, J. S., Zalewska, A., Butterworth, J., & Migliore, A. (2013). *Trends in Employment Outcomes of Young Adults With Intellectual and Developmental Disabilities in Eight States, 2004–2011*. Boston, MA: University of Massachusetts Boston, Institute for Community Inclusion.

Tarazi, R., Mahone, E. M., & Zabel, T. A. (2007). Self-care independence in children with neurological disorders: An interactional model of adaptive demands and executive dysfunction. *Rehabilitation Psychology*, *52*(2), 196–205.

Tarazi, R. A., Zabel, T. A., & Mahone, E. M. (2008). Age-related differences in executive function among children with spina bifida/hydrocephalus based on parent behavior ratings. *The Clinical Neuropsychologist*, *22*(4), 585–602. doi: 10.1080/13854040701425940

Treble-Barna, A., Kulesz, P. A., Dennis, M., & Fletcher, J. M. (2014). Covert orienting in three etiologies of congenital hydrocephalus: The effect of midbrain and posterior fossa dysmorphology. *Journal of the International Neuropsychological Society*, *20*(3), 268–277. doi: 10.1017/S1355617713001501

Trotter Ross, W., & Olsen, M. (2014). Care of the adult patient with Down syndrome. *Southern Medical Journal*, *107*(11), 715–721. doi: 10.14423/SMJ.0000000000000193

Truscott, S. D., & Frank, A. J. (2001). Does the Flynn effect affect IQ scores of students classified as LD? *Journal of School Psychology*, *39*(4), 319–334. doi: 10.1016/S0022-4405(01)00071-1

Vohr, B. R. (2014). Neurodevelopmental outcomes of extremely preterm infants. *Clinics in Perinatology*, *41*(1), 241–255. doi: 10.1016/j.clp.2013.09.003

Wang, P. P., Woodin, M. F., Kreps-Falk, R., & Moss, E. M. (2000). Research on behavioral phenotypes: Velocardiofacial syndrome (deletion 22q11.2). *Developmental Medicine & Child Neurology*, *42*(6), 422–427. doi: 10.1111/j.1469-8749.2000.tb00125.x

Warf, B. C., & Campbell, J. W. (2008). Combined endoscopic third ventriculostomy and choroid plexus cauterization as primary treatment of hydrocephalus for infants with myelomeningocele: long-term results of a prospective intent-to-treat study in 115 East African infants. *Journal of Neurosurgery: Pediatrics*, *2*(5), 310–316. doi: 10.3171/PED.2008.2.11.310

Wehmeyer, M. L., Buntinx, W., Lachapelle, Y., Luckasson, R. A., Schalock, R. L., Verdugo, M. A., . . . Yeager, M. H. (2008). The intellectual disability construct and its relation to human functioning. *Intellectual and Developmental Disabilities*, *46*(4), 311–318.

Willsey, A. J., & State, M. W. (2015). Autism spectrum disorders: From genes to neurobiology. *Current Opinion in Neurobiology*, *30*, 92–99. doi: 10.1016/j.conb.2014.10.015

Woodin, M., Wang, P. P., Aleman, D., McDonald-McGinn, D., Zackai, E., & Moss, E. (2001). Neuropsychological profile of children and adolescents with the 22q11.2 microdeletion. *Genetics in Medicine*, *3*, 34–39. doi: 10.1097/00125817-200101000-00008

Zabel, T. A., Jacobson, L. A., Zachik, C., Levey, E., Kinsman, S., & Mahone, E. M. (2011). Parent- and self-ratings of executive functions in adolescents and young adults with spina bifida. *The Clinical Neuropsychologist*, *25*(6), 926–941. doi: 10.1080/13854046.2011.586002

Zabel, T. A., & Schmidt, A. T. (2011). A case of cerebral palsy (spastic diplegia). In J. E. Morgan, I. S. Baron, & J. H. Ricker (Eds.), *Casebook of Clinical Neuropsychology* (pp. 87–96). New York: Oxford University Press.

Zigman, W. B. (2013). Atypical aging in Down syndrome. *Developmental Disabilities Research Reviews*, *18*, 51–67. doi: 10.1002/ddrr.1128

11 Traumatic Brain Injury in Children and Adolescents

Keith Owen Yeates and Brian L. Brooks

Traumatic brain injuries (TBIs) arising from closed-head trauma in children are the most common source of acquired brain injury among children and adolescents, and represent a major public health problem, with total annual health care costs exceeding $1 billion in the United States (Schneier, Shields, Hostetler, Xiang, & Smith, 2006). Our understanding of the neuropsychological outcomes of pediatric TBI has increased significantly over the last two decades, as reflected in multiple recent reviews (Anderson & Yeates, 2014; Bodin & Yeates, 2010; Kirkwood, Peterson, & Yeates, 2013; Taylor, 2010; Yeates, 2010). Nevertheless, much remains to be learned (Anderson & Yeates, 2010; Kochanek, 2006). In the present chapter, we summarize current knowledge regarding pediatric TBI. We then critique existing research, and highlight recent conceptual and methodological advances. We next provide a clinical case illustration. Finally, we conclude by discussing new directions for future investigation.

Epidemiology

Incidence and Prevalence

Epidemiological studies of pediatric TBI vary widely in their methodologies (Kraus, 1995). The most recent and complete data for the United States comes from the Centers for Disease Control (CDC; Faul, Xu, Wald, & Coronado, 2010), which estimated nearly 700,000 TBIs annually for children ages 0–19, based on deaths, hospitalizations, and emergency department visits, with an overall incidence of 857 per 100,000.

Incidence varies as a function of injury severity. Using data from a 14-state surveillance system, the CDC estimated that 71%–77% of hospital discharges for TBI across youth ages 0–19 years were classified as mild, 7%–11% as moderate, and 8%–12% as severe (Langlois et al., 2003). This is consistent with estimates based on international statistics indicating that 80%–90% of all pediatric TBI fall in the mild range (Cassidy et al., 2004). Both the incidence of pediatric TBI and the proportion that are mild in severity are almost certainly underestimated, because many injuries are treated in outpatient settings and do not result in hospital visits, or go unreported entirely (Sosin, Sniezek, & Thurman, 1996).

Cause of Injury

The most common causes of TBI involve transportation, falls, and blunt trauma (i.e., unintentionally being struck by or against another object, such as colliding with another player during sport). Together, those three causes account for approximately 80% of all pediatric TBI (Faul et al., 2010). The distribution of causes varies significantly as a function of age (Keenan & Bratton, 2006). Infants are especially likely to sustain TBI through falls. School-age children are most likely to be injured through falls or blunt trauma. Adolescents are increasingly likely to be injured in motor vehicle collisions, although falls and blunt trauma remain significant causes among youth.

Demographic Variation

Boys are more likely to sustain TBI than girls, although the ratio is lower in infants and young children than during older childhood and adolescence (Faul et al., 2010). Children ages 0–4 years are most likely to visit emergency departments for evaluation of TBI, with an annual incidence of about 1,256 per 100,000, suggesting that milder injuries may be especially common among younger children. In contrast, older adolescents ages 15–19 show the highest rates of hospitalizations and deaths, with a combined annual incidence of about 139 per 100,000, likely reflecting the increasing severity of TBI in that age group as a function of transportation-related injuries.

Incidence rates also appear to vary as a function of race and socioeconomic status. According to the CDC, Blacks demonstrate higher rates of emergency department visits for TBI than Whites among children 0–14 years of age and higher rates of hospitalization and death for motor vehicle–related TBI among children 0–9 years of age (Faul et al., 2010; Langlois, Rutland-Brown, & Thomas, 2005). The risk of TBI, particularly those linked to motor vehicles, is also substantially higher for children of lower socioeconomic status (Brown, 2010; Howard, Joseph, & Natale, 2005).

Mortality

Unintentional injuries are the leading cause of death among children and adolescents in the United States, and about

40%–50% of the deaths resulting from trauma are associated with TBI (Kraus, 1995). Mortality rates are higher among adolescents and adults than among children, likely because of the increasing rates of transportation-related injuries at later ages. The CDC estimates an annual mortality rate around 3.6 per 100,000 for children 0–14 years of age, but a rate of about 19 per 100,000 for 15–19 year olds (Faul et al., 2010). The mortality rate is highest among children with severe TBI, and very low among children with mild to moderate injuries (Kraus, 1995).

Neuropathology and Pathophysiology

TBI involves multiple forms of neuropathology, ranging from overt damage to brain tissue to disruptions in brain function at a cellular level (see Table 11.1). The pathophysiology of TBI involves interwoven processes that begin at the time of impact but continue for an extended period of time (Farkas & Povlishock, 2007; Giza & Hovda, 2001; Povlishock & Katz, 2005). Thus, TBI can result in protracted neurodegenerative changes in children (Keightley et al., 2014), and is best understood as a disease process and chronic health condition rather than an isolated event (Corrigan & Hammond, 2013; Masel & DeWitt, 2010).

Children's brains respond differently to trauma than do adult brains (Giza, Mink, & Madikians, 2007). For example, children are more likely than adults to display posttraumatic brain swelling, hypoxic-ischemic insult, and other diffuse injuries, but less likely to have focal mass lesions. The biomechanical properties of the young brain may explain at least some of these differences. Compared to adults, children have a larger head-to-body ratio, less myelination, and higher relative proportion of water content and cerebral blood volume. During adolescence, TBI-related pathology begins to more closely resemble that seen in adults.

Table 11.1 Neuropathology of TBI

Type of Insult	*Neuropathology*
Primary	Skull fracture
	Focal contusions and lacerations
	Shear/strain injury
Secondary	Brain swelling
	Cerebral edema
	Elevated intracranial pressure
	Hypoxia-ischemia
	Mass lesions (e.g., epidural hematoma)
Neurochemical and Neurometabolic	Excessive production of free radicals
	Excessive release of excitatory neurotransmitters
	Alterations in glucose metabolism
	Traumatic axonal injury
Late/Delayed	Cerebral atrophy
	Posttraumatic hydrocephalus
	Posttraumatic epilepsy

Primary and Secondary Injuries

Observable injuries resulting from closed-head trauma can be classified into two broad categories: *primary* and *secondary*. Primary injuries result directly from the impact to the head itself. They include skull fractures, contusions and lacerations, and mechanical injuries to nerve fibers and blood vessels. Secondary injuries arise indirectly from the trauma and include brain swelling and edema, hypoxia and hypotension, increased intracranial pressure, and mass lesions.

The biomechanics of TBI are not fully understood in children (Margulies & Coats, 2010). TBI often involve acceleration/deceleration forces that can result in both translational and rotational trauma. Translational trauma can result in deformation of the skull or skull fractures, as well as contusions at the site of impact. Rotational trauma results in the tearing or bruising of blood vessels that gives rise to focal contusions or hemorrhage, as well as in shearing or straining of nerve fibers associated with traumatic axonal injury. Focal lesions are especially likely to occur in the frontal and temporal cortex, because of its proximity to the bony prominences in the anterior and middle fossa of the skull (Bigler, 2007; Wilde et al., 2005). Traumatic axonal injury is most common at the boundaries between gray and white matter.

Medical management of TBI tends to focus less on primary injuries than on the secondary injuries that can arise indirectly following the initial trauma (Kochanek, Carney, Adelson, & Warden, 2012). Brain swelling and cerebral edema are two major secondary complications of TBI and are especially common in children (Kochanek, 2006). They can result in decreased cerebral blood flow, increased cerebral blood volume, and increased intracranial pressure (i.e., intracranial hypertension), which combined can give rise to hypoxic-ischemic injury, as well as to brain herniation and death.

Neurochemical and Neurometabolic Mechanisms

The mechanical forces involved in TBI do not account for the majority of traumatic axonal injury. Instead, traumatic axonal injury likely results from a cascade of biochemical and metabolic reactions that occur after the initial trauma, including the overproduction of free radicals and excitatory neurotransmitters, the disruption of normal calcium homeostasis, and changes in glucose metabolism (Farkas & Povlishock, 2007; Giza & Hovda, 2001; Novack, Dillon, & Jackson, 1996). Despite considerable promise in animal research, clinical trials designed to reduce brain injury by altering neurochemical and neurometabolic mechanisms have been uniformly disappointing in humans (Narayan & Michel, 2002).

Late Effects

TBI can be associated with a variety of late effects. Neurodegenerative processes can result in cerebral atrophy and ventricular enlargement (Ghosh et al., 2009; Keightley et al., 2014). Ventricular dilatation may also be the result of posttraumatic hydrocephalus, although this typically develops only after severe injuries associated with certain predisposing factors, such as subarachnoid hemorrhage (McLean et al., 1995). Early posttraumatic seizures, defined as occurring within the first week after TBI, occur frequently and can involve focal status epilepticus (Statler, 2006). Early posttraumatic seizures do not clearly place children at risk for later epilepsy, which occurs in about 10%–20% of children with severe TBI. Posttraumatic epilepsy is more common in children with penetrating or inflicted injuries, or injuries associated with depressed skull fractures.

Outcomes

Cognitive Abilities

The cognitive consequences of pediatric TBI have been the subject of several reviews and meta-analyses (Babikian & Asarnow, 2009; Taylor, 2010; Yeates, 2010). Overall, research indicates that TBI, especially when severe, can produce deficits across a variety of cognitive domains. In comparison, mild TBI is unlikely to result in long-term cognitive deficits (Belanger, Spiegel, & Vanderploeg, 2010).

Orientation and alertness are often disturbed following TBI, particularly during the initial phase of recovery. Most children with TBI, especially those that are moderate or severe, experience acute fluctuations in arousal, as well as disorientation, confusion, and memory loss after the injury, a constellation typically referred to as posttraumatic amnesia (Ewing-Cobbs, Levin, Fletcher, Miner, & Eisenberg, 1990).

Children with TBI often demonstrate deficits in sensory and motor skills. Approximately 25% of children with severe TBI display deficits in stereognosis, finger localization, and graphesthesia (Levin & Eisenberg, 1979). Deficits are also common in fine-motor skills, especially on timed tasks (Bawden, Knights, & Winogron, 1985). Disturbances in gait and gross motor skills are also common (Kuhtz-Buschbeck et al., 2003).

Children with TBI tend to display both verbal and nonverbal intellectual deficits, as measured by traditional IQ tests, and the magnitude of the deficits is related to injury severity (Anderson, Morse, Catroppa, Haritou, & Rosenfeld, 2004, 2005b; Taylor et al., 1999). IQ scores tend to increase over time following TBI, with the most rapid increases occurring immediately after injury and among children with more severe injuries (Yeates et al., 2002). Persistent deficits in IQ are more likely among children with severe TBI and those injured early in life (Anderson et al., 2004, 2005a).

Spontaneous mutism and expressive language deficits are common immediately after TBI (Levin et al., 1983), but overt aphasic disorders rarely persist. Language deficits typically improve over time, with the greatest gains seen following severe TBI (Catroppa & Anderson, 2004), although long-term deficits have been identified in a variety of basic linguistic skills (Ewing-Cobbs & Barnes, 2002). The most pronounced difficulties, though, occur in the pragmatic aspects of language, particularly narrative discourse (Chapman et al., 2004; Dennis & Barnes, 1990).

Long-term deficits in nonverbal skills are a relatively frequent consequence of pediatric TBI. Deficits have been reported on a variety of constructional tasks (Thompson et al., 1994; Yeates et al., 2002). Deficits also occur on measures of perceptual or spatial skills that do not involve motor output (Lehnung et al., 2001), although they tend to be less pronounced than those in other domains (Babikian & Asarnow, 2009).

Complaints about attention problems are very common following childhood TBI (Yeates et al., 2005), as are deficits on formal tests of attention. On continuous performance tests, children with TBI display poorer response modulation, especially in the presence of distraction, as well as slower reaction times (Dennis, Wilkinson, Koski, & Humphreys, 1995). Children with TBI also show deficits on measures of sustained, selective, shifting, and divided attention, particularly on more complex and timed measures (Catroppa & Anderson, 2005; Catroppa, Anderson, Morse, Haritou, & Rosenfeld, 2007; Ewing-Cobbs et al., 1998b).

Childhood TBI frequently results in concerns about memory deficits (Ward, Shum, Dick, McKinaly, & Baker-Tweney, 2004). Deficits also have been reported on a wide variety of tasks assessing explicit memory, particularly in children with severe TBI (Catroppa & Anderson, 2002, 2007; Yeates, Blumenstein, Patterson, & Deils, 1995). Children with TBI may be less likely to display deficits in implicit memory, which involves demonstrations of learning or facilitation of performance in the absence of conscious recollection (Ward, Shum, Wallace, & Boon, 2002; Yeates & Enrile, 2005). In contrast, children with TBI do display deficits in prospective memory (McCauley & Levin, 2004; Ward, Shum, McKinaly, Baker, & Wallace, 2007).

Deficits in executive functions occur frequently after childhood TBI (Levin & Hanten, 2005) and can persist for years after injury (Nadebaum, Anderson, & Catroppa, 2007). Young children and those with severe injuries are particularly vulnerable to executive deficits following TBI (Anderson & Catroppa, 2005; Ewing-Cobbs, Prasad, Landry, Kramer, & DeLeon, 2004b). Children with TBI also display executive deficits in everyday settings (Mangeot, Armstrong, Colvin, Yeates, & Taylor, 2002; Sesma, Slomine, Ding, & McCarthy, 2008) that have been linked to broader difficulties with social and behavioral adjustment (Ganesalingam, Sanson, Anderson, & Yeates, 2007).

Functional Outcomes

Childhood TBI is frequently associated with declines in school classroom performance (Ewing-Cobbs et al., 2004a; Taylor et al., 2002) and other academic difficulties (Ewing-Cobbs,

Fletcher, Levin, Iovino, & Miner, 1998a; Taylor et al., 2003). Deficits on formal achievement testing are more likely in children injured at a young age (Ewing-Cobbs et al., 2004a, 2006). Academic difficulties are predicted by factors such as premorbid classroom performance (Catroppa & Anderson, 2007), postinjury neuropsychological functioning (Kinsella et al., 1997; Miller & Donders, 2003), and postinjury behavioral adjustment (Yeates & Taylor, 2006). The family environment also moderates academic performance, such that more supportive and functional homes lessen the impact of TBI (Taylor et al., 2002). Surprisingly, standardized achievement testing is not always a strong predictor of academic outcomes after TBI (Yeates & Taylor, 2006).

Childhood TBI also often results in problems with social functioning (Rosema, Crowe, & Anderson, 2012; Yeates et al., 2007). Following TBI, children display deficits in theory of mind (Dennis et al., 2013), as well as in social problem solving (Hanten et al., 2008; Janusz, Kirkwood, Yeates, & Taylor, 2002). Deficits in executive functions and social information processing are linked to poor social outcomes after TBI (Yeates et al., 2004; Robinson et al., 2014). Although frontal lobe injury in association with TBI has been linked in some studies to poor social outcomes (Dennis, Guger, Roncadin, Barnes, & Schachar, 2001a; Hanten et al., 2008; Levin et al., 2004), the relationship of regional brain injury to social functioning after TBI is quite variable (Bigler et al., 2013; Yeates et al., 2014).

TBI in children increases the risk for a wide range of emotional and behavioral problems (Li & Liu, 2013; Taylor et al., 2002). In contrast to cognitive deficits, behavioral problems are more likely to show a stable or even worsening pattern over time (Fay et al., 2009). Indeed, behavioral functioning does not appear to be closely related to cognitive outcomes of TBI (Fletcher, Ewing-Cobbs, Miner, Levin, & Eisenberg, 1990). The determinants of cognitive and behavioral outcomes also may be somewhat independent. Cognitive outcomes are related more strongly to injury-related variables, whereas behavioral outcomes are related more strongly to measures of preinjury family functioning (Yeates et al., 1997).

Childhood TBI is associated with an increased risk of formal psychiatric disorder (Bloom et al., 2001). The most common diagnoses following childhood TBI are oppositional defiant disorder (ODD; Max et al., 1998a), attention deficit/hyperactivity disorder (ADHD; Levin et al., 2007; Max et al., 2005b; Yeates et al., 2005), and personality change due to TBI (Max et al., 2000, 2005a). Internalizing disorders also occur, including obsessive-compulsive symptoms, generalized anxiety, separation anxiety, and depression (Grados et al. 2008; Luis & Mittenberg, 2002; Vasa et al., 2002). Symptoms of posttraumatic stress disorder (PTSD) are also elevated following childhood TBI, although relatively few children meet full diagnostic criteria for PTSD (Gerring et al., 2002; Levi et al., 1999).

Moderate or severe TBI is followed by persistent deficits in adaptive behavior, including poorer communication, socialization, and daily living skills (Fay et al., 2009; Max et al., 1998c). Children with TBI also demonstrate significant declines in their overall quality of life, although differences are more pronounced based on parent reports than when based on children's self-reports (DiBattista, Soo, Catroppa, & Anderson, 2012; Stancin et al., 2002).

Although few studies of long-term adult outcomes following childhood TBI have been conducted, the existing research clearly documents an increased risk of persistent functional deficits. As adults, children with severe TBI are likely to demonstrate less educational attainment, reduced employment and occupational status, poorer socialization, increased psychiatric disorder, and reductions in functional independence and perceived quality of life (Anderson, Brown, Newitt, & Holie, 2009, 2011; Beauchamp, Dooley, & Anderson, 2010).

Predictors of Outcomes

Most research on the outcomes of pediatric TBI has focused on group comparisons (e.g., severe TBI versus orthopedic injuries). Although such comparisons are informative, they fail to capture the substantial heterogeneity that characterizes the outcomes of TBI, even when stratified by injury severity. These individual differences in outcomes reflect a complex interplay among injury characteristics, non-injury related influences, and developmental factors. Research nowadays more often focuses on factors that predict individual differences in outcome, partly in hope of identifying fruitful avenues for intervention.

Injury Characteristics

Injury severity is a major determinant of the consequences of TBI, with more severe injuries resulting in poorer outcomes. Injury severity can be assessed using a variety of clinical metrics, including level of consciousness, duration of impaired consciousness, and length of posttraumatic amnesia. Other specific medical indicators of severity include brain stem abnormalities (e.g., pupillary reactivity) and elevated intracranial pressure. The Glasgow Coma Scale (GCS; Teasdale & Jennett, 1974) is probably the most frequent metric of injury severity.

The motor scale on the GCS can be used to assess duration of impaired consciousness, often defined as the number of days from an injury until a child is able to follow commands consistently (i.e., the number of days that the score on the GCS motor scale falls below 6). Duration of impaired consciousness is an indirect indicator of rate of recovery, because it reflects the speed with which a child's mental status improves post injury. The length of posttraumatic amnesia also reflects the child's rate of recovery. In comparative studies, duration of coma (i.e., GCS score < 9), impaired consciousness, and posttraumatic amnesia have generally been better predictors of outcome than static measures such as the lowest postresuscitation GCS score (Ewing-Cobbs, Fletcher, Levin, Hastings, & Francis, 1996; McDonald et al., 1994).

The classification of injury severity using the GCS and other clinical metrics has begun to give way to more sophisticated indices that are linked more directly to the pathophysiology of TBI (Saatman et al., 2008). Neuroimaging allows much better characterization of underlying neuropathology. Computed tomography (CT) is preferred acutely after TBI because it is widely available and relatively inexpensive, and also sensitive to lesions that may necessitate neurosurgical intervention (Poussaint & Moeller, 2002). However, magnetic resonance imaging (MRI) is superior to CT in documenting most pathology associated with TBI (Sigmund et al., 2007).

A variety of advanced imaging procedures have been developed to assess both structural and functional brain abnormalities in childhood TBI (see Ashwal, Holshouser, & Tong, 2006b, 2010; Munson, Schroth, & Ernst, 2006). Newer MRI sequences that show increased sensitivity to the structural effects of pediatric TBI include susceptibility-weighted MR imaging (Ashwal et al., 2006a; Beauchamp et al., 2011) and diffusion tensor imaging (Yuan et al., 2007). Brain function can be assessed directly using techniques such as functional MRI (Kramer et al., 2008), proton magnetic resonance spectroscopy (Ashwal et al., 2006a; Babikian et al., 2006), positron emission tomography, and single-photon emission CT (Munson et al., 2006).

Neuroimaging studies in children with TBI generally indicate that the greater the structural or functional abnormalities, the greater the morbidity (Brenner, Freier, Holshouser, Burley, & Ashwal, 2003). In some cases, studies have shown predictable brain-behavior relationships in children with TBI (e.g., Levin et al., 2004; Newsome et al., 2008), although expectations based on adult models are not necessarily applicable after childhood TBI. For instance, frontal lesion volume does not consistently predict attention or executive function (Power, Catroppa, Coleman, Ditchfield, & Anderson, 2007; Slomine et al., 2002), and fronto-temporal lesions do not predict memory performance better than lesions outside those regions (Salorio et al., 2005). A major challenge for neuroimaging studies is that the lesions associated with pediatric TBI are extremely heterogeneous, with relatively little overlap in lesion location from one child to the next (Bigler et al., 2013).

Non-Injury-Related Influences

Because injury severity fails to account for most of the variance in postinjury outcomes after TBI, research has begun to focus on non-injury-related influences. For instance, children's premorbid functioning appears to be an important determinant of the outcomes of childhood TBI (Fay et al., 2010; Yeates et al., 2005), consistent with theories of cognitive and brain reserve capacity suggesting that vulnerability to neurological insults varies as a function of preinjury cognitive abilities and brain integrity (Dennis, Yeates, Taylor, & Fletcher, 2007).

Environmental influences also help to account for outcomes following TBI. General measures of socioeconomic status and family demographics predict outcomes, as do more specific aspects of family status and parenting. Indeed, the family environment actually moderates the impact of TBI, by buffering or exacerbating its adverse consequences (Taylor et al., 2002; Yeates et al., 1997, 2004). Thus, the effects of TBI are more pronounced for children from dysfunctional families.

The treatments and interventions that children with TBI receive are also likely to be critical environmental influences on recovery. Unfortunately, treatment research is very sparse. Guidelines for acute medical management of childhood TBI lack a firm evidence base (Adelson, 2010; Kochanek et al., 2012). Comprehensive reviews of inpatient and outpatient rehabilitation also highlight the relative paucity of research in that domain (Anderson & Catroppa, 2006; Slomine & Locascio, 2009; Tal & Tirosh, 2013; Ylvisaker et al., 2005), and even less is known about the effectiveness of educational interventions (Ylvisaker et al., 2001). Cognitive remediation programs have been developed for pediatric TBI, but research provides little evidence that their effects generalize to everyday environments (Catroppa & Anderson, 2006; Laatsch et al., 2007; Robinson, Kaizar, Catroppa, Godfrey, & Yeates, 2014).

Research regarding treatment for the psychosocial sequelae of pediatric TBI is also relatively limited (Donders, 2007; Ross, Dorris, & McMillan, 2011), although some support exists for certain treatments of behavioral and social problems (Warschausky, Kewman, & Kay, 1999; Ylvisaker, Turkstra, & Coelho, 2005, Ylvisaker et al., 2007). Family based interventions that promote better communication and problem solving, and that incorporate parent training, have shown particular promise in promoting better psychosocial outcomes for children with TBI and their families (Brown, Whittingham, Boyd, & Sofronoff, 2013; Wade, 2010).

Developmental Considerations

The outcomes of childhood TBI vary as a function of three distinct but interrelated developmental dimensions: age at the time of injury, the amount of time that has passed since the injury, and age at the time of outcome assessment (Taylor & Alden, 1997). Injuries sustained during infancy or early childhood are associated with more persistent deficits than those occurring during later childhood and adolescence (Anderson et al., 2005a; Ewing-Cobbs et al., 2006). Younger children demonstrate a slower rate of change over time and more significant residual deficits than do older children, particularly after more severe injuries (Catroppa, Anderson, Morse, Haritou, & Rosenfeld, 2008; Koskiniemi, Kyyka, Nybo, & Jarho, 1995).

Children with TBI generally display a gradual recovery after injury, with the most rapid improvement occurring soon after the injury (Yeates et al., 2002). The initial rate of recovery is most rapid among children with severe TBI, although severe injuries are more likely to be associated with persistent deficits after recovery slows (Fay et al., 2009). Studies of long-term outcomes show little evidence that children with TBI show progressive deterioration in cognitive functioning after their initial recovery (Jonsson, Horneman, & Emanuelson, 2004; Klonoff, Clark, & Klonoff, 1995), although deterioration can occur in behavioral functioning (Fay et al., 2009).

The influence of age at testing has not been a major focus of research. The effects of age at testing would be reflected in latent or delayed sequelae resulting from children's failure to meet new developmental demands following a TBI. Although such sequelae are sometimes suspected in individual cases (Baron, 2008), they are difficult to detect in research because the effects of age at testing are difficult to disentangle from those of age at injury and time since injury (Taylor & Alden, 1997).

Methodological Critique

Sample Selection, Recruitment, and Attrition

Shortcomings in the selection and recruitment of participants characterize many studies of TBI. Children with TBI are sometimes selected retrospectively, based on admission to a rehabilitation facility or referral for neuropsychological evaluation (e.g., Yeates et al., 1995). Samples selected in this way are likely to be less representative than those that are recruited prospectively from consecutive admissions to a hospital or trauma center.

Even when samples are recruited prospectively, they may not be representative of the larger population from which they are drawn or they may become unrepresentative because of selective attrition. The agreement to participate in scientific research is not a random decision, nor is the decision to discontinue participation. Unfortunately, few studies report participation rates or compare participants and nonparticipants in terms of demographics or clinical characteristics, to determine if study participation has introduced bias into sample selection. Similarly, few studies compare children who complete follow-up to those who drop out, to determine if attrition biases their results (Blaha et al., 2015). Statistical procedures such as pattern-mixture analysis can be used to determine whether attrition has biased study results (Hedeker & Gibbons, 1997).

The selection of comparison groups in research on TBI also can be problematic. Children with mild TBI have sometimes been used as a comparison group, despite ongoing controversy regarding the outcomes associated with mild TBI (Satz, 2001; Yeates et al., 2009). In other cases, noninjured children matched for age, gender, and other demographic variables have been used as a comparison group (Jaffe, Polissar, Fay, & Liao, 1995). However, noninjured children are not equated to children with TBI in terms of the experience of a traumatic injury or ensuing medical treatment. Moreover, they may also differ from children with TBI in a variety of premorbid characteristics that are not controlled by matching on demographic factors alone. Children who sustain injuries frequently display more preexisting behavioral, developmental, and learning problems than children who are not injured (Asarnow et al., 1995; Bijur & Haslum, 1995), and also are more likely to come from families that are socially disadvantaged and dysfunctional (Christoffel, Donovan, Schofer, Wills, & Lavigne, 1996; Howard et al., 2005; Parslow, Morris, Tasker, Forsyth, & Hawley, 2005). Although background differences are not reported between children with TBI and noninjured controls or between children with TBI of varying severity in all studies (Catroppa et al., 2015), comparison groups consisting of children who have sustained injuries not involving the head and who have undergone comparable medical treatment are often desirable.

Measurement

Injury characteristics

The literature on TBI suffers from a lack of consistency in the characterization of injury severity. Greater uniformity in the assessment of severity would allow more meaningful cross-study comparisons (Saatman et al., 2008). Future studies are likely to need to incorporate multidimensional approaches to classifying severity that incorporate clinical indicators, neuroimaging, and other biomarkers.

Specific criticisms can be raised about traditional clinical indices of injury severity. The GCS is problematic when used with infants and young children, despite attempts to make suitable modifications (Durham et al., 2000). The duration of impaired consciousness can be difficult to assess reliably, because it is often measured retrospectively, based on clinical assessments by nursing staff or physicians. Similarly, post-traumatic amnesia is often assessed based on retrospective reports from caretakers, despite the availability of standardized instruments such as the Children's Orientation and Amnesia Test (COAT; Ewing-Cobbs et al., 1990) that can provide more reliable and objective measurement.

As noted earlier, neuroimaging allows characterization of injury severity based on underlying neuropathology. The advent of more advanced neuroimaging techniques, such as susceptibility-weighted imaging, diffusion tensor imaging, functional MRI, and proton magnetic resonance spectroscopy, will provide more precise measures of both the diffuse and focal neuropathology associated with TBI, which can in turn be used to predict neurobehavioral outcomes (Levin et al., 2004; Newsome et al., 2008).

Research suggests that serum biomarkers may also provide a more precise characterization of injury severity by assessing biochemical and protein indicators of the neurochemical cascade that occurs in TBI (Berger, Adelson, Richichi, & Kochanek, 2006, 2010; Papa et al., 2013). Biomarkers may be particularly important for diagnosing TBI in young children, for whom conventional indices such as the GCS are often invalid, and for children with inflicted TBI, who may suffer head trauma that is not disclosed (Berger, Ta'Asan, Rand, Lokshin, & Kochanek, 2009; Shore et al., 2007).

Non-injury-related influences

Measures of children's premorbid status are likely to moderate the effects of TBI (Catroppa et al., 2015), and hence should be incorporated into future research. In this regard, a substantial opportunity exists to explore the association of genetics with outcomes. Aside from a small literature on the apolipoprotein (APOE) gene, little is known about genetic influences on recovery from TBI, despite their critical role in neural plasticity and inflammatory responses (Kurowski, Martin, & Wade, 2012).

Research also needs to incorporate more precise measures of children's environments to determine the mechanisms by which the environment moderates the outcomes of childhood TBI. A recent study of parenting skills in preschool children with TBI provides an example of such an approach (Wade et al., 2008).

Future research is also badly needed on the effectiveness of the interventions used to manage TBI. Clinical trials in children with TBI are challenging (Adelson, 2010; Natale et al., 2005), but are badly needed to evaluate the efficacy and effectiveness of potential medical treatments such as hypothermia. The benefits of postacute medical interventions such as psychotropic or anticonvulsant medications, rehabilitative and educational programs, and psychological and behavioral interventions targeted to children and their families also require further investigation.

In recent years, concerns have been raised about relying on randomized clinical trials for assessing treatment effectiveness in TBI, partly because of the difficulties inherent in conducting such trials, but also because of their repeated failures to advance treatment of TBI (Adelson, 2010). These concerns have led to calls for comparative effectiveness studies, which rely on natural variations in care across multiple sites and large numbers of patients to detect the effectiveness of specific interventions (Maas & Menon, 2012; Maas et al., 2012; Powell, Temkin, Machamer, & Dikmen, 2002). Several studies based on this approach are under way in the United States and internationally.

Outcomes

Limitations characterize many of the outcome measures used in studies of pediatric TBI. Clinical judgments, such as those reflected in the Glasgow Outcome Scale (Jennett & Bond, 1975), often lack sensitivity to subtle differences in outcomes. Psychometric tests generally provide more sensitive outcome measures, but their interpretation is complicated by the multifactorial nature of test performance. Tests designed to assess specific skill deficits or that employ experimental manipulations of task demands may yield more precise information about the cognitive sequelae of TBI (Taylor, 2010).

Psychometric testing is not always feasible for measuring critical functional outcomes following TBI, including social competence, behavioral adjustment, and adaptive functioning. The latter outcomes are typically assessed using rating scales and interviews, although many commonly used rating scales were not developed for use with children with TBI and may prove insensitive in that population (Drotar, Stein, & Perrin, 1995; Perrin, Stein, & Drotar, 1991). The use of rating scales that are specifically targeted to children with TBI may be more informative (Yeates et al., 2001).

The range of outcomes assessed in previous research has also been limited, although more attention is beginning to be paid to important outcomes such as social functioning (Yeates et al., 2007), family functioning (Wade et al., 2006), school performance (Taylor et al., 2003), or quality of life (Di Battista et al., 2012). Notably, these functional outcomes are more likely to be moderated by environmental factors than are children's cognitive abilities.

A lack of consistency in outcome measures across studies is also a problem, because it hampers the comparison of results and pooling of data for the purpose of systematic reviews and meta-analyses. The lack of standards or guidelines in this regard has been problematic, but researchers are now being encouraged to use common outcome measures, such as those recommended by the National Institutes of Health (NIH) Common Data Elements Project (McCauley, Wilde, Anderson, Bedell, & Yeates, 2012).

Mechanisms Underlying Recovery

Few studies have attempted to explain the mechanisms that underlie the sequelae of TBI in children (Taylor, 2010). The causal mechanisms that underlie recovery from brain injury may be especially amenable to research in nonhuman animals (Kamper et al., 2013). For instance, although we do not know why younger children display less recovery from TBI than older children, research on nonhuman animals suggests important differences in neural plasticity may play a role (Bittigau et al., 1999; Giza & Prins, 2006). Research on nonhuman animals is not limited to understanding the neural mechanisms that affect recovery from brain injury, but also provides a platform for understanding non-injury-related mechanisms, such as the rearing environment (Bondi, Klitsch, Leary, & Kline, 2014).

Analysis of Change

Cross-sectional designs have been used in many studies of childhood TBI, but they preclude investigation of the process of postinjury recovery. Longitudinal studies are needed to determine the relative importance of injury characteristics, non-injury-related influences, and developmental factors as predictors of outcomes across time (Taylor & Alden, 1997). Most previous longitudinal studies have followed children for relatively brief periods; investigations of much longer duration are needed to document the long-term, adult outcomes of childhood TBI (Anderson et al., 2009, 2011; Beauchamp et al., 2010).

Existing longitudinal studies also have not consistently adopted a developmental approach to modeling recovery. Traditional approaches to data analysis in longitudinal designs, such as repeated-measures analysis of variance, treat individual differences in change as error variance. However, recovery from TBI inherently involves change that is heterogeneous in nature, and individual differences in developmental change should represent a major focus in studies of childhood TBI. Growth curve modeling and related statistical approaches permit the investigation of change at an individual level (Francis, Fletcher, Stuebing, Davidson, & Thompson, 1991). Mixture modeling is another approach that can be used to examine intraindividual change. It empirically identifies latent classes of individuals based on different developmental trajectories (Nagin, 1999). In a study using that technique (Yeates et al., 2009), children with mild TBI were more likely than those with orthopedic injuries to demonstrate trajectories involving high acute levels of symptoms, especially if their acute clinical presentation reflected more severe injury.

Prediction of Individual Outcomes

Clinicians involved in the care of children with TBI want to know whether a given child is likely to recovery fully or demonstrate persistent difficulties. Research can help to address this question by focusing more on individual outcomes. For instance, children with TBI can be divided into subgroups based on injury characteristics or environmental factors to determine if outcomes are different for the different subgroups. Alternatively, individuals with a given outcome can be identified, and then the risk factors linked to this outcome can be determined. The latter method has the advantage of permitting the study of combinations of risk factors associated with the outcome. Analyses of reliable change provide one means of identifying individual children who display unusual decrements in functioning compared to pre-injury estimates and examining the risk factors associated with such increases (McCrea et al., 2005; Yeates et al., 2012).

In the long run, prognostic models and decision rules are needed that can predict which children with TBI will demonstrate poor versus good outcomes. Research along these lines has been very successful at identifying children with mild TBI who are at risk of clinically significant lesions on neuroimaging (Kuppermann et al., 2009; Osmond, Klassen, Wells, Correll, & Stiell, 2010). To be clinically useful, research on outcome prediction must meet a variety of methodological prerequisites, such as large sample sizes, that are likely to necessitate multisite cooperative studies (Mushkudiani et al., 2008). A study along these lines, examining the prediction of postconcussive symptoms in children with mild TBI from acute clinical characteristics in the emergency department setting, was recently completed in Canada (Zemek, Osmond, & Barrowman, 2013).

Case Illustration

To illustrate a fairly typical clinical case of childhood TBI, we have chosen to present Jane, an 11-year-old girl who was struck by a motor vehicle. Her premorbid birth, developmental, school, and psychosocial histories were unremarkable. She sustained multiple internal and orthopedic injuries, and required surgery for a depressed skull fracture. At the scene, her GCS score was 5 out of 15; it increased to 11 en route to the hospital, but dropped to 5 upon arrival, at which time she was intubated and sedated.

MRI of the brain eight days postinjury revealed multiple focal lesions in the right parietal region, inferior portion of the left frontal lobe, bilateral anterior temporal lobe, and left posterior temporal lobe (see Figure 11.1). Multifocal hemorrhages also were apparent, along with traumatic axonal

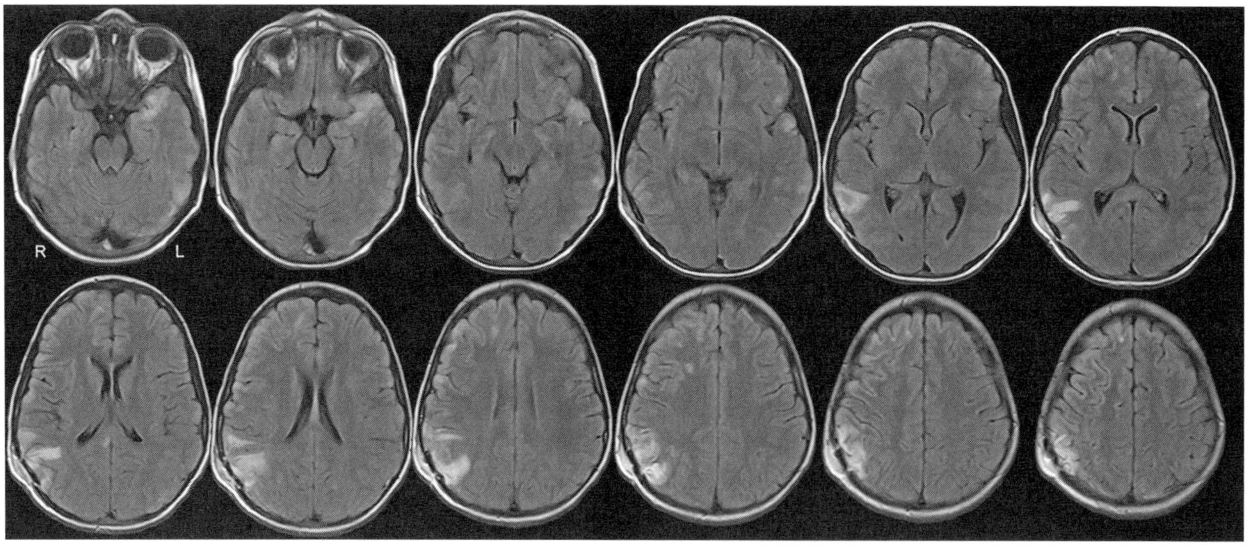

Figure 11.1 MRI of TBI case illustration 12 contiguous axial images obtained on a 1.5T magnetic resonance scanner at eight days postinjury using a fluid attenuated inversion recovery (FLAIR) sequence

injury. Based on formal assessments using the Children's Orientation and Amnesia Test (Ewing-Cobbs et al., 1990), Jane demonstrated posttraumatic amnesia for 21 days postinjury. Her mother reported a period of retrograde amnesia of at least eight hours.

Jane completed a brief neuropsychological evaluation 24 days postinjury. Her performance on a measure of word reading, which provided an indicator of premorbid functioning, was average. She demonstrated clear deficits in reaction time and psychomotor speed, cognitive flexibility, and memory. Jane was subsequently referred for a follow-up neuropsychological evaluation six months postinjury.

On interview, Jane's mother reported gradual improvements in Jane's cognition, personality, mood, and behavior, which were characterized as largely back to baseline. However, she described ongoing concerns regarding poor concentration, forgetfulness, hyperactivity and fidgetiness, reduced speed of mental processing, and increased fatigue. She also reported difficulties remembering multistep directions, comprehending new or complex concepts, making simple decisions of everyday life, independently initiating activities, and transitioning between activities. She denied sleep problems, pain, mood problems, social difficulties, or psychological adjustment problems.

Jane was polite and cooperative during the assessment. She did not display overt hyperactivity or inattention, and her expressive language, motor, hearing, and vision skills appeared intact. Her mood was flat, and she appeared indifferent to success or failure on the tests. She did not initiate conversations or other forms of social interactions with the examiner. Over time, she displayed increasing fatigue.

Jane understood very simple test instructions, but was visibly confused by multistep or complex instructions. Despite multiple repetitions, simplification of test instructions, extended practice, and demonstrations, she was not able to follow some instructions. Her comprehension difficulties may have affected her performance on some tests. However, she displayed adequate performance on a formal measure of performance validity.

On formal testing (see Table 11.2), Jane's overall intellectual functioning was somewhat below average. She showed a moderate difference, found in less than 16% of her peers,

Table 11.2 Summary of assessment results

Test Domain/Measures	*Standard Score*	*Percentile*
Intellectual Abilities		
WISC-IV General Ability Index	Index = 76	5
WISC-IV Verbal Comprehension Index	Index = 87	19
WISC-IV Perceptual Reasoning Index	Index = 72	3
Language Skills		
NEPSY-II Comprehension of Instructions	SS = 4	2
WISC-IV Vocabulary	SS = 6	9
Visuospatial Abilities		
WISC-IV Block Design	SS = 5	5
Learning and Memory		
CVLT-C Trials 1–5 Total Recall	T = 47	38
CVLT-C Long Delay Free Recall	Z = –1.0	16
CVLT-C Recognition Discriminability	Z = –1.5	7
Continuous Visual Memory Test Total	Raw = 54	<3
Continuous Visual Memory Test Delayed Recognition	Raw = 2	<10
Information Processing Speed		
WISC-IV Processing Speed Index	Index = 78	7
NEPSY-II Inhibition-Naming Combined	SS = 4	2
CNS Vital Signs Reaction Time	Index = 87	19
TOVA Response Time	Index = 58	0.3
Attention and Concentration		
TOVA Omission Errors	Index = 40	<1
TOVA Commission Errors	Index = 113	81
Executive Functioning		
CNS Vital Signs Stroop Commission Errors	Index = 78	7
NEPSY-II Inhibition-Inhibition Combined	SS = 5	5
Motor Abilities		
CNS Vital Signs Finger Tapping, Right Hand	Index = 88	21
CNS Vital Signs Finger Tapping, Left Hand	Index = 86	18

Table note: Index = index score, which has a mean = 100 and standard deviation = 15. SS = scaled score, which has a mean = 10 and standard deviation = 3. T = t score, which has a mean = 50 and standard deviation = 10. Z = z score, which has a mean = 0 and standard deviation = 1.0.

favoring her verbal comprehension over her perceptual organization. Reasoning and concept formation were below average on a visual task, but average on a verbal test.

In the language domain, Jane's ability to follow simple instructions was well below average. She also performed below average when defining words. Her visuospatial skills, as reflected in block construction, were also below average. Verbal learning and memory were largely intact, but nonverbal memory fell below average. Ratings by Jane's mother suggested significant deficits in daily memory skills.

Jane's processing speed was below average, although her reaction time was average on a relatively brief measure. Jane's sustained attention was below average, and declined over time. Ratings of her day-to-day attention reflected significant deficits. Inhibitory control was variable, ranging from below average to average. Jane's cognitive flexibility was below average. Ratings of her everyday executive skills suggest significant problems in initiation, working memory, and planning and organization.

Parent ratings of Jane's psychological adjustment were largely within normal limits, although they suggested limited emotional resiliency and ability to cope with emotional problems. She was reported to show mild to moderate postconcussive symptoms. Her mother rated Jane's adaptive skills from below average to average. Jane perceived her adaptive functioning as similar to before her injury, but reported clinically significant symptoms of depression and anxiety.

In summary, despite improvements in reaction time and memory compared to the postacute assessment, Jane displayed persistent and widespread deficits that encompassed language and nonverbal skills, memory, processing speed, attention, and executive functions. She was described as displaying many features of ADHD, presumably secondary to her TBI (i.e., school records and parent report did not suggest that this was a preinjury problem). She also reported significant mood problems. Her neuropsychological profile was consistent with the severity of her injury and with the widespread neuropathology documented on neuroimaging.

Jane was recommended for ongoing special education services, especially to address her difficulties with response speed, attention, and executive functions. She also was referred for ongoing behavioral health services, including psychotherapy and psychiatric consultation to consider psychotropic medication. She was fortunate to have a supportive, well-functioning family, and an unremarkable premorbid history. Both of the latter features increased her chances of ongoing recovery.

Future Directions

Future research on the outcomes of childhood TBI will be shaped by a number of conceptual advances. Our understanding of the underlying biological mechanisms associated with recovery will be enhanced by research on genetic influences, as well as by the search for serum and neuroimaging biomarkers of injury. Biological research also may suggest treatment approaches that minimize the secondary injuries that occur after TBI. At the same time, a growing appreciation that the environment affects recovery should lead to closer study of the ways in which family functioning and parenting affect outcomes, as well as to the translation of such research into psychosocial interventions designed to promote recovery. Ultimately, research is needed that examines the interplay of both biological and environmental influences on recovery.

Methodological improvements will also characterize future research. These will include the study of a broader range of outcomes, moving beyond cognitive abilities to broader aspects of children's functioning, such as friendships and peer relationships, health care utilization, and overall quality of life. Shared outcome measures, based on common data elements, will facilitate the comparison of studies and the pooling of data across studies. Additionally, prospective, longitudinal research designs will provide a better understanding of individual recovery and the variability in outcomes that characterize children with TBI. Combined with statistical techniques that focus on the prediction of individual outcomes, such studies will also promote more accurate prognostic judgments in clinical settings. The advent of comparative effectiveness studies may provide us with more insights into treatment effectiveness than have resulted from randomized clinical trials to date.

In the long run, to truly understand the outcomes of pediatric TBI, research will need to occur outside of traditional academic silos. Research is needed that is integrative, cutting across domains or disciplines, as well as translational, promoting the application of knowledge to clinical care. Scientific advances within specific domains are not likely to yield significant progress in the clinical management of children with TBI until they become the topic of collaborative research that cuts across multiple levels of analysis. The time is ripe for interdisciplinary efforts that promote translational research aimed at improving the lives of children with TBI and their families (Anderson & Yeates, 2010).

Acknowledgement

The authors acknowledge and thank Nicole Ullrich, MD for contributing some of the images presented here.

References

Adelson, P. D. (2010). Clinical trials for pediatric TBI. In V. A. Anderson & K. O. Yeates (Eds.), *Pediatric Traumatic Brain Injury: New Frontiers in Clinical and Translational Research* (pp. 54–67). New York: Cambridge University Press.

Anderson, V., Brown, S., Newitt, H., & Hoile, H. (2009). Educational, vocational, psychosocial, and quality of life outcomes for adult survivors of childhood traumatic brain injury. *Journal of Head Trauma Rehabilitation*, *24*, 303–312.

Anderson, V., Brown, S., Newitt, H., & Hoile, H. (2011). Long-term outcome from childhood traumatic brain injury: Intellectual ability, personality, and quality of life. *Neuropsychology*, *25*, 176–184.

Anderson, V., & Catroppa, C. (2005). Recovery of executive skills following paediatric traumatic brain injury (TBI): A 2 year follow-up. *Brain Injury*, *19*, 459–470.

Anderson, V., & Catroppa, C. (2006). Advances in postacute rehabilitation after childhood acquired brain injury: A focus on cognitive, behavioral, and social domains. *American Journal of Physical Medicine and Rehabilitation*, *85*, 767–778.

Anderson, V. A., Catroppa, C., Morse, S., Haritou, F., & Rosenfeld, J. (2005a). Functional plasticity or vulnerability after early brain injury? *Pediatrics*, *116*, 1374–1382.

Anderson, V. A., Catroppa, C., Morse, S., Haritou, F., & Rosenfeld, J. (2005b). Identifying factors contributing to child and family outcome at 30 months following traumatic brain injury in children. *Journal of Neurology, Neurosurgery & Psychiatry*, *76*, 401–408.

Anderson, V. A., Morse, S., Catroppa, C., Haritou, F., & Rosenfeld, J. (2004). Thirty month outcome from early childhood head injury: A prospective analysis of neurobehavioural recovery. *Brain*, *127*, 2608–2620.

Anderson, V. A., & Yeates, K. O. (Eds.). (2010). *Pediatric Traumatic Brain Injury: New Frontiers in Clinical and Translational Research*. New York: Cambridge University Press.

Anderson, V. A., & Yeates, K. O. (2014). Children and adolescents. In H. Levin, D. Shum, & R. Chan (Eds.), *Understanding Traumatic Brain Injury: Current Research and Future Directions* (pp. 333–355). New York: Oxford University Press.

Asarnow, R. F., Satz, P., Light, R., Zaucha, K., Lewis, R., & McCleary, C. (1995). The UCLA study of mild closed head injuries in children and adolescents. In S. H. Broman & M. E. Michel (Eds.), *Traumatic Head Injury in Children* (pp. 117–146). New York: Oxford University Press.

Ashwal, S., Tong, K. A., Obenaus, A., & Holshouser, B. A. (2010). Advanced neuroimaging techniques in children with traumatic brain injury. In V. A. Anderson & K. O. Yeates (Eds.), *Pediatric Traumatic Brain Injury: New Frontiers in Clinical and Translational Research* (pp. 68–93). New York: Cambridge University Press.

Ashwal, S., Babikian, T., Gardner-Nichols, J., Freier, M. C., Tong, K. A., & Holshouser, B. A. (2006a). Susceptibility-weighted imaging and proton magnetic resonance spectroscopy in assessment of outcome after pediatric traumatic brain injury. *Archives of Physical Medicine and Rehabilitation*, *87*, 50–58.

Ashwal, S., Holshouser, B. A., & Tong, K. A. (2006b). Use of advanced neuroimaging techniques in the evaluation of pediatric traumatic brain injury. *Developmental Neuroscience*, *28*, 309–326.

Babikian, T., & Asarnow, R. (2009). Neurocognitive outcomes and recovery after pediatric TBI: Meta-analytic review of the literature. *Neuropsychology*, *23*, 283–296.

Babikian, T., Freier, M. C., Ashwal, S., Riggs, M. L., Burley, T., & Holshouser, B. A. (2006). MR spectroscopy: Predicting long-term neuropsychological outcome following pediatric TBI. *Journal of Magnetic Resonance Imaging*, *24*, 801–811.

Baron, I. S. (2008). Maturation into impairment: The merit of delayed settlement in pediatric forensic neuropsychology cases. In R. L. Heilbronner (Ed.), *Neuropsychology in the Courtroom: Expert Analysis of Reports and Testimony* (pp. 66–78). New York: Guilford Press.

Bawden, H. N., Knights, R. M., & Winogron, H. W. (1985). Speeded performance following head injury in children. *Journal of Clinical Neuropsychology*, *7*, 39–54.

Beauchamp, M., Dooley, J., & Anderson, V. (2010). Adult outcomes of pediatric traumatic brain injury. In J. Donders & S. J. Hunter (Eds.), *Principles and Practice of Developmental Neuropsychology* (pp. 315–328). Cambridge: Cambridge University Press.

Beauchamp, M. H., Ditchfield, M., Babl, F. E., Kean, M., Catroppa, C., Yeates, K. O., & Anderson, V. (2011). Detecting traumatic brain lesions in children: CT vs MRI vs susceptibility weighted imaging (SWI). *Journal of Neurotrauma*, *28*, 915–927.

Belanger, H. G., Spiegel, E., & Vanderploeg, R. D. (2010). Neuropsychological performance following a history of multiple self-reported concussions: A meta-analysis. *Journal of the International Neuropsychological Society*, *16*, 262–267.

Berger, R. P., Adelson, P. D., Richichi, R., & Kochanek, P. M. (2006). Serum biomarkers after traumatic and hypoxemic brain injuries: Insights into the biochemical response of the pediatric brain to inflicted brain injury. *Developmental Neuroscience*, *28*, 327–335.

Berger, R. P., Hayes, R. L., Wang, K.K.W., & Kochanek, P. (2010). Using serum biomarkers to diagnose, assess, treat and predict outcome after pediatric TBI. In V. A. Anderson & K. O. Yeates (Eds.), *Pediatric Traumatic Brain Injury: New Frontiers in Clinical and Translational Research* (pp. 36–53). New York: Cambridge University Press.

Berger, R. P., Ta'Asan, S., Rand, R., Lokshin, A., & Kochanek, P. (2009). Multiplex assessment of serum biomarker concentrations in well-appearing children with inflicted brain injury. *Pediatric Research*, *65*, 97–102.

Bigler, E. D. (2007). Anterior and middle cranial fossa in traumatic brain injury: Relevant neuroanatomy and neuropathology in the study of neuropsychological outcome. *Neuropsychology*, *21*, 515–531.

Bigler, E. D., Abildskov, T. J., Petrie, J., Farrer, T. J., Farrer, T. J., Dennis, M., . . . Yeates, K. O. (2013). Heterogeneity of brain lesions in pediatric traumatic brain injury. *Neuropsychology*, *27*, 438–451.

Bijur, P. E., & Haslum, M. (1995). Cognitive, behavioral, and motoric sequelae of mild head injury in a national birth cohort. In S. H. Broman & M. E. Michel (Eds.), *Traumatic Head Injury in Children* (pp. 147–164). New York: Oxford University Press.

Bittigau, P., Sifringer, M., Pohl, D., Stadrhaus, D., Ishimaru, M., Shimizu, H., . . . Ikonomidou, C. (1999). Apoptotic neurodegeneration following trauma is markedly enhanced in the immature brain. *Annals of Neurology*, *45*, 724–735.

Blaha, R. Z., Arnett, A. B., Kirkwood, M. W., Taylor, H. G., Stancin, T., Brown, T., & Wade, S. L. (2015). Factors influencing attrition in a multisite, randomized, clinical trial following traumatic brain injury in adolescence. *Journal of Head Trauma Rehabilitation*, *30*, E33–40.

Bloom, D. R., Levin, H. S., Ewing-Cobbs, L., Saunders, A. E., Song, J., Fletcher, J. M., & Kowatch, R. A. (2001). Lifetime and novel psychiatric disorders after pediatric traumatic brain injury. *Journal of the American Academy of Child and Adolescent Psychiatry*, *40*, 572–579.

Bodin, D., & Yeates, K. O. (2010). Traumatic brain injury. In R. J. Shaw & D. R. DeMaso (Eds.), *Textbook of Pediatric Psychosomatic Medicine: Consultation on Physically Ill Children* (pp. 405–419). Washington, DC: American Psychiatric Publishing, Inc.

Bondi, C. O., Klitsch, K. C., Leary, J. B., & Kline, A. E. (2014). Environmental enrichment as a viable neurorehabilitation strategy for experimental traumatic brain injury. *Journal of Neurotrauma*, *31*, 873–888.

Brenner, T., Freier, M. C., Holshouser, B. A., Burley, T., & Ashwal, S. (2003). Predicting neuropsychologic outcome after traumatic brain injury in children. *Pediatric Neurology*, *28*, 104–114.

Brown, F. L., Whittingham, K., Boyd, R., & Sofronoff, K. (2013). A systematic review of parenting interventions for traumatic brain injury: Child and parent outcomes. *Journal of Head Trauma Rehabilitation*, *28*, 349–360.

Brown, R. L. (2010). Epidemiology of injury and the impact of health disparities. *Current Opinion in Pediatrics*, *22*, 321–325.

Cassidy, J. D., Carroll, L. J., Peloso, P. M., Borg, J., von Holst, H., Holm, L., . . . Coronado, V. G. (2004). Incidence, risk factors and prevention of mild traumatic brain injury: Results of the WHO collaborating centre task force on mild traumatic brain injury. *Journal of Rehabilitation Medicine*, *43*(Suppl), 28–60.

Catroppa, C., & Anderson, V. (2002). Recovery in memory function in the first year following TBI in children. *Brain Injury*, *16*, 369–384.

Catroppa, C., & Anderson, V. (2004). Recovery and predictors of language skills two years following pediatric traumatic brain injury. *Brain and Language*, *88*, 68–78.

Catroppa, C., & Anderson, V. (2005). A prospective study of the recovery of attention from acute to 2 years post pediatric traumatic brain injury. *Journal of the International Neuropsychological Society*, *11*, 84–98.

Catroppa, C., & Anderson, V. (2006). Planning, problem-solving, and organizational abilities in children following traumatic brain injury: Intervention techniques. *Pediatric Rehabilitation*, *9*, 89–97.

Catroppa, C., & Anderson, V. (2007). Recovery in memory function, and its relationship to academic success, at 24 months following pediatric TBI. *Child Neuropsychology*, *13*, 240–261.

Catroppa, C., Anderson, V. A., Morse, S. A., Haritou, F., & Rosenfeld, J. V. (2007). Children's attentional skills 5 years post-TBI. *Journal of Pediatric Psychology*, *32*, 354–369.

Catroppa, C., Anderson, V. A., Morse, S. A., Haritou, F., & Rosenfeld, J. V. (2008). Outcome and predictors of functional recovery 5 years following pediatric traumatic brain injury. *Journal of Pediatric Psychology*, *33*, 707–718.

Catroppa, C., Crossley, L., Hearps, S.J.C., Yeates, K. O., Beauchamp, M., Rogers, K., & Anderson, V. (2015). Social and behavioral outcomes: Pre-injury to 6 months following childhood traumatic brain injury. *Journal of Neurotrauma*, *32*, 109–115.

Chapman, S. B., Sparks, G., Levin, H. S., Dennis, M., Roncadin, C., Zhang, L., & Song, J. (2004). Discourse macrolevel processing after severe pediatric traumatic brain injury. *Developmental Neuropsychology*, *25*, 37–60.

Christoffel, K., Donovan, M., Schofer, J., Wills, K., & Lavigne, J. (1996). Psychosocial factors in childhood pedestrian injury: A matched case-control study. *Pediatrics*, *97*, 33–42.

Corrigan, J. D., & Hammond, F. M. (2013). Traumatic brain injury as a chronic health condition. *Archives of Physical Medicine and Rehabilitation*, *94*, 1199–1201.

Dennis, M., & Barnes, M. A. (1990). Knowing the meaning, getting the point, bridging the gap, and carrying the message: Aspects of discourse following closed head injury in childhood and adolescence. *Brain and Language*, *39*, 428–446.

Dennis, M., Guger, S., Roncadin, C., Barnes, M., & Schachar, R. (2001a). Attentional-inhibitory control and social-behavioral regulation after childhood closed head injury: Do biological, developmental, and recovery variables predict outcome? *Journal of the International Neuropsychological Society*, *7*, 683–692.

Dennis, M., Simic, N., Bigler, E. D., Abildskov, T., Agostino, A., Taylor, H. G., . . Yeates, K. O. (2013). Cognitive, affective, and conative theory of mind (ToM) in children with traumatic brain injury. *Developmental Cognitive Neuroscience*, *5*, 25–39.

Dennis, M., Wilkinson, M., Koski, L., & Humphreys, R. P. (1995). Attention deficits in the long term after childhood head injury. In S. H. Broman & M. E. Michel (Eds.), *Traumatic Head Injury in Children* (pp. 165–187). New York: Oxford University Press.

Dennis, M., Yeates, K. O., Taylor, H. G., & Fletcher, J. M. (2007). Brain reserve capacity, cognitive reserve capacity, and age-based functional plasticity after congenital and acquired brain injury in children. In Y. Stern (Ed.), *Cognitive Reserve* (pp. 53–83). New York: Taylor & Francis.

Di Battista, A., Soo, C., Catroppa, C., & Anderson, V. (2012). Quality of life in children and adolescents post-TBI: A systematic review and meta-analysis. *Journal of Neurotrauma*, *29*, 1717–1727.

Donders, J. (2007). Traumatic brain injury. In S. J. Hunter & J. Donders (Eds.), *Pediatric Neuropsychological Intervention* (pp. 91–111). New York: Cambridge University Press.

Drotar, D., Stein, R.E.K., & Perrin, E. C. (1995). Methodological issues in using the child behavior checklist and its related instruments in clinical child psychology research. *Journal of Clinical Child Psychology*, *24*, 184–192.

Durham, S. R., Clancy, R. R., Leuthardt, E., Sun, P., Kamerling, S., Dominquez, T., & Duhaime, A. C. (2000). CHOP Infant Coma Scale ('Infant Face Scale'): A novel coma scale for children less than two years of age. *Journal of Neurotrauma*, *17*, 729–737.

Ewing-Cobbs, L., & Barnes, M. (2002). Linguistic outcomes following traumatic brain injury in children. *Seminars in Pediatric Neurology*, *9*, 209–217.

Ewing-Cobbs, L., Barnes, M., Fletcher, J. M., Levin, H. S., Swank, P. R., & Song, J. (2004a). Modeling of longitudinal academic achievement scores after pediatric traumatic brain injury. *Developmental Neuropsychology*, *25*, 107–133.

Ewing-Cobbs, L., Fletcher, J. M., Levin, H. S., Hastings, P. Z., & Francis, D. J. (1996). Assessment of injury severity following closed head injury in children: Methodological issues. *Journal of the International Neuropsychological Society*, *2*, 39.

Ewing-Cobbs, L., Fletcher, J. M., Levin, H. S., Iovino, I., & Miner, M. E. (1998a). Academic achievement and academic placement following traumatic brain injury in children and adolescents: A two-year longitudinal study. *Journal of Clinical and Experimental Neuropsychology*, *20*, 769–781.

Ewing-Cobbs, L., Levin, H. S., Fletcher, J. M., Miner, M. E., & Eisenberg, H. M. (1990). The children's orientation and amnesia test: Relationship to severity of acute head injury and to recovery of memory. *Neurosurgery*, *27*, 683–691.

Ewing-Cobbs, L., Prasad, M., Fletcher, J. M., Levin, H. S., Miner, M. E., & Eisenberg, H. M. (1998b). Attention after pediatric traumatic brain injury: A multidimensional assessment. *Child Neuropsychology*, *4*, 35–48.

Ewing-Cobbs, L., Prasad, M. R., Kramer, L., Cox, C .S., Jr., Baumgartner, J., Fletcher, S., . . . Swank, P. (2006). Late intellectual and academic outcomes following traumatic brain injury sustained during early childhood. *Journal of Neurosurgery, 105*, 2887–2896.

Ewing-Cobbs, L., Prasad, M. R., Landry, S. H., Kramer, L., & DeLeon, R. (2004b). Executive functions following traumatic brain injury in young children: A preliminary analysis. *Developmental Neuropsychology, 26*, 487–512.

Farkas, O., & Povlishock, J. T. (2007). Cellular and subcellular change evoked by diffuse traumatic brain injury: A complex web of change extending far beyond focal damage. *Progress in Brain Research, 161*, 43–59.

Faul, M., Xu, L., Wald, M. M., & Coronado, V. (2010). *Traumatic Brain Injury in the United States: Emergency Department Visits, Hospitalizations and Deaths, 2002–2006*. Atlanta, GA: Centers for Disease Control and Prevention, National Center for Injury Prevention and Control.

Fay, T. B., Yeates, K. O., Taylor, H. G., Bangert, B., Dietrich, A., Nuss, K. E., . . . Wright, M. (2010). Cognitive reserve as a moderator of postconcussive symptoms in children with complicated and uncomplicated mild traumatic brain injury. *Journal of the International Neuropsychological Society, 16*, 94–105.

Fay, T. B., Yeates, K. O., Wade, S. L., Drotar, D., Stancin, T., & Taylor, H. G. (2009). Predicting longitudinal patterns of functional deficits in children with traumatic brain injury. *Neuropsychology, 23*, 271–282.

Fletcher, J. M., Ewing-Cobbs, L., Miner, M. E., Levin, H. S., & Eisenberg, H. M. (1990). Behavioral changes after closed head injury in children. *Journal of Consulting and Clinical Psychology, 58*, 93–98.

Francis, D. J., Fletcher, J. M., Stuebing, K. K., Davidson, K. C., & Thompson, N. M. (1991). Analysis of change: Modeling individual growth. *Journal of Consulting and Clinical Psychology, 59*, 27–37.

Ganesalingam, K., Sanson, A., Anderson, V., & Yeates, K. O. (2007). Self-regulation as a mediator of the effects of childhood traumatic brain injury on social and behavioral functioning. *Journal of the International Neuropsychological Society, 13*, 298–311.

Gerring, J. P., Slomine, B., Vasa, R. A., Grados, M., Chen, A., Rising, W., . . . Ernst, M. (2002). Clinical predictors of posttraumatic stress disorder after closed head injury in children. *Journal of the American Academy of Child and Adolescent Psychiatry, 41*, 157–165.

Ghosh, A., Wilde, E. A., Hunter, J. V., Bigler, E. D., Chu, Z., Li, X., . . . Levin, H. S. (2009). The relation between Glasgow Coma Scale score and later cerebral atrophy in pediatric traumatic brain injury. *Brain Injury, 23*, 228–233.

Giza, C. C., & Hovda, D. (2001). The neurometabolic cascade of concussion. *Journal of Athletic Training, 36*, 228–235.

Giza, C. C., Mink, R. B., & Madikians, A. (2007). Pediatric traumatic brain injury: Not just little adults. *Current Opinions in Critical Care, 13*, 143–152.

Giza, C. C., & Prins, M. L. (2006). Is being plastic fantastic? Mechanisms of altered plasticity after developmental traumatic brain injury. *Developmental Neuroscience, 28*, 364–379.

Grados, M. A., Vasa, R. A., Riddle, M. A., Slomine, B. S., Salorio, C., Christensen, J., & Gerring, J. P. (2008). New onset obsessive-compulsive symptoms in children and adolescents with severe traumatic brain injury. *Depression and Anxiety, 25*, 398–407.

Hanten, G., Wilde, E. A., Menefee, D. S., Li, X., Lane, S., Vasquez, C., . . Levin, H. S. (2008). Correlates of social problem solving during the first year after traumatic brain injury in children. *Neuropsychology, 22*, 357–370.

Hedeker, D., & Gibbons, R. D. (1997). Application of random-effects pattern-mixture models for missing data in longitudinal studies. *Psychological Methods, 2*, 64–78.

Howard, I., Joseph, J. G., & Natale, J. E. (2005). Pediatric traumatic brain injury: Do racial/ethnic disparities exist in brain injury severity, mortality, or medical disposition? *Ethnicity & Disease, 15*, S551–S556.

Jaffe, K. M., Polissar, N. L., Fay, G. C., & Liao, S. (1995). Recovery trends over three years following pediatric traumatic brain injury. *Archives of Physical Medicine and Rehabilitation, 76*, 17–26.

Janusz, J. A., Kirkwood, M. W., Yeates, K. O., & Taylor, H. G. (2002). Social problem-solving skills in children with traumatic brain injury: Long-term outcomes and prediction of social competence. *Child Neuropsychology, 8*, 179–194.

Jennett, B., & Bond, M. (1975). Assessment of outcome after severe brain damage: A practical scale. *Lancet, 1*, 480–484.

Jonsson, C. A., Horneman, G., & Emanuelson, I. (2004). Neuropsychological progress during 14 years after severe traumatic brain injury in childhood and adolescence. *Brain Injury, 18*, 921–934.

Kamper, J. E., Pop, V., Fukuda, A. M., Ajao, D. O., Hartman, R. E., & Badaut, J. (2013). Juvenile traumatic brain injury evolves into a chronic brain disorder: Behavioral and histological changes over 6 months. *Experimental Neurology, 250*, 8–19.

Keenan, H. T., & Bratton, S. L. (2006). Epidemiology and outcomes of pediatric traumatic brain injury. *Developmental Neuroscience, 28*, 256–263.

Keightley, M. L., Sinopoli, K. J., Davis, K. D., Mikulis, D. J., Wennberg, R., Tartaglia, M. C., . . . Tator, C. H. (2014). Is there evidence for neurodegenerative change following traumatic brain injury in children and youth? A scoping review. *Frontiers in Human Neuroscience, 8*(Article 139), 1–6. doi: 10.3389/fnhum.2014.00139

Kinsella, G., Prior, M., Sawyer, M., Ong, B., Murtagh, D., Eisenmajer, R., . . . Klug, G. (1997). Predictors and indicators of academic outcome in children 2 years following traumatic brain injury. *Journal of the International Neuropsychological Society, 3*, 608–616.

Kirkwood, M. W., Peterson, R. L., & Yeates, K. O. (2013). Traumatic brain injury. In I. S. Baron, PhD & C. Rey-Casserly (Eds.), *Pediatric Neuropsychology: Medical Advances and Lifespan Outcomes* (pp. 302–320). New York: Oxford University Press.

Klonoff, H., Clark, C., & Klonoff, P. S. (1995). Outcomes of head injuries from childhood to adulthood: A twenty-three year follow-up study. In S. H. Broman & M. E. Michel (Eds.), *Traumatic Head Injury in Children* (pp. 219–234). New York: Oxford University Press.

Kochanek, P. M. (2006). Pediatric traumatic brain injury: Quo vadis? *Developmental Neuroscience, 28*, 244–255.

Kochanek, P. M., Carney, N., Adelson, P. D., . . .Warden, C. R. (2012). Guidelines for the acute medical management of severe traumatic brain injury in infants, children, and adolescents: Second edition. *Pediatric Critical Care Medicine, 13*(1 Suppl.), 1–82.

Koskiniemi, M., Kyykka, T., Nybo, T., & Jarho, L. (1995). Long-term outcome after severe brain injury in preschoolers is worse than expected. *Archives of Pediatric Adolescent Medicine, 149*, 249–254.

Kramer, M. E., Chiu, C.Y.P., Walz, N. C., Holland, S. K., Yuan, W., Karunanayaka, P., & Wade, S. L. (2008). Long-term neural processing of attention following early childhood traumatic brain injury: FMRI and neurobehavioral outcomes. *Journal of the International Neuropsychological Society*, *14*, 424–235.

Kraus, J. F. (1995). Epidemiological features of brain injury in children: Occurrence, children at risk, causes and manner of injury, severity, and outcomes. In S. H. Broman & M. E. Michel (Eds.), *Traumatic Head Injury in Children* (pp. 22–39). New York: Oxford University Press.

Kuhtz-Buschbeck, J. P., Hoppe, B., Golge, M., Dreesmann, M., Damm-Stunitz, U., & Ritz, A. (2003). Sensorimotor recovery in children after traumatic brain injury: Analyses of gait, gross motor, and fine motor skills. *Developmental Medicine & Child Neurology*, *12*, 821–828.

Kuppermann, N., Holmes, J. F., Dayan, P. S., Hoyle, J. D., . . . Wooten-Gorges, S. L. (2009). Identification of children at very low risk of clinically-important brain injuries after head trauma: A prospective cohort study. *Lancet*, *374*, 1160–1170.

Kurowski, B., Martin, L. J., & Wade, S. L. (2012). Genetics and outcomes after traumatic brain injury (TBI): What do we know about pediatric TBI? *Journal of Pediatric Rehabilitation Medicine*, *5*, 217–231.

Laatsch, L., Harrington, D., Hotz, G., Marcantuono, J., Mozzoni, M. P., Walsh, V., & Hersey, K. P. (2007). An evidence-based review of cognitive and behavioral rehabilitation treatment studies in children with acquired brain injury. *Journal of Head Trauma Rehabilitation*, *22*, 248–256.

Langlois, J. A., Kegler, S. R., Butler, J. A., Gotsch, K. E., Johnson, R. L., Reichard, A. A., . . . Thurman, D. J. (2003). Traumatic brain injury-related hospital discharges: Results from a 14-state surveillance system, 1997. *MMWR Surveillance Summaries*, *52*, 1–18.

Langlois, J. A., Rutland-Brown, W., & Thomas, K. E. (2005). The incidence of traumatic brain injury among children in the United States: Differences by race. *Journal of Head Trauma Rehabilitation*, *20*, 229–238.

Lehnung, M., Leplow, B., Herzog, A., Benz, B., Ritz, A., Stolze, H., . . . Ferstl, R. (2001). Children's spatial behavior is differentially affected after traumatic brain injury. *Child Neuropsychology*, *7*, 59–71.

Levi, R. B., Drotar, D., Yeates, K. O., & Taylor, H. G. (1999). Posttraumatic stress symptoms in children following orthopedic or traumatic brain injury. *Journal of Clinical Child Psychology*, *28*, 232–243.

Levin, H. S., & Eisenberg, H. M. (1979). Neuropsychological impairment after closed head injury in children and adolescents. *Journal of Pediatric Psychology*, *4*, 389–402.

Levin, H. S., & Hanten, G. (2005). Executive functions after traumatic brain injury in children. *Pediatric Neurology*, *33*, 79–93.

Levin, H., Hanten, G., Max, J., Li, X., Swank, P., Ewing-Cobbs, L., . . . Schachar, R. (2007). Symptoms of attention-deficit/hyperactivity disorder following traumatic brain injury in children. *Journal of Developmental & Behavioral Pediatrics*, *28*, 108–118.

Levin, H. S., Madison, C. F., Bailey, C. B., Meyers, C. A., Eisenberg, H. M., & Guinto, F. C. (1983). Mutism after closed head injury. *Archives of Neurology*, *40*, 601–606.

Levin, H. S., Zhang, L., Dennis, M., Ewing-Cobbs, L., Schachar, R., Max, J., . . . Hunter, J. V. (2004). Psychosocial outcome of TBI in children with unilateral frontal lesions. *Journal of the International Neuropsychological Society*, *10*, 305–316.

Li, L., & Liu, J. (2013). The effect of pediatric traumatic brain injury on behavioral outcomes: A systematic review. *Developmental Medicine & Child Neurology*, *55*, 37–45.

Luis, C. A., & Mittenberg, W. (2002). Mood and anxiety disorders following pediatric traumatic brain injury: A prospective study. *Journal of Clinical and Experimental Neuropsychology*, *24*, 270–279.

Maas, A. I., & Menon, D. K. (2012). Traumatic brain injury: Rethinking ideas and approaches. *Lancet Neurology*, *11*, 12–13.

Maas, A. I., Menon, D. K., Lingsma, H. F., Pineda, J. A., Sandel, M. E., & Manley, G. T. (2012). Re-orientation of clinical research in traumatic brain injury: Report of an international workshop on comparative effectiveness research. *Journal of Neurotrauma*, *29*, 32–46.

Mangeot, S., Armstrong, K., Colvin, A. N., Yeates, K. O., & Taylor, H. G. (2002). Long-term executive function deficits in children with traumatic brain injuries: Assessment using the Behavior Rating Inventory of Executive Function (BRIEF). *Child Neuropsychology*, *8*, 271–284.

Margulies, S., & Coats, B. (2010). Biomechanics of pediatric TBI. In V. A. Anderson & K. O. Yeates (Eds.), *Pediatric Traumatic Brain Injury: New Frontiers in Clinical and Translational Research* (pp. 7–17). New York: Cambridge University Press.

Masel, B. E., & DeWitt, D. S. (2010). Traumatic brain injury: A disease process, not an event. *Journal of Neurotrauma*, *27*, 1529–1540.

Max, J. E., Castillo, C. S., Bokura, H., Robin, D. A., Lindgren, S. D., Smith, W. L., . . . Mattheis, P. J. (1998a). Oppositional defiant disorder symptomatology after traumatic brain injury: A prospective study. *Journal of Nervous and Mental Disease*, *186*, 325–332.

Max, J. E., Koele, S. L., Castillo, C. C., Lindgren, S. D., Arndt, S., Bokura, H., . . . Sato, Y. (2000). Personality change disorder in children and adolescents following traumatic brain injury. *Journal of the International Neuropsychological Society*, *6*, 279–289.

Max, J. E., Koele, S. L., Lindgren, S. D., Robin, D. A., Smith, W. L., Jr., Sato, Y., & Arndt, S. (1998c). Adaptive functioning following traumatic brain injury and orthopedic injury: A controlled study. *Archives of Physical Medicine and Rehabilitation*, *79*, 893–899.

Max, J. E., Levin, H. S., Landis, J., Schachar, R., Saunders, A., Ewing-Cobbs, L., . . . Dennis, M. (2005a). Predictors of personality change due to traumatic brain injury in children and adolescents in the first six months after injury. *Journal of the American Academy of Child & Adolescent Psychiatry*, *44*, 434–442.

Max, J. E., Schachar, R. J., Levin, H. S., Ewing-Cobbs, L., Chapman, S. B., Dennis, M., . . . Landis, J. (2005b). Predictors of secondary attention-deficit/hyperactivity disorder in children and adolescents 6 to 24 months after traumatic brain injury. *Journal of the American Academy of Child & Adolescent Psychiatry*, *44*, 1041–1049.

McCauley, S. R., & Levin, H. S. (2004). Prospective memory in pediatric traumatic brain injury: A preliminary study. *Developmental Neuropsychology*, *25*, 5–20.

McCauley, S. R., Wilde, E. A., Anderson, V. A., Bedell, G., . . . Yeates, K. O. (2012). Recommendations for the use of common outcome measures in pediatric traumatic brain injury research. *Journal of Neurotrauma*, *29*, 678–705.

McCrea, M., Barr, W. B., Guskiewicz, K., Randolph, C., Marshall, S. W., Cantu, R., . . . Kelly, J. P. (2005). Standard regression-based methods for measuring recovery after sport-related concussion. *Journal of the International Neuropsychological Society*, *11*, 58–69.

McDonald, C. M., Jaffe, K. M., Fay, G. C., Polissar, N. L., Martin, K. M., Liao, S., & Rivara, J. B. (1994). Comparison of indices of TBI severity as predictors of neurobehavioral outcomes in children. *Archives of Physical Medicine and Rehabilitation, 75*, 328–337.

McLean, D. E., Kaitz, E. S., Kennan, C. J., Dabney, K., Cawley, M. F., & Alexander, M. A. (1995). Medical and surgical complications of pediatric brain injury. *Journal of Head Trauma Rehabilitation, 10*, 1–12.

Miller, L. M., & Donders, J. (2003). Prediction of educational outcome after pediatric traumatic brain injury. *Rehabilitation Psychology, 48*, 237–241.

Munson, S., Schroth, E., & Ernst, M. (2006). The role of functional neuroimaging in pediatric brain injury. *Pediatrics, 117*, 1372–1381.

Mushkudiani, N. A., Hukkelhoven, C.W.P.M., Hernandez, A. V., Murray, G. D., Choi, S. C., Maas, A.I.R., & Steyerberg, E. W. (2008). A systematic review finds methodological improvements necessary for prognostic models in determining traumatic brain injury outcomes. *Journal of Clinical Epidemiology, 61*, 331–343.

Nadebaum, C., Anderson, V., & Catroppa, C. (2007). Executive function outcomes following traumatic brain injury in young children: A five year follow-up. *Developmental Neuropsychology, 32*, 703–728.

Nagin, D. S. (1999). Analyzing developmental trajectories: A semi-parametric, group-based approach. *Psychological Methods, 4*, 129–177.

Narayan, R. K., & Michel, M. E. (2002). Clinical trials in head injury. *Journal of Neurotrauma, 19*, 503–557.

Natale, J. E., Joseph, J. G., Pretzlaff, R. K., Silber, T. J., & Guerguerian, A.-M. (2005). Clinical trials in pediatric traumatic brain injury: Unique challenges and potential responses. *Developmental Neuroscience, 28*, 276–290.

Newsome, M. R., Steinberg, J. L., Scheibel, R. S., Troyanskaya, M., Chu, Z., Hanten, G., . . . Levin, H. S. (2008). Effects of traumatic brain injury on working memory-related brain activation in adolescents. *Neuropsychology, 22*, 419–425.

Novack, T. A., Dillon, M. C., & Jackson, W. T. (1996). Neurochemical mechanisms in brain injury and treatment: A review. *Journal of Clinical and Experimental Neuropsychology, 18*, 685–706.

Osmond, M. H., Klassen, T. R., Wells, G. A., Correll, R., . . . Stiell, I. G. (2010). Catch: A clinical decision rule for the use of computed tomography in children with minor head injury. *Canadian Medical Association Journal, 182*, 341–348.

Papa, L., Ramia, M. M., Kelly, J. M., Burks, S. S., Pawlowicz, A., & Berger, R. P. (2013). Systematic review of clinical research on biomarkers for pediatric traumatic brain injury. *Journal of Neurotrauma, 30*, 324–338.

Parslow, R. C., Morris, K. P., Tasker, R. C., Forsyth, R. J., & Hawley, C. A. (2005). Epidemiology of traumatic brain injury in children receiving intensive care in the UK. *Archives of Disease in Childhood, 90*, 1182–1187.

Perrin, E. C., Stein, R. E., & Drotar, D. (1991). Cautions in using the child behavior checklist: Observations based on research about children with a chronic illness. *Journal of Pediatric Psychology, 16*, 411–421.

Poussaint, T. Y., &, Moeller, M. D. (2002). Imaging of pediatric head trauma. *Neuroimaging Clinics of North America, 12*, 271–294.

Povlishock, J. T., & Katz, D. I. (2005). Update of neuropathology and neurological recovery after traumatic brain injury. *Journal of Head Trauma Rehabilitation, 20*, 76–94.

Power, T., Catroppa, C., Coleman, L., Ditchfield, M., & Anderson, V. (2007). Do lesion site and severity predict deficits in attentional control after preschool traumatic brain injury (TBI)? *Brain Injury, 21*, 279–292.

Powell, J. M., Temkin, N. R., Machamer, J. E., & Dikmen, S. S. (2002). Nonrandomized studies of rehabilitation for traumatic brain injury: Can they determine effectiveness? *Archives of Physical Medicine and Rehabilitation, 83*, 1235–1244.

Robinson, K. E., Fountain-Zaragoza, S., Taylor, H. G., Bigler, E. D., Rubin, K., Vannatta, K., . . . Yeates, K. O. (2014). Executive functions and theory of mind as predictors of social adjustment in childhood traumatic brain injury. *Journal of Neurotrauma, 31*, 1835–1842.

Robinson, K. E., Kaizar, E., Catroppa, C., Godfrey, C., & Yeates, K. O. (2014). A systematic review and meta-analysis of cognitive interventions for children with central nervous system disorders and neurodevelopmental disorders. *Journal of Pediatric Psychology, 39*, 846–865.

Rosema, S., Crowe, L., & Anderson, V. (2012). Social function in children and adolescents after traumatic brain injury: A systematic review 1989–2011. *Journal of Neurotrauma, 29*, 1277–1291.

Ross, K. A., Dorris, L., & McMillan, T. (2011). A systematic review of psychological interventions to alleviate cognitive and psychosocial problems in children with acquired brain injury. *Developmental Medicine & Child Neurology, 53*, 692–701.

Saatman, K. E., Duhaime, A.-C., Bullock, R., Mass, A.I.R., Valadka, A., Manley, G. T., & Workshop Scientific Team and Advisory Panel Members. (2008). Classification of traumatic brain injury for targeted therapies. *Journal of Neurotrauma, 25*, 719–738.

Salorio, C. F., Slomine, B. S., Grados, M. A., Vasa, R. A., Christensen, J. R., & Gerring, J. P. (2005). Neuroanatomic correlates of CVLT-C performance following pediatric traumatic brain injury. *Journal of the International Neuropsychological Society, 11*, 686–696.

Satz, P. (2001). Mild head injury in children and adolescents. *Current Directions in Psychological Science, 10*, 106–109.

Schneier, A. J., Shields, B. J., Hostetler, S. G., Xiang, H., & Smith, G. A. (2006). Incidence of pediatric traumatic brain injury and associated hospital resource utilization in the United States. *Pediatrics, 118*, 483–492.

Sesma, H. W., Slomine, B. S., Ding, R., & McCarthy, M. L. (2008). Executive functioning in the first year after pediatric traumatic brain injury. *Pediatrics, 121*, e1686–e1695.

Shore, P. M., Berger, R. P., Varma, S., Janesko, K. L., Wisniewski, S. R., Clark, R. S., . . . Kochanek, P. M. (2007). Cerebrospinal fluid biomarkers versus Glasgow Coma Scale and Glasgow Outcome Scale in pediatric traumatic brain injury: The role of young age and inflicted injury. *Journal of Neurotrauma, 24*, 75–86.

Sigmund, G. A., Tong, K. A., Nickerson, J. P., Wall, C. J., Oyoyo, U., & Ashwal, S. (2007). Multimodality comparison of neuroimaging in pediatric traumatic brain injury. *Pediatric Neurology, 36*, 217–226.

Slomine, B. S., Gerring, J. P., Grados, M. A., Vasa, R., Brady, K. D., Christensen, J. R., & Denckla, M. B. (2002). Performance on measures of executive function following pediatric traumatic brain injury. *Brain Injury, 16*, 759–772.

Slomine, B. S., & Locascio, G. (2009). Cognitive rehabilitation for children with acquired brain injury. *Developmental Disabilities Research Reviews, 15*, 133–143.

Sosin, D. M., Sniezek, J. E., & Thurman, D. J. (1996). Incidence of mild and moderate brain injury in the United States, 1991. *Brain Injury, 10*, 47–54.

Stancin, T., Drotar, D., Taylor, H. G., Yeates, K. O., Wade, S. L., & Minich, N. M. (2002). Health-related quality of life of children and adolescents after traumatic brain injury. *Pediatrics, 109*. Retrieved from www.pediatrics.org/cgi/content/full/109/2/e34

Statler, K. D. (2006). Pediatric posttraumatic seizures: Epidemiology, putative mechanisms of epileptogenesis and promising investigational progress. *Developmental Neuroscience, 28*, 354–363.

Tal, G., & Tirosh, E. (2013). Rehabilitation of children with traumatic brain injury: A review. *Pediatric Neurology, 48*, 424–431.

Taylor, H. G. (2010). Neurobehavioral outcomes of pediatric traumatic brain injury. In V. A. Anderson & K. O. Yeates (Eds.), *Pediatric Traumatic Brain Injury: New Frontiers in Clinical and Translational Research* (pp. 145–168). New York: Cambridge University Press.

Taylor, H. G., & Alden, J. (1997). Age-related differences in outcome following childhood brain injury: An introduction and overview. *Journal of the International Neuropsychological Society, 3*, 555–567.

Taylor, H. G., Yeates, K. O., Wade, S. L., Drotar, D., Klein, S. K., & Stancin, T. (1999). Influences on first-year recovery from traumatic brain injury in children. *Neuropsychology, 13*, 76–89.

Taylor, H. G., Yeates, K. O., Wade, S. L., Drotar, D., Stancin, T., & Minich, N. (2002). A prospective study of long- and short-term outcomes after traumatic brain injury in children: Behavior and achievement. *Neuropsychology, 16*, 15–27.

Taylor, H. G., Yeates, K. O., Wade, S. L., Drotar, D., Stancin, T., & Montpetite, M. (2003). Long-term educational interventions after traumatic brain injury in children. *Rehabilitation Psychology, 48*, 227–236.

Teasdale, G., & Jennett, B. (1974). Assessment of coma and impaired consciousness: A practical scale. *Lancet, 2*, 81–84.

Thompson, N. M., Francis, D. J., Stuebing, K. K., Fletcher, J. M., Ewing-Cobbs, L., Miner, M. E., . . . Eisenberg, H. (1994). Motor, visual-spatial, and somatosensory skills after TBI in children and adolescents: A study of change. *Neuropsychology, 8*, 333–342.

Vasa, R. A., Gerring, J. P., Grados, M., Slomine, B., Christensen, J. R., Rising, W., . . . Riddle, M. A. (2002). Anxiety after severe pediatric closed head injury. *Journal of the American Academy of Child and Adolescent Psychiatry, 41*, 148–156.

Wade, S. L. (2010). Psychosocial interventions. In V. A. Anderson & K. O. Yeates (Eds.), *Pediatric Traumatic Brain Injury: New Frontiers in Clinical and Translational Research* (pp. 179–191). New York: Cambridge University Press.

Wade, S. L., Taylor, H. G., Walz, N. C., Salisbury, S., Stancin, T., Bernard, L. A., . . . Yeates, K. O. (2008). Parent-child interactions during the initial weeks following brain injury in young children. *Rehabilitation Psychology, 53*, 180–190.

Wade, S. L., Taylor, H. G., Yeates, K. O., Drotar, D., Stancin, T., Minich, N. M., & Schluchter, M. (2006). Long-term parental and family adaptation following pediatric brain injury. *Journal of Pediatric Psychology, 31*, 1072–1083.

Ward, H., Shum, D., Dick, B., McKinlay, L., & Baker-Tweney, S. (2004). Interview study of the effects of paediatric traumatic brain injury on memory. *Brain Injury, 18*, 471–495.

Ward, H., Shum, D., McKinlay, L., Baker, S., & Wallace, G. (2007). Prospective memory and pediatric traumatic brain injury: Effects of cognitive demand. *Child Neuropsychology, 13*, 219–239.

Ward, H., Shum, D., Wallace, G., & Boon, J. (2002). Pediatric traumatic brain injury and procedural memory. *Journal of Clinical and Experimental Neuropsychology, 24*, 458–470.

Warschausky, S., Kewman, D., & Kay, J. (1999). Empirically supported psychological and behavioral therapies in pediatric rehabilitation of TBI. *Journal of Head Trauma Rehabilitation, 14*, 373–383.

Wilde, E. A., Hunter, J. V., Newsome, M. R., Scheibel, R. S., Bigler, E. D., Johnson, J. L., . . . Levin, H. S. (2005). Frontal and temporal morphometric findings on MRI in children after moderate to severe traumatic brain injury. *Journal of Neurotrauma, 22*, 333–344.

Yeates, K. O. (2010). Traumatic brain injury. In K. O. Yeates, M. D. Ris, H. G. Taylor, & B. F. Pennington (Eds.), *Pediatric Neuropsychology: Research, Theory, and Practice* (2nd ed., pp. 112–146). New York: Guilford Press.

Yeates, K. O., Armstrong, K., Janusz, J., Taylor, H. G., Wade, S., Stancin, T., & Drotar, D. (2005). Long-term attention problems in children with traumatic brain injury. *Journal of the American Academy of Child and Adolescent Psychiatry, 44*, 574–584.

Yeates, K. O., Bigler, E. D., Abildskov, T., Dennis, M., Gerhardt, C. A., Vannatta, K., . . . Taylor, H. G. (2014). Social competence in pediatric traumatic brain injury: From brain to behavior. *Clinical Psychological Science, 2*, 97–107.

Yeates, K. O., Bigler, E. D., Dennis, M., Gerhardt, C. A., Rubin, K. H., Stancin, T., . . . Vannatta, K. (2007). Social outcomes in childhood brain disorder: A heuristic integration of social neuroscience and developmental psychology. *Psychological Bulletin, 133*, 535–556.

Yeates, K. O., Blumenstein, E., Patterson, C. M., & Delis, D. C. (1995). Verbal learning and memory following pediatric TBI. *Journal of the International Neuropsychological Society, 1*, 78–87.

Yeates, K. O., & Enrile, B. G. (2005). Implicit and explicit memory in children with congenital and acquired brain disorder. *Neuropsychology, 19*, 618–628.

Yeates, K. O., Kaizar, E., Rusin, J., Bangert, B., Dietrich, A., Nuss, K., . . . Taylor, H. G. (2012). Reliable change in post-concussive symptoms and its functional consequences among children with mild traumatic brain injury. *Archives of Pediatrics & Adolescent Medicine, 166*, 585–684.

Yeates, K. O., Swift, E., Taylor, H. G., Wade, S. L., Drotar, D., Stancin, T., & Minich, N. (2004). Short- and long-term social outcomes following pediatric traumatic brain injury. *Journal of the International Neuropsychological Society, 10*, 412–426.

Yeates, K. O., & Taylor, H. G. (2006). Behavior problems in school and their educational correlates among children with traumatic brain injury. *Exceptionality, 14*, 141–154.

Yeates, K. O., Taylor, H. G., Barry, C. T., Drotar, D., Wade, S. L., & Stancin, T. (2001). Neurobehavioral symptoms in childhood closed-head injuries: Changes in prevalence and correlates during the first year post-injury. *Journal of Pediatric Psychology, 26*, 79–91.

Yeates, K. O., Taylor, H. G., Drotar, D., Wade, S., Klein, S., & Stancin, T. (1997). Premorbid family environment as a predictor of neurobehavioral outcomes following pediatric TBI. *Journal of the International Neuropsychological Society, 3*, 617–630.

Yeates, K. O., Taylor, H. G., Rusin, J., Bangert, B., Dietrich, A., Nuss, K., . . . Jones, B. L. (2009). Longitudinal trajectories of post-concussive symptoms in children with mild traumatic brain injuries and their relationship to acute clinical status. *Pediatrics, 123*, 735–743.

Yeates, K. O., Taylor, H. G., Wade, S. L., Drotar, D., Stancin, T., & Minich, N. (2002). A prospective study of short-and long-term neuropsychological outcomes after traumatic brain injury in children. *Neuropsychology*, *16*, 514–523.

Ylvisaker, M., Adelson, D., Braga, L. W., Burnett, S. M., Glang, A., Feeney, T., . . . Todis, B. (2005). Rehabilitation and ongoing support after pediatric TBI: Twenty years of progress. *Journal of Head Trauma Rehabilitation*, *20*, 90–104.

Ylvisaker, M., Todis, B., Glang, A., Urbanczyk, B., Franklin, C., DePompei, R., . . . Tyler, J. S. (2001). Educating students with TBI: Themes and recommendations. *Journal of Head Trauma Rehabilitation*, *16*, 76–93.

Ylvisaker, M., Turkstra, L. S., & Coelho, C. (2005). Behavioral and social interventions for individuals with traumatic brain injury: A summary of the research with clinical implications. *Seminars in Speech and Language*, *26*, 256–267.

Ylvisaker, M., Turkstra, L. S., Coehlo, C., Yorkston, K., Kennedy, M., Sohlberg, M. M., & Avery, J. (2007). Behavioural interventions for children and adults with behaviour disorders after TBI: A systematic review of the evidence. *Brain Injury*, *21*, 769–805.

Yuan, W., Holland, S. K., Schmithorst, V. J., Walz, N. C., Cecil, K. M., Jones, B. V., . . . Wade, S. L. (2007). Diffusion tensor MR imaging reveals persistent white matter alteration after traumatic brain injury experienced during early childhood. *American Journal of Neuroradiology*, *28*, 1919–1925.

Zemek, R., Osmond, M. H., Barrowman, N., & Pediatric Emergency Research Canada (PERC) Concussion Team. (2013). *BMJ Open*, e003550, 1–10. doi: 10.1136/bmjopen-2013-003550

12 Pediatric Cancer

Celiane Rey-Casserly and Brenda J. Spiegler

Pediatric oncology has been a productive and rewarding field for neuropsychologists, both because of the remarkable successes in medical care and survival achieved over the past generation and because of the important contributions made by our profession to scientific advances and clinical care. As survival rates for childhood cancer have improved, pediatric neuropsychologists have become increasingly involved in efforts to foster optimal outcomes through participation in interdisciplinary care teams, assessment, and intervention. Childhood cancer was a fatal diagnosis in the 1950s; today more than 80% of children with some forms of cancer (e.g., acute lymphoblastic leukemia, or ALL) will survive (Pui, Carroll, Meshinchi, & Arceci, 2011). Ten-year survival for children with malignant brain tumors has improved from 46% (1973–1976) to 69% (2002–2006) (Ostrom et al., 2015). This remarkable increase in survival is true for many pediatric cancer diagnoses and was achieved with increased intensity of treatment and multimodality therapy (surgery, if warranted; multiagent and multiroute chemotherapy; radiation therapy). Figure 12.1 plots five-year survival rates for brain tumors and ALL from the mid-1970s when central nervous system directed treatment was introduced for ALL. Intense treatment and the resulting increase in survival have come at a cost: Late effects on various organs (heart, lung, kidney, bone, brain), early aging, and second malignant neoplasms affect nearly two-thirds of survivors, with up to one quarter reporting severe or life-threatening conditions (Oeffinger et al., 2006). Many of these adverse late effects are more prevalent in survivors of childhood leukemia treated with cranial radiation therapy (CRT) (Hudson et al., 2013) and survivors of central nervous system (CNS) tumors (Armstrong et al., 2009). As a result, quality of survival has become central to the cost-benefit analysis—and here both health psychologists and neuropsychologists have played a prominent role. In fact, it was early neuropsychological research that first documented the fact that CRT administered to the developing brain was associated with cognitive impairments affecting IQ and academic achievement (Eiser, 1978; Eiser & Lansdown, 1977; Meadows, Massari, Fergusson, Gordon, & Moss, 1981; Waber & Tarbell, 1997; Waber et al., 1995). Later studies began to focus more narrowly on core neuropsychological processes underlying these cognitive impairments. With increasingly effective techniques to image white matter in the brain and advances in the understanding of genetic factors, the study of brain-behavior relations in pediatric oncology has taken on new energy and is an exciting, dynamic area of study with new implications for changes in treatment and care of the child with cancer.

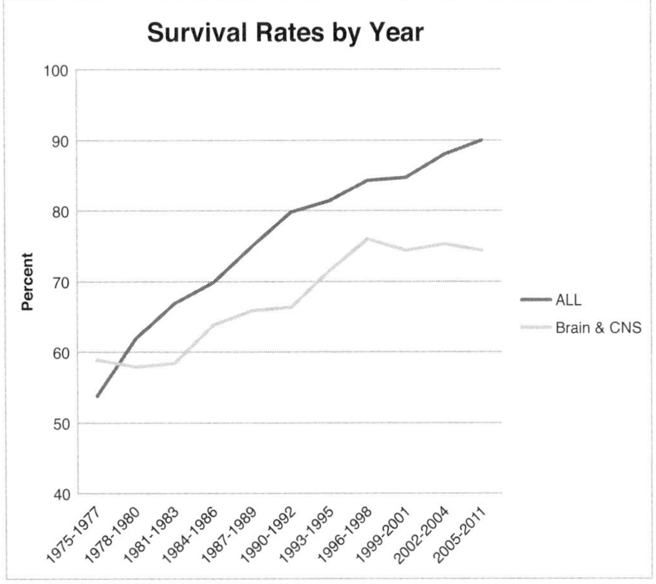

Figure 12.1 Five–year survival rates by year for ALL and brain tumors (Howlader et al., 2015; these data are based on November 2014 SEER data submission, posted to the SEER web site, April 2015)

In this chapter, we will present the historical perspective on incidence, treatments, and survival in childhood cancer, and then focus on the neuropsychological complications and late effects associated with leukemia and brain tumors. These two most common forms of childhood cancer account for approximately 50% of cases and have differing incidence through childhood (Figure 12.2). We will discuss some of the rarer, but particularly interesting, populations (e.g., infants and adolescents/young adults), forms of cancer, and developmental/neuropsychological complications. Finally, we will outline future directions for research and clinical care in this dynamic medical specialty.

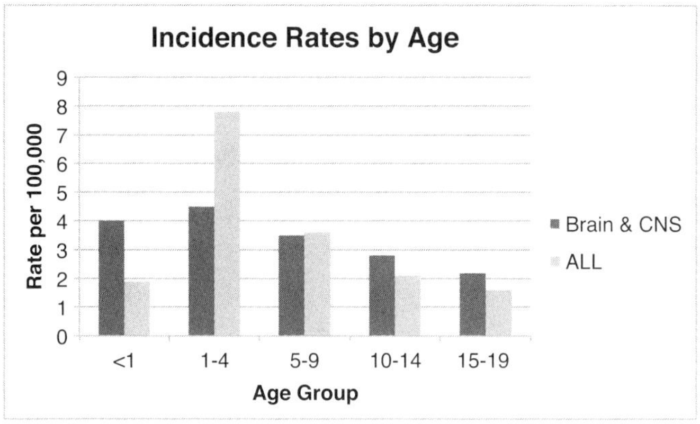

Figure 12.2 Incidence rates by age group for ALL and brain tumor (U.S. Cancer Statistics Working Group, 2014)

Acute Lymphoblastic Leukemia

Leukemia is the most common form of cancer in childhood, with one form, ALL, comprising nearly 25% of all new cancer diagnoses in children under the age of 15 (Kaatsch, 2010). ALL develops when the precursors of white blood cells in the bone marrow proliferate, crowding out healthy and functional cells, impairing formation of normal white blood cells, and causing infiltration of leukemic cells into the bloodstream. ALL is most commonly diagnosed during the preschool years, with peak incidence between 2 and 5 years of age (Inaba, Greaves, & Mullighan, 2013). Boys are 20% more likely to be diagnosed with ALL than girls (Pizzo & Poplack, 2006).

Before the advent of modern multimodal treatments and multiagent chemotherapy, children with ALL survived only a few months (Simone, 2006). The increase in survival from this previously fatal disease is one of the great medical success stories of the past 50 years (Hudson, Link, & Simone, 2014). Even after early chemotherapy regimens allowed short periods of survival, patients invariably relapsed, with disease invading the CNS. This realization led to the recognition that leukemia cells cross the blood-brain barrier and are present in the meninges early in the course of the disease. Subsequently, the addition of craniospinal radiation and CNS-directed chemotherapy dramatically improved long-term survival.

Once high survival rates were achieved, the problem of neuropsychological morbidity and other adverse late effects began to take on greater importance. As the cohort of childhood ALL survivors began to expand in the late 1970s, the significant associated neuropsychological deficits were documented (Eiser, 1978; Eiser & Lansdown, 1977; Meadows & Evans, 1976; Meadows et al., 1981). Neuropsychology as a discipline has been central in identifying the role of CRT and, more recently, high-dose methotrexate and steroids on the neurodevelopmental trajectories of ALL survivors. Documenting the relations among host, treatment factors, and neurocognitive outcome has helped shape modifications in treatment, which highlights the central role of neuropsychology in the specialty of pediatric oncology.

Treatment Protocols

Early protocols utilized 24 Gy of CRT as CNS-directed therapy; while this was effective in eradicating leukemic cells that infiltrated the CNS, neuropsychological studies documented that intellectual level and academic skills declined after treatment, particularly in arithmetic (Eiser, 1978; Meadows et al., 1981; Moss, Nannis, & Poplack, 1981). An early meta-analysis documented an IQ loss of 9 to 10 points relative to controls and population norms (Cousens, Waters, Said, & Stevens, 1988). Beyond IQ, Dowell and colleagues reported effects on tests of memory and attention that were negatively correlated with radiation dose (Dowell, Copeland, Francis, Fletcher, & Stovall, 1991).

In the 1990s, CRT doses were reduced from 24 Gy to 18 Gy in an effort to mitigate neuropsychological late effects. This was achieved without affecting survival by increasing the intensity of chemotherapy. A dose effect was demonstrated in that intellectual outcomes were generally better after 18 Gy than 24 Gy (Halberg et al., 1992; Moore, Kramer, Wara, Halberg, & Ablin, 1991; Smibert, Anderson, Godber, & Ekert, 1996) although this was not a consistent finding (Mulhern, Ochs, & Kun, 1991; Rodgers, Britton, Kernahan, & Craft, 1991; Waber et al., 1995). But even at 18 Gy, CRT was associated with intellectual and academic declines in survivors (Rubenstein, Varni, & Katz, 1990). Declines in neuropsychological functions, including visual-motor integration, processing speed, attention, and short-term memory are most often reported in children treated with 18–24 Gy (Brouwers & Poplack, 1990; Reddick et al., 2006a; Schatz, Kramer, Ablin, & Matthay, 2000; Taylor, Albo, Phebus, Sachs, & Bierl, 1987) while verbal and language abilities are less frequently affected (Ciesielski et al., 1994). In the past decade, the customary dose of CRT, when necessary at all, has been reduced to 12 Gy, but long-term neuropsychological outcomes have yet to be reported.

With contemporary chemotherapy protocols, well over 80% of children with standard risk ALL can expect to survive for the long-term (Pui, Carroll, Meshinchi, & Arceci, 2011; Pui & Evans, 2006; Pui, Relling, & Downing, 2004). Current ALL treatment is designed to minimize adverse late effects while maintaining high survival rates. Late effects are less global and less severe in children treated with chemotherapy-only protocols (Buizer, de Sonneville, & Veerman, 2009; Harila, Winqvist, Lanning, Bloigu, & Harila-Saari, 2009; Janzen & Spiegler, 2008; Spiegler et al., 2006). For this reason, current protocols omit CRT whenever possible. Patients are stratified according to risk of relapse: Low- and standard-risk patients typically receive chemotherapy-only regimens, while CRT is reserved for the 2%–20% of patients considered at high risk for CNS relapse on the basis of presentation or genetic factors (Pui & Howard, 2008). Still, many patients treated with chemotherapy show some degree of neuropsychological impairment (Anderson & Kunin-Batson, 2009; Cheung & Krull, 2015; Conklin et al., 2012; Moleski, 2000). The literature on neuropsychological outcomes after treatment for childhood leukemia with chemotherapy suffers from small sample sizes and variations in sample characteristics, comparison groups, outcome measures, and length of follow-up. In a recent systematic review, Cheung and Krull (2015) confirmed that outcomes are better among this population compared to historical cohorts treated with CRT. But they also showed that cognitive impairments remain measureable, clustering in the domains of attention, executive function, memory, and motor function. In some cases, even when group mean differences do not attain statistical significance, the proportion of ALL survivors with scores below a predetermined cutoff (e.g., 2 SD below the mean) is significantly higher than expected in the normal population, indicating that the rate of significant impairment in the treatment group is increased.

Attention and working memory impairments are most commonly documented among children treated for ALL with chemotherapy only (Ashford et al., 2010; Conklin et al., 2012; Krull, Bhojwani et al., 2013). For example, when tested 120 weeks after completion of consolidation therapy, patients treated with chemotherapy only did not differ from general population means in the domains of cognitive development, academic abilities, learning, and memory. However, sustained attention was impaired, with a full 40% of the sample scoring below the predefined cutoff of 1 SD below the mean (Conklin et al., 2012). Executive function and processing speed (both motor and cognitive processing speed) are other commonly documented areas of impairment (Jansen et al., 2008; Kahalley et al., 2013; Mennes et al., 2005; Winter et al., 2014). Measures of general cognitive development (IQ) are often in the average range and not significantly different from population norms (Conklin et al., 2012; Jansen et al., 2006; Schatz et al., 2000). Several studies have shown that the intensity of chemotherapy, as reflected by the number and cumulative dose of methotrexate (MTX), is related to particular aspects of attention (Conklin et al., 2012; Krull, Bhojwani, et al., 2013). Further study of the factors and mechanisms associated with neuropsychological impairment in survivors treated with chemotherapy for ALL may lead to additional adjustments to treatment protocols and concomitant improvements in outcome.

Risk Factors in Neuropsychological Outcomes

In addition to treatment factors, such as history and dose of CRT, a number of host factors have been shown to moderate outcomes. Girls (Bleyer, 1990; Iuvone et al., 2002; Waber, Tarbell, Kahn, Gelber, & Sallan, 1992; Waber et al., 1990) and children radiated at a younger age are at greater risk for poor outcome (Bleyer, 1990; Cousens et al., 1988; Edelstein, D'Agostino, et al., 2011; Jankovic et al., 1994; Jannoun, 1983; Kingma, Mooyaart, Kamps, Nieuwenhuizen, & Wilmink, 1993; Moss et al., 1981). Longer time since treatment is also associated with lower scores on intelligence and neuropsychological tests of speed and accuracy for survivors treated with CRT (Edelstein, D'Agostino, et al., 2011; Moore et al., 1991; Rubenstein et al., 1990). Some of the same moderators appear to be related to outcome for children treated with chemotherapy only. When an effect is found, it is usually in the same direction: Poorer outcomes are noted for girls and children who are younger at diagnosis and treatment (Buizer et al., 2009; Conklin et al., 2012). Time since diagnosis/treatment does not appear to moderate chemotherapy only treatment effects as it does for CRT (see Janzen & Spiegler, 2008 for review).

Because of the considerable variability in outcome for children treated with chemotherapy only, even after considering the known host and treatment factors, recent studies have investigated genetic polymorphisms and concepts such as brain and cognitive reserve as factors related to neuropsychological outcome. Genetic susceptibility to folate cycle dysfunction, which may be exaggerated by the antifolate MTX, has been suggested as a risk factor for chemotherapy-related neuropsychological deficits. That is, specific genetic polymorphisms may put children at more or less risk for poor neurocognitive outcome if it makes them more or less sensitive to the effects of particular chemotherapeutic agents. Krull and colleagues documented a relationship between folate pathway genetic polymorphisms and the development of attention and processing speed deficits after treatment for ALL in childhood (Kamdar et al., 2011; Krull et al., 2008). Children with specific 5,10-methylenetetrahydrofolatereductase (MTHFR) and methionine synthase (MS) polymorphisms scored more poorly on tests of attention and processing speed and the risk was greater in children who had more risk alleles in the folate pathway. This pattern was confirmed and extended in a more recent study in which children with a specific polymorphism in MS were more likely to show performance deficits in attention and response speed, while parent-reported attention problems were more common in children with a specific polymorphism in apolipoprotein E4 (Krull, Bhojwani, et al., 2013). As more is learned about genetic and epigenetic patterns in relation to neuropsychological outcomes in survivors of ALL, risk stratification may begin to incorporate individualized risk of neuropsychological and other late effects into personalized approaches to treatment.

Methotrexate-Related Neurotoxicity

Methotrexate is a core agent in the successful treatment of childhood leukemia. Intravenous and intrathecal routes of administration can be associated, in a minority of patients, with clinical neurological toxicities that are usually transient and reversible, but can be severe, and more rarely lead to coma and/or death (Tufekci et al., 2011). Toxicities can be acute (hours after administration), subacute (days to weeks after administration), or chronic (months to years after administration). Acute toxicity may present with symptoms such as headache, nausea, vomiting, dizziness, confusion, and somnolence. Seizures may also occur. Subacute toxicity may be characterized by a stroke-like syndrome (SLS) including aphasia, dysarthria, dysphagia, diplopia, hemiparesis, and hemisensory deficits. In one series, the clearest risk factor for SLS was concomitant administration of IV cyclophosphamide and cytarabine (ara-C) (Bond et al., 2013). Chronic toxicity is usually characterized by leukoencephalopathy and disturbances of higher cognitive function (Mahadeo, Dhall, Panigrahy, Lastra, & Ettinger, 2010).

Case reports have described acute chorea (Necioglu Orken et al., 2009) delirium, agitation and encephalopathy (Summers, Abramowsky, & Cooper, 2014), SLS with hemiparesis, dysarthria, and emotional lability (Brugnoletti et al., 2009), generalized tonic-clonic seizures followed by right hemiparesis, aphasia, altered mental status, persistent seizures, and progressive neurological deterioration (Mahadeo et al., 2010). Most patients recover completely and the clinical deficits most often do not recur after further administration of MTX (Bhojwani et al., 2014; Bond et al., 2013).

A characteristic imaging pattern, reflecting leukoencephalopathy (LE), consists of white matter hyperintensities on diffusion weighted and T2 weighted MR images (Figure 12.3). The longitudinal prevalence of LE is related to dose and number of MTX exposures (Bhojwani et al., 2014; Reddick, Glass, Helton, et al., 2005), and can reach up to 85% after seven courses of MTX (Reddick, Glass, Helton, et al., 2005). The prevalence of LE declined by about half when the patients were scanned at week 120 of therapy, about 1.5 years after the last MTX treatment (Reddick, Glass, Helton, et al., 2005). Although this constitutes a significant reduction over

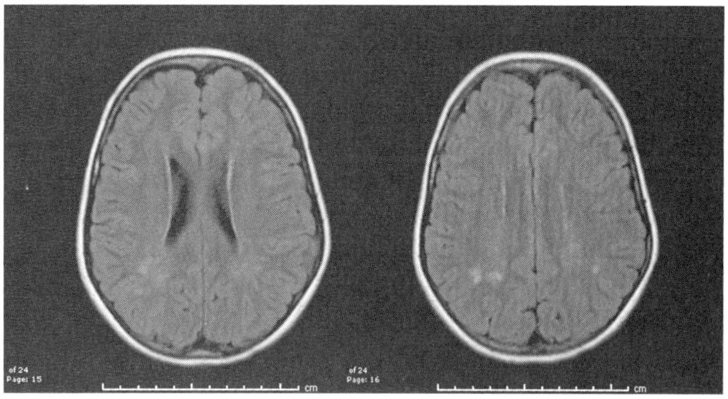

Figure 12.3 A 12-year-old male diagnosed age 2 years with ALL and treated with chemotherapy and radiation (18Gy); periventricular deep white matter changes

time, about 40% of patients continued to show LE at this time point and it is unknown whether further normalization occurs over time.

Posterior reversible encephalopathy syndrome (PRES) is an uncommon MTX-associated toxicity (Dicuonzo et al., 2009) characterized by headaches, seizures, and focal neurological signs. Altered mental status and visual disturbances are also reported (de Laat et al., 2011). High blood pressure precedes symptom onset and the syndrome is thought to be associated with dysregulation of the cerebral vasculature, endothelial damage, capillary leakage and vasogenic edema (Figure 12.4). Some studies find that clinical and radiological recovery is the norm (de Laat et al., 2011), although this is not universal (Lucchini et al., 2008; Morris, Laningham, Sandlund, & Khan, 2007). Morris et al. (2007) found the majority of their 11 patients with PRES had irreversible sequelae in the form of abnormal electroencephalogram (EEG) with or without clinical seizures or radiographic abnormalities. Neurological evaluation was normal in all cases. Long-term

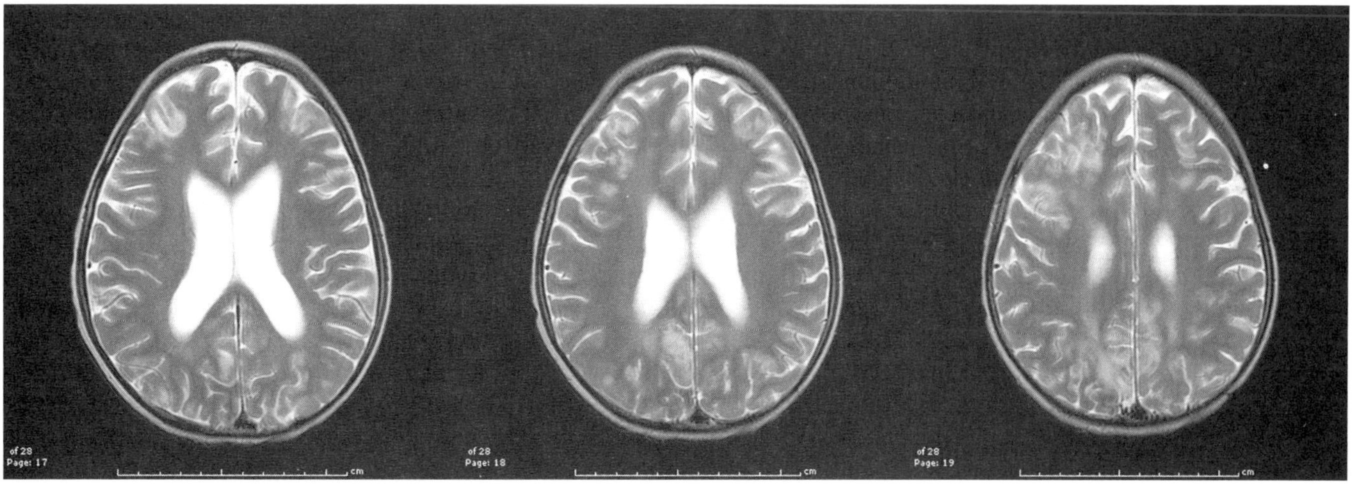

Figure 12.4 Posterior reversible encephalopathy syndrome in a 4-year-old female being treated for ALL with intrathecal chemotherapy and developed seizures. MRI shows scattered areas of signal abnormality in the subcortical white matter at the posterior temporal lobes bilaterally, inferior right frontal lobe and both cerebellar hemispheres (cerebellum not shown in these images).

neuropsychological, cognitive, or developmental outcomes have not been described.

Steroid Treatment

Corticosteroids are a mainstay of treatment for ALL; either dexamethasone or prednisone is incorporated into every modern chemotherapy protocol. During the weeks of active steroid treatment, behavioral and emotional changes are frequently reported by families. Children are described as more emotional and harder to control, and significant sleep problems are noted. In a prospective design, Pound and colleagues (2012) demonstrated higher rates of externalizing disorders as described by parents of children older than 5 who were receiving steroids during maintenance therapy for ALL. Treatment with dexamethasone was associated with greater behavioral impairment than treatment with prednisone (Pound et al., 2012).

With respect to neuropsychological outcomes, Kadan-Lottick et al. (2009) found no significant differences between survivors who had been randomized to receive dexamethasone versus prednisone. However, another research group found that adult survivors of ALL who had been treated with dexamethasone exhibited weaker memory performance on multiple tests, than those treated with prednisone (Edelmann et al., 2013).

Brain Tumors

Brain tumors are the second most common malignancy in childhood and the most common solid tumor. Survival rates have increased substantially over the past 20 years, although brain tumors continue to have the highest mortality of all childhood cancers (Ostrom et al., 2015). Overall five-year survival rates are 73.3% for children diagnosed between birth and 19 years; survival rates vary by tumor type and location: 95% for pilocytic astrocytoma, 65% for medulloblastoma and primitive neuroectodermal tumors, and 28.4% for high-grade glioma (Ostrom et al., 2015). Survival rates also vary by age group, with infants (< 1 year) having the lowest survival rates.

Risk factors for developing brain tumors in childhood include some genetic predisposition syndromes (e.g., Li-Fraumeni, Gorlin's syndrome, neurofibromatosis) and exposure to ionizing radiation (Hottinger & Khakoo, 2009; Preston-Martin, 1996). Other environmental risk factors (e.g., parental exposure to pesticides, advanced parental age, maternal intake of nitrosamines, maternal medications) have been investigated but research findings in these areas have been only suggestive or inconclusive (Grill & Owens, 2013; Johnson et al., 2014).

Brain tumors in children differ from adult onset disease in many respects. The brain is the primary site for intracranial malignancies in childhood, whereas for adults, brain tumors are more likely to be metastatic (originating in other primary sites in the context of melanoma, or cancer of lung, breast, colon, etc.). The same histological type of tumor can carry a very different prognosis and respond to a different treatment depending on whether it occurs in the child or adult setting. Overall, survival rates for pediatric brain tumors are much more favorable than for adult-onset tumors. These findings support the notion that the childhood brain functions very differently with respect to brain tumor biology due to factors affecting the unique microcellular environment of the developing brain. It may be that in the near future, childhood brain tumors will be classified in a different manner than adult neoplasms, incorporating biologic, molecular genetic, and brain maturation factors, not just histology and location. Advances in developmental neuroscience and in the understanding of brain development in childhood are contributing to a more nuanced appreciation of why certain brain tumors emerge at different periods in development and how factors that regulate the sculpting of the brain contribute to tumorigenesis. Furthermore, concepts of selective vulnerability and plasticity are critical in evaluating the emergence and impact of brain insult at different epochs in development and in predicting late effects.

Treatment Protocols

Treatment for pediatric brain tumors varies by age, type of tumor, and location. Surgery is the first-line intervention in most cases if the tumor is in a resectable location; in general, extent of resection is a valuable prognostic indicator for event-free survival. Childhood brain tumors are often associated with hydrocephalus due to blockage of circulation of cerebral spinal fluid at the level of the third ventricle for sellar/suprasellar tumors and the fourth ventricle for posterior fossa tumors. Resection of the tumor can often treat the hydrocephalus but in some instances other procedures are needed such as placement of an external ventricular drain before surgery, ventriculostomy, or ventricular-peritoneal shunt.

Radiation therapy is required in the context of malignant tumors, incomplete resection, or progression. Radiation is avoided in very young children and in tumors associated with neurofibromatosis-1 as this is associated with unacceptable neuropsychological compromise in the former and with increased risk of second tumors or cerebrovascular abnormalities in the latter. Advances in radiation therapy include proton beam therapy that avoids the exit dose to normal brain tissue, thus sparing or lowering the dose to vital structures such as the medial temporal lobe, cochlea, and hypothalamus (Greenberger et al., 2014; MacDonald et al., 2008).

Chemotherapy has become an important tool in the management of childhood brain tumors, allowing for reduction of radiation dose and for targeting unique aspects of certain tumors. Chemotherapy regimens vary as a function of type of tumor. Cytotoxic chemotherapy was incorporated into treatment protocols and found to be effective for medulloblastoma and low-grade gliomas. Currently, innovative and targeted therapies are being studied in clinical trials and used in treatment protocols; these include agents targeting angiogenesis (Kieran, 2005), immune response (Pollack, Jakacki, Butterfield, & Okada, 2013), and tumor-signaling pathways (Gerber et al., 2014; Nageswara Rao & Packer, 2012). The long-term effects of these therapies is as yet unknown and the basis of these treatments center on interrupting biologic mechanisms that may also support essential brain developmental processes. Consequently, monitoring of neuropsychological outcomes and late effects will need to be included in the ongoing study of these therapies.

Risk Factors in Neuropsychological Outcomes

Children treated for brain tumors are at substantial risk for developing cognitive, academic, adaptive, and psychosocial impairments. For children treated with craniospinal radiation, particularly at a younger age, progressive decline in abilities occurs (Palmer et al., 2003; Palmer et al., 2001; Ris, Packer, Goldwein, Jones-Wallace, & Boyett, 2001). Contributing factors are multiple and interrelated, and have ongoing impact across development (Reimers et al., 2003). These factors include tissue damage related to location, brain response to injury, radiation field and intensity, surgical complications, hydrocephalus, and chemotherapy treatments. Direct impact of endocrine and motor/sensory deficits related to the tumor and its treatment can also compromise neuropsychological function. Host factors—such as age at diagnosis, time since treatment, psychosocial and family circumstances, socioeconomic status, and specific genetic vulnerabilities—are also critical variables. An individualized approach to understanding the role and relationships among these factors is needed in the long-term management of these children.

Advances in surgical techniques have the potential to improve long-term neuropsychological outcomes; MRI-guided surgery allows for more complete resections and can limit possible neurological injury (Choudhri, Klimo, Auschwitz, Whitehead, & Boop, 2014). Surgical sequelae remain challenging and these include perioperative stroke, neurological deficits, changes in physical appearance, and damage to pituitary/hypothalamic structures. Posterior fossa syndrome (PFS), also referred to as *cerebellar mutism,* is a complication of posterior fossa surgery that occurs more commonly in children than adults. The incidence reported in the literature varies, but clusters in the range of 25% following resection of posterior fossa tumors in children (Pollack, 1997; Robertson et al., 2006). Symptoms develop 12 to 48 hours after surgery and can include mutism or limited speech, dysarthria, ataxia, emotional lability, and personality changes. Cranial nerve deficits are also commonly seen. Treatment in a rehabilitation hospital is often needed to address speech/language, motor, and emotional dysfunction. PFS used to be referred to as a "transient" complication since symptoms improve over time; however, long-term neurobehavioral sequelae persist. Impact on speech fluency and processing speed tends to be long lasting (Huber, Bradley, Spiegler, & Dennis, 2006). With respect to etiology, PFS appears to have increased in frequency over recent years and has been associated with more extensive tumor resection (Pitsika & Tsitouras, 2013). Various theories have been proposed related to the etiology of PFS: disruption of cerebellar (dentate nuclei)-thalamo-cortical pathways, incision/splitting of cerebellar vermis, and brain stem involvement are implicated as risk factors (Law et al., 2012; Pitsika & Tsitouras, 2013; Reed-Berendt et al., 2014). From a neuropsychological perspective, children who have PFS require ongoing follow-up and intervention. Persistent difficulties in speed of processing and production compromise functioning in academic, social, and emotional domains. In neuropsychological outcome studies of children treated for medulloblastoma, those who had PFS consistently demonstrate poorer performance (Knight et al., 2014; Palmer et al., 2010).

Hydrocephalus is a significant risk factor for compromise in neuropsychological functioning. Many brain tumors are associated with symptoms of increased intracranial pressure related to obstruction of cerebral spinal fluid flow. Cognitive and motor/sensory complications can ensue, often secondary to damage to periventricular white matter pathways. In a group of children with ependymoma, hydrocephalus at diagnosis was associated with increased risk of neuropsychological deficits, even after the effects of the tumor and treatment were accounted for (von Hoff et al., 2008). In a study of medical complications in children treated for posterior fossa tumors (cerebellar astrocytoma and medulloblastoma), Roncadin et al. (2008) noted that medical complications, such as increased intracranial pressure, affect long-term outcome, even in children who do not require additional tumor-directed treatment after surgery.

Radiation therapy is an essential modality of treatment for many pediatric brain tumors and doses are much higher in this context than for prophylactic treatment in ALL. For malignant embryonal tumors such as medulloblastoma, standard protocols include 24.3 Gy craniospinal to control disease across the neuroaxis, with a focal boost to the posterior fossa up to 54 Gy. Younger age at treatment is a critical risk factor for more severe neuropsychological late effects that can manifest years after treatment. Other important factors include dose, field, and critical brain structures involved. Radiation dose above the range of 20 Gy is likely to cause late effects in children (Thorp & Taylor, 2014): These include neuropsychological deficits, endocrine dysfunction including compromised fertility, hearing loss (particularly in the context of platinum-based chemotherapy agents), vision problems (cataracts), bone growth issues, vasculopathies, and increased risk of second malignancies (Fossati, Ricardi, & Orecchia, 2009; Shih, Loeffler, & Tarbell, 2009).

The pathophysiology of neuropsychological late effects after CRT in children treated for brain tumors is related to the increased vulnerability of rapidly developing brain processes to toxicity. CRT can disrupt the blood-brain barrier through damage to cerebral vascular endothelium, selectively injure oligodendrocyte progenitor cells critical for myelination, and affect the microcellular environment that supports neurogenesis in the hippocampal region (Dietrich, Monje, Wefel, & Meyers, 2008; Gibson & Monje, 2012). Consequently, psychological processes such as working memory, processing speed, and attention, are commonly affected in children treated with CRT for brain tumors and contribute to declines in ability over time (Mabbott, Penkman, Witol, Strother, & Bouffet, 2008). Decline in intellectual ability is related to failure to acquire new skills at the expected rate for age, rather than loss of skills or developmental regression (Palmer, 2008). Studies have documented decreased volume of white matter in survivors of childhood brain tumors that is correlated with reduced neuropsychological function (Merchant, Kiehna, Li, Xiong, & Mulhern, 2005; Reddick, Glass, Palmer, et al., 2005; Reddick et al., 2006b; Reddick et al., 2003a; Reddick et al., 2003b). Processing speed is particularly vulnerable in children treated for brain tumors. In a prospective study that examined change in these processes over time, scores on processing speed tests declined following treatment for medulloblastoma with surgery, CRT, and chemotherapy (Palmer et al., 2013). Younger age at diagnosis, more intensive treatment and higher radiation dose due to high-risk disease, and higher baseline scores contributed to a steeper decline in processing speed. Similar findings were found for working memory and broad attention, but processing speed scores were the lowest. These same factors (younger age at diagnosis and higher intensity treatment) are associated with reduced white matter volume relative to peers; the discrepancy in white matter volume as compared to peers increases over time (Reddick et al., 2014).

Chemotherapy has become increasingly useful in the treatment of childhood brain tumors. It is an important component of protocols for malignant embryonal tumors, for young children, and for low-grade glioma. The late effects of chemotherapy in the treatment of brain tumors need to be considered in the context of other factors such as type and location of tumor, complications, and combination with other therapies. Various types of chemotherapy agents are used in the treatment of brain tumors that have different side-effect and long-term risk profiles (Gururangan, 2009). As described on p. 160, antimetabolites such as MTX affect white matter integrity. Vinca alkaloids (vincristine) can cause peripheral neuropathy that can persist after treatment. Sensorineural hearing loss is associated with the use of platinum-based agents such as carboplatin and cisplatin. CRT exacerbates the risk of hearing loss, which needs to be monitored periodically over time as the loss can be progressive and does not necessarily emerge during or immediately after treatment. The late effects of newer chemotherapy treatments on the developing child are as yet unknown.

Types of Brain Tumors and Neuropsychological Outcomes

Low-grade glioma

Low-grade gliomas are common brain tumors in childhood; they vary in histology and location. Pilocytic astrocytoma is the most frequently diagnosed pediatric low-grade glioma, often occurring in the cerebellum (Figure 12.5) (Bergthold et al., 2014). Survival rates are very high: A recent review of outcomes from 1973 to 2008 demonstrated a long-term (20 year) survival rate of 87% (Bandopadhayay et al., 2014). Surgery, if possible, is the primary treatment and often the only treatment needed. For tumors in the optic pathway, hypothalamus, or brain stem, surgery may not be an option or be incomplete due to risk of neurological complications. Chemotherapy is often used to treat progression seen on imaging or exacerbation of symptoms. Despite excellent survival and more limited use of CRT in this population, neurobehavioral outcomes can be compromised due to effects of the tumor and treatment. In a study of survivors of low-grade gliomas treated with surgery only, medical late effects were common. Overall intellectual ability for this cohort is generally in the average range, though investigators find that a larger proportion of the group performs in the below average range on measures of intelligence, executive function,

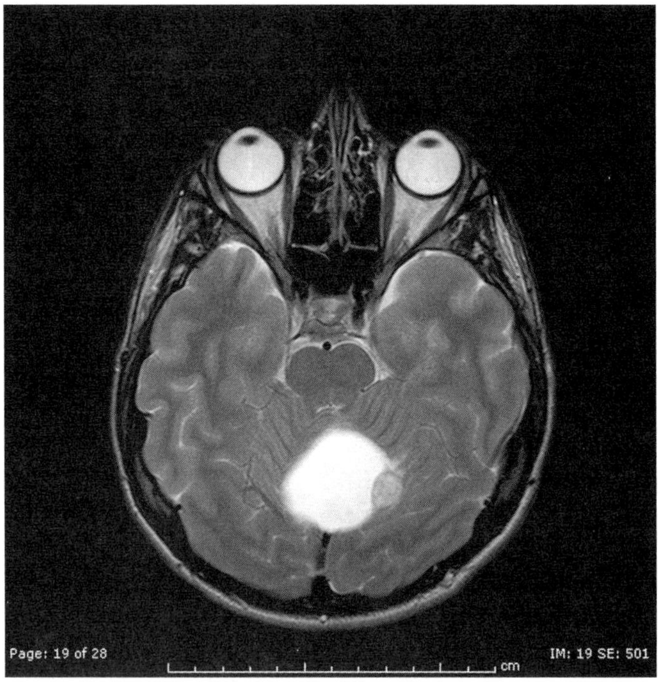

Figure 12.5 Juvenile pilocytic astrocytoma in the cerebellum: T2-weighted MRI shows astrocytoma in cerebellum with cystic and solid components

and adaptive skills (Beebe & Ris, 2001; Ris et al., 2008; Turner et al., 2009). In this group with normal intelligence, compromise in executive function had a greater impact on overall adaptive skills and level of independence than intellectual ability.

Craniopharyngioma

Craniopharyngioma is a relatively rare tumor of the sellar/suprasellar region that accounts for 4% of brain tumors in children less than 14 years of age (Ostrom et al., 2015). It arises from remnants of Rathke's pouch, from which the pituitary develops in embryological development. Though technically a benign tumor, it often recurs and its location near to and invasion of critical brain structures such as the optic nerves and chiasm, hypothalamus, pituitary, and vascular structures of the circle of Willis contribute to its significant morbidity (Figure 12.6). Although survival rates are high, neuropsychological, psychosocial, and medical late effects significantly compromise quality of life (Lo et al., 2014). There is considerable controversy regarding treatment strategies for craniopharyngioma; extent of surgical resection is associated with risk of recurrence, though more aggressive surgery is believed to cause more extensive damage to the hypothalamic-pituitary-axis (Müller, 2014; Zygourakis et al., 2014). Radiation therapy is used in the context of incomplete resection and progression. Studies from St. Jude Children's Research Hospital note more favorable outcomes with respect to intellectual ability in those treated with more limited surgery plus radiation as compared to gross total resection (Merchant et al., 2002). Children diagnosed with craniopharyngioma often present with headaches as well as evidence of neuroendocrine dysfunction and vision changes (Müller, 2014; Ullrich, Scott, & Pomeroy, 2005). Endocrine dysfunction continues postsurgery and most survivors have pituitary hormone deficiencies (diabetes insipidus, hypothyroidism, adrenal insufficiency, growth hormone deficiency, and sex hormone deficiency). Hypothalamic dysfunction causes obesity, daytime sleepiness, sleep disturbance, circadian rhythm irregularities, and problems regulating body temperature. Visual acuity as well as visual fields can be affected due to the pressure effects of the tumor and hydrocephalus, or surgical damage to the optic pathway or vascular supply (Ullrich et al., 2005). Specific neurobehavioral sequelae are seen in memory, executive function (initiation, inhibitory control, organization), and emotional regulation (Carpentieri et al., 2001; Ullrich et al., 2005; Waber et al., 2006). Memory problems affect the child's ability to encode and retrieve material as well as to track everyday activities and are likely a consequence of disturbance in limbic pathways secondary to the tumor and surgery. The combination of complex medical issues and neuropsychological dysfunction contributes to adverse quality of life despite generally average intellectual ability. Hypothalamic obesity is a significant health and psychosocial problem. Survivors of cranipharyngioma can have symptoms similar to Prader-Willi syndrome, with unremitting food-seeking behaviors and limited regulation of affect and aggression. In severe cases, specialized residential programming can be required. A recent systematic review of psychological and social outcomes found a high incidence of school problems, emotional and behavioral difficulties, and social isolation in survivors of pediatric craniopharyngioma (Zada, Kintz, Pulido, & Amezcua, 2013).

Medulloblastoma

Medulloblastoma is a malignant embryonal tumor that occurs in the cerebellum (Figure 12.7). It can occur at all ages in childhood and is rarely seen in adults; the incidence is highest between the ages of 4 and 7 years. Since it has the propensity to disseminate across the neuroaxis, multimodality treatment including surgery, CRT, and chemotherapy is

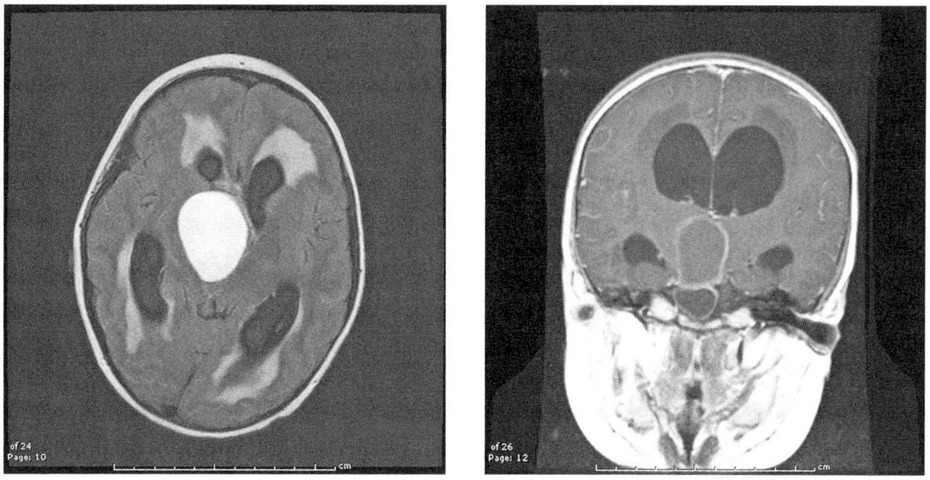

Figure 12.6 Craniopharyngioma: MRI shows tumor in region of third ventricle and evidence of transependymal flow secondary to obstructive hydrocephalus (image 1); dilated ventricles (image 2)

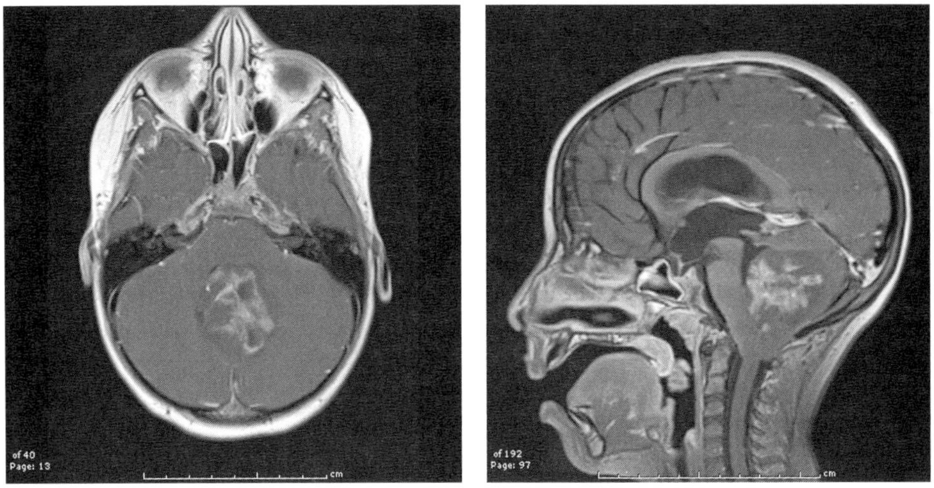

Figure 12.7 Medulloblastoma: MRI shows large, enhancing midline cerebellar tumor (image 1) and tumor obstructing fourth ventricle and associated obstructive hydrocephalus (image 2)

given in most cases. Presenting symptoms often are related to increased intracranial pressure due to hydrocephalus or signs of cerebellar dysfunction. Surgical resection and management of hydrocephalus are the first steps in treatment. Children with medulloblastoma have been traditionally classified into standard or high risk based on clinical factors such as age at diagnosis, degree of dissemination/metastasis, and extent of residual disease postsurgery. Advances in molecular biology now demonstrate that medulloblastoma is a much more heterogeneous disease than previously thought. Gene expression patterns are now used to distinguish four different subgroups, each having different profiles of incidence in specific groups, neurodevelopmental origin, response to treatment, and clinical implications (Gibson et al., 2010; Northcott, Korshunov, Pfister, & Taylor, 2012; Northcott et al., 2011; Taylor et al., 2012). Based on these stratification variables, future treatment protocols will be able to treat specific subgroups with less intense regimens that will reduce toxicity and late effects. In addition, targeted therapies can be developed based on gene expression and signaling pathways.

Survival rates for standard-risk medulloblastoma are now quite high but late effects compromising health status and neuropsychological and adaptive function are common. Tumor location in the cerebellum is an important factor given the now-accepted notion that the cerebellum is critically involved in cognitive as well as motor function in the brain. Associated hydrocephalus and other complications as well as high-dose CRT are associated with adverse neuropsychological outcomes. Studies consistently demonstrate a decline in IQ over time, and this decline is more pronounced in survivors who were younger at diagnosis and who had higher functioning at baseline; decline in IQ is estimated at 2 to 4 points per year (Palmer et al., 2001; Ris et al., 2001; Spiegler et al., 2006). This pattern of decline in intellectual and academic abilities is seen even when CRT dose is reduced (Ris et al., 2013).

Working memory, attention, and processing speed are believed to be core deficits in children treated for medulloblastoma that in turn compromise neuropsychological and academic progress over time (Mabbott et al., 2008; Palmer et al., 2013). In our clinical experience, children, adolescents, and young adults treated for medulloblastoma often encounter difficulties with higher-order integrative skills that emerge over time, even in the context of normal intellectual ability. Progressive decline in abilities is presumed to be related to volume reductions in white matter (Palmer, 2008) and in the hippocampus (Nagel et al., 2004). Recent studies using diffusion tensor imaging reveal damage to cerebro-cerebellar pathways in children treated for medulloblastoma (Law et al., 2015), as well as reductions in fractional anisotropy associated with decreased intellectual ability (Khong et al., 2006; Mabbott, Noseworthy, Bouffet, Rockel, & Laughlin, 2006; Rueckriegel et al., 2010). These findings support the notion that children treated for medulloblastoma have an evolving brain injury that affects development in a dynamic and interactive way throughout development.

Adult Outcomes, Cognitive Reserve, and Early Aging in Childhood Cancer Survivors

There were 388,501 survivors of childhood cancer alive in the United States as of 2011 and this number is expected to increase in coming years (Phillips et al., 2015). Survival into adulthood is now the expectation. In 2011 there were more than twice as many adult survivors of childhood CNS cancer than ALL in the over-40 age group; however, the number of ALL survivors is expected to increase substantially as current childhood/young adult survivors move into later adulthood. The quality of adult survivorship is an area of active research efforts with findings that are relevant for adult and pediatric neuropsychology practice. The Childhood Cancer Survivor Study (CCSS) is an important resource for understanding adult outcomes of childhood cancers. The study uses periodic surveys to track the outcomes of approximately 14,000 participants treated for childhood cancer between 1970 and 1986, comparing findings to sibling controls (Robison et al., 2005; Robison et al., 2002). Participants were recruited from cancer centers across North America and represent a geographically and socioeconomically diverse cohort. The CCSS is a rich source of information regarding the long-term quality of life, health, and social outcomes of survivors. In general, adult survivors of childhood cancer are more likely to have chronic health-related problems and the prevalence of these problems increases with age (Hudson et al., 2015; Oeffinger et al., 2006). Adverse health outcomes experienced by childhood cancer survivors include increased risk of infertility (Barton et al., 2013), physical performance limitations (Rueegg et al., 2012), endocrine and cardiovascular problems (Gurney et al., 2003), higher hospitalization rates (Kurt et al., 2011), and pulmonary complications (Huang et al., 2014). Additionally, the risk of second neoplasms is substantially higher in survivors of childhood cancer compared to siblings; those treated with radiation, treated in an earlier era, of female sex, and with diagnosis of Hodgkin lymphoma were more likely to develop a subsequent malignancy (Friedman et al., 2010).

In most of these adult outcome studies, survivors treated with CRT were more likely to experience adverse health and quality of life outcomes (Armstrong, Stovall, & Robison, 2010), including stroke and sensory-motor impairments (Bowers et al., 2006; Packer et al., 2003). A dose-dependent relationship exists between risk of stroke in adulthood and prior treatment with CRT (Mueller et al., 2013).

Psychosocial and adaptive outcomes are notable for increased likelihood of special education, lower employment status, and decreased rate of marriage and college attendance; these outcomes were more common in survivors with cancers or treatment affecting the CNS (Gurney et al., 2009). Employment limitations (likelihood of lower-skill occupations) were more likely in survivors who were Black, of younger age at diagnosis, or treated with high-dose CRT (Kirchhoff et al., 2011).

The CCSS provides valuable insights into the life span outcomes of childhood cancer survivors. The outcomes of children currently undergoing treatment for ALL and CNS tumors may be moderated somewhat given the marked changes and refinements in treatment protocols that are now being used. Nevertheless, the combined impact of CNS-directed treatment and chronic health conditions will continue to affect long-term adult outcomes and we need to be increasingly concerned with how survivors navigate the developmental challenges of later adulthood (Ris & Hisock, 2013).

Cognitive reserve represents the idea that an individual's ability to cope with brain injury of any type is related to genetic, environmental, and/or experiential factors that can mediate brain or cognitive resources. A person with higher cognitive reserve can theoretically maintain better cognitive function than a person with lower cognitive reserve, after sustaining a comparable degree of brain injury (Stern, 2009). Kesler et al. (2010) explored the concept of cognitive reserve, as indexed by maternal education, as a moderator of outcome in children treated for ALL with chemotherapy only. Their index of cognitive reserve was directly related to cognitive performance on tests of verbal learning and working memory for ALL survivors. Furthermore, as predicted, cognitive reserve was inversely related to brain white matter volume of ALL survivors, suggesting that children with higher cognitive reserve could withstand more WM damage before exhibiting cognitive changes.

Another way to think about the contribution of cognitive reserve in this population is to study outcome in children treated for ALL who come into their diagnosis with premorbid developmental vulnerabilities, another expression of reduced cognitive reserve. Children with preexisting developmental vulnerabilities comprise up to 25% of new ALL diagnoses (Janzen et al., 2015) yet are systematically excluded from neuropsychological outcome studies. A recent study of children with Down syndrome (DS) who were also survivors of ALL documented a pattern of deficits in multiple neuropsychological domains and in overall adaptive function, in comparison to children with DS who had not been treated for cancer (Roncadin et al., 2014).

Recently, several studies of 20–25 year outcomes have been published, comparing adult survivors treated for ALL in childhood with CRT to those treated with chemotherapy only. Without exception, adults treated with CRT in childhood fare more poorly on a variety of measures than those treated with chemotherapy. Among nearly 2,000 adult survivors of ALL in the CCSS, self-reported neurocognitive function was worse than sibling controls on measures of task efficiency, memory, and emotional regulation for the subgroup that had been treated with CRT. Higher dose of CRT (>18 Gy) was associated with greater risk of impairment than lower dose (Kadan-Lottick et al., 2010).

Similar findings are seen for the 2,000 survivors of CNS tumors in the CCSS cohort who consistently reported more problems in neurocognitive function than survivors of other types of childhood cancer. Impairments in neurocognitive functioning were correlated with CRT dose; impairments in memory were associated with higher CRT dose to the temporal brain regions, with CRT to the frontal regions associated with more health problems and physical disabilities (Armstrong et al., 2010). The types of neuropsychological problems noted in adult survivors that affect working memory and information processing (Ellenberg et al., 2009) mirror the cognitive difficulties associated with aging.

The concept of accelerated aging was framed in the context of biological and cognitive reserve by Dennis, Spiegler, and Hetherington (2000). This concept is now being discussed in the context of adult survivors of childhood cancer (Armstrong, 2013). Data supporting accelerated aging have been reported for adult survivors of ALL treated with CRT in childhood who have now reached middle adulthood (Schuitema et al., 2013). Changes in spectral power on MEG imaging that are characteristic of the aging brain were demonstrated in adult survivors of ALL treated with CRT in childhood, but not in survivors treated with chemotherapy only (Daams et al., 2012). The documented pattern of change in white matter integrity (decreased fractional anisotropy-FA) with increasing age in ALL survivors 25 years after treatment with CRT mimics aging in its pattern and progression. However, the rate of decline was accelerated when compared to healthy controls. Lower FA was correlated with both cumulative radiation dose and younger age at treatment. Lower FA was also correlated with performance on tests of visual-motor function on a computerized test battery. In contrast, survivors treated with chemotherapy only did not show the pattern of white matter changes characteristic of accelerated aging.

Early aging was also suggested by the high rate of impairment in a range of neuropsychological outcome measures in another group of ALL survivors a mean of 25 years post-diagnosis. Increasing risk of impaired executive function was associated with longer time from diagnosis. Compared to a group of survivors treated with chemotherapy only, patients treated with 24 Gy CRT were at six times the risk for impaired executive function after 45 years (Krull, Brinkman, et al., 2013).

Perhaps of most concern is the finding that adult survivors of ALL who were treated with 24 Gy CRT and tested in their early 40s, with a median time since treatment of 30 years, demonstrated very high rates of immediate and delayed memory impairment. The mean performance on a test of delayed story memory was comparable to population expectations for adults over the age of 69! On tests of word pair recall and visual reproduction, performance was comparable to expectations for the 55–64 year old group in the general population. Early onset of delayed memory impairment but without functional impairment (employment rates did not differ among the groups) is suggestive of mild cognitive impairment and may reflect the reduced cognitive reserve induced by CRT in childhood. In support of this argument is the finding that the group of survivors with memory impairment also showed changes on structural and functional imaging in patterns similar to that seen in older adults with mild cognitive impairment (Armstrong et al., 2013).

Adult survivors of childhood brain tumors are at increased risk of a number of late effects, many of which compromise neurological and neuropsychological function. Long-term follow-up studies continue to clarify the quality of survival for these patients. Similar to research with the CCSS, findings from European studies of survivors of childhood brain tumors reveal lower educational achievement, more restricted employment opportunities, lower income, and lower likelihood of living independently (Boman, Lindblad, & Hjern, 2010; Koch et al., 2006; Kuehni et al., 2012). Marriage, employment, income level, participation in physical activities, and social engagement are all protective factors relative to quality of life and decline in older adults; survivors of childhood brain tumors may be at increased risk of early aging due to multiple sources of reduced brain and cognitive reserve.

Signs of early aging are seen in adult survivors of medulloblastoma in declining working memory performance over time (Edelstein, Spiegler, et al., 2011). Ris and colleagues (Ris, 2014) are currently studying adult outcomes of survivors of childhood low-grade gliomas in a multisite study using the CCSS cohort (NIH/NCI R01 CA132899–01). Preliminary findings reveal more survivors relative to controls with more limited education and at the lower extremes of income, particularly for those treated with surgery and CRT. Motor, sensory, and neurological impairments were more common in the brain tumor survivor group as compared to a sibling control group. With respect to neuropsychological outcomes, the proportion of survivors scoring below the expected range was much higher than expected on measures sensitive to the effects of aging and in attention. The goal of this study is to identify factors that contribute to accelerated cognitive aging in this population and the role of cognitive reserve in mitigating cognitive decline.

A proportion of emerging adult survivors of brain tumors may have significant compromise of cognitive, physical, and social skills. Consequently, degree of independence with respect to major financial, social, and medical decision making needs to be assessed in order to provide optimal care and guidance to patients and their families and health care providers. Neuropsychologists play a unique role in the care team at this time of developmental transition.

Special Issues

Adolescence/Young Adulthood

When an adolescent or young adult (AYA) is diagnosed with cancer, an entirely different set of treatment, adaptive, and psychosocial challenges require individualized management that recognizes the unique needs of this population as they transition to adulthood. During this phase of "emerging adulthood," promoting a sense of normalcy is crucial to health-related quality of life. Developmental challenges at this stage involve enhancing and increasing social and financial autonomy, increasing independence from parents, developing personal and unique values and identity, focusing on peer relationships—including intimate and sexual relationships—and preparing to join the workforce. Optimal care requires flexibility on the part of the care team, because dealing with illness and following through with treatment regimens can be challenging (Windebank & Spinetta, 2008). The team must develop sensitivity to the unique developmental needs of the AYA population; they must learn to provide information in a respectful and open manner, openly address issues of sexuality and fertility, and address academic, vocational, and financial concerns (D'Agostino, Penney, & Zebrack, 2011).

The survival rates for the AYA population continue to lag behind younger children for several reasons. The psychosocial and biological changes that are characteristic of the AYA population contribute to delays in diagnosis and also relate to the types of cancer seen and treatment outcomes. Presenting symptoms may be difficult to distinguish from normal maturational changes at this time. Once diagnosed, patients in this age group are less likely to participate in clinical trials, which can limit advances in knowledge and treatment outcomes (Ferrari, Montello, Budd, & Bleyer, 2008). Treatment compliance can suffer when the AYA patient is not under the full-time care of a parent; managing issues of independence and complex treatment protocols can be challenging. Longer-term longitudinal studies are often not undertaken and lack of coordination from pediatric to adult health care can contribute to poor continuity in follow-up and management. Because the types of cancer most commonly diagnosed in the AYA population differ from both the pediatric and the older adult population, different treatments and clinical trial recruitment strategies are required if survival rates are to improve (Burke, Albritton, & Marina, 2007).

For the AYA patient diagnosed with ALL, poorer outcomes are likely due to a combination of biological factors (higher incidence of Philadelphia chromosome, higher incidence of high risk (T-cell) ALL), treatment with adult rather than pediatric-like regimens, and poorer compliance with treatment (Figure 12.8) (Pui et al., 2011; Pui & Howard, 2008).

In the AYA age group, both brain tumor location and histology differ from younger children: Embryonal tumors become much less common, and pituitary and germ cell tumors increase in frequency, suggesting that processes associated with puberty have an impact on the brain environment and tumorigenesis such that different biological mechanisms are involved (Bleyer et al., 2008). Outcomes for the same tumor type can vary whether it is diagnosed in adolescence or early adulthood; for example, prognosis for low-grade gliomas varies by age, and adolescents are more likely to respond to chemotherapy regimens that may not be as effective in adulthood.

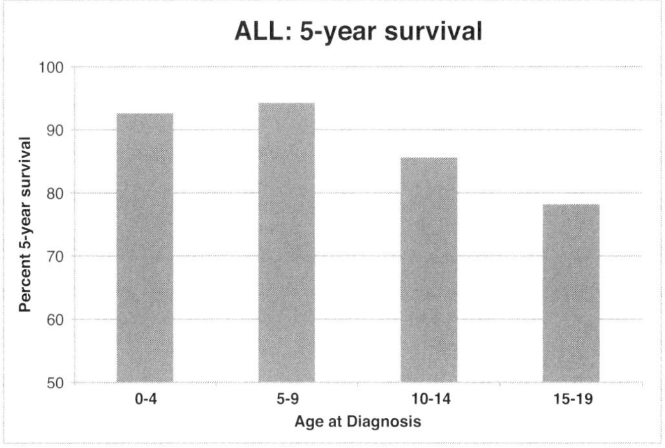

Figure 12.8 5 Year survival Rrates for ALL and age at diagnosis

Opsoclonus Myoclonus Ataxia Syndrome

Opsoclonus myoclonus ataxia syndrome (OMA) is a rare autoimmune disorder that occurs as a paraneoplastic phenomenon in a small proportion (2%–3%) of children diagnosed with neuroblastoma (Hayward et al., 2001; Mitchell et al., 2002; Rudnick et al., 2001). The mechanism is thought to be cross-reactive autoimmunity between neuroblastoma cells and nervous system cells, particularly affecting cells in the cerebellum. Children with neuroblastoma and OMA generally have lower-stage disease and excellent outcomes of their cancer diagnosis (Russo, Cohn, Petruzzi, & de Alarcon, 1997). This may be explained by the hypothesis that higher autoimmune response limits tumor growth, and thus is associated with lower-stage disease. This higher autoimmune response then also attacks healthy neurons, leading to OMA.

Presentation

Children often present with symptoms of OMA before the diagnosis of neuroblastoma is made. Presentation is characterized by a unique constellation of neurological, cognitive, and behavioral features. Neurological symptoms include involuntary conjugate eye movements (opsoclonus), ataxia, and involuntary jerking of limbs and trunk (myoclonus). Sleep disturbance is common, with more than 90% of parents reporting sleep disturbance in their children with OMA (Pranzatelli et al., 2005). Cognitive or neuropsychological features include regression and impairments in speech and language, attention, and fine and gross motor skills. Behavior often becomes highly disruptive, with irritability, aggression, and rage attacks quite unlike the child's premorbid personality (Pranzatelli et al., 2005; Turkel, Brumm, Mitchell, & Tavare, 2006). Children are described as inconsolable, aggressive (biting, kicking, hair pulling, head banging) and set off by minor frustrations, not getting their way, trivial provocations, or no apparent reason. These episodes are easily distinguished from normal tantrums by severity and duration, with rage attacks lasting from 20 minutes to several hours. They are more frequent in children with disrupted sleep. These marked changes in sleep and behavior can be especially distressing and difficult to manage. Treatment with trazodone improved sleep and behavior in 95% of those treated, with a 72% increase in total sleep time and a 33% reduction in rage attacks (Pranzatelli et al., 2005).

Treatment

Treatment is aimed at reducing autoimmune reactivity, and commonly involves oral corticosteroids, adrenocorticotropic hormone, intravenous immunoglobulin, chemotherapy, or some combination of these. More recently, rituximab (anti-CD20 monoclonal antibody) has shown promising preliminary efficacy (Brunklaus, Pohl, Zuberi, & de Sousa, 2011). Children often require treatment for months to years as most tend to relapse with attempts to wean treatment or as a function of intercurrent infection.

Long-term outcome

Unlike the neuropsychological late effects associated with treatment for pediatric cancers, OMA is associated with long-term speech and language impairment and behavioral disorders, as well as significant cognitive deficits (Mitchell et al., 2002). The neurological symptoms of OMA (opsoclonus, myoclonus, and ataxia) tend to respond to treatment and improve slowly over time, but other symptoms are long-lasting, even if small improvements are achieved (Catsman-Berrevoets et al., 2009; Mitchell et al., 2005; Russo et al., 1997). General cognitive development can remain well below average, often in the borderline range (Brunklaus et al., 2011; Catsman-Berrevoets et al., 2009; Mitchell et al., 2002; Papero, 1995; Turkel, 2006). Speech impairment is characterized by low intelligibility associated with motor features of oral, phonatory, and respiratory incoordination (Brunklaus et al., 2011; Catsman-Berrevoets et al., 2009; Mitchell et al., 2002; Papero et al., 1995). Expressive language is generally more impaired than receptive language (De Grandis et al., 2009; Papero et al., 1995). Psychiatric and behavioral features persist in about 70% of cases (De Grandis et al., 2009) with attention deficit, irritability, dysphoric mood, and poor affective regulation (Brunklaus et al., 2011; Catsman-Berrevoets et al., 2009; Mitchell et al., 2002; Turkel et al., 2006). Quality of life estimates from parents reveal impairments in autonomy, and cognitive and social function. This pattern of neurobehavioral symptoms may represent an extreme example of cerebellar cognitive affective syndrome (Schmahmann & Sherman, 1998).

Prognosis

The most consistent prognostic feature is course of illness. A minority of patients have a monophasic course (they can be tapered from treatment without relapse) and these children tend to have a better cognitive outcome than those who have multiple relapses (Brunklaus et al., 2011; De Grandis et al., 2009; Klein, Schmitt, & Boltshauser, 2007). Although numbers are small, Mitchell et al. (2005) showed that the majority of children with a monophasic course can achieve normal range performance on cognitive, behavioral, and adaptive measures.

Children with initially more severe OMA symptoms tended to have a chronic relapsing course more often than those with mild initial symptoms which, in turn, predict cognitive problems in the long term (Brunklaus et al., 2011). Treatment type or length was not associated with differences in cognitive, adaptive, or motor outcome (Catsman-Berrevoets et al., 2009; Mitchell et al., 2002). When followed over a period of years, it appears that small improvements can be documented (Brunklaus et al., 2011; Mitchell et al., 2005); in any event, the prognosis is not one of progressive deterioration. Longer length of follow-up has been associated with better outcomes (Hayward et al., 2001), another piece of evidence that the condition tends to slowly improve over time. One study suggested that younger children improve more than older children (Mitchell et al., 2005) while another showed that children who were younger at diagnosis and had more severe initial symptoms were more likely to have cognitive problems in the long run (Brunklaus et al., 2011). Russo et al. (1997) did not find an association between age at diagnosis and outcome or persistence of symptoms.

Time between symptom onset and diagnosis/treatment, or *diagnostic delay,* has been explored as a prognostic factor. In one study, longer diagnostic delay was associated with worse outcome on measures of memory, motor function, and behavior (De Grandis et al., 2009). More often, however, no differences in cognitive, adaptive, or motor outcome were documented as a function of diagnostic delay (Catsman-Berrevoets et al., 2009; Hayward et al., 2001; Koh et al., 1994; Mitchell et al., 2002; Russo et al., 1997). Degree of response to initial treatment did not consistently predict outcome (Brunklaus et al., 2011; Russo et al., 1997).

Paradoxically, Rudnick and colleagues (2001) showed that patients with more advanced stage neuroblastoma and OMA had better neurological outcomes, perhaps due to a diminished immune response to tumor in these patients (leading to more aggressive tumor growth/spread) and also sparing normal neurons. The effect of steroid treatment on the development of the young brain has not been directly addressed in these studies.

Infant ALL and Brain Tumors

Survival rates for infants (defined as under 1 year of age at diagnosis) with ALL have historically been far lower than for older children, and even in a recent trial, the 4-year event-free survival (EFS) for infant ALL was only 47%. This is due in part to a more aggressive biology in a vulnerable host (Brown, 2013). This rare condition often presents with high white blood cell counts, CNS involvement, hepatosplenomegaly, and skin infiltration.

MLL gene rearrangements (MLL-r) occur in 5% of childhood ALL cases overall, but in 70% to 80% of infant ALL. The presence of this genetic signature is associated with poorer outcomes. In CCG-1953, the five-year EFS for MLL-r infants was 34% compared with 60% with germline MLL (MLL-g) (Brown, 2013). Younger age and higher white blood count at diagnosis were independent predictors of poor outcome. A common pattern of response to chemotherapy is to achieve rapid complete remission, but then to relapse in the first year, suggesting the emergence of chemo-resistant cell populations. Another risk for these young patients is that infants are more vulnerable to complications and toxicities than are older children. They are particularly vulnerable to infection, and early mortality from treatment-related complications is much more common among infants.

For those infants who do survive, cognitive outcomes are poor, especially for survivors of CRT at such a young age. Babies under the age of 2 treated with 18–24 Gy displayed significant deficits in overall intellectual ability, math, and memory when tested five to ten years after diagnosis and compared to cancer controls (Mulhern et al., 1992). Longer time since treatment was correlated with lower IQ and poorer performance on tests of auditory long-term memory and math achievement. Therefore, all efforts are made to avoid CRT in infants with ALL. When chemotherapy-only regimens are used, neurodevelopmental outcomes improve dramatically. Infants treated with an intense chemotherapy protocol and without CRT had mean developmental estimates in the average range at four to five years postdiagnosis (Kaleita, Reaman, MacLean, Sather, & Whitt, 1999). At a median of 13 years postdiagnosis, specialized tutoring or special education placement was reported for 10% of infant ALL survivors treated with chemotherapy only; 59% of those treated with chemotherapy and CRT; and 86% of those treated with chemotherapy, CRT, and bone marrow transplant. For every month younger a child was at CRT, the estimated odds of academic problems increased by 18% (Leung et al., 2000).

Brain tumors that present in infancy are also particularly challenging to treat. Similar to ALL, tumors in this age group tend to be more aggressive and these children are more vulnerable to brain injury. Given the unacceptable side effects of radiotherapy at this young age, treatment options are limited. Delay in diagnosis, as well as increased vulnerability to surgical complications in this age group, also present challenges for management (Bishop, McDonald, Chang, & Esiashvili, 2010; Van Poppel et al., 2011).

New treatment protocols for young children with malignant brain tumors are showing some promise of improved survival and disease control (Rutkowski et al., 2005). Use of CRT in young children has declined and is typically deferred to the extent possible (Bishop et al., 2010). Innovative strategies include use of high-dose chemotherapy that can be followed by autologous stem cell transplant (Dhall et al., 2008). In European protocols for malignant brain tumors in infants, intraventricular methotrexate is used during induction and high-dose chemotherapy treatment (Friedrich et al., 2013; Rutkowski et al., 2010). Overall survival has been favorable for children with medulloblastoma (93%) and less favorable for children with other malignant tumor types (Friedrich et al., 2013). In children who do not respond to induction or who have progressive disease, radiation therapy is then used as a salvage treatment.

Studies of neuropsychological outcomes in this group are limited due to small numbers, changes in treatment (some children go on to receive CRT), use of historical controls for comparison, and lack of longer-term follow-up. Imaging studies show evidence of leukoencephalopathy during and after treatment that improves in some patients over time; the long-term implications of these findings are unclear (Rutkowski et al., 2010). In a study of children treated with high-dose myeloablative therapy and autologous stem cell transplantation, neuropsychological outcomes remained fairly stable over a 12-year follow up period (Guerry, Finlay, & Sands, 2014). This is in marked contrast to the findings of decline in neuropsychological function seen in children treated with CRT for medulloblastoma.

Intervention and Treatment

Even after decades of studying and documenting neuropsychological late effects in survivors of childhood cancer, and relating them to host and treatment factors, much still remains to be understood. As reviewed in this chapter, efforts to reduce late effects of ALL treatment have taken the form of reducing dose and field of radiation or eliminating CRT entirely, especially in young children, and by replacing CRT with more intense and multimodal chemotherapy. For children with brain tumors, reduction of radiation dose or field, or elimination of CRT, has been achieved though refinements in risk stratification strategies and the addition of chemotherapy. These efforts have been successful in reducing the frequency and severity of neuropsychological deficits. Nonetheless, many are now turning to the study of interventions to prevent or ameliorate neuropsychological late effects when they do occur (Askins & Moore, 2008). Intervention efforts take several forms: pharmacological, behavioral, cognitive, educational, and social (Castellino, Ullrich, Whelen, & Lange, 2014).

Pharmacological

Pharmacological interventions are used to address specific cognitive or emotional symptoms. Because the attention deficits exhibited by survivors of pediatric cancers treated with CNS-direct chemotherapy and CRT are reminiscent of children with ADHD, methylphenidate (MPH) has been used in an attempt to treat those symptoms. Early reports were observational in nature and variable in outcome (DeLong, Friedman, Friedman, Gustafson, & Oakes, 1992): Eight of 12 patients with ALL or brain tumor showed a "good" response; two a "fair" response and two a "poor" response to treatment with MPH. In another early study, treatment did not have an effect on attention and memory deficits in children with malignant brain tumors (Torres et al., 1996). Acute efficacy was documented in randomized, double-blind, placebo-controlled trials (Thompson et al., 2001) and patients showed a significant improvement on a test of sustained attention after 90 minutes, but not on tests of verbal memory or learning (N = 32). Longer term effects were documented in a randomized, double-blind, three-week crossover trial of low versus moderate dose MPH compared to a placebo control group. While there was no difference between the low and medium dose treatment groups, they were both rated as improved compared to the placebo group on parent and teacher ratings of attention, and teacher ratings of social skills. No direct measures of performance or achievement were included in this trial (Mulhern et al., 2004) A third study in this series (N = 122) added measures of attention, memory and academic achievement in a two-day double-blind crossover trial -comparing moderate dose MPH with placebo (Conklin et al., 2007). Results documented significant improvement on a test of cognitive flexibility and processing speed (Stroop), but no effect on tests of academic achievement, verbal learning, or attention. The authors point out that study participants with lower IQs (<70) were less likely to show a positive response to the MPH than did participants with average IQs and this factor should be considered in clinical settings. Furthermore, use of performance versus parent/teacher report measures may also affect the ability to document positive responses to MPH as an intervention for neuropsychological late effects in survivors of childhood cancer.

Because fewer children who have been treated for cancer have a positive response to MPH than do children with developmental ADHD, Conklin et al. (2010) studied factors that predicted a positive response to MPH in this population (N = 106). Teacher report of changes in the ADHD Index of the Conners Teacher Rating Scale was used as the definition of positive clinical response, and this outcome was documented for nearly half the subjects in the moderate-dose group (45%). This is significantly lower than the reported response rate in developmental ADHD populations (75%). Unlike in their 2007 study, Conklin and her colleagues did *not* find that higher global cognitive level was associated with a positive response. Rather, only parent and teacher reports of attention and behavior problems at screening were predictive of a positive medication response.

Conklin and her colleagues studied longer-term efficacy of MPH treatment in a group of brain tumor and ALL survivors (Conklin, Reddick, et al., 2010). Over the course of one year, treatment benefits were documented by performance and observational measures, at home and at school, affecting both attention and behavioral variables. No effects were observed on measures of cognitive function or academic skills. Similar findings were noted in a systematic review of controlled trials of stimulant medication to address cognitive late effects in children treated for brain tumors; attention processes appear to improve but impact on academic progress is not evident (Smithson, Phillips, Harvey, & Morrall, 2013).

Researchers have also investigated medications used to treat dementia symptoms in adults. Donezepil, an acetylcholinesterase inhibitor, was used in a small pilot study with survivors of childhood brain tumors. Some improvements in executive functions on the D-KEFS Tower and on the Plan/Organize scale of the Behavior Rating Inventory of Executive Function (BRIEF) were documented. A large multisite trial has been undertaken but no findings have been released to date. Modafanil, a stimulant medication, is used to treat fatigue and daytime sleepiness in children treated for brain tumors. A multicenter clinical trial sponsored by Children's Oncology Group (ACCL0922) is under way to evaluate if a six-week course of modafanil can improve neuropsychological function (attention, working memory, processing speed) in children treated for brain tumors. The study will also evaluate the medication's effect on fatigue and domains of executive function.

Psychopharmacological treatment is used clinically to address emotional adjustment issues seen in children treated for cancer. These problems can include anxiety and depression, as well as significant behavioral/emotional regulation deficits. In these instances, traditional psychopharmacological and psychotherapeutic interventions are indicated.

Behavioral

The role of exercise and physical fitness in promoting health as well as mood and cognitive function is being elucidated in a number of populations. In animal and human studies, physical activity has been associated with neurogenesis in the hippocampus (Pereira et al., 2007). Exercise as a form of intervention for survivors of childhood cancer has been found to be feasible (Keats & Culos-Reed, 2008) and safe (Baumann, Bloch, & Beulertz, 2013). Positive outcomes have been demonstrated on level of fatigue (Chang, Mu, Jou, Wong, & Chen, 2013) and quality of life (Baumann et al., 2013; Rodgers, Trevino, Zawaski, Gaber, & Leasure, 2013). Exercise represents a potential treatment that may help mitigate the adverse effects of radiation therapy on brain plasticity. Preliminary evidence suggests that cognitive late effects can be traced to CRT induced suppression of hippocampal cell proliferation and that exercise may be effective as an independent or adjuvant therapy (Rodgers et al., 2013). Mabbott and colleagues have shown that an aerobic exercise intervention may be effective for repairing neural damage following CRT in survivors of brain tumors (Riggs et al., 2014). Results suggest that aerobic exercise may not only promote white matter repair and hippocampal growth, but also improve reaction time in these patients.

Cognitive

Cognitive interventions, based on rehabilitation strategies developed for patients with traumatic brain injury, are being increasingly applied to survivors of childhood cancer. Butler and colleagues (2008), developed and evaluated a cognitive rehabilitation intervention program that draws upon techniques from three disciplines: brain injury rehabilitation, educational psychology, and clinical psychology. The intervention, delivered individually by a trained therapist, was programmatic but individualized as necessary to meet the child's needs. Twenty two-hour weekly sessions were conducted over a four- to five-month period and incorporated techniques to improve attention, concentration, and processing speed; metacognitive strategies to improve study skills; and cognitive behavioral strategies to address executive function. In a randomized, multicenter clinical trial, changes in attention, memory/learning, academic achievement and parent and self-reports of attention, self-esteem, and quality of life were assessed and compared to a wait list control group. Although significant improvements were documented for several variables (academic achievement, metacognitive strategy use, parent report of attention) there were no significant changes in neuropsychological function and effect sizes were small.

Because the time, effort, and cost of the Butler approach was large in comparison to demonstrated outcomes, home-based computerized intervention programs have been explored for feasibility and efficacy. Hardy and colleagues (Hardy, Willard, & Bonner, 2011) demonstrated good acceptability and variable compliance with a home-based computerized cognitive training program in a small group of brain tumor and ALL survivors ($N = 9$) with documented attention and working memory problems. Preliminary evidence suggested some degree of efficacy, with significant improvements at posttest for digit span forward and parent reported attention problems, but not for digit span backward or number letter sequencing. In this pilot study, there was no control group, and so the authors could not rule out parent reporting bias or practice effects on performance measures.

Kesler and colleagues tested the feasibility and efficacy of an internet-based cognitive rehabilitation program with 23 survivors of childhood posterior fossa brain tumors or ALL (Kesler, Lacayo, & Jo, 2011). The intervention was aimed at ameliorating deficits in executive function, including cognitive flexibility, attention, and working memory, and was designed as an eight-week course with five sessions per week, 20 minutes per session. They assessed neuropsychological function and conducted fMRI studies before and after the intervention. Results were encouraging and demonstrated excellent compliance with 83% of the group completing the course. Significant improvements were documented on tests of processing speed, cognitive flexibility and memory, but not on direct measures of working memory or attention. fMRI showed significant increases in dorsolateral prefrontal cortex activation following the intervention compared to baseline.

In an effort to specifically target working memory deficits, Hardy and colleagues (2011) tested the feasibility and preliminary efficacy of Cogmed Working Memory Training (Cogmed) as an at-home rehabilitation program for 20 survivors of childhood brain tumor and ALL. Two-thirds of the sample was assigned to the intervention arm, which consisted of 25 sessions over five to eight weeks in which difficulty was adapted to performance. The remaining one-third of the sample was assigned to an active "control" condition wherein the same exercises were presented but the difficulty level remained static. Feasibility was good with 85%, of subjects completing at least 80% of training sessions. Participants' ratings of ease of use and acceptability were also good. When the groups were compared with respect to efficacy of treatment, significant post active intervention increases were noted on performance measures of visual working memory and parent-rated learning problems. No effects were documented on tests of verbal working memory or attention; children with higher baseline IQ demonstrated greater improvements after training.

Educational

Educational interventions are delivered at various levels. School consultation and reintegration programs support survivors of childhood cancer in the school setting and provide a valuable educational component, helping teachers and school personnel understand cognitive and psychological late effects. Pediatric neuropsychologists work with schools to help implement interventions needed to address the impact of cancer and its treatment on learning and adjustment. An intervention specifically aimed at ameliorating the common deficits in math performance was tested by Moore et al. (Moore et al., 2000). Using a two-group longitudinal design, eight children treated for ALL received an active math intervention; seven children comparably treated for ALL received no intervention. The intervention group received 40–50 hours of math tutoring, which was skill and concept–based and was individualized to student needs. At follow-up, the treatment group showed improvement in math achievement compared to their baseline, while the control group did not.

The investigators then asked whether it was possible to prevent declines in math skills by intervening early, during active treatment (Moore, Hockenberry, Anhalt, McCarthy, & Krull, 2012). Fifty-seven children treated for ALL with chemotherapy only were enrolled at diagnosis and 60% (32 subjects) completed all assessments. The baseline assessment was conducted 12 months after completion of induction therapy. Post intervention assessment was conducted one year later, soon after completion of the one-year math intervention. The final assessment was conducted one year thereafter. Patients were randomized to math intervention or standard care. After completion of the intervention, the intervention group showed significant improvement on tests of calculation and applied math. One year later, visual working memory was significantly better than at baseline in the intervention group only. Improvements were specific to math and visual working memory, as they were not apparent on test of reading or spelling. The standard care group did not improve over time on any measure; however, neither did that group decline as predicted.

Social

Social competence is significantly affected, particularly in survivors of brain tumors. Reviews of the literature on social development in this group found that both social adjustment and competence are compromised (Hocking et al., 2015; Schulte & Barrera, 2010). Research findings and our clinical experience reveal that the social problems experienced by survivors of childhood brain tumors are characterized by social isolation, lack of sustaining peer friendships, and lack of peer acceptance. Studies of friendship quality in children treated for brain tumors note lack of integration and involvement in activities by peers (Vannatta et al., 2008; Vannatta, Gartstein, Short, & Noll, 1998; Vannatta, Gerhardt, Wells, & Noll, 2007). Compromise in executive functions may underlie these problems as well as limited opportunities to expand and refine social skills across development (Wolfe et al., 2012). Interventions to address social problems include support groups and structured events for adolescent and young adult survivors. Schulte and colleagues have developed a group social skills program consisting of eight weekly sessions focused on friendship making, cooperation, managing social cruelty, conflict resolution, empathy, and assertiveness (Schulte, Bartels, & Barrera, 2014; Schulte, Vannatta, & Barrera, 2014). Sessions use cognitive behavioral problem-solving strategies, role modeling, and cooperative activities. Following the intervention, improvements were noted in teacher and parent ratings of social skills, as well as in observed social performance, but there was no effect noted on a measure of social problem solving. These pilot studies are helpful in identifying targets for guiding social skill intervention programs.

Future Directions

The field of oncology is moving toward individualized and targeted therapies. Advances in understanding molecular genetics, disease processes in patients, and types of neoplasms foster refinements in treatment protocols that are adapted to the unique combination of specific disease within a particular host or context. Risk stratification strategies are much more sophisticated. In ALL, protocols now incorporate information regarding the individual's specific vulnerability to toxicity of treatment agents and chemotherapy doses are adjusted accordingly (Cheok & Evans, 2006). Similarly, now that we understand specific subgroups of medulloblastoma, less-intensive treatment can be considered for some patients to reduce neurotoxicity. These techniques have the potential to reduce the neurobehavioral impact of cancer therapies on the developing child.

Efforts to mitigate or prevent late effects may be advanced through the study of neuroprotective factors (Albers, Cavaletti, & Donehower, 2014; Avan et al., 2015). This area of investigation is still in its early stages but the focus of this research is to identify ways of protecting healthy cells, sparing cells in stages of active neurodevelopment, or replacing damaged cells to preserve cognitive development and function (Gibson & Monje, 2012).

Ongoing research in childhood cancer must continue to incorporate long-term follow-up of neuropsychological outcomes. In neuropsychology, the focus is on understanding how specific cognitive processes are affected and the related downstream effects of disruptions in brain development in childhood. A more nuanced understanding of plasticity, injury, and dynamic developmental processes will contribute to these approaches (Dennis et al., 2013; Johnston, 2009). Plasticity has been described as a double-edged sword: Less developed systems have more capacity for growth and development, yet the same developmental processes that support brain development also contribute to the developing brain's exquisite vulnerability to injury or insult and carry lifelong consequences.

Neuropsychologists working in childhood cancer have incorporated lessons learned from the study of traumatic brain injury in children in research and clinical care. Although the pathophysiology of the insult to the brain is different, similar neuropsychological processes are affected in both conditions. Intervention efforts in childhood cancer are based on cognitive rehabilitation techniques used to treat brain injury. In addition, studies of risk and resilience can assist with identifying targets for intervention. The field needs to move toward addressing modifiable risk factors over the short and long term. For example, we know that family and psychosocial factors have a significant impact on response to and outcome of any type of brain injury. Intervention efforts need to be individualized as well as comprehensive, addressing family functioning in subgroups at increased risk of adverse outcomes (Ach et al., 2013). As the transition to adulthood is considered, addressing health behaviors, social integration, and independence needs to be included in the scope of neuropsychological care.

Future research into intervention strategies will need to identify the active elements of effective interventions and their impact at different stages in development. As we learn more about how brain systems and neuropsychological processes of attention, working memory, and information processing speed are affected by childhood cancer and treatment, preventive educational or training strategies may be incorporated early in the treatment course, before these issues are manifest and compromise functioning; a similar strategy is proposed for addressing emerging working memory problems in children born very prematurely (Pascoe et al., 2013).

Clinical care and research endeavors need to be comprehensive and interdisciplinary, with active interchange of ideas that integrate physiological, developmental, and psychological systems. In order to truly advance the field, research methodologies will need to incorporate all of these factors, yet retain an individualized focus. Identifying the factors that contribute to resilience in some children as well as those involved in the selective vulnerability of others is of critical importance.

References

Ach, E., Gerhardt, C. A., Barrera, M., Kupst, M. J., Meyer, E. A., Patenaude, A. F., & Vannatta, K. (2013). Family factors associated with academic achievement deficits in pediatric brain tumor survivors. *Psycho-Oncology*, *22*(8), 1731–1737. doi: 10.1002/pon.3202

Albers, J. W., Chaudhry, V., Cavaletti, G., & Donehower, R. C. (2014). Interventions for preventing neuropathy caused by cisplatin and related compounds. *Cochrane Database Systematic Reviews*, *3*, CD005228. doi: 10.1002/14651858.CD005228.pub4

Anderson, F. S., & Kunin-Batson, A. S. (2009). Neurocognitive late effects of chemotherapy in children: The past 10 years of research on brain structure and function. *Pediatric Blood & Cancer*, *52*(2), 159–164. doi: 10.1002/pbc.21700

Armstrong, F. D. (2013). Implications of 25-year follow-up of white matter integrity and neurocognitive function of childhood leukemia survivors: A wake-up call. *Journal of Clinical Oncology*, *31*(27), 3309–3311. doi: 10.1200/JCO.2013.50.8879

Armstrong, G. T., Jain, N., Liu, W., Merchant, T. E., Stovall, M., Srivastava, D. K., . . . Krull, K. R. (2010). Region-specific radiotherapy and neuropsychological outcomes in adult survivors of childhood CNS malignancies. *Neuro-Oncology*, *12*(11), 1173–1186. doi: 10.1093/neuonc/noq104

Armstrong, G. T., Liu, Q., Yasui, Y., Huang, S., Ness, K. K., Leisenring, W., . . . Packer, R. J. (2009). Long-term outcomes among adult survivors of childhood central nervous system malignancies in the childhood cancer survivor study. *Journal of the National Cancer Institute*, *101*(13), 946–958. doi: 10.1093/jnci/djp148

Armstrong, G. T., Reddick, W. E., Petersen, R. C., Santucci, A., Zhang, N., Srivastava, D., . . . Krull, K. R. (2013). Evaluation of memory impairment in aging adult survivors of childhood acute lymphoblastic leukemia treated with cranial radiotherapy. *Journal of the National Cancer Institute*, *105*(12), 899–907.

Armstrong, G. T., Stovall, M., & Robison, L. L. (2010). Long-term effects of radiation exposure among adult survivors of childhood cancer: Results from the childhood cancer survivor study. *Radiation Research*, *174*(6), 840–850. doi: 10.1667/rr1903.1

Ashford, J., Schoffstall, C., Reddick, W. E., Leone, C., Laningham, F. H., Glass, J. O., . . . Conklin, H. M. (2010). Attention and working memory abilities in children treated for acute lymphoblastic leukemia. *Cancer*, *116*(19), 4638–4645. doi: 10.1002/cncr.25343

Askins, M. A., & Moore, B. D., 3rd. (2008). Preventing neurocognitive late effects in childhood cancer survivors. *Journal of Child Neurology*, *23*(10), 1160–1171. doi: 23/10/1160 [pii] 10.1177/0883073808321065 [doi]

Avan, A., Postma, T. J., Ceresa, C., Cavaletti, G., Giovannetti, E., & Peters, G. J. (2015). Platinum-induced neurotoxicity and preventive strategies: Past, present, and future. *The Oncologist*, *20*(4), 411–432. doi: 10.1634/theoncologist.2014-0044

Bandopadhayay, P., Bergthold, G., London, W. B., Goumnerova, L. C., Morales La Madrid, A., Marcus, K. J., . . . Manley, P. E. (2014). Long-term outcome of 4,040 children diagnosed with pediatric low-grade gliomas: An analysis of the surveillance epidemiology and end results (SEER) database. *Pediatric Blood & Cancer*, *61*(7), 1173–1179. doi: 10.1002/pbc.24958

Barton, S. E., Najita, J. S., Ginsburg, E. S., Leisenring, W. M., Stovall, M., Weathers, R. E., . . . Diller, L. (2013). Infertility, infertility treatment, and achievement of pregnancy in female survivors of childhood cancer: A report from the Childhood Cancer Survivor Study cohort. *Lancet Oncology*, *14*(9), 873–881. doi: 10.1016/s1470-2045(13)70251-1

Baumann, F. T., Bloch, W., & Beulertz, J. (2013). Clinical exercise interventions in pediatric oncology: A systematic review. *Pediatric Research*, *74*(4), 366–374. doi: 10.1038/pr.2013.123

Beebe, D., & Ris, M. D. (2001). Contributors to neuropsychological outcome in low grade astrocytoma. *Journal of the International Neuropsychological Society*, *7*(2), 214.

Bergthold, G., Bandopadhayay, P., Bi, W. L., Ramkissoon, L., Stiles, C., Segal, R. A., . . . Kieran, M. W. (2014). Pediatric low-grade gliomas: How modern biology reshapes the clinical field. *Biochimica et Biophysica Acta*, *1845*(2), 294–307. doi: 10.1016/j.bbcan.2014.02.004

Bhojwani, D., Sabin, N. D., Pei, D., Yang, J. J., Khan, R. B., Panetta, J. C., . . . Relling, M. V. (2014). Methotrexate-induced neurotoxicity and leukoencephalopathy in childhood acute lymphoblastic leukemia. *Journal of Clinical Oncology*, *32*(9), 949–959.

Bishop, A. J., McDonald, M. W., Chang, A. L., & Esiashvili, N. (2010). Infant brain tumors: Incidence, survival, and the role of radiation based on surveillance, epidemiology, and end results (SEER) data. *International Journal of Radiation Oncology, Biology, Physics*, *82*(1), 341–347. doi: S0360-3016(10)03066-X [pii] 10.1016/j.ijrobp.2010.08.020

Bleyer, A. (1990). Acute lymphoblastic leukemia in children. Advances and prospectus. *Cancer*, *65*(3 Suppl), 689–695.

Bleyer, A., Barr, R., Hayes-Lattin, B., Thomas, D., Ellis, C., & Anderson, B. (2008). The distinctive biology of cancer in adolescents and young adults. *Nature Reviews: Cancer*, *8*(4), 288–298. doi: 10.1038/nrc2349

Boman, K. K., Lindblad, F., & Hjern, A. (2010). Long-term outcomes of childhood cancer survivors in Sweden: A population-based study of education, employment, and income. *Cancer*, *116*(5), 1385–1391. doi: 10.1002/cncr.24840

Bond, J., Hough, R., Moppett, J., Vora, A., Mitchell, C., & Goulden, N. (2013). 'Stroke-like syndrome' caused by intrathecal methotrexate in patients treated during the ukall 2003 trial. *Leukemia*, *27*(4), 954–956.

Bowers, D. C., Liu, Y., Leisenring, W., McNeil, E., Stovall, M., Gurney, J. G., . . . Oeffinger, K. C. (2006). Late-occurring stroke among long-term survivors of childhood leukemia and brain tumors: A report from the childhood cancer survivor study. *Journal of Clinical Oncology*, *24*(33), 5277–5282. doi: 10.1200/JCO.2006.07.2884

Brouwers, P., & Poplack, D. (1990). Memory and learning sequelae in long-term survivors of acute lymphoblastic leukemia: Association with attention deficits. *American Journal of Pediatric Hematology Oncology*, *12*(2), 174–181.

Brown, P. (2013). Treatment of infant leukemias: Challenge and promise. *ASH Education Program Book*, *2013*(1), 596–600. doi: 10.1182/asheducation-2013.1.596

Brugnoletti, F., Morris, E. B., Laningham, F. H., Patay, Z., Pauley, J. L., Pui, C. H., . . . Inaba, H. (2009). Recurrent intrathecal methotrexate induced neurotoxicity in an adolescent with acute lymphoblastic leukemia: Serial clinical and radiologic findings. *Pediatric Blood & Cancer*, *52*(2), 293–295.

Brunklaus, A., Pohl, K., Zuberi, S. M., & de Sousa, C. (2011). Outcome and prognostic features in opsoclonus-myoclonus syndrome from infancy to adult life. *Pediatrics*, *128*(2), e388–394. doi: 10.1542/peds.2010-3114

Buizer, A. I., de Sonneville, L. M., & Veerman, A. J. (2009). Effects of chemotherapy on neurocognitive function in children with acute lymphoblastic leukemia: A critical review of the literature. *Pediatric Blood & Cancer*, *52*(4), 447–454.

Burke, M. E., Albritton, K., & Marina, N. (2007). Challenges in the recruitment of adolescents and young adults to cancer clinical trials. *Cancer*, 110(11), 2385–2393. doi: 10.1002/cncr.23060

Butler, R. W., Copeland, D. R., Fairclough, D. L., Mulhern, R. K., Katz, E. R., Kazak, A. E., . . . Sahler, O.J.Z. (2008). A multicenter, randomized clinical trial of a cognitive remediation program for childhood survivors of a pediatric malignancy. *Journal of Consulting and Clinical Psychology*, *76*(3), 367–378.

Carpentieri, S. C., Waber, D. P., Scott, R. M., Goumnerova, L. C., Kieran, M. W., Cohen, L. E., . . . Pomeroy, S. L. (2001). Memory deficits among children with craniopharyngiomas. *Neurosurgery*, *49*(5), 1053–1057; discussion 1057–1058.

Castellino, S. M., Ullrich, N. J., Whelen, M. J., & Lange, B. J. (2014). Developing interventions for cancer-related cognitive dysfunction in childhood cancer survivors. *Journal of the National Cancer Institute*, *106*(8), 1–6. doi: 10.1093/jnci/dju186

Catsman-Berrevoets, C. E., Aarsen, F. K., van Hemsbergen, M. L., van Noesel, M. M., Hakvoort-Cammel, F. G., & van den Heuvel-Eibrink, M. M. (2009). Improvement of neurological status and quality of life in children with opsoclonus myoclonus syndrome at long-term follow-up. *Pediatric Blood & Cancer*, *53*(6), 1048–1053. doi: 10.1002/pbc.22226

Chang, C. W., Mu, P. F., Jou, S. T., Wong, T. T., & Chen, Y. C. (2013). Systematic review and meta-analysis of nonpharmacological interventions for fatigue in children and adolescents with cancer. *Worldviews on Evidence-Based Nursing/Sigma Theta Tau International, Honor Society of Nursing*, *10*(4), 208–217. doi: 10.1111/wvn.12007

Cheok, M. H., & Evans, W. E. (2006). Acute lymphoblastic leukaemia: A model for the pharmacogenomics of cancer therapy. *Nature Reviews: Cancer*, *6*(2), 117–129. doi: 10.1038/nrc1800

Cheung, Y. T., & Krull, K. R. (2015). Neurocognitive outcomes in long-term survivors of childhood acute lymphoblastic leukemia treated on contemporary treatment protocols: A systematic review. *Neuroscience and Biobehavioral Reviews*, *53*, 108–120. doi: 10.1016/j.neubiorev.2015.03.016

Choudhri, A. F., Klimo, P., Auschwitz, T. S., Whitehead, M. T., & Boop, F. A. (2014). 3t intraoperative mri for management of pediatric CNS neoplasms. *American Journal of Neuroradiology*, *35*(12), 2382–2387. doi: 10.3174/ajnr.A4040

Ciesielski, K. T., Yanofsky, R., Ludwig, R. N., Hill, D. E., Hart, B. L., Astur, R. S., & Snyder, T. (1994). Hypoplasia of the cerebellar vermis and cognitive deficits in survivors of childhood leukemia. *Archives of Neurology*, *51*, 985–993.

Conklin, H. M., Helton, S., Ashford, J., Mulhern, R. K., Reddick, W. E., Brown, R., . . . Khan, R. B. (2010). Predicting methylphenidate response in long-term survivors of childhood cancer: A randomized, double-blind, placebo-controlled, crossover trial. *Journal of Pediatric Psychology*, *35*(2), 144–155. doi: 10.1093/jpepsy/jsp044

Conklin, H. M., Khan, R. B., Reddick, W. E., Helton, S., Brown, R. T., Howard, S. C., . . . Mulhern, R. K. (2007). Acute neurocognitive response to methylphenidate among survivors of childhood cancer: A randomized, double-blind, cross-over trial. *Journal of Pediatric Psychology*, *32*(9), 1127–1139.

Conklin, H. M., Krull, K. R., Reddick, W. E., Pei, D., Cheng, C., & Pui, C. H. (2012). Cognitive outcomes following contemporary treatment without cranial irradiation for childhood acute lymphoblastic leukemia. *Journal of the National Cancer Institute*, *104*(18), 1386–1395.

Conklin, H. M., Reddick, W. E., Ashford, J., Ogg, S., Howard, S. C., Morris, E. B., . . . Khan, R. B. (2010). Long-term efficacy of methylphenidate in enhancing attention regulation, social skills, and academic abilities of childhood cancer survivors. *Journal of Clinical Oncology*, *28*(29), 4465–4472. doi: 10.1200/jco.2010.28.4026

Cousens, P., Waters, B., Said, J., & Stevens, M. (1988). Cognitive effects of cranial irradiation in leukaemia: A survey and meta-analysis. *Journal of Child: Psychology and Psychiatry*, *29*(6), 839–852.

Daams, M., Schuitema, I., van Dijk, B. W., van Dulmen-den Broeder, E., Veerman, A. J., van den Bos, C., & de Sonneville, L. M. (2012). Long-term effects of cranial irradiation and intrathecal chemotherapy in treatment of childhood leukemia: A MEG study of power spectrum and correlated cognitive dysfunction. *BMC Neurology*, *12*(84). doi: 10.1186/1471-2377-12-84

D'Agostino, N. M., Penney, A., & Zebrack, B. (2011). Providing developmentally appropriate psychosocial care to adolescent and young adult cancer survivors. *Cancer*, *117*(10 Suppl), 2329–2334. doi: 10.1002/cncr.26043

De Grandis, E., Parodi, S., Conte, M., Angelini, P., Battaglia, F., Gandolfo, C., . . . Veneselli, E. (2009). Long-term follow-up of neuroblastoma-associated opsoclonus-myoclonus-ataxia syndrome. *Neuropediatrics*, *40*(3), 103–111. doi: 10.1055/s-0029-1237723

de Laat, P., Te Winkel, M. L., Devos, A. S., Catsman-Berrevoets, C. E., Pieters, R., & van den Heuvel-Eibrink, M. M. (2011). Posterior reversible encephalopathy syndrome in childhood cancer. *Annals of Oncology: Official Journal of the European Society for Medical Oncology/ESMO*, *22*(2), 472–478. doi: 10.1093/annonc/mdq382

DeLong, R., Friedman, H., Friedman, N., Gustafson, K., & Oakes, J. (1992). Methylphenidate in neuropsychological sequelae of radiotherapy and chemotherapy of childhood brain tumors and leukemia. *Journal of Child Neurology*, *7*(4), 462–463.

Dennis, M., Spiegler, B. J., & Hetherington, R. (2000). New survivors for the new millennium: Cognitive risk and reserve in adults with childhood brain insults. *Brain and Cognition*, *42*(1), 102–105. doi: 10.1006/brcg.1999.1174

Dennis, M., Spiegler, B. J., Juranek, J. J., Bigler, E. D., Snead, O. C., & Fletcher, J. M. (2013). Age, plasticity, and homeostasis in childhood brain disorders. *Neuroscience and Biobehavioral Reviews*, *37*(10 Pt 2), 2760–2773. doi: 10.1016/j.neubiorev.2013.09.010

Dhall, G., Grodman, H., Ji, L., Sands, S., Gardner, S., Dunkel, I. J., . . . Finlay, J. L. (2008). Outcome of children less than three years old at diagnosis with non-metastatic medulloblastoma treated with chemotherapy on the "Head Start" I and II protocols. *Pediatric Blood & Cancer*, *50*(6), 1169–1175. doi: 10.1002/pbc.21525

Dicuonzo, F., Salvati, A., Palma, M., Lefons, V., Lasalandra, G., De Leonardis, F., & Santoro, N. (2009). Posterior reversible encephalopathy syndrome associated with methotrexate neurotoxicity: Conventional magnetic resonance and diffusion-weighted imaging findings. *Journal of Child Neurology*, *24*(8), 1013–1018.

Dietrich, J., Monje, M., Wefel, J., & Meyers, C. (2008). Clinical patterns and biological correlates of cognitive dysfunction associated with cancer therapy. *The Oncologist, 13*(12), 1285–1295. doi: 10.1634/theoncologist.2008-0130

Dowell, R. E., Copeland, D. R., Francis, D. J., Fletcher, J. M., & Stovall, M. (1991). Absence of synergistic effects of CNS treatments on neuropsychologic test performance among children. *Journal of Clinical Oncology, 9*(6), 1029–1036.

Edelmann, M. N., Ogg, R. J., Scoggins, M. A., Brinkman, T. M., Sabin, N. D., Pui, C. H., . . . Krull, K. R. (2013). Dexamethasone exposure and memory function in adult survivors of childhood acute lymphoblastic leukemia: A report from the sjlife cohort. *Pediatric Blood & Cancer, 60*(11), 1778–1784. doi: 10.1002/pbc.24644

Edelstein, K., D'Agostino, N., Bernstein, L. J., Nathan, P. C., Greenberg, M. L., Hodgson, D. C., . . . Spiegler, B. J. (2011). Long-term neurocognitive outcomes in young adult survivors of childhood acute lymphoblastic leukemia. *Journal of Pediatric Hematology/Oncology, 33*(6), 450–458.

Edelstein, K., Spiegler, B. J., Fung, S., Panzarella, T., Mabbott, D. J., Jewitt, N., . . . Hodgson, D. C. (2011). Early aging in adult survivors of childhood medulloblastoma: Long-term neurocognitive, functional, and physical outcomes. *Neuro-Oncology, 13*(5), 536–545. doi: 10.1093/neuonc/nor015

Eiser, C. (1978). Intellectual abilities among survivors of childhood leukaemia as a function of CNS irradiation. *Archives of Disease of Childhood, 53*, 391–395

Eiser, C., & Lansdown, R. (1977). Retrospective study of intellectual development in children treated for acute lymphoblastic leukaemia. *Archives of Disease in Childhood, 52*, 525–529.

Ellenberg, L., Liu, Q., Gioia, G., Yasui, Y., Packer, R. J., Mertens, A., . . . Zeltzer, L. K. (2009). Neurocognitive status in long-term survivors of childhood CNS malignancies: A report from the Childhood Cancer Survivor Study. *Neuropsychology, 23*(6), 705–717. doi: 10.1037/a0016674

Ferrari, A., Montello, M., Budd, T., & Bleyer, A. (2008). The challenges of clinical trials for adolescents and young adults with cancer. *Pediatric Blood & Cancer, 50*(5 Suppl), 1101–1104. doi: 10.1002/pbc.21459

Fossati, P., Ricardi, U., & Orecchia, R. (2009). Pediatric medulloblastoma: Toxicity of current treatment and potential role of protontherapy. *Cancer Treatment Reviews, 35*(1), 79–96.

Friedman, D. L., Whitton, J., Leisenring, W., Mertens, A. C., Hammond, S., Stovall, M., . . . Neglia, J. P. (2010). Subsequent neoplasms in 5-year survivors of childhood cancer: The Childhood Cancer Survivor Study. *Journal of the National Cancer Institute, 102*(14), 1083–1095. doi: 10.1093/jnci/djq238

Friedrich, C., von Bueren, A. O., von Hoff, K., Gerber, N. U., Ottensmeier, H., Deinlein, F., . . . Rutkowski, S. (2013). Treatment of young children with CNS-primitive neuroectodermal tumors/pineoblastomas in the prospective multicenter trial HIT 2000 using different chemotherapy regimens and radiotherapy. *Neuro-Oncology, 15*(2), 224–234. doi: 10.1093/neuonc/nos292

Gerber, N. U., Mynarek, M., von Hoff, K., Friedrich, C., Resch, A., & Rutkowski, S. (2014). Recent developments and current concepts in medulloblastoma. *Cancer Treatment Reviews, 40*(3), 356–365. doi: http://dx.doi.org/10.1016/j.ctrv.2013.11.010

Gibson, E., & Monje, M. (2012). Effect of cancer therapy on neural stem cells: Implications for cognitive function. *Current Opinion in Oncology, 24*(6), 672–678. doi: 10.1097/CCO.0b013e3283571a8e

Gibson, P., Tong, Y., Robinson, G., Thompson, M. C., Currle, D. S., Eden, C., . . . Gilbertson, R. J. (2010). Subtypes of medulloblastoma have distinct developmental origins. *Nature, 468*(7327), 1095–1099. doi: 10.1038/nature09587

Greenberger, B. A., Pulsifer, M. B., Ebb, D. H., MacDonald, S. M., Jones, R. M., Butler, W. E., . . . Yock, T. I. (2014). Clinical outcomes and late endocrine, neurocognitive, and visual profiles of proton radiation for pediatric low-grade gliomas. *International Journal of Radiation Oncology, Biology, Physics, 89*(5), 1060–1068. doi: 10.1016/j.ijrobp.2014.04.053

Grill, J., & Owens, C. (2013). Central nervous system tumors. *Handbook of Clinical Neurology, 112*, 931–958. doi: 10.1016/B978-0-444-52910-7.00015-5

Guerry, L., Finlay, J., & Sands, S. (2014). *Neruopsychological follow-up of head start ii survivors: An update.* Paper presented at the 16th International Symposium on Pediatric Neuro-Oncology, Singapore.

Gurney, J. G., Kadan-Lottick, N. S., Packer, R. J., Neglia, J. P., Sklar, C. A., Punyko, J. A., . . . Robison, L. L. (2003). Endocrine and cardiovascular late effects among adult survivors of childhood brain tumors: Childhood Cancer Survivor Study. *Cancer, 97*(3), 663–673.

Gurney, J. G., Krull, K. R., Kadan-Lottick, N., Nicholson, H. S., Nathan, P. C., Zebrack, B., . . . Ness, K. K. (2009). Social outcomes in the Childhood Cancer Survivor Study cohort. *Journal of Clinical Oncology, 27*(14), 2390–2395. doi: 10.1200/JCO.2008.21.1458

Gururangan, S. (2009). Late effects of chemotherapy. In S. Goldman & C. D. Turner (Eds.), *Late Effects of Treatment for Brain Tumors* (pp. 43–65). New York: Springer.

Halberg, F. E., Kramer, J. H., Moore, I. M., Wara, W. M., Matthay, K. K., & Ablin, A. R. (1992). Prophylactic cranial irradiation dose effects on late cognitive function in children treated for acute lymphoblastic leukemia. *International Journal of Radiation Oncology, Biology, Physics, 22*(1), 13–16.

Hardy, K. K., Willard, V. W., & Bonner, M. J. (2011). Computerized cognitive training in survivors of childhood cancer: A pilot study. *Journal of Pediatric Oncology Nursing, 28*(1), 27–33. doi: 10.1177/1043454210377178

Harila, M. J., Winqvist, S., Lanning, M., Bloigu, R., & Harila-Saari, A. H. (2009). Progressive neurocognitive impairment in young adult survivors of childhood acute lymphoblastic leukemia. *Pediatric Blood & Cancer, 53*(2), 156–161.

Hayward, K., Jeremy, R. J., Jenkins, S., Barkovich, A. J., Gultekin, S. H., Kramer, J., . . . Matthay, K. K. (2001). Long-term neurobehavioral outcomes in children with neuroblastoma and opsoclonus-myoclonus-ataxia syndrome: Relationship to MRI findings and anti-neuronal antibodies. *The Journal of Pediatrics, 139*(4), 552–559. doi: 10.1067/mpd.2001.118200

Hocking, M. C., McCurdy, M., Turner, E., Kazak, A. E., Noll, R. B., Phillips, P., & Barakat, L. P. (2015). Social competence in pediatric brain tumor survivors: Application of a model from social neuroscience and developmental psychology. *Pediatric Blood & Cancer, 62*(3), 375–384. doi: 10.1002/pbc.25300

Hottinger, A. F., & Khakoo, Y. (2009). Neurooncology of familial cancer syndromes. *Journal of Child Neurology, 24*(12), 1526–1535. doi: 10.1177/0883073809337539

Howlader, N., Noone, A., Krapcho, M., Garshell, J., Miller, D., Altekruse, S., . . . Cronin, K. (2015). *SEER Cancer Statistics Review, 1975–2012.* Retrieved from http://seer.cancer.gov/csr/1975_2012/

Huang, T. T., Chen, Y., Dietz, A. C., Yasui, Y., Donaldson, S. S., Stokes, D. C., . . . Ness, K. K. (2014). Pulmonary outcomes in survivors of childhood central nervous system malignancies: A report from the Childhood Cancer Survivor Study. *Pediatric Blood & Cancer*, *61*(2), 319–325. doi: 10.1002/pbc.24819

Huber, J. F., Bradley, K., Spiegler, B. J., & Dennis, M. (2006). Long-term effects of transient cerebellar mutism after cerebellar astrocytoma or medulloblastoma tumor resection in childhood. *Child's Nervous System*, *22*(2 (Print)), 132–138.

Hudson, M. M., Link, M. P., & Simone, J. V. (2014). Milestones in the curability of pediatric cancers. *Journal of Clinical Oncology*, *32*(23), 2391–2397. doi: 10.1200/JCO.2014.55.6571

Hudson, M. M., Ness, K. K., Gurney, J. G., Mulrooney, D. A., Chemaitilly, W., Krull, K. R., . . . Robison, L. L. (2013). Clinical ascertainment of health outcomes among adults treated for childhood cancer. *Journal of the American Medical Association*, *309*(22), 2371–2381. doi: 10.1001/jama.2013.6296

Hudson, M. M., Oeffinger, K. C., Jones, K., Brinkman, T. M., Krull, K. R., Mulrooney, D. A., . . . Ness, K. K. (2015). Age-dependent changes in health status in the childhood cancer survivor cohort. *Journal of Clinical Oncology*, *33*(5), 479–491. doi: 10.1200/JCO.2014.57.4863

Inaba, H., Greaves, M., & Mullighan, C. G. (2013). Acute lymphoblastic leukaemia. *The Lancet*, *381*(9881), 1943–1955. doi: http://dx.doi.org/10.1016/S0140-6736(12)62187-4

Iuvone, L., Mariotti, P., Colosimo, C., Guzzetta, F., Ruggiero, A., & Riccardi, R. (2002). Long-term cognitive outcome, brain computed tomography scan, and magnetic resonance imaging in children cured for acute lymphoblastic leukemia. *Cancer*, *95*(12), 2562–2570.

Jankovic, M., Brouwers, P., Valsecchi, M. G., Van Veldhuizen, A., Huisman, J., Kamphuis, R., . . . et al. (1994). Association of 1800 cgy cranial irradiation with intellectual function in children with acute lymphoblastic leukaemia. ISPACC. International study group on psychosocial aspects of childhood cancer. *Lancet*, *344*(8917), 224–227.

Jannoun, L. (1983). Are cognitive and educational development affected by age at which prophylactic therapy is given in acute lymphoblastic leukaemia? *Archives of Disease in Childhood*, *58*(12), 953–958.

Janzen, L. A., David, D., Walker, D., Hitzler, J., Zupanec, S., Jones, H., & Spiegler, B. J. (2015). Pre-morbid developmental vulnerabilities in children with newly diagnosed acute lymphoblastic leukemia (all). *Pediatric Blood Cancer*, *62*(12), 2183–2188. doi: 10.1002/pbc.25692

Jansen, N. C., Kingma, A., Schuitema, A., Bouma, A., Huisman, J., Veerman, A. J., & Kamps, W. A. (2006). Post-treatment intellectual functioning in children treated for acute lymphoblastic leukaemia (all) with chemotherapy-only: A prospective, sibling-controlled study. *European Journal of Cancer*, *42*(16), 2765–2772. doi: 10.1016/j.ejca.2006.06.014

Jansen, N. C., Kingma, A., Schuitema, A., Bouma, A., Veerman, A. J., & Kamps, W. A. (2008). Neuropsychological outcome in chemotherapy-only treated children with acute lymphoblastic leukemia. *Journal of Clinical Oncology*, *26*(18), 3025–3030. doi: 10.1200/JCO.2007.12.4149

Janzen, L. A., & Spiegler, B. J. (2008). Neurodevelopmental sequelae of pediatric acute lymphoblastic leukemia and its treatment. *Developmental Disabilities Research Reviews*, *14*(3), 185–195.

Johnson, K. J., Cullen, J., Barnholtz-Sloan, J. S., Ostrom, Q. T., Langer, C. E., Turner, M. C., . . . Scheurer, M. E. (2014). Childhood brain tumor epidemiology: A brain tumor epidemiology consortium review. *Cancer Epidemiology, Biomarkers & Prevention*, *23*(12), 2716–2736. doi: 10.1158/1055-9965.EPI-14-0207

Johnston, M. V. (2009). Plasticity in the developing brain: Implications for rehabilitation. *Developmental Disabilities Research Reviews*, *15*(2), 94–101. doi: 10.1002/ddrr.64

Kaatsch, P. (2010). Epidemiology of childhood cancer. *Cancer Treatment Reviews*, *36*(4), 277–285. doi: 10.1016/j.ctrv.2010.02.003

Kadan-Lottick, N. S., Brouwers, P., Breiger, D., Kaleita, T., Dziura, J., Liu, H., . . . Neglia, J. P. (2009). A comparison of neurocognitive functioning in children previously randomized to dexamethasone or prednisone in the treatment of childhood acute lymphoblastic leukemia. *Blood*, *114*(9), 1746–1752. doi: 10.1182/blood-2008-12-186502

Kadan-Lottick, N. S., Zeltzer, L. K., Liu, Q., Yasui, Y., Ellenberg, L., Gioia, G., . . . Krull, K. R. (2010). Neurocognitive functioning in adult survivors of childhood non-central nervous system cancers. *Journal of the National Cancer Institute*, *102*(12), 881–893. doi: 10.1093/jnci/djq156

Kahalley, L. S., Conklin, H. M., Tyc, V. L., Hudson, M. M., Wilson, S. J., Wu, S., . . . Hinds, P. S. (2013). Slower processing speed after treatment for pediatric brain tumor and acute lymphoblastic leukemia. *Psycho-Oncology*, *22*(9), 1979–1986. doi: 10.1002/pon.3255

Kaleita, T. A., Reaman, G. H., MacLean, W. E., Sather, H. N., & Whitt, J. K. (1999). Neurodevelopmental outcome of infants with acute lymphoblastic leukemia: A Children's Cancer Group report. *Cancer*, *85*(8), 1859–1865.

Kamdar, K. Y., Krull, K. R., El-Zein, R. A., Brouwers, P., Potter, B. S., Harris, L. L., . . . Okcu, M. F. (2011). Folate pathway polymorphisms predict deficits in attention and processing speed after childhood leukemia therapy. *Pediatric Blood & Cancer*, *57*(3), 454–460.

Keats, M. R., & Culos-Reed, S. N. (2008). A community-based physical activity program for adolescents with cancer (project trek): Program feasibility and preliminary findings. *Journal of Pediatric Hematology/Oncology*, *30*(4), 272–280. doi: 10.1097/MPH.0b013e318162c476

Kesler, S. R., Lacayo, N. J., & Jo, B. (2011). A pilot study of an online cognitive rehabilitation program for executive function skills in children with cancer-related brain injury. *Brain Injury*, *25*(1), 101–112. doi: 10.3109/02699052.2010.536194

Kesler, S. R., Tanaka, H., & Koovakkattu, D. (2010). Cognitive reserve and brain volumes in pediatric acute lymphoblastic leukemia. *Brain Imaging & Behavior*, *4*(3–4), 256–269.

Khong, P.-L., Leung, L.H.T., Fung, A.S.M., Fong, D.Y.T., Qiu, D., Kwong, D.L.W., . . . Chan, G.C.F. (2006). White matter anisotropy in post-treatment childhood cancer survivors: Preliminary evidence of association with neurocognitive function. *Journal of Clinical Oncology*, *24*(6), 884–890. doi: 10.1200/jco.2005.02.4505

Kieran, M. W. (2005). Anti-angiogenic therapy in pediatric neuro-oncology. *Journal of Neuro-Oncology*, *75*(3), 327–334.

Kingma, A., Mooyaart, E. L., Kamps, W. A., Nieuwenhuizen, P., & Wilmink, J. T. (1993). Magnetic resonance imaging of the brain and neuropsychological evaluation in children treated for acute lymphoblastic leukemia at a young age. *The American Journal of Pediatric Hematology/Oncology*, *15*(2), 231–238.

Kirchhoff, A. C., Krull, K. R., Ness, K. K., Park, E. R., Oeffinger, K. C., Hudson, M. M., . . . Leisenring, W. (2011). Occupational outcomes of adult childhood cancer survivors: A report from the Childhood Cancer Survivor Study. *Cancer*, *117*(13), 3033–3044. doi: 10.1002/cncr.25867

Klein, A., Schmitt, B., & Boltshauser, E. (2007). Long-term outcome of ten children with opsoclonus-myoclonus syndrome. *European Journal of Pediatrics*, *166*(4), 359–363. doi: 10.1007/s00431-006-0247-4

Knight, S. J., Conklin, H. M., Palmer, S. L., Schreiber, J. E., Armstrong, C. L., Wallace, D., . . . Gajjar, A. (2014). Working memory abilities among children treated for medulloblastoma: Parent report and child performance. *Journal of Pediatric Psychology*, *39*(5), 501–511. doi: 10.1093/jpepsy/jsu009

Koch, S. V., Kejs, A.M.T., Engholm, G., Møller, H., Johansen, C., & Schmiegelow, K. (2006). Leaving home after cancer in childhood: A measure of social independence in early adulthood. *Pediatric Blood & Cancer*, *47*(1), 61–70. doi: 10.1002/pbc.20827

Koh, P. S., Raffensperger, J. G., Berry, S., Larsen, M. B., Johnstone, H. S., Chou, P., . . . Cohn, S. L. (1994). Long-term outcome in children with opsoclonus-myoclonus and ataxia and coincident neuroblastoma. *The Journal of Pediatrics*, *125*(5 Pt 1), 712–716.

Krull, K. R., Bhojwani, D., Conklin, H. M., Pei, D., Cheng, C., Reddick, W. E., . . . Pui, C. H. (2013). Genetic mediators of neurocognitive outcomes in survivors of childhood acute lymphoblastic leukemia. *Journal of Clinical Oncology*, *31*(17), 2182–2188. doi: 10.1200/JCO.2012.46.7944

Krull, K. R., Brinkman, T. M., Li, C., Armstrong, G. T., Ness, K. K., Srivastava, D. K., . . . Hudson, M. M. (2013). Neurocognitive outcomes decades after treatment for childhood acute lymphoblastic leukemia: A report from the St Jude Lifetime Cohort Study. *Journal of Clinical Oncology*, *31*(35), 4407–4415. doi: 10.1200/JCO.2012.48.2315

Krull, K. R., Brouwers, P., Jain, N., Zhang, L., Bomgaars, L., Dreyer, Z., . . . Okcu, M. F. (2008). Folate pathway genetic polymorphisms are related to attention disorders in childhood leukemia survivors. *Journal of Pediatrics*, *152*(1), 101–105.

Kuehni, C. E., Strippoli, M.-P. F., Rueegg, C. S., Rebholz, C. E., Bergstraesser, E., Grotzer, M., . . . for the Swiss Pediatric Oncology, G. (2012). Educational achievement in Swiss childhood cancer survivors compared with the general population. *Cancer*, *118*(5), 1439–1449. doi: 10.1002/cncr.26418

Kurt, B. A., Nolan, V. G., Ness, K. K., Neglia, J. P., Tersak, J. M., Hudson, M. M., . . . Arora, M. (2011). Hospitalization rates among survivors of childhood cancer in the Childhood Cancer Survivor Study cohort. *Pediatric Blood & Cancer*, *59*(1), 126–132. doi: 10.1002/pbc.24017

Law, N., Greenberg, M., Bouffet, E., Laughlin, S., Taylor, M. D., Malkin, D., . . . Mabbott, D. (2015). Visualization and segmentation of reciprocal cerebrocerebellar pathways in the healthy and injured brain. *Human Brain Mapping*, *36*(7), 2615–2628. doi: 10.1002/hbm.22795

Law, N., Greenberg, M., Bouffet, E., Taylor, M. D., Laughlin, S., Strother, D., . . . Mabbott, D. J. (2012). Clinical and neuroanatomical predictors of cerebellar mutism syndrome. *Neuro-Oncology*, *14*(10), 1294–1303. doi: 10.1093/neuonc/nos160

Leung, W., Hudson, M., Zhu, Y., Rivera, G. K., Ribeiro, R. C., Sandlund, J. T., . . . Pui, C. H. (2000). Late effects in survivors of infant leukemia. *Leukemia*, *14*(7), 1185–1190.

Lo, A. C., Howard, A. F., Nichol, A., Sidhu, K., Abdulsatar, F., Hasan, H., & Goddard, K. (2014). Long-term outcomes and complications in patients with craniopharyngioma: The British Columbia cancer agency experience. *International Journal of Radiation Oncology, Biology, Physics*, *88*(5), 1011–1018. doi: 10.1016/j.ijrobp.2014.01.019

Lucchini, G., Grioni, D., Colombini, A., Contri, M., De Grandi, C., Rovelli, A., . . . Jankovic, M. (2008). Encephalopathy syndrome in children with hemato-oncological disorders is not always posterior and reversible. *Pediatric Blood & Cancer*, *51*(5), 629–633. doi: 10.1002/pbc.21688

Mabbott, D. J., Noseworthy, M. D., Bouffet, E., Rockel, C., & Laughlin, S. (2006). Diffusion tensor imaging of white matter after cranial radiation in children for medulloblastoma: Correlation with IQ. *Neuro-Oncology*, *8*(3), 244–252.

Mabbott, D. J., Penkman, L., Witol, A., Strother, D., & Bouffet, E. (2008). Core neurocognitive functions in children treated for posterior fossa tumors. *Neuropsychology*, *22*(2), 159–168.

MacDonald, S. M., Safai, S., Trofimov, A., Wolfgang, J., Fullerton, B., Yeap, B. Y., . . . Yock, T. (2008). Proton radiotherapy for childhood ependymoma: Initial clinical outcomes and dose comparisons. *International Journal of Radiation Oncology, Biology, Physics*, *71*(4), 979–986. doi: S0360-3016(07)04758-X [pii] 10.1016/j.ijrobp.2007.11.065

Mahadeo, K. M., Dhall, G., Panigrahy, A., Lastra, C., & Ettinger, L. J. (2010). Subacute methotrexate neurotoxicity and cerebral venous sinus thrombosis in a 12-year-old with acute lymphoblastic leukemia and methylenetetrahydrofolate reductase (MTHFR) C677T polymorphism: Homocysteine-mediated methotrexate neurotoxicity via direct endothelial injury. *Pediatric Hematology & Oncology*, *27*(1), 46–52.

Meadows, A. T., & Evans, A. E. (1976). Effects of chemotherapy on the central nervous system: A study of parenteral methotrexate in long-term survivors of leukemia and lymphoma in childhood. *Cancer*, *37*(2 Suppl), 1079–1085.

Meadows, A. T., Massari, D. J., Fergusson, J., Gordon, J., P., L., & Moss, K. (1981). Declines in IQ scores and cognitive dysfunctions in children with acute lymphocytic leukaemia treated with cranial irradiation. *The Lancet*, *2*, 1015–1018.

Mennes, M., Stiers, P., Vandenbussche, E., Vercruysse, G., Uyttebroeck, A., Meyer, G. D., & Van Gool, S. W. (2005). Attention and information processing in survivors of childhood acute lymphoblastic leukemia treated with chemotherapy only. *Pediatric Blood & Cancer*, *44*(5), 479–486. doi: 10.1002/pbc.20147

Merchant, T. E., Kiehna, E. N., Li, C., Xiong, X., & Mulhern, R. K. (2005). Radiation dosimetry predicts IQ after conformal radiation therapy in pediatric patients with localized ependymoma. *International Journal of Radiation Oncology, Biology, Physics*, *63*(5 (Print)), 1546–1554.

Merchant, T. E., Kiehna, E. N., Sanford, R. A., Mulhern, R. K., Thompson, S. J., Wilson, M. W., . . . Kun, L. E. (2002). Craniopharyngioma: The St. Jude Children's Research Hospital experience 1984–2001. *International Journal of Radiation Oncology, Biology, Physics*, *53*(3), 533–542.

Mitchell, W. G., Brumm, V. L., Azen, C. G., Patterson, K. E., Aller, S. K., & Rodriguez, J. (2005). Longitudinal neurodevelopmental evaluation of children with opsoclonus-ataxia. *Pediatrics*, *116*(4), 901–907. doi: 10.1542/peds.2004-2377

Mitchell, W. G., Davalos-Gonzalez, Y., Brumm, V. L., Aller, S. K., Burger, E., Turkel, S. B., . . . Padilla, S. (2002). Opsoclonus-ataxia caused by childhood neuroblastoma: Developmental and neurologic sequelae. *Pediatrics*, *109*(1), 86–98.

Moleski, M. (2000). Neuropsychological, neuroanatomical, and neurophysiological consequences of CNS chemotherapy for acute lymphoblastic leukemia. *Archives of Clinical Neuropsychology*, *15*(7), 603–630.

Moore, I. M., Espy, K. A., Kaufmann, P., Kramer, J., Kaemingk, K., Miketova, P., . . . Matthay, K. (2000). Cognitive consequences and central nervous system injury following treatment for childhood leukemia. *Seminars in Oncology Nursing*, *16*(4), 279–290; discussion 291–279.

Moore, I. M., Hockenberry, M. J., Anhalt, C., McCarthy, K., & Krull, K. R. (2012). Mathematics intervention for prevention of neurocognitive deficits in childhood leukemia. *Pediatric Blood & Cancer*, *59*(2), 278–284. doi: 10.1002/pbc.23354

Moore, I. M., Kramer, J. H., Wara, W., Halberg, F., & Ablin, A. R. (1991). Cognitive function in children with leukemia:Effect of radiation dose and time since irradiation. *Cancer*, *68*, 1913–1917.

Morris, E. B., Laningham, F. H., Sandlund, J. T., & Khan, R. B. (2007). Posterior reversible encephalopathy syndrome in children with cancer. *Pediatric Blood & Cancer*, *48*(2), 152–159. doi: 10.1002/pbc.20703

Moss, H. A., Nannis, E. D., & Poplack, D. G. (1981). The effects of prophylactic treatment of the central nervous system on the intellectual functioning of children with acute lymphocytic leukemia. *American Journal of Medicine*, *71*, 47–52.

Mueller, S., Fullerton, H. J., Stratton, K., Leisenring, W., Weathers, R. E., Stovall, M., . . . Krull, K. R. (2013). Radiation, atherosclerotic risk factors, and stroke risk in survivors of pediatric cancer: A report from the childhood cancer survivor study. *International Journal of Radiation Oncology, Biology, Physics*, *86*(4), 649–655. doi: 10.1016/j.ijrobp.2013.03.034

Mulhern, R. K., Khan, R. B., Kaplan, S., Helton, S., Christensen, R., Bonner, M., . . . Reddick, W. E. (2004). Short-term efficacy of methylphenidate: A randomized, double-blind, placebo-controlled trial among survivors of childhood cancer. *Journal of Clinical Oncology*, *22*(23), 4795–4803. doi: 10.1200/JCO.2004.04.128

Mulhern, R. K., Kovnar, E., Langston, J., Carter, M., Fairclough, D., Leigh, L., & Kun, L. E. (1992). Long-term survivors of leukemia treated in infancy: Factors associated with neuropsychologic status. *Journal of Clinical Oncology*, *10*(7), 1095–1102.

Mulhern, R. K., Ochs, J., & Kun, L. E. (1991). Changes in intellect associated with cranial radiation therapy. In P. H. Gutin, S. A. Leibel, & G. E. Sheline, (Eds.), *Radiation Injury to the Nervous System* (pp. 325–340). New York: Raven Press.

Müller, H. L. (2014). Chapter 16: Craniopharyngioma. In M. K. Eric Fliers & A. R. Johannes (Eds.), *Handbook of Clinical Neurology*, *124*, 235–253. doi: 10.1016/B978-0-444-59602-4.00016-2

Nagel, B. J., Palmer, S. L., Reddick, W. E., Glass, J. O., Helton, K. J., Wu, S., . . . Mulhern, R. K. (2004). Abnormal hippocampal development in children with medulloblastoma treated with risk-adapted irradiation. *AJNR: American Journal of Neuroradiology*, *25*(9), 1575–1582. doi: 25/9/1575 [pii]

Nageswara Rao, A. A., & Packer, R. J. (2012). Impact of molecular biology studies on the understanding of brain tumors in childhood. *Current Oncology Reports*, *14*(2), 206–212. doi: 10.1007/s11912-012-0214-3

Necioglu Orken, D., Yldrmak, Y., Kenangil, G., Kandraloglu, N., Forta, H., & Celik, M. (2009). Intrathecal methotrexate-induced acute chorea. *Journal of Pediatric Hematology/Oncology*, *31*(1), 57–58.

Northcott, P. A., Korshunov, A., Pfister, S. M., & Taylor, M. D. (2012). The clinical implications of medulloblastoma subgroups. *Nature Reviews: Neurology*, *8*(6), 340–351. doi: 10.1038/nrneurol.2012.78

Northcott, P. A., Korshunov, A., Witt, H., Hielscher, T., Eberhart, C. G., Mack, S., . . . Taylor, M. D. (2011). Medulloblastoma comprises four distinct molecular variants. *Journal of Clinical Oncology*, *29*(11), 1408–1414. doi: 10.1200/JCO.2009.27.4324

Oeffinger, K. C., Mertens, A. C., Sklar, C. A., Kawashima, T., Hudson, M. M., Meadows, A. T., . . . Robison, L. L. (2006). Chronic health conditions in adult survivors of childhood cancer. *The New England Journal of Medicine*, *355*(15), 1572–1582. doi: 10.1056/NEJMsa060185

Ostrom, Q. T., de Blank, P. M., Kruchko, C., Petersen, C. M., Liao, P., Finlay, J. L., . . . Barnholtz-Sloan, J. S. (2015). Alex's Lemonade Stand Foundation infant and childhood primary brain and central nervous system tumors diagnosed in the United States in 2007–2011. *Neuro-Oncology*, *16*(Suppl 10), x1–x36. doi: 10.1093/neuonc/nou327

Packer, R. J., Gurney, J. G., Punyko, J. A., Donaldson, S. S., Inskip, P. D., Stovall, M., . . . Robison, L. L. (2003). Long-term neurologic and neurosensory sequelae in adult survivors of a childhood brain tumor: Childhood Cancer Survivor Study. *Journal of Clinical Oncology*, *21*(17 (Print)), 3255–3261.

Palmer, S. L. (2008). Neurodevelopmental impact on children treated for medulloblastoma: A review and proposed conceptual model. *Developmental Disabilities Research Reviews*, *14*(3), 203–210. doi: 10.1002/ddrr.32

Palmer, S. L., Armstrong, C., Onar-Thomas, A., Wu, S., Wallace, D., Bonner, M. J., . . . Gajjar, A. (2013). Processing speed, attention, and working memory after treatment for medulloblastoma: An international, prospective, and longitudinal study. *Journal of Clinical Oncology*, *31*(28), 3494–3500. doi: 10.1200/JCO.2012.47.4775

Palmer, S. L., Gajjar, A., Reddick, W. E., Glass, J. O., Kun, L. E., Wu, S., . . . Mulhern, R. K. (2003). Predicting intellectual outcome among children treated with 35–40 Gy craniospinal irradiation for medulloblastoma. *Neuropsychology*, *17*(4), 548–555.

Palmer, S. L., Goloubeva, O., Reddick, W. E., Glass, J. O., Gajjar, A., Kun, L., . . . Mulhern, R. K. (2001). Patterns of intellectual development among survivors of pediatric medulloblastoma: A longitudinal analysis. *Journal of Clinical Oncology*, *19*(8), 2302–2308.

Palmer, S. L., Hassall, T., Evankovich, K., Mabbott, D. J., Bonner, M., Deluca, C., . . . Gajjar, A. (2010). Neurocognitive outcome 12 months following cerebellar mutism syndrome in pediatric patients with medulloblastoma. *Neuro-Oncology*, *12*(12), 1311–1317. doi: 10.1093/neuonc/noq094

Papero, P. H., Pranzatelli, M. R., Margolis, L. J., Tate, E., Wilson, L. A., & Glass, P. (1995). Neurobehavioral and psychosocial functioning of children with opsoclonus-myoclonus syndrome. *Developmental Medicine and Child Neurology*, *37*(10), 915–932.

Pascoe, L., Roberts, G., Doyle, L. W., Lee, K. J., Thompson, D. K., Seal, M. L., . . . Anderson, P. J. (2013). Preventing academic difficulties in preterm children: A randomised controlled trial of an adaptive working memory training intervention—imprint study. *BMC Pediatrics*, *13*, 144. doi: 10.1186/1471-2431-13-144

Pereira, A. C., Huddleston, D. E., Brickman, A. M., Sosunov, A. A., Hen, R., McKhann, G. M., . . . Small, S. A. (2007). An in vivo correlate of exercise-induced neurogenesis in the adult dentate gyrus. *Proceedings of the National Academy of Sciences of the United States of America*, *104*(13), 5638–5643. doi: 10.1073/pnas.0611721104

Phillips, S. M., Padgett, L. S., Leisenring, W. M., Stratton, K. K., Bishop, K., Krull, K. R., . . . Mariotto, A. B. (2015). Survivors of childhood cancer in the United States: Prevalence and burden of morbidity. *Cancer Epidemiology, Biomarkers & Prevention: A Publication of the American Association for Cancer Research, Cosponsored by the American Society of Preventive Oncology*, *24*(4), 653–663. doi: 10.1158/1055-9965.EPI-14-1418

Pitsika, M., & Tsitouras, V. (2013). Cerebellar mutism. *Journal of Neurosurgery: Pediatrics*, *12*(6), 604–614. doi: 10.3171/2013.8.PEDS13168

Pizzo, P. A., & Poplack, D. G. (2006). *Principles and Practice of Pediatric Oncology* (5th ed.). Philadelphia, PA: Lippincott Williams & Wilkins.

Pollack, I. F. (1997). Posterior fossa syndrome. *International Review of Neurobiology*, *41*, 411–432.

Pollack, I. F., Jakacki, R. I., Butterfield, L. H., & Okada, H. (2013). Ependymomas: Development of immunotherapeutic strategies. *Expert Review of Neurotherapeutics*, *13*(10), 1089–1098. doi: 10.1586/14737175.2013.840420

Pound, C. M., Clark, C., Ni, A., Athale, U., Lewis, V., & Halton, J. M. (2012). Corticosteroids, behavior, and quality of life in children treated for acute lymphoblastic leukemia; a multicentered trial. *Journal of Pediatric Hematology/Oncology*, *34*(7), 517–523. doi: 10.1097/MPH.0b013e318257fdac

Pranzatelli, M. R., Tate, E. D., Dukart, W. S., Flint, M. J., Hoffman, M. T., & Oksa, A. E. (2005). Sleep disturbance and rage attacks in opsoclonus-myoclonus syndrome: Response to trazodone. *The Journal of Pediatrics*, *147*(3), 372–378. doi: 10.1016/j.jpeds.2005.05.016

Preston-Martin, S. (1996). Epidemiology of primary CNS neoplasms. *Neurologic Clinics*, *14*(2), 273–290.

Pui, C. H., Carroll, W. L., Meshinchi, S., & Arceci, R. J. (2011). Biology, risk stratification, and therapy of pediatric acute leukemias: An update. *Journal of Clinical Oncology*, *29*(5), 551–565. doi: 10.1200/JCO.2010.30.7405

Pui, C. H., & Evans, W. E. (2006). Treatment of acute lymphoblastic leukemia. *The New England Journal of Medicine*, *354*(2), 166–178. doi: 10.1056/NEJMra052603

Pui, C. H., & Howard, S. C. (2008). Current management and challenges of malignant disease in the CNS in paediatric leukaemia. [review] [83 refs]. *Lancet Oncology*, *9*(3), 257–268.

Pui, C. H., Relling, M. V., & Downing, J. R. (2004). Acute lymphoblastic leukemia. *The New England Journal of Medicine*, *350*(15), 1535–1548. doi: 10.1056/NEJMra023001

Reddick, W. E., Glass, J. O., Helton, K. J., Langston, J. W., Xiong, X., Wu, S., & Pui, C. H. (2005). Prevalence of leukoencephalopathy in children treated for acute lymphoblastic leukemia with high-dose methotrexate. *AJNR: American Journal of Neuroradiology*, *26*(5), 1263–1269.

Reddick, W. E., Glass, J. O., Palmer, S. L., Wu, S., Gajjar, A., Langston, J. W., . . . Mulhern, R. K. (2005). Atypical white matter volume development in children following craniospinal irradiation. *Neuro-Oncology*, *7*(1), 12–19.

Reddick, W. E., Shan, Z. Y., Glass, J. O., Helton, S., Xiong, X., Wu, S., . . . Mulhern, R. K. (2006a). Smaller white-matter volumes are associated with larger deficits in attention and learning among long-term survivors of acute lymphoblastic leukemia. *Cancer*, *106*(4), 941–949.

Reddick, W. E., Shan, Z. Y., Glass, J. O., Helton, S., Xiong, X., Wu, S., . . . Mulhern, R. K. (2006b). Smaller white-matter volumes are associated with larger deficits in attention and learning among long-term survivors of acute lymphoblastic leukemia. *Cancer*, *106*(4), 941–949.

Reddick, W. E., Taghipour, D. J., Glass, J. O., Ashford, J., Xiong, X., Wu, S., . . . Conklin, H. M. (2014). Prognostic factors that increase the risk for reduced white matter volumes and deficits in attention and learning for survivors of childhood cancers. *Pediatric Blood & Cancer*, *61*(6), 1074–1079. doi: 10.1002/pbc.24947

Reddick, W. E., White, H., Glass, J. O., Wheeler, G., Thompson, S., Gajjar, A., . . . Mulhern, R. K. (2003a). Neurodevelopmental model relating white matter volume to neurocognitive deficits in pediatric brain tumor survivors. *Cancer Chemotherapy and Pharmacology*, *97*, 2512–2519.

Reddick, W. E., White, H. A., Glass, J. O., Wheeler, G. C., Thompson, S. J., Gajjar, A., . . . Mulhern, R. K. (2003b). Developmental model relating white matter volume to neurocognitive deficits in pediatric brain tumor survivors. *Cancer*, *97*(10), 2512–2519.

Reed-Berendt, R., Phillips, B., Picton, S., Chumas, P., Warren, D., Livingston, J., . . . Morrall, M.H.J. (2014). Cause and outcome of cerebellar mutism: Evidence from a systematic review. *Child's Nervous System*, *30*(3), 375–385. doi: 10.1007/s00381-014-2356-0

Reimers, T. S., Ehrenfels, S., Mortensen, E. L., Schmiegelow, M., Sonderkaer, S., Carstensen, H., . . . Muller, J. (2003). Cognitive deficits in long-term survivors of childhood brain tumors: Identification of predictive factors. *Medical and Pediatric Oncology*, *40*(1), 26–34.

Riggs, L., Piscione, J., Bouffet, E., Timmons, B., Laughlin, S., Cunningham, T., . . . Mabbott, D. J. (2014). *Exercise increases hippocampal volume in children treated with cranial radiation.* Paper presented at the 16th International Symposium on Pediatric Neuro-Oncology, Singapore.

Ris, M. D. (2014). Personal communication.

Ris, M. D., Beebe, D. W., Armstrong, F. D., Fontanesi, J., Holmes, E., Sanford, R. A., & Wisoff, J. H. (2008). Cognitive and adaptive outcome in extracerebellar low-grade brain tumors in children: A report from the children's oncology group. *Journal of Clinical Oncology*, *26*(29), 4765–4770. doi: JCO.2008.17.1371 [pii] 10.1200/JCO.2008.17.1371

Ris, M. D., & Hisock, M. (2013). Modeling cognitive aging following early CNS injury: Reserve and the Flynn effect. In I. S. Baron & C. Rey-Casserly (Eds.), *Pediatric Neuropsychology: Medical Advances and Lifespan Outcomes* (pp. 395–422). New York: Oxford University Press.

Ris, M. D., Packer, R. J., Goldwein, J., Jones-Wallace, D., & Boyett, J. M. (2001). Intellectual outcome after reduced-dose radiation therapy plus adjuvant chemotherapy for medulloblastoma: A Children's Cancer Group study. *Journal of Clinical Oncology*, *19*(15), 3470–3476.

Ris, M. D., Walsh, K., Wallace, D., Armstrong, F. D., Holmes, E., Gajjar, A., . . . Packer, R. J. (2013). Intellectual and academic outcome following two chemotherapy regimens and radiotherapy for average-risk medulloblastoma: COG A9961. *Pediatric Blood & Cancer*, *60*(8), 1350–1357. doi: 10.1002/pbc.24496

Robertson, P. L., Muraszko, K. M., Holmes, E. J., Sposto, R., Packer, R. J., Gajjar, A., . . . Allen, J. C. (2006). Incidence and severity of postoperative cerebellar mutism syndrome in children with medulloblastoma: A prospective study by the children's oncology group. *Journal of Neurosurgery*, *105*(6), 444–451.

Robison, L. L., Green, D. M., Hudson, M., Meadows, A. T., Mertens, A. C., Packer, R. J., . . . Zeltzer, L. K. (2005). Long-term outcomes of adult survivors of childhood cancer. *Cancer*, *104*(11 Suppl (Print)), 2557–2564.

Robison, L. L., Mertens, A. C., Boice, J. D., Breslow, N. E., Donaldson, S. S., Green, D. M., . . . Zeltzer, L. K. (2002). Study design and cohort characteristics of the childhood cancer survivor study: A multi-institutional collaborative project. *Medical & Pediatric Oncology*, *38*(4), 229–239.

Rodgers, J., Britton, P. G., Kernahan, J., & Craft, A. W. (1991). Cognitive function after two doses of cranial irradiation for acute lymphoblastic leukaemia. *Archives of Disease in Childhood*, *66*, 1245–1246.

Rodgers, S. P., Trevino, M., Zawaski, J. A., Gaber, M. W., & Leasure, J. L. (2013). Neurogenesis, exercise, and cognitive late effects of pediatric radiotherapy. *Neural Plasticity*, *2013*, 12. doi: 10.1155/2013/698528

Roncadin, C., Dennis, M., Greenberg, M. L., & Spiegler, B. J. (2008). Adverse medical events associated with childhood cerebellar astrocytomas and medulloblastomas: Natural history and relation to very long-term neurobehavioral outcome. *Child's Nervous System*, *24*(9), 995–1002; discussion 1003. doi: 10.1007/s00381-008-0658-9

Roncadin, C., Hitzler, J., Downie, A., Montour-Proulx, I., Alyman, C., Cairney, E., & Spiegler, B. J. (2014). Neuropsychological late effects of treatment for acute leukemia in children with Down syndrome. *Pediatric Blood & Cancer*, *62*(5), 854–858. doi: 10.1002/pbc.25362

Rubenstein, C. L., Varni, J. W., & Katz, E. R. (1990). Cognitive functioning in long-term survivors of childhood leukemia: A prospective analysis. *Journal of Developmental and Behavioral Pediatrics*, *11*(6), 301–305.

Rudnick, E., Khakoo, Y., Antunes, N. L., Seeger, R. C., Brodeur, G. M., Shimada, H., . . . Matthay, K. K. (2001). Opsoclonus-myoclonus-ataxia syndrome in neuroblastoma: Clinical outcome and antineuronal antibodies-a report from the children's cancer group study. *Medical and Pediatric Oncology*, *36*(6), 612–622. doi: 10.1002/mpo.1138

Rueckriegel, S. M., Driever, P. H., Blankenburg, F., Lüdemann, L., Henze, G., & Bruhn, H. (2010). Differences in supratentorial damage of white matter in pediatric survivors of posterior fossa tumors with and without adjuvant treatment as detected by magnetic resonance diffusion tensor imaging. *International Journal of Radiation Oncology, Biology, Physics*, *76*(3), 859–866. doi: 10.1016/j.ijrobp.2009.02.054

Rueegg, C. S., Michel, G., Wengenroth, L., von der Weid, N. X., Bergstraesser, E., & Kuehni, C. E. (2012). Physical performance limitations in adolescent and adult survivors of childhood cancer and their siblings. *PLoS One*, *7*(10), e47944. doi: 10.1371/journal.pone.0047944

Russo, C., Cohn, S. L., Petruzzi, M. J., & de Alarcon, P. A. (1997). Long-term neurologic outcome in children with opsoclonus-myoclonus associated with neuroblastoma: A report from the pediatric oncology group. *Medical and Pediatric Oncology*, *28*(4), 284–288.

Rutkowski, S., Bode, U., Deinlein, F., Ottensmeier, H., Warmuth-Metz, M., Soerensen, N., . . . Kuehl, J. (2005). Treatment of early childhood medulloblastoma by postoperative chemotherapy alone. *The New England Journal of Medicine*, *352*(10), 978–986.

Rutkowski, S., Cohen, B., Finlay, J., Luksch, R., Ridola, V., Valteau-Couanet, D., . . . Grill, J. (2010). Medulloblastoma in young children. *Pediatric Blood & Cancer*, *54*(4), 635–637. doi: 10.1002/pbc.22372

Schatz, J., Kramer, J. H., Ablin, A., & Matthay, K. (2000). Processing speed, working memory, and IQ: A developmental model of cognitive deficits following cranial radiation therapy. *Neuropsychology*, *14*(2), 189–200.

Schmahmann, J. D., & Sherman, J. C. (1998). The cerebellar cognitive affective syndrome. *Brain*, *121*(4), 561–579. doi: 10.1093/brain/121.4.561

Schuitema, I., Deprez, S., Van Hecke, W., Daams, M., Uyttebroeck, A., Sunaert, S., . . . de Sonneville, L. M. (2013). Accelerated aging, decreased white matter integrity, and associated neuropsychological dysfunction 25 years after pediatric lymphoid malignancies. *Journal of Clinical Oncology*, *31*(27), 3378–3388.

Schulte, F., & Barrera, M. (2010). Social competence in childhood brain tumor survivors: A comprehensive review. *Supportive Care in Cancer: Official Journal of the Multinational Association of Supportive Care in Cancer*, *18*(12), 1499–1513. doi: 10.1007/s00520-010-0963-1

Schulte, F., Bartels, U., & Barrera, M. (2014). A pilot study evaluating the efficacy of a group social skills program for survivors of childhood central nervous system tumors using a comparison group and teacher reports. *Psycho-Oncology*, *23*(5), 597–600. doi: 10.1002/pon.3472

Schulte, F., Vannatta, K., & Barrera, M. (2014). Social problem solving and social performance after a group social skills intervention for childhood brain tumor survivors. *Psycho-Oncology*, *23*(2), 183–189. doi: 10.1002/pon.3387

Shih, H. A., Loeffler, J. S., & Tarbell, N. (2009). Late effects of CNS radiation therapy. In S. Goldman & C. D. Turner (Eds.), *Late Effects of Treatment for Brain Tumors* (pp. 23–41). New York: Springer.

Simone, J. V. (2006). History of the treatment of childhood ALL: A paradigm for cancer cure. *Best Practice & Research: Clinical Haematology*, *19*(2), 353–359. doi: 10.1016/j.beha.2005.11.003

Smibert, E., Anderson, V., Godber, T., & Ekert, H. (1996). Risk factors for intellectual and educational sequelae of cranial irradiation in childhood acute lymphoblastic leukaemia. *British Journal of Cancer*, *73*, 825–830.

Smithson, E. F., Phillips, R., Harvey, D. W., & Morrall, M. C. (2013). The use of stimulant medication to improve neurocognitive and learning outcomes in children diagnosed with brain tumours: A systematic review. *European Journal of Cancer*, *49*(14), 3029–3040. doi: 10.1016/j.ejca.2013.05.023

Spiegler, B. J., Kennedy, K., Maze, R., Greenberg, M. L., Weitzman, S., Hitzler, J. K., & Nathan, P. C. (2006). Comparison of long-term neurocognitive outcomes in young children with acute lymphoblastic leukemia treated with cranial radiation or high-dose or very high-dose intravenous methotrexate. *Journal of Clinical Oncology*, *24*(24), 3858–3864. doi: 10.1200/JCO.2006.05.9055

Stern, Y. (2009). Cognitive reserve. *Neuropsychologia*, *47*(10), 2015–2028. doi: 10.1016/j.neuropsychologia.2009.03.004

Summers, R. J., Abramowsky, C. R., & Cooper, T. M. (2014). Correlating pathology with the clinical symptoms of methotrexate-induced leukoencephalopathy in a child with relapsed T-cell acute lymphoblastic leukemia. *Journal of Pediatric Hematology/Oncology*, *36*(1), e19–e22.

Taylor, H. G., Albo, V. C., Phebus, C. K., Sachs, B. R., & Bierl, P. G. (1987). Postirradiation treatment outcomes for children with acute lymphocytic leukemia: Clarification of risks. *Journal of Pediatric Psychology*, *12*(3), 395–411.

Taylor, M. D., Northcott, P. A., Korshunov, A., Remke, M., Cho, Y. J., Clifford, S. C., . . . Pfister, S. M. (2012). Molecular subgroups of medulloblastoma: The current consensus. *Acta Neuropathologica*, *123*(4), 465–472. doi: 10.1007/s00401-011-0922-z

Thompson, S. J., Leigh, L., Christensen, R., Xiong, X., Kun, L. E., Heideman, R. L., . . . Mulhern, R. K. (2001). Immediate neurocognitive effects of methylphenidate on learning-impaired survivors of childhood cancer. *Journal of Clinical Oncology*, *19*(6), 1802–1808.

Thorp, N. J., & Taylor, R. E. (2014). Management of central nervous system tumours in children. *Clinical Oncology*, *26*(7), 438–445. doi: 10.1016/j.clon.2014.04.029

Torres, C. F., Korones, D. N., Palumbo, D. R., Wissler, K. H., Valdasz, E., & Cox, C. (1996). Effect of methylphenidate in the post-radiation attention and memory deficits in children. *Annals of Neurology*, *40*, 331–332.

Tufekci, O., Yilmaz, S., Karapinar, T. H., Gozmen, S., Cakmakci, H., Hiz, S., . . . Oren, H. (2011). A rare complication of intrathecal methotrexate in a child with acute lymphoblastic leukemia. *Pediatric Hematology & Oncology*, *28*(6), 517–522.

Turkel, S. B., Brumm, V. L., Mitchell, W. G., & Tavare, C. J. (2006). Mood and behavioral dysfunction with opsoclonus-myoclonus ataxia. *The Journal of Neuropsychiatry and Clinical Neurosciences*, *18*(2), 239–241. doi: 10.1176/appi.neuropsych.18.2.239

Turner, C. D., Chordas, C. A., Liptak, C. C., Rey-Casserly, C., Delaney, B. L., Ullrich, N. J., . . . Kieran, M. W. (2009). Medical, psychological, cognitive and educational late-effects in pediatric low-grade glioma survivors treated with surgery only. *Pediatric Blood & Cancer*, *53*(3), 417–423. doi: 10.1002/pbc.22081

Ullrich, N. J., Scott, R. M., & Pomeroy, S. L. (2005). Craniopharyngioma therapy: Long-term effects on hypothalamic function. *The Neurologist*, *11*(1 (Print)), 55–60.

U.S. Cancer Statistics Working Group. (2014). *U.S. Cancer Statistics: 1999–2011 Incidence and Mortality Web-Based Report.* Retrieved from www.cdc.gov/uscs.

Van Poppel, M., Klimo, P., Jr., Dewire, M., Sanford, R. A., Boop, F., Broniscer, A., . . . Gajjar, A. J. (2011). Resection of infantile brain tumors after neoadjuvant chemotherapy: The St. Jude experience. *Journal of Neurosurgery: Pediatrics*, *8*(3), 251–256. doi: 10.3171/2011.6.PEDS11158

Vannatta, K., Fairclough, F., Farkas-Patenaude, A., Gerhardt, C., Kupst, M., Olshefski, R., . . . Turner, C. (2008). *Peer relationships of pediatric brain tumor survivors.* Paper presented at 13th International Symposium on Pediatric Neuro-Oncology, Chicago, IL.

Vannatta, K., Gartstein, M. A., Short, A., & Noll, R. B. (1998). A controlled study of peer relationships of children surviving brain tumors: Teacher, peer, and self ratings. *Journal of Pediatric Psychology*, *23*(5), 279–287.

Vannatta, K., Gerhardt, C. A., Wells, R. J., & Noll, R. B. (2007). Intensity of CNS treatment for pediatric cancer: Prediction of social outcomes in survivors. *Pediatric Blood & Cancer*, *49*(5), 716–722. doi: 10.1002/pbc.21062

von Hoff, K., Kieffer, V., Habrand, J. L., Kalifa, C., Dellatolas, G., & Grill, J. (2008). Impairment of intellectual functions after surgery and posterior fossa irradiation in children with ependymoma is related to age and neurologic complications. *BMC Cancer*, *8*, 15. doi: 10.1186/1471-2407-8-15

Waber, D. P., Pomeroy, S. L., Chiverton, A. M., Kieran, M. W., Scott, R. M., Goumnerova, L. C., & Rivkin, M. J. (2006). Everyday cognitive function after craniopharyngioma in childhood. *Pediatric Neurology*, *34*(1), 13–19.

Waber, D. P., & Tarbell, N. J. (1997). Toxicity of CNS prophylaxis for childhood leukemia. *Oncology*, *11*(2), 259–264; discussion 264–255.

Waber, D. P., Tarbell, N. J., Fairclough, D., Atmore, K., Castro, R., Isquith, P., . . . Schiller, M.E.A. (1995). Cognitive sequelae of treatment in childhood acute lymphoblastic leukemia: Cranial radiation requires an accomplice. *Journal of Clinical Oncology*, *13*(10), 2490–2496.

Waber, D. P., Tarbell, N. J., Kahn, C. M., Gelber, R. D., & Sallan, S. E. (1992). The relationship of sex and treatment modality to neuropsychologic outcome in childhood acute lymphoblastic leukemia. *Journal of Clinical Oncology*, *10*(5), 810–817.

Waber, D. P., Urion, D. K., Tarbell, N. J., Niemeyer, C., Gelber, R., & Sallan, S. E. (1990). Late effects of central nervous system treatment of acute lymphoblastic leukemia in childhood are sex-dependent. *Developmental Medicine and Child Neurology*, *32*(3), 238–248.

Windebank, K. P., & Spinetta, J. J. (2008). Do as I say or die: Compliance in adolescents with cancer. *Pediatric Blood & Cancer*, *50*(5 Suppl), 1099–1100. doi: 10.1002/pbc.21460

Winter, A. L., Conklin, H. M., Tyc, V. L., Stancel, H., Hinds, P. S., Hudson, M. M., & Kahalley, L. S. (2014). Executive function late effects in survivors of pediatric brain tumors and acute lymphoblastic leukemia. *Journal of Clinical and Experimental Neuropsychology*, *36*(8), 818–830. doi: 10.1080/13803395.2014.943695

Wolfe, K. R., Walsh, K. S., Reynolds, N. C., Mitchell, F., Reddy, A. T., Paltin, I., & Madan-Swain, A. (2012). Executive functions and social skills in survivors of pediatric brain tumor. *Child Neuropsychology*, *19*(4), 370–384. doi: 10.1080/09297049.2012.669470

Zada, G., Kintz, N., Pulido, M., & Amezcua, L. (2013). Prevalence of neurobehavioral, social, and emotional dysfunction in patients treated for childhood craniopharyngioma: A systematic literature review. *PloS One*, *8*(11), e76562. doi: 10.1371/journal.pone.0076562

Zygourakis, C. C., Kaur, G., Kunwar, S., McDermott, M. W., Madden, M., Oh, T., & Parsa, A. T. (2014). Modern treatment of 84 newly diagnosed craniopharyngiomas. *Journal of Clinical Neuroscience: Official Journal of the Neurosurgical Society of Australasia*, *21*(9), 1558–1566. doi: 10.1016/j.jocn.2014.03.005

13 Autism Spectrum Disorder

Gerry A. Stefanatos and Deborah Fein

Introduction and Definition

Although the behaviors associated with autism have been noted for centuries (Houston & Frith, 2002; Wolff, 2004), its recognition as a discrete disorder occurred only decades ago, based on Leo Kanner's (1943) seminal description of 11 children evaluated at Johns Hopkins University clinics. Kanner meticulously outlined a behavioral symptom-complex shared by these children that he felt differentiated their condition from other recognized forms of childhood psychopathology. The predominant characteristic was *marked difficulties in relating to other people and situations in a normal manner*. This was reflected in striking limitations of social awareness and a relative disregard for the people around them. The children often acted "as if people weren't there," (p. 223) seemed "happiest when left alone," (p. 218) or displayed an inordinate interest in objects and pictures that seemed to eclipse their interest in people. Indeed, Kanner remarked that one 5-year-old "did not pay even the slightest attention to Santa Claus in full regalia." (p. 218) Secondly, the children demonstrated an *anxiously obsessive desire for the maintenance of sameness*, manifested in repetitive and stereotyped behaviors, and negative reactions to changes in routines or their environment. A third core feature, *unusual or impaired use of language for interpersonal communication*, was reflected in verbal communications that were marked by echolalic utterances, stereotyped language, and a tendency to reverse personal pronouns ("I" for "you"). By parent history, behavioral anomalies had been evident in infancy and toddlerhood and had persisted through subsequent stages of development. Kanner recognized that the extreme aloneness, obsessiveness, stereotyped behaviors and echolalia resembled childhood-onset schizophrenia. However, he reasoned that his cohort did not fit this diagnosis because their symptoms were evident "from the very beginning of life" (p. 248). He therefore conjectured that their symptom-complex represented a separate disorder which he subsequently dubbed *early infantile autism* (Kanner, 1944).

Characterizations of the core features of autism have varied considerably since its initial description, and establishing reliable diagnostic criteria has proven difficult. The development of an acceptable diagnostic algorithm and classification scheme has entailed a reiterative process of formulation, evaluation, and revision that has continued to the present day (Wing, Gould, & Gillberg, 2011). Accordingly, the nomenclature and diagnostic criteria outlined in the current American Psychiatric Association's *Diagnostic and Statistical Manual*, fifth edition (DSM-5; APA, 2013) differs in substantive ways from previous iterations. Autism is no longer presented as a categorical designation diagnosis with defined boundaries to separate it from similar diagnostic entities such as Asperger's disorder, childhood disintegrative disorder, and pervasive developmental disorder–not otherwise specified. Instead, DSM-5 has merged these subtypes into a single category called *autism spectrum disorder* (ASD). This somewhat controversial reframing reflects an ongoing "revolution" (Rutter, 2013) in conceptualizing autism, its diverse manifestations, and its diagnosis. Explicit in this integrated view is the notion that ASD is not a single, unified disorder but is instead a collection of disorders that reflect the diverse consequences of functional compromise of neural networks involved in the development of social communication, and appropriately flexible and diverse thinking and behavior.

A prodigious amount of research has been directed towards ASD in recent years. The search for a simple etiology has been abandoned in the face of overwhelming evidence of multiple pathogenetic pathways, with many or most involving a complex interplay of several genetic and environmental risk factors. Neurodevelopmental anomalies have been identified at numerous levels of neural structure and function, from cytoarchitecture and neurochemistry to gross neuroanatomy, electrophysiology, and regional cerebral metabolism. Efforts to understand these alterations and their association to potential etiopathogenetic mechanisms now span numerous scientific disciplines, from molecular genetics to immunology and gastroenterology. The extant literature on ASD is enormous, remarkably diverse and expanding at a formidable and somewhat daunting rate.

In this chapter, we constrain our discussion of ASD to a selective review of topics of greatest relevance to theory and practice in neuropsychology. We begin with a brief review of the changes in the diagnostic criteria set forth in DSM-5 and their implications for clinical practice. This is followed by a cursory overview of the epidemiology of ASD in which we survey evidence suggesting an alarming increase in prevalence. Sections on etiology summarize some of the complex and diverse factors thought to increase risk for the diagnosis. We then consider the latest advances in our understanding of the neurobiological basis and neuropsychological correlates of the disorder. More comprehensive coverage of ASD is available to the interested reader in edited volumes by Amaral, Geschwind, and Dawson (2011); Volkmar (2013); Patel, Preedy, and Martin (2014), each more than 1,400 pages in length. Alternatively, Reber (2012) provides a concise discussion of the biological foundations of the disorder and practical discussions regarding its treatment. In addition, excellent reviews of the neuroscience and neuropsychology of autism are available in volumes edited by Fein (2011) and Buxbaum and Hof (2012).

Comparative Nosology—Refining the Diagnosis of ASD

Autism has proven to be one of the most complex and enigmatic forms of developmental psychopathology to define, in part because of the substantial diversity in its expression. Given that it emerges in infancy or early childhood and is a lifelong disorder, the symptoms vary considerably in their manifestations, severity, specificity, and developmental course, resulting in marked variation across individuals and within individuals over time. Furthermore, the diversity in early clinical presentation does not map in any straightforward way onto the heterogeneity in genetic findings, family history, outcome, or neuroimaging results. Even the heterogeneity in one area of function, such as language, does not seem to map easily onto heterogeneity in other areas, such as social functioning (Rapin, 2014; Waterhouse, 2013).

This diversity has greatly complicated the development of a widely accepted and broadly applicable classification scheme and diagnostic algorithm to identify the disorder and differentiate it from other similar disorders (Wing et al., 2011). Kanner waited more than a decade after his original description before he delineated the facets of the disorder that he believed all patients had in common and could be used for diagnostic purposes. He settled on "extreme self-isolation" and "obsessive insistence on the preservation of sameness" as the two key features of the disorder (Eisenberg & Kanner, 1956, p. 557). However, from a diagnostic standpoint, these characteristics failed to define a unique or homogeneous population, and disagreements regarding the definition and validity of infantile autism as a distinct clinical entity ensued for over two decades.

Rutter (1978) and Wing and Gould (1979) conceptualized three core areas of deficit in autism often referred to as the *autism triad*: (a) social interaction, (b) communication, and (c) rigid and repetitive activities and interests. These formulations guided the delineation of the diagnostic criteria for *infantile autism* when it was first incorporated as a distinct diagnosis in the American Psychiatric Association's *Diagnostic and Statistical Manual of Mental Disorders, Third Edition* (DSM-III; APA, 1980). The Diagnostic Statistical Manual-III criteria were associated with high sensitivity but low specificity, while revisions implemented in DSM-III-R (APA, 1987) resulted in the opposite pattern.

Modifications incorporated in the *Diagnostic and Statistical Manual of Mental Disorders, Fourth Edition* (DSM-IV; APA, 1994) and carried over to the *Diagnostic and Statistical Manual of Mental Disorders, Fourth Edition, Text Revision* (DSM-IV-TR; APA, 2000) marked a substantial change over previous iterations. Autistic disorder (AD) was conceived as one of five diagnoses in a broader category entitled *Pervasive Developmental Disorder* (PDD). The inception of the PDD category was intended to provide a supraordinate framework within which the heterogenous clinical presentations of AD and closely related disorders could be parsed into distinguishable, clinically meaningful diagnostic entities on the basis of differences in patterns of behavioral symptoms, their severity, and age of presentation. Besides AD, the category included Asperger's Disorder (AspD), Childhood Disintegrative Disorder (CDD), Rett's Disorder (RD), and a nonspecific diagnosis entitled *Pervasive Developmental Disorder–Not Otherwise Specified* (PDD-NOS).

The diagnostic criteria for AD were based on 12 separate symptoms spanning the three domains of the autism triad. To meet criteria for the disorder, a child needed to exhibit six or more of these symptoms, with at least two symptoms involving impairments in the *social interaction* domain and at least one symptom from each of the remaining two domains (*communication, restrictive/stereotyped behaviors and interests*). The onset of symptoms had to occur before 3 years of age in at least one of these three areas. This schema resulted in good sensitivity (.91) and specificity (.53) for the AD diagnosis. However, it was criticized as being too static, of questionable help in diagnosing infants, young children, and adults, and difficult to apply consistently across different clinical practices and treatment centers (Leekam, Libby, Wing, Gould, & Gillberg, 2000; Wing et al., 2011). These shortcomings were largely related to the failure of the scheme to adequately accommodate differences in the clinical picture that occurred as a function of age, gender, or different environments.

In addition, problems surrounded the definition and criteria used for the other disorders comprising the PDD category. Specifically, RD (a progressive disorder) did not seem to fit the category, while others such as AspD and PDD-NOS had relatively poor specificity (0.34 and 0.24, respectively). Moreover, the boundaries differentiating the disorders sometimes seemed arbitrary with no clear guidelines on how to operationalize them. Miller and Ozonoff (1997), for example, pointed out that none of the original cases described by Asperger (1944) met DSM-IV criteria for AspD, but instead would be diagnosed with AD. Similarly, questions arose as to whether the proposed criteria could reliably distinguish CDD from AD because of issues concerning the age of onset (Hendry, 2000). In view of clinician dissatisfaction with the DSM-IV scheme and a perceived lack of robust, replicated evidence to support some of the diagnostic distinctions, the term *autistic spectrum disorder* (Allen, 1988) came into increasingly common usage to refer collectively to AD and the closely related disorders such as AspD and PDD-NOS.

Current Criteria for Diagnosis and Classification

The diagnostic framework recently outlined in DSM-5 (APA, 2013) differs from previous iterations in several important respects. In order to avert some of the diagnostic boundary issues discussed in the last section, DSM-5 eliminated the supraordinate category of (PDD) and its associated subtypes (AD, AspD, CDD, PDD-NOS), and instead, defined a single category: ASD. RD has been excluded entirely from this new category due to recognition of its clear genetic basis (Amir et al., 1999).

This reorganization has been accompanied by a restructuring of the domains of behavior covered by the symptom checklist. While DSM-IV-TR treated social and communication impairments as separate domains, DSM-5 has combined them into a single domain entitled *social communication.* Accordingly, children must demonstrate persistent impairment from early childhood in two domains: (a) social communication (SC) and (b) restricted, repetitive patterns of behaviors and interests or activities (RRBIA). Factor analytic studies have shown that these domains emerge as separable factors (Frazier et al., 2012; Mandy, Charman, & Skuse, 2012).

An important aspect of this reorganization is that disorders of language development are treated as separate from ASD. Correspondingly, an individual can have ASD with or without a coexisting language disorder. If present, the language disorder is coded separately. Deficiencies in particular aspects of language use that have long been strongly associated with AD continue to be reflected in the new diagnostic criteria, but have been reallocated to the most appropriate SC or RRBIA symptom category. For example, the inability to have a normal conversation, which reflect problems with the pragmatic or social use of language, is included under SC. By contrast, stereotyped language, such as pedantic speech and echolalia, is now found under RRBIA. Other common comorbid disorders where separate coding is now permitted include Attention Deficit/Hyperactivity Disorder (ADHD) and Intellectual Disability (ID).

The symptom list has also been consolidated so that the number of symptoms required to meet the diagnostic criteria has been reduced from the twelve in DSM-IV-TR to seven in DSM-5. Some of these describe more general principles and behaviors. In addition, the age of onset criteria have been relaxed. While symptoms should be present early in childhood, it is recognized that they may not fully manifest until demand characteristics increase later in development. Endorsement of symptoms on the diagnostic checklist can be made on the basis of current presentation or by history so that symptoms are scored on the basis of lifetime occurrence.

Symptoms must be present across multiple contexts and be clearly atypical from a developmental perspective. Hand flapping, for example, would not necessarily be considered atypical if seen only between 6 to 9 months of age or within a somewhat later temporal window in a child with general developmental delays. In general, the same behavior should not be utilized as an exemplar to satisfy two criteria. In order to mitigate overly strict application, the DSM-5 manual explicitly states that the given examples are illustrative and not exhaustive, and that some symptoms may be masked by strategies learned later in life. Finally, and importantly, in recognition of the dimensional nature of ASD, the diagnostic criteria are accompanied by a severity scale in order to capture the substantial variation in the degree of impairment that characterizes this population. This is operationalized in a three-point classification system according to the level of support a child requires : “support,” “substantial support,” or “very substantial support.” As these indicators are new and were not evaluated prior to their inclusion in DSM-5, it remains unclear how well they will function in clinical practice (Lord & Bishop, 2015).

Interestingly, there is less flexibility allowed in scoring the diagnostic checklist in DSM-5. Within each behavioral domain, the symptom checklist is divided into subdomains: there are three subdomains of SC and four subdomains of RRBIA. In order to meet criteria for the diagnosis, a child must demonstrate symptoms in all three of the SC subdomains and in at least two of the four subdomains of RRBIA. An outline of the key domains of impairment, subdomain symptoms, and criteria is provided in the left-hand column of Table 13.1; the right column lists some of the corresponding early behavioral markers that have been identified in infancy and childhood. A narrative description relevant to the contents of the table is provided in next section.

Social Communication

SC has long been recognized as a cardinal area of impairment in ASD. The DSM-5 criteria pertaining to SC require that individuals demonstrate impairment in social-emotional reciprocity that is persistent and apparent across multiple contexts. Impairment must be evident in *each* of the following three subdomains: (a) deficits in social approach, (b) deficits in nonverbal communicative behaviors used for social interaction, and (b) deficits in developing and maintaining relationships (see Table 13.1, section A, subsections 1, 2, and 3 respectively in the left column).

Deficits in the first subdomain, social approach, can include abnormal social initiation, approach, and responsiveness. Children may fail to approach other individuals to engage them socially or may be inappropriately disinhibited or indiscriminative in approach (e.g., with strangers). Similarly, they may fail to respond appropriately to social overtures. Deficits may also be apparent in an inability to maintain normal back-and-forth conversation (poor pragmatics), reduced or absent social interest, or a lack in sharing thoughts, interests, and emotions/affect.

Table 13.1 DSM-5 diagnostic criteria for ASD with extension to infants and toddlers

Must meet DSM-5 diagnostic criteria A, B, C, and D

A. *Persistent deficits in social communication and social interaction across multiple contexts, as manifested by the following, currently or by history (examples are illustrative, not exhaustive, see text).*

DSM-5 criteria (SC) (must include problems in all three areas)	*Behaviors at 2 Years or Earlier*
1. Deficits in social-emotional reciprocity, ranging, for example, from abnormal social approach and failure of normal back-and-forth conversation; to reduced sharing of interests, emotions, or affect; to failure to initiate or respond to social interactions. 2. Deficits in nonverbal communicative behaviors used for social interaction ranging, for example, from poorly integrated verbal and nonverbal communication, to abnormalities in eye contact and body language or deficits in understanding and use of gestures, to a total lack of facial expressions and nonverbal communication. 3. Deficits in developing, maintaining, and understanding relationships ranging, for example, from difficulties adjusting behavior to suit various social contexts, to difficulties in sharing imaginative play or in making friends, to absence of interest in peers.	• Poor eye contact • Failure to follow gaze • Lack of directed vocalizations (e.g., social babbling) • A lack of pointing to express interest or a lack of spontaneous pointing • Does not follow pointing by others • Failure to produce or understand gestures (e.g., head nodding, waving, pointing, showing) • Lack of initiation of joint attention (e.g., look at what I have, look at what I'm doing) • Ignores activities of others • Failure to respond to name being called • Failure to produce or understand facial expressions • Limited social smiling • Failure to show an interest in others and in sharing enjoyment (e.g., tickling) • Lack of social overtures (e.g., showing things of interest, requesting) • Atypical response to others' emotions, facial affect, unusual reactivity • Limited social play (e.g., peekaboo, pat-a-cake) • Poor rapport, appears disinterested or disconnected in social interactions • Lack of interest in other toddlers • No interest in simple pretend play (e.g., pretending to talk into a toy telephone, put a baby doll in bed, feed a stuffed animal)

B. *Restricted, repetitive patterns of behavior, interests, or activities, as manifested by at least two of the following, currently or by history (examples are illustrative, not exhaustive; see text).*

DSM-5 criteria (RRBIA) (must have problems in at least two areas)	*Behaviors at 2 Years or Earlier*
1. Stereotyped or repetitive motor movements, use of objects, or speech (e.g., simple motor stereotypies, lining up toys or flipping objects, echolalia, idiosyncratic phrases). 2. Insistence on sameness, inflexible adherence to routines, or ritualized patterns or verbal nonverbal behavior (e.g., extreme distress at small changes, difficulties with transitions, rigid thinking patterns, greeting rituals, need to take same route or eat food every day). 3. Highly restricted, fixated interests that are abnormal in intensity or focus (e.g., strong attachment to or preoccupation with unusual objects, excessively circumscribed or perseverative interests). 4. Hyper or hyporeactivity to sensory input or unusual interests in sensory aspects of the environment (e.g., apparent indifference to pain/temperature, adverse response to specific sounds or textures, excessive smelling or touching of objects, visual fascination with lights or movement).	• Excess of repetitive play (e.g., lining up cars, spinning wheels) • Excessive adverse reaction to changes in routines or environment (e.g., resists changing clothing as weather changes, insists on particular foods, seating arrangements, wearing certain clothing) • Motor mannerisms or stereotyped behavior (e.g., hand flapping, unusual finger movements, toe walking, rocking) • Unusual interests, interest in nonfunctional elements of play material (e.g., spinning tires on a toy car) • Unusual sensory interests (e.g., excessive interest in spinning objects or particular textures, explores objects from the corner of eyes rather than central vision, constantly sniffs objects, seeks out deep pressure stimulation) • Produces unusual complex mannerisms • Immediate echolalia • Stereotyped language • Hypersensitivity to certain forms of visual, auditory, tactile, olfactory input (e.g., bright lighting, sound of vacuum cleaner, blender, certain food textures, clothing fabrics, seams, tags, noxious reactions to certain smells) • Hyposensitivity to sensory input (e.g., at times appears deaf, unconcerned by extreme temperatures or painful events such as ear infection)

C. *Symptoms must be present in early childhood (but may not become fully manifest until social demands exceed limited capacities).*

D. *Symptoms together limit and impair everyday functioning.*

The left column presents the DSM-5 criteria for ASD. The diagnosis requires that a child demonstrate a minimum of seven symptoms of impaired function across two domains. A child must demonstrate symptoms in all three of the SC subdomains and in at least two of the four subdomains of RRBIA. The right column lists some of the corresponding early behavioral markers that have been identified in infancy and childhood.

Deficits in the second subdomain, nonverbal communicative behaviors, involve a lack of integration of verbal and nonverbal communication that is normally intrinsic to social interaction. Problems can include anomalies in eye contact and body language, and deficits in understanding and using nonverbal communications. Problems with gesture and nonverbal communication may be evident in simple failures to utilize head or hand gestures such as pointing, waving, or nodding, and a lack of facial expression. Correspondingly, impairment may also be reflected in difficulties reading and responding appropriately to gestural communications. Symptoms affecting particular language-related behaviors may be included in this category if they are fundamentally related to underlying problems with social communication and interaction.

The third subdomain involves deficits in developing and maintaining relationships appropriate to the child's developmental level. This may be evident in difficulties adjusting behavior so that it is appropriate and in keeping with different social contexts. Children may demonstrate a lack of imaginative play with peers, interest in developing peer relationships (friendships) or social imitation (e.g., during social games). If severe, these difficulties may entail an absence of interest in others, significant withdrawal and aloofness, and a strong preference for solitary activity.

Restricted and Repetitive Patterns of Behavior Interests and Activities

The second broad domain in which impairment must be evident to be diagnosed with ASD relates to RRBIAs. These behaviors are also diverse in their manifestations and have been divided into the following four subdomains: (a) stereotyped or repetitive speech, motor movements, or use of objects; (a) excessive adherence to routines and rituals and resistance to change; (c) highly restricted interests and preoccupations; and (d) hyper- or hyporeactivity to sensory input. An individual must demonstrate impairment in at least two of these four RRBIA areas (see Table 13.1, section B, subsections 1, 2, 3 and 4 respectively in the left column). The manifestations of these behaviors can vary over the course of development. For example, "lower-order" hand and finger mannerisms or unusual sensory interests are fairly common (~87.5%) by age 2, while "higher-order" behaviors such as compulsions and unusual preoccupations are less common at this age but evolve over time (Lord et al., 2006; Richler, Huerta, Bishop, & Lord, 2010).

The first subdomain includes a variety of complex stereotyped behaviors such as lining up objects and intricate mannerisms (e.g., tapping the teeth before ingesting food). It also encompasses a number of "lower-order" behaviors including simple sensory-motor stereotypies (e.g., facial grimacing, finger flicking, hand flapping, toe walking) and unusual sensory interests (e.g., watching ceiling fans). In addition, it incorporates utilization of stereotyped or ritualized forms of language such as echolalia, idiosyncratic speech, and pronoun reversal (e.g., using "you" when referring to self), repetitive questioning, and pedantic speech.

The second subdomain concerns insistence on sameness, resistance to change, and inflexible adherence to routines or ritualistic behaviors. These "higher-order" RRBIAs encompass compulsions and rituals such as having unusual attachments to particular objects or a needing to perform certain activities in a rigid or heavily prescribed manner. The subdomain also subsumes inordinate reactions to small changes in the environment, an insistence on strict adherence to rules, greeting rituals, difficulties transitioning from one activity to another, and rigid or perseverative thinking patterns (e.g., failure to understand idioms, irony, humor). Behaviors comprising this subdomain load as a separate factor from the repetitive sensorimotor behaviors described in the previous subdomain and appear to become more salient with increasing age (Cuccaro et al., 2003; Leekam, Tandos, et al., 2007).

The third subdomain concerns manifestations of highly restricted or circumscribed interests that are fixated or of unusual intensity. This can include preoccupation with unusual objects, excessive, perseverative areas of circumscribed interests (e.g., intense interest in train schedules, lawn mowers), and perfectionism. It can also consist of preoccupations or obsessions, and may entail the development of unusual fears (e.g., fear of bananas). These behaviors may also become more evident with increasing age.

Sensory hypersensitivities and hyposensitivities comprise the fourth subdomain. Long recognized in ASD, these symptoms were excluded from the diagnostic criteria in earlier versions of DSM, presumably because they can occur in a variety of neurodevelopmental disorders (e.g., ADHD, Fragile X, schizophrenia) (Reynolds & Lane, 2008). Their inclusion in DSM-5 therefore marks a significant addition to the new criteria. In the context of ASD, hypersensitivity refers to either increased sensory acumen (e.g., lowered sensory thresholds) or to exaggerated or inappropriate responses to sensory stimuli that, in a typical person, would yield unremarkable sensory responses.

Hypersensitivity in the auditory domain is often referred to as "hyperacusis" (Klein, Armstrong, Greer, & Brown, 1990). In children with ASD, everyday sounds (e.g., vacuum cleaner or food blender) that are neither threatening nor uncomfortably loud to a typical person may cause children with hyperacusis to cover their ears, undertake avoidant measures, and demonstrate considerable distress and dysphoria. These same children may tolerate other similar noises without difficulty. Often, the oversensitivity cannot be simply attributed to sound levels or the presence of particular frequencies.

In the somatosensory realm, tactile hypersensitivities may be reflected in "tactile defensiveness," in which children respond negatively to being touched or held, or display an aversion to social touch as may occur when in crowded situations. These hypersensitivities can cause a dislike to particular articles of clothing or fabrics (e.g., tags), certain foods because of their texture (e.g., creamy liquids), or specific activities (e.g., having their hair cut, brushing teeth). It may influence toy preferences (e.g., hard objects) or unusual attachments to particular objects or situations. Alternatively, children may seek out particular forms of somatosensory stimulation (e.g., deep pressure) that they may find calming, or perform self-stimulatory activities (e.g., rubbing certain textured objects), which may be reinforcing.

In the visual domain, children can show a particular fascination with reflections and brightly colored objects or alternatively demonstrate avoidant responses to them. Children may prefer to look at objects only out of the corner of their eyes, from unusual angles, or when squinting. Hypersensitivity can also be evident to particular smells or tastes and may therefore influence food preferences and aversions. Unusual or idiosyncratic exploratory behavior can occur in any of these modalities as part of this propensity to demonstrate RRBIAs.

As with hypersensitivity, hyposensitivity may also be evident in any of the five senses. In the auditory domain, for example, hypoacusis may be evident in diminished or inconsistent responses to sounds in the environment. This may occur to an extent that it raises concerns of possible hearing impairment. Children with ASD may demonstrate diminished or absent startle reflex to loud sounds in the environment, such as a loud clap produced behind them. Examples of hyposensitivity in the somatosensory domain include reduced sensitivity to cold temperatures (e.g., walking barefoot in snow) or high pain thresholds. Sensory regulatory anomalies can emerge as early as the first year (Baranek, 1999; DeGangi, Breinbauer, Roosevelt, Porges, & Greenspan, 2000).

Implications of Changes in DSM-5

Several preliminary studies revealed that the merging of the subgroups of PDD into a single diagnosis of ASD in the DSM-5 has resulted in significant improvements in several psychometric indices. Field trials using criteria close to those adopted in the final DSM-5 version have shown good test-retest reliability (kappa = 0.69) and improved specificity (0.74), indicating a reduced number of false-positive diagnoses (Regier et al., 2013). However, the higher degree of specificity may have come at a cost of lowered sensitivity. Although some studies have found no substantial change in sensitivity (0.89 to 0.93; see Huerta, Bishop, Duncan, Hus, & Lord, 2013) others claim a reduction in diagnosis as high as 88% in selected subgroups (Barton, Robins, Jashar, Brennan, & Fein, 2013; Mayes et al., 2014; McPartland, Reichow, & Volkmar, 2012; Taheri & Perry, 2012). The reduced sensitivity appears to particularly affect the diagnosis of older children, adolescents, adults, individuals without intellectual impairment, and individuals who previously met criteria for AspD and PDD-NOS. In addition, the new criteria may also have reduced sensitivity when diagnosing low-functioning adults (Matson, Belva, Horovitz, Kozlowski, & Bamburg, 2012) and at-risk toddlers (Matson, Kozlowski, Hattier, Horovitz, & Sipes, 2012).

Questions have arisen as to whether the observations of lower sensitivity of the DSM-5 criteria could be an artifact of the methodology used in these preliminary studies. In most, the data used were collected using DSM-IV-TR criteria and then mapped onto the DSM-5 descriptions, so these data may not provide sufficient information to adequately assess the full range of behaviors delineated in the DSM-5 criteria (Swedo et al., 2012). However, a prospective study by Gibbs, Aldridge, Chandler, Witzlsperger, and Smith (2012) provided evidence supporting the view that the new criteria may be overly stringent. Clearly, more experience is needed with the new criteria to address these questions.

One of the primary reasons that children diagnosed with a PDD using DSM-IV-TR criteria failed to meet the DSM-5 diagnosis for ASD is that they did not demonstrate sufficient evidence of deficits in nonverbal social communication. It has therefore been suggested that "relaxing" the number of social communication subdomain symptoms required to meet criteria from three to two might increase sensitivity (Frazier et al., 2012; Matson, Hattier, & Williams, 2012; Mayes et al., 2014). Empirical evaluation has confirmed that this approach results in an increase in sensitivity. However, the relaxation also caused a decrease in specificity relative to the original criteria (Taheri & Perry, 2012), although in many cases this was minimal (Mayes et al., 2014).

An additional concern with toddlers is that repetitive behaviors and resistance to change may not appear until age 3–4 years or even later for some children, while the social communication impairments of ASD appear as early as the first or second year of life (Garon et al., 2009; Osterling, Dawson, & Munson, 2002; Stone et al., 1999). Therefore, Barton et al. (2013) suggested that, at least as applied to toddlers, reducing the required number of repetitive behaviors to one would prevent unduly lowered sensitivity.

One of the more sensitive and heated criticisms of the changes in DSM-5 is that the new criteria will threaten delivery of services to some individuals. Since the inception of the Individuals with Disability Act in 1990, individuals receiving the diagnosis of autism have been eligible for special education services. Given changes in the sensitivity of the DSM-5 criteria, it is likely that a proportion of individuals (estimated from 10% to 47%) diagnosed with a PDD such as AspD or PDD-NOS according to DSM-IV-TR may no longer meet criteria for ASD using the new criteria (Huerta, Bishop, Duncan, Hus, & Lord, 2012; Matson, Kozlowski, et al., 2012; McPartland et al., 2012).

Epidemiology

Data from developed countries have shown consistent increases in ASD prevalence over the past 20 to 30 years (Davidovitch, Hemo, Manning-Courtney, & Fombonne,

2013; Elsabbagh et al., 2012; Kogan et al., 2009; Parner et al., 2011; Russell, Rodgers, Ukoumunne, & Ford, 2014). Numerous social and methodological issues have complicated the interpretation of this trend. Factors thought to contribute to the higher estimates include: (a) increased public and professional awareness of AD; (b) improvements in case-finding methods (e.g., higher estimates from studies that utilize repeated developmental checks); (c) heightened awareness of the full spectrum of the disorder; (d) increased recognition that AD can be associated with other developmental, physical, or psychiatric disorders; (e) earlier age of recognition; (f) better diagnostic tools; (g) diagnostic substitution (e.g., with intellectual deficiency); (h) rise of advocacy and disability rights; (i) better access to services and surveillance mechanisms (e.g., state-wide screening programs and national screening mandates (Plauché Johnson & Myers, 2007); and (j) broadened criteria and greater sensitivity of more recent diagnostic criteria (DSM-IV/DSM-IV-TR) in comparison to earlier formulations (DSM-III-R) (Elsabbagh et al., 2012; Fombonne, Quirke, & Hagen, 2009; Wing & Potter, 2002). However, prevalence rates have continued to show increases despite use of the same diagnostic criteria (Keyes et al., 2012).

The magnitude of the increase has been cause for serious concern. Based on studies published from 1966 to 2008, Fombonne (2009) suggested that prevalence rates for children diagnosed with an ASD were in the range of 60–70 per 10,000, corresponding to approximately one child in about 150 children. By contrast, recent large-scale surveys have yielded substantially higher prevalence estimates, in the range of 1%–2% (Baron-Cohen et al., 2009; Blumberg et al., 2013; Russell et al., 2014). Figures recently released by the Centers for Disease Control and Prevention (CDC) in the United States suggested that one in 88 children (11.3 per 1,000 8-year-olds) sampled in 2008 from multiple communities across the United States were identified with ASD (Baio, 2014). Overall, these recent figures mark an apparent continuation of a significant increase in prevalence estimates in the United States with approximately 36,500 cases added each year (Wingate et al., 2014). Increases have also been noted in Asia (Chien, Lin, Chou, & Chou, 2011; Kim et al., 2011), Europe (Baron-Cohen et al., 2009), and Australia (Williams, MacDermott, Ridley, Glasson, & Wray, 2008). Some data from the United Kingdom suggests that these incremental changes may be reaching a plateau (Taylor, Jick, & MacLaughlin, 2013).

One finding to possibly temper the alarming increase in prevalence observed worldwide is a study of autism prevalence in adults of different ages in the United Kingdom (Brugha et al., 2011). This study found no difference in prevalence for adults in different age bands, and adult prevalence was similar to that reported recently for children. These findings suggest that apparent increases may relate, at least in part, to case definitions and ascertainment methods. Nevertheless, ASD currently ranks as one of the most common forms of developmental disability. It is also one of the most costly disabilities, with an estimated lifetime cost of $3.2 million for an individual and family, resulting in approximately $34.8 billion in societal costs (Ganz, 2006).

Adopting the DSM-5 diagnostic criteria may complicate the continued monitoring of prevalence over time (Maenner et al., 2014; Mattila et al., 2011). The decreased sensitivity of the DSM-5 criteria would result in exclusion of some individuals classified with an ASD according to DSM-IV-TR or the International Classification of Diseases – 10th Edition (ICD-10) diagnostic criteria (Gibbs et al., 2012; Wing et al., 2011). This shift in diagnostic bias could potentially result in stasis or a lowering of future prevalence estimates.

Gender

ASD is four to five times more common in males compared to females (Brugha et al., 2011; Fombonne, 2009). This gender difference increases to approximately 6:1 in individuals with normal-range intelligence (Fombonne, 1999) and decreases to approximately 2:1 in individuals with severe ID (Mattila et al., 2011). The gender difference may increase to 11:1 when individuals with milder variants (e.g., Asperger's disorder) are included (Gillberg, Cederlund, Lamberg, & Zeijlon, 2006). Variability in male/female ratios may, in part, reflect gender differences in expression. Males are more likely to come to attention because they demonstrate externalizing behaviors such as aggression, hyperactivity, and stereotypies. Females are more likely to demonstrate internalizing symptoms such as anxiety, depression, or other mood disorder (Solomon, Miller, Taylor, Hinshaw, & Carter, 2012; Szatmari et al., 2012). In addition, females tend to exhibit better adaptive strategies or behaviors that "camouflage" behaviors associated with the diagnosis (Attwood, 2007; Dworzynski, Ronald, Bolton, & Happe, 2012; Kopp & Gillberg, 2011). Because of these differences in presentation, girls may need to have more cognitive or behavioral difficulties than males to be clinically diagnosed with ASD. Indeed, empirical studies have suggested that girls who receive the diagnosis are likely to be more severely affected. When the severity of autistic traits is held constant, boys remain more likely to get an ASD diagnosis, but the gender disparity is substantially reduced (Giarelli et al., 2010; Russell, Steer, & Golding, 2011).

Several lines of evidence have suggested that gender differences may also reflect the influence of protective factors in females that may mitigate, to some extent, the effects of genetic influences on the expression of ASD (Robinson, Lichtenstein, Anckarsater, Happe, & Ronald, 2013). In the circumstances of comparable genetic risk, males are more likely to exhibit symptoms of ASD, such as repetitive behaviors (Szatmari et al., 2012), and are more likely to receive a diagnosis of ASD than are females (Sato et al., 2012). It is unclear whether this effect is related to genetic factors (i.e., sex chromosomes), hormonal influences, or both. Given that individuals at the high end of the spectrum have a reduced likelihood of meeting the DSM-5 criteria for ASD, it is possible that fewer girls will be given the diagnosis.

Social Class

Kanner's (1943) original cohort came mainly from highly intelligent families with upper socioeconomic status. Parents and grandparents included physicians, lawyers, scientists, and writers. While subsequent studies have described an excess of college-educated professionals in parents of children with ASD, the findings have not been consistent. It has been hypothesized that the "systematizing" tendencies that are believed to form a latent trait of individuals within the broader autism spectrum may be advantageous in certain professional activities. Systematizing, according to Baron-Cohen, Richler, Bisarya, Gurunathan, and Wheelwright (2003), refers to the drive to analyze how systems work, how they can be built, and how they can be controlled. In support of this hypothesis, several studies have observed that relatives of children with ASD are overrepresented in a number of technically-oriented occupations in which systematizing tendencies would be particularly advantageous (Windham, Fessel, & Grether, 2009). This includes engineering (Baron-Cohen, Wheelwright, Stott, Bolton, & Goodyer, 1997; Turner, Stone, Pozdol, & Coonrod, 2006), mathematics (Baron-Cohen, Wheelwright, Burtenshaw, & Hobson, 2007), and computer or information technology sciences (Roelfsema et al., 2012).

Race

ASDs have similar prevalence in many countries around the world and different cultures or ethnicities (Fombonne, 2009). However, several recent reports have suggested that Caucasian children were more likely than African American or Hispanic children to be identified with ASD. In recent estimates from the CDC, ASD was identified in 1 of 63 White children, one in 81 African American children, and one in 93 Hispanic children. Furthermore, children with ASD from minority, low socioeconomic status, or rural families are likely to be screened and diagnosed later than others (Mandell, Listerud, Levy, & Pinto-Martin, 2002; Mandell & Novak, 2005).

Parental Age

Recent epidemiological studies have disclosed a possible association between advancing parental age and risk of autism (Croen, Najjar, Fireman, & Grether, 2007; Grether, Anderson, Croen, Smith, & Windham, 2009; Parner et al., 2012). However, the nature of this effect has been somewhat inconsistent across studies. Some reports have found modest independent effects of both maternal and paternal age, while others have observed that the age of only one (Reichenberg et al., 2006) or neither parent (Lauritsen, Pedersen, & Mortensen, 2005) was associated with risk of ASD in offspring (Lauritsen et al., 2005; Reichenberg et al., 2006).

A meta-analysis conducted by Hultman, Sandin, Levine, Lichtenstein, and Reichenberg (2011) in an attempt to resolve these disparities revealed a strong monotonic relationship between paternal age and risk of autism. The underlying mechanisms, however, remain unclear. One possible explanation is deferred paternity; paternal traits related to the broader ASD phenotype, such as shyness and aloofness, may delay success when searching for prospective mates and thus result in older paternal age (Puleo et al., 2012). This deferred paternity may increase risk of spontaneous genetic mutations due to either biological or environmental factors. Spermatogonial stem cell divisions, for example, are prone to higher mutation rates and cytogenetic abnormalities with advancing age (Buwe, Guttenbach, & Schmid, 2005; Crow, 2000). In addition, the longer the timeframe to conception, the greater the risk of exposure to potentially harmful environmental events (Yauk et al., 2008). This increased risk for spontaneous genetic mutations may combine with heritable genetic factors to increase the probability of penetrance of the ASD phenotype. This explanation is of considerable interest given growing evidence of the contribution of de novo mutations to the disorder (discussed in the next section). These possibilities are depicted schematically in Figure 13.1 (upper left) among a variety of other potential genetic, epigenetic, and environmental contributions to the risk of ASD, which will also be discussed in more detail in the following section.

Etiology

Genetic Influences

Dysmorphogenesis in ASD

Gross and minor physical anomalies can provide clues to identifying genetic factors contributing to abnormalities in embryonic or postnatal development. Although Kanner (1943) remarked on the absence of gross dysmorphic features in his original cohort of 11 children, he noted in passing that five of the children had "relatively large heads." (p. 248) In the absence of correlated signs or symptoms (e.g., other physical stigmata, raised intracranial pressure, hyperostosis), this physical feature was likely of uncertain significance. While it was recognized at that time that an unusually large head or *macrocephaly* was potentially indicative of excessive growth (hypertrophy) of the brain (Wilson, 1934), it was also well-established that benign forms of macrocephaly existed. Outcome was known to be quite diverse, from supranormal intelligence (e.g., Lord Byron, Oliver Cromwell, see Lawson, 1875) to severe developmental retardation and seizures (Campbell, 1895; Fletcher, 1900; Middlemass, 1895).

Subsequent investigations have revealed that children with ASD do indeed exhibit more dysmorphic features than the general population (Dufour-Rainfray et al., 2011; Miles &

Hillman, 2000; Ozgen, Hop, Hox, Beemer, & van Engeland, 2010). These anomalies tend to be minor and manifest in four body areas: the head, ears, mouth, and hands (Tripi et al., 2008). They include low-settled ears, adherent ear lobes, posteriorly rotated ears, hypertelorism, macrocephaly, furrowed tongue, large hands, two-to-three toe syndactyly, and small feet (Rodier, Bryson, & Welch, 1997; Walker, 1977). Some of these slight morphological deviations have been taken as evidence of genetic contributions to the development of ASD (Miles et al., 2005). A recent meta-analysis confirmed a robust effect of increased minor physical anomalies in ASD and suggested that this resulted from shared genetic vulnerability involving genes that play a role in shaping body morphology (Ozgen et al., 2010).

Macrocephaly and its association with ASD has received considerable attention in recent years. Macrocephaly may occur for a variety of nongenetic reasons such as hydrocephalus, neonatal intraventricular hemorrhage, or infection. From a genetic viewpoint, a large number of syndromes have been associated with macrocephaly, some with identified genetic determinants (e.g., neurofibromatosis, PTEN hamartoma syndromes, Soto's syndrome, Fragile X syndrome, Alexander disease). Macrocephaly occurs in about 15%–35% of children with ASD. Family studies have suggested that 35%–45% of children with ASD who have macrocephaly have a parent with a similarly elevated head size (Lainhart et al., 2006; Miles, Hadden, Takahashi, & Hillman, 2000). Younger siblings of children with ASD also appear to demonstrate this trait with higher than expected frequency (Elder, Dawson, Toth, Fein, & Munson, 2008), although this finding has not been consistently found. Familial forms of macrocephaly are generally benign and asymptomatic. In these cases, increased head size is attributable to increased cerebrospinal fluid (CSF) space (in early development) and not increased brain volume. In ASD, macrocephaly appears to be correlated with increased brain volume in early development and therefore meets criteria for *megencephaly*. Megencephaly is discussed at some length in the "Neuroscience of ASD" section.

Heritability

Initial descriptions of ASD noted the presence of behavioral peculiarities or idiosyncrasies in many of the parents of affected children (Asperger, 1944; Kanner, 1943). Kanner commented, "For the most part, the parents, grandparents, and collaterals are persons strongly preoccupied with abstractions of a scientific, literary, or artistic nature, and limited in genuine interest in people" (p. 250). However, in the absence of major mental illness in parents, it was generally concluded that genetic factors were not a relevant feature of the clinical picture (Judd & Mandell, 1968). This seemed to be supported by family pedigree data that suggested that the recurrence rate in families was fairly low, in the order of ~3% (Hanson & Gottesman, 1976; Smalley, Asarnow, & Spence, 1988). However, beginning in the late 1950s, case reports pointed to a high concordance in monozygotic (Campbell, Dominijanni, & Schneider, 1977; Chapman, 1957; McQuaid, 1975) and dizygotic twins (Kotsopoulos, 1976). A subsequent multifamily study showed a significantly higher concordance rate in monozygotic (36%) compared to dizygotic (0%) twins (Folstein & Rutter, 1977). Given that monozygotic (MZ) twins share ~100% of their DNA while dizygotic (DZ) twins share ~50%, it was concluded that genetic factors may indeed play an important role in increasing risk for the disorder.

Subsequent studies have generally confirmed higher concordance estimates in monozygotic (43%–95%) relative to dizygotic (0%–25%) twins (Nordenbaek, Jorgensen, Kyvik, & Bilenberg, 2014; Ritvo, Freeman, Mason-Brothers, Mo, & et al., 1986). On the basis of such differences, heritability was estimated to be as high as 80%–90% (Bailey, Le Couteur, Gottesman, & Bolton, 1995; Farley et al., 2009; Folstein & Rutter, 1988), placing ASD among the most heritable of child psychiatric disorders (Lichtenstein, Carlstrom, Rastam, Gillberg, & Anckarsater, 2010). However, some investigators have expressed caution regarding these estimates and their interpretation. The basic underlying premise that the quality of the pre- and postnatal environment in the two types of twin is comparable has been called into question (Carlier & Spitz, 1999). Greenberg, Hodge, Sowinski, and Nicoll (2001), for example, pointed out that complications arising from the twinning process itself (e.g., restriction of growth, risk of placental dysfunction) may be an important factor in increasing risk and inflating concordance for ASD in twins. Other problems with twin studies of ASD include low sample size and limitations or inconsistencies in case definition (Anderson, 2012). While some recent twin studies have supported a high heritability rate (Nordenbaek et al., 2014), others have yielded substantially lower estimates, ranging from 38% (Hallmayer et al., 2011) to 50% (Sandin et al., 2014), suggesting an equally important role for shared environmental influences in the expression of the disorder (Deth, Muratore, Benzecry, Power-Charnitsky, & Waly, 2008). Methodologically, the lower recent estimates may be due, in part, to the stricter cutoffs used for autism. Relatedly, while ASD may show high heritability in childhood, estimates drop in adulthood due to different assessment strategies or to complex gene-environment interactions (Posthuma & Polderman, 2013).

Broader Autism Phenotype

The heritable contribution to risk for ASD is also evidenced to some degree by observations of recurrence within families. If a family has a child with ASD, the likelihood that an additional child will also receive the diagnosis is significantly increased. Recent estimates of this recurrence risk range from 10%–20% (Constantino, Zhang, Frazier, Abbacchi, & Law, 2010; Ozonoff et al., 2011), substantially higher than previously thought. This represents as much as a 20-fold increase in risk compared to the general population (~1%) (Baird, Simonoff, et al., 2006). These high recurrence rates may underestimate the true risk of recurrence due to "reproductive stoppage rules," whereby parents of a child with a severe disability choose not have further children.

Heritability may also contribute to observations that similar but milder behavioral anomalies occur in 10%–20% of the nontwin siblings of children with ASD (Bolton, Macdonald, Pickles, Rios, & et al., 1994; Piven, Palmer, Jacobi, Childress, & Arndt, 1997). These irregularities in social communication and RRBIAs are mild or subtle, generally do not warrant clinical concern (subclinical), and tend to aggregate more often in male relatives compared to female relatives (Wheelwright, Auyeung, Allison, & Baron-Cohen, 2010). Similar if less pronounced anomalies may also be evident in grandparents, uncles/aunts, and first cousins (Pickles et al., 2000; Szatmari et al., 2000). These observations have argued for the existence of a "broader autism phenotype" (BAP) comprised of relatives (parents, siblings and to a lesser degree more distant relatives) who share some of the traits of autism present in the family member diagnosed with ASD (Piven, Palmer, et al., 1997). When twins meeting criteria for ASD are pooled with twins possessing traits of BAP, then concordance among monozygotic twins rises to 82% compared with approximately 10% in dizygotic twins.

Recent twin and BAP studies have suggested that the inherited liability for ASD is associated with some trait specificity (Ronald, Larsson, Anckarsater, & Lichtenstein, 2010). For example, children with ASD who show a high frequency of repetitive behaviors are nine times more likely to have parents with obsessive-compulsive disorder compared to children with ASD who demonstrate lesser repetitive behaviors (Hollander, King, Delaney, Smith, & Silverman, 2003). Comparable effects have also been observed for communicative abilities (Alarcon, Cantor, Liu, Gilliam, & Geschwind, 2002; Chen, Kono, Geschwind, & Cantor, 2006) and social aspects of ASD (Liu et al., 2011; Sasson, Nowlin, & Pinkham, 2013). Similarly, a recent study has also implicated specific genetic influences on sensory atypicalities such as tactile sensitivity (GABRB3, which influences GABA metabolism) (Tavassoli, Auyeung, Murphy, Baron-Cohen, & Chakrabarti, 2012). A few studies have suggested that the BAP may also share cognitive difficulties (e.g., executive function) (Hughes, Plumet, & Leboyer, 1999) and dysmorphic features (e.g., megencephaly) (Elder et al., 2008). Together, the twin and BAP findings could potentially be due to family genetic influences or shared genetic and environmental influences but is unlikely to be accounted for by environmental influences alone. Some have inferred from this body of evidence that ASD may result from anomalies of multiple genes where each contributes to specific traits that form part of the larger constellation of symptoms comprising ASD.

The schematic shown in Figure 13.1 is a hypothetical representation of the variety of genetic, epigenetic, and environmental factors implicated in the etiopathogenesis of ASD. The influence of these factors on neurodevelopment is complex and often dynamic. They have the potential, usually when occurring in combination, to cause alterations in neurodevelopment that lead to neuropsychological impairments and neurobehavioral anomalies. The resulting constellation of behavioral symptoms, if sufficient in number, breadth and severity, can lead to a diagnosis of ASD. For example, TSC1 and TSC2 are genes that encode for Hamartin and Tuberin respectively and are believed to be involved in tumor suppression. Mutations of these genes can lead to tuberous sclerosis complex (TSC) which can sometimes result in a co-diagnosis of ASD. Mutations of these and other genes (eg., NF1, FMR1) account for a number of the syndromic forms of ASD. Lesser genetic anomalies such as single nucleotide polymorphisms (SNPs) and copy number variations (CNVs) can also result in perturbations of neurodevelopment, affecting processes such as cell differentiation, proliferation, adhesion, migration and apoptosis. As conceptualized in Figure 13.1, when these anomalies are sufficient in number and/or their impact on neurodevelopment, they can contribute to behavioral differences and delays that can increase risk for a diagnosis of ASD. While a comprehensive discussion of the genetic contributions to ASD is well beyond the scope of this chapter, we attempt to summarize some of this extremely complex and rapidly expanding literature in the sections that follow. Table 13.2 (p. 198) lists a number of the genes that have been tentatively linked to ASD in recent years along with their impact on neurodevelopment.

Syndromic Forms of ASD

Despite compelling evidence for genetic contributions to ASD, early cytogenetic studies failed to identify consistent and specific anomalies associated with the full spectrum of the disorder. These studies were able only to detect anomalies large enough to be resolved through microscopic cytogenetic analysis. Analyses of the karyotypes of children with ASD established that only a small, albeit significant, number of children diagnosed with an ASD demonstrated visible cytological abnormalities (Gillberg, Winnergard, & Wahlstroem, 1984; Mariner et al., 1986). Anomalies included assorted sex chromosome abnormalities such as 45X (Turner syndrome), 47XYY, and 47XXY. Other rare chromosomal disorders associated with ASD include trisomy 21 and abnormalities of chromosome 15 (Wassink, Piven, & Patil, 2001). A

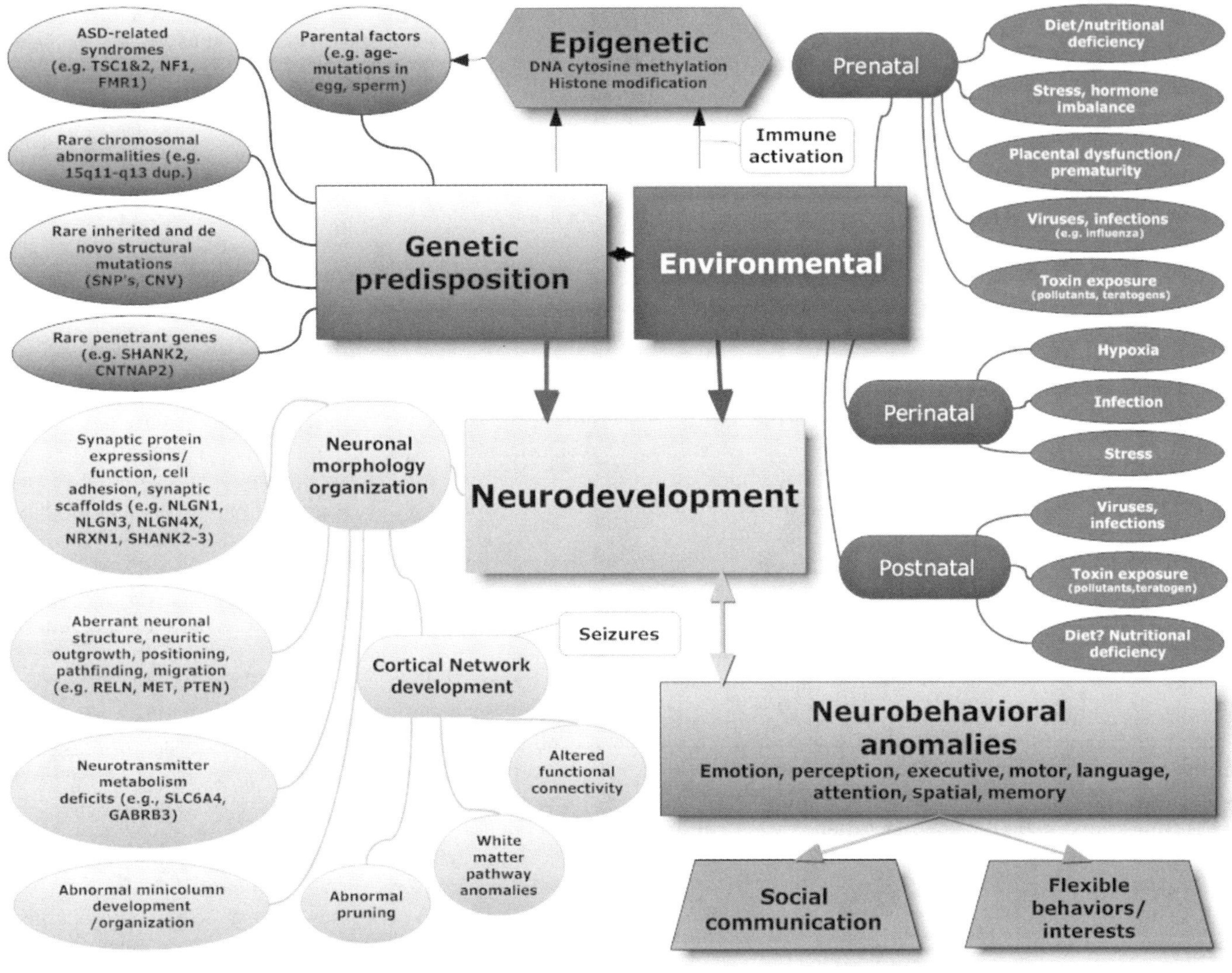

Figure 13.1 Etiopathogenetic pathways in ASD

number of anomalies associated with Mendelian modes of inheritance were also identified, including Fragile X (~1%–2%), tuberous sclerosis (~1%), neurofibromatosis (<1%) and Rett syndrome (~0.5%). Overall, rare chromosomal abnormalities were found in approximately 5% of ASD samples. One of the most common cytogenetic anomalies, identified in 1%–3% of individuals diagnosed with ASD, has been a 15q11-q13 duplication of the maternal allele associated with Prader-Willi/Angelman syndrome (Muhle, Trentacoste, & Rapin, 2004).

Subsequently, a number of other uncommon single gene defects and rare marker deletions associated with genetic syndromes have been found in populations of children with ASD. This includes but is not limited to Williams-Beuren, Sotos, Moebius, Smith-Lemli-Opitz, Cowden, Potocki-Lupski and Timothy syndromes (Johansson, Gillberg, & Rastam, 2010). Taken as a whole, approximately 1%–20% of cases of ASD are associated with medical and genetic conditions (Barton & Volkmar, 1998; Bauman, 2010). Individuals with these so-called syndromic forms of ASD are commonly but not uniformly excluded from genetic studies, which typically focus on exploring the genetic correlates of idiopathic forms of ASD. Systematic cytogenetically-visible anomalies in idiopathic ASD have been observed in 2.2% (Xu, Zwaigenbaum, Szatmari, & Scherer, 2004) to 5.8% (Marshall et al., 2008) of cases.

Genomic Perspectives on ASD: From Microscopic to Molecular

Advances in molecular genetics in the last 15 years have enabled in-depth examination of the molecular structure of the genome. While this has significantly enhanced efforts to identify the genetic factors that confer increased susceptibility for the disorder, this area of investigation is extremely complicated and fraught with methodological issues and challenges in interpreting the data. It is beyond the scope of this chapter to comprehensively review this complex and rapidly changing literature, but we offer here an abbreviated discussion of this material to provide the reader with a sense of the state-of-the-art. For the sake of brevity, this treatment assumes some basic knowledge of genetic principles and provides only a cursory coverage of those essential aspects of molecular genetics required for understanding terminology and concepts relevant to the literature on ASD. To provide a foundation for the material to follow, we first discuss some fundamental concepts.

FUNDAMENTALS CONCEPTS OF MOLECULAR GENETICS

DNA is a nucleic acid present in the nucleus of every cell. The DNA molecule is a polymer made up of (monomer) units referred to as *nucleotides*. Each nucleotide consists of a nitrogenous base—adenine (A) thymine (T), cytosine (C) or guanine (G)—connected to a sugar (deoxyribose) and a phosphate group. The sugar and phosphate of each nucleotide is linked to the sugar-phosphate molecules of adjacent nucleotides, forming a linear chain referred to as the *backbone*. The nitrogenous bases extend from the backbone like the teeth of a zipper. The DNA molecule consists of two long parallel strands of these nucleotides held together in the middle by weak bonds linking specific nitrogenous bases into pairs (A with T and G with C). Because these pairings are specific, knowing the order of nucleotides in one strand allows precise knowledge of the order in the opposing strand. These strands wind around together to form a spiral staircase-like double-helix structure. Approximately 6 billion nucleotides make up each DNA molecule. Genetic information—the genetic blueprint used to assemble the entire body—is coded in the sequence of the bases along either strand.

Genes are the basic physical and functional unit of heredity. Genes consist of a specific sequence of nucleotide bases at a given position on the DNA molecule. They vary in size from just a few thousand pairs of nucleotides to more than2 million base pairs. Genes are packaged into 46 chromosomes, which are divided into two sets of 23 chromosomes, one set inherited from each parent. Approximately 20–25 thousand genes collectively comprise the human genome. Chromosomes vary enormously in size and are numbered from largest to smallest (1–22). While chromosome 22 was originally thought to be the smallest, it was subsequently discovered that chromosome (21) was actually smaller, containing 447 to 635 genes, which corresponds to approximately 48 million nucleotide base pairs. The numbering was not changed because mutations of chromosome 21 had become known to possibly lead to Down syndrome. The largest chromosome (1) contains approximately 2,000 to 2,100 genes, spanning about 249 million base pairs. The sex chromosomes make up the 23rd chromosome pair (XX or XY). Only about a third of genes are expressed (active) primarily in the brain.

Genes consist of three types of nucleotide sequences: coding regions, noncoding regions, and regulatory sequences. The genetic code present in DNA instructs the cell how to assemble amino acids in order to make different proteins. Proteins are involved in virtually every aspect of cell growth and function, from the physical structure of the cell to the enzymes involved in neurotransmission. Each gene provides the code for the synthesis of specific proteins. The actual synthesis of proteins takes place outside of the nucleus of the cell. Code present in the DNA must therefore be transcripted and conveyed by messenger RNA (mRNA) to ribosomes, where it is translated to create amino acid chains that will be folded to create a protein.

Genes are biologically programmed to turn on and off in a prescribed manner over the course of development. Their expression can function as catalysts in the timing of important chemical and physiological events. However, the results of gene activity in the brain are incorporated into the dynamic and ever-changing molecular and cellular physiology of the brain, which is heavily influenced by experience. As a consequence, experience plays a large part in determining the extent to which genetic influences are expressed. Environmental events can result in molecular interactions that can impede the transcription of information stored in DNA. Epigenetic mechanisms such as DNA methylation, RNA-associated silencing, and histone modification can inhibit and even prevent the implementation of genetic instructions. Alterations in development can therefore result from anomalies of genetic structure, environmental influences, gene-environment interactions, gene-gene interactions and epigenetic factors. (These issues are discussed at length in the sections on genetic factors that follow.)

Comparing any two unrelated individuals reveals that 99.9% of the genome is identical, although the DNA sequence comprising the same chromosome may vary between the two versions. Numerous studies have now shown that significant variations in the sequencing structure of the genome occur in ASD. One type of genetic variation, termed *single nucleotide polymorphisms* (SNP), involves an alteration in DNA sequence in which there is a substitution of one nucleotide for another in the base pairs comprising the molecule (e.g., substitution of C with T so that DNA fragments differ between individuals (e.g., AAGC*C*TA vs. AAGC*T*TA). SNPs are not an uncommon feature of normal variation: from the approximately 3 billion base pairs comprising the human genome, roughly 10 million SNPs may occur in coding or noncoding areas. Variations can be transmitted or acquired through de novo mutations. While most of these alterations have no effect on health or brain development, it is believed that some of the SNPs that occur in individuals with ASD may play a direct or indirect role in risk for the disorder.

While SNPs affect a single nucleotide base, *copy number variation* is an anomaly affecting relatively large regions of the genome in which sections have been deleted or duplicated more than the usual number of times. Normally, an individual inherits two copies of every gene, one from each parent. However, in some regions in the genome, there are deviations from the two-copy rule, resulting in copy number variants (CNV). In these regions, the number of copies may vary from 0 to more than 14 copies of a gene. CNVs may range in size from about 1 kilobase (1,000 nucleotide bases) to as many as several megabases. They can be limited to a single gene and have implications similar to a SNP, or they can involve several genes (Lee & Scherer, 2010).

These structural variations contribute to our uniqueness, influencing traits that include susceptibility to diseases and disorders. CNVs, for example, account for some of the differences distinguishing so-called identical twins. They also account for some of the phenotypic variability associated within a disorder (due to differences in gene dosage). It is thought that rare de novo and inherited CNVs contribute to genetic vulnerability for ASD in as many as 10% of cases (Abrahams & Geschwind, 2008).

CANDIDATE GENE AND LINKAGE STUDIES

CNV screening and direct sequencing have provided rapid and useful methods to identify both large and small genetic variations that merit further characterization in relation to ASD. Given the large number of base pairs comprising the human genome and the fact that SNPs are not an uncommon feature of normal variation, discriminating those SNPs and CNVs that are specifically related to ASD from random variants or anomalies related to other traits poses a daunting task. Traditionally, efforts to identify genes related to a specific disorder begin with studies that attempt to identify the rough location of a candidate gene. These studies often try to localize the search to a region of the genome that is deemed etiologically relevant by virtue of its association with a specific syndrome or disorder. A number of early initiatives focused on linkages between the diagnosis of ASD and anomalies at loci in regions that had been implicated in prior cytogenetic studies as related to particular phenotypes, deficits, or diseases. Additionally, the search for candidate loci also guided by hypotheses regarding the biological origins of ASD. Once a locus has been identified, linkage and association studies can then attempt to identify which genes in that region may have a specific association to ASD. For example, given that duplications in chromosome 15 had been identified in previous cytological studies (Wassink et al., 2001), molecular studies have explored associations between ASD and anomalies in the region of chromosome 15, which spans more than 102 million base pairs. These efforts ultimately resulted in the identification of anomalies involving a gene in chromosome 15 that influences glutamate metabolism (GABRG3; Martin et al., 2000; Menold et al., 2001; Yang & Pan, 2013). In a similar vein, motivated by numerous studies demonstrating anomalies of serotonin metabolism in ASD, early molecular genetic studies identified polymorphisms in genes involved in 5-HT metabolism (e.g., SLC6A4, which codes for a serotonin transporter protein; see Betancur et al., 2002; Cook et al., 1997; Huang & Santangelo, 2008; Sutcliffe et al., 2005).

GENOME-WIDE ASSOCIATION STUDIES (GWAS)

Advances in molecular genetics in the last decade have made it possible for researchers interested in ASD to perform scans of the entire genome in search of the SNPs that contribute to risk for developing the disorder. In genome-wide association studies (GWAS), large numbers of individuals with ASD are assayed (i.e., genotyped) to obtain a comprehensive catalog of genetic markers distributed across the coding regions of the genome. Using techniques such as *logistic regression analysis,* control family members who have never met criteria for the disorder are compared to members of families with at least two affected relatives (typically siblings). Ideally, dense pedigrees (3+) are optimal, but these are often difficult to recruit in the ASD population given the reduced fecundity of individuals with ASD (Power et al., 2013) and the tendency for reproductive stoppage after parents have given birth to an affected child (Jones & Szatmari, 1988). The aim of the analysis is to identify those structural DNA variations or markers that may predispose individuals to develop ASD. From these analyses, it is possible to distinguish multiple genetic risk factors and discern inherited from de novo structural variations.

Overall, however, complications (i.e., heterogeneity, reproductive stoppage, insufficient sample size) have contributed to slow progress in showing definitive correspondences between specific genetic anomalies and risk for idiopathic ASD. A recent review of the literature catalogued 103 disease genes and 44 genomic loci that may potentially be associated with AD or autistic behavior (Betancur, 2010). This underscores the substantial heterogeneity of the genetic determinants of ASD. In their review, Abrahams and Geschwind (2010) nicely conveyed the greater complexities of this area of investigation, suggesting that 20% of autism cases may be attributable to a mutation involving a known risk gene, but no single region within the genome can account for more than 1%–2% of cases. This has led to a discussion of the "missing heritability problem," which relates to the observation that loci detected by GWAS explain such a small amount of the inferred genetic variants associated with ASD.

RARE AND COMMON VARIANTS

Both rare and common genetic variants underlie risk for most complex disorders. The twin studies of ASD prompted speculation that the genetic liability for ASD may be conferred by anomalies in a small number of genes that had large effects. A number of rare SNPs and CNVs have been identified in ASD, each with a frequency of occurrence of less than 1%. These rare variants include NLGN3, NLGN4, NRXN1, SHANK2, SHANK3, PTCHD1, 1q21.1, maternally inherited duplication of 15q11-q13, 16p11.2, CDH8, ASTN2, and CNTNAP2 among others. A number of these anomalies can have significant influences on neurodevelopment, sufficient enough to be monogenic causes of ASD. (For more details, see the "Genetic Influences on Neurodevelopment in ASD" section). However, these rare variants account for only a small proportion of individuals diagnosed with ASD.

More recent reconsideration of the available evidence has suggested that liability for ASD may more generally arise from the influence of many genes with small to modest effects on the traits associated with ASD. A recent population-based study from Sweden used statistical models to partition the heritable risk of ASD from rare and common variants (Gaugler et al., 2014). Gaugler and colleagues estimated that more than 90% of the heritable risk was likely to be due to common variants. While several hundred structural variants have been identified in families of individuals with ASDs (Marshall et al., 2008), GWASs have largely failed to identify common CNVs and SNPs that can account for the expected degree of transmitted variation (Cook & Scherer, 2008; Devlin & Scherer, 2012; Freitag, Staal, Klauck, Duketis, & Waltes, 2010). Some of the difficulty is that, given the large number of statistical comparisons (~1 million) and the small effect sizes, many of the studies have relatively low power, resulting in a paucity of consistently replicated results (Lee et al., 2013). For example, a meta-analysis by Anney et al. (2010) of three previously identified SNPs (on 5p14.1, 5p15, and 20p12.1) failed to support consistent effects on any of the identified loci. Due in part to power issues, associations identified in GWAS may represent the "low-hanging fruit" that reached statistical significance for a variety of reasons and are thus not consistent between studies (Anney, 2013).

DE NOVO MUTATIONS

In view of the inconsistency in the genes identified in association studies, a number of recent studies have underscored the potential contribution of de novo (not inherited) genetic variations in the risk for ASD (Ronemus, Iossifov, Levy, & Wigler, 2014). It has been suggested that between 10% and 30% of the genetic liability for ASD can be traced to de novo CNVs, point mutations, insertions, or deletions (Devlin & Scherer, 2012; Iossifov et al., 2014; Neale et al., 2012). New mutations are fairly common (~100 per child) but very few (~1%) fall within coding regions of the genome (Awadalla et al., 2010). De novo mutations have been observed in approximately 7% of families with ASD and are more likely to account for ASD in singleton families (since one family member is affected, the child is compared to his or her parents). There is a two- to fourfold increase in de novo mutations among ASD individuals (Neale et al., 2012; Sanders et al., 2012). While some of these mutations can potentially have large effects (Gilman et al., 2011; Iossifov et al., 2012; Sebat et al., 2007), affected individuals more often have multiple sequence variants and CNVs with presumed small-to-medium effects. These findings suggest that the high incidence of autism in some families could best be explained by structural variants at multiple loci. Factors that may contribute to risk for de novo mutations are multifold, including a variety of potential environmental and biological (e.g., aging) risk factors. The effects of advancing parental age, for example, may be related to either or both, insofar as aging both increases the risk for spontaneous mutations as well as provides more opportunity for exposure to possible mutagenic environmental influences (Lee & McGrath, 2015).

A number of the genes that have been identified in studies examining de novo mutations have been previously implicated as candidate genes. Some of the identified de novo variants include FMRP, CNTNAP2, SHANK 2, PTEN, CHD2, CHD8, SYNGAP1, DYRK1A, GRI, SCN2A, and TBR1. Among these, CHD8, SCN2A, and DYRK1A, have been most consistently implicated (Neale et al., 2012, p. 6; O'Roak et al., 2012; Sanders et al., 2012). Many of these genes play a significant role in signaling and synaptic function during neurodevelopment, some by influencing the action of other genes that have been implicated directly or indirectly in ASD (e.g., PTEN; see Devlin & Scherer, 2012; Krumm, O'Roak, Shendure, & Eichler, 2014). A full appreciation of the genetic determinants of ASD requires an understanding of gene networks and how anomalies of particular genes may affect the expression of other genes. Some examples of this are illustrated in the following discussion on "Genetic Influences on Neurodevelopment in ASD." Such considerations also relate to the important role that epigenetic factors play in the risk for ASD. Epigenetic factors refer to those influences that affect gene expression that are not due to structural alterations in DNA. This is briefly discussed in a separate section on "Epigenetics."

Genetic Influences on Neurodevelopment in ASD

The genes that have been implicated in ASD impact a variety of physiological processes including chromatin remodeling, transcription and translation, and metabolic function. A significant number of them have an impact on synaptic function. A selection of these genes and their function are illustrated in Table 13.2.

Several of the more penetrant genes fall within the neurexin and cadherin (calcium-dependent adhesion) superfamilies of genes (Pardo & Eberhart, 2007; Redies, Hertel, & Hubner, 2012; Sudhof, 2008). The neurexin genes (e.g., NRXN1, NRXN2, NRXN4) code for proteins that facilitate the formation of neuronal trans-synaptic cell adhesion complexes (Lise & El-Husseini, 2006; Varoqueaux et al., 2006). The activity of these genes can influence axonal and dendritic growth, synaptic formation, and neural plasticity. Anomalies have the potential to result in broad effects on brain development and function, influencing neurotransmission, particularly glutamatergic and GABAergic synapses, as

Table 13.2 Genes implicated in risk for ASD

Gene Family	*Gene Name*	*Locus*	*Function*	*Comorbidities*
SYN (Synapsin)	SYN1 SYN2	Xp11.23 3p25	Synaptic vesicle cycling	ASD, epilepsy
RIM (Regulating synaptic membrane exocytosis)	RIMS3	1p34.2	Synaptic vesicle cycling	ASD
CACN (Calcium channels, voltage-dependent)	CACNA1E CACNB2	1q25.3 10p12	Neurotransmission	ASD
SCN (Sodium channels voltage-gated)	SCN1A SCN2A SCN3A	2q24.3 2q24.3 2q24	Neuronal excitability	Dravet syndrome, ASD, epilepsy
KCNM (Potassium channels, calcium activated)	KCNMA1 KCNMB4	10q22.3 12q	Neuronal excitability	ASD
KCN (Potassium channels)	KCNQ3 KCNQ5 KCND2	8q24 6q14 7q31	Neuronal excitability	ASD, epilepsy
NRXN (Neurexin)	NRXN1 NRXN2	2p16.3 11q13	Cell adhesion	ASD, schizophrenia
NLGN (Neuroligin)	NLGN3 NLGN4X	Xq13.1 Xp22.32-p22.31	Cell adhesion	ASD, ID
CNTNAP (Contactin-associated protein-like 2)	CNTNAP2 (aka NRXN4) CNTNAP4	7q35 16q23.1	Cell adhesion	ASD, ID, language impairment, schizophrenia, epilepsy
CDH (Cadherin)	CDH5 CDH8 CDH9 CDH10 CDH11 CDH13 CDH15	16q22.1 16q22.1 5p14 5p14.2 16q21 16q23.3 16q24.3	Cell adhesion	ASD, ID
PCDH (Protocadherin)	PCDHB4 PCDH10 PCDH19	5q31 4q28.3 Xq22.1	Cell adhesion	ASD, ID
CNTN (Contactin)	CNTN4 CNTN5 CNTN6	3p26.3 11q22.1 3p26-p25	Cell adhesion	ASD, ID
IL1RAPL (Interleukin 1 receptor accessory protein-like 1)	IL1RAPL1	Xp22.121.3	Cell adhesion	ASD, ID
SHANK (SH3 and multiple ankyrin repeat domains)	SHANK1 SHANK2 SHANK3	19q13.3 11q13.3 22q13.3	Glutamate receptor signaling	ASD
SYNGAP (Synaptic Ras GTPase activating protein)	SYNGAP1	6p21.3	Glutamate receptor signaling	ASD
GABRG (Gamma subunits of GABA-A receptor)	GABRB3	15q12	Neurotransmission	ASD
FMR1 (Fragile X mental retardation 1)	FMRP	Xq27.3	Synaptic Plasticity	Fragile X syndrome, ASD, Fragile X–associated tremor/ataxia syndrome
RELN (Reelin)	Reelin	7q22	Neuronal migration	ASD, schizophrenia, bipolar disorder, major depression, temporal lobe epilepsy, lissencephaly with cerebellar hyperplasia
PTEN (Phosphatase and tensin homolog)	PTEN	10q23	Neuron, positioning, dendritic development, synapse formation	ASD
CHRNA7 (Cholinergic receptor, nicotinic, alpha 7)	CHRNA7	15q13. 3	Signal transmission	ASD, schizophrenia
UBE3A (Ubiquitin protein ligase E3A)	UBE3A	15q11.2	Protein degradation targeting	Angelman's syndrome
MECP2 (Methyl CpG binding protein 2)	MECP2	Xq28	DNA methylation, transcription repressor	Rett's syndrome, ID

This table provides information regarding some of the genes implicated in risk for ASD, their known or suspected role in neurodevelopment, and the clinical conditions that have been associated with mutations. (Adapted and expanded from Giovedi et al. 2014) well as resulting in neuronal migration abnormalities. They have been implicated in a variety of other neuropsychiatric disorders, including epilepsy. Genes that code for neuroligands (NLGN3, NLGN4X) have also been implicated in ASD (Freitag et al., 2010; Volaki et al., 2013), although the evidence has been mixed (Gauthier et al., 2005).

Relatedly, both common and rare variants of the contactin associated protein-like 2 gene (CNTNAP2, CNTNAP4 also known as Caspr2 and Caspr4 respectively) have been implicated in ASD (Bakkaloglu et al., 2008; Burbach & van der Zwaag, 2009; Penagarikano & Geschwind, 2012). CNTNAP2 is located on chromosome 7 (7q35) and was first connected to ASD as a recessive mutation associated to a syndromic form of ASD known as *cortical dysplasia-focal epilepsy syndrome* (CDFE; see Strauss et al., 2006). CNTNAP2 codes for a cell adhesion protein that mediates neuron-glia interactions and the clustering of potassium channels in myelinated axons (Poliak et al., 2003). Nearly two-thirds of individuals with this anomaly demonstrate epileptic seizures, language regression, intellectual impairment, and ADHD symptoms. CNTNAP2 has since been linked to increased risk of ASD and ASD-like endophenotypes comprised of four key features: ID, seizures, autistic characteristics, and language problems (Scott-Van Zeeland et al., 2010). The associated language impairments range from dysarthric speech and language delay to the absence of speech. Nearly half of affected individuals demonstrate evidence of a neuromigrational disorder on structural neuroimaging.

Other disorders associated with CNTNAP2 include schizophrenia, developmental delay, and ADHD. In addition, SNPs and CNVs in the CNTNAP2 region have also been linked to specific language impairment (SLI) and dyslexia (Newbury et al., 2011; Simpson et al., 2015). CNTNAP2's location on the chromosome is near the FOXP2 gene (7q31), which has also been implicated in developmental disorders affecting speech and language. Interestingly, FOXP2, a gene associated with verbal dyspraxia and impaired linguistic processing (Vargha-Khadem, Gadian, Copp, & Mishkin, 2005), has not been implicated in ASD.

A number of genes in the cadherin family (e.g., CDH9, CDH10, CDH13, CDH15, PCDH19) have also been implicated in ASD (Chapman et al., 2010; Pagnamenta et al., 2011; Sanders et al., 2012; Wang et al., 2009). These genes code for cadherins, which are proteins that play an important role in cell adhesion, forming and remodeling of synaptic junctions, and mediating aspects of intracellular signaling (Giagtzoglou, Ly, & Bellen, 2009; Hirano, Suzuki, & Redies, 2003). They also play an important role in neural tube regionalization, neural migration, and gray matter differentiation (Hirano & Takeichi, 2012; Redies et al., 2012).

Other genes implicated in risk for ASD include the SHANK family (e.g., SHANK2 and SHANK3) of genes (Berkel et al., 2010; Boccuto et al., 2013; Moessner et al., 2007). The SHANK genes code for proteins that are involved in the process of synaptic development by scaffolding and connecting neurotransmitter receptors, ion channels, and other membrane proteins to the neuronal cytoskeleton. They therefore play an important role in the formation, maturation, and maintenance of synapses and dendritic spines (Blundell et al., 2009; Guilmatre, Huguet, Delorme, & Bourgeron, 2014; Uchino & Waga, 2013). SHANK3, located on chromosome 22, seems to be associated with more common, milder variants of ASD (Boccuto et al., 2013). While some genes may begin to be expressed during fetal brain development, the SHANK genes may have the greatest impact on changes that occur in the postnatal period during critical periods of proliferation of neural processes (axons and dendrites) and the formation of synapses (Gutierrez et al., 2009; Yamakawa et al., 2007). They are thought to play an important role in specifying synaptic functions and interactions with other proteins to localize neurotransmitter receptors on postsynaptic neurons as they mature. Other genes thought to potentially influence neurotransmission include SYNGAP1 (which codes for a protein largely localized to dendritic spines and neocortical pyramidal neurons, where it suppresses NMDA receptor mediated synaptic plasticity), GABRG1 (which codes a protein that plays a role in GABAergic neurotransmission), and CHRNA7 (which codes for a protein involved in acetylcholinergic signal transmission).

RELN is a gene that encodes an extracellular protein, reelin, that is involved in cell-to-cell interactions critical for cell positioning and neuronal migration during brain development (Fatemi et al., 2005). Decreased levels of reelin have been identified in cerebellar tissue obtained from postmortem examination of individuals with autism (Persico & Bourgeron, 2006). Interestingly, findings in mice have linked reelin pathway anomalies to prenatal infection with influenza virus or other causes of activation of the immune system during pregnancy (Fatemi, Emamian, et al., 2002). These findings form part of a larger literature connecting ASD to both genetic and environmental influences on immune system function (see "Immunological Factors" in the following section for more information).

The synapsin family of genes (SYN1, SYN2) has also been implicated in ASD. These comprise a family of genes that act as regulators in synaptic development and plasticity (Giovedi, Corradi, Fassio, and Benfenati et al., 2014). Interestingly, these genes are expressed at low levels at birth but their expression increases progressively in the course of early development, reaching a plateau at about 2 months coinciding with the beginning of a period of increasing synaptogenesis. This window also coincides with one of the peak periods of epileptogenesis in ASD. Mutations in SYN1 have been identified in individuals with both epilepsy and ASD while SYN2 mutations have been observed in ASD without epilepsy.

When considered individually, the contribution of these genes to ASD appears relatively small (Huguet, Ey, & Bourgeron, 2013). Overall, the genetic anomalies that have been associated with ASD do not appear to be specific to the ASD phenotype, but rather are associated with a range of phenotypes, many of which are characterized by symptoms that are often comorbid in ASD. This includes epilepsy (Mefford et al., 2010; Penagarikano et al., 2011), ADHD (Rommelse, Franke, Geurts, Hartman, & Buitelaar, 2010; Ronald, Simonoff, Kuntsi, Asherson, & Plomin, 2008; Semrud-Clikeman, Fine, Bledsoe, & Zhu, 2014), developmental language disorders (Bartlett et al., 2014; Nudel et al., 2014; Stefanatos & Postman-Caucheteaux, 2010), and schizophrenia (Stefansson et al., 2014; Sullivan et al., 2012). It has therefore been argued that, like schizophrenia, ASD liability arises from the cumulative effect of genetic variation involving multiple mutations. Individual mutations, whether inherited or de novo, may exert a small effect, but collectively they can exert a major influence on ASD risk (Klei et al., 2012; Pinto et al., 2010).

Epigenetics

A variety of factors influence how the genotype is transformed into the phenotype in the course of development of ASD. These include interactions between genes and the environment, interactions between genes themselves, or from unknown events or influences. Through diverse mechanisms, "epigenetic" factors result in alterations in gene expression through mechanisms other than changes in DNA sequence (Elia, Laracy, Allen, Nissley-Tsiopinis, & Borgmann-Winter, 2012). Epigenetic mechanisms include chromosome organization, DNA methylation, and effects of transcriptional factors. For example, animal models have demonstrated that environmental insults such as prenatal stress or maternal deprivation can influence DNA methylation. This can result in sustained hypersensitivity to stress, which in turn can affect mood, cognition, and reactivity later in life. Environmental influences that have been specifically implicated in ASD include exposure to environmental toxins, parental age, and teratogenic effects such as the maternal use of valproic acid during pregnancy. Epigenetic pathways are varied, and in many cases are not very well understood. However, in the case of valproic acid, it appears that maternal use can inhibit histone deacetylase, which has downstream effects on the production of GABAergic inhibitory neurons (Stodgell, Gnall, & Rodier, 2001) and glutamate metabolism (Kim et al., 2013).

Several genes implicated in autism may be influenced by epigenetic factors, including GABRB3, UBE3A, and MECP2. These genes have decreased expression in the brain of individuals with ASD, and are known to have a significant impact on neurodevelopment. As mentioned earlier, GABRB3 is a gene located on 15q11–13 and is important to the development of $GABA_A$ receptors, which are known to be underexpressed in the brains of individuals with ASD. Animal models have shown that when this gene is no longer able to exert its effects, it results in seizures and autistic-like behaviors, including impaired social ability and anxiety (DeLorey, 2005). UBE3A has been implicated in Angelman's syndrome and appears to play a role in maintaining synaptic plasticity and experience-dependent changes in the brain (Yashiro et al., 2009). MECP2 is a gene on the X chromosome that is important in a number of epigenetic processes critical to synaptogenesis and long-term synaptic plasticity (Kavalali, Nelson, & Monteggia, 2011). While anomalies of a gene that codes for protein called MECP2 is highly associated with Rett syndrome, recent studies have shown significant reductions in MECP2 protein expression also occurs in a substantial proportion of individuals with ASD (Gonzales & LaSalle, 2010). In individuals without Rett syndrome, MECP2 gene mutations appear to be associated with global developmental delay with obsessive-compulsive disorder and ADHD (Suter, Treadwell-Deering, Zoghbi, Glaze, & Neul, 2014).

Some of the other genes implicated in ASD may also have an epigenetic role in the expression of the disorder. This includes RELN (discussed on p. 193), the FMR1 gene related to Fragile X syndrome and the oxytocin receptor gene (OXTR). Oxytocin is a hormone produced in the hypothalamus that acts as a neuromodulator in the brain. It has effects on affiliative behavior and has been implicated in deficits in social relatedness and repetitive behavior in ASD (Bakermans-Kranenburg & van Ijzendoorn, 2014; LoParo & Waldman, 2015).

Endophenotypes

It appears that structural genetic variants associated with ASD may play a role in determining risk for particular symptoms or symptom clusters rather than exerting influences that are specific to the disorder itself. As noted in the previous section on heritability, it appears that different behavioral characteristics associated with ASD may have distinctive underlying genetic determinants (Happé & Ronald, 2008). Familiality effects have been observed for repetitive behaviors (Hollander et al., 2003), communicative abilities (Alarcon et al., 2002; Chen et al., 2006), and social aspects of ASD (Liu et al., 2011; Sasson et al., 2013). These observations have prompted a strategic shift in genetic research on ASD that emphasizes the importance of delineating endophenotypes. Endophenotypes are defined by key or fundamental deficits that underlie a disorder and contribute to its expression in a significant way (Gottesman & Gould, 2003). An underlying assumption of this approach is that these fundamental problems may more directly reflect or index the influence of genetic factors than does symptomatic behavior. Interest has recently grown in identifying cognitive endophenotypes of ASD—patterns of cognitive ability or disability that may provide a more direct expression of genetic variation in ASD (Charman, Jones, et al., 2011; Happé, Briskman, & Frith, 2001; Hughes et al., 1999; Tager-Flusberg & Joseph, 2003). Recent studies have utilized language endophenotypes or levels of impairment, for example, to help strengthen signal and reduce variability in genome-wide studies (Bartlett et al., 2014; Spence et al., 2006). A visual endophenotype has been defined, characterized by deficits in sensitivity to visual stimuli that are low in spatial frequency and high in temporal frequency (Goodbourn et al., 2014). An endophenotype based on executive function deficits has also been proposed (Delorme et al., 2007).

Summary and Broader Implications

Overall, studies of SNPs, CNVs, sequence-level changes, and other variants in seemingly noncoding regions of the genome have implicated potentially hundreds of genes in the expression of the ASD phenotype (Neale et al., 2012; Persico & Napolioni, 2013; Stein, Parikshak, & Geschwind, 2013). The genetic contribution to ASD is likely to be polygenic, possibly involving as few to as many as 15 genes in various combinations. The mechanisms appear to include both inherited genetic influences and de novo mutations. An X-linked genetic or epigenetic contribution has been suggested given that males are more likely to be diagnosed with the disorder (Jiang et al., 2013; Piton et al., 2010). Some of the anomalies have fairly direct influences on brain development because they code for the expression of structures involved in cellular development, positioning, or migration. Other genetic influences may act on neurodevelopment indirectly through their influence on immune or hormonal function or through epigenetic pathways.

Given the diversity of the genetic anomalies that have been associated with ASD, and given their often broad impact on neurodevelopment, it is perhaps not surprising that some of the genes that confer risk for ASD also confer risk for conditions that are often comorbid in ASD. Among these, ADHD ranks among the most common comorbid conditions, with approximately 50% of children with ASD also meeting criteria for ADHD (Rommelse et al., 2010). Indeed, there is growing evidence to suggest that individuals diagnosed with ADHD also demonstrate some characteristics commonly associated with ASD (Demopoulos, Hopkins, & Davis, 2013). This relationship suggests that the two disorders may share some common neurobiological risk factors, possibly because the same gene or genes may contribute to different phenotypes. Such pleiotropic relationships are often mediated by gene effects on a metabolic pathway that contributes to different behavioral phenotypes. Pathways implicated in both ASD and ADHD include both the dopamine (Swanson et al., 2007) and GABA neurotransmitter systems (Fatemi et al., 2012). A few studies that have examined the shared genetic risk between the two conditions found that it is modest and that there are also some common environmental influences explaining their covariation (Polderman, Hoekstra, Posthuma, & Larsson, 2014; Ronald, Edelson, Asherson, & Saudino, 2010). Interestingly, Polderman et al. found that stronger genetic correlations (from .22 to .64) occurred when symptoms associated with restricted repetitive and stereotyped behaviors and interests were compared to dimensions of ADHD. Other conditions commonly comorbid in ASD, possibly through pleiotropic effects, include epilepsy, language impairment, depression, and anxiety disorders. More comprehensive discussions of comorbidity in ASD are provided by Mannion and Leader (2013) and (Bauman, 2010).

Environmental Influences

Given the high estimates of heritability for ASD by twin studies, environmental factors were until fairly recently thought to play a relatively minor causative role in ASD (Burd, Severud, Kerbeshian, & Klug, 1999). However, as mentioned on p. 192, some recent genetic studies have suggested that the heritability of autism may not be as great as previously believed (Hallmayer et al., 2011; Ronald & Hoekstra, 2011). Moreover, recent increases in ASD prevalence cannot readily be explained on the basis of heritability. Individuals with autism and their siblings demonstrate reduced fecundity (Power et al., 2013). The lower probability of reproducing in these individuals seems incompatible with the rise in prevalence due to heritable genetic factors alone. In addition, growing recognition of the importance of de novo genetic mutations in determining risk for ASD has necessitated a closer look at identifying potential environmental determinants of these mutations. These factors have led to increased interest in elucidating potential gene–environment interactions that could have implications for neurodevelopment and thereby increase risk for autism (Herbert, 2010; Stamou, Streifel, Goines, & Lein, 2013).

Adverse Pre-and Perinatal Events

Numerous studies have established an association between adverse pre- and perinatal events and risk for ASD (Juul-Dam, Townsend, & Courchesne, 2001; Piven, Simon, Chase, Wzorek, & et al., 1993; Wilkerson, Volpe, Dean, & Titus, 2002). Some of the more commonly implicated factors include low birth weight, multiple gestation, prematurity, vaginal bleeding, threatened abortion, poor fetal growth, prolonged labor, hypoxia, a need for resuscitation at birth, and a five-minute Apgar score below 7 (Hultman, Sparen, & Cnattingius, 2002). A review by Kolevzon, Gross, and Reichenberg (2007) identified low birth weight and intrapartum hypoxia as two of the more consistent obstetric risk factors for autism.

Schieve et al. (2011) examined multiple perinatal factors associated with obstetric risk (e.g., preterm, very preterm, low and very low birth weight, multiple birth, cesarean delivery, breech presentation, and assisted reproductive technology use) and evaluated their contribution to increases in prevalence of ASD identified in recent population studies. Their analysis suggested that these factors alone or in combination accounted for a very small proportion (less than 1%) of the observed increase in ASD prevalence. Given that most children born under conditions of obstetric risk do not develop ASD, it has been suggested that decreased obstetric optimality may be an epiphenomenon of ASD that derives from preexisting abnormality of the fetus, rather than being a causative agent at delivery (Zwaigenbaum et al., 2002).

Others have pointed to a variety of pre-and perinatal environmental exposures as potentially increasing risk for ASD. This includes maternal cigarette smoking during early pregnancy (Hultman et al., 2002), exposure to certain drugs (e.g., sodium valproate, thalidomide, cocaine), and psychological stress during pregnancy (Dawson, Ashman, & Carver, 2000) as potential risk factors for adverse outcomes. The data supporting some of these assertions has been mixed.

Events such as hypoxia result in a cascade of immune responses, including neuroinflammation. In prenatal development, the fetus is highly vulnerable to a broad range of events or environmental exposures that can potentially elicit an innate or adaptive immune response (Onore, Careaga, & Ashwood, 2012; Rossignol & Frye, 2012; Stigler, Sweeten, Posey, & McDougle, 2009). Numerous studies have identified abnormalities of immune function in individuals with ASD (Depino, 2013; Noriega & Savelkoul, 2014). Some have suggested anomalies of the blood-brain barrier (Noriega & Savelkoul, 2014), while others have proposed that some of the genetic contributions to ASD may involve genes that influence immune system activation and regulation (Campbell, Li, Sutcliffe, Persico, & Levitt, 2008; Torres, Westover, & Rosenspire, 2012).

Immunological Factors

One obvious mechanism by which immune system dysfunction can increase risk for ASD involves prenatal susceptibility or inadequate protection against viruses or other pathogens. It has long been recognized that direct viral infection (e.g., herpes encephalitis, congenital rubella) of the developing brain can have devastating neurodevelopmental consequences that increase risk for ASD (Chess, 1971; Ghaziuddin, Al-Khouri, & Ghaziuddin, 2002; Gillberg, 1986).

Recent interest has turned to the possibility that milder infectious episodes may also increase risk for ASD. Approximately one in every six brains of individuals with ASD demonstrates some evidence of immune-mediated reactions (lymphocytic infiltrates) in postmortem brain tissue samples (Bailey, Luthert, et al., 1998; Guerin et al., 1996). Some of the findings have implicated anomalies occurring during fetal development. The presence of lymphocytes in brain tissue is indicative of an adaptive immune response to infection. While maternal infection with mild common infectious diseases or febrile episodes is not associated with ASD, Atladottir, Henriksen, Schendel, and Parner (2012) have suggested that maternal influenza infection during pregnancy may double the risk for autism, and episodes causing prolonged fever can triple the risk. Although these results are preliminary and require replication, there is compelling data from animal studies associating both maternal fever (Edwards, 2006) and maternal influenza infection (Fatemi, Earle, et al., 2002; Fatemi, Folsom, Reutiman, Huang, et al., 2009) with alterations in fetal and postnatal development.

The underlying mechanisms for the anomalies in brain development in offspring remain unclear, but potential mediators include increased placental cytokines and oxidative stress. Animal models of the effects of influenza have shown that maternal immune activation results in elevations of pro-inflammatory cytokines and activation of astrocytes and microglia that may especially affect particular areas of the fetus's developing brain. Cytokines are proteins that regulate the nature, duration, and intensity of immune reactions and are involved in multiple aspects of neurodevelopment. Immune cytokines can influence neurodevelopment, specifically impacting progenitor cell differentiation, neural migration, and synaptic network formation (Deverman & Patterson, 2009).

Cytokine dysregulation can potentially have widespread effects on neurodevelopment (Goines & Ashwood, 2013). Animal studies have shown that areas of the brain showing evidence of cytokine activation include frontal and cingulate cortices, the hippocampus (Garay, Hsiao, Patterson, & McAllister, 2013), the cerebellum (Fatemi, Folsom, Reutiman, Abu-Odeh, et al., 2009) and the brain stem (Miller et al., 2013). Fatemi et al. (2008) found that prenatal exposure to influenza in mice resulted in reduced brain volumes at birth, but macrocephaly in later development. Fatemi and colleagues have suggested that maternal infection leads to abnormal gene regulation with consequent effects on brain development. These findings are of particular interest given evidence of a higher than expected incidence of macrocephaly in ASD (Barnard-Brak, Sulak, & Hatz, 2011; Davidovitch, Patterson, & Gartside, 1996; Deutsch, Folstein, Tager-Flusberg, & Gordon-Vaughn, 1999; Lainhart et al., 2006; Woodhouse et al., 1996). (See the section on "Head Circumference, Macrocephaly, and Megalencephaly.") Antineuronal antibodies can be found in the sera of children with ASD and as well as their mothers (Zimmerman et al., 2007) and are correlated with the autism severity (Piras et al., 2014). These findings appear to dovetail with several population-based cohort studies in humans which have identified maternal immune activation (MIA) as a risk factor in ASD (Atladottir et al., 2012; Zerbo et al., 2013).

Several studies have found abnormal immunoglobulin profiles in children with autism, although the evidence for this has been variable. Serum IgG, for example, has been described as increased, decreased, or both (Stigler et al., 2009). A recent animal study has also demonstrated some of the effects that immunoglobulins can have on brain development. When macaque mothers were administered immunoglobulins (IgG), and then isolated from mothers of children with ASD, their offspring not only showed abnormal social behavior during development but also demonstrated structural differences in brain development, particularly involving white matter in the frontal lobe (Bauman et al., 2013). Relatedly, studying humans has shown that parenteral autoimmune disease status was significantly associated with autism in offspring (Keil et al., 2010; Lyall, Ashwood, Van de Water, & Hertz-Picciotto, 2014).

Evidence of another type of immune response, one involving the production of microglia and astroglia, has also been observed in postmortem studies of ASD brains. Microglia are indigenous macrophages of the brain and are activated as part of the innate immune system's response in order to scavenge the brain for damaged neurons and infectious agents, which are then removed. They play a particularly important role in protecting the brain due to the unavailability of antibodies from other parts of the body that are too big to cross the blood-brain barrier. Microglia must therefore be sensitive to extremely small pathological changes in order to prevent fatal damage. Their activation is typically followed by the activation of pro-inflammatory and anti-inflammatory cytokines. Microglia and astroglia are also involved in repair and restoration following neuronal loss and produce growth factors to help maintain normal function within the CNS. Vargas, Nascimbene, Krishnan, Zimmerman, and Pardo (2005) examined postmortem brain tissue samples from individuals with ASD and observed evidence of widespread microglial and astroglial activation that was most common in cerebellum (present in 9 out of 10 brains). Laurence and Fatemi (2005) found increased levels of a protein marker of astroglial activation in the cerebellum, cingulate cortex and frontal lobe in postmortem samples from ten individuals with ASD. Morgan et al. (2010) examined postmortem tissue samples from dorsolateral frontal cortex (Brodmann area 9/46) of 13 individuals with autism and found evidence of microglial activation and increased microglial density in 38% of their sample. Zimmerman and colleagues have also demonstrated the presence of neuroglia and innate immune system activation in brain tissue of individuals with autism, supporting the view that neuroimmune abnormalities may contribute to the autism phenotype (Pardo, Vargas, & Zimmerman, 2006).

The circumstances prompting microglia and astroglia activation in the brains of autistic individuals remain unclear. Given that microglia activation is the main cellular response to CNS dysfunction, it could potentially reflect an innate autoimmune response to synaptic or neural network disturbances. Similar responses are evident in a number of neurodegenerative diseases such as Alzheimer's disease and Parkinson's disease. This contrasts with the findings of an adaptive immune response (e.g., lymphocyte and/or antibody-mediated reactions) observed in other neuropathological studies of the brain in ASD (Bailey, Luthert, et al., 1998; Guerin et al., 1996), which signify a response to infection.

Numerous reports have speculated on possible autoimmune factors that may prompt the production of autoantibodies that attack the brain (Braunschweig et al., 2013; Connolly, Streif, & Chez, 2003; Singer et al., 2008; see Stefanatos, Kinsbourne, & Wasserstein, 2002b for discussion). Data from diverse samples have suggested that anti-brain autoantibodies have been identified in about 30% to 70% of autistic children (Singh & Rivas, 2004; Singh, Warren, Averett, & Ghaziuddin, 1997; Todd, Hickok, Anderson, & Cohen, 1988). This includes but is not limited to autoantibodies to serotonin receptors, alpha-2 adrenergic binding sites, brain endothelial cells, myelin basic protein, and nerve growth factor (Ashwood & Van de Water, 2004; Hsiao, 2013; Krause, He, Gershwin, & Shoenfeld, 2002). In addition, there have been scattered reports of elevated anti-brain antibodies in the serum of mothers of children diagnosed with ASD (Zimmerman et al., 2007), suggesting that maternal antibodies might cross the placenta and affect prenatal brain development of their offspring. To further complicate interpretation, some of the observed cytokine elevations are similar to those associated with inflammation caused by epileptic spikes and may perhaps be suggestive of excessive glutamate excitotoxic effects (Pickering, Cumiskey, & O'Connor, 2005). Alternatively, the increased cytokines may represent a heightened immune response possibly associated with chronic brain inflammation and tissue necrosis (Li et al., 2009). The production of cytokines can have a significant impact on gene expression and neurodevelopment related to ASD (Cohly & Panja, 2005; Crespi & Thiselton, 2011; Gesundheit et al., 2013).

One of the first suggestions that autoimmune dysfunction may play a role in etiology of ASD emanated from a case report describing a child with ASD and a strong family history of autoimmune disorder (Money, Bobrow, & Clarke, 1971). This has since been followed by several studies indicating that autoimmune disorders cluster in the families of ASD children. Comi, Zimmerman, Frye, Law, and Peeden (1999) found that 46% of families with an autistic child had two or more members with autoimmune disorders. Common conditions were Type 1 diabetes, adult rheumatoid arthritis, hypothyroidism, and systemic lupus erythematosus. It is noteworthy that immune function is mediated by similar genes to those implicated in brain development (Warren et al., 1996).

Together, these findings suggest that different immune-mediated mechanisms may be operative in ASD. In some cases, the activation could possibly represent an abnormal neuroimmune response to some unspecified infection, while in others it could reflect an innate reaction to CNS dysfunction (Morgan et al., 2010; Vargas et al., 2005).

Genetic/Environmental Interactions

It has been suggested that some variants of ASD may occur as a result of genetically-related susceptibility to environmental stressors and exposures such as air pollution, heavy metals, insecticides, ethyl alcohol, food contaminants, and maternal smoking early in pregnancy (Geier & Geier, 2007; Kalia, 2008; Roberts et al., 2013; Roberts & English, 2013; Volk, Lurmann, Penfold, Hertz-Picciotto, & McConnell,

2013). In addition, a number of teratogenic influences have been implicated (e.g., thimerosal, thalidomide, valproic acid, ultrasound) (Landrigan, 2010; Williams & Casanova, 2010; Young, Geier, & Geier, 2008).

Some forms of exposure can potentially result in de novo genetic mutations that could potentially lead to deleterious phenotypes in the next generation. Others may result in oxidative stress, neuroinflammation, or mitochondrial dysfunction that could increase risk of consequences related to obstetric suboptimality (Rose et al., 2012; Zerbo et al., 2014). To date, there have been no large-population, cohort, or case-control studies that have definitely identified a specific toxic agent as a specific risk factor.

Stress

It has been argued that stressful life events and hardships should also be included among the pre- and perinatal risk events, since these events can potentially have biological effects on the pregnancy, delivery, and the neonatal phase (Dawson et al., 2000; Kinney, Barch, Chayka, Napoleon, & Munir, 2010). Ward (1990) previously reported that mothers of children with ASD described significantly higher family discord and psychiatric problems during pregnancy than mothers of children without ASD. The causal mechanisms underlying this association are ambiguous. However, Kinney, Miller, Crowley, Huang, and Gerber (2008) noted an increase in prevalence of ASD in Louisiana that was related, in a dose-response fashion, to the severity of storm exposure in the prenatal period, especially with exposures near the middle or end of gestation. Further exploration of this hypothesis in a large study examining the impact of multiple stressful life events failed to find an association between prenatal exposure and risk for ASD (Rai et al., 2012). This may relate to difficulties in operationalizing stress effects at the individual level.

Summary

Overall, there is reasonably compelling evidence connecting immune dysfunction to autism, but much of it remains indirect and fragmented. The mechanisms by which immune mechanism may alter brain anatomy and physiology of the specific pathways that are involved in autism are complex and remain to be fully elucidated. Further explorations in this area holds the promise of potentially leading to new avenues to treat or prevent the disorder (Chez, Memon, & Hung, 2004; Zerbo et al., 2014).

To date, evidence that immune-based therapy is beneficial in autism remains sparse. Groundbreaking reports by Buitelaar et al. (1992) and Stefanatos, Grover, and Geller (1995) described isolated successes of this approach in specific cases. These have been followed by additional case studies (Matarazzo, 2002; Mordekar, Prendergast, Chattopadhyay, & Baxter, 2009; Shenoy, Arnold, & Chatila, 2000) and small group studies (Plioplys, 1998; Stefanatos, Kollros, & Rabinovich, 1996). A recent retrospective study by Duffy et al. (2014) compared 20 children with regressive autism spectrum disorder (RASD) treated with corticosteroids to 24 children with ASD not treated with steroids (NSA). They described significant improvements in both clinical function as well as in the steady-state auditory evoked responses as described by Stefanatos (1993) and (Stefanatos, Foley, Grover, & Doherty, 1997). This research provides a rationale for a randomized trial with steroid therapy to determine the longer-term benefits and complications of steroids in this population (Golla & Sweeney, 2014).

Neuroscience of ASD

Diverse anomalies involving neural structure and function (cytoarchitecture, gross neuroanatomy, electrophysiology, regional cerebral metabolism, and neurochemistry) have been identified in children with autism. Here, we selectively review this literature with a view to providing sufficient background to understand current neuropsychological conceptualizations of ASD and its biological basis.

Head Circumference, Macrocephaly, and Megalencephaly

As noted earlier, Kanner's observation of "relatively large heads" in five of the children in his original cohort was likely of uncertain significance given the diverse developmental sequelae of macrocephaly. In order to differentiate the benign from the more neurologically-involved cases, Fletcher (1900) adopted the term *megalencephaly* to specifically denote head-size enlargement associated with pathological brain growth that resulted in impairment of function. In his defining postmortem investigation of megalencephaly, Fletcher described an overtly well-formed brain of increased volume and weight that on microscopic inspection revealed a variety of cytoarchitectural anomalies, the main one being excess density and number of glial cells. Kinnier Wilson (1934), one of the preeminent neurologists of the 1920s and 1930s, described diverse abnormalities of neural structure and organization in megalencephaly, including irregularities in cellular shape and size, heterotopias, perturbations in the laminar composition of the cortex and "disharmonic" distribution of gray and white matter (e.g., small corpus callosum, "packed" appearance of cerebral gyri). A case presented by McGrath (1935) is of particular interest given Kanner's observations. McGrath described a 32-year-old gentleman who, like many previously-reported cases of megalencephaly, was extremely low-functioning (mental age of 5 years, 11 months) and had a seizure disorder. The case is noteworthy because this gentleman displayed an unusual talent for remembering dates—a savant skill. He could correctly name the day of the week of any given date and could remember the precise date of significant events that occurred to himself or others on his ward (e.g., deaths, promotions, job start dates, blood draws, spinal taps, etc). While Kanner (1943) recognized special talents in his original 11 cases of infantile autism, he regarded them as "unquestionably endowed with good cognitive potentialities," and only one (Case 10) had a childhood history of seizures.

Kanner's observation regarding head size was overlooked for a half a century until Bailey et al. (1993) reported heavier than normal brain weight in a handful of cases of ASD who had come to postmortem investigation. These findings extended an earlier postmortem report of increased brain weight in one of two individuals with ASD (Williams, Hauser, Purpura, DeLong, & Swisher, 1980). Though the number of cases was small, Bailey et al. (1993) underscored the significance of this observation by pointing to findings from an epidemiological twin study showing a curiously high percentage of boys (42%) with autistic disorder (> 16 years) with unusually large occipital-frontal head circumference (OFHC) measurements (> 97th percentile) (Bailey et al., 1995). As evidence that this increased rate of macrocephaly was unrelated to twinning, Bailey et al. (1995) noted that a separate family genetic study showed a very similar elevation (37%) of macrocephaly in singletons with ASD (Bolton, Macdonald, Pickles, Rios, & et al., 1994). Given the established high correlation between OFHC and both brain weight (Lemons, Schreiner, & Gresham, 1981) and volume (Bray, Shields, Wolcott, & Madsen, 1969), Bailey et al. (1993) conjectured that a substantial proportion of cases of ASD were related to megalencephaly.

Numerous reports subsequently confirmed a significantly higher frequency of macrocephaly (9.5%–31.1%) in children and adults with ASD (Courchesne & Pierce, 2005a; Davidovitch et al., 1996; Fidler, Bailey, & Smalley, 2000; Fombonne, Roge, Claverie, Courty, & Fremolle, 1999; Gillberg & de Souza, 2002; Lainhart et al., 1997; Sacco et al., 2007a) compared to the general population (~3%). Indeed, this was, for a time, one of the most replicated anatomical findings concerning ASD (Lainhart, 2003). However, estimates of the proportion of affected individuals varied considerably from one study to the next, with relatively few studies matching the high rates observed by Bailey and colleagues Bailey et al., 1993; Bailey et al., 1995; Bolton, Macdonald, Pickles, Rios, & et al., 1994; Woodhouse et al., 1996). Pooling data from several sources, Fombonne et al. (1999) estimated that approximately 20% of individuals with ASD met criteria for frank macrocephaly. However, many subsequent studies have reported somewhat lower prevalence estimates (Deutsch et al., 1999; Lainhart et al., 1997; Torrey, Dhavale, Lawlor, & Yolken, 2004), and a few have failed to find that the frequency of macrocephaly in ASD was significantly different from reference populations (Cederlund, Miniscalco, & Gillberg, 2014; Constantino, Majmudar, et al., 2010; Davidovitch, Golan, Vardi, Lev, & Lerman-Sagie, 2011).

The age at which head circumference measurements are taken was identified as an important factor influencing the frequency of observations of macrocephaly in ASD. Mason-Brothers et al. (1987) examined birth records of children with ASD and found that the rate of macrocephaly (2%) was unremarkable. Subsequent studies have yielded similarly low estimates (typically 1%–6%), and most have concluded that the rate of macrocephaly at birth in ASD is not significantly different from that seen in the general population (Courchesne et al., 2001; Dementieva et al., 2005; Dissanayake, Bui, Huggins, & Loesch, 2006; Lainhart et al., 1997; Mraz, Green, Dumont-Mathieu, Makin, & Fein, 2007; Stevenson, Schroer, Skinner, Fender, & Simensen, 1997; Torrey et al., 2004; Whitehouse, Hickey, Stanley, Newnham, & Pennell, 2011). Interestingly, a couple of studies retrospectively examined prenatal ultrasound images and found a low frequency of macrocephaly in the fetal brain of children later diagnosed with ASD (Hobbs et al., 2007; Whitehouse et al., 2011). When observed, it was usually transient and normalized by birth. Indeed, anomalies in head size at birth in children with ASD may as likely be reflected in unusually small head circumference or *microcephaly* (defined as an OFHC < 3rd percentile) (Courchesne, Carper, & Akshoomoff, 2003; Fombonne et al., 1999; Grandgeorge, Lemonnier, & Jallot, 2013; Mason-Brothers et al., 1990; Miles et al., 2000; Torrey et al., 2004). Given these findings, it was reasoned that the higher rates of macrocephaly observed in young children and adults must be associated with developmental changes that occur some time after birth.

Although the number of children with ASD meeting criteria for macrocephaly is relatively small, it has been argued that this finding may have broader significance in understanding the neurobiological basis of ASD insofar as this subgroup may represent the extreme of a more general positive shift in the distribution of head size in children with ASD (Davidovitch et al., 2011; Dementieva et al., 2005; Fombonne et al., 1999). Considerable effort has therefore been devoted to gaining a better understanding of the mechanisms and time course associated with the emergence of macrocephaly in ASD. Given that neurogenesis is mostly complete by the end of the second trimester (Bystron, Blakemore, & Rakic, 2008), excess neurogenesis during fetal development seems an unlikely direct cause of subsequent observations of brain enlargement in ASD. Rather, the postnatal onset of macrocephaly more likely implicates a period of exuberant growth that occurs in the first few years of life (Huttenlocher, 1999; Koenderink & Uylings, 1995), although proliferative events in utero could possibly predispose children to exhibit anomalies at this later point in neurodevelopment. The first few years are a remarkably important period of brain development during which there is rapid growth of axons and apical dendrites, expansion of cortical synaptogenesis and interneuronal connectivity, and significant local proliferation and differentiation of glial cells (Ge, Miyawaki, Gage, Jan, & Jan, 2012). While all major sulci and gyri are established by the end of the third trimester of gestation (Chi, Dooling, & Gilles, 1977), brain volume and cortical surface at birth are only one-third of the adult brain (Hill et al., 2010; Thompson et al., 2007). In the first year alone, growth results in a near doubling (1.8x) of the cortical surface (Li et al., 2013) and is associated with an increase in head circumference at rates of approximately 0.4 cm per week (Lorber & Priestley, 1981). By 24 months of life, head size has grown to two-thirds of its eventual adult size.

Development of the cortex is a highly dynamic process, unfolding according to genetic code but influenced by experiential and epigenetic factors. The growth of connections between neighboring aggregations of cortical neurons located in different layers of cortex gives rise to the formation of *minicolumns,* the basic processing units of the cerebral cortex (Casanova, Buxhoeveden, Switala, & Roy, 2002; Mountcastle, 1997). This process begins at about the 20th gestational week and continues until about the second year of postnatal life. A spurt of growth at around 7 to 10 months involves lengthening of dendritic terminal segments and bifurcations, particularly in layers III and V (Koenderink, Uylings, & Mrzljak, 1994), which are the source of associational and projectional connections, respectively (Mrzljak, Uylings, Vaneden, & Judas, 1990). While cortical synaptogenesis begins at about 25 weeks gestation (Zecevic, 1998), peak periods occur in the first few years of postnatal life (Bianchi et al., 2013; Huttenlocher, 1999). Periods of proliferation are typically followed by subtractive phases during which there is pruning of superfluous axons, dendrites and synapses as well as programmed cell death (apoptosis). This pruning occurs in order to fine-tune and increase the efficiency of developing neural networks and is a particularly protracted process continuing into the third decade of life (Petanjek et al., 2011). As a consequence of these subtractive influences, the adult brain possesses approximately half the number of synapses as an average 2-year-old brain.

Given this extended postnatal timetable for neurodevelopment, numerous studies have attempted to identify when in childhood macrocephaly emerges. Early studies of macrocephaly in ASD defined a window for onset between 2 and 12 years (Aylward, Minshew, Field, Sparks, & Singh, 2002; Lainhart et al., 1997), during which there appeared to be a linear increase in the rate of macrocephaly with age (Fombonne et al., 1999). However, more than a dozen systematic retrospective and prospective studies subsequently demonstrated that most children with ASD show unusual enlargement in head size in the first two to three years of postnatal life (Courchesne et al., 2003; Courchesne et al., 2001; Dawson, Munson, et al., 2007; Dementieva et al., 2005; Mraz et al., 2007; Torrey et al., 2004; Webb et al., 2007). These studies have characterized an atypical head growth trajectory in ASD marked by an accelerated rate of increase in head circumference beginning around the fourth through sixth months (Courchesne & Pierce, 2005a; Dawson, Munson, et al., 2007; Gillberg & de Souza, 2002) that continues until just after the first year and then plateaus or decelerates (Courchesne et al., 2003; Dawson, Munson, et al., 2007; Sacco et al., 2007b). The accelerated rate of growth occurs independently of increases in body weight or length. While some studies report normalization of brain volume by adolescence (Aylward et al., 2002; Courchesne et al., 2001) and a lower frequency of macrocephaly (Bailey et al., 1995), others have reported that macrocephaly was more common in adolescents and adults with ASD than in younger children (Fombonne et al., 1999; Lainhart et al., 1997).

According to Courchesne et al. (2001), accelerated brain growth can be observed in the majority (~70%) of 2- to 3-year-old children with ASD, whether or not they eventually meet criteria for macrocephaly. It has been suggested that this accelerated early head growth trajectory may be a more important risk factor than macrocephaly for the later development of ASD (Dementieva et al., 2005; Elder et al., 2008). Others have suggested that the abnormal brain growth trajectories may be present in only a subpopulation of individuals with ASD. Suren, Stoltenberg, et al. (2013), for example, reported that accelerated head growth was not evident in girls with ASD and suggested that it may be a gender-specific phenomena. A few recent studies reported that accelerated head growth was limited to children with ASD who had a history of developmental regression (Chaste et al., 2013; Nordahl et al., 2011), although other studies have failed to find any such association (Webb et al., 2007) (see extended discussion of regression phenomena in the "Clinical Features and Developmental Course" section). Some investigators have suggested that macrocephaly may be a marker of more severe involvement, evidenced by significant correlations between macrocephaly and psychological characteristics such as low intelligence (Deutsch & Joseph, 2003; Miles et al., 2000), and greater severity of some of the core diagnostic features of autism (Lainhart et al., 2006). Others have reported that individuals with macrocephaly have higher levels of adaptive and social functioning (Dementieva et al., 2005).

It also remains unclear to what extent this pattern of early accelerated growth is specific to autism. Several studies have noted that it cuts across the autism spectrum to include Asperger syndrome and PDD-NOS (Dissanayake et al., 2006; Gillberg & de Souza, 2002). A few studies have observed that the prevalence of macrocephaly was also higher in relatives of macrocephalic children with ASD (Biran-Gol et al., 2010; Constantino, Majmudar, et al., 2010; Fidler et al., 2000; Miles et al., 2000), suggesting that it may be related to familial or endophenotypic factors. Elder et al. (2008) found that siblings of children with ASD who exhibited larger head circumference at 12 months with a subsequent deceleration of head growth between 12 and 24 months were more likely to demonstrate symptoms of autism than those siblings with more typical head growth trajectories. Rommelse et al. (2011) have argued that abnormal head growth may actually occur in other psychiatric disorders such as ADHD, oppositional defiant disorder, and communication disorders. Others have also noted a connection to ADHD symptomology (Ghaziuddin, Zaccagnini, Tsai, & Elardo, 1999; Gillberg & de Souza, 2002; Shinawi et al., 2010).

Genetic investigations have observed an association between macrocephaly and the gene PTEN (Buxbaum et al., 2007; Herman et al., 2007; Klein, Sharifi-Hannauer, & Martinez-Agosto, 2013; Marchese et al., 2014; McBride et al., 2010), which regulates a signaling pathway involved in controlling cellular growth, proliferation, and survival (Zhou & Parada, 2012). As a consequence of this relationship, screening PTEN has become a standard part of genetic screening in patients who present with autism and macrocephaly. In addition, mutations in the GLIALCAM gene can also result in megalencephaly and developmental delays and are sometimes associated with ASD and seizures (van der Knaap et al., 2010). Polymorphisms in the HOXA1 gene (Conciatori et al., 2004) and CNVs in the 16p interval (Luo et al., 2012) have also been associated with risk for an abnormally large head. These genes, like many others that have been implicated in ASD, may confer susceptibility to ASD by their role in multiple aspects of gene expression affecting morphogenesis and differentiation, influencing neuronal growth, migration, and the formation of neural connections. Behavioral anomalies associated with these mutations can span the autism spectrum and are certainly not specific to it.

The study of macrocephaly in ASD has remained an intense area of interest, in part because the measurement of OFHC offers an inexpensive, effective, and widely available means of monitoring brain growth early in development. The inconsistency in the findings may stem in part from relatively small sample size in many of the studies. Other factors potentially contributing to the variability in results include differences in recruitment methods (e.g., clinic, community, epidemiological), sample demographic characteristics (e.g., gender distribution, age), diagnostic criteria (e.g., strictly autistic disorder vs. ASD), and variations in the definition of macrocephaly. While most studies have defined macrocephaly as an OFHC of more than two standard deviations above the mean (Fishman, 1990), this has been interpreted slightly differently (e.g., ≥ 97th percentile vs. > 97th percentile vs. ≥ 98th vs. > 98th percentile). A related procedural difference concerns the choice of normative databases used to determine the empirical cutoff for classification of macrocephaly. Studies completed in the United States have utilized norms from Roche, Guo, Wholihan, and Casey (1997); Nellhaus (1968); or the CDC (Kuczmarski et al., 2002; Rollins, Collins, & Holden, 2010). Studies from the United Kingdom have often utilized norms compiled by Tanner (1978) or the World Health Organization (WHO, 2007), while Scandinavian studies (e.g., Cederlund et al., 2014; Gillberg & de Souza, 2002) have utilized national and local population norms. The choice of normative database has become a critical issue given recent observations that different norm sources describe substantially different distributions especially at the upper percentiles (Daymont, Hwang, Feudtner, & Rubin, 2010). Indeed, Raznahan et al. (2013) have argued that many of the observations of accelerated head growth in ASD reflect biases in the head circumference norms used. Specifically, they cite several recent studies suggesting that utilization of norms from the CDC (Kuczmarski et al., 2002) can lead to observations of abnormal growth trajectories in the first year in samples of healthy neurotypical children. Relatedly, given secular increases in population head circumference measurements that have apparently occurred over time (Ounsted, Moar, & Scott, 1985), it has been argued that norms widely used in the United Kingdom (Tanner, Gairdner-Pearson, 1978) are obsolete. While new norm sources are available, problems also exist with these alternatives at least beyond the age of 2 years (Rollins et al., 2010; Wright et al., 2002).

A recent study by Muratori et al. (2012) is illustrative of some of the procedural issues and problems inherent in a number of these investigations. These investigators retrospectively analyzed serial head circumference measurements from birth to 12 months in 50 preschoolers who had been diagnosed with ASD following assessment at a second-level autism center. These measurements were then compared to measurements obtained from 100 healthy typically developing children seen in pediatric practices in the same metropolitan area (Pisa, Italy). Measurements were collected at four time points for each child: birth, 1–2 months, 3–5 months, and 6–12 months of age. Consistent with some previous reports, there were no group differences in head circumference at birth, but by the third to fifth months, mean head size was significantly larger in the ASD group. When referenced to the CDC norms at the 6–12 month interval, 18% of the children with ASD had macrocephaly compared to 9% of the controls. These results were interpreted as demonstrating that the accelerated growth in head circumference in children with ASD begins in the first few months of life, a conclusion that is consistent with some other reports (e.g., Dementieva et al., 2005). However, it is noteworthy that the rate of macrocephaly reported in the neurotypical controls in this study matched or exceeded the rate found in ASD in some other studies (e.g., 4%, see Cederlund et al., 2014; 4.4%, see Davidovitch et al., 2011; 6%, see Grandgeorge et al., 2013; 9%, see Suren, Bakken, et al., 2013). In light of the lower prevalence of macrocephaly observed in these studies and the methodological concerns discussed on p. 206, questions have arisen as to whether there is a special connection between head size or macrocephaly and ASD (Cederlund et al., 2014; Davidovitch et al., 2011).

Neuropathological Studies

Several early studies attempted to identify neuroanatomic substrates underlying ASD through histological analysis of postmortem brain specimens (Schain & Yannet, 1960; Williams et al., 1980) or biopsy material (Aarkrog, 1968). Although Schain and Yannet alluded to the "dropping out of cells in the hippocampal formation" (1960, p. 565), due to the subtle nature of the underlying pathophysiology and given technological limitations of the time, these studies had limited yield. However, the emergence of rigorous computer-facilitated stereological analytic methods to examine the cytoarchitecture of the brain in the 1970s proved to be a significant technical advance for comparing brain development in neurotypical individuals to individuals with ASD.

Limbic and Paralimbic Structures

In a pioneering study, Bauman and Kemper (1985) compared postmortem specimens obtained of a 29-year-old man with autism to that of an age -and sex-matched control. While they observed no differences in myelination or in the cellular architecture of several subcortical structures (basal forebrain, thalamus, hypothalamus, and basal ganglia), anomalies were apparent in the cerebellum, limbic, and paralimbic structures. Neurons in the hippocampus and amygdala were smaller in size and showed higher cell-packing density (increased number of neurons per-unit volume). Similar findings were evident in samples taken from the subiculum, entorhinal cortex, mammillary bodies, and medial septal nucleus. Further analysis revealed that hippocampal neurons from layers CA1 and CA4 showed evidence of limitations in intercellular connectivity and communication, which were apparent in diminished complexity and extent of dendritic arbors. They did not find evidence of substantial gliosis and overall regarded the observed changes as characteristic of neural architecture at an early stage of brain maturation rather than brain damage. While the results from this case were potentially confounded by a premorbid history of epilepsy (Amaral, Bauman, & Schumann, 2003), similar anomalies were evident in five additional cases by the same investigators (reviewed in Kemper & Bauman, 1993) and in an independent sample of two subjects (Raymond, Bauman, & Kemper, 1996). However, others have suggested that this is not a consistent finding (Bailey, Luthert, et al., 1998). Amaral, Schumann, and Nordahl (2008), for example, failed to observe anomalies in neuronal size in amygdala, but did find significant overall reductions in neuron counts.

Wegiel et al. (2010) recently reported the presence of heterotopias in hippocampus as well as in periventricular areas in 4 of 13 individuals (31%) with ASD. Irregular organization of neurons has also been identified in posterior cingulate gyrus (Kemper & Bauman, 1993; Oblak, Rosene, Kemper, Bauman, & Blatt, 2011). These findings are suggestive of problems in neural migration.

Cerebellum

A more consistent finding, initially observed by Bauman and Kemper (1985) and subsequently replicated by several other investigators (Bailey, Luthert, et al., 1998; Fatemi, Emamian, et al., 2002; Kemper & Bauman, 1998; Lee et al., 2002; Ritvo & et al., 1986; Wegiel et al., 2010), concerns a decrease in the number and size of Purkinje cells and, to a lesser degree, granule cells in the neocerebellar cortex and the inferior olivary nucleus of the brain stem. Kemper and Bauman (1998) commented that, in their experience, these anomalies occurred in the absence of glial cell hyperplasia and therefore likely emerged early in the prenatal period (prior to 30 weeks gestation) when glial cells are unable to proliferate. The cerebellum and the inferior olivary nucleus develop reciprocal connections during fetal development that are fairly well established by 28–30 weeks gestation. Loss of Purkinje cells after this period generally results in retrograde degeneration of neurons in the inferior olive. Given that neurons in the inferior olivary nucleus appeared small, but not diminished in number, Bauman and Kemper (2005) argued that it is likely that the Purkinje cells loss in ASD occurs early in neurodevelopment before the functional coupling with the inferior olive. Others, however (e.g., Bailey, Luthert, et al., 1998), have observed that Purkinje cell loss may sometimes be accompanied by gliosis, allowing the possibility that postmortem anomalies in some cases reflect peri- or postnatal factors. Purkinje cells have an exceptionally high metabolic demand and are susceptible to multiple pathogenic influences. Some of these influences may be associated with birth trauma (ischemia, hypoxia, excitotoxicity), while others may be related to adverse events during fetal development such as viral infections, thiamine deficiency, and exposure to heavy metals and toxins (Kern, 2003). While loss of Purkinje cells has been reported in nearly three-quarters of known autopsy cases (Palmen, van Engeland, Hof, & Schmitz, 2004), the neurodevelopmental significance of this finding remains to be fully elucidated.

Cortex

Although early studies reported no anomalies of the cerebral neocortex (Bauman & Kemper, 2005; Coleman, Romano, Lapham, & Simon, 1985; Guerin et al., 1996), more recent studies have identified subtle disturbances of cortical development in a proportion of cases (Bailey, Luthert, et al., 1998; Casanova, 2007; Hof, Knabe, Bovier, & Bouras, 1991). Anomalies include cortical thickening, increased neuronal density, irregular patterns of cortical lamination, small and unusually-oriented pyramidal cells, and heterotopias (Bailey, Luthert, et al., 1998; Coleman et al., 1985; Kemper & Bauman, 1998). However, the number of subjects in these studies was often small, and there is typically considerable interindividual variability. These issues continue to be evident in more recent studies. Jacot-Descombes et al. (2012) studied eight postmortem brains of individuals with ASD and identified decreased size of pyramidal neurons in areas 44 and 45 (Broca's area), although there was no difference in neuron number or layer volumes. By contrast, Courchesne et al. (2012) examined seven postmortem brains and found 67% more neurons in the prefrontal cortex (PFC) and 75% more neurons in dorsolateral prefrontal cortex compared to controls. This was accompanied by an increase in brain weight. Given the atypical developmental trajectories of brain growth in ASD, the difference in findings may be attributable to the younger age at which the specimens became available for study in the Courchesne study (6–16 years vs. 4–48 years). However, (Stoner et al., 2014) recently reported that the brains of individuals with ASD demonstrated focal patches of cytoarchitectural abnormalities, which showed some degree of regional variation across individuals. Specifically, they observed abnormal laminar cytoarchitecture and cortical disorganization of neurons in most patches of tissue from prefrontal and temporal cortex, but not in tissue from occipital cortex. Glial cells were unaffected. Anomalies were most clearly evident in layers 4 and 5, although no layer was spared. These findings point to disturbances of cortical layer formation and neuronal differentiation that typically occurs during prenatal brain development. While these findings may reflect a migrational defect, they could also possibly arise from early anomalies of genetic transcriptional changes that sequentially specify distinct cell fates of progenitor cells.

Additional anomalies in corticogenesis have been identified by Casanova et al. (2002), who reported that cortical minicolumns were unusually configured in the brains of individuals with ASD in at least three areas of cortex: (a) Brodmann area 9 (BA 9) of prefrontal cortex, (b) BA 21 in the temporal lobe, and (c) BA 22 in posterior temporal cortex. Columns were smaller and there was less of the space between cells that normally contains dendrites, axons, and synapses (neuropil). Minicolumns were abnormally narrow in frontal and temporal cortex but not in occipital cortex. It was suggested that the resulting circuitry may lack the inhibitory influences that minicolumns typically exert on adjacent columns. This lack of lateral inhibition may potentially result in diminished ability to discriminate sensory information due to an increase in "neural noise," which may account for the hypersensitivity seen in many children with ASD. In addition, islands of excessive excitatory activity could potentially develop into seizure foci (Casanova, 2006). The factors underlying the emergence of this atypical architecture remain unclear. Since the number of minicolumns in developing cortex is related to the number of cells produced in the subventricular proliferative zone (Kornack & Rakic, 1998), the apparent migrational disturbances may indirectly relate to excessive proliferation of neurons earlier in development.

A few studies have provided evidence indicating that individuals with ASD also demonstrate an excess of dendritic spines on apical dendrites of pyramidal cells in cortical layer 2 of frontal, temporal, and parietal cortex (Hutsler & Zhang, 2010; Phillips & Pozzo-Miller, 2015). This excess potentially implicates problems during embryogenesis, or alternatively, these observations may reflect a failure of pruning processes that normally follow exuberant growth. In contrast to these excesses, significant reductions in neuronal density (van Kooten et al., 2008) and decreases in $GABA_A$ and $GABA_B$ receptor density have been observed in the fusiform gyrus (FG), an area thought to play a special role in face perception. Similarly, significant reductions in $GABA_A$ receptor density have been observed in anterior and posterior cingulate cortex (PCC; see Oblak, Gibbs, & Blatt, 2009; Oblak, Gibbs, & Blatt, 2010), structures involved in cognitive control that have been implicated in restricted or repetitive behaviors in ASD. Fatemi, Reutiman, Folsom, and Thuras (2009) observed reductions in $GABA_A$ receptor subunits in the cerebellum, superior frontal cortex (BA9), and parietal cortex. These areas have often been implicated in ASD utilizing a variety of methods of investigation. Several studies have recently confirmed anomalies in GABA concentration in vivo utilizing ^1H magnetic resonance spectroscopy (^1H MRS). These are discussed in a later section, "Magnetic Resonance Spectroscopy and Positron Emission Tomography."

Summary

The interpretation of histopathological studies in ASD is complicated by a large number of potential confounding variables. The very small number of cases comprising each of these studies is a serious problem that is exacerbated by inconsistencies in the quantitative histopathological techniques used and the tremendous heterogeneity of the disorder itself. Most of the studies have involved the examination of human pathological material obtained from deceased older children and adults, so the results are inevitably also confounded by an enormous number of potential epigenetic and environmental effects. Given the manner in which specimens come under study, important variables such as the presence of intellectual disability, seizure disorders, medical complications, and use of medications have remained uncontrolled. It could therefore be argued that the findings described in these reports reflect the effects of having autism as much as the neurobiological circumstances that increase risk for developing the disorder.

Other findings such as increased neuronal density and number, variations in cortical thickness, disturbances of laminar structure, the presence of ectopic neurons, and the anomalies of minicolumn formation implicate anomalies in neural proliferation and migration probably occurring in the first six months of gestation (Bailey, Palferman, Heavey, & Le Couteur, 1998; Gillberg, 1999; Piven, Berthier, Starkstein, Nehme, et al., 1990). Other anomalies implicate disturbances of program cell death (apoptosis), cell fate specification, pruning, and neuronal connectivity that could reflect anomalies in the postnatal neurodevelopment. As already discussed, recent advances in genetics have implicated the possible role of a number of genes that have a direct impact on neurodevelopment after birth, towards the second half of the first year. These anomalies can lead to a number of disturbances identifiable at the macrostructural level such as atypical formation of the cortex (e.g., polymicrogyria or macrogyria) and cortical heterotopias.

Structural Neuroimaging

Head circumference has provided an easy and important window to study early brain growth in ASD. However, approximately 90% of adult total brain volume occurs by 5 years of age, so that an increasing proportion of variance in subsequent head growth is accounted for by growth of non-neural tissue (Tate, Bigler, McMahon, & Lainhart, 2007). As a result, the strong correlation (.88–.93) that exists between head circumference and total brain volume in young children (Bartholomeusz, Courchesne, & Karns, 2002; Hazlett et al., 2005) decreases with age to about .67 (Piven, Arndt, Bailey, & Andreasen, 1996). Recognizing these limitations, an increasing number of investigators have undertaken a more direct approach to examining brain growth using high-resolution structural neuroimaging. This approach offers an opportunity to examine brain development in vivo with exquisite anatomic resolution and independently of other aspects of physical growth. On the assumption that symptoms of ASD must arise from anomalies of neural function that arise prior to the end of toddlerhood, a growing number of these studies have been directed to examining brain growth in the first few years of life at a time when symptoms of autism are unfolding.

Overall, structural MRI studies have generally confirmed that young children with ASD (2–4 years) demonstrate larger whole-brain volumes of gray and white matter than controls (Aylward et al., 2002; Piven et al., 1995; Sparks et al., 2002) than controls. Differences were identified in the first 6 to 12 months after birth, and by 2 to 4 years of age, whole-brain volumes in ASD were approximately 10% larger than neurotypical controls (Hazlett et al., 2005; Redcay & Courchesne, 2005). By 4 to 5 years of age, brain size in individuals with ASD approached maximum volume, which was comparable to the volume of typically developing adolescents (Courchesne et al., 2001). Some studies have suggested the total brain volume in adolescents are within normal limits (Courchesne et al., 2001; Stanfield et al., 2008), while others have reported that elevated total brain volume can persist into adolescence and adulthood (Freitag et al., 2009; Hazlett, Poe, Gerig, Smith, & Piven, 2006).

While differences in brain size in ASD have been most reliably indexed by total volume measures, a number of studies have suggested differential involvement of various regions of cortex (Piven et al., 1996). Several reports have described an anterior-to-posterior gradient, with most enlargement in frontal lobes and temporal lobes (Courchesne et al., 2007), followed by parietal areas (Amaral et al., 2008), and least enlargement in the occipital lobes (Brun et al., 2009; Carper & Courchesne, 2005; Hazlett et al., 2006). A number of studies have explored this further, utilizing methods to parcellate whole-brain images into smaller reliably-defined regions of interest. Several studies have identified enlargement in dorsolateral prefrontal and medial frontal cortex and noted that these volumetric increases were apparent in the first couple of years and changed less over time compared to typically-developing children. (Carper & Courchesne, 2005; Carper, Moses, Tigue, & Courchesne, 2002).

Other areas of enlargement noted in the first 2 to 4 years includes the temporal and parietal lobes (Hazlett et al., 2011; Schumann et al., 2010), the cingulate (Schumann et al., 2010), cerebellum (Bloss & Courchesne, 2007; Courchesne et al., 2001), and the amygdala (Mosconi et al., 2009; Schumann, Barnes, Lord, & Courchesne, 2009; Sparks et al., 2002). Relatively few studies have examined differences in subcortical structures in young children with ASD. A few studies have reported decreased volumes in the brain stem (Hashimoto et al., 1995) and cerebellar vermis relative to controls (Bloss & Courchesne, 2007; Hashimoto et al., 1995; Webb et al., 2009). However, conclusions derived from the results of these studies must be tempered with recognition of the often small sample sizes. Other studies have found no evidence of early abnormalities in brain structure in ASD (Zeegers et al., 2009).

A meta-analysis by Stanfield et al. (2008) of 43 structural imaging studies largely involving children greater than 7 years of age, adolescents, and adults, confirmed that the total brain volume in individuals with ASD was larger than controls. In addition, the analysis revealed increased volume of both left and right cerebral hemispheres, the cerebellum and the caudate. By contrast, decreased volumes were evident in midbrain, cerebellar vermis, and parts of the corpus callosum. Overall, the results reveal a complex pattern of regional overdevelopment and underdevelopment within more general effects related to overall brain volume. Because of the continual changes that occur in brain development from infancy through adulthood, longitudinal studies are required to assess the reliability of obtained and cross-sectional studies. Some preliminary longitudinal studies recently described increased volume in amygdala and hippocampus in children with ASD between 2 and 4 years (Mosconi et al., 2009; Nordahl et al., 2012) and also in 8–12 year olds (Barnea-Goraly et al., 2014). One of the largest longitudinal studies followed 41 children diagnosed with ASD examining multiple scans that had been collected from 1.5 years up to 5 years of age. Significant enlargement in both cerebral gray and white matter were evident by 2.5 years of age, with the most severe enlargement occurring in frontal, temporal, and cingulate cortices (Schumann et al., 2010).

Gray Matter Versus White Matter

Questions arose as to whether this excess growth primarily affected gray or white matter, or both. A meta-analysis by Via, Radua, Cardoner, Happe, and Mataix-Cols (2011) focused on a small number of studies utilizing voxel-based morphometry (VBM), a method that is well-suited to detecting regional differences in gray and white matter throughout the brain. The analysis failed to find differences in global gray matter volumes between individuals with ASD and controls, although small increases in gray matter volume were evident in left middle inferior frontal gyrus (BA 46 and BA 10). These areas in rostral and adjacent dorsolateral prefrontal cortex are thought to be involved in executive function. By contrast, robust gray matter reductions in the ASD group were evident in the amygdala/hippocampus (particularly on the right side) and medial parietal areas (precuneus-BA 7). A meta-analysis by Cauda et al. (2011) revealed rather more extensive gray matter increases involving the cerebellum, middle temporal gyrus, cingulate cortex, regions around the junction of the occipital, temporal and parietal lobes, and several subcortical structures including the caudate head and the insula. Decreases in gray matter were evident bilaterally in the cerebellar tonsils, inferior parietal lobule, right amygdala, insula, and middle temporal gyrus, as well as the caudate tail and precuneus. Together, these analyses revealed a very mixed pattern of over- and underdevelopment in highly-distributed areas of frontal, temporal, and parietal cortex, as well as in several subcortical structures including the cerebellum, amygdala, and parts of the basal ganglia.

A few studies have shown an accelerated decrease in cortical thickness in temporal, parietal, and occipital cortex during late childhood and early adolescence (Hardan, Libove, Keshavan, Melhem, & Minshew, 2009; Raznahan et al., 2010; Scheel et al., 2011; Wallace, Dankner, Kenworthy, Giedd, & Martin, 2010). These changes then appear to abate in adulthood (Zielinski et al., 2014). Cortical thinning has been noted in several studies of adults with ASD (Hadjikhani, Joseph, Snyder, & Tager-Flusberg, 2006; Hardan, Muddasani, Vemulapalli, Keshavan, & Minshew, 2006) involving areas critical to both communication and social function (inferior frontal cortex, superior temporal sulcus) as well as regions that may be more specifically involved in social perception and interaction (FG, cingulate gyrus, inferior parietal lobule). By contrast, gray matter increases have been noted in primary and associative auditory and visual cortex, providing a potential structural correlate to observations of enhanced auditory and visual processing skills (Hyde, Samson, Evans, & Mottron, 2010).

Analysis of white matter differences also revealed a complex pattern of anomalies. Some studies have reported increased whole-brain white matter volume (Bigler et al., 2010; Hazlett et al., 2005), while others have observed no difference. Reports of increased volume in specific regions, particularly areas underlying frontal and temporal cortex, have been inconsistent (Ke et al., 2009). There has been greater agreement regarding areas of diminished white matter volume. One of the more consistently reported structural neuroimaging findings in individuals with ASD is decreased volume of segments of the corpus callosum (CC), although there is inconsistency as to which sections (genu, body, or splenium) are mainly affected (Hardan, Pabalan, et al., 2009; Piven, Bailey, Ranson, & Arndt, 1997; Uddin et al., 2011; Waiter et al., 2005). Both anterior and posterior connections may potentially have a major influence on neuropsychological functions that require integration of information between the hemispheres and may have a particular impact on social development and social communication (Rosema, Crowe, & Anderson, 2012).

Several studies have suggested that long-range fibers comprising cortico-cortical pathways may also be compromised in ASD. While short U-shaped association fibers provide connections between adjacent gyri, these long association fibers mediate the communication of information between widely distributed areas of cortex. Several studies have identified anomalies of fibers linking frontal cortex to other areas in the brain (Courchesne & Pierce, 2005b; Just, Cherkassky, Keller, Kana, & Minshew, 2007; Just, Cherkassky, Keller, & Minshew, 2004). Herbert et al. (2004) suggested that the timing of myelination is a primary contributor to regional variations in white matter enlargement. Consistent with this, Carper and Courchesne (2005) observed a rapid increase in white matter volume in dorsolateral and medial frontal cortex in children with ASD between 2 and 5 years of age. Dorsolateral prefrontal cortex subsequently showed decreased development with increasing age from 2 to 11 years. Overall, the results add to growing evidence of patterns of local overconnectivity and long-distance underconnectivity in ASD (Belmonte et al., 2004; Wass, 2011).

Decreased white matter volume has also been identified in the cerebellum (Brun et al., 2009; Lotspeich et al., 2004; McAlonan et al., 2005). Given that the results that many of these studies are based on a small number of subjects, Radua, Via, Catani, and Mataix-Cols (2011) performed a meta-analysis combining information from 13 data sets. This analysis failed to find global volumetric differences in white matter. However, increased white matter volumes were evident in the right arcuate fasciculus, and left uncinate and inferior fronto-occipital fasciculi. The left external and extreme capsule were also moderately enlarged. Small decreases in white matter volume were evident in right anterior cingulate and corpus callosum.

Summary

The reliability of a number of the identified differences in brain structure and function remains uncertain given the relatively small number of studies incorporated into the analyses and the broad age range of the combined sample. Since brain development is a dynamic and nonlinear process, it is possible that changes in ASD that are particular to early childhood are not currently appreciated. Importantly, a number of recent longitudinal studies have been completed focusing on young children with ASD (<4 years). These have generally found significant enlargement in gray and, to a lesser extent, white matter volumes compared with other clinical samples and typical controls (Carper et al., 2002; Hazlett et al., 2005; Hoeft et al., 2011; Schumann et al., 2010; Sparks et al., 2002). Schumann et al. (2010) found enlargement in frontal, temporal, and cingulate cortices starting by age 2.5 years. Hazlett et al. (2011) noted generalized cortical enlargement that was particularly evident in temporal white matter. There was no significant increase in the rate of cerebral growth across multiple brain regions from 2 to 4 years of age, suggesting that volumetric differences had emerged earlier in life. No between-group differences were found for cortical thickness, but there were significant increases in estimates of cortical surface area. Overall, they concluded that the overgrowth was most likely related to increased cortical surface area. Overgrowth tends to be observed in association areas more consistently than in primary sensory or motor cortex (Carper & Courchesne, 2005).

Diffusion Tensor Imaging

The significance of anomalies of white matter development in ASD also been examined utilizing diffusion tensor imaging (DTI). By tracking local water molecule displacement patterns, DTI provides measures of the integrity of axons: fractional anisotropy (FA); mean diffusivity (MD); and the degree of myelination, which is inversely related to radial diffusion (RD). Several recent DTI studies have disclosed anomalies in the microintegrity of subsections of the corpus callosum (Brito et al., 2009; Noriuchi et al., 2010; Shukla, Keehn, Lincoln, & Muller, 2010; Thomas, Humphreys, Jung, Minshew, & Behrmann, 2011; Weinstein et al., 2011). In addition, a number of studies have fairly consistently implicated anomalies of the internal capsule (Brito et al., 2009; Ingalhalikar, Parker, Bloy, Roberts, & Verma, 2011; Keller, Kana, & Just, 2007; Shukla, Keehn, & Muller, 2011) and cerebellar white matter pathways, particularly the middle cerebellar peduncle (Brito et al., 2009; Cheng et al., 2010; Shukla et al., 2010; Sivaswamy et al., 2010). There are also numerous reports of abnormal diffusivities involving long tracts that mediate cortico-cortical connectivity including the cingulum (Bloemen et al., 2010; Noriuchi et al., 2010), arcuate and superior longitudinal fasciculus (Fletcher et al., 2010; Ingalhalikar et al., 2011; Knaus et al., 2010; Kumar et al., 2009), uncinate fasciculus (Poustka et al., 2012), occipital-frontal fasciculus, and inferior longitudinal fasciculus (in the region of the right FG) (Jou et al., 2011; Mills et al., 2013).

Overall, these studies suggest widespread microstructural anomalies of the axonal membranes and/or myelin in multiple long white matter tracts involved in cortical-subcortical connectivity and both intrahemispheric and interhemispheric transmission of information (Vissers, Cohen, & Geurts, 2012). Given the plasticity of the nervous system, and the important role of use-dependent connectivity, it is perhaps not surprising that anomalies of white matter would follow from perturbations of cellular structure and function. A study by Wolff et al. (2012) suggests that these anomalies are present early in life. They measured FA starting at 6 months until 2 years of age in high-risk siblings of children with ASD. Out of 15 fiber pathway trajectories, 12 showed significant differences between children who eventually demonstrated ASD at 2 years relative to those that did not. FA was higher at 6 months, but changed over time and was lower by age 2 years in those children with ASD. Low FA remains low across development into adolescence with ASD. These findings are of interest since they suggest that altered neural circuitry antedates the clinical onset of ASD. The significance of the higher than typical FA early in the first year of development may represent dampened axonal elimination during the pruning that occurs during this period (Cascio et al., 2013; de Graaf-Peters & Hadders-Algra, 2006).

Given particular involvement of multiple long pathways, some have suggested that ASD should be conceptualized as a disconnection syndrome (Frith, 2004; Geschwind & Levitt, 2007; Melillo & Leisman, 2009). According to this viewpoint, many symptoms of ASD may reflect dysfunction of distributed functional networks resulting from anomalies of white matter affecting association and commissural fibers rather than from localized impairment. Due to the widespread distribution of identified white matter anomalies, the functional implications may be many and diverse. Abnormalities of the corpus callosum would suggest inefficiencies in the interhemispheric transfer of information between homologous areas of cortex. These anomalies can potentially impact many aspects of higher-order cognition requiring bihemisphere integration of information and may affect patterns of cerebral organization and modes of processing (Conturo et al., 2008; Fletcher et al., 2010; Travers et al., 2012). Widespread involvement of association fibers may pose problems both in intrahemispheric communication and in cortical-subcortical transfer of information, potentially compromising the function of neural networks distributed in frontal, temporal, and parietal cortex that mediate language, social perception, and behavioral regulation (Langen et al., 2012). Sensory and perceptual processing may also be affected. For example, anomalies of the microstructure (low FA) of inferior longitudinal fasciculus and the splenium of the corpus callosum have been implicated in atypical sensory processing in ASD, including "tactile defensiveness" (Pryweller et al., 2014). Subcortical tracts that appear to be compromised include cortico-subcortical connections between the prefrontal cortex and the thalamus, cingulate, and cerebrocerebellar circuits. Compromise of these white matter tracts can potentially impede memory and motor function (Shukla et al., 2010). They may also affect communication with subcortical structures involved in emotional regulation and attentional divestment such as the amygdala, basal ganglia, and cingulate cortex (Mike et al., 2013; Zikopoulos & Barbas, 2010). Although some studies have also shown compromise of short-distance tracts (Shukla, Keehn, Smylie, & Muller,

2011), local white matter fibers appear to be less affected and some studies have suggested that they may be overdeveloped (Courchesne & Pierce, 2005b).

Metabolic neuroimaging

Magnetic Resonance Spectroscopy

Proton magnetic resonance spectroscopy (MRS) is a very useful neuroimaging method for examining cerebral metabolism in autism. Early studies utilized MRS to inspect metabolic markers of neuronal integrity. Contrary to some expectations based on ana observations of excessive proliferation, concentrations of metabolites of neural activity derived from MRS (NAA, Cr, Cho, mI, and Glx) have been noted to widespread reductions rather than an increase in neuronal or synaptic activity. Metabolite levels have been noted to fluctuate in an age-dependent manner across the whole brain, and in some areas, increases were evident. Overall, these studies have implicated reductions of gray matter integrity in cortex, amygdala, hippocampus, cerebellum, thalamus, cingulate gyrus, and in subregions of the frontal, temporal, and parietal lobes (DeVito et al., 2007; Endo et al., 2007; Hardan et al., 2008; Suzuki et al., 2009). Recent meta-analyses have shown that the metabolic abnormalities tend to decrease and normalize with age (Baruth, Wall, Patterson, & Port, 2013; Ipser et al., 2012). More recently, emphasis has turned to measurement of glutamate metabolism due to postmortem studies that have disclosed evidence of glutamate dysfunction in ASD (Purcell, Jeon, Zimmerman, & Pevsner, 2001). MRS is the only tool available for noninvasive nonradioactive in vivo assessments of glutamate neurotransmission. These studies have revealed alterations of glutamate metabolism in the frontal and temporal lobes and the cingulate gyrus, but not in the cerebellum (Brown, Singel, Hepburn, & Rojas, 2013; Harada et al., 2011; Joshi et al., 2013; Tebartz van Elst et al., 2014). Significant reductions have also been noted in GABA in motor and auditory areas of frontal and temporal lobes, respectively (Gaetz et al., 2014; Harada et al., 2010; Rojas, Singel, Steinmetz, Hepburn, & Brown, 2014). Since GABA is the major inhibitory neurotransmitter in the central nervous system, these findings are compatible with the notion that an imbalance between excitatory and inhibitory influences on neurotransmission is a fundamental aspect of the problems in brain function associated with ASD (Rubenstein, 2010).

Positron Emission Tomography

Positron emission tomography (PET) has allowed the examination of serotonergic metabolism in ASD. The serotonergic system has long been implicated in autism due to observations that approximately 25%–30% of individuals with ASD demonstrate whole blood serotonin levels that are 25% higher than average. Given that serotonin is involved in regulating mood, sleep, and a form of behavioral inhibition, these findings were considered to have etiologic significance. In addition, serotonin is known to play an important role in neurodevelopment, having important neurotrophic properties during neural migration as well as influencing aspects of neuronal differentiation, myelination, dendritic maturation, and synaptogenesis (Vitalis, Ansorge, & Dayer, 2013; Whitaker-Azmitia, 2001). Several PET studies have found evidence of deficient serotonin metabolism in the brain, specifically in frontal cortex, thalamus, and dentate nucleus (Beversdorf et al., 2012; Chugani et al., 1997). Given cytoarchitectonic evidence of anomalous dendritic development in ASD, it is noteworthy that serotonin influences overall dendritic length, spine formation, and arborization in the hippocampus and cerebral cortex (Sikich, Hickok, & Todd, 1990).

Functional Neuroimaging and Connectivity

While DTI discloses information regarding the microstructural integrity of white matter pathways, these data do not necessarily speak to the functional and effective connectivity of distributed neural networks (Damoiseaux & Greicius, 2009). Examination of functional and effective connectivity is generally addressed in investigations of temporal synchrony or coherence in electrophysiological signals (e.g., Electroencephalogram, Magnetoencephalogram, Event-Related Potentials) or through the analysis of coactivation patterns in blood oxygenation level dependent responses (BOLD) as measured with functional magnetic resonance imaging. This area of investigation is one of the most rapidly growing areas of functional neuroimaging (Friston, 2011) and arguably has particular relevance to the study of ASD given the identified anomalies of white matter development discussed in the previous section. We now briefly review studies of functional and effective connectivity in ASD, leaving discussion of more traditional functional neuroimaging findings to later sections of this chapter where it is interwoven into discussions of neuropsychological and cognitve neuroscience aspects of ASD.

Contemporary models of human brain function posit that the brain is organized into multiple large-scale neural networks distributed in anatomically segregated areas of the cortex, each having distinctive roles in mediating perceptual, motor, and cognitive processing. The function, distribution, and interaction of these networks can be inferred from the analysis of correlated patterns of neural activation either during performance of behavioral tasks or during the resting state. *Functional connectivity* is inferred from statistical dependencies among physiological responses measured from different regions of cortex. Since this method does not account for the direction of information flow, it cannot be used to infer causality. By contrast, *effective connectivity* applies methods such as dynamic causal modeling and independent component analysis to the same kind of data to evaluate the influence that one neural system may exert or cause in another.

Based on these methods, several large-scale intrinsic brain networks have been identified with specialized roles in processing information (Menon, 2011; Seeley et al., 2007; Yeo et al., 2011). These networks demonstrate consistent spatial and temporal patterns of coactivation across markedly different tasks. They include a sensory-motor network, a visual cortex network, a limbic network, dorsal and ventral attention networks, a frontal-parietal network involved in executive control, and a default mode network (DMN). With the exception of the DMN, the existence of each of these networks had been recognized previously through multiple areas of investigation. By contrast, the DMN was discovered through observations in functional imaging studies that certain brain regions became active when an individual was not performing a task, but was in a state of wakeful rest, unfocused on the outside world. Key nodes of the network are located in medial prefrontal cortex, anterior and PCC, middle temporal gyrus, and precuneous (Buckner, Andrews-Hanna, & Schacter, 2008). These nodes become active during mind wandering but also during self-referential thinking. They are fairly consistently deactivated in normal controls during cognitive and attention-demanding tasks (Greicius, Supekar, Menon, & Dougherty, 2009). Various subnetworks exist within the DMN, including one for memory (e.g., autobiographical memories of places or experiences) centered in the medial temporal lobe and one for social cognition (e.g., theory of mind – ToM) in prefrontal cortex.

Task-based functional and effective connectivity studies of ASD have identified anomalies in interregional connectivity during performance of tasks examining language (Jones et al., 2010; Just et al., 2004), visual motor coordination (Villalobos, Mizuno, Dahl, Kemmotsu, & Muller, 2005), working memory (Koshino et al., 2008), executive function and cognitive control (Agam, Joseph, Barton, & Manoach, 2010; Just et al., 2007), and social cognition (Di Martino et al., 2009; Kleinhans et al., 2008), among others (see Schipul, Keller, & Just, 2011 for a review). The patterns of coactivation observed in ASD have suggested underconnectivity of long-range connections (Hughes, 2007; Muller, 2007) while short-range connections are either within normal limits or show overconnectivity (Keown et al., 2013; Rippon, Brock, Brown, & Boucher, 2007). It has been argued that this pattern reflects a failure in the fine-tuning of neural networks during development. Some have suggested that underconnectivity is global (Just et al., 2007; Just et al., 2004), although the evidence for this has not been entirely consistent. For example, several studies have shown hyper-connectivity of some long-range thalamocortical connections (Mizuno, Villalobos, Davies, Dahl, & Muller, 2006) and cortico-cortical connections (Noonan, Haist, & Muller, 2009; Shih et al., 2011). Inconsistencies may reflect inherent complexities of brain connectivity, although a variety of other factors can also influence the pattern of results in these studies. This includes variations in task demands, analytic methods, and whether or not movement artifact was adequately addressed (Maximo, Cadena, & Kana, 2014; Muller et al., 2011; Nair et al., 2014). Most of these studies were completed on higher-functioning adolescents and adults because of the need to comply with task demands. For this and other reasons, the results are not readily generalizable to the broader ASD population.

In order to circumvent some of these issues, a number of investigators have turned to utilization of resting-state functional MRI (rs-fMRI). In this paradigm, participants are instructed to rest for 5 to 8 minutes, during which BOLD signals are collected. Strong correlations in spontaneous low-frequencies (< 0.1 Hz) in the BOLD signal in distinct but functionally-related regions of cortex disclose the shared spontaneous neural activity of intrinsically connected networks (Biswal, Yetkin, Haughton, & Hyde, 1995). In the normal course of development, correlations between distant brain regions increase with age, presumably reflecting the strengthening of connections between nodes of distributed networks (integration) (Fair et al., 2007). Simultaneously, there is an increase in segregation from other networks, although short-range functional connections may also increase reflecting improvements in local communication. The results from rs-fMRI have been shown to correlate with neuropsychological performance on measures of higher cortical function such as language (Waites, Briellmann, Saling, Abbott, & Jackson, 2006) and memory (Bettus et al., 2008) in conditions where neural network function has been compromised. The relative merits of utilizing rs-fMRI to examine brain connectivity are that data can be acquired in a shorter space of time than task-based BOLD studies and it requires minimal cooperation (e.g., lying still, stay awake), thus reducing or eliminating some state-related and task-related sources of variability that can be difficult to control without introducing other potential confounds (e.g., cooperation, performance levels, strategies, etc). In addition, the data derived from this paradigm show good test-retest reliability (Shehzad et al., 2009) and are reportedly sufficiently stable that the results can be collected and compared across different imaging facilities (Fair et al., 2012). These attributes make it possible to assess a broader range of individuals (in both age and level of function) (Yerys, Jankowski, et al., 2009), potentially increasing the generalizability of obtained results.

Many studies of functional connectivity in ASD have focused on the DMN, in part because of its role in mediating self-directed thinking and aspects of social cognition. In keeping with task-related studies of connectivity, rs-fMRI studies of adults with ASD demonstrate hypoconnectivity between nodes of the DMN (Assaf et al., 2010; Kennedy & Courchesne, 2008; Weng et al., 2010), particularly between anterior and posterior components (Cherkassky, Kana, Keller, & Just, 2006; Monk et al., 2009; Starck et al., 2013), while overconnectivity is apparent within local DMN nodes (Washington et al., 2014). These in vivo findings are consistent with postmortem brain tissue studies that have demonstrated decreased long-distance and increased short-distance axonal connections in frontal cortex of adults with ASD (Zikopoulos & Barbas, 2013). Observations of decreased long-range connectivity between the precuneus and medial prefrontal cortex/anterior cingulate have suggested anomalies in circuitry involved in self-reflective thinking and ToM, and were inversely correlated with the severity of social and communication deficits (Assaf et al., 2010). Weak long-range connections have also been identified in interhemispheric pathways, specifically the corpus callosum (Anderson et al., 2010; Hahamy, Behrmann, & Malach, 2015). Anomalies of the corpus callosum, including agenesis, have been noted for some time in ASD (Piven, Bailey, et al., 1997). More recently, it has been argued that these disturbances potentially increase risk for the development of ASD (Paul, Corsello, Kennedy, & Adolphs, 2014). These anomalies may be associated with perturbations in the development of hemispheric asymmetries of function in ASD (Floris et al., 2013).

Overall, the findings from functional and effective connectivity studies have been taken as evidence in support of developmental disconnection models of ASD (Belmonte et al., 2004; Just et al., 2004). Related speculations have suggested that these patterns of abnormal connectivity may be a consequence of widespread anomalies of synaptic elimination or formation (Sporns, Tononi, & Edelman, 2000). However, a number of recent studies have complicated the picture, prompting caution against simplistic interpretation regarding general patterns of functional under- or overconnectivity, their behavioral significance, and broader implications. Some studies, for example, have suggested that anomalies of connectivity are not evident in young children (6–9 years) but become apparent in older children and adolescents (Washington et al., 2014). This potentially casts doubt on the primacy of the observed underconnectivity problems and seems inconsistent with some of the structural white matter studies suggesting that problems arise earlier in development. Some have suggested that the connectivity differences in ASD may reflect a maturational lag. However, patterns of functional connectivity are highly idiosyncratic in children and adolescents with ASD, and this may also be true of adults (Hahamy et al., 2015; Uddin, 2015). Age-related changes in connectivity of the DMN are evident in both neurotypical controls and individuals with ASD, but the developmental trajectories and regional expression of the changes differ substantially between groups and show particular variability in the ASD group (Doyle-Thomas et al., 2015; Nomi & Uddin, 2015). The current literature highlights inconsistencies that make generalizations difficult to draw at this point. Nevertheless, it does seem that functional connectivity measures are sensitive to differences in brain function between normal controls and individuals with ASD.

Other intrinsic large-scale networks with particular relevance to the study of ASD include the salience network (SN) and the central executive network (CEN). The SN responds when individuals evaluate the degree of subjective salience of a stimulus, which depends on many factors, including past experience, stimulus attributes, top-down attention, cognitive control processes, and visceral/autonomic responses, among others. This network is likely involved in determinations of the emotional and social significance of environmental stimuli and is thought to play a role in regulating and switching between endogenous and exogenous attention to relevant stimuli that guide our behavior. It may accordingly also function like a switch between the DMN and the CEN (Goulden et al., 2014). Key nodes of this network are distributed in the anterior cingulate cortex (ACC) and anterior insula. Some recent studies have suggested that in ASD this network is overconnected within itself and spatially occupies a more restricted distribution (Zielinski et al., 2012). Uddin et al. (2013) also identified hyperconnectivity of the SN in ASD and indicated that this was the best discriminator of ASD among all the large-scale networks they examined. They and others have suggested that dysfunction of this network is associated with the severity of socioemotional impairment as well as RRBIAs (Ebisch et al., 2010; Nielsen et al., 2013; Uddin et al., 2013).

In summary, examination of the functional connectivity of these large-scale neural networks provides a useful complement to other areas of investigation of the neural correlates of ASD. Poor connectivity can potentially introduce disruptive levels of imprecision into the complex neural computations underlying both simple sensory and higher-order information processing, as well as in organizing appropriate behavioral responses (Pajevic, Basser, & Fields, 2014). The repeated coactivation between regions of the brain that underlie development of network relationships is also important for experiential learning. Problems at this level can thus contribute to anomalous or atypical development of social and communicative behavior. The determinants of the problems observed at a functional connectivity level are unclear but may possibly relate to structural differences such as the degree of myelination (Deoni et al., 2015; Nair, Treiber, Shukla, Shih, & Mueller, 2013) or anomalies at the cellular or molecular level. A possible genetic contribution to the underconnectivity picture was recently raised by Scott-Van Zeeland et al. (2010), who identified reduced functional connectivity in medial prefrontal cortex in carriers of the CNTNAP2 gene. In addition, frontal lobe connectivity is also compromised in individuals with 16p11.2 deletion (Ottet et al., 2013). However, there has been growing recognition that white matter pathways exhibit experience-dependent plasticity (Lovden et al., 2010; Yogarajah et al., 2010), so it also seems possible that underconnectivity may be subject to experiential factors. A better understanding of functional and effective connectivity in ASD has the potential to greatly deepen our understanding of individuals with ASD and to advance progress in other areas of investigation.

Implications and Limitations

Variability has become a hallmark of neuroimaging findings in ASD. Brain volumes can vary according to a number of subject-related variables, such as the age of the child, gender, clinical characteristics (e.g., severity of social impairment,

IQ), and genetic dispositions (Lenroot & Yeung, 2013; Stanfield et al., 2008). Without closer control over these variables, caution is warranted in interpreting the results of the volumetric imaging studies to elucidate the neurobiological basis of ASD. Overall, however, the findings suggest that there are multiple facets and phases to the abnormal cortical development that occurs in individuals with ASD. Accelerated expansion of brain volume of multiple regions involving both gray and white matter occurs in early childhood. These changes do not appear to be regionally-specific, although they appear evident in some areas more than others and follow a different developmental course in various areas of the brain. This is followed by accelerated thinning of cortex in later childhood and adolescence. Finally, there is a deceleration of cortical thinning that occurs in adulthood (Zielinski et al., 2014). These findings are suggestive of anomalies in the normal course of subtractive processes (i.e., dendritic pruning) during postnatal neurodevelopment.

Despite initial overgrowth of white matter in the first two years of life, individuals with ASD later show widespread but idiosyncratic patterns of hypoconnectivity and hyperconnectivity, particularly with regions of the frontal and the fusiform face area (Abrams et al., 2013; Courchesne, Redcay, Morgan, & Kennedy, 2005; Just et al., 2007). Questions remain unanswered as to what is driving the idiosyncratic patterns in ASD and what their significance is in understanding behaviors associated with ASD. Longitudinal studies and better-controlled large-scale replications of cross-sectional data are needed to confirm and extend existing results.

Many of the studies suffer from small numbers of subjects. Researchers are often faced with difficult choices in designing appropriate controls, particularly when functional tasks are used. The vast majority of the functional studies in ASD have recruited high-functioning individuals with ASD (IQ greater than 70) (Stanfield et al., 2008), a selection bias motivated by the need to optimize the probability that participants will be sufficiently cooperative and adaptive to the high constraints of imaging protocols. While this makes pragmatic sense, observed differences may not be generalizable to the broader ASD population. When lower-functioning groups of children with ASD have been studied, their data have often been compared to higher-functioning normal controls. Riva et al. (2011) for example, examined brain volumes in a low-functioning group of ASD children (aged 3–10 years) with a mean IQ of 52 and contrasted the data from this group against neurotypical controls with normal range IQ. Given this design, the pattern of observed gray matter volumetric difference may simply be related to IQ rather than the diagnosis of ASD (Rutter, 2013). It is clear that future neuroimaging studies need to better specify and control for various neuropsychological variables, including age, handedness, gender, general cognitive level, language ability, nature and severity of social impairment, and the presence and severity of RRBIA.

Clinical Features and Developmental Course

Kanner's contention that autism was an "inborn" or congenital condition was based on his interpretation of retrospective reports by parents who recounted various atypical behaviors they had observed in their child's interpersonal interactions in the first year. It has become apparent that most parents (~80%) become aware of developmental anomalies or delays in their children with AD by two years of age (De Giacomo & Fombonne, 1998) and nearly 50% harbor concerns in the first year (Young, Brewer, & Pattison, 2003); parents with an older affected child tend to have earlier concerns than those with an older unaffected child or no older children (Herlihy, Knoch, Vibert, & Fein, 2013). Despite these suspicions, a definitive diagnosis of AD is often not made until children are 3–4 years of age, due to the difficulties in ruling out developmental delays or other similar conditions such as cognitive deficiency in very young children (Howlin & Moore, 1997; Mandell, Novak, & Zubritsky, 2005).

Given the importance of early intervention (Webb, Jones, Kelly, & Dawson, 2014; Wong & Kwan, 2010; Zachor, Ben-Itzchak, Rabinovich, & Lahat, 2007), considerable effort has been devoted to identifying the earliest behavioral signs that are predictive of a later diagnosis of ASD. Given the delays in recognition during ontogeny, initial investigations of the developmental precursors or early manifestations relied on retrospective analyses and were largely limited to parental reports. Detailed and accurate information is difficult to abstract from retrospective parental reports, given that it relies upon recollection of behaviors their child exhibited at an earlier age of development. Bias in memory recall can greatly influence responses to structured interviews and questionnaires (Zwaigenbaum et al., 2007). However, the rise in availability of home video recording and playback equipment that occurred in the 1980s (from 1% of U.S American households in 1980 to more than 75% in 1992) afforded an opportunity to supplement parental histories with systematic examination of the child's behavior as captured on home videos taken by parents at family events (e.g., birthday parties) before the recognition of their child's ASD. The coding of behaviors such as eye contact, attention to communications, motor abilities, emotional reactivity, and expression, provided a remarkably useful window to explore the extent to which children demonstrated anomalies in the first couple of years of life (Adrien, Faure, et al., 1991; Werner & Dawson, 2005). While this approach has inherent methodological limitations (Saint Georges et al., 2010), it has yielded substantial insights into the early development of children with ASD.

The task of delineating those behaviors that can reliably predict later development of ASD is complex and requires very careful analysis of the dynamics of behaviors and an appreciation of the developmental and social context. Given the limitations of these retrospective methods, a number of studies have adopted prospective designs that involve screening and developmental surveillance methods. These studies attempt to identify children as early as 12–18 months through systematic screening and then follow their development over the next few years to ascertain their eventual diagnosis (e.g., Barbaro & Dissanayake, 2010; Bryson et al., 2007; Landa & Garrett-Mayer, 2006; Ozonoff et al., 2010). In addition, some prospective studies have explored even earlier developmental precursors by systematically monitoring from infancy the development of siblings of children with ASD who are at elevated risk for the development of autism due to the shared genetic liability.

In the following sections, we provide a brief overview of the key symptoms associated with ASD from infancy to adolescence, with particular emphasis on recent advances in understanding the early markers and identifying ASD in the first couple of years of life. To contextualize this discussion, we begin with a brief synopsis of our current understanding of typical development of the "social brain." We then provide a cursory overview of changes that may occur over the life span with particular emphasis on the early years. This overview is divided into "Social Communication" and " Restricted and Repetitive Patterns of Behavior Interests and Activities" subsections, which correspond to the "autistic dyad" outlined in the DSM-5 framework for defining ASD (see Table 13.1). The correspondence between the early signs and the behaviors considered diagnostic of ASD is a loose one, given that some developmental precursors or predictors may have broad developmental impact and relate to several later emerging problems that may span more than one domain. Table 13.1 represents an effort to map these early signs with the corresponding behavioral domain as identified in DSM-5.

Social Communication

Impairments in social relatedness and communication are the hallmark features of autism. Parent reports have long suggested that critical social behaviors are often slow or limited in their development in children with ASD. Eye gaze has received considerable attention as a potential early behavioral marker of ASD. Eye contact is regarded as a foundation for early social interaction and communication, and humans demonstrate a preference for direct eye gaze very early in life (Csibra & Gergely, 2006; Itier & Batty, 2009). Kanner (1943) noted anomalies of eye contact in his original description of ASD, and deficient "eye-to-eye gaze" is a specific example of impaired use of nonverbal behaviors to regulate social interaction and communication in the DSM-5. A variety of anomalies of gaze have been described in infants and toddlers, including so-called empty gaze (Dahlgren & Gillberg, 1989), abnormal intensity of eye contact (Wimpory, Hobson, Williams, & Nash, 2000), and unpredictable eye gaze such as inconsistently following another person's eye gaze. A recent paper by Jones and Klin (2013) found that infants at risk for ASD who later received the diagnosis showed an overall decline in eye fixation from normal levels at 2 months of age to lower than normal levels at 6 months of age. These findings suggested that that eye tracking measures as early as 6 months might be useful in detecting children at particular risk for autism.

Additionally, impairments are evident in other early emerging social behaviors seen in typical infants, such as social smiling, interest in faces and facial expressions, strong motivation to have caregivers pay attention to their activities, directing facial affect toward caregivers, and responding to their own name when called. Studies combining the retrospective analysis of videotape with interviews revealed that children diagnosed with ASD tended to show lower frequency of looking at others, diminished orienting to being called by name, a lack of interest in sharing interests or showing objects to others, and a lack of pointing (Mars, Mauk, & Dowrick, 1998; Osterling & Dawson, 1994). Some behavioral differences were identifiable as early as the first 12 months of life (Adrien, Perrot, Hameury, Martineau, & et al., 1991; Baranek, 1999; Clifford & Dissanayake, 2008; Goldberg, Thorsen, Osann, & Spence, 2008; Werner, Dawson, Osterling, & Dinno, 2000). A number of these behaviors seemed useful in distinguishing the behavior of infants with ASD from infants later diagnosed with ID without ASD. While both ID and ASD groups demonstrated more repetitive and stereotyped behaviors compared to typically-developing infants, infants who later developed an ASD looked at other individuals less and failed to orient to their names as often (Osterling et al., 2002).

Overall, these findings underscore the importance of examining social attention and communication in identifying the best early indicators of ASD. A very important feature in early childhood, perhaps the most discriminating feature between autism and other developmental disabilities, is the delayed or absent development of joint attention. Joint attention is reflected in a child's motivation to coordinate his or her attention to an object with that of another person. It can be seen in acts the child initiates (e.g., pointing to show, holding up an object to show) or in responding to the parents' initiation (e.g., following the parent's gaze, following the parent's pointing). Parents often report such behaviors, but when questioned closely, the objects the child brings to them are ones with which he or she needs help (e.g., read me this book, open this box of cookies), not ones being shown for the simple joy of shared attention. Other early signs of ASD are not noticing others' emotions unless they are very obvious, and showing inappropriate reactions, such as laughing if another child is crying.

By the second year of life, typical children show substantial interest in other children. They generally have no cooperative play skills, but are very interested in watching other children or playing near them. Children developing ASD are often minimally interested in other children and are happy when left to play alone. In general, the social interactions of the young child developing ASD are more need-oriented (e.g., they may come to mom for food, tickles, help with a toy, or when distressed) and they show much less than typical interest in simple social play or social contact (e.g., babbling back and forth, sharing facial expressions). Since facial expressions are less meaningful to them, they usually show less than typical social referencing—that is, looking to a caregiver when confronted with an unfamiliar stimulus to see if they look calm and reassuring or worried. Emergence of simple motor imitation is usually delayed in emerging autism. Delays in the simplest forms of ToM can be seen in the fact that some children with emerging autism will make some communicative efforts with parents but without making sure they have the adult's attention or gaze first.

In the later preschool period (ages 2–4), some children continue to have severe delays in all of these areas. Others will develop simple imitation and pretend play but generally remain delayed or impaired in interest in peers and in joint attention. In a preschool, they may be able to join a social group with adult facilitation, but otherwise tend to remain on the margins of the group. If pretend play develops, it tends to be quite simplified and repetitive, unless guided by a peer or sibling. Pretend play scenarios, instead of being a complex series of actions around a theme, tend to remain simple one- or two-act schemas, or acting out of perseverative themes often taken from favorite games or movies.

As the child moves into later childhood and adolescence, a great deal depends on the child's cognitive level and degree of language impairment. With functional language, conversational ability is usually quite impaired, with conversation possible only on preferred topics or reliant on the conversational partner to keep it going. Children with autism are often strongly motivated to ask questions perseveratively to which they already know the answers. Immediate echolalia (repeating what they just heard) and delayed echolalia (quoting extensively from familiar scripts) are very common, although they tend to abate as functional language develops. Pronoun reversals are common; this used to be interpreted as indicating poor sense of self and other, but is now regarded as cognitive difficulty with relational terms. In later childhood and adolescence, a key feature of autism is poor ToM, in which the individual has a poor grasp on what others are thinking, feeling, expecting, or remembering, or on what different information people are able to access.

Restricted and Repetitive Patterns of Behavior Interests and Activities

These features fall into two broad categories: repetitive activities and resistance to change. A third category, that of sensory over- and underreactivity, has been added to this group in DSM-5. Except for this third category (to which we will return shortly), many very young children with emerging autism have few of these behaviors; it may not be until the third or fourth birthday that clear repetitive behaviors and resistance to change emerge (Barton et al., 2013; Turner et al., 2006). Many very young children, especially with cognitive delays, are insufficiently aware of routines to be distressed when they are violated, and may not have the cognitive ability to develop their own routines or their own preoccupying interests. When symptoms in this domain are present in very early childhood, they are usually repetitive motor behaviors such as rocking, toe walking, or hand flapping (although hand flapping with excitement is often seen in normal toddlers as well).

However, sensory symptoms are often seen in toddlers with ASD. On one hand, they may be oblivious to verbal input from others and may ignore auditory, visual, tactile, or even painful stimuli. On the other hand, they may be overreactive, showing distress by crying or covering their ears in response to certain noises, such as vacuum cleaners, washing machines, and the hum of fluorescent lights. They may find it hard to tolerate tactile input such as haircuts, cuffs, or tags—and especially light touch—and prefer deeper input such as being squeezed or being under a heavy blanket. Visual fascinations are very common, especially after age 2. Some of the most common of these are squinting; looking at things out of the corner of the eye; staring at shadows, mirrors, or credits going by on a TV; creating or finding lines (lining up toys or trains, or staring at the junction of two walls) and staring at them at eye level; or moving objects back and forth in the periphery of vision.

In later childhood, repetitive activities extend to verbal and play routines, where they prefer to reenact the same scenes over and over or repeat phrases. Frank obsessions and compulsions may appear, with a drive to complete activities and great distress if routines are violated, environments are changed, or expectations are violated (e.g., even to taking a different route to get somewhere). Older children and adolescents tend to develop very strong preoccupying interests; the nature of these will depend on the cognitive level of the child. At the lowest level, they may be demonstrated by such activities as carrying around things of a certain color, or unusual objects (e.g., paper clips). At higher cognitive levels, such if the child is verbal, he or she may want to talk about a certain topic to the exclusion of most others (e.g., *National Geographic* collection, favorite video game), and they may be fascinated by unusual stimuli such as toilets flushing. Older children and adolescents may have large collections of favorite objects. In the best cases, these interests can actually lead to constructive interests (e.g., dinosaurs, astronomy), although the depth of social disability often prevents these interests from developing into useful activities or pastimes.

Patterns of Onset

In his original description, Kanner (1943) contended that children with autism demonstrated symptoms from the "very beginning of life." (Kanner, 1943, p. 242) While Kanner conveyed that this pattern of early onset was seen uniformly across the group, one child may have demonstrated a somewhat different developmental trajectory—one associated with a loss of previously acquired skills. By parent report, Richard (Case 3) had exhibited some proficiency in imitating words and sounds early in his development but subsequently lost this ability. When seen at age 3 years, 3 months, his mother stated that, "It seems that he has gone backward mentally gradually for the last two years" (Kanner, 1943, p. 225). Kanner did not comment on the significance of this parent's observation beyond mentioning it. However, over a decade later, and after having diagnosed more than 120 children with autism, he noted that some cases developed normally until 18 to 20 months and then demonstrated a "loss of language function, failure to progress socially, and the gradual giving up of interest in normal activities" (Eisenberg & Kanner, 1956, p. 558).

As experience with early infantile autism increased, reports of developmental regression or setbacks became more commonplace. In the first epidemiological study of ASD, Lotter (1966) reported that 31.3% of children with autism had a history of developmental setback comprised either a "loss of some ability" or "a failure to progress after a satisfactory beginning." (Lotter, 1996, p. 130) Rutter and Lockyer (1967) noted that 15% of their cohort of children with ASD regressed after a period of "reasonably definite normal development" (p. 1172). However, the phenomena received scant attention for almost two decades. Kurita (1985) then reported on a cohort of 261 children with ASD, of which more than one-third (37.2%) had demonstrated speech loss. Similar observations were made in a subsequent study in a Japanese cohort (Hoshino et al., 1987). Despite the significant number of affected individuals, the phenomena continued to receive little mention until Rogers and DiLalla (1990) underscored regression as one of a few possible developmental trajectories in ASD, and reports by Deonna, Ziegler, Moura-Serra, and Innocenti (1993); Rapin (1995) and Stefanatos et al. (1995) highlighted that regression may imply distinctive etiologic pathways that differed from nonregressive forms of autism.

Parental reports and clinical observations suggest at least three distinguishable patterns of onset in ASD (Rogers & DiLalla, 1990). In the most common "congenital" or "early onset" pattern of onset, behavioral manifestations of ASD emerge generally in the first year of life. Both retrospective studies of children with ASD and prospective studies of children at high risk for the disorder suggest that symptoms tend to become evident in the latter half first year, although sometimes problems may manifest in the first six months (Jones, Gliga, Bedford, Charman, & Johnson, 2014; Ozonoff, Heung, Byrd, Hansen, & Hertz-Picciotto, 2008; Zwaigenbaum, Bryson, & Garon, 2013). Developmental differences gradually become apparent in impairments of joint attention, eye contact, anticipatory behavior, motility, communication, social interest/responsiveness, and emotional modulation (Maestro et al., 2005; Osterling & Dawson, 1994; Werner et al., 2000). The saliency of these developmental delays or deviations increases with time due to the increasing divergence from a normal trajectory (Dawson, Munson, et al., 2007) to the point where they trigger parental concerns. While 36% (Short & Schopler, 1988) to 55% (Volkmar, Stier, & Cohen, 1985) of parents report noticing problems in the first year, the nature and potential significance of the difficulties are often not appreciated until the second or third year, resulting in a mean age of recognition of 18–19 months (De Giacomo & Fombonne, 1998; Stone et al., 1999).

In a second scenario, children may show normal or near normal early growth and then demonstrate a developmental arrest or "stasis" that is unexpected given the preceding developmental trajectory (Siperstein & Volkmar, 2004). Many of the children fitting this picture may show timely onset of early language milestones and progress normally from babbling to production of proto-words, but then fail to show the usual rapid expansion in their inventory of speech sounds (e.g., consonants) or progress to the production of words, word combinations, phrases and sentences. Recent prospective studies of children with ASD suggest that individuals in this subgroup are later diagnosed because their "plateau" in development tends to occur in the second year of life (Landa & Garrett-Mayer, 2006; Landa, Holman, & Garrett-Mayer, 2007).

Regression

The third pattern of onset entails a developmental regression or setback characterized by loss of skills in one or more domains of behavior. The onset of regression usually occurs between 14 and 30 months (Barger, Campbell, & McDonough, 2013; Fombonne & Chakrabarti, 2001) and is generally characterized by a conspicuous loss of previously-acquired language abilities. Children cease to use words that were previously part of their vocabulary, produce fewer verbal communications, and may manifest a deterioration in their articulation of speech (Kurita, 1985; Lord, Shulman, & DiLavore, 2004; Rogers & DiLalla, 1990). These changes can eventuate in a child who is nonverbal at least for a period of time. The loss of speech is often, but not invariably, accompanied by noteworthy decrements in receptive language (Stefanatos et al., 1995). Children may fail to respond to their name being called or have trouble following directions they were previously able to understand. A concomitant deterioration in social behavior is frequently observed, manifested in reductions in eye contact, social engagement, and play skills (Bernabei, Cerquiglini, Cortesi, & D'Ardia, 2007; Goldberg et al., 2003; Meilleur & Fombonne, 2009; Ozonoff, Williams, & Landa, 2005). Restricted, repetitive or stereotyped behaviors may also emerge, but are often overshadowed by the deterioration in communicative and social domains at this stage of development. Some loss of adaptive skills (e.g., feeding, dressing, toileting) and motor abilities (fine or gross motor) can occur around this time, although these areas of function are typically relatively preserved in comparison to the loss of communication and social skills.

In the majority of cases, both language and social skills are affected, although the loss of language is often more salient and is usually one of the primary cues prompting parental concerns. Some children appear to demonstrate more selective loss that seems to disproportionately affect language or social skills (Goldberg et al., 2003; Hansen et al., 2008; Luyster et al., 2005). The selective deterioration of social function may be difficult to recognize due to problems differentiating the alterations in behavior from changes in behavior resulting from events such as minor illnesses, trauma, adversity in the family, sibling rivalry, and other stresses. Changes in behavior may also be misinterpreted as reflecting the moodiness, negativity, and temperament changes associated with the characteristically difficult stage of social development referred to as the "terrible twos." Consideration of the complexities surrounding the identification of regression prompted Volkmar et al. (1985) to question the existence of regression in ASD. However, the phenomenon has been validated, in part by comparison of pre- and post-regression videotaped material (Goldberg, Thorsen, et al., 2008; Werner & Dawson, 2005).

Alterations in behavior can manifest over the course of a few days to months. Regression can occur in children who were demonstrating seemingly normal or near-normal development or in children with preexisting problems or developmental delays (Kurita, 1985; Ozonoff, Williams, et al., 2005; Richler et al., 2006). The proportion of children showing some preexisting problems varies between studies (Hoshino et al., 1987; Kurita, 1985; Ozonoff, Williams, et al., 2005). Loss of skills may be apparent in a variety of other behaviors in addition to those that define ASD. Changes can include onset of sleep problems (Giannotti, Cortesi, Cerquiglini, Vagnoni, & Valente, 2011), gastrointestinal symptoms (Valicenti-McDermott, McVicar, Cohen, Wershil, & Shinnar, 2008), increases in behavioral disturbances, tantrums, aggressive behavior, and sensory disturbances (Stefanatos, 2008; Thurm, Manwaring, Luckenbaugh, Lord, & Swedo, 2014a).

A recent meta-analysis of 85 studies reported the overall prevalence rate of regressive ASD (RASD) as 32.1%, although estimates have ranged from 12.5% to 50% (Barger et al., 2013). This wide variance has been attributed, in part, to inconsistencies over the operational definition of regression (Hansen et al., 2008; Stefanatos, 2008). Defining regression is problematic as it can occur in disparate domains, to varying degrees, and over different temporal courses. Language regression has traditionally been considered to be a defining feature of RASD but definitions have varied in terms how much language needs to be acquired before regression occurs, the extent of delays that can exist before regression, the magnitude of the loss, the duration of the loss, and whether a loss of babbling and/or nonverbal communication is considered language regression (Ozonoff, Williams, et al., 2005).

It is noteworthy that regression with speech loss is relatively uncommon in children with forms of developmental disability other than ASD. It is comparatively rare both in specific developmental language disorders (Pickles et al., 2009) and in children with general intellectual disabilities (1%–3%) or other developmental problems (Baird, Charman, et al., 2008; Kurita, 1996; Wilson, Djukic, Shinnar, Dharmani, & Rapin, 2003). Like ASD, RASD appears to cut across all socioeconomic strata (Christopher, Sears, Williams, Oliver, & Hersh, 2004). Unlike ASD, there appear to be no significant gender differences in the prevalence of RASD (Lord et al., 2004; Luyster et al., 2005).

Since the late 1990s, there has been a considerable increase in interest in understanding the context and potential etiological basis of regression in ASD. Preliminary studies of possible genetic contributions have provided some evidence of familiality. Lainhart et al. (2002) reported that features of the BAP were equally present in ASD and RASD, raising the possibility of shared genetic liability. Parr et al. (2011) found that only 14 out of 74 affected pairs of ASD siblings were concordant for regression. This concordance rate for regression (18.9%) is not significantly different from the base-rate for regression (estimated to be 23.9%) in ASD. They therefore concluded that there was no separate familial influence on regression other than that related to ASD. However, a linkage study by Molloy, Keddache, and Martin (2005) identified genetic loci that they speculated conferred susceptibility to autism, but possibly with a modified presentation in the group with regression. In particular, the strongest linkage was evident at candidate regions on chromosomes 21 and chromosome 7. Several of the genes mapping to these locations are involved in various aspects of fetal development such as cell differentiation, adhesion, and apoptosis.

The genetic analysis of RASD is especially intriguing given that, as a group, children with RASD show normal or near normal development and attainment of developmental milestones. They produce their first words earlier than children with nonregressive ASD (Baird, Charman, et al., 2008), and at 24 months they show greater skill attainment than children in a nonregressive group (Luyster et al., 2005). Despite the more promising early course, it has been suggested that children with RASD are more likely to demonstrate in long-term severe speech difficulties (Hoshino et al., 1987; Kurita, Uchiyama, & Takesada, 1985), difficulties in initiating conversation, asking or answering questions, or conveying information verbally (Brown & Prelock, 1995), and intelligence estimates in the cognitively deficient range (Hoshino et al., 1987; Kurita et al., 1985; Meilleur & Fombonne, 2009). Thus, notwithstanding evidence of higher levels of cognitive development prior to the regression, these children may have poorer long-term developmental trajectories, particularly in the area of communication (Bernabei et al., 2007; Goin-Kochel, Esler, Kanne, & Hus, 2014; Hansen et al., 2008; Rogers, 2004). In addition, they also demonstrate a higher frequency of comorbid psychiatric conditions and challenging behaviors (Matson, Wilkins, & Fodstad, 2010).

These findings may possibly be explained by postulating either additional or differential genetic liability in RASD compared to nonregressive ASD. Alternatively, individuals with RASD may experience a second biological "hit" or predisposition that is stimulated by environmental or developmental factors and that causes derailment of language and social function (Lainhart et al., 2002; Stefanatos et al., 2002b). Proposed associations with vaccination (Baird, Pickles, et al., 2008), gastrointestinal problems (Baird, Charman, et al., 2008), mitochondrial disease (Shoffner et al., 2010), and low birthweight (Christopher et al., 2004; Lampi et al., 2012; Mann, McDermott, Bao, Hardin, & Gregg, 2010) have not been substantial enough to differentiate this group from children with nonregressive ASD. In addition, traditional risk factors in ASD—such as pre-, peri- or postnatal complications or intrauterine exposure to viruses or other immune challenges—have not been causally linked to the emergence of RASD (Christopher et al., 2004).

The emergence of epilepsy and epileptiform disorders has been considered as related to a potential "second hit" mechanism. Numerous studies have noted that the prevalence of epilepsy is higher in both ASD and RASD (~5% to 38%) compared to population estimates in children (2%–3%) (Danielsson, Gillberg, Billstedt, Gillberg, & Olsson, 2005; Spence & Schneider, 2009). The prevalence of epileptiform abnormalities with or without seizures is also substantially higher in children with ASD (6%–60%) compared to healthy children (1%–4%). The evidence overall does not appear to disclose consistent differences between RASD and ASD in either the prevalence or form of epilepsy or epileptiform abnormalities (Hansen et al., 2008; Luyster et al., 2005). However, a couple of studies have found a twofold increase in epileptiform EEG abnormalities in RASD compared to ASD (Baird, Robinson, Boyd, & Charman, 2006; Tuchman & Rapin, 1997). Such observations have prompted continuing conjecture on a potential causal relationship between these symptoms.

While regression is rare in developmental disorders other than ASD, it is a hallmark of a newly defined category of disorders termed *epileptic encephalopathies* (Nabbout & Dulac, 2003) in which epileptiform activity is thought to be responsible for cognitive and behavioral deterioration. The exemplar for this group of disorders is epileptic aphasia, commonly referred to as Landau-Kleffner syndrome (LKS) (Landau & Kleffner, 1957). In its classic form, children with LKS develop language normally until 2 and 10 years of age and then demonstrate an acute or insidious loss of language accompanied by epileptiform EEG abnormalities. Overt seizures may not be evident, but if they occur, they are only loosely related to the onset of regression and are typically infrequent and easily managed. The regression results in a profound aphasia, affecting both the production and comprehension of language. This language loss is considered to result from "functional ablation" of eloquent cortex caused by the seizures or persistent epileptiform discharges (Landau & Kleffner, 1957). Severe forms of the disorder tend to be associated with near continuous spike-and-wave activity during sleep (CSWS) (Dulac, 2001; Van Hirtum-Das et al., 2006). Behavioral disturbances commonly co-occur, ranging from ADHD symptomology to behaviors associated with ASD (Deonna & Roulet-Perez, 2010; Stefanatos & DeMarco, 2010). Though rare, this disorder has become the most frequently described form of acquired aphasia in children (Stefanatos, 2011). Given some similarities in the natural history and symptomology of RASD and LKS, it has been speculated that similar mechanisms of action may underlie both disorders (Nass, Gross, & Devinsky, 1998; Nass & Petrucha, 1990).

The relationship between LKS and RASD has long been discussed (Deonna & Roulet-Perez, 2010; Stefanatos et al., 2002b; Tuchman, 2006) and continues to attract interest and debate, particularly given recent studies suggesting that the prevalence of regression in autism may be considerably higher than previously thought (Ozonoff et al., 2010; Thurm, Manwaring, Luckenbaugh, Lord, & Swedo, 2014b). The epileptic encephalopathy explanation has some superficial appeal, in view of the high rates of both epilepsy and epileptiform activity in ASD (Parmeggiani et al., 2010) and the twofold increase in epileptiform abnormalities in children with RASD. However, given that cognitive outcome is poorer in children with regression (Hoshino et al., 1987), these increases may, in part, reflect a more general relationship between epilepsy/epileptiform activity and lower cognitive ability (Viscidi et al., 2013). Canitano, Luchetti, and Zappella (2005) found no evidence to support a causal relationship between regression rate in children with RASD and the presence or absence of epilepsy/epileptiform abnormalities. Relatedly, while CSWS can be observed in RASD, it is relatively uncommon (Tuchman, 2009). At best, epileptiform abnormalities may play a minor role in the emergence of RASD, perhaps exerting an effect in a small number of special cases like CSWS or when particular neurologic circumstances exist (Deonna, Roulet-Perez, Chappuis, & Ziegler, 2007). Overall then, the weight of evidence does not support a general causal relationship between epilepsy or epileptiform abnormalities and regression in ASD (Deonna & Roulet, 2006; Rapin, 1995).

Early in this line of inquiry, Stefanatos et al. (1995) suggested that alternative mechanisms would be needed to account for regression in ASD, possibly involving immunologic/inflammatory mechanisms. Implied in this view is that epileptiform activity can largely be considered an epiphenomenon of the pathophysiological anomalies that underlie RASD. A variety of intriguing correspondences related to evidence of immunologic dysfunction shared by these conditions has since some to light (Braunschweig et al., 2013; Connolly et al., 2003; Singer et al., 2008; see Stefanatos et al., 2002b for discussion). Links between RASD and abnormal immune or autoimmune function have been observed in a variety of reports (Jyonouchi, Sun, & Le, 2001; Molloy et al., 2006; Shenoy et al., 2000; Stefanatos et al., 1995), including rare conditions such as NMDA receptor encephalitis (Gonzalez-Toro et al., 2013; Scott et al., 2014). Regression has been shown to be significantly associated with a family history of autoimmune disorders (Molloy et al., 2006; Valicenti-McDermott et al., 2008). One gene implicated by Molloy et al. (2005) is a member of the immunoglobulin superfamily, which may possibly relate to speculations that regression is associated with abnormal immune responses to viruses. Relatedly, a couple of recent studies have implicated immunoglobulin imbalances, particularly in children with regressive forms of ASD (Braunschweig et al., 2013; Wasilewska, Kaczmarski, Stasiak-Barmuta, Tobolczyk, & Kowalewska, 2012).

Interestingly, associations have been noted between large head size and a positive history of allergic/immune disorders in parents of affected offspring (Sacco et al., 2007a). A number of investigations have suggested that increased head circumference is more likely to occur in RASD (Chaste et al., 2013; Nordahl et al., 2011) and that the timing of regression coincides with a period in development when macrocephaly is most likely to emerge in ASD (Courchesne & Pierce, 2005a). Animal models have shown that maternal immune challenge during pregnancy can result a cascade of events that can influence the expression of genes in offspring and cause alterations in brain function and development, including larger brain size and regression (Fatemi, Earle, et al., 2002).

Correspondences between LKS and RASD have also prompted the recent discovery of similarities at the genetic level (Lesca et al., 2012). Comparative genomic assays revealed that individuals with LKS demonstrate a large number of anomalies involving genomic regions that have also been associated with ASD. Implicated genes include CDH9, CDH13, CNTNAP2, and SHANK3. The investigators suggested that CNVs encoding cell adhesion proteins (cadherins, protocadherins, contactins, and catenins) were particularly evident. The effect of these anomalies may be particularly important during periods of rapid synaptic development. Rapid brain growth is typically followed by a period of subtractive changes that refine circuitry by pruning inefficient neural elements. A related hypothesis derived from computational modelling has suggested that regression may be the result of overly aggressive synaptic pruning (Thomas, Knowland, & Karmiloff-Smith, 2011).

In summary, there are no a priori reasons to suspect that a common causal agent can account for all or most cases of RASD. There is emerging evidence that multiple phenotypes of RASD exist and may relate to diverse pathways of etiopathogenesis (Ozonoff et al., 2010; Rapin, 2006; Stefanatos & Baron, 2011). These pathways may entail the combined influence of genetic susceptibility and abnormal immune responses during pre- or postnatal life (Fatemi et al., 2008; Needleman & McAllister, 2012; Wei, Alberts, & Li, 2013). At present, our knowledge of the diverse manner in which immune function can influence brain development remains rudimentary, so how exactly these factors may play a role in risk for RASD needs to be explored.

Assessment

It is now appreciated that most parents (~80%) recognize developmental anomalies or delays in their children with ASD by 2 years of age (De Giacomo & Fombonne, 1998), and 30%–50% harbor concerns as early as the first year of life (Harrington, Rosen, & Garnecho, 2006; Young et al., 2003). Despite this, a definitive diagnosis of ASD is often not made until children are 3–4 years of age (Howlin & Moore, 1997; Mandell et al., 2005; Yeargin-Allsopp et al., 2003). Recognizing and validating the critical earliest behaviors that are predictive of a later diagnosis of ASD has been a major concentration of recent research, motivated in part by recognition that availability of reliable tools for early identification would permit more timely initiation of intervention (Bryson, Rogers, & Fombonne, 2003). In addition, more precise specification of the earliest signs and subsequent evolution of the disorder would also potentially facilitate a better understanding of the diverse underlying pathogenic mechanisms, guide the identification of endophenotypes, and possibly inform subtyping of the disorder (e.g., early vs. late onset vs. regressive; Shumway et al., 2011; Stefanatos, Kinsbourne, & Wasserstein, 2002a). Given evidence that the risk of having a second child with autism is considerably increased (>25 times) over that of the general population (Abrahams & Geschwind, 2008; Smalley, 1991), early detection and diagnosis can also have a substantial impact on family planning.

Screening, Early Identification, and Diagnosis

Baron-Cohen, Cox, Baird, Sweettenham, and Nightingale (1996) conducted one of the first prospective studies of ASD in order to assess the validity of an observational tool called the Checklist for Autism and Toddlers (CHAT), which can be used in primary health care settings to identify 18-month-old children at risk for an ASD (Baron-Cohen et al., 2000). The CHAT, while highly specific, has limited sensitivity (Baird et al., 2000). A modified version of the CHAT, the Modified Checklist for Autism in Toddlers (M-CHAT; Robins, Fein, Barton, & Green, 2001), is now the most widely used instrument for early ASD screening; a recent revision (Robins et al., 2014) detects more cases and has better psychometric properties. These instruments are for children 16–30 months and have been endorsed by the American Academy of Pediatrics. Preliminary data suggest the utility of screening for autism as early as 12 months for some children (Pierce et al., 2011; Turner-Brown, Baranek, Reznick, Watson, & Crais, 2013), although some symptoms are clearly not prevalent until after 12 months (Ozonoff et al., 2010). It is recommended that all children be screened specifically for ASD during well-child doctor visits at 18 and 24 months. Some children do not show frank symptoms until the second or even occasionally the third year, so additional screening in the second year and later is also needed. A summary of measures designed to assist in the early identification of at risk children is presented in Table 13.3.

When screening measures suggest significant risk for the development of ASD, a second, more detailed level of evaluation may be indicated. These "Level 2" evaluations are typically multidisciplinary, involving pediatricians and pediatric specialists in psychology, psychiatry, developmental pediatrics, or neurology, as well as a variety of other medical (e.g., genetics) and allied health specialties (e.g., speech-language pathology, audiology, occupational therapists). Pediatric psychologists and neuropsychologists are integral members of this team, often taking charge of assessing the cognitive and behavioral functioning of children with a known or suspected ASD. Information obtained from these evaluations assist in the diagnostic assessment but are also instrumental in formulating the team's treatment recommendations.

The structure of such an evaluation is often tailored to address the referral issues, the presentation of the child, and the goals of the assessment. The form of the evaluations may vary substantially depending on the age and level of functioning of the child. Primary efforts are directed to gathering information relevant to behaviors included in the DSM-5 diagnostic criteria. This is usually accomplished by a thorough and comprehensive interview, in addition to observing and interacting with the child in both structured and unstructured interactions. A number of instruments have been specifically developed in order to assist the diagnostic process. A summary of selected measures is briefly presented in Tables 13.3 and 13.4. Unfortunately, at present, there are relatively few unbiased sources to guide clinicians in the choice of these instruments (Norris & Lecavalier, 2010).

Neuropsychologists may also perform more comprehensive assessments of children with ASD. They are particularly well-suited for this due to their training and expertise in assessing and integrating information across multiple cognitive and behavioral domains relevant to ASD. Neuropsychological evaluations can provide useful information

Table 13.3 Diagnostic screening measures for ASD during infancy and toddlerhood

Screening Measures for ASD			
Measure	*Parent*	*Clinician*	*Comments*
Autism Observation Scale for Infants (Bryson, Zwaigenbaum, McDermott, Rombough, & Brian, 2008)		X	Developed to detect and monitor early signs of autism as they emerge in high-risk infants at 6, 12, and 18 months. Uses structured activities to elicit 18 behaviors including visual tracking, disengaging attention, orienting to name, reciprocal smiling, differential response to facial emotion, imitation and social anticipation. Early data suggested potential to distinguish high- from low-risk infants as early as 12 months (Zwaigenbaum et al., 2005).
Infant-Toddler Checklist (ITC) (Wetherby & Prizant, 2002)	X		Comprised of 25 questions from the Communication and Symbolic Behavior Scales and Developmental Profile (Wetherby & Prizant, 2002) that can be used as a broadband screener for ASD (2008). Positive predictive values above 70% for children age 9–24 months for communication delays, and 93.3% sensitivity for ASD in particular, but does not discriminate ASD from other communication delays unless social competence score is less than the 10th percentile.
First Year Inventory (FYI) (Reznick, Baranek, Reavis, Watson, & Crais, 2007)	X		Developed to assess behaviors in 12-month-olds suggestive of an eventual diagnosis of AD. Large-scale longitudinal study has not yet been reported to evaluate predictive validity.
Modified Checklist for Autism in Toddlers (M-CHAT) (Robins et al., 2001):	X	X	A 23-item parent questionnaire completed at 18 months. Good estimates of specificity and sensitivity when follow-up interview with clinician is added to review failed items. Positive predictive value reported as .68–.74 after interview (Kleinman et al., 2008). Does not allow good differentiation of ASD, language delays and global delays.
Pervasive Developmental Disorders Screening Test-II (PDDST-II) (Siegel, 2004)	X		A three-stage screening questionnaire completed by parent. Stage 1 completed by pediatricians has high sensitivity (.92) and specificity (.91). Useful as a Stage 2 screener with children in developmental clinics (but see McQuistin & Zieren, 2006).
Parent Observation of Early Markers Scale (Feldman et al., 2011)	X		Developed to allow parents to prospectively monitor 61 possible early behavioral manifestations of ASD in 1- to 24-month-old infants. Overall specificity and sensitivity were .74 and .73, respectively.
Screening Tool for Autism in Two-year-olds (STAT) (Stone, Coonrod, & Ousley, 2000)		X	A 12-item, 20-minute interactive test administered by trained professionals measuring play, requesting behavior, directing attention and motor imitation. Good sensitivity (.93) and specificity (.83). Designed to differentiate toddlers with autism from those with other developmental disabilities.

Instruments used to screen for signs of ASD in the first two years of life. These measures are broadly aimed at identifying atypical development of social communication, social orienting, imitation, use of gestures, joint attention, repetitive behaviors, anomalies of play and reciprocal affective behavior. (Adapted and expanded from Stefanatos, 2012.)

Table 13.4 Diagnostic screening measures for ASD in older children and adolescents

Diagnostic Assessment Measures for ASD	
Measure	*Comments*
Autism Diagnostic Interview-Revised (ADI-R; Rutter, LeCouteur, & Lord, 2003)	Semi-structured interview that elicits information from a parent or caregiver regarding behaviors required to make an ICD-10 or DSM-IV-TR diagnosis of autism (social interaction, communication skills, repetitive activities, stereotyped interests). Designed to distinguish developmental delays, qualitative impairments, and behaviors that would be regarded as deviant at any age. Interrater reliability is excellent. Gold standard measure for research because of high interrater reliability. Not advised for use for children with IQs below 20 or mental age below 20 months (Cox et al., 1999).
Autism Diagnostic Observation Schedule Second Edition (ADOS-2; Lord et al., 2012) c	A semi-structured, interactive observation widely accepted as a "gold standard" diagnostic instrument developed for children from 2 to 9 years of age. It is a Level C measure that should be administered and interpreted only by appropriately-credentialed professionals from psychology, medicine, or a related discipline. It can be administered in approximately 40 to 60 minutes. The revisions have expanded diagnostic algorithms in Modules 1 to 4 (Hus & Lord, 2014) and added a Toddler Module for children 12 to 30 months.
Autism Spectrum Screening Questionnaire (ASSQ; Ehlers, Gillberg, & Wing, 1999; Luyster et al., 2009)	Designed as a screening tool for older children (6–17 years of age) with mild to no intellectual impairment. Comprised of 27 yes/no questions addressing social interaction (11 items), communication (6 items), restricted behavior and interest (6 items), and associated symptoms (5 items). Psychometric properties vary depending on the sample and the respondent (parent or teacher). A cutoff score of 19 for parent respondents in a clinical setting yielded a sensitivity of .62 and specificity of .91. Their scores can be used to help differentiate high-functioning ASD from other behavior and learning disorders.
Autism Spectrum Rating Scale (ASRS; Goldstein & Naglieri, 2012)	Comprised of questionnaires to be completed in about 20 minutes by parents and teachers to rate ASD behaviors. Separate forms for ages 2–5 and 6–18 for both parent and teacher ratings. Short screening forms (five minutes) are available. The normative and clinical samples for the ASRS are large. Recent updates are available to score protocols according to DSM-5 criteria. In addition, a scoring updates is available for scoring nonverbal individuals or individuals who speak infrequently.
Child Autism Rating Scale–Second Edition (CARS-2; Schopler & Van Bourgondien, 2010)	This update of the CARS remains the single most widely used standardized instrument specifically designed for the diagnosis of autism. CARS-2 retains the original CARS form for use with younger or lower functioning individuals (renamed the CARS2-ST for "Standard Form"). Has a new separate rating scale for use with higher-functioning individuals (named the CARS2-HF for "High-Functioning"). Designed as a clinician rating scale to be completed after a direct observation of the child by a trained professional familiar with autism. Information from parents can be obtained with the CARS2-QPC (Questionnaire of Parent Concerns).
Gilliam Autism Rating Scale–third Edition (GARS-3; Gilliam, 2013)	GARS-3 consists of 56 items based on the DSM-5 diagnostic criteria for ASD. Items are grouped into six subscales: Restrictive, Repetitive Behaviors, Social Interaction, Social Communication, Emotional Responses, Cognitive Style, and Maladaptive Speech. Yields standard scores, percentile ranks, severity level, and probability of autism.
Parent Interview for Autism–Clinical Version (PIA-CV; Stone, Coonrod, Pozdol, & Turner, 2003)	A 118-item semi-structured interview provides information about the presence and severity of autistic symptomology across several behavioral domains. Good psychometric properties and sensitive to symptomology present in younger samples. Good sensitivity to behavioral change in 2-year-olds.
PDD Behavior Inventory (PDDBI; Cohen, Schmidt-Lackner, Romanczyk, & Sudhalter, 2003)	Comprised of rating scales completed by caregivers or teachers assessing both adaptive and nonadaptive behaviors. Sensitive to change in maladaptive behaviors. Assesses joint attention skills, pretend play, and referential gesture. Good internal consistency and test-retest reliability.
Social Communication Questionnaire (SCQ; Rutter, Bailey, & Lord, 2003)	Utilizes 40 critical questions from the ADI-R and the same diagnostic algorithm. Items are arranged in four subscales: Social Interaction, Communication, Abnormal Language, and Stereotyped Behaviors. Applicable in children from 4 years (or mental age of 2 years) to adulthood. Not advised for use with profound ID.
Social Responsiveness Scale (SRS; Constantino et al., 2003)	Comprised of 65 items using a 4-point Likert response scale measuring reciprocal social behavior. Yields a single score that indexes the severity of impairment in reciprocal social behaviors. Psychometric properties are acceptable (sensitivity of .78 and a specificity of .77). The SRS is a highly focused measure of social impairment that may not be appropriate for children with moderate to profound intellectual disability.

A selection of instruments developed for use in diagnostic assessments of children to support the diagnosis of ASD. Some measures such as the ADI-R, ADOS and the CARS are intended to be administered by experienced clinicians with expertise in the diagnosis of ASD and who have undergone training on the use of these instruments. The other measures are questionnaires to be completed by parents and teachers and are designed to solicit observations regarding the presence of behaviors indicative of impairments of social communication and manifestations of restricted and repetitive behaviors, interests and activities. (Adapted and expanded from Stefanatos, 2012) regarding areas of strength or weakness that can guide the provision of services and facilitate the task of educators and therapists in designing and implementing appropriate interventions. A comprehensive discussion of the role of the neuropsychologist in the evaluation of ASD is beyond the scope of this chapter. For more extensive discussions the reader is referred to Black and Stefanatos (2000); Ozonoff, Goodlin-Jones, and Solomon (2005) and Kanne, Randolph, and Farmer (2008). In the next section, we provide a brief summary of the neuropsychological correlates of ASD.

Neuropsychological correlates

Intelligence

Intelligence estimates span an enormous range in ASD, from severe ID to the very superior range of intelligence. Decades ago, several studies suggested that about 25% of children with ASD had IQs of 70 or above and were thus classified as high-functioning. Correspondingly, approximately 75% were considered to function in a range indicative of intellectual handicap (<70). These proportions have become outdated due to changes in diagnostic criteria in DSM-IV and DSM-IV TR, such that less than half (~45%) of children with ASD were considered to fall within the range of ID (Chakrabarti & Fombonne, 2005; Charman, Pickles, et al., 2011; Fombonne, Quirke, & Hagen, 2011). It remains to be seen how these proportions will change with the new diagnostic criteria in DSM-5. However, as mentioned earlier in this chapter, preliminary studies suggest that high-functioning individuals are less likely to receive the diagnosis. As a result, a higher proportion of individuals who receive the diagnosis may function in the range indicative of intellectual handicap.

Several investigators have attempted to identify patterns of performance on IQ measures to index the etiological heterogeneity of ASD and provide a basis for subtyping (Bolton, Macdonald, Pickles, Rios, Goode, et al., 1994; Fein et al., 1999; Zwaigenbaum et al., 2000). Performance on the Comprehension and Vocabulary subtests are often relatively weak, reflecting difficulties with language skills and a poor appreciation of social norms and expectations (Dawson, Soulieres, Gernsbacher, & Mottron, 2007). By contrast, individuals with ASD tend to score significantly better on some nonverbal subtests, specifically Block Design (BD) (Dawson, Estes, et al., 2007). A peak on BD, while not uniformly found (Charman, Jones, et al., 2011), is present in the subtest profile of almost half (47%) of individuals with ASD compared to only 2% of the typical population (Caron, Mottron, Berthiaume, & Dawson, 2006). The strong performance on BD is thought to be related to relatively enhanced ability to perceive figure-ground relationships (Dawson, Estes, et al., 2007). This forms part of a larger pattern whereby individuals with ASD tend to struggle with verbal tasks and do better on visuospatial tasks (Bolte, Dziobek, & Poustka, 2009). Strong performance is also frequently evident on Matrix Reasoning and Picture Concepts (Mayes & Calhoun, 2008), in part because of relatively preserved or even enhanced visual perceptual functioning (see reviews by Mottron, Dawson, Soulieres, Hubert, & Burack, 2006; Simmons et al., 2009) and visual imagery (Soulieres, Zeffiro, Girard, & Mottron, 2011). However, low scores are often apparent on Symbol Search and Coding, in part because of relative deficiencies in visual motor skills (Green et al., 2009). Dawson, Estes, et al. (2007) suggested intelligence in ASD is often underestimated, and the low estimate should be regarded to reflect atypical rather than dysfunctional cognition.

While IQ appears to be as steady and predictable in ASD as it is in other clinical populations, the temporal stability of specific patterns of subtest or index scores is generally poor (Borsuk, Watkins, & Canivez, 2006). This may be related to interactions between the child's stage of development and the demand characteristics of tasks. Subtests requiring verbal information processing tend to produce lower estimates of intelligence than those dependent on spatial reasoning and this may be especially true early in development. Mayes and Calhoun (2003) observed that 67% of a cohort of children with ASD demonstrated relatively depressed Verbal IQ estimates (compared to Performance IQ) throughout their preschool years, reflecting delayed language development. As language improved with increasing age, this gap diminished, resulting in higher overall IQ estimates. Given the intersubtest variability, it has been argued that the use of short-form IQ tests or abridged administration may be associated with some reductions in the predictive validity. However, these declines do not seem disproportionate to those seen in neurotypical individuals, according to Minshew, Turner, and Goldstein (2005). Nevertheless, it is important to bear in mind that the specific content of the short form used can have a significant impact on an individual's score.

Some have argued that the use of IQ tests in the ASD population is of questionable utility, since the results do not reveal diagnostically-relevant traits (Zander & Dahlgren, 2010). The measure is not a sensitive marker of genetic risk factors associated with ASD (LeCouteur et al., 1996), in as much as autistic traits appear to be genetically independent of intellectual functioning (Hoekstra, Happé, Baron-Cohen, & Ronald, 2010). Others highlight the utility of IQ as a stable measure of general cognitive function that is also a reasonably good predictor of long-term outcome (Bolte et al., 2009; Gillberg & Steffenburg, 1987; Howlin, Goode, Hutton, & Rutter, 2004) and academic achievement (Mayes & Calhoun, 2008). A Performance IQ of less than 70 appears to be associated with much poorer prognosis in adulthood (Howlin et al., 2004). Overall, independent living is a possibility for individuals with ASD who have an IQ in the normal range (> 70), although outcome can still be variable at this level (Howlin et al., 2004).

Motor

Among the neurological comorbidities of ASD, motor impairment is among the most common. Indeed, Kanner (1943) noted that several of the children in his initial cohort were "somewhat clumsy in gait and gross motor performance." Impairments may become apparent early in life in delays in attaining motor milestones such as righting, sitting, crawling, and walking, as well as a failure to demonstrate protective motor responses when falling (Baranek, 1999; Teitelbaum, Teitelbaum, Nye, Fryman, & Maurer, 1998). In toddlerhood, sensory motor deficits such as hypotonia are common (~50%), although this may dissipate over time (Ming, Brimacombe, & Wagner, 2007). Children with ASD tend to walk 1.6 months later than their age peers (Sheat-Klein, Shinnar, & Rapin, 2014) and often demonstrate gait abnormalities. Periods of toe walking may also be observed in a smaller number of children with ASD (Ming et al., 2007). Disturbances in both fine and gross motor coordination, gait (Jansiewicz et al., 2006; Rinehart et al., 2006), balance (Jansiewicz et al., 2006; Whyatt & Craig, 2012), motor planning (Dowd, McGinley, Taffe, & Rinehart, 2012; Hughes, 1996), and spontaneous imitation of actions (Rogers, Young, Cook, Giolzetti, & Ozonoff, 2008; Stephens, 2008) become apparent in the course of development and cannot be attributed to motor weakness, sensory loss, or general intellectual deficiency (Vivanti, Trembath, & Dissanayake, 2014). Some of these early problems are predictive of future diagnosis of autism (Teitelbaum et al., 1998), the presence of coexisting communication difficulties (Bhat, Galloway, & Landa, 2012; Gernsbacher, Sauer, Geye, Schweigert, & Hill Goldsmith, 2008), and pragmatic language skills (Miniscalco, Rudling, Rastam, Gillberg, & Johnels, 2014), and whether or not the child will retain the diagnosis of ASD later in life (Sutera et al., 2007). On standardized assessment batteries, individuals with ASD between 7 and 32 years of age demonstrate poor upper limb coordination during tasks requiring manual dexterity and visual motor coordination. In addition, they exhibit poor performance on tasks requiring balance, agility, speed, and coordination of the lower limbs (Dewey, Cantell, & Crawford, 2007; Ghaziuddin & Butler, 1998). These difficulties were initially thought to be limited to children with lower IQ scores, but in more recent studies, it has become evident that impairment exists in children with normal range intelligence as well. Deficits may even be evident in specific fairly common tasks such as reaching to grasp (Mari, Castiello, Marks, Marraffa, & Prior, 2003). Motor issues persisting into adulthood can also include features of an ataxic gait characterized by constrained range of motion of the ankle, increased variability in stride distance, and instability (Hallett et al., 1993).

One of the most consistent findings is that individuals with autism are impaired in their ability to imitate skilled gestures. Early theories postulated that these difficulties were related to disturbances in the perceptual organization of movements that limit their ability to develop representations of the sequence of movements to be imitated (Smith & Bryson, 1994). Numerous studies have suggested that children with ASD may be limited in their capacity to build internal representations of actions and use them to organize, plan, and execute movements (Dowd et al., 2012; Dowell, Mahone, & Mostofsky, 2009; Haswell, Izawa, Dowell, Mostofsky, & Shadmehr, 2009). According to this view, the ability to perform skilled actions is contingent upon the formation of internal models of the complex movement sequences required to execute actions. This process is thought to entail a system of correlating executed motor programs with proprioceptive and visual feedback obtained during self-generated attempts to perform and evaluate the success of a given action. Learning involves generalization based on both proprioceptive and visual feedback as well as watching others perform the same or similar actions. Building upon knowledge gained from the discovery of mirror neurons (Rizzolatti & Fabbri-Destro, 2008), some have speculated that these difficulties may be rooted, at least in part, in failure of the mirror neuron system. According to some recent findings, individuals with ASD may discount visual cues during the process of performing motor actions and build stronger than normal associations between self-generated motor commands and proprioceptive feedback (Haswell et al., 2009). This would place them at a significant disadvantage in imitating movements and understanding other people's actions.

Given evidence of difficulties with movement sequencing, gestural imitation, production of gesture to command, and disturbances in the use of objects and tools (Mostofsky et al., 2006; Williams, Whiten, & Singh, 2004), it has been proposed that individuals with ASD may have a generalized praxis deficit (Dewey et al., 2007; Miller, Chukoskie, Zinni, Townsend, & Trauner, 2014; Mostofsky et al., 2006). It has been suggested that a variety of dyspraxic forms may exist in ASD, including ideational, limb kinetic and buccal-facial forms (Dewey et al., 2007; Miller et al., 2014). While some studies have found an association between impairment of basic motor skills and dyspraxic difficulties (Dowell et al., 2009; Dziuk et al., 2007), the problems with dyspraxia cannot simply be attributed to the more basic problems (Miller et al., 2014). Potential underlying difficulties range from problems with motor pre-programming to deficient meta-knowledge regarding the properties and motor execution of complex actions. Explanations invoking general deficiencies of the mirror neuron system seem incompatible with the prevalence of echopraxia and echolalia in this population as well as the results of a recent neuroimaging study (Spengler, Bird, & Brass, 2010). Conceptually, the findings broadly implicate deficiencies in top-down control of motor actions that are contingent upon integrating proprioceptive, visual, and motor information with conceptual representations of action and the intent of actions (e.g., mental state considerations). The level(s) and precise nature of the underlying processing impairment(s) remain to be more fully explored in future research.

Attention

Attention functioning in ASD has been a topic of clinical and research interest since the publication of Rimland's landmark book (1964) in which he pointed out many of the attentional abnormalities commonly seen in this population. Abnormally prolonged attention for preferred activities along with great distractibility and difficulty engaging mental effort for nonpreferred activities is a common clinical observation. Starting in Britain in the 1960s and 70s and accelerating in the 1980s, experimental studies of various aspects of attention have attempted to pinpoint the underlying sources of these clinical observations. A recent source of interest in attention in ASD is studies of the emergence of symptoms in infant siblings of affected children, in which difficulty disengaging social inattention can be seen as early as 6 months of age in some children (Bhat, Galloway, & Landa, 2010), and problems disengaging visual attention become evident by 12–14 months or even earlier (Elsabbagh et al., 2013; Zwaigenbaum et al., 2005). Whether attentional findings in ASD reflect primary abnormalities in attention system(s) or stem from a different motivational structure from whatever comparison group is being used is unclear, since most studies do not manipulate or attempt to maximize motivation (for informative exceptions, see Garretson, Fein, & Waterhouse, 1990; Ozonoff, 1995). There is a large literature on ASD and the many components of attention; the reader is referred to recent reviews (Ames & Fletcher-Watson, 2010; Sanders, Johnson, Garavan, Gill, & Gallagher, 2008) for a more comprehensive discussion.

EXOGENOUS AND ENDOGENOUS ORIENTING

Exogenous orienting refers to involuntary orienting in which attention is pulled to an external stimulus, often in the periphery; this system develops within the first few months of life (Johnson, Posner, & Rothbart, 1991). Using a Posner-type orienting task, several studies have found relative deficiency in exogenous orienting in individuals with ASD (Greenaway & Plaisted, 2005; but see Minshew, Luna, & Sweeney, 1999; Renner, Grofer Klinger, & Klinger, 2006; Townsend et al., 1999). Furthermore, the components of exogenous orienting have been identified as *disengaging* from the current focus of attention, *moving* attention to the new location, and *re-engaging attention* on the new stimulus, each of which have been correlated with activity of relatively distinct brain systems (Posner & Fan, 2004). Several studies suggest that individuals with high-functioning ASD have relative impairment in the *disengaging* component of exogenous orienting (Landry & Bryson, 2004; Pascualvaca, Fantie, Papageorgiou, & Mirsky, 1998; Wainwright-Sharp & Bryson, 1993), which has been suggested to rely heavily on parietal functioning (Posner & Fan, 2004). In contrast, the later-developing endogenous orienting system, in which attention is voluntarily and intentionally moved to a new location (e.g., in response to a task instruction such as an arrow appearing at central fixation pointing to where attention should be reallocated), is found to be relatively intact in ASD (Landry, Mitchell, & Burack, 2009). However, when the time between the cue and target is very short, results are more mixed (Landry et al., 2009; Senju, Tojo, Dairoku, & Hasegawa, 2004).

Townsend et al. (1999) suggest that attentional shifting in ASD is generally slowed and is similar to performance of patients with cerebellar lesions (Courchesne et al., 1994), while Renner et al. (2006) propose that attentional shifting in ASD requires more effortful, endogenous processing, which is slower than normal exogenous shifting. Minshew et al. (1999) demonstrated that oculomotor functioning in automatic shifts of attention is normal while volitional eye movements (e.g., antisaccades) are inefficient, and argue that this implicates frontal-parietal circuitry and not cerebellar circuitry.

Furthermore, even when performance on selective visuospatial attention tasks is normal, activation of neural systems is not. Belmonte and Yurgelun-Todd (2003) found abnormal patterns of activation in a small group of autistic individuals, including more activation in occipital and subcortical areas and less activation in frontal, parietal, and temporal areas than typically-developing controls. Haist, Adamo, Westerfield, Courchesne, and Townsend (2005) also found reduced activation in a spatial cuing task in parietal and especially in frontal regions and occipital regions, and a virtual lack of activation in the cerebellar vermis.

FOCUS OF ATTENTION

Literature going back to the early 1970s has demonstrated overselective attention to specific details in ASD (Fein, Tinder, & Waterhouse, 1979; Lovaas & Schreibman, 1971). In fact, a detail-oriented perceptual style in which elements are not integrated into more holistic percepts and concepts was originally suggested in Rimland's (1964) groundbreaking book on autism. Enhanced perceptual analysis of elementary aspects of stimuli has been demonstrated in a series of studies by Mottron and colleagues (Mottron et al., 2006) and confirmed by others (Eigsti & Fein, 2013); findings are generally consistent in showing a local over global perceptual bias in ASD (Wang, Mottron, Peng, Berthiaume, & Dawson, 2007). Manjaly et al. (2007), in looking at activation during a local visual search task, confirmed behavioral superiority in autism in local processing and found not only enhanced occipital activation in adolescents with ASD, but more right-lateralized activation compared to controls.

Various theoretical models have been proposed in which this enhanced local processing and orientation to detail form a central explanatory concept of autism referred to as *central coherence*. According to this conception, individuals with ASD suffer from weak central coherence in which a detail-oriented bias prevails, with mixed evidence on whether global processing is impaired or simply not preferred. Weak central coherence has been evoked to explain perceptual performance as well as social deficits (Happé & Frith, 2006). This conception is somewhat similar to Rimland's (1964) proposal. Other theoretical models of autism have related attention deficits, including the overfocused and perseverative interest in details, to both overarousal (Dawson & Lewy, 1989; Hutt, Hutt, Lee, & Ounsted, 1964) and to unstable arousal (Hiscock & Kinsbourne, 2011).

Some attentional abnormalities seen in ASD are core diagnostic features of the diagnosis in both DSM-IV and DSM-5. This includes the repetitive and unusual sensory-rather-than-meaning-oriented visual examination of objects, especially visual displays with straight lines, shadows, lights, or objects that can be moved in the visual periphery. There is some inconsistency in reports about when these behaviors tend to emerge, with some arguing that they generally emerge later than social deficits (Stone et al., 1999), while others have found them in infant siblings, who later received an ASD diagnosis, as early as 12 months (Ozonoff, Heung, et al., 2008).

In addition to detail orientation, and on more elementary perceptual elements, the content of attentional focus has been repeatedly shown to be abnormal in autism. In particular, there is avoidance of social stimuli, starting at an early age (Bhat et al., 2010), and in particular, avoidance of the eye region of others' faces, which starts to decline in the initial half of the first year and continues to decline over the first two years or so (Jones & Klin, 2013). Children with autism show selective deficits in orienting to social information, such as a parent calling their name (Dawson, Meltzoff, Osterling, Rinaldi, & Brown, 1998). A study of source memory showed that memory for origins of information was impaired only in aspects of the source related to the face of the speaker (O'Shea, Fein, Cillessen, Klin, & Schultz, 2005), and Goldberg, Mostow, et al. (2008) showed that direction of eye gaze was difficult for individuals with ASD to use as an endogenous orienting cue. One striking example of this avoidance of the face can be seen in a fascinating set of drawings by a 3-year-old girl with autism, in which there are some beautifully done drawings of human figures up to the neck, with the head represented by a tiny circle (Selfe, 1995).

INHIBITION

Individuals with ASD, both high-functioning and with ID, appear to be relatively intact in their capacity to inhibit prepotent responses, when compared to typical individuals or those with mild intellectual disability and no autism (Happé, Booth, Charlton, & Hughes, 2006; Ozonoff & Jensen, 1999; Ozonoff & Strayer, 1997; Raymaekers, Antrop, van der Meere, Wiersema, & Roeyers, 2007; Russell, Jarrold, & Hood, 1999). However, at least two studies suggest that while children with ASD may perform similarly to mental-age-matched peers, adolescents and adults with ASD may be deficient relative to typical controls (Raymaekers, Van der Meere, & Roeyers, 2004; Solomon, Ozonoff, Cummings, & Carter, 2008). Despite good behavioral performance, neuroimaging suggests that individuals with ASD may need to employ different levels of activation in inhibitory areas to achieve the same behaviors (Kana, Keller, Minshew, & Just, 2007; Schmitz et al., 2006).

SUSTAINED ATTENTION

The ability of individuals with ASD to *sustain attention* has been examined with variations on the Continuous Performance Task. Garretson et al. (1990) found that children with ASD sustained attention comparably to mental-age-matched typical children, as long as motivation was maximized with tangible reinforcers, and the task difficulty was kept to a moderate level (slow rather than fast stimulus presentation). Several other studies using a variety of paradigms and test batteries have also found relatively strong ability to sustain attention (Goldstein, Johnson, & Minshew, 2001; Johnson et al., 2007; Pascualvaca et al., 1998) although, as with other aspects of attention, functioning neuroimaging reveals different patterns of activation underlying normal behavioral performance. Christakou et al. (2013) examined neural activation in groups of typically-developing boys with ADHD and ASD in a sustained attention task with varying cognitive loads, and reported shared abnormalities in fronto-striato-parietal activation and suppression of the default mode network, but an autism-specific fronto-striato-cerebellar dysregulation. Kennedy and Courchesne (2008), however, present evidence that resting state functional connectivity is abnormal in the large-scale neural networks responsible for social-emotional processing, but essentially normal on the large-scale network underlying sustained attention and goal-directed activity.

Therefore, overall, evidence is fairly consistent that sustained attention seems to be an area of spared functioning in autism, as long as the exertion of mental effort required is moderate and motivation is present, although different neural activation patterns probably underlie this performance.

SET-SHIFTING

Set-shifting differs from endogenous and exogenous shifts in that the former is a general change in cognitive strategy, which may be spatial or along some other dimension, while the latter has most often been studied in the context of shifts of spatial attention. In addition, set-shifting is usually initiated by the subject in response to changes in some environmental condition, rather than being specifically instructed or elicited by the stimulus material, and is taken as an index of cognitive flexibility. Set-shifting has most often been examined with the

Wisconsin Card Sorting Test or a similar task. Most studies show deficits in set-shifting in autism (Goldstein et al., 2001; Tsuchiya, Oki, Yahara, & Fujieda, 2005), with particular tendencies to perseveration, and, as with exogenous shifts of attention, a particular problem with disengaging from a previously reinforced strategy (Pascualvaca et al., 1998), although the deficits are sometimes mild (Kaland, Smith, & Mortensen, 2008). Although the majority of studies do find tendencies to perseveration and poorer set-shifting in ASD, Ozonoff (1995) and Pascualvaca et al. (1998) demonstrated that a computer version of a set-shifting task showed attenuated deficits in set-shifting over standard administration with social feedback, implicating a motivational component to the deficit.

SUMMARY

In general, inhibition, sustained attention, and endogenous shifts of attention are relatively spared in individuals with ASD, while exogenous shifts, set-shifting, and focus of attention are abnormal. However, there are many individual exceptions to these generalizations and much inconsistency among studies, depending on specific tasks and subject characteristics. In fact, it is a significant shortcoming in most studies that they report group-level performance rather than focusing on variability within clinical groups or correlations between attention measures and clinical phenomena. Functional imaging studies are much more recent and less numerous, and show, if anything, more variability and inconsistency in results than behavioral studies. Variability is undoubtedly driven not only by differences in samples and in task parameters, but in imaging and analysis methods.

Memory

As with other neuropsychological functions, the study of memory in high-functioning individuals with autism has to be considered separately from that of memory in low-functioning individuals, in whom separating memory deficits from their general ID is very difficult. Most of what we know about selective memory impairments in autism, therefore, comes from the study of high-functioning groups. The literature on memory impairment also overlaps with the literature on attention, executive functions, and material-specific processes such as verbal memory. We will focus here on studies that specifically identify themselves as memory research. For more detailed reviews, see Boucher, Mayes, and Bigham (2012) and Shalom et al. (2003).

One conclusion that can be drawn about memory research in autism is that mixed and contradictory findings abound, more so than in some other areas of cognitive research. For example, despite some contradictions in the literature on language, there is a general body of consistent research on basic functions (e.g., phonology, syntax). This may be due in part to the fact that language impairments form part of the definition of autism in some diagnostic and descriptive systems, while memory impairment does not. The further one gets from definitional features, the more inconsistency is found in the body of research, and this is certainly true for memory. This is probably due in part to sensitivity of findings to method variation among studies of recall and recognition, and perhaps even more to the heterogeneity of relatively small samples in these studies. For these reasons, there are few general conclusions about memory functioning in autism, but there are several areas that show some fairly consistent findings.

MEMORY PROCESSES

Profiles of ability on the Wechsler Memory Scale-III (WMS-III) in high-functioning autism (HFA) were characterized by Williams, Goldstein, Carpenter, and Minshew (2005). Performance was unimpaired on immediate and delayed memory for paired associates and stories, and on a verbal working memory task. Autistic performance was impaired on immediate and delayed recall of faces and of family scenes as well as spatial working memory; the latter was attributed to the computational demands of this particular task, and the former to a deficit in memory for social material, which directly impacts functioning in daily life (Williams, Goldstein, Carpenter, et al., 2005; Williams, Goldstein, & Minshew, 2005, 2006).

Working memory has been confirmed as impaired by some groups (Williams, Goldstein, et al., 2006), while others have found intact verbal working memory in HFA (Ozonoff & Strayer, 2001); as with other areas, it is likely that differences among studies rest on heterogeneity of samples and subtle or not-so-subtle differences in task procedures and motivational conditions. Rather surprisingly, given the general superiority of visuospatial over linguistic processes in autism, verbal working memory has been found to be more intact in autism than visuospatial working memory (Steele, Minshew, Luna, & Sweeney, 2007). Luna et al. (2002) examined neural activation during a spatial working memory task and reported that individuals with autism showed less task-related activation in dorsolateral prefrontal cortex and PCC but not in other regions related to spatial working memory, including the cortical eye fields, ACC, insula, basal ganglia, thalamus, and lateral cerebellum.

Renner, Klinger, and Klinger (2000) directly addressed the idea that autism might involve an amnesia comparable to that of medial temporal lobe patients, in which explicit but not implicit memory would be expected to be deficient. Their findings did not support this idea: They showed, instead, that both explicit and implicit memory functions were intact, but that the strategy for explicit recall was different in participants with autism. These participants did not show the usual pattern developing of primacy and recency effects, but recalled words mainly from the end of the recall list, a finding that can be interpreted as suggesting a passive rather than an active encoding approach, or shallow encoding. Reduced primacy effects were also reported by Toichi and Kamio (2003). Other studies have confirmed the generalized sparing of implicit learning. For example, implicit learning of spatial context (Barnes et al., 2008), perceptual priming (Gardiner, Bowler, & Grice, 2003), and implicit category formation (Molesworth, Bowler, & Hampton, 2005) were all found to be unimpaired in HFA. (Brown, Aczel, Jimenez, Kaufman, & Grant, 2010) examined autistic performance on four implicit learning tasks (contextual cueing, serial reaction time, artificial grammar learning, and probabilistic classification learning) and found them all to be unimpaired in individuals with autism.

Within the explicit memory domain, recognition memory for a variety of types of material has generally been found to be normal or even superior in autism, while various forms of free and cued recall produce much more mixed findings. Recognition memory for shapes, words, and objects (but not faces) has been consistently comparable to controls or even superior (e.g., Barth, Fein, & Waterhouse, 1995; Brian & Bryson, 1996; Hillier, Campbell, Keillor, Phillips, & Beversdorf, 2007; Renner et al., 2000; Toichi & Kamio, 2002).

Free recall is generally reported as less intact in autism than cued recall, although this varies to some extent with stimulus materials, and is often interpreted as a strategic deficit in activating appropriate recall strategies without a degree of "task support" (Bowler, Gardiner, & Berthollier, 2004). For example, Gaigg, Gardiner, and Bowler (2008) tested the hypothesis that memory for relational information rather than item-specific information is impaired in autism and concluded that while the former is impaired in spontaneous memory, it can be deployed when environmental support is provided. In general, free recall of unrelated items is less impaired than recall of related items, presumably because the individuals with autism essentially treat the semantically related items as unrelated; this seems to hold for both immediate (Smith & Gardiner, 2008) and delayed recall (Renner et al., 2000). For example, Fein et al., 1996, reported that performance in HFA was comparable to that of matched individuals with specific language impairment for memory for sentences, but superior for digit memory and inferior for story memory. Minshew and Goldstein (2001) also found impaired autistic performance on the California Verbal Learning Test (CVLT) and on a story memory task. Bennetto, Pennington, and Rogers (1996) presented a detailed analysis of performance of individuals with ASD on the CVLT. The ASD group showed less free recall of the word list on Trials 3–5, but did not forget more words than controls over short or long delay periods. However, overall, they showed increased intrusions. Additionally, while they correctly endorsed an equivalent numbers of words on a recognition trial, they demonstrated increased false positives that were from the interfering list or other words that were semantically related to the target words. Phelan, Filliter, and Johnson (2010), in contrast, found unimpaired overall list learning ability on the CVLT in HFA, but reported that cued recall was superior to free recall (relative to norms). (Bowler, Gaigg, & Gardiner, 2009) also showed that although autistic participants did use semantic clustering to aid recall, the categories they formed were idiosyncratic, in contrast to the word groupings of typical controls.

With regard to episodic and autobiographical memory, Bowler, Gaigg, & Gardiner, 2008, reported that the experiences of remembering events by individuals with autism are qualitatively similar to those of controls, although they report fewer such memories. Reduced recall of autobiographical episodes in the context of normal recall of autobiographical and other facts (Crane & Goddard, 2008; Klein, Chan, & Loftus, 1999; Minshew et al., 2005) confirms this impaired retention or reporting of meaningful personal episodes. This impairment is difficult to reconcile with the often-reported extremely detailed memory of some autistic individuals for specific, distant episodes, complete with details that are not viewed as central or memorable by others, and suggests that only certain episodes capture the attention of these individuals sufficiently for these details to be retained. For interesting discussions of the relationship between episodic memory and the concept of the self in autism, see Toichi and Kamio (2002); Lind and Bowler (2010) and Lombardo and Baron-Cohen (2010).

A few studies have examined various aspects of source memory (memory for time, place, or other aspects of situation in which the event occurred) in autism, including source monitoring (attributing a remembered event to one's own thoughts, words, or actions [internal source] or to another's actions or words [external source]). Generally intact identification of the source of memories has been found in HFA, especially when recognition tasks are used (Bowler et al., 2004; Gaigg et al., 2008; Williams, Goldstein, & Minshew, 2005). Bowler, Gardiner, and Grice (2000) showed intact recognition of words in autism, but recognition was more often present when subjects reported "knowing" that they had seen the word rather than "remembering" the actual event; Bowler et al. interpret this finding as indicating deficit in self-aware (autonoetic), episodic memories. O'Shea et al. (2005) reported intact recognition of impersonal contextual information (e.g., the color of the wall behind the speaker), but impaired recognition of social contextual information (e.g., the face of the speaker). Hala, Rasmussen, and Henderson (2005) also found source monitoring to be less efficient in autism than in controls, although the pattern of difficulty of different types of source monitoring (e.g., self vs. other, real vs. imagined) was the same in both groups.

MATERIAL-SPECIFIC DEFICITS

A series of studies by Gaigg and Bowler (Gaigg & Bowler, 2008; Gaigg et al., 2008) examined the effect of emotionally arousing stimuli on conditioning and found that fear conditioning was impaired in autism, and although emotionally arousing words were learned more readily than neutral words, as in typical controls, such words were not as resistant to forgetting in the autism group as they were in the controls. Gaigg and Bowler argue that these and other results support the idea that amygdala–cortical connections are underrepresented in autism, leading to abnormal conditioning of arousing stimuli. Illusory memories are less likely in controls when stimuli are emotionally charged than when they are neutral, while subjects with ASD are less affected by the emotionality of the stimuli (Gaigg & Bowler, 2009).

As mentioned on p. 230, incidental source memory was found to be normal on all aspects of the context in which stories were heard, except for a specifically social aspect of the learning context (e.g., the face of the speaker; see O'Shea et al., 2005), confirming a memory deficit for social information, possibly secondary to reduced attention to this aspect of the environment. A material-specific deficit in memory for faces has been confirmed in direct tests of face memory (Dawson et al., 2002; Hauck, Fein, Maltby, Waterhouse, & Feinstein, 1998; Klin et al., 1999; Williams, Goldstein, & Minshew, 2005). Howard et al. (2000) also found poor recognition memory for faces, and found it to be associated with enlarged amygdala volume and abnormal processing of fear expressions. Koshino et al. (2008) examined brain activation and functional connectivity in a working memory task involving faces. There was reduced activation in the autism group in the left inferior prefrontal and right posterior temporal areas and a slightly different location for fusiform activation. The results were interpreted as reflecting impacted working memory, ToM processing, and a tendency to analyze faces as nonsocial stimuli.

MEMORY AS SECONDARY TO OTHER COGNITIVE PROCESSES

Some theorists have argued that memory deficits in autism are secondary to other cognitive deficits. In particular, Minshew and Goldstein (2001) have maintained that apparent memory impairments are not amnestic deficits per se, nor are they material-specific, but rather are secondary to impaired deployment of organizing strategies to improve memory efficiency. They administered a battery of memory tests to a group of high-functioning adolescents and young adults with autism; memory deficits were directly related to the complexity of the material being remembered (e.g., complex vs. simple mazes, paired-associates vs. list and story recall). Williams, Goldstein, et al. (2006) confirmed this complexity effect and also found deficits in working memory, which depends on strategy utilization. In addition, they established that memory factor structure was different in autistic and control groups.

Similarly, Bennetto et al. (1996) found specific impairment in an HFA group in temporal order memory, source memory, supraspan free recall, and working memory, but not on short- and long-term recognition, cued recall, or new learning. They interpreted this pattern of findings as consistent with a primary executive dysfunction, which contributed to the memory impairments.

Compensation for poor semantic encoding with the use of rote memory strategies or phonological encoding has also been suggested. For most populations, semantic strategies assist memory more than phonological ones, but Toichi and Kamio (2002) found a lack of superiority of semantic cuing over phonological cuing in HFA. Mottron, Morasse, and Belleville (2001) suggest that in autism, phonological processing of language cues is enhanced (rather than suggesting semantic deficits).

SUMMARY

Memory findings in autism are extremely mixed and contradictory. The most consistent findings are probably the material-specific abnormality in memory for social stimuli, especially faces, and the lack of differential memory for emotionally arousing versus neutral stimuli. Free recall is often reported as abnormal, both in total amount of material recalled and in strategies spontaneously deployed to aid recall (reduced or idiosyncratic semantic encoding and clustering, reduced primacy but reliance on recency effects). Cued recall seems to boost memory in participants with autism more than in controls. Just as cued recall is better than free recall, recognition memory is better yet, but there is a tendency towards endorsing related false positives. Once learned, forgetting over immediate and longer-term retention intervals is not generally reported. Findings on source memory and source monitoring is mixed, but there is some evidence that episodic memory, and particularly autobiographical remembering, is impoverished in HFA, despite clinical accounts of some remarkable event memory. When functional imaging is performed during memory tasks, areas of activation are often abnormal, even in the context of normal-level behavioral performance.

Perceptual abilities

Sensory and perceptual abnormalities in autism have been in the literature since Kanner's original paper in 1943, where he described such classic sensory autistic behaviors as a child looking at objects while shaking or spinning them, and showing pleasure at watching spinning items. Early researchers such as Ornitz, Rimland, and the Hutts wrote extensively about sensory phenomena and theories in the 1960s and 70s (Ornitz, 1973). Following these descriptions and simple experiments, sensory phenomena rather fell out of favor among mainstream autism researchers, who were focusing on language, other cognitive processes, and initial attempts at biological research, followed by an upsurge in interest in social behavior and social cognition. In the last 10–15 years, however, there has been a resurgence of interest in sensory and perceptual processing in autism, perhaps best indicated by the inclusion of sensory abnormalities as a diagnostic criterion in the recently published DSM-5. For more extensive reviews of sensory and perceptual research, see Rogers and Ozonoff

(2005); Leekam, Nieto, Libby, Wing, and Gould (2007), and Fine, Musielak, and Semrud-Clikeman (2014), which also has an interesting historical perspective. The piecemeal perceptual style of most individuals with autism (Happé & Frith, 2006) has been variously viewed as a deficit in integrative processes leading to poor gestalt perception and intact perception of detail, or as a processing style or preference in which the inclination is to process detail, but in which integrative processing of gestalts is not impaired when the motivation for it exists (see discussion by Bolte et al., 2012).

CLINICAL PHENOMENA AND DIAGNOSTIC CRITERIA

Rogers and Ozonoff (2005) include in their review of sensory features of autism over-or underresponsiveness, preoccupations with sensory features of objects, and unusual reactions to sensory stimuli. Overresponsiveness might include such behaviors as covering the ears in response to loud sounds, oversensitivity to smells that other don't notice, overly picky food choices based on texture or temperature, or resistance to being touched. Underresponsiveness might include ignoring loud sounds, ignoring others' voices, insensitivity to painful experiences (such as minor injuries or blood draws), and insensitivity to being hot or cold. Preoccupations with sensory features of objects might include visual fascinations with things like shadows, water dripping, objects spinning, movie or TV credits scrolling, and straight lines. Unusual reactions could encompass all of the above, and usually refer to specific isolated sensitivities or fascinations, like being fearful of vacuum cleaners. It could also include sensory-seeking behavior, where the individual engages in behaviors that appear to be intended to provide to provide unusual sensory input, like wiggling fingers in the visual periphery or looking at things upside down.

Although DSM-IV does not mention sensory abnormalities per se, it includes two criteria under "restricted and repetitive behaviors" that can include abnormal responses to sensory input: first, "encompassing preoccupation with one or more stereotyped and restricted patterns of interest that is abnormal either in intensity or focus," and second, "persistent preoccupation with parts of objects" (APA, 2000, p. 71). Although the first of these is often applied mainly to objects that the individual with autism wants to talk about, collect, or play with, it can also apply to fixations on sensory qualities, such as wanting to carry around yellow things. The second relates more directly to sensory abnormalities, an example being a child who persistently stares at or spins the wheels on a toy rather than playing with the toy functionally. Since the DSM-IV is polythetic, allowing for a selection among symptoms, it permits a diagnosis of PDD-NOS with *no* repetitive behaviors, including the two types just mentioned. A diagnosis of autistic disorder can be made with just one of these types of restricted and repetitive behavior. DSM-5 is more nomothetic, that is, it requires all three of the social-communication symptoms to be present, although it allows more flexibility in the domain of repetitive behaviors, requiring two of the four such symptoms. One of these is explicitly sensory: "Hyper- or hypo-reactivity to sensory input or unusual interests in sensory aspects of the environment (e.g., apparent indifference to pain/temperature, adverse response to specific sounds or textures, excessive smelling or touching of objects, visual fascination with lights or movement)" (APA, 2013).

The inclusion of explicitly sensory symptoms in the DSM-5 has not drawn a lot of criticism, since the presence of these symptoms in many affected individuals has been well-established for so long, but the requirement of at least two repetitive behaviors has raised concerns about individuals who met DSM-IV-TR criteria for an ASD losing the diagnosis. Leekam, Nieto, et al. (2007), using the Diagnostic Interview for Social and Communication Disorders (DISCO; Leekam, Libby, Wing, Gould, & Taylor, 2002) found that more than 90% of children with autism had sensory abnormalities. Furthermore, sensory symptoms were shown in multiple domains (including atypical responses to auditory, visual, tactile and olfactory stimuli, and insensitivity to pain), with the biggest differences between children with autism and those with other clinical conditions being in the specific domains of smell/taste and vision. They also found that symptoms persist across time, but can manifest differently at various ages, and with different levels of cognitive functioning.

Despite this high prevalence of abnormal responsiveness to sensory stimuli in autism, some empirical data have suggested that a not-insubstantial number of individuals with autism may not meet the DSM-5 requirement of two RRBIA symptoms. McPartland et al. (2012) found reduced sensitivity of DSM-5 relative to DSM-IV-TR, with a significant number of cases failing to meet two of the four RRBIA criteria. Barton et al. (2013) investigated the sensitivity and specificity of the DSM-5 criteria with specific reference to toddlers, raising the concern that although sensory over- and underresponsiveness and fascinations may be present in many toddlers, other repetitive behaviors such as obsessive interests, repetitive movements and speech, and resistance to change in routines and environments may not appear until later. Therefore a significant number of toddlers may lose the diagnosis. In fact, they found that sensitivity of DSM-5 for toddlers previously diagnosed was inadequate unless the criteria were relaxed to two-thirds of the social symptoms and one-fourth of the repetitive symptoms.

Methodological issues abound in the domain of sensory and perceptual research. First is the problem that plagues autism research in general: the heterogeneity of subject samples, in terms of age, cognitive functioning, social relationships, biological features, and sensory abnormalities themselves. As Waterhouse (2013) repeatedly points out, grouping together a set of individuals who meet some criteria for autism and investigating their sensory functioning, when they vary tremendously on multiple dimensions, presents many problems and uninterpretable results. Second is the measurement issue. Many studies rely on parent report, some by interview using instruments like the ADI or the DISCO, and some with questionnaires such as the various version of Dunn's Sensory Profile. Valuable as parent report is, especially since it can encompass behavior across time and in multiple situations, it needs validation with more objective measures and cannot reveal anything about underlying mechanisms. In recent years, EEG, ERP, functional imaging, and psychophysical experiments have greatly supplemented the reliance on clinical observation and parent report. However, these suffer from the problem of taking a (usually) one-time measurement in a group in which attention and motivation can greatly impact performance on sensory tasks.

PARENT REPORTS

Much of the literature to the present day has relied on various versions of Winnie Dunn's Sensory Profile (Dunn & Westman, 1997). Ninety-five percent of the sample of children with ASD demonstrated some degree of sensory processing dysfunction on the Short Sensory Profile Total Score, showing differences from controls on 92% of items and across all domains (Tomchek & Dunn, 2007). The greatest differences from controls were found on the Underresponsive/Seeks Sensation, Auditory Filtering, and Tactile Sensitivity sections. Rogers, Hepburn, and Wehner (2003) also used the Sensory Profile in comparing three clinical groups and controls. The group with autism had poor auditory filtering and showed elevated scores on the Seeks Stimulation/Underresponsive sections (that is, seeking stimulation with such activities as wiggling objects and fingers in front of eyes but failing to respond to caregiver-presented stimuli). While they were comparable in overall abnormality to children with Fragile X, the autistic group had the highest rates of irregularity in taste and smell specifically. This and other studies conclude that sensory deficits are not specific to autism, but that certain behaviors—particularly involving taste, smell, and tactile input—may be more specific to autism than more general categories like underresponsiveness.

Similar results were reported by Wiggins, Robins, Bakeman, and Adamson (2009), who explored the sensory functioning of very young children with autism at the time of diagnosis. They found that these young children with ASD had more tactile and taste/smell sensitivities and difficulties with auditory filtering than age-matched children with other developmental disorders. In addition, sensory abnormalities were associated with stereotyped interests and behaviors. These findings were taken as supportive of the inclusion of sensory abnormalities in diagnostic criteria for autism. The relationship of sensory abnormalities—in particular tactile defensiveness—was also reported by Baranek, Foster, and Berkson (1997), who showed that individuals with higher levels of tactile defensiveness were more likely to display rigid or repetitive behaviors in other domains, such as stereotyped speech.

Also using the Sensory Profile, Kern and Jones (2006) confirmed that a wide age range of individuals with autism were abnormal across all domains. Their results suggest that sensory abnormalities in autism are global in nature (involving several modalities) but have the potential to improve with age, except for low threshold for tactile input, which was consistent across age and could lead to tactile defensiveness.

Liss, Saulnier, Fein, and Kinsbourne (2006) looked at a large group of individuals with ASDs to examine the relationship of sensory reactions to Kinsbourne's hypothesized "overfocused attention" style (Kinsbourne, 1991). They assessed whether children with unstable arousal systems who might overreact to sensations would overfocus on preferred topics and develop extraordinary memory for selected material. They added items to the Sensory Profile to cover some specific autistic behaviors, resulting in a 103-item expanded Sensory Profile. Parents of children with ASD rated items in the areas of "sensory overreactivity," "sensory underreactivity," "sensory seeking behaviors," "overselective attention" and "exceptional memory," and completed the Vineland Adaptive Behavior Scales. On one hand, overreactivity in the whole group was significantly associated with social symptoms and delays, perseveration and overfocusing, and with reports of exceptional memory. Underreactivity, on the other hand, was strongly related to all domains of autism symptomatology and to lower cognitive and adaptive functioning, but not to exceptional memory. Sensory seeking was also found to be related to all domains of autism symptomatology and lower adaptive skills, and sensory seeking and underreactivity were the most strongly intercorrelated of the three reaction patterns. Cluster analysis showed one large group of children with the predicted overfocused pattern of attention who demonstrated overreactivity, perseverative behaviors and interests, and exceptional memory. A second clear cluster was underreactive and sensory seeking, with prominent autism symptoms and low adaptive skills. The conclusion, therefore, was that overreactivity was associated with unstable arousal with consequent defensive overfocusing on selected interests, resulting in exceptional memory for this material. In contrast, underreactivity and sensory seeking were more strongly associated with severe autism and low adaptive skills.

LABORATORY STUDIES

A very useful review of controlled laboratory studies was conducted by Rogers and Ozonoff (2005). They conclude, unlike some of the studies cited earlier, that although sensory symptoms are commonplace in children with autism and more frequent than in typical children, they also appear with equal or greater frequency in other developmentally challenged groups, such as those with Fragile X and deaf-blind children. They also considered the overarousal and underarousal theories to explain abnormal sensory responses and concluded that the overarousal theory had little support. Children with autism, in their view, are more likely to be underaroused and underresponsive, but the methodological limitations, lack of replications, different subject samples, different sensory modalities, and different assessment methods leave this matter unresolved.

A number of studies have attempted to shed light on the social deficits characteristic of ASD by examining basic sensory and perceptual abilities that may come into play when processing social stimuli. Perception of nonbiological motion (such as randomly moving dots) triggers activity in an area of extrastriate cortex known as visual area MT (V5). One class of studies examined the percentage of dots that must move in the same direction for perceived motion to occur. Studies are consistent in finding that in autism, as in dyslexia, the threshold for perceiving motion is higher than in controls (Pellicano, Gibson, Maybery, Durkin, & Badcock, 2005). This finding has been interpreted as suggesting an impairment in dorsal visual stream processing in ASD. Furthermore, the deficit appears to lie primarily in later parts of the dorsal stream. Kenet et al. (2012), however, reviewed other evidence suggesting that these findings do not reflect a difficulty in the dorsal stream processing per se, but rather a more general deficit in perception of motion *or* complex stationery stimuli, possibly based in a broad signal-to-noise problem. For example, a variant on the movement paradigm, where dot coherence is needed to perceive a shape (rather than motion), also showed that individuals in the HFA group were impaired (needing higher dot coherence), while individuals with dyslexia or Asperger syndrome were not impaired (Tsermentseli, O'Brien, & Spencer, 2008). Bertone, Mottron, Jelenic, and Faubert (2003) found deficits in specific motion perception paradigms but not others and concluded that these results support a deficit in perception of complex stimuli rather than a deficit in the motion-detection magnocellular pathway per se. Similar conclusions were reached by Sanchez-Marin and Padilla-Medina (2008), who found impaired perception of a vertical line embedded in visual noise, whether moving or stationery. Vandenbroucke, Scholte, van Engeland, Lamme, and Kemner (2008) suggest that deficits are found in studies using high spatial frequency, whether they involved motion or not (see Kenet, 2011, for more discussion and interpretation of these studies).

Perception of biological motion has been localized to a small area in the superior temporal sulcus, with more activity generally on the right side (Grossman, Klin, Carter, & Volkmar, 2000). In the last ten years, a number of studies have examined both behavioral and neurological responses to biological motion perception tasks in autism. Blake, Turner, Smoski, Pozdol, and Stone (2003) compared performance on a biological motion task (point-light animated figures) to a static visual perception task (perception of a gestalt from fragments) and found specific deficits on perception of biological motion. Freitag (2008) found that a group of adolescents and adults with autism showed abnormal neural activation and slowed reaction time in response to a biological motion detection task. However, they unexpectedly showed deficits in perception and recognition of spatially-moving point lights even in nonbiological motion. They also found a correlation of the biological motion task with difficulties in hand/finger imitation; these combined results suggest the possibility that difficulties with perception of biological motion may be part of a larger class of visual-perceptual deficits but specifically impact social development.

In an effort to identify more precisely where in the processing stream of biological motion the autistic impairment is found, Kroger et al. (2014) studied ERPs in children and adolescents watching human motion stimuli. Like Freitag (2008), they unexpectedly found diminished amplitude of early response components; specifically, the P100 amplitude was decreased in response to both random and biological motion, suggesting deficits in visual processing that were not specific to biological motion stimuli. Furthermore, the N200 component showed abnormal lateralization, and a later human-motion-specific activation also appeared reduced and more diffuse in autism. Results of this study were taken to support the idea that abnormal early sensory processing abnormalities contribute to higher-order, later components specific to perception of biological motion.

Finally, Klin, Lin, Gorrindo, Ramsay, and Jones (2009) examined the preferential-looking behaviors of 2-year-olds with diagnosed autism to point-light displays of adults playing children's games such as peek-a-boo, with a control condition where the display was played upside down and backwards, out of sync with the audio of the actor. Comparison groups were typically-developing and developmentally delayed toddlers. The group with autism showed no preference for either stimulus type, while both comparison groups preferred the (upright) biological motion with synced voice. Further analysis showed that the group with autism was strongly influenced by concordance of audio change in amplitude with velocity change in each light point, attending preferentially to the more synchronized display, while the control groups were not influenced by the audio-visual synchrony but consistently preferred the upright moving figures. Klin et al. interpreted this as indicating that the attention of toddlers with ASD was captured by the coincidence of physical audio and visual stimuli, rather than the social input associated with the true biological motion. They also suggested that this could explain the child's preference for looking at the mouth rather than the eyes of a speaker, because the mouth has more synchrony with the sound produced than the eyes.

SUPERIOR PERCEPTUAL ABILITY

Both in the visual and auditory domains, it has been suggested that perceptual acuity is actually superior in autism and might drive the attention-to-detail processing style that impairs perception of gestalts and extraction of meaning. A recent study by Ashwin, Ashwin, Rhydderch, Howells, and Baron-Cohen (2009) showed that individuals with ASD have superior visual acuity, extending even into the acuity range of birds of prey. However, Bolte et al. (2012) and others have questioned this finding and have not replicated it. Keita, Mottron, and Bertone (2010) failed to find better visual acuity in individuals with autism but did observe a lack of visual crowding effect, suggestive of altered local lateral connectivity in early perceptual processing streams underlying spatial information processing, which might lead to downstream processing abnormalities.

However, in the auditory domain, there is replicated evidence of normal or even superior performance in ASD for pitch discrimination and musical ability (Bonnel et al., 2003; Lepisto et al., 2005; Mottron et al., 2006). The Lepisto et al. study documented enhanced ERP response to small differences in pitch to nonspeech stimuli, but this response was attenuated to differences in speech sounds.

Eigsti and Fein (2013) studied individuals diagnosed with ASD before age 5, who later have no autism symptoms (e.g., having optimal outcomes). As in previous studies, the non-optimal ASD comparison group showed heightened pitch discrimination. By contrast, the optimal outcome group's abilities did not differ from those of typical controls. Furthermore, enhanced pitch discrimination was associated with current autism symptomatology and with delayed early language onset. They suggest that exceptional pitch discrimination may lead to overdevelopment of low-level perceptual processes in general (Bonnel et al., 2003), consistent with local neural overconnectivity (Belmonte et al., 2004), which in turn may impede the formation of phonological categories and lead to inability to extract words from acoustic signals.

Mismatch negativity response on EEG to a deviant frequency or duration sound reflects behavioral discrimination ability and is a preattentive process. This is important to study in autism, since poor attention to language may cause (rather than result from) poor auditory discrimination of language sounds. Kenet (2011) reviewed studies of preattentive auditory discrimination using mismatch negativity and concluded that the findings are extremely heterogeneous among studies. Response latency has been variously described as shortened, lengthened, or normal, while one study found no mismatch negativity response at all.

The tactile modality is the least studied of the major sensory systems, but clinical observations of tactile oversensitivity and defensiveness abound. One tactile perception study (Cascio et al., 2008) showed that adults with ASD were more sensitive than controls to vibrations on their forearm, and to thermal pain on both the forearm and the palm. In contrast, there were no differences between groups in detection of light touch or innocuous thermal stimuli. Cascio et al. (2012) examined psychophysical ratings and fMRI responses to tactile stimuli in adults with autism and controls. They found that while ratings were fairly similar, the autism group gave more extreme ratings. In addition, the BOLD responses were quite different, with the autism group showing more extreme responses to unpleasant textures in PCC and the insula. This suggested that an exaggerated limbic response to unpleasant touch might mediate some of the social avoidance.

Taste/smell sensitivity, resulting in picky eating and aversion to certain people and environments, is very commonly reported. Taste/smell sensitivity seems to be more specific to autism than abnormalities in other modalities, as mentioned on p. 233. Very little laboratory investigation has occurred in this domain, but behavioral reports are thoroughly reviewed by Cermak, Curtin, and Bandini (2010).

THEORETICAL ACCOUNTS AND RELATIONSHIP TO CORE AUTISM CRITERIA

Rogers and Ozonoff (2005) reviewed the leading theories that attempt to account for abnormal responses to sensory stimuli. Most of these are variants of theories that go back into the 1960s, 1970s, and 1980s and comprise ideas of overarousal, underarousal, unstable arousal, and poor cross-modal integration. Waterhouse, Fein, and Modahl (1996) and Brock, Brown, Boucher, and Rippon (2002) suggest that failure to bind sensory elements together into cross-modal percepts or to perceive events in association with their context lead to focus on individual perceptual elements of a stimulus, with a consequent impairment in perception of meaning, similar to the lack of central coherence theory. The focus on individual elements leads to emphasis on parts of objects rather than wholes, in addition to a focus on the physical characteristics of stimuli. Hiscock and Kinsbourne (2011) suggests that unstable arousal leads to a defensive focus on narrow and perseverative aspects of stimuli, as well as avoidance of social stimuli and engagement in repetitive movements. This linking of putative unstable arousal with a focus on unusual aspects of stimuli also posits avoidance of social stimuli because they are unpredictable and thus potentially arousing. This idea is also presented by Dawson and Lewy (1989), who described social stimuli as more novel and complex and therefore more arousing. Kenet (2011) suggested that imbalance in overall excitatory-inhibitory control over early cortical activity could be produced by abnormalities in GABA or glutamate. This could lead to abnormal signal-to-noise ratio, which in turn may lead to heightened perceptual response to sensory input. It might also relate to other aspects of autism, such as vulnerability to seizures. Kenet elaborated on how these "hypersensitivities, distortions, and altered pathways for responding to sensory stimuli" (p. 216) can have downstream effects on higher cognitive functions.

SUMMARY

As with other areas of neuropsychological function, there are inconsistencies and contradictions in this literature. However, a few sensory/perceptual findings have been replicated: in the auditory domain, hyperacusis and increased discriminability are often found and are related to impaired language development. In visual and tactile domains, there are abundant reports of behavioral abnormalities, but no consistent electrophysiological findings. There are sufficient findings of EEG and ERP abnormalities at early cortical levels to suggest that preattentive processes in early sensory processing are abnormal for most individuals with autism, and cannot be attributed to different states of attention or motivation. The weight of the evidence is that the attention-to-detail processing style is just that, a processing preference, rather than a deficiency in the ability to form gestalts, once motivation is maximized and task demands are clear. It seems plausible that early processing abnormality and an overfocus on physical characteristics of stimuli could lead to many of the downstream cognitive style attributes of autism, as well as deficiency in language comprehension and social interaction. Biological suggestions related to arousal differences, signal-to-noise ratio differences, poor processing related to complexity or spatial frequency of stimuli, or differences in cortical under- and overconnectivity, are just beginning to be seriously investigated. The extent to which the nature of social interaction and social input leads to avoidance of social stimuli, costing proficiency in social learning, is not yet known.

Language

While many individuals with ASD have little-to-no speech, a significant proportion have no delay in language development (Wilkinson, 1998). Language difficulties were one of the three defining categories of autism symptoms in DSM-IV-TR. Within this category, the three symptoms were delayed language (no words by 18 months, no phrases by 24 months), difficulty having a reciprocal conversation (when sufficient language was present), and repetitive or echolalic language. A fourth symptom placed in this category was absent, delayed, or repetitive pretend play. With the advent of DSM-V, language symptoms have been folded into the other two categories: poor conversational ability is covered in the social communication category, and repetitive speech and play are covered in the repetitive behavior category. Language delay per se is no longer present as a symptom, but the presence of language impairment is coded as a separate dimension. Some autism researchers, especially those who deal with young children, regret the deletion of language delay as a defining symptom since this is consistently shown to be the most common first concern of parents of children with autism (Herlihy et al., 2013). Furthermore, the age of first words is a powerful predictor not only of later language, but also of cognitive and adaptive skills (Mayo, Chlebowski, Fein, & Eigsti, 2013).

Language impairments are virtually universal in autism, but vary tremendously among individuals, ranging from subtle pragmatic difficulties to essentially no language, either receptive or expressive. The prior estimate of as many as 50% of children with autism being totally mute has given way to a less pessimistic estimate, although language impairments are often severe (Lord & Paul, 1997). This decrease in nonverbal children is probably due to more effective and successful early intervention, as well as increasing numbers of high-functioning, verbal individuals being diagnosed with some form of autism (Kelley, 2011). In general, pragmatics and prosody tend to be consistent areas of difficulty (Lord & Paul, 1997), while syntax, phonology, and semantics tend to be spared relative to overall verbal level, with many individual exceptions (Condouris, Meyer, & Tager-Flusberg, 2003; Kjelgaard & Tager-Flusberg, 2001; Swensen, Kelley, Fein, & Naigles, 2007).

PHONOLOGY

Phonological ability, that is, the ability to discriminate and produce basic speech sounds, has been generally thought not to be an area of a specific deficit in autism (Bartolucci, Pierce, Streiner, & Eppel, 1976; Kjelgaard & Tager-Flusberg, 2001; Tager-Flusberg, 1981), although low-functioning children with significant intellectual deficiency often do have significant difficulties with both receptive and expressive phonology, consistent with their overall impairment in language and cognitive functioning. In addition, some individuals with HFA or Asperger syndrome show distortions of articulation (Shriberg et al., 2001). It has been argued that phonological impairments, when they exist, are secondary to a more general motor disability (Gernsbacher et al., 2008). However, a fascinating glimpse into the social nature of phonological functioning was provided by Baron-Cohen and Staunton (1994), who showed that the majority of children with autism raised in England by non–native-speaking mothers acquired their mothers' accents, while typical children in the same situation acquired the accent of their English peers. Furthermore, relatives of individuals with autism often share the social communication difficulties in milder form (BAP), but do not share the phonological difficulties, suggesting that these difficulties are characteristic only of those with the full-blown syndrome and not the prodromic form (Bishop et al., 2004).

PROSODY

Prosody is another acoustic characteristic of speech. The term refers to the melody of speech that conveys both grammatical and emotional information. Prosodic abnormality, both expressive and receptive, has often been noted as one of the most pervasive areas of autistic language impairment, but is also very difficult to characterize (Kelley, 2011; McCann & Peppe, 2003). Adults with ASD tend to place stress in the wrong place in a sentence or display unusual melodic contour (Shriberg et al., 2001). Not only do they produce abnormal prosody, but they have difficulty in using it to disambiguate meaning from a speaker; for example, Diehl, Bennetto, Watson, Gunlogson, and McDonough (2008) showed that individuals with ASD did not use prosody to decide between different possible meanings of a sentence, and individuals with ASD have particular difficulty with producing and understanding stressed words (Paul, Augustyn, Klin, & Volkmar, 2005). Peppe, McCann, Gibbon, O'Hare, and Rutherford (2007) also showed that receptive and expressive prosody were highly correlated to verbal mental age, and were both delayed and deviant in autism. In an fMRI study of comprehension of prosody in autism, Eigsti, Schuh, Mencl, Schultz, and Paul (2012) found several more brain areas recruited in the group with autism; this widespread activation was taken as evidence of multiple cognitive strategies being employed to comprehend what is a relatively simple and automatic task in typical individuals. A study of irony comprehension in high-functioning children with autism (Wang, Lee, Sigman, & Dapretto, 2006, 2007), using both contextual and prosodic cues, showed similar results: the autistic group's neural activation included areas recruited by typical controls, but was much more widespread, indicating greater effortful processing needed. Overall, it is clear that prosodic information is difficult for individuals with autism to both produce and comprehend, although the deficient components of this complex set of processes remains to be identified and quantified.

GRAMMAR

Grammar is usually defined to include syntax (word order to convey meaning) and morphology (combining basic units of meaning, such as a noun plus "s" to convey plural or possessive). Until fairly recently, syntax was considered to be an aspect of speech and language, like phonology, that was relatively preserved in autism and consistent with overall language level (Kelley, 2011; Swensen et al., 2007). Some recent findings, however, suggest that syntax in HFA may be somewhat repetitive and simplified, and use forms that place less load on working memory (Eigsti, Bennetto, & Dadlani, 2007). Despite a roughly normal progression of emergence of grammatical morphemes (Waterhouse & Fein, 1982), children with ASD do show some specific difficulty with relational terms, including pronouns, prepositions, and tense (Bartolucci, Pierce, & Streiner, 1980; Lord & Paul, 1997). In a study that received a good deal of attention, Kjelgaard and Tager-Flusberg (2001) described a subset of verbal autistic children whose language was quite similar to that of children with specific language impairment (SLI), including difficulties with syntax. They were also found to have delays or abnormalities in morphology (Roberts, Rice, & Tager-Flusberg, 2004). Tager-Flusberg has argued that specific impairments in structural aspects of language, such as syntax and morphology, is not a characteristic of all individuals with autism, but of a subset of affected children who may share genetic risk with individuals with SLI. Kelley (2011) discussed the performance-competence distinction in relation to grammar in ASD; for many children, they may have mastered syntax and morphology, but because their language is used more for need fulfillment than social communication, language samples may fail to capture their competence. In addition, the tendency to produce perseverative and repetitive language, which is a defining characteristic of ASD in DSM-IV, may lead to perseveration of simple language forms, even if complex ones are within their repertoire.

SEMANTICS

Semantics, or word meanings, has been well studied in autism over the last 40 years. In general, semantics is another area of language that is considered to be relatively preserved in autism, especially when tested as single-word receptive and expressive vocabulary (Kjelgaard & Tager-Flusberg, 2001; Swensen et al., 2007). However, there are a few exceptions to this generalization. First, despite scores on standardized tests of vocabulary that tend to be a high point in their language profiles, children with ASD may show somewhat reduced fluency when asked to quickly produce words in response to semantic or phonemic cues (Turner, 1999b), and the words they produce may be less paradigmatic of the category than words produced by controls (Dunn, Gomes, & Sebastian, 1996). Klinger and Dawson (2001) found that children with ASD as well as those with Down syndrome had relative difficulty in categorizing new information by forming prototypes, but performed normally when given explicit rules about a category. Kamio and colleagues (Kamio, Robins, Kelley, Swainson, & Fein, 2007; Kamio & Toichi, 2000) documented impaired semantic priming in a lexical decision task in individuals with ASD and normal verbal IQ. Though children with ASD and typical speakers have difficulty in using semantic categories, individuals with ASD seem to have particular difficulty with mental state words, words that convey specific information about processes such as knowing, guessing, expecting, and estimating (Akechi, Kikuchi, Tojo, Osanai, & Hasegawa, 2014; Baron-Cohen et al., 1994b; Dennis, Lazenby, & Lockyer, 2001; Kelley, Paul, Fein, & Naigles, 2006; Tager-Flusberg, 1992). As with studies of other aspects of language, beginning research on neural activation with semantic processing suggests that even when behavior performance is spared, activation patterns are different. In one case, semantic processing shifted activation from Broca's to Wernicke's area (Brodmann Area 22) in children with autism relative to controls, with less sensitivity to concrete versus abstract word differences (Harris et al., 2006). Overall, therefore, semantics is a spared area of function in autism, depending on overall language and cognitive level, but with some abnormality in specific semantic classes, in fluency and in semantic priming.

Verbal memory has also been examined in ASD; in general, verbal memory is worse than visuospatial memory and suffers from less automatic processing for meaning than in typical development. Compared to children with other language impairments, Fein et al. (1996) found that children with autism were superior in remembering digits, showed equivalent performance with sentences, and were inferior in recalling stories. They interpreted these findings as supporting the idea that children with autism relied on rote memory and did not tend to automatically encode the material for meaning or use that meaning to aid recall. These findings were consistent with those of Gabig (2008), who also found difficulty in autism with recalling material of greater complexity or semantic structure. This interpretation has been generally supported by tests of list learning, such as the CVLT, where children with ASD may have difficulty using semantic information to recall lists of words (Bennetto et al., 1996; Minshew & Goldstein, 1993; but see Phelan et al., 2010 who found no difference between TD and ASD children and adolescents). A recent study by Tyson et al. (2014) confirmed the poorer use of semantic cues to aid recall, as well as more perseverations and intrusions, in a group with HFA, although their scores were still mostly within the average range. Furthermore, Tyson et al. (2014) examined the performance of a group of optimal outcome children on this task and found no differences from the typical group on any learning characteristics.

PRAGMATICS

Pragmatics, or the social use of language, is abnormal in autism, almost by definition. As summarized by Kelley (2011), pragmatics includes taking the perspective of the listener; maintaining the topic of interest; giving enough (but not too much) information to the listener; using humour, sarcasm, metaphor, and idiom; and using nonverbal communication (e.g., facial expressions and gesture). In addition, constructing narratives is often included in discussions of pragmatics. If all aspects of pragmatic function are normal, then autism is unlikely. Degree of pragmatic difficulties are correlated to severity of autism symptoms (Volden, Coolican, Garon, White, & Bryson, 2009), and subtle pragmatic difficulties are often found in the BAP that are sometimes apparent in unaffected relatives (Landa, Folstein, & Isaacs, 1991; Whitehouse, Barry, & Bishop, 2008). Expressive pragmatic language impairments cause a great deal of stigmatization of individuals with ASD, and receptive difficulties impair their ability to understand the conversational intent of others (Landa, 2000). High-functioning adolescents and young adults with ASD have particular difficulty during conversation in maintaining eye contact with their partner, intonation, and appropriately staying on topic (Paul, Orlovski, Marcinko, & Volkmar, 2009). In fact, inability to hold a reciprocal conversation, insensitivity to cues from the listener, and the improper word selection for the social context (e.g., not being overly formal) is so pervasive that difficulty with conversation is a symptom of autism in the DSM-IV. Individuals with ASD have difficulty with nonliteral language, especially figures of speech and idioms (Dennis et al., 2001; MacKay & Shaw, 2004), and also with making inferences about incomplete verbal information (Dennis et al., 2001; Norbury & Bishop, 2002). Although comprehension and recall of stories was good in high-functioning individuals with autism, their retelling was less coherent, and they tended to neglect causal connections among events as well as the psychological states of the main characters (Capps, Losh, & Thurber, 2000; Diehl, Bennetto, & Young, 2006; Ge & Han, 2008). Kelley et al. (2006) found some persisting similar deficits in constructing narratives in a group of optimal outcome (OO) children with a history of autism (i.e., those who no longer met diagnostic criteria), despite normal scores in semantic and grammatical language measures. Suh et al. (2013) confirmed the presence of multiple deficits in story-constructing in high-functioning adolescents with autism (including fewer "gist" elements, more ambiguous pronouns, speech dysfluency, and not naming characters). Although their OO adolescents did not show most of these features and were average or above on almost all measures of language (Tyson et al., 2014), they demonstrated subtle persisting signs of dysfluency and idiosyncratic language. Overall, therefore, pragmatic deficits in the social use of language as well as in constructing or retelling narratives are ubiquitous in autism, present in relatives without autism, and persist in subtle form even when almost all other language abnormalities and delays have resolved.

SUMMARY

Language was one of the first areas of autism functioning to be studied, and the literature on this topic is enormous. By and large, the generalizations made in the 1980s and 1990s that individuals with autism show almost universal abnormality in prosody and pragmatics has been supported. Language development in other domains such as phonology and syntax are more variably impaired, and for the most part, semantics is often relatively spared. However, many exceptions both in individual children and in components of these "spared" processes have been found. More sophisticated theory and methodology—such as correlations with genetic subtypes, studies of language deficits in unaffected relatives, use of preferential looking to test comprehension without the necessity of test responses (Naigles, Kelty, Jaffery, & Fein, 2011), and functional activation on language tasks—will no doubt further our understanding of this very complex set of questions, and help the design of more effective therapies.

Executive Function

One of the more long-standing neuropsychological theories of autism proposes that key aspects of the disorder are based in disturbances of executive function. Propounding this viewpoint, Damasio and Maurer (1978) remarked that the disturbances of attention, repetitive/stereotyped behaviors, and cognitive flexibility seen in autism were remarkably similar to problems typical of patients with acquired frontal lesions. Restricted and repetitive patterns of behavior, interests, and activities are cardinal features of ASD and thus are seen with regularity in school-aged children through to adults

(Hughes & Ensor, 2007; Sachse et al., 2013). Speculations that these symptoms may reflect a breakdown in executive function is compatible with observations that, throughout this age range, a positive association exists between rigidity/stereotyped behavior and executive function deficits (Bramham et al., 2009; Yerys, Wallace, et al., 2009). Also in keeping with this notion are claims by some investigators that executive function is profoundly and pervasively impaired in ASD (Corbett, Constantine, Hendren, Rocke, & Ozonoff, 2009; Verte, Geurts, Roeyers, Oosterlaan, & Sergeant, 2006). However, there is also sufficient contradictory evidence to call into question the strength of this association: first, numerous studies have shown that many aspects of executive function are relatively intact or only mildly impaired in ASD (Goldberg et al., 2005; Happé et al., 2006; Losh et al., 2009). Second, it has been reported that significant deficiencies in executive function occur in only a minority of children with ASD (Geurts, Sinzig, Booth, & Happe, 2014).

The inconsistencies between studies may, in part, relate to inherent difficulties in defining and operationalizing elements of executive function and in devising appropriate measures to assess these aspects of cognitive function in this population. Pennington and Ozonoff (1996) outlined six domains of executive function, including working memory, contextual memory, inhibition, planning, generativity (or fluency), and cognitive flexibility or set-shifting. Of these, the most commonly implicated problems in ASD include inhibitory and inference control (Adams & Jarrold, 2009; Christ, Kester, Bodner, & Miles, 2011; Happé et al., 2006), and set-shifting/cognitive flexibility (Corbett, Constantine, et al., 2009; Van Eylen et al., 2011). The findings related to these specific aspects of executive ability are again inconsistent, with some studies demonstrating intact function in many aspects of inhibitory control (Brian, Tipper, Weaver, & Bryson, 2003; Christ et al., 2011) and relatively unimpaired performance on measures of set shifting and cognitive flexibility (for reviews, see Pellicano, 2012; Russo et al., 2007).

It has become apparent through these investigations that relatively minor variations in task demands or administration can have a significant influence on whether or not performance in individuals with ASD is impaired (Kaland et al., 2008; Ozonoff, 1995; Rinehart, Bradshaw, Moss, Brereton, & Tonge, 2000). Other neuropsychological measures (e.g., Trail Making), hybrid neuropsychological/experimental measures (e.g., CANTAB), and experimental test-switching paradigms have also yielded somewhat inconsistent findings. Many of the formal measures of executive function are highly contrived and structured, yet deficits in ASD may be more likely to be evident in everyday situations that are unstructured, unpredictable or uncontrolled, or when open-ended questions are used (Mackinlay, Charman, & Karmiloff-Smith, 2006; Van Eylen, Boets, Steyaert, Wagemans, & Noens, 2015). Investigations have been further complicated by the fact that different aspects of executive function emerge at various points in development and unfold at different rates. Preschoolers are relatively unimpaired on measures of executive function appropriate to that age group (Yerys, Hepburn, Pennington, & Rogers, 2007), while greater divergence from normative levels of performance may occur in ASD with increasing age. Differences may therefore be particularly evident for metacognitive executive abilities (Rosenthal et al., 2013). Overall, a clear understanding of the relationship between RRBIAs and executive function requires more precise and ecologically valid measurement tools (Geurts, Corbett, & Solomon, 2009; Van Eylen et al., 2015).

There has long been a debate over the relationship of executive function to ToM (Ozonoff, Pennington, & Rogers, 1991; Pellicano, 2010). ToM refers to the cognitive capacity to make inferences regarding the mental states of others, their feelings, beliefs, and intents (Baron-Cohen, 2001; Premack & Woodruff, 1978). This ability to successfully and accurately "mentalize" or "mind read" another person and respond appropriately is thought to play an important role in multiple aspects of social communication, including the establishment of a common ground or frame of reference for the exchange of information and the sharing of interests (Sperber & Wilson, 2002). Deficits in ToM have been advanced to account for many of the core problems associated with ASD, including but not limited to deficiencies in joint attention, social relatedness, and empathy. The neural substrate mediating the development of ToM, and relatedly empathy, appears to involve medial PFC, superior temporal sulcus (STS), and the temporal parietal junction (TPJ), along with the precuneous (Dodell-Feder, Koster-Hale, Bedny, & Saxe, 2011).

Some have argued that poor ToM can be understood in terms of problems with executive function or language processing (de Villiers, 2000; Fine, Lumsden, & Blair, 2001; Russell, Saltmarsh, & Hill, 1999). It has become apparent that difficulties with ToM are not unique to ASD—similar if less severe problems in performing ToM tasks have been observed in children with hearing impairment, language disorder, and intellectual handicap (Harris et al., 2008; Lecciso, Petrocchi, & Marchetti, 2013; Li et al., 2014; Peterson, Wellman, & Liu, 2005). Given this, it has been suggested that linguistic and executive abilities may be important precursors to the development of ToM (Dahlgren, Sandberg, & Hjelmquist, 2003; Fisher, Happe, & Dunn, 2005) or are at least moderating factors in the performance on ToM tasks. In order to address this question and gain a clearer perspective on the relationship between ToM and executive function, Iao and Leekam (2014) recently reported a study that utilized a nonverbal ToM task that was specifically devised to circumvent the language and executive function confounds of more traditional ToM tasks (e.g., false belief). As predicted, children with ASD performed worse than typically-developing children on this task. While Iao and Leekam (2014) contended that this performance deficit could not be explained by problems with executive functioning or language problems, they further concluded it may not be adequately accounted for by a specific ToM deficit either. They instead related the poor performance to representational demands inherent in performance of ToM tasks.

ASD: A Developmental Cognitive Neuroscience Perspective

A fundamental assumption in neuropsychology is that developmental and learning disorders reflect functional compromise of domain-specific neural systems that mediate various aspects of cognition and behavior (e.g., attention, memory, perceptual skills, motor abilities, language, executive function). Each system is conceptualized as having specialized processing components (modules, nodes), interconnected in distributed networks in the brain, resulting in localization or regional specialization of cerebral functions. These networks are thought to be sufficiently independent in their organization that the development of a particular system or subsystem may be arrested, delayed, or otherwise impaired in a fairly selective manner, causing delays or differences in development in the respective domain of behavior. The possible sources of such disruptions are diverse since alterations can occur at various levels (structural, metabolic, electrophysiological, neurochemical) that are often interrelated.

As reviewed in this chapter, there is now overwhelming evidence that ASD represents a collection of disorders that are fundamentally rooted in alterations in neural structure and function. Anomalies have been identified at multiple levels of analysis, from neuronal morphology and organization to neural pathway development and functional connectivity. A primary manifestation of these differences in neurodevelopment is compromised ontogeny of one of the most important aspects of human behavior: social communication (see Stefanatos & Baron, 2011 for a review).

There has been much discussion in recent years in the fields of social and communication neuroscience suggesting that specialized neural networks evolved in the human brain to mediate the highly complex and specialized computational demands underlying our capacity to communicate with each other (Berwick, Friederici, Chomsky, & Bolhuis, 2013; Tomasello, 2008). Given that communication is intrinsically a social act, related and overlapping systems evolved in tandem, one to process language and the other to mediate intersubjectivity which is existing between conscious minds, and the ability to make inferences about the intentions, feelings, and thoughts of another person (Baron-Cohen & Ring, 1994; Brothers, 1990; Frith & Frith, 2010). From an evolutionary viewpoint, the requisite neural architecture likely emerged both through exaptation (exploiting, redeploying existing neural circuits without necessarily compromising their original functions) and through substantial expansion of neural substrate, including but not limited to areas of frontal and temporal neocortex (Dunbar, 2012; Schoenemann, 2009). This circuitry is necessarily intimately connected with other cortical systems normally engaged in social communication (e.g., motor control, hearing, vision) as well as with subcortical structures involved in processing socially relevant information and interactions, particularly the amygdala, thalamus, basal ganglia, and cerebellum.

The resulting neural circuitry involves a collection of parallel, highly-distributed, sometimes overlapping neural networks with critical components distributed cortically in the frontal, temporal, and, to a lesser degree, parietal lobes. Components involved in communication are mainly distributed in perisylvian cortex of the left cerebral hemisphere, including inferior frontal lobe, middle and superior temporal gyrus, STS, anterior temporal lobe, supramarginal gyrus, and insula (Aboitiz et al., 1995; Catani, Jones, & ffytche, 2005; Friederici, 2011). Recent reconceptions of ASD have placed greater emphasis on the system sometimes referred to as the "social brain" (Adolphs, 2009; Brothers, 1990), which evolved to mediate social awareness, intersubjectivity, social attunement, and mentalizing another person's mental or emotional state. This system involves components in ventromedial prefrontal cortex (BA10), intraparietal sulcus, medial parietal cortex (precuneous), posterior superior STS, and TPJ, ACC, anterior temporal cortex, and the amygdala (Adolphs, 2009; Brothers, 1990; Lewis, Rezaie, Brown, Roberts, & Dunbar, 2011; Mills, Lalonde, Clasen, Giedd, & Blakemore, 2014). In the following sections, we provide a brief synopsis of how this conceptual understanding of these networks, their function and evolution, bear on and enrich our conceptualizations of the neural basis for the chief problems associated with ASD.

Social Communication

Social communication is such an important aspect of human behavior that infants appear to be born with native biases and predispositions to attend to, observe, and process socially-relevant information. Within hours of birth, newborns demonstrate preferential responses to the voice of their mother and face-like visual configurations (Johnson, Dziurawiec, Ellis, & Morton, 1991). Within days of birth, infants prefer direct eye gaze (Farroni, Menon, Rigato, & Johnson, 2007) and show sensitivity to facial geometry and expressions (Leppanen & Nelson, 2009; Parr, Modi, Siebert, & Young, 2013) and patterns of biological motion (Bardi, Regolin, & Simion, 2011). These nascent capacities likely reflect genetic predispositions, and form the foundations for the development of the highly complex system that will unfold across the course of development to mediate social cognition. Evidence from diverse sources suggests that some of these early dispositions are mediated via subcortical mechanisms (e.g., Johnson, 2005), and that cerebral specialization for processing the human voice, faces, and emotion begins to emerge in the first days of life and continues to evolve in the following months as new components of the system come "online" (Cheng, Lee, Chen, Wang, & Decety, 2012; Johnson, Grossmann, & Farroni, 2008; Simion, Leo, Turati, Valenza, & Dalla Barba, 2007)

A large body of research has linked face recognition problems with ASD (Sasson, 2006), and it has been proposed that face processing difficulties are an essential aspect of the disorder (Dawson, Webb, & McPartland, 2005; Schultz, 2005; Weigelt, Koldewyn, & Kanwisher, 2013). It has long been recognized that individuals with ASD often avoid direct eye contact, have poor eye-to-eye gaze (Itier & Batty, 2009), and are poor at judging direction of eye gaze. Reduced attention to the eyes contributes to and is often accompanied by deficiencies in face processing in children and adults with ASD (Dalton et al., 2005; Spezio, Adolphs, Hurley, & Piven, 2007; Sterling et al., 2008). Early face recognition problems, evident at 7 months of age, have recently been observed to be predictive of an ASD diagnosis at 3 years (Gliga, Jones, Bedford, Charman, & Johnson, 2014). Similar, if milder, difficulties can also be observed in unaffected family members, suggesting that problems with face recognition may represent a cognitive endophenotype of the disorder (Dawson, Webb, Wijsman, et al., 2005; Wallace, Sebastian, Pellicano, Parr, & Bailey, 2010).

The FG, located in the ventral temporal lobe, has received wide attention for its seemingly special role in processing faces (Corbett, Carmean, et al., 2009; Critchley et al., 2000; Schultz, 2005). Functional neuroimaging studies of face processing have revealed that older children and adults with ASD do not show the usual pattern of activation of the amygdala and the FG that is seen in neurotypical individuals. Some have suggested that these anomalies may relate, at least in part, to a lack of the attentional bias for faces that is generally evident from an early age in typically-developing infants (Chawarska, Volkmar, & Klin, 2010). Others have contended that the difficulties with face recognition are neither related to the perceptual nor attentional issues but are contingent upon the memory demands of the task (Weigelt et al., 2014). Interestingly, normal patterns of activation of FG have been observed when participants with ASD were explicitly directed to fixate on the eye region (Hadjikhani et al., 2004; Hadjikhani, Joseph, Snyder, & Tager-Flusberg, 2007) or when pictures of personally familiar individuals were presented (Pierce, Haist, Sedaghat, & Courchesne, 2004; Pierce & Redcay, 2008). Given these findings, it has been suggested that anomalous activations may be related to social motivational deficiencies (Dawson, Webb, & McPartland, 2005) or the allocation of visual attention (Hadjikhani et al., 2004). It may be that evaluative and interpretive processes mediated by the amygdala (e.g., emotional significance, unfamiliarity) determine deployment of visual attention to stimuli, and this in turn influences the likelihood of anomalous patterns of activation in FG (Adolphs, 2010). Despite ongoing disagreements regarding the nature of the underlying processing difficulties and the significance of the anomalous activations of FG (Gauthier, Curran, Curby, & Collins, 2003), there seems to be compelling evidence from behavioral, event-related potential, and functional neuroimaging studies suggesting that individuals with ASD, from a very early age, spend less time and therefore have less experience processing faces. This may impede social interactions by the effect it has on their ability to utilize information derived from the face in social interactions (Pelphrey, Shultz, Hudac, & Wyk, 2011).

Areas in posterior STS also play a critical and varied role in social cognition (Zilbovicius et al., 2006 for a review). Like the amygdala, the STS is commonly activated during the processing of facial expressions (Hadjikhani et al., 2007; Humphreys, Hasson, Avidan, Minshew, & Behrmann, 2008) and the perception of eye gaze (Materna, Dicke, & Thier, 2008; Pelphrey, Morris, & McCarthy, 2005). Direct eye gaze improves facial recognition of another individual (Itier & Batty, 2009). The STS also plays a special role in processing biologically-based motion (Castelli, Happe, Frith, & Frith, 2000; Freitag et al., 2008 ; Pelphrey & Carter, 2008) and has been implicated as part of a network involved in the perception of action, the analysis of gesture, and the ability to understand and attribute the intentions of others (Vollm et al., 2006). The STS often fails to show normal patterns of activation in individuals with ASD during performance of these tasks (Grezes, Wicker, Berthoz, & de Gelder, 2009; Hirai & Hiraki, 2005; Klin & Jones, 2008; Klin et al., 2009; Pelphrey, Morris, McCarthy, & Labar, 2007). Interestingly, STS is also an area that normally becomes active during voice recognition, and studies have shown that individuals with ASD fail to show this activation, despite their having normal activation of STS in response to nonvocal sounds (Gervais et al., 2004).

Evidence from structural and functional imaging studies have confirmed long-held beliefs that ASD is associated with alterations of functioning of the amygdala (Nordahl et al., 2012; Paul, Corsello, Tranel, & Adolphs, 2010). These findings provide anatomical and functional correlates to the cytoarchitectural anomalies (e.g., reduced neuron counts, smaller size) identified in clinicopathological studies (Amaral & Schumann, 2003; Bauman & Kemper, 2005). From an evolutionary standpoint, the amygdala has long been a hub in neural systems mediating communication. Its volume increased greatly in size (especially the lateral portion) in conjunction with the rapid expansion of the human cortex that occurred approximately 100,000 years ago. Wired to rapidly process social information, it has intimate connections with neighboring structures involved in memory (hippocampus) and more remote structures involved in processing socially-relevant information including the FG, both auditory and somatosensory systems, and prefrontal cortex. The amygdala emerges as a key component in the development of the social brain in the first several months of life. It is widely known for its involvement in fear processing and emotional regulation, but it has also been implicated in later emerging problems of social interaction in ASD, particularly in deficits in the development of empathy and systematizing (Baron-Cohen, 2009). As previously discussed in this chapter, these capacities are mediated by a complex and distributed neural network involving the amygdala, cingulate gyrus, medial frontal cortex, orbital frontal cortex, inferior frontal gyrus, and the superior temporal sulcus (Baron-Cohen et al., 1994a; Happé et al., 1996; Schulte-Ruether et al., 2011; Vollm et al., 2006). Individuals with ASD perform poorly on ToM tasks, and on functional imaging, they do not demonstrate typical patterns of activation during tasks requiring mentalizing and ToM (Kana, Keller, Cherkassky, Minshew, & Just, 2009; Schulte-Ruether et al., 2011; Williams, Waiter, et al., 2006). The distribution of this network overlaps substantially with the mirror neuron system, and it has been suggested that dysfunction of the mirror neuron system may contribute to problems with empathy and some other social deficits experienced by individuals with ASD (Dapretto et al., 2006; Iacoboni & Dapretto, 2006). Others have suggested that these systems are dissociable (Marsh & Hamilton, 2011).

Over the course of development, the amygdala comes under the increasing control of orbital and medial prefrontal cortex, which are also essential components of the social brain. The relationship between these structures is such that it is difficult to consider the function of one without reference to the other. Areas in the PFC are responsible for conscious deliberation and rational decision-making. These structures work dynamically with the amygdala to evaluate the significance of environmental events and to formulate an appropriate response. Serving a regulatory role over the amygdala, the PFC incorporates and integrates information from internal bodily sensations, external information, and past experience and knowledge, and incorporates this information to temper responses of the rapidly reactive amygdala. Pathological changes have been identified in the PFC of individuals with ASD, including increased neuron numbers (Courchesne et al., 2011), increased glial cell numbers (Edmonson, Ziats, & Rennert, 2014), and abnormalities of minicolumn development (Casanova, 2008). At a macrostructural level, documented differences include frontal lobe overgrowth in childhood evident in increased brain volume and cortical thickness (Carper & Courchesne, 2005; Ecker et al., 2013; Keller et al., 2007; Mundy, Sullivan, & Mastergeorge, 2009).

The frontal cortex also interacts closely with the cingulate gyrus, which seems to play an intermediary role in evaluating information and organizing appropriate responses. The exact functions of the cingulate are incompletely understood but appear to be diverse. Circuitry in the frontal cortex and ACC form part of a larger fronto-striato-thalamo-parietal network involved in inhibitory controls and conflict detection (Solomon et al., 2014). This will be discussed in the next section. The PCC, on the other hand, seems to be involved in supporting internally-directed cognition, forming part of the default mode network, but also in directing attention (Leech & Sharp, 2014). In addition, the PCC forms part of a circuit including the medial frontal cortex and lateral temporal cortex that is involved in mentalizing. Damage to the PCC affects the function of this system and decreases empathy, emotional expressiveness, and motivation (Dennis et al., 2013; Kiehl, 2006). Relatedly, a recent study has identified cytoarchitectural abnormalities in the PCC, evident in irregularly-distributed neurons, poor laminar organization in layers IV and V, and increased presence of neurons in white matter (Oblak et al., 2011).

Perhaps the most discussed subcortical structure implicated in autism is the cerebellum. The cerebellum has long been known to play a major role in motor planning and control, but in recent years, there has been growing recognition of its involvement in various cognitive and language processes, including procedural and working memory, attentional control, speech production, aspects of language acquisition, and behavioral planning (O'Halloran, Kinsella, & Storey, 2011; Schmahmann, 2010; Strick, Dum, & Fiez, 2009). Emerging evidence suggests that early cerebellar injury may influence remote cortical development causing functional compromise of a fronto-cerebellar pathway extending from lateral regions of each cerebellar hemisphere (crus I and II) to contralateral areas of neocortex including dorsolateral prefrontal cortex (PFC), premotor and sensorimotor cortex, and mid-temporal region (Limperopoulos et al., 2014). This was correlated with scores on measures of gross motor skill and expressive language. Relatedly, Skefos et al. (2014) reported decreases in Purkinje cell density in crus I and II in ASD and suggested that this may cause dysfunction of a prefrontal cortical network involved in modulating aspects of social behavior and behavioral planning (Schmahmann, 2010). Other studies have also implicated fronto-cerebellar networks in impaired expressive language, working memory, attention, and aspects of gross motor function (Hodge et al., 2010; Rogers et al., 2011; Townsend et al., 2001). Loss of vermis volume has been tentatively associated with more global impairments of development (Bolduc et al., 2011). Overall, this body of literature is theoretically of importance, particularly in highlighting that early damage or dysfunction to a particular node in a distributed network can have substantial remote effects on other parts of the network.

Restricted and Repetitive Patterns of Behavior Interests and Activities

Restricted and repetitive patterns of behavior, interests, and activities are among the earliest signs of ASD (Wolff et al., 2014). They can be seen in infants and toddlers (Kim & Lord, 2010; Morgan, Wetherby, & Barber, 2008), supporting their status as a core diagnostic feature. However, some have questioned their diagnostic utility in children younger than 3 years, in part because repetitive behaviors are also seen in other disorders and indeed in the normal course of early development (Moore & Goodson, 2003). In infants with ASD, these behaviors include atypical patterns of object exploration (Ozonoff, Macari, et al., 2008), sensory self-stimulation (Zwaigenbaum et al., 2005), preferential attending to nonsocial stimuli (Bhat et al., 2010), and difficulty shifting attention away from objects (Zwaigenbaum et al., 2005).

Despite their considerable clinical importance, these behaviors have received less research attention, and as a consequence less is known about their nature and basis. In recent years, interest has focused on the possibility that restricted interests and stereotyped behaviors may reflect underlying deficits in aspects of executive function, particularly cognitive flexibility (Lopez, Lincoln, Ozonoff, & Lai, 2005). Cognitive flexibility refers to the ability to shift thoughts or actions depending on situational demands and contingencies (Monsell, 2003). While a relationship between impaired cognitive flexibility and RRBIAs seems to have face validity, it has proven difficult to prove or disprove. Confusions stem both from inherent difficulties in operationalizing and quantifying problems in cognitive flexibility, as well as in the diversity of the ASD population. For example, one of the more frequently cited findings pointing to deficits in cognitive flexibility in ASD is impaired set-shifting (often indexed as perseverative errors on the Wisconsin Card Sorting Test). While several studies have shown that individuals with ASD are impaired in set-shifting (Corbett, Constantine, et al., 2009; South, Ozonoff, & McMahon, 2007), others using the same or similar measures have found that set-shifting is relatively spared (Goldberg et al., 2005; Kaland et al., 2008; Minshew, Goldstein, & Siegel, 1997; Rinehart, Bradshaw, Moss, Brereton, & Tonge, 2001). Some of the discrepancies in results may relate to participant characteristics (e.g., IQ, age, severity of ASD symptomology, comorbid conditions).

In this context, rigidity and stereotyped behavior in ASD have been shown to be positively associated with set-shifting deficits in school-aged children and adults (Bramham et al., 2009; Yerys, Wallace, et al., 2009). In addition, increased severity of repetitive and stereotyped behaviors have been related to difficulties in maintaining set (Miller, Ragozzino, Cook, Sweeney, & Mosconi, 2015). Given the variability that characterizes such investigations, the strength of these associations and their basis remains to be firmly established through further studies. Progress in this area will depend upon development of more finely tuned paradigms (Geurts et al., 2009; Van Eylen et al., 2015).

Recently, a number of neuroimaging studies have provided evidence supporting the notion that restricted and repetitive behaviors may be related to pathophysiology of neural networks subserving executive function. As already discussed, it is well-established from both structural and functional neuroimaging and postmortem studies that frontal lobe development proceeds in an atypical fashion in ASD. In addition, frontal lobe connectivity is abnormal, with overconnectivity via short fiber connections but poor connectivity through long fibers, such as those connecting it to striatal structures (Courchesne & Pierce, 2005b; Lee et al., 2009). A number of studies have linked dysfunction of this circuitry to stereotypic and repetitive behaviors in ASD changes in activation patterns that involve frontal lobe and the frontal-striatal system (Philip et al., 2012). Shafritz, Dichter, Baranek, and Belger (2008), for example, noted that individuals with ASD showed reduced activation in frontal, striatal, and parietal regions during performance on a task requiring shifts in cognitive set. The severity of repetitive or restricted behaviors in ASD was associated with decreased activation of anterior cingulate and posterior parietal regions. Anomalies of cingulate cortex have also been implicated in studies of response inhibition (Agam et al., 2010) and cognitive control (Solomon et al., 2014) in individuals with ASD. The connectivity between ACC and other components of the fronto-striatal network also appears to be compromised. Thakkar et al. (2008) found reduced integrity of white matter (indexed by fractional anisotropy on DTI) in the region of the anterior cingulate was associated with higher ratings of repetitive behavior.

Structures in the basal ganglia, particularly the caudate, have also been implicated in ASD. In a recent longitudinal study, Langen et al. (2014) observed that the volume of caudate nucleus in children (~9–12 years of age) with ASD increased at double the rate seen in the normal controls. The faster growth rate was correlated with more severe repetitive behaviors seen during their preschool years. Interestingly, Langen et al. (2014) speculated that this increased growth rate was a secondary consequence of the presence of repetitive and restricted behaviors, rather than related to some underlying causal factor.

Overall, these lines of evidence implicate dysfunction of the fronto-striato-thalamo-parietal network that is thought to be involved in aspects of self-regulatory behavior such as response monitoring, cognitive flexibility, inhibitory controls, and conflict detection (Solomon et al., 2014; Turner, 1999a; Verte, Geurts, Roeyers, Oosterlaan, & Sergeant, 2005). The central role that the cingulate and caudate appear to play in RRBIA remains to be more clearly specified. Both structures play key roles in attention, response selection, inhibition, and cognitive control, and both have also been consistently implicated in ADHD. Additionally, the anterior cingulate plays a special role in error detection. It forms part of a cortical limbic component to fronto-striatal circuitry, having connections to both lateral prefrontal and parietal cortex as well as the amygdala nucleus, accumbens, thalamus, and insula. It is therefore well-positioned to coordinate response monitoring and error detection with structures involved with in emotional responses and reward.

Summary

Despite substantial research effort, the etiological basis and precise mechanisms that lead to autism remain incompletely understood. Risk factors appear to be multifactorial, involving complex interactions between environmental factors, genetic predispositions, epigenetic mechanisms, and other biological variables (Abrahams & Geschwind, 2008; Grafodatskaya, Chung, Szatmari, & Weksberg, 2010; Herbert, 2010). Figure 13.1 presents in schematic form the enormous complexities involved in teasing these various factors apart.

While many of the genes implicated in ASD may have fairly direct effects on neurodevelopment, others may influence risk for ASD through their role in increasing risk for disease states or conditions or through epigenetic pathways that can have neurodevelopmental implications.

As depicted in Figure 13.1, the final common pathway of the diverse risk factors—whether genetic, environmental, or epigenetic—is that they directly or indirectly affect neurodevelopment. Happé and Ronald (2008) have cogently argued that the symptom complex defining ASD is fractionable and that deficits in each domain (social communication, restricted activities and interests) are likely related to largely independent genetic influences. While some evidence supports this notion (Gotts et al., 2012), the majority of the genes currently implicated in risk for ASD have rather broad effects on neurodevelopment. It is possible that by virtue of their specific functional implications and timeline for expression, some may influence the behaviors associated with ASD more than others. However, none has effects that are specific to the manifestation of the cardinal features of the disorder, and it is likely that multiple variations of mutations can result in the complex behavioral constellations associated with ASD.

Genetic propensities may lay out biological constraints on behavioral potentialities, but it is through experience—through attending, perceiving, remembering and responding to sensory inputs—that infants ultimately learn to read emotions, decipher intentions, and understand and share interests with others. Impairments in the development of neuropsychological systems can be viewed as intermediary influences in the causal links between brain dysfunction and the overt behaviors that comprise the manifest disorder of ASD. How neuropsychological systems are affected and how this relates to the broader symptom complex associated with ASD remains to be fully detailed.

Evidence from a variety of sources has suggested that the developing brain may not possess the same degree of functional localization as the adult brain. Specifically, the immature brain is thought to be anatomically less differentiated and more interconnected (Neville, 2006), but becomes progressively modularized in its organization over the course of development (Johnson, 2001; Karmiloff-Smith, 2010). Given the highly dynamic and interactive processes underlying these changes, dysfunction emerging early in neurodevelopment can interfere with this modularization and differentiation process, with the result that additional brain regions may be recruited to subserve developing cognitive or behavioral processes. Early dysfunction can result in a cascading influence on subsequent growth and function. Disturbances of lower level structures and functions can impede the function of upstream structures and later developing processes. However, it is also plausible, given the interconnectivity and functional dependence of each component on exposure to appropriate experience, that dysfunction at higher level systems can also result in faulty development of downstream processes. Supporting the position cogently outlined by Brothers (1997) Franks (2010) reinforces the assertion that "The functioning brain is social in the sense that any given brain is completely dependent on other brains for its development" (p. 39). A potential functional consequence of the less optimal organization stemming from early damage or dysfunction is that it can result in more generalized patterns of cognitive and behavioral impairment.

Overall, there is compelling evidence to suggest that several aspects of social and self-regulatory functions that normally emerge early in development are derailed in individuals with ASD. Our understanding of the development of these systems is currently rudimentary, and available data is often inconsistent, so the determination of precise causal pathways remains open for speculation. Such considerations provide a strong and continuing rationale to examine ASD from a neuropsychological standpoint and attempt to tease apart the various processing deficits that may underlie the problems observed in social communication and behavioral flexibility. A major area for future expansion of the field, both from a neuropsychological and neuroimaging viewpoint, will be to understand factors influencing brain development in the first two years of life and to further explore genetic-environmental interactions and their relation to identified anomalies in brain structure and function.

Acknowledgements

We would like to thank Harry Zobel, Rachel Taormina, Ben Sargent, Maura Lunney, and Meredith Benner for their assistance in tracking down references and editing previous drafts. Harry Zobel also created the tables and flow chart, and Arianna K. Stefanatos proofread the entire manuscript and provided helpful suggestions. In addition, we are grateful to Temple University and the University of Connecticut for their support during its preparation.

References

Aarkrog, T. (1968). Organic factors in infantile psychoses and borderline psychoses: Retrospective study of 45 cases subjected to pneumoencephalography. *Danish Medical Bulletin*, *15*, 283–288.

Aboitiz, F., Ide, A., Navarrete, A., Pena, M., Rodriguez, E., Wolff, V., & Zaidel, E. (1995). The anatomical substrates for language and hemispheric specialization. *Biological Research*, *28*(1), 45–50.

Abrahams, B. S., & Geschwind, D. H. (2008). Advances in autism genetics: On the threshold of a new neurobiology. *Nature Review Genetics*, *9*(5), 341–355.

Abrahams, B. S., & Geschwind, D. H. (2010). Connecting genes to brain in the autism spectrum disorders. *Archives of Neurology*, *67*(4), 395–399.

Abrams, D. A., Lynch, C. J., Cheng, K. M., Phillips, J., Supekar, K., Ryali, S., . . . Menon, V. (2013). Underconnectivity between voice-selective cortex and reward circuitry in children with autism. *Proceedings of the National Academy of Sciences of the United States of America*, *110*(29), 12060–12065.

Adams, N. C., & Jarrold, C. (2009). Inhibition and the validity of the Stroop task for children with autism. *Journal of Autism and Developmental Disorders*, *39*(8), 1112–1121.

Adolphs, R. (2009). The social brain: Neural basis of social knowledge. *Annual Review of Psychology*, *60*, 693–716.

Adolphs, R. (2010). What does the amygdala contribute to social cognition? *Annals of the New York Academy of Sciences*, *1191*, 42–61.

Adrien, J. L., Faure, M., Perrot, A., Hameury, L., Garreau, B., Barthelemy, C., & Sauvage, D. (1991). Autism and family home movies: Preliminary findings. *Journal of Autism and Developmental Disorders*, *21*(1), 43–49.

Adrien, J.L., Lenoir, P., Martineau, J., Perrot, A., Hameury, L., Larmande, C., & Sauvage, D. (1991). Family home movies: Identification of early autistic signs in infants later diagnosed as autistics. *Brain Dysfunction*, *4*(6), 355–362.

Agam, Y., Joseph, R. M., Barton, J.J.S., & Manoach, D. S. (2010). Reduced cognitive control of response inhibition by the anterior cingulate cortex in autism spectrum disorders. *Neuroimage*, *52*(1), 336–347.

Akechi, H., Kikuchi, Y., Tojo, Y., Osanai, H., & Hasegawa, T. (2014). Neural and behavioural responses to face-likeness of objects in adolescents with autism spectrum disorder. *Scientific Reports*, *4*, 3874.

Alarcon, M., Cantor, R. M., Liu, J., Gilliam, T. C., & Geschwind, D. H. (2002). Evidence for a language quantitative trait locus on chromosome 7q in multiplex autism families. *American Journal of Medical Genetics*, *70*(1), 60–71.

Allen, D. A. (1988). Autistic spectrum disorders: Clinical presentation in preschool children. *Journal of Child Neurology*, *3*(Suppl), S48–56.

Amaral, D. G., Bauman, M. D., & Schumann, C. M. (2003). The amygdala and autism: Implications from non-human primate studies. *Genes Brain and Behavior*, *2*(5), 295–302.

Amaral, D. G., Geschwind, D., & Dawson, G. (Eds.). (2011). *Autism Spectrum Disorders*. Oxford: Oxford University Press.

Amaral, D. G., & Schumann, C. M. (2003). MRI and postmortem stereological investigation of the amygdala in autism. *FASEB Journal*, *17*(4), A379–A379.

Amaral, D. G., Schumann, C. M., & Nordahl, C. W. (2008). Neuroanatomy of autism. *Trends in Neuroscience*, *31*(3), 137–145.

Ames, C., & Fletcher-Watson, S. (2010). A review of methods in the study of attention in autism. *Developmental Review*, *30*(1), 52–73.

Amir, R. E., Van den Veyver, I. B., Wan, M., Tran, C. Q., Francke, U., & Zoghbi, H. Y. (1999). Rett syndrome is caused by mutations in X-linked MECP2, encoding methyl-CpG-binding protein 2. *Nature Genetics*, *23*(2), 185–188.

Anderson, G. M. (2012). Twin studies in autism: What might they say about genetic and environmental influences. *Journal of Autism and Developmental Disorders*, *42*(7), 1526–1527.

Anderson, J. S., Druzgal, T. J., Froehlich, A., Dubray, M. B., Lange, N., Alexander, A. L., . . . Lainhart, J. E. (2010). Decreased interhemispheric functional connectivity in autism. *Cerebral Cortex*, *21*(5), 1134–1146.

Anney, R. (2013). Common genetic variants in autism spectrum disorders. In J. D. Buxbaum & P. R. Hof (Eds.), *The Neuroscience of Autism Spectrum Disorders* (pp. 155–167). New York: Elsevier.

Anney, R., Klei, L., Pinto, D., Regan, R., Conroy, J., Magalhaes, T. R., . . . Hallmayer, J. (2010). A genome-wide scan for common alleles affecting risk for autism. *Human Molecular Genetics*, *19*(20), 4072–4082.

APA. (1980). *Diagnostic and Statistical Manual of Mental Disorders* (3rd ed.). Washington, DC: American Psychiatric Association.

APA. (1987). *Diagnostic and Statistical Manual of Mental Disorders* (3rd ed.-rev.). Washington, DC: American Psychiatric Association.

APA. (1994). *Diagnostic and Statistical Manual of Mental Disorders* (4th ed.). Washington, DC: American Psychiatric Association.

APA. (2000). *Diagnostic and Statistical Manual of Mental Disorders* (4th ed.-text rev.). Washington, DC: American Psychiatric Association.

APA. (2013). *Diagnostic and Statistical Manual of Mental Disorders* (5th ed.). Arlington, VA: American Psychiatric Publishing.

Ashwin, E., Ashwin, C., Rhydderch, D., Howells, J., & Baron-Cohen, S. (2009). Eagle-eyed visual acuity: An experimental investigation of enhanced perception in autism. *Biological Psychiatry*, *65*(1), 17–21.

Ashwood, P., & Van de Water, J. (2004). Is autism an autoimmune disease? *Autoimmunology Review*, *3*(7–8), 557–562.

Asperger, H. (1944). Die autistischen Psychopathen im Kindersalter. *Archiv fuer Psychiatrie und Nervenkrankheiten*, *117*, 76–136.

Assaf, M., Jagannathan, K., Calhoun, V. D., Miller, L., Stevens, M. C., Sahl, R., . . . Pearlson, G. D. (2010). Abnormal functional connectivity of default mode sub-networks in autism spectrum disorder patients. *Neuroimage*, *53*(1), 247–256.

Atladottir, H. O., Henriksen, T. B., Schendel, D. E., & Parner, E. T. (2012). Autism after infection, febrile episodes, and antibiotic use during pregnancy: An exploratory study. *Pediatrics*, *130*(6), E1447–E1454.

Attwood, T. (2007). *The Complete Guide to Asperger's Syndrome*. London: Jessica Kingsley Publishers.

Awadalla, P., Gauthier, J., Myers, R. A., Casals, F., Hamdan, F. F., Griffing, A. R., . . . Rouleau, G. A. (2010). Direct measure of the de novo mutation rate in autism and schizophrenia cohorts. *American Journal of Medical Genetics*, *87*(3), 316–324.

Aylward, E. H., Minshew, N. J., Field, K., Sparks, B. F., & Singh, N. (2002). Effects of age on brain volume and head circumference in autism. *Neurology*, *59*(2), 175–183.

Bailey, A., Le Couteur, A., Gottesman, I., & Bolton, P. (1995). Autism as a strongly genetic disorder: Evidence from a British twin study. *Psychological Medicine*, *25*(1), 63–77.

Bailey, A., Luthert, P., Bolton, P., Le Couteur, A., Rutter, M., & Harding, B. (1993). Autism and megalencephaly. *Lancet*, *341*(8854), 1225–1226.

Bailey, A., Luthert, P., Dean, A., Harding, B., Janota, I., Montgomery, M., . . . Lantos, P. (1998). A clinicopathological study of autism. *Brain*, *121*, 889–905.

Bailey, A., Palferman, S., Heavey, L., & Le Couteur, A. (1998). Autism: The phenotype in relatives. *Journal of Autism and Developmental Disorders*, *28*(5), 369–392.

Baio, J. (2014). Prevalence of Autism spectrum disorder among children aged 8 years: Autism and developmental disabilities monitoring network, 11 sites, United States, 2010. *Surveillance Summaries: Centers for Disease Control*, *March 28*(63(SS02)), 1–21.

Baird, G., Charman, T., Baron-Cohen, S., Cox, A., Swettenham, J., Wheelwright, S., & Drew, A. (2000). A screening instrument for autism at 18 months of age: A 6-year follow-up study. *Journal of the American Academy of Child and Adolescent Psychiatry*, *39*(6), 694–702.

Baird, G., Charman, T., Pickles, A., Chandler, S., Loucas, T., Meldrum, D., . . . Simonoff, E. (2008). Regression, developmental trajectory and associated problems in disorders in the autism spectrum: The SNAP study. *Journal of Autism and Developmental Disorders*, *38*(10), 1827–1836.

Baird, G., Pickles, A., Simonoff, E., Charman, T., Sullivan, P., Chandler, S., . . . Brown, D. (2008). Measles vaccination and antibody response in autism spectrum disorders. *Archives of Disease in Childhood*, *93*(10), 832–837.

Baird, G., Robinson, R. O., Boyd, S., & Charman, T. (2006). Sleep electroencephalograms in young children with autism with and without regression. *Developmental Medicine and Child Neurology*, *48*(7), 604–608.

Baird, G., Simonoff, E., Pickles, A., Chandler, S., Loucas, T., Meldrum, D., & Charman, T. (2006). Prevalence of disorders of the autism spectrum in a population cohort of children in South Thames: The Special Needs and Autism Project (SNAP). *Lancet*, *368*(9531), 210–215.

Bakermans-Kranenburg, M. J., & van Ijzendoorn, M. H. (2014). A sociability gene? Meta-analysis of oxytocin receptor genotype effects in humans. *Psychiatric Genetics*, *24*(2), 45–51.

Bakkaloglu, B., O'Roak, B. J., Louvi, A., Gupta, A. R., Abelson, J. F., Morgan, T. M., . . . State, M. W. (2008). Molecular cytogenetic analysis and resequencing of contactin associated protein-like 2 in autism spectrum disorders. *American Journal of Medical Genetics*, *82*(1), 165–173.

Baranek, G. T. (1999). Autism during infancy: A retrospective video analysis of sensory-motor and social behaviors at 9–12 months of age. *Journal of Autism and Developmental Disorders*, *29*(3), 213–224.

Baranek, G. T., Foster, L. G., & Berkson, G. (1997). Tactile defensiveness and stereotyped behaviors. *American Journal of Occupational Therapy*, *51*(2), 91–95.

Barbaro, J., & Dissanayake, C. (2010). Infancy and toddlerhood using developmental surveillance: The social attention and communication study. *Developmental Pediatrics*, *31*(5), 376–385.

Bardi, L., Regolin, L., & Simion, F. (2011). Biological motion preference in humans at birth: Role of dynamic and configural properties. *Developmental Science*, *14*(2), 353–359.

Barger, B. D., Campbell, J. M., & McDonough, J. D. (2013). Prevalence and onset of regression within autism spectrum disorders: A meta-analytic review. *Journal of Autism and Developmental Disorders*, *43*(4), 817–828.

Barnard-Brak, L., Sulak, T., & Hatz, J. K. (2011). Macrocephaly in children with autism spectrum disorders. *Pediatric Neurology*, *44*(2), 97–100.

Barnea-Goraly, N., Frazier, T. W., Piacenza, L., Minshew, N. J., Keshavan, M. S., Reiss, A. L., & Hardan, A. Y. (2014). A preliminary longitudinal volumetric MRI study of amygdala and hippocampal volumes in autism. *Progress in Neuro-Psychopharmacology and Biological Psychiatry*, *48*, 124–128.

Barnes, K. A., Howard, J. H., Jr., Howard, D. V., Gilotty, L., Kenworthy, L., Gaillard, W. D., & Vaidya, C. J. (2008). Intact implicit learning of spatial context and temporal sequences in childhood autism spectrum disorder. *Neuropsychology*, *22*(5), 563–570.

Baron-Cohen, S. (2001). Theory of mind and autism: A review. In L.M. Glidden (ED). *International Review of Research in Mental Retardation* (Vol. 23, pp. 169–184). Cambridge, MA: Elsevier. San Diego, CA: Academic Press.

Baron-Cohen, S. (2009). Autism: The empathizing-systemizing (E-S) theory. *Annals of the New York Academy of Sciences*, *1156*, 68–80.

Baron-Cohen, S., Cox, A., Baird, G., Sweettenham, J., & Nightingale, N. (1996). Psychological markers in the detection of autism in infancy in a large population. *British Journal of Psychiatry*, *168*(2), 158–163.

Baron-Cohen, S., Richler, J., Bisarya, D., Gurunathan, N., & Wheelwright, S. (2003). The systemizing quotient: An investigation of adults with Asperger syndrome or high-functioning autism, and normal sex differences. *Philosophical Transactions of the Royal Society of London: Series B: Biological Sciences*, *358*(1430), 361–374.

Baron-Cohen, S., & Ring, H. (1994). A model of the mindreading system: Neuropsychological and neurobiological perspectives. In C. Lewis & P. Mitchell (Eds.), *Children's Early Understanding of Mind: Origins and Development* (pp. 183–207, xvi, 493). East Sussex, UK. Hove: Erlbaum.

Baron-Cohen, S., Ring, H., Moriarty, J., Schmitz, B., Costa, D., & Ell, P. (1994a). Recognition of mental state terms: Clinical findings in children with autism and a functional neuroimaging study of normal adults. *British Journal of Psychiatry*, *165*, 640–649.

Baron-Cohen, S., Ring, H., Moriarty, J., Schmitz, B., Costa, D., & Ell, P. (1994b). Recognition of mental state terms: Clinical findings in children with autism and a functional neuroimaging study of normal adults. *British Journal of Psychiatry*, *165*(5), 640–649.

Baron-Cohen, S., Scott, F. J., Allison, C., Williams, J., Bolton, P., Matthews, F. E., & Brayne, C. (2009). Prevalence of autism-spectrum conditions: UK school-based population study. *British Journal of Psychiatry*, *194*(6), 500–509.

Baron-Cohen, S., & Staunton, R. (1994). Do children with autism acquire the phonology of their peers? An examination of group identification through the window of bilingualism. *First Language*, *14*, 241–248.

Baron-Cohen, S., Wheelwright, S., Burtenshaw, A., & Hobson, E. (2007). Mathematical talent is linked to autism. *Human Nature-an Interdisciplinary Biosocial Perspective*, *18*(2), 125–131.

Baron-Cohen, S., Wheelwright, S., Cox, A., Baird, G., Charman, T., Swettenham, J., . . . Doehring, P. (2000). Early identification of autism by the CHecklist for Autism in Toddlers (CHAT). *Journal of the Royal Society of Medicine*, *93*(10), 521–525.

Baron-Cohen, S., Wheelwright, S., Stott, C., Bolton, P., & Goodyer, I. (1997). Is there a link between engineering and autism? *Autism*, *1*, 101–109.

Barth, C., Fein, D., & Waterhouse, L. (1995). Delayed match-to-sample performance in autistic-children. *Developmental Neuropsychology*, *11*(1), 53–69.

Bartholomeusz, H. H., Courchesne, E., & Karns, C. M. (2002). Relationship between head circumference and brain volume in healthy normal toddlers, children, and adults. *Neuropediatrics*, *33*(5), 239–241.

Bartlett, C. W., Hou, L. P., Flax, J. F., Hare, A., Cheong, S. Y., Fermano, Z., . . . Brzustowicz, L. M. (2014). A genome scan for loci shared by autism spectrum disorder and language impairment. *American Journal of Psychiatry*, *171*(1), 72–81.

Bartolucci, G., Pierce, S. J., & Streiner, D. (1980). Cross-sectional studies of grammatical morphemes in autistic and mentally retarded children. *Journal of Autism and Developmental Disorders*, *10*(1), 39–50.

Bartolucci, G., Pierce, S. J., Streiner, D., & Eppel, P. (1976). Phonological investigation of verbal autistic and mentally retarded subjects. *Journal of Autism and Childhood Schizophrenia*, *6*, 303–316.

Barton, M. L., Robins, D. L., Jashar, D., Brennan, L., & Fein, D. (2013). Sensitivity and specificity of proposed DSM-5 criteria for autism spectrum disorder in toddlers. *Journal of Autism and Developmental Disorders*, *43*(5), 1184–1195.

Barton, M. L., & Volkmar, F. (1998). How commonly are known medical conditions associated with autism? *Journal of Autism and Developmental Disorders*, *28*(4), 273–278.

Baruth, J. M., Wall, C. A., Patterson, M. C., & Port, J. D. (2013). Proton magnetic resonance spectroscopy as a probe into the pathophysiology of autism spectrum disorders (ASD): A review. *Autism Research*, *6*(2), 119–133.

Bauman, M. D., Iosif, A. M., Ashwood, P., Braunschweig, D., Lee, A., Schumann, C. M., . . . Amaral, D. G. (2013). Maternal antibodies from mothers of children with autism alter brain growth and social behavior development in the rhesus monkey. *Translational Psychiatry*, *3*(7), E278.

Bauman, M. L. (2010). Medical comorbidities in autism: Challenges to diagnosis and treatment. *Neurotherapeutics*, *7*(3), 320–327.

Bauman, M. L., & Kemper, T. L. (1985). Histoanatomic observations of the brain in early infantile autism. *Neurology*, *35*(6), 866–874.

Bauman, M. L., & Kemper, T. L. (2005). Neuroanatomic observations of the brain in autism: A review and future directions. *International Journal of Developmental Neuroscience*, *23*(2–3), 183–187.

Belmonte, M. K., Allen, G., Beckel-Mitchener, A., Boulanger, L. M., Carper, R. A., & Webb, S. J. (2004). Autism and abnormal development of brain connectivity. *Journal of Neuroscience*, *24*(42), 9228–9231.

Belmonte, M. K., & Yurgelun-Todd, D. A. (2003). Functional anatomy of impaired selective attention and compensatory processing in autism. *Cognitive Brain Research*, *17*(3), 651–664.

Bennetto, L., Pennington, B. F., & Rogers, S. J. (1996). Intact and impaired memory functions in autism. *Child Development*, *67*(4), 1816–1835.

Berkel, S., Marshall, C. R., Weiss, B., Howe, J., Roeth, R., Moog, U., . . . Rappold, G. A. (2010). Mutations in the SHANK2 synaptic scaffolding gene in autism spectrum disorder and mental retardation. *Nature Genetics*, *42*(6), 489–491.

Bernabei, P., Cerquiglini, A., Cortesi, F., & D'Ardia, C. (2007). Regression versus no regression in the autistic disorder: Developmental trajectories. *Journal of Autism & Developmental Disorders*, *37*(3), 580–588.

Bertone, A., Mottron, L., Jelenic, P., & Faubert, J. (2003). Motion perception in autism: A "complex" issue. *Journal of Cognitive Neuroscience*, *15*(2), 218–225.

Berwick, R. C., Friederici, A. D., Chomsky, N., & Bolhuis, J. J. (2013). Evolution, brain, and the nature of language. *Trends in Cognitive Sciences*, *17*(2), 89–98.

Betancur, C. (2010). Etiological heterogeneity in autism spectrum disorders: More than 100 genetic and genomic disorders and still counting. *Brain Research Bulletin*, *1380*, 42–77.

Betancur, C., Corbex, M., Spielewoy, C., Philippe, A., Laplanche, J. L., Launay, J. M., . . . Leboyer, M. (2002). Serotonin transporter gene polymorphisms and hyperserotonemia in autistic disorder. *Molecular Psychiatry*, *7*(1), 67–71.

Bettus, G., Wendling, F., Guye, M., Valton, L., Regis, J., Chauvel, P., & Bartolomei, F. (2008). Enhanced EEG functional connectivity in mesial temporal lobe epilepsy. *Epilepsy Research*, *81*(1), 58–68.

Beversdorf, D. Q., Nordgren, R. E., Bonab, A. A., Fischman, A. J., Weise, S. B., Dougherty, D. D., . . . Bauman, M. L. (2012). 5-HT2 receptor distribution shown by [18F] setoperone PET in high-functioning autistic adults. *Journal of Neuropsychiatry and Clinical Neurosciences*, *24*(2), 191–197.

Bhat, A. N., Galloway, J. C., & Landa, R. J. (2010). Social and non-social visual attention patterns and associative learning in infants at risk for autism. *Journal of Child Psychology and Psychiatry*, *51*(9), 989–997.

Bhat, A. N., Galloway, J. C., & Landa, R. J. (2012). Relation between early motor delay and later communication delay in infants at risk for autism. *Infant Behavior & Development*, *35*(4), 838–846.

Bianchi, S., Stimpson, C. D., Duka, T., Larsen, M. D., Janssen, W.G.M., Collins, Z., . . . Sherwood, C. C. (2013). Synaptogenesis and development of pyramidal neuron dendritic morphology in the chimpanzee neocortex resembles humans. *Proceedings of the National Academy of Sciences of the United States of America*, *110*, 10395–10401.

Bigler, E. D., Abildskov, T. J., Petrie, J. A., Johnson, M., Lange, N., Chipman, J., . . . Lainhart, J. E. (2010). Volumetric and voxel-based morphometry findings in autism subjects with and without macrocephaly. *Developmental Neuropsychology*, *35*(3), 278–295.

Biran-Gol, Y., Malinger, G., Cohen, H., Davidovitch, M., Lev, D., Lerman-Sagie, T., & Schweiger, A. (2010). Developmental outcome of isolated fetal macrocephaly. *Ultrasound in Obstetrics and Gynecology*, *36*(2), 147–153.

Bishop, D. V., Maybery, M., Wong, D., Maley, A., Hill, W., & Hallmayer, J. (2004). Are phonological processing deficits part of the broad autism phenotype? *American Journal of Medical Genetics*, *128B*(1), 54–60.

Biswal, B., Yetkin, F. Z., Haughton, V. M., & Hyde, J. S. (1995). Functional connectivity in the motor cortex of resting human brain using echo-planar MRI. *Magnetic Resonance in Medicine*, *34*(4), 537–541.

Black, L., & Stefanatos, G. A. (2000). Neuropsychological assessment of developmental and learning disorders. In S. I. Greenspan & S. Weider (Eds.), *Interdisciplinary Council on Developmental and Learning Disorders: Clinical Practice Guidelines* (pp. 425–488). Bethesda, MD: ICDL Press.

Blake, R., Turner, L. M., Smoski, M. J., Pozdol, S. L., & Stone, W. L. (2003). Visual recognition of biological motion is impaired in children with autism. *Psychological Science*, *14*(2), 151–157.

Bloemen, O. J., Deeley, Q., Sundram, F., Daly, E. M., Barker, G. J., Jones, D. K., . . . Murphy, D. G. (2010). White matter integrity in Asperger syndrome: A preliminary diffusion tensor magnetic resonance imaging study in adults. *Autism Research: Official Journal of the International Society for Autism Research*, *3*(5), 203–213.

Bloss, C. S., & Courchesne, E. (2007). MRI neuroanatomy in young girls with autism: A preliminary study. *Journal of the American Academy of Child and Adolescent Psychiatry*, *46*(4), 515–523.

Blumberg, S. J., Bramlett, M. D., Kogan, M. D., Schieve, L. A., Jones, J. R., & Lu, M. C. (2013). *Changes in Prevalence of Parent-Reported Autism Spectrum Disorder in School-Aged U.S. Children: 2007 to 2011–2012*. Hyattsville, MD: National Center for Health Statistics.

Blundell, J., Tabuchi, K., Bolliger, M. F., Blaiss, C. A., Brose, N., Liu, X., . . . Powell, C. M. (2009). Increased anxiety-like behavior in mice lacking the inhibitory synapse cell adhesion molecule neuroligin 2. *Genes Brain & Behavior*, *8*(1), 114–126.

Boccuto, L., Lauri, M., Sarasua, S. M., Skinner, C. D., Buccella, D., Dwivedi, A., . . . Schwartz, C. E. (2013). Prevalence of SHANK3 variants in patients with different subtypes of autism spectrum disorders. *European Journal of Human Genetics*, *21*(3), 310–316.

Bolduc, M. E., du Plessis, A. J., Sullivan, N., Guizard, N., Zhang, X., Robertson, R. L., & Limperopoulos, C. (2012). Regional cerebellar volumes predict functional outcome in children with cerebellar malformations. *Cerebellum 11*(2), 531–542.

Bolte, S., Dziobek, I., & Poustka, F. (2009). Brief report: The level and nature of autistic intelligence revisited. *Journal of Autism and Developmental Disorders*, *39*(4), 678–682.

Bolte, S., Schlitt, S., Gapp, V., Hainz, D., Schirman, S., Poustka, F., . . . Walter, H. (2012). A close eye on the eagle-eyed visual acuity hypothesis of autism. *Journal of Autism and Developmental Disorders*, *42*(5), 726–733.

Bolton, P., Macdonald, H., Pickles, A., Rios, P., Goode, S., Crowson, M., Bailey, A., & Rutter, M. (1994). A case-control family history study of autism. *Journal of Child Psychology and Psychiatry and Allied Disciplines*, *35*(5), 877–900.

Bolton, P., Macdonald, H., Pickles, A., Rios, P., Goode, S., Crowson, M., . . . Rutter, M. (1994). A case-control family history study of autism. *Journal of Child Psychology and Psychiatry and Allied Disciplines*, *35*(5), 877–900.

Bonnel, A., Mottron, L., Peretz, I., Trudel, M., Gallun, E., & Bonnel, A. M. (2003). Enhanced pitch sensitivity in individuals with autism: A signal detection analysis. *Journal of Cognitive Neuroscience*, *15*(2), 226–235.

Borsuk, E. R., Watkins, M. W., & Canivez, G. L. (2006). Long-term stability of membership in a Weschler Intelligence Scale for Children-Third Edition (WISC-III) subtest core profile taxonomy. *Journal of Psychoeducational Assessment*, *24*, 52–68.

Boucher, J., Mayes, A., & Bigham, S. (2012). Memory in autistic spectrum disorder. *Psychological Bulletin*, *138*(3), 458–496.

Bowler, D. A., Gaigg, S. B., & Gardiner, J. M. (2008). Effects of related and unrelated context on recall and recognition by adults with high-functioning autism spectrum disorder. *Neuropsychologia*, *46*(4), 993–999.

Bowler, D. M., Gaigg, S. B., & Gardiner, J. M. (2009). Free recall learning of hierarchically organised lists by adults with Asperger's syndrome: Additional evidence for diminished relational processing. *Journal of Autism and Developmental Disorders*, *39*(4), 589–595.

Bowler, D. M., Gardiner, J. M., & Berthollier, N. (2004). Source memory in adolescents and adults with Asperger's syndrome. *Journal of Autism and Developmental Disorders*, *34*(5), 533–542.

Bowler, D. M., Gardiner, J. M., & Grice, S. J. (2000). Episodic memory and remembering in adults with Asperger syndrome. *Journal of Autism and Developmental Disorders*, *30*(4), 295–304.

Bramham, J., Ambery, F., Young, S., Morris, R., Russell, A., Xenitidis, K., . . . Murphy, D. (2009). Executive functioning differences between adults with attention deficit hyperactivity disorder and autistic spectrum disorder in initiation, planning and strategy formation. *Autism*, *13*(3), 245–264.

Braunschweig, D., Krakowiak, P., Duncanson, P., Boyce, R., Hansen, R. L., Ashwood, P., . . . Van de Water, J. (2013). Autism-specific maternal autoantibodies recognize critical proteins in developing brain. *Translational Psychiatry*, *3*(7), 277.

Bray, P. F., Shields, W. D., Wolcott, G. J., & Madsen, J. A. (1969). Occipitofrontal head circumference: An accurate measure of intracranial volume. *Journal of Pediatrics*, *75*(2), 303.

Brian, J. A., & Bryson, S. E. (1996). Disembedding performance and recognition memory in autism/PDD. *Journal of Child Psychology and Psychiatry*, *37*(7), 865–872.

Brian, J. A., Tipper, S. P., Weaver, B., & Bryson, S. E. (2003). Inhibitory mechanisms in autism spectrum disorders: Typical selective inhibition of location versus facilitated perceptual processing. *Journal of Child Psychology and Psychiatry*, *44*(4), 552–560.

Brito, A. R., Vasconcelos, M. M., Domingues, R. C., Hygino da Cruz, L. C., Jr., Rodrigues Lde, S., Gasparetto, E. L., & Calcada, C. A. (2009). Diffusion tensor imaging findings in school-aged autistic children. *Journal of Neuroimaging*, *19*(4), 337–343.

Brock, J., Brown, C. C., Boucher, J., & Rippon, G. (2002). The temporal binding deficit hypothesis of autism. *Development and Psychopathology*, *14*(2), 209–224.

Brothers, L. (1990). The social brain: A project for integrating primate behavior and neurophysiology in a new domain. *Conceptual Neuroscience*, *1*, 27–51.

Brothers, L. (1997). *Friday's Footprint: How Society Shapes the Human Mind*. New York: Oxford University Press.

Brown, J., Aczel, B., Jimenez, L., Kaufman, S. B., & Grant, K. P. (2010). Intact implicit learning in autism spectrum conditions. *Quarterly Journal of Experimental Psychology*, *63*(9), 1789–1812.

Brown, J., & Prelock, P. A. (1995). Brief report: The impact of regression on language development in autism. *Journal of Autism and Developmental Disorders*, *25*(3), 305–309.

Brown, M. S., Singel, D., Hepburn, S., & Rojas, D. C. (2013). Increased glutamate concentration in the auditory cortex of persons with autism and first-degree relatives: A (1)H-MRS study. *Autism Research: Official Journal of the International Society for Autism Research*, *6*(1), 1–10.

Brugha, T. S., McManus, S., Bankart, J., Scott, F., Purdon, S., Smith, J., . . . Meltzer, H. (2011). Epidemiology of autism spectrum disorders in adults in the community in England. *Archives of General Psychiatry*, *68*(5), 459–465.

Brun, C. C., Nicolson, R., Lepore, N., Chou, Y. Y., Vidal, C. N., DeVito, T. J., . . . Thompson, P. M. (2009). Mapping brain abnormalities in boys with autism. *Human Brain Mapping*, *30*(12), 3887–3900.

Bryson, S. E., Rogers, S. J., & Fombonne, E. (2003). Autism spectrum disorders: Early detection, intervention, education, and psychopharmacological management. *Canadian Journal of Psychiatry-Revue Canadienne De Psychiatrie*, *48*(8), 506–516.

Bryson, S. E., Zwaigenbaum, L., Brian, J., Roberts, W., Szatmari, P., Rombough, V., & McDermott, C. (2007). A prospective case series of high-risk infants who developed autism. *Journal of Autism and Developmental Disorders*, *37*(1), 12–24.

Bryson, S. E., Zwaigenbaum, L., McDermott, C., Rombough, V., & Brian, J. (2008). The autism observation scale for infants: Scale development and reliability data. *Journal of Autism and Developmental Disorders*, *38*(4), 731–738.

Buckner, R. L., Andrews-Hanna, J. R., & Schacter, D. L. (2008). The brain's default network: Anatomy, function, and relevance to disease. *Annals of the New York Academy of Sciences*, *1124*, 1–38.

Buitelaar, J. K., Van Engeland, H., de Kogel, K. H., de Vries, H., Van Hooff, J., & Van Ree, J. M. (1992). The use of adrenocorticotrophic hormone (4–9) analog ORG 2766 in autistic children: Effects on the organization of behavior. *Biological Psychiatry*, *31*(11), 1119–1129.

Burbach, J. P., & van der Zwaag, B. (2009). Contact in the genetics of autism and schizophrenia. *Trends in Neurosciences*, *32*(2), 69–72.

Burd, L., Severud, R., Kerbeshian, J., & Klug, M. G. (1999). Prenatal and perinatal risk factors for autism. *Journal of Perinatal Medicine*, *27*(6), 441–450.

Buwe, A., Guttenbach, M., & Schmid, M. (2005). Effect of paternal age on the frequency of cytogenetic abnormalities in human spermatozoa. *Cytogenetic and Genome Research*, *111*(3–4), 213–228.

Buxbaum, J. D., Cai, G. Q., Chaste, P., Nygren, G., Goldsmith, J., Reichert, J., . . . Betancur, C. (2007). Mutation screening of the PTEN gene in patients with autism spectrum disorders and macrocephaly. *American Journal of Medical Genetics Part B-Neuropsychiatric Genetics*, *144B*(4), 484–491.

Buxbaum, J. D., & Hof, P. R. (Eds.). (2012). *The Neuroscience of Autism Spectrum Disorders* (Vol. 1). New York: Academic Press.

Bystron, I., Blakemore, C., & Rakic, P. (2008). Development of the human cerebral cortex: Boulder Committee revisited. *Nature Reviews Neuroscience*, *9*(2), 110–122.

Campbell, D. B., Li, C., Sutcliffe, J. S., Persico, A. M., & Levitt, P. (2008). Genetic evidence implicating multiple genes in the MET receptor tyrosine kinase pathway in autism spectrum disorder. *Autism Research*, *1*(3), 159–168.

Campbell, J. A. (1895). Heavy brains. *The Lancet*, *1*, 1511.

Campbell, M., Dominijanni, C., & Schneider, B. (1977). Monozygotic twins concordant for infantile autism: Follow-up. *British Journal of Psychiatry*, *131*, 616–622.

Canitano, R., Luchetti, A., & Zappella, M. (2005). Epilepsy, electroencephalographic abnormalities, and regression in children with autism. *Journal of Child Neurology*, *20*(1), 27–31.

Capps, L., Losh, M., & Thurber, C. (2000). "The frog ate the bug and made his mouth sad": Narrative competence in children with autism. *Journal of Abnormal Child Psychology*, *28*(2), 193–204.

Carlier, M., & Spitz, E. (1999). The twin method. In P. Mormède & B. Jones (Eds.), *Cellular and Quantitative Methods in Neurogenetics* (pp. 187–197). Boca Raton, FL: CRC Press LLC.

Caron, M. J., Mottron, L., Berthiaume, C., & Dawson, M. (2006). Cognitive mechanisms, specificity and neural underpinnings of visuospatial peaks in autism. *Brain*, *129*(Pt 7), 1789–1802.

Carper, R. A., & Courchesne, E. (2005). Localized enlargement of the frontal cortex in early autism. *Biological Psychiatry*, *57*(2), 126–133.

Carper, R. A., Moses, P., Tigue, Z. D., & Courchesne, E. (2002). Cerebral lobes in autism: Early hyperplasia and abnormal age effects. *Neuroimage*, *16*(4), 1038–1051.

Casanova, M. F. (2006). Neuropathological and genetic findings in autism: The significance of a putative mini columnopathy. *Neuroscientist*, *12*(5), 435–441.

Casanova, M. F. (2007). The neuropathology of autism. *Brain Pathology*, *17*(4), 422–433.

Casanova, M. F. (2008). The minicolumnopathy of autism: A link between migraine and gastrointestinal symptoms. *Medical Hypotheses*, *70*(1), 73–80.

Casanova, M. F., Buxhoeveden, D. P., Switala, A. E., & Roy, E. (2002). Minicolumnar pathology in autism. *Neurology*, *58*(3), 428–432.

Cascio, C., Gribbin, M., Gouttard, S., Smith, R. G., Jomier, M., Field, S., . . . Piven, J. (2013). Fractional anisotropy distributions in 2-to 6-year-old children with autism. *Journal of Intellectual Disability Research*, *57*(11), 1037–1049.

Cascio, C., McGlone, F., Folger, S., Tannan, V., Baranek, G., Pelphrey, K., & Essick, G. (2008). Tactile perception in adults with autism: A multidimensional psychophysical study. *Journal of Autism and Developmental Disorders*, *38*(1), 127–137.

Cascio, C. J., Moana, E. J., Guest, S., Nebel, M. B., Weisner, J., Baranek, G. T., & Essick, G. K. (2012). Perceptual and neural response to affective tactile texture stimulation in adults with autism spectrum disorders. *Autism Research*, *5*(4), 231–244.

Castelli, F., Happe, F., Frith, U., & Frith, C. (2000). Movement and mind: A functional imaging study of perception and interpretation of complex intentional movement patterns. *Neuroimage*, *12*(3), 314–325.

Catani, M., Jones, D. K., & ffytche, D. H. (2005). Perisylvian language networks of the human brain. *Annals of Neurology*, *57*(1), 8–16.

Cauda, F., Geda, E., Sacco, K., D'Agata, F., Duca, S., Geminiani, G., & Keller, R. (2011). Grey matter abnormality in autism spectrum disorder: An activation likelihood estimation meta-analysis study. *Journal of Neurology, Neurosurgery and Psychiatry*, *82*(12), 1304–1313.

Cederlund, M., Miniscalco, C., & Gillberg, C. (2014). Pre-school-children with autism spectrum disorders are rarely macrocephalic: A population study. *Research in Developmental Disabilities*, *35*(5), 992–998.

Cermak, S. A., Curtin, C., & Bandini, L. G. (2010). Food selectivity and sensory sensitivity in children with autism spectrum disorders. *Journal of the American Dietetic Association*, *110*(2), 238–246.

Chakrabarti, S., & Fombonne, E. (2005). Pervasive developmental disorders in preschool children: Confirmation of high prevalence. *The American Journal of Psychiatry*, *162*(6), 1133–1141.

Chapman, A. H. (1957). Early infantile autism in identical twins; report of a case. *A.M.A. Archives of Neurology and Psychiatry*, *78*(6), 621–623.

Chapman, N. H., Estes, A., Munson, J., Bernier, R., Webb, S. J., Rothstein, J. H., . . . Wijsman, E. M. (2010). Genome-scan for IQ discrepancy in autism: Evidence for loci on chromosomes 10 and 16. *Human Genetics*, *129*(1), 59–70.

Charman, T., Jones, C. R., Pickles, A., Simonoff, E., Baird, G., & Happé, F. (2011). Defining the cognitive phenotype of autism. *Brain Research*, *1380*, 10–21.

Charman, T., Pickles, A., Simonoff, E., Chandler, S., Loucas, T., & Baird, G. (2011). IQ in children with autism spectrum disorders: Data from the special needs and autism project (SNAP). *Psychologial Medicine*, *41*, 619–627.

Chaste, P., Klei, L., Sanders, S. J., Murtha, M. T., Hus, V., Lowe, J. K., . . . Kim, S. J. (2013). Adjusting head circumference for covariates in autism: Clinical correlates of a highly heritable continuous trait. *Biological Psychiatry*, *74*(8), 576–584.

Chawarska, K., Volkmar, F., & Klin, A. (2010). Limited attentional bias for faces in toddlers with autism spectrum disorders. *Archives of General Psychiatry*, *67*(2), 178–185.

Chen, G. K., Kono, N., Geschwind, D. H., & Cantor, R. M. (2006). Quantitative trait locus analysis of nonverbal communication in autism spectrum disorder. *Molecular Psychiatry*, *11*(2), 214–220.

Cheng, Y. W., Chou, K. H., Chen, I. Y., Fan, Y. T., Decety, J., & Lin, C. P. (2010). Atypical development of white matter microstructure in adolescents with autism spectrum disorders. *Neuroimage*, *50*(3), 873–882.

Cheng, Y. W., Lee, S.-Y., Chen, H.-Y., Wang, P.-Y., & Decety, J. (2012). Voice and emotion processing in the human neonatal brain. *Journal of Cognitive Neuroscience*, *24*(6), 1411–1419.

Cherkassky, V. L., Kana, R. K., Keller, T. A., & Just, M. A. (2006). Functional connectivity in a baseline resting-state network in autism. *Neuroreport*, *17*(16), 1687–1690.

Chess, S. (1971). Autism in children with congenital rubella. *Journal of Autism and Childhood Schizophrenia*, *1*(1), 33–47.

Chez, M. G., Memon, S., & Hung, P. C. (2004). Neurologic treatment strategies in autism: An overview of medical intervention strategies. *Seminars in Pediatric Neurology*, *11*(3), 229–235.

Chi, J. G., Dooling, E. C., & Gilles, F. H. (1977). Gyral development of human brain. *Annals of Neurology*, *1*(1), 86–93.

Chien, I. C., Lin, C. H., Chou, Y. J., & Chou, P. (2011). Prevalence and incidence of autism spectrum disorders among national health insurance enrollees in Taiwan from 1996 to 2005. *Journal of Child Neurology*, *26*(7), 830–834.

Christ, S. E., Kester, L. E., Bodner, K. E., & Miles, J. H. (2011). Evidence for selective inhibitory impairment in individuals with autism spectrum disorder. *Neuropsychology*, *25*(6), 690–701.

Christakou, A., Murphy, C. M., Chantiluke, K., Cubillo, A. I., Smith, A. B., Giampietro, V., . . . Rubia, K. (2013). Disorder-specific functional abnormalities during sustained attention in youth with Attention Deficit Hyperactivity Disorder (ADHD) and with autism. *Molecular Psychiatry*, *18*(2), 236–244.

Christopher, J. A., Sears, L. L., Williams, P. G., Oliver, J., & Hersh, J. (2004). Familial, medical and developmental patterns of children with autism and a history of language regression. *Journal of Developmental and Physical Disabilities*, *16*(2), 163–170.

Chugani, D. C., Muzik, O., Rothermel, R., Behen, M., Chakraborty, P., Mangner, T., . . . Chugani, H. T. (1997). Altered serotonin synthesis in the dentatothalamocortical pathway in autistic boys. *Annals of Neurology*, *42*(4), 666–669.

Clifford, S. M., & Dissanayake, C. (2008). The early development of joint attention in infants with autistic disorder using home video observations and parental interview. *Journal of Autism and Developmental Disorders*, *38*(5), 791–805.

Cohen, I. L., Schmidt-Lackner, S., Romanczyk, R., & Sudhalter, V. (2003). The PDD Behavior Inventory: A rating scale for assessing response to intervention in children with pervasive developmental disorder. *Journal of Autism and Developmental Disorders*, *33*(1), 31–45.

Cohly, H. H., & Panja, A. (2005). Immunological findings in autism. *International Review of Neurobiology*, *71*, 317–341.

Coleman, P. D., Romano, J., Lapham, L., & Simon, W. (1985). Cell counts in cerebral cortex of an autistic patient. *Journal of Autism and Developmental Disorders*, *15*(3), 245–255.

Comi, A. M., Zimmerman, A. W., Frye, V. H., Law, P. A., & Peeden, J. N. (1999). Familial clustering of autoimmune disorders and evaluation of medical risk factors in autism. *Journal of Child Neurology*, *14*(6), 388–394.

Conciatori, M., Stodgell, C. J., Hyman, S. L., O'Bara, M., Militerni, R., Bravaccio, C., . . . Persico, A. M. (2004). Association between the HOXA1 A218G polymorphism and increased head circumference in patients with autism. *Biological Psychiatry*, *55*(4), 413–419.

Condouris, K., Meyer, E., & Tager-Flusberg, H. (2003). The relationship between standardized measures of language and measures of spontaneous speech in children with autism. *American Journal of Speech-Language Pathology*, *12*(3), 349–358.

Connolly, A. M., Streif, E. M., & Chez, M. G. (2003). Brain-derived neurotrophic factor and antibodies to brain-derived neurotrophic factor are elevated in children with autism, autism with regression, and epilepsy. *Annals of Neurology*, *54*, S146–S147.

Constantino, J. N., Davis, S. A., Todd, R. D., Schindler, M. K., Gross, M. M., Brophy, S. L., . . . Reich, W. (2003). Validation of a brief quantitative measure of autistic traits: Comparison of the social responsiveness scale with the autism diagnostic interview-revised. *Journal of Autism and Developmental Disorders*, *33*(4), 427–433.

Constantino, J. N., Majmudar, P., Bottini, A., Arvin, M., Virkud, Y., Simons, P., & Spitznagel, E. L. (2010). Infant head growth in male siblings of children with and without autism spectrum disorders. *Journal of Neurodevelopmental Disorders*, *2*(1), 39–46.

Constantino, J. N., Zhang, Y., Frazier, T., Abbacchi, A. M., & Law, P. (2010). Sibling recurrence and the genetic epidemiology of autism. *American Journal of Psychiatry*, *167*(11), 1349–1356.

Conturo, T. E., Williams, D. L., Smith, C. D., Gultepe, E., Akbudak, E., & Minshew, N. J. (2008). Neuronal fiber pathway abnormalities in autism: An initial MRI diffusion tensor tracking study of hippocampo-fusiform and amygdalo-fusiform pathways. *Journal of the International Neuropsychological Society*, *14*(6), 933–946.

Cook, E. H., Courchesne, R., Lord, C., Cox, N. J., Yan, S., Lincoln, A., . . . Leventhal, B. L. (1997). Evidence of linkage between the serotonin transporter and autistic disorder. *Molecular Psychiatry*, *2*(3), 247–250.

Cook, E. H., Jr., & Scherer, S. W. (2008). Copy-number variations associated with neuropsychiatric conditions. *Nature*, *455*(7215), 919–923.

Corbett, B. A., Carmean, V., Ravizza, S., Wendelken, C., Henry, M. L., Carter, C., & Rivera, S. M. (2009). A functional and structural study of emotion and face processing in children with autism. *Psychiatry Research*, *173*(3), 196–205.

Corbett, B. A., Constantine, L. J., Hendren, R., Rocke, D., & Ozonoff, S. (2009). Examining executive functioning in children with autism spectrum disorder, attention deficit hyperactivity disorder and typical development. *Psychiatry Research*, *166*(2–3), 210–222.

Courchesne, E., Carper, R., & Akshoomoff, N. (2003). Evidence of brain overgrowth in the first year of life in autism. *Jama-Journal of the American Medical Association*, *290*(3), 337–344.

Courchesne, E., Karns, C. M., Davis, H. R., Ziccardi, R., Carper, R. A., Tigue, Z. D., . . . Courchesne, R. Y. (2001). Unusual brain growth patterns in early life in patients with autistic disorder: An MRI study. *Neurology*, *57*(2), 245–254.

Courchesne, E., Mouton, P. R., Calhoun, M. E., Semendeferi, K., Ahrens-Barbeau, C., Hallet, M. J., . . . Pierce, K. (2011). Neuron number and size in prefrontal cortex of children with autism. *Journal of the American Medical Association*, *306*(18), 2001–2010.

Courchesne, E., Mouton, P. R., Calhoun, M. E., Semendeferi, K., Ahrens-Barbeau, C., Hallet, M. J., . . . Pierce, K. (2012). Neuron number and size in prefontal cortex of children with autism. *Archives of Neurology*, *69*(7), 906–906.

Courchesne, E., & Pierce, K. (2005a). Brain overgrowth in autism during a critical time in development: Implications for frontal pyramidal neuron and interneuron development and connectivity. *International Journal of Developmental Neuroscience*, *23*(2–3), 153–170.

Courchesne, E., & Pierce, K. (2005b). Why the frontal cortex in autism might be talking only to itself: Local over-connectivity but long-distance disconnection. *Current Opinion in Neurobiology*, *15*(2), 225–230.

Courchesne, E., Pierce, K., Schumann, C. M., Redcay, E., Buckwalter, J. A., Kennedy, D. P., & Morgan, J. (2007). Mapping early brain development in autism. *Neuron*, *56*(2), 399–413.

Courchesne, E., Redcay, E., Morgan, J. T., & Kennedy, D. P. (2005). Autism at the beginning: Microstructural and growth abnormalities underlying the cognitive and behavioral phenotype of autism. *Development and Psychopathology*, *17*(3), 577–597.

Courchesne, E., Townsend, J., Akshoomoff, N. A., Saitoh, O., Yeung-Courchesne, R., Lincoln, A. J., . . . Lau, L. (1994). Impairment in shifting attention in autistic and cerebellar patients. *Behavioral Neuroscience*, *108*(5), 848–865.

Cox, A., Klein, K., Charman, T., Baird, G., Baron-Cohen, S., Swettenham, J., . . . Wheelwright, S. (1999). Autism spectrum disorders at 20 and 42 months of age: Stability of clinical and ADI-R diagnosis. *Journal of Child Psychology and Psychiatry*, *40*(5), 719–732.

Crane, L., & Goddard, L. (2008). Episodic and semantic autobiographical memory in adults with autism spectrum disorders. *Journal of Autism and Developmental Disorders*, *38*(3), 498–506.

Crespi, B. J., & Thiselton, D. L. (2011). Comparative immunogenetics of autism and schizophrenia. *Genes, Brain & Behavior*, *10*(7), 689–701.

Critchley, H. D., Daly, E. M., Bullmore, E. T., Williams, S. C., Van Amelsvoort, T., Robertson, D. M., . . . Murphy, D. G. (2000). The functional neuroanatomy of social behaviour: Changes in cerebral blood flow when people with autistic disorder process facial expressions. *Brain*, *123*(Pt 11), 2203–2212.

Croen, L. A., Najjar, D. V., Fireman, B., & Grether, J. K. (2007). Maternal and paternal age and risk of autism spectrum disorders. *Archives of Pediatrics and Adolescent Medicine*, *161*(4), 334–340.

Crow, J. F. (2000). The origins, patterns and implications of human spontaneous mutation. *Nature Reviews Genetics*, *1*(1), 40–47.

Csibra, G., & Gergely, G. (2006). Social learning and social cognition: The case for pedagogy. In Y. Munakata & M. H. Johnson (Eds.), *Processes of Change in Brain and Cognitive Development* (pp. 249–274). Oxford: Oxford University Press.

Cuccaro, M. L., Shao, Y., Grubber, J., Slifer, M., Wolpert, C. M., Donnelly, S. L., . . . Pericak-Vance, M. A. (2003). Factor analysis of restricted and repetitive behaviors in autism using the Autism Diagnostic Interview-R. *Child Psychiatry and Human Development*, *34*(1), 3–17.

Dahlgren, S. O., & Gillberg, C. (1989). Symptoms in the first two years of life: A preliminary population study of infantile autism. *European Archives of Psychiatry and Neurological Sciences*, *238*(3), 169–174.

Dahlgren, S. O., Sandberg, A. D., & Hjelmquist, E. (2003). The non-specificity of theory of mind deficits: Evidence from children with communicative disabilities. *European Journal of Cognitive Psychology*, *15*(1), 129–155.

Dalton, K. M., Nacewicz, B. M., Johnstone, T., Schaefer, H. S., Gernsbacher, M. A., Goldsmith, H. H., . . . Davidson, R. J. (2005). Gaze fixation and the neural circuitry of face processing in autism. *Nature Neuroscience*, *8*(4), 519–526.

Damasio, A. R., & Maurer, R. G. (1978). A neurological model for childhood autism. *Archives of Neurology*, *35*(12), 777–786.

Damoiseaux, J. S., & Greicius, M. D. (2009). Greater than the sum of its parts: A review of studies combining structural connectivity and resting-state functional connectivity. *Brain Structure & Function*, *213*(6), 525–533.

Danielsson, S., Gillberg, I. C., Billstedt, E., Gillberg, C., & Olsson, I. (2005). Epilepsy in young adults with autism: A prospective population-based follow-up study of 120 individuals diagnosed in childhood. *Epilepsia*, *46*(6), 918–923.

Dapretto, M., Davies, M. S., Pfeifer, J. H., Scott, A. A., Sigman, M., Bookheimer, S. Y., & Iacoboni, M. (2006). Understanding emotions in others: Mirror neuron dysfunction in children with autism spectrum disorders. *Nature Neuroscience*, *9*(1), 28–30.

Davidovitch, M., Golan, D., Vardi, O., Lev, D., & Lerman-Sagie, T. (2011). Israeli children with autism spectrum disorder are not macrocephalic. *Journal of Child Neurology*, *26*(5), 580–585.

Davidovitch, M., Hemo, B., Manning-Courtney, P., & Fombonne, E. (2013). Prevalence and incidence of autism spectrum disorder in an Israeli population. *Journal of Autism and Developmental Disorders*, *43*(4), 785–793.

Davidovitch, M., Patterson, B., & Gartside, P. (1996). Head circumference measurements in children with autism. *Journal of Child Neurology*, *11*(5), 389–393.

Dawson, G., Ashman, S. B., & Carver, L. J. (2000). The role of early experience in shaping behavioral and brain development and its implications for social policy. *Development and Psychopathology*, *12*(4), 695–712.

Dawson, G., Carver, L., Meltzoff, A. N., Panagiotides, H., McPartland, J., & Webb, S. J. (2002). Neural correlates of face and object recognition in young children with autism spectrum disorder, developmental delay, and typical development. *Child Development*, *73*(3), 700–717.

Dawson, G., Estes, A., Munson, J., Schellenberg, G., Bernier, R., & Abbott, R. (2007). Quantitative assessment of autism symptom-related traits in probands and parents: Broader phenotype autism symptom scale. *Journal of Autism and Developmental Disorders*, *37*(3), 523–536.

Dawson, G., & Lewy, A. (1989). Reciprocal subcortical-cortical influences in autism: The role of attentional mechanisms. In G. Dawson (Ed.), *Autism: Nature, Diagnosis, and Treatment* (pp. 144–173, xxv, 417). New York: Guilford Press.

Dawson, G., Meltzoff, A. N., Osterling, J., Rinaldi, J., & Brown, E. (1998). Children with autism fail to orient to naturally occurring social stimuli. *Journal of Autism and Developmental Disorders*, *28*(6), 479–485.

Dawson, G., Munson, J., Webb, S. J., Nalty, T., Abbott, R., & Toth, K. (2007). Rate of head growth decelerates and symptoms worsen in the second year of life in autism. *Biological Psychiatry*, *61*(4), 458–464.

Dawson, G., Webb, S. J., & McPartland, J. (2005). Understanding the nature of face processing impairment in autism: Insights from behavioral and electrophysiological studies. *Developmental Neuropsychology*, *27*(3), 403–424.

Dawson, G., Webb, S. J., Wijsman, E., Schellenberg, G., Estes, A., Munson, J., & Faja, S. (2005). Neurocognitive and electrophysiological evidence of altered face processing in parents of children with autism: Implications for a model of abnormal development of social brain circuitry in autism. *Developmental Psychopathology*, *17*(3), 679–697.

Dawson, M., Soulieres, I., Gernsbacher, M. A., & Mottron, L. (2007). The level and nature of autistic intelligence. *Psychological Science*, *18*(8), 657–662.

Daymont, C., Hwang, W. T., Feudtner, C., & Rubin, D. (2010). Head-circumference distribution in a large primary care network differs from CDC and WHO curves. *Pediatrics*, *126*(4), e836–842.

De Giacomo, A., & Fombonne, E. (1998). Parental recognition of developmental abnormalities in autism. *European Child and Adolescent Psychiatry*, *7*(3), 131–136.

de Graaf-Peters, V. B., & Hadders-Algra, M. (2006). Ontogeny of the human central nervous system: What is happening when? *Early Human Development*, *82*(4), 257–266.

de Villiers, J. (2000). Language and theory of mind: What are the developmental relationships? In S. Baron-Cohen, H. Tager-Flusberg, & D. J. Cohen (Eds.), *Understanding Other Minds: Perspectives From Developmental Cognitive Neuroscience* (pp. 83–123). Oxford, UK: Oxford University Press.

DeGangi, G. A., Breinbauer, C., Roosevelt, J. D., Porges, S., & Greenspan, S. (2000). Prediction of childhood problems at three years in children experiencing disorders of regulation during infancy. *Infant Mental Health Journal*, *21*(3), 156–175.

DeLorey, T. M. (2005). GABRB3 gene deficient mice: A potential model of autism spectrum disorder. *International Review of Neurobiology*, *71*, 359–382.

Delorme, R., Gousse, V., Roy, I., Trandafir, A., Mathieu, F., Mouren-Simeoni, M. C., . . . Leboyer, M. (2007). Shared executive dysfunctions in unaffected relatives of patients with autism and obsessive-compulsive disorder. *European Psychiatry*, *22*(1), 32–38.

Dementieva, Y. A., Vance, D. D., Donnelly, S. L., Elston, L. A., Wolpert, C. M., Ravan, S. A., . . . Cuccaro, M. L. (2005). Accelerated head growth in early development of individuals with autism. *Pediatric Neurology*, *32*(2), 102–108.

Demopoulos, C., Hopkins, J., & Davis, A. (2013). A comparison of social cognitive profiles in children with autism spectrum disorders and attention-deficit/hyperactivity disorder: A matter of quantitative but not qualitative difference? *Journal of Autism and Developmental Disorders*, *43*(5), 1157–1170.

Dennis, M., Lazenby, A. L., & Lockyer, L. (2001). Inferential language in high-function children with autism. *Journal of Autism and Developmental Disorders*, *31*(1), 47–54.

Dennis, M., Simic, N., Bigler, E. D., Abildskov, T., Agostino, A., Taylor, H. G., . . . Yeates, K. O. (2013). Cognitive, affective, and conative Theory of Mind (ToM) in children with traumatic brain injury. *Developmental Cognitive Neuroscience*, *5*, 25–39.

Deoni, S.C.L., Zinkstok, J. R., Daly, E., Ecker, C., Williams, S.C.R., Murphy, D.G.M., & Consortium, M. A. (2015). White-matter relaxation time and myelin water fraction differences in young adults with autism. *Psychological Medicine*, *45*(4), 795–805.

Deonna, T., & Roulet, E. (2006). Autistic spectrum disorder: Evaluating a possible contributing or causal role of epilepsy. *Epilepsia*, *47*(Suppl 2), 79–82.

Deonna, T., & Roulet-Perez, E. (2010). Early onset acquired epileptic aphasia (Landau-Kleffner syndrome, LKS) and regressive autistic disorders with epileptic EEG abnormalities: The continuing debate. *Brain and Development*, *32*(9), 746–752.

Deonna, T., Roulet-Perez, E., Chappuis, H., & Ziegler, A. L. (2007). 'Autistic regression associated with seizure onset in an infant with tuberous sclerosis'. *Developmental Medicine and Child Neurology*, *49*(4), 320.

Deonna, T., Ziegler, A. L., Moura-Serra, J., & Innocenti, G. (1993). Autistic regression in relation to limbic pathology and epilepsy: Report of two cases. *Developmental Medicine and Child Neurology*, *35*(2), 166–176.

Depino, A. M. (2013). Peripheral and central inflammation in autism spectrum disorders. *Molecular and Cellular Neuroscience*, *53*, 69–76.

Deth, R., Muratore, C., Benzecry, J., Power-Charnitsky, V. A., & Waly, M. (2008). How environmental and genetic factors combine to cause autism: A redox/methylation hypothesis. *Neurotoxicology*, *29*(1), 190–201.

Deutsch, C. K., Folstein, S., Tager-Flusberg, H., & Gordon-Vaughn, K. G. (1999). Macrocephaly in autism pedigrees. *American Journal of Human Genetics*, *65*(4), A147–A147.

Deutsch, C. K., & Joseph, R. M. (2003). Brief report: Cognitive correlates of enlarged head circumference in children with autism. *Journal of Autism and Developmental Disorders*, *33*(2), 209–215.

Deverman, B. E., & Patterson, P. H. (2009). Cytokines and CNS development. *Neuron*, *64*(1), 61–78.

DeVito, T. J., Drost, D. J., Neufeld, R.W.J., Rajakumar, N., Pavlosky, W., Williamson, P., & Nicolson, R. (2007). Evidence for cortical dysfunction in autism: A proton magnetic resonance spectroscopic imaging study. *Biological Psychiatry*, *61*(4), 465–473.

Devlin, B., & Scherer, S. W. (2012). Genetic architecture in autism spectrum disorder. *Current Opinion in Genetics and Development*, *22*(3), 229–237.

Dewey, D., Cantell, M., & Crawford, S. G. (2007). Motor and gestural performance in children with autism spectrum disorders, developmental coordination disorder, and/or attention deficit hyperactivity disorder. *Journal of the International Neuropsychological Society*, *13*(2), 246–256.

Diehl, J. J., Bennetto, L., Watson, D., Gunlogson, C., & McDonough, J. (2008). Resolving ambiguity: A psycholinguistic approach to understanding prosody processing in high-functioning autism. *Brain and Language*, *106*(2), 144–152.

Diehl, J. J., Bennetto, L., & Young, E. C. (2006). Story recall and narrative coherence of high-functioning children with autism spectrum disorders. *Journal of Abnormal Child Psychology*, *34*(1), 87–102.

Di Martino, A., Ross, K., Uddin, L. Q., Sklar, A. B., Castellanos, F. X., & Milham, M. P. (2009). Functional brain correlates of social and nonsocial processes in autism spectrum disorders: An activation likelihood estimation meta-analysis. *Biological Psychiatry*, *65*(1), 63–74.

Dissanayake, C., Bui, Q. M., Huggins, R., & Loesch, D. Z. (2006). Growth in stature and head circumference in high-functioning autism and Asperger disorder during the first 3 years of life. *Development and Psychopathology*, *18*(2), 381–393.

Dodell-Feder, D., Koster-Hale, J., Bedny, M., & Saxe, R. (2011). fMRI item analysis in a theory of mind task. *Neuroimage*, *55*(2), 705–712.

Dowd, A. M., McGinley, J. L., Taffe, J. R., & Rinehart, N. J. (2012). Do planning and visual integration difficulties underpin motor dysfunction in autism? A kinematic study of young children with autism. *Journal of Autism and Developmental Disorders*, *42*(8), 1539–1548.

Dowell, L. R., Mahone, E. M., & Mostofsky, S. H. (2009). Associations of postural knowledge and basic motor skill with dyspraxia in autism: Implication for abnormalities in distributed connectivity and motor learning. *Neuropsychology*, *23*(5), 563–570.

Doyle-Thomas, K. A., Lee, W., Foster, N. E., Tryfon, A., Ouimet, T., Hyde, K. L., . . . NeuroDevNet, A.S.D.I.G. (2015). Atypical functional brain connectivity during rest in autism spectrum disorders. *Annals of Neurology*, *77*(5), 866–876.

Duffy, F. H., Shankardass, A., McAnulty, G. B., Eksioglu, Y. Z., Coulter, D., Rotenberg, A., & Als, H. (2014). Corticosteroid therapy in regressive autism: A retrospective study of effects on the Frequency Modulated Auditory Evoked Response (FMAER), language, and behavior. *BMC Neurology*, *14*, 70.

Dufour-Rainfray, D., Vourc'h, P., Tourlet, S., Guilloteau, D., Chalon, S., & Andres, C. R. (2011). Fetal exposure to teratogens: Evidence of genes involved in autism. *Neuroscience and Biobehavioral Reviews*, *35*(5), 1254–1265.

Dulac, O. (2001). Epileptic encephalopathy. *Epilepsia*, *42*(Suppl 3), 23–26.

Dunbar, R.I.M. (2012). The social brain meets neuroimaging. *Trends in Cognitive Sciences*, *16*(2), 101–102.

Dunn, M., Gomes, H., & Sebastian, M. (1996). Prototypicality of responses in autistic, language-disordered, and normal children in a word fluency task. *Child Neuropsychology*, *2*, 99–108.

Dunn, W., & Westman, K. (1997). The sensory profile: The performance of a national sample of children without disabilities. *American Journal of Occupational Therapy*, *51*(1), 25–34.

Dworzynski, K., Ronald, A., Bolton, P., & Happe, F. (2012). How different are girls and boys above and below the diagnostic threshold for autism spectrum disorders? *Journal of the American Academy of Child and Adolescent Psychiatry*, *51*(8), 788–797.

Dziuk, M. A., Gidley Larson, J. C., Apostu, A., Mahone, E. M., Denckla, M. B., & Mostofsky, S. H. (2007). Dyspraxia in autism: Association with motor, social, and communicative deficits. *Developmental Medicine and Child Neurology*, *49*(10), 734–739.

Ebisch, S. J., Gallese, V., Willems, R. M., Mantini, D., Groen, W. B., Romani, G. L., . . . Bekkering, H. (2010). Altered intrinsic functional connectivity of anterior and posterior insula regions in high-functioning participants with autism spectrum disorder. *Human Brain Mapping*, *32*(7), 1013–1028.

Ecker, C., Ronan, L., Feng, Y., Daly, E., Murphy, C., Ginestet, C. E., . . . Murphy, D. G. (2013). Intrinsic gray-matter connectivity of the brain in adults with autism spectrum disorder. *Proceedings of the National Academy of Sciences of the United States of America*, *110*(32), 13222–13227.

Edmonson, C., Ziats, M. N., & Rennert, O. M. (2014). Altered glial marker expression in autistic post-mortem prefrontal cortex and cerebellum. *Molecular Autism*, *5*(1), 3.

Edwards, M. J. (2006). Review: Hyperthermia and fever during pregnancy. *Birth Defects Research Part a-Clinical and Molecular Teratology*, *76*(7), 507–516.

Ehlers, S., Gillberg, C., & Wing, L. (1999). A screening questionnaire for Asperger syndrome and other high-functioning autism spectrum disorders in school age children. *Journal of Autism and Developmental Disorders*, *29*(2), 129–141.

Eigsti, I. M., Bennetto, L., & Dadlani, M. B. (2007). Beyond pragmatics: Morphosyntactic development in autism. *Journal of Autism and Developmental Disorders*, *37*(6), 1007–1023.

Eigsti, I. M., & Fein, D. A. (2013). More is less: Pitch discrimination and language delays in children with optimal outcomes from autism. *Autism Research: Official Journal of the International Society for Autism Research*, *6*(6), 605–613.

Eigsti, I. M., Schuh, J., Mencl, E., Schultz, R. T., & Paul, R. (2012). The neural underpinnings of prosody in autism. *Child Neuropsychology*, *18*(6), 600–617.

Eisenberg, L., & Kanner, L. (1956). Early infantile autism, 1943–55, Childhood Schizophrenia Symposium, 1955. *American Journal of Orthopsychiatry*, *26*(3), 556–566.

Elder, L. M., Dawson, G., Toth, K., Fein, D., & Munson, J. (2008). Head circumference as an early predictor of autism symptoms in younger siblings of children with autism spectrum disorder. *Journal of Autism and Developmental Disorders*, *38*(6), 1104–1111.

Elia, J., Laracy, S., Allen, J., Nissley-Tsiopinis, J., & Borgmann-Winter, K. (2012). Epigenetics: Genetics versus life experiences. *Current Topics in Behavioral Neurosciences*, *9*, 317–340.

Elsabbagh, M., Divan, G., Koh, Y. J., Kim, Y. S., Kauchali, S., Marcin, C., . . . Fombonne, E. (2012). Global prevalence of autism and other pervasive developmental disorders. *Autism Research: Official Journal of the International Society for Autism Research*, *5*(3), 160–179.

Elsabbagh, M., Fernandes, J., Jane Webb, S., Dawson, G., Charman, T., & Johnson, M. H. (2013). Disengagement of visual attention in infancy is associated with emerging autism in toddlerhood. *Biological Psychiatry*, *74*(3), 189–194.

Endo, T., Shioiri, T., Kitamura, H., Kimura, T., Endo, S., Masuzawa, N., & Someya, T. (2007). Altered chemical metabolites in the amygdala-hippocampus region contribute to autistic symptoms of autism spectrum disorders. *Biological Psychiatry*, *62*(9), 1030–1037.

Fair, D. A., Dosenbach, N. U., Church, J. A., Cohen, A. L., Brahmbhatt, S., Miezin, F. M., . . . Schlaggar, B. L. (2007). Development of distinct control networks through segregation and integration. *Proceedings of the National Academy of Sciences*, *104*(33), 13507–13512.

Fair, D. A., Nigg, J. T., Iyer, S., Bathula, D., Mills, K. L., Dosenbach, N. U., . . . Milham, M. P. (2012). Distinct neural signatures detected for ADHD subtypes after controlling for micro-movements in resting state functional connectivity MRI data. *Frontiers in Systems Neuroscience*, *6*, 80.

Farley, M. A., McMahon, W. M., Fombonne, E., Jenson, W. R., Miller, J., Gardner, M., . . . Coon, H. (2009). Twenty-year outcome for individuals with autism and average or near-average cognitive abilities. *Autism Research: Official Journal of the International Society for Autism Research*, *2*(2), 109–118.

Farroni, T., Menon, E., Rigato, S., & Johnson, M. H. (2007). The perception of facial expressions in newborns. *European Journal of Developmental Psychology*, *4*(1), 2–13.

Fatemi, S. H., Aldinger, K. A., Ashwood, P., Bauman, M. L., Blaha, C. D., Blatt, G. J., . . . Welsh, J. P. (2012). Consensus paper: Pathological role of the cerebellum in autism. *Cerebellum*, *11*(3), 777–807.

Fatemi, S. H., Earle, J., Kanodia, R., Kist, D., Emamian, E. S., Patterson, P. H., . . . Sidwell, R. (2002). Prenatal viral infection leads to pyramidal cell atrophy and macrocephaly in adulthood: Implications for genesis of autism and schizophrenia. *Cellular and Molecular Neurobiology*, *22*(1), 25–33.

Fatemi, S. H., Emamian, E. S., Sidwell, R. W., Kist, D. A., Stary, J. M., Earle, J. A., & Thuras, P. (2002). Human influenza viral infection in utero alters glial fibrillary acidic protein immunoreactivity in the developing brains of neonatal mice. *Molecular Psychiatry*, *7*(6), 633–640.

Fatemi, S. H., Folsom, T. D., Reutiman, T. J., Abu-Odeh, D., Mori, S., Huang, H., & Oishi, K. (2009). Abnormal expression of myelination genes and alterations in white matter fractional anisotropy following prenatal viral influenza infection at E16 in mice. *Schizophrenia Research*, *112*(1–3), 46–53.

Fatemi, S. H., Folsom, T. D., Reutiman, T. J., Huang, H., Oishi, K., & Mori, S. (2009). Prenatal viral infection of mice at E16 causes changes in gene expression in hippocampi of the offspring. *European Neuropsychopharmacology*, *19*(9), 648–653.

Fatemi, S. H., Reutiman, T. J., Folsom, T. D., Huang, H., Oishi, K., Mori, S., . . . Juckel, G. (2008). Maternal infection leads to abnormal gene regulation and brain atrophy in mouse offspring: Implications for genesis of neurodevelopmental disorders. *Schizophrenia Research*, *99*(1–3), 56–70.

Fatemi, S. H., Reutiman, T. J., Folsom, T. D., & Thuras, P. D. (2009). GABA(A) receptor downregulation in brains of subjects with autism. *Journal of Autism and Developmental Disorders*, *39*(2), 223–230.

Fatemi, S. H., Snow, A. V., Stary, J. M., Araghi-Niknam, M., Reutiman, T. J., Lee, S., . . . Pearce, D. A. (2005). Reelin signaling is impaired in autism. *Biological Psychiatry*, *57*(7), 777–787.

Fein, D. (Ed.). (2011). *The Neuropsychology of Autism*. New York: Oxford University Press.

Fein, D., Dunn, M., Allen, D. A., Aram, D. M., Hall, N., Morris, R., & Wilson, B. C. (1996). Neuropsychological and language data. In I. Rapin (Ed.), *Preschool Children with Inadequate Communication: Developmental Language Disorder, Autism, Low IQ* (pp. 123–154). London: Mac Keith Press.

Fein, D., Stevens, M., Dunn, M., Waterhouse, L., Allen, D., Rapin, I., & Feinstein, C. (1999). Subtypes of pervasive developmental disorder: Clinical characteristics. *Child Neuropsychology*, *5*(1), 1–23.

Fein, D., Tinder, P., & Waterhouse, L. (1979). Stimulus generalization in autistic and normal children. *Journal of Child Psychology and Psychiatry*, *20*(4), 325–335.

Feldman, M. A., Ward, R. A., Savona, D., Regehr, K., Parker, K., Hudson, M., . . . Holden, J. J. (2011). Development and initial validation of a parent report measure of the behavioral development of infants at risk for autism spectrum disorders. *Journal of Autism and Developmental Disorders, 42*(1), 13–22.

Fidler, D. J., Bailey, J. N., & Smalley, S. L. (2000). Macrocephaly in autism and other pervasive developmental disorders. *Developmental Medicine and Child Neurology*, *42*(11), 737–740.

Fine, C., Lumsden, J., & Blair, R. J. (2001). Dissociation between 'theory of mind' and executive functions in a patient with early left amygdala damage. *Brain*, *124*(Pt 2), 287–298.

Fine, J. G., Musielak, K. A., & Semrud-Clikeman, M. (2014). Smaller splenium in children with nonverbal learning disability compared to controls, high-functioning autism and ADHD. *Child Neuropsychology: A Journal on Normal and Abnormal Development in Childhood and Adolescence*, *20*(6), 641–661.

Fisher, N., Happe, F., & Dunn, J. (2005). The relationship between vocabulary, grammar, and false belief task performance in children with autistic spectrum disorders and children with moderate learning difficulties. *Journal of Child Psychology and Psychiatry*, *46*(4), 409–419.

Fishman, M. A. (1990). *Developmental Defects*. Philadelphia, PA: Lippincott.

Fletcher, H. M. (1900). A case of megalencephaly. *Transactions of a Pathological Society of London*, *51*, 230–232.

Fletcher, P. T., Whitaker, R. T., Tao, R., DuBray, M. B., Froehlich, A., Ravichandran, C., . . . Lainhart, J. E. (2010). Microstructural connectivity of the arcuate fasciculus in adolescents with high-functioning autism. *Neuroimage*, *51*(3), 1117–1125.

Floris, D. L., Chura, L. R., Holt, R. J., Suckling, J., Bullmore, E. T., Baron-Cohen, S., & Spencer, M. D. (2013). Psychological correlates of handedness and corpus callosum asymmetry in autism: The left hemisphere dysfunction theory revisited. *Journal of Autism and Developmental Disorders*, *43*(8), 1758–1772.

Folstein, S. E., & Rutter, M. L. (1977). Infantile autism: A genetic study of 21 twin pairs. *Journal of Child Psychology and Psychiatry and Allied Disciplines*, *18*(4), 297–321.

Folstein, S. E., & Rutter, M. L. (1988). Autism: Familial aggregation and genetic implications. *Journal of Autism and Developmental Disorders*, *18*(1), 3–30.

Fombonne, E. (1999). The epidemiology of autism: A review. *Psychological Medicine*, *29*(4), 769–786.

Fombonne, E. (2009). Epidemiology of pervasive developmental disorders. *Pediatric Research*, *65*(6), 591–598.

Fombonne, E., & Chakrabarti, S. (2001). No evidence for a new variant of measles-mumps-rubella-induced autism. *Pediatrics*, *108*(4), E58.

Fombonne, E., Quirke, S., & Hagen, A. (2009). Prevalence and interpretation of recent trends in rates of pervasive developmental disorders. *McGill Journal of Medicine*, *12*(2), 73.

Fombonne, E., Quirke, S., & Hagen, A. (2011). Epidemiology of pervasive developmental disorders. In D. G. Amaral, G. Dawson, & D. H. Geschwind (Eds.), *Autism Spectrum Disorders* (pp. 90–111). New York: Oxford University Press.

Fombonne, E., Roge, B., Claverie, J., Courty, S., & Fremolle, J. (1999). Microcephaly and macrocephaly in autism. *Journal of Autism and Developmental Disorders*, *29*(2), 113–119.

Franks, D. D. (2010) Neurosociology: The Nexus Between Neuroscience and Social Psychology, New York, NY: Springer Press.

Frazier, T. W., Youngstrom, E. A., Speer, L., Embacher, R., Law, P., Constantino, J., . . . Eng, C. (2012). Validation of proposed DSM-5 criteria for autism spectrum disorder. *Journal of the American Academy of Child and Adolescent Psychiatry*, *51*(1), 28–40 e23.

Freitag, C. M. (2008). [The genetics of autistic disorders]. *Zeitschrift fur Kinder-und Jugendpsychiatrie und Psychotherapie*, *36*(1), 7–14; quiz 14–15.

Freitag, C. M., Konrad, C., Haberlen, M., Kleser, C., von Gontard, A., Reith, W., . . . Krick, C. (2008). Perception of biological motion in autism spectrum disorders. *Neuropsychologia*, *46*(5), 1480–1494.

Freitag, C. M., Luders, E., Hulst, H. E., Narr, K. L., Thompson, P. M., Toga, A. W., . . . Konrad, C. (2009). Total brain volume and corpus callosum size in medication-naive adolescents and young adults with autism spectrum disorder. *Biological Psychiatry*, *66*(4), 316–319.

Freitag, C. M., Staal, W., Klauck, S. M., Duketis, E., & Waltes, R. (2010). Genetics of autistic disorders: Review and clinical implications. *European Journal of Child and Adolescent Psychiatry*, *19*(3), 169–178.

Friederici, A. D. (2011). The brain basis of language processing: From structure to function. *Physiological Reviews*, *91*(4), 1357–1392.

Friston, K. J. (2011). Functional and effective connectivity: A review. *Brain Connectivity*, *1*(1), 13–36.

Frith, C. D. (2004). Is autism a disconnection disorder? *Lancet Neurology*, *3*(10), 577.

Frith, U., & Frith, C. (2010). The social brain: Allowing humans to boldly go where no other species has been. *Philosophical Transactions of the Royal Society of London Series B-Biological Sciences*, *365*(1537), 165–176.

Gabig, C. S. (2008). Verbal working memory and story retelling in school-age children with autism. *Language, Speech, and Hearing Services in Schools*, *39*(4), 498–511.

Gaetz, W., Bloy, L., Wang, D. J., Port, R. G., Blaskey, L., Levy, S. E., & Roberts, T.P.L. (2014). GABA estimation in the brains of children on the autism spectrum: Measurement precision and regional cortical variation. *Neuroimage*, *86*, 1–9.

Gaigg, S. B., & Bowler, D. M. (2008). Free recall and forgetting of emotionally arousing words in autism spectrum disorder. *Neuropsychologia*, *46*(9), 2336–2343.

Gaigg, S. B., & Bowler, D. M. (2009). Illusory memories of emotionally charged words in autism spectrum disorder: Further evidence for atypical emotion processing outside the social domain. *Journal of Autism and Developmental Disorders*, *39*(7), 1031–1038.

Gaigg, S. B., Gardiner, J. M., & Bowler, D. A. (2008). Free recall in autism spectrum disorder: The role of relational and item-specific encoding. *Neuropsychologia*, *46*(4), 983–992.

Ganz, M. (2006). The costs of autism. In S. O. Moldin & J. L. Rubenstein (Eds.), *Understanding Autism* (pp. 475–502). Boca Raton, FLA: Taylor and Francis.

Garay, P. A., Hsiao, E. Y., Patterson, P. H., & McAllister, A. K. (2013). Maternal immune activation causes age-and region-specific changes in brain cytokines in offspring throughout development. *Brain Behavior and Immunity*, *31*, 54–68.

Gardiner, J. M., Bowler, D. M., & Grice, S. J. (2003). Further evidence of preserved priming and impaired recall in adults with Asperger's syndrome. *Journal of Autism and Developmental Disorders*, *33*(3), 259–269.

Garon, N., Bryson, S. E., Zwaigenbaum, L., Smith, I. M., Brian, J., Roberts, W., & Szatmari, P. (2009). Temperament and its relationship to autistic symptoms in a high-risk infant sib cohort. *Journal of Abnormal Child Psychology*, *37*(1), 59–78.

Garretson, H. B., Fein, D., & Waterhouse, L. (1990). Sustained attention in children with autism. *Journal of Autism and Developmental Disorders*, *20*(1), 101–114.

Gaugler, T., Klei, L., Sanders, S. J., Bodea, C. A., Goldberg, A. P., Lee, A. B., . . . Buxbaum, J. D. (2014). Most genetic risk for autism resides with common variation. *Nature Genetics*, *46*(8), 881–885.

Gauthier, I., Curran, T., Curby, K. M., & Collins, D. (2003). Perceptual interference supports a non-modular account of face processing. *Nature Neuroscience*, *6*(4), 428–432.

Gauthier, J., Bonnel, A., St-Onge, J., Karemera, L., Laurent, S., Mottron, L., . . . Rouleau, G. A. (2005). NLGN3/NLGN4 gene mutations are not responsible for autism in the Quebec population. *American Journal of Medical Genetics Part B-Neuropsychiatric Genetics*, *132B*(1), 74–75.

Ge, J. Q., & Han, S. H. (2008). Distinct neurocognitive strategies for comprehensions of human and artificial intelligence. *PLoS One*, *3*(7), E3797.

Ge, W. P., Miyawaki, A., Gage, F. H., Jan, Y. N., & Jan, L. Y. (2012). Local generation of glia is a major astrocyte source in postnatal cortex. *Nature*, *484*(7394), 376–U381.

Geier, D. A., & Geier, M. R. (2007). A prospective study of mercury toxicity biomarkers in autistic spectrum disorders. *Journal of Toxicology and Environmental Health: Part A*, *70*(20), 1723–1730.

Gernsbacher, M. A., Sauer, E. A., Geye, H. M., Schweigert, E. K., & Hill Goldsmith, H. (2008). Infant and toddler oral-and manual-motor skills predict later speech fluency in autism. *Journal of Child Psychology and Psychiatry*, *49*(1), 43–50.

Gervais, H., Belin, P., Boddaert, N., Leboyer, M., Coez, A., Ignacio, S., . . . Zilbovicius, M. (2004). Abnormal cortical voice processing in autism. *Nature Neuroscience*, *7*(8), 801–802.

Geschwind, D. H., & Levitt, P. (2007). Autism spectrum disorders: Developmental disconnection syndromes. *Current Opinion in Neurobiology*, *17*(1), 103–111.

Gesundheit, B., Rosenzweig, J. P., Naor, D., Lerer, B., Zachor, D. A., Prochazka, V., . . . Ashwood, P. (2013). Immunological and autoimmune considerations of autism spectrum disorders. *Journal of Autoimmunity*, *44*, 1–7.

Geurts, H., Sinzig, J., Booth, R., & Happe, F. (2014). Neuropsychological heterogeneity in executive functioning in autism spectrum disorders. *International Journal of Developmental Disabilities*, *60*(3), 155–162.

Geurts, H. M., Corbett, B., & Solomon, M. (2009). The paradox of cognitive flexibility in autism. *Trends in Cognitive Sciences*, *13*(2), 74–82.

Ghaziuddin, M., Al-Khouri, I., & Ghaziuddin, N. (2002). Autistic symptoms following herpes encephalitis. *European Child and Adolescent Psychiatry*, *11*(3), 142–146.

Ghaziuddin, M., & Butler, E. (1998). Clumsiness in autism and Asperger syndrome: A further report. *Journal of Intellectual Disability Research*, *42*(Pt 1), 43–48.

Ghaziuddin, M., Zaccagnini, J., Tsai, L., & Elardo, S. (1999). Is megalencephaly specific to autism? *Journal of Intellectual Disability Research*, *43*, 279–282.

Giagtzoglou, N., Ly, C. V., & Bellen, H. J. (2009). Cell adhesion, the backbone of the synapse: "Vertebrate" and "invertebrate" perspectives. *Cold Spring Harbor Perspectives in Biology*, *1*(4), a003079.

Giannotti, F., Cortesi, F., Cerquiglini, A., Vagnoni, C., & Valente, D. (2011). Sleep in children with autism with and without autistic regression. *Journal of Sleep Research*, *20*(2), 338–347.

Giarelli, E., Wiggins, L. D., Rice, C. E., Levy, S. E., Kirby, R. S., Pinto-Martin, J., & Mandell, D. (2010). Sex differences in the evaluation and diagnosis of autism spectrum disorders among children. *Disability and Health Journal*, *3*(2), 107–116.

Gibbs, V., Aldridge, F., Chandler, F., Witzlsperger, E., & Smith, K. (2012). Brief report: An exploratory study comparing diagnostic outcomes for autism spectrum disorders under DSM-IV-TR with the proposed DSM-5 revision. *Journal of Autism and Developmental Disorders*, *42*(8), 1750–1756.

Gillberg, C. (1986). Brief report: Onset at age 14 of a typical autistic syndrome: A case report of a girl with herpes simplex encephalitis. *Journal of Autism and Developmental Disorders*, *16*(3), 369–375.

Gillberg, C. (1999). Prevalence of disorders in the autism spectrum. *Infants and Young Children*, *12*(2), 64–74.

Gillberg, C., Cederlund, M., Lamberg, K., & Zeijlon, L. (2006). Brief report: "The autism epidemic": The registered prevalence of autism in a Swedish urban area. *Journal of Autism and Developmental Disorders*, *36*(3), 429–435.

Gillberg, C., & de Souza, L. (2002). Head circumference in autism, Asperger syndrome, and ADHD: A comparative study. *Developmental Medicine and Child Neurology*, *44*(5), 296–300.

Gillberg, C., & Steffenburg, S. (1987). Outcome and prognostic factors in infantile autism and similar conditions: A population-based study of 46 cases followed through puberty. *Journal of Autism and Developmental Disorders*, *17*(2), 273–287.

Gillberg, C., Winnergard, I., & Wahlstroem, J. (1984). The sex chromosomes-one key to autism? An XYY case of infantile autism. *Applied Research in Mental Retardation*, *5*(3), 353–360.

Gilliam, J. E. (2013). *Gilliam Autism Rating Scale, Third Edition (GARS-3)*. Torrance, CA: Western Psychological Services.

Gilman, S. R., Iossifov, I., Levy, D., Ronemus, M., Wigler, M., & Vitkup, D. (2011). Rare de novo variants associated with autism implicate a large functional network of genes involved in formation and function of synapses. *Neuron*, *70*(5), 898–907.

Giovedi, S., Corradi, A., Fassio, A., & Benfenati, F. (2014). Involvement of synaptic genes in the pathogenesis of autism spectrum disorders: The case of synapsins. *Frontiers in Pediatrics*, *2*, 94.

Gliga, T., Jones, E. J., Bedford, R., Charman, T., & Johnson, M. H. (2014). From early markers to neuro-developmental mechanisms of autism. *Developmental Review*, *34*(3), 189–207.

Goin-Kochel, R. P., Esler, A. N., Kanne, S. M., & Hus, V. (2014). Developmental regression among children with autism spectrum disorder: Onset, duration, and effects on functional outcomes. *Research in Autism Spectrum Disorders*, *8*(7), 890–898.

Goines, P. E., & Ashwood, P. (2013). Cytokine dysregulation in autism spectrum disorders (ASD): Possible role of the environment. *Neurotoxicology and Teratology*, *36*, 67–81.

Goldberg, M. C., Mostofsky, S. H., Cutting, L. E., Mahone, E. M., Astor, B. C., Denckla, M. B., & Landa, R. J. (2005). Subtle executive impairment in children with autism and children with ADHD. *Journal of Autism and Developmental Disorders*, *35*(3), 279–293.

Goldberg, M. C., Mostow, A. J., Vecera, S. P., Larson, J. C., Mostofsky, S. H., Mahone, E. M., & Denckla, M. B. (2008). Evidence for impairments in using static line drawings of eye gaze cues to orient visual-spatial attention in children with high functioning autism. *Journal of Autism and Developmental Disorders*, *38*(8), 1405–1413.

Goldberg, W. A., Osann, K., Filipek, P. A., Laulhere, T., Jarvis, K., Modahl, C., . . . Spence, M. A. (2003). Language and other regression: Assessment and timing. *Journal of Autism and Developmental Disorders*, *33*(6), 607–616.

Goldberg, W. A., Thorsen, K. L., Osann, K., & Spence, M. A. (2008). Use of home videotapes to confirm parental reports of regression in autism. *Journal of Autism and Developmental Disorders*, *38*(6), 1136–1146.

Goldstein, G., Johnson, C. R., & Minshew, N. J. (2001). Attentional processes in autism. *Journal of Autism and Developmental Disorders*, *31*(4), 433–440.

Goldstein, S., & Naglieri, J. A. (2012). *Autism Spectrum Rating Scales (ASRS)*. Torrance, CA: Western Psychological Services.

Golla, S., & Sweeney, J. A. (2014). Corticosteroid therapy in regressive autism: Preliminary findings from a retrospective study. *Bmc Medicine*, *12*, 79.

Gonzales, M. L., & LaSalle, J. M. (2010). The role of MeCP2 in brain development and neurodevelopmental disorders. *Current Psychiatry Reports*, *12*(2), 127–134.

Gonzalez-Toro, M. C., Jadraque-Rodriguez, R., Sempere-Perez, A., Martinez-Pastor, P., Jover-Cerda, J., & Gomez-Gosalvez, F. (2013). Anti-NMDA receptor encephalitis: Two paediatric cases. *Revista de Neurologia*, *57*(11), 504–508.

Goodbourn, P. T., Bosten, J. M., Bargary, G., Hogg, R. E., Lawrance-Owen, A. J., & Mollon, J. D. (2014). Variants in the 1q21 risk region are associated with a visual endophenotype of autism and schizophrenia. *Genes Brain and Behavior*, *13*(2), 144–151.

Gottesman, II, & Gould, T. D. (2003). The endophenotype concept in psychiatry: Etymology and strategic intentions. *American Journal of Psychiatry*, *160*(4), 636–645.

Gotts, S. J., Simmons, W. K., Milbury, L. A., Wallace, G. L., Cox, R. W., & Martin, A. (2012). Fractionation of social brain circuits in autism spectrum disorders. *Brain*, *135*, 2711–2725.

Goulden, N., Khusnulina, A., Davis, N. J., Bracewell, R. M., Bokde, A. L., McNulty, J. P., & Mullins, P. G. (2014). The salience network is responsible for switching between the default mode network and the central executive network: Replication from DCM. *Neuroimage*, *99*, 180–190.

Grafodatskaya, D., Chung, B., Szatmari, P., & Weksberg, R. (2010). Autism spectrum disorders and epigenetics. *Journal of the American Academy of Child and Adolescent Psychiatry*, *49*(8), 794–809.

Grandgeorge, M., Lemonnier, E., & Jallot, N. (2013). Autism spectrum disorders: Head circumference and body length at birth are both relative. *Acta Paediatrica*, *102*(9), 901–907.

Green, D., Charman, T., Pickles, A., Chandler, S., Loucas, T., Simonoff, E., & Baird, G. (2009). Impairment in movement skills of children with autistic spectrum disorders. *Developmental Medicine and Child Neurology*, *51*(4), 311–316.

Greenaway, R., & Plaisted, K. (2005). Top-down attentional modulation in autistic spectrum disorders is stimulus-specific. *Psychological Science*, *16*(12), 987–994.

Greenberg, D. A., Hodge, S. E., Sowinski, J., & Nicoll, D. (2001). Excess of twins among affected sibling pairs with autism: Implications for the etiology of autism. *American Journal of Medical Genetics*, *69*(5), 1062–1067.

Greicius, M. D., Supekar, K., Menon, V., & Dougherty, R. F. (2009). Resting-state functional connectivity reflects structural connectivity in the default mode network. *Cerebral Cortex*, *19*(1), 72–78.

Grether, J. K., Anderson, M. C., Croen, L. A., Smith, D., & Windham, G. C. (2009). Risk of autism and increasing maternal and paternal age in a large north American population. *American Journal of Epidemiology*, *170*(9), 1118–1126.

Grezes, J., Wicker, B., Berthoz, S., & de Gelder, B. (2009). A failure to grasp the affective meaning of actions in autism spectrum disorder subjects. *Neuropsychologia*, *47*(8–9), 1816–1825.

Grossman, J. B., Klin, A., Carter, A. S., & Volkmar, F. R. (2000). Verbal bias in recognition of facial emotions in children with Asperger syndrome. *Journal of Child Psychology and Psychiatry*, *41*(3), 369–379.

Guerin, P., Lyon, G., Barthelemy, C., Sostak, E., Chevrollier, V., Garreau, B., & Lelord, G. (1996). Neuropathological study of a case of autistic syndrome with severe mental retardation. *Developmental Medicine and Child Neurology*, *38*(3), 203–211.

Guilmatre, A., Huguet, G., Delorme, R., & Bourgeron, T. (2014). The emerging role of SHANK genes in neuropsychiatric disorders. *Developmental Neurobiology*, *74*(2), 113–122.

Gutierrez, R. C., Hung, J., Zhang, Y., Kertesz, A. C., Espina, F. J., & Colicos, M. A. (2009). Altered synchrony and connectivity in neuronal networks expressing an autism-related mutation of neuroligin 3. *Neuroscience*, *162*(1), 208–221.

Hadjikhani, N., Joseph, R. M., Snyder, J., Chabris, C. F., Clark, J., Steele, S., . . . Tager-Flusberg, H. (2004). Activation of the fusiform gyrus when individuals with autism spectrum disorder view faces. *Neuroimage*, *22*(3), 1141–1150.

Hadjikhani, N., Joseph, R. M., Snyder, J., & Tager-Flusberg, H. (2006). Anatomical differences in the mirror neuron system and social cognition network in autism. *Cerebral Cortex*, *16*(9), 1276–1282.

Hadjikhani, N., Joseph, R. M., Snyder, J., & Tager-Flusberg, H. (2007). Abnormal activation of the social brain during face perception in autism. *Human Brain Mapping*, *28*(5), 441–449.

Hahamy, A., Behrmann, M., & Malach, R. (2015). The idiosyncratic brain: Distortion of spontaneous connectivity patterns in autism spectrum disorder. *Nature Neuroscience*, *18*(2), 302–309.

Haist, F., Adamo, M., Westerfield, M., Courchesne, E., & Townsend, J. (2005). The functional neuroanatomy of spatial attention in autism spectrum disorder. *Developmental Neuropsychology*, *27*(3), 425–458.

Hala, S., Rasmussen, C., & Henderson, A. M. (2005). Three types of source monitoring by children with and without autism: The role of executive function. *Journal of Autism and Developmental Disorders*, *35*(1), 75–89.

Hallett, M., Lebiedowska, M. K., Thomas, S. L., Stanhope, S. J., Denckla, M.B., & Rumsey, J. (1993). Locomotion of autistic adults. *Archives of Neurology*, *50*(12), 1304–1308.

Hallmayer, J., Cleveland, S., Torres, A., Phillips, J., Cohen, B., Torigoe, T., . . . Risch, N. (2011). Genetic heritability and shared environmental factors among twin pairs with autism. *Archives of General Psychiatry*, *68*(11), 1095–1102.

Hansen, R. L., Ozonoff, S., Krakowiak, P., Angkustsiri, K., Jones, C., Deprey, L. J., . . . Hertz-Picciotto, I. (2008). Regression in autism: Prevalence and associated factors in the CHARGE study. *Ambulatory Pediatrics*, *8*(1), 25–31.

Hanson, D. R., & Gottesman, II. (1976). The genetics, if any, of infantile autism and childhood schizophrenia. *Journal of Autism and Childhood Schizophrenia*, *6*(3), 209–234.

Happé, F., Booth, R., Charlton, R., & Hughes, C. (2006). Executive function deficits in autism spectrum disorders and attention-deficit/hyperactivity disorder: Examining profiles across domains and ages. *Brain and Cognition*, *61*(1), 25–39.

Happé, F., Briskman, J., & Frith, U. (2001). Exploring the cognitive phenotype of autism: Weak "central coherence" in parents and siblings of children with autism: I. Experimental tests. *Journal of Child Psychology and Psychiatry*, *42*(3), 299–307.

Happé, F., Ehlers, S., Fletcher, P., Frith, U., Johansson, M., Gillberg, C., . . . Frith, C. (1996). 'Theory of mind' in the brain: Evidence from a PET scan study of Asperger syndrome. *Neuroreport*, *8*(1), 197–201.

Happé, F., & Frith, U. (2006). The weak coherence account: Detail-focused cognitive style in autism spectrum disorders. *Journal of Autism and Developmental Disorders*, *36*(1), 5–25.

Happé, F., & Ronald, A. (2008). The 'fractionable autism triad': A review of evidence from behavioural, genetic, cognitive and neural research. *Neuropsychology Review*, *18*(4), 287–304.

Harada, M., Taki, M. M., Nose, A., Kubo, H., Mori, K., Nishitani, H., & Matsuda, T. (2010). Non-invasive evaluation of the GABAergic/glutamatergic system in autistic patients observed by MEGA-editing proton MR spectroscopy using a clinical 3 tesla instrument. *Journal of Autism and Developmental Disorders*, *41*(4), 447–454.

Harada, M., Taki, M. M., Nose, A., Kubo, H., Mori, K., Nishitani, H., & Matsuda, T. (2011). Non-invasive evaluation of the GABAergic/glutamatergic system in autistic patients observed by MEGA-editing proton MR spectroscopy using a clinical 3 tesla instrument. *Journal of Autism and Developmental Disorders*, *41*(4), 447–454.

Hardan, A. Y., Libove, R. A., Keshavan, M. S., Melhem, N. M., & Minshew, N. J. (2009). A preliminary longitudinal magnetic resonance imaging study of brain volume and cortical thickness in autism. *Biological Psychiatry*, *66*(4), 320–326.

Hardan, A. Y., Minshew, N. J., Melhem, N. M., Srihari, S., Jo, B., Bansal, R., . . . Stanley, J. A. (2008). An MRI and proton spectroscopy study of the thalamus in children with autism. *Psychiatry Research: Neuroimaging Section*, *163*(2), 97–105.

Hardan, A. Y., Muddasani, S., Vemulapalli, M., Keshavan, M. S., & Minshew, N. J. (2006). An MRI study of increased cortical thickness in autism. *American Journal of Psychiatry*, *163*(7), 1290–1292.

Hardan, A. Y., Pabalan, M., Gupta, N., Bansal, R., Melhem, N. M., Fedorov, S., . . . Minshew, N. J. (2009). Corpus callosum volume in children with autism. *Psychiatry Research: Neuroimaging Section*, *174*(1), 57–61.

Harrington, J. W., Rosen, L., & Garnecho, A. (2006). Parental perceptions and use of complementary and alternative medicine practices for children with autistic spectrum disorders in private practice. *Journal of Developmental and Behavioral Pediatrics*, *27*(2), S156–S161.

Harris, G. J., Chabris, C. F., Clark, J., Urban, T., Aharon, I., Steele, S., . . . Tager-Flusberg, H. (2006). Brain activation during semantic processing in autism spectrum disorders via functional magnetic resonance imaging. *Brain and Cognition*, *61*(1), 54–68.

Harris, J. M., Best, C. S., Moffat, V. J., Spencer, M. D., Philip, R. C., Power, M. J., & Johnstone, E. C. (2008). Autistic traits and cognitive performance in young people with mild intellectual impairment. *Journal of Autism and Developmental Disorders*, *38*(7), 1241–1249.

Hashimoto, T., Tayama, M., Murakawa, K., Yoshimoto, T., Miyazaki, M., Harada, M., & Kuroda, Y. (1995). Development of the brainstem and cerebellum in autistic patients. *Journal of Autism and Developmental Disorders*, *25*(1), 1–18.

Haswell, C. C., Izawa, J., Dowell, L. R., Mostofsky, S. H., & Shadmehr, R. (2009). Representation of internal models of action in the autistic brain. *Nature Neuroscience*, *12*(8), 970–972.

Hauck, M., Fein, D., Maltby, N., Waterhouse, L., & Feinstein, C. (1998). Memory for faces in children with autism. *Child Neuropsychology*, *4*(3), 187–198.

Hazlett, H. C., Poe, M. D., Gerig, G., Smith, R. G., & Piven, J. (2006). Cortical gray and white brain tissue volume in adolescents and adults with autism. *Biological Psychiatry*, *59*(1), 1–6.

Hazlett, H. C., Poe, M. D., Gerig, G., Smith, R. G., Provenzale, J., Ross, A., . . . Piven, J. (2005). Magnetic resonance imaging and head circumference study of brain size in autism: Birth through age 2 years. *Archives of General Psychiatry*, *62*(12), 1366–1376.

Hazlett, H. C., Poe, M. D., Gerig, G., Styner, M., Chappell, C., Smith, R. G., . . . Piven, J. (2011). Early brain overgrowth in autism associated with an increase in cortical surface area before age 2 years. *Archives of General Psychiatry*, *68*(5), 467–476.

Hendry, C. N. (2000). Childhood disintegrative disorder: Should it be considered a distinct diagnosis? *Clinical Psychology Review*, *20*(1), 77–90.

Herbert, M. R. (2010). Contributions of the environment and environmentally vulnerable physiology to autism spectrum disorders. *Current Opinion in Neurology*, *23*(2), 103–110.

Herbert, M. R., Ziegler, D. A., Makris, N., Filipek, P. A., Kemper, T. L., Normandin, J. J., . . . Caviness, V. S., Jr. (2004). Localization of white matter volume increase in autism and developmental language disorder. *Annals of Neurology*, *55*(4), 530–540.

Herlihy, L., Knoch, K., Vibert, B., & Fein, D. (2013). Parents' first concerns about toddlers with autism spectrum disorder: Effect of sibling status. *Autism 19*(1), 20–28.

Herman, G. E., Butter, E., Enrile, B., Pastore, M., Prior, T. W., & Sommer, A. (2007). Increasing knowledge of PTEN germline mutations: Two additional patients with autism and macrocephaly. *American Journal of Medical Genetics Part A*, *143*(6), 589–593.

Hill, J., Dierker, D., Neil, J., Inder, T., Knutsen, A., Harwell, J., . . . Van Essen, D. (2010). A surface-based analysis of hemispheric asymmetries and folding of cerebral cortex in term-born human infants. *Journal of Neuroscience*, *30*(6), 2268–2276.

Hillier, A., Campbell, H., Keillor, J., Phillips, N., & Beversdorf, D. Q. (2007). Decreased false memory for visually presented shapes and symbols among adults on the autism spectrum. *Journal of Clinical and Experimental Neuropsychology*, *29*(6), 610–616.

Hirai, M., & Hiraki, K. (2005). An event-related potentials study of biological motion perception in human infants. *Cognitive Brain Research*, *22*, 301–304.

Hirano, S., Suzuki, S. T., & Redies, C. (2003). The cadherin superfamily in neural development: Diversity, function and interaction with other molecules. *Frontiers in Bioscience*, *8*, d306–355.

Hirano, S., & Takeichi, M. (2012). Cadherins in brain morphogenesis and wiring. *Physiological Reviews*, *92*(2), 597–634.

Hiscock, M., & Kinsbourne, M. (2011). Attention and the right-ear advantage: What is the connection? *Brain and Cognition*, *76*(2), 263–275.

Hobbs, K., Kennedy, A., Dubray, M., Bigler, E. D., Petersen, P. B., McMahon, W., & Lainhart, J. E. (2007). A retrospective fetal ultrasound study of brain size in autism. *Biological Psychiatry*, *62*(9), 1048–1055.

Hodge, S. M., Makris, N., Kennedy, D. N., Caviness, V. S., Jr., Howard, J., McGrath, L., . . . Harris, G. J. (2010). Cerebellum, language, and cognition in autism and specific language impairment. *Journal of Autism and Developmental Disorders*, *40*(3), 300–316.

Hoeft, F., Walter, E., Lightbody, A. A., Hazlett, H. C., Chang, C., Piven, J., & Reiss, A. L. (2011). Neuroanatomical differences in toddler boys with fragile x syndrome and idiopathic autism. *Archives of General Psychiatry*, *68*(3), 295–305.

Hoekstra, R. A., Happé, F., Baron-Cohen, S., & Ronald, A. (2010). Limited genetic covariance between autistic traits and intelligence: Findings from a longitudinal twin study. *American Journal of Medical Genetics Part B-Neuropsychiatric Genetics*, *153B*(5), 994–1007.

Hof, P. R., Knabe, R., Bovier, P., & Bouras, C. (1991). Neuropathological observations in a case of autism presenting with self-injury behavior. *Acta Neuropathologica*, *82*(4), 321–326.

Hollander, E., King, A., Delaney, K., Smith, C. J., & Silverman, J. M. (2003). Obsessive-compulsive behaviors in parents of multiplex autism families. *Psychiatry Research*, *117*(1), 11–16.

Hoshino, Y., Kaneko, M., Yashima, Y., Kumashiro, H., Volkmar, F. R., & Cohen, D. J. (1987). Clinical features of autistic children with setback course in their infancy. *Japanese Journal of Psychiatry and Neurology*, *41*(2), 237–245.

Houston, R., & Frith, U. (2002). Autism in history: The case of Hugh Blair of Borgue. *History of Science*, *40*(127), 119–119.

Howard, M. A., Cowell, P. E., Boucher, J., Broks, P., Mayes, A., Farrant, A., & Roberts, N. (2000). Convergent neuroanatomical and behavioural evidence of an amygdala hypothesis of autism. *Neuroreport*, *11*(13), 2931–2935.

Howlin, P., Goode, S., Hutton, J., & Rutter, M. (2004). Adult outcome for children with autism. *Journal of Child Psychology and Psychiatry*, *45*(2), 212–229.

Howlin, P., & Moore, A. (1997). Diagnosis in autism: A survey of over 12,000 patients in the UK. *Autism*, *1*, 135–162.

Hsiao, E. Y. (2013). Immune dysregulation in autism spectrum disorder. In G. Konopka (Ed.), *Neurobiology of Autism* (Vol. 113, pp. 269–302). San Diego: Elsevier Academic Press Inc.

Huang, C. H., & Santangelo, S. L. (2008). Autism and serotonin transporter gene polymorphisms: A systematic review and meta-analysis. *American Journal of Medical Genetics Part B-Neuropsychiatric Genetics*, *147B*(6), 903–913.

Huerta, M., Bishop, S. L., Duncan, A., Hus, V., & Lord, C. (2012). Application of DSM-5 criteria for autism spectrum disorder to three samples of children with DSM-IV diagnoses of pervasive developmental disorders. *American Journal of Psychiatry*, *169*(10), 1056–1064.

Huerta, M., Bishop, S. L., Duncan, A., Hus, V., & Lord, C. (2013). Commentary on the application of DSM-5 criteria for autism spectrum disorder response. *American Journal of Psychiatry*, *170*(4), 445–446.

Hughes, C. (1996). Brief report: Planning problems in autism at the level of motor control. *Journal of Autism and Developmental Disorders*, *26*(1), 99–107.

Hughes, C., & Ensor, R. (2007). Executive function and theory of mind: Predictive relations from ages 2 to 4. *Developmental Psychology*, *43*(6), 1447–1459.

Hughes, C., Plumet, M. H., & Leboyer, M. (1999). Towards a cognitive phenotype for autism: Increased prevalence of executive dysfunction and superior spatial span amongst siblings of children with autism. *Journal of Child Psychology and Psychiatry*, *40*(5), 705–718.

Hughes, J. R. (2007). Autism: The first firm finding = underconnectivity? *Epilepsy & Behavior*, *11*(1), 20–24.

Huguet, G., Ey, E., & Bourgeron, T. (2013). The genetic landscapes of autism spectrum disorders. In A. Chakravarti & E. Green (Eds.), *Annual Review of Genomics and Human Genetics* (Vol. 14, pp. 191–213). Palo Alto: Annual Reviews.

Hultman, C. M., Sandin, S., Levine, S. Z., Lichtenstein, P., & Reichenberg, A. (2011). Advancing paternal age and risk of autism: New evidence from a population-based study and a meta-analysis of epidemiological studies. *Molecular Psychiatry*, *16*(12), 1203–1212.

Hultman, C. M., Sparen, P., & Cnattingius, S. (2002). Perinatal risk factors for infantile autism. *Epidemiology*, *13*(4), 417–423.

Humphreys, K., Hasson, U., Avidan, G., Minshew, N., & Behrmann, M. (2008). Cortical patterns of category-selective activation for faces, places and objects in adults with autism. *Autism Research*, *1*(1), 52–63.

Hutsler, J. J., & Zhang, H. (2010). Increased dendritic spine densities on cortical projection neurons in autism spectrum disorders. *Brain Research*, *1309*, 83–94.

Hus, V., & Lord, C. (2014) The Autism Diagnostic Observation Schedule, Module 4: Revised algorithm and standardized severity scale. *Journal of Autism and Developmental Disorders*, 44: 1996–2012.

Hutt, C., Hutt, S. J., Lee, D., & Ounsted, C. (1964). Arousal and childhood autism. *Nature*, *204*, 908–909.

Huttenlocher, P. R. (1999). Dendritic and synaptic development in human cerebral cortex: Time course and critical periods. *Developmental Neuropsychology*, *16*(3), 347–349.

Hyde, K. L., Samson, F., Evans, A. C., & Mottron, L. (2010). Neuroanatomical differences in brain areas implicated in perceptual and other core features of autism revealed by cortical thickness analysis and voxel-based morphometry. *Human Brain Mapping*, *31*(4), 556–566.

Iacoboni, M., & Dapretto, M. (2006). The mirror neuron system and the consequences of its dysfunction. *Nature Reviews Neuroscience*, *7*(12), 942–951.

Iao, L. S., & Leekam, S. R. (2014). Nonspecificity and theory of mind: New evidence from a nonverbal false-sign task and children with autism spectrum disorders. *Journal of Experimental Child Psychology*, *122*, 1–20.

Ingalhalikar, M., Parker, D., Bloy, L., Roberts, T. P., & Verma, R. (2011). Diffusion based abnormality markers of pathology: Toward learned diagnostic prediction of ASD. *Neuroimage*, *57*(3), 918–927.

Iossifov, I., O'Roak, B. J., Sanders, S. J., Ronemus, M., Krumm, N., Levy, D., . . . Wigler, M. (2014). The contribution of de novo coding mutations to autism spectrum disorder. *Nature*, *515*(7526), 216–221.

Iossifov, I., Ronemus, M., Levy, D., Wang, Z., Hakker, I., Rosenbaum, J., . . . Wigler, M. (2012). De novo gene disruptions in children on the autistic spectrum. *Neuron*, *74*(2), 285–299.

Ipser, J. C., Syal, S., Bentley, J., Adnams, C. M., Steyn, B., & Stein, D. J. (2012). 1H-MRS in autism spectrum disorders: A systematic meta-analysis. *Metabolic Brain Disease*, *27*(3), 275–287.

Itier, R. J., & Batty, M. (2009). Neural bases of eye and gaze processing: The core of social cognition. *Neuroscience and Biobehavioral Reviews*, *33*(6), 843–863.

Jacot-Descombes, S., Uppal, N., Wicinski, B., Santos, M., Schmeidler, J., Giannakopoulos, P., . . . Hof, P. R. (2012). Decreased pyramidal neuron size in Brodmann areas 44 and 45 in patients with autism. *Acta Neuropathologica*, *124*(1), 67–79.

Jansiewicz, E. M., Goldberg, M. C., Newschaffer, C. J., Denckla, M. B., Landa, R., & Mostofsky, S. H. (2006). Motor signs distinguish children with high functioning autism and Asperger's syndrome from controls. *Journal of Autism and Developmental Disorders*, *36*(5), 613–621.

Jiang, Y. H., Yuen, R.K.C., Wang, M. B., Jin, X., Chen, N., Wu, X. L., . . . Scherer, S. W. (2013). Detection of clinically relevant genetic variants in autism spectrum disorder by whole-genome sequencing. *American Journal of Human Genetics*, *93*(2), 249–263.

Johansson, M., Gillberg, C., & Rastam, M. (2010). Autism spectrum conditions in individuals with Mobius sequence, CHARGE syndrome and oculo-auriculo-vertebral spectrum: Diagnostic aspects. *Research in Developmental Disabilities*, *31*(1), 9–24.

Johnson, K. A., Robertson, I. H., Kelly, S. P., Silk, T. J., Barry, E., Daibhis, A., . . . Bellgrove, M. A. (2007). Dissociation in performance of children with ADHD and high-functioning autism on a task of sustained attention. *Neuropsychologia*, *45*(10), 2234–2245.

Johnson, M. H. (2001). Functional brain development in humans. *Nature Reviews Neurology*, *2*(7), 475–483.

Johnson, M. H. (2005). Subcortical face processing. *Nature Reviews Neuroscience*, *6*(10), 766–774.

Johnson, M. H., Dziurawiec, S., Ellis, H., & Morton, J. (1991). Newborns' preferential tracking of face-like stimuli and its subsequent decline. *Cognition*, *40*(1–2), 1–19.

Johnson, M. H., Grossmann, T., & Farroni, T. (2008). The social cognitive neuroscience of infancy: Illuminating the early development of social brain functions. In R. V. Kail (Ed.), *Advances in Child Development and Behavior* (Vol. 36, pp. 331–372). New York: Elsevier.

Johnson, M. H., Posner, M. I., & Rothbart, M. K. (1991). Components of visual orienting in early infancy: Contingency learning, anticipatory looking, and disengaging. *Journal of Cognitive Neuroscience*, *3*(4), 335–344.

Jones, E.J.H., Gliga, T., Bedford, R., Charman, T., & Johnson, M. H. (2014). Developmental pathways to autism: A review of prospective studies of infants at risk. *Neuroscience and Biobehavioral Reviews*, *39*, 1–33.

Jones, M. B., & Szatmari, P. (1988). Stoppage rules and genetic studies of autism. *Journal of Autism and Developmental Disorders*, *18*(1), 31–40.

Jones, T. B., Bandettini, P. A., Kenworthy, L., Case, L. K., Milleville, S. C., Martin, A., & Birn, R. M. (2010). Sources of group differences in functional connectivity: An investigation applied to autism spectrum disorder. *Neuroimage*, *49*(1), 401–414.

Jones, W., & Klin, A. (2013). Attention to eyes is present but in decline in 2–6-month-old infants later diagnosed with autism. *Nature*, *504*(7480), 427–431.

Joshi, G., Biederman, J., Wozniak, J., Goldin, R. L., Crowley, D., Furtak, S., . . . Gonenc, A. (2013). Magnetic resonance spectroscopy study of the glutamatergic system in adolescent males with high-functioning autistic disorder: A pilot study at 4T. *European Archives of Psychiatry and Clinical Neuroscience*, *263*(5), 379–384.

Jou, R. J., Jackowski, A. P., Papademetris, X., Rajeevan, N., Staib, L. H., & Volkmar, F. R. (2011). Diffusion tensor imaging in autism spectrum disorders: Preliminary evidence of abnormal neural connectivity. *Australian and New Zealand Journal of Psychiatry*, *45*(2), 153–162.

Judd, L. L., & Mandell, A. J. (1968). Chromosome studies in early infantile autism. *Archives of General Psychiatry*, *18*(4), 450–457.

Just, M. A., Cherkassky, V. L., Keller, T. A., Kana, R. K., & Minshew, N. J. (2007). Functional and anatomical cortical underconnectivity in autism: Evidence from an FMRI study of an executive function task and corpus callosum morphometry. *Cerebral Cortex*, *17*(4), 951–961.

Just, M. A., Cherkassky, V. L., Keller, T. A., & Minshew, N. J. (2004). Cortical activation and synchronization during sentence comprehension in high-functioning autism: Evidence of underconnectivity. *Brain*, *127*(Pt 8), 1811–1821.

Juul-Dam, N., Townsend, J., & Courchesne, E. (2001). Prenatal, perinatal, and neonatal factors in autism, pervasive developmental disorder–not otherwise specified, and the general population. *Pediatrics*, *107*(4), E63.

Jyonouchi, H., Sun, S. I., & Le, H. (2001). Innate and adaptive immune responses in children with regression autism: Evaluation of the effects of environmental factors including vaccination. *Journal of Allergy and Clinical Immunology*, *107*(2), S274–S274.

Kaland, N., Smith, L., & Mortensen, E. L. (2008). Brief report: Cognitive flexibility and focused attention in children and adolescents with Asperger syndrome or high-functioning autism as measured on the computerized version of the Wisconsin Card Sorting Test. *Journal of Autism and Developmental Disorders*, *38*(6), 1161–1165.

Kalia, M. (2008). Brain development: Anatomy, connectivity, adaptive plasticity, and toxicity. *Metabolism: Clinical and Experimental*, *57*(Suppl 2), S2–S5.

Kamio, Y., Robins, D., Kelley, E., Swainson, B., & Fein, D. (2007). Atypical lexical/semantic processing in high-functioning autism spectrum disorders without early language delay. *Journal of Autism and Developmental Disorders*, *37*(6), 1116–1122.

Kamio, Y., & Toichi, M. (2000). Dual access to semantics in autism: Is pictorial access superior to verbal access? *Journal of Child Psychology and Psychiatry*, *41*(7), 859–867.

Kana, R. K., Keller, T. A., Cherkassky, V. L., Minshew, N. J., & Just, M. A. (2009). Atypical frontal-posterior synchronization of theory of mind regions in autism during mental state attribution. *Social Neuroscience*, *4*(2), 135–152.

Kana, R. K., Keller, T. A., Minshew, N. J., & Just, M. A. (2007). Inhibitory control in high-functioning autism: Decreased activation and underconnectivity in inhibition networks. *Biological Psychiatry*, *62*(3), 198–206.

Kanne, S. M., Randolph, J. K., & Farmer, J. E. (2008). Diagnostic and assessment findings: A bridge to academic planning for children with autism spectrum disorders. *Neuropsychology Review*, *18*(4), 367–384.

Kanner, L. (1943). Autistic disturbances of affective contact. *Nervous Child*, *2*, 217–250.

Kanner, L. (1944). Early infantile autism. *Pediatrics*, *25*(3), 211–217.

Karmiloff-Smith, A. (2010). A developmental perspective on modularity. In B. M. Glatzeder, V. Goel, & A. VonMuller (Eds.), *Towards a Theory of Thinking: Building Blocks for a Conceptual Framework* (pp. 179–187). Berlin: Springer-Verlag Berlin.

Kavalali, E. T., Nelson, E. D., & Monteggia, L. M. (2011). Role of MeCP2, DNA methylation, and HDACs in regulating synapse function. *Journal of Neurodevelopmental Disorders*, *3*(3), 250–256.

Ke, X., Tang, T., Hong, S., Hang, Y., Zou, B., Li, H., . . . Liu, Y. (2009). White matter impairments in autism, evidence from voxel-based morphometry and diffusion tensor imaging. *Brain Research*, *1265*, 171–177.

Keil, A., Daniels, J. L., Forssen, U., Hultman, C., Cnattingius, S., Soderberg, K. C., . . . Sparen, P. (2010). Parental autoimmune diseases associated with autism spectrum disorders in offspring. *Epidemiology*, *21*(6), 805–808.

Keita, L., Mottron, L., & Bertone, A. (2010). Far visual acuity is unremarkable in autism: Do we need to focus on crowding? *Autism Research: Official Journal of the International Society for Autism Research*, *3*(6), 333–341.

Keller, T. A., Kana, R. K., & Just, M. A. (2007). A developmental study of the structural integrity of white matter in autism. *Neuroreport*, *18*(1), 23–27.

Kelley, E. (2011). Language in ASD. In D. Fein (Ed.), *The Neuropsychology of Autism* (pp. 123–138). New York: Oxford University Press.

Kelley, E., Paul, J. J., Fein, D., & Naigles, L. R. (2006). Residual language deficits in optimal outcome children with a history of autism. *Journal of Autism and Developmental Disorders*, *36*(6), 807–828.

Kemper, T. L., & Bauman, M. L. (1993). The contribution of neuropathologic studies to the understanding of autism. *Neurologic Clinics*, *11*(1), 175–187.

Kemper, T. L., & Bauman, M. L. (1998). Neuropathology of infantile autism. *Journal of Neuropathology and Experimental Neurology*, *57*(7), 645–652.

Kenet, T. (2011). Sensory functions in ASD. In D. Fein (Ed.), *The Neuropsychology of Autism* (pp. 215–224). New York: Oxford University Press.

Kenet, T., Orekhova, E. V., Bharadwaj, H., Shetty, N. R., Israeli, E., Lee, A. K., . . . Manoach, D. S. (2012). Disconnectivity of the cortical ocular motor control network in autism spectrum disorders. *Neuroimage*, *61*(4), 1226–1234.

Kennedy, D. P., & Courchesne, E. (2008). Functional abnormalities of the default network during self-and other-reflection in autism. *Social Cognitive and Affective Neuroscience*, *3*(2), 177–190.

Keown, C. L., Shih, P., Nair, A., Peterson, N., Mulvey, M. E., & Muller, R. A. (2013). Local functional overconnectivity in posterior brain regions is associated with symptom severity in autism spectrum disorders. *Cell Reports*, *5*(3), 567–572.

Kern, J. K. (2003). Purkinje cell vulnerability and autism: A possible etiological connection. *Brain and Development*, *25*(6), 377–382.

Kern, J. K., & Jones, A. M. (2006). Evidence of toxicity, oxidative stress, and neuronal insult in autism. *Journal of Toxicology and Environmental Health-Part B-Critical Reviews*, *9*(6), 485–499.

Keyes, K. M., Susser, E., Cheslack-Postava, K., Fountain, C., Liu, K., & Bearman, P. S. (2012). Cohort effects explain the increase in autism diagnosis among children born from 1992 to 2003 in California. *International Journal of Epidemiology*, *41*(2), 495–503.

Kiehl, K. A. (2006). A cognitive neuroscience perspective on psychopathy: Evidence for paralimbic system dysfunction. *Psychiatry Research*, *142*(2–3), 107–128.

Kim, K. C., Kim, P., Go, H. S., Choi, C. S., Park, J. H., Kim, H. J., . . . Shin, C. Y. (2013). Male-specific alteration in excitatory postsynaptic development and social interaction in pre-natal valproic acid exposure model of autism spectrum disorder. *Journal of Neurochemistry*, *124*(6), 832–843.

Kim, S. H., & Lord, C. (2010). Restricted and repetitive behaviors in toddlers and preschoolers with autism spectrum disorders based on the Autism Diagnostic Observation Schedule (ADOS). *Autism Research: Official Journal of the International Society for Autism Research*, *3*(4), 162–173.

Kim, Y. S., Leventhal, B. L., Koh, Y. J., Fombonne, E., Laska, E., Lim, E. C., . . . Grinker, R. R. (2011). Prevalence of autism spectrum disorders in a total population sample. *American Journal of Psychiatry*, *168*(9), 904–912.

Kinney, D. K., Barch, D. H., Chayka, B., Napoleon, S., & Munir, K. M. (2010). Environmental risk factors for autism: Do they help cause de novo genetic mutations that contribute to the disorder? *Medical Hypotheses*, *74*(1), 102–106.

Kinney, D. K., Miller, A. M., Crowley, D. J., Huang, E., & Gerber, E. (2008). Autism prevalence following prenatal exposure to hurricanes and tropical storms in Louisiana. *Journal of Autism and Developmental Disorders*, *38*(3), 481–488.

Kinsbourne, M. (1991). Overfocusing: An apparent subtype of attention deficit hyperactivity disorder. In N. Amir, I. Rapin, & D. Branski (Eds.), *Pediatric Neurology: Behavior and Cognition of the Child with Brain Dysfunction* (Vol. 1, pp. 18–35). Basel: Karger.

Kjelgaard, M. M., & Tager-Flusberg, H. (2001). An investigation of language impairment in autism: Implications for genetic subgroups. *Language and Cognitive Processes*, *16*(2–3), 287–308.

Klei, L., Sanders, S. J., Murtha, M. T., Hus, V., Lowe, J. K., Willsey, A. J., . . . Devlin, B. (2012). Common genetic variants, acting additively, are a major source of risk for autism. *Molecular Autism*, *3*:9.

Klein, A. J., Armstrong, B. L., Greer, M. K., & Brown, F. R. (1990). Hyperacusis and otitis media in individuals with Williams syndrome. *Journal of Speech and Hearing Disorders*, *55*, 339–334.

Klein, S. B., Chan, R. L., & Loftus, J. (1999). Independence of episodic and semantic self-knowledge: The case from autism. *Social Cognition*, *17*(4), 413–436.

Klein, S. B., Sharifi-Hannauer, P., & Martinez-Agosto, J. A. (2013). Macrocephaly as a clinical indicator of genetic subtypes in autism. *Autism Research: Official Journal of the International Society for Autism Research*, *6*(1), 51–56.

Kleinhans, N. M., Richards, T., Sterling, L., Stegbauer, K. C., Mahurin, R., Johnson, L. C., . . . Aylward, E. (2008). Abnormal functional connectivity in autism spectrum disorders during face processing. *Brain*, *131*(Pt 4), 1000–1012.

Kleinman, J. M., Robins, D. L., Ventola, P. E., Pandey, J., Boorstein, H. C., Esser, E. L., . . . Fein, D. (2008). The modified checklist for autism in toddlers: A follow-up study investigating the early detection of autism spectrum disorders. *Journal of Autism and Developmental Disorders*, *38*(5), 827–839.

Klin, A., & Jones, W. (2008). Altered face scanning and impaired recognition of biological motion in a 15-month-old infant with autism. *Developmental Science*, *11*(1), 40–46.

Klin, A., Lin, D. J., Gorrindo, P., Ramsay, G., & Jones, W. (2009). Two-year-olds with autism orient to non-social contingencies rather than biological motion. *Nature*, *459*(7244), 257–261.

Klin, A., Sparrow, S. S., de Bildt, A., Cicchetti, D. V., Cohen, D. J., & Volkmar, F. R. (1999). A normed study of face recognition in autism and related disorders. *Journal of Autism and Developmental Disorders*, *29*(6), 499–508.

Klinger, L. G., & Dawson, G. (2001). Prototype formation in autism. *Development and Psychopathology*, *13*(1), 111–124.

Knaus, T. A., Silver, A. M., Kennedy, M., Lindgren, K. A., Dominick, K. C., Siegel, J., & Tager-Flusberg, H. (2010). Language laterality in autism spectrum disorder and typical controls: A functional, volumetric, and diffusion tensor MRI study. *Brain and Language*, *112*(2), 113–120.

Koenderink, M.J.T., & Uylings, H.B.M. (1995). Postnatal maturation of layer v pyramidal neurons in the human prefrontal cortex: A quantitative golgi analysis. *Brain Research*, *678*(1–2), 233–243.

Koenderink, M.J.T., Uylings, H.B.M., & Mrzljak, L. (1994). Postnatal maturation of the layer-III pyramidal neurons in the human prefrontal cortex: A quantitative golgi analysis. *Brain Research*, *653*(1–2), 173–182.

Kogan, M. D., Blumberg, S. J., Schieve, L. A., Boyle, C. A., Perrin, J. M., Ghandour, R. M., . . . van Dyck, P. C. (2009). Prevalence of parent-reported diagnosis of autism spectrum disorder among children in the US, 2007. *Pediatrics*, *124*(5), 1395–1403.

Kolevzon, A., Gross, R., & Reichenberg, A. (2007). Prenatal and perinatal risk factors for autism: A review and integration of findings. *Archives of Pediatrics and Adolescent Medicine*, *161*(4), 326–333.

Kopp, S., & Gillberg, C. (2011). The Autism Spectrum Screening Questionnaire (ASSQ)-Revised Extended Version (ASSQ-REV): An instrument for better capturing the autism phenotype in girls? A preliminary study involving 191 clinical cases and community controls. *Research in Developmental Disabilities*, *32*(6), 2875–2888.

Kornack, D. R., & Rakic, P. (1998). Changes in cell-cycle kinetics during the development and evolution of primate neocortex. *Proceedings of the National Academy of Sciences of the United States of America*, *95*(3), 1242–1246.

Koshino, H., Kana, R. K., Keller, T. A., Cherkassky, V. L., Minshew, N. J., & Just, M. A. (2008). fMRI investigation of working memory for faces in autism: Visual coding and underconnectivity with frontal areas. *Cerebral Cortex*, *18*(2), 289–300.

Kotsopoulos, S. (1976). Infantile autism in dizygotic twins: A case report. *Journal of Autism and Childhood Schizophrenia*, *6*(2), 133–138.

Krause, I., He, X. S., Gershwin, M. E., & Shoenfeld, Y. (2002). Brief report: Immune factors in autism: A critical review. *Journal of Autism and Developmental Disorders*, *32*(4), 337–345.

Kroger, A., Bletsch, A., Krick, C., Siniatchkin, M., Jarczok, T. A., Freitag, C. M., & Bender, S. (2014). Visual event-related potentials to biological motion stimuli in autism spectrum disorders. *Social Cognitive and Affective Neuroscience*, *9*(8), 1214–1222.

Krumm, N., O'Roak, B. J., Shendure, J., & Eichler, E. E. (2014). A de novo convergence of autism genetics and molecular neuroscience. *Trends in Neurosciences*, *37*(2), 95–105.

Kuczmarski, R. J., Ogden, C. L., Guo, S. S., Grummer-Strawn, L. M., Flegal, K. M., Mei, Z., . . . Johnson, C. L. (2002). 2000 CDC growth charts for the United States: Methods and development. *Vital and Health Statistics: Series 11: Data from the National Health Survey*(246), 1–190.

Kumar, A., Sundaram, S. K., Sivaswamy, L., Behen, M. E., Makki, M. I., Ager, J., . . . Chugani, D. C. (2009). Alterations in frontal lobe tracts and corpus callosum in young children with autism spectrum disorder. *Cerebral Cortex*, *20*(9), 2103–2113.

Kurita, H. (1985). Infantile autism with speech loss before the age of thirty months. *Journal of the American Academy of Child Psychiatry*, *24*(2), 191–196.

Kurita, H. (1996). Specificity and developmental consequences of speech loss in children with pervasive developmental disorders. *Psychiatry and Clinical Neurosciences*, *50*(4), 181–184.

Kurita, H., Uchiyama, T., & Takesada, M. (1985). Tokyo child development schedule I: Test-retest reliability and concurrent validity. *Folia Psychiatrica et Neurologica Japonica*, *39*(2), 129–137.

Lainhart, J. E. (2003). Increased rate of head growth during infancy in autism. *Jama-Journal of the American Medical Association*, *290*(3), 393–394.

Lainhart, J. E., Bigler, E. D., Bocian, M., Coon, H., Dinh, E., Dawson, G., . . . Volkmar, F. (2006). Head circumference and height in autism: A study by the collaborative program of excellence in autism. *American Journal of Medical Genetics Part A*, *140*(21), 2257–2274.

Lainhart, J. E., Ozonoff, S., Coon, H., Krasny, L., Dinh, E., Nice, J., & McMahon, W. (2002). Autism, regression, and the broader autism phenotype. *American Journal of Medical Genetics*, *113*(3), 231–237.

Lainhart, J. E., Piven, J., Wzorek, M., Landa, R., Santangelo, S. L., Coon, H., & Folstein, S. E. (1997). Macrocephaly in children and adults with autism. *Journal of the American Academy of Child and Adolescent Psychiatry*, *36*(2), 282–290.

Lampi, K. M., Lehtonen, L., Tran, P. L., Suominen, A., Lehti, V., Banerjee, P. N., . . . Sourander, A. (2012). Risk of autism spectrum disorders in low birth weight and small for gestational age infants. *Journal of Pediatrics*, *161*(5), 830–836.

Landa, R. (2000). Social language use in Asperger syndrome and high-functioning autism. In A. Klin, F. R. Volkmar, & S. S. Sparrow (Eds.), *Asperger Syndrome* (pp. 125–155). New York: Guilford Press.

Landa, R. J., Folstein, S. E., & Isaacs, C. (1991). Spontaneous narrative-discourse performance of parents of autistic individuals. *Journal of Speech and Hearing Research*, *34*(6), 1339–1345.

Landa, R. J., & Garrett-Mayer, E. (2006). Development in infants with autism spectrum disorders: A prospective study. *Journal of Child Psychology and Psychiatry*, *47*(6), 629–638.

Landa, R. J., Holman, K. C., & Garrett-Mayer, E. (2007). Social and communication development in toddlers with early and later diagnosis of autism spectrum disorders. *Archives of General Psychiatry*, *64*(7), 853–864.

Landau, W. M., & Kleffner, F. R. (1957). Syndrome of acquired aphasia with convulsive disorder in children. *Neurology*, *7*, 523–530.

Landrigan, P. J. (2010). What causes autism? Exploring the environmental contribution. *Current Opinion in Pediatrics*, *22*(2), 219–225.

Landry, O., Mitchell, P. L., & Burack, J. A. (2009). Orienting of visual attention among persons with autism spectrum disorders: Reading versus responding to symbolic cues. *Journal of Child Psychology and Psychiatry*, *50*(7), 862–870.

Landry, R., & Bryson, S. E. (2004). Impaired disengagement of attention in young children with autism. *Journal of Child Psychology and Psychiatry*, *45*(6), 1115–1122.

Langen, M., Bos, D., Noordermeer, D. S., Nederveen, H., van Engeland, H., & Durston, S. (2014). Changes in the development of striatum are involved in repetitive behavior in autism. *Biological Psychiatry*, *76*(5), 405–411.

Langen, M., Leemans, A., Johnston, P., Ecker, C., Daly, E., Murphy, C. M., . . . Consortium, A. (2012). Fronto-striatal circuitry and inhibitory control in autism: Findings from diffusion tensor imaging tractography. *Cortex*, *48*(2), 183–193.

Laurence, J. A., & Fatemi, S. H. (2005). Glial fibrillary acidic protein is elevated in superior frontal, parietal and cerebellar cortices of autistic subjects. *Cerebellum*, *4*(3), 206–210.

Lauritsen, M. B., Pedersen, C. B., & Mortensen, P. B. (2005). Effects of familial risk factors and place of birth on the risk of autism: A nationwide register-based study. *Journal of Child Psychology and Psychiatry*, *46*(9), 963–971.

Lawson, R. (1875). Brains and intellect. *The Lancet*, *August 28*, 306–308.

Lecciso, F., Petrocchi, S., & Marchetti, A. (2013). Hearing mothers and oral deaf children: An atypical relational context for theory of mind. *European Journal of Psychology of Education*, *28*(3), 903–922.

LeCouteur, A., Bailey, A., Goode, S., Pickles, A., Robertson, S., Gottesman, I., & Rutter, M. (1996). A broader phenotype of autism: The clinical spectrum in twins. *Journal of Child Psychology and Psychiatry and Allied Disciplines*, *37*(7), 785–801.

Le Couteur, A., Lord, C., & Rutter, M. (2003). The autism diagnostic interview-revised (ADI-R). Los Angeles, CA: Western Psychological Services.

Lee, B. K., & McGrath, J. J. (2015). Advancing parental age and autism: Multifactorial pathways. *Trends in Molecular Medicine*, *21*(2), 118–125.

Lee, C., & Scherer, S. W. (2010). The clinical context of copy number variation in the human genome. *Expert Reviews in Molecular Medicine*, *12*.

Lee, M., Martin-Ruiz, C., Graham, A., Court, J., Jaros, E., Perry, R., . . . Perry, E. (2002). Nicotinic receptor abnormalities in the cerebellar cortex in autism. *Brain*, *125*(Pt 7), 1483–1495.

Lee, P. S., Yerys, B. E., Della Rosa, A., Foss-Feig, J., Barnes, K. A., James, J. D., . . . Kenworthy, L. E. (2009). Functional connectivity of the inferior frontal cortex changes with age in children with autism spectrum disorders: A fcMRI study of response inhibition. *Cerebral Cortex*, *19*(8), 1787–1794.

Lee, S. H., Ripke, S., Neale, B. M., Faraone, S. V., Purcell, S. M., Perlis, R. H., . . . Int Inflammatory Bowel Dis, G. (2013). Genetic relationship between five psychiatric disorders estimated from genome-wide SNPs. *Nature Genetics*, *45*(9), 984–994.

Leech, R., & Sharp, D. J. (2014). The role of the posterior cingulate cortex in cognition and disease. *Brain*, *137*, 12–32.

Leekam, S., Libby, S., Wing, L., Gould, J., & Gillberg, C. (2000). Comparison of ICD-10 and Gillberg's criteria for Asperger syndrome. *Autism*, *1*(4), 11–28.

Leekam, S., Tandos, J., McConachie, H., Meins, E., Parkinson, K., Wright, C., . . . Le Couteur, A. (2007). Repetitive behaviours in typically developing 2-year-olds. *Journal of Child Psychology and Psychiatry*, *48*(11), 1131–1138.

Leekam, S. R., Libby, S. J., Wing, L., Gould, J., & Taylor, C. (2002). The diagnostic interview for social and communication disorders: Algorithms for ICD-10 childhood autism and Wing and Gould autistic spectrum disorder. *Journal of Child Psychology and Psychiatry*, *43*(3), 327–342.

Leekam, S. R., Nieto, C., Libby, S. J., Wing, L., & Gould, J. (2007). Describing the sensory abnormalities of children and adults with autism. *Journal of Autism and Developmental Disorders*, *37*(5), 894–910.

Lemons, J. A., Schreiner, R. L., & Gresham, E. L. (1981). Relationship of brain weight to head circumference in early infancy. *Human Biology*, *53*(3), 351–354.

Lenroot, R. K., & Yeung, P. K. (2013). Heterogeney within autism spectrum disorders: What have we learned from neuroimaging studies? *Frontiers in Human Neuroscience*, *7*, 733.

Lepisto, T., Kujala, T., Vanhala, R., Alku, P., Huotilainen, M., & Naatanen, R. (2005). The discrimination of and orienting to speech and non-speech sounds in children with autism. *Brain Research*, *1066*(1–2), 147–157.

Leppanen, J. M., & Nelson, C. A. (2009). Tuning the developing brain to social signals of emotions. *Nature Reviews Neuroscience*, *10*(1), 37–47.

Lesca, G., Rudolf, G., Labalme, A., Hirsch, E., Arzimanoglou, A., Genton, P., . . . Szepetowski, P. (2012). Epileptic encephalopathies of the Landau-Kleffner and continuous spike and waves during slow-wave sleep types: Genomic dissection makes the link with autism. *Epilepsia*, *53*(9), 1526–1538.

Lewis, P. A., Rezaie, R., Brown, R., Roberts, N., & Dunbar, R.I.M. (2011). Ventromedial prefrontal volume predicts understanding of others and social network size. *Neuroimage*, *57*(4), 1624–1629.

Li, G., Nie, J. X., Wang, L., Shi, F., Lin, W. L., Gilmore, J. H., & Shen, D. G. (2013). Mapping region-specific longitudinal cortical surface expansion from birth to 2 years of age. *Cerebral Cortex*, *23*(11), 2724–2733.

Li, X. M., Chauhan, A., Sheikh, A. M., Patil, S., Chauhan, V., Li, X. M., . . . Malik, M. (2009). Elevated immune response in the brain of autistic patients. *Journal of Neuroimmunology*, *207*(1–2), 111–116.

Li, X. M., Wang, K., Wu, J. X., Hong, Y. F., Zhao, J. P., Feng, X. J., . . . Zhang, X. C. (2014). The link between impaired theory of mind and executive function in children with cerebral palsy. *Research in Developmental Disabilities*, *35*(7), 1686–1693.

Lichtenstein, P., Carlstrom, E., Rastam, M., Gillberg, C., & Anckarsater, H. (2010). The genetics of autism spectrum disorders and related neuropsychiatric disorders in childhood. *American Journal of Psychiatry*, *167*(11), 1357–1363.

Limperopoulos, C., Chilingaryan, G., Sullivan, N., Guizard, N., Robertson, R. L., & du Plessis, A. J. (2014). Injury to the premature cerebellum: Outcome is related to remote cortical development. *Cerebral Cortex*, *24*(3), 728–736.

Lind, S. E., & Bowler, D. M. (2010). Episodic memory and episodic future thinking in adults with autism. *Journal of Abnormal Psychology*, *119*(4), 896–905.

Lise, M. F., & El-Husseini, A. (2006). The neuroligin and neurexin families: From structure to function at the synapse. *Cellular and Molecular Life Sciences*, *63*(16), 1833–1849.

Liss, M., Saulnier, C., Fein, D., & Kinsbourne, M. (2006). Sensory and attention abnormalities in autistic spectrum disorders. *Autism: The International Journal of Research & Practice*, *10*(2), 155–172.

Liu, X. Q., Georgiades, S., Duku, E., Thompson, A., Devlin, B., Cook, E. H., . . . Szatmari, P. (2011). Identification of genetic loci underlying the phenotypic constructs of autism spectrum disorders. *Journal of the American Academy of Child and Adolescent Psychiatry*, *50*(7), 687–696 e613.

Lombardo, M. V., & Baron-Cohen, S. (2010). Unraveling the paradox of the autistic self. *Wiley Interdisciplinary Reviews-Cognitive Science*, *1*(3), 393–403.

LoParo, D., & Waldman, I. D. (2015). The oxytocin receptor gene (OXTR) is associated with autism spectrum disorder: A meta-analysis. *Molecular Psychiatry*, *20*(5), 640–646.

Lopez, B. R., Lincoln, A. J., Ozonoff, S., & Lai, Z. (2005). Examining the relationship between executive functions and restricted, repetitive symptoms of autistic disorder. *Journal of Autism and Developmental Disorders*, *35*(4), 445–460.

Lorber, J., & Priestley, B. L. (1981). Children with large heads: A practical approach to diagnosis in 557 children, with special reference to 109 children with megalencephaly. *Developmental Medicine and Child Neurology*, *23*(4), 494–504.

Lord, C., & Bishop, S. L. (2015). Recent advances in autism research as reflected in DSM-5 criteria for autism spectrum disorder. *Annual Review of Clinical Psychology*, *11*, 53–70.

Lord, C., & Paul, R. (1997). Language and communication and autism. In D. J. Cohen & F. R. Volkmar (Eds.), *Handbook of Autism and Pervasive Developmental Disorders* (pp. 195–225). New York: John Wiley & Sons.

Lord, C., Risi, S., DiLavore, P. S., Shulman, C., Thurm, A., & Pickles, A. (2006). Autism from 2 to 9 years of age. *Archives of General Psychiatry*, *63*(6), 694–701.

Lord, C., Rutter, M., DiLavore, P. C., Risi, S., Gotham, K., & Bishop, S. (2012). *Autism Diagnostic Observation Schedule, Second Edition Manual*. Los Angeles: Western Psychological Services.

Lord, C., Shulman, C., & DiLavore, P. (2004). Regression and word loss in autistic spectrum disorders. *Journal of Child Psychology and Psychiatry*, *45*(5), 936–955.

Losh, M., Adolphs, R., Poe, M. D., Couture, S., Penn, D., Baranek, G. T., & Piven, J. (2009). Neuropsychological profile of autism and the broad autism phenotype. *Archives of General Psychiatry*, *66*(5), 518–526.

Lotspeich, L. J., Kwon, H., Schumann, C. M., Fryer, S. L., Goodlin-Jones, B. L., Buonocore, M. H., . . . Reiss, A. L. (2004). Investigation of neuroanatomical differences between autism and Asperger syndrome. *Archives of General Psychiatry*, *61*(3), 291–298.

Lotter, V. (1966). Epidemiology of autistic conditions in young children. *Psychiatry*, *1*, 124–137.

Lovaas, O. I., & Schreibman, L. (1971). Stimulus overselectivity of autistic children in a two stimulus situation. *Behaviour Research and Therapy*, *9*(4), 305–310.

Lovden, M., Bodammer, N. C., Kuhn, S., Kaufmann, J., Schutze, H., Tempelmann, C., . . . Lindenberger, U. (2010). Experience-dependent plasticity of white-matter microstructure extends into old age. *Neuropsychologia*, *48*(13), 3878–3883.

Luna, B., Minshew, N. J., Garver, K. E., Lazar, N. A., Thulborn, K. R., Eddy, W. F., & Sweeney, J. A. (2002). Neocortical system abnormalities in autism: An fMRI study of spatial working memory. *Neurology*, *59*(6), 834–840.

Luo, R., Sanders, S. J., Tian, Y., Voineagu, I., Huang, N., Chu, S. H., . . . Geschwind, D. H. (2012). Genome-wide transcriptome profiling reveals the functional impact of rare de novo and recurrent CNVs in autism spectrum disorders. *American Journal of Medical Genetics*, *91*(1), 38–55.

Luyster, R., Gotham, K., Guthrie, W., Coffing, M., Petrak, R., Pierce, K., . . . Lord, C. (2009). The autism diagnostic observation schedule-toddler module: A new module of a standardized diagnostic measure for autism spectrum disorders. *Journal of Autism and Developmental Disorders*, *39*(9), 1305–1320.

Luyster, R., Richler, J., Risi, S., Hsu, W. L., Dawson, G., Bernier, R., . . . Lord, C. (2005). Early regression in social communication in autism spectrum disorders: A CPEA study. *Developmental Neuropsychology*, *27*(3), 311–336.

Lyall, K., Ashwood, P., Van de Water, J., & Hertz-Picciotto, I. (2014). Maternal immune-mediated conditions, autism spectrum disorders, and developmental delay. *Journal of Autism and Developmental Disorders*, *44*(7), 1546–1555.

MacKay, G., & Shaw, A. (2004). A comparative study of figurative language in children with autism spectrum disorders. *Child Language Teaching and Therapy*, *20*, 13–32.

Mackinlay, R., Charman, T., & Karmiloff-Smith, A. (2006). High functioning children with autism spectrum disorder: A novel test of multitasking. *Brain and Cognition*, *61*(1), 14–24.

Maenner, M. J., Rice, C. E., Arneson, C. L., Cunniff, C., Schieve, L. A., Carpenter, L. A., . . . Durkin, M. S. (2014). Potential impact of DSM-5 criteria on autism spectrum disorder prevalence estimates. *Jama Psychiatry*, *71*(3), 292–300.

Maestro, S., Muratori, F., Cesari, A., Cavallaro, M. C., Paziente, A., Pecini, C., . . . Sommario, C. (2005). Course of autism signs in the first year of life. *Psychopathology*, *38*(1), 26–31.

Mandell, D. S., Listerud, J., Levy, S. E., & Pinto-Martin, J. A. (2002). Race differences in the age at diagnosis among medicaid-eligible children with autism. *Journal of the American Academy of Child and Adolescent Psychiatry*, *41*(12), 1447–1453.

Mandell, D. S., & Novak, M. M. (2005). The role of culture in families' treatment decisions for children with autism spectrum disorders. *Mental Retardation and Developmental Disabilities Research Reviews*, *11*(2), 110–115.

Mandell, D. S., Novak, M. M., & Zubritsky, C. D. (2005). Factors associated with age of diagnosis among children with autism spectrum disorders. *Pediatrics*, *116*(6), 1480–1486.

Mandy, W.P.L., Charman, T., & Skuse, D. H. (2012). Testing the construct validity of proposed criteria for DSM-5 autism spectrum disorder. *Journal of the American Academy of Child and Adolescent Psychiatry*, *51*(1), 41–50.

Manjaly, Z. M., Bruning, N., Neufang, S., Stephan, K. E., Brieber, S., Marshall, J. C., . . . Fink, G. R. (2007). Neurophysiological correlates of relatively enhanced local visual search in autistic adolescents. *Neuroimage*, *35*(1), 283–291.

Mann, J. R., McDermott, S., Bao, H., Hardin, J., & Gregg, A. (2010). Pre-eclampsia, birth weight, and autism spectrum disorders. *Journal of Autism and Developmental Disorders*, *40*(5), 548–554.

Mannion, A., & Leader, G. (2013). Comorbidity in autism spectrum disorder: A literature review. *Research in Autism Spectrum Disorders*, *7*(12), 1595–1616.

Marchese, M., Conti, V., Valvo, G., Moro, F., Muratori, F., Tancredi, R., . . . Sicca, F. (2014). Autism-epilepsy phenotype with macrocephaly suggests PTEN, but not GLIALCAM, genetic screening. *BMC Medical Genetics*, *15*, 26.

Mari, M., Castiello, U., Marks, D., Marraffa, C., & Prior, M. (2003). The reach-to-grasp movement in children with autism spectrum disorder. *Philosophical Transactions of the Royal Society of London: Series B: Biological Sciences*, *358*(1430), 393–403.

Mariner, R., Jackson, A. W., 3rd, Levitas, A., Hagerman, R. J., Braden, M., McBogg, P. M., . . . Berry, R. (1986). Autism, mental retardation, and chromosomal abnormalities. *Journal of Autism and Developmental Disorders*, *16*(4), 425–440.

Mars, A. E., Mauk, J. E., & Dowrick, P. W. (1998). Symptoms of pervasive developmental disorders as observed in prediagnostic home videos of infants and toddlers. *Journal of Pediatrics*, *132*(3), 500–504.

Marsh, L. E., & Hamilton, A. F. (2011). Dissociation of mirroring and mentalising systems in autism. *Neuroimage*, *56*(3), 1511–1519.

Marshall, C. R., Noor, A., Vincent, J. B., Lionel, A. C., Feuk, L., Skaug, J., . . . Scherer, S. W. (2008). Structural variation of chromosomes in autism spectrum disorder. *American Journal of Human Genetics*, *82*(2), 477–488.

Martin, E. R., Menold, M. M., Wolpert, C. M., Bass, M. P., Donnelly, S. L., Ravan, S. A., . . . Pericak-Vance, M. A. (2000). Analysis of linkage disequilibrium in gamma-aminobutyric acid receptor subunit genes in autistic disorder. *American Journal of Medical Genetics*, *96*(1), 43–48.

Mason-Brothers, A., Ritvo, E. R., Guze, B., Mo, A., Freeman, B. J., Funderburk, S. J., & Schroth, P. C. (1987). Pre-, peri-, and postnatal factors in 181 autistic patients from single and multiple incidence families. *Journal of the American Academy of Child and Adolescent Psychiatry*, *26*(1), 39–42.

Mason-Brothers, A., Ritvo, E. R., Pingree, C., Petersen, P. B., Jenson, W. R., McMahon, W. M., Freeman, B. J., Jorde, L., & Mo, A. (1990). The UCLA-University of Utah epidemiologic survey of autism: Prenatal, perinatal, and postnatal factors. *Pediatrics*, *86*(4), 514–519.

Matarazzo, E. B. (2002). Treatment of late onset autism as a consequence of probable autommune processes related to chronic bacterial infection. *The World Journal of Biological Psychiatry*, *3*(3), 162–166.

Materna, S., Dicke, P. W., & Thier, P. (2008). The posterior superior temporal sulcus is involved in social communication not specific for the eyes. *Neuropsychologia*, *46*(11), 2759–2765.

Matson, J. L., Belva, B. C., Horovitz, M., Kozlowski, A. M., & Bamburg, J. W. (2012). Comparing symptoms of autism spectrum disorders in a developmentally disabled sdult population using the current DSM-IV-TR diagnostic criteria and the proposed DSM-5 diagnostic criteria. *Journal of Developmental and Physical Disabilities*, *24*(4), 403–414.

Matson, J. L., Hattier, M. A., & Williams, L. W. (2012). How does relaxing the algorithm for autism affect DSM-V prevalence rates? *Journal of Autism and Developmental Disorders*, *42*(8), 1549–1556.

Matson, J. L., Kozlowski, A. M., Hattier, M. A., Horovitz, M., & Sipes, M. (2012). DSM-IV vs. DSM-5 diagnostic criteria for toddlers with autism. *Developmental Neurorehabilitation*, *15*(3), 185–190.

Matson, J. L., Wilkins, J., & Fodstad, J. C. (2010). Children with autism spectrum disorders: A comparison of those who regress vs. those who do not. *Developmental Neurorehabilitation*, *13*(1), 37–45.

Mattila, M. L., Kielinen, M., Linna, S. L., Jussila, K., Ebeling, H., Bloigu, R., . . . Moilanen, I. (2011). Autism spectrum disorders according to DSM-IV-TR and comparison with DSM-5 draft criteria: An epidemiological study. *Journal of the American Academy of Child and Adolescent Psychiatry*, *50*(6), 583–592 e511.

Maximo, J. O., Cadena, E. J., & Kana, R. K. (2014). The implications of brain connectivity in the neuropsychology of autism. *Neuropsychology Review*, *24*(1), 16–31.

Mayes, S. D., & Calhoun, S. L. (2003). Ability profiles in children with autism: Influence of age and IQ. *Autism*, *7*(1), 65–80.

Mayes, S. D., & Calhoun, S. L. (2008). WISC-IV and WIAT-II profiles in children with high-functioning autism. *Journal of Autism and Developmental Disorders*, *38*(3), 428–439.

Mayes, S. D., Calhoun, S. L., Murray, M. J., Pearl, A., Black, A., & Tierney, C. D. (2014). Final DSM-5 under-identifies mild autism spectrum disorder: Agreement between the DSM-5, CARS, CASD, and clinical diagnoses. *Research in Autism Spectrum Disorders*, *8*(2), 68–73.

Mayo, J., Chlebowski, C., Fein, D. A., & Eigsti, I. M. (2013). Age of first words predicts cognitive ability and adaptive skills in children with ASD. *Journal of Autism and Developmental Disorders*, *43*(2), 253–264.

McAlonan, G. M., Cheung, V., Cheung, C., Suckling, J., Lam, G. Y., Tai, K. S., . . . Chua, S. E. (2005). Mapping the brain in autism: A voxel-based MRI study of volumetric differences and intercorrelations in autism. *Brain*, *128*(Pt 2), 268–276.

McBride, K. L., Varga, E. A., Pastore, M. T., Prior, T. W., Manickam, K., Atkin, J. F., & Herman, G. E. (2010). Confirmation study of PTEN mutations among individuals with autism or developmental delays/mental retardation and macrocephaly. *Autism Research: Official Journal of the International Society for Autism Research*, *3*(3), 137–141.

McCann, J., & Peppe, S. (2003). Prosody in autism spectrum disorders: A critical review. *International Journal of Language and Communication Disorders*, *38*(4), 325–350.

McGrath, W. M. (1935). A case of megalencephaly showing an unusual talent for calculating dates. *British Medical Journal*, *1935*, 699–701.

McPartland, J. C., Reichow, B., & Volkmar, F. R. (2012). Sensitivity and specificity of proposed DSM-5 diagnostic criteria for autism spectrum disorder. *Journal of the American Academy of Child and Adolescent Psychiatry*, *51*(4), 368–383.

McQuaid, P. E. (1975). Infantile autism in twins. *British Journal of Psychiatry*, *127*, 530–534.

McQuistin, A., & Zieren, C. (2006). Clinical experiences with the PDDST-II. *Journal of Autism and Developmental Disorders*, *36*(4), 577–578.

Mefford, H. C., Muhle, H., Ostertag, P., von Spiczak, S., Buysse, K., Baker, C., . . . Eichler, E. E. (2010). Genome-wide copy number variation in epilepsy: Novel susceptibility loci in idiopathic generalized and focal epilepsies. *PLoS Genetics*, *6*(5), e1000962.

Meilleur, A. A., & Fombonne, E. (2009). Regression of language and non-language skills in pervasive developmental disorders. *Journal of Intellectual Disability Research*, *53*(2), 115–124.

Melillo, R., & Leisman, G. (2009). Autistic spectrum disorders as functional disconnection syndrome. *Reviews in the Neurosciences*, *20*(2), 111–131.

Menold, M. M., Shao, Y. J., Wolpert, C. M., Donnelly, S. L., Raiford, K. L., Martin, E. R., . . . Gilbert, J. R. (2001). Association analysis of chromosome 15 GABA(A) receptor subunit genes in autistic disorder. *Journal of Neurogenetics*, *15*(3–4), 245–259.

Menon, V. (2011). Large-scale brain networks and psychopathology: A unifying triple network model. *Trends in Cognitive Sciences*, *15*(10), 483–506.

Middlemass, J. (1895, June). A heavy brain. *Lancet*, *8*, 1432–1434.

Mike, A., Strammer, E., Aradi, M., Orsi, G., Perlaki, G., Hajnal, A., . . . Illes, Z. (2013). Disconnection mechanism and regional cortical atrophy contribute to impaired processing of facial expressions and theory of mind in multiple sclerosis: A structural MRI study. *PLoS One*, *8*(12), E82422.

Miles, J. H., Hadden, L. L., Takahashi, T. N., & Hillman, R. E. (2000). Head circumference is an independent clinical finding associated with autism. *American Journal of Medical Genetics*, *95*(4), 339–350.

Miles, J. H., & Hillman, R. E. (2000). Value of a clinical morphology examination in autism. *American Journal of Medical Genetics*, *91*(4), 245–253.

Miles, J. H., Takahashi, T. N., Bagby, S., Sahota, P. K., Vaslow, D. F., Wang, C. H., . . . Farmer, J. E. (2005). Essential versus complex autism: Definition of fundamental prognostic subtypes. *American Journal of Medical Genetics Part A*, *135*(2), 171–180.

Miller, H. L., Ragozzino, M. E., Cook, E. H., Sweeney, J. A., & Mosconi, M. W. (2015). Cognitive set shifting deficits and their relationship to repetitive behaviors in autism spectrum disorder. *Journal of Autism and Developmental Disorders*, *45*(3), 805–815.

Miller, J. N., & Ozonoff, S. (1997). Did Asperger's cases have Asperger disorder? A research note. *Journal of Child Psychology and Psychiatry*, *38*(2), 247–251.

Miller, M., Chukoskie, L., Zinni, M., Townsend, J., & Trauner, D. (2014). Dyspraxia, motor function and visual-motor integration in autism. *Behavioural Brain Research*, *269*, 95–102.

Miller, V. M., Zhu, Y., Bucher, C., McGinnis, W., Ryan, L. K., Siegel, A., & Zalcman, S. (2013). Gestational flu exposure induces changes in neurochemicals, affiliative hormones and brainstem inflammation, in addition to autism-like behaviors in mice. *Brain, Behavior, and Immunity*, *33*, 153–163.

Mills, B. D., Lai, J., Brown, T. T., Erhart, M., Halgren, E., Reilly, J., . . . Moses, P. (2013). White matter microstructure correlates of narrative production in typically developing children and children with high functioning autism. *Neuropsychologia*, *51*(10), 1933–1941.

Mills, K. L., Lalonde, F., Clasen, L. S., Giedd, J. N., & Blakemore, S. J. (2014). Developmental changes in the structure of the social brain in late childhood and adolescence. *Social Cognitive and Affective Neuroscience*, *9*(1), 123–131.

Ming, X., Brimacombe, M., & Wagner, G. C. (2007). Prevalence of motor impairment in autism spectrum disorders. *Brain and Development*, *29*(9), 565–570.

Miniscalco, C., Rudling, M., Rastam, M., Gillberg, C., & Johnels, J. A. (2014). Imitation (rather than core language) predicts pragmatic development in young children with ASD: A preliminary longitudinal study using CDI parental reports. *International Journal of Language and Communication Disorders*, *49*(3), 369–375.

Minshew, N. J., & Goldstein, G. (1993). Is autism an amnesic disorder? Evidence from the California Verbal Learning Test. *Neuropsychology*, *7*(2), 209–216.

Minshew, N. J., & Goldstein, G. (2001). The pattern of intact and impaired memory functions in autism. *Journal of Child Psychology and Psychiatry*, *42*(8), 1095–1101.

Minshew, N. J., Goldstein, G., & Siegel, D. J. (1997). Neuropsychologic functioning in autism: Profile of a complex information processing disorder. *Journal of the International Neuropsychological Society*, *3*(4), 303–316.

Minshew, N. J., Luna, B., & Sweeney, J. A. (1999). Oculomotor evidence for neocortical systems but not cerebellar dysfunction in autism. *Neurology*, *52*(5), 917–922.

Minshew, N. J., Turner, C. A., & Goldstein, G. (2005). The application of short forms of the Wechsler intelligence scales in adults and children with high functioning autism. *Journal of Autism and Developmental Disorders*, *35*(1), 45–52.

Mizuno, A., Villalobos, M. E., Davies, M. M., Dahl, B. C., & Muller, R. A. (2006). Partially enhanced thalamocortical functional connectivity in autism. *Brain Research*, *1104*(1), 160–174.

Moessner, R., Marshall, C. R., Sutcliffe, J. S., Skaug, J., Pinto, D., Vincent, J., . . . Scherer, S. W. (2007). Contribution of SHANK3 mutations to autism spectrum disorder. *American Journal of Medical Genetics*, *81*(6), 1289–1297.

Molesworth, C. J., Bowler, D. M., & Hampton, J. A. (2005). The prototype effect in recognition memory: Intact in autism? *Journal of Child Psychology and Psychiatry*, *46*(6), 661–672.

Molloy, C. A., Keddache, M., & Martin, L. J. (2005). Evidence for linkage on 21q and 7q in a subset of autism characterized by developmental regression. *Molecular Psychiatry*, *10*(8), 741–746.

Molloy, C. A., Morrow, A. L., Meinzen-Derr, J., Dawson, G., Bernier, R., Dunn, M., . . . Lord, C. (2006). Familial autoimmune thyroid disease as a risk factor for regression in children with autism spectrum disorder: A CPEA study. *Journal of Autism and Developmental Disorders*, *36*(3), 317–324.

Money, J., Bobrow, N. A., & Clarke, F. C. (1971). Autism and autoimmune disease: A family study. *Journal of Autism and Childhood Schizophrenia*, *1*(2), 146–160.

Monk, C. S., Peltier, S. J., Wiggins, J. L., Weng, S. J., Carrasco, M., Risi, S., & Lord, C. (2009). Abnormalities of intrinsic functional connectivity in autism spectrum disorders. *Neuroimage*, *47*(2), 764–772.

Monsell, S. (2003). Task switching. *Trends in Cognitive Sciences*, *7*, 134–140.

Moore, V., & Goodson, S. (2003). How well does early diagnosis of autism stand the test of time? Follow-up study of children assessed for autism at age 2 and development of an early diagnostic service. *Autism*, *7*(1), 47–63.

Mordekar, S. R., Prendergast, M., Chattopadhyay, A. K., & Baxter, P. S. (2009). Corticosteroid treatment of behaviour, language and motor regression in childhood disintegrative disorder. *European Journal of Paediatric Neurology*, *13*(4), 367–369.

Morgan, J. T., Chana, G., Pardo, C. A., Achim, C., Semendeferi, K., Buckwalter, J., . . . Everall, I. P. (2010). Microglial activation and increased microglial density observed in the dorsolateral prefrontal cortex in autism. *Biological Psychiatry*, *68*(4), 368–376.

Morgan, L., Wetherby, A. M., & Barber, A. (2008). Repetitive and stereotyped movements in children with autism spectrum disorders late in the second year of life. *Journal of Child Psychology and Psychiatry*, *49*(8), 826–837.

Mosconi, M. W., Cody-Hazlett, H., Poe, M. D., Gerig, G., Gimpel-Smith, R., & Piven, J. (2009). Longitudinal study of amygdala volume and joint attention in 2-to 4-year-old children with autism. *Archives of General Psychiatry*, *66*(5), 509–516.

Mostofsky, S. H., Dubey, P., Jerath, V. K., Jansiewicz, E. M., Goldberg, M. C., & Denckla, M. B. (2006). Developmental dyspraxia is not limited to imitation in children with autism spectrum disorders. *Journal of the International Neuropsychological Society*, *12*(3), 314–326.

Mottron, L., Dawson, M., Soulieres, I., Hubert, B., & Burack, J. (2006). Enhanced perceptual functioning in autism: An update, and eight principles of autistic perception. *Journal of Autism and Developmental Disorders*, *36*(1), 27–43.

Mottron, L., Morasse, K., & Belleville, S. (2001). A study of memory functioning in individuals with autism. *Journal of Child Psychology and Psychiatry*, *42*(2), 253–260.

Mountcastle, V. B. (1997). The columnar organization of the neocortex. *Brain*, *120*, 701–722.

Mraz, K. D., Green, J., Dumont-Mathieu, T., Makin, S., & Fein, D. (2007). Correlates of head circumference growth in infants later diagnosed with autism spectrum disorders. *Journal of Child Neurology*, *22*(6), 700–713.

Mrzljak, L., Uylings, H.B.M., Vaneden, C. G., & Judas, M. (1990). Neuronal development in human prefrontal cortex in prenatal and postnatal stages. *Progress in Brain Research*, *85*, 185–222.

Muhle, R., Trentacoste, S. V., & Rapin, I. (2004). The genetics of autism. *Pediatrics*, *113*(5), e472–486.

Muller, R. A. (2007). The study of autism as a distributed disorder. *Mental Retardation and Developmental Disabilities Research Reviews*, *13*(1), 85–95.

Muller, R. A., Shih, P., Keehn, B., Deyoe, J. R., Leyden, K. M., & Shukla, D. K. (2011). Underconnected, but how? A survey of functional connectivity MRI studies in autism spectrum disorders. *Cerebral Cortex*, *21*(10), 2233–2243.

Mundy, P., Sullivan, L., & Mastergeorge, A. M. (2009). A parallel and distributed-processing model of joint attention, social cognition and autism. *Autism Research*, *2*(1), 2–21.

Muratori, F., Calderoni, S., Apicella, F., Filippi, T., Santocchi, E., Calugi, S., . . . Narzisi, A. (2012). Tracing back to the onset of abnormal head circumference growth in Italian children with autism spectrum disorder. *Research in Autism Spectrum Disorders*, *6*(1), 442–449.

Nabbout, R., & Dulac, O. (2003). Epileptic encephalopathies: A brief overview. *Journal of Clinical Neurophysiology*, *20*(6), 393–397.

Naigles, L. R., Kelty, E., Jaffery, R., & Fein, D. (2011). Abstractness and continuity in the syntactic development of young children with autism. *Autism Research*, *4*(6), 422–437.

Nair, A., Keown, C. L., Datko, M., Shih, P., Keehn, B., & Mueller, R.-A. (2014). Impact of methodological variables on functional connectivity findings in autism spectrum disorders. *Human Brain Mapping*, *35*(8), 4035–4048.

Nair, A., Treiber, J. M., Shukla, D. K., Shih, P., & Mueller, R.-A. (2013). Impaired thalamocortical connectivity in autism spectrum disorder: A study of functional and anatomical connectivity. *Brain*, *136*, 1942–1955.

Nass, R., Gross, A., & Devinsky, O. (1998). Autism and autistic epileptiform regression with occipital spikes. *Developmental Medicine and Child Neurology*, *40*(7), 453–458.

Nass, R., & Petrucha, D. (1990). Acquired aphasia with convulsive disorder: A pervasive developmental disorder variant. *Journal of Child Neurology*, *5*(4), 327–328.

Neale, B. M., Kou, Y., Liu, L., Ma'ayan, A., Samocha, K. E., Sabo, A., . . . Daly, M. J. (2012). Patterns and rates of exonic de novo mutations in autism spectrum disorders. *Nature*, *485*(7397), 242–U129.

Needleman, L. A., & McAllister, A. K. (2012). The major histocompatibility complex and autism spectrum disorder. *Developmental Neurobiology*, *72*(10), 1288–1301.

Nellhaus, G. (1968). Head circumference from birth to 18 years: Practical composite international and interracial graphs. *Pediatrics*, *41*(1P1), 106.

Neville, H. J. (2006). Different profiles of plasticity within human cognition. In Y. Munakata & M. H. Johnson (Eds.), *Processes of Change in Brain and Cognitive Development: Attention and Performance Xxi* (pp. 287–314). New York: Oxford University Press.

Newbury, D. F., Paracchini, S., Scerri, T. S., Winchester, L., Addis, L., Richardson, A. J., . . . Monaco, A. P. (2011). Investigation of dyslexia and SLI risk variants in reading-and language-impaired subjects. *Behavior Genetics*, *41*(1), 90–104.

Nielsen, J. A., Zielinski, B. A., Fletcher, P. T., Alexander, A. L., Lange, N., Bigler, E. D., . . . Anderson, J. S. (2013). Multisite functional connectivity MRI classification of autism: ABIDE results. *Frontiers in Human Neuroscience*, *7*, 599.

Nomi, J. S., & Uddin, L. Q. (2015). Developmental changes in large-scale network connectivity in autism. *NeuroImage: Clinical*, *7*, 732–741.

Noonan, S. K., Haist, F., & Muller, R. A. (2009). Aberrant functional connectivity in autism: Evidence from low-frequency BOLD signal fluctuations. *Brain Research*, *1262*, 48–63.

Norbury, C. F., & Bishop, D. V. (2002). Inferential processing and story recall in children with communication problems: A comparison of specific language impairment, pragmatic language impairment and high-functioning autism. *International Journal of Language and Communication Disorders*, *37*(3), 227–251.

Nordahl, C. W., Lange, N., Li, D. D., Barnett, L. A., Lee, A., Buonocore, M. H., . . . Amaral, D. G. (2011). Brain enlargement is associated with regression in preschool-age boys with autism spectrum disorders. *Proceedings of the National Academy of Sciences of the United States of America*, *108*(50), 20195–20200.

Nordahl, C. W., Scholz, R., Yang, X. W., Buonocore, M. H., Simon, T., Rogers, S., & Amaral, D. G. (2012). Increased rate of amygdala growth in children aged 2 to 4 years with autism spectrum disorders A longitudinal study. *Archives of General Psychiatry*, *69*(1), 53–61.

Nordenbaek, C., Jorgensen, M., Kyvik, K. O., & Bilenberg, N. (2014). A Danish population-based twin study on autism spectrum disorders. *European Child and Adolescent Psychiatry*, *23*(1), 35–43.

Noriega, D. B., & Savelkoul, H.F.J. (2014). Immune dysregulation in autism spectrum disorder. *European Journal of Pediatrics*, *173*(1), 33–43.

Noriuchi, M., Kikuchi, Y., Yoshiura, T., Kira, R., Shigeto, H., Hara, T., . . . Kamio, Y. (2010). Altered white matter fractional anisotropy and social impairment in children with autism spectrum disorder. *Brain Research*, *1362*, 141–149.

Norris, M., & Lecavalier, L. (2010). Screening accuracy of Level 2 autism spectrum disorder rating scales: A review of selected instruments. *Autism*, *14*(4), 263–284.

Nudel, R., Simpson, N. H., Baird, G., O'Hare, A., Conti-Ramsden, G., Bolton, P. F., . . . The, S.L.I.C. (2014). Associations of HLA alleles with specific language impairment. *Journal of Neurodevelopmental Disorders*, *6*(1), 1.

Oblak, A. L., Gibbs, T. T., & Blatt, G. J. (2009). Decreased GABAA receptors and benzodiazepine binding sites in the anterior cingulate cortex in autism. *Autism Research: Official Journal of the International Society for Autism Research*, *2*(4), 205–219.

Oblak, A. L., Gibbs, T. T., & Blatt, G. J. (2010). Decreased GABA(B) receptors in the cingulate cortex and fusiform gyrus in autism. *Journal of Neurochemistry*, *114*(5), 1414–1423.

Oblak, A. L., Rosene, D. L., Kemper, T. L., Bauman, M. L., & Blatt, G. J. (2011). Altered posterior cingulate cortical cyctoarchitecture, but normal density of neurons and interneurons in the posterior cingulate cortex and fusiform gyrus in autism. *Autism Research: Official Journal of the International Society for Autism Research*, *4*(3), 200–211.

O'Halloran, C. J., Kinsella, G. J., & Storey, E. (2011). The cerebellum and neuropsychological functioning: A critical review. *Journal of Clinical and Experimental Neuropsychology, 34*(1), 35–56.

Onore, C., Careaga, M., & Ashwood, P. (2012). The role of immune dysfunction in the pathophysiology of autism. *Brain Behavior and Immunity*, *26*(3), 383–392.

Ornitz, E. M. (1973). Childhood autism: A review of the clinical and experimental literature. *California Medicine*, *118*(4), 21–47.

O'Roak, B. J., Vives, L., Fu, W., Egertson, J. D., Stanaway, I. B., Phelps, I. G., . . . Shendure, J. (2012). Multiplex targeted sequencing identifies recurrently mutated genes in autism spectrum disorders. *Science*, *338*(6114), 1619–1622.

O'Shea, A. G., Fein, D. A., Cillessen, A. H., Klin, A., & Schultz, R. T. (2005). Source memory in children with autism spectrum disorders. *Developmental Neuropsychology*, *27*(3), 337–360.

Osterling, J., & Dawson, G. (1994). Early recognition of children with autism: A study of first birthday home videotapes. *Journal of Autism and Developmental Disorders*, *24*(3), 247–257.

Osterling, J. A., Dawson, G., & Munson, J. A. (2002). Early recognition of 1-year-old infants with autism spectrum disorder versus mental retardation. *Development and Psychopathology*, *14*(2), 239–251.

Ottet, M.-C., Schaer, M., Cammoun, L., Schneider, M., Debbane, M., Thiran, J.-P., & Eliez, S. (2013). Reduced fronto-temporal and limbic connectivity in the 22q11.2 deletion syndrome: Vulnerability markers for developing schizophrenia? *PLoS One*, *8*(3), 1–8.

Ounsted, M., Moar, V. A., & Scott, A. (1985). Head circumference charts updated. *Archives of Disease in Childhood*, *60*, 936–939.

Ozgen, H. M., Hop, J. W., Hox, J. J., Beemer, F. A., & van Engeland, H. (2010). Minor physical anomalies in autism: A meta-analysis. *Molecular Psychiatry*, *15*(3), 300–307.

Ozonoff, S. (1995). Reliability and validity of the Wisconsin Card Sorting Test in studies of autism. *Neuropsychology*, *9*(4), 491–500.

Ozonoff, S., Goodlin-Jones, B. L., & Solomon, M. (2005). Evidence-based assessment of autism spectrum disorders in children and adolescents. *Journal of Clinical Child and Adolescent Psychology*, *34*(3), 523–540.

Ozonoff, S., Heung, K., Byrd, R., Hansen, R., & Hertz-Picciotto, I. (2008). The onset of autism: Patterns of symptom emergence in the first years of life. *Autism Research*, *1*(6), 320–328.

Ozonoff, S., Iosif, A. M., Baguio, F., Cook, I. C., Hill, M. M., Hutman, T., . . . Young, G. S. (2010). A prospective study of the emergence of early behavioral signs of autism. *Journal of the American Academy of Child and Adolescent Psychiatry*, *49*(3), 256–266 e251–252.

Ozonoff, S., & Jensen, J. (1999). Brief report: Specific executive function profiles in three neurodevelopmental disorders. *Journal of Autism and Developmental Disorders*, *29*(2), 171–177.

Ozonoff, S., Macari, S., Young, G. S., Goldring, S., Thompson, M., & Rogers, S. J. (2008). Atypical object exploration at 12 months of age is associated with autism in a prospective sample. *Autism*, *12*(5), 457–472.

Ozonoff, S., Pennington, B. F., & Rogers, S. J. (1991). Executive function deficits in high-functioning autistic individuals: Relationship to theory of mind. *Journal of Child Psychology and Psychiatry*, *32*(7), 1081–1105.

Ozonoff, S., & Strayer, D. L. (1997). Inhibitory function in nonretarded children with autism. *Journal of Autism and Developmental Disorders*, *27*(1), 59–77.

Ozonoff, S., & Strayer, D. L. (2001). Further evidence of intact working memory in autism. *Journal of Autism and Developmental Disorders*, *31*(3), 257–263.

Ozonoff, S., Williams, B. J., & Landa, R. (2005). Parental report of the early development of children with regressive autism: The delays-plus-regression phenotype. *Autism*, *9*(5), 461–486.

Ozonoff, S., Young, G. S., Carter, A., Messinger, D., Yirmiya, N., Zwaigenbaum, L., . . . Stone, W. L. (2011). Recurrence Risk for Autism Spectrum Disorders: A Baby Siblings Research Consortium Study. *Pediatrics, 128*(3), 488–495.

Pagnamenta, A. T., Khan, H., Walker, S., Gerrelli, D., Wing, K., Bonaglia, M. C., . . . Monaco, A. P. (2011). Rare familial 16q21 microdeletions under a linkage peak implicate cadherin 8 (CDH8) in susceptibility to autism and learning disability. *Journal of Medical Genetics*, *48*(1), 48–54.

Pajevic, S., Basser, P. J., & Fields, R. D. (2014). Role of myelin plasticity in oscillations and synchrony of neuronal activity. *Neuroscience*, *276*, 135–147.

Palmen, S., van Engeland, H., Hof, P. R., & Schmitz, C. (2004). Neuropathological findings in autism. *Brain*, *127*, 2572–2583.

Pardo, C. A., & Eberhart, C. G. (2007). The neurobiology of autism. *Brain Pathology*, *17*(4), 434–447.

Pardo, C. A., Vargas, D. L., & Zimmerman, A. W. (2006). Immunity, neuroglia and neuroinflammation in autism. *International Review of Psychiatry*, *17*(6), 485–495.

Parmeggiani, A., Barcia, G., Posar, A., Raimondi, E., Santucci, M., & Scaduto, M. C. (2010). Epilepsy and EEG paroxysmal abnormalities in autism spectrum disorders. *Brain and Development*, *32*(9), 783–789.

Parner, E. T., Baron-Cohen, S., Lauritsen, M. B., Jorgensen, M., Schieve, L. A., Yeargin-Allsopp, M., & Obel, C. (2012). Parental age and autism spectrum disorders. *Annals of Epidemiology*, *22*(3), 143–150.

Parner, E. T., Thorsen, P., Dixon, G., de Klerk, N., Leonard, H., Nassar, N., . . . Glasson, E. J. (2011). A comparison of autism prevalence trends in Denmark and Western Australia. *Journal of Autism and Developmental Disorders*, *41*(12), 1601–1608.

Parr, J. R., Le Couteur, A., Baird, G., Rutter, M., Pickles, A., Fombonne, E., . . . Imgsac. (2011). Early developmental regression in autism spectrum disorder: Evidence from an international multiplex sample. *Journal of Autism and Developmental Disorders*, *41*(3), 332–340.

Parr, L. A., Modi, M., Siebert, E., & Young, L. J. (2013). Intranasal oxytocin selectively attenuates rhesus monkeys' attention to negative facial expressions. *Psychoneuroendocrinology*, *38*(9), 1748–1756.

Pascualvaca, D. M., Fantie, B. D., Papageorgiou, M., & Mirsky, A. F. (1998). Attentional capacities in children with autism: Is there a general deficit in shifting focus? *Journal of Autism and Developmental Disorders*, *28*(6), 467–478.

Patel, V. B., Preedy, V. R., & Martin, C. R. (2014). *Comprehensive Guide to Autism*. New York, New York: Springer.

Paul, L. K., Corsello, C., Kennedy, D. P., & Adolphs, R. (2014). Agenesis of the corpus callosum and autism: A comprehensive comparison. *Brain*, *137*, 1813–1829.

Paul, L. K., Corsello, C., Tranel, D., & Adolphs, R. (2010). Does bilateral damage to the human amygdala produce autistic symptoms? *Journal of Neurodevelopmental Disorders*, *2*(3), 165–173.

Paul, R., Augustyn, A., Klin, A., & Volkmar, F. R. (2005). Perception and production of prosody by speakers with autism spectrum disorders. *Journal of Autism and Developmental Disorders*, *35*(2), 205–220.

Paul, R., Orlovski, C. M., Marcinko, H. C., & Volkmar, F. (2009). Conversational behaviors in youth with high-functioning ASD and Asperger syndrome. *Journal of Autism and Developmental Disorders*, *39*, 115–125.

Pellicano, E. (2010). Individual differences in executive function and central coherence predict developmental changes in theory of mind in autism. *Developmental Psychology*, *46*(2), 530–544.

Pellicano, E. (2012). The development of executive function in autism. *Autism Research and Treatment*, *2012*, 146132.

Pellicano, E., Gibson, L., Maybery, M., Durkin, K., & Badcock, D. R. (2005). Abnormal global processing along the dorsal visual pathway in autism: A possible mechanism for weak visuospatial coherence? *Neuropsychologia*, *43*(7), 1044–1053.

Pelphrey, K. A., & Carter, E. J. (2008). Charting the typical and atypical development of the social brain. *Development and Psychopathology*, *20*(4), 1081–1102.

Pelphrey, K. A., Morris, J. P., & McCarthy, G. (2005). Neural basis of eye gaze processing deficits in autism. *Brain*, *128*(Pt 5), 1038–1048.

Pelphrey, K. A., Morris, J. P., McCarthy, G., & Labar, K. S. (2007). Perception of dynamic changes in facial affect and identity in autism. *Social Cognitive and Affective Neuroscience*, *2*(2), 140–149.

Pelphrey, K. A., Shultz, S., Hudac, C. M., & Wyk, B.C.V. (2011). Research review: Constraining heterogeneity: The social brain and its development in autism spectrum disorder. *Journal of Child Psychology and Psychiatry*, *52*(6), 631–644.

Penagarikano, O., Abrahams, B. S., Herman, E. I., Winden, K. D., Gdalyahu, A., Dong, H., . . . Geschwind, D. H. (2011). Absence of CNTNAP2 leads to epilepsy, neuronal migration abnormalities, and core autism-related deficits. *Cell*, *147*(1), 235–246.

Penagarikano, O., & Geschwind, D. H. (2012). What does CNTNAP2 reveal about autism spectrum disorder? *Trends in Molecular Medicine*, *18*(3), 156–163.

Pennington, B. F., & Ozonoff, S. (1996). Executive functions and developmental psychopathology. *Journal of Child Psychology and Psychiatry*, *37*(1), 51–87.

Peppe, S., McCann, J., Gibbon, F., O'Hare, A., & Rutherford, M. (2007). Receptive and expressive prosodic ability in children with high-functioning autism. *Journal of Speech Language and Hearing Research*, *50*(4), 1015–1028.

Persico, A. M., & Bourgeron, T. (2006). Searching for ways out of the autism maze: Genetic, epigenetic and environmental clues. *Trends in Neurosciences*, *29*(7), 349–358.

Persico, A. M., & Napolioni, V. (2013). Autism genetics. *Behavioural Brain Research*, *251*, 95–112.

Petanjek, Z., Judas, M., Simic, G., Rasin, M. R., Uylings, H. B., Rakic, P., & Kostovic, I. (2011). Extraordinary neoteny of synaptic spines in the human prefrontal cortex. *Proceedings of the National Academy of Sciences of the United States of America*, *108*(32), 13281–13286.

Peterson, C. C., Wellman, H. M., & Liu, D. (2005). Steps in theory-of-mind development for children with deafness or autism. *Child Development*, *76*(2), 502–517.

Phelan, H. L., Filliter, J. H., & Johnson, S. A. (2010). Brief report: Memory performance on the California verbal learning test: Children's version in autism spectrum disorder. *Journal of Autism and Developmental Disorders*, *41*(4), 518–523.

Philip, R.C.M., Dauvermann, M. R., Whalley, H. C., Baynham, K., Lawrie, S. M., & Stanfield, A. C. (2012). A systematic review and meta-analysis of the fMRI investigation of autism spectrum disorders. *Neuroscience and Biobehavioral Reviews*, *36*(2), 901–942.

Phillips, M., & Pozzo-Miller, L. (2015). Dendritic spine dysgenesis in autism related disorders. *Neuroscience Letters*, *601*, 30–40.

Pickering, M., Cumiskey, D., & O'Connor, J. J. (2005). Actions of TNF-alpha on glutamatergic synaptic transmission in the central nervous system. *Experimental Physiology*, *90*(5), 663–670.

Pickles, A., Simonoff, E., Conti-Ramsden, G., Falcaro, M., Simkin, Z., Charman, T., . . . Baird, G. (2009). Loss of language in early development of autism and specific language impairment. *Journal of Child Psychology and Psychiatry*, *50*(7), 843–852.

Pickles, A., Starr, E., Kazak, S., Bolton, P., Papanikolaou, K., Bailey, A., . . . Rutter, M. (2000). Variable expression of the autism broader phenotype: Findings from extended pedigrees. *Journal of Child Psychology and Psychiatry*, *41*(4), 491–502.

Pierce, K., Carter, C., Weinfeld, M., Desmond, J., Hazin, R., Bjork, R., & Gallagher, N. (2011). Detecting, studying, and treating autism early: The one-year well-baby check-up approach. *Journal of Pediatrics*, *159*(3), 458–U326.

Pierce, K., Haist, F., Sedaghat, F., & Courchesne, E. (2004). The brain response to personally familiar faces in autism: Findings of fusiform activity and beyond. *Brain*, *127*(Pt 12), 2703–2716.

Pierce, K., & Redcay, E. (2008). Fusiform function in children with an autism spectrum disorder is a matter of "who." *Biological Psychiatry*, *64*(7), 552–560.

Pinto, D., Pagnamenta, A. T., Klei, L., Anney, R., Merico, D., Regan, R., . . . Betancur, C. (2010). Functional impact of global rare copy number variation in autism spectrum disorders. *Nature*, *466*(7304), 368–372.

Piras, I. S., Haapanen, L., Napolioni, V., Sacco, R., Van de Water, J., & Persico, A. M. (2014). Anti-brain antibodies are associated with more severe cognitive and behavioral profiles in Italian children with autism spectrum disorder. *Brain Behavior and Immunity*, *38*, 91–99.

Piton, A., Gauthier, J., Hamdan, F. F., Lafreniere, R. G., Yang, Y., Henrion, E., . . . Rouleau, G. A. (2010). Systematic resequencing of X-chromosome synaptic genes in autism spectrum disorder and schizophrenia. *Molecular Psychiatry*, *16*(8), 867–880.

Piven, J., Arndt, S., Bailey, J., & Andreasen, N. (1996). Regional brain enlargement in autism: A magnetic resonance imaging study. *Journal of the American Academy of Child and Adolescent Psychiatry*, *35*(4), 530–536.

Piven, J., Arndt, S., Bailey, J., Havercamp, S., Andreasen, N. C., & Palmer, P. (1995). An MRI study of brain size in autism. *American Journal of Psychiatry*, *152*(8), 1145–1149.

Piven, J., Bailey, J., Ranson, B. J., & Arndt, S. (1997). An MRI study of the corpus callosum in autism. *American Journal of Psychiatry*, *154*(8), 1051–1056.

Piven, J., Berthier, M. L., Starkstein, S. E., Nehme, E., Pearlson, G., & Folstein, S. (1990). Magnetic resonance imaging evidence for a defect of cerebral cortical development in autism. *American Journal of Psychiatry*, *147*(6), 734–739.

Piven, J., Palmer, P., Jacobi, D., Childress, D., & Arndt, S. (1997). Broader autism phenotype: Evidence from a family history study of multiple-incidence autism families. *American Journal of Psychiatry*, *154*(2), 185–190.

Piven, J., Simon, J., Chase, G. A., Wzorek, M., Landa, R., Gayle, J., & Folstein, S. (1993). The etiology of autism: Pre-, peri- and neonatal factors. *Journal of the American Academy of Child and Adolescent Psychiatry*, *32*(6), 1256–1263.

Plauché Johnson, C., & Myers, S. M. (2007). Identification and evaluation of children with autism spectrum disorders. *Pediatrics*, *120*, 1183–1215.

Plioplys, A. V. (1998). Intravenous immunoglobulin treatment of children with autism. *Journal of Child Neurology*, *13*(2), 79–82.

Polderman, T.J.C., Hoekstra, R. A., Posthuma, D., & Larsson, H. (2014). The co-occurrence of autistic and ADHD dimensions in adults: An etiological study in 17 770 twins. *Translational Psychiatry*, *4*(9), E435.

Poliak, S., Salomon, D., Elhanany, H., Sabanay, H., Kiernan, B., Pevny, L., . . . Peles, E. (2003). Juxtaparanodal clustering of Shaker-like K+ channels in myelinated axons depends on Caspr2 and TAG-1. *Journal of Cell Biology*, *162*(6), 1149–1160.

Posner, M. I., & Fan, J. (2004). Attention as an organ system. In J. R. Pomerantz & M. C. Crair (Eds.), *Topics in Integrative Neuroscience: From Cells to Cognition*, 31–61. Cambridge: Cambridge University Press.

Posthuma, D., & Polderman, T.J.C. (2013). What have we learned from recent twin studies about the etiology of neurodevelopmental disorders? *Current Opinion in Neurology*, *26*(2), 111–121.

Poustka, L., Jennen-Steinmetz, C., Henze, R., Vomstein, K., Haffner, J., & Sieltjes, B. (2012). Fronto-temporal disconnectivity and symptom severity in children with autism spectrum disorder. *World Journal of Biological Psychiatry*, *13*(4), 269–280.

Power, R. A., Kyaga, S., Uher, R., MacCabe, J. H., Langstrom, N., Landen, M., . . . Svensson, A. C. (2013). Fecundity of patients with schizophrenia, autism, bipolar disorder, depression, anorexia nervosa, or substance abuse vs. their unaffected siblings. *Jama Psychiatry*, *70*(1), 22–30.

Premack, D., & Woodruff, G. (1978). Does the chimpanzee have a "theory of mind"? *Brain and Behavioral Sciences*, *4*, 515–526.

Pryweller, J. R., Schauder, K. B., Anderson, A. W., Heacock, J. L., Foss-Feig, J. H., Newsom, C. R., . . . Cascio, C. J. (2014). White matter correlates of sensory processing in autism spectrum disorders. *Neuroimage: Clinical*, *6*, 379–387.

Puleo, C. M., Schmeidler, J., Reichenberg, A., Kolevzon, A., Soorya, L. V., Buxbaum, J. D., & Silverman, J. M. (2012). Advancing paternal age and simplex autism. *Autism*, *16*(4), 367–380.

Purcell, A. E., Jeon, O. H., Zimmerman, A. W., & Pevsner, J. (2001). Postmortem brain abnormalities of the glutamate neurotransmitter system in autism. *Neurology*, *57*(9), 1618–1628.

Radua, J., Via, E., Catani, M., & Mataix-Cols, D. (2011). Voxel-based meta-analysis of regional white-matter volume differences in autism spectrum disorder versus healthy controls. *Psychological Medicine*, *41*(7), 1539–1550.

Rai, D., Golding, J., Magnusson, C., Steer, C., Lewis, G., & Dalman, C. (2012). Prenatal and early life exposure to stressful life events and risk of autism spectrum disorders: Population-based studies in Sweden and England. *PLoS One*, *7*(6), e38893.

Rapin, I. (1995). Autistic regression and disintegrative disorder: How important the role of epilepsy? *Seminars in Pediatric Neurology*, *2*(4), 278–285.

Rapin, I. (2006). Language heterogeneity and regression in the autism spectrum disorders: Overlaps with other childhood language regression syndromes. *Clinical Neuroscience Research*, *6*(3–4), 209–218.

Rapin, I. (2014). Classification of behaviorally defined disorders: Biology versus the DSM. *Journal of Autism and Developmental Disorders*, *44*(10), 2661–2666.

Raymaekers, R., Antrop, I., van der Meere, J. J., Wiersema, J. R., & Roeyers, H. (2007). HFA and ADHD: A direct comparison on state regulation and response inhibition. *Journal of Clinical and Experimental Neuropsychology*, *29*(4), 418–427.

Raymaekers, R., Van der Meere, J., & Roeyers, H. (2004). Event-rate manipulation and its effect on arousal modulation and response inhibition in adults with high functioning autism. *Journal of Clinical and Experimental Neuropsychology*, *26*(1), 74–82.

Raymond, G. V., Bauman, M. L., & Kemper, T. L. (1996). Hippocampus in autism: A golgi analysis. *Acta Neuropathologica*, *91*(1), 117–119.

Raznahan, A., Toro, R., Daly, E., Robertson, D., Murphy, C., Deeley, Q., . . . Murphy, D.G.M. (2010). Cortical anatomy in autism spectrum disorder: An in vivo MRI study on the effect of age. *Cerebral Cortex*, *20*(6), 1332–1340.

Raznahan, A., Wallace, G. L., Antezana, L., Greenstein, D., Lenroot, R., Thurm, A., . . . Giedd, J. N. (2013). Compared to what? Early brain overgrowth in autism and the perils of population norms. *Biological Psychiatry*, *74*(8), 563–575.

Reber, M. (Ed.). (2012). *The Autism Spectrum: Scientific Foundations and Treatment*. New York: Cambridge University Press.

Redcay, E., & Courchesne, E. (2005). When is the brain enlarged in autism? A meta-analysis of all brain size reports. *Biological Psychiatry*, *58*, 1–9.

Redies, C., Hertel, N., & Hubner, C. A. (2012). Cadherins and neuropsychiatric disorders. *Brain Research*, *1470*, 130–144.

Regier, D. A., Narrow, W. E., Clarke, D. E., Kraemer, H. C., Kuramoto, S. J., Kuhl, E. A., & Kupfer, D. J. (2013). DSM-5 field trials in the United States and Canada, part II: Test-retest reliability of selected categorical diagnoses. *American Journal of Psychiatry*, *170*(1), 59–70.

Reichenberg, A., Gross, R., Weiser, M., Bresnahan, M., Silverman, J., Harlap, S., . . . Susser, E. (2006). Advancing paternal age and autism. *Archives of General Psychiatry*, *63*(9), 1026–1032.

Renner, P., Grofer Klinger, L., & Klinger, M. R. (2006). Exogenous and endogenous attention orienting in autism spectrum disorders. *Child Neuropsychology*, *12*(4–5), 361–382.

Renner, P., Klinger, L. G., & Klinger, M. R. (2000). Implicit and explicit memory in autism: Is autism an amnesic disorder? *Journal of Autism and Developmental Disorders*, *30*(1), 3–14.

Reynolds, S., & Lane, S. J. (2008). Diagnostic validity of sensory over-responsivity: A review of the literature and case reports. *Journal of Autism and Developmental Disorders*, *38*(3), 516–529.

Reznick, J. S., Baranek, G. T., Reavis, S., Watson, L. R., & Crais, E. R. (2007). A parent-report instrument for identifying one-year-olds at risk for an eventual diagnosis of autism: The first year inventory. *Journal of Autism and Developmental Disorders*, *37*(9), 1691–1710.

Richler, J., Huerta, M., Bishop, S. L., & Lord, C. (2010). Developmental trajectories of restricted and repetitive behaviors and interests in children with autism spectrum disorders. *Development and Psychopathology*, *22*(1), 55–69.

Richler, J., Luyster, R., Risi, S., Hsu, W. L., Dawson, G., Bernier, R., . . . Lord, C. (2006). Is there a 'regressive phenotype' of autism spectrum disorder associated with the measles-mumps-rubella vaccine? A CPEA study. *Journal of Autism and Developmental Disorders*, *36*(3), 299–316.

Rimland, B. (1964). *Infantile Autism: The Syndrome and Its Implications for a Neural Theory of Behavior*. New York: Appleton-Century-Crofts.

Rinehart, N. J., Bradshaw, J. L., Moss, S. A., Brereton, A. V., & Tonge, B. J. (2000). A comparison of executive functioning in high-functioning autism and Asperger disorder using tasks sensitive to inhibitory and set-shifting deficits. *Journal of Intellectual Disability Research*, *44*, 442–442.

Rinehart, N. J., Bradshaw, J. L., Moss, S. A., Brereton, A. V., & Tonge, B. J. (2001). A deficit in shifting attention present in high-functioning autism but not Asperger's disorder. *Autism*, *5*(1), 67–80.

Rinehart, N. J., Tonge, B. J., Iansek, R., McGinley, J., Brereton, A. V., & Enticott, P. G. (2006). Gait function in newly diagnosed children with autism: Cerebellar and basal ganglia related motor disorder. *Developmental Medicine and Child Neurology*, *48*, 819–824.

Rippon, G., Brock, J., Brown, C., & Boucher, J. (2007). Disordered connectivity in the autistic brain: Challenges for the "new psychophysiology." *International Journal of Psychophysiology*, *63*(2), 164–172.

Ritvo, E. R., Freeman, B. J., Scheibel, A. B., Duong, T., Robinson, H., Guthrie, D., & Ritvo, A (1986). Lower Purkinje cell counts in the cerebella of four autistic subjects: Initial findings of the UCLA-NSAC research report. *American Journal of Psychiatry*, *143*(7), 862–866.

Ritvo, E. R., Freeman, B., Mason-Brothers, A., Mo, A., & Ritvo, A. M. (1986). Concordance for the syndrome of autism in 40 pairs of afflicted twins. *Annual Progress in Child Psychiatry & Child Development*, *142*, 74–77.

Riva, D., Bulgheroni, S., Aquino, D., Di Salle, F., Savoiardo, M., & Erbetta, A. (2011). Basal forebrain involvement in low-functioning autistic children: A voxel-based morphometry study. *AJNR: American Journal of Neuroradiology*, *32*(8), 1430–1435.

Rizzolatti, G., & Fabbri-Destro, M. (2008). The mirror system and its role in social cognition. *Current Opinion in Neurobiology*, *18*(2), 179–184.

Roberts, A. L., Lyall, K., Hart, J. E., Laden, F., Just, A. C., Bobb, J. F., . . . Weisskopf, M. G. (2013). Perinatal air pollutant exposures and autism spectrum disorder in the children of nurses' health study II participants. *Environmental Health Perspectives*, *121*(8), 978–984.

Roberts, E. M., & English, P. B. (2013). Bayesian modeling of time-dependent vulnerability to environmental hazards: An example using autism and pesticidedata. *Statistics in Medicine*, *32*(13), 2308–2319.

Roberts, J. A., Rice, M. L., & Tager-Flusberg, H. (2004). Tense marking in children with autism. *Applied Psycholinguistics*, *25*, 429–448.

Robins, D. L., Casagrande, K., Barton, M., Chen, C. M., Dumont-Mathieu, T., & Fein, D. (2014). Validation of the modified checklist for autism in toddlers, revised with follow-up (M-CHAT-R/F). *Pediatrics*, *133*(1), 37–45.

Robins, D. L., Fein, D., Barton, M. L., & Green, J. A. (2001). The modified checklist for autism in toddlers: An initial study investigating the early detection of autism and pervasive developmental disorders. *Journal of Autism and Developmental Disorders*, *31*(2), 131–144.

Robinson, E. B., Lichtenstein, P., Anckarsater, H., Happe, F., & Ronald, A. (2013). Examining and interpreting the female protective effect against autistic behavior. *Proceedings of the National Academy of Sciences of the United States of America*, *110*(13), 5258–5262.

Roche, A. F., Guo, S. S., Wholihan, K., & Casey, P. H. (1997). Reference data for head circumference-for-length in preterm low-birth-weight infants. *Archives of Pediatrics and Adolescent Medicine*, *151*(1), 50–57.

Rodier, P. M., Bryson, S. E., & Welch, J. P. (1997). Minor malformations and physical measurements in autism: Data from Nova Scotia. *Teratology*, *55*(5), 319–325.

Roelfsema, M. T., Hoekstra, R. A., Allison, C., Wheelwright, S., Brayne, C., Matthews, F. E., & Baron-Cohen, S. (2012). Are autism spectrum conditions more prevalent in an information-technology region? A school-based study of three regions in the Netherlands. *Journal of Autism and Developmental Disorders*, *42*(5), 734–739.

Rogers, S. J. (2004). Developmental regression in autism spectrum disorders. *Mental Retardation and Developmental Disabilities Research Reviews*, *10*(2), 139–143.

Rogers, S. J., & DiLalla, D. L. (1990). Age of symptom onset in young children with pervasive developmental disorders. *Journal of the American Academy of Child and Adolescent Psychiatry*, *29*(6), 863–872.

Rogers, S. J., Hepburn, S., & Wehner, E. (2003). Parent reports of sensory symptoms in toddlers with autism and those with other developmental disorders. *Journal of Autism and Developmental Disorders*, *33*(6), 631–642.

Rogers, S. J., & Ozonoff, S. (2005). Annotation: What do we know about sensory dysfunction in autism? A critical review of the empirical evidence. *Journal of Child Psychology and Psychiatry*, *46*(12), 1255–1268.

Rogers, S. J., Young, G. S., Cook, I., Giolzetti, A., & Ozonoff, S. (2008). Deferred and immediate imitation in regressive and early onset autism. *Journal of Child Psychology and Psychiatry*, *49*(4), 449–457.

Rogers, T. D., Dickson, P. E., Heck, D. H., Goldowitz, D., Mittleman, G., & Blaha, C. D. (2011). Connecting the dots of the cerebro-cerebellar role in cognitive function: Neuronal pathways for cerebellar modulation of dopamine release in the prefrontal cortex. *Synapse*, *65*(11), 1204–1212.

Rojas, D. C., Singel, D., Steinmetz, S., Hepburn, S., & Brown, M. S. (2014). Decreased left perisylvian GABA concentration in children with autism and unaffected siblings. *Neuroimage*, *86*, 28–34.

Rollins, J. D., Collins, J. S., & Holden, K. R. (2010). United States head circumference growth reference charts: Birth to 21 years. *Journal of Pediatrics*, *156*(6), 907–913.

Rommelse, N.N.J., Franke, B., Geurts, H. M., Hartman, C. A., & Buitelaar, J. K. (2010). Shared heritability of attention-deficit/hyperactivity disorder and autism spectrum disorder. *European Child and Adolescent Psychiatry*, *19*(3), 281–295.

Rommelse, N.N.J., Peters, C.T.R., Oosterling, I. J., Visser, J. C., Bons, D., van Steijn, D. J., . . . Buitelaar, J. K. (2011). A pilot study of abnormal growth in autism spectrum disorders and other childhood psychiatric disorders. *Journal of Autism and Developmental Disorders*, *41*(1), 44–54.

Ronald, A., Edelson, L. R., Asherson, P., & Saudino, K. J. (2010). Exploring the relationship between autistic-like traits and ADHD behaviors in early childhood: Findings from a community twin study of 2-year-olds. *Journal of Abnormal Child Psychology*, *38*(2), 185–196.

Ronald, A., & Hoekstra, R. A. (2011). Autism spectrum disorders and autistic traits: A decade of new twin studies. *American Journal of Medical Genetics Part B-Neuropsychiatric Genetics*, *156*(3), 255–274.

Ronald, A., Larsson, H., Anckarsater, H., & Lichtenstein, P. (2010). A twin study of autism symptoms in Sweden. *Molecular Psychiatry*, *16*, 1039–1047.

Ronald, A., Simonoff, E., Kuntsi, J., Asherson, P., & Plomin, R. (2008). Evidence for overlapping genetic influences on autistic and ADHD behaviours in a community twin sample. *Journal of Child Psychology and Psychiatry*, *49*(5), 535–542.

Ronemus, M., Iossifov, I., Levy, D., & Wigler, M. (2014). The role of de novo mutations in the genetics of autism spectrum disorders. *Nature Reviews Genetics*, *15*(2), 133–141.

Rose, S., Melnyk, S., Pavliv, O., Bai, S., Nick, T. G., Frye, R. E., & James, S. J. (2012). Evidence of oxidative damage and inflammation associated with low glutathione redox status in the autism brain. *Translational Psychiatry*, *2*(7), E134.

Rosema, S., Crowe, L., & Anderson, V. (2012). Social function in children and adolescents after traumatic brain injury: A systematic review 1989–2011. *Journal of Neurotrauma*, *29*(7), 1277–1291.

Rosenthal, M., Wallace, G. L., Lawson, R., Wills, M. C., Dixon, E., Yerys, B. E., & Kenworthy, L. (2013). Impairments in real-world executive function increase from childhood to adolescence in autism spectrum disorders. *Neuropsychology*, *27*(1), 13–18.

Rossignol, D. A., & Frye, R. E. (2012). A review of research trends in physiological abnormalities in autism spectrum disorders: Immune dysregulation, inflammation, oxidative stress, mitochondrial dysfunction and environmental toxicant exposures. *Molecular Psychiatry*, *17*(4), 389–401.

Rubenstein, J.L.R. (2010). Three hypotheses for developmental defects that may underlie some forms of autism spectrum disorder. *Current Opinion in Neurology*, *23*(2), 118–123.

Russell, G., Rodgers, L. R., Ukoumunne, O. C., & Ford, T. (2014). Prevalence of parent-reported ASD and ADHD in the UK: Findings from the Millennium Cohort Study. *Journal of Autism and Developmental Disorders*, *44*(1), 31–40.

Russell, G., Steer, C., & Golding, J. (2011). Social and demographic factors that influence the diagnosis of autistic spectrum disorders. *Social Psychiatry and Psychiatric Epidemiology*, *46*(12), 1283–1293.

Russell, J., Jarrold, C., & Hood, B. (1999). Two intact executive capacities in children with autism: Implications for the core executive dysfunctions in the disorder. *Journal of Autism and Developmental Disorders*, *29*(2), 103–112.

Russell, J., Saltmarsh, R., & Hill, E. (1999). What do executive factors contribute to the failure on false belief tasks by children with autism? *Journal of Child Psychology and Psychiatry and Allied Disciplines*, *40*(6), 859–868.

Russo, N., Flanagan, T., Iarocci, G., Berringer, D., Zelazo, P. D., & Burack, J. A. (2007). Deconstructing executive deficits among persons with autism: Implications for cognitive neuroscience. *Brain and Cognition*, *65*(1), 77–86.

Rutter, M. (1978). Diagnosis and definitions of childhood autism. *Journal of Autism and Childhood Schizophrenia*, *8*(2), 139–161.

Rutter, M. (2013). Changing concepts and findings on autism. *Journal of Autism and Developmental Disorders*, *43*(8), 1749–1757.

Rutter, M., Bailey, A., & Lord, C. (2003). *Social Communication Questionnaire (SCQ) Manual*. Los Angeles: Western Psychological Services. Autism Diagnostic Interview-Revised Manual. (Western Psychological Services 2003).

Rutter, M., Le Couteur, A., & Lord, C. (2003) Autism Diagnostic Interview Revised (ADI-R). Los Angeles, Western Psychological Services.

Rutter, M., & Lockyer, L. (1967). A 5 to 15 year follow-up study of infantile psychosis I: Description of sample. *British Journal of Psychiatry*, *113*(504), 1169.

Sacco, R., Militerni, R., Frolli, A., Bravaccio, C., Gritti, A., Elia, M., . . . Persico, A. M. (2007a). Clinical, morphological, and biochemical correlates of head circumference in autism. *Biological Psychiatry*, *62*(9), 1038–1047.

Sacco, R., Militerni, R., Frolli, A., Bravaccio, C., Gritti, A., Elia, M., . . . Persico, A. M. (2007b). Clinical, morphological, and biochemical correlates of head circumference in autism. *Biological Psychiatry*, *62*(9), 1038–1047.

Sachse, M., Schlitt, S., Hainz, D., Ciaramidaro, A., Schirman, S., Walter, H., . . . Freitag, C. M. (2013). Executive and visuo-motor function in adolescents and adults with autism spectrum disorder. *Journal of Autism and Developmental Disorders*, *43*(5), 1222–1235.

Saint Georges, C., Cassel, R. S., Cohen, D., Chetouani, M., Laznik, M. C., Maestro, S., & Muratori, F. (2010). What studies of family home movies can teach us about autistic infants: A literature review. *Research in Autism Spectrum Disorders*, *4*, 355–366.

Sanchez-Marin, F. J., & Padilla-Medina, J. A. (2008). A psychophysical test of the visual pathway of children with autism. *Journal of Autism and Developmental Disorders*, *38*(7), 1270–1277.

Sanders, J., Johnson, K. A., Garavan, H., Gill, M., & Gallagher, L. (2008). A review of neuropsychological and neuroimaging research in autistic spectrum disorders: Attention, inhibition and cognitive flexibility. *Research in Autism Spectrum Disorders*, *2*(1), 1–16.

Sanders, S. J., Murtha, M. T., Gupta, A. R., Murdoch, J. D., Raubeson, M. J., Willsey, A. J., . . . State, M. W. (2012). De novo mutations revealed by whole-exome sequencing are strongly associated with autism. *Nature*, *485*(7397), 237–U124.

Sandin, S., Lichtenstein, P., Kuja-Halkola, R., Larsson, H., Hultman, C. M., & Reichenberg, A. (2014). The familial risk of autism. *JAMA*, *311*(17), 1770–1777.

Sasson, N. J. (2006). The development of face processing in autism. *Journal of Autism and Developmental Disorders*, *36*(3), 381–394.

Sasson, N. J., Nowlin, R. B., & Pinkham, A. E. (2013). Social cognition, social skill, and the broad autism phenotype. *Autism*, *17*(6), 655–667.

Sato, D., Lionel, A. C., Leblond, C. S., Prasad, A., Pinto, D., Walker, S., . . . Scherer, S. W. (2012). SHANK1 deletions in males with autism spectrum disorder. *American Journal of Medical Genetics*, *90*(5), 879–887.

Schain, R. J., & Yannet, H. (1960). Infantile autism: An analysis of 50 cases and a consideration of certain relevant neurophysiologic concepts. *Journal of Pediatrics*, *57*(4), 560–567.

Scheel, C., Rotarska-Jagiela, A., Schilbach, L., Lehnhardt, F. G., Krug, B., Vogeley, K., & Tepest, R. (2011). Imaging derived cortical thickness reduction in high-functioning autism: Key regions and temporal slope. *Neuroimage*, *58*(2), 391–400.

Schieve, L. A., Rice, C., Devine, O., Maenner, M. J., Lee, L. C., Fitzgerald, R., . . . Durkin, M. (2011). Have secular changes in perinatal risk factors contributed to the recent autism prevalence increase? Development and application of a mathematical assessment model. *Annals of Epidemiology*, *21*(12), 930–945.

Schipul, S. E., Keller, T. A., & Just, M. A. (2011). Inter-regional brain communication and its disturbance in autism. *Frontiers in Systems Neuroscience*, *5*, 10.

Schmahmann, J. D. (2010). The role of the cerebellum in cognition and emotion: Personal reflections since 1982 on the dysmetria of thought hypothesis, and its historical evolution from theory to therapy. *Neuropsychology Review*, *20*(3), 236–260.

Schmitz, N., Rubia, K., Daly, E., Smith, A., Williams, S., & Murphy, D. G. (2006). Neural correlates of executive function in autistic spectrum disorders. *Biological Psychiatry*, *59*(1), 7–16.

Schoenemann, P. T. (2009). Brain evolution relevant to language. In J. W. Minett & W. S.-Y. Wang (Eds.), *Language, Evolution, and the Brain* (pp. 191–223). Hong Kong: University of Hong Kong Press.

Schopler, E., & Van Bourgondien, M. E. (2010). *Childhood Autism Rating Scale, Second Edition (CARS-2)*. Torrance, CA: Western Psychological Services.

Schulte-Ruether, M., Greimel, E., Markowitsch, H. J., Kamp-Becker, I., Remschmidt, H., Fink, G. R., & Piefke, M. (2011). Dysfunctions in brain networks supporting empathy: An fMRI study in adults with autism spectrum disorders. *Social Neuroscience*, *6*(1), 1–21.

Schultz, R. T. (2005). Developmental deficits in social perception in autism: The role of the amygdala and fusiform face area. *International Journal of Developmental Neuroscience*, *23*(2/3), 125–141.

Schumann, C. M., Barnes, C. C., Lord, C., & Courchesne, E. (2009). Amygdala enlargement in toddlers with autism related to severity of social and communication impairments. *Biological Psychiatry*, *66*(10), 942–949.

Schumann, C. M., Bloss, C. S., Barnes, C. C., Wideman, G. M., Carper, R. A., Akshoomoff, N., . . . Courchesne, E. (2010). Longitudinal magnetic resonance imaging study of cortical development through early childhood in autism. *Journal of Neuroscience*, *30*(12), 4419–4427.

Scott, O., Richer, L., Forbes, K., Sonnenberg, L., Currie, A., Eliyashevska, M., & Goez, H. R. (2014). Anti-N-Methyl-D-Aspartate (NMDA) receptor encephalitis an unusual cause of autistic regression in a toddler. *Journal of Child Neurology*, *29*(5), 691–694.

Scott-Van Zeeland, A. A., Abrahams, B. S., Alvarez-Retuerto, A. I., Sonnenblick, L. I., Rudie, J. D., Ghahremani, D., . . . Bookheimer, S. Y. (2010). Altered functional connectivity in frontal lobe circuits is associated with variation in the autism risk gene CNTNAP2. *Science Translational Medicine*, *2*(56), 56ra80.

Sebat, J., Lakshmi, B., Malhotra, D., Troge, J., Lese-Martin, C., Walsh, T., . . . Wigler, M. (2007). Strong association of de novo copy number mutations with autism. *Science*, *316*(5823), 445–449.

Seeley, W. W., Menon, V., Schatzberg, A. F., Keller, J., Glover, G. H., Kenna, H., . . . Greicius, M. D. (2007). Dissociable intrinsic connectivity networks for salience processing and executive control. *Journal of Neuroscience*, *27*(9), 2349–2356.

Selfe, L. (1995). *Nadia Reconsidered*. Hillsdale, NJ: Lawrence Erlbaum.

Semrud-Clikeman, M., Fine, J. G., Bledsoe, J., & Zhu, D. C. (2014). Regional volumetric differences based on structural MRI in children with two subtypes of ADHD and controls. *Journal of Attention Disorders*, *21*(12), 1040–1049.

Senju, A., Tojo, Y., Dairoku, H., & Hasegawa, T. (2004). Reflexive orienting in response to eye gaze and an arrow in children with and without autism. *Journal of Child Psychology and Psychiatry*, *45*(3), 445–458.

Shafritz, K. M., Dichter, G. S., Baranek, G. T., & Belger, A. (2008). The neural circuitry mediating shifts in behavioral response and cognitive set in autism. *Biological Psychiatry*, *63*(10), 974–980.

Shalom, D. B., Mostofsky, S. H., Hazlett, R. L., Goldberg, M. C., McLeod, D. R., & Hoehn-Saric, R. (2003). Intact galvanic skin responses and impaired self-reports in response to emotional pictures in high-functioning autism. *Annals of the New York Academy of Sciences*, *985*, 501–504.

Sheat-Klein, M., Shinnar, S., & Rapin, I. (2014). Abnormalities of joint mobility and gait in children with autism spectrum disorders. *Brain and Development*, *36*(2), 91–96.

Shehzad, Z., Kelly, A. M., Reiss, P. T., Gee, D. G., Gotimer, K., Uddin, L. Q., . . . Milham, M. P. (2009). The resting brain: Unconstrained yet reliable. *Cerebral Cortex*, *19*(10), 2209–2229.

Shenoy, S., Arnold, S., & Chatila, T. (2000). Response to steroid therapy in autism secondary to autoimmune lymphoproliferative syndrome. *Journal of Pediatrics*, *136*(5), 682–687.

Shih, P., Keehn, B., Oram, J. K., Leyden, K. M., Keown, C. L., & Muller, R. A. (2011). Functional differentiation of posterior superior temporal sulcus in autism: A functional connectivity magnetic resonance imaging study. *Biological Psychiatry*, *70*(3), 270–277.

Shinawi, M., Liu, P. F., Kang, S.H.L., Shen, J., Belmont, J. W., Scott, D. A., . . . Lupski, J. R. (2010). Recurrent reciprocal 16p11.2 rearrangements associated with global developmental delay, behavioural problems, dysmorphism, epilepsy, and abnormal head size. *Journal of Medical Genetics*, *47*(5), 332–341.

Shoffner, J., Hyams, L., Langley, G. N., Cossette, S., Mylacraine, L., Dale, J., . . . Hyland, K. (2010). Fever plus mitochondrial disease could be risk factors for autistic regression. *Journal of Child Neurology*, *25*(4), 429–434.

Short, A. B., & Schopler, E. (1988). Factors relating to age of onset in autism. *Journal of Autism and Developmental Disorders*, *18*(2), 207–216.

Shriberg, L. D., Paul, R., McSweeny, J. L., Klin, A. M., Cohen, D. J., & Volkmar, F. R. (2001). Speech and prosody characteristics of adolescents and adults with high-functioning autism and Asperger syndrome. *Journal of Speech, Language, and Hearing Research*, *44*(5), 1097–1115.

Shukla, D. K., Keehn, B., Lincoln, A. J., & Muller, R. A. (2010). White matter compromise of callosal and subcortical fiber tracts in children with autism spectrum disorder: A diffusion tensor imaging study. *Journal of the American Academy of Child and Adolescent Psychiatry*, *49*(12), 1269–1278, 1278 e1261–e1262.

Shukla, D. K., Keehn, B., & Muller, R. A. (2011). Tract-specific analyses of diffusion tensor imaging show widespread white matter compromise in autism spectrum disorder. *Journal of Child Psychology and Psychiatry*, *52*(3), 286–295.

Shukla, D. K., Keehn, B., Smylie, D. M., & Muller, R. A. (2011). Microstructural abnormalities of short-distance white matter tracts in autism spectrum disorder. *Neuropsychologia*, *49*(5), 1378–1382.

Shumway, S., Thurm, A., Swedo, S. E., Deprey, L., Barnett, L. A., Amaral, D. G., . . . Ozonoff, S. (2011). Brief report: Symptom onset patterns and functional outcomes in young children with autism spectrum disorders. *Journal of Autism and Developmental Disorders*, *41*(12), 1727–1732.

Siegel, B. (2004). *Pervasive Developmental Disorders Screening Test—II*. San Antonio, TX: Harcourt.

Sikich, L., Hickok, J. M., & Todd, R. D. (1990). 5-HT1A receptors control neurite branching during development. *Brain Research: Developmental Brain Research*, *56*, 269–274.

Simion, F., Leo, I., Turati, C., Valenza, E., & Dalla Barba, B. (2007). How face specialization emerges in the first months of life. *Progress in Brain Research*, *164*, 169–185.

Simmons, D. R., Robertson, A. E., McKay, L. S., Toal, E., McAleer, P., & Pollick, F. E. (2009). Vision in autism spectrum disorders. *Vision Research*, *49*(22), 2705–2739.

Simpson, N. H., Ceroni, F., Reader, R. H., Covill, L. E., Knight, J. C., the, S.L.I.C., . . . the, S.L.I.C. (2015). Genome-wide analysis identifies a role for common copy number variants in specific language impairment. *European Journal of Human Genetics*, *23*(10), 1370–1377.

Singer, H. S., Morris, C. M., Gause, C. D., Gillin, P. K., Crawford, S., & Zimmerman, A. W. (2008). Antibodies against fetal brain in sera of mothers with autistic children. *Journal of Neuroimmunology*, *194*(1–2), 165–172.

Singh, V. K., & Rivas, W. H. (2004). Prevalence of serum antibodies to caudate nucleus in autistic children. *Neuroscience Letters*, *355*(1/2), 53.

Singh, V. K., Warren, R., Averett, R., & Ghaziuddin, M. (1997). Circulating autoantibodies to neuronal and glial filament proteins in autism. *Pediatric Neurology*, *17*(1), 88–90.

Siperstein, R., & Volkmar, F. (2004). Brief report: Parental reporting of regression in children with pervasive developmental disorders. *Journal of Autism and Developmental Disorders*, *34*(6), 731–734.

Sivaswamy, L., Kumar, A., Rajan, D., Behen, M., Muzik, O., Chugani, D., & Chugani, H. (2010). A diffusion tensor imaging study of the cerebellar pathways in children with autism spectrum disorder. *Journal of Child Neurology*, *25*(10), 1223–1231.

Skefos, J., Cummings, C., Enzer, K., Holiday, J., Weed, K., Levy, E., . . . Bauman, M. (2014). Regional alterations in Purkinje cell density in patients with autism. *PLoS One*, *9*(2), 1–12.

Smalley, S. L. (1991). Genetic influences in autism. *Psychiatric Clinics of North America*, *14*(1), 125–139.

Smalley, S. L., Asarnow, R. F., & Spence, M. A. (1988). Autism and genetics: A decade of research. *Archives of General Psychiatry*, *45*(10), 953–961.

Smith, B., & Gardiner, J. (2008). Rehearsal and directed forgetting in Asperger syndrome. In J. Boucher & D. M. Bowler (Eds.), *Memory in Autism: Theory and Evidence* (pp. 249–267). Cambridge, UK: Cambridge University Press.

Smith, I. M., & Bryson, S. E. (1994). Imitation and action in autism: A critical review. *Psychological Bulletin*, *116*(2), 259–273.

Solomon, M., Miller, M., Taylor, S. L., Hinshaw, S. P., & Carter, C. S. (2012). Autism symptoms and internalizing psychopathology in girls and boys with autism spectrum disorders. *Journal of Autism and Developmental Disorders*, *42*(1), 48–59.

Solomon, M., Ozonoff, S. J., Cummings, N., & Carter, C. S. (2008). Cognitive control in autism spectrum disorders. *International Journal of Developmental Neuroscience*, *26*(2), 239–247.

Solomon, M., Yoon, J. H., Ragland, J. D., Niendam, T. A., Lesh, T. A., Fairbrother, W., & Carter, C. S. (2014). The development of the neural substrates of cognitive control in adolescents with autism spectrum disorders. *Biological Psychiatry*, *76*(5), 412–421.

Soulieres, I., Zeffiro, T. A., Girard, M. L., & Mottron, L. (2011). Enhanced mental image mapping in autism. *Neuropsychologia*, *49*(5), 848–857.

South, M., Ozonoff, S., & McMahon, W. M. (2007). The relationship between executive functioning, central coherence, and repetitive behaviors in the high-functioning autism spectrum. *Autism: The International Journal of Research & Practice*, *11*(5), 437–451.

Sparks, B. F., Friedman, S. D., Shaw, D. W., Aylward, E. H., Echelard, D., Artru, A. A., . . . Dager, S. R. (2002). Brain structural abnormalities in young children with autism spectrum disorder. *Neurology*, *59*(2), 184–192.

Spence, S. J., Cantor, R. M., Chung, L., Kim, S., Geschwind, D. H., & Alarcon, M. (2006). Stratification based on language-related endophenotypes in autism: Attempt to replicate reported linkage. *American Journal of Medical Genetics Part B-Neuropsychiatric Genetics*, *141B*(6), 591–598.

Spence, S. J., & Schneider, M. T. (2009). The role of epilepsy and epileptiform EEGs in autism spectrum disorders. *Pediatric Research*, *65*(6), 599–606.

Spengler, S., Bird, G., & Brass, M. (2010). Hyperimitation of actions is related to reduced understanding of others' minds in autism spectrum conditions. *Biological Psychiatry*, *68*(12), 1148–1155.

Sperber, D., & Wilson, D. (2002). Pragmatics, modularity and mindreading. *Mind & Language*, *17*, 3.

Spezio, M. L., Adolphs, R., Hurley, R. S., & Piven, J. (2007). Abnormal use of facial information in high-functioning autism. *Journal of Autism and Developmental Disorders*, *37*(5), 929–939.

Sporns, O., Tononi, G., & Edelman, G. M. (2000). Theoretical neuroanatomy: Relating anatomical and functional connectivity in graphs and cortical connection matrices. *Cerebral Cortex*, *10*(2), 127–141.

Stamou, M., Streifel, K. M., Goines, P. E., & Lein, P. J. (2013). Neuronal connectivity as a convergent target of gene x environment interactions that confer risk for autism spectrum disorders. *Neurotoxicology and Teratology*, *36*, 3–16.

Stanfield, A. C., McIntosh, A. M., Spencer, M. D., Philip, R., Gaur, S., & Lawrie, S. M. (2008). Towards a neuroanatomy of autism: A systematic review and meta-analysis of structural magnetic resonance imaging studies. *European Psychiatry*, *23*(4), 289–299.

Starck, T., Nikkinen, J., Rahko, J., Remes, J., Hurtig, T., Haapsamo, H., . . . Kiviniemi, V. J. (2013). Resting state fMRI reveals a default mode dissociation between retrosplenial and medial prefrontal subnetworks in ASD despite motion scrubbing. *Frontiers in Human Neuroscience*, *7*, 802.

Steele, S. D., Minshew, N. J., Luna, B., & Sweeney, J. A. (2007). Spatial working memory deficits in autism. *Journal of Autism and Developmental Disorders*, *37*(4), 605–612.

Stefanatos, G., Kinsbourne, M., & Wasserstein, J. (2002a). Acquired epileptiform aphasia: A dimensional view of landau-kleffner syndrome and the relation to regressive autistic spectrum disorders. *Child Neuropsychology*, *8*(3), 195–228.

Stefanatos, G. A. (1993). Frequency modulation analysis in children with Landau-Kleffner syndrome. *Annals of the New York Academy of Sciences*, *682*, 412–414.

Stefanatos, G. A. (2008). Regression in autistic spectrum disorders. *Neuropsychology Review*, *18*(4), 305–319.

Stefanatos, G. A. (2011). Changing perspectives on Landau-Kleffner syndrome. *The Clinical Neuropsychologist*, *25*(6), 963–988.

Stefanatos, G. A. (2012). Autism spectrum disorder. In C. Noggle & R. Dean (Eds.), *The Neuropsychology of Psychopathology* (pp. 97–170). New York: Springer Press.

Stefanatos, G. A., & Baron, I. S. (2011). The ontogenesis of language impairment in autism: A neuropsychological perspective. *Neuropsychology Review*, *21*(3), 252–270.

Stefanatos, G. A., & DeMarco, A. T. (2010). Landau-Kleffner syndrome. In J. E. Morgan, I. S. Baron & J. H. Ricker (Eds.), *Casebook of Clinical Neuropsychology* (pp. 136–163). New York: Oxford University Press.

Stefanatos, G. A., Foley, C., Grover, W., & Doherty, B. (1997). Steady-state auditory evoked responses to pulsed frequency modulations in children. *Electroencephalography and Clinical Neurophysiology*, *104*(1), 31–42.

Stefanatos, G. A., Grover, W., & Geller, E. (1995). Case-study: Corticosteroid treatment of language regression in pervasive developmental disorder. *Journal of the American Academy of Child and Adolescent Psychiatry*, *34*(8), 1107–1111.

Stefanatos, G. A., Kinsbourne, M., & Wasserstein, J. (2002b). Acquired epileptiform aphasia: A dimensional view of Landau-Kleffner syndrome and the relation to regressive autistic spectrum disorders. *Child Neuropsychology: A Journal on Normal and Abnormal Development in Childhood and Adolescence*, *8*(3), 195–228.

Stefanatos, G. A., Kollros, P. R., & Rabinovich, H. (1996). Childhood idiopathic language deterioration: Positive treatment responses associated with improved steady state auditory evoked potentials. *Annals of Neurology*, *40*(2), 61–61.

Stefanatos, G. A., & Postman-Caucheteaux, W. A. (2010). Genetics of language. In G. F. Koob, M. Le Moal, & R. F. Thompson (Eds.), *Encyclopedia of Behavioral Neuroscience* (Vol. 1, pp. 583–588). Oxford, UK: Academic Press.

Stefansson, H., Meyer-Lindenberg, A., Steinberg, S., Magnusdottir, B., Morgen, K., Arnarsdottir, S., . . . Stefansson, K. (2014). CNVs conferring risk of autism or schizophrenia affect cognition in controls. *Nature*, *505*(7483), 361–366.

Stein, J. L., Parikshak, N. N., & Geschwind, D. H. (2013). Rare inherited variation in autism: Beginning to see the forest and a few trees. *Neuron*, *77*(2), 209–211.

Stephens, C. E. (2008). Spontaneous imitation by children with autism during a repetitive musical play routine. *Autism*, *12*(6), 645–671.

Sterling, L., Dawson, G., Webb, S., Murias, M., Munson, J., Panagiotides, H., & Aylward, E. (2008). The role of face familiarity in eye tracking of faces by individuals with autism spectrum disorders. *Journal of Autism and Developmental Disorders*, *38*(9), 1666–1675.

Stevenson, R. E., Schroer, R. J., Skinner, C., Fender, D., & Simensen, R. J. (1997). Autism and macrocephaly. *Lancet*, *349*(9067), 1744–1745.

Stigler, K. A., Sweeten, T. L., Posey, D. J., & McDougle, C. J. (2009). Autism and immune factors: A comprehensive review. *Research in Autism Spectrum Disorders*, *3*(4), 840–860.

Stodgell, C. J., Gnall, S., & Rodier, P. (2001). Valproic acid exposure alters gene expression in rat embryos: Mechanism of teratogenicity and relationship to autism spectrum disorders. *American Journal of Human Genetics*, *69*(4), 584–584.

Stone, W. L., Coonrod, E. E., & Ousley, O. Y. (2000). Brief report: Screening tool for autism in two-year-olds (STAT): Development and preliminary data. *Journal of Autism and Developmental Disorders*, *30*(6), 607–612.

Stone, W. L., Coonrod, E. E., Pozdol, S. L., & Turner, L. M. (2003). The Parent Interview for Autism-Clinical Version (PIA-CV): A measure of behavioral change for young children with autism. *Autism*, *7*(1), 9–30.

Stone, W. L., Lee, E. B., Ashford, L., Brissie, J., Hepburn, S. L., Coonrod, E. E., & Weiss, B. H. (1999). Can autism be diagnosed accurately in children under 3 years? *Journal of Child Psychology and Psychiatry and Allied Disciplines*, *40*(2), 219–226.

Stoner, R., Chow, M. L., Boyle, M. P., Sunkin, S. M., Mouton, P. R., Roy, S., . . . Courchesne, E. (2014). Patches of disorganization in the neocortex of children with autism. *New England Journal of Medicine*, *370*(13), 1209–1219.

Strauss, K. A., Puffenberger, E. G., Huentelman, M. J., Gottlieb, S., Dobrin, S. E., Parod, J. M., . . . Morton, D. H. (2006). Recessive symptomatic focal epilepsy and mutant contactin-associated protein-like 2. *New England Journal of Medicine*, *354*(13), 1370–1377.

Strick, P. L., Dum, R. P., & Fiez, J. A. (2009). Cerebellum and nonmotor function. *Annual Review of Neuroscience*, *32*, 413–434.

Sudhof, T. C. (2008). Neuroligins and neurexins link synaptic function to cognitive disease. *Nature*, *455*(7215), 903–911.

Suh, J., Eigsti, I., Naigles, L., Barton, M., Kelley, E., & Fein, D. A. (2013). Narrative competence and pragmatic language abilities of optimal outcome children with a history of autism spectrum disorders as evaluated by Peer ratings. *Clinical Neuropsychologist*, *27*(4), 642–642.

Sullivan, P. F., Magnusson, C., Reichenberg, A., Boman, M., Dalman, C., Davidson, M., . . . Lichtenstein, P. (2012). Family history of schizophrenia and bipolar disorder as risk factors for autism. *Archives of General Psychiatry*, *69*(11), 1099–1103.

Suren, P., Bakken, I. J., Lie, K. K., Schjolberg, S., Aase, H., Reichborn-Kjennerud, T., . . . Stoltenberg, C. (2013). Differences across counties in the registered prevalence of autism, ADHD, epilepsy and cerebral palsy in Norway. *Tidsskrift for Den Norske Laegeforening*, *133*(18), 1929–1934.

Suren, P., Stoltenberg, C., Bresnahan, M., Hirtz, D., Lie, K. K., Lipkin, W. I., . . . Hornig, M. (2013). Early growth patterns in children with autism. *Epidemiology*, *24*(5), 660–670.

Sutcliffe, J. S., Delahanty, R. J., Prasad, H. C., McCauley, J. L., Han, Q., Jiang, L., . . . Blakely, R. D. (2005). Allelic heterogeneity at the serotonin transporter locus (SLC6A4) confers susceptibility to autism and rigid-compulsive behaviors. *American Journal of Medical Genetics*, *77*(2), 265–279.

Suter, B., Treadwell-Deering, D., Zoghbi, H. Y., Glaze, D. G., & Neul, J. L. (2014). Brief report: MECP2 mutations in people without Rett syndrome. *Journal of Autism and Developmental Disorders*, *44*(3), 703–711.

Sutera, S., Pandey, J., Esser, E. L., Rosenthal, M. A., Wilson, L. B., Barton, M., . . . Fein, D. (2007). Predictors of optimal outcome in toddlers diagnosed with autism spectrum disorders. *Journal of Autism and Developmental Disorders*, *37*(1), 98–107.

Suzuki, K., Nishimura, K., Sugihara, G., Nakamura, K., Tsuchiya, K. J., Matsumoto, K., . . . Mori, N. (2009). Metabolite alterations in the hippocampus of high-functioning adult subjects with autism. *International Journal of Neuropsychopharmacology*, *13*(4), 529–534.

Swanson, J. M., Kinsbourne, M., Nigg, J., Lanphear, B., Stefanatos, G. A., Volkow, N., . . . Wadhwa, P. D. (2007). Etiologic subtypes of attention-deficit/hyperactivity disorder: Brain imaging, molecular genetic and environmental factors and the dopamine hypothesis. *Neuropsychology Review*, *17*(1), 39–59.

Swedo, S. E., Baird, G., Cook, E. H., Happe, F. G., Harris, J. C., Kaufmann, W. E., . . . Wright, H. H. (2012). Commentary from the DSM-5 workgroup on neurodevelopmental disorders. *Journal of the American Academy of Child and Adolescent Psychiatry*, *51*(4), 347–349.

Swensen, L. D., Kelley, E., Fein, D., & Naigles, L. R. (2007). Processes of language acquisition in children with autism: Evidence from preferential looking. *Child Development*, *78*(2), 542–557.

Szatmari, P., Liu, X.-Q., Goldberg, J., Zwaigenbaum, L., Paterson, A. D., Woodbury-Smith, M., . . . Thompson, A. (2012). Sex differences in repetitive stereotyped behaviors in autism: Implications for genetic liability. *American Journal of Medical Genetics Part B-Neuropsychiatric Genetics*, *159B*(1), 5–12.

Szatmari, P., MacLean, J. E., Jones, M. B., Bryson, S. E., Zwaigenbaum, L., Bartolucci, G., . . . Tuff, L. (2000). The familial aggregation of the lesser variant in biological and nonbiological relatives of PDD probands: A family history study. *Journal of Child Psychology and Psychiatry*, *41*(5), 579–586.

Tager-Flusberg, H. (1981). On the nature linguistic functioning in early infantile autism. *Journal of Autism and Developmental Disorders*, *11*(1), 45–56.

Tager-Flusberg, H. (1992). Autistic children's talk about psychological states: Deficits in the early acquisition of a theory of mind. *Child Development*, *63*(1), 161–172.

Tager-Flusberg, H., & Joseph, R. M. (2003). Identifying neurocognitive phenotypes in autism. *Philosophical Transactions of the Royal Society of London: Series B: Biological Sciences*, *358*(1430), 303–314.

Taheri, A., & Perry, A. (2012). Exploring the proposed DSM-5 criteria in a clinical sample. *Journal of Autism and Developmental Disorders*, *42*(9), 1810–1817.

Tanner, J. M. (1978). *Girls: Birth-16 Years: Head Circumference*. Welwyn Garden City, Herts: Castlemead Publications.

Tate, D. F., Bigler, E. D., McMahon, W., & Lainhart, J. (2007). The relative contributions of brain, cerebrospinal fluid-filled structures and non-neural tissue volumes to occipital-frontal head circumference in subjects with autism. *Neuropediatrics*, *38*(1), 18–24.

Tavassoli, T., Auyeung, B., Murphy, L. C., Baron-Cohen, S., & Chakrabarti, B. (2012). Variation in the autism candidate gene GABRB3 modulates tactile sensitivity in typically developing children. *Molecular Autism*, *3*(1), 6.

Taylor, B., Jick, H., & MacLaughlin, D. (2013). Prevalence and incidence rates of autism in the UK: Time trend from 2004–2010 in children aged 8 years. *Bmj Open*, *3*(10), E003219.

Tebartz van Elst, L., Maier, S., Fangmeier, T., Endres, D., Mueller, G. T., Nickel, K., . . . Perlov, E. (2014). Disturbed cingulate glutamate metabolism in adults with high-functioning autism spectrum disorder: Evidence in support of the excitatory/inhibitory imbalance hypothesis. *Molecular Psychiatry*, *19*(12), 1314–1325.

Teitelbaum, P., Teitelbaum, O., Nye, J., Fryman, J., & Maurer, R. G. (1998). Movement analysis in infancy may be useful for early diagnosis of autism. *Proceedings of the National Academy of Sciences of the United States of America*, *95*(23), 13982–13987.

Thakkar, K. N., Polli, F. E., Joseph, R. M., Tuch, D. S., Hadjikhani, N., Barton, J. J., & Manoach, D. S. (2008). Response monitoring, repetitive behaviour and anterior cingulate abnormalities in autism spectrum disorders (ASD). *Brain*, *131*(Pt 9), 2464–2478.

Thomas, C., Humphreys, K., Jung, K. J., Minshew, N., & Behrmann, M. (2011). The anatomy of the callosal and visual-association pathways in high-functioning autism: A DTI tractography study. *Cortex*, *47*(7), 863–873.

Thomas, M. S., Knowland, V. C., & Karmiloff-Smith, A. (2011). Mechanisms of developmental regression in autism and the broader phenotype: A neural network modeling approach. *Psychological Review*, *118*(4), 637–654.

Thompson, D. K., Warfield, S. K., Carlin, J. B., Pavlovic, M., Wang, H. X., Bear, M., . . . Inder, T. E. (2007). Perinatal risk factors altering regional brain structure in the preterm infant. *Brain*, *130*, 667–677.

Thurm, A., Manwaring, S. S., Luckenbaugh, D. A., Lord, C., & Swedo, S. E. (2014a). Patterns of skill attainment and loss in young children with autism. *Development and Psychopathology*, *26*(1), 203–214.

Thurm, A., Manwaring, S. S., Luckenbaugh, D. A., Lord, C., & Swedo, S. E. (2014b). Patterns of skill attainment and loss in young children with autism. *Development and Psychopathology*, *26*(1), 203–214.

Todd, R. D., Hickok, J. M., Anderson, G. M., & Cohen, D. J. (1988). Antibrain antibodies in infantile autism. *Biological Psychiatry*, *23*(6), 644–647.

Toichi, M., & Kamio, Y. (2002). Long-term memory and levels-of-processing in autism. *Neuropsychologia*, *40*(7), 964–969.

Toichi, M., & Kamio, Y. (2003). Long-term memory in high-functioning autism: Controversy on episodic memory in autism reconsidered. *Journal of Autism and Developmental Disorders*, *33*(2), 151–161.

Tomasello, M. (2008). *Origins of Human Communication*. Cambridge, MA: MIT Press.

Tomchek, S. D., & Dunn, W. (2007). Sensory processing in children with and without autism: A comparative study using the short sensory profile. *American Journal of Occupational Therapy*, *61*(2), 190–200.

Torres, A. R., Westover, J. B., & Rosenspire, A. J. (2012). HLA immune function genes in autism. *Autism Research and Treatment*, *2012*, 959073.

Torrey, E. F., Dhavale, D., Lawlor, J. P., & Yolken, R. H. (2004). Autism and head circumference in the first year of life. *Biological Psychiatry*, *56*(11), 892–894.

Townsend, J., Courchesne, E., Covington, J., Westerfield, M., Harris, N. S., Lyden, P., . . . Press, G. A. (1999). Spatial attention deficits in patients with acquired or developmental cerebellar abnormality. *Journal of Neuroscience*, *19*(13), 5632–5643.

Townsend, J., Westerfield, M., Leaver, E., Makeig, S., Jung, T. P., Pierce, K., & Courchesne, E. (2001). Event-related brain response abnormalities in autism: Evidence for impaired cerebello-frontal spatial attention networks. *Cognitive Brain Research*, *11*(1), 127–145.

Travers, B. G., Adluru, N., Ennis, C., Tromp, D.P.M., Destiche, D., Doran, S., . . . Alexander, A. L. (2012). Diffusion tensor imaging in autism spectrum disorder: A review. *Autism Research*, *5*(5), 289–313.

Tripi, G., Roux, S., Canziani, T., Brithault, F. B., Barthelemy, C., & Canziani, F. (2008). Minor physical anomalies in children with autism spectrum disorder. *Early Human Development*, *84*(4), 217–223.

Tsermentseli, S., O'Brien, J. M., & Spencer, J. V. (2008). Comparison of form and motion coherence processing in autistic spectrum disorders and dyslexia. *Journal of Autism and Developmental Disorders*, *38*(7), 1201–1210.

Tsuchiya, E., Oki, J., Yahara, N., & Fujieda, K. (2005). Computerized version of the Wisconsin card sorting test in children with high-functioning autistic disorder or attention-deficit/hyperactivity disorder. *Brain and Development*, *27*(3), 233–236.

Tuchman, R. (2006). Autism and epilepsy: What has regression got to do with it? *Epilepsy Currents*, *6*(4), 107–111.

Tuchman, R. (2009). CSWS-related autistic regression versus autistic regression without CSWS. *Epilepsia, 50* (Suppl 7), 18–20.

Tuchman, R. F., & Rapin, I. (1997). Regression in pervasive developmental disorders: Seizures and epileptiform electroencephalogram correlates. *Pediatrics*, *99*(4), 560–566.

Turner, L. M., Stone, W. L., Pozdol, S. L., & Coonrod, E. E. (2006). Follow-up of children with autism spectrum disorders from age 2 to age 9. *Autism*, *10*(3), 243–265.

Turner, M. (1999a). Annotation: Repetitive behaviour in autism: A review of psychological research. *Journal of Child Psychology and Psychiatry and Allied Disciplines*, *40*(6), 839–849.

Turner, M. A. (1999b). Generating novel ideas: Fluency performance in high-functioning and learning disabled individuals with autism. *Journal of Child Psychology and Psychiatry*, *40*(2), 189–201.

Turner-Brown, L. M., Baranek, G. T., Reznick, J. S., Watson, L. R., & Crais, E. R. (2013). The first year inventory: A longitudinal follow-up of 12-month-old to 3-year-old children. *Autism*, *17*(5), 527–540.

Tyson, K., Kelley, E., Fein, D., Orinstein, A., Troyb, E., Barton, M., . . . Rosenthal, M. (2014). Language and verbal memory in individuals with a history of autism spectrum disorders who have achieved optimal outcomes. *Journal of Autism and Developmental Disorders*, *44*(3), 648–663.

Uchino, S., & Waga, C. (2013). SHANK3 as an autism spectrum disorder-associated gene. *Brain and Development*, *35*(2), 106–110.

Uddin, L. Q. (2015). Idiosyncratic connectivity in autism: Developmental and anatomical considerations. *Trends in Neurosciences*, *38*(5), 261–263.

Uddin, L. Q., Menon, V., Young, C. B., Ryali, S., Chen, T., Khouzam, A., . . . Hardan, A. Y. (2011). Multivariate searchlight classification of structural magnetic resonance imaging in children and adolescents with autism. *Biological Psychiatry*, *70*(9), 833–841.

Uddin, L. Q., Supekar, K., Lynch, C. J., Khouzam, A., Phillips, J., Feinstein, C., . . . Menon, V. (2013). Salience network-based classification and prediction of symptom severity in children with autism. *Jama Psychiatry*, *70*(8), 869–879.

Valicenti-McDermott, M. D., McVicar, K., Cohen, H. J., Wershil, B. K., & Shinnar, S. (2008). Gastrointestinal symptoms in children with an autism spectrum disorder and language regression. *Pediatric Neurology*, *39*(6), 392–398.

van der Knaap, M. S., Lai, V., Kohler, W., Salih, M. A., Fonseca, M. J., Benke, T. A., . . . Scheper, G. C. (2010). Megalencephalic leukoencephalopathy with cysts without MLC1 defect. *Annals of Neurology*, *67*(6), 834–837.

Van Eylen, L., Boets, B., Steyaert, J., Evers, K., Wagemans, J., & Noens, I. (2011). Cognitive flexibility in autism spectrum disorder: Explaining the inconsistencies? *Research in Autism Spectrum Disorders*, *5*, 1590–1401.

Van Eylen, L., Boets, B., Steyaert, J., Wagemans, J., & Noens, I. (2015). Executive functioning in autism spectrum disorders: Influence of task and sample characteristics and relation to symptom severity. *European Child and Adolescent Psychiatry*, *24*(11), 1399–1417.

Van Hirtum-Das, M., Licht, E. A., Koh, S., Wu, J. Y., Shields, W. D., & Sankar, R. (2006). Children with ESES: Variability in the syndrome. *Epilepsy Research*, *70*(Suppl 1), S248–258.

van Kooten, I. A., Palmen, S. J., von Cappeln, P., Steinbusch, H. W., Korr, H., Heinsen, H., . . . Schmitz, C. (2008). Neurons in the fusiform gyrus are fewer and smaller in autism. *Brain*, *131*(Pt 4), 987–999.

Vandenbroucke, M. W., Scholte, H. S., van Engeland, H., Lamme, V. A., & Kemner, C. (2008). A neural substrate for atypical low-level visual processing in autism spectrum disorder. *Brain*, *131*(Pt 4), 1013–1024.

Vargas, D. L., Nascimbene, C., Krishnan, C., Zimmerman, A. W., & Pardo, C. A. (2005). Neuroglial activation and neuroinflammation in the brain of patients with autism. *Annals of Neurology*, *57*(1), 67–81.

Vargha-Khadem, F., Gadian, D. G., Copp, A., & Mishkin, M. (2005). FOXP2 and the neuroanatomy of speech and language. *Nature Reviews Neuroscience*, *6*(2), 131–138.

Varoqueaux, F., Aramuni, G., Rawson, R. L., Mohrmann, R., Missler, M., Gottmann, K., . . . Brose, N. (2006). Neuroligins determine synapse maturation and function. *Neuron*, *51*(6), 741–754.

Verte, S., Geurts, H. M., Roeyers, H., Oosterlaan, J., & Sergeant, J. A. (2005). Executive functioning in children with autism and Tourette syndrome. *Developmental Psychopathology*, *17*(2), 415–445.

Verte, S., Geurts, H. M., Roeyers, H., Oosterlaan, J., & Sergeant, J. A. (2006). Executive functioning in children with an autism spectrum disorder: Can we differentiate within the spectrum? *Journal of Autism and Developmental Disorders*, *36*(3), 351–372.

Via, E., Radua, J., Cardoner, N., Happe, F., & Mataix-Cols, D. (2011). Meta-analysis of gray matter abnormalities in autism spectrum disorder: Should Asperger disorder be subsumed under a broader umbrella of autistic spectrum disorder? *Archives of General Psychiatry*, *68*(4), 409–418.

Villalobos, M. E., Mizuno, A., Dahl, B. C., Kemmotsu, N., & Muller, R. A. (2005). Reduced functional connectivity between V1 and inferior frontal cortex associated with visuomotor performance in autism. *Neuroimage*, *25*(3), 916–925.

Viscidi, E. W., Triche, E. W., Pescosolido, M. F., McLean, R. L., Joseph, R. M., Spence, S. J., & Morrow, E. M. (2013). Clinical characteristics of children with autism spectrum disorder and co-occurring epilepsy. *PLoS One*, *8*(7), e67797.

Vissers, M. E., Cohen, M. X., & Geurts, H. M. (2012). Brain connectivity and high functioning autism: A promising path of research that needs refined models, methodological convergence, and stronger behavioral links. *Neuroscience and Biobehavioral Reviews*, *36*(1), 604–625.

Vitalis, T., Ansorge, M. S., & Dayer, A. G. (2013). Serotonin homeostasis and serotonin receptors as actors of cortical construction: Special attention to the 5-HT3A and 5-HT6 receptor subtypes. *Frontiers in Cellular Neuroscience*, *7*, 93.

Vivanti, G., Trembath, D., & Dissanayake, C. (2014). Mechanisms of imitation impairment in autism spectrum disorder. *Journal of Abnormal Child Psychology*, *42*(8), 1395–1405.

Volaki, K., Pampanos, A., Kitsiou-Tzeli, S., Vrettou, C., Oikonomakis, V., Sofocleous, C., & Kanavakis, E. (2013). Mutation screening in the Greek population and evaluation of NLGN3 and NLGN4X genes causal factors for autism. *Psychiatric Genetics*, *23*(5), 198–203.

Volden, J., Coolican, J., Garon, N., White, J., & Bryson, S. (2009). Brief report: Pragmatic language in autism spectrum disorder: Relationships to measures of ability and disability. *Journal of Autism and Developmental Disorders*, *39*(2), 388–393.

Volk, H. E., Lurmann, F., Penfold, B., Hertz-Picciotto, I., & McConnell, R. (2013). Traffic-related air pollution, particulate matter, and autism. *Jama Psychiatry*, *70*(1), 71–77.

Volkmar, F. R. (2013). *Encyclopedia of Autism Spectrum Disorders*. New York: Springer Press.

Volkmar, F. R., Stier, D. M., & Cohen, D. J. (1985). Age of recognition of pervasive developmental disorder. *American Journal of Psychiatry*, *142*(12), 1450–1452.

Vollm, B. A., Taylor, A. N., Richardson, P., Corcoran, R., Stirling, J., McKie, S., . . . Elliott, R. (2006). Neuronal correlates of theory of mind and empathy: A functional magnetic resonance imaging study in a nonverbal task. *Neuroimage*, *29*(1), 90–98.

Wainwright-Sharp, J. A., & Bryson, S. E. (1993). Visual orienting deficits in high-functioning people with autism. *Journal of Autism and Developmental Disorders*, *23*(1), 1–13.

Waiter, G. D., Williams, J.H.G., Murray, A. D., Gilchrist, A., Perrett, D. I., & Whiten, A. (2005). Structural white matter deficits in high-functioning individuals with autistic spectrum disorder: A voxel-based investigation. *Neuroimage*, *24*(2), 455–461.

Waites, A. B., Briellmann, R. S., Saling, M. M., Abbott, D. F., & Jackson, G. D. (2006). Functional connectivity networks are disrupted in left temporal lobe epilepsy. *Annals of Neurology*, *59*(2), 335–343.

Walker, H. A. (1977). Incidence of minor physical anomaly in autism. *Journal of Autism and Childhood Schizophrenia*, *7*(2), 165–176.

Wallace, G. L., Dankner, N., Kenworthy, L., Giedd, J. N., & Martin, A. (2010). Age-related temporal and parietal cortical thinning in autism spectrum disorders. *Brain*, *133*(Pt 12), 3745–3754.

Wallace, S., Sebastian, C., Pellicano, E., Parr, J., & Bailey, A. (2010). Face processing abilities in relatives of individuals with ASD. *Autism Research: Official Journal of the International Society for Autism Research*, *3*(6), 345–349.

Wang, A. T., Lee, S. S., Sigman, M., & Dapretto, M. (2006). Neural basis of irony comprehension in children with autism: The role of prosody and context. *Brain*, *129*(Pt 4), 932–943.

Wang, A. T., Lee, S. S., Sigman, M., & Dapretto, M. (2007). Reading affect in the face and voice: Neural correlates of interpreting communicative intent in children and adolescents with autism spectrum disorders. *Archives of General Psychiatry*, *64*(6), 698–708.

Wang, K., Zhang, H., Ma, D., Bucan, M., Glessner, J. T., Abrahams, B. S., . . . Hakonarson, H. (2009). Common genetic variants on 5p14.1 associate with autism spectrum disorders. *Nature*, *459*(7246), 528–533.

Wang, L., Mottron, L., Peng, D., Berthiaume, C., & Dawson, M. (2007). Local bias and local-to-global interference without global deficit: A robust finding in autism under various conditions of attention, exposure time, and visual angle. *Cognitive Neuropsychology*, *24*(5), 550–574.

Ward, A. J. (1990). A comparison and analysis of the presence of family problems during pregnancy of mothers of "autistic" children and mothers of normal children. *Child Psychiatry and Human Development*, *20*(4), 279–288.

Warren, R. P., Odell, J. D., Warren, W. L., Burger, R. A., Maciulis, A., Daniels, W. W., & Torres, A. R. (1996). Strong association of the third hypervariable region of HLA-DR beta 1 with autism. *Journal of Neuroimmunology*, *67*(2), 97–102.

Washington, S. D., Gordon, E. M., Brar, J., Warburton, S., Sawyer, A. T., Mease-Ference, E. R., Girton, L., Hailu, A., Mbwana, J., Gaillard, W. D., Kalbfleisch, M. L., & VanMeter, J. W. (2014). Dysmaturation of the default mode network in autism. *Human Brain Mapping*, *35*(4), 1284–1296.

Wasilewska, J., Kaczmarski, M., Stasiak-Barmuta, A., Tobolczyk, J., & Kowalewska, E. (2012). Low serum IgA and increased expression of CD23 on B lymphocytes in peripheral blood in children with regressive autism aged 3–6 years old. *Archives of Medical Science*, *8*(2), 324–331.

Wass, S. (2011). Distortions and disconnections: Disrupted brain connectivity in autism. *Brain and Cognition*, *75*(1), 18–28.

Wassink, T. H., Piven, J., & Patil, S. R. (2001). Chromosomal abnormalities in a clinic sample of individuals with autistic disorder. *Psychiatric Genetics*, *11*(2), 57–63.

Waterhouse, L. (2013). *Rethinking Autism: Variation and Complexity*. New York: Elsevier.

Waterhouse, L., & Fein, D. (1982). Language skills in developmentally disabled children. *Brain and Language*, *15*(2), 307–333.

Waterhouse, L., Fein, D., & Modahl, C. (1996). Neurofunctional mechanisms in autism. *Psychological Review*, *103*(3), 457–489.

Webb, S. J., Jones, E.J.H., Kelly, J., & Dawson, G. (2014). The motivation for very early intervention for infants at high risk for autism spectrum disorders. *International Journal of Speech-Language Pathology*, *16*(1), 36–42.

Webb, S. J., Nalty, T., Munson, J., Brock, C., Abbott, R., & Dawson, G. (2007). Rate of head circumference growth as a function of autism diagnosis and history of autistic regression. *Journal of Child Neurology*, *22*(10), 1182–1190.

Webb, S. J., Sparks, B. F., Friedman, S. D., Shaw, D.W.W., Giedd, J., Dawson, G., & Dager, S. R. (2009). Cerebellar vermal volumes and behavioral correlates in children with autism spectrum disorder. *Psychiatry Research-Neuroimaging*, *172*(1), 61–67.

Wegiel, J., Kuchna, I., Nowicki, K., Imaki, H., Marchi, E., Ma, S. Y., . . . Wisniewski, T. (2010). The neuropathology of autism: Defects of neurogenesis and neuronal migration, and dysplastic changes. *Acta Neuropathol*, *119*(6), 755–770.

Wei, H., Alberts, I., & Li, X. (2013). Brain IL-6 and autism. *Neuroscience*, *252*, 320–325.

Weigelt, S., Koldewyn, K., Dilks, D. D., Balas, B., McKone, E., & Kanwisher, N. (2014). Domain-specific development of face memory but not face perception. *Developmental Science*, *17*(1), 47–58.

Weigelt, S., Koldewyn, K., & Kanwisher, N. (2013). Face recognition deficits in autism spectrum disorders are both domain specific and process specific. *PLoS One*, *8*(9), 1–8.

Weinstein, M., Ben-Sira, L., Levy, Y., Zachor, D. A., Ben Itzhak, E., Artzi, M., . . . Ben Bashat, D. (2011). Abnormal white matter integrity in young children with autism. *Human Brain Mapping*, *32*(4), 534–543.

Weng, S. J., Wiggins, J. L., Peltier, S. J., Carrasco, M., Risi, S., Lord, C., & Monk, C. S. (2010). Alterations of resting state functional connectivity in the default network in adolescents with autism spectrum disorders. *Brain Research*, *1313*, 202–214.

Werner, E., & Dawson, G. (2005). Validation of the phenomenon of autistic regression using home videotapes. *Archives of General Psychiatry*, *62*(8), 889–895.

Werner, E., Dawson, G., Osterling, J., & Dinno, N. (2000). Brief report: Recognition of autism spectrum disorder before one year of age: A retrospective study based on home videotapes. *Journal of Autism and Developmental Disorders*, *30*(2), 157–162.

Wetherby, A. M., & Prizant, B. M. (2002). *Communication and Symbolic Behavior Scales and Developmental Profile*. Baltimore, MD: Brookes.

Wheelwright, S., Auyeung, B., Allison, C., & Baron-Cohen, S. (2010). Defining the broader, medium and narrow autism phenotype among parents using the Autism Spectrum Quotient (AQ). *Molecular Autism*, *1*(1), 10.

Whitaker-Azmitia, P. M. (2001). Serotonin and brain development: Role in human developmental diseases. *Brain Research Bulletin*, *56*(5), 479–485.

Whitehouse, A. J., Barry, J. G., & Bishop, D. V. (2008). Further defining the language impairment of autism: Is there a specific language impairment subtype? *Journal of Communication Disorders*, *41*(4), 319–336.

Whitehouse, A.J.O., Hickey, M., Stanley, F. J., Newnham, J. P., & Pennell, C. E. (2011). Brief report: A preliminary study of fetal head circumference growth in autism spectrum disorder. *Journal of Autism and Developmental Disorders*, *41*(1), 122–129.

WHO. (2007). *Multicentre Growth Reference Study Group: WHO Child Growth Standards: Head Circumference-for-Age, Arm Circumference-for-Age, Triceps Skinfold-for-Age and Subscapular Skinfold-for-Age. Methods and Development*. Geneva, Vol. World Health Organization Press.

Whyatt, C. P., & Craig, C. M. (2012). Motor skills in children aged 7–10 years, diagnosed with autism spectrum disorder. *Journal of Autism and Developmental Disorders*, *42*(9), 1799–1809.

Wiggins, L. D., Robins, D. L., Bakeman, R., & Adamson, L. B. (2009). Brief report: Sensory abnormalities as distinguishing symptoms of autism spectrum disorders in young children. *Journal of Autism and Developmental Disorders*, *39*(7), 1087–1091.

Wilkerson, D. S., Volpe, A. G., Dean, R. S., & Titus, J. B. (2002). Perinatal complications as predictors of infantile autism. *International Journal of Neuroscience*, *112*(9), 1085–1098.

Wilkinson, K. M. (1998). Profiles of language and communication skills in autism. *Mental Retardation and Developmental Disabilities Research Reviews*, *4*(2), 73–79.

Williams, D. L., Goldstein, G., Carpenter, P. A., & Minshew, N. J. (2005). Verbal and spatial working memory in autism. *Journal of Autism and Developmental Disorders*, *35*(6), 747–756.

Williams, D. L., Goldstein, G., & Minshew, N. J. (2005). Impaired memory for faces and social scenes in autism: Clinical implications of memory dysfunction. *Archives of Clinical Neuropsychology*, *20*(1), 1–15.

Williams, D. L., Goldstein, G., & Minshew, N. J. (2006). The profile of memory function in children with autism. *Neuropsychology*, *20*(1), 21–29.

Williams, E. L., & Casanova, M. F. (2010). Autism and dyslexia: A spectrum of cognitive styles as defined by minicolumnar morphometry. *Medical Hypotheses*, *74*(1), 59–62.

Williams, J. H., Waiter, G. D., Gilchrist, A., Perrett, D. I., Murray, A. D., & Whiten, A. (2006). Neural mechanisms of imitation and 'mirror neuron' functioning in autistic spectrum disorder. *Neuropsychologia*, *44*(4), 610–621.

Williams, J. H., Whiten, A., & Singh, T. (2004). A systematic review of action imitation in autistic spectrum disorder. *Journal of Autism and Developmental Disorders*, *34*(3), 285–299.

Williams, K., MacDermott, S., Ridley, G., Glasson, E. J., & Wray, J. A. (2008). The prevalence of autism in Australia: Can it be established from existing data? *Journal of Paediatrics and Child Health*, *44*(9), 504–510.

Williams, R. S., Hauser, S. L., Purpura, D. P., DeLong, G. R., & Swisher, C. N. (1980). Autism and mental retardation: Neuropathologic studies performed in four retarded persons with autistic behavior. *Archives of Neurology*, *37*(12), 749–753.

Wilson, S., Djukic, A., Shinnar, S., Dharmani, C., & Rapin, I. (2003). Clinical characteristics of language regression in children. *Developmental Medicine and Child Neurology*, *45*(8), 508–514.

Wilson, S.A.K. (1934). Megalencephaly. *Journal of Neurology and Psychopathology*, *14*(55), 193–216.

Wimpory, D. C., Hobson, R. P., Williams, J. M., & Nash, S. (2000). Are infants with autism socially engaged? A study of recent retrospective parental reports. *Journal of Autism and Developmental Disorders*, *30*(6), 525–536.

Windham, G. C., Fessel, K., & Grether, J. K. (2009). Autism spectrum disorders in relation to parental occupation in technical fields. *Autism Research: Official Journal of the International Society for Autism Research*, *2*(4), 183–191.

Wing, L., & Gould, J. (1979). Severe impairments of social interaction and associated abnormalities in children: Epidemiology and classification. *Journal of Autism and Developmental Disorders*, *9*(1), 11–29.

Wing, L., Gould, J., & Gillberg, C. (2011). Autism spectrum disorders in the DSM-V: Better or worse than the DSM-IV? *Research in Developmental Disabilities*, *32*(2), 768–773.

Wing, L., & Potter, D. (2002). The epidemiology of autistic spectrum disorders: Is the prevalence rising? *Mental Retardation and Developmental Disabilities Research Reviews*, *8*(3), 151–161.

Wingate, M., Kirby, R. S., Pettygrove, S., Cunniff, C., Schulz, E., Ghosh, T., . . . Autism Dev Disabilities, M. (2014). Prevalence of autism spectrum disorder among children aged 8 years: Autism and developmental disabilities monitoring network, 11 sites, United States, 2010. *Mmwr Surveillance Summaries*, *63*(2), 1–21.

Wolff, J. J., Botteron, K., Dager, S. R., Elison, J., Estes, A., Gu, H., Hazlett, H. C., Pandey, J., Paterson, S. J., Schultz, R. T., Zwaigenbaum, L., Piven, J., & The IBIS Network (2014). Longitudinal patterns of repetitive behavior in toddlers with autism. *Journal of Child Psychology and Psychiatry*, *55*(8), 945–953.

Wolff, J. J., Gu, H. B., Gerig, G., Elison, J. T., Styner, M., Gouttard, S., . . . Network, I. (2012). Differences in white matter fiber tract development present from 6 to 24 months in infants with autism. *American Journal of Psychiatry*, *169*(6), 589–600.

Wolff, S. (2004). The history of autism. *European Child and Adolescent Psychiatry*, *13*(4), 201–208.

Wong, V. C., & Kwan, Q. K. (2010). Randomized controlled trial for early intervention for autism: A pilot study of the autism

1–2–3 project. *Journal of Autism and Developmental Disorders*, *40*(6), 677–688.

Woodhouse, W., Bailey, A., Rutter, M., Bolton, P., Baird, G., & Le Couteur, A. (1996). Head circumference in autism and other pervasive developmental disorders. *Journal of Child Psychology and Psychiatry*, *37*(6), 665–671.

Woodhouse, W., Bailey, A., Rutter, M., Bolton, P., Baird, G., & LeCouteur, A. (1996). Head circumference in autism and other pervasive developmental disorders. *Journal of Child Psychology and Psychiatry and Allied Disciplines*, *37*(6), 665–671.

Wright, C. M., Booth, I. W., Buckler, J.M.H., Cameron, N., Cole, T. J., Healy, M.J.R., . . . Williams, A. F. (2002). Growth reference charts for use in the United Kingdom. *Archives of Disease in Childhood*, *86*(1), 11–14.

Xu, J., Zwaigenbaum, L., Szatmari, P., & Scherer, S. W. (2004). Molecular cytogenetics of autism. *Current Genomics*, *5*, 347–364.

Yamakawa, H., Oyama, S., Mitsuhashi, H., Sasagawa, N., Uchino, S., Kohsaka, S., & Ishiura, S. (2007). Neuroligins 3 and 4X interact with syntrophin-gamma2, and the interactions are affected by autism-related mutations. *Biochemical and Biophysical Research Communications*, *355*(1), 41–46.

Yang, Y., & Pan, C. H. (2013). Role of metabotropic glutamate receptor 7 in autism spectrum disorders: A pilot study. *Life Sciences*, *92*(2), 149–153.

Yashiro, K., Riday, T. T., Condon, K. H., Roberts, A. C., Bernardo, D. R., Prakash, R., . . . Philpot, B. D. (2009). Ube3a is required for experience-dependent maturation of the neocortex. *Nature Neuroscience*, *12*(6), 777–783.

Yauk, C., Polyzos, A., Rowan-Carroll, A., Somers, C. M., Godschalk, R. W., Van Schooten, F. J., . . . Kovalchuk, O. (2008). Germ-line mutations, DNA damage, and global hypermethylation in mice exposed to particulate air pollution in an urban/industrial location. *Proceedings of the National Academy of Sciences of the United States of America*, *105*(2), 605–610.

Yeargin-Allsopp, M., Rice, C., Karapurkar, T., Doernberg, N., Boyle, C., & Murphy, C. (2003). Prevalence of autism in a U.S. metropolitan area. *JAMA*, *289*(1), 49–55.

Yeo, B. T., Krienen, F. M., Sepulcre, J., Sabuncu, M. R., Lashkari, D., Hollinshead, M., . . . Buckner, R. L. (2011). The organization of the human cerebral cortex estimated by intrinsic functional connectivity. *Journal of Neurophysiology*, *106*(3), 1125–1165.

Yerys, B. E., Hepburn, S. L., Pennington, B. F., & Rogers, S. J. (2007). Executive function in preschoolers with autism: Evidence consistent with a secondary deficit. *Journal of Autism and Developmental Disorders*, *37*(6), 1068–1079.

Yerys, B. E., Jankowski, K. F., Shook, D., Rosenberger, L. R., Barnes, K. A., Berl, M. M., . . . Gaillard, W. D. (2009). The fMRI success rate of children and adolescents: Typical development, epilepsy, attention deficit/hyperactivity disorder, and autism spectrum disorders. *Human Brain Mapping*, *30*(10), 3426–3435.

Yerys, B. E., Wallace, G. L., Harrison, B., Celano, M. J., Giedd, J. N., & Kenworthy, L. E. (2009). Set-shifting in children with autism spectrum disorders reversal shifting deficits on the intradimensional/extradimensional shift test correlate with repetitive behaviors. *Autism*, *13*(5), 523–538.

Yogarajah, M., Focke, N. K., Bonelli, S. B., Thompson, P., Vollmar, C., McEvoy, A. W., . . . Duncan, J. S. (2010). The structural plasticity of white matter networks following anterior temporal lobe resection. *Brain*, *133*(Pt 8), 2348–2364.

Young, H. A., Geier, D. A., & Geier, M. R. (2008). Thimerosal exposure in infants and neurodevelopmental disorders: An assessment of computerized medical records in the vaccine safety datalink. *Journal of the Neurological Sciences*, *271*(1–2), 110–118.

Young, R. L., Brewer, N., & Pattison, C. (2003). Parental identification of early behavioural abnormalities in children with autistic disorder. *Autism*, *7*(2), 125–143.

Zachor, D. A., Ben-Itzchak, E., Rabinovich, A. L., & Lahat, E. (2007). Change in autism core symptoms with intervention. *Research in Autism Spectrum Disorders*, *1*(4), 304–317.

Zander, E., & Dahlgren, S. O. (2010). WISC-III index score profiles of 520 Swedish children with pervasive developmental disorders. *Psychological Assessment*, *22*(2), 213–222.

Zecevic, N. (1998). Synaptogenesis in layer I of the human cerebral cortex in the first half of gestation. *Cerebral Cortex*, *8*(3), 245–252.

Zeegers, M., Pol, H. H., Durston, S., Nederveen, H., Schnack, H., van Daalen, E., . . . Buitelaar, J. (2009). No differences in MR-based volumetry between 2- and 7-year-old children with autism spectrum disorder and developmental delay. *Brain and Development*, *31*(10), 725–730.

Zerbo, O., Iosif, A. M., Walker, C., Ozonoff, S., Hansen, R. L., & Hertz-Picciotto, I. (2013). Is maternal influenza or fever during pregnancy associated with autism or developmental delays? Results from the CHARGE (CHildhood Autism Risks from Genetics and Environment) study. *Journal of Autism and Developmental Disorders*, *43*(1), 25–33.

Zerbo, O., Yoshida, C., Grether, J. K., Van de Water, J., Ashwood, P., Delorenze, G. N., . . . Croen, L. A. (2014). Neonatal cytokines and chemokines and risk of autism spectrum disorder: The Early Markers for Autism (EMA) study: A case-control study. *Journal of Neuroinflammation*, *11*, 113.

Zhou, J., & Parada, L. F. (2012). PTEN signaling in autism spectrum disorders. *Current Opinion in Neurobiology*, *22*(5), 873–879.

Zielinski, B. A., Anderson, J. S., Froehlich, A. L., Prigge, M.B.D., Nielsen, J. A., Cooperrider, J. R., . . . Lainhart, J. E. (2012). scMRI reveals large-scale brain network abnormalities in autism. *PLoS One*, *7*(11), 1–14.

Zielinski, B. A., Prigge, M. B., Nielsen, J. A., Froehlich, A. L., Abildskov, T. J., Anderson, J. S., . . . Lainhart, J. E. (2014). Longitudinal changes in cortical thickness in autism and typical development. *Brain*, *137*(Pt 6), 1799–1812.

Zikopoulos, B., & Barbas, H. (2010). Changes in prefrontal axons may disrupt the network in autism. *Journal of Neuroscience*, *30*(44), 14595–14609.

Zikopoulos, B., & Barbas, H. (2013). Altered neural connectivity in excitatory and inhibitory cortical circuits in autism. *Frontiers in Human Neuroscience*, *7*, 1–24.

Zilbovicius, M., Meresse, I., Chabane, N., Brunelle, F., Samson, Y., & Boddaert, N. (2006). Autism, the superior temporal sulcus and social perception. *Trends in Neurosciences*, *29*(7), 359–366.

Zimmerman, A. W., Connors, S. L., Matteson, K. J., Lee, L. C., Singer, H. S., Castaneda, J. A., & Pearce, D. A. (2007). Maternal antibrain antibodies in autism. *Brain, Behavior, and Immunity*, *21*(3), 351–357.

Zwaigenbaum, L., Bryson, S., & Garon, N. (2013). Early identification of autism spectrum disorders. *Behavioural Brain Research*, *251*, 133–146.

Zwaigenbaum, L., Bryson, S., Rogers, T., Roberts, W., Brian, J., & Szatmari, P. (2005). Behavioral manifestations of autism in the first year of life. *International Journal of Developmental Neuroscience*, *23*(2–3), 143–152.

Zwaigenbaum, L., Szatmari, P., Goldberg, J., Bryson, S., Mahoney, W., & Bartolucci, G. (2000). The broader autism phenotype: Defining genetically informative dimensions. *American Journal of Human Genetics*, *67*(4), 213–213.

Zwaigenbaum, L., Szatmari, P., Jones, M. B., Bryson, S. E., MacLean, J. E., Mahoney, W. J., . . . Tuff, L. (2002). Pregnancy and birth complications in autism and liability to the broader autism phenotype. *Journal of the American Academy of Child and Adolescent Psychiatry*, *41*(5), 572–579.

Zwaigenbaum, L., Thurm, A., Stone, W., Baranek, G., Bryson, S., Iverson, J., . . . Sigman, M. (2007). Studying the emergence of autism spectrum disorders in high-risk infants: Methodological and practical issues. *Journal of Autism and Developmental Disorders*, *37*(3), 466–480.

14 Neurodevelopmental Disorders of Attention and Learning

ADHD and LD Across the Life Span

Jeanette Wasserstein, Gerry A. Stefanatos, Robert L. Mapou, Yitzchak Frank, and Josephine Elia

Introduction

Although learning disability (LD) and attention deficit/hyperactivity disorder (ADHD) are commonly intertwined in clinical presentation, their recognition as separate clinical entities followed rather distinctive historical paths. On one hand, the origins of the concept of LD are closely tied to notions of localization of cognitive function in the human brain that emerged in the late 19th century. Broca's (1861) association of circumscribed deficits in speech production to acquired damage of inferior frontal gyrus prompted speculation that specific language impairments in children may have a similar anatomic basis (Vaisse, 1866). While this was soon dispelled by Cotard (1868), the notion remained that some children demonstrated fairly specific cognitive impairments that may be based in dysfunction or maldevelopment of particular areas of the brain. On the other hand, problems related to ADHD, have a rather different and more varied conceptual history, originally having been considered a defect of moral control (Still, 1902), and then a disorder of excessive movement (hyperkinesis) (Laufer, Denhoff, & Solomons, 1957), before eventually being conceptualized as a neurodevelopmental disorder (ADHD) that particularly affected neural systems mediating attention (Douglas, 1972, Cantwell, 1983).

From a public health perspective, both LD and ADHD are among the most common neurobehavioral disorders of childhood (DHHS, 2003, Wallman, 2008). Educators have reported a rise in the number of children diagnosed with these disorders (Education, 2007) with concomitant increases in the number of children requiring special education services (Wagner, Kutash, Duchnowski, Epstein, & Sumi, 2005). Both disorders are associated with increased risk for a range of emotional, behavioral, and psychosocial issues (Murphy, Barkley, & Bush, 2002; Daniel, Walsh, et al., 2006; Goldston, Walsh, et al., 2007) and pediatricians have recorded increases in outpatient visits to address these related problems (Kelleher, McInerny, Gardner, Childs, & Wasserman, 2000). While the disorders emerge in childhood, associated difficulties often persist in some form into adulthood, resulting in occupational concerns ranging from performance issues and underemployment (Halmoy, Fasmer, et al., 2009; Barkley & Fischer, 2011) to increased injury risk (Breslin & Pole, 2009). Long-term outcome can be significantly improved with continuing treatment and support, resulting in significant public health costs that often persist beyond childhood and adolescence (Schnoes, Reid, et al., 2006).

The high rate of comorbidity of these disorders has long been recognized both in clinical samples (Semrud-Clikeman et al., 1992) and in nonreferred samples recruited from the community (Fergusson & Horwood, 1992; Pastor & Reuben, 2008). The actual observed degree of overlap has varied broadly across studies. For example, the prevalence of LD in the ADHD population has reportedly ranged from a quarter or less (Pliszka, 1998), to two-thirds (e.g., Mayes, et al., 2000) or more (Semrud-Clikeman et al., 1992). According to a recent report by the Centers for Disease Control (Pastor & Reuben, 2008), approximately 5% of school-aged children in the United States are diagnosed with ADHD without LDs and approximately 5% have LDs without ADHD. An additional 4% are diagnosed with both conditions (i.e., roughly 30% comorbidity in this sample). All three groups require special education services, and are likely to have other health conditions and neurobehavioral dysfunction of varying degrees through much of the life span.

Numerous factors have been proposed to explain the comorbidity between these disorders, ranging from shared genetic and environmental risk factors (Fisher & DeFries, 2002, Gayan et al., 2005) and shared underlying processing deficits (e.g., Denckla, 1993, Seidman, Biederman, Monuteaux, Doyle, & Faraone, 2001) to interactions between the disorders whereby the existence of one disorder influences the diagnosis and course of the other (see Boada, Willcutt, & Penningtone, 2012 for a review). Given the complex interweaving of these disorders, they are presented together in this chapter. We review the historical roots of conceptualization and nosological classifications of each disorder, their clinical presentations over the life span, current neuroscientific understanding, assessment highlights and emerging or controversial issues.

Historical Roots of LD and ADHD

One of the first recognized accounts of LD was a description of a specific reading disorder published, in 1896, by the English pediatrician W. P. Morgan. He described a bright and intelligent 14-year-old boy who was quick with games and intellectually no weaker than any of his peers (Morgan, 1896). His singular great difficulty was his inability to learn to read despite the utmost effort. Morgan referred to the disorder as "congenital word-blindness" because, in his view, the pattern of impairment resembled adult acquired cases of "word-blindness" or alexia that had been previously described by Kussmaul (1877) and others. Word blindness referred to loss of the ability to interpret written or printed language despite normal vision and the ability to see words and letters distinctly. It was thought to occur from acquired damage to the left angular gyrus, which functionally compromised a center for the processing of a construct termed *optic images of letters* (Dejerine, 1892).

Morgan's report represented an attempt to utilize these concepts to explain congenital forms of reading impairment that he ascribed to defective development of that same region of the brain. Due to confusions arising from the term *word-blindness* (Broadbent, 1895), it was slowly replaced by *dyslexia* (Hinshelwood, 1896), which had been coined a decade earlier by the German ophthalmologist Rudolph Berlin (1887). Dyslexia came to refer to an inability to learn to read despite adequate vision, intelligence, motivation, and instruction. For many years, it was considered related to difficulty in the visual analysis and representation of written or printed symbols (Hinshelwood, 1917, Orton, 1925), although later research implicated subtle language-processing abnormalities as the major determinant (Myklebust & Johnson, 1962).

Over several decades, additional forms of LD affecting the acquisition of other academic and even social skills were eventually delineated. This includes dyscalculia (math LD) (Cohn, 1968; Kosc, 1974), dysgraphia (writing LD) (Ohare, Brown, & Aitken, 1991), and nonverbal LD (NVLD, primarily social LD) (Johnson, 1987; Rourke, 1989). More recently, clinicians have posited an LD based upon executive dysfunction, although this has not yet been recognized as a separate entity (see Wasserstein & Denckla, 2009 for review). Dyslexia remains the most common and best understood LD (see Frank, 2014 for review). Over time, the acronym *LD* has been transmuted to meaning *learning disorder* and/or *learning difference.* These terms are essentially synonymous, although the latter sometimes implies lesser degree of challenge or deficit.

The delineation of ADHD started earlier and followed a rather different history. Sir Alexander Crichton alluded to children with attention problems in a chapter entitled "On Attention and Its Diseases" (Crichton, 1798), in which he noted that such problems likely resulted from "an unnatural morbid sensibility of the nerves" that may be either "born with the person, or may be the effect of accidental diseases." Heinrich Hoffman, a German physician, later depicted two characters—Zappel-Philipp (i.e., Fidgety Philip) and Hans Kuck-in-die-Luft (i.e., Hans Look-in-the-Air)—who demonstrated characteristics of ADHD in an illustrated children's book of short moral fables entitled *Der Struwwelpeter* (1845). Fidgety Philip demonstrated behaviors consistent with the impulsive/hyperkinetic subtype or presentation, while Hans demonstrated behaviors consistent with the inattentive presentation. The first scientific discussion of the disorder is often credited to Sir George Still, a British pediatrician who discussed similar children that he described as having "defect of moral control . . .without general impairment of intellect" (Still, 1902, p. 1079). While his portrayals spanned many types of disruptive behavior disorders, he placed particular emphasis on impulsivity and poor capacity for sustained attention, which he linked to possible brain damage. This correlation between early brain damage and subsequent behavior problems and/or learning difficulties was reified on a global scale by the encephalitis lethargica epidemic from 1917 to 1928 (Lange, et al., 2010)—surviving children often became hyperactive, distractible, and unmanageable in school (Hohman, 1922; Ebaugh, 1923).

In 1932 two German physicians, Franz Kramer and Hans Pollnow, coined the term *hyperkinetic disease* to denote children with probable brain damage who showed marked motor restlessness and many other currently recognized symptoms of ADHD. Subsequently, theoreticians like Strauss and Lehtinen (1947) collapsed the multiple cognitive and behavioral disorders seen in childhood into one entity, "minimal brain dysfunction" (MBD). The term carried the implication that brain damage existed in children who demonstrated these behaviors, even though it may not be detectable because of the fallibility of neurological examinations. However, the moderating role of environmental factors became apparent in observations that postencephalitic children who were successfully treated in special residential treatment centers commonly relapsed when they returned to maladjusted parents (Bond & Smith, 1935). As evidence accrued, it became apparent that the full spectrum of causality in cognitive and behavior disorders needed to consider multiple factors, including genetic influences, gestational and perinatal experiences, and the stresses and trauma of later life (Clements & Peters, 1962).

Such observations, along with recognition that brain dysfunction was in fact only being inferred (Kessler, 1980), shifted the emphasis away from a focus on structural brain damage (i.e., MBD) toward a focus on symptoms or behavior, such as excessive activity and inattention. The terms *hyperactivity* and/or *hyperkinesis* gained popularity in the 1960s when excess motor activity was emphasized (Chess, 1960; Laufer, Denhoff, & Solomons, 2011). Subsequently, the role of attention deficits was highlighted based on observations that these children performed poorly on laboratory measures of attention (Douglas, 1972; Douglas, 1976), and *attention deficit disorder (ADD), with or without hyperactivity* emerged in the 1980s. Finally ADHD was adopted (Sommers, Fragapane, & Schmock, 1994), an acknowledgment of the diverse manifestations of disordered behavior (i.e., activity level vs. attention). Three possible subtypes were delineated: predominantly inattentive, predominantly hyperactive/impulsive, and a combined subtype. These changes completed the segregation of this disorder from specific disorders of learning (i.e., LDs).

Changing Concepts and Nosology

ADHD

The American Psychiatric Association's (APA) *Diagnostic and Statistical Manual of Mental Disorders* (DSM) initiated the first systematic effort to categorize and define the full gamut of behavioral disorders now associated with ADHD. In its second edition, DSM-II (APA, 1968), the disorder was termed *Hyperkinetic Reaction of Childhood* with the clear focus on the high levels of motor activity as the primary deficit. The third edition of the DSM, the DSM-III (APA, 1968) marked a turning point when it explicitly incorporated into the disorder's symptomology deficits of attention and impulse control, as well as the long-observed hyperactivity. Accordingly, the disorder was renamed *attention deficit disorder,* with two subtypes (with and without hyperactivity). The DSM-III also introduced the category of ADD-Residual Type, recognizing that some adolescents and adults outgrew hyperactivity yet still exhibited other symptoms of inattention and impulsivity without remission. While this category acknowledged that the condition could persist, in a partial form, into an older age group, there was still no recognized adult version of the full disorder. By regrouping symptoms into subtypes with and without hyperactivity, DSM-III (APA, 1980) made motor activity a secondary symptom of the disorder. DSM-III R (APA, 1987) then shifted to a global conception that unified the three core symptoms into a single entity (with one symptom list). The DSM-IV (APA, 2000) returned to a dichotomous conception of ADHD, and reframed it as a multidimensional spectrum disorder based on the primary symptom clusters of inattention and/or hyperactivity/impulsivity (i.e., predominantly hyperactive/impulsive type, predominantly inattentive type, and combined type). Interestingly, while acknowledging in the text that ADHD may be diagnosed in adults (e.g., "In . . . adults, symptoms of hyperactivity take the form of feelings of restlessness" (APA, 2000, p. 79) and "a minority experience the full complement of symptoms . . . into mid-adulthood" (p. 82), no formal anchors were established. Thus, the description and criteria remained oriented towards children and adolescents (ages 4–17 years) and offered few practical guidelines for diagnosing adults.

Criteria for ADHD in the most recent fifth edition of the DSM (APA, 2013) are very similar to those in the DSM-IV, except that ADHD in adults is now formally acknowledged and requires a lower number of symptoms (i.e., five symptoms from either the Inattention cluster or the Hyperactivity and Impulsivity cluster). While this new symptom threshold is less than the six symptoms required for children, it is still higher than the four symptoms suggested by the only two existing empirical studies of diagnostic thresholds for adults (Barkley, 2010; Solanto, Wasserstein, Marks, & Mitchell, 2012). Another change is the use of "presentation" as opposed to "type" when referring to the predominant symptom cluster(s). This semantic shift recognizes the empirical reality that the primary areas of problem behaviors often change in the same individual over time. That is, the child who shows excessive hyperactive/impulsive or combined type symptoms can, and often does, become mainly inattentive as an adult.

LD

Samuel A. Kirk (1963), a clinical psychologist who is often regarded as the father of special education, introduced the term "learning disabilities" at a conference devoted to the problems of perceptually handicapped children. His statement captures the essence of a diagnosis by exclusion:

> I have used the term 'learning disabilities' to describe a group of children who have disorders in development in language, speech, reading, and associated communication skills needed for social interaction. In this group I do not include children who have sensory handicaps such as blindness or deafness, because we have methods of managing and training the deaf and the blind. I also exclude from this group children who have generalized mental retardation.
>
> (Kirk, 1963, p. 6)

His conceptualization had a significant impact on the field and on social policy. Subsequently a number of legal definitions of LD were created. The first federal definition was established in the late 1960s, and was later included in special education law in the well-known 1975 Education for All Handicapped Children Act (Public Law 94–142). Despite advancing research, this federal definition has remained essentially unchanged in the 1990 Individuals with Disabilities Education Act (IDEA, Public Law 101–476), and its 1997 and 2004 revisions. This definition is also widely used when developing individual education plans (IEPs) and 504 plans for children in public schools. It states:

> Specific learning disability means a disorder in one or more of the basic psychological processes involved in understanding or in using language, spoken or written, that may manifest itself in an imperfect ability to listen, think, speak, read, write, spell, or do mathematical calculations. The term includes such conditions as perceptual handicaps, brain injury, minimal brain dysfunction, dyslexia, and developmental aphasia. The term does not include children who have learning problems that are primarily the result of visual, hearing, or motor handicaps; of mental retardation; of emotional disturbance; or of environmental, cultural, or economic disadvantage.
>
> *(IDEA, 1990)*

Unfortunately, this definition is not well operationalized, is not neuropsychologically based, and does not recognize the persistence of LD into adulthood. The definition also lumps acquired neurological disorders (i.e., brain injury) together with developmental disorders, reflecting the initial focus of special education law on identification and service delivery for children with all types of cognitive disabilities. However, learning in adolescents and adults who developed normally but subsequently experience brain damage is likely different from that of those born with LD. Consequently, a number of other organizations took on the challenge of defining the disorder (disorders).

Following several revisions, the National Joint Committee on Learning Disabilities (1990) proposed another definition:

> *Learning Disabilities* is a general term that refers to a heterogeneous group of disorders manifested by significant difficulties in the acquisition and use of listening, speaking, reading, writing, reasoning, or mathematical abilities. These disorders are intrinsic to the individual and presumed to be due to central nervous system dysfunction, and may occur across the life span. Problems in self-regulatory behaviors, social perception, and social interaction may exist with the learning disabilities, but do not, by themselves, constitute a learning disability. Although learning disabilities may occur concomitantly with other disabilities (e.g., sensory impairment, mental retardation, serious emotional disturbance), or with extrinsic influences (such as cultural differences, insufficient or inappropriate instruction), they are not the result of those conditions or influences.

While recognizing that LDs persist across the life span and are brain-based, this definition excludes problems with self-regulatory behaviors, social perception, and social interaction. This is problematic for individuals with NVLDs, for whom difficulties with social perception and social interaction often define the disorder and lead to its initial identification (Tsatsanis & Rourke, 2008; Wasserstein, Vadhan, Barboza, & Stefanatos, 2008, but see and subsequent sections in this chapter for contrary views). It is also problematic for individuals who have disorders of executive functioning and self-regulatory behavior, but who do not meet strict diagnostic criteria for attention-deficit/ hyperactivity disorder (Cutting & Denckla, 2003).

A third definition, oriented toward rehabilitation of adults with LDs, was established by the Rehabilitation Services Administration (RSA) in 1985, following their acceptance of learning disabilities as a medically recognized disability (Katz, Goldstein, & Beers, 2001):

> A specific learning disability is a disorder in one or more of the central nervous system processes involved in perceiving, understanding, and/or using concepts through verbal (spoken or written) language or nonverbal means. This disorder manifests itself with a deficit in one or more of the following areas: attention, reasoning, processing, memory, communication, reading, writing, spelling, calculation, coordination, social competence, and emotional maturity.
>
> (Rehabilitation Services Administration, 1985, January 24)

From a neuropsychological standpoint, this definition is the best of the three. It is also better suited for adults. However, the definition is not widely known to many working in the LD field or used very often. The first two definitions, via IDEA and NJC, have been disseminated far more broadly.[1] Although definitions of specific LDs that are based on empirical research using specific criteria, i.e., evidence-based, would be desirable, there is just one close approximation, for dyslexia. It states:

> Dyslexia is a specific learning disability that is neurobiological in origin. It is characterized by difficulties with accurate and/or fluent word recognition and by poor spelling and decoding abilities. These difficulties typically result from a deficit in the phonological component of language that is often unexpected in relation to other cognitive abilities and the provision of effective classroom instruction. Secondary consequences may include problems in reading comprehension and reduced reading experience that can impede growth of vocabulary and background knowledge.
>
> (Lyon, Shaywitz, & Shaywitz, 2003)

Unfortunately, there are no evidence-based definitions of specific LDs in mathematics or written expression. Nonetheless, research has identified some core skills affected by these disorders (Fletcher, Lyon, Fuchs, & Barnes, 2007). These have been incorporated into the new DSM-5, wherein LDs are now classified as neurodevelopmental disorders. Key characteristics include the following (APA, 2013: 67):

- Symptoms must persist for six months, despite intervention.
- Academic skills are "substantially and quantifiably below those expected for the individual's chronological age" and cause "significant interference" with academic, occupational, or everyday functioning.
- Difficulties are confirmed by "individually administered standardized achievement measures and comprehensive clinical assessment."
- For individuals 17 or older, a documented history of impairing learning difficulties may be substituted for the standardized assessment.
- Onset is during school years, but effects may not become fully obvious until learning demands increase.
- Difficulties are not better accounted for by another disorder, lack of language proficiency, or inadequate instruction.

In contrast to the DSM-IV, there is only a single category for LD in DSM-5, specific learning disorder, with specifiers for the types of academic domains affected: reading, written expression, and/or mathematics. For each academic skill domain there are subdomains that have been supported by research, although these subdomains are best established for reading disorders. Specific skill areas and their subdomains are shown below. Full diagnosis includes the level of severity of the specific LD (i.e., mild, moderate, and severe) and the subdomains affected.

315.00 (F81.0) with impairment in reading:

- Word reading accuracy
- Reading rate or fluency
- Reading comprehension

315.2 (F81.81) with impairment in written expression:

- Spelling accuracy
- Grammar and punctuation accuracy
- Clarity or organization of written expression

315.1 (F81.2) with impairment in mathematics:

- Number sense
- Memorization of arithmetic facts
- Accurate or fluent calculation
- Accurate math reasoning

Thus, the DSM-5 recognizes considerable differences in the presentation of the LDs. This allows identification and research in even more subcategories, with potentially different underlying neuropsychological deficits. For example, poor oral word reading may reflect the well-established phonemic processing deficit, or an oral dyspraxia, and/or even a subset of visual agnosia. However, in contrast to the DSM-IV, which included a category for unspecified LD, the DSM-5 restricts the Specific LD category to only academic skill deficits. As a result, people with what was called nonverbal/social/visual-perceptual LD (i.e., NVLD or NLD) may no longer meet criteria for any specific form of LD, despite having executive and other deficits that globally impede their academic and social learning (Wasserstein et al., 2008; Wasserstein & Denckla, 2009). Historically, the actual existence of LD had been operationalized by using defined statistical discrepancies between aptitude and achievement test scores, e.g., −1.5 SD or greater in DSM-IV (APA, 1994). More recently, however, some researchers argue the approach is not empirically supported (Fletcher et al., 2007; see Siegel and Smythe, 2008 for review). There is ongoing controversy on this issue, especially in identification of LD in the high-IQ individual. In such cases, most or all of the achievement scores may fall within normal ranges but well below expectations for aptitude. Arguably, reliance on on the DSM V criteria of "a documented history of impairing learning difficulties" could be used.

Clinical Profiles

Clinical profiles of ADHD and LD are complex and change over time, in part as a function of developmental demands (Mapou, 2009a) and successful remediation and/or learning. It is also emphasized that both ADHD and LDs are "continuum disorders," that is, disorders that exist at the extremes of the normal distribution (e.g., (Shaywitz, Escobar, et al., 1992). Thus many qualitative descriptions apply to most people to varying degrees. However, there is no consensus regarding where to draw the line regarding where "normal" ends and disorder begins. Opinions differ greatly (e.g., psychometrically defined 95th or 98th percentiles for age-cohorts, arbitrary symptom cutoffs applied across all most ages). Finally, while ADHD and LD clearly coexist, they are separate conditions that are often mistaken for each other and can be difficult to disentangle, both conceptually and clinically.

ADHD: Presentations and Possible Underlying Deficits

ADHD is characterized by a pattern of persistent problems related to inattention and/or hyperactivity-impulsivity, which are more frequent and severe than typically seen in individuals at similar levels of development (i.e., age inappropriate). The behavioral manifestations are diverse and can include excessive motor activity (Kinsbourne, 1977; Halperin, Matier, Bedi, Sharma, & Newcorn, 1992); poor inhibitory control over behavior (Chelune, Ferguson, Koon, & Dickey, 1986; Barkley, 1997a, 1997b; Nigg, 2001); and difficulties focusing, sustaining, and shifting attention (Douglas, 1972; Levine et al., 1982; Seidel & Joschko, 1990, Epstein, Conners, Ehrhardt, March, & Swanson, 1997; Cepeda et al., 2000). The performance of individuals with ADHD is notoriously inconsistent and context dependent, suggesting that motivational factors and reinforcement contingencies are also important considerations in neuropsychological conceptualizations of the disorder (Sonuga-Barke & Coghill, 2014).

Symptoms of the disorder commonly emerge in the preschool years (Campbell, 1995; Connor, 2002) and often persist in altered form into adolescence and adulthood (Faraone, Biederman, & Friedman, 2000; Barkley, Fischer, Smallish, & Fletcher, 2002). The changes in the manifestations reflect mixed influences related to biological maturational changes, as well as successful application of self-applied or formal treatment interventions (Hechtman & Weiss, 1983; Wender, 1998). Hyperkinesis decreases most consistently while problems with inattention and executive function may persist or even become more apparent (e.g., Wolf & Wasserstein, 2001).

The exact prevalence of ADHD is difficult to specify. Depending on the criteria used for "abnormal" (e.g., above 95th to 98th percentile for same-age peers), ADHD would be expected to exist in about 2% –5% of the population. However, a recent (2011) Centers for Disease Control (CDC) survey found that roughly one in five male high school students and one in ten females had ever been given this diagnosis. These data argue that base rates during childhood range from 10% to 20%, depending on the child's sex (i.e., boys twice as high as girls). Even allowing for the uncertainty regarding diagnostic criteria used, ADHD is clearly extremely common in children. Similarly, the exact prevalence of ADHD in adults is also unknown.

There is a continuing controversy around the persistence of ADHD into adulthood. It is estimated that 50%–75% of ADHD children will have significant symptoms by adolescence (Barkley, Fischer, et al., 2002) while anywhere from 4%–60% will still have significant symptoms during adulthood (Weiss, Hechtman, Milroy, & Perlman, 1985; Barkley, Fischer, et al., 2002). Conservative estimates now converge at around 50% persistence in clinical samples (Pary et al., 2002). From a different perspective, community studies place the adult prevalence rate between 4% and 5% (Murphy & Barkley, 1996; Heiligenstein, Conyers, Berns, & Miller, 1998). Combining clinical outcome data and epidemiological studies, the prevalence estimate would be between 2% and 4% of the general adult population (Pary et al., 2002). Notably, however, the standards used to define excessive levels of residual symptoms in these studies relied on criteria set for children aged 7–17. Since adults should be compared with adults, and not with children or teenagers, utilization of the existing child-oriented criteria may result in underestimation of base rates for adults.[2]

The gender ratio in children is approximately 4:1 in favor of males (Wolraich, Hannah, Pinnock, Baumgaertel, & Brown, 1996) but appears to be a more balanced 3:2 in adults (Biederman et al., 1994; Murphy& Tsuang, 1995). Thus, ADHD females may be underidentified during childhood, and/or the later higher ratio may indicate adult ADHD females are more inclined to pursue services (Wilens et al., 2002). Overall, gender differences in prevalence are confounded by gender biases in diagnostic criteria. Gender differences also vary according to ADHD type (see Stefanatos and Baron, 2007, for a fuller discussion of gender issues in the diagnosis of ADHD).

Disruptive behavior and poor school performance are the most typical referral reasons for children with ADHD. By contrast, many ADHD adults refer themselves for evaluation due to difficulties in day-to-day functioning, at home and/or at work, many of whom have not been diagnosed (Faraone, Spencer, Montano, & Biederman, 2004). Time management (e.g., not paying bills or filing taxes) and organizational problems (e.g., not finishing or tracking long-term projects, running a household) become especially more apparent during the teen years and adulthood. Many adults also self-refer after the diagnosis of a child or other family member triggers their own recognition of the symptoms (Faraone et al., 2004). In addition, they seek consultation after learning about the condition through the media, or when seeking accommodations in school or work settings (Wolf & Wasserstein, 2001). Some are referred by spouses or other medical professionals (Faraone et al., 2004). Irrespective of the referral source, adults with ADHD fall into two broad categories: those who were originally diagnosed as children and those who were never diagnosed. The first group often includes those who were hyperactive and/or oppositional as children. The second group may be more difficult to recognize and frequently show an inattentive presentation and/or variable levels of compensation skills.

ADHD is diagnosed when one or more of the three core symptoms lead to significant functional deficits at home, school, and/or work. Children with ADHD may be unable to sit through, or to focus on, classes or reading material. They may touch objects compulsively, make excessive noise while playing or studying, and otherwise be "disruptive." Adults with ADHD may be unable to sit through a meeting or persevere on projects, and/or may be disorganized at work or in their homes. Sources of distraction for either age group can be external, like ambient noises or visual data, or internal, like thoughts. Although no one person shows all problems, individuals with ADHD, irrespective of age, often perform inconsistently or below expectations. It is emphasized that ADHD is seen at all intellectual and professional levels. Contrary to lay conceptions, having a JD, MD or PhD does not rule it out. The distinguishing feature is significant underperformance and/or underachievement relative to apparent aptitude and/or education. Such aptitude/achievement discrepancies can create a diagnostic quagmire around ADHD and the specific LDs, which contributes to the frequent conflation of these different and sometimes-discrete neurodevelopmental conditions. This ambiguity also sometimes makes it difficult to disentangle the two—ADHD or LD—in a given individual.

Approximately two-thirds (50%–70%) of ADHD individuals demonstrate academic learning difficulties (Barry, Lyman, & Klinger, 2002; Mayes et al., 2000). These problems reflect comorbid specific LD (e.g., dyslexia, dyscalculia, dysgraphia), the disruptive impact of core ADHD symptoms on learning, or both. Learning problems can appear as early as the preschool years when acquisition of preacademic skills can become disrupted by poor impulse control, motor overactivity, and difficulties attending to instruction (DuPaul, McGoey, Eckert, & VanBrakle, 2001; Barkley, Shelton, et al., 2002). Over time, deficiencies in attention (Aaron, Joshi, Palmer, Smith, & Kirby, 2002), working memory (Martinussen & Tannock, 2006), and executive function (Samuelsson et al., 2004; Miranda et al., 2006) play a greater role in academic performance and productivity, and detract from the child's ability to benefit from explicit learning experiences. These factors ultimately can also have a subtle impact on general intellectual development and acquisition of early reading and listening comprehension skills. In fact, difficulty with basic prereading and arithmetic skills are often evident during the first school year (Mariani & Barkley, 1997). By late childhood (~11 years), as many as 80% of children with ADHD have fallen behind grade level in one or several of these areas (Baker & Cantwell, 1992). Dysgraphia is also common, particularly among children with ADHD combined presentation (Marcotte & Stern, 1997).

Compared to controls, adults with ADHD are more likely to have dropped out of school, received below average grades, and/or performed below their potential. Such academic deficits certainly explain the well-documented lower occupational status of probands compared to controls

(Mannuzza, Klein, Bessler, Malloy, & LaPadula, 1993). Retrospective studies of scholastic dysfunction are consistent with the prospective studies discussed earlier. These show that adults with ADHD have a greater lifetime prevalence of academic remediation, grade repetition, and special education placement (Biederman et al., 1993). Murphy and Barkley (1996) and others (Crozier et al., 1999) also found that, relative to controls, clinic-referred adults with ADHD had more academic underachievement with higher rates of subsequent occupational impairment.

A number of different etiological models have been proposed regarding the core deficits underlying ADHD (see Swanson et al., 2007). Most frequently emphasized are various aspects of executive dysfunction, including impaired inhibitory control (Barkley, 1997a, 1997b) and impaired executive working memory (Rapport, VanVoorhis, Tzelepis, Friedman, 2001). Somewhat paradoxically, Halperin and Schulz (2006) focus on the role of intact executive functioning in compensating for a proposed core subcortical dysfunction in arousal. See Table 14.1 for a summary of the principal current models and their associated seminal papers. As can be seen, there is as yet no clear consensus, and details of the debates are beyond the scope of this chapter. This literature is extensive and interested readers may want to consult relevant books and review articles (e.g., Solanto, 2011; Barkley, 2012).

Common Types of Comorbidity in ADHD

PSYCHIATRIC DISORDERS

While the symptoms of ADHD decline with increasing age, the probability of having a comorbid psychiatric diagnosis increases (Biederman, Mick, & Faraone, 2000). By adulthood, only 13% of individuals with ADHD are free of comorbid diagnosis (McGough et al., 2005). Moreover, ADHD adults and children differ in their comorbidity patterns. Children more consistently show acting-out behaviors and learning issues, while adults more commonly show mood and anxiety disorders, in addition to well-known tendencies for substance use and antisocial behavior. Considerable variability has also been reported with regard to psychiatric comorbidity rates in adults, likely reflecting use of prospective versus retrospective/cross-sectional designs, as well as other methodological differences between studies. That is, retrospective and cross-sectional studies typically report higher rates of diagnostic overlap, because participants are on average ten years older than those in longitudinal studies and have had greater opportunity to receive a psychiatric diagnosis. Their elevated rates of reported psychiatric comorbidity may further reflect a referral bias whereby patients who sought psychiatric services may distort (typically inflate) their level of impairment.

There are a number of explanations for the high rates of psychiatric comorbidity among ADHD individuals (Marks, Newcorn, & Halperin, 2001). Some researchers suggest that comorbidities reflect similar genetic and/or environmental underpinnings. For example, Biederman and colleagues have repeatedly shown elevated rates for psychiatric diagnoses in the first-degree relatives of ADHD probands, including antisocial behavior (Faraone & Biederman, 1997), mood (Biederman, Newcorn, & Sprich, 1991; Faraone & Biederman, 1997), and anxiety (Biederman et al., 1992) disorders. Others argue that comorbid disorders might constitute the psychiatric sequelae of living with ADHD (see discussion in Marks et al., 2001). Still others have intimated that the syndromes might be linked such that ADHD might be seen as a risk factor or developmental precursor for subsequent externalizing behaviors (e.g., Faraone & Biederman, 1997; Caron & Rutter, 1991).

Taken together, such findings are consistent with both the psychological impact of lifelong struggles, as well as structural or genetic overlap with other psychiatric disorders. Biological and environmental factors during development also play a role (see reviews by Swanson et al., 2007). Relative to their childhood counterparts, adults with ADHD have more mature brains, but also have endured a longer period of psychosocial stressors (e.g., protracted academic underachievement, increased rates of divorce, occupational instability, etc.). Behaviors that were viewed as developmentally appropriate during childhood may have become increasingly maladaptive over time (e.g., task avoidance, dependence on others to provide structure). Accordingly, when considering comorbidities in ADHD across the life span, one must consider the developmental and environmental context. Wasserstein and Stefanatos (2016) have posited that the high frequency of comorbidities, as well as their variability, may reflect structural or functional abnormalities (or disruptions) in different regions (and levels) of frontal corticostriatal pathways. This perspective builds on the work of Cummings (1993) who argued for a pivotal role of these pathways in many forms of psychopathology. While reductionist, this perspective may be worth keeping in mind. The following sections review the more common comorbidities.

ANTISOCIAL BEHAVIOR AND SUBSTANCE USE

In their 15-year prospective investigation of hyperactive children, Weiss and colleagues (1985) found that antisocial personality disorder was approximately ten times more common among young ADHD adults (23%) relative to controls (2.4%). In two independent longitudinal investigations, Mannuzza et. al. (1993, 1998), also found elevated rates of adult antisocial behavior in formerly ADHD children without comorbid conduct disorder. One study (Mannuzza et al., 1993) closely approximated the elevated (i.e., nearly ten-times higher risk profile) found by found by Weiss et al. (1985), and the second (Mannuzza et al., 1998) documented a fourfold increase in antisocial behavior relative to age-matched controls. Among adult probands, Satterfield and Schell (1997) observed a 21-fold increase in rates of felony offenses and a significantly higher rate of incarceration (12% of probands vs. 0% of controls). Murphy and Barkley (Crozier et al.,

Table 14.1 ADHD etiological models with testable predictions regarding neurocognitive training

Model	*Model description of ADHD*	*Probable Neurocognitive Intervention Targets*	*Representative publications*
Attentional Lapse Models	Models vary from DSM-5 Clinical Model (core attention deficit in ADHD) to attention deficits attributable to alternate processes/mechanisms.	One or more attention processes	Leth-Steensen, Elbaz, and Douglas (2000)
Behavioral Inhibition Model	A core deficit model wherein deficits in behavioral inhibition (stopping pre-potent/ongoing responses and interference control) result in four areas of executive dysfunction that collectively result in ADHD behavioral symptoms.	Behavioral inhibition	Barkley (1997a, 1997b)
Cognitive Neuroenergetic/ State Regulation Deficit Model	Decreased ATP production and inadequate lactate supply from deficient astrocyte functioning cause depletions in energetic resources associated with activation and effort. These depletions result in performance variability, which in turn impacts performance on executive functioning tasks. Executive functions interact with primary impairments in effort and activation via both top-down and bottom-up processes to result in the behavioral features of ADHD.	Response variability; information processing efficiency; attention; inhibition, due to association with energetic dysfunction; activation and/or effort	Russell et al. (2006, 2014); Sergeant (2005)
Default Mode Network Model	A multiple pathway model that hypothesizes that disruptions in cortico-striato-thalamo-cortical neuroanatomical circuitry—consisting of "hot" and "cool" regions—contribute to functional behavioral and cognitive differences in ADHD. Rhythmic, periodic interruption of resting state ("default mode") brain waves into task-positive networks during task engagement result in ADHD inattentive behavior.	Unclear; response variability?	Castellanos et al. (2005); Castellanos and Tannock (2002); Sonuga-Barke and Castellanos (2007)
Dynamic Developmental Model	A core deficit model that hypothesizes that reduced dopaminergic functioning causes narrower reinforcement gradients and altered extinction processes in normal behavior-consequence relationships. These deficient dual processes contribute to core ADHD symptoms and behavioral variability, which vary based on context, task, and function. Executive dysfunction, particularly disinhibition, is viewed as an outcome of these altered reinforcement and extinction processes.	Unclear; training to widen reinforcement gradients?	Sagvolden, Johansen, Aase, and Russell (2005)
Subcortical Deficit Model	A developmental model that hypothesizes that ADHD is caused by subcortical neural dysfunction that manifests early in ontogeny, remains relatively static throughout life, and is not associated with the remission of symptomatology. Executive dysfunction does not cause ADHD symptoms, but developmental growth in executive functions facilitates recovery.	Working memory manipulation. Note: Expected to benefit only patients with major allele homozygosity in two DRD1 polymorphisms; may be more beneficial later in development.	Halperin and Schulz (2006)
Tripartite Pathway Model	A multiple pathway/equifinality model in which ADHD symptoms are caused by deficits in one or more dissociable cognitive (behavioral inhibition, temporal processing) and/or motivational (delay aversion) processes.	Behavioral inhibition, temporal processing, and/or delay aversion dependent on patient's particular pattern of impairments	Sonuga-Barke et al. (2010)
Working Memory Model	A core deficit model that views inattention, hyperactivity, and impulsivity as phenotypic/behavioral expressions of the interaction between neurobiological vulnerability and environmental demands that overwhelm these children's impaired working memory. Associated features of ADHD arise through direct effects of impaired working memory, or indirect effects of impaired working memory through its impact on core behavioral symptoms.	Central executive (CE) and working memory (WM; i.e., updating, dual-task/ manipulation, serial reordering). Note: Expected to benefit ~80% of children with ADHD with CE WM deficits.	Rapport, Chung, Shore, and Isaacs (2001); Rapport et al., 2008) Rapport, Orban, Kofler, and Friedman (2013)

Reprinted from Chacko, Kofler, and Jarrett (2014).

1999) found that adults with ADHD were 17 times more likely than controls to have received a lifetime diagnosis of conduct disorder (CD), and five times more likely to have received a diagnosis of oppositional defiant disorder (ODD). Nevertheless, from a clinical perspective, in our experience as practitioners, most ADHD adults seen in outpatient practice do not share this outcome.

It is unclear how much the persistence of ADHD symptoms into adolescence or adulthood is a risk factor for substance abuse. Results of scientific studies have varied with methodological technique. A retrospective study reported alcohol abuse to be two to three times greater among ADHD adults than among controls (Shekim et al., 1990). By contrast, neither of the longitudinal studies conducted thus far has found differences in rate of alcohol abuse between probands and controls (Hechtman & Weiss, 1986; Mannuzza et al., 1993; Mannuzza, Klein, Bessler, Malloy, & LaPadula, 1998). However, studies consistently find that ADHD adults are more than twice as likely to meet criteria for tobacco dependence (Lambert & Hartsough, 1998), and two to four times as likely to have a lifetime history of non-alcohol-related substance use (Mannuzza et al., 1993; Biederman et al., 1995; Mannuzza et al., 1998). Encouraging data suggest that effective psychopharmacological treatment of ADHD may mitigate this increased risk for substance-use disorders (Wilens, Faraone, et al., 2003).

MOOD AND ANXIETY DISORDERS

In all age groups, the overlap between many symptoms of ADHD and affective disorders complicates differential diagnosis for both conditions (Marks et al., 2001). For example, unrecognized (and thus untreated) ADHD was associated with "treatment failure" in adults originally diagnosed with depression (Ratey, Greenberg, Bemporad, & Lindem, 1992). Yet empirical findings are inconsistent. Prospective investigations of ADHD have not found group differences in lifetime rates of mood disorders (Mannuzza et al., 1998; Weiss et al., 1985), while cross-sectional and retrospective studies have found higher rates of comorbidity. For example, Biederman and colleagues reported that 31% of probands versus 5% of adult controls met criteria for major depression (Biederman et al., 1993). These differences in rates of mood disorders may reflect sampling differences. That is, the longitudinal studies disproportionately included children with acting out behaviors, while the cross sectional studies disproportionately included adults seeking help because of a lifetime of struggles.

Murphy et al. (2002) found that, relative to controls, young adults with ADHD had significantly higher rates of dysthymia. Thus, as noted previously, ADHD can be both difficult to differentiate from mood disorder and/or they may coexist.

PERSONALITY DISORDERS

Enduring ADHD symptoms, and their psychosocial impact, are associated with maladaptive personality traits. Fisher and colleagues (2002) measured the prevalence of DSM-IV Axis II disorders as part of their prospective follow-up of hyperactive children. Compared to community controls, more ADHD adult probands met criteria for passive-aggressive (18%), borderline (14%), and histrionic (12%) personality disorders. Notably, however, these elevations in risk are explained mostly by the presence of child conduct problems and adolescent conduct disorder rather than ADHD per se. Addressing this confound, May and Bos (2000) compared the prevalence of Axis II personality disorders in a cohort of adults classified by the persistence of ODD or other (unspecified) comorbid diagnoses. According to these investigators, ADHD-only adults evinced mild histrionic traits, while ADHD-comorbid participants displayed predominantly avoidant and dependent characteristics. In particular, ADHD-ODD adults exhibited histrionic, narcissistic, aggressive-sadistic, and negativistic qualities, while the ADHD-ODD-comorbid group demonstrated avoidant, narcissistic, antisocial, aggressive-sadistic, negativistic, and self-defeating personality features. It may therefore be the case that comorbid psychiatric phenomena may aggregate in an additive fashion to increase the risk of maladaptive characterological features in ADHD.

From a psychodynamic perspective, Bemporad (2001. p 306) proposed that core symptoms of ADHD lead to development of "characteristic defensive operations" that are built upon neurologically based tendencies. Thus, for example, hyperactive impulsive traits may predispose to "apparent neglect of feelings or intensions of others," and both "their tendency to escape into action" and inattention enable "systematic denial . . . by diverting their attention to less threatening subjects or activities." By extension, such "characteristic defensive operations" could be argued to underlie narcissism and hysteria, respectively. While not fully developed, this approach provides interesting alternative formulations for personality disorder in ADHD. That is, some neurological tendencies due to ADHD may predispose to the development of certain personality pathologies.

LANGUAGE DISORDERS AND AUTISM

ADHD co-occurs with numerous other neurodevelopmental disorders in addition to the specific LDs (see Stefanatos & Baron, 2007). Of these, speech and language disorders are particularly common in children diagnosed with ADHD (Baker & Cantwell, 1992; Baird et al., 2000; Cohen, Vallance, et al., 2000; Bruce, Thernlund, & Nettelbladt, 2006). Some clinical samples find that 40%–64% have speech and language difficulties of sufficient magnitude to require evaluation and/or therapeutic intervention (Taylor, Sandberg, Thorley, & Giles, 1991; Humphries, Koltun, Malone, & Roberts, 1994). Since children with speech and language disorders also have higher-than-expected prevalence of ADHD (30%–58%) some regard this as a two-way comorbidity (e.g., Tannock & Brown, 2000).

A percentage of children with or without concomitant language problems demonstrate particular difficulty understanding what they hear despite normal hearing sensitivity. Problems may be particularly apparent when material is unfamiliar or if it is presented in a noisy or distracting environment, such as a classroom. If comprehension problems become apparent during school, children may be referred to an audiologist to determine if they have a hearing problem or central auditory processing disorder (CAPD; see Riccio, Hynd, Cohen, Hall, & Molt, 1994; Gomez & Condon, 1999; Breier, Gray, Klaas, Fletcher, & Foorman, 2002). CAPD is thought to arise when central neural processes underlying the analysis of auditory information by the brain are functionally compromised. The disorder encompasses deficits in one or more of the following auditory behaviors: sound localization and lateralization, auditory discrimination, auditory pattern recognition, and auditory temporal processing (e.g., resolution, integration). Although recognized for more than 50 years, there is poor agreement on when a CAPD diagnosis should be made and on its significance. The clinical presentation of CAPD includes a variety of symptoms that overlap with ADHD, including poor concentration, distractibility, fidgetiness, and poor academic achievement (Stefanatos & DeMarco, 2012). Consequently, a child diagnosed with ADHD by a physician or mental health provider may possibly have received a diagnosis of CAPD if first seen by an audiologist or speech/language pathologist. The relative presence of ADHD and/or CAPD is not clear, in part because each exists in different nosology systems. In short, ADHD and CAPD may be different conditions that are sometimes comorbid, or the same condition assessed by different disciplines.

ADHD is also very common in children with autism spectrum disorder (ASD). While DSM-IV did not permit comorbid diagnosis of ADHD and ASD, 30%–50% of children diagnosed with ASD demonstrated symptoms consistent with ADHD (Lee & Ousley, 2006; Leyfer et al., 2006; Simonoff et al., 2013; Mannion & Leader, 2014). In addition, studies have shown that as much as 20% with a diagnosis of ADHD demonstrate symptomology associated with ASD (e.g., Clark, Feehan, et al., 1999). A more recent study examining this relationship found that when mothers had a diagnosis of ADHD, their first-born offspring were at increased risk of ADHD alone (sixfold increase) or ASD alone (2.5-fold increase). Given the high rate of comorbidity and the fact that both disorders are highly heritable, it has been suggested that both disorders may share some familial transmission and including genetic risk factors (van der Meer et al., 2012) and partially overlapping diathesis (Musser et al., 2014). Both disorders are highly represented in populations of institutionalized children, perhaps pointing to a contribution of experience (Nelson, 2015). Regardless of these complex issues, the DSM-5 now recognizes that the two conditions can coexist.

GENETIC DISORDERS

ADHD is commonly diagnosed in several genetic disorders, including Klinefelter syndrome (Ross et al., 2008), Turner syndrome (Zinn et al., 2007), neurofibromatosis, tuberous sclerosis, Fragile X, and Williams syndrome (Lo-Castro, D'Agati, & Curatolo, 2011; Cederlof et al., 2014). A recent study indicated that ADHD was the most frequent disorder in children (37.10%) with chromosome 22q11.2 deletion syndrome (Schneider et al., 2014), a neurogenetic disorder that occurs in one of 2,000–4,000 live births and is commonly also referred to as *DiGeorge syndrome* or *velocardiofacial syndrome.* The neurocognitive profile in these children generally includes low average to deficient intelligence, learning difficulties, motor delay, and attention/executive problems. This syndrome has emerged as a genetic model for the development of schizophrenia, given that 23%–43% of individuals with a schizophrenia spectrum disorder demonstrate the deletion (Monks et al., 2014). However, the study of this condition also has implications for understanding the ADHD behavioral phenotype. The deletion in chromosome 22 leaves only one copy of about 60 genes, among them COMT, a gene that codes an enzyme that participates in the inactivation of catecholamines such as dopamine. Interestingly, this enzyme particularly affects dopamine metabolism in prefrontal cortex and has significant effects on executive function and working memory (Magalona et al., 2013). Individuals with 22q11.2 deletion syndrome have only a single allele (Val or Met) whereas normal individuals have two alleles (Val/Val, Met/Met, or Val/Met). The Met variant has significantly lower COMT activity, presumably resulting in slower degradation of dopamine in the synapse. Carriers of a single Val allele perform worse on measures of intelligence and executive control (Carmel et al., 2014).

MOTOR DISORDERS

Among the neurodevelopmental disorders, motor and tic disorders have among the highest rates of comorbidity with ADHD. Approximately half of children diagnosed with a tic disorder also meet criteria for ADHD (Kurlan et al., 2002). Conversely, approximately 20% of children with ADHD are also diagnosed with a tic disorder (Kadesjo & Gillberg, 2001; Robertson, 2006). Both disorders appear to be related to diminished dopaminergic function that fails to modulate amino acid-based signal transmission (primarily glutamate in GABA). This particularly affects the nigrostriatal dopamine branch, which is involved in modulating motor function and also plays a role in mediating aspects of impulse control, procedural learning, and working memory (Sagvolden et al., 2005). While these conditions appear to share some common neurobiological correlates such as reduced volume of caudate nuclei and corpus callosum (Hynd et al., 1991; Giedd et al., 1996; Plessen et al., 2006), there also appear to be neuroimaging findings that differ between these entities. For example, children who demonstrate ADHD show reduced volumes in prefrontal cortex only (Castellanos, Giedd, et al., 2001), while children with Tourette Syndrome and Tourette

Syndrome+ADHD show larger dorsal prefrontal volume (Peterson et al., 2001).

Motor problems and neurological soft signs have long been associated with ADHD. Several studies have reported that as many as 50% of children diagnosed with developmental coordination disorder (DCD) demonstrate comorbid ADHD (Gillberg, 2003; Watemberg, Waiserberg, Zuk, & Lerman-Sagie, 2007). Aside from sharing some motor symptoms, there is significant overlap in cognitive symptoms. Children with DCD have difficulties performing a variety of visuospatial processing tasks that do not have a motor component (Wilson & McKenzie, 1998), suggesting that visuospatial processing deficits are closely associated with DCD and exist independent of the contribution of motor deficits. Similar visuospatial difficulties can be observed in a subgroup of children with ADHD (Voeller & Heilman, 1988; Stefanatos & Wasserstein, 2001; Dobler et al., 2005; Kalanthroff, Naparstek, & Henik, 2013; Jung, Woo, Kang, Choi, & Kim, 2014). These findings have implicated right-hemisphere pathophysiology in ADHD and this has been supported by numerous structural (Semrud-Clikeman et al., 2000) and functional neuroimaging studies (Overmeyer et al., 2001; Courvoisie, Hooper, Fine, Kwock, & Castillo, 2004; Rubia, Halari, et al., 2009). Very few neuroimaging investigations have been conducted in children with DCD independent of a comorbid ADHD. However, a recent study examining functional connectivity in a small group of children with DCD found similar neurophysiological anomalies to those observed in children with ADHD in children with both DCD and ADHD (McLeod, Langevin, Goodyear, & Dewey, 2014). Some studies have suggested that they may share genetic etiology (Martin, Piek, & Hay, 2006).

SEIZURE DISORDERS

Children with epilepsy have increased risk of comorbid ADHD, with approximately 12%–17% receiving the diagnosis (Davies, Heyman, & Goodman, 2003; Reilly, 2011). In tertiary care centers, however, ADHD is even more common, affecting approximately one-third of preschoolers and almost two-thirds of school-aged children with epilepsy (Thome-Souza et al., 2004). Although in most cases the diagnosis of epilepsy precedes the diagnosis of ADHD, in some cases ADHD symptoms predate the onset of epilepsy. Children with epilepsy are most likely to receive a diagnosis of the predominantly inattentive subtype of ADHD, followed by the hyperactive impulsive subtype (McDermott, Mani, & Krishnaswami, 1995; Williams, Griebel, Dykman, 1998). Attentional problems have often been attributed to the seizure disorder or to its treatment. However, a history of attention problems is twice as common in children seen after their first seizure compared to controls (Austin et al., 2001; Hesdorffer et al., 2004), suggesting that a common antecedent may exist for both conditions.

LD: Presentations and Possible Underlying Deficits

Presentations of the specific LDs vary with the type of LD, stage in life, and level of remediation. Each type of LD can occur alone or in combination with other types, or with comorbidities, especially ADHD (e.g., Greven, Kovas, et al., 2014).

Delays in meeting early developmental milestones can be risk signs for future LD. Language delays are particularly noteworthy indicators for potential dyslexia (Chilosi et al., 2009; Nash et al., 2013), while difficulty with visual-motor tasks such as scribbling and puzzle assembly may indicate risk for nonverbal/spatial deficits seen in dyscalculia and/or NVLD (Rourke, 1993). By definition, school-age children with LD have difficulty learning basic skills out of proportion to their age-peers and/or intellectual endowment. For dyslexic children this may be seen in slow acquisition of letter names and/or letter sounds, look-say vocabulary, and later in spelling. For children with dyscalculia this may be seen in slow acquisition of number facts, such as automatic recall of single-digit addition or memorizing the times tables. Later, children with dyscalculia may have struggles learning/recalling math operations and/or appreciation of quantity and spatial relations. Difficulties with word problems can be seen with either dyslexia and/or dyscalculia. School-age children with LD may also show behavioral signs of underlying academic distress in the form of avoidance, withdrawal, and/or disruptive behavior. In addition, they tend to be less well liked by peers, because of frank deficits in social processing (as seen in NVLD) and/or because of linguistic processing deficits (i.e., pragmatic dysfunction), either of which make it difficult for the child to participate in reciprocal relationships. All of these problems translate into high likelihood of low self-esteem, as well as many other forms of psychological comorbidity (both internalizing and externalizing). Similar to children with ADHD, the later presumably reflects reactions to their struggles as well as to underlying structural overlap between syndromes.

Having LD can have negative impact throughout adulthood. For example, Witte, Philips, and Kakelaet al. (1998) reported that college graduates with LD reported less satisfaction with pay, promotional opportunities, and their job overall, in addition to educational impact, such as taking longer to graduate and lower college GPA. Many other studies have found that adults with LD are at increased risk for psychosocial difficulties (e.g.,Gregg, Hoy, King, Moreland, & Jagota, 1992; Hooper & Olley, 1996; Hoy & Manglitz, 1996; Vogel & Forness, 1992; Katz et al., 2001). This was the case for both those with NVLD, which is commonly associated with difficulty processing emotional information (Ahmad, Rourke, & Drummond, 2002; Cleaver & Whitman, 1998), as well as for those with other types of LD. Notably, while NVLD has been associated with pronounced psychosocial dysfunction, a more recent naturalistic study reported wide and varied outcomes (Wasserstein et al., 2008).

Anecdotally, the authors of this chapter have found that once LD children reach adulthood, many will have reached a functional level in basic academic skills. Most can learn, albeit laboriously and to varying levels of proficiency: i.e., they have "disabilities," not inabilities. Nevertheless, qualitative (e.g., slow fluency) and even quantitative (i.e., both normative and ipsative) deficits can remain. Thus, LDs in adults may be subtle and implied, rather than overt and obvious.

Dyslexia and/or Reading Disorders

Dyslexia is the prototypical form of LD and is the most common type. It usually manifests in slow and inaccurate single word recognition, despite adequate intelligence and instruction, and the absence of gross sensory or motor problems. While characterized by inordinate difficulties with accurate or fluent word decoding, spelling is commonly also affected and often to a similar degree. Different types of dyslexia have been proposed, including dysphonetic, dyseidetic, neglect, and semantic forms (i.e., phonological, visual, attentional, and comprehension basis, respectively). Hulme and Snowling (2013) provide a review of current thinking about dyslexia and its underlying cognitive deficits, which can subsume most types. Briefly, reading is argued to develop via a "triangle model" composed of interactions between orthography, phonology, and semantics. *Orthography* refers to writing systems and their codes (i.e., spelling and other rules of written language). *Phonology* refers to the fundamental elements of the linguistic system or smallest units of sound, phonemes. *Semantics* refers to meaning in whatever form. In alphabetic orthography systems, such as English, auditory phonemes are represented by visual graphemes (i.e., the smallest units in written language, or letters). In learning to decode words, a reader has to initially segment the word into its underlying auditory elements, the phonemes (i.e., units of sound), or fundamental elements of the linguistic system. In written material the phonemes have been translated into graphemes, reflecting direct connections between phonological and orthographic codes (Plaut, McClelland, Seidenberg, & Patterson, 1996). Semantic representations, the third leg of the triangle model of reading, are thought to activate a word's meaning and pronunciation, and ultimately contribute to understanding as well as to decoding in context.

Given the diversity of deficits found in the neuropsychological profiles of reading impaired patients, the implications of the triangle model of reading are compelling. Logically, disturbances in any of the three legs could lead to a reading disorder that is not necessarily based on deficits in phonetic processing. For example, visual and attention dysfunction could disrupt the orthography unit of reading skill acquisition, while receptive language disorders could disrupt the semantic leg. Notably, early classification of reading disorders separated children into those who could not read due to difficulties with word sounds (dysphonetic) and those who had difficulties with visual processing of words (dyseidetic) (see Greenblatt & Greenblatt, 1997 for discussion). Thus, dysfunction in processing of orthographic information (due to visual-perceptual, attentional, and/or nonverbal memory dysfunction) could also lead to dysfluent single-word decoding, as was originally described for dyseidetic dyslexia. Dysfunction in the semantic leg of the triangle model could lead to deficits in reading comprehension rather than word decoding. The latter would create a type of reading disability comprised of individuals who show accurate phonological decoding, but poor understanding of material that is read. Some researchers reserve the term *dyslexia* solely for individuals with phonological reading disorders. Thus poor readers who do not have phonetic processing deficits may not be regarded as having dyslexia, but may still be diagnosed with a "reading disability." Others use the terms *dyslexia* and *reading disability* interchangeably, thereby implicitly accepting a more complicated model of reading and component abilities.

Despite such ambiguity, abnormal phonetic awareness and processing has been found in the majority of studies of reading disabled children (e.g., de Gelder & Vrooman, 1996; Elbro, 1998; Katz et al., 2001; Birch & Chase, 2004), in line with the emphasis on phonology in the triangle model. Such deficits have also been found cross-culturally (e.g., Paulesu et al., 2001). For example, Birch and Chase (2004) found that adults with stronger phonological skills were better readers, while better orthographic skills did not predict better reading. There also does not appear to be a pure orthographic deficit group in adults (e.g., Osmon, Braun, & Plambeck, 2005). Consequently, a reading disorder is currently thought to usually reflect inadequate processing/representation of phonemic units, resulting in a difficulty with single word decoding in reading, writing, and spelling. To the extent that word recognition in dyslexia is slow and labored, comprehension can also be affected, although typically this is more intact. Nevertheless, multiple neuropsychological deficits have been associated with reading dysfunction; a review of these follows.

One of the first neuropsychological deficits found to be predictive of dyslexia was a weak ability to rapidly name objects, colors, letters, and/or numbers, which is referred to as rapid automatic naming (RAN). Originally developed and reported by Denckla and Rudel (1976), they characterized RAN as a "deficit in the automatization of verbal responses to visual stimuli, not restricted to symbols." Subsequently RAN was found to be one of the best predictors of later reading achievement in children with and without reading disabilities, independent of their level of phonemic awareness (e.g., Blachman, 1984; Scarbough, 1998; Manis, Seidenberg, & Doi, 1999) and dissociated from ADHD (e.g., Semrud-Clikeman, Guy, et al., 2000). The basis for this predictive ability for reading skill acquisition is not yet understood, although it has been suggested that RAN tasks assess speed of linguistic processing rather than general processing speed (Neuhaus, Foorman, Francis, & Carlson, 2001). The possibility of a double-deficit in RAN, as well as in phonological awareness, has been proposed, and is supported to some degree (Birch & Chase, 2004; Vukovic, Wilson, & Nash, 2004; Cirino, Israelian, Morris, & Morris, 2005). For example, Laasonen and collegues (Laasonen, Lehtinen, Leppämäki, Tani, & Hokkanen, 2010), in a study of Finish dyslexic adults, reported deficits in phonological awareness and phonological memory, as well as deficits in rapid naming. They also had deficits in arithmetic accuracy, showing the co-occurrence of math and reading problems often found in children with dyslexia. In any case, RAN clearly taps into a key component of fluent reading, which deserves further understanding and research.

Broader problems in auditory-verbal attention, working memory, vocabulary, spoken language comprehension, and general knowledge are also frequent in people with reading disabilities (Isaki & Plante, 1997; Katz et al., 2001; Ransby & Swanson, 2003; Birch & Chase, 2004; Braze, Tabor, Shankweiler, & Mencl, 2007). Furthermore, phonological awareness may be more important for reading acquisition than for reading comprehension, where language skills and general knowledge may make a more important contribution. For example, in the Laasonen et al. (2010) study, controlling for IQ enhanced the findings on the phonological measures, but attenuated the findings on the reading measures. The latter result suggests that brighter adults with dyslexia compensate more effectively for reading difficulties, a theme that is common in studies of LD. Thus, when their language and metalinguistic skills are stronger, those with dyslexia can compensate more effectively for underlying difficulties with phonological awareness. Similarly, Stothers and Klein (2010) found that phonological deficits, which persist in adults with reading disabilities, can affect reading speed, but not necessarily comprehension. With relevance to compensation, they also found that stronger vocabulary and nonverbal processes (i.e., Perceptual Organization Index) were associated with stronger comprehension.

Berninger et al. (2006), who studied families of children and adults with dyslexia, found a complex picture of contributing deficits in three working memory components (phonological and orthographic word-form storage), a time-sensitive phonological loop that involves naming orthographic stimuli, and executive functions (focusing and shifting attention) involving phonology. They found that phonologic, orthographic, morphologic, rapid naming and switching, verbal fluency, and inhibition acted in combination to determine reading and writing skills in adults. A second study from this group showed how impairment in executive functioning can also affect strategic coordination of the phonologic, orthographic, and morphologic demands of reading, even when the individual skills are not impaired (Amtmann, Abbott, & Berninger, 2007). The inability of individuals with LDs to apply skills strategically is echoed by the dysexecutive type of LD discussed by Wasserstein and Denckla (2009). These studies illustrate how broad assessment of spoken language, attention, executive functions, and general knowledge are all-important when evaluating reading problems.

Some dyslexic individuals have weaknesses in visual perceptual skills (Graves, Frerichs, & Cook, 1999; Iles, Walsh, Richardson, 2000; Ben-Yehudah, Sackett, Malchi-Ginzberg, & Ahissar, 2001; Mano & Osmon, 2008) and orthographic skills (Osmon et al., 2005), and have visual hemi-attention (Gabay et al., 2013). Nevertheless, studies have not found clear evidence that deficits in visual skills are causal in reading disorder (Vellutino, Fletcher, Snowling, & Scanlon, 2004), or that remediation of visual skills improves reading (Handler et al., 2011). Nevertheless, Stothers and Klein (2010) found that stronger visuospatial skills are associated with better reading comprehension. Similarly, Bacon and Handley (2010), using a reasoning measure that required transitive inference, found that college students with dyslexia were more likely than controls to use a visual rather than an abstract verbal strategy. Unlike subjects without dyslexia, they also did not show interference from visual information and visual memory predicted reasoning accuracy. Bacon and Handley (2010) concluded that rather than cause dyslexia, visual processes could help offset weaknesses in phonological awareness and verbal memory.

More recently, Swanson (2012) attempted to parse out the relative contributions of various neuropsyhcological functions through a meta-analysis of 52 studies. His overall sample consisted of 1,793 adults with reading disabilities and 1,893 adults without reading disabilities. They ranged in age from 18 to 44, and 55% were male. The overall effect size on all measures was 0.72, most with nonreading impaired adults performing better. As expected, for the reading-impaired group, effect sizes were largest for word attack, reading recognition, reading comprehension, and spelling. Effect sizes also were large for writing and math, reflecting the frequent co-occurrence of written expression and math disabilities with reading disabilities. Regarding the component skills needed for reading, effect sizes were largest for phonological processing, processing speed (including rapid naming), vocabulary, verbal intelligence, general information, and verbal memory. Unlike the studies by Berninger and colleagues, effect sizes for executive functioning skills (problem solving and reasoning, cognitive monitoring) were small. The effect size for social and personal skills also was small, as was the effect size for overall intelligence. Interestingly, effect sizes for perceptual motor skills and visuospatial memory were moderate and favored adults with reading disabilities. This intriguing finding again suggests strength in visual memory can be used to compensate. It is not clear why the small effect size for auditory-perceptual skills favored the adults with reading disabilities, but most likely reflects basic auditory-perceptual skills separate from phonological awareness.

These observations likely apply to children as well, although replication is needed.

Dyscalculia and/or Math Disorders

Developmental dyscalculia (DD) is a specific LD affecting mathematical skills and numerical competence that is found in children and adults with normal intelligence and without acquired neurological injuries (American Psychiatric Association, 1987). People with DD have mixed combinations of problems in mathematics, including difficulty with learning and retrieving number facts (e.g., times tables), executing calculation procedures/operations (e.g., long division, adding mixed numbers), understanding mathematical concepts (e.g., fractions, percents, or negative numbers) (Geary & Hoard, 2001), and developing problem-solving strategies (Shalev & Gross-Tsur, 2001). They also have long solution times and high error rates (Geary, 1993), presumably due to all of the previously listed challenges.

The prevalence of DD across countries is relatively uniform, with estimates of 3%–7% (range 1.3% –10.3%) in the normal population, similar to that of dyslexia and ADHD (Kucian et al., 2006). Girls and boys seem to be affected equally (Devine, Soltesz, Nobes, Goswami, & Szucs, 2013), and like other LDs, DD has a significant familial aggregation, suggesting a role for genetics (Alarcon, Pennington, et al., 2000). While DD may in some cases occur as a stand-alone LD (Rourke, 1993), it is frequently (but not always) present in association with other learning impediments, especially a reading/spelling disability or ADHD (Gross-Tsur, Manor, & Shalev, 1996; Shalev & Gross-Tsur, 2001).

Early references to DD were by Henschen (1920); Berger (1926); and Gerstmann (1940). Later, Kinsbourne and Warrington (1963) noted that dyscalculia existed in children without acquired brain damage, but Cohn (1968) was the first to employ the term *developmental dyscalculia.* Regarding the neural basis of arithmetic skills and disorders, Henschen (1920) wrote, "the calculation ability is a highly composite cerebral function that results from the collaboration of various posterior areas of the left hemisphere." Twenty years later, Gerstmann (1940) described the Gerstmann syndrome, which consists of dyscalculia, finger agnosia, left-right confusion and dysgraphia, and was attributed to damage to the left angular gyrus region. Around that same time, Luria (1946) noted that dyscalculia was common in diffuse high cortical impairment. However, after years of additional study of brain-damaged individuals, he later subdivided dyscalculia into three types: spatial, verbal, and operational, reflecting at least three corresponding regions of brain dysfunction (i.e., posterior right hemisphere, posterior left hemisphere, and frontal, respectively; see Luria, 1966). Over the years there have been other attempts to classify the neurocognitive abnormalities that underlie dyscalculia, in addition to the three-system typology of Luria. Kosc (1974) distinguished six types: verbal, apractognostic, lexical, graphic, ideognostic, and operational. Later Rourke (1993) proposed two types, either due to visuospatial or verbal/auditory perceptual dysfunction.

The education literature noted that mathematics is particularly complex, involving language and other symbols, understanding of space and quantity, and recall and use of operations. An important conceptual distinction was made between "primary dyscalculia," where the deficit reflects abnormality in underlying numerical cognition (i.e., domain specific), as well as cases wherein the dyscalculia is "secondary" to other more general cognitive impairments, such as deficits in memory, attention or visual-perceptual and spatial understanding (i.e., domain-general impairments) (Rosenberger, 1989; Henik, Rubinsten, & Ashkenazi, 2011). Domain general research has examined the association of DD/dyscalculia with other nonnumeric deficits, such as poor working memory (Luculano, Moro, et al., 2011; Geary, 1993; David, 2012), inattention (Ashkenazi & Henik, 2012), disorders of visual-spatial functioning (Venneri et al., 2003), impaired memory retrieval, and executive function deficits (Szucs et al., 2013). Domain-specific research has examined abilities more specifically related to numerical understanding and abilities.

Overall, the weight of evidence has revealed involvement of combinations of general cognitive capacities (i.e., domain general). For example, in two studies of college students referred for assessment of LDs, Cirino, Morris, and Morris (2002, 2007) found that written calculation and math problem-solving skills were predicted by retrieval of semantic knowledge, executive functioning, and visuospatial skills. Osmon and colleagues (Osmon, Smerz, et. al., 2006), using academic and cognitive measures from the Woodcock-Johnson tests and standard neuropsychological tests, also found that college students with DD showed impairment in visuospatial skills and executive functioning. Those who were impaired in both areas (i.e., double deficit) had the most impaired skills. More recently, and also using the Woodcock-Johnson tests in DD college students, Proctor (2012) found that the Math Calculation score was predicted by the Processing Speed and Working Memory scores, and the Math Reasoning score was predicted by the Comprehension-Knowledge, Fluid Reasoning, and Working Memory scores. This, too, showed the importance of attention, working memory, processing speed, and reasoning and acquired knowledge for math skills.

Another strand of education research has focused on more domain-specific abilities, such as the role of lower-level "building blocks of numerical cognition" (Ansari & Karmiloff-Smith, 2002) or "foundational numerical capacities" (Butterworth, 2010), which may underlie DD. *Numerical cognition* is one of such domain-specific ability categories, which include subitizing and counting, comparative judgments and distance effect, and automaticity of numerical processing (see Henik, Rubinsten, et al., 2011, for review). Subitizing refers to the number of objects the mind can simultaneously process without counting and averages around four to five in adults (e.g., immediate recognition of dice). A number of studies have reported slower processing speed and smaller subitizing ranges among those with DD (e.g., (Landerl, Bevan, & Butterworth, 2004). For example, Koontz and Berch (1996) asked DD children to decide whether two stimuli (using mixtures of dots and/or digits) were the same or not, and found slower times. Such findings are not universal among those with DD. For example, Desoete and Gregoire (2007) found that only 33% of school-aged DD children had subitizing deficits. *Comparative judgment* refers to tasks wherein subjects are asked to decide which of two numbers is larger, and is thought to utilize an internalized number line. Most variations on this approach have found that DD children show a "distance effect." That is, it takes them longer than controls to decide relative differences between two numbers, which is thought to reflect less well-differentiated representations of numbers on their mental number line (see Henik, Rubinsten, et al., 2011, for review)

There are a number of other proposed domain specific abilities that may be compromised in DD. Children with DD also show deficits in their *automaticity of numerical processing*, which refers to the rapid subjective understanding of the numerical symbol system, e.g., the meaning of digits. Multiple group studies, using various procedures, have found automaticity deficits in both children and adults with DD (see Henik, Rubinsten et al., 2011, for review). This is thought to reflect a deficiency in the association of symbols with quantities and sizes.

According to recent conceptualizations, elementary numerical processing is dependent upon fundamental numerical systems. A Small Number System mediates the exact representations for numbers under 4, while larger numbers require an Approximate Number System (ANS) that enables children to develop representations and make comparisons approximate magnitudes/amounts of objects, events, and time (Dehaene, Molko, Cohen, & Wilson, 2004; Feigenson, Dehaene, & Spelke, 2004). Some research has found correlation between ANS deficits and mathematical ability in DD children (Piazza, Facoetti, et al., 2010). However, Butterworth (2010) has argued that a deficit in numerosity coding (i.e., capacity to quantify sets and operations upon them), rather than the ANS, was central to DD.

A number of studies have suggested that numerical sense deficits and weakness in particular domain-general abilities may combine in particular constellations to impede mathematical skill development (Fuchs, Geary, et al., 2010). For example, problems in basic aspects of number sense representation were found to exist in combination with deficits in working memory and visual spatial processing (Geary, Hoard, Nugent, & Bailey, 2012). Another research group (Rubinstein & Henik, 2005) examined both domain general (i.e., attention) and domain specific numerical processing in DD college students. First, using a Stroop task in which digits of differing numerical value were presented in different physical sizes, Rubinstein and Henik found a smaller interference effect in the DD students. They interpreted this finding as showing a lack of automaticity in activation of numerical value, both thought to be domain-specific skills. In a second study they found that DD students had difficulty recruiting attention to numerical information (Ashkenazi, Rubinsten, & Henik, 2009), thereby replicating and extending their intial study. In a third study, using a Posner-type task, they found broader deficits in the alertness and executive functioning networks in DD college students (Ashkenazi & Henik, 2010a). Finally, they found that attention training improved attention in college students with DD, but had no effect on numerical processing (Ashkenazi & Henik, 2012). Examining attention in a different way, Ashkenazi and Henik (2010b) administered standard line and number line bisection tasks to college students with DD. Those with DD did not show the usual leftward bias on the line bisection task, but showed a more pronounced leftward bias on the number bisection task, implying that they had an internal logarithmic representation of numerical value that is more typical of younger children. Performance on the two tasks was unrelated. These studies showed deficits in both attention and numerical processing, reflecting underlying dysfunctions in both domain general and domain specific skills. Consequently, these authors argued that DD is a heterogeneous disorder with both domain general and domain specific determinants.

A final consideration is the role of anxiety in math dysfunction (Katz, Goldstein, et al., 2001), as it can either worsen and/or even simulate DD. Although early difficulties in math may dissipate over time, adults may remain highly anxious and thus dysfunctional when attempting computations. For example, Buelow and Frakey (2013) found that math anxiety affected performance on the Arithmetic subtest of the Wechsler Adult Intelligence Scale-Fourth Edition but did not affect performance on other Working Memory subtests that did not require arithmetic.

Dysgraphia

Dysgraphia denotes a failure in the normal development of writing skills despite adequate intelligence, motivation, and instruction (Gubbay & Deklerk, 1995). Writing is a complex task requiring the mastery and integration of a number of subskills, including fine motor control, visual and tactile perception, language, memory, and executive functioning. The term itself is derived from conjoining the Greek words *dys* meaning "impaired" with *graphia* meaning "making letterforms by hand" (De Ajuriaguerra et al., 1979). Some children or adults have difficulties in one aspect of the process, such as producing legible handwriting or spelling, whereas others have difficulty organizing and sequencing their ideas. Difficulties in one area can delay skill development in the other areas. Some regard dysgraphia to include problems with spelling and other writing mechanics (such as punctuation and grammar), while others maintain the more narrow view that regards the disorder as an abnormality of complex motor skill or handwriting (Berninger & May, 2011). Thus the scope and limits of this disorder are not well-defined and there is considerable confusion regarding what is being described with this diagnosis.

Due to the extreme differences in definition, and the lack of a "gold standard" measurement instrument, prevalence estimates vary greatly, ranging from 5% to 27% of school-aged children (van Hartingsveldt, de Groot, Aarts, & Nijhuis-van der Sanden, 2011). Future studies will be further complicated by the trend to deemphasize handwriting in favor of keyboarding skills. As a consequence, increasing numbers of students are not receiving formal instruction in cursive handwriting, despite its continuing importance in many academic endeavors (Christensen, 2009). Handwriting difficulties usually manifest during early schooling. By contrast, problems with spelling and other writing mechanics, and/or with composition, become more apparent during middle school. Absent intervention, both can persist throughout life.

Similar to the other academic skills, handwriting is a complex task that engages a variety of cognitive processes including attention, memory, proprioception, and linguistic processing (Graham & Weintraub, 1996; Bara & Gentaz, 2011), as well as the more obvious fine-motor skills. It requires access to both mental representations of letters and words, as well as access to the motor programs for executing selected letters and letter sequences. In addition, execution must be constrained by the spatial arrangement of the page. Letter shape, size, spacing, sequencing, slant, direction, trajectory, and allographic considerations must all be taken into account, while implementing the motor program, which must be accomplished with the potential for online correction in order to maintain consistency with previously written letters. Thus, the task also engages multiple executive processes (Graham, Struck, Santoro, & Berninger, 2006).

Problems with written expression denote difficulties with writing, writing mechanics (like spelling and/or grammer and punctuation), and/or with execution of text (like organization, initiation, and completion). Given the broad clinical profile, it is no surprize that dysgraphia is often seen with other neurodevelopmental disorders. Poor writing mechanics, especially spelling, are among the more common comorbid problems of dyslexia. For example, Connelly, Campbell, MacLean, and Barnes (2006) found that college students with dyslexia wrote poorer-quality essays, with the best predictors of essay quality being handwriting speed and spelling errors, similar to conclusions drawn by Peverly (2006) in a review. Dyslexic college students also made more spelling errors in their essays than expected based on a separate spelling test, suggesting that the dual demands for spelling and writing may have overloaded their processing systems. Berninger, Nielsen, Abbott, Wijsman and Raskind (2008), in their family study of dyslexia, found that male adults with dyslexia were more impaired in handwriting, spelling, orthographic, and composing skills than female adults with dyslexia. They also reported that the males were more impaired in reading rate and accuracy. They concluded that reading and writing difficulties were confounded by gender differences, and that over time, men with dyslexia may fall behind women with dyslexia in the development of their writing skills. Finally, while spelling dysgraphia is most frequently associated with dyslexia, clinically we have found that poor handwriting and/or poor composition are often seen in the context of ADHD. Nevertheless, dysgraphia can also exist alone.

Nonverbal Learning Disability

First described in the latter half of the 20th century by Johnson and Myklebust (1967), NVLD is one of the most recently recognized forms of LD. Originally it was described as a social learning disorder that grew out of poor "reading" of nonverbal social and emotional cues (due to poor spatial and perceptual processing). Only later did Johnson and Myklebust (1971) report that this social LD often, but not always, was associated with dyscalculia. Myklebust eventually coined the term "nonverbal learning disabilities" and attributed it to dysfunction of the right cerebral hemisphere (1975). Rourke, through studying neuropsychological deficits in dyslexic and dyscalculic children, subsequently popularized awareness of this LD and more tightly intertwined dyscalculia and social processing LD, along with deficits in visuospatial skills, motor skills, and complex problem solving (e.g., Rourke, Young, Strang, & Russell, 1986; Tsatsanis & Rourke, 2008). Similar to Myklebust, he attributed this deficit profile to right-hemisphere dysfunction, but primarily of white matter. The suggestion of almost universal co-occurrance between dyscalculia and NVLD may be an overgeneralization from the LD samples Rourke originally studied, which consisted of children with either dyslexia, dyscalculia, or both. Different comorbidity patterns were seen in a retrospective chart review study by two coauthors of this chapter and other colleagues (Wasserstein et al., 2008). Consistent with Rourke's model, most of these people had deficits in visuospatial-constructional skills, visual memory, and fine motor skills. As expected, 80% also reported impairment in social functioning. However, while 50% had (or reported) math disorder, another 50% showed (or reported) reading disability, with and without dyscalculia. Interestingly, 85% showed inattention and executive dysfunction, and were diagnosed with ADHD. Thus, NVLD often occurred with reading disorder, was not universally associated with dyscalculia, and was most commonly associated with executive dysfunction and/or ADHD.

Not surprisingly, there is controversy over whether NVLD is a specific LD separate from other disorders, such as math disabilities, ADHD, developmental coordination disorders, and ASDs (Pennington, 2008). Fletcher, Lyon, Fuchs, and Barnes (2007) do not include NVLD in their model of specific LDs, because there is not always impact on a specific academic skill. More damaging to the concept is Spreen's

(2011) critical review of the extant research on NVLD. He made the following arguments:

- NVLD has been accepted as a viable diagnosis without sufficient support.
- Studies of NVLD have not sufficiently researched and demonstrated reliability and validity of the diagnosis.
- The characteristics of subjects defined as having NVLD vary from study to study.
- NVLD occurs rarely, despite unsupported prevalence estimates of 10%–29%.
- Support for associated socioemotional disorders has been mixed.
- Unlike dyslexia, for which there is neuroimaging support, there is no neuroimaging support showing that NVLD is due to white matter dysfunction or focal right hemisphere dysfunction, as hypothesized.
- The NVLD profile is not found universally in childhood disorders with which it has been proposed to be associated.

In summarizing the literature, Spreen (2011) concluded that:

> The concept of NVLD has been discussed and investigated for more than 30 years. Yet, no firm data are available on the frequency of occurrence of NLD, its socioemotional features, or its hypothetical neurological basis. At this point, it must be concluded that NVLD remains a hypothesis, but that it should not be used in clinical practice unless it is supported by solid research findings.
>
> (p. 435)

Thus while each of the specific LDs appear to be multifaceted and likely represent a number of subtypes, NVLD may be the most so. Until there is more definitive research, the NVLD category has to be considered tentative and evolving. With appropriate caveats, however, it can be helpful in conceptualization of some neuropsychological profiles, and as an explanatory vehicle for both patient/parent.

Neuroscience of ADHD and LD

Neurobiological theories of ADHD and LD have been developed in addition to the clinical and psychological descriptions reviewed previously. Such theories were originally based on similarities between problems resulting from various forms of acquired brain damage and the problems seen in children with either disorder. However, neurobiological theories were historically met with skepticism, which persists in some circles to this day (e.g., Timimi & Taylor, 2004; Visser & Jehan, 2009). Advances in genetics, and structural and functional neuroimaging, have provided unprecedented perspectives on the neural correlates of ADHD and LD. For example, structural magnetic resonance imaging (MRI) can differentiate, in exquisite anatomic detail, the spatial location, extent, and boundaries of different forms of tissue (gray matter, white matter), enabling quantification of the physical characteristics of various brain structures such as the volume, thickness, or surface area. This capacity has allowed investigators to examine rates and patterns of growth of various brain structures in individuals with ADHD or LD, and compare them to typically developing individuals. In addition, functional neuroimaging and electrophysiological methods, such as quantitative EEG and event-related potentials (ERP), have provided useful methods to evaluate the functional implications of structural differences.

There is more research regarding the genetics of ADHD versus LD, and the following reviews are weighted accordingly. There is also more research with children than with adults, and some findings likely change with development. Where possible such distinctions are made. Finally, disorders of reading represent the LD for which there is the most research and are consequently the emphasis of the LD section. Dyscalculia, dysgraphia, and NVLD are considered but not as extensively discussed.

Neurobiology of ADHD

Genetics of ADHD

ADHD is strongly familial, with higher rates reported in siblings of ADHD probands (20.8% vs. 5.6% in controls) (Biederman et al., 1992), first-degree family members of ADHD males (Lombroso, Pauls, & Leckman, 1994) and females (Faraone et al., 1991; Faraone et al., 1995), second-degree relatives (Faraone et al., 1994), and biological parents (18% ADHD in biological vs. 6% in adoptive parents) (Sprich, Biederman, Crawford, Mundy, & Faraone, 2000). In a recent study of adopted children and their adoptive and biologically related mothers, the biological mothers' ADHD symptoms significantly predicted the child's ADHD symptoms at age 6 (Harold et al., 2013), further supporting the existence of shared genes responsible for the increased familial aggregation. There are a number of different approaches to researching the genetics of any condition including studies of heritability, candidate genes, genome-wide association studies, epigenetic modulators, and animal models.

HERITABILITY STUDIES

Twin studies attempt to distinguish genetic and environmental risk factors by comparing phenotypes of monozygotic (100% genetically identical) and dizygotic (sharing about 50% of genes) twins. These have reported heritability rates in the 70% range in childhood ADHD (Nikolas & Burt, 2010) for both severe and subthreshold levels (Larsson, Anckarsater, Rastam, Chang, & Lichtenstein, 2012). Lower heritability estimates, in the range of 30%–40%, have been reported in ADHD adults (Posthuma & Polderman, 2013).

Data from the few ongoing longitudinal studies provide greater understanding of heritability estimates across the life span. Results from the Twins Early Development Study in the United Kingdom suggest that some of the same genes may confer risk for hyperactive-impulsive symptoms, while a different set of genes may confer risk for the inattentive symptoms (McLoughlin, Rijsdijk, Asherson, & Kuntsi, 2011). Similarly, a Swedish longitudinal study of ADHD twin pairs, followed from childhood to adolescence, noted a decrease in hyperactivity-impulsivity and increase in inattentive symptoms across development, with both trajectories being highly heritable (Larsson, Dilshad, Lichtenstein, & Barker, 2011). In this sample attention problems were investigated from childhood to young adulthood using multiple informants rather than just self-report. Results showed that the genetic effects operating at ages 8–9 continued to explain 41%, 34%, and 24% of the total variance at ages 13–14, 16–17 and 19–20 years, respectively. Rater variance was considered to be playing a role in another longitudinal study, the Netherland Twin Registry, where heritability of ADHD was estimated to be 70%–74% during childhood based on maternal ratings, followed by lower estimates (i.e., 51%–56% in adolescence and 40%–54% in adulthood) based on self-ratings (Kan et al., 2013). Importantly, new sets of genetic risk factors have been noted to emerge in adolescence and young adulthood (Chang, Lichtenstein, Asherson, & Larsson, 2013), suggesting that different genes may be relevant at different developmental stages. For example, in adolescence there is accelerated development of dorsolateral prefrontal and temporal brain regions, areas with the highest DRD4 expression. Thus this gene may confer greater risk during this time period (Meador-Woodruff et al., 1996). Epigenetics may also be contributing as seen by decreased DAT mRNA expression reported with age (Bannon & Whitty, 1997).

CANDIDATE GENE STUDIES

The high heritability reported in the twin studies prompted the search for genes involved in neurotransmission. The initial approach had been to focus on genetic variation within *prespecified genes* (i.e., candidates) and phenotypes or diseases. This approach assumed that variations in these candidate genes, which were involved in neurotransmission, would occur at greater frequencies in individuals with ADHD versus those without ADHD. Observed differences would lead to the identification of the common genes conferring a higher level of risk for the disorder. Numerous studies were performed, but the predicted variants were not consistently found in most ADHD subjects and also occurred at high frequencies in controls. As reviewed by Chiyoko and colleagues (Akutagava-Martins, Salatino-Oliveira, Kieling, Rohde, & Hutz, 2013) and Gizer and colleagues (Gizer, Ficks, & Waldman, 2009), the strongest support emerged for gene variants in dopaminergic genes (e.g., DAT1(SLC6A3), DRD4, DRD5, DBH, DDC), noradrenergic (NET1(SLC6A2), ADRA2A, ADRA2c), serotonergic (5-HTT(SLC6A4), HTR1B, HTR2A, TPH2) and others (SNAP-25, CHRNA4, NMDA, BDNF, NGF). However, in humans, variations in these genes were found to confer minimal risk (Gizer et al., 2009).

Numerous methodological issues further confounded candidate gene studies, including sample size and complex phenotypes derived from various age ranges. An example is the seven-repeat (7R) allele of DRD4, one of ADHD candidate genes thought to confer decreasing sensitivity to dopamine (Asghari et al., 1995, Schoots & Van Tol, 2003). A longitudinal study of ADHD subjects and their nonaffected siblings (from childhood through adolescence) (Altink et al., 2012) indicated that the proposed effect may differ across the developmental trajectory. In this study, non-ADHD adolescents who were DRD4 7R carriers performed worse than noncarriers on neurocognitive function. However, the effect was not observed in the younger children, suggesting there was varying brain susceptibility during the different developmental stages. Such developmental differences may reflect increased sensitivity in the adolescent brain due to global changes that occur during this period, such as decrease in gray matter and increase in white matter density (Krain & Castellanos, 2006), shifts in cortical thickness (Polderman et al., 2007) and, as noted previously, accelerated development of dorsolateral prefrontal and temporal brain regions (i.e., areas with the highest DRD4 expression; see Meador-Woodruff et al., 1996). Increased vulnerability during adolescence may also be conferred by the decreasing dopamine receptor density (Thompson, Pogue-Geile, & Grace, 2004), rendering carriers of DRD4 7R, known to produce fewer or less responsive D4 receptors to dopamine stimulation (Asghari et al., 1995), even more vulnerable. By contrast, the state of brain development in younger children may render them less vulnerable to DRD4 variants.

Despite such considerations, data from current genetic studies have not usually taken into account developmental stages, making it difficult to associate the phenotypic data with genetic data. Developmental variations in gene expression may also be especially important in ongoing discussions about the possibility of later onset ADHD.

GENOME-WIDE ASSOCIATION STUDIES

Advances in bioinformatics (i.e., an interdisciplinary field that develops methods and software for understanding biological date) and genotyping technology (i.e., determining the genetic make-up of an individual) allow extensive exploration across the whole genome. Unlike the candidate gene method, these methods provided the opportunity to discover variants not otherwise considered since genes were not chosen with any a priori hypothesis. At this time no "common variant" has been identified (Neale et al., 2010; Hinney et al., 2011; Williams et al. 2012; Yang et al., 2013). This refers to a similar genetic variation that confers risk in many individuals (Casals & Bertranpetit, 2012). However the technology has led to the discovery of "structural variants" in ADHD cohorts. What are structural genetic variants? Human DNA consists of more than 3 billion base pairs, which are not always arranged in the same order. In contrast to single nucleotide variations (referred to as single-nucleotide polymorphisms, or SNPs), more than 13% of the DNA consists of large sections (ranging from 1,000 to 1 million nucleotides) that are repeated (once or a number of times) or that may be deleted (Stankiewicz & Lupski, 2010). These are called *structural variations,* and are thought to play a significant role in: (a) phenotypic variability (i.e., by changing gene dosage), (b) complex behavioral characteristics such as those seen in ADHD, as well as in (c) disease susceptibility (Zhang, Gu, Hurles, & Lupski, 2009).

Inherited rare structural variations conferring risk in ADHD were fairly recently reported by Elia and colleagues (Elia et al., 2010), discovered in genes known to be important in learning, behavior, and synaptic transmission. Additional inherited and de novo variants have been reported by other groups (Williams et al., 2010; Lesch et al., 2011; Lionel et al., 2011; Elia, Glessner, et al., 2012; Stergiakouli et al., 2012; Williams et al., 2012; Jacob et al., 2013; Yang et al., 2013). Rare variants, by definition, are identified in only a few individuals and therefore are not usually replicable. However, as would be expected, different rare variants impacting on similar genes in ADHD samples are now also being reported, seen for example, in the BCHE gene (Elia et al., 2010; Lesch et al., 2011; Lionel et al., 2011; Jacob et al., 2013), which is expressed in cholinergic neurons and is involved in regulating vigilance (Darvesh, Hopkins, & Geula, 2003). Genetic variants associated with conferring risk for ADHD have also been reported in other neuropsychiatric disorders such as autism (Lionel et al., 2011). This suggests that rare variants may be symptom- and not syndrome-specific and associated with numerous comorbid syndromes.

EPIGENETICS

While gene sequence remains the same throughout life, the regulation of gene activity and gene expression can be changed by a number of nongenetic factors, referred to as *epigenetics*. Animal studies have led research in this area, implicating factors influencing prenatal development, such as malnutrition, maternal stress, infection, and toxicity, in altered brain function and behavior in the offspring. For example, dopaminergic and serotonergic deficiencies were reported in young adult rats that were prenatally exposed to bacterial lipopolysaccharide (Wang, Yan, Lo, Carvey, & Ling, 2009). Other examples include the following: low-dose prenatal and neonatal bisphenol exposure resulted in deficits in development of synaptic plasticity in rat dorsal striatum (Zhou, Zhang, Zhu, Chen, & Sokabe, 2009), and size and distribution of midbrain dopaminergic populations were permanently altered by perinatal glucocorticoid exposure in a sex-region and time-specific manner (McArthur, McHale, & Gillies, 2007). Hyperactivity and alteration of the midbrain dopaminergic system were reported in maternally stressed male mice offspring (Son et al., 2007).

Reviews of human studies (Archer, Oscar-Berman, & Blum, 2011; Elia, Laracy, Allen, Nissley-Tsiopinis, & Borgmann-Winter, 2012; Latimer et al., 2012; Thapar, Cooper, Eyre, & Langley, 2013) also indicate a number of suspected prenatal, perinatal, and postnatal potential risk factors for ADHD, such as prematurity, maternal smoking, family adversity, and exposure to toxins and low birth weight. For example, low birth weight has consistently been associated with ADHD (Szatmari, Saigal, Rosenbaum, Campbell, & King, 1990; Breslau & Chilcoat, 2000). Further supporting its role is the lower birth weight associated with ADHD in monozygotic birth weight-discordant twin pairs (Sharp et al., 2003; Asbury, Dunn, & Plomin, 2006; Lehn et al., 2007) where the lighter twin from both the monozygotic and dizygotic birth weight–discordant twins also showed higher ADHD ratings (Hultman et al., 2007). Elucidating the impact of such risk factors in humans is complicated since it's often difficult to separate confounding factors. For example, the role of prenatal nicotine and alcohol exposure in ADHD is less clear than that of low birth weight since exposure to these substances also increases risk for low birth weight (Mick, Biederman, Prince, Fischer, & Faraone, 2002). Studies in larger cohorts that allow data analyses in subgroups are providing further clarification. For example, genetic variations within latrophilin (LPHN3), a gene that codes for G-protein coupled receptors that are involved in the regulation of neurotransmitter transmission (Silva, Suckling, & Ushkaryov, 2009) and neurodegeneration following hypoxia (Bin Sun, Ruan, Xu, & Yokota, 2002) have been reported to be associated with ADHD in several independent studies. Further investigation indicates that this association appears primarily in the subgroup of mothers exposed to minimal but not significant stress during pregnancy, regardless of whether they smoked (Choudhry et al., 2012). Studies are also showing that some of the well-known mechanisms implicated in increasing or decreasing gene expression (i.e., DNA methylation, (Robertson, 2005), histone modifications (Berger, 2007), transcription factors (Latchman, 1997), miRNAs (Pasquinelli, 2012) may be playing a role in ADHD.

The 3 billion base pairs of the human genome are formed by adenine-thymine (ApT) and cytosine-guanine (CpG) nucleotides bound by a phosphate. Methylation of cytosine (mCpG) occurs in about 2%–6% of the CpG dinucleotide pairs and usually results in transcriptional repression or silencing (Robertson, 2005). Differences have also been reported in human brain where methylation in non-CpG nucleotides (G is replaced by A, C, or T) accounts for 53% versus 47% CpG in neurons (Lister et al., 2013) and these forms are also thought to inhibit transcription (Varley et al., 2013). Cortical neuronal methylation increases during the first two years after birth and continues up to adolescence (Lister et al., 2013), overlapping the same time frame for synaptogenesis and synaptic pruning (Huttenlocher &

Dabholkar, 1997) rendering this time frame particularly vulnerable to environmental factors that could confer risk for ADHD. Methylation differences between monozygotic and dizygotic twins on several genes implicated in ADHD (i.e., DRD4, SLC6A/SERT, MAOA) have already been reported (Wong et al., 2010). Also, lower DNA methylation of several genes, including DRD4, derived from cord-blood leucocytes at birth was associated with higher ADHD symptoms during early childhood (van Mil et al., 2014).

Inside the nucleus, DNA is coiled around histone proteins that when condensed prevent transcription. DNA can open to an active state by various mechanisms including methylation, acetylation, phosphorylation, ubiquitylation, and sumoylation (Berger, 2007). The transcription of DNA to RNA is mediated by regulatory proteins called *transcription factors* that bind to specific regions of the DNA and stimulate or inhibit transcription (Karin, 1990). Several transcription factors, including sp1 have been reported to mediate hormone-dependent gene activation for DAT, known to play a role in ADHD (Shumay, Fowler, & Volkow, 2010). More recently, a group of small molecules (20–22 nucleotides) referred to as *miRNAs* (micro RNAs) have been identified that suppress the translation process, or effect mRNA degradation. These control the activity of about 50% of protein-encoding genes, indicating a potentially significant role in neuropsychiatric disorders (Tardito, Mallei, & Popoli, 2013). Sequence variants at a miRNA affecting serotonin receptor genes have been associated with ADHD in adulthood (Sanchez-Mora et al., 2013).

Most epigenetic changes are limited to an individual over the course of an individual's lifetime. However epigenetic changes that cause DNA mutations in progeny cells are inherited from one generation to the next (Chandler, 2007) adding another layer of complexity in deciphering the underlying genetic and epigenetic factors in ADHD. Taken together, any environmental processes which disrupt DNA expression in somatic (Wong et al., 2010; van Mil et al., 2014; Shumay et al., 2010) or germ-lines (Chandler, 2007) could precipitate or worsen the clinical picture, for either the individual and/or his or her progeny.

Neural Correlates of ADHD

THE FRONTO-STRIATAL SYSTEM

Guided by models derived from clinical neuropsychological studies of the effects of frontal lobe lesions (Mattes, 1980), as well as preliminary functional neuroimaging findings (Lou, Hendrickson, et al., 1989), early structural neuroimaging studies found reduced volume in fronto-striatal brain structures of ADHD probands compared to age-matched controls, specifically the caudate and globus pallidus. Some studies reported that this effect was greater in the left hemisphere (Hynd et al., 1993; Aylward et al., 1996; Filipek et al., 1997) while others described larger reductions in the right (Castellanos et al., 1994; Castellanos et al., 1996; Casey et al., 1997). Supplementing their findings with functional neuroimaging, Casey et al. (1997) noted that diminished volumes in the right caudate nucleus and inferior frontal cortex were correlated with poorer task performance on measures of response inhibition, and suggested that deficiencies in right fronto-striatal circuitry may be particularly related to poor inhibitory controls in ADHD.

With some exceptions (Hill et al., 2003), subsequent studies have generally confirmed volume reductions in striatal structures in ADHD individuals. However, the findings have been inconsistent regarding which basal ganglia structures are affected and whether the diminished volume is apparent predominantly in the right or left hemisphere, or both (Mataro et al., 1997; Garrett et al., 2008; Nakao, Radua, Rubia, & Mataix-Cols, 2011; Proal et al., 2011; Seidman et al., 2011; Onnink et al., 2014; Semrud-Clikeman, Pliszka, Bledsoe, & Lancaster, 2014). Studies using a *regions of interest* (ROI) approach, have most consistently implicated the caudate, although diminished volume of globus pallidus (Aylward et al., 1996; Castellanos et al., 1996; Qiu et al., 2009) and the putamen (Lopez-Larson et al., 2009; Qiu et al., 2009) have also been described. Two meta-analyses seem to provide partial resolution of these inconsistencies. Both demonstrated greater volume reductions in right striatal structures, with one showing diminished caudate volume (Valera, Faraone, Murray, & Seidman, 2007) and the other pointing to reductions in the putamen/globus pallidus region (Ellison-Wright, Ellison-Wright, & Bullmore, 2008). To some extent, these inconsistencies may relate to a variety of factors, including subjective judgments in manually tracing structures on MRI that are inherent in the ROI methodology.

Subsequently, a number of studies have utilized whole-brain voxel-based morphometry (VBM), which employs an automatized segmentation algorithm and does not require a priori hypotheses regarding which regions are of interest. A recent meta-analysis of VBM studies in children demonstrated reduced right globus pallidus and putamen volumes, but differences in caudate volumes failed to remain significant (Frodl & Skokauskas, 2012). The results also confirmed suggestions (from a number of previous reports) that the observed differences in basal ganglia volume diminished over time from childhood to adulthood. However, an independent meta-analysis suggested that the volume reductions in basal ganglia—specifically right caudate and globus pallidus/putamen—continue to be a robust finding in adulthood (Nakao et al., 2011). Despite some inconsistency, reductions in basal ganglia volume remain one of the more prominent and replicable structural abnormalities in ADHD.

Prefrontal and premotor cortex volume has also been reported as relatively diminished in individuals with ADHD. Most studies have shown that these reductions are apparent in both gray and white matter (Mostofsky, Cooper, Kates, Denckla, & Kaufmann, 2002; Seidman et al., 2006; Narr et al., 2009; Mahone et al., 2011). Subsequent investigations examined whether the biological basis for these volumetric differences was driven by differences in cortical thickness or surface area, or a combination of both. Cortical thinning was identified in medial, dorsolateral, orbital frontal, and inferior frontal cortex (Shaw et al., 2006; Makris et al., 2007; Gilliam, et al., 2011; Ducharme et al., 2012), particularly in the right hemisphere (Makris et al., 2007; Narr et al., 2009; Proal et al., 2011; Gilliam, et al., 2011; Langevin, MacMaster, et al., 2014). These decreases in cortical thickness were correlated with key symptoms of ADHD such as hyperactivity and impulsivity (Shaw, Malek, et al., 2012). In addition, the right anterior cingulate also appears smaller and thinner in ADHD compared to age-matched controls (Pliszka et al., 2006; Bledsoe, Semrud-Clikeman, & Pliszka, 2013). Notably, the anterior cingulate forms part of a cortico-limbic component to fronto-striatal circuitry, having connections to both lateral prefrontal and parietal cortex as well as to the amygdala, nucleus accumbens, hypothalamus, and insula.

Mahone et al. (2011) reported that in school-aged (8 to 13 years) children with ADHD, the left supplementary motor cortex (SMC) was also reduced in volume, and was evident in both boys and girls. This difference, which was evident in both gray and white matter volumes, was associated with significantly higher commission rates on a go/no-go task, providing an important and relevant functional correlate to the anatomical findings. Given other evidence that the SMC, particularly the rostral portion, is critical to response control and selection (Mostofsky & Simmonds, 2008), it was argued that abnormal fronto-striatal development including SMC may underlie one of the key impairments in ADHD: inhibitory control (Wodka et al., 2007). More broadly, deficits in response inhibition may reflect abnormal function of a circuit that includes SMC and its connections to basal ganglia, which are critically involved in inhibiting competing motor programs and disinhibiting intended behaviors (Mink, 2003).

Overall, these findings implicate dysfunction of multiple structures in fronto-striatal brain regions in the etiology of ADHD. Key components appear to include ventromedial, dorsolateral and orbital prefrontal cortex, premotor and supplementary motor cortex, the basal ganglia and cingulate gyrus. Given that the caudate nucleus, globus pallidus, and prefrontal cortex contain a high density of dopaminergic receptors, pathophysiology of this network is consistent with evidence from other sources (neuropsychological, and genetic, neurochemical, and neuroimaging) implicating dysfunction of dopamine pathways in ADHD (Seidman, Valera, & Bush, 2004; Durston et al., 2005; Kieling, Goncalves, Tannock, & Castellanos, 2008). Studies that are more recent have raised alternative pharmacologic mechanisms, specifically a polymorphism in a noradrenalin transporter gene (Chamberlain, Hampshire, et al., 2009). The neuroanatomical findings may relate to decreased $GABA_A$ mediated short-term inhibitory influences that frontal motor regions exert on functions of the basal ganglia (Gilbert, Isaacs, Augusta, MacNeil, & Mostofsky, 2011). Particular anomalies do remain evident in adulthood and in some cases appear to be predictive of neuropsychological impairment in specific functions. For example, Depue, Burgess, Bidwell, Willcutt, & Banich (2010) observed that in young adults, decreased frontal gray matter volume was correlated with poor processing speed and difficulties with response inhibition.

Together these data provide some support for previous speculation that the inhibitory and attentional difficulties experienced by individuals with ADHD may particularly relate to right-sided dysfunction of the fronto-striatal system (Heilman, Voeller, & Nadeu, 1991; Stefanatos & Wasserstein, 2001). Anatomical evidence compatible with this assertion includes the greater volume reductions in right basal ganglia (Castellanos et al., 1994; Casey et al., 1997), right cingulate (Makris et al., 2010), and cortical thinning in right inferior frontal areas in ADHD (Makris et al., 2007; Gilliam, et al., 2011). In addition, recent meta-analyses of both structural and functional MRI (fMRI) studies have supported the view that dysfunction of the right fronto-striatal system as a key role in ADHD (Nakao et al., 2011; Hart, Radua, Mataix-Cols, & Rubia, 2012).

PARIETAL LOBE

Right-hemispheric involvement in ADHD is also consistent with several studies demonstrating that individuals with ADHD can show subtle signs of inattention to the left side of space (Voeller & Heilman, 1988; Dobler et al., 2005). Manifestations include disproportionately slow reaction time to left-sided targets on computerized target detection tasks (Nigg, Swanson, & Hinshaw, 1997), reduced attention in the left hemifield on Posner's valid/invalid cueing task (Carter, Krener, Chaderjian, Northcutt, & Wolfe, 1995), increased left-sided omissions on cancellation tasks (Malone, Couitis, Kershner, & Logan, 1994), and a rightward bias on line bisection tasks (Sheppard, Bradshaw, Purcell, & Pantelis, 1999; Boles, Adair, & Joubert, 2009). These anomalies are reminiscent of the spatial neglect problems commonly seen in patients with acquired lesions of right parietal cortex. It has therefore been suggested that these anomalies may reflect parietal lobe dysfunction in ADHD. Alternatively, the problems with spatial attention may simply reflect a spatial bias arising from deficiencies in more general attentional processes such as sustained attention and vigilance for which the right hemisphere also plays a crucial role (Robertson, 1989). Aman, Roberts, and Pennington (1998) have suggested that performance is more impaired on frontal than parietal tasks in ADHD, although improvements are evident on both in response to medication.

Right parietal involvement in ADHD is consistent with a number of recent structural neuroimaging findings that have shown volume reductions and cortical thinning in the parietal lobe, particularly on the right side (Makris et al., 2007; McAlonan, Cheung, et al., 2007; Narr et al., 2009). In addition, white matter anomalies have been identified in right inferior parietal occipital cortex, suggestive of decreased neural branching (Silk et al., 2009). Tractography suggested that these anomalies involved pathways connecting parietal cortex to basal ganglia and a larger neural network including the cerebellum. Several recent fMRI studies have demonstrated that individuals with ADHD exhibit reduced activation of parietal association cortex during performance of tasks requiring relational reasoning (Silk et al., 2008) and fluid intelligence (Tamm & Juranek, 2012).

CEREBELLUM

It has become increasingly clear that differences in brain structure and function in individuals with ADHD exists beyond the fronto-striatal and parietal systems just described. Volumetric reductions have been identified in the thalamus and cerebellum (posterior inferior cerebellar vermis; see Proal et al., 2011). These observations have coincided with a dramatic increase in our understanding of the role of the cerebellum in regulating the speed, consistency, and appropriateness of various aspects of cognitive processes (e.g., complex reasoning, judgment, attention, working memory, and language) (1991, Schmahmann; 2004 #3676; Schmahmann & Pandya, 1997). The influence of the cerebellum on cortical functioning is thought to be mediated through major fiber tracts connecting multiple areas in the prefrontal and parietal association cortex to the pons and through feedback loops mediated via the thalamus and basal ganglia. These findings add an additional layer of complexity to models of the pathophysiology associated with ADHD since reductions in volume of the basal ganglia could be shaped by modulatory influences from the cerebellum (Giedd, Blumenthal, Molloy, & Castellanos, 2001; Seidman, Valera, & Makris, 2005).

WHITE MATTER

Some of the earliest structural neuroimaging studies identified reductions in the anterior portions of the corpus callosum (Hynd, Semrud-Clikeman, et al., 1991; Giedd et al., 1994), the major fiber tract connecting orbital regions of the left and right frontal cortex. This finding has been replicated, although not consistently (Overmeyer et al., 2000). Nevertheless, it is regarded as one of the more replicable findings in ADHD, having shown significant results in two independent meta-analyses (Valera et al., 2007; Hutchinson, Mathias, & Banich, 2008). The study of white matter in ADHD expanded to implicate other major white fiber tracts. A picture has now emerged that neural anomalies associated with ADHD are more widespread than had previously been considered. Some propose these neural anomalies may best be conceptualized in terms of a breakdown of widely distributed large-scale brain networks, including the default mode network (DMN; see e.g.,Castellanos & Proal, 2012).

Recent advances in diffusion tensor imaging (DTI) have allowed more detailed exploration of changes in white matter. The most commonly cited index of anomalies of white matter is fractional anisotropy (FA), which reflects a combination of tissue properties including axonal density, ordering, and myelination. While FA does not directly measure white matter integrity, it does reflect physical differences in white matter structure. DTI studies of individuals with ADHD have disclosed reduced white matter connectivity in subregions of the corpus callosum (Ashtari et al., 2005; Langevin, MacMaster, et al., 2014). The corpus callosum itself may undergo an abnormal growth trajectory in ADHD, particularly in its anterior extent (Gilliam et al., 2011). White matter anomalies have also been identified in the right external and internal capsules, right premotor and striatal regions (Adisetiyo et al., 2014), insula, and bilateral frontal (Mostofsky et al., 2002) and parietal lobes (Filipek, Semrud-Clikeman, et al., 1997), particularly in deep white matter. Involvement of deep white matter suggests anomalies in long association and projection fiber bundles. Interestingly, some areas in prefrontal cortex show decreased connectivity, while other areas, specifically orbitofrontal-striatal circuitry, show increased connectivity. The decreased connectivity in the left prefrontal circuitry has been found to be significantly correlated with inattention, while the increased connectivity of orbitofrontal-striatal circuitry was correlated with hyperactivity/impulsivity (Cao et al., 2013). In keeping with such observations, a recent review article by Konrad and Eickhoff (2010) noted a major shift in the research on the neuroscience of ADHD, from focus on abnormalities in isolated brain regions to abnormalities in organization and functioning of distributed brain regions.

van Ewijk, Heslenfeld, Zwiers, Buitelaar, and Oosterlaan (2012) recently reported the results of a meta-analysis of nine studies using a voxel white whole-brain analysis (VBA), which utilizes an automatized segmentation of the whole brain. This analysis yielded five significant clusters, suggesting disturbances of white matter integrity. This included the uncinate fasciculus (which connects anterior and mid temporal lobe to inferior frontal cortex) as well as widespread changes in the right corona radiata, which likely included fibers of the superior longitudinal fasciculus. The second-largest cluster was found in the left cerebellar white matter and smaller clusters were identified in the internal capsule bilaterally and in an area close to the genu of the corpus callosum. These findings only partially map onto results obtained in various ROI analyses. This again underscores some of the difficulties in evaluating the significance of structural correlates of neurodevelopmental disorders, including the possibility that some variation in results may relate to differences in the methods used. This general issue underscores the need to obtain corollary evidence from neuropsychological, neurophysiological and functional neuroimaging studies.

Functional Implications

Overall, this area of research has made significant headway in identifying the distinct functional role of the structures comprising the fronto-striatal system and their contribution to symptomology associated with ADHD. The basal ganglia form a highly interconnected network within the forebrain that interacts with and influences multiple neural systems through large-scale loops (Alexander, DeLong, & Strick, 1986; Utter & Basso, 2008). The caudate, putamen, and nucleus accumbens receive excitatory input from the entire cortex and interlaminar nuclei of the thalamus. In contrast to the putamen, which receives input from primary somatosensory and motor cortex, the caudate head receives input mainly from prefrontal, premotor, and supplementary motor areas. The caudate body receives parietal-occipital cortex projections and temporal lobe connects to the caudate tail. This pattern of connectivity suggests that the putamen is primarily concerned with motor control, while the caudate appears more involved in higher-order aspects of motor programming and cognitive control. Outputs of the basal ganglia project mainly from the substantia nigra and the globus pallidus that in turn connect indirectly and directly to the thalamus, which then influences cortical activity. This circuitry is thought to play a fundamental role in action selection, motor control, and sequence learning, but is also critically involved in cognitive function, supporting executive processes such as response inhibition and cognitive control, and the allocation of attention and timing functions (Rubia, Halari, et al., 2009; Aron, Robbins, & Poldrack, 2014; Botvinick & Cohen, 2014).

Functional neuroimaging studies in healthy adults have recently suggested that different aspects of inhibition may be mediated by distinguishable neural circuits. Motor response inhibition appears to be mediated by overlapping fronto-striato-thalamo-parietal networks involving predominantly right inferior frontal cortex, supplementary motor area, anterior cingulate cortex, caudate, thalamus, and inferior parietal regions (Miller, Nigg, & Miller, 2009). By contrast, interference inhibition tasks, which typically have a higher cognitive load due to the need for some aspect of conflict detection and inhibition from distraction, tend to be associated with greater activation of left hemisphere activation (Bernal & Altman, 2009) particularly in AAC and left IFC (Nigg et al., 1997).

When there is the need for high levels of mental effort, the anterior cingulate appears to be involved in coordinating with prefrontal cortex in evaluating how and when to exert cognitive controls, determining the significance of outcomes, and anticipating a course of action (Carter, Botvinick, & Cohen, 1999; Bush, 2011). It is not only involved in executive processes, but also its connections to limbic structures and the nucleus accumbens point to its role in incorporating information regarding emotional and motivational or reinforcement significance of actions or outcomes (Williams, Bush, Rauch, Cosgrove, & Eskandar, 2004; Makris et al., 2009). The result is a highly complex system that plays a role in dynamically and adaptively parsing and evaluating incoming information, suppressing responses to salient but irrelevant events, and choosing the most appropriate motor, cognitive or emotional response or action.

Several studies have noted that individuals with ADHD have fairly consistent deficits in various behaviors contingent on timing (Rubia, Taylor, Taylor, & Sergeant, 1999; Levy & Swanson, 2001; Smith, Taylor, Rogers, Newman, & Rubia, 2002; Toplak & Tannock, 2005). This is evident in relatively poor performance on simple tasks requiring maintenance of information regarding temporal order or duration (Radonovich & Mostofsky, 2004; Toplak & Tannock, 2005; Himpel et al., 2009). In addition, it is also been argued that timing issues may underlie the tendency of individuals with ADHD to demonstrate premature or poorly timed responses, difficulties in delaying gratification, and inadequate consideration of future implications of their actions (Rubia, Halari, et al., 2009). In a recent meta-analysis of time related implications (Hart et al., 2012), the most reliable deficits in ADHD individuals relative to controls were reduced fMRI activations in areas commonly associated in timing aspects of cognitive operations. During cognitive tasks requiring timing, the left fronto-parieto-cerebellar areas showed less activation. By contrast, right fronto-striatal anomalies were evident during tasks requiring inhibitory and attention functions.

Overall, a picture has emerged suggesting that ADHD deficits may partially represent the effects of a maturational lag in brain development (e.g., El-Sayed, Larsson, Persson, Santosh, & Rydelius, 2003). From a developmental perspective, the volume reductions of whole-brain gray and white matter, frontal cortex, caudate nucleus, and anterior cingulate have been observed in childhood and adolescence, while the reductions in some of these areas ceased to differentiate individuals with ADHD from controls in adolescence (Swanson, Castellanos, Murias, LaHoste, & Kennedy, 1998; Castellanos et al., 2002). In addition, a number of studies appear to suggest that individuals with ADHD have performance patterns or brain responses that appear very similar to patterns produced by younger neurotypical individuals. This hypothesis has received some support from behavioral (Berger, Slobodin, Aboud, Melamed, & Cassuto, 2013), electrophysiological (Clarke, Barry, McCarthy, Selikowitz, & Brown, 2002), and neuroimaging data (Shaw, Eckstrand, et al., 2007; Shaw, Gogtay, et al., 2010; Sato, Hoexter, Castellanos, & Rohde, 2012). In most cases, however, the developmental data are cross-sectional rather than longitudinal. Given considerable individual differences in responses and often small sample sizes, these studies are not ideally suited to identify maturational changes. By contrast, Doehnert, Brandeis, Imhof, Drechsler, and Steinhausen (2010) conducted a longitudinal study examining electrophysiological markers considered to assess the integrity of anterior and posterior attentional brain networks. While the behavioral data appeared to support a maturational lag, the ERP data suggested that these effects were unrelated to variations in neural activation. In other words, the anomalies evident on the ERPs did not resemble responses evident in younger control children. Similarly, Shaw and colleagues (2006, 2012) followed ADHD and normal control children into early adulthood using longitudinal MRIs. They found delays in regional cortical maturation that appeared to be correlated with key symptoms of ADHD such as hyperactivity and impulsivity (Shaw, Malek, et al., 2012). Notably, lag in the maturation of many cortical surface areas, sometimes as large as two to three years, was especially evident in the right frontal lobe. By extension, children with ADHD are often many years behind their peers in inhibitory control and self-regulation. This finding may again point to a differential importance of right hemisphere dysfunction in the condition (Stefanatos & Wasserstein, 2001). Other anomalies, nevertheless, do remain evident in adulthood and in some cases appear to be predictive of neuropsychological impairment in specific functions. For example, Depue et al. (2010) observed that decreased gray matter volume was correlated with poor processing speed and difficulties with response inhibition in young adults.

An exciting thread in the neuroscience of ADHD concerns evidence suggesting that to some extent, the neural correlates of ADHD can be altered by treatment. A meta-analysis by Hart et al. (2012) confirmed findings from previous studies suggesting that diminished activation in right dorsolateral prefrontal cortex can potentially normalize with long-term psychostimulant treatment. In addition, Ivanov, Murrough, Bansal, Hao, and Peterson (2014) recently found that stimulant use was associated with greater neural development in the left cerebellum.

It has been suggested that the neuroanatomical findings may relate to decreased $GABA_A$ mediated short-term inhibitory influences that frontal motor regions exert on functions of the basal ganglia (Gilbert et al., 2011; Wu, Gilbert, Shahana, Huddleston, & Mostofsky, 2012). Earlier functional brain imaging studies pointed to hypoperfusion of frontal cortex (Zametkin et al., 1990) and basal ganglia, particularly the caudate nucleus (Lou et al., 1984), and considered this related to reductions in the density of dopamine receptors. Treatment with methylphenidate resulted in increased activity in basal ganglia but decreases in frontal motor areas. More recent functional neuroimaging studies have implicated right inferior frontal cortex in impulse control and its disorders (Aron et al., 2014) and have raised alternative pharmacologic mechanisms, specifically a polymorphism in a noradrenalin transporter gene (Chamberlain, Hampshire, et al., 2009).

Neurobiology of LD—Dyslexia

Genetics of Dyslexia

Genetic factors are probably the single most important factor in the etiology of dyslexia (Pennington, Gilger, et al., 1991; Gayan & Olson, 1999). Early familial studies suggested that inheritance of reading disability is autosomal dominant (Hallgren, 1950; Finucci, Guthric, et al., 1976) with genetic heterogeneity. Early on, the Colorado Family Reading study found that the reading performance of the relatives of children with dyslexia was substantially lower than in controls (DeFries, Singer, Fich, & Lewitter, 1978). In later twin studies, a higher concordance rate for reading disability was noted for monozygotic (68%–100%) compared with dizygotic (20%–38%) twins (DeFries & Alarcon, 1996; DeFries, Alarcon, & Olson, 1997). Taken together, estimates of the risk to first-degree relatives are 35%–45%. Genetic transmission is probably complex and nonexclusive.

Molecular genetic linkage studies in families with dyslexia have identified chromosome regions in which the presence of dyslexia susceptibility genes is suspected, including links on chromosomes 15, 6 (Grigorenko et al., 1997; Fisher et al., 1999; Gayan et al., 1999), and 2 (Fagerheim et al., 1999). Similarly, complete quantitative trait loci analysis based on genome-wide scans for dyslexia in two large independent sets of families found linkage for chromosome 6, 2, 3, and 18 (Fisher et al., 2002). Altogether, linkage analyses in families with dyslexia have reported nine chromosomal regions where the presence of susceptibility genes is suspected: dyslexia susceptibility 1 (DYX1) to dyslexia susceptibility 9 (DYX9), on chromosomes 1, 2, 3, 6, 15, and 18 (Schumacher, Hoffmann, Schmäl, Schulte-Körne, & Nöthen, 2007). The most significant dyslexia candidate genes are DCDC2 and K1AA0319, both identified within DYX2 on chromosome 6p22. DCDC2, associated with reading disability, contains a double cortin homology domain, modulates neuronal development in the brain, is possibly involved in cortical neuron migration, and is expressed in the fetal and adult central nervous system. ROBO1 (i.e., roundabout Drosophila homolog1) was discovered through mapping of a translocation in a Finnish family. Another candidate gene, DYX1C1 was cloned in a two-generation Finish family with a translocation, in a region on chromosome 15. It is expressed in the brain and may be involved in the functional cell state. Almost all these candidate genes are implicated in global brain development processes such as neural migration and axonal guidance. DCDC2, DYX1C1, and KIAA0319 are involved in cell migration.

Importantly, early on, the contribution of phonological coding to the heritability of reading deficit, tested by single-word reading, was established to be high in a twin study, whereas orthographic coding did not contribute to this heritability (Reynolds et al., 1996). In a similar vein, shortly thereafter Grigorenko et al. (1997) demonstrated linkage between phonological awareness, single-word reading and two different chromosomal regions on chromosomes 6 and 15 respectively. The chromosome 6 locus had a role in phonological awareness, and to a lesser extent in single-word reading, whereas the locus on chromosome 15 affected single-word reading only. Other genetic studies with phenotyping support these findings, with a positive linkage between dyslexia and measures of phonological processing with genetic markers on chromosomes 1, 2, 3, 6, 15, and 18 (Cardon et al., 1994; Grigorenko, Wood, Meyer, & Pauls, 2000).

A few studies have implicated shared genetic risk in dyslexia and ADHD. Specifically, twin studies have pointed to evidence that genetic influences that are associated with increased risk for dyslexia also increase risk for inattention symptoms of ADHD (Gayan et al., 2005; Willcutt et al., 2007). However, the specific genetic mutations or variants involved in both disorders have not yet been identified (Smith, 2007).

Neural Correlates of Dyslexia

EARLIEST STRUCTURAL FINDINGS

Discovery of structural anatomical asymmetries in the region of the Sylvain fissure and the planum temporale represents some of the earliest research in the neuroscience of dyslexia. Path-breaking work by Geschwind and Levitsky (1968) found the planum temporale to be larger on the left in most people, but not in dyslexics. This loss of the usual hemispheric asymmetry in dyslexia was thought to reflect a failure of the postulated asymmetrical cell loss during gestation. Later, Hynd and colleagues demonstrated reversal of the usual planum temporale asymmetry seen in two-thirds of normal adult brains (Hynd et al., 1995), and found correlations between planum temporale asymmetry patterns and measures of language processing and reading. While such findings were not universal (e.g., Best & Demb, 1999), together these observations led to one of the first theories of dyslexia based on neuroscience: That is, the observed developmental abnormality of the left hemisphere led to loss of dominance for language, developmental language processing abnormality, reading abnormality, a shift of motor dominance from the left to the right hemisphere, and left handedness (Geschwind & Galaburda, 1985; Habib, 2000). Other early studies reported differences in size of the corpus callosum between dyslexics and normally reading individuals (Duara et al., 1991), including a smaller anterior part (genu) in dyslexic children (Hynd et al., 1995).

CYTOARCHITECTURAL ABNORMALITIES IN DYSLEXIA

Pathological studies of the brains of people who had developmental dyslexia are uncommon. Nevertheless, three types of neuroanatomic abnormalities have been described: absence of the normal cerebral asymmetries, the presence of cortical developmental abnormalities including microdysgenesis (ectopias and cell loss), and abnormalities of the visual pathways. For example, Geschwind and Galaburda (1985) found abnormalities in (a) the arrangement of neurons from one cortical layer to another or in the same layer, and (b) a high frequency of microdysgenesis (including focal microgyria, neuronal nests, missing or duplicated gyri, and fewer layers and primitive orientation of neurons), in addition to loss of the usual hemispheric asymmetry in the planum temporale. Cohen, Campbell and Yaghmai (1989) also found gliosis. Generally, such microstructure abnormalities are most frequently seen in the temporal lobes, especially on the left. Ectopias and dysplasias suggest anomalous migration during stages of brain development when neurons migrate from their place of birth, in the subcortical periventricular areas, to their appropriate location in the cortex. The second type of brain pathology (i.e., the presence of glial scars) suggests potential injury to the brain and neuronal loss during a later part of brain development in utero.

CEREBELLAR ABNORMALITIES IN DYSLEXIA

The cerebellum was traditionally thought to only have a role in motor coordination, motor planning, and motor learning. Recent evidence, however, points to a broader role that includes perceptual and cognitive processes. Functional neuroimaging studies of unimpaired subjects report cerebellar activation during a variety of cognitive tasks, including problem solving, working memory, verb generation, attention tasks, and nonword reading (e.g., Fulbright et al., 1990). Anatomic connections between the cerebellum and the cerebral cortex include connections to the frontal, temporal, and parietal lobes (Middleton & Strick, 1994; Schmahmann, 1996), thereby providing extensive structural underpinning for a role in cognition. These regions are all also areas that are well-known to be engaged during reading. The cerebellum may be affected in both dyslexic adults and children (Zeffiro & Eden, 2001). Notably, a volumetric MRI study of dyslexic children reported significantly smaller brain volume and right anterior lobe of the cerebellum, pars triangularis bilaterally. These anomalies correctly classified 72% of the dyslexic subjects and 88% of controls, and were significantly correlated with reading, spelling, and language measures related to dyslexia (Eckert et al., 2003). Taken together, such findings are consistent with Nicolson, Fawcett and Dean's cerebellar deficit hypothesis of dyslexia (Nicolson, Fawcett, & Dean, 2001). This model proposes that through its role in motor control during the articulation of speech, the cerebellum contributes to the phonological processing deficits, which often cause dyslexia. They also proposed that weakness of the cerebellum can disrupt learning of grapheme-phoneme relationships, and that it contributes to automatization of learned behaviors (Nicolson, Fawcett, & Dean, 2001).

However, considering that the structural anomalies in dyslexia are not isolated to the cerebellum, and that the tasks used in functional imaging studies involved a much broader distributed network, the findings cannot be considered to specifically implicate the cerebellum. Many, if not most, individuals with dyslexia do not have cerebellar signs and most cerebellar patients do not have reading problems. It seems that the effects on cerebellum may reflect a more general pattern of anomalies involving the distributed reading network, so impaired cerebellar function is unlikely a primary causal factor in dyslexia (Stoodley & Stein, 2013).

STRUCTURAL NEUROIMAGING

VBM is an MRI technique measuring regional cerebral volume and tissue concentration. VBM studies have found decreased brain gray matter in dyslexics—in cerebral, cerebellar, and basal ganglia areas—and at least one study demonstrated smaller total brain volume in the dyslexic subjects (Eckert et al., 2003; Brambati et al., 2004). Anatomical variables that differentiated dyslexic from normal readers were correlated with real word reading, pseudoword reading, and spelling, the same three language skills on which the dyslexic children were reliably different from the controls.

As described previously, DTI is an MRI method that provides information about integrity of white matter tracts. DTI studies have found that, compared with good readers, poor readers had lower white matter diffusion anisotropy (i.e., FA) in a region of the temporo-parietal lobe. This was seen bilaterally in adults and in the left parietal occipital area in children. Dyslexics also had white matter abnormalities in the region of the supramarginal gyrus. The FA values correlated with reading skills (e.g., Klingberg et al., 2000; Deutsch et al., 2005). Finally, a recent DTI study of children who were poor readers showed functional improvements after intense remediation (Feldman, Yeatmen, Lee, Barde, & Gaman-Bean, 2010). DTI results imply structural abnormalities in the connections between various cortical regions in dyslexia.

FUNCTIONAL NEUROIMAGING

As phonological processing appears to be a main cause for dyslexia, much of the functional neuroimaging research, both positron emission tomography (PET) and fMRI, has focused on letter- and word-reading tasks that involve phonological processing. Results of such studies, performed mostly in adults, point to reduction of brain activation in response to reading- or language-related tasks. That is, compared with normal readers, dyslexics generally underactivate brain regions, mostly in the left hemisphere and especially in the temporal lobe, inferior parietal cortex (near angular/supramarginal gyrus), and frontal operculum (Brunswick, McCrory, Price, Frith, & Frith, 1999; Rumsey et al., 1997). The studies vary in the exact location and the type of alteration, and presence of activation in corresponding areas of the right hemisphere.

The classic neurologic model for reading—based on studies of patients with acquired alexia—hypothesizes functional linkages between the angular gyrus in the left hemisphere and visual association areas in the occipital and temporal lobes. A number of studies indicate disruption of this system in dyslexia. For example, an early PET study during single-word reading showed strong connectivity between left angular gyrus and other left hemisphere regions in normal controls, but not in dyslexics. This suggested a functional disconnection of the left angular gyrus from visual areas, Wernicke's area, and the inferior frontal cortex (Horwitz, Rumsey, et al., 1998). Similarly, regional cerebral blood flow (rCBF) in the left angular gyrus, during single-word reading, has been positively correlated with level of reading skill in normal readers. By contrast, these same correlations were negative in dyslexic men, also suggesting an important role for this region in developmental reading disorder (Rumsey et al., 1997). In addition, despite their inherent differences in language systems, dyslexics in French-, Italian-, and English-speaking countries all show less activity than controls at the occipito-temporal junction of the left hemisphere during word processing (Paulesu et al., 2001). Based on such observations, Demonet, Taylor, and Chaixet (2004) suggested that the left inferior temporal region, at the junction between lateral and mesial aspect, is possibly an interface between regions associated with processing visual features of written words, regions involved in complex visual processing, and more dorsal language areas in the middle and superior temporal gyri. Thus it may mediate the visual entry into the linguistic system (Demonet et al., 2004).

fMRI research has identified cortical areas, mostly in the posterior part of the left hemisphere—especially temporal and parietal lobes—that are activated during different stages of "normal" reading. Notably, different regions in the left hemisphere, termed *pathways* (but subsuming both gray and underlying white matter), are engaged at different stages of reading development. The left "dorsal" parietal-attention pathway is activated during reading in children who are learning to read. It includes the angular and supramarginal gyri, which were typically underactive in dyslexic children during PET studies, and mediates a slow, phonologically based, assembly process. There is evidence also for a faster "posterior/ventral" pathway. This left occipital-temporal pathway is centered in the posterior fusiform gyrus, activating a "visual word form" area. The ventral pathway is involved with the development of fluent reading, when word recognition skills become more automatic and direct visual access to the mental lexicon is the predominant reading strategy (Pugh et al., 2000; Shaywitz et al., 2002). It is a rapid whole-word system (McCandliss, Cohen, & Dehaene, 2003) and brain activation in this region increases as reading skill increases (Shaywitz et al., 2002). Activation during reading-related activity can also be found less frequently in the left inferior frontal gyrus connected to the two posterior pathways, implicated in the output of phonological and articulatory aspects (Demonet et al., 2004). Taken together, the left angular, supramarginal, fusiform, and inferior frontal gyri, as well as the "where" and "what" visual pathways, appear essential in reading acquisition and fluent reading.

Consistent with the discussion so far, fMRI and magnetoencephalographic studies of dyslexics have shown reduced activity of multiple left hemisphere brain systems during reading (Horwitz, Rumsey, et al., 1998; Brunswick,

McCrory, Price, Frith, & Frith, 1999; Helenius, Tarkiainen, Cornelissen, Hansen, & Salmelin, 1999; Paulesu et al., 2001). Reduced activation is seen in both the parietotemporal region (including the posterior aspects of the superior and middle temporal gyri, and the supramarginal and the angular gyri) and in the occipital-temporal region of the left hemisphere, including the left fusiform gyrus (Brunswick et al., 1999; Paulesu et al., 2001; Shaywitz et al., 2002). For example, Shaywitz and associates (1998) carried out a detailed investigation of regional metabolic activity in 29 dyslexic adults and 32 controls. fMRI demonstrated significant group-task interactions in four regions: the posterior superior temporal gyrus (Wernicke's area), angular gyrus, striate cortex, and inferior frontal gyrus (Broca's area). Unlike normal readers, dyslexics did not show an increase in activation as phonologic coding demands increased. In addition, differences between the two groups were present also in anterior brain areas where dyslexics showed a pattern of over activation. Meaning Shaywitz et al. (1998) proposed a general explanation of posterior hypo-activation in dyslexics during phonological processing, suggesting a disruption of this system. Similar results were found later in a similar fMRI study done with a large group of normally reading children and dyslexic children (Shaywitz et al., 2002). Activation of left inferior frontal area in dyslexics is more variable—less active in some studies and higher than normal activation in other studies (Brunswick et al., 1999; Paulesu et al., 2001; Pugh et al., 2000). Higher than normal activation suggests the presence of compensatory engagement. Similarly, activation of areas in the right hemisphere during reading related tasks in dyslexics is variable and may be the result of compensation (Demonet et al., 2004).

Another line of research grows out of therapy for reading disorders. A number of studies found that successful reading remediation is accompanied by increased activity in multiple brain areas, bringing activation in these regions closer to that seen in normal readers. For example, Eden and colleagues (2004) described differences in brain activity of adult dyslexic subjects during a phonological manipulation task, before and after behavioral intervention. They found that behavioral improvements were associated with signal increases in left-hemisphere regions usually activated by normal readers (i.e., left parietal cortex and left fusiform cortex), as well as in areas in the right perisylvian. Another fMRI study, in dyslexic children during phonemic processing, demonstrated brain plasticity in response to remediation. Activation in parietal, temporal, frontal, and cerebellar areas partially normalized after treatment. Remediation may also produce additional compensatory activation in other brain regions (Temple, Deutsch, et al., 2003). Thus, successful reading therapy can produce both normalization of brain regions usually involved in reading and compensatory overactivation in other brain changes in other brain areas. Compensatory systems may recruit areas around the inferior frontal gyrus in both hemispheres and perhaps the right-hemisphere homologue of the left occipital-temporal word form area as well.

ELECTROENCEPHALOGRAPHY, EVENT-RELATED POTENTIALS, VISUAL EVOKED POTENTIALS AND MAGNETOENCEPHALOGRAPHY

In general, regular clinical EEG does not reveal specific abnormalities in dyslexic people. Quantitative EEG studies, however, demonstrate increased amount of slower background frequencies, in the theta and delta range, and reduced amount of alpha frequency waves (Harmony et al., 1995). Similarly, Brain Electrical Activity Mapping (BEAM), which provides regional quantitative EEG power spectra, recorded during resting and during cognitive activity, has demonstrated electrophysiological differences between dyslexic and nondyslexic boys. Similar to findings from other methodologies, differences have been found in the left temporal and left posterior quadrant regions and in the frontal areas bilaterally. Findings suggest aberrant neurophysiology is present in dyslexia in a number of cortical areas, anteriorly and posteriorly, and in the right as well as the left hemispheres (Duffy, Denckla, Bartels, Sandini, & Kiessling, 1980).

ERPs are brain electrical responses to specific stimuli, recorded over the scalp at characteristic times after stimulus onset. Mismatch negativity (MMN) is a frontal central negativity that appears when a deviant physical stimulus occurs within a group of ongoing stimuli. It is an automatic change-detecting response, is preattentive, and appears 150–200 milliseconds after the event. Using speech stimuli (i.e., /da//ba /wa) it was found that dyslexic children could not discriminate speech sounds as well as normal readers. Impaired discrimination was associated with diminished MMN, and differences between dyslexics and controls were found for language stimuli but not for pure tone discrimination (Leppanen & Lyytinen, 1997). In another electrophysiological study, dyslexics showed increased latency and smaller amplitude in the P3 wave, an ERP response to an "odd ball" cognitive stimulus (Frank, Seiden, & Napolitano, 1996). Studies using word presentations, including nonsense words and rhyming, demonstrated ERP abnormalities in dyslexics compared with slow readers and ADHD children who read normally. This pattern was manifested mostly in N450 (Ackermann, Riecker, et al., 2001). ERP elicited when words are presented usually include a later surface negative late wave (N400–450). The characteristics of this wave depend on the subject's phonetic skills. Together such findings clearly indicate processing differences in dyslexics which occur at a very fundamental level. Moreover, results are also are entirely in line with phonemic processing models of dyslexia.

Magnetoencephalography (MEG) records the magnitude and topography of spontaneous or evoked brain electrical activity. Although it has lesser resolution and lower ability to precisely localize brain activity than fMRI, it has the advantage of ability to time electrical brain activities in response to stimuli. MEG studies of pseudo-word reading in normal readers show early activity in lateral occipito-temporal regions bilaterally; after a delay, this is followed by near-simultaneous peaks of activity in the fusiform, angular, and middle temporal gyri. Subsequent activity peaks are seen in the right inferior frontal gyrus and later in left inferior frontal gyrus. By contrast, dyslexics failed to activate the left inferior temporo-occipital region, suggesting either an inability to achieve early operations of global word form perception or inefficient immediate phonological extraction (Salmelin, Service, Kiesila, Uutela, & Salonen, 1996; Simos et al., 2008). Furthermore, a left inferior frontal area was activated within 400 milliseconds in dyslexics but not in normal readers, a finding interpreted as a compensatory activity in the dyslexic subjects. Abnormalities in the degree and timing of cortical activation associated with phonological decoding in dyslexics were also found.

Finally, studies using visual evoked potentials (VEP) have also found evidence for visual system abnormalities in dyslexia. VEP is primarily used to assess functional integrity of visual pathways and refers to electrical potentials initiated by presentation of brief visual stimuli and extracted from the EEG. A number of VEP studies suggest that dyslexics generally process visual information more slowly than normal readers. Starting in the retina, the visual system divides into major pathways that can be distinguished based on the kind of information that the pathways conveyed to visual cortex. Two of the major pathways are the magnocellular pathway, which rapidly conveys low contrast information that is important for processing motion (but not color), and the parvocellular system, which conveys high contrast information about color and fine detail. This division continues in the lateral geniculate nucleus, the primary visual cortex, and higher-order visual cortices. The parvocellular system contributes to the ventral or "what" pathway from visual cortex to inferotemporal cortex that is involved in object recognition. The magnocellular system predominantly contributes to the dorsal or "where" pathway from visual cortex to inferior parietal lobule, which is involved in motion analysis and spatial processing. Livingstone, Rosen, Drislane, and Galaburda (1991) found abnormalities in dyslexics' response to low contrast, high frequency stimuli, which would correspond to letters. The same dyslexic children responded normally to targets of lower frequencies and higher contrast (Livingstone et al., 1991). The pattern of results suggested an abnormality specifically affecting the magnocellular pathway of the visual system. Histological measurement of neurons of the magnocellular and parvocellular layers of the lateral geniculate nucleus in five dyslexic and five control brains also revealed that the usually larger magnocellular cells were smaller in this dyslexic group, complementing the physiological findings. The parvocellar layers in the same brains were normal. However, these findings have not been replicated, and the evidence for these abnormalities as the basis of dyslexia has not been consistent (Kubova, Kuba, Peregrin, & Novakova, 1996).

Neurobiology of LD—Dyscalculia

Genetics of Dyscalculia

Substantially fewer studies have been directed to understanding genetic contributions to the acquisition of arithmetic skills compared to reading disability. Several molecular genetic studies have shown that certain genetic disorders (e.g., Williams syndrome) are associated with particular deficits in math performance (Mazzocco, 2011). In addition, several family studies have suggested that there is a high prevalence of developmental dyscalculia among siblings (Alarcon, DeFries et al., 1997). Heritability estimates have ranged from .2 to .9 (Oliver & Plomin, 2007). This enormous variability may be explained by the fact that different aspects of mathematic ability may have different genetic contributions. However, according to recent multivariate genetic analyses, the genetic correlation between various aspects of mathematics is .91, suggesting that the same set of genes are largely responsible in different areas of mathematics performance (Kovas, Harlaar, et al., 2005). These genetic influences appear to covary with general cognitive ability and reading skills as well as with other genetic influences. Finally, a number of recent studies have suggested that there is significant longitudinal stability in math performance (Jordan, Hanich, et al., 2003). Shalev et al. (2005), for example found that 95% of children diagnosed with dyscalculia in the fifth grade continued to perform poorly in arithmetic in the 11th grade. This implies likely underlying genetic control.

Neural Correlates of Dyscalculia

INTRAPARIETAL SULCUS AND UNDERSTANDING QUANTITY AND SPACE

Behavioral studies in animals reveal number perception, discrimination, and elementary calculation abilities in chimpanzees, showing that a sense of numerosity (the number of objects in a set) exists even in animals. Similar core numerical skills also develop in infants without formal schooling. These types of observations led Dehaene and Cohen (1997) to propose that "number sense" is a basic capacity of the primate brain with dedicated built-in brain circuits, which are engaged in recognizing numerosity. From this perspective, the pathophysiology of dyscalculia is explained by the presence of a selective deficit in the fundamental representation of numerosities (Piazza, Facoetti, et al., 2010). Both human and monkey studies relate the processing of quantity information to the posterior parietal cortex, especially the intraparietal sulcus (IPS; see Dehaene et al., 2004). Electrophysiological recordings from monkey parietal cortex reveal that neurons in the lateral intraparietal cortex respond more when more objects are presented. Similarly, the human IPS is activated in most neuroimaging studies of number processing and may therefore constitute a central nervous system region for amodal representation of quantity (Dehaene, Piazza, Pinel, & Cohen, 2003). Notably, the IPS activates whether the numbers are spoken or written, and is independent of the form in which numbers appear (Nacchache & Dehaene, 2001; Eger, Sterzer, Russ, Giraud, & Kleinschmidt, 2003).

fMRI studies further demonstrate that the IPS is involved in various aspects of calculation, including processing of numerical quantities, number detection, magnitude comparison, number comparison, and simple quantity manipulations (Dehaene, Dehaene-Lambertz, & Cohen, 1998; Dehaene et al., 2003). Notably, the IPS is more strongly activated in approximate calculation than in exact calculation, and more strongly activated in subtraction than in multiplication (Stanescu-Cosson et al., 2000). Research using fMRI has found that children with DD have less gray matter in the left IPS (e.g., Kucian et al., 2006). Such observations led to the proposal that the IPS, bilaterally, is the crucial area for the representation of quantities (Piazza, Pinel, LeBihan, & Dehaene, 2007), as well as for understanding of some arithmetic operations. Consistent with this, a more recent study has shown that electrical activity in a particular group of IPS nerve cells spiked only when subjects were performing calculations, in the laboratory or outside (Dastjerdi, Ozker, Foster, Rangarajan, & Parvizi, 2013). Quantitative stimuli included simple arithmetic and even quantitative references such as *some more, many,* or *bigger than the other one* (Dastjerdi et al., 2013).

ANGULAR GYRUS AND MATH FACTS AND CALCULATION

The left angular gyrus belongs to the language system, is critical in reading, and may relate more to linguistic than to quantity processing. Yet it is activated during some arithmetic tasks such as retrieval of arithmetic facts, multiplication, and exact calculation (Grabner et al., 2009). Additionally, stronger left angular gyrus activation has been seen on fMRI in mathematically more competent subjects (Grabner, Reishofer, Koschutnig, Ebner, & Parvizi, 2011). Since some arithmetic operations are more dependent on language-based fact retrieval (and thus more on the angular gyrus) and others on quantity processing (and thus on the IPS) (Piazza et al., 2007), it has been proposed that the left angular gyrus supports the retrieval of previously learned and verbally stored arithmetic facts (like multiplication tables) from memory (Grabner et al., 2011). By contrast, in a PET study, multiplication activated a number of brain areas, including the left and right inferior parietal gyri, the left fusiform and lingual gyri, and the right cuneus, as well as preferentially left lenticular nucleus, and precentral and inferior frontal gyri (Dehaene et al., 1996). This suggests that multiplication and comparison may rest on a number of distinct and differing neural and functional networks.

INFERIOR PREFRONTAL CORTEX

Neurons in the lateral prefrontal cortex of the monkey are also selectively tuned to numerical rank and numerical quantity, but typically later than IPS neurons (Nieder, Freedman, & Miller, 2002; Nieder, Diester, & Tudusciuc, 2006). In humans, the inferior prefrontal cortex (Stanescu-Cosson et al., 2000) has a function in more demanding mathematical calculations. For example, learning to solve new and complex arithmetic problems which require reasoning and working memory leads to greater activation in the inferior prefrontal gyrus. By contrast the IPS is required for the representation of the magnitudes of the numbers involved, and when comparing them to previously learned facts (Delazar et al., 2003; (Krueger et al., 2008). Developmental changes when performing routine calculations include shifting from frontal areas to parietal and temporal-occipital regions.

The IPS, therefore, appears to be pivotal in fundamental appreciation of quantity, irrespective of modality. As such it holds a format-independent representation of numerical magnitude and is systematically engaged in any task drawing on magnitude manipulations—from basic number comparison to complex calculations (Dehaene, Piazza, Pinel, & Cohen, 2003, 2004). By contrast, the left angular gyrus is pivotal in retrieval and/or understanding of verbal mathematical information. Thus the language-based left angular gyrus verbal system and the posterior parietal attention system most probably mediate different aspects of mathematical thinking. For example, the left angular gyrus, as well as the left prefrontal regions, may be mainly implicated in retrieval of arithmetic facts and in exact verbal-memory based and language-dependent calculation, while the IPS is the place for understanding of quantity, relative size and position of figures. Prefrontal regions are likely involved in the more executively demanding aspects of all of the above. Dyscalculia may consequently be the result of a structural brain abnormality in either the size or cellular composition of one of these areas specific to mathematics—or in its connectivity. Similar to dyslexia, compensation may require either recovery of weakened regions or recruitment of other regions.

DEVELOPMENTAL ASPECTS AND THE DYSCALCULIC BRAIN

Developmental studies reveal that in tasks involving numerical symbols normal children rely more than adults on prefrontal regions (Rotzer et al., 2008). As children grow up, however, the IPS and the left temporal-parietal cortex become more specialized for numerical magnitude processing and calculation (Ansari, 2008), with a concomitant decrease of reliance on general purpose (frontal) areas. Thus during the process of normal learning of calculation skills, neural organization shifts from one network to the other, similar to that which occurs in learning to read. Developmental changes include the shifting from frontal areas to parietal and temporal-occipital areas. Learning new arithmetic facts involves primarily the frontal lobes and the IPS, while using previously learned facts involves the left angular gyrus.

Morphometric studies in subjects with developmental dyscalculia have shown reduced gray matter in the left, right, and bilateral IPS and frontal regions (Mazzocco, 2011; Isaacs et al., 2001; Rotzer et al., 2009). Reduced connectivity between parietal areas involved in numerosity, and between these areas and occipito-temporal areas involved in the processing of symbolic number forms, has been demonstrated using DTI (Zhou, Zhang, Zhu, Chen, & Sokabe, 2009). Brain activation studies in dyscalculic children have revealed reduced activation in neural networks, including the IPS, and the middle and inferior frontal gyrus of both hemispheres. Notably, the left IPS, the left inferior frontal gyrus, and the right middle frontal gyrus often seemed to play crucial roles during comparison of numerosities, comparison of number symbols, and arithmetic, since brain activation correlated with accuracy rate in these regions (Price et al., 2007; Mussolin, De Volder et al., 2010). Consequently it has been suggested children with dyscalculia suffer from deficient recruitment of neural resources when processing analog magnitudes of numbers (Kucian et al., 2006). Other studies have shown abnormal brain function and structure in the parietal cortex, especially in the interparietal sulcus (Rubinstein & Henik, 2009; Butterworth, Varma, & Laurilland, 2011).

MEG revealed that, compared to controls with normal mathematical ability, students with dyscalculia had increased neurophysiological activity in inferior and superior parietal regions in the right hemisphere, as well as increased early engagement of prefrontal cortices, while the left hemisphere activity was delayed and did not show the expected task-related changes (Simos et al., 2008). Finally, differences in the IPS region, in isolation or as a part of a more extensive brain abnormality, are also found in a number of genetic conditions associated with mathematical dysfunction, including Turner syndrome, FFragile X syndrome, and velocardiofacial syndrome (Rivera, Menon, White, Glaser, & Reiss, 2002), and Williams syndrome (Hoeft et al., 2007).

Summary of Neuroscience and Concluding Thoughts

Despite being extremely heritable, the search for genes conferring risk for ADHD, has proven challenging. Conclusions vary depending on the symptoms chosen and the raters used, although hyperkinesis/impulsivity and inattention are generally dissociated. Importantly, ADHD in most individuals is not due to a single gene variant but is more likely due to potentially thousands of rare variants that disrupt neuronal pathway function. There may also be a few not-yet-identified common genetic variants that disrupt similar regions. Gene expression likely fluctuates with age, sometimes decreasing and at other points increasing. Both genetic and epigenetic variables contribute to the fluctuation. This temporal variation in genetic expression may account for instances of later onset of this neurodevelopmental disorder.

The posited disruption in neuronal pathway function, in turn, produces a similar endophenotype (i.e., characteristic cognitive, neurophysiological, biochemical, neuroanatomical, and/or neuropsychological profiles) that translates into core traits of the diagnosis. Thus, ADHD is the result of cumulative and complex genetically mediated dysfunction in multiple neural regions or pathways. In addition, expression of some genes can vary with development, which can further complicate clinical presentations and course.

Given the diversity of the genetics associated with the ADHD endophenotype, it is not surprising that similarly diverse neural regions and systems have been identified as correlates. Early structural imaging research used a ROI method that introduces biases in the choice of brain volumes to investigate. Many of these studies focused on frontal regions and failed to provide evidence that observed volumetric differences correlated with specific behaviors evident in the ADHD individuals studied. The importance of obtaining direct behavioral correlates to observed anatomical differences grew as further studies revealed other areas in which volumetric differences existed in individuals with ADHD. These areas expanded to include the basal ganglia, corpus callosum, and cerebellum. Furthermore, differences in the age and the gender composition of the groups contributed to inconsistencies that undermined a consensus regarding which volumetric differences are associated with ADHD (Valera et al., 2007). Later studies incorporated independent and unbiased markers of neurodevelopmental anomalies in ADHD, such as anomalies of cortical density and thickness. More recent functional neuroimaging studies have generally confirmed that behavioral deficits associated with ADHD are most frequently related to poor activation and functional connectivity of circuits in dorsolateral frontal cortex that regulate attention, planning, and working memory. Areas of inferior frontal cortex that mediate cognitive control, including inhibitory control, interference control, and cognitive flexibility also show lack of activation (Pliszka et al., 2006; Cubillo et al., 2010). Lateral orbital and ventromedial prefrontal cortex circuitry is involved in emotional regulation and emotion (Price, Carmichael, & Drevets, 1996; Best, Williams, & Coccaro, 2002). These areas have strong connections with subcortical structures involved in processing emotion such as the amygdala, hippocampus, and nucleus accumbens. Default mode network dysregulation, or differential right hemisphere dysfunction, are other proposed neural correlates of ADHD.

Continuing limitations of this body of research exist. Firstly, the vast majority of studies have predominantly or exclusively studied males with ADHD (Yang et al., 2008). Given known gender differences in brain development (Lenroot et al., 2007), it is unclear whether the morphological anomalies identified in these reports are apparent or differ in substantial ways in females with ADHD. Qiu et al. (2009), for example, it is recently reported that volumetric decreases in specific regions of putamen and caudate observed in males were not apparent in females with ADHD. It has also been noted that frontal lobe volumetric differences observed in males with ADHD were equivocal among females with ADHD (Castellanos, Giedd, et al., 2001). Secondly, concerns have also been raised that the observed structural differences may be epiphenomena of the behavioral symptoms. Some of the identified structural changes may reflect the effects of having problems with attention and impulse control. While it is no doubt important to consider the environmental effects, several lines of evidence suggest that these factors cannot be a full account of the findings. A study by Durston et al. (2004), for example, allayed these concerns to some extent by showing that affected first-degree relatives exhibited similar but more subtle volumetric differences in both gray and white matter volume. This suggested that observed morphological differences in ADHD were based more in genetic than epigenetic factors. Similarly, Ent et al. (2007) contrasted volume loss in concordant and discordant twins and found that the concordant high-risk pairs showed volume loss in orbitofrontal subdivisions. High-risk members from the discordant twin pairs exhibited volume reduction in the right inferior dorsolateral prefrontal cortex. In addition, the posterior corpus callosum was compromised in concordant high-risk pairs only. Ent et al.'s findings indicated that different components of the distributed action-attentional network system are differentially affected by genetic versus environmental influences.

There are similar concerns regarding LD. Genes that affect a quantitatively measured trait such as reading are termed *quantitative trait loci* (QTL). Because reading is a complex construct, reading disability may have a polygenetic and multifactorial etiology and no single QTL is either necessary, nor sufficient, to cause the disorder (McGrath et al., 2006). A number of QTL genes likely underlie the transmission of both the normal variations in reading skill and dyslexia. Different genes may be implicated in different aspects of the reading disorder, with the final result being a deficit in the ability to integrate the information needed for learning to read (Mitchell, 2011). However, those genes that affect various aspects of phonological processing (e.g., coding, awareness, discrimination, or expression) show the most consistent linkage with dyslexia. Finally, since dyscalculia is associated with some genetic conditions, general heritability of this LD is also likely.

Dyslexia is associated with both macroscopic and microscopic structural abnormalities, preferentially evident in the left hemisphere. The earliest findings implicated gross anatomical asymmetries in the planum temporale in superior posterior temporal cortex, as well as cytoarchitectural abnormalities in structure and/or cell migration. Subsequently, other abnormalities have been observed in white matter tracts such as the cerebellum and/or the corpus callosum. Functional neuroimaging has supplemented this research and most consistently identified dysfunction in the left hemisphere fusiform gyrus, angular gyrus, and supramarginal gyrus, and bilaterally in inferior frontal gyri. These regions are part of two posterior visual pathways (i.e., dorsal or ventral, where or what, slow effortful or whole word), which engage differentially depending on the stage of learning to read and/or the fluency/automaticity of decoding. Electrophysiological studies document disturbances in either phonemic processing (via MEG) and/or visual processing (VEP), consistent with both linguistic and visual vulnerabilities. Notably, remediation/compensation is associated with normalization of regional brain activation, as well as engagement of ancillary regions, including on the right.

The neurocognitive deficits in dyscalculia include impaired understanding of quantity and space, impaired recall of math facts and calculation, and general attention to execution and sequencing. Correlated with these are the left IPS, the left anterior gyrus, and the inferior prefrontal cortex, respectively. Given the overlap between some of these regions and those implicated in dyslexia (e.g., left angular gyrus, inferior prefrontal cortex) and the close proximity between others (IPS and supramarginal gyrus), comorbidity between dyscalculia seems highly probable but not inevitable. Moreover, since (as in dyslexia) different neural pathways are activated or required at different times or for different stages, it is not surprising that clinical manifestations and even diagnoses change over time.

This chapter has reviewed the history of conceptualization and diagnosis of these extremely common neurodevelopmental disorders, their presentations across the lifespan, and the underlying neuroscience. When possible threatment options have been discussed, a number of issues are especially challenging. For example, diagnosis of LD in the high aptitude individual remains controversial. In addition, many of these conditions co-exist, leading to shifting diagnosis over time, depending on the developmental challenges the individual is faced with as well as their underlying neural maturation. Research in dyslexia, dyscalculia and dysgraphia is greatly limited by poor consensus regarding diagnosis. Such complications make generalization between studies extraordinarily difficult. With coordinated work between disciplines and researchers, presumably these complicated issues will become clearer.

Notes

1 One of the authors of this chapter, R. Mapou, has proposed a definition for LD (2009a) that responds to the different needs of adults and attempts to incorporate concepts from neuropsychology and the 1990 Americans with Disabilities Act.
2 The DSM-5 recognized this concern and lowered the number of required symptoms for adults.
3 Thanks to Jessica Moriah Dean for technical assistance.

References

Aaron, P. G., Joshi, R. M., Palmer, H., Smith, N., & Kirby, E. (2002). Separating genuine cases of reading disability from reading deficits caused by predominantly inattentive ADHD behavior. *Journal of Learning Disabilities*, *35*(5), 425–435, 447.

Ackermann, H., Riecker, A., Mathiak, K., Erb, M., Grodd, W., & Wildgruber, D. (2001). Rate-dependent activation of a prefrontal-insular-cerebellar network during passive listening to trains of click stimuli: *An fMRI Study. Neuroreport*, *12*, 4087–4092.

Adisetiyo, V., Tabesh, A., Di Martino, A., Falangola, M. F., Castellanos, F. X., Jensen, J. H., & Helpern, J. A. (2014). Attention-deficit/hyperactivity disorder without comorbidity is associated with distinct atypical patterns of cerebral microstructural development. *Human Brain Mapping*, *35*(5), 2148–2162.

Ahmad, S. A., Rourke, B. P., & Drummond, C. (2002). A comparison of older children and adults with BPPD and NLD. *Journal of the International Neuropsychological Society*, *8*, 298.

Akutagava-Martins, G. C., Salatino-Oliveira, A., Kieling, C. C., Rohde, L. A., & Hutz, M. H. (2013). Genetics of attention-deficit/hyperactivity disorder: Current findings and future directions. *Expert Review of Neurotherapeutics*, *13*, 435–445.

Alarcón, M., DeFries, J. C., Light, J. G., & Pennington, B. F. (1997). A twin study of mathematics disability. *Journal of Learning Disabilities*, *30*(6), 617–623.

Alarcon, M., Pennington, B., Filipek, P.A., & DeFries, J. (2000). Etiology of neuroanatomical correlates of reading disability. *Developmental Neuropsychology*, *17*(3), 339–360.

Alexander, G. E., DeLong, M. R., & Strick, P. L. (1986). Parallel organization of functionally segregated circuits linking basal ganglia and cortex. (Research support, non-U.S. gov't research support, U.S. gov't, non-P.H.S. research support, U.S. gov't, P.H.S. review). *Annual Review of Neuroscience*, *9*, 357–381.

Altink, M. E., Rommelse, N. N., Slaats-Willemse, D. I., Vasquez, A. A., Franke, B., Buschgens, C. J., & Buitelaar, J. K. (2012). The dopamine receptor D4 7-repeat allele influences neurocognitive functioning, but this effect is moderated by age and ADHD status: An exploratory study. *The Official Journal of the World Federation of Societies of Biological Psychiatry*, *13*, 293–305.

Aman, C. J., Roberts, R. J., & Pennington, B. F. (1998). A neuropsychological examination of the underlying deficit in attention deficit hyperactivity disorder: Frontal lobe versus right parietal lobe theories. *Developmental Psychology*, *34*(5), 956–969.

American Psychiatric Association. (1968). *Diagnostic and Statistical Manual of Mental Disorders (DSM)* (2nd ed.). Washington, DC: American Psychiatric Association.

American Psychiatric Association. (1980). *Diagnostic and Statistical Manual of Mental Disorders (DSM)* (3rd ed.). Washington, DC: American Psychiatric Association.

American Psychiatric Association. (1987). *Diagnostic and Statistical Manual of Mental Disorders (DSM)* (3rd ed.—revised). Washington, DC: American Psychiatric Association.

American Psychiatric Association. (2000). *Diagnostic and Statistical Manual of Mental Disorders*. Text Revision/Edition 4. Washington, DC: American Psychiatric Publishing, Inc.

American Psychiatric Association. (1994). *Diagnostic and Statistical Manual of Mental Disorders (DSM)* (4th ed.). Washington, DC: American Psychological Association, 1792–1798.

American Psychiatric Association. (2013). *Diagnostic and Statistical Manual of Mental Disorders (DSM)* (5th ed.). Arlington, VA: American Psychiatric Publishing.

Amtmann, D., Abbott, R. D., & Berninger, V. W. (2007). Mixture growth models of RAN and RAS row by row: Insight into the reading system at work over time. *Reading and Writing*, *20*, 785–813.

Ansari, D. (2008). Effect of development and enculturation on number representation in the brain. *Nature Review of Neuroscience*, *9*, 278–291.

Ansari, D., & Karmiloff-Smith, A. (2002). Atypical trajectories of number development: A neuroconstructivist perspective. *Trends in Cognitive Sciences*, *6*(12), 511–516.

Archer, T., Oscar-Berman, M., & Blum, K. (2011). Epigenetics in developmental disorder: ADHD and endophenotypes. *Journal of Genetic Syndrome & Gene Therapy*, *2*(104), 1–33.

Aron, A. R., Robbins, T. W., & Poldrack, R. A. (2014). Inhibitrion and the right inferior frontal cortex: One decade on. *Trends in Cognitive Sciences*, *18*(4), 177–185.

Asbury, K., Dunn, J. F., & Plomin, R. (2006). Birthweight-discordance and differences in early parenting relate to monozygotic twin differences in behaviour problems and academic achievement at age 7. *Developmental Science*, *9*, F22–F31.

Asghari, V., Sanyal, S., Buchwaldt, S., Paterson, A., Jovanovic, V., & Van Tol, H. H. (1995). Modulation of intracellular cyclic AMP levels by different human dopamine D4 receptor variants. *Journal of Neurochemistry*, *65*, 1157–1165.

Ashkenazi, S., & Henik, A. (2010a). Attentional networks in developmental dyscalculia. *Behavioral and Brain Functions*, *6*(2), 1–12.

Ashkenazi, S., & Henik, A. (2010b). A dissociation between physical and mental number bisection in developmental dyscalculia. *Neuropsychologia*, *48*, 2861–2868.

Ashkenazi, S., & Henik, A. (2012). Does attentional training improve numerical processing in developmental dyscalculia? *Neuropsychology*, *26*, 45–56.

Ashkenazi, S., Rubinstein, O., & Henik, A. (2009). Attention, automaticity, and developmental dyscalculia. *Neuropsychology*, *23*, 535–540.

Ashtari, M., Kumra, S., Bhaskar, S. L., Clarke, T., Thaden, E., Cervellione, K. L., . . . Ardekani, B. A. (2005). Attention-deficit/hyperactivity disorder: A preliminary diffusion tensor imaging study. *Biological Psychiatry*, *57*(5), 448–455.

Austin, J. K., Harezlak, J., Dunn, D. W., Huster, G. A., Rose, D. F., & Ambrosius, W. T. (2001). Behavior problems in children before first recognized seizures. *Pediatrics*, *107*(1), 115–122.

Aylward, E. H., Reiss, A. L., Reader, M. J., Singer, H. S., Brown, J. E., & Denckla, M. B. (1996). Basal ganglia volumes in children with attention-deficit hyperactivity disorder. *Journal of Child Neurology*, *11*(2), 112–115.

Aylward, E. H., Richards, T., Berninger, V., Nagy, W., Field, K., Grimme, A., & Cramer, S. C. (2003). Instructional treatment associated with changes in brain activation in children with dyslexia. *Neurology*, *61*, 212–219.

Bacon, A. M., & Handley, S. J. (2010). Dyslexia and reasoning: The importance of visual processes. *British Journal of Psychology*, *101*, 433–452.

Baker, L., & Cantwell, D. P. (1992). Attention deficit disorder and speech/language disorders. *Comprehensive Mental Health Care*, *2*, 3–16.

Baird, J., Stevenson, J. C., & Williams, D. C. (2000). The evolution of ADHD: A disorder of communication? *Quarterly Review of Biology*, *75*(1), 17–35.

Bannon, M. J., & Whitty, C. J. (1997). Age-related and regional differences in dopamine transporter mRNA expression in human midbrain. *Neurology*, *48*, 969–977.

Bara, F., & Gentaz, E. (2011). Haptics in teaching handwriting: The role of perceptual and visuo-motor skills. *Human Movement Science*, *30*(4), 745–759.

Barkley, R. A. (1997a). *ADHD and the Nature of Self-Control.* New York: The Guilford Press.

Barkley, R. A. (1997b). Behavioral inhibition, sustained attention, and executive functions: Constructing a unifying theory of ADHD. *Psychological Bulletin, 121*, 65–94.

Barkley, R. A. (2006a). ADHD in adults: Developmental course and outcome of children with ADHD, and ADHD in clinic-referred adults. In R. A. Barkley (Ed.), *Attention-Deficit/Hyperactivity Disorder: A Handbook for Diagnosis and Treatment* (3rd ed., pp. 248–296). New York: Guilford Press.

Barkley, R. A. (2006b). A theory of ADHD. In R. A. Barkley (Ed.), *Attention-Deficit/Hyperactivity Disorder: A Handbook for Diagnosis and Treatment* (3rd ed., pp. 297–334). New York: Guilford Press.

Barkley, R. A. (2010). Against the status quo: Revising the diagnostic criteria for ADHD. *Journal of the American Academy of Child and Adolescent Psychiatry, 49*(3), 205–206.

Barkley, R. A. (2011a). *Barkley Adult ADHD Rating Scale-IV (BAARS-IV).* New York: Guilford Press.

Barkley, R. A. (2011b). *Barkley Deficits in Executive Functioning Scale (BDEFS).* New York: Guilford Press.

Barkley, R. A. (2012). *Executive Functions: What They Are, How They Work, and Why They Evolved.* New York: The Guilford Press.

Barkley, R. A., & Benton, C. M. (2010). *Taking Charge of Adult ADHD.* New York: Guilford Press.

Barkley, R. A., & Fischer, M. (2011). Predicting impairment in major life activities and occupational functioning in hyperactive children as adults: Self-reported executive function (EF) deficits vs. EF tests. *Developmental Neuropsychology, 36*, 137–161.

Barkley, R. A., Fischer, M., Smallish, L., & Fletcher, K. (2002). The persistence of attention-deficit/hyperactivity disorder into young adulthood as a function of reporting source and definition of disorder. *Journal of Abnormal Psychology, 111*, 279–289.

Barkley, R. A., Knouse, L., & Murphy, K. R. (2011). Correspondence and disparity in the self- and other ratings of current and childhood ADHD symptoms and impairment in adults with ADHD. *Psychological Assessment, 23*, 437–446.

Barkley, R. A., & Murphy, K. R. (2010). Impairment in occupational functioning and adult ADHD: The predictive utility of executive function (EF) ratings versus EF tests. *Archives of Clinical Neuropsychology, 25*, 157–173.

Barkley, R. A., & Murphy, K. R. (2011). The nature of executive function (EF) deficits in daily life activities in adults with ADHD and their relationship to performance on EF tests. *Journal of Psychopathology and Behavioral Assessment, 33*, 137–158.

Barkley, R. A., Murphy, K. R., & Fischer, M. (2008). *ADHD in Adults: What the Science Says.* New York: Guilford.

Barkley, R. A., Shelton, T. L., Crosswait, C., Moorehouse, M., Fletcher, K., Barrett, S., . . . Metevia, L. (2002). Preschool children with disruptive behavior: Three-year outcome as a function of adaptive disability. *Developmental Psychopathology, 14*(1), 45–67.

Barry, T. D., Lyman, R. D., & Klinger, L. G. (2002). Academic underachievement and attention-deficit/hyperactivity disorder: The negative impact of symptom severity on school performance. *Journal of School Psychology, 40*(3), 259–283.

Bemporad, J. R. (2001). Aspects of psychotherapy with adults with attention deficit disorder. In J. S. Wasserstein, L. E. Wolf, & F. F. Lefever (Eds.), *Adult Attention Deficit Disorder: Brain Mechanisms and Outcomes* (Vol. 931, pp. 302–309). Annals of the New York Academy of Sciences.

Ben-Yehudah, G., Sackett, E., Malchi-Ginzberg, L., & Ahissar, M. (2001). Impaired temporal contrast sensitivity in dyslexics specific to retain-and-compare paradigms. *Brain, 124*, 1381–1395.

Berger, H. (1926). Uber rechenstorunger bei herderkraunkunger des grosshirns. *Archives of Psychiatry and Neurology, 78*, 236–263.

Berger, I., Slobodin, O., Aboud, M., Melamed, J., & Cassuto, H. (2013). Maturational delay in ADHD: Evidence from CPT. *Frontiers in Human Neuroscience, 7.*

Berger, S. L. (2007). The complex language of chromatin regulation during transcription. *Nature, 447*, 407–412.

Berlin, J. (1887). *Eine besondere art der Wortblindhert. Dyslexie.* Neuer Medicinischer, Verlaz Von J. F. Bergman in Weisbaden.

Bernal, B., & Altman, N. (2009). Neural networks of motor and cognitive inhibition are dissociated between brain hemispheres: An fMRI study. *International Journal of Neuroscience, 119*(10), 1848–1880.

Berninger, V. W., Abbott, R. D., Thomson, J., Wagner, R., Swanson, H. L., Wijsman, E. M., & Raskind, W. (2006). Modeling phonological core deficits within a working memory architecture in children and adults with developmental dyslexia. *Scientific Studies of Reading, 10*, 165–198.

Berninger, V. W., & May, M. O. (2011). Evidence-based diagnosis and treatment for specific learning disabilities involving impairments in written and/or oral language. *Journal of Learning Disabilities, 44*(2), 167–183.

Berninger, V. W., Nielsen, K. H., Abbott, R. D., Wijsman, E. M., & Raskind, W. (2008). Gender differences in severity of writing and reading disabilities. *Journal of School Psychology, 46*, 151–172.

Best, M., & Demb, J. B. (1999). Normal planum temporale asymmetry in dyslexics with a magnocellular pathway deficit. *Neuroreport, 10*, 607–612.

Best, M., Williams, J. M., & Coccaro, E. F. (2002). Evidence for a dysfunctional prefrontal circuit in patients with an impulsive aggressive disorder. *Proceedings of the National Academy of Sciences, 99*(12), 8448–8453.

Biederman, J., Faraone, S. V., Keenan, K., Benjamin, J., Krifcher, B., Moore, C., & Tsuang, M. T. (1992). Further evidence for family-genetic risk factors in attention deficit hyperactivity disorder: Patterns of comorbidity in probands and relatives psychiatrically and pediatrically referred samples. *Archives of General Psychiatry, 49*, 728–738.

Biederman, J., Faraone, S. V., Mick, E., Wozniak, J., Chen, L., Ouellette, C., & Lelon, E. (1996). Attention-deficit hyperactivity disorder and juvenile mania: An overlooked comorbidity? *Journal of the American Academy of Child and Adolescent Psychiatry, 34*, 867–876.

Biederman, J., Faraone, S. V., Monuteaux, M. C., Bober, M., & Cadogen, E. (2004). Gender effects on attention-deficit/hyperactivity disorder in adults, revisited. *Biological Psychiatry, 55*, 692–700.

Biederman, J., Faraone, S. V., Spencer, T., Wilens, T., Mick, E., & Lapey, K. A. (1994). Gender differences in a sample of adults with attention deficit hyperactivity disorder. *Psychiatry Research, 53*, 13–29.

Biederman, J., Faraone, S. V., Spencer, T., Wilens, T., Norman, D., Lapey, K. A., . . . Doyle, A. (1993). Patterns of psychiatric comorbidity, cognition, and psychosocial functioning in adults with attention deficit hyperactivity disorder. *American Journal of Psychiatry, 150*, 1792–1798.

Biederman, J., Mick, E., & Faraone, S. V. (2000). Age dependent decline of ADHD symptoms revisited: Impact of remission definition and symptom subtype. *American Journal of Psychiatry*, *157*, 816–818.

Biederman, J., Monuteaux, M. C., Mick, E., Spencer, T., Wilens, T. E., Silva, J. M., . . . Faraone, S. V. (2006). Young adult outcome of attention deficit hyperactivity disorder: A controlled 10-year follow-up study. *Psychological Medicine*, *36*, 167–179.

Biederman, J., Newcorn, J., & Sprich, S. (1991). Comorbidity of attention deficit hyperactivity disorder with conduct, depressive, anxiety, and other disorders. *American Journal of Psychiatry*, *148*, 564–577.

Biederman, J., Wilens, T., Mick, E., Milberger, S., Spencer, T. J., & Faraone, S. V. (1995). Psychoactive substance use disorders in adults with attention deficit hyperactivity disorder (ADHD): Effects of ADHD and psychiatric comorbidity. *American Journal of Psychiatry*, *152*, 1652–1658.

Bin Sun, H., Ruan, Y., Xu, Z. C., & Yokota, H. (2002). Involvement of the calcium-independent receptor for alpha-latrotoxin in brain ischemia. *Brain Research*, *104*, 246–249.

Birch, S., & Chase, C. (2004). Visual and language processing deficits in compensated and uncompensated college students with dyslexia. *Journal of Learning Disabilities*, *37*, 389–410.

Blachman, B. (1984). Relationship of rapid naming ability and language analysis skills to kindergarten and first-grade reading achievement. *Journal of Educational Psychology*, *76*, 610–622.

Bledsoe, J. C., Semrud-Clikeman, M., & Pliszka, S. R. (2013). Anterior cingulate cortex and symptom severity in attention-deficit/hyperactivity disorder. (Article). *Journal of Abnormal Psychology*, *122*(2), 558–565.

Boada, R., Willcutt, E. G., & Pennington, B. F. (2012). Understanding the comorbidity between dyslexia and attention-deficit/hyperactivity disorder. *Topics in Language Disorders*, *32*(3), 264–284.

Boles, D. B., Adair, L. P., & Joubert, A. M. (2009). A preliminary study of lateralized processing in attention-deficit/hyperactivity disorder. *Journal of General Psychology*, *136*(3), 243–258.

Bond, E. D., & Smith, L. H. (1935). Post-encephalitic behavior disorders: A ten year review of the Franklin school. *American Journal of Psychiatry*, *92*(1), 17–33.

Botvinick, M. M., & Cohen, J. D. (2014). The computational and neural basis of cognitive control: Charted territory and new frontiers. *Cognitive Science*, *38*(6), 1249–1285

Brambati, S. M., Termine, C., Ruffino, M., Stella, M. G., Fazio, F., Cappa, S. F., & Perani, D. (2004). Regional reductions of gray matter volume in familial dyslexia. *Neurology*, *63*, 742–745.

Braze, D., Tabor, W., Shankweiler, D. P., & Mencl, W. E. (2007). Speaking up for vocabulary: Reading skill differences in young adults. *Journal of Learning Disabilities*, *40*, 226–243.

Breier, J. I., Gray, L. C., Klaas, P., Fletcher, J. M., & Foorman, B. (2002). Dissociation of sensitivity and response bias in children with attention-deficit/hyperactivity disorder during central auditory masking. *Neuropsychology*, *16*(1), 28–34.

Breslau, N., & Chilcoat, H. D. (2000). Psychiatric sequelae of low birth weight at 11 years of age. *Biological Psychiatry*, *47*, 1005–1011.

Breslin, F. C., & Pole, J. D. (2009). Work injury risk among young people with learning disabilities and attention-deficit/hyperactivity disorder in Canada. *American journal of public health*, *99*(8), 1423–1430.

Broadbent, W. H. (1895). Note on Dr. Hinshelwood's communication on word-blindness and visual memory. *Lancet*, *1*, 18.

Broca, P. (1861). Nouvelle observation d'aphemie produite par une lesion de la motie posterieure des deuxieme et troisieme circonvolutions frontales. *Bulletin de la Societe d'Anatomiqu3*, *6*, 398–407.

Broen, P. A., Moller, K. T., Carlstrom, J., Doyle, S. S., Devers, M., & Keenan, K. M. (1996). Comparison of the hearing histories of children with and without cleft palate. *The Cleft Palate-Craniofacial Journal*, *33*(2), 127-133.

Brooks, B. L. (2010). Seeing for forest for the trees: Prevalence of low scores on the wechsler intelligence scale for children, fourth edition (WISC-IV). *Psychological Assessment*, *22*, 650–656.

Bruce, B., Thernlund, G., & Nettelbladt, U. (2006). ADHD and language impairment. *European Child & Adolescent Psychiatry*, *15*(1), 52–60.

Brunswick, N., McCrory, E., Price, C. J., Frith, C. D., & Frith, U. (1999). Explicit and implicit processing of words and pseudowords by adult developmental dyslexics: A search for Wernicke's Wortschatz? *Brain*, *122*, 1901–1917.

Buelow, M. T., & Frakey, L. L. (2013). Math anxiety differentially affects WAIS-IV arithmetic performance in undergraduates. *Archives of Clinical Neuropsychology*, *28*, 356–362.

Bush, G. (2011). Cingulate, frontal, and parietal cortical dysfunction in attention-deficit/hyperactivity disorder. *Biological Psychiatry*, *69*(12), 1160–1167.

Butterworth, B. (2010). Foundational numerical capacities and the origins of dyscalculia. *Trends in Cognitive Sciences*, *14*(12), 534–541

Butterworth, B., Varma, S., & Laurilland, D. (2011). Dyscalculia: From brain to education. *Science*, *332*, 1049–1053.

Campbell, S. B. (1995). Behavior problems in the preschool child: A review of the recent literature. *Journal of Child Psychology and Psychiatry*, *36*, 113–149.

Cantwell, D. P. (1983). Diagnostic validity of the hyperactive-child (attention deficit disorder with hyperactivity) syndrome. *Psychiatric Developments*, *1*(3), 277–300.

Cao, Q. J., Shu, N., An, L., Wang, P., Sun, L., Xia, M. R., & He, Y. (2013). Probabilistic diffusion tractography and graph theory analysis reveal abnormal white matter structural connectivity networks in drug-naive boys with attention deficit/hyperactivity disorder. *Journal of Neuroscience*, *33*(26), 10676–10687.

Cardon, L. R., Smith, S. D., Fulker, D. W., Kimberling, W. J., Pennington, B. F., & DeFries, J. C. (1994). Quantitative trait locus for reading disability on chromosome 6. *Science*, *266*, 276–279.

Carmel, M., Zarchi, O., Michaelovsky, E., Frisch, A., Patya, M., Green, T., & Weizman, A. (2014). Association of COMT and PRODH gene variants with intelligence quotient (IQ) and executive functions in 22q11.2DS subjects. *Journal of Psychiatric Research*, *56*, 28–35.

Caron, C., & Rutter, M. (1991). Comorbidity in child psychopathology: Concepts, issues, and research strategies. *Journal of Child Psychology and Psychiatry*, *32*, 1063–1080.

Carter, C. S., Botvinick, M. M., & Cohen, J. D. (1999). The contribution of the anterior cingulate cortex to executive processes in cognition. *Reviews in the Neurosciences*, *10*(1), 49–57.

Carter, C. S., Krener, P., Chaderjian, M., Northcutt, C., & Wolfe, V. (1995). Abnormal processing of irrelevant information in attention-deficit hyperactivity disorder. *Psychiatry Research*, *56*(1), 59–70.

Casals, F., & Bertranpetit, J. (2012). Genetics: Human genetic variation, shared and private. *Science*, *337*, 39–40.

Casey, B. J., Castellanos, F. X., Giedd, J. N., Marsh, W. L., Hamburger, S. D., Schubert, A. B., & Rapport, J. L. (1997). Implication of right frontostriatal circuitry in response inhibition and attention-deficit/hyperactivity disorder. *Journal of the American Academy of Child and Adolescent Psychiatry*, *36*(3), 374–383.

Castellanos, F. X., Giedd, J. N., Berquin, P. C., Walter, J. M., Sharp, W., Tran, T., & Rapport, J. L. (2001). Quantitative brain magnetic resonance imaging in girls with attention-deficit/hyperactivity disorder. *Archives of General Psychiatry*, *58*(3), 289–295.

Castellanos, F. X., Giedd, J. N., Eckburg, P., Marsh, W. L., Vaituzis, A. C., Kaysen, D., . . . Rapoport, J. L. (1994). Quantitative morphology of the caudate-nucleus in attention-deficit hyperactivity disorder. *American Journal of Psychiatry*, *151*(12), 1791–1796.

Castellanos, F. X., Giedd, J. N., Marsh, W. L., Hamburger, S. D., Vaituzis, A. C., Dickstein, D. P., . . . Rapoport, J. L. (1996). Quantitative brain magnetic resonance imaging in attention-deficit hyperactivity disorder. *Archives of General Psychiatry*, *53*(7), 607–616.

Castellanos, F. X., Lee, P. P., Sharp, W., Jeffries, N. O., Greenstein, D. K., Clasen, L. S., . . . Rapport, J. L. (2002). Developmental trajectories of brain volume abnormalities in children and adolescents with attention-deficit/hyperactivity disorder. *Journal of the American Medical Association*, *288*, 1740–1748.

Castellanos, F. X., & Proal, E. (2012). Large-scale brain systems in ADHD: Beyond the prefrontal-striatal model. *Trends in Cognitive Science*, *16*, 17–26.

Castellanos, F. X., Sonuga-Barle, E. J. S., Scheres, A., Di Martino, A., Hyde, C., & Walters, J. R. (2005). Varieties of ADHD-related intra-individual variability. *Biological Psychiatry*, *57*, 1416–1423.

Castellanos, F. X., & Tannock, R. (2002). Neuroscience of attention-deficit/hyperactivity disorder: The search for endophenotypes. *Nature Reviews Neuroscience*, *3*, 617–628.

Cederlof, M., Ohlsson Gotby, A., Larsson, H., Serlachius, E., Boman, M., Langstrom, N., & Lichtenstein, P. (2014). Klinefelter syndrome and risk of psychosis, autism and ADHD. *Journal of Psychiatric Research*, *48*(1), 128–130.

Cederlöf, M., Gotby, A. O., Larsson, H., Serlachius, E., Boman, M., Långström, N., . . . Lichtenstein, P. (2014). *Klinefelter Syndrome and Risk of Psychosis, Autism and ADHD.*

Cepeda, N. J., Cepeda, M. L., & Kramer, A. F. (2000). Task switching and attention deficit hyperactivity disorder. *Journal of Abnormal Chid Psychology*, *28*(3): 213–226.

Chamberlain, S. R., Hampshire, A., Müller, U., Rubia, K., Del Campo, N., Craig, K., . . . Sahakian, B. J. (2009). Atomoxetine modulates right inferior frontal activation during inhibitory control: A pharmacological functional magnetic resonance imaging study. *Biological Psychiatry*, *65*(7), 550–555.

Chandler, V. L. (2007). Paramutation: From maize to mice. *Cell*, *128*, 641–645.

Chang, Z., Lichtenstein, P., Asherson, P. J., & Larsson, H. (2013). Developmental twin study of attention problems: High heritabilities throughout development. *JAMA Psychiatry*, *70*, 311–318.

Chelune, G. J., Ferguson, W., Koon, R., & Dickey, T. O. (1986). Frontal lobe disinhibition in attention deficit disorder. *Child Psychiatry & Human Development*, *16*(4), 221–234.

Chess, S. (1960). Diagnosis and treatment of the hyperactive child. *New York State Journal of Medicine*, *60*, 2379–2385.

Chilosi, A. M., Brizzolara, D., Lami, L., Pizzoli, C., Gasperini, C., Pecini, C., & Zoccolotti, P. (2009). Reading and spelling disabilities in children with and without a history of early language delay: A neuropsychological and linguistic study. *Child Neuropsychology*, *15*(6), 582–604.

Choudhry, Z., Sengupta, S. M., Grizenko, N., Fortier, M. E., Thakur, G. A., Bellingham, J., & Joober, R. (2012). LPHN3 and attention-deficit/hyperactivity disorder: Interaction with maternal stress during pregnancy. *Journal of Child Psychology and Psychiatry*, *53*, 892–902.

Christensen, C. A. (2009). The critical role handwriting plays in the ability to produce high-quality written text. In R. Beard, D. Myhill, J. Riley, & M. Nystrand (Eds.), *The Sage Handbook of Writing Development*. London: Sage.

Cirino, P. T., Israelian, M. K., Morris, M. K., & Morris, R. D. (2005). Evaluation of the double-deficit hypothesis in college students referred for learning difficulties. *Journal of Learning Disabilities*, *38*, 29–44.

Cirino, P. T., Morris, M. K., & Morris, R. D. (2002). Neuropsychological concomitants of calculation skills in college students referred for learning difficulties. *Developmental Neuropsychology*, *21*, 201–218.

Cirino, P. T., Morris, M. K., & Morris, R. D. (2007). Semantic, executive, and visuospatial abilities in mathematical reasoning of referred college students. *Assessment*, *14*, 94–104.

Clarke, A. R., Barry, R. J., McCarthy, R., Selikowitz, M., & Brown, C. R. (2002). EEG evidence for a new conceptualisation of attention deficit hyperactivity disorder. *Clinical Neurophysiology*, *113*(7), 1036–1044.

Clark, T., Feehan, C., Tinline, C.,& Vostanis, P. (1999). Autistic symptoms in children with attention deficit-hyperactivity disorder. *European Child & Adolescent Psychiatry*, *8*(1), 435–445.

Cleaver, R. L., & Whitman, R. D. (1998). Right hemisphere, white matter learning disabilities associated with depression in an adolescent and young adult psychiatric population. *Journal of Nervous and Mental Disease*, *186*, 561–565.

Clements, S., & Peters, J. E. (1962). Minimal brain dysfunctions in the school-aged child: Diagnosis and treatment. *Archives of General Psychiatry*, *6*, 185–197.

Cohen, M., Campbell, R., & Yaghmai, F. (1989). Neuropathological abnormalities in developmental dysphasia. *Annals of Neurology*, *25*(6), 567–570.

Cohen, N.J., Vallance, D.D., Barwick, M., Im, N., Menna, R., Horodezky, N.B., & Isaacson, L. (2000). The interface between ADHD and language impairment: An examination of language, achievement, and cognitive processing. *The Journal of Child Psychology and Psychiatry and Allied Disciplines*, *41*(3), 353–362.

Cohn, R. (1968). Developmental dyscalculia. *Pediatric Clinicians of North America*, *15*(3), 651–658.

Connelly, V., Campbell, S., MacLean, M., & Barnes, J. (2006). Contribution of lower order skills to the written composition of college students with and without dyslexia. *Developmental Neuropsychology*, *29*, 175–196.

Connor, D. F. (2002). Preschool attention deficit hyperactivity disorder: A review of prevalence, diagnosis, neurobiology, and stimulant treatment. *Journal of Developmental Behavior Pediatrics*, *23*, S1–S9.

Cotard, J. (1868). *Etude sur l'atrophie cerebrale*. Paris: A. Parent.

Courvoisie, H., Hooper, S. R., Fine, C., Kwock, L., & Castillo, M. (2004). Neurometabolic functioning and neuropsychological correlates in children with ADHD-H: Preliminary findings. (Article). *Journal of Neuropsychiatry and Clinical Neurosciences*, *16*(1), 63–69

Crichton, A. (1798). *On Attention, and Its Diseases* (Reprinted by AMS Press, New York, 1976 ed.). London: Caddell, Junior and Davies.

Crozier, S., Sirigu, A., Lehericy, S., van de Moortele, P. F., Pillon, B., Grafman, J., & LeBihan, D. (1999). Distinct prefrontal activations in processing sequence at the sentence and script level: An fMRI study. *Neuropsychologia*, *37*, 1469–1476.

Cubillo, A., Halari, R., Ecker, C., Giampietro, V., Taylor, E., & Rubia, K. (2010). Reduced activation and inter-regional functional connectivity of fronto-striatal networks in adults with childhood attention-deficit hyperactivity disorder (ADHD) and persisting symptoms during tasks of motor inhibition and cognitive switching. *Journal of Psychiatry Research*, *44*(10), 629–639.

Cummings, J. L. (1993). Frontal-subcortical circuits and human behavior. *Archives of Neurology*, *50*, 873–880.

Cutting, L. E., & Denckla, M. B. (2003). Attention: Relationships between attention-deficit hyperactivity disorder and learning disabilities. In H. L. Swanson, K. R. Harris, & S. Graham (Eds.), *Handbook of Learning Disabilities* (pp. 125–139). New York: Guilford Press.

Daniel, S. S., Walsh, A. K., Goldston, D. B., Arnold, E. M., Reboussin, B. A., & Wood, F. B. (2006). Suicidality, school dropout, and reading problems among adolescents. *Journal of Learning Disabilities*, *39*(6), 507–514.

Darvesh, S., Hopkins, D. A., & Geula, C. (2003). Neurobiology of butyrylcholinesterase. *Nature Reviews*, *4*, 131–138.

Dastjerdi, M., Ozker, M., Foster, B. L., Rangarajan, V., & Parvizi, J. (2013). Numerical processing in the human parietal cortex during experimental and natural conditions. *Nature Communications*, *4*(2528), 1–11.

David, C. V. (2012). Working memory deficits in Math learning difficulties: A meta-analysis. *International Journal of Developmental Disabilities*, *58*(2), 67–84.

Davies, S., Heyman, I., & Goodman, R. (2003). A population survey of mental health problems in children with epilepsy. [Article]. *Developmental Medicine and Child Neurology*, *45*(5), 292–295.

De Ajuriaguerra, J., Auzias, M., Coumes, F., Denner A., Lavondes-Monod V., Perron R., & Stambak M. (1979). *Children's Writing: The Evolution of Writing and Its Difficulties* (3rd ed.). Paris: Delachaux & Niestle.

DeFries, J. C., & Alarcon, M. (1996). Genetic of specific reading disability. *Mental Retardation and Developmental Disabilities Research Reveiws*, *2*, 39–47.

DeFries, J. C., Alarcon, M., & Olson, R. K. (1997). Genetics and dyslexia: Developmental differences in the etiologies of reading and spelling deficits. In C. Hulme & M. Snowling (Eds.), *Dyslexia: Biological Bases Identification and Intervention* (pp. 20–37). London: Whurr Publishing.

DeFries, J. C., Singer, S. M., Foch, T. T., & Lewitter, F. I. (1978). Familial nature of reading disability. *British Journal of Psychiatry*, *132*, 361–367.

de Gelder, B., & Vrooman, J. (1996). Auditory illusions as evidence for a role of the syllable in adult developmental dyslexics. *Brain and Language*, *52*, 373–385.

Dehaene, S., & Cohen, L. (1997). Cerebral pathways for calculation: Double dissociation between rote verbal and quantitative knowledge of arithmetic. *Cortex*, *33*, 219–250.

Dehaene, S., Dehaene-Lambertz, G., & Cohen, L. (1998). Abstract representations of numbers in the animal and human brain. *Trends in Neuroscience*, *21*, 355–361.

Dehaene, S., Piazza, M., Pinel, P., & Cohen, L. (2003). Three parietal circuits for number processing. *Cognitive Neuropsychology*, *20*, 487–506.

Dehaene, S., Molko, N., Cohen, L., & Wilson, A. (2004). Arithmetic and the brain. *Current Opinion in Neurobiology*, *14*, 218–224.

Dehaene, S., Tzourio, N., Frak, V., Reynaud, L., Cohen, L., Mehler, J., & Mazoyer, B. (1996). Cerebral activation during number multiplication and comparison: A PET study. *Neuropsychologia*, *34*, 1097–1106.

Dejerine, J. J. (1892). Contribution a l'etude anatomo-pathologique et clinique des differentes varietes de cecute verbale. *Memoires Societe Biologique*, *4*, 61–90.

Delazar, M., Domahs, F., Bartha, L., Brenneis, C., Lochy, A., Trieb, T., & Benke, T. (2003). Learning complex arithmetic: An fMRI study. *Cognitive Brain Research*, *18*, 76–88.

Demonet, J. F., Taylor, M. J., & Chaix, Y. (2004). Developmental dyslexia. *The Lancet*, *363*, 1451–1452.

Denckla, M. B. (1993). The child with developmental disabilities grown up: Adult residua of childhood disorders. *Neurological Clinics*, *11*(1), 105–125.

Denckla, M. B., & Rudel, R. G. (1976). Rapid "automatized" naming (R.A.N): Dyslexia differentiated from other learning disabilities. *Neuropsychologia*, *14*(4), 471–479.

Depue, B. E., Burgess, G. C., Bidwell, L. C., Willcutt, E. G., & Banich, M. T. (2010). Behavioral performance predicts grey matter reductions in the right inferior frontal gyrus in young adults with combined type ADHD. [Article]. *Psychiatry Research-Neuroimaging*, *182*(3), 231–237.

Desoete, A., & Gregoire, J. (2007). Numerical competence in young children and in children with mathematical learning disabilities. *Learning and Individual Differences*, *16*, 351–367.

Deutsch, G. K., Dougherty, R. F., Bammer, R., Siok, W. T., Gabrieli, J. D., & Wandell, B. (2005). Children's reading performance is correlated with white matter structure measured by diffusion tensor imaging. *Cortex*, *41*, 354–363.

Devine, A., Soltesz, F., Nobes, A., Goswami, & Szucs, D. (2013). Gender differences in developmental dyscalculia depend on diagnostic criteria. *Learning and Instruction*, *27*, 31–39.

DHHS. (2003). *New Freedom Commission on Mental Health. Achieving the promise: Transforming mental health care in America*. Final report. Rockville, MD.

Dobler, V. B., Anker, S., Gilmore, J., Robertson, I. H., Atkinson, J., & Manly, T. (2005). Asymmetric deterioration of spatial awareness with diminishing levels of alertness in normal children and children with ADHD. (Review). *Journal of Child Psychology and Psychiatry*, *46*(11), 1230–1248.

Doehnert, M., Brandeis, D., Imhof, K., Drechsler, R., & Steinhausen, H. C. (2010). Mapping attention-deficit/hyperactivity disorder from childhood to adolescence-no neurophysiologic evidence for a developmental lag of attention but some for inhibition. *Biological Psychiatry*, *67*(7), 608–616.

Douglas, V. I. (1972). Stop, look, and listen: The problem of sustained attention and impulse control in hyperactive and normal children. *Canadian Journal of Behavioral Science*, *4*, 259–282.

Douglas, V. I. (1976). Research on hyperactivity: Stage two. *Journal Abnormal Child Psychology*, *4*(4), 307–308.

Duara, R., Kushch, A., Gross-Glen, K., Barker, W. W., Jallad, B., Pascal, S., & Loewenstein, D. A. (1991). Neuroanatomic differences between dyslexic and normal readers on magnetic resonance imaging scans. *Archives of Neurology*, *48*, 410–416.

Ducharme, S., Hudziak, J. J., Botteron, K. N., Albaugh, M. D., Nguyen, T. V., Karama, S., . . . Brain Dev Cooperative, G. (2012). Decreased regional cortical thickness and thinning rate are associated with inattention symptoms in healthy children. *Journal of the American Academy of Child and Adolescent Psychiatry*, *51*(1), 18–27.

Duffy, F. H., Denckla, M. B., Bartels, P. H., Sandini, G., & Kiessling, L. S. (1980). Dyslexia: Automated diagnosis by computerized classification of brain electrical activity. *Annals of Neurology*, *7*, 421–428.

DuPaul, G. J., McGoey, K. E., Eckert, T. L., & VanBrakle, J. (2001). Preschool children with attention-deficit/hyperactivity disorder: Impairments in behavioral, social, and school functioning. *Journal of the American Academy of Child Adolescent Psychiatry*, *40*(5), 508–515.

Durston, S., Fossella, J. A., Casey, B. J., Pol, H. E. H., Galvan, A., Schnack, H. G., . . . van Engeland, H. (2005). Differential effects of DRD4 and DAT1 genotype on fronto-striatal gray matter volumes in a sample of subjects with attention deficit hyperactivity disorder, their unaffected siblings, and controls. *Molecular Psychiatry*, *10*(7), 678–685.

Durston, S., Pol, H. E. H., Schnack, H. G., Buitelaar, J. K., Steenhuis, M. P., Minderaa, R. B., . . . van Engeland, H. (2004). Magnetic resonance imaging of boys with attention-deficit/hyperactivity disorder and their unaffected siblings. *Journal of the American Academy of Child and Adolescent Psychiatry*, *43*(3), 332–340.

Ebaugh, F. G. (1923). Neuropsychiatric sequelae of acute epidemic encephalitis in children. *American Journal of Diseases of Children*, *25*, 89–97.

Eckert, M. A., Leonard, C. M., Richards, T. L., Aylwards, E. H., Thompson, J., & Berninger, V. W. (2003). Anatomical correlations of dyslexia: Frontal and cerebellar findings. *Brain*, *126*(2), 482–494.

Eden, G. F., Jones, K. M., Cappell, K., Gareau, L., Wood, F. B., Zeffiro, T. A., . . . Flowers, D. L. (2004). Neuronal changes following remediation in adult developmental dyslexia. *Neuron*, *44*, 411–422.

Education for All Handicapped Children Act of 1975. Public Law 94–142, 89 Stat. 773 (1975).

Education, U. S. D. o. (2007). *2005 Report to Congress on the Implementation of the Individuals With Disabilities Education Act* (Vol. 1). Washington, DC: U.S. DoED.

Eger, E., Sterzer, P. P., Russ, M. O., Giraud, A. L., & Kleinschmidt, A. (2003). A supramodal number representation in human intraparietal cortex. *Neuron*, *37*, 719–725.

Elbro, C. (1998). When reading is "readn" or somthn: Distinctiveness of phonological representations of lexical items in normal and disabled readers. *Scandinavian Journal of Psychology*, *39*, 149–153.

Elia, J., Gai, X., Xie, H. M., Perin, J. C., Geiger, E., Glessner, J. T., . . . D'Arcy, M. (2010). Rare structural variants found in attention-deficit hyperactivity disorder are preferentially associated with neurodevelopmental genes. *Molecular Psychiatry*, *15*, 637–646.

Elia, J., Glessner, J. T., Wang, K., Takahashi, N., Shtir, C. J., Hadley, D., . . . Hakonarson, H. (2012). Genome-wide copy number variation study associates metabotropic glutamate receptor gene networks with attention deficit hyperactivity disorder. *Nature Genetics*, *44*, 78–84.

Elia, J., Laracy, S., Allen, J., Nissley-Tsiopinis, J., & Borgmann-Winter, K. (2012). Epigenetics: Genetics versus life experiences. *Current Topics in Behavioral Neuroscience*, *9*, 317–340.

Ellison-Wright, I., Ellison-Wright, Z., & Bullmore, E. (2008). Structural brain change in attention deficit/ hyperactivity disorder identified by meta-analysis. *BMC Psychiatry*, *8*(1), 51.

El-Sayed, E., Larsson, J. O., Persson, H. E., Santosh, P. J., & Rydelius, P. A. (2003). "Maturational lag" hypothesis of attention deficit hyperactivity disorder: An update. *Acta Paediatrica*, *92*(7), 776–784.

Ent, D. V., Lehn, H., Derks, E. M., Hudziak, J. J., Van Strien, N. M., Veltman, D. J., . . . Boomsma, D. I. (2007). A structural MRI study in monozygotic twins concordant or discordant for attention/hyperactivity problems: Evidence for genetic and environmental heterogeneity in the developing brain. *Neuroimage*, *35*(3), 1004–1020.

Epstein, J. N., Conners, C. K., Ehrhardt, D., March, J. S., & Swanson, J. M. (1997). Asymmetrical hemispheric control of visual-spatial attention in adults with attention deficit hyperactivity disorder. *Neuropsychology*, *11*, 467–473.

Fagerheim, T., Raeymaekers, P., Tonnessen, F. E., Pedersen, M., Tranebjaerg, L., & Lubs, H. A. (1999). A new gene (DYX3) for dyslexia is located on chromosome 2. *Journal of Medical Genetics*, *1*, 664–669.

Faraone, S. V., & Biederman, J. (1997). Do attention deficit hyperactivity disorder and major depression share familial risk factors? *Journal of Nervous & Mental Disease*, *185*, 533–541.

Faraone, S. V., Biederman, J., Chen, W. J., Milberger, S., Warburton, R., & Tsuang, M. T. (1995). Genetic heterogeneity in attention-deficit hyperactivity disorder (ADHD): Gender, psychiatric comorbidity, and maternal ADHD. *Journal of Abnormal Psychology*, *104*, 334–345.

Faraone, S. V., Biederman, J., & Friedman, D. (2000). Validity of DSM-IV subtypes of attention-deficit/hyperactivity disorder: A family study perspective. *Journal of the American Academy of Child & Adolescent Psychiatry*, *39*, 300–307.

Faraone, S. V., Biederman, J., Keenan, K., & Tsuang, M. T. (1991). A family-genetic study of girls with DSM-III attention deficit disorder. *American Journal of Psychiatry*, *148*, 112–117.

Faraone, S. V., Biederman, J., & Mick, E. (2006). The age-dependent decline of attention-deficit hyperactivity disorder: A meta-analysis of follow-up studies. *Psychological Medicine*, *36*, 159–165.

Faraone, S. V., Biederman, J., & Milberger, S. (1994). An exploratory study of ADHD among second-degree relatives of ADHD children. *Biological Psychiatry*, *35*, 398–402.

Faraone, S. V., Spencer, T. J., Montano, C. B., & Biederman, J. (2004). Attention-deficit/hyperactivity disorder in adults: A survey of current practice in psychiatry and primary care. *Archives of Internal Medicine*, *164*(11), 1221–1226.

Feigenson, L., Dehaene, S., & Spelke, E. (2004). Core systems of number. *Trends in Cognitive Sciences*, *8*(7), 307–314.

Feldman, H., Yeatmen, J., Lee, E. S., Barde, L. H., & Gaman-Bean, S. (2010). Diffusion tensor imaging: A review for pediatric researchers and clinicians. *Journal of Developmental and Behavioral Pediatrics*, *31*, 346–356.

Fergusson, D. M., & Horwood, L. J. (1992). Attention deficit and reading achievement. *Journal of Child Psychology and Psychiatry*, *33*(2), 375–385.

Filipek, P. A., Semrud-Clikeman, M., Steingard, R. J., Renshaw, P. F., Kennedy, D. N., & Biederman, J. (1997). Volumetric MRI analysis comparing subjects having attention-deficit hyperactivity disorder with normal controls. *Neurology*, *48*(3), 589–601.

Finucci, J. M., Guthric, J. T., Childs, A. L., Abbey, H., & Childs, B. (1976). The genetics of specific reading disability. *Annals of Human Genetics*, *40*, 1–23.

Fisher, S. E., & DeFries, J. C. (2002). Developmental dyslexia: Genetic dissection of a complex cognitive trait. *Nature Reviews Neuroscience*, *3*(10), 767–780.

Fisher, S. E., Francks, C., Marlow, A. J., MacPhie, I. L., Newbury, D. F., Cardon, L. R., . . . Monaco, A. P. (2002). Independent genome-wide scans identify a chromosome 18 quantitative-trait locus influencing dyslexia. *Nature Genetics*, *30*, 86–91.

Fisher, S. E., Marlow, A. J., Lamb, J., Maestrini, E., Williams, D. F., Richardson, A. J., . . . Weeks, D. E. (1999). A quantitative-trait locus on chromosome 6p influences different aspects of developmental dyslexia. *American Journal of Human Genetics*, *64*, 146–156.

Fletcher, J. M., Lyon, G. R., Fuchs, L. S., & Barnes, M. A. (2007). *Learning Disabilities: From Identification to Intervention*. New York: Guilford Press.

Frank, Y. (2014). *Specific Learning Disabilities*. New York: Oxford University Press.

Frank, Y., Seiden, J., & Napolitano, B. (1996). Visual event related potentials and reaction time in normal adults, normal children and children with attention deficit hyperactivity disorder: Differences in short term memory processing. *International Journal of Neuroscience*, *88*, 109–124.

Frodl, T., & Skokauskas, N. (2012). Meta-analysis of structural MRI studies in children and adults with attention deficit hyperactivity disorder indicates treatment effects. (Article). *Acta Psychiatrica Scandinavica*, *125*(2), 114–126.

Fuchs, L. S., Geary, D. C., Compton, D. L., Fuchs, D., Hamlett, L., Seethaler, P. M., . . . Schatschneider, C. (2010). Do different types of school mathematics development depend on different constellations of numerical versus general cognitive abilities? *Developmental Psychology*, *46*(6), 1731–1746.

Fulbright, R. K., Jenner, A. R., Mencl, W. E., Pugh, K. R., Shaywitz, B. A., Shaywitz, S. E., . . . Frost, S. J. (1990). The cerebellum's role in reading: A functional MR imaging study. *American Journal of Neuroradiology*, *20*(10), 1925–1930.

Gabay, Y., Gabay, S., Schiff, R., Ashkenazi, S., & Henik, A. (2013). Visuospatial deficits in developmental dyslexia: Evidence from visual and mental number line bisection tasks. *Archives of Clinical Neuropsychology*, *28*, 829–836.

Garrett, A., Penniman, L., Epstein, J. N., Casey, B. J., Hinshaw, S. P., Glover, G., & Reiss, A. L. (2008). Neuroanatomical abnormalities in adolescents with attention-deficit/hyperactivity disorder. *Journal of the American Academy of Child and Adolescent Psychiatry*, *47*(11), 1321–1328.

Gayan, J., & Olson, R. K. (1999). Reading disability: evidence for a genetic etiology. *European Child & Adolescent Psychiatry*, *8*, S52–S55.

Gayan, J., Smith, S. D., Cherny, S. S., Cardon, L. R., Fulker, D. W., Brower, A. M., & DeFries, J. C. (1999). Quantitative-trait locus for specific language and reading deficits on chromosome 6p. *American Journal of Human Genetics*, *64*, 157–164.

Gayan, J., Willcutt, E. G., Fisher, S. E., Francks, C., Cardon, L. R., Olson, R. K., & DeFries, J. C. (2005). Bivariate linkage scan for reading disability and attention-deficit/hyperactivity disorder localizes pleiotropic loci. *Journal of Child Psychology and Psychiatry*, *46*(10), 1045–1056.

Geary, D. C. (1993). Mathematical disabilities: Cognitive, neuropsychological, and genetic components. *Psychological Bulletin*, *114*, 345–362.

Geary, D. C., & Hoard, M. K. (2001). Numerical and arithmetical deficits in learning-disabled children: Relation to dyscalculia and dyslexia. *Aphasiology*, *15*(7), 635–647.

Geary, D. C., Hoard, M. K., Nugent, L., & Bailey, D. H. (2012). Mathematical cognition deficits in children with learning disabilities and persistent low achievement: A five-year prospective study. *Journal of Educational Psychology*, *104*(1), 206–223.

Gerstmann, J. (1940). Syndrome of finger agnosia, disorientation for left and right, agraphia and acalculia. *Archives of Neurology and Psychiatry*, *44*, 398–408.

Geschwind, N., & Galaburda, A. M. (1985). Cerebral lateralization: Biological mechanisms, associations, and pathology. *Archives of Neurology*, *42*, 428–458.

Geschwind, N., & Levitsky, W. (1968). Human brain: Left-right asymmetries in temporal speech region. *Science*, *161*, 186–187.

Giedd, J. N., Blumenthal, J., Molloy, E., & Castellanos, F. X. (2001). Brain imaging of attention deficit/hyperactivity disorder. *Annals of the New York Academy of Sciences*, *931*, 33–49.

Giedd, J. N., Castellanos, F. X., Casey, B. J., Kozuch, P., King, A. C., Hamburger, S. D., & Rapoport, J. L. (1994). Quantitative morphology of the corpus callosum in attention deficit hyperactivity disorder. *American Journal of Psychiatry*, *151*(5), 665–669.

Giedd, J. N., Rumsey, J. M., Castellanos, F. X., Rajapakse, J. C., Kaysen, D., Vaituzis, A. C., & Rapoport, J. L. (1996). A quantitative MRI study of the corpus callosum in children and adolescents. [Article]. *Developmental Brain Research*, *91*(2), 274–280.

Gilbert, D. L., Isaacs, K. M., Augusta, M., MacNeil, L. K., & Mostofsky, S. H. (2011). Motor cortex inhibition: A marker of ADHD behavior and motor development in children. *Neurology*, *76*(7), 615–621.

Gillberg, C. (2003). Deficits in attention, motor control, and perception: A brief review. *Archives of Disease in Childhood*, *88*(10), 904–910.

Gilliam, M., Stockman, M., Malek, M., Sharp, W., Greenstein, D., Lalonde, F., . . . Shaw, P. (2011). Developmental trajectories of the corpus callosum in attention-deficit/hyperactivity disorder. *Biological Psychiatry*, *69*(9), 839–846.

Gizer, I. R., Ficks, C., & Waldman, I. D. (2009). Candidate gene studies of ADHD: A meta-analytic review. *Human Genetics*, *126*, 51–90.

Gomez, R., & Condon, M. (1999). Central auditory processing ability in children with ADHD with and without learning disabilities. *Journal of Learning Disabilities*, *32*(2), 150–158.

Goldston, D., Walsh, A., Mayfield, A., Reboussin, B., Sergent, D., Erkanli, A., et al. (2007). Reading problems, psychiatric disorders, and functional impairment from mid- to late adolescence. *Journal of the American Academy of Child and Adolescent Psychiatry*, *46*(1), 25–32.

Grabner, R. H., Ansari, D., Koschutnig, K., Reishofer, G., Ebner, F., & Neuper, C. (2009). To retrieve or to calculate? Left angular gyrus mediates the retrieval of arithmetic facts during problem solving. *Neuropsychologia*, *47*, 604–608.

Grabner, R. H., Reishofer, G., Koschutnig, K., Ebner, F., & Parvizi, J. (2011). Competence in processing mathematical representations. *Frontiers in Human Neuroscience*, *5*, 1–11.

Graham, S., Struck, M., Santoro, J., & Berninger, V. W. (2006). Dimensions of good and poor handwriting legibility in first and second graders: Motor programs, visual-spatial arrangement, and letter formation parameter setting. *Developmental Neuropsychology*, *29*(1), 43–60.

Graham, S., & Weintraub, N. (1996). A review of handwriting research: Progress and prospects from 1980 to 1994. *Educational Psychology Review*, *8*(1), 7–87.

Graves, R. E., Frerichs, R. J., & Cook, J. A. (1999). Visual localization in dyslexia. *Neuropsychology*, *13*, 575–581.

Greenblatt, E., & Greenblatt, R. M. (1997). Learning disabilities and developmental disorders. In J. D. Noshitz, P. Kernberg, & J. Bemporad. (Eds.), *The Handbook of Child and Adolescent Psychiatry* (Vol. 2, pp. 235–252). New York: John Wiley & Sons.

Gregg, N., Coleman, C., Davis, M., & Chalk, J. C. (2007). Timed essay writing: Implications for high-stakes tests. *Journal of Learning Disabilities*, *40*, 306–318.

Gregg, N., Hoy, C., & Gay, A. F. (Eds.). (1996). *Adults with Learning Disabilities*. New York: Guilford.

Gregg, N., Hoy, C., King, W. M., Moreland, C. M., & Jagota, M. (1992). The MMPI-2 profile of adults with learning disabilities in university and rehabilitation settings. *Journal of Learning Disabilities*, *25*, 386–395.

Greven, C. U., Kovas, Y., Willcutt, E. G., Petrill, S. A., & Plomin, R. (2014). Evidence for shared genetic risk between ADHD symptoms and reduced mathematics ability: a twin study. *The Journal of Child Psychology and Psychiatry*, *55*, 39–48.

Grigorenko, E. (2001). Developmental dyslexia: An update on genes, brains and environments. *Journal of Child Psychology and Psychiatry*, *42*, 91–125.

Grigorenko, E. (2008). Developmental dyslexia in adults. In L. E. Wolf, H. Schreiber, & J. Wasserstein (Eds.), *Adult Learning Disorders: Contemporary Issues* (pp. 83–109). New York: Psychology Press.

Grigorenko, E. L., Wood, F. B., Meyer, M. S., Hart, L. A., Speed, W. C., Shuster, A., & Pauls, D. L. (1997). Susceptibility loci for distinct components of developmental dyslexia on chromosomes 6 and 15. *American Journal of Human Genetics*, *60*, 27–39.

Grigorenko, E. L., Wood, F. B., Meyer, M. S., & Pauls, D. L. (2000). Chromosome 6p influences on different dyslexia-related cognitive processes: Further confirmation. *American Journal of Human Genetics*, *66*, 715–723.

Grodzinsky, G. M., & Diamond, R. (1992). Frontal lobe functioning in boys with attention deficit hyperactivity disorder. *Developmental Neuropsychology*, *8*(4), 427–445.

Gross-Tsur, V., Manor, O., & Shalev, R. (1996). Developmental dyscalculia: Prevalence and demographic features. *Developmental Medicine in Child Neurology*, *38*, 25–33.

Gubbay, S. S., & Deklerk, N. H. (1995). A study and review of developmental dysgraphia in relation to acquired dysgraphia. *Brain & Development*, *17*(1), 1–8.

Habib, M. (2000). The neurological basis of developmental dyslexia: An overview and working hypothesis. *Brain*, *123*, 2373–2399.

Hallgren, B. (1950). Specific dyslexia ('congenital word-blindness'): a clinical and genetic study. *Acta Psychiatry Neurology Scandinavia*, *65*, 1–287.

Halmoy, A., Fasmer, O. B., Gillberg, C., & Haavik, J. (2009). Occupational outcome in adult ADHD: Impact of symptom profile, comorbid psychiatric problems, and treatment: A cross-sectional study of 414 clinically diagnosed adult ADHD patients. *Journal of Attention Disorders*, *13*(2), 175–187.

Halperin, J. M., Matier, K., Bedi, G., Sharma, V., & Newcorn, J. (1992). Specificity of inattention, impulsivity, and hyperactivity to the diagnosis of attention-deficit hyperactivity disorder. *Journal of the American Academy of Child and Adolescent Psychiatry*, *31*(2), 190–196.

Halperin, J. M., & Schulz, K. P. (2006). Revisiting the role of the prefrontal cortex in the pathophysiology of attention-deficit/hyperactivity disorder. *Psychological Bulletin*, *132*, 560–581.

Handler, S. M., Fierson, W. M., American Academic of Pediatrics, Section on Ophthalmology, Council on Children with Disabilities, American Society of Ophthalmology, American Association of Ophthalmology, American Association for Pediatric Ophthalmology and Strabismus, & American Association of Certified Orthoptists. (2011). Joint Statement: Learning disabilities, dyslexia, and vision. *Pediatrics*, *127*, e818–e8585.

Harmony, T., Marosi, E., Becker, J., Rodriguez, M., Reyes, A., Fernandez, T., . . . Bernal, J. (1995). Longitudinal quantitative EEG study of children with different performances on a reading-writing test. *Electroencephalogry Clinical Neurophysiology*, *95*, 426–433.

Harold, G. T., Leve, L. D., Barrett, D., Elam, K., Neiderhiser, J. M., Natsuaki, M. N., & Thapar, A. (2013). Biological and rearing mother influences on child ADHD symptoms: Revisiting the developmental interface between nature and nurture. *Journal of Child Psychology and Psychiatry*, *54*, 1038–1046.

Harrison, A. G., Edwards, M. J., Armstrong, C. D., & Parker, K. C. H. (2010). An investigation of methods to detect feigned reading disabilities. *Archives of Clinical Neuropsychology*, *25*, 89–98.

Harrison, A. G., & Holmes, A. (2012). Easier said than done: Operationalizing the diagnosis of learning disability for use at the postsecondary level in Canada. *Canadian Journal of School Psychology*, *27*, 12–34.

Hart, H., Radua, J., Mataix-Cols, D., & Rubia, K. (2012). Meta-analysis of fMRI studies of timing in attention-deficit hyperactivity disorder (ADHD). *Neuroscience and Biobehavioral Reviews*, *36*(10), 2248–2256.

Hechtman, L. (1996). Families of children with attention deficit disorder: A review. *Canadian Journal of Psychiatry*, *4*, 350–360.

Hechtman, L., & Weiss, G. (1983). Long-term outcome of hyperactive children. *American Journal of Orthopsychiatry*, *53*(3), 532–541.

Hechtman, L., & Weiss, G. (1986). Controlled prospective fifteen year follow-up of hyperactives as adults: non-medical drug and alcohol use and antisocial behavior. *Canadian Journal of Psychiatry*, *31*, 557–567.

Heiligenstein, E., Conyers, L. M., Berns, A. R., & Miller, M. A. (1998). Preliminary normative data on DSM-IV attention deficit hyperactivity disorder in college students. *Journal of American College Health*, *46*(4), 185–188.

Heilman, K. M., Voeller, K. K. S., & Nadeau, S. E. (1991). A possible pathophysiologic substrate of attention-deficit hyperactivity disorder. *Journal of Child Neurology*, *6*, S76–S81.

Helenius, P., Tarkiainen, A., Cornelissen, P., Hansen, P. C., & Salmelin, R. (1999). Dissociation of normal feature analysis and deficient processing of letter-strings in dyslexic adults. *Cerebral Cortex*, *4*, 476–483.

Henik, A., Rubinsten, O., & Ashkenazi, S. (2011). The "where" and "what" of developmental dyscalculia. *Clinical Neuropsychologist*, *25*(6), 989–1008.

Henschen, S. E. (1920). *Klinishe und Pathologische Beitrage zur Pathologiedes Gehirns*. Stockholm: Nordiske Bokhandeln.

Hervey, A. S., Epstein, J. N., Curry, J. F., & Dreer, L. (2003). The neuropsychology of adults with ADHD: A meta-analytic review. *Journal of the International Neuropsychological Society*, *9*, 179.

Hesdorffer, D. C., Ludvigsson, P., Olafsson, E., Gudmundsson, G., Kjartansson, O., & Hauser, W. A. (2004). ADHD as a risk factor for incident unprovoked seizures and epilepsy in children. *Archives of General Psychiatry*, *61*(7), 731–736.

Hill, D. E., Yeo, R. A., Campbell, R. A., Hart, B., Vigil, J., & Brooks, W. (2003). Magnetic resonance imaging correlates of attention-deficit/hyperactivity disorder in children. *Neuropsychology*, *17*(3), 496–506.

Himpel, S., Banaschewski, T., Gruttner, A., Becker, A., Heise, A., Uebel, H., & Rammsayer, T. (2009). Duration discrimination in the range of milliseconds and seconds in children with ADHD and their unaffected siblings. *Psychology Medicine*, *39*(10), 1745–1751.

Hinney, A., Scherag, A., Jarick, I., Albayrak, O., Putter, C., Pechlivanis, S., & Hebebrand, J. (2011). Genome-wide association study in German patients with attention deficit/hyperactivity disorder. *American Journal of Medical Genetics B Neuropsychiatry Genetics*, *156B*, 888–897.

Hinshelwood, J. (1896). A case of dyslexia: A peculiar form of word blindness. *Lancet*, *1*, 1451–1454.

Hinshelwood, J. (1917). Congenital word-blindness. *Lancet*, *2*, 980–980.

Hoeft, F., A. Meyler, A. Hernandez, A., Juel, C., Taylor-Hill, H., Martindale, J. L., . . . Gabrieli, J. D. (2007). Functional and morphometric brain dissociation between dyslexia and reading ability. *Proceedings of the National Academy of Sciences*, *104*(10), 4234–4239.

Hohman, L. B. (1922). Post-encephalitic behavior disorders in children. *Bulletin of the Johns Hopkins Hospital*, *33*, 372–375.

Hooper, S. R., & Olley, J. G. (1996). Psychological comorbidity in adults with learning disabilities. In N. Gregg, C. Hoy, & A. F. Gay (Eds.), *Adults With Learning Disabilities* (pp. 162–183). New York: Guilford.

Horwitz, B., Rumsey, J. M., & Donohue, B. C. (1998). Functional connectivity of the angular gyrus in normal reading and dyslexia. *Proceedings of the National Academy of Sciences*, *95*, 8939–8944.

Hoy, C., & Manglitz, E. (1996). Social and affective adjustment of adults with learning disabilities: A life-span perspective. In N. Gregg, C. Hoy, & A. F. Gay (Eds.), *Adults With Learning Disabilities* (pp. 208–231). New York: Guilford.

Hulme, C., & Snowling, M. J. (2013). Learning to read: What we know and what we need to understand better. *Child Development Perspectives*, *7*(1), 1–5.

Hultman, C. M., Torrang, A,. Tuvblad, C., Cnattingius, S., Larsson, J. O., & Lichtenstein, P. (2007). Birth weight and attention-deficit/hyperactivity symptoms in childhood and early adolescence: A prospective Swedish twin study. *Journal of the American Academy of Child and Adolescent Psychiatry*, *46*, 370–377.

Humphries, T., Koltun, H., Malone, M., & Roberts, W. (1994). Teacher-identified oral language difficulties among boys with attention problems. *Developmental and Behavioral Pediatrics*, *15*, 92–98.

Hutchinson, A. D., Mathias, J. L., & Banich, M. T. (2008). Corpus callosum morphology in children and adolescents with attention deficit hyperactivity disorder: A meta-analytic review. *Neuropsychology*, *22*(3), 341–349.

Huttenlocher, P. R., & Dabholkar, A. S. (1997). Regional differences in synaptogenesis in human cerebral cortex. *The Journal of Comparative Neurology*, *387*, 167–178.

Hynd, G. W., Hall, J., Novey, E. S., Eliopulos, D., Black, K., Gonzalez, J. J., & Cohen, M. (1995). Dyslexia and corpus callosum morphology. *Archives of Neurology*, *52*, 32–38.

Hynd, G. W., Hern, K. L., Novey, E. S., Eliopulos, D., Marshall, R., Gonzalez, J. J., & Voeller, K. K. (1993). Attention deficit hyperactivity disorder and asymmetry of the caudate nucleus. *Journal of Child Neurology*, *8*(4), 339–347.

Hynd, G. W., Semrud-Clikeman, M., Lorys, A. R., Novey, E. S., & Eliopulos, D. (1990). Brain morphology in developmental dyslexia and attention deficit disorder hyperactivity. *Archives of Neurology*, *47*(8), 919–926.

Hynd, G. W., Semrud-Clikeman, M., Lorys, A. R., Novey, E. S., Eliopulos, D., & Lyytinen, H. (1991). Corpus callosum morphology in attention deficit hyperactivity disorder: Morphometric analysis of MRI. *Journal of Learning Disabilities*, *24*(3), 141–146.

Iles, J., Walsh, V., & Richardson, A. (2000). Visual search performance in dyslexia. *Dyslexia*, *6*, 163–177.

Individuals with Disabilities Education Act (IDEA) of 1990, Public Law 101–476, 104 Stat. 1142 (1990).

Individuals with Disabilities Education Act (IDEA) of 2004, Public Law 108–446, 118 Stat. 2647 (2004).

Isaacs, E. B., Edmonds, C. J., Lucas, A., & Gadian, D. G. (2001). Calculation difficulties in children of very low birthweight: A neural correlate. *Brain*, *124*, 1701–1707.

Isaki, E., & Plante, E. (1997). Short-term and working memory differences in language/learning disabled and normal adults. *Journal of Communication Disorders*, *30*, 427–437.

Ivanov, I., Murrough, J. W., Bansal, R., Hao, X., & Peterson, B. S. (2014). Cerebellar morphology and the effects of stimulant medications in youths with attention deficit-hyperactivity disorder. *Neuropsychopharmacology*, *39*(3), 718–726.

Jacob, C. P., Weber, H., Retz, W., Kittel-Schneider, S., Heupel, J., Renner, T., . . . Reif, A. (2013). Acetylcholine-metabolizing butyrylcholinesterase (BCHE) copy number and single nucleotide polymorphisms and their role in attention-deficit/hyperactivity syndrome. *Journal of Psychiatric Research*, *47*, 1902–1908.

Johnson, D. E., Epstein, J. N., Waid, L. R., Latham, P. K., Voronin, K. E., & Anton, R. F. (2001). Neuropsychological performance deficits in adults with attention-deficit/hyperactivity disorder. *Archives of Clinical Neuropsychology*, *16*, 587–604.

Johnson, D. J. (1987). Nonverbal learning disabilities. *Pediatric Annals*, *16*(2), 133–141.

Johnson, D. J., & Myklebust, H. R. (1967). *Learning Disabilities: Educational Principles and Practices*. New York: Grune & Stratton.

Johnson, D. J., & Myklebust, H. R. (1971). *Learning Disabilities*. New York: Grune & Stratton.

Jordan, N. C., Hanich, L. B., & Kaplan, D. (2003). A longitudinal study of mathematical competencies in children with specific mathematics difficulties versus children with comorbid mathematics and reading difficulties. *Child Development*, *74*(3), 834–850.

Jung, H., Woo, Y. J., Kang, J. W., Choi, Y. W., & Kim, K. M. (2014). Visual perception of ADHD children with sensory processing disorder. *Psychiatry Investigation*, *11*(2), 119–123.

Kadesjo, B., & Gillberg, C. (2001). The comorbidity of ADHD in the general population of Swedish school-age children. *Journal of Child Psychology and Psychiatry and Allied Disciplines*, *42*(4), 487–492.

Kalanthroff, E., Naparstek, S., & Henik, A. (2013). Spatial processing in adults with Attention Deficit Hyperactivity Disorder. [Article]. *Neuropsychology*, *27*(5), 546–555.

Kan, K. J., Dolan, C. V., Nivard, M. G., Middeldorp, C. M., van Beijsterveldt, C. E., Willemsen, G., & Boomsma, D. I. (2013). Genetic and environmental stability in attention problems across the lifespan: Evidence from the Netherlands twin register. *Journal of the American Academy of Child and Adolescent Psychiatry*, *52*, 12–25.

Karin, M. (1990). Too many transcription factors: Positive and negative interactions. *New Biology*, *2*, 126–131.

Katz, L. J., Goldstein, G., & Beers, S. R. (2001). *Learning Disabilities in Older Adolescents and Adults*. New York: Kluwer Academic/Plenum Publishers.

Kelleher, K. J., McInerny, T. K., Gardner, W. P., Childs, G. E., & Wasserman, R. C. (2000). Increasing identification of psychosocial problems: 1979–1996. *Pediatrics International*, *105*(6), 1313–1321.

Kessler, J. W. (1980). History of minimal brain dysfunction. In E. Rie & H. Rie (Eds.), *Handbook of Minimal Brain Dysfunction: A Critical Review* (pp. 18–52). New York: Wiley Press.

Kieling, C., Goncalves, R. R. F., Tannock, R., & Castellanos, F. X. (2008). Neurobiology of attention deficit hyperactivity disorder. *Child and Adolescent Psychiatric Clinics of North America*, *17*(2), 285–307.

Kinsbourne, M. (1977). The mechanism of hyperactivity. In M. Blau, I. I. Rapin, & M. Kinsbourne (Eds.), *Topics in Child Neurology*. New York, Spectrum.

Kinsbourne, M., & Warrington, E. K. (1963). The developmental Gerstmann syndrome. *Archives of Neurology*, *8*, 490–501.

Kirk, S. A. (1963). Behavioral diagnosis and remediation of learning disabilities. In *Proceedings of the annual meeting: Conference on exploration into the problems of the perceptually handicapped child* (Vol. 1, pp. 1–7). Evanston, IL.

Klingberg, T., Hedehus, M., Temple, E., Salz, T., Gabrieli, J., Moseley, M., & Poldrack, R. A. (2000). Microstructure of temporoparietal white matter as a basis for reading ability: Evidence from diffusion tensor magnetic resonance imaging. *Neuron*, *25*, 493–500.

Konrad, K., & Eickhoff, S. B. (2010). Is the ADHD brain wired differently? A review on structural and functional connectivity in attention deficit hyperactivity disorder. *Human Brain Mapping*, *31*, 904–916.

Koontz, K. L., & Berch, D. B. (1996). Identifying simple numerical stimuli: Processing inefficiencies exhibited by arithmetic learning disabled children. *Mathematical Cognition*, *2*, 1–23.

Kosc, L. (1974). Developmental dyscalculia. *Journal of Learning Disabilities*, *7*(3), 164–177.

Kovas, Y., Harlaar, N., Petrill, S. A., & Plomin, R. (2005). 'Generalist genes' and mathematics in 7-year-old twins. *Intelligence*, *33*(5), 473–489.

Krain, A. L., & Castellanos, F. X. (2006). Brain development and ADHD. *Clinical Psychology Review*, *26*, 433–444.

Kramer, F., & Pollnow, H. (1932). Über eine hyperkinetische erkrankung im kindesalter. *Monatsschrift für Psychiatrie und Neurologie*, *82*, 1–40.

Krueger, F., Spampinato, M. V., Pardini, M., Pajevic, S., Wood, J. N., Weiss, J. S., & Grafman, J. (2008). Integral calculus problem solving: An fMRI investigation. *Neuroreport*, *19*(11), 1095–1099.

Kubova, Z., Kuba, M., Peregrin, J., & Novakova, V. (1996). Visual evoked potential evidence for magnocellular system deficit in dyslexia. *Physiological Research*, *45*, 87–89.

Kucian, K., Loenneker, T., Dietrich, T., Dosch, M. Martin, E., & von Aster, M. (2006). Impaired neural networks for approximate calculation in dyscalculic children: A functional MRI study. *Behavior and Brain Function*, *2*, 31.

Kucian, K., von Aster, M., Loenneker, T., Dietrich, T., & Martin, E. (2008). Development of neural networks for exact and approximate calculation: An FMRI study. *Developmental Neuropsychology*, *33*, 447–473.

Kurlan, R., Como, P. G., Miller, B., Palumbo, D., Deeley, C., Andresen, E. M., & McDermott, M. P. (2002). The behavioral spectrum of tic disorders: A community-based study. [Comparative Study Research Support, U.S. Gov't, P.H.S.]. *Neurology*, *59*(3), 414–420.

Kussmaul, A. (1877). Disturbance of speech. In H. von Ziemssen (Ed.), *Cyclopaedia of the Practice of Medicine* (Vol. 14, pp. 581–875). New York: William Wood.

Laasonen, M., Lehtinen, M., Leppämäki, S., Tani, P., & Hokkanen, L. (2010). Project DyADD: Phonological processing, reading, spelling, and arithmetic in adults with dyslexia or ADHD. *Journal of Learning Disabilities*, *43*, 3–14.

Lambert, N., & Hartsough, C. S. (1998). Prospective study of tobacco smoking and substance dependencies among samples of ADHD and non-ADHD participants. *Journal of Learning Disabilities*, *31*, 533–544.

Landerl, K., Bevan, A., & Butterworth, B. (2004). Developmental dyscalculia and basic numerical capacities: A study of 8–9-year-old students. *Cognition*, *93*, 99–125.

Lange, K. W., Reichl, S., Lang, K. M., Tucha, L., & Tucha, O. (2010). The history of attention deficit hyperactivity disorder. *Attention Deficit Hyperactivity Disorder*, *2*, 241–255.

Langevin, L. M., MacMaster, F. P., Crawford, S., Lebel, C., & Dewey, D. (2014). Common white matter microstructure alterations in pediatric motor and attention disorders. *Journal of Pediatrics*, *164*(5), 1157–1164.

Larochette, A.-C., & Harrison, A. G. (2012). Word Memory Test: Performance in Canadian adolescents with learning disabilities: A preliminary study. *Applied Neuropsychology: Child*, *1*, 38–47.

Larsson, H., Anckarsater, H., Rastam, M., Chang, Z., & Lichtenstein, P. (2012). Childhood attention-deficit hyperactivity disorder as an extreme of a continuous trait: A quantitative genetic study of 8,500 twin pairs. *Journal of Child Psychology and Psychiatry*, *53*, 73–80.

Larsson, H., Dilshad, R., Lichtenstein, P., & Barker, E. D. (2011). Developmental trajectories of DSM-IV symptoms of attention-deficit/hyperactivity disorder: Genetic effects, family risk and associated psychopathology. *Journal of Child Psychology and Psychiatry*, *52*, 954–963.

Latchman, D. S. (1997). Transcription factors: An overview. *International Journal of Biochemical Cell Biology*, *29*(12), 1305–1312.

Latimer, K., Wilson, P., Kemp, J., Thompson, L., Sim, F., Gillberg, C., & Minnis, H. (2012). Disruptive behaviour disorders: A systematic review of environmental antenatal and early years risk factors. *Child: Care, Health and Development*, *38*, 611–628.

Laufer, M. W., Denhoff, E. H., & Solomons, G. T. (1957). Hyperkinetic impulse disorder in children's behavior problems. *Psychosomatic Medicine*, *19*, 38–49.

Laufer, M. W., Denhoff, E., & Solomons, G. T. (2011). Hyperkinetic impulse disorder in children's behavior problems. [Editorial Material]. *Journal of Attention Disorders*, *15*(8), 620–625.

Lee, D. O., & Ousley, O. Y. (2006). Attention-deficit hyperactivity disorder symptoms in a clinic sample of children and adolescents with pervasive developmental disorders. *Journal of Child and Adolescent Psychopharmacology*, *16*(6), 737–746.

Lehn, H., Derks, E. M., Hudziak, J. J., Heutink, P., van Beijsterveldt, T. C., & Boomsma, D. I. (2007). Attention problems and attention-deficit/hyperactivity disorder in discordant and concordant monozygotic twins: Evidence of environmental mediators. *Journal of the American Academy of Child and Adolescent Psychiatry*, *46*, 83–91.

Lenroot, R. K., Gogtay, N., Greenstein, D. K., Wells, E. M., Wallace, G. L., Clasen, L. S., . . . Giedd, J. N. (2007). Sexual dimorphism of brain developmental trajectories during childhood and adolescence. *Neuroimage*, *36*(4), 1065–1073.

Leppanen, P. H., & Lyytinen, H. (1997). Auditory event related potentials in the study of developmental language related disoreders. *Audiology and Neurotology*, *2*, 308–340.

Lesch, K. P., Selch, S., Renner, T. J., Jacob, C., Nguyen, T. T., Hahn, T., & Ullmann, R. (2011). Genome-wide copy number variation analysis in attention-deficit/hyperactivity disorder: Association with neuropeptide Y gene dosage in an extended pedigree. *Molecular Psychiatry*, *16*, 491–503.

Leth-Steensen, C., Elbaz, Z. K., & Douglas, V. I. (2000). Mean response times, variability, and skew in the responding of ADHD children: A response time distributional approach. *Acta Psychologica*, *104*, 167–190.

Levine, M. D., Busch, B., & Aufseeser, C. (1982). The dimension of inattention among children with school problems. *Pediatrics*, *70*(3), 387–395.

Levy, F., & Swanson, J. M. (2001). Timing, space and ADHD: The dopamine theory revisited. *Australian and New Zealand Journal of Psychiatry*, *35*(4), 504–511.

Leyfer, O. T., Folstein, S. E., Bacalman, S., Davis, N. O., Dinh, E., Morgan, J., & Lainhart, J. E. (2006). Comorbid psychiatric disorders in children with autism: Interview development and rates of disorders. *Journal of Autism and Developmental Disorders*, *36*(7), 849–861

Lionel, A. C., Crosbie, J., Barbosa, N., Goodale, T., Thiruvahindrapuram, B., Rickaby, J., . . . Scherer, S. W. (2011). Rare copy number variation discovery and cross-disorder comparisons identify risk genes for ADHD. *Science Translational Medicine*, *3*, 95ra75.

Lister, R., Mukamel, E. A., Nery, J. R., Urich, M., Puddifoot, C. A., Johnson, N. D., & Ecker, J. R. (2013). Global epigenomic reconfiguration during mammalian brain development. *Science*, *341*(6146), 1237905.

Livingstone, M. S., Rosen, G. D., Drislane, F. W., & Galaburda, A. M. (1991). Physiological and anatomical evidence for a magnocellular defect in developmental dyslexia. *Proceedings of the National Academy of Sciences, USA*, *88*, 7943–7947.

Lo-Castro, A., D'Agati, E., & Curatolo, P. (2011). ADHD and genetic syndromes. [Review]. *Brain & Development*, *33*(6), 456–461.

Lombroso, P. J., Pauls, D. L., & Leckman, J. F. (1994). Genetic mechanisms in childhood psychiatric disorders. *Journal of the American Academy of Child and Adolescent Psychiatry*, *33*, 921–938.

Lopez-Larson, M., Michael, E. S., Terry, J. E., Breeze, J. L., Hodge, S. M., Tang, L., & Frazier, J. A. (2009). Subcortical differences among youths with attention-deficit/hyperactivity disorder compared to those with bipolar disorder with and without attention-deficit/hyperactivity disorder. *Journal of Child and Adolescent Psychopharmacology*, *19*(1), 31–39.

Lou, H. C., Hendrickson, L., & Bruhn, P. (1989). Striatal dysfunction in attention deficit and hyperkinetic disorder. *Archives of Neurology*, *46*, 48–52.

Lou, H. C., Henriksen, L., & Bruhn, P. (1984). Focal cerebral hypoperfusion in children with dysphasia and or attention deficit disorder. *Archives of Neurology*, *41*(8), 825–829.

Luculano, T., Moro, R., & Butterworth, B. (2011). Updating working memory and arithmetical attainment in school. *Learning and Individual Differences*, *21*(6), 655–661.

Luria, A. R. (1946). On the pathology of computational operations. *Proceedings of the Academy of Pedagogical Science of the RSRSR*, *3*, 181–207.

Luria, A. R. (1966). *Higher Cortical Functions in Man*. New York: Basic Books.

Lyon, G. R., Shaywitz, S. E., & Shaywitz, B. A. (2003). A definition of dyslexia. *Annals of Dyslexia*, *53*, 1–14.

Magalona, S. C., Rasetti, R., Chen, J., Chen, Q., Gold, I., Decot, H., & Mattay, V. S. (2013). Effect of tolcapone on brain activity during a variable attentional control task: A double-blind, placebo-controlled, counter-balanced trial in healthy volunteers. *CNS Drugs*, *27*(8), 663–673.

Mahone, E. M., & Mapou, R. L. (2014). Learning disabilities. In K. Stucky, M. Kirkwood, & J. Donders (Eds.), *American Academy of Clinical Neuropsychology Study Guide and Board Review* (pp. 184–201). New York: Oxford University Press.

Mahone, E. M., Ranta, M. E., Crocetti, D., O'Brien, J., Kaufmann, W. E., Denckla, M. B., & Mostofsky, S. H. (2011). Comprehensive examination of frontal regions in boys and girls with attention-deficit/hyperactivity disorder. *Journal of the International Neuropsychological Society*, *17*(6), 1047–1057.

Makris, N., Biederman, J., Valera, E. M., Bush, G., Kaiser, J., Kennedy, D. N., & Seidman, L. J. (2007). Cortical thinning of the attention and executive function networks in adults with attention-deficit/hyperactivity disorder. *Cerebral Cortex*, *17*(6), 1364–1375.

Makris, N., Biederman, J., Monuteaux, M. C., & Seidman, L. J. (2009). Towards conceptualizing a neural systems-based anatomy of attention-deficit/hyperactivity disorder. *Developmental Neuroscience*, *31*(1–2), 36–49.

Makris, N., Seidman, L. J., Valera, E. M., Biederman, J., Monuteaux, M. C., Kennedy, D. N., & Faraone, S. V. (2010). Anterior cingulate volumetric alterations in treatment-naive adults with ADHD: a pilot study. *Journal of Attention Disorders*, *13*(4), 407–413.

Malone, M. A., Couitis, J., Kershner, J. R., & Logan, W. J. (1994). Right-hemisphere dysfunction and methylphenidate effects in children with attention-deficit/hyperactivity disorder (ADHD). *Journal of Child and Adolescent Psychopharmacology*, *4*(4), 245–253.

Manis, F. R., Seidenberg, M. S., & Doi, L. M. (1999). See Dick RAN: Rapid naming and the longitudinal prediction of reading subskills in first and second graders. *Scientific Studies of Reading*, *3*, 129–157.

Mannion, A., & Leader, G. (2014). Attention-deficit/hyperactivity disorder (AD/HD) in autism spectrum disorder. *Research in Autism Spectrum Disorders*, *8*(4), 432–439.

Mannuzza, S., Klein, R. G., Bessler, A., Malloy, P., & LaPadula, M. (1993). Adult outcome of hyperactive boys: Educational achievement, occupational rank, and psychiatric status. *Archives of General Psychiatry*, *50*, 565–576.

Mannuzza, S., Klein, R. G., Bessler, A., Malloy, P., & LaPadula, M. (1998). Adult psychiatric status of hyperactive boys grown up. *American Journal of Psychiatry*, *155*, 493–498.

Mano, Q. R., & Osmon, D. C. (2008). Visuoperceptual-orthographic reading abilities: A confirmatory factor analysis study. *Journal of Clinical and Experimental Neuropsychology*, *2008*, 421–434.

Mapou, R. L. (2009a). *Adult Learning Disabilities and ADHD: Research-Informed Assessment*. p. 8. New York: Oxford University Press.

Marcotte, A. C., & Stern, C. (1997). Qualitative analysis of graphomotor output in children with attentional disorders. *Child Neuropsychology*, *3*, 147–153.

Mariani, M. A., & Barkley, R. A. (1997). Neuropsychological and academic functioning in preschool boys with attention deficit hyperactivity disorder. *Developmental Neuropsychology*, *13*(1), 111–129.

Marks, D. J., Newcorn, J. H., & Halperin, J. M. (2001). Comorbidity in adult ADHD. *Annals of the New York Academy of Sciences*, *931*, 216–238.

Martin, N. C., Piek, J. P., & Hay, D. (2006). DCD and ADHD: A genetic study of their shared aetiology. *Human Movement Science*, *25*(1), 110–124.

Martinussen, R., & Tannock, R. (2006). Working memory impairments in children with attention-deficit hyperactivity disorder with and without comorbid language learning disorders. *Journal of Clinical and Experimental Neuropsychology*, *28*(7), 1073–1094.

Mataro, M., GarciaSanchez, C., Junque, C., Estévez-González, A., & Pujol, J. (1997). Magnetic resonance imaging measurement of the caudate nucleus in adolescents with attention-deficit hyperactivity disorder and its relationship with neuropsychological and behavioral measures. *Archives of Neurology*, *54*(8), 963–968.

Mattes, J. A. (1980). The role of frontal lobe dysfunction in childhood hyperkinesis. *Comprehensive Psychiatry*, *21*, 358–369.

Manis, F. R., Seidenberg, M. S., Doi, L. M. (1999). See Dick RAN: Rapid naming and the longitudinal prediction of reading subskills in first and second graders. *Scientific Studies of reading*, *3*(2), 129–157.

May, B., & Bos, J. (2000). Personality characteristics of ADHD adults assessed with the Millon Clinical Multiaxial Inventory-II: Evidence of four distinct subtypes. *Journal of Personality Assessment*, *75*, 237–248.

Mayes, S. D., Calhoun, S. L., & Crowell, E. W. (2000). Learning disabilities and ADHD: Overlapping spectrum disorders. *Journal of learning disabilities*, *33*(5), 417–424.

Mazzocco, M. M. (2011). Defining and differentiating mathematical learning disabilities and difficulties. In D. B. Berch, M. M.& Mazzocco (Eds.), *Why Is Math So Hard for Some Children? The Nature and Origins of Mathematical Learning Difficulties and Disabilities* (pp. 29–47). Baltimore, MD: Paul H. Brookes.

McArthur, S., McHale, E., & Gillies, G. E. (2007). The size and distribution of midbrain dopaminergic populations are permanently altered by perinatal glucocorticoid exposure in a sex-region- and time-specific manner. *Neuropsychopharmacology*, *32*, 1462–1476.

McCandliss, B. D., Cohen, L., & Dehaene, S. (2003). The visual word form area: Expertise for reading in the fusiform gyrus. *Trends in Cognitive Science*, *7*, 293–299.

McAlonan, G. M., Cheng, V., Cheung, C., Chua, S. E., Murphy, D. G. M., Suckling, J., Tai, K-S., Yip, L. K. C., Leung, P., & Ho, T. P. (2007). Mapping brain structure in attention deficit-hyperactivity disorder: a voxel-based MRI study of regional grey and white matter volume. *Psychiatry Research: Neuroimaging*, *154*(2), 171–180.

McCann, B. S., Scheele, L., Ward, N., & Roy-Byrne, P. (2000). Discriminant validity of the Wender Utah Rating Scale for attention-deficit/hyperactivity disorder in adults. *Journal of Neuropsychiatry and Clinical Neurosciences*, *12*, 240–245.

McDermott, S., Mani, S., & Krishnaswami, S. (1995). A population-based analysis of specific behavior problems associated with childhood seizures. *Journal of Epilepsy*, *8*(2), 110–118.

McGough, J. J., Smalley, S. L., McCracken, J. T., Yang, M., Del'Homme, M., Lynn, D. E., & Loo, S. (2005). Psychiatric comorbidity in adult attention deficit hyperactivity disorder: Findings from multiplex families. *Americal Journal of Psychiatry*, *162*(9), 1621–7.

McGrath, L. M., Smith, S. D., & Penington, B. F. (2006). Breakthroughs in the search for dyslexia genes. *Trends in Molecular Medicine*, *12*, 333–341.

McLeod, K. R., Langevin, L. M., Goodyear, B. G., & Dewey, D. (2014). Functional connectivity of neural motor networks is disrupted in children with developmental coordination disorder and attention-deficit/hyperactivity disorder. *Neuroimage: Clinical*, *4*, 566–575.

McLoughlin, G., Rijsdijk, F., Asherson, P., & Kuntsi, J. (2011). Parents and teachers make different contributions to a shared perspective on hyperactive-impulsive and inattentive symptoms: A multivariate analysis of parent and teacher ratings on the symptom domains of ADHD. *Behavior Genetics*, *41*, 668–679.

Meador-Woodruff, J. H., Damask, S. P., Wang, J., Haroutunian, V., Davis, K. L., & Watson, S. J. (1996). Dopamine receptor mRNA expression in human striatum and neocortex. *Neuropsychopharmacology: Official Publication of the American College of Neuropsychopharmacology*, *15*, 17–29.

Mick, E., Biederman, J., Prince, J., Fischer, M. J., & Faraone, S. V. (2002). Impact of low birth weight on attention-deficit hyperactivity disorder. *Journal of Developmental and Behavioral Pediatrics*, *23*(1), 16–22.

Middleton, F. A., & Strick, P. L. (1994). Anatomical evidence for cerebellar and basal ganglia involvement in higher cognitive function. *Science*, *266*, 458–461.

Miller, T. W., Nigg, J. T., & Miller, R. L. (2009). Attention deficit hyperactivity disorder in African American children: What can be concluded from the past ten years? *Clinical Psychology Review*, *29*(1), 77–86.

Mink, J. W. (2003). The basal ganglia and involuntary movements: Impaired inhibition of competing motor patterns. [Review]. *Archives of Neurology*, *60*(10), 1365–1368.

Miranda, A., Soriano, M., Miranda, A., & García, R. (2006). Reading comprehension and written composition problems of children with ADHD: Discussion of research and methodological considerations. In *Applications of Research Methodology* (pp. 237–256). Bingley, UK: Emerald Group Publishing Limited.

Mitchell, K. G. (2011). Curious and curiouser: Genetic disorders of cortical specialization. *Current Opinion in Genetics & Development*, *21*, 271–277.

Monks, S., Niarchou, M., Davies, A. R., Walters, J. T. R., Williams, N., Owen, M. J., . . . Murphy, K. C. (2014). Further evidence for high rates of schizophrenia in 22q11.2 deletion syndrome. *Schizophrenia Research*, *153*(1–3), 231–236.

Morgan, W. P. (1896). A case of congenital word blindness. *British Medical Journal*, *2*(1871), 1378.

Mostofsky, S. H., Cooper, K. L., Kates, W. R., Denckla, M. B., & Kaufmann, W. E. (2002). Smaller prefrontal and premotor volumes in boys with attention-deficit/hyperactivity disorder. *Biological Psychiatry*, *52*(8), 785–794.

Mostofsky, S. H., & Simmonds, D. J. (2008). Response inhibition and response selection: Two sides of the same coin. *Journal of Cognitive Neuroscience*, *20*(5), 751–761.

Murphy, K. R., & Barkley, R. A. (1996). Attention deficit hyperactivity disorder adults: Comorbidities and adaptive impairments. *Comprehensive Psychiatry*, *37*, 393–401.

Murphy, K. R., & Barkley, R. A. (2006). Assessment of adults with ADHD. In R. A. Barkley (Ed.), *Attention-Deficit/Hyperactivity Disorder: A Handbook for Diagnosis and Treatment* (3rd ed. pp. 425–450). New York: Guilford Press.

Murphy, K. R., Barkley, R. A., & Bush, T. (2002). Young adults with attention deficit hyperactivity disorder: Subtype differences in comorbidity, educational, and clinical history. *Journal of Nervous and Mental Disease*, *190*, 147–157.

Murphy, J., & Tsuang, M. T. (1995). Attention deficit hyperactivity disorder and comorbid disorders: issues of overlapping symptoms. *American Journal of Psychiatry*, *152*, 1793–1799.

Musser, E. D., Hawkey, E., Kachan-Liu, S. S., Lees, P., Roullet, J. B., Goddard, K., & Nigg, J. T. (2014). Shared familial transmission of autism spectrum and attention-deficit/hyperactivity disorders. *Journal of Child Psychology and Psychiatry*, *55*(7), 819–827.

Mussolin, C., De Volder, A., Grandin, C., Schlögel, X., Nassogne, M. C., & Noël, M. P. (2010). Neural correlates of symbolic number comparison in developmental dyscalculia. *Journal of Cognitive Neuroscience*, *22*(5), 860–874.

Myklebust, H. R., & Johnson, D. (1962). Dyslexia in children. *Exceptional Children*, *29*(1), 14–25.

Naccache, L., & Dehaene, S. (2001). The priming method: Imaging unconscious repetition priming reveals an abstract representation of number in the parietal lobes. *Cerebral Cortex*, *11*, 966–974.

Nakao, T., Radua, J., Rubia, K., & Mataix-Cols, D. (2011). Gray matter volume abnormalities in ADHD: Voxel-based meta-analysis exploring the effects of age and stimulant medication. *American Journal of Psychiatry*, *168*(11), 1154–1163.

Narr, K. L., Woods, R. P., Lin, J., Kim, J., Phillips, O. R., Del'Homme, M., & Levitt, J. G. (2009). Widespread cortical thinning is a robust anatomical marker for attention-deficit/hyperactivity disorder. *Journal of the American Academy of Child and Adolescent Psychiatry*, *48*(10), 1014–1022.

Nash, H. M., Hulme, C., Gooch, D., & Snowling, M. J. (2013). Preschool language profiles of children at family risk of dyslexia: continuities with specific language impairment. *Journal of Child Psychology and Psychiatry*, *54*(9), 958–968.

National Joint Committee on Learning Disabilities (NJCLD). (1990). Operationalizing the NJCLD definition of learning disabilities for ongoing assessment in schools: A report from the National Joint Committee on Learning Disabilities. Perspectives: *The International Dyslexia Association*, *23*(4), 29.

Neale, B. M., Medland, S. E., Ripke, S., Asherson, P., Franke, B., Lesch, K. P., & Daly, M. (2010). Meta-analysis of genome-wide association studies of attention-deficit/hyperactivity disorder. *Journal of the American Academy of Child & Adolescent Psychiatry*, *49*(9), 884–897.

Nelson, C. A. (2015). Commentary: Developmental origins of autism and ADHD: A commentary on Johnson et al. (2015). *Journal of Child Psychology and Psychiatry and Allied Disciplines*, *56*(3), 248–250.

Neuhaus, G., Foorman, B. R., Francis, D. J., & Carlson, C. D. (2001). Measures of information processing in rapid automatized naming (RAN) and their relation to reading. *Journal of Experimental Child Psychology*, *78*, 359–373.

Nicolson, R. I., Fawcett, A. J., & Dean, P. (2001). Developmental dyslexia: The cerebellar deficit hypothesis. *Trends in Neuroscience*, *24*(9), 508–511.

Nieder, A., Diester, I., & Tudusciuc, O. (2006). Temporal and spatial enumeration process in the primate parietal cortex. *Science*, *313*, 1431–1435.

Nieder, A., Freedman, D. J., & Miller, E. K. (2002). Representation of the quantity of visual items in the primate prefrontal cortex. *Science*, *297*, 1708–1711.

Nigg, J. T. (2001). Is ADHD a disinhibitory disorder? *Psychological Bulletin*, *127*(5), 571–598.

Nigg, J. T., Swanson, J. M., & Hinshaw, S. P. (1997). Covert visual spatial attention in boys with attention deficit hyperactivity disorder: Lateral effects, methylphenidate response and results for parents. *Neuropsychologia*, *35*(2), 165–176.

Nikolas, M. A., & Burt, S. A. (2010). Genetic and environmental influences on ADHD symptom dimensions of inattention and hyperactivity: A meta-analysis. *Journal of Abnormal Psychology*, *119*, 1–17.

Ohare, A. E., Brown, J. K., & Aitken, K. (1991). Dyscalculia in children. *Developmental Medicine and Child Neurology*, *33*(4), 356–361.

Oliver, B. R., & Plomin, R. (2007). Twins' Early Development Study (TEDS): A multivariate, longitudinal genetic investigation of language, cognition and behavior problems from childhood through adolescence. *Twin Research and Human Genetics*, *10*(1), 96–105.

Onnink, A. M. H., Zwiers, M. P., Hoogman, M., Mostert, J. C., Kan, C. C., Buitelaar, J., & Franke, B. (2014). Brain alterations in adult ADHD: effects of gender, treatment and comorbid depression. *European Neuropsychopharmacology*, *24*(3), 397–409.

Orton, S. (1925). Word blindness in school children. *Archives of Neurology and Psychiatry*, *14*, 581–615.

Osmon, D. C., Braun, M. M., & Plambeck, E. A. (2005). Processing abilities associated with phonologic and orthographic skills in adult learning disability. *Journal of Clinical and Experimental Neuropsychology*, *27*, 544–554.

Osmon, D. C., Plambeck, E. A., Klein, L., & Mano, Q. (2006). The word reading test of effort in adult learning disability: A simulation study. *The Clinical Neuropsychologist*, *20*, 315–324.

Osmon, D. C., Smerz, J. M., Braun, M. M., & Plambeck, E. A. (2006). Processing abilities associated with math skills in adult learning disability. *Journal of Clinical and Experimental Neuropsychology*, *28*, 84–95.

Overmeyer, S., Bullmore, E. T., Suckling, J., Simmons, A., Williams, S. C. R., Santosh, P. J., & Taylor, E. (2001). Distributed grey and white matter deficits in hyperkinetic disorder: MRI evidence for anatomical abnormality in an attentional network. *Psychological Medicine*, *31*(8), 1425–1435.

Overmeyer, S., Simmons, A., Santosh, J., Andrew, C., Williams, S. C. R., Taylor, A., & Taylor, E. (2000). Corpus callosum may be similar in children with ADHD and siblings of children with ADHD. *Developmental Medicine and Child Neurology*, *42*(1), 8–13.

Pary, R., Lewis, S., Matuschka, P. R., Rudzinskiy, P., Safi, M., & Lippmann, S. (2002). Attention deficit disorder in adults. *Annals of Clinical Psychiatry*, *14*(2), 105–111.

Pasquinelli, A. E. (2012). MicroRNAs and their targets: Recognition, regulation and an emerging reciprocal relationship. *Nature Reviews Genetics*, *13*, 271–282.

Pastor, P. N., & Reuben, C. A. (2008). *Diagnosed attention deficit hyperactivity disorder and learning disability: United States*, 2004–2006. Centers for Disease Control, Vital and Health Statistics, Series 10 (Number 237).

Paulesu, E., Demonet, J. F., Fazio, F., McCrory, E., Chanoine, V., Brunswick, N., . . . Frith, U. (2001). Dyslexia: Cultural diversity and biological unity. *Science*, *291*, 2165–2167.

Pennington, B. F. (2008). *Diagnosing Learning Disorders: A Neuropsychological Framework* (2nd ed.). New York: The Guilford Press.

Pennington, B. F., Gilger, J. W., Pauls, D., Smith, S. A., Smith, S. D., & DeFries, J. C. (1991). Evidence for major gene transmission of developmental dyslexia. *Jama*, *266*(11), 1527–1534.

Peterson, B. S., Staib, L., Scahill, L., Zhang, H., Anderson, C., Leckman, J. F., & Webster, R. (2001). Regional brain and ventricular volumes in Tourette syndrome. *Archives of General Psychiatry*, *58*(5), 427–440.

Peverly, S. (2006). The importance of handwriting speed in adult writing. *Developmental Neuropsychology*, *29*, 197–216.

Piazza, M., Pinel, P., LeBihan, D., & Dehaene, S. (2007). A magnitude code common to neumerosities and number symbols in human intraparietal cortex. *Neuron*, *53*, 293–305.

Plaut, D. C., McClelland, J. L., Seidenberg, M. S., & Patterson, K. (1996). Understanding normal and impaired word reading: Computational principles in quasi-regular domains. *Psychological Review*, *103*, 56–115.

Plessen, K. J., Gruner, R., Lundervold, A., Hirsch, J. G., Xu, D. R., Bansal, R., et al. (2006). Reduced white matter connectivity in the corpus callosum of children with Tourette syndrome. *Journal of Child Psychology and Psychiatry*, *47*(10), 1013–1022.

Pliszka, S. R. (1998). Comorbidity of attention-deficit/hyperactivity disorder with psychiatric disorder: An overview. *Journal of Clinical Psychiatry*, *59*, 50–58.

Pliszka, S. R., Glahn, D. C., Semrud-Clikeman, M., Franklin, C., Perez, R., & Xiong, J. J. (2006). Neuroimaging of inhibitory control areas in children with attention deficit hyperactivity disorder who were treatment naive or in long-term treatment. *American Journal of Psychiatry*, *163*(6), 1052–1060.

Piazza, M., Facoetti, A., Trussardi, A. N., Berteletti, I., Conte, S., Lucangeli, D., & Zorzi, M. (2010). Developmental trajectory of number acuity reveals a severe impairment in developmental dyscalculia. *Cognition*, *116*(1), 33–41.

Polderman, T. J., Posthuma, D., De Sonneville, L. M., Stins, J. F., Verhulst, F. C., & Boomsma, D. I. (2007). Genetic analyses of the stability of executive functioning during childhood. *Biological Psychology*, *76*, 11–20.

Posthuma, D., & Polderman, T. J. (2013). What have we learned from recent twin studies about the etiology of neurodevelopmental disorders? *Current Opinion in Neurology*, *26*, 111–121.

Price, G, R., Holloway, I., Rasanen, P., Vesterinen, M., & Ansari, D. (2007). Impaired parietal magnitude processing in developmental dyscalculia. *Current Biology*, *17*, R1042–R1043.

Price, J. L., Carmichael, S. T., & Drevets, W. C. (1996). Networks related to the orbital and medial prefrontal cortex; a substrate for emotional behavior? *Progressive Brain Research*, *107*, 523–536.

Proal, E., Reiss, P. T., Klein, R. G., Mannuzza, S., Gotimer, K., Ramos-Olazagasti, M. A., . . . Castellanos, F. X. (2011). Brain gray matter deficits at 33-year follow-up in adults with attention-deficit/hyperactivity disorder established in childhood. *Archives of General Psychiatry*, *68*(11), 1122–1134.

Proctor, B. (2012). Relationships between Cattell-Horn-Carroll (CHC) cognitive abilities and math achievement within a sample of college students with learning disabilities. *Journal of Learning Disabilities*, *45*, 278–287.

Pugh, K. R., Mencl, W. E., Shaywitz, B. A., Shaywitz, S. E., Fulbright, R. K., Constable, R. T., & Liberman, A. M. (2000). The angular gyrus in developmental dyslexia: task-specific differences in functional connectivity within posterior cortex. *Psychological science*, *11*(1), 51–56.

Qiu, A. Q., Crocetti, D., Adler, M., Mahone, E. M., Denckla, M. B., Miller, M. I., & Mostofsky, S. H. (2009). Basal ganglia volume and shape in children with attention deficit hyperactivity disorder. *American Journal of Psychiatry*, *166*(1), 74–82.

Radonovich, K. J., & Mostofsky, S. H. (2004). Duration judgments in children with ADHD suggest deficient utilization of temporal information rather than general impairment in timing. *Child Neuropsychology*, *10*(3), 162–172.

Ramsay, J. R. (2010). *Nonmedication Treatments for Adult ADHD*. Washington, DC: American Psychological Association.

Ransby, M. J., & Swanson, H. L. (2003). Reading comprehension skills of young adults with childhood diagnoses of dyslexia. *Journal of Learning Disabilities*, *36*, 538–555.

Rapport, L. J., Van Voorhis, A., Tzelepis, A., & Friedman, S. R. (2001). Executive functioning in adult attention-deficit hyperactivity disorder. *The Clinical Neuropsychologist*, *15*, 479–491.

Rapport, M. D., Alderson, R. M., Kofler, M. J., Sarver, D. E., Bolden, J., & Sims, V. (2008). Working memory deficits in boys with attention-deficit/hyperactivity disorder (ADHD): The contribution of central executive and subsystem processes. *Journal of Abnormal Child Psychology*, *36*, 825–837.

Rapport, M. D., Chung, K., Shore, G., & Isaacs, P. (2001). A conceptual model of child psychopathology: Implications for understanding attention deficit hyperactivity disorder and treatment efficacy. *Journal of Clinical Child Psychology*, *30*, 48–58.

Rapport, M. D., Orban, S. A., Kofler, M. J., & Friedman, L. M. (2013). Do programs designed to train working memory, other executive functions, and attention benefit children with ADHD: A meta-analytic review of cognitive, academic, and behavioral outcomes. *Clinical Psychology Review*, *33*, 1237–1252.

Ratey, J., Greenberg, M. S., Bemporad, J. R., & Lindem, K. J. (1992). Unrecognized attention-deficit hyperactivity disorder in adults presenting for outpatient psychotherapy. *Journal of Child and Adolescent Psychopharmacology*, *2*, 267–75.

Rehabilitation Services Administration. (1985). *Program Policy Directive*. Washington, DC: U.S. Office of Special Education and Rehabilitation Services.

Reilly, C. J. (2011). Attention deficit hyperactivity disorder (ADHD) in childhood epilepsy. *Research in Developmental Disabilities*, *32*(3), 883–893.

Reynolds, C. A., Hewitt, J. K., Erickson, M. T., Silberg, J. L., Rutter, M., Simonoff, E., & Eaves, L. J. (1996). The genetics of children's oral reading performance. *Journal of Child Psychology and Psychiatry*, *37*(4), 425–434.

Riccio, C. A., Hynd, G. W., Cohen, M. J., Hall, J., & Molt, L. (1994). Comorbidity of central auditory processing disorder and attention-deficit hyperactivity disorder. *Journal of the American Academy of Child and Adolescent Psychiatry*, *33*(6), 849–857.

Rivera, S. M., Menon, V., White, C. D., Glaser, B., & Reiss, A. L. (2002). Functional brain activation during arithmetic processing in females with Fragile X syndrome is related to FMR1 protein expression. *Human Brain Mapping*, *16*, 206–218.

Robertson, I. (1989). Anomalies in the laterality of omissions in unilateral left visual neglect: Implications for an attentional theory of neglect. *Neuropsychologia*, *27*(2), 157–165.

Robertson, K. D. (2005). DNA methylation and human disease. *National Review of Genetics*, *6*(8), 597–610.

Robertson, M. M. (2006). Attention deficit hyperactivity disorder, tics and Tourette's syndrome: The relationship and treatment implications. *European Child & Adolescent Psychiatry*, *15*(1), 1–11.

Rosenberger, P. B. (1989). Perceptual-motor and attentional correlates of developmental dyscalculia. *Annals of Neurology*, *26*(2), 216–220.

Ross, J. L., Roeltgen, D. P., Stefanatos, G., Benecke, R., Zeger, M. P. D., Kushner, H., & Zinn, A. R. (2008). Cognitive and motor development during childhood in boys with Klinefelter syndrome. *American Journal of Medical Genetics Part A*, *146A*(6), 708–719.

Rotzer, S., Kucian, K., Martin, E., von Aster, M., Klaver, P., & Loenneker, T. (2008). Optimized voxel-based morphometry in children with developmental dyscalculia. *Neuroimage*, *39*(1), 417–422.

Rotzer, S., Loenneker, T., Kucina, K., Martin, E., Klaver, P., & Von Aster, M. (2009). Dysfunctional neural network of spatial working memory contributes to developmental dyscalculia. *Neuropsychologia*, *47*(13), 2859–2865.

Rourke, B. P. (1989). Nonverbal learning disabilities, socioemotional disturbance, and suicide: A reply. *Journal of Learning Disabilities*, *22*(3), 186–187.

Rourke, B. P. (1993). Arithmetic disabilities, specific and otherwise: A neuropsychological perspective. *Journal of Learning Disabilities*, *26*(4), 214–226.

Rourke, B. P., Young, G. C., Strang, J. D., & Russell, D. L. (1986). Adult outcomes of childhood central processing deficiencies. In I. Grant & K. M. Adams (Eds.), *Neuropsychological Assessment of Neuropsychiatric Disorders* (pp. 244–267). New York: Oxford University Press.

Rubia, K. (2011). "Cool" inferior frontostriatal dysfunction in attention-deficit/hyperactivity disorder versus "hot" ventromedial orbitofrontal-limbic dysfunction in conduct disorder: A review. *Biological Psychiatry*, *69*(12), E69–E87.

Rubia, K., Halari, R., Christakou, A., & Taylor, E. (2009). Impulsiveness as a timing disturbance: Neurocognitive abnormalities in attention-deficit hyperactivity disorder during temporal processes and normalization with methylphenidate. *Philosophical Transactions of the Royal Society of Biological Sciences*, *364*(1525), 1919–1931.

Rubia, K., Taylor, A., Taylor, E., & Sergeant, J. A. (1999). Synchronization, anticipation, and consistency in motor timing of children with dimensionally defined attention deficit hyperactivity behaviour. *Perceptual Motor Skills*, *89*(3), 1237–1258.

Rubinstein, O., & Henik, A. (2005). Automatic activation of internal magnitudes: A study of developmental dyscalculia. *Neuropsychology*, *19*, 641–648.

Rubinstein, O., & Henik, A. (2009). Developmental dyscalculia: Heterogeneity might not mean different mechanisms. *Trends in Cognitive Sciences*, *13*, 92–99.

Rumsey, J. M., Nace, K., Donohue, B., Wise, D., Maisog, J. M., & Andreason, P. (1997). A positron emission tomographic study of impaired word recognition and phonological processing in dyslexic men. *Archives of Neurology*, *54*, 562–573.

Russell, G., Rodgers, L. R., Ukoumunne, O. C., & Ford, T. (2014). Prevalence of parent-reported ASD and ADHD in the UK: Findings from the Millennium Cohort Study. *Journal of Autism and Developmental Disorders*, *44*(1), 31–40.

Russell, V. A., Oades, R. D., Tannock, R., Killeen, P. R., Auerbach, J. G., & Sagvolden, T. (2006). Response variability in ADHD: A neuronal and glial energetics hypothesis. *Behavior & Brain Functions*, *2*, 30–45.

Sagvolden, T., Johansen, E. B., Aase, H., & Russell, V. A. (2005). A dynamic developmental theory of attention-deficit/hyperactivity disorder (ADHD) predominantly hyperactive/impulsive and combined subtypes. *Behavioral Brain Research*, *28*(3), 397–419.

Salmelin, R., Service, E., Kiesila, P., Uutela, K., & Salonen, O. (1996). Impaired visual word processing in dyslexia revealed with magnetoencephalography. *Annals of Neurology*, *40*, 157–162.

Samuelsson, S., Lundberg, I., & Herkner, B. (2004). ADHD and reading disability in male adults: Is there a connection? *Journal of Learning Disabilities*, *37*(2), 155–168.

Sanchez-Mora, C., Ramos-Quiroga, J. A., Garcia-Martinez, I., Fernandez-Castillo, N., Bosch, R., Richarte, V., & Martínez-Luna, N. (2013). Evaluation of single nucleotide polymorphisms in the miR-183–96–182 cluster in adulthood attention-deficit and hyperactivity disorder (ADHD) and substance use disorders (SUDs). *European Neuropsychopharmacology*, *23*(11), 1463–1473.

Sato, J. R., Hoexter, M. Q., Castellanos, X. F., & Rohde, L. A. (2012). Abnormal brain connectivity patterns in adults with ADHD: A coherence study. *PloS One*, *7*(9).

Satterfield, J. H., & Schell, A. (1997). A prospective study of hyperactive boys with conduct problems and normal boys: Adolescent and adult criminality. *Journal of the American Academy of Child and Adolescent Psychiatry*, *36*, 1726–1735.

Scarborough, H. S. (1998). Early identification of children at risk for reading disabilities: Phonological awareness and some other promising predictors. *Specific Reading Disability: A View of the Spectrum*, 75–119.

Schmahmann, J. D. (1991). An emerging concept: The cerebellar contribution to higher function. *Archives of Neurology*, *48*(11), 1178–1187.

Schmahmann, J. D. (1996). From movement to thought: Anatomic substrates of the cerebellar contribution to cognitive processing. *Human Brain Mapping*, *4*, 174–198.

Schmahmann, J. D. (1998). Dysmetria of thought: Clinical consequences of cerebellar dysfunction on cognition and affect. *Trends in Cognitive Science*, *2*(9), 362–371.

Schmahmann, J. D. (2004). Disorders of the cerebellum: Ataxia, dysmetria of thought, and the cerebellar cognitive affective syndrome. [Review]. *Journal of Neuropsychiatry Clinical Neuroscience*, *16*(3), 367–378.

Schmahmann, J. D., & Pandya, D. N. (1997). Anatomic organization of the basilar pontine projections from prefrontal cortices in rhesus monkey. *Journal of Neuroscience*, *17*(1), 438–458.

Schneider, M., Debbane, M., Bassett, A. S., Chow, E. W. C., Fung, W. L. A., van den Bree, M. B. M. (2014). Psychiatric disorders from childhood to adulthood in 22q11.2 deletion syndrome: Results from the International Consortium on Brain and Behavior in 22q11.2 deletion syndrome. *American Journal of Psychiatry*, *171*(6), 627–639.

Schnoes, C., Reid, R., Wagner, M., & Marder, C. (2006). ADHD among students receiving special education services: A national survey. *Exceptional Children*, *72*(4), 483–496.

Schoots, O., & Van Tol, H. H. (2003). The human dopamine D4 receptor repeat sequences modulate expression. *The Pharmacogenomics Journal*, *3*, 343–348.

Schumacher, J., Hoffmann, P., Schmäl, C., Schulte-Körne, G., & Nöthen, M. M. (2007). Genetics of dyslexia: The evolving landscape. *Journal of Medical Genetics*, *44*(5), 289–297.

Seidel, W. T., & Joschko, M. (1990). Evidence of difficulties in sustained attention in children with ADDH. *Journal of Abnormal Child Psychology*, *18*(2), 217–229.

Seidman, L. J., Biederman, J., Monuteaux, M., Doyle, A., & Faraone, S. V. (2001). Learning disabilities and executive dysfunction in boys with attention-deficit/hyperactivity disorder. *Neuropsychology*, *15*, 544–556.

Seidman, L. J., Biederman, J., Liang, L., Valera, E. M., Monuteaux, M. C., Brown, A., & Makris, N. (2011). Gray matter alterations in adults with attention-deficit/hyperactivity disorder identified by voxel based morphometry. *Biological psychiatry*, *69*(9), 857–866.

Seidman, L. J., Valera, E. M., & Bush, G. (2004). Brain function and structure in adults with attention-deficit/hyperactivity disorder. *Psychiatric Clinics of North America*, *27*(2), 323–347.

Seidman, L. J., Valera, E. M., & Makris, N. (2005). Structural brain imaging of attention-deficit/hyperactivity disorder. *Biological Psychiatry*, *57*(11), 1263–1272.

Seidman, L. J., Valera, E. M., Makris, N., Monuteaux, M. C., Boriel, D. L., Kelkar, K., . . . Biederman, J. (2006). Dorsolateral prefrontal and anterior cingulate cortex volumetric abnormalities in adults with attention-deficit/hyperactivity disorder identified by magnetic resonance imaging. *Biological Psychiatry*, *60*(10), 1071–1080.

Semrud-Clikeman, M., Biederman, J., Sprich-Buckminster, S., Lehman, B. K., Faraone, S. V., & Norman, D. (1992). Comorbidity between ADDH and learning disability: A review and report in a clinically referred sample. *Journal of the American Academy of Child and Adolescent Psychiatry*, *31*(3), 439–448.

Semrud-Clikeman, M., Guy, K., Griffin, J. D., & Hynd, G. W. (2000). Rapid naming deficits in children and adolescents with reading disabilities and attention deficit hyperactivity disorder. *Brain and Language*, *74*(1), 70–83.

Semrud-Clikeman, M., Pliszka, S. R., Bledsoe, J., & Lancaster, J. (2014). Volumetric MRI differences in treatment naive and chronically treated adolescents with ADHD-combined type. *Journal of Attention Disorders*, *18*(6), 511–520.

Semrud-Clikeman, M., Steingard, R. J., Filipek, P., Biederman, J., Bekken, K., & Renshaw, P. F. (2000). Using MRI to examine brain-behavior relationships in males with attention deficit disorder with hyperactivity. *Journal of the American Academy of Child and Adolescent Psychiatry*, *39*(4), 477–484.

Sergeant, J. A. (2005). Modeling attention deficit/hyperactivity disorder: A critical appraisal of the cognitive-energetic model. *Biological Psychiatry*, *57*, 1248–1255.

Shalev, R. S., & Gross-Tsur, V. (2001). Developmental dyscalculia. *Pediatric Neurology*, *24*, 337–342.

Shalev, R. S., Manor, O., & Gross-Tsur, V. (2005). Developmental dyscalculia: a prospective six-year follow-up. *Developmental Medicine and Child Neurology*, *47*(2), 121–125.

Sharp, W. S., Gottesman, R. F., Greenstein, D. K., Ebens, C. L., Rapoport, J. L., & Castellanos, F. X. (2003). Monozygotic twins discordant for attention-deficit/hyperactivity disorder: Ascertainment and clinical characteristics. *Journal of the American Academy of Child and Adolescent Psychiatry*, *42*, 93–97.

Shaw, P., Eckstrand, K., Sharp, W., Blumenthal, J., Lerch, J. P., Greenstein, D., Rapoport, J. L. (2007). Attention-deficit/hyperactivity disorder is characterized by a delay in cortical maturation. *Proceedings of the National Academy of Sciences of the United States*, *104*(49), 19649–19654.

Shaw, P., Gogtay, N., & Rapoport, J. (2010). Childhood psychiatric disorders as anomalies in neurodevelopmental trajectories. *Human Brain Mapping*, *31*(6), 917–925.

Shaw, P., Lerch, J., Greenstein, D., Sharp, W., Clasen, L., Evans, A., Rapoport, J. (2006). Longitudinal mapping of cortical thickness and clinical outcome in children and adolescents with attention-deficit/hyperactivity disorder. *Archives of General Psychiatry*, *63*(5), 540–549.

Shaw, P., Malek, M., Watson, B., Sharp, W., Evans, A., Greenstein, D. (2012). Development of cortical surface area and gyrification in attention-deficit/hyperactivity disorder. *Biological Psychiatry*, *72*(3), 191–197.

Shaywitz, S., Escober, M. D., Shaywitz, B. A., Fletcher, J. M., & Makach, R. (1992). Evidence that dyslexia may represent the lower tail of a normal distribution of reading ability. *The New England Journal of Medicine*, *326*, 145–150.

Shaywitz, S. E., Shaywitz, B. A., Pugh, K. R., Fulbright, R. K., Constable, R. T., Mencl, W. E., . . . & Katz, L. (1998). Functional disruption in the organization of the brain for reading in dyslexia. *Proceedings of the National Academy of Sciences*, *95*(5), 2636–2641.

Shaywitz, B. A., Shaywitz, S. E., Pugh, K. R., Mencl, E. W., Fulbright, R. K., Skudlarski, P., . . . Gore, J. C. (2002). Disruption of posterior brain systems for reading in children with developmental dyslexia. *Biological Psychiatry*, *52*, 101–110.

Shaywitz, S. E., & Shaywitz, B. A. (2005). Dyslexia (specific reading disability). *Biological Psychiatry*, *57*, 1301–1309.

Shekim, W., Asarnow, R. F., Hess, E., Zaucha, K., & Wheeler, N. (1990). A clinical and demographic profile of a sample of adults with attention deficit hyperactivity disorder, residual state. *Comprehensive Psychiatry*, *31*, 416–425.

Sheppard, D. M., Bradshaw, J. L., Purcell, R., & Pantelis, C. (1999). Tourette's and Comorbid syndromes: Obsessive compulsive and attention deficit hyperactivity disorder: A common etiology? *Clinical Psychology Review*, *19*(5), 531–552.

Shumay, E., Fowler, J. S., & Volkow, N. D. (2010). Genomic features of the human dopamine transporter gene and its potential epigenetic states: Implications for phenotypic diversity. *PloS One*, *5*, e11067.

Siegel, L. S., & Smythe, I. S. (2008). The importance of phonological processing rather than IQ discrepancy in understanding adults with reading disorders. In L. E. Wolf, H. Schreiber, & J. Wasserstein (Eds.), *Adult Learning Disorders: Contemporary Issues* (pp. 275–300). New York: Psychology Press.

Silk, T. J., Vance, A., Rinehart, N., Bradshaw, J. L., & Cunnington, R. (2008). Dysfunction in the fronto-parietal network in attention deficit hyperactivity disorder (ADHD): an fMRI study. *Brain Imaging and Behavior*, *2*(2), 123–131.

Silk, T. J., Vance, A., Rinehart, N., Bradshaw, J. L., & Cunnington, R. (2009). White-matter abnormalities in attention deficit hyperactivity disorder: a diffusion tensor imaging study. *Human Brain Mapping*, *30*(9), 2757–2765.

Silva, J. P., Suckling, J., & Ushkaryov, Y. (2009). Penelope's web: Using alpha-latrotoxin to untangle the mysteries of exocytosis. *Journal of Neurochemistry*, *111*, 275–290.

Simonoff, E., Jones, C. R. G., Baird, G., Pickles, A., Happe, F., & Charman, T. (2013). The persistence and stability of psychiatric problems in adolescents with autism spectrum disorders. *Journal of Child Psychology and Psychiatry*, *54*(2), 186–194.

Simos, P. G., Kanatsouli, K., Fletcher, J. M., Juranek, J., Cirino, P., & Papanicolaou, A. C. (2008). Aberrant spatiotemporal activation profiles associated with math difficulties in children: a magnetic source imaging study. *Neuropsychology*, *22*(5), 571.

Sitlington, P. L. (1996). Transition to living: The neglected component of transition programming for individuals with learning disabilities. *Journal of Learning Disabilities*, *29*, 31–39, 52.

Smith, A., Taylor, E., Rogers, J. W., Newman, S., & Rubia, K. (2002). Evidence for a pure time perception deficit in children with ADHD. *Journal of Child Psychology and Psychiatry*, *43*(4), 529–542.

Smith, S. D. (2007). Genes, language development, and language disorders. *Mental Retardation and Developmental Disabilities Research Review*, *13*(1), 96–105.

Schnoes, C. J., Kuhn, B. R., Workman, E. F., & Ellis, C. R. (2006). Pediatric prescribing practices for clonidine and other pharmacologic agents for children with sleep disturbance. *Clinical Pediatrics (Phila)*, *45*(3), 229–238.

Solanto, M. V. (2011). *Cognitive-Behavioral Therapy for Adult ADHD: Targeting Executive Dysfunction*. New York: Guilford Press.

Solanto, M. V., Wasserstein, J., Marks, D. J., & Mitchell, K. J. (2012). Diagnosis of ADHD in adults: What is the appropriate DSM-5 symptom threshold for hyperactivity-impulsivity? *Journal of Attention Disorders*, *16*, 631–634.

Sommers, R. K., Fragapane, L., & Schmock, K. (1994). Changes in maternal attitudes and perceptions and children's communication skills. *Perceptual Motor Skills*, *79*(2), 851–861.

Son, G. H., Chung, S., Geum, D., Kang, S. S., Choi, W. S., Kim, K., & Choi, S. (2007). Hyperactivity and alteration of the midbrain dopaminergic system in maternally stressed male mice offspring. *Biochemical and Biophysical Research Communications*, *352*, 823–829.

Sonuga-Barke, E., Bitsakou, P., & Thompson, M. (2010). Beyond the dual pathway model: Evidence for the dissociation of timing, inhibitory, and delay-related impairments in attention-deficit/hyperactivity disorder. *Journal of the American Academy of Child and Adolescent Psychiatry*, *49*(4), 345–355.

Sonuga-Barke, E., & Castellanos, F. X. (2007). Spontaneous attentional fluctuations in impaired states and pathological conditions: A neurological hypothesis. *Neuroscience and Biobehavioral Reviews*, *31*, 977–986.

Sonuga-Barke, E. J., & Coghill, D. (2014). The foundations of next generation attention-deficit/hyperactivity disorder neuropsychology: Building on progress during the last 30 years. *Journal of Child Psychology and Psychiatry*, *55*(12), e1–e5.

Sparks, R. L., Javorsky, J., & Philips, L. (2004). College students classified with ADHD and the foreign language requirement. *Journal of Learning Disabilities*, *37*, 169–178.

Sparks, R. L., Philips, L., & Javorsky, J. (2003). Students classified as LD who petitioned for or fulfilled the college foreign language requirement: Are they different? *Journal of Learning Disabilities*, *36*, 348–362.

Spreen, O. (2011). Nonverbal learning disabilities: A critical review. *Child Neuropsychology*, *17*, 418–443.

Sprich, S., Biederman, J., Crawford, M. H., Mundy, E., & Faraone, S. V. (2000). Adoptive and biological families of children and adolescents with ADHD. *Journal of the American Academy of Child and Adolescent Psychiatry*, *39*, 1432–1437.

Stanescu-Cosson, R., Pinel, P., van de Moortele, P. F., Le Bihan, D., Cohen, L., & Dehaene, S. (2000). Understanding dissociations in dyscalculia: A brain imaging study of the impact of number size on the cerebral networks for exact and approximate calculation. *Brain*, *123*, 2240–2255.

Stankiewicz, P., & Lupski, J. R. (2010). Structural variation in the human genome and its role in disease. *Annual Review of Medicine*, *61*, 437–455.

Stefanatos, G. A., & Baron, I. S. (2007). Attention-deficit/hyperactivity disorder: A neuropsychological perspective towards DSM-V. *Neuropsychology Review*, *17*(1), 5–38.

Stefanatos, G. A., & DeMarco, A. T. (2012). Central auditory processing disorders. In V. S. Ramachandran (Ed.), *Encyclopedia of Human Behavior* (2nd ed., Vol. 2, pp. 441–453). Oxford: Academic Press.

Stefanatos, G. A., & Wasserstein, J. (2001). Attention deficit/hyperactivity disorder as a right hemisphere syndrome: Selective literature review and detailed neuropsychological case studies. *Annals of the New York Academy of Science*, *931*, 172–195.

Stergiakouli, E., Hamshere, M., Holmans, P., Langley, K., Zaharieva, I., Hawi, Z., & Thapar, A. (2012). Investigating the contribution of common genetic variants to the risk and pathogenesis of ADHD. *American Journal of Psychiatry*, *169*, 186–194.

Still, G. F. (1902). The goulstonian lectures on some abnormal psychical conditions in children. *Lancet*, *1*, 1008–1012.

Stothers, M., & Klein, P. (2010). Perceptual organization, phonological awareness, and reading comprehension in adults with and without learning disabilities. *Annals of Dyslexia*, *60*(2), 209–237.

Stoodley, C. J., & Stein, J. F. (2013). Cerebella function in developmental dyslexia. *Cerebellum*, *12*, 267–276.

Strauss, A. A., & Lehtinen, L. E. (1947). *Psychopathology and Education of the Brain-Injured Child*. New York: Grune & Stratton.

Swanson, H. L. (2012). Adults with reading disabilities: Converting a meta-analysis to practice. *Journal of Learning Disabilities*, *45*, 17–30.

Swanson, J., Castellanos, F. X., Murias, M., LaHoste, G., & Kennedy, J. (1998). Cognitive neuroscience of attention deficit hyperactivity disorder and hyperkinetic disorder. *Current Opinion in Neurobiology*, *8*(2), 263–271.

Swanson, J. M., Kinsbourne, M., Nigg, J., Lanphear, B., Stefanatos, G. A., Volkow, N., . . . Wadhwa, P. D. (2007). Etiologic subtypes of attention-deficit/hyperactivity disorder: Brain imaging, molecular genetic and environmental factors and the dopamine hypothesis. *Neuropsychology Review*, *17*(1), 39–59.

Szatmari, P., Saigal, S., Rosenbaum, P., Campbell, D., & King, S. (1990). Psychiatric disorders at five years among children with birthweights less than 1000g: A regional perspective. *Developmental Medicine and Child Neurology*, *32*, 954–962.

Szucs, D., Devine, A., Soltesz, F., Nobes, A., & Gabriel, F. (2013). Developmental dyscalculia is related to visuo-spatial memory and inhibition impairment. *Cortex*, *49*(10), 2674–2688.

Tamm, L., & Juranek, J. (2012). Fluid reasoning deficits in children with ADHD: Evidence from fMRI. *Brain Research*, *1465*, 48–56.

Tannock, R., & Brown, T. E. (2000). Attention-deficit disorders with learning disorders in children and adolescents. In T. E. Brown (Ed.), *Attention Deficit Disorders and Comorbidities and Children, Adolescents and Adults* (pp. 231–296). Washington, DC: American Psychiatric Press.

Tardito, D., Mallei, A., & Popoli, M. (2013). Lost in translation: New unexplored avenues for neuropsychopharmacology: Epigenetics and microRNAs. *Expert Opinion on Investigational Drugs*, *22*, 217–233.

Taylor, E., Sandberg, S., Thorley, G., & Giles, S. (1991). *The Epidemiology of Childhood Hyperactivity*. London: Oxford University Press.

Temple, E., Deeutsch, G. K., & Poldrack, R. A. (2003). Neural deficits in children with dyslexia ameliorated by behavioral remediation: evidence from functional MRI. *Proceedings of the National Academy of Science*, *100*, 2860–2865.

Thapar, A., Cooper, M., Eyre, O., & Langley, K. (2013). What have we learnt about the causes of ADHD? *Journal of Child Psychology and Psychiatry, and Allied Disciplines*, *54*, 3–16.

Thome-Souza, S., Kuczynski, E., Assumpcao, F., Jr., Rzezak, P., Fuentes, D., Fiore, L., & Valente, K. D. (2004). Which factors may play a pivotal role on determining the type of psychiatric disorder in children and adolescents with epilepsy? *Epilepsy & Behavior*, *5*(6), 988–994.

Thompson, J. L., Pogue-Geile, M. F., & Grace, A. A. (2004). Developmental pathology, dopamine, and stress: A model for the age of onset of schizophrenia symptoms. *Schizophrenia Bulletin*, *30*, 875–900.

Timimi, S., & Taylor, E. (2004). ADHD is best understood as a cultural construct. *British Journal of Psychiatry*, *184*, 8–9.

Toplak, M. E., & Tannock, R. (2005). Time perception: Modality and duration effects in attention-deficit/hyperactivity disorder (ADHD). *Journal of Abnormal Child Psychology*, *33*(5), 639–654.

Tsatsanis, K. D., & Rourke, B. P. (2008). Syndrome of Nonverbal Learning Disabilities in Adults. In L. E. Wolf, H. Schreiber, & J. Wasserstein (Eds.), *Adult Learning Disorders: Contemporary Issues* (pp. 159–190). New York: Psychology Press. London: Taylor & Francis.

Utter, A. A., & Basso, M. A. (2008). The basal ganglia: An overview of circuits and function. *Neuroscience and Biobehavioral Reviews*, *32*(3), 333–342.

Vaisse, L. (1866). Des sourds-muets et de certains cas d'aphasie congenitale. *Bulletins de la Société d'anthropologie* (Paris), *1*, 146–150.

Valera, E. M., Faraone, S. V., Murray, K. E., & Seidman, L. J. (2007). Meta-analysis of structural imaging findings in attention-deficit/hyperactivity disorder. *Biological Psychiatry*, *61*(12), 1361–1369.

van der Meer, J. M. J., Oerlemans, A. M., van Steijn, D. J., Lappenschaar, M. G. A., de Sonneville, L. M. J., Buitelaar, J. K., & Rommelse, N. N. J. (2012). Are autism spectrum disorder and attention-deficit/hyperactivity disorder different manifestations of one overarching disorder? Cognitive and symptom evidence from a clinical and population-based sample. *Journal of the American Academy of Child and Adolescent Psychiatry*, *51*(11), 1160–1172.

van Ewijk, H., Heslenfeld, D. J., Zwiers, M. P., Buitelaar, J. K., & Oosterlaan, J. (2012). Diffusion tensor imaging in attention deficit/hyperactivity disorder: A systematic review and meta-analysis. *Neuroscience and Biobehavioral Reviews*, *36*(4), 1093–1106.

van Hartingsveldt, M. J., de Groot, I. J. M., Aarts, P. B. M., & Nijhuis-van der Sanden, M. W. G. (2011). Standardized tests of handwriting readiness: A systematic review of the literature. *Developmental Medicine and Child Neurology*, *53*(6), 506–515.

van Mil, N. H., Steegers-Theunissen, R. P., Bouwland-Both, M. I., Verbiest, M. M., Rijlaarsdam, J., Hofman, A., . . . & Stolk, L. (2014). DNA methylation profiles at birth and child ADHD symptoms. *Journal of Psychiatric Research*, *49*, 51–59.

Varley, K. E., Gertz, J., Bowling, K. M., Parker, S. L., Reddy, T. E., Pauli-Behn, F., & Absher, D. M. (2013). Dynamic DNA methylation across diverse human cell lines and tissues. *Genome Research*, *23*(3), 555–567.

Vellutino, F. R., Fletcher, J. M., Snowling, M. J., & Scanlon, D. M. (2004). Specific reading disability (dyslexia): What have we learned in the past four decades? *Journal of Child Psychology and Psychiatry*, *45*, 2–40.

Venneri, A., Cornoldi, C., & Garuti, M. (2003). Arithmetic difficulties in children with visuospatial learning disability (VLD). *Child Neuropsychology*, *9*(3), 175–183.

Visser, J., & Jehan, Z. (2009). ADHD: A scientific fact or a factual opinion? A critique of the veracity of attention deficit hyperactivity disorder. *Emotional and Behavioral Difficulties*, *14*(2), 127–140.

Voeller, K. K., & Heilman, K. M. (1988). Attention deficit disorder in children: A neglect syndrome? *Neurology*, *38*(5), 806–808.

Vogel, S., & Forness, S. R. (1992). Social functioning in adults with learning disabilities. *School Psychology Review*, *21*, 275–286.

Vukovic, R. K., Wilson, A. M., & Nash, K. K. (2004). Naming speed deficits in adults with reading disabilities: A test of the double-deficit hypothesis. *Journal of Learning Disabilities*, *37*, 440–450.

Wagner, M., Kutash, K., Duchnowski, A. J., Epstein, M. H., & Sumi, W. C. (2005). The children and youth we serve: A national picture of the characteristics of students with emotional disturbances receiving special education. *Journal of Emotional and Behavioral Disorders*, *13*, 79–96.

Wallman, K. K. (2008). Federal interagency forum on child and family statistics. *America's Children in Brief: Key National Indicators of Well-Being*.

Wang, S., Yan, J. Y., Lo, Y. K., Carvey, P. M., & Ling, Z. (2009). Dopaminergic and serotoninergic deficiencies in young adult rats prenatally exposed to the bacterial lipopolysaccharide. *Brain Research*, *1265*, 196–204.

Wasserstein, J., & Denckla, M. B. (2009). ADHD and learning disabilities in adults: Overlap with executive dysfunction. In T. E. Brown (Ed.), *ADHD Comorbidities: Handbook for ADHD Complications in Children and Adults* (pp. 267–285). Washington, DC: American Psychiatric Publishing.

Wasserstein, J., & Stefanatos, G. A. (2000). The right hemisphere and psychopathology. Neuroscience and Psychoanalysis, *Special Edition of the Journal of the American Academy of Psychoanalysis*, *28*, 371–393.

Wasserstein, J., & Stefanatos, G. A. (2016). Re-examining ADHD as corticostriatal disorder: Implications for understanding common comorbidities. *The ADHD Report*, *24*(4), 1–10.

Wasserstein, J., Vadhan, N. P., Barboza, K., & Stefanatos, G. A. (2008). Outcomes in probable nonverbal learning disabled (NLD) adults: A naturalistic study. In L. E. Wolf, H. Schreiber, & J. Wasserstein (Eds.), *Adult Learning Disorders: Contemporary Issues* (pp. 462–491). New York: Psychology Press.

Wasserstein, J., Wasserstein, A., & Wolf, L. (2001). *Attention Deficit Disorder in Adults*. Online publication by Education Resources Information Center (ERIC), ERIC Digest Number ED461959. National Library of Education.

Watemberg, N., Waiserberg, N., Zuk, L., & Lerman-Sagie, T. (2007). Developmental coordination disorder in children with attention-deficit-hyperactivity disorder and physical therapy intervention. *Developmental Medicine & Child Neurology*, *49*(12), 920–925.

Weiss, G. L., Hechtman, L., Milroy, T., & Perlman, T. (1985). Psychiatric status of hyperactives as adults: A controlled prospective 15-year follow-up of 63 hyperactive children. *Journal of the American Academy of Child and Adolescent Psychiatry*, *24*, 211–220.

Wender, P. H. (1998). Attention-deficit hyperactivity disorder in adults. *Psychiatric Clinics of North America*, *21*(4), 761–774.

Wilens, T. E. (2004). Impact of ADHD and its treatment on substance abuse in adults. *Journal of Clinical Psychiatry*, *65*(Suppl 3), 38–45.

Wilens, T. E., Biederman, J., & Spencer, T. (2002). Attention deficit/hyperactivity disorder across the life span. *Annual Review of Medicine*, *53*, 113–131.

Wilens, T. E., Faraone, S. V., Biederman, J., & Gunawardene, S. (2003). Does stimulant therapy of attention-deficit/hyperactivity disorder beget later substance abuse? A meta-analytic review of the literature. *Pediatrics*, *111*(1), 179–185.

Willcutt, E. G., Betjemann, R. S.,Wadsworth, S. J., Samuelsson, S., Corley, R., DeFries, J. C., . . . Olson, R. K. (2007). Preschool twin study of the relation between attention-deficit/hyperactivity disorder and prereading skills. *Reading and Writing*, *20*(1–2), 103–125.

Willcutt, E. G., Doyle, A. E., Nigg, J. T., Faraone, S. V., & Pennington, B. F. (2005). Validity of the executive function theory of attention-deficit/hyperactivity disorder: A meta-analytic review. *Biological Psychiatry*, *57*(11), 1336–1346.

Williams, J., Griebel, M. L., & Dykman, R. A. (1998). Neuropsychological patterns in pediatric epilepsy. [Article]. *Seizure-European Journal of Epilepsy*, *7*(3), 223–228. 1311(98)80040-x.

Williams, N. M., Zaharieva, I., Martin, A., Langley, K., Mantripragada, K., Fossdal, R., . . . Thapar, A. (2010). Rare chromosomal deletions and duplications in attention-deficit hyperactivity disorder: A genome-wide analysis. *Lancet*, *376*, 1401–1408.

Williams, N. M., Franke, B., Mick, E., Anney, R. J., Freitag, C. M., Gill, M., . . . Faraone, S. V. (2012). Genome-wide analysis of copy number variants in attention deficit hyperactivity disorder: The role of rare variants and duplications at 15q13.3. *American Journal of Psychiatry*, *169*, 195–204.

Williams, Z. M., Bush, G., Rauch, S. L., Cosgrove, G. R., & Eskandar, E. N. (2004). Human anterior cingulate neurons and the integration of monetary reward with motor responses. *Nature Neuroscience*, *7*(12), 1370–1375.

Wilson, A. M., Armstrong, C. D., Furrie, A., & Walcot, E. (2009). The mental health of Canadians with self-reported learning disabilities. *Journal of Learning Disabilities*, *42*, 24–40.

Wilson, H. K., Cox, D. J., Merkel, R. L., Moore, M., & Coghill, D. (2006). Effect of extended release stimulant-based medications on neuropsychological functioning among adolescents with attention-deficit/hyperactivity disorder. *Archives of Clinical Neuropsychology*, *21*, 797–807.

Wilson, P. H., & McKenzie, B. E. (1998). Information processing deficits associated with developmental coordination disorder: A meta-analysis of research findings. *Journal of Child Psychology and Psychiatry*, *39*(6), 829–840.

Witte, R. H., Philips, L., & Kakela, M. (1998). Job satisfaction of college students with learning disabilities. *Journal of Learning Disabilities*, *31*, 259–265.

Wodka, E. L., Mahone, E. M., Blankner, J. G., Larson, J. C., Fotedar, S., Denckla, M. B., & Mostofsky, S. H. (2007). Evidence that response inhibition is a primary deficit in ADHD. *Journal of Clinical Experience in Neuropsychology*, *29*(4), 345–356.

Wolf, L. E., Schreiber, H., & Wasserstein, J. (Eds.). (2008). *Adult Learning Disorders: Contemporary Issues*. New York: Psychology Press.

Wolf, L. E., & Wasserstein, J. (2001). Adult ADHD: Concluding thoughts. *Annals of the New York Academy of Sciences*, *931*, 396–408.

Wolraich, M, Hannah, J. N., Pinnock, T. Y., Baumgaertel, A., & Brown, J. (1996). Comparison of diagnostic criteria for attention-deficit hyperactivity disorder in a county-wide sample. *Journal of the American Academy of Child and Adolescent Psychiatry*, *35*, 319–324.

Wong, C. C., Caspi, A., Williams, B., Craig, I. W., Houts, R., Ambler, A., . . . Mill, J. (2010). A longitudinal study of epigenetic variation in twins. *Epigenetics: Official Journal of the DNA Methylation Society*, *5*, 516–526.

Wu, S. W., Gilbert, D. L., Shahana, N., Huddleston, D. A., & Mostofsky, S. H. (2012). Transcranial Magnetic Stimulation measures in attention-deficit/hyperactivity disorder. *Pediatric Neurology*, *47*(3), 177–185.

Yang, L., Neale, B. M., Liu, L., Lee, S. H., Wray, N. R., Ji, N., . . . Hu, X. (2013). Polygenic transmission and complex neuro developmental network for attention deficit hyperactivity disorder: Genome-wide association study of both common and rare variants. *American Journal of Medical Genetics Part B*, *162B*, 419–430.

Yang, P. C., Wang, P. N., Chuang, K. H., Jong, Y. J., Chao, T. C., & Wu, M. T. (2008). Absence of gender effect on children with attention-deficit/hyperactivity disorder as assessed by optimized voxel-based morphometry. *Psychiatry Research-Neuroimaging*, *164*(3), 245–253.

Zametkin, A. J., Nordahl, T. E., Gross, M., King, A. C., Semple, W. E., Rumsey, J., & Cohen, R. M. (1990). Cerebral glucose metabolism in adults with hyperactivity of childhood onset. *New England Journal of Medicine*, *323*(20), 1361–1366.

Zametkin, A. J., Nordahl, T. E., Gross, M., King, A. C., Semple, W. E., Rumsey, J., & Cohen, R. M. (1990). Cerebral glucose metabolism in adults with hyperactivity of childhood onset. *New England Journal of Medicine*, *323*(20), 1361–1366.

Zeffiro, T., & Eden, G. (2001). The cerebellum and dyslexia: Perpetrator or innocent bystander? *Trends in Neuroscience*, *24*, 512–513.

Zhang, F., Gu, W., Hurles, M. E., & Lupski, J. R. (2009). Copy number variation in human health, disease, and evolution. *Annual Review of Genomics and Human Genetics*, *10*, 451–481.

Zhou, R., Zhang, Z., Zhu, Y., Chen, L., & Sokabe, M. (2009). Deficits in development of synaptic plasticity in rat dorsal striatum following prenatal and neonatal exposure to low-dose bisphenol. *Annals of Neuroscience*, *159*, 161–171.

Zinn, A. R., Roeltgen, D., Stefanatos, G., Ramos, P., Elder, F. F., Kushner, H., & Ross, J. L. (2007). A Turner syndrome neurocognitive phenotype maps to Xp22.3. *Behavioral and Brain Functions*, *3*(1), 24.

15 Consciousness

Disorders, Assessment, and Intervention

Kathleen T. Bechtold and Megan M. Hosey

I think therefore I am.

—Descartes

Human consciousness is a complex and relatively poorly understood process of the brain. The majority of clinical attention has been given to the disorders of consciousness that occur most commonly with severe brain trauma leading to severe arousal/vigilance issues. However, consciousness extends well beyond basic arousal to some of the most

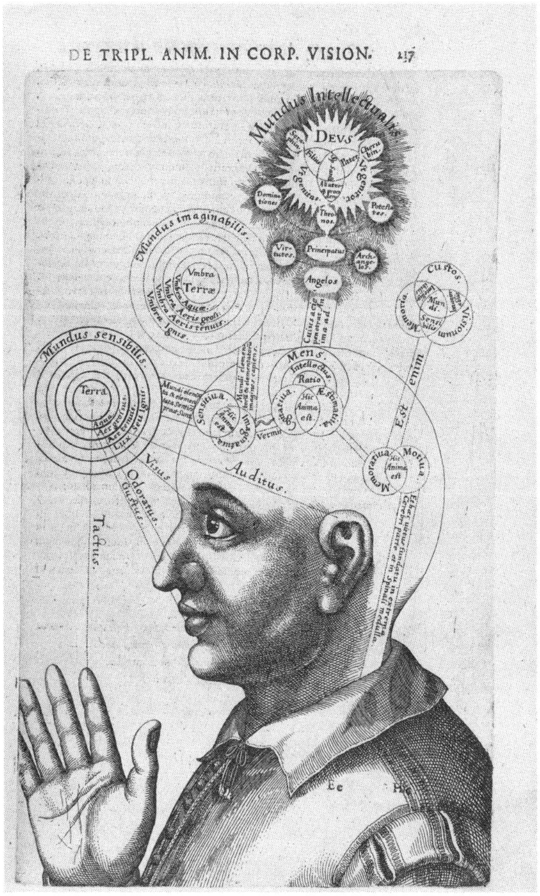

Figure 15.1 17th century conceptualization of consciousness

Source: Wellcome Images (http://wellcomeimages.org/indexplus/obf_images/58/ea/0f84202fa8ff58b9bc4819f8fe04.jpg)

complex abilities of the brain to understand the self in ways that are possibly unique to humans. Consciousness is not only the basic level of alertness, but also the ability of the brain to have a concept of self, a personal past and future, and an awareness of one's strengths and weaknesses.

When one delves into the cognitive psychology and neuroscience literature, a rich tapestry unfolds to reveal the many colors and textures of consciousness. However, digesting the theoretical models, the comparative animal studies, and the human case studies leads to many more questions than answers about consciousness and how we need to address impairments in consciousness clinically. To begin the discussion, we must define what we are talking about by establishing our terminology. It may appear obvious at first glance what consciousness is, but once one steps back to truly contemplate consciousness, the complexities arise and one's philosophical and religious biases may sneak in. Although the contemplation of consciousness is firmly rooted historically in philosophy and religion (see Figure 15.1), this is not for discussion in this text. The nod to Descartes at the beginning of this chapter is more in acknowledgement of the long history in which humans have contemplated their own selves, than any foreshadowing of a philosophical bent to the discussion to come. Nor will we delve into theoretical physics and the attempts to apply quantum theory to the understanding of consciousness. The interested reader is encouraged to see Hameroff and Penrose (2013) for a discussion of Orch-OR theory and Pribram (1991) for a discussion of holonomic brain theory. For the sake of the current discussion, we will restrict our digestion to the realm of cognitive science, neuroscience, neuropsychology, and rehabilitation with the goal of trying to understand consciousness enough (given the state of the field) to guide clinical practice with individuals with neuropathology.

Once we have defined our terminology and taken a brief walk through both evolution and human development, then we can discuss what we know about the variety of disorders of consciousness and how as neuropsychologists we can attempt to assess and intervene to assist individuals in truly engaging in life after the onset of neuropathology. Finally, we will make some suggestions about where the field should go from here to push the envelope of our understanding of human consciousness in order to broaden our understanding of the brain and how we can better address the needs of our patients clinically.

Consciousness and Its Elements

Consciousness is a very complex and somewhat abstruse subject that challenges us all to think about our ability to conceive, plot, plan, reflect, to be "on-line." Consciousness broadly defined for the current discussion is the state of being aware of one's thinking and being. It has been defined by terms such as *sentience*, *awareness*, *subjectivity*, and *selfhood* (Farthing, 1992). In an attempt to capture the essence of consciousness, in his *Search after Truth*, Descartes refers to consciousness as *internal testimony* (Heinämaa, Lähteenmäki, & Remes, 2007). It is likely that all these terms are accurate as they each capture some aspect of consciousness: the human ability to have a sense of self; to be aware and experience the world around through our senses; and to think about ourselves, our past, and our future.

In order to define consciousness, particularly for understanding disorders of consciousness, one must identify the underlying processes. There is somewhat a forest for the trees issue though, and so the reader is asked to keep in mind that we know so little about consciousness that we get caught up in mostly focusing on the elements of consciousness rather than understanding the overarching construct. With that said, we may not be thwarted in our aim of understanding how disorders of consciousness manifest and thus still be able to establish a framework to guide our discussion. Such a framework incorporates the elements of consciousness and captures the interrelationship among the elements, which we propose is hierarchical in nature with the elements building upon one another such that higher order, more complex processes are reliant on intact (at least to some degree) lower-level processes (see Figure 15.2).

Arousal/Vigilance

Consciousness at its birth relies upon a certain level of arousal. Where does consciousness begin? It is not known, or more accurately, it is open for debate. What is known is that neuropathology and chemical and mechanical effects on the brain can render a human *unconscious* or to lack sufficient arousal and the ability to have a sense of self, to be aware and experience the world around through the senses, and to think about his or herself, past, and future. There is a threshold level of neuronal excitement that must be crossed for consciousness to be birthed. *Vigilance* refers to this level of excitement in cortical and thalamic networks that is the foundational element of consciousness. It is a state with many gradations and thus has been referred to as *intransitive consciousness* (for a review, see Dehaene, 2014).

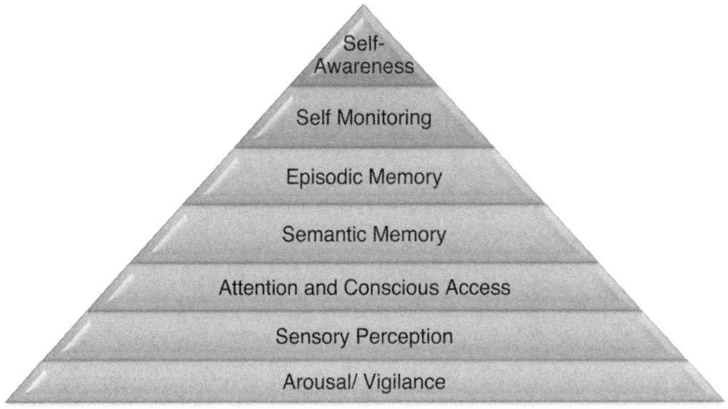

Figure 15.2 Hierarchical model of the elements of consciousness

Sensory Perception

Our senses are our gateway to experiencing the world around us. They allow us to compare what we see to what we tactilely feel to what we hear to what we taste and smell. However, we think one would be hard pressed to argue that an individual who has impairment in one or more of the senses has an impairment in consciousness. With that said, the senses are needed to some degree in order for the individual to develop a sense of self that is based upon experiencing and interacting in the world. Molyneux's problem—a thought experiment posed to John Locke by William Molyneux (Locke, 1690)—gives us a chance to consider sensory input in light of our ability to experience the world around us (see Table 15.1).

Table 15.1 Molyneux's problem (Locke, 1690)

I shall here insert a problem of that very ingenious and studious promoter of real knowledge, the learned and worthy Mr. Molyneux, which he was pleased to send me in a letter some months since; and it is this:—"Suppose a man born blind, and now adult, and taught by his touch to distinguish between a cube and a sphere of the same metal, and nighly of the same bigness, so as to tell, when he felt one and the other, which is the cube, which the sphere. Suppose then the cube and sphere placed on a table, and the blind man be made to see: quaere, whether by his sight, before he touched them, he could now distinguish and tell which is the globe, which the cube?" To which the acute and judicious proposer answers, "Not. For, though he has obtained the experience of how a globe, how a cube affects his touch, yet he has not yet obtained the experience, that what affects his touch so or so, must affect his sight so or so; or that a protuberant angle in the cube, that pressed his hand unequally, shall appear to his eye as it does in the cube."—I agree with this thinking gentleman, whom I am proud to call my friend, in his answer to this problem; and am of opinion that the blind man, at first sight, would not be able with certainty to say which was the globe, which the cube, whilst he only saw them; though he could unerringly name them by his touch, and certainly distinguish them by the difference of their figures felt. This I have set down, and leave with my reader, as an occasion for him to consider how much he may be beholden to experience, improvement, and acquired notions, where he thinks he had not the least use of, or help from them. And the rather, because this observing gentleman further adds, that "having, upon the occasion of my book, proposed this to divers very ingenious men, he hardly ever met with one that at first gave the answer to it which he thinks true, till by hearing his reasons they were convinced."

Molyneux was highlighting the difference between our perceptions and true understanding of what we are perceiving. Research has demonstrated that Molyneux and Locke were indeed correct in the sense that individuals who are blind and then gain sight have no understanding of what they are perceiving through sight (Held et al., 2011). However, there is greater complexity here because our brains do not operate based solely on unimodal information. The adaptivity of human behavior is rooted in the integration of sensory information to finely tune our behavior. Our senses not only allow us to *access* the world around us, they allow us to have feedback in-the-moment, which can guide our behavior. Without information from our senses, information from our world around us cannot be perceived and thus cannot inform our conscious concept of that world and ourselves. There is no information to guide behavior or sense of self. Is it possible that if a child is restricted in his or her experiences or incurs injury to the brain during key developmental periods leading to sensory impairment that he or she may be impaired in some aspects of consciousness? Is autism a disorder of consciousness because of the limitations imposed by the impairments in processing sensory information? It is clear that how individuals with autism experience the world around them differently from individuals without autism. Again, we have no clear answers, but for understanding how to approach assessment and interventions of individuals that have suffered an insult to the brain or have a developmental disorder, we must consider the possible impact of sensory impairment on consciousness. One might argue that in order to have awareness of being, one must have a concept of the relationship between others and the world around her- or himself. Without sensory input, that would not be possible. Thus for the current discussion, we assume that intact sensory input in some way shape or form is needed in order for the human being to gain information about his or her environment and to interact with that environment in meaningful ways and have a sense of self.

Attention and Conscious Access

In order to process information in our internal environment (in our minds) and our external environment (the world around us), we need to attend to that internal or external environment. When we focus our mental resources on a particular object or thought, we can bring that information into our awareness and report it to others. Attention is controlled by the individual. The focus of attention depends upon what that individual is drawn to. There can be incredible occurrences that pass right before our eyes that do not gain our attention and thus do not enter consciousness. Absorption of our consciousness on one point leads to blindness, of sorts, to the rest of the external world, which has been dubbed *inattentional blindness* (for a larger discussion, see Dehaene, 2014). A classic demonstration of inattentional blindness is the "invisible gorilla experiment" (Simons & Chabris, 1999), which everyone should experience at least once (www.theinvisiblegorilla.com/gorilla_experiment.html). This is one of many reasons that humans are not good eyewitnesses. What information is processed consciously depends upon where we have focused our attention, what information we have accessed. It is the *access* of the information into awareness that allows one to perceive it, contemplate it, talk about it, act in response to it. This process of *conscious access* relies upon sufficient arousal of the system and attention of cognitive resources onto the information (Dehaene, 2014). Without conscious access, the ability to process information is extremely limited.

Knowing (Semantic Memory)

The role of memory in consciousness has been theorized for centuries. The sense of self is bound to the continuity of self even with changes in the physical body through development and aging and the evolution of personality, skills, and abilities across time (Locke, 1690; Searle, 2005). For continuity of self, we must have memory to record the events, to record what we *know* about ourselves and the world around us and to update the knowledge as needed across time. That which is *known* is mentally experienced and can be behavioral expressed, although behavioral expression is not necessary. This catalogue of information is the semantic (declarative) memory system, which is a large, complex, multimodal system capable of fast, single-trial encoding (Squire, 1992). The information from this system has truth value, is accessible, and can form the basis for inferences about other objects and events in the world; however, it is not time-linked and is not dependent on any sense of self, although self-relevant information is stored in this system (Tulving, 2005).

Remembering (Episodic Memory)

Remembering is the ability to link the episodes of life with time and place such that one can think about past experiences (whether thought about or directly experienced) and possible future experiences (Tulving, 1985). As far as we know, no other species has the ability to mentally travel into the past and into the future. Tulving has long grappled with the potential uniqueness of the human episodic memory system and how it affords us the ability to conceptualize self in light of having a past and a future (for in-depth discussion, see Tulving, 1985). He argues that episodic memory allows mental time travel, which gives each of us a sense of *self*; we are the *owner* of our past and future experiences. Conscious recollection of personal happenings is the essence of autonoesis and what Tulving calls *autonoetic consciousness* (Tulving, 1985). Episodic memory is reliant upon semantic knowing (e.g., knowledge of ourselves and the world), but it has the distinct process of remembering the events, the episodes in the context of time and place. Without remembering, an individual does not have the capacity to think in terms of his or her past or the future and understand the implications of the past for the future.

Inner Speech and Self-Monitoring

As humans traverse daily life experiences, there is a running internal monologue. We think through problems, analyze the situation at hand, think about what has happened, and muse to ourselves—all without others knowing what is going on inside our heads. From time to time, we may even vocalize the "voice in our heads" but most frequently, we mentally process what has caught our attention. This "inner speech" is the silent production of words in one's mind and is argued to play a key role in human consciousness at the interchange between language and thought (Morin, 2011). There is evidence that inner speech plays a notable role in various cognitive functions, including working memory (Marvel & Desmond, 2012), episodic memory retrieval (Morin, 2011), planning (Sokolov, 1972), and self-awareness (Morin & Michaud, 2007). The inner monologue may be a foundational aspect of our ability to self-monitor and direct behavior, such as for planning of behavior (Agnati et al., 2012), problem solving (Baldo et al., 2005), and task switching (Emerson & Miyake, 2003). However, it also can be maladaptive by distracting cognitive resources and mental energy from behaviors that are productive, such is the case in depressive rumination (Davis & Nolen-Hoeksema, 2000) or the inner voices of schizophrenia (Farrer & Franck, 2007).

Searle (2005) argues that one element of consciousness that underlies our sense of self is our ability to guide/determine our own behavior, our *free will*, our inner voice that guides our behavior. When I consciously engage in a voluntary action, I am choosing to do this action versus another. Thus, I am mindfully directing my behavior. In the field of psychology, there has been increased interest in *mindfulness* with the goal of guiding humans to think before they act and be aware of how thoughts and feelings drive behavior and to develop more healthy response patterns. When impairments in working memory, episodic memory, or awareness are present, it is likely that the individual is going to be challenged in his or her ability to be mindful. The individual's inner voice may not have access to accurate, up-to-date information. That is not to say that individuals with neurodevelopmental disorders or acquired brain injuries cannot be mindful. However, how they are likely to be challenged in being mindful and self-monitoring their behavior.

Self-Awareness

The ability to know oneself, one's abilities, strengths, weaknesses is deeply reliant upon all the other elements of consciousness, from the very basic understanding of our own motor and sensory functioning to the very complex comprehension of our cognitive-behavioral abilities, idiosyncrasies, foibles, and talents. Without feedback through our sensory systems of our interactions with the world around us, we would know very little about ourselves or even have a sense of self. And what we *know* about ourselves is stored in our semantic memory system (e.g., "I know how to play volleyball." "I am the mother of two children." "I have tasted Coche-Dury Meursault Chardonnay from the Burgundy region of France"). But in order to judge meaning of one's abilities, to determine whether something is a strength or weakness, to determine personal likes and dislikes, the individual must have the ability to review the past for episodes of success and failure and project into the future consequences of behavior ("I play volleyball well because I remembering playing in many leagues and winning quite frequently." "I am a mother because I remember birthing and taking care of my daughters over the years and will do so for many years to come." "I remember going to Beaune, France, and tasting the beautiful nutty, creamy, buttery flavor of the Meursault Chardonnay, which I very much enjoyed"). Although the individual may have a distorted view of her or his strengths or weaknesses, likes and dislikes, these judgments are still grounded in what the individual *knows*, *remembers*, and *predicts* about her or his own behavior and experiences. The meaningfulness of behavior for that person influences her or his interpretation of the behavior on a continuum of strengths to weaknesses. If one does not find meaning in a behavior, then she will not incorporate that behavior into her self-definition and sense of self. That does not imply that she cannot answer the question can she do X activity or does she have Y skill, but rather that in her self-conceptualization and self-description, she will not include those skills and attributes and note them as strengths or weaknesses or likes or dislikes.

A Little Bit About the Neuroscience of Consciousness

There is little to no consensus on how the brain produces consciousness. For the interested reader who would like to grapple a little more in depth how a biologic process can result in the production of *self*, the experience of *me*, the ability to time travel from one's past and into the future, there have been a number of conferences that have resulted in summary works (Boly et al., 2013; Feinberg & Keenan, 2005; Terrace & Metcalfe, 2005). However, at least a cursory understanding of the possible neuroscience of consciousness will assist in the understanding of how disorders of consciousness develop with the onset of neuropathology.

There have been some critical findings over the last three decades that help us ground consciousness in brain functioning (rather than some philosophical or religious conceptualization of a soul). As the basis of consciousness, arousal is related to the functioning of the reticular formation, specific brain stem nuclei, and thalamo-cortical projections.

However, as we consider the broader conceptualization of consciousness, the overarching evidence supports that consciousness is not "located" somewhere in the brain (hearken back to Descartes' thought of the pineal gland being the seat of the soul), but rather is the product of integration of information from across the brain. It is produced by the brain's ability to integrate sensory, memory, emotional information from both hemispheres of the brain to create a unified experience. As argued by Searle (2005), consciousness has a unified field that allows the individual to incorporate the whole experience (forest) rather than just experience the constituent parts (trees). To make this more tangible, consider a daily life experience, such as eating a delicious meal in a restaurant and carrying on a conversation with your dinner companion. The unified field of consciousness allows you to experience the taste of the food while experiencing the conversation within the beautiful setting (forest) as opposed to sitting in a restaurant, eating the food, and having the conversation (trees). The unified field allows humans to have a higher level, integrated experience.

Sperry (1984) also saw human consciousness and unified sense of self as the product of the sum rather than the constituent parts and argued that consciousness is not in the nerve cells or in the molecules or the atoms of brain processing. He concluded that consciousness is the product of the dynamic emergence of brain activity and to be the "crowning achievement . . . of evolution" (Sperry, 1977). There is interesting evidence of this unified sense of self in the split-brain experiments of Sperry and Gazzaniga (for a review, see Gazzaniga, 1985), who demonstrated that cutting the corpus callosum leads to patients to demonstrating behaviors of having two separate conscious fields.

This type of advanced higher order integration of information would need to be subserved by the phylogenetically most advanced regions of the brain. Evolutionarily, rostral migration of functions fostered the forebrain—and in humans, the cerebral cortex—to become those regions (Sanides, 1975) with the prefrontal cortex subserving the highest order behavior (Mesulam, 2002). The human frontal system is a heteromodal brain region, which is the most well integrated, most complex, and least reflexive and hard wired (Mesulam, 2002). The human frontal systems are ontologically developed later (Lebel, Walker, Leemans, Phillips, & Beaulieu, 2008), are the most well developed in humans (Semendeferi, Lu, Schenker, & Damásio, 2002), and when damage occurs, it leads to the impairments in the elements of consciousness.

Researchers have attempted to identify the circuitry by conducting innovative studies of self-awareness of own mental states, first-perspective, self-concept, autobiographical memory, and sense of agency (for a review, see Gillihan & Farah, 2005). Overall, research on the underlying neural circuitry of consciousness consistently reveals an integration between limbic regions and the frontal systems. There are neuronal subtypes in these regions (anterior cingulate and insular cortex) called *Von Economo neurons* (VENs) that are found in the greatest numbers in the human brain, but also have been identified in great apes (Allman et al., 2010), cetaceans (Butti et al., 2009), and elephants (Hakeen et al., 2009)—all species that have been shown to have some level of self-awareness (Byrne & Bates, 2010; Craig, 2009). Investigations of clinical populations have revealed that individuals with fronto-temporal dementia (FTD) have a significantly reduced number of VENs. The behavioral variant of this dementia is characterized by social deterioration and impaired self-monitoring of behavior (Seeley et al., 2010), whereas individuals with autism have a larger number of VENs and this disorder is characterized by dysfunctional social interactions and impaired self-awareness (Santos et al., 2010). Although further work needs to be conducted, there are interesting findings implicating the role of the anterior cingulate (e.g., Lane, Fink, Chau, & Donlan, 1997) and frontal operculum (e.g., Gusnard, Akbudak, Shulman, & Raichle, 2001). As noted previously, it is unlikely that consciousness resides in one location in the brain. A conscious sense of self and thinking about one's thinking, past, and future is not a combination of any brain regions per se, but an integration of information not only in the moment of processing, but also in the amalgamation of information stored in the brain over time, which combines to create a unity of selfness (Pinker, 1997).

Clinical Disorders of Consciousness

Within the field of neuropsychology, we have applied the greatest efforts to understanding and creating clinical assessments and interventions for the least sophisticated but foundational elements of consciousness (i.e., arousal, conscious access, sensory perception, attention), whereas there is a relative dearth of information regarding the higher level, more complex elements of episodic memory, self-monitoring, and self-awareness. It is true that if our patients are not able to maintain a sufficient level of arousal or attend well to the world around them, then it is challenging for those patients to interact in meaningful ways. It is also true that these more foundational elements of consciousness are more tangible and behaviorally manifested. Thus, it has been of great importance, interest, and to some degree, relative ease to study and develop assessments and interventions to address impairments in arousal, sensory perception, conscious access, and attention. However, one might argue that the human ability to navigate daily life successfully is highly reliant upon the higher order elements of consciousness and so the relative inattention to these elements is somewhat surprising. Of course, the complexity of these elements and their inherent subjectivity has made objective experimentation of them challenging, to say the least (Dehaene, 2014). The reader should be mindful of this state of the field when digesting the following discussion of assessment and intervention for disorders of consciousness.

Arousal Disorders

After brain trauma, there are a range of disorders of impaired consciousness that are characterized by reduced arousal and ability to process external and internal stimuli at the basic level (for a review, see Laureys & Schiff, 2012). The three main types of arousal disorders are coma, vegetative state (VS), and minimally conscious state (MCS). Within the last two decades, work groups and conferences have been assembled to aggregate diagnostic and intervention guidelines for the appropriate treatment of individuals with persistent arousal disorders of consciousness, including VS and MCS. The International Working Party on the Management of the Vegetative State (Andrews, 1996), the American Academy of Neurology (The Multi-Society Task Force on PVS, 1994), and the American Congress of Rehabilitation Medicine (Giacino et al., 1995) each published position statements about nomenclature, diagnosis, and management of these two persistent arousal disorders. In an attempt to rectify the differences in recommendations among these position statements for VS and MCS and provide evidence-based guidelines, the Aspen Neurobehavioral Conference was organized (Giacino et al., 1997; Giacino et al., 2002). The participants concluded that there is a paucity of research regarding assessment and intervention, thus precluding the development of evidence-based guidelines. Instead, they developed consensus-based guidelines identifying behaviors consistent with those in MCS or VS (see Table 15.2).

It is important to consider that initial studies examining the functional outcomes and mortality of individuals with severe arousal disorders were bleak. These studies reported high death rates, short windows of recovery before reaching "plateau," and minimal need for rehabilitation in patients with minimal or vegetative consciousness. However, recent studies with larger sample sizes reveal that many patients admitted to the hospital with severe arousal disorders can benefit from rehabilitation interventions, and can regain higher levels of consciousness and continue to demonstrate gains for at least two years (Whyte & Nakase-Richardson, 2013; Whyte et al. 2013). These recent findings highlight the importance of proper diagnosis and treatment in arousal disorders, so that families can be adequately prepared to make decisions for loved ones and so that patients receive the treatment they need to achieve maximal recovery. Additionally, every clinician should bear in mind that there is so little that is known about recovery from severe arousal disorders that we cannot conclude the outcome for any one person based upon the existing literature. The interested reader is referred to a *New York Times* article documenting the recovery course of Terry Willis, a man who had remained in an MCS for 19 years when he began to spontaneously and consistently communicate with family members (Carey, 2006).

Table 15.2 Characteristics of disorders of arousal and attention and conscious access

Diagnosis	*Arousal*	*Attention*	*Conscious Access*	*Sleep Cycles*	*Communication*	*Sensory-Motor Function*	*Auditory Processing*	*Visual Processing*
Coma	None	None	None	No	None	Postural responses	None	None
VS	None	None	None	Yes	None; vocalizations but no language	Nonpurposeful, posturing, withdrawal from noxious stimuli	Startle response, brief orienting to sound	None
MCS	Partial	Partial	Minimal	Yes	Inconsistent, intelligible, stimulus reliant	Localize noxious stimuli, reach for objects, automatic movements	Localize sound location, inconsistent response to commands	Visual fixation, visual pursuit
Post-Confusional State	Extended periods of wakefulness	Inconsistent, waxing/ waning	Variable	Yes	Speaks in sentences intelligibly, reveals disorganized thinking, sometimes perseverative	Use of objects, may be slowed or hyperactive	Easily orient and recognize sounds, consistent one-step command following	Object recognition
Delirium	Extended periods of wakefulness	Inconsistent, waxing/ waning	Variable	Yes	Intelligible, may be disorganized and difficult to interpret	Use of objects, May be slowed or hyperactive	Easily orient and recognize sounds, reductions in multi-step command following	Fixation, pursuit, potential for presence of hallucinations

Coma

Coma refers to a state in which individuals maintain neither arousal nor awareness. Eyes are closed during coma, and patients do not demonstrate periods of arousal or wakefulness in response to even noxious stimuli. Additionally, there is no evidence of sleep/wake cycle on electroencephalogram. This state must persist for at least one hour, lest it be categorized as concussion or another transitory change in consciousness. After several days or weeks of survival in this state, individuals with a coma diagnosis usually progress to improved levels of consciousness. See Table 15.2 for general diagnostic criteria and behaviors exhibited during coma. For additional clinical diagnostic coma criteria, refer to Plum and Posner (1982), which is a seminal article with the most widely regarded criterion.

Vegetative State

It should first be noted that a current trend in discussions of disorders of consciousness, the term *vegetative state* is increasingly considered a depreciatory term. Although providers initially coined the term to be consistent with patients' behavior during this state (i.e., "to vegetate"), patients, their families and sensitive clinicians have been aware of the fact that it may be confused with or used as a noun (e.g., "my loved one is a vegetable"). New terminology has been brought to the fore by the European Task Force on Disorders of Consciousness and *unresponsive wakefulness syndrome* is under consideration (Laureys et al., 2010). For the current discussion, we will persist with the use of VS.

VS refers to the state of consciousness in which an individual displays some signs of arousal, but demonstrates no signs of awareness of self or the environment. In this state, patients will open their eyes, have intact sleep-wake cycles, have preserved autonomic and hypothalamic function, and maintain cranial nerve reflexes, but make no reproducible or voluntary response to environmental stimuli, demonstrate no ability to interact with others, and demonstrate no language comprehension or expression. These patients may demonstrate some behavioral signs of arousal, including blinking, eye movement, sound utterance, poorly sustained visual pursuit, yawn, swallowing of saliva, nonpurposeful movement, startle myoclonus, auditory startle, withdrawal from painful stimuli, and facial expressions (Jennett & Plum, 1972; Bernat, 2006).

Minimally Conscious State

MCS involves partial recovery of awareness (sensory processing and attention) and arousal (Giacino et al., 2002, 2014). Generally, individuals in MCS are able to demonstrate purposeful behaviors, but are unable to consistently communicate effectively. One working group has suggested still further subcategorization of individuals in MCS. Depending on the individual's behaviors, they may be categorized as MCS plus (MCS+) or MCS minus (MCS; see Bruno, Vanhaudenhuyse, Thibaut, Moonen, & Laureys, 2011). Individuals who engage in nonreflexive movement, orient to noxious stimuli, smile or cry in response to relevant stimuli, or track visual stimuli in the environment are categorized as MCS–. Alternatively, individuals who would be diagnosed MCS+ are inconsistently able to follow simple commands, speak intelligibly, and can provide yes/no responses.

Assessment in Coma, VS, and MCS

As one may have gathered, proper assessment and diagnosis of individuals with severe arousal disorders can be challenging as it relies almost entirely on behavioral observation of the patient. As of yet, there is no "gold standard" in this type of evaluation. Nevertheless, accurately characterizing an individual's level of consciousness through evaluation of the individual's awareness of self and the environment, and ability to interact with others and the environment, is a critical aspect of care and recovery. For thorough guidelines and review of clinical criteria and measures most useful in assessment and diagnosis of arousal disorders, the reader is referred to the most recent State of the Science review (Giacino, Fins, Laureys, & Schiff, 2014).

Assessment of severe arousal disorders includes behavioral assessment that is guided by structured instruments, such as neurobehavioral rating scales and individualized quantitative behavioral assessment (IQBA). There are several neurobehavioral rating scales with acceptable levels of reliability and validity. However, there has not been extensive research to yield information about sensitivity, specificity, or predictive outcome. The most widely used measure continues to be the Glasgow Coma Scale (Teasdale & Jennett, 1974). This is a 15-point scale that assesses motor, verbal, and eye motor responses to determine level of functioning for each. Researchers have attempted to raise caution about this measure, as all-too-often practitioners use the total score, rather than scores for each of the three areas of function. This can be highly misleading, particularly regarding patients who are unable to respond sufficiently for reasons other than brain stem injury. For example, those who are ventilated, sedated, when eyes are swollen shut, or when they have been paralyzed during injury are unable to mount sufficient responses, but they may not meet criteria for coma or VS (Majerus, Gill-Thwaites, Andrews, & Laureys, 2005). Other promising and specified neurobehavioral rating scales include the Coma Recovery Scale–Revised (CRS-R; Giacino, Kalmar, & Whyte, 2004) and the Sensory Modality Assessment and Rehabilitation Technique (Gill-Thwaites & Munday, 2004). Each of these measures allows for more careful examination of recovery of consciousness by accounting for auditory function, communication, and eye-opening to stimulus. Honed assessment of an individual's ability to respond to external stimulus is a key means of differentiation in diagnosis.

In addition to rating scales, IQBA is another means of assessing recovery from coma and vegetative state and is typically used in combination with neurobehavioral rating scales. In IQBA, trained staff members conduct single-subject experimental designs to determine the level of volition a patient exerts to complete a behavior. Such methods require providers to document a behavior after commands, in response to multiple sources of stimulation (sound, touch, visual), and at rest. Statistical methods are employed to determine whether the behavior is exhibited at random chance, or in response to a given stimulus.

In addition to behavioral study, measurement of electrophysiology through electroencephalography (EEG) and measurement of event-related potentials (ERPs) have been used to capture brain activity as a window on level of brain functioning. EEG provides a means of visually investigating spontaneous electrical activity generated by the brain. ERPs refer to averaged EEG responses that are time-referenced to external stimuli. Using EEG or ERPs for differential diagnosis between VS or MCS is not yet possible (Giacino et al., 2014); however, these techniques may assist in other ways. For example, in patients with coma, EEG can be useful for identifying seizure activity. In individuals in VS or MCS, EEG can identify global electrical slowing. ERPs may be used to predict longer-term outcome. In patients in a coma, the dearth of electrical response to stimulation of median nerves corresponds to poor longer term outcomes (Wijdicks et al., 2006). The more far reaching utility of EEG and ERPs remains to be determined.

Structural and/or functional neuroimaging—computed tomography (CT), magnetic resonance imaging (MRI), functional MRI (fMRI), positron emission tomography (PET)—is increasingly being considered in the diagnosis and treatment of individuals with disorders of arousal. CT and MRI scanning are used to localize and determine the degree of structural damage in the brain. This guides treatment teams in their understanding of how impairments may present over the recovery process. There have been some interesting studies using functional neuroimaging attempting to capture cerebral response to stimulation when verbal and motor responses are not possible (see Giacino et al., 2014, for a review). Although there are only preliminary findings, there is some evidence to suggest that functional neuroimaging can detect the ability to follow commands without verbalization or motor activity as brain regions have been found to "light up" in response to yes/no questions. It should be stated that all studies of this nature have small sample sizes and the preliminary findings need further investigation.

Treatment of Coma, VS, and MCS

Treatment strategies may vary based on the level of acuity of injury, duration of symptoms of arousal disorders, and availability of institutional resources. In the earliest stages of arousal disorders (i.e., during acute treatment), adequate medical management is a paramount concern (Seel et al., 2013). Because multiple physiologic systems are likely to be affected by the brain injury, proper monitoring and treatment of respiratory, cardiac, renal, and musculoskeletal functions are essential. During this time, it is also important to monitor for infection, behaviors that endanger the patient (e.g., self-extubation), behaviors that suggest the patient is experiencing pain, and proper positioning to avoid skin breakdown. This type of management will involve observation from all members of the interdisciplinary team. Additionally, proper monitoring requires various types of imaging, proper administration of medications, and interventional strategies including respiratory support (e.g., intubation) and dietary administration (e.g., Percutaneous endoscopic gastrostomy (PEG) tube placement). Risk of medical complications trend down as the patient becomes more aroused and ambulatory. Patients who remain in a vegetative or minimally conscious state or with reduced mobility for an extended period of time will require ongoing monitoring.

Interventions to assist the patient in regaining consciousness are all based in provision of stimulation. When not contraindicated, medications may be administered to promote stimulation (e.g., amantadine or hydrochloride; Giacino et al., 2012). Stimulation to the body through movement and sensory input as well as direct stimulation of the brain are the main approaches.

Sensorimotor Regulation

Several clinicians and researchers have noted the importance of sensory processing in recovery of consciousness. There is some literature—mostly in the form of case study and retrospective data analysis—that suggests assessment of frequency, duration, intensity of sensory stimuli, with gradual and scheduled exposure to sensory information assists patients as they become more aroused and begin to regain awareness of themselves and their surroundings (Giacino, Katz, & Whyte, 2013; Seel et al., 2013). This method of rehabilitation requires observation of patient's ability to process sights, smells, visual information, and auditory cues, as well as documentation and attentiveness for proper execution. In an article detailing the rehabilitation program for arousal disorders at Sheperd Center in Atlanta, Georgia, Seel and colleagues (2013) outlined their strategies for scheduled sensory stimulation. Strategies include repeated, consistent use of same type of stimulation across therapies to increase the likelihood of habitual responding and incorporation of visual information, such as mirrors, pictures of family, computer programs, and bright objects (e.g., flashing mirrors). Auditory simulation includes familiar sounds, such as music and familiar voices. Tactile stimulation may include laying the patient on his or her side or seating the patient on a mat. Careful attention must be paid to the time of day and level of stimulation applied, given that level of stimulation varies across the day based upon biorhythms and light exposure. Balance of the stimulation is key so that the patient is not over- or understimulated. When patients are able, and not prone to overstimulation, early mobilization has been demonstrated to be helpful in the recovery process (Seel et al., 2013).

Brain Stimulation

Recent research has begun to examine the utility of both invasive and noninvasive methods of neural regulation through the application of stimulators. An invasive approach, deep brain stimulation (DBS), involves surgical implantation of electrodes that generate electrical impulses into prespecified areas of the brain. Generally, this type of treatment is reserved for patients who continue to present with arousal disorders some years after their injury (it is generally thought that DBS for patients in acute states of brain injury may disrupt the recovery process). DBS is thought to improve patients' behavioral control by reactivating cortical structures that were previously down-regulated after injury. This treatment remains in investigational stages, but shows early promise for individuals with persistent arousal disorders (Giacino et al., 2013; Lemaire et al., 2014).

In terms of noninvasive neural stimulation, case examples and small case studies have provided some evidence that application of repetitive transcranial magnetic stimulation (rTMS) may be another useful tool for assisting patients in improvements of level of awareness and arousal. rTMS involves the use of electromagnets to induce weak electrical currents in the brain. The magnetic energy passes through the skull and is thought to create electrical pulses in specified regions of the brain. This type of stimulation is theorized to assist in either up-regulation or down-regulation of affected neurons to assist patients in increasing arousal and awareness (Giacino et al., 2013; Louise-Bender Pape et al., 2009). This treatment continues to be in the early stages of research and is not without risk. Risks include induction of seizure, transient headache, and transient changes in hearing.

Disorders Involving Global Impairment of Attention and Conscious Access

Brain trauma, infections, metabolic disturbances, and/or exposure to anesthesia or certain types of medications often results in persistent impairments in ability to focus, sustain attention, and consciously access information about oneself and the environment. These disorders are characterized by intact arousal periods punctuated by confusion secondary to impairments in the ability to attend, process, and encode information (see Table 15.2).

Delirium

Delirium is characterized by disturbed consciousness with a waxing and waning course, disruption of the sleep/wake cycle, global cognitive dysfunction, and psychomotor disturbances (Maldonado, 2008). There are many causes of delirium and it is generally conceptualized as a transitional status of neurologic functioning secondary to acute metabolic disturbances, intoxication, and structural brain lesions (Maldonado, 2008; Ouimet, Kavanagh, Gottfried, & Skrobik, 2007).

Research suggests that there are two main behavioral patterns in delirium: a hypoactive subtype and a hyperactive subtype (Maldonado, 2008). The hypoactive subtype is characterized by withdrawal, decreased responsiveness, apathy (poor initiation), staring, and sparse or slowed speech. Alternatively, the hyperactive subtype is notable for agitation, restlessness, nightmares, wandering, combativeness, and emotional lability. However, it should be noted that some patients can display a mixed behavioral pattern notable for symptoms of both hypo- and hyperactivity. All types can be characterized by hallucinations and delusions (Maldonado, 2008; Meagher et al., 2011). However, the cardinal feature of delirium is attention impairment, not hallucinations or delusions (Meagher et al., 2011). Delirium is a particularly salient concern in hospitals, as the incidence rate ranges from 11% to 80% of patients in intensive care and acute medicine units (Ouimet et al., 2007). Not surprisingly, hyperactive delirium is detected and diagnosed more frequently than hypoactive delirium (Maldonado, 2008). Hypoactive is the most common, but is frequently missed because its behavioral features do not draw clinical attention as readily (McNicoll et al., 2003).

There are several medical markers and demographic characteristics that make individuals more prone to experience of delirium. These include very young or very old age (particularly in those with dementia), neurotransmitter imbalance, inflammation and infection, hypertension/hypotension, hearing/vision impairment, changes in sodium level, placement of restraints, impaired oxygen metabolism, and deliriogenic medications including opiates and benzodiazepines (Girard, Pandharipande, & Ely, 2008). Risky health behaviors that predispose individuals to delirium include poor hydration, smoking, and alcohol use (Ouimet et al., 2007). Careful evaluation of each of these factors is important to assist with resolution of symptoms. The presence of delirium during hospitalization has been associated with increased institutionalization after discharge in elderly patients (Neufeld et al., 2013) and the development of persistent cognitive impairments many years after the delirium has "resolved" (Jackson, Gordon, Hart, Hopkins, & Ely, 2004; Neufeld et al., 2013; Ouimet et al., 2007).

Posttraumatic Confusional State

Traditionally, the state of confusion that follows moderate to severe traumatic brain injury in which the individual has gross impairments in attention and encoding new information has been referred to as *posttraumatic amnesia*. However, this label captures only one of the neurobehavioral impairments that persons present with following TBI. More recently, this state—which occurs in persons with moderate to severe TBI—has been thought of as a subtype of delirium and labeled *posttraumatic confusional state* (PTCS) (Sherer, Nakase-Richardson, Yablon, & Gontkovsky, 2005). There are a wide variety of behavioral disturbances associated with this state, including impulsivity, sleep disturbance, agitation, and disorientation to place and situation, which all can lead to safety concerns for patients and the staff who are caring for them. Additionally, up to 40% of patients with confusion have psychotic-type symptoms (e.g., hallucinations; Sherer, Yablon, Nakase-Richardson, & Nick, 2008). The individual's ability to focus, sustain, and shift attention is consistently impaired, similarly to the pattern of impairment found in early phase of recovery from delirium. Awareness of changes in motor, sensory, cognitive, and behavioral functioning is impaired and these patients do not readily take these impairments into consideration when making decisions. Consequently, their ability to plan, problem-solve, and guide their behavior in appropriate ways is markedly impaired.

Stuss and his colleagues (1999) were among the first to decipher cognitive recovery patterns in individuals after TBI and noted that the primary cognitive impairment in PTCS is in the realm of attention. They observed that simple and complex attentional processes typically recovered prior to efficient memory encoding and retrieval, which tend to linger the longest in the impaired range. Thus, the individual begins to attend to and process information in the environment and about him- or herself prior to being able to consistently encode that information. In similar findings, Sherer and colleagues (Sherer et al., 2008) found that with variability in PTCS symptoms, there does appear to be a predictable pattern of resolution of symptoms of confusion, with psychotic-type symptoms and sleep disturbance resolving first and the attentional impairments taking longer to resolve. Importantly, posttraumatic confusional state symptom severity and course have been shown to be independent predictors of important functional outcomes and community reintegration. For example, Nakase-Richardson, Yablon, and Sherer (2007) found that severity of confusion after brain injury was more strongly associated with one-year employment outcome than duration of the confusional state. Additionally, the presence of psychotic-type symptoms (e.g., hallucinations) has been found to be an independent predictor of poorer recovery (Sherer, Yablon, & Nick, 2014). These findings suggest that clinical attention to the characteristics of the PTCS, such as severity, not just its presence and duration of cognitive symptoms may assist the clinical team in predicting longer term care needs and assistance.

Assessment and Interventions for Delirium

Assessments of delirium and PTCS typically include behavioral ratings that are conducted by hospital staff. In acute care settings, the Confusion Assessment Metrics (CAM) is often employed, particularly in the intensive care unit (i.e., CAM-ICU). The CAM-ICU is designed to capture data about acute changes in mental status, inattention, disorganized thinking, and altered level of consciousness (i.e., somnolence, sleep/wake disruption; Ely et al., 2001). The Confusion Assessment Protocol (CAP) was developed by Scherer and colleagues (Scherer et al., 2005) for assessing PTCS in particular. Key symptoms assessed with the CAP are orientation to time and situation, attention, vigilance, and working memory (complex attention), waxing and waning of symptoms, agitation, reversal of sleep-wake cycle (night-time arousal and decreased daytime arousal), and psychotic symptoms (e.g., suspiciousness, hallucinations).

The most important method for management of delirium is to identify and treat underlying pathophysiologic factors that perpetuate symptoms. In many cases, management of infection, correction of sedating medications, proper hydration and nutrition, and assessment and regulation of basic metabolic factors are critical in resolution of delirium. Pain is a frequent instigator of agitation and aggression in patients with delirium and PTCS; thus, pain management strategies are critical in resolution of confusion. Similarly, management of sensory deficits has also been shown to reduce symptoms of delirium and aid recovery. For example, ensuring that patients have their glasses and/or hearing aids dramatically reduces confusion (Inouye et al., 1999). Psychopharmacological interventions may be employed to improve safety of patients and staff and to ease the recovery course. However, pharmacological management of delirium is somewhat controversial, as several medications prescribed to alleviate agitation, sleep disruption, and symptoms can result in oversedation and circumstances that worsen confusion. In general, the current trend in the literature and recent clinical practice is to minimize the use of sedating medications. However, when necessary for the safety of patients and staff, randomized controlled clinical trials suggest that quetiapine (Devlin et al., 2010; Kim, Bader, Kotlyar, & Gropper, 2003) and haloperidol (Devlin et al., 2010) may be successfully used in hospitalized patients.

In treatment of delirium and PTCS, environmental support for symptoms is paramount. As in treatment for individuals in VS and MCS, management of stimulation and sensory input is important. When patients are able, and not prone to overstimulation, early mobilization has been demonstrated to be helpful in the recovery process (Seel et al., 2013). The primary tenets of environmental/behavioral management of delirium include training staff about how to modulate their own behavior to avoid stimulating agitation in patients, adapting the environment to avoid over- or understimulating the patient, and providing salient orientation cues so that the patient can begin to attend, process, and encode relevant information (Inouye et al., 1999). For a list of behavioral strategies for management of delirium and PTCS, see Table 15.3.

Table 15.3 Behavioral and environmental interventions for confusional states

Patient Symptom/Behavior	*Staff/Environmental Intervention*
Agitation/Aggression	• Take on a calm, caring and soothing tone. • Listen patiently. • Instruct the patient. Do not ask "Do you want to. . ." • Use simple, concrete language. • Reduce noise in the room (e.g., TV turned off). • Clear clutter. • Limit visitors and visitor conversation in the room. • Allow plenty of personal space for the patient. • Attempt to avoid or discontinue use of restraints. • Monitor medical equipment, which can be agitating (e.g., beeping monitors, leads or lines that pull at the body). • Mobilize and assistance with ambulation, when possible.
Hallucinations/Delusions	• Avoid correcting the patient or telling them their experience is not real. • Acknowledge that you have heard the patient. • Reassure patient of their safety and your concern.
Disorientation	• Provide orientation cues in close proximity (clock, calendar, location, reason for hospitalization). • Provide gentle reorientation cues in conversation (e.g., "Now that it is noon, we will have lunch," "Now that it is April, the flowers are blooming"). • Create consistent schedule in patient cares and activities.
Anxiety/Emotional Lability	• Lower yourself to patient's eye level and take an open stance. • Provide frequent reassurance of care and concern. • Provide frequent, time-contingent checks. • Provide easy, distracting activities.
Sleep Disruption	• Regulate sleep/wake cycles (avoid allowing the patient to nap for significant portions of the day). • Curtains/blinds open during the day, closed at night. • Lights on during the day/ off at night.

Memory Impairments (Semantic vs. Episodic)

Memory provides the individual with a history and a future that is foundational to his or her sense of self. Consequently, impairments in memory can thwart the individual accessing past and current information about self and environment and situation and obstruct construction of an accurate sense of the present and the future.

Assessment and Intervention of Memory's Role in Consciousness

The field of neuropsychology has focused primarily on semantic memory because breakdowns in *knowing* information have been linked to specific pathologies depending on whether the breakdown was in encoding, storage, and/or retrieval. Assessment of semantic memory has been traditionally structured to capture the encoding of verbal information (rote or within a context) or visual information and the later retrieval of that information within cued and uncued formats. For understanding consciousness, it is important for the clinician to realize that when there are impairments in *knowing*, then the individual will have difficulty with *remembering*. The breakdown may be in that information was never encoded in the first place or that the information cannot be retrieved efficiently from memory stores when needed. Either way, the individual will have limited or no access to up-to-date information about daily life experiences to incorporate that knowledge in what she or he knows about her or himself (e.g., orientation to self) and her or his life (e.g., orientation to situation) and the world (e.g., orientation to time and place).

However, there has been much less attention to the assessment of *remembering*. Human success in daily life is highly reliant upon understanding the consequences of past behavior and anticipating, thinking about, and planning for the personal future (Atance & O'Neill, 2001; Kwan et al. 2013). Individuals with impairments in episodic memory will be impaired in their ability to act on the basis of their knowledge of the past and their expectations for the future (Tulving, 2005). The loss of awareness of future time means that the individual will be impaired in predicting what is to come, planning and goal-setting, and differentiating right from wrong. Without the ability to mentally time travel to their own personal futures, there is no basis for moral judgment. We then start to understand the potential reasons for the high rates of social disturbance, substance abuse, criminality, and risk-taking behavior in individuals with brain injury. Individuals without autonoetic episodic memory cannot think about their futures, anticipate the challenges and rewards that may come depending on their behavior, and take action now to influence the future. Consequently, the rules guiding behavior are not future oriented; they are focused on the here and now. One might label those behaviors as pleasure seeking, impulsive, or disinhibited. Behavior is reactive based upon in-the-moment thoughts and environmental cues and is likely the root of responses that are deemed "impulsive."

Proactive behavior is not possible because there is no thought of down-the-road implications. The individual may be described as having a change in his or her personality because he or she behaves in ways that are more linked to the here-and-now. Behavior is no longer guided by accurate information in-the-moment nor information to plan for the future.

The core interventions for memory impairments are founded in using external strategies and equipment to document scheduled activities and tasks to be completed so that the individual can follow a written schedule rather than rely upon an impaired memory system to recall what needs to be done. For a review of such strategies, see Haskins' and colleagues' (Haskins et al., 2012) *Cognitive Rehabilitation Manual.* However, the effectiveness of such a system for successful life management requires that the individual also considers what did not get accomplished yesterday, any changes in schedule given unexpected life situations, and planning for more infrequent life activities that may disrupt the routines of day-to-day life. With impairments in episodic memory, the individual will have difficulty pulling into consciousness information that is relevant about what was accomplished yesterday, what is planned for over the longer term, and the relevance of unexpected life situation to the daily life schedule. Compensation for these impairments in episodic memory again are rooted in using external aids to track the episodes of daily life that are of importance and to prompt the individual to review what has been accomplished and what still needs to get done in the day. However, because of the impairments in retrieving information in-the-moment from memory stores, the individual will also have to learn strategies for planning ahead, problem solving, and decision making. The best synopsis of cognitive rehabilitation strategies and approaches to address these types of breakdowns in cognitive functioning can be found in the *Cognitive Rehabilitation Manual* (Haskins et al., 2012).

Impairments in Self-Monitoring

Self-monitoring in the moment brings the activity, and to some extent, its elements, to conscious awareness and thus control. When we do not consciously self-monitor, we "lose track of time." We go into "autopilot." We rely upon overlearned behavior patterns. These overlearned skills and tasks have become so routinized that they do not require a high level of cognitive oversight. Our efficiency in daily life is linked to our ability to take certain tasks and activities out of conscious control. Multitasking, the holy grail of cognitive efficiency, is reliant upon certain complex action sequences becoming automatic, habitual, routinized. We can conceptualize consciousness as an ability of the brain to modulate how much monitoring is required to complete the task. When we are learning a new skill, we must focus on each step, practice the skill over and over, and are quite distracted by interruptions. However, with practice and repetition, the brain learns the steps so well that it no longer needs to put conscious energy to it and then we are freed to do two tasks at once.

Conscious oversight can be a bit of a double-edged sword, though. When we self-monitor our behavior, then our error rate is reduced, but our efficiency, resistance to distraction, and ability to multitask is also reduced. One tangible example is learning to walk. Infants learn the patterned motor movements (and proprioceptive and vestibular sense) for bipedal ambulation and these patterns become overlearned through practice. Over time, we humans become so skilled on our feet that we can perform other complex acts while walking without any degradation in our walking pattern or efficiency per se. However, with cerebral damage leading to motor, sensory, vestibular, or motor planning impairments, walking becomes disordered. When learning to walk again, patients must apply conscious oversight. In the clinical setting, in which most environmental factors are controlled, an individual may successfully be able to regain safe, efficient ambulation. However, out in the community where the individual is barraged with information, the patient's conscious oversight of safe ambulation is now competing with conscious oversight of where to walk, following directions, monitoring foot and car traffic, and processing a conversation with a companion, for example. Walking pattern and efficiency suffers.

Assessment and Interventions of Self-Monitoring

There are no distinct assessments for self-monitoring per se. As neuropsychologists, we focus more on the cognitive elements that underlie our abilities to self-monitor our own behavior, including working memory, attention, and speed of information processing. It is likely that patients who have impairments in these areas of cognitive functioning will have difficulty with self-monitoring and will complain of difficulties with multitasking. Interventions have focused on allocating attention resources and managing the rate of information processing in order to assist the patient in self-monitoring multiple task demands despite interruptions (Cicerone, 2002; Fasotti, Kovacs, Eling, & Brouwer, 2000; Sohlberg, McLaughlin, Pavese, Heidrich, & Posner, 2000; Sohlberg, Johnson, Paule, Raskin, & Mateer, 2001).

There is mounting evidence that *mindfulness*, the application of conscious oversight to a behavior, thinking pattern, or emotions, can assist in compensating and possibly even reducing the actual symptoms of certain disorders and cognitive impairments. In brief, interventions for increasing mindfulness are focused on teaching the individual skills for sustaining attention in the face of competing distractors on the task at hand. Mindfulness may be viewed as a type of sustained attention training and is proposed to be effective because of the skills influence on attention regulation, emotional regulation, somatic awareness, and distancing from a self-focused perspective (Hölzel et al., 2011). Interventions have been found to be effective in improving attention and self-regulation in attention deficit/hyperactivity disorder (Schoenberg et al., 2014). There is some evidence to suggest that mindfulness techniques such as meditation can offset age-related cognitive decline (for a review, see Gard, Britta, Hölzel, & Lazar, 2014; Prakash, De Leon, Patterson, Schirda, & Janssen, 2014). Interestingly, there is one study that has found that mindfulness meditation techniques may positively affect cellular longevity by reducing cognitive stress and stress arousal and increasing positive states of mind and hormonal factors (Epel, Daubenmier, Moskowitz, Folkman, & Blackburn, 2009). Mindfulness training has also been shown to have positive effects on psychological health by increasing subjective well-being, reducing psychological symptoms and emotional reactivity, and improving behavioral regulation (Keng, Smoski, & Robins, 2011). A mindfulness stress reduction intervention has been found to reduce depression and the experience of pain and increase energy levels following traumatic brain injury (Bédard et al., 2012) and to reduce depression and anxiety in individuals with autism (Spek, van Ham, & Nyklíček, 2013). Overall, there is burgeoning evidence that mindfulness training may be a viable intervention technique for improving some aspects of self-monitoring in both healthy individuals as well as those with a range of cognitive disorders.

Impaired Awareness (Anosognosia) and Denial of Illness, Impairments, or Disability

Self-awareness is reliant upon three functions: (1) memory functioning to update the data about strengths and weaknesses and how these impact task completion and activity engagement, (2) sensory and proprioceptive functioning to provide feedback about how the system is operating (which is most key for motor functioning), and (3) emotional functioning to note the meaningfulness of the change for the individual. Through life experiences and learned behaviors, an individual learns to interpret the meaning of certain attributes, abilities, and skills in the context of others and society as a whole. The value that the individual puts on these, how the individual defines him- or herself, and how the individual copes with perceived weaknesses can all play a role in how the individual adapts and adjusts to the onset of impairment or disability.

As argued by Stuss and colleagues (Stuss, Rosenbaum, Malcom, Christiana, & Keenan, 2005), self-awareness is born from our experiences, which lead to the construction of a model, with each of us having our own concept of ourselves and the world around us. Our current experiences are then processed and conceptualized within the context of our model, thus facilitating efficient processing and reinforcement of the parameters of the model. However, the model becomes more rigid and less malleable after time, thus hindering modification when needed (Stuss et al., 2005). When the clinician considers this conceptualization of awareness, then the implications of neuropathology start to become clearer. The rigidity of the model makes incorporation of new information that is discrepant with the long-standing model difficult. Additionally, if there is damage that hinders the brain from integrating new information (e.g., memory impairments) or getting feedback about changes in functioning (e.g., anosognosia for hemiplegia), then the individual's model does not change. So new information that is quite different is rejected as not possible, plausible. If the information is not deemed as meaningful (the deficit is seen as minor or not present at all), then the impact on functioning is not realized or perhaps accepted.

There are two main classes of awareness disorders: anosognosia, which is rooted in a neurological dysfunction, and denial, which is rooted in psychological response (Kortte & Wegener, 2004; Prigatano, 1999). The overarching element of both of these is a degradation in the self-understanding of illness, impairment, or disability. Although there is some aspect of the individual that has been affected (health, longevity, functioning, abilities), she or he does not appear to recognize the effect. For a thorough discussion of awareness disorders, the reader should refer to the edited works of Prigatano and Schacter (1991) and Prigatano (2010).

Assessment and Intervention of Awareness Disorders

Assessment of awareness disorder depends upon the type of awareness problem that is present. An individual can be impaired in his or level of awareness of illness, disease, injury (e.g., schizophrenia, Alzheimer's disease, traumatic brain injury), an impairment in any realm of functioning (i.e., motor functioning, sensory, cognitive, behavioral, emotional), and/or the impact of that illness or impairment on daily life functioning. For clinical assessment, the clinician should focus in on assessing two levels of unawareness: what realm is impaired (motor, sensory, cognitive, behavioral, emotional), and is the individual taking into consideration the functional implications. See Table 15.4 for examples of tools for assessing these different realms in which awareness may be impaired. For a summary of the measurement of awareness syndromes, the reader is encouraged to read Orfei, Caltagirone, and Spalletta (2010).

Intervention During Impaired Arousal or Attention

As noted previously, all disorders of consciousness that are subsequent to impaired arousal and/or attention also have a strong unawareness component to the behavioral presentation. Clinicians should take the unawareness component into consideration when making decisions on modifying the environment to maintain safety for the individual. Without in-the-moment understanding of areas of impairment, individuals may attempt tasks that put them at risk for additional harm. Individuals with reduced arousal may attempt to pull out tubes or IVs, or may scratch themselves. Use of the lowest level of restraint, such as hand mitts, will help to reduce the chance for inadvertent injury. Individuals with delirium are at risk for injury secondary to attempting activities without consideration of their motor, sensory, and/or cognitive impairments on their abilities. Consequently, these individuals have higher incidence

Table 15.4 Assessment of impairments of awareness

Realm of Impaired Awareness	*Example Assessment Tools*
Motor	• Bisiach Scale (Bisiach, Vallar, Perani, Papagno & Berti, 1986) • Anosognosia Questionnaire (Starkstein, Fedoroff, Price, Leiguarda, & Robinson, 1992)
Sensory	• Bisiach Scale (Bisiach et al., 1986)
Cognitive	• Self-Awareness of Deficit Interview (Fleming, Strong & Ashton, 1996)
Emotional/Behavioral	• Awareness Questionnaire (Sherer, Bergloff, Boake, High, & Levin, 1998)
Functional Implications	• Patient Competency Rating Scale (Prigatano et al., 1986) • Self-Awareness of Deficit Interview (Fleming et al., 1996)
Denial	• Clinician's Ratings Scale for Evaluating Impaired Self-Awareness and Denial of Disability After Brain Injury (Prigatano & Klonoff, 1998)

of falls and attempts at elopement. Additionally, because they do not understand their impairments and possibly their need for hospitalization, these individuals may also become agitated in response to attempts to restrict their activities. It is important that these individuals receive frequent reassurance and reorientation to their current situation. Clinicians should take a errorless learning approach in order to both evaluate the patients current level of orientation to place and situation, but also to provide the needed reorientation to the accurate information (see Haskins, et al., 2012 for discussion of use of errorless learning techniques). With impairments in attention, memory, and awareness, it is critical that the patient not be allowed to make mistakes on which he or she may perseverate, thus reinforcing confabulated misinformation. With provision of a safe environment and feedback regarding the current situation, the individual will begin to incorporate new information about his or her situation and functioning as levels of arousal and attention improves. Once the individual is able to consistently lay down new memories, then intervention specifically aimed at enhancing awareness can be employed.

Interventions for Enhancing Awareness

Given that awareness syndromes are rooted in a reduced understanding of the illness, injury, impairments, functional implications, a multilevel approach should be undertaken to improve the level of awareness. The interplay between neuropathology and the experience and reaction of the individual to the resulting impairments cannot be teased apart easily and so interventions must include elements to address both underlying causes. A variety of approaches have been developed for addressing deficits in self-awareness, including feedback approaches (e.g., verbal, audiovisual, experiential), activity-based approaches, anticipation/predictive performance approaches, self-evaluation approaches, and adaptation/generalization approaches (for reviews, see Schrijnemaekers, Smeets, Ponds, van Heugten, & Rasquin, 2014; Tate et al., 2014). In addition to the approaches that are focused on improving the neurologically based impairments in awareness, there is the need to always keep in mind the more psychological coping aspects of awareness. Techniques should be incorporated for developing a strong therapeutic alliance through a trusting therapeutic relationship with the individual who is supported in engaging fully in collaborative goal setting and selection of activities that are relevant and motivating (Lucas & Fleming, 2005). Additionally, there must be ongoing monitoring of the individual's emotional status so that interventions are guided by the individual's level of acceptance of current abilities (Lucas & Fleming, 2005). Finally, therapeutic tasks should be emotional neutral, nonthreatening, focused on the application of strategies, and allow for the demonstration of improvements (Lucas & Fleming, 2005).

This class of interventions is rooted in a set of theoretical models of self-awareness, including the *pyramid model of awareness*, the *self-determination approach to enhance self-awareness*, and the *Comprehensive Dynamic Interactional Model* of awareness (for a review of these models and discussion of awareness interventions in greater detail, see Fleming & Ownsworth, 2006). The key components (although somewhat different terminology is used among the three models; Crosson et al., 1989) are:

- *intellectual awareness,* in which the individual has a basic knowledge of the deficits and the implications;
- *emergent awareness,* in which the individual can recognize the impact of the deficits while performing a task; and
- *anticipatory awareness,* in which the individual is able to predict how she or he will perform on a particular task and/or whether a problem will occur given the deficits.

Interventional approaches target each of these three key components (see Table 15.5). Preliminary research suggests that interventions targeting all of these components within a comprehensive rehabilitation program that affords the individual to learn and practice skills within multiple contexts are effective (Goverover, Johnston, Toglia, & Deluca, 2007; Lundqvist, Linnros, Orlenius, & Samuelsson, 2010; Toglia, Johnston, Goverover, & Dain, 2010; Zlotnik, Sachs, Rosenblum, Shpasser, & Josman, 2009). Future research needs to expand upon these findings and replicate the results with larger sample sizes, but this line of research suggests that a multicontextual approach that targets the three components

Table 15.5 Key elements of awareness interventions

Element	*Target*	*Therapeutic Approach*
Intellectual	Educational	Aimed at patients learning about the types of deficits that they have following brain injury and how they impact daily life functioning. Assumed that the individual does not have information about themselves due to a lack of access and/or understanding of the problem.
Emergent	Feedback	Aimed at provision of cues and tangible feedback regarding performance on tasks (i.e., videotaped, observer feedback, self appraisal, timing feedback). Assumed that the individual cannot glean on his or her own the implications of the information about his or her deficits.
Anticipatory	Predictive	Aimed at the patient predicting his or her performance on a task taking into consideration all of his or her strengths and weaknesses. Assumed that individual bases prediction on past knowledge of self and so must "recalibrate" expectations and self-knowledge.

of complete awareness may offer a foundation for interventions for awareness syndromes.

Final Thoughts About Neuropsychology's Role in Understanding Consciousness

There is much work left to be done to understand consciousness, which is both incredibly exciting as well as daunting. We spent the time writing this chapter frequently thinking about our own thinking, pondering that our brains were grappling with understanding themselves, and relishing our conscious thoughts about consciousness. As neuropsychologists, we should never forget that we are explorers of the relationships between the physical (brain) and the manifestation of its functioning (behavior) and not become complaisant or resistant to exploring more complex, nebulous constructs, particularly to how these relate to our clinical work. The challenge at our feet as scientists and clinicians is to not avoid the uncharted territory, but to take one step at a time exploring the entire landscape of consciousness, developing tools and techniques to chart it, capture it, and do something about impairment: treat it. Although there are neuroscientists who are grappling with the underlying mechanisms of consciousness—comparing humans to animals in an attempt to understand whether humans' conscious self is unique, and exploring how our brain *creates* consciousness—there is a relatively small number of scientists trying to apply what we know to the clinical realm. We need to continue our work towards understanding how impairments in the elements of consciousness affect our ability to be completely conscious human beings. What are the implications for impairments in consciousness for our ability to traverse the complex human relationships, plan for the future, understand the implication and consequences of our own behavior, and establish a goal and march out the steps accomplishing it? When we can unravel consciousness at these levels, then we will be better able to understand how injury to the brain can lead to criminal behavior, increased substance abuse, and failed intimate relationships in individuals who before injury had no history of social impropriety. Within the field of rehabilitation, we are quite good at addressing the biomechanical impairments that arise with injury to the brain. However, the complex social, interpersonal, and self-defining implications of brain dysfunction are left unaddressed to a large extent. The field of clinical neuropsychology is well-poised to assist in better understanding the complexities of human consciousness and how to assess it most particularly. We should apply our expertise to better assessing the elements of consciousness with an eye towards the implications of the impairments on ability of the brain to have a concept of self, a personal past and future, and an awareness of one's strengths and weaknesses. This knowledge will be foundational to further refining and developing new interventions to assist in the recovery from brain injury and the adaptation in the face of neurodevelopmental disorders that impact consciousness.

References

Agnati, L. F., Barlow, P., Ghidoni, R., Borroto-Escuela, D. O., Guidolin, D., & Fuxe, K. (2012). Possible genetic and epigenetic links between human inner speech, schizophrenia and altruism. *Brain Research*, *1476*, 38–57.

Allman, J. M., Tetreault, N. A., Hakeem, A. Y., Manaye, K. F., Semenderferi, K., Erwin, J. M., Park, S., Goubert, V., Hof, P. R. (2010). The von Economo neurons in frontoinsular and anterior cingulate cortex in great apes and humans. *Brain Structure and Function*, *214*, 495–517.

Andrews, K. (1996). International working party on the management of the vegetative state: Summary report. *Brain Injury*, *10*(11), 797–806.

Atance, C.M., & O'Neill, D.K. (2001). Episodic future thinking. *Trends in Cognitive Science*, *5*(12), 533–539.

Baldo, J. V., Dronkers, N. F., Wilkins, D., Ludy, C., Raskin, P., & Kim, J. (2005). Is problem solving dependent on language? *Brain and Language*, *92*(3), 240–250.

Bédard, M., Felteau, M., Marshall, S., Dubois, S., Gibbons, C., Klein, R., & Weaver, B. (2012). Mindfulness-based cognitive therapy: Benefits in reducing depression following a traumatic brain injury. *Advances In Mind Body Medicine*, *26*, 14–20.

Bernat, J. L. (2006). Chronic disorders of consciousness. *The Lancet*, *367*(9517), 1181–1192.

Bisiach, E., Vallar, G., Perani, D., Papagno, C., & Berti, A. (1986). Unawareness of disease following lesions of the right hemisphere:

Anosognosia for hemiplegia and anosognosia for hemianopia. *Neuropsychologia, 24*, 471–482.

Boly, M., Seth, A., Wilke, M., Ingmundson, P., Baars, B., Laureys, S., Edelman, D., & Tsuchiya, N. (2013). Consciousness in humans and non-human animals: Recent advances and future directions. *Frontiers in Psychology, 4*, 1–20.

Bruno, M., Vanhaudenhuyse, A., Thibaut, A., Moonen, G., & Laureys, S. (2011). From unresponsive wakefulness to minimally conscious PLUS and functional locked-in syndromes: Recent advances in our understanding of disorders of consciousness. *Journal of Neurology, 258*(7), 1373–1384.

Butti, C., Sherwood, C. C., Hakeem, A. Y., Allman, J. M., & Hof, P. R. (2009). Total number and volume of von Economo neurons in the cerebral cortex of cetaceans. *Journal of Comparative Neurology, 515*(2), 243–259

Byrne, R. W., & Bates, L. A. (2010). Primate social cognition: Uniquely primate, uniquely social, or just unique? *Neuron, 65*, 815–830.

Carey, B. (2006, July 4). Mute 19 years, he helps reveal brain's mysteries. *The New York Times*.

Cicerone, K. (2002). Remediation of working attention in mild traumatic brain injury. *Brain Injury, 16*, 185–195.

Crosson, B., Barco, P., Velezo, C., Bolesta, M., Cooper, P., Werts, D., & Brobeck, T. (1989). Awareness of compensation in postacute head injury rehabilitation. *Journal of Head Trauma Rehabilitation, 4*, 46–54.

Davis, R. N., & Nolen-Hoeksema, S. (2000). Cognitive inflexibility among ruminators and nonruminators. *Cognitive Therapy and Research, 24*(6), 699–711.

Dehaene, S. (2014). *Consciousness and the Brain: Deciphering How the Brain Codes Our Thoughts*. New York: Penguin.

Devlin, J. W., Roberts, R. J., Fong, J. J., Skrobik, Y., Riker, R. R., Hill, N. S., Robbins, T., Garpestad, E. (2010). Efficacy and safety of quetiapine in critically ill patients with delirium: A prospective, multicenter, randomized, double-blind, placebo-controlled pilot study. *Critical Care Medicine, 38*(2), 419–427.

Ely, E. W., Margolin, R., Francis, J., May, L., Truman, B., Dittus, R., et al. (2001). Evaluation of delirium in critically ill patients: Validation of the confusion assessment method for the intensive care unit (CAM-ICU). *Critical Care Medicine, 29*(7), 1370–1379.

Emerson, M. J., & Miyake, A. (2003). The role of inner speech in task switching: A dual-task investigation. *Journal of Memory and Language, 48*(1), 148–168.

Epel, E., Daubenmier, J., Moskowitz, J., Folkman, S., & Blackburn, E. (2009). Can meditation slow rate of cellular aging? Cognitive stress, mindfulness, and telomeres. *Annals of the New York Academy of Sciences, 1172*, 34–53.

Farrer, C., & Franck, N. (2007). Self-monitoring in schizophrenia. *Current Psychiatry Reviews, 3*(4), 243–251.

Farthing, G. W. (1992). *The Psychology of Consciousness*. Englewood Cliffs, NJ: Prentice-Hall, Inc.

Fasotti, L., Kovacs, F., Eling, P., & Brouwer, W. (2000). Time pressure management as a compensatory strategy training after closed head injury. *Neuropsychological Rehabilitation, 10*, 47–65.

Feinberg, T.E., & Keenan, J.P. (2005). Where in the brain is self? *Consciousness and Cognition, 14*, 661–678.

Fleming, J. M., & Ownsworth, T. (2006). A review of awareness interventions in brain injury rehabilitation. *Neuropsychological Rehabilitation, 16*(4), 474–500.

Fleming, J. M., Strong, J., & Ashton, R. (1996). Self-awareness of deficits in adults with traumatic brain injury: How best to measure? *Brain Injury, 10*, 1–15.

Gard, T., Hölzel, B., & Lazarl, S. (2014). The potential effects of meditation on age-related cognitive decline: A systematic review. *Annals of the New York Academy of Sciences, 1307*, 89–103.

Gazzangia, M. S. (1985). *The Social Brain*. New York: Basic Books.

Giacino, J. T., Ashwal, S., Childs, N., Cranford, R., Jennett, B., Katz, D. I., et al. (2002). The minimally conscious state: Definition and diagnostic criteria. *Neurology, 58*(3), 349–353.

Giacino, J. T., Fins, J. J., Laureys, S., & Schiff, N. D. (2014). Disorders of consciousness after acquired brain injury: The state of the science. *Nature Reviews Neurology, 10*(2), 99–114.

Giacino, J. T., Kalmar, K., & Whyte, J. (2004). The JFK coma recovery scale-revised: Measurement characteristics and diagnostic utility. *Archives of Physical Medicine and Rehabilitation, 85*(12), 2020–2029.

Giacino, J. T., Katz, D. I., & Whyte, J. (2013). Neurorehabilitation in disorders of consciousness. *Seminars in Neurology, 33*(2), 142–156.

Giacino, J. T., Whyte, J., Bagiella, E., Kalmar, K., Childs, N., Khademi, A., et al. (2012). Placebo-controlled trial of amantadine for severe traumatic brain injury. *New England Journal of Medicine, 366*(9), 819–826.

Giacino, J. T., Zasler, N. D., Katz, D. I., Kelly, J. P., Rosenberg, J. H., & Filley, C. M. (1997). Development of practice guidelines for assessment and management of the vegetative and minimally conscious states. *The Journal of Head Trauma Rehabilitation, 12*(4), 79–89.

Giacino, J. T., Zasler, N., Whyte, J., Katz, D., Glen, M., & Andary, M. (1995). Recommendations for use of uniform nomenclature pertinent to patients with severe alterations in consciousness. *Archives of Physical Medicine and Rehabilitation, 76*(2), 205–209.

Gill-Thwaites, H., & Munday, R. (2004). The sensory modality assessment and rehabilitation technique (SMART): A valid and reliable assessment for vegetative state and minimally conscious state patients. *Brain Injury, 18*(12), 1255–1269.

Gillihan, S. J. Farah, & M. J. (2005). Is self special: A critical review of evidence from experimental psychology and cognitive neuroscience. *Psychological Bullentin, 131*(1), 76–97.

Girard, T. D., Pandharipande, P. P., & Ely, E. W. (2008). Delirium in the intensive care unit. *Critical Care (London, England), 12*(Suppl 3), S3.

Goverover, Y., Johnston, M. V., Toglia, J., & Deluca, J. (2007). Treatment to improve self-awareness in persons with acquired brain injury. *Brain Injury, 21*, 913–923.

Gusnard, D.A., Akbudak, E., Shulman, G.L., & Raichle, M.E. (2001). Medial prefrontal cortex and self-referential mental activity: relation to a default mode of brain function. *Proceedings of the National Academy of Sciences, 98*(7), 4259–4264.

Hakeen, A. Y., Sherwood, C. C., Bonar, C. J., Butti, C., Hof, P. R., Allman, & J. M. (2009). Von Economo neurons in the elephant brain. *Anatomical Record, 292*(2), 242–248.

Hameroff, S., & Penrose, R. (2014). Consciousness in the universe: A review of the "Orch OR" theory. *Physics of Life Reviews, 11*(1), 39–78.

Haskins, E. C., Cicerone, K, Dams-O'Connor, K., Eberle, R., Langenbahn, D., & Shapiro-Rosenbaum, A. (Eds.). (2012). *Cognitive Rehabilitation Manual: Translating Evidence-Based Recommendations Into Practice*. Reston, VA: American Congress of Rehabilitation Medicine Publishing.

Heinämaa, S., Lähteenmäki, V., & Remes, P. (2007). *Consciousness: From Perception to Reflection in the History of Philosophy*. Dordrecht: Springer.

Held, R., Ostrovsky, Y., de Gelder, B., Gandhi, T., Ganesh, S., Mathur, U., et al. (2011). The newly sighted fail to match seen with felt. *Nature Neuroscience, 14*(5), 551–553.

Hölzel, B. K., Lazar, S. W., Gard, T., Schuman-Olivier, Z., Vago, D. R., & Ott, U. (2011). How does mindfulness meditation work? Proposing mechanisms of action from a conceptual and neural perspective. *Perspectives on Psychological Science*, *6*, 537–559.

Inouye, S. K., Bogardus, S. T., Jr., Charpentier, P. A., Leo-Summers, L., Acampora, D., Holford, T. R., Cooney, L.M., Jr (1999). A multicomponent intervention to prevent delirium in hospitalized older patients. *New England Journal of Medicine*, *340*(9), 669–676.

Jackson, J. C., Gordon, S. M., Hart, R. P., Hopkins, R. O., & Ely, E. W. (2004). The association between delirium and cognitive decline: A review of the empirical literature. *Neuropsychology Review*, *14*(2), 87–98.

Jennett, B., & Plum, F. (1972). Persistent vegetative state after brain damage: A syndrome in search of a name. *The Lancet*, *299*(7753), 734–737.

Keng, S., Smoski, M., & Robins, C. (2011). Effects of mindfulness on psychological health: A review of empirical studies. *Clinical Psychology Review*, *31*, 1041–1056.

Kim, K. Y., Bader, G. M., Kotlyar, V., & Gropper, D. (2003). Treatment of delirium in older adults with quetiapine. *Journal of Geriatric Psychiatry and Neurology*, *16*(1), 29–31.

Kortte, K. B., & Wegener, S. T. (2004). Denial of illness in medical rehabilitation populations: Theory, research, and definition. *Rehabilitation Psychology*, *49*, 187–199.

Kwan, D., Craver, C.F., Green, L., Myerson, J., Rosenbaum, & R.S. (2013). Dissociations in future thinking following hippocampal damage: evidence from discounting and time perspective in episodic amnesia. *Journal of Experimental Psychology*, *142*(4), 1355–1369.

Lane, R. D., Fink, G. R., Chau, P. M., & Dolan, R. J. (1997). Neural activation during selective attention to subjective emotional responses. *Neuroreport*, *8*(18), 3969–3972.

Laureys, S., Celesia, G. G., Cohadon, F., Lavrijsen, J., Leon-Carrion, J., Sannita, W. G., et al. (2010). Unresponsive wakefulness syndrome: A new name for the vegetative state or apallic syndrome. *BMC Medicine*, *8*, 68-7015-8-68.

Laureys, S., & Schiff, N. D. (2012). Coma and consciousness: Paradigms (re) framed by neuroimaging. *Neuroimage*, *61*(2), 478–491.

Lebel, C., Walker, L., Leemans, A., Phillips, L., & Beaulieu, C. (2008). Microstructural maturation of the human brain from childhood to adulthood. *Neuroimage*, *40*(3), 1044–1055.

Lemaire, J., Sontheimer, A., Nezzar, H., Pontier, B., Luauté, J., Roche, B., Gillart, T., Gabrillargues, J., Rosenberg, S.,Sarret, C., Feschet, F.,Vassal, F., Fontaine D, Coste (2014). Electrical modulation of neuronal networks in brain-injured patients with disorders of consciousness: A systematic review. *Annales Francaises d'Anesthesie Et De Reanimation*, *33*(2), 88–97.

Locke, J. (1690). An essay concerning human understanding: In four books. Book II, Chapter 9, London: Thomas Bassett.

Louise-Bender Pape, T., Rosenow, J., Lewis, G., Ahmed, G., Walker, M, Guernon, A., Roth, H., & Patil, V. (2008). Repetitive transcranial magnetic stimulation-associated neurobehavioral gains during coma recovery. *Brain Stimulation*, *2*(1), 22–35.

Lucas, S. E., & Fleming, J. M. (2005). Interventions for improving self awareness following acquired brain injury. *Australian Occupational Therapy Journal*, *52*, 160–170.

Lundqvist, A., Linnros, H., Orlenius, H., & Samuelsson, K. (2010). Improved self-awareness and coping strategies for patients with acquired brain injury: A group therapy programme. *Brain Injury*, *24*(6), 823–832.

Majerus, S., Gill-Thwaites, H., Andrews, K., & Laureys, S. (2005). Behavioral evaluation of consciousness in severe brain damage. *Progress in Brain Research*, *150*, 397–413.

Maldonado, J. R. (2008). Delirium in the acute care setting: Characteristics, diagnosis and treatment. *Critical Care Clinics*, *24*(4), 657–722.

Marvel, C. L., & Desmond, J. E. (2012). From storage to manipulation: How the neural correlates of verbal working memory reflect varying demands on inner speech. *Brain and Language*, *120*(1), 42–51.

McNicoll, L., Pisani, M. A., Zhang, Y., Ely, E., Siegel, M. D., & Inouye, S. K. (2003). Delirium in the intensive care unit: Occurrence and clinical course in older patients. *Journal of the American Geriatrics Society*, *51*(5), 591–598.

Meagher, D. J., Leonard, M., Donnelly, S., Conroy, M., Adamis, D., & Trzepacz, P. T. (2011). A longitudinal study of motor subtypes in delirium: Relationship with other phenomenology, etiology, medication exposure and prognosis. *Journal of Psychosomatic Research*, *71*(6), 395–403.

Mesulam, M. (2002). The human frontal lobes: Transcending the default mode through contingent encoding. *Principles of Frontal Lobe Function*, New York: Oxford University Press, pp. 8–30.

Morin, A. (2011). Inner speech. In W. Hirstein (Ed.), *Encyclopedia of Human Behavior* (2nd ed.). London: Elsevier, pp. 436–443.

Morin, A., & Michaud, J. (2007). Self-awareness and the left inferior frontal gyrus: Inner speech use during self-related processing. *Brain Research Bulletin*, *74*(6), 387–396.

The Multi-Society Task Force on PVS. (1994). Medical aspects of the persistent vegetative state. *New England Journal Medicine*, *330*, 1499–1508.

Nakase-Richardson, R., Yablon, S. A., & Sherer, M. (2007). Prospective comparison of acute confusion severity with duration of post-traumatic amnesia in predicting employment outcome after traumatic brain injury. *Journal of Neurology, Neurosurgery, and Psychiatry*, *78*(8), 872–876.

Neufeld, K. J., Leoutsakos, J. M., Sieber, F. E., Wanamaker, B. L., Gibson Chambers, J. J., Rao, V., et al. (2013). Outcomes of early delirium diagnosis after general anesthesia in the elderly. *Anesthesia and Analgesia*, *117*(2), 471–478.

Orfei, M. D., Caltagirone, C., & Spalletta, G. (2010). The behavioral measurement of anosognosia as a multifaceted phenomenon. In G. P. Prigatano (Ed.), *The Study of Anosognosia* (pp. 429–452). New York: Oxford University Press.

Ouimet, S., Kavanagh, B. P., Gottfried, S. B., & Skrobik, Y. (2007). Incidence, risk factors and consequences of ICU delirium. *Intensive Care Medicine*, *33*(1), 66–73.

Pinker, S. (1997). *How the Mind Works*. New York: Norton.

Plum, F., & Posner, J. B. (1982). *The Diagnosis of Stupor and Coma*. Oxford: Oxford University Press.

Prakash, R., De Leon, A., Patterson, B., Schirda, B., & Janssen, A. (2014). Mindfulness and the aging brain: A proposed paradigm shift. *Frontiers in Aging Neuroscience*, *6*, 1–17.

Pribram, K. H. (1991). *Brain and Perception: Holonomy and Structure in Figural Processing*. New York: Psychology Press.

Prigatano, G. P. (1999). *Principles of Neuropsychological Rehabilitation* (pp. 265–293). New York: Oxford University Press.

Prigatano, G. P. (2010). *The Study of Anosognosia*. New York: Oxford University Press.

Prigatano, G. P., Fordyce, D. J., Zeiner, H. K., Roueche, J. R., Pepping, M., & Wood, B. C. (1986). *Neuropsychological Rehabilitation After Brain Injury*. Baltimore, MD: Johns Hopkins University Press.

Prigatano, G. P., & Klonoff, P. S. (1998). A clinician's rating scale for evaluating impaired self-awareness and denial of disability after brain injury. *The Clinical Neuropsychologist*, *12*, 56–67.

Prigatano, G. P., & Schacter, D. L. (1991). *Awareness of Deficit after Brain Injury: Clinical and Theoretical Issues*. New York: Oxford University Press.

Sanides, F. (1975). Comparative neurology of the temporal lobe in primates including man with reference to speech. *Brain and Language*, *2*, 396–416.

Santos, M., Uppal, N., Butti, Wicinski, B., Schmeidler, J., Giannakopoulos, P., Heinsen, H., Schmitz, C., & Hof, P. R. (2011). Von Economo neurons in autism: a stereologic study of the frontoinsular cortex in children. *Brain Research*, *1380*, 206–217.

Schoenberg, P., Hepark, S., Kan, C., Barendregt, H., Buitelaar, J., & Speckens, A. (2014). Effects of mindfulness-based cognitive therapy on neurophysiological correlates of performance monitoring in adult attention-deficit/hyperactivity disorder. *Clinical Neurophysiology*, *125*, 1407–1416.

Schrijnemaekers, A., Smeets, S., Ponds, R., van Heugten, C. M., & Rasquin, S. (2014). Treatment of unawareness of deficits in patients with acquired brain injury: A systematic review. *Journal of Head Trauma Rehabilitation*.

Searle, J. R. (2005). The self as a problem in philosophy and neurobiology. In T. E. Feinberg & J. P. Keenan (Eds.), *The Lost Self: Pathologies of Brain and Identity* (pp. 7–19). New York: Oxford University Press.

Seel, R. T., Douglas, J., Dennison, A. C., Heaner, S., Farris, K., & Rogers, C. (2013). Specialized early treatment for persons with disorders of consciousness: Program components and outcomes. *Archives of Physical Medicine and Rehabilitation*, *94*(10), 1908–1923.

Seeley, W. W., Carlin, D. A., Allman, J. M., Macedo, M. N., Miller, B. L., Dearmond, S. L. (2006). Early frontotemporal dementia targets neurons unique to apes and humans. *Annals of Neurology*, *60*(6), 660–667.

Semendeferi, K., Lu, A., Schenker, N., & Damásio, H. (2002). Humans and great apes share a large frontal cortex. *Nature Neuroscience*, *5*(3), 272–276.

Sherer, M., Bergloff, P., Boake, C., High, W., & Levin, E. (1998). The Awareness Questionnaire: Factor structure and internal consistency. *Brain Injury*, *12*, 63–68.

Sherer, M., Nakase-Thompson, R., Yablon, S. A., & Gontkovsky, S. T. (2005). Multidimensional assessment of acute confusion after traumatic brain injury. *Archives of Physical Medicine and Rehabilitation*, *86*(5), 896–904.

Sherer, M., Yablon, S. A., Nakase-Richardson, R., & Nick, T. G. (2008). Effect of severity of post-traumatic confusion and its constituent symptoms on outcome after traumatic brain injury. *Archives of Physical Medicine and Rehabilitation*, *89*(1), 42–47.

Sherer, M., Yablon, S. A., & Nick, T. G. (2014). Psychotic symptoms as manifestations of the posttraumatic confusional state: Prevalence, risk factors, and association with outcome. *Journal of Head Trauma Rehabilitation*, *29*, 11–18.

Simons D., & Chabris C. (1999). Gorillas in our mist: Sustained inattentive blindness for dynamic events. *Perception*, *28*, (9), 1059–1074.

Sohlberg, M., Johnson, L., Paule, L., Raskin, S., & Mateer, C. (2001). *Attention Process Training II: A Program to Address Attentional Deficits for Persons With Mild Cognitive Dysfunction*. Puyallup, WA: Lash & Associates Publishing/Training, Inc.

Sohlberg, M., McLaughlin, K., Pavese, A., Heidrich, A., & Posner, M. (2000). Evaluation of attention process training and brain injury education in persons with acquired brain injury. *Journal of Clinical and Experimental Neuropsychology*, *22*, 656–676.

Sokolov, A. N. (1975). *Inner Speech and Thought*. New York: Springer Science & Business.

Spek, A. A., van Ham, N. C., & Nyklíček, I. (2013). Mindfulness-based therapy in adults with an autism spectrum disorder: A randomized controlled trial. *Research on Developmental Disabilities*, *34*, 246–53.

Sperry, R. W. (1977). Forebrain commissurotomy and conscious awareness. *Journal of Medicine and Philosophy*, *2*(2), 101–126.

Sperry, R. W. (1984). Consciousness, personal identity and the divided brain. *Neuropsychologia*, *22*(6), 661–673.

Squire, L. R. (1992). Memory and the hippocampus: A synthesis from findings with rats, monkeys, and humans. *Psychological Review*, *99*(2), 195.

Starkstein, S. E., Fedoroff, J. P., Price, T. R., Leiguarda, R., & Robinson, R. G. (1992). Anosognosia in patients with cerebrovascular lesions: A study of causative factors. *Stroke*, *23*, 1446–1453.

Stuss, D. T., Binns, M. A., Carruth, F. G., Levine, B., Brandys, C. E., Moulton, R. J., et al. (1999). The acute period of recovery from traumatic brain injury: Posttraumatic amnesia or posttraumatic confusional state? *Journal of Neurosurgery*, *90*(4), 635–643.

Stuss, D. T., Rosenbaum, S., Malcom, S., Christiana, W., & Keenan, J. P. (2005) The frontal lobes and self-awareness. In T. E. Feinberg and J. P. Keenan (Eds.), *The Lost Self: Pathologies of the Brain and Identity*. New York: Oxford University Press.

Tate, R., Kennedy, M., Ponsford, J., Douglas, J., Velikonja, D., Bayley, M., & Stergiou-Kita, M. (2014). INCOG recommendations for management of cognition following traumatic brain injury, Part III: Executive function and self-awareness. *Journal of Head Trauma Rehabilitation*, *29*, 338–352.

Teasdale, G., & Jennett, B. (1974). Assessment of coma and impaired consciousness: A practical scale. *The Lancet*, *304*(7872), 81–84.

Terrace, H.S., & Metcalf, J. (2005). *The Missing Link in Cognition: Origins of Self-Reflective Consciousness*. Oxford, UK: Oxford University Press.

Toglia, J., Johnston, M. V., Goverover, Y., & Dain, B. (2010). A multicontext approach to promoting transfer of strategy use and self regulation after brain injury: An exploratory study. *Brain Injury*, *24*(4), 664–677.

Tulving, E. (1984). Relations among components and processes of memory. *Behavioral and Brain Sciences*, *7*(2), 257–268.

Tulving, E. (1985). *Elements of Episodic Memory*. New York: Oxford University Press.

Tulving, E. (2005). Episodic memory and autonoesis: Uniquely human? In H. S. Terrace, and J. Metcalf (Eds.), *The Missing Link in Cognitive* (pp. 4-56). New York: Oxford University Press.

Whyte, J., & Nakase-Richardson, R. (2013). Disorders of consciousness: Outcomes, comorbidities, and care needs. *Archives of Physical Medicine and Rehabilitation*, *94*(10), 1851–1854.

Wijdicks, E. F., Hijdra, A., Young, G. B., Bassetti, C. L., Wiebe, S., & Quality Standards Subcommittee of the American Academy of Neurology. (2006). Practice parameter: Prediction of outcome in comatose survivors after cardiopulmonary resuscitation (an evidence-based review): Report of the quality standards subcommittee of the American academy of neurology. *Neurology*, *67*(2), 203–210.

Whyte, J., Nakase-Richardson, R., Hammond, F.M., McNamee, S., Giacino, J.T., Kalmar, K., Greenwald, B.D., Yablon, S.A., & Horn, L.J. (2013). Functional outcomes in traumatic disorders of consciousness: 5-year outcomes from the National Institute on Disability and Rehabilitation Research Traumatic Brain Injury Model Systems. *Archives of Physical Medicine and Rehabilitation*, *94*(10), 1855–1860.

Zlotnik, S., Sachs, D., Rosenblum, S., Shpasser, R., & Josman, N. (2009). Use of the Dynamic Interactional Model in self-care and motor intervention after traumatic brain injury: Explanatory case studies. *American Journal of Occupational Therapy*, *63*(5), 549–558.

16 Cerebrovascular Disease

C. Munro Cullum, Heidi C. Rossetti, Hunt Batjer, Joanne R. Festa, Kathleen Y. Haaland, and Laura H. Lacritz

Introduction

The acute and long-term clinical picture of cerebrovascular disease varies depending on underlying neuropathology, nature of onset, course, location, duration, and extent of lesion. These factors in turn contribute to differences in symptom presentation, intervention options, and prognosis. The intent of this chapter is to provide a resource for the clinical neuropsychologist on the diagnosis, evaluation, and management of stroke and related disorders. We will provide a review of relevant terminology, epidemiology, pathology and etiology, summarize current diagnostic work-up and treatment approaches, and discuss the current and future role of neuropsychology in relation to cerebrovascular disease.

General Terminology

Cerebrovascular disease encompasses a wide array of neurologic conditions that compromise the function of brain blood vessels. Multiple pathophysiologic processes result in or contribute to cerebrovascular disease, including processes that are intrinsic to the vessel (e.g., atherosclerosis, inflammation, amyloid deposition, venous thrombosis), remote processes (e.g., embolism), inadequate blood flow (e.g., reduced perfusion or high blood viscosity), or vessel rupture. Each of these processes can result in a *stroke*, also known by the older term *cerebrovascular accident* (CVA). Stroke is typically defined as the abrupt onset of a focal neurologic deficit that is consistent with a vascular distribution and lasts more than 24 hours with or without positive imaging results or less than 24 hours with a positive imaging result. *Ischemia* refers to partially reduced blood supply that may lead to *infarction*, causing tissue death. A *lacune*, or *lacunar infarct*, is a small cavity caused by a stroke. A *transient ischemic attack* (TIA) is a brief episode of neurologic dysfunction caused by focal brain or retinal ischemia, with clinical symptoms typically lasting less than one hour but as long as 24 hours and without evidence of tissue death. *Silent stroke* refers to the presence of vascular-related brain injury seen on neuroimaging without associated clinical symptoms. Consensus recommendation advocates the use of *brain attack/stroke* as the best umbrella term to raise public awareness of cerebrovascular disease, including TIA and stroke (Albers et al., 2002).

Epidemiology of Cerebrovascular Disease

From 1999 to 2009, the actual number of stroke deaths declined by 23% (Go et al., 2013). However, stroke remains the most common serious neurologic problem in the world and continues to be a major cause of morbidity and mortality. In the United States, the lifetime risk of stroke for middle-aged and older individuals is one in six (Seshadri et al., 2006). Cognitive impairment is present in up to 64% of individuals with a history of stroke, and nearly one-third develop frank dementia (Jin, Di Legge, Ostbye, Feightner, & Hachinski, 2006). Stroke costs the nation nearly $40 billion annually, including the cost of health care services, medications, and lost productivity (Heidenreich et al., 2011), in addition to the emotional costs and impact upon quality of life. Stroke is the fourth leading cause of death in the United States. On average, every 40 seconds, someone in the United States has a stroke, with resultant death approximately every four minutes. Each year, nearly 800,000 people experience a new or recurrent stroke. Approximately 610,000 of these are first attacks, and 185,000 are recurrent attacks. Although mortality due to stroke is on the decline, a 22% increase in stroke prevalence is expected by 2030 due to changing demographics such as the aging of the population and increased number of ethnic minorities (Go et al., 2013).

Stroke is more prevalent in older adults, African Americans, individuals with lower education, and in the southeastern United States (see Figure 16.1). In this "stroke belt" region, stroke mortality is approximately 20% higher than the rest of the nation (Go et al., 2013).

Women have lower stroke risk than men until late life, when that association reverses. Lifetime risk for incident stroke appears to be decreasing in Caucasians but similar declines have not been observed for African Americans, and among Mexican Americans rates may be increasing (Carandang et al., 2006; Kleindorfer et al., 2010; Morgenstern et al., 2004). Approximately 15% of all strokes are heralded by a TIA, the majority of which occurred within 30 days of the first stroke (Sacco, 2004). The estimated prevalence of self-reported physician-diagnosed TIA was 2.3% or approximately 5 million individuals (Johnston et al., 2003), and this is certainly an underestimate given that many TIAs go unreported. Of all strokes, 87% are ischemic, 10%

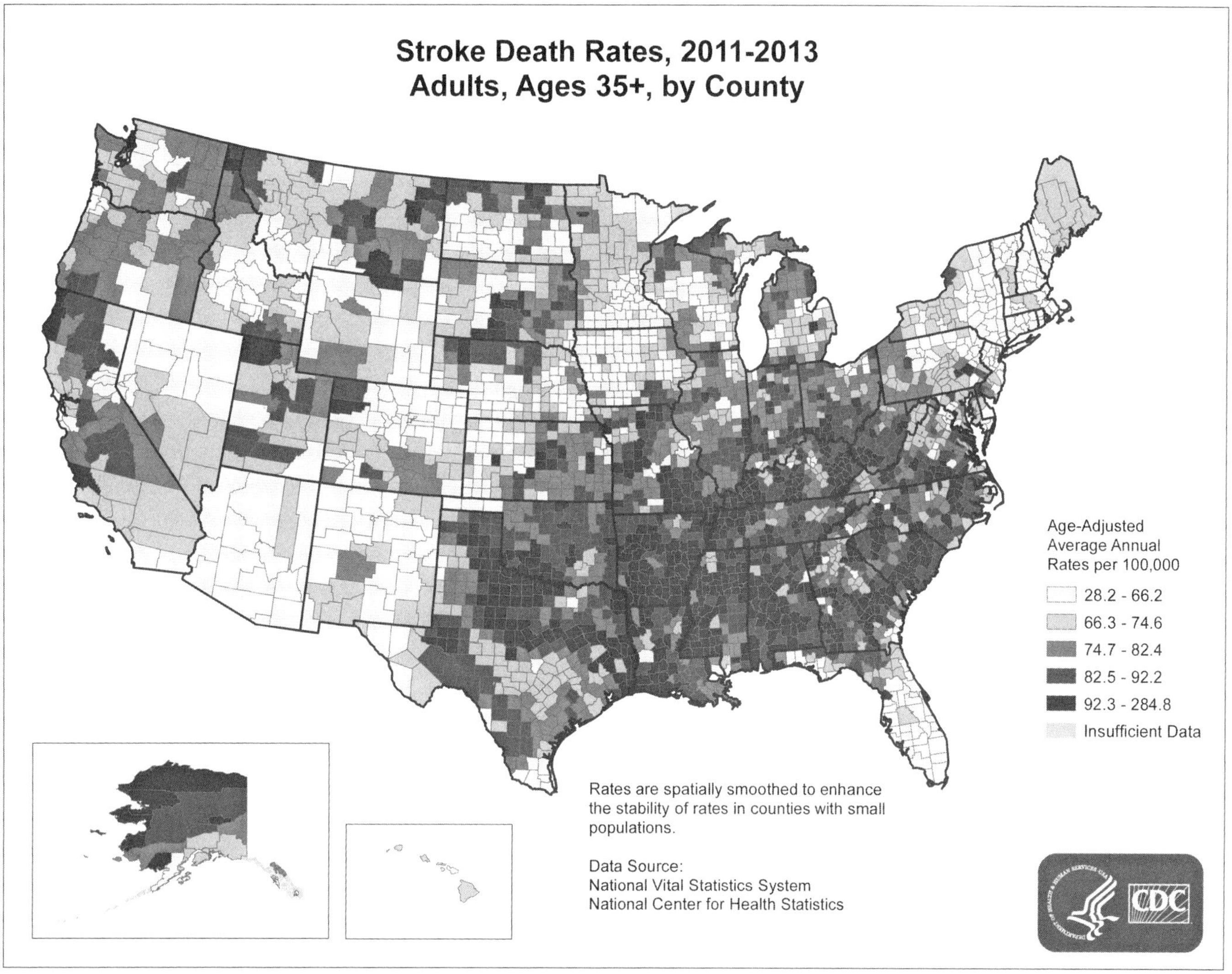

Figure 16.1 Centers of Disease Control stroke death rates, 2011–2013. *A color version of this figure can be found in Plate section 2.*

are intracerebral hemorrhagic, and 3% are subarachnoid hemorrhagic.

Web Resource: CDC Interactive Atlas of Heart Disease and Stroke

This application (available at www.cdc.gov/dhdsp/maps/atlas/index.htm) allows users to view county-level maps of heart disease and stroke, along with maps of social environmental conditions and health services for the entire United States or for a chosen state or territory.

Cerebral Vasculature

The arterial supply to the brain consists primarily of two pairs of arteries: the internal carotid arteries and the vertebral arteries (see Figure 16.2). The internal carotid arteries give rise to the anterior circulation, and the vertebral arteries to the posterior circulation (see Figure 16.3). The vertebral arteries join to form the basilar artery, which converges with the two internal carotid arteries, thus forming the *circle of Willis,* a complete arterial ring at the base of the brain connecting the anterior and posterior circulation systems. The circle of Willis gives rise to all major cerebral blood vessels, including the three main arteries that supply the cerebral hemispheres: the anterior cerebral arteries (ACAs), the middle cerebral arteries (MCAs), and the posterior cerebral arteries (PCAs). The ACAs and MCAs are connected by the anterior communicating artery (ACom) and comprise the anterior circulation system, supplying most of the anterior medial cortex, from the frontal lobes to the anterior parietal lobes, as well as the majority of cortex along the dorsolateral convexity. The PCAs constitute the posterior circulation system and

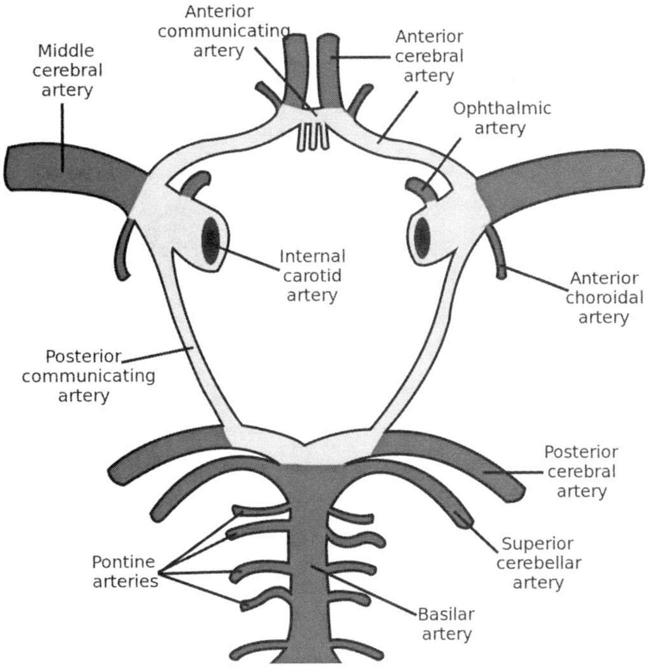

Figure 16.2 Cerebral vasculature: major arteries

supply the inferior and medial temporal lobes and the medial occipital cortex. The anterior and posterior circulations are joined by the posterior communicating arteries (PCom). The distinction between anterior and posterior circulation events is routinely made on clinical grounds during an initial emergency room evaluation for stroke. Aphasia, visual field cuts, hemi-neglect, and sensory-motor deficits typically suggest hemispheric regions; while vertigo, nausea and vomiting, and ataxia usually imply vertebrobasilar territory.

The venous system of the brain is essentially comprised of three groups of vessels that allow for drainage: the superficial cortical veins, the deep or central veins, and the venous sinuses in the dura. The cerebral cortex is primarily drained by the superficial cortical veins. Most cerebral venous blood eventually drains into the dural sinuses. With the exception of venous rupture leading to subdural hematoma, arterial disease has been considered more significant than venous disease.

Hemodynamics

The brain accounts for a mere 2% of adult body weight but utilizes 20% of cardiac output and accounts for nearly 25% of resting total body oxygen consumption. Since the brain

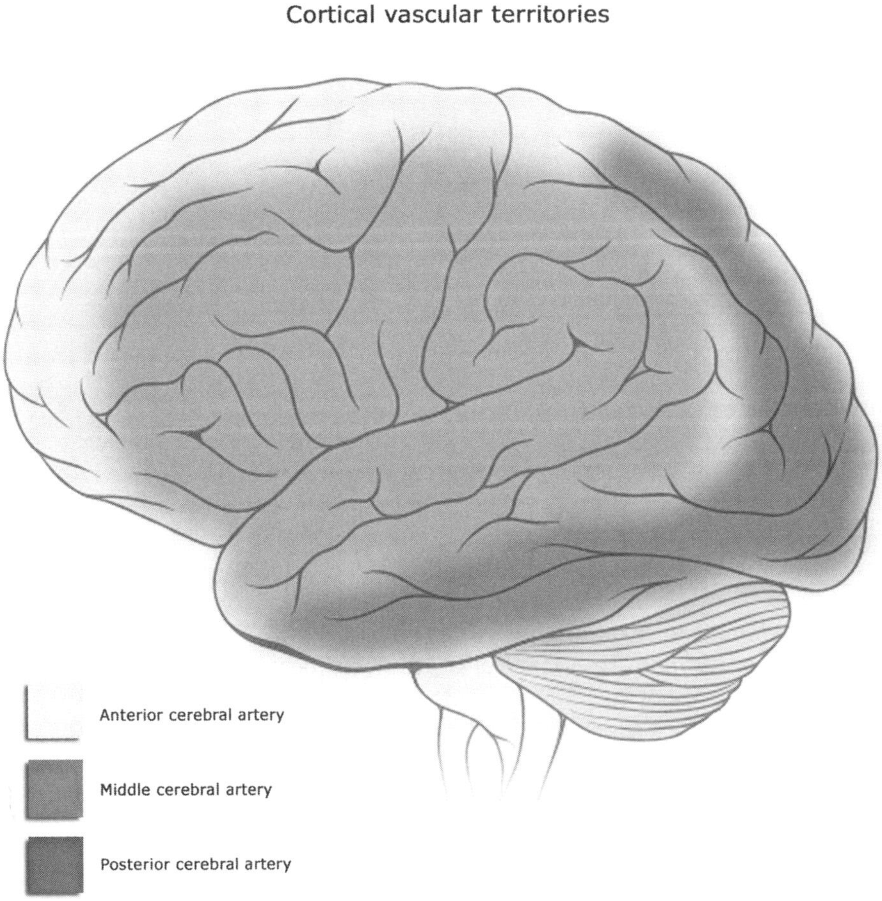

Figure 16.3 Vascular circulation territories. *A color version of this figure can be found in Plate section 2.*

does not store nutrients, it requires an uninterrupted supply of oxygen and glucose. The brain can function for only six to eight minutes if oxygen and glucose fall below critical levels, and complete blockage of blood flow will typically result in loss of consciousness within seconds. Physiologic mechanisms that regulate cerebral circulation are designed to meet metabolic demand in the face of disrupted supply. The delicate physiologic balance among cerebral blood flow (CBF), metabolism, and neuronal activity is governed by an array of functional mechanisms.

CBF is the volume of blood delivered to a defined mass of tissue per unit time, which under normal conditions is maintained at approximately 50 ml/100 g/minute. This consistent rate of blood flow is achieved by virtue of the process of autoregulation. The autoregulation of blood flow that is present in most vascular beds throughout the body is particularly well developed in the brain. Hemodynamic autoregulation involves changes in cerebral vascular resistance via vasodilation of cerebral arterioles when peripheral blood pressure is reduced or vasoconstriction when blood pressure is elevated. Metabolic autoregulation results in increased oxygen extraction fraction (OEF; the percentage of oxygen removed from blood as it passes through the capillary labyrinth), and as such is an additional mechanism that can increase the amount of oxygen extracted from blood (see Figure 16.4). The state of maximal arteriolar vasodilation is referred to as Stage I hemodynamic failure, which indicates that the brain is delivering all of the available oxygenated blood. Maximal vasodilation in addition to increased OEF is termed Stage II hemodynamic failure. Further loss of perfusion pressure and CBF falling below 15 to 20 ml/110 g/min will lead to ischemia and infarction, the hallmark of which is the combination of low flow with subnormal OEF, resulting in loss of functional tissue integrity due to cessation of electrical function and transfer of energy metabolism from aerobic to anaerobic glycolysis. Chronically suppressed global cerebral perfusion, as caused by underlying heart disease or carotid artery stenosis, can impair cognitive function independent of infarction (Marshall, 2012).

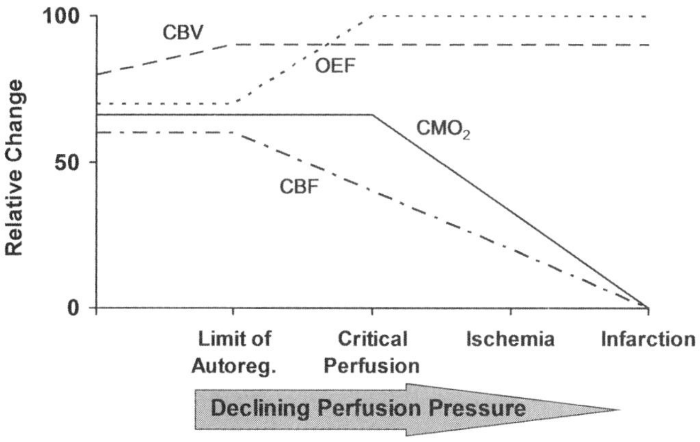

Figure 16.4 Cerebral response to hypoperfusion

Note. CBV= Cerebral Blood Volume; OEF= Oxygen Extraction Fraction; CMO_2= Cerebral Metabolic Rate; CBF= Cerebral Blood Flow

In addition to autoregulation, collateral distribution is another mechanism for brain protection. It enables disruption of flow in one vessel to be compensated by distribution from an alternate supply. This built-in redundancy allows proper neuronal functioning to continue in face of a certain degree of vascular disruption. For example, an occluded carotid artery may have no measurable effect on distal cerebral perfusion if collateral flow through the circle of Willis is adequate. This is not true for the whole of brain vasculature, however, as small arteries and arterioles lack collateral mechanisms and have few interconnections. For example, the basal ganglia comprise an end-arterial region without extensive collateral circulation, which thus increases its vulnerability to ischemia and infarction.

Finally, the concept of *diaschisis* is relevant for understanding downstream effects of stroke pathology. Diaschisis refers to areas of reduced flow and metabolism at sites remote from the infarction site. This results from "stealing" of blood flow to distal brain regions. It is therefore possible to see clinical deficits corresponding to deafferentation of remote and/or ipsilateral cortical structures following a subcortical infarct. Accordingly, cognitive symptoms may also arise in functions not directly associated with the site of infarction. Because of the organization of cerebrovasculature and underlying cerebral organization, it is also important to keep in mind that small subcortical strokes may mimic cortical strokes in terms of clinical symptoms.

Mechanisms and Pathology

Ischemic Stroke

Ischemia, a reduction or loss of blood flow, can be focal or global. Global ischemia is the loss or reduction of blood flow to the entire brain, as seen in cardiac arrest. Focal ischemia refers to the loss of or reduction of blood flow to a specific vascular territory. Ischemic stroke results in two zones of injury known as the *core* and the *penumbra*. The core is the center of the infarct where blood flow is essentially absent, leading to tissue necrosis and the most severe area of damage. The area surrounding the core that has not yet been infarcted is the penumbra. The penumbra reflects the pathophysiologic state of viable brain tissue for which restored perfusion may restore both metabolism and function. The degree of tissue damage depends on a variety of factors, including the location and duration of ischemia, individual variations in vascular structure and collateral blood supply, edema of the surrounding tissue, and type and timing of therapeutic intervention. Secondary insults such as hypotension and hypoxia are devastating in this setting and usually result in a completed territorial infarction.

Ischemic stroke is the most common type of stroke, accounting for nearly 90% of cases (Go et al., 2013). Focal brain ischemia typically results from three primary mechanisms: large vessel atherothrombosis, embolism, and small vessel disease. Small vessel disease is usually attributable to hypertension, which over time damages vessel walls and may lead to ischemia or infarction.

Thrombosis is an obstruction of blood flow due to a blood clot, which narrows or occludes the lumen of a vessel most commonly due to underlying atherosclerosis. Atherosclerosis involves the formation of fatty plaques along an arterial interior wall, which results in the deposition of fibrin, thrombin, and clots. Large vessels (e.g., middle cerebral artery) are particularly common sites for atherosclerosis, predisposing them to thrombotic infarcts. Other pathologies can lead to thrombosis as well, including hematologic conditions such as polycythemia or systemic hypercoagulable state. Obstruction of large vessels can also occur in vasculitis, arteritis, and fibromuscular dysplagia. Thrombotic infarcts often develop slowly and painlessly with a fluctuating course.

Embolism occurs when material from a distant site lodges in a cerebral vessel and occludes blood flow. Emboli are often fragments of a thrombus but could also be composed of fat, plaque, air, bacteria, tumor cells, or particles from an injection. Emboli most commonly originate from the heart, but may arise from the carotid or vertebral arteries, or from systemic veins, and typically cause the sudden onset of neurological symptoms (Caplan, 1993). Emboli may break up as they travel upstream and hit several areas of the brain, causing widespread and varying symptoms (known as *embolic shower*).

Clinical Presentation

Symptom presentation of ischemic stroke varies by individual; however, there are classic syndromes that can be expected following occlusions within a specific vascular territory (see Table 16.1). In general, left hemisphere strokes are associated with aphasia and apraxia, while right hemisphere strokes are associated with neglect, constructional dyspraxia, and dysprosody. Motor and sensory impairments typically occur contralateral to the involved hemisphere though there is evidence of subtle ipsilateral deficits (Schaefer, Haaland, & Sainburg, 2009). This more detailed snapshot of clinical syndromes associated with specific territories is also useful (Haaland & Yeates, 2014)

Aphasia has received the greatest study, in part because few other higher cognitive functions demonstrate such predictable associations with underlying tissue damage, and aphasia syndromes are useful for localization. However, very few patients present with "classic" aphasia syndromes that fit neatly into the classification schemes that are studied by all neuropsychology and medical students. The nature and degree of language impairment will vary, for example, by lesion size, precise location, and tracts involved. As such, the neurobehavioral sequelae of the same injury may differ by individual, much like the anatomical organization of language and underlying brain topography varies. A summary of aphasic syndromes is provided in Table 16.2 and we refer the reader to "Domains of Neuropsychological Function and Related Neurobehavioral Disorders" and "Aphasia: A Clinical Perspective" for a review of aphasia classification (Benson & Ardila, 1996; L. Schaefer & Hebben, 2014) as well as a proposed reinterpretation and reclassification of aphasic syndromes (Ardila, 2010).

Transient Ischemic Attack

TIA has historically been defined as a sudden, focal neurologic deficit of presumed vascular origin lasting less than 24 hours. Until the 1970s, events lasting 24 hours to seven days were termed *reversible ischemic neurologic deficit* (RIND) and only symptoms lasting more than seven days were labeled "stroke." However, present-day imaging techniques show that the majority of events between 24 hours and seven days in fact represent infarction. High-resolution computed tomography (CT) and diffusion-weighted magnetic resonance imaging (MRI) have demonstrated that the 24-hour duration criterion misclassified up to one-third of patients with actual infarction (Easton et al., 2009). Symptom duration does not appear to have a significant relationship to the 24-hour criterion, since 60% of classically labeled TIAs resolve within one hour, 70% in less than two hours, and only 14% last more than six hours (Shah, Kleckner, & Edlow, 2008). TIA has been reconceptualized as a brief episode of neurologic dysfunction caused by focal brain or retinal ischemia, with clinical symptoms lasting less than one hour, and without evidence of acute infarction on imaging (Albers et al., 2002). More recent consensus dropped the one-hour criterion in order to reflect that no single time threshold accurately distinguishes between patients with or without acute cerebral infarction, and to encourage tissue-based, rather than temporally based, definitions that serve to focus clinical attention on diagnosis and treatment of underlying pathology. The American Heart Association and the American Academy of Neurology now define TIA as a transient episode of neurologic dysfunction resulting from focal brain, spinal cord, or retinal ischemia, without acute infarction. The typical duration is less than one or two hours, but prolonged episodes may occur (Easton et al., 2009).

Diagnosis

CT or MRI imaging was employed in more than 70% of emergency room TIA evaluations in 2001 (Edlow, Kim, Pelletier, & Camargo, 2006), and all TIA patients should undergo imaging studies as soon as possible. The preferred technique is MRI with diffusion-weighted imaging (DWI). Noninvasive vascular imaging (carotid ultrasound, transcranial doppler, magnetic resonance angiography, or CT angiography) to assess extracranial and intracranial circulation is also recommended. Finally, echocardiography is useful to rule out emboli of cardiac origin.

Table 16.1 Major clinical syndromes of MCA, ACA, and PCA territories

Nonfluent, or Broca's aphasia, and right face and arm weakness of the upper motor neuron type. In some cases there may also be some right face and arm cortical-type sensory loss.	Left MCA superior division	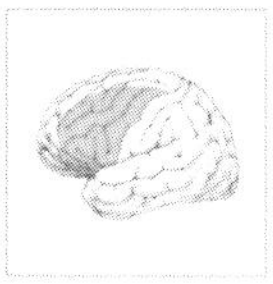	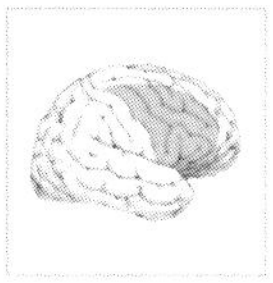	Right MCA superior division	Left face and arm weakness of the upper motor neuron type. Left hemineglect is present to a variable extent. In some cases there may also be some left face and arm corticaltype sensory loss.
Fluent, or Wernicke's, aphasia and a right visual field deficit. There may be some right face and arm cortical-type sensory loss. Motor findings are usually absent. Patients may initially seem confused or crazy, but otherwise intact, unless carefully examined. Some mild right-sided weakness may be present, especially at the onset of symptoms.	Left MCA inferior division	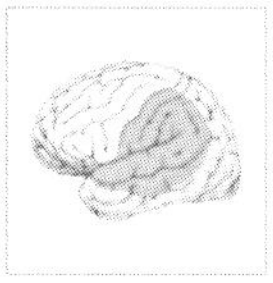	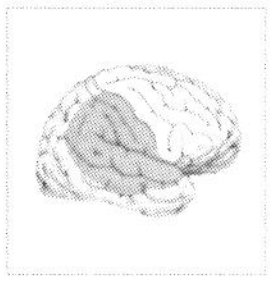	Right MCA inferior division	Profound left hemineglect. Left visual field and somatosensory deficits often present (these may be difficult to test due to neglect). Motor neglect with decreased voluntary or spontaneous initiation of movements on the left side can occur. Patients with left motor neglect usually have normal strength on the left side. Some mild right-sided weakness may be present. There is often a right gaze preference, especially at the onset.
Right pure motor hemiparesis of the upper motor neuron type. Larger infarcts may produce cortical deficits as well, such as aphasia.	Left MCA deep territory	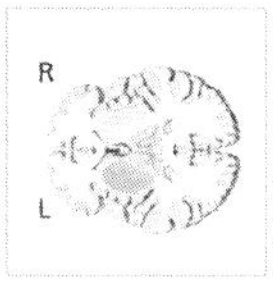	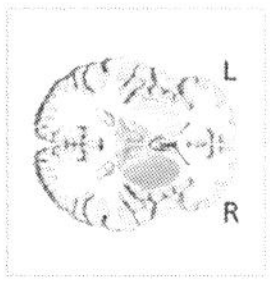	Right MCA deep territory	Left pure motor hemiparesis of the upper motor neuron type. Larger infarcts may produce "cortical" deficits as well, such as left hemineglect.
Combination of the above, with right hemiplegia, right hemianesthesia, right homonymous hemianopia, and global aphasia. There is often a left gaze preference, especially at the onset, caused by damage to left hemisphere cortical areas important for driving the eyes to the right.	Left MCA stem	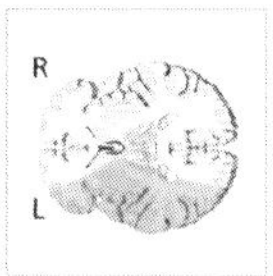	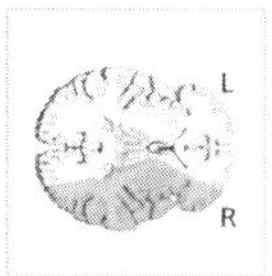	Right MCA stem	Combination of the above with left hemiplegia, left hemianesthesia, left homonymous hemianopia, and profound left hemineglect. There is usually a right gaze preference, especially at the onset, caused by damage to the right hemisphere cortical areas important.
Right leg weakness of the upper motor neuron type and right leg cortical-type sensory loss. Grasp reflex, frontal lobe behavioral abnormalities, and transcortical aphasia can also be seen. Larger infarcts may cause right hemiplegia.	Left ACA	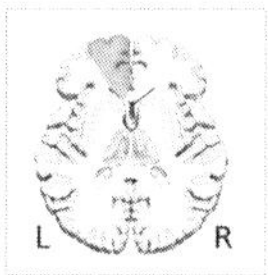	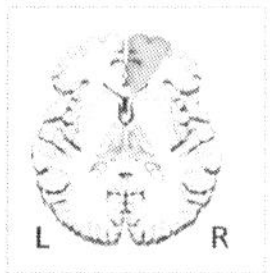	Right ACA	Left leg weakness of the upper motor neuron type and left leg cortical-type sensory loss. Grasp reflex, frontal lobe behavioral abnormalities, and left hemineglect can also be seen. Larger infarcts may cause hemiplegia.
Right homonymous hemianopia. Extension to the splenium of the corpus collosum can cause alexia without agraphia. Larger infarcts including thalamus and internal capsule may cause aphasia, right hemisensory and right hemiparesis.	Left PCA	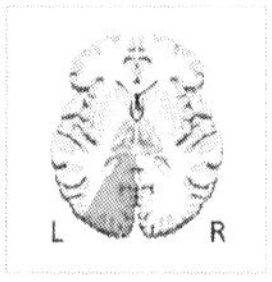	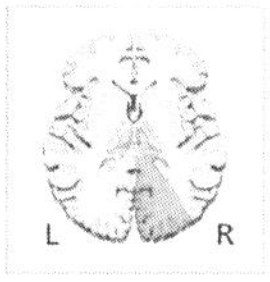	Right PCA	Left PCA Right PCA Left homonymous hemianopia. Larger infarcts including the thalamus and internal capsule may cause left hemisensory loss and left hemiparesis.

Table 16.2 Classic aphasia syndromes and associated language impairments

	Broca's aphasia (motor)	*Wernicke's aphasia (sensory)*	*Global aphasia*	*Conduction aphasia*	*TCMA*	*TCSA*	*MTCA*
Fluency	Impaired	Intact	Impaired	Intact	Dysfluent	Intact	Dysfluent
Content	Impaired	Impaired	Impaired	Mildly affected	Limited	Impaired, empty	Impaired
Naming	Impaired	Severely impaired	Severely impaired	Impaired	Impaired	Impaired	Impaired
Repetition	Impaired	Impaired	Impaired	Severely impaired	Intact	Intact	Intact
Comprehension	Intact	Impaired	Impaired	Intact	Intact	Impaired	Impaired
Reading	Intact	Impaired	Impaired	Intact	Intact	Impaired	Impaired
Writing	Poor, grammatical errors	Impaired	Impaired	Intact	Impaired	Impaired	Impaired

Note. TCMA = transcortical motor aphasia; TCSA = transcortical sensory aphasia; MTCA = mixed transcortical aphasia.

Treatment

Historically, TIAs were often considered relatively benign; however, with increased understanding of TIA and associated risks, there is greater emphasis on identifying TIAs and initiating treatment of the underlying cerebrovascular pathology (Rothwell et al., 2007). Given that between 10% and 50% of patients have a stroke within three months of TIA, with half of those occurring within 48 hours, there is great impetus for early evaluation and treatment. Early carotid endarterectomy following TIA has become an increasingly common means to decrease recurrence and risk of stroke with favorable cost-benefit outcomes (Ferrero et al., 2014). Fewer than one in six patients with symptom duration of at least one hour will demonstrate full resolution of symptoms by 24 hours (Levy, 1988), further highlighting the need for prompt stroke intervention, rather than a wait-and-see approach.

Neuropsychological Implications

Aside from classic neuroanatomical correlates of TIA that can be seen with other focal lesion effects, relatively little is known about cognitive changes in the first few days following TIA or whether such symptoms have prognostic value. In patients who underwent brief cognitive screening with the Mini-mental State Exam (MMSE) either within one to seven days or after seven days following TIA or minor stroke (defined as a National Institutes of Health Stroke Scale ≤ 3), nearly 40% of the acute group (vs. 19% of the 7+ day group) showed "transient cognitive impairment" as defined by a baseline MMSE score ≥ 2 points lower than follow-up MMSE scores obtained one month later. These patients also demonstrated higher five-year risk of subsequent cognitive impairment, suggesting that even minor stroke can result in subtle cognitive changes and are a risk for further decline over time (Pendlebury, Wadling, Silver, Mehta, & Rothwell, 2011). This conclusion is supported by data from the Geographic and Racial Differences in Stroke (REGARDS) Study, which showed higher Framingham Stroke Risk Scores and greater risk (up to twofold) of cognitive impairment on a cognitive screening measure in those with history of stroke-like symptoms or TIA compared to those without such a history in an otherwise stroke-free sample (Kelley et al., 2013). Additionally, diffusion tensor imaging (DTI) has been shown to detect microstructural abnormalities that correlated with performance on the Montreal Cognitive Assessment (MoCA) in patients with TIA and carotid artery disease (Guo et al., 2014). Given that many of the large-scale studies in this area have tended to rely upon brief omnibus screening tests to assess cognitive outcome, it is likely that greater impairments would be detected through the use of more sensitive and detailed neuropsychological procedures.

Hemorrhagic Stroke

Spontaneous intracerebral hemorrhage (ICH) is the second most common subtype of stroke and accounts for approximately 10%–20% of all strokes (Ikram, Wieberdink, & Koudstaal, 2012). *Hemorrhage* is defined as the spontaneous bleeding within the brain or subarachnoid space as the result of vessel leakage or rupture. Primary brain damage from ICH occurs from interruption of blood supply, direct mechanical injury from the expanding clot, increased intracranial pressure (ICP), and/or herniation through the tentorium secondary to mass effect. In addition, the secondary effect of an ICH is a powerful inflammatory reaction triggered by toxic elements in the blood clot. Hemorrhagic stroke damage is manifested within the primary vascular territory affected by the disrupted perfusion, and also in overlapping or shared areas, referred to as watershed zones. There are numerous causes of intracranial hemorrhage (see Table 16.3). The majority of hemorrhagic strokes are attributable to hypertension, vascular malformations, and aneurysms.

Table 16.3 Causes of nontraumatic intracranial hemorrhage

Chronic hypertension
Vascular malformation
Arterial aneurysm
Hemorrhagic infarction (including venous sinus thrombosis)
Septic embolism, mycotic aneurysm
Brain tumor
Bleeding disorders, anticoagulants, thrombolytic therapy
Central nervous system infection (eg, herpes simplex encephalitis)
Moyamoya
Vasculitis
Drugs (cocaine, amphetamines)

The most common etiology of spontaneous ICH is the chronic effect of hypertension. Bleeding related to hypertension usually involves small penetrating vessels that branch directly off major intracerebral arteries at up to 90-degree angles. It is thought that penetrating arteries are more vulnerable to effects of hypertension because they are directly exposed to the larger vessel's pressure, which is ordinarily reduced by a gradual decrease in the size of other branching vessels. The territory of these vessels is the basal ganglia, thalamus, pons, and subcortical white matter. Many hypertensive hemorrhages begin as slow leaks, and in contrast to subarachnoid hemorrhage or embolic stroke, neurologic symptoms often do not begin abruptly and are not maximal at the onset. Rather, the major bleed may be preceded for weeks to months by fluctuating neurologic signs or seizure, and at onset, symptoms typically increase gradually over minutes or hours. Classic symptoms include severe headache, vomiting, decreased level of consciousness, oculomotor disturbance, and nuchal rigidity (neck stiffness). However, clinical signs will vary based on the size and location of the bleed (see Table 16.4).

Cerebrovascular malformations include congenital and acquired lesions and their rupture constitutes a major cause of devastating hemorrhagic stroke, particularly in young people. Arteriovenous malformations and cavernomas are

Table 16.4 Clinical presentation of intracranial hemorrhage by location

ICH Type	*Site*	*Symptoms*
Lobar	Most often affects the parietal and occipital lobes. Associated with a higher incidence of seizures.	Parietal: contralateral sensory impairment. Occipital: dense contralateral homonymous hemianopsia. Frontal: contralateral plegia or paresis of the leg with relative sparing of the arm.
Putamenal	Commonly occurs along white matter fiber tracts.	Hemiplegia, hemisensory loss, homonymous hemianopsia, gaze palsy, stupor, and coma.
Cerebellar	Originates in the dentate nucleus, extends into the hemisphere and fourth ventricle, and possibly into the pontine tegmentum.	Imbalance, vomiting, headache, neck stiffness, gaze palsy, and facial weakness. May become stuporous due to brain stem compression if the hemorrhage is unrecognized or untreated.
Thalamic	May extend in a transverse direction to the posterior limb of the internal capsule, downward to put pressure on the tectum of the midbrain, or may rupture into the third ventricle.	Hemiparesis, hemisensory loss, occasionally transient homonymous hemianopsia or quadrantanopsia. May be an upgaze palsy with miotic pupils that are unreactive, peering at the tip of the nose, skewed, or "wrong way eyes" toward the weak side. Aphasia if dominant hemisphere; neglect or anosognosia in nondominant hemisphere.
Pontine	Medial hematoma that extends into the base of the pons, disruption of the reticular activating system.	Deep coma within first few minutes, total paralysis, pinpoint pupils, absent horizontal eye movements, facial palsy, deafness, and/or dysarthria if awake.

common causes of ICH but conditions such as developmental venous anomalies, and capillary telangiectasias do not typically bleed.

Arteriovenous Malformation

An arteriovenous malformation (AVM) is a tangle of blood vessels that form an abnormal connection between arteries and veins without an intervening capillary network (see Figure 16.5). AVMs have historically been considered congenital developmental vascular lesions because of their unusual angioarchitecture, but the pathogenesis is not well understood. It is likely that many are acquired during life, related to a two-hit hypothesis in which an inborn genetic mutation followed by a second mutation or another type of inflammatory insult results in the development of an AVM (Walker et al., 2011). They can vary in size from a few millimeters to several centimeters in diameter, and may grow over time (Soderman, Andersson, Karlsson, Wallace, & Edner, 2003). Increasing AVM mass can compress neighboring structures and result in the gradual onset of neurologic symptoms. Regional brain perfusion can be compromised due to the brain AVM "stealing" flow from normal surrounding tissue. Focal symptoms can occur if the AVM forms a pathway in which blood flows away from the site and causes hypoperfusion of brain tissue. AVMs are susceptible to spontaneous rupture because of their thin vessel walls. Supratentorial lesions account for 90% of AVMs; the remainder are in the posterior fossa. AVMs account for 1%–2% of all strokes, 3% of strokes in young adults, and 9% of subarachnoid hemorrhages, and are responsible for 4% of ICH cases overall (Al-Shahi & Warlow, 2001). In addition to traditional angiography to assist in identification and illustration of AVMs and associated blood vessel involvement (see Figure 16.5), advances in neuroimaging and computer software now allow for sophisticated interface between structural and functional techniques (see Figure 16.6) to help plan and guide surgical treatments (see Figures 16.7 and 16.8).

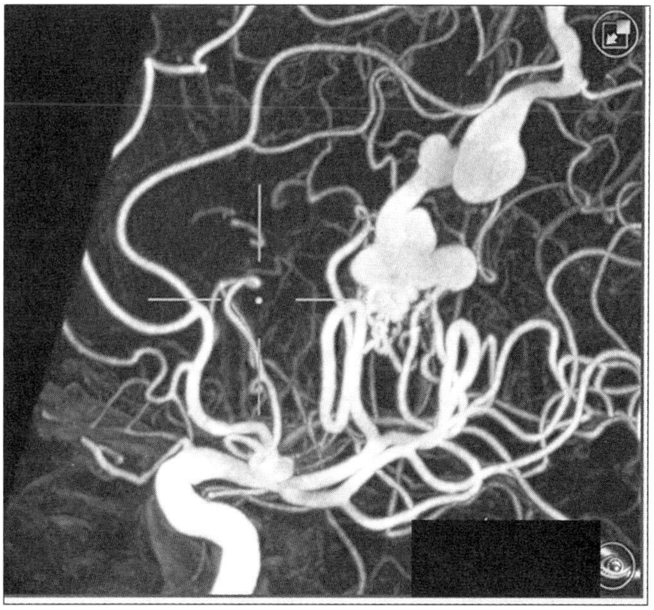

Figure 16.5 Angiographic image of superficial peri-Rolandic AVM with dysplastic venous drainage

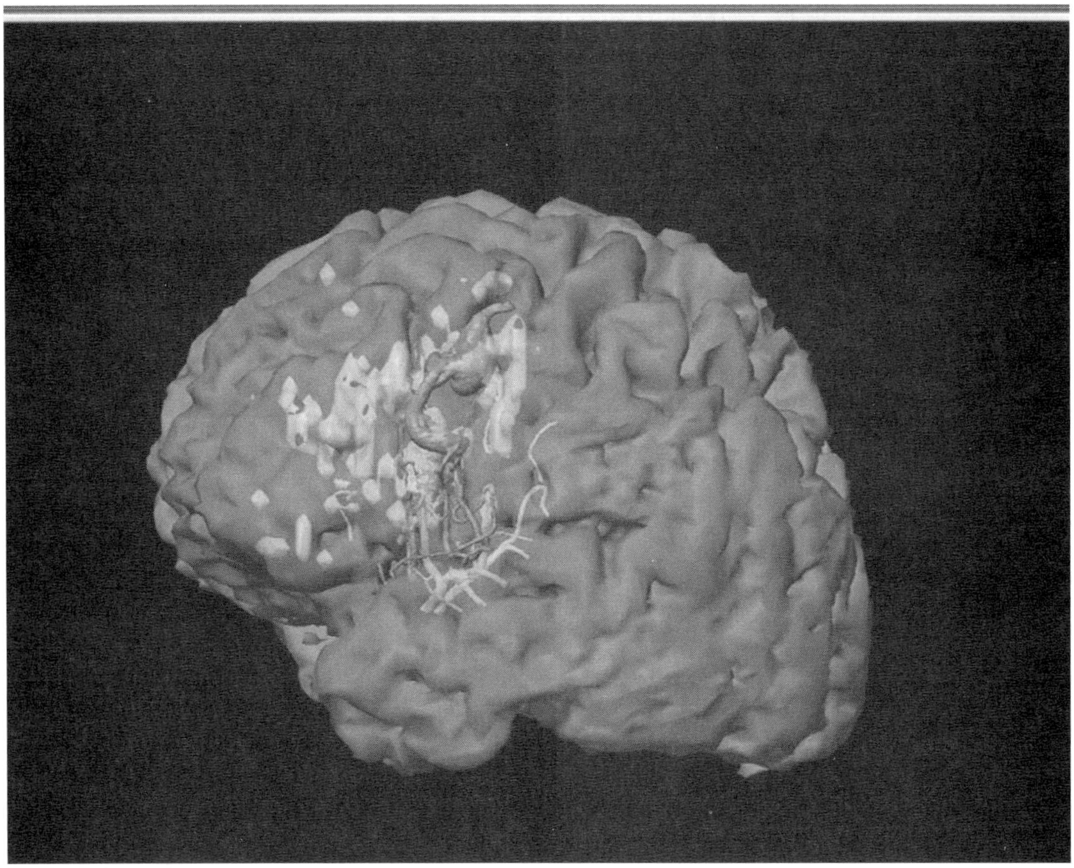

Figure 16.6 Merger of CT, MRI, and fMRI to illustrate the location of AVM (arterial phase, orange; venous phase, red; and functional activation for expressive language, purple) *A color version of this figure can be found in Plate section 2.*

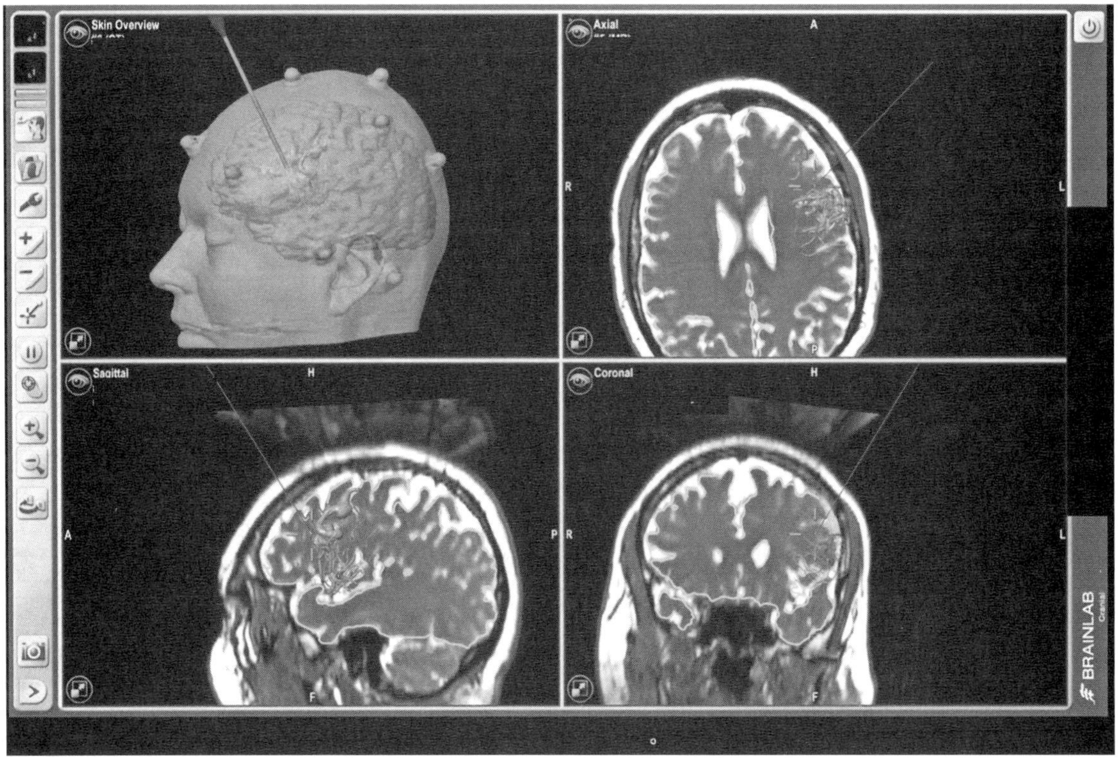

Figure 16.7 Intraoperative navigation technique to localize lesion and plan AVM resection. *A color version of this figure can be found in Plate section 2.*

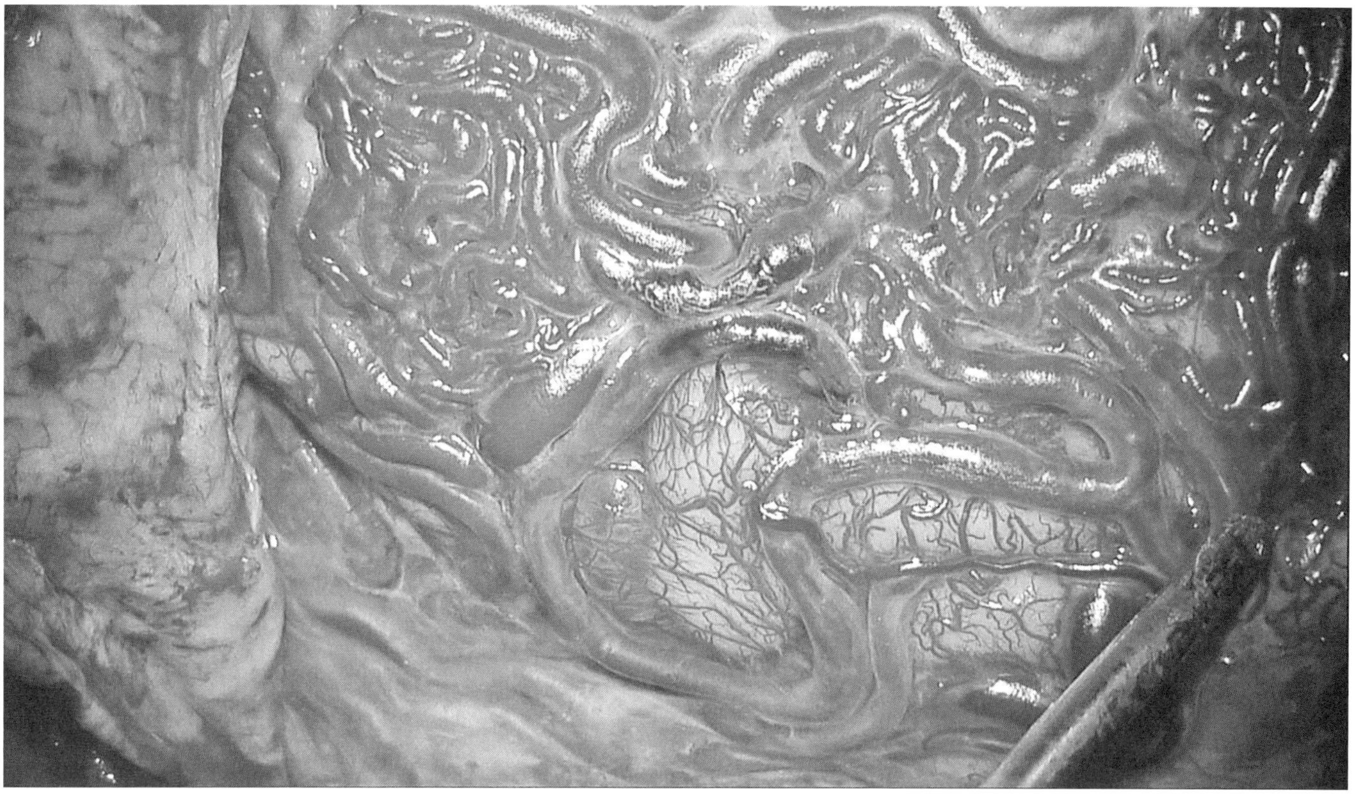

Figure 16.8 Actual appearance of a large left frontal AVM at craniotomy. *A color version of this figure can be found in Plate section 2.*

Clinical Presentation

Patients with AVMs may be asymptomatic until later in life, though symptom onset is often between the ages of 10 and 40. ICH is the most common clinical presentation (between 40% to 80% of AVM cases). Prior to rupture, headaches and seizures are common. The rate of hemorrhage in untreated cases is approximately 4% per year, with up to 2.4% causing sudden death (Huang & van Gelder, 2002). Over 90% of patients survive the initial hemorrhage and risk of recurrent bleeds is 1%–4% per year if untreated.

Treatment

Mainstay treatment techniques for AVM include surgical excision, radiosurgery, or endovascular techniques. Stereotactic radiosurgery deploys high-energy beams to progressively destroy the AVM. The latency period (e.g., the time between treatment and obliteration) is typically one to three years. Once the lesion is completely obliterated, the hemorrhage risk is low. Complications after radiosurgery include radiation necrosis with new neurologic deficits and seizures. In contrast to standard cranial irradiation, radiosurgery may have a lesser impact on cognitive function, although comparative data are limited (Blonder, Hodes, Ranseen, & Schmitt, 1999). Endovascular embolization, often an adjunct to surgery, has relatively low risk of disabling complications. Embolization prior to radiosurgery is employed to reduce size of large brain AVMs and to occlude vessels prior to surgical excision whose bleeding may be difficult to control during surgery. About 5%–10% of AVMs can be completely obliterated by endovascular methods (Yu, Chan, Lam, Tam, & Poon, 2004).

The long-term benefit of treatment for unruptured AVMs is unclear. A systematic review and meta-analysis of observational studies concluded that all available treatments were associated with considerable risks, including a 5%–7% median rate of permanent neurologic complications or death, and incomplete efficacy of 13%–96% (van Beijnum et al., 2011). The first multisite, randomized control trial comparing medical management to invasive treatments found the event rate in the intervention group was more than three times higher than in the medical management group after a mean follow-up of 33 months, suggesting that on average, medical management and careful monitoring are superior to intervention in patients with unruptured AVMs (Mohr et al., 2014). Extended follow-up is planned to determine whether the disparity in event rates will persist over time, however.

Neuropsychological Implications

AVMs less consistently result in well-lateralized or focal neuropsychological impairments compared to ischemic stroke. The variability in neuropsychological outcome may be due to AVM pathology resulting in differences in the development of cerebral (re-)organization, as well as variation in site and rate of expansion. When asymmetrical neuropsychological findings are present, the AVM laterality can be predicted as accurately as in embolic stroke. Interestingly, developmental learning disorders have been found in adults with AVMs at a rate four times that of the general population (Lazar et al., 1999). Neuropsychological functioning has been shown to improve postsurgery and may be attributable to the reduced mass effect of the AVM or surrounding edema. Alternatively, improvement may be related to eliminating the "steal effect" in which shunting through the AVM results in decreased cerebral perfusion in the surrounding area (Malik, Seyfried, & Morgan, 1996). Outcomes may also differ by age, given that executive dysfunction has been observed in adolescents, while performance on executive function tests improved in adults following AVM excision (Whigham & O'Toole, 2007). Understanding of cognitive deficit in AVM is commonly hampered by studies with comingled samples of unruptured and ruptured AVM, with incidence estimates of neuropsychological impairment ranging from 7% to 48% (Lantz & Meyers, 2008). It is possible that hemorrhage itself accounts for this wide difference among AVM patients, rather than the actual AVM, although combining patients with AVMs in various locations may also contribute to neuropsychological outcome heterogeneity.

Cavernous Malformation

Cavernous malformations consist of a large vascular lumen with collagenous walls lined with a layer of endothelial cells and may vary in size from 2 mm to several centimeters. These vascular anomalies are typically sporadic though there are familial occurrences, particularly among individuals of Mexican descent (Morrison & Akers, 1993). In contrast to AVMs, cavernous malformations affect veins with trivial arterial connections. The majority of cavernous malformations are located in the supratentorial white matter. About a quarter of cases occur infratentorially, most often in the pons, followed by cerebellum, midbrain, and medulla. Rare cases of spinal cord cavernous malformations have been reported. Incidence estimates range from 0.02% to 0.9% in the general population, though this may be an underestimate, as many patients may remain asymptomatic throughout life. The risk of hemorrhage from a cavernous malformation may be comparable to AVMs, but most events tend to be small, clinically silent, and may not be detected on standard angiogram due to minimal blood flow through the lesion (Lobato, Perez, Rivas, & Cordobes, 1988). The MRI signature of a cavernoma is classic and is the ideal technique by which to follow patients over time (see Figure 16.9).

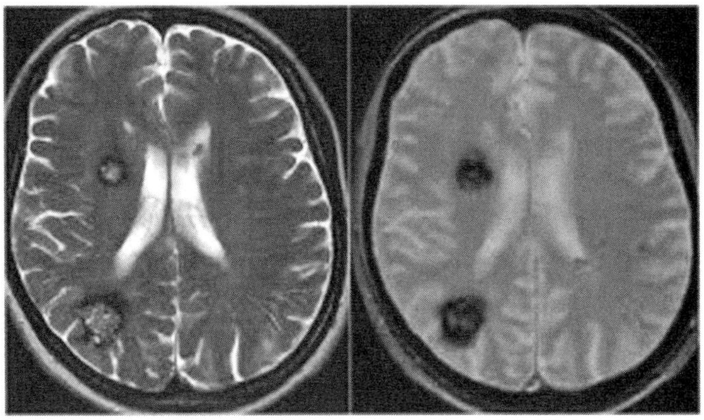

Figure 16.9 Classic MRI appearance of cavernoma with T2 (left) and Gradient (right) sequences

Clinical Presentation

The mean age of symptom onset is 30–40. Cavernous malformations can be associated with headache, focal neurologic signs, and elevated ICP, though symptom manifestation varies greatly. Supratentorial lesions commonly present with hemorrhage, recurrent and intractable seizures, and progressive neurologic deficits. Seizure disorder is nearly twice as common in patients with cavernous malformations as AVM cases. The hemorrhage rate is estimated at 0.25%–1.1%. Infratentorial cavernous malformations commonly present with hemorrhage and progressive neurologic deficits. The annual bleeding rate for brain stem lesions is 2%–3% per year, with recurrent hemorrhage rates up to 20%. Brain stem lesions may produce a syndrome of waxing and waning neurologic symptoms (e.g., dysconjugate gaze, nystagmus, ataxia; see Vrethem, Thuomas, & Hillman, 1997).

Treatment

Management of cavernous malformations may include routine clinical monitoring, antiepileptic medications, or surgical excision, the latter being most successful with superficial lesions. Stereotactic radiosurgery has not been shown to be beneficial. Regardless of location, asymptomatic lesions are typically closely monitored rather than treated. Expanding brain stem lesions may be treated if the malformation can be accessed without damaging critical tissue. Symptomatic cavernous malformations that are entirely surrounded by "eloquent" tissue (areas of cortex that if removed would result in loss of sensory processing, language or other cognitive abilities, or motor impairment, such as Rolandic cortex, brain stem, thalamus/basal ganglia) are usually untreated despite the poor prognosis of untreated brain stem and thalamic lesions. Stereotactic radiosurgery may be used for such surgically inaccessible lesions. However, radiosurgery for deep lesions remains controversial due to high rates of radiation-related complications including posttreatment hemorrhage and the unclear impact on future hemorrhage risk.

Neuropsychological Implications

Systematic studies of cavernous malformations are generally lacking, as these cases are often included with AVM and other focal lesion samples. As with AVMs, neuropsychological deficits typically are not as "focal" or lateralized as stroke, but often disrupt associated local systems and result in more generalized deficits, particularly when leading to hemorrhagic stroke. Persistent seizures associated with cavernous malformations can lead to additional cognitive morbidity. Case reports of cavernous malformations involving the thalamus have mentioned memory disturbance being common, but have lacked formal testing. A case study of cavernous malformation of the mammillary bodies reported preoperative learning and retention impairment on the Wechsler Memory Scale–Revised and Rey Auditory Verbal Learning Test (Loesch, Gilman, Del Dotto, & Rosenblum, 1995), suggesting that focal deficits may occur.

Aneurysm

The most common cause of nontraumatic subarachnoid hemorrhage (SAH) is aneurysmal rupture. An aneurysm is a saccular outpouching of a blood vessel at a site of local weakness in the elastic membrane. There are three major types of aneurysm (see Table 16.5), the most common of which is round in shape and known as a *berry aneurysm* (see Figure 16.10). Saccular aneurysms tend to form at the bifurcation or branching of a vessel, and the majority (approximately 85%) develop within the anterior circulation at the ACom (30%) though other common sites include the PCom (25%), MCA (20%), and the vertebrobasilar apex (15%). Aneurysms range in size from 2 mm to 3 cm in diameter, with an average of 7 mm. Those larger than 2.5 cm are termed *giant aneurysms* (see Figures 16.11–16.13). As an aneurysm grows, the vessel wall stretches, thins, and becomes increasingly vulnerable to rupture. For example, aneurysms < 7 mm in diameter have an annual rupture rate of 0.05%–2%, aneurysms > 12 mm and less than 25 mm have an annual rupture rate of 7%–10%, and aneurysms >25 mm have a five year mortality rate of

Table 16.5 Types of aneurysms

Type	*Description*
Saccular	Berry-shaped with a narrow stem. Most commonly located in the anterior circulation.
Dissecting	Caused by a tear along the innermost layer of the vessel wall, with blood subsequently leaking in between layers of the wall. Often result of traumatic brain injury.
Fusiform	Bulges out on all sides (circumferentially), forming a dilated artery. Often associated with atherosclerosis.

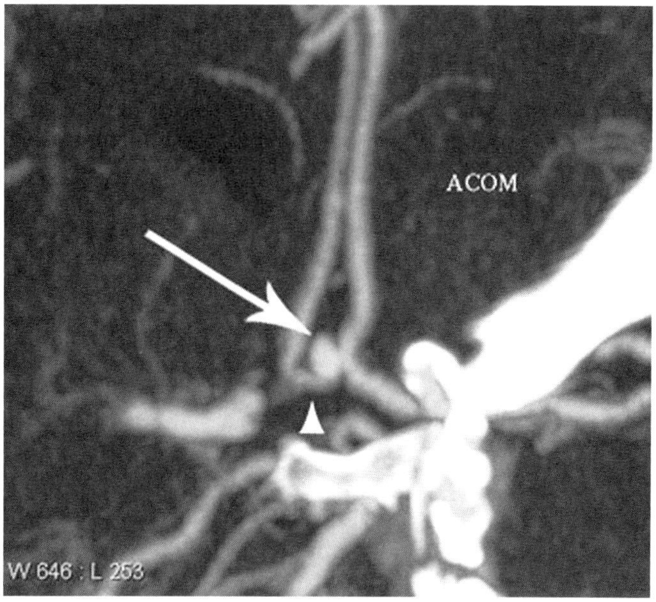

Figure 16.10 Small unruptured anterior communicating artery aneurysm

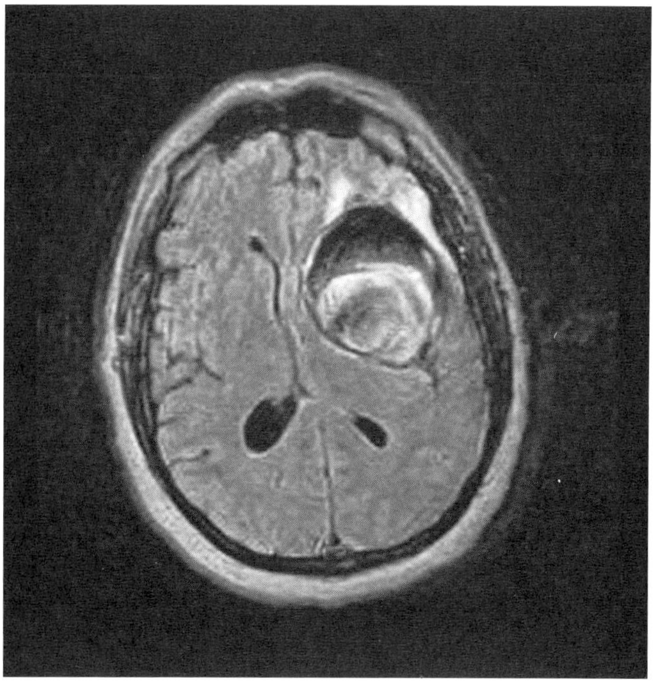

Figure 16.11 MRI of giant partially thrombotic middle cerebral aneurysm

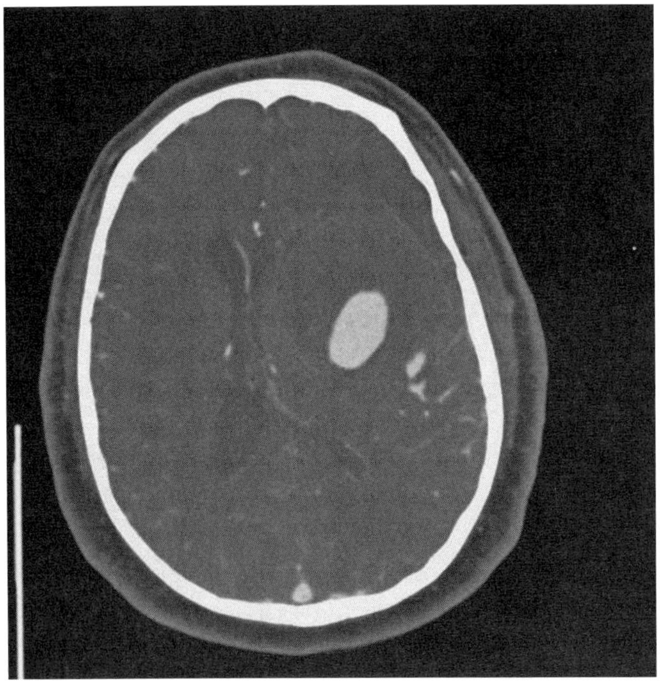

Figure 16.12 Computed tomography angiography (CTA) appearance of aneurysm from Figure 16.11

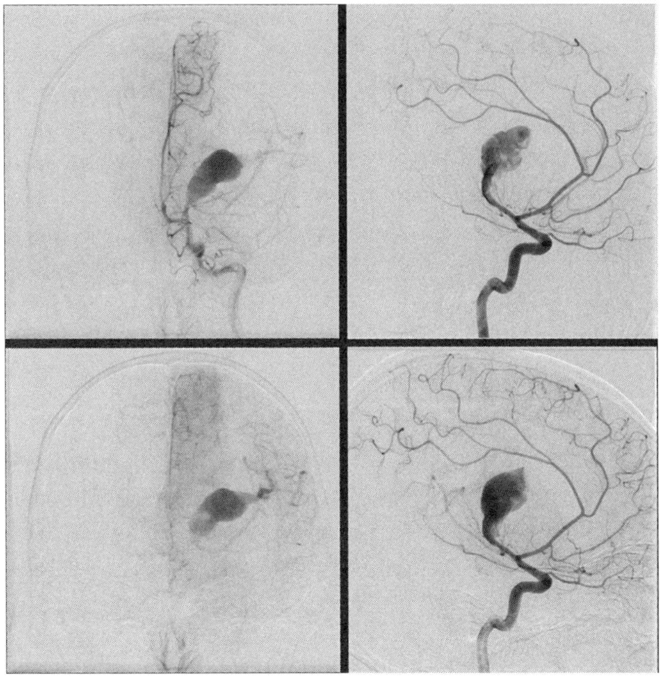

Figure 16.13 Angiographic appearance of MCA giant aneurysm seen in Figures 16.11 and 16.12

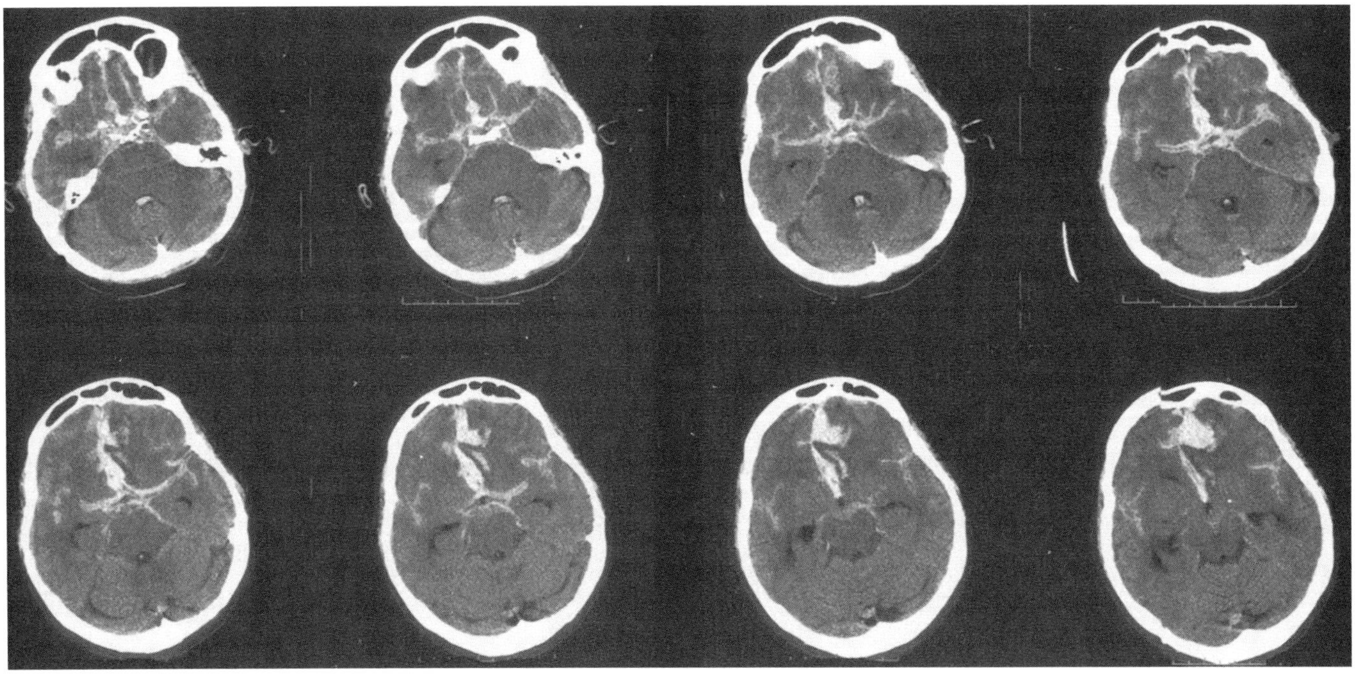

Figure 16.14 CT without contrast demonstrating diffuse SAH and some intracerebral hemorrhage from ruptured anterior communicating artery aneurysm

80% if untreated (see Figure 16.14). In addition to size, risk of rupture and SAH is heightened by age, hypertension, atherosclerosis, alcohol use, and cigarette smoking, the latter of which has been shown to double the rate of SAH from aneurysms (Weir et al., 1998).

Aneurysms are typically considered a developmental or acquired vascular defect, though genetic factors may play a role. For example, individuals with two or more first- or second-degree relatives with a history of aneurysm or SAH (known as *familial intracranial aneurysm*) are up to four times more likely to have an unruptured aneurysm compared to the general population (Ronkainen et al., 1998). Genetic diseases such as neurofibromatosis type I, Marfan's syndrome, Ehlers-Danlos Type IV, and autosomal dominant polycystic kidney disease carry higher risk of aneurysm and SAH but account for less than 5% of intracranial aneurysm cases (Gieteling & Rinkel, 2003).

Clinical Presentation

Most aneurysms are asymptomatic; however, symptoms can manifest with localized head pain related to compression of cranial nerves or stretching of arteries, and transient symptoms of headache, speech disturbance, and unilateral weakness or numbness may be experienced. At the time of rupture, the classic symptom is the abrupt onset of sharp, excruciating headache often described as the "worst headache of my life" resulting from the sudden release of blood into the subarachnoid space and increased ICP. In awake and alert patients, severe headache at onset is nearly invariable, and vomiting is also a common symptom. Unlike intracerebral hemorrhage, SAH usually does not present with focal neurologic symptoms, although "suspicious" neurologic signs may occur, including Kernig's sign (inability to straighten the leg when the hip is flexed to 90 degrees due to severe hamstring pain), Brudzinki's sign (neck flexion causes hip flexion), and oculomotor palsy (Blumenfeld, 2010). In contrast to vascular malformations, aneurysms are more likely to hemorrhage during exertion. SAH accounts for approximately 5% of all strokes. Approximately 10% of patients die prior to reaching the hospital, and mortality within the first 30 days approaches 50%, mostly due to the effects of initial and recurrent bleeding. Rebleeding is associated with an estimated 70% mortality.

Treatment

The risk of rebleeding is high in aneurysmal SAH, with estimated rates of 3%–4% in the first 24 hours. Anticoagulants and antiplatelet agents are typically discontinued until the aneurysm is repaired. After SAH, treatment of the offending aneurysm is an immediate priority due to the high risk of early rebleeding, as well as the extreme risk of induced hypotension to manage vasospasm if the aneurysm has not been secured. Considerable progress has been made in the endovascular treatment of aneurysms in the past decade, including coiling, stent-assisted coiling, balloon remodeling of coil mass, and more recently, flow diversion. These treatments are subject to surgical risks just as is open craniotomy for aneurysm clip reconstruction. The decision to select either modality is best accomplished by experienced, multidisciplinary teams of neurosurgeons and neurointerventionists. The decisions are based on aneurysmal location and morphology, severity of neurological dysfunction, presence of vasospasm, patient age, and other factors. In general, endovascular strategies are somewhat lower-risk on the day of treatment but pose a 10%–20% risk of recurrence that is not seen with clipping. Operative risks associated with aneurysm treatment include new or worsened neurologic deficits caused by brain retraction, temporary arterial occlusion, and intraoperative hemorrhage (Fridriksson et al., 2002). As might be expected, better outcomes are seen at specialized neurosurgical centers performing high volumes of cerebral aneurysm procedures compared with treatment at lower volume centers (Berman, Solomon, Mayer, Johnston, & Yung, 2003).

An alternative to surgical clipping is endovascular occlusion, in which a tiny platinum coil is inserted into the lumen of the aneurysm, forming a thrombus that then obliterates the aneurysmal sac. Endovascular techniques are generally safe and effective, although coil embolization is associated with high rate of recurrence (approximately 20% of patients). Attempts to combine endovascular treatment with gene therapies (to enhance aneurysm thrombosis) hold promise for improved outcomes (Ribourtout & Raymond, 2004).

Neuropsychological Implications

Cognitive dysfunction is common after subarachnoid hemorrhage (Mayer et al., 2002). In a case study series of 217 patients treated for aneurysm rupture, 21.7% showed cognitive impairment on a telephone screening measure (von Vogelsang, Svensson, Wengstrom, & Forsberg, 2013). Neuropsychological deficits following hemorrhage are less focal or lateralized than following ischemic stroke, although the primary site of the bleed may lead to symptoms based upon associated functional brain regions. After SAH, patients may demonstrate a range of neuropsychological deficits that often do not correlate well with aneurysm location (Stabell, 1991). ACom aneurysms are often overrepresented in neuropsychological studies of aneurysm, and sequelae may manifest as broad cognitive decline, more prominent executive function deficit, an amnestic syndrome with associated frontal dysfunction, or no neuropsychological impairment (DeLuca & Diamond, 1995). Cognitive impairment ranging from mild to severe has been identified in several domains, including intellect, memory, visuospatial abilities, processing speed, and concept formation, even in patients with otherwise good surgical outcomes and up to several years after hemorrhage. Gross cognitive impairment, as measured by the MMSE, has been observed at one-year follow-up in patients who underwent aneurysm clipping (Gupta et al., 2014). In a study of patients who underwent surgery for aneurysm rupture and repair, 65% were impaired in at least one cognitive domain six months later, with 19% showing executive impairments alone, 14% showing memory impairments alone, and 32% showing deficits in both domains (Tidswell, Dias, Sagar, Mayes, & Battersby, 1995). Neuropsychological performance did not differ based on aneurysm location, but cognitive outcome was influenced by postoperative complications such as vasospasm. The risk of cognitive impairment may be greater in those treated surgically versus endovascularly, though this issue remains unsettled, as both interventions carry risks. It is likely that neuropsychologic sequelae relate more to the site and volume of SAH rather than the mode of treatment. An increasing number of unruptured intracranial aneurysms are treated prophylactically, and a prospective comparison of patients who underwent surgical treatment of unruptured and ruptured MCA aneurysms found that 12 months after surgery, those treated for unruptured aneurysm performed at preoperative levels on a neuropsychological battery and those with ruptured aneurysms showed reduced verbal memory but otherwise mostly normal cognitive functions (Haug et al., 2009).

Cerebral Amyloid Angiopathy

Cerebral amyloid angiopathy (CAA) refers to the deposition of the protein beta amyloid in small and midsized blood vessels of the brain and leptomenginges, weakening the vessel walls and making them vulnerable to rupture. CAA is an important cause of both large hemorrhages and microbleeds, typically in the cortex (Auriel & Greenberg, 2012). The incidence of CAA increases with age and is relatively uncommon before 60 years of age. The prevalence of CAA is estimated at 2.3% between the ages of 65 and 74, 8% between 75 and 84, and 12% over the age of 85 (Greenberg & Vonsattel, 1997). Unlike the much more common forms of intracerebral hemorrhage, CAA is not associated with hypertension. CAA is attributable to genetic mutations of amyloid precursor protein (APP), with heritable forms of the disease seen in specific Dutch, Iowan, Italian, and Arctic populations. Apolipoprotein (ApoE) is a protein that helps transport blood cholesterol and fat. The three common polymorphisms of the gene for this protein are ApoE2, ApoE3, and ApoE4. Individuals with ApoE2 or ApoE 4 polymorphism appear to be at greater risk for CAA-related hemorrhage than those with the more common ApoE3 allele (Maxwell et al., 2011). Although ApoE 4 is most strongly associated with a risk of Alzheimer's disease, it has been associated with other cognitive disorders as well. CAA is found in more than 90% of Alzheimer's disease cases but has also been observed in 20%–40% of elderly nondemented people (Charidimou, Gang, & Werring, 2012).

Clinical Presentation

CAA is often asymptomatic but can occur in association with Alzheimer's disease, certain familial syndromes, or more rarely as transient neurologic symptoms. It is an important cause of spontaneous lobar hemorrhage in the elderly. Definitive CAA diagnosis relies on pathological examination, but probable clinical diagnosis may be made with MRI evidence of two or more hemorrhages or microhemorrhages in the cortex and sparing of sites typically affected by hypertensive hemorrhage (basal ganglia, thalamus, and pons) (see Figure 16.15).

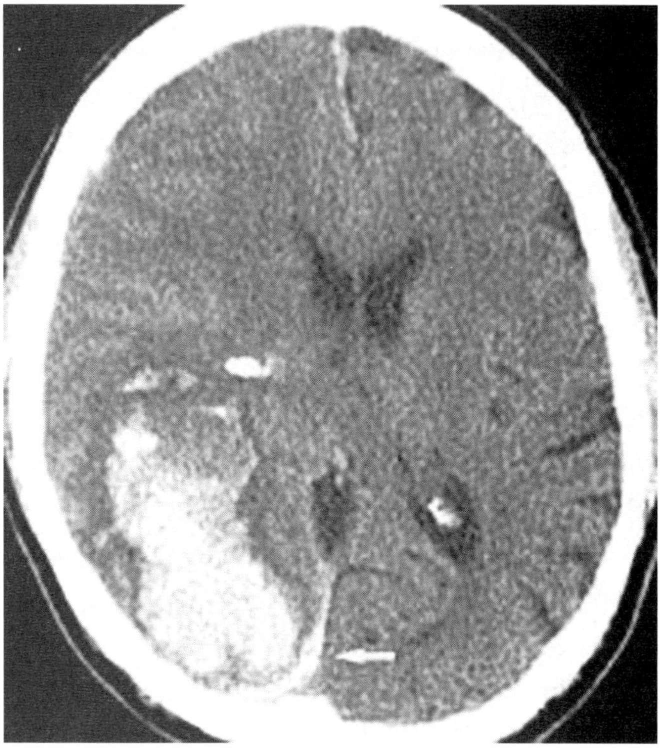

Figure 16.15 Classical CT example of a parietal-occipital hemorrhage from cerebral amyloid angiopathy

Treatment

Acute treatment of CAA hemorrhage is the same as for other forms of hemorrhage. Surgical hematoma evacuation may be performed. CAA bleeds often recur and anticoagulant and antiplatelet agents are avoided. There is some evidence that rare inflammatory forms of CAA may be responsive to immunosuppressive therapy (Chung, Anderson, Hutchinson, Synek, & Barber, 2011).

Neuropsychological Implications

Cognitive impairment has been observed in severe CAA independent of major hemorrhagic stroke and in the absence of extensive Alzheimer's disease pathology. The potential role of asymptomatic CAA in cognitive dysfunction has been highlighted by autopsy studies in which severe CAA yielded an elevated odds ratio for dementia of 7.7 (Neuropathology Group, Medical Research Council Cognitive & Aging, 2001).

Moderate-to-very severe CAA, but not mild CAA, was associated with lower perceptual speed and episodic memory but not semantic memory, working memory, or visuospatial skills in a sample of 400 individuals in the Religious Orders study (Arvanitakis et al., 2011). These effects were observed after controlling for age, sex, education, and autopsy findings of Alzheimer's disease pathology, infarcts, and the presence of neocortical Lewy bodies.

Cerebral Autosomal Dominant Arteriopathy With Subcortical Infarcts and Leukoencephalopathy

Cerebral autosomal dominant arteriopathy with subcortical infarcts and leukoencephalopathy (CADASIL) is an autosomal dominantly inherited angiopathy caused by mutations in the NOTCH3 gene on chromosome 19 (Joutel et al., 1996). Earlier terminology referring to CADASIL included familial subcortical dementia, hereditary multiinfarct dementia, and chronic familial vascular encephalopathy. The pathology of CADASIL involves amyloid-negative angiopathy involving small arteries and capillaries primarily in the brain, which result in loss of the periventricular subcortical white matter, lacunar infarcts in the basal ganglia, thalamus, and brain stem, and chronic ischemia (see Figure 16.16). CADASIL usually manifests in adulthood and is an important cause of stroke in the young (Chabriat, Joutel, Dichgans, Tournier-Lasserve, & Bousser, 2009). CADASIL has been reported to account for 2% of lacunar strokes with leukoaraiosis in patients younger than 65 years and for 11% of cases in those younger than 50 years (Dong et al., 2003). Ischemic stroke and TIA occur in approximately 85% of symptomatic individuals (Chabriat et al., 2009). In a large retrospective study, the age at onset for ischemic stroke ranged from 19 to 67 years, and the median age for ischemic stroke onset in men and women was 51 and 53 years, respectively (Opherk, Peters, Herzog, Luedtke, & Dichgans, 2004).

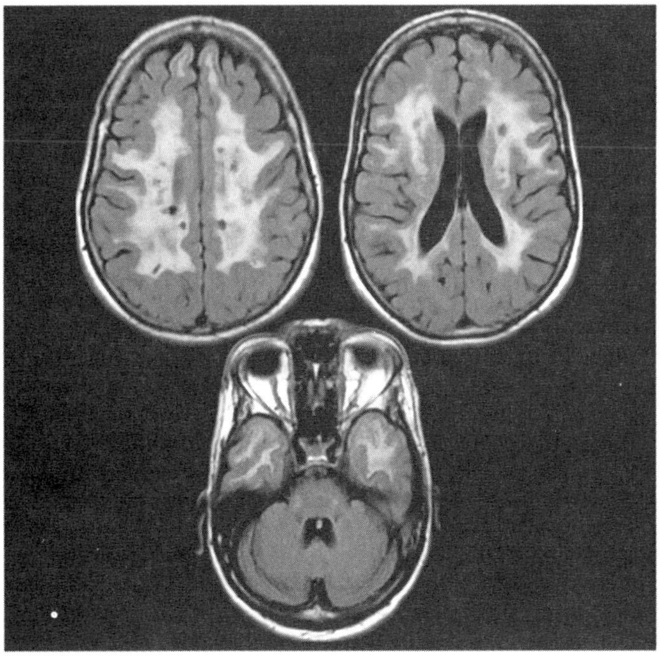

Figure 16.16 Characteristic MRI of a patient with CADASIL; note extensive white matter injury

Clinical Presentation

CADASIL typically manifests with ischemic episodes, migraine with aura, cognitive impairment, or psychiatric disturbance. Ischemic episodes are nearly always subcortical with a classic lacunar syndrome presentation (pure motor stroke, ataxic-hemiparesis, dysarthria–clumsy hand syndrome, sensorimotor deficit). Strokes are often recurrent, leading to gait disturbance, urinary incontinence, and pseudobulbar palsy. Migraine with aura occurs in about 30% of CADASIL cases and is usually an early symptom (Liem, Oberstein, van der Grond, Ferrari, & Haan, 2010). The rate of migraine with aura is five times greater than in the general population, but rates of migraine without aura do not differ (Chabriat et al., 2009). The average age at onset of migraine with aura is approximately 30 years. Aura symptoms tend to involve the visual and sensory system. Some episodes involve hemiplegic migraine, basilar migraine, or prolonged aura, which may be difficult to differentiate from ischemic episodes. Less commonly, manifestations may include acute reversible encephalopathy or seizures.

Treatment

There is no specific disease-modifying treatment for CADASIL. Management is predominantly symptomatic, with a focus on controlling headache, depression, and urinary incontinence. Acute TIA and stroke in CADASIL patients is managed by general stroke guidelines. Secondary prevention involves basic risk reduction strategies (e.g., weight management, smoking cessation, etc.); treatment of hypertension may be of particular benefit in patients with CADASIL. Asymptomatic adult family members may undergo testing for the NOTCH3 mutation and possibly a skin biopsy for specific structural deposits within the small blood vessels.

Neuropsychological Implications

Cognitive impairment is a common clinical manifestation of CADASIL and approximately 75% of carriers eventually develop dementia (Opherk et al., 2004). Onset may be insidious and deficits may appear well before the first TIA or stroke. Cognitive decline tends to be slowly progressive with superimposed stepwise deterioration due to strokes. Predictors of cognitive impairment include older age, lesion location, lesion volume, and global brain atrophy on brain MRI. The cognitive syndrome typically involves deficits in multiple domains with early executive dysfunction and impaired processing speed. In a series of 42 patients between 35 and73 years of age, executive impairment was present in all individuals, and attention and memory were also affected (Buffon et al., 2006). Verbal fluency, ideational praxis, and error monitoring have also been described (Peters et al., 2005). Recognition memory, verbal episodic memory, and visuospatial skills may be relatively spared and severe aphasia and agnosia are rare, though the cognitive pattern becomes more homogeneous and diffuse late in the course of CADASIL. Major depression and apathy related to executive dysfunction occur in about 20%–30% of patients with CADASIL. Other manifestations include severe mood swings, panic disorder, visual hallucinations, and transient delusions. These episodes can precede other signs of CADASIL pathology or MRI findings. Overall, CADASIL cases may initially present with psychiatric dysfunction that is followed by pervasive cognitive impairment later in disease course (Harris & Filley, 2001).

Moyamoya Disease

Moyamoya disease is most commonly reported in Japan and other Asian countries. It is a chronic progressive cerebrovascular disease characterized by bilateral stenosis or occlusion of the arteries around the circle of Willis with prominent arterial collateral circulation. *Moyamoya* is a Japanese word meaning *puffy, obscure,* or *hazy*—like a puff of smoke in the air. The term was applied to this condition to describe the smoky angiographic appearance of the vascular collateral network (see Figure 16.17). Moyamoya vessels can be seen in a number of other medical conditions; therefore, the term *moyamoya phenomenon* or *moyamoya syndrome* is used to differentiate from idiopathic moyamoya disease. Classic angiographic moyamoya findings without known risk factors are designated as moyamoya disease, while individuals with a recognized associated condition are classified as having moyamoya syndrome (Roach et al., 2008). A few of the many conditions associated with moyamoya include sickle cell disease, Graves' disease, neurofibromatosis type 1, Down syndrome, and polycystic kidney disease. Estimated incidence in Japan is 0.35–0.94 per 100,000 (vs. 0.086 in the United States), with an approximate 1:2 male-to-female ratio and a family history found in 10%–15% of cases. Moyamoya disease can occur at any age and there may be a bimodal distribution with peaks during middle childhood and mid-adulthood (Duan et al., 2012).

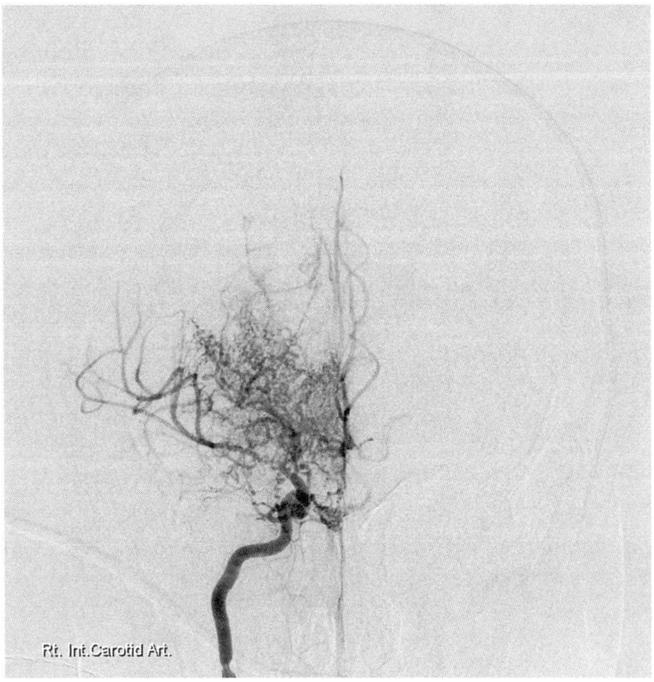

Figure 16.17 The angiographic hallmark of Moyamoya includes proximal occlusive lesions as well as deep basal gangliar collateralization

Clinical Presentation

The clinical manifestations of moyamoya can include TIA, ischemic stroke, hemorrhagic stroke, and epilepsy. Children present most commonly with TIA or infarction (up to 77% of cases) while hemorrhagic stroke (up to 70% of cases) is more common in adults with moyamoya. Hemorrhagic stroke in moyamoya disease often presents as intraventricular hemorrhage with or without intraparenchymal hemorrhage (Nah et al., 2012). The majority of these data come from Asian samples, and research in Caucasian populations suggests that clinical expression of idiopathic moyamoya disease may differ between Asians and Caucasians. For example, in a small German study (N = 21) including 16 adults all cases presented with ischemic events (Kraemer, Heienbrok, & Berlit, 2008). The course of moyamoya may be different in North America, where moyamoya has a later onset and is less likely to involve hemorrhagic stroke. Common initial symptoms of moyamoya are motor disturbance, speech disturbance, migraine-like headache, seizures, and impaired consciousness. Uncommon presentations include dystonia, chorea, or dyskinesia (Baik & Lee, 2010). Ischemic episodes in children can be triggered by exercise, coughing, crying, fever, or hyperventilation (Hung, Tu, Su, Lin, & Shih, 1997). Epilepsy is also more frequent in children than in adults (25% vs. 5%).

Treatment

Moyamoya is a progressive disease with no known cure. Stroke prevention typically involves surgical revascularization for moyamoya patients with progressive symptoms due to infarction or ischemia. Revascularization may include anastomosis of the superficial temporal artery to the middle cerebral artery, encephalomyosynangiosis, and encephaloduro-arteriosynangiosis, and as yet no one method of revascularization surgery has been shown to be more effective than another. Surgical revascularization for hemorrhagic moyamoya is controversial given concerns about increased risk of recurrent hemorrhage; however, one report found that the risk of rebleeding after seven years was lower in hemorrhagic patients treated with revascularization than those who received conservative therapy (7% vs. 43%) (Liu et al., 2013). The conceptual argument for direct or indirect revascularization in hemorrhagic moyamoya is that providing augmentation of distal blood flow may reduce flow through the fragile deep collateral bed within the basal ganglia, which is the typical source of bleeding. There have been no randomized, controlled studies to determine the effectiveness of surgical revascularization treatment for moyamoya. A systematic review of retrospective case series and case reports identified 55 studies with data for 1,156 children (mainly from Japan) who underwent surgical revascularization (Fung, Thompson, & Ganesan, 2005). Over approximately five years, 87% of children had symptomatic benefit, defined as disappearance or reduction in symptomatic cerebral ischemia. Revascularization surgery may be more effective in children than in adults (Ueki, Meyer, & Mellinger, 1994), although treatment guidelines in the latter are lacking. Furthermore, there are no controlled studies directly comparing medical and surgical therapy for moyamoya, and antiplatelet therapy is generally contraindicated given the risk of hemorrhage.

Acute treatment is primarily symptomatic with the goal of reducing elevated ICP, improving CBF, and preventing seizures. Intraparenchymal hemorrhage may require ventricular drainage and/or hematoma removal. In children with moyamoya hospitalized for acute stroke, management includes precautions to minimize crying and hyperventilation as these can cause vasoconstriction and thus induce or worsen ischemia (Parray, Martin, & Siddiqui, 2011).

Neuropsychological Implications

Relatively little is known about the neuropsychology of moyamoya. The disease course tends to be progressive, with stepwise cognitive changes due to repeated ischemic stroke or hemorrhage. In studies with long-term follow-up of untreated patients, progressive neurologic deficits and poor outcome were reported in 50%–66%. Most research on cognitive effects of moyamoya has been limited to children in Japan, focused on intelligence, or conducted only postsurgically. In the first adult study, moyamoya disease had an impact on cognition, but it was not severe or pervasive (Karzmark et al., 2008). On measures of intelligence and other cognitive abilities, group performance was within normal limits. Cognitive impairment was present in approximately one-third of patients, and judged to be moderate to severe in only 11%. Executive functioning was the most common area of difficulty. These results contrast with typical pediatric findings of significant loss of intellectual capacity (Matsushima, Aoyagi, Masaoka, Suzuki, & Ohno, 1990). More recently, a report of a moyamoya patients from three centers demonstrated at least moderate cognitive impairment (>2 SD beneath the mean) in two-thirds of the sample (Festa et al., 2010). The most common deficits were in delayed word list recall (31%), processing speed (29%), letter fluency (26%), and executive dysfunction (25%), in addition to significant decrements in grip strength and fine motor dexterity (36%–58%). Moderate to severe symptoms of depression were observed in 28% of cases, although depression was unrelated to cognitive impairment.

Vascular Cognitive Impairment and Vascular Dementia

Broadly, dementias in which vascular mechanisms play a pathologic role are considered vascular dementias (VaD). VaD is thought to be responsible for at least 20% of cases of dementia, second only to Alzheimer's disease (Gorelick et al., 2011). Progress on VaD has been complicated by varying diagnostic principles and a lack of defined pathologic criteria, which have proved challenging given that cerebrovascular disease itself encompasses a wide variety of pathophysiologic mechanisms and clinical manifestations. Further, a diagnosis of VaD does not exclude the presence of Alzheimer pathology. In fact, the presence of vascular pathology increases the risk of Alzheimer's disease (Sahathevan, Brodtmann, & Donnan, 2012). This could be related to evidence that Alzheimer's disease and vascular dementia may share some of the same biological causes (Breteler, 2000) or to the fact that combined pathologies might increase dementia severity or clinical emergence. Furthermore, up to one-third of all-cause late-life dementia cases show significant vascular pathology at postmortem (Kalaria, 2002). Given that vascular risk factors are treatable, and thus VaD is theoretically preventable or modifiable, the development of satisfactory diagnostic standards is critical. The designation of VaD is perhaps currently best conceptualized as a heterogeneous syndrome rather than a distinct disorder.

Diagnosis

There are four widely used independent diagnostic criteria for VaD; the National Institute of Neurological Disorders and Stroke–Association International pour la Recherche et l'Enseignement en Neurosciences (NINDS-AIREN) for possible and probable VaD (Roman et al., 1993), the State of California Alzheimer Disease Diagnostic and Treatment Centers (ADDTC) criteria for possible and probable ischemic VaD (Chui et al., 1992), the *International Classification of Diseases,* tenth edition (ICD-10) criteria for VaD (WHO, 1993), and the *Diagnostic and Statistical Manual for Mental Disorders,* fifth edition (DSM-5) for major or mild vascular neurocognitive disorder (APA, 2013).

These four diagnostic approaches vary based on how dementia is defined, what types of cerebrovascular disease are included, what disorders must be specifically excluded, whether focal findings are required, whether the presence of vascular disease must be corroborated by neuroimaging, and whether a temporal relationship between stroke event and cognitive decline is required. The different criteria identify different patients and are not interchangeable, contributing to variations in epidemiologic estimates. For example, in a sample of 167 persons who met criteria for dementia, only five met criteria for VaD using all four classification systems (Wetterling, Kanitz, & Borgis, 1996). A thorough review of the various clinical diagnostic criteria for vascular dementia highlighted the marked variability among reported sensitivities and specificities, incidence, and prevalence rates as well as substantial differences in the clinical classification of cases of dementia, and found that none of the available criteria distinguished mixed dementia from vascular dementia or recognized early vascular cognitive changes (Wiederkehr, Simard, Fortin, & van Reekum, 2008a, 2008b). More recently, a fifth approach was proposed by a joint American Heart Association and American Stroke Association statement that provided diagnostic criteria for probable and possible VaD, and probable, possible, and unstable vascular cognitive impairment (VCI) (Gorelick et al., 2011). VCI is presently conceptualized as "a syndrome with evidence of clinical stroke or subclinical vascular brain injury and cognitive impairment affecting at least one cognitive domain" (Gorelick et al., 2011: 2677).

The National Institute of Neurological Disorders and Stroke–Canadian Stroke Network Vascular Cognitive Impairment Harmonization Standards proposed a set of common data elements to help in common clinical practice or large research studies (Hachinski et al., 2006). This workgroup provided recommendations in several areas, including neuropathology, imaging, and neuropsychology. For example, the Neuropsychological Working Group proposed three separate protocols for use of research investigations related to VCI (Table 16.6) with particular attention to tasks involving information processing speed, set-shifting, and working memory, based on the generally accepted notion that executive dysfunction is a key aspect of VCI.

Pathology

At least three common pathologies contribute substantively to VaD. These include large artery infarctions, small artery subcortical infarctions or lacunes, and chronic subcortical ischemia (Kalaria, 2012). Lacunar infarctions and chronic ischemic changes in the white matter share a common primary vascular pathology—the lipohyalinosis or microatheroma of small penetrating arteries—and therefore tend to occur together and are particularly common in individuals with hypertension or diabetes and in the elderly. Other clinical manifestations attributed to small-artery disease and associated with VCI are retinopathy and the presence of cerebral microbleeds in the deep hemispheric and infratentorial

Table 16.6 NINDS VCI harmonization standards proposed neuropsychological protocols

60-Minute Test Protocol	*30-Minute Test Protocol*	*5-Minute Protocol*
Executive/Activation	Semantic Fluency (Animal Naming)	MoCA subtests:
Semantic Fluency (Animal Naming)	Phonemic Fluency (Controlled Oral Word Association Test)	Five-Word Memory Task (registration, recall, recognition)
Phonemic Fluency (Controlled Oral Word Association Test)	WAIS-III Digit Symbol-Coding	Six-Item Orientation
WAIS-III Digit Symbol-Coding	Hopkins Verbal Learning Test–Revised	One-Letter Phonemic Fluency
Trail Making Test	Center for Epidemiologic Studies-Depression Scale (CESD)	**Supplemental**
List Learning Test Strategies	Neuropsychiatric Inventory Questionnaire Version (NPI-Q)	Remainder of the MoCA
Future Use: Simple and Choice Reaction Time	**Supplemental**	Semantic Fluency (Animal Naming)
Language/Lexical Retrieval	MMSE	Trail Making Test
Boston Naming Test, second Edition, Short Form	Trail Making Test	MMSE
Visuospatial		
Rey-Osterrieth Complex Figure Copy		
Supplemental: Complex Figure Memory		
Memory		
Hopkins Verbal Learning Test-Revised		
Alternate: California Verbal Learning Test–2		
Supplemental: Boston Naming Test Recognition		
Supplemental: Digit Symbol Coding Incidental Learning		
Neuropsychiatric/Depressive Symptoms		
Neuropsychiatric Inventory–Questionnaire Version (NPI-Q)		
Center for Epidemiological Studies-Depression Scale (CESD)		
Other		
Informant Questionnaire for Cognitive Decline in the Elderly, Short Form		
MMSE		

regions (Qiu et al., 2010). In contrast to cortical stroke, there is evidence of diffuse blood-brain barrier dysfunction throughout the white matter with lacunar infarction. Chronic subcortical microischemia can result in cognitive impairment even in the absence of ischemic lesions (Balestrini et al., 2013) and is a more frequent clinical-pathologic correlate of VCI and VaD than multiple large infarcts (Hulette et al., 1997; Jellinger, 2013). Deep white matter tracts are particularly susceptible to vascular pathology, in part because white matter is marginally perfused and particularly vulnerable to alterations in CBF and disruption of the blood-brain barrier, both of which contribute to oxidative stress, inflammation, and subsequent demyelination.

The role of vascular insults as initiator, stimulator, or additive contributor to VaD is significantly related to lesion volume, number, and location. Areas of strategic importance for deficits may be cortical (i.e., hippocampus, angular gyrus, frontal lobe) or subcortical (i.e., thalamus, caudate, genu of the internal capsule). Thalamic damage may be a particularly important contributor to cognitive impairment (Stebbins et al., 2008). Even a single stroke in so-called strategic areas can result in prominent cognitive impairment. This is sometimes referred to as "strategic infarct dementia," though these cases generally have a static presentation rather than a degenerative course. Similarly, other vascular events may cause significant cognitive impairment (e.g., subarachnoid hemorrhage, impairment after cardiac bypass surgery, watershed infarction) but are not generally considered with VaD because of the lack of expected progression.

Neuropsychological Implications

In contrast to the classic clinical picture of Alzheimer's disease, which generally involves the insidious onset of cognitive impairments, vascular dementia classically is associated with an acute onset and fluctuating intensity of symptoms and a stepwise decline in cognitive functioning combined with evidence of cerebrovascular disease (e.g., focal neurological signs). However, the stepwise trajectory is typically expected with frank strokes rather than chronic microischemic insults that may have a more slowly progressive course. Alzheimer's disease is typically associated with greater memory dysfunction and fewer executive deficits than VaD in early stages; however, the reverse is not always true (Reed et al., 2007). Despite extensive study, there remains no clear consensus of which cognitive functions or neuropsychological tests best discriminate between VaD and Alzheimer's disease (Looi & Sachdev, 1999; Mathias & Burke, 2009). White matter pathology and subsequent disruption of fronto-subcortical networks, particularly associated with chronic subcortical microischemia, are thought to lead to slowed information processing speed, the neurocognitive symptom most commonly associated with VCI/VaD. In general, other symptoms associated with VaD include attention deficits, executive dysfunction, reduced phonemic verbal fluency, and impaired motor programming. In terms of memory findings, relatively less prominent impairment is expected than in Alzheimer's disease, and recognition memory performance tends to be better than free recall. However, the neuropsychological profile will depend on location and degree of the underlying cerebrovascular pathology. Gait disturbance, parkinsonism, urinary incontinence, and depression are more frequently implicated in VaD, relative to other dementias.

Mixed Dementia

Mixed dementia, or Alzheimer's disease with cerebrovascular disease, is recognized as a separate entity due to the common co-occurrence of Alzheimer's disease and VaD pathology. Approximately 30% of patients with a clinical diagnosis of VaD demonstrate Alzheimer's disease pathology at autopsy (Kalaria, 1993) and up to 50% of those with Alzheimer's disease diagnoses will show vascular pathology at autopsy (Kalaria, 2012). Elderly patients with dementia may in fact be more likely to have mixed pathology (e.g., amyloid plaques, neurofibrillary tangles, and ischemic lesions) than Alzheimer's disease or VaD alone (Launer, Petrovitch, Ross, Markesbery, & White, 2008) (Schneider, Arvanitakis, Bang, & Bennett, 2007). Furthermore, there is evidence that Alzheimer's disease and VaD may have common etiologies and influence each other's course. For example, after controlling for Alzheimer's disease pathology in autopsied subjects (Schneider, 2007), cortical infarcts increased the odds of dementia fivefold. After subsequently controlling for the effect of cortical infarct, subcortical infarcts carried fourfold increased odds of dementia and were associated with lower performance on tasks of episodic, semantic, and working memory. Vascular risk factors such as hypertension, hyperlipidemia, diabetes, smoking, and coronary artery disease have been linked to both VaD and Alzheimer's disease. The ApoE4 genotype has been associated with both Alzheimer's disease and cardiovascular disease, though as with other central nervous system disorders, the association between ApoE4 and VaD remains unclear (Slooter et al., 2004). In part because of the common overlap of Alzheimer's disease and VaD symptoms and shared risk factors, it has been posited that sporadic Alzheimer's disease may in fact be a primary vascular disorder rather than a neurodegenerative disorder (de la Torre, 2002). Additional support for this view comes from studies showing the important role of cerebral perfusion in Alzheimer's disease, including that Alzheimer's disease risk factors reduce perfusion, medications employed in Alzheimer's disease treatment improve cerebral perfusion, and neuroimaging evidence of regional cerebral hypoperfusion in preclinical Alzheimer's disease. Alternatively, the hypoperfusion associated with cerebrovascular disease may impair beta-amyloid clearance. However, the interaction between cerebrovascular factors and Alzheimer's disease remains poorly understood, as some studies find no relationship between Alzheimer's disease pathology and infarctions

(Schneider, Wilson, Bienias, Evans, & Bennett, 2004). Alzheimer's disease pathology can overwhelm the impact of vascular or other forms of pathology (Chui et al., 2006), and cardiovascular risk profiles and white matter hyperintensities are not associated with Alzheimer's disease-specific pathology such as hippocampal atrophy and cerebrospinal fluid-derived biomarkers (Lo & Jagust, 2012).

Cerebrovascular Risk Factors

> **Web Resource**
>
> The National Stroke association offers an interactive guide (www.stroke.org/site/PageServer?pagename=riskfactors) that explains 26 of the more common risk factors for stroke.

Cerebrovascular disease is typically due to a chronic, systemic process such as atherosclerosis or hypertension. Numerous risk factors exist and many individuals have more than one. Most risk factors have independent effects as well as interaction effects and may be more common in different disease processes. Prevention, identification, and treatment of risk factors are critical to decrease morbidity of these conditions.

Hypertension

Hypertension is the single most important risk factor for both hemorrhagic and ischemic stroke, with approximately 77% of individuals presenting with first stroke having blood pressures higher than 140/90 (Go et al., 2013) and about 50% having a history of hypertension (Britton, Carlsson, & de Faire, 1986). Blood pressure ordinarily increases with age. Elevation of blood pressure above standard norms for age occurs in approximately a third of the general adult population and prevalence increases with age. High blood pressure places stress on blood vessel walls and subsequent morphologic changes result in cerebrovascular remodeling, impaired vasodilation and autoregulation, amyloid angiopathy, the accumulation of atherosclerotic plaque, white matter changes, and cognitive changes ranging from mild cognitive impairment to dementia (Faraco & Iadecola, 2013). There is compelling evidence that the control of high blood pressure contributes to the prevention of stroke. Numerous studies have found an association between antihypertensive drug treatment and lowered risk of dementia, presumably via the resulting reduction in subsequent major cardiovascular events and recurrent strokes (Furie et al., 2011).

Diabetes

Diabetes mellitus, both Type I (absence of pancreatic insulin production) and Type II (insulin resistance; low production of insulin) cause elevation of blood sugar to above 100 mg/dL, and cause microvascular (retinopathy, neuropathy) and macrovascular complications (peripheral, coronary, and cerebral atherothrombotic). Diabetes affects approximately 5% of the population, with Type II accounting for 85% of cases. Patients with diabetes have a threefold increase in risk for all cardiovascular diseases. Diabetes increases stroke risk in all ages, but particularly for African Americans younger than 55 years of age and Caucasians younger than 65 years (Go et al., 2013). This heightened risk relates to ischemic stroke while hemorrhagic stroke risk is comparable to those without diabetes (Bell, 1994). For those with a history of TIA, impaired glucose tolerance has been associated with twice the risk of stroke compared to those with normal blood glucose (Vermeer et al., 2006). Brain damage may be more severe and extensive if glucose is high at stroke onset because hyperglycemia is associated with increased edema and lesion size as well as decreased CBF (Capes, Hunt, Malmberg, Pathak, & Gerstein, 2001) .

Dyslipidemia

Three major classes of lipoproteins are found in the serum of fasting individuals: low density lipoproteins (LDL), high density lipoproteins (HDL), and very low density lipoproteins (VLDL), which together are referred to as total cholesterol. LDL augments plaque build-up and can raise the risk of ischemic stroke and TIA. HDL may reduce stroke risk. An estimated 100 million adults in the United States have total cholesterol values of 200 mg/dL and higher, and about a third of those have levels of 240 (< 200 is now established as the desirable level) or above. LDL cholesterol levels above 100 mg/dL appear to be atherogenic. The relationship between high cholesterol and neuropsychological function has been widely studied but remains inconsistent, with some studies showing a link between mid-life hypercholesterolemia and later dementia. The mechanisms underlying the relationship between cholesterol and cognitive decline remain to be clarified, though suggested processes include altered cholesterol metabolism in the brain (van den Kommer et al., 2009), increased beta amyloid production (Sparks et al., 1994), or blood-brain barrier compromise (Bjorkhem, Cedazo-Minguez, Leoni, & Meaney, 2009).

Metabolic Syndrome

Metabolic syndrome is defined as the presence of ≥ three of the following factors: (a) abdominal obesity as determined by waist circumference > 102 cm or > 40 inches for men and > 88 cm or > 35 inches for women; (b) triglycerides ≥ 150 mg/dL; (c) HDL cholesterol < 40 mg/dL for men and < 50 mg/dL for women; (d) blood pressure ≥ 130 / ≥ 85 mm Hg; and (e) fasting blood glucose ≥ 110 mg/dL (Goldstein et al., 2006). The World Health Organization modified the definition with the addition of hyperinsulinemia. Obesity, a sedentary lifestyle, and other factors seem to interact to produce the metabolic syndrome. Metabolic syndrome may be an independent risk factor for ischemic stroke beyond the sum of its individual components. For example, in a prospective study of middle-aged subjects who were stroke-free at baseline, metabolic syndrome was present in 39% and a dose-response relationship was observed between the number of metabolic syndrome components and risk of ischemic stroke (Rodriguez-Colon et al., 2009). Elevated blood pressure and elevated fasting glucose were the two components that conveyed the highest risk. However, presence of metabolic syndrome may not be more effective for prediction of stroke than traditional assessments such as the Framingham Risk Score, a well-established algorithm used to estimate the ten-year stroke risk of an individual (Wannamethee, Shaper, Lennon, & Morris, 2005; Wolf, D'Agostino, Belanger, & Kannel, 1991).

Heart Disease

Heart disease and impaired cardiac function are well-known precursors and comorbidities of stroke, including coronary artery disease, congestive heart failure, left ventricular hypertrophy, and atrial fibrillation (AF), which leads to the formation of intraventricular blood clots. AF is associated with nearly half of strokes with a cardiac origin (Force, 1989), and it increases stroke risk across the life span, with a nearly fivefold independent increase in risk. Given that AF is often clinically silent, this risk estimate may be underestimated (Elijovich, Josephson, Fung, & Smith, 2009).

Atherosclerosis

Atherosclerosis, the principal cause of cardiovascular disease in adults, progresses over time and commonly manifests in mid-to-late life as heart attack or stroke. Atherosclerosis is thought to be related to chronic inflammation and subtle injury to artery walls from hypertension and high cholesterol. In response to the injured arterial wall, certain types of white blood cells migrate into the endothelium and are transformed into fat-laded foam cells that build up and form patchy deposits, or *plaques*, that are vulnerable to rupture into the arterial lumen. If a plaque ruptures, it initiates the clotting mechanism, which in turn leads to the formation of a thrombus and acute obstruction of the vessel.

ApoE4

The epsilon4 allele of the apolipoprotein E gene (ApoE) is a risk factor for atherosclerosis, myocardial infarction, stroke, and Alzheimer's disease. ApoE4 polymorphism is linked to the development of small vessel pathology and enhances the extent of neuronal damage from cerebral ischemia. Amyloid beta peptide levels are associated with increased risk for lacunar stroke in carriers of the ApoE4 allele (van Dijk et al., 2004). Hypertensive ApoE4 carriers are at increased risk for the development of subcortical white matter lesions (de Leeuw et al., 2004). The combined presence of ApoE4 and other cerebrovascular risk factors may diminish later-life cognitive performance significantly more than expected from the independent effects of ApoEe4 or cerebrovascular disease alone.

Homocysteine

Homocysteine is a sulfhydryl-containing amino acid derived from dietary methionine. Fasting plasma levels of homocysteine $\geq$ 16 µmol/L indicate hyperhomocysteinemia. The exact mechanism of its atherogenic effect is unknown, but it is thought to contribute to endothelial damage, irregular vascular contraction, and coagulation abnormalities (Christopher, Nagaraja, & Shankar, 2007). Elevated total plasma homocysteine levels are related to several well-established stroke risk factors, including age, male sex, smoking, hypertension, and atherosclerosis. It is also has an independent relationship with stroke incidence. High levels of homocysteine may increase stroke risk from 1.2 to 4.7 odds ratio. Vitamin B supplementation (folic acid, B_{12}, and B_6) lowers serum homocysteine levels and has been associated with a reduction in atherosclerotic plaque progression (Ji et al., 2013).

Inflammatory Biomarkers

C-reactive protein (CRP) is an acute phase-reactant that increases in response to inflammatory stimuli and is a known mediator of adhesion molecule production and thrombogenic factor release. Elevated CRP levels have been associated with both cardiovascular and cerebrovascular events. CRP elevations confer a two- and threefold increase in stroke risk in healthy men and women, respectively. Risk of ischemic stroke is significantly increased at CRP levels of > 4.19 mg/L. Numerous other inflammatory markers are emerging as identifiable factors associated with atherosclerotic plaque instability. For example, the CD40/CD40 ligand system plays a role in the activation of inflammatory mediators. CD40L was significantly elevated in patients with noncardioembolic stroke and remained elevated in both stroke and TIA after three months. Interleukin-18 (IL-18), a cytokine with proatherogenic properties, and monocyte chemotactic protein-1 (MCP-1), are among other proinflammatory markers of interest. The impact on stroke of inflammatory markers such as CRP is not yet clear, and these biomarkers have not yet been recommended for routine clinical use.

Smoking

Cigarette smoking increases heart rate and blood pressure, and decreases arterial distensibility. Individuals who smoke cigarettes have two to four times the risk of stroke compared to nonsmokers, and risk increases with the number of cigarettes smoked per day (Go et al., 2013). Smoking is linked to both ischemic and hemorrhagic stroke. Exposure to environmental tobacco smoke is also a substantial stroke risk factor. Second-hand smoke has been shown to compromise endothelial function in healthy young people in a manner indistinguishable from that of active smokers and has been associated with increased inflammatory markers including CRP protein and homocysteine (Panagiotakos et al., 2004). Fortunately, smoking cessation results in reduced stroke risk across demographic groups: Within five years, stroke risk is no greater than in those who never smoked.

Obstructive Sleep Apnea

Obstructive sleep apnea (OSA) is a treatable form of disordered breathing characterized by the intermittent cessation or reduction of airflow during sleep due to complete or partial upper airway obstruction. OSA prevalence among patients with stroke exceeds 60%, compared with 4% in the middle-aged adult population. OSA is intertwined with many cardiovascular burdens, but is also an independent risk factor for stroke, nearly doubling its risk (Redline et al., 2010). There is also a dose-response effect: Individuals with severe OSA have three to four times increased risk (Yaggi et al., 2005). Proposed mechanisms include acute hemodynamic changes during episodes of OSA, decreased CBF, hypercoagulability, and hypoxia. The main medical therapy for OSA is airway pressurization, which has been shown to reverse hemodynamic changes and even reduce the risk of cardiovascular events.

Obesity

Obesity is associated with an array of atherogenic risk factors, including sleep apnea, hypertension, and diabetes, and it is also an independent stroke risk factor. The pattern of fat deposition appears meaningful. Abdominal deposition of fat has been linked to atherosclerotic disease, but not weight carried in the hips and thighs. Abdominal obesity is defined by a waist circumference > 102 cm (40 in) in men and 88 cm (35 in) in women. It is a stronger risk factor for vascular and metabolic disease than total body obesity, even for individuals who are not overweight, perhaps due to greater metabolic activity in visceral adiposity. Abdominal obesity has implications for cognitive dysfunction, as obesity in midlife has been associated with a threefold increased risk of dementia, independent of diabetes and cardiovascular comorbidities (Whitmer et al., 2008).

Psychiatric Considerations in Cerebrovascular Disease

Depression is the most common psychiatric sequela of stroke. One-third of all stroke survivors develop poststroke depression at some point during recovery. Depression is significantly more likely after stroke than other illnesses with comparable disability and cannot be accounted for by the existence or extent of physical symptoms. Following a stroke, individuals have approximately a sixfold higher risk of developing depression even two or more years after the stroke event, compared to age-matched controls (Whyte, Mulsant, Vanderbilt, Dodge, & Ganguli, 2004). Major depression is particularly common in individuals with left frontal or left basal ganglia lesions. Importantly, poststroke depression can adversely affect recovery and rehabilitation. At two years follow-up, depressed poststroke patients showed less recovery of physical and language functions than comparably treated nondepressed patients (Parikh et al., 1990). Furthermore, patients with poststroke depression show greater cognitive impairment even after controlling for age, education, and lesion size and location (Starkstein, Robinson, & Price, 1988). A number of psychosocial risk factors appear to increase the likelihood of developing poststroke depression. These include premorbid major depression and poststroke social isolation. Other variables—including degree of cognitive impairment, age, and gender—have not been consistently associated with the development of poststroke depression, although the presence of depression may complicate and delay cognitive recovery. Last, risk of death is three times higher over the next decade in depressed stroke survivors compared to survivors without depression, further underscoring the importance of depression screening in this population.

The clinical manifestation of poststroke depression varies, and some symptoms overlap with cognitive sequelae (e.g., anhedonia, loss of initiative). It can also be overlooked in the presence of physical symptoms such as limb paralysis, but as noted, it occurs irrespective of physical disability. Acute symptoms are often characterized by sad or apathetic mood, tearfulness, feelings of guilt, poor appetite and sleep, and pessimism about the future. Effective treatment of poststroke depression can be accomplished using conventional psychopharmacologic and/or psychotherapeutic interventions (Broomfield et al., 2011; Mikami et al., 2013; Robinson et al., 2008).

Anxiety following stroke is also common, but is assessed and reported less frequently than depression. Approximately one-fourth of poststroke patients meet criteria (except for the duration criterion) for generalized anxiety disorder at some point during recovery. As with depression, poststroke anxiety is also associated with poorer or delayed functional recovery, which can persist for years after stroke. Patients with generalized anxiety in the acute poststroke period have also been noted to show a decreased ability to perform activities of daily living (ADLs) when compared to poststroke patients without anxiety (Astrom, 1996).

Less common than depression and anxiety, psychotic symptoms may occur following stroke. Visual hallucinations are most common in poststroke delirium, but may occur later as well. Factors predisposing to hallucinations include lesions of the right temporo-parieto-occipital area, seizures, and subcortical atrophy. Visual hallucinations have also been associated with auditory hallucinations, delusions, and depression, all more common after right-hemisphere lesions.

Pseudobulbar affect, a clinical syndrome involving frequent and easily provoked emotion (typically manifested by involuntary laughing and/or crying unrelated to mood), is seen in approximately 10%–15% of poststroke patients. Poststroke mania occurs in less than 1% of patients, although hypomanic, "euphoric," or indifferent reactions and symptoms are more frequent in patients with right-hemisphere stroke.

Structural, Metabolic, and Functional Neuroimaging

Computed Tomography

CT is widely available, inexpensive, and remains the most commonly used imaging method in the initial evaluation of stroke. CT effectively detects acute bleeds and excludes many other processes such as neoplasm. CT signs of acute stroke include edema, loss of gray–white matter distinction, and blurring of the internal capsule and insular cortex. These changes result from cellular injury due to fluid influx; however, they are often subtle, and up to 60% of CT scans are normal in the first hours after insult (Mehta, 1997). After the acute period, most large vessel infarcts manifest on CT as wedge-shaped areas of attenuation, with increasing mass effect up to a few days after insult. Edema can cause midline shift, effacement of ventricles and sulci, ventriculomegaly, and transtentorial herniation. Later stages of stroke will manifest on CT generally at three to four weeks with shrunken gyri, glial scars, resolved edema, regional or global ventricular dilation, and reabsorption of necrotic tissue.

Magnetic Resonance Imaging

MRI has greater sensitivity and specificity than CT for ischemic lesions. In contrast to CT, more than 80% of magnetic resonance scans are sensitive to acute infarcts within the first 24 hours (Bryan et al., 1991). DWI images are more precise for ischemic damage detection than standard CT or MRI (Easton et al., 2009). MRI with diffusion sequences is now considered superior to noncontrast CT and a preferred diagnostic technique for acute stroke or suspected TIA (Schellinger et al., 2010). DWI may also be useful for predicting late clinical outcome. Early MRI changes in stroke include gray matter swelling and increased signal intensity. With use of contrast agents, early enhancement surrounding the lesion (due to slow flow) and meningeal enhancement (due to irritation of overlying meninges) may be seen. Contrast MRI also helps differentiate strokes of indeterminate age, with subacute lesions showing enhancement that is often ring-like that typically resolves by eight weeks (up to three months) and meningeal enhancement resolving within two to four days. In later stages, enhancement and mass effect tend to abate. Subacute MRI changes become more prominent with time due to edema and mass effect, and enlargement of T2 hyperintensities, though this can also reflect late effects of regional atrophy and/or ventricular dilation. Other MRI-based techniques include DTI, which can depict abnormalities of white matter tracts. Functional MRI (fMRI) allows for analysis of small blood flow changes in response to cognitive challenge tasks. Resting-state fMRI examines spontaneous synchronous activation of various brain regions and circuits. These latter techniques remain largely investigative at this point, but show promise in terms of depicting structural and functional brain changes following stroke. Because it involves a strong magnetic field, MRI is not possible in patients with pacemakers and internal defibrillators.

Cerebral Angiography

Cerebral angiography is the technique to measure intracranial vascular disease (Citron et al., 2003). It involves the insertion of a catheter into an artery in the arm or thigh, which is then threaded through the circulatory system to the carotid artery where a contrast agent is injected. A series of radiographs are taken as the contrast agent spreads through the brain's arterial system, and a second series as it reaches the venous system. Cerebral angiography provides information about collateral flow and perfusion status, determines degree of arterial stenosis, and detects dissection, or lesions such as vascular malformations. Conventional angiography carries a low risk of stroke (0.14%–1%), transient ischemia (0.4%–3%), and clinically silent embolism (up to 25%). The procedure has been made safer and easier with advances in catheter technology, nonionic contrast media, and digital image three-dimensional reconstruction. This technique remains more sensitive than noninvasive methods in cases of suspected large-vessel occlusion though continued advances in noninvasive neuroimaging techniques may eventually replace cerebral angiography. Conventional angiography is also utilized for planning neurosurgical and endovascular interventions.

Magnetic Resonance Angiography

Magnetic resonance angiography (MRA) is a noninvasive technique for assessing vascular flow. MRA sensitivity and specificity for detection and degree of stenosis is 80%–95%, with 5% of exams being nondiagnostic due to patient motion artifact (Mehta, 1997). Contrast-enhanced MRA may be more accurate than standard time-of-flight studies and has replaced the use of catheter angiography in some areas (Phan, Huston, Bernstein, Riederer, & Brown, 2001). An initial screen of the carotid bifurcation is performed with ultrasound, MRA, or CTA, and if the study is abnormal a second noninvasive test or catheter angiography is conducted prior to endarterectomy. Prompt testing in symptomatic persons is critical in order to quickly identify patients with severe disease for whom endarterectomy would be beneficial.

Magnetic Resonance Spectroscopy

Magnetic resonance spectroscopy (MRS) is a complement to MRI as a noninvasive method for chemical tissue characterization. In contrast to MRI, which uses hydrogen protons to form anatomic images, MRS determines the concentration of brain metabolites such as choline, creatine, and lactate. MRS allows for in vivo localized measurements of selected metabolite levels from focal lesions deep within the brain. Its utility in the evaluation of cerebrovascular disease has been limited by long scan times and limited spatial resolution, but faster imaging sequences have been developed. The earliest spectroscopic abnormality in stroke is an increase in lactate (Gujar, Maheshwari, Bjorkman-Burtscher, & Sundgren, 2005).

Positron Emission Tomography

PET is a functional imaging test that measures CBF and local metabolism using a radioactive tracer. The method is based on the assumption that CBF directly reflects neuronal activity. PET scans obtained in acute stroke have been shown to help predict prognosis at two months (Marchal et al., 1993). PET may prove particularly useful in monitoring therapeutic interventions aimed at improving cerebral oxygenation and blood flow in acute stroke, as it is currently the only accurate method for assessing regional CBF and oxygen levels.

Single Photon Emission Computed Tomography

Single photon emission computed tomography (SPECT) utilizes cerebral flood flow measurement, which can be used to detect and characterize remaining viable tissue, and demonstrate reperfusion. SPECT is similar to PET in its use of radioactive tracer material and detection of gamma ray, but uses radioisotopes that are longer-lived and more easily obtainable. It is therefore less expensive, though it offers lower resolution than PET. SPECT scans show the entire low-flow area, including the ischemic core and surrounding penumbra, and unlike CT, occlusive damage is visible on SPECT immediately. Lesions in the cortex are more easily identified by SPECT than are deep lesions. SPECT is inexpensive, repeatable, and typically safe, though there are concerns about exposure to the ionizing radiation. However, SPECT does not assess cerebral metabolism. Other limitations of SPECT include limited image resolution compared to MRI or CT, variable interrater reliability, and the lack of standardized SPECT acquisition/analysis protocols, which make it difficult to compare results from different centers.

Transcranial Doppler Sonography

Transcranial Doppler sonography (TCD) is a noninvasive bedside technique that that uses a pulsed Doppler transducer to measure CBF velocity. It is used to detect gross abnormalities in intracranial cerebral hemodynamics and is relatively quick and inexpensive. TCD can help diagnosis emboli and vasospasm, detect severe stenosis, assess extent of collateral circulation, evaluate suspected brain death, and assist in the diagnosis of AVM. TCD can detect recanalization following thrombolytic therapy and may guide treatment following tPA intervention.

Web Resource

Transcranial Doppler Simulator Educational Software (www.transcranial.com/edu/index.html) introduces the transcranial Doppler investigation technique, includes a tour of the cerebral arteries with a three-dimensional simulation of the ultrasound approaches used in the clinical setting, and includes simulation of compression maneuvers to observe the activation of collateral flow.

Acute Management and Treatment

The primary goals of initial stroke management are to diagnose the likely cause and extent of stroke, quickly initiate treatment, identify other potential contributing factors, and anticipate and prevent potential complications. Immediate focus is on ensuring medical stability, with particular attention to airway, breathing, and circulation, and determining if patients with acute ischemic stroke are candidates for thrombolytic therapy. The importance of immediate assessment of patient eligibility for thrombolytics or other treatment cannot be overstated, given that for each minute in which a large vessel ischemic stroke is untreated, an estimated 1.9 million neurons, 13.8 billion synapses, and seven miles of axonal fibers are lost, and for each hour the brain experiences a neuronal loss equivalent to approximately three years of normal aging (Saver, 2006).

A general overview of an initial stroke work-up is provided in Table 16.7. All patients with a possible TIA or stroke should undergo neuroimaging. Routine blood tests include a complete blood count, chemistry panel, and basic blood coagulation studies (e.g., prothrombin time), and specialized coagulation tests for young, healthy individuals. Cardiac and vascular imaging tests will be ordered based on brain imaging results. Noninvasive tests such as ultrasound or MRA usually precede catheter angiography, which is done when a lesion is suspected but not otherwise evident in prior testing. Cardiac studies, including electrocardiogram and chest x-ray, are a routine part of the workup and useful for detecting a heart or aortic source of embolization or comorbid coronary artery disease. Other key acute management issues that arise

Table 16.7 Initial stroke workup

Laboratory Studies
Hematology: CBC, Platelet Count, Prothrombin Time, Partial Thromboplastin Time
Chemistry: Electrolytes, BUN, Creatinine, Glucose
Toxicology Screen (suspected drug abuse)
Arterial Blood Gas (suspected hypoxia)
Electrocardiogram
Chest x-ray
Neuroimaging/Neurophysiologic Studies
CT, MRI, Transcranial Doppler, SPECT, PET, angiography, EEG
Lumbar Puncture (if CT negative and SAH suspected)

include blood pressure control, swallowing assessment, management of abnormal blood glucose levels, and treatment of fever and infection.

Most strokes are caused by intra-arterial occlusion from clots. Timely restoration of blood flow using thrombolytic therapy is the most effective means of salvaging ischemic brain tissue that is not already infarcted. The efficacy of intravenous tissue plasminogen activator (tPA or alteplase) therapy is well established for reducing neurologic damage in selected patients with acute ischemic stroke. Once it has been determined that the patient has an acute ischemic stroke and hemorrhagic stroke has been ruled out, consideration should be given to the use of thrombolysis. However, eligible patients may be treated with intravenous thrombolysis if neurovascular imaging is not readily available or if obtaining imaging would significantly delay therapy. There is a narrow window during which this can be accomplished, and the sooner tPA is administered, the greater the efficacy (Hacke et al., 2004). The conventional accepted treatment time window for administration of tPA is within 3 to 4.5 hours after clearly defined symptom onset and potentially between 3 and 6 hours. Symptomatic intracranial hemorrhage is the most important complication of thrombolytic therapy. Other interventions for ischemic stroke associated with better outcomes include antithrombotic therapy initiated within 48 hours of stroke onset, prophylaxis for deep venous thrombosis and pulmonary embolism, antithrombotic therapy at discharge, and initiation of lipid-lowering therapy. In addition to thrombolysis, two major classes of antithrombotic drugs—antiplatelet agents and anticoagulants—can be used to treat acute ischemic stroke. In terms of prophylaxis, low-dose aspirin (81 mg) is the most commonly used antiplatelet agent and has proven value as a risk reducer of stroke and stroke mortality.

Acute treatment of hemorrhagic stroke involves a combination of medical and surgical interventions, the latter depending on the site of the bleed. Surgical removal of blood clots is particularly indicated in patients with cerebellar hemorrhages, brain stem compression, and/or hydrocephalus due to ventricular obstruction, typically via posterior fossa decompression. Surgical hematoma evacuation for supratentorial ICH is controversial, and suggested primarily for large bleeds that are near the surface. Other features that increase the likelihood of surgical intervention include clinical deterioration, stuporous arousal, and involvement of the nondominant hemisphere. Open craniotomy is the most common technique for supratentorial ICH; other methods include endoscopic hemorrhage aspiration, use of fibrinolytic therapy to dissolve the clot followed by aspiration, and CT-guided stereotactic aspiration. Ventriculostomy can be used in the setting of ventricular enlargement, particularly of the third and fourth ventricles. Balloon angioplasty may be used in the management of vasospasm after subarachnoid hemorrhage.

Telestroke

There are various important developments in modern technology utilization for stroke management. Although a full review is beyond the scope of this chapter, telemedicine applications to stroke are increasingly commonplace. In fact, the implementation and evaluation of mobile telemedicine systems in emergency medical services has been recommended by the American Heart Association. Only a small fraction (< 1.5% nationally) of acute stroke victims receives thrombolytic intervention and few benefit from the expertise and experience of dedicated stroke units. Telemedicine technology for stroke management, or *telestroke*, has the potential to greatly reduce geographic disparities in stroke care and rapidly link underserved areas to stroke expertise anywhere in the country or across the world.

Telestroke programs are typically employed for emergency department consultation, patient triage, and inpatient consultation. The American Heart Association and American Stroke Association (AHA/ASA) support the use of telemedicine in the acute stroke setting when local stroke expertise is not available. Quality videoconferencing systems are useful for patient evaluation, review of neuroimaging results, and thrombolysis decision making. The utility of telemedicine for remote intravenous tPA treatment decisions before transfer to a stroke unit is a subject of ongoing debate. The use of telemedicine-equipped ambulances has been explored as a means of providing advance patient information and improving time management, referral of patients to specialized hospitals, and identification of patients eligible for thrombolysis (Liman et al., 2012). Data to suggest that telemedicine is cost-effective for acute stroke care are accumulating, particularly given that telestroke costs are short-lived and improved stroke care has lifelong benefits (Nelson, Saltzman, Skalabrin, Demaerschalk, & Majersik, 2011). Important barriers to program growth include lack of program funds, low insurance reimbursement rates, high equipment costs, liability, and credentialing in out-of-state situations. Teleneuropsychology is an emerging area with demonstrated feasibility in areas such as dementia assessment (Cullum, Weiner, Gehrmann, & Hynan, 2006) and clear potential utility for subacute stroke evaluation. Preliminary practical and ethical considerations for neuropsychologists are provided by Grosch, Gottlieb, and Cullum (2011).

Complications

Preventing medical complications is an important aspect of stroke management. These include hypoxemia, metabolic acidosis, and hyperglycemia. Other complications that may develop in the acute or subacute phase of stroke include heart failure, dysphagia, aspiration pneumonia, deep vein thrombosis, pulmonary embolism, and urinary tract infection. Common complications are discussed in detail in this section.

Edema and Increased Intracranial Pressure

Life-threatening complications of edema and ICP may occur in as many as 10% of all strokes. Large supratentorial infarcts are particularly associated with edema. Early clinical signs include decreased level of consciousness, asymmetric pupils, and changes in breathing pattern. Edema associated with infratentorial stroke, particularly cerebellar hemorrhage, can result in hydrocephalus, brain stem compression, and death. Mortality rates rise to more than 50% once there is elevated ICP and significant mass effect. Surgical interventions to improve the chance of survival include infarct resection or hemicraniectomy. Resection of edematous tissue typically employs temporal and frontal lobectomies of the right hemisphere. In hemicraniectomy, a large bone flap is removed and the dura is opened to allow the brain to expand, with a cranioplasty performed at a later date.

Vasospasm

Clinically significant vasospasm occurs in approximately 20%–30% of patients with aneurysmal SAH, and is the leading cause of death and disability after aneurysm rupture. Vasospasm may occur because nearby vessels are irritated by the blood from the ruptured aneurysm, which generates spasmogenic substances during the lysis (breakdown) of the clots. It typically presents around day five after hemorrhage and peaks at days seven to eight. Vasospasm manifests with a decline in neurologic status including the onset of focal neurologic abnormalities. Vasospasm can sometimes be visualized on MRI or MRA, though treatment can be difficult.

Hydrocephalus

Hydrocephalus (i.e., expansion of the cerebral ventricles) is a common complication of SAH, occurring in up to 20% of cases. Ventricular drainage via shunt placement is considered for patients who develop hydrocephalus and experience a deteriorating level of consciousness and for those in whom no improvement in hydrocephalus occurs within 24 hours. Delayed enlargement of the ventricles can also occur.

Hemorrhagic Conversion and Cerebral Hyperperfusion Syndrome

Hemorrhagic conversion or transformation (secondary bleeding) is a potential complication of ischemic infarction that occurs in approximately 10% of cases and is usually asymptomatic. The current classification of hemorrhagic transformation encompasses a broad spectrum of secondary bleeding, ranging from small areas of petechial hemorrhage to large space-occupying hematomas. The former often appear as patchy areas of bleeding with indistinct margins within the vascular territory of the infarction, representing movement of blood cells through capillaries without frank vessel rupture. Parenchymal hematomas are discrete, dense collections of blood that may exert mass effects associated with rupture of an ischemic vessel that has been subject to reperfusion pressures. This hemorrhagic conversion is also known as *cerebral hyperperfusion syndrome.* Though relatively uncommon, this is a well-described complication of revascularization surgery. Revascularization restores blood flow to a normal or elevated pressure in the area that was previously hypoperfused with compensatory dilation of cerebral vessels. These vessels are unable to vasoconstrict quickly, causing breakthrough perfusion pressure. Cerebral hyperperfusion syndrome may manifest with headache, seizures, reversible focal neurologic deficits, cerebral edema, and rarely intracerebral hemorrhage.

Seizures

Seizures are a relatively common complication of hemorrhagic stroke, occurring in 4%–29% of patients with acute spontaneous ICH and more commonly in lobar bleeds than in deep hemorrhage. Antiepileptic drugs (AEDs) are usually continued for approximately six months in patients who experience an acute seizure (i.e., within seven days) following SAH, although there are no strict guidelines. The most commonly used agents include phenytoin and carbamazepine. The use of AEDs to prevent seizures in patients with SAH has been widely debated (Naval, Stevens, Mirski, & Bhardwaj, 2006). Many experts favor seizure prophylaxis in the setting of an unsecured aneurysm because of the relatively low risk of AEDs compared to the potential damage from seizures in a compromised brain. However, AED exposure may be associated with worse neurologic and cognitive outcome after SAH, and current guidelines indicate that AEDs for seizure prophylaxis after SAH should be minimized. The incidence of late epilepsy (more than two weeks after surgery) is unclear. In a retrospective report of 472 patients with aneurysmal SAH who underwent surgical clipping and were followed for at least 12 months, late epilepsy occurred in only 5% (Buczacki, Kirkpatrick, Seeley, & Hutchinson, 2004).

Cognitive Impairment

Cognitive impairment is a very common outcome of stroke that often is unrecognized or underappreciated by clinicians and patients. In contrast to the routine inclusion of screening measures of quality of life, large randomized stroke-treatment trials traditionally have unfortunately failed to include neuropsychological measures of stroke morbidity. A systematic review of 51 randomized studies of acute stroke drug intervention studies involving more than 50,000 participants (Duncan, Jorgensen, & Wade., 2000) found only two that measured cognitive deficit—both using the MMSE, which is insensitive to many cognitive deficits and provides only cursory insight into cognitive status. Furthermore, only one study reviewed used a brief neuropsychological battery that included measures of aphasia, perceptual discrimination, sustained concentration, and processing speed (Duncan et al., 2000). A more recent review of 190 acute stroke treatment trials found similarly poor examination of neuropsychological outcomes, with only three studies incorporating specific measures of cognitive function, specifically the Trail Making Test, Boston Naming Test, Visual Form Discrimination Test, and Line Cancellation Test (Anderson, Arciniegas, & Filley, 2005). The MoCA, another global cognitive screening tool that is slightly more sensitive than the MMSE in some populations, was included as a three-month outcome measure in a multicenter trial of earlier and more frequent mobilization after stroke, and preliminary results indicated the feasibility of the MoCA in stroke trials as a complement to existing efficacy outcomes (Cumming, Bernhardt, & Linden, 2011). Future studies of stroke treatment and outcome should address the dearth of more sensitive and detailed neuropsychological outcome data.

Rehabilitation

Stroke is a leading cause of disability in the United States (Centers for Disease and Prevention, 2009). Among Medicare patients with stroke, 45% are discharged home (32% of these utilize home health care services), 24% enter inpatient rehabilitation facilities, and 31% go to skilled nursing facilities (Buntin, Colla, Deb, Sood, & Escarce, 2010). In the Framingham Heart Study, the following disabilities were observed after six months in ischemic stroke survivors over age 65: 50% had some hemiparesis, 46% had cognitive deficits, 35% had depressive symptoms, 19% had aphasia, and 26% were institutionalized (Kelly Hayes et al., 2003).

Neurologic recovery is most rapid during the first three months and tends to plateau around 6–12 months poststroke, though continued improvements can continue over the coming months and even years following stroke. Stroke rehabilitation efforts should begin immediately. The overall goal of stroke rehabilitation is to help patients regain and relearn the skills of everyday living, adapt to new limitations, prevent secondary complications, and educate the patient and family members in appropriate supports. Rehabilitation programs are generally directed toward improving motor function, speech, and performance of daily activities. A rehabilitation team is typically multidisciplinary and often includes physiatrists, neuropsychologists, speech and language therapists, physical therapists, occupational therapists, and social workers. Interventions may include physical therapy to address strength and ambulation, occupational therapy to increase functional independence, speech therapy to improve dysphasia and dysphagia, and group or individual psychotherapy to combat discouragement, manage mood symptoms, and help patients to develop realistic expectations. As noted earlier, it is particularly important to identify mood disorders, as they can complicate and protract cognitive and functional recovery. Although large-scale studies are limited, cognitive rehabilitation programs have shown efficacy in enhancing neurobehavioral function and quality of life (Cumming, Marshall, & Lazar, 2013).

Cerebral plasticity, important in the developing nervous system, persists to some degree throughout life and is a fundamental factor in stroke recovery. Neuroimaging studies in stroke patients indicate altered poststroke activation patterns, which suggest some functional reorganization. Many of these changes may be explained by the well-established compensatory process known as *functional reorganization* or *functional adaptation;* however, modern views acknowledge that recovery of function may also be accounted for by partial restitution of the impaired neuropsychological processes themselves via experience-dependent brain plasticity (Robertson & Murre, 1999; Rossini et al., 2007). Enhanced understanding of brain plasticity will likely improve stroke rehabilitation efforts, particularly as targeted therapies are developed.

Innovative Technologies

Although specific technologies are beyond the scope of this chapter, we want to mention several technologic innovations that have implications for stroke rehabilitation. The use of virtual reality and video games is being explored as a means of promoting exercise, social interaction, and rehabilitation (Laver, George, Thomas, Deutsch, & Crotty, 2015). This type of therapy uses computer-based programs designed to simulate real-life objects and events and may be more motivating for patients (see Figure 16.18). Transcranial magnetic stimulation (TMS) and transcranial direct-current stimulation are noninvasive methods that can improve motor and language function (Naeser et al., 2012). TMS instruments consist of a high-voltage capacitor that can be discharged through an insulated coil of wires and the magnetic field passes through the skull and induces an electrical current in brain tissue. In healthy individuals, TMS can produce a contralateral evoked response in the muscle and a movement when the coil is placed on the scalp over the motor cortex. Such stimulation over the damaged motor cortex may be used

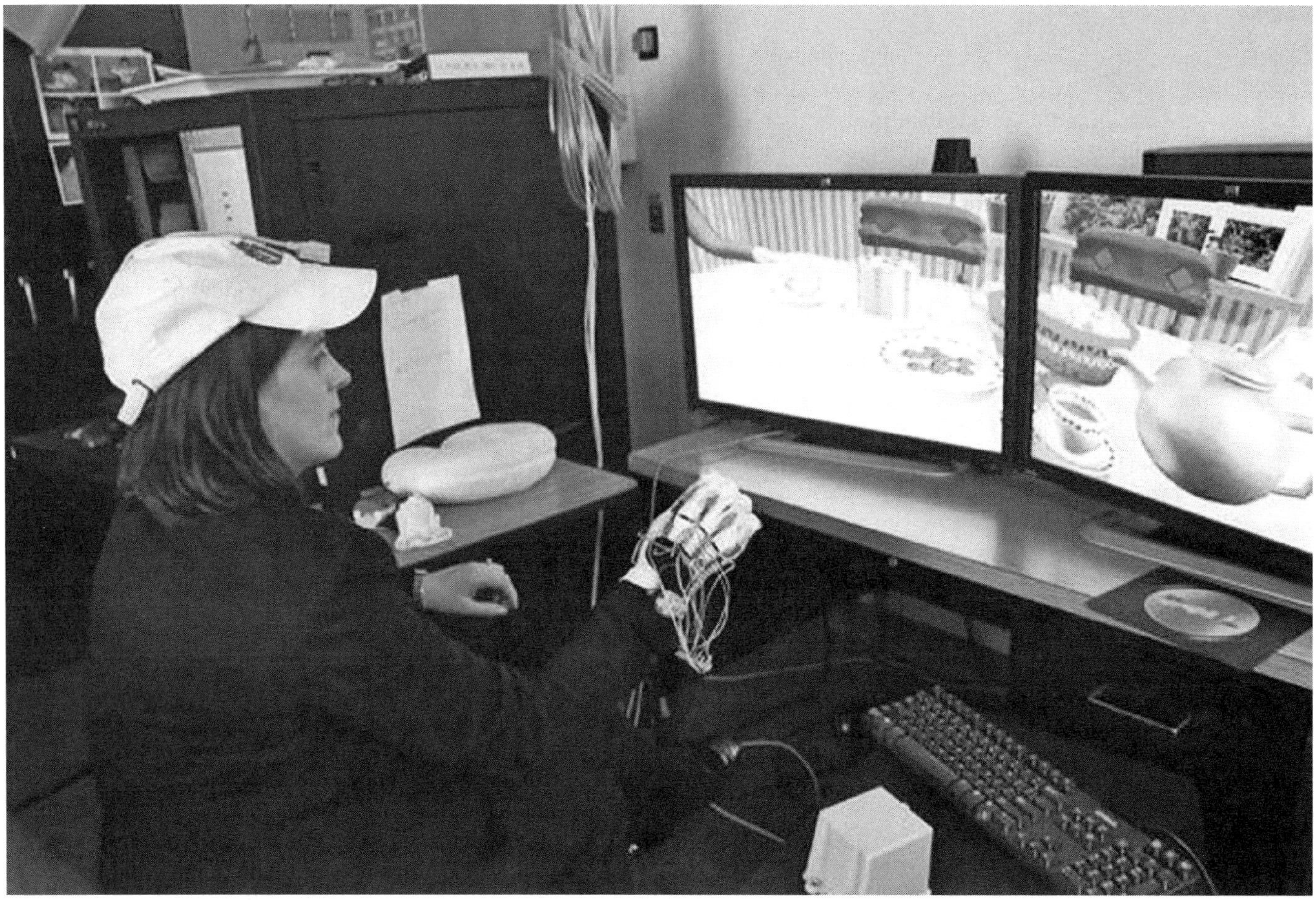

Figure 16.18 Virtual reality (VR) system assisting poststroke hand rehabilitation. The user wears a custom pneumatic glove, which assists finger extension. Magnetic trackers provide information regarding head orientation and hand location; the virtual scene is updated accordingly. Reproduced with permission from D. Tsoupikova, Electronic Visualization Laboratory. *A color version of this figure can be found in Plate section 2.*

to increase poststroke motor-evoked potentials with associated functional improvements (Dimyan & Cohen, 2010). Brainwave technology known as brain–computer interfaces (BCI) and brain–machine interfaces (BMI) stimulate cortical activity at the level of neuronal action potentials and may facilitate recovery by normalizing neurophysiologic activity (Wang et al., 2010). These brain training devices facilitate motor relearning to help patients control external devices (such as a computer cursor or arm prosthesis) and move paretic limbs (Meng et al., 2009). Other promising noninvasive rehabilitation methods include robotic therapies, such as robot-assisted physical therapy with robotic manipulation of impaired limbs. Home telerehabilitation programs will also likely play an important future role in stroke treatment (Chumbler et al., 2012; McCue, Fairman, & Pramuka, 2010).

Prevention

Secondary stroke prevention interventions include anticoagulants, platelet inhibitors, carotid endarterectomy, and stenting. Carotid endarterectomy, the removal of plaque to correct stenosis, is the most frequently performed surgical procedure to prevent stroke, with about 100,000 inpatient procedures performed in the United States in 2010 (Go et al., 2013). Carotid artery stenting is a relatively newer and less-invasive procedure that involves threading a stent and expanding a small protective device in the artery to widen the blocked area and capture any dislodged plaque. A large randomized stroke prevention trial over nine years found that safety and effectiveness between carotid endarterectomy and carotid stenting were generally equal, with stenting being slightly better in younger patients (Timaran et al., 2013).

Advances in acute stroke therapy will continue; however, primary prevention will remain the most important and effective strategy for reducing mortality and morbidity from stroke. Primary prevention includes both education and management of risk profiles. In 2009, 51% of a sample of approximately 20,000 individuals was aware of five stroke warning symptoms and would call 911 if they thought someone was having a stroke. This awareness was higher among Caucasians, women, and individuals with higher education (Go et al., 2013). In a study of individuals with a history of stroke, only 55% were able to identify one stroke symptom. The median time from symptom onset to emergency room admission was 16 hours, and only 32% entered an emergency room in less than two hours (Zerwic, Hwang, & Tucco, 2007). In a UK study of TIA, approximately 70% of patients did not correctly recognize their TIA or minor stroke; 30% delayed seeking medical attention for > 24 hours, regardless of age, sex, social class, or educational level; and approximately 30% of early recurrent strokes occurred prior to receiving medical attention (Chandratheva, Lasserson, Geraghty, & Rothwell, 2010). It is helpful for the public to develop heart-healthy habits and estimate stroke risk. Risk-assessment tools can be used to identify persons at elevated risk and to guide appropriate use of further diagnostic testing. Public awareness campaigns with phrases such as "F.A.S.T." (face, arms, speech, and time) and "Time Is Brain" seek to emphasize that brain tissue is rapidly lost as a stroke progresses and that rapid treatment is urgently needed.

Most strokes are the outcome of pathologic processes, such as atherosclerosis, that are typically set into motion many years prior and are preceded by a number of risk factors that are common across all stroke types. Preventive care should include reduction of individual risk factors, such as the components of the metabolic syndrome. Preventive care for vascular risk reduction should include lifestyle modification (diet, exercise, smoking cessation, and avoiding weight gain). Regular physical activity has well-established benefits for reducing the risk of premature death and cardiovascular disease (Nelson et al., 2007; Sattelmair et al., 2011). At least 30 minutes of moderate intensity exercise, defined as vigorous activity sufficient to break a sweat or noticeably raise the heart rate (e.g., walking briskly, riding a bicycle or exercise bicycle) one to three times a week may significantly reduce risk factors and comorbid conditions associated with an increased likelihood of recurrent stroke. There are no data to confirm that weight reduction directly reduces the risk of recurrent stroke for overweight persons; however, weight loss is beneficial for improved control of other important parameters, including blood pressure, glucose, and lipid levels. Current guidelines for stroke prevention include intake of folic acid (400 μg/d), B_6 (1.7 mg/d), and B_{12} (2.4 μg/d) either by supplementation or by dietary means (Furie et al., 2011).

> **Web Resource**
>
> For examples of patient educational tools, please refer to the National Stroke Association's website (www.stroke.org/site/DocServer/Scorecard.Q._08.pdf?docID=601).

Conclusion

Cerebrovascular disease represents an array of related disorders and pathophysiologic processes that often result in neuropsychological and functional morbidities. The focal lesion model provided by patients with strokes and related disorders helped propel the field of neuropsychological assessment forward. These patients can sometimes be extremely challenging to evaluate because of deficits, such as aphasia, which can confound the accurate characterization of other neuropsychological deficits. Although stroke research often includes only brief indices of global cognitive function, there is growing recognition of the importance of neuropsychological outcomes in clinical trials, patient recovery, and quality of life in patients with cerebrovascular disorders. Because significant cognitive and mood disorders may go undetected or underappreciated in standard clinical settings, there is a need for routine and efficient neuropsychological assessment procedures in such populations in clinical and research settings. Furthermore, the residual neuropsychological sequelae of cerebrovascular disease can vary greatly by individual, and as such, there is more to be learned about clinical phenotypes and multimodal prediction models of outcome that incorporate neuropsychologic, neuroimaging, clinical, and biomarker measurement techniques.

Acknowledgements

We are grateful to Myron Weiner, M.D. who kindly contributed his medical expertise and editorial guidance.

References

Albers, G. W., Caplan, L. R., Easton, J. D., Fayad, P. B., Mohr, J. P., Saver, J. L., & Sherman, D. G. (2002). Transient ischemic attack: Proposal for a new definition. *New England Journal of Medicine*, *347*(21), 1713–1716. doi: 10.1056/NEJMsb020987, 347/21/1713 [pii]

Al-Shahi, R., & Warlow, C. (2001). A systematic review of the frequency and prognosis of arteriovenous malformations of the brain in adults. *Brain*, *124*(Pt 10), 1900–1926.

Anderson, C., Arciniegas, D., & Filley, C. (2005). Treatment of acute ischemic stroke: Does it impact neuropsychiatric outcome? *The Journal of Neuropsychiatry and Clinical Neurosciences*, *17*(4), 486–488. doi: 10.1176/appi.neuropsych.17.4.486

APA. (2013). *Diagnostic and Statistical Manual of Mental Disorders* (5th ed.). Arlington, VA: American Psychiatric Publishing.

Ardila, A. (2010). A proposed reinterpretation and reclassification of aphasic syndromes. *Aphasiology*, *24*(3), 363–394.

Arvanitakis, Z., Leurgans, S. E., Wang, Z., Wilson, R. S., Bennett, D. A., & Schneider, J. A. (2011). Cerebral amyloid angiopathy pathology and cognitive domains in older persons. *Annals of Neurology*, *69*(2), 320–327. doi: 10.1002/ana.22112

Astrom, M. (1996). Generalized anxiety disorder in stroke patients: A 3-year longitudinal study. *Stroke*, *27*(2), 270–275.

Auriel, E., & Greenberg, S. M. (2012). The pathophysiology and clinical presentation of cerebral amyloid angiopathy. *Current Atherosclerosis Reports*, *14*(4), 343–350. doi: 10.1007/s11883-012-0254-z

Baik, J. S., & Lee, M. S. (2010). Movement disorders associated with moyamoya disease: A report of 4 new cases and a review of literatures. *Movement Disorders*, *25*(10), 1482–1486. doi: 10.1002/mds.23130

Balestrini, S., Perozzi, C., Altamura, C., Vernieri, F., Luzzi, S., Bartolini, M., . . . Silvestrini, M. (2013). Severe carotid stenosis and impaired cerebral hemodynamics can influence cognitive deterioration. *Neurology*, *80*(23), 2145–2150. doi: 10.1212/WNL.0b013e318295d71a

Bell, D. S. (1994). Stroke in the diabetic patient. *Diabetes Care*, *17*(3), 213–219.

Benson, D. F., & Ardila, A. (1996). *Aphasia: A Clinical Perspective* (1st ed.). Oxford: Oxford University Press.

Berman, M. F., Solomon, R. A., Mayer, S. A., Johnston, S. C., & Yung, P. P. (2003). Impact of hospital-related factors on outcome after treatment of cerebral aneurysms. *Stroke*, *34*(9), 2200–2207. doi: 10.1161/01.STR.0000086528.32334.06

Bjorkhem, I., Cedazo-Minguez, A., Leoni, V., & Meaney, S. (2009). Oxysterols and neurodegenerative diseases. *Molecular Aspects of Medicine*, *30*(3), 171–179. doi: 10.1016/j.mam.2009.02.001

Blonder, L. X., Hodes, J. E., Ranseen, J. D., & Schmitt, F. A. (1999). Short-term neuropsychological outcome following Gamma Knife radiosurgery for arteriovenous malformations: A preliminary report. *Applied Neuropsychology*, *6*(3), 181–186. doi: 10.1207/s15324826an0603_7

Blumenfeld, H. (2010). *Neuroanatomy Through Clinical Cases* (2nd ed.). Sunderland, MA: Sinauer Associates.

Breteler, M. M. (2000). Vascular involvement in cognitive decline and dementia: Epidemiologic evidence from the Rotterdam Study and the Rotterdam Scan Study. *Annals of the New York Academy of Sciences*, *903*, 457–465.

Britton, M., Carlsson, A., & de Faire, U. (1986). Blood pressure course in patients with acute stroke and matched controls. *Stroke*, *17*(5), 861–864.

Broomfield, N. M., Laidlaw, K., Hickabottom, E., Murray, M. F., Pendrey, R., Whittick, J. E., & Gillespie, D. C. (2011). Post-stroke depression: The case for augmented, individually tailored cognitive behavioural therapy. *Clinical Psychology & Psychotherapy*, *18*(3), 202–217. doi: 10.1002/cpp.711

Bryan, R. N., Levy, L. M., Whitlow, W. D., Killian, J. M., Preziosi, T. J., & Rosario, J. A. (1991). Diagnosis of acute cerebral infarction: Comparison of CT and MR imaging. *American Journal of Neuroradiology*, *12*(4), 611–620.

Buczacki, S. J., Kirkpatrick, P. J., Seeley, H. M., & Hutchinson, P. J. (2004). Late epilepsy following open surgery for aneurysmal subarachnoid haemorrhage. *The Journal of Neurology, Neurosurgery, and Psychiatry*, *75*(11), 1620–1622. doi: 10.1136/jnnp.2003.026856

Buffon, F., Porcher, R., Hernandez, K., Kurtz, A., Pointeau, S., Vahedi, K., . . . Chabriat, H. (2006). Cognitive profile in CADASIL. *The Journal of Neurology, Neurosurgery, and Psychiatry*, *77*(2), 175–180. doi: 10.1136/jnnp.2005.068726, 77/2/175 [pii]

Buntin, M. B., Colla, C. H., Deb, P., Sood, N., & Escarce, J. J. (2010). Medicare spending and outcomes after postacute care for stroke and hip fracture. *Medical Care*, *48*(9), 776–784. doi: 10.1097/MLR.0b013e3181e359df

Capes, S. E., Hunt, D., Malmberg, K., Pathak, P., & Gerstein, H. C. (2001). Stress hyperglycemia and prognosis of stroke in nondiabetic and diabetic patients: A systematic overview. *Stroke*, *32*(10), 2426–2432.

Caplan, L. R. (1993). Brain embolism, revisited. *Neurology*, *43*(7), 1281–1287.

Carandang, R., Seshadri, S., Beiser, A., Kelly-Hayes, M., Kase, C. S., Kannel, W. B., & Wolf, P. A. (2006). Trends in incidence, lifetime risk, severity, and 30-day mortality of stroke over the past 50 years. *JAMA*, *296*(24), 2939–2946. doi: 10.1001/jama.296.24.2939, 296/24/2939 [pii]

Centers for Disease Control & Prevention. (2009). Prevalence and most common causes of disability among adults: United States, 2005. *Morbidity and Mortality Weekly Report*, *58*(16), 421–426.

Chabriat, H., Joutel, A., Dichgans, M., Tournier-Lasserve, E., & Bousser, M. G. (2009). Cadasil. *The Lancet Neurology*, *8*(7), 643–653. doi: 10.1016/S1474-4422(09)70127-9 [pii]

Chandratheva, A., Lasserson, D. S., Geraghty, O. C., & Rothwell, P. M. (2010). Population-based study of behavior immediately after transient ischemic attack and minor stroke in 1000 consecutive patients: Lessons for public education. *Stroke*, *41*(6), 1108–1114. doi: 10.1161/STROKEAHA.109.576611 [pii]

Charidimou, A., Gang, Q., & Werring, D. J. (2012). Sporadic cerebral amyloid angiopathy revisited: Recent insights into pathophysiology and clinical spectrum. *The Journal of Neurology, Neurosurgery, and Psychiatry*, *83*(2), 124–137. doi: 10.1136/jnnp-2011-301308

Christopher, R., Nagaraja, D., & Shankar, S. K. (2007). Homocysteine and cerebral stroke in developing countries. *Current Medicinal Chemistry*, *14*(22), 2393–2401.

Chui, H. C., Victoroff, J. I., Margolin, D., Jagust, W., Shankle, R., & Katzman, R. (1992). Criteria for the diagnosis of ischemic vascular dementia proposed by the State of California Alzheimer's Disease Diagnostic and Treatment Centers. *Neurology*, *42*(3 Pt 1), 473–480.

Chui, H. C., Zarow, C., Mack, W. J., Ellis, W. G., Zheng, L., Jagust, W. J., . . . Vinters, H. V. (2006). Cognitive impact of subcortical vascular and Alzheimer's disease pathology. *Annals of Neurology*, *60*(6), 677–687. doi: 10.1002/ana.21009

Chumbler, N. R., Quigley, P., Li, X., Morey, M., Rose, D., Sanford, J., . . . Hoenig, H. (2012). Effects of telerehabilitation on physical function and disability for stroke patients: A randomized, controlled trial. *Stroke*, *43*(8), 2168–2174. doi: 10.1161/STROKEAHA.111.646943

Chung, K. K., Anderson, N. E., Hutchinson, D., Synek, B., & Barber, P. A. (2011). Cerebral amyloid angiopathy related inflammation: Three case reports and a review. *The Journal of Neurology, Neurosurgery, and Psychiatry*, *82*(1), 20–26. doi: 10.1136/jnnp.2009.204180

Citron, S. J., Wallace, R. C., Lewis, C. A., Dawson, R. C., Dion, J. E., Fox, A. J., . . . American Society of Neuroradiology. (2003). Quality improvement guidelines for adult diagnostic neuroangiography: Cooperative study between ASITN, ASNR, and SIR. *Journal of Vascular and Interventional Radiology*, *14*(9 Pt 2), S257–S262.

Cullum, C. M., Weiner, M. F., Gehrmann, H. R., & Hynan, L. S. (2006). Feasibility of telecognitive assessment in dementia. *Assessment*, *13*(4), 385–390. doi: 10.1177/1073191106289065

Cumming, T. B., Bernhardt, J., & Linden, T. (2011). The montreal cognitive assessment: Short cognitive evaluation in a large stroke trial. *Stroke*, *42*(9), 2642–2644. doi: 10.1161/STROKEAHA.111.619486

Cumming, T. B., Marshall, R. S., & Lazar, R. M. (2013). Stroke, cognitive deficits, and rehabilitation: Still an incomplete picture. *International Journal of Stroke*, *8*(1), 38–45. doi: 10.1111/j.1747-4949.2012.00972.x

de la Torre, J. C. (2002). Alzheimer disease as a vascular disorder: Nosological evidence. *Stroke*, *33*(4), 1152–1162.

de Leeuw, F. E., Richard, F., de Groot, J. C., van Duijn, C. M., Hofman, A., Van Gijn, J., & Breteler, M. M. (2004). Interaction between hypertension, apoE, and cerebral white matter lesions. *Stroke, 35*(5), 1057–1060. doi:10.1161/01.STR.0000125859.71051.83

DeLuca, J., & Diamond, B. J. (1995). Aneurysm of the anterior communicating artery: A review of neuroanatomical and neuropsychological sequelae. *Journal of Clinical and Experimental Neuropsychology*, *17*(1), 100–121. doi: 10.1080/13803399508406586

Dimyan, M. A., & Cohen, L. G. (2010). Contribution of transcranial magnetic stimulation to the understanding of functional recovery mechanisms after stroke. *Neurorehabilitation and Neural Repair*, *24*(2), 125–135. doi: 10.1177/1545968309345270

Dong, Y., Hassan, A., Zhang, Z., Huber, D., Dalageorgou, C., & Markus, H. S. (2003). Yield of screening for CADASIL mutations in lacunar stroke and leukoaraiosis. *Stroke*, *34*(1), 203–205.

Duan, L., Bao, X. Y., Yang, W. Z., Shi, W. C., Li, D. S., Zhang, Z. S., . . . Feng, J. (2012). Moyamoya disease in China: Its clinical features and outcomes. *Stroke*, *43*(1), 56–60. doi: 10.1161/STROKEAHA.111.621300

Duncan, P. W., Jorgensen, H. S., & Wade, D. T. (2000). Outcome measures in acute stroke trials: A systematic review and some recommendations to improve practice. *Stroke*, *31*(6), 1429–1438.

Easton, J. D., Saver, J. L., Albers, G. W., Alberts, M. J., Chaturvedi, S., Feldmann, E., . . . Sacco, R. L. (2009). Definition and evaluation of transient ischemic attack: A scientific statement for healthcare professionals from the American Heart Association and American Stroke Association Stroke Council; Council on Cardiovascular Surgery and Anesthesia; Council on Cardiovascular Radiology and Intervention; Council on Cardiovascular Nursing; and the Interdisciplinary Council on Peripheral Vascular Disease. The American Academy of Neurology affirms the value of this statement as an educational tool for neurologists. *Stroke*, *40*(6), 2276–2293. doi: 10.1161/STROKEAHA.108.192218 [pii]

Edlow, J. A., Kim, S., Pelletier, A. J., & Camargo, C. A., Jr. (2006). National study on emergency department visits for transient ischemic attack, 1992–2001. *Academic Emergency Medicine*, *13*(6), 666–672. doi: 10.1197/j.aem.2006.01.014 [pii]

Elijovich, L., Josephson, S. A., Fung, G. L., & Smith, W. S. (2009). Intermittent atrial fibrillation may account for a large proportion of otherwise cryptogenic stroke: A study of 30-day cardiac event monitors. *Journal of Stroke and Cerebrovascular Diseases*, *18*(3), 185–189. doi: 10.1016/j.jstrokecerebrovasdis.2008.09.005

Faraco, G., & Iadecola, C. (2013). Hypertension: A harbinger of stroke and dementia. *Hypertension*, *62*(5), 810–817. doi: 10.1161/HYPERTENSIONAHA.113.01063

Ferrero, E., Ferri, M., Viazzo, A., Labate, C., Berardi, G., Pecchio, A., . . . Nessi, F. (2014). A retrospective study on early carotid endarterectomy within 48 hours after transient ischemic attack and stroke in evolution. *Annals of Vascular Surgery*, *28*(1), 227–238. doi: 10.1016/j.avsg.2013.02.015

Festa, J. R., Schwarz, L. R., Pliskin, N., Cullum, C. M., Lacritz, L., Charbel, F. T., . . . Lazar, R. M. (2010). Neurocognitive dysfunction in adult moyamoya disease. *Journal of Neurology*, *257*(5), 806–815. doi: 10.1007/s00415-009-5424-8

Force, C.E.T. (1989). Cardiogenic brain embolism: The second report of the Cerebral Embolism Task Force. *Archives of Neurology*, *46*(7), 727–743.

Fridriksson, S., Saveland, H., Jakobsson, K. E., Edner, G., Zygmunt, S., Brandt, L., & Hillman, J. (2002). Intraoperative complications in aneurysm surgery: A prospective national study. *Journal of Neurosurgery*, *96*(3), 515–522. doi: 10.3171/jns.2002.96.3.0515

Fung, L. W., Thompson, D., & Ganesan, V. (2005). Revascularisation surgery for paediatric moyamoya: A review of the literature. *Child's Nervous System*, *21*(5), 358–364. doi: 10.1007/s00381-004-1118-9

Furie, K. L., Kasner, S. E., Adams, R. J., Albers, G. W., Bush, R. L., Fagan, S. C., . . . Outcomes, R. (2011). Guidelines for the prevention of stroke in patients with stroke or transient ischemic attack: A guideline for healthcare professionals from the American Heart Association and American Stroke Association. *Stroke*, *42*(1), 227–276. doi: 10.1161/STR.0b013e3181f7d043

Garcia, J. H., & Ho, K. L. (1992). Pathology of hypertensive arteriopathy. *Neurosurgery Clinics of North America*, *3*(3), 497–507.

Gieteling, E. W., & Rinkel, G. J. (2003). Characteristics of intracranial aneurysms and subarachnoid haemorrhage in patients with polycystic kidney disease. *Journal of Neurology*, *250*(4), 418–423. doi: 10.1007/s00415-003-0997-0

Go, A. S., Mozaffarian, D., Roger, V. L., Benjamin, E. J., Berry, J. D., Borden, W. B., . . . Turner, M. B. (2013). Heart disease and stroke statistics: 2013 update: A report from the American Heart Association. *Circulation*, *127*(1), e6–e245. doi: 10.1161/CIR.0b013e31828124ad [pii]

Goldstein, L. B., Adams, R., Alberts, M. J., Appel, L. J., Brass, L. M., Bushnell, C. D., . . . American Academy of Neurology. (2006). Primary prevention of ischemic stroke: A guideline from the American Heart Association and American Stroke Association Stroke Council: Cosponsored by the Atherosclerotic Peripheral Vascular Disease Interdisciplinary Working Group; Cardiovascular Nursing Council; Clinical Cardiology Council; Nutrition, Physical Activity, and Metabolism Council; and the Quality of Care and Outcomes Research Interdisciplinary Working Group: The American Academy of Neurology affirms the value of this guideline. *Stroke*, *37*(6), 1583–1633. doi: 10.1161/01.STR.0000223048.70103.F1

Gorelick, P. B., Scuteri, A., Black, S. E., Decarli, C., Greenberg, S. M., Iadecola, C., . . . Anesthesia. (2011). Vascular contributions to cognitive impairment and dementia: A statement for healthcare professionals from the American Heart Association/American Stroke Association. *Stroke*, *42*(9), 2672–2713. doi: 10.1161/STR.0b013e3182299496

Greenberg, S. M., & Vonsattel, J. P. (1997). Diagnosis of cerebral amyloid angiopathy. Sensitivity and specificity of cortical biopsy. *Stroke*, *28*(7), 1418–1422.

Grosch, M. C., Gottlieb, M. C., & Cullum, C. M. (2011). Initial practice recommendations for teleneuropsychology. *The Clinical Neuropsychologist*, *25*(7), 1119–1133. doi: 10.1080/13854046.2011.609840

Gujar, S. K., Maheshwari, S., Bjorkman-Burtscher, I., & Sundgren, P. C. (2005). Magnetic resonance spectroscopy. *Journal of Neuro-Ophthalmology*, *25*(3), 217–226.

Guo, J., Wang, S., Li, R., Chen, N., Zhou, M., Chen, H., . . . He, L. (2014). Cognitive impairment and whole brain diffusion in patients with carotid artery disease and ipsilateral transient ischemic attack. *Neurological Research*, *36*(1), 41–46. doi: 10.1179/1743132813Y.0000000255

Gupta, S. K., Chhabra, R., Mohindra, S., Sharma, A., Mathuriya, S. N., Pathak, A., . . . Khosla, V. K. (2014). Long-term outcome in surviving patients after clipping of intracranial aneurysms. *World Neurosurgery, 81*(2), 316–321. doi:10.1016/j.wneu.2013.01.034

Haaland, K. Y., & Yeates, K. O. (2014). *Table 25.2: Neuropsychology Study Guide and Board Review*. New York: Oxford University Press.

Hachinski, V., Iadecola, C., Petersen, R. C., Breteler, M. M., Nyenhuis, D. L., Black, S. E., . . . Leblanc, G. G. (2006). National Institute of Neurological Disorders and Stroke-Canadian Stroke Network vascular cognitive impairment harmonization standards. *Stroke, 37*(9), 2220–2241. doi: 10.1161/01.STR.0000237236.88823.47 [pii]

Hacke, W., Donnan, G., Fieschi, C., Kaste, M., von Kummer, R., Broderick, J. P., . . . Investigators, N. r.-P.S.G. (2004). Association of outcome with early stroke treatment: pooled analysis of ATLANTIS, ECASS, and NINDS rt-PA stroke trials. *Lancet, 363*(9411), 768–774. doi:10.1016/S0140-6736(04)15692-4

Harris, J. G., & Filley, C. M. (2001). CADASIL: Neuropsychological findings in three generations of an affected family. *Journal of the International Neuropsychological Society, 7*(6), 768–774.

Haug, T., Sorteberg, A., Sorteberg, W., Lindegaard, K. F., Lundar, T., & Finset, A. (2009). Surgical repair of unruptured and ruptured middle cerebral artery aneurysms: Impact on cognitive functioning and health-related quality of life. *Neurosurgery, 64*(3), 412–420; discussion 421–412. doi: 10.1227/01.NEU.0000338952.13880.4E

Heidenreich, P. A., Trogdon, J. G., Khavjou, O. A., Butler, J., Dracup, K., Ezekowitz, M. D., . . . Woo, Y. J. (2011). Forecasting the future of cardiovascular disease in the United States: A policy statement from the American Heart Association. *Circulation, 123*(8), 933–944. doi: 10.1161/CIR.0b013e31820a55f5 [pii]

Huang, J., & van Gelder, J. M. (2002). The probability of sudden death from rupture of intracranial aneurysms: A meta-analysis. *Neurosurgery, 51*(5), 1101–1105; discussion 1105–1107.

Hulette, C., Nochlin, D., McKeel, D., Morris, J. C., Mirra, S. S., Sumi, S. M., & Heyman, A. (1997). Clinical-neuropathologic findings in multi-infarct dementia: A report of six autopsied cases. *Neurology, 48*(3), 668–672.

Hung, C. C., Tu, Y. K., Su, C. F., Lin, L. S., & Shih, C. J. (1997). Epidemiological study of moyamoya disease in Taiwan. *Clinical Neurology and Neurosurgery, 99*(Suppl 2), S23–S25.

Ikram, M. A., Wieberdink, R. G., & Koudstaal, P. J. (2012). International epidemiology of intracerebral hemorrhage. *Current Atherosclerosis Report, 14*(4), 300–306. doi:10.1007/s11883-012-0252-1

Jellinger, K. A. (2013). Pathology and pathogenesis of vascular cognitive impairment—a critical update. *Frontiers in Aging Neuroscience, 5*, 17. doi: 10.3389/fnagi.2013.00017

Ji, Y., Tan, S., Xu, Y., Chandra, A., Shi, C., Song, B., . . . Gao, Y. (2013). Vitamin B supplementation, homocysteine levels, and the risk of cerebrovascular disease: A meta-analysis. *Neurology, 81*(15), 1298–1307. doi: 10.1212/WNL.0b013e3182a823cc

Jin, Y. P., Di Legge, S., Ostbye, T., Feightner, J. W., & Hachinski, V. (2006). The reciprocal risks of stroke and cognitive impairment in an elderly population. *Alzheimers Dement, 2*(3), 171–178. doi: 10.1016/j.jalz.2006.03.006, S1552-5260(06)00071-9 [pii]

Johnston, S. C., Fayad, P. B., Gorelick, P. B., Hanley, D. F., Shwayder, P., van Husen, D., & Weiskopf, T. (2003). Prevalence and knowledge of transient ischemic attack among US adults. *Neurology, 60*(9), 1429–1434.

Joutel, A., Corpechot, C., Ducros, A., Vahedi, K., Chabriat, H., Mouton, P., . . . Tournier-Lasserve, E. (1996). Notch3 mutations in CADASIL, a hereditary adult-onset condition causing stroke and dementia. *Nature, 383*(6602), 707–710. doi: 10.1038/383707a0

Kalaria, R. N. (1993). The immunopathology of Alzheimer's disease and some related disorders. *Brain Pathology, 3*(4), 333–347.

Kalaria, R. N. (2002). Small vessel disease and Alzheimer's dementia: Pathological considerations. *Cerebrovascular Diseases, 13*(Suppl 2), 48–52. doi: 49150

Kalaria, R. N. (2012). Cerebrovascular disease and mechanisms of cognitive impairment: Evidence from clinicopathological studies in humans. *Stroke, 43*(9), 2526–2534. doi: 10.1161/STROKEAHA.112.655803 [pii]

Karzmark, P., Zeifert, P. D., Tan, S., Dorfman, L. J., Bell-Stephens, T. E., & Steinberg, G. K. (2008). Effect of moyamoya disease on neuropsychological functioning in adults. *Neurosurgery, 62*(5), 1048–1051; discussion 1051–1042. doi: 10.1227/01.neu.0000325866.29634.4c

Kelley, B. J., McClure, L. A., Letter, A. J., Wadley, V. G., Unverzagt, F. W., Kissela, B. M., . . . Howard, G. (2013). Report of stroke-like symptoms predicts incident cognitive impairment in a stroke-free cohort. *Neurology, 81*(2), 113–118. doi: 10.1212/WNL.0b013e31829a352e

Kelly-Hayes, M., Beiser, A., Kase, C. S., Scaramucci, A., D'Agostino, R. B., & Wolf, P. A. (2003). The influence of gender and age on disability following ischemic stroke: The Framingham study. *Journal of Stroke and Cerebrovascular Diseases, 12*(3), 119–126. doi: 10.1016/S1052-3057(03)00042-9

Kleindorfer, D. O., Khoury, J., Moomaw, C. J., Alwell, K., Woo, D., Flaherty, M. L., . . . Kissela, B. M. (2010). Stroke incidence is decreasing in whites but not in blacks: A population-based estimate of temporal trends in stroke incidence from the Greater Cincinnati/Northern Kentucky Stroke Study. *Stroke, 41*(7), 1326–1331. doi: 10.1161/STROKEAHA.109.575043 [pii]

Kraemer, M., Heienbrok, W., & Berlit, P. (2008). Moyamoya disease in Europeans. *Stroke, 39*(12), 3193–3200. doi: 10.1161/STROKEAHA.107.513408

Lantz, E. R., & Meyers, P. M. (2008). Neuropsychological effects of brain arteriovenous malformations. *Neuropsychology Review, 18*(2), 167–177. doi: 10.1007/s11065-008-9060-3

Launer, L. J., Petrovitch, H., Ross, G. W., Markesbery, W., & White, L. R. (2008). AD brain pathology: Vascular origins? Results from the HAAS autopsy study. *Neurobiology of Aging, 29*(10), 1587–1590. doi: 10.1016/j.neurobiolaging.2007.03.008

Laver, K. E., George, S., Thomas, S., Deutsch, J. E., & Crotty, M. (2015). Virtual reality for stroke rehabilitation. *Cochrane Database of Systematic Reviews, 2.* doi:ARTN CD00834910.1002/14651858.CD008349.pub3

Lazar, R. M., Connaire, K., Marshall, R. S., Pile-Spellman, J., Hacein-Bey, L., Solomon, R. A., . . . Mohr, J. P. (1999). Developmental deficits in adult patients with arteriovenous malformations. *Archives of Neurology, 56*(1), 103–106.

Levy, D. E. (1988). How transient are transient ischemic attacks? *Neurology, 38*(5), 674–677.

Liem, M. K., Oberstein, S. A., van der Grond, J., Ferrari, M. D., & Haan, J. (2010). CADASIL and migraine: A narrative review. *Cephalalgia, 30*(11), 1284–1289.

Liman, T. G., Winter, B., Waldschmidt, C., Zerbe, N., Hufnagl, P., Audebert, H. J., & Endres, M. (2012). Telestroke ambulances in prehospital stroke management: Concept and pilot feasibility study. *Stroke*, *43*(8), 2086–2090. doi: 10.1161/STROKEAHA.112.657270

Liu, X., Zhang, D., Shuo, W., Zhao, Y., Wang, R., & Zhao, J. (2013). Long term outcome after conservative and surgical treatment of haemorrhagic moyamoya disease. *Journal of Neurology, Neurosurgery & Psychiatry*, *84*(3), 258–265. doi: 10.1136/jnnp-2012-302236

Lo, R. Y., & Jagust, W. J. (2012). Vascular burden and Alzheimer disease pathologic progression. *Neurology*, *79*(13), 1349–1355. doi: 10.1212/WNL.0b013e31826c1b9d [pii]

Lobato, R. D., Perez, C., Rivas, J. J., & Cordobes, F. (1988). Clinical, radiological, and pathological spectrum of angiographically occult intracranial vascular malformations: Analysis of 21 cases and review of the literature. *Journal of Neurosurgery*, *68*(4), 518–531. doi: 10.3171/jns.1988.68.4.0518

Loesch, D. V., Gilman, S., Del Dotto, J., & Rosenblum, M. L. (1995). Cavernous malformation of the mammillary bodies: Neuropsychological implications. [Case Report]. *Journal of Neurosurgery*, *83*(2), 354–358. doi: 10.3171/jns.1995.83.2.0354

Looi, J. C., & Sachdev, P. S. (1999). Differentiation of vascular dementia from AD on neuropsychological tests. *Neurology*, *53*(4), 670–678.

Malik, G. M., Seyfried, D. M., & Morgan, J. K. (1996). Temporal lobe arteriovenous malformations: Surgical management and outcome. *Surgical Neurology*, *46*(2), 106–114; discussion 114–105.

Marchal, G., Serrati, C., Rioux, P., Petit-Taboue, M. C., Viader, F., de la Sayette, V., . . . et al. (1993). PET imaging of cerebral perfusion and oxygen consumption in acute ischaemic stroke: Relation to outcome. *Lancet*, *341*(8850), 925–927.

Marshall, R. S. (2012). Effects of altered cerebral hemodynamics on cognitive function. *Journal of Alzheimer's Disease*, *32*(3), 633–642. doi: 10.3233/JAD-2012-120949

Mathias, J. L., & Burke, J. (2009). Cognitive functioning in Alzheimer's and vascular dementia: A meta-analysis. *Neuropsychology*, *23*(4), 411–423. doi: 10.1037/a0015384

Matsushima, Y., Aoyagi, M., Masaoka, H., Suzuki, R., & Ohno, K. (1990). Mental outcome following encephaloduroarteriosynangiosis in children with moyamoya disease with the onset earlier than 5 years of age. *Child's Nervous System*, *6*(8), 440–443.

Maxwell, S. S., Jackson, C. A., Paternoster, L., Cordonnier, C., Thijs, V., Al-Shahi Salman, R., & Sudlow, C. L. (2011). Genetic associations with brain microbleeds: Systematic review and meta-analyses. *Neurology*, *77*(2), 158–167. doi:10.1212/WNL.0b013e318224afa3

Mayer, S. A., Kreiter, K. T., Copeland, D., Bernardini, G. L., Bates, J. E., Peery, S., . . . Connolly, E. S., Jr. (2002). Global and domain-specific cognitive impairment and outcome after subarachnoid hemorrhage. *Neurology*, *59*(11), 1750–1758.

McCue, M., Fairman, A., & Pramuka, M. (2010). Enhancing quality of life through telerehabilitation. *Physical Medicine & Rehabilitation Clinics of North America*, *21*(1), 195–205. doi: 10.1016/j.pmr.2009.07.005

Mehta, B. (1997). Cerebral arteriography. In K.M.A. Welch, L. Caplan, D. Reis, B. Siesjo, & B. Weir (Eds.), *Primer on Cerebrovascular Diseases* (pp. 611–614). San Diego, CA: Academic Press.

Meng, F., Tong, K. Y., Chan, S. T., Wong, W. W., Lui, K. H., Tang, K. W., . . . Gao, S. (2009). Cerebral plasticity after subcortical stroke as revealed by cortico-muscular coherence. *Transactions on Neural Systems and Rehabilitation Engineering*, *17*(3), 234–243. doi: 10.1109/TNSRE.2008.2006209

Mikami, K., Jorge, R. E., Moser, D. J., Arndt, S., Jang, M., Solodkin, A., . . . Robinson, R. G. (2013). Prevention of poststroke apathy using escitalopram or problem-solving therapy. *The American Journal of Geriatric Psychiatry*, *21*(9), 855–862. doi: 10.1016/j.jagp.2012.07.003

Mohr, J. P., Parides, M. K., Stapf, C., Moquete, E., Moy, C. S., Overbey, J. R., . . . international, A. i. (2014). Medical management with or without interventional therapy for unruptured brain arteriovenous malformations (ARUBA): a multicentre, non-blinded, randomised trial. *Lancet*, *383*(9917), 614–621. doi:10.1016/S0140-6736(13)62302-8

Morgenstern, L. B., Hemphill, J. C., 3rd, Anderson, C., Becker, K., Broderick, J. P., Connolly, E. S., Jr., . . . Tamargo, R. J. (2004). Guidelines for the management of spontaneous intracerebral hemorrhage: A guideline for healthcare professionals from the American Heart Association/American Stroke Association. *Stroke*, *41*(9), 2108–2129. doi: 10.1161/STR.0b013e3181ec611b [pii]

Morrison, L., & Akers, A. (1993). Cerebral cavernous malformation, familial. In R. A. Pagon, M. P. Adam, T. D. Bird, C. R. Dolan, C. T. Fong, & K. Stephens (Eds.), *GeneReviews*. Seattle, WA: University of Seattle.

Naeser, M. A., Martin, P. I., Ho, M., Treglia, E., Kaplan, E., Bashir, S., & Pascual-Leone, A. (2012). Transcranial magnetic stimulation and aphasia rehabilitation. *Archives of Physical Medicine and Rehabilitation*, *93*(Suppl 1), S26–S34. doi: 10.1016/j.apmr.2011.04.026

Nah, H. W., Kwon, S. U., Kang, D. W., Ahn, J. S., Kwun, B. D., & Kim, J. S. (2012). Moyamoya disease-related versus primary intracerebral: Hemorrhage location and outcomes are different. *Stroke*, *43*(7), 1947–1950. doi: 10.1161/STROKEAHA.112.654004

Naval, N. S., Stevens, R. D., Mirski, M. A., & Bhardwaj, A. (2006). Controversies in the management of aneurysmal subarachnoid hemorrhage. *Critical Care Medicine*, *34*(2), 511–524.

Nelson, M. E., Rejeski, W. J., Blair, S. N., Duncan, P. W., Judge, J. O., King, A. C., . . . American Heart Association. (2007). Physical activity and public health in older adults: Recommendation from the American College of Sports Medicine and the American Heart Association. *Circulation*, *116*(9), 1094–1105. doi: 10.1161/CIRCULATIONAHA.107.185650

Nelson, R. E., Saltzman, G. M., Skalabrin, E. J., Demaerschalk, B. M., & Majersik, J. J. (2011). The cost-effectiveness of telestroke in the treatment of acute ischemic stroke. *Neurology*, *77*(17), 1590–1598. doi: 10.1212/WNL.0b013e318234332d

Neuropathology Group, Medical Research Council Cognitive Function & Aging Study. (2001). Pathological correlates of late-onset dementia in a multicentre, community-based population in England and Wales. [Neuropathology Group of the Medical Research Council Cognitive Function and Ageing Study (MRC CFAS)]. *Lancet*, *357*(9251), 169–175.

Opherk, C., Peters, N., Herzog, J., Luedtke, R., & Dichgans, M. (2004). Long-term prognosis and causes of death in CADASIL: A retrospective study in 411 patients. *Brain*, *127*(Pt 11), 2533–2539. doi: 10.1093/brain/awh282 [pii]

Panagiotakos, D. B., Pitsavos, C., Chrysohoou, C., Skoumas, J., Masoura, C., Toutouzas, P., . . . ATTICA Study. (2004). Effect of exposure to secondhand smoke on markers of inflammation: The ATTICA study. *The American Journal of Medicine*, *116*(3), 145–150.

Parikh, R. M., Robinson, R. G., Lipsey, J. R., Starkstein, S. E., Fedoroff, J. P., & Price, T. R. (1990). The impact of poststroke depression on recovery in activities of daily living over a 2-year follow-up. *Archives of Neurology*, *47*(7), 785–789.

Parray, T., Martin, T. W., & Siddiqui, S. (2011). Moyamoya disease: A review of the disease and anesthetic management. *Journal of Neurosurgical Anesthesiology*, *23*(2), 100–109. doi: 10.1097/ANA.0b013e3181f84fac

Pendlebury, S. T., Wadling, S., Silver, L. E., Mehta, Z., & Rothwell, P. M. (2011). Transient cognitive impairment in TIA and minor stroke. *Stroke*, *42*(11), 3116–3121. doi: 10.1161/STROKEAHA.111.621490 [pii]

Peters, N., Opherk, C., Danek, A., Ballard, C., Herzog, J., & Dichgans, M. (2005). The pattern of cognitive performance in CADASIL: A monogenic condition leading to subcortical ischemic vascular dementia. *The American Journal of Psychiatry*, *162*(11), 2078–2085. doi: 10.1176/appi.ajp.162.11.2078, 162/11/2078 [pii]

Phan, T., Huston, J., 3rd, Bernstein, M. A., Riederer, S. J., & Brown, R. D., Jr. (2001). Contrast-enhanced magnetic resonance angiography of the cervical vessels: Experience with 422 patients. *Stroke*, *32*(10), 2282–2286.

Qiu, C., Cotch, M. F., Sigurdsson, S., Jonsson, P. V., Jonsdottir, M. K., Sveinbjrnsdottir, S., . . . Launer, L. J. (2010). Cerebral microbleeds, retinopathy, and dementia: The AGES-Reykjavik Study. *Neurology*, *75*(24), 2221–2228. doi: 10.1212/WNL.0b013e3182020349, 75/24/2221 [pii]

Redline, S., Yenokyan, G., Gottlieb, D. J., Shahar, E., O'Connor, G. T., Resnick, H. E., . . . Punjabi, N. M. (2010). Obstructive sleep apnea-hypopnea and incident stroke: The sleep heart health study. *American Journal of Respiratory and Critical Care Medicine*, *182*(2), 269–277. doi: 10.1164/rccm.200911-1746OC

Reed, B. R., Mungas, D. M., Kramer, J. H., Ellis, W., Vinters, H. V., Zarow, C., . . . Chui, H. C. (2007). Profiles of neuropsychological impairment in autopsy-defined Alzheimer's disease and cerebrovascular disease. *Brain*, *130*(Pt 3), 731–739. doi: 10.1093/brain/awl385

RiboURtout, E., & Raymond, J. (2004). Gene therapy and endovascular treatment of intracranial aneurysms. *Stroke*, *35*(3), 786–793. doi: 10.1161/01.STR.0000117577.94345.CC

Roach, E. S., Golomb, M. R., Adams, R., Biller, J., Daniels, S., Deveber, G., . . . Council on Cardiovascular Disease in the Young. (2008). Management of stroke in infants and children: A scientific statement from a Special Writing Group of the American Heart Association Stroke Council and the Council on Cardiovascular Disease in the Young. *Stroke*, *39*(9), 2644–2691. doi: 10.1161/STROKEAHA.108.189696

Robertson, I. H., & Murre, J. M. (1999). Rehabilitation of brain damage: Brain plasticity and principles of guided recovery. *Psychological Bulletin*, *125*(5), 544–575.

Robinson, R. G., Jorge, R. E., Moser, D. J., Acion, L., Solodkin, A., Small, S. L., . . . Arndt, S. (2008). Escitalopram and problem-solving therapy for prevention of poststroke depression: A randomized controlled trial. *JAMA*, *299*(20), 2391–2400. doi: 10.1001/jama.299.20.2391

Rodriguez-Colon, S. M., Mo, J., Duan, Y., Liu, J., Caulfield, J. E., Jin, X., & Liao, D. (2009). Metabolic syndrome clusters and the risk of incident stroke: The atherosclerosis risk in communities (ARIC) study. *Stroke*, *40*(1), 200–205. doi: 10.1161/STROKEAHA.108.523035

Roman, G. C., Tatemichi, T. K., Erkinjuntti, T., Cummings, J. L., Masdeu, J. C., Garcia, J. H., . . . Scheinberg, P. (1993). Vascular dementia: Diagnostic criteria for research studies. [Report of the NINDS-AIREN International Workshop]. *Neurology*, *43*(2), 250–260.

Ronkainen, A., Miettinen, H., Karkola, K., Papinaho, S., Vanninen, R., Puranen, M., & Hernesniemi, J. (1998). Risk of harboring an unruptured intracranial aneurysm. *Stroke*, *29*(2), 359–362.

Rossini, P. M., Altamura, C., Ferreri, F., Melgari, J. M., Tecchio, F., Tombini, M., . . . Vernieri, F. (2007). Neuroimaging experimental studies on brain plasticity in recovery from stroke. *Europa Medicophysica*, *43*(2), 241–254.

Rothwell, P. M., Giles, M. F., Chandratheva, A., Marquardt, L., Geraghty, O., Redgrave, J. N., . . . Mehta, Z. (2007). Effect of urgent treatment of transient ischaemic attack and minor stroke on early recurrent stroke (EXPRESS study): A prospective population-based sequential comparison. *Lancet*, *370*(9596), 1432–1442. doi: 10.1016/S0140-6736(07)61448-2 [pii]

Sacco, R. L. (2004). Risk factors for TIA and TIA as a risk factor for stroke. *Neurology*, *62*(8 Suppl 6), S7–S11.

Sahathevan, R., Brodtmann, A., & Donnan, G. A. (2012). Dementia, stroke, and vascular risk factors; a review. *International Journal of Stroke*, *7*(1), 61–73. doi: 10.1111/j.1747-4949.2011.00731.x

Sattelmair, J., Pertman, J., Ding, E. L., Kohl, H. W., 3rd, Haskell, W., & Lee, I. M. (2011). Dose response between physical activity and risk of coronary heart disease: A meta-analysis. *Circulation*, *124*(7), 789–795. doi: 10.1161/CIRCULATIONAHA.110.010710

Saver, J. L. (2006). Time is brain: Quantified. *Stroke*, *37*(1), 263–266. doi: 10.1161/01.STR.0000196957.55928.ab

Schaefer, L., & Hebben, N. (2014). Domains of neuropsychological function and related neurobehavioral disorders. In K. J. Stucky, M. W. Kirkwood, & J. Donders (Eds.), *Neuropsychology Study Guide and Board Review* (pp. 54–60). New York: Oxford University Press.

Schaefer, S. Y., Haaland, K. Y., & Sainburg, R. L. (2009). Hemispheric specialization and functional impact of ipsilesional deficits in movement coordination and accuracy. *Neuropsychologia*, *47*(13), 2953–2966. doi: 10.1016/j.neuropsychologia.2009.06.025

Schellinger, P. D., Bryan, R. N., Caplan, L. R., Detre, J. A., Edelman, R. R., Jaigobin, C., . . . Technology Assessment Subcommittee of the American Academy of Neurology. (2010). Evidence-based guideline: The role of diffusion and perfusion MRI for the diagnosis of acute ischemic stroke: Report of the Therapeutics and Technology Assessment Subcommittee of the American Academy of Neurology. *Neurology*, *75*(2), 177–185. doi: 10.1212/WNL.0b013e3181e7c9dd

Schneider, J. A., Arvanitakis, Z., Bang, W., & Bennett, D. A. (2007). Mixed brain pathologies account for most dementia cases in community-dwelling older persons. *Neurology*, *69*(24), 2197–2204. doi: 10.1212/01.wnl.0000271090.28148.24

Schneider, J. A., Wilson, R. S., Bienias, J. L., Evans, D. A., & Bennett, D. A. (2004). Cerebral infarctions and the likelihood of dementia from Alzheimer disease pathology. *Neurology*, *62*(7), 1148–1155.

Seshadri, S., Beiser, A., Kelly Hayes, M., Kase, C. S., Au, R., Kannel, W. B., & Wolf, P. A. (2006). The lifetime risk of stroke: Estimates from the Framingham Study. *Stroke*, *37*(2), 345–350. doi: 10.1161/01.STR.0000199613.38911.b2 [pii]

Shah, K. H., Kleckner, K., & Edlow, J. A. (2008). Short-term prognosis of stroke among patients diagnosed in the emergency department with a transient ischemic attack. *Annals of Emergency Medicine*, *51*(3), 316–323. doi: 10.1016/j.annemergmed.2007.08.016, S0196-0644(07)01445-X [pii]

Slooter, A. J., Cruts, M., Hofman, A., Koudstaal, P. J., van der Kuip, D., de Ridder, M. A., . . . van Duijn, C. M. (2004). The impact of APOE on myocardial infarction, stroke, and dementia: The Rotterdam Study. *Neurology*, *62*(7), 1196–1198.

Soderman, M., Andersson, T., Karlsson, B., Wallace, M. C., & Edner, G. (2003). Management of patients with brain arteriovenous malformations. *European Journal of Radiology*, *46*(3), 195–205. doi: S0720048X03000913 [pii]

Sparks, D. L., Scheff, S. W., Hunsaker, J. C., 3rd, Liu, H., Landers, T., & Gross, D. R. (1994). Induction of Alzheimer-like beta-amyloid immunoreactivity in the brains of rabbits with dietary cholesterol. *Experimental Neurology*, *126*(1), 88–94. doi: 10.1006/exnr.1994.1044

Stabell, K. (1991). *Neuropsychological Investigation of Patients With Surgically Treated Aneurysm Rupture at Different Cerebral Sites*. Oslo, Norway: Institute of Psychology.

Starkstein, S. E., Robinson, R. G., & Price, T. R. (1988). Comparison of patients with and without poststroke major depression matched for size and location of lesion. *Archives of General Psychiatry*, *45*(3), 247–252.

Stebbins, G. T., Nyenhuis, D. L., Wang, C., Cox, J. L., Freels, S., Bangen, K., . . . Gorelick, P. B. (2008). Gray matter atrophy in patients with ischemic stroke with cognitive impairment. *Stroke*, *39*(3), 785–793. doi:10.1161/STROKEAHA.107.507392

Tidswell, P., Dias, P. S., Sagar, H. J., Mayes, A. R., & Battersby, R. D. (1995). Cognitive outcome after aneurysm rupture: Relationship to aneurysm site and perioperative complications. *Neurology*, *45*(5), 875–882.

Timaran, C. H., Mantese, V. A., Malas, M., Brown, O. W., Lal, B. K., Moore, W. S., . . . CREST Investigators. (2013). Differential outcomes of carotid stenting and endarterectomy performed exclusively by vascular surgeons in the Carotid Revascularization Endarterectomy versus Stenting Trial (CREST). *Journal of Vascular Surgery*, *57*(2), 303–308. doi: 10.1016/j.jvs.2012.09.014

Ueki, K., Meyer, F. B., & Mellinger, J. F. (1994). Moyamoya disease: The disorder and surgical treatment. *Mayo Clinic Proceedings*, *69*(8), 749–757.

van Beijnum, J., van der Worp, H. B., Buis, D. R., Al-Shahi Salman, R., Kappelle, L. J., Rinkel, G. J., . . . Klijn, C. J. (2011). Treatment of brain arteriovenous malformations: A systematic review and meta-analysis. *JAMA*, *306*(18), 2011–2019. doi: 10.1001/jama.2011.1632, 306/18/2011 [pii]

van den Kommer, T. N., Dik, M. G., Comijs, H. C., Fassbender, K., Lutjohann, D., & Jonker, C. (2009). Total cholesterol and oxysterols: Early markers for cognitive decline in elderly? *Neurobiology of Aging*, *30*(4), 534–545. doi: 10.1016/j.neurobiolaging.2007.08.005

van Dijk, E. J., Prins, N. D., Vermeer, S. E., Hofman, A., van Duijn, C. M., Koudstaal, P. J., & Breteler, M. M. (2004). Plasma amyloid beta, apolipoprotein E, lacunar infarcts, and white matter lesions. *Annals of Neurology*, *55*(4), 570–575. doi: 10.1002/ana.20050

Vermeer, S. E., Sandee, W., Algra, A., Koudstaal, P. J., Kappelle, L. J., Dippel, D. W., & Dutch, T.I.A.T.S.G. (2006). Impaired glucose tolerance increases stroke risk in nondiabetic patients with transient ischemic attack or minor ischemic stroke. *Stroke*, *37*(6), 1413–1417. doi: 10.1161/01.STR.0000221766.73692.0b

von Vogelsang, A. C., Svensson, M., Wengstrom, Y., & Forsberg, C. (2013). Cognitive, physical, and psychological status after intracranial aneurysm rupture: A cross-sectional study of a Stockholm case series 1996 to 1999. *World Neurosurgery*, *79*(1), 130–135. doi: 10.1016/j.wneu.2012.03.032

Vrethem, M., Thuomas, K. A., & Hillman, J. (1997). Cavernous angioma of the brain stem mimicking multiple sclerosis. *New England Journal of Medicine*, *336*(12), 875–876. doi: 10.1056/NEJM199703203361213

Walker, E. J., Su, H., Shen, F., Choi, E. J., Oh, S. P., Chen, G., . . . Young, W. L. (2011). Arteriovenous malformation in the adult mouse brain resembling the human disease. *Annals of Neurology*, *69*(6), 954–962. doi: 10.1002/ana.22348

Wang, W., Collinger, J. L., Perez, M. A., Tyler-Kabara, E. C., Cohen, L. G., Birbaumer, N., . . . Weber, D. J. (2010). Neural interface technology for rehabilitation: Exploiting and promoting neuroplasticity. *Physical Medicine & Rehabilitation Clinics of North America*, *21*(1), 157–178. doi: 10.1016/j.pmr.2009.07.003

Wannamethee, S. G., Shaper, A. G., Lennon, L., & Morris, R. W. (2005). Metabolic syndrome vs Framingham Risk Score for prediction of coronary heart disease, stroke, and type 2 diabetes mellitus. *Archives of Internal Medicine*, *165*(22), 2644–2650. doi: 10.1001/archinte.165.22.2644

Weir, B. K., Kongable, G. L., Kassell, N. F., Schultz, J. R., Truskowski, L. L., & Sigrest, A. (1998). Cigarette smoking as a cause of aneurysmal subarachnoid hemorrhage and risk for vasospasm: A report of the Cooperative Aneurysm Study. *Journal of Neurosurgery*, *89*(3), 405–411. doi: 10.3171/jns.1998.89.3.0405

Wetterling, T., Kanitz, R. D., & Borgis, K. J. (1996). Comparison of different diagnostic criteria for vascular dementia (ADDTC, DSM-IV, ICD-10, NINDS-AIREN). *Stroke*, *27*(1), 30–36.

Whigham, K. B., & O'Toole, K. (2007). Understanding the neuropsychologic outcome of pediatric AVM within a neurodevelopmental framework. *Cognitive and Behavioral Neurology*, *20*(4), 244–257. doi: 10.1097/WNN.0b013e31815e6224

Whitmer, R. A., Gustafson, D. R., Barrett-Connor, E., Haan, M. N., Gunderson, E. P., & Yaffe, K. (2008). Central obesity and increased risk of dementia more than three decades later. *Neurology*, *71*(14), 1057–1064. doi: 10.1212/01.wnl.0000306313.89165.ef

WHO. (1993). *The ICD-10 Classification of Mental and Behavioral Disorders: Diagnostic Criteria for Research*. Geneva, Switzerland: World Health Organization.

Whyte, E. M., Mulsant, B. H., Vanderbilt, J., Dodge, H. H., & Ganguli, M. (2004). Depression after stroke: A prospective epidemiological study. *Journal of the American Geriatrics Society*, *52*(5), 774–778. doi: 10.1111/j.1532-5415.2004.52217.x, JGS52217 [pii]

Wiederkehr, S., Simard, M., Fortin, C., & van Reekum, R. (2008a). Comparability of the clinical diagnostic criteria for vascular dementia: A critical review: Part I. *Journal of Neuropsychiatry and Clininical Neurosciences*, *20*(2), 150–161. doi: 10.1176/appi.neuropsych.20.2.150

Wiederkehr, S., Simard, M., Fortin, C., & van Reekum, R. (2008b). Validity of the clinical diagnostic criteria for vascular dementia: A critical review: Part II. *The Journal of Neuropsychiatry and Clinical Neurosciences*, *20*(2), 162–177. doi: 10.1176/appi.neuropsych.20.2.162

Wolf, P. A., D'Agostino, R. B., Belanger, A. J., & Kannel, W. B. (1991). Probability of stroke: A risk profile from the Framingham Study. *Stroke*, *22*(3), 312–318.

Yaggi, H. K., Concato, J., Kernan, W. N., Lichtman, J. H., Brass, L. M., & Mohsenin, V. (2005). Obstructive sleep apnea as a risk factor for stroke and death. *New England Journal of Medicine*, *353*(19), 2034–2041. doi: 10.1056/NEJMoa043104

Yu, S. C., Chan, M. S., Lam, J. M., Tam, P. H., & Poon, W. S. (2004). Complete obliteration of intracranial arteriovenous malformation with endovascular cyanoacrylate embolization: Initial success and rate of permanent cure. *American Journal of Neuroradiology*, *25*(7), 1139–1143.

Zerwic, J., Hwang, S. Y., & Tucco, L. (2007). Interpretation of symptoms and delay in seeking treatment by patients who have had a stroke: Exploratory study. *Heart Lung*, *36*(1), 25–34. doi: 10.1016/j.hrtlng.2005.12.007

17 Moderate and Severe Traumatic Brain Injury

Tresa Roebuck-Spencer and Mark Sherer

Traumatic brain injury (TBI) has been defined by the Centers for Disease Control and Prevention (CDC) as an injury to the head that involves at least one of the following: (a) decreased level of consciousness, (b) amnesia, (c) skull fracture, or (d) objective neurological or neuropsychological abnormality or diagnosed intracranial lesion (Marr & Coronado, 2004). TBI severity is classified on a continuum from mild to moderate to severe, with treatment, recovery course, and ultimate outcome varying widely across these groups. Neuropsychological assessment and intervention are frequently requested for patients with TBI at all levels of injury severity and across multiple time points in the treatment and recovery course.

Individuals with moderate to severe TBI often have persisting impairments that impact their ability to return to their previous level of functioning. These patients are much more likely than patients with mild injuries to require inpatient or postacute rehabilitation and subsequently may be followed for ongoing outpatient care related to their injuries (Harrison-Felix, Newton, Hall, & Kreutzer, 1996; Malec & Moessner, 2000). Neuropsychologists in both inpatient and outpatient settings may be asked to evaluate and treat patients with moderate and severe TBI to address referral questions including, but not limited to, stage of recovery, supervision/guardianship needs, ability to return to work or school, and effectiveness of psychotropic medication or other interventions.

This chapter will provide a review of neuropsychological issues relevant to moderate and severe TBI. Specifically, this chapter will cover (a) incidence/prevalence and risk factors, (b) classification of TBI severity, (c) neuroanatomical effects of TBI, (d) course of recovery, (e) neuropsychological and neurobehavioral effects of TBI, (f) neuropsychological assessment, and (g) outcome following moderate and severe TBI.

Incidence/Prevalence and Risk Factors for TBI

TBI is a serious public health issue that affects all ages, genders, and ethnicities. In its most recent report on TBI in the United States spanning the years 2002–2006, the CDC reported an estimated 1,691,481 people (576.8 per 1000,000) sustain a TBI annually (Faul, Xu, Wald, & Coronado, 2010). Of this number, nearly 80% are treated in the emergency department (ED) and released, with approximately 275,000 individuals hospitalized for further care. In addition, 52,000 individuals are reported to die as a result of their injuries with TBI identified as a contributing factor in a third of all injury-related deaths.

Comparison of incidence rates over time revealed increases in TBI-related ED visits and hospitalizations (Faul et al., 2010; Langlois, Rutland-Brown, & Thomas, 2006), particularly in children and older adults (Faul et al., 2010), likely due to increases in population and increases in falls. However, this increase may also represent increased public awareness of TBI. TBI-related deaths decreased as much as 8.2% over time (Coronado et al., 2011; Faul et al., 2010; Langlois et al., 2006), potentially related to increased preventive measures such as seat belt and helmet use (Braver, Ferguson, Greene, & Lund, 1997; Thompson, Rivara, & Thompson, 1989) and better overall treatment for severe TBI (Faul, Wald, Rutland-Brown, Sullivent, & Sattin, 2007).

Incidence of new-onset disability from TBI has been estimated to be 80,000 to 90,000 new cases each year (Thurman, Alverson, Dunn, Guerrero, & Sniezek, 1999) and more than a million Americans live with disability due to TBI (Thurman, 1999). A more recent projected estimate indicated that incidence of new onset disability may actually be higher, at the rate of more than 124,626 new cases per year, or 43.3% of all hospitalized TBI survivors (Selassie et al., 2008).

Regarding severity, CDC estimates from the year 2000 documented that, of patients hospitalized due to TBI, more than 50% had mild injuries, 21% had moderate injuries, and 19% had severe injuries (Thurman & Guerrero, 1999). Other estimates indicate that mild TBI makes up 75% of the TBIs in the United States each year (National Center for Injury Prevention and Control, 2003). The actual incidence of mild TBI in the United States is difficult to determine because many individuals with mild TBI do not seek treatment or are not hospitalized for their injuries. Further, CDC estimates of TBI incidence are limited because they do not include individuals treated in outpatient settings or who do not present for treatment at all (Coronado et al., 2011) with estimates that up to one-fourth of all persons who sustain a TBI do not seek medical care (Sosin, Sniezek, & Thurman, 1996). Further, incidence varies widely across studies from 92 cases per 100,000 persons (Thurman & Guerrero, 1999) to 618 per

100,000 (Sosin et al., 1996) most likely due to methodological differences such as populations sampled and case definitions of TBI used. Additionally, the most recent CDC data do not include military personnel who sustained a TBI abroad or who received care for TBI in federal, military, or Veterans Administration hospitals (Faul et al., 2010).

The leading causes of TBI in the U.S. civilian population are falls (35.2%), followed by motor-vehicle-related injuries (17.3%), a strike or blow to the head from or against objects (16.5%), assaults (10%), and other or unknown causes (21%) (Faul et al., 2010). Fall-related TBIs are greatest at the extremes of the life span (i.e., children less than 4 and adults over 75 years), and motor-vehicle-related injuries are the leading cause of TBIs in late adolescence (ages 15–19) and early adulthood (ages 20–24). Assault-related TBIs are also highly represented in the 20–24 year age group (Faul et al., 2010; Rutland-Brown, Langlois, Thomas, & Xi, 2006).

Risk factors for TBI vary greatly, with some specific groups at higher risk than others. Age is a risk factor, with children under 4, adolescents between the ages of 15 and 19, and adults over 65 years of age showing the highest rates of brain injury (Faul et al., 2010). A disproportionate number of elderly individuals sustained brain injuries as a result of falls and there is evidence that elderly individuals are at risk for worse outcome from TBI than younger individuals (Howard, Gross, Dacey, & Winn, 1989; Rothweiler, Temkin, & Dikmen, 1998). Additionally, probability of TBI-related long-term disability has been shown to increase with age (Selassie et al., 2008). Sex also represents a risk factor for TBI, with males accounting for approximately 59% of all TBI cases in the United States (Faul et al., 2010). Probability of long-term disability following TBI is significantly higher for females (49.5% compared to 39.9%) (Selassie et al., 2008), whereas death rates from TBI are three times higher among males (Coronado et al., 2011). Alcohol use and intoxication have long been documented as risk factors for TBI, with 23% to 56% of individuals sustaining TBIs documented as intoxicated at injury (Cherner, Temkin, Machamer, & Dikmen, 2001; Dikmen, Machamer, Donovan, Winn, & Temkin, 1995; Parry-Jones, Vaughan, & Miles Cox, 2006). Further, a preinjury history of alcohol and substance abuse has been shown to increase risk for TBI and negative outcome across a variety of domains (Corrigan, 1995; Corrigan, Bogner, & Holloman, 2012; Graham & Cardon, 2008; Parry-Jones et al., 2006; Taylor, Kreutzer, Demm, & Meade, 2003). Prior brain injury poses a separate risk for TBI (Salcido & Costich, 1992; Saunders et al., 2009), with the risk of a second TBI for those with past injuries being approximately three times that of the general noninjured population. Rates for a third injury given two prior injuries increase even further (Annegers, Grabow, Kurland, & Laws, 1980). A recent study found that 20% of patients in the TBI Model Systems database had a prior TBI, with 80% of these prior injuries being the mild range and 40% occurring prior to the age of 16 (Corrigan et al., 2013). Finally, there is evidence that lower socioeconomic status and inclusion in a minority racial/ethnic group may increase risk for TBI and poorer overall psychosocial and functional outcome following TBI (Arango-Lasprilla et al., 2011; Arango-Lasprilla & Kreutzer, 2010; Cooper et al., 1983; Kraus, Fife, Ramstein, Conroy, & Cox, 1986; Langlois et al., 2006; Sosin et al., 1996; Whitman, Coonley-Hoganson, & Desai, 1984; Williams, Arango-Lasprilla, & Stevens, 2009).

Classification of TBI Severity

Initial presentation of TBI varies greatly across patients and has significant implications for ultimate outcome. Thus, classification of injury severity has become one of the most important predictors for immediate and long-term outcome. Severity of TBI can be measured in a variety of ways, but is generally determined by depth of coma, duration of coma or unconsciousness, and duration of acute confusion following injury.

The most commonly used index of injury severity is the Glasgow Coma Scale (GCS; see Teasdale & Jennett, 1974), which measures depth of coma by determining a patient's responsiveness level in eye opening, motor movement, and verbal communication. Scores range from 3 to 15, with higher scores indicating more intact functioning. Patients with postresuscitation GCS scores of 3 to 8 are classified as having had severe TBI and those with scores from 9 to 12 are classified as having had moderate injuries (Clifton, Hayes, Levin, Michel, & Choi, 1992; Hannay & Sherer, 1996; Levin & Eisenberg, 1991). Some researchers further divide the severe group into severe (GCS 6 to 8) and very severe (GCS 3 to 5) (Zhang, Jiang, Zhong, Yu, & Zhu, 2001). Patients with GCS scores between 13 and 15 are classified as having had mild injuries. Outcomes of these patients can differ drastically depending on the presence or absence of findings on the initial neuroimaging and, thus, they are often subdivided into complicated and uncomplicated mild TBI. Patients with GCS scores between 13 and 15 with no intracranial abnormalities on neuroimaging (uncomplicated mild TBI) typically have very favorable outcomes with resolution of clinical symptoms within three months (Belanger, Curtiss, Demery, Lebowitz, & Vanderploeg, 2005; Belanger, Spiegel, & Vanderploeg, 2010; Dikmen, Machamer, Powell, & Temkin, 2003; Rohling et al., 2011; Schretlen & Shapiro, 2003; Williams, Levin, & Eisenberg, 1990). In contrast, patients with initial GCS scores between 13 and 15 who also demonstrate depressed skull fractures or other intracranial abnormalities (complicated mild TBI) have outcomes more similar to patients with moderate TBI (Dikmen et al., 2003; Kashluba, Hanks, Casey, & Millis, 2008; Williams et al., 1990). See Table 17.1 for the association between GCS scores and injury severity.

The advantages of using GCS scores to classify injury severity are that these scores can be determined in the first 24 hours and are predictive of early important outcomes, such as survival (Wardlaw, Easton, & Statham, 2002), and later functional outcomes, such as employment (Dikmen et al., 1994). However, there is disagreement about which time point GCS should be collected (Marion & Carlier, 1994). Many use GCS scores obtained immediately postresuscitation or at admission to the ED for classification of TBI severity, whereas others suggest that the best or worst GCS within the first 24 hours of injury are better options. GCS scores at early time points may underestimate severity for patients whose responsiveness deteriorates due to intracranial hematomas or other complications within the first 24 hours. In contrast, GCS taken at early time points may overestimate severity level for patients who are under the influence of alcohol or other substances at the time of injury. GCS scores may also be affected by early management such as intubation or sedating and paralyzing medications, and the use of GCS scores is limited in patients with aphasia or facial injuries that limit eye opening or verbalization.

A recent study by Barker and colleagues (2014) examined the impact of changes in emergency management from 1987 to 2012 on the relationship between GCS scores and functional outcome, and found that the predictive utility of GCS did not decline over time. Rates of intubation did not change over time, whereas the use of chemical paralytics or heavy sedatives increased. Paralyzed and sedated patients performed slightly better on average than those with severe TBI, raising the possibility that the paralyzed group may contain people with less-severe brain injuries. Thus, caution should be taken when interpreting studies that classify all medically sedated patients as having severe TBI.

Injury severity can also be determined by the length of time it takes an individual to return to a conscious or responsive state, which is most often indicated by the ability to follow simple commands, indicate yes/no responses reliably through words or gestures, give intelligible verbalizations, or other purposeful behaviors (Giacino et al., 2002). Studies typically use time to follow commands as the indicator for when a patient has returned to a conscious state, but others have specifically used spontaneous eye opening (Ariza et al., 2004; Eisenberg & Weiner, 1987) or withdrawal from a painful stimulus (Levin, 1995; Whyte, Cifu, Dikmen, & Temkin, 2001). Thus, it is important to specifically determine the criteria used for duration of unconsciousness before comparing results across studies. The interval from injury to recovery of ability to follow commands, corresponding to a GCS motor score of 6, has proven to be a more useful index in determining injury severity when compared to the interval between injury and time to motor localization (GCS motor score of 5) (Whyte et al., 2001). Some authors substitute the term *duration of unconsciousness, coma duration,* or *length of coma* for this variable. A classification scheme for this index reported by Lezak and colleagues (Lezak, 1995; Lezak, Howieson, Loring, Hannay, & Fischer, 2004) classified an interval of < 20 minutes coma duration as a mild injury, an interval of < six hours as a moderate injury, and > six hours as a severe injury. (See Table 17.1); however, it should be noted that across studies authors tend to use different cut points for this variable when assigning severity levels. Importantly, time to follow commands has been shown to be predictive of global outcome, neuropsychological functioning, personal independence, and employment outcome after TBI (Dikmen & Machamer, 1995; Dikmen, McLean, Temkin, & Wyler, 1986; Dikmen et al., 1994; Dikmen, Ross, Machamer, & Temkin, 1995).

Advantages of using time to follow commands for determining injury severity are that this index takes into account early complications and can be obtained during relatively early stages of recovery. However, this interval can be affected by early sedation and the patient must be closely monitored for an extended period of time. This index is also limited by difficult to interpret behaviors and fluctuations in patient's mental status. Further, this index is not immediately available for early prediction of outcome, there is no commonly agreed upon classification scheme, and it is often not available to later treating clinicians because of lack of availability of initial medical records.

The duration of posttraumatic amnesia (PTA) has also commonly been used to classify TBI severity. PTA refers to the phase of recovery following TBI during which the patient is responsive, but acutely confused, disoriented and unable to form and retain new memories (Russell, 1932; Symonds,

Table 17.1 Comparison of different methods of injury severity classification

	Classification Method			
Injury Severity	Glasgow Coma Scale (GCS)[1]	Time to Follow Commands[2]	Posttraumatic Amnesia (PTA)[3]	Mississippi PTA Classification Scheme[4]
Mild	13–15	< 20 minutes	< 1 hour	
Moderate	9–12	< 6 hours	1 to 24 hours	0–14 days
Moderate Severe				15–28 days
Severe	6–8	> 6 hours	1–7 days	29–70 days
Very Severe	3–5		> 7 days	> 70 days

[1](Clifton et al., 1992; Hannay & Sherer, 1996; Levin & Eisenberg, 1991)
[2](Lezak, 1995; Lezak et al., 2004)
[3](Russell & Smith, 1961)
[4](Nakase-Richardson et al., 2009; Nakase-Richardson et al., 2011)

1937). Duration of PTA can be assessed retrospectively by waiting until the patient is no longer confused and asking him or her to report the first memory that he or she can recall following brain injury (Symonds & Russell, 1943). More commonly, duration of PTA is determined prospectively by serial assessment of the patient's degree of disorientation using measures such as the Galveston Orientation and Amnesia Scale (GOAT) (Levin, O'Donnell, & Grossman, 1979), the Orientation Log (Jackson, Novack, & Dowler, 1998), the Oxford Scale (Fortuny, Briggs, Newcombe, Ratcliff, & Thomas, 1980), and the Westmead Scale (Shores, Marosszeky, Sandanam, & Batchelor, 1986).

While disorientation and memory disturbance are hallmarks of this phase of recovery, recent researchers have noted the similarity of this state to delirium and have recommended use of the term Posttraumatic Confusional State (PTCS) (Nakase-Thompson, Sherer, Yablon, Nick, & Trzepacz, 2004; Sherer, Nakase-Thompson, Yablon, & Gontkovsky, 2005; Stuss et al., 1999). As with time to follow commands, the usefulness of duration of PTA as an index of TBI severity is limited by the lack of commonly agreed-upon criteria for intervals indicating severe, moderate, and mild injuries. One of the most commonly used criteria, developed by Russell and Smith (1961), classifies patients with PTA < one hour as having had slight concussion, patients with PTA of one to 24 hours as having had moderate concussion, patients with PTA of one to seven days as having had severe concussion, and patients with PTA of greater than seven days as having had very severe concussion (see Table 17.1). Numerous studies have shown that duration of PTA is predictive of various aspects of outcome after TBI including neuropsychological outcome, independent living status, and return to work (Dikmen et al., 1994; Ellenberg, Levin, & Saydjari, 1996; Sherer et al., 2002). However, this measure is limited in that it may not be available for an extended period of time following injury; requires close monitoring of the patient over time; and is affected by fluctuations in behavior, aphasia, intubation, and other issues preventing effective communication.

It is not uncommon for patients in rehabilitation settings to have PTA durations well beyond one week postinjury. Thus, PTA as a classification system reaches ceiling levels for patients at the more severe end of the severity spectrum, resulting in decreased prognostic value for this index as defined by Russell and Smith (1961). Newer classification systems for PTA duration have been proposed, demonstrating that PTA durations of four and eight weeks are better threshold points for predicting functional outcome (Walker et al., 2010). Likewise, a new Mississippi PTA classification scheme examined and validated by Nakase-Richardson and colleagues (Nakase-Richardson et al., 2009; Nakase-Richardson et al., 2011) shows improved prediction of later outcome compared with the original Russell classification system.

There are clear pros and cons of using each of these indices to determine injury severity. Further complicating the issue is that classification using these indices independently does not always correspond to the same injury severity level within a given patient. Thus, a given patient's injury can be assigned different severity levels depending on which of these indices is considered. To illustrate this point, Sherer, Struchen, Nakase-Thompson, and Yablon (2005) compared these three indices of TBI severity in a sample of 259 consecutive admissions to an acute rehabilitation setting and found significant discrepancies in classification depending on which index was used. When GCS scores were used, 63% of patients were classified as severe, 19% of patients were classified as moderate, and 18% of patients were classified as mild. Of note, 88% of "mild" patients had pathology on initial CT. Using GCS as the standard, the time to follow commands criteria reported by Lezak and colleagues (Lezak, 1995; Lezak et al., 2004) misclassified as severe 84% of patients with a moderate level of injury and 72% of patients with a mild level of injury. Russell and Smith's PTA criteria (1961) misclassified as severe 100% of patients with a moderate level of injury and 87% of patients with a mild level of injury. Thus, studies using a combination of these indices to assign subjects to severity levels should be interpreted with caution. Additional caution should be taken when relying on a patient's self-report of duration of coma and PTA to estimate severity of injury, given recent findings that individuals with a history of TBI consistently overestimate coma duration by approximately ten days (Sherer Sander, Maestas, Pastorek, Nick & Li, 2015).

Neuroanatomical Findings Following TBI

Although the circumstances under which the brain can be injured are diverse, two principal mechanisms have been described. First, contact injuries occur either when an object strikes the head or when the brain comes into contact with the skull. Second, acceleration/deceleration injuries result from unrestricted movement of the head resulting in shear, tensile, and compressive strain on brain tissues (Gennarelli & Graham, 2005). Similarly, categorization of injury can be described as focal, affecting a circumscribed region(s) of the brain, or diffuse, affecting the brain in a widespread pattern (Graham, Gennarelli, & McIntosh, 2002).

Mechanism of injury determines to a large extent the nature of the resulting pathology to the brain. That is, the pathology resulting from a contact injury tends to be focal in nature and may include injury to the scalp, skull fracture, surface contusions, and associated intracerebral hematomas. Pathology resulting from acceleration/deceleration injuries often includes tearing of bridging veins, subdural hematomas, diffuse axonal injury, and diffuse vascular injury (Gennarelli & Graham, 2005). In addition to the primary brain changes that occur as a direct result of the injury itself, secondary or delayed complications can also occur, leading to further neuropathologic damage. Secondary factors can include swelling/edema, hypoxia/ischemia, raised intracranial pressure, associated vascular changes, meningitis, and abscess (Gennarelli & Graham, 2005). Secondary factors—particularly raised intracranial pressure, hypoxia, and hypotensive events—have been found to be predictive of later outcome (Andrews et al., 2002; Jiang, Gao, Li, Yu, & Zhu, 2002; King, Carlier, & Marion, 2005).

Lesions of the scalp, skull, and dura provide a clue to the site and nature of the injury. For instance, bruising at the back of the head is often associated with severe frontal contusions as a result of coup contra coup injuries (Gennarelli & Graham, 2005). Whereas the presence of a skull fracture does not necessarily indicate underlying brain damage (Williams et al., 1990), the absence of skull fracture does not mean that the brain has not been injured. In fact 20% of fatal cases do not have skull fracture (Jennett & Teasdale, 1981). There is a strong association, however, between the presence of a skull fracture and development of an intracranial hematoma (Mendelow et al., 1983).

Contusions have been considered the hallmark of brain damage following TBI, with a characteristic distribution involving the frontal and temporal poles, the lateral and inferior aspects of the frontal and temporal lobes, and less commonly the inferior aspects of the cerebellum (Adams, Graham, Scott, Parker, & Doyle, 1980; Gennarelli & Graham, 2005; Holbourn, 1943; Levin, Amparo, et al., 1987; Levin, Williams, Eisenberg, High, & Guinto, 1992). This pattern of findings is most likely due to friction caused between the brain and the bony ridges on the surface of the skull in these areas (Ommaya & Gennarelli, 1974). These parenchymal contusions often result in focal signs and symptoms and have been blamed in some studies for the frontal executive behavioral deficits following TBI (Levin, Amparo, et al., 1987; Levin et al., 1993). However, other studies have found no differences in neuropsychological functioning between groups of TBI patients with and without lesions confined to the frontal lobes on tests of executive functioning (Anderson, Bigler, & Blatter, 1995).

Intracranial hematomas are commonly seen following TBI and are the most common cause of serious clinical deterioration in patients who initially present well (Reilly, Graham, Adams, & Jennett, 1975; Rockswold, Leonard, & Nagib, 1987). Subarachnoid hemorrhage is frequent in moderate to severe TBI and typically occurs in conjunction with surface contusions. When present, subarachnoid hemorrhage is related to worse outcome at time of discharge from acute hospitalization and worse neuropsychological and vocational outcome at one year postinjury (Hanlon, Demery, Kuczen, & Kelly, 2005). An epidural hematoma consists of a convex-shaped collection of clotted blood between the skull and the dura. Most commonly, this type of hematoma results from temporal bone fracture and tearing of the middle meningeal artery, but it can also occur in relation to the frontal or parietal aspects of the brain. Because the source of bleeding is arterial, the hematoma develops rapidly, causing mass effect. If they are not treated quickly, epidural hematomas can be life-threatening, but in many cases there is little associated underlying brain damage (Gennarelli & Graham, 2005).

Subdural hematoma (SDH) results from rupture to bridging veins between the upper surface of the brain to the sagittal sinus (Gennarelli & Thibault, 1982). Because this blood can spread freely throughout the subdural space, SDHs tend to cover a large area and often appear crescent-shaped on neuroimaging. SDHs are often large enough to act as significant mass lesions and have been reported in between 26% to 63% of blunt head injuries (Freytag, 1963; Maloney & Whatmore, 1969). The incidence of SDH may be higher in patients sustaining fall injuries than other types of injuries (Gennarelli & Thibault, 1982). While in a small percentage of cases (8%–13%) these hematomas are not associated with other brain damage, most are associated with considerable brain damage, resulting in relatively greater mortality and morbidity compared with epidural hematomas (Gennarelli & Graham, 2005). Although early reports describe overall mortality rates from acute subdural hematomas ranging from 40% to 90%, with poor outcomes observed in all age groups, more recent studies indicate mortality rates are more than four times higher in older patients than in younger ones (74% vs. 18%) despite similar treatment (Howard et al., 1989). SDH may take longer to cause a marked decrease in level of consciousness in older adults as compared to younger adults due to a greater amount of cortical atrophy and slower time to midline shift, thus initial GCS may be a less-sensitive indicator in older adults (Rothweiler et al., 1998).

In acceleration/deceleration injuries, the brain is at particular risk for diffuse axonal injury (DAI) (Gennarelli, 1983; Gennarelli & Graham, 2005). DAI refers to a number of pathologies including hemorrhages and tissue tears seen throughout the brain. The cerebral commissures and other white matter tracts of the brain stem are vulnerable to stretching and shearing as a result of mechanical forces (Gennarelli, 1983). The extent of DAI may be the principal pathological substrate responsible for the range of neurological deficit from mild to severe brain injury (Gennarelli et al., 1982). For instance, DAI was determined to be the cause of death in a group of individuals with fatal TBI without associated intracranial mass lesion (Gennarelli, 1983). Evidence from animal models suggests that extensive DAI in the brain stem may play a contributory role in posttraumatic coma (Gennarelli, 1994). Further, clusters of microglia have been found even in patients with mild brain injury who died of unrelated causes (Oppenheimer, 1968).

DAI is generally not readily apparent on traditional MRI scans but can be seen microscopically with the histological appearance depending on the length of survival after injury. Diffusion tensor imaging (DTI), which allows visualization of disruptions in white matter pathways, has been proposed to indicate DAI in acute recovery from mild TBI (Arfanakis et al., 2002; Inglese et al., 2005; Wilde et al., 2008; Yallampalli et al., 2013). Although some studies demonstrate relationships between abnormal DTI findings and severity of postconcussion symptoms and cognitive functioning in acute mild TBI (Wilde et al., 2008; Yallampalli et al., 2013), other studies have not replicated these findings (Lange, Iverson, Brubacher, Madler, & Heran, 2012; Waljas et al., 2014). DTI abnormalities have also been proposed as a marker for chronic white matter changes years after injury in individuals with moderate to severe TBI (Kennedy et al., 2009; Kraus et al., 2007; Wilde et al., 2006) with abnormal DTI findings showing relationships with impaired cognitive functioning (Kraus et al., 2007). White matter changes seen on DTI in chronic TBI samples may represent multiple injury processes including direct primary mechanisms such as DAI shearing, hemorrhages, and contusions; secondary mechanisms such as swelling; and tissue atrophy from Wallerian degeneration (Kennedy et al., 2009).

DTI studies to date demonstrate evidence that white matter changes exist on a continuum corresponding to severity of injury with greater white matter abnormality seen in more severe TBI and related to greater cognitive deficits (Kraus et al., 2007). Other studies have shown that DTI shows promise in tracking recovery in patients with severe TBI, with improved DTI indices related to more favorable outcome over time (Sidaros et al., 2008). Although further study is warranted to improve specificity, particularly with mild TBI, this technology is showing promise in detecting DAI and may ultimately become an early prognostic indicator in patients with TBI.

Course of Recovery from TBI

Individuals who sustain a moderate to severe brain injury typically pass through a series of predictable stages as they recover from injury to the brain. Almost all patients will pass through at least one of the stages described below. See Figure 17.1 for stages of recovery. While progression through these stages is fairly constant, specific stages and length of time spent in each varies significantly from patient to patient.

Impaired consciousness has been described as the hallmark of severe TBI, with coma representing the most extreme end of the spectrum (Levin, 1992; Ommaya & Gennarelli, 1974). Coma is a temporary nonresponsive state in which the patient has closed eyes, follows no instructions, gives no communication, and shows no purposeful movements (Teasdale & Jennett, 1974). Patients with severe injuries are often

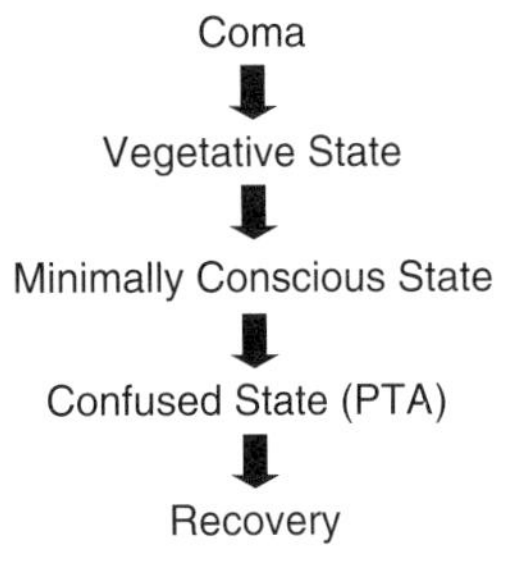

Figure 17.1 Stages of recovery

in coma for some period of time immediately following their injury. While 23%–49% of patients in coma do not recover from this state, those that do survive almost always recover to a more responsive state (Lippert-Gruner, Wedekind, & Klug, 2003; Murray et al., 1999; Zhang et al., 2001).

Following resolution of coma, a small percentage of surviving patients remain in a nonresponsive vegetative state (Lippert-Gruner et al., 2003; Murray et al., 1999), characterized by a complete absence of behavioral evidence for self or environmental awareness. These patients demonstrate recovery of some brain stem functioning and have return of sleep/wake cycles with periods of eye opening. Only a few patients remain in the vegetative state as their ultimate outcome. At three months postinjury, less than 10% of patients are in a vegetative state (Choi & Barnes, 1996; Choi et al., 1994) and by six months, only 4% remain vegetative (Murray et al., 1999). Of those who are vegetative at three months, 50% improve, 25% expire, and 25% remain in a vegetative state so that, by one year postinjury, the incidence of vegetative state ranges from less than 1% (Jiang et al., 2002) to 2% or 3% (Choi & Barnes, 1996; Choi et al., 1994) of severe TBI survivors.

Surviving, nonvegetative patients who go on to recover a limited degree of responsiveness to the environment may be classified as being in a minimally conscious state. Patients in this state show minimal, but definite, evidence of awareness of self or the environment, such as localized motor responses to noxious stimuli or sounds, sustained visual fixation, vocalization in response to a stimulus, smiling or crying in response to a stimulus, and inconsistent command following (Giacino et al., 2002). Resolution of the minimally conscious state is indicated by consistent command following, verbal or gestural yes/no responding, intelligible verbalization, or some other evidence of consistent purposeful behavior such as functional use of objects. This state is generally temporary but may be permanent in a small subset of patients.

In many cases, resolution of coma is followed by a responsive, but markedly confused state (bypassing vegetative and minimially conscious states). Likewise, patients with moderate TBI who have lost consciousness at the time of injury typically evolve directly into a responsive but confused state once consciousness is regained. This confused phase of recovery manifests in a variety of neurobehavioral impairments that were described by early writers (Russell, 1932; Symonds, 1937) as deficits in arousal, memory, orientation, attention, language, behavior, mood, and perception. This stage is generally referred to as PTA, but it has also been referred to as *acute traumatic psychosis, after effects of concussion, traumatic confusion,* and *delirium.*

The term *posttraumatic amnesia* is reflective of the fact that early investigations of this period of confusion after TBI primarily focused on disorientation and poor memory encoding (Russell, 1932; Symonds, 1937). These authors described PTA as the period of time between onset of injury and return of a patient's orientation and ability to encode and retain memories from day to day. High, Levin, and Gary (1990) confirmed the high rate of disorientation following TBI and found that orientation after TBI recovers sequentially with initial recovery of orientation to person followed by orientation to place and time. Memory disturbance after head trauma is characterized by some loss of ability to recall events immediately preceding injury (retrograde amnesia) as well as a period of inability to encode and later recall new memories (anterograde amnesia) (Levin, 1992). Complicating the concept of PTA is the presence of islands of intact memory within an otherwise amnestic period, a lucid interval with delayed amnesia, and progressive shrinkage in the temporal extent of retrograde amnesia (Russell, 1971).

While disorientation and memory disturbance are hallmarks of this phase of recovery, recent researchers have noted the similarity of this state to delirium rather than an amnestic state (Nakase-Thompson et al., 2004; Sherer, Nakase-Thompson, et al., 2005; Stuss et al., 1999). Specifically, Stuss and colleagues (1999) argued that attentional disturbance is a key aspect of impaired consciousness after TBI, with recovery of attention happening in an orderly manner prior to resolution of PTA based on GOAT scores. These authors noted the similarity of this state to delirium and proposed the term "posttraumatic confusional state" (PTCS) to replace the more commonly used PTA.

Providing further support of this conceptualization, Nakase-Thompson, Sherer, Yablon, and colleagues (2004) found that 59 (69%) of 85 consecutive TBI patients admitted for inpatient rehabilitation met diagnostic criteria for delirium (American Psychiatric Association, 1994) at some point during their hospitalizations, and the presence of delirium was associated with poorer functional outcome at discharge from inpatient rehabilitation (Nakase-Thompson, Sherer, Yablon, Kennedy, & Nick, 2002). Sherer and colleagues (Sherer, Yablon, & Nick, 2014) found that seven key symptoms characterize the confused state after TBI, including (a) disorientation, (b) impaired cognition, (c) restlessness, (d) fluctuation of symptom presentation, (e) sleep disturbance, (f) decreased daytime level of arousal, and (g) psychotic-type symptoms. PTA (or PTCS) presents in a heterogeneous fashion but has been shown to have a predictable pattern of symptom resolution, such that psychotic-type symptoms, decreased daytime arousal, and nighttime sleep disturbance resolve the earliest and fluctuation and cognitive impairment remain the most persistent (Sherer, Yablon, & Nakase-Richardson, 2009). Sherer, Yablon, Nakase-Richardson, and Nick (2008) showed that presence of psychotic-type symptoms (e.g., hallucinations or delusions) during inpatient rehabilitation was associated with poorer long-term outcome, even though all patients showed resolution of these symptoms and none showed new onset of a persistent psychotic disorder. In a follow-up study, shorter time postinjury, more severe cognitive impairment, and presence of sleep disturbance were associated with a greater likelihood for psychotic-type symptoms with the presence of psychotic-type symptoms early in recovery from TBI serving as a negative prognostic indicator (Sherer, Yablon, & Nick, 2014).

For some, recovery may be compromised by late (greater than two weeks postinjury) complications such as posttraumatic seizures or posttraumatic hydrocephalus. The incidence of late seizures is lower in survivors of nonpenetrating TBI (4%–7%), compared to survivors of penetrating TBI (up to 50%) (Annegers, Hauser, Coan, & Rocca, 1998; Yablon, 1996). The incidence of posttraumatic hydrocephalus is less well known due to variation in the degree of monitoring for this condition. One prospective series in which all patients with moderate or severe TBI admitted for inpatient rehabilitation received head CT scans found an incidence of hydrocephalus of 13% (Yu, Yablon, Ivanhoe, & Boake, 1995).

After resolution of PTA, patients continue to show progressive resolution of physical, cognitive, and behavioral impairments. Impaired performances are consistently seen soon after injury on tests of reasoning, concept formation, cognitive flexibility, and psychomotor speed, and are inconsistently seen on tests of attention, concentration, and incidental memory (Dikmen, Reitan, & Temkin, 1983). Improvement over time appears to be the rule, with general agreement that recovery continues for up to 18–24 months after moderate or severe TBI (Dikmen et al., 1983; Finnanger et al., 2013; Levin, 1995; Tabaddor, Mattis, & Zazula, 1984). There is evidence that some cognitive functions may continue to recover beyond this time frame (Millis et al., 2001; van Zomeren & Deelman, 1978).

Persistent motor impairments, including spasticity, dysphagia (impaired swallowing), dysarthria, balance disturbances, or hemiparesis, may be present in TBI patients with large focal hemispheric lesions or certain subcortical, brain stem, or cerebellar lesions (Bontke, Zasler, & Boake, 1996; Horn & Sherer, 1999). Most patients with moderate or severe TBI, however, show good resolution of motor impairments and (when present) motor impairments are less likely than cognitive and emotional impairments to interfere with return to independent functioning and productive activity (Brooks, McKinlay, Symington, Beattie, & Campsie, 1987).

When considering very long-term outcome, the link between moderate to severe TBI and risk for dementia later in life has been repeatedly established (Fleminger, Oliver, Lovestone, Rabe-Hesketh, & Giora, 2003; Guo et al., 2000; Jellinger, Paulus, Wrocklage, & Litvan, 2001; Lee et al., 2013; Lye & Shores, 2000; Mortimer et al., 1991; Plassman et al., 2000; Rasmusson, Brandt, Martin, & Folstein, 1995; Salib & Hillier, 1997; Schofield et al., 1997; Starkstein & Jorge, 2005; van Duijn et al., 1992; Wang et al., 2012). Systematic reviews (Bazarian, Cernak, Noble-Haeusslein, Potolicchio, & Temkin, 2009; Institute of Medicine, 2009) conclude an increased risk of dementia in individuals with a previous history of at least one moderate to severe TBI compared to those with no TBI history. Some studies provide evidence that history of TBI accelerates dementia onset by a few years (Gedye, Beattie, Tuokko, Horton, & Korsarek, 1989; Nemetz et al.,

1999; Schofield et al., 1997) and that risk for developing dementia increases with increasing severity of TBI (Guo et al., 2000; Plassman et al., 2000). Explanations for the risk of dementia following TBI focus on a presumed neuropathological trigger at the time of injury that persists and evolves over time, ultimately resulting in progression to dementia. Both human studies and animal models have convincingly demonstrated that multiple proteins associated with neurodegenerative disorders accumulate as a result of TBI (Uryu et al., 2007) particularly within axons damaged by trauma (Johnson, Stewart, & Smith, 2010).

Neuropsychological and Neurobehavioral Functioning After Moderate and Severe TBI

The magnitude and pattern of cognitive and neurobehavioral impairments resulting from moderate and severe TBI vary widely across patients. This heterogeneity in outcome is caused by many factors, including patient variables such as premorbid level of functioning, type and severity of injury, and representativeness of the sample being studied. Risk for persistent cognitive impairment is related to initial injury severity as indicated by postresuscitation GCS score or time to follow commands, with more significant cognitive impairment seen in those with the most severe initial injuries (Dikmen & Machamer, 1995; Tabaddor et al., 1984). Furthermore, the extent and pattern of cognitive impairment depends to a great extent on severity of injury and timing of the assessment relative to injury, with recovery seen across almost all areas of cognitive functioning (Dikmen et al., 1983; Finnanger et al., 2013; Millis et al., 2001).

At one month postinjury, Dikmen and colleagues (1986) found that brain injury resulted in deficits on almost all measures of neuropsychological functioning included in a comprehensive battery of tests when compared to a matched control group. Specifically, these authors found that the degree of neuropsychologic impairment depended on the severity of head injury, with those with the most severe injuries showing impairments on most measures including motor speed, attention, cognitive flexibility, processing speed, memory, and reasoning skills. Impairments in less severely injured groups (time to follow commands between one and 24 hours) were more selective, occurring most frequently on tests of memory, cognitive flexibility, and psychomotor speed.

Lasting cognitive impairment is not uncommon in patients with moderate to severe TBI, with those with the most severe injuries demonstrating the widest range of cognitive impairment. At one year postinjury, all patients with very severe TBI (time to follow commands > 14 days) have residual cognitive impairments, while more than one half of those with time to follow commands between one hour and 13 days have residual deficits (Dikmen & Machamer, 1995). This pattern remains in more recent studies, showing executive functioning deficits in patients with moderate and severe TBI, whereas patients with severe TBI demonstrated a much broader range of cognitive deficits in areas of motor function, processing speed, and memory (Finnanger et al., 2013).

Improvement is the general rule, with evidence of improved cognitive functioning from three to 12 months across multiple cognitive domains for both moderate and severe TBI (Finnanger et al., 2013). Continuing improvements are seen for 12–24 months postinjury (Dikmen, Machamer, Temkin, & McLean, 1990; Dikmen et al., 1983; Tabaddor et al., 1984). Tasks requiring more complex functions, such as problem solving and complex attention, appear to recover more slowly than tests with more simple cognitive demands (Dikmen et al., 1983). Although a subgroup of patients shows improvement beyond the typically reported 18–24 month follow-up (Millis et al., 2001), there is limited evidence that another subgroup of patients may show late decline (Millis et al., 2001; Ruff et al., 1991). Age at time of injury appears to be a risk factor for late decline, with older age at time of injury indicating greater risk for late decline.

Overall, the typical pattern of impairments after blunt head trauma includes slowed fine motor movements, decreased attention, decreased cognitive speed, memory impairment, impaired complex language skills and discourse, and impaired executive functions. Severe persistent aphasia or visual perceptual impairment are uncommon after diffuse injuries but may occur in patients with focal injuries (Levin, 1993). Tate and colleagues (1991) followed a consecutive series of 100 patients with severe blunt head injuries for up six years after trauma to examine potential patterns of cognitive impairment. Principal component analyses were applied to 85 of these patients to examine the incidence of impairment in specific neuropsychological domains, including classical neuropsychological syndromes, learning and memory, rate of information processing, and personality change. Seventy percent of patients showed cognitive impairment, and isolated cognitive findings were common. Although no single functional area was consistently impaired, the most frequent area of impairment was learning and memory, occurring in 56.5% of patients. When premorbid functioning is accounted for using tests of reading recognition, patients with TBI show the greatest decline in performance on tests of information processing speed and cognitive flexibility, followed by less significant declines on tests of immediate and delayed memory. Overall intellectual level is only minimally affected (Johnstone, Hexum, & Ashkanazi, 1995).

Although discrete cognitive findings may be seen in patients with focal injuries, these are generally superimposed on global cognitive dysfunction resulting from diffuse injury. While there is great variability in the pattern of cognitive dysfunction in individual patients with moderate to severe TBI, the most commonly affected areas of cognition include attention, memory, language and communication, and executive functioning.

Attention

Impaired attentional processes and information processing speed are prevalent after TBI across all levels of injury severity. Specifically, patients with TBI consistently demonstrate impairments on tests of simple and choice reaction-time, color naming and word reading, symbol digit coding, and divided attention (Finnanger et al., 2013; Ponsford & Kinsella, 1992; Stuss, Stethem, Hugenholtz, et al., 1989; Stuss, Stethem, Picton, Leech, & Pelchat, 1989). Even patients with supposed good recovery continue to show impairments on tests of complex attention and higher level reasoning skills (Stuss et al., 1985). While many studies have described a primary deficit in attention, others have suggested that deficits in information processing speed underlie these attentional impairments (Ponsford & Kinsella, 1992).

Memory

Memory dysfunction is also common after TBI, even in postacute phases, with a dose–response relationship such that greater impairments in memory are seen with increasing levels of injury severity (Carlozzi, Grech, & Tulsky, 2013). In patients with moderate to severe TBI, dysfunction in memory often persists even after normalization of other areas of cognition (Ruff et al., 1991). Investigators report that memory problems occur across different aspects of memory processing including encoding, consolidation, and retrieval (Curtiss, Vanderploeg, Spencer, & Salazar, 2001; Wright & Schmitter-Edgecombe, 2011) while others suggest that patients with TBI have specific problems in the consolidation of newly learned information leading to poor recall of information over time (Vanderploeg, Crowell, & Curtiss, 2001; Vanderploeg, Donnell, Belanger, & Curtiss, 2014). While memory performance tends to improve in most TBI patients over time (Finnanger et al., 2013), a select group fails to show improvement or may even show decline. It has been speculated that the presence of injury-related factors such as hypoxia may contribute to a failure for performance to improve over time, and patient-related factors such as depression may contribute to declines in performance (Ruff et al., 1991). Further research is needed to better understand this observed heterogeneity of performance on memory measures and to determine if distinct memory problems characterize subgroups of patients. Specific deficits have also been noted on tasks of prospective memory, or the ability to remember one's future intentions (Huang et al., 2014; Kinsella et al., 1996; Mathias & Mansfield, 2005), episodic and autobiographical memory (Rasmussen & Berntsen, 2014), and meta-memory or the awareness of memory efficiency (Kennedy & Yorkston, 2000).

Language and communication

Although persisting classic aphasia syndromes are rare following TBI, impairments in language are common, including deficits in naming, verbal fluency, and comprehension of complex commands (Levin, Grossman, & Kelly, 1976; Sarno, Buonaguro, & Levita, 1986). Traditional neuropsychological tests may be insensitive to language and communication problems observed in patients with TBI, especially at postacute stages. For instance, studies of naturalistic language have shown that patients with TBI demonstrate less productive speech, convey less content with longer utterances, and have generally more fragmented language than their peers (Hartley & Jensen, 1991). Difficulties in pragmatic language have also been reported in patients with TBI, including problems initiating and maintaining a conversation and interpreting indirect communication (Snow & Douglas, 2000). Similarly, deficits in social cognition (emotion recognition, theory of mind, empathy) have been specifically reported following TBI (Spikman, Timmerman, Milders, Veenstra, & van der Naalt, 2012). These problems in language functioning and social cognition likely contribute to impairments in psychosocial functioning.

Executive function

Executive dysfunction is common following TBI and may be one of the critical cognitive determinants of independent functioning and return to occupational functioning (Crepeau & Scherzer, 1993; Finnanger et al., 2013; Hart et al., 2003; Sherer, Nick, Millis, & Novack, 2003). Patients with moderate to severe TBI show a wide range of executive function deficits, with reported impairments on tests of verbal and design fluency (Millis et al., 2001; Ruff, Evans, & Marshall, 1986), conceptual reasoning/flexibility (Millis et al., 2001; Sherer, Nick, Millis, et al., 2003; Stuss et al., 1985), working memory (Stuss et al., 1985; Stuss, Stethem, Hugenholtz, et al., 1989), response inhibition (Rochat, Beni, Annoni, Vuadens, & Van der Linden, 2013), application of clustering strategies on verbal memory testing (Levin & Goldstein, 1986), time discrimination (Mioni, Stablum, & Cantagallo, 2013), and planning (Leon-Carrion et al., 1998). However, performance on formal neuropsychological tasks may fail to capture the executive-based neurobehavioral deficits seen in social functioning and self-regulation frequently seen in patients with TBI (Levine, Dawson, Boutet, Schwartz, & Stuss, 2000).

Persistent neurobehavioral impairments and impaired psychosocial functioning are common in patients with TBI. Specifically, patients are noted to have increased irritability, headache, anxiety and depression, difficulty concentrating, fatigue, restlessness, and impulsivity/aggression (Bhalerao et al., 2013; O'Dell, Barr, Spanier, & Warnick, 1998; Satz et al., 1998). Patients and family members are more distressed by these neurobehavioral impairments, particularly personality change and threats of violence, than either cognitive or physical impairments (Brooks, Campsie, Symington, Beattie, & McKinlay, 1986; Kaitaro, Koskinen, & Kaipio, 1995; Lezak, 1987, 1988). There is some evidence that family member report of these symptoms may actually increase with the passage of time (Brooks et al., 1986), but it is unclear whether this is due to an actual increase in behavioral problems or to greater sensitivity to these problems.

Limited awareness of cognitive and psychosocial problems is common after TBI and may play a role in family member stress associated with residual neurobehavioral impairments (Prigatano, Altman, & O'Brien, 1990; Sherer, Boake, et al., 1998). Impaired self-awareness is common after moderate and severe TBI both in the acute (Sherer, Hart, et al., 2003) and the postacute periods (Sherer, Bergloff, et al., 1998; Vanderploeg, Belanger, Duchnick, & Curtiss, 2007). Although self-awareness improves over time, impairments in self-awareness have been shown to persist five years or more following injury (Kelley et al., 2014). Self-awareness of cognitive impairment is related to employability and employment outcomes (Sherer, Bergloff, et al., 1998; Sherer, Hart, et al., 2003), presumably because awareness of cognitive impairments is needed in order for an individual to appreciate the need for and learn compensatory strategies needed to maintain employment (Kelley et al., 2014). Patients with poor self-awareness have poor motivation to change, as they do not perceive the need to change. Some authors have suggested the decreased ability to recognize and acknowledge changes in one's functioning may be related to impaired executive functions and abstract reasoning (Malec & Moessner, 2000). Life satisfaction has been shown to be higher for individuals who *perceive* higher levels of neurological impairment, even when this perception is discrepant from that reported by their significant others (Kelley et al., 2014). In return, there is evidence that distress and symptoms of depression increase with increasing self-awareness (Godfrey, Partridge, Knight, & Bishara, 1993).

Neuropsychological Assessment of Patients with Moderate and Severe TBI

Given the range of cognitive and neurobehavioral impairments resulting from TBI and their impact on functional outcome, psychosocial functioning, and family functioning, neuropsychologists are poised to make significant contributions to the care of persons with moderate and severe TBI. Evaluations of neuropsychological functioning can provide documentation of cognitive, behavioral, and emotional status that may ultimately assist with determination of patients' ability to function independently (Sherer & Novack, 2003). Specifically, neuropsychologists are asked to determine functional abilities, such as decision-making capacity, capacity for safe and independent home functioning, driving capacity, and ability to return to work. Additionally, documentation of neuropsychological functioning is useful to provide feedback to family members, improve patient self-awareness, guide treatment efforts, assess the effectiveness of medication trials, and assist with discharge planning.

The focus of neuropsychological assessment is determined both by the goals of the assessment and the stage of recovery of the patient. Early neuropsychological assessment may focus on determining level of responsiveness and documenting changes in level of responsiveness in minimally conscious patients. Measures such as the Coma Recovery Scale–Revised (Giacino, Kalmar, & Whyte, 2004) assess arousal and attention, auditory perception, visual perception, motor function, oromotor ability, communication, and initiation, and provide a structured repeatable protocol for assessing low-level patients. With responsive but confused patients, assessment focuses on orientation, attentional skills, ability to form new memories, and level of agitation. Measures such as the GOAT (Levin et al., 1979) or Orientation Log (Jackson et al., 1998) are well suited to assess orientation, while the Toronto Test of Acute Recovery After TBI (Stuss et al., 1999) includes simple measures of attentional skills and the ability to form and retain new memories. The Agitated Behavior Scale (Corrigan, 1989) is the most commonly used measure of agitation after TBI. The Confusion Assessment Protocol (Sherer, Nakase-Thompson, et al., 2005) includes elements of all these areas, and findings indicate that it may be useful in assessing a wide range of symptoms of confusion after TBI.

There is some disagreement about when to first administer traditional neuropsychological tests. Some recommend delaying administration of formal neuropsychological tests until the patient has emerged from PTA (Clifton et al., 1992), due to the assumption that confused, disoriented patients will perform poorly on all tests resulting in limited information regarding profile of cognitive strengths and weaknesses. In contrast, there is evidence that administration of selected neuropsychological measures to patients still in PTA is feasible (Kalmar et al., 2008) and can result in useful data that are predictive of later functional status (Hannay & Sherer, 1996; Pastorek, Hannay, & Contant, 2004). In an attempt to provide some guidance regarding timing of neuropsychological evaluations for patients with TBI, Sherer and Novack (2003) conducted a survey of neuropsychologists who were selected based on board certification, extensive clinical experience with TBI, published research on TBI, and current participation in TBI research. Guidelines for timing of assessments based on this survey were contingent on severity of injury and period of time since injury. For instance, respondents recommended preliminary testing at resolution of PTA for all levels of TBI severity. Early testing between one week and one month postinjury was recommended for patients with mild TBI with repeat assessment at one year. In contrast, respondents recommended that the initial follow up testing not occur until three months for patients with moderate to severe injury, with subsequent repeat assessments as needed at six months, one year, and two years postinjury. Importantly, these guidelines provide general suggestions only, and timing of testing for any specific patient should be determined by clinician judgment based on factors unique to that patient.

Although several different neuropsychological batteries have been used in the literature to assess the cognitive effects of TBI, no specific battery of tests for TBI has been proposed or widely accepted. However, batteries such as the NIH Toolbox (Weintraub et al., 2013), a computerized battery of cognitive tests designed for longitudinal cognitive assessment, are being used in large-scale longitudinal studies of TBI and may show promise as an effective TBI outcome measure in the future. There is also emerging evidence supporting the use of the Neuropsychological Assessment Battery (NAB) for assessment of cognitive impairment following TBI (Donders & Levitt, 2012). Regardless of battery chosen, neuropsychological evaluations of persons with moderate or severe TBI should assess a wide range of cognitive abilities including orientation, fine motor skills, divided and sustained attention, cognitive speed, learning and memory, language skills, visual-perceptual skills, and executive functions (Hannay & Sherer, 1996). Despite the presence of clear-cut evidence that a patient has sustained a brain injury (i.e., neuroimaging reports, medical documentation of loss of consciousness or coma, and operative reports), some patients may either consciously or unconsciously exaggerate symptoms when seen for follow-up evaluations. This possibility is even stronger for those engaged in litigation or with other secondary gain issues. Consequently, symptom validity measures should be included in assessment batteries when appropriate. Further, comparison of current performance with past neuropsychological reports may be helpful to document expected trajectory of recovery over time. With no other intervening factors, it would be unusual and unexpected for neuropsychological performance to decline significantly over time.

In addition to cognition, neurobehavioral problems such as mental flexibility, planning, unusual thought content, agitation, disinhibition, emotional withdrawal, hostility, depression, anxiety, and motor slowing should also be assessed (McCauley et al., 2001). Such neurobehavioral impairments are frequently assessed with measures such as the Neurobehavioral Rating Scale (Levin, High, et al., 1987) and the Neurobehavioral Functioning Inventory (Kreutzer, Marwitz, Seel, & Serio, 1996).

Functional status is a separate but important factor to consider in a neuropsychological evaluation. Thus, it is often beneficial to assess functional status separately from traditional neuropsychological measures. There are a number of instruments that can be used to directly rate a given patient's functional status. The Disability Rating Scale (DRS) (Rappaport, Hall, Hopkins, Belleza, & Cope, 1982) was developed to track patient progress after TBI from coma to return to community activities (Gouvier, Blanton, LaPorte, & Nepomuceno, 1987; Rappaport et al., 1982). It has been shown to be sensitive to improvements in functioning between two and six months postinjury, as well as between six months and one year (Hall, Cope, & Rappaport, 1985). The Supervision Rating Scale (SRS) (Boake, 1996) can be used to quantify the level of personal independence. SRS scores are related to patient living arrangement and to skills in activities of daily living. Additionally, assessment of participation in community activities and societal roles is crucial to understanding the long-term impact of TBI. The Community Integration Questionnaire (CIQ) (Willer, Rosenthal, Kreutzer, Gordon, & Rempel, 1993) was developed to assess degree of community integration after TBI across three areas, including home integration, social integration, and productive activity. More recently, items from previously validated measures of participation were combined to create the Participation Assessment with Recombined Tools—Objective (PART-O). The PART-O measures important aspects of participation such as involvement in productive activities, degree of social integration, and community involvement (Bogner, Bellon, Kolakowsky-Hayner, & Whiteneck, 2013; Whiteneck et al., 2011).

Outcome After Moderate and Severe TBI

Outcome after moderate and severe TBI can be assessed in many ways and at many time points postinjury. Neurosurgical studies generally focus on early survival, with the Glasgow Outcome Scale (GOS; see Jennett & Bond, 1975) being the most commonly used measure of overall outcome after TBI. Table 17.2 presents a breakdown of the five different GOS categories. Table 17.3 provides a summary of global outcome for patients with moderate and severe TBI over time intervals ranging from three months to one year using the GOS as an outcome variable. As expected, global outcome varies significantly depending on the time point examined

Table 17.2 Description of individual categories for the Glasgow Outcome Scale (GOS)

GOS Category	*Description*
Death	
Vegetative State	Unable to follow commands or communicate.
Severe Disability	Conscious but requiring assistance to meet basic physical and cognitive needs such as feeding, toileting, grooming, or personal safety.
Moderate Disability	Able to meet basic physical and cognitive needs and use public transportation and work in a sheltered workshop, but unable to return to nonsheltered work or resume other major societal roles.
Good Recovery	Able to return to nonsheltered work though perhaps in a decreased capacity and resume social roles, though some neurologic or psychologic impairments may remain.

Table 17.3 Global outcome based on the Glasgow Outcome Scale for TBI Patients with Severe and Moderate Injuries. Numbers represent percentage of TBI patients in each category.

Severe TBI				*Moderate TBI*
	3 months postinjury	6 months postinjury	1 year postinjury	6 months postinjury
Death	23%–50% [1,2,3,4,5]			< 10% [3,8]
Vegetative State	< 10% [6,7]	4% [3]	< 1% [5]–3% [6,7]	
Severe Disability	31%–32% [6,7]	22% [3,6,7]	17% [6,7]	0% [8]–14% [3,9]
Moderate Disability	30% [3,6,7]	30% [3,6,7]	17%–22% [4,6]	25% [8,9,10]
Good Recovery	22% [6,7]	35% [3,6]	46%–54% [4,6]	53% [9]–73% [10]

[1] Braakman, Gelpke, Habbema, Maas, and Minderhoud (1980)
[2] Marion (1996)
[3] Murray et al. (1999)
[4] Zhang et al. (2001)
[5] Jiang et al. (2002)
[6] Choi, et al., 1994
[7] Choi et al. (1996)
[8] Stein (1996)
[9] Williams et al. (1990)
[10] Jain, Layton and Murray (2000)

postinjury with a general trend toward better outcome with passing time.

Death is a relatively common outcome for patients sustaining a severe TBI, occurring in approximately 40% of hospitalized patients. Specific death rates range from 23% to 50% (Braakman et al., 1980; Jiang et al., 2002; Marion, 1996; Murray et al., 1999; Zhang et al., 2001). Causes of early death after severe TBI include brain swelling, diffuse axonal injury, increased intracranial pressure, and intracranial hematomas (Graham, Adams, & Gennarelli, 1993; Marion, 1996). In contrast, death is a rare outcome after moderate TBI, occurring in fewer than 10% of cases (Murray et al., 1999; Stein, 1996). When death does occur, it is likely to be due to associated trauma or medical complications (Signorini, Andrews, Jones, Wardlaw, & Miller, 1999).

Factors most predictive of death after TBI are those that directly indicate neurologic and physiologic status early after injury. Such factors include: (a) level of responsiveness as indicated by admission GCS score (Eisenberg & Weiner, 1987; Mosenthal et al., 2002), (b) pupillary responses (Andrews et al., 2002; Jiang et al., 2002; Wardlaw et al., 2002), (c) initial CT scan findings (particularly presence of subarachnoid blood or mass lesion such as subdural hematoma) (Eisenberg & Weiner, 1987; Mataro et al., 2001; Wardlaw et al., 2002), (d) elevated temperature (Andrews et al., 2002; Jiang et al., 2002), (e) electrophysiologic findings (Claassen & Hansen, 2001; Vespa et al., 2002), (f) elevated intracranial pressure (Eisenberg & Weiner, 1987; Jiang et al., 2002), and (g) hypoxia (Andrews et al., 2002; Eisenberg & Weiner, 1987; Jiang et al., 2002). Of demographic variables, age is most predictive of death, with older age being associated with greater risk of death (Jiang et al., 2002; Mosenthal et al., 2002; Susman et al., 2002). Early neurosurgical management also affects death rates. Centers that managed patients aggressively, as indicated by intracranial monitor placement, had 40% lower mortality rates than centers with less aggressive management (Bulger et al., 2002).

Vegetative state is a rare outcome after severe and moderate TBI, with between 1% and 3% of severe TBI patients remaining in this state at one year and reports of no cases in patients with moderate TBI in large trauma series (Murray et al., 1999). Approximately 31%–32% of surviving patients initially hospitalized with severe TBI were categorized as having Severe Disability (Choi & Barnes, 1996; Choi et al., 1994) at three months postinjury, compared with 30% of patients categorized as having Moderate Disability (Choi & Barnes, 1996; Choi et al., 1994; Murray et al., 1999) and 22% with Good Recovery (Choi & Barnes, 1996; Choi et al., 1994). Percentages of individuals with Severe Disability tend to decrease over time (Choi & Barnes, 1996; Choi et al., 1994; Murray et al., 1999) in conjunction with these patients progressing to higher levels of functioning. Improved functioning for those patients categorized in the Moderate Disability range at three months was masked by the fact that some patients progressed to Good Recovery while patients with Severe Disability improved to the Moderate Disability range. Thus, an overall trend is seen in which patients with severe TBI show gains in general functioning over time, evidenced by increases in the percentage of individuals categorized as having Good Recovery at six months and at one year (Choi et al., 1994; Zhang et al., 2001). However, it is important to note that these patients may remain with significant cognitive or neurobehavioral problems even though they have recovered well enough to return to work.

For patients with moderate TBI, few patients remain in Severe Disability at six months (Murray et al., 1999; Stein, 1996; Williams et al., 1990) and only 25% of patients remained in Moderate Disability at six months postinjury (Jain et al., 2000; Stein, 1996; Williams et al., 1990). Good Recovery is by far the most common outcome for patients with moderate TBI with 53% (Murray et al., 1999) to 73% (Williams et al., 1990) of cases showing Good Recovery by six months postinjury. As with severe TBI patients, Good Recovery cannot be taken to mean the absence of lasting impairments or functional disability.

The outcome studies discussed so far focus on survival and global disability but do not provide specific information about functional status, such as whether a patient will return to work, community activities, and/or independent living. In fact, it is this functional information that is often of most concern to clinicians, families, and patients, particularly in the inpatient rehabilitation setting where neuropsychologists are most likely to encounter these patients.

Disorders of consciousness (DOC)—including coma, vegetative state, and minimally conscious state— following TBI have gained increasing attention in the literature. While many individuals with DOC recover quickly, others remain with impaired consciousness for prolonged periods or even permanently. A recent large longitudinal study by Nakase-Richardson and colleagues (2012) examined the recovery course of patients who were admitted to acute inpatient rehabilitation with DOC. During inpatient rehabilitation, 68% regained consciousness and 23% emerged from PTA. Outcome was assessed at one, two, and five years postinjury and found that 8% had died within an average of two years after discharge. Of survivors, 21% improved to the point of living without in-house supervision, and 20% improved to the point of having employment potential based on the Disability Rating Scale. Importantly, despite a perception that patients with posttraumatic DOC have a poor prognosis regarding functional outcome, this study demonstrated substantial recovery among patients with DOC relatively early following injury with continuing recovery for two to five years postinjury.

There is a large body of literature examining employment outcomes and prediction of employment in patients with moderate and severe TBI with reported return to work rates ranging from 22% to 66% (Sander, Kreutzer, Rosenthal, Delmonico, & Young, 1996). The wide range of rates is contributed to by interstudy differences in injury classification, populations sampled, time from injury to follow-up, and definition of employment. An early study by Brooks and colleagues (1987) reported on a series of patients with severe TBI seen on an acute neurosurgical service with follow-up evaluations ranging from two to seven years postinjury. The employment rate dropped from 86% before injury to 29% after injury. Younger patients and those with technical/managerial jobs before injury were more likely to return to work than those over 45 years of age or in unskilled occupations. Physical deficits were less related to return to work than was the presence of cognitive, behavioral, and personality changes.

In their seminal study, Dikmen and colleagues (1994) reported on a series of 366 previously employed patients with TBI who were admitted to a trauma center. At one year postinjury, 26% of patients with severe injuries had returned to work and 56% of patients with moderate injuries had returned to work. By two years postinjury, 37% of patients with severe injuries were working while 64% of patients with moderate injuries were working. Age, education, stability of preinjury work history, and injury severity were all strongly related to the amount of time it took patients to return to work. Specifically, individuals over the age of 50, those with less than high school education, and those with an unstable preinjury work history were less likely to return to work and took longer to go back to work than those in other groups. Further, individuals with milder injuries went back to work more frequently and sooner than those with more severe injuries. Only 8% of those in the most severely injured group (time to follow commands > 29 days) returned to work by two years and those with the best neuropsychological abilities at one month postinjury had the highest return to work rates (96% by one year).

Doctor and colleagues (2005) examined unemployment rates among individuals with TBI one year postinjury after adjusting for risk of unemployment in the general population. This study found that 42% of individuals with TBI were unemployed at one year compared with a 9% expected unemployment rate based on demographically similar persons in the general population. Relative risk for unemployment was higher for males, those with higher levels of education, those with more severe injuries, and those with greater impairment on early neuropsychological and functional status. Specifically, greater risk for unemployment at one year was associated with poor performance on Trailmaking Test Part B, Performance IQ, and the Digit Symbol subtest of the Wechsler Adult Intelligence Scale administered at one month. Those that were unable to complete testing at one month showed the greatest risk of unemployment.

The studies just reviewed focused on consecutive cases seen at trauma centers. In contrast, many other studies of outcome focus on patients recruited from inpatient rehabilitation settings. While both populations are important to study, results from one population cannot necessarily be generalized to the other. Specifically, patients admitted for inpatient rehabilitation may exclude those with very poor outcomes such as vegetative patients or very good outcomes that might preclude them from entering inpatient rehabilitation programs. Such samples may be most representative of patients evaluated by neuropsychologists. One such study conducted by Sherer, Nick, Sander, and colleagues (2003) reported on 1615 patients with TBI who were admitted to 17 TBI Model Systems sites for inpatient rehabilitation. Of this population, 72% were employed at time of injury. Of the 1,083 patients with employment data available at one year, 63% had severe injuries, 16% had moderate injuries, and 20% had complicated mild injuries. The postinjury employment rate for these patients combined was 35%. However, patients available at follow-up had a higher preinjury employment rate (76%) than those lost to follow-up (68%). Thus, this postinjury employment rate is likely an overestimate.

Independent living outcomes have been studied less often than employment outcome, perhaps because of the greater difficulty in characterizing personal independence compared to employment status. Hart and colleagues (2003) examined predictors of supervision level using a series of 563 patients with TBI who were seen for inpatient rehabilitation. Patients who could not complete a neuropsychological evaluation during inpatient rehabilitation were excluded from study, meaning that patients with more severe injuries might be underrepresented in the study sample. Sixty-nine percent of this sample received no supervision at one-year follow-up, 24% received varying degrees of part-time supervision, and 7% received full-time supervision. Amount of supervision received at follow-up was generally related to initial injury severity as determined by GCS rating, such that individuals with more impaired GCS ratings received more supervision at follow-up. However, initial GCS scores ranged from 3 to 15 for those who were independent as well as for those receiving the highest levels of supervision at follow-up. Furthermore, in an analysis of a subgroup of patients who were able to complete neuropsychological testing, supervision at one year was predicted by educational level and scores on the Trail Making Test Part B and Digit Span Backward from the Wechsler Memory Scale–Revised.

Factors predictive of functional outcome (return to work and independent living) can be categorized as preinjury factors (preinjury employment status and demographic variables), injury severity variables, cognitive and neurobehavioral impairments, and environmental supports. As time from injury to outcome becomes greater, injury characteristics become less important and other factors such as premorbid functioning and environmental supports become more important. Interpretation of the literature predicting outcome following TBI is complicated by the wide variety of populations sampled, time frames of outcomes, potential predictors selected, and outcomes studied. Factors predictive of a given outcome in a particular population over a specified time frame may not be at all predictive of apparently related outcomes in a different population over a different time frame. This is particularly the case for subpopulations that are highly selected (e.g., patients admitted for postacute rehabilitation services). A review of studies using these variables to predict functional outcome is presented in Table 17.4.

Table 17.4 Factors predictive of functional outcome after TBI

Predictors	*References*
Preinjury factors	
Age	Brown et al., 2005; Keyser-Marcus et al., 2002; Poon, Zhu, Ng, & Wong, 2005; Ruff et al., 1993; Sherer, Nick, Sander, et al., 2003; Testa, Malec, Moessner, & Brown, 2005
Race/minority status	Arango-Lasprilla et al., 2011; Arango-Lasprilla & Kreutzer, 2010
Years of education	Hart et al., 2003; Ponsford, Draper, & Schonberger, 2008; Sherer, Bergloff, High, & Nick, 1999; Sherer et al., 2002
Pre-injury employment	Davis et al., 2012; Keyser-Marcus et al., 2002; Sherer et al., 2002
Pre-injury psychiatric status	Davis et al., 2012
Substance use	Davis et al., 2012; MacMillan, Hart, Martelli, & Zasler, 2002; Sherer et al., 1999
Injury severity variables	
Initial GCS	Dikmen et al., 1994; Levin et al., 1990; Poon et al., 2005
Time to follow commands	Dikmen et al., 1994; Hart et al., 2003; Ruff et al., 1993
Duration of PTA	Boake et al., 2001; Brown et al., 2005; Nakase-Richardson et al., 2009; Nakase-Richardson et al., 2011; Ponsford et al., 2008; Sherer et al., 2002; Walker et al., 2010
Neuroanatomical variables	Hanlon et al., 2005; Teasdale & Engberg, 2005; Wedekind & Lippert-Gruner, 2005
CT Scan Findings	Nelson et al., 2010; Williams et al., 2013
Physical Impairments	Brown et al., 2005
Cognitive and neurobehavioral impairments	
Early cognitive status	Boake et al., 2001; Dikmen et al., 1994; Hanks et al., 2008; Sherer et al., 2002; M. W. Williams et al., 2013
Attention & Executive Functioning	Finnanger et al., 2013
Postinjury depression/anxiety	Ponsford et al., 2008; Ruff et al., 1993; Seel et al., 2003
Impaired self-awareness	Kelley et al., 2014; Sherer, Bergloff, et al., 1998; Trudel, Tryon, & Purdum, 1998
Early functional status	Gollaher et al., 1998; Ponsford, Olver, Curran, & Ng, 1995
Environmental supports	
Family support	Prigatano et al., 1994; Sady et al., 2010
Postacute brain injury rehabilitation	Altman, Swick, Parrot, & Malec, 2010; Malec & Basford, 1996
Caregiver distress	Sady et al., 2010; Sander, Maestas, Sherer, Malec, & Nakase-Richardson, 2012

Determination of prognosis for favorable outcomes and potential ability to return to previous activities is a common referral question for neuropsychologists being asked to evaluate an individual with a history of TBI. In a review, Sherer and Novack (2003) reported that results from neuropsychological evaluations are generally predictive of personal safety, independent living, driving safety, and return to work. Neuropsychological testing has been shown to be predictive of later productivity even when controlling for demographic and injury severity variables (Sherer et al., 2002). There is also evidence that a brief battery of neuropsychological tests administered early in the recovery course is predictive of handicap, functional outcome, supervision needs, and employability at one year (Hanks et al., 2008). This battery was able to predict functional outcome at one year above and beyond functional and injury severity variables, providing strong support for the incremental validity of neuropsychological testing in moderate to severe TBI. A recent study found that early evaluation of neuropsychological functioning was predictive of long-term functional disability at one to two years postinjury even after considering demographic variables, injury severity, and CT findings. Both CT findings and neuropsychological evaluations were predictive of return to work at two years (Williams, Rapport, Hanks, Millis, & Greene, 2013). Regarding specific areas of functioning, there is evidence that measures of attention and executive functioning are predictive of independent living and employment status at one year (Finnanger et al., 2013).

While individual factors may be independently related to outcome after TBI, more recent research indicates the importance of considering multifactorial models of outcome. Bush and colleagues (2003) used structural equation modeling to validate a model using premorbid variables, injury severity indices, cognitive abilities, and functional status to predict functional outcome as measured by the CIQ and DRS at one year postinjury, and then cross-validated their findings on a larger national prospectively collected sample. Both samples were followed longitudinally from injury through acute rehabilitation to one year postinjury. Results generally replicated an earlier path analysis study (Novack, Bush, Meythaler, & Canupp, 2001) showing that premorbid characteristics and cognitive and functional status were better predictors of outcome at one year than were injury severity variables. Results further indicated that although injury severity indices had a significant causal impact on functional skills and cognitive status, they did not independently influence one-year outcome. Premorbid status (particularly preinjury employment) had a positive influence on functional skills, cognition, and outcome. Further, both cognitive and functional status strongly influenced outcome. These findings indicate that understanding recovery requires consideration of multiple factors and cannot be achieved by evaluating injury severity alone. Based on these results, Novack and colleagues (2001) assert that interventions to improve outcome after TBI must continue to focus on rehabilitation of cognitive and functional skills in combination with amelioration of the effects of premorbid factors on postinjury functional and cognitive status.

In closing, this chapter illustrates that mortality and morbidity due to TBI are major public health problems in the United States. Although a large percentage of individuals with moderate and severe TBI have lasting physical, cognitive, and neurobehavioral impairments, the course of recovery, pattern of resulting impairments, and ultimate functional outcome of these individuals is highly variable and dependent on a combination of potential predictive factors that often differ across populations studied. When encountering these patients, the neuropsychologist is challenged with the task of not only evaluating current cognitive and neurobehavioral functioning but also making recommendations regarding expectations of ultimate outcome. Thus, neuropsychologists are well poised to help patients and their families understand and adjust to injury-related cognitive and emotional changes while helping them to make realistic plans for the future. Finally, future research is needed determine which specific rehabilitation and neuropsychological interventions are most beneficial in helping patients with moderate to severe TBI reach their optimal recovery potential.

Acknowledgments

Completion of this chapter was partially supported by U.S. Department of Education National Institute on Disability and Rehabilitation Research (NIDRR) Grant #H133A120020.

References

Adams, J. H., Graham, D. I., Scott, G., Parker, L. S., & Doyle, D. (1980). Brain damage in fatal non-missile head injury. *Journal of Clinical Pathology*, *33*(12), 1132–1145.

Altman, I. M., Swick, S., Parrot, D., & Malec, J. F. (2010). Effectiveness of community-based rehabilitation after traumatic brain injury for 489 program completers compared with those precipitously discharged. *Archives of Physical Medicine and Rehabilitation*, *91*(11), 1697–1704. doi: 10.1016/j.apmr.2010.08.001

American Psychiatric Association. (1994). *Diagnostic and Statistical Manual of Mental Disorders* (4th ed.). Washington, DC: American Psychiatric Association.

Anderson, C. V., Bigler, E. D., & Blatter, D. D. (1995). Frontal lobe lesions, diffuse damage, and neuropsychological functioning in traumatic brain-injured patients. *Journal of Clinical and Experimental Neuropsychology*, *17*(6), 900–908.

Andrews, P. J., Sleeman, D. H., Statham, P. F., McQuatt, A., Corruble, V., Jones, P. A., . . . Macmillan, C. S. (2002). Predicting recovery in patients suffering from traumatic brain injury by using admission variables and physiological data: A comparison between decision tree analysis and logistic regression. *Journal of Neurosurgery*, *97*(2), 326–336.

Annegers, J. F., Grabow, J. D., Kurland, L. T., & Laws, E. R., Jr. (1980). The incidence, causes, and secular trends of head trauma in Olmsted County, Minnesota, 1935–1974. *Neurology*, *30*(9), 912–919.

Annegers, J. F., Hauser, W. A., Coan, S. P., & Rocca, W. A. (1998). A population-based study of seizures after traumatic brain injuries. *New England Journal of Medicine*, *338*(1), 20–24.

Arango-Lasprilla, J. C., Ketchum, J. M., Lewis, A. N., Krch, D., Gary, K. W., & Dodd, B. A., Jr. (2011). Racial and ethnic disparities in employment outcomes for persons with traumatic brain injury: A longitudinal investigation 1–5 years after injury. *P M R: The Journal of Injury, Function and Rehabilitation*, *3*(12), 1083–1091. doi: 10.1016/j.pmrj.2011.05.023

Arango-Lasprilla, J. C., & Kreutzer, J. S. (2010). Racial and ethnic disparities in functional, psychosocial, and neurobehavioral outcomes after brain injury. *Journal of Head Trauma Rehabilitation*, *25*(2), 128–136. doi: 10.1097/HTR.0b013e3181d36ca3

Arfanakis, K., Haughton, V. M., Carew, J. D., Rogers, B. P., Dempsey, R. J., & Meyerand, M. E. (2002). Diffusion tensor MR imaging in diffuse axonal injury. *American Journal of Neuroradiology*, *23*(5), 794–802.

Ariza, M., Mataro, M., Poca, M. A., Junque, C., Garnacho, A., Amoros, S., & Sahuquillo, J. (2004). Influence of extraneurological insults on ventricular enlargement and neuropsychological functioning after moderate and severe traumatic brain injury. *Journal of Neurotrauma*, *21*(7), 864–876.

Barker, M. D., Whyte, J., Pretz, C. R., Sherer, M., Temkin, N., Hammond, F. M., . . . Novack, T. (2014). Application and clinical utility of the Glasgow coma scale over time: A study employing the NIDRR traumatic brain injury model systems database. *Journal of Head Trauma Rehabilitation*, *29*(5), 400–406. doi: 10.1097/HTR.0b013e31828a0a45

Bazarian, J. J., Cernak, I., Noble-Haeusslein, L., Potolicchio, S., & Temkin, N. (2009). Long-term neurologic outcomes after traumatic brain injury. *Journal of Head Trauma Rehabilitation*, *24*(6), 439–451. doi: 10.1097/HTR.0b013e3181c15600

Belanger, H. G., Curtiss, G., Demery, J. A., Lebowitz, B. K., & Vanderploeg, R. D. (2005). Factors moderating neuropsychological outcomes following mild traumatic brain injury: A meta-analysis. *Journal of the International Neuropsychological Society*, *11*(3), 215–227. doi: S1355617705050277 [pii] 10.1017/S135561 7705050277

Belanger, H. G., Spiegel, E., & Vanderploeg, R. D. (2010). Neuropsychological performance following a history of multiple self-reported concussions: A meta-analysis. *Journal of the International Neuropsychological Society*, *16*(2), 262–267. doi: 10.1017/S1355617709991287

Bhalerao, S. U., Geurtjens, C., Thomas, G. R., Kitamura, C. R., Zhou, C., & Marlborough, M. (2013). Understanding the neuropsychiatric consequences associated with significant traumatic brain injury. *Brain Injury*, *27*(7–8), 767–774. doi: 10.3109/02699052.2013.793396

Boake, C. (1996). Supervision rating scale: A measure of functional outcome from brain injury. *Archives of Physical Medicine and Rehabilitation*, *77*(8), 765–772.

Boake, C., Millis, S. R., High, W. M., Jr., Delmonico, R. L., Kreutzer, J. S., Rosenthal, M., . . . Ivanhoe, C. B. (2001). Using early neuropsychologic testing to predict long-term productivity outcome from traumatic brain injury. *Archives of Physical Medicine and Rehabilitation*, *82*(6), 761–768.

Bogner, J., Bellon, K., Kolakowsky-Hayner, S. A., & Whiteneck, G. (2013). Participation assessment with recombined tools-objective (PART-O). *Journal of Head Trauma Rehabilitation*, *28*(4), 337–339. doi: 10.1097/HTR.0b013e31829af969

Bontke, C. F., Zasler, N. D., & Boake, C. (1996). Rehabilitation of the head-injured patient. In R. K. Naravan, J. E. Wilberger, & J. T. Povlishock (Eds.), *Neurotrauma* (pp. 841–858). New York: McGraw-Hill.

Braakman, R., Gelpke, G. J., Habbema, J. D., Maas, A. I., & Minderhoud, J. M. (1980). Systematic selection of prognostic features in patients with severe head injury. *Neurosurgery*, *6*(4), 362–370.

Braver, E. R., Ferguson, S. A., Greene, M. A., & Lund, A. K. (1997). Reductions in deaths in frontal crashes among right front passengers in vehicles equipped with passenger air bags. *JAMA*, *278*(17), 1437–1439.

Brooks, N., Campsie, L., Symington, C., Beattie, A., & McKinlay, W. (1986). The five year outcome of severe blunt head injury: A relative's view. *Journal of Neurology, Neurosurgery and Psychiatry*, *49*(7), 764–770.

Brooks, N., McKinlay, W., Symington, C., Beattie, A., & Campsie, L. (1987). Return to work within the first seven years of severe head injury. *Brain Injury*, *1*(1), 5–19.

Brown, A. W., Malec, J. F., McClelland, R. L., Diehl, N. N., Englander, J., & Cifu, D. X. (2005). Clinical elements that predict outcome after traumatic brain injury: A prospective multicenter recursive partitioning (Decision-Tree) analysis. *Journal of Neurotrauma*, *22*(10), 1040–1051.

Bulger, E. M., Nathens, A. B., Rivara, F. P., Moore, M., MacKenzie, E. J., & Jurkovich, G. J. (2002). Management of severe head injury: Institutional variations in care and effect on outcome. *Critical Care Medicine*, *30*(8), 1870–1876.

Bush, B. A., Novack, T. A., Malec, J. F., Stringer, A. Y., Millis, S. R., & Madan, A. (2003). Validation of a model for evaluating outcome after traumatic brain injury. *Archives of Physical Medicine and Rehabilitation*, *84*(12), 1803–1807.

Carlozzi, N. E., Grech, J., & Tulsky, D. S. (2013). Memory functioning in individuals with traumatic brain injury: An examination of the Wechsler Memory Scale-Fourth Edition (WMS-IV). *Journal of Clinical and Experimental Neuropsychology*, *35*(9), 906–914. doi: 10.1080/13803395.2013.833178

Cherner, M., Temkin, N. R., Machamer, J. E., & Dikmen, S. S. (2001). Utility of a composite measure to detect problematic alcohol use in persons with traumatic brain injury. *Archives of Physical Medicine and Rehabilitation*, *82*(6), 780–786. doi: 10.1053/apmr.2001.23263

Choi, S. C., & Barnes, T. Y. (1996). Predicting Outcome in the head-injured patient. In R. K. Naravan, J. E. Wilberger, & J. T. Povlishock (Eds.), *Neurotrauma* (pp. 779–792). New York: McGraw-Hill.

Choi, S. C., Barnes, T. Y., Bullock, R., Germanson, T. A., Marmarou, A., & Young, H. F. (1994). Temporal profile of outcomes in severe head injury. *Journal of Neurosurgery*, *81*(2), 169–173.

Claassen, J., & Hansen, H. C. (2001). Early recovery after closed traumatic head injury: Somatosensory evoked potentials and clinical findings. *Critical Care Medicine*, *29*(3), 494–502.

Clifton, G. L., Hayes, R. L., Levin, H. S., Michel, M. E., & Choi, S. C. (1992). Outcome measures for clinical trials involving traumatically brain-injured patients: Report of a conference. *Neurosurgery*, *31*(5), 975–978.

Cooper, K. D., Tabaddor, K., Hauser, W. A., Shulman, K., Feiner, C., & Factor, P. R. (1983). The epidemiology of head injury in the Bronx. *Neuroepidemiology*, *2*, 70–88.

Coronado, V. G., Xu, L., Basavaraju, S. V., McGuire, L. C., Wald, M. M., Faul, M. D., . . . Hemphill, J. D. (2011). Surveillance for traumatic brain injury: Related deaths—United States, 1997–2007. *Centers for Disease Control and Prevention Morbidity and Mortality Weekly Report*, *60*(5), 1–32.

Corrigan, J. D. (1989). Development of a scale for assessment of agitation following traumatic brain injury. *Journal of Clinical and Experimental Neuropsychology*, *11*(2), 261–277.

Corrigan, J. D. (1995). Substance abuse as a mediating factor in outcome from traumatic brain injury. *Archives of Physical Medicine and Rehabilitation*, *76*(4), 302–309.

Corrigan, J. D., Bogner, J., & Holloman, C. (2012). Lifetime history of traumatic brain injury among persons with substance use disorders. *Brain Injury*, *26*(2), 139–150. doi: 10.3109/02699052.2011.648705

Corrigan, J. D., Bogner, J., Mellick, D., Bushnik, T., Dams-O'Connor, K., Hammond, F. M., . . . Kolakowsky-Hayner, S. (2013). Prior history of traumatic brain injury among persons in the Traumatic Brain Injury Model Systems National Database. *Archives of Physical Medicine and Rehabilitation*, *94*(10), 1940–1950. doi: 10.1016/j.apmr.2013.05.018

Crepeau, F., & Scherzer, P. (1993). Predictors and indicators of work status after traumatic brain injury: A meta-analysis. *Neuropsychological Rehabilitation*, *3*, 5–35.

Curtiss, G., Vanderploeg, R. D., Spencer, J., & Salazar, A. M. (2001). Patterns of verbal learning and memory in traumatic brain injury. *Journal of the International Neuropsychological Society*, *7*(5), 574–585.

Davis, L. C., Sherer, M., Sander, A. M., Bogner, J. A., Corrigan, J. D., Dijkers, M. P., . . . Seel, R. T. (2012). Preinjury predictors of life satisfaction at 1 year after traumatic brain injury. [Research Support, U.S. Gov't, Non-P.H.S.]. *Archives of Physical Medicine and Rehabilitation*, *93*(8), 1324–1330. doi: 10.1016/j.apmr.2012.02.036

Dikmen, S., & Machamer, J. (1995). Neurobehavioral outcomes and their determinants. *Journal of Head Trauma Rehabilitation*, *10*, 74–86.

Dikmen, S., Machamer, J., Temkin, N., & McLean, A. (1990). Neuropsychological recovery in patients with moderate to severe head injury: 2 year follow-up. *Journal of Clinical and Experimental Neuropsychology*, *12*(4), 507–519.

Dikmen, S., Machamer, J. E., Donovan, D. M., Winn, H. R., & Temkin, N. R. (1995). Alcohol use before and after traumatic head injury. *Annals of Emergency Medicine*, *26*(2), 167–176.

Dikmen, S., Machamer, J. E., Powell, J. M., & Temkin, N. R. (2003). Outcome 3 to 5 years after moderate to severe traumatic brain injury. *Archives of Physical Medicine and Rehabilitation*, *84*(10), 1449–1457.

Dikmen, S., McLean, A., Jr., Temkin, N. R., & Wyler, A. R. (1986). Neuropsychologic outcome at one-month postinjury. *Archives of Physical Medicine and Rehabilitation*, *67*(8), 507–513.

Dikmen, S., Reitan, R. M., & Temkin, N. R. (1983). Neuropsychological recovery in head injury. *Archives of Neurology*, *40*(6), 333–338.

Dikmen, S., Temkin, N. R., Machamer, J. E., Holubkov, A. L., Fraser, R. T., & Winn, H. R. (1994). Employment following traumatic head injuries. *Archives of Neurology*, *51*(2), 177–186.

Dikmen, S. S., Ross, B. L., Machamer, J. E., & Temkin, N. R. (1995). One year psychosocial outcome in head injury. *Journal of the International Neuropsychological Society*, *1*(1), 67–77.

Doctor, J. N., Castro, J., Temkin, N. R., Fraser, R. T., Machamer, J. E., & Dikmen, S. S. (2005). Workers' risk of unemployment after traumatic brain injury: A normed comparison. *Journal of the International Neuropsychological Society*, *11*(6), 747–752.

Donders, J., & Levitt, T. (2012). Criterion validity of the neuropsychological assessment battery after traumatic brain injury. *Archives of Clinical Neuropsychology*, *27*(4), 440–445. doi: 10.1093/arclin/acs043

Eisenberg, H. M., & Weiner, R. L. (1987). Input variables: How information from the acute injury can be used to characterize groups of patients for studies of outcome. In H. S. Levin, J. Grafman & H. M. Eisenberg (Eds.), *Neurobehavioral Recovery from Head Injury* (pp. 13–29). New York: Oxford University Press.

Ellenberg, J. H., Levin, H. S., & Saydjari, C. (1996). Posttraumatic Amnesia as a predictor of outcome after severe closed head injury: Prospective assessment. *Archives of Neurology*, *53*(8), 782–791.

Faul, M., Wald, M. M., Rutland-Brown, W., Sullivent, E. E., & Sattin, R. W. (2007). Using a cost-benefit analysis to estimate outcomes of a clinical treatment guideline: Testing theBrain Trauma Foundation guidelines for the treatment of severe traumatic brain injury. *Journal of Trauma*, *63*(6), 1271–1278. doi: 10.1097/TA.0b013e3181493080

Faul, M., Xu, L. S., Wald, M. M., & Coronado, V. G. (2010). *Traumatic Brain Injury in the United States: Emergency Department Visits, Hospitalizations and Deaths 2002–2006*. Atlanta, GA: Centers for Disease Control and Prevention, National Center for Injury Prevention and Control.

Finnanger, T. G., Skandsen, T., Andersson, S., Lydersen, S., Vik, A., & Indredavik, M. (2013). Differentiated patterns of cognitive impairment 12 months after severe and moderate traumatic brain injury. *Brain Injury*, *27*(13–14), 1606–1616. doi: 10.3109/02699052.2013.831127

Fleminger, S., Oliver, D. L., Lovestone, S., Rabe-Hesketh, S., & Giora, A. (2003). Head injury as a risk factor for Alzheimer's disease: The evidence 10 years on: A partial replication. *Journal of Neurology, Neurosurgery and Psychiatry*, *74*(7), 857–862.

Fortuny, L. A., Briggs, M., Newcombe, F., Ratcliff, G., & Thomas, C. (1980). Measuring the duration of post traumatic amnesia. *Journal of Neurology, Neurosurgery and Psychiatry*, *43*(5), 377–379.

Freytag, E. (1963). Autopsy findings in head injuries from blunt forces: Statistical evaluation of 1,367 cases. *Archives of Pathology*, *75*, 402–413.

Gedye, A., Beattie, B. L., Tuokko, H., Horton, A., & Korsarek, E. (1989). Severe head injury hastens age of onset of Alzheimer's disease. *Journal of the American Geriatrics Society*, *37*(10), 970–973.

Gennarelli, T. A. (1983). Head injury in man and experimental animals: Clinical aspects. *Acta Neurochirurgica Supplementum*, *32*, 1–13.

Gennarelli, T. A. (1994). Animate models of human head injury. *Journal of Neurotrauma*, *11*(4), 357–368.

Gennarelli, T. A., & Graham, D. I. (2005). Neuropathology. In J. M. Silver, T. W. McAllister, & S. C. Yudofsky (Eds.), *Textbook of Traumatic Brain Injury* (pp. 27–50). Washington, DC: American Psychiatric Publishing, Inc.

Gennarelli, T. A., & Thibault, L. E. (1982). Biomechanics of acute subdural hematoma. *Journal of Trauma*, *22*(8), 680–686.

Gennarelli, T. A., Thibault, L. E., Adams, J. H., Graham, D. I., Thompson, C. J., & Marcincin, R. P. (1982). Diffuse axonal injury and traumatic coma in the primate. *Annals of Neurology*, *12*(6), 564–574.

Giacino, J. T., Ashwal, S., Childs, N., Cranford, R., Jennett, B., Katz, D. I., . . . Zasler, N. D. (2002). The minimally conscious state: Definition and diagnostic criteria. *Neurology*, *58*(3), 349–353.

Giacino, J. T., Kalmar, K., & Whyte, J. (2004). The JFK coma recovery scale-revised: Measurement characteristics and diagnostic utility. *Archives of Physical Medicine and Rehabilitation*, *85*(12), 2020–2029.

Godfrey, H. P., Partridge, F. M., Knight, R. G., & Bishara, S. (1993). Course of insight disorder and emotional dysfunction following closed head injury: A controlled cross-sectional follow-up study. *Journal of Clinical and Experimental Neuropsychology*, *15*(4), 503–515.

Gollaher, K., High, W., Sherer, M., Bergloff, P., Boake, C., Young, M. E., & Ivanhoe, C. (1998). Prediction of employment outcome one to three years following traumatic brain injury (TBI). *Brain Injury*, *12*(4), 255–263.

Gouvier, W. D., Blanton, P. D., LaPorte, K. K., & Nepomuceno, C. (1987). Reliability and validity of the Disability Rating Scale and the Levels of Cognitive Functioning Scale in monitoring recovery from severe head injury. *Archives of Physical Medicine and Rehabilitation*, *68*(2), 94–97.

Graham, D. I., Adams, J. H., & Gennarelli, T. A. (1993). Pathology of brain damage in head injury. In P. R. Cooper (Ed.), *Head Injury* (pp. 133–154). Baltimore: Williams & Wilkins.

Graham, D. I., Gennarelli, T. A., & McIntosh, T. K. (2002). Trauma. In D. I. Graham & P. L. Lantos (Eds.), *Greenfield's Neuropathology* (p. 823). London: Arnold.

Graham, D. P., & Cardon, A. L. (2008). An update on substance use and treatment following traumatic brain injury. *Annals of the New York Academy of Sciences*, *1141*, 148–162. doi: 10.1196/annals.1441.029

Guo, Z., Cupples, L. A., Kurz, A., Auerbach, S. H., Volicer, L., Chui, H., . . . Farrer, L. A. (2000). Head injury and the risk of AD in the MIRAGE study. *Neurology*, *54*(6), 1316–1323.

Hall, K., Cope, D. N., & Rappaport, M. (1985). Glasgow outcome scale and disability rating scale: Comparative usefulness in following recovery in traumatic head injury. *Archives of Physical Medicine and Rehabilitation*, *66*(1), 35–37.

Hanks, R. A., Millis, S. R., Ricker, J. H., Giacino, J. T., Nakese-Richardson, R., Frol, A. B., . . . Gordon, W. A. (2008). The predictive validity of a brief inpatient neuropsychologic battery for persons with traumatic brain injury. *Archives of Physical Medicine and Rehabilitation*, *89*(5), 950–957. doi: S0003-9993(08)00167-6 [pii] 10.1016/j.apmr.2008.01.011

Hanlon, R. E., Demery, J. A., Kuczen, C., & Kelly, J. P. (2005). Effect of traumatic subarachnoid haemorrhage on neuropsychological profiles and vocational outcome following moderate or severe traumatic brain injury. *Brain Injury*, *19*(4), 257–262.

Hannay, H. J., & Sherer, M. (1996). Assessment of outcome from head injury. In R. K. Narayan, J. E. Wilberger, & J. T. Povlishock (Eds.), *Neurotrauma* (pp. 723–747). New York: McGraw-Hill.

Harrison-Felix, C., Newton, C. N., Hall, K. M., & Kreutzer, J. S. (1996). Descriptive findings from the traumatic brain injury model systems national database. *Journal of Head Trauma Rehabilitation*, *11*(5), 1–14.

Hart, T., Millis, S., Novack, T., Englander, J., Fidler-Sheppard, R., & Bell, K. R. (2003). The relationship between neuropsychologic function and level of caregiver supervision at 1 year after traumatic brain injury. *Archives of Physical Medicine and Rehabilitation*, *84*(2), 221–230.

Hartley, L. L., & Jensen, P. J. (1991). Narrative and procedural discourse after closed head injury. *Brain Injury*, *5*(3), 267–285.

High, W. M., Jr., Levin, H. S., & Gary, H. E., Jr. (1990). Recovery of orientation following closed-head injury. *Journal of Clinical and Experimental Neuropsychology*, *12*(5), 703–714.

Holbourn, A. (1943). Mechanics of head injury. *Lancet*, *2*, 438–441.

Horn, L. J., & Sherer, M. (1999). Rehabilitation of traumatic brain injury. In M. Grabois, S. J. Garrison, K. A. Hart, & L. D. Lehmkuhl (Eds.), *Physical Medicine and Rehabilitation: The Complete Approach* (pp. 1281–1304). Cambridge, MA: Blackwell Science.

Howard, M. A., 3rd, Gross, A. S., Dacey, R. G., Jr., & Winn, H. R. (1989). Acute subdural hematomas: An age-dependent clinical entity. *Journal of Neurosurgery*, *71*(6), 858–863.

Huang, J., Fleming, J., Pomery, N. L., O'Gorman, J. G., Chan, R. C., & Shum, D. H. (2014). Perceived importance of prospective memory failures in adults with traumatic brain injury. *Neuropsychol Rehabil*, *24*(1), 61–70. doi: 10.1080/09602011.2013.854723

Inglese, M., Makani, S., Johnson, G., Cohen, B. A., Silver, J. A., Gonen, O., & Grossman, R. I. (2005). Diffuse axonal injury in mild traumatic brain injury: A diffusion tensor imaging study. *Journal of Neurosurgery*, *103*(2), 298–303.

Institute of Medicine. (2009). *Gulf War and Health. Vol. 7: Long-Term Consequences of Traumatic Brain Injury*. Washington, DC: The National Academies Press.

Jackson, W. T., Novack, T. A., & Dowler, R. N. (1998). Effective serial measurement of cognitive orientation in rehabilitation: The Orientation Log. *Archives of Physical Medicine and Rehabilitation*, *79*(6), 718–720.

Jain, N. S., Layton, B. S., & Murray, P. K. (2000). Are aphasic patients who fail the GOAT in PTA? A modified Galveston Orientation and Amnesia Test for persons with aphasia. *Clinical Neuropsychologist*, *14*(1), 13–17.

Jellinger, K. A., Paulus, W., Wrocklage, C., & Litvan, I. (2001). Traumatic brain injury as a risk factor for Alzheimer disease: Comparison of two retrospective autopsy cohorts with evaluation of ApoE genotype. *BMC Neurology*, *1*, 3.

Jennett, B., & Bond, M. (1975). Assessment of outcome after severe brain damage. *Lancet*, *1*(7905), 480–484.

Jennett, B., & Teasdale, G. (1981). *Management of Head Injuries*. Philadelphia, PA: Davis.

Jiang, J. Y., Gao, G. Y., Li, W. P., Yu, M. K., & Zhu, C. (2002). Early indicators of prognosis in 846 cases of severe traumatic brain injury. *Journal of Neurotrauma*, *19*(7), 869–874.

Johnson, V. E., Stewart, W., & Smith, D. H. (2010). Traumatic brain injury and amyloid-beta pathology: A link to Alzheimer's disease? *Nature Reviews Neuroscience*, *11*(5), 361–370. doi: 10.1038/nrn2808

Johnstone, B., Hexum, C. L., & Ashkanazi, G. (1995). Extent of cognitive decline in traumatic brain injury based on estimates of premorbid intelligence. *Brain Injury*, *9*(4), 377–384.

Kaitaro, T., Koskinen, S., & Kaipio, M.-L. (1995). Neuropsychological problems in everyday life: A 5-year follow-up study of young severely closed-head-injured patients. *Brain Injury*, *9*(7), 713–727.

Kalmar, K., Novack, T. A., Nakase-Richardson, R., Sherer, M., Frol, A. B., Gordon, W. A., . . . Ricker, J. H. (2008). Feasibility of a brief neuropsychologic test battery during acute inpatient rehabilitation after traumatic brain injury. *Archives of Physical Medicine and Rehabilitation*, *89*(5), 942–949. doi: 10.1016/j.apmr.2008.01.008

Kashluba, S., Hanks, R. A., Casey, J. E., & Millis, S. R. (2008). Neuropsychologic and functional outcome after complicated mild traumatic brain injury. *Archives of Physical Medicine and Rehabilitation*, *89*(5), 904–911. doi: S0003-9993(08)00070-1 [pii] 10.1016/j.apmr.2007.12.029

Kelley, E., Sullivan, C., Loughlin, J. K., Hutson, L., Dahdah, M. N., Long, M. K., . . . Poole, J. H. (2014). Self-awareness and neurobehavioral outcomes, 5 years or more after moderate to severe brain injury. *Journal of Head Trauma Rehabilitation*, *29*(2), 147–152. doi: 10.1097/HTR.0b013e31826db6b9

Kennedy, M. R., Wozniak, J. R., Muetzel, R. L., Mueller, B. A., Chiou, H. H., Pantekoek, K., & Lim, K. O. (2009). White matter and neurocognitive changes in adults with chronic traumatic brain injury. *Journal of the International Neuropsychological Society*, *15*(1), 130–136. doi: 10.1017/S1355617708090024

Kennedy, M. R., & Yorkston, K. M. (2000). Accuracy of metamemory after traumatic brain injury: Predictions during verbal learning. *Journal of Speech, Language, and Hearing Research*, *43*(5), 1072–1086.

Keyser-Marcus, L. A., Bricout, J. C., Wehman, P., Campbell, L. R., Cifu, D. X., Englander, J., . . . Zafonte, R. D. (2002). Acute predictors of return to employment after traumatic brain injury: A longitudinal follow-up. *Archives of Physical Medicine and Rehabilitation*, *83*(5), 635–641.

King, J. T., Carlier, P. M., & Marion, D. W. (2005). Early Glasgow outcome scale scores predict long-term functional outcome in patients with severe traumatic brain injury. *Journal of Neurotrauma*, *22*(9), 947–954.

Kinsella, G., Murtagh, D., Landry, A., Homfray, K., Hammond, M., O'Beirne, L., . . . Ponsford, J. (1996). Everyday memory following traumatic brain injury. *Brain Injury*, *10*(7), 499–507.

Kraus, J. F., Fife, D., Ramstein, K., Conroy, C., & Cox, P. (1986). The relationship of family income to the incidence, external causes, and outcomes of serious brain injury, San Diego County, California. *American Journal of Public Health*, *76*(11), 1345–1347.

Kraus, M. F., Susmaras, T., Caughlin, B. P., Walker, C. J., Sweeney, J. A., & Little, D. M. (2007). White matter integrity and cognition in chronic traumatic brain injury: A diffusion tensor imaging study. *Brain*, *130*(Pt 10), 2508–2519.

Kreutzer, J. S., Marwitz, J. H., Seel, R., & Serio, C. D. (1996). Validation of a neurobehavioral functioning inventory for adults with traumatic brain injury. *Archives of Physical Medicine and Rehabilitation*, *77*(2), 116–124.

Lange, R. T., Iverson, G. L., Brubacher, J. R., Madler, B., & Heran, M. K. (2012). Diffusion tensor imaging findings are not strongly associated with postconcussional disorder 2 months following mild traumatic brain injury. *Journal of Head Trauma Rehabilitation*, *27*(3), 188–198. doi: 10.1097/HTR.0b013e318217f0ad

Langlois, J. A., Rutland-Brown, W., & Thomas, K. E. (2006). *Traumatic Brain Injury in the United States: Emergency Department Visits, Hospitalizations, and Deaths*. Atlanta, GA: Centers for Disease Control and Prevention, National Center for Injury Prevention and Control.

Lee, Y. K., Hou, S. W., Lee, C. C., Hsu, C. Y., Huang, Y. S., & Su, Y. C. (2013). Increased risk of dementia in patients with mild traumatic brain injury: A nationwide cohort study. *PLoS One*, *8*(5), e62422. doi: 10.1371/journal.pone.0062422

Leon-Carrion, J., Alarcon, J. C., Revuelta, M., Murillo-Cabezas, F., Dominguez-Roldan, J. M., Dominguez-Morales, M. R., . . . Forastero, P. (1998). Executive functioning as outcome in patients after traumatic brain injury. *International Journal of Neuroscience*, *94*(1–2), 75–83.

Levin, H. S. (1992). Neurobehavioral recovery. *Journal of Neurotrauma*, *9*(Suppl 1), S359–373.

Levin, H. S. (1993). Neurobehavioral sequelae of closed head injury. In P. R. Cooper (Ed.), *Head Injury* (pp. 525–551). Baltimore: Williams & Wilkins.

Levin, H. S. (1995). Prediction of recovery from traumatic brain injury. *Journal of Neurotrauma*, *12*(5), 913–922.

Levin, H. S., Amparo, E., Eisenberg, H. M., Williams, D. H., High, W. M., Jr., McArdle, C. B., & Weiner, R. L. (1987). Magnetic resonance imaging and computerized tomography in relation to the neurobehavioral sequelae of mild and moderate head injuries. *Journal of Neurosurgery*, *66*(5), 706–713.

Levin, H. S., Culhane, K. A., Mendelsohn, D., Lilly, M. A., Bruce, D., Fletcher, J. M., . . . Eisenberg, H. M. (1993). Cognition in relation to magnetic resonance imaging in head-injured children and adolescents. *Archives of Neurology*, *50*(9), 897–905.

Levin, H. S., & Eisenberg, H. M. (1991). Management of head injury: Neurobehavioral outcome. *Neurosurgery Clinics of North America*, *2*(2), 457–472.

Levin, H. S., Gary, H. E., Jr., Eisenberg, H. M., Ruff, R. M., Barth, J. T., Kreutzer, J., . . . Jane, J. A. (1990). Neurobehavioral outcome 1 year after severe head injury: Experience of the Traumatic Coma Data Bank. *Journal of Neurosurgery*, *73*(5), 699–709.

Levin, H. S., & Goldstein, F. C. (1986). Organization of verbal memory after severe closed-head injury. *Journal of Clinical and Experimental Neuropsychology*, *8*(6), 643–656.

Levin, H. S., Grossman, R. G., & Kelly, P. J. (1976). Aphasic disorder in patients with closed head injury. *Journal of Neurology, Neurosurgery and Psychiatry*, *39*(11), 1062–1070.

Levin, H. S., High, W. M., Goethe, K. E., Sisson, R. A., Overall, J. E., Rhoades, H. M., . . . Gary, H. E. (1987). The neurobehavioural rating scale: Assessment of the behavioural sequelae of head injury by the clinician. *Journal of Neurology, Neurosurgery and Psychiatry*, *50*(2), 183–193.

Levin, H. S., O'Donnell, V. M., & Grossman, R. G. (1979). The Galveston Orientation and Amnesia Test: A practical scale to assess cognition after head injury. *Journal of Nervous and Mental Disease*, *167*(11), 675–684.

Levin, H. S., Williams, D. H., Eisenberg, H. M., High, W. M., Jr., & Guinto, F. C., Jr. (1992). Serial MRI and neurobehavioural findings after mild to moderate closed head injury. *Journal of Neurology, Neurosurgery and Psychiatry*, *55*(4), 255–262.

Levine, B., Dawson, D., Boutet, I., Schwartz, M. L., & Stuss, D. T. (2000). Assessment of strategic self-regulation in traumatic brain injury: Its relationship to injury severity and psychosocial outcome. *Neuropsychology*, *14*(4), 491–500.

Lezak, M. D. (1987). Relationships between personality disorder, social disturbances, and physical disability following traumatic brain injury. *Journal of Head Trauma Rehabilitation*, *2*, 57–69.

Lezak, M. D. (1988). Brain damage is a family affair. *Journal of Clinical and Experimental Neuropsychology*, *10*(1), 111–123.

Lezak, M. D. (1995). *Neuropsychological Assessment* (3rd ed.). New York: Oxford University Press.

Lezak, M. D., Howieson, D. B., Loring, D. W., Hannay, H. J., & Fischer, J. S. (2004). *Neuropsychological Assessment* (4th ed.). New York: Oxford University Press.

Lippert-Gruner, M., Wedekind, C., & Klug, N. (2003). Outcome of prolonged coma following severe traumatic brain injury. *Brain Injury*, *17*(1), 49–54.

Lye, T. C., & Shores, E. A. (2000). Traumatic brain injury as a risk factor for Alzheimer's disease: A review. *Neuropsychology Review*, *10*(2), 115–129.

MacMillan, P. J., Hart, R. P., Martelli, M. F., & Zasler, N. D. (2002). Pre-injury status and adaptation following traumatic brain injury. *Brain Injury*, *16*(1), 41–49.

Malec, J. F., & Basford, J. S. (1996). Postacute brain injury rehabilitation. *Archives of Physical Medicine and Rehabilitation*, *77*, 198–207.

Malec, J. F., & Moessner, A. M. (2000). Self-awareness, distress, and postacute rehabilitation outcome. *Rehabilitation Psychology*, *45*, 227–241.

Maloney, A. F., & Whatmore, W. J. (1969). Clinical and pathological observations in fatal head injuries: A 5-year study of 173 cases. *British Journal of Surgery*, *56*, 23–31.

Marion, D. W. (1996). Outcome from severe head injury. In R. K. Narayan, J. E. Wilberger, & J. T. Povlishock (Eds.), *Neurotrauma* (pp. 767–777). New York: McGraw-Hill.

Marion, D. W., & Carlier, P. M. (1994). Problems with initial Glasgow Coma Scale assessment caused by prehospital treatment of patients with head injuries: Results of a national survey. *Journal of Trauma*, *36*(1), 89–95.

Marr, A., & Coronado, V. (Eds.). (2004). *Central Nervous System Injury Surveillance Data Submission Standards-2002*. Atlanta GA: Centers for Disease Control and Prevention, National Center for Injury Prevention and Control.

Mataro, M., Poca, M. A., Sahuquillo, J., Pedraza, S., Ariza, M., Amoros, S., & Junque, C. (2001). Neuropsychological outcome in relation to the traumatic coma data bank classification of computed tomography imaging. *Journal of Neurotrauma*, *18*(9), 869–879.

Mathias, J. L., & Mansfield, K. M. (2005). Prospective and declarative memory problems following moderate and severe traumatic brain injury. *Brain Injury*, *19*(4), 271–282.

McCauley, S. R., Levin, H. S., Vanier, M., Mazaux, J. M., Boake, C., Goldfader, P. R., . . . Clifton, G. L. (2001). The neurobehavioural rating scale-revised: Sensitivity and validity in closed head injury assessment. *Journal of Neurology, Neurosurgery and Psychiatry*, *71*(5), 643–651.

Mendelow, A. D., Teasdale, G., Jennett, B., Bryden, J., Hessett, C., & Murray, G. (1983). Risks of intracranial haematoma in head injured adults. *British Medical Journal (Clinical Research Edition)*, *287*(6400), 1173–1176.

Millis, S. R., Rosenthal, M., Novack, T. A., Sherer, M., Nick, T. G., Kreutzer, J. S., . . . Ricker, J. H. (2001). Long-term neuropsychological outcome after traumatic brain injury. *Journal of Head Trauma Rehabilitation*, *16*(4), 343–355.

Mioni, G., Stablum, F., & Cantagallo, A. (2013). Time discrimination in traumatic brain injury patients. *Journal of Clinical and Experimental Neuropsychology*, *35*(1), 90–102. doi: 10.1080/13803395.2012.755151

Mortimer, J. A., van Duijn, C. M., Chandra, V., Fratiglioni, L., Graves, A. B., Heyman, A., Jorm, A. F., Kokmen, E., Kondo, K., Rocca, W.A., Shalat, S.L., Soininen, H., Hofman, A. for the Eurodem Risk Factors Research Group (1991). Head trauma as a risk factor for Alzheimer's disease: A collaborative re-analysis of case-control studies: EURODEM Risk Factors Research Group. *International Journal of Epidemiology*, *20*(Suppl 2), S28–35.

Mosenthal, A. C., Lavery, R. F., Addis, M., Kaul, S., Ross, S., Marburger, R., . . . Livingston, D. H. (2002). Isolated traumatic brain injury: Age is an independent predictor of mortality and early outcome. *Journal of Trauma*, *52*(5), 907–911.

Murray, G. D., Teasdale, G. M., Braakman, R., Cohadon, F., Dearden, M., Iannotti, F., . . . Unterberg, A. (1999). The European Brain Injury Consortium survey of head injuries. *Acta Neurochirurgica Supplementum*, *141*(3), 223–236.

Nakase-Richardson, R., Sepehri, A., Sherer, M., Yablon, S. A., Evans, C., & Mani, T. (2009). Classification schema of posttraumatic amnesia duration-based injury severity relative to 1-year outcome: Analysis of individuals with moderate and severe traumatic brain injury. *Archives of Physical Medicine and Rehabilitation*, *90*(1), 17–19. doi: S0003-9993(08)01542-6 [pii] 10.1016/j.apmr.2008.06.030

Nakase-Richardson, R., Sherer, M., Seel, R. T., Hart, T., Hanks, R., Arango-Lasprilla, J. C., . . . Hammond, F. (2011). Utility of post-traumatic amnesia in predicting 1-year productivity following traumatic brain injury: Comparison of the Russell and Mississippi PTA classification intervals. *Journal of Neurology, Neurosurgery, and Psychiatry*, *82*(5), 494–499. doi: jnnp.2010.222489 [pii] 10.1136/jnnp.2010.222489

Nakase-Richardson, R., Whyte, J., Giacino, J. T., Pavawalla, S., Barnett, S. D., Yablon, S. A., . . . Walker, W. C. (2012). Longitudinal outcome of patients with disordered consciousness in the NIDRR TBI Model Systems Programs. *Journal of Neurotrauma*, *29*(1), 59–65. doi: 10.1089/neu.2011.1829

Nakase-Thompson, R., Sherer, M., Yablon, S., Kennedy, R., & Nick, T. G. (2002). Persistent delirium and outcome following TBI. *Journal of the International Neuropsychological Society*, *8*, 219.

Nakase-Thompson, R., Sherer, M., Yablon, S. A., Nick, T. G., & Trzepacz, P. T. (2004). Acute confusion following traumatic brain injury. *Brain Injury*, *18*(2), 131–142.

National Center for Injury Prevention and Control. (2003). *Report to Congress on Mild Traumatic Brain Injury in the United States: Steps to Prevent a Serious Public Health Problem*. Atlanta, GA: Centers for Disease Control and Prevention.

Nelson, D. W., Nystrom, H., MacCallum, R. M., Thornquist, B., Lilja, A., Bellander, B. M., . . . Weitzberg, E. (2010). Extended analysis of early computed tomography scans of traumatic brain injured patients and relations to outcome. *Journal of Neurotrauma*, *27*(1), 51–64. doi: 10.1089/neu.2009.0986

Nemetz, P. N., Leibson, C., Naessens, J. M., Beard, M., Kokmen, E., Annegers, J. F., & Kurland, L. T. (1999). Traumatic brain injury and time to onset of Alzheimer's disease: A population-based study. *American Journal of Epidemiology*, *149*(1), 32–40.

Novack, T. A., Bush, B. A., Meythaler, J. M., & Canupp, K. (2001). Outcome after traumatic brain injury: Pathway analysis of contributions from premorbid, injury severity, and recovery variables. *Archives of Physical Medicine and Rehabilitation*, *82*(3), 300–305.

O'Dell, M. W., Barr, K., Spanier, D., & Warnick, R. E. (1998). Functional outcome of inpatient rehabilitation in persons with brain tumors. *Archives of Physical Medicine and Rehabilitation*, *79*(12), 1530–1534.

Ommaya, A. K., & Gennarelli, T. A. (1974). Cerebral concussion and traumatic unconsciousness: Correlation of experimental and clinical observations of blunt head injuries. *Brain*, *97*(4), 633–654.

Oppenheimer, D. R. (1968). Microscopic lesions in the brain following head injury. *Journal of Neurology, Neurosurgery and Psychiatry*, *31*(4), 299–306.

Parry-Jones, B. L., Vaughan, F. L., & Miles Cox, W. (2006). Traumatic brain injury and substance misuse: A systematic review of prevalence and outcomes research (1994–2004). [Review]. *Neuropsychol Rehabilitation*, *16*(5), 537–560. doi: 10.1080/09602010500231875

Pastorek, N. J., Hannay, H. J., & Contant, C. S. (2004). Prediction of global outcome with acute neuropsychological testing following closed-head injury. *Journal of the International Neuropsychological Society*, *10*(6), 807–817.

Plassman, B. L., Havlik, R. J., Steffens, D. C., Helms, M. J., Newman, T. N., Drosdick, D., . . . Breitner, J. C. (2000). Documented head injury in early adulthood and risk of Alzheimer's disease and other dementias. *Neurology*, *55*(8), 1158–1166.

Ponsford, J., Draper, K., & Schonberger, M. (2008). Functional outcome 10 years after traumatic brain injury: Its relationship with demographic, injury severity, and cognitive and emotional status. *Journal of the International Neuropsychological Society*, *14*(2), 233–242.

Ponsford, J., & Kinsella, G. (1992). Attentional deficits following closed-head injury. *Journal of Clinical and Experimental Neuropsychology*, *14*(5), 822–838.

Ponsford, J., Olver, J. H., Curran, C., & Ng, K. (1995). Prediction of employment status 2 years after traumatic brain injury. *Brain Injury*, *9*(1), 11–20.

Poon, W. S., Zhu, X. L., Ng, S. C., & Wong, G. K. (2005). Predicting one year clinical outcome in traumatic brain injury (TBI) at the beginning of rehabilitation. *Acta Neurochirurgica Supplementum*, *93*, 207–208.

Prigatano, G. P., Altman, I. M., & O'Brien, K. P. (1990). Behavioral limitations that traumatic-brain-injured patients tend to underestimate. *The Clinical Neuropsychologist*, *4*(2), 163–176.

Prigatano, G. P., Klonoff, P. S., O'Brien, K. P., Altman, I. M., Amin, K., Chiapello, D., . . . Mora, M. (1994). Productivity after neuropsychologically oriented milieu rehabilitation. *Journal of Head Trauma Rehabilitation*, *9*(1), 91–102.

Rappaport, M., Hall, K. M., Hopkins, K., Belleza, T., & Cope, D. N. (1982). Disability Rating Scale for severe head trauma: Coma to community. *Archives of Physical Medicine and Rehabilitation*, *63*, 118–123.

Rasmussen, K. W., & Berntsen, D. (2014). Autobiographical memory and episodic future thinking after moderate to severe traumatic brain injury. *Journal of Neuropsychology*, *8*(1), 34–52. doi: 10.1111/jnp.12003

Rasmusson, D. X., Brandt, J., Martin, D. B., & Folstein, M. F. (1995). Head-injury as a risk factor in Alzheimers-disease. *Brain Injury*, *9*(3), 213–219. doi: 10.3109/02699059509008194

Reilly, P. L., Graham, D. I., Adams, J. H., & Jennett, B. (1975). Patients with head injury who talk and die. *Lancet*, *2*(7931), 375–377.

Rochat, L., Beni, C., Annoni, J. M., Vuadens, P., & Van der Linden, M. (2013). How inhibition relates to impulsivity after moderate to severe traumatic brain injury. *Journal of the International Neuropsychological Society*, *19*(8), 890–898. doi: 10.1017/s1355617713000672

Rockswold, G. L., Leonard, P. R., & Nagib, M. G. (1987). Analysis of management in thirty-three closed head injury patients who "talked and deteriorated." *Neurosurgery*, *21*(1), 51–55.

Rohling, M. L., Binder, L. M., Demakis, G. J., Larrabee, G. J., Ploetz, D. M., & Langhinrichsen-Rohling, J. (2011). A meta-analysis of neuropsychological outcome after mild traumatic brain injury: Re-analyses and reconsiderations of Binder et al. (1997), Frencham et al. (2005), and Pertab et al. (2009). [Meta-Analysis]. *Clinical Neuropsychologist*, *25*(4), 608–623. doi: 10.1080/13854046.2011.565076

Rothweiler, B., Temkin, N. R., & Dikmen, S. S. (1998). Aging effect on psychosocial outcome in traumatic brain injury. *Archives of Physical Medicine and Rehabilitation*, *79*(8), 881–887.

Ruff, R. M., Evans, R., & Marshall, L. F. (1986). Impaired verbal and figural fluency after head injury. *Archives of Clinical Neuropsychology*, *1*(2), 87–101.

Ruff, R. M., Marshall, L. F., Crouch, J., Klauber, M. R., Levin, H. S., Barth, J., . . . Marmarou, A. (1993). Predictors of outcome following severe head trauma: Follow-up data from the Traumatic Coma Data Bank. *Brain Injury*, *7*(2), 101–111.

Ruff, R. M., Young, D., Gautille, T., Marshall, L. F., Barth, J., Jane, J. A., . . . Foulkes, M. A. (1991). Verbal learning deficits following severe head injury: Heterogeneity in recovery over 1 year. *Journal of Neurosurgery*, *75*, S50–S58.

Russell, W. R. (1932). Cerebral involvement in head injury: A study on the examination of two hundred cases. *Brain*, *55*, 549–603.

Russell, W. R. (1971). *The Traumatic Amnesias*. New York: Oxford University Press.

Russell, W. R., & Smith, A. (1961). Post-traumatic amnesia in closed head injury. *Archives of Neurology*, *5*, 4–17.

Rutland-Brown, W., Langlois, J. A., Thomas, K. E., & Xi, Y. L. (2006). Incidence of traumatic brain injury in the United States, 2003. *Journal of Head Trauma Rehabilitation*, *21*(6), 544–548.

Sady, M. D., Sander, A. M., Clark, A. N., Sherer, M., Nakase-Richardson, R., & Malec, J. F. (2010). Relationship of preinjury caregiver and family functioning to community integration in adults with traumatic brain injury. *Archives of Physical Medicine and Rehabilitation*, *91*(10), 1542–1550. doi: 10.1016/j.apmr.2010.07.012

Salcido, R., & Costich, J. F. (1992). Recurrent traumatic brain injury. *Brain Injury*, *6*(3), 293–298.

Salib, E., & Hillier, V. (1997). Head injury and the risk of Alzheimer's disease: A case control study. *International Journal of Geriatric Psychiatry*, *12*(3), 363–368.

Sander, A. M., Kreutzer, J., Rosenthal, M., Delmonico, R., & Young, M. E. (1996). A multicenter longitudinal investigation of return to work and community integration following traumatic brain injury. *Journal of Head Trauma Rehabilitation*, *11*(5), 70–84.

Sander, A. M., Maestas, K. L., Sherer, M., Malec, J. F., & Nakase-Richardson, R. (2012). Relationship of caregiver and family functioning to participation outcomes after postacute rehabilitation for traumatic brain injury: A multicenter investigation. *Archives of Physical Medicine and Rehabilitation*, *93*(5), 842–848. doi: 10.1016/j.apmr.2011.11.031

Sarno, M. T., Buonaguro, A., & Levita, E. (1986). Characteristics of verbal impairment in closed head injured patients. *Archives of Physical Medicine and Rehabilitation*, *67*(6), 400–405.

Satz, P., Zaucha, K., Forney, D. L., McCleary, C., Asarnow, R. F., Light, R., . . . Becker, D. (1998). Neuropsychological, psychosocial and vocational correlates of the Glasgow Outcome Scale at 6 months post-injury: A study of moderate to severe traumatic brain injury patients. *Brain Injury*, *12*(7), 555–567.

Saunders, L. L., Selassie, A. W., Hill, E. G., Nicholas, J. S., Horner, M. D., Corrigan, J. D., & Lackland, D. T. (2009). A population-based study of repetitive traumatic brain injury among persons with traumatic brain injury. *Brain Injury*, *23*(11), 866–872. doi: 10.1080/02699050903283213

Schofield, P. W., Tang, M., Marder, K., Bell, K., Dooneief, G., Chun, M., . . . Mayeux, R. (1997). Alzheimer's disease after remote head injury: An incidence study. *Journal of Neurology, Neurosurgery and Psychiatry*, *62*(2), 119–124.

Schretlen, D. J., & Shapiro, A. M. (2003). A quantitative review of the effects of traumatic brain injury on cognitive functioning. *International Review of Psychiatry*, *15*(4), 341–349. doi: 10.1080/09540260310001606728

Seel, R. T., Kreutzer, J. S., Rosenthal, M., Hammond, F. M., Corrigan, J. D., & Black, K. (2003). Depression after traumatic brain injury: A National Institute on Disability and Rehabilitation Research Model Systems multicenter investigation. *Archives of Physical Medicine and Rehabilitation*, *84*(2), 177–184.

Selassie, A. W., Zaloshnja, E., Langlois, J. A., Miller, T., Jones, P., & Steiner, C. (2008). Incidence of long-term disability following traumatic brain injury hospitalization, United States, 2003. *Journal of Head Trauma Rehabilitation*, *23*(2), 123–131. doi: 10.1097/01.HTR.0000314531.30401.39. [pii] 00001199-200803000-00007

Sherer, M., Bergloff, P., High, W., Jr., & Nick, T. G. (1999). Contribution of functional ratings to prediction of longterm employment outcome after traumatic brain injury. *Brain Injury*, *13*(12), 973–981.

Sherer, M., Bergloff, P., Levin, E., High, W. M., Jr., Oden, K. E., & Nick, T. G. (1998). Impaired awareness and employment outcome after traumatic brain injury. *Journal of Head Trauma Rehabilitation*, *13*(5), 52–61.

Sherer, M., Boake, C., Levin, E., Silver, B. V., Ringholz, G., & High, W. M., Jr. (1998). Characteristics of impaired awareness after traumatic brain injury. *Journal of the International Neuropsychological Society*, *4*(4), 380–387.

Sherer, M., Hart, T., Nick, T. G., Whyte, J., Thompson, R. N., & Yablon, S. A. (2003). Early impaired self-awareness after traumatic brain injury. *Archives of Physical Medicine and Rehabilitation*, *84*(2), 168–176.

Sherer, M., Nakase-Thompson, R., Nick, T. G., & Yablon, S. (2003). Patterns of neurobehavioral deficits in TBI patients at rehabilitation admission. *Journal of the International Neuropsychological Society*, *9*, 251–252.

Sherer, M., Nakase-Thompson, R., Yablon, S. A., & Gontkovsky, S. T. (2005). Multidimensional assessment of acute confusion after traumatic brain injury. *Archives of Physical Medicine and Rehabilitation*, *86*(5), 896–904.

Sherer, M., Nick, T. G., Millis, S. R., & Novack, T. A. (2003). Use of the WCST and the WCST-64 in the assessment of traumatic brain injury. *Journal of Clinical and Experimental Neuropsychology*, *25*(4), 512–520.

Sherer, M., Nick, T. G., Sander, A. M., Hart, T., Hanks, R., Rosenthal, M., . . . Yablon, S. A. (2003). Race and productivity outcome after traumatic brain injury: Influence of confounding factors. *Journal of Head Trauma Rehabilitation*, *18*(5), 408–424.

Sherer, M., & Novack, T. (2003). Neuropsychological assessment after traumatic brain injury in adults. In G. P. Prigatano & N. H. Pliskin (Eds.), *Clinical Neuropsychology and Cost Outcome Research* (pp. 39–60). New York: Psychology Press, Inc.

Sherer, M., Sander, A.M., Maestas, K.L., Pastorek, N.J., Nick, T.G., & Li, J. (2015). Accuracy of self-reported length of coma and posttraumatic amnesia in persons with medically verified traumatic brain injury. *Archives of Physical Medicine and Rehabilitation*, *96*(4), 652–8. doi: 10.1016/j.apmr.2014.10.024

Sherer, M., Sander, A. M., Nick, T. G., High, W. M., Jr., Malec, J. F., & Rosenthal, M. (2002). Early cognitive status and productivity outcome after traumatic brain injury: Findings from the TBI model systems. *Archives of Physical Medicine and Rehabilitation*, *83*(2), 183–192.

Sherer, M., Struchen, M. A., Nakase-Thompson, R., & Yablon, S. A. (2005). Comparison of indices of severity of traumatic brain injury. *Journal of the International Neuropsychological Society*, *11*(S1), 48.

Sherer, M., Yablon, S. A., & Nakase-Richardson, R. (2009). Patterns of recovery of posttraumatic confusional state in neurorehabilitation admissions after traumatic brain injury. *Archives of Physical Medicine and Rehabilitation*, *90*(10), 1749–1754. doi: 10.1016/j.apmr.2009.05.011

Sherer, M., Yablon, S. A., Nakase-Richardson, R., & Nick, T. G. (2008). Effect of severity of post-traumatic confusion and its constituent symptoms on outcome after traumatic brain injury. *Archives of Physical Medicine and Rehabilitation*, *89*(1), 42–47. doi: S0003-9993(07)01610-3 [pii] 10.1016/j.apmr.2007.08.128

Sherer, M., Yablon, S. A., & Nick, T. G. (2014). Psychotic symptoms as manifestations of the posttraumatic confusional state: Prevalence, risk factors, and association with outcome. *Journal of Head Trauma Rehabilitation*, *73*(14). doi: 10.1097/HTR.0b013e318287f894

Shores, E. A., Marosszeky, J. E., Sandanam, J., & Batchelor, J. (1986). Preliminary validation of a clinical scale for measuring the duration of post-traumatic amnesia. *Medical Journal of Australia*, *144*(11), 569–572.

Sidaros, A., Engberg, A. W., Sidaros, K., Liptrot, M. G., Herning, M., Petersen, P., . . . Rostrup, E. (2008). Diffusion tensor imaging during recovery from severe traumatic brain injury and relation to clinical outcome: A longitudinal study. *Brain*, *131*(Pt 2), 559–572.

Signorini, D. F., Andrews, P. J., Jones, P. A., Wardlaw, J. M., & Miller, J. D. (1999). Predicting survival using simple clinical variables: A case study in traumatic brain injury. *Journal of Neurology, Neurosurgery and Psychiatry*, *66*(1), 20–25.

Snow, P. C., & Douglas, J. M. (2000). Conceptual and methodological challenges in discourse assessment with TBI speakers: Towards an understanding. *Brain Injury*, *14*(5), 397–415.

Sosin, D. M., Sniezek, J. E., & Thurman, D. J. (1996). Incidence of mild and moderate brain injury in the United States, 1991. *Brain Injury*, *10*(1), 47–54.

Spikman, J. M., Timmerman, M. E., Milders, M. V., Veenstra, W. S., & van der Naalt, J. (2012). Social cognition impairments in relation to general cognitive deficits, injury severity, and prefrontal lesions in traumatic brain injury patients. *Journal of Neurotrauma*, *29*(1), 101–111. doi: 10.1089/neu.2011.2084

Starkstein, S. E., & Jorge, R. (2005). Dementia after traumatic brain injury. *International Psychogeriatrics*, *17*(Suppl 1), S93–107.

Stein, S. C. (1996). Outcome from moderate head injury. In R. K. Narayan, J. E. Wilberger, & J. T. Povlishock (Eds.), *Neurotrauma* (pp. 755–765). New York: McGraw-Hill.

Stuss, D. T., Binns, M. A., Carruth, F. G., Levine, B., Brandys, C. E., Moulton, R. J., . . . Schwartz, M. L. (1999). The acute period of recovery from traumatic brain injury: Posttraumatic amnesia or posttraumatic confusional state? *Journal of Neurosurgery*, *90*(4), 635–643.

Stuss, D. T., Ely, P., Hugenholtz, H., Richard, M. T., LaRochelle, S., Poirier, C. A., & Bell, I. (1985). Subtle neuropsychological deficits in patients with good recovery after closed head injury. *Neurosurgery*, *17*(1), 41–47.

Stuss, D. T., Stethem, L. L., Hugenholtz, H., Picton, T., Pivik, J., & Richard, M. T. (1989). Reaction time after head injury: Fatigue, divided and focused attention, and consistency of performance. *Journal of Neurology, Neurosurgery and Psychiatry*, *52*(6), 742–748.

Stuss, D. T., Stethem, L. L., Picton, T. W., Leech, E. E., & Pelchat, G. (1989). Traumatic brain injury, aging and reaction time. *Canadian Journal of Neurological Sciences*, *16*(2), 161–167.

Susman, M., DiRusso, S. M., Sullivan, T., Risucci, D., Nealon, P., Cuff, S., . . . Benzil, D. (2002). Traumatic brain injury in the elderly: Increased mortality and worse functional outcome at discharge despite lower injury severity. *Journal of Trauma*, *53*(2), 219–223; discussion 223–214.

Symonds, C. P. (1937). Mental disorder following head injury. *Proceedings of the Royal Society of Medicine*, *30*, 1081–1094.

Symonds, C. P., & Russell, W. R. (1943). Accidental head injuries: Prognosis in service patients. *Lancet*, *241*(6227), 7–10.

Tabaddor, K., Mattis, S., & Zazula, T. (1984). Cognitive sequelae and recovery course after moderate and severe head injury. *Neurosurgery*, *14*(6), 701–708.

Tate, R. L., Fenelon, B., Manning, M. L., & Hunter, M. (1991). Patterns of neuropsychological impairment after severe blunt head injury. *Journal of Nervous and Mental Disease*, *179*(3), 117–126.

Taylor, L. A., Kreutzer, J. S., Demm, S. R., & Meade, M. A. (2003). Traumatic brain injury and substance abuse: A review and analysis of the literature. *Neuropsychological Rehabilitation*, *13*(1–2), 165–188. doi: 10.1080/09602010244000336

Teasdale, G., & Jennett, B. (1974). Assessment of coma and impaired consciousness: A practical scale. *Lancet*, *2*(7872), 81–84.

Teasdale, T. W., & Engberg, A. W. (2005). Subjective well-being and quality of life following traumatic brain injury in adults: A long-term population-based follow-up. *Brain Injury*, *19*(12), 1041–1048.

Testa, J. A., Malec, J. F., Moessner, A. M., & Brown, A. W. (2005). Outcome after traumatic brain injury: Effects of aging on recovery. *Archives of Physical Medicine and Rehabilitation*, *86*(9), 1815–1823.

Thompson, R. S., Rivara, F. P., & Thompson, D. C. (1989). A case-control study of the effectiveness of bicycle safety helmets. *New England Journal of Medicine*, *320*(21), 1361–1367. doi: 10.1056/NEJM198905253202101

Thurman, D. J. (1999). *Traumatic Brain Injury in the United States: A Report to Congress*. Atlanta, GA: Centers for Disease Control and Prevention.

Thurman, D. J., Alverson, C., Dunn, K. A., Guerrero, J., & Sniezek, J. E. (1999). Traumatic brain injury in the United States: A public health perspective. *Journal of Head Trauma Rehabilitation*, *14*(6), 602–615.

Thurman, D. J., & Guerrero, J. (1999). Trends in hospitalization associated with traumatic brain injury. *Journal of the American Medical Association*, *282*(10), 954–957.

Trudel, T. M., Tryon, W. W., & Purdum, C. M. (1998). Awareness of disability and long-term outcome after traumatic brain injury. *Rehabilitation Psychology*, *53*, 267–281.

Uryu, K., Chen, X. H., Martinez, D., Browne, K. D., Johnson, V. E., Graham, D. I., . . . Smith, D. H. (2007). Multiple proteins implicated in neurodegenerative diseases accumulate in axons after brain trauma in humans. *Experimental Neurology*, *208*(2), 185–192.

Vanderploeg, R. D., Belanger, H. G., Duchnick, J. D., & Curtiss, G. (2007). Awareness problems following moderate to severe traumatic brain injury: Prevalence, assessment methods, and injury correlates. *Journal of Rehabilitation Research & Development*, *44*(7), 937–950.

Vanderploeg, R. D., Crowell, T. A., & Curtiss, G. (2001). Verbal learning and memory deficits in traumatic brain injury: Encoding, consolidation, and retrieval. *Journal of Clinical and Experimental Neuropsychology*, *23*(2), 185–195.

Vanderploeg, R. D., Donnell, A. J., Belanger, H. G., & Curtiss, G. (2014). Consolidation deficits in traumatic brain injury: The core and residual verbal memory defect. *Journal of Clinical and Experimental Neuropsychology*, *36*(1), 58–73. doi: 10.1080/13803395.2013.864600

van Duijn, C. M., Tanja, T. A., Haaxma, R., Schulte, W., Saan, R. J., Lameris, A. J., . . . Hofman, A. (1992). Head trauma and the risk of Alzheimer's disease. [Research Support, Non-U.S. Gov't]. *American Journal of Epidemiology*, *135*(7), 775–782.

van Zomeren, A. H., & Deelman, B. G. (1978). Long-term recovery of visual reaction time after closed head injury. *Journal of Neurology, Neurosurgery and Psychiatry*, *41*(5), 452–457.

Vespa, P. M., Boscardin, W. J., Hovda, D. A., McArthur, D. L., Nuwer, M. R., Martin, N. A., . . . Becker, D. P. (2002). Early and persistent impaired percent alpha variability on continuous electroencephalography monitoring as predictive of poor outcome after traumatic brain injury. *Journal of Neurosurgery*, *97*(1), 84–92.

Waljas, M., Lange, R., Hakulinen, U., Huhtala, H., Dastidar, P., Hartikainen, K., . . . Iverson, G. (2014). Biopsychosocial outcome following uncomplicated mild traumatic brain injury. *Journal of Neurotrauma*, *31*(1), 108–124. doi: 10.1089/neu.2013.2941

Walker, W. C., Ketchum, J. M., Marwitz, J. H., Chen, T., Hammond, F., Sherer, M., & Meythaler, J. (2010). A multicentre study on the clinical utility of post-traumatic amnesia duration in predicting global outcome after moderate-severe traumatic brain injury. *Journal of Neurology, Neurosurgery, and Psychiatry*, *81*(1), 87–89. doi: 81/1/87 [pii] 10.1136/jnnp.2008.161570

Wang, H. K., Lin, S. H., Sung, P. S., Wu, M. H., Hung, K. W., Wang, L. C., . . . Tsai, K. J. (2012). Population based study on patients with traumatic brain injury suggests increased risk of dementia. *Journal of Neurology, Neurosurgery and Psychiatry*, *83*(11), 1080–1085. doi: 10.1136/jnnp-2012-302633

Wardlaw, J. M., Easton, V. J., & Statham, P. (2002). Which CT features help predict outcome after head injury? *Journal of Neurology, Neurosurgery and Psychiatry*, *72*(2), 188–192; discussion 151.

Wedekind, C., & Lippert-Gruner, M. (2005). Long-term outcome in severe traumatic brain injury is significantly influenced by brainstem involvement. *Brain Injury*, *19*(9), 681–684.

Weintraub, S., Dikmen, S. S., Heaton, R. K., Tulsky, D. S., Zelazo, P. D., Bauer, P. J., . . . Gershon, R. C. (2013). Cognition assessment using the NIH Toolbox. *Neurology*, *80*(11, Suppl 3), S54–S64. doi: 10.1212/WNL.0b013e3182872ded

Whiteneck, G. G., Dijkers, M. P., Heinemann, A. W., Bogner, J. A., Bushnik, T., Cicerone, K. D., . . . Millis, S. R. (2011). Development of the participation assessment with recombined tools-objective for use after traumatic brain injury. *Archives of Physical Medicine and Rehabilitation*, *92*(4), 542–551. doi: 10.1016/j.apmr.2010.08.002

Whitman, S., Coonley-Hoganson, R., & Desai, B. T. (1984). Comparative head trauma experiences in two socioeconomically different Chicago-area communities: A population study. *American Journal of Epidemiology*, *119*(4), 570–580.

Whyte, J., Cifu, D., Dikmen, S., & Temkin, N. (2001). Prediction of functional outcomes after traumatic brain injury: A comparison of 2 measures of duration of unconsciousness. *Archives of Physical Medicine and Rehabilitation*, *82*(10), 1355–1359.

Wilde, E. A., Chu, Z., Bigler, E. D., Hunter, J. V., Fearing, M. A., Hanten, G., . . . Levin, H. S. (2006). Diffusion tensor imaging in the corpus callosum in children after moderate to severe traumatic brain injury. *Journal of Neurotrauma*, *23*(10), 1412–1426.

Wilde, E. A., McCauley, S. R., Hunter, J. V., Bigler, E. D., Chu, Z., Wang, Z. J., . . . Levin, H. S. (2008). Diffusion tensor imaging of acute mild traumatic brain injury in adolescents. *Neurology*, *70*(12), 948–955. doi: 10.1212/01.wnl.0000305961.68029.54

Willer, B. S., Rosenthal, M., Kreutzer, J. S., Gordon, W. A., & Rempel, R. (1993). Assessment of community integration following rehabilitation for traumatic brain injury. *Journal of Head Trauma Rehabilitation*, *8*(2), 75–87.

Williams, D. H., Levin, H. S., & Eisenberg, H. M. (1990). Mild head injury classification. *Neurosurgery*, *27*(3), 422–428.

Williams, G. K., Arango-Lasprilla, J. C., & Stevens, L. F. (2009). Do racial/ethnic differences exist in post-injury outcomes after TBI? A comprehensive review of the literature. *Brain Injury*, *23*(10), 775–789.

Williams, M. W., Rapport, L. J., Hanks, R. A., Millis, S. R., & Greene, H. A. (2013). Incremental validity of neuropsychological evaluations to computed tomography in predicting long-term outcomes after traumatic brain injury. *Clinical Neuropsychologist*, *27*(3), 356–375. doi: 10.1080/13854046.2013.765507

Wright, M. J., & Schmitter-Edgecombe, M. (2011). The impact of verbal memory encoding and consolidation deficits during recovery from moderate-to-severe traumatic brain injury. [Research Support, N.I.H., Extramural]. *Journal of Head Trauma Rehabilitation*, *26*(3), 182–191. doi: 10.1097/HTR.0b013e318218dcf9

Yablon, S. (1996). Posttraumatic seizures. In L. J. Horn & N. D. Zasler (Eds.), *Medical Rehabilitation of Traumatic Brain Injury* (pp. 363–394). Philadelphia, PA: Hanley & Belfus, Inc.

Yallampalli, R., Wilde, E. A., Bigler, E. D., McCauley, S. R., Hanten, G., Troyanskaya, M., . . . Levin, H. S. (2013). Acute white matter differences in the fornix following mild traumatic brain injury using diffusion tensor imaging. *Journal of Neuroimaging*, *23*(2), 224–227. doi: 10.1111/j.1552-6569.2010.00537.x

Yu, E. J., Yablon, S., Ivanhoe, C., & Boake, C. (1995). Posttraumatic hydrocephalus: Incidence and outcome following screening of consecutive admissions. *Archives of Physical Medicine and Rehabilitation*, *76*, 1041.

Zhang, J., Jiang, J. Y., Zhong, T., Yu, M., & Zhu, C. (2001). Outcome of 2,284 cases with acute traumatic brain injury. *Chinese Journal of Traumatology*, *4*, 152–155.

18 Concussion and Mild Traumatic Brain Injury

Heather G. Belanger, David F. Tate, and Rodney D. Vanderploeg

Definition of Mild TBI

Mild traumatic brain injury (or mild TBI) is typically defined as disrupted brain functioning from any force to the head as evidenced by altered or lost consciousness that is of shorter duration than more severe TBI. There are somewhat divergent diagnostic criteria, which will be briefly discussed in the next section, that detail the specifics of the duration of the altered state of consciousness. Some diagnostic criteria allow for diagnosis of mild TBI or "possible'" mild TBI with the mere presence of symptoms post-event and do not require altered or lost consciousness (Malec et al., 2007; Smits et al., 2007). The term *concussion,* is sometimes used to refer to a milder subcategory of mild TBI (McCrory et al., 2013), but is more typically used synonymously with mild TBI (and will be in this chapter).

Pathophysiology of Mild TBI

Mechanical forces cause injury to the brain in two phases: an immediate phase in which damage occurs as a direct result of the mechanical impact, and a later phase of altered biochemical events that may result in delayed tissue damage. While posttraumatic increases in cellular calcium do not inevitably lead to cell death, cell death can occur due to a variety of mechanisms (see Giza & Hovda, 2001) that lead to free-radical overproduction, cytoskeletal reorganization, and activation of apoptotic genetic signals.

Axons in the brain may stretch and twist due to mild TBI. The resulting damage should be considered a "process rather than an event" (Gennarelli & Graham, 1998: 163; see also Gaetz, 2004). Following a head insult in animal models of mild TBI, scattered axons swell slightly and become misaligned, but unlike moderate TBI, there is no altered axolemmal permeability (Pettus, Christman, Giebel, & Povlishock, 1994). Contrary to the widely held "shearing hypothesis," in which axonal injury was thought to be the result of axons being disconnected at the time of impact (i.e., primary axotomy), there is no physical tearing or shearing of the axon cylinder (Gaetz, 2004). Several terms are used to describe the secondary axonal injury resulting from closed head injury, including *traumatic axonal injury* (TAI), *diffuse axonal injury* (DAI), or *multifocal axonal injury*. In most cases, TAI is most accurately understood as a relatively short-duration event in which axonal alterations evolve through a complex cytochemical cascade which can lead to axonal disconnection. Importantly, disconnection does not necessarily lead to rapid cell death (Singleton, Zhu, Stone, & Povlishock, 2002). Due to mild TBI, scattered axons may swell and disconnect, while others remain intact (Greer, Povlishock, & Jacobs, 2012). Animal models show that mild TBI uncomplicated by contusion can cause perturbation with electrophysiological changes, in the form of increased excitability, even in some intact neurons, that return largely to normal within a day or two (Greer, et al., 2012). Disconnection can be followed by various processes that lead to atrophy in some neurons and neuroinflammation, as has been demonstrated one month postinjury in moderate TBI animal models (Kelley, Lifshitz, & Povlishock, 2007; Lifshitz, Witgen, & Grady, 2007).

By definition, there is disruption to the functioning of the brain with mild TBI. Some structural injury may also occur. Borg et al. (2004) reported on the prevalence of abnormalities on computed tomography (CT) scans, for those who go to the hospital following mild TBI, as follows: 5% for those with a Glasgow Coma Score (GCS) of 15, 20% with GCS score of 14, and 30% with GCS score of 13. Clearly, when abnormalities are present on neuroimaging, cellular damage is present. Indeed, this is corroborated by studies demonstrating metabolic changes in the vicinity of brain injury seen on scans (Govindaraju et al., 2004; Son et al., 2000).

However, the vast majority of mild TBI cases are normal on clinical neuroimaging (i.e., CT and structural magnetic resonance imaging, or MRI). Indeed some clinical diagnostic criteria require normal acute neuroimaging (e.g., U.S. Department of Defense and Veterans Administration [VA] criteria). The question then becomes whether "invisible" persistent structural injury is present. An autopsy study of five people with history of mild TBI with loss of consciousness (LOC), who died of other causes 2 to 99 days postinjury, revealed evidence of axonal injury in all cases, particularly in the corpus callosum and fornices (Blumbergs et al., 1994). Recent studies using more advanced imaging methods—i.e., susceptibility weighted imaging (SWI) and diffusion tensor imaging (DTI)—have also begun to demonstrate imaging abnormalities previously unseen in mild TBI patients (see "Current Clinical Imaging Findings" section later in this chapter). SWI has been shown to be up to six times more sensitive than other more traditional MRI modalities (i.e., T2, fluid attenuated inversion recovery, or FLAIR) commonly employed in TBI to detect small lesions and discrete vascular changes (Tong et al., 2003). In our own sample of mild TBI patients (*N* = 74), 13.6% have SWI abnormalities while other imaging modalities appear to demonstrate no abnormalities (Tate, Gusman, Kini, et al., 2013). These findings are similar to reports from other groups (Haacke, Raza, Bo, & Kou, 2013). These studies may indicate pathology previously undetected and may have relatively unexplored clinical implications.

Epidemiology of Mild TBI

TBI is a leading cause of death and disability in the United States. Data from emergency room visits, hospitalizations, and deaths suggest that 1.7 million TBIs occur each year (Faul, Xu, Wald, & Coronado, 2010). It is estimated that approximately 70%–90% of all TBIs are mild in severity. While the incidence of TBI-related hospital admissions decreased between 1993/1994 and 2006/2007, most hospitalized adult TBI patients were classified as mild in both time periods (Farhad et al., 2013). Some individuals who sustained a mild TBI may not have that diagnosis recorded in their list of ER discharge diagnoses, thereby resulting in under-estimates of incidence (Powell, Ferraro, Dikmen, Temkin, & Bell, 2008; Puljula et al., 2012). Extrapolating from the 1.7 million estimated annual TBIs, and assuming that 80%–90% of those are mild, we can conclude that about 1.36 million of annual TBIs are mild. However, this is likely an underestimate, as these were hospital data and many people likely seek no treatment at all, or consult their primary care physician or some other provider (e.g., military health care system). Methodological limitations in estimating the incidence and prevalence of mild TBI also include variability in definition/diagnostic criteria and ascertainment methods (i.e., self-report, discharge diagnoses based on medical records/billing, emergency medical records, survey, etc.). These limitations must be considered when examining epidemiological studies, as well as variances based on context (i.e., sports vs. military vs. general population).

Diagnosis and Diagnostic Criteria

There is disagreement about what criteria should be used to identify mild TBI, and it is important to realize that different criteria have been used in research studies of mild TBI. The most common diagnostic criteria utilized are those proposed by the American Congress of Rehabilitation Medicine (1993). These criteria are delineated in Table 18.1.

Severity of TBI is determined at the time of injury, and not by level of functioning at some later point in time. Though severity level has prognostic value, it does not necessarily predict a patient's likelihood of functional recovery. Severity of TBI is a continuum and the particular classification used to designate a patient as having mild, moderate, or severe injury is somewhat arbitrary.

Table 18.1 American Congress of Rehabilitation Medicine criteria for mild TBI

Diagnostic Criteria for Mild Traumatic Brain Injury

I. Traumatically induced physiologic disruption of brain function as indicated by at least one of the following:
   A. Any loss of consciousness
   B. Any loss of memory for events immediately before or after the accident
   C. Any alteration in mental state at the time of the accident (e.g., feeling dazed, disoriented, or confused)
   D. Focal neurologic deficit(s) that may or may not be transient
II. Severity of the injury does not exceed:
   A. Loss of consciousness (LOC) of 30 minutes or less
   B. After 30 minutes, an initial Glasgow Coma Scale (GCS) score of 13–15
   C. Posttraumatic amnesia (PTA) not greater than 24 hours

Source: American Congress of Rehabilitation Medicine(1993)

In 2004 the World Health Organization published a review paper on the various diagnostic criteria for mild TBI and concluded that the degree of variance was impeding progress in the field (Carroll, Cassidy, Holm, Kraus, & Coronado, 2004). So, for example, some research studies on mild TBI included participants with a GCS score between 13 and 15, while others included only those with GCS of 14 or 15. The authors proposed a set of diagnostic criteria that they acknowledged was based largely on the ACRM criteria but allowed for later assessment of GCS ("upon presentation for healthcare"), eliminated the word "dazed" from description of altered consciousness, and noted "transient neurological abnormalities such as focal signs, seizure, and intracranial lesion not requiring surgery" (p. 115) may be present.

Because knowing whether or not a person has sustained a mild TBI is in some cases impossible, some argue that broad and inclusive criteria should be used to identify those at greater risk, to ensure proper evaluation and treatment (e.g., McCrory, et al., 2013; Scholten, Cernich, Hurley, & Helmick, 2013). For example, a recently published consensus statement on concussion in the sports arena encourages assessment and management of athletes showing "features" of concussion, which includes symptoms such as headache and emotional lability, and sleep disturbance (McCrory, et al., 2013). However, inclusion of possible mild TBI would not suffice in a legal setting where injury and attribution of symptoms to a particular etiology is part and parcel of what cases are about.

Unlike moderate to severe TBI, diagnosis of mild TBI often cannot be corroborated with objective diagnostic tools or medical personnel. First, not all traumatic injurious events are witnessed and often there is no documentation or corroboration of the person's immediate status following the injurious event. Any period of disturbed consciousness may resolve before it can be assessed and documented by medical personnel. Second, a person may mildly injure his or her brain and not report it or seek medical care. Because of reliance on self-report and because emergency and other personnel may not ask (Powell, et al., 2008), mild TBI is likely under- or overdiagnosed, depending on the setting.

When neuroimaging findings or positive signs on an acute neurological examination are present following what otherwise would be classified as a mild TBI, the classification changes to "complicated mild TBI." Complicated mild TBIs have a six-month outcome more similar to moderate TBI than to an uncomplicated mild TBI (Borgaro, Prigatano, Kwasnica, & Rexer, 2003; Goldstein & Levin, 2001; Kashluba, Hanks, Casey, & Millis, 2008; Williams, Levin, & Eisenberg, 1990). Although several studies have failed to demonstrate this difference in outcome (see bolded studies in Table 18.2), as can be seen in Table 18.2, these studies utilized less-sensitive outcome measures (i.e., not cognitive performance) or involved chronic, clinical samples that likely do not represent the mild TBI population at large (i.e., sample bias). Of note, in some diagnostic criteria, abnormal imaging that is attributed to the injury (i.e., typically, in the acute phase) results in the patient being considered to have greater than mild injury.(Department of Veterans Affairs and Department of Defense, April, 2009)

To complicate matters, the term *concussion* is sometimes used synonymously with mild TBI but may also be used to denote a less serious injury. The term *concussion* tends to be used in the sports arena, while the term *mild TBI* tends to be used more in medical settings. It has been suggested that the term *concussion* should be used, rather than *mild TBI,* due to the potentially iatrogenic effects of being told one has a "brain injury" (Hoge, Goldberg, & Castro, 2009). Indeed,

Table 18.2 Mild TBI outcomes in adults in relation to neuroimaging findings

Study	*Mild TBI Participants*	*Mild TBI criteria*	*Time Since Injury*	*Outcome Measure(s)*	*Performance Validity Assessed?*	*Caveats*	*Did CT/ MRI+ Have Worse Outcome?*
Borgaro et al. 2003	28 patients recruited in emergency room	GCS	13 days	Cognitive performance	No	No differences based on affective disturbance	Yes
de Guise et al. (2010)	**167 symptomatic outpatient clinic referrals**	**ACRM**	**3 weeks**	**Cognitive performance PCS GOS-R Mood**	**No**	**No data on % involved in litigation**	**No**
Dagher et al. (2013)	2,127 hospitalized patients	ACRM	?	GOS-E FIM	No	No data on % involved in litigation	Yes
Goldstein and Levin (2001)	35 patients	GCS 13–15, LOC < 20 min	28 days	Cognitive performance	No	4 of the "complicated mild" group met GCS criteria for moderate TBI	Yes
Hanlon, Demery, Martinovich, and Kelly 1999	**100 consecutive referrals to concussion clinic**	**ACRM**	**5.9 months**	**Cognitive performance**	**No**	**48% of CT negative cases were legal cases (vs. 18% of CT positive)**	**No**
Hofman et al. (2001)	21 consecutive patients under age 50 presenting at emergency room	GCS 14–15 LOC < 20 min PTA < 6hrs	Baseline 2 months 6 months	Cognitive performance Mood	No	No data on % involved in litigation	Yes (cognitive)
Hsiang et al. (Hsiang, Yeung, Yu, & Poon, 1997)	1,360 consecutive admissions to neurosurgery	GCS	6 months	GOS	No	No data on % involved in litigation	Yes
Hughes et al. (2004)	271 consecutive emergency department	ACRM	72 hours	Cognitive performance PCS Return to work	No	None	Yes*
Iverson (2006)	100 patients seen in trauma service	GCS	4 days	Cognitive performance	No	None	Yes
Iverson, Franzen, and Lovell (1999)	546 patients seen in trauma service	GCS	Within a week	Cognitive performance	No	None	Yes

(*Continued*)

Table 18.2—continued

Study	*Mild TBI Participants*	*Mild TBI criteria*	*Time Since Injury*	*Outcome Measure(s)*	*Performance Validity Assessed?*	*Caveats*	*Did CT/ MRI+ Have Worse Outcome?*
Iverson et al. (2012)	**47 patients seen in emergency department**	**ACRM**	**25.7 days**	**Cognitive performance PCS Return to work Mood**	**No**	**None**	**No****
Jacobs et al. (2010)	1,069 consecutive patients admitted to hospital	GCS	6 months	GOSE	No	No data on % involved in litigation	Yes
Kashluba et al. (2008)	102 patients at trauma hospital within 24 hours of injury and received rehab	GCS	Discharge 1 year	Cognitive performance	No	No difference between complicated mild and moderate TBI	Yes
Kurca Sivak, and Kucera (2006)	30 patients undergoing clinical evaluation	ACRM	96 hours	Cognitive performance	No	None	Yes
Lange, Iverson, and Zakrzewski, Ethel-King, andFranzen (2005)	531 patients seen in trauma service	GCS	Within a week	Cognitive performance	No	None	Yes
Lange, Iverson, and Franzen (2009)	167 patients seen in trauma service	GCS	3.5 days	Cognitive performance	No	None	Yes
Lange et al. (2012)	41 patients seen after medical evacuation from combat referred for clinical evaluation	PTA < 24 hours; LOC < 15 min	2.4 months	Cognitive performance Mood	Yes	No data on % disability ratings	No
Lee et al. (2008)	36 consecutive patients seen in emergency room	GCS LOC	2 weeks, 1 month, 1 year	Cognitive performance	No	No data on % involved in litigation	No
McCauley et al. (2001)	95 patients recruited in emergency room or inpatient unit	GCS 13–15, LOC < 20 min	3 months	DSM-IV Postconcussion disorder	No	CT/MRI+ group includes 20 with moderate TBI; No data on % involved in litigation	No
McMahon et al. (McMahon et al., 2014)	375 patients in emergency room	GCS	3, 6, and 12 months	GOSE PCS Mood	No	No data on % involved in litigation	No***
Mooney, Speed, and Sheppard (2005)	67 outpatients from clinic	ACRM	15 months	Subjective disability	Yes	All involved in worker's comp and/or litigation	No****
Muller et al. (2009)	59 patients admitted to neurosurgery	GCS (had to have LOC)	Discharge 6 months	Cognitive performance	No	No data on % involved in litigation	Yes
Panenka et al. (2015)	62 patients from emergency room (< 50 years and no excessive drinking)	ACRM (but only those in more severe range)	47 days	Cognitive performance PCS Mood	Yes	Complicated mild group had greater duration PTA	No
Sadowski-Cron et al. (2006)	205 consecutive patients presenting to emergency room	GCS	2 hours, 1 year	Cognitive performance acutely, PCS at one year	No	No data on % involved in litigation	Yes*****

Study	*Mild TBI Participants*	*Mild TBI criteria*	*Time Since Injury*	*Outcome Measure(s)*	*Performance Validity Assessed?*	*Caveats*	*Did CT/ MRI+ Have Worse Outcome?*
Sigurdardottir, Andelic, Roe, Jerstad, and Schanke (2009)	40 consecutive referrals to trauma hospital	GCS	3 months, 1 year	GOSE	Yes	No data on % involved in litigation	No
Smits et al. (2008)	312 consecutive patients at hospital within 24 hours of injury who had positive CT scans	GCS	15 months	GOSE	N/A	Parenchymal damage significantly predicted GOSE	Yes
Stulemeijer, Van der Werf, Borm, and Vos (2008)	Consecutive patients to emergency room	GCS LOC PTA	6 months	PCS Return to work	No	No data on % involved in litigation or other variables	No
Temkin, Machamer, and Dikmen (2003)	Consecutive patients to trauma hospital	GCS	3–5 years	FSE	N/A	No difference between complicated mild and moderate TBI	Yes
van der Naalt, Hew, Van Zomeren, Sluiter, and Minderhoud (1999)	43 patients admitted to hospital	GCS	1 year	GOSE DOS	N/A	No data on % involved in litigation	Yes
Williams et al. (1990)	155 consecutive patients admitted to neurosurgery service	GCS	12 days 6 months	Cognitive performance, GOS	No	Complicated mild group included some with depressed skull fractures	Yes
Yuh et al. (2013)	Consecutive patients to emergency room	GCS	3 months	GOSE	No	No data on % involved in litigation or other variables	Yes

Note: Studies with null findings are in bold. CT/MRI+ = abnormalities seen on CT and/or MRI images; LOC = loss of consciousness; PTA = posttraumatic amnesia; ACRM = American Congress of Rehabilitation Medicine criteria (1993) such that LOC < 30 minutes, PTA < 24 hours and GCS 13–15; GOSE = Glasgow Outcome Scale–Extended (Wilson, Pettigrew, & Teasdale, 1998); FIM = Functional Independence Measure; DOS = Differential Outcome Scale (van der Naalt et al., 1999); GCS = diagnosis of mild TBI based only on Glasgow Coma Scale

*Groups did not differ on severity of postconcussion symptoms (PCS) or return to work at 6 months.
**Group with +MRI/CT did have better return to work outcome.
***No differences only once those with positive medical histories (e.g., prior TBI, drug use, etc.) and incomplete data removed.
****It's unclear how many patients had neuroimaging findings—only a nonsignificant chi-square is reported suggesting no relationship between disability grouping and neuroimaging findings.
*****No difference between the groups acutely on cognitive performance, just on chronic PCS.

there is empirical evidence to suggest that poorer outcomes and greater symptoms of posttraumatic stress disorder (PTSD) are expected following "mild TBI" as opposed to "concussion" when these labels are used to describe the same injury (Dematteo et al., 2010; Sullivan, Edmed, & Kempe, 2014; Weber & Edwards, 2010). Within the sports literature, diagnosis and management of concussion is typically multidimensional and includes assessment of signs and symptoms, as well as objective assessment of cognitive functioning, balance and other functional capacities.(McCrea & Guskiewicz, 2014). Please see Chapter 27 for more details about mild TBI sustained in sports.

Outcomes

The lay public and sometimes even the "experts" have a tendency to lump any type of TBI together, as though all TBIs are the same. As the recovery trajectories can vary widely depending on severity (as well as other factors), it is important to differentiate between mild and more severe forms of TBI. Likewise, when discussing outcomes, it is important to specify what type of outcome. As people recover from injuries (of any kind), they do so in different domains, at different rates, and at different rates based on the domain. Outcomes of interest may include the experience of unpleasant or debilitating postconcussive symptoms (PCS) such as headaches, fatigue, and dizziness; psychiatric sequelae; cognitive performance; utilization of health care services; or return to work or other activities. These different outcomes may or may not be correlated with one another, hence the need to consider the particular outcome of interest. So, for example, subjective experience of cognitive impairment is typically not correlated with objective performance on cognitive tests (Drag, Spencer, Walker, Pangilinan, & Bieliauskas, 2012; Spencer, Drag, Walker, & Bieliauskas, 2010).

Cognitive Outcomes

Many individuals with mild TBI experience cognitive decline immediately after injury (Landre, Poppe, Davis, Schmaus, & Hobbs, 2006). In population-based studies of mild TBI, there are acute/subacute cognitive difficulties in virtually all aspects of neuropsychological functioning. Individuals with mild TBI perform about half a standard deviation ($d = 0.57$) more poorly than demographic-matched controls in the initial weeks following a mild TBI (Belanger, Curtiss, Demery, Lebowitz, & Vanderploeg, 2005). For the overwhelming majority of individuals, several independent meta-analytic studies suggest a favorable prognosis, with recovery of function over the course of several days to no more than a few months (Belanger, et al., 2005; Binder, Rohling, & Larrabee, 1997; Frencham, Fox, & Maybery, 2005; Rohling et al., 2011; Schretlen & Shapiro, 2003). Indeed, the effect size associated with mild TBI becomes essentially zero by one to three months postinjury (Belanger et al., 2005; Schretlen & Shapiro, 2003). Similar to the studies in meta-analytic reviews, Himanen et al. (2006) found no evidence of cognitive decline in those with mild to moderate TBI, relative to controls, an average of 30 years postinjury. Likewise, Hessen et al. (2007) found neuropsychological test scores in the average range in those with mild TBI sustained 23 years prior.

In contrast to this typical pattern of excellent recovery following mild TBI in the population at large (i.e., prospective or population-based studies), individuals with mild TBI who present to clinics in the chronic phase for medical or neuropsychological evaluation or who are in litigation (i.e., groups composed of individuals reporting ongoing symptoms and problems) represent a different subsample of patients. At least a portion of these individuals perform more poorly on neuropsychological measures, but in a manner not associated with any specific pattern. In contrast to the expected recovery, worse neuropsychological performance is seen across time (Belanger et al., 2005). See Table 18.3 for the effect sizes associated with different samples.

It may be that typical neuropsychological batteries are not sensitive to subtle, long-term impact of mild TBI, or it may be that there generally is no long-term impact on cognitive performance measures. A few studies have demonstrated differences between those with a history of mild TBI and controls on experimental tasks. Table 18.4 summarizes

Table 18.3 Time since injury by cognitive domain by participant selection context

	Litigation-Based	*Clinic-Based*	*Population-Based*
Cognitive Domain	*Studies*	*Studies*	*Studies*
Time Since Injury	*d (k)*	*d (k)*	*d (k)*
Averaged Across Domains			
< 90 Days	0.52* (2)	No Studies	0.63* (23)
≥ 90 Days	0.78* (6)	0.74* (11)	0.04 (8)

Note: These are meta-analytic results from Belanger et al. (2005). *d is the effect size; k is the number of studies that contributed to the effect size.*

* indicates significant at $p < .05$.

those nonclinical studies (e.g., studies using population-based recruiting such as from introductory psychology courses, veterans of the Vietnam War, etc.) that have found differences between mild TBI participants and controls at long-term follow-up. These studies have the advantage of a relative lack of diagnosis threat (though see caveats noted in Table 18.4) and relative lack of external incentives to perform poorly. One common denominator between the studies in Table 18.4 is that the tasks that elicit differences tend to be "experimental" and/or the differences occur on portions of standard tests not typically examined. Given that impairments tend not to occur on standard neuropsychological batteries, the question becomes one of ecological validity. That is, are these subtle differences (found in some studies but not others) meaningful in the real world? Might they account for subjective complaints many months after injury in a small subset of patients? Given the limitations of these studies (e.g., sample selection issues, the role of expectation due to diagnosis threat, etc.) and the potentially futile philosophical arguments about "importance," it is impossible to answer these questions. Perhaps a next step is correlating these subtle "impairments" with functional limitations and/or psychological distress. Vanderploeg and colleagues (2007) attempted to do that and found that of those with a mild TBI and subtle neuropsychological attention problems, 40% reported a complex of postconcussion symptoms. Of patients with mild TBI and major depression, 69% had the postconcussion complex of symptoms. In contrast, PCS was unlikely to predict other adverse outcomes.

Structural/Functional Outcomes

In recent years, there has been a growing interest in mild TBI neuroimaging research, summarized in detail elsewhere (Koerte et al., 2015; Lin et al., 2012; McDonald, Saykin, & McAllister, 2012; Shenton et al., 2012; Wilde et al., 2015). Findings can be summarized into two major categories:

Table 18.4 Studies using nonclinical samples demonstrating some decline in mild TBI participants at long-term follow-up

Study	*Time Post Injury*	*Sample Size*	*Main Finding*	*Caveats*
Bernstein 2002	8 years	13 mild TBI 10 controls	No differences on standard battery except Digit Symbol; mild TBI worse on dual task of visual and tone discrimination	• 7/13 had > 1 mild TBI • Diagnosis based on self-report
Ozen 2012	6.8 years	26 mild TBI 31 controls	No differences on standard battery; mild TBI slower despite comparable or superior accuracy on working memory	• All mild TBI had LOC • Mild TBI group more anxious • Unknown if more than one mild TBI
Segalowitz, Bernstein, and Lawson, 2001	6.4 years	10 mild TBI 12 controls	No differences on standard battery; mild TBI worse only on most difficult experimental sustained attention task	• Diagnosis Threat • 7/10 had > 1 mild TBI • 3/10 had been hospitalized • 8/10 had LOC
Sterr, Herron, Hayward, and Montaldi, 2006	6.8 years	11 mild TBI + PCS 27 mild TBI − PCS 38 controls	Poorer performance by mild TBI + PCS but not mild TBI − PCS on some but not all measures of attention and working memory	• Diagnosis Threat • Diagnosis based on self-report
Vanderploeg, Curtiss, and Belanger, 2005	8 years	254 mild TBI 539 MVA controls 3,214 controls	No differences on standard battery; Mild TBI greater proactive interference and discontinuation on PASAT	• Mild TBI severity inferred • Unknown if more than one mild TBI

Note: LOC = loss of consciousness; PCS = postconcussive symptoms; diagnosis threat possible based on either recruitment method or instructions/tasks; MVA = motor vehicle accident.

current clinical imaging findings and advanced experimental imaging findings.

Current Clinical Imaging Findings

Since the advent of in vivo imaging methods, clinicians and researchers have examined patients with TBI. In the case of mild TBI, there is limited utility in acquiring imaging, as it is often found to be negative. This is especially true of CT imaging, which is extremely useful in detecting lesions or bleeds that might require neurosurgical interventions but poor at imaging soft tissue, uses radiation, and offers limited contrast between tissue types (e.g., gray and white matter). For these reasons, there are guidelines that govern the use of CT in emergency room settings (Haydel et al., 2000; Papa et al., 2012; Stiell et al., 2001). In the absence of clinical red flags (i.e., progressive declining level of consciousness, worsening neurologic exam, focal neurologic deficit, disorientation, etc.), no medical imaging is recommended by most criteria.

In contrast, there are a growing number of structural MRI research studies examining the effects of mild TBI. MRI has several advantages over CT imaging, including improved contrast between tissue types, submillimeter resolution, and no radiation exposure. It is sensitive to small contusions and white matter damage when examining mild TBI patients. In fact, direct comparison of CT and MRI findings in mild TBI demonstrates that as many as 30% of the mild TBI patients with a negative CT scan will have hemorrhagic and non-hemorrhagic diffuse axonal abnormalities on MRI (Mittl & Yousem, 1994). However, these imaging abnormalities are not always related to functional changes in mild TBI patients (Slobounov, Gay, Johnson, & Zhang, 2012). To date, the majority of quantitative structural MRI studies in TBI have included mixed samples of patients across the range of severity, vary in chronicity of injury, are cross-sectional in nature, and have limited evidence of relationships between imaging and functional outcomes.

Regardless, there are a few important conclusions that can be gleaned from structural MRI studies to date. First, it is clear from studies that include the full range of severity that several regions of the brain tend to be more vulnerable to the effects of TBI, including the frontal and temporal poles, medial temporal lobe structures (including the hippocampus), and inferior frontal gyri (Bigler & Tate, 2001; Levin et al., 2004). In addition, overall brain volume loss seems to be a common finding in TBI patients, with the moderate and severe TBI patients experiencing the most volume loss (Bigler et al., 2013; Gale, Baxter, Roundy, & Johnson, 2005). However, mild TBI patients also demonstrate volume loss compared to healthy controls that may become evident only when examined in a prospective fashion (Levine et al., 2008; MacKenzie et al., 2002). More sophisticated postprocessing methods of structural MRI (e.g., cortical thickness, hippocampal shape, etc.) demonstrate diffuse abnormalities in TBI (Bigler, et al., 2013; Merkley et al., 2008; Tate et al., 2013) though many of these studies often include a range in injury severity, making it more difficult to know what types of atrophy may occur in mild TBI. Only a few studies have demonstrated relationships between structural imaging abnormalities and cognitive outcomes (Bergeson et al., 2004;

Monti et al., 2013; Wilde et al., 2011) and once again often include a range of injury severity before any relationship is noted. Thus, the clinical utility of structural imaging studies has been limited when trying to understand the clinical significance of any abnormalities that might be observed in mild TBI patients.

Advanced Experimental Imaging Findings

In contrast to standard clinical imaging, recent advances in experimental neuroimaging techniques promise new insights into the diagnosis, functional outcomes, and treatment of mild TBI patients. Advances include new techniques for acquiring MRI data (i.e., DTI, SWI), and new postprocessing analytic methods/statistics (i.e., machine learning, finite-element models, etc.). Current research is also emphasizing prospective MRI data to begin tracking the evolution and progression of changes resulting from mild TBI. Though these advanced MRI methods require additional research before the pathological and functional relevance of findings are fully understood, there is accumulating evidence that these methods have additional sensitivity in detecting important features associated with injury.

DTI has been touted by many as an imaging method that could provide unique pathological and functional insight into the changes associated with mild TBI. DTI differs from conventional structural MRI in that it is sensitive to the microstructural changes in white matter that may be the primary locus of injury in mild TBI (Basser, Mattiello, & LeBihan, 1994; Pierpaoli & Basser, 1996). Because this sequence is tuned to the orientation and degree of water movement in living tissue, the local changes in these measurements can provide important information regarding microstructure of the underlying tissue. In healthy brain parenchyma, white matter is highly organized (often linear), making tracking of white matter pathways easier and improving the sensitivity of this measure to white matter injury across a variety of neurologic disorders.

In mild TBI, there is growing evidence of compromised DTI metrics—e.g., mean diffusivity (MD), fractional anisotropy (FA), etc.—when comparing controls (typically orthopedic-injured controls) and mild TBI patients. These differences have been noted across several brain regions, including the corpus callosum (Matsushita, Hosoda, Naitoh, Yamashita, & Kohmura, 2011; Mayer et al., 2010), internal capsule (Grossman et al., 2012), cerebellar peduncles (Mac Donald et al., 2011), corona radiata (Matthews et al., 2011), forceps major/minor (Messe et al., 2011), and several major white matter pathways including the inferior longitudinal fasciculus, cingulum bundle, and corticospinal tracts (Messe et al., 2011; Smits et al., 2011; Wilde et al., 2012; Wu et al., 2010). Importantly, there are also studies that do not demonstrate differences in DTI metrics between mild TBI patients and controls (Arfanakis et al., 2002; Lange, Iverson, Brubacher, Madler, & Heran, 2012) though there are often methodological differences between these studies including sample differences (i.e., time since injury), scanner differences, and/or analysis methods (i.e., voxel wise, tract based, region of interest) that require further examination before these disparate results can be better understood.

Critically, DTI metrics appear to explain additional functional variance in mild TBI patients compared to volumetric MRI studies. For example, several studies have demonstrated significant relationships between DTI metrics in the white matter and subtle changes in cognitive function including reaction time deficits (Arenth, Russell, Scanlon, Kessler, & Ricker, 2013; Niogi et al., 2008; Wu et al., 2010), executive functions (Hartikainen et al., 2010), attention (Kraus et al., 2007), memory (Tate et al., 2013), and measures of global cognitive function (Lipton et al., 2008). In addition, mild TBI patients who report postconcussive symptoms six months postinjury also demonstrate significantly worse (i.e., reduced FA) global DTI metric differences compared to mild TBI patients not reporting postconcussive symptoms (Messe et al., 2012). Combined, these studies appear to demonstrate the utility of DTI findings as a potential biomarker for functional deficits in mild TBI subjects. However, it is clear that additional research is needed to fully understand the pathological underpinnings of these findings (Bigler & Maxwell, 2012) and/or the complex evolution and progression of the metrics over time (Lipton et al., 2008; Rosenbaum & Lipton, 2012; Wilde et al., 2012).

Recent DTI efforts appear to be focused on developing methods to examine the individual mild TBI patient (Bouix et al., 2013; Lipton et al., 2008; Shenton et al., 2012). Conceptually, this may prove to be a huge advantage both pathologically and functionally. Due to spatial variation in injury location across patients, group analyses may obscure potential findings, especially in mild TBI patients (Shenton et al., 2012). For example, Bouix and colleagues (2013) demonstrated unique subject-specific abnormal DTI profiles in mild TBI patients experiencing persistent postconcussive symptoms in spite of nonsignificant group difference findings. Identifying these unique spatial locations of injury in individual patients may not only improve diagnosis, but also provide unique insights into patient-specific functional changes leading to improved prognostication and treatment recommendations not available currently.

SWI has also demonstrated additional sensitivity to injury in mild TBI patients not available in conventional MRI techniques. One of the main clinical applications of SWI to date is the detection of micro-hemorrhages, shearing, and DAI in TBI (Haacke, Tang, Neelavalli, & Cheng, 2010). In fact, SWI is extremely sensitive (up to six times more sensitive) to injury after TBI, detecting subtle lesions (i.e., small punctate lesions typically located at the gray/white matter boundaries) and venous changes (i.e., venous undulations/bulbs) previously unobserved using conventional MRI technique. In our own sample of mild TBI patients, SWI detects previously unobserved lesions in 22% of mild TBI patients with persistent cognitive symptoms. Importantly, there is a clear relationship between the number/volume of SWI lesions and functional outcomes of TBI patients (Beauchamp et al., 2013; Spitz et al., 2013; Tong et al., 2004). More specifically, an increase in the number and/or volume of SWI lesions is related to worse functional outcomes in these patients, including clinical measures such as GCS, length of hospital stay, and intellectual function (Tong et al., 2004).

In summary, CT and structural MR imaging have broadened our understanding of mild TBI in important ways, though these methods leave many unanswered questions. Currently, CT remains the clinical standard, though in the case of mild TBI or concussion, CT has very little benefit and, if indeed imaging is required, MRI should be considered given its markedly improved sensitivity. Determining the imaging biomarkers that are predictive of long-term outcome in mild TBI will be an important emphasis in future clinical and academic research as accurate identification of these markers will improve our ability to differentially diagnose (i.e., PTSD vs. TBI), treat, and prognosticate (i.e., why some mild TBI patients experience persistent symptoms), as well as evaluate and develop new treatment options.

Psychological Outcomes/Mood Disorders

Prevalence of a psychiatric disorder in the first year following a mild TBI is elevated compared to the general population (Fann et al., 2004). Those with prior psychiatric history are at greater risk. Depression is the most common psychiatric diagnosis following TBI of any severity. The prevalence of depression following mild TBI (as opposed to moderate to severe TBI) has not been as well studied. Nonetheless, those who sustain a mild TBI are at greater risk of depression than noninjured controls but not injured controls (Levin et al., 2001; McCauley, Boake, Levin, Contant, & Song, 2001; Vanderploeg, Curtiss, Luis, and Salazar, 2007). Indeed, depression is relatively common following mild TBI, with a prevalence of 14%–35% (Busch & Alpern, 1998; McCauley et al., 2001; Rao et al., 2010; Rapoport, McCullagh, Streiner, & Feinstein, 2003). Older age and abnormal neuroimaging are predictors of new-onset depression following mild TBI (Levin et al., 2005; Rao et al., 2010). It is unclear whether the new onset depression following mild TBI is due to psychological reaction to the injury or brain dysfunction due to neurotransmitter dysfunction. It is clear that those who develop depression have poorer outcomes than those who do not (Mooney et al., 2005; Rapoport et al., 2003; Silver, McAllister, & Arciniegas, 2009).

There is notably less research on the prevalence of anxiety disorders and mild TBI, with the possible exception of PTSD with the recent wars (see Chapter 32 for a discussion of PTSD and mild TBI). The estimated prevalence of new-onset anxiety disorders is approximately 24%–33% in mild TBI patients (Mooney & Speed, 2001). Significantly higher percentages of psychiatric inpatients have a reported history of mild TBI than the 13%–19% in a nonpsychiatric comparison group (McGuire, Burright, Williams, & Donovick, 1998). The prevalence of acute stress disorder is roughly 15% in those with a history of mild TBI (Harvey & Bryant, 1998), while the prevalence of generalized anxiety disorder is 16% (Vanderploeg et al., 2007). Once psychiatric and demographic comparisons are made, these rates are likely not elevated compared to non-TBI controls (Vanderploeg et al., 2007). The prevalence of PTSD among noncombat mild TBI patients ranges from 12% to 24% (Bryant & Harvey, 1999; Levin et al., 2001; McCauley et al., 2001; Vanderploeg et al., 2007), again not elevated relative to trauma controls. The rate of PTSD tends to hold steady when reassessed two years later (Harvey & Bryant, 1998).

A few important caveats are in order when considering new-onset psychiatric disorders following mild TBI. The first is that patients may experience symptoms of a disorder without meeting full diagnostic criteria. So, for example, depressed mood is a frequently cited postconcussive symptom that may interfere with cognitive functioning. Depressed mood may or may not be indicative of a depressive disorder. Second, it is of course also important to realize that depression and anxiety often co-occur. For example, one small study of a mixed TBI sample found that every TBI patient diagnosed with generalized anxiety disorder also had clinical depression (Jorge et al., 2004). Another small sample found that 18% of mild TBI patients had both PTSD and depression (Levin et al., 2001). Finally, for the most part, it is currently unclear to what extent a mild TBI affects the prevalence of specific psychiatric disorders. However, prevalence of any psychiatric disorder in the first year following a mild TBI is elevated compared to the general population, with those with prior psychiatric history at greatest risk.

Symptom-Related Outcomes

Postconcussive Syndrome refers to a set of symptoms that can arise after mild TBI, consisting of physical/somatic (e.g., headache, dizziness, photophobia, fatigue), cognitive (e.g., impaired memory, decreased concentration), and emotional (e.g., depression, irritability) symptoms (Hall & Chapman, 2005). In the *Diagnostic and Statistical Manual of Mental Disorders*, fourth edition (DSM-IV; American Psychiatric Association, 1994) postconcussional disorder (PCD) is listed as a proposed diagnostic criteria for investigation, whereas Postconcussive Syndrome is listed as an actual diagnosis in the *International Statistical Classification of Disease and Related Health Problems*, tenth edition (ICD-10; World Health Organization, 1992). Criteria differed between the DSM-IV and ICD-10 in that only the DSM-IV requires neuropsychological evidence of attention or memory difficulty and only the ICD-10 indicates that Postconcussive Syndrome may be accompanied by hypochondriacal preoccupation. The ICD-10 lack of requirement for evidence of neuropsychological impairment results in a sixfold increase in the prevalence of a Postconcussive Syndrome diagnosis over the DSM-IV

PCD diagnosis (ICD-10 = 64% vs. DSM-IV = 11%) at three months postinjury in one study (Boake et al., 2005). PCD has been eliminated altogether in the recent *Diagnostic and Statistical Manual of Mental Disorders,* fifth edition (DSM-V). Indeed, prospective studies of symptom complexes have cast doubt on the clinical utility of Postconcussive Syndrome (Arciniegas, Anderson, Topkoff, & McAllister, 2005; Ettenhofer & Barry, 2012). By definition, a syndrome constitutes a compilation of symptoms that tend to occur together and/or resolve together over time. This has not been the case with Postconcussive Syndrome symptoms. Studies of Postconcussive Syndrome symptom trajectories over time do not support the syndrome construct.

By definition, mild TBI results in some initial brief loss or alteration of consciousness. Shortly after a concussion, several symptoms tend to predominate. The initial alteration of consciousness is experienced as confusion and some disorientation to one's immediate environment. Individuals may describe feeling "confused," "fuzzy," or "slowed down." Although a variety of other symptoms can be associated with TBI, they are not part of the definition of TBI, and other than loss or clear alteration of consciousness (i.e., immediate confusion and disorientation), there are no pathognomonic symptoms or signs. Symptoms should not be attributed to the mild TBI if they are better explained by preexisting conditions or other medical, neurological, or psychological causes—except in cases of an immediate postinjury exacerbation of a preexisting condition (Department of Veterans Affairs and Department of Defense, April, 2009). Within days of injury, patients with mild TBI do not differ from controls in their report of postconcussion-like symptoms (Landre et al., 2006; McCrea et al., 2003). See Figure 18.1 for symptom recovery in college football players.

When patients are initially examined in the emergency room after a mild TBI, one study found the most commonly reported symptoms to be headaches (61%), nausea (27%), dizziness (18%), and vomiting (6%) (De Kruijk et al., 2002). However, as with acute onset cognitive impairments described earlier, these initial symptoms resolve quickly in most individuals. In the sports concussion literature, both cognitive problems and symptom reports resolve in parallel over seven days (McCrea et al., 2003).

In another study, the most frequently reported symptoms within the first 14 days were fatigue (45%), insomnia (32%), headaches (28%), dizziness (24%), and irritability (24%) (Meares et al., 2011). However, the frequency and severity of these symptoms did not differ between a mild TBI and a trauma control group, either during the initial 14 days or at three-month follow-up. Similarly, using a criteria of three or more postconcussive-like symptoms to define Postconcussive Syndrome, the mild TBI and trauma control groups had comparable findings during the first 14 days (mild TBI = 40.3% vs. trauma controls = 50.0%) and again at three-month follow-up (mild TBI = 46.8% vs. trauma controls = 48.3%). These findings replicated an earlier study in which mild TBI (43.3%) and trauma control (43.5%) groups did not differ in the frequency of PCS at five days postinjury (Meares et al., 2008). However, findings in prospective studies have not been entirely consistent. Although Boake and colleagues (2005) found comparable rates for DSM-IV PCD at three-months postinjury for a mild TBI (11%) and an extracranial control group (7%), they found higher rates for the ICD-10 criteria of Postconcussion Syndrome in the mild TBI group (64%) compared to the extracranial control group (40%). McCauley and colleagues (2013) also found that a diagnosis of mild TBI compared to an orthopedic injury was associated with PCS at one week and one month, over and above demographic characteristics and preinjury depression and resilience. Participants with a mild TBI had greater levels of PCS, as well as acute anxiety and PTSD symptoms, than did the orthopedic control group.

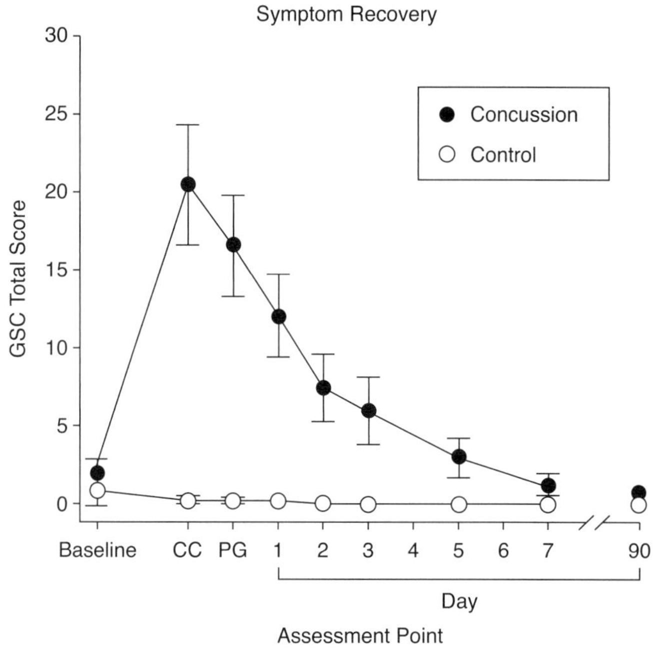

Figure 18.1 Symptom recovery in college football players

Note: CC = time of concussion. PG = postgame/postpractice. GCS = Graded Symptom Checklist; higher scores on the GCS indicate more severe symptoms. Error bars represent the 95% confidence interval. Baseline is preinjury. Figure reproduced with permission, McCrea, Iverson, McAllister, Hammeke, Powell, Barr, & Kelly (2009).

Although some individuals with mild TBI report symptoms months and even years following a concussion, the available longitudinal literature indicates that these symptoms are less likely to be related to the mild TBI as time goes by (Losoi et al., 2015; Meares et al., 2008; Meares et al., 2011; Ponsford et al., 2012) and that the natural course of mild TBI is recovery (Meares et al., 2011). As might be expected with nonspecific symptoms (e.g., headaches, fatigue, insomnia, concentration problems, irritability) in the general population postconcussion-like symptoms following mild TBI wax and wane over time (Meares et al., 2011). Further, these studies show that these symptoms are generally not related to mild TBI, particularly as time goes by, but instead are associated with accompanying acute posttraumatic stress, and depression or anxiety disorders (Boake et al., 2005; Meares et al., 2008; Meares et al., 2011; Ponsford et al., 2012). As such, the prevailing viewpoint appears to be that while neurological factors contribute to acute symptoms, psychological factors likely account for ongoing symptoms. Longitudinal studies with appropriate injured controls are critical in understanding etiology and time course of symptom complaints.

Regardless of etiology, a minority of individuals complain of cognitive difficulty and other distressing symptoms months (Alves, Macciocchi, & Barth, 1993; Dikmen, Machamer, Fann, & Temkin, 2010; Dikmen, McLean, & Temkin, 1986; McCrea et al., 2013; Powell, Collin, & Sutton, 1996) or years postinjury (Alexander, 1992; Boake et al., 2005; Deb, Lyons, & Koutzoukis, 1999; Dikmen et al., 2010; Hartlage, Durant-Wilson, & Patch, 2001) after having a concussion. Some have suggested that these are symptoms are due to subtle neurological dysfunction allegedly beneath the detection threshold of routine diagnostic procedures such as CT, MRI, and EEG (see Hayes & Dixon, 1994). However, as discussed on pp. 417–419, as well as in a review of the neuroimaging literature (Belanger, Vanderploeg, Curtiss, & Warden, 2007), even more sensitive imaging modalities (such as functional MRI) have yet to explain chronic symptom complaints in a convincing way.

At the present time, most research suggests that postconcussion-like symptoms are indistinguishable from the diffuse, nonspecific symptoms experienced by many normal healthy individuals and symptoms that are at increased rates following physical injury or periods of stress, or associated with a variety of mental health conditions (Gunstad & Suhr, 2004; Smith-Seemiller, Fow, Kant, & Franzen, 2003). In fact, a recent study demonstrates that the frequency of this cluster of symptoms is higher in a variety of psychiatric disorders than it is in the chronic phase of mild TBI (Donnell, Kim, Silva, & Vanderploeg, 2012).

Therefore, it is safe to conclude, as suggested by Silver and Kay (2013), that if symptoms persist for more than a few months, increase over time, spread into multiple domains, and become associated with global functional impairment, it is no longer reasonable to speak of a Postconcussion Syndrome or PCS. Instead it is more accurate to say that there is a problem of persistent symptoms that occurred surrounding a concussion but in which multiple factors play a role. The original concussion is no longer the force driving the symptoms and resulting dysfunction.

Dementia

The association between mild TBI and the development of Alzheimer's disease has been thoroughly reviewed, with mixed findings (Bazarian, Cernak, Noble-Haeusslein, Potolicchio, & Temkin, 2009; Jellinger, 2004; Plassman et al., 2000). One such review (Bazarian et al., 2009) concluded that dementia of the Alzheimer's type was associated with moderate and severe TBI, but not with mild TBI unless there was loss of consciousness, though the evidence for the latter was limited. Most epidemiological studies suggest an increased risk of dementia/Alzheimer's disease following severe TBI, relative to the general population, though again the evidence regarding mild TBI is limited and inconclusive. A recent, retrospective analysis of a national insurance administrative database in Taiwan (Lee et al., 2013) found a relationship between a mild TBI diagnosis (gleaned from ICD-9 codes) and a dementia diagnosis (with an odds ratio of 3.26) after controlling for age, gender, and various other demographic and health status variables. However, the average duration between mild TBI diagnosis and the dementia diagnosis was only one year, calling into question how generalizable these findings might be.

Selected Factors Affecting Outcomes

There are a myriad of factors that can affect outcomes following concussion. Variability on these factors likely account for individual differences in outcome. A model is proposed to depict the various factors that have been associated with outcomes across time (see Figure 18.2). This model is an amalgamation of previously proposed models (Silverberg & Iverson, 2011; Vanderploeg, Belanger, & Curtiss, 2006) and is based on existing literature, which will be briefly summarized in this section. As can be seen in Figure 18.2, it is hypothesized that predisposing factors and causal factors, as well as perpetuating and mitigating factors, have both direct and indirect effects on one another and on outcome. In addition, factors may interact in complex ways to adversely affect outcome. So, for example, the presence of pain may adversely affect sleep which in turn might adversely affect cognition or may exacerbate other symptoms (e.g., Gosselin et al., 2012; Khoury et al., 2013). Despite the complexities in any one person, however, the general rule is one of recovery over time following a single concussion, regardless of the outcome of interest.

Injury Severity

It would seem intuitive that greater injury severity might be associated with worse outcome. In a prospective study of emergency department patients, those with recent mild TBI and PTA or LOC were more likely to have neurocranial traumatic findings on CT but were not any more likely to require neurosurgical intervention than those without PTA/LOC (Smits et al., 2007). In this study, those with GCS of 15 and certain symptoms (such as vomiting, headache, seizure, etc.) constituted the "without PTA/LOC" group.

Generally speaking, the strongest predictors of outcome in moderate to severe TBI are injury severity variables (i.e., GCS, PTA, LOC). However, within an exclusively mild TBI

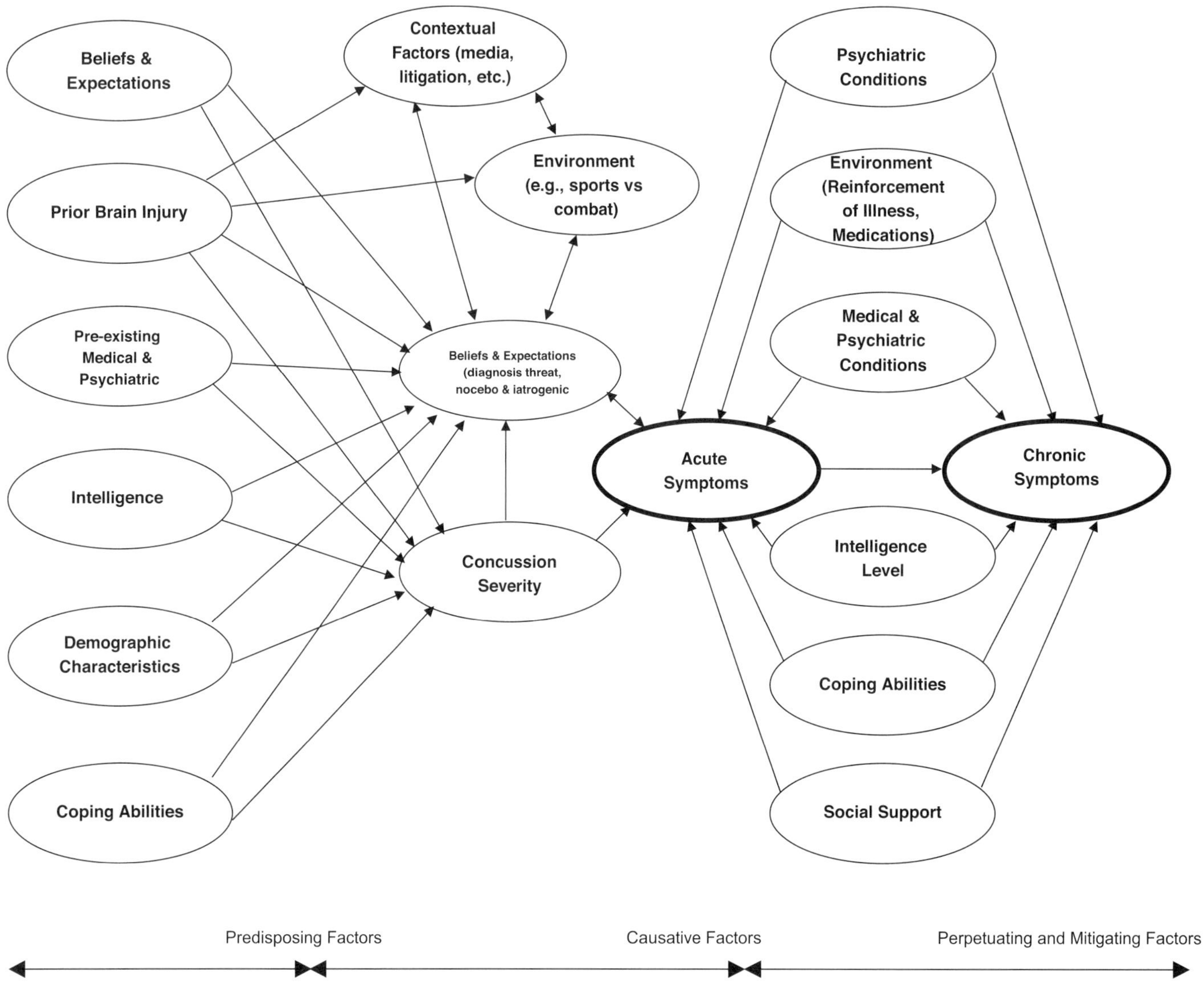

Figure 18.2 A proposed model of factors related to concussion outcome

population, the data are mixed. This may be because we often do not have medical records that give us good estimates of these injury severity indices following a mild TBI, or it may be because injury severity is predictive acutely but that psychological factors play a more prominent role in the long run. So, for example, prospective study in children postconcussion has shown that while injury characteristics like LOC predict symptoms in the first months following mild TBI, there is decreasing contribution over time (McNally et al., 2013).

One way to examine the contribution of TBI severity to the presence and duration of PCS is to compare mild TBI with moderate to severe TBI. In a mixed sample of patients admitted to the hospital for acute TBI, Sigurdardottir et al. (2009) found that those with mild TBI were more likely to meet ICD-10 symptom criteria for Postconcussion Syndrome at three months. However, this difference disappeared by one year, when mild, moderate, and severe TBI patients all had similar rates of Postconcussion Syndrome and similar symptom severity level (Sigurdardottir, et al., 2009). These findings are consistent with cross-sectional data in a chronic sample of veterans showing no differences in PCS severity reporting across TBI severity levels, once PTSD symptom severity is controlled for in analyses (Belanger, Kretzmer, Vanderploeg, & French, 2010). Dikmen et al. (Dikmen et al., 2010) found differences by TBI severity only on memory complaints one year following injury, with a greater percentage of severely injured TBI patients reporting memory problems. However, there were no differences with other symptoms.

Another way to examine the contribution of TBI severity to the presence and duration of PCS within mild TBI is to examine the presence or absence of LOC. On one hand, some investigators have found no relationship between LOC and outcomes in adults with a history of mild TBI. Chrisman et al. (2013) found no difference between those with LOC and no LOC in terms of symptoms lasting more than a week in athletes. Kennedy (Kennedy et al., 2012) similarly found that LOC was not a predictor of return-to-duty amongst a sample of 337 service members seen for acute concussion evaluation following medical evacuation from the battlefield. Whittaker, Kemp, and House (2007) found that measures of severity (GCS, PTA, and LOC) were not associated with Postconcussion Syndrome three months postinjury, nor were they associated with functional outcome. On the other hand, McCrea (McCrea et al., 2013) found that LOC was a predictor of prolonged recovery (defined as a lack of relative improvement on symptom reporting compared to controls within seven days) in a small sample of athletes, as was duration of PTA and greater symptom severity acutely. Finally, in a sample of 47 athletes who sustained concussion and were followed by Erlanger et al. (2003) with Internet-based symptom assessments until resolution of symptoms, the presence of LOC, dizziness, nausea, or headache at the first assessment was predictive of the total number of symptoms reported. However, LOC was not associated with the number of symptoms reported at the first follow-up an average of two days later, nor was it associated with the overall duration of symptoms.

In terms of cognitive performance measures, studies have consistently found no association with LOC or PTA duration. Lovell et al. (Lovell, Iverson, Collins, McKeag, & Maroon, 1999) found no differences on neuropsychological measures between those with and without LOC in a large sample of patients seen in an emergency department and assessed within seven days postinjury. Similarly, Hanlon et al. (Hanlon et al. 1999) found no differences on comprehensive neuropsychological measures or on vocational outcome between those with LOC and without LOC in 100 consecutive referrals to a concussion care clinic in patients who were three to 40 months postinjury. Drag et al. (2012) found no relationship between self-reported injury characteristics and cognitive functioning in their chronic sample of veterans. This is similar to findings from Ruff et al. (1999) in a sample of civilian, mixed medical/legal cases an average of 14 months postinjury. There was no relationship between groups based on LOC/PTA duration and performance on neuropsychological measures.

Beyond LOC, another way to examine the contribution of TBI severity to the presence and duration of PCS within mild TBI is to examine the duration of PTA as well as the presence of retrograde amnesia. Prospective study of 71 patients with mild TBI and 60 orthopedic controls followed longitudinally after being seen in the Emergency Department with mild TBI revealed that presence of retrograde and anterograde amnesia was predictive of DSM-defined PCD at three months, but not six months (Bazarian et al., 1999). Meares et al. (Meares et al., 2008) found no relationship between duration of PTA and ICD-10 diagnosis of Postconcussion Syndrome in those who were admitted to a hospital for mild TBI and assessed an average of 4.9 days later. Ponsford et al. (Ponsford et al., 2000) likewise found no relationship between PTA duration and symptom reporting at three months postinjury in their prospective study of consecutive mild TBI patients presenting to emergency departments. Overall, there does not seem to be a reliable association between PTA duration and PCS. Presence of retrograde amnesia may be predictive in the postacute stage but not longer-term.

Studies conducted with veterans and military samples have examined the relationship between injury severity variables and outcomes within mild TBI samples that were examined a year or more postinjury. In these chronic samples, LOC has been found to be related to greater symptom reporting in some studies (Drag et al., 2012; Walker, McDonald, Ketchum, Nichols, & Cifu, 2013). In such studies, however, it is important to note that the presence or absence of LOC is typically determined through self-report and the patient's retrospective recall. This is obviously problematic, as symptomatic patients are likely in distress and may be more apt to have a negative recall bias about their injury. It's unclear that people can accurately report LOC, or any other presumed injury severity indicator. Furthermore, these studies are typically conducted in clinical samples (i.e., those having difficulties) and therefore are not representative of mild TBI in general. VA samples in particular typically rely on the VA's TBI screening and evaluation process to recruit patients and as such exclude nonsymptomatic patients with history of mild TBI. Hoge et al. (2008) reported an association between LOC and PCS, but controlling for PTSD symptoms nullified the relationship except for headaches. Psychiatric distress also mediated the relationship between injury severity variables (PTA and/or LOC) and PCS in the Drag et al. sample (2012) as well.

One study of civilians presenting to an emergency department followed them into the postacute and chronic stages (Bazarian et al., 1999). This was a prospective, observational, case-control study of 71 patients who met very conservative criteria for mild TBI (i.e., LOC < 10 minutes or the presence of amnesia, GCS of 15, not admitted to the hospital, clean neuroimaging, etc.). In this study, LOC, when entered collectively into a model with other clinical variables, was not predictive of DSM-defined PCS at any time point. Retrograde and anterograde amnesia were predictive at one and three months (though the effects were very small), but not at six months.

In summary, it appears as though injury severity variables are not associated with cognitive performance or other performance-based variables like return-to-duty or vocational status in mild TBI patients. There is greater inconsistency of findings related to symptom reporting, particularly whether or not there is increased symptom reporting associated with the presence of LOC. There does not seem to be a reliable association between PTA duration and PCS. Presence of retrograde amnesia may be predictive in the postacute stage but not in more chronic stages.

Comorbidities

The presence of a mood disorder and/or mood symptoms following mild TBI may adversely impact outcome. Vasterling et al. (2012) found, for example, that while history of mild TBI was not predictive of cognitive decline postdeployment, current depressive and PTSD symptoms were predictive of cognitive decline. Specifically, greater severity of PTSD and depression symptom reporting was associated with pre- to postdeployment decrements in reaction time, learning efficiency, and recall. In addition, PTSD and depression symptoms were associated with self-reported decrements in health and cognitive functioning. So, both performance-based and subjective outcomes were associated with psychiatric variables, but not mild TBI. These findings are similar to other prospective studies, underscoring the importance of psychiatric status on outcomes (Meares et al., 2008; Ponsford et al., 2012) and with other studies that were not longitudinal but similarly found psychiatric variables to be more predictive of symptom reporting than mild TBI in military and veteran samples (Donnell et al., 2012; Fear et al., 2009; Hoge et al., 2008; Schneiderman, Braver, & Kang, 2008; Vanderploeg et al., 2012). It is important to note that the presence of *premorbid* mood disorder/symptoms are also predictive of outcome (Dikmen et al., 2010; Luis, Vanderploeg, & Curtiss, 2003; Meares et al., 2011; Ponsford et al., 2012; Ponsford et al., 2000). In the Vasterling et al. study (2012), premorbid psychiatric symptom severity was controlled for in the analyses, suggesting that the relationship between cognitive performance and current mood symptoms was not due to premorbid mood factors.

In summary, the presence of anxiety and depressive symptomatology can adversely affect outcomes, both cognitive and subjective, following a mild TBI. Iverson (2005) compared meta-analytic studies of the neuropsychological impact of mild TBI vis-à-vis various disorders. By putting different disorders on the same neuropsychologic metric, he demonstrated that mild TBI, particularly in the chronic phase, has virtually no effect on cognitive outcomes, whereas moderate to severe TBI, depression, malingering, and chronic benzodiazepine use have much greater effects.

Pain and sleep problems are also common comorbidities that can affect outcome in those with mild TBI. In samples recruited from emergency departments, estimates of opioid administration acutely to mild TBI patients are 61%–63% (Meares et al., 2008; Ponsford et al., 2012), and 34% within 14 days postinjury (Meares et al., 2011), with minimal use at longer term follow-up (Ponsford et al., 2012). In their prospective study, Ponsford et al. (2012) found that pain severity at one week postinjury was a significant predictor of ongoing PCS three months postinjury, as was concurrent pain severity at three months. Similarly, Meares et al. (2008) found that while mild TBI was not predictive of ICD-10-defined Postconcussion Syndrome acutely (i.e., within five days postinjury), the presence of an anxiety or affective disorder and pain severity were predictive. In prospective studies, Sheedy and colleagues (Sheedy, Geffen, Donnelly, & Faux, 2006; Sheedy, Harvey, Faux, Geffen, & Shores, 2009) have found that although there were no differences in levels of reported pain in the emergency department between those with mild TBI versus those with orthopedic injury, acute pain at the time of injury was significantly associated with PCS severity at one and three months postinjury. These findings are similar to cross-sectional studies with more chronic patients, in which PCS severity is associated with pain, even when controlling for depression (Gasquoine, 2000; Mooney et al., 2005; Smith-Seemiller et al., 2003). Opioid analgesia administered on the day of assessment is not related to performance on cognitive tasks or psychological distress (Meares et al., 2008). Opioid use in the more chronic phase is associated with slowed reaction time (Meares et al., 2011). Interestingly, each unit increase in pain for mild TBI patients is associated with increased odds of acute PCS, whereas for trauma controls, each unit increase in pain actually *reduces* the likelihood of acute PCS (Meares et al., 2008). Studies investigating the role of pain on cognitive performance have found no effect within 4.5 days of injury (Landre et al., 2006) though the general consensus is that chronic pain can adversely impact neurocognitive performance independently of TBI (Block & Cianfrini, 2013; Hart, Martelli, & Zasler, 2000).

Sleep is obviously another variable to consider when thinking about outcome following mild TBI, given its known impact on cognitive performance (Fortier-Brochu, Beaulieu-Bonneau, Ivers, & Morin, 2012). Most studies have found that mild TBI patients report significantly more sleep problems than patients with moderate to severe TBI (Beetar, Guilmette, & Sparadeo, 1996; Clinchot, Bogner, Mysiw, Fugate, & Corrigan, 1998; Fichtenberg, Millis, Mann, Zafonte, & Millard, 2000; Mahmood, Rapport, Hanks, & Fichtenberg, 2004; Ouellet, Beaulieu-Bonneau, & Morin, 2006; Parcell, Ponsford, Rajaratnam, & Redman, 2006) though other studies have found no differences in sleep complaints by TBI severity (Hou et al., 2013; Ponsford, Parcell, Sinclair, Roper, & Rajaratnam, 2013). These different findings are likely due to sample differences such as the presence of mood symptoms, pain, and other factors that have a demonstrated relationship with sleep. Fichtenberg et al. (2000) did a logistic regression on their postacute outpatient rehabilitation TBI sample and found that only depression and GCS scores made unique contributions to insomnia (and not pain or litigation status).

Unfortunately, the prevalence of objective sleep difficulties following mild TBI has not been well studied. In a pediatric sample, 18% complained of at least one sleep symptom an average of three years postinjury (Kaufman et al., 2001). Further, sleep difficulties were objectively found using polysomnography and actigraphy at a rate that exceeded age and gender-matched controls. Unfortunately, there are currently no prospective studies with concomitant objective assessment of sleep in mild TBI. Self-reported sleep disturbance in individuals with a history of mild TBI is estimated to be between 32% and 38% (Ouellet et al., 2006; Segalowitz & Lawson, 1995). After controlling for gender, age, and depression, having a self-reported history of mild TBI is associated with self-reported sleep disturbance (Segalowitz & Lawson, 1995). When sleep complaints differentiate mild TBI groups from controls initially, this difference disappears at long-term follow-up (Dikmen et al., 1986). Using polysomnography, Schreiber et al. (2008) found abnormal sleep architecture and excessive daytime episodes of sleep in clinical samples of mild TBI. Due to sample bias and lack of a control group, the specific role of mild TBI cannot be determined.

Finally, alcohol and substance abuse represent comorbidities that may be problematic. Estimates suggest that between 36% and 51% of individuals who present with TBI are intoxicated at the time of injury (Corrigan, 1995; Parry-Jones, Vaughan, & Miles Cox, 2006). While it makes intuitive sense that substance abuse might adversely affect outcomes, the data suggest otherwise. Specifically, Sigurdardottir et al. (2009) found no effect of current alcohol/drug consumption on functional outcome (as measured by the GOSE) one year postinjury. Similarly, Meares et al. (2008) found that preinjury substance abuse was not predictive of ICD-10-defined Postconcussion Syndrome in the first five days postinjury. Studies conducted with all TBI severity levels have also produced mixed results, with some studies suggesting that alcohol may be neuroprotective, while others suggest increased morbidity. More research is needed.

Premorbid Factors: Demographics and Mental/Physical Health

Demographic variables such as age, education, and gender are known to be associated with outcomes, both in terms of cognitive performance and symptom reporting. In general, for adults, female gender, older age, and less education are associated with worse outcomes following a mild TBI (Alves, Macciocchi, &Barth, 1993; Bazarian et al., 1999; Covassin, Elbin, Harris, Parker, & Kontos, 2012; Dougan, Horswill, & Geffen, 2013; Jacobs et al., 2010; Lannsjo, Backheden, Johansson, Af Geijerstam, & Borg, 2013; Meares et al., 2008; Ponsford et al., 2012; Ponsford et al., 2000). Bazarian et al. (1999) observe that different mechanisms of injury may underlie some of the gender differences, as females are more likely to be injured in car accidents and males in sports, at least in their sample, the latter of which is associated with fewer symptoms and better outcomes more generally. Gender differences in neuropsychological functioning may not be apparent at longer-term follow-up (Tsushima, Lum, & Geling, 2009).

Some investigators have found an interaction between gender and age such that women who sustain TBI at age 30 or older have poorer outcomes than men and women younger than 30 (Kirkness, Burr, Mitchell, & Newell, 2004; Tsushima et al., 2009). However, sampling and methodological issues such as participant involvement in litigation, lack of control group, etc., make these studies somewhat difficult to interpret.

Preexisting physical injuries/disease and psychiatric disorders tend to have an adverse impact on outcome following concussion. So, for example, Ponsford et al. (2012) found that pre-injury physical and psychiatric problems were predictive of PCS at both one week and three months postconcussion. Similarly, those with premorbid alcohol abuse and psychiatric histories tended to report more symptoms at one year postinjury (Dikmen et al., 2010). Luis et al. (2003) found that early life psychiatric difficulties, limited social support, lower intelligence, and the interactions among these variables predicted ICD-10 and DSM-IV diagnosis of Postconcussion Syndrome in a large sample of Vietnam veterans. These findings are similar to a prospective study (Meares et al., 2008) that found female gender, preinjury psychiatric diagnosis, estimated IQ, performance on the Symbol Digits Modalities Test, and acute stress to be predictive of Postconcussion Syndrome within two weeks of injury. Being diagnosed with concussion versus some other trauma was not predictive of Postconcussion Syndrome. Finally, recent work suggests that constructs such as "anxiety sensitivity," defined as sensitivity to one's own bodily sensations with a tendency to misinterpret autonomic arousal, may have utility in predicting PCS severity (Wood, O'Hagan, Williams, McCabe, & Chadwick, 2014).

Luis et al. (2003) examined the association between a remote history of mild TBI and current Postconcussion Syndrome in a large epidemiological sample of veterans who, following their military service, suffered a civilian mild TBI an average of six years prior to assessment. Demographic factors accounted for 9.2% unique variance in predicting current Postconcussion Syndrome, and preexisting psychiatric conditions accounted for 6.3% unique variance, but history of concussion still accounted for 1.3% unique variance in current postconcussion symptom complex. Similarly, in a university sample, concussion was associated with modestly elevated mean level of PCS reporting for somatic and cognitive symptoms, relative to orthopedic controls (Ettenhofer & Barry, 2012), but not affective symptoms. In a follow-up study (Ettenhofer, Reinhardt, & Barry, 2013) examining factors associated with posconcussion-like symptoms, female gender, and a history of depression and anxiety were the most potent predictors, followed by other mental health issues and learning problems. A lifetime history of mild TBI was also a significant predictor, but accounted for far less variance.

Beliefs/Expectations

It is important to realize that beliefs, expectations, and attributions have an impact on recovery from mild TBI. Calling attention to a person's history of mild TBI can adversely affect both cognitive performance (Ozen & Fernandes, 2011; Pavawalla, Salazar, Cimino, Belanger, & Vanderploeg, 2013; Suhr & Gunstad, 2002) and symptom reporting (Ozen & Fernandes, 2011). This is presumably because people associate a mild TBI with negative outcomes and experience a type of "diagnosis threat." As Sullivan and Edmed (2012b) demonstrated, even a very mild TBI vignette among nonconcussed undergraduates can elicit expectations of significant PCS. Hou and colleagues (2012) found that negative perceptions of mild TBI were the best predictor of PCS at six months postinjury.

People may also underestimate the extent to which they experienced "postconcussion symptoms" prior to their TBI (Gunstad & Suhr, 2001; Mittenberg, DiGiulio, Perrin, & Bass, 1992). This finding is called the "expectation as etiology" principle (Mittenberg et al., 1992). In other words, some percentage of PCS reporting is likely due to (potentially false) attributions to mild TBI. Snell, Hay-Smith, Surgenor, and Siegert (2013) found that those individuals endorsing (a) stronger injury identity beliefs (i.e., the extent to which symptoms are attributed to mild TBI), (b) expectations of lasting severe consequences following injury, and (c) greater distress at three months post-mild TBI had greater odds of poor outcome at six months postinjury.

"Postconcussion" symptoms, particularly in the chronic phase, are not specific to TBI. However, people may nonetheless attribute their current symptoms and difficulties to having sustained a brain injury. Indeed, Larson and colleagues (2012) reported that attribution to concussion was associated with more severe PCS reporting in their sample of veterans. Similarly, Belanger, Barwick, Kip, Kretzmer, and Vanderploeg (2013) found that the most potent predictor of PCS severity was attribution—that is, the extent to which one attributed symptoms to mild TBI versus other potential causes. Importantly, work in other specialties suggests that attributional styles are mutable and can be modified (Peters, Constans, & Mathews, 2011).

It's important to note that method of assessment has an impact on symptom reporting as well, most likely because method of assessment has an impact on perception of the construct. So, for example, asking about symptoms in an open-ended manner tends to elicit fewer symptoms than using checklists or structured interviews (Sullivan & Edmed, 2012a). Suggesting symptoms to an examinee may make the examinee more likely to endorse them. Iverson, Brooks, Ashton, and Lange (2010) found, for example, that participants endorsed an average of 3.3 symptoms when queried in an open-ended manner versus 9.1 symptoms when queried via standardized questionnaire.

In an interesting longitudinal study, Whittaker et al. (2007) found that PCS at three months postinjury was not related to injury severity or psychological distress but rather was related to what they termed "consequences" and "timeline." "Consequences" was the extent to which people believed that a mild TBI would have a negative impact on their lives, while "timeline" was the extent to which people believed concussion-related symptoms would last. In a regression analysis, only "consequences" was a significant predictor of outcome. Patients who believed that the symptoms they experienced following a mild TBI have serious negative consequences on their lives, and likely will continue to do so, were at heightened risk of experiencing enduring symptoms. Interpreting symptoms as serious and enduring puts patients at risk of chronic PCS. However, initial severity of PCS was not an independent predictor of persisting symptoms. Furthermore, anxiety, depression, and PTSD symptom severity did not significantly improve the predictive model of chronic PCS. In summary, what people believe about mild TBI plays an important role in outcome, suggesting the need to assess and manage patient perceptions and beliefs.

Number of Injuries

While the long-term effect of a single concussion on cognitive measures has been relatively well studied and with consistent findings, much less is known about the long-term impact of multiple concussions, and there has been more inconsistency in findings. For instance, while some studies have found adverse long-term effects on cognitive performance (Collins, Lovell, & McKeag, 1999; Moser & Schatz, 2002; Moser, Schatz, & Jordan, 2005; Wall et al., 2006), others have not (Gaetz, Goodman, & Weinberg, 2000; Iverson, Brooks, Collins, & Lovell, 2006; Iverson, Brooks, Lovell, & Collins, 2006; Macciocchi, Barth, Littlefield, & Cantu, 2001). Furthermore, some studies have found that athletes with two prior concussions recover more slowly (Guskiewicz et al., 2003; Wrightson & Gronwall, 1981) from a concussion, while other studies find no such relationship between recovery time and prior concussion history (Iverson, 2007). We (Belanger, Spiegel, & Vanderploeg, 2010) conducted a meta-analysis that found that the overall effect of multiple mild TBIs on neuropsychological functioning was minimal and not significant ($d = 0.06$). However, follow-up analyses in each cognitive domain revealed that multiple concussions (vs. a single concussion) were associated with poorer performance on measures of delayed memory and executive functioning.

The extent to which there may be a "threshold effect" has yet to be determined. (A threshold effect would be the minimum number of concussions or amount of accumulated brain damage that is sufficient to produce long-term cognitive deficit or to start some type of neurodegenerative cascade.) In sports, age may be associated with worse outcomes to the extent that it serves as a proxy for exposure. That is, older participants in a risky sport are likely to have participated in it longer and therefore will have had more opportunity for TBI. So, for example, in boxing, one of the risk factors for dementia pugilistica is boxing for longer than ten years (Rabadi & Jordan, 2001).

In a meta-analysis of the effect of mild TBI on cognition in athletes, Belanger and Vanderploeg (2005) found that athletes involved in risky sports (i.e., soccer and boxing), as compared to control participants in less risky sports (e.g., track and field), had significantly worse performance on cognitive measures ($d = 0.31$). The overall effect (d) of "exposure" as measured by examining the correlation between length of participation and neuropsychological functioning was .71 ($p < .05$) based on four effect-size estimates. In these studies, exposure was determined by number of boxing bouts and/or length of career, or frequency of heading in soccer. The largest effects were noted in the domains of delayed memory, executive functions, and language. Finally, there is evidence from retrospective research that late adult, former athletes with a history of concussion do more poorly on neuropsychological assessment than age-similar former athletes with no concussion history (De Beaumont et al., 2009; Tremblay et al., 2012). In addition, they exhibit abnormal enlargement of the ventricles, cortical thinning, and various neurometabolic and neuroelectrical abnormalities.

As with cognitive performance outcomes, findings related to the presence and severity of PCS and number of concussions is mixed. Among rugby players, concussion exposure is associated with an increase in symptom severity, but not diminished neurocognitive functioning (Hollis et al., 2009). More specifically, extent of concussion exposure (i.e., greater number of concussions) is associated with increased memory complaints and overall PCS endorsements in a dose-dependent manner for retired and older recreational players, but not for those who are younger (Thornton, Cox, Whitfield, & Fouladi, 2008).

In general samples seen in concussion clinics, the data are mixed with regard to PCS. Silverberg et al., in a cross-sectional retrospective study (2013), found no relationship between number of concussions and PCS reporting. However, a longitudinal study found that those who had not recovered by three months postinjury in terms of PCS were more likely to have a history of prior TBI (Ponsford, et al., 2000). Other cross-sectional studies also suggest greater PCS severity with multiple concussions (Iverson, Gaetz, Lovell, & Collins, 2004; Schatz, Moser, Covassin, & Karpf, 2011).

Limited neuroimaging data suggest that a history of two or more concussions is not associated with changes in brain activation (via Blood-Oxygen-Level Dependent fMRI) during working memory tasks, relative to those with no concussion histories (Elbin et al., 2012; Terry et al., 2012). However, Tremblay et al. (2012) found that relative to athlete controls with no concussion history, those with a history of concussion(s) decades earlier (average of two concussions) had abnormal ventricular enlargement, greater cortical thinning, various neurometabolic anomalies, and episodic memory and verbal fluency decline. There remains much to be understood about how multiple concussive events might affect the evolution and progression of any medical imaging brain abnormalities observed in this population.

Finally, the association between repeated mild TBIs and the development of dementia has been investigated with mostly mixed findings. Guskiewicz et al. (2005) found an association between a history of repeat concussion and clinically diagnosed mild cognitive impairment (MCI) in a large sample of retired National Football League (NFL) football players. Retired players with three or more reported concussions had a fivefold prevalence of MCI diagnosis and a threefold prevalence of reported significant memory problems compared with retirees without a history of concussion. There was a trend of earlier onset of Alzheimer's disease in the retirees as compared to the general U.S. male population, though there was no overall association between a history of repetitive concussion and Alzheimer's disease. This study was retrospective and therefore susceptible to recall bias of participants. A recent mortality study of retired NFL players (Lehman, Hein, Baron, & Gersic, 2012) found a significantly increased risk of death from Alzheimer's disease and amyotrophic lateral sclerosis (ALS). Further analysis found that non-line players were at higher risk than line players, possibly because of an increased risk of concussion. As has been pointed out by Karantzoulis and Randolph (2013), however, the overall rate of death is significantly lower among retired NFL players, as compared to the general male population, and so the conclusions that can be rendered are limited (there were only six deaths due to ALS and two deaths due to Alzheimer's disease out of 334 deaths). Finally, a retrospective analysis of high school football players between 1946 to 1956 (when headgear was less protective than current headgear) revealed no increased risk of dementia, Parkinson's disease, or ALS among the 438 football players compared with the 140 non-football-playing male classmate controls (Savica, Parisi, Wold, Josephs, & Ahlskog, 2012).

Rather than simple "black and white" answers regarding multiple injuries, it is likely that there is some threshold after which adverse outcomes may occur. This threshold may vary by an individual's genetic make-up, demographics, premorbid intelligence, general health, and other factors, as well as injury-related factors, such as the number of concussions, severity of concussions, time interval between concussions, etc. Recent animal work suggests, for example, that increasing the time interval between concussions to one month versus one day or one week attenuates adverse cognitive outcomes following multiple injuries (Meehan, Zhang, Mannix, & Whalen, 2012). Similar findings have been reported in humans such that the impact of multiple concussions on PCS lessens as time between concussions increases (Silverberg et al., 2013).

Context

Sports

The CDC estimates that 173,285 sports-related concussion among children and adolescents present to U.S. emergency departments each year (Centers for Disease Control, 2011). Many probably do not receive medical attention, so this number is likely an underestimate. In fact, it has been estimated that there are 1.6 million to 3.8 million sports-related concussions a year in the United States (Langlois, Rutland-Brown, & Wald,

2006). Football and ice hockey are associated with the highest percentage of concussions each year (Giza et al., 2013; Lincoln et al., 2011). For females, the greatest concussion risk is associated with soccer (Giza et al., 2013; Lincoln et al., 2011).

The majority of athletes recover from a mild TBI within seven days (Belanger & Vanderploeg, 2005), with parallel recovery of initial symptoms, cognitive impairment, and postural instability (McCrea et al., 2003). Importantly, nonconcussive bodily injuries can cause acute cognitive impairment (Hutchison, Comper, Mainwaring, & Richards, 2011) emphasizing the importance of using injured controls in prospective studies of concussion. In general, those who sustain mild TBI from sports report fewer symptoms than those injured via other mechanisms (Bazarian et al., 1999). More prolonged recovery in terms of PCS (i.e., greater than seven days of symptoms) occurs in about 10% of concussed athletes and is predicted by LOC, PTA, more severe acute symptoms (McCrea et al., 2013), and the presence of dizziness (Lau, Kontos, Collins, Mucha, & Lovell, 2011). Neuropsychological assessment, as well as symptom scales, and balance testing are recommended for repeated assessment following concussion in athletes and are included in well-established guidelines for evaluation and clinical management following a sports-related concussion (Giza et al., 2013). However, there is some controversy surrounding the utility of baseline and follow-up neuropsychological testing in particular, given the lack of sensitivity to change and lack of incremental utility beyond symptom resolution (Randolph, 2011; Randolph, McCrea, & Barr, 2005). Please see Chapter 27 for more details about mild TBI sustained in sports.

Forensic

Research has shown that compensation and litigation factors are the single most stable predictor of prolonged PCS in mild TBI samples (Carroll et al., 2004). This is based in part on a meta-analysis by Binder and Rohling (1996) that found financial compensation was a strong risk factor for long-term disability, symptoms, and poorer cognitive performance after mild TBI. Importantly, financial incentives appeared to play a more powerful role in patients with mild versus moderate/severe head injuries. Subsequent to that meta-analysis, Paniak and colleagues (Paniak et al., 2002; Paniak, Toller-Lobe, Reynolds, Melnyk, & Nagy, 2000) found that compensation-seeking strongly predicted delayed return to work, more long-term symptoms and greater symptom severity, independent of mild TBI injury severity. Similarly, Cassidy and colleagues (2004) found that making tort claims following motor vehicle accidents was one of the strongest factors associated with slower recovery. In another meta-analysis, Belanger et al. (2005) also found greater neuropsychological impairment in the late stage of recovery among concussion samples who were involved in litigation compared to prospectively followed samples. Secondary gain factors clearly negatively affect both subjective PCS reporting and objective neuropsychological performance.

Although important in all evaluation settings, validity assessment is crucial in forensic settings. Larrabee (2012) has suggested the use of the terms "performance validity testing" (PVT) and "symptom validity testing" (SVT) to be more accurate and descriptive than terms such as *tests of effort* or *response bias*. Performance validity refers to the extent to which a person's cognitive or neuropsychological test performance reflects their actual level of ability. In contrast, symptom validity refers to the accuracy of symptom reporting on self-report symptom measures. Tests such as the MMPI-2 and Personality Assessment Inventory have scales of symptom exaggeration and these can be considered symptom validity indices. Both performance validity and symptom validity are significant issues of concern in the evaluation of mild TBI, particularly in forensic settings where secondary gain issues can be prominent (e.g., personal injury legal suits, disability determination evaluations, workers' compensation evaluations, and veterans' compensation and pension examinations).

It should not be surprising that base rates of performance validity test failure are increased among compensation-seeking individuals (Heilbronner, Sweet, Morgan, Larrabee, & Millis, 2009). Larrabee (2003) reviewed the literature up to 2003 and found 11 studies yielding 548/1363 subjects (40%) that were identified with motivated performance deficits suggestive of malingering. The frequency of invalid performance ranged from 15% (Trueblood & Schmidt, 1993) to 64% (Heaton, Smith, Lehman, & Vogt, 1978). These base rates are similar to those found by Mooney and colleagues (2005) in a sample of mild TBI patients with poor recovery from PCS (i.e., base rates ranging from 28% to 59% across performance validity indices). Similarly, evidence of noncredible somatic disability presentation (i.e., exaggeration of somatic symptoms) shows base rates of 30%–40% in secondary gain contexts (Greve, Ord, Bianchini, & Curtis, 2009; Meyers, Millis, & Volkert, 2002; Mittenberg, Patton, Canyock, & Condit, 2002).

Importantly, however, failure on performance validity measures also occurs in nonforensic settings. For example, in one longitudinal study that followed people with mild TBI after attending an emergency department in the Netherlands, 110 people were asked to participate in neuropsychological evaluations an average of six months postinjury. In that nonreferred sample, 27% failed performance validity measures. Failure was associated with lower education, changes in work status, psychological distress, fatigue, and negative affect, but not with litigation (Stulemeijer, Andriessen, Brauer, Vos, & Van Der Werf, 2007).

Military

Mild TBI may occur in as many as 20% of combatants (Hoge et al., 2008; Tanielian & Jaycox, 2008; Terrio et al., 2009) and has been called the "signature injury" of recent wars. Identifying and treating mild TBI has been a high priority within both the U.S. Department of Defense (DoD) and the VA since the onset of operations Enduring Freedom (OEF), Iraqi Freedom (OIF), and more recently New Dawn (OND). Being injured via an explosion or other event in a combat zone, often in the midst of a firefight, is an emotionally charged event. Given such circumstances, it is difficult to know whether any reported "alteration" in consciousness is due to a brain concussion, emotional trauma, adrenaline rush, pain related to other bodily injuries, or some other cause. A TBI-induced alteration of consciousness (i.e., confusion, disorientation, incoherency at the scene of the event) is different from a psychologically induced alteration of consciousness, although they may be difficult to distinguish, particularly if information is being obtained months later.

However, the role of expectation must be considered in the military context. The media attention of concussion as a "signature injury" of deployment, and the discussion of PTSD, depression, suicidality, and cognitive impairment in the same context, brings to the fore the adverse effects of beliefs, expectations and attributions on outcomes. Secondary gain is also relevant, both in the potential avoidance of further deployments and in possible disability or compensation benefits. However, these factors may be partially offset by the warrior mentality and sense of duty and unit cohesion similar to the sports concussion context. Please see the "Political/Media" section to follow, as well as Chapter 33, for more details about mild TBI sustained in combat.

Political/Media

It is important to realize and appreciate the power of expectation and the role that media coverage plays in this regard. To experimentally investigate the effects of media messages on health outcomes, Witthoft and Rubin (2013) randomly assigned healthy university research volunteers (i.e., students and staff) to watch a real television report that promoted a link between exposure to Wi-Fi and symptoms (n = 76) or a control film about the security of mobile phone data transmission (n = 71). After watching their respective films, participants received a 15-minute sham exposure to a Wi-Fi signal. More than half of the television Wi-Fi report participants (54%) reported symptoms that they attributed to the sham exposure. These included: tingling in fingers, hands, and feet; pressure and tingling in the head; stomachaches; and trouble concentrating. Two of the participants found the experience so unpleasant that they had to stop the sham Wi-Fi exposure before their time was up. Simply watching the television report about potential effects of Wi-Fi exposure increased health worries. Sham Wi-Fi exposure subsequently increased symptom levels, more so in those with higher pre-exposure anxiety who were also more likely to attribute their symptoms to the sham Wi-Fi exposure.

Sensational media attention in recent years regarding the adverse effects of sports-concussions (and resulting chronic traumatic encephalopathy, or CTE) and concussions in military personnel exposed to blasts is the same scenario as the media Wi-Fi study described. These repeated media messages likely create a heightened and biased perception about adverse health outcomes following mild TBI. DoD and VA postdeployment screening for concussion within this context sets the stage for negative expectancies to exert an adverse influence on the patient's belief system and to attribute many or all difficulties to TBI (Mittenberg et al., 1992). The work of Suhr and Gunstad (Suhr & Gunstad, 2002, 2005) has been particularly illustrative of the effects of the context of the evaluation on cognitive performance outcomes, a situation they refer to as "diagnosis threat." They have demonstrated that calling attention to one's brain injury diagnosis tends to increase symptom reporting and decrease cognitive performance.

Given the disparagement experienced by many returning Vietnam Era veterans, there currently is a very strong desire to "do the right thing" for OEF/OIF/OND war-injured veterans. If there is any indication of exposure to or injury from blasts, or having sustained a mild TBI, there may be unwitting pressure to assume that current symptoms and complaints are valid and related to deployment-related events like TBI and further to favor physical diagnoses over psychological diagnoses.

Furthermore, with the advent of population-based screening and evaluation for concussion in the military and VA, as well as increased media attention on concussion, there is likely much more evaluation and treatment following concussion than ever before. In such a context, there is greater potential for diagnosis threat (discussed on p., 426), nocebo effects, iatrogenic effects, and "good old day" bias (Gunstad & Suhr, 2001; Vanderploeg & Belanger, 2013).

Not only are individuals with a history of mild TBI affected by expectations, but clinicians can be as well. The explosion of media attention surrounding mild TBI, both in the sports and postcombat arenas, can create a biased perception (perhaps even subconsciously) of poor recovery rates following a mild TBI, even in the most astute clinician. Additionally, with the increased presence of clinical neuropsychology in the forensic arena over the past decade (Sweet, Meyer, Nelson, & Moberg, 2011), there may be financial incentives (again, possibly subconscious) to overestimate the likelihood of chronic disability in any given case of mild TBI. In contrast, group studies suggesting recovery may obscure a clinician's ability to appreciate the possibility of continued difficulties in individual patients.

Treatment

For individuals who have sustained a mild TBI and experience PCS, research has shown the benefit of acute, brief psychological treatment for significantly reducing the severity and duration of symptoms. Several standardized, empirically supported treatment manuals are available (Mittenberg, Tremont, Zielinski, Fichera, & Rayls, 1996; Mittenberg, Zielinski, & Fichera, 1993). Mittenberg et al. (1996) demonstrated that a psychoeducational intervention, which included giving the patient a printed manual and having them meet with a therapist for one hour prior to hospital discharge, resulted in significantly shorter symptom duration and significantly fewer symptoms at six month follow-up compared to a matched control group who received routine hospital care. This one hour meeting included reviewing the nature and incidence of expected symptoms, providing a cognitive-behavioral model of symptom maintenance and treatment, providing symptom-specific strategies, and providing instructions for gradual resumption of activities.

Table 18.5 summarizes the studies published to date with regard to nonmedication interventions following mild TBI. The right-most column details whether or not there was a positive outcome with regard to symptom reduction. First, it is important to realize that not all these studies were designed with the goal of symptom reduction. For example, Hinkle et al. (1986) conducted a trial with the goal of "restoring social competence." Nonetheless, as can be seen from the table, in the acute phase (studies in bold), brief treatment has demonstrated efficacy in reducing symptoms at follow-up in patients following mild TBI in most but not all studies (78% of studies conducted within the first seven to ten days show positive impact). Closer examination of those studies conducted within this time frame is illustrative. The three studies with prospective recruitment within one week of injury (i.e., Mittenberg et al., 1996; Ponsford et al., 2002; Wade, King, Wenden, Crawford, & Caldwell, 1998) all demonstrated significantly reduced symptoms at follow-up secondary to

Table 18.5 Nonmedication intervention studies with mild TBI patients

First Author	*Year Published*	*Design*	*Intervention(s) Tested*	*Study Sample*	*Tx and Control Groups*	*Follow-Up*	*Tx Effect?*
Alves	**1993**	**RCT**	**1. Information + reassurance of recovery 2. Information only 3. Control**	**Hospitalized after mild TBI**	**$N = 201$ $N = 176$ $N = 210$**	**3, 6, 12 months**	**Yes***
Azulay	2013	Pre-Post	Mindfulness training	7 to 36 months postinjury	$N = 22$	Posttreatment	No
Belanger	2015	RCT	1.Web-based information 2.Control	< 1 month, 1 month–1 year, > 1 year	$N = 69$ $N = 70$	7 days, 6 months	No
Bell	**2008**	**RCT**	**1. Handout + telephone counsel (4–5 calls over 12 weeks) providing education and reassurance and individualized plans for symptom management 2. Handout in ED**	**Within 48 hours of injury**	**$N = 146$ $N = 166$**	**6 months**	**Yes**
Bryant	2003	RCT	1.CBT 2.Supportive Counseling	Within 2 weeks of injury	$N = 12$ $N = 12$	6 months	Yes**
Chin	2015	Pre-post	Aerobic Exercise	Average of 4 years postinjury	$N = 7$	Posttreatment	No***
Cicerone	2002	Prospective case comparison	Attention strategy training hourly for 11 to 27 weeks	Average of 7.6 months postinjury with cognitive impairment	$N = 4$ $N = 4$	Posttreatment (roughly 16 weeks)	Yes
Elgmark	2007	RCT	Information, support by multiple disciplines (mostly OT)	Median of 3 weeks postinjury	$N = 264$ $N = 131$	12 months	No
Ferguson as reported in Miller	1996	Pre-Post	12-session manualized cognitive-behavioral treatment	Referrals to outpatient clinic	$N = 4$	12 weeks	Yes
Ghaffar	**2006**	**RCT**	**Multidisciplinary treatment**	**Within 1 week of injury**	**$N = 97$ $N = 94$**	**6 months**	**No**
Gronwall	1986	Not randomized	Information booklet	Within 2 weeks of injury	$N = 34$ $N = 54$	3 months	No
Hanna-Pladdy	2001	RCT	Relaxation	Less than 1 to multiple years postinjury	$N = 44$ $N = 44$	Post-stress induction or none	Yes
Hinkle	**1986**	**RCT**	**1. Education + reassurance 2. Control (return to normal activity)**	**Hospitalized after mild TBI**	**$N = 166$ $N = 75$**	**3 months**	**No******
Kjeldgaard	2014	RCT	CBT	27 months postinjury	$N = 35$ $N = 37$	6.5 months	No

First Author	*Year Published*	*Design*	*Intervention(s) Tested*	*Study Sample*	*Tx and Control Groups*	*Follow-Up*	*Tx Effect?*
Leddy	2013	Quasi-random assignment with matched control	1. Exercise 2. Stretching 3. Healthy Control	Average of 117 days postinjury with PCS	*N* = 4 *N* = 4 *N* = 4	Posttreatment (roughly 17 weeks)	Yes
Matuseviciene	2013	RCT	1. Assessment + verbal education + printed education + gradual return to activity 2. Printed information	Recruited in ED and symptomatic at 10 days; intervention at 14–21 days postinjury	*N* = 39 *N* = 41	3 months	No
Minderhoud	**1980**	**Retrospective comparison**	**Printed + verbal education + activity encouraged after week of bed rest.**	**Hospitalized after mild TBI**	***N* = 180** ***N* = 352**	**6 months**	**Yes**
Mittenberg	**1996**	**RCT**	**Printed manual + one-hour session**	**Hospitalized after mild TBI**	***N* = 29** ***N* = 29**	**6 months**	**Yes**
Paniak	1998, 2000	RCT	1. Assessment and feedback + treatment as needed for symptoms 2. Single session education + brochure	Hospital emergency room (12 days postinjury)	*N* = 53 *N* = 58	3 to 4 months, 12 months	No
Ponsford	**2002**	**Alternate assignment to group**	**Information booklet**	**Hospital emergency room (within a week)**	***N* = 79** ***N* = 123**	**3 months**	**Yes**
Relander	**1972**	**RCT**	**Seen daily at hospital + encouragement to get out of bed + physical therapy**	**Within 36 hours of hospital admission (not all milds)**	***N* = 82** ***N* = 96**	**12 months postinjury**	**No****
Silverberg	2013	RCT	1. CBT 2. Printed education + 3-hour educational session	Less than 6 weeks postinjury (average of 24 days); symptomatic	*N* = 13 *N* = 11	3 months postinjury	Yes
Suffoletto	**2013**	**RCT**	**Text messaging assessment with self-care support messages**	**In emergency room**	***N* = 43** ***N* = 25**	**14 days**	**No**
Tiersky	2005	RCT with multiple baselines	CBT + cognitive treatment for 11 weeks	Average of 5 years postinjury	*N* = 7 (milds) *N* = 9	1 and 3 months	Yes
Wade	**1998**	**RCT**	**Printed and verbal education + continued support as needed**	**7 to 10 days postinjury**	***N* = 132** ***N* = 86**	**6 months**	**Yes**
Wolf	2012	RCT	Hyperbaric oxygen	3–71 months postinjury	*N* = 24 *N* = 24	6 weeks	No

Notes: Studies in **bold** font are studies with participants in the acute phase postinjury.

*For reassurance treatment group only, assuming that patients not seen at follow-up are asymptomatic.
** Outcome measures were depression, PTSD, and impact of event.
***Exercise group improved cognitive performance but not mood or sleep.
****No difference in symptom reporting but treatment groups returned to work sooner. RCT = randomized controlled trial; CBT = cognitive behavioral therapy; Tx = Treatment; LOC = loss of consciousness; CBT = cognitive behavioral therapy.

educational interventions. These studies all involved interventions that were psychoeducational in nature (e.g., providing an informational booklet that outlined common symptoms, as well as their likely time course and suggested coping strategies) with a varying degree of additional support.

One study conducted in the acute phase that did not find a positive impact of intervention was the Relander et al. (1972) study. However, they did not use a standardized measure of PCS and did report improvements in return to work in their intervention group. This study was conducted in the 1970s with hospitalized patients and did not provide much detail about the intervention other than participants were seen daily, were encouraged to get out of bed, and participated in physical therapy. Additionally, one study (Ghaffar, McCullagh, Ouchterlony, & Feinstein, 2006) found that multidisciplinary treatment in the acute phase was not useful in reducing PCS.

Taken together, these studies suggest that providing education in the acute phase is useful in reducing PCS. Examination of findings related to interventions administered during the postacute to chronic stages does not provide as much clarity. Differences between interventions, samples studied, and methodologies make comparisons difficult. For example, one study by Hanna-Pladdy et al. 2001, was a test of relaxation training, rather than an educational/supportive intervention. It is also notable that most of the studies with null findings used frequency counts of symptoms as the dependent measure, rather than symptom severity. It may be that the effect of these interventions in the postacute to chronic phases is small and that nonparametric statistics are less likely to reveal treatment effects.

It is also notable that Paniak and colleagues (Paniak, Toller–Lobe, Durand, and Nagy, 1998; Paniak et al., 2000), in their randomized controlled trial in the postacute phase, found that there was no added benefit in providing more extensive treatment (as is typically provided following more severe TBI) as compared to a single informational meeting during which patients' post-TBI experiences were legitimized, education was provided about common symptoms and coping strategies, and reassurance of positive outcomes was provided. Given the present literature, it is unknown if patients seen more chronically (i.e., months or more postinjury) can benefit from brief psychoeducational interventions. Positive results (Huckans et al., 2010; Tiersky et al., 2005) observed during the time frame included much more involved interventions than the studies conducted on patients evaluated soon after injury.

In summary, careful review of the extant literature suggests a positive impact of psychoeducational interventions provided in the acute care setting (i.e., in the emergency room or within one week of injury). Beyond that, results are less clear. Indeed, providing education about mild TBI in the chronic phase may actually "neurologize" (Paniak et al., 1998) difficulties that are due to psychological issues such as posttraumatic stress, chronic pain, or other factors. Furthermore, it is notable that the presence of financial compensation significantly inflates symptom reporting regardless of time since injury (Paniak et al., 2002). It is worth noting that there is evidence that treating comorbid psychological conditions in those with a history of mild TBI is effective; in other words, there is no evidence that psychological interventions should be withheld in those with a history of mild TBI. Bryant, Moulds, Guthrie, and Nixon (2003), for example, found that PTSD was much more likely to be prevented in those individuals with acute stress disorder following mild TBI who were treated with five sessions of cognitive behavioral therapy.

Controversies and Future Directions

Biomarkers

In recent years, owing to the frustration surrounding the lack of objective markers of the milder forms of brain injury, interest in biomarkers of TBI has increased. A biomarker is a physiological indicator of disease or injury and may include neuroimaging or blood-based markers. As reviewed on pp. 418–419, newer neuroimaging techniques, such as DTI, have demonstrated sensitivity to mild TBI in tissue that appears normal on standard clinical scans. The question of longer-term utility remains, however, as there has yet to be any demonstration that subtle injury found in the acute or postacute stages has any long-term prognostic utility.

In terms of blood-borne biomarkers, investigators have examined various proteins in the hopes that a low-cost blood test might prove useful in deciding which patients might need neuroimaging in the emergency room. The most widely studied biomarker is S100B, which is a protein predominantly expressed by astrocytes; levels of S100B increase during the acute phase of brain damage and decrease later on. It has excellent sensitivity to injury but poor specificity. Indeed, the utility of S100B lies in its negative predictive value, meaning its ability to confirm the absence of injury that might require neurosurgical intervention. As such, the American College of Emergency Physicians issued a "Level C" guideline stating that a CT scan is optional in patients without significant extracranial injury if serum S100B is less than 0.1 ng/mL within the first four hours of injury (Jagoda et al., 2008). It is thought that the negative predictive value of S100B is due to the fact that serum S100B levels reflect blood-brain barrier permeability changes (Jeter et al., 2013). In other words, because S100B does not cross the blood-brain barrier, there is poor correlation between its values in the CSF versus the blood.

Many other biomarkers have been explored, including other proteins, microRNAs, and metabolites. None have sufficient sensitivity and specificity to serve as stand-alone diagnostic tests for mild TBI (see Jeter et al., 2013, for review), nor have any been able to provide a means of early identification of those cases that will have long-term functional difficulties. However, a recent study by Siman et al. (2011) suggests that a neurodegeneration biomarker called *calpain-cleaved αll-spectrin N-terminal fragment* (SNTF) may hold promise. SNTF is released from neurons upon plasma membrane disruption. The researchers assessed three groups of participants within 24 hours of injury: 17 with CT-negative mild TBI, 13 with orthopedic injury, and 8 normal, uninjured controls. Elevated SNTF in a subset of 7 mild TBI cases and 3 orthopedic injury cases was related to DTI-assessed abnormalities in the corpus callosum and uncinate fasciculus and with cognitive impairment that persisted for three months. The elevation of SNTF in the three orthopedic injury cases, coupled with neurocognitive dysfunction and microstructural abnormalities, raises the possibility that SNTF on the day of injury may be helpful in diagnosing heretofore "unknown" cases of mild TBI. Additional, larger studies are needed to validate these findings.

Genetics

Interest in the relationship between genetics and mild TBI stems largely from a desire to explain the heterogeneity and individual differences apparent in outcome. Genetic make-up may influence not only response and recovery from injury, but also proclivity to injury, extent of injury, and extent of cognitive reserve, among other factors (McAllister, 2010). Though there is very little study of genetic influence specific to mild TBI, this is likely to change with the recent mapping of the human genome and trends in personalized medicine.

The most commonly studied genetic influence to TBI outcome is that of the apolipoprotein E (APOE) gene, located on chromosome 19, which is responsible for lipid transport in the brain and may have a role in recovery after neurological injury. Of the three alleles (ε2, ε3, and ε4), APOE-ε4 is implicated in Aβ pathology in Alzheimer's disease. There has been general acceptance that carriers of the ε4 allele have increased risk of Alzheimer's disease compared to those without this allele (Bookheimer et al., 2000). In those with a history of TBI, the ε4 allele is associated with unfavorable cognitive and functional recovery (Crawford et al., 2002; Friedman et al., 1999) in samples of primarily moderate to severe TBI. Nonetheless, the extent to which the ε4 allele may moderate increased risk for Alzheimer's disease following TBI is controversial, with conflicting findings (Lye & Shores, 2000). Few studies have specifically examined this question in mild TBI alone. In a study that specifically examined mild TBI, Sundstrom et al. (2007) found that among 543 community-dwelling participants, those with prior mild TBI without APOE ε4 status had no increased risk of dementia at five years after baseline whereas those with the ε4 allele had a significantly increased risk of dementia.

In a prospective study of mild to moderate TBI, Chamelian, Reis, and Feinstein (2004) found no association between the presence of APOE-ε4 and neurocognitive performance, emotional distress, global functioning (as measured by the Glasgow Outcome Scale), psychosocial outcome, or post-concussion symptom severity six months postinjury. These findings were consistent with an earlier study (Liberman, Stewart, Wesnes, & Troncoso, 2002) of 87 patients also with mild to moderate TBI, which failed to find a relationship between APOE-ε4 status and neuropsychological recovery at six weeks postinjury. Likewise, Terrell et al. (2008) failed to find a relationship between APOE-ε4 status and risk for concussion in their exclusively mild TBI sample. However, they did find a nearly threefold increase in risk of self-reported concussion for those with the APOE promoter G-219T TT genotype compared to those with the GG genotype. They did not find any association between concussion risk and tau protein genotypes. A large, prospective study will be needed to confirm these findings, as well as to determine whether there is any association between APOE promoter G-219T TT genotype and clinical outcome following mild TBI.

In sum, the relationship between mild TBI, APOE status, and dementia requires further study. There is evidence that APOE allele status does affect clinical outcome following TBI broadly, although this does not appear to be the case in those studies that look solely at mild TBI. Specifically, APOE–ε4 status does not seem to be related to cognitive or functional recovery in those with mild TBI. Research in genetic influence on TBI outcome is in its infancy and has yet to examine many of the potential candidates, let alone their interactions with each other and with environmental factors. Given the small effect sizes and frequency of different alleles in the population, very large prospective studies are likely needed (McAllister, 2010).

Chronic Traumatic Encephalopathy (CTE)

There is growing concern that repetitive head trauma can lead to the pathologic findings associated with CTE, a histopathologically defined condition that is hypothesized to be secondary to repetitive head trauma and to represent a degenerative condition that leads to pronounced behavior and cognitive dysfunction (McKee et al., 2009). Historically, the term "dementia pugilistica" or "punch drunk syndrome" was used to denote a similar entity, described in boxers with repetitive head trauma (Bazarian et al., 2009). Pathologically, CTE is most commonly described to include: presence of perivascular foci of p-tau immunoreactive astrocytic tangles and neurofibrillary tangles, irregular cortical distribution of p-tau immunoreactive neurofibrillary tangles and astrocytic tangles with a predilection for the depth of cerebral sulci, clusters of subpial and periventricular astrocytic tangles in the cerebral cortex, diencephalon, basal ganglia and brain stem, and neurofibrillary tangles in the cerebral cortex located preferentially in the superficial layers (McKee et al., 2013). The hallmark of CTE is the neurofibrillary tangles. Unlike in Alzheimer's disease, the neurofibrillary tangles are unevenly distributed with a predilection for the depths of the sulci and around blood vessels (Mez, Stern, & McKee, 2013), particularly early in the disease. Deposition of beta-amyloid (Aß) plaques, a hallmark of Alzheimer's disease along with tangles, occurs in fewer than half the cases of traumatic encephalopathy (McKee et al., 2009).

There are no consensus criteria for the neuropathology of CTE. The two prominent labs in this line of research have promulgated different criteria. Omalu et al. (2011a) propose four distinct phenotypes based on the varying histopathological features and distribution of neurofibrillary tangles and neuritic threads, while McKee et al. (2013) describe four pathological criteria they deem necessary to CTE. One key difference is that Omalu et al. have not described marked accumulation and/or prominent perivascular distribution of tau immunoreactive astrocytes. The discrepancies between these labs illustrate the central conundrum of CTE. The broad and heterogeneous pathological criteria become rather nonspecific. Indeed, neurofibrillary tangles, the hallmark of CTE, are present in some elderly people with no cognitive impairment (Bennett et al., 2006), and they are present in 11 of the 18 control brains (or 61%) described in McKee et al. (2013) and absent in 17 of the 85 (or 20%) individuals with repetitive head trauma. Additionally, Hazrati et al. (2013) reported a case series in which the *absence* of CTE was notable in several retired Canadian football players who had sustained multiple mild TBIs and significant cognitive decline. As Wortzel, Brenner, and Arciniegas (2013) argue, establishment of the sensitivity and specificity of the core histopathological features is critical.

Further complicating the picture are the broad clinical phenotypes described to date. Clinical features described have included depression, anxiety, PTSD, alcohol/substance abuse/dependence, dysarthria, dysphagia, gaze disturbance, chronic pain, anabolic steroid use, coronary artery disease, headaches, suicide, aggression, dementia, poor impulse control, gait instability/parkinsonism, ocular deficits, cognitive difficulties, paranoid ideations, poor insight, disinhibition, inappropriate sexual behavior, apathy, and risk taking. Furthermore, the clinical symptoms begin an average of eight to ten years after the proposed causal traumatic injury(ies) (McKee et al., 2013). As with fronto-temporal dementia, CTE reportedly begins most typically in midlife with behavior and personality changes (McKee et al., 2013), though Stern et al. (2013) suggest different clinical subtypes based on symptom presentation and onset, with a "behavioral/mood" group having earlier onset (mean age of onset of 35) than a "cognitive" group (mean age of onset of 59). Nonetheless, the time lag makes tying the repetitive (often temporally spaced out) trauma to the behavior and ultimately the neuropathology difficult. Though a recent report detailing CTE in a "blast-exposed" veteran with PTSD who committed suicide has received attention (Omalu et al., 2011b) as suggesting the possibility that CTE might be caused by mere blast exposure or possibly PTSD, review of the case description details a complex history that includes premilitary substance abuse, acting-out behaviors prior to reported concussive events, and possibly several concussions.

Importantly, it is impossible to estimate the incidence and prevalence of CTE due to the ascertainment bias inherent in autopsy studies. That is, families of individuals with significant cognitive and/or behavioral difficulties are more likely to initiate and participate in brain donation. Prospective studies are needed to determine what causes CTE. Post hoc associations between behavioral disturbances and histopathology are an important first step in advancing science. However, they are inherently biased and self-selecting. Additionally, while retrospective case studies from autopsy cases have revealed some commonalities (such as irritability, impulsivity, aggression, depression, suicidality, memory impairment), there are presently no clinical criteria for CTE.

The highly publicized accounts of these high-profile cases can give the public a biased perception of recovery rates expected following a concussion, even a single concussion. Sensational media attention in recent years on individual cases who have exhibited drastic behavior (e.g., suicide) in association with pathological findings consistent with CTE at autopsy also tends to create a biased perception among the public. However, as Iverson notes (Iverson, 2014), there are no published cross-sectional, epidemiological or prospective studies showing a relation between contact sports and risk of suicide. One published epidemiological study (Baron, Hein, Lehman, & Gersic, 2012) suggests that retired NFL players have decreased mortality compared to the general population and are actually less likely to die by suicide. In a case series reported by McKee et al. (2013), six out of the ten former athletes who committed suicide were in the control (i.e., non-CTE pathology) group. Clearly, as Iverson cogently observes, "there is a mature body of evidence suggesting that the causes of suicide are complex, multifactorial and difficult to predict in individual cases" (Iverson, 2014: 163).

In sum, the broad and nonspecific clinical and histopathological phenomenology of CTE, as currently conceptualized, is problematic and is currently based on samples of convenience. The described pathology could be secondary to a host of factors, repetitive brain trauma being one of them. The described clinical presentation likewise is probably broadly determined. Even a behavioral correlate like "cognitive impairment," seemingly both objectively determined and somewhat clear-cut, is determined by a complex set of factors. In two large epidemiological clinical-pathologic studies, brain pathology accounted for only 40% of the variance in cognitive decline (Boyle et al., 2013). Prospective epidemiological study is needed to clarify the incidence of prevalence of CTE and its associated risk factors. Additionally, controlled prospective study of the clinical features with blinded neuropathological study will be needed.

Subconcussions

Animal models suggest that repetitive, subthreshold force, which typically does not cause cellular death, can nonetheless cause damage when repeated several times within short periods (Slemmer & Weber, 2005). As such, it is possible that this happens in human beings. The questions then become: how frequent, what is the minimal force required, how close in time must they occur, and how many are needed to sustain this damage? Additionally, what might the long-term consequences be?

A "subconcussive" blow is one that does not meet the clinical diagnosis of concussion, yet may have an adverse long-term effect, particularly via repetitive occurrences. A recent review of the subconcussion literature (Bailes, Petraglia, Omalu, Nauman, & Talavage, 2013) concludes that subconcussive blows may have a deleterious neurological effect over time. Not surprisingly, human data comes primarily from football players, who endure an average of 652 impacts to the helmet per season at the high school level (Broglio et al., 2010). Pellman, Viano, Tucker, Casson (2003) found that a force in excess of 98*g*s is 75% specific to concussion in the NFL while Schnebel, Gwin, Anderson, and Gatlin (2007) reported a range of 90–120*g*s in collegiate players. Perhaps surprisingly, the magnitude of impacts to the helmet does not necessarily correlate with the probability of sustaining a concussion (Guskiewicz & Mihalik, 2011) suggesting that there may not be a "threshold effect" for concussion with respect to force. Clinical studies of the neurological/neuropsychological impact of subconcussive blows have been mixed.

Gysland et al. (2012) studied 46 collegiate football players by assessing them with neuropsychological, sensory, balance, and symptom-based measures both before and after a single season during which a head impact telemetry system recorded head impacts. Changes in performance were mostly independent of prior concussion history, and the total number, magnitude, and location of sustained impacts over one season. Specifically, head impact variables (including the total number of impacts, the total number of impacts greater than 90*gs*, the total cumulative magnitude of impacts, and the total number of impacts to the top of the head) did not predict neurocognitive performance over time, nor did they predict changes in balance on the Sensory Organization Test or total symptom severity. On another measure of balance (the Balance Error Scoring System), they found somewhat contradictory findings. That is, a higher number of impacts and higher number of prior concussions was predictive of improved balance over the course of the season, while a higher cumulative magnitude of head impacts predicted declining balance. Finally, while total symptom severity was not related to head impact variables, an increase in the total number of symptoms reported was related to having a higher number of severe head impacts (over 90*gs*) and a higher number of impacts to the top of the head. This study of course does not address the potential effects of lifetime dose, though it did find that the amount of college football exposure (based on number of years played) was associated with poorer balance and increased symptom reporting. Miller, Adamson, Pink, and Sweetet al. (2007) similarly assessed 76 collegiate football players at preseason, midseason, and postseason on neuropsychological measures and found no significant declines throughout the season despite likely repeated subconcussive impacts. Of note, these researchers did not measure head impacts, so the relationship between magnitude and number of blows was not directly assessed. Finally, McAllister et al. (2012) followed 214 collegiate football and hockey players from pre- to postseason and compared them to 45 noncontact-sport athletes assessed at the same intervals. They found no significant between-athlete group differences by time on a variety of neuropsychological measures, despite the contact athletes sustaining an average of 469 head impacts over the season with an average acceleration of 132 *g*s. They concluded that the number of head impacts does not have a widespread short-term detrimental effect. These authors did additional analyses to examine if there were a subset of individuals who did worse than expected at postseason, based on the noncontact athletes' preseason performance and test-retest interval. After conducting multiple comparisons, they found that a statistically significantly higher percentage (24% vs. 3.6%) of athletes in the contact sport group performed below predicted performance on the California Verbal Learning Test (CVLT), a verbal memory measure. However, performance on the CVLT was not significantly correlated with head impact exposure, though Trails B and reaction time were.

Overall, studies employing neuropsychological assessment within a single season have failed to demonstrate any consistent relationship between number and severity of subconcussive blows and cognitive change. Further prospective study is needed to determine if there is a lifetime dose effect. However, recent studies that have included a neuroimaging component have demonstrated a potential cumulative effect of subconcussive blows, at least in a subset of individuals. Specifically, in a prospective study of 21 high school football players during the 2009 season who were assessed pre- and postseason (with some assessed in-season as well), it was found that four of the eight non-concussed players who were reassessed in-season had significant reductions on verbal and/or visual memory scores and significantly decreased fMRI activation levels in the dorsolateral prefrontal cortex and cerebellum (Talavage et al., 2013) during working memory tasks. Furthermore, these players' cognitive and fMRI data were similar to those three players who sustained a concussion during the season. This group also had a greater total number of collision events throughout the season. The number of impacts experienced in the week immediately preceding in-season assessment was significantly correlated with changes in fMRI activation. It was further demonstrated that while the total number of blows differentiated the groups, the median peak linear acceleration did not (Breedlove et al., 2012). Oddly, these authors did not report pre-post season comparisons, nor did they report whether total season impact variables correlated with functional variables. Thus, while there may be a subset of individuals who show acute clinical changes related to recent subconcussive impacts, the longer-term (or even season-specific) implications are unclear.

Recent work has also employed DTI to investigate subconcussive blows. In a prospective cohort of nine football/ice hockey high school athletes and six controls (some injured, some not), changes in white matter, as detected using DTI, were most apparent in the one concussed athlete, followed by the nonconcussed athletes (with subconcussive blows), followed by the controls (Bazarian, Zhu, Blyth, Borrino, & Zhong, 2012). However, the changes in fractional anisotropy and mean diffusivity were in both directions (both increased and decreased), making interpretation difficult. Additionally, the "subconcussive group" did not report more symptoms than the control group and did not perform any differently than the control group on cognitive measures (and in fact outperformed them on visual motor speed and reaction time). So the subconcussive-relevant findings seem restricted to white matter changes of unclear meaning. Unfortunately, this study relied on retrospective self-reported diaries for its assessment of subconcussive blows, further limiting its interpretability. Again, given that this study followed the athletes for only one season, the longer-term implications are unclear.

In summary, while it seems as though the magnitude of impacts does not correlate with the probability of sustaining a concussion, there is recent interest in the potential cumulative impact of repeated subconcussive blows. Clinical studies of the neurological/neuropsychological impact of subconcussive blows have been mixed, however. Studies relying on cognitive measures have failed to demonstrate a relationship with head impact variables. Though some findings related to balance and symptoms have been reported, they are inconsistent and the sheer number of comparisons made in these studies suggests the need for replication in other samples. Studies conducted with neuroimaging modalities hold promise, but the long-term implications are unclear at present.

Summary and Conclusions

Despite decades of research suggesting minimal long-term sequelae associated with a single mild TBI (and to a much lesser extent, even two mild TBIs), there continues to be intense controversy about long-term sequelae of concussion. We now have multiple, independent meta-analyses, as well as seminal, prospective studies (e.g., Dikmen, Machamer, Winn, & Temkin, 1995; Levin et al., 1987; Meares et al., 2011) that suggest significant impairment due to mild TBI is unlikely to persist more than a month. This ongoing controversy is probably due to several factors, including increased forensic work in this area as well as increased media attention.

The etiology of PCS has been hypothesized to be due to neural damage, pre- and postinjury psychological factors, somatization, malingering, etc. Nonetheless, trying to determine the extent to which any given patient's difficulties are "biologically based" may be misguided. Overly focusing on biological or physiological etiology leads to "black and white" thinking, when most clinical phenomena are determined by multiple factors that may have independent and interactive effects. Given emerging, highly sensitive neuroimaging techniques and the existence of some patients who have chronic symptoms, it may be more productive to try to tease apart the many possible factors that may be related to ongoing difficulties: e.g., (a) genetic predisposition; (b) subtle brain changes; (c) psychological factors such as beliefs, expectations, and premorbid and comorbid conditions; and (d) media, medical, and legal messages conveyed either overtly or covertly. This would lay the foundation for developing algorithms for use in identifying who is at risk (Stulemeijer et al., 2008), and then test targeted intervention strategies.

The long-term impact of repeated mild TBI is less clear. The importance of large, prospective studies with appropriate, orthopedically injured controls, as well as well-defined and characterized injuries, cannot be overstated as science moves forward in this arena.

References

Alexander, M. P. (1992). Neuropsychiatric correlates of persistant postconcussive syndrome. *Journal of Head Trauma Rehabilitation*, *8*, 60–69.

Alves, W. M., Macciocchi, S. N., & Barth, J. T. (1993). Postconcussive symptoms after uncomplicated mild head injury. *Journal of Head Trauma Rehabilitation*, *8*(3), 48–59.

American Congress of Rehabilitation Medicine. (1993). Report of the mild traumatic brain injury committee of the head injury interdisciplinary special interest group. *Journal of Head Trauma Rehabilitation*, *8*, 86–87.

American Psychiatric Association. (1994). *Diagnostic and Statistical Manual of Mental Disorders* (4th ed.). Washington, DC: Author.

Arciniegas, D. B., Anderson, C. A., Topkoff, J., & McAllister, T. W. (2005). Mild traumatic brain injury: A neuropsychiatric approach to diagnosis, evaluation, and treatment. *Neuropsychiatric Disease and Treatment*, *1*(4), 311–327.

Arenth, P. M., Russell, K. C., Scanlon, J. M., Kessler, L. J., & Ricker, J. H. (2013). Corpus callosum integrity and neuropsychological performance after traumatic brain injury: A diffusion tensor imaging study. *The Journal of Head Trauma Rehabilitation*, *29*(2), E1–E10. doi: 10.1097/HTR.0b013e318289ede5

Arfanakis, K., Haughton, V. M., Carew, J. D., Rogers, B. P., Dempsey, R. J., & Meyerand, M. E. (2002). Diffusion tensor MR imaging in diffuse axonal injury. *AJNR American Journal of Neuroradiology*, *23*(5), 794–802.

Azulay, J., Smart, C. M., Mott, T., & Cicerone, K. D. (2013). A pilot study examining the effect of mindfulness-based stress reduction on symptoms of chronic mild traumatic brain injury/postconcussion syndrome. *Journal of Head Trauma Rehabilitation*, *28*(4), 323–331. doi: 10.1097/HTR.0b013e318250ebda.

Bailes, J. E., Petraglia, A. L., Omalu, B. I., Nauman, E., & Talavage, T. (2013). Role of subconcussion in repetitive mild traumatic brain injury. *Journal of Neurosurgery*, *119*(5), 1235–1245. doi: 10.3171/2013.7.JNS121822

Baron, S. L., Hein, M. J., Lehman, E., & Gersic, C. M. (2012). Body mass index, playing position, race, and the cardiovascular mortality of retired professional football players. *American Journal of Cardiology*, *109*(6), 889–896. doi: 10.1016/j.amjcard.2011.10.050 S0002-9149(11)03387-X [pii]

Basser, P. J., Mattiello, J., & LeBihan, D. (1994). MR diffusion tensor spectroscopy and imaging. *Biophysical Journal*, *66*(1), 259–267.

Bazarian, J. J., Cernak, I., Noble-Haeusslein, L., Potolicchio, S., & Temkin, N. (2009). Long-term neurologic outcomes after traumatic brain injury. *Journal of Head Trauma Rehabilitation*, *24*(6), 439–451.

Bazarian, J. J., Wong, T., Harris, M., Leahey, N., Mookerjee, S., & Dombovy, M. (1999). Epidemiology and predictors of post-concussive syndrome after minor head injury in an emergency population. *Brain Injury*, *13*(3), 173–189.

Bazarian, J. J., Zhu, T., Blyth, B., Borrino, A., & Zhong, J. (2012). Subject-specific changes in brain white matter on diffusion tensor imaging after sports-related concussion. *Magnetic Resonance Imaging*, *30*(2), 171–180. doi: 10.1016/j.mri.2011.10.001

Beauchamp, M. H., Beare, R., Ditchfield, M., Coleman, L., Babl, F. E., Kean, M., . . . Anderson, V. (2013). Susceptibility weighted imaging and its relationship to outcome after pediatric traumatic brain injury. *Cortex*, *49*(2), 591–598. doi: 10.1016/j.cortex.2012.08.015

Beetar, J. T., Guilmette, T. J., & Sparadeo, F. R. (1996). Sleep and pain complaints in symptomatic traumatic brain injury and neurologic populations. *Archives of Physical Medicine & Rehabilitation*, *77*(12), 1298–1302. doi: S0003-9993(96)90196-3 [pii]

Belanger, H. G., Barwick, F. H., Kip, K. E., Kretzmer, T., & Vanderploeg, R. D. (2013). Postconcussive symptom complaints and potentially malleable positive predictors. *Clinical Neuropsychologist*, *27*(3), 343–355. doi: 10.1080/13854046.2013.774438.

Belanger, H. G., Barwick, F., Silva, M. A., Kretzmer, T., Kip, K. E., & Vanderploeg, R. D. (2015). Web-based psychoeducational intervention for postconcussion symptoms: A randomized trial. *Military Medicine*, *180*(2), 192–200. doi: 10.7205/MILMED-D-14-00388

Belanger, H. G., Curtiss, G., Demery, J. A., Lebowitz, B. K., & Vanderploeg, R. D. (2005). Factors moderating neuropsychological outcome following mild traumatic brain injury: A meta-analysis. *Journal of the International Neuropsychological Society*, *11*(3), 215–227.

Belanger, H. G., Kretzmer, T., Vanderploeg, R., & French, L. M. (2010). Symptom complaints following combat-related TBI: Relationship to TBI severity and PTSD. *Journal of the International Neuropsychological Society*, *16*(1), 194–199.

Belanger, H. G., Spiegel, E., & Vanderploeg, R. D. (2010). Neuropsychological performance following a history of multiple self-reported concussions: A meta-analysis. *Journal of the International Neuropsychological Society*, *16*(2), 262–267.

Belanger, H. G., & Vanderploeg, R. D. (2005). The neuropsychological impact of sports-related concussion: A meta-analysis. *Journal of the International Neuropsychological Society*, *11*(4), 345–357.

Belanger, H. G., Vanderploeg, R. D., Curtiss, G., & Warden, D. (2007). Recent neuroimaging techniques in mild traumatic brain injury: A critical review. *Journal of Neuropsychiatry and Clinical Neurosciences*, *19*(1), 5–20.

Bell, K. R., Hoffman, J. M., Temkin, N. R., Powell, J. M., Fraser, R. T., Esselman, P. C., . . . Dikmen, S. (2008). The effect of telephone counselling on reducing post-traumatic symptoms after mild traumatic brain injury: A randomised trial. *Journal of Neurology, Neurosurgery & Psychiatry*, *79*(11), 1275–1281.

Bennett, D. A., Schneider, J. A., Arvanitakis, Z., Kelly, J. F., Aggarwal, N. T., Shah, R. C., & Wilson, R. S. (2006). Neuropathology of older persons without cognitive impairment from two community-based studies. *Neurology*, *66*(12), 1837–1844.

Bergeson, A. G., Lundin, R., Parkinson, R. B., Tate, D. F., Victoroff, J., Hopkins, R. O., & Bigler, E. D. (2004). Clinical rating of cortical atrophy and cognitive correlates following traumatic brain injury. *Clinical Neuropsychologist*, *18*(4), 509–520. doi: 10.1080/1385404049052414

Bernstein, D. M. (2002). Information processing difficulty long after self-reported concussion. *Journal of the International Neuropsychological Society*, *8*(5), 673–682.

Bigler, E. D., Abildskov, T. J., Petrie, J., Farrer, T. J., Dennis, M., Simic, N., . . . Owen Yeates, K. (2013). Heterogeneity of brain lesions in pediatric traumatic brain injury. *Neuropsychology*, *27*(4), 438–451. doi: 10.1037/a0032837

Bigler, E. D., & Maxwell, W. L. (2012). Neuropathology of mild traumatic brain injury: Relationship to neuroimaging findings. [Review]. *Brain Imaging and Behavior*, *6*(2), 108–136. doi: 10.1007/s11682-011-9145-0

Bigler, E. D., & Tate, D. F. (2001). Brain volume, intracranial volume, and dementia. *Investigative Radiology*, *36*(9), 539–546.

Binder, L. M., & Rohling, M. L. (1996). Money matters: A meta-analytic review of the effects of financial incentives on recovery after closed-head injury. *American Journal of Psychiatry*, *153*(1), 7–10.

Binder, L. M., Rohling, M. L., & Larrabee, J. (1997). A review of mild head trauma. Part I: Meta-analytic review of neuropsychological studies. *Journal of Clinical and Experimental Neuropsychology*, *19*(3), 421–431.

Block, C., & Cianfrini, L. (2013). Neuropsychological and neuroanatomical sequelae of chronic non-malignant pain and opioid analgesia. *NeuroRehabilitation*, *33*(2), 343–366.

Blumbergs, P. C., Scott, G., Manavis, J., Wainwright, H., Simpson, D. A., & McLean, A. J. (1994). Staining of amyloid precursor protein to study axonal damage in mild head injury. *Lancet*, *344*(8929), 1055–1056.

Boake, C., McCauley, S. R., Levin, H. S., Pedroza, C., Contant, C. F., Song, J. X., . . . Diaz-Marchan, P. J. (2005). Diagnostic criteria for postconcussional syndrome after mild to moderate traumatic brain injury. *Journal of Neuropsychiatry and Clinical Neurosciences*, *17*(3), 350–356.

Bookheimer, S. Y., Strojwas, M. H., Cohen, M. S., Saunders, A. M., Pericak-Vance, M. A., Mazziotta, J. C., & Small, G. W. (2000). Patterns of brain activation in people at risk for Alzheimer's disease. *New England Journal of Medicine*, *343*(7), 450–456.

Borg, J., Holm, L., Cassidy, J. D., Peloso, P. M., Carroll, L. J., von Holst, H., & Ericson, K. (2004). Diagnostic procedures in mild traumatic brain injury: Results of the WHO Collaborating Centre Task Force on Mild Traumatic Brain Injury. *Journal of Rehabilitation Medicine*, *43*(Suppl), 61–75.

Borgaro, S. R., Prigatano, G. P., Kwasnica, C., & Rexer, J. L. (2003). Cognitive and affective sequelae in complicated and uncomplicated mild traumatic brain injury. *Brain Injury*, *17*(3), 189–198.

Bouix, S., Pasternak, O., Rathi, Y., Pelavin, P. E., Zafonte, R., & Shenton, M. E. (2013). Increased gray matter diffusion anisotropy in patients with persistent post-concussive symptoms following mild traumatic brain injury. *PLoS One*, *8*(6), e66205. doi: 10.1371/journal.pone.0066205

Boyle, P. A., Wilson, R. S., Yu, L., Barr, A. M., Honer, W. G., Schneider, J. A., & Bennett, D. A. (2013). Much of late life cognitive decline is not due to common neurodegenerative pathologies. *Annals of Neurology*, *74*(3), 478–489. doi: 10.1002/ana.23964

Breedlove, E. L., Robinson, M., Talavage, T. M., Morigaki, K. E., Yoruk, U., O'Keefe, K., . . . Nauman, E. A. (2012). Biomechanical correlates of symptomatic and asymptomatic neurophysiological impairment in high school football. *Journal of Biomechanics*, *45*(7), 1265–1272.

Broglio, S. P., Schnebel, B., Sosnoff, J. J., Shin, S., Fend, X., He, X., & Zimmerman, J. (2010). Biomechanical properties of concussions in high school football. *Medicine and Science in Sports and Exercise*, *42*(11), 2064–2071. doi: 10.1249/MSS.0b013e3181dd9156

Bryant, R. A., & Harvey, A. G. (1999). The influence of traumatic brain injury on acute stress disorder and post-traumatic stress disorder following motor vehicle accidents. *Brain Injury*, *13*(1), 15–22.

Bryant, R. A., Moulds, M., Guthrie, R., & Nixon, R. D. (2003). Treating acute stress disorder following mild traumatic brain injury. *American Journal of Psychiatry*, *160*(3), 585–587.

Busch, C. R., & Alpern, H. P. (1998). Depression after mild traumatic brain injury: A review of current research. *Neuropsychology Review*, *8*(2), 95–108.

Carroll, L. J., Cassidy, J. D., Holm, L., Kraus, J., & Coronado, V. G. (2004). Methodological issues and research recommendations for mild traumatic brain injury: The WHO Collaborating Centre Task Force on Mild Traumatic Brain Injury. *Journal of Rehabilitation Medicine*, *43*(Suppl), 113–125.

Carroll, L. J., Cassidy, J. D., Peloso, P. M., Borg, J., von Holst, H., Holm, L., . . . Pepin, M. (2004). Prognosis for mild traumatic brain injury: Results of the WHO Collaborating Centre Task Force on Mild Traumatic Brain Injury. *Journal of Rehabilitation Medicine*, *43*(Suppl), 84–105.

Cassidy, J. D., Carroll, L., Cote, P., Holm, L., & Nygren, A. (2004). Mild traumatic brain injury after traffic collisions: A population-based inception cohort study. *Journal of Rehabilitation Medicine, Suppl 43*, 28–60.

Centers for Disease Control. (2011). Take concussions out of play: Learn to prevent, recognize, and respond to concussions. Retrieved April 23, 2013, from www.cdc.gov/Features/ProtectYoungAthletes/

Chamelian, L., Reis, M., & Feinstein, A. (2004). Six-month recovery from mild to moderate Traumatic Brain Injury: The role of APOE-epsilon4 allele. *Brain*, *127*(Pt 12), 2621–2628.

Chin, L. M., Keyser, R. E., Dsurney, J., & Chan, L. (2015). Improved cognitive performance following aerobic exercise training in people with traumatic brain injury. *Archives of Physical Medicine and Rehabilitation*, *96*(4), 754–759. doi: 10.1016/j.apmr.2014.11.009

Chrisman, S. P., Rivara, F. P., Schiff, M. A., Zhou, C., & Comstock, R. D. (2013). Risk factors for concussive symptoms 1 week or longer in high school athletes. *Brain Injury*, *27*(1), 1–9.

Cicerone, K.D. (2002). Remediation of "working attention" in mild traumatic brain injury. *Brain Injury*, *16*(3), 185–195.

Clinchot, D. M., Bogner, J., Mysiw, W. J., Fugate, L., & Corrigan, J. (1998). Defining sleep disturbance after brain injury. *American Journal of Physical Medicine and Rehabilitation*, *77*(4), 291–295.

Collins, M. W., Lovell, M. R., & McKeag, D. B. (1999). Current issues in managing sports-related concussion. *JAMA*, *282*(24), 2283–2285.

Cooper, D. B., Bowles, A. O., Kennedy, J. E., Curtiss, G., French, L. M., Tate, D. F., & Vanderploeg, R. D. (2017). Cognitive rehabilitation for military service members with mild traumatic brain injury: A randomized clinical trial. *Journal of Head Trauma Rehabilitation*, *32*(3), E1–E15. doi: 10.1097/HTR.0000000000000254

Corrigan, J. D. (1995). Substance abuse as a mediating factor in outcome from traumatic brain injury. *Archives of Physical Medicine and Rehabilitation*, *76*(4), 302–309. doi: S0003-9993(95) 80654-7

Covassin, T., Elbin, R. J., Harris, W., Parker, T., & Kontos, A. (2012). The role of age and sex in symptoms, neurocognitive performance, and postural stability in athletes after concussion. *American Journal of Sports Medicine*, *40*(6), 1303–1312.

Crawford, F. C., Vanderploeg, R. D., Freeman, M. J., Singh, S., Waisman, M., Michael, L., . . . Mullan, M. J. (2002). APOE genotype influences acquisition and recall following traumatic brain injury. *Neurology*, *58*, 1115–1118.

Dagher, J. H., Richard-Denis, A., Lamoureux, J., de Guise, E., & Feyz, M. (2013). Acute global outcome in patients with mild uncomplicated and complicated traumatic brain injury. *Brain Injury*, *27*(2), 189–199. doi: 10.3109/02699052.2012.729288

De Beaumont, L., Theoret, H., Mongeon, D., Messier, J., Leclerc, S., Tremblay, S., . . . Lassonde, M. (2009). Brain function decline in healthy retired athletes who sustained their last sports concussion in early adulthood. *Brain*, *132*(Pt 3), 695–708.

de Guise, E., Lepage, J. F., Tinawi, S., LeBlanc, J., Dagher, J., Lamoureux, J., & Feyz, M. (2010). Comprehensive clinical picture of patients with complicated vs uncomplicated mild traumatic brain injury. *Clinical Neuropsychologist*, *24*(7), 1113–1130.

De Kruijk, J. R., Leffers, P., Menheere, P. P., Meerhoff, S., Rutten, J., & Twijnstra, A. (2002). Prediction of post-traumatic complaints after mild traumatic brain injury: Early symptoms and biochemical markers. *Journal of Neurology, Neurosurgery and Psychiatry*, *73*(6), 727–732.

Deb, S., Lyons, I., & Koutzoukis, C. (1999). Neurobehavioural symptoms one year after a head injury. *British Journal of Psychiatry*, *174*, 360–365.

Dematteo, C. A., Hanna, S. E., Mahoney, W. J., Hollenberg, R. D., Scott, L. A., Law, M. C., . . . Xu, L. (2010). "My child doesn't have a brain injury, he only has a concussion." *Pediatrics*, *125*(2), 327–334.

Department of Veterans Affairs and Department of Defense. (April, 2009). VA/DOD clinical practice guideline for management of concussion/mild traumatic brain injury Retrieved November, 2012, from www.healthquality.va.gov/mtbi/concussion_mtbi_full_1_0.pdf

Dikmen, S., Machamer, J., Fann, J. R., & Temkin, N. R. (2010). Rates of symptom reporting following traumatic brain injury. *Journal of the International Neuropsychological Society*, *16*(3), 401–411.

Dikmen, S. S., Machamer, J. E., Winn, R., & Temkin, N. (1995). Neuropsychological outcome at 1-year post head injury. *Neuropsychology*, *9*(1), 80–90.

Dikmen, S., McLean, A., & Temkin, N. (1986). Neuropsychological and psychosocial consequences of minor head injury. *Journal of Neurology, Neurosurgery & Psychiatry*, *49*(11), 1227–1232.

Donnell, A. J., Kim, M. S., Silva, M. A., & Vanderploeg, R. D. (2012). Incidence of postconcussion symptoms in psychiatric diagnostic groups, mild traumatic brain injury, and comorbid conditions. *Clinical Neuropsychologist*, *26*(7), 1092–1101.

Dougan, B. K., Horswill, M. S., & Geffen, G. M. (2013). Athletes' Age, Sex, and Years of Education Moderate the Acute Neuropsychological Impact of Sports-Related Concussion: A Meta-analysis. *Journal of the International Neuropsychological Society*, 1–17.

Drag, L. L., Spencer, R. J., Walker, S. J., Pangilinan, P. H., & Bieliauskas, L. A. (2012). The contributions of self-reported injury characteristics and psychiatric symptoms to cognitive functioning in OEF/OIF veterans with mild traumatic brain injury. *Journal of the International Neuropsychological Society*, *18*(3), 576–584.

Elbin, R. J., Covassin, T., Hakun, J., Kontos, A. P., Berger, K., Pfeiffer, K., & Ravizza, S. (2012). Do brain activation changes persist in athletes with a history of multiple concussions who are asymptomatic? *Brain Injury*, *26*(10), 1217–1225.

Elgmark Andersson, E., Emanuelson, I., Bjorklund, R., & Stalhammar, D. A. (2007). Mild traumatic brain injuries: The impact of early intervention on late sequelae. A randomized controlled trial. *Acta Neurochir (Wien)*, *149*(2), 151–159; discussion 160.

Erlanger, D., Kaushik, T., Cantu, R., Barth, J. T., Broshek, D. K., Freeman, J. R., & Webbe, F. M. (2003). Symptom-based assessment of the severity of a concussion. *Journal of Neurosurgery, 98*(3), 477–484.

Ettenhofer, M. L., & Barry, D. M. (2012). A comparison of long-term postconcussive symptoms between university students with and without a history of mild traumatic brain injury or orthopedic injury. *Journal of the International Neuropsychological Society, 18*(3), 451–460.

Ettenhofer, M. L., Reinhardt, L. E., & Barry, D. M. (2013). Predictors of neurobehavioral symptoms in a university population: A multivariate approach using a postconcussive symptom questionnaire. *Journal of the International Neuropsychological Society, 19*(9), 977–985.

Fann, J. R., Burington, B., Leonetti, A., Jaffe, K., Katon, W. J., & Thompson, R. S. (2004). Psychiatric illness following traumatic brain injury in an adult health maintenance organization population. *Archives of General Psychiatry, 61*(1), 53–61.

Farhad, K., Khan, H. M., Ji, A. B., Yacoub, H. A., Qureshi, A. I., & Souayah, N. (2013). Trends in outcomes and hospitalization costs for traumatic brain injury in adult patients in the United States. *Journal of Neurotrauma, 30*(2), 84–90. doi: 10.1089/neu.2011.2283

Faul, M, Xu, L., Wald, M. M., & Coronado, V. G. (2010). Traumatic brain injury in the United States: Emergency department visits, hospitalizations, and deaths. In *National Center for Injury Prevention and Control Centers for Disease Control and Prevention* (pp. 1–74). Atlanta, GA: Centers for Disease Control.

Fear, N. T., Jones, E., Groom, M., Greenberg, N., Hull, L., Hodgetts, T. J., & Wessely, S. (2009). Symptoms of post-concussional syndrome are non-specifically related to mild traumatic brain injury in UK Armed Forces personnel on return from deployment in Iraq: An analysis of self-reported data. [Psychol Med]. *Psychological Medicine, 39*(8), 1379–1387.

Ferguson, R. J., & Mittenberg, W. (1996). Cognitive-behavioral treatment of postconcussion syndrome: A therapist's manual. In V. B. Van Hasselt & M. Hersen (Eds.), *Sourcebook of Psychological Treatment Manuals for Adult Disorders* (pp. 615–655). New York: Plenum Press.

Fichtenberg, N. L., Millis, S. R., Mann, N. R., Zafonte, R. D., & Millard, A. E. (2000). Factors associated with insomnia among post-acute traumatic brain injury survivors. *Brain Injury, 14*(7), 659–667.

Fortier-Brochu, E., Beaulieu-Bonneau, S., Ivers, H., & Morin, C. M. (2012). Insomnia and daytime cognitive performance: A meta-analysis. *Sleep Medicine Review, 16*(1), 83–94.

Frencham, K. A., Fox, A. M., & Maybery, M. T. (2005). Neuropsychological studies of mild traumatic brain injury: A meta-analytic review of research since 1995. *Journal of Clinical and Experimental Neuropsychology, 27*(3), 334–351.

Friedman, G., Froom, P., Sazbon, L., Grinblatt, I., Shochina, M., Tsenter, J., . . . Groswasser, Z. (1999). Apolipoprotein E-epsilon4 genotype predicts a poor outcome in survivors of traumatic brain injury. *Neurology, 52*(2), 244–248.

Gaetz, M. (2004). The neurophysiology of brain injury. *Clinical Neurophysiology, 115*(1), 4–18.

Gaetz, M., Goodman, D., & Weinberg, H. (2000). Electrophysiological evidence for the cumulative effects of concussion. *Brain Injury, 14*(12), 1077–1088.

Gale, S. D., Baxter, L., Roundy, N., & Johnson, S. C. (2005). Traumatic brain injury and grey matter concentration: A preliminary voxel based morphometry study. *Journal of Neurology, Neurosurgery & Psychiatry, 76*(7), 984–988. doi: 10.1136/jnnp.2004.036210

Gasquoine, P. G. (2000). Postconcussional symptoms in chronic back pain. *Applied Neuropsycholog, 7*(2), 83–89. doi: 10.1207/S15324826AN0702_3

Gennarelli, T. A., & Graham, D. I. (1998). Neuropathology of the head injuries. *Seminars in Clinical Neuropsychiatry, 3*(3), 160–175.

Ghaffar, O., McCullagh, S., Ouchterlony, D., & Feinstein, A. (2006). Randomized treatment trial in mild traumatic brain injury. *Journal of Psychosomatic Research, 61*(2), 153–160.

Giza, C. C., & Hovda, D. A. (2001). The neurometabolic cascade of concussion. *Journal of Athletic Training, 36*(3), 228–235.

Giza, C. C., Kutcher, J. S., Ashwal, S., Barth, J., Getchius, T. S., Gioia, G. A., . . . Zafonte, R. (2013). Summary of evidence-based guideline update: Evaluation and management of concussion in sports: Report of the Guideline Development Subcommittee of the American Academy of Neurology. *Neurology*.

Goldstein, F. C., & Levin, H. S. (2001). Cognitive outcome after mild and moderate traumatic brain injury in older adults. *Journal of Clinical & Experimental Neuropsychology, 23*(6), 739–753.

Gosselin, N., Chen, J. K., Bottari, C., Petrides, M., Jubault, T., Tinawi, S., . . . Ptito, A. (2012). The influence of pain on cerebral functioning after mild traumatic brain injury. *Journal of Neurotrauma, 29*(17), 2625–2634. doi: 10.1089/neu.2012.2312

Govindaraju, V., Gauger, G. E., Manley, G. T., Ebel, A., Meeker, M., & Maudsley, A. A. (2004). Volumetric proton spectroscopic imaging of mild traumatic brain injury. *AJNR American Journal of Neuroradiology, 25*(5), 730–737.

Greer, J. E., Povlishock, J. T., & Jacobs, K. M. (2012). Electrophysiological abnormalities in both axotomized and nonaxotomized pyramidal neurons following mild traumatic brain injury. *Journal of Neuroscience, 32*(19), 6682–6687.

Greve, K. W., Ord, J. S., Bianchini, K. J., & Curtis, K. L. (2009). Prevalence of malingering in patients with chronic pain referred for psychologic evaluation in a medico-legal context. *Archives of Physical Medicine & Rehabilitation, 90*(7), 1117–1126.

Gronwall, D. (1986). Rehabilitation programs for patients with mild head injury: Components, problems, and evaluation. *Journal of Head Trauma Rehabilitation, 1*, 53–63.

Grossman, E. J., Ge, Y., Jensen, J. H., Babb, J. S., Miles, L., Reaume, J., . . . Inglese, M. (2012). Thalamus and cognitive impairment in mild traumatic brain injury: A diffusional kurtosis imaging study. *Journal of Neurotrauma, 29*(13), 2318–2327. doi: 10.1089/neu.2011.1763

Gunstad, J., & Suhr, J. A. (2001). "Expectation as etiology" versus "the good old days": Postconcussion syndrome symptom reporting in athletes, headache sufferers, and depressed individuals. *Journal of the International Neuropsychological Society, 7*(3), 323–333.

Gunstad, J., & Suhr, J. A. (2004). Cognitive factors in Postconcussion Syndrome symptom report. *Archives of Clinical Neuropsychology, 19*(3), 391–405.

Guskiewicz, K. M., Marshall, S. W., Bailes, J., McCrea, M., Cantu, R. C., Randolph, C., & Jordan, B. D. (2005). Association between recurrent concussion and late-life cognitive impairment in retired professional football players. *Neurosurgery, 57*(4), 719–726; discussion 719–726.

Guskiewicz, K. M., McCrea, M., Marshall, S. W., Cantu, R. C., Randolph, C., Barr, W., . . . Kelly, J. P. (2003). Cumulative effects associated with recurrent concussion in collegiate football players: The NCAA Concussion Study. *Journal of the American Medical Association*, *290*(19), 2549–2555.

Guskiewicz, K. M., & Mihalik, J. P. (2011). Biomechanics of sport concussion: Quest for the elusive injury threshold. *Exercise and sport sciences reviews*, *39*(1), 4–11. doi: 10.1097/JES.0b013e318201f53e

Gysland, S. M., Mihalik, J. P., Register-Mihalik, J. K., Trulock, S. C., Shields, E. W., & Guskiewicz, K. M. (2012). The relationship between subconcussive impacts and concussion history on clinical measures of neurologic function in collegiate football players. *Annals of Biomedical Engineering*, *40*(1), 14–22. doi: 10.1007/s10439-011-0421-3

Haacke, E. M., Raza, W., Bo, W., & Kou, Z. (Eds.). (2013). *The Presence of Venous Damage and Microbleeds in Traumatic Brain Injury and the Potential Future Role of Angiographic and Perfusion Magnetic Resonance Imaging*. New York: Springer.

Haacke, E. M., Tang, J., Neelavalli, J., & Cheng, Y. C. (2010). Susceptibility mapping as a means to visualize veins and quantify oxygen saturation. *Journal of Magnetic Resonance Imaging: JMRI*, *32*(3), 663–676. doi: 10.1002/jmri.22276

Hall, R. C., & Chapman, M. J. (2005). Definition, diagnosis, and forensic implications of postconcussional syndrome. *Psychosomatics*, *46*(3), 195–202.

Hanlon, R. E., Demery, J. A., Martinovich, Z., & Kelly, J. P. (1999). Effects of acute injury characteristics on neurophysical status and vocational outcome following mild traumatic brain injury. *Brain Injury*, *13*(11), 873–887.

Hanna-Pladdy, B., Berry, Z. M., Bennett, T., Phillips, H. L., & Gouvier, W. D. (2001). Stress as a diagnostic challenge for postconcussive symptoms: Sequelae of mild traumatic brain injury or physiological stress response. *Clinical Neuropsychologist*, *15*(3), 289–304.

Hart, R. P., Martelli, M. F., & Zasler, N. D. (2000). Chronic pain and neuropsychological functioning. *Neuropsychology Review*, *10*(3), 131–149.

Hartikainen, K. M., Waljas, M., Isoviita, T., Dastidar, P., Liimatainen, S., Solbakk, A. K., . . . Ohman, J. (2010). Persistent symptoms in mild to moderate traumatic brain injury associated with executive dysfunction. *Journal of Clinical and Experimental Neuropsychology*, *32*(7), 767–774.

Hartlage, L. C., Durant-Wilson, D., & Patch, P. C. (2001). Persistent neurobehavioral problems following mild traumatic brain injury. *Archives of Clinical Neuropsychology*, *16*(6), 561–570.

Harvey, A. G., & Bryant, R. A. (1998). Predictors of acute stress following mild traumatic brain injury. *Brain Injury*, *12*(2), 147–154.

Haydel, M. J., Preston, C. A., Mills, T. J., Luber, S., Blaudeau, E., & DeBlieux, P. M. (2000). Indications for computed tomography in patients with minor head injury. *New England Journal of Medicine*, *343*(2), 100–105.

Hayes, R. L., & Dixon, C. E. (1994). Neurochemical changes in mild head injury. *Seminars in Neurology*, *14*(1), 25–31.

Hazrati, L. N., Tartaglia, M. C., Diamandis, P., Davis, K. D., Green, R. E., Wennberg, R., . . . Tator, C. H. (2013). Absence of chronic traumatic encephalopathy in retired football players with multiple concussions and neurological symptomatology. *Frontiers in Human Neuroscience*, *7*, 222.

Heaton, R. K., Smith, H. H., Jr., Lehman, R. A., & Vogt, A. T. (1978). Prospects for faking believable deficits on neuropsychological testing. *Journal of Consulting and Clinical Psychology*, *46*(5), 892–900.

Heilbronner, R. L., Sweet, J. J., Morgan, J. E., Larrabee, G. J., & Millis, S. R. (2009). American Academy of Clinical Neuropsychology Consensus Conference Statement on the neuropsychological assessment of effort, response bias, and malingering. *Clinical Neuropsychologist*, *23*(7), 1093–1129.

Hessen, E., Nestvold, K., & Anderson, V. (2007). Neuropsychological function 23 years after mild traumatic brain injury: A comparison of outcome after paediatric and adult head injuries. *Brain Injury*, *21*(9), 963–979.

Himanen, L., Portin, R., Isoniemi, H., Helenius, H., Kurki, T., & Tenovuo, O. (2006). Longitudinal cognitive changes in traumatic brain injury: A 30-year follow-up study. *Neurology*, *66*(2), 187–192.

Hinkle, J. L., Alves, W. M., Rimell, R. W., & Jane, J. A. (1986). Restoring social competence in minor head-injury patients. *Journal of Neuroscience Nursing*, *18*(5), 268–271.

Hofman, P. A., Stapert, S. Z., van Kroonenburgh, M. J., Jolles, J., de Kruijk, J., & Wilmink, J. T. (2001). MR imaging, single-photon emission CT, and neurocognitive performance after mild traumatic brain injury: *AJNR American Journal of Neuroradiology*, *22*(3), 441–449.

Hoge, C. W., Goldberg, H. M., & Castro, C. A. (2009). Care of war veterans with mild traumatic brain injury-flawed perspectives. *New England Journal of Medicine*, *360*(16), 1588–1591.

Hoge, C. W., McGurk, D., Thomas, J. L., Cox, A. L., Engel, C. C., & Castro, C. A. (2008). Mild traumatic brain injury in U.S. Soldiers returning from Iraq. *New England Journal of Medicine*, *358*(5), 453–463.

Hollis, S. J., Stevenson, M. R., McIntosh, A. S., Shores, E. A., Collins, M. W., & Taylor, C. B. (2009). Incidence, risk, and protective factors of mild traumatic brain injury in a cohort of Australian nonprofessional male rugby players. *American Journal of Sports Medicine*, *37*(12), 2328–2333.

Hou, L., Han, X., Sheng, P., Tong, W., Li, Z., Xu, D., . . . Dong, Y. (2013). Risk Factors Associated with Sleep Disturbance following Traumatic Brain Injury: Clinical Findings and Questionnaire Based Study. *Public Library of Science One*, *8*(10), e76087.

Hou, R., Moss-Morris, R., Peveler, R., Mogg, K., Bradley, B. P., & Belli, A. (2012). When a minor head injury results in enduring symptoms: A prospective investigation of risk factors for postconcussional syndrome after mild traumatic brain injury. *Journal of Neurology, Neurosurgery and Psychiatry*, *83*(2), 217–223.

Hsiang, J. N., Yeung, T., Yu, A. L., & Poon, W. S. (1997). High-risk mild head injury. *Journal of Neurosurgery*, *87*(2), 234–238. doi: 10.3171/jns.1997.87.2.0234

Huckans, M., Pavawalla, S., Demadura, T., Kolessar, M., Seelye, A., Roost, N., . . . Storzbach, D. (2010). A pilot study examining effects of group-based Cognitive Strategy Training treatment on self-reported cognitive problems, psychiatric symptoms, functioning, and compensatory strategy use in OIF/OEF combat veterans with persistent mild cognitive disorder and history of traumatic brain injury. *Journal of Rehabilitation Research & Development*, *47*(1), 43–60.

Hughes, D. G., Jackson, A., Mason, D. L., Berry, E., Hollis, S., & Yates, D. W. (2004). Abnormalities on magnetic resonance imaging seen acutely following mild traumatic brain injury: Correlation with neuropsychological tests and delayed recovery. *Neuroradiology*, *46*(7), 550–558. doi: 10.1007/s00234-004-1227-x

Hutchison, M., Comper, P., Mainwaring, L., & Richards, D. (2011). The influence of musculoskeletal injury on cognition: Implications for concussion research. *American Journal of Sports Medicine*, *39*(11), 2331–2337.

Iverson, G. L. (2005). Outcome from mild traumatic brain injury. *Current Opinions in Psychiatry*, *18*(3), 301–317.

Iverson, G. L. (2006). Complicated vs. uncomplicated mild traumatic brain injury: Acute neuropsychological outcome. *Brain Injury*, *20*(13–14), 1335–1344.

Iverson, G. L. (2007). Predicting slow recovery from sport-related concussion: The new simple-complex distinction. *Clinical Journal of Sport Medicine*, *17*(1), 31–37.

Iverson, G. L. (2014). Chronic traumatic encephalopathy and risk of suicide in former athletes. *British Journal of Sports Medicine*, *48*(2), 162–165.

Iverson, G. L., Brooks, B. L., Ashton, V. L., & Lange, R. T. (2010). Interview versus questionnaire symptom reporting in people with the postconcussion syndrome. *Journal of Head Trauma Rehabilitation*, *25*(1), 23–30.

Iverson, G. L., Brooks, B. L., Collins, M. W., & Lovell, M. R. (2006). Tracking neuropsychological recovery following concussion in sport. *Brain Injury*, *20*(3), 245–252.

Iverson, G. L., Brooks, B. L., Lovell, M. R., & Collins, M. W. (2006). No cumulative effects for one or two previous concussions. *British Journal of Sports Medicine*, *40*(1), 72–75.

Iverson, G. L., Franzen, M. D., & Lovell, M. R. (1999). Normative comparisons for the controlled oral word association test following acute traumatic brain injury. *Clinical Neuropsychologist*, *13*(4), 437–441.

Iverson, G. L., Gaetz, M., Lovell, M. R., & Collins, M. W. (2004). Cumulative effects of concussion in amateur athletes. *Brain Injury*, *18*(4), 1.

Iverson, G. L., Lange, R. T., Waljas, M., Liimatainen, S., Dastidar, P., Hartikainen, K. M., . . . Ohman, J. (2012). Outcome from complicated versus uncomplicated mild traumatic brain injury. *Rehabilitation Research and Practice*, *415740*. doi: 10.1155/2012/415740

Jacobs, B., Beems, T., Stulemeijer, M., van Vugt, A. B., van der Vliet, T. M., Borm, G. F., & Vos, P. E. (2010). Outcome prediction in mild traumatic brain injury: Age and clinical variables are stronger predictors than CT abnormalities. *Journal of Neurotrauma*, *27*(4), 655–668.

Jagoda, A. S., Bazarian, J. J., Bruns, J. J., Jr., Cantrill, S. V., Gean, A. D., Howard, P. K., . . . Whitson, R. R. (2008). Clinical policy: Neuroimaging and decisionmaking in adult mild traumatic brain injury in the acute setting. *Annals of Emergency Medicine*, *52*(6), 714–748.

Jellinger, K. A. (2004). Head injury and dementia. *Current Opinion in Neurology*, *17*(6), 719–723. doi: 00019052-200412000-00012 [pii]

Jeter, C. B., Hergenroeder, G. W., Hylin, M. J., Redell, J. B., Moore, A. N., & Dash, P. K. (2013). Biomarkers for the diagnosis and prognosis of mild traumatic brain injury/concussion. *Journal of Neurotrauma*, *30*(8), 657–670. doi: 10.1089/neu.2012.2439

Jorge, R. E., Robinson, R. G., Moser, D., Tateno, A., Crespo-Facorro, B., & Arndt, S. (2004). Major depression following traumatic brain injury. *Archives of General Psychiatry*, *61*(1), 42–50.

Karantzoulis, S., & Randolph, C. (2013). Modern chronic traumatic encephalopathy in retired athletes: What is the evidence? *Neuropsychology Review*, *23*(4), 350–360.

Kashluba, S., Hanks, R. A., Casey, J. E., & Millis, S. R. (2008). Neuropsychologic and functional outcome after complicated mild traumatic brain injury. *Archives of Physical Medicine & Rehabilitation*, *89*(5), 904–911.

Kaufman, Y., Tzischinsky, O., Epstein, R., Etzioni, A., Lavie, P., & Pillar, G. (2001). Long-term sleep disturbances in adolescents after minor head injury. *Pediatric Neurology*, *24*(2), 129–134. doi: S0887-8994(00)00254-X [pii]

Kelley, B. J., Lifshitz, J., & Povlishock, J. T. (2007). Neuroinflammatory responses after experimental diffuse traumatic brain injury. *Journal of Neuropathology and Experimental Neurology*, *66*(11), 989–1001.

Kennedy, C. H., Porter Evans, J., Chee, S., Moore, J. L., Barth, J. T., & Stuessi, K. A. (2012). Return to combat duty after concussive blast injury. *Archives of Clinical Neuropsychology*, *27*(8), 817–827.

Khoury, S., Chouchou, F., Amzica, F., Giguere, J. F., Denis, R., Rouleau, G. A., & Lavigne, G. J. (2013). Rapid EEG activity during sleep dominates in mild traumatic brain injury patients with acute pain. *Journal of Neurotrauma*, *30*(8), 633–641. doi: 10.1089/neu.2012.2519

Kirkness, C. J., Burr, R. L., Mitchell, P. H., & Newell, D. W. (2004). Is there a sex difference in the course following traumatic brain injury? *Biological Research for Nursing*, *5*(4), 299–310.

Kjeldgaard, D., Forchhammer, H. B., Teasdale, T. W., & Jensen, R. H. (2014). Cognitive behavioural treatment for the chronic post-traumatic headache patient: A randomized controlled trial. *The Journal of Headache and Pain*, *15*, 81. doi: 10.1186/1129-2377-15-81

Koerte, I. K., Lin, A. P., Willems, A., Muehlmann, M., Hufschmidt, J., Coleman, M. J., . . . Shenton, M. E. (2015). A review of neuroimaging findings in repetitive brain trauma. *Brain Pathology*, *25*(3), 318–349. doi: 10.1111/bpa.12249

Kraus, M. F., Susmaras, T., Caughlin, B. P., Walker, C. J., Sweeney, J. A., & Little, D. M. (2007). White matter integrity and cognition in chronic traumatic brain injury: A diffusion tensor imaging study. *Brain*, *130*(Pt 10), 2508–2519. doi: 10.1093/brain/awm216

Kurca, E., Sivak, S., & Kucera, P. (2006). Impaired cognitive functions in mild traumatic brain injury patients with normal and pathologic magnetic resonance imaging. *Neuroradiology*, *48*(9), 661–669. doi: 10.1007/s00234-006-0109-9

Landre, N., Poppe, C. J., Davis, N., Schmaus, B., & Hobbs, S. E. (2006). Cognitive functioning and postconcussive symptoms in trauma patients with and without mild TBI. *Archives of Clinical Neuropsychology*, *21*(4), 255–273.

Lange, R. T., Brickell, T. A., French, L. M., Merritt, V. C., Bhagwat, A., Pancholi, S., & Iverson, G. L. (2012). Neuropsychological outcome from uncomplicated mild, complicated mild, and moderate traumatic brain injury in US military personnel. *Archives of Clinical Neuropsychology*, *27*(5), 480–494.

Lange, R. T., Iverson, G. L., Brubacher, J. R., Madler, B., & Heran, M. K. (2012). Diffusion tensor imaging findings are not strongly associated with postconcussional disorder 2 months following mild traumatic brain injury. *Journal of Head Trauma Rehabilitation*, *27*(3), 188–198. doi: 10.1097/HTR.0b013e318217f0ad

Lange, R. T., Iverson, G. L., & Franzen, M. D. (2009). Neuropsychological functioning following complicated vs. uncomplicated mild traumatic brain injury. *Brain Injury*, *23*(2), 83–91.

Lange, R. T., Iverson, G. L., Zakrzewski, M. J., Ethel-King, P. E., & Franzen, M. D. (2005). Interpreting the trail making test following traumatic brain injury: Comparison of traditional time scores and derived indices. *Journal of Clinical and Experimental Neuropsychology*, *27*(7), 897–906.

Langlois, J. A., Rutland-Brown, W., & Wald, M. M. (2006). The epidemiology and impact of traumatic brain injury: A brief overview. *Journal of Head Trauma Rehabilitation*, *21*(5), 375–378.

Lannsjo, M., Backheden, M., Johansson, U., Af Geijerstam, J. L., & Borg, J. (2013). Does head CT scan pathology predict outcome after mild traumatic brain injury? *European Journal of Neurology*, *20*(1), 124–129.

Larrabee, G. J. (2003). Detection of malingering using atypical performance patterns on standard neuropsychological tests. *Clinical Neuropsychologist*, *17*(3), 410–425. doi: 10.1076/clin.17.3.410.18089

Larrabee, G. J. (2012). Performance validity and symptom validity in neuropsychological assessment. *Journal of the International Neuropsychological Society*, *18*(4), 625–630.

Larson, E. B., Kondiles, B. R., Starr, C. R., & Zollman, F. S. (2012). Postconcussive Complaints, Cognition, Symptom Attribution and Effort among Veterans. *Journal of the International Neuropsychological Society*, 1–8.

Lau, B. C., Kontos, A. P., Collins, M. W., Mucha, A., & Lovell, M. R. (2011). Which on-field signs/symptoms predict protracted recovery from sport-related concussion among high school football players? *American Journal of Sports Medicine*, *39*(11), 2311–2318.

Leddy, J. J., Cox, J. L., Baker, J. G., Wack, D. S., Pendergast, D. R., Zivadinov, R., & Willer, B. (2013). Exercise treatment for postconcussion syndrome: a pilot study of changes in functional magnetic resonance imaging activation, physiology, and symptoms. *The Journal of Head Trauma Rehabilitation*, *28*(4), 241–249.

Lee, Y. K., Hou, S. W., Lee, C. C., Hsu, C. Y., Huang, Y. S., & Su, Y. C. (2013). Increased risk of dementia in patients with mild traumatic brain injury: A nationwide cohort study. *PLoS One*, *8*(5), e62422.

Lee, H., Wintermark, M., Gean, A. D., Ghajar, J., Manley, G. T., & Mukherjee, P. (2008). Focal lesions in acute mild traumatic brain injury and neurocognitive outcome: CT versus 3T MRI. *Journal of Neurotrauma*, *25*(9), 1049–1056. doi: 10.1089/neu.2008.0566

Lehman, E. J., Hein, M. J., Baron, S. L., & Gersic, C. M. (2012). Neurodegenerative causes of death among retired National Football League players. *Neurology*, *79*(19), 1970–1974.

Levin, H. S., Brown, S. A., Song, J. X., McCauley, S. R., Boake, C., Contant, C. F., . . . Kotrla, K. J. (2001). Depression and posttraumatic stress disorder at three months after mild to moderate traumatic brain injury. *Journal of Clinical and Experimental Neuropsychology*, *23*(6), 754–769.

Levin, H. S., Mattis, S., Ruff, R. M., Eisenberg, H. M., Marshall, L. F., Tabaddor, K., . . . Frankowski, R. F. (1987). Neurobehavioral outcome following minor head injury: A three-center study. *Journal of Neurosurgery*, *66*(2), 234–243.

Levin, H. S., McCauley, S. R., Josic, C. P., Boake, C., Brown, S. A., Goodman, H. S., . . . Brundage, S. I. (2005). Predicting depression following mild traumatic brain injury. *Archives of General Psychiatry*, *62*(5), 523–528.

Levin, H. S., Zhang, L., Dennis, M., Ewing-Cobbs, L., Schachar, R., Max, J., . . . Hunter, J. V. (2004). Psychosocial outcome of TBI in children with unilateral frontal lesions. *Journal of the International Neuropsychological Society*, *10*(3), 305–316. doi: 10.1017/S1355617704102129

Levine, B., Kovacevic, N., Nica, E. I., Cheung, G., Gao, F., Schwartz, M. L., & Black, S. E. (2008). The Toronto traumatic brain injury study: Injury severity and quantified MRI. *Neurology*, *70*(10), 771–778.

Liberman, J. N., Stewart, W. F., Wesnes, K., & Troncoso, J. (2002). Apolipoprotein E epsilon 4 and short-term recovery from predominantly mild brain injury. *Neurology*, *58*(7), 1038–1044.

Lifshitz, J., Witgen, B. M., & Grady, M. S. (2007). Acute cognitive impairment after lateral fluid percussion brain injury recovers by 1 month: Evaluation by conditioned fear response. *Behavioral Brain Research*, *177*(2), 347–357.

Lin, A. P., Liao, H. J., Merugumala, S. K., Prabhu, S. P., Meehan, W. P., 3rd, & Ross, B. D. (2012). Metabolic imaging of mild traumatic brain injury. *Brain Imaging and Behavior*, *6*(2), 208–223. doi: 10.1007/s11682-012-9181-4

Lincoln, A. E., Caswell, S. V., Almquist, J. L., Dunn, R. E., Norris, J. B., & Hinton, R. Y. (2011). Trends in concussion incidence in high school sports: A prospective 11-year study. *American Journal of Sports Medicine*, *39*(5), 958–963.

Lipton, M. L., Gellella, E., Lo, C., Gold, T., Ardekani, B. A., Shifteh, K., . . . Branch, C. A. (2008). Multifocal white matter ultrastructural abnormalities in mild traumatic brain injury with cognitive disability: A voxel-wise analysis of diffusion tensor imaging. *Journal of Neurotrauma*, *25*(11), 1335–1342.

Losoi, H., Silverberg, N. D., Waljas, M., Turunen, S., Rosti-Otajarvi, E., Helminen, M., . . . Iverson, G. L. (2015). Recovery from Mild Traumatic Brain Injury in Previously Healthy Adults. *Journal of Neurotrauma*. doi: 10.1089/neu.2015.4070

Lovell, M. R., Iverson, G. L., Collins, M. W., McKeag, D., & Maroon, J. C. (1999). Does loss of consciousness predict neuropsychological decrements after concussion? *Clinical Journal of Sport Medicine*, *9*(4), 193–198.

Luis, C. A., Vanderploeg, R. D., & Curtiss, G. (2003). Predictors for a postconcussion symptom complex in community dwelling male veterans. *Journal of the International Neuropsychology Society*, *9*, 1001–1015.

Lye, T. C., & Shores, E. A. (2000). Traumatic brain injury as a risk factor for Alzheimer's disease: A review. *Neuropsychology Review*, *10*(2), 115–129.

Macciocchi, S. N., Barth, J. T., Littlefield, L., & Cantu, R. C. (2001). Multiple Concussions and Neuropsychological Functioning in Collegiate Football Players. *Journal of Athletic Training*, *36*(3), 303–306.

Mac Donald, C. L., Johnson, A. M., Cooper, D., Nelson, E. C., Werner, N. J., Shimony, J. S., . . . Brody, D. L. (2011). Detection of blast-related traumatic brain injury in U.S. military personnel. *New England Journal of Medicine*, *364*(22), 2091–2100. doi: 10.1056/NEJMoa1008069

MacKenzie, J. D., Siddiqi, F., Babb, J. S., Bagley, L. J., Mannon, L. J., Sinson, G. P., & Grossman, R. I. (2002). Brain atrophy in mild or moderate traumatic brain injury: A longitudinal quantitative analysis. *American Journal of Neuroradiology*, *23*(9), 1509–1515.

Mahmood, O., Rapport, L. J., Hanks, R. A., & Fichtenberg, N. L. (2004). Neuropsychological performance and sleep disturbance following traumatic brain injury. *Journal of Head Trauma Rehabilitation*, *19*(5), 378–390. doi: 00001199-200409000-00003 [pii]

Malec, J. F., Brown, A. W., Leibson, C. L., Flaada, J. T., Mandrekar, J. N., Diehl, N. N., & Perkins, P. K. (2007). The mayo classification system for traumatic brain injury severity. *Journal of Neurotrauma*, *24*(9), 1417–1424.

Matsushita, M., Hosoda, K., Naitoh, Y., Yamashita, H., & Kohmura, E. (2011). Utility of diffusion tensor imaging in the acute stage of mild to moderate traumatic brain injury for detecting white matter lesions and predicting long-term cognitive function in adults. *Journal of neurosurgery*, *115*(1), 130–139. doi: 10.3171/2011.2.JNS101547

Matthews, S. C., Strigo, I. A., Simmons, A. N., O'Connell, R. M., Reinhardt, L. E., & Moseley, S. A. (2011). A multimodal imaging study in U.S. veterans of Operations Iraqi and Enduring Freedom with and without major depression after blast-related concussion. *Neuroimage*, *54*(Suppl 1), S69–S75. doi: 10.1016/j.neuroimage.2010.04.269

Mayer, A. R., Ling, J., Mannell, M. V., Gasparovic, C., Phillips, J. P., Doezema, D., . . . Yeo, R. A. (2010). A prospective diffusion tensor imaging study in mild traumatic brain injury. *Neurology*, *74*(8), 643–650. doi: 10.1212/WNL.0b013e3181d0ccdd

McAllister, T. W. (2010). Genetic factors modulating outcome after neurotrauma. *Physical Medicine & Rehabilitation*, *2*(12 Suppl 2), S241–252.

McAllister, T. W., Flashman, L. A., Maerlender, A., Greenwald, R. M., Beckwith, J. G., Tosteson, T. D., . . . Turco, J. H. (2012). Cognitive effects of one season of head impacts in a cohort of collegiate contact sport athletes. *Neurology*, *78*(22), 1777–1784.

McCauley, S. R., Boake, C., Levin, H. S., Contant, C. F., & Song, J. X. (2001). Postconcussional disorder following mild to moderate traumatic brain injury: Anxiety, depression, and social support as risk factors and comorbidities. *Journal of Clinical & Experimental Neuropsychology*, *23*(6), 792–808. doi: 10.1076/jcen.23.6.792.1016

McCauley, S. R., Wilde, E. A., Miller, E. R., Frisby, M. L., Garza, H. M., Varghese, R., . . . McCarthy, J. J. (2013). Preinjury resilience and mood as predictors of early outcome following mild traumatic brain injury. *Journal of Neurotrauma*, *30*(8), 642–652. doi: 10.1089/neu.2012.2393

McCrea, M., & Guskiewicz, K. (2014). Evidence-based management of sport-related concussion. *Progress in Neurological Surgery*, *28*, 112–127. doi: 10.1159/000358769

McCrea, M., Guskiewicz, K. M., Marshall, S. W., Barr, W., Randolph, C., Cantu, R. C., . . . Kelly, J. P. (2003). Acute effects and recovery time following concussion in collegiate football players: The NCAA Concussion Study. *Journal of the American Medical Association*, *290*(19), 2556–2563.

McCrea, M., Guskiewicz, K., Randolph, C., Barr, W. B., Hammeke, T. A., Marshall, S. W., . . . Kelly, J. P. (2013). Incidence, clinical course, and predictors of prolonged recovery time following sport-related concussion in high school and college athletes. *Journal of the International Neuropsychological Society*, *19*(1), 22–33.

McCrea, M., Iverson, G. L., McAllister, T. W., Hammeke, T. A., Powell, M. R., Barr, W. B., & Kelly, J. P. (2009). An integrated review of recovery after mild traumatic brain injury (MTBI): Implications for clinical management. *The Clinical Neuropsychologist*, *23*(8), 1368–1390.

McCrory, P., Meeuwisse, W. H., Aubry, M., Cantu, B., Dvorak, J., Echemendia, R. J., . . . Turner, M. (2013). Consensus statement on concussion in sport: The 4th International Conference on Concussion in Sport held in Zurich, November 2012. *British Journal of Sports Medicine*, *47*(5), 250–258.

McDonald, B. C., Saykin, A. J., & McAllister, T. W. (2012). Functional MRI of mild traumatic brain injury (mTBI): Progress and perspectives from the first decade of studies. *Brain Imaging and Behavior*, *6*(2), 193–207. doi: 10.1007/s11682-012-9173-4

McGuire, L. M., Burright, R. G., Williams, R., & Donovick, P. J. (1998). Prevalence of traumatic brain injury in psychiatric and non-psychiatric subjects. *Brain Injury*, *12*(3), 207–214.

McKee, A. C., Cantu, R. C., Nowinski, C. J., Hedley-Whyte, E. T., Gavett, B. E., Budson, A. E., . . . Stern, R. A. (2009). Chronic traumatic encephalopathy in athletes: Progressive tauopathy after repetitive head injury. *Journal of Neuropathology and Experimental Neurology*, *68*(7), 709–735.

McKee, A. C., Stern, R. A., Nowinski, C. J., Stein, T. D., Alvarez, V. E., Daneshvar, D. H., . . . Cantu, R. C. (2013). The spectrum of disease in chronic traumatic encephalopathy. *Brain*, *136*(Pt 1), 43–64.

McMahon, P., Hricik, A., Yue, J. K., Puccio, A. M., Inoue, T., Lingsma, H. F., . . . Investigators, Track-Tbi. (2014). Symptomatology and functional outcome in mild traumatic brain injury: Results from the prospective TRACK-TBI study. *Journal of Neurotrauma*, *31*(1), 26–33.

McNally, K. A., Bangert, B., Dietrich, A., Nuss, K., Rusin, J., Wright, M., . . . Yeates, K. O. (2013). Injury versus noninjury factors as predictors of postconcussive symptoms following mild traumatic brain injury in children. *Neuropsychology*, *27*(1), 1–12.

Meares, S., Shores, E. A., Taylor, A. J., Batchelor, J., Bryant, R. A., Baguley, I. J., . . . Marosszeky, J. E. (2008). Mild traumatic brain injury does not predict acute postconcussion syndrome. *Journal of Neurology, Neurosurgery, & Psychiatry*, *79*(3), 300–306.

Meares, S., Shores, E. A., Taylor, A. J., Batchelor, J., Bryant, R. A., Baguley, I. J., . . . Marosszeky, J. E. (2011). The prospective course of postconcussion syndrome: The role of mild traumatic brain injury. *Neuropsychology*, *25*(4), 454–465.

Meehan, W. P., 3rd, Zhang, J., Mannix, R., & Whalen, M. J. (2012). Increasing recovery time between injuries improves cognitive outcome after repetitive mild concussive brain injuries in mice. *Neurosurgery*, *71*(4), 885–891.

Merkley, T. L., Bigler, E. D., Wilde, E. A., McCauley, S. R., Hunter, J. V., & Levin, H. S. (2008). Diffuse changes in cortical thickness in pediatric moderate-to-severe traumatic brain injury. *Journal of Neurotrauma*, *25*(11), 1343–1345. doi: 10.1089/neu.2008.0615

Messe, A., Caplain, S., Paradot, G., Garrigue, D., Mineo, J. F., Soto Ares, G., . . . Leherícy, S. (2011). Diffusion tensor imaging and white matter lesions at the subacute stage in mild traumatic brain injury with persistent neurobehavioral impairment. *Human Brain Mapping*, *32*(6), 999–1011. doi: 10.1002/hbm.21092

Messe, A., Caplain, S., Pelegrini-Issac, M., Blancho, S., Montreuil, M., Levy, R., . . . Benali, H. (2012). Structural integrity and postconcussion syndrome in mild traumatic brain injury patients. *Brain Imaging and Behavior*, *6*(2), 283–292. doi: 10.1007/s11682-012-9159-2

Meyers, J. E., Millis, S. R., & Volkert, K. (2002). A validity index for the MMPI-2. *Archives of Clinical Neuropsychology*, *17*(2), 157–169. doi: S0887617700001074 [pii]

Mez, J., Stern, R. A., & McKee, A. C. (2013). Chronic traumatic encephalopathy: Where are we and where are we going? *Current Neurology and Neuroscience Reports*, *13*(12), 407. doi: 10.1007/s11910-013-0407-7

Miller, J. R., Adamson, G. J., Pink, M. M., & Sweet, J. C. (2007). Comparison of preseason, midseason, and postseason neurocognitive scores in uninjured collegiate football players. *American Journal of Sports Medicine*, *35*(8), 1284–1288.

Miller, L. J., & Mittenberg, W. (1998). Brief cognitive behavioral interventions in mild traumatic brain injury. *Applied Neuropsychology*, *5*(4), 172–183.

Minderhoud, J. M., Boelens, M. E., Huizenga, J., & Saan, R. J. (1980). Treatment of minor head injuries. *Clinical Neurology and Neurosurgery*, *82*(2), 127–140.

Mittenberg, W., DiGiulio, D. V., Perrin, S., & Bass, A. E. (1992). Symptoms following mild head injury: Expectation as aetiology. *Journal of Neurology, Neurosurgery & Psychiatry*, *55*(3), 200–204.

Mittenberg, W., Patton, C., Canyock, E. M., & Condit, D. C. (2002). Base rates of malingering and symptom exaggeration. *Journal of Clinical and Experimental Neuropsychology*, *24*(8), 1094–1102. doi: 10.1076/jcen.24.8.1094.8379

Mittenberg, W., Tremont, G., Zielinski, R. E., Fichera, S., & Rayls, K. R. (1996). Cognitive-behavioral prevention of postconcussion syndrome. *Archives of Clinical Neuropsychology*, *11*(2), 139–145.

Mittenberg, W., Zielinski, R. E., & Fichera, S. (1993). Recovery from mild head injury: A treatment manual for patients. *Psychotherapy in Private Practice*, *12*, 37–52.

Mittl, R. L., Jr., & Yousem, D. M. (1994). Frequency of unexplained meningeal enhancement in the brain after lumbar puncture. *American Journal of Neuroradiology*, *15*(4), 633–638.

Monti, J. M., Voss, M. W., Pence, A., McAuley, E., Kramer, A. F., & Cohen, N. J. (2013). History of mild traumatic brain injury is associated with deficits in relational memory, reduced hippocampal volume, and less neural activity later in life. *Frontiers in Aging Neuroscience*, *5*, 41. doi: 10.3389/fnagi.2013.00041

Mooney, G., & Speed, J. (2001). The association between mild traumatic brain injury and psychiatric conditions. *Brain Injury*, *15*(10), 865–877.

Mooney, G., Speed, J., & Sheppard, S. (2005). Factors related to recovery after mild traumatic brain injury. *Brain Injury*, *19*(12), 975–987.

Moser, R. S., & Schatz, P. (2002). Enduring effects of concussion in youth athletes. *Archives of Clinical Neuropsychology*, *17*(1), 91–100.

Moser, R. S., Schatz, P., & Jordan, B. D. (2005). Prolonged effects of concussion in high school athletes. *Neurosurgery*, *57*(2), 300–306; discussion 300–306.

Muller, K., Ingebrigtsen, T., Wilsgaard, T., Wikran, G., Fagerheim, T., Romner, B., & Waterloo, K. (2009). Prediction of time trends in recovery of cognitive function after mild head injury. *Neurosurgery*, *64*(4), 698–704; discussion 704. doi: 10.1227/01.NEU.0000340978.42892.78

Niogi, S. N., Mukherjee, P., Ghajar, J., Johnson, C., Kolster, R. A., Sarkar, R., . . . McCandliss, B. D. (2008). Extent of microstructural white matter injury in postconcussive syndrome correlates with impaired cognitive reaction time: A 3T diffusion tensor imaging study of mild traumatic brain injury. *AJNR. American Journal of Neuroradiology*, *29*(5), 967–973. doi: 10.3174/ajnr.A0970

Omalu, B., Bailes, J., Hamilton, R. L., Kamboh, M. I., Hammers, J., Case, M., & Fitzsimmons, R. (2011a). Emerging histomorphologic phenotypes of chronic traumatic encephalopathy in American athletes. *Neurosurgery*, *69*(1), 173–183; discussion 183. doi: 10.1227/NEU.0b013e318212bc7b

Omalu, B., Hammers, J. L., Bailes, J., Hamilton, R. L., Kamboh, M. I., Webster, G., & Fitzsimmons, R. P. (2011b). Chronic traumatic encephalopathy in an Iraqi war veteran with posttraumatic stress disorder who committed suicide. *Neurosurgical Focus*, *31*(5), E3. doi: 10.3171/2011.9.FOCUS11178

Ouellet, M. C., Beaulieu-Bonneau, S., & Morin, C. M. (2006). Insomnia in patients with traumatic brain injury: Frequency, characteristics, and risk factors. *Journal of Head Trauma Rehabilitation*, *21*(3), 199–212. doi: 00001199-200605000-00001 [pii]

Ozen, L. J., & Fernandes, M. A. (2011). Effects of "diagnosis threat" on cognitive and affective functioning long after mild head injury. *Journal of the International Neuropsychological Society*, *17*(2), 219–229.

Ozen, L. J., & Fernandes, M. A. (2012). Slowing down after a mild traumatic brain injury: A strategy to improve cognitive task performance? *Archives of Clinical Neuropsychology*, *27*(1), 85–100.

Panenka, W. J., Lange, R. T., Bouix, S., Shewchuk, J. R., Heran, M. K., Brubacher, J. R., . . . Iverson, G. L. (2015). Neuropsychological outcome and diffusion tensor imaging in complicated versus uncomplicated mild traumatic brain injury. *PLoS One*, *10*(4), e0122746. doi: 10.1371/journal.pone.0122746

Paniak, C., Reynolds, S., Toller-Lobe, G., Melnyk, A., Nagy, J., & Schmidt, D. (2002). A longitudinal study of the relationship between financial compensation and symptoms after treated mild traumatic brain injury. *Journal of Clinical & Experimental Neuropsychology*, *24*(2), 187–193. doi: 10.1076/jcen.24.2.187.999

Paniak, C., Toller-Lobe, G., Durand, A., & Nagy, J. (1998). A randomized trial of two treatments for mild traumatic brain injury. *Brain Injury*, *12*(12), 1011–1023.

Paniak, C., Toller-Lobe, G., Reynolds, S., Melnyk, A., & Nagy, J. (2000). A randomized trial of two treatments for mild traumatic brain injury: 1 year follow-up. *Brain Injury*, *14*(3), 219–226.

Papa, L., Stiell, I. G., Clement, C. M., Pawlowicz, A., Wolfram, A., Braga, C., . . . Wells, G. A. (2012). Performance of the Canadian CT Head Rule and the New Orleans Criteria for predicting any traumatic intracranial injury on computed tomography in a United States Level I trauma center. *Academy of Emergency Medicine*, *19*(1), 2–10. doi: 10.1111/j.1553–2712.2011.01247.x

Parcell, D. L., Ponsford, J. L., Rajaratnam, S. M., & Redman, J. R. (2006). Self-reported changes to nighttime sleep after traumatic brain injury. *Archives of Physical Medicine and Rehabilitation*, *87*(2), 278–285.

Parry-Jones, B. L., Vaughan, F. L., & Miles Cox, W. (2006). Traumatic brain injury and substance misuse: A systematic review of prevalence and outcomes research (1994–2004). *Neuropsychological Rehabilitation*, *16*(5), 537–560.

Pavawalla, S. P., Salazar, R., Cimino, C., Belanger, H. G., & Vanderploeg, R. D. (2013). An exploration of diagnosis threat and group identification following concussion injury. *Journal of the International Neuropsychological Society*, *19*(3), 305–313.

Pellman, E. J., Viano, D. C., Tucker, A. M., & Casson, I. R. (2003). Concussion in professional football: Location and direction of helmet impacts-Part 2. *Neurosurgery*, *53*(6), 1328–1340; discussion 1340–1321.

Peters, K. D., Constans, J. I., & Mathews, A. (2011). Experimental modification of attribution processes. *Journal of Abnormal Psychology*, *120*(1), 168–173.

Pettus, E. H., Christman, C. W., Giebel, M. L., & Povlishock, J. T. (1994). Traumatically induced altered membrane permeability:

Its relationship to traumatically induced reactive axonal change. *Journal of Neurotrauma, 11*(5), 507–522.

Pierpaoli, C., & Basser, P. J. (1996). Toward a quantitative assessment of diffusion anisotropy. *Magnetic Resonance in Medicine, 36*(6), 893–906.

Plassman, B. L., Havlik, R. J., Steffens, D. C., Helms, M. J., Newman, T. N., Drosdick, D., . . . Breitner, J. C. (2000). Documented head injury in early adulthood and risk of Alzheimer's disease and other dementias. *Neurology, 55*(8), 1158–1166.

Ponsford, J., Cameron, P., Fitzgerald, M., Grant, M., Mikocka-Walus, A., & Schonberger, M. (2012). Predictors of postconcussive symptoms 3 months after mild traumatic brain injury. *Neuropsychology, 26*(3), 304–313.

Ponsford, J. L., Parcell, D. L., Sinclair, K. L., Roper, M., & Rajaratnam, S. M. (2013). Changes in sleep patterns following traumatic brain injury: A controlled study. *Neurorehabilitation and Neural Repair, 27*(7), 613–621.

Ponsford, J., Willmott, C., Rothwell, A., Cameron, P., Kelly, A. M., Nelms, R., & Curran, C. (2002). Impact of early intervention on outcome following mild head injury in adults. *Journal of Neurology, Neurosurgery and Psychiatry, 73*(3), 330–332.

Ponsford, J., Willmott, C., Rothwell, A., Cameron, P., Kelly, A. M., Nelms, R., . . . Ng, K. (2000). Factors influencing outcome following mild traumatic brain injury in adults. *Journal of the International Neuropsychological Society, 6*(5), 568–579.

Powell, T. J., Collin, C., & Sutton, K. (1996). A follow-up study of patients hospitalized after minor head injury. *Disability and Rehabilitation, 18*(5), 231–237.

Powell, J. M., Ferraro, J. V., Dikmen, S. S., Temkin, N. R., & Bell, K. R. (2008). Accuracy of mild traumatic brain injury diagnosis. *Archives of Physical Medicine & Rehabilitation, 89*(8), 1550–1555.

Puljula, J., Cygnel, H., Makinen, E., Tuomivaara, V., Karttunen, V., Karttunen, A., & Hillbom, M. (2012). Mild traumatic brain injury diagnosis frequently remains unrecorded in subjects with craniofacial fractures. *Injury, 43*(12), 2100–2104.

Rabadi, M. H., & Jordan, B. D. (2001). The cumulative effect of repetitive concussion in sports. *Clinical Journal of Sport Medicine, 11*(3), 194–198.

Randolph, C. (2011). Baseline neuropsychological testing in managing sport-related concussion: Does it modify risk? *Current Sports Medicine Reports, 10*(1), 21–26.

Randolph, C., McCrea, M., & Barr, W. B. (2005). Is neuropsychological testing useful in the management of sport-related concussion? *Journal of Athletic Training 40*(3), 139–152.

Rao, V., Bertrand, M., Rosenberg, P., Makley, M., Schretlen, D. J., Brandt, J., & Mielke, M. M. (2010). Predictors of new-onset depression after mild traumatic brain injury. *Journal of Neuropsychiatry and Clinical Neurosciences, 22*(1), 100–104.

Rapoport, M. J., McCullagh, S., Streiner, D., & Feinstein, A. (2003). The clinical significance of major depression following mild traumatic brain injury. *Psychosomatics, 44*(1), 31–37.

Relander, M., Troupp, H., & Bjorkesten, G. (1972). Controlled trial of treatment for cerebral concussion. *British Medical Journal, 4*, 777–779.

Rohling, M. L., Binder, L. M., Demakis, G. J., Larrabee, G. J., Ploetz, D. M., & Langhinrichsen-Rohling, J. (2011). A meta-analysis of neuropsychological outcome after mild traumatic brain injury: Re-analyses and reconsiderations of Binder et al. (1997), Frencham et al. (2005), and Pertab et al. (2009). *Clinical Neuropsychologist, 25*(4), 608–623.

Rosenbaum, S. B., & Lipton, M. L. (2012). Embracing chaos: The scope and importance of clinical and pathological heterogeneity in mTBI. [Review]. *Brain Imaging and Behavior, 6*(2), 255–282. doi: 10.1007/s11682-012-9162-7

Ruff, R. M., & Jurica, P. (1999). In search of a unified definition for mild traumatic brain injury. *Brain Injury, 13*(12), 943–952.

Sadowski-Cron, C., Schneider, J., Senn, P., Radanov, B. P., Ballinari, P., & Zimmermann, H. (2006). Patients with mild traumatic brain injury: Immediate and long-term outcome compared to intra-cranial injuries on CT scan. *Brain Injury, 20*(11), 1131–1137.

Savica, R., Parisi, J. E., Wold, L. E., Josephs, K. A., & Ahlskog, J. E. (2012). High school football and risk of neurodegeneration: A community-based study. [Mayo Clin Proc]. *Mayo Clinic Proceedings, 87*(4), 335–340.

Schatz, P., Moser, R. S., Covassin, T., & Karpf, R. (2011). Early indicators of enduring symptoms in high school athletes with multiple previous concussions. *Neurosurgery, 68*(6), 1562–1567; discussion 1567. doi: 10.1227/NEU.0b013e31820e382e

Schnebel, B., Gwin, J. T., Anderson, S., & Gatlin, R. (2007). In vivo study of head impacts in football: A comparison of National Collegiate Athletic Association Division I versus high school impacts. *Neurosurgery, 60*(3), 490–495; discussion 495–496.

Schneiderman, A. I., Braver, E. R., & Kang, H. K. (2008). Understanding sequelae of injury mechanisms and mild traumatic brain injury incurred during the conflicts in Iraq and Afghanistan: Persistent postconcussive symptoms and posttraumatic stress disorder. *American Journal of Epidemiology, 167*(12), 1446–1452.

Scholten, J., Cernich, A., Hurley, R. A., & Helmick, K. (2013). Department of Veterans Affairs's traumatic brain injury screening and evaluation program: Promoting individualized interdisciplinary care for symptomatic veterans. *Journal of Head Trauma Rehabilitation, 28*(3), 219–222.

Schreiber, S., Barkai, G., Gur-Hartman, T., Peles, E., Tov, N., Dolberg, O. T., & Pick, C. G. (2008). Long-lasting sleep patterns of adult patients with minor traumatic brain injury (mTBI) and non-mTBI subjects. *Sleep Medicine, 9*(5), 481–487.

Schretlen, D. J., & Shapiro, A. M. (2003). A quantitative review of the effects of traumatic brain injury on cognitive functioning. *International Review of Psychiatry, 15*, 341–349.

Segalowitz, S. J., Bernstein, D. M., & Lawson, S. (2001). P300 event-related potential decrements in well-functioning university students with mild head injury. *Brain and Cognition, 45*(3), 342–356.

Segalowitz, S. J., & Lawson, S. (1995). Subtle symptoms associated with self-reported mild head injury. *Journal of Learning Disabilities, 28*(5), 309–319.

Sheedy, J., Geffen, G., Donnelly, J., & Faux, S. (2006). Emergency department assessment of mild traumatic brain injury and prediction of post-concussion symptoms at one month post injury. *Journal of Clinical and Experimental Neuropsychology, 28*(5), 755–772.

Sheedy, J., Harvey, E., Faux, S., Geffen, G., & Shores, E. A. (2009). Emergency department assessment of mild traumatic brain injury and the prediction of postconcussive symptoms: A 3-month prospective study. *Journal of Head Trauma Rehabilitation, 24*(5), 333–343.

Shenton, M. E., Hamoda, H. M., Schneiderman, J. S., Bouix, S., Pasternak, O., Rathi, Y., . . . Zafonte, R. (2012). A review of magnetic resonance imaging and diffusion tensor imaging findings in mild traumatic brain injury. *Brain Imaging and Behavior*, *6*(2), 137–192.

Sigurdardottir, S., Andelic, N., Roe, C., Jerstad, T., & Schanke, A. K. (2009). Post-concussion symptoms after traumatic brain injury at 3 and 12 months post-injury: A prospective study. *Brain Injury*, *23*(6), 489–497.

Silver, J. M., & Kay, T. (2013). Persistent symptoms after a concussion. In N. D. Zasler, D. B. Arciniegas, R. D. Vanderploeg, & M. S. Jaffee (Eds.), *Management of Adults With Traumatic Brain* (pp. 475–500). Washington, DC: American Psychiatric Publishing.

Silver, J. M., McAllister, T. W., & Arciniegas, D. B. (2009). Depression and cognitive complaints following mild traumatic brain injury. *American Journal of Psychiatry*, *166*(6), 653–661.

Silverberg, N. D., & Iverson, G. L. (2011). Etiology of the post-concussion syndrome: Physiogenesis and Psychogenesis revisited. *NeuroRehabilitation*, *29*(4), 317–329.

Silverberg, N. D., Lange, R. T., Millis, S. R., Rose, A., Hopp, G., Leach, S., & Iverson, G. L. (2013). Post-concussion symptom reporting after multiple mild traumatic brain injuries. *Journal of Neurotrauma*, *30*(16), 1398–1404. doi: 10.1089/neu.2012.2827

Siman, R., Giovannone, N., Toraskar, N., Frangos, S., Stein, S. C., Levine, J. M., & Kumar, M. A. (2011). Evidence that a panel of neurodegeneration biomarkers predicts vasospasm, infarction, and outcome in aneurysmal subarachnoid hemorrhage. *PLoS One*, *6*(12), e28938.

Singleton, R. H., Zhu, J., Stone, J. R., & Povlishock, J. T. (2002). Traumatically induced axotomy adjacent to the soma does not result in acute neuronal death. *Journal of Neuroscience*, *22*(3), 791–802. doi: 22/3/791 [pii]

Slemmer, J. E., & Weber, J. T. (2005). The extent of damage following repeated injury to cultured hippocampal cells is dependent on the severity of insult and inter-injury interval. *Neurobiology of Disease*, *18*(3), 421–431.

Slobounov, S., Gay, M., Johnson, B., & Zhang, K. (2012). Concussion in athletics: Ongoing clinical and brain imaging research controversies. *Brain Imaging and Behavior*, *6*(2), 224–243.

Smith-Seemiller, L., Fow, N. R., Kant, R., & Franzen, M. D. (2003). Presence of post-concussion syndrome symptoms in patients with chronic pain vs. mild traumatic brain injury. *Brain Injury*, *17*(3), 199–206.

Smits, M., Houston, G. C., Dippel, D. W., Wielopolski, P. A., Vernooij, M. W., Koudstaal, P. J., . . . van der Lugt, A. (2011). Microstructural brain injury in post-concussion syndrome after minor head injury. *Neuroradiology*, *53*(8), 553–563. doi: 10.1007/s00234-010-0774-6

Smits, M., Hunink, M. G., Nederkoorn, P. J., Dekker, H. M., Vos, P. E., Kool, D. R., . . . Dippel, D. W. (2007). A history of loss of consciousness or post-traumatic amnesia in minor head injury: "conditio sine qua non" or one of the risk factors? *Journal of Neurology, Neurosurgery & Psychiatry*, *78*(12), 1359–1364.

Smits, M., Hunink, M. G., van Rijssel, D. A., Dekker, H. M., Vos, P. E., Kool, D. R., . . . Dippel, D. W. (2008). Outcome after complicated minor head injury. *AJNR American Journal of Neuroradiology*, *29*(3), 506–513.

Snell, D. L., Hay-Smith, E. J., Surgenor, L. J., & Siegert, R. J. (2013). Examination of outcome after mild traumatic brain injury: The contribution of injury beliefs and Leventhal's Common Sense Model. *Neuropsychological Rehabilitation*, *23*(3), 333–362.

Son, B. C., Park, C. K., Choi, B. G., Kim, E. N., Choe, B. Y., Lee, K. S., . . . Kang, J. K. (2000). Metabolic changes in pericontusional oedematous areas in mild head injury evaluated by 1H MRS. *Acta neurochirurgica. Supplement.*, *76*, 13–16.

Spencer, R. J., Drag, L. L., Walker, S. J., & Bieliauskas, L. A. (2010). Self-reported cognitive symptoms following mild traumatic brain injury are poorly associated with neuropsychological performance in OIF/OEF veterans. *Journal of Rehabilitation Research & Development*, *47*(6), 521–530.

Spitz, G., Maller, J. J., Ng, A., O'Sullivan, R., Ferris, N. J., & Ponsford, J. L. (2013). Detecting lesions after traumatic brain injury using susceptibility weighted imaging: A comparison with fluid-attenuated inversion recovery and correlation with clinical outcome. *Journal of Neurotrauma*, *30*(24), 2038–2050. doi: 10.1089/neu.2013.3021

Stern, R. A., Daneshvar, D. H., Baugh, C. M., Seichepine, D. R., Montenigro, P. H., Riley, D. O., . . . McKee, A. C. (2013). Clinical presentation of chronic traumatic encephalopathy. *Neurology*, *81*(13), 1122–1129.

Sterr, A., Herron, K. A., Hayward, C., & Montaldi, D. (2006). Are mild head injuries as mild as we think? Neurobehavioral concomitants of chronic post-concussion syndrome. *BMC Neurology*, *6*, 7.

Stiell, I. G., Wells, G. A., Vandemheen, K., Clement, C., Lesiuk, H., Laupacis, A., . . . Worthington, J. (2001). The Canadian CT Head Rule for patients with minor head injury. *Lancet*, *357*(9266), 1391–1396. doi: S014067360004561X [pii]

Stulemeijer, M., Andriessen, T. M., Brauer, J. M., Vos, P. E., & Van Der Werf, S. (2007). Cognitive performance after mild traumatic brain injury: The impact of poor effort on test results and its relation to distress, personality and litigation. *Brain Injury*, *21*(3), 309–318.

Stulemeijer, M., van der Werf, S., Borm, G. F., & Vos, P. E. (2008). Early prediction of favorable recovery 6 months after mild traumatic brain injury. *Journal of Neurology, Neurosurgery and Psychiatry*, *79*(8), 936–942.

Suffoletto, B., Wagner, A. K., Arenth, P. M., Calabria, J., Kingsley, E., Kristan, J., & Callaway, C. W. (2013). Mobile phone text messaging to assess symptoms after mild traumatic brain injury and provide self-care support: A pilot study. *The Journal of Head Trauma Rehabilitation*, *28*(4), 302–312. doi: 10.1097/HTR.0b013e3182847468

Suhr, J. A., & Gunstad, J. (2002). "Diagnosis Threat": The effect of negative expectations on cognitive performance in head injury. *Journal of Clinical and Experimental Neuropsychology*, *24*(4), 448–457.

Suhr, J. A., & Gunstad, J. (2005). Further exploration of the effect of "diagnosis threat" on cognitive performance in individuals with mild head injury. *Journal of the International Neuropsychological Society*, *11*(1), 23–29.

Sullivan, K. A., & Edmed, S. L. (2012a). An examination of the expected symptoms of postconcussion syndrome in a nonclinical sample. *Journal of Head Trauma Rehabilitation*, *27*(4), 293–301. doi: 10.1097/HTR.0b013e31822123ce

Sullivan, K. A., & Edmed, S. L. (2012b). Systematic variation of the severity of motor vehicle accident-related traumatic brain injury vignettes produces different post-concussion symptom reports. *Clinical Neuropsychologist*, *26*(8), 1255–1277.

Sullivan, K. A., Edmed, S. L., & Kempe, C. (2014). The effect of injury diagnosis on illness perceptions and expected postconcussion syndrome and posttraumatic stress disorder symptoms. *Journal of Head Trauma Rehabilitation, 29*(1), 54–64. doi: 10.1097/HTR.0b013e31828c708a

Sundstrom, A., Nilsson, L. G., Cruts, M., Adolfsson, R., Van Broeckhoven, C., & Nyberg, L. (2007). Increased risk of dementia following mild head injury for carriers but not for non-carriers of the APOE epsilon4 allele. *International Psychogeriatrics, 19*(1), 159–165.

Sweet, J. J., Meyer, D. G., Nelson, N. W., & Moberg, P. J. (2011). The TCN/AACN 2010 "salary survey": Professional practices, beliefs, and incomes of U.S. neuropsychologists. *Clinical Neuropsychologist, 25*(1), 12–61.

Talavage, T. M., Nauman, E. A., Breedlove, E. L., Yoruk, U., Dye, A. E., Morigaki, K. E., . . . Leverenz, L. J. (2013). Functionally-detected cognitive impairment in high school football players without clinically-diagnosed concussion. *Journal of Neurotrauma, 31*(4), 327–338. doi: 10.1089/neu.2010.1512

Tanielian, T., & Jaycox, L. H. (Eds.). (2008). *Invisible Wounds of War: Psychological and Cognitive Injuries, Their Consequences, and Services to Assist Recovery*. Santa Monica, CA: Rand Corporation.

Tate DF, Gusman M, Kini J, et al. 2017 Susceptibility weighted imaging and white matter abnormality findings in service members with persistent cognitive symptoms following mild traumatic brain injury. *Military Medicine, 182*(3):e1651–e1658. doi:10.7205/MILMED-D-16-00132.

Tate, D. F., York, G. E., Reid, M. W., Cooper, D. B., Jones, L., Robin, D. A., . . . Lewis, J. (2013). Preliminary findings of cortical thickness abnormalities in blast injured service members and their relationship to clinical findings. *Brain Imaging and Behavior*. doi: 10.1007/s11682-013-9257-9

Temkin, N. R., Machamer, J. E., & Dikmen, S. S. (2003). Correlates of functional status 3–5 years after traumatic brain injury with CT abnormalities. *Journal of Neurotrauma, 20*(3), 229–241. doi: 10.1089/089771503321532815

Terrell, T. R., Bostick, R. M., Abramson, R., Xie, D., Barfield, W., Cantu, R., . . . Ewing, T. (2008). APOE, APOE promoter, and Tau genotypes and risk for concussion in college athletes. *Clinical Journal of Sports Medicine, 18*(1), 10–17.

Terrio, H., Brenner, L. A., Ivins, B. J., Cho, J. M., Helmick, K., Schwab, K., . . . Warden, D. (2009). Traumatic brain injury screening: Preliminary findings in a US Army Brigade Combat Team. *Journal of Head Trauma Rehabilitation, 24*(1), 14–23.

Terry, D. P., Faraco, C. C., Smith, D., Diddams, M. J., Puente, A. N., & Miller, L. S. (2012). Lack of long-term fMRI differences after multiple sports-related concussions. *Brain Injury, 26*(13–14), 1684–1696.

Thornton, A. E., Cox, D. N., Whitfield, K., & Fouladi, R. T. (2008). Cumulative concussion exposure in rugby players: Neurocognitive and symptomatic outcomes. *Journal of Clinical & Experimental Neuropsychology, 30*(4), 398–409.

Tiersky, L. A., Anselmi, V., Johnston, M. V., Kurtyka, J., Roosen, E., Schwartz, T., & Deluca, J. (2005). A trial of neuropsychologic rehabilitation in mild-spectrum traumatic brain injury. *Archives of Physical Medicine and Rehabilitation, 86*(8), 1565–1574.

Tong, K. A., Ashwal, S., Holshouser, B. A., Nickerson, J. P., Wall, C. J., Shutter, L. A., . . . Kido, D. (2004). Diffuse axonal injury in children: Clinical correlation with hemorrhagic lesions. *Annals of Neurology, 56*(1), 36–50. doi: 10.1002/ana.20123

Tong, K. A., Ashwal, S., Holshouser, B. A., Shutter, L. A., Herigault, G., Haacke, E. M., & Kido, D. K. (2003). Hemorrhagic shearing lesions in children and adolescents with posttraumatic diffuse axonal injury: Improved detection and initial results. *Radiology, 227*(2), 332–339.

Tremblay, S., De Beaumont, L., Henry, L. C., Boulanger, Y., Evans, A. C., Bourgouin, P., . . . Lassonde, M. (2012). Sports concussions and aging: A neuroimaging investigation. *Cerebral Cortex, 23*(5), 1159–1166.

Trueblood, W., & Schmidt, M. (1993). Malingering and other validity considerations in the neuropsychological evaluation of mild head injury. *Journal of Clinical and Experimental Neuropsychology, 15*(4), 578–590. doi: 10.1080/01688639308402580

Tsushima, W. T., Lum, M., & Geling, O. (2009). Sex differences in the long-term neuropsychological outcome of mild traumatic brain injury. *Brain Injury, 23*(10), 809–814.

van der Naalt, J., Hew, J. M., van Zomeren, A. H., Sluiter, W. J., & Minderhoud, J. M. (1999). Computed tomography and magnetic resonance imaging in mild to moderate head injury: Early and late imaging related to outcome. *Annals of Neurology, 46*(1), 70–78.

van der Naalt, J., van Zomeren, A. H., Sluiter, W. J., & Minderhoud, J. M. (1999). One year outcome in mild to moderate head injury: The predictive value of acute injury characteristics related to complaints and return to work. *Journal of Neurology, Neurosurgery, and Psychiatry, 66*(2), 207–213.

Vanderploeg, R. D., & Belanger, H. G. (2013). Screening for a remote history of mild traumatic brain injury: When a good idea is bad. *Journal of Head Trauma Rehabilitation, 28*(3), 211–218.

Vanderploeg, R. D., Belanger, H. G., & Curtiss, G. (2006). Mild traumatic brain injury: Medical and legal causality considerations. In G. Young, A. Kane, & K. Nicholson (Eds.), *Psychological Knowledge in Court: PTSD, Pain and TBI* (pp. 279–307). New York: Springer.

Vanderploeg, R. D., Belanger, H. G., Horner, R. D., Spehar, A. M., Powell-Cope, G., Luther, S. L., & Scott, S. G. (2012). Health outcomes associated with military deployment: Mild traumatic brain injury, blast, trauma, and combat associations in the Florida National Guard. *Archives of Physical Medicine & Rehabilitation, 93*(11), 1887–1895.

Vanderploeg, R. D., Curtiss, G., & Belanger, H. G. (2005). Adverse long-term neuropsychological outcomes following mild traumatic brain injury. *Journal of the International Neuropsychological Society, 11*, 228–236.

Vanderploeg, R. D., Curtiss, G., Luis, C. A., & Salazar, A. M. (2007). Long-term morbidities following self-reported mild traumatic brain injury. *Journal of Clinical & Experimental Neuropsychology, 29*(6), 585–598.

Vasterling, J. J., Brailey, K., Proctor, S. P., Kane, R., Heeren, T., & Franz, M. (2012). Neuropsychological outcomes of mild traumatic brain injury, post-traumatic stress disorder and depression in Iraq-deployed US Army soldiers. *British Journal of Psychiatry, 201*(3), 186–192.

Wade, D. T., King, N. S., Wenden, F. J., Crawford, S., & Caldwell, F. E. (1998). Routine follow up after head injury: A second randomised controlled trial. *Journal of Neurology, Neurosurgery and Psychiatry, 65*(2), 177–183.

Walker, W. C., McDonald, S. D., Ketchum, J. M., Nichols, M., & Cifu, D. X. (2013). Identification of transient altered consciousness induced by military-related blast exposure and its relation to postconcussion symptoms. *Journal of Head Trauma Rehabilitation, 28*(1), 68–76. doi: 10.1097/HTR.0b013e318255dfd0

Wall, S. E., Williams, W. H., Cartwright-Hatton, S., Kelly, T. P., Murray, J., Murray, M., . . . Turner, M. (2006). Neuropsychological dysfunction following repeat concussions in jockeys. *Journal of Neurology, Neurosurgery and Psychiatry*, *77*(4), 518–520.

Weber, M., & Edwards, M. G. (2010). The effect of brain injury terminology on university athletes' expected outcome from injury, familiarity and actual symptom report. *Brain Injury*, *24*(11), 1364–1371. doi: 10.3109/02699052.2010.507110

Whittaker, R., Kemp, S., & House, A. (2007). Illness perceptions and outcome in mild head injury: A longitudinal study. *Journal of Neurology, Neurosurgery & Psychiatry*, *78*(6), 644–646.

Wilde, E. A., Bouix, S., Tate, D. F., Lin, A. P., Newsome, M. R., Taylor, B. A., . . . York, G. (2015). Advanced neuroimaging applied to veterans and service personnel with traumatic brain injury: State of the art and potential benefits. *Brain Imaging and Behavior*, *9*(3), 367–402. doi: 10.1007/s11682-015-9444-y

Wilde, E. A., Merkley, T. L., Bigler, E. D., Max, J. E., Schmidt, A. T., Ayoub, K. W., . . . Levin, H. S. (2012). Longitudinal changes in cortical thickness in children after traumatic brain injury and their relation to behavioral regulation and emotional control. *International Journal of Developmental Neuroscience*, *30*(3), 267–276. doi: 10.1016/j.ijdevneu.2012.01.003

Wilde, E. A., Newsome, M. R., Bigler, E. D., Pertab, J., Merkley, T. L., Hanten, G., . . . Levin, H. S. (2011). Brain imaging correlates of verbal working memory in children following traumatic brain injury. *International Journal of Psychophysiology*, *82*(1), 86–96. doi: 10.1016/j.ijpsycho.2011.04.006

Williams, D. H., Levin, H. S., & Eisenberg, H. M. (1990). Mild head injury classification. *Neurosurgery*, *27*(3), 422–428.

Wilson, J. T., Pettigrew, L. E., & Teasdale, G. M. (1998). Structured interviews for the Glasgow Outcome Scale and the extended Glasgow Outcome Scale: Guidelines for their use. *Journal of Neurotrauma*, *15*(8), 573–585.

Witthoft, M., & Rubin, G. J. (2013). Are media warnings about the adverse health effects of modern life self-fulfilling? An experimental study on idiopathic environmental intolerance attributed to electromagnetic fields (IEI-EMF). *Journal of Psychosomatic Research*, *74*(3), 206–212.

Wolf, G., Cifu, D., Baugh, L., Carne, W., & Profenna, L. (2012). The effect of hyperbaric oxygen on symptoms after mild traumatic brain injury. *Journal of Neurotrauma*, *29*(17), 2606–2612. doi: 10.1089/neu.2012.2549

Wood, R. L., O'Hagan, G., Williams, C., McCabe, M., & Chadwick, N. (2014). Anxiety sensitivity and alexithymia as mediators of postconcussion syndrome following mild traumatic brain injury. *Journal of Head Trauma Rehabilitation*, *29*(1), E9-E17. doi: 10.1097/HTR.0b013e31827eabba

World Health Organization. (1992). *International Statistical Classification of Diseases and Related Health Problems* (10th ed.). Geneva, Switzerland: Author.

Wortzel, H. S., Brenner, L. A., & Arciniegas, D. B. (2013). Traumatic Brain Injury and Chronic Traumatic Encephalopathy: A Forensic Neuropsychiatric Perspective. *Behavioral Sciences and the Law*, *31*(6), 721–738. doi: 10.1002/bsl.2079

Wrightson, P., & Gronwall, D. (1981). Time off work and symptoms after minor head injury. *Injury*, *12*(6), 445–454.

Wu, T. C., Wilde, E. A., Bigler, E. D., Yallampalli, R., McCauley, S. R., Troyanskaya, M., . . . Levin, H. S. (2010). Evaluating the relationship between memory functioning and cingulum bundles in acute mild traumatic brain injury using diffusion tensor imaging. *Journal of Neurotrauma*, *27*(2), 303–307. doi: 10.1089/neu.2009.1110

Yuh, E. L., Mukherjee, P., Lingsma, H. F., Yue, J. K., Ferguson, A. R., Gordon, W. A., . . . Investigators, Track-Tbi. (2013). Magnetic resonance imaging improves 3-month outcome prediction in mild traumatic brain injury. *Annals of Neurology*, *73*(2), 224–235. doi: 10.1002/ana.23783

19 Neurocognitive Assessment in Epilepsy

Advances and Challenges

Joseph I. Tracy and Jennifer R. Tinker

The pathophysiology of seizures is closely linked to the formation of networks subserving cognition. Epilepsy research has provided us with landmark insights into amnesia and set the foundation for our understanding of episodic memory. H.M., who suffered severe anterograde amnesia as a result of bilateral medial temporal lobe resection to control seizures, is likely the best known, and most studied, patient in the history of neuroscience (Squire, 2009). Many of the fundamental principles of episodic memory owe a great debt to lesional epilepsy, particularly early models focused on the temporal stages of processing. Seizure activity, however, induces neuroplasticity, and our conceptualization of the cognitive effects of epilepsy is expanding beyond the focal/modular approach common to early lesional models towards more dynamic network models of dysfunction.

In this chapter, we will present evidence for cognitive network dysfunction in epilepsy, emphasizing seizure-induced neuroplasticity, and its broad effects on cognition and brain network organization. We will present data from functional imaging and other sources, demonstrating that even focal epilepsies can induce more widespread neuropsychological changes than originally thought. We will briefly discuss models of network organization in the setting of seizures, noting how these help explain the complex nonfocal deficit patterns that are often observed. In line with the notion that ongoing seizures create a dynamic, not static, cognitive profile, we review the evidence for cognitive reorganization, and describe the impact of variables with cognitive impacts that vary with age or development (e.g., age of onset, chronicity, hemispheric dominance, and medication). We will also examine the changing algorithm for presurgical assessments in epilepsy, and the impact these changes have on our methods for predicting neuropsychological and emotional/behavioral status postsurgery. The advent of technologies that can more directly link cognition to underlying neurobiologic mechanisms (e.g., structural and functional neuroimaging, electrocorticography) will both challenge and enhance the role of neuropsychologists who work in surgical epilepsy centers. Our use of these technologies to refine and improve our understanding of brain-behavior relationships will make neuropsychologists particularly well-suited to contribute to surgical decision-making, and greatly advance our understanding of epilepsy's cognitive effects. Throughout this chapter, we emphasize that only by understanding the neuroplasticity initiated by seizures will we be able to effectively identify cognitive status and predict cognitive outcomes in epilepsy, as it is these neuroplastic responses that govern the status of both neurocognitive and epileptogenic networks.

Seizures, Neuroplasticity, and Cognition

The key to grasping the paradigm shift from a focal, modular approach to that of a network approach is to understand that the neural mechanisms underlying network development (i.e., neuroplasticity) and the neuropathology of seizures are similar. Indeed, little separates the neurobiology of learning and of seizures. Many of the neural mechanisms of learning are key factors in the regulation of seizures, and the highly plastic brain regions specialized for learning and memory are particularly susceptible to seizures. More than characterizing the effects of seizures or predicting outcomes after surgery, there are fundamental cognitive neuroscience reasons for neuropsychologists to study epilepsy.

Epilepsy is an electrical disorder characterized by neural cell hypersynchrony. The origin of this hypersynchrony can vary as epilepsy is the end state of a wide range of pathologic mechanisms (e.g., trauma, stroke, genetic, tumor, atrophy, dysplasia, infection). Epileptogenesis can begin with a single neuron. A seizing neuron recruits adjacent neurons into a hypersynchronous process until a critical mass of tissue transforms into a single active unit whose components no longer respond to existing functional network connections. Therefore, the process of epileptogenesis provides us with an avenue for studying the development of favored neural pathways that are distinct from developmentally and adaptively formed neural networks. The degree to which these maladaptive seizure networks overlap and interact with either established or developing cognitive networks is what neuropsychologists must determine when conducting their evaluations.

Broadly speaking, the ramifications of epileptic activity in the brain include: (a) intracellular changes (i.e., expression of cellular proteins or alterations in calcium channels, signaling molecules, or neurotransmitters such as GABA), (b) injury to cortical pyramidal neurons that make membrane ion channels more amenable to excitatory input, (c) mossy fiber and axonal sprouting within pyramidal cells that enhance excitatory connections, (d) hyperinnervation, (e) failure to prune immature connections when occurring early in life, and (f) changes in glial cells and in the organization of axons and dendrites to favor hypersynchrony (Ben-Ari, Crepel, & Represa, 2008; Jacobs, Graber, Kharazia, Parada, & Prince, 2000; Somera-Molina et al., 2007; Sutula & Dudek, 2007). These neuroplastic changes are most evident within the hippocampus, but have been observed in the neocortex as well (Schwartzkroin, 2001). All constitute mechanisms of neuroplasticity at different levels of organization, working in a single or combined way to restructure surviving synapses, leading to reorganization of surviving neuronal networks.

Both seizures and plasticity are controlled and regulated by complex molecular mechanisms and recent research has focused largely on inhibitory processes (Brooks-Kayal, 2011; Kullmann, Moreau, Bakiri, & Nicholson, 2012). GABAa receptors mediate most fast synaptic inhibition and are crucial in regulating both neuronal excitability and the impact of excitatory synapses. There is increasing evidence that GABAergic synapses are plastic and demonstrate long-term, bidirectional changes in connectivity strength throughout the brain (Castillo, Chiu, & Carroll, 2011). Studies examining GABAa subunit alterations have uncovered seizure-induced pathways that contribute to epileptogenesis, with several transcription factors regulating GABAa in a way that leads to chronic epilepsy (Grabenstatter, Russek, & Brooks-Kayal, 2012). These transcription factors and cell modulators (e.g., brain-derived neurotrophic factor, cAMP response element binding protein, inducible cAMP early repressor, and early growth response factors) are the focus of intense investigation in epilepsy as potential targets for antiepileptic drugs.

Mesial temporal lobe epilepsy (MTL) is the best-characterized type of epilepsy, due to its high relative incidence and relatively homogenous etiology (e.g., hippocampal sclerosis). The temporal lobe is particularly vulnerable to epileptogenesis due to the neuroanatomic and neurochemical properties that support learning and memory. Regions specialized for learning and memory in the brain, such as the hippocampus, appear most prone to seizures. The main neurotransmitters associated with seizures are GABA and NMDA. NMDA receptor density is high in the CA1 and CA3 regions of the hippocampus (Coultrap, Nixon, Alvestad, Valenzuela, & Browning, 2005). In fact, NMDA receptor density predicts both the probability of Hebbian learning and epileptogenicity (McClelland, 2001; Nicoll & Malenka, 1999). Hebbian learning mechanisms of long-term potentiation (LTP) and long-term depression (LTD) are the primary mechanisms of neural network development and underlie the processes of learning and remembering. The immature brain exhibits greater plasticity potential than the adult brain. Ironically, the plasticity that makes the immature brain quite responsive to environmental stimulation and facile at learning also means that the environment, stress, injury, and illness (i.e., seizures) can have a more profound and devastating effect. Some have argued that epilepsy, along with other conditions (e.g., intellectual disabilities, autism spectrum disorders), may be best understood as disorders of synaptic plasticity that result in a developmental imbalance of excitation and inhibition (Brooks-Kayal, 2011).[1]

Given the cellular and synaptic transmission modifications at work, one can see that there are ample opportunities for cognitive deficits to emerge in regions outside the primary epileptogenic focus. When cells in these remote sites seize (i.e., display abnormal spiking patterns) following initial activity in the original epileptic focus, these intense epileptic dynamics can force the abnormal integration of these remote cells into the epileptogenic network (Schneider-Mizell et al., 2010). After joining the hypersynchronous activity of the ictal focus, these remote cells may eventually come to initiate seizures independently (Morrell & deToledo-Morrell, 1999), potentially forcing both functional and structural connectivity changes. Thus, the ictal focus of a seizure can be seen as initiating a neural circuit, a circuit that if instantiated repeatedly by ongoing seizures leads to frequent aberrant neural "communication" with other regions of the brain. Cells downstream from the seizure generator will respond to the excitation of seizures as if learning has occurred. From this perspective, epileptogenesis appears to be a process similar to LTP (Shimizu et al., 2000; Tracy et al., 2009), with these aberrant networks active not just during ictal stimulation but also during cognitive stimulation of one or more seizure network nodes, ultimately disrupting the underlying cognition. Eventually, through a process that reduces action potential thresholds similar to neural kindling (Goddard, 1967; Wada & Mizoguchi, 1984), these epileptogenic pathways create a biased, favored network that is both maladaptive to cognition and pathologic to otherwise healthy neural tissue, as it now has to bear the burden of periodic epileptiform activity. In this way, seizures produce a dysfunctional, maladaptive cognitive network by linking brain areas randomly through seizure propagations and secondary epileptogenesis, rather than through normal adaptive learning and experience driven plasticity and connectivity. Accordingly, the development of normal neural networks, through the LTP or LTD associated with normal learning, appears to bear a striking resemblance to epileptogenesis. More specifically, injury, pathology, or genetically driven abnormal excitability (and inhibition) induces neuronal neuroplastic responses, causing cognitive network dysfunction both directly and indirectly through the formation of seizure/epileptiform networks. Interventions such as resective surgery, ablation, or medication can also trigger cognitive reorganization adaptively through seizure control, or maladaptively by allowing seizure recurrence. Figure 19.1 illustrates a pathway depicting the development of seizure networks, maladaptive to cognition triggering reorganization, carried through to additional potential cognitive reorganization related to intervention such as temporal lobe surgery.

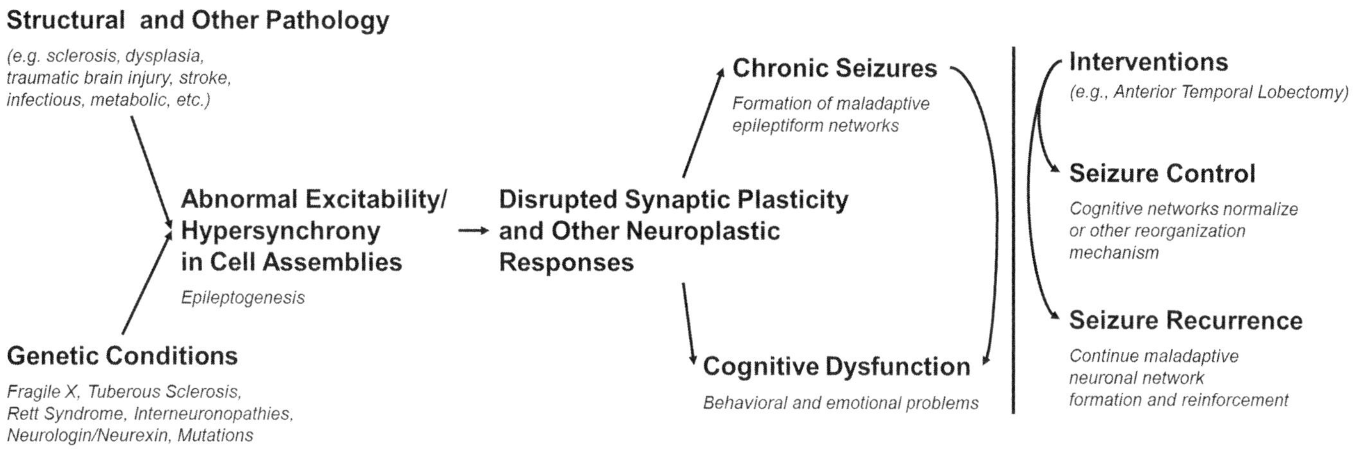

Figure 19.1 Pathway depicting the development of seizure networks, maladaptive to cognition but triggering reorganization, carried through to intervention by anterior temporal lobectomy (ATL). More specifically, pathology or genetically driven abnormal excitability induces neuronal neuroplastic responses contributing both directly and indirectly (through seizure/epileptiform networks) to cognitive network dysfunction. Interventions such as ATL can also trigger cognitive reorganization adaptively through seizure control, or maladaptively through seizure recurrence.

Seizure-Induced Reorganization of Cognitive Networks

The central nervous system in adults continues to adjust and adapt over the course of the lifetime. These adaptations generally occur in two contexts: neuroplastic processes operating in a normal brain as part of development or in response to experience, and those that operate in the abnormal or pathologic brain creating an atypical historical environment for the organism (injury-induced plasticity). Brain plasticity is evident in the normal brain and occurs with normal learning (May, 2011; Tracy et al., 2003). Injury-induced plasticity has been demonstrated in acute brain injury (Demirtas-Tatlidede, Vahabzadeh-Hagh, Bernabeu, Tormos, & Pascual-Leone, 2012; Xiong, Mahmood, & Chopp, 2010), stroke (Meinzer, Harnish, Conway, & Crosson, 2011), and resective surgery (McCormick, Quraan, Cohn, Valiante, & McAndrews, 2013). In this section, we discuss the evidence for cognitive reorganization in epilepsy.[2]

Neuropsychological, intracarotid amobarbital (popularly known as the *Wada test*), functional magnetic resonance imaging (fMRI), and functional connectivity (FC) studies have all provided evidence that the brain representation of cognitive functions in patients with temporal lobe epilepsy (TLE), for a variety of tasks, can reorganize to regions not seen in matched control samples. Neuropsychological and intracarotid amobarbital studies, particularly in early onset left TLE, provided the initial evidence for reorganization of verbal memory and expressive language skills, with indications of either a left-to-right interhemispheric or anterior-to-posterior intrahemispheric reorganization pattern (Jokeit, Ebner, Holthausen, Markowitsch, & Tuxhorn, 1996; Seidenberg et al., 1997).

Task-driven fMRI studies have demonstrated that TLE patients show altered organization of major cognitive networks such as those involved in expressive language. An fMRI study by Wilke et al. (2011), using narrative and letter sound processing tasks in epileptic children and matched controls, found a high rate of atypical language organization, with the homotopic contralateral region the most common site of reorganization, though the distribution of left hemisphere representations (frontal and temporal regions) also showed alterations from normative locations (e.g., classical Broca's and Wernicke's areas). Cousin, Baciu, Pichat, Kahane, and Le Bas (2008) found that the asymmetry of typical language lateralization was significantly lower in left TLE patients than controls, with early onset patients showing stronger signs of right temporal and parietal reorganization than late-onset patients, in addition to a tendency toward intrahemispheric reorganization involving the frontal lobe. They also found that hippocampal sclerosis increased the probability of interhemispheric shift of the temporal lobe activation. Rosenberger and colleagues (2009) looked at fMRI language activation patterns in left TLE patients during a lexical decision task (e.g., correct/incorrect definitions provided auditorily) and found an increased frequency of atypical language representations involving right hemisphere language areas, homologs of left hemisphere Broca and Wernicke's areas. Interestingly, they found little evidence for intrahemispheric reorganization in patients with left hemisphere epilepsy who remained left language dominant by fMRI, and these effects did not vary by age at epilepsy onset, duration of epilepsy, or pathology. Hamberger and Cole (2011) reviewed the area of language reorganization and found that preserved naming ability in the setting of hippocampal sclerosis was associated with intrahemispheric (i.e., more posterior temporal) reorganization in response to early disease in the mesial temporal region. They noted that this pattern makes sense given the known bias of TLE seizure discharges to proceed anteriorly. It remains unclear how large the epileptogenic region (or lesion) has to be to force contralateral language reorganization. Also unclear is the degree to which interhemispheric reorganization is dependent on the particular brain region housing the pathology. There is, however, some evidence that damage to the hippocampus may be the crucial structure compelling contralateral, as opposed to ipsilateral, language reorganization (for review see Tracy & Boswell, 2008).

Memory also appears to reorganize in the face of intractable seizures. Figueiredo et al. (2008) utilized a visual episodic memory fMRI task, and found that, relative to controls, right TLE patients with hippocampal sclerosis demonstrated functional reorganization through the transfer of function from the right to the left hemisphere, with preserved visual memory performance. Richardson, Strange, Duncan, and Dolan (2003) utilized a verbal encoding fMRI task and found that successful encoding was associated with activation of the left hippocampus in nonpatients, but the right hippocampus and parahippocampal gyrus in left TLE patients. A study of verbal semantic memory by Koylu et al. (2006) showed that, compared to controls, left TLE patients showed a shift in activation from the typical left frontal and medial temporal areas to homologs in the right hemisphere. The left TLE patients also recruited subcortical structures such as the thalamus and putamen to accomplish the task. In contrast, the right TLE patients more closely resembled healthy controls, though they did exhibit bilateral frontal hypoactivation. Alessio et al. (2013) studied verbal and visual memory in patients with hippocampal sclerosis, and found that left hippocampal sclerosis (HS) patients produced more bilateral or right-lateralized verbal encoding-related activations, suggesting reorganization in reaction to a dysfunctional mesial temporal lobe. For the visual memory encoding task in this study, the left and right HS groups, in addition to the controls, recruited widespread cortex bilaterally. The right HS group was the only group recruiting the left inferior temporal cortex, interpreted by the authors to reflect material-specific memory compensation of right mesial temporal dysfunction. Finally, in a FC study from our lab, examining memory, we found significant FC reductions in both left and right TLE localized in angular gyri, thalami, posterior cingulum, and medial frontal cortex. We found that the FC between the left non-pathologic MTL and the medial frontal cortex was positively correlated with the delayed recall score of a nonverbal memory test in right MTLE patients, suggesting potential adaptive changes to preserve this memory function (see Figure 19.2). In contrast, we observed a negative correlation between a verbal memory test and the FC between the left pathologic MTL and posterior cingulum in left MTLE patients, suggesting potential functional maladaptative changes in the pathologic hemisphere. Overall, this study provided some indication that left MTLE may be more impairing than right MTLE patients to normative functional connectivity. The data also indicated that the pattern of extratemporal FC might vary as a function of episodic memory material and each hemisphere's capacity for cognitive reorganization.

Interestingly, there is evidence from task-based fMRI studies of memory that reorganization may not always be adaptive. For instance, a study by Vannest, Szaflarski, Privitera, Schefft, and Holland (2008) demonstrated that intractable epilepsy (mixed pathology, some mesial temporal sclerosis, or MTS) influenced the functional neuroanatomy of a scene-encoding task, with both left and right epilepsy patients showing a pattern of increased contralateral medial temporal activation, within the setting of broader bilateral activation compared to healthy controls. This contralateral activation was associated with decreased memory performance, potentially providing evidence that not all reorganization is necessarily adaptive. It is important to note, however, that when unique (nonnormative) fMRI activation patterns are associated with lower cognitive performance, this could still represent adaptive compensation, emerging from incomplete or flawed compensation efforts.

Whole-brain network alterations have been observed in TLE relative to healthy controls in several specific functional networks including the well-known default mode network (DMN), in addition to attention, perceptual, and language networks (Liao et al., 2010; Waites, Briellmann, Saling, Abbott, & Jackson, 2006; Zhang, Lu, Zhong, Tan, Liao et al., 2009; Zhang et al., 2010; Zhang, Lu, Zhong, Tan, Yang, et al., 2009). These studies provide strong evidence that epileptic activity causes functional changes in complex and widespread resting-state networks (RSNs), putting at risk a wide range of neurocognitive and affective functions.

Most studies of resting-state FC in mesial TLE have focused on FC emerging from the ictal hippocampus (Doucet, Osipowicz, Sharan, Sperling, & Tracy, 2013; Morgan, Rogers, Sonmezturk, Gore, & Abou-Khalil, 2011; Pereira et al., 2010; Z. Zhang et al., 2010). The findings suggest that, compared to controls, there is increased connectivity with the contralateral hippocampus, as well as other contralateral limbic structures, with this interpreted as a form of compensatory connectivity (Bettus et al., 2010; Bettus et al., 2009; Doucet, Osipowicz, et al., 2013; Pittau, Grova, Moeller, Dubeau, & Gotman, 2012). Finally, resting-state FC work from our lab (Tracy et al., 2014) has shown that highly focal, unilateral TLE, with no evidence of interictal activity outside the ictal temporal lobe, is associated with a strong inhibitory surround (i.e., anticorrelated activity) in the contralateral hemisphere (see Figure 19.3). In contrast, TLE patients who display extratemporal interictal activity lack this surrounding anti-correlated activity. Thus, large regions of healthy cortex seem to respond, through contralateral anticorrelated activity, even to focal seizures, representing a form of protective and adaptive inhibition, helping to constrain epileptiform activity to the pathologic temporal lobe. The cognitive cost of maintaining such an inhibitory surround is unknown, but clearly this could put a variety of functions

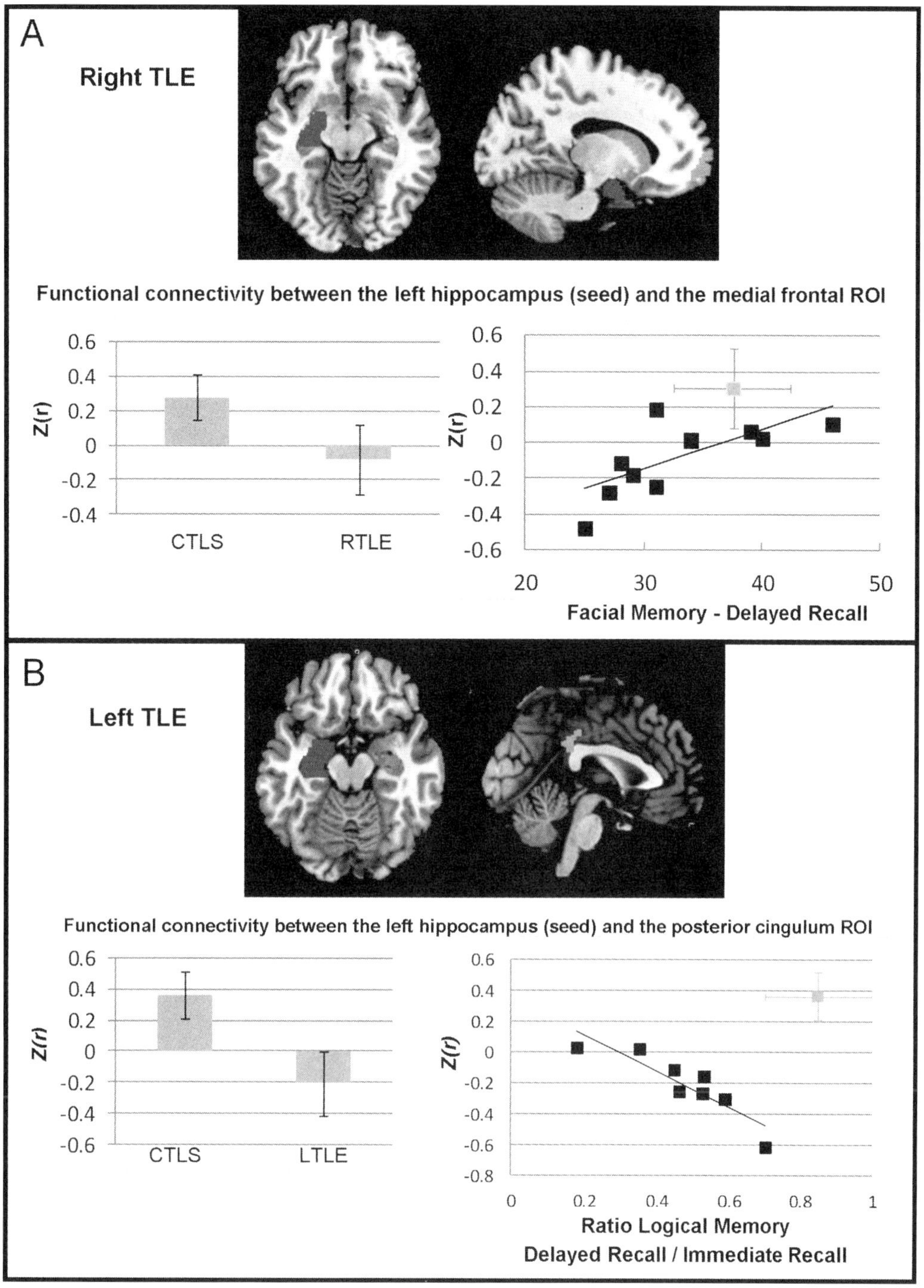

Figure 19.2 Correlation between FC values with the left hippocampal seed in right mesial TLE (RTLE), Panel A, and in left mesial TLE (LTLE), Panel B, with episodic memory scores. *A color version of this figure can be found in Plate section 2*

Modified and reprinted with permission from Human Brain Mapping, Doucet et al., (2013a), John Wiley and Sons.

Panel A: reduced FC between the left hippocampal seed (blue) and medial frontal cortex (green, $x = -14$, $y = 56$, $z = -10$; also see Table 3) in right mesial TLE patients compared with controls (*left bottom plot*); positive correlation between FC values between these two regions and the Facial Memory II Delayed Recall scores (*right bottom plot*, Spearman correlation, r = 0.78; p = 0.0045). The normative values of the controls on the right bottom plot are shown by the green data point where the *y-axis* indicates the average FC value of the controls' data and the *x-axis* is the normative value of age-matched healthy controls of the Facial Memory II Delayed Recall scores II score. Bars indicate standard deviation.

Panel B: reduced FC between the left seed (blue) and posterior cingulate cortex (green, $x = 2$, $y = -36$, $z = 32$; also see Table 3) in left mesial TLE patients compared with controls (*left bottom plot*); negative correlation between the FC values between these two regions and the ratio Logical Memory II Delayed Recall scores/ Logical memory I Immediate Recall scores (*right bottom plot*, Spearman correlation, r = −0.93; p = 0.001). The normative values of the controls are shown through the green data point where the *y-axis* indicates the average FC value of the controls' data and the *x-axis* is the normative value of age-matched healthy controls of the Logical Memory ration (II/I) score. Bars indicate standard deviation.

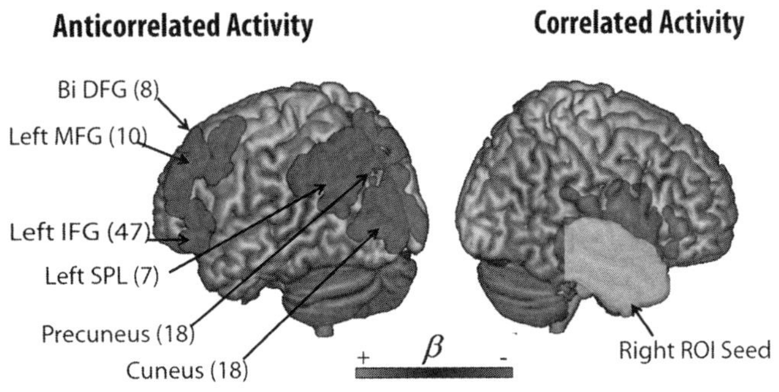

Figure 19.3 Positive (+) and negative (–) functional connectivity with the right temporal lobe ROI (*) in right unilateral TLE patients. DFG = medial part of superior frontal gyrus; MFG = middle frontal gyrus; IFG = inferior frontal gyrus; SPL = superior parietal lobule. *A color version of this figure can be found in Plate section 2*

Modified and reprinted with permission from Human Brain Mapping, Tracy et al. (2014), John Wiley and Sons.

at risk. Even lesional epilepsy with focal seizures appears to cause reactions throughout large regions of the brain, potentially impacting multiple cognitive functions and networks.

Importantly, these changes in network organization and FC appear related to actual cognitive performance, raising the possibility that episodic memory deficits in TLE are associated with changes in neocortical-hippocampal communication or interactions (i.e., changes in the excitatory/inhibitory balance) (Bartolomei et al., 2004; Liao et al., 2010; Tracy et al., 2014; Waites et al., 2006). For instance, Wagner and colleagues (2007) showed that stronger FC between the hippocampus and neocortical regions (e.g., inferior frontal and superior temporal cortices) was associated with better performance in right and left TLE patients during a verbal encoding and recognition memory task composed of concrete and highly imaginable word-pairs. Work from our lab (Doucet, Osipowicz, et al., 2013) has found the FC between the left non-pathologic mesial TL and the medial frontal cortex was positively correlated with delayed recall scores on a nonverbal memory task in right TLE patients, suggesting adaptive connectivity changes took place to preserve this memory function. In contrast, we observed a negative correlation between verbal memory performance and the level of FC between the left pathologic mesial TL and posterior cingulate cortex in left TLE patients, suggesting potential maladaptative changes in the pathologic hemisphere.

White matter (WM) connectivity can also be used to address issues of network reorganization. Fractional anisotropy (FA), which reflects microstructural integrity of WM, has shown that tracts proximal to the ictal focus have reduced FA in chronic TLE patients, i.e., the uncinate, the parahippocampal fasciculus, and the inferior longitudinal fasciculus (Ahmadi et al., 2009; Concha, Beaulieu, Collins, & Gross, 2009; Liacu, Idy-Peretti, Ducreux, Bouilleret, & de Marco, 2012). In addition, there is evidence that WM tracts in areas remote from the pathology have reduced FA as well, i.e., the corpus callosum, the internal/external capsules, and the arcuate fasciculus (Arfanakis et al., 2002; Otte et al., 2012). FA reductions, at least in part, appear to depend on the side of epilepsy, with left TLE associated with more extensive FA reductions bilaterally, whereas those with right TLE have more limited reductions often restricted to ipsilateral tracts (Kemmotsu et al., 2011; Pustina, Doucet, Skidmore, Sperling, & Tracy, 2014; Voets et al., 2009). These FA reductions in some instances correlate with diminished memory performance (Diehl et al., 2008; Yogarajah et al., 2008). Recent pilot data from our lab, however, suggest that the relationship between FA and seizures is mediated by other factors. We compared healthy controls with unilateral (ictal) TLE patients who had either bilateral or unilateral interictal spikes on EEG. Unexpectedly, patients with bilateral interictal spikes had more normative FA values in tracts connecting the two hemispheres, suggesting that the spread of epileptic pathology occurs in the context of better WM structural connectivity (Osipowicz et al., under review). Thus, impaired WM connectivity indexed by an FA decrease may have the benefit of isolating the ictal focus from the rest of the brain, mitigating or delaying the effect of epileptic activity on remote healthy areas. In other work from our lab we examined several WM tracts to determine which, in the setting of TLE, might be most associated with seizure spread. Our results indicated that the tapetum was associated with contralateral epileptiform activity, implicating this structure in seizures and possible secondary epileptogenesis. We describe two mechanisms that might explain this association (the interruption of inhibitory signals or the toxic effect of carrying epileptiform signals toward the healthy hemisphere), but also acknowledge other rival factors that may be at work. In this study, we also report that TLE patients with bilateral spikes had increased lateral bitemporal lobe functional connectivity. This study brought together important functional and structural data to elucidate the basis of contralateral interictal activity in focal, unilateral epilepsy. Finally, in our lab (Pustina et al., 2014a) we examined right and left anterior temporal lobectomy (ATL) patients, and found that in left ATL patients, preexisting low FA values in right superior longitudinal and uncinate fasciculi normalized after surgery. Preoperative verbal fluency correlated with FA values in all areas that later increased FA in left TLE patients, but postoperative verbal fluency correlated only with FA of the right superior longitudinal fasciculus. The results demonstrated that genuine reorganization occurs in nondominant language tracts after dominant hemisphere resection, a process that may help implement the interhemispheric shift of language activation found in fMRI studies. Moreover, the results indicate that left TLE patients, despite showing more initial WM damage, have the potential for greater adaptive changes postoperatively than right TLE patients.

Based on all the previously discussed work on cognitive network reorganization in TLE, it is tempting to conclude that recruiting regions of the healthy hemisphere into the network is an adaptive response to seizures, perhaps following the logic of material specificity (e.g., verbal memory shows a left-to-right hemisphere shift and recruitment in the setting of left temporal pathology and left language dominance). The evidence, however, is still too mixed, and other influential factors in terms of seizure type, strength of hemispheric dominance, education, chronological age, and variations in brain reserve have yet to be adequately explored. Indeed, when altered networks in TLE are discovered it is very difficult to know whether the pattern is innate and premorbid, or one that was initially organized normally and then reorganized in response to emergent and ongoing seizures, with the latter being the working assumption of most studies.

Multifocal Deficits in Focal Epilepsies

Given the clear evidence for pathological mechanisms and reorganization effects operating outside the epileptogenic zone, it is no surprise that patients with intractable, long-standing focal epilepsy exhibit greater cognitive dysfunction than would be expected solely on the basis of their focal epileptogenic pathology (Hermann, Seidenberg, Schoenfeld, & Davies, 1997). While it is readily known that generalized tonic-clonic (Wang et al., 2011) and absence seizures (Luo et al., 2011) can cause widespread disruptions of neural connectivity patterns and lead to diffuse cognitive dysfunction, well beyond the regions considered most likely to be the ictal generator (i.e., the thalamus), there is also evidence that such remote effects emerge from focal epilepsies such as TLE (Liao et al., 2010; Waites et al., 2006), with both ictal and interictal activity playing a role (Fahoum, Lopes, Pittau, Dubeau, & Gotman, 2012). For instance, Oyegbile and colleagues (2004) demonstrated that, in comparison to a group of healthy controls, patients with TLE exhibited not only worse memory performance, but also inferior performance on measures of intelligence, language, executive function, and motor speed, highlighting the extratemporal and sometimes widespread neurocognitive deficits associated with a focal epilepsy syndrome. One of the most difficult challenges for neuropsychologists is the variability in cognitive outcome in individual epilepsy patients. While relatively robust effects of memory impairment have been demonstrated, there is also a persistent finding of interindividual variability among epilepsy patients, both among those who demonstrate a good response to medication and those who remain refractory to medical or surgical treatment. Hermann, Seidenberg, Lee, Chan, and Rutecki (2007) utilized a taxonomic approach to predict cognitive and behavioral outcome by identifying distinct cognitive phenotypes based solely on classification by cognitive profile. By utilizing cluster analysis techniques to identify demographic, seizure, and neurobiological features associated with different cognitive phenotypes, the authors highlighted the multifocal nature of cognitive deficits in TLE patients (see Figure 19.4). In an examination of 96 patients

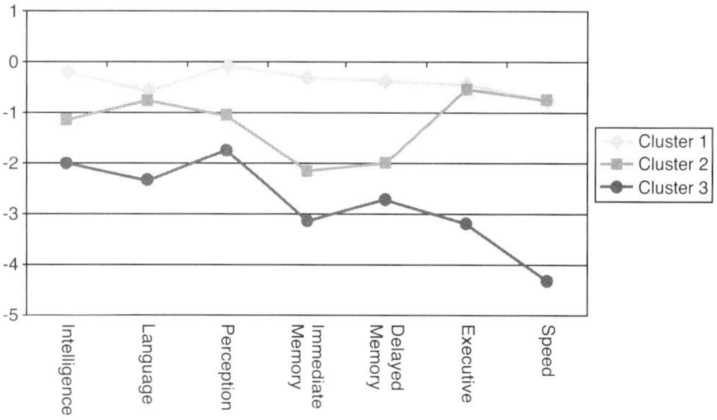

Figure 19.4 Mean cluster performance across cognitive domains. Cluster 1 = minimally impaired group; Cluster 2 = memory impaired group; Cluster 3 = memory, executive, and speed impaired group.

Modified and reprinted with permission from Journal of the International Neuropsychological Society, Hermann et al. (2006), Cambridge University Press.

with TLE and 82 healthy controls, three distinct cognitive profile types emerged: minimally impaired (47%); memory impaired (24%); and memory, executive, and speed impaired (29%). The more globally impaired group was older, had a longer duration of epilepsy, was prescribed more medications, and demonstrated abnormal WM and CSF volume. The authors concluded that this group was most likely to have incurred an early neurodevelopmental insult, and a more protracted and severe course of epilepsy that led to greater overall neurocognitive dysfunction. The search for cognitive phenotypes may yield greater understanding of the variability within epilepsy groups. Before turning to summarize some of the major neuropsychological findings within the most commonly encountered examples of focal epilepsy, it important to consider the factors that cause multifocal deficit patterns.

Several mechanisms appear to offer a more specific explanation for deficits in cognitive functions not typically associated with region of ictal focus. These include: undiagnosed seizure activity elsewhere in the brain, diaschisis (downstream impact on functioning), seizure propagation (spread, secondary generalization, interictal activity), secondary epileptogenesis (new neural connections built up by seizures), or the neuronal burden of maintaining an inhibitory surround to control seizures (see Tracy, Osipowicz, Stamos, and Berman, 2010 for further exploration of these processes). While areas proximal to the epileptogenic zone may be most strongly affected, more remote regions relying on either long or indirect pathway connections could be susceptible to these processes (Eliashiv, Dewar, Wainwright, Engel, & Fried, 1997; Weiser, 2004). These extratemporal effects are not considered truly random, as they likely take advantage of relative differences in the breakdown of protective/inhibitory neuronal processes in other brain areas. For instance, ipsilateral frontal cortex seems to be a common dispersion pathway for temporal lobe seizures, spreading through the uncinate fasciculus, with the contralateral temporal lobe (Morrell & deToledo-Morrell, 1999) being another common spread path. Neuropsychological testing can be sensitive to these extratemporal effects, but no current method exists to distinguish between deficits caused by the ictal focus versus those emerging from these other mechanisms. The hope is that by better integration of the neuropsychological data with techniques that can distinguish between these mechanisms (electrocorticography, functional connectivity analyses) finer-grained linkages between the neuropsychological data to specific epileptogenic processes can be made.

Temporal Lobe Epilepsy

Neuropsychological deficits within the episodic memory domain are well established in patients with MTLE (Bonilha, Alessio, et al., 2007; Helmstaedter & Kockelmann, 2006; Marques et al., 2007). Such impairments can be logically correlated with underlying medial temporal lobe pathology. However, patients with focal, lesional TLE have consistently demonstrated neurocognitive impairments in intelligence, language, visuospatial, executive, or motor function—impairments that cannot be solely explained by the underlying focal mesial neuropathology (Hermann, Seidenberg, & Jones, 2008). Several studies have documented that cognitive dysfunction in mesial TLE can, in particular, extend to domains such as language (e.g., naming and fluency) and executive functioning (Bartha et al., 2004; Corcoran & Thompson, 1993; Grant, Henry, Fernandez, Hill, & Sathian, 2005; Hermann, Wyler, & Richey, 1988; Howell, Saling, Bradley, & Berkovic, 1994; Martin et al., 2000; Schefft, Marc Testa, Dulay, Privitera, & Yeh, 2003; Shulman, 2000; Strauss, Hunter, & Wada, 1993; Tracy & Boswell, 2008; Trenerry, Jack, & Ivnik, 1993). For instance, Rzezak and colleagues (2007) identified significant executive dysfunction in 84% of a cohort of children and adolescents with TLE.

With regard to these deficits, it is likely extensive anatomic and functional connectivity between the frontal and temporal lobes that allows the temporal epileptogenic focus to impact frontal and prefrontal regions (Braakman et al., 2011). Evidence of the extratemporal seizure impact can be found in remote nonictal gray matter. For instance, structural neuroimaging studies have consistently shown atrophy in an extensive bilateral extratemporal network in unilateral TLE patients, most reliably in thalami, parietal, cerebellar, and contralateral temporal cortex including the contralateral hippocampus and parahippocampal gyrus (Bonilha, Rorden, et al., 2007; see review of Keller & Roberts, 2008; Riederer et al., 2008; Staba et al., 2012). Also, patients with a mesial temporal epileptogenic focus demonstrate ipsilateral reductions in extratemporal regions, including the thalamus, posterior cingulate cortex, cerebellum, and frontal and parietal opercular cortex (Cormack et al., 2005). Research with magnetic resonance imaging (MRI) using voxel-based morphometry (VBM) found hippocampal atrophy correlated with a reduction of gray matter concentrations in extra-hippocampal limbic regions, lateral temporal lobe, and orbito-frontal cortex (Bonilha et al., 2006; Duzel et al., 2006; Guerreiro et al., 1999).

This extratemporal seizure burden also appears in WM, with diffusivity abnormalities in TLE patients not restricted to the known epileptogenic temporal lobe (Gross, 2011), but extending to regions such as the posterior corpus callosum (Arfanakis et al., 2002), cerebellum, and the contralateral WM near the healthy (i.e., nonsclerotic) hippocampus, amygdala, and temporal pole (Thivard et al., 2005). Yu et al. (2008) found WM reductions in both temporal lobes, bilateral frontal lobes, and the corpus callosum. Even more distant from the epileptogenic region, cerebellar atrophy in the cerebellum has also been noted (Sandok, O'Brien, Jack, & So, 2000). In our lab (Pustina et al., 2014b), we examined right and left ATL lobectomy patients, and found that left ATL patients had lower FA values in tracts outside the pathologic temporal lobe (e.g., right superior longitudinal and uncinate fasciculi). In terms of still other measures, metabolic compromise appears to emerge both in the ipsilateral (ictal) and contralateral hemisphere in TLE patients, consisting of abnormal N-acetyl aspartate/choline ratios as derived from magnetic resonance spectroscopy. Blumenfeld and colleagues (2004) found increased cerebral blood flow (CBF) in the ipsilateral temporal lobe associated with seizure activity and simultaneously diminished CBF in frontal and parietal cortical regions. Arnold et al. (1996) reported suppressed regional cerebral glucose metabolism in the hippocampus, parahippocampal gyrus, and middle temporal gyrus, all ipsilateral to the epileptogenic focus. Blumenfeld et al. (2004) reported prominent slow-wave EEG activity in extratemporal areas during temporal lobe seizures, most notably the bilateral frontal and ipsilateral parietal association regions. Clearly, distinguishing the cognitive effects of these different seizure-related impacts and the time frame of their effects would be ideal, but is currently beyond reach by standard neuropsychological testing.

Frontal Lobe Epilepsy

Frontal lobe epilepsy (FLE) is the second most common localization-related or focal epilepsy. However, there are relatively few systematic studies examining the effect of FLE on cognition, and there are no known group studies examining neuropsychological functioning in nonlesional FLE cases. It has been more difficult to establish a "cognitive profile" of FLE due to the functional heterogeneity of the frontal lobes, the strong interconnections between prefrontal regions and associated brain regions, and the rapid propagation of frontal lobe seizures both bilaterally and to other cortical regions (Elger, Helmstaedter, & Kurthen, 2004; Lee, 2010; Yu et al., 2008). That said, there is good evidence suggesting the cognitive dysfunction in FLE is characterized by impairments similar to those seen in other frontal lobe diseases, with prominent behavioral changes and deficits in motor skills, attention, working memory, psychomotor speed, response inhibition, concept formation, and fluency (Exner et al., 2002; Helmstaedter, Kemper, & Elger, 1996). In a review of childhood FLE, attention, visuospatial organization, verbal search, mental flexibility, impulse control, working memory, complex motor sequences and coordination, and executive function (planning ability, response inhibition) deficits were the primary deficits, but there was significant interindividual variability. General reductions in IQ, language impairment, and memory deficits have also been reported (Braakman et al., 2011).

Emerging evidence from resting-state fMRI of altered network organization and connectivity patterns supports the network model of cognitive dysfunction in FLE. Vaessen and colleagues (2014) revealed whole-brain resting-state network abnormalities in children with FLE. In their cohort, children with more isolated functional brain subnetworks demonstrated greater cognitive impairment, suggesting less efficient interregional transfer. The authors concluded that decreased coupling between large-scale functional network modules is a hallmark for impaired cognition in childhood FLE. This line of research is in its infancy, with other data suggesting both high local and remote connectivity abnormalities compared to healthy controls (Luo, An, Yao, & Gotman, 2014). Centeno and colleagues (2014) reported evidence from structural MRI of increased gray matter volume in the piriform cortex, amygdala, and parahippocampal gyrus bilaterally, as well as the left mid-temporal gyrus of patients relative to controls, suggesting involvement of these areas in the epileptogenic network of FLE. Braakman et al. (2014) conducted diffusion tensor imaging (DTI) examining cerebral WM properties in children with FLE and healthy controls and revealed WM abnormalities predominantly in posterior brain regions beyond the epileptogenic focus. Importantly, the extent of WM abnormalities correlated with the severity of cognitive impairment. Abnormal structural network connectivity is increasingly being associated with impaired neurocognitive function (Widjaja, Zamyadi, Raybaud, Snead, & Smith, 2013).

Parietal and Occipital Lobe Epilepsy

Parietal lobe epilepsy (PLE) is rare even in large specialty centers, and few investigational series of PLE patients have been reported. The parietal lobe is comprised of large areas of association cortex and an extensive synaptic network that lends itself towards multiple seizure spread patterns, particularly to the frontal and temporal lobes (Foldvary et al., 2001; Williamson et al., 1992). Electrophysiological studies suggest that the interictal epileptiform discharges in PLE are widespread and multifocal, and often bilateral, suggesting an irritative zone that extends well beyond the epileptogenic focus (Binder et al., 2009). In addressing the frequent mislocalization of parietal lobe seizures on EEG, Ristic, Alexopoulos, So, Wong, and Najm (2012) refer to PLE as the "great imitator" among focal epilepsies due to greater variability in interictal and ictal EEG findings compared to FLE or TLE. Aura and ictal phenomena associated with PLE are often somatosensory in nature, and include paresthesias and dysesthesias, but ictal spread to the frontal lobe often transmutes ictal and postictal symptoms (Jokeit & Schacher, 2004). There have been very few studies exclusively examining cognition in PLE, likely due to the low frequency of such cases. Lesions in the parietal lobe have been associated with visual associative agnosia; attentional dysfunction, including hemineglect; visuospatial deficits; apraxia; and linguistic deficits. There is some evidence suggesting cognitive impairment extending beyond the epileptogenic zone, as children with PLE demonstrate diminished IQ, poor memory, inattention, and executive dysfunction (Gleissner, Kuczaty, Clusmann, Elger, & Helmstaedter, 2008).

Regarding occipital lobe epilepsy (OLE), ictal spread into frontal and temporal regions is quite frequent. Knopman and colleagues (2014) examined the cognitive profile of presurgical OLE patients with functional neuroimaging and neuropsychological assessment. Mild impairments in IQ, speed attention, and executive functioning were identified. In this sample, OLE was associated with widespread cognitive comorbidity, suggesting cortical dysfunction beyond the occipital lobe, another example of remote cortical dysfunction in focal epilepsy. Further, the investigators found that verbal memory impairment was associated with left temporal lobe hypometabolism, supporting the relationship between neuropsychological dysfunction and remote hypometabolism in focal epilepsy. Bilo et al. (2013) identified impairments in complex visuospatial and executive skills in a group of normal IQ patients with cryptogenic and idiopathic OLE, again suggesting that frontal and visuospatial cognitive deficits may reflect epileptic activity spreading within a neural network that extends beyond the occipital lobe.

Factors Mediating Cognitive Network Reorganization in Epilepsy

Age of Onset and Chronological Age

The best substantiated cases of cognitive reorganization involve individuals with early onset epilepsy (Springer et al., 1999). While seizures at an early age put individuals at risk for the effects of chronicity, the young brain exhibits greater plasticity, making it both more hyperexcitable and prone to seizures (Raol, Budreck, & Brooks-Kayal, 2003), but also better suited for cognitive reorganization. Left-sided hemispherectomy patients can display reorganization of language to the right side, though these children still have significant language deficits. This is particularly evident when removal of the dominant hemisphere occurs after age 6, a critical period for language acquisition (Hertz-Pannier et al., 2002;

Vargha-Khadem et al., 1997). Approximately 30% of children with epilepsy have intellectual and developmental disabilities (Tuchman, Moshe, & Rapin, 2009).

Atypical language networks in pediatric populations have been established through both intracarotid amobarbital studies (Rasmussen & Milner, 1977) and an abundant fMRI literature (Anderson et al., 2006; Yuan et al., 2006), with good evidence that patients with symptomatic and cryptogenic left TLE demonstrate varying evidence of language reorganization. In nonpatients, the natural developmental course of language shows a trend of increasingly left hemispheric lateralization from childhood to adulthood, with language lateralization in the dominant hemisphere increasing between the ages of 5–20, plateauing between ages 20–25, and slowly decreasing between ages 25–70 (Szaflarski, Holland, Schmithorst, & Byars, 2006). In order to disentangle the effect of pure epilepsy from lesional epilepsy in the pediatric population, Datta and colleagues (2013) examined the rates of atypical language dominance in children with benign epilepsy with centrotemporal spikes (BECTS), a common idiopathic pediatric epilepsy variant. While BECTS patients did not differ neurocognitively (perhaps due to the relatively mild nature of cognitive deficits associated with BECTS), patients demonstrated significantly lower language laterality indices than controls, with greater bilateral or right hemispheric activations during a sentence generation task. Notably, this finding persisted when controlled for duration of epilepsy and medication side effects.

At both a neuronal and cognitive level, neurocognitive reorganization can come at a cost. Animal studies have suggested a concomitant depletion in neural progenitor cells associated with neural repair. For instance, Dallison and Kolb (2003) found that when rats suffered early brain damage, hippocampal neurogenesis in adulthood was far below that of controls. The concept of "crowding effects" also demonstrates this phenomenon. The reduction of typically right hemisphere functions in favor of dominant hemisphere verbal memory processing implies that language can reorganize to the right hemisphere in left hemisphere epilepsy; however, there is often a cost in terms of material-specific memory loss or conflicts in information processing—disabling, for instance, simultaneous verbal and visual-spatial processing (Elger et al., 2004).

Impact of Chronicity

Factors such as the temporal pattern of the brain insult (i.e., slow vs. rapid) change the likelihood of both reorganization and the restoration of function. "Slow growing" pathologies (e.g., intractable seizures) increase the probability and efficiency of reorganization processes (Braun et al., 2008), particularly in regions more remote from the "at risk" skill or function. Interestingly, the initial brain insult that might produce a seizure is often followed by a latency period of epileptogenesis, which can take up to years before a clinically observable seizure occurs. Likewise, cognitive problems are often not demonstrated until after this latency period. Yet, once seizures begin, the disease and cognitive problems can progress even during the nonsymptomatic interictal state, although very little is known about the potentially unique cognitive impact of this interictal period.

Cognitive network reorganization is dynamic and there is an inherent constant evolution of these networks in response to chronic, intractable seizures. Consequently, the cognitive impact of seizures must be conceptualized with this underlying framework in mind, as well as interplay between cognitive network reorganization and the effects of advancing age. Resting-state FC research has begun to disambiguate these complex interactions. For instance, a resting-state study by Morgan et al. (2011) showed that cross-hippocampal connectivity varied with TLE duration. In the first ten years of seizures, connectivity was variable and often diminished, but beyond that point interhemispheric connectivity appeared to increase. Wang et al. (2011) investigated generalized tonic-clonic seizure (GTCS) patients at rest, and found that the degree of FC within key regions of either the DMN (the right medial prefrontal cortex), or the dorsal attention network (e.g., left intraparietal sulcus) were negatively correlated with epilepsy duration, suggesting damage accrues to these networks in association with more chronic GTCS. FC data from our lab (Doucet, Osipowicz, et al., 2013; Doucet et al., 2014) suggest that the characteristics of whole-brain organization (e.g., measures of segregation such as clustering coefficient, or CC) vary as an interaction between age of seizure onset and lesional status in TLE. For instance, when TLE onset comes early in life, the impact of MTS, the most common etiology for TLE, on whole-brain organization may be mitigated. In our data the late-onset MTS group, who had more perturbed whole-brain organization relative to matched controls, had an illness duration three times shorter than the early onset group, suggesting that the adult injured brain may need more time to develop compensatory responses to adult MTS pathology. Interestingly, we found very few differences between the late- and early onset groups in non-lesional TLE (i.e., no evidence of a structural lesion), suggesting that age of onset has little progressive impact on FC when no focal lesion is detectable.

Little is known about the effect of chronic seizures on the temporal stability of large-scale brain networks, such as those known to be involved in key cognitive function such as memory (i.e., the ventral default mode network, or vDMN). In our lab, we devised a measure of temporal stability of functional resting-state connectivity, capturing temporal variations of BOLD correlations between brain regions. In a comparison of TLE patients and matched, healthy controls, we found that temporal stability in the vDMN involving the temporal lobe does characterize the healthy brain, but that such functional connectivity in TLE patients shows instability (Robinson et al., 2014). It was unclear whether such instability arose as a pathologic mechanism from the impact of seizures or as a protective mechanism to ensure functional integrity and prevent seizure spread (Tracy et al., 2014). Given the link of the vDMN network with episodic memory, the findings raise the possibility that the episodic memory disorder observed in TLE may be related to instability of the vDMN network. Electrophysiology research is beginning to address the dynamic changes that occur in networks over various time scales (Honey, Kotter, Breakspear, & Sporns, 2007). As this knowledge increases, we will be able to distinguish the more transient acute effects (i.e., ictal or temporary interictal effects) from the initial and more drawn-out effects of chronic seizures.

Impact of Cerebral Dominance

There is strong evidence that early onset epilepsy is associated with higher rates of atypical language representation involving either bilateral or more complete language representation in the right hemisphere. In an intracarotid amobarbital study of TLE from our lab (Tracy et al., 2009), we found that 40.3% of left TLE patients (n = 124) displayed atypical language organization (i.e., stronger right hemisphere representation) on at least one language skill (e.g., repetition, naming, comprehension, reading, and speech quality/dysarthria; see Figure 19.5). While the majority (60%) of patients showing atypical language representation do so on more than one language skill, the proportion showing atypicality on all five skills was low, only 5.6% of the left TLE sample. These data clearly show atypical hemispheric dominance is not an "all-or-nothing" phenomenon, with all aspects of language reorganizing together in a monolithic fashion. Thus, hemispheric language dominance and its reorganization is a heterogeneous, complex process, with distinct language systems showing independence, making clear that the pressures compelling atypical reorganization in TLE do not work with equal force on all language functions.

Finally, it is worth noting that there is some evidence that gray matter extra-temporal damage is more widespread in left compared to right-sided TLE (Riederer et al., 2008), raising the possibility that regional seizure network growth may be influenced by brain function properties such as the presence of language dominance.

Cognitive and Behavioral Impact of Medications

Antiepileptic drugs (AEDs) are frequently associated with cognitive side effects. While the newer AEDs typically exhibit less-adverse neurocognitive profiles, medication must be considered when distinguishing the multiple forces influencing a patient's cognition. Medication side effects can negatively affect medication compliance, everyday functioning, and quality of life (Witt & Helmstaedter, 2013). Side effects are generally based on four factors: dose concentration, inherent side effects, idiosyncratic effects, and drug load (i.e., additive or interactive effects of multiple medications). While a comprehensive review is beyond the scope of this chapter, a basic knowledge of AED side effect profiles is necessary for neuropsychological evaluation of patients with seizure disorders.

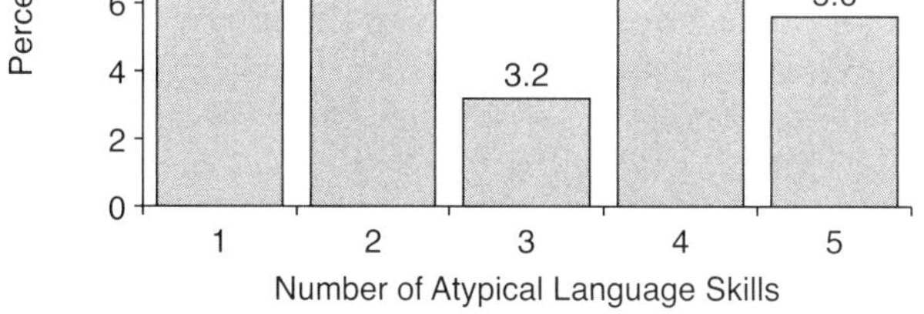

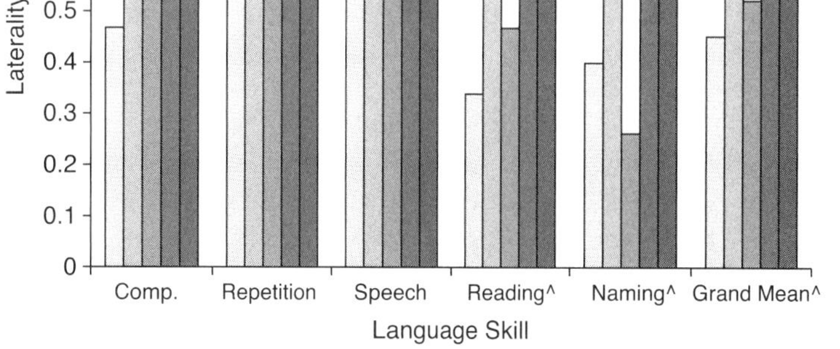

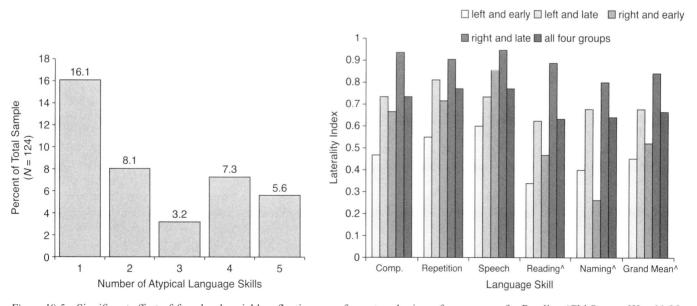

Figure 19.5 Significant effect of four level variable reflecting age of onset and seizure focus groups for Reading (Chi Square [3] = 11.95, $p < 0.01$), and the Grand Mean (Chi Square [3] = 9.7, $p < 0.05$).

Panel A, left chart. Percent of total sample (N = 124) showing atypical dominance for one, two, three, four, or all five language skills.

Panel B, right chart. Mean Laterality Index of five language skills for left and early, left and late, right and early, right and late, and all four groups.

Table 19.1 Overview of affected domains by different antiepileptic medications

Antiepileptic agent	*Affected Domains*		
Carbamazepine	↓	↓	
Clobazam	↓	0	↓
Felbamate	(↓)		
Gabapentin	↓	0	0
Lamotrigine	0	0	0
Oxcarbazepine	0	0	
Phenobarbital	↓ / ↑	0	
Phenytoin	↓	↓	↓
Tiagabine	↓	↓	
Topiramate	0	0	0
Valproic Acid	↓	↓	↓
Vigabatrin	↓	↓	0
Zonisamide	0	0	0

↓, negative effect; ↑, positive effect; ( ): possible effect; 0: no deficits.
Modified and reprinted with permission from Epilepsy & Behavior, *Witt & Helmstaedter (2013).*

Table 19.1 depicts in general terms the cognitive profile associated with the major current antiepileptic medications.

Importantly, while much of the literature compares and contrasts the relative cognitive impact of AEDs, the majority of medications have some, albeit sometimes subtle, impact on cognitive functioning, particularly attention and memory (Witt & Helmstaedter, 2013). Of the traditional AEDs, benzodiazepines and phenobarbital are more commonly associated with negative cognitive side effects in comparison to phenytoin, valproic acid, or carbamazepine. Phenobarbital has been linked to lower IQ (Farwell et al., 1990), slowed psychomotor speed, impaired attention, and reduced processing speed (Manni, Ratti, Perucca, Galimberti, & Tartara, 1993). While relatively less impactful, phenytoin has been associated with declines in visuomotor function (Pulliainen & Jokelainen, 1995) and carbamazepine has been associated with reductions in information processing speed, attention, memory, and verbal fluency (Wesnes, Edgar, Dean, & Wroe, 2009). Valproic acid has consistently demonstrated minimal cognitive interference (Eddy, Rickards, & Cavanna, 2011), but has been associated with Parkinsonism in a very small subset of patients (Ristic, Vojvodic, Jankovic, Sindelic, & Sokic, 2006).

In large part, second-generation AEDs have a superior cognitive profile, with the exceptions of topiramate and, potentially, zonisamide. Topirimate is notorious among AEDs for cognitive side effects, and while attention and a specific verbal fluency deficit are most common, impaired concentration, cognitive slowing, psychomotor slowing, short-term memory, and working memory have all been reported (Coppola et al., 2002; Fritz et al., 2005; Froscher et al., 2005; Gomer et al., 2007). There is evidence of improvement in cognitive functions following topiramate withdrawal (Kockelmann, Elger, & Helmstaedter, 2003). There is also emerging evidence of cognitive dysfunction associated with zonisamide. A prospective, randomized trial of the long-term effects of zonisamide monotherapy demonstrated good seizure control and minimal increase in psychiatric symptomatology but significant reductions in aspects of memory, verbal fluency, and information processing speed (Park et al., 2008).

Amongst the second-generation AEDs, levetiracetam and lamotrigine demonstrate the most appealing neurocognitive profiles. Studies have consistently shown no cognitive impact for these AEDs (Bootsma et al., 2008; Huang, Pai, & Tsai, 2008; Levisohn et al., 2009; Pressler, Binnie, Coleshill, Chorley, & Robinson, 2006). In fact, both have been shown to have positive effects on cognition. For instance, a randomized, double-blind, placebo-controlled examination of levetiracetam reported improvements in cognitive set-shifting, attention, and verbal memory in patients with complex partial seizures in comparison to healthy controls (Zhou et al., 2008). As a result of such work, levetiracetam is being evaluated for broader use as a cognitive enhancer. Similarly, few adverse cognitive effects have been associated with tiagabine (Aikia, Jutila, Salmenpera, Mervaala, & Kalviainen, 2006) and there is some evidence of improvement in motor speed, concentration, and verbal fluency with tiagabine therapy (Dodrill et al., 1998). Unstudied aspects of antiepileptic medications remain the effects of shorter versus longer term use, and the way particular medications may interact with aging.

Are Cognitive Deficits Progressive?

There are somewhat mixed results in the literature when trying to determine if cognitive deficits in epilepsy worsen with continued seizures. Some studies suggest a relative stability in cognitive status over time (Dodrill & Wilensky, 1992), whereas most others suggest that when seizures remain intractable there is steady damage to hippocampal circuitry, with progressive and cumulative adverse cognitive effects (Bernhardt, Chen, He, Evans, & Bernasconi, 2011; Sutula, 2004). Several studies of TLE have suggested that neuropsychological deficits increase with epilepsy duration (Helmstaedter, 2002; B. Hermann, Seidenberg, & Bell, 2002; Jokeit & Ebner, 2002). A longitudinal study of ATL patients post-surgery revealed progressive cognitive decline with ongoing intractable seizures (Helmstaedter, Kurthen, Lux, Reuber, & Elger, 2003). There does appear to be a mild accumulating and deteriorative effect on IQ in TLE (Dodrill, 2004), with some cross-sectional studies suggesting IQ declines after about three decades (Jokeit & Ebner, 2002). Other longitudinal studies make clear that TLE causes a slow and steady decline in episodic memory that cannot strictly be accounted for by age (Hamberger & Cole, 2011; Jokeit & Ebner, 1999; Rausch et al., 2003). It may be that duration of active epilepsy is a better predictor of the severity of cognitive deficits than type or even location of the seizures (Farwell, Dodrill, & Batzel, 1985). Fortunately, there is some data that suggests memory decline in epilepsy can be stopped, if not reversed, if seizures are fully controlled (C. Helmstaedter et al., 2003).

There are clear neuroanatomical differences in chronic TLE patients in comparison to healthy controls. Dabbs and colleagues (2012) reported extensive anatomic abnormalities in a group of adults ($N = 55$) with childhood/adolescent onset epilepsy. The authors identified significant abnormalities in subcortical structures, cerebral gray matter, and WM, in terms of both total volume and thickness in temporal and extratemporal lobes (frontal and parietal). In comparison to healthy controls, however, age-accelerated changes were identified in the third and lateral ventricles only, suggesting that brain changes occurring in epilepsy progressed in a largely age-appropriate manner, with the exception of age-accelerated ventricular expansion.

Helmstaedter et al. (2014) suggest a developmental hindrance effect, such that the majority of cognitive deficits evolve at the onset of, if not before, the first seizure, and interfere with normal cognitive development. Critical phases for episodic memory are at work throughout childhood and young adulthood; when these critical periods are interfered upon, the risk for premature cognitive decline increases. This notion is supported by a Helmstaedter and Elger (2009) study examining cross-sectional comparisons of age-related regressions on verbal learning and memory in a large TLE sample ($n = 1,156$) compared to healthy controls ($n = 1,000$). The authors identified critical phases during which epilepsy interfered with normal cognitive development during childhood and in adolescence. The learning/memory curve for TLE patients peaked earlier (ages 16–17 vs. 23–24 in healthy controls), but was then comparable to the normal group. However, due to the initial discrepancy between groups, TLE patients reached levels of impairment significantly earlier. The implications of this model highlight the importance of early control of epilepsy, and the value of examining the interaction between the life course of epilepsy and aging/developmental effects.

Interaction Between Cognitive and Emotional/Behavioral Disruptions

The comorbidity of epilepsy and depression is well established (Fuller-Thomson & Brennenstuhl, 2009; Tellez-Zenteno, Patten, Jette, Williams, & Wiebe, 2007). Depression and anxiety represent the most commonly reported comorbid symptoms by TLE patients (Tracy, Dechant, Sperling, Cho, & Glosser, 2007; Tracy, Lippincott, et al., 2007). Lifetime prevalence estimates of depression in epilepsy range from 13% to 35%, with much of the variability accounted for by the heterogeneity in depression ascertainment methods (Fiest et al., 2013). Depression is the strongest predictor of diminished quality of life in epilepsy, not seizure frequency, nor age of epilepsy onset (Boylan et al., 2004; Tracy, Dechant, et al., 2007).

Historically, patients with TLE were thought to experience more depressive symptoms than patients with generalized epilepsy or extra-temporal foci (Harden, 2002), although this finding has not been consistently replicated. There are multiple cumulative factors that contribute to depression in epilepsy, including seizure frequency, age of onset, laterality of temporal lobe focus, and concomitant frontal lobe dysfunction (Garcia, 2012).

More recently, we have begun to understand the neurobiology behind the comorbidity of psychiatric symptoms and TLE, with some arguing that depression emerges from epileptic activity (Reuber, Andersen, Elger, & Helmstaedter, 2004). Given the major role of the amygdala in the processing of fear and related emotions (LeDoux, 2000; Phelps & LeDoux, 2005), several studies have suggested this structure plays a role in the expression of comorbid emotional conditions (see review of Kondziella, Alvestad, Vaaler, & Sonnewald, 2007). A positive correlation has been described between the left amygdala volume and depression severity in left TLE patients (Tebartz van Elst, Woermann, Lemieux, & Trimble, 2000, 1999), with the authors suggesting the amygdala is hyperactive in anxiety and mood disorders (Tebartz van Elst et al., 1999). Physiologic studies have demonstrated a positive correlation between the density of neuropeptide Y-positive neurons in the amygdala and depression scores in MTLE patients (Frisch et al., 2009). Also, studies in psychiatric samples have revealed a direct relation between atypical amygdala responsiveness and either anxiety (Killgore & Yurgelun-Todd, 2005; Thomas et al., 2001) or depression levels (Abercrombie et al., 1998; Roberson-Nay et al., 2006). The amygdala, and more generally the limbic system, of the right hemisphere is more highly involved in emotional processing (see reviews of Davidson, 2003; Gainotti, 2012), and is associated with higher levels of panic and other emotional disorders than the left hemisphere (Sazgar, Carlen, & Wennberg, 2003).

As was the case with cognition, neuroimaging techniques are providing a growing body of evidence that the functional abnormalities in MTLE associated with their psychiatric status are not limited to the epileptogenic region. For instance, task (i.e., emotion-driven) fMRI imaging has provided evidence of amygdala abnormalities in MTLE. Bonelli et al. (2009) showed that left MTLE patients had significantly reduced activation in left and right amygdala compared to controls and right MTLE patients during the viewing of fearful and neutral faces. In addition, these authors demonstrated that in right but not left MTLE patients, bilateral amygdala activation was significantly related to the level of anxiety and depression reported. Data from our lab showed that FC emerging from subdivisions of the amygdala are distinct and vary with the side of the epileptic pathology. Right MTLE patients show more functional network impairments involving the amygdala compared to controls than left MTLE patients, with these impairments associated with increased psychiatric symptomatology (see Figure 19.6; see also Doucet, Skidmore et al., 2013).

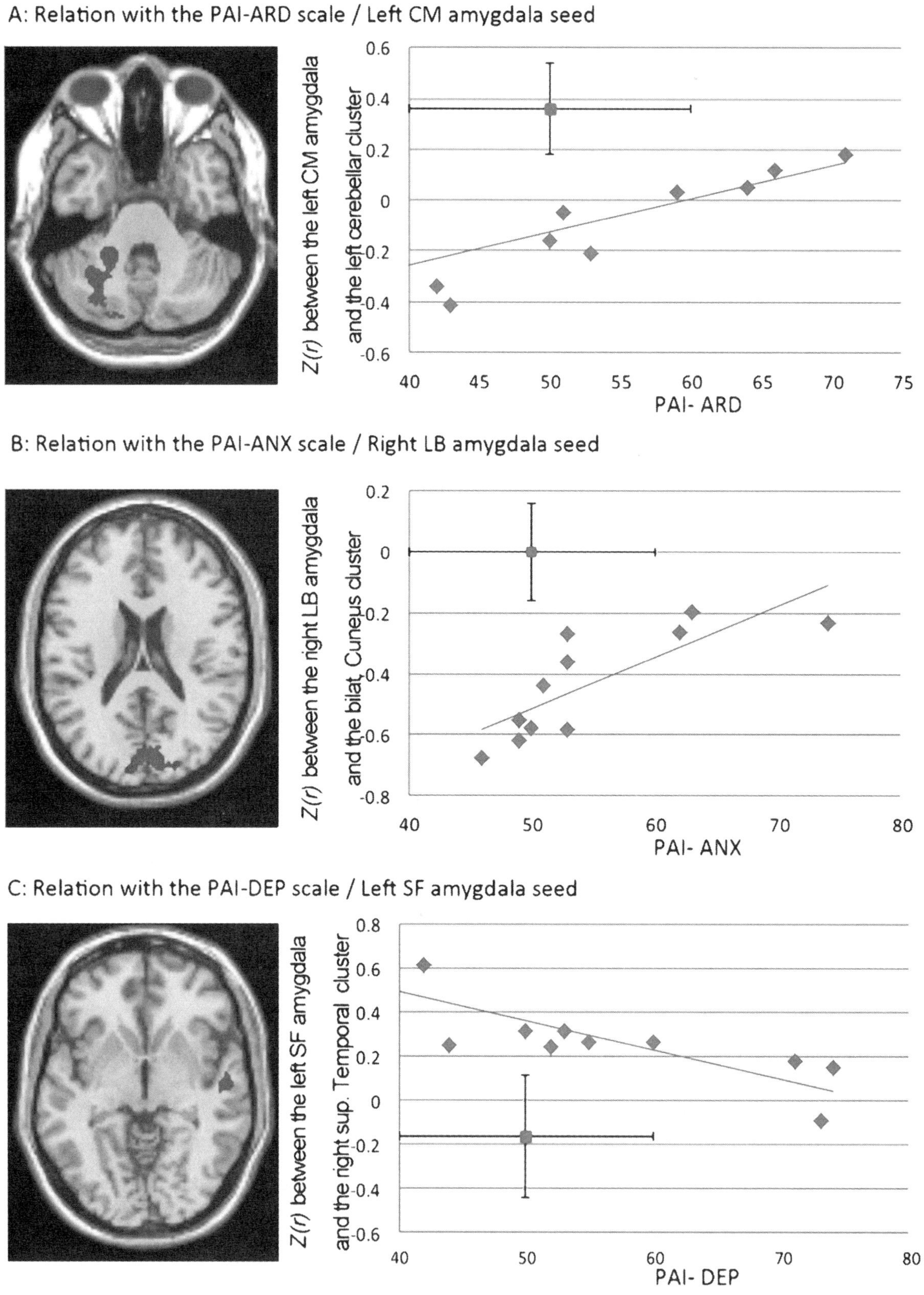

Figure 19.6 Significant relationships between abnormal reduced FC in the RMTLE group. Panel A: with the anxiety-related disorder level scale (PAI-ARD). Panel B: with the anxiety level scale (PAI-ANX). C: Panel with the Depression level scale (PAI-DEP). The mean FC value for normal controls (with standard deviation [SD] as vertical line) and the PAI-manual referenced value for normals (with SD as horizontal line) is displayed in red. *A color version of this figure can be found in Plate section 2*

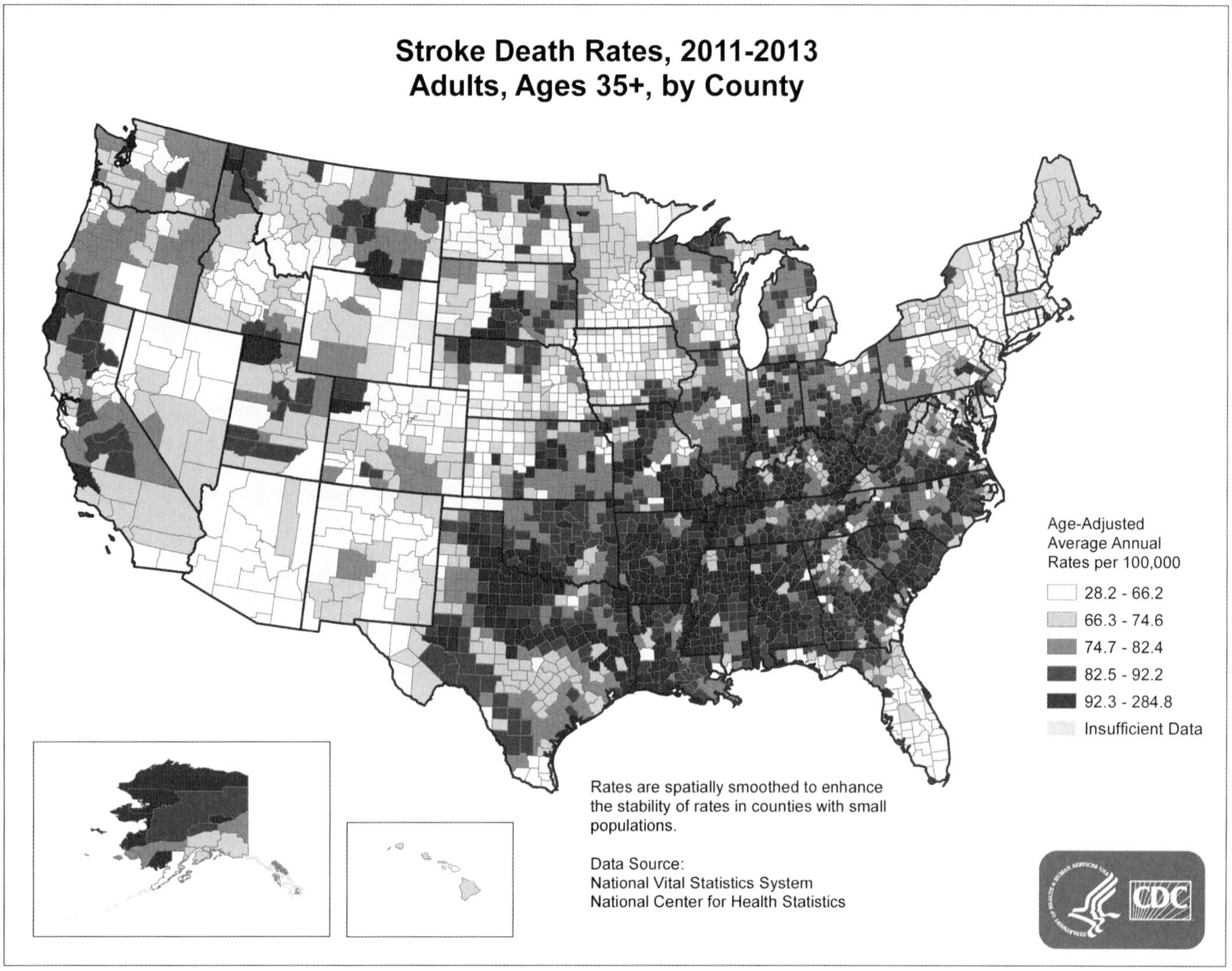
Stroke Death Rates, 2011-2013
Adults, Ages 35+, by County
Age-Adjusted
Average Annual
Rates per 100,000
28.2 - 66.2
66.3 - 74.6
74.7 - 82.4
82.5 - 92.2
92.3 - 284.8
Insufficient Data
Rates are spatially smoothed to enhance the stability of rates in counties with small populations.
Data Source:
National Vital Statistics System
National Center for Health Statistics
CDC

Figure 16.1

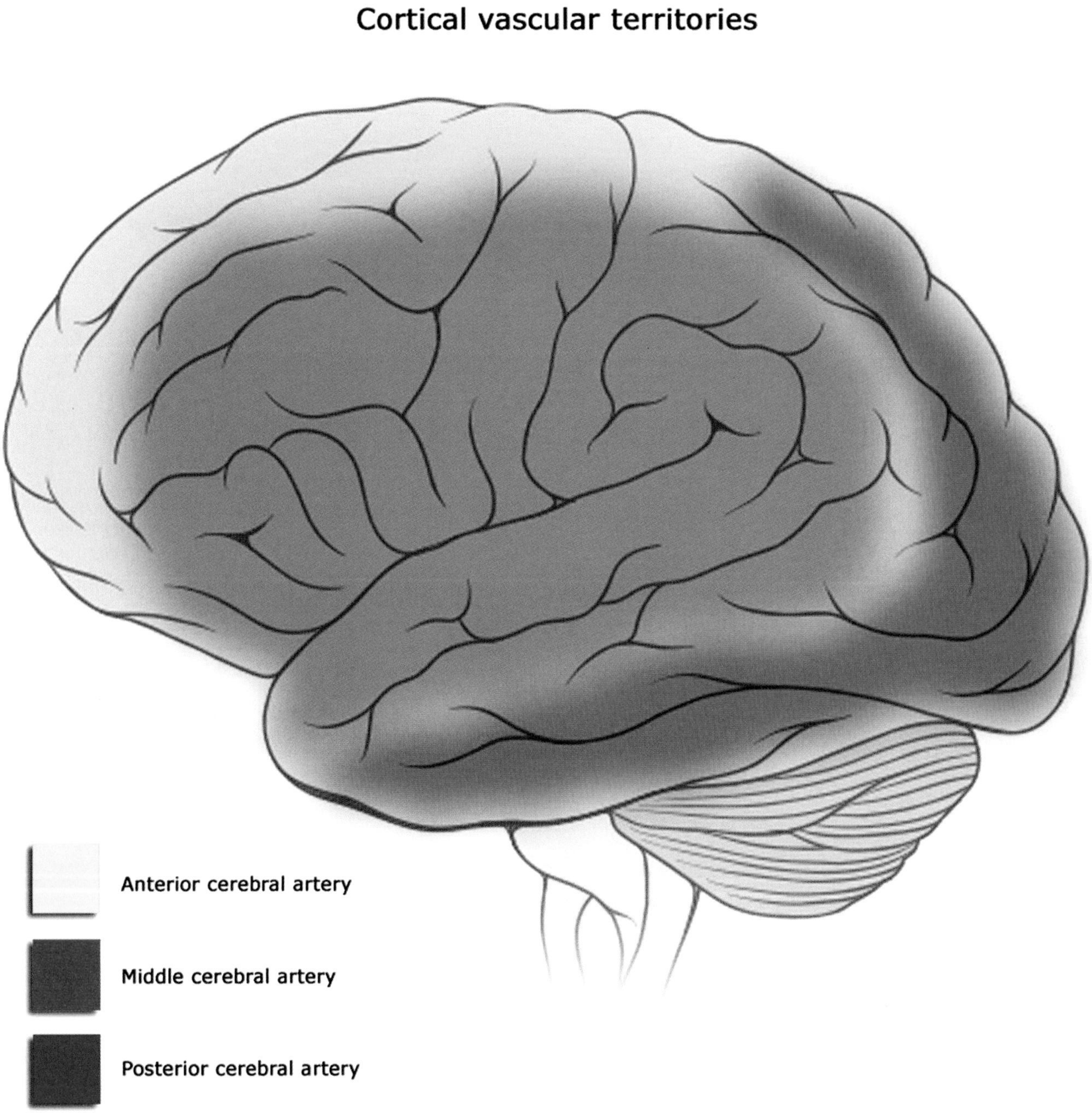
Cortical vascular territories
Anterior cerebral artery
Middle cerebral artery
Posterior cerebral artery

Figure 16.3

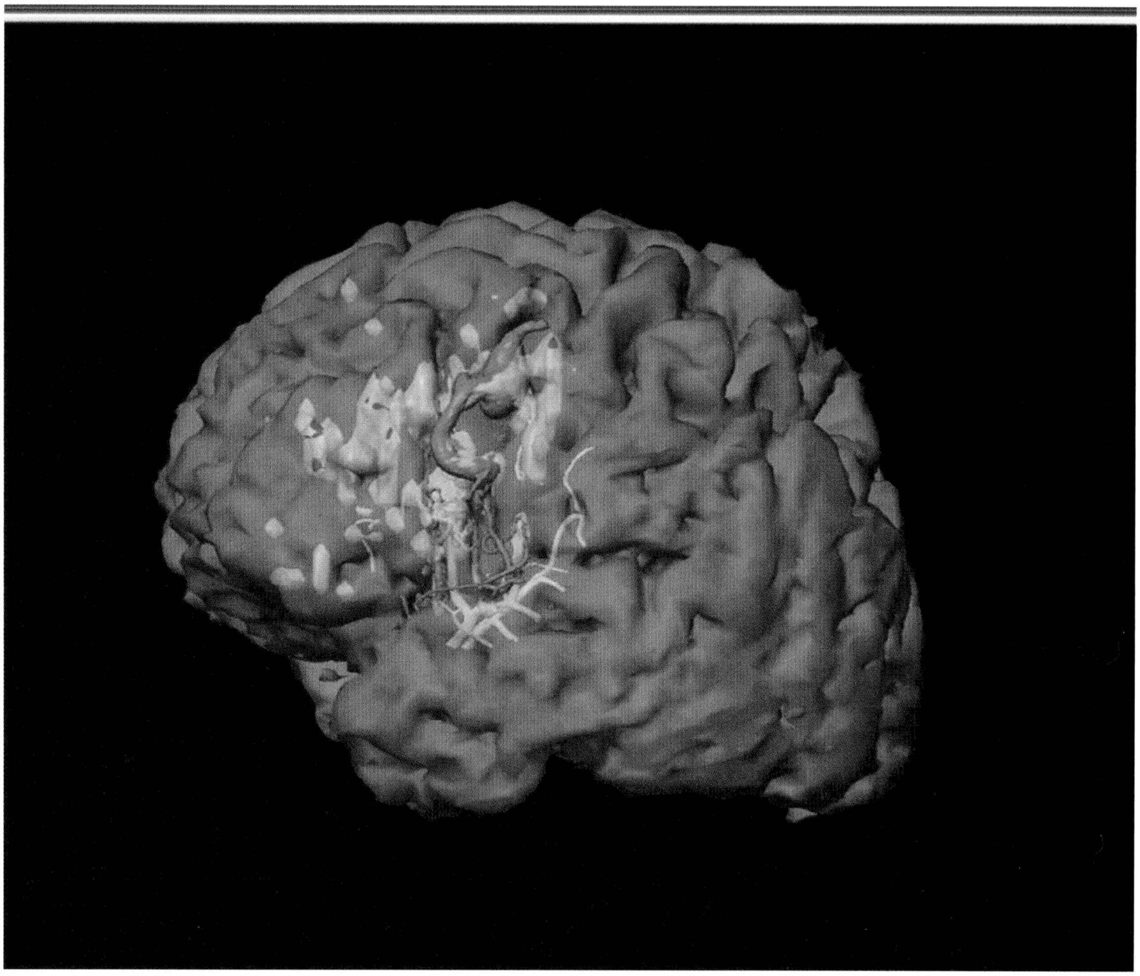

Figure 16.6

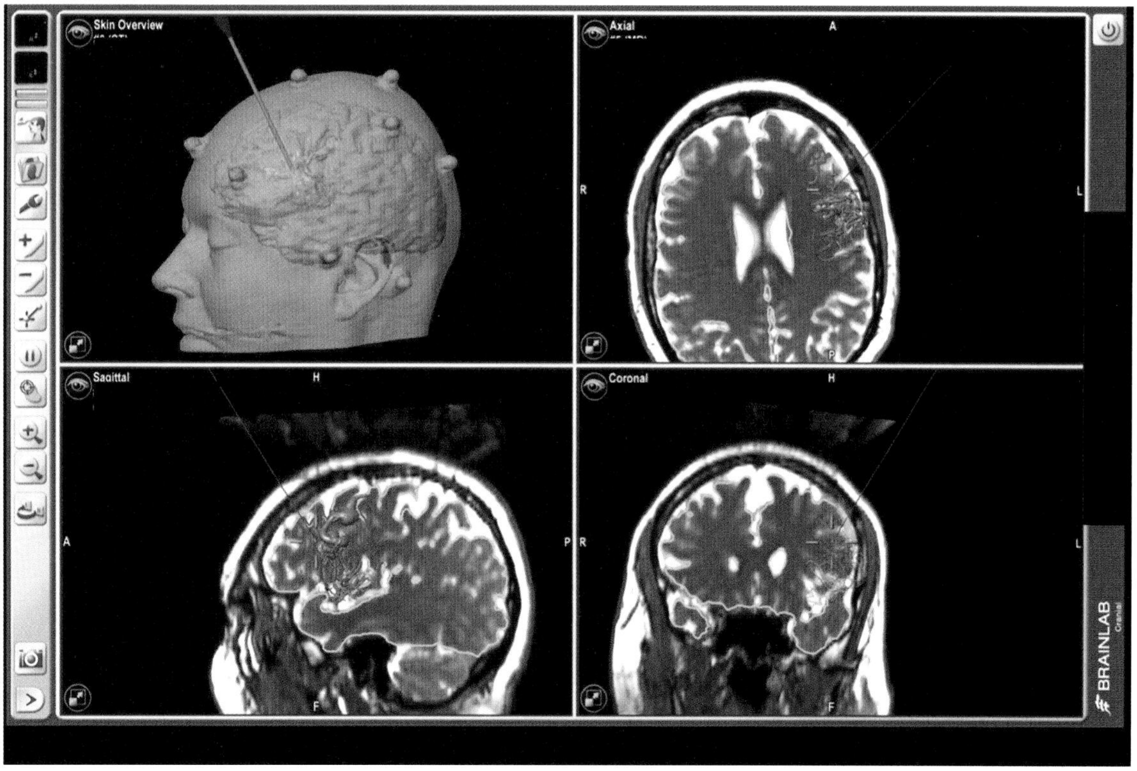

Figure 16.7

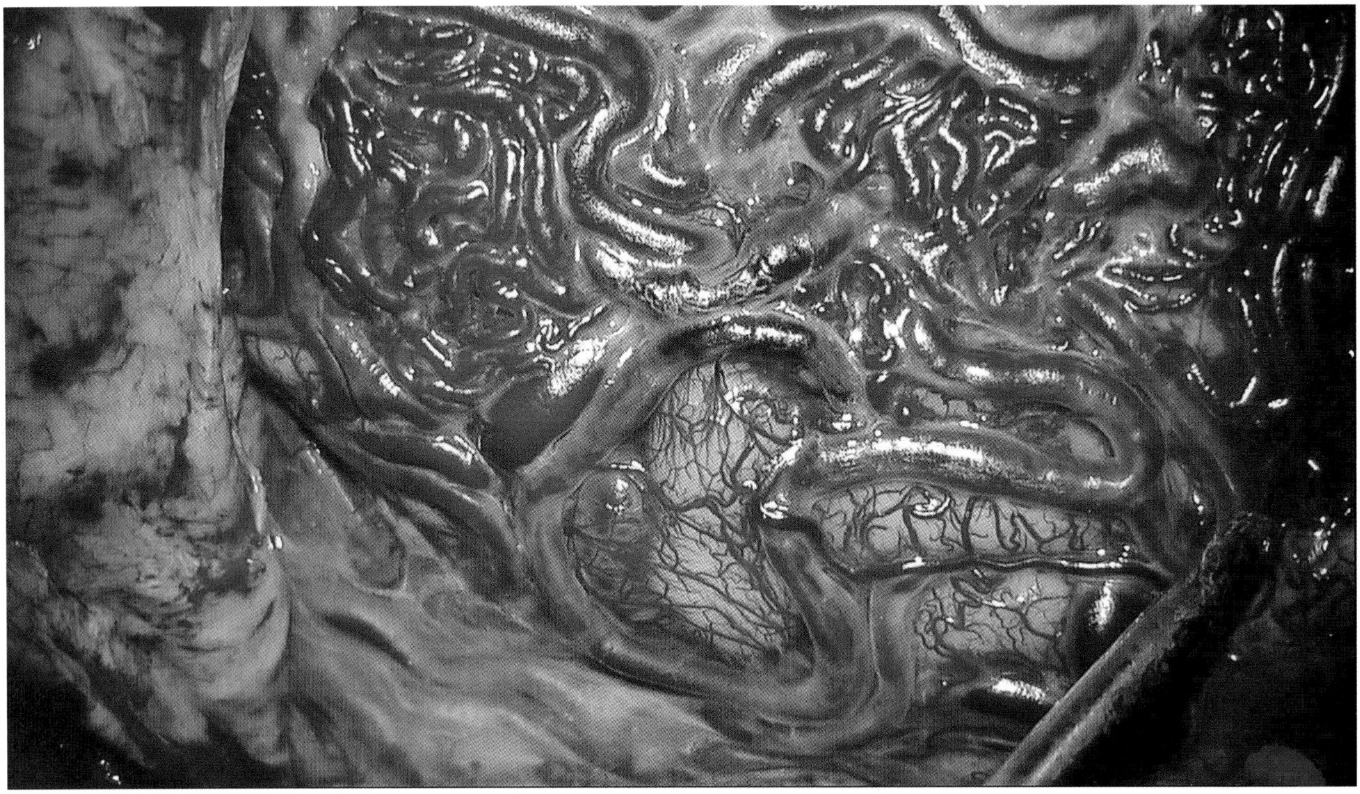

Figure 16.8

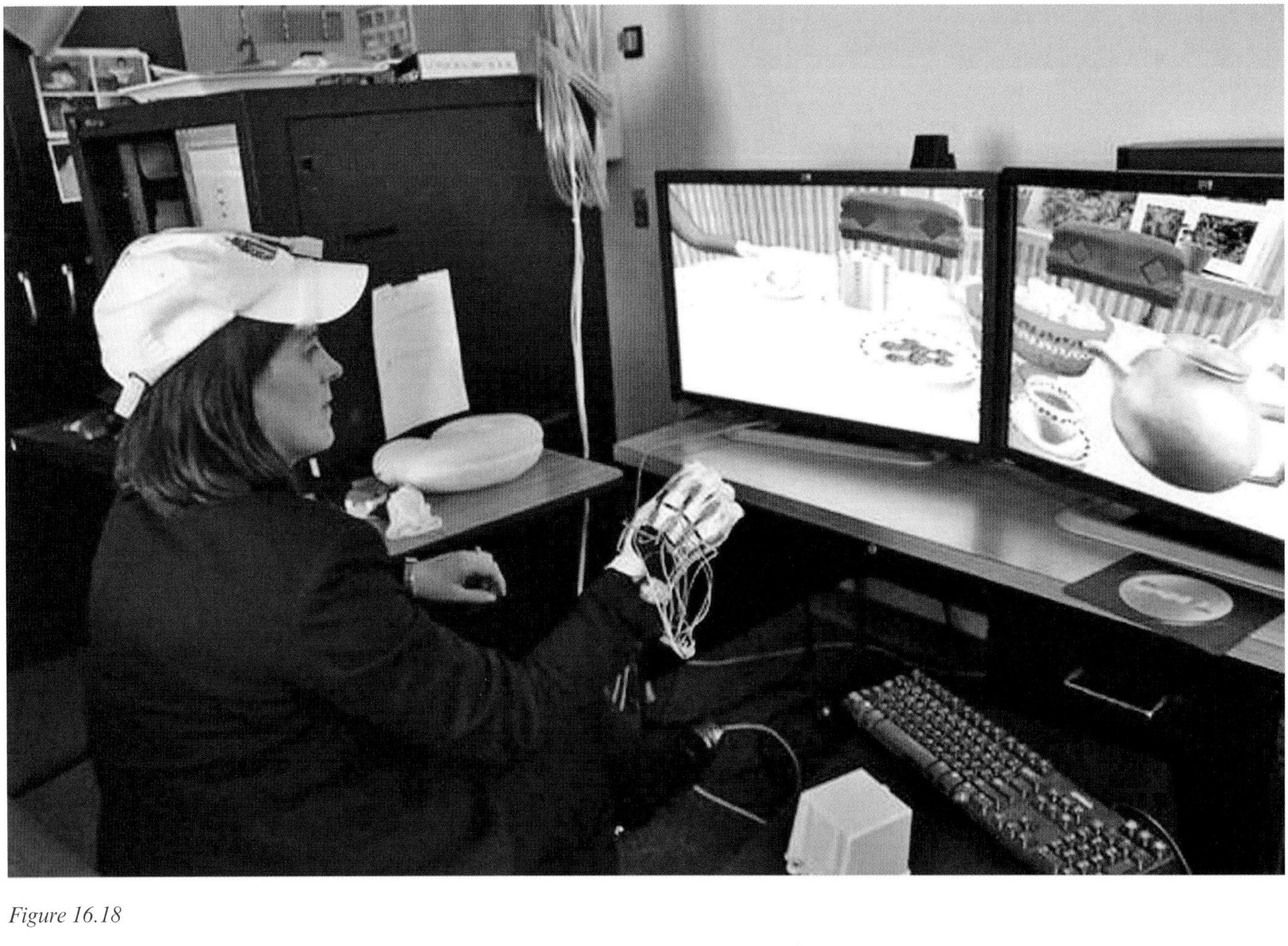

Figure 16.18

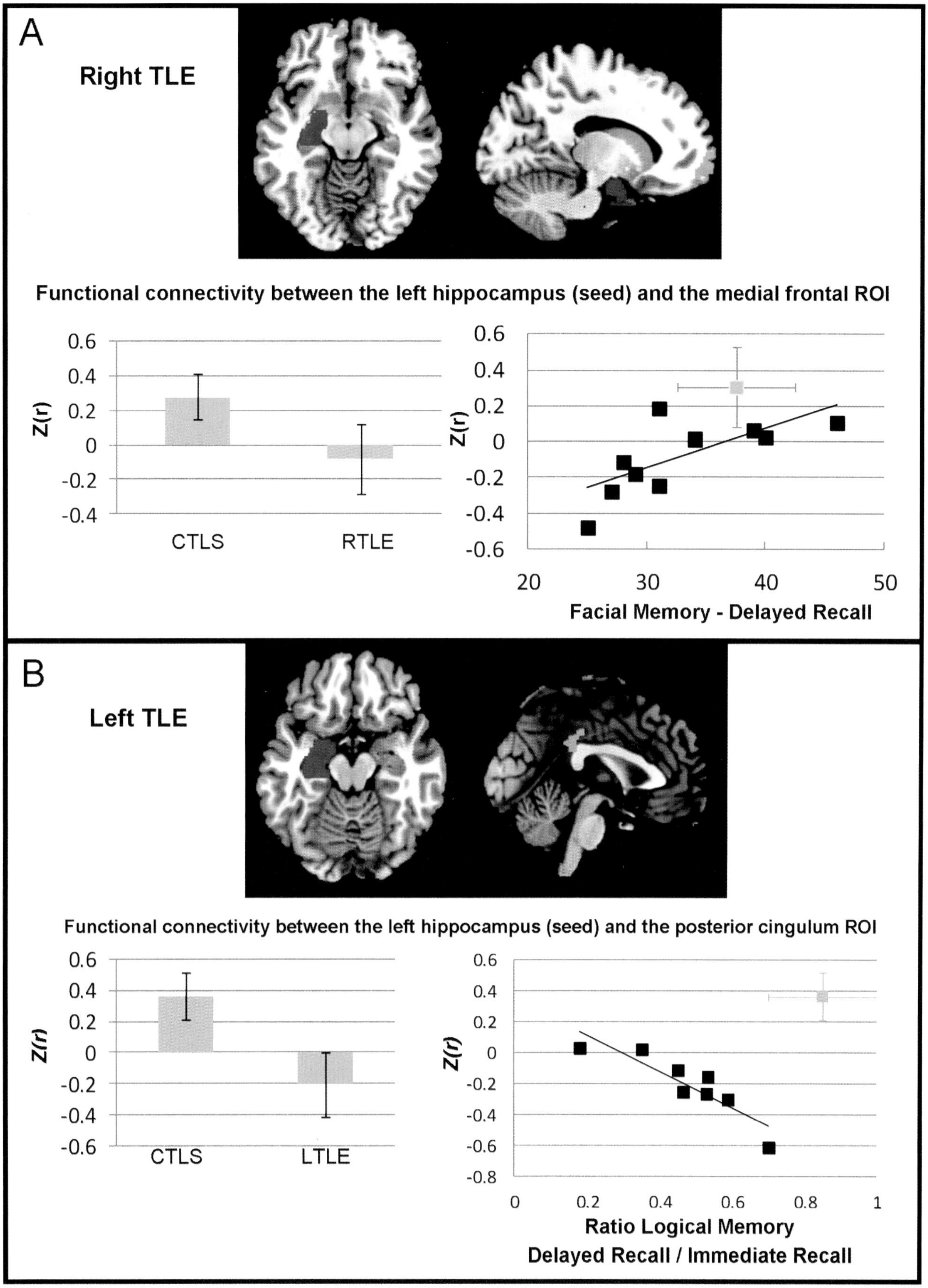
A
Right TLE
Functional connectivity between the left hippocampus (seed) and the medial frontal ROI
0.6
0.4
0.2
0
-0.2
-0.4
Z(r)
CTLS
RTLE
0.6
0.4
0.2
0
-0.2
-0.4
-0.6
Z(r)
20
30
40
50
Facial Memory - Delayed Recall
B
Left TLE
Functional connectivity between the left hippocampus (seed) and the posterior cingulum ROI
0.6
0.4
0.2
0
-0.2
-0.4
-0.6
Z(r)
CTLS
LTLE
0.6
0.4
0.2
0
-0.2
-0.4
-0.6
-0.8
Z(r)
0
0.2
0.4
0.6
0.8
1
Ratio Logical Memory
Delayed Recall / Immediate Recall

Figure 19.2

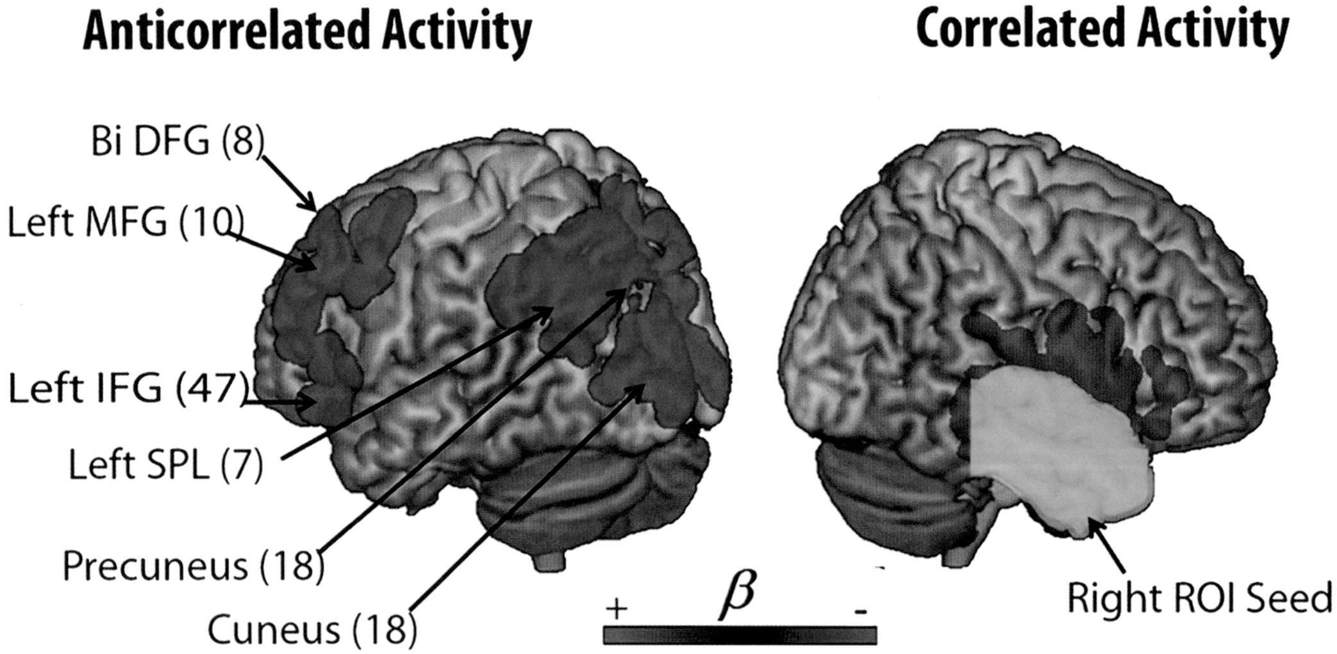
Anticorrelated Activity
Correlated Activity
Bi DFG (8)
Left MFG (10)
Left IFG (47)
Left SPL (7)
Precuneus (18)
Cuneus (18)
+
β
-
Right ROI Seed

Figure 19.3

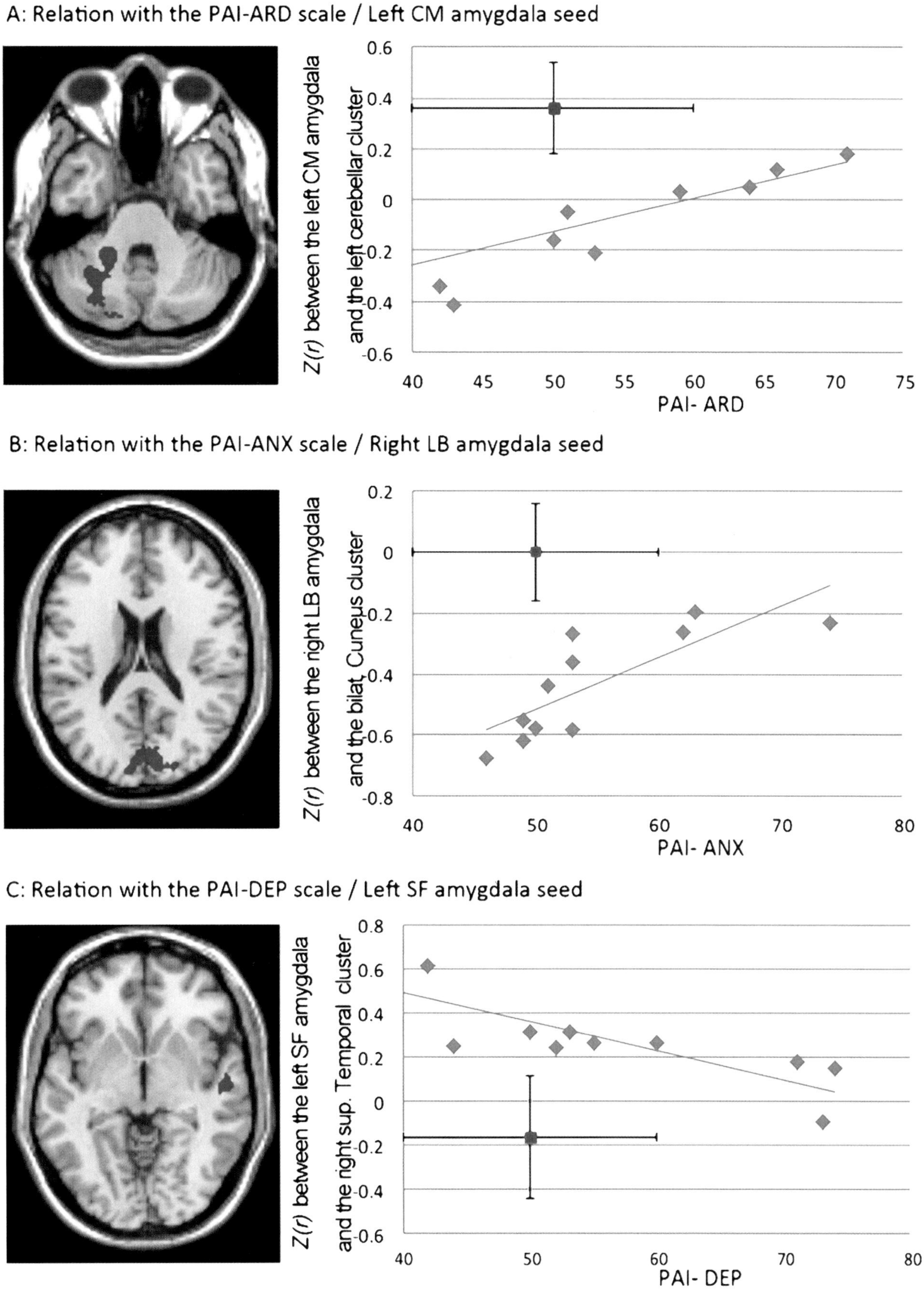
A: Relation with the PAI-ARD scale / Left CM amygdala seed
Z(r) between the left CM amygdala
and the left cerebellar cluster
0.6
0.4
0.2
0
-0.2
-0.4
-0.6
40
45
50
55
60
65
70
75
PAI- ARD
B: Relation with the PAI-ANX scale / Right LB amygdala seed
Z(r) between the right LB amygdala
and the bilat. Cuneus cluster
0.2
0
-0.2
-0.4
-0.6
-0.8
40
50
60
70
80
PAI- ANX
C: Relation with the PAI-DEP scale / Left SF amygdala seed
Z(r) between the left SF amygdala
and the right sup. Temporal cluster
0.8
0.6
0.4
0.2
0
-0.2
-0.4
-0.6
40
50
60
70
80
PAI- DEP

Figure 19.6

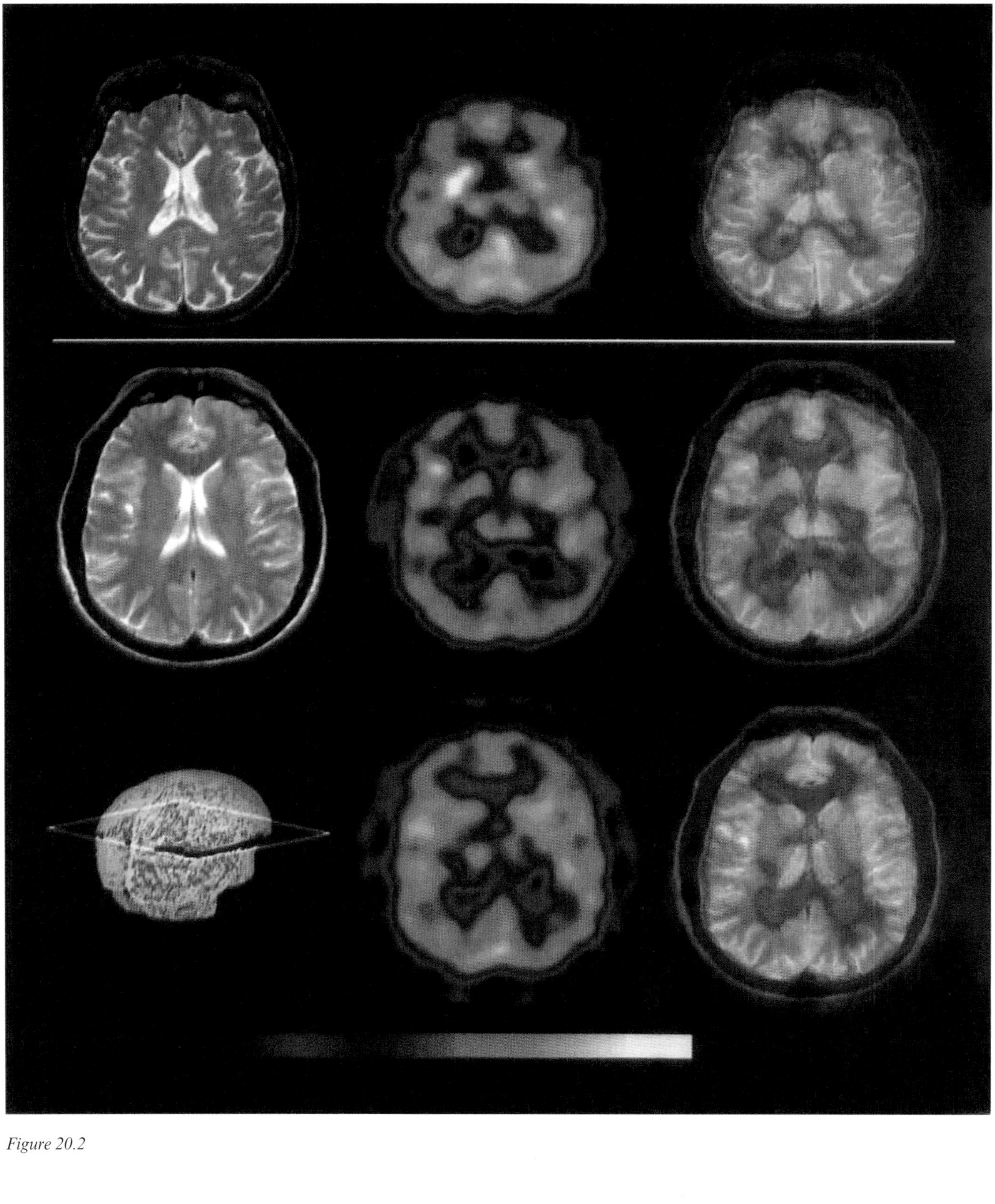

Figure 20.2

As these findings vary by amygdala subregions, they suggest that lateralized epileptic pathology may disturb specific emotional processes and psychiatric symptoms, with indications that different symptoms are subserved by different functional connectivity networks. Thus, epileptic pathology in the emotion-dominant right hemisphere appears to negatively impact the expression of emotion-related networks. Our data highlight opposite functional connectivity relations between anxiety, depression, and brain functioning in right and left MTLE, arguing against a simple or highly general conceptualization of reorganization in unilateral TLE. There may be several types of reorganization, with right hemisphere pathology playing a crucial role in the reorganization of emotion functions. Thus, hemispheric function and dominance may have a large impact on the nature of seizure-related reorganization, with left MTLE patients showing more hippocampal-based disruptions in association with verbal memory (Doucet, Osipowicz, Sharan, Sperling, & Tracy, 2012), and right MTLE patients showing more amygdala-based disruptions in association with emotional states and emotion processing.

Another recent pilot study from our lab identified psychiatric changes postsurgically in both left (LTLE) and right TLE (RTLE). However, the direction of the effects differed in the groups such that the LTLE group consistently demonstrated a worsening of symptoms postsurgery, whereas the RTLE group had lower levels of anxiety/stress in association with the decreases in right amygdala volume that came with the right temporal lobe resection (see Figure 19.7). In combination, these data may suggest the catalyst of postsurgical psychiatric symptom change differs in the two ATL groups, with the left group more susceptible to causes less related to brain structure and more related to diminished dominant hemisphere functions (e.g., language/memory), and the impact of these deficits on communication or vocational skills. In contrast, psychiatric symptom change in right ATL appeared more closely aligned with structural change (i.e., loss) in the ipsilateral amygdala, reducing pathologic emotion processing (Moadel et al., 2014).

The functional consequences of these potential amygdala effects most clearly manifest in emotion processing and psychiatric symptoms, but limbic system effects involving depression and emotional status may also have a deleterious impact on cognitive performance in TLE (Tracy, Lippincott, et al., 2007).

Predicting Neuropsychological Status After Resective or Ablative Surgery

Improved seizure control is the driving factor in epilepsy surgical decision making, but preservation of cognitive function is also important. The potential for cognitive decline following surgery is balanced by the competing need to remove all of the potential epileptogenic tissue; however, exact identification is uncertain, as even the best imaging and electrocorticography techniques leave uncertain the epileptogenicity of areas surrounding the epileptic focus. The role of functional neuroimaging (both task driven and resting-state BOLD) has expanded to help inform surgical planning and strategy, while neuropsychology has also improved its ability to identify cognitive functions at risk and is beginning to contribute more strongly to predictive algorithms. The gold standard for good outcome remains strong seizure control, and this is the case for both clinicians and patients. For example, an examination of health-related quality of life (HRQOL) in patients undergoing epilepsy surgery found an improvement in HRQOL in those patients who were seizure-free postsurgically, despite memory declines (Langfitt et al., 2007). HRQOL among the patients who were not in seizure remission at two and five year intervals remained stable when there

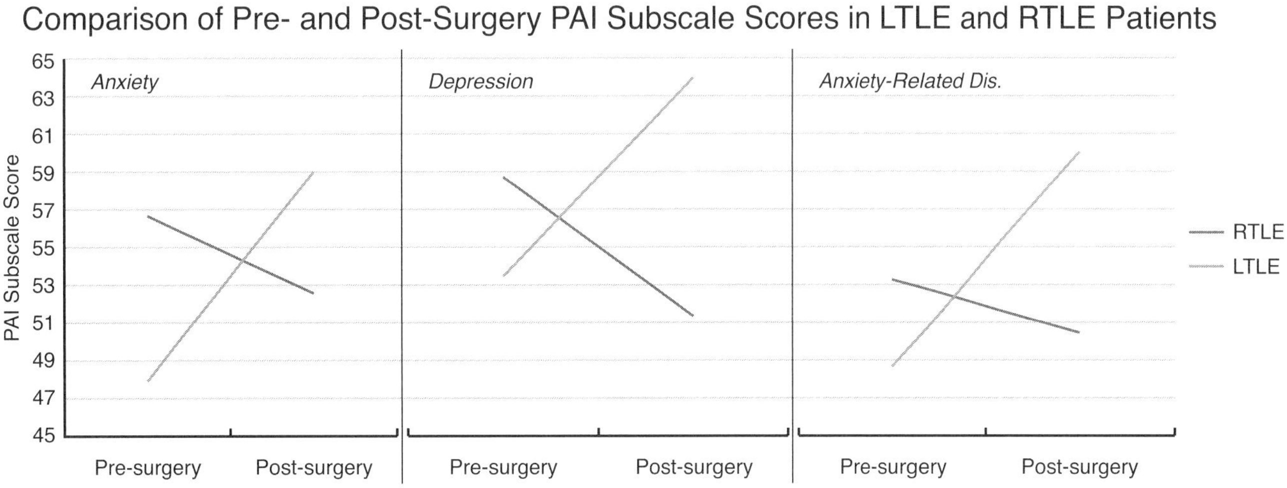

Figure 19.7 Average pre- and post-surgical PAIANX, PAIDEP, and PAIARD scores plotted pre- and postsurgery. Psychiatric scores tend to decrease in RTLE patients postsurgery, whereas scores tend to increase postsurgery in LTLE patients.

was no change in memory, but HRQOL was significantly lower at these intervals when memory declined. Thus, while seizure freedom is often paramount, in the face of continued seizures, cognitive changes are particularly distressing and debilitating.

Most of the data predicting cognitive outcome postsurgically comes from ATL patients. In this group, up to 80% of patients experience significant seizure reduction postsurgery (Engel, 1993; McLachlan et al., 1997; Sperling, O'Conner, Saykin, & Plummer, 1996). While it is intuitive to suggest that reduced seizure freedom will lead to improved cognitive functioning, there is evidence that what accounts for this effect is the improved status of nonresected regions related to the release from seizure burden (Rausch, 1987; Rausch & Crandall, 1982).

The abundant postsurgical literature has identified clear risk factors for significant cognitive decline postsurgically. Factors associated with worse cognitive outcomes are, most notably: good structural and functional integrity of the to-be-resected tissue, bilateral or multifocal epileptogenic focus, dominant hemisphere resection, cerebral volume loss, and earlier age of onset. Each factor tends to emphasize either the role played by the functional adequacy of the to be resected tissue, or the functional reserve of nonresected tissue, to generate potential cognitive reorganization and the underlying neuroplastic processes associated with the maintenance and/or recovery of function. It is interesting to note that the predictors of good surgical outcome are similar (though not identical) to those that predict a good cognitive outcome: namely, a lesional MRI (e.g., MTS), unilateral temporal lobe spikes, concordant EEG, and a history of febrile seizures (Spencer, 2005). Approximately 30%–60% of dominant ATL patients experience substantive decline in verbal memory (Hamberger & Drake, 2006; McCormick et al., 2013). While identifying a discrete pattern of visual memory decline in nondominant ATL patients has been more elusive, there is some evidence that spatial memory and learning are affected more by right than left hemisphere surgery (Dulay et al., 2009). Faced with such group data, the challenge and question for neuropsychologists becomes how to predict decline in the individual case.

Memory declines are more likely if there is evidence that the to-be-resected temporal lobe is structurally and functionally intact and contributes to normal memory function (Bell, Lin, Seidenberg, & Hermann, 2011; Chelune, Naugle, & Luders, 1991; Harvey et al., 2008). High preoperative verbal memory scores results in greater cognitive risk. For instance, Chelune et al. (1991) found that 67% of MTL patients with average memory scores presurgery had a decline of at least 10% six months after surgery, whereas only 12% of those with borderline or poor preoperative memory showed a 10% decline postsurgery. This risk has been replicated in visual memory in RATL patients. Dulay and colleagues (2009) demonstrated declines in spatial location memory in RATL patients, with a particular vulnerability evident in patients with stronger presurgical spatial memory. Studies examining hippocampal pyramidal cell density (Sass et al., 1990), hippocampal neuron loss (Rausch & Babb, 1993), and the pathological status of the mesial temporal lobe (Hermann, Wyler, Somes, Berry, & Dohan, 1992) have consistently demonstrated that the risk of postoperative memory change is greatest in those with less hippocampal cell volume loss and presumably a more functionally intact hippocampus. Conversely, a lack of hippocampal integrity, as seen in unilateral, circumscribed lesions (e.g., MTS) have better postsurgical cognitive outcomes (Clusmann et al., 2002). Severe hippocampal sclerosis (HS), as determined in the preoperative MRI, is thought to indicate a low risk for memory decline following ATL as compared to mild HS (Martin et al., 2002). Figure 19.8 illustrates the difference in verbal memory changes in relation to hippocampal pathology.

Neurocognitive risk following nondominant hemisphere surgery is lower than surgery to the language dominant hemisphere (Chelune et al., 1991; Ivnik, Sharvrough, & Laws, 1988; Lee, Loring, & Thompson, 1989; Milner, 1975; Morris, Mueller, Swanson, & Inglese, 2005; Ojemann & Dodrill, 1985; Saykin, Gur, Sussman, O'Connor, & Gur, 1989; Seidenberg et al., 1998) (Bell, Davies, Haltiner, & Walter, 2000; Meador, 2002; Sabsevitz et al., 2003). In contrast, studies have found that removal of the language-dominant

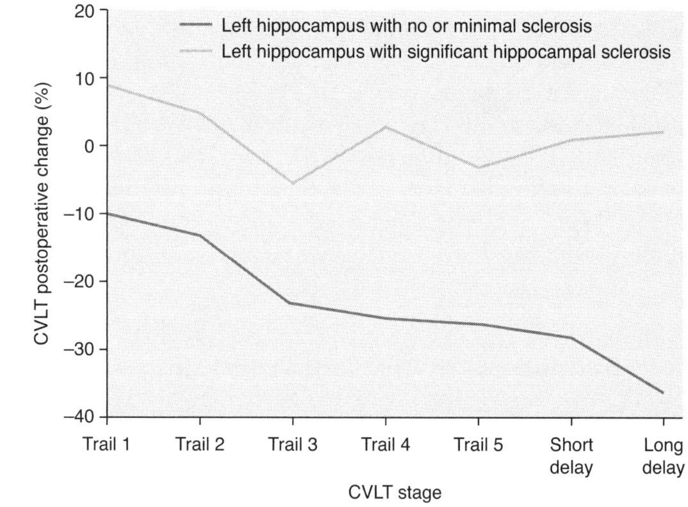

Figure 19.8 Verbal memory change following left ATL in relation to hippocampal pathology. Resection of left hippocampus with no or minimal sclerosis results in significant preoperative to postoperative decline in trial-to-trial learning. Long-delay recall is ≈ 35% lower compared with preoperative performance. Resection of left hippocampus with significant hippocampal sclerosis has a minimal effect on postoperative trial-to-trial learning compared to preoperative performance. All patients were confirmed to be left-hemisphere-speech dominant by the Wada test. Abbreviation: CVLT, California Verbal Learning Test.

Modified and reprinted with permission from Nature Reviews Neurology, *Bell et al. (2011).*

temporal lobe, high preoperative verbal memory scores, and intact memory with contralateral injection on the IAP, all present with high risk for cognitive deficit. These predictors of outcome appear to hold regardless of whether the patient remains seizure-free following surgery. Chelune et al. (1991) found in a multivariate regression model predicting cognitive (memory) outcome that side of surgery was the best single predictor, with the nondominant hemisphere associated with a better outcome.

As might be expected, bilateral temporal lobe damage (e.g., MTS contralateral to the side of surgery) presents greater risk than unilateral, focal damage for postoperative memory impairment, if memory still appears functional. Other identified cognitive risk factors include age of onset and cerebral volume loss. Earlier age of onset is associated with poorer presurgical memory but less decline after ATL (Saykin et al., 1989), likely secondary to the increased probability of focal hippocampal pathology in early onset forms of temporal lobe disease (Bell et al., 2011; Davies et al., 1996). MR volume loss is related to hippocampal loss (Casino, Jack, & Parisi, 1991; Cendes, Leproux, & Melanson, 1993; Kuzniecky, de la Sayette, & Ethier, 1987; Lencz, McCarthy, & Bronen, 1992) and individuals with more extensive pathology show worse memory preoperatively and more declines postoperatively (Trenerry et al., 1993; Trennery, Jack, & Ivnik, 1991), although several studies have not observed a reliable relationship between those variables (Hermann, Wyler, & Somes, 1993; Leonard, 1991; Loring, Lee, & Meador, 1991). Studies examining long-term outcome following ATL have revealed hemisphere-specific patterns of cognitive change over time. Alpherts and colleagues (2006) demonstrated a dynamic decline in verbal memory in LTLE patients for the first two years following surgery, followed by a stabilization of verbal memory. LTLE patients showed an ongoing memory decline for acquisition and consolidation of verbal material at six-month and two-year time points, with this remaining stable six years postsurgery. Interestingly, RTLE patients demonstrated initial improvement in learning and memory that did not persist long-term. Notably, as demonstrated elsewhere, mesial temporal sclerosis was predictive of poorer verbal memory performance, but the degree of decline was greater for the LTLE patients with MTS in comparison to those without MTS. Arguing against the notion that temporal lobe resection can exert delayed effects, Andersson-Roswall, Engman, Samuelsson, and Malmgren (2010) demonstrated cognitive stability in memory functions from two to ten years after temporal lobe resection. Dominant hemisphere resection patients exhibited expected declines in postsurgical verbal memory that was present two years postoperatively, but remained stable at a ten-year interval.

While much has been learned from studies identifying individual predictors of cognitive and behavioral outcome postsurgically, the most promising research focuses on multivariate prediction that can utilize multiple information sources (Bell et al., 2011). Stroup et al. (2003) developed a multivariate risk factor model to predict postoperative verbal memory decline utilizing routine pre-surgical data, including side of resection, preoperative memory testing, IAP performance, and extent of hippocampal sclerosis, each of which provided independent outcome information. Binder and colleagues (2008) examined a group of 60 LATL patients in order to determine whether preoperative language mapping using fMRI could contribute to the prediction of verbal memory decline following LATL. In the 30% of the cohort that experienced verbal memory decline, good preoperative memory performance, late age of epilepsy onset, left hemisphere language dominance on fMRI, and left hemisphere dominance on preoperative intracarotid amobarbital testing were each predictive of postsurgical memory decline. Presurgical memory performance and age of onset collectively accounted for 50% of the variance, with an additional 10% of the variance explained by the fMRI language index.

The Changing Surgical Algorithm and Neuroimaging

At most centers the procedure followed for selecting patients for temporal lobe surgery involves an algorithm that includes scalp/sphenoidal ictal EEG (rhythmic 3–8Hz over the temporal lobe within the first seconds of seizure onset), scalp interictal EEG (state dependent localized spikes or focal slow wave activity), and MRI with evidence of mesial temporal sclerosis or gliosis (hippocampal atrophy and increased T2 signal). Additional criteria include FDG positron emission tomography (PET) interictal hypometabolism in the temporal lobe, asymmetric language and memory findings from both neuropsychological testing and the IAP implicating deficits on the surgery target side along with integrity in the contralateral side, semiology and EEG findings consistent with temporal lobe seizures, ictal single photon emission computed tomography (SPECT) hypoperfusion in the temporal lobe, and localized background EEG abnormalities in the temporal lobe. If the localization of seizures is equivocal, then cortical surface and possibly depth electrodes and electrocorticography procedures are used to better localize the epileptogenic zone. With implants in place—often as part of the same surgical procedure—electrocortical stimulation (ECS) is undertaken through a "knock out" test paradigm to determine the cognitive functionality of the neural tissue adjacent to the implanted electrode (Zangaladze et al., 2008).

fMRI and other functional imaging modalities are becoming an essential part of the surgical algorithm. In fact, at our center, we have all but replaced the IAP with fMRI, with only a handful of exceptional cases each year warranting Wada testing. The literature supports this transition, given the strong concordance rates between fMRI and the IAP for both language (Woermann et al., 2003) and memory (Jokeit, Okujava, & Woermann, 2001), and the safer and less invasive nature of fMRI. Emerging technologies, including functional connectivity MRI (fcMRI) and DTI (or more advanced diffusion techniques such as Neurite Orientation Dispersion and Density Imaging; see Zhang, Schneider, Wheeler-Kingshott, & Alexander, 2012), are now being utilized to enhance the visual rendering of the underlying neuroanatomy. Diffusion imaging can be seen as a means of verifying the anatomical connection between the gray matter regions. fcMRI can be viewed as a means of verifying that the relevant gray matter regions are indeed communicating and signaling each other. In this context, fMRI can then be viewed as a means of determining the content or nature of the signal (i.e., what the regions are communicating about).

fMRI

fMRI is a safer and cheaper alternative to the IAP, and is capable of providing a depiction of the full circuit of regions involved in a task. This technique measures changes in cerebral blood flow, specifically changes in the concentration of deoxyhemoglobin in local vasculature following regional brain activation, to map neural activity. Functional MRI has the advantage of giving a picture of the full neural circuit that is actually used, but it does not test the necessity of any one particular region for carrying out the relevant cognitive activity. This broad sensitivity to brain functional status shares similarity with neuropsychological testing, and for both procedures it is a quality that lessens their ability to conclusively point to specific areas of the brain that are impaired. The BOLD signal is best associated with local field potentials, not multiunit potentials, and thus it reflects local synaptic and not spiking neurons (Logothetis & Pfeuffer, 2004). Nevertheless, fMRI can show neocortical regional involvement in a task with millimeter resolution. Particularly advantageous for clinical populations, fMRI does not require the use of endogenous contrast and repeated scanning sessions in the same individual and can be conducted even over a short time interval. fMRI in epilepsy has been used to determine hemispheric representation of language and memory, to predict outcomes after temporal lobectomy, to predict the side of seizure focus and seizure outcome, and to verify the functional reorganization of skills such as language.

Diffusion Imaging

DTI takes advantage of the directionality created by structural constraints on the diffusion of water in the brain (i.e., anisotropic diffusion), allowing it to measure the structural orientation and density of WM tracts. In the context of epilepsy, it has been shown previously that hippocampal sclerosis confirmed on MRI is often associated with creation of a seizure focus (Brooks et al., 1990). Using DTI, the WM regions neighboring these epileptogenic zones have demonstrated reduced anisotropy. Further, these abnormal areas appear to extend into regions of the brain that appear normal on MRI. Hence, DTI may serve to enhance presurgical evaluation by providing corroborating evidence of the epileptogenic region, and its impact on connected afferent and efferent WM structural networks.

The most important current use of DTI in presurgical mapping involves delineation of important sensory and motor tracts that need to be avoided during surgery. Damage to Meyers loop, the most anterior part of the optic radiation, results in a visual field deficit (VFD) in 50%–100% of patients (Barton, Hefter, Chang, Schomer, & Drislane, 2005; Nilsson, Malmgren, Rydenhag, & Frisen, 2004). Given that a primary motivation for surgery is the ability to drive, limiting VFD is fundamental in improving quality of life outcomes. In a cohort of 21 patients who underwent anterior temporal lobe resection, Winston and colleagues (2014) demonstrated that the use of preoperative optic radiation tractography and intraoperative MRI (iMRI) improved outcome. The severity of VFD in the contralateral superior quadrant was significantly reduced with tractography and iMRI guidance. Supporting the importance of integrating such techniques into neuronavigation technologies, none of the patients in the iMRI cohort developed a VFD that precluded driving, whereas 13% of the non-iMRI cohort failed to meet driving criteria. Tracts that connect gray matter regions would, of course, form important neurocognitive circuits for memory and language, which could potentially become reliably depicted by DTI, but this research is in its infancy (Zhang et al., 2012).

Functional Connectivity MRI

fcMRI utilizes the temporal correlation of neurophysiological activity in different brain regions to assess functional connections between brain areas (i.e., neural communication and potential information sharing), and characterizes their organization in terms of participation in integrated or segregated neural network. Functional connectivity has been previously defined as the temporal correlation of a neurophysiological index measured in different brain areas (Friston, Frith, Liddle, & Frackowiak, 1993). Low-frequency hemodynamic fluctuations constitute such a neurophysiological index, and functional connectivity maps can be created based on these fluctuations. In healthy persons, there is a high degree of co-occurrence between the functional connectivity maps (using resting-state image time series) and functional activation maps obtained in cognitive task studies. This suggests that generating functional connectivity maps using correlated low frequency oscillation of cerebral hemodynamic parameters (i.e., perfusion, oxygenation) represent a robust approach for brain functional imaging. Functional synchrony in particular brain areas can be quantified by means of cross-correlation coefficients of low-frequency spontaneous oscillation of the BOLD signal in different areas. Great advances have also been made in utilizing resting-state fMRI data for development of a whole-brain connectome and using graph theory statistics of connectivity to understand the organization and function of brain networks instantiated during both rest and a variety of cognitive activities. Resting state functional connectivity has distinct advantages over task-driven fMRI and Wada. Such data can be collected with only a five-minute scanning period. Resting-state FC methods have an advantage over task-based fMRI methods as they allow for more careful individual analysis of the role played by the strength of particular regional connections in the determination of language dominance. Resting state FC also offers advantages in terms of testing impaired patient populations who cannot otherwise cooperate or respond effectively to the demands of either fMRI or IAP.

Electrocorticography

When the localization of the epileptogenic focus remains equivocal after all noninvasive measures have been exhausted, extraoperative and/or intraoperative subdural electrocorticography is often used to identify the epileptogenic zone and to guide surgical resection, with a focus on sparing eloquent cortex. The patient undergoes a craniotomy, followed by surgical implantation of strip and grid electrodes on the surface of the cortex based on the information collected during the preoperative evaluation. With implants in place, often as part of the same surgical procedure, electro-cortical stimulation mapping (ESM) is undertaken to map out functions associated with the neural tissue adjacent to the implanted electrode, with the goal of preserving function postoperatively. When current is applied to a functional cortical area, a positive response may be elicited or a specific function may be disabled. Depth electrode placements in areas such as the hippocampus are done routinely to locate seizure foci through passive EEG recordings. Depth electrodes are typically used when patients have a suspected focal seizure onset but surface EEG is not definitive.

Electrical stimulation of these electrodes provides the means to demonstrate the necessity of a particular pool of neurons for carrying a specific cognitive task. In contrast, fMRI has the ability to provide a complete map of the brain regions implementing a given task. In this sense, ESM and fMRI are complementary. ESM can indicate the structures necessary for a task, while fMRI can depict the full neural circuit that is sufficient for its successful completion.

Summary

In terms of functional assessments, fMRI and fcMRI as brain-mapping techniques will likely become as common an early step as neuropsychological testing, reducing the need for the IAP, which, due to its inherent risks, would be the last to use of the functional techniques. The hope is that techniques such as diffusion imaging and fcMRI will yield important information about structural and functional connectivity of networks that implement cognitive functions, and give better functional and anatomical grounding to the network of activation implied by fMRI.

To render all these sources of information (functional neurocognitive maps, WM tracts, vascular structures, implanted electrodes stimulated during ESM) into a single multimodal image that can be imported into a probe-based neuronavigation system is the goal. However, numerous registration problems exist as each imaging modality and its related information brings with it its own set of distortions. For instance, at our center we currently utilize the functional data from neuropsychological testing, IAP, fMRI, rsfMRI, and ECS with structural information from MRI, diffusion, and CT (which contains the exact location of the electrodes used during ECS), but improvement is needed to integrate these into a seamless multimodal rendering that captures all structural and functional components together in one image that can be used during surgery for neuronavigation.

It is likely these emergent technologies will transform the daily activities of the neuropsychologist. As the ultimate goal is to obtain an integrated model of brain structure and function, the field of neuropsychology will be forced to adapt in order to make continued contributions to the presurgical assessment algorithms. Just as the relative contributions of the neuropsychologist to make localization and lateralization decisions have improved with the advent of functional neuroimaging, neuropsychology will need to shift again as the integration of technologies advances. Future neuropsychologists will need to accommodate and integrate cognitive tests with techniques that have better temporal (e.g., surface and depth electrocorticography; brain electrical stimulation) or spatial resolutions (fMRI, fcMRI, diffusion) in order to provide a more robust method for capturing the strength, location, and organization of specific cognitive functions and network connectivity. This integrative shift has the goal of improving neuronavigation during the resective, stimulation, or ablative techniques aimed at stopping seizures. It is likely that future neuropsychological assessments in the setting of epilepsy will require the development of new assessment procedures and protocols that are uniquely suited to easy integration with these other functional and structural technologies.

Notes

1 That said, it is not clear that the neural mechanisms involved in epileptogenesis, particularly in the hippocampus, can fully account for the cognitive and behavioral deficits associated with temporal lobe epilepsy. Early life seizures are not generally associated with cell loss or mossy fiber sprouting, despite the presence of cognitive deficits (Toth, Yan, Haftoglou, Ribak, & Baram, 1998). Also, experimental rats that kindle rapidly do not necessarily learn rapidly (Leech & McIntyre, 1976). More generally, cell death, synaptic reorganization, and altered neurogenesis do not appear the most likely explanation of cognitive deficits in epilepsy. Mechanisms related to increased inhibitory neurotransmission (e.g., increased postsynaptic inhibition of GABAa receptor changes, increased presynaptic inhibition involving HCN changes), decreased excitatory neurotransmission (decreased dendritic spine density, reduced NMDA receptor expression), and altered regulatory and neuromodulatory pathways (CREB, CHN) appear to be much more likely causes of cognitive dysfunction (Brooks-Kayal, 2005).

2 In Tracy and Osipowicz (2011) we defined several mechanisms of cognitive reorganization. These included functional redundancy,

functional substitution, cognitive control, cognitive reserve, and normalization. We view these types of reorganization as occurring in the setting of a complex network, with the particular task function or cognitive component that is redundant, substituted, etc., varying not just with the nature of task, but in accord with the clinical pathology, disease duration, chronological age, and a host of other factors. We define functional redundancy as the presence of duplicate representation of a function, which gets unmasked and recruited into a network, and is then used to successfully implement the task following acquired injury (i.e., resective surgery). Functional substitution utilizes a new, previously unincorporated neural region to substitute for the function of a lost node, a node that lacked redundant representation in the brain. Cognitive control utilizes supervisory systems to alter the affected or impaired network by increasing attentional resources, facilitating information exchange, improving sensory filtering/suppression, or increasing executive monitoring. Cognitive reserve is a general mechanism of resiliency, utilizing the remaining healthy brain to withstand injury and protect against a loss of function. Finally, the normalization mechanism is defined, based on evidence that patients with surgically relieved seizure burden can undergo cognitive reorganization of language function or other cognitive functions that returns functional neuroanatomical representations to their more normative locations (Lutz, Clusmann, Elger, Schramm, & Helmstaedter, 2004; Martin et al., 2000; Takaya et al., 2009). Importantly, normalization, which takes into account the potential abnormal functional organization presurgery, highlights the fact that the new area(s) recruited may be normative for the task. In the context of neuroimaging, normalization involves the reorganization of cognitive networks not through the formation of atypical, compensatory networks, as is the case with the other mechanisms noted earlier, but by the emergence of a network that better resembles the normative, age appropriate network implementing a task. In this sense, the first four cognitive mechanisms appear more suited to explaining neuroplastic compensation following acute injury, such as traumatic brain injury or stroke. One must be careful in applying them to chronic disorders, such as epilepsy, which may have the propensity to disrupt functional neuroanatomy early on, altering or perhaps never even allowing for normative patterns to develop (for a review see Cadotte et al., 2009; Elger et al., 2004).

References

Abercrombie, H. C., Schaefer, S. M., Larson, C. L., Oakes, T. R., Lindgren, K. A., Holden, J. E., . . . Davidson, R. J. (1998). Metabolic rate in the right amygdala predicts negative affect in depressed patients. *Neuroreport*, *9*(14), 3301–3307.

Ahmadi, M. E., Hagler, D. J., Jr., McDonald, C. R., Tecoma, E. S., Iragui, V. J., Dale, A. M., & Halgren, E. (2009). Side matters: Diffusion tensor imaging tractography in left and right temporal lobe epilepsy. *AJNR American Journal of Neuroradiology*, *30*(9), 1740–1747. doi: 10.3174/ajnr.A1650

Aikia, M., Jutila, L., Salmenpera, T., Mervaala, E., & Kalviainen, R. (2006). Comparison of the cognitive effects of tiagabine and carbamazepine as monotherapy in newly diagnosed adult patients with partial epilepsy: Pooled analysis of two long-term, randomized, follow-up studies. *Epilepsia*, *47*(7). doi: 10.1111/j.1528-1167.2006.00545.x 16886974

Alessio, A., Pereira, F. R., Sercheli, M. S., Rondina, J. M., Ozelo, H. B., Bilevicius, E., . . . Cendes, F. (2013). Brain plasticity for verbal and visual memories in patients with mesial temporal lobe epilepsy and hippocampal sclerosis: An fMRI study. *Human Brain Mapping*, *34*(1), 186–199. doi: 10.1002/hbm.21432

Alpherts, W. C., Vermeulen, J., van Rijen, P. C., da Silva, F. H., van Veelen, C. W., & Dutch Collaborative Epilepsy Surgery, P. (2006). Verbal memory decline after temporal epilepsy surgery? A 6-year multiple assessments follow-up study. *Neurology*, *67*(4), 626–631. doi: 10.1212/01.wnl.0000230139.45304.eb

Anderson, D. P., Harvey, A. S., Saling, M. M., Anderson, V., Kean, M., Abbott, D. F., . . . Jackson, G. D. (2006). FMRI lateralization of expressive language in children with cerebral lesions. *Epilepsia*, *47*(6), 998–1008. doi: 10.1111/j.1528-1167.2006.00572.x

Andersson-Roswall, L., Engman, E., Samuelsson, H., & Malmgren, K. (2010). Cognitive outcome 10 years after temporal lobe epilepsy surgery: A prospective controlled study. *Neurology*, *74*(24), 1977–1985. doi: 10.1212/WNL.0b013e3181e39684

Arfanakis, K., Hermann, B. P., Rogers, B. P., Carew, J. D., Seidenberg, M., & Meyerand, M. E. (2002). Diffusion tensor MRI in temporal lobe epilepsy. *Magnetic Resonance Imaging*, *20*(7), 511–519.

Arnold, S., Schlaug, G., Niemann, H., Ebner, A., Luders, H., Witte, O. W., & Seitz, R. J. (1996). Topography of interictal glucose hypometabolism in unilateral mesiotemporal epilepsy. *Neurology*, *46*(5), 1422–1430.

Bartha, L., Trinka, E., Ortler, M., Donnemiller, E., Felber, S., Bauer, G., & Benke, T. (2004). Linguistic deficits following left selective amygdalohippocampectomy: A prospective study. *Epilepsy & Behavior*, *5*(3), 348–357. doi: 10.1016/j.yebeh.2004.02.004

Bartolomei, F., Wendling, F., Regis, J., Gavaret, M., Guye, M., & Chauvel, P. (2004). Pre-ictal synchronicity in limbic networks of mesial temporal lobe epilepsy. *Epilepsy Research*, *61*(1–3), 89–104. doi: 10.1016/j.eplepsyres.2004.06.006

Barton, J. J., Hefter, R., Chang, B., Schomer, D., & Drislane, F. (2005). The field defects of anterior temporal lobectomy: A quantitative reassessment of Meyer's loop. *Brain*, *128*(Pt 9), 2123–2133. doi: 10.1093/brain/awh544

Bell, B., Davies, A., Haltiner, A., & Walter, R. (2000). Intracarotid amobarbital procedure and prediction of postoperative memory in patients with temporal lobe epilepsy and hippocampal sclerosis. *Epilepsia*, *41*, 992–997.

Bell, B., Lin, J. J., Seidenberg, M., & Hermann, B. (2011). The neurobiology of cognitive disorders in temporal lobe epilepsy. *Nat Rev Neurol*, *7*(3), 154–164. doi: 10.1038/nrneurol.2011.3

Ben-Ari, Y., Crepel, V., & Represa, A. (2008). Seizures beget seizures in temporal lobe epilepsies: The boomerang effects of newly formed aberrant kainatergic synapses. *Epilepsy Currents*, *8*(3), 68–72. doi: 10.1111/j.1535-7511.2008.00241.x

Bernhardt, B. C., Chen, Z., He, Y., Evans, A. C., & Bernasconi, N. (2011). Graph-theoretical analysis reveals disrupted small-world organization of cortical thickness correlation networks in temporal lobe epilepsy. *Cereb Cortex*, *21*(9), 2147–2157. doi: 10.1093/cercor/bhq291

Bettus, G., Bartolomei, F., Confort-Gouny, S., Guedj, E., Chauvel, P., Cozzone, P. J., . . . Guye, M. (2010). Role of resting state functional connectivity MRI in presurgical investigation of mesial temporal lobe epilepsy. *Journal of Neurology, Neurosurgery, and Psychiatry*, *81*(10), 1147-1154. doi: 10.1136/jnnp.2009.191460

Bettus, G., Guedj, E., Joyeux, F., Confort-Gouny, S., Soulier, E., Laguitton, V., . . . Guye, M. (2009). Decreased basal fMRI functional connectivity in epileptogenic networks and contralateral compensatory mechanisms. *Human Brain Mapping*, *30*(5), 1580–1591. doi: 10.1002/hbm.20625

Bilo, L., Santangelo, G., Improta, I., Vitale, C., Meo, R., & Trojano, L. (2013). Neuropsychological profile of adult patients with nonsymptomatic occipital lobe epilepsies. *Journal of Neurol*, *260*(2), 445–453. doi: 10.1007/s00415-012-6650-z

Binder, D. K., Podlogar, M., Clusmann, H., Bien, C., Urbach, H., Schramm, J., & Kral, T. (2009). Surgical treatment of parietal lobe epilepsy. *Journal of Neurosurg*, *110*(6), 1170–1178. doi: 10.3171/2008.2.17665

Binder, J. R., Sabsevitz, D. S., Swanson, S. J., Hammeke, T. A., Raghavan, M., & Mueller, W. M. (2008). Use of preoperative functional MRI to predict verbal memory decline after temporal lobe epilepsy surgery. *Epilepsia*, *49*(8), 1377–1394. doi: 10.1111/j.1528-1167.2008.01625.x

Blumenfeld, H., Rivera, M., McNally, K., Davis, K. D., Spencer, D., & Spencer, S. (2004). Ictal neocortical slowing in temporal lobe epilepsy. *Neurology*, *62*, 1015–1021.

Bonelli, S. B., Powell, R., Yogarajah, M., Thompson, P. J., Symms, M. R., Koepp, M. J., & Duncan, J. S. (2009). Preoperative amygdala fMRI in temporal lobe epilepsy. *Epilepsia*, *50*(2), 217–227. doi: 10.1111/j.1528-1167.2008.01739.x

Bonilha, L., Alessio, A., Rorden, C., Baylis, G., Damasceno, B. P., Min, L. L., & Cendes, F. (2007). Extrahippocampal gray matter atrophy and memory impairment in patients with medial temporal lobe epilepsy. *Human Brain Mapping*, *28*(12), 1376–1390. doi: 10.1002/hbm.20373

Bonilha, L., Montenegro, M. A., Rorden, C., Castellano, G., Guerreiro, M. M., Cendes, F., & Li, L. M. (2006). Voxel-based morphometry reveals excess gray matter concentration in patients with focal cortical dysplasia. *Epilepsia*, *47*(5), 908–915. doi: 10.1111/j.1528-1167.2006.00548.x

Bonilha, L., Rorden, C., Halford, J. J., Eckert, M., Appenzeller, S., Cendes, F., & Li, L. M. (2007). Asymmetrical extra-hippocampal grey matter loss related to hippocampal atrophy in patients with medial temporal lobe epilepsy. *Journal of Neurology, Neurosurgery & Psychiatry*, *78*(3), 286–294.

Bootsma, H. P., Ricker, L., Diepman, L., Gehring, J., Hulsman, J., Lambrechts, D., . . . Aldenkamp, A. P. (2008). Long-term effects of levetiracetam and topiramate in clinical practice: A head-to-head comparison. *Seizure*, *17*(1), 19–26. doi: 10.1016/j.seizure.2007.05.019

Boylan, L. S., Flint, L. A., Labovitz, D. L., Jackson, S. C., Starner, K., & Devinsky, O. (2004). Depression but not seizure frequency predicts quality of life in treatment-resistant epilepsy. *Neurology*, *62*(2), 258–261.

Braakman, H. M., Vaessen, M. J., Hofman, P. A., Debeij-van Hall, M. H., Backes, W. H., Vles, J. S., & Aldenkamp, A. P. (2011). Cognitive and behavioral complications of frontal lobe epilepsy in children: A review of the literature. *Epilepsia*, *52*(5), 849–856. doi: 10.1111/j.1528-1167.2011.03057.x

Braakman, H. M., Vaessen, M. J., Jansen, J. F., Debeij-van Hall, M. H., de Louw, A., Hofman, P. A., . . . Backes, W. H. (2014). Pediatric frontal lobe epilepsy: White matter abnormalities and cognitive impairment. *Acta Neurologica Scandinavica*, *129*(4), 252–262. doi: 10.1111/ane.12183

Braun, M., Finke, C., Ostendorf, F., Lehmann, T. N., Hoffmann, K. T., & Ploner, C. J. (2008). Reorganization of associative memory in humans with long-standing hippocampal damage. *Brain*, *131*(Pt 10), 2742–2750.

Brooks, B., King, D., el Gammal, T., Meador, K., Yaghmai, F., Gay, J., . . . Flanigin, H. (1990). MR imaging in patients with intractable complex partial epileptic seizures. *American Journal of Roentgenology*, *154*(3), 577–583.

Brooks-Kayal, A. (2005). *Behavioral and cognitive comorbidities in pediatric epilepsy: Recognition, mechanisms, assesment and treatment*. Paper presented at the American Epilepsy Society, Annual Meeting, Washington DC.

Brooks-Kayal, A. (2011). Molecular mechanisms of cognitive and behavioral comorbidities of epilepsy in children. *Epilepsia*, *52*(Suppl 1), 13–20. doi: 10.1111/j.1528-1167.2010.02906.x

Casino, G., Jack, C., & Parisi, J. (1991). Magnetic resonance imaging volume studies in temporal lobe epilepsy: Pathological correlations. *Annals of Neurology*, *29*, 1–36.

Castillo, P. E., Chiu, C. Q., & Carroll, R. C. (2011). Long-term plasticity at inhibitory synapses. *Current Opinion in Neurobiology*, *21*(2), 328–338. doi: 10.1016/j.conb.2011.01.006

Cendes, F., Leproux, F., & Melanson, D. (1993). MRI of amygdala and hippocampus in temporal lobe epilepsy. *Journal of Computer Assisted Tomography*, *17*, 206–210.

Centeno, M., Vollmar, C., Stretton, J., Symms, M. R., Thompson, P. J., Richardson, M. P., . . . Koepp, M. J. (2014). Structural changes in the temporal lobe and piriform cortex in frontal lobe epilepsy. *Epilepsy Research*, *108*(5), 978–981. doi: 10.1016/j.eplepsyres.2014.03.001

Chelune, G., Naugle, R., & Luders, H. (1991). Prediction of cognitive change as a function of preoperative ability status among temporal lobectomy patients seen at 6-month follow-up. *Neurology*, *41*, 399–404.

Clusmann, H., Schramm, J., Kral, T., Helmstaedter, C., Ostertun, B., Fimmers, R., . . . Elger, C. E. (2002). Prognostic factors and outcome after different types of resection for temporal lobe epilepsy. *Journal of Neurosurgery*, *97*(5), 1131–1141.

Concha, L., Beaulieu, C., Collins, D. L., & Gross, D. W. (2009). White-matter diffusion abnormalities in temporal-lobe epilepsy with and without mesial temporal sclerosis. *Journal of Neurology, Neurosurgery, and Psychiatry*, *80*(3), 312–319. doi: 10.1136/jnnp.2007.139287

Coppola, G., Caliendo, G., Veggiotti, P., Romeo, A., Tortorella, G., De Marco, P., & Pascotto, A. (2002). Topiramate as add-on drug in children, adolescents and young adults with Lennox-Gastaut syndrome: An Italian multicentric study. *Epilepsy Research*, *51*(1–2), 147–153.

Corcoran, R., & Thompson, P. (1993). Epilepsy and poor memory: Who complains and what do they mean? *British Journal of Clinical Psychology*, *32*, 199–208.

Cormack, F., Gadian, D. G., Vargha-Khadem, F., Cross, J. H., Connelly, A., & Baldeweg, T. (2005). Extra-hippocampal grey matter density abnormalities in paediatric mesial temporal sclerosis. *Neuroimage*, *27*(3), 635–643. doi: 10.1016/j.neuroimage.2005.05.023

Coultrap, S. J., Nixon, K. M., Alvestad, R. M., Valenzuela, C. F., & Browning, M. D. (2005). Differential expression of NMDA receptor subunits and splice variants among the CA1, CA3 and dentate gyrus of the adult rat. *Brain Research Molecular Brain Research*, *135*(1–2), 104–111. doi: 10.1016/j.molbrainres.2004.12.005

Cousin, E., Baciu, M., Pichat, C., Kahane, P., & Le Bas, J. F. (2008). Functional MRI evidence for language plasticity in adult epileptic patients: Preliminary results. *Neuropsychiatric Disease and Treatment*, *4*(1), 235–246.

Dabbs, K., Becker, T., Jones, J., Rutecki, P., Seidenberg, M., & Hermann, B. (2012). Brain structure and aging in chronic temporal lobe epilepsy. *Epilepsia*, *53*(6), 1033–1043. doi: 10.1111/j.1528-1167.2012.03447.x

Dallison, A., & Kolb, B. (2003). Recovery from infant medial frontal cortical lesions in rats is reversed by cortical lesions in adulthood. *Behavioural Brain Research*, *146*(1–2), 57–63.

Datta, A. N., Oser, N., Bauder, F., Maier, O., Martin, F., Ramelli, G. P., . . . Penner, I. K. (2013). Cognitive impairment and cortical reorganization in children with benign epilepsy with centrotemporal spikes. *Epilepsia*, *54*(3), 487–494. doi: 10.1111/epi.12067

Davidson, R. J. (2003). Darwin and the neural bases of emotion and affective style. *Annals of the New York Academy of Sciences*, *1000*, 316–336.

Davies, K. G., Hermann, B. P., Dohan, F. C., Jr., Foley, K. T., Bush, A. J., & Wyler, A. R. (1996). Relationship of hippocampal sclerosis to duration and age of onset of epilepsy, and childhood febrile seizures in temporal lobectomy patients. *Epilepsy Research*, *24*(2), 119–126.

Demirtas-Tatlidede, A., Vahabzadeh-Hagh, A. M., Bernabeu, M., Tormos, J. M., & Pascual-Leone, A. (2012). Noninvasive brain stimulation in traumatic brain injury. *Journal of Head Trauma Rehabilitation*, *27*(4), 274–292. doi: 10.1097/HTR.0b013e318217df55

Diehl, B., Busch, R. M., Duncan, J. S., Piao, Z., Tkach, J., & Luders, H. O. (2008). Abnormalities in diffusion tensor imaging of the uncinate fasciculus relate to reduced memory in temporal lobe epilepsy. *Epilepsia*, *49*(8), 1409–1418. doi: 10.1111/j.1528-1167.2008.01596.x

Dodrill, C. B. (2004). Neuropsychological effects of seizures. *Epilepsy Behav*, *5*(Suppl 1), S21–24.

Dodrill, C. B., Arnett, J. L., Shu, V., Pixton, G. C., Lenz, G. T., & Sommerville, K. W. (1998). Effects of tiagabine monotherapy on abilities, adjustment, and mood. *Epilepsia*, *39*(1), 33–42.

Dodrill, C. B., & Wilensky, A. J. (1992). Neuropsychological abilities before and after 5 years of stable antiepileptic drug therapy. *Epilepsia*, *33*(2), 327–334.

Doucet, G., Osipowicz, K., Sharan, A., Sperling, M. R., & Tracy, J. I. (2012). Extratemporal functional connectivity impairments at rest are related to memory performance in mesial temporal epilepsy. *Human Brain Mapping*. doi: 10.1002/hbm.22059. doi: 10.1002/hbm.22059

Doucet, G., Osipowicz, K., Sharan, A., Sperling, M. R., & Tracy, J. I. (2013). Extratemporal functional connectivity impairments at rest are related to memory performance in mesial temporal epilepsy. *Human Brain Mapping*, *34*(9), 2202–2216. doi: 10.1002/hbm.22059

Doucet, G., Skidmore, C., Evans, A., Sharan, A., Sperling, M., Pustina, D., & Tracy, J. (2014). Temporal lobe epilepsy and surgery selectively alter the dorsal, not the ventral, default-mode network. *Frontiers in Neurology*, *5*, 23. doi: 10.3389/fneur.2014.00023

Doucet, G., Skidmore, C., Pustina, D., Sharan, A., Sperling, M., & Tracy, J. (2013). *Effect of age of seizure onset and mesial temporal sclerosis on brain functional organization in temporal lobe epilepsy*. Paper presented at the American Epilepsy Society, Washington, DC.

Dulay, M. F., Levin, H. S., York, M. K., Mizrahi, E. M., Verma, A., Goldsmith, I., . . . Yoshor, D. (2009). Predictors of individual visual memory decline after unilateral anterior temporal lobe resection. *Neurology*, *72*(21), 1837–1842. doi: 10.1212/WNL.0b013e3181a71132

Duzel, E., Schiltz, K., Solbach, T., Peschel, T., Baldeweg, T., Kaufmann, J., . . . Heinze, H. J. (2006). Hippocampal atrophy in temporal lobe epilepsy is correlated with limbic systems atrophy. *Journal of Neurology*, *253*(3), 294–300. doi: 10.1007/s00415-005-0981-y

Eddy, C. M., Rickards, H. E., & Cavanna, A. E. (2011). The cognitive impact of antiepileptic drugs. *Therapeutic Advances in Neurological Disorders*, *4*(6), 385–407. doi: 10.1177/1756285611417920

Elger, C. E., Helmstaedter, C., & Kurthen, M. (2004). Chronic epilepsy and cognition. *Lancet Neurology*, *3*(11), 663–672.

Eliashiv, S. D., Dewar, S., Wainwright, I., Engel, J., Jr., & Fried, I. (1997). Long-term follow-up after temporal lobe resection for lesions associated with chronic seizures. *Neurology*, *48*(5), 1383–1388.

Engel, J. (1993). *Surgical Treatment of the Epilepsies* (2nd ed.). New York: Raven Press.

Exner, C., Boucsein, K., Lange, C., Winter, H., Weniger, G., Steinhoff, B. J., & Irle, E. (2002). Neuropsychological performance in frontal lobe epilepsy. *Seizure*, *11*(1), 20–32. doi: 10.1053/seiz.2001.0572

Fahoum, F., Lopes, R., Pittau, F., Dubeau, F., & Gotman, J. (2012). Widespread epileptic networks in focal epilepsies: EEG-fMRI study. *Epilepsia*, *53*(9), 1618–1627. doi: 10.1111/j.1528-1167.2012.03533.x

Farwell, J. R., Dodrill, C. B., & Batzel, L. W. (1985). Neuropsychological abilities of children with epilepsy. *Epilepsia*, *26*(5), 395–400.

Farwell, J. R., Lee, Y. J., Hirtz, D. G., Sulzbacher, S. I., Ellenberg, J. H., & Nelson, K. B. (1990). Phenobarbital for febrile seizures: Effects on intelligence and on seizure recurrence. *New England Journal of Medicine*, *322*(6), 364–369. doi: 10.1056/NEJM199002083220604

Fiest, K. M., Dykeman, J., Patten, S. B., Wiebe, S., Kaplan, G. G., Maxwell, C. J., . . . Jette, N. (2013). Depression in epilepsy: A systematic review and meta-analysis. *Neurology*, *80*(6), 590–599. doi: 10.1212/WNL.0b013e31827b1ae0

Figueiredo, P., Santana, I., Teixeira, J., Cunha, C., Machado, E., Sales, F., . . . Castelo-Branco, M. (2008). Adaptive visual memory reorganization in right medial temporal lobe epilepsy. *Epilepsia*, *49*(8), 1395–1408. doi: 10.1111/j.1528-1167.2008.01629.x

Foldvary, N., Klem, G., Hammel, J., Bingaman, W., Najm, I., & Luders, H. (2001). The localizing value of ictal EEG in focal epilepsy. *Neurology*, *57*(11), 2022–2028.

Frisch, C., Hanke, J., Kleineruschkamp, S., Roske, S., Kaaden, S., Elger, C. E., . . . Helmstaedter, C. (2009). Positive correlation between the density of neuropeptide y positive neurons in the amygdala and parameters of self-reported anxiety and depression in mesiotemporal lobe epilepsy patients. *Biological Psychiatry*, *66*(5), 433–440. doi: 10.1016/j.biopsych.2009.03.025

Friston, K., Frith, C., Liddle, P., & Frackowiak, R. (1993). Cereb blood flow. *Metabolism*, *12*, 491–499.

Fritz, N., Glogau, S., Hoffmann, J., Rademacher, M., Elger, C. E., & Helmstaedter, C. (2005). Efficacy and cognitive side effects of tiagabine and topiramate in patients with epilepsy. *Epilepsy & Behavior*, *6*(3). doi: 10.1016/j.yebeh.2005.01.002 15820346

Froscher, W., Schier, K. R., Hoffmann, M., Meyer, A., May, T. W., Rambeck, B., & Rosche, J. (2005). Topiramate: A prospective study on the relationship between concentration, dosage and adverse events in epileptic patients on combination therapy. *Epileptic Disord*, *7*(3), 237–248.

Fuller-Thomson, E., & Brennenstuhl, S. (2009). The association between depression and epilepsy in a nationally representative sample. *Epilepsia*, *50*(5), 1051–1058. doi: 10.1111/j.1528-1167.2008.01803.x

Gainotti, G. (2012). Unconscious processing of emotions and the right hemisphere. *Neuropsychologia*, *50*(2), 205–218. doi: 10.1016/j.neuropsychologia.2011.12.005

Garcia, C. S. (2012). Depression in temporal lobe epilepsy: A review of prevalence, clinical features, and management considerations. *Epilepsy Research and Treatment*, *2012*, 809843. doi: 10.1155/2012/809843

Gleissner, U., Kuczaty, S., Clusmann, H., Elger, C. E., & Helmstaedter, C. (2008). Neuropsychological results in pediatric patients with epilepsy surgery in the parietal cortex. *Epilepsia*, *49*(4), 700–704. doi: 10.1111/j.1528-1167.2007.01497.x

Goddard, G. V. (1967). Development of epileptic seizures through brain stimulation at low intensity. *Nature*, *214*(5092), 1020–1021.

Gomer, B., Wagner, K., Frings, L., Saar, J., Carius, A., Harle, M., . . . Schulze-Bonhage, A. (2007). The influence of antiepileptic drugs on cognition: A comparison of levetiracetam with topiramate. *Epilepsy & Behavior*, *10*(3). doi: 10.1016/j.yebeh.2007.02.007

Grabenstatter, H. L., Russek, S. J., & Brooks-Kayal, A. R. (2012). Molecular pathways controlling inhibitory receptor expression. *Epilepsia*, *53*(Suppl 9), 71–78. doi: 10.1111/epi.12036

Grant, A. C., Henry, T. R., Fernandez, R., Hill, M. A., & Sathian, K. (2005). Somatosensory processing is impaired in temporal lobe epilepsy. *Epilepsia*, *46*(4), 534–539. doi: 10.1111/j.0013-9580.2005.54604.x

Gross, D. W. (2011). Diffusion tensor imaging in temporal lobe epilepsy. *Epilepsia*, *52*(Suppl 4), 32–34. doi: 10.1111/j.1528-1167.2011.03149.x

Guerreiro, C., Cendes, F., Li, L. M., Jones-Gotman, M., Andermann, F., Dubeau, F., . . . Feindel, W. (1999). Clinical patterns of patients with temporal lobe epilepsy and pure amygdalar atrophy. *Epilepsia*, *40*(4), 453–461.

Hamberger, M. J., & Cole, J. (2011). Language organization and reorganization in epilepsy. *Neuropsychology Review*, *21*(3), 240–251. doi: 10.1007/s11065-011-9180-z

Hamberger, M. J., & Drake, E. B. (2006). Cognitive functioning following epilepsy surgery. *Current Neurology and Neuroscience Reports*, *6*(4), 319–326.

Harden, C. L. (2002). Depression and anxiety in epilepsy patients. *Epilepsy & Behavior*, *3*(3), 296.

Harvey, D. J., Naugle, R. I., Magleby, J., Chapin, J. S., Najm, I. M., Bingaman, W., & Busch, R. M. (2008). Relationship between presurgical memory performance on the Wechsler Memory Scale-III and memory change following temporal resection for treatment of intractable epilepsy. *Epilepsy & Behavior*, *13*(2), 372–375. doi: 10.1016/j.yebeh.2008.04.024

Helmstaedter, C. (2002). Effects of chronic epilepsy on declarative memory systems. *Brain Research*, *135*, 439–453.

Helmstaedter, C., Aldenkamp, A. P., Baker, G. A., Mazarati, A., Ryvlin, P., & Sankar, R. (2014). Disentangling the relationship between epilepsy and its behavioral comorbidities—the need for prospective studies in new-onset epilepsies. *Epilepsy & Behavior*, *31*, 43–47. doi: 10.1016/j.yebeh.2013.11.010

Helmstaedter, C., Kemper, B., & Elger, C. E. (1996). Neuropsychological aspects of frontal lobe epilepsy. *Neuropsychologia*, *34*(5), 399–406.

Helmstaedter, C., & Kockelmann, E. (2006). Cognitive outcomes in patients with chronic temporal lobe epilepsy. *Epilepsia*, *47*(Suppl 2), 96–98. doi: 10.1111/j.1528-1167.2006.00702.x

Helmstaedter, C., Kurthen, M., Lux, S., Reuber, M., & Elger, C. E. (2003). Chronic epilepsy and cognition: A longitudinal study in temporal lobe epilepsy. *Annals of Neurology*, *54*(4), 425–432. doi: 10.1002/ana.10692

Hermann, B., Seidenberg, M., & Bell, B. (2002). The neurodevelopmental impact of childhood onset temporal lobe epilepsy on brain structure and function and the risk of progressive cognitive effects. *Progress in Brain Research*, *135*, 428–438.

Hermann, B., Seidenberg, M., & Jones, J. (2008). The neurobehavioural comorbidities of epilepsy: Can a natural history be developed? *Lancet Neurology*, *7*(2), 151–160. doi: 10.1016/S1474-4422(08)70018-8

Hermann, B., Seidenberg, M., Lee, E. J., Chan, F., & Rutecki, P. (2007). Cognitive phenotypes in temporal lobe epilepsy. *Journal of the International Neuropsychological Society*, *13*(1), 12–20. doi: 10.1017/S135561770707004X

Hermann, B., Wyler, A., & Somes, G. (1993). Memory loss following left anterior temporal lobectomy is associated with hippocampal pathology and not extent of hippocampal resection. *Journal of Clinical and Experimental Neuropsychology*, *6*, 350.

Hermann, B. P., Seidenberg, M., Schoenfeld, J., & Davies, K. (1997). Neuropsychological characteristics of the syndrome of mesial temporal lobe epilepsy. *Archives of Neurolology*, *54*(4), 369–376.

Hermann, B. P., Wyler, A. R., & Richey, E. T. (1988). Wisconsin Card Sorting Test performance in patients with complex partial seizures of temporal-lobe origin. *Journal of Clinical & Experimental Neuropsychology*, *10*(4), 467–476.

Hermann, B. P., Wyler, A. R., Somes, G., Berry, A. D., 3rd, & Dohan, F. C., Jr. (1992). Pathological status of the mesial temporal lobe predicts memory outcome from left anterior temporal lobectomy. *Neurosurgery*, *31*(4), 652–656; discussion 656–657.

Hertz-Pannier, L., Chiron, C., Jambaque, I., Renaux-Kieffer, V., Van de Moortele, P. F., Delalande, O., . . . Le Bihan, D. (2002). Late plasticity for language in a child's non-dominant hemisphere: A pre- and post-surgery fMRI study. *Brain*, *125*(Pt 2), 361–372.

Honey, C. J., Kotter, R., Breakspear, M., & Sporns, O. (2007). Network structure of cerebral cortex shapes functional connectivity on multiple time scales. *Proceedings of the National Academy of Sciences*, *104*(24), 10240–10245. doi: 10.1073/pnas.0701519104

Howell, R. A., Saling, M. M., Bradley, D. C., & Berkovic, S. F. (1994). Interictal language fluency in temporal lobe epilepsy. *Cortex*, *30*(3), 469–478.

Huang, C. W., Pai, M. C., & Tsai, J. J. (2008). Comparative cognitive effects of levetiracetam and topiramate in intractable epilepsy. *Psychiatry and Clinical Neurosciences*, *62*(5), 548–553. doi: 10.1111/j.1440-1819.2008.01848.x

Ivnik, R., Sharvrough, F., & Laws, E. (1988). Anterior temporal lobectomy for the control of partial complex seizures: Information for counseling patients. *Mayo Clinic Proceedings*, *63*, 783–793.

Jacobs, K. M., Graber, K. D., Kharazia, V. N., Parada, I., & Prince, D. A. (2000). Postlesional epilepsy: The ultimate brain plasticity. *Epilepsia*, *41*(Suppl 6), S153–S161.

Jokeit, H., & Ebner, A. (1999). Long term effects of refractory temporal lobe epilepsy on cognitive abilities: A cross sectional study. *Journal of Neurology, Neurosurgery, and Psychiatry*, *67*(1), 44–50.

Jokeit, H., & Ebner, A. (2002). Effects of chronic epilepsy on intellectual functions. *Progress in Brain Research*, *135*, 455–463.

Jokeit, H., Ebner, A., Holthausen, H., Markowitsch, H. J., & Tuxhorn, I. (1996). Reorganization of memory functions after human temporal lobe damage. *Neuroreport*, *7*(10), 1627–1630.

Jokeit, H., Okujava, M., & Woermann, F. G. (2001). Memory fMRI lateralizes temporal lobe epilepsy. *Neurology*, *57*(10), 1786–1793.

Jokeit, H., & Schacher, M. (2004). Neuropsychological aspects of type of epilepsy and etiological factors in adults. *Epilepsy & Behavior*, *5*(Suppl 1), S14–20.

Keller, S. S., & Roberts, N. (2008). Voxel-based morphometry of temporal lobe epilepsy: An introduction and review of the literature. *Epilepsia*, *49*(5), 741–757. doi: 10.1111/j.1528-1167.2007.01485.x

Kemmotsu, N., Girard, H. M., Bernhardt, B. C., Bonilha, L., Lin, J. J., Tecoma, E. S., . . . McDonald, C. R. (2011). MRI analysis in temporal lobe epilepsy: Cortical thinning and white matter disruptions are related to side of seizure onset. *Epilepsia*, *52*(12), 2257–2266. doi: 10.1111/j.1528-1167.2011.03278.x

Killgore, W. D., & Yurgelun-Todd, D. A. (2005). Social anxiety predicts amygdala activation in adolescents viewing fearful faces. *Neuroreport*, *16*(15), 1671–1675.

Knopman, A. A., Wong, C. H., Stevenson, R. J., Homewood, J., Mohamed, A., Somerville, E., . . . Bleasel, A. F. (2014). The cognitive profile of occipital lobe epilepsy and the selective association of left temporal lobe hypometabolism with verbal memory impairment. *Epilepsia*. doi: 10.1111/epi.12623

Kockelmann, E., Elger, C., & Helmstaedter, C. (2003). Significant improvement in frontal lobe associated neuropsychological functions after withdrawl of topiramate in epilepsy patients. *Epilepsy Research*, *54*, 171–178.

Kondziella, D., Alvestad, S., Vaaler, A., & Sonnewald, U. (2007). Which clinical and experimental data link temporal lobe epilepsy with depression? *Journal of Neurochemistry*, *103*(6), 2136–2152. doi: 10.1111/j.1471-4159.2007.04926.x

Koylu, B., Trinka, E., Ischebeck, A., Visani, P., Trieb, T., Kremser, C., . . . Benke, T. (2006). Neural correlates of verbal semantic memory in patients with temporal lobe epilepsy. *Epilepsy & Research*, *72*(2–3), 178–191. doi: 10.1016/j.eplepsyres.2006.08.002

Kullmann, D. M., Moreau, A. W., Bakiri, Y., & Nicholson, E. (2012). Plasticity of inhibition. *Neuron*, *75*(6), 951–962. doi: 10.1016/j.neuron.2012.07.030

Kuzniecky, R., de la Sayette, V., & Ethier, R. (1987). Magnetic resonance imaging in temporal lobe epilepsy. *Annals of Neurology*, *22*, 341–347.

Langfitt, J. T., Westerveld, M., Hamberger, M. J., Walczak, T. S., Cicchetti, D. V., Berg, A. T., . . . Spencer, S. S. (2007). Worsening of quality of life after epilepsy surgery: Effect of seizures and memory decline. *Neurology*, *68*(23). doi: 10.1212/01.wnl.0000264000.11511.30 17548548

LeDoux, J. E. (2000). Emotion circuits in the brain. *Annual Review of Neuroscience*, *23*, 155–184. doi: 10.1146/annurev.neuro.23.1.155

Lee, G. (2010). *Neuropsychology of Epilepsy and Epilepsy Surgery*. New York: Oxford University Press.

Lee, G. P., Loring, D., & Thompson, J. L. (1989). Construct validity of material specific memory measures following unilateral temporal lobe ablations. *Psychological Assessment: Journal of Consulting and Clinical Psychology*, *3*, 192–197.

Leech, C., & McIntyre, D. (1976). Kindling rates in inbred mice: An analog to learning. *Behavioral Biology*, *16*, 439–452.

Lencz, T., McCarthy, G., & Bronen, R. (1992). Quantitative magnetic resonance imaging in temporal lobe epilepsy: Relationship to neuropathology and neuropsychological function. *Annals of Neurology*, *31*, 629–637.

Leonard, G. (1991). Temporal lobe surgery for epilepsy: Neuropsychological variables related to surgical outcome. *Canadian Journal of Neurological Sciences*, *18*, 593–597.

Levisohn, P. M., Mintz, M., Hunter, S. J., Yang, H., Jones, J., & Group, N.L.S. (2009). Neurocognitive effects of adjunctive levetiracetam in children with partial-onset seizures: A randomized, double-blind, placebo-controlled, noninferiority trial. *Epilepsia*, *50*(11), 2377–2389. doi: 10.1111/j.1528-1167.2009.02197.x

Liacu, D., Idy-Peretti, I., Ducreux, D., Bouilleret, V., & de Marco, G. (2012). Diffusion tensor imaging tractography parameters of limbic system bundles in temporal lobe epilepsy patients. *Journal of Magnetic Resonance Imaging*, *36*(3), 561–568. doi: 10.1002/jmri.23678

Liao, W., Zhang, Z., Pan, Z., Mantini, D., Ding, J., Duan, X., . . . Chen, H. (2010). Altered functional connectivity and small-world in mesial temporal lobe epilepsy. *PLoS One*, *5*(1), e8525. doi: 10.1371/journal.pone.0008525

Logothetis, N., & Pfeuffer, J. (2004). On the nature of the BOLD fMRI contrast mechanism. *Magnetic Resonance Annual*, *22*, 1517–1531.

Loring, D., Lee, G., & Meador, K. (1991). Hippocampal contribution to verbal recent memory following dominant hemisphere temporal lobectomy. *Journal of Clinical and Experimental Neuropsychology*, *13*, 575–586.

Luo, C., An, D., Yao, D., & Gotman, J. (2014). Patient-specific connectivity pattern of epileptic network in frontal lobe epilepsy. *NeuroImage: Clinical*, *4*, 668–675. doi: 10.1016/j.nicl.2014.04.006

Luo, C., Li, Q., Lai, Y., Xia, Y., Qin, Y., Liao, W., . . . Gong, Q. (2011). Altered functional connectivity in default mode network in absence epilepsy: A resting state fMRI study. *Human Brain Mapping*, *32*(3), 438–439.

Manni, R., Ratti, M. T., Perucca, E., Galimberti, C. A., & Tartara, A. (1993). A multiparametric investigation of daytime sleepiness and psychomotor functions in epileptic patients treated with phenobarbital and sodium valproate: A comparative controlled study. *Electroencephalography and Clinical Neurophysiology*, *86*(5), 322–328.

Marques, C. M., Caboclo, L. O., da Silva, T. I., Noffs, M. H., Carrete, H., Jr., Lin, K., . . . Yacubian, E. M. (2007). Cognitive decline in temporal lobe epilepsy due to unilateral hippocampal sclerosis. *Epilepsy & Behavior*, *10*(3), 477–485. doi: 10.1016/j.yebeh.2007.02.002

Martin, R., Kretzmer, T., Palmer, C., Sawrie, S., Knowlton, R., Faught, E., . . . Kuzniecky, R. (2002). Risk to verbal memory following anterior temporal lobectomy in patients with severe left-sided hippocampal sclerosis. *Archives of Neurology*, *59*, 1895–1901.

Martin, R., Sawrie, S., Edwards, R., Roth, D., Kuzniecky, R., Morawetz, R., & Gilliam, F. (2000). Investigation of executive function change following anterior temporal lobectomy: Selective normalization of verbal fluency. *Neuropsychology*, *14*(4), 501–508.

May, A. (2011). Experience-dependent structural plasticity in the adult human brain. *Trends in Cognitive Sciences*, *15*(10), 475–482. doi: 10.1016/j.tics.2011.08.002

McClelland, J. L. (2001). Failures to learn and their remediation: A Hebbian Account. In J.L.M.A.R.S. Seigler (Ed.), *Mechanisms of Cognitive Development: Behavioral and Neural Perspectives* (pp. 97–121). Mahwah, NJ: Lawrence Erlbaum Associates.

McCormick, C., Quraan, M., Cohn, M., Valiante, T. A., & McAndrews, M. P. (2013). Default mode network connectivity indicates episodic memory capacity in mesial temporal lobe epilepsy. *Epilepsia*, *54*(5), 809–818. doi: 10.1111/epi.12098

McLachlan, R., Rose, K., Derry, P., Bonnar, C., Blume, W. T., & Girvin, J. P. (1997). Health-related quality of life and seizure control in temporal lobe epilepsy. *Annals of Neurology*, *41*, 482–489.

Meador, K. (2002). Cognitive outcomes and predicting factors in epilepsy. *Neurology*, *58*, 21–26.

Meinzer, M., Harnish, S., Conway, T., & Crosson, B. (2011). Recent developments in functional and structural imaging of aphasia recovery after stroke. *Aphasiology*, *25*(3), 271–290. doi: 10.1080/02687038.2010.530672

Milner, B. (1975). Psychological aspects of focal epilepsy and its neurosurgical management. In D. Purpura, P. JK, & R. Walter (Eds.), *Adv Neurol* (pp. 299–321). New York: Raven Press.

Moadel, D., Doucet, G., Pustina, D., Rider, R., Taylor, N., Sperling, M., Sharan, A., & Tracy, J. I. (2014). *Amygdala volume and predictors of psychiatric symptoms after anterior temporal lobectomy*. Paper presented at the 20th Annual Meeting of the Organization for Human Brain Mapping, Hamburg, Germany.

Morgan, V. L., Rogers, B. P., Sonmezturk, H. H., Gore, J. C., & Abou-Khalil, B. (2011). Cross hippocampal influence in mesial temporal lobe epilepsy measured with high temporal resolution functional magnetic resonance imaging. *Epilepsia*, *52*(9), 1741–1749. doi: 10.1111/j.1528-1167.2011.03196.x

Morrell, F., & deToledo-Morrell, L. (1999). From mirror focus to secondary epileptogenesis in man: An historical review. *Advances in Neurol*, *81*, 11–23.

Morris, G., Mueller, W., Swanson, S., & Inglese, C. (2005). *Normal MRI does not afftect seizure free outcomes after epilepsy surgery: Results in 176 surgeries*. Paper presented at the American Epilepsy Society, Annual Meeting, Washington, DC.

Nicoll, R. A., & Malenka, R. C. (1999). Expression mechanisms underlying NMDA receptor-dependent long-term potentiation. *Annals of the New York Academy of Sciences*, *868*, 515–525.

Nilsson, D., Malmgren, K., Rydenhag, B., & Frisen, L. (2004). Visual field defects after temporal lobectomy: Comparing methods and analysing resection size. *Acta Neurologica Scandinavica*, *110*(5), 301–307. doi: 10.1111/j.1600-0404.2004.00331.x

Ojemann, J., & Dodrill, C. B. (1985). Verbal memory deficits after ledt temporal lobectomy for epilepsy. *Journal of Neurosurgery*, *62*, 101–107.

Osipowicz, K., Pajor, N., Sharan, A., Skidmore, C., Sperling, M., & Tracy, J. (under review). The effects of interictal seizure burden on white matter in temporal lobe epilepsy.

Otte, W. M., van Eijsden, P., Sander, J. W., Duncan, J. S., Dijkhuizen, R. M., & Braun, K. P. (2012). A meta-analysis of white matter changes in temporal lobe epilepsy as studied with diffusion tensor imaging. *Epilepsia*, *53*(4), 659–667. doi: 10.1111/j.1528-1167.2012.03426.x

Oyegbile, T., Dow, C., Jones, J., & et al. (2004). The nature and course of neuropsychological morbidity in chronic temporal lobe epilepsy. *Neurology*, *62*, 1736–1742.

Park, S. P., Hwang, Y. H., Lee, H. W., Suh, C. K., Kwon, S. H., & Lee, B. I. (2008). Long-term cognitive and mood effects of zonisamide monotherapy in epilepsy patients. *Epilepsy & Behavior*, *12*(1), 102–108. doi: 10.1016/j.yebeh.2007.08.002

Pereira, F. R., Alessio, A., Sercheli, M. S., Pedro, T., Bilevicius, E., Rondina, J. M., . . . Cendes, F. (2010). Asymmetrical hippocampal connectivity in mesial temporal lobe epilepsy: Evidence from resting state fMRI. *BMC Neuroscience*, *11*, 66. doi: 10.1186/1471-2202-11-66

Phelps, E. A., & LeDoux, J. E. (2005). Contributions of the amygdala to emotion processing: From animal models to human behavior. *Neuron*, *48*(2), 175–187. doi: 10.1016/j.neuron.2005.09.025

Pittau, F., Grova, C., Moeller, F., Dubeau, F., & Gotman, J. (2012). Patterns of altered functional connectivity in mesial temporal lobe epilepsy. *Epilepsia*, *53*(6), 1013–1023. doi: 10.1111/j.1528-1167.2012.03464.x

Pressler, R. M., Binnie, C. D., Coleshill, S. G., Chorley, G. A., & Robinson, R. O. (2006). Effect of lamotrigine on cognition in children with epilepsy. *Neurology*, *66*(10), 1495–1499. doi: 10.1212/01.wnl.0000216273.94142.84

Pulliainen, V., & Jokelainen, M. (1995). Comparing the cognitive effects of phenytoin and carbamazepine in long-term monotherapy: A two-year follow-up. *Epilepsia*, *36*(12), 1195–1202.

Pustina, D., Doucet, G., Evans, J., Sharan, A., Sperling, M., Skidmore, C., & Tracy, J. (2014a). Genuine and artifactual white matter plasticity following anterior temporal lobectomy in epilepsy.

Pustina, D., Doucet,. G., Skidmore, C., Sperling, M., & Tracy, J. (2014b). Contralateral interictal spikes are related to tapetum damage in left temporal lobe epilepsy. *Epilepsia*. doi: 10.1111/epi.12721

Raol, Y. S., Budreck, E. C., & Brooks-Kayal, A. R. (2003). Epilepsy after early life seizures can be independent of hippocampal injury. *Annals of Neurology*, *53*(4), 503–511. doi: 10.1002/ana.10490

Rasmussen, T., & Milner, B. (1977). The role of early left-brain injury in determining lateralization of cerebral speech functions. *Annals of the New York Academy of Sciences*, *299*, 355–369.

Rausch, R. (1987). Psychological evaluation. In J. Engel, Jr. (Ed.), *Surgical Treatment of Epilepsies* (pp. 181–195). New York: Raven Press.

Rausch, R., & Babb, T. L. (1993). Hippocampal neuron loss and memory scores before and after temporal lobe surgery for epilepsy. *Archives of Neurology*, *50*(8), 812–817.

Rausch, R., & Crandall, P. (1982). Psychological status related to surgical control of temporal lobe seizures. *Epilepsia*, *23*, 191–202.

Rausch, R., Kraemer, S., Pietras, C. J., Le, M., Vickrey, B. G., & Passaro, E. A. (2003). Early and late cognitive changes following temporal lobe surgery for epilepsy. *Neurology*, *60*(6), 951–959.

Reuber, M., Andersen, B., Elger, C. E., & Helmstaedter, C. (2004). Depression and anxiety before and after temporal lobe epilepsy surgery. *Seizure*, *13*(2), 129–135.

Richardson, M. P., Strange, B. A., Duncan, J. S., & Dolan, R. J. (2003). Preserved verbal memory function in left medial temporal pathology involves reorganisation of function to right medial temporal lobe. *Neuroimage*, *20*(Suppl 1), S112–119.

Riederer, F., Lanzenberger, R., Kaya, M., Prayer, D., Serles, W., & Baumgartner, C. (2008). Network atrophy in temporal lobe epilepsy. *Neurology*, *71*(6), 419.

Ristic, A. J., Alexopoulos, A. V., So, N., Wong, C., & Najm, I. M. (2012). Parietal lobe epilepsy: The great imitator among focal epilepsies. *Epileptic Disorders*, *14*(1), 22–31. doi: 10.1684/epd.2012.0484

Ristic, A. J., Vojvodic, N., Jankovic, S., Sindelic, A., & Sokic, D. (2006). The frequency of reversible parkinsonism and cognitive decline associated with valproate treatment: A study of 364 patients with different types of epilepsy. *Epilepsia*, *47*(12), 2183–2185. doi: 10.1111/j.1528-1167.2006.00711.x

Roberson-Nay, R., McClure, E. B., Monk, C. S., Nelson, E. E., Guyer, A. E., Fromm, S. J., . . . Pine, D. S. (2006). Increased amygdala activity during successful memory encoding in adolescent major depressive disorder: An FMRI study. *Biological Psychiatry*, *60*(9), 966–973. doi: 10.1016/j.biopsych.2006.02.018

Robinson, L., Barnett, P., Doucet, G., Pustina, D., Ghani, A., & Tracy, J. (2014). The temporal instability of the ventral default mode network connectivity in intractable epilepsy.

Rosenberger, L. R., Zeck, J., Berl, M. M., Moore, E. N., Ritzl, E. K., Shamim, S., . . . Gaillard, W. D. (2009). Interhemispheric and intrahemispheric language reorganization in complex partial epilepsy. *Neurology*, *72*(21), 1830–1836. doi: 10.1212/WNL.0b013e3181a7114b

Rzezak, P., Fuentes, D., Guimaraes, C. A., Thome-Souza, S., Kuczynski, E., Li, L. M., . . . Valente, K. D. (2007). Frontal lobe dysfunction in children with temporal lobe epilepsy. *Pediatr Neurol*, *37*(3), 176–185. doi: 10.1016/j.pediatrneurol.2007.05.009

Sabsevitz, D., Swanson, S., Hammeke, T., Spanaki, M., Possing, E., Morris, G., . . . Binder, J. (2003). Use of preoperative functional neuroimaging to predict language deficits from epilepsy surgery. *Neurology*, *60*, 1788–1792.

Sandok, E. K., O'Brien, T. J., Jack, C. R., & So, E. L. (2000). Significance of cerebellar atrophy in intractable temporal lobe epilepsy: A quantitative MRI study. *Epilepsia*, *41*(10), 1315–1320.

Sass, K. J., Spencer, D. D., Kim, J. H., Westerveld, M., Novelly, R. A., & Lencz, T. (1990). Verbal memory impairment correlates with hippocampal pyramidal cell density. *Neurology*, *40*(11), 1694–1697.

Saykin, A., Gur, R., Sussman, N., O'Connor, M., & Gur, R. (1989). Memory deficits before and after temporal lobectomy: Effect of laterality and age of onset. *Brain and Cognition*, *9*(2), 191–200.

Sazgar, M., Carlen, P. L., & Wennberg, R. (2003). Panic attack semiology in right temporal lobe epilepsy. *Epileptic Disorders*, *5*(2), 93–100.

Schefft, B. K., Marc Testa, S., Dulay, M. F., Privitera, M. D., & Yeh, H. S. (2003). Preoperative assessment of confrontation naming ability and interictal paraphasia production in unilateral temporal lobe epilepsy. *Epilepsy & Behavior*, *4*(2), 161–168.

Schneider-Mizell, C. M., Caboclo, L. O., Parent, J. M., Ben-Jacob, E., Zochowski, M. R., & Sander, L. M. (2010). From network structure to network reorganization: Implications for adult neurogenesis. *Physical Biology*, *7*(4), 046008. doi: 10.1088/1478-3975/7/4/046008

Schwartzkroin, P. A. (2001). Mechanisms of brain plasticity: From normal brain function to pathology. *International Review of Neurobiology*, *45*, 1–15.

Seidenberg, M., Hermann, B., Wyler, A., Davies, K., Dohan, F., & Leveroni, C. (1998). Neuropsychological outcome following anterior temporal lobectomy in patients with and without the syndrome of mesial temporal lobe epilepsy. *Neuropsychology*, *12*, 303–316.

Seidenberg, M., Hermann, B. P., Schoenfeld, J., Davies, K., Wyler, A., & Dohan, F. C. (1997). Reorganization of verbal memory function in early onset left temporal lobe epilepsy. *Brain and Cognition*, *35*(1), 132–148. doi: 10.1006/brcg.1997.0931

Shimizu, T., Nariai, T., Maehara, T., Hino, T., Komori, T., Shimizu, H., . . . Senda, M. (2000). Enhanced motor cortical excitability in the unaffected hemisphere after hemispherectomy. *Neuroreport*, *11*(14), 3077–3084.

Shulman, M. B. (2000). The frontal lobes, epilepsy, and behavior. *Epilepsy & Behavior*, *1*(6), 384–395.

Somera-Molina, K. C., Robin, B., Somera, C. A., Anderson, C., Stine, C., Koh, S., . . . Wainwright, M. S. (2007). Glial activation links early life seizures and long-term neurologic dysfunction: Evidence using a small molecule inhibitor of proinflammatory cytokine upregulation. *Epilepsia*, *48*(9), 1785–1800. doi: 10.1111/j.1528-1167.2007.01135.x

Spencer, S. (2005, Monday, December 5). *Resective epilepsy surgery: Patient selection and outcomes*. Paper presented at the American Epilepsy Society, Annual Meeting, Washington, DC.

Sperling, M., O'Conner, M., Saykin, A., & Plummer, C. (1996). Temporal lobectomy for refractory epilepsy. *JAMA*, *276*, 470–475.

Springer, J. A., Binder, J. R., Hammeke, T. A., Swanson, S. J., Frost, J. A., Bellgowan, P. S., . . . Mueller, W. M. (1999). Language dominance in neurologically normal and epilepsy subjects: A functional MRI study. *Brain*, *122*(Pt 11), 2033–2046.

Squire, L. R. (2009). The legacy of patient H.M. for neuroscience. *Neuron*, *61*(1), 6–9. doi: 10.1016/j.neuron.2008.12.023

Staba, R. J., Ekstrom, A. D., Suthana, N. A., Burggren, A., Fried, I., Engel, J., Jr., & Bookheimer, S. Y. (2012). Gray matter loss correlates with mesial temporal lobe neuronal hyperexcitability inside the human seizure-onset zone. *Epilepsia*, *53*(1), 25–34. doi: 10.1111/j.1528-1167.2011.03333.x

Strauss, E., Hunter, M., & Wada, J. (1993). Wisconsin card sorting performance: Effects of age of onset of damage and laterality of dysfunction. *Journal of Clinical and Experimental Neuropsychology*, *15*, 896–902.

Stroup, E., Langfitt, J., Berg, M., McDermott, J., Pilcher, W., & Como, P. (2003). Predicting verbal memory decline following anterior temporal lobectomy (ATL). *Neurology*, *60*, 1266–1273.

Sutula, T. P. (2004). Mechanisms of epilepsy progression: Current theories and perspectives from neuroplasticity in adulthood and development. *Epilepsy Research*, *60*(2–3), 161–171. doi: 10.1016/j.eplepsyres.2004.07.001

Sutula, T. P., & Dudek, F. E. (2007). Unmasking recurrent excitation generated by mossy fiber sprouting in the epileptic dentate gyrus: An emergent property of a complex system. *Progress in Brain Research*, *163*, 541–563. doi: 10.1016/S0079-6123(07)63029-5

Szaflarski, J. P., Holland, S. K., Schmithorst, V. J., & Byars, A. W. (2006). fMRI study of language lateralization in children and adults. *Human Brain Mapping*, *27*(3), 202–212. doi: 10.1002/hbm.20177

Tebartz van Elst, L., Woermann, F. G., Lemieux, L., & Trimble, M. R. (1999). Amygdala enlargement in dysthymia: A volumetric study of patients with temporal lobe epilepsy. *Biological Psychiatry*, *46*(12), 1614–1623.

Tebartz van Elst, L., Woermann, F. G., Lemieux, L., & Trimble, M. R. (2000). Increased amygdala volumes in female and depressed humans. A quantitative magnetic resonance imaging study. *Neuroscience Letters*, *281*(2–3), 103–106.

Tellez-Zenteno, J. F., Patten, S. B., Jette, N., Williams, J., & Wiebe, S. (2007). Psychiatric comorbidity in epilepsy: A population-based analysis. *Epilepsia*, *48*(12), 2336–2344. doi: 10.1111/j.1528-1167.2007.01222.x

Thivard, L., Lehericy, S., Krainik, A., Adam, C., Dormont, D., Chiras, J., . . . Dupont, S. (2005). Diffusion tensor imaging in medical temporal lobe epilepsy with hippocampal sclerosis. *Neuroimage*.

Thomas, K. M., Drevets, W. C., Dahl, R. E., Ryan, N. D., Birmaher, B., Eccard, C. H., . . . Casey, B. J. (2001). Amygdala response to fearful faces in anxious and depressed children. *Archives of General Psychiatry*, *58*(11), 1057–1063.

Toth, Z., Yan, X., Haftoglou, S., Ribak, C. E., & Baram, T. Z. (1998). Seizure-induced neuronal injury: Vulnerability to febrile seizures in an immature rat model. *Journal of Neuroscience*, *18*(11), 4285–4294.

Tracy, J. I., & Boswell, S. (2008). Modeling the Interaction between Language and Memory: The case of temporal lobe epilepsy. In B.S.H. Whitaker (Ed.), *Handbook of the Neuroscience of Language* (pp. 319–328). San Diego, CA: Academic Press.

Tracy, J. I., Dechant, V., Sperling, M. R., Cho, R., & Glosser, D. (2007). The association of mood with quality of life ratings in epilepsy. *Neurology*, *68*(14), 1101–1107. doi: 10.1212/01.wnl.0000242582.83632.73

Tracy, J. I., Flanders, A., Madi, S., Laskas, J., Stoddard, E., Pyrros, A., . . . DelVecchio, N. (2003). Regional brain activation associated with different performance patterns during learning of a complex motor skill. *Cerebral Cortex*, *13*(9), 904–910.

Tracy, J. I., Lippincott, C., Mahmood, T., Waldron, B., Kanauss, K., Glosser, D., & Sperling, M. R. (2007). Are depression and cognitive performance related in temporal lobe epilepsy? *Epilepsia*, *48*(12), 2327–2335. doi: 10.1111/j.1528-1167.2007.01254.x

Tracy, J. I., Osipowicz, K., Spechler, P., Sharan, A., Skidmore, C., Doucet, G., & Sperling, M. R. (2014). Functional connectivity evidence of cortico-cortico inhibition in temporal lobe epilepsy. *Human Brain Mapping*, *35*(1), 353–366. doi: 10.1002/hbm.22181

Tracy, J. I., Osipowicz, K., Stamos, C., & Berman, A. (2010). Epilepsy and cognitive plasticity. In C. Armstrong & L. Morrow (Eds.), *The Neuropsychology of Medical Disorders*. New York: Springer.

Tracy, J. I., Waldron, B., Glosser, D., Sharan, A., Mintzer, S., Zangaladze, A., . . . Sperling, M. R. (2009). Hemispheric lateralization and language skill coherence in temporal lobe epilepsy. *Cortex*, *45*(10), 1178–1189. doi: 10.1016/j.cortex.2009.01.007

Trenerry, M., Jack, C., & Ivnik, R. (1993). MRI hippocampal volumes and memory function before and after temporal lobectomy. *Neurology*, *43*, 1800–1805.

Trennery, M., Jack, C., & Ivnik, R. (1991). Memory is correlated with presurgical magnetic resonance imaging hippocampal volumes before and after temporal lobectomy for intractable epilepsy. *Epilepsia*, *31*, 73.

Tuchman, R., Moshe, S. L., & Rapin, I. (2009). Convulsing toward the pathophysiology of autism. *Brain and Development*, *31*(2), 95–103. doi: 10.1016/j.braindev.2008.09.009

Vaessen, M. J., Jansen, J. F., Braakman, H. M., Hofman, P. A., De Louw, A., Aldenkamp, A. P., & Backes, W. H. (2014). Functional and structural network impairment in childhood frontal lobe epilepsy. *PLoS One*, *9*(3), e90068. doi: 10.1371/journal.pone.0090068

Vannest, J., Szaflarski, J. P., Privitera, M. D., Schefft, B. K., & Holland, S. K. (2008). Medial temporal fMRI activation reflects memory lateralization and memory performance in patients with epilepsy. *Epilepsy & Behavior*, *12*(3), 410–418. doi: 10.1016/j.yebeh.2007.11.012

Vargha-Khadem, F., Carr, L. J., Isaacs, E., Brett, E., Adams, C., & Mishkin, M. (1997). Onset of speech after left hemispherectomy in a nine-year-old boy. *Brain*, *120*(Pt 1), 159–182.

Voets, N. L., Adcock, J. E., Stacey, R., Hart, Y., Carpenter, K., Matthews, P. M., & Beckmann, C. F. (2009). Functional and structural changes in the memory network associated with left temporal lobe epilepsy. *Human Brain Mapping*, *30*(12), 4070–4081. doi: 10.1002/hbm.20830

Wada, J. A., & Mizoguchi, T. (1984). Limbic kindling in the forebrain-bisected photosensitive baboon, Papio papio. *Epilepsia*, *25*(3), 278–287.

Wagner, K., Frings, L., Halsband, U., Everts, R., Buller, A., Spreer, J., . . . Schulze-Bonhage, A. (2007). Hippocampal functional connectivity reflects verbal episodic memory network integrity. *Neuroreport*, *18*(16), 1719–1723. doi: 10.1097/WNR.0b013e3282f0d3c5

Waites, A. B., Briellmann, R. S., Saling, M. M., Abbott, D. F., & Jackson, G. D. (2006). Functional connectivity networks are disrupted in left temporal lobe epilepsy. *Annals of Neurology*, *59*(2), 335–343.

Wang, Z., Lu, G., Zhang, Z., Zhong, Y., Jiao, Q., Tan, Q., . . . Liu, Y. (2011). Altered resting state networks in epileptic patients with generalized tonic-conic seizures. *Brain Research*, *1374*, 134–141.

Weiser, H. (2004). ILAE commission report: Mesial temporal lobe epilepsy with hippocampal sclerosis. *Epilepsia*, *45*, 695–714.

Wesnes, K. A., Edgar, C., Dean, A. D., & Wroe, S. J. (2009). The cognitive and psychomotor effects of remacemide and carbamazepine in newly diagnosed epilepsy. *Epilepsy & Behavior*, *14*(3), 522–528. doi: 10.1016/j.yebeh.2008.11.012

Widjaja, E., Zamyadi, M., Raybaud, C., Snead, O. C., & Smith, M. L. (2013). Abnormal functional network connectivity among resting-state networks in children with frontal lobe epilepsy. *AJNR American Journal of Neuroradiology*, *34*(12), 2386–2392. doi: 10.3174/ajnr.A3608

Wilke, M., Pieper, T., Lindner, K., Dushe, T., Staudt, M., Grodd, W., . . . Krageloh-Mann, I. (2011). Clinical functional MRI of the language domain in children with epilepsy. *Human Brain Mapping*, *32*(11), 1882–1893. doi: 10.1002/hbm.21156

Williamson, P. D., Boon, P. A., Thadani, V. M., Darcey, T. M., Spencer, D. D., Spencer, S. S., . . . Mattson, R. H. (1992). Parietal lobe epilepsy: Diagnostic considerations and results of surgery. *Annals of Neurology*, *31*(2), 193–201. doi: 10.1002/ana.410310210

Winston, G. P., Daga, P., White, M. J., Micallef, C., Miserocchi, A., Mancini, L., . . . McEvoy, A. W. (2014). Preventing visual field deficits from neurosurgery. *Neurology*. doi: 10.1212/WNL.0000000000000685

Witt, J. A., & Helmstaedter, C. (2013). Monitoring the cognitive effects of antiepileptic pharmacotherapy: Approaching the individual patient. *Epilepsy & Behavior*, *26*(3), 450–456. doi: 10.1016/j.yebeh.2012.09.015

Woermann, F. G., Jokeit, H., Luerding, R., Freitag, H., Schulz, R., Guertler, S., . . . Ebner, A. (2003). Language lateralization by Wada test and fMRI in 100 patients with epilepsy. *Neurology*, *61*(5), 699–701.

Xiong, Y., Mahmood, A., & Chopp, M. (2010). Neurorestorative treatments for traumatic brain injury. *Discovery Medicine*, *10*(54), 434–442.

Yogarajah, M., Powell, H. W., Parker, G. J., Alexander, D. C., Thompson, P. J., Symms, M. R., . . . Duncan, J. S. (2008). Tractography of the parahippocampal gyrus and material specific memory impairment in unilateral temporal lobe epilepsy. *Neuroimage*, *40*(4), 1755–1764. doi: 10.1016/j.neuroimage.2007.12.046

Yu, A., Li, K., Li, L., Shan, B., Wang, Y., & Xue, S. (2008). Whole-brain voxel-based morphometry of white matter in medial temporal lobe epilepsy. *European Journal of Radiology*, *65*(1), 86–90. doi: http://dx.doi.org/10.1016/j.ejrad.2007.04.011

Yuan, W., Szaflarski, J. P., Schmithorst, V. J., Schapiro, M., Byars, A. W., Strawsburg, R. H., & Holland, S. K. (2006). fMRI shows atypical language lateralization in pediatric epilepsy patients. *Epilepsia*, *47*(3), 593–600. doi: 10.1111/j.1528-1167.2006.00474.x

Zangaladze, A., Sharan, A., Evans, J., Wyeth, D. H., Wyeth, E. G., Tracy, J. I., . . . Sperling, M. R. (2008). The effectiveness of low-frequency stimulation for mapping cortical function. *Epilepsia*, *49*(3), 481–487. doi: 10.1111/j.1528-1167.2007.01307.x

Zhang, H., Schneider, T., Wheeler-Kingshott, C. A., & Alexander, D. C. (2012). NODDI: Practical in vivo neurite orientation dispersion and density imaging of the human brain. *Neuroimage*, *61*(4), 1000–1016. doi: 10.1016/j.neuroimage.2012.03.072

Zhang, Z., Lu, G., Zhong, Y., Tan, Q., Liao, W., Chen, Z., . . . Liu, Y. (2009). Impaired perceptual networks in temporal lobe epilepsy revealed by resting fMRI. *Journal of Neurology*, *256*(10), 1705–1713. doi: 10.1007/s00415-009-5187-2

Zhang, Z., Lu, G., Zhong, Y., Tan, Q., Liao, W., Wang, Z., . . . Liu, Y. (2010). Altered spontaneous neuronal activity of the default-mode network in mesial temporal lobe epilepsy. *Brain Research*, *1323*, 152–160. doi: 10.1016/j.brainres.2010.01.042

Zhang, Z., Lu, G., Zhong, Y., Tan, Q., Yang, Z., Liao, W., . . . Liu, Y. (2009). Impaired attention network in temporal lobe epilepsy: A resting FMRI study. *Neuroscience Letters*, *458*(3), 97–101. doi: 10.1016/j.neulet.2009.04.040

Zhou, B., Zhang, Q., Tian, L., Xiao, J., Stefan, H., & Zhou, D. (2008). Effects of levetiracetam as an add-on therapy on cognitive function and quality of life in patients with refractory partial seizures. *Epilepsy & Behavior*, *12*(2), 305–310. doi: 10.1016/j.yebeh.2007.10.003

20 Neurotropic Infections

Herpes Simplex Virus, Human Immunodeficiency Virus, and Lyme Disease

Richard F. Kaplan and Ronald A. Cohen

Introduction

The brain, spinal cord and adjacent structures can become infected by many kinds of microorganisms. The four main categories include bacteria, viruses, fungi, and protozoa. These microorganisms can have acute and chronic effects on brain function and consequently cognitive functioning. Depending on the location of the invading microorganism, different names are given to the diseases. Meningitis is an infection of the meninges, the tough layer of tissue that surrounds the brain and the spinal cord. Meningitis can be caused by bacterial infection, viruses, and fungi. If not treated, meningitis can lead to brain swelling, which could result in coma, permanent disability, and death. Encephalitis is an inflammation of the brain itself. It is usually caused by a viral infection. Viral infections of the brain are typically referred to as aseptic, although this is a misnomer because aseptic literally means an absence of infection. Nevertheless this terminology persists and an aseptic meningitis or encephalitis has come to mean that the inflammation is not caused by a pyogenic bacteria. As it is beyond the scope of this chapter to cover every microorganism capable of invading the nervous system, we will focus on those bacterial and viral infections most common in neuropsychology practice. These will include herpes simplex virus (HSV), human immunodeficiency virus (HIV), and the most common tick-borne bacterial infection, *Borrelia burgdorferi*, the agent responsible for Lyme disease.

Herpes Simplex Encephalitis

A 22-year-old woman was hospitalized after she presented in the emergency room with a high fever (over 104°), nausea, severe headache, and confusion. Herpes simplex encephalitis (HSE) was suspected by history, and viral DNA identification was confirmed by polymerase chain reaction (PCR). She was started on antiviral therapy and was hospitalized for three weeks. Prior to her hospitalization she had been working as a waitress and living independently. After discharge she moved in with her mother and sister, as she was no longer able to care for herself. The mother and sister reported aphasia, memory loss, confusion, and personality change. The relationship with her mother became strained as she became increasingly irritable, paranoid, and aggressive. Her mother noted that she could be "out of control." For example, in one instance, the patient took off in the car and the police were called. She was able to care for her dressing and hygiene but she was unable to cook. She also began "binge eating" and started smoking cigarettes. An EEG was reported to show left hemisphere spike/sharp wave pattern—which had not been seen during her initial hospitalization—and she was started on an anticonvulsant. A second EEG one month later showed left temporo-parieto-occipital delta slowing, but no epileptiform discharges, with normal alpha rhythm in the right hemisphere. Magnetic resonance imaging (MRI) showed abnormalities consistent with HSE such as left temporal encephalomalacia including the hippocampus Figure 20.1 Neuropsychological testing revealed impaired performances in virtually every cognitive domain, with only

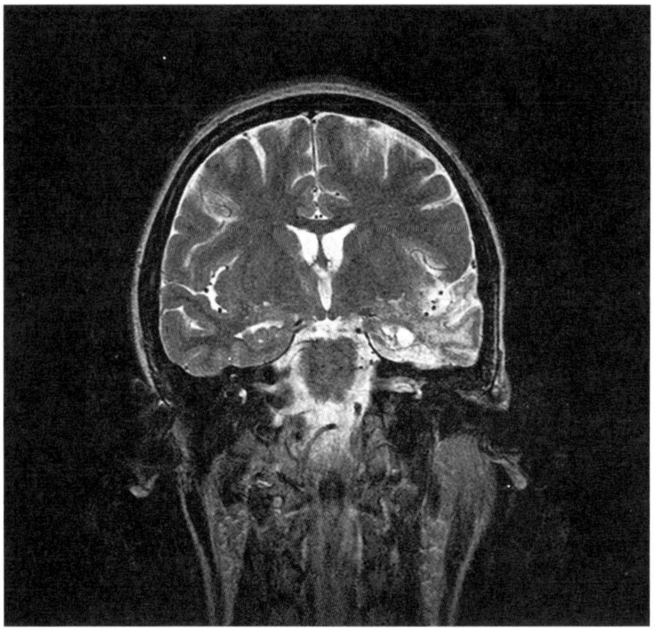

Figure 20.1 Coronal MRI T2-weighted image showing increased signal enhancement in the left temporal lobe including hippocampus and amygdala of a 22-year-old woman with confirmed HSE. The remaining brain parenchyma is unremarkable.

nonverbal skills, nonverbal problem solving, block design, judgment of line orientation, and copying relatively intact. Language testing showed expressive and receptive language deficits indicative of a global aphasia, although she was able to communicate through gesturing.

Neuropathology

HSV Type 1 (HSV1) and Type2 (HSV2), and varicella-zoster virus, are human neurotropic viruses and members of the herpesviridea family of DNA viruses (Steiner, Kennedy, & Pachner, 2007). HSV must contact mucosal surfaces or abraded skin to initiate infection and the type of herpes virus that develops is a function of the host's immune system (Whitley & Roizman, 2001). Infection with HSV1 is thought to occur in childhood with detectable antibodies found in 60%–90% of the adult population. However, recent research shows seroprevalence to be declining among younger people (Bradley, Markowitz, Gibson, & McQuillan, 2014). HSE is primarily caused by HSV1 in adults and HSV2 in neonates via transmission from infected mothers (Whitley & Roizman, 2001). HSV1 is acquired and spread by saliva, and once infected persists for life, albeit in a latent form (Fatahzadeh & Schwartz, 2007). In contrast, HSV2 is typically sexually transmitted. Given the prevalence of HSV in the general population, HSE is a relatively rare disease and occurs in approximately one in 150,000 individuals. A Swedish study showed the incidence of confirmed cases to be 2.2 per million per year (Hjalmarsson, Blomqvist, & Skoldenberg, 2007). Primary infection occurs in the mucosal membranes and is spread by the trigeminal or olfactory tract to the central nervous system (CNS). In patients with recurrent infection leading to HSE, reactivation of the virus peripherally has been suggested as the initial event. After initial infection the virus can remain latent indefinitely (Steiner et al., 2007) and in situ reactivation of a latent infection in the dorsal route ganglion appears to be more likely than retrograde spread along a cranial nerve in at least a third of all patients (Levitz, 1998). What causes the latent virus to become active is not completely clear, but a wide variety of internal and external triggers may lead to reactivation. These include psychological stress, fatigue, fever, immunosuppression, and corticosteroid administration (Fatahzadeh & Schwartz, 2007; Sarrazin, Bonneville, & Martin-Blondel, 2012). Although it is relatively rare, HSE is the most common nonepidemic encephalitis and the most common cause of sporadic lethal encephalitis. Untreated HSE is progressive, with a 70% mortality rate in 7–14 days. Even with antiviral treatment, HSE has a significant rate of mortality, 15%–20%, and morbidity (Karanjia, 1996).

In the brain, HSE has an affinity for the frontal and temporal lobes, which is likely due to the anatomical proximity of these structures to the olfactory nerve. The damage usually begins in the anterior part of the temporal lobe and can include parahippocampal gyrus, amygdala, and head of the hippocampus. It can also extend back and reach the inferior orbital cortex, the cingulate gyrus, and insula. Acute focal, necrotizing encephalitis with inflammation and swelling of the brain is a characteristic feature (Skoldenberg et al., 2006). Disease begins unilaterally, and then spreads to the contralateral temporal lobe. The lesion is clearly hyperintense in the T1 MRI sequence and hypointense in the T2 and fluid attenuated inversion recovery (FLAIR) sequence (Sarrazin et al., 2012) as described earlier and shown in Figure 20.1. The EEG is abnormal in about 85% of all cases, with lateralized epileptiform discharges superimposed on a disorganized background over one or both temporal areas (Karanjia, 1996). Although the pathogenesis of HSE-related brain damage is not completely understood, current thinking is that direct virus mechanisms and indirect immune-mediated factors both play a role (Aurelius, Andersson, Forsgren, Skoldenberg, & Strannegard, 1994). In a recent study, researchers found N-Methyl-D-Aspartate (NMDA) receptor antibodies in 30% of patients with PCR-confirmed HSE cases (Pruss et al., 2012). The NMDA receptors in the hippocampus have been directly linked to synaptic plasticity and memory (Liu et al., 2004), which may explain a potential mechanism causing amnesia in some HSE patients.

Clinical Considerations

The clinical presentation of HSE includes malaise, fever, headache, and nausea, followed by or in combination with acute or subacute onset of an encephalopathy with symptoms that typically include lethargy, confusion, and delirium. There can be seizures and coma during the course of the disease (Sarrazin et al., 2012). The cerebrospinal fluid in HSE is variable, but usually consists of a pleocytosis with both polymorphonuclear leukocytes and monocytes. The protein concentration is characteristically elevated, glucose is usually normal, and red blood cells are frequently present (Karanjia, 1996). The clinical presentation does not reliably distinguish HSE from other types of viral and bacterial encephalitis. In the past a brain biopsy provided the most definitive diagnosis, but this has largely been replaced by MRI and PCR of cerebral spinal fluid (CSF).

Neuropsychology

In his now-classic paper, Cermak (Cermak, 1976) described the profound amnesia that can result from HSE. Patient S.S. was a 44-year-old male physicist when he contracted the disorder that permanently changed his life. A pneumoencephalogram revealed dilated lateral and third ventricles, marked atrophy of the left temporal lobe, some atrophy of the right temporal lobe, and possible atrophy of the thalamus. When evaluated two years later, he had a Wechsler Adult Intelligence Scale (WAIS) IQ score of 133, and Wechsler Memory Scale (WMS) score of 83. Although there was improvement in his performance several years later, and S.S. was able to use his analytical abilities, he could not retain previously learned information in memory (Cermak & O'Connor, 1983). In one of the first studies to utilize magnetic resonance imaging (MRI) Kapur and colleagues (Kapur et al., 1994) reported on a series of ten recovered HSE cases. The extent of pathology and degree of cognitive impairment varied between individuals. Damage to the hippocampus, either unilaterally or bilaterally, was always accompanied by damage to adjacent structures such as the parahippocampal gyrus, anterior and inferior temporal lobe gyri, insula, mammillary bodies, fornix, and the amygdala. As with patient S.S., WAIS subtest scores were mostly normal, with the greatest impairment on Information, which mainly measures general knowledge. Sixty percent of the patients showed a dense amnesia (WMS-R Quotient < 50), 40% showed impairment on picture naming, and 40% were impaired on a modified card-sorting test. Patients with naming deficits were otherwise fluent in conversational language. With the small number of subjects the authors were unable to correlate cognitive deficits with individual brain regions, but did report that the extent of medial temporal involvement was correlated with the severity of memory impairment. A more recent case study (Pimental & Gregor, 2012), did show the pattern of neuropsychological deficits to correspond with MRI and EEG findings. A 66-year-old man was hospitalized after an apparent seizure. PCR analysis of CSF was positive for HSE. An EEG showed abnormal slowing consistent with a generalized cerebral process, while the MRI revealed abnormal signal from the left temporal lobe extending into the left hippocampus and insular cortex. The neuropsychological test results were significant for deficits in memory and language indicative of greater left hemisphere dysfunction.

In addition to amnesia, dysphasia, and other related cognitive disorders, HSE is a known etiology for the human Kluver-Bucy syndrome. The human Kluver-Bucy syndrome is similar to that described in Rhesus monkeys after anterior bilateral temporal lobectomy. The syndrome, first described by Heinrich Kluver and Paul Bucy in 1937 in monkeys included loss of fear, indiscriminate dietary behavior, changes in diet, hypermetamorphosis (a tendency to react to every visual stimulus), hypersexuality, hyperorality (a tendency to examine all objects by mouth), and visual agnosia. The human syndrome was first reported by Terzian and Ore (1955) in a patient with temporal lobectomy, and other cases have since been reported involving damage to deep temporal lobe structure including HSE. Rarely is the full syndrome present in humans and most studies report on a limited number of cases. Moreover, unlike animal studies that are based on circumscribed surgical lesions, the extent and pattern of mesial temporal brain damage in humans afflicted with HSE varies and is related to residual cognitive and psychiatric outcomes (Caparros-Lefebvre et al., 1996). In a report describing the natural history of three HSE cases treated with antiviral agents, all initially showed hypersexuality, increased appetite, and varying degrees of visual agnosia in addition to memory, language, and other cognitive impairments. All three patients showed substantial functional recovery in the weeks to months after treatment (Hart, Kwentus, Frazier, & Hormel, 1986).

Although amnesia can occur with herpetic and nonherpetic encephalitis (Hokkanen, Salonen, & Launes, 1996), the long-term prognosis of patients with HSE appears worse than for patients with acute encephalitis from other etiologies (Hokkanen, Poutiainen, et al., 1996; Pewter, Williams, Haslam, & Kay, 2007).

If HSE is left untreated, only 2%–5% of surviving patients regain normal neurological function (Whitley & Roizman, 2001). Treatment with antivirals clearly reduces morbidity in HSE (Hokkanen & Launes, 1997; Hokkanen, Poutiainen, et al., 1996). Antiviral therapy does not cure the infection, but modifies the clinical course through inhibition of viral replication and prevention of subsequent tissue damage. Diagnosing HSE quickly is critical because the virus multiplies rapidly and the prognosis of the patient is highly dependent on when treatment begins. The use of idoxuridine in the 1960s and 1970s showed some promise in comparison to nontreatment (Nolan, Carruthers, & Lerner, 1970), however, neuropsychological follow-up studies of treated patients showed residual cognitive deficits—particularly memory loss—in most patients (Rennick, Nolan, Bauer, & Lerner, 1973). Currently, acyclovir, a synthetic acyclic purine-nucleoside analogue, is the standard therapy for HSV infections (Whitley & Roizman, 2001). In a retrospective study of the long-term outcome of 42 patients with confirmed HSE who were treated with acyclovir, 70% of the patients survived. Of the survivors, the most frequent residual cognitive deficits were memory impairment, 69%; personality and behavioral abnormalities, 45%; and language deficits, 41% (McGrath, Anderson, Croxson, & Powell, 1997). Of the 45% reported to have personality and behavioral abnormalities, symptoms included depression, anxiety, insomnia, irritability, poor motivation, and emotional lability. It has been suggested that psychiatric symptoms such as depression may be more prevalent in patients who are less awareness of their cognitive impairment, although this finding was based on a relatively small sample (Pewter et al., 2007). Although there is a clear relationship between HSE lesions and the frontal and temporal brain regions, case studies suggest considerable anatomic variability with shorter times between first symptom and the initiation of treatment predicting better outcomes (Kaplan & Bain, 1999).

Acquired Immunodeficiency Syndrome

During a routine visit to the infectious medicine clinic, a 52-year old man with a 25-year history of HIV infection reported that he was experiencing memory problems, episodes of confusion, and difficulty managing his finances. He indicated that he had become cognizant of these difficulties when his partner began complaining about a year ago that he was not remembering their conversations and recent events. His activities of daily living were largely intact. He continued to work in managerial position in a large corporation, but was experiencing some difficulty with multitasking and some of his coworkers were concerned that he was taking longer to complete tasks than in the past. He had experienced some depressive symptoms after his initial diagnosis and following the death of his partner at the time from acquired immunodeficiency syndrome (AIDS), but indicated that he was no longer. He reported some concern about the possibility that his memory was failing.

The patient was first diagnosed with HIV in the late 1980s when a blood test was conducted after his homosexual partner was diagnosed with AIDS. An enzyme-linked immunosorbent assay (ELISA) revealed that he was HIV-seropositive, though was asymptomatic, never having experienced any medical problems associated with AIDS. Subsequent blood tests of immune function indicated a CD4 cell count of 350, which indicated T-cell levels that were below normal. He remained asymptomatic as an adult, though four years after his initial diagnosis his immunological status had worsened (CD4 = 150), and a viral load assay indicated moderately elevated HIV-RNA (24,000 copies/ml). He was started on antiretroviral therapy, which has continued until the present time. After six months his immune function had reconstituted (CD4 = 520) and his viral load was no longer detectable. Combined antiretroviral therapy (CART) was initiated a decade ago after he experienced a sustained drop in his CD4 cell count. His HIV status has been stable since. Five years ago he was diagnosed as having a metabolic syndrome, with prediabetic insulin resistance, moderate obesity, hypertension, and elevated total cholesterol and triglyceride levels. He has no family history of Alzheimer's disease or other neurodegenerative disease.

The patient was referred for a neuropsychological assessment by his physician. He did not exhibit global cognitive dysfunction indicative of dementia, nor was there aphasia, apraxia, agnosia, or other neuropsychological syndrome indicative of a focal lesion. However, he had mild to moderate impairments in processing speed, attention, executive function, working memory, new learning and delayed recall. Delayed recall was impaired on both the Hopkins Verbal Learning Test and Brief Visual Memory Test, with recognition memory intact. Neuroimaging was obtained within two weeks of the neuropsychological evaluation to assess structural brain integrity. Consistent with the neuropsychological findings, there were no focal cortical or subcortical lesions on the T1 images and no signs of opportunistic brain infection. However, there was greater than expected cortical atrophy for his age. Furthermore, FLAIR imaging revealed the presence of white matter hyperintensities (WMH) not normally found in middle-aged adults.

Clinical Considerations

Despite major advances in the treatment and clinical management of HIV, it continues to be very prevalent in this country and to an even greater extent worldwide. The advent of CART led to dramatic reductions in HIV-associated mortality and morbidity. Yet, HIV resides in the body tissues of even effectively treated people once they are infected, as efforts to fully eradicate the virus have not yet been successful. Accordingly, HIV-infected people live with a chronic illness that has the potential to cause severe medical problems, with clinical efforts largely directed at managing the infection by (a) suppressing viral replication, (b) enhancing immune functions, reducing various secondary factors and comorbid conditions that contribute to poor health outcome, and (c) treating opportunistic infections when they occur.

HIV status is determined by laboratory and clinical findings. For most patients, this first involves discovery that their blood contains antibodies to HIV on ELISA. The health of the immune system is then determined by assessing the cluster of differentiation-4 of a specific glycogen protein found on the surface of immune system cells, such as T-cells, macrophages, and monocytes found in blood samples. Healthy people usually have CD4 cell counts in the range of 500–1,000 cells/ml. When otherwise healthy people are actively fighting an infection (e.g., influenza), it is common for white blood cells (T-cells) to increase. However, in people with compromised immune function, CD4 cell count decreases to the point that they are no longer able to effectively combat infections. HIV infection impairs the immune system, resulting in reduced CD4 cell count. Clinical outcome in HIV is associated with immune function integrity as reflected by CD4 cell count (Dragic et al., 1996; Flanigan et al., 1992; Janssen, Nwanyanwu, Selik, & Stehr-Green, 1992; Lillo et al., 1999; Mayer et al., 1992; Nockher, Bergmann, & Scherberich, 1994; Palella et al., 1998; Thieblemont, Weiss, Sadeghi, Estcourt, & Haeffner-Cavaillon, 1995; Veugelers et al., 1997).

A diagnosis of AIDS is made if CD4 levels fall below 200 cells/ml. This cut point is somewhat arbitrary, though there is strong evidence that below this level, people are more likely to experience opportunistic diseases, with risk increasing the closer CD4 is to zero. The lowest CD4 count that a particular patient ever experienced is referred to as the *nadir CD4* and has been shown to be predictive of brain disturbances in a number of studies. Past studies showed a relationship between CD4 and neurocognitive functioning, dementia risk, and EEG and MRI abnormalities (Becker et al., 1997; Bouwman et al., 1998; Brew, Dunbar, Pemberton, & Kaldor, 1996; De Ronchi et al., 2002; Egan, Chiswick, Brettle, & Goodwin, 1993; Ellis, Deutsch, et al., 1997; Gruzelier et al., 1996; Harrison et al., 1998; Heaton et al., 1995; Heaton et al., 2004; S. Letendre, Ances, Gibson, & Ellis, 2007; Marcotte et al., 2003; Wallace et al., 1997; Wallace et al., 1996; Wilkie et al., 2003). This relationship was most obvious prior to CART. The risk of cognitive impairment associated with HIV is clearly greatest among symptomatic patients with AIDS who have very low CD4 cell counts (Clark & Bessinger, 1997; Cohen et al., 2001; Odiase, Ogunrin, & Ogunniyi, 2006) with a three-fold increase in risk among patients with CD4 counts below 200 mm^3, and sevenfold among patients with CD4 counts below 100 cells/ml (Mellors et al., 1997). We previously found strongest associations with neurocognitive performance when CD4 levels fall below 100, with dramatic increases in impairment at this level CD4 (Bornstein et al., 1991). In the early years of the HIV epidemic, AIDS was primarily diagnosed on the basis of the occurrence of opportunistic infection, AIDS-associated disease, or other symptoms. Symptomatic HIV is no longer required for a diagnosis of AIDS, though whether or not a person has experienced AIDS symptoms remains an important clinical consideration. This is particularly true for opportunistic brain infections, which include toxoplasmosis, cytomegalovirus, and JC virus, which cause progressive multifocal leukoencephalopathy.

Today a much more complex relationship exists between CD4 and neurocognitive functioning. Some studies continue to find reduced CD4 levels to be associated with cognitive dysfunction, but others do not (Marcotte et al., 2003; McArthur et al., 1997; Miller et al., 1990; Tozzi et al., 2005; Villa et al., 1996). There are several reasons for differences across studies: (a) The range of CD4 among patients in particular cohorts varies quite dramatically; (b) the CD4 levels used to group patients is often quite different; (c) CD4 nadir (i.e., lowest level of immune function during disease course), duration of CD4 suppression, and duration of infection vary across studies; (d) whether or not symptomatic patients are considered in a study; and (e) what treatments were available at the time a particular study was conducted. In the post–highly active antiretroviral therapy era, the relationship between CD4 cell count and cognitive impairment has become less clear cut. It is possible that plasma levels of HIV RNA and CD4 cell count may or may not fully reflect the degree of viral suppression in the CSF, because of differential penetration of drugs across the blood-brain barrier. While neurocognitive studies of impaired immune function have primarily focused on CD4, other lymphocytes have also been implicated in HIV infection (e.g., CD8, CD16, CD57) (Aronsson, Troye-Blomberg, & Smedman, 2004).

While various issues remain unresolved regarding neurocognitive dysfunction in the context of immune system suppression, several conclusions can be reached:

1. Asymptomatic patients with CD4 levels greater than 400 or 500 cells/ml typically have little cognitive impairment that can be attributed to HIV after other factors are accounted for.
2. Patients with CD4 levels below 100 are much more likely to have impairments.
3. When CD4 drops below 200 cell/ml, a curvilinear relationship seems to exist with the greatest impairments when CD4 levels have fallen below 50.

While CD4 reflects immune system impairment, the burden of HIV is ultimately a function of viral load: i.e., the number of copies of HIV-RNA detected in the blood plasma or CSF (Geskus et al., 2003). Historically, plasma viral load was shown to be associated with the development of symptoms and HIV prognosis. Patients with plasma HIV RNA > 50,000 copies/μl have 12–18 times the risk for developing AIDS and dying. Risk dramatically increases between 500 and 50,000 copies/mL, doubling between 500 and 3,000, with six- to tenfold increases at viral load of 50,000 (Mellors et al., 1997; Mellors, 1997). Both plasma and CSF viral load are associated with neurocognitive dysfunction and HIV-associated dementia (Gonzalez et al., 2003; Vitiello et al., 2007). Plasma viral loads of greater than 50,000 copies/mL were predictive of subsequent dementia, with a relative hazard of 9.1 compared to those patients with viral loads < 500 (Childs et al., 1999). Patients with lower CD4 cell counts at baseline also had increased risk for developing dementia (Childs et al., 1999). Similar findings have been reported by other groups (DalPan et al., 1998). HIV infection of the brain is characterized by replication of viral RNA in the CSF, as well as rapid turnover, suggesting that the CNS effects are caused by rapidly proliferating cells (Eggers, van Lunzen, Buhk, & Stellbrink, 1999). As one might expect, CSF viral load has tended to relate more strongly than plasma viral load with neurocognitive performance and the occurrence of HIV-associated dementia (HAD; Bandaru et al., 2007; Chang, Ernst, Leonido-Yee, Walot, & Singer, 1999; Chang et al., 2003; Christo, Greco, Aleixo, & Livramento, 2005; Cysique et al., 2005; Ellis, Hsia, et al., 1997; Heaton et al., 1995; Krivine et al., 1999; Letendre et al., 2004; Marcotte et al., 1999; Robertson et al., 1998; Vitiello et al., 2007; Wiley et al., 1998).

Following several months of antiretroviral therapy, the majority of patients exhibit undetectable viral loads (e.g., HIV-RNA < 50 copies (Gulick et al., 1997). Yet, HIV continues to replicate despite suppression of free virus, which may create a substantial burden on the system over time (Chun et al., 2005). This is important given the continued prevalence of HIV-associated neurocognitive disorder (HAND) among people with reconstituted immune function and suppressed HIV-RNA secondary to CART, despite a reduced incidence of dementia (Gartner, 2000) Quantitative methods were developed for measuring cell-associated "proviral" HIV-DNA (Coombs, 1998; Panther et al., 1999). A significant relationship has been shown between levels of circulating provirus and HAD (Shiramizu et al., 2005; Shiramizu et al., 2007) and milder cognitive dysfunction as well (Shiramizu et al., 2007).

Complicating the clinical presentation is that HIV typically occurs against the backdrop of other medical and psychiatric comorbidities, as well as various psychosocial factors, all of which contribute to poorer functional outcome. For example, previous exposure to measles seems to have a synergistic effect on HIV (Aronsson et al., 2004). Of particular concern is coinfection with hepatitis C virus (HCV), which is particularly common among people with history of intravenous drug use or sexual contact with infected people. While HCV infection is characterized by chronic inflammation of the liver and development of hepatic cancer in many cases (Moriishi & Matsuura, 2003), it also contributes to cognitive impairments and decline it its own right that cannot be explained by psychiatric symptoms, drug abuse status, or hepatic failure (Hilsabeck, Hassanein, Carlson, Ziegler, & Perry, 2003; Hilsabeck, Perry, & Hassanein, 2002). In fact, we have found that HCV is currently a major contributor to HAND as well as associated brain abnormalities. Cortical electrophysiological changes occur with HCV, including delayed P300 latencies. These correlate with cognitive impairment (Kramer et al., 2002), apart from interferon treatment, which is also known to cause fatigue and affect cognition (Dieperink, Willenbring, & Ho, 2000; Kamei et al., 2002).

Neuropathology

HIV infection affects the brain both directly and indirectly (Clifford, 1997; Price et al., 1988). Damage to axons, myelin, and large astrocytes may occur as either a direct effect of HIV and also may be due to encephalitis or other secondary infections. Vasculitis may develop in patients, and this is associated with increased risk of infarctions secondary to hemorrhage in subcortical regions of the brain. Brain abnormalities are considered to be directly caused by HIV if they can be attributed to neuropathological factors attributable directly to the effects of virus in the brain. Alternatively, secondary brain abnormalities occur due to opportunistic infections and other diseases that develop as HIV infection progresses to AIDS. Evidence of direct CNS effects comes from cases in which there has been no opportunistic infection of the brain, yet there is significant neurocognitive impairment that is not attributable to other neurological brain diseases. Human studies and animal studies have both demonstrated that the virus can be detected in the brain within two weeks of initial infection, where it presumably remains until death (Davis et al., 1992; Goulsmith, DeWolf, & Paul, 1986; Palmer, Hjeelle, & Wiley, 1994). While the mechanisms underlying direct effects of HIV on the brain are still not fully understood, elevated free calcium is thought to occur directly from HIV effects, such as the enveloping of proteins (e.g., gpl20), with calcium influx via ionic channels causing neuronal damage (Price et al., 1988). Excitatory amino acids and receptor antagonists, such as quinolinic acid, also seem to play a direct role or as a secondary response to the presence of the virus or its "immunological footprint" in the brain.

HIV has a predilection for the basal ganglia and white matter pathways (Aylward, Henderer, & McCarthur, 1993; Budka, 1991; Budka et al., 1991; I. Everall, P. Luthert, & P. Lantos, 1993; Everall, P. J. Luthert, & P. L. Lantos, 1993; Navia, Cho, & Petito, 1986; Wiley et al., 1999; Wiley et al., 1991). The reason for this is not fully understood, though it may relate to blood-brain barrier dysfunction of the parenchyma surrounding the basal ganglia facilitating CNS penetration, perhaps secondary to particular glycoproteins (Toneatto, Finco, van der Putten, Abrignani, & Annunziata, 1999). Analysis of autopsies of people with HIV between 1988 and 1996 revealed brain lesions in 79% of patients (Lanjewar, Jain, & Shetty, 1998). Both focal and diffuse brain lesions were evident, with various types of pathology present including multifocal myelin loss (21%), microglial nodules (18%), infarcts-hemorrhage (15%), angiocentric pallor (6%), and calcification (5%). At a cellular level, multinucleated giant cells, macrophagic subcortical infiltration, myelin pallor, and gliosis may occur. Leukoencephalopathy (myelin loss, nucleated macrophages/microglia, reactive astrogliosis) is very common. Vacuolar leukoencephalopathy is associated with deep white matter swelling.

Opportunistic viral and nonviral infections, tumors, and cerebrovascular disturbances can produce severe brain dysfunction among people with HIV (Bernick & Gregorios, 1984; Clifford, 1997; Cysique et al., 2005; Eberwein, Hansen, & Agostini, 2005; Gonzales & Davis, 1988; Koralnik et al., 2005; Lanjewar, Surve, Maheshwari, Shenoy, & Hira, 1998; Lee, Chen, Wang, Yen, & Hsu, 2007; Leport et al., 1988; McMurtray, Nakamoto, Shikuma, & Valcour, 2007; Mobley, Rotterdam, Lerner, & Tapper, 1985; Paul et al., 2007; Post et al., 1983; Price et al., 1988; Ramsey & Geremia, 1988; Schmidbauer et al., 1990; Vago et al., 1996). Opportunistic brain infections (e.g., progressive multifocal leukoencephalopathy) still occur, causing severe cognitive disturbances with very poor prognosis (Lanjewar, Surve, et al., 1998; Reuter, 2005). Fortunately such cases have become relatively uncommon in recent years, and only a small percentage of HIV-infected individuals have secondary brain infections. Moreover, most of these infections are treatable and a majority of patients recover (Leport et al., 1988).

HIV causes structural and functional brain abnormalities on neuroimaging. The most dramatic structural abnormalities occur in patients with opportunistic brain infections, tumors, or cerebrovascular disturbances who are experiencing immunosuppression (Guiloff & Tan, 1992; Mundinger et al., 1992; Steinmetz et al., 1995). For example, toxoplasmosis (a parasitic infection) often produces large brain lesions apparent on CT or MRI. Progressive multifocal leukoencephalopathy produces multifocal white matter lesions that become more extensive over time and are easily seen on FLAIR MRI. However, in the absence of opportunistic infections or symptomatic AIDS, in the current post-CART era, people with chronic HIV tend to exhibit more subtle structural brain abnormalities (Heindel et al., 1994; Jernigan et al., 1993; Stout et al., 1998). While changes in brain structure may be evident through visual analysis of MRI scans over time, more often than not determination of such changes requires quantitative analysis of WMH, and cortical subcortical volume or other indices. Furthermore, these structural abnormalities correspond with clinical factors tied to HIV status, including immunologic and proinflammatory pathophysiology, chronic viral exposure, disease and treatment history, and comorbid medical conditions (Jellinger et al., 2000; Mahadevan et al., 2007; Masliah, DeTeresa, Mallory, & Hansen, 2000; Morgello, Mahboob, Yakoushina, Khan, & Hague, 2002; Neuenburg et al., 2002; Silva et al., 2012; Xing et al., 2009).

Though functional neuroimaging is less commonly conducted as part of routine neurodiagnostic evaluations, when it is done, it reveals abnormalities that are quite robust among HIV-infected people. Disturbances of both resting-state and task-associated functional MRI (fMRI) are relatively easily demonstrated when people with HIV are compared to seronegative controls. Alterations in activation of brain regions known to be involved in working memory, attention, and executive control occur, along with abnormal deactivation of brain regions comprising the default network. HIV causes a reduction in the dynamic range of functional brain response that seems to be associated with cognitive frailty in people with chronic infection.

Cerebral metabolite abnormalities are also well documented among HIV-infected people, using magnetic resonance spectroscopy (MRS). Depletion of certain metabolites that reflect neuronal loss (e.g., N-Acetyl Aspartate, Glutamate) occurs in cortical and subcortical gray and white matter, along with increased concentrations of other metabolites (e.g., choline, myo-inositol) associated with pro-inflammatory processes and cell membrane disturbances. The basal ganglia have been shown to be particularly vulnerable to these metabolite disturbances. MRS abnormalities have been shown to correspond with structural and functional brain abnormalities (via fMRI), and also with HIV clinical factors and cognitive performance.

Neuropsychology

When AIDS was first discovered in the early 1980s, severe cognitive and functional disturbances were very common. Many infected patients experienced dementia (Navia et al., 1986), though most subsequently died given the lack of therapy to combat the virus. The neurocognitive performance of patients with AIDS dementia was similar to that described at the time as a "frontal-subcortical" dementia, which reinforced the idea that HIV had a predilection for the basal ganglia, frontal-striatal systems, and white matter pathways. Of course, not all patients developed dementia, and a milder form of cognitive-motor disturbance was also observed in many infected people. The cognitive problems that occurred in these individuals were similar to that of AIDS dementia, though less severe. The fact that both cognitive and motor disturbance were observed is important as it reflects the dominant finding of cognitive and motor slowing that tended to occur among most patients with neurological symptoms.

Soon after antiretroviral therapy was first introduced, there was a reduction in the incidence of dementia. However, cognitive-motor disturbances continued to be common, although their occurrence tended to be greatest in patients with symptomatic AIDS, and to correspond with severe immune system impairment and elevated viral loads. Between the mid-1980s and late 1990s, people without compromised immune functions, elevated viral load, or AIDS symptomatology tended not to experience significant cognitive dysfunction. Yet, neurocognitive impairments continued to also be observed among people whose HIV infection was not well controlled. Studies during this period reported impairments on tests of working memory, processing speed, focused attention, and certain aspects of executive control. Impairments were commonly found on the Trail Making, Stroop, and Verbal Fluency tests, as well as motor tasks such as Grooved Pegboard. Deficits on symbol coding, sequencing, and other tests with attention-executive and working memory demands also tended to be affected. Learning inefficiencies were also described, though impairments of learning and memory were less consistently reported. Language (e.g., naming), semantics, visual perception, and other core cognitive functions tended to be largely spared. While learning inefficiency and memory recall problems occurred in some patients, severe impairments were uncommon, and primary amnestic disturbances as seen in Alzheimer's and other neurodegenerative diseases were very rare.

The situation continued to improve with the advent of CART, as treated patients exhibited improved cognitive functioning, whereas untreated patients worsened. CART was widely adopted and the incidence of HAD decreased dramatically. This led many in the field to conclude that the neurological manifestations of HIV would cease to be a major problem in the future. Unfortunately, this initial optimism was dashed when studies conducted over the past decade continued to report HAND in as many as 50% of infected people. These impairments were occurring among people whose immune functions were no longer suppressed and without elevated viral load, suggesting that prior HIV history may continue to impact the brain even after the infection is controlled. Of particular concern is the fact that many recent studies still have found problems with learning and memory recall among people with chronic HIV.

There is also growing evidence that HIV is contributing to premature cognitive aging in many people. Whereas healthy adults often exhibit generalized slowing and problems with tasks requiring working memory, focused attention, and executive control as they advance in age into their 70s or 80s, HIV-infected people are exhibiting these changes much earlier in life. A number of studies have reported an increase in age-associated cognitive deficits among people with HIV who are in their 50s, suggesting that HIV and aging may interact to adversely affect the brain and cognition.

Even though mortality and morbidity have been greatly reduced in this country, HIV continues to be rampant around the world, and is particularly prevalent in underdeveloped countries without modern or accessible health care systems. In sum, many challenges remain. It seems likely that HIV will continue to be a significant clinical and public health problem in the foreseeable future and the source of brain dysfunction and concern about impending cognitive and functional decline as people age with this chronic infection.

Lyme Disease and Related Disorders

A 30-year-old man was referred for neuropsychological testing by his internist who reported joint pain, a peripheral neuropathy, arms and legs, and decreased cognitive functioning as symptoms. The patient stated that he had been diagnosed with Lyme disease three years earlier, and was treated with three weeks of oral doxycline, the current standard antibiotic treatment for Lyme. He initially got better, but six months prior to this referral he described recurring symptoms. These included joint pain, a peripheral neuropathy and decreased cognitive functioning as symptoms. He also described problems with concentration, word finding, memory, fatigue and depression. These symptoms have affected his work. A Western Blot Test for Lyme disease was serum-positive for Lyme, but his CSF tests were negative. He was treated as an outpatient with IV antibiotics, but the treatment was discontinued after a month due to a blood clot at the infusion site. After treatment the patient continued to report problems with concentration, word finding, and memory; however, his neuropsychological profile was mostly normal, with above-average memory performances.

Clinical Considerations

Lyme disease is a tick-borne infection caused by the spirochete *Borrelia burgdorferi* (Steere et al., 1983). It is a multisystem disorder that may affect the skin, joints, heart, eyes, and nervous system. The classic neurological symptoms of early stage Lyme disease include meningitis, cranial neuritis, and radiculoneuritis. These may occur alone or in combination in 15% of untreated patients (Pachner & Steere, 1985). Diagnosis is made by pleocytosis, the synthesis of intrathecal antibodies to *Borrelia burgdorferi*, detection by culture, or PCR in CSF (Stanek, Lusa, Ogrinc, Markowicz, & Strle, 2013). For most patients ten days of oral doxycycline, a tetracycline antibiotic, provide an optimal recovery rate at 30 months posttreatment, and additional antibiotics do not improve outcome (Wormser et al., 2003). A small percentage of patients develop a mild to moderate encephalopathy, often following long periods of latent infection. The encephalitic symptoms tend to be diffuse and nonspecific, and typically include memory loss, naming problems, difficulty concentrating, reduced efficiency, somnolence, and fatigue. For patients with these symptoms, it has been proposed (Finkel, Halperin, & Finkel, 1992; Garcia-Monco & Benach, 1995) that those with abnormal CSF, characterized by intrathecal production of antibody to *Borrelia burgdorferi*, increased CSF protein, or both, have a neurological basis to their illness, although the mechanism is not fully understood. There have been case reports of more serious neurological involvement related to Lyme disease (Reik, Smith, Khan, & Nelson, 1985), although documented cases are rare.

Traditional brain neurophysiological and neuroimaging techniques have not been shown to be highly sensitive to the pathophysiology of CNS Lyme disease. The routine EEG is typically normal and although MRI abnormalities have been described in Lyme patients, these are nonspecific and relatively infrequent (Finkel et al., 1992). MRI abnormalities described in patients with Lyme disease suggest an inflammatory process and usually involve the subcortical white matter (Krupp et al., 1991). Even in patients with confirmed CNS involvement, MRI evidence of tissue damage is rare (Agosta et al., 2006). Single photon emission computed tomography (SPECT), a functional imaging technique that measures regional cerebral blood flow to provide information about metabolic activity in specific brain regions, has shown some promise in localizing the neuroanatomic basis for cognitive symptoms in Lyme disease. Logigian et al. (1997) studied a series of 13 patients with objective evidence of Lyme encephalopathy using a quantitative SPECT technique. The Lyme patients showed patterns of multifocal hypoperfusion, most notably in frontal subcortical areas including the basal ganglia and white matter of the cerebral hemispheres, which was not apparent in normal controls. Six months posttreatment with IV ceftriaxone, cerebral perfusion improved in all 13 cases, suggesting that the reduced cerebral perfusion in frontal and temporal lobe structures may be the neuroanatomical basis of Lyme encephalopathy (see Figure 20.2). Moreover, these same white matter regions form the large-scale neurocognitive networks involved in mediating memory and attention (Mesulam, 1990), consistent with the nature of cognitive symptoms. Other studies have similarly reported decreased regional blood flow in white matter in Lyme encephalopathy. Reductions have been linked to deficits in memory (Fallon, Keilp, Prohovnik, Heertum, & Mann, 2003) and some clinicians advocate using this in making a definitive diagnosis. However, while sensitive to brain abnormalities, SPECT hypoperfusion in these brain regions is not specific to Lyme disease and can be found in other conditions such as depression (Ito et al., 1996) and chronic fatigue syndrome (Schwartz et al., 1994), which have overlapping symptoms. Therefore although quantitative SPECT provides an objective and useful measure of cerebral hypoperfusion in Lyme encephalopathy, it cannot be used alone in diagnosing the condition.

Neuropsychology

Neuropsychological studies of individuals with Lyme disease have almost exclusively been comprised treated patients with persistent symptoms. An exception was a

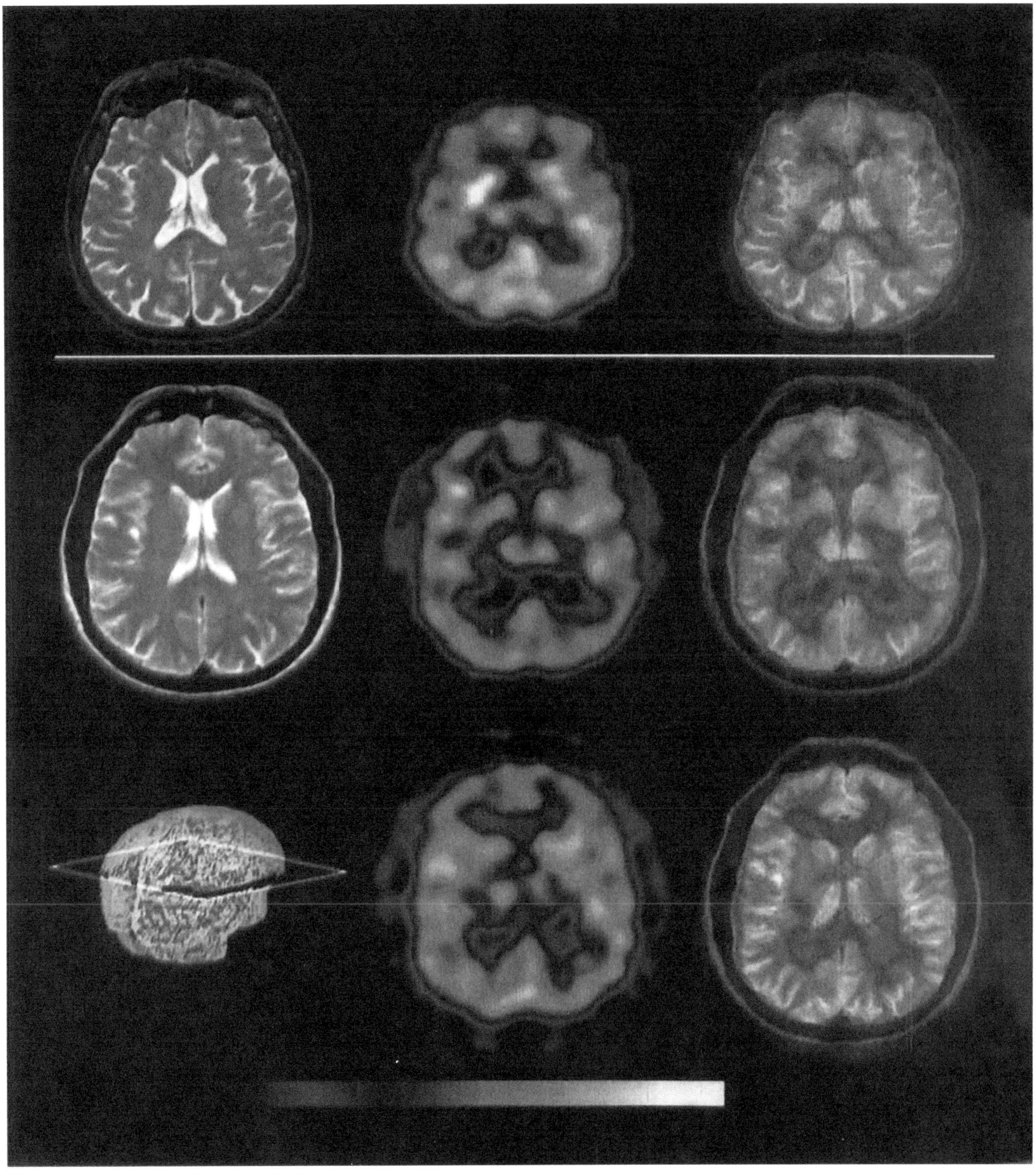

Figure 20.2 Representative MRI (left column) and SPECT images (middle column), and superimposed MRISPECT (right column) in a normal subject (top row) and a patient with objective evidence of Lyme encephalopathy prior to treatment (middle row) and six months after treatment (bottom row). A brain surface rendering demonstrating the slice plane is shown in the lower left. Although the MR images in the patient were normal, there was reduced tracer activity in a multifocal pattern in cortical and subcortical structures in the pretreatment SPECT and a moderately elevated perfusion defect index. In the posttreatment SPECT, the uptake improved, and the defect index declined. Color scale: blue corresponds to lower and orange to higher perfusion. *A color version of this figure can be found in Plate section 2*

group studied by Halperin and colleagues (Halperin, Pass, Anand, Luft, Volkman, & Dattwyler 1988) before and after antibiotic treatment. Although Halperin et al. reported pretreatment cognitive deficits in almost every area examined, the data are difficult to interpret because they did not include a normative comparison group, and because there was no indication of the number of patients whose performance was outside of the normative range. Nevertheless, there were statistically significant improvements following treatment on standardized measures of visuospatial skills, speed of processing, executive functioning, and verbal recall with short-term attention span, verbal fluency, and recognition memory unchanged. Patients also completed the self-administered depression inventory, and while there was no evidence of significant depression before treatment, the average depression score was almost halved following treatment. In a study of treated Lyme patients who still reported memory deficits, Krupp et al. (1991) reported relatively lower scores on several memory tests, and a word fluency test compared to normal controls, but no differences in Wechsler IQ subtest scores or executive functioning tests. List-learning verbal memory tests, such as the California Verbal Learning (CVLT) (Delis, Kramer, Kaplan, & Ober, 1987) and Selective Reminding Test (SRT) (Buschke & Fuld, 1974) have been shown to be the most reliable indicators of neuropsychological impairment in treated Lyme patients (Halperin et al., 1988; Kaplan, Meadows, Vincent, Logigian, & Steere, 1992; Krupp et al., 1991; Ravdin, Hilton, Primeau, Clements, & Barr, 1996; Shadick et al., 1994; Westervelt & McCaffrey, 2002). Because neuropsychological impairment was not correlated with either serum or CSF antibody titers to *Borrelia burgdorferi* in these patients, the Krupp group proposed that cognitive deficits could occur in patients who no longer have evidence of active disease. However, this remains controversial. In a study comparing Lyme patients with evidence of infection in their CSF with Lyme patients without CSF abnormalities and normal controls, Kaplan and colleagues (Kaplan, Jones-Woodward, Workman, Steere, Logigian, & Meadows, 1999) showed that the Lyme disease group with abnormal CSF had significantly lower memory scores than the Lyme patients with normal CSF and normal controls. Memory test performances were not correlated with either greater depression or increased anxiety scores in any of the groups. The nature and magnitude of cognitive problems in the Lyme encephalopathy group were similar to those reported previously (Krupp et al., 1991); namely, lower memory scores on the retrieval measures of the SRT, a word-learning measure. Although the test battery sampled a wide range of cognitive abilities—including measures of attention, executive functioning and language—neither patient group had other deficits in comparison to the controls. However, both Lyme disease groups had higher depression scores than the control subjects, and the Lyme group with normal CSF also showed greater anxiety scores than controls. Objective memory test performances were not correlated with either greater depression or increased anxiety scores in any of the groups.

Some patients report persistent symptoms after the recommended antibiotic treatment (Bujak, Weinstein, & Dornbush, 1996), which has been termed *post–Lyme disease syndrome* or *chronic Lyme disease*. Although the majority of these patients present with cognitive complaints, attempts to provide objective evidence of cognitive impairment, using neuropsychological tests, have been variable and inconclusive. In a study of previously treated patients with Lyme disease who continued to report memory problems three to 12 months following standard antibiotic therapy, the patients performed significantly worse on measures of verbal fluency and memory than healthy controls, but did not differ on tests of attention, psychomotor skills, and executive functioning (Krupp et al., 1991). However, other investigators found virtually no objective evidence of neuropsychological dysfunction in 125 chronic Lyme patients, although 70% reported memory decline as a primary symptom (Kaplan et al., 2003). Self-reported cognitive dysfunction was related to greater self-reported pain, limits in role functioning, and symptoms of depression, and was only weakly related to objective measures of cognitive dysfunction. Although there was a slight improvement in scores on a number of attention and memory tests in follow-up, there was no benefit of antimicrobials over placebo for patients with self-reported neurocognitive symptoms that do not show clear evidence of persisting *Borrelia burgdorferi* infection or evidence of cognitive impairment.

Lyme encephalopathy with the characteristic clinical picture of a positive serology to *Borrelia burgdorferi* and abnormal CSF, is likely due to active infection (Wormser et al., 2006). Neuropsychological testing in these patients typically shows mild, but significant, deficits on memory testing (Kaplan et al., 1992) and reduced cerebral perfusion on SPECT images (Logigian et al., 1997). In addition to demonstrated neuropsychological deficits, Lyme patients have also often shown affective symptoms and fatigue. Although there appears to be little relationship between objective neuropsychological functioning and affective symptoms such as depression, these may be related to the perception of cognitive loss (Kaplan et al., 2003; Westervelt & McCaffrey, 2002). After standard antibiotic therapy, most patients show significant improvements in their cognitive functioning (Halperin et al., 1988; Logigian, Kaplan, & Steere, 1990, 1999) and better cerebral perfusion (Logigian et al., 1997). However, a small minority of Lyme patients without evidence of memory loss on objective testing continues to have memory complaints. This is not unique to Lyme disease. The perception of memory loss has been shown to be weakly related to memory test performance and strongly associated with psychiatric symptoms in a number of disorders (Bolla, Lindgren, Bonaccorsy, & Bleecker, 1991; Broadbent, Cooper, FitzGerald, & Parkes, 1982). Moreover, there is little scientific evidence that chronic Lyme disease without evidence of an active *Borrelia burgdorferi* infection in CSF is the cause of Lyme-related neurological disease (Feder et al., 2007). Unfortunately, some advocates for chronic Lyme continue to argue for an occult latent infection that can respond only to long-term antibiotics, such that the argument has become political rather than scientific (Auwaerter et al., 2011). That patients with previously treated Lyme disease have may have persistent symptoms is not the issue. The issue is whether these symptoms are caused by a *Borrelia burgdorferi* infection, and the available science does not support that. An autoimmune response (Steere, 2001) or coinfections with other tick-borne infections like human granulocytic anaplasmosis (also known as *ehrlichiosis*) and babesiosis remain potential candidates.

Steere, Gross, Meyer, and Huber (2001) proposed a model to explain treatment-resistant Lyme arthritis via an autoimmune response resulting from the initial *Borrelia burgdorferi* infection. Patients with Lyme arthritis who carry the HLA-DR4 or DR2 allele are more vulnerable to developing a chronic antibiotic-resistant arthritis. Chronic Lyme patients also have higher amounts of *Borrelia burgdorferi*–specific foxhead box P3 (FoxP3) than healthy controls, indicating that regulatory T-cells might also play a role, by immunosuppression, in the development of chronic Lyme disease. FoxP3 is a specific marker of regulatory T cells. The signaling pathway P38 mitogen activated protein kinase (p38 MAP kinase) has also been identified as promoting expression of proinflammatory cytokines from *Borrelia burgdorferi*(Jarefors, Janefjord, Forsberg, Jenmalm, & Ekerfelt, 2007). In addition to *Borrelia burgdorferi,* the Ixiodes tick can be coinfected with and transmit other pathogens such as *Anaplasma phagocytophilum* and *Babesia microti*. Human ranulocytic anaplasmosis (HGA) is a rickettsial infection caused by *Anaplasma phagocytophilum,* a gram-negative bacterium that is unusual in its tropism to neurtrophils (Wormser et al., 2006). Clinical manifestations are nonspecific and may include fever, chills, headache, and myalgia. Serologic testing using an indirect fluorescent antibody assay provides the most reliable diagnosis, and doxycycline is the recommended treatment. Chronic HGA infections have not been described in humans, and to our knowledge there have been no neuropsychological sequelae reported in affected patients. However, even without evidence of neurological involvement, encephalitic symptoms probably have been often associated with many types of systemic infections (Halperin, 2008). *Babesia microti*, the primary cause of babesiosis, seems a more likely candidate. It is also tick-borne infection that exists in the same endemic areas as Lyme disease (Wormser et al., 2006). This parasite attacks red blood cells in much the same way as the parasite that causes malaria, and the clinical presentation can be similar (Boustani & Gelfand, 1996). Approximately 10% of patients with Lyme disease in southern New England are coinfected with babesiosis (Mylonakis, 2001). Symptoms develop one to six weeks after tick feeding and often include fever, fatigue, chills, sweats, and headache. Less common are myalgia, anorexia, cough, nausea, vomiting, arthralgia, emotional lability, and depression (Krause, 2002). A combination of atovaquone and azithromycin is currently the treatment of choice for mild to moderate babesiosis (Vannier & Krause, 2012). If left untreated, symptoms may continue for months or even years. Unlike HGA, babesiosis is known to have encephalic symptoms and may be a more likely culprit in some cases of the treatment-resistant "Lyme" encephalopathy since there is known coinfection and babesiosis does not respond to the standard treatments for Lyme.

Conclusion

Neurotropic infectious diseases have long been within the purview of neuropsychology practice. As with other neurobehavioral syndromes, neuropsychological assessment has been an integral part of diagnosis, rehabilitation, and research. With improved diagnostic methods and more effective treatments, neuropsychological methods become even more important in defining the phenotype and natural history of encephalitic disorders, particularly those with previously unknown etiologies. This chapter provided a glimpse into just three neurotropic infections—herpes simplex encephalitis, HIV and Lyme disease—but as noted earlier, there are many other brain infections, each with its own neuropsychological profile, response to treatment, and long-term outcome. While it was beyond the scope of this chapter to review the many infections capable of producing brain disease, it is important for neuropsychologists to stay abreast of the advances in brain infection research and remain relevant by designing assessments to best delineate the cognitive and emotional aspects of these disorders.

References

Agosta, F., Rocca, M. A., Benedetti, B., Capra, R., Cordioli, C., & Filippi, M. (2006). MR imaging assessment of brain and cervical cord damage in patients with neuroborreliosis. *American Journal of Neuroradiology*, *27*(4), 892–894.

Aronsson, B., Troye-Blomberg, M., & Smedman, L. (2004). Increase of circulating CD8+CD57+ lymphocytes after measles infection but not after measles vaccination. *Journal of Clinical & Laboratory Immunology*, *53*, 1–12.

Aurelius, E., Andersson, B., Forsgren, M., Skoldenberg, B., & Strannegard, O. (1994). Cytokines and other markers of intrathecal immune response in patients with herpes simplex encephalitis. [Research Support, Non-U.S. Gov't]. *Journal of Infectious Disease*, *170*(3), 678–681.

Auwaerter, P. G., Bakken, J. S., Dattwyler, R. J., Dumler, J. S., Halperin, J. J., McSweegan, E., . . . Wormser, G. P. (2011). Antiscience and ethical concerns associated with advocacy of Lyme disease. [Research Support, N.I.H., Extramural]. *The Lancet. Infectious Diseases*, *11*(9), 713–719. doi: 10.1016/S1473-3099(11)70034-2

Aylward, E., Henderer, B., & McCarthur, J.E.A. (1993). Reduced basal ganglia volume in HIV-1 associated dementia: Results from quantitative neuroimaging. *Neurology*, *43*, 2099–2104.

Bandaru, V. V., McArthur, J. C., Sacktor, N., Cutler, R. G., Knapp, E. L., Mattson, M. P., & Haughey, N. J. (2007). Associative and predictive biomarkers of dementia in HIV-1-infected patients. *Neurology*, *68*(18), 1481–1487.

Becker, J. T., Sanchez, J., Dew, M. A., Lopez, O. L., Dorst, S. K., & Banks, G. (1997). Neuropsychological abnormalities among HIV-infected individuals in a community-based sample. *Neuropsychology*, *11*(4), 592–601.

Bernick, C., & Gregorios, J. B. (1984). Progressive multifocal leukoencephalopathy in a patient with acquired immune deficiency syndrome. *Archives of Neurology*, *41*(7), 780–782.

Bolla, K. I., Lindgren, K. N., Bonaccorsy, C., & Bleecker, M. L. (1991). Memory complaints in older adults: Fact or fiction? [Research Support, U.S. Gov't, P.H.S.]. *Archives of Neurology*, *48*(1), 61–64.

Bornstein, R. A., Nasrallah, H. A., Para, M. F., Fass, R. J., Whitacre, C. C., & Rice, R. R., Jr. (1991). Rate of CD4 decline and neuropsychological performance in HIV infection. *Archives of Neurology*, *48*(7), 704–707.

Boustani, M. R., & Gelfand, J. A. (1996). Babesiosis. [Review]. *Clinical Infectious Diseases*, *22*(4), 611–615.

Bouwman, F. H., Skolasky, R. L., Hes, D., Selnes, O. A., Glass, J. D., Nance-Sproson, T. E., . . . McArthur, J. C. (1998). Variable progression of HIV-associated dementia. *Neurology*, *50*(6), 1814–1820.

Bradley, H., Markowitz, L. E., Gibson, T., & McQuillan, G. M. (2014). Seroprevalence of herpes simplex virus types 1 and 2--United States, 1999–2010. [Research Support, Non-U.S. Gov't Research Support, U.S. Gov't, P.H.S.]. *Journal of Infectious Disease*, *209*(3), 325–333. doi: 10.1093/infdis/jit458

Brew, B. J., Dunbar, N., Pemberton, L., & Kaldor, J. (1996). Predictive markers of AIDS dementia complex: CD4 cell count and cerebrospinal fluid concentrations of beta 2-microglobulin and neopterin. *Journal of Infectious Disease*, *174*(2), 294–298.

Broadbent, D. E., Cooper, P. F., FitzGerald, P., & Parkes, K. R. (1982). The Cognitive Failures Questionnaire (CFQ) and its correlates. [Research Support, Non-U.S. Gov't]. *British Journal of Clinical Psychology*, *21*(Pt 1), 1–16.

Budka, H. (1991). Neuropathology of human immunodeficiency virus infection. *Brain Pathology*, *1*(3), 163–175.

Budka, H., Wiley, C., Kleihues, P., Artigas, J., Asbury, A., Cho, E., . . . Dickson, D.E.A. (1991). HIV-associated disease of the nervous system: Review of nomenclature and proposal for neuropathology-based terminology. *Brain Pathology*, *1*(3), 143–152.

Bujak, D. I., Weinstein, A., & Dornbush, R. L. (1996). Clinical and neurocognitive features of the post Lyme syndrome. [Research Support, Non-U.S. Gov't Research Support, U.S. Gov't, P.H.S.]. *The Journal of Rheumatology*, *23*(8), 1392–1397.

Buschke, H., & Fuld, P. (1974). Evaluating storage, retention, and retrieval in disordered memory and learning. *Neurology*, *24*, 1019–1025.

Caparros-Lefebvre, D., Girard-Buttaz, I., Reboul, S., Lebert, F., Cabaret, M., Verier, A., . . . Petit, H. (1996). Cognitive and psychiatric impairment in herpes simplex virus encephalitis suggest involvement of the amygdalo-frontal pathways. [Research Support, Non-U.S. Gov't]. *Journal of Neurology*, *243*(3), 248–256.

Cermak, L. S. (1976). The encoding capacity of a patient with amnesia due to encephalitis. [Case Reports Comparative Study Research Support, U.S. Gov't, Non-P.H.S.]. *Neuropsychologia*, *14*(3), 311–326.

Cermak, L. S., & O'Connor, M. (1983). The anterograde and retrograde retrieval ability of a patient with amnesia due to encephalitis. [Case Reports Research Support, U.S. Gov't, Non-P.H.S. Research Support, U.S. Gov't, P.H.S.]. *Neuropsychologia*, *21*(3), 213–234.

Chang, L., Ernst, T., Leonido-Yee, M., Walot, I., & Singer, E. (1999). Cerebral metabolite abnormalities correlate with clinical severity of HIV-1 cognitive motor complex. *Neurology*, *52*(1), 100–108.

Chang, L., Ernst, T., Witt, M. D., Ames, N., Walot, I., Jovicich, J., . . . Miller, E. N. (2003). Persistent brain abnormalities in antiretroviral-naive HIV patients 3 months after HAART. *Antiviral Therapy*, *8*(1), 17–26.

Childs, E. A., Lyles, R. H., Selnes, O. A., Chen, B., Miller, E. N., Cohen, B. A., . . . McArthur, J. C. (1999). Plasma viral load and CD4 lymphocytes predict HIV-associated dementia and sensory neuropathy. *Neurology*, *52*(3), 607–613.

Christo, P. P., Greco, D. B., Aleixo, A. W., & Livramento, J. A. (2005). HIV-1 RNA levels in cerebrospinal fluid and plasma and their correlation with opportunistic neurological diseases in a Brazilian AIDS reference hospital. *Arq Neuropsiquiatr*, *63*(4), 907–913.

Chun, T. W., Nickle, D. C., Justement, J. S., Large, D., Semerjian, A., Curlin, M. E., . . . Fauci, A. S. (2005). HIV-infected individuals receiving effective antiviral therapy for extended periods of time continually replenish their viral reservoir. *The Journal of Clinical Investigation*, *115*(11), 3250–3255.

Clark, R. A., & Bessinger, R. (1997). Clinical manifestations and predictors of survival in older women infected with HIV. *Journal of Acquired Immune Deficiency Syndromes and Human Retrovirology*, *15*(5), 341–345.

Clifford, D. B. (1997). Primary neurologic complications of HIV infection. *International AIDS Society-USA*, *5*, 4–7.

Cohen, R. A., Boland, R., Paul, R., Tashima, K. T., Schoenbaum, E. E., Celentano, D. D., . . . Carpenter, C. C. (2001). Neurocognitive performance enhanced by highly active antiretroviral therapy in HIV-infected women. *AIDS*, *15*(3), 341–345.

Coombs, R. W. (1998). *Preliminary evaluation of HIV-1 proviral DNA quantification assay*. Paper presented at the Conference on the Laboratory Science of HIV.

Cysique, L. A., Brew, B. J., Halman, M., Catalan, J., Sacktor, N., Price, R. W., . . . Romero, C. (2005). Undetectable cerebrospinal fluid HIV RNA and beta-2 microglobulin do not indicate inactive AIDS dementia complex in highly active antiretroviral therapy-treated patients. *Journal of Acquired Immune Deficiency Syndromes*, *39*(4), 426–429.

DalPan, G., Farzadegan, H., Selness, O., Hoover, D., Miller, E., Skolasky, R., . . . McArthur, J. (1998). Sustained cognitive decline in HIV infection: Relationsip to CD4 cell count, plasma viremia & p24 antigenemia. *Journal of Neurovirology*, *4*(1), 95–99.

Davis, L. E., Hjelle, B. L., Miller, V. E., Palmer, D. L., Llewellyn, A. L., Merlin, T. L., . . . Wiley, C. A. (1992). Early viral brain invasion in iatrogenic human immunodeficiency virus infection. *Neurology*, *42*(9), 1736–1739.

Delis, D. C., Kramer, J. H., Kaplan, E., & Ober, B. (1987). *California Verbal Learning Test Manual*. New York: The Psychological Corporation.

De Ronchi, D., Faranca, I., Berardi, D., Scudellari, P., Borderi, M., Manfredi, R., & Fratiglioni, L. (2002). Risk factors for cognitive impairment in HIV-1-infected persons with different risk behaviors. *Archives of Neurology*, *59*(5), 812–818.

Dieperink, E., Willenbring, M., & Ho, S. B. (2000). Neuropsychiatric symptoms associated with hepatitis C and interferon alpha: A review. *American Journal of Psychiatry*, *157*(6), 867–876.

Dragic, T., Litwin, V., Allaway, G. P., Martin, S. R., Huang, Y., Nagashima, K. A., . . . Paxton, W. A. (1996). HIV-1 entry into CD4+ cells is mediated by the chemokine receptor CC-CKR-5. *Nature*, *381*(6584), 667–673.

Eberwein, P., Hansen, L. L., & Agostini, H. T. (2005). Genotypes of JC virus, DNA of cytomegalovirus, and proviral DNA of human immunodeficiency virus in eyes of acquired immunodeficiency syndrome patients. *Journal of Neurovirology*, *11*(1), 58–65.

Egan, V. G., Chiswick, A., Brettle, R. P., & Goodwin, G. M. (1993). The Edinburgh cohort of HIV-positive drug users: The relationship between auditory P3 latency, cognitive function and self-rated mood. *Psychological Medicine*, *23*(3), 613–622.

Eggers, C. C., van Lunzen, J., Buhk, T., & Stellbrink, H. J. (1999). HIV infection of the central nervous system is characterized by rapid turnover of viral RNA in cerebrospinal fluid. *Journal of Acquired Immune Deficiency Syndromes and Human Retrovirology*, *20*(3), 259–264.

Ellis, R. J., Deutsch, R., Heaton, R. K., Marcotte, T. D., McCutchan, J. A., Nelson, J. A., . . . Grant, I. (1997). Neurocognitive impairment is an independent risk factor for death in HIV infection. [San Diego HIV Neurobehavioral Research Center Group]. *Archives of Neurology*, *54*(4), 416–424.

Ellis, R. J., Hsia, K., Spector, S. A., Nelson, J. A., Heaton, R. K., Wallace, M. R., . . . McCutchan, J. A. (1997). Cerebrospinal fluid human immunodeficiency virus type 1 RNA levels are elevated in neurocognitively impaired individuals with acquired immunodeficiency syndrome. [HIV Neurobehavioral Research Center Group]. *Annals of Neurol*, *42*(5), 679–688.

Everall, I., Luthert, P., & Lantos, P. (1993). A review of neuronal damage in human immunodeficiency virus infection: Its assessment, possible mechanism and relationship to dementia. *Journal of Neuropathology & Experimental Neurology*, *52*(6), 561–566.

Everall, I. P., Luthert, P. J., & Lantos, P. L. (1993). Neuronal number and volume alterations in the neocortex of HIV infected individuals. *Journal of Neurology, Neurosurgery, and Psychiatry*, *56*(5), 481–486.

Fallon, B. A., Keilp, J., Prohovnik, I., Heertum, R. V., & Mann, J. J. (2003). Regional cerebral blood flow and cognitive deficits in chronic lyme disease. [Comparative Study Research Support, Non-U.S. Gov't]. *The Journal of Neuropsychiatry and Clinical Neurosciences*, *15*(3), 326–332.

Fatahzadeh, M., & Schwartz, R. A. (2007). Human herpes simplex virus infections: Epidemiology, pathogenesis, symptomatology, diagnosis, and management. [Review]. *Journal of the American Academy of Dermatology*, *57*(5), 737–763; quiz 764–736. doi: 10.1016/j.jaad.2007.06.027

Feder, H. M., Jr., Johnson, B. J., O'Connell, S., Shapiro, E. D., Steere, A. C., Wormser, G. P., . . . Zemel, L. (2007). A critical appraisal of "chronic Lyme disease." [Review]. *New England Journal of Medicine*, *357*(14), 1422–1430. doi: 10.1056/NEJMra072023

Finkel, M. F., Halperin, J. J., & Finkel, M. J. (1992). Nervous system Lyme borreliosis—revisited [corrected; erratum to be published]. [Review]. *Archives of Neurology*, *49*(1), 102–107.

Flanigan, T., Jesdale, B., Zierler, S., Imam, N., Stein, M., Flanagan, K., & Carpenter, C. (1992). Fall in CD4 count among HIV infected women: A comparison of injection drug use and heterosexual transmission groups. [Abstract No. PoC4367]. *International Conference on AIDS*, *8*(2), C306.

Garcia-Monco, J. C., & Benach, J. L. (1995). Lyme neuroborreliosis. [Research Support, U.S. Gov't, P.H.S. Review]. *Annals of Neurology*, *37*(6), 691–702. doi: 10.1002/ana.410370602

Gartner, S. (2000). HIV infection and dementia. *Science*, *287*(5453), 602–604.

Geskus, R. B., Miedema, F. A., Goudsmit, J., Reiss, P., Schuitemaker, H., & Coutinho, R. A. (2003). Prediction of residual time to AIDS and death based on markers and cofactors. *Journal of Acquired Immune Deficiency Syndromes*, *32*(5), 514–521.

Gonzales, M. F., & Davis, R. L. (1988). Neuropathology of acquired immunodeficiency syndrome. *Neuropathology and Applied Neurobiology*, *14*(5), 345–363.

Gonzalez, R., Heaton, R. K., Moore, D. J., Letendre, S., Ellis, R. J., Wolfson, T., . . . Grant, I. (2003). Computerized reaction time battery versus a traditional neuropsychological battery: Detecting HIV-related impairments. *Journal of the International Neuropsychological Society*, *9*(1), 64–71.

Goulsmith, J., DeWolf, F., & Paul, D. A., et al. (1986). Expression of human immunodeficiency virus antigen (HIV-Ag) in serum and cerebrospinal fluid during acute and chronic infection. *Lancet*, *11*, 177–180.

Gruzelier, J., Burgess, A., Baldeweg, T., Riccio, M., Hawkins, D., Stygall, J., . . . Catalan, J. (1996). Prospective associations between lateralised brain function and immune status in HIV infection: Analysis of EEG, cognition and mood over 30 months. *International Journal of Psychophysiology*, *23*(3), 215–224.

Guiloff, R. J., & Tan, S. V. (1992). Central nervous system opportunistic infections in HIV disease: Clinical aspects. *Bailliere's Clinical Neurology*, *1*(1), 103–154.

Gulick, R. M., Mellors, J. W., Havlir, D., Eron, J. J., Gonzalez, C., McMahon, D., . . . Chodakewitz, J. A. (1997). Treatment with indinavir, zidovudine, and lamivudine in adults with human immunodeficiency virus infection and prior antiretroviral therapy. *The New England Journal of Medicine*, *337*(11), 734–739.

Halperin, J. J. (2008). Prolonged Lyme disease treatment: Enough is enough. [Comment Editorial]. *Neurology*, *70*(13), 986–987. doi: 10.1212/01.WNL.0000291407.40667.69

Halperin, J. J., Pass, H. L., Anand, A. K., Luft, B. J., Volkman, D. J., & Dattwyler, R. J. (1988). Nervous system abnormalities in Lyme disease. *Annals of the New York Academy of Sciences*, *539*, 24–34.

Harrison, M. J., Newman, S. P., Hall-Craggs, M. A., Fowler, C. J., Miller, R., Kendall, B. E., . . . Williams, I. (1998). Evidence of CNS impairment in HIV infection: Clinical, neuropsychological, EEG, and MRI/MRS study. *Journal of Neurology, Neurosurgery, and Psychiatry*, *65*(3), 301–307.

Hart, R. P., Kwentus, J. A., Frazier, R. B., & Hormel, T. L. (1986). Natural history of Kluver-Bucy syndrome after treated herpes encephalitis. [Case Reports]. *Southern Medical Journal*, *79*(11), 1376–1378.

Heaton, R. K., Grant, I., Butters, N., White, D. A., Kirson, D., Atkinson, J. H., et al. (1995). The HNRC 500—neuropsychology of HIV infection at different disease stages. [HIV Neurobehavioral Research Center]. *Journal of the International Neuropsychological Society*, *1*(3), 231–251.

Heaton, R. K., Marcotte, T. D., Mindt, M. R., Sadek, J., Moore, D. J., Bentley, H., . . . Grant, I. (2004). The impact of HIV-associated neuropsychological impairment on everyday functioning. *Journal of the International Neuropsychological Society*, *10*(3), 317–331.

Heindel, W. C., Jernigan, T. L., Archibald, S. L., Achim, C. L., Masliah, E., & Wiley, C. A. (1994). The relationship of quantitative brain magnetic resonance imaging measures to neuropathologic indexes of human immunodeficiency virus infection. *Archives of Neurology*, *51*(11), 1129–1135.

Hilsabeck, R. C., Hassanein, T. I., Carlson, M. D., Ziegler, E. A., & Perry, W. (2003). Cognitive functioning and psychiatric symptomatology in patients with chronic hepatitis C. *Journal of the International Neuropsychological Society*, *9*(6), 847–854.

Hilsabeck, R. C., Perry, W., & Hassanein, T. I. (2002). Neuropsychological impairment in patients with chronic hepatitis C. *Hepatology*, *35*(2), 440–446.

Hjalmarsson, A., Blomqvist, P., & Skoldenberg, B. (2007). Herpes simplex encephalitis in Sweden, 1990–2001: Incidence, morbidity, and mortality. [Research Support, Non-U.S. Gov't]. *Clinical Infectious Diseases*, *45*(7), 875–880. doi: 10.1086/521262

Hokkanen, L., & Launes, J. (1997). Cognitive recovery instead of decline after acute encephalitis: A prospective follow up study. [Research Support, Non-U.S. Gov't]. *Journal of Neurology, Neurosurgery, and Psychiatry*, *63*(2), 222–227.

Hokkanen, L., Poutiainen, E., Valanne, L., Salonen, O., Iivanainen, M., & Launes, J. (1996). Cognitive impairment after acute encephalitis: Comparison of herpes simplex and other aetiologies. *Journal of Neurology, Neurosurgery, and Psychiatry*, *61*(5), 478–484.

Hokkanen, L., Salonen, O., & Launes, J. (1996). Amnesia in acute herpetic and nonherpetic encephalitis. *Archives of Neurology*, *53*(10), 972–978.

Ito, H., Kawashima, R., Awata, S., Ono, S., Sato, K., Goto, R., . . . Fukuda, H. (1996). Hypoperfusion in the limbic system and prefrontal cortex in depression: SPECT with anatomic standardization technique. [Comparative Study Research Support, Non-U.S. Gov't]. *Journal of Nuclear Medicine*, *37*(3), 410–414.

Janssen, R. S., Nwanyanwu, O. C., Selik, R. M., & Stehr-Green, J. K. (1992). Epidemiology of human immunodeficiency virus encephalopathy in the United States. *Neurology*, *42*(8), 1472–1476.

Jarefors, S., Janefjord, C. K., Forsberg, P., Jenmalm, M. C., & Ekerfelt, C. (2007). Decreased up-regulation of the interleukin-12Rbeta2-chain and interferon-gamma secretion and increased number of forkhead box P3-expressing cells in patients with a history of chronic Lyme borreliosis compared with asymptomatic Borrelia-exposed individuals. [Comparative Study Research Support, Non-U.S. Gov't]. *Clinical & Experimental Immunology*, *147*(1), 18–27. doi: 10.1111/j.1365-2249.2006.03245.x

Jellinger, K. A., Setinek, U., Drlicek, M., Bohm, G., Steurer, A., & Lintner, F. (2000). Neuropathology and general autopsy findings in AIDS during the last 15 years. *Acta Neuropathologica*, *100*(2), 213–220.

Jernigan, T. L., Archibald, S., Hesselink, J. R., Atkinson, J. H., Velin, R. A., McCutchan, J. A., . . . Grant, I. (1993). Magnetic resonance imaging morphometric analysis of cerebral volume loss in human immunodeficiency virus infection. [The HNRC Group]. *Archives of Neurology*, *50*(3), 250–255.

Kamei, S., Sakai, T., Matsuura, M., Tanaka, N., Kojima, T., Arakawa, Y., . . . Hirayanagi, K. (2002). Alterations of quantitative EEG and mini-mental state examination in interferon-alpha-treated hepatitis C. *European Neurology*, *48*(2), 102–107.

Kaplan, C. P., & Bain, K. P. (1999). Cognitive outcome after emergent treatment of acute herpes simplex encephalitis with acyclovir. [Case Reports Review]. *Brain Injury*, *13*(11), 935–941.

Kaplan, R. F., Jones-Woodward, L., Workman, K., Steere, A. C., Logigian, E. L., & Meadows, M. E. (1999). Neuropsychological deficits in Lyme disease patients with and without other evidence of central nervous system pathology. [Comparative Study Research Support, U.S. Gov't, P.H.S.]. *Applied Neuropsychology*, *6*(1), 3–11. doi: 10.1207/s15324826an0601_1

Kaplan, R. F., Meadows, M. E., Vincent, L. C., Logigian, E. L., & Steere, A. C. (1992). Memory impairment and depression in patients with Lyme encephalopathy: Comparison with fibromyalgia and nonpsychotically depressed patients. [Comparative Study Research Support, U.S. Gov't, P.H.S.]. *Neurology*, *42*(7), 1263–1267.

Kaplan, R. F., Trevino, R. P., Johnson, G. M., Levy, L., Dornbush, R., Hu, L. T., . . . Klempner, M. S. (2003). Cognitive function in post-treatment Lyme disease: Do additional antibiotics help? [Clinical Trial Comparative Study Multicenter Study Randomized Controlled Trial Research Support, U.S. Gov't, P.H.S.]. *Neurology*, *60*(12), 1916–1922.

Kapur, N., Barker, S., Burrows, E. H., Ellison, D., Brice, J., Illis, L. S., . . . Loates, M. (1994). Herpes simplex encephalitis: Long term magnetic resonance imaging and neuropsychological profile. [Research Support, Non-U.S. Gov't]. *Journal of Neurology, Neurosurgery, and Psychiatry*, *57*(11), 1334–1342.

Karanjia, P. N. (1996). Herpes simplex encephalitis. In M. A. Samuels & S. Feske (Eds.), *Office Practice of Neurology* (pp. 404–408). New York: Churchill Livingstone Inc.

Kluver, H., & Bucy, P. C. (1937). Psychic blindness and other symptoms following bilateral temporal lobectomy in rhesus monkeys. *American Journal of Physiology*, *119*, 352–353.

Koralnik, I. J., Wuthrich, C., Dang, X., Rottnek, M., Gurtman, A., Simpson, D., & Morgello, S. (2005). JC virus granule cell neuronopathy: A novel clinical syndrome distinct from progressive multifocal leukoencephalopathy. *Annals of Neurology*, *57*(4), 576–580.

Kramer, L., Bauer, E., Funk, G., Hofer, H., Jessner, W., Steindl-Munda, P., . . . Ferenci, P. (2002). Subclinical impairment of brain function in chronic hepatitis C infection. *Journal of Hepatology*, *37*(3), 349–354.

Krause, P. J. (2002). Babesiosis. [Research Support, U.S. Gov't, P.H.S.Review]. *Medical Clinics of North America*, *86*(2), 361–373.

Krivine, A., Force, G., Servan, J., Cabee, A., Rozenberg, F., Dighiero, L., . . . Lebon, P. (1999). Measuring HIV-1 RNA and interferon-alpha in the cerebrospinal fluid of AIDS patients: Insights into the pathogenesis of AIDS dementia complex. *Journal of NeuroVirology*, *5*(5), 500–506.

Krupp, L. B., Masur, D., Schwartz, J., Coyle, P. K., Langenbach, L. J., Fernquist, S. K., . . . Halperin, J. J. (1991). Cognitive functioning in late Lyme borreliosis. [Research Support, Non-U.S. Gov't]. *Archives of Neurology*, *48*(11), 1125–1129.

Lanjewar, D. N., Jain, P. P., & Shetty, C. R. (1998). Profile of central nervous system pathology in patients with AIDS: An autopsy study from India. *AIDS*, *12*(3), 309–313.

Lanjewar, D. N., Surve, K. V., Maheshwari, M. B., Shenoy, B. P., & Hira, S. K. (1998). Toxoplasmosis of the central nervous system in the acquired immunodeficiency syndrome. *Indian Journal of Pathology and Microbiology*, *41*(2), 147–151.

Lee, M. H., Chen, Y. Z., Wang, L. S., Yen, P. S., & Hsu, Y. H. (2007). Progressive multifocal leukoencephalopathy in an AIDS patient. *Journal of the Formosan Medical Association*, *106*(3 Suppl), S24–S28.

Leport, C., Raffi, F., Matheron, S., Katlama, C., Regnier, B., Saimot, A. G., . . . Vilde, J. L. (1988). Treatment of central nervous system toxoplasmosis with pyrimethamine/sulfadiazine combination in 35 patients with the acquired immunodeficiency syndrome: Efficacy of long-term continuous therapy. *American Journal of Medicine*, *84*(1), 94–100.

Letendre, S., Ances, B., Gibson, S., & Ellis, R. J. (2007). Neurologic complications of HIV disease and their treatment. *Topics in HIV Medicine*, *15*(2), 32–39.

Letendre, S. L., McCutchan, J. A., Childers, M. E., Woods, S. P., Lazzaretto, D., Heaton, R. K., . . . Ellis, R. J. (2004). Enhancing antiretroviral therapy for human immunodeficiency virus cognitive disorders. *Annals of Neurology*, *56*(3), 416–423.

Levitz, R. E. (1998). Herpes simplex encephalitis: A review. [Review]. *Heart & Lung*, *27*(3), 209–212.

Lillo, F. B., Ciuffreda, D., Veglia, F., Capiluppi, B., Mastrorilli, E., Vergani, B., . . . Lazzarin, A. (1999). Viral load and burden modification following early antiretroviral therapy of primary HIV-1 infection. *AIDS*, *13*(7), 791–796.

Liu, L., Wong, T. P., Pozza, M. F., Lingenhoehl, K., Wang, Y., Sheng, M., . . . Wang, Y. T. (2004). Role of NMDA receptor subtypes in governing the direction of hippocampal synaptic plasticity. [In Vitro Research Support, Non-U.S. Gov't]. *Science*, *304*(5673), 1021–1024. doi: 10.1126/science.1096615

Logigian, E. L., Johnson, K. A., Kijewski, M. F., Kaplan, R. F., Becker, J. A., Jones, K. J., . . . Steere, A. C. (1997). Reversible cerebral hypoperfusion in Lyme encephalopathy. [Research Support, U.S. Gov't, P.H.S.]. *Neurology*, *49*(6), 1661–1670.

Logigian, E. L., Kaplan, R. F., & Steere, A. C. (1990). Chronic neurologic manifestations of Lyme disease. [Research Support, U.S. Gov't, P.H.S.]. *The New England Journal of Medicine*, *323*(21), 1438–1444. doi: 10.1056/NEJM199011223232102

Logigian, E. L., Kaplan, R. F., & Steere, A. C. (1999). Successful treatment of Lyme encephalopathy with intravenous ceftriaxone. [Research Support, Non-U.S. Gov't Research Support, U.S. Gov't, P.H.S.]. *The Journal of Infectious Diseases*, *180*(2), 377–383. doi: 10.1086/314860

Mahadevan, A., Shankar, S. K., Satishchandra, P., Ranga, U., Chickabasaviah, Y. T., Santosh, V., . . . Zink, M. C. (2007). Characterization of human immunodeficiency virus (HIV)-infected cells in infiltrates associated with CNS opportunistic infections in patients with HIV clade C infection. *Journal of Neuropathology & Experimental Neurology*, *66*(9), 799–808. doi: 10.1097/NEN.0b013e3181461d3e00005072-200709000 00004 [pii]

Marcotte, T. D., Deutsch, R., McCutchan, J. A., Moore, D. J., Letendre, S., Ellis, R. J., . . . Grant, I. (2003). Prediction of incident neurocognitive impairment by plasma HIV RNA and CD4 levels early after HIV seroconversion. *Archives of Neurology*, *60*(10), 1406–1412.

Marcotte, T. D., Heaton, R. K., Wolfson, T., Taylor, M. J., Alhassoon, O., Arfaa, K., . . . Grant, I. (1999). The impact of HIV-related neuropsychological dysfunction on driving behavior. [The HNRC Group]. *Journal of the International Neuropsychological Society*, *5*(7), 579–592.

Masliah, E., DeTeresa, R. M., Mallory, M. E., & Hansen, L. A. (2000). Changes in pathological findings at autopsy in AIDS cases for the last 15 years. *AIDS*, *14*(1), 69–74.

Mayer, K., Jesdale, B., Flanigan, T., Fiore, T., Bettencourt, F., Stein, M., . . . Carpenter, C. (1992). The prevalence of specific illnesses in HIV-infected US women with associated CD4 counts. [Abstract No. PoC4371]. *International Conference on AIDS*, *8*(2), C306.

McArthur, J. C., McClernon, D. R., Cronin, M. F., Nance-Sproson, T. E., Saah, A. J., St Clair, M., & Lanier, E. R. (1997). Relationship between human immunodeficiency virus-associated dementia and viral load in cerebrospinal fluid and brain. *Annals of Neurology*, *42*(5), 689–698.

McGrath, N., Anderson, N. E., Croxson, M. C., & Powell, K. F. (1997). Herpes simplex encephalitis treated with acyclovir: Diagnosis and long term outcome. [Research Support, Non-U.S. Gov't]. *Journal of Neurology, Neurosurgery, and Psychiatry*, *63*(3), 321–326.

McMurtray, A., Nakamoto, B., Shikuma, C., & Valcour, V. (2007). Small-vessel vascular disease in human immunodeficiency virus infection: The Hawaii aging with HIV Cohort Study. *Cerebrovascular Diseases*, *24*(2–3), 236–241.

Mellors, J., Munoz, A., Giorgi, J., Margolick, J., Tassoni, C., Gupta, P., . . . Rinaldo, C. J. (1997). Plasma viral load and CD4+ lymphocytes as prognostic markers of HIV-1 infection. *Annals of Internal Medicine*, *126*(12), 946–954.

Mellors, J. W. (1997). Viral load and clinical outcome. *International AIDS Society-USA*, *5*, 8–10.

Mesulam, M. M. (1990). Large-scale neurocognitive networks and distributed processing for attention, language, and memory. [Research Support, Non-U.S. Gov't Review]. *Annals of Neurology*, *28*(5), 597–613. doi: 10.1002/ana.410280502

Miller, E. N., Selnes, O. A., McArthur, J. C., Satz, P., Becker, J. T., Cohen, B. A., . . . Visscher, B. (1990). Neuropsychological performance in HIV-1-infected homosexual men: The Multicenter AIDS Cohort Study (MACS). *Neurology*, *40*(2), 197–203.

Mobley, K., Rotterdam, H. Z., Lerner, C. W., & Tapper, M. L. (1985). Autopsy findings in the acquired immune deficiency syndrome. *Pathology Annual*, *20*(Pt 1), 45–65.

Morgello, S., Mahboob, R., Yakoushina, T., Khan, S., & Hague, K. (2002). Autopsy findings in a human immunodeficiency virus-infected population over 2 decades: Influences of gender, ethnicity, risk factors, and time. *Archives of Pathology & Laboratory Medicine*, *126*(2), 182–190. doi: 10.1043/0003-9985(2002)126<0182:AFIAHI>2.0.CO;2

Moriishi, K., & Matsuura, Y. (2003). Mechanisms of hepatitis C virus infection. *Antiviral Chemistry and Chemotherapy*, *14*(6), 285–297.

Mundinger, A., Adam, T., Ott, D., Dinkel, E., Beck, A., Peter, H. H., . . . Schumacher, M. (1992). CT and MRI: Prognostic tools in patients with AIDS and neurological deficits. *Neuroradiology*, *35*(1), 75–78.

Mylonakis, E. (2001). When to suspect and how to monitor babesiosis. *American Family Physician*, *63*(10), 1969–1974.

Navia, B., Cho, E., & Petito, C., et al. (1986). The AIDS dementia complex II. Neuropathology. *Annals of Neurology*, *19*, 525–535.

Neuenburg, J. K., Brodt, H. R., Herndier, B. G., Bickel, M., Bacchetti, P., Price, R. W., . . . Schlote, W. (2002). HIV-related neuropathology, 1985 to 1999: Rising prevalence of HIV encephalopathy in the era of highly active antiretroviral therapy. *Journal of Acquired Immune Deficiency Syndromes*, *31*(2), 171–177.

Nockher, W. A., Bergmann, L., & Scherberich, J. E. (1994). Increased soluble CD14 serum levels and altered CD14 expression of peripheral blood monocytes in HIV-infected patients. *Clinical & Experimental Immunology*, *98*(3), 369–374.

Nolan, D. C., Carruthers, M. M., & Lerner, A. M. (1970). Herpesvirus hominis encephalitis in Michigan. Report of thirteen cases, including six treated with idoxuridine. *The New England Journal of Medicine*, *282*(1), 10–13. doi: 10.1056/NEJM197001012820103

Odiase, F., Ogunrin, O., & Ogunniyi, A. (2006). Effect of progression of disease on cognitive performance in HIV/AIDS. *Journal of the National Medical Association*, *98*(8), 1260–1262.

Pachner, A. R., & Steere, A. C. (1985). The triad of neurologic manifestations of Lyme disease: Meningitis, cranial neuritis, and radiculoneuritis. [Research Support, Non-U.S. Gov't Research Support, U.S. Gov't, P.H.S.]. *Neurology*, *35*(1), 47–53.

Palella, F. J., Jr., Delaney, K. M., Moorman, A. C., Loveless, M. O., Fuhrer, J., Satten, G. A., . . . Holmberg, S. D. (1998). Declining morbidity and mortality among patients with advanced human immunodeficiency virus infection. [HIV Outpatient Study Investigators]. *The New England Journal of Medicine*, *338*(13), 853–860.

Palmer, D., Hjeelle, B., & Wiley, C., et al. (1994). HIV-1 infection despite immediate combination antiretroviral therapy after infusion of contaminated white cells. *American Journal of Medicine*, *97*, 289–295.

Panther, L. A., Coombs, R. W., Aung, S. A., dela Rosa, C., Gretch, D., & Corey, L. (1999). Unintegrated HIV-1 circular 2-LTR proviral DNA as a marker of recently infected cells: Relative effect of recombinant CD4, zidovudine, and saquinavir in vitro. *Journal of Medical Virology*, *58*(2), 165–173.

Paul, R. H., Laidlaw, D. H., Tate, D. F., Lee, S., Hoth, K. F., Gunstad, J., . . . Flanigan, T. (2007). Neuropsychological and neuroimaging outcome of HIV-associated progressive multifocal leukoencephalopathy in the era of antiretroviral therapy. *Journal of Integrative Neuroscience*, *6*(1), 191–203.

Pewter, S. M., Williams, W. H., Haslam, C., & Kay, J. M. (2007). Neuropsychological and psychiatric profiles in acute encephalitis in adults. [Research Support, Non-U.S. Gov't]. *Neuropsychological Rehabilitation*, *17*(4–5), 478–505. doi: 10.1080/09602010701202238

Pimental, P. A., & Gregor, M. M. (2012). Neuropsychological consultation in infectious diseases: Pathogenesis and neuropsychological sequelae in herpes simples encephalitis. *Journal of Neuroparasitology*, *3*.

Post, M. J., Chan, J. C., Hensley, G. T., Hoffman, T. A., Moskowitz, L. B., & Lippmann, S. (1983). Toxoplasma encephalitis in Haitian adults with acquired immunodeficiency syndrome: A clinical-pathologic-CT correlation. *American Journal of Roentgenology*, *140*(5), 861–868.

Price, R. W., Brew, B., Sidtis, J., Rosenblum, M., Scheck, A. C., & Cleary, P. (1988). The brain in AIDS: Central nervous system HIV-1 infection and AIDS dementia complex. *Science*, *239*(4840), 586–592.

Pruss, H., Finke, C., Holtje, M., Hofmann, J., Klingbeil, C., Probst, C., . . . Wandinger, K. P. (2012). N-methyl-D-aspartate receptor antibodies in herpes simplex encephalitis. [Research Support, N.I.H., Extramural Research Support, Non-U.S. Gov't]. *Annals of Neurology*, *72*(6), 902–911. doi: 10.1002/ana.23689

Ramsey, R. G., & Geremia, G. K. (1988). CNS complications of AIDS: CT and MR findings. *AJR American Journal of Roentgenology*, *151*(3), 449–454.

Ravdin, L. D., Hilton, E., Primeau, M., Clements, C., & Barr, W. B. (1996). Memory functioning in Lyme borreliosis. [Comparative Study]. *Journal of Clinical Psychiatry*, *57*(7), 282–286.

Reik, L., Jr., Smith, L., Khan, A., & Nelson, W. (1985). Demyelinating encephalopathy in Lyme disease. [Case Reports]. *Neurology*, *35*(2), 267–269.

Rennick, P. M., Nolan, D. C., Bauer, R. B., & Lerner, A. M. (1973). Neuropsychologic and neurologic follow-up after herpesvirus hominis encephalitis. *Neurology*, *23*(1), 42–47.

Reuter, J. D. (2005). Cytomegalovirus induces T-cell independent apoptosis in brain during immunodeficiency. [Research Support, N.I.H., Extramural Research Support, U.S. Gov't, P.H.S.]. *Journal of Clinical Virology*, *32*(3), 218–223. doi: 10.1016/j.jcv.2004.07.012

Robertson, K., Fiscus, S., Kapoor, C., Robertson, W., Schneider, G., Shepard, R., . . . Hall, C. (1998). CSF, plasma viral load and HIV associated dementia. *Journal of NeuroVirology*, *4*(1), 90–94.

Sarrazin, J. L., Bonneville, F., & Martin-Blondel, G. (2012). Brain infections. [Review]. *Diagnostic and Interventional Imaging*, *93*(6), 473–490. doi: 10.1016/j.diii.2012.04.020

Schmidbauer, M., Budka, H., Okeda, R., Cristina, S., Lechi, A., & Trabattoni, G. R. (1990). Multifocal vacuolar leucoencephalopathy: A distinct HIV-associated lesion of the brain. *Neuropathology and Applied Neurobiology*, *16*(5), 437–443.

Schwartz, R. B., Garada, B. M., Komaroff, A. L., Tice, H. M., Gleit, M., Jolesz, F. A., & Holman, B. L. (1994). Detection of intracranial abnormalities in patients with chronic fatigue syndrome: Comparison of MR imaging and SPECT. [Comparative Study Research Support, U.S. Gov't, P.H.S.]. *AJR American Journal of Roentgenology*, *162*(4), 935–941. doi: 10.2214/ajr.162.4.8141020

Shadick, N. A., Phillips, C. B., Logigian, E. L., Steere, A. C., Kaplan, R. F., Berardi, V. P., . . . Liang, M. H. (1994). The long-term clinical outcomes of Lyme disease: A population-based retrospective cohort study. [Research Support, Non-U.S. Gov't Research Support, U.S. Gov't, P.H.S.]. *Annals of Internal Medicine*, *121*(8), 560–567.

Shiramizu, B., Gartner, S., Williams, A., Shikuma, C., Ratto-Kim, S., Watters, M., . . . Valcour, V. (2005). Circulating proviral HIV DNA and HIV-associated dementia. *AIDS*, *19*(1), 45–52.

Shiramizu, B., Ratto-Kim, S., Sithinamsuwan, P., Nidhinandana, S., Thitivichianlert, S., Watt, G., . . . Valcour, V. (2007). HIV DNA and dementia in treatment-naive HIV-1-infected individuals in Bangkok, Thailand. *International Journal of Medical Sciences*, *4*(1), 13–18.

Silva, A. C., Rodrigues, B. S., Micheletti, A. M., Tostes, S., Jr., Meneses, A. C., Silva-Vergara, M. L., & Adad, S. J. (2012). Neuropathology of AIDS: An autopsy review of 284 cases from Brazil comparing the findings pre- and post-HAART (Highly Active Antiretroviral Therapy) and pre- and postmortem correlation. *AIDS Research and Treatment*, *2012*, 186850. doi: 10.1155/2012/186850

Skoldenberg, B., Aurelius, E., Hjalmarsson, A., Sabri, F., Forsgren, M., Andersson, B., . . . Rosengren, L. (2006). Incidence and pathogenesis of clinical relapse after herpes simplex encephalitis in adults. [Comparative Study]. *Journal of Neurology*, *253*(2), 163–170. doi: 10.1007/s00415-005-0941-6

Stanek, G., Lusa, L., Ogrinc, K., Markowicz, M., & Strle, F. (2013). Intrathecally produced IgG and IgM antibodies to recombinant VlsE, VlsE peptide, recombinant OspC and whole cell extracts in the diagnosis of Lyme neuroborreliosis. *Medical Microbiology and Immunology*. doi: 10.1007/s00430-013-0322-1

Steere, A. C. (2001). Lyme disease. [Research Support, Non-U.S. Gov't Research Support, U.S. Gov't, P.H.S. Review]. *The New England Journal of Medicine*, *345*(2), 115–125. doi: 10.1056/NEJM200107123450207

Steere, A. C., Grodzicki, R. L., Kornblatt, A. N., Craft, J. E., Barbour, A. G., Burgdorfer, W., . . . Malawista, S. E. (1983). The spirochetal etiology of Lyme disease. [Research Support, Non-U.S. Gov't Research Support, U.S. Gov't, P.H.S.]. *The New England Journal of Medicine*, *308*(13), 733–740. doi: 10.1056/NEJM198303313081301

Steere, A. C., Gross, D., Meyer, A. L., & Huber, B. T. (2001). Autoimmune mechanisms in antibiotic treatment-resistant lyme arthritis. [Research Support, Non-U.S. Gov't Research Support, U.S. Gov't, P.H.S. Review]. *Journal of Autoimmunity*, *16*(3), 263–268. doi: 10.1006/jaut.2000.0495

Steiner, I., Kennedy, P. G., & Pachner, A. R. (2007). The neurotropic herpes viruses: Herpes simplex and varicella-zoster. [Research Support, Non-U.S. Gov't Review]. *Lancet Neurology*, *6*(11), 1015–1028. doi: 10.1016/S1474-4422(07)70267-3

Steinmetz, H., Arendt, G., Hefter, H., Neuen-Jacob, E., Dorries, K., Aulich, A., & Kahn, T. (1995). Focal brain lesions in patients with AIDS: Aetiologies and corresponding radiological patterns in a prospective study. *Journal of Neurology*, *242*(2), 69–74.

Stout, J. C., Ellis, R. J., Jernigan, T. L., Archibald, S. L., Abramson, I., Wolfson, T., . . . Grant, I. (1998). Progressive cerebral volume loss in human immunodeficiency virus infection: A longitudinal volumetric magnetic resonance imaging study. [HIV Neurobehavioral Research Center Group]. *Archives of Neurology*, *55*(2), 161–168.

Terzian, H., & Ore, G. D. (1955). Syndrome of Kluver and Bucy; reproduced in man by bilateral removal of the temporal lobes. *Neurology*, *5*(6), 373–380.

Thieblemont, N., Weiss, L., Sadeghi, H. M., Estcourt, C., & Haeffner-Cavaillon, N. (1995). CD14lowCD16high: A cytokine-producing monocyte subset which expands during human immunodeficiency virus infection. *European Journal of Immunology*, *25*(12), 3418–3424.

Toneatto, S., Finco, O., van der Putten, H., Abrignani, S., & Annunziata, P. (1999). Evidence of blood-brain barrier alteration and activation in HIV-1 gp120 transgenic mice. *AIDS*, *13*(17), 2343–2348.

Tozzi, V., Balestra, P., Lorenzini, P., Bellagamba, R., Galgani, S., Corpolongo, A., . . . Narciso, P. (2005). Prevalence and risk factors for human immunodeficiency virus-associated neurocognitive impairment, 1996 to 2002: Results from an urban observational cohort. *Journal of NeuroVirology*, *11*(3), 265–273.

Vago, L., Cinque, P., Sala, E., Nebuloni, M., Caldarelli, R., Racca, S., . . . Costanzi, G. (1996). JCV-DNA and BKV-DNA in the CNS tissue and CSF of AIDS patients and normal subjects: Study of 41 cases and review of the literature. *Journal of Acquired Immune Deficiency Syndromes and Human Retrovirology*, *12*(2), 139–146.

Vannier, E., & Krause, P. J. (2012). Human babesiosis. [Research Support, N.I.H., Extramural Research Support, Non-U.S. Gov't]. *The New England Journal of Medicine*, *366*(25), 2397–2407. doi: 10.1056/NEJMra1202018

Veugelers, P. J., Strathdee, S. A., Kaldor, J. M., Shafer, K. A., Moss, A. R., Schechter, M. T., . . . van Griensven, G. J. (1997). Associations of age, immunosuppression, and AIDS among homosexual men in the Tricontinental Seroconverter Study. *Journal of Acquired Immune Deficiency Syndromes and Human Retrovirology*, *14*(5), 435–441.

Villa, G., Solida, A., Moro, E., Tavolozza, M., Antinori, A., De Luca, A., . . . Tamburrini, E. (1996). Cognitive impairment in asymptomatic stages of HIV infection: A longitudinal study. *European Neurology*, *36*(3), 125–133.

Vitiello, B., Goodkin, K., Ashtana, D., Shapshak, P., Atkinson, J. H., Heseltine, P. N., . . . Lyman, W. D. (2007). HIV-1 RNA concentration and cognitive performance in a cohort of HIV-positive people. *AIDS*, *21*(11), 1415–1422.

Wallace, M. R., Heaton, R. K., McCutchan, J. A., Malone, J. L., Velin, R., Nelson, J., . . . Grant, I. (1997). Neurocognitive impairment in human immunodeficiency virus infection is correlated with sexually transmitted disease history. *Sexually Transmitted Diseases*, *24*(7), 398–401.

Wallace, M. R., Moss, R. B., Beecham, H. J., 3rd, Grace, C. J., Hersh, E. M., Peterson, E., . . . Levine, A. M. (1996). Early clinical markers and CD4 percentage in subjects with human immunodeficiency virus infection. *Journal of Acquired Immune Deficiency Syndromes and Human Retrovirology*, *12*(4), 358–362.

Westervelt, H. J., & McCaffrey, R. J. (2002). Neuropsychological functioning in chronic Lyme disease. [Review]. *Neuropsychology Review*, *12*(3), 153–177.

Whitley, R. J., & Roizman, B. (2001). Herpes simplex virus infections. [Review]. *Lancet*, *357*(9267), 1513–1518. doi: 10.1016/S0140-6736(00)04638-9

Wiley, C. A., Achim, C. L., Christopherson, C., Kidane, Y., Kwok, S., Masliah, E., . . . Soontornniyomkij, V. (1999). HIV mediates a productive infection of the brain. *AIDS*, *13*(15), 2055–2059.

Wiley, C. A., Masliah, E., Morey, M., Lemere, C., DeTeresa, R., Grafe, M., . . . Terry, R. (1991). Neocortical damage during HIV infection. *Annals of Neurology*, *29*(6), 651–657.

Wiley, C. A., Soontornniyomkij, V., Radhakrishnan, L., Masliah, E., Mellors, J., Hermann, S. A., . . . Achim, C. L. (1998). Distribution of brain HIV load in AIDS. *Brain Pathology*, *8*(2), 277–284.

Wilkie, F. L., Goodkin, K., Khamis, I., van Zuilen, M. H., Lee, D., Lecusay, R., . . . Eisdorfer, C. (2003). Cognitive functioning in younger and older HIV-1-infected adults. *Journal of Acquired Immune Deficiency Syndromes*, *33*(Suppl 2), S93–S105.

Wormser, G. P., Dattwyler, R. J., Shapiro, E. D., Halperin, J. J., Steere, A. C., Klempner, M. S., . . . Nadelman, R. B. (2006). The clinical assessment, treatment, and prevention of lyme disease, human granulocytic anaplasmosis, and babesiosis: Clinical practice guidelines by the Infectious Diseases Society of America. [Practice Guideline]. *Clinical Infectious Diseases*, *43*(9), 1089–1134. doi: 10.1086/508667

Wormser, G. P., Ramanathan, R., Nowakowski, J., McKenna, D., Holmgren, D., Visintainer, P., . . . Nadelman, R. B. (2003). Duration of antibiotic therapy for early Lyme disease: A randomized, double-blind, placebo-controlled trial. [Clinical Trial Randomized Controlled Trial Research Support, U.S. Gov't, P.H.S.]. *Annals of Internal Medicine*, *138*(9), 697–704.

Xing, H. Q., Hayakawa, H., Izumo, K., Kubota, R., Gelpi, E., Budka, H., & Izumo, S. (2009). In vivo expression of proinflammatory cytokines in HIV encephalitis: An analysis of 11 autopsy cases. *Neuropathology*, *29*(4), 433–442. doi: 10.1111/j.1440-1789.2008.00996.x NEU996 [pii]

21 Hypoxia of the Central Nervous System

Ramona O. Hopkins

Introduction

More than 424,000 deaths due to cardiac and respiratory arrest occur each year in the United States (Kudenchuk et al., 2015). Improvements in emergency and critical care medicine have resulted an increase in successful cardiopulmonary resuscitation, which has led to a fairly stable mortality rate over the last 20 years (Sandroni, Nolan, Cavallaro, & Antonelli, 2007). However, more than half of all survivors experience significant morbidities such as long-term cognitive impairments that include impairments in memory and executive function and they experience depression, anxiety and reduced quality of life (Moulaert, Verbunt, van Heugten, & Wade, 2009). A significant percent of patients with anoxia (up to 90%) are unable to return to their premorbid level of function (Kaplan, 1999). Patient outcomes vary based on the location (in hospital vs. out of hospital) and the cause of cardiac arrest (Kudenchuk et al., 2015). In addition to cardiac or respiratory arrest, a number of other disorders cause a lack of oxygen to the brain. Anoxia, hypoxia, or ischemia occur in a variety of disorders including asthma, cardiac or respiratory arrest, cardiac disease or surgery, carbon monoxide poisoning, attempted hanging, complications of anesthesia, near downing, obstructive sleep apnea (OSA), chronic obstructive pulmonary disease (COPD), and acute respiratory distress syndrome. Given that a number of disorders result in an anoxic/ischemic event, a substantial number of individuals will subsequently develop hypoxic brain injury along with its associated morbidities.

Hypoxic Brain Injury

The human brain constitutes approximately 2% of the total body mass but utilizes up to 25% of the body's total oxygen consumption (Haddad & Jiang, 1993). Due to a high metabolic demand, the brain requires a constant supply of oxygen and glucose to produce energy and uses aerobic glucose oxidation to produce 95% of the brain's adenosine triphosphate (ATP) (Hicks, 1968). It is essential that the neocortical and subcortical areas receive a continuous supply of oxygen, as neurons are not able to store oxygen and glucose for later use (Hicks, 1968). Slight decreases in oxygen delivery to the brain may lead to permanent biochemical and morphological changes. Both hypoxia and ischemia result in decreased oxygen delivery to the tissues. *Ischemia* is defined as insufficient blood supply to the brain or other organs (ie.e cardiac arrest) due to interruption or reduction of blood delivery, *anoxia* is the absence or near complete absence of oxygen in the arterial blood supply to an organ or tissue, *hypoxia* is diminished availability of oxygen to the tissues, and *hypoxemia* is a condition in which there is reduced oxygenation of the blood (Biagas, 1999; Kuroiwa & Okeda, 1994).

Effects of oxygen deprivation on cognitive function are well known. Early studies found that a decrease in the partial pressure of arterial oxygen (PaO_2) in humans such that PaO_2 is 75% of normal impairs complex task performance; at 65%, memory impairments are manifest; at 50%, judgment is impaired and unconscious may occur; and very low levels (30%–40%) death will occur (Blass & Gibson, 1979). Regional brain oxygen utilization is not homogeneous, as some brain regions are more vulnerable to the effects of hypoxia than are others. Neural structures in the marginal zones of the vascular supply (end arteries), structures with high metabolic rates, or proximity to structures with high levels of excitatory amino acids such as glutamate or aspartate are affected differentially by hypoxia (Miyamoto & Auer, 2000). Vulnerable brain regions include the neocortex, hippocampus, basal ganglia, cerebellar Purkinje cells, primary visual cortex, frontal regions, and the thalamus (Chalela, Wolf, Maldjian, & Kasner, 2001; Oechmichen & Meissner, 2006). The time course of hypoxic-induced neuronal injury varies over time in different brain regions, with lesions of the basal ganglia and cortex occurring in the first few hours following hypoxia, whereas damage to the hippocampus may not occur for days to weeks (Kuroiwa & Okeda, 1994). In rodents who undergo anoxia, cell death in the globus pallidus, thalamus, and dentate gyrus occurred in the first 24 to 48 hours and the rate of neuronal cell death declined rapidly, or alternatively cell death in the cortex, striatum and CA1 subregion of the hippocampus worsen over the first week (Nakajima et al., 2000). Early neuronal injury occurs from acute mechanisms of injury including oxygen deprivation and reduction, ATP, and brain edema, leading to a decline in cerebral perfusion and disruption of the blood-brain barrier (Oechmichen & Meissner, 2006). Delayed neuronal damage is due to mechanisms of secondary neuronal injury, including antiapoptotic growth factor, vulnerability of microtubule-associated protein and tubulin, and disrupted protein synthesis (Bodsch, Barbier, Oehmichen, Grosse Ophoff, & Hossmann, 1986; Miyamoto & Auer, 2000).

Mechanisms of Brain Injury

The mechanisms of hypoxic brain injury have been elucidated over the last several decades, in both in vivo and in vitro models. For detailed reviews of mechanisms of hypoxic brain injury, see Busl and Greer (2010), Guo, Yu, and Ma (2011), and Oechmichen and Meissner (2006). Mechanisms of hypoxic brain injury are divided into several categories: (a) biochemical effects, (b) functional neuronal changes, (c) reperfusion or reoxygenation injury, and (d) neuronal cell death from necrosis and apoptosis (Busl & Greer, 2010).

Biochemical Changes

A brief description of the biochemical changes that occur in hypoxic brain injury follows. Early injury is mediated by prolonged axonal depolarization and subsequent increased calcium influx (approximately a 25% increase via the NMDA receptors), and concomitant intracellular accumulation of calcium due to ionic pump failure (Kass & Lipton, 1986; Schurr, Lipton, West, & Rigor, 1990). Increased intracellular calcium activates calpain, which leads to cell death via apoptosis Busl and Greer (2010). Decreasing ATP production without decreasing ATP utilization results in energy depletion leading to cell death (Lutz & Nilsson, 1994). Energy failure results in ionic pump failure, outflow of K+, and inflow of Ca^{2}+ (Lutz & Nilsson, 1994). Lactic acidosis due to anaerobic metabolism also results in neural injury (Michenfelder & Sundt, 1971). High blood glucose levels and concomitant hypoxia result in elevated brain lactate levels posthypoxia (Siemkowicz & Hansen, 1978; Welsh, Ginsberg, Rieder, & Budd, 1980). The energy failure opens postsynaptic excitatory receptors, especially voltage-gated NMDA glutamate receptors (Gilland, Puka-Sundvall, Hillered, & Hagberg, 1998) and destructive enzymes such as lipases, proteases, and nucleases. Neuronal cell death due to neurotoxicity of excitatory amino acid (EEA) neurotransmitters such as glutamate and aspartate, which are released in relatively large quantities following hypoxia and cause increased neuronal firing, calcium influx, and subsequent neuronal death (Olney, 1969). Excitotoxic-induced neuronal damage occurs in the hippocampus (Kuroiwa & Okeda, 1994), cerebellum (Inage, Itoh, Wada, & Takashima, 1998), cerebral cortex, and basal ganglia (Johnston, Nakajima, & Hagberg, 2002), as well as multiple brain regions depending on the duration of anoxia/hypoxia. Hypoxia also decreases expression of the glutamate transporter EAAT4 expression (i.e., removes glutamate from the synapse) in Purkinje cells and is linked to glutamate toxicity (Inage et al., 1998).

Functional Neuronal Changes

Functional cellular changes include mitochondrial damage, disaggregation of polyribosomes and abnormal Golgi complexes, resulting in a loss of cell structure due to cytoskeletal damage via intracellular calcium accumulation (Busl & Greer, 2010; Petito, Feldmann, Pulsinelli, & Plum, 1987). In hypoxia, depressed protein synthesis is increased by elevated levels of intracellular calcium, aggravating cytoskeletal damage (Raley-Susman & Lipton, 1990). Finally, activation of glutamate receptors actives early gene upregulation (Busl & Greer, 2010).

Reperfusion or Reoxygenation Injury

With the return of oxygenation to the brain, the risk to the brain is not over—reoxygenation and reperfusion injury occurs. The formation of oxygen radicals during reperfusion or reoxygenation can lead to cell death. During hypoxia ATP levels fall and xanthine accumulates and glutamate release can occur along the neural shifts in calcium (Bottiger, Schmitz, Wiessner, Vogel, & Hossmann, 1998). Upon reperfusion and reoxygenation xanthine oxidase catalyzes the conversion of xanthine to uric acid resulting in superoxide, which impairs cell proliferation, gene expression, and disrupts membrane function (Biagas, 1999; Floyd, 1990; Granger, McCord, Parks, & Hollwarth, 1986). Nitric oxide synthase (NOS) is expressed in inflammatory cells (i.e., macrophages) and can be induced by hypoxia. It contributes to brain injury via impaired neurotransmission, impaired protein synthesis, and membrane peroxidation (Biagas, 1999). Thus, hypoxic brain injury results in a cascade of pathophysiological processes that result in cell damage and subsequent neuronal cell death (see Table 21.1).

Apoptosis and Necrosis

Hypoxia and associated biochemical cascades can initiate necrosis and/or apoptosis. Necrosis occurs due to edema and rupture of the cell sending the intracellular contents into the extra cellular space, resulting influx of inflammatory cells and vascular disruption (Biagas, 1999). Cell damage often culminates in necrotic cell death (Hossmann, Oschlies, Schwindt, & Krep, 2001). Apoptosis is programmed cell death with associated cell shrinkage, DNA fragmentation, and cellular changes, and appearance of apoptotic bodies, secondary inflammation, and fibrosis (Steller, 1995). Apoptosis is triggered by hypoxia-induced free radicals, nitric oxide, and reduced mitochondrial function (Busl & Greer, 2010). Neurons in the anoxic-ischemic region die from necrosis, neurons in the penumbra (bordering areas) die due to necrosis and apoptosis, and distant neurons like those in the hippocampus initially survive and then undergo delayed apoptotic cell death (Beilharz, Williams, Dragunow, Sirimanne, & Gluckman, 1995; Li, Powers, Jiang, & Chopp, 1998).

Table 21.1 Mechanisms of neuronal damage and death following hypoxic brain injury

Mechanisms	*Etiology of Cellular Death*
Biochemical Changes	
Decreased ATP production	• Energy failure and ionic outflow
Calcium Induced Neuronal Death	• Calcium influx and release from intracellular stores
Excitotoxicity	• Ionic pump failure ® cell death
	• Release catabolic enzymes ® cellular proteolysis
	• Excessive release of excitatory amino acid neurotransmitters (EAAs) (e.g., glutamate)
	• Calcium influx ® cell death
	• Decreased expression of excitatory amino acid transporter-4 (EAAT4) (glutamate transporter)
Functional Neuronal Changes	
	• Mitochondrial damage
	• Disaggregation of polyribosomes
	• Loss of cell structures ® cytoskeletal damage via calcium
	• Depressed protein synthesis
	• Activation of glutamate receptors via early gene upregulation
Reperfusion or Reoxygenation Injury	
Reperfusion	• Secondary disruption of energy metabolism
Oxidative Injury	• Xanthine catalyzed to uric acid ® reactive oxygen specices such as the hydrogen peroxide, superoxide anion and the hydroxyl radical (OH)
	• Reactive oxygen radicals attack cell membranes.
	• Lipid peroxidation impairs cell proliferation and gene expression
	• Inflammatory mediators (lipid-derived factors, cytokines, neutrophils, platelet adhesion, etc.)
	• Formation of nitric oxide
	• Alters neuronal transmission
	• Disrupts proteins
	• Cause membrane peroxidation
Necrosis and Apoptosis	
Necrosis	• Edema
Apoptosis	• Rupture of cell membrane
	• Influx of inflammatory cells
	• Vascular Disruption
	• Programmed cell death triggered by
	• free radicals
	• nitric oxide
	• reduced mitochondrial function

Neuroimaging Findings

Hypoxic brain injury can result in both focal and diffuse neuropathologic lesions and atrophy. Brain regions are affected differentially based on their selective vulnerability to hypoxia due to their arterial supply and location in the brain, such as in watershed areas (White, Zhang, Helvey, & Omojola, 2013). For example, hypoxia may result profound damage such as in diffuse damage to the cerebral cortex (Bachevalier & Meunier, 1996; Caine & Watson, 2000; Hopkins, Kesner, & Goldstein, 1995a); also see Figure 21.1). Cortical injury can be easily identified on diffusion-weighted imaging and is manifest as hypointense areas in the gray matter (White et al., 2013). Cortical regions that are vulnerable include occipital and perirondalic cortices (Rademakers, van der Knaap, Verbeeten, Barth, & Valk, 1995); primary sensory motor region (Macey et al., 2002); and insula, cingulate, and ventromedial prefrontal cortex (Harper, Kumar, Ogren, & Macey, 2013).

Focal damage occurs in a variety of neural structures, including the basal ganglia and hippocampi, which are more vulnerable to hypoxia compared to adjacent cortical regions such as the parahippocampal gyrus or other temporal lobe gyri (Hopkins et al., 1995; Kesner & Hopkins, 2001; Press, Amaral, & Squire, 1989). Significant hippocampal atrophy occurs following hypoxic brain injury (Hopkins et al., 1995; Kesner & Hopkins, 2001; Manns, Hopkins, Reed, Kitchener, & Squire, 2003; Press et al., 1989), and lesions in the hippocampus (Bayley, Gold, Hopkins, & Squire, 2005; Bayley, Hopkins, & Squire, 2003; Manns et al., 2003) (see Figure 21.2), basal ganglia (see Figure 21.3), and cerebellum are common (Armengol, 2000; Speach, Wong, Cattarin, & Livecchi, 1998). Hypoxic brain injury results in white matter changes including lesions in the cerebellar white matter (Mascalchi, Petruzzi, & Zampa, 1996), subcortical and periventricular white matter lesions (Davies et al., 2001; Parkinson et al., 2002), and corpus callosum atrophy (Porter, Hopkins, Weaver, Bigler, & Blatter, 2002). A study using diffusion tensor imaging found reduced white matter integrity in the cerebellum, basal ganglia, limbic regions, corpus callosum, and within the corona radiata; the changes in white matter integrity were associated with hypoxia (Kumar et al., 2014). In a review of the literature of anoxia, Caine and Watson (2000) reviewed a number of studies in 90 patients with

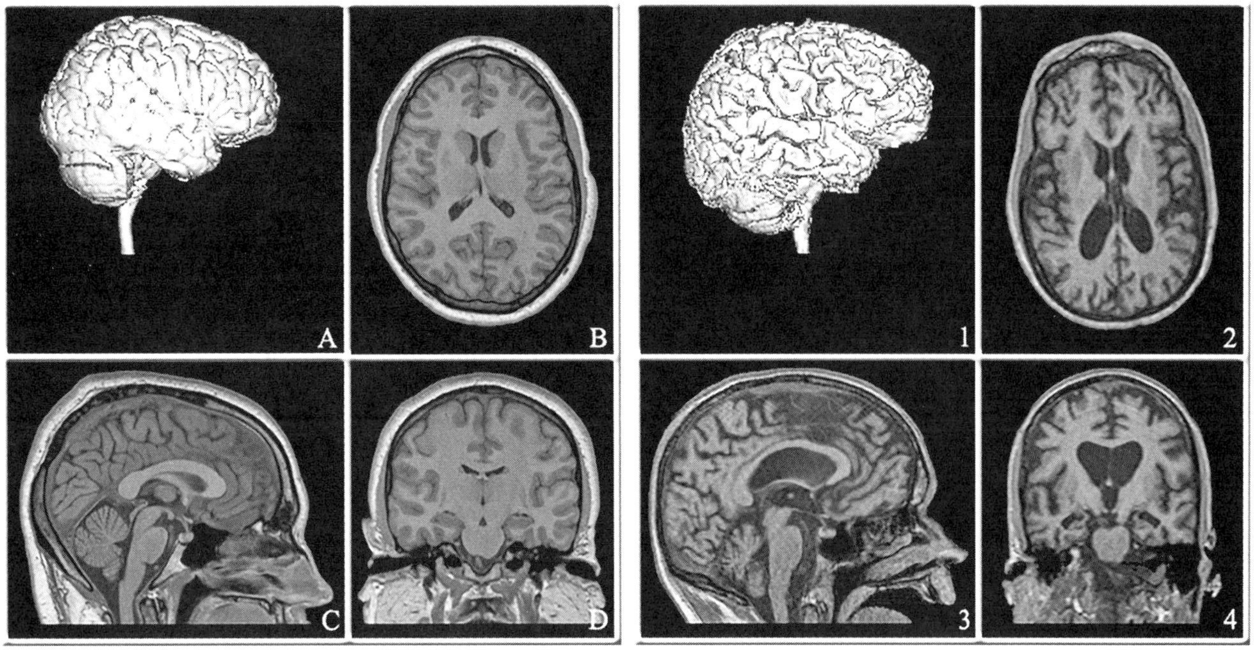

Figure 21.1 This figure shows magnetic resonance imaging of the brain in a normal individual (panels A thru D) and a participant who has had an anoxic brain injury (panels 1 thru 4). For the normal participant, Panel A shows a three-dimensional reconstruction of the brain, Panel B an axial view of the brain thru the body of the lateral ventricles, Panel C the midsagittal slice through the corpus callosum, and Panel D a coronal view though the hippocampus. For the anoxic brain-injured participant; Panel 1 shows a three-dimensional reconstruction with significant gyral atrophy and sulcal widening. Panel 2 shows an axial view thru the body of the lateral ventricles with significant ventricular enlargement and sulcal widening. Panel 3 show the midsagittal view thru the corpus callosum showing significant collosal atrophy. Finally, Panel 4 shows a coronal view thru the hippocampus-showing enlargement of the lateral ventricles, third ventricle, and temporal horns of the lateral ventricles, and bilateral hippocampal atrophy.

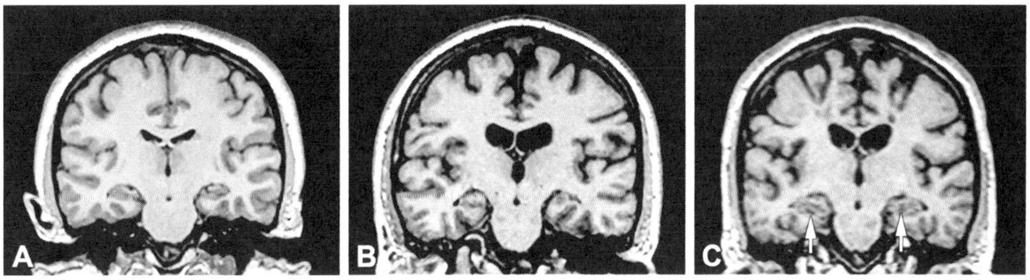

Figure 21.2 This figure shows brain magnetic resonance images in the coronal plane through the hippocampus at the level of the forth ventricle. Panel A shows a brain MRI in a normal individual, Panel B shows a participant with anoxic brain injury who has bilateral hippocampal atrophy, and Panel C shows a second participant with an anoxic brain injury who has bilateral hippocampal lesions.

hypoxia who underwent brain imaging. Of the 90 patients, 44% had cortical edema or atrophy, 33% had cerebellar lesions, 22% had basal ganglia lesions, 21% had hippocampal atrophy, and 3% had thalamic lesions (Caine & Watson, 2000). In a systematic review of near drowning, in 46 cases, 36% had diffuse cerebral atrophy, 15% had infarcts, and 75% had basal ganglia lesions (Nucci-da-Silva & Amaro, 2009). The high prevalence of basal ganglia lesions in near drowning is similar to that found after carbon monoxide poisoning, which occurs in 32% to 86% of individuals (Hopkins, Fearing, Weaver, & Foley, 2006).

During the acute period following hypoxic brain injury, conventional magnetic resonance imaging (MRI) and computed tomography (CT) findings may be normal or exhibit only subtle changes. Imaging techniques such as diffusion-weighted MRI (which measures cytotoxic edema) found more extensive neuropathologic changes in the early acute phase than previously reported. For example, individuals

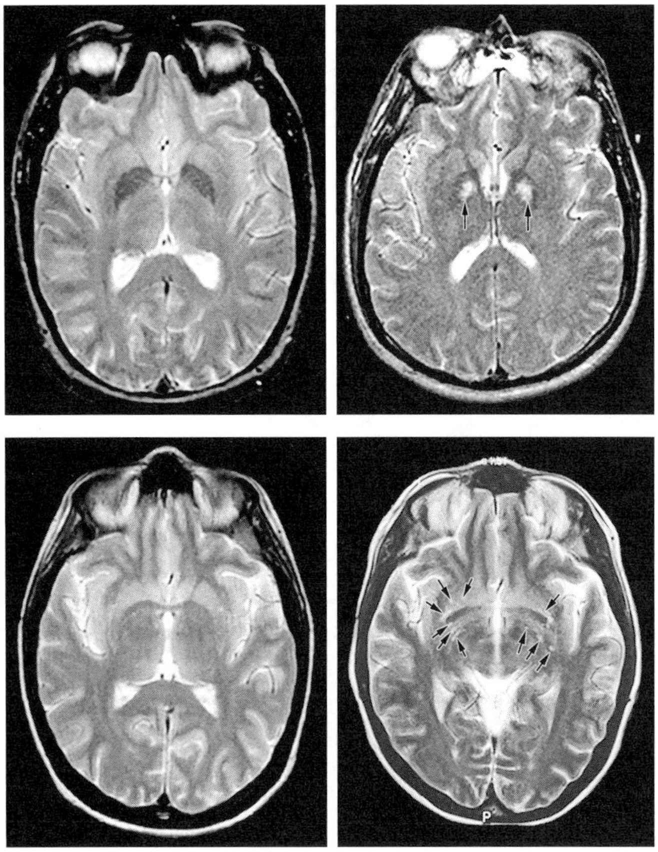

Figure 21.3 This figure shows brain MRI in the axial plane thru the basal ganglia in anoxic participants. The panel in the top left shows an anoxic participant on the day of injury (carbon monoxide poisoning) and the top panel on the right shows the same participant two weeks postinjury with bilateral lesions in the globus pallidus (arrows). The lower left panel shows an anoxic participant (carbon monoxide poisoning) 4.5 weeks post injury and the lower right panel shows the same participant 8 months postinjury with numerous foci of abnormal signal intensity in the deep cerebral white matter and basal ganglia bilaterally and symmetrically.

with hypoxia had early and extensive abnormalities in the basal ganglia, cerebellum and cortex in the acute period and gray and white matter abnormalities in the subacute period on diffusion-weighted MRI (Arbelaez, Castillo, & Mukherji, 1999). Chalela, Wolf, Maldjian, and Kasner (2001) found white matter abnormalities within seven days of hypoxic brain injury on diffusion-weighted MRI. The pattern and extent of brain abnormalities identified on diffusion-weighted MRI may be markers for prognosis following hypoxic brain injury (Singhal, Topcuoglu, & Koroshetz, 2002).

Limbic System

As discussed previously the mesial temporal lobes, in particular the hippocampus, are selectively vulnerable to hypoxic brain injury, which manifests as lesions and atrophy that are associated with memory impairments (Bayley et al., 2005; Bayley et al., 2003; Manns et al., 2003). Because of the hippocampus's distinct anatomy and location in the brain, hippocampal volumes can be readily quantified (Bigler et al., 1997; Bigler & Clement, 1997; White et al., 2013). Hippocampal atrophy is a common finding in OSA (Gale & Hopkins, 2004; Macey et al., 2002; Morrell et al., 2003). The temporal horns of the lateral ventricles are sensitive to temporal lobe damage and neuronal loss, and may indicate temporal lobe and/or hippocampal atrophy (Bigler, 2001). Lesions are also found in the fornix and cingulum (White et al., 2013). Kesler, Hopkins, Blatter, Edge-Booth, and Bigler, (2001) measured cross-sectional surface areas of the fornix in a group of hypoxic brain injury subjects following carbon monoxide poisoning and found mild atrophy of the fornix. Since the fornix is the major output pathway from the hippocampus to the mammillary bodies, it follows that fornix would atrophy due to anterograde degeneration of the hippocampal axons following hippocampal neuronal loss.

Cerebellum

The cerebellum is vulnerable to hypoxic brain injury (lesions can be diffuse or focal in nature) and Purkinje cell death due to excitoxicity results in diffuse and focal injury (Welsh et al., 1980). Both necrotic processes and demyelination occur in the cerebellum (Chang, Han, Kim, Wie, & Han, 1992; Mascalchi et al., 1996). Cerebellar atrophy correlates with low Glasgow coma scores, profound acidosis, and electrocardiograph abnormalities (O'Donnell, Buxton, Pitkin, & Jarvis, 2000). Cerebellar damage occurs in the cerebellar cortex and deep nuclei (Harper et al., 2013), and it results in ataxia or motor incoordination, problems initiating or ending purposeful movements, impaired balance, difficulty maintaining posture, problems with gait, wide-based stance, and a positive Romberg sign (Heimer, 1995). Cognitive deficits secondary to cerebellar pathology include impaired executive function, visuospatial processing, and language, as well as impaired memory and affective changes (Schmahmann & Pandya, 1997).

Brain Stem

While the effects of hypoxic brain injury on the cerebral cortex, cerebellum, hippocampus, and thalamus are well described, less is known about the effects on the brain stem. Lesions in brain stem nuclei following hypoxia (Gilles, 1969; Lindenberg, 1963) occur in widely distributed regions including the midbrain, pons, locus coeruleus, superior olive, inferior colliculi, reticular formation, and cranial nerve nuclei (Revesz & Geddes, 1988). Lesions have been reported in the dorsal, ventral, and ventrolateral medulla in individuals with OSA (Kumar, Macey, Woo, Alger, & Harper, 2008). Functional markers of brain stem integrity include evoked potentials. Abnormal somatosensory evoked potentials (Chen, Bolton, & Young, 1996), and brain stem auditory evoked potentials (Goldberg & Karazim, 1998), are indicators of poor survival following hypoxic brain injury. Alternatively, normal brain stem auditory evoked potentials have been reported in individuals with anoxic coma, indicating sparing of rostral brain stem function.

Neuropsychological Effects

Regardless of the etiology, neuropsychological deficits are a common morbidity following hypoxic brain injury. Neuropsychological impairments include impaired memory (Bigler & Alfano, 1988; Hopkins et al., 1995b; Hopkins, Weaver, et al., 2005; Hopkins & Woon, 2006; Zola-Morgan & Squire, 1990), dysexecutive function (Hopkins et al., 1995; Lezak, Howieson, Bigler, & Tranel, 2012), agnosia (Farah, 1990), visual-spatial deficits (Barat, Blanchard, & Carriet, 1989), and generalized decline in intellectual function (Bigler & Alfano, 1988; Parkin, Miller, & Vincent, 1987; Wilson, 1996). A review of neuropsychological outcomes following hypoxia identified 67 cases of which 54% had amnesia, 46.2% impaired executive function or personality change, 31.3% visuospatial deficits, and 9% language impairments (Caine & Watson, 2000). Motor disturbances are also common following hypoxic brain injury and include difficulties with posture, gait, involuntary movements, Parkinsonian symptoms, and apraxia (Lishman, 1998). Although hypoxic brain injury may result in diffuse neuroanatomical damage (Bachevalier & Meunier, 1996; Hopkins et al., 1995a), in select cases cell death appears limited to (or particularly severe in) the hippocampus (Zola-Morgan, Squire, & Amaral, 1986). A number of studies show that memory impairments are associated with hippocampal atrophy (Hopkins et al., 1995; Manns et al., 2003). The degree of neuropsychological impairment appears to parallel the degree of morphologic abnormalities (Hopkins et al., 1995; Hopkins, Tate, & Bigler, 2005).

Controversy exists in the literature regarding whether hypoxia in the absence of ischemia can result in brain injury (Miyamoto & Auer, 2000). Neurologic sequelae following hypoxia without ischemia in a study of 22 patients with hypoxia without hypotension found that while all patients experienced coma, recovery to their premorbid level of function occurred in only 50% of the patients (Gray & Horner, 1970). In a case study of three patients with hypoxia (PO_2 less than 45 mm Hg) without ischemia, all patients died of cardiac failure due to hypoxia even though they did not have hypotension (Rie & Bernad, 1980). Alternatively, evidence in a variety of pulmonary disorders provide evidence that hypoxia can cause cognitive impairments.

Patients with pulmonary disorders including COPD and OSA with concomitant hypoxia have similar neuropsychological deficits to patients with anoxia. Prigatano Wright, and Levin (1984) found mild impairments in problem solving in patients with COPD who experienced mild hypoxemia. Other COPD studies find impaired memory, impaired executive function including inability to form new concepts, inability to think flexibly (Grant, Heaton, McSweeny, Adams, & Timms, 1982), impaired attention, and slow processing speed (Fix, Golden, Daughton, Kass, & Bell, 1982) that correlated with the severity of the hypoxemia (Hopkins et al., 1995; Hopkins, Weaver, et al., 2005). Studies in patients with OSA find these individuals have impaired memory, executive function, perception, spatial abilities (Kales et al., 1985), attention, memory, and problem solving abilities (Findley et al., 1986). A meta-review of cognitive impairments in OSA found mild to severe cognitive deficits were associated with severity of hypoxemia; specifically, severe groups could be identified based on a higher apnea-hypopnea index score (Bucks, Olaithe, & Eastwood, 2013). The neuropsychological deficits in the OSA patients correlate with the severity of the nocturnal hypoxemia (Bedard, Montplaisir, Richer, Rouleau, & Malo, 1991) and with sleep fragmentation (Naismith, Winter, Gotsopoulos, Hickie, & Cistulli, 2004). It is unclear whether sleep fragmentation or hypoxia is the best predictor of cognitive function in OSA (Naismith et al., 2004; Tsai, 2010); however, the majority of studies in OSA find deficits in attention, memory, visuospatial abilities, and executive function, with sparing of language and psychomotor abilities (Bucks et al., 2013).

Studies in critically ill patients with acute respiratory distress syndrome (ARDS) have demonstrated the relationship between hypoxia and cognitive impairments. A study by Hopkins and colleagues found ARDS survivors had impairments in memory, attention, concentration, and mental processing speed, as well as global cognitive decline (Hopkins, Weaver, Pope, Orme, Bigler, & Larson-Lohr, 1999). At one-year follow-up, 30% of the patients had lower intellectual function and 78% had impaired memory, attention, concentration and/or mental processing speed. The ARDS survivors' average duration of hypoxemia was measured using continuous pulse oximetry during their intensive care treatment. The mean duration of hypoxemia was $< 90\% = 122 \pm 144$ hours, $< 85\% = 13 \pm 18$ hours, and $< 80\% = 1 \pm 3$ hours, and the hypoxemia significantly correlated with neuropsychological impairments (Hopkins et al., 1999). In addition, a subset of ARDS survivors exhibited brain atrophy, significantly enlarged ventricles, and an increased Ventricle-to-Brain Ratio (a measure of generalized atrophy) compared to the matched controls, suggesting that hypoxia results in global brain injury and cognitive impairments (Hopkins, Gale, Pope, Weaver, & Bigler, 2000). The association between lower oxygenation values and cognitive impairment was confirmed in a second study of ARDS survivors with moderate to severe hypoxia (Mikkelsen et al., 2012). Of these patients, 55% had cognitive impairments at 12 months, and patients with cognitive impairments had significantly lower PaO_2 values compared to the ARDS patients who did not develop cognitive impairments. The severity of hypoxemia may serve as a marker of illness severity and risk for developing cognitive impairments (Mikkelsen et al., 2012).

This research suggests that hypoxia and not the etiology of the hypoxic brain injury may be the critical factor in determining the effects on neurocognitive function. There are only a few studies that compare neuropsychological outcome in hypoxic patients with different etiologies. For example, neuropsychological impairments observed with OSA were similar to COPD patients for complex reasoning and memory (Roehrs et al., 1995). Alternatively, Gale and Hopkins (2004) found neuropathologic abnormalities and impaired cognitive impairments in patients with carbon monoxide poisoning and OSA, however the carbon monoxide group consistently performed worse on most cognitive measures while the OSA group had more selective impairments. The variability of these results mirrors the heterogeneity reported neuropsychological outcome following hypoxic brain injury.

Weaver and colleagues (2002) studied individuals with hypoxic brain injury due to acute carbon monoxide poisoning who were compared for cognitive outcome following either hyperbaric oxygen or normobaric oxygen treatment in a randomized double-blind clinical trial. The cognitive impairments were significantly more frequent in the normobaric oxygen group (14.5%) as compared with (3.9%; P=0.03) in the hyperbaric oxygen group (Weaver et al., 2002). Hyperbaric oxygen therapy reduced cognitive impairments by 46% at six-week outcome. Both groups improved with time, but the difference in cognitive impairments between the groups was maintained at 12 months (Weaver et al., 2002). These results suggest that treatments such as hyperbaric oxygen may potentially ameliorate hypoxia-associated cognitive impairments.

Psychiatric and Affective Changes

Psychiatric and behavioral changes following hypoxic brain injury include euphoria, irritability, hostility, depression, and anxiety (Bahrke & Schukitt-Hale, 1993; Li et al., 2000). Studies have shown that exposure to acute hypobaric hypoxia is associated with development of negative moods which progressively worsen with longer duration of exposure and increased severity of the hypoxia (Bahrke & Schukitt-Hale, 1993; Li et al., 2000). Psychiatric disorders are not only common but also vary in type and severity following hypoxic brain injury (Gale et al., 1999; Hopkins, Tate, et al., 2005; Hopkins, Weaver, et al., 2005; Wilson, 1996). The psychiatric disorders include depression (Bruno, Wagner, & Orrison, 1993; Gale et al., 1999; Hopkins, Key, Suchyta, Weaver, & Orme, 2010), anxiety (Bruno et al., 1993), personality changes (Chapel & Husain, 1978), and emotional lability (Chapel & Husain, 1978). Some individuals may show lack of concern for or awareness of their deficits, show little emotional response to their cognitive impairments, or exhibit emotional lability including anger, agitation, and depression on one extreme and laughter or mania on the other (Armengol, 2000). Secondary mania posthypoxic brain injury has been reported; symptoms include irritable mood, hyperactivity, push of speech, flight of ideas, grandiosity, decreased sleep, distractibility, and lack of judgment (Krauthammer & Klerman, 1978; Sullivan & Jenkins, 1995). Finally, patients with basal ganglia lesions may develop obsessive-compulsive disorder with stereotyped behaviors, loss of drive, and flattened affect (Laplane et al., 1989).(Laplane et al., 1989).

Case Study

Adult: Focal Anoxic Brain Injury

Case A1 is a 26-year-old Caucasian male who sustained a full cardiopulmonary arrest and underwent cardiopulmonary resuscitation following a motor-vehicle accident in January 1990. Additionally, he received resuscitation (45 minutes of open cardiac resuscitation) intraoperatively while undergoing exploratory laparotomy and left anterior thoracotomy. The brain CT scan on the same date was incomplete, but read as normal. He was treated in the intensive care unit and was placed on mechanical ventilation after he developed acute respiratory distress syndrome. His blood alcohol on admission was 0.23 mg%. An elecgtroencephalogram (EEG) during his hospital stay was "borderline normal." He was confused and agitated but had no complications or seizures while hospitalized.

Social History: A1 completed high school and one year of college with grades of Bs and Cs. Prior to his injury, he was employed as a carpenter. He had no history of prior learning disabilities, traumatic brain injury, or psychiatric problems. He occasionally drank alcohol (one to two beers per day) with occasional marijuana and cocaine use. He has been drug free since in the years since his injury.

A1's ICU length of stay was 12 days and he was then transferred to an inpatient rehabilitation unit where he remained for 60 days. On admission to the rehabilitation unit he exhibited moderate to severe cognitive and language deficits and lacked insight into his deficits, however he was able to follow simple two-step commands. He exhibited inappropriate and impulsive behavior that improved with administration of carbamazepine. Following his discharge from the rehabilitation unit, he continued to have significant impairments in memory, attention, and judgment. He returned to Utah to live with his parents and receive outpatient rehabilitation services.

Brain MRI showed significant hippocampal atrophy (see Figure 21.2, Panel B). Table 21.2 shows his neuropsychological scores. He continued to have persistent and severe verbal and visual memory impairments. In order to remember things, he writes everything down in a planner or notebook, including what he had for breakfast and any appointments. He has been unemployed for the majority of the time since his injury due to his memory impairments and received disability payments.

Table 21.2 Neuropsychological Test Scores in A1

Neuropsychological Tests	*1990 Age 27*	*1994 Age 31*	*2003 Age 40*	*2014 Age 50*
Intelligence (WAIS-R)			**(WASI)**	
VIQ	92	90	100	103
PIQ	79	93	100	92
FSIQ	85	90	100	106
Information		9		11
Digit Span		5		7
Vocabulary		10		12
Arithmetic		10		8
Comprehension		8		10
Similarities		10		14
Picture Completion		11		10
Picture Arrangement		10		10
Block Design		7		10
Object Assembly		11		10
Digit Symbol		6		9
WMS-R				
Verbal Memory Index	63	65	Logical Memory	68
Visual Memory Index	67	95	I = 28	92
General Memory Index	54	70	II = 5	72
Attention/Concentration Index	87	87		105
Delayed Recall Index	< 50	< 50		60
Rey-Osterrieth Complex Fig.				
Copy		32	36	
Immediate Recall		5	4	
Delayed Recall		5	7	
WRAT3				
Reading		58th percentile		
Spelling		37th percentile		
Arithmetic		39th percentile		
Category Test				
Errors		42		
T-score		43		
Wisconsin Card Sorting Test				
# Completed Categories		3	5	
Perseverative Errors		22	19	
Trail Making Test				
Part A (time in seconds)		43	25	
Part B (time in seconds)		72	58	

The above case illustrates the variable outcome that can occur following anoxic brain injury, with some individuals having diffuse neuropathological abnormalities with diffuse cognitive impairments and other having more focal brain abnormalities and more select cognitive impairments.

Characterization and Treatment of Cognitive Impairment

Outcome following hypoxic brain injury is variable; however, the majority of patients have poor outcome (Bachman & Katz, 1997). Information regarding the effects of rehabilitation on neurocognitive outcome following hypoxic brain injury is limited. For patients with severe anoxia coma (> 24 hours), both survival, if they do survive, and recovery of function is poor (Groswasser, Cohen, & Costeff, 1989). Survival rates following postanoxic coma range from 9% to 40% (Bedell, Delbanco, Cook, & Epstein, 1983; Levy et al., 1985; Snyder et al., 1980). Patients who survived anoxic coma may regain mobility and ability to perform activities of daily living, but they do not return to their preinjury level of cognitive function (Groswasser et al., 1989). Outcome following anoxic coma is not predicted by age, sex, site of resuscitation, cause of anoxia, nor presence of postanoxic seizures (Levy et al., 1985). A single case study suggested that "relatively" good cognitive function in the first month postanoxic coma may indicate improved recovery and benefit from rehabilitation (Kaplan, 1999); however, this is not generally reported.

Groswasser et al. (1989) followed a group of 31 patients following cardiopulmonary arrest with coma. On long-term follow-up, 13 were independent in activities of daily living, two had regained premorbid cognitive function, and four had returned to work, but only one to the same job. Patients who were younger with shorter duration of coma had had somewhat better outcomes but often they did not return to their pre-injury level of functioning. In addition, cognitive and functional recovery was significantly worse in patients with hypoxic brain injury compared to patients with traumatic brain injury with prolonged coma. The differences in recovery may be due to the interaction between diffuse damage and delayed cell death, but was not related to the etiology of the hypoxic brain injury (Groswasser et al., 1989).

Armengol (2000) reported eight individuals with severe anoxia who underwent treatment in a neurobehavioral rehabilitation program. Six of the eight individuals had poor outcome, with significant cognitive impairments including deficits in attention, executive function, memory, reasoning, language, visuospatial, and motor skills. The two remaining patients had mild cognitive impairments. Similar findings of significant cognitive impairments and affective dysregulation that significantly complicated rehabilitation were reported in a single case (Parkin et al., 1987). A study following hypoxic brain injury found that in-patient rehabilitation improved functional status (measured by the Functional Independence Measure, with individuals who had higher scores on admission having the best outcome), however, few of the patients were able to resume their previous jobs and level of function (Schmidt, Drew-Cates, & Dombovy, 1997).

Conclusions

Patients with hypoxic brain injury have both diffuse and focal brain injury, and concomitant neuropsychological impairments. The etiology of hypoxic brain injury is variable, but includes asthma, cardiac or respiratory arrest, cardiac disease or surgery, carbon monoxide poisoning, attempted hanging, complications of anesthesia, near downing, OSA, COPD, and acute respiratory distress syndrome that result in anoxia, hypoxia, or ischemia. Hypoxic brain injury results in focal and diffuse neuropathological lesions and atrophy including hippocampal, basal ganglia, cerebellar, and white matter abnormalities. Cognitive impairments include intellectual decline, memory deficits, decreased attention, visuoperceptual, problem solving, executive dysfunction, and decreased mental processing speed and location of the damage are associated with the cognitive impairments. Hypoxic brain injury results in a high prevalence of psychiatric disorders including new euphoria, irritability, hostility, depression, and anxiety and personality changes. The rate of psychiatric disorders is variable and may depend on the etiology of the hypoxia (e.g., COPD 37%–42%, asthma 24%–42%, OSA40%, and carbon monoxide poisoning 39%–60%), and the prevalence rate is significantly higher than that observed in the general population (2%–9% major depression and 3% generalized anxiety) and the rate observed in medical populations (12%). Hypoxic brain injury results in significant neurological structural and functional abnormalities, as well as neuropsychological impairments—and recovery of function appears limited.

References

Arbelaez, A., Castillo, M., & Mukherji, S. K. (1999). Diffusion-weighted MR imaging of global cerebral anoxia. *American Journal of Neuroradiology*, *20*(6), 999–1007.

Armengol, C. G. (2000). Acute oxygen deprivation: Neuropsychological profiles and implications for rehabilitation. *Brain Injury*, *14*(3), 237–250.

Bachevalier, J., & Meunier, M. (1996). Cerebral ischemia: Are the memory deficits associated with hippocampal cell loss? *Hippocampus*, *6*(5), 553–560.

Bachman, D., & Katz, D. I. (1997). Anoxic-hypotensive brain injury and encephalitis. In V. M. Mills, J. W. Cassidy, & D. I. Katz (Eds.), *Neurologic Rehabilitation: A Guide to Diagnosis, Prognosis, and Treatment Planning* (pp. 145–176). Malden, MA: Blackwell Science Ltd.

Bahrke, M. S., & Schukitt-Hale, B. (1993). Effects of altitude on mood, behaviour, and cognitive functioning: A review. *Journal of Sports Medicine*, *16*, 97–125.

Barat, M., Blanchard, J., & Carriet, D. (1989). Les troubles neuropsychologiques des anozies cerebrales prolongees. *Annales de Readaptation et de Medecine Physique*, *32*, 657–668.

Bayley, P. J., Gold, J. J., Hopkins, R. O., & Squire, L. R. (2005). The neuroanatomy of remote memory. *Neuron*, *46*(5), 799–810.

Bayley, P. J., Hopkins, R. O., & Squire, L. R. (2003). Successful recollection of remote autobiographical memories by amnesic patients with medial temporal lobe lesions. *Neuron*, *38*(1), 135–144.

Bedard, M. A., Montplaisir, J., Richer, F., Rouleau, I., & Malo, J. (1991). Obstructive sleep apnea syndrome: Pathogenesis of neuropsychological deficits. *Journal of Clinical and Experimental Neuropsychology*, *13*(6), 950–964.

Bedell, S. E., Delbanco, T. L., Cook, E. F., & Epstein, F. H. (1983). Survival after cardiopulmonary resuscitation in the hospital. *New England Journal of Medicine*, *309*(10), 569–576. doi: 10.1056/NEJM198309083091001

Beilharz, E. J., Williams, C. E., Dragunow, M., Sirimanne, E. S., & Gluckman, P. D. (1995). Mechanisms of delayed cell death following hypoxic-ischemic injury in the immature rat: Evidence for apoptosis during selective neuronal loss. *Brain Research. Molecular Brain Research*, *29*(1), 1–14.

Biagas, K. (1999). Hypoxic-ischemic brain injury: Advancements in the understanding of mechanisms and potential avenues for therapy. *Current Opinion in Pediatrics*, *11*(3), 223–228.

Bigler, E. D. (2001). Quantitative magnetic resonance imaging in traumatic brain injury. *Journal of Head Trauma Rehabilitaion*, *16*(2), 117–134.

Bigler, E. D., & Alfano, M. (1988). Anoxic encephalopathy: Neuroradiological and neuropsychological findings. *Archives of Clinical Neuropsychology*, *3*, 383–396.

Bigler, E. D., Blatter, D. D., Anderson, C. V., Johnson, S. C., Gale, S. D., Hopkins, R. O., & Burnett, B. (1997). Hippocampal volume in normal aging and traumatic brain injury. *American Journal of Neuroradiology*, *18*(1), 11–23.

Bigler, E. D., & Clement, P. F. (1997). Traumatic disorders of the nervous system. In E. D. Bigler & P. F. Clement (Eds.), *Diagnostic Clinical Neuropsychology* (3rd ed., pp. 126–166). Austin, TX: University of Texas Press.

Blass, J. P., & Gibson, G. E. (1979). Consequences of mild, graded hypoxia. *Advances in Neurology*, *26*, 229–250.

Bodsch, W., Barbier, A., Oehmichen, M., Grosse Ophoff, B., & Hossmann, K. A. (1986). Recovery of monkey brain after prolonged ischemia: II. Protein synthesis and morphological alterations. *Journal of Cerebral Blood Flow and Metabolism*, *6*(1), 22–33. doi: 10.1038/jcbfm.1986.4

Bottiger, B. W., Schmitz, B., Wiessner, C., Vogel, P., & Hossmann, K. A. (1998). Neuronal stress response and neuronal cell damage after cardiocirculatory arrest in rats. *Journal of Cerebral Blood Flow and Metabolism*, *18*(10), 1077–1087. doi: 10.1097/00004647-199810000-00004

Bruno, A., Wagner, W., & Orrison, W. W. (1993). Clinical outcome and brain MRI four years after carbon monoxide intoxication. *Acta Neurologica Scandinavica*, *87*(3), 205–209.

Bucks, R. S., Olaithe, M., & Eastwood, P. (2013). Neurocognitive function in obstructive sleep apnoea: A meta-review. *Respirology*, *18*(1), 61–70. doi: 10.1111/j.1440-1843.2012.02255.x

Busl, K. M., & Greer, D. M. (2010). Hypoxic-ischemic brain injury: Pathophysiology, neuropathology and mechanisms. *NeuroRehabilitation*, *26*(1), 5–13. doi: 10.3233/NRE-2010–0531

Caine, D., & Watson, J. D. (2000). Neuropsychological and neuropathological sequelae of cerebral anoxia: A critical review. *Journal of the International Neuropsychological Society*, *6*(1), 86–99.

Chalela, J. A., Wolf, R. L., Maldjian, J. A., & Kasner, S. E. (2001). MRI identification of early white matter injury in anoxic-ischemic encephalopathy. *Neurology*, *56*(4), 481–485.

Chang, K. H., Han, M. H., Kim, H. S., Wie, B. A., & Han, M. C. (1992). Delayed encephalopathy after acute carbon monoxide intoxication: MR imaging features and distribution of cerebral white matter lesions. *Radiology*, *184*(1), 117–122.

Chapel, J. L., & Husain, A. (1978). The neuropsychiatric aspects of carbon monoxide poisoning. *Psychiatric Opinion*, March, 33–37.

Chen, R., Bolton, C. F., & Young, B. (1996). Prediction of outcome in patients with anoxic coma: A clinical and electrophysiologic study. *Critical Care Medicine*, *24*(4), 672–678.

Davies, C. W., Crosby, J. H., Mullins, R. L., Traill, Z. C., Anslow, P., Davies, R. J., & Stradling, J. R. (2001). Case control study of cerebrovascular damage defined by magnetic resonance imaging in patients with OSA and normal matched control subjects. *Sleep*, *24*(6), 715–720.

Farah, M. (1990). *Visual Agnosia*. Cambridge, MA: MIT Press.

Findley, L. J., Barth, J. T., Powers, D. C., Wilhoit, S. C., Boyd, D. G., & Suratt, P. M. (1986). Cognitive impairment in patients with obstructive sleep apnea and associated hypoxemia. *Chest*, *90*(5), 686–690.

Fix, A. J., Golden, C. J., Daughton, D., Kass, I., & Bell, C. W. (1982). Neuropsychological deficits among patients with chronic obstructive pulmonary disease. *International Journal of Neuroscience*, *16*(2), 99–105.

Floyd, R. A. (1990). Role of oxygen free radicals in carcinogenesis and brain ischemia. *FASEB Journal*, *4*(9), 2587–2597.

Gale, S. D., & Hopkins, R. O. (2004). Effects of hypoxia on the brain: Neuroimaging and neuropsychological findings following carbon monoxide poisoning and obstructive sleep apnea. *Journal of the International Neuropsychological Society*, *10*(1), 60–71. doi: 10.1017/S1355617704101082

Gale, S. D., Hopkins, R. O., Weaver, L. K., Bigler, E. D., Booth, E. J., & Blatter, D. D. (1999). MRI, quantitative MRI, SPECT, and neuropsychological findings following carbon monoxide poisoning. *Brain Injury*, *13*(4), 229–243.

Gilland, E., Puka-Sundvall, M., Hillered, L., & Hagberg, H. (1998). Mitochondrial function and energy metabolism after hypoxia-ischemia in the immature rat brain: Involvement of NMDA-receptors. *Journal of Cerebral Blood Flow and Metabolism*, *18*(3), 297–304.

Gilles, F. H. (1969). Hypotensive brain stem necrosis: Selective symmetrical necrosis of tegmental neuronal aggregates following cardiac arrest. *Archives of Pathology*, *88*(1), 32–41.

Goldberg, G., & Karazim, E. (1998). Application of evoked potentials to the prediction of discharge status in minimally responsive patients: A pilot study. *Journal of Head Trauma Rehabilitation*, *13*(1), 51–68.

Granger, D. N., McCord, J. M., Parks, D. A., & Hollwarth, M. E. (1986). Xanthine oxidase inhibitors attenuate ischemia-induced vascular permeability changes in the cat intestine. *Gastroenterology*, *90*(1), 80–84.

Grant, I., Heaton, R., McSweeny, A., Adams, K., & Timms, R. (1982). Neuropsychological findings in hypoxemic chronic obstructive pulmonary disease. *Archives of Internal Medicine*, *142*, 1470–1476.

Gray, F. D., Jr., & Horner, G. J. (1970). Survival following extreme hypoxemia. *JAMA*, *211*(11), 1815–1817.

Groswasser, Z., Cohen, M., & Costeff, H. (1989). Rehabilitation outcome after anoxic brain damage. *Archives of Physical Medicine and Rehabilitation*, *70*(3), 186–188.

Guo, M. F., Yu, J. Z., & Ma, C. G. (2011). Mechanisms related to neuron injury and death in cerebral hypoxic ischaemia. *Folia Neuropathol*, *49*(2), 78–87.

Haddad, G. G., & Jiang, C. (1993). O2 deprivation in the central nervous system: On mechanisms of neuronal response, differential sensitivity and injury. *Progress in Neurobiology*, *40*(3), 277–318.

Harper, R. M., Kumar, R., Ogren, J. A., & Macey, P. M. (2013). Sleep-disordered breathing: Effects on brain structure and function. *Respiratory Physiology and Neurobiology*, *188*(3), 383–391. doi: 10.1016/j.resp.2013.04.021

Heimer, L. (1995). *Human Brain and Spinal Cord Second Edition* (2nd ed.). New York: Springer-Verlag.

Hicks, S. P. (1968). Vascular pathophysiology and acute and chronic oxygen deprivation. In J. Minckler (Ed.), *Pathology of the Nervous System* (Vol. 1, pp. 341–350). New York: McGraw-Hill.

Hopkins, R. O., Fearing, M. A., Weaver, L. K., & Foley, J. F. (2006). Basal ganglia lesions following carbon monoxide poisoning. *Brain Injury*, *20*(3), 273–281.

Hopkins, R. O., Gale, S. D., Johnson, S. C., Anderson, C. V., Bigler, E. D., Blatter, D. D., & Weaver, L. K. (1995). Severe anoxia with and without concomitant brain atrophy and neuropsychological impairments. *Journal of the International Neuropsychological Society*, *1*(5), 501–509.

Hopkins, R. O., Gale, S. D., Pope, D., Weaver, L. K., & Bigler, E. D. (2000). Ventricular enlargement in patients with acute respiratory distress syndrome. *Journal of the International Neuropsychological Society*, *6*, 229.

Hopkins, R. O., Kesner, R. P., & Goldstein, M. (1995a). Item and order recognition memory in subjects with hypoxic brain injury. *Brain and Cognition*, *27*(2), 180–201.

Hopkins, R. O., Kesner, R. P., & Goldstein, M. (1995b). Memory for novel and familiar spatial and linguistic temporal distance information in hypoxic subjects. *Journal of the International Neuropsychological Society*, *1*(5), 454–468.

Hopkins, R. O., Key, C. W., Suchyta, M. R., Weaver, L. K., & Orme, J. F., Jr. (2010). Risk factors for depression and anxiety in survivors of acute respiratory distress syndrome. *General Hospital Psychiatry*, *32*(2), 147–155. doi: S0163-8343(09)00231-X [pii] 10.1016/j.genhosppsych.2009.11.003

Hopkins, R. O., Tate, D. F., & Bigler, E. D. (2005). Anoxic versus traumatic brain injury: Amount of tissue loss, not etiology, alters cognitive and emotional function. *Neuropsychology*, *19*(2), 233–242.

Hopkins, R. O., Weaver, L. K., Collingridge, D., Parkinson, R. B., Chan, K. J., & Orme, J. F., Jr. (2005). Two-year cognitive, emotional, and quality-of-life outcomes in acute respiratory distress syndrome. *American Journal of Respiratory and Critical Care Medicine*, *171*(4), 340–347.

Hopkins, R. O., Weaver, L. K., Pope, D., Orme, J. F., Jr., Bigler, E. D., & Larson-Lohr, V. (1999). Neuropsychological sequelae and impaired health status in survivors of severe acute respiratory distress syndrome. *American Journal of Respiratory and Critical Care Medicine*, *160*(1), 50–56.

Hopkins, R. O., & Woon, F. L. (2006). Neuroimaging, cognitive, and neurobehavioral outcomes following carbon monoxide poisoning. *Behavioral and Cognitive Neuroscience Reviews*, *5*(3), 141–155.

Hossmann, K. A., Oschlies, U., Schwindt, W., & Krep, H. (2001). Electron microscopic investigation of rat brain after brief cardiac arrest. *Acta Neuropathol*, *101*(2), 101–113.

Inage, Y. W., Itoh, M., Wada, K., & Takashima, S. (1998). Expression of two glutamate transporters, GLAST and EAAT4, in the human cerebellum: Their correlation in development and neonatal hypoxic-ischemic damage. *Journal of Neuropathology and Experimental Neurology*, *57*(6), 554–562.

Johnston, M. V., Nakajima, W., & Hagberg, H. (2002). Mechanisms of hypoxic neurodegeneration in the developing brain. *Neuroscientist*, *8*(3), 212–220.

Kales, A., Caldwell, A., Cadieux, R., Vela-Bueno, A., Ruch, L., & Mayes, S. (1985). Severe obstructive sleep apnea-II: Associated psychopathology and psychosocial consequences. *Journal of Chronic Diseases*, *38*, 427–434.

Kaplan, C. P. (1999). Anoxic-hypotensive brain injury: Neuropsychological performance at 1 month as an indicator of recovery. *Brain Injury*, *13*(4), 305–310.

Kass, I. S., & Lipton, P. (1986). Calcium and long-term transmission damage following anoxia in dentate gyrus and CA1 regions of the rat hippocampal slice. *Journal of Physiology*, *378*, 313–334.

Kesler, S. R., Hopkins, R. O., Blatter, D. D., Edge-Booth, H., & Bigler, E. D. (2001). Verbal memory deficits associated with fornix atrophy in carbon monoxide poisoning. *Journal of the International Neuropsychological Society*, *7*(5), 640–646.

Kesner, R. P., & Hopkins, R. O. (2001). Short-term memory for duration and distance in humans: Role of the hippocampus. *Neuropsychology*, *15*(1), 58–68.

Krauthammer, C., & Klerman, G. L. (1978). Secondary mania: Manic syndromes associated with antecedent physical illness or drugs. *Archives of General Psychiatry*, *35*(11), 1333–1339.

Kudenchuk, P. J., Sandroni, C., Drinhaus, H. R., Bottiger, B. W., Cariou, A., Sunde, K., . . . Laterre, P. F. (2015). Breakthrough in cardiac arrest: Reports from the 4th Paris International Conference. *Annals of Intensive Care*, *5*(1), 22. doi: 10.1186/s13613-015-0064-x

Kumar, R., Macey, P. M., Woo, M. A., Alger, J. R., & Harper, R. M. (2008). Diffusion tensor imaging demonstrates brainstem and cerebellar abnormalities in congenital central hypoventilation syndrome. *Pediatric Research*, *64*(3), 275–280. doi: 10.1203/PDR.0b013e31817da10a

Kumar, R., Pham, T. T., Macey, P. M., Woo, M. A., Yan-Go, F. L., & Harper, R. M. (2014). Abnormal myelin and axonal integrity in recently diagnosed patients with obstructive sleep apnea. *Sleep*, *37*(4), 723–732. doi: 10.5665/sleep.3578

Kuroiwa, T., & Okeda, R. (1994). Neuropathology of cerebral ischemia and hypoxia: Recent advances in experimental studies on its pathogenesis. *Pathology International*, *44*(3), 171–181.

Laplane, D., Levasseur, M., Pillon, B., Dubois, B., Baulac, M., Mazoyer, B., . . . Baron, J. C. (1989). Obsessive-compulsive and other behavioural changes with bilateral basal ganglia lesions: A neuropsychological, magnetic resonance imaging and positron tomography study. *Brain*, *112*(Pt 3), 699–725.

Levy, D. E., Caronna, J. J., Singer, B. H., Lapinski, R. H., Frydman, H., & Plum, F. (1985). Predicting outcome from hypoxic-ischemic coma. *JAMA*, *253*(10), 1420–1426.

Lezak, M. D., Howieson, D. B., Bigler, E. D., & Tranel, D. (2012). *Neuropsychological Assessment* (5th ed.). New York: Oxford University Press.

Li, X. Y., Wu, X. Y., Fu, C., Shen, X. F., Wu, Y. H., & Wang, T. (2000). Effects of acute mild and moderate hypoxia on human mood state. *Space Medicine and Medical Engineering*, *13*(1), 1–5.

Li, Y., Powers, C., Jiang, N., & Chopp, M. (1998). Intact, injured, necrotic and apoptotic cells after focal cerebral ischemia in the rat. *Journal of Neurological Sciences*, *156*(2), 119–132.

Lindenberg, R. (1963). Patterns of CNS vulnerability in acute hypoxaemia, including anaesthetic accidents. In J. P. Schade & W.H.E. McMenemey (Eds.), *Selective Vulnerability of the Brain in Hypoxaemia* (pp. 189–210). Oxford: Blackwell Scientific Publications.

Lishman, W. A. (1998). *Organic Psychiatry: The Psychological Consequences of Cerebral Disorder* (3rd ed.). Oxford: Blackwell Science Ltd.

Lutz, P. L., & Nilsson, G. E. (1994). *The Brain Without Oxygen Causes of Failure and Mechanisms for Survival*. Austin, TX: R. G. Landes Company.

Macey, P. M., Henderson, L. A., Macey, K. E., Alger, J. R., Frysinger, R. C., Woo, M. A., Harper, R. K., Yan-Go, F. L., & Harper, R. M. (2002). Brain morphology associated with obstructive sleep apnea. *American Journal of Respiratory and Critical Care Medicine*, *166*(10), 1382–1387. doi: 10.1164/rccm.200201-050OC

Manns, J. R., Hopkins, R. O., Reed, J. M., Kitchener, E. G., & Squire, L. R. (2003). Recognition memory and the human hippocampus. *Neuron*, *37*(1), 171–180.

Mascalchi, M., Petruzzi, P., & Zampa, V. (1996). MRI of cerebellar white matter damage due to carbon monoxide poisoning: Case report. *Neuroradiology*, *38*(Suppl 1), S73–S74.

Michenfelder, J. D., & Sundt, T. M., Jr. (1971). Cerebral ATP and lactate levels in the squirrel monkey following occlusion of the middle cerebral artery. *Stroke*, *2*(4), 319–326.

Mikkelsen, M. E., Christie, J. D., Lanken, P. N., Biester, R. C., Thompson, B. T., Bellamy, S. L., . . . Angus, D. C. (2012). The adult respiratory distress syndrome cognitive outcomes study: Long-term neuropsychological function in survivors of acute lung injury. *American Journal of Respiratory and Critical Care Medicine*, *185*(12), 1307–1315. doi: 10.1164/rccm.201111-2025OC

Miyamoto, O., & Auer, R. N. (2000). Hypoxia, hyperoxia, ischemia, and brain necrosis. *Neurology*, *54*(2), 362–371.

Morrell, M. J., McRobbie, D. W., Quest, R. A., Cummin, A. R., Ghiassi, R., & Corfield, D. R. (2003). Changes in brain morphology associated with obstructive sleep apnea. *Sleep Medicine*, *4*(5), 451–454.

Moulaert, V. R., Verbunt, J. A., van Heugten, C. M., & Wade, D. T. (2009). Cognitive impairments in survivors of out-of-hospital cardiac arrest: A systematic review. *Resuscitation*, *80*(3), 297–305. doi: 10.1016/j.resuscitation.2008.10.034

Naismith, S., Winter, V., Gotsopoulos, H., Hickie, I., & Cistulli, P. (2004). Neurobehavioral functioning in obstructive sleep apnea: Differential effects of sleep quality, hypoxemia and subjective sleepiness. *Journal of Clinical and Expermental Neuropsychology*, *26*(1), 43–54. doi: 10.1076/jcen.26.1.43.23929

Nakajima, W., Ishida, A., Lange, M. S., Gabrielson, K. L., Wilson, M. A., Martin, L. J., . . . Johnston, M. V. (2000). Apoptosis has a prolonged role in the neurodegeneration after hypoxic ischemia in the newborn rat. *Journal of Neuroscience*, *20*(21), 7994–8004.

Nucci-da-Silva, M. P., & Amaro, E., Jr. (2009). A systematic review of magnetic resonance imaging and spectroscopy in brain injury after drowning. *Brain Injury*, *23*(9), 707–714. doi: 10.1080/02699050903123351

O'Donnell, P., Buxton, P. J., Pitkin, A., & Jarvis, L. J. (2000). The magnetic resonance imaging appearances of the brain in acute carbon monoxide poisoning. *Clinical Radiology*, *55*(4), 273–280.

Oechmichen, M., & Meissner, C. (2006). Cerebral hypoxia and ischemia: The forensic point of view: A review. *Journal of Forensic Sciences*, *51*(4), 880–887. doi: 10.1111/j.1556-4029.2006.00174.x

Olney, J. W. (1969). Brain lesions, obesity, and other disturbances in mice treated with monosodium glutamate. *Science*, *164*(880), 719–721.

Parkin, A. J., Miller, J., & Vincent, R. (1987). Multiple neuropsychological deficits due to anoxic encephalopathy: A case study. *Cortex*, *23*(4), 655–665.

Parkinson, R. B., Hopkins, R. O., Cleavinger, H. B., Weaver, L. K., Victoroff, J., Foley, J. F., & Bigler, E. D. (2002). White matter hyperintensities and neuropsychological outcome following carbon monoxide poisoning. *Neurology*, *58*(10), 1525–1532.

Petito, C. K., Feldmann, E., Pulsinelli, W. A., & Plum, F. (1987). Delayed hippocampal damage in humans following cardiorespiratory arrest. *Neurology*, *37*(8), 1281–1286.

Porter, S. S., Hopkins, R. O., Weaver, L. K., Bigler, E. D., & Blatter, D. D. (2002). Corpus callosum atrophy and neuropsychological outcome following carbon monoxide poisoning. *Archives of Clinical Neuropsychology*, *17*(2), 195–204.

Press, G. A., Amaral, D. G., & Squire, L. R. (1989). Hippocampal abnormalities in amnesic patients revealed by high-resolution magnetic resonance imaging. *Nature*, *341*(6237), 54–57.

Prigatano, G. P., Wright, E. C., & Levin, D. (1984). Quality of life and its predictors in patients with mild hypoxemia and chronic obstructive pulmonary disease. *Archives of Internal Medicine*, *144*(8), 1613–1619.

Rademakers, R. P., van der Knaap, M. S., Verbeeten, B., Jr., Barth, P. G., & Valk, J. (1995). Central cortico-subcortical involvement: A distinct pattern of brain damage caused by perinatal and postnatal asphyxia in term infants. *Journal of Computer Assisted Tomography*, *19*(2), 256–263.

Raley-Susman, K. M., & Lipton, P. (1990). In vitro ischemia and protein synthesis in the rat hippocampal slice: The role of calcium and NMDA receptor activation. *Brain Research*, *515*(1–2), 27–38.

Revesz, T., & Geddes, J. F. (1988). Symmetrical columnar necrosis of the basal ganglia and brain stem in an adult following cardiac arrest. *Clinical Neuropathology*, *7*(6), 294–298.

Rie, M. A., & Bernad, P. G. (1980). Prolonged hypoxia in man without circulatory compromise fail to demonstrate cerebral pathology. *Neurology*, *30*, 433.

Roehrs, T., Merrion, M., Pedrosi, B., Stepanski, E., Zorick, F., & Roth, T. (1995). Neuropsychological function in obstructive sleep apnea syndrome (OSAS) compared to chronic obstructive pulmonary disease (COPD). *Sleep*, *18*(5), 382–388.

Sandroni, C., Nolan, J., Cavallaro, F., & Antonelli, M. (2007). In-hospital cardiac arrest: Incidence, prognosis and possible measures to improve survival. *Intensive Care Medicine*, *33*(2), 237–245. doi: 10.1007/s00134-006-0326-z

Schmahmann, J. D., & Pandya, D. N. (1997). The cerebrocerebellar system. *International Review of Neurobiology*, *41*, 31–60.

Schmidt, J. G., Drew-Cates, J., & Dombovy, M. L. (1997). Anoxic encephalopathy: Outcome after inpatient rehabilitation. *Journal of Neurologic Rehabilitation*, *11*(3), 189–195.

Schurr, A., Lipton, P., West, C. A., & Rigor, B. M. (1990). The role of energy in metabolism and divalent cations in the neurotoxicity of excitatory amino acids in vitro. In J. Krieglstein (Ed.), *Pharmacology of Cerebral Ischemia* (pp. 217–226). Boca Raton, FL: CRC Press LLC.

Siemkowicz, E., & Hansen, A. J. (1978). Clinical restitution following cerebral ischemia in hypo-, normo- and hyperglycemic rats. *Acta Neurologica Scandinavica*, *58*(1), 1–8.

Singhal, A. B., Topcuoglu, M. A., & Koroshetz, W. J. (2002). Diffusion MRI in three types of anoxic encephalopathy. *Journal of the Neurological Sciences*, *196*(1–2), 37–40.

Snyder, B., Loewenson, R. B., Bumnit, R. J., Auser, W. A., Leppik, L. E., & Ramirez-Lassepas, M. (1980). Neurological prognosis after cardiopulmonary arrest: II level of consciousness. *Neurology*, *30*, 52–58.

Speach, D. P., Wong, T. M., Cattarin, J. A., & Livecchi, M. A. (1998). Hypoxic brain injury with motor apraxia following an anaphylactic reaction to hymenoptera venom. *Brain Injury*, *12*(3), 239–244.

Steller, H. (1995). Mechanisms and genes of cellular suicide. *Science*, *267*(5203), 1445–1449.

Sullivan, G., & Jenkins, P. L. (1995). Secondary mania following cerebral hypoxia. *Irish Journal of Psychological Medicine*, *12*, 68–69.

Tsai, J. C. (2010). Neurological and neurobehavioral sequelae of obstructive sleep apnea. *NeuroRehabilitation*, *26*(1), 85–94. doi: 10.3233/NRE-2010-0538

Weaver, L. K., Hopkins, R. O., Chan, K. J., Churchill, S., Elliott, C. G., Clemmer, T. P., . . . Morris, A. H. (2002). Hyperbaric oxygen for acute carbon monoxide poisoning. *New England Journal of Medicine*, *347*(14), 1057–1067.

Welsh, F. A., Ginsberg, M. D., Rieder, W., & Budd, W. W. (1980). Deleterious effect of glucose pretreatment on recovery from diffuse cerebral ischemia in the cat: II. Regional metabolite levels. *Stroke*, *11*(4), 355–363.

White, M. L., Zhang, Y., Helvey, J. T., & Omojola, M. F. (2013). Anatomical patterns and correlated MRI findings of non-perinatal hypoxic-ischaemic encephalopathy. *British Journal of Radiology*, *86*(1021), 20120464. doi: 10.1259/bjr.20120464

Wilson, B. A. (1996). Cognitive functioning of adult survivors of cerebral hypoxia. *Brain Injury*, *10*(12), 863–874.

Zola-Morgan, S., & Squire, L. R. (1990). Neuropsychological investigations of memory and amnesia: Finding from humans and nonhuman primates. In A. Diamond (Ed.), *The Development and Neural Bases of Higher Cognitive Functions* (pp. 434–456). New York: New York Academy of Sciences.

Zola-Morgan, S., Squire, L. R., Amaral, D. G. (1986). Human amnesia and the medial temporal region: enduring memory impairment following a bilateral lesion limited to field CA1 of the hippocampus. *Journal of Neuroscience, 6*(10), 950–967.

22 Parkinson's Disease and Other Movement Disorders

Alexander I. Tröster and Robin Garrett

Introduction

This chapter focuses on Parkinson's disease (PD), an α-synucleinopathy associated primarily with dysfunction of the basal ganglia and fronto-striatal circuits and manifesting as a hypokinetic movement disorder with a constellation of nonmotor symptoms. It describes the epidemiology, genetics, pathology, pathophysiology, and neurobehavioral features of the disease, including the recent concept of mild cognitive impairment (MCI) in PD (PD-MCI). Medical and surgical treatments of PD and their impact on cognition and behavior are also reviewed. Although it remains controversial whether PD with dementia (PDD) and dementia with Lewy bodies (DLB) are distinct entities or two sides of the same coin, similarities and differences between the two conditions are briefly summarized. The chapter then briefly describes neuropsychological aspects of atypical parkinsonian conditions, including one synucleinopathy (multiple system atrophy, or MSA) and two tauopathies (progressive supranuclear palsy, or PSP, and corticobasal syndrome, or CBS). After summarizing neuropsychological aspects of a hyperkinetic movement disorder (Huntington's disease, or HD), the key neuropsychological features of essential tremor and dystonia are briefly described. Brief mention is also made of psychogenic movement disorders (PMDs) to alert the neuropsychologist to possible somatoform disorders among persons with movement disorders. Tourette syndrome, given its vast range of neuropsychological features, is beyond the scope of this chapter and the interested reader is referred to a recent review (Murphy & Eddy, 2013). The chapter also includes a general strategy for the neuropsychological evaluation of persons with movement disorders and some case presentations that highlight some of the information described. While citing recent empirical research, the chapter seeks to provide references especially to recent reviews that permit readers to delve in greater depth into those topics of particular interest to them.

Parkinson's Disease, Parkinson's Disease With Dementia, and Dementia With Lewy Bodies

At the outset it is important to note that PD is not the same as parkinsonism. Whereas the former is a distinct disease, parkinsonism refers to a constellation of four signs (gait instability, rigidity, tremor, and bradykinesia) that are observable in a host of conditions, both neurological and psychogenic. Commonly used to diagnose PD, the UK Brain Bank criteria are listed in **Table 22.1**.

Table 22.1 UK Parkinson's Disease Society Brain Bank (Queen Square) criteria for diagnosis of PD

1 Presence of parkinsonian syndrome evidenced by
- bradykinesia
- at least one of:
  - muscular rigidity,
  - 4–6 Hz resting tremor, or
  - postural instability not related to proprioceptive, vestibular, visual, or cerebellar dysfunction.

2 Exclusion, by history, of:
- repeated strokes,
- repeated head injury,
- use of antipsychotic or dopamine-depleting drugs,
- encephalitis,
- multiple affected relatives,
- no response to levodopa,
- sustained remission of symptoms,
- continued unilateral symptoms after three years,
- gaze palsy,
- early dementia,
- exposure to known neurotoxin,
- evidence on neuroimaging of tumor or communicating hydrocephalus,
- cerebellar signs,
- early dysautonomia, or
- Babinski sign.

3 Definite PD defined by at least three of the following supportive features:
- unilateral onset,
- persistence of symptom asymmetry,
- progression of symptoms,
- excellent response to levodopa,
- levodopa response sustained for five years,
- resting tremor,
- levodopa-induced dyskinesias, or
- clinical course over ten years.

Historical Perspectives

The illness bearing his name was first described by James Parkinson in 1817. In that description of six patients (of whom Parkinson had personally examined three), it was categorically asserted that intellect and senses were preserved, but the author's recognition of depression in these patients is suggested by his use of terms such as *melancholia* (see also Darvesh & Freedman, 1996; Parkinson, 1817). Though the assertion that PD leaves cognition unscathed was challenged by Charcot and Vulpian (1861, 1862), and by isolated reports in the late 19th and early 20th centuries, many outside France remained unconvinced of cognitive compromise in PD probably until the middle of the 20th century (see Goetz, 1992). Naville (1922) introduced the term "bradyphrenia" to capture the phenomena of slowed information processing and diminished attention in postencephalitic parkinsonians without dementia. Dementia was rarely a topic of early medical manuscripts concerned with *paralysis agitans*. Interestingly, Fritz Lewy—whose name the eosinophilic, neuronal inclusion bodies bear since 1918 (see Schiller, 2000)—did not distinguish between depression and dementia when he described the neuropathology and mental alterations of PD (Lewy, 1912, 1923). Furthermore, Lewy apparently did not appreciate the significance of the inclusion bodies he had identified, and the entity of DLB was not recognized until the last 30 years of the 20th century (Holdorff, 2002).

Neuropsychological investigations using standardized, psychometric tests were rarely carried out in early studies of PD, but the likely first published use of such tests can be traced to Shaskin, Yarnell, and Alper (1942) administration of the Wechsler Bellevue Scale, an intelligence scale, to postencephalitic parkinsonians. A further catalyst for neuropsychological evaluation (using projective tests and tests of cognition and intelligence) in PD was the advent in the 1950s of the neurosurgical treatment of parkinsonism (idiopathic, postencephalitic, and vascular; see, for example, Diller, Riklan, & Cooper, 1956). Though the number of surgical interventions for PD declined dramatically after the introduction of levodopa in the late 1960s (Siegfried & Blond, 1997), numerous psychometric studies of the neuropsychological effects of thalamotomy and pallidotomy were carried out both in North America (e.g., Jurko & Andy, 1964; Riklan & Levita, 1969; Shapiro, Sadowsky, Henderson, & Van Buren, 1973) and on the other side of the Atlantic (e.g., Almgren, Andersson, & Kullberg, 1969; Asso, Crown, Russell, & Logue, 1969; Christensen, Juul-Jensen, Malmros, & Harmsen, 1970; Fünfgeld, 1967; McFie, 1960; Vilkki & Laitinen, 1974; Welman, 1971). The clinical focus of early neuropsychological studies of PD was maintained by investigators examining the cognitive effects of levodopa in the 1960s and 1970s (e.g., Beardsley & Puletti, 1971). By the 1980s, clinically oriented studies concerned themselves with the neuropsychological characterization of dementia in PD and its discriminability from other dementias (e.g., Huber, Shuttleworth, Paulson, Bellchambers, & Clapp, 1986; Pillon, Dubois, Lhermitte, & Agid, 1986; Pirozzolo, Hansch, Mortimer, Webster, & Kuskowski, 1982). In parallel, studies increasingly informed by cognitive psychological theory began to provide more detailed and sophisticated descriptions of neuropsychological deficits in PD (e.g., Boller, Mizutani, Roessmann, & Gambetti, 1980; Brown & Marsden, 1988; Cooper, Sagar, Jordan, Harvey, & Sullivan, 1991; Lees & Smith, 1983; Levin, Llabre, & Weiner, 1989; Taylor, Saint-Cyr, & Lang, 1986). Advances in understanding the neural substrates and cognitive mechanisms underlying neuropsychological deficits in PD continued as functional neuroimaging technology matured and became more readily available (e.g., Cools, Stefanova, Barker, Robbins, & Owen, 2002; Dagher, Owen, Boecker, & Brooks, 1999; Feigin et al., 2003; Owen, Doyon, Dagher, Sadikot, & Evans, 1998) and as radioactive tracers became available for specific neurotransmitter systems (Bohnen et al., 2007; Klein et al., 2010; Pfeiffer, Lokkegaard, Zoetmulder, Friberg, & Werdelin, 2014). The 1990s saw a renaissance of neurobehavioral studies of surgical treatments of PD, including deep brain stimulation (DBS), that continues today. Studies in the late 20th and early 21st century examining differences between PDD and DLB, are yet to resolve controversy about whether the conditions are distinct or two sides of one coin (Goldman, Williams-Gray, Barker, Duda, & Galvin, 2014). The difficulty distinguishing these conditions may in part have been an impetus to better understand predementia cognitive impairment in PD and the formulation of MCI criteria (Litvan et al., 2012; Tröster, 2011). Indeed, there is now interest in the possibility that subtle cognitive changes may be present in the premotor phase of the disease, i.e., persons deemed at risk for PD (Hawkins et al., 2010; Thaler et al., 2012) .

Epidemiology

The number of new cases per year (incidence) and the total number of cases at a given time (prevalence) vary as a function of case ascertainment, meaning the methods and criteria by which cases of PD are searched, for, screened, and diagnosed. Generally, reported disease rates are higher when broad rather than when strict diagnostic criteria are applied. Population-based door-to-door survey followed by clinical examination is the most complete case-finding strategy. Because prevalence is impacted by survival, incidence might be a more precise estimate of PD occurrence.

PD rarely occurs before age 50 years, and age-specific prevalence increases until the ninth decade. Reported overall prevalence rates of PD range from 167 to 5,703 per 100,000 persons per year (Wirdefeldt, Adami, Cole, Trichopoulos, & Mandel, 2011). Worldwide, the prevalence of PD in individuals above 50 was between 4.1 and 4.6 million in 2005, with that number projected to rise to between 8.7 and 9.3 million by 2030 (Dorsey et al., 2007). Among studies that report gender differences, a higher prevalence is consistently found among males than females, specifically, twofold in a recent study (Baldereschi et al., 2000). Lower PD prevalence among Blacks than Whites and Hispanics may be an artifact of apparently diminished survival.

Overall, incidence rates for PD among all age groups ranged between 1.5 and 22 per 100,000 person-years (Wirdefeldt et al., 2011). Based on the eight studies deemed to be of the best quality, the median standardized incidence rate in developed countries was estimated to be 14 per 100,000 person-years. This number increases to about 160 per 100,000 person-years among those 65 years and older (Hirtz et al., 2007). Incidence of parkinsonism is obviously higher than that of PD by virtue of including a larger number of conditions: One North American study reported an annual incidence of 26 per 100,000 of *parkinsonism*, and a *PD* incidence of 11 per 100,000 (Bower, Maraganore, McDonnell, & Rocca, 1999).

Dementia prevalence estimates vary from 8% to 93%, depending upon diagnostic criteria, sampling, and case ascertainment methods used, but the most accepted prevalence rates are 20% to 40% (Mohr, Mendis, & Grimes, 1995) with the highest-quality studies yielding a prevalence of 31% (Aarsland, Zaccai, & Brayne, 2005). Dementia incidence is about 3% for persons with PD younger than 60 years and 15% for persons with PD older than 80 years (Biggins et al., 1992; Marder, Tang, Cote, Stern, & Mayeux, 1995; Mayeux et al., 1990). MCI is thought to occur in about a third of patients, though recent criteria have yielded some higher estimates (Goldman et al., 2013).

Genetics

Genetic factors do not play a major role in sporadic PD. Were genetic factors to play a major role in the etiology of PD, then concordance rates for PD ought to be much higher among monozygotic than dizygotic twins, which is not the case. Nonetheless, 10%–15% of patients have a family history of the disease, suggesting a genetic contribution in those patients, particularly in early onset disease. A number of genetic mutations and loci (PARK 1–20, at the time of writing) linked to parkinsonism have been identified (Clarimon & Kulisevsky, 2013). These genetic findings may help identify molecular pathways of therapeutic relevance. The monogenic (or Mendelian) transmission of PD is not entirely straightforward because often there is incomplete penetrance, meaning that a carrier of the mutation may not develop the disease (perhaps because the gene interacts with other genes or the environment). Furthermore, several of the genes identified each may have various alterations (e.g., mutations or variations in copy number) with different clinical expressions or phenotypes (Halliday, Leverenz, Schneider, & Adler, 2014). In addition to monogenic transmission, various genetic polymorphisms (variations common in the population) may increase disease risk, although disease will be expressed only in the presence of other factors. More recently, studies have begun to examine potential genetic contributions to cognitive dysfunction in PD, including genes implicated in other cognition-compromising diseases (e.g., APOE) and in PD per se (e.g., SNCA, LRRK2) (Sharp & Alcalay, 2015). Frequent issues that have plagued these studies are a lack of statistical power and the use of relatively insensitive cognitive screening measures or patient report. Nonetheless, the research with positive findings allows one to raise hypotheses regarding potential genetic contributions to cognitive decline in PD.

Among genes implicated in PD, PARKIN (PARK2), which is linked to autosomal recessive inheritance of PD and early disease onset, seems not to associate with cognitive impairment. Indeed, gene carriers may perform similarly (Caccappolo et al., 2011) or better than early onset PD noncarriers or healthy controls on neuropsychological tests tapping perception, attention, and memory (Alcalay et al., 2014). SNCA, the gene encoding for α-synuclein that is the building block of Lewy bodies, causes autosomal dominant PD by virtue of mutations (PARK1) or copy-number variations (PARK4). However, the expressed phenotype is variable. This gene is of particular neuropsychological interest as the Iowa kindred (PARK4) tends to develop early dementia (Farrer et al., 1999), and the Contursi kindred (PARK1) may show atypical clinical features including fluent aphasia and palilalia (Golbe et al., 1996). Unfortunately, due to rarity (the gene accounts for only 2% of autosomal dominant PD cases) and the lack of sophisticated neuropsychological study, precise cognitive characterizations are lacking. One study did report early perceptual deficit followed by executive and memory dysfunction in one family (Muenter et al., 1998), but another failed to find an association between SNCA and a broad range of neuropsychological tests (Mata et al., 2014).

Studies of potential cognitive differences between carriers of LRRK2 mutations (PARK8), the most frequently mutated gene in PD and inherited in autosomal dominant fashion, have yielded contradictory findings. Whereas some studies report similar performance on cognitive screening measures (Aasly et al., 2005; Alcalay et al., 2010), others have observed poorer performance among LRRK2 carriers than noncarriers (Healy et al., 2008; Lesage et al., 2006). The number of studies addressing cognition and psychiatric features in person with PINK1 (PARK6) are few and generally lack lengthy follow-up, but it is possible that dementia is relatively rare among carriers (Ephraty et al., 2007; Healy et al., 2004). One study found no association between LRRK2, MCI, dementia, and anxiety (Estanga et al., 2014). Similarly, cognitive characteristics of carriers of DJ-1 mutations are rarely described, but one study suggests that the phenotype resembles PD-Dementia-ALS complex and involves dementia within ten years of symptom onset (Annesi et al., 2005).

Cognitive correlates have also been studied for genes related to other neurodegenerative disease (e.g., APOE, MAPT) and dopaminergic function (e.g., COMT and BDNF). The APOE ε4 allele increases risk for Alzheimer's disease (AD) and two meta-analyses have reported this allele to be either associated with greater risk of PDD (Huang, Chen, Kaufer, Troster, & Poole, 2006) or to be overrepresented among those with PDD relative to those without dementia (Williams-Gray, Goris, et al., 2009). Prospective studies have been less apt to find such an association, with two finding no association between the allele and dementia (Kurz et al., 2009) or Mini Mental State Exam (MMSE) score change (Williams-Gray, Goris, et al., 2009), whilst another study reported the allele to be associated with greater change on the Dementia Rating Scale (DRS) (Morley et al., 2012). Among PD patients without dementia, the ε4 allele is associated with poorer memory and semantic fluency (Mata et al., 2014). A combination of polymorphisms referred to as the H1/H1 haplotype of the microtubule-associated protein tau (MAPT) gene are linked to tau formation and have been implicated in AD and progressive supranuclear palsy. The predominance of evidence implicates the haplotype in cognitive decline and dementia risk in PD (Goris et al., 2007; Williams-Gray, Evans, et al., 2009), although this finding may obtain only in those persons developing dementia fairly early in the disease course. In patients with longer disease duration, the haplotype may be associated with impaired memory (Morley et al., 2012), but another study failed to find an association between MAPT and neuropsychological test performance (Mata et al., 2014).

Dopamine is degraded by enzymes including catechol-O-methyl-transferase (COMT). The COMT met/met polymorphism leads to lower enzyme activity (and thus presumably higher synaptic dopamine levels) than the val/val variant and is associated with better performance on the Wisconsin Card Sorting Test (WCST) in healthy persons. Counterintuitively, one study found that an increasing number of met alleles was associated with *poorer* planning performance on the Tower of London (Foltynie, Goldberg, et al., 2004). Although two other studies associated the COMT polymorphism with attention impairment (Morley et al., 2012; Williams-Gray, Hampshire, Barker, & Owen, 2008), a large study using an extensive neuropsychological test battery failed to find any effect (Hoogland et al., 2010). It is possible that the conflicting findings may relate to patients' severity of dopamine depletion and medication. The role of the brain-derived neurotrophic factor (BDNF) gene polymorphisms remains unclear. Dopamine release and dopaminergic cell survival are shown to be activated and enhanced by BDNF. The finding that the low secretion (met) allele of BDNF was associated with better planning on the Tower of London task than the high secretion val allele, like the COMT finding, again seems counterintuitive. Indeed, the finding linking cognition and BDNF in PD has not been replicated (Gao et al., 2010).

Neuropathology and Pathophysiology

PD involves the loss of pigmented cells from the substantia nigra and it is estimated that 70%–80% of this system's neurons have been lost when PD symptoms emerge (Bernheimer, Birkmayer, Hornykiewicz, Jellinger, & Seitelberger, 1973). Dopamine depletion in the striatum is more profound in the putamen than the caudate, and eventual abnormalities in the dopaminergic mesolimbic and mesocortical projection systems contribute to neurobehavioral changes. Dysfunction and pathology in other neurotransmitter systems also contribute to the neurobehavioral features of PD (Halliday et al., 2014). Cell loss in PD is also evident in the locus coeruleus (noradrenergic), the dorsal raphe nuclei (serotonergic), the nucleus basalis of Meynert (cholinergic), and the dorsal vagal nucleus. Dysfunction of these neurotransmitter systems has also been linked especially to executive and affective changes in PD, and imaging studies of dopaminergic (Ito et al., 2002; O'Brien et al., 2009), cholinergic (Bohnen et al., 2007; Bohnen et al., 2006; Hilker et al., 2005; Klein et al., 2010), and noradrenergic systems (Remy, Doder, Lees, Turjanski, & Brooks, 2005) have yielded complementary findings regarding these systems' neuropsychological impact in PD.

An important feature of the neuropathology of PD is the presence of Lewy bodies in the brain stem and/or amygdala and, later in the disease, in neocortex. These Lewy bodies contain the protein α-synuclein. The stages of the evolution of the neuroanatomical pathology of PD was described by Braak and colleagues (2003) (see Table 22.2 and Figure 22.1). Although this description has been challenged because the evolution of clinical features of PD is heterogeneous and sometimes inconsistent with such a systematic evolution of pathology, the model has heuristic value. From a neuropsychological standpoint it is useful to note that by the time a diagnosis of PD is made (Stage 3 or 4), even a relatively

Table 22.2 Braak staging of neuropathology in Parkinson's Disease (after Braak et al., 2003)

Stage	*Primary Brain Region Affected*	*Loci of Pathology*
1	medulla	Dorsal IX/X motor nucleus and/or immediate reticular zone
2	medulla and	Stage 1 + caudal raphe nuclei, gigantocellular reticular pontine tegmentum nucleus and caeruleus-subcaeruleus complex
3	midbrain	Stage 2 + midbrain (esp. pars compacta of substantia nigra)
4	basal prosencephalon	Stage 3 + prosencephalon (confined to transentorhinal and mesocortex region and CA2-plexus)
5	neocortex	Stage 4 + high order sensory association areas of the neocortex and prefrontal cortex
6	neocortex	Stage 5 + first order sensory association neocortical areas and premotor areas; may be some mild changes in primary sensory areas and primary motor field

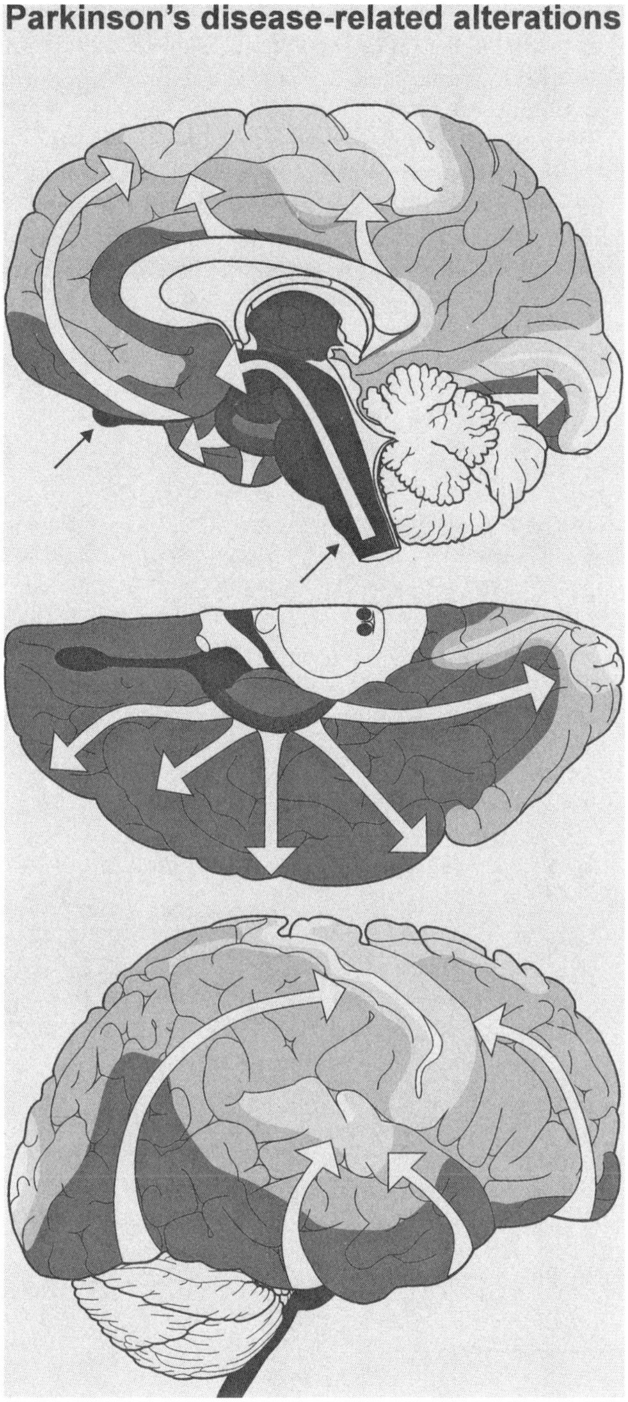

Figure 22.1 Progression of pathology in PD according to the Braak staging system (from allocortex through mesocortex to neocortex)

Figure courtesy of Prof. Dr. Heiko Braak.

insensitive measure such as the MMSE may disclose cognitive impairment in some patients (Braak, Rub, & Del Tredici, 2006; Braak, Rub, Jansen Steur, Del Tredici, & de Vos, 2005), a finding consistent with the observation that as many as one-fifth to one-third of patients may show at least subtle impairments on neuropsychological tests at or near the time of PD diagnosis (Aarsland, Bronnick, Larsen, Tysnes, & Alves, 2009; Elgh et al., 2009; Foltynie, Brayne, Robbins, & Barker, 2004; Muslimovic, Post, Speelman, & Schmand, 2005). Severity of dementia has been associated with cortical Lewy body burden (Hurtig et al., 2000), but there are cases of PDD that lack cortical pathology (Perry et al., 1985; Xuereb et al., 1990) and cases of PD that meet neuropathological criteria for DLB at autopsy but do not have a history of dementia (Colosimo, Hughes, Kilford, & Lees, 2003). Cognitive changes are not simply a manifestation of synuclein pathology, however. Coexisting pathologic AD may be evident in 10%–40% of persons with PDD (Irwin et al., 2012), and AD-like pathology, particularly β-amyloid containing plaques in an even higher proportion, though tau-related tangles are seen less frequently (Apaydin, Ahlskog, Parisi, Boeve, & Dickson, 2002). These pathologic findings are consonant with the association between cerebrospinal fluid (CSF) reductions in β-amyloid and cognition (Leverenz et al., 2011; Montine et al., 2010) and the absence of the elevated tau levels seen in AD CSF. Nonetheless, an association between CSF tau levels and memory and executive decline in PD may be found once dopaminergic therapy is initiated (Liu et al., 2015). Given the consistency of findings implicating β-amyloid in the cognitive decline of PD/PDD, the apparent lack of association between cognitive impairment and imaged brain β-amyloid burden in PD is puzzling (Gomperts et al., 2012). PDD may also be related to vascular pathology (Jellinger & Attems, 2008), as may some cases of PD-MCI (Adler et al., 2010).

The pathology underlying different phenotypes of Lewy body disease may also differ. The prospective Sydney Multicenter Study of PD (Halliday & McCann, 2010), showed three phenotypes of patients: one group with early, prominent dementia and akinetic-rigid PD (clinically resembling DLB); another group of older (> 70 years) patients with widespread alpha-synuclein pathology who develop dementia in three to ten years (clinically resembling PDD); and a final, slightly younger group (disease onset before 70 years) who develop dementia after ten to 15 years and who have brain atrophy with lesser alpha-synuclein deposition. Consistent with the Sydney study, another study reported that PD patients developing dementia late in the disease (after about ten years) have less cortical alpha-synuclein pathology and fewer plaques but greater cholinergic abnormalities than those developing dementia early on, whose pathology resembled more strongly that of DLB (Ballard et al., 2006).

Neurobehavioral changes in PD (and its motor signs) can also be understood by considering the pathophysiology of fronto-striatal circuits (Zgaljardic, Borod, Foldi, & Mattis, 2003). The original model of frontal-basal ganglionic-thalamic-frontal circuits (Alexander, DeLong, & Strick, 1986) has undergone refinement (Wichmann & De Long, 2015). Recent research has shown that the information from limbic circuits may be shared with the associative and motor circuits, that the basal ganglia interact with the cerebellar-cortical circuits, and that several of the subcortical structures may have direct links with cortex, including nonfrontal cortex, and among each other (Middleton & Strick, 2000). For example, animal work has identified a hyperdirect pathway between frontal cortex and subthalamic nucleus (STN; see Haynes & Haber, 2013) that may explain some of the behavioral effects of subthalamic stimulation. According to the simplified model, the frontal cortex, basal ganglia and thalamus are linked by five anatomically and functionally segregated circuits that retain their relative position to each other and share the same neurotransmitters at each point. The circuits, named for their origin (dorsolateral, orbitofrontal, anterior cingulate, motor, and oculomotor), are closed but have open elements to permit communication with cortical regions implicated in functions similar to those of a circuit. The dorsolateral, orbitofrontal, and cingulate circuits are particularly important in the regulation of cognition, affect, and motivation, respectively. The circuits have both direct and indirect pathways linking the striatum with the substantia nigra and internal globus pallidus (GPi), with the indirect pathway involving the external globus pallidus (GPe) and STN (Figure 22.2). In PD, the STN is overactive and excessively activates the GPi. This effect is amplified by the direct pathway's diminished inhibition of the GPi. A result of the of the GPi's overactivity is an excessive braking of the thalamus, and the subsequent dampening of the thalamus' excitatory influence on cortical regions. The pathophysiologic changes in these and other neural circuits probably interact to produce the complex behavioral syndromes observed in PD. Specific cognitive deficits can also be understood in terms of specific neural network dysfunctions and the neurotransmitter abnormalities affecting these networks in different stages of PD (Gratwicke, Jahanshahi, & Foltynie, 2015).

Neurobehavioral Features of Parkinson's Disease

Subtle cognitive alterations may precede PD diagnosis and be evident already at time of diagnosis. As PD progresses, the disease can compromise a variety of cognitive domains along a continuum of severity ranging from subclinical changes to MCI and eventually dementia. Deficits in early PD are most apparent on those tasks demanding of self-initiated information processing strategies (Taylor & Saint-Cyr, 1995), but executive impairments cannot account for the full range of cognitive deficits in PD (Tröster & Fields, 1995). If signs of cortical dysfunction (apraxia, amnesia, aphasia,

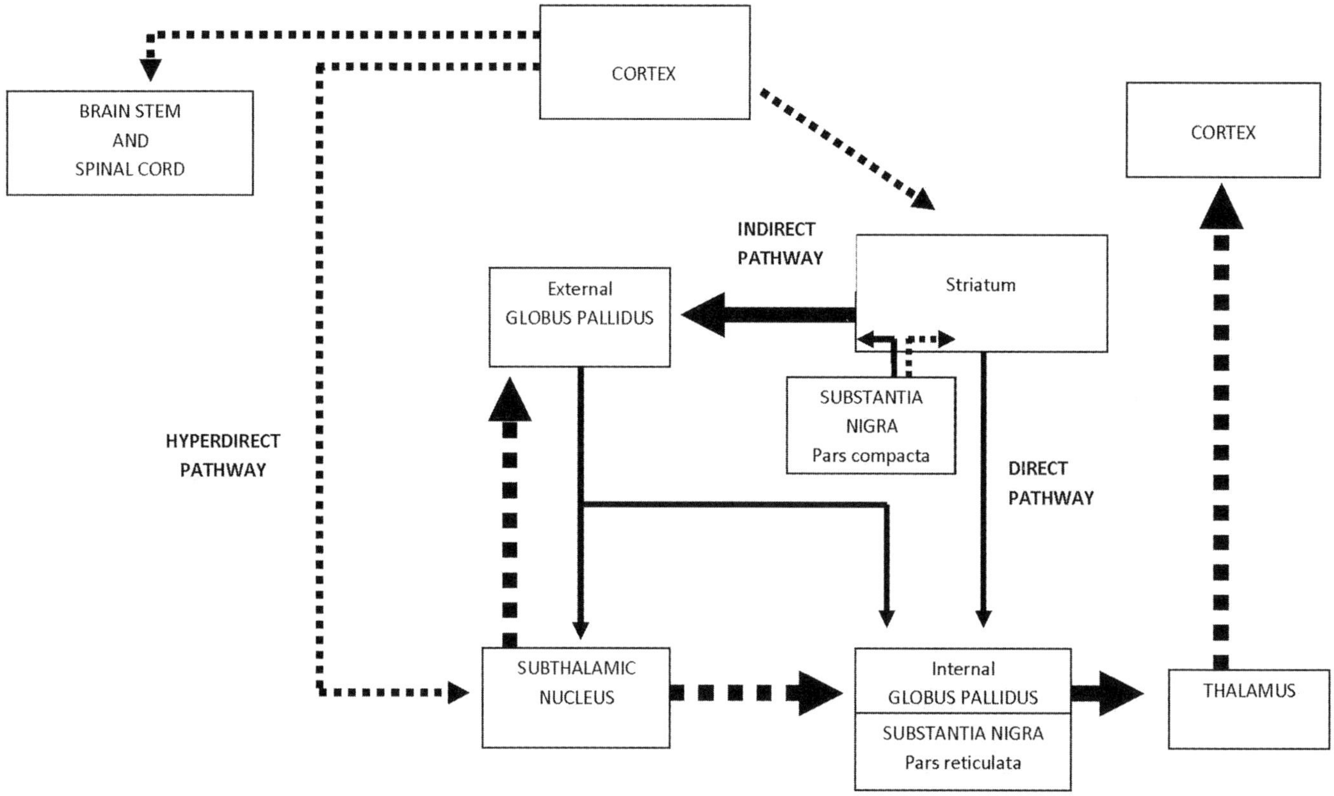

Figure 22.2 Fronto-striatal circuit dysfunction in PD

Key: solid arrows, inhibitory influence; dotted arrows, excitatory influence; narrow arrows, underactive relative to normal; broad arrows, overactive relative to normal

and agnosia) are evident within the first year of motor signs, these deficits suggest the presence of another condition, such as AD, DLB, atypical parkinsonism, or vascular dementia. The vast majority of findings relating to cognitive deficits in PD have led to the postulated existence of two distinct cognitive syndromes: at first, a predominantly dopamine-mediated frontal-subcortical executive syndrome compromising, for example, working memory, planning, and set shifting; and later, another syndrome characterized by compromise of cognitive functions (e.g., memory, visuospatial perception) mediated primarily by posterior cortical regions and related to dysfunction in cholinergic, serotonergic, and noradrenergic systems (Kehagia, Barker, & Robbins, 2010).

Specific Cognitive (Dys)Functions in Parkinson's Disease

The following discussion examines how various cognitive functions are impacted or spared by PD and its treatment, the performance by parkinsonians on clinical neuropsychological tests evaluating these functions, and some of the putative mechanisms underlying deficient task performance.

INTELLIGENCE

Intelligence is preserved in PD until dementia evolves, though even patients without dementia may perform more poorly than expected on Performance Scale subtests of the Wechsler Adult Intelligence Scales (WAIS; Ross et al., 1996). To our knowledge WAIS-IV performance has not been examined in PD, but studies using earlier versions of the Wechsler scales found impoverished performance especially on Digit Symbol, Picture Arrangement, and Object Assembly.

ATTENTION AND WORKING MEMORY

Working memory is a limited-capacity, multicomponent system allowing temporary, online manipulation and storage of information to guide and control action. Consequently, working memory deficits can impact performance on other cognitive tasks. The role of dopaminergic system dysfunction in the PD working memory impairment is well established (Cools, 2006) and dopaminergic medications may transiently improve working memory in early stages of the disease (Kehagia et al., 2010), especially on tasks involving longer delays between presentation and recall (Moustafa, Bell, Eissa, & Hewedi, 2013).

Performance on simple attention tasks, such as digit span and spatial span, is often intact or only very mildly impaired in early PD. Performance, however, becomes increasingly impaired as tasks make greater demands on the manipulation of information within working memory. A meta-analysis of 56 studies reported deficits in PD in tasks tapping verbal simple attention (digit span forward), visual simple attention (Corsi blocks), verbal complex attention (digit span backward), and visual complex attention (CANTAB spatial working memory test) (Siegert, Weatherall, Taylor, & Abernethy, 2008). The impairment was mild for verbal span but moderate for complex verbal as well as simple and complex visual spans. The authors provided several explanations for the more pronounced visual attention impairment: (a) visuospatial impairment is primary in PD; (b) visuospatial span tasks may be more difficult and demanding of central executive resources; (c) more patients in the analysis had left-sided onset and thus, presumably, greater right hemisphere dysfunction; and (e) the role of the right hemisphere in the maintenance and control of attention and working memory storage/recall. Working memory deficits in PD have variously been attributed to reduced capacity of the system (Gabrieli, Singh, Stebbins, & Goetz, 1996), difficulty manipulating information within working memory (Lewis et al., 2003), and difficulty inhibiting responses (Kensinger, Shearer, Locascio, & Growdon, 2003; Rieger, Gauggel, & Burmeister, 2003). Whether deficits updating working memory might be due to increased susceptibility to the entry of irrelevant information or resistance of existing information to deletion has not been resolved.

As regards performance on other working memory and attention tasks, even newly diagnosed patients with PD are impaired on the Digit Ordering Task, during which they are read a randomly ordered string of digits they are then asked to repeat in ascending order (Stebbins, Gabrieli, Masciari, Monti, & Goetz, 1999). Similarly, patients with PD are likely to demonstrate difficulty on tasks requiring divided or selective attention, though impairments may be task dependent (Lee, Wild, Hollnagel, & Grafman, 1999). Both limited attentional resources and attentional set shifting may contribute to patients' poor performance on Stroop-like tasks (Woodward, Bub, & Hunter, 2002). Patients typically show impairments on visual search and cancellation tasks presumably due to impaired selective attention and vigilance rather than motor slowing (Filoteo, Williams, Rilling, & Roberts, 1997).

EXECUTIVE FUNCTIONS

Executive functions—including planning, conceptualization, flexibility of thought, insight, judgment, self-monitoring, and self-regulation—are important to evaluate given that PD affects several of these functions. Consistent with the hypothesis that early executive deficits are linked to dopaminergic dysfunction, a study of more than 300 drug-naive patients revealed that executive function (but not memory or visuospatial) differences between patients and controls were related to nigrostriatal dysfunction as indexed by diminished striatal dopamine transporter binding on DAT-SPECT scan (Siepel et al., 2014). Executive functions are important to assess from a pragmatic standpoint because these functions are linked to the realization of goals, to the capacity to consent to medical treatment (Dymek, Atchison, Harrell, &

Marson, 2001), and to the ability to engage in instrumental activities of daily living (IADLs) (Cahn et al., 1998). Executive dysfunction may also be an early indicator of incipient dementia in PD (Mahieux et al., 1998; Woods & Tröster, 2003), although some find that tests mediated predominantly by posterior brain regions provide a more imminent signal of dementia (Williams-Gray, Evans, et al., 2009; Williams-Gray et al., 2013). In addition, although the driving accident rate in PD as a whole is comparable to that of the rest of the population (Homann et al., 2003), patients with cognitive flexibility and working memory compromise might be at greater risk for accidents (Ranchet et al., 2013).

An important issue in neuropsychological evaluation is whether diminished awareness of deficits (anosognosia) is likely to compromise the validity of information obtained on interview and self-report measures. Advancing PD might involve metacognitive compromise (Seltzer, Vasterling, Mathias, & Brennan, 2001), but PD patients as a group do not have significantly diminished awareness (Seltzer et al., 2001). Brown, MacCarthy, Jahanshahi, and Marsden (1989) found that persons with PD-MCI, even when depressed, validly completed self-report measures. Another study found that patient and caregiver report was related to performance on cognitive tests (Naismith, Pereira, Shine, & Lewis, 2011). However, accuracy of self-report, and presumably awareness, may decline as cognitive impairment advances (Sitek, Soltan, Wieczorek, Robowski, & Slawek, 2011) and patients may demonstrate lack of awareness of motor versus cognitive deficits (Amanzio et al., 2010; Maier et al., 2012), including dyskinesias (Pietracupa et al., 2013). This lack of motor deficit awareness might be related to right hemisphere dysfunction, motor phenotype, and proprioceptive deficits.

Several clinical neuropsychological tests are routinely used to assess executive functions in PD, the most common among them Tower of London, card sorting, verbal fluency, Trail Making and interference tasks. A meta-analysis showed that all five of these tasks reveal differences of medium to large effect size between patients and healthy individuals, but the clinical significance of such findings remains elusive (Kudlicka, Clare, & Hindle, 2011). Numerous studies have evaluated planning in PD using the Tower of Hanoi or variants thereof (e.g., Tower of Toronto, Tower of London). While some studies found PD patients to show normal accuracy (number of moves) but a slowness in problem solving (e.g., Morris et al., 1988), others also observed diminished planning accuracy (Owen et al., 1995; Saint-Cyr, Taylor, & Lang, 1988) and planning deficits associated with decreased motivation (Weintraub et al., 2005). One study reported deficits with problem solving only on tasks with a high visuospatial content (McKinlay et al., 2010). Card-sorting tests evaluate, among other functions, the ability to conceptualize and form, maintain and switch set. Studies using tasks such as the WCST (Heaton, Chelune, Talley, Kay, & Curtiss, 1993) have, with only rare exception, found patients with PD to have difficulty with one or more of set formation, set maintenance, and set shifting. The number of sorts completed on the WCST, indicating indexing concept formation, is often reduced already in early PD (Pillon, Dubois, Ploska, & Agid, 1991). Patients with PD may also be slow to conceptualize, as inferred from an increased number of trials needed to complete the first series of consecutive correct sorts (Taylor et al., 1986); have set-shifting difficulty as revealed by perseverative errors (Cooper et al., 1991); and lose set, especially later in PD, as evident from nonperseverative errors and failures to maintain set (Taylor et al., 1986). The impairment in set shifting may be a critical determinant of whether patients with PD demonstrate difficulty on various executive function tasks (Cronin-Golomb, Corkin, & Growdon, 1994), but is not ubiquitous. Thus, research suggests that patients with PD have difficulty with extradimensional set shifting (i.e., responding to a new stimulus dimension, as when one has to respond to the color of a stimulus instead of its shape), but not intradimensional set shifting (responding to one characteristic of a stimulus dimension instead of another characteristic, as one might when required to respond to yellow rather than blue stimuli); for a very lucid review of this topic, see Robbins, Owen, and Sahakian (1998).

A test evaluating decision making, judgment and impulsivity is the Iowa Gambling Task (IGT; see Bechara, 2007). Examinees are instructed to maximize their gambling winnings by choosing cards from different decks that yield either a high payoff coupled with high risk, or a low payoff at low risk. Over the long run, the low payoff, low-risk decks are advantageous, resulting in net winnings, while the high payoff, high-risk decks are designed to yield net losses. A review of 13 studies did not find a clear relationship between executive functioning or other cognitive functions and performance on the IGT, and concluded that PD patients treated with dopaminergic medications demonstrated preserved IGT performance (Poletti, Cavedini, & Bonuccelli, 2011). Nonetheless, Czernecki et al. (2002) found that patients' performance on the gambling task did not improve across assessments, suggesting a failure to benefit from experience. Deficits on gambling tasks may be observable only when patients are on dopamimetic medications (Cools, Barker, Sahakian, & Robbins, 2003), a finding consistent with the reported association of pathological gambling with dopaminergic therapy in PD (Gschwandtner, Aston, Renaud, & Fuhr, 2001).

LANGUAGE

Motor speech abnormalities (dysarthria, hypophonia) are often evident in advanced PD and may impact performance on some language tasks such as sentence repetition (Matison, Mayeux, Rosen, & Fahn, 1982). Certain aspects of language are compromised in PD patients with dementia, but these patients rarely have a frank aphasia (Levin & Katzen, 1995). Subtle alterations in performance on language tasks are also observed in patients without dementia, but these changes are often attributed to diminished attention, working memory, or inefficient information processing strategy development and deployment.

Visual confrontation naming task performance, requiring naming of pictured or actual objects, is preserved in PD (Levin et al., 1989; Lewis, Lapointe, & Murdoch, 1998), though rare studies report subtle naming impairments in early PD (Globus, Mildworf, & Melamed, 1985). Patients with obvious cognitive impairment, in contrast, do show naming impairments (Beatty & Monson, 1989; Lewis et al., 1998), which are less severe and emerge later than in AD (Stern et al., 1998).

Verbal fluency tasks require patients to orally generate as many words as possible within a time limit that either begin with a given letter of the alphabet, or belong to a category. Patients with dementia perform more poorly on these tasks than those without dementia (Azuma et al., 1997; Cummings, Darkins, Mendez, Hill, & Benson, 1988; Tröster et al., 1998; Troyer, Moscovitch, Winocur, Leach, & Freedman, 1998), and indeed, patients without dementia may demonstrate intact performance (Cohen, Bouchard, Scherzer, & Whitaker, 1994; Lewis et al., 1998). Two verbal fluency tasks especially sensitive to PD are alternating word fluency, requiring retrieval of consecutive words from alternate semantic or letter categories (Kudlicka et al., 2011; Zec et al., 1999); and verb fluency tasks, requiring naming of actions (Piatt, Fields, Paolo, Koller, & Tröster, 1999). Indeed, when asked to generate verbs (action fluency), patients with PD may be even more impaired than those with AD (McDowd et al., 2011). The impairment in action fluency is more pronounced when patients are off than on medication, and when off medication they tend to generate mainly higher-frequency verbs (Herrera, Cuetos, & Ribacoba, 2012).

Research suggests that diminished phonemic and semantic verbal fluency may be related to diminished processing speed (McDowd et al., 2011), semantic memory alterations (Henry & Crawford, 2004), retrieval deficits, or to a deficit in an underlying process such as switching but not clustering (which respectively refer to the processes of disengaging from one category of words to produce those from another category, and the production of consecutive words from the same semantic or phonemic category). Thus, switching impairments are more readily observed among patients with PDD than in AD, while deficits in clustering are more pronounced in AD than PDD (Tröster et al., 1998; Troyer et al., 1998). Even when verbal fluency output is diminished in PD patients without dementia, clustering appears to be preserved (Heiss, Kalbe, & Kessler, 2001).

Other subtle linguistic impairments observed in PD include those in syntactic comprehension and production (Murray, 2000). The mechanisms underlying the subtle sentence comprehension deficits in PD remain controversial, but proposed ones include grammatical processing deficits (Cohen et al., 1994; Ullman et al., 1997), slowed information processing (Grossman et al., 2002), and diminished attention (Lee, Grossman, Morris, Stern, & Hurtig, 2003) or working memory. There may also be mild phonetic and pragmatics impairments in early PD. Grossman, Carvell, Stern, Gollomp, and Hurtig (1992) and Lee et al. (2003) found that patients had difficulty detecting phonetic errors in words. Patients with PD have been reported to have problems in conversational appropriateness, turn taking, prosody, and proxemics (McNamara & Durso, 2003).

VISUOPERCEPTUAL AND SPATIAL FUNCTIONS

Visuospatial deficits may be among the earliest and most readily observable neurobehavioral deficits in PD (Passafiume, Boller, & Keefe, 1986), though the nature of impairments may be a function of disease duration, disease severity, and presence of dementia (Alegret, Pere, Junqué, Valldeoriola, & Tolosa, 2001; Levin et al., 1991). It has also been reported that visuospatial impairments might be more evident in patients with left motor symptom onset (right hemisphere dysfunction), but that such a difference may be evident only in samples with longer disease duration (Karadi et al., 2015) or only in persons in whom symptoms other than tremor are prominent (Seichepine, Neargarder, Davidsdottir, Reynolds, & Cronin-Golomb, 2015). Furthermore, the ability to elicit impairments on drawing tasks (e.g., complex figure, clock) may depend on the scoring method used (Karadi et al., 2015; Seichepine et al., 2015).

Tasks that patients with PD might perform poorly include following a route; assembling blocks to match a pattern; drawing, tracing, or copying complex figures; matching pictures of faces; matching lines of similar spatial orientation; identifying objects from fragmented pictures; and identifying drawings embedded among lines (embedded figures) (Bowen, Hoehn, & Yahr, 1972; Pirozzolo et al., 1982; Stern, Mayeux, & Rosen, 1984). It has been suggested that visuospatial task deficits may be secondary to motor impairments or limitations in information processing resources and executive strategies (Brown & Marsden, 1986; Higginson, Wheelock, Levine, Pappas, & Sigvardt, 2011). However, it is unlikely that motor or executive impairments can fully account for visuoperceptual and spatial deficits in PD, because impairments on visuoperceptual and spatial tasks are also observed when tasks' motor demands are minimized (Lee, Harris, & Calvert, 1998; Levin et al., 1991). Similarly, although impaired saccadic eye movements may contribute to visuoperceptual impairments, they cannot fully account for them (Bodis-Wollner, 2003).

One motor-demand-free visuoperceptual task on which patients with PD may demonstrate difficulty is a facial matching task (Levin et al., 1989). Facial identification relies on perceptual processing of both individual features or components and feature configurations. Cousins, Hanley, Davies, Turnbull, and Playfer (2000) found that the facial recognition impairment in PD was associated with configural (but not componential) visuoperceptual processing difficulties, even after controlling for intelligence, age, and depressive symptoms. Because the two forms of processing are unlikely to differentially tax information processing resources, it appears that PD-associated facial matching difficulties are unlikely to be just a manifestation of limitations in information processing resources and their allocation. Another visuospatial task free of motor demands is one requiring patients to match lines of similar spatial orientation. Alegret et al. (2001) and Finton, Lucas, Graff-Radford, and Uitti (1998) found that PD patients made more serious errors on the Judgment of Line Orientation (JLO) test than control groups. Patients with PD committed more errors that involved confusing an oblique line with one from the same quadrant that was displaced by two or three 18° segments from the target line, and in Alegret et al.'s (2001) study the patients also made more errors than controls involving mismatching of horizontal lines.

Though motor deficits can certainly contribute to PD patient's difficulty with visuo-constructional tasks, an error analysis of drawings of patients with PDD makes it clear that cognitive and visuo-perceptual problems also underlie these patients' drawing difficulties. Specifically, Freeman et al. (2000) compared errors made by patients with PDD on the Rey-Osterrieth Complex Figure test to those made by healthy controls and patients with AD. Compared to these two groups, the PD patients made more placement errors, configural errors, errors of omission, and perseverations, and produced more fragmented drawings that lacked more of the clusters of elements within the figure. In contrast, recognition of the figure after a delay was much better in PD than AD.

MEMORY AND LEARNING

The classic notion holds that the impairment in new learning and memory in PD is due to a retrieval deficit, and the primary evidence for this is the finding of poor immediate recall accompanied by intact (Beatty, Staton, Weir, Monson, & Whitaker, 1989), or at least better (if not completely intact) recognition of memoranda (Whittington, Podd, & Kan, 2000). An issue with this interpretation is that early studies may have assumed rather than demonstrated intact encoding. The preponderance of evidence now suggests that PD anterograde (declarative) memory deficits may be due to either or both of deficient encoding and retrieval. Indeed, shallow encoding may be sufficient to support adequate recognition but not recall. The mild recall impairment in PD without dementia is evident on many tasks: word lists (Buytenhuijs et al., 1994), paired associate learning (Huber, Shuttleworth, & Paulson, 1986), recall of prose passages (Tröster, Stalp, Paolo, Fields, & Koller, 1995), complex figure reproduction (Stefanova, Kostic, Ziropadja, Ocic, & Markovic, 2001), memory for spatial locations on maps (Beatty et al., 1989), and abstract designs (Sullivan & Sagar, 1989). As patients develop more global cognitive impairments both recall and recognition are affected, though in comparison to AD, recognition may still be disproportionately better than recall (Tierney et al., 1994). Memory impairment in PD can also be exacerbated by depression (Tröster et al., 1995).

The learning of new information may be slowed in PD (Faglioni, Saetti, & Botti, 2000). The rate with which a semantic encoding strategy evolves across word list learning trials is slow and diminished in comparison to healthy elderly persons (Berger et al., 1999; Bronnick, Alves, Aarsland, Tysnes, & Larsen, 2011; Buytenhuijs et al., 1994), and if learning of persons with PD and controls is equated on a semantically related word list, recall and recognition are comparable between the groups (Chiaravalloti et al., 2014). In contrast to semantic encoding, serial encoding appears to be preserved (Berger et al., 1999; Buytenhuijs et al., 1994), as are serial position effects (Stefanova et al., 2001). One explanation for these findings is that serial encoding reflects the use of an externally imposed strategy, whereas semantic encoding relies more on self-initiated learning strategies that are diminished in PD (Taylor & Saint-Cyr, 1995). Given this difficulty in spontaneously developing effective encoding strategies, it is not surprising then that patients benefit from externally supported retrieval as provided by cuing (Knoke, Taylor, & Saint-Cyr, 1998) and recognition formats (van Oostrom et al., 2003). However, the finding of similar performance under incidental and intentional recall conditions (Ellfolk, Huurinainen, Joutsa, & Karrasch, 2012) would not be predicted by such an explanation. Some have found that encoding is impaired while the patient is on dopaminergic medication, whilst retrieval is impaired off medication, suggesting encoding to be mediated by ventral striatum but retrieval by dorsal striatum (MacDonald et al., 2013). However, the finding of encoding deficits in never-medicated patients (Bronnick et al., 2011) challenges this hypothesis. Retention of word lists over time is usually normal (Massman, Delis, Butters, Levin, & Salmon, 1990), and intrusion errors (production of nonlist words during recall) are typically semantically related to the words on the list and qualitatively similar to those of normal elderly (Massman et al., 1990).

As more severe cognitive impairment develops in PD, a multiplicity of memory mechanisms become affected, including storage, as suggested by rapid rates of forgetting, though these are not observed in all patients. Given that there are probably multiple neuropathological bases for the cognitive impairment in PD it is not surprising that the memory profiles of patients with PD can be quite heterogeneous, with some patients displaying normal learning and memory, others showing deficits that are reminiscent of those in subcortical dementias such as HD, and yet others showing impairments characteristic of AD (Filoteo, Rilling, et al., 1997).

Recollection of information from the past is typically preserved. Fama et al. (2000) found that patients with PD were as accurate as a normal control group in recalling and recognizing past presidents' and presidential candidates' names, and in identifying them from photographs. Similar findings have been reported by others: Unless demented, patients with PD were as able as healthy elderly people to identify once-famous individuals from photographs and to answer questions about famous persons and well-known public and historical events (Freedman, Rivoira, Butters, Sax, & Feldman, 1984; Huber et al., 1986; Leplow et al., 1997), although one study reported impairments in recalling and dating public events (Venneri et al., 1997). Retrieval of autobiographical memories may be impaired in PD without dementia (Souchay & Smith, 2013). Unlike their nondemented counterparts, patients with PDD do develop impairments in remote memory (Freedman et al., 1984; Huber et al., 1986; Leplow et al., 1997). However, unlike in AD, the impairment in PD is equally severe for information across past decades.

Prospective memory, or memory and execution of intended future actions tends to be impaired in PD, although this impairment may be contingent upon the presence of MCI (Costa et al., 2015). Prospective memory tasks differ in the cues utilized and the nature of the cues may be critical in determining whether or not impairments in PD are evidenced. Specifically, the cues to which memory retrieval and action execution is linked may be time- or event-based, and embedded within the ongoing task (focal) or not (nonfocal). Katai, Maruyama, Hashimoto, and Ikeda (2003) found an impairment on an event-based prospective memory task in PD relative to controls, but others have reported impairments in time-based tasks only, which may relate to the greater executive function demands that these time-based tasks place on the person (Costa, Peppe, Caltagirone, & Carlesimo, 2008; Raskin et al., 2010). Although it has been suggested that prospective memory impairment in PD tends to emerge when strategic monitoring demands of the tasks are high (Kliegel, Altgassen, Hering, & Rose, 2011), impairments can be observed on both focal (low demand) and nonfocal cue (high demand) tasks (Costa et al., 2015). Assessment of prospective memory in clinical settings will likely assume greater importance given the important role of this type of memory in the execution of activities of daily living (Costa et al., 2015).

Findings with respect to nondeclarative memory in PD are inconsistent and this form of memory is rarely assessed in clinical contexts. In general, studies have reported preserved priming in PD without dementia (Filoteo et al., 2003) and even in PDD (Kuzis et al., 1999). Impairments on procedural memory tasks (which require the acquisition of perceptual, motor, or cognitive skills through exposure to an activity that is constrained by certain rules) may be found only in a subset of patients or be task specific, although impairments tend to be found on tasks that require learning from feedback and especially positive feedback or reward (Foerde & Shohamy, 2011).

Mild Cognitive Impairment in Parkinson's Disease

MCI is conceptualized in the traditional sense as a transition state between normal cognition and dementia, but it is important to recall that some patients with MCI never progress to dementia. With the evolution of the concept of MCI from a mild memory impairment to impairment in single or multiple cognitive domains (which may or may not include memory; see Petersen, 2011), the relevance of MCI to PD increased. The notion of a cognitive syndrome such as MCI is of particular relevance when evaluating the presence or absence of cognitive impairments in the individual, rather than differences between various patient or control groups, and in determining risk factors for decline, protective factors against decline, and the efficacy of treatment (Schmand & Tröster, 2015). Early studies of MCI frequently used *mild* as an adjective rather than referring to a specific syndrome, and when referring to a syndrome used inconsistent definitions and ascertainment methods. Consequently, preliminary research criteria (Tröster, 2011) and formal clinical criteria for PD-MCI (see Table 22.3) were proposed. Whereas the research criteria involve two sets of criteria differing on the basis of the probability that the MCI is attributable to PD versus a comorbid condition, the clinical criteria require a judgment that the impairment is due to PD. However, the clinical criteria involve two levels of ascertainment (varying in extent of neuropsychological assessment), with the more extensive Level II assessment allowing subtyping of MCI and greater confidence of MCI presence/absence. It is emphasized that the criteria were intended to lead to research that would address their utility and potential revision. Furthermore, rather than specifying a specific test cutoff score or test for identification of MCI, latitude was incorporated into the criteria as regards extent of deficit (test scores of one to two standard deviations below the mean) and the standard against which the deficit was defined (e.g., normative vs. relative to estimated premorbid functioning) specifically to facilitate clinical use and judgment.

Research evaluating the new criteria has just begun to be published, and findings are exclusively based on retrospective analyses. This initial research suggests that the criteria have good interrater reliability (kappa = 0.91) (Broeders et al., 2013), but often identify a higher rate of MCI (33%–62% using Level II criteria; see Goldman et al., 2013; Marras et al., 2013) and especially multidomain MCI (65%–97% of those with MCI) than might be anticipated on the basis of studies completed prior to publication of the criteria (Broeders et al., 2013; Marras et al., 2013). Concern has been expressed that persons diagnosed with PD-MCI might show a high reversion rate to normal over two years (25% among multidomain PD-MCI) (Loftus et al., 2015) and three years (22%) (Pedersen, Larsen, Tysnes, & Alves, 2013). However, a study carefully applying level II criteria found reversion rates of only 8.5% between baseline and Year 3 and 6% between Year 3 and Year 5 follow-up (Broeders et al., 2013). Furthermore, even in one of the studies reporting high reversion rates, the rate was only 9% if MCI had been consistently diagnosed in consecutive years (Pedersen et al., 2013). Although the criteria will require further study,

Table 22.3 PD-MCI criteria and assessment strategies based on Movement Disorder Society Task Force Guidelines (Litvan et al., 2012)

Inclusion Criteria	*Exclusion Criteria*
• Diagnosis of PD per UK PD Brain Bank Criteria • Gradual cognitive decline reported by patient, informant, or observed by clinician • Cognitive decline evident on neuropsychological testing and/or PD–appropriate cognitive screening instrument or global cognitive measure • Cognitive decline may make activities of daily living more effortful or challenging but does not compromise functional independence	• Diagnosis of dementia • Other potential explanation for impairment (e.g., medication, medical condition) • Conditions comorbid with PD that impact neuropsychological test performance (e.g., motor impairment, fatigue, psychosis)
Level I-Abbreviated assessment	*Level II-Comprehensive assessment*
• Impairment on PD-appropriate global cognitive ability scale (e.g., DRS) • Impairment on at least two neuropsychological tests when a limited set of tests is used (fewer than two tests per domain or fewer than five cognitive domains assessed)	• Neuropsychological testing includes two tests per domain (attention and working memory, executive functions, language, memory, and visuospatial skills) • Impairment on two tests in one domain or impairment on one test in two different domains • Impairment shown by score 1–2 SD below norms, or significant decline on serial testing, or significant decline from estimated premorbid functioning
PD-MCI Subtype classification (comprehensive, Level II assessment required)	
• Single domain: impairment on two tests in one domain • Multiple domain: impairment on at least one test in each of two or more domains	

and the diagnosis of multidomain MCI may benefit from stricter or more conservative criteria (e.g., impairments on two tests in each of two or more domains rather than on only one test in each domain), they do seem to have utility in identifying heightened risk for dementia. Among newly diagnosed patients, 14%–17% of those with MCI developed dementia within two-year epochs across the five-year follow-up (Broeders et al., 2013) and in another study of newly diagnosed, initially drug-naive patients, 27% of MCI developed dementia within three years versus 1% of those without MCI (Pedersen et al., 2013).

Mood, Affect, and Psychiatric Disturbances in Parkinson's Disease

The most recent version of the *Diagnostic and Statistical Manual of Mental Disorders* (DSM-5; American Psychiatric Association, 2013) contains within the categories of depressive, anxiety, and schizophrenia spectrum and other psychotic disorders those caused by another medical condition (such as PD). Adjustment reactions (such as those that might be precipitated by diagnosis of a chronic illness or discrete, related stressors) are classified under trauma and stressor-related disorders. Impulse control disorders, receiving increasing attention in PD, are not formally classified except for gambling. Within the disorders caused by another medical condition, there is within DSM-5 less specification than for the same disorders not attributable to a medical condition. For example, although the DSM-IV criteria for major depression, minor depression, and dysthymia were deemed to be applicable to PD (Starkstein et al., 2008), within DSM-5 depressive disorders due to a medical condition only allow specification of either the presence of depressive features, major depressive-like episode, or mixed features (of mania or hypomania). Similarly, anxiety disorders due to a general medical condition are not subtyped as corresponding to generalized anxiety or one of the phobias, although there is a separate category due to a medical condition within the obsessive-compulsive and related disorders. The impact of these classifications on the accuracy of prevalence and incidence estimates, as well as treatment implications remain to be empirically evaluated. Pre-DSM-5 studies observed that despite a depression prevalence of up to 50% among persons with PD (McDonald, Richard, & DeLong, 2003; Reijnders, Ehrt, Weber, Aarsland, & Leentjens, 2008; Slaughter, Slaughter, Nichols, Holmes, & Martens, 2001) and anxiety in almost 50% (Pontone et al., 2009), these conditions may go underrecognized (Shulman, Taback, Rabinstein, & Weiner, 2002) and undertreated (Weintraub, Moberg, Duda, Katz, & Stern, 2003).

Depression

Incidence and prevalence rates of depression in PD are considerably higher in research centers than in community samples (about 50% vs. 10%). Among patients with depression, about half have a minor mood disturbance while the other half meet diagnostic criteria for major depression. Even among early, still untreated PD patients, significant depressive symptoms may be evident in almost 15% (Weintraub, Simuni, et al., 2015). Nonetheless, suicide is uncommon (below 0.1%), and is tenfold lower in PD than among the elderly in general (Myslobodsky, Lalonde, & Hicks, 2001) per National Center for Health Statistics data, although higher rates have been reported in small cohort studies.

Assessment and diagnosis of depression in PD is complicated by symptom overlap in depression and PD (Marsh & Dobkin, 2015). For example, sleep disturbance, psychomotor retardation, lack of energy, stooped posture, masked facial expression, dry mouth, and sexual dysfunction can be observed in both conditions. Whilst some have suggested that early morning awakening, anergia, and psychomotor slowing not be considered when diagnosing depression in PD (Starkstein, Bolduc, Mayberg, Preziosi, & Robinson, 1990), a National Institutes of Health (NIH) workgroup recommended attribution of overlapping somatic and neurovegetative symptoms to depression rather than PD (Marsh, McDonald, Cummings, & Ravina, 2006). Because depression and PD symptoms overlap, self-report and rating instruments probably overestimate depression in PD. Attempts to address this issue include the evaluation of various depression scales in PD and the development of cutoff scores to screen for and diagnose depression specifically in PD (Table 22.4). A comparison of nine scales using modified cutoffs found that all of the scales using modified cutoffs provided adequate sensitivity and specificity in screening for depression but that the 30-item Geriatric Depression

Table 22.4 Self-report and rating scales with empirically modified cutoff scores to detect depression in PD (Tröster et al., 2013)

Scale (Reference)	*Number of Items; Maximum Score; Traditional Cutoff (*)*	*PD Cutoffs Recommended By:*	*Recommended Cutoff to Distinguish Depressed vs. Nondepressed PD (Sensitivity/Specificity)*	*Recommended Screening Cutoff for PD (Sensitivity/Specificity)*	*Recommended Diagnostic Cutoff for PD (Sensitivity/Specificity)*
Beck Depression Inventory (Beck, Ward, Mendelson, Mock, & Erbaugh, 1961)	21 items; maximum = 63 10 = mild 12 = moderate 30 = severe	Leentjens, Verhey, Luijckx, and Troost (2000)	13/14 (0.67/0.88)	8/9 (0.92/0.59)	16/17 (0.42/0.98)
Hamilton Rating Scale for Depression (17-item) (Hamilton, 1960)	17 items; maximum = 50 8 = mild 14 = moderate 19 = severe 23 = very severe 24 items	Leentjens, Verhey, Lousberg, Spitsbergen, and Wilmink (2000); Naarding, Leentjens, Van Kooten, and Verhey (2002); Dissanayaka et al. (2007); Weintraub, Oehlberg, Katz, and Stern (2006)	13/14 (0.88/0.89) 12/13 (0.80/0.92) 12/13 (0.89/0.93) 9/10 (0.88/0.78)	11/12 (0.94/0.75) 9/10 (0.95/0.98) NA NA	16/17 (0.75/0.98) 15/16 (0.99/0.93) 18/19 (1.00/0.99) NA
Hamilton Depression Inventory (17-item) (Reynolds & Kobak, 1995)	17 items; maximum = 52	Dissanayaka et al. (2007)	13.5/14 (0.78/0.90)	NA	15.5/16 (0.89/0.93)
Geriatric Depression Scale (15-item) (Sheikh & Yesavage, 1986)	15 items; maximum = 15	Weintraub et al. (2006); Dissanayaka et al. (2007);	4/5 (0.88/0.85) 6/7 (0.89/0.87)	NA NA	NA 8/9 (0.89/0.87)
Geriatric Depression Scale (30-item) (Yesavage et al., 1983)	30 items; maximum = 30 10 = mild 20 = severe	Mondolo et al. (2006)	10/11 (1.00/0.76)	10/11 (1.00/0.76)	12/13 (0.80/0.85)
Montgomery-Åsberg Depression Rating Scale (Montgomery & Asberg, 1979)	10 items; maximum = 60 15 = mild 25 = moderate 31 = severe 44 = very severe	Leentjens, Verhey, Lousberg, et al. (2000)	14/15 (0.88/0.89)	14/15 (0.88/0.89)	17/18 (0.63/0.94)
Hospital Anxiety and Depression Scale (Zigmond & Snaith, 1983)	Depression subscale; 7 items; maximum = 21 8 = mild 11 = severe	Mondolo et al. (2006)	10/11 (1.00/0.95)	10/11 (1.00/0.95)	11/12 (0.80/0.98)

Scale (GDS) may be favored given its brevity, psychometric properties, and availability in the public domain (Williams et al., 2012).

The treatment of depression is of great importance in PD given its considerable impact on quality of life of the patient (Hinnell et al., 2012) and caregiver (Aarsland, Larsen, Karlsen, Lim, & Tandberg, 1999), and because depression exacerbates cognitive impairment (Fernandez et al., 2009; Troster et al., 1995; Tröster, Prizer, & Baxley, 2013). Furthermore, depression hastens progression to disability (Cole et al., 1996) and increases health care utilization (Chen et al., 2007). Despite widespread use of selective serotonin reuptake inhibitors in PD, it is only relatively recently that adequately sized, randomized clinical trials have supported the use in PD depression of agents targeting serotonin and/or norepinephrine, such as desipramine (Devos et al., 2008), nortriptyline (Menza et al., 2009), citalopram (Devos et al., 2008), venlafaxine (Richard et al., 2012), and paroxetine (Menza et al., 2009; Richard et al., 2012). Nonetheless, long-term treatment effects remain unknown. Literature concerning the benefit of depression treatment on cognition remains inconclusive per a meta-analysis (Price et al., 2011). However, preliminary evidence suggests that executive dysfunction predicts response to antidepressant treatment (Dobkin et al., 2010). Psychological interventions for depression in PD remain understudied, but preliminary evidence affords support for the effectiveness of cognitive behavioral therapy (Dobkin et al., 2011; Veazey, Cook, Stanley, Lai, & Kunik, 2009), which may also afford modest improvements in verbal memory and executive function (Dobkin et al., 2014). In the case of cognitive behavioral therapy too, baseline executive function may be predictive of treatment response.

Anxiety

Probably about 50% of patients with PD have significant symptoms of anxiety, and as many as 75% of those patients with PD *and* depression may have a comorbid anxiety disorder (Schiffer, Kurlan, Rubin, & Boer, 1988). Among early, untreated patients, questionnaire assessment indicates clinically remarkable anxiety symptoms in about 20% of persons (Weintraub, Simuni, et al., 2015). However, the reported prevalence of actual anxiety disorders (vs. symptoms) in PD ranges from 5% to 40% (Walsh & Bennett, 2001). Stein, Heuser, Juncos, and Uhde (1990) found that almost 20% of PD patients had generalized anxiety and 20% had a social phobia, while 16% to 20% experience significant social anxiety (Bolluk, Ozel-Kizil, Akbostanci, & Atbasoglu, 2010), and recurrent panic attacks may occur in up to 24% of patients treated with levodopa (Vazquez, Jimenez-Jimenez, Garcia-Ruiz, & Garcia-Urra, 1993). Although patients with PD rarely meet the full DSM criteria for obsessive-compulsive disorder (OCD) (about 3%; see Nuti et al., 2004), a considerable number have symptoms of OCD. The severity of OCD symptoms may be greater later in the disease (Alegret, Junqué, et al., 2001) and associated with severity of left-sided motor symptoms (Tomer & Levin, 1993). Such symptoms may be more common in familial parkinsonism (Lauterbach & Duvoisin, 1991).

As was true for depression, diagnosis of an anxiety disorder in PD is hindered by symptom overlap between PD and anxiety disorders. Unfortunately, the validity and reliability of anxiety rating instruments have not been widely studied. In evaluating the Beck Anxiety Inventory (BAI) and Profile of Mood States (POMS), Higginson, Fields, Koller, and Tröster. (2001) found that, among 59 patients, the two instruments yielded scores associated with clinical anxiety in 54% and 63% of patients, respectively. Although these rates are higher than that of the clinical diagnosis of anxiety (38%) based on interview (Stein et al., 1990), elimination of symptom inventory items reflecting manifestations of autonomic and neurophysiologic function was not advised as it was felt that this would lead to underestimation of anxiety in PD. Other symptom inventories that have been used to assess various aspects of anxiety in PD include the State-Trait Anxiety Inventory, Profile of Mood States, Hospital Anxiety and Depression Scale, Maudsley Obsessional-Compulsive Inventory, and the Yale-Brown Obsessive Compulsive Scale. Scales recommended for use in PD by the International Parkinson and Movement Disorders Society are listed in Table 22.5. In addition, a scale for specific use in PD, the Parkinson Anxiety Scale (PAS; see Leentjens et al., 2014) has undergone initial validation (Forjaz et al., 2015).

Apathy

Apathy refers to a diminution of motivation and a reduction in interest, emotion, and goal-directed behavior. Unlike persons with depression, those with apathy typically are not distressed by this condition. Apathy can occur together with depression or cognitive impairment (most often executive deficits), or as an independent phenomenon. A meta-analysis of 23 studies estimated that about 40% of individuals with PD have apathy, but that almost half of those have no associated depression or cognitive compromise (den Brok et al., 2015). The study identified increasing age, disability, depression, more severe motor symptoms, and cognitive impairment to be associated with apathy. One recent model conceives of apathy as involving four domains that in isolation and overlap produce the clinical behavioral syndrome: a reward deficiency component (best treated with dopamine agonists, bupropion, methylphenidate), emotional distress/negative affect (best treated with antidepressants), executive dysfunction (best treated with cholinesterase inhibitors), and an autoactivation deficit or psychic akinesia (responsive to dopamine agonists) (Pagonabarraga, Kulisevsky, Strafella, & Krack, 2015).

Table 22.5 Movement Disorder Society (MDS) recommended and suggested rating scales for the assessment of neuropsychological and psychiatric features of PD

	Recommended Scales (Stronger Evidence)	*Suggested Scales (Weaker Evidence)*
Depression (Schrag et al., 2007)	Screening (and recommended cutoff in PD): Hamilton Depression Rating Scale (HAM-D, 9/10); Beck Depression Inventory (BDI, 13/14); Hospital Anxiety and Depression Scale (HADS, 10/11); Montogomery-Asberg Depression Rating Scale (MADRS; 14/15); Geriatric Depression Scale (GDS-30: 9/10; GDS-15: 4/5)	For patients with dementia (though insufficient evidence): MADRS; GDS; Cornell Scale for Depression in Dementia (CSDD, 5/6)
Anxiety (Leentjens et al., 2008a)	None	Beck Anxiety Inventory (BAI), HADS, Zung Self-Rated Anxiety Scale (Zung SAS), Zung Anxiety Status Inventory (Zung ASI), State-Trait Anxiety Inventory (STAI), Hamilton Anxiety Rating Scale (HARS), Neuropsychiatric Inventory (NPI) anxiety section
Apathy and anhedonia (Leentjens et al., 2008b)	Apathy Scale (Starkstein et al., 1992) (screening cutoff 13/14); Unified Parkinson's Disease Rating Scale (UPDRS) Item 4 (motivation/initiative) (screening cutoff 2/3)	Apathy Evaluation Scale (AES) (Marin, Biedrzycki, & Firinciogullari, 1991) (screening cutoff 38/39); Lille Apathy Rating Scale (LARS) (screening cutoff 16/17); Neuropsychiatric Inventory (NPI) Item 7; Snaith-Hamilton Pleasure Scale (SHAPS) (screening cutoff 2/3)
Psychosis (Fernandez et al., 2008)	Neuropsychiatric Inventory (NPI); Brief Psychiatric Rating Scale (BPRS); Positive and Negative Syndrome Scale (PANNS); Schedule for Assessment of Positive Symptoms (SAPS)	Parkinson Psychosis Rating Scale (PPRS); Parkinson Psychosis Questionnaire (PPQ); Behavioral Pathology in Alzheimer's Disease Rating Scale (Behave-AD); Clinical Global Impression Scale (CGIS)
Sleep disturbances (Hogl et al., 2010)	*Daytime sleepiness*: Epworth Sleepiness Scale (ESS) *Overall sleep impairment*: Parkinson's Disease Sleep Scale (PDSS); Pittsburgh Sleep Quality Index (PSQI); Scales for Outcomes in Parkinson's Disease (SCOPA-Sleep)	*Daytime sleepiness*: Inappropriate Sleep Composite Score (ISCS); Stanford Sleepiness Scale (SSS)
Fatigue (Friedman et al., 2010)	Fatigue Severity Scale (for severity and screening); Multidimensional Fatigue Inventory (for severity); Parkinson's Fatigue Scale (for screening); Functional Assessment of Chronic Illness Therapy—Fatigue Scale (for screening)	Multidimensional Fatigue Inventory (for screening); Fatigue Assessment Inventory (for severity and screening); Functional Assessment of Chronic Illness Therapy—Fatigue Scale (for severity); Parkinson's Fatigue Scale (for severity); Fatigue Impact Scale for Daily Use (for severity)

Impulsive and Related Behaviors

In the DOMINION study, involving more than 3,000 individuals with PD, impulse control disorders (ICDs) were estimated to occur in about 14% (Weintraub et al., 2010). These disorders include excessive gambling, eating, shopping, dopaminergic medication use, and hypersexuality (Voon, 2015; Weintraub, David, Evans, Grant, & Stacy, 2015; Weintraub & Goldman, 2015). Some also include under this rubric compulsive behaviors such as punding (simple prolonged, purposeless, and stereotyped behaviors such as sorting buttons), hobbyism (excessive time spent on complex, goal-directed behaviors such as assembling model airplanes), and walkabout (aimless wandering). The overuse of dopaminergic medications in PD was initially referred to as *hedonistic homeostatic dysregulation syndrome* (Giovannoni, O'Sullivan, Turner, Manson, & Lees, 2000a) but the term *dopaminergic dysregulation syndrome* has also been used (Evans & Lees, 2004). Risk factors for ICDs include use of dopamine agonists (almost threefold risk) or levodopa use (1.5-fold risk) (Weintraub et al., 2010). Other risk factors have been more extensively studied for gambling than other ICDs, but they include being younger, single, male, having a family history of pathological gambling, and having a personal or family history of alcohol use (Voon, 2015). Females seem more likely than males to engage in impulsive eating and buying (Weintraub, David, et al., 2015). A scale has been developed for assessment of ICDs and related behaviors in PD, namely the Questionnaire for Impulsive-Compulsive Disorders in Parkinson's disease (QUIP) (Weintraub et al., 2009) and its derivative, the briefer QUIP-RS (Weintraub et al., 2012). Treatment usually involves withdrawal or reduction of the offending medication, although cognitive behavioral therapy may also be beneficial (Okai et al., 2013).

Several studies have explored neuropsychological functions in patients with PD and impulsive behaviors, and a review indicates that these studies have revealed deficits in executive functions, increased risk taking, novelty seeking, enhanced learning based on gain versus loss, and altered reward–punishment learning (Aarsland, Taylor, & Weintraub, 2014).

Psychosis

Typically, psychosis presents as delusions and hallucinations and occurs in about one-third of persons with PD (although hallucinations are far more common than delusions, the latter affecting only about 5%–10% of treated patients; see Fenelon & Alves, 2010). Most often hallucinations are visual, well-formed, and nonthreatening to the patient, but hallucinations can occur in all sensory modalities, particularly later in the disease course (Goetz, Stebbins, & Ouyang, 2011). Later in the disease course, patients may lose insight that hallucinations are not real. Psychosis impacts patient quality of life, hastens institutionalization, increases risk of mortality, and increases care-partner stress (Weintraub & Goldman, 2015). Furthermore, hallucinators tend to have poorer attention and executive and visuospatial functioning than patients without hallucinations (Tröster et al., 2013; Weintraub & Goldman, 2015).

The proposed criteria for PD-associated psychosis (Ravina et al., 2007) extend the definition of psychosis to include more minor phenomena such as illusions (misperceptions such as perceiving a fire hydrant as a dog) and a sense of presence (someone being close by when there is no one). In addition, passage phenomena (i.e., peripheral visual phenomena of moving persons and animals) are considered minor visual hallucinations. Treatment with dopaminergic medications is neither a necessary nor sufficient condition for psychosis in PD, but in treatment, the most likely offending agent may be tapered. Preferred for treatment of psychosis in PD are atypical antipsychotics (e.g., quetiapine) that act predominantly by serotonergic antagonism rather than dopamine receptor blockade that aggravates the movement disorder. Nonpharmacologic treatment strategies for hallucinations (nightlights, reassurance, coping techniques) have also been suggested (Diederich, Pieri, & Goetz, 2003). Several scales have been recommended by MDS for the assessment of psychosis in PD (see Table 22.5) (Fernandez et al., 2008) although none specifically is designed for use in PD.

Case Examples: Parkinson's Disease and Parkinson's Disease With Dementia

Neuropsychological test results for a PD patient without dementia are presented in Table 22.6. This 74-year-old, White male with 12 years of education had worked full-time as a motorcycle mechanic until he retired at age 65 years, 3 years after being diagnosed with PD. He had continued to work part-time until a year before the evaluation. Medications included levodopa, entacapone, and pramipexole. He acknowledged disability due to physical limitations, but he and his family denied changes in activities of daily living related to cognitive decline. Psychiatric illness was denied.

His neuropsychological test results are chosen for presentation because they are atypical of the traditional "subcortical" profile expected in PD, yet reflect a cognitive profile that is not uncommon (see earlier discussion of heterogeneity of memory profiles in PD). His executive function is intact: indeed, the patient performed very well on the Wisconsin Card Sorting task, and in the average range on the DRS

Table 22.6 Neuropsychological profile of a patient with PD

Test	*Raw Score*	*T-Score or %ile*
WAIS III		
Information	22	60
Similarities	25	60
Digit Span	14	47
Letter-Number Sequencing	11	60
Arithmetic	12	50
Digit Symbol	33	37
Symbol Search	17	43
DRS 2		
Attention	37	60
Initiation/Perseveration	26	27
Construction	6	50
Conceptualization	37	50
Memory	22	43
Total	128	37
Trail Making Test		
Part A	39	50
Part B	118	47
Stroop (Golden)		
Word	90	48
Color	63	46
Color-Word	31	51
Interference	+3	53
WCST (64)		
Total Errors	24	46
Perseverative Responses	6	68
Perseverative Errors	6	68
Categories	2	>16%ile
Trials to Complete First Category	12	>16%ile
Letter Fluency	27	42
Category Fluency	26	66
Boston Naming Test	59	70
Finger Tapping		
Dominant	47	49
Nondominant	44	46
Hopkins Verbal Learning Test–Revised		
Total Recall Trials 1–3	20	44
Delayed Recall	0	19
Percent Retention	0	19
Discrimination Index	7	32
Brief Visuospatial Memory Test–Revised		
Total Recall Trials 1–3	8	29
Delayed Recall	6	43
Percent Retention	150	>16%ile
Discrimination Index	+5	>16%ile
Beck Depression Inventory	9	

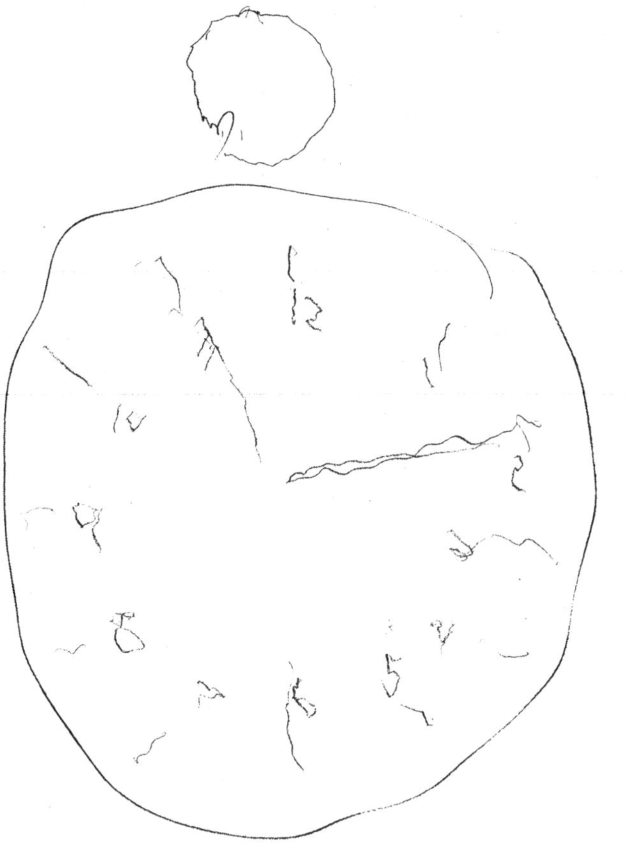

Figure 22.3 Drawing-to-command of a clock by a patient with PD. When asked to draw a clock, to include all the numbers, and set the hands at 10 minutes after 11, the patient initially drew a small circle. The small circle drawn initially may reflect poor foresight and planning. When asked to draw a big clock face, the patient had little difficulty. Although tremor is evident, the numbers are correct, well spaced, and the hands correctly placed allowing for tremor.

Conceptualization scale. Letter fluency is low average and weaker than category fluency (well above average), which is seen in PD. Visual confrontation naming is well preserved, as is praxis (see Figure 22.3). Striking is the patient's poor performance on learning and memory tests. On the list learning task his immediate recall across learning trials is average, but delayed recall is impaired. Though recognition is better than recall it is not intact. In contrast, on a visual learning task, his immediate recall of the figures across trials is poor, yet delayed recall and recognition are intact. Given the intact praxis, category fluency, and visual confrontation naming, coupled with no decline in activities of daily living, the possibility of AD is remote. DLB is unlikely given a lack of fluctuation in cognition, absence of hallucinations, a long course of PD with minimal cognitive impairment and extended employment, and the relative preservation of visuospatial and attentional functions.

Table 22.7 Neuropsychological profile of a patient with PDD

TEST	*Raw Score*	*T-Score or %ile*
WAIS-III		
Information	23	60
Similarities	23	53
Digit Span	18	53
Letter-Number Sequencing	10	53
Arithmetic	9	40
Digit Symbol	44	40
Symbol Search	12	33
DRS-2		
Attention	35	50
Initiation/Perseveration	37	53
Construction	5	40
Conceptualization	30	37
Memory	22	40
Total	129	37
Trail Making Test		
Part A	26	55
Part B	147	35
Stroop (Golden)		
Word	75	38
Color	38	25
Color-Word	20	30
Interference	−3	47
WCST (64)		
Total Errors	33	32
Perseverative Responses	19	37
Perseverative Errors	18	35
Categories	2	11–16%ile
Trials to Complete First Category	14	>16%ile
Letter Fluency	55	62
Animal Naming	20	49
Boston Naming Test	55	
Finger Tapping		
Dominant	55	57
Nondominant	52	57
Hopkins Verbal Learning Test-Rev.		
Total Recall Trials 1–3	14	19
Delayed Recall	7	33
Percent Retention	100	55
Discrimination Index	9	37
Brief Visuospatial Memory Test-Rev.		
Total Recall Trials 1–3	10	24
Delayed Recall	4	26
Percent Retention	80	11–16
Discrimination Index	+6	>16
Beck Depression Inventory	17	

The neuropsychological test results of a patient with PD (early onset) and dementia are presented in Table 22.7. This 55-year-old White male with two years of college education had had symptoms of PD for 11 years and complained of increasing concentration problems and forgetfulness for the two years before evaluation. He acknowledged occasionally failing to pay bills, but denied other distressing memory changes. His wife, in contrast, considered his cognitive deficits as interfering significantly with ability to carry out instrumental ADLs. Though his current mood was described as good, the patient acknowledged past depression with suicidal ideation but without plan or intent. He described improved mood since treated with sertraline. He had a history of treatment for posttraumatic stress disorder in the remote past. Hallucinations, delusions, and fluctuating levels of cognition were denied. Anti-Parkinsonian medications included levodopa and pramipexole. He demonstrated difficulty on tasks demanding of working memory, divided and selective attention, and information processing speed (WAIS-III: Arithmetic, Digit Symbol, Symbol Search, Trail Making Part B, and all parts of the Stroop, though susceptibility to interference was normal). While he demonstrated executive dysfunction (DRS and WCST), more pronounced was his difficulty learning and retaining new information. Visual confrontation naming and verbal fluency were preserved. He also has dramatic difficulty with clock drawing (see Figures 22.4, 22.5, and 22.6). His apparently rapid decline in cognition over two years, coupled with

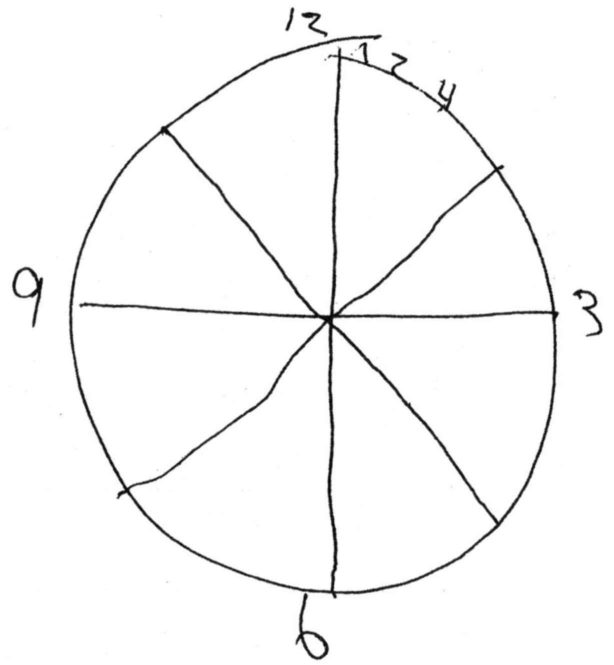

Figure 22.4 Drawing-to-command of a clock by a patient with PD and dementia. When asked to draw a clock, to include all the numbers, and set the hands at 10 minutes after 11, the patient drew a circular clock face and correctly placed the number 3, 6, 9, and 12. Despite guiding his attempt to place other numbers by drawing additional diameter lines, he misplaced the 4, then realized this error and made a new attempt at drawing the clock (see Figure 22.4)

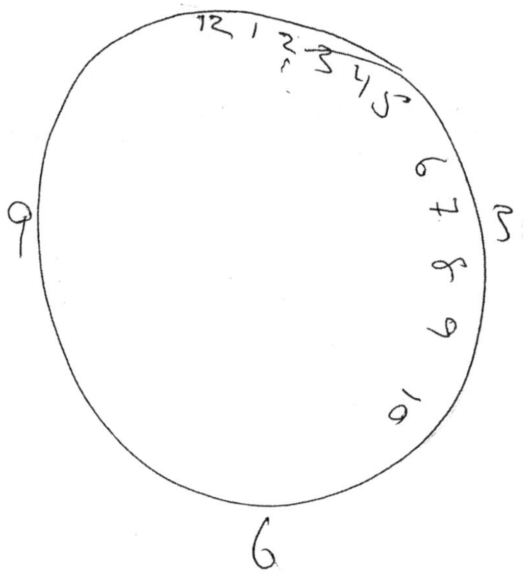

Figure 22.5 The PD with dementia patient's second attempt at drawing a clock to command. After placing the 12 inside the clock face, the patient places the 3, 6, and 9 outside the clock face. Without the guidance of the diameter lines he drew previously (see Figure 22.3), he simply places the remaining numbers incorrectly within the right half of the clock face. This reveals stimulus-bound behavior and loss of a detailed concept of how a clock face looks.

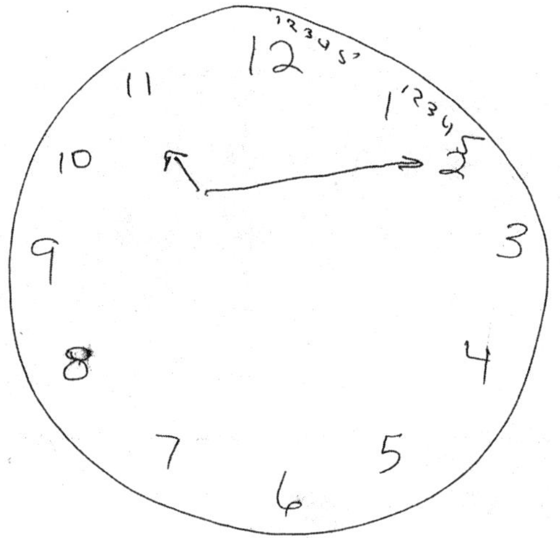

Figure 22.6 Clock drawing of the patient with PDD. Even after the examiner draws the clock face and places the numbers on the clock face, the patient has difficulty setting the hands to show "10 after 11." The hands do not originate in the center of the clock face and the size discrepancy between the big and small hands is excessive. Again, a conceptual loss is evident—the patient no longer "knows," or no longer has a representation of the gestalt, that the big hand at the "2" reflects the passage of 10 minutes past the hour. He compensates for this loss by inserting two five-minute depictions between the numbers 12 and 2 (revealing that he still knows that five minutes elapse when the big hand moves from one number to the next).

pronounced learning and recall, attention, and visuoconstructional deficits superimposed on milder executive dysfunction and bradyphrenia, suggests a possible AD-related dementia superimposed upon the cognitive deficits observed in PD.

Neuropsychological Evaluation in the Differential Diagnosis of Parkinson's Disease With Dementia and Dementia With Lewy Bodies

While group comparisons of cognitive profiles associated with various dementias and movement disorders (e.g., AD, DLB, PDD, and progressive supranuclear palsy) are helpful in highlighting the similarities and differences among these profiles, and thus in suggesting etiologies and neural bases of cognitive disturbances, the diagnostic sensitivity and specificity of cognitive profiles remains largely unknown. Group comparisons of AD and DLB have yielded rather consistent findings, although it should be borne in mind that probably more studies have compared AD and DLB with coexisting AD pathology rather than pure cases of DLB. Generally, these comparisons reveal that AD is characterized by more prominent memory impairment, especially rapid forgetting and poor recognition (Hamilton et al., 2004) whereas DLB is associated with more pronounced visuoperceptual, attentional, and verbal fluency impairments (Aarsland, Litvan, et al., 2003; Connor et al., 1998; Galasko, Katzman, Salmon, & Hansen, 1996; Gnanalingham, Byrne, Thornton, Sambrook, & Bannister, 1997; Sahgal et al., 1992; Salmon & Galasko, 1996; Salmon et al., 1996; Shimomura et al., 1998; Walker, Allen, Shergill, & Katona, 1997). Although sensitivity and specificity of neuropsychological tests in differential diagnosis of AD and DLB has rarely been addressed, one study reported that poor naming (Boston Naming Test) and rapid forgetting (on the Auditory Verbal Learning Test) pointed toward an AD diagnosis, whereas poor Rey-Osterrieth figure copy and poor Trail Making Part A performance (processing speed) pointed to a diagnosis of DLB. These tests in tandem differentiated AD and DLB with 83% sensitivity and 91% specificity (Ferman et al., 2006).

Comparisons between DLB and PDD using neuropsychological rather than cognitive screening measures are rarer. Interpretation of Gnanalingham et al.'s (1997) finding of more pronounced attentional and frontal function impairments in DLB than PD is difficult because the DLB group demonstrated greater overall cognitive impairment than the PD group. However, similar findings were reported by Downes et al. (1998), who matched DLB and PDD groups for age, education, estimated premorbid IQ, and overall severity of cognitive impairment (MMSE score). DLB demonstrated more severe impairments than PDD on tasks involving attention and working memory (WAIS-R Arithmetic, Stroop), and verbal fluency (letter, category, and alternating fluency). Although the greater attention impairment in DLB than PDD may be associated with the fluctuating level of cognition observed in DLB (Walker et al., 2000), not all studies find this attentional impairment. Employing computerized simple and choice reaction time and vigilance tasks, Ballard et al. (2002) failed to demonstrate differences in attention between DLB and PDD. Noe et al. (2004) also failed to observe any neuropsychological differences between PDD and DLB groups equated for overall severity of dementia, though they did replicate others' findings of greater memory impairment in AD than DLB and PDD, and greater attention, visuoperceptual, and constructional deficits in DLB than AD. The similarities between PDD and DLB cognitive and behavioral profiles may be even more accentuated when PDD patients develop cognitive fluctuations (Varanese et al., 2010). Although specific aspects of test performance may differ between DLB and PDD—such as increased perseverations in PDD but more severe overall memory impairment and faster forgetting in DLB on list learning tests (Filoteo et al., 2009)—such findings remain to be replicated, especially in longitudinal studies because the test-retest reliability of more fine grained learning and memory parameters may be less than optimal. Before neuropsychological findings can be used with confidence in differential diagnosis, large prospective studies will need to evaluate their predictive power, sensitivity, and specificity. Although other differences in the clinical phenotypes of PDD and DLB exist to support the separation of these disorders (Goldman et al., 2014), it appears that neuropsychological features are less helpful in supporting the distinction between DLB and PDD, except perhaps for showing differences in the time course when cognitive and motor features occur in the two conditions.

Neurobehavioral Impact of Pharmacological Treatments

Table 22.8 lists the medications most often used to treat PD and their possible adverse and beneficial neurobehavioral effects. Agents that augment dopamine (levodopa) or act as dopamine agonists all have the potential to cause psychotic symptoms such as hallucinations and delusions as well as sleep disturbance. The non-ergot-- dopamine agonists in particular may be associated with somnolence. While levodopa does not have a convincing or clinically significant antidepressant effect in PD, it can impact mood, either through its administration or withdrawal. For example, acute infusions of levodopa reduce anxiety and dysphoria in patients with motor fluctuations when they are in the "off" state. In addition, some dopamine agonists have been noted to elevate mood. Hedonistic homeostatic dysregulation syndrome (Giovannoni, O'Sullivan, Turner, Manson, & Lees, 2000b) or dopamine dysregulation syndrome (Lawrence, Evans, & Lees, 2003), is associated with dopamine replacement therapy.

Findings concerning the impact of levodopa on cognition are inconsistent and reveal both positive and negative effects (Cools, 2006). Levodopa probably has at least short-term

Table 22.8 Possible neurobehavioral effects of medications commonly used in the treatment of PD

Drug Category	*Generic Name(s)*	*Trade Name(s)*	*Possible Neurobehavioral Adverse Effects in PD*	*Possible Neurobehavioral Therapeutic Effects in PD*
Dopamine Replacement				
	Levodopa + carbidopa	Sinemet Atamet	Hallucinations, delusions, euphoria, confusion, depression, anxiety, agitation, nightmares; hedonistic homeostatic dysregulation syndrome (Giovannoni et al., 2000b); hypomania/mania (Maier et al., 2014); cognitive ("frontal") effects vary by disease stage	May improve working memory early in disease (Costa et al., 2003); may improve dysphoria; may improve creativity (Faust-Socher, Kenett, Cohen, Hassin-Baer, & Inzelberg, 2014)
		Rytary (combination immediate and delayed release carbidopa + levodopa in 1:4 ratio) Duodopa (enteral suspension)	Anxiety, insomnia, depression, anxiety, confusion	
Combined Dopamine Replacement and Catechol-O-methyl-transferase (***COMT***) ***Inhibitor***				
	levodopa + carbidopa + entacapone	Stalevo	Depression, psychosis, but generally unstudied due to novelty of drug	
Dopamine Agonists				
ergot alkaloids	bromocriptine	Parlodel	As for levodopa, possibly more severe; minimal effect on cognition (Cooper et al., 1993; Piccirilli et al., 1986; Weddell & Weiser, 1995)	
	pergolide	Permax	As for levodopa, possibly more severe somnolence; minimal cognitive effect (Brusa et al., 2005; Stern, Mayeux, Ilson, et al., 1984)	
non–ergot alkaloids	pramipexole	Mirapex	Similar to levodopa; fatigue, somnolence, impulse control disorder; may impair cognition (Brusa et al., 2003)	As for levodopa; antidepressant effect (Barone et al., 2006)
	ropinirole rotigotine	Requip Neupro	Similar to levodopa; fatigue, somnolence, impulse control disorder;as for other agonists	As for levodopa
COMT-Inhibitors				
	entacapone	Comtan	Hallucinations	
	tolcapone (rarely used due to liver toxicity)	Tasmar		Possible attention and memory improvement when used as adjunct to levodopa (Gasparini, Fabrizio, Bonifati, & Meco, 1997)
MAO-Inhibitors	selegiline rasagiline	Eldepryl Deprenyl Azilect	Rare confusion or hallucinations; sleepiness, depressed mood	Small, uncontrolled studies suggest possible cognitive benefits (Finali, Piccirilli, & Piccinin, 1994; Hietanen, 1991) but not confirmed in large prospective study (Kieburtz et al., 1994)
Anticholinergics	trihexyphenidyl biperiden benztropine	Artane Akineton Cogentin	Sedation, delirium, memory impairment, executive dysfunction (Bedard et al., 1999; Koller, 1984; Meco et al., 1984; Reid et al., 1992)	
Antiglutamatergics	amantadine	Symmetrel	Cognitive deficits	

effects on selected aspects of memory (specifically working memory) and executive functions in the early disease stages, and it may differentially impair functions (e.g., stimulus–stimulus associations) mediated by ventral striatum, but facilitate functions (e.g., decision making in ambiguous contexts) mediated by dorsal striatum (MacDonald et al., 2011). Kulisevsky and colleagues (2000) reported short-term improvements in learning and memory, visual perception, and select executive functions with dopamine replacement in drug-naive patients, but these improvements were not maintained. Owen et al. (1995) reported that planning accuracy was improved by levodopa therapy early in the disease, while response latency on planning tasks were unaffected. Studies of the effects of levodopa withdrawal also show only very selective and limited cognitive alterations, for example, declines in working memory (Fournet, Moreaud, Roulin, Naegele, & Pellat, 2000; Lange et al., 1992). These selective cognitive effects of levodopa may be related to its alteration of dorsolateral frontal cortical blood flow during executive task performance (Cools et al., 2002). Dopamine agonists such as pergolide (Stern, Mayeux, Ilson, et al., 1984) and bromocriptine (Cooper, Sagar, & Sullivan, 1993; Piccirilli et al., 1986; Weddell & Weiser, 1995) have limited if any cognitive effects at therapeutic doses, acutely or after chronic administration.

Catechol-O-methyl-transferase (COMT) inhibitors are used to reduce peripheral breakdown of levodopa and thereby increase the amount of levodopa reaching the brain. COMT in the brain is principally found in nonneuronal cells such as glia and is thought to be especially important in intrasynaptic dopamine regulation in the prefrontal cortex (Winterer & Goldman, 2003). One study has found that after six months of treatment with the COMT-inhibitor tolcapone (and gradually decreasing doses of levodopa) patients demonstrated better attention, memory, and constructional skills (Gasparini et al., 1997). It remains to be determined whether these cognitive improvements relate to COMT therapy directly, increased brain availability of levodopa, or a reduction in possible adverse effects of levodopa therapy.

Anticholinergic medications used to treat motor symptoms (e.g., benztropine and trihexyphenidyl) can adversely affect executive functions (Bedard et al., 1999) and memory (Koller, 1984; Meco et al., 1984; Reid et al., 1992). Anticholinergic-induced memory impairments are most likely to occur in patients with preexisting cognitive impairment (Saint-Cyr et al., 1993), and anticholinergics are to be avoided in elderly patients susceptible to confusion (Pondal, Del Ser, & Bermejo, 1996). The profound impact that anticholinergics can have on memory in PD is illustrated by the memory test results shown in Table 22.9. This patient had notable memory deficits but atypical in quality for PD (impaired delayed recall and recognition of a word list). He was tapered off anticholinergic medication (trihexyphenidyl, 2 mg, four times daily) prescribed to control tremor and reevaluated six weeks later. Memory scores improved well beyond the extent expected by practice effects alone.

Table 22.9 Cognitive screening, language, and memory test results in a patient with PD before and one month after discontinuation of anticholinergic medication

TEST	*Baseline*		*Post Medication Change*	
	Raw Score	*T-Score/ %ile*	*Raw Score*	*T-Score/ %ile*
WASI				
Full Scale IQ	89	23%ile		
DRS-2				
Attention	36	53	35	50
Initiation/Perseveration	35	43	36	50
Construction	4	33	6	50
Conceptualization	31	37	30	37
Memory	20	33	23	50
Total Score	126	33	130	40
Letter Fluency	32	49		
Animal Naming	20	59		
Boston Naming Test	55			
Wechsler Memory Scale III				
Working Memory Index	88	99		
Logical Memory I Immediate Recall	17	4	34	10
Logical Memory II Delayed Recall	8	5	20	11
Logical Memory % Retained	57	8	95	14
Facial Recognition Immediate Recall	28	7		
Facial Recognition Delayed Recall	29	8		
Facial Recognition % Retained	100	12		
California Verbal Learning Test-II				
Total Trials 1–5	27	38	32	45
Short Delay Free Recall	4	40	5	40
Long Delay Free Recall	3	35	6	40
Recognition Hits	10	25	9	25
Recognition Discriminability	.9	30	2	45

While cholinesterase inhibitors are widely used in the treatment of AD, they were initially used cautiously in PDD and DLB because they might exacerbate motor symptoms (Richard, Justus, Greig, Marshall, & Kurlan, 2002). Subsequent studies, however, suggest that cholinesterase inhibitors such as donepezil, rivastigmine, and galantamine can be safely used to ameliorate the neuropsychiatric, and to lesser extent, the cognitive symptoms in PDD and DLB (Bullock & Cameron, 2002; Kaufer, 2002; McKeith et al., 2000; Reading, Luce, & McKeith, 2001). A recent meta-analysis of the efficacy and safety of cholinesterase inhibitors and memantine in PD, PDD, and DLB concluded that memantine and cholinesterase inhibitors improve Clinician Global Impression of Change ratings, but only cholinestersase inhibitors produce positive results on the MMSE (Wang et al., 2015). Unfortunately, the analysis was based on only ten trials (four of them with 28 or fewer subjects) using different agents, outcome measures, and patient populations that limit the conclusions that can be drawn. Only one small trial included PD patients with MCI, and indeed, a Cochrane review indicated inadequate support for the use of these agents in PD without dementia, although it too supported use of cholinesterase inhibitors in PDD based on positive effects on cognition, behavior, and activities of daily living (Rolinski, Fox, Maidment, & McShane, 2012). At this time, in the United States, the only FDA-approved medication for PDD is rivastigmine.

Neurobehavioral Impact of Neurosurgical Treatments

Surgical treatments of PD, like drug treatments, are symptomatic rather than curative and fall into four broad categories: ablation, DBS, tissue transplantation, and gene therapy. Though ablative operations such as pallidotomy, thalamotomy, and subthalamotomies were carried out for PD in the 1940s and 1950s, the use of these treatments declined dramatically after the introduction of levodopa in the 1960s (Siegfried & Blond, 1997). Realization of the limitations of drug treatments, accompanied by advances in neurosurgery, radiology, and knowledge about basal ganglia physiology, prompted a renaissance of surgical treatments in the 1990s. Possible neurobehavioral consequences of various surgical procedures are summarized in Table 22.10.

Ablative procedures are far less frequently done in the United States or Europe since the advent of DBS, but retain a place in the surgical armamentarium. Early ablative interventions were associated with considerable cognitive morbidity (for review, see Tröster & Woods, 2003). Although modern unilateral ablative interventions targeting the thalamus (Hugdahl & Wester, 2000), STN (Alvarez et al., 2001; Patel et al., 2003), or GPi appear relatively safe from a cognitive perspective they are not without occasional complications affecting verbal fluency, attention, memory, and executive functions. Putative risk factors for cognitive decline after unilateral pallidotomy include cognitive impairment, age, and side of surgery (dominant hemisphere). Bilateral pallidotomy has been variously associated with minimal cognitive change, purported gains in memory, and marked cognitive deterioration. Given the perceived risk of cognitive dysfunction, bilateral pallidotomy is typically not advocated by experts, particularly since the advent of DBS.

DBS involves unilateral or bilateral implantation of electrodes and the application of high frequency electrical stimulation from an implanted pulse generator to the thalamus, GPi, or STN. Unilateral thalamic DBS appears to be well tolerated (Woods et al., 2001), but it is rarely done for PD

Table 22.10 Possible neurobehavioral effects of modern surgical interventions for PD

Procedure Type	*Target*	*Possible Adverse Effects in PD*	*Possible Beneficial Effects in PD*
Ablation			
	GPi	Confusion, depression, dypomania, cognitive, impairment (esp. after bilateral procedure)	Reduction in obsessive-compulsive symptoms
	Ventralintermediate nucleus of Thalamus (Vim)	Confusion, rare cognitive impairment	Reduction in depressive and obsessive symptoms
	STN (modern target)	Mild cognitive deficits	Not reported
DBS	GPi	Rare cognitive dysfunction, hypomania, depression	Mildly improved performance on some memory tests (probably not a true memory improvement), reduced anxiety and depressive symptoms
	Vim		Reduction in depressive symptoms, mild naming improvement
	STN	Apathy, depression (incl. suicidality), (hyypo)mania, psychosis, euphoria/mirth, impulse control disorders, cognitive impairment	Improved psychomotor speed, reduced depressive and anxiety symptoms
Transplantation	Putamen and/or caudate	Psychosis, depression, cognitive dysfunction	Transient memory improvement

given that its principal effect is on tremor and other targets provide relief of a wider range of symptoms. Unilateral GPi and STN DBS are relatively safe from a neurobehavioral standpoint, although postoperative declines in verbal fluency are possible. Debate persists regarding the comparative safety of bilateral GPi and STN DBS. Although studies using small samples and a limited range of tests have suggested that GPi DBS may be cognitively safer (Williams, Foote, & Okun, 2014) and result in greater reduction in Beck Depression Inventory scores (Liu et al., 2014), two large, randomized trials have failed to establish any large or clinically meaningful differences in the cognitive or behavioral outcomes of the two procedures (Odekerken et al., 2015; Odekerken et al., 2013; Rothlind et al., 2015). Although the trials yield somewhat different estimates of cognitive and behavioral risk, it seems reasonable to conclude that declines on multiple cognitive tests, sufficient to be associated with quality of life change, are evident in 11% or more of patients 6–12 months after DBS. Older patients with cognitive deficits may be at higher risk of adverse outcomes after DBS (Fields, 2015). Dementia is a contraindication for DBS, but the role of MCI in surgical outcome remains unclear. Two retrospective analyses (one using Level I criteria, the other Level II criteria) reported no difference in outcome after STN DBS between those with and without MCI (Abboud et al., 2014; Merola et al., 2014), but the exact nature of cognitive impairment may have important consequences. For example, attentional impairment has been shown to increase risk of postoperative confusion and length of hospitalization (Abboud et al., 2014), and together with preoperative levodopa response and age might predict cognitive outcome after STN DBS (Smeding, Speelman, Huizenga, Schuurman, & Schmand, 2011).

Despite the relative cognitive safety of STN DBS, numerous psychiatric issues have been identified as associated with STN DBS (although disease progression, medication changes, and psychosocial factors may also play a role). Such psychiatric issues include suicidality; apathy; hypomania, hypersexuality, and other impulse control phenomena; depression; anxiety; disinhibition; and psychosis (Mosley & Marsh, 2015; Volkmann, Daniels, & Witt, 2010).

Fetal mesencephalic cell transplantation is not currently being pursued given disappointing outcomes in initial trials, but the use of induced pluripotent and embryonic stem cells may be brought from bench to clinic in the not-too-distant future (Buttery & Barker, 2014). In addition, clinical trials are under way evaluating gene therapies that seek to replace dopamine, although a trial seeking to inhibit the STN via glutamic acid decarboxylase yielded disappointing results (LeWitt et al., 2011).

Cognitive Rehabilitation

Very little data are available regarding nonpharmacologic treatment of cognition in PD, and particularly about cognitive rehabilitation (Hindle, Petrelli, Clare, & Kalbe, 2013). Two reviews concluded that there was insufficient empirical evidence to recommend the use of such interventions in PD (Calleo et al., 2012; Langenbahn, Ashman, Cantor, & Trott, 2013). Nonetheless, several studies, many with only small samples, at least hint at patient acceptability of attention training in PD (Mohlman, Chazin, & Georgescu, 2011) and the feasibility of improving attention, memory, and executive functions by using cognitive rehabilitation. One study described gains on a Stroop-like task after approximately six months of training with Sudoku-like puzzles (Nombela et al., 2011) . Another study, albeit with inadequately described cognitive and motor interventions, reported that a six-week training program lead to improvements in verbal fluency, executive functions, and memory (Sinforiani, Banchieri, Zucchella, Pacchetti, & Sandrini, 2004), whilst another reported gains in executive functions after as little as ten 30-minute sessions of cognitive training compared to standard physical and occupational therapy (Sammer, Reuter, Hullmann, Kaps, & Vaitl, 2006). A recent randomized trial of integrated cognitive training versus occupational activities for three weekly sessions for three months showed that cognitive training produced significantly greater gains in visual memory, theory of mind task performance, processing speed, and functional disability (Pena et al., 2014). Another study using a wait-list control group showed that a program encompassing psychoeducation and cognitive training, and also targeting mood and health behaviors, delivered for two hours, twice weekly, for seven weeks, yielded gains on the Logical Memory paragraphs in the treatment group (Naismith, Mowszowski, Diamond, & Lewis, 2013). Finally, one study showed gains in a wide range of cognitive functions, including visuospatial, executive, verbal fluency, attention, and processing speed after four weeks of three weekly 45-minute sessions of computerized and pencil-and-paper tasks training versus speech therapy. However, these gains did not translate into patient perceptions of improvements in quality of life or day-to-day cognition (Paris et al., 2011). In addition to raising the issue of whether gains on tests translate into better functioning, another study questioned the specificity of the effect of cognitive training, noting that nonspecific computerized sports games produced as much gain as cognition-specific computerized training (Zimmermann et al., 2014).

Atypical Parkinsonian Disorders

Progressive Supranuclear Palsy (Steele-Richardson-Olszewski Syndrome)

Epidemiology and Genetics

The prevalence and incidence of progressive supranuclear palsy (PSP) is understudied. While a survey in New Jersey reported an age-adjusted prevalence of PSP of about 1.4 per 100,000 (Golbe, Davis, Schoenberg, & Duvoisin, 1988), epidemiologic studies using strict diagnostic criteria reveal an age-adjusted prevalence of about five per 100,000 (Nath et al., 2001; Schrag, Ben-Shlomo, & Quinn, 1999). Average annual incidence across ages 50–99 years has also been estimated at per 100,000 (Bower, Maraganore, McDonnell, & Rocca, 1997), with a marked increase in incidence with age (from 1.7 per 100,000 at ages 50–59 years to 14.7 per 100,000 at ages 80–99 years).

Most cases of PSP are sporadic. Some forms of familial PSP (usually atypical in presentation) may relate to tau gene mutations though some refer to such cases as familial tauopathies rather than PSP (Wszolek et al., 2001). Nonetheless, polymorphisms in the tau gene may be associated with PSP (Conrad et al., 1997).

Neuropathology

Unlike in PD, the pathology of PSP includes the entire substantia nigra, and dopaminergic depletion is comparable in caudate and putamen. There is neuronal loss and gliosis in the whole globus pallidus, subthalamic nuclei, red nuclei, dentate, superior colliculi, and periaqueductal gray matter. Neurofibrillary tangles different from those seen in AD, and they, along with neuropil threads, are readily observed in the basal ganglia, brain stem, dentate, and nucleus basalis of Meynert, the latter of which is associated with cholinergic depletion. Figures 22.7a, b and 22.8a, b show the brain changes visible in magnetic resonance imaging (MRI) in a patient with PSP over a two year span.

Neurobehavioral Features of Progressive Supranuclear Palsy

When first described in eight cases by Richardson, Steele, and Olszewski in the early 1960s, PSP was said to involve dementia (Colosimo, Bak, Bologna, & Berardelli, 2014). Almost ten years later Albert, Feldman, and Willis (1974) more precisely characterized the PSP neurobehavioral syndrome as a *subcortical dementia* (a term originated by von Stockert in 1932 but described by Naville in 1922). Dementia, estimated to occur in 50%–80% of persons with PSP, is argued by some to reflect an overestimate given the severe bradyphrenia (as well as emotional and visual dysfunction) often seen in PSP. The presence of neurobehavioral dysfunction varies by PSP phenotype. Whereas the traditional Richardson syndrome[1] frequently involves early cognitive and psychiatric alterations (frontal dysfunction in more than 50% of cases within two years), the parkinsonian variant does not (Williams et al., 2005). Parkinsonian signs predominate in this variant and it may at least transiently respond to dopaminergic therapy. Recent analysis of 100 pathologically verified cases suggests even greater phenotypic heterogeneity of PSP: possibly seven phenotypes with many cases showing overlapping features (Respondek et al., 2014). Nonetheless, it is generally accepted that PSP often involves a pattern of neurobehavioral deficits reminiscent of the prototypical subcortical dementia, involving bradyphrenia and executive dysfunction (Dubois, Deweer, & Pillon, 1996; Grafman, Litvan, & Stark, 1995;

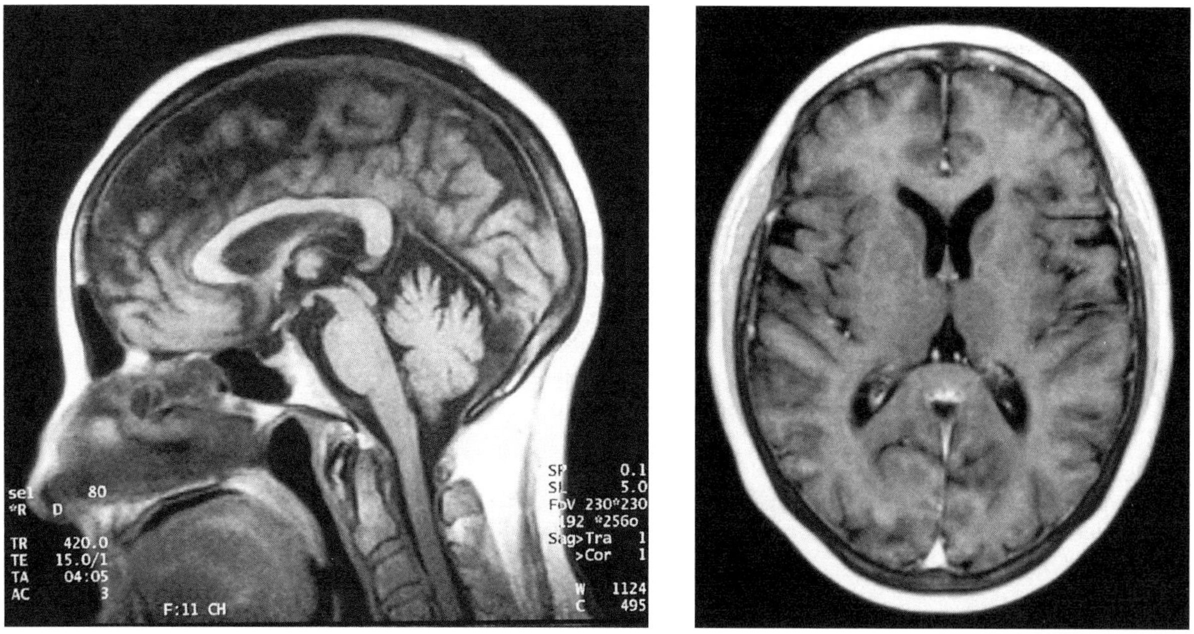

Figures 22.7 Baseline sagittal and axial MRI scans of a patient with presumed PSP. The 67-year-old patient, a right-handed, White female, noticed insidious onset of an upgoing right toe and gait difficulty. She was diagnosed as having right-sided dystonia and brain MRI was read as revealing mild cortical atrophy.

(Images courtesy of Xuemei Huang, MD, PhD).

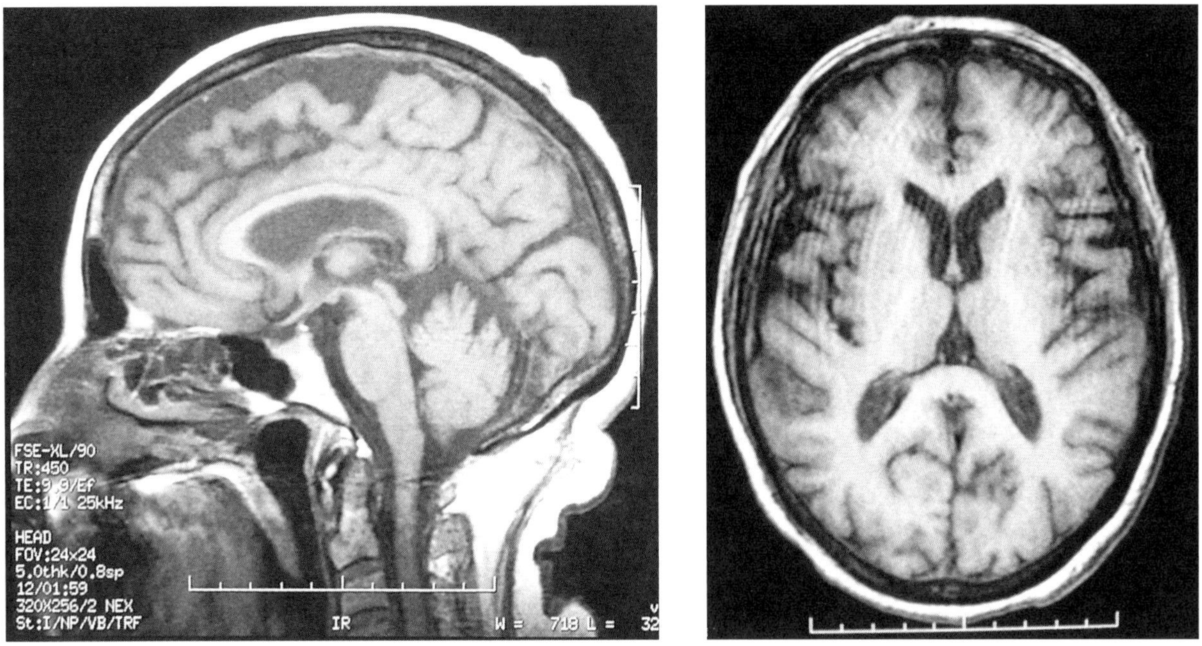

Figures 22.8 Repeat sagittal and axial MRIs of the patient with PSP (about three years after baseline MRI). The patient's gait and cognitive status continued to deteriorate and she became wheelchair bound about two years after initial evaluation. After three years she was not orientated to year, and date, could not spell "WORLD" backwards, had pseudobulbar affect, supranuclear gaze palsy, and severe axial (greater than distal) rigidity and bradykinesia. The repeat brain MRI reveals thinning of the anterior-posterior diameter of the midbrain tectum and tegmentum with atrophy of the colliculi and disproportionate enlargement of the Sylvian fissures and posterior third ventricle.

(Images courtesy of Xuemei Huang, MD, PhD)

Maher, Smith, & Lees, 1985). This executive dysfunction was long thought to reflect a frontal deafferentation or the downstream frontal cortical effects of basal ganglia pathology. One study (Cordato et al., 2002), however, found that MRI-measured frontal gray matter volume was strongly related to the "frontal" behavioral symptoms of PSP, suggesting that frontal lobe pathology contributes directly to neurobehavioral deficits.

Patients with PSP frequently have early and prominent executive dysfunction (Gerstenecker, Mast, et al., 2013). Patients perform more poorly than patients with PD on tests sensitive to frontal lobe dysfunction, such as card sorting, verbal fluency, and execution of graphic sequences (Dubois, Pillon, Legault, Agid, & Lhermitte, 1988; Pillon, Gouider-Khouja, et al., 1995). In addition, visual search and card-sorting task performance may decline more rapidly in PSP than PD (Soliveri et al., 2000). Episodic memory impairments (e.g., in prose recall, list learning, and paired-associate learning) are observed in PSP (Litvan, Grafman, Gomez, & Chase, 1989; Pillon et al., 1986; Pillon, Gouider-Khouja, et al., 1995). The severity of the episodic memory impairment may be comparable to that in PD, and less severe than that in AD (Aarsland, Hutchinson, & Larsen, 2003; Pillon et al., 1986; Pillon et al., 1991), but more severe than that in striatonigral degeneration (SND) corresponding to the parkinsonian form of multiple system atrophy (MSA-P) (Pillon, Gouider-Khouja, et al., 1995). Nondeclarative memory performance is task-dependent—generally, patients with PSP do poorly on procedural learning tasks, but show intact priming (Grafman et al., 1995). Though language and semantic memory have been held to be intact in PSP, van der Hurk and Hodges (1995) found PSP patients to show similar impairments to AD on a visual confrontation naming test (Boston Naming Test), with 44% of the PSP patients scoring in the impaired range, and more profound impairment in determining whether members of word pairs have similar or different meanings. In addition, on rare occasion, PSP can present resembling primary progressive aphasia (PPA) (Boeve et al., 2003; Mochizuki et al., 2003).

From a psychiatric standpoint, patients with PSP frequently report apathy and to lesser extent (but in a third or more of cases) depression and disinhibition (Aarsland, Litvan, & Larsen, 2001; Gerstenecker, Duff, Mast, Litvan, & Group, 2013; Litvan, Mega, Cummings, & Fairbanks, 1996).

Case Example

The patient, a 78-year-old male with a doctorate in engineering, with history of lower extremity radiculopathy, over the course of almost a year became slower in mobility and developed severe hoarseness, dysarthria, cognitive decline, and gait problems. The disorder responded minimally to levodopa. Blood tests were unremarkable and brain MRI, aside from revealing mild volume loss and presumed small vessel disease, was also unremarkable. Neurological exam revealed difficulty executing a two-step command and word-finding difficulty for more complex words. Extraocular movements were markedly abnormal: Smooth pursuit had broken down and saccadic eye movements were slow. Up- and downgaze were limited. Facial animation was reduced, but sensation was not. Speech was severely dysarthric and hypophonic and tongue movements were slowed. Neck muscle tone was increased. Rigidity was mild and symmetrical in the upper extremities, somewhat greater in the lower extremities. There was no tremor. Bradykinesia was moderate to severe and symmetrical. Sensory exam was abnormal in the distal lower extremities, with vibratory sense absent in the toes bilaterally. Tendon reflexes were normal in the upper extremities, brisk in the knees, and absent at the ankles.

Neuropsychological evaluation (see Table 22.11) revealed diminished intelligence from estimated premorbid levels, impaired visual confrontation naming, lower than expected (but not impaired) written word and design fluency (both average), borderline information processing speed, poor visuomotor speed and dexterity (greater impairment on the right than left), executive dysfunction, and generally below-average memory. Attention and praxis were intact (see Figures 22.9 and 22.10).

Table 22.11 Neuropsychological test scores in a patient with presumed PSP

Test	*Raw Score*	*T-Score or %ile*
WASI		
Vocabulary	34	31
Block Design	12	41
Similarities	13	31
Matrix Reasoning	10	44
Verbal IQ	73	4 %ile
Performance IQ	88	21 %ile
Full-Scale IQ	78	7 %ile
DRS-2		
Attention	34	47
Initiation/Perseveration	24	27
Construction	6	50
Conceptualization	28	33
Memory	21	40
Total	113	27
Symbol Digit Modalities Test		
Written	23	38
Oral	28	36
Ruff Figural Fluency Test	68	47
Written Word Fluency	54	51
Boston Naming Test (/60)	36	12
Grooved Pegboard		
Dominant	159"	28
Nondominant	167"	39
Wechsler Memory Scale-3rd ed.		
Subtest Scores		
Logical Memory I	15	33
Faces I	34	50
Family Pictures I	16	37
Letter-Number Sequencing	3	30
Spatial Span	12	47
Logical Memory II	8	40
Faces II	31	47
Family Pictures II	19	37
Logical Memory % Retention	89	63
Index Scores (%ile)		
Visual Immediate	88	21 %ile
Visual Delayed	84	14 %ile
Working Memory	81	74–93 %ile
Geriatric Depression Scale	11	

Multiple System Atrophy

MSA is a sporadic, progressive neurodegenerative condition with a clinical picture that involves a variable combination of cerebellar ataxia, autonomic dysfunction, and both pyramidal and extrapyramidal (parkinsonian) motor signs. The combination of three conditions previously thought to be distinct—SND, Shy-Drager syndrome (SDS), and olivopontocerebellar atrophy (OPCA)—into the single MSA category was largely a result of the recognition that all three conditions are multisystem degenerations with unique oligodendroglial cytoplasmic inclusions (Wenning, Colosimo, Geser, & Poewe, 2004). These inclusions were later shown reactive to alpha-synuclein immunostaining, and thus MSA, like PD and DLB, is considered an alpha-synucleinopathy. Recently, it has been suggested that neuron-to-oligodendrocyte transfer of alpha-synuclein by a prion-like spread may induce myelin and oligodendritic dysfunction and system neurodegeneration in MSA (Jellinger, 2014). There are two predominant motor presentations of MSA: the parkinsonian subtype (MSA-P) in about 80% of cases, and the cerebellar ataxia subtype (MSA-C) in approximately 20% of cases. These subtypes closely correspond to SND and OPCA both clinically and neuropathologically.

Unfortunately, given the changes in terminology over time, it is difficult to compare previous epidemiological and neurobehavioral studies' results, because it is often unclear to what extent OPCA, SND, and SDS were represented within MSA samples. Although consensual probabilistic criteria for MSA have been revised (Gilman et al., 2008), the utility of these diagnostic criteria remains to be evaluated in prospective studies. Given poor diagnostic accuracy in the past (25%–50%, depending on disease stage) (Wenning, Seppi, Scherfler, Stefanova, & Puschban, 2001), it is unclear how

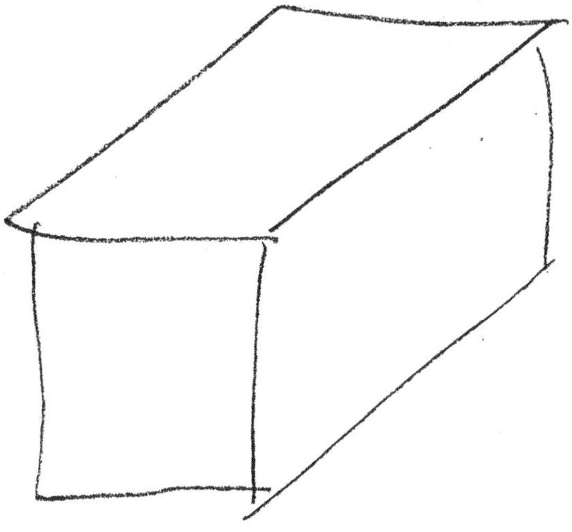

Figure 22.9 Drawing-to-command of a cube by a patient with PSP. When asked to draw a cube so that the top and two sides are visible, the patient has no difficulty, indicating an absence of constructional apraxia.

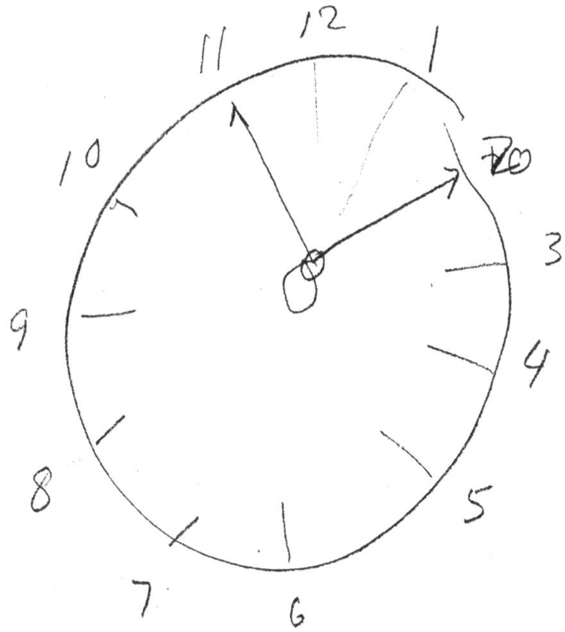

Figure 22.10 Drawing-to-Command of a Clock by the Patient with Presumed Progressive Supranuclear Palsy (PSP). Though the patient clearly retains the general concept of a clock and knows how to set the hands to show a time of "10 after 11," stimulus-bound behavior is evident. He draws the clock face and sets the hands at positions he indicates by the numbers "11" and "10" (after correctly starting with a "2" and then overwriting the incorrect "10" with the "2"). Subtle errors are evident from his drawing the numbers outside the clock face and from big and small hands that are indistinguishable in size.

accurate the neurobehavioral characterizations of clinically diagnosed (rather than pathologically confirmed) MSA are.

Epidemiology and Genetics

Bower et al. (1997), examining MSA incidence in Olmsted County, Minnesota, found an annual incidence of three per 100,000 among persons aged 50–99 years. Prevalence estimates range from about two to five per 100,000 (see Wenning et al. 2004). Although there are familial cases of OPCA, MSA is considered a sporadic disorder.

Neuropathology

Cell loss and gliosis are seen in the striatum (especially the caudal and dorsolateral aspects of the putamen), substantia nigra pars compacta, and the basis pontis. There is a loss of pontocerebellar transverse fibers and the middle cerebellar peduncle appears shrunken. The relative brunt of the pathology is nigrostriatal in MSA-P, and olivopontocerebellar in MSA-C. Figure 22.11 shows an MRI revealing the marked pontine and cerebellar atrophy in a case of MSA-C. As noted, glial cytoplasmic inclusions are a hallmark of MSA, and these inclusions, as well as neuronal inclusions are a result of alpha-synuclein aggregation.

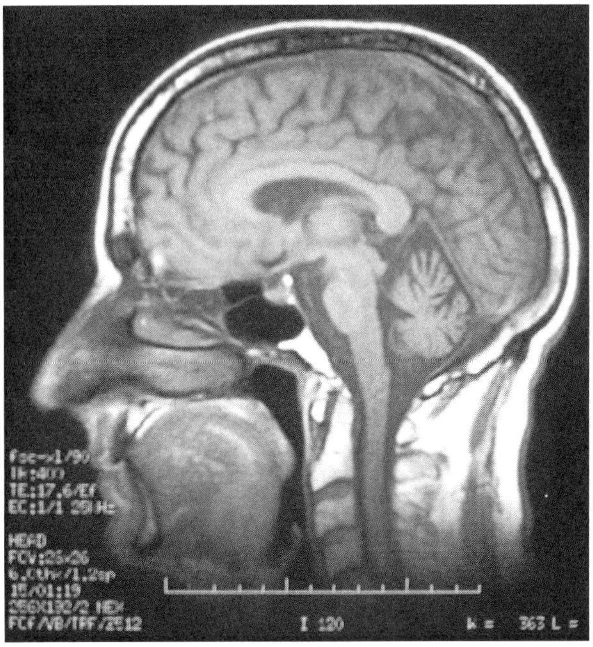

Figure 22.11 Sagittal MRI of a patient with presumed MSA-C (olivopontocerebellar atrophy) showing severe pontine and cerebellar atrophy. The 63-year-old, right-handed, White male noticed insidious onset of shuffling gait, slurred speech, and falls. Neurological examination revealed greater axial than distal rigidity, bradykinesia, left Babinski sign, left greater than right dysmetria, and gait ataxia. Movement disorder was unresponsive to medications.

(Scan courtesy of Xuemei Huang, MD, PhD.)

Neurobehavioral Features of Multiple System Atrophy

Consensus diagnostic criteria considered severe cognitive disorder as not supporting an MSA diagnosis (Gilman et al., 2008). In 2014, the Neuropsychology Task Force of the MDS Multiple System Atrophy (MODIMSA) Study Group, based on an extensive literature review, concluded that MSA-P and MSA-C often impair executive functions (including verbal fluency) and sometimes impair attention, visuospatial functions, and aspects of memory (recall and/or recognition) (Stankovic et al., 2014). Furthermore, it was recognized that cognitive impairment can span a full spectrum of severity, and that depression and anxiety are common.

In MSA-P impairments have been noted relative to healthy persons in verbal fluency, visual search and attention, executive functions, and verbal memory (Dujardin, Defebvre, Krystkowiak, Degreef, & Destee, 2003; Monza et al., 1998). Though there may be some subtle differences in the cognitive profiles of PD and MSA, there are many similarities (Pillon, Gouider-Khouja, et al., 1995; Robbins et al., 1992; Robbins et al., 1994), and commonalities appear to exceed differences. Verbal fluency may be more impaired in MSA than PD (even when the groups are equated for overall level of cognitive impairment and disease severity indexed) (Dujardin et al., 2003; Monza et al., 1998; Soliveri et al., 2000), though this is not a uniform finding (Lange et al., 2003; Testa et al., 1993). Similarly, attention may be more impaired in MSA than PD (Meco, Gasparini, & Doricchi, 1996; Pirtosek, Jahanshahi, Barrett, & Lees, 2001).

Impairment on detailed cognitive screening measures is more common in PSP than MSA (57% vs. 20%) (Brown et al., 2010). Cognitive impairments are probably also less severe in MSA than PSP. Lange et al. (2003) and Monza et al. (1998) found that verbal fluency deficits are less pronounced in MSA than PSP. In addition, using a broader test battery than Lange et al. (2003) and Monza et al. (1998) also found executive, visuospatial and attention impairments to be less severe in MSA than PSP, findings consistent with those of Pillon, Gouider-Khouja et al. (1995) and Soliveri et al. (2000). In comparison to persons with MSA-C, those with MSA-P may have more severe recognition memory and verbal fluency deficits (Berent et al., 2002). However, dementia may be more prevalent in familial than sporadic MSA-C (Berciano, 1982). With regard to affective disturbance, PD patients may be more anxious and depressed than those with MSA, but emotional blunting (unresponsive to levodopa therapy) may be more evident in MSA than PD (Fetoni, Soliveri, Monza, Testa, & Girotti, 1999). However, psychiatric complaints are common in MSA, perhaps reported by 50%–80% of patients (Colosimo et al., 2010).

Corticobasalganglionic Degeneration: Distinction Between Corticobasal Syndrome and Corticobasal Degeneration

First described as corticodentatonigral degeneration with neuronal achromasia (Rebeiz, Kolodny, & Richardson, 1968), corticobasal ganglionic degeneration (CBGD) was long thought to be predominantly a motor disorder. The motor presentation most often involves a progressive, asymmetric, akinetic-rigid parkinsonism of insidious onset that is poorly responsive to levodopa and is sometimes accompanied by dystonia or myoclonus. Cortical signs that are common in CBGD include apraxia and alien hand sign. This mixture of motor and cortical and subcortical signs are hallmarks of CBGD. However, the recognition of CBGD as a tauopathy that has heterogeneous presentations, including PSP, progressive aphasia, and fronto-temporal dementia (Kertesz, Martinez-Lage, Davidson, & Munoz, 2000), has led some to argue that CBD is a member of the "Pick complex" of disorders, including primary progressive aphasia, progressive supranuclear palsy, and fronto-temporal dementia (Kertesz, 2003). Given the clinically heterogeneous presentation of CBGD, and the fact that the core features of CBGD can be produced by other conditions, it was recommended that the term *corticobasal syndrome* (CBS) be applied to the core clinical features of CBD regardless of etiology. In contrast, the term *corticobasal degeneration* (CBD) should be reserved for the distinctive neuropathological condition of corticobasal ganglionic degeneration, regardless of its clinical presentation (Lang, 2003).

Initial findings were inconsistent about whether neurobehavioral abnormalities are presenting features of CBD and how frequently they occur in the later disease stages (Grimes, Lang, & Bergeron, 1999; Rinne, Lee, Thompson, & Marsden, 1994). It is now widely accepted that neurobehavioral abnormalities occur in most if not all patients already early in the disease course (Burrell, Hodges, & Rowe, 2014). Indeed, new diagnostic criteria based on clinical material, and case and literature review, recognize not only that cognitive compromise is evident in more than 50% of cases at presentation, but also that it characterizes two of four CBD phenotypes on the basis of neurobehavioral disturbances (i.e., the frontal behavioral-spatial syndrome and the nonfluent/agrammatic variant of primary progressive aphasia) (Armstrong et al., 2013).

Epidemiology and Genetics

Prevalence and incidence of CBD are unknown; poor diagnostic accuracy (Litvan et al., 1997), even of the new diagnostic criteria (Alexander et al., 2014), no doubt contributes to this. Although the H1/H1 tau haplotype has been identified as heightening susceptibility to both CBD and PSP, no clear genetic etiology has been identified. Disease onset is usually in the sixth decade of life, and mean time to death from diagnosis is about seven years.

Neuropathology

Among cortical regions, the frontal and fronto-parietal cortices show asymmetric atrophy. The pons, medulla, and dentate are also atrophied, and the caudate may appear flattened. The substantia nigra shows decreased pigmentation and cell loss. Neuronal loss and gliosis, in addition to being evident in fronto-parietal cortex, is seen in basal ganglia, thalamus, STN, dentate, and red nucleus. Ballooned and achromatic neurons, hallmark of CBD, are most numerous usually in fronto-parietal cortex, but are also seen in the anterior cingulate, amygdala, and insular cortex. Neuronal and glial inclusions are immunoreactive for tau but not alpha synuclein. Imaging of CBS reveals especially primary motor cortex atrophy. Imaging also shows more variable involvement of supplementary motor, inferior parietal, and posterior temporal regions, perhaps related to heterogeneity of underlying pathology (Burrell et al., 2014).

Neurobehavioral Features of Corticobasal Degeneration

CBD involves an asymmetric apraxia, typically of the ideomotor variety, with ideational and limb kinetic apraxias occurring more rarely (Leiguarda, Lees, Merello, Starkstein, & Marsden, 1994; Pharr et al., 2001; Pillon, Blin, et al., 1995; Soliveri et al., 1999). Thus, patients most often have difficulty demonstrating the use of tools. Poor drawing (constructional apraxia) is also commonly seen. CBD can present as a primary progressive aphasia. Graham, Bak, and Hodges (2003) noted in their review of published cases mentioning aphasia in CBD, that the aphasia is most often nonfluent (about 56% of cases), followed in frequency by anomic aphasia (30%). Fluent and mixed cases were quite rare: each about 5%–7% of cases. The pattern of performance on language tests in patients with the traditional CBD presentation is somewhat inconsistent across studies, but it has been suggested that phonological impairments may be a key feature of the language problems in CBD (Graham, Bak, Patterson, & Hodges, 2003). In general, performance on verbal fluency tasks is impaired (Graham, Bak, Patterson, et al., 2003; Pillon, Blin, et al., 1995) probably in large part due to the executive demands of those tasks rather than aphasia (Hohler, Ransom, Chun, Tröster, & Samii, 2003). Performance on semantic memory tasks such as conceptual matching and visual confrontation naming (Graham, Bak, Patterson, et al., 2003), and on expressive vocabulary (Massman, Kreiter, Jankovic, & Doody, 1996; Mimura, White, & Albert, 1997), is relatively preserved and impaired in a minority of patients. When naming is impaired, disproportionate benefit is derived from cuing suggesting a retrieval rather than semantic memory deficit (Beatty, Scott, Wilson, Prince, & Williamson, 1995; Massman et al., 1996). Patients also may have agraphia with both central and peripheral components (Riley & Lang, 1996).

Executive dysfunction, as indicated by poor performance on tasks such as the WCST (Pillon, Blin, et al., 1995; Soliveri et al., 1999) and Trail Making test (Beatty et al., 1995; Mimura et al., 1997), is common. The episodic memory impairments in CBD are more pronounced than in AD, and appear to involve both encoding and retrieval deficits (Massman et al., 1996; Pillon, Blin, et al., 1995). Remote memory impairment may be attributable to retrieval deficits given poor recall but intact recognition on remote memory tasks (Beatty et al., 1995). Visuospatial impairments have been observed (Graham, Bak, & Hodges, 2003; Soliveri et al., 1999).

With respect to emotional and neuropsychiatric issues, Litvan et al. (1998), using the Neuropsychiatric Inventory (NPI) found depression in 73% of CBD patients, with apathy (40%), irritability (20%), and agitation (20%) also occurring at notable rates. In comparison to PSP patients, CBD patients have less apathy, but more depression and irritability. Changes in personality and social cognition may resemble those seen in fronto-temporal dementia (Burrell, Hornberger, Villemagne, Rowe, & Hodges, 2013). We have previously described in detail the neurologic and neuropsychological features of a case of CBS (Tröster & Browner, 2013).

The Use of Neuropsychological Tests in Differentiating Among Atypical Parkinsonisms

Although many tests are useful in detecting cognitive impairments in PD and atypical parkinsonisms relative to normal, there is overlap in the test performances of these groups. Thus, although group comparison studies among PD and atypical parkinsonism sometimes reveal statistically significant differences in mean scores, their utility in differential diagnosis in the individual case is unknown. A meta-analysis (Lee, Williams, & Storey, 2012) identified 19 of 1,038 articles meeting inclusion criteria. Test utility was then defined on the basis of effect size of the difference between group means (Cohen's *d*) or positive likelihood ratio (ratio of posttest to pretest probability of the condition of interest given a positive test result). The larger the effect size, the less the overlap in test score distributions, and the higher the diagnostic utility. For discussion here, only tests deemed moderately (20%–29% overlap) to very useful (less than 20% overlap) in differentiating between two or more groups are presented in Table 22.12. In brief, neuropsychological tests appear more helpful in differentiating PD from atypical parkinsonisms than in differentiating among atypical parkinsonisms. Tests of praxis seem especially useful in identifying CBD, whereas

Table 22.12 Neuropsychological tests deemed moderately to very useful (Lee et al., 2012) in distinguishing between PD and atypical Parkinsonian disorders

Conditions Differentiated	*PD*	*PSP*	*MSA*	*CBS*
PD	–	Semantic fluency, phonemic fluency alternating semantic fluency, Wisconsin Card Sorting (categories, errors, perseverative errors), trail Making A, frontal assessment battery, Digit Span, JOL, orientation choice reaction time, (all worse in PSP)	Trail Making B, Stroop (both worse in MSA)	Orofacial and ideomotor apraxia (both worse in CBS)
PSP	–	–	Semantic fluency, phonemic Fluency, alternating phonemic fluency, semantic fluency, alternating semantic fluency, Wisconsin Card Sorting (categories and errors), addenbrooke's cognitive examination (ACE), JOL (all worse in PSP)	None
MSA	–	–	–	Orofacial apraxia (worse in CBS)

Abbreviations: PD: PD, PSP: Progressive Supranuclear Palsy, MSA: Multiple System Atrophy, CBS: Corticobasal Syndrome

verbal fluency tests are useful in identifying PSP, a conclusion confirmed by the findings that this task had sensitivity and specificity of 0.90 or higher in differentiating PSP from PD (Rittman et al., 2013) and of a recent meta-analysis (Lee, Williams, & Anderson, 2016).

Huntington's Disease

Unlike the other neurodegenerative conditions discussed in this chapter, the cause of HD (Huntington, 1872) is well established: It is an autosomal dominantly inherited condition. HD is a hyperkinetic movement disorder characterized by choreiform movements and dystonias early on, but bradykinesia and incoordination also occur later on. Cognitive and psychiatric disturbance is almost invariable and may predate motor symptom onset. It is likely that the triad of cognitive, emotional, and motor symptoms contributes to functional disability, but it has been difficult to disentangle the impact of motor and cognitive dysfunction (Fink et al., 2014). Diagnosis remains clinical and is based on the finding of an extrapyramidal movement disorder in the context of a positive genetic test for the HD CAG expansion or a positive family history of HD. Despite evidence that cognitive changes such as psychomotor speed and executive functions can progress prior to motor symptom onset (Paulsen & Long, 2014), cognitive variables are not considered among biomarkers of premanifest HD (Ross & Tabrizi, 2011). Cognitive variables are, however, considered to be relevant clinical trial outcomes (Papoutsi, Labuschagne, Tabrizi, & Stout, 2014; Tabrizi et al., 2012; Tabrizi et al., 2013).

Epidemiology and Genetics

Prevalence of HD ranges from 4–10 per 100,000 in the Western world. The most common age at onset is in the 40s, though juvenile and senescent onset occurs, and disease duration is about 15–20 years (Ross & Tabrizi, 2011). One estimate indicates that 38% of prodromal HD individuals have deficits on neuropsychological testing (Repeatable Battery for the Assessment of Neuropsychological Status, or RBANS; see Duff, Beglinger, Theriault, Allison, & Paulsen, 2010).

An expansion of the CAG triplet in the Huntington gene on chromosome 4 results in the misfolding of the protein coded in this sequence, and its accumulation in the cell body leads to cell death. HD is inherited in an autosomal dominant manner, meaning if one parent carries the gene, the offspring has a 50% chance of inheriting it. Usually the number of CAG repeats is reported for each of the two alleles. The normal number of CAG repeats ranges from 10 to 35: Those with an allele with 36–39 repeats may or may not develop symptoms, whereas those with 40 or more repeats almost always do. Penetrance is age dependent and is almost 100% by age 65. Although the relationship between CAG repeat length and age at disease onset is not linear, a greater number of repeats are generally associated with earlier onset but not rate of progression. The phenomenon of anticipation refers to the observation that as the altered HTT gene is passed from generation to generation, the number of CAG trinucleotide repeats increases and symptom onset is earlier (esp. when transmission is paternal).

Neuropathology

Although the cellular functions of the HTT protein are not yet known, it is likely that HD arises largely from a gain of toxic function from an abnormal conformation of mutant HTT. Even though HTT is expressed in the body and throughout the brain, it relatively selectively affects the striatum early on, perhaps due to an interaction of HTT with the Rhes protein in the striatum, glutamate excitotoxicity, or loss of BDNF. Specifically, there is an early decline in the GABAergic medium spiny neurons of the striatum, especially in the caudate, and on imaging there is evidence of striatal atrophy and abnormality in the white matter tracts connecting striatum and cortex (Tabrizi et al., 2012; Tabrizi et al., 2013). Eventually more widespread atrophy occurs, which manifests in a wide range of neurocognitive deficits (Papoutsi et al., 2014).

From a pathophysiologic standpoint, HD can be understood from the model of cortico-striatal-thalamic dysfunction used to explain PD. However, unlike in PD, in which the thalamus is underactive, HD involves hyperactivity of the thalamus related to a decrease in the GABAergic inhibitory control exerted over it by the GPi and substantia nigra pars reticulata. The underactivity of GPi is atttributable to its excessive inhibition via the direct pathway and the insufficient excitatory influence of the STN via the indirect pathway.

Neurobehavioral Features of Huntington's Disease

Studies in the 1980s and 1990s often compared neuropsychological features of HD and either AD or PD to highlight differences among prototypical cortical and subcortical dementias and to infer cognitive functions of the striatum. More recent studies have focused on which cognitive changes emerge before disease diagnosis and whether these have clear neuroimaging correlates. In manifest HD, the neuropsychological changes have been well described (Brandt, 2009), and an increasing number of studies have documented the tests on which persons estimated to be within ten years of manifest disease have deficits (Paulsen, 2011). In the prodrome, many tests tapping processing speed, motor speed, attention, and executive functions are sensitive to deficits. One study outlined the effect sizes associated with differences in test performance in persons within 9 years, 9–15 years, and more than 15 years of HD diagnosis relative to controls (Stout et al., 2011). Although tests of emotional recognition revealed deficits in those 15 or more years from diagnosis, it is generally acknowledged that there is little evidence for measurable or meaningful cognitive deficits ten years or more before diagnosis (Papoutsi et al., 2014). Test revealing medium to large effect sizes in the 9–15 and less than 9 years prediagnosis groups included motor tasks (e.g., finger tapping), Symbol Digit Modalities, smell test, Hopkins Verbal Learning Test total learning, Trail Making Part B, Stroop, and phonemic verbal fluency among others.

Patients with manifest HD are impaired on attention tasks demanding of vigilance and response flexibility and executive tasks such as Trail Making, Wisconsin Card Sorting, Stroop, and verbal fluency (Brandt, 2009). Visuospatial perception and visuomotor integration may also be compromised, and this likely reflects posterior cortical dysfunction (Wolf et al., 2014). Memory impairments are characterized by impoverished encoding and retrieval deficits (Montoya et al., 2006). If remote memory is affected, it is less so than in AD and characterized by lack of temporal gradient likely due to general retrieval difficulties (Beatty, Salmon, Butters, Heindel, & Granholm, 1988). Language is relatively intact, although as the disease progresses speech problems and processing speed/multitasking deficits can compromise communication (Paulsen, 2011). At this time, the limited studies of treatment of cognitive dysfunction in HD have yielded disappointing findings regarding the use of antidepressants, atypical stimulants (e.g., modafinil), and cholinesterase inhibitors (Killoran & Biglan, 2014).

In addition to cognitive changes, psychiatric conditions are common in HD, and it has been estimated that psychiatric symptoms occur in 30%–70% of those with HD (van Duijn, Kingma, & van der Mast, 2007). Unlike the time course shown in HD for motor and cognitive symptoms, there is no predictable time course for psychiatric features. The most common behavioral symptom in HD is irritability (40%–80%) (van Duijn et al., 2007) which is often accompanied by aggression. One study reported that at first HD clinic visit, 60% of caregivers reported aggression by the patient (Marder et al., 2000). Also, apathy occurs in about 50% of patients. Suicide risk is fourfold that of the general population: Whilst completed suicide rates are 3%–7%, attempts have been reported among as many as 25% of patients during the course of illness (Weintraub, Siderowf, Troster, & Anderson, 2011). Psychosis is rarer, most often involving delusions and occurring most often among those with early disease onset.

Case Example of Huntington's Disease

Neuropsychological test results for a patient with HD are presented in Table 22.13. The 58-year-old man with 18 years of education was diagnosed with HD three years prior to the neuropsychological evaluation (roughly one year after his wife had noticed his mild abnormal facial and shoulder movements) on the basis of clinical examination, genetic testing (42 CAG repeats), and family history. Cognitively, the patient reported problems with speech (slow and slurred at times), occasional word-finding difficulty, short-term memory problems, attentional problems, decreased problem-solving ability (difficulty multitasking and requiring checklists to complete complex tasks), and visuo-perceptual changes (requiring more room to

Table 22.13 Neuropsychological test scores of a patient with Huntington's Disease

Test	*Raw Score*	*T-Score or %ile*
Wechsler Test of Adult Reading (WTAR)	31	98
WAIS IV		
Digit Span	20	SS = 7
Arithmetic	14	SS = 10
Symbol Search	16	SS = 5
Coding	45	SS = 7
Similarities	26	SS = 10
Information	14	SS = 10
Matrix Reasoning	9	SS = 6
Visual Puzzles	7	SS = 6
Verbal Comprehension Index	31	102
Perceptual Reasoning Index	19	79
Working memory Index	17	92
Processing Speed Index	12	79
Full Scale IQ	79	85
Trail Making Test		
Part A	45"/ 1 err.	T = 21
Part B	151"/1 err.	T = 18
Stroop Neuropsychological Screening Test		
Color Task	112/0 err.	
Color-Word Task	53/0 err	2–4 %ile
WCST-64		
Number of Categories Correct	4/6	> 16 %ile
Trials to Complete 1st Category	11	> 16 %ile
Failure to Maintain Set	0	
Total Errors	13	T = 49
Perseverative Responses	8	T = 41
Perseverative Errors	8	T = 40
Conceptual Level Responses	49	T = 47
Controlled Oral Word Association Test		
Lexical/Phonemic Fluency (FAS)	28	T = 30
Semantic/Category Fluency (Animals)	14	T = 24
Benton Judgment of Line orientation-Short Form V		
Corrected Raw	18	4 %ile
Hopkins Verbal Learning Test—Revised (Form 1)		
Trial 1	5	
Trial 2	5	
Trial 3	7	
Total	17	T = 24
Delayed Recall	6	T = 28
% Retained	86%	T = 44
Discrimination Index	10	T = 44
True Positives(Hits)	12	
False Positives	2	
WMS-IV Logical Memory		
Logical Memory I	21	SS = 8
Logical memory II	16	SS = 8
Recognition	24/30	26–50 %ile
Brief Visuospatial Memory Test-Revised (Form 1)		
Trial 1	3	T = 37
Trial 2	4	T = 30
Trial 3	3	T = <20
Total Recall	10	T = 26
Learning	1	T = 35
Delayed Recall	4	T = 28
% Retention	100%	> 16 %ile
Hits	5	> 16 %ile
False Positives	0	
Finger Tapping Test		
Dominant Hand (Right)	34.67	T = 18
Nondominant Hand	25.33	T = 13
Beck Depression Inventory II		7/63
Starkstein Apathy Scale		6/42

Note: SS = scaled score

park a car and causing several minor car accidents). The patient's wife noted that his information processing and verbal response speed had slowed, and that he was less able to complete small home repairs. Cognitive changes had caused difficulty in his work as a corporation's chief financial officer, including several costly financial errors. Psychiatric history was notable for depression without suicidality, the onset of which coincided with his HD diagnosis and initially involved low mood, anergia, and sleep disturbance. Although mood improved with the use of citalopram, he attributed mild, recent dysphoria and worry to difficulty performing his job.

He ambulated independently and without unsteadiness or imbalance, but had mild truncal and limb choreiform movements. Neuropsychological tests disclosed impairments in the areas of processing speed, visual-spatial perception and judgment, and learning and memory. Learning and memory impairment was characterized by slow learning and retrieval deficits on recall, but relatively adequate recognition. Memory was better for externally structured material (e.g., prose). Some of his executive function test scores fell into the low average to mildly impaired range, possibly also related to slow processing speed. Finger tapping speed was impaired bilatreally. Self-report scales relating to mood and personality were valid for interpretation and did not disclose clinical psychopathology. Overall, findings of multiple cognitive impairments impacting occupational functioning were deemed consistent with mild dementia secondary to HD.

A Bird's-Eye View of Some Other Movement Disorders: Essential Tremor, Dystonia, and Psychogenic Movement Disorders

Essential Tremor

Essential tremor (ET) is one of the most common movement disorders, with prevalence estimates averaging 4.6% among those 65 years and older (Louis & Ferreira, 2010). The condition is characterized by postural tremor when the limb is held against gravity, or kinetic tremor during actions which can affect a range of ADLs including writing, eating, grooming, and dressing. Despite its moniker of "benign" tremor, ET can significantly disrupt social and occupational functioning and quality of life (Troster, Pahwa, Fields, Tanner, & Lyons, 2005). In about half of cases the tremor is hereditary, although mutations identified in two genes impact only a small minority of patients (Zeuner & Deuschl, 2012).

Given the role of the cerebellum in cognition (Schmahmann, 2001; Schmahmann & Sherman, 1998), and the putative cerebello-thalamo-cortical basis of ET (Deuschl & Bergman, 2002), it is not surprising that ET, once thought exclusively a motor disorder, might have neurobehavioral manifestations. Visuospatial and executive dysfunction have also been linked to fronto-parietal white matter abnormalities by mean, radial, and axial diffusivity on diffusion tensor imaging (Bhalsing et al., 2015). The cognitive characteristics of ET were first studied among patients with family histories of ET versus PD (Gasparini et al., 2001) and candidates for thalamic DBS (Lacritz, Dewey, Giller, & Cullum, 2002; Lombardi, Woolston, Roberts, & Gross, 2001; Tröster et al., 2002). These studies most frequently identify problems with executive functions, complex attention, verbal fluency, and to lesser extent memory (Janicki, Cosentino, & Louis, 2013; Lyons & Tröster, 2015). ET may involve increased risk for MCI (Benito-Leon, Louis, Mitchell, & Bermejo-Pareja, 2011) and dementia (Benito-Leon, Louis, & Bermejo-Pareja, 2006) but the concept of neurodegeneration in ET remains controversial (Rajput, Adler, Shill, & Rajput, 2012). When MCI is identified, it is most often nonamnestic in nature (Park et al., 2015). Executive problems impact quality of life and functioning in ET (Woods, Scott, Fields, Poquette, & Troster, 2008), and the cognitive problems are independent of psychiatric comorbidity (Janicki et al., 2013). Patients with ET have increased rates of anxiety and social phobia, and often feel embarrassed and stigmatized (Tröster & Tucker, 2005). Because tremor may be alcohol-responsive, neuropsychological interview should routinely cover possible alcohol abuse. Treatments for ET most often employ beta-blockers or antiepileptic drugs. Some of these drugs (e.g., gabapentin, topiramate) may affect cognition (e.g., attention or word finding). Thalamic DBS is relatively safe, and the most common cognitive risk involves declines in verbal fluency (Fields, 2015; Fields et al., 2003).

Dystonia

Dystonia, with a prevalence of about 15 per 100,000 is the third most common movement disorder (after essential tremor and PD) and involves sustained or intermittent muscle contractions causing abnormal movements (twisting, tremor) or postures. A proposed dystonia classification system uses two axes: clinical characteristics (age at onset, body distribution, temporal pattern) and associated features (additional movement disorders or neurological features) along one axis, and etiology (nervous system pathology and inheritance) on the other (Albanese et al., 2013). The exact pathophysiology of dystonia has not been specified, but the basal ganglia and cerebellum have been clearly implicated (Torkamani & Jahanshahi, 2015).

Whereas primary dystonias (i.e., idiopathic or genetic) are less often associated with cognitive deficits, dystonia plus syndromes (mycoclonus dystonia, dopa-responsive dystonia, and X-linked parkinsonism dystonia), though rarely studied, are more often associated with cognitive changes (executive function and memory). When cognitive changes are identified in primary dystonia, they most often involve attention (shifting, sustained, divided), working memory, or executive functions (e.g., verbal fluency, perseverations on the WCST) (Jahanshahi, Rowe, & Fuller, 2003; Scott et al., 2003; Torkamani & Jahanshahi, 2015). DBS treatment appears relatively safe from a cognitive standpoint. Changes observed in individual patients are difficult to interpret given possible practice effects and confounds of motor improvement and anticholinergic medicine reduction (Jahanshahi, Czernecki, & Zurowski, 2011).

Psychogenic Movement Disorders

Psychogenic counterparts may be seen for almost all movement disorders, though psychogenic tremor and dystonia are estimated to account for almost three quarters of all PMDs (Lang, 2011). One classification of PMD (Gupta & Lang, 2009) is based on diagnostic certainty. A *documented* PMD is a condition that remits with suggestion, placebo, physiotherapy, psychotherapy, or when the person is "unobserved." A *clinically established* diagnosis is based on observation that the movement disorder is inconsistent over time, incongruent with a clinical condition, and has other features such as false neurological signs and multiple somatizations with or without obvious psychiatric disturbance. A *clinically definite* diagnosis requires both the documented and clinically established criteria to be met, whilst a *laboratory-supported definite* diagnosis require electrophysiologic confirmation of psychogenicity.

Neuropsychological studies of cognition in PMD are virtually nonexistent. A preliminary study found that two of eight patients with PMD who had low scores on a test of effort (the Test of Memory Malingering, or TOMM), also had variable performance across neuropsychological tests. However, it was concluded that tests probably lack adequate sensitivity and specificity to characterize volition in individual cases (Nahan & Levin, 2011). Even psychological assessment has been rarely reported and studies have more often used psychiatric interviews (Anderson, 2011), or documented outcomes of psychotherapy or antidepressant treatment with anxiety and depression scales (Hinson, Weinstein, Bernard, Leurgans, & Goetz, 2006; Voon & Lang, 2005). Depression and anxiety are common in psychogenic tremor, dystonia, and myoclonus, occurring in about half or more of cases in small sample studies (Koller, Marjama, & Tröster, 2002). One report based on DSM diagnoses via interview (Feinstein, Stergiopoulos, Fine, & Lang, 2001), but was likely marred by a strong self-selection bias (42 of 88 PMD patients agreed to be interviewed), found point prevalence being 38% for anxiety disorders, 19% for major depression, and 12% for comorbid anxiety and depression. 45% of patients were deemed to have a personality disorder. In another study (Kranick et al., 2011), patients with PMD relative to age- and sex-matched controls and hand dystonia patients had higher rates of childhood trauma (emotional abuse and physical neglect, but not physical or sexual abuse). However, unlike the former study this study did not find PMD patients to have higher rates of psychiatric diagnoses. In addition, the groups did not differ in personality traits or dissociative experiences. Although direct empirical evidence appears lacking, the PAI, by virtue of the structure of the Somatic Complaints subscale and provision of clinical correlates for conversion and somatization, has been recommended in the assessment of PMD and suspected malingering (Rogers & Wooley, 2011). Psychotherapy (Morgante, Edwards, & Espay, 2013) and physical therapy/rehabilitation (Jordbru, Smedstad, Klungsoyr, & Martinsen, 2014) may both be beneficial in treating PMD, although outcome studies are limited. Clearly, given the prevalence of PMD, further neuropsychological research is much needed.

Practical Clinical Issues in the Neuropsychological Evaluation of Patients With Movement Disorders

Utility of Clinical Neuropsychological Evaluation in Persons With Movement Disorders

Tröster and Woods (2003) outlined several ways in which neuropsychological evaluation informs and potentially enriches the management of the patient with PD, and these utilities of neuropsychological evaluation apply to the other movement disorders and associated dementias as well. Specifically, neuropsychological evaluation can:

- provide information about the likely etiology of recent cognitive deterioration;
- yield objective data in the assessment of competence to consent to medical treatment;
- facilitate financial, legal, and living situation decision making by patient and family;
- provide a profile of cognitive and behavioral strengths and weaknesses, thereby
    - informing adaptive changes in the home or work environment to minimize handicap,
    - guiding development of strategies that minimize the impact of cognitive changes on day-to-day functioning, and
    - suggesting rehabilitation services such as speech therapy and psychotherapy;
- serve as an aid in adjudicating the appropriateness of certain medical and surgical interventions for a given patient with a movement disorder such as PD (e.g., Saint-Cyr & Trépanier, 2000; Tröster & Fields, 2003) and to document neurobehavioral and quality of life outcomes of such treatments; and
- help identify persons with PMDs (see Koller et al., 2002).

Selecting Neuropsychological Test Batteries for Movement Disorders and Possible Test Modifications

Specific test batteries have been proposed for evaluating patients with PD and other movement disorders. While these efforts are well-intentioned, there is probably greater agreement about the domains one should assess than about the specific tests best used. Test selection should rest on the referral question(s), patient and caregiver questions, the clinician's competence in using specific tests, the normative and psychometric properties of the tests (e.g., availability of alternate forms, test-retest reliability, validity for use in movement disorders), the patient's ability to tolerate and cooperate with the tests, and a thorough awareness of how manifestations of PD and other movement disorders can impact evaluation (e.g., motor "on-off" fluctuations, wearing off and freezing, sleep disturbance and fatigability, choreiform and dystonic dyskinesias, gaze palsy, apraxia, dysarthria, and hypersalivation). Thus, neuropsychologists should conduct a careful interview with the patient that asks about his or her symptoms, their time course, and his or her medication schedule. This allows planning of a successful evaluation. Examples of tests often used in the evaluation of PD and other movement disorders are presented in Table 22.14.

Standard administration methods may sometimes have to be modified for test use with patients with movement disorders. Patients with PSP, for example, often have downward gaze palsy, making it difficult for them to voluntarily look down at test forms. In such cases, stimuli may be held up for the patient to see. When impediments such as slurred speech are evident, patients may be asked to repeat responses if they are unclear, although it need be borne in mind that this is often frustrating and tiring to the patient, perhaps necessitating testing over multiple brief sessions. Patients with

Table 22.14 Commonly used neuropsychological tests by cognitive domain assessed

Cognitive Domain	*Test*
Premorbid Estimates	North American Adult Reading Test (NAART); Wechsler Test of Adult Reading (WTAR); Wide Range Achievement Test (WRAT); Advanced Clinical Solutions Test of Premorbid Functioning (TOPF)
Neuropsychological Screening	Mattis DRS; MMSE; Repeatable Battery for the Assessment of Neuropsychological Status (RBANS); Montreal Cognitive Assessment; Parkinson's Disease–Cognitive Rating Scale; Frontal Assessment Battery
Intelligence	Raven's Progressive Matrices; Wechsler Abbreviated Scale of Intelligence (WASI); Wechsler Adult Intelligence Scale (WAIS) (recent editions)
Attention and Working Memory	Auditory Consonant Trigrams (ACT); Brief Test of Attention (BTA); Continuous Performance Tests (CPT); Digit and Visual Spans; Paced Auditory Serial Addition Test (PASAT); Stroop Test *
Executive Function	Cognitive Estimation Test (CET); Delis-Kaplan Executive Function Scale (DKEFS); Halstead Category Test; Trailmaking Test (TMT)*; WCST; Tower of Toronto; Tower of London
Memory	Benton Visual Retention Test (BVRT-R); California Verbal Learning Test (CVLT-II); Rey Auditory Verbal Learning Test (RAVLT); Selective Reminding Test; Rey Complex Figure Test (RCFT) *; Wechsler Memory Scale (WMS) (recent editions) *
Language	Boston Naming Test (BNT); Controlled Oral Word Association Test (COWAT); Sentence Repetition; Token Test; Complex Ideational Material
Visuoperception	Benton Facial Recognition Test; Benton Judgment of Line Orientation (JLO); Hooper Visual Organization Test (VOT); Visual Object and Space Perception Battery
Motor and Sensory-Perception	Finger Tapping*; Grooved Pegboard*; Hand Dynamometer*; Sensory-Perceptual Examination
Mood State and Personality	Beck Anxiety Inventory (BAI); Beck Depression Inventory (BDI); Hamilton Depression Scale (HDS) or Inventory (HDI); The Neuropsychiatric Inventory (NPI); Minnesota Multiphasic Personality Inventory (MMPI) (recent editions); Profile of Mood States (POMS); State-Trait Anxiety Inventory (STAI); Maudsley Obsessional-Compulsive Inventory; Yale-Brown Obsessive Compulsive Scale; Hospital Anxiety and Depression Scale (HADS), Montgomery–Åsberg Depression Rating Scale
Quality of Life, Coping, and Stressors	Parkinson's Disease Questionnaire (PDQ); Medical Outcomes Study 36-item short form (SF-36); Sickness Impact Profile (SIP); Coping Responses Inventory (CRI); Ways of Coping Questionnaire; Life Stressors and Social Resources Inventory (LISRES)

(*Test may not be appropriate for patients with marked motor impairment)

hypophonia may be provided an amplification device to minimize the number of times they are asked to repeat answers. A patient with tremor, choreiform dyskinesias or dystonia who is to be administered tests or questionnaires requiring writing, circling of alternatives, or filling in of "multiple choice "bubbles" will probably require the examiner to make the motor responses corresponding to the patient's oral verbal response. Similarly, on some tasks, such as card sorting or tower tests, it may behoove the examiner to hold and move the cards or blocks/beads as instructed by the patient. In contrast, tests requiring pointing rather than oral responses may be more appropriate for patients with speech impairment. In general, tests with significant motor demands are better avoided with patients who have movement disorders. In parkinsonians with fatigability, severe motor "off" periods, or frequent fluctuations, breaks will need to be taken. Though nonmotor tasks might be administered when patients have dyskinesias, the patient may still be distracted by these movements and this needs to be considered in interpreting the test results. Although there may occasionally be a need to compare performances in the "on" and "off" medications, it is recommended that patients be tested while on their medications. Some have found that similarities outweigh differences when test performances are compared in motor "on" and "off" states (Delis & Massman, 1992), but this may only be true earlier in the disease when the difference between motor "on" and "off" is much smaller than later in the disease, when this difference is pronounced. In more advanced PD, testing during the "off" state can be unnecessarily challenging for patient and test administrator, and the patient may also experience increased dysphoria and anxiety, further complicating test interpretation.

Note

1 The traditional Richardson syndrome is equivalent to what is commonly understood to be PSP.

References

Aarsland, D., Bronnick, K., Larsen, J. P., Tysnes, O. B., & Alves, G. (2009). Cognitive impairment in incident, untreated Parkinson disease: The Norwegian ParkWest study. *Neurology*, *72*(13), 1121–1126. doi: 01.wnl.0000338632.00552.cb [pii] 10.1212/01.wnl.0000338632.00552.cb

Aarsland, D., Hutchinson, M., & Larsen, J. P. (2003). Cognitive, psychiatric and motor response to galantamine in Parkinson's disease with dementia. *International Journal of Geriatric Psychiatry*, *18*(10), 937–941.

Aarsland, D., Larsen, J. P., Karlsen, K., Lim, N. G., & Tandberg, E. (1999). Mental symptoms in Parkinson's disease are important contributors to caregiver distress. *International Journal of Geriatric Psychiatry*, *14*(10), 866–874.

Aarsland, D., Litvan, I., & Larsen, J. P. (2001). Neuropsychiatric symptoms of patients with progressive supranuclear palsy and Parkinson's disease. *Journal of Neuropsychiatry and Clinical Neurosciences*, *13*(1), 42–49.

Aarsland, D., Litvan, I., Salmon, D., Galasko, D., Wentzel-Larsen, T., & Larsen, J. P. (2003). Performance on the Dementia Rating Scale in Parkinson's disease with dementia and dementia with Lewy bodies: Comparison with progressive supranuclear palsy and Alzheimer's disease. *Journal of Neurology, Neurosurgery, and Psychiatry*, *74*, 1215–1220.

Aarsland, D., Taylor, J. P., & Weintraub, D. (2014). Psychiatric issues in cognitive impairment. *Movement Disorders*, *29*(5), 651–662. doi: 10.1002/mds.25873

Aarsland, D., Zaccai, J., & Brayne, C. (2005). A systematic review of prevalence studies of dementia in Parkinson's disease. *Movement Disorders*, *20*(10), 1255–1263.

Aasly, J. O., Toft, M., Fernandez-Mata, I., Kachergus, J., Hulihan, M., White, L. R., & Farrer, M. (2005). Clinical features of LRRK2-associated Parkinson's disease in central Norway. *Annals of Neurology*, *57*(5), 762–765. doi: 10.1002/ana.20456

Abboud, H., Floden, D., Thompson, N. R., Genc, G., Oravivattanakul, S., Alsallom, F., . . . Fernandez, H. H. (2014). Impact of mild cognitive impairment on outcome following deep brain stimulation surgery for Parkinson's disease. *Parkinsonism and Related Disorders*, *21*, 249–253. doi: 10.1016/j.parkreldis.2014.12.018

Adler, C. H., Caviness, J. N., Sabbagh, M. N., Shill, H. A., Connor, D. J., Sue, L., . . . Beach, T. G. (2010). Heterogeneous neuropathological findings in Parkinson's disease with mild cognitive impairment. *Acta Neuropathologica*, *120*(6), 827–828. doi: 10.1007/s00401-010-0744-4

Albanese, A., Bhatia, K., Bressman, S. B., Delong, M. R., Fahn, S., Fung, V. S., . . . Teller, J. K. (2013). Phenomenology and classification of dystonia: A consensus update. *Movement Disorders*, *28*(7), 863–873. doi: 10.1002/mds.25475

Albert, M. L., Feldman, R. G., & Willis, A. L. (1974). The 'subcortical dementia' of progressive supranuclear palsy. *Journal of Neurology Neurosurgery and Psychiatry*, *37*(2), 121–130.

Alcalay, R. N., Caccappolo, E., Mejia-Santana, H., Tang, M. X., Rosado, L., Orbe Reilly, M., . . . Marder, K. S. (2014). Cognitive and motor function in long-duration PARKIN-associated Parkinson disease. *JAMA Neurology*, *71*(1), 62–67. doi: 10.1001/jamaneurol.2013.4498

Alcalay, R. N., Mejia-Santana, H., Tang, M. X., Rakitin, B., Rosado, L., Ross, B., . . . Caccappolo, E. (2010). Self-report of cognitive impairment and mini-mental state examination performance in PRKN, LRRK2, and GBA carriers with early onset Parkinson's disease. *Journal of Clinical and Experimental Neuropsychology*, *32*(7), 775–779. doi: 10.1080/13803390903521018

Alegret, M., Junqué, C., Valldeoriola, F., Vendrell, P., Marti, M. J., & Tolosa, E. (2001). Obsessive-compulsive symptoms in Parkinson's disease. *Journal of Neurology, Neurosurgery, and Psychiatry*, *70*(3), 394–396.

Alegret, M., Pere, V., Junqué, C., Valldeoriola, F., & Tolosa, E. (2001). Visuospatial deficits in Parkinson's disease assessed by Judgment of Line Orientation Test: Error analyses and practice effects. *Journal of Clinical and Experimental Neuropsychology*, *23*(5), 592–598.

Alexander, G. E., DeLong, M. R., & Strick, P. L. (1986). Parallel organization of functionally segregated circuits linking basal ganglia and cortex. *Annual Review of Neuroscience*, *9*, 357–381.

Alexander, S. K., Rittman, T., Xuereb, J. H., Bak, T. H., Hodges, J. R., & Rowe, J. B. (2014). Validation of the new consensus criteria for the diagnosis of corticobasal degeneration. *Journal of Neurology, Neurosurgery, and Psychiatry*, *85*(8), 925–929. doi: 10.1136/jnnp-2013-307035

Almgren, P. E., Andersson, A. L., & Kullberg, G. (1969). Differences in verbally expressed cognition following left and right ventrolateral thalamotomy. *Scandinavian Journal of Psychology*, *10*(4), 243–249.

Alvarez, L., Macias, R., Guridi, J., Lopez, G., Alvarez, E., Maragoto, C., . . . Obeso, J. A. (2001). Dorsal subthalamotomy for Parkinson's disease. *Movement Disorders*, *16*(1), 72–78.

Amanzio, M., Monteverdi, S., Giordano, A., Soliveri, P., Filippi, P., & Geminiani, G. (2010). Impaired awareness of movement disorders in Parkinson's disease. *Brain and Cognition*, *72*(3), 337–346. doi: 10.1016/j.bandc.2009.10.011

American Psychiatric Association. (2013). *Diagnostic and Statistical Manual of Mental Disorders (DSM-5)* (5th ed.). Washington, DC: American Psychiatric Association.

Anderson, K. E. (2011). Psychiatric testing. In M. Hallett, A. E. Lang, J. Jankovic, S. Fahn, P. W. Halligan, V. Voon, & C. R. Cloninger (Eds.), *Psychogenic Movement Disorders and Other Conversion Disorders* (pp. 235–239). Cambridge, UK: Cambridge University Press.

Annesi, G., Savettieri, G., Pugliese, P., D'Amelio, M., Tarantino, P., Ragonese, P., . . . Quattrone, A. (2005). DJ-1 mutations and parkinsonism-dementia-amyotrophic lateral sclerosis complex. *Annals of Neurology*, *58*(5), 803–807. doi: 10.1002/ana.20666

Apaydin, H., Ahlskog, J. E., Parisi, J. E., Boeve, B. F., & Dickson, D. W. (2002). Parkinson disease neuropathology: Later-developing dementia and loss of the levodopa response. *Archives of Neurology*, *59*(1), 102–112.

Armstrong, M. J., Litvan, I., Lang, A. E., Bak, T. H., Bhatia, K. P., Borroni, B., . . . Weiner, W. J. (2013). Criteria for the diagnosis of corticobasal degeneration. *Neurology*, *80*(5), 496–503. doi: 10.1212/WNL.0b013e31827f0fd1

Asso, D., Crown, S., Russell, J. A., & Logue, V. (1969). Psychological aspects of the stereotactic treatment of parkinsonism. *British Journal of Psychiatry*, *115*(522), 541–553.

Azuma, T., Bayles, K. A., Cruz, R. F., Tomoeda, C. K., Wood, J. A., McGeagh, A., & Montgomery, E. B., Jr. (1997). Comparing the difficulty of letter, semantic, and name fluency tasks for normal elderly and patients with Parkinson's disease. *Neuropsychology*, *11*(4), 488–497.

Baldereschi, M., Di Carlo, A., Rocca, W. A., Vanni, P., Maggi, S., Perissinotto, E., . . . Inzitari, D. (2000). Parkinson's disease and parkinsonism in a longitudinal study: Two-fold higher incidence in men: Italian longitudinal study on aging. *Neurology*, *55*(9), 1358–1363.

Ballard, C. G., Aarsland, D., McKeith, I., O'Brien, J., Gray, A., Cormack, F., . . . Tovee, M. (2002). Fluctuations in attention: PD dementia vs DLB with parkinsonism. *Neurology*, *59*(11), 1714–1720.

Ballard, C. G., Ziabreva, I., Perry, R., Larsen, J. P., O'Brien, J., McKeith, I., . . . Aarsland, D. (2006). Differences in neuropathologic characteristics across the Lewy body dementia spectrum. *Neurology*, *67*(11), 1931–1934. doi: 10.1212/01.wnl.0000249130.63615.cc

Barone, P., Scarzella, L., Marconi, R., Antonini, A., Morgante, L., Bracco, F., . . . Musch, B. (2006). Pramipexole versus sertraline in the treatment of depression in Parkinson's disease: A national multicenter parallel-group randomized study. *Journal of Neurology*, *253*(5), 601–607.

Beardsley, J., & Puletti, F. (1971). Personality (MMPI) and cognitive (WAIS) changes after L-DOPA treatment. *Archives of Neurology*, *25*, 145–150.

Beatty, W. W., & Monson, N. (1989). Lexical processing in Parkinson's disease and multiple sclerosis. *Journal of Geriatric Psychiatry and Neurology*, *2*(3), 145–152.

Beatty, W. W., Salmon, D. P., Butters, N., Heindel, W. C., & Granholm, E. L. (1988). Retrograde amnesia in patients with Alzheimer's disease or Huntington's disease. *Neurobiology of Aging*, *9*(2), 181–186.

Beatty, W. W., Scott, J. G., Wilson, D. A., Prince, J. R., & Williamson, D. J. (1995). Memory deficits in a demented patient with probable corticobasal degeneration. *Journal of Geriatric Psychiatry and Neurology*, *8*(2), 132–136.

Beatty, W. W., Staton, R. D., Weir, W. S., Monson, N., & Whitaker, H. A. (1989). Cognitive disturbances in Parkinson's disease. *Journal of Geriatric Psychiatry and Neurology*, *2*(1), 22–33.

Bechara, A. (2007). *Iowa Gambling Task Professional Manual*. Lutz, FL: Psychological Assessment Resources.

Beck, A. T., Ward, C. H., Mendelson, M., Mock, J., & Erbaugh, J. (1961). An inventory for measuring depression. *Archives of General Psychiatry*, *4*, 53–63.

Bedard, M. A., Pillon, B., Dubois, B., Duchesne, N., Masson, H., & Agid, Y. (1999). Acute and long-term administration of anticholinergics in Parkinson's disease: Specific effects on the subcortico-frontal syndrome. *Brain and Cognition*, *40*(2), 289–313.

Benito-Leon, J., Louis, E. D., & Bermejo-Pareja, F. (2006). Elderly-onset essential tremor is associated with dementia. *Neurology*, *66*(10), 1500–1505. doi: 66/10/1500 [pii] 10.1212/01.wnl.0000216134.88617.de

Benito-Leon, J., Louis, E. D., Mitchell, A. J., & Bermejo-Pareja, F. (2011). Elderly-onset essential tremor and mild cognitive impairment: A population-based study (NEDICES). *Journal of Alzheimer's Disease*, *23*(4), 727–735. doi: 10.3233/JAD-2011-101572

Berciano, J. (1982). Olivopontocerebellar atrophy: A review of 117 cases. *Journal of the Neurological Sciences*, *53*(2), 253–272.

Berent, S., Giordani, B., Gilman, S., Trask, C. L., Little, R. J., Johanns, J. R., . . . Koeppe, R. A. (2002). Patterns of neuropsychological performance in multiple system atrophy compared to sporadic and hereditary olivopontocerebellar atrophy. *Brain and Cognition*, *50*(2), 194–206.

Berger, H. J., van Es, N. J., van Spaendonck, K. P., Teunisse, J. P., Horstink, M. W., van 't Hof, M. A., & Cools, A. R. (1999). Relationship between memory strategies and motor symptoms in Parkinson's disease. *Journal of Clinical and Experimental Neuropsychology*, *21*(5), 677–684.

Bernheimer, H., Birkmayer, W., Hornykiewicz, O., Jellinger, K., & Seitelberger, F. (1973). Brain dopamine and the syndromes of Parkinson and Huntington. *Journal of the Neurological Sciences*, *20*, 415–455.

Bhalsing, K. S., Kumar, K. J., Saini, J., Yadav, R., Gupta, A. K., & Pal, P. K. (2015). White matter correlates of cognitive impairment in essential tremor. *American Journal of Neuroradiology*, *36*(3), 448–453. doi: 10.3174/ajnr.A4138

Biggins, C. A., Boyd, J. L., Harrop, F. M., Madeley, P., Mindham, R.H.S., Randall, J. I., & Spokes, E.G.S. (1992). A controlled, longitudinal study of dementia in Parkinson's disease. *Journal of Neurology, Neurosurgery, and Psychiatry*, *55*(7), 566–571.

Bodis-Wollner, I. (2003). Neuropsychological and perceptual defects in Parkinson's disease. *Parkinsonism and Related Disorders*, *9*, S83–S89.

Boeve, B., Dickson, D., Duffy, J., Bartleson, J., Trenerry, M., & Petersen, R. (2003). Progressive nonfluent aphasia and subsequent aphasic dementia associated with atypical progressive supranuclear palsy pathology. *European Neurology*, *49*(2), 72–78.

Bohnen, N. I., Kaufer, D. I., Hendrickson, R., Constantine, G. M., Mathis, C. A., & Moore, R. Y. (2007). Cortical cholinergic denervation is associated with depressive symptoms in Parkinson's disease and parkinsonian dementia. *Journal of Neurology, Neurosurgery, and Psychiatry*, *78*(6), 641–643.

Bohnen, N. I., Kaufer, D. I., Hendrickson, R., Ivanco, L. S., Lopresti, B. J., Constantine, G. M., . . . Dekosky, S. T. (2006). Cognitive correlates of cortical cholinergic denervation in Parkinson's disease and parkinsonian dementia. *Journal of Neurology*, *253*(2), 242–247.

Boller, F., Mizutani, T., Roessmann, U., & Gambetti, P. (1980). Parkinson disease, dementia, and Alzheimer disease: Clinicopathological correlations. *Annals of Neurology*, *7*(4), 329–335.

Bolluk, B., Ozel-Kizil, E. T., Akbostanci, M. C., & Atbasoglu, E. C. (2010). Social anxiety in patients with Parkinson's disease. *The Journal of Neuropsychiatry and Clinical Neurosciences*, *22*(4), 390–394. doi: 10.1176/appi.neuropsych.22.4.390

Bowen, F. P., Hoehn, M. M., & Yahr, M. D. (1972). Parkinsonism: Alterations in spatial orientation as determined by a route-walking test. *Neuropsychologia*, *10*(3), 355–361.

Bower, J. H., Maraganore, D. M., McDonnell, S. K., & Rocca, W. A. (1997). Incidence of progressive supranuclear palsy and multiple system atrophy in Olmsted County, Minnesota, 1976 to 1990. *Neurology*, *49*(5), 1284–1288.

Bower, J. H., Maraganore, D. M., McDonnell, S. K., & Rocca, W. A. (1999). Incidence and distribution of parkinsonism in Olmsted County, Minnesota, 1976–1990. *Neurology*, *52*(6), 1214–1220.

Braak, H., Rub, U., & Del Tredici, K. (2006). Cognitive decline correlates with neuropathological stage in Parkinson's disease. *Journal of Neurological Sciences*, *248*(1–2), 255–258.

Braak, H., Rub, U., Jansen Steur, E. N., Del Tredici, K., & de Vos, R. A. (2005). Cognitive status correlates with neuropathologic stage in Parkinson disease. *Neurology*, *64*(8), 1404–1410.

Braak, H., Tredici, K. D., Rüb, U., de Vos, R. A., Jansen Steur, E. N., & Braak, E. (2003). Staging of brain pathology related to sporadic Parkinson's disease. *Neurobiology of Aging*, *24*(2), 197–211.

Brandt, J. (2009). Huntington's disease. In I. Grant & K. M. Adams (Eds.), *Neuropsychological Assessment of Neuropsychiatric and Neuromedical Disorders* (3rd ed., pp. 223–240). New York: Oxford University Press.

Broeders, M., de Bie, R. M., Velseboer, D. C., Speelman, J. D., Muslimovic, D., & Schmand, B. (2013). Evolution of mild cognitive impairment in Parkinson disease. *Neurology*, *81*(4), 346–352. doi: 10.1212/WNL.0b013e31829c5c86

Bronnick, K., Alves, G., Aarsland, D., Tysnes, O. B., & Larsen, J. P. (2011). Verbal memory in drug-naive, newly diagnosed Parkinson's disease: The retrieval deficit hypothesis revisited. *Neuropsychology*, *25*(1), 114–124. doi: 10.1037/a0020857

Brown, R. G., Lacomblez, L., Landwehrmeyer, B. G., Bak, T., Uttner, I., Dubois, B., . . . Leigh, N. P. (2010). Cognitive impairment in patients with multiple system atrophy and progressive supranuclear palsy. *Brain: A Journal of Neurology*, *133*(Pt 8), 2382–2393. doi: 10.1093/brain/awq158

Brown, R. G., MacCarthy, B., Jahanshahi, M., & Marsden, C. D. (1989). Accuracy of self-reported disability in patients with parkinsonism. *Archives of Neurology*, *46*(9), 955–959.

Brown, R. G., & Marsden, C. D. (1986). Visuospatial function in Parkinson's disease. *Brain*, *109*(Pt 5), 987–1002.

Brown, R. G., & Marsden, C. D. (1988). Internal versus external cues and the control of attention in Parkinson's disease. *Brain*, *111*(Pt 2), 323–345.

Brusa, L., Bassi, A., Stefani, A., Pierantozzi, M., Peppe, A., Caramia, M. D., . . . Stanzione, P. (2003). Pramipexole in comparison to l-dopa: A neuropsychological study. *Journal of Neural Transmission*, *110*(4), 373–380. doi: 10.1007/s00702-002-0811-7

Brusa, L., Tiraboschi, P., Koch, G., Peppe, A., Pierantozzi, M., Ruggieri, S., & Stanzione, P. (2005). Pergolide effect on cognitive functions in early-mild Parkinson's disease. *Journal of Neural Transmission*, *112*(2), 231–237.

Bullock, R., & Cameron, A. (2002). Rivastigmine for the treatment of dementia and visual hallucinations associated with Parkinson's disease: A case series. *Current Medical Research and Opinion*, *18*(5), 258–264.

Burrell, J. R., Hodges, J. R., & Rowe, J. B. (2014). Cognition in corticobasal syndrome and progressive supranuclear palsy: A review. *Movement Disorders*, *29*(5), 684–693. doi: 10.1002/mds.25872

Burrell, J. R., Hornberger, M., Villemagne, V. L., Rowe, C. C., & Hodges, J. R. (2013). Clinical profile of PiB-positive corticobasal syndrome. *PloS One*, *8*(4), e61025. doi: 10.1371/journal.pone.0061025

Buttery, P. C., & Barker, R. A. (2014). Treating Parkinson's disease in the 21st century: Can stem cell transplantation compete? *Journal of Comparative Neurology*, *522*(12), 2802–2816. doi: 10.1002/cne.23577

Buytenhuijs, E. L., Berger, H. J., Van Spaendonck, K. P., Horstink, M. W., Borm, G. F., & Cools, A. R. (1994). Memory and learning strategies in patients with Parkinson's disease. *Neuropsychologia*, *32*(3), 335–342.

Caccappolo, E., Alcalay, R. N., Mejia-Santana, H., Tang, M. X., Rakitin, B., Rosado, L., . . . Marder, K. S. (2011). Neuropsychological profile of Parkin mutation carriers with and without Parkinson disease: The CORE-PD study. *Journal of the International Neuropsychological Society*, *17*(1), 91–100. doi: 10.1017/S1355617710001190

Cahn, D. A., Sullivan, E. V., Shear, P. K., Pfefferbaum, A., Heit, G., & Silverberg, G. (1998). Differential contributions of cognitive and motor component processes to physical and instrumental activities of daily living in Parkinson's disease. *Archives of Clinical Neuropsychology*, *13*, 575–583.

Calleo, J., Burrows, C., Levin, H., Marsh, L., Lai, E., & York, M. K. (2012). Cognitive rehabilitation for executive dysfunction in Parkinson's disease: Application and current directions. *Parkinsons Disease*, *2012*, 512892. doi: 10.1155/2012/512892

Charcot, J. M., & Vulpian, A. (1861). De la paralysie agitante. *Gazette Hebdomadaire de Medicine et Chirurgie*, *8*, 765–767.

Charcot, J. M., & Vulpian, A. (1862). De la paralysie agitante. *Gazette Hebdomadaire de Medicine et Chirurgie*, *9*, 54–59.

Chen, P., Kales, H. C., Weintraub, D., Blow, F. C., Jiang, L., Ignacio, R. V., & Mellow, A. M. (2007). Depression in veterans with Parkinson's disease: Frequency, co-morbidity, and healthcare utilization. *International Journal of Geriatric Psychiatry*, *22*(6), 543–548. doi: 10.1002/gps.1712

Chiaravalloti, N. D., Ibarretxe-Bilbao, N., DeLuca, J., Rusu, O., Pena, J., Garcia-Gorostiaga, I., & Ojeda, N. (2014). The source of the memory impairment in Parkinson's disease: Acquisition versus retrieval. *Movement Disorders*, *29*(6), 765–771. doi: 10.1002/mds.25842

Christensen, A. L., Juul-Jensen, P., Malmros, R., & Harmsen, A. (1970). Psychological evaluation of intelligence and personality in parkinsonism before and after stereotaxic surgery. *Acta Neurologica Scandanavica*, *46*(4), 527–537.

Clarimon, J., & Kulisevsky, J. (2013). Parkinson's disease: From genetics to clinical practice. *Current Genomics*, *14*(8), 560–567. doi: 10.2174/13892029146661312102123O5

Cohen, H., Bouchard, S., Scherzer, P., & Whitaker, H. (1994). Language and verbal reasoning in Parkinson's disease. *Neuropsychiatry, Neuropsychology, and Behavioral Neurology*, *7*(3), 166–175.

Cole, S. A., Woodard, J. L., Juncos, J. L., Kogos, J. L., Youngstrom, E. A., & Watts, R. L. (1996). Depression and disability in Parkinson's disease. *Journal of Neuropsychiatry and Clinical Neuroscience*, *8*(1), 20–25.

Colosimo, C., Bak, T. H., Bologna, M., & Berardelli, A. (2014). Fifty years of progressive supranuclear palsy. *Journal of Neurology, Neurosurgery, and Psychiatry*, *85*(8), 938–944. doi: 10.1136/jnnp-2013-305740

Colosimo, C., Hughes, A. J., Kilford, L., & Lees, A. J. (2003). Lewy body cortical involvement may not always predict dementia in Parkinson's disease. *Journal of Neurology, Neurosurgery, and Psychiatry*, *74*, 852–856.

Colosimo, C., Morgante, L., Antonini, A., Barone, P., Avarello, T. P., Bottacchi, E., . . . Priamo Study, G. (2010). Non-motor symptoms in atypical and secondary parkinsonism: The PRIAMO study. *Journal of Neurology*, *257*(1), 5–14. doi: 10.1007/s00415-009-5255-7

Connor, D. J., Salmon, D. P., Sandy, T. J., Galasko, D., Hansen, L. A., & Thal, L. J. (1998). Cognitive profiles of autopsy-confirmed Lewy body variant vs pure Alzheimer disease. *Archives of Neurology*, *55*(7), 994–1000.

Conrad, C., Andreadis, A., Trojanowski, J. Q., Dickson, D. W., Kang, D., Chen, X., . . . Saitoh, T. (1997). Genetic evidence for the involvement of tau in progressive supranuclear palsy. *Annals of Neurology*, *41*(2), 277–281.

Cools, R. (2006). Dopaminergic modulation of cognitive function-implications for L-DOPA treatment in Parkinson's disease. *Neuroscience and Biobehavioral Reviews*, *30*(1), 1–23.

Cools, R., Barker, R. A., Sahakian, B. J., & Robbins, T. W. (2003). L-Dopa medication remediates cognitive inflexibility, but increases impulsivity in patients with Parkinson's disease. *Neuropsychologia*, *41*, 1431–1441.

Cools, R., Stefanova, E., Barker, R. A., Robbins, T. W., & Owen, A. M. (2002). Dopaminergic modulation of high-level cognition in Parkinson's disease: The role of the prefrontal cortex revealed by PET. *Brain*, *125*(Pt 3), 584–594.

Cooper, J. A., Sagar, H. J., Jordan, N., Harvey, N. S., & Sullivan, E. V. (1991). Cognitive impairment in early, untreated Parkinson's disease and its relationship to motor disability. *Brain*, *114*(Pt 5), 2095–2122.

Cooper, J. A., Sagar, H. J., & Sullivan, E. V. (1993). Short-term memory and temporal ordering in early Parkinson's disease: Effects of disease chronicity and medication. *Neuropsychologia*, *31*(9), 933–949.

Cordato, N. J., Pantelis, C., Halliday, G. M., Velakoulis, D., Wood, S. J., Stuart, G. W., . . . Morris, J. G. (2002). Frontal atrophy correlates with behavioural changes in progressive supranuclear palsy. *Brain*, *125*(Pt 4), 789–800.

Costa, A., Peppe, A., Caltagirone, C., & Carlesimo, G. A. (2008). Prospective memory impairment in individuals with Parkinson's disease. *Neuropsychology*, *22*(3), 283–292. doi: 2008-05020-001 [pii] 10.1037/0894-4105.22.3.283

Costa, A., Peppe, A., Dell'Agnello, G., Carlesimo, G. A., Murri, L., Bonuccelli, U., & Caltagirone, C. (2003). Dopaminergic modulation of visual-spatial working memory in Parkinson's disease. *Dementia and Geriatric Cognitive Disorders*, *15*(2), 55–66.

Costa, A., Peppe, A., Zabberoni, S., Serafini, F., Barban, F., Scalici, F., . . . Carlesimo, G. A. (2015). Prospective memory performance in individuals with Parkinson's disease who have mild cognitive impairment. *Neuropsychology, 29*, 782–791. doi: 10.1037/neu0000184

Cousins, R., Hanley, J. R., Davies, A. D., Turnbull, C. J., & Playfer, J. R. (2000). Understanding memory for faces in Parkinson's disease: The role of configural processing. *Neuropsychologia*, *38*(6), 837–847.

Cronin-Golomb, A., Corkin, S., & Growdon, J. H. (1994). Impaired problem solving in Parkinson's disease: Impact of a set-shifting deficit. *Neuropsychologia*, *32*(5), 579–593.

Cummings, J. L., Darkins, A., Mendez, M., Hill, M. A., & Benson, D. F. (1988). Alzheimer's disease and Parkinson's disease: Comparison of speech and language alterations. *Neurology*, *38*(5), 680–684.

Czernecki, V., Pillon, B., Houeto, J. L., Pochon, J. B., Levy, R., & Dubois, B. (2002). Motivation, reward, and Parkinson's disease: Influence of dopatherapy. *Neuropsychologia*, *40*, 2257–2267.

Dagher, A., Owen, A. M., Boecker, H., & Brooks, D. J. (1999). Mapping the network for planning: A correlational PET activation study with the Tower of London task. *Brain*, *122*(Pt 10), 1973–1987.

Darvesh, S., & Freedman, M. (1996). Subcortical dementia: A neurobehavioral approach. *Brain and Cognition*, *31*(2), 230–249.

Delis, D. C., & Massman, P. J. (1992). The effects of dopamine fluctuation on cognition and affect. In S. J. Huber & J. L. Cummings (Eds.), *Parkinson's Disease: Neurobehavioral Aspects* (pp. 288–302). New York: Oxford University Press.

den Brok, M. G., Dalen, J. W., van Gool, W. A., Moll van Charante, E. P., de Bie, R. M., & Richard, E. (2015). Apathy in Parkinson's disease: A systematic review and meta-analysis. *Movement Disorders*, *30*, 759–769. doi: 10.1002/mds.26208

Deuschl, G., & Bergman, H. (2002). Pathophysiology of nonparkinsonian tremors. *Movement Disorders*, *17*(Suppl. 3), S41–S48.

Devos, D., Dujardin, K., Poirot, I., Moreau, C., Cottencin, O., Thomas, P., . . . Defebvre, L. (2008). Comparison of desipramine and citalopram treatments for depression in Parkinson's disease: A double-blind, randomized, placebo-controlled study. *Movement Disorders*, *23*(6), 850–857. doi: 10.1002/mds.21966

Diederich, N. J., Pieri, V., & Goetz, C. G. (2003). Coping strategies for visual hallucinations in Parkinson's disease. *Movement Disorders*, *18*(7), 831–832. doi: 10.1002/mds.10450

Diller, L., Riklan, M., & Cooper, I. S. (1956). Preoperative response to stress as a criterion of the response to neurosurgery in Parkinson's disease. *Journal of the American Geriatrics Society*, *4*, 1301–1308.

Dissanayaka, N. N., Sellbach, A., Matheson, S., Marsh, R., Silburn, P. A., O'Sullivan, J. D., . . . Mellick, G. D. (2007). Validity of Hamilton depression inventory in Parkinson's disease. *Movement Disorders*, *22*(3), 399–403.

Dobkin, R. D., Menza, M., Allen, L. A., Gara, M. A., Mark, M. H., Tiu, J., . . . Friedman, J. (2011). Cognitive-behavioral therapy for depression in Parkinson's disease: A randomized, controlled trial. *American Journal of Psychiatry*, *168*(10), 1066–1074. doi: 10.1176/appi.ajp.2011.10111669

Dobkin, R. D., Menza, M., Bienfait, K. L., Gara, M., Marin, H., Mark, M. H., . . . Troster, A. (2010). The impact of antidepressant treatment on cognitive functioning in depressed patients with Parkinson's disease. *The Journal of Neuropsychiatry and Clinical Neurosciences*, *22*(2), 188–195. doi: 10.1176/appi.neuropsych.22.2.188

Dobkin, R. D., Troster, A. I., Rubino, J. T., Allen, L. A., Gara, M. A., Mark, M. H., & Menza, M. (2014). Neuropsychological outcomes after psychosocial intervention for depression in Parkinson's disease. *The Journal of Neuropsychiatry and Clinical Neurosciences*, *26*(1), 57–63. doi: 10.1176/appi.neuropsych.12120381

Dorsey, E. R., Constantinescu, R., Thompson, J. P., Biglan, K. M., Holloway, R. G., Kieburtz, K., . . . Tanner, C. M. (2007). Projected number of people with Parkinson disease in the most populous nations, 2005 through 2030. *Neurology*, *68*(5), 384–386. doi: 10.1212/01.wnl.0000247740.47667.03

Downes, J. J., Priestley, N. M., Doran, M., Ferran, J., Ghadiali, E., & Cooper, P. (1998). Intellectual, mnemonic, and frontal functions in dementia with Lewy bodies: A comparison with early and advanced Parkinson's disease. *Behavioural Neurology*, *11*(3), 173–183.

Dubois, B., Deweer, B., & Pillon, B. (1996). The cognitive syndrome of progressive supranuclear palsy. *Advances in Neurology*, *69*, 399–403.

Dubois, B., Pillon, B., Legault, F., Agid, Y., & Lhermitte, F. (1988). Slowing of cognitive processing in progressive supranuclear palsy: A comparison with Parkinson's disease. *Archives of Neurology*, *45*(11), 1194–1199.

Duff, K., Beglinger, L. J., Theriault, D., Allison, J., & Paulsen, J. S. (2010). Cognitive deficits in Huntington's disease on the repeatable battery for the assessment of neuropsychological status. *Journal of Clinical and Experimental Neuropsychology*, *32*(3), 231–238. doi: 10.1080/13803390902926184

Dujardin, K., Defebvre, L., Krystkowiak, P., Degreef, J. F., & Destee, A. (2003). Executive function differences in multiple system atrophy and Parkinson's disease. *Parkinsonism and Related Disorders*, *9*, 205–211.

Dymek, M. P., Atchison, P., Harrell, L., & Marson, D. C. (2001). Competency to consent to medical treatment in cognitively impaired patients with Parkinson's disease. *Neurology*, *56*(1), 17–24.

Elgh, E., Domellof, M., Linder, J., Edstrom, M., Stenlund, H., & Forsgren, L. (2009). Cognitive function in early Parkinson's disease: A population-based study. *European Journal of Neurology*, *16*(12), 1278–1284. doi: ENE2707 [pii] 10.1111/j.1468-1331.2009.02707.x

Ellfolk, U., Huurinainen, S., Joutsa, J., & Karrasch, M. (2012). The effect of encoding condition on free recall in Parkinson's disease:

Incidental and intentional memory are equally affected. *The Clinical Neuropsychologist*, *26*(6), 909–925. doi: 10.1080/13854046.2012.697192

Ephraty, L., Porat, O., Israeli, D., Cohen, O. S., Tunkel, O., Yael, S., . . . Hassin-Baer, S. (2007). Neuropsychiatric and cognitive features in autosomal-recessive early parkinsonism due to PINK1 mutations. *Movement Disorders*, *22*(4), 566–569. doi: 10.1002/mds.21319

Estanga, A., Rodriguez-Oroz, M. C., Ruiz-Martinez, J., Barandiaran, M., Gorostidi, A., Bergareche, A., . . . Marti-Masso, J. F. (2014). Cognitive dysfunction in Parkinson's disease related to the R1441G mutation in LRRK2. *Parkinsonism Relat Disord*, *20*(10), 1097–1100. doi: 10.1016/j.parkreldis.2014.07.005

Evans, A. H., & Lees, A. J. (2004). Dopamine dysregulation syndrome in Parkinson's disease. *Current Opinion in Neurology*, *17*(4), 393–398.

Faglioni, P., Saetti, M. C., & Botti, C. (2000). Verbal learning strategies in Parkinson's disease. *Neuropsychology*, *14*(3), 456–470.

Fama, R., Sullivan, E. V., Shear, P. K., Stein, M., Yesavage, J. A., Tinklenberg, J. R., & Pfefferbaum, A. (2000). Extent, pattern, and correlates of remote memory impairment in Alzheimer's disease and Parkinson's disease. *Neuropsychology*, *14*(2), 265–276.

Farrer, M., Gwinn-Hardy, K., Muenter, M., DeVrieze, F. W., Crook, R., Perez-Tur, J., . . . Hardy, J. (1999). A chromosome 4p haplotype segregating with Parkinson's disease and postural tremor. *Human Molecular Genetics*, *8*(1), 81–85.

Faust-Socher, A., Kenett, Y. N., Cohen, O. S., Hassin-Baer, S., & Inzelberg, R. (2014). Enhanced creative thinking under dopaminergic therapy in Parkinson disease. *Annals of Neurology*, *75*(6), 935–942. doi: 10.1002/ana.24181

Feigin, A., Ghilardi, M. F., Carbon, M., Edwards, C., Fukuda, M., Dhawan, V., . . . Eidelberg, D. (2003). Effects of levodopa on motor sequence learning in Parkinson's disease. *Neurology*, *60*, 1744–1749.

Feinstein, A., Stergiopoulos, V., Fine, J., & Lang, A. E. (2001). Psychiatric outcome in patients with a psychogenic movement disorder: A prospective study. *Neuropsychiatry Neuropsychology and Behavioral Neurology*, *14*(3), 169–176.

Fenelon, G., & Alves, G. (2010). Epidemiology of psychosis in Parkinson's disease. *Journal of the Neurological Sciences*, *289*(1–2), 12–17. doi: 10.1016/j.jns.2009.08.014

Ferman, T. J., Smith, G. E., Boeve, B. F., Graff-Radford, N. R., Lucas, J. A., Knopman, D. S., . . . Dickson, D. W. (2006). Neuropsychological differentiation of dementia with Lewy bodies from normal aging and Alzheimer's disease. *The Clinical Neuropsychologist*, *20*(4), 623–636.

Fernandez, H. H., Aarsland, D., Fenelon, G., Friedman, J. H., Marsh, L., Troster, A. I., . . . Goetz, C. G. (2008). Scales to assess psychosis in Parkinson's disease: Critique and recommendations. *Movement Disorders*, *23*(4), 484–500. doi: 10.1002/mds.21875

Fernandez, H. H., See, R. H., Gary, M. F., Bowers, D., Rodriguez, R. L., Jacobson, C. T., & Okun, M. S. (2009). Depressive symptoms in Parkinson disease correlate with impaired global and specific cognitive performance. *Journal of Geriatric Psychiatry and Neurology*, *22*(4), 223–227. doi: 10.1177/0891988709335792

Fetoni, V., Soliveri, P., Monza, D., Testa, D., & Girotti, F. (1999). Affective symptoms in multiple system atrophy and Parkinson's disease: Response to levodopa therapy. *Journal of Neurology, Neurosurgery, and Psychiatry*, *66*(4), 541–544.

Fields, J. A. (2015). Effects of deep brain stimulation in movement disorders on cognition and behavior. In A. I. Tröster (Ed.), *Clinical Neuropsychology and Cognitive Neurology of Parkinson's Disease and Other Movement Disorders* (pp. 332–375). New York: Oxford University Press.

Fields, J. A., Tröster, A. I., Woods, S. P., Higginson, C. I., Wilkinson, S. B., Lyons, K. E., . . . Pahwa, R. (2003). Neuropsychological and quality of life outcomes 12 months after unilateral thalamic stimulation for essential tremor. *Journal of Neurology, Neurosurgery, and Psychiatry*, *74*(3), 305–311.

Filoteo, J. V., Friedrich, F. J., Rilling, L. M., Davis, J. D., Stricker, J. L., & Prenovitz, M. (2003). Semantic and cross-case identity priming in patients with Parkinson's disease. *Journal of Clinical and Experimental Neuropsychology*, *25*(4), 441–456.

Filoteo, J. V., Rilling, L. M., Cole, B., Williams, B. J., Davis, J. D., & Roberts, J. W. (1997). Variable memory profiles in Parkinson's disease. *Journal of Clinical and Experimental Neuropsychology*, *19*(6), 878–888.

Filoteo, J. V., Salmon, D. P., Schiehser, D. M., Kane, A. E., Hamilton, J. M., Rilling, L. M., . . . Galasko, D. R. (2009). Verbal learning and memory in patients with dementia with Lewy bodies or Parkinson's disease with dementia. *Journal of Clinical and Experimental Neuropsychology*, *31*(7), 823–834. doi: 908749749 [pii] 10.1080/13803390802572401

Filoteo, J. V., Williams, B. J., Rilling, L. M., & Roberts, J. W. (1997). Performance of Parkinson's disease patients on the visual search and attention test: Impairment in single-feature but not dual-feature visual search. *Archives of Clinical Neuropsychology*, *12*(7), 621–634.

Finali, G., Piccirilli, M., & Piccinin, G. L. (1994). Neuropsychological correlates of L-deprenyl therapy in idiopathic parkinsonism. *Progress in Neuro-Psychopharmacology and Biological Psychiatry*, *18*(1), 115–128.

Fink, K. D., Crane, A. T., Leveque, X., Dues, D. J., Huffman, L. D., Moore, A. C., . . . Dunbar, G. L. (2014). Intrastriatal transplantation of adenovirus-generated induced pluripotent stem cells for treating neuropathological and functional deficits in a rodent model of Huntington's disease. *Stem Cells Translational Medicine*, *3*(5), 620–631. doi: 10.5966/sctm.2013-0151

Finton, M. J., Lucas, J. A., Graff-Radford, N. R., & Uitti, R. J. (1998). Analysis of visuospatial errors in patients with Alzheimer's disease or Parkinson's disease. *Journal of Clinical and Experimental Neuropsychology*, *20*, 186–193.

Foerde, K., & Shohamy, D. (2011). The role of the basal ganglia in learning and memory: Insight from Parkinson's disease. *Neurobiology of Learning and Memory*, *96*(4), 624–636. doi: 10.1016/j.nlm.2011.08.006

Foltynie, T., Brayne, C. E., Robbins, T. W., & Barker, R. A. (2004). The cognitive ability of an incident cohort of Parkinson's patients in the UK: The CamPaIGN study. *Brain*, *127*(Pt 3), 550–560.

Foltynie, T., Goldberg, T. E., Lewis, S. G., Blackwell, A. D., Kolachana, B. S., Weinberger, D. R., . . . Barker, R. A. (2004). Planning ability in Parkinson's disease is influenced by the COMT val158met polymorphism. *Movement Disorders*, *19*(8), 885–891.

Forjaz, M. J., Ayala, A., Martinez-Martin, P., Dujardin, K., Pontone, G. M., Starkstein, S. E., . . . Leentjens, A. F. (2015). Is the Parkinson anxiety scale comparable across raters? *Movement Disorders*, *30*(4), 545–551. doi: 10.1002/mds.26111

Fournet, N., Moreaud, O., Roulin, J. L., Naegele, B., & Pellat, J. (2000). Working memory functioning in medicated Parkinson's disease patients and the effect of withdrawal of dopaminergic medication. *Neuropsychology*, *14*(2), 247–253.

Freedman, M., Rivoira, P., Butters, N., Sax, D. S., & Feldman, R. G. (1984). Retrograde amnesia in Parkinson's disease. *Canadian Journal of Neurological Sciences*, *11*(2), 297–301.

Freeman, R. Q., Giovannetti, T., Lamar, M., Cloud, B. S., Stern, R. A., Kaplan, E., & Libon, D. J. (2000). Visuoconstructional problems in dementia: Contribution of executive systems functions. *Neuropsychology*, *14*(3), 415–426.

Friedman, J. H., Alves, G., Hagell, P., Marinus, J., Marsh, L., Martinez-Martin, P., . . . Schrag, A. (2010). Fatigue rating scales critique and recommendations by the Movement Disorders Society task force on rating scales for Parkinson's disease. *Movement Disorders: Official Journal of the Movement Disorder Society*, *25*(7), 805–822. doi: 10.1002/mds.22989

Fünfgeld, E. W. (1967). *Psychopathologie und Klinik des Parkinsonismus vor und nach Stereotaktischen Operationen*. Berlin: Springer Verlag.

Gabrieli, J.D.E., Singh, J., Stebbins, G., & Goetz, C. G. (1996). Reduced working memory span in Parkinson's disease: Evidence for the role of a frontostriatal system in working and strategic memory. *Neuropsychology*, *10*, 322–332.

Galasko, D., Katzman, R., Salmon, D. P., & Hansen, L. (1996). Clinical and neuropathological findings in Lewy body dementias. *Brain and Cognition*, *31*(2), 166–175.

Gao, L., Diaz-Corrales, F. J., Carrillo, F., Diaz-Martin, J., Caceres-Redondo, M. T., Carballo, M., . . . Mir, P. (2010). Brain-derived neurotrophic factor G196A polymorphism and clinical features in Parkinson's disease. *Acta Neurologica Scandinavica*, *122*(1), 41–45. doi: 10.1111/j.1600-0404.2009.01253.x

Gasparini, M., Bonifati, V., Fabrizio, E., Fabbrini, G., Brusa, L., Lenzi, G. L., & Meco, G. (2001). Frontal lobe dysfunction in essential tremor: A preliminary study. *Journal of Neurology*, *248*(5), 399–402.

Gasparini, M., Fabrizio, E., Bonifati, V., & Meco, G. (1997). Cognitive improvement during Tolcapone treatment in Parkinson's disease. *Journal of Neural Transmission*, *104*(8–9), 887–894.

Gerstenecker, A., Duff, K., Mast, B., Litvan, I., & Group, E.-P. S. (2013). Behavioral abnormalities in progressive supranuclear palsy. *Psychiatry Research*, *210*(3), 1205–1210. doi: 10.1016/j.psychres.2013.08.045

Gerstenecker, A., Mast, B., Duff, K., Ferman, T. J., Litvan, I., & Group, E.-P. S. (2013). Executive dysfunction is the primary cognitive impairment in progressive supranuclear palsy. *Archives of Clinical Neuropsychology*, *28*(2), 104–113. doi: 10.1093/arclin/acs098

Gilman, S., Wenning, G. K., Low, P. A., Brooks, D. J., Mathias, C. J., Trojanowski, J. Q., . . . Vidailhet, M. (2008). Second consensus statement on the diagnosis of multiple system atrophy. *Neurology*, *71*(9), 670–676. doi: 10.1212/01.wnl.0000324625.00404.15

Giovannoni, G., O'Sullivan, J. D., Turner, K., Manson, A. J., & Lees, A. J. (2000a). Hedonistic homeostatic dysregulation in patients with Parkinson's disease on dopamine replacement therapies. *Journal of Neurology, Neurosurgery, and Psychiatry*, *68*(4), 423–428.

Giovannoni, G., O'Sullivan, J. D., Turner, K., Manson, A. J., & Lees, A. J. (2000b). Hedonistic homeostatic dysregulation in patients with Parkinson's disease on dopamine replacement therapies. *Journal of Neurology, Neurosurgery, and Psychiatry*, *68*(4), 423–428.

Globus, M., Mildworf, B., & Melamed, E. (1985). Cerebral blood flow and cognitive impairment in Parkinson's disease. *Neurology*, *35*(8), 1135–1139.

Gnanalingham, K. K., Byrne, E. J., Thornton, A., Sambrook, M. A., & Bannister, P. (1997). Motor and cognitive function in Lewy body dementia: Comparison with Alzheimer's and Parkinson's diseases. *Journal of Neurology, Neurosurgery, and Psychiatry*, *62*(3), 243–252.

Goetz, C. G. (1992). The historical background of behavioral studies in Parkinson's disease. In S. J. Huber & J. L. Cummings (Eds.), *Parkinson's Disease: Neurobehavioral Aspects* (pp. 3–9). New York: Oxford University Press.

Goetz, C. G., Stebbins, G. T., & Ouyang, B. (2011). Visual plus nonvisual hallucinations in Parkinson's disease: Development and evolution over 10 years. *Movement Disorders*, *26*(12), 2196–2200. doi: 10.1002/mds.23835

Golbe, L. I., Davis, P. H., Schoenberg, B. S., & Duvoisin, R. C. (1988). Prevalence and natural history of progressive supranuclear palsy. *Neurology*, *38*(7), 1031–1034.

Golbe, L. I., Di Iorio, G., Sanges, G., Lazzarini, A. M., La Sala, S., Bonavita, V., & Duvoisin, R. C. (1996). Clinical genetic analysis of Parkinson's disease in the Contursi kindred. *Annals of Neurology*, *40*(5), 767–775.

Goldman, J. G., Holden, S., Bernard, B., Ouyang, B., Goetz, C. G., & Stebbins, G. T. (2013). Defining optimal cutoff scores for cognitive impairment using Movement Disorder Society Task Force criteria for mild cognitive impairment in Parkinson's disease. *Movement Disorders*, *28*(14), 1972–1979. doi: 10.1002/mds.25655

Goldman, J. G., Williams-Gray, C., Barker, R. A., Duda, J. E., & Galvin, J. E. (2014). The spectrum of cognitive impairment in Lewy body diseases. *Movement Disorders*, *29*(5), 608–621. doi: 10.1002/mds.25866

Gomperts, S. N., Locascio, J. J., Marquie, M., Santarlasci, A. L., Rentz, D. M., Maye, J., . . . Growdon, J. H. (2012). Brain amyloid and cognition in Lewy body diseases. *Movement Disorders*, *27*(8), 965–973. doi: 10.1002/mds.25048

Goris, A., Williams-Gray, C. H., Clark, G. R., Foltynie, T., Lewis, S. J., Brown, J., . . . Sawcer, S. J. (2007). Tau and alpha-synuclein in susceptibility to, and dementia in, Parkinson's disease. *Annals of Neurology*, *62*(2), 145–153. doi: 10.1002/ana.21192

Grafman, J., Litvan, I., & Stark, M. (1995). Neuropsychological features of progressive supranuclear palsy. *Brain and Cognition*, *28*(3), 311–320.

Graham, N. L., Bak, T. H., & Hodges, J. R. (2003). Corticobasal degeneration as a cognitive disorder. *Movement Disorders*, *18*(11), 1224–1232.

Graham, N. L., Bak, T. H., Patterson, K., & Hodges, J. R. (2003). Language function and dysfunction in corticobasal degeneration. *Neurology*, *61*(4), 493–499.

Gratwicke, J., Jahanshahi, M., & Foltynie, T. (2015). Parkinson's disease dementia: A neural networks perspective. *Brain, 138,* 1454–1476. doi: 10.1093/brain/awv104

Grimes, D. A., Lang, A. E., & Bergeron, C. B. (1999). Dementia as the most common presentation of cortical-basal ganglionic degeneration. *Neurology*, *53*(9), 1969–1974.

Grossman, M., Carvell, S., Stern, M. B., Gollomp, S., & Hurtig, H. I. (1992). Sentence comprehension in Parkinson's disease: The role of attention and memory. *Brain and Language*, *42*(4), 347–384.

Grossman, M., Zurif, E., Lee, C., Prather, P., Kalmanson, J., Stern, M. B., & Hurtig, H. I. (2002). Information processing speed and sentence comprehension in Parkinson's disease. *Neuropsychology*, *16*(2), 174–181.

Gschwandtner, U., Aston, J., Renaud, S., & Fuhr, P. (2001). Pathologic gambling in patients with Parkinson's disease. *Clinical Neuropharmacology*, *24*(3), 170–172.

Gupta, A., & Lang, A. E. (2009). Psychogenic movement disorders. *Current Opinion in Neurology*, *22*(4), 430–436. doi: 10.1097/WCO.0b013e32832dc169

Halliday, G. M., Leverenz, J. B., Schneider, J. S., & Adler, C. H. (2014). The neurobiological basis of cognitive impairment in Parkinson's disease. *Movement Disorders*, *29*(5), 634–650. doi: 10.1002/mds.25857

Halliday, G. M., & McCann, H. (2010). The progression of pathology in Parkinson's disease. *Annals of the New York Academy of Sciences*, *1184*, 188–195. doi: NYAS5118 [pii] 10.1111/j.1749-6632.2009.05118.x

Hamilton, J. M., Salmon, D. P., Galasko, D., Delis, D. C., Hansen, L. A., Masliah, E., . . . Thal, L. J. (2004). A comparison of episodic memory deficits in neuropathologically confirmed Dementia with Lewy bodies and Alzheimer's disease. *Journal of the International Neuropsychological Society*, *10*(5), 689–697.

Hamilton, M. (1960). A rating scale for depression. *Journal of Neurology, Neurosurgery, and Psychiatry*, *23*, 56–62.

Hawkins, K., Jennings, D., Marek, K., Siderowf, A., Stern, M., & PARS Study Investigators. (2010). Cognitive deficits associated with dopamine transporter loss in the pre-motor subjects in the PARS cohort. *Movement Disorders*, *25*(Suppl 3), S690–S691.

Haynes, W. I., & Haber, S. N. (2013). The organization of prefrontal-subthalamic inputs in primates provides an anatomical substrate for both functional specificity and integration: Implications for Basal Ganglia models and deep brain stimulation. *Journal of Neuroscience*, *33*(11), 4804–4814. doi: 10.1523/JNEUROSCI.4674-12.2013

Healy, D. G., Abou-Sleiman, P. M., Gibson, J. M., Ross, O. A., Jain, S., Gandhi, S., . . . Lynch, T. (2004). PINK1 (PARK6) associated Parkinson disease in Ireland. *Neurology*, *63*(8), 1486–1488.

Healy, D. G., Falchi, M., O'Sullivan, S. S., Bonifati, V., Durr, A., Bressman, S., . . . International, L. C. (2008). Phenotype, genotype, and worldwide genetic penetrance of LRRK2-associated Parkinson's disease: A case-control study. *Lancet Neurology*, *7*(7), 583–590. doi: 10.1016/S1474-4422(08)70117-0

Heaton, R. K., Chelune, G. J., Talley, J. L., Kay, G. G., & Curtiss, G. (1993). *Wisconsin Card Sorting Test Manual*. Odessa: Psychological Assessment Resources.

Heiss, C., Kalbe, E., & Kessler, J. (2001). Quantitative und qualitative Analysen von verbalen Flüssigkeitsaufgaben bei Parkinsonpatienten. *Zeitschrift für Neuropsychologie*, *12*(3), 188–199.

Henry, J. D., & Crawford, J. R. (2004). Verbal fluency deficits in Parkinson's disease: A meta-analysis. *Journal of the International Neuropsychological Society*, *10*(4), 608–622.

Herrera, E., Cuetos, F., & Ribacoba, R. (2012). Verbal fluency in Parkinson's disease patients on/off dopamine medication. *Neuropsychologia*, *50*(14), 3636–3640. doi: 10.1016/j.neuropsychologia.2012.09.016

Hietanen, M. H. (1991). Selegiline and cognitive function in Parkinson's disease. *Acta Neurologica Scandanavica*, *84*(5), 407–410.

Higginson, C. I., Fields, J. A., Koller, W. C., & Tröster, A. I. (2001). Questionnaire assessment potentially overestimates anxiety in Parkinson's disease. *Journal of Clinical Psychology in Medical Settings*, *8*(2), 95–99.

Higginson, C. I., Wheelock, V. L., Levine, D., Pappas, C. T., & Sigvardt, K. A. (2011). Predictors of HVOT performance in Parkinson's disease. *Applied Neuropsychology*, *18*(3), 210–215. doi: 10.1080/09084282.2011.595447

Hilker, R., Thomas, A. V., Klein, J. C., Weisenbach, S., Kalbe, E., Burghaus, L., . . . Heiss, W. D. (2005). Dementia in Parkinson disease: Functional imaging of cholinergic and dopaminergic pathways. *Neurology*, *65*(11), 1716–1722. doi: 65/11/1716 [pii] 10.1212/01.wnl.0000191154.78131.f6

Hindle, J. V., Petrelli, A., Clare, L., & Kalbe, E. (2013). Nonpharmacological enhancement of cognitive function in Parkinson's disease: A systematic review. *Movement Disorders*, *28*(8), 1034–1049. doi: 10.1002/mds.25377

Hinnell, C., Hurt, C. S., Landau, S., Brown, R. G., Samuel, M., & Group, P.-P. S. (2012). Nonmotor versus motor symptoms: How much do they matter to health status in Parkinson's disease? *Movement Disorders*, *27*(2), 236–241. doi: 10.1002/mds.23961

Hinson, V. K., Weinstein, S., Bernard, B., Leurgans, S. E., & Goetz, C. G. (2006). Single-blind clinical trial of psychotherapy for treatment of psychogenic movement disorders. *Parkinsonism and Related Disorders*, *12*(3), 177–180. doi: 10.1016/j.parkreldis.2005.10.006

Hirtz, D., Thurman, D. J., Gwinn-Hardy, K., Mohamed, M., Chaudhuri, A. R., & Zalutsky, R. (2007). How common are the "common" neurologic disorders? *Neurology*, *68*(5), 326–337. doi: 10.1212/01.wnl.0000252807.38124.a3

Hogl, B., Arnulf, I., Comella, C., Ferreira, J., Iranzo, A., Tilley, B., . . . Goetz, C. G. (2010). Scales to assess sleep impairment in Parkinson's disease: Critique and recommendations. *Movement Disorders*, *25*(16), 2704–2716. doi: 10.1002/mds.23190

Hohler, A. D., Ransom, B. R., Chun, M. R., Tröster, A. I., & Samii, A. (2003). The youngest reported case of corticobasal degeneration. *Parkinsonism and Related Disorders*, *10*, 47–50.

Holdorff, B. (2002). Friedrich Heinrich Lewy (1885–1950) and his work. *Journal of the History of the Neurosciences*, *11*(1), 19–28.

Homann, C. N., Suppan, K., Homann, B., Crevenna, R., Ivanic, G., & Ruzicka, E. (2003). Driving in Parkinson's disease—a health hazard? *Journal of Neurology*, *250*(12), 1439–1446.

Hoogland, J., de Bie, R. M., Williams-Gray, C. H., Muslimovic, D., Schmand, B., & Post, B. (2010). Catechol-O-methyltransferase val158met and cognitive function in Parkinson's disease. *Movement Disorders*, *25*(15), 2550–2554. doi: 10.1002/mds.23319

Huang, X., Chen, P., Kaufer, D. I., Troster, A. I., & Poole, C. (2006). Apolipoprotein E and dementia in Parkinson disease: A meta-analysis. *Archives of Neurology*, *63*(2), 189–193.

Huber, S. J., Shuttleworth, E. C., & Paulson, G. W. (1986). Dementia in Parkinson's disease. *Archives of Neurology*, *43*(10), 987–990.

Huber, S. J., Shuttleworth, E. C., Paulson, G. W., Bellchambers, M. J., & Clapp, L. E. (1986). Cortical vs subcortical dementia: Neuropsychological differences. *Archives of Neurology*, *43*(4), 392–394.

Hugdahl, K., & Wester, K. (2000). Neurocognitive correlates of stereotactic thalamotomy and thalamic stimulation in Parkinsonian patients. *Brain and Cognition*, *42*(2), 231–252.

Huntington, G. (1872). On chorea. *Advances in Neurology*, *1*, 33–35.

Hurtig, H. I., Trojanowski, J. Q., Galvin, J., Ewbank, D., Schmidt, M. L., Lee, V. M.-Y., . . . Arnold, S. E. (2000). Alpha-synuclein cortical Lewy bodies correlate with dementia in Parkinson's disease. *Neurology*, *54*(10), 1916–1921.

Irwin, D. J., White, M. T., Toledo, J. B., Xie, S. X., Robinson, J. L., Van Deerlin, V., . . . Trojanowski, J. Q. (2012). Neuropathologic substrates of Parkinson disease dementia. *Annals of Neurology*, *72*(4), 587–598. doi: 10.1002/ana.23659

Ito, K., Nagano-Saito, A., Kato, T., Arahata, Y., Nakamura, A., Kawasumi, Y., . . . Brooks, D. J. (2002). Striatal and extrastriatal dysfunction in Parkinson's disease with dementia: A 6-[18F]fluoro-L-dopa PET study. *Brain*, *125*(Pt 6), 1358–1365.

Jahanshahi, M., Czernecki, V., & Zurowski, A. M. (2011). Neuropsychological, neuropsychiatric, and quality of life issues in DBS for dystonia. *Movement Disorders*, *26*(Suppl 1), S63–S78. doi: 10.1002/mds.23511

Jahanshahi, M., Rowe, J., & Fuller, R. (2003). Cognitive executive function in dystonia. *Movement Disorders*, *18*(12), 1470–1481.

Janicki, S. C., Cosentino, S., & Louis, E. D. (2013). The cognitive side of essential tremor: What are the therapeutic implications? *Therapeutic Advances in Neurological Disorders*, *6*(6), 353–368. doi: 10.1177/1756285613489591

Jellinger, K. A. (2014). Neuropathology of multiple system atrophy: New thoughts about pathogenesis. *Movement Disorders*, *29*(14), 1720–1741. doi: 10.1002/mds.26052

Jellinger, K. A., & Attems, J. (2008). Prevalence and impact of vascular and Alzheimer pathologies in Lewy body disease. *Acta Neuropathologica*, *115*(4), 427–436. doi: 10.1007/s00401-008-0347-5

Jordbru, A. A., Smedstad, L. M., Klungsoyr, O., & Martinsen, E. W. (2014). Psychogenic gait disorder: A randomized controlled trial of physical rehabilitation with one-year follow-up. *Journal of Rehabilitation Medicine*, *46*(2), 181–187. doi: 10.2340/16501977-1246

Jurko, M. F., & Andy, O. J. (1964). Psychological aspects of diencephalotomy. *Journal of Neurology, Neurosurgery, and Psychiatry*, *27*, 516–521.

Karadi, K., Lucza, T., Aschermann, Z., Komoly, S., Deli, G., Bosnyak, E., . . . Kovacs, N. (2015). Visuospatial impairment in Parkinson's disease: The role of laterality. *Laterality*, *20*(1), 112–127. doi: 10.1080/1357650X.2014.936444

Katai, S., Maruyama, T., Hashimoto, T., & Ikeda, S. (2003). Event based and time based prospective memory in Parkinson's disease. *Journal of Neurology, Neurosurgery, and Psychiatry*, *74*(6), 704–709.

Kaufer, D. I. (2002). Pharmacologic therapy of dementia with Lewy bodies. *Journal of Geriatric Psychiatry and Neurology*, *15*(4), 224–232.

Kehagia, A. A., Barker, R. A., & Robbins, T. W. (2010). Neuropsychological and clinical heterogeneity of cognitive impairment and dementia in patients with Parkinson's disease. *Lancet Neurology*, *9*(12), 1200–1213. doi: 10.1016/S1474-4422(10)70212-X

Kensinger, E. A., Shearer, D. K., Locascio, J. J., & Growdon, J. H. (2003). Working memory in mild Alzheimer's disease and early Parkinson's disease. *Neuropsychology*, *17*(2), 230–239.

Kertesz, A. (2003). Pick complex: An integrative approach to frontotemporal dementia: Primary progressive aphasia, corticobasal degeneration, and progressive supranuclear palsy. *Neurologist*, *9*(6), 311–317.

Kertesz, A., Martinez-Lage, P., Davidson, W., & Munoz, D. G. (2000). The corticobasal degeneration syndrome overlaps progressive aphasia and frontotemporal dementia. *Neurology*, *55*(9), 1368–1375.

Kieburtz, K., McDermott, M., Como, P., Growdon, J., Brady, J., Carter, J., . . . Group, T.P.S. (1994). The effect of deprenyl and tocopherol on cognitive performance in early untreated Parkinson's disease. *Neurology*, *44*(9), 1756–1759.

Killoran, A., & Biglan, K. M. (2014). Current therapeutic options for Huntington's disease: Good clinical practice versus evidence-based approaches? *Movement Disorders*, *29*(11), 1404–1413. doi: 10.1002/mds.26014

Klein, J. C., Eggers, C., Kalbe, E., Weisenbach, S., Hohmann, C., Vollmar, S., . . . Hilker, R. (2010). Neurotransmitter changes in dementia with Lewy bodies and Parkinson disease dementia in vivo. *Neurology*, *74*(11), 885–892. doi: WNL.0b013e3181d55f61 [pii] 10.1212/WNL.0b013e3181d55f61

Kliegel, M., Altgassen, M., Hering, A., & Rose, N. S. (2011). A process-model based approach to prospective memory impairment in Parkinson's disease. *Neuropsychologia*, *49*(8), 2166–2177. doi: 10.1016/j.neuropsychologia.2011.01.024

Knoke, D., Taylor, A. E., & Saint-Cyr, J. A. (1998). The differential effects of cueing on recall in Parkinson's disease and normal subjects. *Brain and Cognition*, *38*(2), 261–274.

Koller, W. C. (1984). Disturbance of recent memory function in parkinsonian patients on anticholinergic therapy. *Cortex*, *20*(2), 307–311.

Koller, W. C., Marjama, J., & Tröster, A. I. (2002). Psychogenic movement disorders. In J. Jankovic & E. Tolosa (Eds.), *Parkinson's Disease and Movement Disorders* (4th ed., pp. 546–552). Philadelphia, PA: Lippincott, Williams & Wilkins.

Kranick, S., Ekanayake, V., Martinez, V., Ameli, R., Hallett, M., & Voon, V. (2011). Psychopathology and psychogenic movement disorders. *Movement Disorders*, *26*(10), 1844–1850. doi: 10.1002/mds.23830

Kudlicka, A., Clare, L., & Hindle, J. V. (2011). Executive functions in Parkinson's disease: Systematic review and meta-analysis. *Movement Disorders*, *26*(13), 2305–2315. doi: 10.1002/mds.23868

Kulisevsky, J., Garcia-Sanchez, C., Berthier, M. L., Barbanoj, M., Pascual-Sedano, B., Gironell, A., & Estevez-Gonzalez, A. (2000). Chronic effects of dopaminergic replacement on cognitive function in Parkinson's disease: A two-year follow-up study of previously untreated patients. *Movement Disorders*, *15*, 613–626.

Kurz, M. W., Dekomien, G., Nilsen, O. B., Larsen, J. P., Aarsland, D., & Alves, G. (2009). APOE alleles in Parkinson disease and their relationship to cognitive decline: A population-based, longitudinal study. *Journal of Geriatric Psychiatry and Neurology*, *22*(3), 166–170. doi: 10.1177/0891988709332945

Kuzis, G., Sabe, L., Tiberti, C., Merello, M., Leiguarda, R., & Starkstein, S. E. (1999). Explicit and implicit learning in patients with Alzheimer disease and Parkinson disease with dementia. *Neuropsychiatry, Neuropsychology, and Behavioral Neurology*, *12*(4), 265–269.

Lacritz, L. H., Dewey, R., Jr., Giller, C., & Cullum, C. M. (2002). Cognitive functioning in individuals with "benign" essential tremor. *Journal of the International Neuropsychological Society*, *8*(1), 125–129.

Lang, A. E. (2003). Corticobasal degeneration: Selected developments. *Movement Disorders*, *18*(Suppl 6), S51–S56.

Lang, A. E. (2011). Phenomenology of psychogenic movement disorders. In M. Hallett, A. E. Lang, J. Jankovic, S. Fahn, P. W.

Halligan, V. Voon, & C. R. Cloninger (Eds.), *Psychogenic Movement Disorders and Other Conversion Disorders* (pp. 6–13). Cambridge, UK: Cambridge University Press.

Lange, K. W., Robbins, T. W., Marsden, C. D., James, M., Owen, A. M., & Paul, G. M. (1992). L-dopa withdrawal in Parkinson's disease selectively impairs cognitive performance in tests sensitive to frontal lobe dysfunction. *Psychopharmacology*, *107*(2–3), 394–404.

Lange, K. W., Tucha, O., Alders, G. L., Preier, M., Csoti, I., Merz, B., . . . Naumann, M. (2003). Differentiation of parkinsonian syndromes according to differences in executive functions. *Journal of Neural Transmission*, *110*(9), 983–995.

Langenbahn, D. M., Ashman, T., Cantor, J., & Trott, C. (2013). An evidence-based review of cognitive rehabilitation in medical conditions affecting cognitive function. *Archives of Physical Medicine and Rehabilitation*, *94*(2), 271–286. doi: 10.1016/j.apmr.2012.09.011

Lauterbach, E. C., & Duvoisin, R. C. (1991). Anxiety disorders in familial parkinsonism. *American Journal of Psychiatry*, *148*(2), 274.

Lawrence, A. D., Evans, A. H., & Lees, A. J. (2003). Compulsive use of dopamine replacement therapy in Parkinson's disease: Reward systems gone awry? *Lancet Neurology*, *2*, 595–604.

Lee, A. C., Harris, J. P., & Calvert, J. E. (1998). Impairments of mental rotation in Parkinson's disease. *Neuropsychologia*, *36*(1), 109–114.

Lee, C., Grossman, M., Morris, J., Stern, M. B., & Hurtig, H. I. (2003). Attentional resource and processing speed limitations during sentence processing in Parkinson's disease. *Brain and Language*, *85*(3), 347–356.

Lee, S. S., Wild, K., Hollnagel, C., & Grafman, J. (1999). Selective visual attention in patients with frontal lobe lesions or Parkinson's disease. *Neuropsychologia*, *37*(5), 595–604.

Lee, W., Williams, D. R., & Storey, E. (2012). Cognitive testing in the diagnosis of parkinsonian disorders: A critical appraisal of the literature. *Movement Disorders*, *27*(10), 1243–1254. doi: 10.1002/mds.25113

Lee, Y. E., Williams, D. R., & Anderson, J. F. (2016). Frontal deficits differentiate progressive supranuclear palsy from Parkinson's disease. *Journal of Neuropsychology*, *10*, 1–14. doi: 10.1111/jnp.12053

Leentjens, A. F., Dujardin, K., Marsh, L., Martinez-Martin, P., Richard, I. H., Starkstein, S. E., . . . Goetz, C. G. (2008a). Anxiety rating scales in Parkinson's disease: Critique and recommendations. *Movement Disorders*, *23*(14), 2015–2025. doi: 10.1002/mds.22233

Leentjens, A. F., Dujardin, K., Marsh, L., Martinez-Martin, P., Richard, I. H., Starkstein, S. E., . . . Goetz, C. G. (2008b). Apathy and anhedonia rating scales in Parkinson's disease: Critique and recommendations. *Movement Disorders*, *23*(14), 2004–2014. doi: 10.1002/mds.22229

Leentjens, A. F., Dujardin, K., Pontone, G. M., Starkstein, S. E., Weintraub, D., & Martinez-Martin, P. (2014). The Parkinson Anxiety Scale (PAS): Development and validation of a new anxiety scale. *Movement Disorders*, *29*(8), 1035–1043. doi: 10.1002/mds.25919

Leentjens, A. F., Verhey, F. R., Lousberg, R., Spitsbergen, H., & Wilmink, F. W. (2000). The validity of the Hamilton and Montgomery-Asberg depression rating scales as screening and diagnostic tools for depression in Parkinson's disease. *International Journal of Geriatric Psychiatry*, *15*(7), 644–649.

Leentjens, A. F., Verhey, F. R., Luijckx, G. J., & Troost, J. (2000). The validity of the Beck Depression Inventory as a screening and diagnostic instrument for depression in patients with Parkinson's disease. *Movement Disorders*, *15*(6), 1221–1224.

Lees, A. J., & Smith, E. (1983). Cognitive deficits in the early stages of Parkinson's disease. *Brain*, *106*(Pt 2), 257–270.

Leiguarda, R., Lees, A. J., Merello, M., Starkstein, S., & Marsden, C. D. (1994). The nature of apraxia in corticobasal degeneration. *Journal of Neurology, Neurosurgery, and Psychiatry*, *57*(4), 455–459.

Leplow, B., Dierks, C., Herrmann, P., Pieper, N., Annecke, R., & Ulm, G. (1997). Remote memory in Parkinson's disease and senile dementia. *Neuropsychologia*, *35*(4), 547–557.

Lesage, S., Durr, A., Tazir, M., Lohmann, E., Leutenegger, A. L., Janin, S., . . . French Parkinson's Disease Genetics Study, G. (2006). LRRK2 G2019S as a cause of Parkinson's disease in North African Arabs. *New England Journal of Medicine*, *354*(4), 422–423. doi: 10.1056/NEJMc055540

Leverenz, J. B., Watson, G. S., Shofer, J., Zabetian, C. P., Zhang, J., & Montine, T. J. (2011). Cerebrospinal fluid biomarkers and cognitive performance in non-demented patients with Parkinson's disease. *Parkinsonism and Related Disorders*, *17*(1), 61–64. doi: 10.1016/j.parkreldis.2010.10.003

Levin, B. E., & Katzen, H. L. (1995). Early cognitive changes and nondementing behavioral abnormalities in Parkinson's disease. In W. J. Weiner & A. E. Lang (Eds.), *Advances in Neurology: Vol 65. Behavioral Neurology of Movement Disorders* (pp. 85–95). New York: Raven Press.

Levin, B. E., Llabre, M. M., Reisman, S., Weiner, W. J., Sanchez-Ramos, J., Singer, C., & Brown, M. C. (1991). Visuospatial impairment in Parkinson's disease. *Neurology*, *41*(3), 365–369.

Levin, B. E., Llabre, M. M., & Weiner, W. J. (1989). Cognitive impairments associated with early Parkinson's disease. *Neurology*, *39*(4), 557–561.

Lewis, F. M., Lapointe, L. L., & Murdoch, B. E. (1998). Language impairment in Parkinson's disease. *Aphasiology*, *12*, 193–206.

Lewis, S. J., Cools, R., Robbins, T. W., Dove, A., Barker, R. A., & Owen, A. M. (2003). Using executive heterogeneity to explore the nature of working memory deficits in Parkinson's disease. *Neuropsychologia*, *41*(6), 645–654.

LeWitt, P. A., Rezai, A. R., Leehey, M. A., Ojemann, S. G., Flaherty, A. W., Eskandar, E. N., . . . Feigin, A. (2011). AAV2-GAD gene therapy for advanced Parkinson's disease: A double-blind, sham-surgery controlled, randomised trial. *Lancet Neurology*, *10*(4), 309–319. doi: 10.1016/S1474-4422(11)70039-4

Lewy, F. H. (1912). Paralysis agitans I: Pathologische anatomie. In M. Lewandowsky (Ed.), *Handbuch Der Neurologie, Band 3* (pp. 920–933). Berlin: Springer Verlag.

Lewy, F. H. (1923). *Die Lehre vom Tonus und der Bewegung. Zugleich Systmatische Untersuchungen zur Klinik, Physiologie, Pathologie und Pathogenese der Paralysis Agitans*. Berlin: Julius Springer.

Litvan, I., Agid, Y., Goetz, C., Jankovic, J., Wenning, G. K., Brandel, J. P., . . . Bartko, J. J. (1997). Accuracy of the clinical diagnosis of corticobasal degeneration: A clinicopathologic study. *Neurology*, *48*(1), 119–125.

Litvan, I., Cummings, J. L., & Mega, M. (1998). Neuropsychiatric features of corticobasal degeneration. *Journal of Neurology, Neurosurgery, and Psychiatry*, *65*(5), 717–721.

Litvan, I., Goldman, J. G., Troster, A. I., Schmand, B. A., Weintraub, D., Petersen, R. C., . . . Emre, M. (2012). Diagnostic criteria for mild cognitive impairment in Parkinson's disease: Movement disorder society task force guidelines. *Movement Disorders*, *27*(3), 349–356. doi: 10.1002/mds.24893

Litvan, I., Grafman, J., Gomez, C., & Chase, T. N. (1989). Memory impairment in patients with progressive supranuclear palsy. *Archives of Neurology*, *46*(7), 765–767.

Litvan, I., Mega, M. S., Cummings, J. L., & Fairbanks, L. (1996). Neuropsychiatric aspects of progressive supranuclear palsy. *Neurology*, *47*(5), 1184–1189.

Liu, C., Cholerton, B., Shi, M., Ginghina, C., Cain, K. C., Auinger, P., . . . Zhang, J. (2015). CSF tau and tau/Abeta predict cognitive decline in Parkinson's disease. *Parkinsonism and Related Disorders*. doi: 10.1016/j.parkreldis.2014.12.027

Liu, Y., Li, W., Tan, C., Liu, X., Wang, X., Gui, Y., . . . Chen, L. (2014). Meta-analysis comparing deep brain stimulation of the globus pallidus and subthalamic nucleus to treat advanced Parkinson disease. *Journal of Neurosurgery*, *121*(3), 709–718. doi: 10.3171/2014.4.JNS131711

Loftus, A. M., Bucks, R. S., Thomas, M., Kane, R., Timms, C., Barker, R. A., & Gasson, N. (2015). Retrospective assessment of movement disorder society criteria for mild cognitive impairment in Parkinson's disease. *Journal of the International Neuropsychological Society*, *21*(2), 137–145. doi: 10.1017/S1355617715000041

Lombardi, W. J., Woolston, D. J., Roberts, J. W., & Gross, R. E. (2001). Cognitive deficits in patients with essential tremor. *Neurology*, *57*(5), 785–790.

Louis, E. D., & Ferreira, J. J. (2010). How common is the most common adult movement disorder? Update on the worldwide prevalence of essential tremor. *Movement Disorders*, *25*(5), 534–541. doi: 10.1002/mds.22838

Lyons, K. E., & Tröster, A. I. (2015). Essential tremor. In A. I. Tröster (Ed.), *Clinical Neuropsychology and Cognitive Neurology of Parkinson's Disease and Other Movement Disorders* (pp. 484–500). New York: Oxford University Press.

MacDonald, A. A., Seergobin, K. N., Owen, A. M., Tamjeedi, R., Monchi, O., Ganjavi, H., & MacDonald, P. A. (2013). Differential effects of Parkinson's disease and dopamine replacement on memory encoding and retrieval. *PloS One*, *8*(9), e74044. doi: 10.1371/journal.pone.0074044

MacDonald, P. A., MacDonald, A. A., Seergobin, K. N., Tamjeedi, R., Ganjavi, H., Provost, J. S., & Monchi, O. (2011). The effect of dopamine therapy on ventral and dorsal striatum-mediated cognition in Parkinson's disease: Support from functional MRI. *Brain*, *134*(Pt 5), 1447–1463. doi: 10.1093/brain/awr075

Maher, E. R., Smith, E. M., & Lees, A. J. (1985). Cognitive deficits in the Steele-Richardson-Olszewski syndrome (progressive supranuclear palsy). *Journal of Neurology, Neurosurgery, and Psychiatry*, *48*(12), 1234–1239.

Mahieux, F., Fenelon, G., Flahault, A., Manifacier, M. J., Michelet, D., & Boller, F. (1998). Neuropsychological prediction of dementia in Parkinson's disease. *Journal of Neurology, Neurosurgery, and Psychiatry*, *64*(2), 178–183.

Maier, F., Merkl, J., Ellereit, A. L., Lewis, C. J., Eggers, C., Pedrosa, D. J., . . . Timmermann, L. (2014). Hypomania and mania related to dopamine replacement therapy in Parkinson's disease. *Parkinsonism and Related Disorders*, *20*(4), 421–427. doi: 10.1016/j.parkreldis.2014.01.001

Maier, F., Prigatano, G. P., Kalbe, E., Barbe, M. T., Eggers, C., Lewis, C. J., . . . Timmermann, L. (2012). Impaired self-awareness of motor deficits in Parkinson's disease: Association with motor asymmetry and motor phenotypes. *Movement Disorders*, *27*(11), 1443–1447. doi: 10.1002/mds.25079

Marder, K., Tang, M. X., Cote, L., Stern, Y., & Mayeux, R. (1995). The frequency and associated risk factors for dementia in patients with Parkinson's disease. *Archives of Neurology*, *52*(7), 695–701.

Marder, K., Zhao, H., Myers, R. H., Cudkowicz, M., Kayson, E., Kieburtz, K., . . . Shoulson, I. (2000). Rate of functional decline in Huntington's disease: Huntington study group. *Neurology*, *54*(2), 452–458.

Marin, R. S., Biedrzycki, R. C., & Firinciogullari, S. (1991). Reliability and validity of the apathy evaluation scale. *Psychiatry Research*, *38*(2), 143–162.

Marras, C., Armstrong, M. J., Meaney, C. A., Fox, S., Rothberg, B., Reginold, W., . . . Duff-Canning, S. (2013). Measuring mild cognitive impairment in patients with Parkinson's disease. *Movement Disorders*, *28*(5), 626–633. doi: 10.1002/mds.25426

Marsh, L., & Dobkin, R. D. (2015). Depression and anxiety in Parkinson's disease. In A. I. Tröster (Ed.), *Clinical Neuropsychology and Cognitive Neurology of Parkinson's Disease and Other Movement Disorders* (pp. 265–290). New York: Oxford University Press.

Marsh, L., McDonald, W. M., Cummings, J., & Ravina, B. (2006). Provisional diagnostic criteria for depression in Parkinson's disease: Report of an NINDS/NIMH work group. *Movement Disorders*, *21*(2), 148–158. doi: 10.1002/mds.20723

Massman, P. J., Delis, D. C., Butters, N., Levin, B. E., & Salmon, D. P. (1990). Are all subcortical dementias alike? Verbal learning and memory in Parkinson's and Huntington's disease patients. *Journal of Clinical and Experimental Neuropsychology*, *12*(5), 729–744.

Massman, P. J., Kreiter, K. T., Jankovic, J., & Doody, R. S. (1996). Neuropsychological functioning in cortical-basal ganglionic degeneration: Differentiation from Alzheimer's disease. *Neurology*, *46*(3), 720–726.

Mata, I. F., Leverenz, J. B., Weintraub, D., Trojanowski, J. Q., Hurtig, H. I., Van Deerlin, V. M., . . . Zabetian, C. P. (2014). APOE, MAPT, and SNCA genes and cognitive performance in Parkinson disease. *JAMA Neurology*, *71*(11), 1405–1412. doi: 10.1001/jamaneurol.2014.1455

Matison, R., Mayeux, R., Rosen, J., & Fahn, S. (1982). "Tip-of-the-tongue" phenomenon in Parkinson disease. *Neurology*, *32*(5), 567–570.

Mayeux, R., Chen, J., Mirabello, E., Marder, K., Bell, K., Dooneief, G., . . . Stern, Y. (1990). An estimate of the incidence of dementia in idiopathic Parkinson's disease. *Neurology*, *40*(10), 1513–1517.

McDonald, W. M., Richard, I. H., & DeLong, M. R. (2003). Prevalence, etiology, and treatment of depression in Parkinson's disease. *Biological Psychiatry*, *54*(3), 363–375.

McDowd, J., Hoffman, L., Rozek, E., Lyons, K. E., Pahwa, R., Burns, J., & Kemper, S. (2011). Understanding verbal fluency in healthy aging, Alzheimer's disease, and Parkinson's disease. *Neuropsychology*, *25*(2), 210–225. doi: 10.1037/a0021531

McFie, J. (1960). Psychological effects of stereotaxic operations for the relief of parkinsonian symptoms. *Journal of Mental Science*, *106*, 1512–1517.

McKeith, I., Del Ser, T., Spano, P., Emre, M., Wesnes, K., Anand, R., . . . Spiegel, R. (2000). Efficacy of rivastigmine in dementia with Lewy bodies: A randomised, double-blind, placebo-controlled international study. *Lancet*, *356*(9247), 2031–2036.

McKinlay, A., Grace, R. C., Dalrymple-Alford, J. C., & Roger, D. (2010). Characteristics of executive function impairment in Parkinson's disease patients without dementia. *Journal of the International Neuropsychological Society*, *16*, 268–277. doi: 10.1017/S1355617709991299

McNamara, P., & Durso, R. (2003). Pragmatic communication skills in patients with Parkinson's disease. *Brain and Language*, *84*(3), 414–423.

Meco, G., Casacchia, M., Lazzari, R., Franzese, A., Castellana, F., Carta, A., . . . Agnoli, A. (1984). Mental impairment in Parkinson's disease: The role of anticholinergic drugs. *Acta Psychiatrica Belgique*, *84*(4), 325–335.

Meco, G., Gasparini, M., & Doricchi, F. (1996). Attentional functions in multiple system atrophy and Parkinson's disease. *Journal of Neurology, Neurosurgery and Psychiatry*, *60*(4), 393–398.

Menza, M., Dobkin, R. D., Marin, H., Mark, M. H., Gara, M., Buyske, S., . . . Dicke, A. (2009). A controlled trial of antidepressants in patients with Parkinson disease and depression. *Neurology*, *72*(10), 886–892. doi: 01.wnl.0000336340.89821.b3 [pii] 10.1212/01.wnl.0000336340.89821.b3

Merola, A., Rizzi, L., Artusi, C. A., Zibetti, M., Rizzone, M. G., Romagnolo, A., . . . Lopiano, L. (2014). Subthalamic deep brain stimulation: Clinical and neuropsychological outcomes in mild cognitive impaired parkinsonian patients. *Journal of Neurology*, *261*(9), 1745–1751. doi: 10.1007/s00415-014-7414-8

Middleton, F. A., & Strick, P. L. (2000). Basal ganglia output and cognition: Evidence from anatomical, behavioral, and clinical studies. *Brain and Cognition*, *42*(2), 183–200.

Mimura, M., White, R. F., & Albert, M. L. (1997). Corticobasal degeneration: Neuropsychological and clinical correlates. *Journal of Neuropsychiatry and Clinical Neurosciences*, *9*(1), 94–98.

Mochizuki, A., Ueda, Y., Komatsuzaki, Y., Tsuchiya, K., Arai, T., & Shoji, S. (2003). Progressive supranuclear palsy presenting with primary progressive aphasia-clinicopathological report of an autopsy case. *Acta Neuropathologica (Berlin)*, *105*(6), 610–614.

Mohlman, J., Chazin, D., & Georgescu, B. (2011). Feasibility and acceptance of a nonpharmacological cognitive remediation intervention for patients with Parkinson disease. *Journal of Geriatric Psychiatry and Neurology*, *24*(2), 91–97. doi: 10.1177/0891988711402350

Mohr, E., Mendis, T., & Grimes, J. D. (1995). Late cognitive changes in Parkinson's disease with an emphasis on dementia. *Advances in Neurology*, *65*, 97–113.

Mondolo, F., Jahanshahi, M., Grana, A., Biasutti, E., Cacciatori, E., & Di Benedetto, P. (2006). The validity of the hospital anxiety and depression scale and the geriatric depression scale in Parkinson's disease. *Behavioural Neurology*, *17*(2), 109–115.

Montgomery, S. A., & Asberg, M. (1979). A new depression scale designed to be sensitive to change. *British Journal of Psychiatry*, *134*, 382–389.

Montine, T. J., Shi, M., Quinn, J. F., Peskind, E. R., Craft, S., Ginghina, C., . . . Zhang, J. (2010). CSF Abeta(42) and tau in Parkinson's disease with cognitive impairment. *Movement Disorders*, *25*(15), 2682–2685. doi: 10.1002/mds.23287

Montoya, A., Pelletier, M., Menear, M., Duplessis, E., Richer, F., & Lepage, M. (2006). Episodic memory impairment in Huntington's disease: A meta-analysis. *Neuropsychologia*, *44*(10), 1984–1994. doi: S0028-3932(06)00027-3 [pii] 10.1016/j.neuropsychologia.2006.01.015

Monza, D., Soliveri, P., Radice, D., Fetoni, V., Testa, D., Caffarra, P., . . . Girotti, F. (1998). Cognitive dysfunction and impaired organization of complex motility in degenerative parkinsonian syndromes. *Archives of Neurology*, *55*(3), 372–378.

Morgante, F., Edwards, M. J., & Espay, A. J. (2013). Psychogenic movement disorders. *Continuum (Minneap Minn)*, *19*(5 Movement Disorders), 1383–1396. doi: 10.1212/01.CON.0000436160.41071.79

Morley, J. F., Xie, S. X., Hurtig, H. I., Stern, M. B., Colcher, A., Horn, S., . . . Siderowf, A. (2012). Genetic influences on cognitive decline in Parkinson's disease. *Movement Disorders*, *27*(4), 512–518. doi: 10.1002/mds.24946

Morris, R. G., Downes, J. J., Sahakian, B. J., Evenden, J. L., Heald, A., & Robbins, T. W. (1988). Planning and spatial working memory in Parkinson's disease. *Journal of Neurology, Neurosurgery, and Psychiatry*, *51*(6), 757–766.

Mosley, P. E., & Marsh, R. (2015). The psychiatric and neuropsychiatric symptoms after subthalamic stimulation for Parkinson's disease. *Journal of Neuropsychiatry and Clinical Neurosciences*, *27*(1), 19–26. doi: 10.1176/appi.neuropsych.14040069

Moustafa, A. A., Bell, P., Eissa, A. M., & Hewedi, D. H. (2013). The effects of clinical motor variables and medication dosage on working memory in Parkinson's disease. *Brain and Cognition*, *82*(2), 137–145. doi: 10.1016/j.bandc.2013.04.001

Muenter, M. D., Forno, L. S., Hornykiewicz, O., Kish, S. J., Maraganore, D. M., Caselli, R. J., . . . Calne, D. B. (1998). Hereditary form of parkinsonism-dementia. *Brain and Cognition*, *43*(6), 768–781. doi: 10.1002/ana.410430612

Murphy, T., & Eddy, C. M. (2013). Neuropsychological assessment in Tourette syndrome. In D. Martino & J. F. Leckam (Eds.), *Tourette Syndrome* (pp. 439–484). New York: Oxford University Press.

Murray, L. L. (2000). Spoken language production in Huntington's and Parkinson's diseases. *Journal of Speech, Language, and Hearing Research*, *43*(6), 1350–1366.

Muslimovic, D., Post, B., Speelman, J. D., & Schmand, B. (2005). Cognitive profile of patients with newly diagnosed Parkinson disease. *Neurology*, *65*(8), 1239–1245.

Myslobodsky, M., Lalonde, F. M., & Hicks, L. (2001). Are patients with Parkinson's disease suicidal? *Journal of Geriatric Psychiatry and Neurology*, *14*(3), 120–124.

Naarding, P., Leentjens, A. F., Van Kooten, F., & Verhey, F. R. (2002). Disease-specific properties of the Hamilton Rating Scale for depression in patients with stroke, Alzheimer's dementia, and Parkinson's disease. *Journal of Neuropsychiatry and Clinical Neurosciences*, *14*(3), 329–334.

Nahan, F. B., & Levin, B. E. (2011). Characterizing and assessing the spectrum of volition in psychogenic movement disorders. In M. Hallett, A. E. Lang, J. Jankovic, S. Fahn, P. W. Halligan, V. Voon, & C. R. Cloninger (Eds.), *Psychogenic Movement Disorders and Other Conversion Disorders* (pp. 217–224). Cambridge, UK: Cambridge University Press.

Naismith, S. L., Mowszowski, L., Diamond, K., & Lewis, S. J. (2013). Improving memory in Parkinson's disease: A healthy brain ageing cognitive training program. *Movement Disorders*, *28*(8), 1097–1103. doi: 10.1002/mds.25457

Naismith, S. L., Pereira, M., Shine, J. M., & Lewis, S. J. (2011). How well do caregivers detect mild cognitive change in Parkinson's disease? *Movement Disorders*, *26*(1), 161–164. doi: 10.1002/mds.23331

Nath, U., Ben-Shlomo, Y., Thomson, R. G., Morris, H. R., Wood, N. W., Lees, A. J., & Burn, D. J. (2001). The prevalence of progressive supranuclear palsy (Steele-Richardson-Olszewski syndrome) in the UK. *Brain*, *124*(Pt 7), 1438–1449.

Naville, F. (1922). Les complications et let sequelles mentales de l'encephalite epidemique. *Encephale*, *17*, 369–375, 423–336.

Noe, E., Marder, K., Bell, K. L., Jacobs, D. M., Manly, J. J., & Stern, Y. (2004). Comparison of dementia with Lewy bodies to Alzheimer's disease and Parkinson's disease with dementia. *Movement Disorders*, *19*(1), 60–67.

Nombela, C., Bustillo, P. J., Castell, P. F., Sanchez, L., Medina, V., & Herrero, M. T. (2011). Cognitive rehabilitation in Parkinson's disease: Evidence from neuroimaging. *Frontiers in Neurology*, *2*, 82. doi: 10.3389/fneur.2011.00082

Nuti, A., Ceravolo, R., Piccinni, A., Dell'Agnello, G., Bellini, G., Gambaccini, G., . . . Bonuccelli, U. (2004). Psychiatric comorbidity in a population of Parkinson's disease patients. *European Journal of Neurology*, *11*(5), 315–320. doi: 10.1111/j.1468-1331.2004.00781.x

O'Brien, J. T., McKeith, I. G., Walker, Z., Tatsch, K., Booij, J., Darcourt, J., . . . Group, D.L.B. S. (2009). Diagnostic accuracy of 123I-FP-CIT SPECT in possible dementia with Lewy bodies. *British Journal of Psychiatry*, *194*(1), 34–39. doi: 10.1192/bjp.bp.108.052050

Odekerken, V. J., Boel, J. A., Geurtsen, G. J., Schmand, B. A., Dekker, I. P., de Haan, R. J., . . . Group, N. S. (2015). Neuropsychological outcome after deep brain stimulation for Parkinson disease. *Neurology*, *84*(13), 1355–1361. doi: 10.1212/WNL.0000000000001419

Odekerken, V. J., van Laar, T., Staal, M. J., Mosch, A., Hoffmann, C. F., Nijssen, P. C., . . . de Bie, R. M. (2013). Subthalamic nucleus versus globus pallidus bilateral deep brain stimulation for advanced Parkinson's disease (NSTAPS study): A randomised controlled trial. *Lancet Neurology*, *12*(1), 37–44. doi: 10.1016/S1474-4422(12)70264-8

Okai, D., Askey-Jones, S., Samuel, M., O'Sullivan, S. S., Chaudhuri, K. R., Martin, A., . . . David, A. S. (2013). Trial of CBT for impulse control behaviors affecting Parkinson patients and their caregivers. *Neurology*, *80*(9), 792–799. doi: 10.1212/WNL.0b013e3182840678

Owen, A. M., Doyon, J., Dagher, A., Sadikot, A., & Evans, A. C. (1998). Abnormal basal ganglia outflow in Parkinson's disease identified with PET: Implications for higher cortical functions. *Brain*, *121*(Pt 5), 949–965.

Owen, A. M., Sahakian, B. J., Hodges, J. R., Summers, B. A., Polkey, C. E., & Robbins, T. W. (1995). Dopamine-dependent fronto-striatal planning deficits in early Parkinson's disease. *Neuropsychology*, *9*, 126–140.

Pagonabarraga, J., Kulisevsky, J., Strafella, A. P., & Krack, P. (2015). Apathy in Parkinson's disease: Clinical features, neural substrates, diagnosis, and treatment. *Lancet Neurology*, *14*(5), 518–531. doi: 10.1016/S1474-4422(15)00019-8

Papoutsi, M., Labuschagne, I., Tabrizi, S. J., & Stout, J. C. (2014). The cognitive burden in Huntington's disease: Pathology, phenotype, and mechanisms of compensation. *Movement Disorders*, *29*(5), 673–683. doi: 10.1002/mds.25864

Paris, A. P., Saleta, H. G., de la Cruz Crespo Maraver, M., Silvestre, E., Freixa, M. G., Torrellas, C. P., . . . Bayes, A. R. (2011). Blind randomized controlled study of the efficacy of cognitive training in Parkinson's disease. *Movement Disorders*, *26*(7), 1251–1258. doi: 10.1002/mds.23688

Park, I. S., Oh, Y. S., Lee, K. S., Yang, D. W., Song, I. U., Park, J. W., & Kim, J. S. (2015). Subtype of mild cognitive impairment in elderly patients with essential tremor. *Alzheimer Disease and Associated Disorders*, *29*(2), 141–145. doi: 10.1097/WAD.0000000000000054

Parkinson, J. (1817). *An Essay on the Shaking Palsy*. London: Sherwood, Neely & Jones.

Passafiume, D., Boller, F., & Keefe, M. C. (1986). Neuropsychological impairment in patients with Parkinson's disease. In I. Grant & K. M. Adams (Eds.), *Neuropsychological Assessment of Neuropsychiatric Disorders* (pp. 374–383). New York: Oxford University Press.

Patel, N. K., Heywood, P., O'Sullivan, K., McCarter, R., Love, S., & Gill, S. S. (2003). Unilateral subthalamotomy in the treatment of Parkinson's disease. *Brain*, *126*(Pt 5), 1136–1145.

Paulsen, J. S. (2011). Cognitive impairment in Huntington disease: Diagnosis and treatment. *Current Neurology and Neuroscience Reports*, *11*(5), 474–483. doi: 10.1007/s11910-011-0215-x

Paulsen, J. S., & Long, J. D. (2014). Onset of Huntington's disease: Can it be purely cognitive? *Movement Disorders*, *29*(11), 1342–1350. doi: 10.1002/mds.25997

Pedersen, K. F., Larsen, J. P., Tysnes, O. B., & Alves, G. (2013). Prognosis of mild cognitive impairment in early Parkinson disease: The Norwegian ParkWest study. *JAMA Neurology*, *70*(5), 580–586. doi: 10.1001/jamaneurol.2013.2110

Pena, J., Ibarretxe-Bilbao, N., Garcia-Gorostiaga, I., Gomez-Beldarrain, M. A., Diez-Cirarda, M., & Ojeda, N. (2014). Improving functional disability and cognition in Parkinson disease: Randomized controlled trial. *Neurology*, *83*(23), 2167–2174. doi: 10.1212/WNL.0000000000001043

Perry, E. K., Curtis, M., Dick, D. J., Candy, J. M., Atack, J. R., Bloxham, C. A., . . . Perry, R. H. (1985). Cholinergic correlates of cognitive impairment in Parkinson's disease: Comparisons with Alzheimer's disease. *Journal of Neurology, Neurosurgery, and Psychiatry*, *48*(5), 413–421.

Petersen, R. C. (2011). Clinical practice; Mild cognitive impairment. *The New England Journal of Medicine*, *364*(23), 2227–2234. doi: 10.1056/NEJMcp0910237

Pfeiffer, H. C., Lokkegaard, A., Zoetmulder, M., Friberg, L., & Werdelin, L. (2014). Cognitive impairment in early-stage non-demented Parkinson's disease patients. *Acta Neurologica Scandinavica*, *129*(5), 307–318. doi: 10.1111/ane.12189

Pharr, V., Uttl, B., Stark, M., Litvan, I., Fantie, B., & Grafman, J. (2001). Comparison of apraxia in corticobasal degeneration and progressive supranuclear palsy. *Neurology*, *56*(7), 957–963.

Piatt, A. L., Fields, J. A., Paolo, A. M., Koller, W. C., & Tröster, A. I. (1999). Lexical, semantic, and action verbal fluency in Parkinson's disease with and without dementia. *Journal of Clinical and Experimental Neuropsychology*, *21*(4), 435–443.

Piccirilli, M., Piccinin, G. L., D'Alessandro, P., Finali, G., Piccolini, C., Scarcella, M. G., & Testa, A. (1986). Cognitive performances in parkinsonians before and after bromocriptine therapy. *Acta Neurologica (Napoli)*, *8*(3), 167–172.

Pietracupa, S., Fasano, A., Fabbrini, G., Sarchioto, M., Bloise, M., Latorre, A., . . . Berardelli, A. (2013). Poor self-awareness of levodopa-induced dyskinesias in Parkinson's disease: Clinical features and mechanisms. *Parkinsonism and Related Disorders*, *19*(11), 1004–1008. doi: 10.1016/j.parkreldis.2013.07.002

Pillon, B., Blin, J., Vidailhet, M., Deweer, B., Sirigu, A., Dubois, B., & Agid, Y. (1995). The neuropsychological pattern of corticobasal degeneration: Comparison with progressive supranuclear palsy and Alzheimer's disease. *Neurology*, *45*(8), 1477–1483.

Pillon, B., Dubois, B., Lhermitte, F., & Agid, Y. (1986). Heterogeneity of cognitive impairment in progressive supranuclear palsy, Parkinson's disease, and Alzheimer's disease. *Neurology*, *36*(9), 1179–1185.

Pillon, B., Dubois, B., Ploska, A., & Agid, Y. (1991). Severity and specificity of cognitive impairment in Alzheimer's, Huntington's, and Parkinson's diseases and progressive supranuclear palsy. *Neurology*, *41*(5), 634–643.

Pillon, B., Gouider-Khouja, N., Deweer, B., Vidailhet, M., Malapani, C., Dubois, B., & Agid, Y. (1995). Neuropsychological pattern of striatonigral degeneration: Comparison with Parkinson's disease and progressive supranuclear palsy. *Journal of Neurology, Neurosurgery, and Psychiatry*, *58*(2), 174–179.

Pirozzolo, F. J., Hansch, E. C., Mortimer, J. A., Webster, D. D., & Kuskowski, M. A. (1982). Dementia in Parkinson disease: A neuropsychological analysis. *Brain and Cognition*, *1*(1), 71–83.

Pirtosek, Z., Jahanshahi, M., Barrett, G., & Lees, A. J. (2001). Attention and cognition in bradykinetic-rigid syndromes: An event-related potential study. *Annals of Neurology*, *50*(5), 567–573.

Poletti, M., Cavedini, P., & Bonuccelli, U. (2011). Iowa gambling task in Parkinson's disease. *Journal of Clinical and Experimental Neuropsychology*, *33*(4), 395–409. doi: 10.1080/13803395.2010.524150

Pondal, M., Del Ser, T., & Bermejo, F. (1996). Anticholinergic therapy and dementia in patients with Parkinson's disease. *Journal of Neurology*, *243*(7), 543–546.

Pontone, G. M., Williams, J. R., Anderson, K. E., Chase, G., Goldstein, S. A., Grill, S., . . . Marsh, L. (2009). Prevalence of anxiety disorders and anxiety subtypes in patients with Parkinson's disease. *Movement Disorders*, *24*(9), 1333–1338. doi: 10.1002/mds.22611

Price, A., Rayner, L., Okon-Rocha, E., Evans, A., Valsraj, K., Higginson, I. J., & Hotopf, M. (2011). Antidepressants for the treatment of depression in neurological disorders: A systematic review and meta-analysis of randomised controlled trials. *Journal of Neurology, Neurosurgery and Psychiatry*, *82*(8), 914–923. doi: 10.1136/jnnp.2010.230862

Rajput, A. H., Adler, C. H., Shill, H. A., & Rajput, A. (2012). Essential tremor is not a neurodegenerative disease. *Neurodegenerative Disease Management*, *2*(3), 259–268. doi: 10.2217/nmt.12.23

Ranchet, M., Paire-Ficout, L., Uc, E. Y., Bonnard, A., Sornette, D., & Broussolle, E. (2013). Impact of specific executive functions on driving performance in people with Parkinson's disease. *Movement Disorders, 28,* 1941–1948. doi: 10.1002/mds.25660

Raskin, S. A., Woods, S. P., Poquette, A. J., McTaggart, A. B., Sethna, J., Williams, R. C., & Troster, A. I. (2010). A differential deficit in time-versus event-based prospective memory in Parkinson's disease. *Neuropsychology, 25,* 201–209. doi: 10.1037/a0020999

Ravina, B., Marder, K., Fernandez, H. H., Friedman, J. H., McDonald, W., Murphy, D., . . . Goetz, C. (2007). Diagnostic criteria for psychosis in Parkinson's disease: Report of an NINDS, NIMH work group. *Movement Disorders*, *22*(8), 1061–1068. doi: 10.1002/mds.21382

Reading, P. J., Luce, A. K., & McKeith, I. G. (2001). Rivastigmine in the treatment of parkinsonian psychosis and cognitive impairment: Preliminary findings from an open trial. *Movement Disorders*, *16*(6), 1171–1174.

Rebeiz, J. J., Kolodny, E. H., & Richardson, E. P., Jr. (1968). Corticodentatonigral degeneration with neuronal achromasia. *Archives of Neurology*, *18*(1), 20–33.

Reid, W. G., Broe, G. A., Morris, J. G., Hely, M. A., Moss, N. G., Genge, S. A., . . . Williamson P. M. (1992). The role of cholinergic deficiency in neuropsychological deficits in idiopathic Parkinson's disease. *Dementia and Geriatric Cognitive Disorders*, *3*, 114–120.

Reijnders, J. S., Ehrt, U., Weber, W. E., Aarsland, D., & Leentjens, A. F. (2008). A systematic review of prevalence studies of depression in Parkinson's disease. *Movement Disorders*, *23*(2), 183–189; quiz 313. doi: 10.1002/mds.21803

Remy, P., Doder, M., Lees, A., Turjanski, N., & Brooks, D. (2005). Depression in Parkinson's disease: Loss of dopamine and noradrenaline innervation in the limbic system. *Brain*, *128*(Pt 6), 1314–1322. doi: 10.1093/brain/awh445

Respondek, G., Stamelou, M., Kurz, C., Ferguson, L. W., Rajput, A., Chiu, W. Z., . . . Movement Disorder Society-endorsed, P.S.P.S.G. (2014). The phenotypic spectrum of progressive supranuclear palsy: A retrospective multicenter study of 100 definite cases. *Movement Disorders*, *29*(14), 1758–1766. doi: 10.1002/mds.26054

Reynolds, W. M., & Kobak, K., A. (1995). *Hamilton Depression Inventory—A Self-Report Version of the Hamilton Depression Rating Scale (HDRS)*. Odessa, FL: Psychological Assessment Resources.

Richard, I. H., Justus, A. W., Greig, N. H., Marshall, F., & Kurlan, R. (2002). Worsening of motor function and mood in a patient with Parkinson's disease after pharmacologic challenge with oral rivastigmine. *Clinical Neuropharmacology*, *25*(6), 296–299.

Richard, I. H., McDermott, M. P., Kurlan, R., Lyness, J. M., Como, P. G., Pearson, N., . . . Group, S.-P. S. (2012). A randomized, double-blind, placebo-controlled trial of antidepressants in Parkinson disease. *Neurology*, *78*(16), 1229–1236. doi: 10.1212/WNL.0b013e3182516244

Rieger, M., Gauggel, S., & Burmeister, K. (2003). Inhibition of ongoing responses following frontal, nonfrontal, and basal ganglia lesions. *Neuropsychology*, *17*(2), 272–282.

Riklan, M., & Levita, E. (1969). *Subcortical Correlates of Human Behavior: A Psychological Study of Thalamic and Basal Ganglia Surgery*. Baltimore: Williams & Wilkins.

Riley, D. E., & Lang, A. E. (1996). Non-Parkinson akinetic-rigid syndromes. *Current Opinion in Neurology*, *9*(4), 321–326.

Rinne, J. O., Lee, M. S., Thompson, P. D., & Marsden, C. D. (1994). Corticobasal degeneration: A clinical study of 36 cases. *Brain*, *117*(Pt 5), 1183–1196.

Rittman, T., Ghosh, B. C., McColgan, P., Breen, D. P., Evans, J., Williams-Gray, C. H., . . . Rowe, J. B. (2013). The Addenbrooke's cognitive examination for the differential diagnosis and longitudinal assessment of patients with parkinsonian disorders. *Journal of Neurology, Neurosurgery and Psychiatry*, *84*(5), 544–551. doi: 10.1136/jnnp-2012-303618

Robbins, T. W., James, M., Lange, K. W., Owen, A. M., Quinn, N. P., & Marsden, C. D. (1992). Cognitive performance in multiple system atrophy. *Brain*, *115*(Pt 1), 271–291.

Robbins, T. W., James, M., Owen, A. M., Lange, K. W., Lees, A. J., Leigh, P. N., . . . Summers, B. A. (1994). Cognitive deficits in progressive supranuclear palsy, Parkinson's disease, and multiple system atrophy in tests sensitive to frontal lobe dysfunction. *Journal of Neurology, Neurosurgery, and Psychiatry*, *57*(1), 79–88.

Robbins, T. W., Owen, A. M., & Sahakian, B. J. (1998). The neuropsychology of basal ganglia disorders: An integrative cognitive and comparative approach. In M. A. Ron & A. S. David (Eds.), *Disorders of Brain and Mind* (pp. 57–83). Cambridge, UK: Cambridge University Press.

Rogers, R., & Wooley, C. (2011). Diagnostic considerations for the assessment of malingering within the context of psychogenic movement disorders. In M. Hallett, A. E. Lang, J. Jankovic, S. Fahn, P. W. Halligan, V. Voon, & C. R. Cloninger (Eds.), *Psychogenic Movement Disorders and Other Conversion Disorders* (pp. 240–247). Cambridge, UK: Cambridge University Press.

Rolinski, M., Fox, C., Maidment, I., & McShane, R. (2012). Cholinesterase inhibitors for dementia with Lewy bodies, Parkinson's disease dementia and cognitive impairment in Parkinson's disease. *Cochrane Database Systematic Reviews*, *3*, CD006504. doi: 10.1002/14651858.CD006504.pub2

Ross, C. A., & Tabrizi, S. J. (2011). Huntington's disease: From molecular pathogenesis to clinical treatment. *Lancet Neurology*, *10*(1), 83–98. doi: 10.1016/S1474-4422(10)70245-3

Ross, H. F., Hughes, T. A., Boyd, J. L., Biggins, C. A., Madeley, P., Mindham, R.H.S., & Spokes, E.G.S. (1996). The evolution and profile of dementia in Parkinson's disease. In L. Battistin, G. Scarlato, T. Caraceni, & S. Ruggieri (Eds.), *Advances in Neurology* (Vol. 69, pp. 343–347). Philadelphia, PA: Lippincott-Raven Publishers.

Rothlind, J. C., York, M. K., Carlson, K., Luo, P., Marks, W. J., Jr., Weaver, F. M., . . . Group, C.S.P.S. (2015). Neuropsychological changes following deep brain stimulation surgery for Parkinson's disease: Comparisons of treatment at pallidal and subthalamic targets versus best medical therapy. *Journal of Neurology, Neurosurgery and Psychiatry*, *86*(6), 622–629. doi: 10.1136/jnnp-2014-308119

Sahgal, A., Galloway, P. H., McKeith, I. G., Lloyd, S., Cook, J. H., Ferrier, I. N., & Edwardson, J. A. (1992). Matching-to-sample deficits in patients with senile dementias of the Alzheimer and Lewy body types. *Archives of Neurology*, *49*(10), 1043–1046.

Saint-Cyr, J. A., Taylor, A. E., & Lang, A. E. (1988). Procedural learning and neostriatal dysfunction in man. *Brain*, *111*(Pt 4), 941–959.

Saint-Cyr, J. A., Taylor, A. E., & Lang, A. E. (1993). Neuropsychological and psychiatric side effects in the treatment of Parkinson's disease. *Neurology*, *43*(Suppl. 6)(12), S47–S52.

Saint-Cyr, J. A., & Trépanier, L. L. (2000). Neuropsychologic assessment of patients for movement disorder surgery. *Movement Disorders*, *15*(5), 771–783.

Salmon, D. P., & Galasko, D. (1996). Neuropsychological aspects of Lewy body dementia. In R. Perry, I. McKeith, & E. Perry (Eds.), *Dementia with Lewy Bodies: Clinical, Pathological, and Treatment Issues* (pp. 99–113). Cambridge, UK: Cambridge University Press.

Salmon, D. P., Galasko, D., Hansen, L. A., Masliah, E., Butters, N., Thal, L. J., & Katzman, R. (1996). Neuropsychological deficits associated with diffuse Lewy body disease. *Brain and Cognition*, *31*(2), 148–165.

Sammer, G., Reuter, I., Hullmann, K., Kaps, M., & Vaitl, D. (2006). Training of executive functions in Parkinson's disease. *Journal of the Neurological Sciences*, *248*(1–2), 115–119. doi: S0022-510X(06)00224-3 [pii] 10.1016/j.jns.2006.05.028

Schiffer, R. B., Kurlan, R., Rubin, A., & Boer, S. (1988). Evidence for atypical depression in Parkinson's disease. *American Journal of Psychiatry*, *145*(8), 1020–1022.

Schiller, F. (2000). Fritz Lewy and his bodies. *Journal of the History of the Neurosciences*, *9*, 148–151.

Schmahmann, J. D. (2001). The cerebrocerebellar system: Anatomic substrates of the cerebellar contribution to cognition and emotion. *International Review of Psychiatry*, *13*, 247–260.

Schmahmann, J. D., & Sherman, J. C. (1998). The cerebellar cognitive affective syndrome. *Brain*, *121*(Pt 4), 561–579.

Schmand, B., & Tröster, A. I. (2015). Earliest cognitive changes and mild cognitive impairment in Parkinson's disease. In A. I. Tröster (Ed.), *Clinical Neuropsychology and Cognitive Neurology of Parkinson's Disease and Other Movement Disorders* (pp. 205–238). New York: Oxford University Press.

Schrag, A., Barone, P., Brown, R. G., Leentjens, A. F., McDonald, W. M., Starkstein, S., . . . Goetz, C. G. (2007). Depression rating scales in Parkinson's disease: Critique and recommendations. *Movement Disorders*, *22*(8), 1077–1092.

Schrag, A., Ben-Shlomo, Y., & Quinn, N. P. (1999). Prevalence of progressive supranuclear palsy and multiple system atrophy: A cross-sectional study. *Lancet*, *354*(9192), 1771–1775.

Scott, R. B., Gregory, R., Wilson, J., Banks, S., Turner, A., Parkin, S., . . . Aziz, T. (2003). Executive cognitive deficits in primary dystonia. *Movement Disorders*, *18*(5), 539–550.

Seichepine, D. R., Neargarder, S., Davidsdottir, S., Reynolds, G. O., & Cronin-Golomb, A. (2015). Side and type of initial motor symptom influences visuospatial functioning in Parkinson's disease. *Journal of Parkinsons Disease*, *5*(1), 75–83. doi: 10.3233/JPD-140365

Seltzer, B., Vasterling, J. J., Mathias, C. W., & Brennan, A. (2001). Clinical and neuropsychological correlates of impaired awareness of deficits in Alzheimer disease and Parkinson disease: A comparative study. *Neuropsychiatry, Neuropsychology, and Behavioral Neurology*, *14*(2), 122–129.

Shapiro, D. Y., Sadowsky, D. A., Henderson, W. G., & Van Buren, J. M. (1973). An assessment of cognitive function in postthalamotomy Parkinson patients. *Confinia Neurologica*, *35*(3), 144–166.

Sharp, M. E., & Alcalay, R. N. (2015). Genetics and cognition in Parkinson's disease. In A. I. Tröster (Ed.), *Clinical Neuropsychology and Cognitive Neurology of Parkinson's Disease and Other Movement Disorders* (pp. 179–204). New York: Oxford University Press.

Shaskin, D., Yarnell, H., & Alper, K. (1942). Physical, psychiatric, and psychometric studies of post-encephalitic parkinsonism. *Journal of Nervous and Mental Disease*, *96*, 652–662.

Sheikh, J. I., & Yesavage, J. A. (1986). Geriatric Depression Scale (GDS): Recent evidence and development of a shorter version. *Clinical Gerontologist*, *5*, 165–173.

Shimomura, T., Mori, E., Yamashita, H., Imamura, T., Hirono, N., Hashimoto, M., . . . Hanihara, T. (1998). Cognitive loss in dementia with Lewy bodies and Alzheimer disease. *Archives of Neurology*, *55*(12), 1547–1552.

Shulman, L. M., Taback, R. L., Rabinstein, A. A., & Weiner, W. J. (2002). Non-recognition of depression and other non-motor symptoms in Parkinson's disease. *Parkinsonism and Related Disorders*, *8*, 193–197.

Siegert, R. J., Weatherall, M., Taylor, K. D., & Abernethy, D. A. (2008). A meta-analysis of performance on simple span and more complex working memory tasks in Parkinson's disease. *Neuropsychology*, *22*(4), 450–461. doi: 10.1037/0894-4105.22.4.450

Siegfried, J., & Blond, S. (1997). *The Neurosurgical Treatment of Parkinson's Disease and Other Movement Disorders*. London: Williams & Wilkins Europe Ltd.

Siepel, F. J., Bronnick, K. S., Booij, J., Ravina, B. M., Lebedev, A. V., Pereira, J. B., . . . Aarsland, D. (2014). Cognitive executive impairment and dopaminergic deficits in de novo Parkinson's disease. *Movement Disorders*, *29*(14), 1802–1808. doi: 10.1002/mds.26051

Sinforiani, E., Banchieri, L., Zucchella, C., Pacchetti, C., & Sandrini, G. (2004). Cognitive rehabilitation in Parkinson's disease. *Archives of Gerontology and Geriatrics Supplements* (9), 387–391.

Sitek, E. J., Soltan, W., Wieczorek, D., Robowski, P., & Slawek, J. (2011). Self-awareness of memory function in Parkinson's disease in relation to mood and symptom severity. *Aging and Mental Health*, *15*(2), 150–156. doi: 10.1080/13607863.2010.508773

Slaughter, J. R., Slaughter, K. A., Nichols, D., Holmes, S. E., & Martens, M. P. (2001). Prevalence, clinical manifestations, etiology, and treatment of depression in Parkinson's disease. *Journal of Neuropsychiatry and Clinical Neurosciences*, *13*(2), 187–196.

Smeding, H. M., Speelman, J. D., Huizenga, H. M., Schuurman, P. R., & Schmand, B. (2011). Predictors of cognitive and psychosocial outcome after STN DBS in Parkinson's Disease. *Journal of Neurology, Neurosurgery, and Psychiatry*, *82*(7), 754–760. doi: 10.1136/jnnp.2007.140012

Soliveri, P., Monza, D., Paridi, D., Carella, F., Genitrini, S., Testa, D., & Girotti, F. (2000). Neuropsychological follow up in patients with Parkinson's disease, striatonigral degeneration-type multisystem atrophy, and progressive supranuclear palsy. *Journal of Neurology, Neurosurgery, and Psychiatry*, *69*(3), 313–318.

Soliveri, P., Monza, D., Paridi, D., Radice, D., Grisoli, M., Testa, D., . . . Girotti, F. (1999). Cognitive and magnetic resonance imaging aspects of corticobasal degeneration and progressive supranuclear palsy. *Neurology*, *53*(3), 502–507.

Souchay, C., & Smith, S. J. (2013). Autobiographical memory in Parkinson's disease: A retrieval deficit. *Journal of Neuropsychology*, *7*(2), 164–178. doi: 10.1111/jnp.12014

Stankovic, I., Krismer, F., Jesic, A., Antonini, A., Benke, T., Brown, R. G., . . . Movement Disorders Society, M.S.A.S.G. (2014). Cognitive impairment in multiple system atrophy: A position statement by the Neuropsychology Task Force of the MDS Multiple System Atrophy (MODIMSA) study group. *Movement Disorders*, *29*(7), 857–867. doi: 10.1002/mds.25880

Starkstein, S. E., Bolduc, P. L., Mayberg, H. S., Preziosi, T. J., & Robinson, R. G. (1990). Cognitive impairments and depression in Parkinson's disease: A follow up study. *Journal of Neurology, Neurosurgery, and Psychiatry*, *53*(7), 597–602.

Starkstein, S. E., Mayberg, H. S., Preziosi, T. J., Andrezejewski, P., Leiguarda, R., & Robinson, R. G. (1992). Reliability, validity, and clinical correlates of apathy in Parkinson's disease. *Journal of Neuropsychiatry and Clinical Neurosciences*, *4*(2), 134–139.

Starkstein, S. E., Merello, M., Jorge, R., Brockman, S., Bruce, D., Petracca, G., & Robinson, R. G. (2008). A validation study of depressive syndromes in Parkinson's disease. *Movement Disorders*, *23*(4), 538–546. doi: 10.1002/mds.21866

Stebbins, G. T., Gabrieli, J. D., Masciari, F., Monti, L., & Goetz, C. G. (1999). Delayed recognition memory in Parkinson's disease: A role for working memory? *Neuropsychologia*, *37*(4), 503–510.

Stefanova, E. D., Kostic, V. S., Ziropadja, L. J., Ocic, G. G., & Markovic, M. (2001). Declarative memory in early Parkinson's disease: Serial position learning effects. *Journal of Clinical and Experimental Neuropsychology*, *23*(5), 581–591.

Stein, M. B., Heuser, I. J., Juncos, J. L., & Uhde, T. W. (1990). Anxiety disorders in patients with Parkinson's disease. *American Journal of Psychiatry*, *147*(2), 217–220.

Stern, Y., Mayeux, R., Ilson, J., Fahn, S., & Cote, L. (1984). Pergolide therapy for Parkinson's disease: Neurobehavioral changes. *Neurology*, *34*(2), 201–204.

Stern, Y., Mayeux, R., & Rosen, J. (1984). Contribution of perceptual motor dysfunction to construction and tracing disturbances in Parkinson's disease. *Journal of Neurology, Neurosurgery, and Psychiatry*, *47*(9), 983–989.

Stern, Y., Tang, M. X., Jacobs, D. M., Sano, M., Marder, K., Bell, K., . . . Côté, L. (1998). Prospective comparative study of the evolution of probable Alzheimer's disease and Parkinson's disease dementia. *Journal of the International Neuropsychological Society*, *4*(3), 279–284.

Stout, J. C., Paulsen, J. S., Queller, S., Solomon, A. C., Whitlock, K. B., Campbell, J. C., . . . Aylward, E. H. (2011). Neurocognitive signs in prodromal Huntington disease. *Neuropsychology*, *25*(1), 1–14. doi: 10.1037/a0020937

Sullivan, E. V., & Sagar, H. J. (1989). Nonverbal recognition and recency discrimination deficits in Parkinson's disease and Alzheimer's disease. *Brain*, *112*(Pt 6), 1503–1517.

Tabrizi, S. J., Reilmann, R., Roos, R. A., Durr, A., Leavitt, B., Owen, G., . . . Investigators, T.-H. (2012). Potential endpoints for clinical trials in premanifest and early Huntington's disease in the TRACK-HD study: Analysis of 24 month observational data. *Lancet Neurology*, *11*(1), 42–53. doi: 10.1016/S1474-4422(11)70263-0

Tabrizi, S. J., Scahill, R. I., Owen, G., Durr, A., Leavitt, B. R., Roos, R. A., . . . Investigators, T.-H. (2013). Predictors of phenotypic progression and disease onset in premanifest and early-stage Huntington's disease in the TRACK-HD study: Analysis of 36-month observational data. *Lancet Neurology*, *12*(7), 637–649. doi: 10.1016/S1474-4422(13)70088-7

Taylor, A. E., & Saint-Cyr, J. A. (1995). The neuropsychology of Parkinson's disease. *Brain and Cognition*, *28*(3), 281–296.

Taylor, A. E., Saint-Cyr, J. A., & Lang, A. E. (1986). Frontal lobe dysfunction in Parkinson's disease: The cortical focus of neostriatal outflow. *Brain*, *109*(Pt 5), 845–883.

Testa, D., Fetoni, V., Soliveri, P., Musicco, M., Palazzini, E., & Girotti, F. (1993). Cognitive and motor performance in multiple system atrophy and Parkinson's disease compared. *Neuropsychologia*, *31*(2), 207–210.

Thaler, A., Mirelman, A., Gurevich, T., Simon, E., Orr-Urtreger, A., Marder, K., . . . Giladi, N. (2012). Lower cognitive performance in healthy G2019S LRRK2 mutation carriers. *Neurology*, *79*(10), 1027–1032. doi: 10.1212/WNL.0b013e3182684646

Tierney, M. C., Nores, A., Snow, W. G., Fisher, R. H., Zorzitto, M. L., & Reid, D. W. (1994). Use of the Rey Auditory Verbal Learning Test in differentiating normal aging from Alzheimer's and Parkinson's dementia. *Psychological Assessment*, *6*(2), 129–134.

Tomer, R., & Levin, B. E. (1993). Differential effects of aging on two verbal fluency tasks. *Perceptual and Motor Skills*, *76*(2), 465–466.

Torkamani, M., & Jahanshahi, M. (2015). Neuropsychological and neuropsychiatric features of dystonia and the impact of medical and surgical treatment. In A. I. Tröster (Ed.), *Clinical*

Neuropsychology and Cognitive Neurology of Parkinson's Disease and Other Movement Disorders (pp. 455–483). New York: Oxford University Press.

Tröster, A. I. (2011). A precis of recent advances in the neuropsychology of mild cognitive impairment(s) in Parkinson's disease and a proposal of preliminary research criteria. *Journal of the International Neuropsychological Society*, *17*, 393–406. doi: 10.1017/S1355617711000257

Tröster, A. I., & Browner, N. (2013). Movement disorders with dementia in older adults. In L. D. Ravdin & H. L. Katzen (Eds.), *Handbook on the Neuropsychology of Aging and Dementia* (pp. 333–361). New York: Springer.

Tröster, A. I., & Fields, J. A. (1995). Frontal cognitive function and memory in Parkinson's disease: Toward a distinction between prospective and declarative memory impairments? *Behavioural Neurology*, *8*, 59–74.

Tröster, A. I., & Fields, J. A. (2003). The role of neuropsychological evaluation in the neurosurgical treatment of movement disorders. In D. Tarsy, J. L. Vitek, & A. M. Lozano (Eds.), *Surgical Treatment of Parkinson's Disease and Other Movement Disorders* (pp. 213–240). Totowa, NJ: Humana Press.

Tröster, A. I., Fields, J. A., Testa, J. A., Paul, R. H., Blanco, C. R., Hames, K. A., . . . Beatty, W. W. (1998). Cortical and subcortical influences on clustering and switching in the performance of verbal fluency tasks. *Neuropsychologia*, *36*(4), 295–304.

Troster, A. I., Pahwa, R., Fields, J. A., Tanner, C. M., & Lyons, K. E. (2005). Quality of life in Essential Tremor Questionnaire (QUEST): Development and initial validation. *Parkinsonism Relat Disord*, *11*(6), 367–373.

Troster, A. I., Paolo, A. M., Lyons, K. E., Glatt, S. L., Hubble, J. P., & Koller, W. C. (1995). The influence of depression on cognition in Parkinson's disease: A pattern of impairment distinguishable from Alzheimer's disease. *Neurology*, *45*(4), 672–676.

Tröster, A. I., Prizer, L. P., & Baxley, A. (2013). Parkinson's disease: Secondary influences on cognition. In P. A. Arnett (Ed.), *Secondary Influences on Neuropsychological Test Performance* (pp. 259–291). New York: Oxford University Press.

Tröster, A. I., Stalp, L. D., Paolo, A. M., Fields, J. A., & Koller, W. C. (1995). Neuropsychological impairment in Parkinson's disease with and without depression. *Archives of Neurology*, *52*(12), 1164–1169.

Tröster, A. I., & Tucker, K. A. (2005). Impact of essential tremor and its medical and surgical treatment on neuropsychological functioning, activities of daily living, and quality of life. In K. E. Lyons & R. Pahwa (Eds.), *Handbook of Essential Tremor and Other Tremor Disorders* (pp. 117–131). Boca Raton, FL: Taylor and Francis.

Tröster, A. I., & Woods, S. P. (2003). Neuropsychological aspects of Parkinson's disease and parkinsonian syndromes. In R. Pahwa, K. E. Lyons, & W. C. Koller (Eds.), *Handbook of Parkinson's Disease* (3rd ed., pp. 127–157). New York: Marcel Dekker.

Tröster, A. I., Woods, S. P., Fields, J. A., Lyons, K. E., Pahwa, R., Higginson, C. I., & Koller, W. C. (2002). Neuropsychological deficits in essential tremor: An expression of cerebello-thalamo-cortical pathophysiology? *European Journal of Neurology*, *9*(2), 143–151.

Troyer, A. K., Moscovitch, M., Winocur, G., Leach, L., & Freedman, M. (1998). Clustering and switching on verbal fluency tests in Alzheimer's and Parkinson's disease. *Journal of the International Neuropsychological Society*, *4*(2), 137–143.

Ullman, M. T., Corkin, S., Coppola, M., Hickok, G., Growdon, J. H., Koroshetz, W. J., & Pinker, S. (1997). A neural dissociation within language: Evidence that the mental dictionary is part of declarative memory, and that grammatical rules are processed by the procedural system. *Journal of Cognitive Neuroscience*, *9*, 266–276.

van der Hurk, P. R., & Hodges, J. R. (1995). Episodic and semantic memory in Alzheimer's disease and progressive supranuclear palsy: A comparative study. *Journal of Clinical and Experimental Neuropsychology*, *17*(3), 459–471.

van Duijn, E., Kingma, E. M., & van der Mast, R. C. (2007). Psychopathology in verified Huntington's disease gene carriers. *Journal of Neuropsychiatry and Clinical Neurosciences*, *19*(4), 441–448. doi: 19/4/441 [pii] 10.1176/appi.neuropsych.19.4.441

van Oostrom, I., Dollfus, S., Brazo, P., Abadie, P., Halbecq, I., Théry, S., & Marié, R.-M. (2003). Verbal learning and memory in schizophrenic and Parkinson's disease patients. *Psychiatry Research*, *117*, 25–34.

Varanese, S., Perfetti, B., Monaco, D., Thomas, A., Bonanni, L., Tiraboschi, P., & Onofrj, M. (2010). Fluctuating cognition and different cognitive and behavioural profiles in Parkinson's disease with dementia: Comparison of dementia with Lewy bodies and Alzheimer's disease. *Journal of Neurology*, *257*(6), 1004–1011. doi: 10.1007/s00415-010-5453-3

Vazquez, A., Jimenez-Jimenez, F. J., Garcia-Ruiz, P., & Garcia-Urra, D. (1993). "Panic attacks" in Parkinson's disease: A long-term complication of levodopa therapy. *Acta Neurologica Scandanavica*, *87*(1), 14–18.

Veazey, C., Cook, K. F., Stanley, M., Lai, E. C., & Kunik, M. E. (2009). Telephone-administered cognitive behavioral therapy: A case study of anxiety and depression in Parkinson's disease. *Journal of Clinical Psychology in Medical Settings*, *16*(3), 243–253. doi: 10.1007/s10880-009-9167-6

Venneri, A., Nichelli, P., Modonesi, G., Molinari, M. A., Russo, R., & Sardini, C. (1997). Impairment in dating and retrieving remote events in patients with early Parkinson's disease. *Journal of Neurology, Neurosurgery, and Psychiatry*, *62*(4), 410–413.

Vilkki, J., & Laitinen, L. V. (1974). Differential effects of left and right ventrolateral thalamotomy on receptive and expressive verbal performances and face-matching. *Neuropsychologia*, *12*(1), 11–19.

Volkmann, J., Daniels, C., & Witt, K. (2010). Neuropsychiatric effects of subthalamic neurostimulation in Parkinson disease. *Nature Reviews Neurology*, *6*(9), 487–498. doi: 10.1038/nrneurol.2010.111

Voon, V. (2015). Impulse control disorders. In H. Reichmann (Ed.), *Neuropsychiatric Symptoms of Movement Disorders* (pp. 79–98). Cham, Switzerland: Springer.

Voon, V., & Lang, A. E. (2005). Antidepressant treatment outcomes of psychogenic movement disorder. *Journal of Clinical Psychiatry*, *66*(12), 1529–1534.

Walker, M. P., Ayre, G. A., Perry, E. K., Wesnes, K., McKeith, I. G., Tovee, M., . . . Ballard, C. G. (2000). Quantification and characterisation of fluctuating cognition in dementia with Lewy bodies and Alzheimer's disease. *Dementia and Geriatric Cognitive Disorders*, *11*(6), 327–335.

Walker, Z., Allen, R. L., Shergill, S., & Katona, C. L. (1997). Neuropsychological performance in Lewy body dementia and Alzheimer's disease. *British Journal of Psychiatry*, *170*, 156–158.

Walsh, K., & Bennett, G. (2001). Parkinson's disease and anxiety. *Postgraduate Medical Journal*, *77*(904), 89–93.

Wang, H. F., Yu, J. T., Tang, S. W., Jiang, T., Tan, C. C., Meng, X. F., . . . Tan, L. (2015). Efficacy and safety of cholinesterase inhibitors and memantine in cognitive impairment in Parkinson's disease, Parkinson's disease dementia, and dementia with Lewy bodies: Systematic review with meta-analysis and trial sequential analysis. *Journal of Neurology Neurosurgery and Psychiatry*, *86*(2), 135–143. doi: 10.1136/jnnp-2014-307659

Weddell, R. A., & Weiser, R. (1995). A double-blind cross-over placebo-controlled trial of the effects of bromocriptine on psychomotor function, cognition, and mood in de novo patients with Parkinson's disease. *Behavioural Pharmacology*, *6*, 81–91.

Weintraub, D., David, A. S., Evans, A. H., Grant, J. E., & Stacy, M. (2015). Clinical spectrum of impulse control disorders in Parkinson's disease. *Movement Disorders*, *30*(2), 121–127. doi: 10.1002/mds.26016

Weintraub, D., & Goldman, J. G. (2015). Impulse control disorders, apathy, and psychosis. In A. I. Tröster (Ed.), *Clinical Neuropsychology and Cognitive Neurology of Parkinson's Disease and Other Movement Disorders* (pp. 291–331). New York: Oxford University Press.

Weintraub, D., Hoops, S., Shea, J. A., Lyons, K. E., Pahwa, R., Driver-Dunckley, E. D., . . . Voon, V. (2009). Validation of the questionnaire for impulsive-compulsive disorders in Parkinson's disease. *Movement Disorders*, *24*, 1461–1467 doi: 10.1002/mds.22571

Weintraub, D., Koester, J., Potenza, M. N., Siderowf, A. D., Stacy, M., Voon, V., . . . Lang, A. E. (2010). Impulse control disorders in Parkinson disease: A cross-sectional study of 3090 patients. *Archives of Neurology*, *67*(5), 589–595. doi: 10.1001/archneurol.2010.65

Weintraub, D., Mamikonyan, E., Papay, K., Shea, J. A., Xie, S. X., & Siderowf, A. (2012). Questionnaire for impulsive-compulsive disorders in Parkinson's disease-rating scale. *Movement Disorders*, *27*(2), 242–247. doi: 10.1002/mds.24023

Weintraub, D., Moberg, P. J., Culbertson, W. C., Duda, J. E., Katz, I. R., & Stern, M. B. (2005). Dimensions of executive function in Parkinson's disease. *Dementia and Geriatric Cognitive Disorders*, *20*, 140–144.

Weintraub, D., Moberg, P. J., Duda, J. E., Katz, I. R., & Stern, M. B. (2003). Recognition and treatment of depression in Parkinson's disease. *Journal of Geriatric Psychiatry and Neurology*, *16*(3), 178–183.

Weintraub, D., Oehlberg, K. A., Katz, I. R., & Stern, M. B. (2006). Test characteristics of the 15-item geriatric depression scale and Hamilton depression rating scale in Parkinson disease. *American Journal of Geriatric Psychiatry*, *14*(2), 169–175.

Weintraub, D., Siderowf, A. D., Tröster, A. I., & Anderson, K. E. (2011). Parkinson's disease and movement disorders. In C. E. Coffey, J. L. Cummings, M. S. George, & D. Weintraub (Eds.), *Textbook of Geriatric Neuropsychiatry* (3rd ed., pp. 569–597). Washington, DC: American Psychiatric Press.

Weintraub, D., Simuni, T., Caspell-Garcia, C., Coffey, C., Lasch, S., Siderowf, A., . . . The Parkinson's Progression Markers, I. (2015). Cognitive performance and neuropsychiatric symptoms in early, untreated Parkinson's disease. *Movement Disorders*, *30*, 919–927. doi: 10.1002/mds.26170

Welman, A. J. (1971). Neuropsychologische Untersuchung von Parkinsonpatienten (Vor und nach Thalomotomie). *Schweizer Archiv für Neurologie, Neurochirurgie und Psychiatrie*, *108*(1), 175–188.

Wenning, G. K., Colosimo, C., Geser, F., & Poewe, W. (2004). Multiple system atrophy. *Lancet Neurology*, *3*, 93–103.

Wenning, G. K., Seppi, K., Scherfler, C., Stefanova, N., & Puschban, Z. (2001). Multiple system atrophy. *Seminars in Neurology*, *21*(1), 33–40.

Whittington, C. J., Podd, J., & Kan, M. M. (2000). Recognition memory impairment in Parkinson's disease: Power and meta-analyses. *Neuropsychology*, *14*(2), 233–246.

Wichmann, T., & De Long, M. R. (2015). Basal ganglia circuits: Structure, function and dysfunction. In A. I. Tröster (Ed.), *Clinical Neuropsychology and Cognitive Neurology of Parkinson's Disease and Other Movement Disorders* (pp. 3–26). New York: Oxford University Press.

Williams, D. R., de Silva, R., Paviour, D. C., Pittman, A., Watt, H. C., Kilford, L., . . . Lees, A. J. (2005). Characteristics of two distinct clinical phenotypes in pathologically proven progressive supranuclear palsy: Richardson's syndrome and PSP-parkinsonism. *Brain*, *128*(Pt 6), 1247–1258.

Williams, J. R., Hirsch, E. S., Anderson, K., Bush, A. L., Goldstein, S. R., Grill, S., . . . Marsh, L. (2012). A comparison of nine scales to detect depression in Parkinson disease: Which scale to use? *Neurology*, *78*(13), 998–1006. doi: 10.1212/WNL.0b013e31824d587f

Williams, N. R., Foote, K. D., & Okun, M. S. (2014). STN vs. GPi Deep brain stimulation: Translating the rematch into clinical practice. *Movement Disorders: Clinical Practice*, *1*(1), 24–35. doi: 10.1002/mdc3.12004

Williams-Gray, C. H., Evans, J. R., Goris, A., Foltynie, T., Ban, M., Robbins, T. W., . . . Barker, R. A. (2009). The distinct cognitive syndromes of Parkinson's disease: 5 year follow-up of the CamPaIGN cohort. *Brain*, *132*(Pt 11), 2958–2969. doi: awp245 [pii] 10.1093/brain/awp245

Williams-Gray, C. H., Goris, A., Saiki, M., Foltynie, T., Compston, D. A., Sawcer, S. J., & Barker, R. A. (2009). Apolipoprotein E genotype as a risk factor for susceptibility to and dementia in Parkinson's disease. *Journal of Neurology*, *256*(3), 493–498. doi: 10.1007/s00415-009-0119-8

Williams-Gray, C. H., Hampshire, A., Barker, R. A., & Owen, A. M. (2008). Attentional control in Parkinson's disease is dependent on COMT val 158 met genotype. *Brain*, *131*(Pt 2), 397–408. doi: awm313 [pii] 10.1093/brain/awm313

Williams-Gray, C. H., Mason, S. L., Evans, J. R., Foltynie, T., Brayne, C., Robbins, T. W., & Barker, R. A. (2013). The CamPaIGN study of Parkinson's disease: 10-year outlook in an incident population-based cohort. *Journal of Neurology, Neurosurgery and Psychiatry*, *84*(11), 1258–1264. doi: 10.1136/jnnp-2013-305277

Winterer, G., & Goldman, D. (2003). Genetics of human prefrontal function. *Brain Research. Brain Research Reviews*, *43*(1), 134–163.

Wirdefeldt, K., Adami, H. O., Cole, P., Trichopoulos, D., & Mandel, J. (2011). Epidemiology and etiology of Parkinson's disease: A review of the evidence. *European Journal of Epidemiology*, *26*(Suppl 1), S1–S58. doi: 10.1007/s10654-011-9581-6

Wolf, R. C., Sambataro, F., Vasic, N., Baldas, E. M., Ratheiser, I., Bernhard Landwehrmeyer, G., . . . Orth, M. (2014). Visual system integrity and cognition in early Huntington's disease. *European Journal of Neuroscience*, *40*(2), 2417–2426. doi: 10.1111/ejn.12575

Woods, S. P., Fields, J. A., Lyons, K. E., Koller, W. C., Wilkinson, S. B., Pahwa, R., & Tröster, A. I. (2001). Neuropsychological and quality of life changes following unilateral thalamic deep brain stimulation in Parkinson's disease: A 12-month follow-up. *Acta Neurochirurgica*, *143*, 1273–1278.

Woods, S. P., Scott, J. C., Fields, J. A., Poquette, A., & Troster, A. I. (2008). Executive dysfunction and neuropsychiatric symptoms predict lower health status in essential tremor. *Cognitive and Behavioral Neurology*, *21*(1), 28–33.

Woods, S. P., & Tröster, A. I. (2003). Prodromal frontal/executive dysfunction predicts incident dementia in Parkinson's disease. *Journal of the International Neuropsychological Society*, *9*, 17–24.

Woodward, T. S., Bub, D. N., & Hunter, M. A. (2002). Task switching deficits associated with Parkinson's disease reflect depleted attentional resources. *Neuropsychologia*, *40*(12), 1948–1955.

Wszolek, Z. K., Tsuboi, Y., Uitti, R. J., Reed, L., Hutton, M. L., & Dickson, D. W. (2001). Progressive supranuclear palsy as a disease phenotype caused by the S305S tau gene mutation. *Brain*, *124*(Pt 8), 1666–1670.

Xuereb, J. H., Tomlinson, B. E., Irving, D., Perry, R. H., Blessed, G., & Perry, E. K. (1990). Cortical and subcortical pathology in Parkinson's disease: Relationship to parkinsonian dementia. *Advances in Neurology*, *53*, 35–40.

Yesavage, J., Brink, T. L., Rose, T. L., Lum, O., Huang, V., Adey, M., & Leirer, V. O. (1983). Development and validation of a geriatric depression screening scale. *Journal of Psychiatric Research*, *17*, 37–49.

Zec, R. F., Landreth, E. S., Fritz, S., Grames, E., Hasara, A., Fraizer, W., . . . Manyam, B. (1999). A comparison of phonemic, semantic, and alternating word fluency in Parkinson's disease. *Archives of Clinical Neuropsychology*, *14*(3), 255–264.

Zeuner, K. E., & Deuschl, G. (2012). An update on tremors. *Current Opinion in Neurology*, *25*(4), 475–482. doi: 10.1097/WCO.0b013e3283550c7e

Zgaljardic, D. J., Borod, J. C., Foldi, N. S., & Mattis, P. (2003). A review of the cognitive and behavioral sequelae of Parkinson's disease: Relationship to frontostriatal circuitry. *Cognitive and Behavioral Neurology*, *16*(4), 193–210.

Zigmond, A. S., & Snaith, R. P. (1983). The hospital anxiety and depression scale. *Acta Psychiatrica Scandinavica*, *67*(6), 361–370.

Zimmermann, R., Gschwandtner, U., Benz, N., Hatz, F., Schindler, C., Taub, E., & Fuhr, P. (2014). Cognitive training in Parkinson disease: Cognition-specific vs nonspecific computer training. *Neurology*, *82*(14), 1219–1226. doi: 10.1212/WNL.0000000000000287

23 Cognitive Functions in Adults With Central Nervous System and Non-Central Nervous System Cancers

Denise D. Correa and James C. Root

Introduction

Cognitive dysfunction is common in many cancer patients and can be related to the disease and to treatment with chemotherapy and/or radiotherapy (RT). The neuropsychological domains affected and the severity of the deficits may vary as a result of disease and treatment type, but difficulties in executive functions, motor speed, and learning, and retrieval of information are the most prevalent. In a significant number of cancer patients, changes in cognitive functions interfere with their ability to resume work and social activities at prediagnosis levels.

There has been an increase in the number of studies and clinical trials that incorporate standardized cognitive outcome measures for the assessment of patients with cancer of the central nervous system (CNS; see Correa, 2006; Taphoorn & Klein, 2004). New developments have been described in the study of the cognitive side effects of chemotherapy for non-CNS cancers (Correa & Ahles, 2008). These lines of research have provided valuable information about the incidence of cognitive dysfunction in patients with various cancers, and the contribution of treatments involving different regimens and modalities. Studies have also begun to investigate the underlying mechanisms that may contribute to the neurotoxicity of RT and chemotherapy (Dietrich, Han, Yang, Mayer-Proschel, & Noble, 2006; Nordal & Wong, 2005) and interventions to minimize or prevent both structural and functional damage associated with these regimens have been proposed (Gehring, Sitskoorn, Aaronson, & Taphoorn, 2008).

The current chapter reviews studies involving patients with brain tumors and breast cancer, considering that most of the research has been conducted in these patient groups. Of note, other emerging areas of study include cognitive dysfunction associated with androgen ablation for prostate cancer (Jamadar, Winters, & Maki, 2012; Nelson, Lee, Gamboa, & Roth, 2008), chemotherapy for ovarian cancer (Correa & Hess, 2012; Correa et al., 2012; Correa, Zhou, Thaler, Maziarz, Hurley, & Hensley, 2010), and high-dose chemotherapy and stem cell transplantation for hematological cancers (Correa et al., 2013; Syrjala et al., 2011; Syrjala, Dikmen, Langer, Roth-Roemer, & Abrams, 2004).

Brain Tumors

Primary brain tumors are classified by their predominant histologic appearance and location; they account for less than 2% of all cancers. Gliomas are the most common primary tumors accounting for approximately 40% of all CNS neoplasms (Greenberg, Chandler, & Sandler, 1999). High-grade gliomas (WHO Grade III-IV) include glioblastoma multiforme, anaplastic astrocytomas, anaplastic oligodendrogliomas, and anaplastic mixed gliomas. Low-grade gliomas (WHO Grade I-II) include astrocytomas, oligodendrogliomas, and mixed gliomas. Other less frequent brain tumors are primary CNS lymphoma (PCNSL), ependymomas, meningiomas, and medulloblastomas (Bondy, El-Zein, Wrench, 2005). Brain metastases are also common intracranial tumors in adults (Mehta & Tremont-Lukas, 2004)

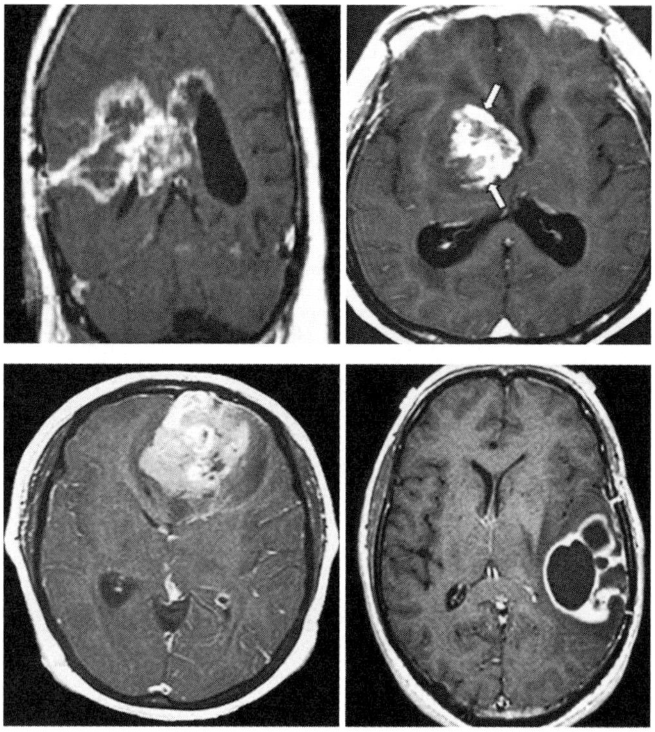

Figure 23.1 Coronal and axial MRIs showing a brain tumor involving cortical and subcortical regions

As effective treatment interventions have increased survival, there has been greater awareness that many brain tumor patients experience cognitive dysfunction, despite adequate disease control (Poortmans et al., 2003). This dysfunction can be related to both the disease and its treatment including surgery, RT, and chemotherapy. The side effects of medications such as corticosteroids and antiepileptics often contribute to or exacerbate these cognitive difficulties. The relevance of including cognitive and quality of life (QoL) evaluations as outcome variables in neuro-oncology research has been increasingly recognized (Johnson & Wefel, 2013; Meyers & Brown, 2006) and the National Cancer Institute (NCI) Brain Tumor Progress Review Group report has recommended that routine cognitive and QoL assessment become the standard care for patients with brain tumors (BTPRG, 2000). Meyers and Brown (2006) published guidelines for the neuropsychological assessment of patients with brain tumors within the context of clinical trials. The suggested core neuropsychological test batteries include standardized instruments with demonstrated sensitivity to the neurotoxic effects of cancer treatment and include tests of attention, executive functions, learning, and retrieval of new information, and graphomotor speed (Correa et al., 2004; Wefel, Kayl, & Meyers, 2004). The feasibility of incorporating a relatively brief cognitive test battery in multi-institutional clinical trials within the context of the Radiation Therapy Oncology Group (RTOG) has also been demonstrated (Meyers et al., 2004; Regine et al., 2004).

Recent longitudinal studies documented that along with age, histology, and performance status, cognitive functioning is a sensitive and important factor in clinical trials involving patients with high-grade tumors (Reardon et al., 2011; Wefel et al., 2011). Performance on a test of verbal memory was independently and strongly related to survival after accounting for age, performance status, histology, extent of resection, number of recurrences, and time since diagnosis in patients with glioblastoma or anaplastic astrocytoma (Meyers, Hess, Yung, & Levin, 2000). Neuropsychological test performance predicted survival in patients with metastases and leptomeningeal disease (Meyers et al., 2004), and glioblastomas (Johnson, Sawyer, Meyers, O'Neill, & Wefel, 2012; Klein et al., 2003). Cognitive decline preceded radiographic evidence of tumor progression by several weeks in glioma patients (Armstrong, Goldstein, Shera, Ledakis, & Tallent, 2003; Brown et al., 2006; Meyers & Hess, 2003). However, these results are interpreted with caution considering that some studies had missing data, lacked a control group, and did not account for the possible effects of medications (Mauer et al., 2007).

Disease and Treatment Effects

Seizures, headaches, increased intracranial pressure, focal neurological signs, and cognitive impairment are common presenting symptoms in patients with brain tumors. Several studies documented cognitive impairment at diagnosis and prior to RT or chemotherapy in patients with high-grade gliomas (Klein et al., 2001), low-grade gliomas (Klein et al., 2002), and PCNSLs (Correa, DeAngelis, & Shi, 2007). Cognitive difficulties present at the time of diagnosis are often related to the location of the tumor (Klein et al., 2001), but a diffuse pattern of deficits has also been reported (Crossen, Goldman, Dahlborg, & Neuwelt, 1992). Rate of tumor growth is a predictor of cognitive impairment, as slow-growing tumors (e.g., low-grade gliomas) are often associated with less severe cognitive dysfunction than rapidly growing tumors (e.g., high-grade gliomas) (Anderson, Damasio, & Tranel, 1990; Hom & Reitan, 1984). Tumor type or volume has not been found to predict cognitive performance (Kayl & Meyers, 2003).

Surgical resection can be associated with transient neurological and cognitive deficits due to damage to tumor-surrounding tissue and edema (Bosma et al., 2007; Duffau, 2005), with impairments often consistent with tumor location (Klein, 2012). Intraoperative stimulation mapping has been used in patients undergoing surgical resection for gliomas, and a recent meta-analysis (De Witt Hamer, Robles, Zwinderman, Duffau, & Berger, 2012) showed that the procedure was associated with fewer neurological deficits and allowed for more extensive resections. However, the incidence and extent of cognitive dysfunction related to tumor surgical resection is unknown, given the relatively limited number of studies including pre- and postsurgical neuropsychological evaluations. In addition, the specific contribution of the tumor to cognitive performance is difficult to ascertain considering that the majority of patients receive corticosteroids and antiepileptic medications following diagnosis and perioperatively. Steroids may improve cognitive deficits due to resolution of edema (Klein et al., 2001), but can also be associated with transient mood disturbance and working memory difficulties (Bosma et al., 2007; Lupien, Gillin, & Hauger, 1999). Antiepileptics can disrupt some aspects of cognitive functions in brain tumor patients, particularly graphomotor speed and executive abilities (van Breemen, Wilms, & Vecht, 2007).

Whole-Brain and Conformal Radiotherapy

MECHANISMS OF CNS INJURY

The pathophysiological mechanisms of radiation injury involve interactions between multiple cell types within the brain including astrocytes, endothelial cells, microglia, neurons, and oligodendrocytes (Greene-Schloesser, Moore, & Robbins, 2013; Greene-Schloesser et al., 2012). Suggested mechanisms include depletion of glial progenitor cells and perpetuation of oxidative stress (Tofilon & Fike, 2000). Radiation may diminish the reproductive capacity of the O-2A progenitors of oligodendrocytes, disrupting the normal turnover of myelin. Blood-vessel dilatation and wall thickening with hyalinization, increased blood-brain barrier

(BBB) permeability due to endothelial cell loss and apoptosis, and a decrease in vessel density have also been hypothesized to lead to white matter necrosis (Nordal & Wong, 2005; Warrington et al., 2013). The extent to which radiation damage is due to direct toxicity on cells or secondary to deleterious effects on the vasculature remains to be elucidated (Noble & Dietrich, 2002). Progressive demyelination may take months to cause symptoms because of the slow turnover of oligodendrocytes, contributing to the latency in onset of neurotoxicity and its progressive nature. In addition, RT achieves therapeutic effects in part through DNA damage by introducing interstrand DNA and DNA-protein crosslinks, single- and double-stranded DNA breaks, methylation, oxidation, and by increasing formation of reactive oxygen species (ROS). Increased numbers of reactive astrocytes and microglia have been shown to produce ROS, proinflammatory cytokines, and growth factors that may cause progressive inflammatory injury (Kim, Brown, Jenrow, & Ryu, 2008). The accumulation of DNA damage in neuronal cells, when unrepaired, can lead to the transcription of defective proteins, apoptosis, and neurodegeneration (Fishel, Vasko, & Kelley, 2007). Recent animal and human studies have documented that RT, chemotherapy, and corticosteroids can disrupt hippocampal neurogenesis (Dietrich et al., 2006; Fike, Rosi, & Limoli, 2009; Monje & Dietrich, 2012; Monje et al., 2007). RT produces elevation of inflammatory cytokines in the brain (Lee, Sonntag, Mitschelen, Yan, & Lee, 2010), and inflammation surrounding neural stem cells may contribute to neurogenesis inhibition (Monje, Toda, & Palmer, 2003). RT-induced apoptosis and a decline in neurogenesis in the subgranular zone of the dentate gyrus were associated with deficits in hippocampal-dependent tasks in some studies (Madsen, Kristjansen, Bolwig, & Wortwein, 2003; Raber et al., 2004).

CLINICAL FINDINGS

Radiation encephalopathy has been classified into three phases according to the time between the administration of RT and the development of symptoms (DeAngelis & Posner, 2009). These are described as acute, early delayed, and late delayed. Acute encephalopathy develops within days of RT and the most common symptoms are nausea, headache, and worsening of neurological signs. Disruption of the BBB by endothelial apoptosis, increased cerebral edema, and intracranial pressure have been suggested as underlying mechanisms. Early delayed effects occur within a few weeks to six months following RT and are reversible in most cases. Lethargy, somnolence, and resurgence of neurological signs, and a transient decline in cognitive functioning may occur, but these factors are not predictive of delayed cognitive deficits. Transient white matter hyperintensity suggesting demyelination may be seen on magnetic resonance imaging (MRI), and are thought to be related to BBB disruption or injury to oligodendrocytes.

The late-delayed effects of RT become apparent a few months to many years after treatment, and often produce irreversible and progressive damage to the CNS (Sheline, Wara, & Smith, 1980). Risk factors for developing delayed RT-induced brain injury include greater volume of radiated tissue, higher total dose of RT (> 2 Gy dose per fraction), concomitant administration of chemotherapy, age greater than 60 years, and presence of comorbid vascular risk factors (Behin, 2003; Constine, Konski, Ekholm, McDonald, & Rubin, 1988; DeAngelis & Posner, 2009). MRI typically shows hyperintensities in periventricular and subcortical white matter, and these changes are often more pronounced in older patients (see Figure 23.2). Radiation-induced microbleeds were recently described in patients with gliomas treated with external-beam RT (Bian, Hess, Chang, Nelson, & Lupo, 2013). In a diffusion tensor imaging (DTI) study, there was evidence of early dose-dependent progressive demyelination and axonal degeneration after RT, and subsequent diffuse dose-independent demyelination (Chapman et al., 2013; Nagesh et al., 2008). Chapman et al. (2013) used DTI to study 14 patients with brain metastases before and after whole-brain RT ± chemotherapy. The results showed regional variation in white matter changes post-RT, with a significant decrease in fractional anisotropy in the cingulate and fornix. A study using positron emission tomography (PET) in a small cohort of brain tumor patients reported dose-dependent reduction in glucose metabolism in brain regions that received greater than 40 Gy at three- and six-month follow-ups; these changes correlated with decreased performance on tests of problem solving and cognitive flexibility (Hahn et al., 2009).

A substantial number of brain tumor patients treated with RT experience cognitive dysfunction that varies from mild to severe, and it is currently considered the most frequent complication among long-term survivors (Behin, 2003). The peak of neurocognitive difficulties resulting from RT occurs

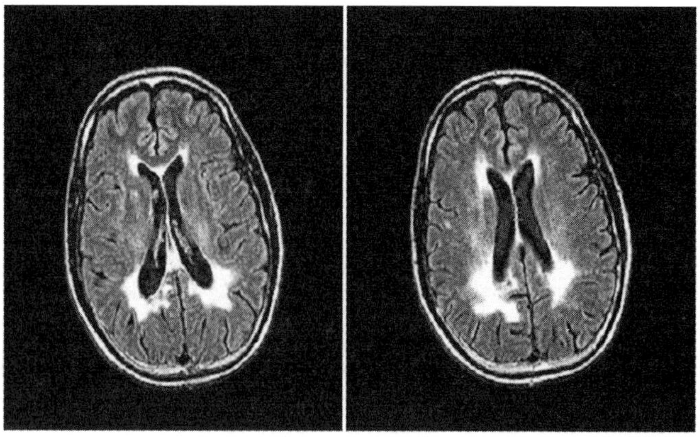

Figure 23.2 T1-weighted axial MRIs showing periventricular white matter abnormalities in a 50-year-old man six years post treatment with high-dose chemotherapy and whole-brain radiotherapy

approximately six months to two years after treatment completion, and its incidence is proportional to the percentage of patients with disease-free survival (DeAngelis, Yahalom, Thaler, & Kher, 1992). The variability in the documented frequency of RT-induced cognitive deficits may be partially associated with the insensitivity of the methods of assessment used, duration of follow-up, retrospective nature of many studies, inclusion of patients treated with different regimens, and population discrepancies. In addition, the high incidence of tumor recurrence and short-term survival in patients with high-grade malignancies have often been considered confounding variables that hampered the ability to quantify the frequency, onset, and course of the delayed cognitive effects of RT (Crossen, Garwood, Glatstein, & Neuwelt, 1994). A review of the literature suggests that the pattern of neuropsychological impairments associated with the delayed effects of whole-brain RT is diffuse (Duffey, Chari, Cartlidge, & Shaw, 1996), and most consistent with frontal-subcortical dysfunction with deficits in attention, executive functions, learning and retrieval of new information, and graphomotor speed (Archibald et al., 1994; Crossen et al., 1994; Salander, Karlsson, Bergenheim, & Henriksson, 1995; Scheibel, Meyers, & Levin, 1996; Taphoorn & Klein, 2004; Wefel, Kayl, et al., 2004; Weitzner & Meyers, 1997).

In recent years, conformal RT that includes the area of the tumor and surrounding margin has supplanted whole-brain RT in the treatment of gliomas due to equivalent efficacy and reduced neurotoxicity (DeGroot, Aldape, & Colman, 2005). Some studies suggest that conformal RT is associated with less severe cognitive dysfunction than whole-brain RT (Torres et al., 2003), but most studies were retrospective and revealed variable outcomes ranging from no morbidity to marked cognitive deficits (Armstrong et al., 2000; Armstrong et al., 2002; Postma et al., 2002; Surma-aho et al., 2001; Taphoorn et al., 1994). Recent research reported that radiation dose to specific regions, such as the right temporal lobes and the hippocampi, may be more predictive of cognitive impairment than total RT dose (Peiffer et al., 2013). Similarly, a prospective study of patients with low-grade or benign tumors treated with fractionated stereotactic RT reported a dose-response relationship, with higher RT doses to the hippocampi showing an association with impairment in word-list delayed recall (Gondi, Hermann, Mehta, & Tome, 2013).

Chemotherapy Alone or Combined WithRadiotherapy

The pathophysiological mechanisms of chemotherapy-induced CNS damage are not well understood. Candidate mechanisms include demyelination, secondary inflammatory response, oxidative stress, and DNA damage; immune dysregulation; and microvascular injury (Ahles & Saykin, 2007). There is increasing evidence that chemotherapy has direct toxic effects on progenitor cells, oligodendrocytes, white matter, gliogenesis, and neurogenesis (Dietrich, 2010). Increased cell death and decreased cell division in the subventricular zone and in the dentate gyrus of the hippocampus have been reported in mice (Dietrich et al., 2006; Dietrich, Monje, Wefel, & Meyers, 2008); neural progenitor cells and oligodendrocytes are particularly vulnerable.

Neurotoxicity has been reported after high-dose regimens with procarbazine, lomustine, and vincristine (PCV) chemotherapy (Postma et al., 1998), and after high-dose methotrexate (HD-MTX) and high-dose cytarabine, particularly if RT is administered before or during chemotherapy (DeAngelis & Shapiro, 1991; see Figure 23.2). Chemotherapy administered intrathecally is more likely to cause CNS toxicity than when it is applied systemically. Combined treatment with RT and chemotherapy may have a synergistic effect (Keime-Guibert, Napolitano, & Delattre, 1998), as chemotherapy agents may interfere with the same cellular structures as radiation and may act as a radiosensitizer. Radiation may alter the distribution kinetics of chemotherapeutic agents in the CNS by increasing the permeability of the BBB, affecting the ability of arachnoid granulations or choroid plexus to clear the drug, or interrupting the ependymal barrier to allow drugs in the cerebrospinal fluid to enter the white matter. Finally, RT-induced cellular changes may allow greater amounts of the drug to enter nontumor cells or less of it to exit. The interactions between RT and HD-MTX are the most clearly demonstrated (Keime-Guibert et al., 1998), and nonenhancing, confluent lesions in the periventricular and subcortical white matter have been documented on MRI studies (Correa et al., 2004; Keime-Guibert et al., 1998). Decrease in white matter density in the corpus callosum, hippocampal cell death, and memory impairments were reported in rats treated with HD-MTX (Seigers et al., 2009). Carmustine, cyclophosphamide, cisplatin, cytarabine, thiotepa, and methotrexate were found to be associated with neurotoxicity, with changes in cortical and subcortical brain regions (Rzeski et al., 2004). Deficits in spatial and nonspatial memory have been described after administration of methotrexate and 5-fluorouracil in mice (Winocur, Vardy, Binns, Kerr, & Tannock, 2006). However, the cognitive side-effects of chemotherapy are often difficult to determine in brain tumor patients as most also receive RT in the course of their treatment.

Variation in genetic polymorphisms may increase the susceptibility to cognitive dysfunction following RT ± chemotherapy. In a recent cross-sectional study (Correa, et al., 2013), brain tumor patients with at least one Apolipoprotein E (APOE) ϵ-4 allele had significantly lower scores in verbal learning and delayed recall, and marginally significant lower scores in executive function, in comparison to non-carriers of a ϵ-4 allele.

Neuropsychological Studies

High-Grade Tumors

Patients with high-grade gliomas often present with symptoms of increased intracranial pressure, seizures or focal neurological signs (Greenberg et al., 1999). The majority of patients undergo surgical tumor resection and receive a combined modality regimen of RT and chemotherapy; recent trials involving glioblastoma patients have also included anti-angiogenic therapy with bevacizumab (Gilbert et al., 2014). The median survival time is less than two years for patients with glioblastomas, and two to three years for anaplastic astrocytomas (Carson, Grossman, Fisher, & Shaw, 2007; Stupp et al., 2005). Cognitive impairment in patients with high-grade gliomas is multifactorial and includes the tumor and the adverse effects of treatment. Disease recurrence and short-term survival have been considered confounding variables that limit the ability to quantify the frequency, onset, and course of the delayed cognitive effects of RT and chemotherapy. Several studies have suggested that tumor progression contributes significantly to cognitive decline, and that relatively stable performance is seen in patients without recurrent disease (Brown et al., 2006).

Klein et al. (2001) studied cognitive functioning in 61 patients with high-grade gliomas following surgery or biopsy, and included comparison groups of 50 patients with lung cancer and age-matched healthy controls. As compared to healthy controls, cognitive impairment (i.e., attention and executive functions) was evident in all glioma patients and 52% of lung cancer patients. The use of antiepileptic medication was associated with working memory deficits. Patients with tumors in the right hemisphere had greater difficulties in visuospatial tests, and patients with left hemisphere tumors showed greater susceptibility to interference and slower visual scanning. Bosma et al. (2007) assessed cognitive functions at eight- and 16-month intervals after RT in 32 and 18 high-grade glioma patients, respectively. Patients with tumor progression had a more pronounced cognitive decline (i.e., psychomotor speed, executive functions) than patients who remained stable; however, the decline was also considered to be in part related to the side effects of antiepileptics and corticosteroids. However, in a recent study of patients with high-grade tumors (de Groot et al., 2013) treated with levetiracetam (n = 35), valproic acid or phenytoin (n = 38), or no antiepileptics (n = 44), there were no significant differences on cognitive test performance between patients on newer compared to older antiepileptics and patients receiving no medication six weeks postsurgery; there was a beneficial effect of both antiepileptics on verbal memory.

Hilverda et al. (2010) studied 13 patients with glioblastoma multiforme treated with RT and temozolomide with no evidence of disease progression. Neurocognitive evaluations were performed after surgery, six weeks post-RT and concomitant temozolomide, and after three cycles of adjuvant temozolomide in progression-free patients. The results showed that at baseline, 11 patients had impaired attention, information processing speed, and executive functions in comparison to healthy controls. At the first follow-up, four patients improved, four deteriorated, and the others were relatively stable. At the last follow-up, cognitive performance remained stable in all domains for 11 patients, with one patient improving and one patient declining in the interim. The authors concluded that cognitive functions are likely to be relatively stable in the absence of disease progression. Froklage and colleagues (2013) assessed cognitive functions and radiological abnormalities in patients with newly diagnosed high-grade gliomas treated with chemoradiation followed by adjuvant temozolomide. Neuropsychological assessments were conducted before treatment and prior to adjuvant temozolomide (n = 33), during and after temozolomide (n = 25 and 17, respectively), and three and seven months post treatment completion (n = 9 and 5, respectively); patient dropout was primarily due to disease progression. In comparison to matched healthy controls, 63% of patients had deficits in executive functions, processing speed. and working memory at baseline. Approximately 70% of the patients remained stable during the follow-up period, and most of the patients who declined had tumor progression. Cerebral atrophy and white matter hyperintensities developed or worsened in approximately 45% of patients during follow-up.

Brown et al. (2006) reported the results of prospective Mini-Mental Status Examinations (MMSE) in 1, 244 high-grade tumor patients who participated in the North Central Cancer Treatment Group treatment trials, which used radiation and nitrosurea-based chemotherapy. The proportion of patients without tumor progression who had significant cognitive deterioration ranged from 13% to 18%, and remained stable over the 24-month follow-up period; a decline in MMSE scores was a predictor of more rapid time to tumor progression and preceded radiographic changes. Corn et al. (2009) examined QoL and mental status in 203 patients with glioblastoma multiforme within the context of a Phase I/II study of the RTOG to assess the impact of dose escalation conformal RT. Patients were administered the MMSE at the start and at the end of radiation, and at four-month intervals subsequently. The results showed a decline in the MMSE over the follow-up period, and this was considered to be at least in part related to RT. However, considering the demonstrated low sensitivity of cognitive screening measures (e.g., MMSE) to detect cognitive dysfunction in brain tumor patients (Meyers & Wefel, 2003), the findings of these two large studies may represent an underestimation.

A Phase II trial evaluated cognitive functioning in 167 patients with recurrent glioblastoma treated with bevacizumab-based therapy (Wefel et al., 2011). Patients with objective response to treatment or progression free survival greater than six months had stable median cognitive test scores across the 24-month follow-up, but patients with evidence of progressive disease exhibited cognitive decline. In a prospective study of newly diagnosed glioblastoma patients treated with temozolomide, hypofractionated stereotactic RT and bevacizumab, 37 patients underwent longitudinal neuropsychological evaluations (Correa et al., 2011). Linear mixed model analyses showed a significant decline in set-shifting and verbal learning ($p < 0.05$) from baseline to the four-month follow-up, and performance remained stable or improved slightly at subsequent intervals. Visuospatial memory was stable at four months, but showed a trend toward a decline at subsequent follow-ups. The decline in executive functions and memory in the early phase of treatment was thought to be related to the acute effects of RT. In a recent, large clinical trial for patients with newly diagnosed glioblastoma comparing the efficacy of standard chemo-radiation, maintenance temozolomide, and placebo or bevacizumab, cognitive evaluations were performed longitudinally in patients without disease progression (Gilbert et al., 2014). The initial results suggested that patients randomized to bevacizumab, compared to placebo, experienced greater decline over time in executive functions and information processing speed, suggesting either bevacizumab-related neurotoxicity or unrecognized tumor progression. In a recent study of long-term survivors of anaplastic oligodendrogliomas treated with RT versus RT and procarbazine, lomustine and vincristine (Habets et al., 2014), a variable pattern of cognitive impairment was seen in 75% of patients who were progression free, regardless of initial treatment type.

Low-Grade Tumors

Low-grade gliomas are slow-growing infiltrative tumors most common in young and middle-aged adults, and the majority of patients present with seizures and headaches (Greenberg et al., 1999). The median survival ranges from five to ten years, and these tumors invariably progress to more aggressive high-grade gliomas (Shaw et al., 2002). Treatment interventions remain controversial regarding the optimal timing of surgical intervention, RT, and chemotherapy (Cairncross, 2000; Kiebert et al., 1998; Shaw et al., 2002; Soffietti et al., 2010). Several studies that documented cognitive dysfunction in low-grade glioma patients found that the tumor itself, rather than RT, was the primary contributing factor (Laack et al., 2003; Taphoorn et al., 1994; Torres et al., 2003). However, studies including long-term survivors reported that both partial and whole-brain RT was associated with cognitive dysfunction several years after treatment completion (Douw et al., 2009), and a decline in nonverbal memory was evident in some studies. Tumor-related epilepsy and the side effects of antiepileptic medications also contribute to cognitive dysfunction in these patients (Klein, 2012). Methodological problems including differences in the sensitivity of the neuropsychological measures administered, retrospective designs, and the inclusion of patients with high- and low-grade tumors, and patients treated with partial and whole-brain RT (Imperato, Paleologos, & Vick, 1990; Kleinberg, Wallner, & Malkin, 1993; Torres et al., 2003) may account for some of the variability of the findings in the literature. A recent report by the Response Assessment in Neuro-Oncology group (RANO), recommended that standardized assessments of cognitive functions and QoL be incorporated in clinical trials involving low-grade glioma patients (van den Bent et al., 2011). The characterization of tumor- and treatment-related cognitive dysfunction in patients with low-grade tumors is particularly relevant given the relatively prolonged survival and the controversy in the effectiveness of early treatment.

A cross-sectional study assessed cognitive outcome in 195 low-grade glioma patients (104 treated with RT 1–22 years prior to enrollment) compared to 100 low-grade hematological cancer patients, and 194 healthy controls (Taphoorn et al., 1994). Glioma patients completed the cognitive evaluation at a mean of six years after diagnosis, and obtained lower test scores than the cancer control group on psychomotor speed, visual memory, and executive functions. Although the authors concluded that the tumor had the most detrimental effects on cognition, decreased verbal and visual memory was evident in patients who received RT in daily fractions exceeding 2 Gy, and some of the cognitive test scores declined over time only among those treated with RT. Antiepileptic treatment was associated with more pronounced cognitive dysfunction. A follow-up study (Douw et al., 2009) included 65 of these patients who underwent a neuropsychological re-evaluation at a mean of 12 years (range 6–28 years) after the initial assessment. Patients who received RT showed a decline in attention, executive function, and information processing speed, regardless of fraction dose. White matter hyperintensities and cortical atrophy correlated with worse cognitive test performance. Surma-aho et al.(2001) assessed cognitive functioning in low-grade glioma patients approximately seven years post-RT ± chemotherapy ($n = 28$) or surgical resection alone ($n = 23$); 19 patients had whole-brain RT and nine had focal RT. The results showed that patients treated with RT had significantly lower scores in percent retention of visual materials and estimated Performance IQ, and more extensive periventricular white matter abnormalities on MRI, in comparison to patients who did not receive RT. The authors concluded that RT increased the risk for cognitive impairment and leukoencephalopathy in patients with low-grade tumors.

Correa et al. (2007) studied cognitive functions in 40 patients with low-grade gliomas: 24 patients had surgery only, and 16 had conformal RT ± chemotherapy. Patients treated with RT ± chemotherapy had lower scores in attention and executive functions, psychomotor speed, verbal and nonverbal memory, and naming than untreated patients. In addition, patients who completed treatment at intervals greater than three years had significantly lower scores in nonverbal memory. Antiepileptic polytherapy, treatment history, and disease duration contributed to reduced psychomotor speed; 62% of treated patients had white matter disease on MRI, whereas only 10% of the untreated patients had such changes. In a subsequent study (Correa et al., 2008), 25 of these patients completed additional cognitive follow-ups. The results showed a mild decline in nonverbal memory 12 months after the initial evaluation regardless of treatment status; scores remained one standard deviation below normative values in other cognitive domains. Among the 16 patients who completed a subsequent evaluation (12–27 months later), there was improvement in untreated patients, but a decline in some aspects of executive function in patients treated with RT ± chemotherapy. Disease duration and treatment history were thought to contribute to the pattern of findings.

Armstrong et al. (2000) assessed cognitive functions prospectively in 20 patients with low-grade tumors treated with conformal RT. A decrement in verbal memory retrieval was evident during the early delayed period following RT with improvement at longer intervals. The long-term effects of RT on cognition were examined in a subsequent study involving 26 patients with low-grade tumors (Armstrong, Stern, & Corn, 2001). A selective decline in learning and recall of visual information five years post-RT was detected despite continued improvement up to that point. Long-term improvements were noted on tests of attention, executive functions, and verbal recall. The authors concluded that partial RT was not associated with significant delayed cognitive impairments in this population. In a recent study (Gondi et al., 2013), 18 patients with low-grade or benign tumors treated with fractionated stereotactic RT completed a neuropsychological evaluation at baseline and 18 months following treatment. The results suggested that RT dose greater than 7.3 Gy to 40% of the bilateral hippocampi was associated with impairment on a list-learning delayed recall test. Alterations in functional connectivity using magnetoencephalography have also been described recently in patients with low-grade gliomas (Bosma et al., 2008).

Primary Central Nervous System Lymphoma (PCNSL)

PCNSL is a rare infiltrative tumor that develops most frequently in the subcortical periventricular white matter, with single lesions occurring in 60%–70% of patients and multifocal lesions in 30%–40%. It is a disease of middle and late adult life with a mean age at diagnosis of 60 years, and it is slightly more common in men. Focal neurological signs are the most common presentation followed by psychiatric symptoms, headaches, and seizures (Batchelor et al., 2012; Rubenstein, Ferreri, & Pittaluga, 2008). The standard treatment for PCNSL often includes HD-MTX regimens and whole-brain RT. Although this treatment approach is effective, with a median survival of 30 to 60 months (DeAngelis et al., 2002), it is associated with delayed neurotoxicity in most patients (Correa et al., 2012; Poortmans et al., 2003; Thiel et al., 2010). Delayed treatment-related cognitive dysfunction has been recognized as a frequent complication among long-term survivors, and may interfere with QoL (Correa et al., 2007). Recent studies suggest that HD-MTX without RT can be efficacious in the treatment of PCNSL and diminish the risk for delayed neurotoxicity (Juergens et al., 2010; Rubenstein et al., 2013; Thiel et al., 2010). However, since disease relapse is relatively common and some patients require salvage therapy, the optimal induction and consolidative therapy for PCNSL remains controversial. The importance of assessing the incidence and extent of cognitive dysfunction associated with HD-MTX regimens with and without WBRT has been recognized by the International Primary CNS Lymphoma Collaborative Group (IPCG; (Abrey et al., 2005; Ferreri, Zucca, Armitage, Cavalli, & Batchelor, 2013) and guidelines for standardized cognitive assessments to be incorporated in clinical trials have been developed (Correa et al., 2007). A literature review indicated that cognitive function was evaluated systematically in a relatively limited number of studies, and methodological problems limited the understanding of the contribution of disease and treatments (Correa et al., 2007).

RT AND CHEMOTHERAPY REGIMENS

Studies involving patients treated with whole-brain RT and HD-MTX, or with whole-brain RT and chemotherapy with BBB disruption reported significant cognitive impairment. The pattern of cognitive deficits was diffuse and the domains disrupted included attention and executive functions, psychomotor speed, and learning and retrieval of new information. Harder et al. (2004) studied cognitive functions in 19 PCNSL patients at a mean of 23 months after treatment with HD-MTX followed by whole-brain RT. In comparison to a non-CNS-cancer control group, PCNSL patients had lower scores on verbal and nonverbal memory, attention, executive function, and motor speed. Correa et al. (2012) studied 50 PCNSL treated with whole-brain RT and HD-MTX ($n = 24$), or HD-MTX alone ($n = 26$) between three and 54 months posttreatment. Patients treated with whole-brain RT and HD-MTX had impairments in selective attention and executive functions, verbal memory, and graphomotor speed across most cognitive domains; these were of sufficient severity to interfere with QoL as more than 50% were not working due to their illness. Patients treated with HD-MTX alone had significantly higher scores on tests of selective attention and memory than patients treated with the combined modality regimen. Patients with more extensive white matter disease on MRIs had lower scores on tests of set-shifting and memory. Thirty-three patients completed an additional follow-up cognitive evaluation at a mean of 14–16 months after the initial visit. The results suggested no significant changes on any of the cognitive tests among patients treated with whole-brain RT and HD-MTX, but patients who received HD-MTX alone obtained a significantly higher score on auditory attention. Doolittle, Korfel, et al. (2013) studied neuropsychological functions and neuroimaging outcomes in 80patients with PCNSL evaluated at a median of 5.5 years (range: 2 to 26 years) after diagnosis. Treatment modalities included: HD-MTX ($n = 32$), HD-MTX (intra-arterial) in conjunction with BBB disruption ($n = 25$), HD-MTX followed by high-dose chemotherapy and autologous stem cell transplant (ASCT) (n = 8), and HD-MTX followed by whole-brain RT (n = 15); five of these patients also received high-dose chemotherapy and ASCT prior to whole-brain RT. Patients treated with HD-MTX and whole-brain RT had significantly lower mean scores in attention, executive function, and motor speed than patients treated with HD-MTX in conjunction with BBB disruption, and all patients treated without WBRT combined. Among patients treated with BBB disruption chemotherapy, there was a significant improvement in executive functions and no evidence of decline in other domains (Doolittle, Dosa, et al., 2013). White matter abnormalities were more extensive in the patients treated with RT. The findings were consistent with other studies, suggesting increased risk for delayed neurotoxicity following combined modality regimens. However, the retrospective nature of these studies limited the ability to examine the specific contributions of the tumor and the delayed effects of treatment.

In a recent prospective study (Correa et al., 2009; Morris et al., 2013), PCNSL patients treated with induction rituximab, methotrexate, procarbazine, and vincristine (R-MPV) followed by consolidation reduced-dose whole-brain RT (23.4 Gy) and cytarabine underwent cognitive evaluations prior to treatment and up to four years after treatment completion. At baseline, impairments in selective attention, memory, and motor speed were evident. After induction chemotherapy, there was a significant improvement in executive function and memory. There was no evidence of significant cognitive decline during the follow-up period, except for motor speed. The preliminary findings were interpreted as evidence that cognitive dysfunction was primarily related to the disease, and that the new treatment approach with low-dose RT may not be associated with progressive cognitive decline.

CHEMOTHERAPY REGIMENS

The studies that reported cognitive outcome in PCNSL patients treated with HD-MTX alone or with BBB disruption chemotherapy without RT were mostly prospective (Correa et al., 2007). Several studies documented cognitive impairment prior to therapy in attention, executive functions, memory, graphomotor speed, and language. Posttreatment follow-up intervals were variable across studies, but several reported either stable or improved cognitive performance. Methodological problems in several of these studies, however, limited the ability to discern the specific contributions of the disease and chemotherapy alone regimens to cognitive dysfunction.

Pels et al. (2003) performed cognitive evaluations in 22 patients between four and 82 months after completion of treatment with HD-MTX. There was no evidence of decline in attention, verbal memory, visual memory, word fluency, or visual-construction abilities in patients who had either a partial or a complete response to treatment. Fliessbach et al. (2005) assessed cognitive functions in 23 patients prior to and up to a median of 44 months after treatment with HD-MTX (all patients were in disease remission). At the pretreatment baseline, impairments were evident in attention and executive functions, verbal and nonverbal memory, and word fluency; these were classified as mild ($z \leq -1.5$) in three patients, moderate ($z \leq -2$ and > -3) in ten, and severe ($z \leq -3$) in six patients. At the last follow-up, impairment (in at least one domain) was mild in five patients, moderate in five, and severe in one; 12 patients had no deficits. Twenty-one patients improved, but scores remained in the low average range on tests of attention, non-verbal memory, and word fluency. The authors concluded that the cognitive deficits were associated primarily with tumor and there was no treatment-related cognitive decline. The most sensitive domains were attention, executive functions, and memory.

McAllister et al. (2000) studied a cohort of 23 prior to and post BBB disruption chemotherapy (mean =16.5 months, SD = 10.9). The results showed significantly improved cognitive functioning posttreatment (summary z-score). When examining individual tests, there was evidence of improvement in intellectual functioning, learning, memory, attention, and visuospatial skills, with a nonsignificant trend demonstrated for executive functioning; seven patients had cognitive decline, mostly in motor speed. Neuwelt et al. (1991) studied 15patients before and one year after BBB disruption chemotherapy; nine patients were also seen for long-term follow-up (mean of 3.5 years after diagnosis). Focus of data analysis was on the summary z-score, which ranged at baseline from −2.59 to 0.46 with a mean of −1.1 (SD = 1.1). At the end of treatment, the summary score ranged from −1.45 to 0.26 with a mean of 0.35 (SD = 0.52), suggesting a significant improvement in cognitive functioning from baseline. As reported recently by Doolittle, Dosa, et al. (2013), long-term follow-up of PCNSL patients at a median of 12years after BBB disruption chemotherapy indicated either stable or improved cognitive functions.

Metastatic Brain Tumors

Brain metastases are common and develop most often in patients with lung cancer (50%), followed by breast cancer (15%–20%) and melanoma (10%), and less frequently in other cancers (e.g., colorectal, kidney) (Lassman & DeAngelis, 2003). Patients may present with headaches, focal weakness, altered mental status, and seizures. Standard treatment has involved surgical resection and external beam whole-brain RT; the median survival is four to six months (Lassman & DeAngelis, 2003). Recent randomized trials comparing stereotactic radiosurgery plus whole-brain RT versus whole-brain RT alone reported improvement in survival with the addition of radiosurgery in patients with solitary metastases (Andrews et al., 2004; Ayoma et al., 2006). Temozolomide and radiosensitizers have also been added to the regimen recently (Abrey et al., 2001). Although whole-brain RT has been shown to improve tumor control across several studies (Brown, Asher, & Farace, 2008) and to reduce the development of subsequent metastases (Kocher et al., 2011), the neurotoxicity of whole-brain RT, including cognitive dysfunction, has been a concern. A recent report by RANO supports the inclusion of standardized assessments of cognitive functions and QoL in clinical trials involving patients with brain metastases (Lin et al., 2013).

Deficits in memory and motor speed have been documented in patients with newly diagnosed or recurrent metastases evaluated either during or after whole-brain RT (Herman et al., 2003; Platta, Khuntia, Mehta, & Suh, 2010). Several studies also documented cognitive dysfunction prior to therapy, and Meyers et al. (2004) reported that baseline cognitive performance predicted survival in patients with brain metastases. A pilot study including 15 patients treated with stereotactic radiosurgery alone (Chang et al., 2007) documented impaired executive function, manual dexterity, and memory at baseline; 13 patients declined on one or more tests at the one-month follow-up, and the five long-term survivors had stable or improved cognitive performance. Welzel et al. (2008) studied memory functions prospectively in 44 patients treated with prophylactic RT for small-cell lung cancer and in patients with brain metastases treated with whole-brain RT. At baseline, lung cancer patients had lower memory scores than patients with brain metastasis. Verbal memory decline was evident during RT in patients with metastases only, but at the eight-week post-RT follow-up both groups had memory impairment.

Meyers et al. (2004) studied cognitive outcome in the context of a Phase II randomized trial involving 400 patients with brain metastases treated with whole-brain RT alone or in combination with motexafin gadolinium. At baseline, 91% of patients had impairment in one or more cognitive domains, and 42% had impairment in four of eight tests. Optimal tumor control following treatment correlated with preservation of cognitive function, and in a small group of long-term survivors there was stable or improved performance. In a Phase III trial involving 554 patients with brain metastasis (Mehta et al., 2009), the interval to neurocognitive decline was prolonged in the group treated with whole-brain RT and motexafin gadolinium. Serial neurocognitive assessments were performed in the context of a randomized trial involving patients with one to three brain metastases treated with radiosurgery (n = 30) versus radiosurgery plus whole-brain-RT (n = 28) (Chang et al., 2009). Patients treated with radiosurgery plus whole-brain RT were significantly more likely to show a decline in verbal learning at four months posttreatment than patients treated with radiosurgery alone. In a study of 208 brain metastases patients treated with whole-brain RT (30 Gy) (Li, Bentzen, Renschler, & Mehta, 2007), the median time to decline in executive and motor functions was longer in patients with a poor response to treatment (i.e., less tumor shrinkage). In patients surviving more than 15 months, reduced tumor size was correlated with preserved executive and motor functions, but not with memory performance; a significant decline in memory at four months posttreatment was noted. In addition, the risk of delayed leukoencephalopathy was found to be significantly higher for patients with brain metastases treated with radiosurgery and whole-brain RT relative to patients who had radiosurgery alone (Monaco et al., 2013). A recent review of randomized controlled studies involving patients treated with prophylactic RT, radiosurgery, and radiosurgery and whole-brain RT suggested that whole-brain RT, particularly high-dose regimens (36 vs. 25 Gy), was associated with a deleterious effect in memory, executive functions, and processing speed (McDuff et al., 2013).

Preventive or Treatment Interventions

There are no established preventive or therapeutic interventions for cancer-treatment-related cognitive dysfunction. Ghia et al. (2007) developed a hippocampal-sparing intensity-modulated approach to whole-brain RT that limits the radiation dose to the hippocampus with the intent of reducing the neurocognitive sequelae of RT. Preliminary results from a clinical trial involving 113 patients with brain metastases (Gondi et al., 2013) showed that sparing the subgranular zone of the hippocampus during whole-brain RT was associated with more preserved memory function at the four- and six-month posttreatment follow-ups, in comparison to historical controls treated with standard whole-brain RT; however, only 28 patients were available for the six-month assessment (Brown et al., 2013). In a randomized study, the potential protective effects of memantine versus placebo on cognitive function were evaluated in 508 patients with brain metastases receiving whole-brain RT (Brown et al., 2013). The results showed that patients treated with memantine had significantly longer time to cognitive decline, and a reduced rate of decline in memory, executive function, and processing speed compared to placebo; however, attrition may have limited statistical power as only 29% of patients completed the 24-week assessment.

Treatments that target the vascular mechanism of RT damage including hyperbaric oxygenation, anticoagulation, and aspirin have been attempted, but without clear benefits (DeAngelis & Posner, 2009). There is preliminary evidence suggesting that bevacizumab may reduce abnormal enhancement associated with necrosis, possibly through the removal of VEGF-induced reactive vascularization (Torcuator et al., 2009). In a placebo-controlled, randomized study of bevacizumab for the treatment of RT necrosis in 14 brain tumor patients (Levin et al., 2011), there was a decrease in MRI enhancement and improvement in neurological symptoms in all patients treated with bevacizumab. A decrease in radiation necrosis on MRI following bevacizumab was also reported in 11 patients with brain metastases treated with stereotactic radiosurgery (Boothe et al., 2013). However, a recent review of the use of bevacizumab for the treatment of RT necrosis suggested that although most studies reported a reduction in radiographic volume of necrosis-associated edema, a high rate of serious complications raised concerns about this treatment approach (Lubelski, Abdullah, Weil, & Marko, 2013).

Pharmacological treatments for RT-induced cognitive dysfunction have been based primarily on therapies used for other neurological disorders that cause similar symptoms (Kim et al., 2008). Agents such as psychostimulants and acetylcholinesterase inhibitors have been used to treat cognitive dysfunction in patients with brain tumors. Comprehensive reviews of studies on interventions for this clinical population indicated that there are several completed and ongoing trials using these and other medications, as well as cognitive rehabilitation and behavioral interventions (Gehring, Aaronson, Taphoorn, & Sitskoorn, 2010; Wefel, Kayl, et al., 2004). A prospective open-label Phase II study was conducted to assess the efficacy of donepezil in the treatment of cognitive dysfunction in 24 patients with primary brain tumors (Shaw et al., 2006). After 24 weeks of treatment there was evidence of improvement in attention, verbal and visual memory, in mood, and QoL. A recent open-label randomized pilot study examined the efficacy of four weeks of methylphenidate and modafanil in 24 brain tumor patients either during or following treatment with RT or chemotherapy (Gehring et al., 2012). The results showed a beneficial effect of stimulant treatment in speed of processing and executive functions requiring divided attention, and on patient-reported fatigue and QoL, regardless of the medication used. However, the results were interpreted with caution give the small sample size and large proportion of dropouts. A recent multicenter double-blind placebo-controlled study including 37 patients with primary brain tumors treated with modafinil for six weeks showed no beneficial effects on cognitive function, fatigue, or mood in comparison to placebo (Boele et al., 2013).

The small number of studies using cognitive rehabilitation in brain tumor patients suggests some beneficial effects, but problems with accrual and attrition and methodological problems limit the evaluation of its efficacy (Gehring et al., 2010). In a study involving 13 brain tumor patients (Sherer, Meyers, & Bergloff, 1997), there was a significant increase in functional independence in approximately half of the patients following three to 12 weeks of training in the use of compensatory strategies. Locke et al. (2008) compared the feasibility of memory and problem solving training in dyads of primary brain tumor patients and caregivers versus a no-intervention control group. At the three-month follow-up 50% of patients reported using the strategies, but there was no significant intervention effect on QoL and functional capacity and not enough patients completed the neuropsychological assessment. Gehring et al. (2008) conducted a randomized controlled trial to assess the efficacy of computer-based attention training and compensatory skills training in 140 patients with gliomas; patients were randomly assigned to the intervention group or to a wait list control group. There was a significant improvement in self-reported cognitive function but not on neuropsychological test performance immediately after completion of the seven-week program. Conversely, at the six-month follow-up patients showed an improvement in attention and verbal memory, but not on self-reported cognitive function. The prevention of cognitive deficits with agents that may protect neurons from treatment-induced damage is an area of growing interest (Kim et al., 2008), and the potential neuroprotective effects of lithium and other agents are under investigation (Gehring et al., 2010; Khasraw, Ashley, Wheeler, & Berk, 2012; Wefel, Kayl, et al., 2004).

Non-CNS Cancers

Beyond the effects of primary CNS cancers on cognition, non-CNS cancer diagnosis and treatment has also been found to be associated with cognitive dysfunction. Among primary cancers, breast cancer is relatively common, with approximately 124 per 100,000 new cases diagnosed each year, and a prevalence of approximately 2.8 million women currently diagnosed in the United States alone (http://seer.cancer.gov/statfacts/html/breast.html), with 89% survival rates of five years or more. Given its prevalence and survival rates, cognitive changes associated with breast cancer diagnosis and treatment have been most widely studied. In this section we review cross-sectional and longitudinal studies assessing neuropsychological outcome and self-reported cognitive dysfunction in individuals diagnosed with breast cancer. Contributions of structural and functional imaging that may help to clarify the underlying changes in brain structure and function following treatment are then discussed, followed by potential mechanisms by which treatments may exert an effect on the brain and cognition.

While terms such as *chemo-brain* and *chemo-fog* would indicate a primary role for chemotherapy, recent research has questioned whether chemotherapy exposure alone is either necessary or sufficient for cognitive decline following treatment (Hurria, Somlo, & Ahles, 2007). Treatment varies with stage of disease but includes surgical resection potentially in combination with radiation treatment to the breast, adjuvant chemotherapy in later stages, and endocrine therapies depending on receptor characteristics of tumor cells. Surgical resection alone (lumpectomy or mastectomy) may be performed in early stage disease in cases in which the tumor is relatively small and there is no evidence of extended disease either to the lymph nodes or other anatomical sites. Adjuvant chemotherapy treatment, in which chemotherapy drugs are delivered following surgical resection, may be used to prevent recurrence or in cases in which the disease is found to extend, i.e., to have metastasized, beyond the primary site. Radiation may be used to reduce the size of a tumor prior to resection, and to prevent recurrence following resection, as well as in later stages of the disease. Hormonal therapies may be used following primary treatment on an extended basis in cases in which tumor cells are found to have a high receptor count for either progesterone or estrogen; these therapies work by reducing availability of estrogen and so lower the promotion of tumor cells.

Self-Reported Cognitive Changes Following Treatment

Changes in cognitive function following treatment, including slowing, inattention, distraction, forgetfulness, difficulties in multitasking, and language function, are commonly reported by cancer survivors. Early research found that approximately half of cancer patients reported some change in cognition at one point in their treatment (Cull, Stewart, & Altman, 1995). Six or more months following treatment, 30% of lymphoma patients reported concentration difficulties and 52% reported forgetfulness (Cull et al., 1996). Schagen et al. (1999) described persistent self-reported difficulties in concentration (31%) and memory (21%) in breast cancer survivors at longer intervals. Ahles et al. (2002) described self-reported difficulties in concentration and complex attention in survivors of breast cancer and lymphoma up to ten years after chemotherapy. Incidence of self-reported cognitive dysfunction at similar intervals was found in other studies surveying the effects of treatment of diverse cancers on cognition (Castellon et al., 2004; Downie, Mar Fan, Houede-Tchen, Yi, & Tannock, 2006; Hermelink et al., 2007; Jansen, Dodd, Miaskowski, Dowling, & Kramer, 2008; Mehnert et al., 2007; Poppelreuter et al., 2004; Schagen et al., 2008; Shilling & Jenkins, 2007; van Dam et al., 1998).

Cross-Sectional Neuropsychological Studies—Posttreatment

The first studies to examine cognitive effects of treatment were generally cross-sectional, comparing cancer patients and healthy control groups, or comparing cancer patients stratified by treatment regimen. In an early study comparing high-dose chemotherapy, low-dose chemotherapy, and healthy control groups two years after completion of treatment, individuals treated with high-dose chemotherapy performed significantly worse in measures of attention, psychomotor speed, visual memory, and motor function than healthy controls, while the high-dose group performed significantly worse than the low-dose group only on a measure of reaction time (van Dam et al., 1998). In a study examining breast cancer survivors approximately two years following completion of cyclophosphamide, methotrexate, and 5-fluorouracil (CMF) chemotherapy treatment compared with survivors treated with surgery and radiation only, significantly greater impairment was found in the chemotherapy group in domains of psychomotor speed, motor function, attention, mental flexibility, and visual memory (Schagen et al., 1999). Evidence for cognitive effects at longer intervals was found by Ahles et al. (2002) at approximately five years postdiagnosis, between chemotherapy and no-chemotherapy groups in the domains of verbal memory and psychomotor speed. While other studies found similar differences between treatment groups and healthy controls (Yamada, Denburg, Beglinger, & Schultz, 2010), a subset found significant differences only between cancer-diagnosed (regardless of treatment) and healthy control groups or normative data (Jim et al., 2009; Scherwath et al., 2006), while a minority failed to find any difference between treatments or health status (Donovan et al., 2005; Inagaki et al., 2007; Yoshikawa et al., 2005). The most recent and largest study (N = 196) of long-term effects of chemotherapy exposure (mean = 20 years) found significantly lower performance on measures of immediate and delayed verbal memory, psychomotor speed, and executive functioning in chemotherapy-treated subjects compared to healthy controls (Koppelmans et al., 2012).

The interpretation of these crosssectional studies and later ones is limited due to the absence of a pretreatment, baseline time point. This is a significant limitation since work following initial cross-sectional studies suggests that significant cognitive differences exist prior to treatment. Wefel et al. (2004) found that 35% of women exhibited cognitive impairment prior to cancer treatment, specifically in verbal learning (18%) and memory function (25%). Ahles et al. (2008) investigated pretreatment cognitive ability in healthy controls, and patients diagnosed with invasive (Stages 1–3) and noninvasive (Stage 0) breast cancer, and found significantly slowed reaction time in the invasive group compared to healthy controls, and lower overall performance in the invasive group compared to the healthy and noninvasive patient groups. While pretreatment, baseline differences remain poorly understood in regard to mechanism or etiology, that differences are present prior to treatment between groups requires that longitudinal assessments be conducted to delineate specific treatment-related contributions to cognitive dysfunction.

Longitudinal Neuropsychological Studies: Pre- and Posttreatment

Given the potential for pretreatment cognitive dysfunction, longitudinal studies generally find more modest declines in cognitive dysfunction than cross-sectional, posttreatment studies have reported. These studies have generally found that a subset of patients are affected following treatment within a larger cohort of unaffected individuals; as a result, rates of impairment or decline are more useful in assessing putative effects of treatment than reliance on group mean differences, since group means will tend to obscure subgroup differences. Also problematic are widely varying assessment batteries and screening instruments, making aggregation of numerous studies in systematic reviews or meta-analyses difficult. Despite these issues, available data do suggest significant treatment related effects found in longitudinal studies, although a subset of studies have reported null results.

In an early longitudinal study using published normative data for comparison, Wefel et al. (2004) found that 61% of chemotherapy treated patients exhibited a decline in one or more cognitive domains, mainly consisting of psychomotor speed, attention, and learning three weeks following completion of treatment. Shilling, Jenkins, Morris, Deutsch, and Bloomfield (2005) found significant reliable change (declines on at least two or more measures) from pretreatment baseline to six months posttreatment compared to healthy controls in 34% of patients (18.6% in healthy controls); they also found significant declines (time X group interactions) in the patient group as compared to controls were found in selective attention, working memory, and delayed verbal memory measures. Schagen et al. (2006) found a greater proportion of high-dose chemotherapy patients declined from baseline to six-months posttreatment time points (25%) compared with healthy control subjects (6.7%), while standard-dose and cancer-diagnosed subjects not treated with chemotherapy did not exhibit any significant difference. Stewart et al. (2008) found a greater proportion of chemotherapy-treated patients exhibited a reliable decline (31%) than patients not treated with chemotherapy (12%) with working memory the most affected. Collins et al. (2009) found significant declines in working memory and visual memory for chemotherapy treated patients from baseline to six months posttreatment compared to patients treated with hormonal therapies. Quesnel, Savard, and Ivers (2009) compared groups treated with combination chemotherapy/RT to RT alone and to healthy controls before and after treatment, and three months posttreatment; significant pretreatment attentional differences were noted in the patient group compared to healthy controls, with significant posttreatment verbal memory declines in both patient groups and significantly greater verbal fluency decline in the chemotherapy treated group. Vearncombe et al. (2009) compared groups treated with chemotherapy with or without hormonal and RT to a group not treated with adjuvant therapies at baseline and four weeks following completion of treatment: 16.9% of the chemotherapy group exhibited decline in verbal learning and memory, abstract reasoning, and motor function following treatment, with an association of decreased hemoglobin and increased anxiety to impairment.

Ahles et al. (2010) compared performance of patients treated with chemotherapy, patients not treated with chemotherapy, and healthy controls at baseline, one month, and six months following treatment. The chemotherapy group failed to improve in verbal ability at the one-month time point compared to the other groups, and a significant contribution of age and baseline cognitive reserve to chemotherapy-related cognitive decline in processing speed was found; performance in the chemotherapy group was similar to no-chemotherapy and healthy controls at the six-month time point. Wefel et al. (2010) examined performance in a single group of chemotherapy-treated patients at pretreatment, during treatment, and approximately one month following completion of treatment: 21% exhibited dysfunction predominantly in learning and memory, executive function, and psychomotor speed at the pretreatment time point; 65% of patients exhibited significant decline in the same domains during or shortly after treatment compared to baseline. Hedayati, Alinaghizadeh, Schedin, Nyman, and Albertsson (2012) compared chemotherapy, hormone therapy, no therapy, and healthy controls prior to surgery, prior to adjuvant treatment, six months after start of adjuvant treatment, and three months after completion of treatment; results indicated significantly worse memory performance for breast cancer diagnosed subjects regardless of treatment, and lower memory and processing speed performance following chemotherapy treatment compared with the pretreatment time point. Jansen, Cooper, Dodd, and Miaskowski (2011) examined cognitive changes in patients treated with doxorubicin and cyclophosphamide combination (referred to as *AC*) therapy alone and AC therapy followed by taxane before treatment, one week and six months following completion of treatment. Prior to therapy, 23% of patients exhibited cognitive impairment with significant declines in visuospatial ability, attention, and delayed memory immediately following treatment, and general improvement after six months. Biglia et al. (2012) examined cognitive functioning in a single group of women diagnosed with breast cancer before and immediately after completion of chemotherapy treatment, and reported a significant decline in attention. Collins, Mackenzie, Tasca, Scherling, and Smith (2013b) compared chemotherapy and healthy control groups shortly after completion of treatment and one year following completion of treatment: Results suggested significantly improved global cognition performance at one year with a specific improvement in working memory; however, approximately one-third of patients exhibited persistent cognitive dysfunction at the one-year time point. In a novel study examining dose-response in chemotherapy treatment, Collins, MacKenzie, Tasca, Scherling, and Smith (2013a) conducted serial assessments in women undergoing active treatment with chemotherapy and compared these to seven yoked time points in a healthy control group; declines in global cognitive performance as well as specific declines in working memory, psychomotor speed, verbal and visual memory performance were exhibited with increasing frequency over the seven assessment points (chemotherapy group impairment time 1 = 11.7% and at time 7 = 37%; control group impairment time 1 = 10% and at time 7 = 15.2%).

Other studies examining cognitive abilities at short intervals following treatment have failed to find significant effects. Jenkins et al. (2006) found no significant differences between groups treated with chemotherapy, endocrine/RT, and healthy controls from pretreatment baseline to six months posttreatment, but did find a potential effect of treatment-related menopause initiation on attention and memory measures. Hermelink et al. (2007) assessed a single group of patients before and toward the end of active treatment and found mean performance before treatment to be significantly below normative values in five out of 12 neuropsychological measures. At the second time point, approximately equal proportions of patients exhibited reliable improvement (28%) or decline (27%) from pretreatment performance, although interpretation is limited given that no control group was available for comparison. Mehlsen, Pedersen, Jensen, and Zachariae (2009) compared patients treated with chemotherapy, cardiac patients, and healthy controls, but failed to find any increased rate of impairment or decline in the chemotherapy group. Debess, Riis, Pedersen, and Ewertz (2009) compared chemotherapy, chemotherapy and hormonal therapy, no-chemotherapy, and healthy control groups and found no significant differences six months following completion of treatment in any cognitive domain. Tager et al. (2010) compared chemotherapy and no-chemotherapy groups at baseline and at six months and one year following treatment; while no significant cognitive effect was exhibited, women not treated with chemotherapy improved in motor functioning compared to those treated with chemotherapy, which was interpreted as being potentially related to improvement in treatment-related peripheral neuropathy.

Several studies have examined longer-term cognitive effects of treatment at one-year time points and beyond. At one year posttreatment, Wefel et al. (2004) found improvement in approximately 50% of affected patients, and persistent dysfunction was evident in the remaining half of the sample. In a study with baseline assessment during active treatment, one-year, and two-year time points, Mar Fan et al. (2008) found 16% of patients on active treatment exhibited moderate to severe impairment on the High Sensitivity Cognitive Screen (compared with 5% in the healthy control group). These effects appeared to decline in severity at one- and two-year time points, with 4.4% exhibiting moderate to severe dysfunction in the chemotherapy group at one year (3.6% in healthy controls), and 3.8% at two years (0% in healthy controls), although significant practice effects for this screening measure are implicated. In a single group of chemotherapy-treated patients using normative data as comparison, Wefel et al. (2010) found that 61% of patients exhibited either new or persistent decline at one year posttreatment with most frequent decline in learning and memory. In contrast, in a study with pretreatment, six-month, and one-year time points, Collins et al. (2009) found no difference in impairment in chemotherapy-treated and hormone-treated patients (11% and 10% respectively) at one year, although, significantly, those patients treated with chemotherapy and on active hormonal treatments at one year exhibited decreased psychomotor speed and verbal memory. Similarly, Ahles et al. (2010) found no significant difference in performance for chemotherapy, no-chemotherapy, and healthy control groups at one year following treatment.

Summary of Neuropsychological Findings

Based on the literature reviewed, cognitive dysfunction following diagnosis and treatment of breast cancer is a significant concern in the immediate to intermediate periods following active treatment, with a subset of studies finding persistent cognitive dysfunction at one year and greater time points, and even at 20 years posttreatment. Contextualization of these findings is important as several factors influence interpretation of these results. First, estimates of self-reported dysfunction would suggest much higher rates of cognitive difficulties (up to 50%) than are found in either cross-sectional or longitudinal studies employing objective measures. Disagreement between self-report and objective assessment is a well-known and typical finding in several other neurocognitive syndromes (Reid & Maclullich, 2006). Sources of disagreement that lead to overestimates of cognitive dysfunction include emotional factors that lead to negative perceptions of functioning, and priming as a result of knowledge of potential effects of treatment (Schagen, Das, & van Dam, 2009). Factors that potentially lead to underestimates of cognitive dysfunction following treatment include insensitivity of objective measures to subtle cognitive dysfunction, assessment of performance in the rarefied environment of the consulting office that limits distraction and competing demands, and potentially poor ecological validity of objective measures resulting in poor approximation of real-world cognitive demands.

Second, cross-sectional objective studies would also suggest higher rates of cognitive dysfunction than similar longitudinal studies. As discussed in the previous section, this may be due to preexisting cognitive dysfunction in patients prior to treatment as has been found in a subset of studies. It is important to note that "pretreatment" in this case is before adjuvant chemotherapy treatment but not necessarily before surgical resection. In the study by Ahles et al. (2008), all patients were postsurgery at baseline, and in Wefel et al. (2004) 50% of patients had already undergone either lumpectomy or mastectomy at baseline. Underscoring the importance of this observation, Wefel et al. reported that patients who underwent surgical resection were approximately twice as likely to have cognitive impairment compared to biopsy alone ($p = 0.03$), although this did not meet the a priori significance level specified by the authors ($p = 0.01$). Another potential influence on cognitive function prior to chemotherapy treatment is the stress related to cancer diagnosis and treatment. In general, in those studies that formally assessed mood symptoms, cognitive performance was not associated with self-reported anxiety, although direct effects of chronic stress and hypothalamic-pituitary-adrenal axis (HPA) dysregulation may be one promising future research direction that so far had been only minimally studied. Regardless of etiology, effects of other variables—e.g., stress of diagnosis and treatment, surgical stress and potential inflammatory dysregulation, and anesthetic exposure, all of which precede chemotherapy treatment—may play a role in addition to specific effects of adjuvant therapies that follow.

Finally, longitudinal studies suggest that cognitive dysfunction following treatment may be subtle and exhibited in only a subset of patients. Several potential mechanisms and risk factors for posttreatment cognitive dysfunction have been proposed (Ahles, Root, & Ryan, 2012; Ahles & Saykin, 2007) that may predispose individuals to decline. Age and cognitive reserve have been found to be associated with significantly greater declines in processing speed from pre- to posttreatment in older individuals with lower cognitive reserve (Ahles et al., 2010). Genetic contributions have also been identified, including interaction of the COMT-Val (Val+; Val/Val; Val/Met) genotype with treatment regimen on cognition (Small et al., 2011), as well as the APOE-e4 genotype (Ahles et al., 2003). To the extent that diagnosis and treatment may interact with specific risk factors prior to treatment, averaging cognitive test performance within a given treatment group may obscure significant patient subgroups in whom risk for cognitive dysfunction may be heightened. In addition to clarifying the longitudinal course of cognitive dysfunction in survivors following treatment, potential mechanisms of cognitive dysfunction have received increasing attention. Principal among these has been research investigating underlying brain structure and function and potential changes due to cancer diagnosis and treatment.

Structural and Functional Imaging Studies

Imaging studies investigating potential effects of cancer and treatment on brain structure and function have accumulated in recent years, and multiple reviews are available summarizing these findings (Ahles et al., 2012; de Ruiter & Schagen, 2013; Deprez, Billiet, Sunaert, & Leemans, 2013; McDonald & Saykin, 2013; Reuter-Lorenz & Cimprich, 2013; see also Tables 23.1 and 23.2). Following a similar trajectory as in neuropsychological studies, early structural and functional research focused on cross-sectional designs posttreatment, limiting the interpretability of results given no pretreatment baseline comparisons. Cross-sectional, posttreatment studies using MRI (Abraham et al., 2008; Dale, Fischl, & Sereno, 1999; de Ruiter, Reneman, Boogerd, Veltman, Caan, et al., 2011; Deprez et al., 2011; Inagaki et al., 2007) have documented reductions in gray matter, primarily in frontal cortex and the hippocampus, and white matter integrity in cancer survivors treated with chemotherapy, although negative results have also been reported. In the most recent study utilizing DTI methods, while no group difference was reported, significant associations of white matter integrity with time since treatment were found within a breast cancer cohort at mean interval of 20 years since treatment (Koppelmans et al., 2014).

Longitudinal studies have reported similar results: First, decreased gray matter density in bilateral frontal, temporal (including hippocampus), and cerebellar regions and right thalamus at one month postchemotherapy, with only partial recovery at one year postchemotherapy in several structures, compared with no significant changes in gray matter over time in the no-chemotherapy cancer group or the healthy controls (McDonald et al., 2010); and second, decreased frontal, parietal, and occipital white matter integrity in chemotherapy-exposed patients, with no changes in the no-chemotherapy group or healthy controls posttreatment (Deprez et al., 2012). Gray matter density alterations were replicated by McDonald, Conroy, Smith, West, and Saykin (2013), who found reduced gray matter density one month after completion of treatment, which was associated with greater self-reported executive dysfunction.

Cross-sectional studies of cancer survivors using functional imaging techniques, including functional MRI (fMRI) (de Ruiter, Reneman, Boogerd, Veltman, van Dam, et al., 2011; Ferguson, McDonald, Saykin, & Ahles, 2007; Kesler et al., 2009; Kesler et al., 2011) and functional positron emission tomography (fPET) (Silverman et al., 2007), have demonstrated areas of increased and decreased activation during performance, primarily in working memory and executive functioning tasks, in survivors exposed to chemotherapy, as compared with controls, in areas similar to the structural differences described. McDonald et al. (2012) conducted a longitudinal study using fMRI and found frontal lobe hyperactivation to support a working memory task before treatment, decreased activation one month postchemotherapy, and a return to pretreatment hyperactivation at one year posttreatment. Interestingly, two other studies reported hyperactivation during a memory task before treatment in patients with cancer compared with healthy controls, consistent with the reports of neuropsychological deficits at pretreatment (Cimprich et al., 2010; Scherling et al., 2011). One interpretation is that pretreatment hyperactivation represents an attempt to compensate for preexisting deficits; however, over years, patients lose the ability for compensatory activation as a result of exposure to cancer treatments and/or age-associated changes in the brain. More recent work has found associations of functional recruitment with verbal working memory (Lopez Zunini et al., 2013). In a novel pilot-study, reductions in functional connectivity shortly after treatment were found in the dorsal attention network and default mode network, with partial resolution in the dorsal attention network at one year but persistent reduced connectivity in the default mode network (Dumas et al., 2013).

The most recent imaging work has investigated putative mechanisms of structural and functional alterations following treatment. A potential role of proinflammatory cytokines is suggested by recent work finding an association of inflammatory biomarkers (IL-1ra; sTNF-RI) with regional brain metabolism (Pomykala et al., 2013) utilizing fPET. Similarly, hippocampal volumes and verbal memory performance have

Table 23.1 Structural imaging studies

Authors	*Design/ Modality*	*Assessment schedule*	*Participants*	*Outcomes*
Yoshikawa et al. (2005)	Cross-sectional MRI	t1: 12 months post-tx	CTX+: *n* = 44 CTX−: *n* = 31	No difference in hippocampal volume or memory performance between CTX+ and CTX− at 12 months posttreatment.
Inagaki et al. (2007)	Cross-sectional MRI	t1: > 12 months post-tx	CTX+: *n* = 51 CTX−: *n* = 54 HC: *n* =55	Smaller gray and white matter in prefrontal, parahippocampal, cingulate, and precuneus in CTX+ compared to CTX− at 12 months posttreatment.
Inagaki et al. (2007)	Cross-sectional MRI	t1: > 36 months post-tx	CTX+: *n* = 73 CTX−: *n* = 59 HC: *n* =37	No difference between CTX+ and CTX− at 36 months posttreatment.
Abraham et al. (2008)	Cross-sectional DTI	t1: 22 months post-tx	CTX+: *n* = 10 HC: *n* =9	Lower FA in genu and slower processing speed in CTX+ compared with healthy controls at 22 months posttreatment.
McDonald, Conroy, Ahles, West, and Saykin (2010)	Longitudinal MRI	t1: pre-tx t2: one month post-tx t3: 12 months post-tx	CTX+: *n* = 17 CTX−: *n* = 12 HC: *n* = 18	Decreased gray matter density in both CTX+ and CTX− compared with healthy controls at one month posttreatment. Decreased frontal, temporal, thalamic, and cerebellar gray matter density in CTX+ at one month posttreatment compared with pretreatment. Gray matter density recovered in the CTX+ group with areas of reduced density remaining at one year posttreatment.
Koppelmans et al. (2011)	Cross-sectional MRI	t1: 21 years post-tx	CTX+: *n* = 184 HC: *n* = 368	Smaller total brain volume and gray matter volume in CTX+ compared with health controls at 21 years posttreatment.
Deprez et al. (2011)	Cross-sectional MRI DTI	t1: 80–160 days post-tx	CTX+ *n* = 18 CTX− *n* = 10 HC *n* = 18	Decreased frontal and temporal FA and increased frontal MD in CTX+ compared to CTX− and healthy controls 80–160 days posttreatment.
Deprez et al. (2012)	Longitudinal MRI, DTI	t1: pre-tx t2: 3–4 months post-tx	CTX+ *n* =34 CTX− *n* =16 HC *n* =19	Decreased frontal, parietal, and occipital FA in CTX+ with no changes in either CTX− or healthy controls at three to four months —posttreatment.
de Ruiter and Schagen (2013)	Cross-sectional MRI, DTI, MRS	t1: > 9 years post-tx	CTX+: *n* = 17 CTX−: *n* = 15	Reduced white matter integrity in CTX+ compared with CTX− > 9 years −posttreatment. Reduced N-acetylasparate/creatine in left centrum semiovale in CTX+ compared with CTX− > 9 years −posttreatment. Smaller posterior parietal volume in CTX+ compared with CTX− > 9 years —posttreatment
McDonald et al. (2013)	Longitudinal MRI	t1: pre-tx t2: 1 month post-tx	CTX+ *n* = 27 CTX− *n* = 28 HC *n* =24	Reduced gray matter density in the chemotherapy treated group at one month post-completion of treatment.
Kesler et al. (2013)	Cross-sectional MRI	t1: average 5 years post-tx	CTX+ *n* = 42 HC *n* = 35	Left hippocampal volume reduced in chemotherapy treated group. IL-6 and TNFa increased in chemotherapy group. Hippocampal volume positively correlated with TNFa and negatively correlated with IL-6.
Conroy et al. (2013)	Cross-sectional MRI	t1: average 6 years post-tx	CTX+ *n* = 24 HC *n* = 23	CTX+ group exhibited regional reductions in gray matter density compared to HC. Time since treatment was associated with greater gray matter density in CTX+ group. Oxidative DNA damage was negatively correlated with gray matter density.
Koppelmans et al. (2014)	Cross sectional DTI	t1: average 20 years post-tx	CTX+ *n* = 187 HC *n* = 374	No significant difference in global or regional white matter integrity. Time since treatment was associated with declining white matter integrity.

Notes: CTX+ = chemotherapy; CTX− = no chemotherapy; MRS = magnetic resonance spectroscopy; HC = healthy controls; FA = fractional anisotropy; MD = mean diffusivity

Table 23.2 Functional imaging studies

Authors	*Design/ Modality*	*Assessment Schedule*	*Participants*	*In-Scanner Task*	*Outcomes*
Pretreatment					
Cimprich et al. (2010)	Cross-sectional fMRI	t1: pre-tx only	BC: n = 10 HC: n = 9	Verbal working memory	Greater bilateral activation during verbal working memory task in breast cancer diagnosed subjects compared to healthy controls pretreatment.
Scherling, Collins, Mackenzie, Bielajew, and Smith (2011)	Cross-sectional fMRI	t1: pre-tx only	BC: n = 23 HC: n = 23	Visual N-back	Greater inferior frontal gyrus, insula, thalamus and midbrain activations during working memory task in breast cancer diagnosed subjects compared with healthy controls pretreatment.
Posttreatment					
Ferguson et al. (2007)	Cross-sectional MRI; fMRI	t1: 22 months post-tx	CTX+: n = 1 HC: n = 1	Auditory N-back	Greater WM hyperintensities and greater spatial extent of frontal activation during working memory in the CTX+ case compared with twin healthy control case.
Silverman et al. (2007)	Cross-sectional PET	t1: 5–10 years post-tx	CTX+: n = 5 CTX+Tam: n =7 CTX−: n = 5 HC: n = 3	Paired word memory task 10-minute delay, 1-day delay	Lower inferior frontal gyrus metabolism in CTX+ compared to CTX- and healthy controls 5to 10years posttreatment. Lower basal ganglia metabolism in CTX+Tam treated subjects compared to CTX+, CTX−, and healthy controls 5to 10years posttreatment.
Kesler, Bennett, Mahaffey, and Spiegel (2009)	Cross-sectional fMRI	t1: 3 years post-tx	CTX+: n = 14 HC: n = 14	Verbal declarative encoding Verbal declarative recognition	Lower prefrontal cortex activation during encoding in CTX+ compared to healthy controls 3years posttreatment. Greater regional activations during recall in CTX+ compared to healthy controls 3years posttreatment.
Kesler, Kent, and O'Hara (2011)	Cross-sectional fMRI	t1: 5 years post-tx	CTX+: n = 25 CTX−: n = 19	Card sorting task	Lower left middle dorsolateral prefrontal cortex activation and premotor cortex activation in breast cancer diagnosed subjects compared to healthy controls. Lower left caudal lateral prefrontal cortex activation in CTX+ compared with CTX− and healthy controls 5years posttreatment.
de Ruiter et al. (2011)	Cross-sectional fMRI	t1: 10 years post-tx	CTX+: n = 19 CTX−: n = 15	Tower of London, Paired Associates	Lower dorsolateral prefrontal cortex activity during Tower of London task, lower parahippocampal gyrus activity during paired associates task in CTX+ compared to CTX− 10 years posttreatment.
McDonald et al. (2012)	Longitudinal fMRI	t1: pre-tx t2: 1 month post-tx t3: 1 year post-tx	CTX+: n = 16 CTX−: n = 12 HC: n = 15	N-Back Task	Greater frontal activation and lower parietal activation at baseline in BC diagnosed patients relative to controls. Lower frontal activation in BC-diagnosed patients relative to healthy controls immediately following treatment. Greater frontal activation in BC diagnosed patients relative to healthy controls one year following treatment.
Lopez Zunini et al. (2013)	Longitudinal fMRI	t1: pre-tx t2: 1 month post-tx	CTX+: n =21 HC: n = 21	Verbal recall task	At pre-tx, CTX+ exhibited reduced recruitment in anterior cingulated compared to controls. At one month post-tx, CTX+ exhibited reduced recruitment in bilateral insula, left inferior orbitofrontal cortex and left middle temporal gyrus compared to controls. Fatigue, depression, and anxiety were associated with a subset of difference in recruitment.
Dumas et al. (2013)	Longitudinal fMRI	T1: pre-tx T2: 1 month post-tx T3: 1 year post-tx	CTX+ n =9	Resting state functional connectivity	Reductions in functional connectivity shortly after treatment were found in the dorsal attention network and default mode network, with partial resolution in the dorsal attention network at one year but persistent reduced connectivity in the default mode network.
Pomykala et al. (2013)	Longitudinal PET	T1: post-tx T2: 1 year post-tx	CTX+ n = 23 CTX− n = 10	Resting FDG PET	Association of inflammatory biomarkers (IL-1ra; sTNF-RI) with regional brain metabolism utilizing PET.

Key: Ctx+ = chemotherapy; Ctx- = no chemotherapy; fMRI = functional magnetic resonance imaging been found to be associated with serum inflammatory cytokines (TNFa; IL6) following treatment (Kesler, Janelsins, et al., 2013). A potential role of DNA damage and its association with cortical gray matter was recently suggested in a study by Conroy et al. (2013) that found higher oxidative DNA damage in a sample of breast cancer survivors than in healthy controls and associations of oxidative DNA damage with gray matter density.

Treatment Interventions

Treatment of cognitive dysfunction in breast cancer patients is a challenging clinical need and newly expanding area of research. One particularly challenging aspect with regard to rehabilitation in this cohort is the often significant but subtle cognitive dysfunction exhibited in these patients. In contrast to rehabilitation programs in traumatic brain injury or primary CNS tumors, the target of cognitive rehabilitation in non-CNS cancers may be difficult to discern, and multiple diffusc processes may be affected. Treatment has generally taken the form of both compensatory and direct (restitutive) rehabilitation, as well as cognitive behavioral therapy, and pharmacologic treatment. Although it is not the focus of this brief review, mindfulness-based programs and exercise regimens have also been considered either as alternatives to cognitive rehabilitation programs or as parts of a multitreatment strategy. Generally, outcomes of treatment are promising but the research on which they are based is still in the early stage of development and no definitive conclusions can be drawn from the handful of studies that have been conducted.

In an early, single-arm study to address treatment strategies for cognitive dysfunction following treatment (Ferguson, Ahles, et al., 2007), a program of Memory and Attention Adaptation Training (MAAT) was tested that included (a) education on memory and attention; (b) self-awareness training; (c) self-regulation via relaxation training; and (d) compensatory strategy training. Improved self-reported and objective cognitive function was found, along with adequate feasibility and patient satisfaction, although no comparison arm is available for assessing placebo and practice effects. In a later, two-arm trial (Ferguson et al., 2012), patients were randomized to receive either MAAT or assigned to a wait-list control group. Patients treated with MAAT exhibited significantly improved verbal memory as compared to the wait list control group, as well as significantly improved self-reported "spiritual well-being," although no significant effect was found for other cognitive domains or for other self-reported cognitive outcomes. Poppelreuter, Weis, and Bartsch (2009) compared the effectiveness of computer-based training, and a rehabilitation program to a control group at baseline, at end of rehabilitation, and at six months, although no specific effect of intervention was found, with all groups improving over time on measures of cognitive function. Von Ah et al. (2012) studied effects of memory or processing speed training versus a wait list control group at baseline, shortly following training, and two months after completion of the intervention, with significant effects for processing speed at both the immediate and two month follow-up evaluation, and significant memory effects at the two month follow-up evaluation; interpretation of delayed effects are complicated by no significant effect immediately following training. Cherrier et al. (2013) examined the effectiveness of a compensatory and mindfulness rehabilitation program versus control at baseline and following training and found improvement on self-reported cognitive function as well as in objective attention functioning. In a cognitive-training rehabilitation study, Kesler et al. (2013) utilized online training software to examine remediation of executive functioning skills and found significant improvements on the Wisconsin Card Sorting Test, Symbol Search, and letter fluency in the active treatment group versus controls, together with improved self-reported cognitive functioning in the active treatment group.

In addition to direct and compensatory rehabilitation programs, pharmacologic treatments have also been investigated including modafanil and dexymethylphenidate. Results are mixed regarding efficacy of dexymethylphenidate, with a subset of studies finding significant improvement in fatigue and cognition (Lower et al., 2009) while others find no beneficial effect (Mar Fan et al., 2008). Modafinil has received increasing attention for its efficacy in treating cognitive dysfunction following treatment, again specifically with regard to treatment of attentional dysfunction and fatigue, with promising results (Kohli et al., 2009; Lundorff, Jonsson, & Sjogren, 2009).

Conclusion

The recent literature suggests that both brain tumor and the adverse effects of treatment contribute to cognitive dysfunction in a significant number of brain tumor patients. The studies reviewed indicated that whole-brain RT alone or in combination with chemotherapy result in more pronounced cognitive dysfunction than either partial RT or chemotherapy alone. Antiepileptics and corticosteroids, often used in the treatment of these patients, may also further disrupt cognitive functioning. The cognitive domains suggested to be particularly sensitive to treatment-induced cognitive dysfunction include several aspects of attention and executive functions, learning and retrieval of new information, and graphomotor speed.

Advancements in the field include the development of guidelines for the use of standardized neuropsychological tests in the context of clinical trials, and the inclusion of cognitive outcome measures in several recent and ongoing multi-center studies and clinical trials in neuro-oncology. The findings from such studies would improve our understanding of the toxicity of various treatment modalities, and enable both physicians and patients to make decisions regarding treatment based not only on survival rates and time to disease progression, but also on QoL.

In non-CNS cancers, the body of literature on self-reported cognitive dysfunction, cross-sectional and longitudinal objective cognitive assessments before and after treatment, and structural and functional imaging findings strongly support the occurrence of neuropsychological dysfunction associated with diagnosis and treatment for breast cancer. Cognitive changes may appear early in the posttreatment course but may become more apparent after physical/medical factors and concerns have resolved or when patients attempt to return to prediagnosis responsibilities (school, work, household demands). Currently, long-term effects are poorly understood, with the majority of studies suggesting persistent cognitive problems and another subset suggesting relative resolution of difficulties over time.

Recent studies have begun to describe the pathophysiological mechanisms that may underline the adverse effects of RT and chemotherapy, and additional research is necessary to identify contributing factors for the development of treatment-related cognitive dysfunction (e.g., genetic susceptibility). The efficacy of pharmacological and behavioral interventions to improve cognitive function is increasingly being investigated in studies involving patients with brain tumors and non-CNS cancers.

References

Abraham, J., Haut, M. W., Moran, M. T., Filburn, S., Lemiuex, S., & Kuwabara, H. (2008). Adjuvant chemotherapy for breast cancer: Effects on cerebral white matter seen in diffusion tensor imaging. *Clinical Breast Cancer*, *8*(1), 88–91. doi: 10.3816/CBC.2008.n.007

Abrey, L. E., Batchelor, T. T., Ferreri, A. J., Gospodarowicz, M., Pulczynski, E. J., Zucca, E., . . . International Primary, C.N.S.L.C.G. (2005). Report of an international workshop to standardize baseline evaluation and response criteria for primary CNS lymphoma. *Journal of Clinical Oncology*, *23*(22), 5034–5043. doi: 10.1200/JCO.2005.13.524

Abrey, L. E., Olson, J. D., Raizer, J. J., Mack, M., Rodavitch, A., Boutros, D. Y., & Malkin, M. G. (2001). A phase II trial of temozolomide for patients with recurrent or progressive brain metastases. *Journal of Neuro-Oncology*, *53*(3), 259–265.

Ahles, T. A., Root, J. C., & Ryan, E. L. (2012). Cancer- and cancer treatment-associated cognitive change: An update on the state of the science. *Journal of Clinical Oncology*, *30*(30), 3675–3686. doi: 10.1200/JCO.2012.43.0116

Ahles, T. A., & Saykin, A. J. (2007). Candidate mechanisms for chemotherapy-induced cognitive changes. *Nature Reviews Cancer*, *7*(3), 192–201. doi: 10.1038/nrc2073

Ahles, T. A., Saykin, A. J., Furstenberg, C. T., Cole, B., Mott, L. A., Skalla, K., . . . Silberfarb, P. M. (2002). Neuropsychologic impact of standard-dose systemic chemotherapy in long-term survivors of breast cancer and lymphoma. *Journal of Clinical Oncology*, *20*(2), 485–493.

Ahles, T. A., Saykin, A. J., McDonald, B. C., Furstenberg, C. T., Cole, B. F., Hanscom, B. S., . . . Kaufman, P. A. (2008). Cognitive function in breast cancer patients prior to adjuvant treatment. *Breast Cancer Research and Treatment*, *110*(1), 143–152.

Ahles, T. A., Saykin, A. J., McDonald, B. C., Li, Y., Furstenberg, C. T., Hanscom, B. S., . . . Kaufman, P. A. (2010). Longitudinal assessment of cognitive changes associated with adjuvant treatment for breast cancer: Impact of age and cognitive reserve. *Journal of Clinical Oncology*, *28*(29), 4434–4440. doi: 10.1200/JCO.2009.27.0827

Ahles, T. A., Saykin, A. J., Noll, W. W., Furstenberg, C. T., Guerin, S., Cole, B., & Mott, L. A. (2003). The relationship of APOE genotype to neuropsychological performance in long-term cancer survivors treated with standard dose chemotherapy. *Psychooncology*, *12*(6), 612–619. doi: 10.1002/pon.742

Anderson, S. W., Damasio, H., & Tranel, D. (1990). Neuropsychological impairments associated with lesions caused by tumor or stroke. *Archives of Neurology*, *47*(4), 397–405.

Andrews, D. W., Scott, C. B., Sperduto, P. W., Flanders, A. E., Gaspar, L. E., Schell, M. C., . . . Curran, W. J., Jr. (2004). Whole brain radiation therapy with or without stereotactic radiosurgery boost for patients with one to three brain metastases: Phase III results of the RTOG 9508 randomised trial. *Lancet*, *363*(9422), 1665–1672. doi: 10.1016/S0140-6736(04)16250-8

Archibald, Y. M., Lunn, D., Ruttan, L. A., Macdonald, D. R., Del Maestro, R. F., Barr, H. W., . . . Cairncross, J. G. (1994). Cognitive functioning in long-term survivors of high-grade glioma. *Journal of Neurosurgery*, *80*(2), 247–253. doi: 10.3171/jns.1994.80.2.0247

Armstrong, C. L., Corn, B. W., Ruffer, J. E., Pruitt, A. A., Mollman, J. E., & Phillips, P. C. (2000). Radiotherapeutic effects on brain function: Double dissociation of memory systems. *Neuropsychiatry, Neuropsychology, and Behavioral Neurology*, *13*(2), 101–111.

Armstrong, C. L., Goldstein, B., Shera, D., Ledakis, G. E., & Tallent, E. M. (2003). The predictive value of longitudinal neuropsychologic assessment in the early detection of brain tumor recurrence. *Cancer*, *97*(3), 649–656. doi: 10.1002/cncr.11099

Armstrong, C. L., Hunter, J. V., Ledakis, G. E., Cohen, B., Tallent, E. M., Goldstein, B. H., . . . Phillips, P. (2002). Late cognitive and radiographic changes related to radiotherapy: Initial prospective findings. *Neurology*, *59*(1), 40–48.

Armstrong, C. L., Stern, C. H., & Corn, B. W. (2001). Memory performance used to detect radiation effects on cognitive functioning. *Applied Neuropsychology*, *8*(3), 129–139. doi: 10.1207/S15324826AN0803_1

Ayoma, H., Shirato, H., Tago, M., et al. (2006). Stereotactic radiosurgery plus whole-brain radiation therapy vs. stereotactic radiosurgery alone for treatment of brain metastases: A randomized controlled trial. *Journal of the American Medical Association*, *295*, 2483–2491.

Batchelor, T. T., Neuwelt, E., Wang, D. L., et al. (2012). Clinical and diagnostic considerations in primary central nervous system lymphoma. In T. Batchelor & L. DeAngelis (Eds.), *Lymphoma and Leukemia of the Nervous System* (pp. 113–128). New York: Springer.

Behin, A., & Delattre, J.-Y. (2003). Neurologic sequelae of radiotherapy on the nervous system. In D. Schiff & P. Y. Wen (Eds.), *Cancer Neurology in Clinical Practice* (pp. 173–191). Totowa, NJ: Humana Press.

Bian, W., Hess, C. P., Chang, S. M., Nelson, S. J., & Lupo, J. M. (2013). Computer-aided detection of radiation-induced cerebral microbleeds on susceptibility-weighted MR images. *NeuroImage: Clinical*, *2*, 282–290. doi: 10.1016/j.nicl.2013.01.012

Biglia, N., Bounous, V. E., Malabaila, A., Palmisano, D., Torta, D. M., D'Alonzo, M., . . . Torta, R. (2012). Objective and self-reported cognitive dysfunction in breast cancer women treated with chemotherapy:

A prospective study. *European Journal of Cancer Care (English)*, *21*(4), 485–492. doi: 10.1111/j.1365-2354.2011.01320.x

Boele, F. W., Douw, L., de Groot, M., van Thuijl, H. F., Cleijne, W., Heimans, J. J., . . . Klein, M. (2013). The effect of modafinil on fatigue, cognitive functioning, and mood in primary brain tumor patients: A multicenter randomized controlled trial. *Neuro Oncology*, *15*(10), 1420–1428. doi: 10.1093/neuonc/not102

Bondy, M. L., El-Zein, R., Wrench, M. (2005). Epidemiology of brain cancer. In D. Schiff & B. P. O'Neill (Eds.), *Principles of Neuro-Oncology* (pp. 3–16). New York: McGraw-Hill.

Boothe, D., Young, R., Yamada, Y., Prager, A., Chan, T., & Beal, K. (2013). Bevacizumab as a treatment for radiation necrosis of brain metastases post stereotactic radiosurgery. *Neuro Oncology*, *15*(9), 1257–1263. doi: 10.1093/neuonc/not085

Bosma, I., Douw, L., Bartolomei, F., Heimans, J. J., van Dijk, B. W., Postma, T. J., . . . Klein, M. (2008). Synchronized brain activity and neurocognitive function in patients with low-grade glioma: A magnetoencephalography study. *Neuro Oncology*, *10*(5), 734–744. doi: 10.1215/15228517-2008-034

Bosma, I., Vos, M. J., Heimans, J. J., Taphoorn, M. J., Aaronson, N. K., Postma, T. J., . . . Klein, M. (2007). The course of neurocognitive functioning in high-grade glioma patients. *Neuro Oncology*, *9*(1), 53–62. doi: 10.1215/15228517-2006-012

Brown, P. D., Asher, A. L., & Farace, E. (2008). Adjuvant whole brain radiotherapy: Strong emotions decide but rational studies are needed. *International Journal of Radiation Oncology Biology Physics*, *70*(5), 1305–1309. doi: 10.1016/j.ijrobp.2007.11.047

Brown, P. D., Jensen, A. W., Felten, S. J., Ballman, K. V., Schaefer, P. L., Jaeckle, K. A., . . . Buckner, J. C. (2006). Detrimental effects of tumor progression on cognitive function of patients with high-grade glioma. *Journal of Clinical Oncology*, *24*(34), 5427–5433. doi: 10.1200/JCO.2006.08.5605

Brown, P. D., Pugh, S., Laack, N. N., Wefel, J. S., Khuntia, D., Meyers, C., . . . Radiation Therapy Oncology, G. (2013). Memantine for the prevention of cognitive dysfunction in patients receiving whole-brain radiotherapy: A randomized, double-blind, placebo-controlled trial. *Neuro Oncology*, *15*(10), 1429–1437. doi: 10.1093/neuonc/not114

BTPRG. (2000). *Report of the Brain Tumor Progress Review Group*. Baltimore: National Institutes of Health.

Cairncross, J. G. (2000). Understanding low-grade glioma: A decade of progress. *Neurology*, *54*(7), 1402–1403.

Carson, K. A., Grossman, S. A., Fisher, J. D., & Shaw, E. G. (2007). Prognostic factors for survival in adult patients with recurrent glioma enrolled onto the new approaches to brain tumor therapy CNS consortium phase I and II clinical trials. *Journal of Clinical Oncology*, *25*(18), 2601–2606. doi: 10.1200/JCO.2006.08.1661

Castellon, S. A., Ganz, P. A., Bower, J. E., Petersen, L., Abraham, L., & Greendale, G. A. (2004). Neurocognitive performance in breast cancer survivors exposed to adjuvant chemotherapy and tamoxifen. *Journal of Clinical and Experimental Neuropsychology*, *26*(7), 955–969.

Chang, E. L., Wefel, J. S., Hess, K. R., Allen, P. K., Lang, F. F., Kornguth, D. G., . . . Meyers, C. A. (2009). Neurocognition in patients with brain metastases treated with radiosurgery or radiosurgery plus whole-brain irradiation: A randomised controlled trial. *Lancet Oncology*, *10*(11), 1037–1044. doi: 10.1016/S1470-2045(09)70263-3

Chang, E. L., Wefel, J. S., Maor, M. H., Hassenbusch, S. J., 3rd, Mahajan, A., Lang, F. F., . . . Meyers, C. A. (2007). A pilot study of neurocognitive function in patients with one to three new brain metastases initially treated with stereotactic radiosurgery alone. *Neurosurgery*, *60*(2), 277–283; discussion 283–274. doi: 10.1227/01.NEU.0000249272.64439.B1

Chapman, C. H., Nazem-Zadeh, M., Lee, O. E., Schipper, M. J., Tsien, C. I., Lawrence, T. S., & Cao, Y. (2013). Regional variation in brain white matter diffusion index changes following chemoradiotherapy: A prospective study using tract-based spatial statistics. *PLoS One*, *8*(3), e57768. doi: 10.1371/journal.pone.0057768

Cherrier, M. M., Anderson, K., David, D., Higano, C. S., Gray, H., Church, A., & Willis, S. L. (2013). A randomized trial of cognitive rehabilitation in cancer survivors. *Life Sciences*, *93*(17), 617–622. doi: 10.1016/j.lfs.2013.08.011

Cimprich, B., Reuter-Lorenz, P., Nelson, J., Clark, P. M., Therrien, B., Normolle, D., . . . Welsh, R. C. (2010). Prechemotherapy alterations in brain function in women with breast cancer. *Journal of Clinical and Experimental Neuropsychology*, *32*(3), 324–331. doi: 10.1080/13803390903032537

Collins, B., Mackenzie, J., Stewart, A., Bielajew, C., & Verma, S. (2009). Cognitive effects of chemotherapy in post-menopausal breast cancer patients 1 year after treatment. *Psychooncology*, *18*(2), 134–143. doi: 10.1002/pon.1379

Collins, B., MacKenzie, J., Tasca, G. A., Scherling, C., & Smith, A. (2013a). Cognitive effects of chemotherapy in breast cancer patients: A dose-response study. *Psychooncology*, *22*(7), 1517–1527. doi: 10.1002/pon.3163

Collins, B., MacKenzie, J., Tasca, G. A., Scherling, C., & Smith, A. (2013b). Persistent cognitive changes in breast cancer patients 1 year following completion of chemotherapy. *Journal of the International Neuropsychological Society*, 1–10. doi: 10.1017/S1355617713001215

Conroy, S. K., McDonald, B. C., Smith, D. J., Moser, L. R., West, J. D., Kamendulis, L. M., . . . Saykin, A. J. (2013). Alterations in brain structure and function in breast cancer survivors: Effect of post-chemotherapy interval and relation to oxidative DNA damage. *Breast Cancer Research and Treatment*, *137*(2), 493–502. doi: 10.1007/s10549-012-2385-x

Constine, L. S., Konski, A., Ekholm, S., McDonald, S., & Rubin, P. (1988). Adverse effects of brain irradiation correlated with MR and CT imaging. *International Journal of Radiation Oncology Biology Physics*, *15*(2), 319–330.

Corn, B. W., Wang, M., Fox, S., Michalski, J., Purdy, J., Simpson, J., . . . Movsas, B. (2009). Health related quality of life and cognitive status in patients with glioblastoma multiforme receiving escalating doses of conformal three dimensional radiation on RTOG 98–03. *Journal of Neuro-Oncology*, *95*(2), 247–257. doi: 10.1007/s11060-009-9923-3

Correa, D. D. (2006). Cognitive functions in brain tumor patients. *Hematology/Oncology Clinics of North America*, *20*(6), 1363–1376. doi: 10.1016/j.hoc.2006.09.012

Correa, D. D., & Ahles, T. A. (2008). Neurocognitive changes in cancer survivors. *Cancer Journal*, *14*(6), 396–400. doi: 10.1097/PPO.0b013e31818d8769

Correa, D. D., Baser, R., Beal, K., et al. (2011). Longitudinal cognitive follow-up in newly diagnosed glioblastoma patients treated with bevacizumab, temozolomide and hypofractionated stereotactic radiotherapy. *Neuro Oncology*, *15*, 92.

Correa, D. D., DeAngelis, L. M., & Shi, W. (2007). Cognitive functions and APOE genotype in low grade glioma patients. *Neuro Oncology*, *81*, 175–184.

Correa, D. D., DeAngelis, L. M., Shi, W., Thaler, H., Glass, A., & Abrey, L. E. (2004). Cognitive functions in survivors of primary central nervous system lymphoma. *Neurology*, *62*(4), 548–555.

Correa, D. D., & Hess, L. M. (2012). Cognitive function and quality of life in ovarian cancer. *Gynecologic Oncology*, *124*(3), 404–409. doi: 10.1016/j.ygyno.2011.11.005

Correa, D. D., Maron, L., Harder, H., Klein, M., Armstrong, C. L., Calabrese, P., . . . Schiff, D. (2007). Cognitive functions in primary central nervous system lymphoma: Literature review and assessment guidelines. *Annals of Oncology*, *18*(7), 1145–1151. doi: 10.1093/annonc/mdl464

Correa, D. D., Rocco-Donovan, M., DeAngelis, L. M., Dolgoff-Kaspar, R., Iwamoto, F., Yahalom, J., & Abrey, L. E. (2009). Prospective cognitive follow-up in primary CNS lymphoma patients treated with chemotherapy and reduced-dose radiotherapy. *Journal of Neuro-Oncology*, *91*(3), 315–321. doi: 10.1007/s11060-008-9716-0

Correa, D. D., Root, J. C., Baser, R., Moore, D., Peck, K. K., Lis, E., . . . Relkin, N. (2013). A prospective evaluation of changes in brain structure and cognitive functions in adult stem cell transplant recipients. *Brain Imaging and Behavior*, *7*(4), 478–490. doi: 10.1007/s11682-013-9221-8

Correa, D. D., Satagopan, J., Baser, R. E., Cheung, K., Lin, M., Karimi, S., . . . Orlow, I. (2013). APOE genotype and cognitive outcome in patients with brain tumors. *Neuro Oncology*, *15*, 93.

Correa, D. D., Shi, W., Abrey, L. E., Deangelis, L. M., Omuro, A. M., Deutsch, M. B., & Thaler, H. T. (2012). Cognitive functions in primary CNS lymphoma after single or combined modality regimens. *Neuro Oncology*, *14*(1), 101–108. doi: 10.1093/neuonc/nor186

Correa, D. D., Shi, W., Thaler, H. T., Cheung, A. M., DeAngelis, L. M., & Abrey, L. E. (2008). Longitudinal cognitive follow-up in low grade gliomas. *Journal of Neuro-Oncology*, *86*(3), 321–327. doi: 10.1007/s11060-007-9474-4

Correa, D. D., Zhou, Q., Thaler, H. T., Maziarz, M., Hurley, K., & Hensley, M. L. (2010). Cognitive functions in long-term survivors of ovarian cancer. *Gynecologic Oncology*, *119*(2), 366–369. doi: 10.1016/j.ygyno.2010.06.023

Crossen, J. R., Garwood, D., Glatstein, E., & Neuwelt, E. A. (1994). Neurobehavioral sequelae of cranial irradiation in adults: A review of radiation-induced encephalopathy. *Journal of Clinical Oncology*, *12*(3), 627–642.

Crossen, J. R., Goldman, D. L., Dahlborg, S. A., & Neuwelt, E. A. (1992). Neuropsychological assessment outcomes of nonacquired immunodeficiency syndrome patients with primary central nervous system lymphoma before and after blood-brain barrier disruption chemotherapy. *Neurosurgery*, *30*(1), 23–29.

Cull, A., Hay, C., Love, S. B., Mackie, M., Smets, E., & Stewart, M. (1996). What do cancer patients mean when they complain of concentration and memory problems? *British Journal of Cancer*, *74*(10), 1674–1679.

Cull, A., Stewart, M., & Altman, D. G. (1995). Assessment of and intervention for psychosocial problems in routine oncology practice. *British Journal of Cancer*, *72*(1), 229–235.

Dale, A. M., Fischl, B., & Sereno, M. I. (1999). Cortical surface-based analysis: I. Segmentation and surface reconstruction. *Neuroimage*, *9*(2), 179–194.

DeAngelis, L. M., & Posner, J. B. (2009). Side effects of radiation therapy. In L. M. DeAngelis & J. B. Posner (Eds.), *Neurologic Complications of Cancer* (2nd ed., pp. 551–555). New York: Oxford University Press.

DeAngelis, L. M., Seiferheld, W., Schold, S. C., Fisher, B., Schultz, C. J., & Radiation Therapy Oncology Group, S. (2002). Combination chemotherapy and radiotherapy for primary central nervous system lymphoma: Radiation Therapy Oncology Group Study 93–10. *Journal of Clinical Oncology*, *20*(24), 4643–4648.

DeAngelis, L. M., & Shapiro, W. R. (1991). Drug/radiation interactions and central nervous system injury. In P. H. Gutin, S. A. Leibel, & G. E. Sheline (Eds.), *Radiation Injury to the Nervous System* (pp. 361–382). New York: Raven Press.

DeAngelis, L. M., Yahalom, J., Thaler, H. T., & Kher, U. (1992). Combined modality therapy for primary CNS lymphoma. *Journal of Clinical Oncology*, *10*(4), 635–643.

Debess, J., Riis, J. O., Pedersen, L., & Ewertz, M. (2009). Cognitive function and quality of life after surgery for early breast cancer in North Jutland, Denmark. *Acta Oncologica*, *48*(4), 532–540. doi: 906989492 [pii] 10.1080/02841860802600755

DeGroot, J. F., Aldape, K. D., & Colman, H. (2005). High-grade astrocytomas. In D. Schiff & B. P. O'Neill (Eds.), *Principles of Neuro-Oncology* (pp. 259–288). New York: McGraw-Hill.

de Groot, M., Douw, L., Sizoo, E. M., Bosma, I., Froklage, F. E., Heimans, J. J., . . . Reijneveld, J. C. (2013). Levetiracetam improves verbal memory in high-grade glioma patients. *Neuro Oncology*, *15*(2), 216–223. doi: 10.1093/neuonc/nos288

Deprez, S., Amant, F., Smeets, A., Peeters, R., Leemans, A., Van Hecke, W., . . . Sunaert, S. (2012). Longitudinal assessment of chemotherapy-induced structural changes in cerebral white matter and its correlation with impaired cognitive functioning. *Journal of Clinical Oncology*, *30*(3), 274–281. doi: 10.1200/JCO.2011.36.8571

Deprez, S., Amant, F., Yigit, R., Porke, K., Verhoeven, J., Van den Stock, J., . . . Sunaert, S. (2011). Chemotherapy-induced structural changes in cerebral white matter and its correlation with impaired cognitive functioning in breast cancer patients. *Human Brain Mapping*, *32*(3), 480–493. doi: 10.1002/hbm.21033

Deprez, S., Billiet, T., Sunaert, S., & Leemans, A. (2013). Diffusion tensor MRI of chemotherapy-induced cognitive impairment in non-CNS cancer patients: A review. *Brain Imaging and Behavior*, *7*(4), 409–435. doi: 10.1007/s11682-012-9220-1

de Ruiter, M. B., Reneman, L., Boogerd, W., Veltman, D. J., Caan, M., Douaud, G., . . . Schagen, S. B. (2011). Late effects of high-dose adjuvant chemotherapy on white and gray matter in breast cancer survivors: Converging results from multimodal magnetic resonance imaging. *Human Brain Mapping*. doi: 10.1002/hbm.21422

de Ruiter, M. B., Reneman, L., Boogerd, W., Veltman, D. J., van Dam, F. S., Nederveen, A. J., . . . Schagen, S. B. (2011). Cerebral hyporesponsiveness and cognitive impairment 10 years after chemotherapy for breast cancer. *Human Brain Mapping*, *32*(8), 1206–1219. doi: 10.1002/hbm.21102

de Ruiter, M. B., & Schagen, S. B. (2013). Functional MRI studies in non-CNS cancers. *Brain Imaging and Behavior*, *7*(4), 388–408. doi: 10.1007/s11682-013-9249-9

De Witt Hamer, P. C., Robles, S. G., Zwinderman, A. H., Duffau, H., & Berger, M. S. (2012). Impact of intraoperative stimulation brain mapping on glioma surgery outcome: A meta-analysis. *Journal of Clinical Oncology*, *30*(20), 2559–2565. doi: 10.1200/JCO.2011.38.4818

Dietrich, J. (2010). Chemotherapy associated central nervous system damage. In R. B. Raffa & R. J. Tallarida (Eds.), *Chemo Fog: Cancer Chemotherapy-Related Cognitive Impairment* (pp. 77–85). Austin, TX: Landes Bioscience and Springer Science and Business Media.

Dietrich, J., Han, R., Yang, Y., Mayer-Proschel, M., & Noble, M. (2006). CNS progenitor cells and oligodendrocytes are targets of chemotherapeutic agents in vitro and in vivo. *Journal of Biology*, *5*(7), 1–23. doi: 10.1186/jbiol50

Dietrich, J., Monje, M., Wefel, J., & Meyers, C. (2008). Clinical patterns and biological correlates of cognitive dysfunction associated with cancer therapy. *Oncologist*, *13*(12), 1285–1295. doi: 10.1634/theoncologist.2008-0130

Donovan, K. A., Small, B. J., Andrykowski, M. A., Schmitt, F. A., Munster, P., & Jacobsen, P. B. (2005). Cognitive functioning after adjuvant chemotherapy and/or radiotherapy for early-stage breast carcinoma. *Cancer*, *104*(11), 2499–2507. doi: 10.1002/cncr.21482

Doolittle, N. D., Dosa, E., Fu, R., Muldoon, L. L., Maron, L. M., Lubow, M. A., . . . Neuwelt, E. A. (2013). Preservation of cognitive function in primary CNS lymphoma survivors a median of 12 years after enhanced chemotherapy delivery. *Journal of Clinical Oncology*, *31*(31), 4026–4027. doi: 10.1200/JCO.2013.52.7747

Doolittle, N. D., Korfel, A., Lubow, M. A., Schorb, E., Schlegel, U., Rogowski, S., . . . Neuwelt, E. A. (2013). Long-term cognitive function, neuroimaging, and quality of life in primary CNS lymphoma. *Neurology*, *81*(1), 84–92. doi: 10.1212/WNL.0b013e318297eeba

Douw, L., Klein, M., Fagel, S. S., van den Heuvel, J., Taphoorn, M. J., Aaronson, N. K., . . . Heimans, J. J. (2009). Cognitive and radiological effects of radiotherapy in patients with low-grade glioma: Long-term follow-up. *Lancet Neurology*, *8*(9), 810–818. doi: 10.1016/S1474-4422(09)70204-2

Downie, F. P., Mar Fan, H. G., Houede-Tchen, N., Yi, Q., & Tannock, I. F. (2006). Cognitive function, fatigue, and menopausal symptoms in breast cancer patients receiving adjuvant chemotherapy: Evaluation with patient interview after formal assessment. *Psychooncology*, *15*(10), 921–930. doi: 10.1002/pon.1035

Duffau, H. (2005). Lessons from brain mapping in surgery for low-grade glioma: Insights into associations between tumour and brain plasticity. *Lancet Neurology*, *4*(8), 476–486. doi: 10.1016/S1474-4422(05)70140-X

Duffey, P., Chari, G., Cartlidge, N. E., & Shaw, P. J. (1996). Progressive deterioration of intellect and motor function occurring several decades after cranial irradiation: A new facet in the clinical spectrum of radiation encephalopathy. *Archives of Neurology*, *53*(8), 814–818.

Dumas, J. A., Makarewicz, J., Schaubhut, G. J., Devins, R., Albert, K., Dittus, K., & Newhouse, P. A. (2013). Chemotherapy altered brain functional connectivity in women with breast cancer: A pilot study. *Brain Imaging and Behavior*, *7*(4), 524–532. doi: 10.1007/s11682-013-9244-1

Fan, H. G., Houede-Tchen, N., Yi, Q. L., Chemerynsky, I., Downie, F. P., Sabate, K., & Tannock, I. F. (2005). Fatigue, menopausal symptoms, and cognitive function in women after adjuvant chemotherapy for breast cancer: 1- and 2-year follow-up of a prospective controlled study. *Journal of Clinical Oncology*, *23*(31), 8025–8032. doi: 10.1200/JCO.2005.01.6550

Ferguson, R. J., Ahles, T. A., Saykin, A. J., McDonald, B. C., Furstenberg, C. T., Cole, B. F., & Mott, L. A. (2007). Cognitive-behavioral management of chemotherapy-related cognitive change. *Psychooncology*, *16*(8), 772–777. doi: 10.1002/pon.1133

Ferguson, R. J., McDonald, B. C., Rocque, M. A., Furstenberg, C. T., Horrigan, S., Ahles, T. A., & Saykin, A. J. (2012). Development of CBT for chemotherapy-related cognitive change: Results of a waitlist control trial. *Psychooncology*, *21*(2), 176–186. doi: 10.1002/pon.1878

Ferguson, R. J., McDonald, B. C., Saykin, A. J., & Ahles, T. A. (2007). Brain structure and function differences in monozygotic twins: Possible effects of breast cancer chemotherapy. *Journal of Clinical Oncology*, *25*(25), 3866–3870.

Ferreri, A. J., Zucca, E., Armitage, J., Cavalli, F., & Batchelor, T. T. (2013). Ten years of international primary CNS lymphoma collaborative group studies. *Journal of Clinical Oncology*, *31*(27), 3444–3445.

Fike, J. R., Rosi, S., & Limoli, C. L. (2009). Neural precursor cells and central nervous system radiation sensitivity. *Seminars in Radiation Oncology*, *19*(2), 122–132. doi: 10.1016/j.semradonc.2008.12.003

Fishel, M. L., Vasko, M. R., & Kelley, M. R. (2007). DNA repair in neurons: So if they don't divide what's to repair? *Mutation Research*, *614*(1–2), 24–36. doi: 10.1016/j.mrfmmm.2006.06.007

Fliessbach, K., Helmstaedter, C., Urbach, H., Althaus, A., Pels, H., Linnebank, M., . . . Schlegel, U. (2005). Neuropsychological outcome after chemotherapy for primary CNS lymphoma: A prospective study. *Neurology*, *64*(7), 1184–1188. doi: 10.1212/01.WNL.0000156350.49336.E2

Froklage, F. E., Oosterbaan, L. J., Sizoo, E. M., de Groot, M., Bosma, I., Sanchez, E., . . . Postma, T. J. (2013). Central neurotoxicity of standard treatment in patients with newly diagnosed high-grade glioma: A prospective longitudinal study. *Journal of Neuro-Oncology*, *116*(2), 387–394.

Gehring, K., Aaronson, N. K., Taphoorn, M. J., & Sitskoorn, M. M. (2010). Interventions for cognitive deficits in patients with a brain tumor: An update. *Expert Review of Anticancer Therapy*, *10*(11), 1779–1795. doi: 10.1586/era.10.163

Gehring, K., Patwardhan, S. Y., Collins, R., Groves, M. D., Etzel, C. J., Meyers, C. A., & Wefel, J. S. (2012). A randomized trial on the efficacy of methylphenidate and modafinil for improving cognitive functioning and symptoms in patients with a primary brain tumor. *Journal of Neuro-Oncology*, *107*(1), 165–174. doi: 10.1007/s11060-011-0723-1

Gehring, K., Sitskoorn, M. M., Aaronson, N. K., & Taphoorn, M. J. (2008). Interventions for cognitive deficits in adults with brain tumours. *Lancet Neurology*, *7*(6), 548–560. doi: 10.1016/S1474-4422(08)70111-X

Ghia, A., Tome, W. A., Thomas, S., Cannon, G., Khuntia, D., Kuo, J. S., & Mehta, M. P. (2007). Distribution of brain metastases in relation to the hippocampus: Implications for neurocognitive functional preservation. *International Journal of Radiation Oncology Biology Physics*, *68*(4), 971–977. doi: 10.1016/j.ijrobp.2007.02.016

Gilbert, M. R., Dignam, J. J., Armstrong, T. S., Wefel, J. S., Blumenthal, D. T., Vogelbaum, M. A., . . . Mehta, M. P. (2014). A randomized trial of bevacizumab for newly diagnosed glioblastoma. *The New England Journal of Medicine*, *370*(8), 699–708.

Gondi, V., Hermann, B. P., Mehta, M. P., & Tome, W. A. (2013). Hippocampal dosimetry predicts neurocognitive function impairment after fractionated stereotactic radiotherapy for benign or low-grade adult brain tumors. *International Journal of Radiation Oncology Biology Physics*, *85*(2), 348–354. doi: 10.1016/j.ijrobp.2012.11.031

Gondi, V., Mehta, M., Pugh, S., et al. (2013). Memory preservation with conformal avoidance of the hippocampus during whole-brain radiotherapy (WBRT) for patients with brain metastases: Preliminary results of RTOG 0933. *Neuro Oncology*, *15*, 94.

Greenberg, H. S., Chandler, W. F., & Sandler, H. M. (1999). Brain tumor classification, grading and epidemiology. In W. Chandler,

H. S. Greenberg, & H. M. Sandler (Eds.), *Brain Tumors* (p. 1026). New York: Oxford University Press.

Greene-Schloesser, D., Moore, E., & Robbins, M. E. (2013). Molecular pathways: Radiation-induced cognitive impairment. *Clinical Cancer Research, 19*(9), 2294–2300. doi: 10.1158/1078-0432.CCR-11-2903

Greene-Schloesser, D., Robbins, M. E., Peiffer, A. M., Shaw, E. G., Wheeler, K. T., & Chan, M. D. (2012). Radiation-induced brain injury: A review. *Frontiers in Oncology, 2*, 1–18. doi: 10.3389/fonc.2012.00073

Habets, E. J., Taphoorn, M. J., Nederend, S., Klein, M., Delgadillo, D., Hoang-Xuan, K., . . . Reijneveld, J. C. (2014). Health-related quality of life and cognitive functioning in long-term anaplastic oligodendroglioma and oligoastrocytoma survivors. *Journal of Neuro-Oncology, 116*(1), 161–168. doi: 10.1007/s11060-013-1278-0

Hahn, C. A., Zhou, S. M., Raynor, R., Tisch, A., Light, K., Shafman, T., . . . Marks, L. B. (2009). Dose-dependent effects of radiation therapy on cerebral blood flow, metabolism, and neurocognitive dysfunction. *International Journal of Radiation Oncology Biology Physics, 73*(4), 1082–1087. doi: 10.1016/j.ijrobp.2008.05.061

Harder, H., Holtel, H., Bromberg, J. E., Poortmans, P., Haaxma-Reiche, H., Kluin-Nelemans, H. C., . . . van den Bent, M. J. (2004). Cognitive status and quality of life after treatment for primary CNS lymphoma. *Neurology, 62*(4), 544–547.

Hedayati, E., Alinaghizadeh, H., Schedin, A., Nyman, H., & Albertsson, M. (2012). Effects of adjuvant treatment on cognitive function in women with early breast cancer. *European Journal of Oncology Nursing, 16*(3), 315–322. doi: 10.1016/j.ejon.2011.07.006

Herman, M. A., Tremont-Lukats, I., Meyers, C. A., Trask, D. D., Froseth, C., Renschler, M. F., & Mehta, M. P. (2003). Neurocognitive and functional assessment of patients with brain metastases: A pilot study. *American Journal of Clinical Oncology, 26*(3), 273–279. doi: 10.1097/01.COC.0000020585.85901.7C

Hermelink, K., Untch, M., Lux, M. P., Kreienberg, R., Beck, T., Bauerfeind, I., & Munzel, K. (2007). Cognitive function during neoadjuvant chemotherapy for breast cancer: Results of a prospective, multicenter, longitudinal study. *Cancer, 109*(9), 1905–1913. doi: 10.1002/cncr.22610

Hilverda, K., Bosma, I., Heimans, J. J., Postma, T. J., Peter Vandertop, W., Slotman, B. J., . . . Klein, M. (2010). Cognitive functioning in glioblastoma patients during radiotherapy and temozolomide treatment: Initial findings. *Journal of Neuro-Oncology, 97*(1), 89–94. doi: 10.1007/s11060-009-9993-2

Hom, J., & Reitan, R. M. (1984). Neuropsychological correlates of rapidly vs. slowly growing intrinsic cerebral neoplasms. *Journal of Clinical Neuropsychology, 6*(3), 309–324.

Hurria, A., Somlo, G., & Ahles, T. (2007). Renaming "chemobrain." *Cancer Investigation, 25*(6), 373–377. doi: 782023378 [pii] 10.1080/07357900701506672

Imperato, J. P., Paleologos, N. A., & Vick, N. A. (1990). Effects of treatment on long-term survivors with malignant astrocytomas. *Annals of Neurology, 28*(6), 818–822. doi: 10.1002/ana.410280614

Inagaki, M., Yoshikawa, E., Matsuoka, Y., Sugawara, Y., Nakano, T., Akechi, T., . . . Uchitomi, Y. (2007). Smaller regional volumes of brain gray and white matter demonstrated in breast cancer survivors exposed to adjuvant chemotherapy. *Cancer, 109*(1), 146–156.

Jamadar, R. J., Winters, M. J., & Maki, P. M. (2012). Cognitive changes associated with ADT: A review of the literature. *Asian Journal of Andrology, 14*(2), 232–238. doi: 10.1038/aja.2011.107

Jansen, C. E., Cooper, B. A., Dodd, M. J., & Miaskowski, C. A. (2011). A prospective longitudinal study of chemotherapy-induced cognitive changes in breast cancer patients. *Support Care Cancer, 19*(10), 1647–1656. doi: 10.1007/s00520-010-0997-4

Jansen, C. E., Dodd, M. J., Miaskowski, C. A., Dowling, G. A., & Kramer, J. (2008). Preliminary results of a longitudinal study of changes in cognitive function in breast cancer patients undergoing chemotherapy with doxorubicin and cyclophosphamide. *Psychooncology, 17*(12), 1189–1195. doi: 10.1002/pon.1342

Jenkins, V., Shilling, V., Deutsch, G., Bloomfield, D., Morris, R., Allan, S., . . . Winstanley, J. (2006). A 3-year prospective study of the effects of adjuvant treatments on cognition in women with early stage breast cancer. *British Journal of Cancer, 94*(6), 828–834. doi: 10.1038/sj.bjc.6603029

Jim, H. S., Donovan, K. A., Small, B. J., Andrykowski, M. A., Munster, P. N., & Jacobsen, P. B. (2009). Cognitive functioning in breast cancer survivors: A controlled comparison. *Cancer, 115*(8), 1776–1783. doi: 10.1002/cncr.24192

Johnson, D. R., Sawyer, A. M., Meyers, C. A., O'Neill, B. P., & Wefel, J. S. (2012). Early measures of cognitive function predict survival in patients with newly diagnosed glioblastoma. *Neuro Oncology, 14*(6), 808–816. doi: 10.1093/neuonc/nos082

Johnson, D. R., & Wefel, J. S. (2013). Relationship between cognitive function and prognosis in glioblastoma. *CNS Oncology, 2*, 195–201.

Juergens, A., Pels, H., Rogowski, S., Fliessbach, K., Glasmacher, A., Engert, A., . . . Schlegel, U. (2010). Long-term survival with favorable cognitive outcome after chemotherapy in primary central nervous system lymphoma. *Annals of Neurology, 67*(2), 182–189. doi: 10.1002/ana.21824

Kayl, A. E., & Meyers, C. A. (2003). Does brain tumor histology influence cognitive function? *Neuro Oncology, 5*(4), 255–260. doi: 10.1215/S1152851703000012

Keime-Guibert, F., Napolitano, M., & Delattre, J. Y. (1998). Neurological complications of radiotherapy and chemotherapy. *Journal of Neurology, 245*(11), 695–708.

Kesler, S. R., Bennett, F. C., Mahaffey, M. L., & Spiegel, D. (2009). Regional brain activation during verbal declarative memory in metastatic breast cancer. *Clinical Cancer Research, 15*(21), 6665–6673. doi: 10.1158/1078-0432.CCR-09-1227

Kesler, S. R., Hadi Hosseini, S. M., Heckler, C., Janelsins, M., Palesh, O., Mustian, K., & Morrow, G. (2013). Cognitive training for improving executive function in chemotherapy-treated breast cancer survivors. *Clinical Breast Cancer, 13*(4), 299–306. doi: 10.1016/j.clbc.2013.02.004

Kesler, S. R., Janelsins, M., Koovakkattu, D., Palesh, O., Mustian, K., Morrow, G., & Dhabhar, F. S. (2013). Reduced hippocampal volume and verbal memory performance associated with interleukin-6 and tumor necrosis factor-alpha levels in chemotherapy-treated breast cancer survivors. *Brain Behavior and Immunity*, (Suppl 30), S109–S116. doi: 10.1016/j.bbi.2012.05.017

Kesler, S. R., Kent, J. S., & O'Hara, R. (2011). Prefrontal cortex and executive function impairments in primary breast cancer. *Archives of Neurology, 68*(11), 1447–1453. doi: 10.1001/archneurol.2011.245

Khasraw, M., Ashley, D., Wheeler, G., & Berk, M. (2012). Using lithium as a neuroprotective agent in patients with cancer. *BMC Medicine, 10*, 131. doi: 10.1186/1741-7015-10-131

Kiebert, G. M., Curran, D., Aaronson, N. K., Bolla, M., Menten, J., Rutten, E. H., . . . Karim, A. B. (1998). Quality of life after radiation therapy of cerebral low-grade gliomas of the adult: Results of a randomised phase III trial on dose response (EORTC trial 22844). EORTC Radiotherapy Co-operative Group. *European Journal of Cancer*, *34*(12), 1902–1909.

Kim, J. H., Brown, S. L., Jenrow, K. A., & Ryu, S. (2008). Mechanisms of radiation-induced brain toxicity and implications for future clinical trials. *Journal of Neuro-Oncology*, *87*(3), 279–286. doi: 10.1007/s11060-008-9520-x

Klein, M. (2012). Neurocognitive functioning in adult WHO grade II gliomas: Impact of old and new treatment modalities. *Neuro Oncology*, *14*(Suppl 4), iv17–24. doi: 10.1093/neuonc/nos161

Klein, M., Heimans, J. J., Aaronson, N. K., van der Ploeg, H. M., Grit, J., Muller, M., . . . Taphoorn, M. J. (2002). Effect of radiotherapy and other treatment-related factors on mid-term to long-term cognitive sequelae in low-grade gliomas: A comparative study. *Lancet*, *360*(9343), 1361–1368.

Klein, M., Postma, T. J., Taphoorn, M. J., Aaronson, N. K., Vandertop, W. P., Muller, M., . . . Heimans, J. J. (2003). The prognostic value of cognitive functioning in the survival of patients with high-grade glioma. *Neurology*, *61*(12), 1796–1798.

Klein, M., Taphoorn, M. J., Heimans, J. J., van der Ploeg, H. M., Vandertop, W. P., Smit, E. F., . . . Aaronson, N. K. (2001). Neurobehavioral status and health-related quality of life in newly diagnosed high-grade glioma patients. *Journal of Clinical Oncology*, *19*(20), 4037–4047.

Kleinberg, L., Wallner, K., & Malkin, M. G. (1993). Good performance status of long-term disease-free survivors of intracranial gliomas. *International Journal of Radiation Oncology Biology Physics*, *26*(1), 129–133.

Kocher, M., Soffietti, R., Abacioglu, U., Villa, S., Fauchon, F., Baumert, B. G., . . . Mueller, R. P. (2011). Adjuvant whole-brain radiotherapy versus observation after radiosurgery or surgical resection of one to three cerebral metastases: Results of the EORTC 22952–26001 study. *Journal of Clinical Oncology*, *29*(2), 134–141. doi: 10.1200/JCO.2010.30.1655

Kohli, S., Fisher, S. G., Tra, Y., Adams, M. J., Mapstone, M. E., Wesnes, K. A., . . . Morrow, G. R. (2009). The effect of modafinil on cognitive function in breast cancer survivors. *Cancer*, *115*(12), 2605–2616. doi: 10.1002/cncr.24287

Koppelmans, V., Breteler, M. M., Boogerd, W., Seynaeve, C., Gundy, C., & Schagen, S. B. (2012). Neuropsychological performance in survivors of breast cancer more than 20 years after adjuvant chemotherapy. *Journal of Clinical Oncology*, *30*(10), 1080–1086. doi: 10.1200/JCO.2011.37.0189

Koppelmans, V., de Groot, M., de Ruiter, M. B., Boogerd, W., Seynaeve, C., Vernooij, M. W., . . . Breteler, M. M. (2014). Global and focal white matter integrity in breast cancer survivors 20 years after adjuvant chemotherapy. *Human Brain Mapping*, *35*(3), 889–899. doi: 10.1002/hbm.22221

Koppelmans, V., de Ruiter, M. B., van der Lijn, F., Boogerd, W., Seynaeve, C., van der Lugt, A., . . . Schagen, S. B. (2011). Global and focal brain volume in long-term breast cancer survivors exposed to adjuvant chemotherapy. *Breast Cancer Research and Treatment*. doi: 10.1007/s10549-011-1888-1

Laack, N. N., Brown, P. D., Furth, A., et al. (2003). Neurocognitive function after radiotherapy (RT) for supratentorial low-grade gliomas (LGG): Results of a north central cancer treatment group (NCCTG) prospective study. *International Journal of Radiation Oncology Biology Physics*, *57*, S134.

Lassman, A. B., & DeAngelis, L. M. (2003). Brain metastases. *Neurologic Clinics*, *21*(1), 1–23, vii.

Lee, W. H., Sonntag, W. E., Mitschelen, M., Yan, H., & Lee, Y. W. (2010). Irradiation induces regionally specific alterations in pro-inflammatory environments in rat brain. *International Journal of Radiation Biology*, *86*(2), 132–144. doi: 10.3109/09553000903419346

Levin, V. A., Bidaut, L., Hou, P., Kumar, A. J., Wefel, J. S., Bekele, B. N., . . . Jackson, E. F. (2011). Randomized double-blind placebo-controlled trial of bevacizumab therapy for radiation necrosis of the central nervous system. *International Journal of Radiation Oncology Biology Physics*, *79*(5), 1487–1495. doi: 10.1016/j.ijrobp.2009.12.061

Li, J., Bentzen, S. M., Renschler, M., & Mehta, M. P. (2007). Regression after whole-brain radiation therapy for brain metastases correlates with survival and improved neurocognitive function. *Journal of Clinical Oncology*, *25*(10), 1260–1266. doi: 10.1200/JCO.2006.09.2536

Lin, N. U., Wefel, J. S., Lee, E. Q., et al. (2013). Challenges relating to solid tumour brain metastases in clinical trials, part 2: Neurocognitive, neurological, and quality-o-life outcomes: A report from the RANO group. *Lancet Oncology*, *14*, e407–416.

Locke, D. E., Cerhan, J. H., Wu, W., Malec, J. F., Clark, M. M., Rummans, T. A., & Brown, P. D. (2008). Cognitive rehabilitation and problem-solving to improve quality of life of patients with primary brain tumors: A pilot study. *The Journal of Supportive Oncology*, *6*(8), 383–391.

Lopez Zunini, R. A., Scherling, C., Wallis, N., Collins, B., MacKenzie, J., Bielajew, C., & Smith, A. M. (2013). Differences in verbal memory retrieval in breast cancer chemotherapy patients compared to healthy controls: A prospective fMRI study. *Brain Imaging and Behavior*, *7*(4), 460–477. doi: 10.1007/s11682-012-9213-0

Lower, E. E., Fleishman, S., Cooper, A., Zeldis, J., Faleck, H., Yu, Z., & Manning, D. (2009). Efficacy of dexmethylphenidate for the treatment of fatigue after cancer chemotherapy: a randomized clinical trial. *Journal of Pain and Symptom Management*, *38*, 650–662.

Lubelski, D., Abdullah, K. G., Weil, R. J., & Marko, N. F. (2013). Bevacizumab for radiation necrosis following treatment of high grade glioma: A systematic review of the literature. *Journal of Neuro-Oncology*, *115*(3), 317–322. doi: 10.1007/s11060-013-1233-0

Lundorff, L. E., Jonsson, B. H., & Sjogren, P. (2009). Modafinil for attentional and psychomotor dysfunction in advanced cancer: A double-blind, randomised, cross-over trial. *Palliative Medicine*, *23*(8), 731–738. doi: 10.1177/0269216309106872

Lupien, S. J., Gillin, C. J., & Hauger, R. L. (1999). Working memory is more sensitive than declarative memory to the acute effects of corticosteroids: A dose-response study in humans. *Behavioral Neuroscience*, *113*(3), 420–430.

Madsen, T. M., Kristjansen, P. E., Bolwig, T. G., & Wortwein, G. (2003). Arrested neuronal proliferation and impaired hippocampal function following fractionated brain irradiation in the adult rat. *Neuroscience*, *119*(3), 635–642.

Mar Fan, H. G., Clemons, M., Xu, W., Chemerynsky, I., Breunis, H., Braganza, S., & Tannock, I. F. (2008). A randomised, placebo-controlled, double-blind trial of the effects of d-methylphenidate on fatigue and cognitive dysfunction in women undergoing adjuvant chemotherapy for breast cancer. *Support Care Cancer*, *16*(6), 577–583. doi: 10.1007/s00520-007-0341-9

Mauer, M., Stupp, R., Taphoorn, M. J., Coens, C., Osoba, D., Marosi, C., . . . Bottomley, A. (2007). The prognostic value of health-related quality-of-life data in predicting survival in glioblastoma cancer patients: Results from an international randomised phase III EORTC Brain Tumour and Radiation Oncology Groups, and NCIC Clinical Trials Group study. *British Journal of Cancer*, *97*(3), 302–307. doi: 10.1038/sj.bjc.6603876

McAllister, L. D., Doolittle, N. D., Guastadisegni, P. E., Kraemer, D. F., Lacy, C. A., Crossen, J. R., & Neuwelt, E. A. (2000). Cognitive outcomes and long-term follow-up results after enhanced chemotherapy delivery for primary central nervous system lymphoma. *Neurosurgery*, *46*(1), 51–60; discussion 60–51.

McDonald, B. C., Conroy, S. K., Ahles, T. A., West, J. D., & Saykin, A. J. (2010). Gray matter reduction associated with systemic chemotherapy for breast cancer: A prospective MRI study. *Breast Cancer Research and Treatment*.

McDonald, B. C., Conroy, S. K., Ahles, T. A., West, J. D., & Saykin, A. J. (2012). Alterations in brain activation during working memory processing associated with breast cancer and treatment: A prospective functional magnetic resonance imaging study. *Journal of Clinical Oncology*, *30*(20), 2500–2508. doi: 10.1200/JCO.2011.38.5674

McDonald, B. C., Conroy, S. K., Smith, D. J., West, J. D., & Saykin, A. J. (2013). Frontal gray matter reduction after breast cancer chemotherapy and association with executive symptoms: A replication and extension study. *Brain Behavior and Immunity*, (Suppl 30), S117–125. doi: 10.1016/j.bbi.2012.05.007

McDonald, B. C., & Saykin, A. J. (2013). Alterations in brain structure related to breast cancer and its treatment: Chemotherapy and other considerations. *Brain Imaging and Behavior*, *7*(4), 374–387. doi: 10.1007/s11682-013-9256-x

McDuff, S. G., Taich, Z. J., Lawson, J. D., Sanghvi, P., Wong, E. T., Barker, F. G., 2nd, . . . Chen, C. C. (2013). Neurocognitive assessment following whole brain radiation therapy and radiosurgery for patients with cerebral metastases. *Journal of Neurology, Neurosurgery, and Psychiatry*, *84*(12), 1384–1391. doi: 10.1136/jnnp-2013-305166

Mehlsen, M., Pedersen, A. D., Jensen, A. B., & Zachariae, R. (2009). No indications of cognitive side-effects in a prospective study of breast cancer patients receiving adjuvant chemotherapy. *Psychooncology*, *18*(3), 248–257. doi: 10.1002/pon.1398

Mehnert, A., Scherwath, A., Schirmer, L., Schleimer, B., Petersen, C., Schulz-Kindermann, F., . . . Koch, U. (2007). The association between neuropsychological impairment, self-perceived cognitive deficits, fatigue and health related quality of life in breast cancer survivors following standard adjuvant versus high-dose chemotherapy. *Patient Education and Counseling*, *66*(1), 108–118. doi: 10.1016/j.pec.2006.11.005

Mehta, M. P., Shapiro, W. R., Phan, S. C., Gervais, R., Carrie, C., Chabot, P., . . . Renschler, M. F. (2009). Motexafin gadolinium combined with prompt whole brain radiotherapy prolongs time to neurologic progression in non-small-cell lung cancer patients with brain metastases: Results of a phase III trial. *International Journal of Radiation Oncology Biology Physics*, *73*(4), 1069–1076. doi: 10.1016/j.ijrobp.2008.05.068

Mehta, M. P., & Tremont-Lukas, I. (2004). *Radiosurgery for Single and Multiple Metastases*. Malden, MA: Blackwell.

Meyers, C. A., & Brown, P. D. (2006). Role and relevance of neurocognitive assessment in clinical trials of patients with CNS tumors. *Journal of Clinical Oncology*, *24*(8), 1305–1309. doi: 10.1200/JCO.2005.04.6086

Meyers, C. A., & Hess, K. R. (2003). Multifaceted end points in brain tumor clinical trials: Cognitive deterioration precedes MRI progression. *Neuro Oncology*, *5*(2), 89–95. doi: 10.1215/S1522-8517-02-00026-1

Meyers, C. A., Hess, K. R., Yung, W. K., & Levin, V. A. (2000). Cognitive function as a predictor of survival in patients with recurrent malignant glioma. *Journal of Clinical Oncology*, *18*(3), 646–650.

Meyers, C. A., Smith, J. A., Bezjak, A., Mehta, M. P., Liebmann, J., Illidge, T., . . . Renschler, M. F. (2004). Neurocognitive function and progression in patients with brain metastases treated with whole-brain radiation and motexafin gadolinium: Results of a randomized phase III trial. *Journal of Clinical Oncology*, *22*(1), 157–165. doi: 10.1200/JCO.2004.05.128

Meyers, C. A., & Wefel, J. S. (2003). The use of the mini-mental state examination to assess cognitive functioning in cancer trials: No ifs, ands, buts, or sensitivity. *Journal of Clinical Oncology*, *21*(19), 3557–3558. doi: 10.1200/JCO.2003.07.080

Monaco, E. A., 3rd, Faraji, A. H., Berkowitz, O., Parry, P. V., Hadelsberg, U., Kano, H., . . . Lunsford, L. D. (2013). Leukoencephalopathy after whole-brain radiation therapy plus radiosurgery versus radiosurgery alone for metastatic lung cancer. *Cancer*, *119*(1), 226–232. doi: 10.1002/cncr.27504

Monje, M. L., & Dietrich, J. (2012). Cognitive side effects of cancer therapy demonstrate a functional role for adult neurogenesis. *Behavioural Brain Research*, *227*(2), 376–379. doi: 10.1016/j.bbr.2011.05.012

Monje, M. L., Toda, H., & Palmer, T. D. (2003). Inflammatory blockade restores adult hippocampal neurogenesis. *Science*, *302*(5651), 1760–1765. doi: 10.1126/science.1088417

Monje, M. L., Vogel, H., Masek, M., Ligon, K. L., Fisher, P. G., & Palmer, T. D. (2007). Impaired human hippocampal neurogenesis after treatment for central nervous system malignancies. *Annals of Neurology*, *62*(5), 515–520. doi: 10.1002/ana.21214

Morris, P. G., Correa, D. D., Yahalom, J., Raizer, J. J., Schiff, D., Grant, B., . . . Omuro, A. (2013). Rituximab, methotrexate, procarbazine, and vincristine followed by consolidation reduced-dose whole-brain radiotherapy and cytarabine in newly diagnosed primary CNS lymphoma: Final results and long-term outcome. *Journal of Clinical Oncology*, *31*(31), 3971–3979. doi: 10.1200/JCO.2013.50.4910

Nagesh, V., Tsien, C. I., Chenevert, T. L., Ross, B. D., Lawrence, T. S., Junick, L., & Cao, Y. (2008). Radiation-induced changes in normal-appearing white matter in patients with cerebral tumors: A diffusion tensor imaging study. *International Journal of Radiation Oncology Biology Physics*, *70*(4), 1002–1010. doi: 10.1016/j.ijrobp.2007.08.020

Nelson, C. J., Lee, J. S., Gamboa, M. C., & Roth, A. J. (2008). Cognitive effects of hormone therapy in men with prostate cancer: A review. *Cancer*, *113*(5), 1097–1106. doi: 10.1002/cncr.23658

Neuwelt, E. A., Goldman, D. L., Dahlborg, S. A., Crossen, J., Ramsey, F., Roman-Goldstein, S., . . . Dana, B. (1991). Primary CNS lymphoma treated with osmotic blood-brain barrier disruption: Prolonged survival and preservation of cognitive function. *Journal of Clinical Oncology*, *9*(9), 1580–1590.

Noble, M., & Dietrich, J. (2002). Intersections between neurobiology and oncology: Tumor origin, treatment and repair of treatment-associated damage. *Trends in Neurosciences*, *25*(2), 103–107.

Nordal, R. A., & Wong, C. S. (2005). Molecular targets in radiation-induced blood-brain barrier disruption. *International Journal of Radiation Oncology Biology Physics*, *62*(1), 279–287. doi: 10.1016/j.ijrobp.2005.01.039

Peiffer, A. M., Leyrer, C. M., Greene-Schloesser, D. M., Shing, E., Kearns, W. T., Hinson, W. H., . . . Chan, M. D. (2013).

Neuroanatomical target theory as a predictive model for radiation-induced cognitive decline. *Neurology*, *80*(8), 747–753. doi: 10.1212/WNL.0b013e318283bb0a

Pels, H., Schmidt-Wolf, I. G., Glasmacher, A., Schulz, H., Engert, A., Diehl, V., . . . Schlegel, U. (2003). Primary central nervous system lymphoma: Results of a pilot and phase II study of systemic and intraventricular chemotherapy with deferred radiotherapy. *Journal of Clinical Oncology*, *21*(24), 4489–4495. doi: 10.1200/JCO.2003.04.056

Platta, C. S., Khuntia, D., Mehta, M. P., & Suh, J. H. (2010). Current treatment strategies for brain metastasis and complications from therapeutic techniques: A review of current literature. *American Journal of Clinical Oncology*, *33*(4), 398–407. doi: 10.1097/COC.0b013e318194f744

Pomykala, K. L., Ganz, P. A., Bower, J. E., Kwan, L., Castellon, S. A., Mallam, S., . . . Silverman, D. H. (2013). The association between pro-inflammatory cytokines, regional cerebral metabolism, and cognitive complaints following adjuvant chemotherapy for breast cancer. *Brain Imaging and Behavior*, *7*(4), 511–523. doi: 10.1007/s11682-013-9243-2

Poortmans, P. M., Kluin-Nelemans, H. C., Haaxma-Reiche, H., Van't Veer, M., Hansen, M., Soubeyran, P., . . . Treatment of Cancer Lymphoma, G. (2003). High-dose methotrexate-based chemotherapy followed by consolidating radiotherapy in non-AIDS-related primary central nervous system lymphoma: European Organization for Research and Treatment of Cancer Lymphoma Group Phase II Trial 20962. *Journal of Clinical Oncology*, *21*(24), 4483–4488. doi: 10.1200/JCO.2003.03.108

Poppelreuter, M., Weis, J., & Bartsch, H. H. (2009). Effects of specific neuropsychological training programs for breast cancer patients after adjuvant chemotherapy. *Journal of Psychosocial Oncology*, *27*(2), 274–296. doi: 10.1080/07347330902776044

Poppelreuter, M., Weis, J., Kulz, A. K., Tucha, O., Lange, K. W., & Bartsch, H. H. (2004). Cognitive dysfunction and subjective complaints of cancer patients: A cross-sectional study in a cancer rehabilitation centre. *European Journal of Cancer*, *40*(1), 43–49.

Postma, T. J., Klein, M., Verstappen, C. C., Bromberg, J. E., Swennen, M., Langendijk, J. A., . . . Heimans, J. J. (2002). Radiotherapy-induced cerebral abnormalities in patients with low-grade glioma. *Neurology*, *59*(1), 121–123.

Postma, T. J., van Groeningen, C. J., Witjes, R. J., Weerts, J. G., Kralendonk, J. H., & Heimans, J. J. (1998). Neurotoxicity of combination chemotherapy with procarbazine, CCNU and vincristine (PCV) for recurrent glioma. *Journal of Neuro-Oncology*, *38*(1), 69–75.

Quesnel, C., Savard, J., & Ivers, H. (2009). Cognitive impairments associated with breast cancer treatments: Results from a longitudinal study. *Breast Cancer Research and Treatment*, *116*(1), 113–123. doi: 10.1007/s10549-008-0114-2

Raber, J., Rola, R., LeFevour, A., Morhardt, D., Curley, J., Mizumatsu, S., . . . Fike, J. R. (2004). Radiation-induced cognitive impairments are associated with changes in indicators of hippocampal neurogenesis. *Radiation Research*, *162*(1), 39–47.

Reardon, D. A., Galanis, E., DeGroot, J. F., Cloughesy, T. F., Wefel, J. S., Lamborn, K. R., . . . Wen, P. Y. (2011). Clinical trial end points for high-grade glioma: The evolving landscape. *Neuro Oncology*, *13*(3), 353–361. doi: 10.1093/neuonc/noq203

Regine, W. F., Schmitt, F. A., Scott, C. B., Dearth, C., Patchell, R. A., Nichols, R. C., Jr., . . . Mehta, M. P. (2004). Feasibility of neurocognitive outcome evaluations in patients with brain metastases in a multi-institutional cooperative group setting: Results of Radiation Therapy Oncology Group trial BR-0018. *International Journal of Radiation Oncology Biology Physics*, *58*(5), 1346–1352. doi: 10.1016/j.ijrobp.2003.09.023

Reid, L. M., & Maclullich, A. M. (2006). Subjective memory complaints and cognitive impairment in older people. *Dementia and Geriatric Cognitive Disorders*, *22*(5–6), 471–485. doi: 10.1159/000096295

Reuter-Lorenz, P. A., & Cimprich, B. (2013). Cognitive function and breast cancer: Promise and potential insights from functional brain imaging. *Breast Cancer Research and Treatment*, *137*(1), 33–43. doi: 10.1007/s10549-012-2266-3

Rubenstein, J. L., Ferreri, A. J., & Pittaluga, S. (2008). Primary lymphoma of the central nervous system: Epidemiology, pathology and current approaches to diagnosis, prognosis and treatment. *Leuk Lymphoma*, *49*(Supplement), 43–51.

Rubenstein, J. L., Hsi, E. D., Johnson, J. L., Jung, S. H., Nakashima, M. O., Grant, B., . . . Kaplan, L. D. (2013). Intensive chemotherapy and immunotherapy in patients with newly diagnosed primary CNS lymphoma: CALGB 50202 (Alliance 50202). *Journal of Clinical Oncology*, *31*(25), 3061–3068. doi: 10.1200/JCO.2012.46.9957

Rzeski, W., Pruskil, S., Macke, A., Felderhoff-Mueser, U., Reiher, A. K., Hoerster, F., . . . Ikonomidou, C. (2004). Anticancer agents are potent neurotoxins in vitro and in vivo. *Annals of Neurology*, *56*(3), 351–360. doi: 10.1002/ana.20185

Salander, P., Karlsson, T., Bergenheim, T., & Henriksson, R. (1995). Long-term memory deficits in patients with malignant gliomas. *Journal of Neuro-Oncology*, *25*(3), 227–238.

Schagen, S. B., Boogerd, W., Muller, M. J., Huinink, W. T., Moonen, L., Meinhardt, W., & Van Dam, F. S. (2008). Cognitive complaints and cognitive impairment following BEP chemotherapy in patients with testicular cancer. *Acta Oncologica*, *47*(1), 63–70. doi: 10.1080/02841860701518058

Schagen, S. B., Das, E., & van Dam, F. S. (2009). The influence of priming and pre-existing knowledge of chemotherapy-associated cognitive complaints on the reporting of such complaints in breast cancer patients. *Psychooncology*, *18*(6), 674–678. doi: 10.1002/pon.1454

Schagen, S. B., Muller, M. J., Boogerd, W., Mellenbergh, G. J., & van Dam, F. S. (2006). Change in cognitive function after chemotherapy: A prospective longitudinal study in breast cancer patients. *Journal of the National Cancer Institute*, *98*(23), 1742–1745. doi: 98/23/1742 [pii] 10.1093/jnci/djj470

Schagen, S. B., van Dam, F. S., Muller, M. J., Boogerd, W., Lindeboom, J., & Bruning, P. F. (1999). Cognitive deficits after postoperative adjuvant chemotherapy for breast carcinoma. *Cancer*, *85*(3), 640–650. doi: 10.1002/(SICI)1097-0142(19990201)85:3<640::AID-CNCR14>3.0.CO;2-G [pii]

Scheibel, R. S., Meyers, C. A., & Levin, V. A. (1996). Cognitive dysfunction following surgery for intracerebral glioma: Influence of histopathology, lesion location, and treatment. *Journal of Neuro-Oncology*, *30*(1), 61–69.

Scherling, C., Collins, B., Mackenzie, J., Bielajew, C., & Smith, A. (2011). Pre-chemotherapy differences in visuospatial working memory in breast cancer patients compared to controls: An FMRI study. *Frontiers in Human Neuroscience*, *5*, 122. doi: 10.3389/fnhum.2011.00122

Scherwath, A., Mehnert, A., Schleimer, B., Schirmer, L., Fehlauer, F., Kreienberg, R., . . . Koch, U. (2006). Neuropsychological function in high-risk breast cancer survivors after stem-cell supported high-dose therapy versus standard-dose chemotherapy: Evaluation of long-term treatment effects. *Annals of Oncology, 17*(3), 415–423. doi: mdj108 [pii] 10.1093/annonc/mdj108

Seigers, R., Schagen, S. B., Coppens, C. M., van der Most, P. J., van Dam, F. S., Koolhaas, J. M., & Buwalda, B. (2009). Methotrexate decreases hippocampal cell proliferation and induces memory deficits in rats. *Behavioural Brain Research, 201*(2), 279–284. doi: 10.1016/j.bbr.2009.02.025

Shaw, E. G., Arusell, R., Scheithauer, B., O'Fallon, J., O'Neill, B., Dinapoli, R., . . . Abrams, R. (2002). Prospective randomized trial of low- versus high-dose radiation therapy in adults with supratentorial low-grade glioma: Initial report of a North Central Cancer Treatment Group/Radiation Therapy Oncology Group/Eastern Cooperative Oncology Group study. *Journal of Clinical Oncology, 20*(9), 2267–2276.

Shaw, E. G., Rosdhal, R., D'Agostino, R. B., Jr., Lovato, J., Naughton, M. J., Robbins, M. E., & Rapp, S. R. (2006). Phase II study of donepezil in irradiated brain tumor patients: Effect on cognitive function, mood, and quality of life. *Journal of Clinical Oncology, 24*(9), 1415–1420. doi: 10.1200/JCO.2005.03.3001

Sheline, G. E., Wara, W. M., & Smith, V. (1980). Therapeutic irradiation and brain injury. *International Journal of Radiation Oncology Biology Physics, 6*(9), 1215–1228.

Sherer, M., Meyers, C. A., & Bergloff, P. (1997). Efficacy of postacute brain injury rehabilitation for patients with primary malignant brain tumors. *Cancer, 80*(2), 250–257.

Shilling, V., & Jenkins, V. (2007). Self-reported cognitive problems in women receiving adjuvant therapy for breast cancer. *European Journal of Oncology Nursing, 11*(1), 6–15. doi: 10.1016/j.ejon.2006.02.005

Shilling, V., Jenkins, V., Morris, R., Deutsch, G., & Bloomfield, D. (2005). The effects of adjuvant chemotherapy on cognition in women with breast cancer–preliminary results of an observational longitudinal study. *Breast, 14*(2), 142–150. doi: S0960-9776(04)00215-2 [pii] 10.1016/j.breast.2004.10.004

Silverman, D. H., Dy, C. J., Castellon, S. A., Lai, J., Pio, B. S., Abraham, L., . . . Ganz, P. A. (2007). Altered frontocortical, cerebellar, and basal ganglia activity in adjuvant-treated breast cancer survivors 5–10 years after chemotherapy. *Breast Cancer Research and Treatment, 103*(3), 303–311. doi: 10.1007/s10549-006-9380-z

Small, B. J., Rawson, K. S., Walsh, E., Jim, H. S., Hughes, T. F., Iser, L., . . . Jacobsen, P. B. (2011). Catechol-O-methyltransferase genotype modulates cancer treatment-related cognitive deficits in breast cancer survivors. *Cancer, 117*(7), 1369–1376. doi: 10.1002/cncr.25685

Soffietti, R., Baumert, B. G., Bello, L., von Deimling, A., Duffau, H., Frenay, M., . . . European Federation of Neurological, S. (2010). Guidelines on management of low-grade gliomas: Report of an EFNS-EANO Task Force. *European Journal of Neurology, 17*(9), 1124–1133. doi: 10.1111/j.1468-1331.2010.03151.x

Stewart, A., Collins, B., Mackenzie, J., Tomiak, E., Verma, S., & Bielajew, C. (2008). The cognitive effects of adjuvant chemotherapy in early stage breast cancer: A prospective study. *Psychooncology, 17*(2), 122–130. doi: 10.1002/pon.1210

Stupp, R., Mason, W. P., van den Bent, M. J., Weller, M., Fisher, B., Taphoorn, M. J., . . . Mirimanoff, R. O. (2005). Radiotherapy plus concomitant and adjuvant temozolomide for glioblastoma. *The New England Journal of Medicine, 352*(10), 987–996. doi: 10.1056/NEJMoa043330

Surma-aho, O., Niemela, M., Vilkki, J., Kouri, M., Brander, A., Salonen, O., . . . Jaaskelainen, J. (2001). Adverse long-term effects of brain radiotherapy in adult low-grade glioma patients. *Neurology, 56*(10), 1285–1290.

Syrjala, K. L., Artherholt, S. B., Kurland, B. F., Langer, S. L., Roth-Roemer, S., Elrod, J. B., & Dikmen, S. (2011). Prospective neurocognitive function over 5 years after allogeneic hematopoietic cell transplantation for cancer survivors compared with matched controls at 5 years. *Journal of Clinical Oncology, 29*(17), 2397–2404. doi: 10.1200/JCO.2010.33.9119

Syrjala, K. L., Dikmen, S., Langer, S. L., Roth-Roemer, S., & Abrams, J. R. (2004). Neuropsychologic changes from before transplantation to 1 year in patients receiving myeloablative allogeneic hematopoietic cell transplant. *Blood, 104*(10), 3386–3392. doi: 10.1182/blood-2004-03-1155

Tager, F. A., McKinley, P. S., Schnabel, F. R., El-Tamer, M., Cheung, Y. K., Fang, Y., . . . Hershman, D. L. (2010). The cognitive effects of chemotherapy in post-menopausal breast cancer patients: A controlled longitudinal study. *Breast Cancer Research and Treatment, 123*(1), 25–34. doi: 10.1007/s10549-009-0606-8

Taphoorn, M. J., & Klein, M. (2004). Cognitive deficits in adult patients with brain tumours. *Lancet Neurology, 3*(3), 159–168. doi: 10.1016/S1474-4422(04)00680-5

Taphoorn, M. J., Schiphorst, A. K., Snoek, F. J., Lindeboom, J., Wolbers, J. G., Karim, A. B., . . . Heimans, J. J. (1994). Cognitive functions and quality of life in patients with low-grade gliomas: The impact of radiotherapy. *Annals of Neurology, 36*(1), 48–54. doi: 10.1002/ana.410360111

Thiel, E., Korfel, A., Martus, P., Kanz, L., Griesinger, F., Rauch, M., . . . Weller, M. (2010). High-dose methotrexate with or without whole brain radiotherapy for primary CNS lymphoma (G-PCNSL-SG-1): A phase 3, randomised, non-inferiority trial. *Lancet Oncology, 11*(11), 1036–1047. doi: 10.1016/S1470-2045(10)70229-1

Tofilon, P. J., & Fike, J. R. (2000). The radioresponse of the central nervous system: A dynamic process. *Radiation Research, 153*(4), 357–370.

Torcuator, R., Zuniga, R., Mohan, Y. S., Rock, J., Doyle, T., Anderson, J., . . . Mikkelsen, T. (2009). Initial experience with bevacizumab treatment for biopsy confirmed cerebral radiation necrosis. *Journal of Neuro-Oncology, 94*(1), 63–68. doi: 10.1007/s11060-009-9801-z

Torres, I. J., Mundt, A. J., Sweeney, P. J., Llanes-Macy, S., Dunaway, L., Castillo, M., & Macdonald, R. L. (2003). A longitudinal neuropsychological study of partial brain radiation in adults with brain tumors. *Neurology, 60*(7), 1113–1118.

van Breemen, M. S., Wilms, E. B., & Vecht, C. J. (2007). Epilepsy in patients with brain tumours: Epidemiology, mechanisms, and management. *Lancet Neurology, 6*(5), 421–430. doi: 10.1016/S1474-4422(07)70103-5

van Dam, F. S., Schagen, S. B., Muller, M. J., Boogerd, W., vd Wall, E., Droogleever Fortuyn, M. E., & Rodenhuis, S. (1998). Impairment of cognitive function in women receiving adjuvant treatment for high-risk breast cancer: High-dose versus standard-dose chemotherapy. *Journal of the National Cancer Institute, 90*(3), 210–218.

van den Bent, M. J., Wefel, J. S., Schiff, D., Taphoorn, M. J., Jaeckle, K., Junck, L., . . . Jacobs, A. H. (2011). Response assessment in neuro-oncology (a report of the RANO group): Assessment of outcome in trials of diffuse low-grade gliomas. *Lancet Oncology, 12*(6), 583–593. doi: 10.1016/S1470-2045(11)70057-2

Vearncombe, K. J., Rolfe, M., Wright, M., Pachana, N. A., Andrew, B., & Beadle, G. (2009). Predictors of cognitive decline after chemotherapy in breast cancer patients. *Journal of the International Neuropsychological Society*, *15*(6), 951–962. doi: 10.1017/S1355617709990567

Von Ah, D., Carpenter, J. S., Saykin, A., Monahan, P., Wu, J., Yu, M., . . . Unverzagt, F. (2012). Advanced cognitive training for breast cancer survivors: A randomized controlled trial. *Breast Cancer Research and Treatment*, *135*(3), 799–809. doi: 10.1007/s10549-012-2210-6

Warrington, J. P., Ashpole, N., Csiszar, A., Lee, Y. W., Ungvari, Z., & Sonntag, W. E. (2013). Whole brain radiation-induced vascular cognitive impairment: Mechanisms and implications. *Journal of Vascular Research*, *50*(6), 445–457. doi: 10.1159/000354227

Wefel, J. S., Cloughesy, T., Zazzali, J. L., Zheng, M., Prados, M., Wen, P. Y., . . . Friedman, H. S. (2011). Neurocognitive function in patients with recurrent glioblastoma treated with bevacizumab. *Neuro Oncology*, *13*(6), 660–668. doi: 10.1093/neuonc/nor024

Wefel, J. S., Kayl, A. E., & Meyers, C. A. (2004). Neuropsychological dysfunction associated with cancer and cancer therapies: A conceptual review of an emerging target. *British Journal of Cancer*, *90*(9), 1691–1696. doi: 10.1038/sj.bjc.6601772

Wefel, J. S., Lenzi, R., Theriault, R. L., Buzdar, A. U., Cruickshank, S., & Meyers, C. A. (2004). 'Chemobrain' in breast carcinoma? A prologue. *Cancer*, *101*(3), 466–475. doi: 10.1002/cncr.20393

Wefel, J. S., Lenzi, R., Theriault, R. L., Davis, R. N., & Meyers, C. A. (2004). The cognitive sequelae of standard-dose adjuvant chemotherapy in women with breast carcinoma: Results of a prospective, randomized, longitudinal trial. *Cancer*, *100*(11), 2292–2299. doi: 10.1002/cncr.20272

Wefel, J. S., Saleeba, A. K., Buzdar, A. U., & Meyers, C. A. (2010). Acute and late onset cognitive dysfunction associated with chemotherapy in women with breast cancer. *Cancer*, *116*(14), 3348–3356. doi: 10.1002/cncr.25098

Weitzner, M. A., & Meyers, C. A. (1997). Cognitive functioning and quality of life in malignant glioma patients: A review of the literature. *Psycho-Oncology*, *6*(3), 169–177. doi: 10.1002/(SICI)1099-1611(199709)6:3<169::AID-PON269>3.0.CO;2-#

Welzel, G., Fleckenstein, K., Schaefer, J., Hermann, B., Kraus-Tiefenbacher, U., Mai, S. K., & Wenz, F. (2008). Memory function before and after whole brain radiotherapy in patients with and without brain metastases. *International Journal of Radiation Oncology Biology Physics*, *72*(5), 1311–1318. doi: 10.1016/j.ijrobp.2008.03.009

Winocur, G., Vardy, J., Binns, M. A., Kerr, L., & Tannock, I. (2006). The effects of the anti-cancer drugs, methotrexate and 5-fluorouracil, on cognitive function in mice. *Pharmacology Biochemistry and Behavior*, *85*(1), 66–75. doi: 10.1016/j.pbb.2006.07.010

Yamada, T. H., Denburg, N. L., Beglinger, L. J., & Schultz, S. K. (2010). Neuropsychological outcomes of older breast cancer survivors: Cognitive features ten or more years after chemotherapy. *The Journal of Neuropsychiatry and Clinical Neurosciences*, *22*(1), 48–54.

Yoshikawa, E., Matsuoka, Y., Inagaki, M., Nakano, T., Akechi, T., Kobayakawa, M., . . . Uchitomi, Y. (2005). No adverse effects of adjuvant chemotherapy on hippocampal volume in Japanese breast cancer survivors. *Breast Cancer Research and Treatment*, *92*(1), 81–84. doi: 10.1007/s10549-005-1412-6

24 Toxins in the Central Nervous System

Marc W. Haut, Jennifer Wiener Hartzell, and Maria T. Moran

Introduction

In this chapter, we review a variety of substances that are toxic to the brain. It is beyond the scope of this chapter to cover all toxins; thus, we focus on the most common, most well-studied, and those which we believe are the most interesting. We refer readers to more comprehensive reviews when greater depth is warranted. We begin with toxins occurring most commonly in the workplace, including heavy metals and solvents, and then discuss carbon monoxide poisoning, which may occur at work or at home. We then discuss substances of abuse and complete our review with a description of the neurotoxic effects of chemotherapy for non–central nervous system (CNS) cancers. Although chemotherapy is not typically discussed in chapters related to toxic exposure, it is a toxin to both cancerous and healthy cells, and there is a growing body of literature highlighting the cognitive, neuroanatomical, and functional changes that substantiate the phenomenon of "chemo-brain." For each toxin, we address common neuropsychological deficits, relevant emotional and behavioral changes, and structural magnetic resonance imaging (MRI) findings. Less frequently, we incorporate functional imaging findings to illustrate particular points related to toxic exposure.

There are a few themes to keep in mind while reading. The vast majority of studies in this area are cross-sectional. When longitudinal data are available, they are generally collected after the onset of abuse or exposure and then during the course of continued abuse, exposure, abstinence, or cessation. Cross-sectional data create quite a "chicken or the egg" problem: Are cognitive and structural brain differences in exposed individuals the direct consequence of abuse or exposure or, instead, do they represent preexisting differences that render individuals vulnerable to the effects of toxic exposure or substance abuse? For example, in one study comparing stimulant-dependent subjects to their stimulant-naive siblings and normal controls, the sibling pairs demonstrated the same abnormalities in fronto-striatal brain systems relative to controls (Ersche et al., 2012). Of course, cognitive and structural deficits observed with toxic exposure may represent a combination of preexisting and predisposing deficits, as well as the direct consequences of exposure or abuse. There are some exceptions in studies that are prospective in nature that we will highlight.

There are two other common limitations inherent to the majority of studies on toxic exposure. First, data regarding exposure or abuse are frequently based on self-report. Thus, there are limitations in establishing a dose-response effect. Second, many individuals are poly-substance abusers or exposed to multiple toxins, which makes it challenging to obtain a clean or homogenous sample to investigate the specific effects of neurotoxins. These issues impact the *quality* of the data at hand.

With specific regard to substance abuse, there are occasions when the available data do not fully support a long-term toxic effect of certain substances; however, we believe it is reasonable to assume that there are consequences of chronic substance abuse on brain structure and function. Substances are abused to begin with because they alter how individuals feel or experience the world, which occurs through neural processes. While it is reasonable to assume that, at a certain level of exposure, toxins will produce permanent changes to the CNS, the science must catch up to prove this assumption true. Regardless of whether the deficits associated with toxic exposure are a cause or effect of the exposure, such deficits impact one's ability to participate in and benefit from available treatment options. This concept, in particular, is of great importance when considering the societal effects.

Heavy Metals

The impact of heavy metals on the human brain has been recognized and studied for centuries, dating as far back as the second century B.C. (Needleman, 2004). Loosely, the term *heavy metals* refers to a subset of naturally occurring elements with metallic properties that exert a toxic effect on the environment and living organisms (Duruibe, Ogwuegbu, & Egwurugwu, 2007). Industry and the environment constitute the primary mechanisms of neurotoxic exposure.

Lead

The neurotoxic effects of lead were recognized as far back as antiquity among metal workers and wine drinkers. Centuries ago, the use of lead in wine making was banned, but industry remained a viable source of toxicity (Needleman, 2004; Sandstead, 1986). By the early 1900s, leaded paints and gasoline became major sources of environmental pollution. In 1970s, the U.S. government banned residential and public use of lead-based paints and began phasing out leaded gasoline because of scientific studies demonstrating neurotoxic effects on children (Ibrahim, Froberg, Wolf, & Rusyniak, 2006; Needleman, 1975).

Lead permeates the blood-brain barrier and alters neural activity (Khalil et al., 2009). Children are especially susceptible to lead toxicity during fetal and early development as lead is more easily absorbed by the developing CNS. Lead may be transmitted from mother to child through the umbilical cord and breast milk (Needleman, 2004; Sanders, Liu, Buchner, & Tchounwou, 2009). Prenatal lead exposure has been liked with developmental, cognitive, and neurobehavioral effects. Elevated lead levels were found in children with encephalopathy, mental retardation, learning disabilities, and hyperactivity (Moore, Meredith, & Goldberg, 1977; Marlowe et al., 1982; Needleman, 2004). Relative to children with low lead concentrations, children with high levels of lead were found to have lower intelligence (Landrigan et al., 1975; Needleman, Gunnoe, Leviton, & Peresie, 1978; Needleman, Geiger, & Frank, 1985).

There is a clear dose-response effect, but adverse effects are observed in children with low levels of lead exposure (Needleman, 2009; Needleman et al., 1979). Studies conducted by Herbert Needleman in the late 1970s and 1980s demonstrated intellectual and cognitive deficits in children who did not show overt clinical signs of lead intoxication (Ibrahim et al., 2006; Needleman, 2004; Needleman et al., 1978; Needleman et al., 1979). Specific deficits in overall intelligence, verbal abilities, attention, reaction time, and behavior were identified (Needleman et al., 1979). In a follow-up 11 years later, the same cognitive deficits persisted and higher childhood lead levels were associated with worse academic performance and increased absenteeism in high school (Needleman, Schell, Bellinger, Leviton, & Allred, 1990). This significant and persistent inverse relationship between childhood lead exposure and intellectual functioning has been well-replicated (Bellinger, Stiles, & Needleman, 1992; Lanphear et al., 2005; Mazumdar et al., 2011; Needleman et al., 1985; Needleman & Landrigan, 1981; Tong, Baghurst, McMichael, Sawyer, & Mudge, 1996).

Childhood lead exposure has also been linked with significant social and behavioral problems, including aggression, hyperactivity, impulsivity, delinquency, conduct problems, and antisocial behavior (Dietrich, Ris, Succop, Berger, & Bornshein, 2001; Carpenter, 2001; Marcus, Fulton, & Clarke, 2010; Needleman et al., 1996). A meta-analysis found that lead burden was associated with attention deficit/hyperactivity disorder (ADHD) symptoms; the effect size was similar to the effect sizes between lead and intelligence, as well as lead and conduct problems (Goodlad, Marcus, & Fulton, 2013).

Occupational lead exposure represents the most common route of lead poisoning in adults. There is a high risk of occupational toxicity among miners, welders, smelters, battery plant workers, painters, and construction workers (Ibrahim et al., 2006). Neurologic symptoms of acute lead toxicity include headache, fatigue, emotional lability, tremor, neuropathy, ataxia, and, rarely, encephalopathy (Ibrahim et al., 2006; Järup, 2003; Kim & Kim, 2012). The bilateral wrist drop is a pathognomonic sign (Ibrahim et al., 2006). Behaviorally, lead-exposed workers display increased rates of depression, anxiety, irritability, anger, and hallucinations (Baker, Feldman, White, & Harley, 1983; Flora, Gupta, & Tiwari, 2012; Jeyaratnam, Boey, Ong, Chia, & Phoon, 1986). Workers exposed to lead demonstrate significant and long-term deficits in general intellect, spatial ability, memory, motor speed, and reaction time relative to controls (Baker et al., 1983; Hogstedt, Hane, Agrell, & Bodin, 1983; Jeyaratnam et al., 1986; Khalil et al., 2009).

There is mounting evidence that cognitive deficits associated with lead toxicity progress over time. In old age, former lead-exposed workers demonstrate poorer performance on measures of visuospatial ability, learning and memory, executive functions, and manual dexterity (Needleman, 2004; Schwartz et al., 2000; Shih et al., 2006). Some researchers assert that lead plays a role in the development of neurodegenerative disorders, such as Alzheimer's disease and amyotrophic lateral sclerosis (ALS), although a direct causal link has not been identified (Johnson & Atchison, 2009; Liu, Hao, Zeng, Dai, & Gu, 2013; Vinceti, Bottecchi, Fan, Finkselstein, & Mandrioll, 2012; Weiss, 2011).

On structural neuroimaging, adults exposed to lead during childhood or early adulthood demonstrate white matter lesions, total brain atrophy, and region-specific declines in gray matter volume, particularly in the frontal lobes (Brubaker, Dietrich, Lanphear, & Cecil, 2010; Cecil et al., 2008;Schwartz et al., 2010; Stewart et al., 2006). There is evidence of a longitudinal association between cumulative lead dose and cognitive dysfunction, white matter lesions, and brain volume loss (Schwartz et al., 2010). Similarly, diffusion tensor imaging (DTI) studies illustrate that childhood lead exposure alters early brain myelination and produces long-term, persistent deficits in axonal integrity (Brubaker et al., 2009).

Unfortunately, the toxic effects of lead are nearly impossible to treat or reverse. Although chelation therapy successfully lowers blood lead levels through accelerating the excretion of heavy metals, it does not reduce lead-related morbidity and mortality in children or adults (Dietrich et al., 2004; Kosnett, 2010; Rogan et al., 2001). Other than simply terminating the exposure, efforts are geared toward primary prevention (Flora & Pachauri, 2010; Needleman, 2004).

Mercury

Mercury has been used in industry and medicine for centuries. The toxic properties of mercury were initially recognized in the 1800s, during which time hat makers used mercury to treat animal skins and produce felt for hats. The saying "mad as a hatter" comes from the observed toxic effects among hat makers. The main feature of Mad Hatter's disease, as the condition was labeled, was *erethism*: a behavioral presentation characterized by shyness, social anxiety, paranoia, irritability, and mood lability. Accompanying fatigue, tremor, ataxia, and cognitive changes were also reported (Haut et al., 1999; O'Carroll, Masterton, Dougall, Ebmeier, & Goodwing, 1995).

In the 1950s, the neurotoxic effects of mercury gained more serious global attention. A Japanese chemical plant discharged methyl mercury and contaminated the water and aquatic life of Minamata Bay. The first outbreak of Minamata disease, as mercury poisoning came to be called, occurred in 1953 and has affected thousands since then, primarily through consumption of contaminated fish (Ekino, Susa, Ninomiya, Imamura, & Kitamura, 2007; O'Carroll et al., 1995).

Accidental and occupational mercury exposure still occurs today by way of inhalation of mercury vapor, oral ingestion of liquid mercury (e.g., quicksilver), or cutaneous exposure (Haut et al., 1999; Ibrahim et al., 2006). The most common routes of modern exposure include fish consumption, dental amalgams, and vaccines (Clarkson, Magos, & Myers, 2003; Risher, Murray, & Prince, 2002). Mercury crosses the blood-brain barrier and concentrates within neurons, thus interfering with normal cell function (Ibrahim et al., 2006). Neuropathological studies indicate that occipital and cerebellar neurons are prime targets of mercury-related degeneration (Clarkson et al., 2003; Davidson, Myers, & Weiss, 2004; Ekino et al., 2007).

Prenatal mercury exposure has been correlated with developmental delays and widespread cognitive deficits (Davidson et al., 2004; Grandjean et al., 1997). Beginning in the 1990s, the U.S. Food and Drug Administration (FDA) began issuing advisories on limiting fish consumption during pregnancy (Counter & Buchanan, 2004). Studies conducted in the Faroe Islands, where whale meat was heavily consumed, found long-term deficits affecting motor functions, attention, visuospatial skills, language, and memory among prenatally exposed children (Counter & Buchanan, 2004; Davidson et al., 2004; Grandjean et al., 1997). The Seychelles Child Development Study investigated the effects of lower levels of prenatal mercury exposure from consuming fish and did not find cognitive deficits (Davidson et al., 2004; Davidson et al., 2010; Davidson, Myers, Weiss, Shamlaye, & Cox, 2006).

Among adults, acute mercury poisoning is associated with an array of clinical symptoms. Cerebellar dysfunction is common with gait ataxia, tremor, dysmetria, dysarthria, or gaze nystagmus. Primary visual disturbance is reflected through constriction of the visual fields. Hearing impairment, olfactory and gustatory disturbances, and somatosensory dysfunction are also observed. Behaviorally, erethism remains characteristic of mercury intoxication. Personality change may manifest as disinhibition, emotional lability, emotional hypersensitivity, paranoia, or social anxiety (Ekino et al., 2007; Haut et al., 1999; Kim & Kim, 2012). Clinical symptoms of acute toxicity may present within hours of exposure. Although symptoms of chronic, lower-level mercury poisoning develop more gradually, the same domains are affected (Haut et al., 1999; Ibrahim et al., 2006; Järup, 2003; Risher et al., 2002). The timing of onset, rate of progression, and overall severity of symptoms are contingent upon the level of exposure (Ibrahim et al., 2006).

Neuropsychological deficits associated with mercury toxicity are widespread and nonspecific, but executive dysfunction is a strong theme. Cognitive deficits affecting motor functions, attention and concentration, processing speed, verbal memory, cognitive flexibility, and abstraction have been documented in cases of acute and chronic mercury exposure (Haut et al., 1999; Neghab, Norouzi, Choobineh, Kardaniyan, & Zadeh, 2012; O'Carroll et al., 1995). The severity of cognitive deficits, however, is relatively mild. In a meta-analysis examining the effects of occupational mercury exposure on neuropsychological function, a mild effect size was found, there was no dose-response relationship, and cessation of exposure led to cognitive recovery (Rohling & Demakis, 2006).

Mercury intoxication causes changes to the cerebrum and cerebellum. At autopsy, atrophy of the cerebellar vermis and hemispheres, calcarine cortex, precentral gyrus, postcentral gyrus, and transverse temporal gyri are noted (Eto, 1997). These structural findings correlate with the cerebellar, visual, motor, and various sensory changes observed clinically. In patients with known mercury poisoning, atrophy of the calcarine and cerebellar cortices are most striking on computed tomography (CT) and MRI, and decreased cerebellar blood flow has been demonstrated with single photon emission computed tomography (SPECT) (Eto, 1997; Eto, 2000; Eto, Marumoto, & Takeya, 2010; Farina, Avila, da Rocha, & Aschner, 2012; Itoh et al., 2001; Kim & Kim, 2012; Korogi, Takahashi, Okajima & Eto, 1998). Functional imaging studies suggest a dose-response effect. In one study conducted with the prenatally exposed Faroe Islanders, higher mercury exposure correlated with more widespread brain activation on visual and motor tasks (White et al., 2011).

Theories about the pathogenic role of mercury in neurodegenerative diseases, such as Alzheimer's disease, have also been put forth. Although mercury and other heavy metals may contribute to the onset or progression of neurodegenerative conditions, we emphasize that no causal link has been identified (Carpenter, 2001; Johnson & Atchison, 2009; Mutter, Naumann, Sadaghiani, Schneider, & Walach, 2004; Weiss, 2011).

As with lead toxicity, prevention of mercury intoxication is superior to treatment. Modern preventative efforts include removing amalgam fillings and avoiding high intake of certain fish, such as shark, tuna, and swordfish (Järup, 2003). Antioxidants show promise as potential therapeutic agents, but their efficacy remains unclear. Chelating therapies may partially remove mercury from the body, but cannot reverse CNS damage (Clarkson et al., 2003; Farina et al., 2012). Ultimately, mercury exerts an enduring toxic effect upon living organisms.

Organic Solvents

Organic solvents are used in a wide range of industries in manufacturing and cleaning processes. Exposure may occur through inhalation, dermal absorption, oral routes, or through a combination of these. Acute effects of solvent exposure are similar to the acute effects of alcohol (which is also a solvent), such as feelings of intoxication, dizziness, discoordination, and headache. There is an ever-growing body of research on the effects of chronic exposure to solvents. The reader is referred to prior reviews for details, but the cognitive deficits typically observed after solvent exposure affect attention, memory, motor skills, and visual perception. Processing speed, working memory, and other executive functions may also be impaired (Baker, 1994; Jin et al., 2004; Morrow, Muldoon, & Sandstrom, 2001; van Valen et al., 2012; White & Proctor, 1993). Some studies do not report cognitive deficits following exposure and there has been speculation that chronic low-level exposure does not result in permanent deficits (Dick et al., 2010); however, several well-controlled studies, including a twin study and prospective studies, have documented deficits (Hanninen, Antti-Poika, Juntunen, Koskenvuo, 1991; Morrow, Steinhauer, Condray, & Hodgson, 1997). A meta-analysis of solvent-exposed individuals compared to nonexposed controls reported significant effect sizes. Measures of attention, processing speed, and response inhibition showed particularly strong effects. It should be noted that the meta-analysis failed to document a dose-response relationship, which the authors attributed to the incomplete descriptions of exposure in the studies examined. Individual studies, however, have reported dose-response relationships, such that a greater severity and longer duration of exposure is associated with a greater degree of cognitive deficit (Morrow et al., 2001; Nilson, Bäckman, Sällsten, Hagberg, Barregård, 2003). Indeed, despite the well-demonstrated cognitive effects of solvent exposure, variability in study methodology and individual exposure factors do exist and result in inconsistent findings. In addition, the precise amount and duration of exposure necessary to produce symptoms has not been determined and there is no specific biologic marker that is critical to document exposure. Individuals are also frequently exposed to more than one substance.

The long-term outcome of cognitive deficits following solvent exposure is also debated. Deficits are reversible in some individuals (Morrow et al., 1997), while other studies suggest that aging may exacerbate cognitive deficits (Nilson et al., 2003). It has been hypothesized that solvent-exposed individuals are at increased risk of dementia, but this is not consistently supported in the literature (Berr et al., 2010; Dick et al., 2010). Cognitive reserve may also play a role in the expression of cognitive deficits following solvent exposure, as lower educational attainment was associated with greater cognitive dysfunction in solvent-exposed workers (Sabbath et al., 2012).

Emotional changes are also common, with high rates of depression, anxiety, and personality disturbance in those exposed to solvents (Condray, Morrow, Steinhauer, Hodgson, & Kelley, 2000; Morrow et al., 2000; Visser et al., 2011). Up to 71% of a solvent-exposed sample may meet criteria for an active Axis I condition (Morrow et al., 2000). A positive association has been demonstrated between psychiatric symptoms and the severity and duration of exposure (Condray et al., 2000; Morrow et al., 2000); however, emotional symptoms do not fully account for resultant cognitive deficits (Perrson, Osterberg, Karlson, & Orbaek, 2000; Morrow et al., 2001).

Neuroimaging studies have provided some elucidation of the underlying structural effects of solvent-related cognitive deficits but there are few studies, thus limiting conclusions. There is evidence of white matter change based on proton magnetic resonance spectroscopy (MRS), DTI, and volumetric measurement of the corpus callosum, with an association between degree of white matter change and severity of exposure (Alkan et al., 2004; Haut et al., 2006; Visser et al., 2008). The lipophilic properties of organic solvents are thought to account for their affinity for white matter, as myelin has a high fat content. Changes to gray matter may be expected as well, but have been less thoroughly examined. There is evidence of brain atrophy based on readings of individual clinical scans (Keski-Santti, Mantyla, Lamminen, Hyvarinen, & Sainio, 2009). Functional imaging studies using positron emission tomography (PET) and functional magnetic resonance imaging (fMRI) have documented alterations in frontal lobe activation during working memory tasks (Haut et al., 2000; Tang et al., 2011).

Carbon Monoxide

Carbon monoxide (CO) is a colorless, odorless gas, produced by incomplete combustion of carbons. The affinity of CO for hemoglobin is more than 200 times that of oxygen, displacing oxygen from hemoglobin. Carboxyhemoglobin is formed and interferes with the transport of oxygen to tissue, leading to hypoxia. Common mechanisms of exposure include motor vehicle exhaust, heating units, and generators. Poisoning may be intentional (suicide attempt) or unintentional (fire or faulty heating). There are increases in unintentional exposures with cold temperatures in the winter months and with incorrect use of generators during power outages from natural disasters (CDC, 2009; Iqbal et al., 2012). CO is the most common cause of death by poisoning in the United States (Prockop & Chichkova, 2007). In 2007 alone, there were more than 21,000 visits to emergency departments and 2,300 hospitalizations from confirmed cases of CO poisoning (Iqbal et al., 2012). Because of the nonspecific nature of symptoms, exposures may go unnoticed and, therefore, rates may be underestimated. The literature regarding CO exposure focuses primarily on acute CO poisoning, as it is more readily identified and more frequently comes to clinical attention. The rate of chronic, long-term CO exposure is unknown and its effects are poorly understood. Unless otherwise stated, the findings discussed in this section refer to acute CO poisoning.

The symptoms of exposure range from flu-like symptoms of headache, dizziness, weakness, and nausea to more severe symptoms of syncope, coma, and death. Cardiac symptoms, such as angina and arrhythmias, may occur. Individuals in the same CO exposure event may display different clinical presentations, and the severity of exposure can differ between individuals in the same location (Prockop, 2005). There may be complicating factors of substance intoxication with both accidental exposure and suicide attempts.

CO poisoning is associated with impairments in memory, attention, processing speed, visual-spatial skills, executive functions, and intellect (Chambers, Hopkins, Weaver, & Key, 2008; Gale et al., 1999; Kesler et al., 2001; Parkinson et al., 2002; Porter, Hopkins, Weaver, Bigler, & Blatter, 2002; Prockop, 2005). There is wide individual variability in cognitive deficits and long-term outcome following acute CO exposure (Hopkins & Woon, 2006). This variability may be explained by severity of exposure, but not consistently so. For example, Chambers and colleagues (2008) prospectively examined the neuropsychological performance of 256 individuals with CO poisoning, stratified by severity of exposure (55 less severe, 201 more severe), at serial intervals following the initial exposure. The two groups did not differ in prevalence of cognitive deficits at six weeks, six months, or 12 months postexposure. At six weeks, rates of exposure were 39% and 35% for the less and more severe groups respectively.

Behavioral and emotional symptoms following CO poisoning include depression, anxiety, and mood lability (Chambers et al., 2008; Gale et al., 1999; Jasper, Hopkins, Duker, Waver, 2005). Psychiatric disturbance may predate CO exposure (i.e., depression in individuals with CO poisoning from suicide attempts) and may persist. In general, individuals with CO poisoning due to suicide attempts show higher rates of depression and anxiety relative to individuals who were accidentally exposed (Jasper et al., 2005). Interestingly, depression and anxiety may actually be more common in less-severely poisoned patients early in the course of recovery (Chambers et al., 2008). There are also rare case reports of new-onset obsessive-compulsive disorder (OCD) and symptoms associated with Kluver-Bucy syndrome (Hopkins & Woon, 2006). While behavioral and emotional symptoms may influence cognitive deficits, they do not fully account for cognitive dysfunction in individuals exposed to CO (Porter et al., 2002).

Some individuals experience a delayed-onset neuropsychiatric syndrome with symptoms emerging 7–14 days after exposure, and after an apparent recovery from acute symptoms. The syndrome is typically characterized by parkinsonian symptoms including bradykinesia, masked facies, and gait disturbance. Prevalence estimates range from 0.06% to 40% of CO-exposed individuals (Hopkins & Woon, 2006), and there may be increased risk of the delayed syndrome with increasing age, longer duration of coma, and prolonged anoxia (Min, 1986). The structural neuroimaging findings and clinical symptoms associated with the delayed syndrome may or may not resolve (Choi, 2002; Cocito et al., 2005; Min, 1986; Sohn, Jeong, Kim, Im, & Kim, 2000).

Neuroimaging findings have revealed atrophy in the brains of individuals who have been exposed to CO. In addition to whole-brain atrophy, regional atrophic changes may affect the fornix, hippocampus, corpus callosum, and basal ganglia (Gale et al., 1999; Kesler et al., 2001; Porter et al., 2002; Pulsipher, Hopkins, & Weaver, 2006). Atrophy of the corpus callosum was identified in 80% of patients within six months of exposure (Porter et al., 2002), but there was no correlation with cognitive performance. Infarcts in the bilateral hippocampi have been reported and associated with amnesia (Bourgeois, 2000; Gottfried & Chatterjee, 2001). Voxel-based morphometry reveals lower gray matter volumes in the basal ganglia, claustrum, amygdala, hippocampus, and frontal and parietal regions, as well as a correlation between lower gray matter volume and slower psychomotor speed (Chen, Chen et al., 2013).

Basal ganglia structures, particularly the globus pallidus, have known susceptibility to CO exposure; however, basal ganglia lesions are not universally identified and may even be absent in the presence of parkinsonian symptoms (Cocito et al., 2005; O'Donnell, Buxton, Pitkin, & Jarvis, 2000; Prockop, 2005). For example, following the same exposure event, one individual experienced parkinsonian symptoms without a lesion in the globus pallidus, while another individual had pallidal lesions without parkinsonian symptoms (Sohn et al., 2000). Reliance on individual case reports of observable lesions may be misleading, as other neuroimaging methods have revealed structural compromise in the absence of observable lesions. Pulsipher and colleagues (2006) found decreased basal ganglia volume in 28% of a prospective sample of patients with CO at six months postexposure, with an observable lesion in only one individual.

Damage to white matter, particularly in periventricular regions, is commonly reported following CO exposure and white matter may be more sensitive than gray matter in the acute phases of exposure (Prockop & Chichkova, 2007; Sener, 2003). White matter hyperintensities on MRI have remained stable at six-month follow-up (Parkinson et al., 2002). Using diffusion-weighted imaging, Chen, Huang and colleagues (2013) documented elevations in apparent diffusion coefficient (ADC, a marker of tissue injury) in the globus pallidus and corpus callosum acutely (< two weeks), subacutely (two weeks to six months), and chronically (> one year) following CO exposure. ADC values correlated with cognitive performance. The delayed neuropsychiatric syndrome that may follow CO exposure has also been associated with changes in gray and white matter (Chu et al., 2004; Cocito et al., 2005; Lo et al., 2007). DTI studies have revealed white matter disruption in normal appearing white matter that correlates with cognitive performance and persists after hyperbaric oxygen treatment (Lin et al., 2009; Lo et al., 2007).

Treatment of CO poisoning involves administration of oxygen. Guidelines typically suggest normobaric treatment for lower levels of exposure and less severe symptoms, while hyperbaric treatment is generally utilized in more severe exposures; however, it can be difficult to initially determine the exposure severity (Prockop & Chichkova, 2007). There is also some debate about whether hyperbaric treatment yields a better outcome than normobaric treatment (Stoller, 2007; Weaver et al., 2002; Wolf, Levonas, Sloan, & Jagoda, 2008).

Substances of Abuse

Cannabis

Cannabis use has increased in recent years across the United States. This trend may be, in part, due to the legalization of marijuana's medicinal use in 20 states and recreational use in two states. While there are clear, acute affects of cannabis use on cognition, hence its propensity for use, there are very few prospective studies examining the long-term cognitive effects of cannabis use. One study conducted through the Dunedin Multidisciplinary Health and Development Study seems to provide strong evidence for long-term effects of cannabis on intellect and cognition, at least at first glance (Meier et al., 2012). In this study, a cohort of 1037 individuals was followed from birth to age 38, with cannabis use documented at ages 18, 21, 26, 32, and 38 years. Participants were evaluated at age 13, before cannabis use began, and then again at age 38. Intelligence was reassessed at multiple time points, but more comprehensive neuropsychological evaluations occurred at age 38 only; therefore, true prospective longitudinal data are available only for intelligence. Results illustrated a decline in intelligence in cannabis users, as well as a pattern of increasing intellectual decline with increasing use. The effect was general and impacted all aspects of intelligence, including all four Wechsler Adult Intelligence Scale–IV (WAIS-IV) indices (Verbal Comprehension, Perceptual Reasoning, Working Memory, and Processing Speed). Cognitive deficits were associated with adolescent-onset use, but less so with adult-onset use, and cessation of cannabis use did not fully reverse the cognitive effects. Despite the strengths of this study, including the prospective design and large sample size, there are several potential confounds, such as personality and socioeconomic status, that may account for intellectual changes independent of cannabis use (Daly, 2013; Rogeberg, 2013).

If one carefully examines the Meier study (Meier et al., 2012) and other studies, there are indications that cannabis exerts a long-term impact on variety of neuropsychological functions. The most common deficits observed affect learning and memory and secondary deficits involve working memory, reasoning/judgment, and inhibitory control (Crane et al., 2013; Gonzalez, 2007). Neurodevelopment factors and sex differences are also important variables to consider. Adolescent-onset cannabis use appears to have a more detrimental impact on cognition relative to adult-onset use. Additionally, males appear to have more problems with reasoning/judgment, whereas females have more problems with memory (Crane et al., 2013).

In terms of the structural underpinnings of cannabis-related cognitive deficits, the evidence points to changes in the prefrontal cortex, subcortical striatal structures, and the limbic system (Mata et al., 2010; Smith et al., 2013; Yucel et al., 2008). There is some evidence that heavy use is not associated with differences in brain volume between users and controls although, within users, the volumes of the amygdala and hippocampus varied negatively with use (Cousijn et al., 2012). One particular study of interest examined memory performance using the California Verbal Learning Test-II (CVLT-II) in adolescents who were abstinent for at least six months and correlated their performance with hippocampal volume (Ashtari et al., 2011). Performance was lower in users relative to controls, and correlated with smaller right hippocampal volumes. This structure-function correlation is important, but does not provide definitive evidence linking cannabis use to impaired learning and memory as a result of changes in the hippocampus.

Along the same lines, there is evidence of an association between cannabis use and reduced medial orbital frontal volume, as well as correlation between volume reductions and decision-making deficits (Churchwell, Lopez-Larson, & Yurgelun-Todd, 2010). These findings were accompanied by a dose-response effect. Smith and colleagues (2013) found differences in striatal and thalamic shape among cannabis users, and these differences in brain structure shape correlated with working memory deficits.

Amphetamines and MDMA

Both amphetamines and MDMA (3,4-Methylenedioxymethamphetamine) have high rates of abuse and, in particular, heavy use on college campuses. This brief review will focus most on MDMA. Other amphetamines (speed and methamphetamine) are associated with cognitive deficits affecting attention, inhibition, executive functions, visual spatial skills, and learning and memory (Ersche & Sahakian, 2007; Scott et al., 2007). Methamphetamine abuse is hypothesized to impact fronto-striatal systems, in particular (Scott et al., 2007). Changes are noted in the frontal gray and white matter (Daumann et al., 2011; Koester et al., 2012; Nakam et al., 2011; Tobia et al., 2010), and there is some suggestion that frontal lobe deficits may predate abuse and then worsen secondary to abuse (Winhusen et al., 2013). Questions also remain about the permanency of the deficits, thus it is important to consider moderator variables with individual cases (Dean, Groman, Morales, & London, 2013). Additionally, there are some data to support a causal link between abstinence and improved cognition (Iudicello et al., 2010). It has also been shown that abstinent users are dopamine-deficient and experience memory deficits that are associated with striatal dopamine reductions (McCann et al., 2008).

We chose to focus on MDMA in this review because of its cultural popularity among young adults and the availability of prospective data. In one prospective study of 188 MDMA-naive users who had a high likelihood of use, de Win and colleagues (2008) employed a variety of structural (MRS, DTI) and functional imaging techniques (SPECT to study serotonin transporters and perfusion-weighted imaging to study blood volume). Changes were observed in blood flow in the putamen and globus pallidus and fractional anisotropy in the fronto-parietal white matter and thalamus, with no changes observed in the serotonin system or brain metabolites measured by MRS. These changes occurred after an average use of six tablets. Unfortunately, cognitive data were not provided. A recent review suggests that, while not all aspects of cognition are affected by MDMA abuse, memory and executive functions are most commonly affected (Parrot, 2013). Indeed, some studies report minimal differences between users and controls (Halpern et al., 2010), but there are prospective cognitive data to support memory impairment in MDMA users (Wagner, Becker, Koester, Gouzoulis-Mayfrank, & Daumann, 2012).

Opiates

Opiate use has resurged in recent years with abuse of prescription-based opiate pain medications, which is a particular problem here in Appalachia, and with heroin use and celebrity overdoses making national news. Neuropsychological deficits in long-term opiate users include visual spatial deficits, impaired attention and memory, and more prominent frontal lobe dysfunction (Gruber, Silveri, & Yurgelun-Todd, 2007). Some of these deficits may be related to personality characteristics that actually lead individuals to become users in the first place (Prosser et al., 2008). It is of particular interest that the treatments used for opiate addiction, namely methadone and buprenorphine, are opiates themselves and thus may also have a negative impact on cognition (Prosser et al., 2006; Rapeli, Fabritius, Kalska, & Alho, 2009, 2011). Some data suggest that the effect of methadone is greater (van Holst & Schilt, 2011), but such findings are tentative due to methodological limitations.

Neuroimaging studies suggest that changes in gray matter volume are present immediately after abstinence and that, while some areas may improve over time (i.e., superior frontal gyrus), differences between users and controls remain in the middle frontal gyrus and cingulate (Wang et al., 2012). White matter changes are also present using DTI, with fractional anisotropy (FA) reductions observed in the parahippocampus correlating with memory performance and FA reductions in the orbital frontal white matter correlating with performance on the Iowa Gambling Task (Lin et al., 2012; Qiu et al., 2013).

Alcohol

From a neuropsychological perspective, alcohol is the most widely and thoroughly studied substance of abuse. There are many excellent reviews (e.g., Parsons, 1994; Parsons, 1998; Parsons & Nixon, 1998; Rourke and Loberg, 1993), so we will just briefly summarize the knowledge as we understand it. Cognitive deficits occur in a wide range of areas, including memory, attention, processing, visual spatial skills and frontal lobe/executive functions. Some deficits may improve with abstinence, but some individuals with a sufficiently long duration and intensity of abuse experience persistent deficits. Cognitive deficits can be mild, and in some cases reversible, but may also rise to the level of a dementia syndrome. In those cases, some level of residual cognitive impairment is likely even with prolonged abstinence. Mild cognitive deficits can be detected in social drinkers or those with alcohol dependence (Parsons, 1998). Of course, Korsakoff's amnesia may also present in individuals who abuse alcohol and have concurrent nutritional deficits. We refer readers to a recent series of review articles on this subject published in *Neuropsychology Review* (2012, Volume 22).

Neuroimaging deficits associated with alcohol abuse and dependence affect a wide range of brain structures, including both gray and white matter. MRI demonstrates reduction in the volume of frontal gray and white matter, as well as the cerebellum (Rosenbloom & Pfefferbaum, 2008). As with cognitive deficits, structural brain changes may at least partially reverse with abstinence, and improvements in brain structure are related to improvements in brain function (Sullivan, Harris, & Pfefferbaum, 2010). Consistent with other substances of abuse, there is evidence of preexisting, genetically linked structural deficits that may predispose certain individuals to alcohol abuse (Gierski et al., 2013). In addition, use and abuse during adolescence, when the brain is exceedingly vulnerable to insult, may have particularly negative effects on brain structure (Lisdahl, Gilbart, Wright, Shollenbarger, 2013). There are also some prospective data noting declines in white matter integrity in adolescents who use both alcohol and cannabis, but not in those who use alcohol alone (Jacobus, Squeglia, Bava, & Taper, 2013).

Chemotherapy

Alkylating agents were first introduced as anticancer therapies following World War II. The cytotoxic effects of nitrogen mustards became evident secondary to chemical warfare and, thereafter, mustine or "HN2" became the first chemotherapy drug. Although toxic effects to human tissue were recognized early in the introduction of nitrogen mustard therapy, it was presumed that anticancer agents did not cross the blood-brain barrier and that any cognitive changes occurring in the context of non-CNS tumors were secondary to other factors (Ahles & Saykin, 2007a; Goodman et al., 1946; Karnofsky, 1958; Rhoads, 1946; Silberfarb, Philibert, & Levine, 1980). The neurotoxic effects of chemotherapy were not discussed until the 1980s, when researchers at Dartmouth put forth that cognitive impairment in chemotherapy-treated cancer patients was independent of affective disturbance (Nelson & Suls, 2013; Oxman & Silberfarb, 1980; Silberfarb, 1983; Silberfarb et al., 1980). In the late 1990s, chemotherapy-related cognitive impairment gained more substantial scientific attention and the phenomenon of "chemo-brain" was born (Ahles, 2012; Ahles & Whedon, 1999; van Dam et al., 1998).

Chemo-brain, alternatively known as "chemo-fog" and "chemotherapy-related cognitive impairment," refers to cognitive changes caused by chemotherapy itself (Raffa et al., 2006; Hodgson, Hutchinson, Wilson, & Nettelbeck, 2013). Although high-dose chemotherapy exerts a more potent effect on cognition than standard-dose chemotherapy, both are sufficient to produce cognitive deficits (van Dam et al., 1998). The bulk of research on chemo-brain has been derived from studies of patients having undergone standard-dose chemotherapy for breast cancer, lymphoma, and other non-CNS cancers (Abrey, 2012; Saykin, Ahles, & McDonald, 2003). The precise mechanisms underlying chemotherapy-induced neurotoxicity are not well understood, although the integrity of the blood-brain barrier and oxidative stress are believed to play a role (Saykin et al., 2003; Seigers, Schagen, Tellingen, & Dietrich, 2013).

Between 15% and 75% of cancer patients report at least mild cognitive impairment at some point during or after treatment, while up to 61% may experience persistent post-treatment cognitive deficits (Ahles, 2012; Ahles & Saykin, 2007b; Janelsins et al., 2011; Wefel, Lenzi, Theriault, Davis, & Meyers, 2004). Cognitive deficits in attention, concentration, processing speed, verbal and visual memory, and multitasking are commonly reported following treatment (Ahles & Saykin, 2002; Wefel et al., 2004). A recent meta-analysis of chemotherapy-related cognitive impairment found that the domains of memory and executive function are most consistently affected on neuropsychological testing (Hodgson et al., 2013). Although some cancer patients experience resolution of cognitive symptoms following treatment, others face more persistent cognitive difficulties for up to 20 years following treatment (de Ruiter et al., 2011; Koppelmans et al., 2012).

Mood disturbance is common among cancer patients and may at least partially fuel subjective cognitive complaints (Koppelmans et al., 2012). The prevalence of major depression in cancer survivors has been estimated at between 10% and 25% (Fann et al., 2008), which is fairly consistent with recent estimates from the U.S. adult population (9% as reported by CDC, 2010). Most cancer survivors do not meet clinical criteria for major depression and actually experience fewer depression symptoms relative to normal controls (Koppelmans et al., 2012). There is also evidence that cancer patients experience clinical depression and anxiety prior to cancer treatment (Linden, Vodermaier, MacKenzie, & Greig, 2012). Thus, it does not appear that chemotherapy triggers mood disturbance in the same way that it leads to cognitive deficits, but rather that preexisting depression and anxiety and treatment effects, such as fatigue, contribute to the cognitive sequelae known as chemo-brain.

Some propose that the effects of chemo-brain cannot be fully captured through neuropsychological measures (Reuter-Lorenz & Cimprich, 2013). When cognitive complaints exceed objective deficits, clinicians frequently write the discrepancy off to stress, fatigue, or mood disturbance (Scherling & Smith, 2013). Neuroimaging offers an alternative mechanism to explore the effect of chemotherapy on cognition and the brain.

Structural imaging studies applying tensor-based and voxel-based morphometry demonstrate reductions in total brain volume and gray matter volume in chemotherapy-exposed patients relative to healthy controls (Conroy et al., 2013; Inagaki et al., 2007; Koppelmans et al., 2012; McDonald, Conroy, Ahles, West, & Saykin, 2010). These changes have been documented shortly after treatment and at long-term follow-up, mainly in cross-sectional designs and at least one prospective study (McDonald et al., 2010).

Significant reductions in white matter integrity are consistently reported in DTI studies of patients receiving chemotherapy (Abraham et al., 2008; Deprez, Billiet, Sunaert, & Leemans, 2013; Deprez et al., 2011; Deprez et al., 2012). Decreased FA in various white matter tracts has been found to correlate with neuropsychological performance on measures of processing speed, attention and short-term memory (Abraham et al., 2008; Deprez et al., 2011; Deprez et al., 2012).

Functional imaging studies suggest that chemotherapy influences the way cancer patients use their brains during cognitive tasks (Haut, Wiener, Marano, & Abraham, 2013). As early as one month after chemotherapy, patients demonstrate decreased frontal activation on working memory tasks relative to healthy controls (de Ruiter & Schagen, 2013; McDonald et al., 2012). Some report a return to neurofunctional baseline at one year after treatment, while others report persistent changes in brain activation. In an fMRI study conducted ten years after chemotherapy, breast cancer survivors showed task-specific hyporesponsiveness of the dorsolateral prefrontal cortex and parahippocampal gyrus, in addition to generalized hyporesponsivenss of the bilateral posterior parietal cortex (de Ruiter et al., 2011). Other follow-up studies suggest similar activation patterns and a correlation between frontal activation and cognitive performance (Conroy et al., 2013; Kesler, Kent, & O'Hara, 2011; Simó, Rifa-Ros, Rodriguez-Fornells, & Bruna, 2013).

Functional imaging studies have also documented significantly increased cortical activation in chemotherapy-treated cancer patients relative to healthy controls (Kesler, Bennett, Mahaffey, & Spiegel, 2009). In one study comparing two monozygotic twins, only one of whom received chemotherapy for breast cancer, the chemotherapy-treated twin demonstrated a wider extent of spatial activation during an *n-back* working memory task, but no difference in performance (Ferguson, McDonald, Saykin, & Ahles, 2007). Similarly, one study using ^{18}fluorodeoxygluose-PET found lower resting metabolism in the inferior frontal cortex of patients treated with chemotherapy 5–10 years earlier relative to controls, but then increased frontal activation during a memory task (Silverman et al., 2007). These findings may stem from decreased cognitive efficiency or some sort of compensatory mechanism.

Although cognitive deficits resulting from standard-dose systemic chemotherapy are usually mild, the effect on quality of life may be more substantial (Saykin et al., 2003). Cognitive complaints have been associated with poorer functional outcome (Reid-Arndt et al., 2010). Chemo-brain can influence basic functioning, self-esteem, social relationships, educational goals, and career decisions (Ahles & Saykin, 2001; Ahles & Whedon, 1999; Voh Ah et al., 2013). Social support and fatigue are also important predictors of quality of life (Reid-Arndt, Hsieh, & Perry, 2010). Thus, preventative efforts or treatment are important.

In the last few years, cognitive-behavioral interventions targeting chemo-brain have been developed and researched. Preliminary findings from two recent randomized controlled trials suggest that brief cognitive behavioral therapy (CBT) or cognitive rehabilitation improves cognitive performance and overall life satisfaction in chemotherapy-treated cancer patients relative to no-treatment controls (Cherrier et al., 2013; Ferguson et al., 2012). These results are very promising. Other treatment options include pharmacological interventions targeting attention/alertness, sleep, mood, diet, and physical activity, which mitigate chemotherapy-induced cognitive deficits. The utility of cholinesterase inhibitors and herbal supplements, such as Ginkgo biloba, is unknown (Fardell, Vardy, Johnston, & Winocur, 2011).

Assessment and Other Issues

Although cognitive symptoms vary depending upon the toxin, attention and executive functions are almost universally affected and should be assessed thoroughly as part of a neuropsychological examination. In cases of occupational toxic exposure, issues of secondary gain and malingering must be considered. A substantial portion of patients with suspected chronic toxic encephalopathy demonstrates suboptimal effort on cognitive tests (Greve et al., 2006; van Hout, Schmand, Wekking, & Deelman, 2006; van Hout, Schmand, Wekking, Hageman, & Deelman, 2003) and, therefore, inclusion of performance/symptom validity measures is recommended.

Conclusions

There is clearly individual variability in the effects and sequelae associated with exposure to CNS toxins. From a cognitive perspective, executive dysfunction is a common theme across the toxins discussed in this chapter. Hand-in-hand with this, emotional lability is a frequent behavioral consequence. Apart from alcohol, the threshold for neurotoxicity is poorly understood across toxins. Additionally, because longitudinal data are lacking, the persistence of resultant symptoms is unclear and it is challenging to determine if the deficits observed are, in fact, a consequence of toxic exposure, or a predisposition. There is increasing evidence of structural brain predispositions to substance abuse, in particular. Further research that takes into account genetic and structural vulnerabilities to the effects of toxins is necessary to elucidate threshold and permanency issues.

References

Abraham, J., Haut, M. W., Moran, M., Filburn, S., Lemiuex, S., & Kuwabara, H. (2008). Adjuvant chemotherapy for breast cancer: Effects on cerebral white matter seen in diffusion tensor imaging. *Clinical Breast Cancer*, *8*, 88–91.

Abrey, L. (2012). The impact of chemotherapy on cognitive outcomes in adults with primary brain tumors. *Journal of Neurooncology*, *108*, 285–290.

Ahles, T. (2012). Brain vulnerability to chemotherapy toxicities. *Psycho-Oncology*, *21*, 1141–1148.

Ahles, T., & Saykin, A. (2001). Cognitive effects of standard-dose chemotherapy in patients with cancer. *Cancer Investigation*, *19*, 812–820.

Ahles, T., & Saykin, A. (2002). Breast cancer chemotherapy-related cognitive dysfunction. *Clinical Breast Cancer*, *3*, S84–S90.

Ahles, T., & Saykin, A. (2007a). Breast cancer chemotherapy-related cognitive dysfunction. *Clinical Breast Cancer*, *3*, S84–S90.

Ahles, T., & Saykin, A. (2007b). Candidate mechanisms for chemotherapy-induced cognitive changes. *Nature*, *7*, 192–201.

Ahles, T., & Whedon, M. (1999). "Chemo-Brain": Cognitive impact of systemic chemotherapy. *Coping with Cancer* (July/August), 48.

Alkan, A., Kutlu, R., Hallac, T., Sigirci, A., Emul, M., Pala, N., Altinok, T., Aslan, M., Sarac, K., & Ozcan, C. (2004). Occupational prolonged organic solvent exposure in shoemakers: brain MR spectroscopy findings. *Magnetic Resonance Imaging*, *22*, 707–713.

Ashtari, M., Avants, B., Cyckowski, L., Cervellione, K. L., Roofeh, D., Cook, P., . . . Kumra, S. (2011). Medial temporal lobe structures and memory functions in adolescents with heavy cannabis use. *Journal of Psychiatric Research*, *45*, 1055–1066.

Baker, E. L. (1994). A review of recent research on health effects of human occupational exposure to organic solvents: A critical review. *Journal of Occupational Medicine*, *6*, 1079–1092.

Baker, E. L., Feldman, R., White, R., & Harley, J. (1983). The role of occupational lead exposure in the genesis of psychiatric and behavioral disturbances. *Acta Psychiatrica Scandinavica*, *67*, 38–48.

Bellinger, D., Stiles, K., & Needleman, H. (1992). Low-level lead exposure, intelligence and academic achievement: A long-term follow-up study. *Pediatrics*, *90*, 855–861.

Berr, C., Vercambre, M. N., Bonenfant, S., Manoux, A. S., Zins, M., & Goldberg, M. (2010). Occupational exposure to solvents and cognitive performance in the GAZEL cohort: Preliminary findings. *Dementia and Geriatric Cognitive Disorders*, *30*, 12–19.

Bourgeois, J. A. (2000). Amnesia after carbon monoxide poisoning. *American Journal of Psychiatry*, *157*, 1884–1885.

Brubaker, C., Dietrich, K., Lanphear, B., & Cecil, K. (2010). The influence of age of lead exposure of adult gray matter volume. *Neurotoxicology*, *31*, 259–266.

Brubaker, C., Schmithorst, V., Haynes, E., Dietrich, K., Egelhoff, J., Lindquist, D., . . . Cecil, K. (2009). Altered myelination and axonal integrity in adults with childhood lead exposure: A diffusion tensor imaging study. *Neurotoxicology*, *30*, 867–875.

Carpenter, D. (2001). Effect of metals on the nervous system of humans and animals. *International Journal of Occupational Medicine and Environmental Health*, *14*, 209–218.

Cecil, K., Brubaker, C., Adler, C., Dietrich, K., Altaye, M., Egelhoff, J., . . . Lanphear, B. (2008). Decreased brain volume in adults with childhood lead exposure. *PLoS Medicine*, *5*, e112.

Centers for Disease Control and Prevention. (2009). Carbon monoxide exposures after hurricane Ike—Texas, September 2008. *Morbidity and Mortality Weekly Report*, *58*, 845–849.

Centers for Disease Control and Prevention. (2010). Current depression among adults—United States, 2006 and 2008. *Morbidity and Mortality Weekly Report*, *59*, 1229–1260.

Chambers, C. A., Hopkins, R. O., Weaver, L. K., & Key, C. (2008). Cognitive and affective outcomes of more severe compared to less severe carbon monoxide poisoning. *Brain Injury*, *22*, 387–395.

Chen, H. L., Chen, P. C., Lu, C. H., Hsu, N. W., Chou, K. H., Lin, C. P., . . . Lin, W. C. (2013). Structural and cognitive deficits in chronic carbon monoxide intoxication: A voxel-based morphometry study. *BMC Neurology*, *13*, 129.

Chen, N. C., Huang, C. W., Lui, C. C., Lee, C. C., Chang, W. N., Huang, S. H., . . . Chang, C. C. (2013). Diffusion-weighted imaging improves prediction in cognitive outcome and clinical phases in patients with carbon monoxide intoxication. *Neuroradiology*, *55*, 107–115.

Cherrier, M., Anderson, K., Higano, C., Gray, H., Church, A., & Willis, S. (2013). A randomized trial of cognitive rehabilitation in cancer survivors. *Life Sciences*, *93*, 617–622.

Choi, I. S. (2002). Parkinsonism after carbon monoxide poisoning. *European Neurology*, *48*, 30–33.

Chu, K., Jung, K. H., Kim, H. J., Jeong, S. W., Kang, D. W., & Roh, J. K. (2004). Diffusion-weighted MRI and ^{99m}Tc-HMPAO SPECT in delayed relapsing type of carbon monoxide poisoning: Evidence of delayed cytoxic edema. *European Neurology*, *51*, 98–103.

Churchwell, J. C., Lopez-Larson, M., & Yurgelun-Todd, D. A. (2010). Altered frontal cortical volume and decision making in adolescent cannabis users. *Frontiers in Psychology*, *1*, 225. doi: 10.3389/fpsyg.2010.00225.

Clarkson, T., Magos, L., & Myers, G. (2003). The toxicology of mercury—current exposures and clinical manifestations. *The New England Journal of Medicine*, *349*, 1731–1737.

Cocito, L., Biagioli, M., Fontana, P., Inglese, M. L., Pizzorno, M., Spigno, F., & Volpe, S. (2005). Cognitive recovery after delayed carbon monoxide encephalopathy. *Clinical Neurology and Neurosurgery*, *107*, 347–350.

Conroy, S., McDonald, B., Smith, D., Moser, L., West, J., Kamendulis, L., Klaunig, J., Champion, V., Unverzagt, F., & Saykin, A. (2013). Alterations in brain structure and function in breast cancer survivors: Effect of post-chemotherapy interval and relation to oxidative DNA damage. *Breast Cancer Research and Treatment*, *137*, 493–502.

Condray, R., Morrow, L. A., Steinhauer, S. R., Hodgson, M., & Kelley, M. (2000). Mood and behavioral symptoms in individuals with chronic solvent exposure. *Psychiatry Research*, *97*, 191–206.

Counter, S., & Buchanan, L. (2004). Mercury exposure in children: A review. *Toxicology and Applied Pharmacology*, *198*, 209–230.

Cousijn, J., Wiers, R. W., Ridderinkhof, K. R., van den Brink, W., Veltman, D. J., & Goudriaan, A. E. (2012). Grey matter alterations associated with cannabis use: Results of a VBM study in cannabis users and healthy controls. *NeuroImage*, *59*, 3845–3851.

Crane, N. A., Schuster, R. M., Fusar-Poli, P., & Gonzalez, R. (2013). Effects of cannabis on neurocognitive functioning: Recent advances, neurodevelopmental influences and sex differences. *Neuropsychological Review*, *23*, 117–137.

Crane, N. A., Schuster, R. M., & Gonzalez, R. (2013). Preliminary evidence for a sex-specific relationship between amount of cannabis use and neurocognitive performance in young cannabis users. *The Journal of the International Neuropsychological Society*, *19*, 1009–1015.

Daly, M. (2013). Personality may explain the association between cannabis use and neuropsychological impairment. *Proceedings of the National Academy of Sciences*, *110*, E979.

Daumann, J., Koster, P., Becker, B., Wagner, D., Imperati, D., Gouzoulis-Mayfrank, E., & Tittgemeyer, M. (2011). Medial prefrontal gray matter volume reductions in users of amphetamine-type stimulants revealed by combined tract-based spatial statistics and voxel-based morphometry. *NeuroImage*, *54*, 794–801.

Davidson, P., Leste, A., Benstrong, E., Burns, C., Valentin, J., Sloane-Reeves, J., . . . Myers, G. (2010). Fish consumption, mercury exposure, and their associations with scholastic achievement in the Seychelles Child Development Study. *NeuroToxicology*, *31*, 439–447.

Davidson, P., Myers, G., & Weiss, B. (2004). Mercury exposure and child development outcomes. *Pediatrics*, *113*, 1023–1029.

Davidson, P., Myers, G., Weiss, B., Shamlaye, C., & Cox, C. (2006). Prenatal methyl mercury exposure from fish consumption and child development: A review of evidence and perspectives form the Seychelles Child Development Study. *NeuroToxicology*, *27*, 1106–1109.

Dean, A., Groman, S. M., Morales, A. M., & London, E. D. (2013). An evaluation of the evidence that methamphetamine abuse causes cognitive decline in humans. *Neuropsychopharmacology*, *38*, 259–274.

Deprez, S., Amant, F., Smeets, A., Peeters, R., Leemans, A., Van Hecke, W., . . . Sunaert, S. (2012). Longitudinal assessment of chemotherapy-induced structural changes in cerebral white matter and its correlation with impaired cognitive functioning. *Journal of Clinical Oncology*, *30*, 274–281.

Deprez, S., Amant, F., Yigit, R., Porke, K., Verhoeven, J., Van den Stock, J., . . . Sunaert, S. (2011). Chemotherapy-induced structural changes in cerebral white matter and its correlation with impaired cognitive functioning in breast cancer patients. *Human Brain Mapping*, *32*, 480–493.

Deprez, S., Billiet, T., Sunaert, S., & Leemans, A. (2013). Diffusion tensor MRI of chemotherapy-induced cognitive impairment in non-CNS cancer patients: A review. *Brain Imaging and Behavior*, *7*, 409–435.

de Ruiter, M., Reneman, L., Boogerd, W., Veltman, D., van Dam, F., Nederveen, A., . . . Schagen, S. (2011). Cerebral hyporesponsiveness and cognitive impairment 10 years after chemotherapy for breast cancer. *Human Brain Mapping*, *32*, 1206–1219.

de Ruiter, M., & Schagen, S. (2013). Functional MRI studies in non-CNS cancers. *Brain Imaging and Behavior*, *7*, 388–408.

de Win, M.M.L., Jager, G., Boonj, J., Reneman, L., Schilt, T., Lavini, C., . . . van den Brink, W. (2008). Sustained effects of ecstasy on the human brain: A prospective neuroimaging study in novel users. *Brain*, *131*, 2936–2945.

Dick, F. D., Bourne, V. J., Semple, S. E., Fox, H. C., Miller, B. G., Deary, I. J., & Whalley, L. J. (2010). Solvent exposure and cognitive ability at age 67: A follow-up study of the 1947 Scottish Mental Survey. *Occupational and Environmental Medicine*, *67*, 401–407.

Dietrich, D., Ware, J., Salganik, M., Radcliffe, J., Rogan, W., Rhoads, G., . . . Jones, R. (2004). Effect of chelation therapy of the neuropsychological and behavioral development of lead-exposed children after school entry. *Pediatrics*, *114*, 19–26.

Dietrich, K., Ris, M., Succop, P., Berger, O., & Bornschein, R. (2001). Early exposure to lead and juvenile delinquency. *Neurotoxicology and Teratology*, *23*, 511–518.

Duruibe, J., Ogwuegbu, M., & Egwurugwu, J. (2007). Heavy metal pollution and human biotoxic effects. *International Journal of Physical Sciences*, *2*, 112–118.

Ekino, S., Susa, M., Ninomiya, T., Imamura, K., & Kitamura, T. (2007). Minamata disease revisited: An update on the acute and chronic manifestations of methyl mercury poisoning. *Journal of the Neurological Sciences*, *262*, 131–144.

Ersche, K. D., & Sahakian, B. J. (2007). The neuropsychology of amphetamine and opiate dependence: Implications for treatment. *Neuropsychological Review*, *17*, 317–336.

Ersche, K. E., Jones, P. S., Williams, G. B., Turton, A. J., Robbins, T. W., & Bullmore, E. T. (2012). Abnormal brain structure implicated in stimulant drug addiction. *Science*, *335*, 601–604.

Eto, K. (1997). Pathology of Minamata disease. *Toxicologic Pathology*, *25*, 614–623.

Eto, K. (2000). Minamata disease. *Neuropathology*, *20*, S14–S19.

Eto, K., Marumoto, M., & Takeya, M. (2010). The pathology of methylmercury poisoning (Minamata disease). *Neuropathology*, *30*, 471–479.

Fann, J., Thomas-Rich, A., Katon, W., Cowley, D., Pepping, M., McGregor, B., & Gralow, J. (2008). Major depression after breast cancer: A review of epidemiology and treatment. *General Hospital Psychiatry*, *30*, 112–126.

Fardell, J., Vardy, J., Johnston, I., & Winocur, G. (2011). Chemotherapy and cognitive impairment: Treatment options. *Nature*, *90*, 366–376.

Farina, M., Avila, D., da Rocha, J., & Aschner, M. (2012). Metals, oxidative stress and neurodegeneration: A focus on iron, manganese, and mercury. *Neurochemistry International*, *62*, 575–594.

Ferguson, R., McDonald, B., Rocque, M., Furstenberg, C., Horrigan, S., Ahles, T., & Saykin, A. (2012). Development of CBT for chemotherapy-related cognitive change: Results of a waitlist control trial. *Psycho-Oncology*, *21*, 176–186.

Ferguson, R., McDonald, B., Saykin, A., & Ahles, T. (2007). Brain structure and function differences in monozygotic twins: Possible effects of breast cancer chemotherapy. *Journal of Clinical Oncology*, *25*, 3866–3870.

Flora, G., Gupta, D., & Tiwari, A. (2012). Toxicity of lead: A review with recent updates. *Interdisciplinary Toxicology*, *5*, 47–58.

Flora, S., & Pachauri, V. (2010). Chelation in metal intoxication. *International Journal of Environmental Research and Public Health*, *7*, 2745–2788.

Gale, S. D., Hopkins, R. O., Weaver, L. K., Bigler, E. D., Booth, E. J., & Blatter, D. D. (1999). MRI, quantitative MRI, SPECT, and neuropsychological findings following carbon monoxide poisoning. *Brain Injury*, *13*, 229–243.

Gierski, F., Hubsch, B., Stefania, N., Benexerouk, F., Cuervo-Lombard, C., Bera-Potelle, C., . . . Limosin, F. (2013). Executive functions in adult offspring of alcohol dependent probands: Toward a cognitive endophenotype? *Alcoholism: Clinical and Experimental Research*, *51*, E356–E363.

Gonzalez, R. (2007). Acute and non-acute effects of cannabis on brain functioning and neuropsychological performance. *Neuropsychological Review*, *17*, 347–361.

Goodlad, J., Marcus, D., & Fulton, J. (2013). Lead and attention-deficit/hyperactivity disorder (ADHD) symptoms: A meta-analysis. *Clinical Psychology Review*, *33*, 417–425.

Goodman, L. S., Wintrobe, M. M., Dameshek, W., Goodman, M. J., Gilman, A., & McLennan, M. T. (1946). Nitrogen mustard therapy: Use of methyl-bis (beta-chloroethyl) amine hydrochloride and tris (beta-chloroethyl) amine hydrochloride for Hodgkin's Disease, lymphosarcoma, leukemia and certain allied and miscellaneous disorders. *Journal of the American Medical Association*, *132*, 126–132.

Gottfried, J. A., & Chatterjee, A. (2001). Carbon monoxide-mediated hippocampal injury. *Neurology*, *57*, 17.

Grandjean, P., Weihe, P., White, R., Debes, F., Araki, S., Yokoyama, K., . . . Jørgensen, P. (1997). Cognitive deficit in 7-year-old children with prenatal exposure to methylmercury. *Neurotoxicology and Teratology*, *19*, 417–428.

Greve, K., Bianchini, K., Black, F., Heinly, M., Love, J., Swift, D., & Ciota, M. (2006). The prevalence of cognitive malingering in persons reporting exposure to occupational and environmental substances. *NeuroToxicology*, *27*, 940–950.

Gruber, S. A., Silveri, M. M., & Yurgelun-Todd, D. A. (2007). Neuropsychological consequences of opiate use. *Neuropsychology Review*, *17*, 299–315.

Halpern, J. H., Sherwood, A., Hudson, J. I., Gruber, S., Kozin, D., & Pope, H. G. (2010). Residual neurocognitive features of long-term ecstasy users with minimal exposure to other drugs. *Addiction*, *106*, 777–786.

Hanninen, H., Antti-Poika, M., Juntunen, J., & Koskenvuo, M. (1991). Exposure to organic solvents and neuropsychological dysfunction: A study on monozygotic twins. *British Journal of Industrial Medicine*, *48*, 18–25.

Haut, M. W., Kuwabara, H., Ducatman, A. M., Hatfiled, G., Parsons, M. W., Scott, A., . . . Morrow, L. A. (2006). Corpus callosum volume in railroad workers with chronic exposure to solvents. *Journal of Occupational and Environmental Medicine*, *48*, 615–624.

Haut, M. W., Leach, S., Kuwabara, H., Whyte, S., Callahan, T., Ducatman, A., . . . Gupta, N. (2000). Verbal working memory and solvent exposure: A positron emission tomography study. *Neuropsychology*, *14*, 551–558.

Haut, M. W., Morrow, L., Pool, D., Callahan, T., Haut, J., & Franzen, M. (1999). Neurobehavioral effects of acute exposure to inorganic mercury vapor. *Applied Neurospychology*, *6*, 193–200.

Haut, M. W., Wiener, J., Marano, G., & Abraham, J. (2013). Exploring the biology of "chemo brain": How was PET/CT helped us? *Imaging in Medicine*, *5*, 199–202.

Hodgson, K., Hutchinson, A., Wilson, C., & Nettelbeck, T. (2013). A meta-analysis of the effects of chemotherapy on cognition in patients with cancer. *Cancer Treatment Reviews*, *39*, 297–304.

Hogstedt, C., Hane, M., Agrell, A., & Bodin, L. (1983). Neuropsychological test results and symptoms among workers with well-defined long-term exposure to lead. *British Journal of Industrial Medicine*, *40*, 99–105.

Hopkins, R. O., & Woon, F. L. (2006). Neuroimaging, cognitive, and neurobehavioral outcomes following carbon monoxide poisoning. *Behavioral and Cognitive Neuroscience Reviews*, *5*, 141–156.

Ibrahim, D., Froberg, B., Wolf, A., & Rusyniak, D. (2006). Heavy metal poisoning: Clinical presentations and pathophysiology. *Clinics in Laboratory Medicine*, *26*, 67–97.

Inagaki, M., Yoshikawa, E., Matsuoka, Y., Sugawara, Y., Nakano, T., Akechi, T., . . . Uchitomi, Y. (2007). Smaller regional volumes of brain gray and white matter demonstrated in breast cancer survivors exposed to adjuvant chemotherapy. *Cancer*, *109*, 146–156.

Iqbal, S., Clower, J. H., King, M., Bell, J., & Yip, F. Y. (2012). National carbon monoxide poisoning surveillance framework and recent estimates. *Public Health Reports*, *127*, 486–496.

Itoh, K., Korogi, Y., Tomiguchi, S., Takahashi, M., Okajima, T., & Sato, H. (2001). Cerebellar blood flow in methylmercury poisoning (Minamata disease). *Neuroradiology*, *43*, 279–284.

Iudicello, J. E., Woods, S. P., Vigil, O., Cobb-Scott, J., Cherner, M., Heaton, R. K., . . . Grant, I. (2010). Longer term improvement in neurocognitive functioning and affective distress among methamphetamine users who achieve stable abstinence. *Journal of Clinical and Experimental Neuropsychology*, *32*, 704–718.

Jacobus J., Squeglia, L. M., Bava S., & Tapert S. F. (2013). White matter characterization of adolescent binge drinking with and without co-occurring marijuana use: A 3-year investigation. *Psychiatry Research: Neuroimaging*, *214*, 374–381.

Janelsins, M., Kohli, S., Mohile, S., Usuki, K., Ahles, T., & Morrow, G. (2011). An update on cancer- and chemotherapy-related cognitive dysfunction: Current status. *Seminars in Oncology*, *38*, 431–438.

Järup, L. (2003). Hazards of heavy metal contamination. *British Medical Bulletin*, *68*, 167–182.

Jasper, B. W., Hopkins, R. O., Duker, H. V., & Waver, L. K. (2005). Affective outcome following carbon monoxide poisoning: A prospective longitudinal study. *Cognitive and Behavioral Neurology*, *18*, 127–134.

Jeyaratnam, J., Boey, K., Ong, C., Chia, C., & Phoon, W. (1986). Neuropsychological studies on lead workers in Singapore. *British Journal of Industrial Medicine*, *43*, 626–629.

Jin, C. F., Haut, M. W., Ducatman, A. (2004). Industrial solvents and psychological effects. *Clinics in Occupational and Environmental Medicine*, *4*, 597–620.

Johnson, F., & Atchison, W. (2009). The role of environmental, mercury, lead and pesticide exposure in development of amyotrophic lateral sclerosis. *Neurotoxicology*, *30*, 761–765.

Karnofsky, D. (1958). Summary of results obtained with nitrogen mustard in the treatment of neoplastic disease. *Annals of the New York Academy of Science*, *68*, 899–914.

Keski-Santti, P., Mantyla, R., Lamminen, A., Hyvarinen, H. K., & Sainio, M. (2009). Magnetic resonance imaging in occupational chronic solvent encephalopathy. *International Archives of Occupational and Environmental Health*, *82*, 595–602.

Kesler, S. R., Bennett, C., Mahaffey, M., & Spiegel, D. (2009). Regional brain activation during verbal declarative memory in metastatic breast cancer. *Clinical Cancer Research*, *15*, 6665–6673.

Kesler, S. R., Hopkins, R. O., Weaver, L. K., Blatter, D. D., Edge-Booth, H., & Bigler, E. (2001). Verbal memory deficits associated with fornix atrophy in carbon monoxide poisoning. *Journal of the International Neuropsychological Society*, *7*, 640–646.

Kesler, S. R., Kent, J., & O'Hara, R. (2011). Prefrontal cortex and executive function impairments in primary breast cancer. *Archives of Neurology*, *68*, 1447–1453.

Khalil, N., Morrow, L., Needleman, H., Talbott, E., Wilson, J., & Cauley, J. (2009). Association of cumulative lead and neurocognitive function in an occupational cohort. *Neuropsychology*, *23*, 10–19.

Kim, Y., & Kim, J. (2012). Toxic encephalopathy. *Safety and Health at Work*, *3*, 243–256.

Koester, P., Tittgemeyer, M., Wagner, D., Becker, B., Gouzoulis-Mayfrank, E., & Daumann, J. (2012). Cortical thinning in amphetamine-type stimulant use. *Neuroscience*, *221*, 182–192.

Koppelmans, V., Breteler, M., Boogerd, W., Seynaeve, C., Gundy, C., & Schagen, S. (2011 or 2012). Neuropsychological performance in survivors of breast cancer more than 20 years after adjuvant chemotherapy. *Journal of Clinical Oncology*, *30*, 1080–1086.

Koppelmans, V., de Ruiter, M., van der Lijn, F., Boogerd, W., Seynaive, C., van der Lugt, A., . . . Schagen, S. (2011 or 2012). Global and focal brain volume in long-term breast cancer survivors exposed to adjuvant chemotherapy. *Breast Cancer Research and Treatment*, *132*, 1099–1106.

Korogi, Y., Takahashi, M., Okajima, T., & Eto, K. (1998). MR findings of Minamata disease—organic mercury poisoning. *Journal of Magnetic Resonance Imaging*, *8*, 308–316.

Kosnett, M. (2010). Chelation for heavy metals (arsenic, lead, and mercury): Protective or perilous? *Clinical Pharmacology & Therapeutics*, *88*, 412–415.

Landrigan, P., Whitworth, R., Baloh, R., Staehling, N., Barthel, W., & Rosenblum, B. (1975). Neuropsychological dysfunction in children with chronic low-level lead absorption. *The Lancet*, *305*, 708–712.

Lanphear, B., Hornung, R., Khoury, J., Yolton, K., Baghurst, P., Bellinger, D., . . . Roberts, R. (2005). Low-level environmental lead exposure and children's intellectual function: An international pooled analysis. *Environmental Health Perspectives*, *113*, 894–899.

Lin, W. C., Chou, K. H., Chen, C. C., Huang, C. C., Chen, H. L., Lu, C. H., . . . Lin, C. P. (2012). White matter abnormalities correlating with memory and depression in heroin users under methadone maintenance treatment. *PLoS One*, *7*, e33809.

Lin, W. C., Lu, C. H., Lee, Y. C., Wang, H. C., Lui, C. C., Cheng, Y. F., & Lin, C. P. (2009). White matter damage in carbon monoxide intoxication assessed in vivo using diffusion tensor MR imaging. *American Journal of Neuroradiology*, *30*, 1248–1255.

Linden, W., Vodermaier, A., MacKenzie, R., & Greig, D. (2012). Anxiety and depression after cancer diagnosis: Prevalence rates by cancer type, gender, and age. *Journal of Affective Disorders*, *141*, 343–351.

Lisdahl, K. M., Gilbart, E. R., Wright, N. E., & Shollenbarger, S. (2013). Dare to delay? The impacts of adolescent alcohol and marijuana use onset on cognition, brain structure and function. *Frontiers in Psychiatry*, *4*, 1–19.

Liu, K., Hao, J., Zeng, Y., Dai, F., & Gu, P. (2013). Neurotoxicity and biomarkers of lead exposure: A review. *Chinese Medical Sciences Journal*, *28*, 178–188.

Lo, C. P., Chen, S. Y., Chou, M. C., Wang, C. Y., Lee, K. W., Hsueh, C. J., . . . Huang, G. S. (2007). Diffusion-tensor MR imaging for evaluation of the efficacy of hyperbaric oxygen therapy in patients with delayed neuropsychiatric syndrome cause by carbon monoxide inhalation. *European Journal of Neurology*, *14*, 777–782.

Marcus, D., Fulton, J., & Clarke, E. (2010). Lead and conduct problems: A meta-analysis. *Journal of Clinical Child & Adolescent Psychology*, *39*, 234–241.

Marlowe, M., Folio, R., Hall, D., & Errera, J. (1982). Increased lead burdens and trace-mineral status in mentally retarded children. *The Journal of Special Education*, *16*, 87–99.

Mata, I., Prez-Iglesias, R., Rois-Santianez, R., Tordesillas-Gutierrez, D., Pazos, A., Gutierrez, A., Vazquez-Barquero., J. L., & Crespo-Facorro, B. (2010). Gyrification brain abnormalities associated with adolescence and early adulthood cannabis use. *Brain Research*, *1317*, 297–304.

Mazumdar, M., Bellinger, D., Gregas, M., Abanilla, K., Bacic, J., & Needleman, H. (2011). Low-level environmental lead exposure in childhood and adult intellectual function: A follow-up study. *Environmental Health*, *10*, 24.

McCann, U. D., Kuwabara, H., Kumar, A., Palermo, M., Abbey, R., Brasic, J., . . . Ricaurte, G. A. (2008). Persistent cognitive and dopamine transporter deficits in abstinent methamphetamine users. *Synapse*, *62*, 91–100.

McDonald, B., Conroy, S., Ahles, T., West, J., & Saykin, A. (2010). Gray matter reduction associated with systemic chemotherapy for breast cancer: A prospective MRI study. *Breast Cancer Research and Treatment*, *123*, 819–828.

McDonald, B., Conroy, S., Ahles, T., West, J., & Saykin, A. (2012). Alterations in brain activation during working memory processing associated with breast cancer and treatment: A prospective functional magnetic resonance imaging study. *Journal of Clinical Oncology*, *30*, 2500–2508.

Meier, M. H., Caspi, A., Ambler, A., Harrington, H. L., Houts, R., Keefe, R.S.E., . . . Moffitt, T. E. (2012). Persistent cannabis users show neuropsychological decline from childhood to midlife. *Proceedings of the National Academy of Sciences*, *109*, E2657–E2664.

Min, S. K. (1986). A brain syndrome associated with delayed neuropsychiatric sequelae following acute carbon monoxide intoxication. *Acta Psychiatrica Scandinavica*, *73*, 80–86.

Moore, M., Meredith, P., & Goldberg, A. (1977). A retrospective analysis of blood-lead in mentally retarded children. *The Lancet*, *309*, 717–719.

Morrow, L. A., Gibson, C., Bagovich, G. R., Stein, L., Condray, R., & Scott, A. (2000). Increased incidence of anxiety and depressive disorders in persons with organic solvent exposure. *Psychosomatic Medicine*, *62*, 746–750.

Morrow, L. A., Muldoon, S. B., & Sandstrom, D. J. (2001). Neuropsychological sequelae associated with occupational and environmental exposure to chemicals. In R. Tarter, M. Butters, & S. Beers (Eds.), *Medical Neuropsychology: Impact of Disease on Behavior* (2nd ed., pp. 199–245). New York: Kluwer Academic/Plenum Publishers.

Morrow, L. A., Steinhauer, S. R., Condray, R., & Hodgson, M. (1997). Neuropsychological performance of journeyman painters under acute solvent exposure and exposure-free conditions. *Journal of the International Neuropsychological Society*, *3*, 269–275.

Mutter, J., Naumann, J., Sadaghiani, C., Schneider, R., & Walach, H. (2004). Alzheimer disease: Mercury as a pathogenetic factor and apolipprotein E as a moderator. *Neuroendocrinology Letters*, *25*, 331–339.

Nakam, H., Chang, O., Fein, G., Shimotsu, R., Jiang, C. S., & Ernst, T. (2011). Methamphetamine users show greater than normal age-related cortical gray matter loss. *Addiction*, *106*, 1474–1483.

Needleman, H. (1975). Lead-paint poisoning prevention: An opportunity forfeited. *The New England Journal of Medicine*, *292*, 588–589.

Needleman, H. (2004). Lead poisoning. *Annual Review of Medicine*, *55*, 209–222.

Needleman, H. (2009). Low level lead exposure: History and discovery. *Annals of Epidemiology*, *19*, 235–238.

Needleman, H., Geiger, S., & Frank, R. (1985). Lead and IQ scores: A reanalysis. *Science*, *227*, 701–702, 704.

Needleman, H., Gunnoe, C., Leviton, A., & Peresie, H. (1978). Neuropsychological dysfunction in children with "silent" lead exposure. *Pediatric Research*, *12*, 374.

Needleman, H., Gunnoe, C., Leviton, A., Reed, R., Peresie, H., Maher, C., & Barrett, P. (1979). Deficits in psychologic and classroom performance of children with elevated dentine lead levels. *The New England Journal of Medicine*, *300*, 689–695.

Needleman, H., & Landrigan, P. (1981). The health effects of low level exposure to lead. *Annual Review of Public Health*, *2*, 227–298.

Needleman, H., Reiss, J., Tobin, M., Biesecker, G., & Greenhouse, J. (1996). Bone lead levels and delinquent behavior. *Journal of the American Medical Association*, *275*, 363–369.

Needleman, H., Schell, A., Bellinger, D., Leviton, A., & Allred, E. (1990). The long-term effects of exposure to low doses of lead in children: An 11-year follow-up report. *The New England Journal of Medicine*, *322*, 83–88.

Neghab, M., Norouzi, M., Choobineh, A., Kardaniyan, M., & Zadeh, J. (2012). Health effects associated with long-term occupational exposure of employees of a chlor-alkali plant to mercury. *International Journal of Occupational Safety and Ergonomics*, *18*, 97–106.

Nelson, W., & Suls, J. (2013). New approaches to understand cognitive changes associated with chemotherapy for non-central nervous system tumors. *Journal of Pain and Symptom Management*, *46*, 707–721.

Nilson, L. N., Bäckman, L., Sällsten, G., Hagberg, S., & Barregård, L. (2003). Dose-related cognitive deficits among floor layers with previous heavy exposure to solvents. *Archives of Environmental Health: An International Journal*, *58*, 208–217.

Nilson, L. N., Sällsten, G., Hagberg, S., Bäckman, L., & Barregård, L. (2002). Influence of solvent exposure and aging on cognitive functioning: An 18 year follow up of formerly exposed layers and their controls. *Occupational and Environmental Medicine*, *59*, 49–57.

O'Carroll, R., Masterton, G., Dougall, N., Ebmeier, K., & Goodwin, G. (1995). The neuropsychiatric sequelae of mercury poisoning: The Mad Hatter's disease revisited. *The British Journal of Psychiatry*, *167*, 95–98.

O'Donnell, P., Buxton, P. J., Pitkin, A., & Jarvis, L. J. (2000). The magnetic resonance imaging appearances of the brain in acute carbon monoxide poisoning. *Clinical Radiology*, *55*, 273–280.

Oxman, T., & Silberfarb, P. (1980). Serial cognitive testing in cancer patients receiving chemotherapy. *American Journal of Psychiatry*, *137*, 1263–1265.

Parkinson, R. B., Hopkins, R. O., Cleavinger, H. B., Weaver, L. K., Victoroff, J., Foley, J. F., & Bigler, E. D. (2002). White matter hyperintensities and neuropsychological outcome following carbon monoxide poisoning. *Neurology*, *58*, 1525–1532.

Parrott, A. C. (2013). MDMA, serotonergic neurotoxicity, and the diverse functional deficits of recreational "Ecstasy" users. *Neuroscience and Biobehavioral Reviews*, *27*, 1466–1484.

Parsons, O. A. (1994). Determinants of cognitive deficits in alcoholics: The search continues. *Clinical Neuropsychologist*, *8*, 39–58.

Parsons, O. A. (1998). Neurocognitive deficits in alcoholics and social drinkers: A continuum? *Alcoholism: Clinical and Experimental Research*, *22*, 954–961.

Parsons, O. A., & Nixon, S. J. (1998). Cognitive functioning in sober social drinkers: A review of the research since 1986. *Journal of Studies on Alcohol*, *59*, 180–190.

Persson, R., Osterberg, K., Karlson, B., & Orbaek, P. (2000). Influence of personality traits on neuropsychological test performance in toxic encephalopathy cases and healthy referent subjects. *Neurotoxicology*, *21*, 667–675.

Porter, S. S., Hopkins, R. O., Weaver, L. K., Bigler, E. D., & Blatter, D. D. (2002). Corpus callosum atrophy and neuropsychological outcome following carbon monoxide poisoning. *Archives of Clinical Neuropsychology*, *7*, 195–204.

Prockop, L. D. (2005). Carbon monoxide brain toxicity: Clinical, magnetic resonance imaging, magnetic resonance spectroscopy, and neuropsychological effects in 9 people. *Journal of Neuroimaging*, *15*, 144–149.

Prockop, L. D., & Chichkova, R. I. (2007). Carbon monoxide intoxication: An updated review. *Journal of Neurological Science*, *262*, 122–130.

Prosser, J. M., Eisenberg, D., Davey, E. E., Steinfield, M., Cohen, L. J., London, E. D., & Galynker, I. I. (2008). Character pathology and neuropsychological test performance in remitted opiate dependence. *Substance Abuse Treatment, Prevention, and Policy*, *3*, 23.

Prosser, J. M., Cohen, L. J., Steinfield, M., Eisenberg, D., London, E. D., & Galynker, I. I. (2006). Neuropsychological functioning in opiate-dependent subjects receiving and following methadone maintenance treatment. *Drug and Alcohol Dependence*, *84*, 240–247.

Pulsipher, D. T., Hopkins, R. O., & Weaver, L. K. (2006). Basal ganglia volumes following CO poisoning: A prospective longitudinal study. *Undersea and Hyperbaric Medicine*, *33*, 245–256.

Qiu, Y., Jiang, G., Su, H., Lv, X., Shang, X., Tian, J., & Zhou, F. (2013). Progressive white matter microstructure damage in male chronic heroin dependent individuals: A DTI and TBSS study. *PLoS One*, *8*, e63212.

Raffa, R., Duong, P., Finney, J., Garber, D., Lam, L., Mathew, S., . . . Weng, H. (2006). Is "chemo-fog"/"chemo-brain" caused by cancer chemotherapy? *Journal of Clinical Pharmacy and Therapeutics*, *31*, 129–138.

Rapeli, P., Fabritius, C., Kalska, H., & Alho, H. (2009). Memory function in opioid-dependent patients treated with methadone or buprenorphine along with benzodiazepine: Longitudinal change in comparison to healthy individuals. *Substance Abuse Treatment, Prevention, and Policy*, *4*, 1–16.

Rapeli, P., Fabritius, C., Kalska, H., & Alho, H. (2011). Cognitive functioning in opioid-dependent patients treated with buprenorphine, methadone, and other psychoactive medications: Stability and correlates. *BMC Pharmacology and Toxicology*, *11*, 13.

Reid-Arndt, S., Hsieh, C., & Perry, M. (2010). Neuropsychological functioning and quality of life during the first year after completing chemotherapy for breast cancer. *Psychooncology*, *19*, 535–544.

Reuter-Lorenz, P., & Cimprich, B. (2013). Cognitive function and breast cancer: Promise and potential insights from functional brain imaging. *Breast Cancer Research and Treatment*, *137*, 33–43.

Rhoads, C. (1946). Nitrogen mustards in the treatment of neoplastic disease. *Journal of the American Medical Association*, *131*, 656–658.

Risher, J., Murray, H., & Prince, G. (2002). Organic mercury compounds: Human exposure and its relevance to public health. *Toxicology and Industrial Health*, *18*, 109–160.

Rogan, W., Dietrich, K., Ware, J., Dockery, D., Salganik, M., Radcliffe, J., . . . Rhoads, G. (2001). The effect of chelation therapy with succimer on neuropsychological development in children exposed to lead. *New England Journal of Medicine*, *344*, 1421–1426.

Rogeberg, O. (2013). Correlations between cannabis use and IQ change in the Dunedin cohort are consistent with confounding from socioeconomic status. *Proceedings of the National Academy of Sciences*, *110*, 4251–4254.

Rohling, M., & Demakis, G. (2006). A meta-analysis of the neuropsychological effects of occupational exposure to mercury. *The Clinical Neuropsychologist*, *20*, 108–132.

Rosenbloom, M. J., & Pfefferbaum, A. (2008). Magnetic resonance imaging of the living brain: Evidence for brain degeneration among alcoholics and recovery with abstinence. *Alcohol Research & Health*, *31*, 362–376.

Rourke, S. B., & Loberg, T. (1993). The neurobehavioral correlates of alcoholism. In R. W. Parks, R. F. Zec, & R. S. Wilson (Eds.), *Neuropsychology of Alzheimer's Disease and Other Dementias* (pp. 423–485). Oxford, UK: Oxford University Press.

Sabbath, E. L., Glymour, M. M., Berr, C., Singh-Manoux, A., Zins, M., Goldberg, M., & Beckman, L. F. (2012). Occupational solvent exposure and cognition: Does the association vary by level of education? *Neurology*, *78*, 754–1760.

Sanders, T., Liu, Y., Buchner, V., & Tchounwou, P. (2009). Neurotoxic effects and biomarkers of lead exposure: A review. *Reviews on Environmental Health*, *24*, 15–45.

Sandstead, H. (1986). A brief history of the influence of trace elements on brain function. *The American Journal of Clinical Nutrition*, *43*, 293–298.

Saykin, A., Ahles, T., & McDonald, B. (2003). Mechanisms of chemotherapy-induced cognitive disorders: Neuropsychological, pathophysiological, and neuroimaging perspectives. *Seminars in Clinical Neuropsychology*, *8*, 201–216.

Scherling, C., & Smith, A. (2013). Opening up the window into "chemobrain": A neuroimaging review. *Sensors*, *13*, 3169–3203.

Schwartz, B., Caffo, B., Stewart, W., Hedlin, H., James, B., Yousem, D., & Davatzikos, C. (2010). Evaluation of cumulative lead dose and longitudinal changes in structural MRI in former organolead workers. *Journal of Occupational and Environmental Medicine*, *52*, 407–414.

Schwartz, B., Stewart, W., Bolla, K., Simon, D., Bandeen-Roche, K., Gordon, B., . . . Todd, A. (2000). Past adult lead exposure is associated with longitudinal decline in cognitive function. *Neurology*, *55*, 1144–1150.

Scott, J. C., Woods, S. P., Matt, G. E., Meyer, R. A., Heaton, R. K., Atkinson, J. H., & Grant, I. (2007). Neurocognitive effects of methamphetamine: A critical review and meta-analysis. *Neuropsychology Review*, *17*, 275–297.

Seigers, R., Schagen, S., Tellingen, O., & Dietrich, J. (2013). Chemotherapy-related cognitive dysfunction: Current animal studies and future directions. *Brain Imaging and Behavior*, *7*, 453–459.

Sener, R. H. (2003). Acute carbon monoxide poisoning: Diffusion MR imaging findings. *American Journal of Neuroradiology*, *24*, 1475–1477.

Shih, R., Glass, T., Bandeen-Roche, K., Carlson, M., Bolla, K., Todd, A., & Schwartz, B. (2006). Environmental lead exposure and cognitive function in community-dwelling older adults. *Neurology*, *67*, 1556–1562.

Silberfarb, P. (1983). Chemotherapy and cognitive defects in cancer patients. *Annual Review of Medicine*, *34*, 35–46.

Silberfarb, P., Philibert, D., & Levine, P. (1980). Psychosocial aspects of neoplastic disease: II. Affective and cognitive effects of chemotherapy in cancer patients. *American Journal of Psychiatry*, *137*, 597–601.

Silverman, D., Dy, C., Castellon, S., Lai, J., Pio, B., Abraham, L., . . . Ganz, P. (2007). Altered frontocortical, cerebellar, and basal ganglia activity in adjuvant-treated breast cancer survivors 5–10 years after chemotherapy. *Breast Cancer Research and Treatment*, *103*, 303–311.

Simó, M., Rifà-Ros, X., Rodriguez-Fornells, A., & Bruna, J. (2013). Chemobrain: A systematic review of structural and functional neuroimaging studies. *Neuroscience and Biobehavioral Reviews*, *37*, 1311–1321.

Smith, M. J., Cobia, D. J., Wang, L., Alpert, K. I., Cronenwett, W. J., Goldman, M. B., Mamah D., Barch D. M., & Csernansky, J. G. (2013). Cannabis-related working memory deficits and associated subcortical morphological differences in health individuals and schizophrenia subjects. *Schizophrenia Bulletin*, *40*, 287–299.

Sohn, Y. H., Jeong, Y., Kim, H. S., Im, J. H., & Kim, J. S. (2000). The brain lesion responsible for parkinsonism after carbon monoxide poisoning. *Archives of Neurology*, *57*, 1214–1218.

Stewart, W., Schwartz, B., Davatzikos, D., Shen, D., Liu, D., Wu, X., . . . Youssem, D. (2006). Past adult lead exposure is linked to neurodegeneration measured by brain MRI. *Neurology*, *66*, 1476–1484.

Stoller, K. P. (2007). Hyperbaric oxygen and carbon monoxide poisoning: A critical review. *Neurology Research*, *29*, 146–155.

Sullivan, E. V., Harris, A., & Pfefferbaum, A. (2010). Alcohol's effect on brain and behavior. *Alcohol Research & Health*, *33*, 127–143.

Tang, C. Y., Carpenter, D. M., Eaves, E. L., Ng, J., Ganeshalingam, N., Weisel, C., . . . Fielder, N. L. (2011). Occupational solvent exposure and brain function: An fMRI study. *Environmental Health Perspectives*, *119*, 908–913.

Tobia, M. C., O'Neill, J. O., Hudkins, M., Bartzokis, G., Dean, A. C., & London, E. D. (2010). White-matter abnormalities in brain during early abstinence from methamphetamine abuse. *Psychopharmacology*, *209*, 13–24.

Tong, S., Baghurst, P., McMichael, A., Sawyer, M., & Mudge, J. (1996). Lifetime exposure to environmental lead and children's intelligence at 11–13 years: The Port Pirie cohort study. *British Medical Journal*, *312*, 1569–1575.

van Dam, F., Schagen, S., Muller, M., Boogerd, W., Wall, E., Droogleever Fortuyn, M., & Rodenhuis, S. (1998). Impairment of Cognitive function in women receive adjuvant treatment for high-risk breast cancer: High-dose versus standard-dose chemotherapy. *Journal of the National Cancer Institute*, *90*, 210–218.

van Holst, R. J., & Schilt, T. (2011). Drug-related decrease in neuropsychological functions of abstinent drug users. *Current Drug Abuse Reviews*, *4*, 42–56.

van Hout, M., Schmand, B., Wekking, E., & Deelman, B. (2006). Cognitive functioning in patients with suspected chronic toxic encephalopathy: Evidence for neuropsychological disturbances after controlling for insufficient effort. *Journal of Neurology, Neurosurgery & Psychiatry*, *77*, 296–303.

van Hout, M., Schmand, B., Wekking, E., Hageman, G., & Deelman, B. (2003). Suboptimal performance of neuropsychological tests in patients with suspected chronic toxic encephalopathy. *NeuroToxicology*, *24*, 547–551.

van Valen, E., van Thriel, C., Akila, R., Nilson, L. N., Bast-Pettersen, R., Saino, M., . . . Wekking, E. (2012). Chronic solvent-induced encephalopathy: European consensus of neuropsychological characteristics, assessment, and guidelines for diagnostics. *NeuroToxicology*, *33*, 710–726.

Vinceti, M., Bottecchi, I., Fan, A., Finkselstein, Y., & Mandrioli, J. (2012). Are environmental exposures to selenium, heavy metals, and pesticides risk factors for amyotrophic lateral sclerosis? *Reviews on Environmental Health*, *27*, 19–41.

Visser, L., Lavini, C., Booij, J., Reneman, L., Majoie, C., de Boer, A. G., . . . Schene, A. H. (2008). Cerebral impairment in chronic solvent-induced encephalopathy. *Annals of Neurology*, *63*, 572–580.

Visser, L., Wekking, E. M., de Boer, A.G.E.M., de Joode, E. A., van Hout, M.S.E., van Dorsselaer, S., . . . Schene, A. H. (2011). Prevalence of psychiatric disorders in patients with chronic solvent induced encephalopathy. *NeruoToxicology*, *32*, 916–922.

Voh Ah, D., Habermann, B., Carpenter, J. S., & Schneider, S. L. (2013). Impact of perceived cognitive impairment in breast cancer survivors. *European Journal of Oncology Nursing*, *17*, 236–241.

Wagner, D., Becker, B., Koester, P., Gouzoulis-Mayfrank, E., & Daumann, J. (2012). A prospective study of learning, memory, and executive function in new MDMA users. *Addiction*, *108*, 136–145.

Wang, X., Li, B., Zhou, X., Liao, Y., Tang, J., Liu, T., Hu, D., Hao, W. (2012). Changes in brain gray matter in abstinent heroin addicts. *Drug and Alcohol Dependence*, *126*, 304–308.

Weaver, L. K., Hopkins, R. O., Chan, K. J., Churchill, S., Elliot, C. G., Clemmer, T. P., . . . Morris, A. H. (2002). Hyperbaric oxygen for acute carbon monoxide poisoning. *New England Journal of Medicine*, *347*, 1057–1067.

Wefel, J., Lenzi, R., Theriault, R., Davis, R., & Meyers, C. (2004). The cognitive sequelae of standard-dose adjuvant chemotherapy in women with breast carcinoma. *Cancer*, *100*, 2292–2299.

Weiss, B. (2011). Lead, manganese, and methylmercury as risk factors for neurobehavioral impairment in advanced age. *International Journal of Alzheimer's Disease*. doi: 10.4061/2011/607543

White, R., Palumbo, C., Yugelun-Todd, D., Heaton, K., Weihe, P., Debes, F., & Grandjean, P. (2011). Functional MRI approach to developmental methylmercury and polychlorinated biphenyl neurotoxicity. *NeuroToxicology*, *32*, 975–980.

White, R., & Proctor, S. (1993). Solvent encephalopathy. In R. W. Parks, R. F. Zec, & R. S. Wilson (Eds.), *Neuropsychology of Alzheimer's Disease and Other Dementias* (pp. 350–374). Oxford, UK: Oxford University Press.

Winhusen, T., Somoza, E. C., Lewis, D. F., Kropp, F. B., Origian, V. E., & Adinoff, B. (2013). Frontal systems deficits in stimulant-dependent patients: Evidence of pre-illness dysfunction and relationship to treatment response. *Drug and Alcohol Dependence*, *127*, 94–100.

Wolf, S. J., Lavonas, E. J., Sloan, E. P., & Jagoda, A. S. (2008). Clinical policy: Critical issues in the management of adult patients presenting to the emergency department with acute carbon monoxide poisoning. *Annals of Emergency Medicine*, *51*, 138–152.

Yucel, M., Solowij, N., Respondeh, C., Whittle, S., Fornito, A., Pantelis, C., & Lubman, D. I. (2008). Regional brain abnormalities associated with long-term heavy cannabis use. *Archives of General Psychiatry*, *65*, 694–701.

25 Multiple Sclerosis and Related Disorders

Peter A. Arnett, Jessica E. Meyer, Victoria C. Merritt, and Lauren B. Strober

Introduction

Multiple sclerosis (MS) is the most common nontraumatic neurological condition of early to middle adulthood, and the most common demyelinating condition. Other demyelinating conditions include concentric sclerosis (also known as *Balo's disease*), Schilder's disease, Devic's disease, central pontine myelinolysis, and Marchiafava-Bignami disease. Rarer still are acute disseminated encephalomyelitis and acute hemorrhagic leukoencephalitis. Because MS is the only one of these conditions that has been adequately examined neuropsychologically, the focus of this chapter will be on MS.

Neuropathology

A central feature of MS is demyelination that is presumed to be caused by an autoimmune process, a slow-acting virus, or a delayed reaction to a common virus (Brassington & Marsh, 1998). Multiple discrete plaques at demyelinated sites are formed, in part, by proliferating astrocytes. The plaques are comprised of demyelination, inflammation, gliosis and axonal injury, and myelin sheaths within plaques are swollen and fragmented, or destroyed entirely. When intact, nerves of the central nervous system (CNS) are enclosed in myelin sheaths, which are separated by synaptic gaps from which the nerve impulse fires, facilitating neural conduction. Plaques associated with MS thus interfere with or block neural transmission by limiting this saltatory conduction process. Axons and cell bodies of neurons often remain intact. Lesions are typically found in a random or asymmetrical pattern in the periventricular, juxtacortical, and infratentorial regions.

Plaques occur in both the brain and spinal cord, and the location of plaques is highly heterogeneous among patients. Plaques in the cerebrum are most commonly located near the lateral and third ventricles and the periventricular region. The frontal lobes are next most commonly affected, but plaques in other major lobes of the brain are also frequently seen. Additionally, plaques are commonly seen in the optic nerves, chiasm, or tracts, as well as the corpus callosum, brain stem, and cerebellum. Furthermore, plaques can be found in white matter regions of the thalamus, hypothalamus, and basal ganglia.

Despite long-standing classification as a white matter disease, recent research has suggested significant involvement of gray matter, even early on in the disease (Zivadinov & Pirko, 2012). The most affected gray matter regions include the cingulate, thalamus, basal ganglia, hypothalamus, cerebellum, hippocampus, and frontal and temporal lobes (Horakova, Kalincik, Dusankova, & Dolezal, 2012). This type of cortical demyelination occurs most frequently in Progressive forms of MS and may be indicative of disease progression and potential irreversible disability (Popescu & Lucchinetti, 2012).

Epidemiology

The incidence of MS is lowest in regions close to the equator, with larger numbers of cases in northern and southern latitudes (from about 60 to 300 per 100,000, respectively). There are about 400,000 people with MS in the United States, and 2.5 million people worldwide (National MS Society, 2009). Females are approximately 2.5 times more likely than males to get MS, with some recent work suggesting this disparity is increasing (Koch-Henriksen & Sørensen, 2010), and peak onset for the disease is around age 30 (Chitnis et al., 2011). Those living north of latitude 40 degrees North are about three times as likely to have MS as are those living in the southern United States, a geographic pattern suggesting an environmental contribution to the disease. Still, the 30%–40% concordance rate in identical twins versus only 1%–13% in fraternal twins implicates a substantial genetic contribution, as well. Onset of the disease occurs between age 20 and 40 in 70% of patients (Compston et al., 2005); onset after age 40 is often characterized by quicker progression and greater morbidity. Life expectancy beyond disease onset is approximately 30 years, but there is significant variability around this mean.

Symptom Onset and Diagnosis

Early MS symptoms are variable, but the most common initial symptoms include muscle weakness, paresthesias (i.e., numbness and tingling in the limbs, trunk, or face), gait/balance problems, and visual disturbances. The latter usually involve decreased visual acuity, blurry vision, or diplopia. Urinary disturbance is also common, as are balance difficulties. Cognitive dysfunction, fatigue, and depression are frequently observed, as well. MS symptoms are often transient and unpredictable. For example, visual disturbances and paresthesias may last for seconds or hours. Because of the short-lived and sometimes bizarre nature of the symptoms, it is not uncommon for patients to be diagnosed with hysteric/somatization disorders prior to a formal diagnosis of MS.

The diagnosis of MS is based on guidelines developed by McDonald and colleagues (2001), and these were subsequently revised in 2005 (Polman et al., 2005), and 2010 (Polman et al., 2010). The revision by Polman and colleagues in 2010 was the result of a consensus panel designed to simplify the criteria. Classifications in this new diagnostic system include "MS," "not MS," and "possible MS." Central factors for an MS diagnosis in this new system involve both clinical and paraclinical (e.g., the presence of oligoclonal bands in the cerebral spinal fluid, or CSF) assessments, lesions that are disseminated in space (DIS) and time (DIT), and disease attacks that last at least 24 hours. DIS occurs with the presence of at least one T2 lesion in at least two of four MS-typical regions of the CNS (periventricular, juxtacortical, infratentorial, or spinal cord), or by a clinical attack that implicates a different CNS site. DIT occurs when a new T2 and/or gadolinium-enhancing lesion(s) appears on follow-up MRI after a baseline scan has been conducted; DIT can also be demonstrated by the simultaneous presence of asymptomatic gadolinium-enhancing and nonenhancing lesions.

Per the McDonald et al. (2001) system, MS sometimes presents with an insidious progression rather than via discrete attacks, and is known as Primary Progressive MS. For this to be demonstrated there must be evidence of at least one year of disease progression, as well as at least two of the following: (a) evidence for DIS in the brain, (b) evidence for DIS in the spinal cord based on the presence of at least two T2 spinal cord lesions, or (c) positive CSF findings (isoelectric evidence of oligoclonal bands and/or elevated IgG index).

Prior to the mid-1990s, MS was classified into two major disease course types: Relapsing-Remitting and Chronic Progressive. An updated system was then developed and is now more commonly used (Lublin & Reingold, 1996). Presently, there are four course types in this new system: Relapsing-Remitting, Secondary Progressive, Primary Progressive, and Progressive Relapsing. Relapsing-Remitting is the most common type and affects more than half of all patients. Relapsing-Remitting MS is characterized by clearly defined disease relapses where recovery can be complete or with sequelae and residual deficit; however, there is no progression of disease between relapses. Relapses typically last days to weeks, with a duration of hours or months being less common. The frequency of relapses is highly variable, and can occur weeks or even years apart.

The remaining course types are all progressive in nature and were formerly encompassed by the Chronic Progressive term. The Secondary Progressive course is next most common and always begins as a Relapsing-Remitting course, but is defined by progression occurring even between relapses, and relapses and remissions with this course may or may not occur. The median time to conversion from Relapsing-Remitting to Secondary Progressive course is 15–20 years (Loitfelder et al., 2011). The Primary Progressive type is next most common, and involves an unremitting disease progression from disease onset for most patients with no clear relapses. The least common MS course type is Progressive Relapsing, and this involves disease progression from onset that is punctuated by acute relapses from which patients may or may not fully recover.

Cognitive Functioning

Patterns and Prevalence

Rao, Leo, Bernadin, and Unverzagt's (1991) seminal study remains the definitive examination of prevalence of cognitive dysfunction in MS in a community-based sample, as it compared 100 community-based MS patients with 100 matched healthy controls on an extensive neuropsychological battery. This study showed that individuals with MS demonstrated the greatest impairment on measures of recent memory, sustained attention, verbal fluency, and conceptual reasoning, and were less frequently impaired on measures of language, visuospatial perception, and immediate and remote memory. From this, Rao and colleagues proposed a brief battery—subsequently named the *Brief Repeatable Battery* (BRB) of neuropsychological tests likely to be most sensitive to cognitive impairment in MS, based on the tests that most differentiated MS and normal controls in their study. This initial battery included the Paced Auditory Serial Addition Test (PASAT), Controlled Oral Word Association Test (COWAT), 7/24 Spatial Recall, and the Verbal Selective Reminding Test (SRT). The Symbol Digit Modalities Test (SDMT) was subsequently added for a five-test battery that took about 30 minutes to administer, and included multiple alternate forms for each test (Rao and the Cognitive Function Study Group of the National Multiple Sclerosis Society, 1990). Additionally, the 7/24 Spatial Recall was expanded into a 10/36 Spatial Recall test that required more items to recall to enhance sensitivity. Subsequent studies have generally supported Rao and colleagues' findings about cognitive domains most affected in MS (Benedict et al., 2006; Bobholz & Rao, 2003; Chiaravalloti & DeLuca, 2010). Benedict and colleagues conducted their study on a clinic-based MS sample consisting of 291 MS patients and 56 healthy matched controls. The prevalence rates for cognitive impairment in their MS sample were often higher than Rao et al., though the same general pattern of domains typically affected was found. When discussing the different cognitive domains below, we will primarily reference Rao et al. and Benedict et al.'s studies, with prevalence rates of impairment typical of community-based samples based on the former and rates typical of clinic-based samples based on the latter study. The two studies used similar cutoffs for impairment, with Rao and colleagues defining impairment at the fifth percentile (relative to controls) and Benedict et al. using 1.5 standard deviations below the mean of controls.

SIMPLE AND COMPLEX ATTENTION, INFORMATION PROCESSING SPEED

Simple attention span (as measured by tests such as Digit Span) is usually intact in MS patients, but mild impairments are sometimes found. However, MS patients typically show their greatest difficulty on tasks requiring rapid and complex information processing, including those requiring swift application of working memory operations, attentional switching, or rapid visual scanning. About 25%–30% of community-based MS patients and 25–50% of clinic-based patients show impairments on such tasks of complex attention and processing speed. Some investigators have asserted that slowed information processing is the most fundamental cognitive deficit in MS, noting that such difficulties impact new learning and the ability to perform higher-order cognitive functions (Chiaravalloti & DeLuca, 2010). Working memory and processing speed are typically measured by tasks such as the PASAT and SDMT. The SDMT appears to be more sensitive than the PASAT, perhaps due to its visual nature given that many MS patients have visual problems. Supporting this hypothesis, at least one study (Bruce, Bruce, & Arnett, 2007) has shown that primary visual acuity problems contribute significantly to performance on the SDMT in MS patients, even in patient groups who have been prescreened for significant visual problems. Thus, it appears that even subtle visual anomalies can impact performance on the SDMT, and perhaps inflate sensitivity measures in MS patients. Furthermore, rudimentary oralmotor deficits contribute to group differences on tasks such as the SDMT in MS (Arnett, Smith, Barwick, Benedict, & Ahlstrom, 2008), suggesting that both primary visual and primary oral motor factors may inflate sensitivity measures of the SDMT in MS. In terms of the practical impact of these types of deficits, patients with MS often complain of problems tracking things in conversation, following details of movies or television programs, and quickly and efficiently performing work tasks. Such everyday difficulties may stem from problems with complex attention and speeded information processing.

MEMORY

Memory difficulties in MS are usually manifested as deficits with immediate recall on neuropsychological testing. Although delayed recall is also commonly impaired, this appears to be mostly a function of limited immediate recall, as opposed to actual forgetting. Tests that are most commonly used to measure memory functioning in MS include the California Verbal Learning Test, second edition (CVLT-II), Brief Visuospatial Memory Test–Revised (BVMT-R), 10/36 Spatial Recall, and story memory tests such as Logical Memory from the Wechsler Memory Scale, or the Story Recall test. In community-based MS groups, about 25%–30% of patients have impaired recall, compared with 25% to more than 50% of clinic-based patients. Regarding the upper value for clinic-based patients, this is solely due to MS patients' impairment on the BVMT-R, so this latter test appears to be unusually sensitive to cognitive impairment in clinic-based MS samples. With that said, given the visual-motor problems that are common to MS, it may be that such a test has an inflated sensitivity because it may be affected by noncognitive (i.e., motor, visual) factors in addition to cognitive factors. Consistent with such a hypothesis, Benedict and colleagues (2011) found a high inverse correlation ($r = -0.45$) between BVMT-R performance and upper extremity function (as measured by the 9-Hole Peg Test, or 9-HPT). Their interpretation of such data was different, however, as they suggested that the causal relationship may run in the other direction, with higher-order cognitive functions impacting motor performance and thus accounting for the relationship. Such an interpretation was based, in part, by the fact that the 9-HPT was inversely correlated with performance on a number of other cognitively demanding tests with significant executive components (e.g., Delis-Kaplan Executive Function System [D-KEFS] Sorting Test, PASAT, and SDMT).

The learning curve across repeated trials of memory tests (e.g., CVLT-II, BVMT-R) is typically similar in slope in MS compared with controls, but is lower in magnitude. Working memory, or the ability to maintain and manipulate information "online," is also commonly impaired in MS. However, percent retention, recognition, incidental memory following a delay, remote memory, and semantic memory are usually intact.

Because memory-impaired patients usually display intact recognition memory, MS patients' memory recall problems were initially thought to be due to problems with retrieval (Rao et al., 1991). However, based on additional work finding that patients could recall a normative amount of information if given enough initial learning trials, some investigators asserted that these memory recall problems were primarily due to initial acquisition difficulties (DeLuca, Barbieri-Berger, & Johnson, 1994; Lafosse, Mitchell, Corboy, & Filley, 2013). More recent work has suggested that information processing speed deficits are much more predictive of memory recall problems than working memory deficits, suggesting the primacy of processing speed problems in memory recall tasks (Chiaravalloti, Stojanovic-Radic, & DeLuca, 2014).

In addition to being among the most common cognitive deficits found in MS using objective tests, patients with MS often come to the clinic complaining of memory problems. In practical terms, these get manifested as complaints of difficulty remembering conversations, appointments, and work tasks that are sometimes so debilitating that patients can no longer work at cognitively demanding jobs.

EXECUTIVE FUNCTIONING

The next most common cognitive domain typically affected in MS is executive functioning. Deficits in cognitive flexibility, concept formation, verbal abstraction, problem solving, and planning are very common. Tests most commonly used to measure these cognitive skills include the Wisconsin Card Sorting Test, D-KEFS Sorting Test, Stroop Color-Word Test, Booklet Category Test, and verbal fluency tests, among others. In community-based samples, 15%–20% of individuals with MS show impairments in this domain, whereas the range is between 10% and 25% in clinic-based samples. The range of variability is higher for clinic-based samples because in Benedict and colleagues' (2006) study, they found that very few patients displayed verbal fluency deficits on the COWAT, with more showing impairments on the D-KEFS Sorting Test. In everyday terms, problems in this very broadly defined executive functioning domain can manifest themselves in patients reporting problems planning their day-to-day activities (e.g., job tasks, meals, grocery shopping), organizational difficulties, and problems collecting their thoughts and maintaining the flow of conversation.

VERBAL-LINGUISTIC FUNCTIONING

Depending on the complexity of the task, verbal and linguistic skill deficits can be seen in MS. It is rare (though not unheard of) for patients to have aphasic disorders (Arnett, Hussain, Rao, Swanson, & Hammeke, 1996); mild confrontation naming difficulties are relatively more common, though still usually occur in less than 10% of community-based samples of MS patients. Similarly, alexia, agraphia, and apraxia are very rare. In contrast, speech abnormalities such as dysarthria and hypophonia are common in MS (Arnett, Vargas, Ukueberuwa, & Rabinowitz, 2013). As referred to earlier in the discussion of executive tasks, deficits in verbal fluency are found in 20%–25% of community-based patients, with a surprisingly lower number of clinic-based patients (less than 15% from Benedict et al.'s 2006 study) showing deficits. Still, the latter finding appears somewhat anomalous, as a meta-analysis in more severely affected (Chronic Progressive) patients (who would presumably most closely mirror Benedict and colleagues' clinic-based patients) showed a medium effect size across many studies for verbal fluency tasks in MS relative to healthy controls (Henry & Beatty, 2006). Evidence suggests that impairments in verbal fluency may be as great as impairments in speeded information processing (Henry & Beatty, 2006). This may be due to the fact that performance on verbal fluency tasks requires rapid information processing, so patients' poor performance on such measures may also be reflective of their speeded information processing deficits. It is also important to keep in mind that slowed speech in MS can contribute to patients' verbal fluency deficits (Arnett et al., 2013). In practical terms, patients who have verbal fluency deficits may complain of frequent word-finding problems in conversation, and generally feel as though their ability to readily communicate with others is impacted.

VISUOSPATIAL FUNCTIONING

Visuospatial functioning in neuropsychological terms involves perceiving relationships in space. In MS, visuospatial functioning is commonly screened using tasks such as Judgment of Line Orientation (JLO), with more complex tasks such as the Facial Recognition Test sometimes used. Deficits in this domain are relatively common in MS; in both community- and clinic-based samples, 15%–20% of patients show impairments. It is unclear whether higher order visual deficits are a function of primary visual disturbances involving blurred vision and diplopia (Rao et al., 1991). Patients who report problems in their daily lives with regard to visuospatial functioning may complain of problems running into things frequently while walking (e.g., doorways) or driving (e.g., hitting curbs) because of visual miscalculations.

INTELLECTUAL FUNCTIONING AND ACHIEVEMENT

Intellectual functioning is usually considered to be well-preserved in MS, and is in many patients. Still, in Rao and colleagues' (1991) seminal study, slightly over 20% of patients had deficits in verbal intelligence. Of note, however, few patients (less than 10%) displayed impairments in their fund of knowledge (Information subtest from the Wechsler Adult Intelligence Scale—WAIS), so the Information test may represent a reasonably good index of premorbid cognitive functioning in MS. Finally, there has been little systematic research in how achievement-related skills (e.g., reading, writing, and math) may change with MS progression, but they are generally assumed to be significantly affected in few patients.

Longitudinal Course

Cognitive impairment can occur at any stage of MS and across all disease courses. Even patients with recently diagnosed MS or clinically isolated syndrome (CIS) commonly show deficits, with 45%–49% of individuals with early MS or CIS patients in one study demonstrating impairment on at least one measure (Glanz et al., 2012). Cognitive deficits in and of themselves appear to confer risk for further cognitive decline, even over a two-to-three-year period (Kujala, Portin, & Ruutiainen, 1997). When examined longitudinally, declines in information processing speed, verbal learning and memory, visual memory, and attention/working memory are usually seen in MS, at least over relatively shorter time periods of three to five years (Glanz et al., 2012; Kujala et al., 1997; Nordin & Rorsman, 2012). Verbal fluency and executive function skills also decline during these shorter periods, but this is less common (Glanz et al., 2012; Till et al., 2012).

Longer-term longitudinal investigations (e.g., seven to ten years) reveal declines in long-term verbal memory (Feinstein, 2011), information processing speed, motor speed, reaction time, visuospatial ability, and visual short-term memory (Vattakatuchery, Rickards, & Cavanna, 2011). Amato, Ponziani, Siracusa, and Sorbi (2001) have conducted one of the most comprehensive longitudinal studies to date (spanning ten years). They reported that when individuals with MS are followed from shortly after diagnosis, they show initial deficits on indices of concentration, verbal memory, and abstract reasoning, with the development of later impairments in verbal fluency, verbal comprehension, and short-term verbal and spatial memory/attention. Most strikingly, 26% of patients displayed cognitive impairment at the time of study entry, but this increased to 56% at the ten-year follow-up point.

Relationship to Disease Variables

Studies have consistently shown that patients with a Relapsing-Remitting course type exhibit less severe cognitive impairment than those with Progressive courses. One large meta-analytic study revealed that those patients with a Chronic Progressive course (encompassing all progressive types of MS) were more likely to have frontal-executive impairments, and those with Relapsing-Remitting courses more commonly showed memory-related impairments (Zakzanis, 2000).

Measurement

For cognitive difficulties to be detected in MS, it is important to employ test batteries that assess key areas of cognitive functioning, as the precise pattern of cognitive impairment often varies significantly among individuals. MS patients who show impairment in one domain of cognitive functioning are not necessarily impaired in others (Rao et al., 1991). Optimally, test batteries should be limited to about two to three hours, or less, to circumvent secondary problems (e.g., fatigue) that may compromise performance over a long period of time. There is evidence that MS patients' performance declines more than controls over the course of a long battery (Krupp & Elkins, 2000), and even within the context of a single task, such as the PASAT (Walker, Berard, Berrigan, Rees, & Freedman, 2012). There are at least two well-validated batteries for assessing cognitive impairment in MS, and both will be discussed in the following sections. Additional approaches and considerations will also be discussed.

THE BRIEF REPEATABLE BATTERY (RAO AND THE COGNITIVE FUNCTION STUDY GROUP OF THE NATIONAL MULTIPLE SCLEROSIS SOCIETY, 1990)

This battery consists of five tests that were shown to be most sensitive to cognitive impairments typically seen in MS from Rao's seminal MS study (Rao et al., 1991). As noted earlier, the BRB includes the SDMT, 10/36 Spatial Recall, Six-Trial version of the SRT, PASAT (2s & 3s version), and Word List Generation (WLG). Most of these tests also include 15 alternate forms (in English) to facilitate serial testing. Additionally, a two-form (A and B) version of the BRB has been developed by the European Study Group on Interferon beta-1b in Secondary Progressive MS (Boringa et al., 2001), but with some limitations noted in the comparability of the forms. The BRB has also been shown to have excellent specificity (94%) and adequate sensitivity (71%; see Rao et al., 1991). It has advantages over other batteries in that it has been translated into several languages other than English. The battery, or parts of the battery, have also been explored in Dutch (Boringa et al., 2001), Brazilian (Brooks, 2011), Serbian (Obradovic, Petrovic, Antanasijevic, Marinkovic, & Stojanovic, 2012), Greek (Potagas, Giogkaraki, Koutsis, Mandellos, & Tsirempolou, 2008), and Italian (Goretti et al., 2014) samples, among others. Even an abbreviated version administered in an Italian sample (Portaccio, Goretti, Zipoli, Siracusa, & Sorbi, 2009) showed excellent sensitivity (94%) and specificity (84%) in a group of Relapsing-Remitting patients. Regarding the latter study, the investigators included only the Selective Reminding Test, PASAT (3s version), and SDMT. The BRB takes about 20–30 minutes to administer.

One continuing limitation of the BRB is that adequate norms across the alternate forms of the tests comprising it are generally not available. Boringa and colleagues' study (2001) was a Dutch sample and included only the A and B forms developed by the European Study Group. Even examining only these two forms, the investigators found that scores were higher on the B form for three of the tests (SDMT, WLG, and 10/36 Spatial Recall), so great caution is warranted when using these two forms in repeat testing. Benedict and colleagues (Benedict et al., 2012) developed two alternate forms for the SDMT that were comparable to the original oral form of the SDMT; however, this study was based on a very small sample (25 healthy controls, including six men), so a replication of their findings is warranted before broad clinical application of these new forms takes place. In the absence of good normative data and clear-cut form equivalence for the BRB, one possible solution is to create standardized scores from these authors' control data for each form that could then be compared across different testings.

MINIMAL ASSESSMENT OF COGNITIVE FUNCTION IN MS (MACFIMS; BENEDICT ET AL., 2002)

The MACFIMS was developed as a result of a consensus conference and designed to provide a somewhat more extensive battery than the BRB. The MACFIMS takes about 90 minutes to administer and includes measures of memory (CVLT-II and BVMT-R), Attention and Concentration/Processing Speed (SDMT [Oral Version]), PASAT [2s &

3s]), Verbal-Linguistic Functioning (COWAT), Executive Functioning (D-KEFS Sorting Test), and Visuospatial Skill (JLO). Optional measures were suggested for this battery to measure Premorbid Intellectual Functioning (North American Adult Reading Test, or NAART), Emotional Functioning (BDI– Fast Screen, or BDI-FS), Fatigue (Fatigue Impact Scale, or FIS), Sensorimotor Functioning (9-HPT, Maximum Repetition Rate of Syllables and Multisyllabic Combinations (MRRSMC), and the Rosenbaum Pocket Vision Screener. Depression should be routinely screened in MS because it is so common, and because some research has shown an association between depression and cognitive dysfunction in MS (Arnett, Barwick, & Beeney, 2008).

Besides English (Benedict et al., 2006), the MACFIMS has been validated in Czech (Dusankova, Kalincik, Havrdova, & Benedict, 2012) and Persian (Eshaghi, Riyahi-Alam, Roostaei, Haeri, & Aghsaei, 2012), with reasonably good validity data being reported in these latter languages.

At least two studies recently compared the BRB and the MACFIMS (Goksel Karatepe et al., 2011; Strober et al., 2009), and suggested that the these batteries have comparable sensitivity. The SDMT was shown to be the best predictor of MS status in both studies, but with verbal fluency and verbal memory also contributing independently. Although the SDMT has much appeal, given its high level of sensitivity and ease of administration, performance on it can be compromised by the slowed speech that is common in MS (Arnett et al., 2013), as well as relatively minor rudimentary visual problems (Bruce et al., 2007). In terms of comparing the different verbal and visual learning and memory tasks in these batteries, the SRT and CVLT-II appear to be comparable, but the BVMT-R appears superior to the 10/36 Spatial Recall.

BRIEF INTERNATIONAL COGNITIVE ASSESSMENT FOR MS (BICAMS) (BENEDICT, AMATO, ET AL., 2012)

The BICAMS has yet to be validated, but has been suggested by an international consensus panel of expert neuropsychologists and neurologists in MS. It was developed in recognition of the fact that many centers where patients with MS are tested have limited resources, and may not have the time or expertise to administer and interpret extensive neuropsychological batteries. With this in mind, this group has recommended the adoption of the following tests as targets for validation across a number of cultures and languages: SDMT, BVMT-R, and CVLT-II. Such a battery would be easier to administer than the BRB and takes only about 15 minutes. However, the validation of this protocol across cultures and languages is still in process.

These approaches to neuropsychological assessment in MS attempt to survey the core cognitive domains typically affected in the disease and differ primarily in their comprehensiveness. Selection of one battery versus another depends upon the goals for the evaluation, in addition to the setting in which the evaluation takes place.

Ecological Validity of Neuropsychological Tests in MS

An important aspect of the validity of any neuropsychological test, especially regarding its clinical applicability, is whether it relates to everyday functioning. There is an emerging literature on the ecological validity of these tests in MS that suggests they are associated with important real-world tasks. We now turn to a brief review of the literature on the association of neuropsychological tests to driving and employment.

Driving

The motor, visual, and cognitive symptoms of MS can all contribute to difficulties with driving. Akinwuntan and colleagues (2013) aimed to determine what tests would best predict driving ability as measured by performance on a road test. Forty-four mostly female, middle-aged individuals with Relapsing-Remitting MS completed a comprehensive battery of cognitive, physical, and visual tests. Although 12 cognitive and 3 visual tests were moderately correlated (r = 0.31–0.63) with performance on the road test, multiple regression revealed that a model containing the following five tests accounted for the most variance (R^2 = 0.59) of performance on the road driving test: time to complete the Stroop Color-Word test; the Stroke Driver Screening Assessment (SDSA) directions, compass, and road sign recognition subtests; and the Useful Field of View speed of processing test.

Schultheis et al. (2010) focused on the cognitive contributors to difficulties with driving by measuring cognitive functioning and driving abilities in community-dwelling participants with MS who had no reported visual impairments. Sixty-six middle-aged, mostly female, and Relapsing-Remitting participants with clinically definite MS were included. Participants underwent comprehensive neuropsychological evaluations and behind-the-wheel driving evaluations, and their state-issued driver history abstracts were obtained from the Department of Motor Vehicles to evaluate recent collision and violation involvement. Logistic regression revealed that information processing speed, as measured by the SDMT, was the strongest predictor of behind-the-wheel driving performance (marginally significant at p = .07) while visuospatial learning and recall, as measured by the 7/24 spatial recall test, was the strongest predictor of collision and violation frequency (marginally significant at p = .06).

Employment

Employment status is a critical aspect of daily functioning and an important area of MS research, as most people with MS are diagnosed well before typical retirement age. Demographic, cognitive, physical, and emotional factors of MS have been evaluated as potential predictors of employment status. Honarmand and colleagues (2011) examined 106 participants with confirmed MS or CIS who completed a battery of neurological, cognitive, and psychological assessments. The sample was comprised of mostly middle-aged female patients who had Relapsing-Remitting or Secondary Progressive course types. A binary logistic regression, with employment status as the dependent variable, revealed that the Multiple Sclerosis Functional Composite (MSFC; 9-HPT, 25-foot Timed Walk Test, and the PASAT) was the most robust predictor of employment status ($R^2 = 0.31$, 68% correctly classified). Although the addition of the Expanded Disability Status Scale (EDSS) to the model did not increase its predictive value, the addition of both the NEO Five Factor Inventory (NEO-FFI) Agreeableness scale and the Hospital Anxiety and Depression Scale Depression (HADS) subscale did; the addition of these variables substantially increased the predictive value of the model to 50% of the variance in employment status accounted for ($R^2 = 0.50$, 83% correctly classified). The robust predictive value of the MSFC may be related to its assessment of both cognitive and motor symptoms of MS.

The utility of the PASAT in the MSFC has been questioned, as its predictive value, independent of the motor tasks in the MSFC, has been inconsistent across studies. Strober and colleagues (2014) examined a sample of 77 mostly female and Relapsing-Remitting or Secondary Progressive MS patients. These investigators administered a comprehensive neuropsychological battery, but only the SDMT emerged as a significant predictor of employment status in a stepwise logistic regression analysis, accounting for 15%–20% of the variance with 67% overall classification accuracy. These researchers asserted that their findings provided support for the addition of the SDMT to the MSFC and the potential replacement of the PASAT with the SDMT, given the high association of SDMT performance and employment status.

For both driving and employment, then, the SDMT appears to provide excellent predictive validity, underscoring its usefulness as a core neuropsychological screening measure.

Remediating Cognitive Impairment in MS

Prospective Memory and Emotional Valence

Deficits in prospective memory (PM), or the memory for future intentions, are often seen in MS. PM is essential for the successful completion of many everyday tasks necessary for independent living and improving PM is therefore a valuable target for intervention in MS. Rendell et al. (2012) investigated the efficacy of the use of emotionally valenced information to improve PM in participants with MS. A group of 30 MS participants with confirmed MS diagnoses and 30 age, sex, and education-matched controls took part in this study. A laboratory measure of PM, Virtual Week (which is designed like a computerized board game), was used to assess PM. The MS group performed significantly worse than controls on both the event-based and time-based emotionally valenced Virtual Week tasks. Positivity and negativity enhancement/impairment indices were calculated and it was found that the MS group's performance on event-based tasks was significantly improved by the use of emotionally positive material in the tasks. These results suggest that the use of positive emotional associations and cuing might help to improve PM performance in individuals with MS.

Self-Generated Learning

O'Brien Chiaravalloti, Arango-Lasprilla, Lengenfelder, and DeLuca (2007) examined the generation effect in MS to assess whether it would improve memory functioning. With the generation effect, material that is produced by an individual is learned and remembered better than information that is provided to that individual. These investigators explored whether even cognitively impaired individuals with MS would benefit from using the generation effect. MS participants were compared with healthy controls and TBI patients. In addition to administering a few standard neuropsychological tests, these authors included a generation effect protocol. This involved 32 sentences presented individually on separate pages. In the Generated Condition, 16 sentences were presented with the last word missing. In the Provided Condition, 16 complete sentences were provided with the last word underlined. The task required participants to read the 32 (alternating) sentences presented individually on separate pages. In the Generated Condition, they had to fill in the blank at the end of the sentence with an appropriate word, and in the Provided Condition, they simply had to read the sentence, including the underlined word. Participants then performed a distractor task, and then were asked to recall the words immediately following this, at a 30-minute delay, and after one week. At both the immediate recall and 30-minute delay, MS participants displayed significantly better recall in the Generated versus Provided condition. These data suggested that MS patients may remember information better when they generate it themselves.

The Testing Effect

Sumowski and colleagues (2010) examined the testing effect in a group of MS patients that included a subgroup with significant memory deficits. The testing effect has been shown to be a robust cognitive phenomenon. It involves practicing recall rather than simply restudying something to be learned. These investigators examined this effect in an MS patient group matched to a healthy control group on a verbal paired associates (VPA) task that included three conditions: massed restudy (MR), spaced restudy (SR), and spaced testing (ST). Recall on the VPA test using cued recall was measured after a 45-minute delay. These investigators found that both MS and controls had better recall on the VPA list after they did spaced testing compared with the MR and SR conditions.

The effect held even for a subgroup of 16 MS patients who had objective memory impairment. These findings were extremely promising, and suggest the possibility that applying such a spaced testing method to rehabilitation of memory problems in MS could be effective.

Cognitive Rehabilitation Interventions

Parisi et al. (2014) sought to examine the effectiveness of a cognitive rehabilitation program in a group of MS patients, and to determine the relationship between functional neuroimaging (functional magnetic resonance imaging, or fMRI) and performance on neuropsychological measures. Their sample was small, consisting of 18 female Relapsing-Remitting MS patients; half of the patients were assigned to the treatment condition and the other half served as controls. Participants were administered a battery of neuropsychological tests at baseline, after completion of the 12-week cognitive rehabilitation program, and then again at six months, and resting state fMRI was acquired at baseline and at 12 weeks. These investigators found that participants who received the treatment displayed significantly better performance on measures of attention and executive function. Furthermore, the treatment group demonstrated significantly lower levels of depression and improved quality of life. With respect to the neuroimaging findings, the authors reported that better test performance was associated with greater resting state functional connectivity within default mode network regions.

Neuroimaging Studies on Cognitive Function in MS

Structural Neuroimaging

Generally, cognitive deficits are proportional to MRI-visualized total lesion load on T2 sequences (Bagert, Camplair, & Bourdette, 2002), and regional associations have been reported as well. Sperling and colleagues (2001) found that frontal and parietal region lesion load were correlated with deficits in processing speed and memory. Some studies have also reported an association between MRI lesion location and particular patterns of dysfunction, with primarily frontal lesion patterns associated with executive task dysfunction (Arnett et al., 1994).

Atrophy measures have proven to be as or more associated with patterns of cognitive impairment in MS than lesion burden. Atrophy measures such as bi-caudate ratio, third ventricular width, and brain parenchymal fraction have all been shown to be significantly associated with cognitive impairment in MS (Tekok-Kilic, Benedict, & Zivadinov, 2006; Zivadinov et al., 2001), with some specificity in terms of brain region affected and the types of cognitive impairments observed. Regional frontal volume has been shown to be correlated with performance on measures assessing executive function, attention, and processing speed, while left temporal atrophy has been shown to be predictive of poor verbal memory and both left and right temporal atrophy associated with visual memory performance (Tekok-Kilic et al., 2006).

Several recent studies have also shown that fiber tract integrity in the brain, as measured by diffusion tensor imaging (DTI), is associated with cognitive impairment in MS. Hulst et al. (2013) compared "Cognitively Impaired" and "Cognitively Preserved" MS patients on common DTI measures. They found that, compared with the Cognitively Preserved patients, the Cognitively Impaired patients demonstrated significantly greater white matter integrity changes in a number of brain regions. Koenig et al. (2013) sought to investigate the relationship between common DTI measures (specifically in the fornix) and cognitive performance in mostly Relapsing-Remitting MS patients and healthy controls. Compared with healthy controls, the MS group showed significantly greater mean diffusivity and longitudinal diffusivity, as well as lower fractional anisotropy, suggesting compromised fiber tract integrity in the MS group. Additionally, the MS group demonstrated significantly worse performance than the healthy controls on a neuropsychological test battery consisting of measures of episodic memory, working memory, and attention. Llufriu et al. (2014) examined the relationship between cognitive performance and structural brain damage using DTI in a sample of Relapsing-Remitting MS patients and healthy controls. They found that MS patients demonstrated widespread abnormalities on DTI indices in both gray matter regions and white matter tracts as compared to control participants. Interestingly, the abnormalities observed within the white matter tracts accounted for more of the variance in cognitive dysfunction.

Functional Neuroimaging

Initial studies using functional neuroimaging measures showed that MS patients displayed *greater* increases in brain activation relative to non-MS controls when performing complex cognitive tasks (Forn et al., 2006; Hillary et al., 2003). More recently, Loitfelder and colleagues (2011) reported similar findings. They examined fMRI activation patterns during a Go/No Go Discrimination Task and found that Relapsing-Remitting and Secondary Progressive patients displayed greater activation increases during task performance compared with controls. Interestingly, the patterns of increased activation were more pronounced in the Secondary Progressive patients who showed more widespread activation, and also less deactivation.

Findings from other studies have supported a general increase in brain activation in MS patients; however, this pattern has not been consistently observed across all brain areas. On the Computerized Test of Information Processing, Smith and colleagues (2012) found that, compared with controls, MS patients displayed a significant increase in activation in the prefrontal cortex (PFC) and right temporal gyrus;

however, the MS patients displayed *decreased* activation in areas of the left temporal gyrus. This study suggested that the broadly greater task activation in MS patients versus controls may not always hold true across brain areas. Additional research is needed to clarify the conditions under which increased versus decreased activation occur in MS during task performance.

Wojtowicz, Mazerolle, Bhan, and Fisk (2014) sought to explore the relationship between performance variability (on measures of processing speed) and resting-state functional connectivity in a sample of age-matched Relapsing-Remitting MS participants and healthy controls. The authors reported that performance variability was greater in MS patients as compared to healthy controls. Furthermore, MS patients were found to have decreased functional connectivity between regions associated with the default mode network. Finally, with respect to MS patients, those exhibiting less performance variability (better performance) showed increased connectivity between the ventral medial prefrontal cortex (PFC) and the frontal pole.

Psychiatric Issues

Depression

The risk for lifetime major depression in MS is approximately 50% (Arnett, Barwick, et al., 2008; Chwastiak et al., 2002; Sadovnick et al., 1996), a figure much higher than the 8% lifetime risk in the general population, but also greater than many other neurological disorders and chronic illnesses.

SCREENING FOR DEPRESSION

A common problem associated with the assessment of depression in MS pertains to the overlap between neurovegetative symptoms of depression and MS disease symptoms. Symptoms such as fatigue, sleep disturbance, sexual dysfunction, and concentration difficulties are all neurovegetative symptoms of depression, but they are also symptoms of MS itself. This makes the assessment of depression in MS complicated, because the meaning of such symptoms in MS is unclear. One solution that has been suggested in the literature is to simply discard such symptoms, focusing instead on mood and negative evaluative depression symptoms. Nyenhuis et al. (1995) developed the Chicago Multiscale Depression Inventory (CMDI) for this purpose. The test consists of three 14-item scales, each measuring a different domain of depression. These investigators suggested using only the Mood subscale of the CMDI, as it was least potentially overlapping with MS disease symptoms.

An alternative to the CMDI is the BDI-FS (Beck, Steer, & Brown, 2000). This measure was explicitly developed with medical patients in mind, and includes only mood and negative evaluative symptoms in its seven-item format. There is much to be said for the BDI-FS as a screening measure for depression in MS. It takes only a few minutes to administer, and has been shown to be valid for detecting depression in MS by Benedict and colleagues (2003). They found that it was highly correlated with other self-report measures of depression, other-report measures of depression, and also distinguished between depressed MS patients in treatment and those not being treated.

Another approach to addressing the neurovegetative depression symptom/MS symptom overlap has been suggested by Strober and Arnett (2010). These investigators proposed a "trunk and branch" model of depression in MS. Rather than disregard neurovegetative symptoms entirely, this model distinguishes between symptoms common to the medical condition ("trunk" symptoms), and those independent of the medical condition that are likely to reflect depression ("branch" symptoms). To test this model, a criterion group of likely depressed MS patients was identified. They were compared to a nondepressed MS group and a group of healthy controls on the BDI (Beck & Steer, 1987). Trunk symptoms were those on which the MS group (depressed and nondepressed combined) endorsed significantly more often than the healthy controls (see Figure 25.1). Branch symptoms were those that were endorsed significantly more often by depressed compared with MS compared with nondepressed MS. The researchers also found that there were some trunk symptoms that were more severe in the depressed compared with nondepressed MS group, so these were also considered core MS depression symptoms. As shown in Figure 25.1, the initial branch symptoms and these latter additional symptoms comprised 12 items from the original BDI.

Strober and Arnett (2015) followed up this study and examined the new 12-item "MS-BDI" relative to existing depression measures commonly used in MS, including the BDI-FS, the CMDI, and the BDI-II. The BDI-FS and the CMDI-Mood subscale had the best sensitivity at 94%. The MS-BDI, however, had the highest specificity and corresponding Positive Likelihood Ratio (PLR) of 12.81. PLR is a measure of the increase in the likelihood an individual has a condition (i.e., depression in this case) if he or she scores above a cutoff. A PLR greater than 10 is almost conclusive for the condition, so the MS-BDI fared extremely well when a cutoff of 7 was used.

Strober and Arnett (2015) examined the validity of the depression measures in another way, by comparing the point prevalence rates they produced with that of the criterion group. When selecting the criterion depressed group from the larger sample of 84 individuals with MS, the point prevalence rate for depression was 20%. Importantly, the MS-BDI also produced a point prevalence rate of 20% when the cutoff of 7 was again used, suggesting that scores on it are tightly linked to more rigorous approaches to diagnosing depression that include clinical interviews. An important caveat to this consideration of the MS-BDI is that the data are based on one study only. With that said, the MS-BDI is appealing because it has the highest PLR of any of the

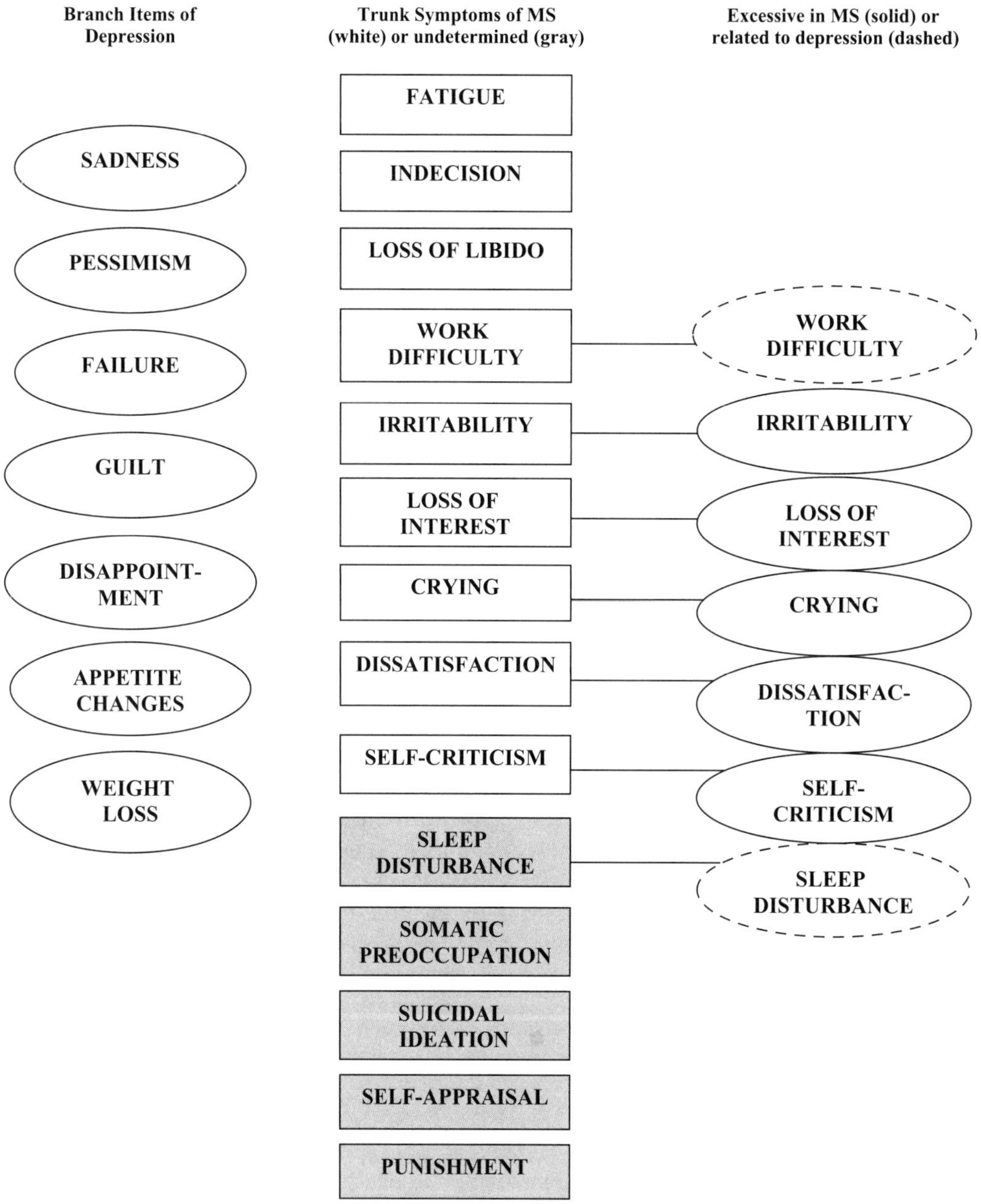

Figure 25.1 Trunk and branch model of depression in MS

Used with permission (Strober & Arnett, 2010)

depression measures assessed, is theoretically driven in relation to MS, incorporates some neurovegetative symptoms, and has prevalence rates comparable to those derived from using a rigorously identified criterion group of depressed MS patients. Still, a cross-validation study on a larger sample will be necessary before clinical application of the MS-BDI would be appropriate.

Another depression measure that has been frequently used in MS is the HADS. This 14-item measure has advantages over the other depression scales already discussed in that it also measures anxiety, which, as will be discussed, is very common in MS. Honarmand and Feinstein (2009) examined the Depression scale of the HADS in an MS sample and found excellent sensitivity (.90) and specificity (.87). Using a cutoff of 8, it also resulted in a point prevalence rate of depression in their sample of 16%, a value close to the 20% for the MS-BDI and the criterion group from Strober and Arnett's (2015) study.

As far as clinical recommendations, at this stage of our knowledge, the BDI-FS clearly appears to be the best screening measure for depression in MS. Its sensitivity is very high, and a cutoff of 4 or above has been demonstrated to be best in at least two studies, a cutoff that is also consistent with what is recommended in the BDI-FS manual for medical patients in general. The sensitivity and specificity of the HADS Depression scale are also excellent; the one caveat is that it has been validated in one MS study only, so greater caution in its use is recommended.

Because of the high prevalence of depression in MS, patients should be routinely screened, with particular optimal approaches for this outlined earlier. Also, it is very treatable through brief and even telephone-based cognitive behavioral therapy (Hind et al., 2014; Mohr et al., 2005; Mohr et al., 2000), as well as group therapy. Still, depression has historically been undertreated in MS, despite the fact that it is unlikely to remit spontaneously.

COPING AND DEPRESSION

Depression in MS has also been consistently found to be associated with the increased use of generally less effective emotion-focused or avoidant-focused coping strategies, and the decreased use of more adaptive active or problem-focused strategies (Arnett, Higginson, Voss, & Randolph, 2002; McCabe, McKern, & McDonald, 2004; Mohr, Goodkin, Gatto, & Van Der Wende, 1997; Pakenham, 1999; Rabinowitz & Arnett, 2009). Despite this, coping strategies are not routinely screened for in clinical evaluations. There is a need for reliable and well-validated coping measures for clinical use, but to our knowledge, none have been fully validated in MS patients. This is unfortunate, because knowledge of coping strategies, especially in psychotherapy contexts, would be useful in guiding therapy. In addition to providing a potential treatment target, and improving quality of life and well-being, altering maladaptive coping strategies in MS patients might also mitigate the impact of cognitive dysfunction on mood (Arnett et al., 2002; Rabinowitz & Arnett, 2009), and fatigue (Ukueberuwa & Arnett, 2014).

OTHER FACTORS ASSOCIATED WITH DEPRESSION

Even though depression is treatable in many MS patients, treatments are effective in reducing depression to remission only about 50% of the time (Ehde et al., 2008; Mohr, Boudewyn, Goodkin, Bostrom, & Epstein, 2001). Depression in MS negatively affects quality of life, adaptive functioning, and well-being (Vargas & Arnett, 2010); interferes with medication adherence (Bruce, Hancock, Arnett, & Lynch, 2010); and may increase mortality (Feinstein, O'Conner, & Feinstein, 2002). There is a need for developing models with greater explanatory power that could result in the development of better treatments to reduce depression in MS.

A history of depression appears to increase risk for future depressive or manic states in MS. Some studies show that depression is associated with cognitive dysfunction, with impairments in complex attention and information processing speed, as well as executive deficits, showing the greatest associations (Arnett, Barwick, et al., 2008; Sundgren, Maurex, Wahlin, Piehl, & Brismar, 2013). These associations are most likely to be seen when depression symptoms contaminated by MS symptomatology (e.g., neurovegetative symptoms) are excluded from the measurement of depression and the focus is on mood and negative evaluative depression symptoms (Arnett, Higginson, & Randolph, 2001; Sundgren et al., 2013). Coping may also be an important moderator between cognitive dysfunction and depression in MS, with cognitive deficits most likely to predict depression if patients rely on avoidant coping or minimally use active coping (Arnett et al., 2002; Rabinowitz & Arnett, 2009). The severity of neurologic disability is inconsistently related to depression in MS (Arnett, Barwick, et al., 2008).

Numerous factors appear to be associated with depression in MS, including high levels of perceived stress, low levels of perceived social support, and disease exacerbation/pharmacological treatment (Arnett, Barwick, et al., 2008). Depression in MS is unlikely to be governed by genetic factors, because studies show that unipolar major depression is not more common in first-degree relatives of depressed MS patients compared with first-degree relatives of non-depressed MS patients. Still, biological factors are clearly associated with depression in MS, as indicated by research showing that depression is predicted by both neuroanatomical and functional neuroimaging parameters.

PHYSICAL ACTIVITY AND DEPRESSION

The mood-boosting effects of physical activity have been observed in healthy controls as well as psychiatric populations, leading it to be studied as a potential cost-effective treatment for depression. Physical activity may be an optimal intervention for those with MS, as this disease is often characterized by high rates of depression and low levels of physical activity. Kratz and colleagues (2014) established physical activity as a successful intervention for depression in MS and additionally evaluated positive and negative affect as mediators for the effects of physical activity counseling on depressive symptoms. Ninety-two individuals with clinically definite MS were randomized into a treatment condition (n = 44) and a waitlist control condition (n = 48). The groups were well-matched in terms of sex and course type. Depressive symptoms and positive and negative affect were evaluated before and after a 12-week motivational interviewing intervention focused on increasing physical activity. Mediational analyses showed that motivational interviewing had significant effects on both positive and negative affect, and these in turn both significantly influenced depressive symptoms. When physical activity, as measured by the 7-day Physical Activity Recall Interview, was included in the model, however, only positive affect mediated the relationship between changes in physical activity and depressive symptoms. These results suggest that physical activity may improve depressive symptoms through an increase in positive affect, and supplementary treatment should be pursued to decrease negative affect and further reduce depressive symptoms.

NEUROPATHOLOGY AND DEPRESSION

Neuropathology has generally been shown to be associated with depression in MS (Feinstein, 2004). Together, lesion load, brain atrophy, and white matter fiber tract integrity account for up to 43% of depression variance in MS (Bakshi et al., 2000; Feinstein et al., 2010), with temporal and frontal brain regions most often implicated (Arnett, Barwick, et al., 2008; Feinstein et al., 2010). However, a study by Gobbi et al. (2013) was not as conclusive. These investigators examined structural neuroanatomical correlates of both depression and fatigue in MS and failed to find any significant relationships between lesion distribution and depression or fatigue. Similarly, there were no significant relationships between white matter atrophy and depression or fatigue. However, gray matter atrophy in several brain regions (including frontal, parietal, and occipital lobes) was significantly related to both depression and fatigue, and the left middle frontal gyrus and right inferior frontal gyrus were associated with depression but not fatigue. With these studies in mind, the mechanisms by which this type of structural brain damage leads to depression in MS are unclear. It may be that such structural changes lead to characteristic functional brain changes that in turn predict depression in MS.

Functional brain variables in relation to emotional functioning in MS have been examined in only a limited way in one study. Passamonti and colleagues (2009) explored emotional processing in a small group ($N = 12$) of Relapsing-Remitting MS participants. They found that, compared with controls, MS participants showed a lack of functional connectivity between the amygdala and the PFC during an emotional processing task involving the matching of affective faces. Although the MS participants in the study were not clinically depressed, they reported significantly higher scores on depression measures than controls. These authors hypothesized that reduced functional connectivity could reflect a disruption in an important affective processing system in the brain of MS patients early in the disease process that might ultimately put them at risk for emotional difficulties such as depression. Clearly, further work examining functional neuroimaging and depression in MS is warranted.

Anxiety

Anxiety has sometimes been shown to be more common than depression in MS, but has been studied far less extensively. The point prevalence of clinically significant anxiety is thought to be about 25%, but lifetime prevalence is unknown. The cause of anxiety in MS is unknown, but it tends to be prominent in the early stages of the disease when the diagnosis and prognosis are most uncertain. Decline in distress is associated with more definitive diagnostic statements by treatment professionals. There are no published studies treating specific anxiety disorders in MS. At least one study has shown that comorbidity of anxiety and depression in MS is more associated with thoughts of self-harm, social dysfunction, and somatic complaints than either alone (Feinstein, O'Connor, Gray, & Feinstein, 1999). The only other emotional disorder occurring with any significant frequency in MS is bipolar disorder, with point prevalence estimated at 0%–2% and lifetime prevalence at 13%–16%. There are no published treatment studies of bipolar disorder in MS.

Conclusion

MS is the most common nontraumatic neurological condition of early to middle adulthood, and the most common demyelinating condition. In this chapter, we have reviewed common sequelae associated with MS, especially focusing on neurocognitive impairments and emotional difficulties including depression and anxiety. We have also included practical suggestions for neuropsychological assessment and for the assessment of depression. Neuropsychologists can play a critical role in the assessment and treatment of cognitive and emotional difficulties in MS. This chapter provides some evidence-based suggestions that can optimize patient care.

References

Akinwuntan, A. E., Devos, H., Stepleman, L., Casillas, R., Rahn, R., Smith, S., & Williams, M. J. (2013). Predictors of driving in individuals with Relapsing-Remitting multiple sclerosis. *Multiple Sclerosis Journal*, *19*, 344–350.

Amato, M. P., Ponziani, G., Siracusa, G., & Sorbi, S. (2001). Cognitive dysfunction in early onset multiple sclerosis: A reappraisal after 10 years. *Archives of Neurology*, *58*, 1602–1606.

Arnett, P. A., Barwick, F. H., & Beeney, J. E. (2008). Depression in multiple sclerosis: Review and theoretical proposal. *Journal of the International Neuropsychological Society*, *14*, 691–724.

Arnett, P. A., Higginson, C. I., & Randolph, J. J. (2001). Depression in multiple sclerosis: Relationship to planning ability. *Journal of the International Neuropsychological Society*, *7*, 665–674.

Arnett, P. A., Higginson, C. I., Voss, W. D., & Randolph, J. J. (2002). Relationship between coping, depression, and cognitive dysfunction in multiple sclerosis. *The Clinical Neuropsychologist*, *16*, 341–355.

Arnett, P. A., Hussain, M., Rao, S., Swanson, S., & Hammeke, T. (1996). Conduction aphasia in Multiple Sclerosis: A case report with MRI findings. *Neurology*, *47*, 576–578.

Arnett, P. A., Rao, S. M., Bernardin, L., Grafman, J., Yetkin, F. Z., & Lobeck, L. (1994). Relationship between frontal lobe lesions and Wisconsin Card Sorting Test performance in patients with multiple sclerosis. *Neurology*, *44*, 420–425.

Arnett, P. A., Smith, M. M., Barwick, F. H., Benedict, R.H.B., & Ahlstrom, B. (2008). Oralmotor slowing in multiple sclerosis: Relationship to complex neuropsychological tasks requiring an oral response. *Journal of the International Neuropsychological Society*, *14*, 454–462.

Arnett, P. A., Vargas, G. A., Ukueberuwa, D., & Rabinowitz, A. R. (2013). The influence of oral motor impairments on cognitive functioning. In P. Arnett (Ed.), *Secondary Influences on Neuropsychological Test Performance* (pp. 166–181). New York: Oxford University Press.

Bagert, B., Camplair, P., & Bourdette, D. (2002). Cognitive dysfunction in multiple sclerosis: Natural history, pathophysiology and management. *CNS Drugs*, *16*, 445–455.

Bakshi, R., Czarnecki, D., Shaikh, Z. A., Priore, R. L., Janardhan, V., Kaliszky, Z., & Kinkel, P. R. (2000). Brain MRI lesions and atrophy are related to depression in multiple sclerosis. *NeuroReport*, *11*(6), 1153–1158.

Beck, A. T., & Steer, R. A. (1987). *BDI: Beck Depression Inventory Manual*. New York: Psychological Corporation.

Beck, A. T., Steer, R. A., & Brown, G. K. (2000). *BDI-Fast Screen for Medical Patients Manual*. San Antonio, TX: The Psychological Corporation.

Benedict, R.H.B., Amato, M. P., Boringa, J., Brochet, B., Foley, F., Fredrikson, S., . . . Langdon, D. (2012). Brief International Cognitive Assessment for MS (BICAMS): International standards for validation. *BMC Neurol*, *12*, 1–8.

Benedict, R.H.B., Cookfair, D., Gavett, R., Gunther, M., Munschauer, F., Garg, N., & Weinstock-Guttman, B. (2006). Validity of the minimal assessment of cognitive function in multiple sclerosis (MACFIMS). *Journal of the International Neuropsychological Society*, *12*, 549–558.

Benedict, R.H.B., Fischer, J. S., Archibald, C. J., Arnett, P. A., Beatty, W. W., Bobholz, J., . . . Munschauer, F. (2002). Minimal neuropsychological assessment of MS patients: A consensus approach. *The Clinical Neuropsychologist*, *16*, 381–397.

Benedict, R.H.B., Fishman, I., McClellan, M. M., Bakshi, R., & Weinstock-Guttman, B. (2003). Validity of the beck depression inventory—fast screen in multiple sclerosis. *Multiple Sclerosis*, *9*, 393–396.

Benedict, R.H.B., Holtzer, R., Motl, R. W., Foley, F. W., Kaur, S., Hojnacki, D., & Weinstock-Guttman, B. (2011). Upper and lower extremity motor function and cognitive impairment in multiple sclerosis. *Journal of the International Neuropsychological Society*, *17*, 643–653.

Benedict, R.H.B., Smerbeck, A., Parikh, R., Rodgers, J., Cadavid, D., & Erlanger, D. (2012). Reliability and equivalence of alternate forms for the Symbol Digit Modalities Test: Implications for multiple sclerosis clinical trials. *Multiple Sclerosis Journal*, *18*, 1320–1325.

Bobholz, J., & Rao, S. M. (2003). Cognitive dysfunction in multiple sclerosis: A review of recent developments. *Current Opinion in Neurology*, *16*, 283–288.

Boringa, J. B., Lazeron, R.H.C., Reuling, I.E.W., Ader, H. J., Pfennings, L., Lindeboom, J., . . . Polman, C. H. (2001). The brief repeatable battery of neuropsychological tests: Normative values allow application in multiple sclerosis clinical practice. *Multiple Sclerosis*, *7*, 263–267.

Brassington, J. C., & Marsh, N. V. (1998). Neuropsychological aspects of multiple sclerosis. *Neuropsychology Review*, *8*, 43–77.

Brooks, J. B., Borela, M.C.M., & Fragoso, Y. D. (2011). Assessment of cognition using the Rao's Brief Repeatable Battery of Neuropsychological Tests on a group of Brazilian patients with multiple sclerosis. *Arquivos de Neuro-Psiquiatria*, *69*, 887–891.

Bruce, J. M., Bruce, A. S., & Arnett, P. A. (2007). Mild visual acuity disturbances are associated with performance on tests of complex visual attention in MS. *Journal of the International Neuropsychological Society*, *13*, 544–548.

Bruce, J. M., Hancock, L. M., Arnett, P. A., & Lynch, S. (2010). Treatment adherence in multiple sclerosis: Association with emotional status, personality, and cognition. *Journal of Behavioral Medicine*, *33*, 219–227.

Chiaravalloti, N. D., & DeLuca, J. (2010). Cognition and multiple sclerosis: Assessment and treatment. In B.C.M.R.E.R.G. Frank (Ed.), *Handbook of Rehabilitation Psychology* (2nd ed., pp. 133–144). Washington, DC: American Psychological Association.

Chiaravalloti, N. D., Stojanovic-Radic, M., & DeLuca, J. (2014). The role of speed versus working memory in predicting learning new information in multiple sclerosis. *Journal of Clinical and Experimental Neuropsychology*, *35*, 180–191.

Chitnis, T., Krupp, L., Yeh, A., Rubin, J., Kuntz, N., Strober, J. B., . . . Waubant, E. (2011). Pediatric multiple sclerosis. *Neurologic Clinics*, *29*, 481–505.

Chwastiak, L., Ehde, D. M., Gibbons, L. E., Sullivan, M., Bowen, J., D., & Kraft, G. H. (2002). Depressive symptoms and severity of illness in multiple sclerosis: Epidemiologic study of a large community sample. *American Journal of Psychiatry*, *159*, 1862–1868.

Compston, A., McDonald, I. R., Noseworthy, J., Lassmann, H., Miller, D. H., Smith, K. J., . . . Confavreux, C. (2005). *McAlpine's Multiple Sclerosis* (4th ed.). London: Churchill Livingstone.

DeLuca, J., Barbieri-Berger, S., & Johnson, S. K. (1994). The nature of memory impairments in multiple sclerosis: Acquisition versus retrieval. *Journal of Clinical and Experimental Neuropsychology*, *16*(2), 183–189.

Dusankova, J. B., Kalincik, T., Havrdova, E., & Benedict, R.H.B. (2012). Cross cultural validation of the Minimal Assessment of Cognitive Function in Multiple Sclerosis (MACFIMS) and the Brief International Cognitive Assessment for Multiple Sclerosis (BICAMS). *The Clinical Neuropsychologist*, *26*, 1186–1200.

Ehde, D. M., Kraft, G. H., Chwastiak, L., Sullivan, M. D., Gibbons, L. E., Bombardier, C. H., & Wadhwani, R. (2008). Efficacy of paroxetine in treating major depressive disorder in persons with multiple sclerosis. *General Hospital Psychiatry*, *30*, 40–48.

Eshaghi, A., Riyahi-Alam, S., Roostaei, T., Haeri, G., & Aghsaei, A. (2012). Validity and reliability of a Persian translation of the Minimal Assessment of Cognitive Function in MS (MACFIMS). *The Clinical Neuropsychologist*, *26*, 975–984.

Feinstein, A. (2004). The neuropsychiatry of multiple sclerosis. *Canadian Journal of Psychiatry*, *49*, 157–163.

Feinstein, A. (2011). Multiple sclerosis and depression. *Multiple Sclerosis*, *17*(11), 1276–1281. doi: 10.1177/1352458511417835

Feinstein, A., O'Connor, P., Akbar, N., Moradzadeh, L., Scott, C.J.M., & Lobaugh, N. J. (2010). Diffusion tensor imaging abnormalities in depressed multiple sclerosis patients. *Multiple Sclerosis*, *16*, 189–196.

Feinstein, A., O'Conner, P., & Feinstein, K. (2002). Multiple sclerosis, interferon beta 1b and depression. *Journal of Neurology*, *24*(9), 815–820.

Feinstein, A., O'Connor, P., Gray, T., & Feinstein, K. (1999). The effects of anxiety on psychiatric morbidity in patients with multiple sclerosis. *Multiple Sclerosis*, *5*, 323–326.

Forn, C., Barros-Loscertales, A., Escudero, J., Belloch, V., Campos, S., Parcet, M. A., & Avila, C. (2006). Cortical reorganization during PASAT task in MS patients with preserved working memory functions. *Neuroimage*, *31*, 686–691.

Glanz, B. I., Degano, I. R., Rintell, D. J., Chitnis, T., Weiner, H. L., & Healy, B. C. (2012). Work productivity in relapsing multiple sclerosis: Associations with disability, depression, fatigue, anxiety, cognition, and health-related quality of life. *Value Health*, *15*(8), 1029–1035. doi: 10.1016/j.jval.2012.07.010

Gobbi, C., Rocca, M., Riccitelli, G., Pagani, E., Messina, R., Preziosa, P., Colombo, B., Rodegher, M., Falini, A., Comi, G. Filippi, M.

(2013). Influence of the topography of brain damage on depression and fatigue in patients with multiple sclerosis. *Multiple Sclerosis, 20*, 192–201.

Goksel Karatepe, A., Kaya, T., Gunaydn, R., Demirhan, A., Ce, P., & Gedizlioglu, M. (2011). Quality of life in patients with multiple sclerosis: The impact of depression, fatigue, and disability. *International Journal of Rehabilitation Research, 34*(4), 290–298. doi: 10.1097/MRR.0b013e32834ad479

Goretti, B., Patti, F., Cilia, S., Mattioli, F., Stampatori, C., Scarpazza, C., . . . Portaccio, E. (2014). The Rao's Brief Repeatable Battery version B: Normative values with age, education and gender corrections in an Italian population. *Neurological Sciences, 35*, 79–82.

Henry, J. D., & Beatty, W. W. (2006). Verbal fluency deficits in multiple sclerosis. *Neuropsychologia, 44*, 1166–1174.

Hillary, F. G., Chiaravalloti, N. D., Ricker, J. H., Steffener, J., Bly, B. M., Liu, W. C., . . . DeLuca, J. (2003). An investigation of working memory rehearsal in multiple sclerosis using fMRI. *Journal of Clinical and Experimental Neuropsychology, 17*, 965–978.

Hind, D., Cotter, J., Thake, A., Bradburn, M., Cooper, C., Isaac, C., & House, A. (2014). Cognitive behavioural therapy for the treatment of depression in people with multiple sclerosis: A systematic review and meta-analysis. *BMC Psychiatry, 14*, 1–30. doi: 10.1186/1471-244X-14-5

Honarmand, K., Akbar, N., Kou, N., & Feinstein, A. (2011). Predicting employment status in multiple sclerosis patients: The utility of the MS functional composite. *Journal of Neurology, 258*, 244–249.

Honarmand, K., & Feinstein, A. (2009). Validation of the Hospital Anxiety and Depression Scale for use with multiple sclerosis patients. *Multiple Sclerosis Journal, 15*, 1518–1524.

Horakova, D., Kalincik, T., Dusankova, J. B., & Dolezal, O. (2012). Clinical correlates of grey matter pathology in multiple sclerosis. *BMC Neurology, 12*, 10.

Hulst, H. E., Steenwijk, M. D., Versteeg, A., Pouwels, P.J.W., Vrenken, H., Uitdehaag, B.M.J., & Barkhof, F. (2013). Cognitive impairment in MS Impact of white matter integrity, gray matter volume, and lesions. *Neurology, 80*, 1025–1032.

Koch-Henriksen, N., & Sørensen, P. S. (2010). The changing demographic pattern of multiple sclerosis epidemiology. *Lancet Neurology, 9*, 520–532.

Koenig, K. A., Sakaie, K. E., Lowe, M. J., Lin, J., Stone, L., Bermel, R. A., & Phillips, M. D. (2013). High spatial and angular resolution diffusion-weighted imaging reveals forniceal damage related to memory impairment. *Magnetic Resonance Imaging, 31*, 695–699.

Kratz, A. L., Ehde, D. M., & Bombardier, C. H. (2014). Affective mediators of a physical activity intervention for depression in multiple sclerosis. *Rehabilitation Psychology, 59*, 57.

Krupp, L. B., & Elkins, L. E. (2000). Fatigue and declines in cognitive functioning in multiple sclerosis. *Neurology, 55*, 934–939.

Kujala, P., Portin, R., & Ruutiainen, J. (1997). The progress of cognitive decline in multiple sclerosis: A controlled 3-year follow-up. *Brain, 120*, 289–297.

Lafosse, J. M., Mitchell, S. M., Corboy, J. R., & Filley, C. M. (2013). The nature of verbal memory impairment in multiple sclerosis: A list-learning and meta-analytic study. *Journal of the International Neuropsychological Society, 19*, 995–1008.

Llufriu, S., Martinez-Heras, E., Fortea, J., Blanco, Y., Berenguer, J., Gabilondo, I., & Sola-Valls, N. (2014). Cognitive functions in multiple sclerosis: Impact of gray matter integrity. *Multiple Sclerosis Journal, 20*, 424–432.

Loitfelder, M., Fazekas, F., Petrovic, K., Fuchs, S., Ropele, S., Wallner-Blazek, M., . . . Enzinger, C. (2011). Reorganization in cognitive networks with progression of multiple sclerosis: Insights from fMRI. *Neurology, 76*, 526–533.

Lublin, F. D., & Reingold, S. C. (1996). Defining the clinical course of multiple sclerosis: Results of an international survey. *Neurology, 46*, 907–911.

McCabe, M. P., McKern, S., & McDonald, E. (2004). Coping and psychological adjustment among people with multiple sclerosis. *Journal of Psychosomatic Research, 56*, 355–361.

McDonald, W. I., Compston, A., Edan, G., Goodkin, D., Hartung, H.-P., Lublin, F. D., . . . Wolinsky, J. S. (2001). Recommended diagnostic criteria for multiple sclerosis: Guidelines from the international panel on the diagnosis of multiple sclerosis. *Annals of Neurology, 50*, 121–127.

Mohr, D. C., Boudewyn, A. C., Goodkin, D. E., Bostrom, A., & Epstein, L. (2001). Comparative outcomes for individual cognitive-behavior therapy, supportive-expressive group psychotherapy, and sertraline for the treatment of depression in multiple sclerosis. *Journal of Consulting and Clinical Psychology, 69*(6), 1–8.

Mohr, D. C., Goodkin, D. E., Gatto, N., & Van Der Wende, J. (1997). Depression, coping and level of neurological impairment in multiple sclerosis. *Multiple Sclerosis, 3*, 254–258.

Mohr, D. C., Hart, S. L., Julian, L., Catledge, C., Honos-Webb, L., Vella, L., & Tasch, E. T. (2005). Telephone-administered psychotherapy for depression *Archives of General Psychiatry, 62*, 1007–1014.

Mohr, D. C., Likosky, W., Bertagnolli, A., Goodkin, D. E., Van Der Wende, J., Dwyer, P., & Dick, L. P. (2000). Telephone-administered cognitive-behavioral therapy for the treatment of depressive symptoms in multiple sclerosis. *Journal of Consulting and Clinical Psychology, 68*(2), 356–361.

National MS Society, (2009). FAQs about MS. Retrieved December 1, 2009, from www.nationalmssociety.org/about-multiple-sclerosis/FAQs-about-MS/index.aspx#whogets

Nordin, L., & Rorsman, I. (2012). Cognitive behavioural therapy in multiple sclerosis: A randomized controlled pilot study of acceptance and commitment therapy. *Journal of Rehabilitation Medicine, 44*(1), 87–90. doi: 10.2340/16501977-0898

Nyenhuis, D. L., Rao, S. M., Zajecka, J., M. D., Luchetta, T., Bernardin, L., & Garron, D. (1995). Mood disturbance versus other symptoms of depression in multiple sclerosis. *Journal of the International Neuropsychological Society, 1*, 291–296.

Obradovic, D., Petrovic, M., Antanasijevic, I., Marinkovic, J., & Stojanovic, T. (2012). The brief repeatable battery: Psychometrics and normative values with age, education and gender corrections in a Serbian population. *Neurological Sciences, 33*, 1369–1374.

O'Brien, A., Chiaravalloti, N., Arango-Lasprilla, J., Lengenfelder, J., & DeLuca, J. (2007). An investigation of the differential effect of self-generation to improve learning and memory in multiple sclerosis and traumatic brain injury. *Neuropsychological Rehabilitation, 17*, 273–292.

Pakenham, K. I. (1999). Adjustment to multiple sclerosis: Application of a stress and coping model. *Health Psychology, 18*, 383–392.

Parisi, L., Rocca, M. A., Mattioli, F., Copetti, M., Capra, R., Valsasina, P., & Filippi, M. (2014). Changes of brain resting state functional connectivity predict the persistence of cognitive rehabilitation effects in patients with multiple sclerosis. *Multiple Sclerosis Journal, 20*, 686–694.

Passamonti, L., Cerasa, A., Liguori, M., Gioia, M. C., Valentino, P., Nistico, R., . . . Fera, F. (2009). Neurobiological mechanisms underlying emotional processing in relapsing-remitting multiple sclerosis. *Brain, 132*, 3380–3391.

Polman, C. H., Reingold, S. C., Banwell, B., Clanet, M., Cohen, J. A., Filippi, M., . . . Wolinsky, J. S. (2010). Diagnostic criteria for multiple sclerosis: 2010 revisions to the McDonald criteria. *Annals of Neurology, 69*, 292–302.

Polman, C. H., Reingold, S. C., Edan, G., Filippi, M., Hartung, H.-P., Kappos, L., . . . Wolinsky, J. S. (2005). Diagnostic criteria for multiple sclerosis: 2005 revisions to the "McDonald Criteria" *Annals of Neurology, 58*, 840–846.

Popescu, B. F., & Lucchinetti, C. F. (2012). Meningeal and cortical grey matter pathology in multiple sclerosis. *BMC Neurology, 12*, 11.

Portaccio, E., Goretti, B., Zipoli, V., Siracusa, G., & Sorbi, S. (2009). A short version of Rao's Brief Repeatable Battery as a screening tool for cognitive impairment in multiple sclerosis. *The Clinical Neuropsychologist, 23*, 268–275.

Potagas, C., Giogkaraki, E., Koutsis, G., Mandellos, D., & Tsirempolou, E. (2008). Cognitive impairment in different MS subtypes and clinically isolated syndromes. *Journal of the Neurological Sciences, 267*, 100–106.

Rabinowitz, A. R., & Arnett, P. A. (2009). A longitudinal analysis of cognitive dysfunction, coping, and depression in multiple sclerosis. *Neuropsychology, 23*, 581–591.

Rao, S. M., & The Cognitive Function Study Group of the National Multiple Sclerosis Society. (1990). *Manual for the Brief Repeatable Battery of Neuropsychological Tests in Multiple Sclerosis*. New York: National Multiple Sclerosis Society.

Rao, S. M., Leo, G. J., Bernardin, L., & Unverzagt, F. (1991). Cognitive dysfunction in multiple sclerosis: 1. Frequency, patterns, and prediction. *Neurology, 41*, 685–691.

Rendell, P. G., Henry, J. D., Phillips, L. H., Garcia, X., Booth, P., Phillips, P., & Kliegel, M. (2012). Prospective memory, emotional valence, and multiple sclerosis. *Journal of Clinical and Experimental Neuropsychology, 34*, 738–749.

Sadovnick, A. D., Remick, R. A., Allen, J., Swartz, E., Yee, I.M.L., Eisen, K., . . . Paty, D. W. (1996). Depression and multiple sclerosis. *Neurology, 46*, 628–632.

Schultheis, M. T., Weisser, V., Ang, J., Elovic, E., Nead, R., Sestito, N., & Millis, S. R. (2010). Examining the relationship between cognition and driving performance in multiple sclerosis. *Archives of Physical Medicine and Rehabilitation, 91*, 465–473.

Smith, A. M., Walker, L.A.S., Freedman, M. S., Berrigan, L. I., St. Pierre, J., Hogan, M. J., & Cameron, I. (2012). Activation patterns in multiple sclerosis on the computerized tests of information processing. *Journal of the Neurological Sciences, 312*, 131–137.

Sperling, R. A., Guttmann, C. R., Hohol, M. J., Warfield, S. K., Jakab, M., & Parente, M. (2001). Regional magnetic resonance imaging lesion burden and cognitive function in multiple sclerosis: A longitudinal study. *Archives of Neurology, 58*, 115–121.

Strober, L. B., & Arnett, P. A. (2010). Assessment of depression in multiple sclerosis: Development of a "trunk and branch" model. *The Clinical Neuropsychologist, 24*, 1146–1166.

Strober, L. B., & Arnett, P. A. (2015). Depression in multiple sclerosis: The utility of common self-report instruments and development of a disease-specific measure. *Journal of Clinical and Experimental Neuropsychology, 37*, 722–732. http://dx.doi.org/10.1080/13803395.2015.1063591.

Strober, L. B., Chiaravalloti, N., Moore, N., & DeLuca, J. (2014). Unemployment in multiple sclerosis (MS): Utility of the MS Functional Composite and cognitive testing. *Multiple Sclerosis Journal, 20*, 112–115.

Strober, L. B., Englert, J., Munschauer, F., Weinstock-Guttman, B., Rao, S., & Benedict, R. (2009). Sensitivity of conventional memory tests in multiple sclerosis: Comparing the Rao brief repeatable neuropsychological battery and the minimal assessment of cognitive function in MS. *Multiple Sclerosis, 15*, 1077–1084.

Sumowski, J. F., Chiaravalloti, N., & DeLuca, J. (2010). Retrieval practice improves memory in multiple sclerosis: Clinical application of the testing effect. *Neuropsychology, 24*, 267–272.

Sundgren, M., Maurex, L., Wahlin, A., Piehl, F., & Brismar, T. (2013). Cognitive impairment has a strong relation to nonsomatic symptoms of depression in relapsing—remitting multiple sclerosis. *Archives of Clinical Neuropsychology, 28*, 144–155.

Tekok-Kilic, A., Benedict, R. H., & Zivadinov, R. (2006). Update on the relationships between neuropsychological dysfunction and structural MRI in multiple sclerosis. *Expert Review in Neurotherapeutics, 6*, 323–331.

Till, C., Udler, E., Ghassemi, R., Narayanan, S., Arnold, D. L., & Banwell, B. L. (2012). Factors associated with emotional and behavioral outcomes in adolescents with multiple sclerosis. *Multiple Sclerosis, 18*(8), 1170–1180. doi: 10.1177/1352458511433918

Ukueberuwa, D. M., & Arnett, P. A. (2014). Evaluating the role of coping style as a moderator of fatigue and risk for future cognitive impairment in multiple sclerosis. *Journal of the International Neuropsychological Society, 20*, 751–755. doi:10.1017/S1355617714000587.

Vargas, G. A., & Arnett, P. A. (2010). Positive everyday experiences interact with social support to predict depression in multiple sclerosis. *Journal of the International Neuropsychological Society, 16*, 1039–1046.

Vattakatuchery, J. J., Rickards, H., & Cavanna, A. E. (2011). Pathogenic mechanisms of depression in multiple sclerosis. *The Journal of Neuropsychiatry and Clinical Neuroscience, 23*(3), 261–276. doi: 10.1176/appi.neuropsych.23.3.261

Walker, L.A.S., Berard, J. A., Berrigan, L. I., Rees, L. M., & Freedman, M. S. (2012). Detecting cognitive fatigue in multiple sclerosis: Method matters. *Journal of the Neurological Sciences, 316*, 86–92.

Wojtowicz, M., Mazerolle, E. L., Bhan, V., & Fisk, J. D. (2014). Altered functional connectivity and performance variability in Relapsing-Remitting multiple sclerosis. *Multiple Sclerosis Journal, 20*, 1453-1463. doi: 10.1177/1352458514524997

Zakzanis, K. (2000). Distinct neurocognitive profiles in multiple sclerosis subtypes. *Archives of Clinical Neuropsychology, 15*, 115–136.

Zivadinov, R., & Pirko, I. (2012). Advances in understanding gray matter pathology in multiple sclerosis: Are we ready to redefine disease pathogenesis? *BMC Neurology, 12*, 9.

Zivadinov, R., Sepcic, J., Nasuelli, D., De Masi, R., Bragadin, L. M., & Tommasi, M. A. (2001). A longitudinal study of brain atrophy and cognitive disturbances in the early phase of relapsing-remitting multiple sclerosis. *Journal of Neurology, Neurosurgery, & Psychiatry, 70*, 773–780.

26 Neuropsychological Functioning in Autoimmune Disorders

Elizabeth Kozora, Andrew Burleson, and Christopher M. Filley

Introduction

Autoimmune disorders represent a spectrum of conditions in which the immune system mistakenly attacks and destroys healthy body tissue. There are more than 80 autoimmune disorders, and the prevalence of autoimmune disease in the United States is about 8%, or approximately 23.5 million people. Women make up an estimated 75% of autoimmune patients, and according to the 2004 U.S. National Women's Health Center, these diseases constitute the fourth largest cause of disability among women. Many autoimmune diseases are characterized by circulating autoantibodies that target healthy tissue, and the brain may be prominently affected. Cognitive dysfunction is one of many manifestations of autoimmune central nervous system (CNS) involvement. Despite an exponential increase in studies over the past ten years, the course, prognosis, neurobiological mechanisms, and optimal treatment of cognitive dysfunction in autoimmune diseases have remained largely elusive.

The most extensive investigation regarding the prevalence and biobehavioral correlates of cognitive dysfunction in disorders of autoimmunity has centered on systemic lupus erythematosus (SLE). However, there is accumulating evidence that other autoimmune disorders such as antiphospholipid syndrome (APS), rheumatoid arthritis (RA), and primary Sjögren's syndrome (PSS) commonly feature cognitive dysfunction that may be directly associated with the autoimmune pathologic process. This chapter will present the basic epidemiology and review the neuropsychological literature in SLE, APS, RA and PSS, four autoimmune disorders that have been the focus of many recent neurobehavioral studies. In addition, the biobehavioral mechanisms and neuroimaging correlates of cognitive dysfunction for these disorders will be discussed.

Systemic Lupus Erythematosus

Definition and Epidemiology

SLE is typified by the production of autoantibodies, and a hallmark of the disease is the presence of serum antibodies directed to nuclear constituents of the cell body. The prevalence of SLE worldwide is approximately 20–150 cases per 100,000, and in women rates vary from 164 (in Caucasians) to 406 (in African Americans) per 100,000 (Chakravarty, Bush, Manzi, Clarke, & Ward, 2007; Lawrence et al., 1998; Pons-Estel, Alarcon, Scofield, Reinlib, & Cooper, 2010). SLE can damage almost any organ of the body, including the brain. Other organ systems prominently affected are the skin, joints, heart, lungs, and kidneys. Epidemiological research estimates that 0.51% of the U.S. population has SLE, or approximately 1.4–1.5 million people. Approximately 90% of SLE patients are women. Patients are most frequently diagnosed with SLE in their 20s and 30s. In the United States, most studies suggest that SLE is more common in African Americans, African Caribbeans, and those with Asian backgrounds in comparison to Caucasians. The diagnosis of SLE is currently based on the presence of at least four out of 11 manifestations (Hochberg, 1997) including malar (butterfly) rash, discoid rash, photosensitivity, oral ulcers, arthritis, serositis (pericarditis or pleuritis), renal dysfunction, neurologic syndromes, hematologic disorder, immunologic disorder, and the presence of an abnormally high titer of antinuclear antibody.

Neuropsychiatric Systemic Lupus Erythematosus

Over 50% of patients with SLE demonstrate psychiatric or neurologic disorders indicating CNS involvement (Bluestein, 1992; West, 2007). Neuropsychiatric (NP) manifestations in SLE are diverse, and may include clinically major overt disorders such as stroke, seizures, and psychotic events, or less dramatic but still significant syndromes such as depression, anxiety, headache, and mild cognitive dysfunction (MCD; see Kozora & Filley, 2011). Estimates of the prevalence of NP manifestations in SLE range from 14% to 75%, a variability that largely reflects differences in classification, assessment tools, subject selection, and attribution of cause (Hanly, 2007).

In SLE patients with NP involvement, pathogenic mechanisms have been distinguished on the basis of NP presentation (West, 1994; West, Emlen, Wener, & Kotzin, 1995). In those with diffuse manifestations (e.g., psychosis and depression), autoantibodies directed to CNS antigens have been proposed as important pathogenic factors. In these cases, immunologically mediated neuronal injury is hypothesized to be caused by a variety of antineuronal autoantibodies

(Bluestein & Woods, 1982; Kelly & Denburg, 1987; Robbins et al., 1988; Temesvari et al., 1983; Wekking, Nossent, van Dam, & Swaak, 1991; Zvaifler & Bluestein, 1982). Anti-ribosomal P antibodies, anti-neuronal antibodies, and, in the cerebrospinal fluid (CSF), elevated IgG index (a major class of immunoglobulins) and oligoclonal bands, have all been regarded as biological markers of diffuse CNS pathology in SLE (West, 1994; West et al., 1995). In contrast to diffuse disease, focal CNS presentations in SLE such as stroke syndromes, seizures (often of focal onset), movement disorders, and myelopathy have been postulated to be due to ischemia (West, 1994; West et al., 1995). These cases appear to be secondary to CNS hypercoagulability (e.g., related to antiphospholipid antibodies) and thrombosis, and less commonly to vasculitis. Focal stroke presentations are typically due to vascular occlusion, and these patients usually have evidence of antiphospholipid antibodies and abnormal brain magnetic resonance imaging (MRI) scans (West et al., 1995). A bland, diffuse, noninflammatory microvasculopathy, sometimes in association with leukocyte plugging, and mediated by complement and endothelial cell activation, is the predominant vascular abnormality in autopsy studies of SLE patients (Belmont, Abramson, & Lie, 1996; Belmont et al., 1986; Ellis & Verity, 1979; Hanly et al., 1992; Johnson & Richardson, 1968). These changes, which appear to be independent of antiphospholipid antibodies, are found in anatomical proximity to cerebral microinfarction, indicating a causative association.

As described in the past (West, 1994; West et al., 1995), altered transport properties of the choroid plexus due to deposition of complement (serum proteins involved in immunoreactivity) in NPSLE are thought to interfere with CNS activity. Inflammatory processes as well as the effects of cytokines (interleuken-1, interleukin-6, and tumor necrosis factor) have also been recognized as potential mediators of CNS alterations. Neuroendocrine and immune system interactions resulting from chronic stress, antioxidative mechanisms, and neuropeptides and endocrine factors also appear to be related to NPSLE. The neuropeptides vasopressin, neuropeptide, and substance P also appear related to NP activity in SLE in animal models (Bracci-Laudiero, Aloe, Lundeberg, Theodorsson, & Stenfors, 1999; Sakic et al., 1999) and human studies (Harle et al., 2006; Lapteva, Yarboro, & Roebuck-Spencer, 2006). Additional mechanisms causing or related to NP symptoms in SLE are diverse and may include infections, medications, hypertension, uremia, electrolyte imbalances, fever, thyroid disease, atherosclerosis, fibromyalgia, and sleep apnea.

In 1999, definitions for 19 NP syndromes were developed, and diagnostic agreement was empirically evaluated by a multidisciplinary committee convened by the American College of Rheumatology (ACR) (1999). Definitions of NPSLE syndromes were developed for CNS and peripheral nervous system (PNS) NP manifestations (Table 26.2), and recommendations for diagnostic testing were produced with input from several disciplines, including neuropsychology. Since none of the syndromes are specific to SLE, relevant factors were listed as "exclusions" if they caused identical symptoms and could be separated from the SLE process (i.e., history of diabetes), and "associations" if the symptoms could be caused by SLE or by another nonmodifiable factor (i.e., drug effects). In a recent review of studies between April 1999 and May of 2008 evaluating classification of the 19 NP syndromes proposed by the ACR, the prevalence of NP syndromes in 2049 SLE patients was estimated to be 56.3%, and the most frequent NP syndromes were headache (28.3%), mood disorders (20.7%), cognitive dysfunction (19.7%), seizures (9.9%), and cerebrovascular disease (8.0%) (Unterman et al., 2011). In another study of 1047 SLE patients between 1999 to 2010, 47.2% of the patients had one or more NP events, and the most frequent NP syndromes were headache (52%), mood disorders (14.4%), seizure disorder (5.8%), anxiety (5.7%), and cerebrovascular disease (5.1%) (Hanly et al., 2011).

Cognitive Dysfunction

The ACR defined the NPSLE syndrome of "cognitive dysfunction" as the presence of "significant deficits in any or all of the following cognitive functions: complex attention, executive skills (e.g., planning, organizing, and sequencing), memory (e.g., learning and recall), visual-spatial processing, language (e.g., verbal fluency) and psychomotor speed." The committee reviewed a number of brief mental status examinations, but because of high false negative rates of these tests, and their failure to detect mild cognitive deficits in many cases (Karzmark, 1997; Nelson, Fogel, & Faust, 1986), the committee concluded that there was no substitute for detailed neuropsychological assessment. Due to the limitations imposed by longer and comprehensive batteries (i.e., time requirements and financial burden), the committee recommended a short one-hour battery. The tests selected for this battery had demonstrated decline in SLE patients in prior studies, and include measures of estimated IQ; complex attention verbal and visual learning and memory; verbal fluency; and complex visuomotor tasks (1999). Cognitive studies subsequent to these recommendations commonly (but not always) included these domains as the minimum to be surveyed. Notably, in the review of studies by Unterman et al. (2011), there was a wide range of cognitive dysfunction prevalence (0%–80%), mostly due to the use of different methods of neuropsychological testing, and in some cases the use of chart-driven self-report methods.

Cognitive deficits using standard neuropsychological tests are well documented in patients with SLE. Deficits in attention, learning and recall, fluency, complex psychomotor functions, visuospatial skills, and motor dexterity have been most commonly identified (Brey et al., 2002; Carbotte, Denburg, & Denburg, 1986; Conti et al., 2012; Denburg, Carbotte, & Denburg, 1997; Ferstl, Niemann, Biehl, Hinrichsen, & Kirch, 1992; Ginsburg et al., 1992; Glanz et al.,

1997; Hanly et al., 1993; Koffler, 1987; Kozora et al., 2008; Kozora et al., 2011; Kozora, Ellison, & West, 2004; Kozora, Filley, et al., 2012; Kozora, Thompson, West, & Kotzin, 1996; Maneeton, Maneeton, & Louthrenoo, 2010; Peretti et al., 2012; Sonies, Klippel, Gerber, & Gerber, 1982; Wekking, Nossent, et al., 1991). Across studies, the incidence of cognitive impairment in SLE patients with overt NP activity such as seizures, stroke, and major depression has ranged from 20% to 87%, with earlier studies demonstrating a higher incidence (Abda et al., 2013; Carbotte et al., 1986; Conti et al., 2012; Denburg et al., 1987a; Glanz, Schur, Lew, & Khoshbin, 2005; Hanly et al., 1992; Hay, Black, Huddy, Creed, Tomenson, Bernstein, & Holt., 1992; Koffler, 1987; Kutner, Busch, Mahmood, Racis, & Krey, 1988; Sonies et al., 1982; Stein, Walters, Dillon, & Schulzer, 1986; Vogel, Bhattacharya, Larsen, & Jacobsen, 2011; Wekking, Nossent, et al., 1991). In the absence of other NP disorders such as seizures and stroke (i.e., non-NPSLE), cognitive dysfunction has been reported in some 20%–60% of SLE patients (Brey et al., 2002; Carbotte et al., 1986; Denburg et al., 1987a; Hanly et al., 1992; Hay et al., 1992; Koffler, 1987; Kozora, Arciniegas, Duggan, West, & Filley, 2013; Kozora & Filley, 2011; Kozora et al., 1996; Kutner et al., 1988; Maneeton et al., 2010; Norwicka-Sauer, Czuszynska, Smolenskda, & Siebert, 2011; Peretti, Peretti, Kozora, Papathanassiou, Chouinard, & Chouinard, 2012; Wekking, Nossent, et al., 1991; Wekking, Vingerhoets, van Dam, Nossent, & Swaak, 1991). For the purposes of this chapter, we continue to use the terms *NPSLE* and *non-NPSLE;* however, we acknowledge the confusion that may be associated with this terminology. As noted earlier, there are 19 NP syndromes in SLE, one of which is cognitive dysfunction. Many SLE investigators, intending to focus on mechanisms and neuroimaging analysis of cognitive dysfunction, exclude patients with any other overt CNS activity such as stroke, seizures, etc. (non-NPSLE) to exclude confounding influence on cognition.

In Figure 26.1 we illustrate the range of cognitive impairment found in studies of NPSLE, non-NPSLE, and (where available) controls. Differences between studies are largely methodological, related to differing characteristics of the SLE sample, selection of tests, and classification of impairment. The classification of impairment is also problematic, as it has been based on several approaches (as outlined at the bottom of Figure 26.1). Some studies compare patient and control groups on tests to assess statistical decline. Other studies utilize norm-referenced criteria and "domain" groups to determine if SLE patients are performing in the "impaired" range. Definitions of impairment frequently refer to one or two standard deviations below the norm on individual tests or domains. Estimated premorbid intellectual levels have also been used to estimate decline in performance across specific cognitive areas.

Despite the recommendations of the ACR to standardize assessment and classification schemes, diversity across study design is prevalent (see Tables 26.1 and 26.2). The ACR proposed a battery of tests, and our group established the reliability and validity of this cognitive battery in relation to a larger SLE battery (Kozora et al., 2004). The inclusion of specific "tests" proposed by the ACR has more consistently emerged across study sites of cognition in SLE (Doninger, Fink, & Utset, 2005; Emori et al., 2005; Julian et al., 2012), but there is still variation in the definition of "cognitive impairment" and no published studies have attempted to compare classification schemes or establish the sensitivity and specificity of the neuropsychological batteries in SLE. In 2007, an Ad Hoc Cognition Sub-committee for the Committee on Lupus Response Criteria further expanded the definition of cognitive dysfunction to include definitions of focal decline (impairment in one or more measures within one domain) and multifocal impairment (decline if impairment exists on measures spanning two or more domains) (Sub-committee, 2007). These definitions, if widely used, may help to standardize cognitive changes over time in SLE patients.

Evidence of Mild Cognitive Dysfunction

Studies over several decades have supported the existence of MCD in SLE (MCD-SLE), although this descriptor was not formally introduced until 2011 (Kozora & Filley, 2011).

Table 26.1 NP syndromes of SLE

Central Nervous System
Acute Confusional State
Cognitive Dysfunction
Psychosis
Mood Disorder
Anxiety Disorder
Headache (including migraine and benign intracranial hypertension)
Cerebrovascular Disease
Myelopathy
Movement Disorder
Demyelinating Syndrome
Seizure Disorders
Aseptic Meningitis
Peripheral Nervous System
Cranial Neuropathy
Polyneuropathy
Plexopathy
Mononeuropathy, single/multiplex
Acute Inflammatory Demyelinating Polyradiculo-Neuropathy (Guillain-Barré Syndrome)
Autonomic Disorder
Myasthenia Gravis

Adapted from ACR Ad Hoc Committee on Neuropsychiatric Lupus Nomenclature. The American College of Rheumatology Nomenclature and Case Definitions for Neuropsychiatric Lupus Syndromes. *Arthritis Rheum* 1999 42(4):599–608.

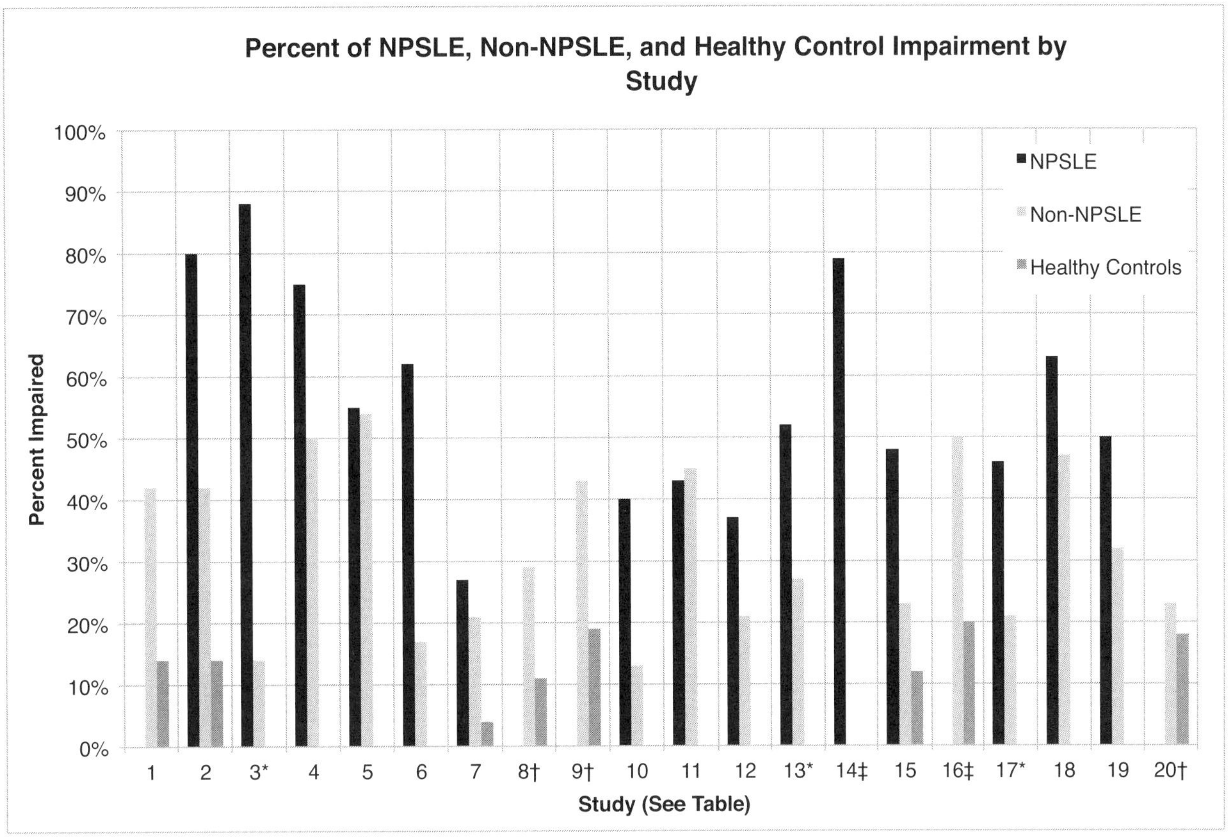

Figure 26.1 Percent of Cognitive Impairment in NPSLE, non-NPSLE and healthy controls

* Study contains healthy controls at 0% impairment
† Study contains only Non-NPSLE (no NPSLE)
‡ SLE only (no division between NP-SLE and Non-NPSLE)

Article	*Authors*	*Participants*	*Cognitive Impairment Classification*
1)	Denburg et al. (1986)	45 NPSLE, 41 Non-NPSLE, 35 HC	≥ 3/17 test scores impaired
2)	Carbotte et al. (1986)	36 NPSLE, 26 Non-NPSLE, 35 HC	> 2/17 test scores impaired
3)	Koffler et al. (1987)	16 NPSLE, 29 Non-NPSLE, 10 HC	3 or more scales below baseline
4)	Kutner et al. (1988)	8 NPSLE, 14 Non-NPSLE	> 4/13 test scores impaired
5)	Wekking et al. (1991)	9 NPSLE, 11 Non-NPSLE	> 3/25 test scores impaired
6)	Hay et al. (1992)	13 NPSLE, 53 Non-NPSLE	> 2/6 test scores impaired
7)	Hanly et al. (1992)	15 NPSLE, 55 Non-NPSLE, 23 HC	> 3/7 domains impaired
8)	Kozora et al. (1996)	51 Non-NPSLE, 27 HC	≥ 2/8 domains impaired
9)	Glanz et al. (1997)	58 Non-NPSLE, 47 HC	≥ 3/18 or more summary scores
10)	Sailer et al. (1997)	20 NPSLE, 15 Non-NPSLE	Mean of all test scores
11)	Sabbadini et al. (1999)	56 NPSLE, 101 Non-NPSLE	> 1/10 test scores impaired
12)	Carlomagno et al. (2000)	27NPSLE, 24 Non-NPSLE	> 3 test scores impaired
13)	Monastero et al. (2001)	23 NPSLE, 52 Non-NPSLE, 27 HC	≥ 2 test scores impaired
14)	Brey et al. (2002)	*67 SLE	Average global impairment rating
15)	Kozora et al. (2004)	31 NPSLE, 22Non-NPSLE, 25 HC	≥ 4/12 test scores impaired
16)	Glanz et al. (2005)	50 SLE, 30 HC	≥ 5/20 test scores impaired
17)	Maneeton et al. (2010)	11 NPSLE, 19 Non-NPSLE, 22 HC	≥ 1 test score impaired
18)	Nowicka-Sauer et al. (2011)	57NPSLE, 36 Non-NPSLE	≥ 1 test scores impaired
19)	Vogel et al. (2011)	20 NPSLE, 37 Non-NPSLE	**Varied classification
20)	Kozora et al. (2012)	84 Non-NPSLE, 37 HC	≥ 4/12 test scores impaired

* Subset of 67 subjects of study's n = 128. Differentiation between NPSLE and Non-NPSLE not made in this subset (frequency of NPSLE in n = 128 was 80%)

** Varied: Three criteria for classifying a patient as cognitively impaired were applied: a) if two (or more) test performances were categorized as "probably impaired," b) if one test score was "probably impaired" and three (or more) were "possibly impaired," c) if four (or more) tests were classified as "possibly impaired."

Table 26.2 Potential biobehavioral mechanisms of cognitive dysfunction in SLE

Disease Characteristics
Duration of Disease
Disease Severity
Organ System Specific
Kidney Damage-Renal Insufficiency
Lung Damage-Pulmonary Abnormalities
Cardiovascular Disease-Hypertension
Other SLE-Related Physical Syndromes
Serositis
Raynaud's Disorder
Obesity
Sleep Apnea
Medication Use
Prednisone
Biological Factors
Vascular Abnormalities
Vasculopathy
Hypercoagulability (see aPL)
Autoantibodies
Antineuronal Antibodies
Cross-reactive Lymphocytoxic Antibodies
Antibodies to N-methyl-D-aspartate (anti-NMDA; NR2a, NR2b)
Antiphospholipid Antibodies (aPL)
Lupus anticoagulant (LAC)
Anticardiolipin (aCL)
Anti-β2-glycoprotein-I antibody (aβ2GPI)
Antibodies to Ribosomal Proteins (anti-P)
Mediators of Inflammation
Proinflammatory Activity
Interluekin-1, 2, 6, 10 (IL-1; IL-2: IL-6; IL-10)
Interferon alpha (IFN-α)
Tumor Necrosis Factor (TNF)
Matrix metalloproteinase (MMP)-9
Additional Biological Factors
Hormones
Neuropeptides
Behavioral Correlates
Psychological Factors
Depression
Anxiety
Pain
Fatigue
Sleep Disorders
Physical Inactivity

Carbotte et al. (1986) reported that 42% of the SLE subjects with no known additional NP activity were cognitively impaired in a wide variety of areas. Kutner et al. (1988) found that 50% of the SLE patients with no known additional NP activity were impaired on their battery. Denburg et al. (1987a) reported that 42% of the SLE patients without any additional NP diagnoses were globally impaired. Wekking, Nossent, et al. (1991) observed that 40% of their SLE patients with no additional NP activity had deficits on three or more cognitive tests. In similar SLE cohorts, cognitive impairment was found in 17% (Hay et al., 1992), 20% (Carlomagno et al., 2000; Hanly et al., 1992), and 27%. (Monastero et al., 2001) of subjects. Finally, Norwicka-Sauer et al., (2011) reported that 47.2% of the non-NPSLE had one to three tests in the impaired range, with none severely impaired.

In our original study (Kozora et al., 1996), 29% of non-NPSLE patients had deficits consistent MCD-SLE (based on two out of eight domain scores considered impaired). Compared to controls, the non-NPSLE patients were impaired on composite domain scores of attention and fluency, which included both verbal and nonverbal modalities. In our 2004 study (with a new cohort of 22 non-NPSLE patients), we reported that 23% of the subjects had deficits consistent with MCD-SLE, including significantly lowered scores in visuomotor speed, attention, and motor functioning in comparison to controls (Kozora et al., 2004). In a third cohort of 84 non-NPSLE patients, 23.8% had MCD-SLE, with lower cognitive performance on measures of visuomotor speed, working memory, verbal learning, and sustained visual attention when compared to controls (Kozora et al., 2012). In a smaller group (n = 20) of non-NPSLE patients in a new geographic site (screened and tested in New York with identical methods and test battery as in our original Denver studies) we found a prevalence of MCD-SLE of 60% (Kozora, Erkan, et al., 2013). Compared to the 84 SLE patients in Denver, these patients had greater deficits in areas of verbal fluency, visuomotor speed, and sequencing skills. To adjust for differences in sample size, we selected 20 SLE patients from the Denver group to match to the New York group. Reanalysis continued to disclose large differences in the frequency of MCD-SLE (60% in New York compared to 25% in Denver). The greater duration of disease and higher prevalence of medical complications in the New York group might have contributed to this difference. Future studies that better evaluate site or selection bias are warranted.

Domains of Cognitive Impairment

A summary of 20 studies that included at least four or more domains of cognitive testing using standardized neuropsychological tests in SLE patients from 1987 through 2014 can be found in Table 26.3. We have reorganized our domain categories from a prior version (Kozora, 2008) and acknowledge that this approach provides only a broad "estimate" of impaired cognitive domains within SLE. Not all the studies investigating a particular domain appear in Table 26.3; sample sizes across studies range from 20 to 93. The columns in the table are ordered based on the number of studies that included tests within a domain. For example, learning and memory was the most commonly studied domain and appears first in the table. Adjusting for the studies that included this domain, 79% of the studies report impairment

Table 26.3 Neuropsychological impairment by domain in SLE: summary of battery-approach Studies

First Author (Date Published)	*# SLE (N)*	*Visual Learning and Memory*	*Verbal Learning and Memory*	*Attention*	*Executive Functions*	*Visuomotor*	*Visuospatial*	*Language*	*Motor and Reaction Time*	*IQ*
Denburg et al(1987)	86	+	+	–	+	+	+	+	–	–
Rummelt et al. (1991)	20	+	+						+	+
Ginsburg et al. (1992)	49	–	–	+			+		+	
Ferstl et al. (1992)	15	+	+	+					+	
Kozora et al. (1996)	51	+	+	+	+	–	–	–		+
Glanz et al. (1997)	58	+	+		–	+		–	+	
Sailer et al. (1997)	35	+		+	+		–			–
Monastero et al. (2001)	75	+	+	–	–		+	–		
Brey et al. (2002)	67	+	+	+	+	+	–	–	–	
Loukkola et al. (2003)	46	–	+	+	+	+	–	–		
Kozora et al. (2004)	53	–	–	+	+	+	+	–	+	+
Glanz et al. (2005)	50	+	+	+	+	+				
Emori et al. (2005)	21	–	+	–	+	+	–			
Vogel et al. (2011)	57	+	–	+	+	–	+	–		–
Norwicka-Saur et al. (2011)	93	+	+	–	+	+	+			
Kozora et al. (2012)	84	–	+	+	–	+	–		–	
Abda et al. (2013)	34	+	+	+	+	+	+			
Conti et al. (2012)	58	–	–	–	–		+			
Peretti et al. (2012)	31	+	+	+		+				
Kozora et al. (2013)	40	+	+	+	+	+	–	+	–	
Total Impairment	**1,023**	**14/20 (70%)**	**15/19 (79%)**	**13 / 18 (72%)**	**12/16 (75%)**	**12/14(86%)**	**8/15 (53%)**	**2/9 (22%)**	**5/9 (56%)**	**3/6 (50%)**

Note: Due to differences in each author's methodology and information available, this table is intended as our interpretation of the literature and should only be considered an overall estimate of cognitive impairment in SLE.

in verbal learning and memory, and 70% in visual learning and memory. Attention (which includes auditory and visual tasks, sustained visual attention, selective attention, and rapid auditory information processing) was impaired in 72% of the studies. Executive functions (measuring problem solving, hypothesis testing, fluency, and sequential visuomotor abilities such as Trail Making Test B) were impaired in 75% of the studies. Motor functions (including motor coordination, speed, and reaction time) were impaired in 56% of the studies. Visuospatial measures (i.e., visuoperceptual and visuoconstructional tasks) were impaired in 53% of the studies. Additional studies not included in the table (because of a focus on one domain or test) clearly suggest that attention and information processing, learning and memory, visuomotor speed, and various measures of executive functions continue to be found impaired in studies from 2005 to 2014 (Conti et al., 2012; Emori et al., 2005; Glanz et al., 2005; Julian et al., 2012; Kozora et al., 2012; Norwicka-Sauer et al., 2011; Paran et al., 2009). Language skills (including auditory and reading comprehension and naming) have been rarely studied in SLE, and, when included, have been found to be impaired in less than 22% of the SLE subjects. Some studies do report deficits in aspects of verbal skills and auditory comprehension (Brey et al., 2002; Maneeton et al., 2010). Although half of the studies suggest lowered overall intelligence (Denburg et al., 1987a; Koffler, 1987; Kozora et al., 1996; Loukkola et al., 2003; Papero, Bluestein, White, & Lipnick, 1990), few studies included this domain (see Table 26.2).

LEARNING AND MEMORY

As illustrated in Table 26.3, a majority of the cognitive studies in SLE have included measures of verbal and nonverbal learning and memory, and deficits using normative data, comparison with control groups, or decline from premorbid levels have been identified (Brey et al., 2002; Carbotte et al., 1986; Denburg et al., 1987a; Emori et al., 2005; Ferstl et al., 1992; Glanz et al., 2005; Glanz et al., 1997; Hanly et al., 1992; Kozora et al., 2004; Kozora et al., 1996; Kutner et al., 1988; Loukkola et al., 2003; Menon et al., 1999; Monastero et al., 2001; Paran et al., 2009; Rummelt et al., 1991; Sailer et al., 1997). In our original study, non-NPSLE patients demonstrated a greater frequency of impairment in a learning domain (combined verbal and visual tasks) compared to controls (Kozora et al., 1996). In a later study, a combined NPSLE and non-NPSLE group showed a greater frequency of impairment in visual memory tasks compared to verbal tasks (Kozora et al., 2004). In our recent study of 64 non-NPSLE patients, we found that more than 20% were impaired in verbal memory, and more than 40% were impaired in visual memory (Kozora et al., 2008). Although some authors studying SLE have suggested that visual memory may be more impaired in SLE compared to verbal memory (Coin-Mejias et al., 2008; Ferstl et al., 1992), a review of studies comparing SLE patients to healthy controls on verbal and nonverbal domains would suggest that most are impaired on both these aspects of memory.

ATTENTION AND INFORMATION PROCESSING

Impairment in sustained attention, complex attention, and information processing are also commonly measured and impaired in SLE (Brey et al., 2002; Ginsburg et al., 1992; Glanz et al., 2005; Hanly et al., 1992; Holliday, Navarete, Escalante, Saklad, & Brey, 2000; Kozora et al., 2004; Loukkola et al., 2003; Maneeton et al., 2010; Norwicka-Sauer et al., 2011; Peretti et al., 2012; Petri, Naqibuddin, Carson, Wallace, et al., 2008; Sailer et al., 1997; Vogel et al., 2011; Wekking, Nossent, et al., 1991). When accounting for all the studies in this area (many not represented in Table 26.2), this may be the most impaired cognitive domain in SLE. A variety of auditory and visual tasks of sustained attention, selective attention, and working memory have been studied in SLE. Several studies have explored more demanding attentional tasks in SLE, including the Paced Auditory Serial Addition Test (PASAT) (Gronwall, 1977), a task that assesses these cognitive processes by requiring attention to auditory input and inhibition of response encoding while attending to the next presented number, and performing at an externally determined pace (Spreen & Strauss, 1991). In 2004, we reported that global PASAT performance was significantly lower in SLE patients with and without NP manifestations compared to controls. SLE patients with NP symptoms performed in the mildly to moderately impaired range while SLE patients without NP activity performed in the mildly impaired range (Kozora et al., 2004). In a study including SLE patients and controls, Shucard, Parrish, Shucard, McCabe, Benedict, and Ambrus (2004) reported higher rates of impaired PASAT performance in relation to the pace of the task: 11.1% of SLE and 7.4% of controls were impaired on the 2.4-second rate, and 17.8% of SLE and 3.7% of controls on the 2.0-second rate. Covey, Shucard, Shucard, Stegen, and Benedict (2012) found that SLE patients performed more poorly than controls on the PASAT total score, and identified the PASAT as the most sensitive measure of SLE-induced cognitive impairment from a larger battery of cognitive tests. In a study with non-NPSLE, 29% of the subjects were impaired on the PASAT (Kozora, Arciniegas, et al., 2013). Several studies have further analyzed the pattern of responses on the PASAT in SLE and show that SLE patients used strategies such as "chunking," suggesting a tendency to use less-demanding working memory strategies to complete the task (Kozora, Arciniegas, et al., 2013; Shucard et al., 2004)

PROBLEM SOLVING AND EXECUTIVE FUNCTIONING

Problem-solving deficits and poor executive function have been identified in many SLE patients. However, classification of tests as specifically assessing executive function, problem solving, and/or attention has varied across studies, an issue that makes generalizations about this domain difficult. Using problem-solving tasks that focus on higher level verbal and nonverbal reasoning as well as hypothesis testing and decision making, deficits were noted in approximately 60% of the studies reviewed (Brey et al., 2002; Conti et al., 2012; Denburg et al., 1987a; Kutner et al., 1988; Papero et al., 1990; Peretti et al., 2012; Sailer et al., 1997; Vogel et al., 2011). Expanding the category to include fluency and visuomotor sequencing tasks increases the number of studies that report impairment in this area (Denburg et al., 1987a; Emori et al., 2005; Glanz et al., 2005; Kozora et al., 1996; Menon et al., 1999; Norwicka-Sauer et al., 2011).

VISUOSPATIAL/VISUOCONSTRUCTION

Fewer than half of the studies in Table 26.3 include this domain, and the findings are somewhat mixed. These differences may be related to the variety of assessment techniques ranging from graphomotor drawings to copy-and-command as well as visuoconstruction with blocks or visuoperception with puzzles (Conti et al., 2012; Ginsburg et al., 1992; Hanly et al., 1992; Koffler, 1987; Kutner et al., 1988; Monastero et al., 2001; Vogel et al., 2011). In several studies, visuoconstruction using blocks was impaired compared to controls (Denburg, Carbotte, Ginsberg, & Denburg, 1997; Kozora et al., 2004) but not in others (Emori et al., 2005; Glanz et al., 2005; Glanz et al., 1997; Kozora & Filley, 2011; Loukkola et al., 2003) Drawings from copy are not commonly impaired compared to controls (Denburg et al., 1987a), although in one study NPSLE and non-NPSLE were more impaired (Monastero et al., 2001). In a recent study of 58 consecutive SLE patients, the visuospatial domain was the most impaired (Conti et al., 2012). Visuomotor functions, including basic psychomotor tasks, are commonly impaired in SLE, as shown in Table 26.3 and as reviewed in the computerized screening section.

LANGUAGE

Disturbances in language are rarely observed in SLE, although it is apparent that they are rarely sought (Table 26.3). The commonplace clinical impression of preserved language in most cases of SLE therefore has some limited support, but more study of this question is needed.

MOTOR FUNCTION AND REACTION TIME

Reaction time (Ferstl et al., 1992; Menon et al., 1999; Sailer et al., 1997) as well as tests measuring psychomotor speed (i.e., motor coordination and motor speed) are also commonly impaired in SLE patients (Brey et al., 2002; Denburg et al., 1987a; Emori et al., 2005; Glanz et al., 2005; Glanz et al., 1997; Hanly et al., 1992; Kozora et al., 2004; Kutner et al., 1988; Loukkola et al., 2003; Rummelt et al., 1991). Many studies using computerized testing further support a decline in reaction time in SLE compared to controls, as reviewed in the next section.

Neuropsychological Screening

The use of brief neuropsychological screening batteries and computer-assisted cognitive testing is increasingly common for generating outcome measures in clinical trials across a range of neurobehavioral disorders. To date, a number of "computerized" assessments have been proposed and used in SLE research, and have the advantages of minimizing patient time and expense. Future studies relevant to scientific advancement in our understanding MCD in SLE may require highly specialized testing, but the increasing need to improve access, reduce financial burden, and provide more immediate and useful information for clinical care in SLE suggest that continued study of brief screening and computerized measures is warranted. The most commonly used computerized assessment in SLE and other autoimmune diseases has been the Automated Neuropsychological Assessment Metrics (ANAM) (Reeves, Kane, & Winter, 1996), a self-administered computerized battery of tests that requires approximately 30–45 minutes to complete. Several studies have found that the ANAM identifies cognitive dysfunction in SLE compared to controls (Holliday et al., 2003; McLaurin, Holliday, Williams, & Brey, 2005; Petri, Naqibuddin, Carson, Sampedro, et al., 2008; Roebuck-Spencer et al., 2006), suggesting that this battery is sufficient for screening cognitive dysfunction in SLE. Roebuck-Spencer et al. (2006) found that in 60 SLE subjects, the ANAM subtests were largely associated with standardized tests requiring psychomotor speed and complex attention. Petri, Naqibuddin, Carson, Wallace, et al. (2008) reported that four of nine subtests measuring sustained attention, working memory, and simple reaction time were impaired in 111 recently diagnosed SLE patients compared to 79 normal controls. Hanly, Omisade, Su, Farewell, and Fisk (2010) clarified the limitations of this tool, and in one study comparing SLE, RA, and multiple sclerosis (MS), they concluded that although the ANAM is sensitive to cognitive impairment as a screening tool it is "lacking specificity as a reliable indicator of impairment of higher cognitive function in SLE patients."

Additional screening measures have been used in SLE studies. As noted earlier, brief mental status examinations appear to be relatively insensitive to cognitive problems in SLE. The popular Mini-mental State Examination (Folstein, Folstein, & McHugh, 1975), for example, did not show good discrimination between SLE and controls (Karzmark, 1997; Nelson et al., 1986) although it did in one later study (Maneeton et al., 2010). The Montreal Cognitive Assessment Scale (MoCA; see Nasreddine et al., 2005), however, may be more useful. Results of MoCA testing have been published in two SLE cohorts. In one study (Adhikari, 2011), the MoCA was administered to 44 SLE patients, and 29.5% were identified as impaired (compared to 25% impaired on the ANAM). In another study, 30 SLE patients scored significantly lower on the MoCA (mean score 14.7) compared to controls (mean score 27.9) (El-Shafey, Abd-El-Geleel, & Soliman, 2012). Self-report measures of cognitive dysfunction are another commonly used screening method to describe SLE patient's perceived cognitive impairments. Our prior study indicated that self-report of cognitive difficulties, measured via lengthy previously established measures, was not related to more objective methods of cognitive assessment in SLE patients (Kozora, Ellison, & West, 2006). Hanly, Su, Omisade, Farewell, and Fisk (2012) reported that a self-reported questionnaire of cognitive symptoms was not associated with an objective measure of cognitive processing in 68 SLE patients; however, self-report complaints were higher in the presence of anxiety and depression. A recent study (Julian et al., 2012) reported that perceived cognitive deficits using a self-report questionnaire yielded lower sensitivity compared to standardized cognitive measures.

Longitudinal Studies of Cognition

Prospective studies of cognition in SLE are limited, and longitudinal evaluation remains understudied. Persistent, emergent, and improved cognition were noted in studies of 28%–59% of SLE patients at one- to five-year intervals, but many methodological issues limit the utility of these findings (Carlomagno et al., 2000; Hanly, Fisk, Sherwood, & Eastwood, 1994; Hay et al., 1994; Holliday, Naqibuddin, Brey, & Petri, 2005; Naqibuddin et al., 2005; Waterloo et al., 2001). Differences in overall findings may relate to subject selection (the presence or absence of NP involvement, varying levels of disease activity, and the presence or absence of control subjects), intervals of retesting (three months to five years), selection of the test battery (comprehensive, brief, or computerized testing) and statistical analyses. In one long-term study (Mikdashi & Handwerger, 2004), 130 unselected SLE patients were followed over seven years, finding that early MRI abnormalities, Caucasian ethnicity, and aPL elevations influenced the emergence of NP disease. Seven years later, half of the 130 patients had not acquired major NP dysfunction; however, cognitive impairment as measured by standardized testing had emerged as the most common NP syndrome (27.3%). Additional studies suggest fluctuating cognitive functioning in SLE patients over time. Hay et al. (1994) reported that the prevalence of cognitive impairment and psychiatric disorder was similar at two time points for 49 SLE patients; however, only one of the nine patients with cognitive impairment at the first interview remained impaired two years later. Additionally, the change in cognitive impairment was associated with improvement in psychiatric status. Hay and colleagues concluded that impaired performance on cognitive testing at one time point does not predict future NP events but the study may have been influenced by the high prevalence of psychiatric SLE events at the start, a high drop-out rate, missing data, and limited test battery. Hanly et al. (1994) followed an SLE cohort and found that significant fluctuations in cognitive function occurred, with 21% of patients impaired at baseline and 12% impaired after one year. Throughout the study period, three patients had persistent impairment, 12 showed resolved impairment, and four others showed emergent dysfunction. In a later study, Hanly, Cassell, and Fisk (1997) reported that among 47 SLE patients examined at three time points over five years, 64% were never impaired, 19% with cognitive impairment at baseline resolved over time, 9% showed emergent cognitive dysfunction, 4% fluctuated, and 4% stayed cognitively impaired. These results suggest that cognitive deficits in SLE may not be "cumulative." The conclusions of this study are similar to those of Hay et al. (1994) in suggesting that the presence of cognitive deficits does not predict later overt NP symptoms or death.

In contrast, other studies have not reported decline, and have even reported improvement in neuropsychological functioning over time in SLE patients. Carlomagno et al. (2000) reported stable cognitive function in 51 SLE patients over one to three year intervals. These findings may be confounded by time points being specifically selected during times of stable neurological functioning; i.e., 27 of the 51 patients had NP symptoms at the first assessment, and these patients were assessed at least four weeks after resolution. Waterloo et al. (2001) examined 28 SLE patients with mild disease at baseline and then five years later. Their results indicated that neuropsychological functions remained unchanged in 78% of the patients and improved in 22%. They reported that a majority of the patients had MCD and remained at this level through follow-up. These findings, however, may be limited by the small sample size, lack of control subjects with whom to compare change over time, and limited level of cognitive testing (eight tests that did not include major areas such as learning and memory). Several recent studies demonstrate cognitive improvement over time in SLE, although practice effects interfere with interpretation. Holliday et al. (2005) reported that of 21 SLE patients tested at baseline and three months later, more than half demonstrated significant improvement in one of the nine subtests. Control subjects who were examined twice in one day also showed significant practice effects on all tests. Holliday et al. (2003) concluded that both SLE and controls had significant practice effects on the computerized battery. In a larger cohort of the same study, Naqibuddin et al. (2005) evaluated cognition using the identical computerized battery in 106 SLE patients and 79 controls at baseline and at three-month intervals for several years. Significant improvement occurred across a majority of subtests at most time sequences, especially during the first three and six months, suggestive of practice effects rather than true clinical change. Overall, the paucity of longitudinal studies in this area exposes the lack of outcome data and highlights an obstacle in our understanding and informed treatment recommendations of cognitive dysfunction in SLE.

Biobehavioral Mechanisms of Cognitive Dysfunction

The mechanisms underlying cognitive abnormalities in SLE remain relatively obscure, and findings across studies remain inconsistent despite improving methodologies. As indicated in Table 26.1, cognitive impairment is now classified as one of 19 NP manifestations of SLE. The mechanisms underlying these cognitive deficits are likely multifactorial, and, as noted in Table 26.2, a variety of disease characteristics, biological abnormalities, and behavioral factors have been studied as potential contributors.

Disease Characteristics

No consistent relationships between duration of disease, disease severity, medication use, and neuropsychological dysfunction have been documented in SLE patients with or without NP activity. Some aspects of SLE disease were related to cognition in some studies of NPSLE patients (Conti et al., 2012; Ferstl et al., 1992; Fisk, Eastwood, Sherwood, & Hanly, 1993; Hanly et al., 1993; Papero et al., 1990; Sailer et al., 1997; Tomietto et al., 2007) but not in a majority of studies (Carbotte et al., 1986; Carbotte, Denburg, & Denburg, 1995; Carlomagno et al., 2000; Ferstl et al., 1992; Ginsburg et al., 1992; Glanz et al., 1997; Hanly et al., 1997; Hanly et al., 1994; Hay et al., 1992; Leritz, Brandt, Minor, Reis-Jensen, & Petri, 2000; Maneeton et al., 2010; Monastero et al., 2001; Norwicka-Sauer et al., 2011; Paran et al., 2009; Sailer et al., 1997; Vogel et al., 2011; Waterloo, Omdal, Husby, & Mellgren, 2002; Waterloo et al., 2001).

DURATION OF DISEASE

Papero et al. (1990) reported that a longer duration of SLE was related to lower cognitive status in adolescents, a finding that could suggest that early onset SLE patients have a higher risk of CNS involvement. A majority of studies of adult onset SLE have not found a strong relationship between duration of disease and cognitive dysfunction (Kozora et al., 1996; Monastero et al., 2001; Maneeton et al., 2010; Vogel et al., 2011; Norwicka-Sauer et al., 2011) A majority of our studies with separate cohorts of non-NPSLE patients found no associations between cognitive dysfunction and duration of disease (Kozora et al., 2008; Kozora, Ellison, et al., 2006; Kozora et al., 1996); however, we recently found a higher duration of disease in 20 non-NPSLE patients in New York compared to 20 non-NPSLE patients (matched demographically and screened in a similar fashion) in Denver (both groups screened with similar procedures), and that higher duration of disease was associated with increased cognitive impairment (Kozora, Erkan, et al., 2013). The New York subjects also had higher levels of serositis and renal failure. Disease duration, especially in relationship to specific SLE symptoms, may continue to play a role in cognitive dysfunction in SLE.

DISEASE ACTIVITY

Aspects of disease activity have been associated with cognitive deficits in SLE, but consistent findings are difficult to identify, likely due to methodological issues (i.e., data not acquired, not analyzed, or not similar across studies). Hanly et al. (1992) reported that a history of serositis was more common in cognitively impaired non-NPSLE patients. Using the same group of SLE patients, Denburg, Denburg, Carbotte, Fisk, and Hanly (1993) further examined the effect of disease activity on cognition by controlling for corticosteroid use and NP status. Results indicated that greater SLE disease activity was associated with impaired immediate memory and attention, suggesting some impact of generalized disease on CNS functioning. Ferstl et al. (1992) also reported a correlation with disease activity and cognition in a group of patients on corticosteroid therapy. Tomietto et al. (2007) found an association between chronic SLE damage and severity of cognitive impairment, and further identified that the presence of hypertension was related to cognitive dysfunction in 52 SLE patients. In addition, the presence of Raynaud's phenomenon and obesity were correlated with the number of cognitive functions impaired. One study found that cognitive dysfunction was correlated with disease activity in 62 SLE patients at time of diagnosis but not at the time of testing (Maneeton et al., 2010) and more recent study reported that cognitive dysfunction was related both to disease severity and cumulative chronic damage in 58 SLE patients(Conti et al., 2012). Recent studies are also suggesting that cardiopulmonary and cardiovascular dysfunction negatively impact cognition in SLE patients (Katz et al., 2012; Kozora, Swigris, et al., 2013). In a pilot study, we reported that SLE patients had worse lung function compared to controls, and that measures of lung function are associated with poor cognition (Kozora, Swigris, et al., 2013).

Some studies have also compared cognition in active and inactive SLE disease states. All of the studies to date indicate a relatively high prevalence of cognitive impairment even in the absence of active disease. Cognitive impairment was noted in 53% of SLE patients without active disease in one study (Carbotte et al., 1995), and measures of global cognitive impairment were not associated with measures of SLE disease activity. Glanz et al. (1997) studied 58 inactive SLE patients, classifying 43% as cognitively impaired. Gladman et al. (2000) reported that 43% of their inactive SLE patients had cognitive impairment; however, based on history, those patients with previously high disease activity or with vasculitis tended to have greater cognitive impairment. There was no relationship between specific organ involvement and cognitive status. Although the majority of studies reporting on disease severity and cognition are negative (Kozora, 2008; Kozora et al., 1996), there is some evidence that aspects of SLE disease activity, organ damage, and related physical impairments may mediate cognitive dysfunction.

MEDICATION USE

The use of prednisone, a mainstay of SLE treatment, has not consistently emerged as an independent factor impacting cognition in SLE (Carbotte et al., 1986; Carlomagno et al., 2000; Denburg et al., 1987; Denburg, Carbotte, & Denburg, 1994; Emori et al., 2005; Fisk et al., 1993; Ginsburg et al., 1992; Gladman et al., 2000; Glanz et al., 1997; Hay et al., 1992; Holliday et al., 2000; Koffler, 1987; Kozora et al., 2008; Kozora, Ellison, et al., 2006; Kozora, Erkan, et al., 2013; Kozora et al., 1996; Maneeton et al., 2010; Monastero et al., 2001; Norwicka-Sauer et al., 2011; Peretti et al., 2012; Waterloo et al., 2001). Few studies have included analyses regarding other medications. Carlomagno et al. (2000) found no relationship between nonsteroidal anti-inflammatory therapy and cognitive impairment, and Waterloo et al. (2001) found no difference in cognitively impaired and nonimpaired SLE patients in terms of the type, presence, or duration of medications. Studies documenting a relationship between cognitive dysfunction and prednisone use in SLE are rare. Ferstl et al. (1992) investigated a small sample of SLE patients, corticosteroid-only patients, and controls. Results in this study suggested that nonverbal memory in SLE may be related to both SLE disease activity and corticosteroid use. Hanly et al. (1992) reported that a higher proportion of SLE patients with cognitive impairment were on prednisone, but did not find a difference in the mean dosage of prednisone between these two groups. Another study reported a relationship between prednisone use and decline in immediate memory and reaction time (Brey et al., 2002). No relationship between cognition and medication has been found longitudinally (Carlomagno et al., 2000; Hanly et al., 1997; Hay et al., 1994; Waterloo et al., 2002). Although group studies do not suggest strong associations between treatment medications in SLE and cognitive impairment, individual SLE patients may often have unique factors impacting cognition that should be considered in a clinical setting.

Autoantibodies

Autoantibody-mediated neuronal injury is thought to be the primary mechanism for some NP syndromes in SLE, including cognitive dysfunction. Autoantibodies are found in serum, CSF (Bluestein, Williams, & Steinberg, 1981), and neural tissue from patients who have died from the disease (Zvaifler & Bluestein, 1982). Autoantibodies associated with general NP activity in SLE to date include antineuronal antibodies, brain cross-reactive lymphocytotoxic antibodies, antibodies to N-methyl-D-aspartate (anti-NMDA) receptors, aPL including lupus anticoagulant (LAC) and anticardiolipin (aCL), antibodies to Anti-β2-glycoprotein-I antibody (aβ2GPI), and antibodies to anti-ribosomal P. Some studies have investigated the relationship between these particular autoantibodies and cognitive functioning.

ANTINEURONAL ANTIBODIES

The relationship between antineuronal antibodies and cognitive dysfunction in SLE has not been strong. Initially, Denburg et al. (1987) reported a relationship between cognition and IgG antineuronal antibody in 97 SLE patients. They found that 84% of the antibody-positive SLE patients were cognitively impaired. Despite the higher incidence of antineuronal antibody in cognitively impaired patients, the finding was not very specific given the high level of impairment (67%) in the antibody negative group. No other studies have reported such an association. Hanly et al. (1993) found that in 70 unselected SLE patients, 34% had elevated antineuronal antibodies; however, there was no difference between the cognitively impaired or unimpaired patients. In another study, antineuronal antibodies were not different between cognitively impaired and unimpaired SLE patients (Sailer et al., 1997). Studies have also examined lymphocytotoxic antibody activity in SLE. Denburg, Carbotte, Long, and Denburg (1988) and Long, Denburg, Carbotte, Singal, and Denburg (1990) studied 98 unselected SLE patients, and reported that 74% of the lymphocytotoxic positive patients and only 48% of the lymphocytotoxic negative SLE patients were cognitively impaired. They further suggested that patterns of visuospatial and cognitive flexibility deficits are associated with elevations of this autoantibody. Interestingly, the SLE patients with a history or presence of NPSLE were not different than the non-NPSLE patients with regard to lymphocytotoxic activity. Hanly et al. (1993) reported elevated lymphocytotoxic antibodies in 47% of their entire SLE group, but found no antibody differences between the cognitively impaired and unimpaired SLE patients.

N-METHYL-D-ASPARTATE (NMDA) RECEPTOR ANTIBODIES

The NMDA receptor is a subtype of glutamate receptor. Antibodies against the NMDA receptor are a subset of pathogenic anti–double stranded DNA (anti-dsDNA) antibodies that cross-react with a consensus peptide sequence of the extracellular, ligand-binding domain of the NMDA receptors NR2a and NR2b (anti-NR2) (DeGiorgio et al., 2001). The NR2 receptors are expressed on neurons in the hippocampus and neocortex, and they bind the neurotransmitter glutamate. These receptors have been postulated to be important in mechanisms underlying learning and memory (Lipton & Rosenberg, 1994). Anti-NR2 antibodies have been demonstrated in the serum and CSF of SLE patients (Rhiannon, 2008). In mouse models, these antibodies can gain access to the CSF through a compromised blood-brain barrier (BBB), after which they can bind to hippocampal neurons, alter hippocampal metabolism, or cause excitotoxic neuronal death by excessive calcium entry into cells, and impair memory and learning (Kowal, DeGiorgio, Nakaoka, Diamond, & Volpe, 2004). Studies to date have not consistently reported a relationship between cognitive functions and the presence of serum markers of anti-NR2 in SLE (Hanly, Robichaud, & Fisk, 2006; Harrison, Ravdin, Volpe, Diamond, & Lockshin, 2004; Kozora et al., 2010; Lapteva, 2004). In one study, poor performance on measures of immediate visual memory, fine motor function, and psychological functioning was associated with elevated levels of anti-NR2 in 57 SLE patients (Omdal et al., 2005), but only two of the 20 cognitive tests showed an association, and all of the tests were within normal limits. Harrison et al. (2004) reported that 25.8% of 93 SLE patients had positive anti-NR2 antibodies; however, no relationship between antibody positivity and cognitive dysfunction, depression, or anxiety was found. Lapteva, Nowak, et al. (2006) reported that 26.6% of 60 SLE patients demonstrated the presence of anti-NR2; no relationship with global or individual cognitive test performance was reported, but a relationship with increased depression levels was found. Hanly et al. (2006) reported that 35% of 65 women with SLE had anti-NR2 antibodies, but they were not associated with cognitive performance at baseline or approximately five years later. These authors also showed that persistence of anti-NR2 antibodies was not related to the development of NP events. Steup-Beekman, Steens, van Buchem, and Huizinga (2007) found no relationship between cognition and NMDA metabolism in SLE. Our group found that the frequency of elevated anti-NR2 was low in 43 non-NPSLE patients (14%), and not significantly different from controls (Kozora et al., 2010). In addition, there was no relationship between the presence of anti-NR2 in serum and global cognitive or memory indices or with level of depression. Taken together, these studies indicate that serum anti-NR2 is not likely related to cognition in non-NPSLE patients. The absence of a relationship between anti-NR2 and cognitive dysfunction suggests that NMDA antibody activity measured in serum is not a fruitful approach to understanding mechanisms of cognitive dysfunction in SLE. Antibody measurement in the CSF, however, may be more productive. A recent study suggested that elevated CSF anti-NR2 was associated with diffuse NP activity in SLE (Arinuma, Yanagida, & Hirohata, 2008); 12.5 % of these patients had cognitive dysfunction. Another study reported a stronger association between NP events and CSF autoantibodies than circulating anti-NR2 (Yoshio, Onda, Nara, & Minota, 2006). In earlier animal models, breakdown of the BBB was necessary for antibodies against the NMDA receptor to alter hippocampal metabolism, cause neuronal death, and produce cognitive dysfunction (Kowal et al., 2004). Continued studies of anti-NR2 and cognitive dysfunction in SLE are warranted using CSF samples to explore compromise of the BBB in more detail.

ANTIPHOSPHOLIPID ANTIBODIES (APL)

Antiphospholipid antibodies including LAC, aCL, and aβ2GPI are common in patients with SLE, and appear to correlate with microvascular thrombosis and other neurologic events (Asherson et al., 1989; Leaven & Welch, 1987). Antiphospholipid antibodies including LAC and aCL are frequently identified as the cause of neurological syndromes such as stroke, seizures, confusional states, and migraine (Gorman & Cummings, 1993). Initial estimates suggested that 30%–40% of SLE patients had positive aPL (Love & Santoro, 1990a), but in a recent multisite study, percentages of aPL were lower with 13.4% for aCL, 15.2% aβ2GPI, and 21.9% LAC (Hanly et al., 2011). In a study of 323 consecutive SLE patients, 39.3% were classified as having aPL, and aPL was significantly higher in SLE patients with overt NP activity (Sanna et al., 2003). Multiple studies have found an association between aPL and cognition in SLE patients, both with and without NP activity (Denburg, Carbotte, Ginsberg, et al., 1997; Hanly, Hong, Smith, & Fisk, 1999; Leritz, Brandt, Minor, Reis-Jensen, & Petri, 2002; Menon et al., 1999; Tomietto et al., 2007). The presence of aPL (via LAC, aCL and aβ2GPI) has been associated with greater impairment in memory, visuomotor speed, and visuoconstruction/visuospatial functions in SLE patients.

A majority of the SLE studies have used LAC and aCL, or both, as markers of aPL. Denburg, Carbotte, Ginsberg, et al. (1997) reported that the 39 LAC-positive SLE patients were two to three times more likely than the 79 LAC-negative group to be defined as cognitively impaired. Further analysis indicated significant differences between these two groups on measures of verbal learning and psychomotor speed. These investigators (Denburg, Carbotte, & Denburg, 1993) also investigated SLE patients who were consistently positive for LAC (over three time periods) and reported that these patients had greater cognitive dysfunction than the patients who were persistently negative, a finding likely related to microvascular thrombosis in the LAC positive group. Sanna et al. (2003) more recently reported that aPL, particularly LAC, was statistically more frequent (15.7%) in SLE patients classified as having a cognitive disorder compared to those who were not (7.6%). Some studies of antiphospholipid activity using the aCL marker have not found a relationship with cognitive dysfunction in SLE (Hanly et al., 2011; Sailer et al., 1997; Waterloo et al., 1999; Waterloo et al., 2001; Sanna et al., 2003). Hanly et al. (1993) reported decreased recognition performance on a verbal memory task in patients with positive aCL, and also reported that patients with persistently elevated IgG aCL had a significant decline in psychomotor speed, and persistently elevated IgA aCL was related to decline in conceptual reasoning and executive ability (Hanly et al., 1999). Menon et al. (1999) studied 45 unselected SLE patients at baseline and at 12–18 month follow-up. The patients who had consistently elevated IgG aCLs over time performed worse on neuropsychological testing. Tomietto et al. (2007), identified a relationship between aPL positivity and impairment in complex attention and executive function over a three-month period. The longitudinal relationship between persistently elevated aCL antibodies and cognitive dysfunction in SLE (Hanly et al., 1999; Menon et al., 1999) indicates the importance of longitudinal designs in exploring the role of aPLs in cognitive dysfunction. More recently, McLaurin et al. (2005) indicated that in 123 patients studied every four months for three years, declining cognitive function was related to the presence of consistently positive aPL. Some studies have not found associations between aPL and cognition in SLE. In our study of 64 non-NPSLE, we reported higher LAC, aCL, and aβ2GPI, but compared to controls these were not significantly different (Kozora et al., 2012). We did not find significant correlations between the aPL measures and a global cognitive score, nor were there differences between cognitively impaired and unimpaired SLE on levels of aPL. This finding is consistent with some prior studies (Carlomagno et al., 2000; Emori et al., 2005; Hanly et al., 1993; Sailer et al., 1997; Waterloo et al., 2001). A minority of SLE patients demonstrated elevated aCL-IgM (5.56%), elevated activated partial thromboplastin time (APTT; 6.56%). These frequencies were relatively low compared to other SLE studies, and may be explained by subject selection (i.e., patients without overt NP activity).

ANTI-RIBOSOMAL P

Several studies have shown that SLE patients with major NP syndromes (i.e., major depression and psychosis) have had elevated serum levels of autoantibodies to ribosomal P proteins (Bonfa et al., 1987; Schneebaum et al., 1991). In a study of 1,047 SLE patients, 9.2% had anti-ribosomal P antibodies, and their presence at baseline was associated with subsequent psychosis (Hanly et al., 2011). Although the question has not extensively investigated, antiribosomal P does not appear to be strongly associated with cognitive impairment in SLE. Hanly et al. (1993) reported the presence of antiribosomal P antibodies in only 17% of SLE patients, and found no difference in the presence of antiribosomal P in cognitively impaired and unimpaired groups. In our prior study, 28% of the SLE patients had elevated antiribosomal P (Kozora et al., 1996), but there were no associations with cognitive dysfunction, or other measures such as psychological functioning and disease activity. Finally, antiribosomal P was not found to be a significant predictor variable along with other demographic and health factors in a model attempting to predict cognitive speed and efficiency in SLE (Holliday et al., 2000).

Mediators of Inflammation

There has been growing evidence that neural, endocrine, and immune cells share common communication molecules and receptors, and are functionally linked to form a brain–endocrine immune axis that integrates physiological responses (DeSouza, 1993; Maier & Watkins, 1998). Studies evaluating inflammation via cytokine activity and other inflammatory measures in SLE suggest they are likely mediators of cognitive dysfunction.

CYTOKINES

Proinflammatory cytokines are elevated in acute anti-inflammatory responses in both animal models and in studies of SLE and RA (al-Janadi, al-Balla, al-Dalaan, & Raziuddin, 1993; Elliott & Maini, 1995; Linker-Israeli et al., 1991; Singh, 1992). Patients with active NPSLE have demonstrated elevations of IL-1, IL-6, IFN-α, and tumor necrosis factor (TNF) in the CSF (Alcocer-Varela, Aleman-Hoey, & Alarcon-Segovia, 1992; Benveniste, 1992; Dellalibera-Joviliano, Dos Reis, Cunha Fde, & Donadi, 2003; Hirohata & Miyamoto, 1990; Shiozawa, Kuroki, Kim, Hirohata, & Ogino, 1992; Tsai et al., 1994; Yeh et al., 1994). Few studies have explored cytokine activity (serum or CSF) in relation to neuropsychological functioning in SLE. Our group did not find that serum IL-6 differed in an early study of 15 non-NPSLE, 15 RA, and 15 healthy control subjects (Kozora, Laudenslager, Lemieux, & West, 2001); however, we did report that IL-6 contributed uniquely to measures of learning beyond the effects of depression, prednisone therapy, and hormonal measures. These findings also suggested that the relationship between IL-6 production and cognitive functioning might be quadratic (as an inverted U-shaped function) whereby moderate levels facilitate, but very low and very high levels disrupt learning capacity. Inflammation measured with c-reactive protein (CRP) was associated with deficits in information processing in SLE patients (Shucard, Gaines, Ambrus, & Shucard, 2007), In a more recent study, IFN-alpha and IL-6 were elevated in 64 non-NPSLE patients compared to controls and lower IFN-alpha was related to a variety of global cognitive scores, memory scores, and individual tests of visuomotor speed and attention (Kozora et al., 2012). These findings were unexpected, as higher IFN-alpha has been associated with NPSLE activity in CSF (Okamoto, Kobayashi, & Yamanaka, 2010), and with other medical disorders such as hepatitis C. IFN-alpha treatment has resulted in cognitive decline (Perry, Hilsabeck, & Hassanein, 2008). Given the relatively weak correlations, our findings remain unremarkable, although they might suggest that peripheral IFN-alpha may act to suppress disease activity in the SLE brain. In contrast to our expectation, elevated IL-6 was not related to a majority of the cognitive summary scores or individual tests in this study. This finding differs from our initial study (Kozora et al., 1998), yet there were no apparent differences in demographics or health characteristics between the subjects included in our current and prior SLE cohorts.

MATRIX METALLOPROTEINASES

Other potentially important inflammatory mediators are matrix metalloproteinases (MMPs), a family of endoperoxidases that degrade extracellular matrix components (Lijnen, 2001). MMP-9 plays a key role in the disruption of the BBB, while its natural inhibitor—tissue inhibitor matrix metalloproteinase-1 (TIMP-1)—is important for stabilizing the BBB. Patients with NPSLE, especially those with cognitive impairment, have elevated levels of MMP-9 in serum (Ainiala et al., 2004), and CSF (Trysberg, Blennow, Zachrisson, & Tarkowski, 2004). The correlation between CSF MMP-9 levels, proinflammatory cytokines, and biomarkers of neuronal and glial degradation in SLE patients (Trysberg et al., 2004) suggests that enhanced production of MMP-9 is linked to CNS damage in SLE and is a likely mediator of cognitive dysfunction in this population.

SERUM VERSUS. CSF STUDIES

Some controversy exists regarding the analysis of serum versus CSF cytokines, and it is possible that reliance on serum cytokine levels explains, at least in part, the relatively limited findings of inflammation related to cognition in SLE studies to date. Trysberg, Carlsten, and Tarkowski (2000) reported that serum IL-6 did not differ between SLE patients with and without NP syndromes, but observed that 86% of the SLE patients with NPSLE demonstrated intrathecal elevations of IL-6. Based on this observation, they suggested that primary systemic production of cytokines with subsequent passage to CSF is not the most likely mechanism by which these cytokines exert their adverse effects on the CNS. As discussed earlier if serum analysis is not useful for understanding the immunopathogenesis of cognitive dysfunction in SLE, it may be more useful to examine the CSF, which will enable assessment of BBB integrity as well as the measurement of intrathecal immune activity including autoantibodies and a variety of soluble cytokines, chemokines, and MMPs. Direct CSF examination may enable more focused investigation or the cascade of molecular changes in the brain that influence cognitive dysfunction in SLE. Several proinflammatory cytokines and chemokines have been detected in the CSF of patients with active NPSLE (Lu et al., 2010; Okamoto et al., 2010), and it is possible that autoantibodies cross a dysfunctional BBB, or are produced intrathecally, to interact with their cognate neuronal antigen and form immune complexes in the CSF. Recent studies have shown that CSF immune complexes can induce CNS microglial cells to produce IFN-α, IL-6, IL-8, and MCP-1 (Santer, Yoshio, Minota, Moller, & Elkon, 2009). IFN-α can cause cognitive difficulties, and can also feed back to further facilitate production of many cytokines and chemokines. IL-8 and MCP-1 can chemoattract immune cells into the CNS that may contribute to intrathecal autoantibody production. There is evidence that IL-6 and IL-8 can upregulate MMP-9 production by resident cells within the CNS. MMP-9 can then contribute to further disruption of the BBB, allowing more influx of autoantibodies into the CSF as well as causing myelin destruction (Trysberg et al., 2004).

Neuropeptide and Hormonal Factors

Dehydroepiandrosterone (DHEA) is the most abundant adrenal steroid hormone in humans, and may relate to cognitive dysfunction in SLE. Interactions of DHEA with the nervous system have been associated with cognitive functions in both animals and human studies (Flood, Morley, & Roberts, 1992; Flood & Roberts, 1988; Melchior & Ritzmann, 1996). Lower DHEA levels have been reported in humans with memory problems (Leblhuber et al., 1993; Nasman et al., 1991) and SLE patients have been found to have lower levels of DHEA (Suzuki, Suzuki, Engleman, Mizushima, & Sakane, 1995). DHEA and DHEA-sulfate were found to be significantly lower in non-NPSLE and RA patients compared to control subjects and lower DHEA-S was related to lowered attention and concentration (Kozora, West, Forrest, & Young, 2001). As noted earlier, several neuropeptides have been linked to behavioral and cognitive changes in animal and human studies, and the role of vasopressin in cognition has been studied extensively (Bennett, Ballard, Watson, & Fone, 1997; Frank & Landgraf, 2008; Ring, 2005). Lapteva, Yarboro, et al. (2006) reported higher serum concentrations of calcitonin gene-related peptide and a trend toward higher concentrations of serum vasopressin in 27 cognitively impaired SLE patients (based on standardized neuropsychological testing) compared to 19 nonimpaired SLE patients. In contrast, oxytocin, vasoactive intestinal peptide, and neuropeptide Y did not differ across their groups. No additional studies have confirmed or disputed the role of hormonal changes or neuropeptides in cognitive dysfunction in SLE, but future studies would be useful in expanding a list of potential mechanistic features of MCD-SLE.

Behavioral Mechanisms

PSYCHOLOGICAL FACTORS

Overall, psychological distress has been found to be elevated in patients with SLE compared to other autoimmune patients and healthy controls (Bluestein, 1992; Carbotte et al., 1986; Denburg et al., 1987a; Giang, 1991; Gladman et al., 2000; Koffler, 1987; Kozora, Ellison, et al., 2006; Kozora et al., 1996; Liang et al., 1984; Liang, Socher, Larson, & Schur, 1989; Monastero et al., 2001; Rummelt et al., 1991; Sabbadini et al., 1999; Sonies et al., 1982; Wekking, Nossent, et al., 1991; West, 1994; West et al., 1995). Several studies further demonstrated that SLE patients with overt NP disorders have stronger associations between psychological distress and cognitive functions (Denburg et al., 1987; Hay et al., 1992; Hay et al., 1994; Kozora, Ellison, et al., 2006; Monastero et al., 2001; Wekking, Nossent, et al., 1991). NPSLE patients with psychiatric histories have been found impaired on motor speed and attention and verbal learning (Sonies et al., 1982), and cognitively impaired SLE patients with psychiatric distress showed greater impairment in short-term retention and verbal fluency when compared to cognitively impaired SLE patients without psychiatric distress (Denburg et al., 1987). In a prospective study, improvement in cognitive abilities paralleled improvement in psychological status, Hay et al. (1994) reported that, at baseline, 26% of their SLE patients had cognitive impairment, whereas two years later, impairment was present in only 17%. Eight-ninths of the non-NPSLE were not impaired at follow-up, a change that mirrored their improvement in psychological status (Glanz et al., 1997).

In contrast, several studies of SLE patients with NPSLE have found no relationship between psychiatric histories, overall psychological function, and cognitive status (Carbotte et al., 1986; Carlomagno et al., 2000; Maneeton et al., 2010; Sailer et al., 1997). Furthermore, SLE patients with inactive disease show little relationship between cognitive and psychological status (Gladman et al., 2000). In most studies with non-NPSLE patients, cognitive deficits have not been related to psychological distress (Carbotte et al., 1986; Denburg et al., 1987; Kozora et al., 2008; Kozora, Ellison, et al., 2006; Rummelt et al., 1991). In a prior study, we did not find our cognitively impaired non-NPSLE patients to have greater psychological distress on any of the six selected scales of the MMPI. However, we found a moderate correlation between a summary cognitive t-score (mean t-score for all eight domains) and the summary psychological t-score (mean of six MMPI-T scores). These correlational findings suggest that a relationship between psychological distress and global cognitive functions might exist even in non-NPSLE patients who have been screened for major psychiatric disorders.

Depression and anxiety as measured by standardized questionnaires of mood and personality are frequently found to be elevated in SLE patients. For example, in our first study, 42% of the non-NPSLE group had psychological distress when six select MMPI-2 scales were analyzed (Kozora et al., 1996), with specific scales indicating higher depression, anxiety, and confused thinking. Depression has been the most frequently documented psychiatric problem in patients with SLE (Giang, 1991; Iverson, 1995, 2002; Iverson & Anderson, 1994; Kozora et al., 1996; Wekking, 1993). Standard questionnaire measures of depression have been related to cognitive dysfunction in SLE (Brey et al., 2002; Holliday et al., 2000; Monastero et al., 2001; Rummelt et al., 1991) but not in others (Denburg et al., 1987; Glanz et al., 2005; Glanz et al., 1997; Kozora, Arciniegas, et al., 2006; Loukkola et al., 2003; Sailer et al., 1997; Vogel et al., 2011). As there is evidence that "depressive" symptoms likely impact cognitive abilities in psychiatric populations (King & Caine, 1996), studies that examine the similarities and differences in cognitive deficits between depressed outpatients and depressed SLE patients may yield important information. Denburg and Denburg (1999) reported that eight depressed SLE patients were more impaired than eight depressed outpatients in tests of verbal fluency, sustained mental effort, verbal and nonverbal fluency, and visuospatial planning. In a larger study on depression in SLE, significant differences between patient self-report using standardized questionnaires, physician ratings, of depression and results of structured psychiatric interviews were noted, suggesting methods may impact findings (Kozora, Arciniegas, et al., 2006; Kozora et al., 2001). Continued studies in this area are necessary to better understand the underlying processes of depression and its relationship to NP and cognitive changes.

FATIGUE AND PAIN

Fatigue and pain have been suggested as mechanisms that may impact cognitive functions in SLE; however, few studies have been published. Fatigue and pain are commonly reported in patients with SLE (Bauman, Barnes, & Schrieber, 1989; Hall & Stickney, 1983; Liang et al., 1984; Middleton, McFarlin, & Lipsky, 1994; Schur, 1989; Taylor et al., 2000; Wysenbeek, Leibovici, Weinberger, & Guedj, 1993), and have been associated with self-report of cognitive problems (Alarcon et al., 2002). Fatigue has been described as the most chronic and debilitating symptom that SLE patients experience (Krupp, LaRocca, Muir, & Steinberg, 1990; Krupp, LaRocca, Muir-Nash, & Steinberg, 1989; Liang et al., 1984; Robb-Nicholson et al., 1989; Schur, 1989), and self-reported fatigue in SLE patients is extremely common, ranging from 46% to 100%. In one of our early pilot studies, declines in sustained attention were strongly associated independently with fatigue and depression in SLE patients (Kozora et al., 2001). In later research (Kozora, Ellison, et al., 2006) we reported a relationship between fatigue and cognitive dysfunction in SLE patients with overt NP manifestations. We have found higher levels of fatigue in SLE patients with and without NPSLE compared to controls using the Fatigue Severity Scale (Krupp et al., 1989), with more than 92% of the SLE patients reporting fatigue. However, only the NPSLE group demonstrated significant correlations between fatigue and measures of verbal learning and verbal recall, immediate and delayed recall of nonverbal material, and complex visuomotor functions. In addition, findings suggested that only the NPSLE group had significant associations between an overall cognitive index and measures of fatigue, pain, and depression. These preliminary findings might suggest that fatigue is related to aspects of cognitive dysfunction in SLE.

Pain has often been reported in SLE patients (Kewman, Vaishampayan, Zald, & Han, 1991) and there is some evidence that pain may reduce overall cognitive efficiency (Grigsby, Rosenberg, & Busenvark, 1994; Schwartz, Barth, & Done, 1987). Relatively few data regarding this relationship are available and sample sizes are small. One of the first studies indicated that in ten SLE patients, pain was associated with cognitive deficits (Denburg, Carbotte, & Denburg, 1997). In our 2004 study, both the group of 29 NPSLE and that with 31 non-NPSLE patients had higher rates of pain on the McGill Pain Severity Scale (Melzak, 1975) compared to controls. Only the NPSLE patients, however, showed a significant correlation between higher self-reported pain and overall cognitive dysfunction. Notably, few studies include measures of pain and fatigue in studies of cognition despite the early positive relationship in SLE. As noted earlier, complex relationships between depression, pain and fatigue likely exist.

SLEEP

Preliminary studies indicate that more than 50% of SLE patients have sleep problems (Chandrasekhara, Jayachandran, Rajasekhar, Thomas, & Narsimulu, 2009; Greenwood, Lederman, & Lindner, 2008; Liang et al., 1984; McKinley, Ouellette, & Winkel, 1995; Palagini et al., 2014; Robb-Nicholson et al., 1989; Tench et al., 2002; Tench, McCurdie, White, & D'Cruz, 2000) that are likely to be related to cognitive dysfunction (Kozora, Zell, Swigris, Duggan, & Make, 2012). Valencia-Flores et al. (1999) reported respiratory and sleep-related movement disorders in 36% of 14 patients using polysomnography (PSG). These sleep disorders also resulted in greater daytime sleepiness. Disease activity was associated with decreases in sleep efficiency and delta sleep, and increases in sleep fragmentation. In a larger study, Laboni, Ibanez, Gladman, Urowitz, and Moldofsky (2006) studied 35 SLE patients complaining of overwhelming tiredness compared to 17 healthy controls. Results indicated that 26% had obstructive sleep apnea (OSA). Compared to controls, SLE patients had significantly impaired sleep efficiency, high arousal frequencies, increased Stage 1 sleep, decreased slow wave sleep and non-REM sleep, and excessive daytime sleepiness. There are a number of other studies in patients with OSA in which cognitive dysfunction, specifically aspects of attention and executive function, have been reported (Felver-Gant et al., 2007; Greenberg, Watson, & Deptula, 1987; Naegele et al., 1995). While sleep disorders are quite common in SLE, they have rarely been studied in relation to objective neuropsychological data. We have some pilot data suggesting a relationship between sleep problems (and sleep apnea) and cognitive dysfunction in SLE (Kozora et al., 2012) and continued assessment may expand our assessment and treatment options.

OBESITY AND EXERCISE ENDURANCE

Additional factors associated with cognition in general, such as obesity and exercise capacity, may be related to cognitive dysfunction in SLE. In one study of 138 SLE patients, self-reported physical inactivity and obesity were associated with decline in cognition, specifically executive functioning (Katz et al., 2012). A recent study of 34 female SLE patients with relatively mild disease activity and no overt NP activity found lower levels of physical activity lower exercise capacity than matched healthy controls (Kozora, Swigris, et al., 2013). Among SLE subjects, there was a moderate association between a physical measure of exercise endurance (six-minute walk test) and cognition. Prior research suggested self-reported physical inactivity in SLE patients may negatively impact cognition, but ours are the first data documenting a relationship between objective measures of physical activity and cognitive dysfunction in this population.

Treatment of Cognitive Dysfunction

Data are limited regarding the treatment of cognitive dysfunction in SLE. Few studies of pharmacologic therapy for SLE-associated cognitive dysfunction have been published. In one study (Denburg et al., 1994) the authors reported improved cognition in five of eight subjects who completed a trial of 0.5-mg/kg prednisone daily. It is not clear whether this beneficial effect was maintained when the corticosteroid was tapered and discontinued. An interesting volumetric MRI study of SLE patients, however, showed that those who received immunosuppressive medications had greater brain white matter (WM) volume than controls, implying a protective effect of standard SLE treatment on WM (Xu et al., 2010). Although there are no clinical trial data to support use of antiplatelet or anticoagulant therapy for cognitive dysfunction in SLE, patients with aPL but without thromboembolic phenomena were found in a longitudinal observational study to have better cognitive performance if they took regular aspirin than if they did not (McLaurin et al., 2005). Agents developed for the treatment of cognitive dysfunction in Alzheimer's disease (AD) (i.e., cholinesterase inhibitors, memantine) and attention deficit disorder (i.e., methylphenidate) are sometimes used, but the lack of trial data and biologic plausibility for such approaches in SLE are problematic. Memantine, a noncompetitive inhibitor of glutamate at the NMDA receptor, does have a more solid rationale in SLE patients, at least those with anti-NR2 antibodies. However, a randomized, double-blind placebo-controlled trial of memantine in 51 SLE patients, using the ANAM computerized battery and an extensive battery of tests recommended by the ACR, found no differences between the groups on the ANAM and a significant improvement on only one ACR test result (verbal fluency), suggesting that memantine produces no significant cognitive improvement in SLE (Petri, Nagibuddin, Asmpedro, Omdal, & Carson, 2011).

Cognitive rehabilitation, which involves intensive retraining of cognitive skills, is an alternative or complementary therapeutic approach. Rehabilitation programs in other conditions (stroke, dementia, traumatic brain injury, MS) teach patients with cognitive dysfunction the means by which they may adapt to their impairments and maintain, if not regain, some level of independence. A novel psychoeducational group intervention targeted specifically at SLE patients with self-perceived cognitive dysfunction (Harrison et al., 2005) demonstrated that participation may result in improvement in memory self-efficacy, memory function, and ability to perform daily activities that require cognitive function. Further study is needed before these kinds of intervention can be recommended.

Neuroimaging

Based on a variety of neuroimaging techniques, damage to both WM and gray matter (GM) of the brain occurs in SLE, and each kind of injury may underlie specific cognitive problems in this population (Appenzeller, Carnevalle, Li, Costallat, & Cendes, 2006; Kozora & Filley, 2011). A summary of neuroimaging abnormalities in SLE will be followed by a review of neuroimaging correlates of cognitive dysfunction in this population.

Neuroimaging Abnormalities

MAGNETIC RESONANCE IMAGING

MRI has largely replaced its predecessor—computed tomography (CT)—and has been the most extensively studied brain imaging modality in SLE. MRI elegantly reveals a wide range of findings in SLE, including WM hyperintensities (WMHI), infarcts, and hemorrhages in either WM or GM, and cerebral atrophy, both in those with and those without NP presentations (Aisen, Gabrielsen, & McCune, 1985; Davie et al., 1995; Fields, Sibbitt, Toubbeh, & Bankhurst, 1990; Ishikawa, Ohnishi, Miyachi, & Ishizaka, 1994; Kozora & Filley, 2011; Kozora & Make, 1998). Whereas not all studies report MRI differences between SLE with and without NP activity (Haider, Zakarya, & Abu-Hegazy, 2012), NPSLE typically involves more florid MRI abnormalities. An important clue to the understanding of cognitive disorders in SLE is that the most common MRI abnormality in NPSLE is the presence of scattered hemispheric WMHIs (Castellino et al., 2008; Graham & Jan, 2003; Karassa et al., 2000; Sailer et al., 1997; Sanna et al., 2003; Sibbitt, Sibbitt, & Brooks, 1999; Toledano, Sarbu, Espinosa, Bargallo, & Cervera, 2013). In several well-designed studies with clearly defined characterizations of NP activity in adult SLE, the number of WMHI has been significantly higher in those patients with overt NP compared to those without (Ainiala et al., 2004; Appenzeller, Pike, & Clarke, 2008; Handa et al., 2003; Zivadinov et al., 2013). NPSLE patients with focal syndromes such as stroke and seizures are of course more likely to have destructive WM lesions, GM lesions, or both (McCune, MacGuire, Aisen, & Gebarski, 1988; Sewell, Livneh, Aranow, & Grayzel, 1989; Stimmler, Coletti, & Quismorio, 1993; West et al., 1995). Even in non-NPSLE, WMHIs occurred in 16% of patients using clinical classification (Jarek, West, Baker, & Rak, 1994), and in up to 35% using quantitative techniques (Kozora & Make, 1998). In other studies, WMHI have been documented in 35%–50% of well-defined SLE patients without overt NP; but data on control subjects were not presented (Abreu et al., 2005; Appenzeller, Vasconcelos Faria, Li, Costallat, & Cendes, 2008). Importantly, however, not all studies have demonstrated MRI abnormalities in SLE patients without NP activity. Using a 3.0T MRI scanner, no differences were noted in total WM or GM volumes, or number and volume of WM lesions in well-defined non-NPSLE patients (Filley, 2009). This study suggested that MRI might not be sensitive to early microstructural WM disease in SLE, and set the stage for more detailed neurometabolic studies whereby the normal-appearing WM (NAWM) could be examined.

The MRI lesions of SLE have a variable course, with some being reversible and others irreversible (Sibbitt, Sibbitt, Griffey, Eckel, & Bankhurst, 1989). This variability reflects the complex nature of SLE, and many additional factors such as treatment effects. Some longitudinal studies in SLE have suggested resolution of WM lesions with high-dose corticosteroid therapy (Aisen et al., 1985; Bell et al., 1991; McCune et al., 1988; Sibbitt et al., 1989), but others have not (Griffey, Brown, Bankhurst, Sibbitt, & Sibbitt, 1990; Stimmler et al., 1993). Gonzalez-Crespo et al. (1995) reported MRI changes over three years in NPSLE, and some, but not all, of the WM lesions disappeared. In another MRI study (Chinn et al., 1997), 32% of SLE patients demonstrated increased atrophy over time, and abnormal MRI findings were more common in patients with a history of CNS events. Some studies have found stable MRI abnormalities over time (Appenzeller, Li, Costallat, & Cendes, 2005; Mortilla, Ermini, Nistri, Dal Pozzo, & Falcini, 2003) while other studies show increase MRI abnormalities. For example, Jennings, Sundgren, Attwood, McCune, and Maly (2004) reported that among 26 NPSLE patients followed for up to five years, eight of these patients had progression of abnormalities, three showed regression, and 15 had no change. Appenzeller et al. (2006) reported hippocampal atrophy in SLE patients at baseline, and after 19 months this volume loss has progressed significantly (43.9% at baseline and 66.7% at follow up); the hippocampal atrophy was associated with cumulative corticosteroid dose and number of CNS manifestations.

MAGNETIC RESONANCE SPECTROSCOPY

Magnetic resonance spectroscopy (MRS) is a neuroimaging technique that identifies and quantifies chemicals in living tissue. Creatine (Cr) is a storage form of high-energy phosphates and is used as a reference marker. N-acetyl aspartate (NAA) is produced by neurons and is a marker of neuronal health; levels decrease markedly with brain insult and axonal loss. Choline (Ch) is a precursor to acetylcholine, an essential chemical for neuronal membrane integrity and synaptic transmission. Elevated Ch/Cr is associated with increased cell production (as occurs with brain tumors), and with increased membrane turnover related to inflammation, demyelination, ischemia, and gliosis. Most SLE studies have focused on NAA/Cr and Ch/Cr in an effort to assess neuronal and myelin integrity. A detailed review of MRS studies of Ch/Cr findings in SLE patients can be found in a recent review (Kozora & Filley, 2011). The studies considered generally reported decreased NAA and increased Ch/Cr in both the NAWM and abnormal-appearing WM (AAWM). The studies differed, however, in their methods, including variation in subject selection, sample size, and neuroimaging techniques. Higher Ch/Cr in SLE is postulated to be more likely due to inflammatory myelinopathy than ischemia or gliosis at this early disease stage (Filley et al., 2009). Studies with carefully characterized non-NPSLE patients suggest that increased Ch/Cr can occur without, and perhaps prior to, lowered NAA/Cr (Appenzeller, Li, Costallat, & Cendes, 2007; Filley et al., 2009; Sundgren et al., 2005). MRS studies have also documented NAA/Cr and Ch/Cr abnormalities before MRI discloses WMHI (Appenzeller, Bonilha, et al., 2007; Castellino et al., 2005) Castellino et al. (2005) found that non-NPSLE patients with high Ch/Cr at baseline had more MRI WM abnormalities at follow-up. Appenzeller, Li, et al. (2007) reported that SLE patients (both NPSLE and non-NPSLE) whose disease activity increased over the course of the study had a concomitant decline in NAA/Cr, that Ch/Cr increased in SLE patients compared to controls, and that patients with elevated Ch/Cr and normal MRI at baseline developed WMHI about one year later.

Studies further suggest that decreased NAA/Cr correlates with cerebral atrophy, focal lesions, aPL, and cognitive dysfunction in SLE, even in the absence of overt NP events (Brooks, Jung, Ford, Greinel, & Sibbitt, 1999; Brooks et al., 1997; Chinn et al., 1997; Davie et al., 1995; Rozell, Sibbitt, & Brooks, 1998; Sabet, Sibbitt, Stidley, Danska, & Brooks, 1998; Sibbitt, Haseler, Griffey, Friedman, & Brooks, 1997; Sibbitt et al., 1994; Sibbitt & Sibbitt, 1993). Reduced NAA in NPSLE may be largely due to microstructural lesions, including microinfarcts too small to discern with MRI (Friedman, Brooks, Jung, Hart, & Yeo, 1998; Sibbitt et al., 1999) that damage axons as well as myelin. NAA has also been found low in NPSLE patients with generalized seizures, psychosis, and confusional states, suggesting that cytotoxic effects of antineuronal antibodies, cytokines, or that small-molecule neurocytotoxins might also be involved (Sibbitt et al., 1999).

DIFFUSION TENSOR IMAGING

DTI provides an index of the structural integrity of WM by using quantitative directional diffusion properties of water molecules for each voxel. The technique is based on the principle of *anisotropy,* a term referring to the propensity for water in the normal state to diffuse along the direction of

WM tracts. Damaged WM, in contrast, is characterized by isotropic diffusion, which is correspondingly less directional and more random. Key DTI measures include fractional anisotropy (FA), mean diffusivity (MD), and the apparent diffusion coefficient (ADC). DTI is particularly sensitive to microstructural WM changes, including both myelin and axonal damage, and is an ideal tool for the study of WM because it can assess the structural integrity of specific tracts in relation to cognitive functions. DTI studies suggest WM damage in well-defined NPSLE patients and compared to controls (Bosma et al., 2004; Hughes et al., 2007; Jung et al., 2010; Zhang et al., 2007). In one controlled study of 37 non-NPSLE patients, no differences in WM, cortical GM, or the hippocampus were observed, but abnormalities were found in the amygdala (Emmer et al., 2006). Another controlled study of 34 NPSLE patients reported increased MD in the frontal lobe and the internal capsule, and decreased FA in the corpus callosum (CC) (Zhang et al., 2007). Abnormal findings were seen in patients with normal MRI scans, supporting the sensitivity of DTI to early WM changes. Use of a 3.0T scanner showed that FA was decreased in fronto-basal and temporal WM tracts of 12 SLE patients (NPSLE and SLE without overt NP; see Emmer et al., 2010), and increased ADC was reported in the frontal lobe as well as the CC splenium and genu in 15 SLE patients without overt NP compared to controls (Ulug et al., 2010). In a study of 26 SLE patients with one or more diffuse NP findings using a 3.0T scanner, increased ADC of NAWM was noted (Zivadinov et al., 2013).

POSITRON EMISSION TOMOGRAPHY AND SINGLE PHOTON EMISSION COMPUTED TOMOGRAPHY

Positron emission tomography (PET) and single photon emission computed tomography (SPECT) are functional brain imaging techniques that examine regional brain glucose metabolism. By their nature, these techniques are useful for the examination of GM areas only, as WM is generally less metabolic than GM. Overall, PET and SPECT studies in SLE patients demonstrate hypoperfusion across the cerebral cortex, and many studies have shown that these functional imaging abnormalities are increased compared to the prevalence of MRI abnormalities in these studies (Chen, Yen, Kao, Lin, & Lee, 2002; Otte et al., 1997; Weiner et al., 2000). Weiner et al. (2000) reported that PET showed hypometabolism in all of their SLE patients with NP manifestations, and also in 40% of the non-NPSLE patients. Studies have also demonstrated more specific hypometabolism in SLE, with abnormalities in the temporal (Csepany et al., 1997), parietal, and parietal-occipital regions (Otte et al., 1997; Weiner et al., 2000). Whereas PET and SPECT have potential utility in the study of cognition in SLE, it should be kept in mind that these techniques are intended primarily to assess cortical metabolism. Because this phenomenon is highly complex, and influenced not only by SLE but by many other unrelated factors, the data gathered from PET and SPECT are relatively nonspecific with respect to the pathogenesis of SLE.

Cognitive Correlates of Neuroimaging Abnormalities in SLE

Across studies, consistent relationships between findings of traditional structural techniques of CT and MRI findings in relation to cognitive abilities have been intriguing but incomplete. Using CT, for example, Denburg et al. (1987) reported abnormalities in only 12% of the patients studied, and found that no CT findings were related to cognitive impairment. However, some of their specific neuropsychological case findings were associated with lateralized CT lesions. MRI has proven far more useful. Waterloo et al. (1999) used MRI in NPSLE and found cerebral atrophy in 47%, which was associated with decreased tactile problem solving, and furthermore, the number of infarcts was associated with impaired motor dexterity. Sailer et al. (1997) reported three or more WM lesions on 57% of their MRI scans in SLE. The number and size of WM lesions on MRI were correlated in this study with the presence of neurological deficits, but not with the severity of cognitive impairment. In contrast, another study showed that the number of WMHI was moderately associated with tests of attention, while cortical atrophy was not (Kozora & Make, 1998). Some studies have not found a relationship between global or specific cognitive dysfunction and WM or GM volume in SLE, either with or without NP activity (Filley et al., 2009; Haider et al., 2012).

Conventional brain imaging with MRI offered important initial information on the origin of cognitive decline in SLE, but findings have indicated that the structural analysis of MRI may not be the most sensitive approach to understanding brain-behavior relationships in this disease. More recent studies have identified more consistent abnormalities when the brain microstructure is examined in detail. The most helpful techniques permitting this kind of study are MRS, which enables measurement of brain neurometabolites; functional MRI (fMRI), which allows assessment of cortical and other GM function; and DTI, which increasingly offers a method of evaluating the microstructure of both WM and GM. The emerging studies using these and other techniques have been reviewed in this section, and important determinants of cognitive decline have been identified in both WM and GM. Rocca et al. (2006), for example, reported increased activation in the contralateral primary sensorimotor cortex, putamen, dentate, and fronto-parietal regions during a motor task in 14 SLE patients compared to 14 controls. In a study of ten pediatric SLE patients (mean age 17.1), working memory tasks resulted in increased activation (Difrancesco et al., 2007), with the pattern of abnormal fMRI activity suggesting disruption of WM connectivity that resulted in neuronal network dysfunction. In a more recent study, these authors examined seven pediatric SLE patients with and 14 without cognitive dysfunction, and noted greater brain activation during tasks of working memory and visuoconstruction (Difrancesco et al., 2013). Fitzgibbon et al. (2008) also examined working memory as well as attention and executive function using a working memory test in nine NPSLE patients compared to RA and healthy control subjects; they reported greater frontal and parietal activation that indicated abnormalities in frontal networks. In another study, a card-sorting task developed to assess executive function (strategic planning and goal directed task performance) indicated higher brain activation in 14 SLE patients compared to demographically matched controls (Mak, Ren, Fu, Cheak, & Ho, 2012).

Several studies further suggest that abnormal fMRI findings may occur in SLE patients with no history of overt NP activity and normal structural MRI. In 33 non-NPSLE patients, resting-state fMRI abnormalities were noted in many brain regions compared to healthy controls, primarily in the posterior cingulate cortex, the precuneus, and the neocerebellum (Lin et al., 2011). In another study of 13 SLE patients with no structural MRI abnormalities and no history of NP activity, greater cortical activation during working memory and emotional response was noted in the amygdala and superior parietal areas, and patients with less than two years of disease had increased activity in the cingulate gyrus, prefrontal cortex, and somatomotor cortex during working memory tasks compared to patients with greater than ten years of disease (Mackay et al., 2011). Another fMRI study, which involved 12 SLE patients with no history of NP activity, indicated increased brain activation in SLE patients during learning in the region of the intraparietal sulcus and around the junction of the precentral and superior frontal sulcus; a relationship between learning efficiency and greater hippocampal functional connectivity was also noted (Shapira-Lichter et al., 2013). Additional studies that suggest hippocampal abnormalities are related to memory impairment in NP and non-NPSLE, and in animal studies declines in learning and memory, as well as dendritic spinal loss in the hippocampal pyramidal neurons, have been reported (Sakic et al., 1998; Tomita, Holman, & Santoro, 2001; Vogelweid, Wright, Johnson, Hewett, & Walker, 1994; Walker et al., 1997). In one study, 35 cognitively impaired SLE patients had reduced hippocampal when compared to 72 SLE patients without cognitive impairment (Appenzeller et al., 2006). In addition, the cognitively impaired SLE patients showed increased hippocampal volume loss over time. We further reported abnormalities of NAA/Cr and glutamate plus glutamine/Cr (Glu+Gln/Cr) in the hippocampus of 64 non-NPSLE patients that were directly related to memory impairment (Kozora et al., 2011).

PET and SPECT studies in SLE including a cognitive component are rare. Carbotte, Denburg, Denburg, Nahmias, and Garnett (1992) reported that in a longitudinal analysis of three SLE patients, PET abnormalities correlated with cognitive deficits. Sailer et al. (1997) did not find cognitive differences in their SLE patients with abnormal global glucose utilization. Komatsu et al. (1999) reported that SLE patients with major psychiatric symptoms had decreased cerebral metabolic rates for glucose in prefrontal inferior parietal and cingulate regions, findings that they related to attentional deficits in this sample of patients. Waterloo et al. (2001) examined 52 SLE patients and reported that 55% had abnormal blood flow on SPECT, and 33% had one to ten focal areas of decreased blood flow. Specific regions of the brain demonstrating decreased blood flow included the frontal, temporal, and parietal regions. Seventy-seven percent of the SLE patients had significant decline in cerebral blood flow in the temporal lobe. These investigators failed to find any correlation between brain region and neuropsychological test findings after controlling for age and cerebral infarcts.

Neuroimaging techniques supporting an association between abnormal WM neuroimaging and cognitive deficits in SLE appear to be some of the strongest findings in the literature. Early MRI investigations demonstrated that the number of WMHI but not cerebral atrophy was associated with attention in 20 non-NPSLE patients, a finding suggesting WM changes associated with MCD-SLE (Kozora & Make, 1998). Subsequently, volumetric WM analyses were conducted, and CC volume was significantly lower in controls, and associated with a decline in measures of visuomotor reasoning and processing speed (Johnson, Pinkston, Bigler, & Blatter, 1996). In another study, CC volumes were significantly smaller (25%) in 115 SLE patients compared to controls (Appenzeller, Rondina, Li, Costallat, & Cendes, 2005); NPSLE had greater CC volume loss than SLE without overt NP. SLE patients with cognitive impairment had reduced CC sizes, but only a third of the patients were cognitively tested and no data were available for review. MRS has further identified WM changes in areas that are normal on MRI. Elevated Ch/Cr associated with cognitive impairment was reported in frontal WM of eight SLE patients without overt NP compared to eight controls (Kozora et al., 2005). In a later study, we did not find cerebral atrophy (based on volumetric analysis) or neuronal damage (based on NAA/Cr measurements) in SLE patients without overt NP compared to controls (Filley et al., 2009). However, higher Ch/Cr was found in the right frontal WM and left frontal WM in the SLE patients without overt NP compared to controls. A composite measure of attention and executive functioning was found to correlate positively with total WM volume and negatively with left frontal WM Ch/Cr (Filley et al., 2009). In a subsequent analysis of these patients, one selected measure (complex auditory information processing) was specifically associated with elevated Ch/Cr, further suggesting that WM changes were related to aspects of cognition (Kozora, Arciniegas, et al., 2013). The available MRS data in SLE indicate that early changes in WM, particularly in myelin, may play an important role in cognitive impairment. Elevated frontal WM Ch/Cr may underlie MCD in SLE, which appears to be a precursor of more obvious brain pathology, advancing cognitive dysfunction, and clinical deterioration.

Summary of Findings

The literature regarding cognitive dysfunction in SLE is extensive, and despite differences in methodology, studies clearly suggest that over 50% of the SLE patients with overt NP activity demonstrate cognitive impairment across a broad range of areas (i.e., memory, attention, executive function visuomotor speed and visuoconstruction). Studies to date further suggest that there is a relatively large group of SLE patients (approximately 30%) where cognitive deficits alone are the primary NP feature. This group of patients, that we label MCD-SLE, has been the focus of multiple studies. Cognitive domains that consistently are impaired in this group include aspects of attention, memory, and executive function. Mechanisms of cognitive dysfunction in SLE continue to be unclear. Studies to date most strongly suggest that aspects of disease severity as well as the presence of specific autoantibodies (i.e., aPLs) and inflammatory markers (pro-inflammatory cytokines) are likely biological mechanisms. There is strong evidence that future studies investigating immune and autoimmune factors within the CSF are necessary to better identify mechanistic pathways. In addition, new studies investigating cardiovascular and cardiopulmonary disorders are promising, and suggest that many systemic aspects of SLE may have an indirect link to cognitive dysfunction. A variety of behavioral factors remain integral to cognitive dysfunction, primarily in the NPSLE subjects. Depression as a mediator of cognitive dysfunction is clear in the NPSLE population; however, few studies have incorporated additional potential factors such as pain, fatigue, sleep disorders, and exercise tolerance. Studies with advanced neuroimaging have allowed a more sophisticated evaluation of brain abnormalities underlying cognitive deficits in the NPSLE and MCD-SLE populations. Although studies continue to explore both GM and WM, it appears that WM abnormalities may occur early in the course of cognitive dysfunction and may be the essential feature underlying MCD-SLE. Studies that have focused on learning and memory dysfunction in SLE also indicate changes in the hippocampus, even in the MCD-SLE group. Although subject selection and descriptors have become more refined, continued controversy regarding assessment and definition of clinical improvement exists. In addition, relatively small sample sizes and lack of longitudinal studies clearly impact the generalizability of current findings and the ability of investigators to empirically model interactions between the various potential biobehavioral factors and cognitive outcomes.

Antiphospholipid Syndrome

Definition and Epidemiology

The Updated Sapporo Classification Criteria define APS as vascular thromboses (arterial, venous, or small vessel) and/or pregnancy morbidity occurring in persons with persistent aPL (LA, aCL (Jain & DeLisa, 1998), and aβ_2GPI (Miyakis et al., 2006). APS may present acutely or run a chronic course affecting multiple organ systems (Stanley & Ghosh, 2013) and is considered primary if no other connective tissue diseases are present (Keeling et al., 2012). Anticoagulation with heparin followed by long-term warfarin is the treatment for APS patients with thrombotic events, while aspirin or anticoagulation is generally used during the pregnancies of APS patients with or without a history of pregnancy morbidities. Risk factors for APS include a variety of genetic markers, race (Black, Hispanic, Asian, Native American), and a diagnosis of SLE, and like SLE and other autoimmune diseases, APS is more prevalent in women than men. It has been estimated that up to 50%–70% of SLE patients may develop APS (Love & Santoro, 1990b; Petri, 2000) when higher levels of aCL and LA are found in these patients (Cervera et al., 2002). Evidence of aPL has been found in between 1% and 5% of otherwise healthy control subjects (Petri, 2000), and, as with other autoimmune diseases, the risk of aPL prevalence increases with age. Any organ in the body can be affected by APS, including the brain, and the range of disorders possible for each system is diverse (Levine, Branch, & Rauch, 2002).

Neuropsychiatric Antiphospholipid Syndrome

The prevalence of NP disorders in APS patients without other autoimmune diseases is unknown. Major overt NP syndromes that occur in aPL-positive patients include stroke, transient ischemic attack, seizures, chorea, Guillain-Barré–like symptoms, headaches including migraine, depression, and cognitive impairment (Brey, Muscal, & Chapman, 2011; Cervera et al., 2002; Rodrigues, Carvalho, & Shoenfeld, 2010; Roldan & Brey, 2007; Sanna et al., 2003). In a European cohort of 1,000 persistently aPL-positive patients, Cervera et al. (2002) found more than 20.2% experience migraine, 19.8% stroke, 11.1% transient ischemic attack, 7% epilepsy, 2.5% multi-infarct dementia, 1.3% chorea, and 0.4% transverse myelopathy. However, in this study it was not clear if the aPL was the cause of the neurological disorder. In the original observations of APS syndrome, Hughes (1988) highlighted the presence of cerebrovascular accident and myelitis in APS; but since the time of this report, neurological manifestations with APS have been noted in the absence of stroke, suggesting that other mechanisms beyond direct vascular thrombosis are active (Carecchio, Cantello, & Comi, 2014). In terms of the mechanism underlying NP activity in APS, aPLs may bind to CNS neurons, leading to permeabilization and depolarization of these cells (Chapman, Cohen-Armon,

Shoenfeld, & Korczyn, 1999). Animal models corroborate that NP performance is affected by aPL independently of the ischemic events (Ziporen, Shoenfeld, Levy, & Korczyn, 1997). In a recent review of the literature, pathological mechanisms by which aPL leads to neurological dysfunction have been summarized as including (a) induction of a proinflammatory or procoagulation state mediated by endothelial cells, and platelet and coagulation cascade activation, and BBB dysfunction that allows for the influx of aPL and cytokines into the brain with toxic impacts on neurons and glial cells; (b) impairment of the normal inhibition of cerebral atherogenesis, leading to an increase in atherosclerotic vascular disease in the brain; and (c) aPL-mediated complement activation leading to CNS toxicity and dysfunction (Brey et al., 2011). Few studies have clearly classified NP events, and the estimates of "cognitive dysfunction" are limited. Although data are limited, a number of clinicians suggest that 25%–50% of patients with APS may have identifiable cognitive dysfunction.

Cognitive Dysfunction

Neuropsychological Studies

Studies in primary APS or in asymptomatic aPL positive patients have shown that cognitive deficits may be present, independent of any history of known CNS involvement, when compared to controls or other patient groups. Jacobson, Rapport, Keenan, Coleman, and Tietjen (1999) examined neuropsychological functioning in 27 nonelderly patients with elevated levels (> 10 IU) of aCL IgG, but without concurrent history of autoimmune disease or any history or report of neurological events. Compared with 27 age- and education-matched controls, there were group differences in domain scores of working memory, executive function, verbal learning, memory and visuospatial functioning. The overall frequency of impaired neuropsychological performance was greater among individuals with aPL than controls (33% vs. 4% respectively), suggesting subtle neurological involvement. Few studies have clearly classified NP events and the estimates of "cognitive dysfunction" are limited. Tektonidou, Varsou, Kotoulas, Antoniou, and Moutsopoulos (2006) examined 39 patients with primary APS, 21 patients with SLE-related APS, and 60 healthy controls using a three-hour neuropsychological battery measuring attention, learning and memory, executive function, visuospatial skills, and depression. In this study, the cutoff limits of aPL positivity are not reported. Results indicated that 42% of the 60 patients with APS (combined primary and SLE-related APS) had cognitive deficits compared with 18% of healthy controls, with deficits most commonly detected in complex attention and verbal fluency. There was no difference in cognitive performance between patients with primary APS and those with SLE-associated APS (although there was a significant association between cognitive dysfunction and WM lesions). In one pilot study of 20 APS patients, 13 out of the 14 APS patients with CNS disorders demonstrated mild cognitive deficits compared to 10 controls (Aharon-Peretz, Brenner, & Amyel, 1995).

Studies to date regarding cognitive dysfunction in primary APS versus those with SLE-associated APS are inconclusive, but tend not to show major differences (Sanna et al., 2003; Tektonidou et al., 2006). In a recent study by our group comparing 20 aPL-positive non-SLE female patients to 20 aPL-negative SLE female patients with no history of overt NP manifestations, 40% of the aPL-positive patients had global cognitive impairment using a comprehensive cognitive battery (compared to 60% of the SLE). The pattern of cognitive difficulties was similar across the two groups, with impaired performance in visual and verbal learning and memory, visuomotor speed, attention and information processing, verbal fluency, and problem solving. This study was consistent with prior studies demonstrating that aPL patients also have a wide range of cognitive impairments, and suggests both have global versus focal cerebral changes. The careful selection and characterization of the two samples further suggests that unique mechanisms underlying cognitive deficits in these autoimmune diseases exist. Future studies that include a third control aPL-positive SLE group at baseline, and evaluate all groups over time, may be necessary to identify the most important risks and mechanisms associated with cognitive impairment in these patients.

Several studies have investigated the role of aPL in relation to dementia or cognitive decline in the aging population. One study reported that 56% of elderly APS patients had dementia based on diagnostic criteria (Chapman et al., 2002), and neuropsychological dysfunction in otherwise normal elderly people was associated with increased levels of aCL (Schmidt, Auer-Grumbach, Fazekas, Offenbacher, & Kapeller, 1995). It is likely that cognitive dysfunction in these patients is due to multiple mechanisms. The underlying pathophysiology may relate to small vessel ischemic events, often involving cerebral WM, or there may be a direct pathogenic role of aPL, which has implications in the treatment.

Biobehavioral Mechanisms of Cognitive Dysfunction in APS

The biobehavioral aspects underlying cognitive dysfunction in APS have not been systematically evaluated, and no studies have examined the potential effects on a large sample of patients. In Tektonidou et al. (2006) a relationship between cognitive dysfunction and one aspect of clinical disease (livedo reticularis) was reported in 39 APS and 21 APS-SLE patients, but no relationship was found with measures of thrombosis, CNS involvement, aCL, LA, aβ2GPI, or depression. Jacobson et al. (1999) did not report any relationship between prior NP history or depression to cognitive dysfunction in 27 APS patients, but also did not present data and duration of disease or other health factors. In our pilot study of 20 APS-only patients, there was no relationship between cognitive impairment and aspects of disease activity, disease duration, medication use, or symptoms of depression (Kozora, Erkan, et al., 2013). Studies suggest that both SLE and APS can result in cognitive dysfunction; however, direct comparison of cognition across these disorders is difficult due to methodological issues. Many prior studies of SLE have not specifically screened out or identified those patients with positive aPL. The prevalence of positive aPL in patients with SLE is approximately 30%–40% (Love & Santoro, 1990b). In SLE studies of cognition, the prevalence of aPL has ranged from 6% to 38% (Conti et al., 2012; Hanly & Harrison, 2005; Maeshima, amada, Yukawa, & Nomoto, 1992; Peretti et al., 2012; Sanna et al., 2003) and the presence of aPL in SLE patients has been associated with greater impairment in memory, visuomotor speed, and visuoconstruction (Conti et al., 2012; Denburg, Carbotte, Ginsberg, et al., 1997; Hanly et al., 1993; Leritz et al., 2002). Our latest study suggests that both SLE patients without aPL and aPL patients with no history of SLE have cognitive dysfunction with no evidence of more overt NP activity. Continued studies that assess and compare biobehavioral characteristics of patients with SLE, aPL and SLE with aPL who experience cognitive decline over time may be the next useful step in understanding these cognitive disorders.

Treatment Studies With APS

No large studies of pharmacological, behavioral, or rehabilitative treatment to improve cognitive function in APS are available. In a retrospective analysis of five aPL-positive patients who tolerated and responded to rituximab (an antibody that binds to CD20 antigen, resulting in a rapid and sustained depletion of peripheral B-lymphocyte lineage), there was some evidence that this drug may be effective for aPL-associated cognitive dysfunction. Four of the five patients showed a decline on the cognitive impairment index, representing cognitive improvement, at 24 weeks (complete response, three; partial response, one; see Erkan, Vega, Ramon, Kozora, & Lockshin, 2013).

Neuroimaging

Neuroimaging abnormalities have been reported in primary APS patients presenting with high levels of overt neurological and psychiatric syndromes, however, even in the absence of NP activity, abnormalities are noted. Infarcts and scattered WM lesions are the most common abnormalities seen on CT and MRI in APS patients. Provenzale, Barboriak, Allen, and Ortel (1996) reported that 54% of aPL patients (with and without SLE) had abnormal studies (large infarcts, cortical infarcts, lacunar infarcts, hyperintense WM foci, or dural sinus thrombosis) in subjects who underwent CT or MRI. Results showed that large infarcts were the most common abnormality (in 22% of patients), followed by hyperintense WM foci (in 17% of patients). The frequency of abnormalities was 57% in the SLE group and 41% in the non-SLE group. Large infarcts were more common in the non-SLE group (26%). In a study of 24 APS patients, 29 SLE patients, and 31 healthy controls undergoing MRI scan, both APS and SLE groups demonstrated greater cortical atrophy and increased WM abnormalities (periventricular and deep WM hyperintensities) compared to controls after controlling for neurological syndromes and other demographic and health variables (Hachulla et al., 1998). Based on a score of two standard deviations below healthy controls, eight APS patients had cortical atrophy and nine had greater WM hyperintensities. Hachulla and colleagues (1998) found only a weak correlation between LAC and cerebral atrophy. Kim, Choi, Choi, Lee, and Suh (2000) also reported that in 11 APS patients with a majority demonstrating overt neurological disease (seven undergoing CT, eight undergoing MRI including some overlap), five had WM abnormalities, four had large infarct of the middle cerebral artery, and two had cortical atrophy. Gomez-Puerta et al. (2005) studied a combined APS/SLE group who underwent CT and/or MRI and reported cortical infarcts in 63% of patients, subcortical infarcts in 30%, basal ganglia infarcts in 23%, and cerebral atrophy in 37%. In the Tektonidou et al. (2006) MRI study, WM lesions were identified as "ill-defined" punctate hyperintensities on T2, proton density, and fluid attenuated inversion recovery (FLAIR) images without prominent T1 hypointensity, and lesions were classified according to location (subcortical, periventricular, and deep) and graded according to size. In 23 APS patients with CNS involvement, they report that 12 (52%) had WM lesions, with 100% in the periventricular regions. Of the 36 APS patients without CNS involvement, eight (22%) had punctate WM lesions, with 88% located in periventricular regions (Tektonidou et al., 2006). In our study of 20 aPL subjects with no other connective tissue disease or NP activity, 50% demonstrated abnormal MRI or incidental MRI findings of WM change or cortical atrophy.

No studies using DTI, fMRI, MRS, PET or SPECT in APS syndrome have been published. Other approaches to studying this disease, however, have been investigated. A recent study of 28 primary APS patients used carotid Doppler ultrasound and echocardiograph evaluations, and reported abnormal function in the middle and anterior cerebral arteries that was associated with LAC, history of stroke, and obesity. Lampropoulos et al. (2005) used EEG to study 57 patients with APS and/or SLE who had NP symptoms (those with a history of stroke, epilepsy, or encephalopathy were excluded). Fourteen patients had APS, 24 were positive for aPL, and 19 patients had SLE without aPL. The frequency of abnormal EEG findings (primarily bitemporal slow activity) of the combined aPL and APS groups was 82%, compared to 32% in the SLE group. An association between abnormal EEG and aPL positivity was found. Of the aPL-positive patients, 82.3% with abnormal EEG results had at least two positive results for aPL, while 28.5% with normal

EEG findings had at least two positive results. Patients with abnormal EEG findings were more likely to report memory problems; however, no formal cognitive testing was applied.

Few studies to date have evaluated cognitive impairment in relation to neuroimaging abnormalities in APS. The use of combined groups of SLE patients with high aPL has disclosed inconsistent relationships. Chapman et al. (2002) reported that only half of their demented APS patients had abnormal CT scans, and suggested that the demented APS patients with normal CT scans may have had micro-lesions or pathology (not necessarily vascular mediated) that might have been detected with MRI or other neuroimaging techniques. In contrast, eight of the nondemented subjects with APS showed diffuse slowing on EEG. Of those with dementia, six had generalized atrophy and seven had focal lesions consistent with vascular pathology. To date, there are only two studies of primary APS patients that report neuroimaging abnormalities in relation to cognitive dysfunction. In a pilot study using clinical procedures, 50% of the MRIs in aPL patients with no history of SLE or NP activity were abnormal, but no association between incidental or major MRI abnormalities and cognitive dysfunction were noted (Kozora, Erkan, et al., 2013). In another study, Tektonidou et al. (2006), of a significant correlation between cognitive deficits and presence of WM lesions was found. In a subgroup of eight APS patients without overt CNS involvement but with WM lesions, cognitive deficits were identified in seven of the patients (Tektonidou et al., 2006). They also noted a positive relationship between WM lesions, livedo reticularis, and cognitive dysfunction, suggesting the presence of microvasculopathy. It is likely that sophisticated neuroimaging techniques such as DTI and MRS, with the capacity to permit better depiction of WM abnormalities, will expand our understanding of cognitive dysfunction in APS (Erkan, Kozora, & Lockshin, 2011).

Summary of Findings

Very few studies of cognitive functioning in APS without overt NP activity and other autoimmune disorders exist. Of those published and available for review, cognitive dysfunction occurred in 33%–42% of the patients. Methodological problems exist that are related to subject selection, test selection, definition of impairment, lack of control subjects, and small sample sizes (less than 30 subjects in largest study). A standardized definition of APS now exists that improves subject selection; however, classification of NP activity in APS is quite varied and may or may not include cognitive dysfunction. As with the early SLE literature, formal studies to facilitate classification of NP in diffuse in focal CNS activity, including cognitive dysfunction, are necessary. The cognitive studies reviewed included a wide range of cognitive domains, and impairments in attention and working memory, learning and memory, executive function, and visuospatial and visuomotor functions were impaired. Standardization and/or adaptation of a test battery would improve future studies. Most existing studies do not include assessment of biobehavioral correlates, and in these studies, aspects of clinical disease and behavior were noted (but not consistently). Finally, the neuroimaging aspects of APS clearly suggest that in addition to the expected cerebral infarcts related to vascular-mediated aPL activity, there is evidence of atrophy as well as multiple WMHI. As with SLE, it is likely that WM abnormalities occur early in APS, are correlated with cognitive dysfunction, and may be detectable well before more obvious structural damage.

Rheumatoid Arthritis

Definition and Epidemiology

RA is an autoimmune disease in which the immune system attacks the body's own tissues, specifically the synovium. The synovium is a smooth, thin membranous lining between joints that produces lubricative synovial fluid. As a result of the body's attacks on the synovium, synovial fluid builds up within joint space and development of fibrous tissue causes systemic pain and inflammation. It may take some time for symptoms to occur, and the rheumatoid factors responsible for pathology are deposited in a different way than in SLE, resulting in inflammation via activated macrophages. Over time, RA can affect several other organ systems, including the integumentary, respiratory, cardiovascular, digestive, and nervous systems, among others. The etiology of RA is not completely known, although it is clear that the disease has a systemic autoimmune component. Risk factors include genetics (accounting for 50% of risk; see van der Woude et al., 2009), and smoking (RA is one to three times as common in smokers than nonsmokers; see Stolt et al., 2003). Once initiated, the disease may worsen over time. For some individuals, the abnormal immune response becomes permanent and chronic. Most people with RA experience intermittent periods of severe disease activity, called *flares,* which are generally treated with glucocorticoids. Otherwise, RA is generally managed with nonsteroidal anti-inflammatory drugs (NSAIDs) and COX-2 inhibitors (NSAIDs targeting the COX-2 enzyme, responsible for inflammation and pain). The prevalence of RA worldwide is surprisingly uniform at approximately 0.5% to 1% (Scott, Wolfe, & Huizinga, 2010), and in the United States the prevalence is approximately 2.5 million, or 0.6% of the population (Helmick et al., 2008). The incidence and prevalence are approximately two to three times greater in women than men. The usual age of onset is between the ages of 30 and 60 for women (with a later onset for men). The prevalence increases with age, with average onset in the third to sixth decade of life.

Neurologic Rheumatoid Arthritis

The neurologic manifestations in RA are thought to be a consequence of local joint changes, extra-articular rheumatoid nodules, and secondary vasculitis (Voss & Stangel, 2012). The most common manifestation in RA is peripheral neuropathy, which can be sensory or sensorimotor in its manifestations. Of particular interest for this chapter, complaints including cognitive dysfunction, depression, and fatigue have also been identified in RA, strongly suggesting the possibility of CNS disease affecting neurobehavioral function (Wolfe & Michaud, 2004).

Cognitive Dysfunction

Several studies indicate that patients with RA may have subtle cognitive dysfunction (Dick, Eccleston, & Crombez, 2002; Kozora et al., 1996; Kutner et al., 1988; Wekking, Nossent, et al., 1991). As with the early studies in cognition in SLE and other autoimmune disorders, methodological issues such as subject inclusion and exclusion, diverse test selection, and varying definitions of cognitive impairment limit the generalizability of studies in RA. Several studies have also shown high rates of cognitive impairment in RA compared to controls. Kutner et al. (1988) indicated that while SLE patients were more impaired than RA patients, the RA group was significantly more impaired than controls on measures of nonverbal reasoning, visuospatial functions, language, and verbal memory. As they also reported impaired motor functioning in RA patients, motor deficits may have impacted some of their other cognitive findings. Wekking, Nossent, et al. (1991) reported that 40% of the RA patients were cognitively impaired and suggested that cognitive impairment may not be specific to SLE but related to autoimmunity in general. In one study of RA (Dick et al., 2002), 20 patients without major NP syndromes (mean age of 62.9) with chronic pain performed worse than pain-free controls on a global score of attention, as well as sustained attention and working memory tasks. In addition, more than 60% of the RA patients had at least one of three scales of attention in the impaired range using demographically corrected scaled scores.

In a study by our group, a high incidence of global cognitive impairment was reported in RA patients (Kozora et al., 1996). We found that 31% of 29 RA patients (carefully screened to exclude all patients with a NP history) were globally impaired (defined as two or more of eight domain scores in the impaired range) with specific deficits in attention and fluency when compared to controls. There was no relationship with disease duration or medication use. Bartolini et al. (2002) studied 30 RA patients (mean age of 55.6) who also had no history of major NP disease including depression, and found that they were impaired on measures of executive function (fluency, reasoning), visuomotor skills (constructive, speed), and learning and memory. Using demographically converted impairment scores, they reported that 71% of the RA patients were impaired in visuospatial construction, 47% in reasoning, 44% in verbal fluency, 50% in visual learning and memory, 38% in mental flexibility, 35% in verbal learning, and 29% in motor function. They further noted that except for attention, disease severity but not duration had a relation to the cognitive profile. In a later study, Appenzeller, Costallat, and Condes (2004) reported cognitive impairment in 30% of RA patients (n = 40) compared to 7.5% of controls (n = 40). Verbal fluency, verbal memory, and short-term memory were significantly impaired in RA compared to controls, and no relationship between cognition, duration of illness, disability, or corticosteroid therapy was noted.

In a study of 55 patients with RA (screened for other autoimmune diseases and major NP symptoms) compared to 48 controls matched for socioeconomic status and education, 71% were impaired, with lower cognitive scores across multiple areas including aspects of memory, attention, reasoning, and verbal skill (Hamed et al., 2012). In addition, these investigators reported that standard measures of disease activity and severity were not related to cognitive dysfunction, and despite high levels of depressive symptoms, there was no correlation between these symptoms and cognition. In a recent well-designed study where 115 RA patients screened for NP completed a comprehensive neuropsychological battery, 31% of the patients were cognitively impaired (based on four of 12 tests in the impaired range; see Shin, Katz, Wallhagen, & Julian, 2012). Twenty percent or more of the RA patients were impaired in aspects of executive function (nonverbal fluency) verbal memory, visual memory, and visuomotor speed, and more than 15% were impaired in working memory. The cognitively impaired RA patients had a greater likelihood of having lower education, low income, use of oral glucocorticoids, and increased cardiovascular risk factor. In a subsequent study of 82 RA patients from this cohort, they report that 15% of the RA group was impaired on a cognitive screening measure (including verbal learning and memory, and phonemic fluency) that was sensitive to the larger comprehensive battery previously described (Julian et al., 2012). Notably, the self-report measure of cognitive functioning yielded low sensitivity.

Several studies have demonstrated that SLE patients performed worse than RA patients on neuropsychological tests (Carbotte et al., 1986; Denburg et al., 1987; Hanly et al., 1993; Julian et al. 2012; Koffler, 1987; Kutner et al., 1988; Yazdany et al., 2011). We also compared SLE and RA patients, and reported that 30% of the 51 non-NPSLE patients and 11% of the 27 healthy controls had global impairment (Kozora et al., 1996). Interestingly, the RA patients were similar to those with SLE, manifesting impairments in attention and fluency compared to controls. Despite global similarities in cognitive dysfunction in SLE and RA, 33% of the non-NPSLE patients had difficulty encoding material compared to 14% in the RA group. These findings might suggest a more general process associated with autoimmunity underlying cognitive dysfunction in RA and SLE, with additional factors specific to SLE (as reviewed earlier). For example, both SLE and RA patients have difficulty with attention and executive function, suggesting that a more general "autoimmune" mechanism may be work and may impact frontal lobe WM.

Biobehavioral Mechanisms of Cognitive Dysfunction in RA

As reviewed on earlier, there are few studies investigating specific biobehavioral mechanisms of cognitive dysfunction, although pain, fatigue, and motor dysfunction have been hypothesized. As with other autoimmune disorders, inconsistent associations between disease parameters in relation to cognitive dysfunction have been reported. In general, few studies have found a relationship between cognitive dysfunction and disease factors such as duration of illness, disease severity, or medication use. One study suggested that motor dysfunction in RA might impact cognitive tasks involving coordination (Kutner et al., 1988). Another study found that cardiovascular risk factors were associated with cognitive dysfunction in RA, and suggested that hypertension, hyperlipidemia, obesity, or current smoking could increase the prevalence of cognitive impairment in RA (Shin et al., 2012). This study also found a relationship between corticosteroids and cognitive dysfunction, and noted that most of the subjects were taking low doses of prednisone (of 115 RA patients, only 14 were taking more than 5 mgs per day). Their findings do suggest that in this population corticosteroid use may increase the risk of cognitive dysfunction. Notably, they did not find that chronic pain or psychological distress was associated with cognitive dysfunction in RA, nor was global disease severity or measures of inflammation such as CRP. Although one study reported an association between pain and cognitive dysfunction in RA (Dick et al., 2002) another study did not find that pain was related to cognitive dysfunction once depression was factored into the analysis of 121 RA patients (Brown, Glass, & Park, 2002). These investigators did report that depressive symptoms remained related to cognitive dysfunction. Notably, many studies reviewed above excluded any RA patients with major depression or psychiatric disorders.

Neuroimaging

There have been several neuroimaging studies in RA patients identifying brain abnormalities. Specifically, preliminary findings are beginning to identify WM abnormalities (increased number of WMHI and abnormal neurometabolic functioning within WM). Some studies also suggest neurometabolic abnormalities of GM. Hamed et al. (2012) reported that seven of 48 MRIs performed on RA patients had WMHI; however when compared to controls, there was no statistically significant difference. A number of studies, however, have indicated increased WMHI occurring in RA patients that correlate with poor scores on attentional, executive, and frontal lobe tasks. Bartolini et al. (2002) performed MRI and SPECT scans on 30 RA patients, and 35% showed "some alterations at the subcortical level in terms of WM hyperintensities (WMHIs) without leukoaraiosis." In addition, the authors report that these 11 patients all had low scores on attentional, executive, and visuospatial tasks. Using SPECT data in particular, they also reported that cognitive deficits in RA were related to hypoperfusion of the frontal (85%) and parietal (40%) lobes.

In a study using MRS of the NAWM, Ch/Cr was elevated in the centrum semiovale of RA patients with active inflammatory disease (Emmer et al., 2009). These authors examined 35 RA patients with active disease and 28 healthy control subjects, none of whom had any neurologic symptoms or signs. Twenty RA patients (79% female, mean age of 51.8, disease duration mean of 7.7 years, mean disease activity score of 28, joint assessment of 4.4) with active disease and elevated erythrocyte sedimentation rates (ESR) had higher Ch/Cr ratio and lower NAA/Cr ratio compared to 20 demographically similar inactive RA patients. No relationships were noted between disease duration or medication use and metabolite ratios in the RA group. Emmer et al. (2009) did not report any difference between the total RA group and controls on neurometabolite values, and suggested that inflammation is the primary mechanism underlying the WM abnormalities. To date there are few studies investigating neuroimaging abnormalities in relation to cognitive functions in RA. One study showed increased WMHI occurring in RA patients with poor scores on attentional, executive, and frontal tasks (Bartolini et al., 2002). No other studies of this nature exist in RA, but the available findings would suggest WM abnormalities likely mediated by inflammation and may underlie cognitive dysfunction in this population.

Summary of Findings

Across many well-designed studies, cognitive deficits have been found to occur in approximately 30% to 40% of RA patients. Notably, deficits in working memory and attention, executive function, learning and memory, visuomotor and visuospatial activity, and motor function were frequently reported. The neuropathology of cognitive deficits in this group of autoimmune patients is unclear. Motor function impairment in RA may impact some, but not all of the cognitive domains. Additional biological mechanisms related to inflammation and possible cardiovascular disease have been noted. Behavioral aspects of pain and depression are also likely mediators, although these have not been consistently noted across studies. Neuroimaging studies in RA indicate that WM abnormalities are the most common finding, and these have been associated with cognitive impairment. Few studies suggest damage to the GM in RA. Although the neuropathology of RA has rarely implicated active CNS disease, a review of the data suggests that there may be biological underpinnings, particularly in relation to inflammation, that impact the brain and contribute to cognitive dysfunction in RA. As with other studies in autoimmunity, limitations exist regarding subject selection, test selection, and definition of impairment, and attention to these issues is likely to improve future studies.

Primary Sjögrens Syndrome

Definition and Epidemiology

PSS is an autoimmune disorder characterized by abnormal proteins in the blood associated with an immune attack against the patient's own tissue. This process causes inflammation and damage primarily involving the exocrine glands, specifically the salivary and lacrimal glands that produce saliva and tears. It is thought that the presence of serum anti-Ro/SSA and/or anti-La/SSB antibodies (specific to PSS) may set in motion a dysfunctional immune response (as evidenced by increased presence of regulatory T cell infiltration) resulting in inflammation, autoreactivity, and tissue destruction (Nocturne & Mariette, 2013). *Primary* Sjögren's syndrome (as opposed to *secondary* Sjögren's syndrome) is not associated with another autoimmune disease such as SLE. The presence of sicca complex (i.e., dryness syndrome) is one of the primary clinical symptoms and typically involves the eyes, mouth, and other mucous membranes. The disorder is marked by a triad of symptoms including keratoconjuctivitis sicca (dry eyes) with or without lacrimal gland enlargement, xerostomia (dry mouth) with or without salivary gland enlargement, and connective tissue disease. Due to relatively benign initial symptoms, PSS may not be considered as a diagnosis for several years. Similar to other autoimmune disorders, PSS can affect many organs, including the kidneys, blood vessels, lungs, liver, pancreas, and nervous system. The etiology of PSS is not well known, although a genetic contribution is thought to exist (Bolstad & Jonsson, 2002) that may make some individuals more susceptible to a distinctive pathogenic process (Voulgarelis & Tzioufas, 2010). Some patients may experience remission or sustained or worsening symptoms that may involve renal disorder development. PSS affects approximately 0.6% of the U.S. population, or approximately 2 million people (Jonsson, Moen, Vestrheim, & Szodoray, 2002). According to the Sjögren's Syndrome Foundation there are upwards of 4 million Americans with this diagnosis and approximately 90% are women (Jonsson et al., 2002). The usual onset of symptoms occurs between 45 and 55 years of age (Borchers, Naguwa, Keen, & Gershwin, 2003), and prevalence generally increases with age (Fox, Stern, & Michelson, 2000).

Neuropsychiatric Primary Sjögren's Syndrome

Patients with PSS have been observed to develop both PNS and CNS disease. The span of overt neurological disorders in PSS includes brain and spinal cord disease that has been described as ranging from transient and reversible to fixed and cumulative. There is no current consensus regarding NP classification in PSS, and the use of different classification criteria, differences in patient populations, and lack of criteria for classification of NP activity are notable (Lauvsnes et al., 2013)—a finding reminiscent to the SLE research prior to the 1980s. CNS involvement may be focal or diffuse, with problems such as strokes, movement disorders, cerebellar and brain stem dysfunction, myelopathy, encephalopathy, aseptic meningitis, seizures, headaches, psychiatric disturbance, and cognitive dysfunction (Fauchais, Magy, & Vidal; Streifler & Molad, 2014; Tobón, Pers, Devasuchelle-Pensec, & Youinou, 2012). The estimated prevalence of CNS manifestations in PSS varies considerably, with some estimates as high as 30% (Alexander, 1986; Tajima et al., 1997; Volk et al., 1994). In Volk et al. (1994), 70% of PSS patients had neurological complications, and PNS changes were twice as frequent as CNS manifestations. Of the 30% with CNS manifestations, cerebral atrophy, hemiparesis, and aseptic meningitis were common. In contrast, CNS manifestations were rare in other studies (Andonopoulos, Lagos, Drosos, & Moutsopoulos, 1990; Binder, Snaith, & Isenberg, 1988; Moutsopoulos, Sarmas, & Taland, 1993). The incidence of more subtle disorders of the CNS such as mood disorders and cognitive dysfunction may be higher, and may be underrepresented due to methodological issues. One review has reported that up to 50% of PSS patients displayed cognitive dysfunction (Vitali et al., 2002). For example, a recent study identified high levels of CNS disorders in carefully screened PSS patients. Of 120 PSS patients, 81 (67%) had evidence of CNS or PNS symptoms, and CNS involvement was more common than PNS dysfunction with the use of neurological, psychological, and psychiatric evaluation (Morreale et al., 2014). These investigators further report that 68 patients (84%) had nonfocal and had 64 focal CNS deficits, and that headache was the most common manifestation (46.9%) followed by cognitive dysfunction (44.4%) and mood disorders (38.3%).

Cognitive Studies

Cognitive dysfunction has been noted in studies to date of PSS patients. As with other studies in autoimmune populations investigating cognitive dysfunction, the methodological problems and variation in subject selection, type of cognitive tests, and definition of impairment have made comparison across studies difficult. Selnes, Gordon, Malinow, and Alexander (1985) reported that 46% of the PSS patients had abnormal cognition primarily in attention and concentration. Malinow et al. (1985) also reported cognitive abnormalities in 44% of 40 PSS patients using similar tests, and reported a correlation with depressive symptoms as well. In another study, incidence of psychiatric and cognitive impairment was found in up to 80% of 131 PSS patients with CNS symptoms (Spezialetti, Bluestein, & Alexander, 1995). Volk et al. (1994) reported cognitive impairment in 70% of 20 PSS patients using measures of intelligence, visual memory, and perceptual speed. Specifically, one-fourth of their patients showed impairment on a visual memory test and up to 70% on a perceptual-motor speed test. Segal et al. (2012) studied 39 PSS (with no NP history) compared to 17 controls similar in premorbid IQ, age, and education and report lower cognitive performance in PSS on measures of psychomotor processing and verbal reasoning. There was no difference between PSS patients with high and low symptoms of depression on cognitive functions except for executive function (which was lower in depressed PSS). Pain also correlated with executive function and working memory dysfunction. Rodrigues et al. (2014) studied 18 PSS patients compared to 18 MS and 18 controls with measures of attention, fluency, visuomotor speed, verbal memory, and visuoconstruction. Group differences between PSS and controls existed on aspects of executive function/flexibility and verbal memory, but not on measures of fluency, visuoconstruction, or visuomotor speed. There was no relationship between depressive symptoms and cognitive functions. Epstein et al. (2014) studied 37 PSS and patients and 37 controls (matched for gender, IQ, education, and past NP history) and found few differences between the groups on measures of attention, visuomotor speed, executive functioning, and memory from a computerized test battery, but did report significantly lower recognition memory and visuomotor speed in PSS patients. Finally, Morreale et al. (2014) reported that 44% of PSS patients had cognitive deficits with abnormal scores reported in aspects of executive functioning (nonverbal reasoning), visuomotor sequencing, and verbal memory.

Biobehavioral Correlates of Cognitive Dysfunction in PSS

To date there are not enough studies to evaluate or comment on potential biobehavioral correlates of cognitive dysfunction in PSS. Most studies do not include correlations between disease factors, medications, and cognitive findings, and of the few that did report depressive symptoms, most detected no significant findings. Interestingly, one group studied 66 PSS patients compared to gender-matched healthy controls and did not report significant differences in performance across the groups on a comprehensive battery of cognitive tests, but did report that the patients with PSS and anti-NR2 antibodies in CSF and serum demonstrated worse performance in learning and memory (Lauvsnes et al., 2013). This study also reported that the patients with depression had serum anti-NR2 antibody levels above the cutoff. These studies suggest that autoimmune antibodies are likely associated with cognitive dysfunction and NP changes in PSS.

Neuroimaging

Neuroimaging studies have demonstrated a range of brain abnormalities in PSS. The major findings include increased number of WMHI, small cerebral strokes, and cerebral volume loss. Alexander et al. (1988) reported that 12 of their 16 PSS patients with active CNS disease had abnormal MRIs (primarily because of focal lesions in the subcortical and periventricular WM) and two out of 22 PSS patients without active CNS disease had similar abnormalities. Notably, seven out of eight PSS patients with psychiatric or cognitive problems (documented with objective evaluations) had abnormal MRIs. In a Medline review of studies through 2003, MRI was found to reveal cerebral tissue damage even in neurologically asymptomatic PSS patients, and periventricular and subcortical WM changes were common. In PSS patients with CNS disease, cortical atrophy was also observed (Morgen, McFarland, & Pillemer, 2004). Compared to controls, higher WMHI numbers were noted in 38 of 53 PSS patients with no history of NP activity, and a relationship was found between disease duration and number of WM lesions (Tzarouchi et al., 2011). This study also reported that PSS patients had decreased GM and WM volume compared to controls, and atrophy of the CC was also significant. In another study, 22 PSS patients with tension headaches had a higher number and size of WMHI compared to 20 age-matched controls with tension headaches (Šarac et al., 2013). These investigators further reported that the increased number of WMHI in the PSS patients was related to disease duration, and with a marker of chronic inflammation.

Few studies using MRS or DTI in PSS exist, but findings to date suggest abnormalities. Of 81 PSS patients in one study, 47 were noted to have decreased NAA/Cr ratios using MRS analysis in subcortical frontal WM and basal ganglia (Morreale et al., 2014). Another study, using DTI analysis in 53 PSS patients with no history of NP activity, reported decreased FA in the corticospinal tract, superior longitudinal fasciculus, anterior thalamic radiation, inferior fronto-occipital fasciculus, uncinate fasciculus, and inferior longitudinal fasciculus (Tzarouchi et al., 2011). This study also found increased MD in many brain fiber tracts in PSS compared to controls.

Studies that integrate cognitive and neuroimaging data in PSS are also rare, but are beginning to emerge. In a study of 321 PSS patients presenting with neurological symptoms, 16% (51 patients) had at least one neuroimaging study, and of that group, 25 had WM abnormalities (Akasbi et al., 2012). WM abnormalities were classified as vascular changes in 21 patients, with ten showing multiple small focal lesions, seven with a confluence of lesions, and four having diffuse involvement. In addition, four patients were classified as having inflammatory/demyelinating lesions that were MS-like in nature. Of the 25 PSS patients, ten had cognitive impairment. Notably, with the subjects without WM abnormalities used as a comparison group, the patients with WM abnormalities were significantly older (mean age 70.3 vs. 58.3), were receiving less antimalarials, had lower leukopenia, lower anti-La/SS-Band, and higher frequency of cardiovascular risk factors (i.e., diabetes, metabolic syndrome, hypertension, and HDL-c levels). Thus, it is unclear if PSS itself is an independent factor contributing to the WM abnormalities found in this study. One study that focused on hippocampal volumes reported that a group of 66 PSS patients had smaller hippocampi (adjusted for total intracerebral volumes) compared to healthy gender-matched controls (Lauvsnes et al., 2013). These investigators also report that higher hippocampal volume was related to higher scores on a majority of the memory tests administered.

Summary of Findings

Although there are relatively few large comparable studies in PSS, findings to date suggest that up to 40% of PSS patients without NP activity or other autoimmune disorders have cognitive dysfunction. Notably, deficits in attention, memory, and executive function are common. As in other autoimmune diseases affecting cognition, methodological issues limit overall the generalizability of findings. Whereas a number of studies and reviews suggest an increasing awareness of NP activity, including cognitive dysfunction in PSS, a standard approach regarding NP classification has not yet emerged. Mediators of cognitive dysfunction in PSS are not consistently evaluated, and to date, clinical disease activity related to PSS has not been associated with cognitive dysfunction. However, there is some evidence that autoimmune activity may be an underlying mechanism for cognitive changes. Most autoantibodies (other than anti-NR2) or inflammatory measures have yet to be studied in this population. Behavioral factors may also be important, but no studies have yet included aspects of depression, pain, fatigue, sleep, and exercise. Neuroimaging abnormalities implicate both GM damage (cortical and hippocampal volume loss) and WM damage (increased WMHI, and MRS and DTI abnormalities).

Conclusion

A thorough review of cognitive dysfunction in four autoimmune diseases for which substantial information is available—SLE, APS, RA and PSS—indicates that cognitive impairment is common. Even in the absence of overt neurologic or psychiatric features, cognitive dysfunction occurs in up to, or more than, 30% of patients with these diseases. SLE remains the most thoroughly studied autoimmune disease, with less information available in APS, RA, and PSS, but in all four diseases, impairments in attention, memory, executive function, and visuomotor/visuospatial functions are typical, suggesting a diffuse pattern of cerebral dysfunction. Underlying mechanisms related to cognitive dysfunction in the autoimmune diseases remain unclear, but there is evidence that biological features, including specific disease characteristics (severity of disease and associated organ involvement) and various autoimmune factors (especially aPL, anti-NMDA antibodies, and proinflammatory cytokines), contribute to the development of cognitive dysfunction. Behavioral features (depression, pain, fatigue, sleep disorders, and physical inactivity) are not always included in studies of these diseases, but findings suggest that these factors also contribute to cognitive impairment, and likely interact with the inflammation that is characteristic of autoimmune diseases. Neuroimaging studies of cognitive dysfunction in these diseases suggest that WM abnormalities are the most common finding, and emerging evidence indicates that both macrostructural lesions (such as WMHIs) and microstructural WM damage are important in the pathogenesis of cognitive dysfunction. In particular, subtle WM damage early in the course of these diseases may be crucial in the early presentation of cognitive dysfunction. In this regard, the term MCD-SLE has been proposed as a descriptor for the insidious cognitive impairment that has been associated with microstructural WM involvement in SLE, and the MCD concept may be applicable to other autoimmune diseases as well, including APS, RA, and PSS. In SLE, APS, and PSS, diffuse GM abnormalities can also be found, and hippocampal volume loss may be important in producing learning and memory deficits. Thus it is clear that both WM and GM deserve study in these complex diseases. The investigation of WM dysfunction, however, offers a novel approach that could help identify a specific neuropathology that is common to all of these diseases. In addition, WM involvement could offer important insights into the processes by which distributed neural networks are disrupted by these diseases. Moreover, early WM injury could prove central to the understanding of the sequence of pathogenic events producing cognitive decline, and point the way toward effective treatments that could reverse or prevent cognitive impairment before more disabling problems develop. Future neuropsychological studies should employ uniform diagnostic criteria for subject selection, standardized classification, and reporting of NP features (for APS and PSS in particular), and standardized, uniform test batteries that at a minimum include attention and working memory, verbal and visual learning and memory, executive and problem solving, and visuomotor/visuospatial tasks. Larger sample sizes, using multisite studies, are also warranted to accommodate longitudinal designs that will lead to better understanding of disease course and potential treatments. The continued application of neuroimaging techniques that focus on WM (i.e., MRS, DTI) as well as GM (i.e., fMRI) will be highly informative, and the use of CSF analysis for measurement of autoimmune and inflammatory markers promises to yield useful data regarding the autoimmune processes underlying brain dysfunction. Whereas the high frequency of cognitive impairment in the autoimmune diseases is distressingly apparent, few treatment options exist for this problem, and future studies focusing on this area will likely improve the outcome for patients with these challenging diseases.

References

Abda, E. A., Selim, Z. I., Radwan, M. E. Mahmoud, N. M., Herdan, O. M., Mohamad, K. A., & Hamed, S. A. (2013). Markers of acute neuropsychiatric systemic lupus erythematosus: A multidisciplinary evaluation. *Rheumatol International, 33*(5), 1243–1253. doi: 10.1007/s00296-012-2531-0

Abreu, M. R., Jakosky, A., Folgerini, M., Brenol, J. C. T., Xavier, R. M., & Kapczinsky, F. (2005). Neuropsychiatric systemic lupus erythematosus: Correlation of brain MR imaging, CT, and SPECT. *Clinical Imaging, 29*(3), 215–221.

Adhikari, T. (2011). Cognitive dysfunction in SLE: Development of a screening tool. *Lupus, 20*, 1142–1146.

Aharon-Peretz, J., Brenner, B., & Amyel, E. (1995). Neurocognitive dysfunction in antiphospholipid syndrome. *Lupus, 4*(Suppl 2), 101.

Ainiala, H., Hietaharju, A., Dastidar, P., Loukkola, J., Lehtimaki, T., Peltola, J., . . . Nikkari, S. T. (2004). Increased serum matrix metalloproteinase 9 levels in systemic lupus erythematosus patients with neuropsychiatric manifestations and brain magnetic resonance imaging abnormalities. *Arthritis and Rheumatism, 50*(3), 858–865.

Aisen, A. M., Gabrielsen, T. O., & McCune, W. J. (1985). MR imaging of systemic lupus erythematosus involving the brain. *American Journal of Roentgenology, 144*, 1027–1031.

Akasbi, M., Berenguer, J., Saiz, A., Brito-Zerón, P., Pérez-De-Lis, M., Bové, A., . . . Ramos-Casals, M. (2012). White matter abnormalities in primary Sjögren syndrome. *QJM: Monthly Journal of the Association of Physicians, 105*(5), 433–443. doi: 10.1093/qjmed/hcr218

Alarcon, G. S., Cianfrini, L., Bradley, L. A., Sanchez, M. L., Brooks, K., Friedman, A. W., . . . Reveille, J. D. (2002). Systemic lupus erythematosus in three ethnic groups: X. Measuring cognitive impairment with the cognitive symptoms inventory. *Arthritis and Rheumatism, 47*(3), 310–319. PMID: 12115162.

Alcocer-Varela, J., Aleman-Hoey, D., & Alarcon-Segovia, D. (1992). Interleukin-1 and interleukin-6 activities are increased in the cerebrospinal fluid of patients with CNS lupus erythematosus and correlate with local late T-cell activation markers. *Lupus, 1*, 111–117.

Alexander, E. L. (1986). Central nervous system (CNS) manifestions of primary Sjogren's syndrome: An overview. *Scandanavian Journal of Rheumatology, 61*(Suppl), 161–165.

Alexander, E. L., Beall, S. S., Gordon, B., Seines, O. A., Yannakakis, G. D., Patronas, N., . . . McFarland, H. F. (1988). Magnetic resonance imaging of cerebral lesions in patients with the Sjogren syndrome. *Annals of Internal Medicine, 108*(6), 815–823.

al-Janadi, M., al-Balla, S., al-Dalaan, A., & Raziuddin, S. (1993). Cytokine profile in systemic lupus erythematosus, rheumatoid arthritis, and other rheumatic diseases. *Journal of Clinical Immunology, 13*(1), 58–67.

American College of Rheumatology. (1999). The American college of rheumatology nomenclature and case definitions for neuropsychiatric lupus syndromes. *Arthritis and Rheumatism, 42*(4), 599–608. PMID: 10211873.

Andonopoulos, A. P., Lagos, G., Drosos, A. A., & Moutsopoulos, H. M. (1990). The spectrum of neurological involvement in Sjogren's syndrome. *British Journal of Rheumatology, 29*(1), 21–23.

Appenzeller, S., Bonilha, L., Rio, P. A., Min Li, L., Costallat, L. T., & Cendes, F. (2007). Longitudinal analysis of gray and white matter loss in patients with systemic lupus erythematosus. *NeuroImage, 34*(2), 694–701. PMID: 17112740.

Appenzeller, S., Carnevalle, A. D., Li, L. M., Costallat, L. T. L., & Cendes, F. (2006). Hippocampal atrophy in systemic lupus erythematosus. *Annals of Rheumatic Disease, 65*(12), 1585–1589. PMID: 16439436.

Appenzeller, S. Costallat, L. T., & Condes, F. (2004, May 9–13). *Analyzing white matter involvement in systemic lupus erythematosus by voxel-based morphometry*. Paper presented at the 7th Annual International Congress of SLE and Related Conditions, New York.

Appenzeller, S., Li, L. M., Costallat, L. T. L., & Cendes, F. (2005). Evidence of reversible axonal dysfunction in systemic lupus erythematosus: A proton MRS study. *Brain: A Journal of Neurology, 128*(Pt 12), 2933–2940.

Appenzeller, S., Li, L. M., Costallat, L. T., & Cendes, F. (2007). Neurometabolic changes in normal white matter may predict appearance of hyperintense lesions in systemic lupus erythematosus. *Lupus, 16*(12), 963–971. PMID: 18042590.

Appenzeller, S., Pike, G. B., & Clarke, A. E. (2008). Magnetic resonance imaging in the evaluation of central nervous system manifestations in systemic lupus erythematosus. *Clinical Reviews in Allergy & Immunology, 34*(3), 361–366. PMID: 18084729. doi: 10.1007/s12016-007-8060-z

Appenzeller, S., Rondina, J. M., Li, L. M., Costallat, L. T. L., & Cendes, F. (2005). Cerebral and corpus callosum atrophy in systemic lupus erythematosus. *Arthritis and Rheumatism, 52*(9), 2783–2789.

Appenzeller, S., Vasconcelos Faria, A., Li, L. M., Costallat, L. T., & Cendes, F. (2008). Quantitative magnetic resonance imaging analyses and clinical significance of hyperintense white matter lesions in systemic lupus erythematosus patients. *Annals of Neurology, 64*(6), 635–643. PMID: 19107986. doi: 10.1002/ana.21483

Arinuma, Y., Yanagida, T., & Hirohata, S. (2008). Association of cerebrospinal fluid anti-NR2 glutamate receptor antibodies with diffuse neuropsychiatric systemic lupus erythematosus. *Arthritis and Rheumatism, 58*(4), 1130–1135.

Asherson, R. A., Khamashata, M. A., Gil, A., Vazquez, J. J., Chan, O., Baguley, E., et al. (1989). Cerebrovascular disease and antiphospholipid antibodies in systemic lupus erythematosus, lupus-like disease and the primary antiphospholipid syndrome. *American Journal of Medicine, 86*(4), 391–399.

Bartolini, M., Candela, M., Brugni, M., Catena, L., Mari, F., Pomponio, G., et al. (2002). Are behavior and motor performances of rheumatoid arthritis patients influenced by subclinical cognitive impairments? A clinical and neuroimaging study. *Clinical and Experimental Rheumatology, 20*, 491–497.

Bauman, A., Barnes, C., & Schrieber, L. (1989). The unmet needs of patients with systemic lupus erythematosus: Planning for patient education. *Patient Education and Counseling, 14*, 235–242.

Bell, C. L., Partington, C., Robbins, M., Graziano, F., Turski, P., & Kornguth, S. (1991). Magnetic resonance imaging of central nervous system lesions in patients with lupus erythematosus: Correlation with clinical remission and antineurofilament and anticardiolipin antibody titers [see comments]. *Arthritis Rheumatology, 34*(4), 432–441.

Belmont, H. M., Abramson, S. B., & Lie, J. T. (1996). Pathology and pathogenesis of vascular injury in systemic lupus erythematosus: Interactions of inflammatory cells and activated endothelium. *Arthritis and Rheumatism, 39*(1), 9–22.

Belmont, H. M., Hopkins, P., Edelson, H. S., Kaplan, H. B., Ludewig, R., Weissmann, G., & Abramson, S. (1986). Complement activation during systemic lupus erythematosus: C3a and C5a anaphylatoxins circulate during exacerbations of disease. *Arthritis and Rheumatism, 29*(9), 1085–1089.

Bennett, G. W., Ballard, T. M., Watson, C. D., & Fone, K. C. (1997). Effect of neuropeptides on cognitive function. *Experimental Gerontology*, *32*(4–5), 451–469.

Benveniste, E. N. (1992). Inflammatory cytokines within the central nervous system: Sources, function, and mechanism of action. *The American Journal of Physiology*, *263*(1 Pt 1), C1–C16.

Binder, A., Snaith, M. L., & Isenberg, D. (1988). Sjorgerns syndrome: A study of its neurological complications. *British Journal of Rheumatology*, *27*, 275–288.

Bluestein, H. G. (1992). The central nervous system in systemic lupus erythematosus. In R. G. Lahita (Ed.), *Systemic Lupus Erythematosus* (2nd ed., pp. 639–655). New York: Churchill Livingstone, Inc.

Bluestein, H. G., Williams, G. W., & Steinberg, A. D. (1981). Cerebrospinal fluid antibodies to neuronal cells: Association with neuropsychiatric manifestations of systemic lupus erythematosus. *American Journal of Medicine*, *70*(2), 240–246.

Bluestein, H. G., & Woods, V. L. (1982). Antineuronal antibodies in systemic lupus erythematosus. *Arthritis & Rheumatology*, *25*(7), 773–778.

Bolstad, A. I., & Jonsson, R. (2002). Genetic aspects of Sjögren's syndrome. *Arthritis Research*, *4*(6), 353–359.

Bonfa, E., Golombek, S. J., Kaufman, L. D., Skelly, S., Weissbach, H., Brot, & Elkon, K. B. (1987). Association between lupus psychosis and anti-ribosomal P protein antibodies. *The New England Journal of Medicine*, *317*(5), 265–271.

Borchers, A. T., Naguwa, S. M., Keen, C. L., & Gershwin, M. E. (2003). Immunopathogenesis of Sjögren's syndrome. *Clinical Reviews in Allergy & Immunology*, *25*(1), 89–104.

Bosma, G. P., Steens, S. C., Petropoulos, H., Admiraal-Behloul, F., van den Haak, A., Doornbos, J., . . . van Buchem, M. A. (2004). Multisequence magnetic resonance imaging study of neuropsychiatric systemic lupus erythematosus. *Arthritis and Rheumatism*, *50*(10), 3195–3202.

Bracci-Laudiero, L., Aloe, L., Lundeberg, T., Theodorsson, E., & Stenfors, C. (1999). Altered levels of neuropeptides characterize the brain of lupus prone mice. *Neuroscience Letters*, *275*(1), 57–60.

Brey, R. L., Holliday, S. L., Saklad, A. R., Navarrete, M. G., Hermosillo-Romo, D., Stallworth, C. L., . . . McGlasson, D. (2002). Neuropsychiatric syndromes in lupus: Prevalence using standardized definitions. *Neurology*, *58*(8), 1214–1220. PMID: 11971089.

Brey, R. L., Muscal, E., & Chapman, J. (2011). Antiphospholipid antibodies and the brain: A consensus report. *Lupus*, *20*(2), 153–157. doi: 10.1177/0961203310396748

Brooks, W. M., Jung, R. E., Ford, C. C., Greinel, E. J., & Sibbitt, W. L., Jr. (1999). Relationship between neurometabolite derangement and neurocognitive dysfunction in systemic lupus erythematosus. *The Journal of Rheumatology*, *26*(1), 81–85. PMID: 9918245.

Brooks, W. M., Sabet, A., Sibbitt, W. L., Jr., Barker, P. B., van Zijl, P. C., Duyn, J. H., & Moonen, C. T. (1997). Neurochemistry of brain lesions determined by spectroscopic imaging in systemic lupus erythematosus. *The Journal of Rheumatology*, *24*(12), 2323–2329. PMID: 9415636.

Brown, S. C., Glass, J. M., & Park, D. C. (2002). The relationship of pain and depression to cognitive function in rheumatoid arthritis patients. *Pain*, *96*(3), 279–284.

Carbotte, R. M., Denburg, S. D., & Denburg, J. A. (1986). Prevalence of cognitive impairment in systemic lupus erythematosus. *Journal of Nervous and Mental Disease*, *174*(6), 357–364. PMID: 3711879.

Carbotte, R. M., Denburg, S. D., & Denburg, J. A. (1995). Cognitive dysfunction in systemic lupus erythematosus is independent of active disease. *The Journal of Rheumatology*, *22*(5), 863–867. PMID: 8587073.

Carbotte, R. M., Denburg, S. D., Denburg, J. A, Nahmias, C., & Garnett, E. S. (1992). Fluctuating cognitive abnormalities and cerebral glucose metabolism in neuropsychiatric lupus erythematosus. *Journal of Neurology, Neurosurgery, and Psychiatry*, *55*, 1054–1059.

Carecchio, M., Cantello, R., & Comi, C. (2014). Revisiting the molecular mechanism of neurological manifestations in antiphospholipid syndrome: Beyond vascular damage. *Journal of Immunology Research*, *2014*(2014), 239398.

Carlomagno, S., Migliaresi, S., Ambrosone, L., Sannino, M., Sanges, G., & Di Iorio, G. (2000). Cognitive impairment in systemic lupus erythematosus: A follow-up study. *Journal of Neurology*, *247*(4), 273–279. PMID: 10836619.

Castellino, G., Govoni, M., Padovan, M., Colamussi, P., Borrelli, M., & Trotta, F. (2005). Proton magnetic resonance spectroscopy may predict future brain lesions in SLE patients: A functional multi-imaging approach and follow up. *Annals of Rheumatic Diseases*, *64*(7), 1022–1027.

Castellino, G., Padovan, M., Bortoluzzi, A., Borrelli, M., Feggi, L., Caniatti, M. L. . . . Govoni, M. (2008). Single photon emission computed tomography and magnetic resonance imaging evaluation in SLE patients with and without neuropsychiatric involvement. *Rheumatology (Oxford)*, *47*(3), 319–323. doi: 10.1093/rheumatology/kem354

Cervera, R., Piette, J. C., Font, J., Khamashta, M. A., Shoenfeld, Y., Camps, M. T., . . . Ingelmo, M. (2002). Antiphospholipid syndrome: Clinical and immunologic manifestations and patterns of disease expression in a cohort of 1,000 patients. *Arthritis and Rheumatism*, *46*(4), 1019–1027.

Chakravarty, E. F., Bush, T. M., Manzi, S., Clarke, A. E., & Ward, M. M. (2007). Prevalence of adult systemic lupus erythematosus in California and Pennsylvania in 2000: Estimates obtained using hospitalization data. *Arthritis and Rheumatism*, *56*(6), 2092–2094. doi: 10.1002/art.22641

Chandrasekhara, P. K., Jayachandran, N. V., Rajasekhar, L., Thomas, J., & Narsimulu, G. (2009). The prevalence and associations of sleep disturbances in patients with systemic lupus erythematosus. *Modern Rheumatology*, *19*(4), 407–415. PMID: 19521744. doi: 10.1007/s10165-009-0185-x

Chapman, J., Abu-Katash, M., Inzelberg, R., Yust, I., Neufeld, M. Y., Vardinon, N., . . . Korczyn, A. D. (2002). Prevalence and clinical features of dementia associated with the antiphospholipid syndrome and circulating anticoagulants. *Journal of the Neurological Sciences*, *203–204*, 81–84.

Chapman, J., Cohen-Armon, M., Shoenfeld, Y., & Korczyn, A. D. (1999). Antiphospholipid antibodies permeabilize and depolarize brain synaptoneurosomes. *Lupus*, *8*(2), 127–133.

Chen, J. J.-H., Yen, R.-F., Kao, A., Lin, C.-C., & Lee, C.-C. (2002). Abnormal regional cerebral blood flow found by technetium-99m ethyl cysteinate dimer brain single photon emission computed tomography in systemic lupus erythematosus patients with normal brain MRI findings. *Clinical Rheumatology*, *21*(6), 516–519.

Chinn, R. J., Wilkinson, I. D., Hall-Craggs, M. A., Paley, M. N., Shortall, E., Carter, S., . . . Harrison, M. J. (1997). Magnetic resonance imaging of the brain and cerebral proton spectroscopy in patients with systemic lupus erythematosus. *Arthritis and Rheumatism*, *40*(1), 36–46. PMID: 9008598.

Coin-Mejias, M. A., Peralta-Ramirez, M. I., Santiago-Ramajo, S., Morente-Soto, G., Ortego-Centeno, N., Rubio, J. L., . . . Perez-Garcia, M. (2008). Alterations in episodic memory in patients with systemic lupus erythematosus. *Archives of Clinical Neuropsychology: The Official Journal of the National Academy of Neuropsychologists*, *23*(2), 157–164.

Conti, F., Alessandri, C., Perricone, C., Scrivo, R., Rezai, S., Ceccarelli, F., . . . Mina, C. (2012). Neurocognitve dysfunction in systemic lupus erythematosus: Association with antiphospholipid antibodies, disease activity and chronic damage. *PloS One*, *7*(3), e33824. doi: 10.1371/journal.pone.0033824

Covey, T. J., Shucard, J. L., Shucard, D. W., Stegen, S., & Benedict, R. H. (2012). Comparison of neuropsychological impairment and vocational outcomes in systemic lupus erythematosus and multiple sclerosis patients. *Journal of the International Neuropsychological Society: JINS*, *18*(3), 530–540. doi: 10.1017/S1355617712000057

Csepany, T., Gulyas, B., Tron, L., Szakall, S., Kiss, E., Kollar, J., . . . Csiba, L. (1997). Cerebral positron emission tomographic study in systemic lupus erytematosus. *Orvosi Hetilap*, *138*, 1947–1952.

Davie, C. A., Feinstein, A., Kartsounis, L. D., Barker, G. J., McHugh, N. J., Walport, M. J., . . . Miller, D. H. (1995). Proton magnetic resonance spectroscopy of systemic lupus erythematosus involving the central nervous system. *Journal of Neurology*, *242*(8), 522–528. PMID: 8530981.

DeGiorgio, L. A., Konstantinov, K. N., Lee, S. C., Hardin, J. A., Volpe, B. T., & Diamond, B. (2001). A subset of lupus anti-DNA antibodies cross-reacts with the NR2 glutamate receptor in systemic lupus erythematosus. *Nature Medicine*, *7*(11), 1189–1193.

Dellalibera-Joviliano, R., Dos Reis, M. L., Cunha Fde, Q., & Donadi, E. A. (2003). Kinins and cytokines in plasma and cerebrospinal fluid of patients with neuropsychiatric lupus. *The Journal of Rheumatology*, *30*(3), 485–492.

Denburg, S. D., Carbotte, R. M., & Denburg, J. A. (1987a). Cognitive impairment in systemic lupus erythematosus: A neuropsychological study of individual and group deficits. *Journal of Clinical and Experimental Neuropsychology*, *9*(4), 323–339.

Denburg, J. A., Carbotte, R. M., & Denburg, S. D. (1987b). Neuronal antibodies and cognitive function in systemic lupus erythematosus. *Neurology*, *37*(3), 464–467. PMID: 3822139.

Denburg, S. D., Carbotte, R. M., & Denburg, J. A. (1993). Cognitive correlates of antiphospholipid antibody positivity in SLE [abstract]. *Arthritis & Rheumatology*, *36*(Suppl 9), S103.

Denburg, S. D., Carbotte, R. M., & Denburg, J. A. (1994). Corticosteroids and neuropsychological functioning in patients with systemic lupus erythematosus. *Arthritis and Rheumatism*, *37*(9), 1311–1320.

Denburg, S. D., Carbotte, R. M., & Denburg, J. A. (1997). Psychological aspects of systemic lupus erythematosus: Cognitive function, mood, and self-report. *The Journal of Rheumatology*, *24*(5), 998–1003. PMID: 9150099.

Denburg, S. D., Carbotte, R. M., Ginsberg, J. S., & Denburg, J. A. (1997). The relationship of antiphospholipid antibodies to cognitive function in patients with systemic lupus erythematosus. *Journal of the International Neuropsychological Society: JINS*, *3*(4), 377–386.

Denburg, S. D., Carbotte, R. M., Long, A. A., & Denburg, J. A. (1988). Neuropsychological correlates of serum lymphocytotoxic antibodies in sysemic lupus erythematosus. *Brain, Behavior, and Immunity*, *2*(3), 222–234. PMID: 3242655.

Denburg, S. D., & Denburg, J. A. (1999). Cognitive dysfunction in systemic lupus erythematosus. In R. G. Lahita (Ed.), *Systemic Lupus Erythematosus* (3rd ed.). New York: Academic Press.

Denburg, S. D., Denburg, J. A., Carbotte, R. M., Fisk, J. D., & Hanly, J. G. (1993). Cognitive deficits in systemic lupus erythematosus. *Rheumatic Disease Clinics of North America*, *19*(4), 815–831.

Dick, B., Eccleston, C., & Crombez, G. (2002). Attentional functioning in fibromyalgia, rheumatoid arthritis, and musculoskeletal pain patients. *Arthritis and Rheumatism*, *47*(6), 639–644.

Difrancesco, M. W., Gitelman, D. R., Klein, M. S., Sagcal-Gironella, A. C., Zelfo, F., Beebe, D., . . . Brunner, H. I. (2013). Functional neuronal network activity differs with dysfunction in childhood-onset systemic lupus erythematosus. *Arthritis Research and Therapy*, *15*(2), R40.

Difrancesco, M. W., Holland, S. K., Ris, M. D., Adler, C. M., Nelson, S., Delbello, M. P., . . . Brunner, H. I. (2007). Functional magnetic resonance imaging assessment of cognitive function in childhood-onset systemic lupus erythematosus: A pilot study. *Arthritis and Rheumatism*, *56*(12), 4151–4163.

Doninger, N. A., Fink, J. W., & Utset, T. O. (2005). Neuropsychologic functioning and health status in systemic lupus erythematosus: Does ethnicity matter? *Journal of Clinical Rheumatology*, *11*(5), 250–256.

Kozora, E., Zell, J., Swigris, J., Duggan, E., & Make, B. (2012). Sleep Abnormalities and Cognitive Dysfunction in Systemic Lupus Erythematosus (SLE). *Journal of the International Neuropsychological Society*, *18*(S1), 129.

Elliott, M. J., & Maini, R. N. (1995). Anti-cytokine therapy in rheumatoid arthritis. *Bailliere's Clinical Rheumatology*, *9*(4), 633–652.

Ellis, S. G., & Verity, M. A. (1979). Central nervous system involvement in systemic lupus erythematosus: A review of neuropathologic findings in 57 cases, 1955–1977. *Seminars in Arthritis and Rheumatism*, *8*(3), 212–221.

El-Shafey, A. M., Abd-El-Geleel, S. M., & Soliman, E. S. (2012). Cognitive impairment in non-neuropsychiatric systemic lupus erythematosus. *The Egyptian Rheumatologist*, *34*(2), 67–73. doi: 10.1016/j.ejr.2012.02.002

Emmer, B. J., Steens, S. C., Steup-Beekman, G. M., van der Grond, J., Admiraal-Behloul, F., Olofsen, H., . . . van Buchem, M. A. (2006). Detection of change in CNS involvement in neuropsychiatric SLE: A magnetization transfer study. *Journal of Magnetic Resonance Imaging*, *24*(4), 812–816.

Emmer, B. J., van der Bijl, A. E., Huizinga, T. W., Breedveld, F. C., Steens, S. C., Th Bosma, G. P., . . . van der Grond, J. (2009). Brain involvement in rheumatoid arthritis: A magnetic resonance spectroscopy study. *Arthritis and Rheumatism*, *60*(11), 3190–3195. doi: 10.1002/art.24932

Emmer, B. J., Veer, I. M., Steup-Beekman, G. M., Huizinga, T. W., van der Grond, J., & van Buchem, M. A. (2010). Tract-based spatial statistics on diffusion tensor imaging in systemic lupus erythematosus reveals localized involvement of white matter tracts. *Arthritis and Rheumatism*, *62*(12), 3716–3721. doi: 10.1002/art.27717

Emori, A., Matsushima, E., Aihara, O., Ohta, K., Koike, R., Miyasaka, N., & Kato, M. (2005). Cognitive dysfunction in systemic lupus erythematosus. *Psychiatry and Clinical Neurosciences*, *59*(5), 584–589.

Epstein, L. C., Masse, G., Harmatz, J. S., Scott, T. M., Papas, A. S., & Greenblatt, D. J. (2014). Characterization of cognitive dysfunction in Sjögren's syndrome patients. *Clinical Rheumatology*, *33*(4), 511–521. doi: 10.1007/s10067-013-2453-6

Erkan, D., Kozora, E., & Lockshin, M. D. (2011). Cognitive dysfunction and white matter abnormalities in antiphospholipid syndrome. *Pathophysiology: The Official Journal of the International Society for Pathophysiology/ISP*, *18*(1), 93–102. doi: 10.1016/j.pathophys.2010.04.010

Erkan, D., Vega, J., Ramon, G., Kozora, E., & Lockshin, M. D. (2013). A pilot open-label phase II trial of rituximab for non-criteria manifestations of antiphospholipid syndrome. *Arthritis and Rheumatism*, *65*(2), 464–471. doi: 10.1002/art.37759

Fauchais, A. L., Magy, L., & Vidal, E. (2012). Central and peripheral neurological complications of primary Sjögren's syndrome. *La Presse Medicale*, *41*. doi: 10.1016/j.lpm.2012.06.002

Felver-Gant, J. C., Bruce, A. S., Zimmerman, M., Sweet, L. H., Millman, R. P., & Aloia, M. S. (2007). Working memory in obstructive sleep apnea: Construct validity and treatment effects. *Journal of Clinical Sleep Medicine*, *3*(6), 589–594. PMID: 17993040.

Ferstl, R., Niemann, T., Biehl, G., Hinrichsen, H., & Kirch, W. (1992). Neuropsychological impairment in auto-immune disease. *European Journal of Clinical Investigation*, 16–20.

Fields, R. A., Sibbitt, W. L., Toubbeh, H., & Bankhurst, A. D. (1990). Neuropsychiatric lupus erythematosus, cerebral infarctions, and anticardiolipin antibodies. *Annals of Rheumatic Diseases*, *49*(2), 114–117.

Filley, C. M. (2009). Exploring white matter microstructure: New insights from diffusion tensor imaging. *Neurology*, *73*(21), 1718–1719. PMID: 19846831. doi: WNL.0b013e3181c2936b

Filley, C. M., Kozora, E., Brown, M. S., Miller, D. E., West, S. G., Arciniegas, D. B., . . . Zhang, L. (2009). White matter microstructure and cognition in non-neuropsychiatric systemic lupus erytematosus. *Cognitive and Behavioral Neurology: Official Journal of the Society for Behavioral and Cognitive Neurology*, *22*(1), 38–44. PMID: 19372769.

Fisk, J. D., Eastwood, B., Sherwood, G., & Hanly, J. G. (1993). Patterns of cognitive impairment in patients with systemic lupus erythematosus. *British Journal of Rheumatology*, *32*(6), 458–462. PMID: 8508281.

Fitzgibbon, B. M., Fairhall, S. L., Kirk, I. J., Kalev-Zylinska, M., Pui, K., Dalbeth, N., . . . McQueen, F. M. (2008). Functional MRI in NPSLE patients reveals increased parietal and frontal brain activation during a working memory task compared with controls. *Rheumatology (Oxford)*, *47*(1), 50–53.

Flood, J. F., Morley, J. E., & Roberts, E. (1992). Memory enhancing effects in male mice of Pregnenolone and steroids metabolically derived from it. *Proceedings of the Natinal Academy of Sciences*, *89*, 1567–1571.

Flood, J. F., & Roberts, E. (1988). Dehydroepiandrosterone sulfate improves memory in aging mice. *Brain Research*, *448*(1), 178–181.

Folstein, M. F., Folstein, S. E., & McHugh, P. R. (1975). "Mini-mental state": A practical method for grading the cognitive state of patients for the clinician. *Journal of Psychiatric Research*, *12*(3), 189–198.

Fox, R. I., Stern, M., & Michelson, P. (2000). Update in Sjögren syndrome. *Current Opinion in Rheumatology*, *12*(5), 391–398.

Frank, E., & Landgraf, R. (2008). The vasopressin system--from antidiuresis to psychopathology. *European Journal of Pharmacology*, *583*(2–3), 226–242.

Friedman, S. D., Brooks, W. M., Jung, R. E., Hart, B. L., & Yeo, R. A. (1998). Proton MR spectroscopic findings correspond to neuropsychological function in traumatic brain injury. *AJNR: American Journal of Neuroradiology*, *19*(10), 1879–1885.

Giang, D. W. (1991). Systemic lupus erythematosus and depression. *Neuropsychiatry Neuropsychology and Behavioral Neurology*, *4*, 78–82.

Ginsburg, K. S., Wright, E. A., Larson, M. G., Fossel, A. H., Albert, M., Schur, P. H., & Liang, M. H. (1992). A controlled study of the prevalence of cognitive dysfunction in randomly selected patients with systemic lupus erythematosus. *Arthritis and Rheumatism*, *35*(7), 776–782. PMID: 1622416.

Gladman, D. D., Urowitz, M. B., Slonim, D., Glanz, B., Carlen, P., Noldy, N., . . . MacKinnon, A. (2000). Evaluation of predictive factors for neurocognitive dysfunction in patients with inactive systemic lupus erythematosus. *The Journal of Rheumatology*, *27*(10), 2367–2371. PMID: 11036831.

Glanz, B. I., Schur, P. H., Lew, R. A., & Khoshbin, S. (2005). Lateralized cognitive dysfunction in patients with systemic lupus erythematosus. *Lupus*, *14*(11), 896–902. PMID: 16335582.

Glanz, B. I., Slonim, D., Urowitz, M. B., Gladman, D. D., Gough, J., & MacKinnon, A. (1997). Pattern of neuropsychologic dysfunction in inactive systemic lupus erythematosus. *Neuropsychiatry Neuropsychology and Behavioral Neurology*, *10*(4), 232–238. PMID 9359119.

Gomez-Puerta, J. A., Cervera, R., Calvo, L. M., Gomez-Anson, B., Espinosa, G., Claver, G., . . . Font, J. (2005). Dementia associated with the antiphospholipid syndrome: Clinical and radiological characteristics of 30 patients. *Rheumatology (Oxford)*, *44*(1), 95–99.

Gonzalez-Crespo, M. R., Blanco, F. J., Ramos, A., Ciruelo, E., Mateo, I., Lopez-Pino, M. A., & Gomez-Reino, J. J. (1995). Magnetic resonance imaging of the brain in systemic lupus erythematosus. *British Journal of Rheumatology*, *34*, 1055–1060.

Gorman, D. G., & Cummings, J. L. (1993). Neurobehavioral presentations of the antiphospholipid antibody syndrome. *The Journal of Neuropsychiatry and Clinical Neurosciences*, *5*(1), 37–42.

Graham, J. W., & Jan, W. (2003). MRI and the brain in systemic lupus erythematosus. *Lupus*, *12*(12), 891–896.

Greenberg, G. D., Watson, R. K., & Deptula, D. (1987). Neuropsychological dysfunction in sleep apnea. *Sleep*, *10*(3), 254–262. PMID: 3629088.

Greenwood, K. M., Lederman, L. L., & Lindner, H. D. (2008). Self-reported sleep in systemic lupus erythematosus. *Clinical Rheumatology*, *27*(9), 1147–1151. PMID: 18408880. doi: 10.1007/s10067-008-0884-2

Griffey, R. H., Brown, M. S., Bankhurst, A. D., Sibbitt, R. R., & Sibbitt, W. L., Jr. (1990). Depletion of high-energy phosphates in the central nervous system of patients with systemic lupus erythematosus, as determined by phosphorus-31 nuclear magnetic resonance spectroscopy. *Arthritis and Rheumatism*, *33*(6), 827–833.

Grigsby, J., Rosenberg, N. L., & Busenvark, D. (1994). Chronic pain adversely effects information processing. *Archive of Clinical Neuropsychology*, *9*, 135–136.

Gronwall, D. M. (1977). Paced auditory serial additional test: A measure of recovery from concussion. *Perceptual and Motor Skills*, *44*(2), 367–373. PMID: 866038.

Hachulla, E., Michon-Pasturel, U., Leys, D., Pruvo, J. P., Queyrel, V., Masy, E., . . . Devulder, B. (1998). Cerebral magnetic resonance imaging in patients with or without antiphospholipid antibodies. *Lupus*, *7*(2), 124–131.

Haider, H., Zakarya, S., & Abu-Hegazy, M. (2012). White matter microstructure and cognitive dysfunction in systemic lupus patients. *Egyptian Journal of Neurology, Psychiatry, & Neurosurgery, 49*(3), 199–206.

Hall, R. C., & Stickney, S. K. (1983). Medical and psychiatric features of systemic lupus erythematosus. *Psychiatric Medicine, 1*(3), 287–301. PMID: 6599852.

Hamed, S. A., Selim, Z. I., Elattar, A. M., Elserogy, Y. M., Ahmed, E. A., & Mohamed, H. O. (2012). Assessment of biocorrelates for brain involvement in female patients with rheumatoid arthritis. *Clinical Rheumatology, 3*(1), 123–132. doi: 10.1007/s10067-011-1795-1

Handa, R., Sahota, P., Kumar, M., Jagannathan, N. R., Bal, C. S., Gulati, M., . . . Wali, J. P. (2003). In vivo proton magnetic resonance spectroscopy (MRS) and single photon emission computerized tomography (SPECT) in systemic lupus erythematosus (SLE). *Magnetic Resonance Imaging, 21*(9), 1033–1037.

Hanly, J. G. (2007). Antineuronal antibodies. In G. C. Tsokos, C. Gordon, & J. S. Smolen (Eds.), *Systemic Lupus Erythematosis: A Companion to Rheumatology* (1st ed., pp. 241–247). Philadelphia, PA: Mosby Elsevier.

Hanly, J. G., Cassell, K., & Fisk, J. D. (1997). Cognitive function in systemic lupus erythematosus: Results of a 5-year prospective study. *Arthritis & Rheumatsim, 40*(8), 1542–1543. PMID: 9259438.

Hanly, J. G., Fisk, J. D., Sherwood, G., & Eastwood, B. (1994). Clinical course of cognitive dysfunction in systemic lupus erythematosus. *Journal of Rheum, 21*(10), 1825–1831. PMID: 7837145.

Hanly, J. G., Fisk, J. D., Sherwood, G., Jones, E., Jones, J. V., & Eastwood, B. (1992). Cognitive impairment in patients with systemic lupus erythematosus. *The Journal of rheumatology, 19*(4), 562–567. PMID: 1593578.

Hanly, J. G., & Harrison, M. J. (2005). Management of neuropsychiatric lupus. *Best Practice and Research Clinical Rheumatology, 19*(5), 799–821.

Hanly, J. G., Hong, C., Smith, S., & Fisk, J. D. (1999). A prospective analysis of cognitive function and anticardiolipin antibodies in systemic lupus erythematosus. *Arthritis & Rheumatolgy, 42*(4), 728–734. PMID: 10211887.

Hanly, J. G., Omisade, A., Su, L., Farewell, V., & Fisk, J. D. (2010). Assessment of cognitive function in systemic lupus erythematosus, rheumatoid arthritis and multiple sclerosis by computerized neuropsychological tests. *Arthritis and Rheumatism, 62*, 1278–1486.

Hanly, J. G., Robichaud, J., & Fisk, J. D. (2006). Anti-NR2 glutamate receptor antibodies and cognitive function in systemic lupus erythematosus. *The Journal of Rheumatology, 33*(8), 1553–1558.

Hanly, J. G., Su, L., Omisade, A., Farewell, V. T., & Fisk, J. D. (2012). Screening for cognitive impairment in systemic lupus erythematosus. *The Journal of Rheumatology, 39*(7), 1371–1377. doi: 10.3899/jrheum.111504

Hanly, J. G., Urowitz, M. B., Su, L., Base, S. C., Gordon, C., Clarke, A., . . . Merrill, J. T. (2011). Autoantibodies as biomarkers for the prediction of neuropsychiatric events isn systemic lupus erythematosus. *Annals of Rheumatic Diseases, 70*(10), 1726–1732. doi: 10.1136/ard.2010.148502

Hanly, J. G., Walsh, N. M., Fisk, J. D., Eastwood, B., Hong, C., Sherwood, G., . . . Elkon, K. (1993). Cognitive impairment and autoantibodies in systemic lupus erythematosus. *British Journal of Rheumatology, 32*(4), 291–296. PMID: 8461922.

Harle, P., Straub, R. H., Wiest, R., Mayer, A., Scholmerich, J., Atzeni, F., . . . Sarzi-Puttini, P. (2006). Increase of sympathetic outflow measured by neuropeptide Y and decrease of the hypothalamic-pituitary-adrenal axis tone in patients with systemic lupus erythematosus and rheumatoid arthritis: Another example of uncoupling of response systems. *Annals of Rheumatic Diseases, 65*(1), 51–56.

Harrison, M. J., Morris, K. A., Horton, R., Toglia, J., Barsky, J., Chait, S., . . . Robbins, L. (2005). Results of intervention for lupus patients with self-perceived cognitive difficulties. *Neurology, 65*(8), 1325–1327.

Harrison, M. J., Ravdin, L., Volpe, B., et al. (2004, May 9–13, 2004). *Anti-NR2 antibody does not identify cognitive dysfunction in a general SLE population.* Paper presented at the The International Congress SLE and Related Conditions: Lupus 2004, New York.

Hay, E. M., Black, D., Huddy, A., Creed, F., Tomenson, B., Bernstein, R. M., & Holt, P. J. (1992). Psychiatric disorder and cognitive impairment in systemic lupus erythematosus. *Arthritis and Rheumatism, 35*(4), 411–416. PMID: 1567490.

Hay, E. M., Huddy, A., Black, D., Mbaya, P., Tomenson, B., Bernstein, R. M., . . . Creed, F. (1994). A prospective study of psychiatric disorder and cognitive function in systemic lupus erythematosus. *Annals of Rheumatic Diseases, 53*(5), 298–303. PMID: 8017982.

Helmick, C. G., Felson, D. T., Lawrence, R. C., Gabriel, S., Hirsch, R., Kwoh, C. K., . . . Stone, J. H. (2008). Estimates of the prevalence of arthritis and other rheumatic conditions in the United States: Part I. *Arthritis and Rheumatism, 58*(1), 15–25. doi: 10.1002/art.23177

Hirohata, S., & Miyamoto, T. (1990). Elevated levels of interleukin-6 in cerebrospinal fluid from patients with systemic lupus erythematosus and central nervous system involvement. *Arthritis and Rheumatism, 33*(5), 644–649.

Hochberg, M. C. (1997). Updating the American College of Rheumatology revised criteria for the classification of systemic lupus erythematosus. *Arthritis & Rheumatolgy, 40*(9), 1725. PMID: 9324032.

Holliday, S., Naqibuddin, M., Brey, R., & Petri, M. (2005). *Change in cognition function over time in newly diagnosed SLE: Brain CONECTIONS.* Paper presented at the Thirty-Third International Neuropsychological Society Conference, St. Louis, MO.

Holliday, S. L., Navarete, G., Escalante, A., Saklad, A. R., & Brey, R. L. (2000, February). Demographic, symptomatic, and serologic predictors of cognitive function in systemic lupus erythematosus: Preliminary results from SALUD: Abstract. *Journal of the International Neuropsychological Society: JINS, 6*, 231–232.

Holliday, S. L.,Navarrete, M. G., Hermosillo-Romo, D., Valdez, C. R., Saklad, A. R., Escalante, A., & Brey, R. L. (2003). Validating a computerized neuropsychological test battery for mixed ethnic lupus patients. *Lupus, 12*(9), 697–703.

Hughes, M. (1988). Systemic lupus erythematosus. *Postgraduate Medical Journal, 64*(753), 517–521.

Hughes, M., Sundgren, P. C., Fan, X., Foerster, B., Nan, B., Welsh, R. C., . . . Gebarski, S. (2007). Diffusion tensor imaging in patients with acute onset of neuropsychiatric systemic lupus erythematosus: A prospective study of apparent diffusion coefficient, fractional anisotropy values, and eigenvalues in different regions of the brain. *Acta radiologica, 48*(2), 213–222. doi: 772612189 [pii] 10.1080/02841850601105825

Ishikawa, O., Ohnishi, K., Miyachi, Y., & Ishizaka, H. (1994). Cerebral lesions in systemic lupus erythematosus detected by magnetic resonance imaging: Relationship to anticardiolipin antibody. *The Journal of Rheumatology, 21*(1), 87–90.

Iverson, G. L. (1995). The need for psychological service for persons with systemic lupus erythematosus. *Rehabilitation Psychology*, *40*, 39–49.

Iverson, G. L. (2002). Screening for depression in systemic lupus erythematosus with the British Columbia Major Depression Inventory. *Psychological Reports*, *90*(3 Pt 2), 1091–1096.

Iverson, G. L., & Anderson, K. (1994). The etiology of psychiatric symptoms in patients with systemic lupus erythematosus. *Scandanavian Journal of Rheumatology*, *23*(5), 277–282.

Jacobson, M. W., Rapport, L. J., Keenan, P. A., Coleman, R. D., & Tietjen, G. E. (1999). Neuropsychological deficits associated with antiphospholipid antibodies. *Journal of Clinical and Experimental Neuropsychology*, *21*(2), 251–264.

Jain, S. S., & DeLisa, J. A. (1998). Chronic fatigue syndrome: A literature review from a physiatric perspective. *American Journal of Physical Medicine and Rehabilitation*, *77*(2), 160–167.

Jarek, M. J., West, S. G., Baker, M. R., & Rak, K. M. (1994). Magnetic resonance imaging in systemic lupus erythematosus patients without a history of neuropsychiatric lupus erythematosus. *Arthritis and Rheumatism*, *37*(11), 1609–1613.

Jennings, J. E., Sundgren, P. C., Attwood, J., McCune, J., & Maly, P. (2004). Value of MRI of the brain in patients with systemic lupus erythematosus and neurologic disturbance. *Neuroradiology*, *46*(1), 15–21.

Johnson, S. C., Pinkston, J. B., Bigler, E. D., & Blatter, D. D. (1996). Corpus callosum morphology in normal controls and traumatic brain injury: Sex differences, mechanisms of injury, and neuropsychological correlates. *Neuropsychology*, *10*(3), 408–415.

Johnson, R. T., & Richardson, E. P. (1968). The neurological manifestations of systemic lupus erythematosus. *Medicine*, *47*(4), 337–369.

Jonsson, R., Moen, K., Vestrheim, D., & Szodoray, P. (2002). Current issues in Sjögren's syndrome. *Oral Diseases*, *8*(3), 130–140.

Julian, L. J., Yazdany, J., Trupin, L., Criswell, L. A., Yelin, E., & Katz, P. P. (2012). Validity of brief screening tools for cognitive impairment in rheumatoid arthritis and systemic lupus erythematosus. *Arthritis Care and Research*, *64*(3), 448954. doi: 10.1002/acr.21566

Jung, R. E., Caprihan, A., Chavez, R. S., Flores, R. A., Sharrar, J., Qualls, C. R., . . . Roldan, C. A. (2010). Diffusion tensor imaging in neuropsychiatric systemic lupus erythematosus. *BMC Neurology*, *10*, 65. doi: 1471-2377-10-65

Karassa, F. B., Ioannidis, J. P., Boki, K. A., Touloumi, G., Argyropoulou, M. I., Strigaris, K. A., & Moutsopoulos, H. M. (2000). Predictors of clinical outcome and radiologic progression in patients with neuropsychiatric manifestations of systemic lupus erythematosus. *The American Journal of Medicine*, *109*(8), 628–634.

Karzmark, P. (1997). Operating characteristics of neurobehavioral cognitive status exam using neuropsychological assessment as the criterion. *Assessment*, *4*, 1–8.

Katz, P., Julian, L., Tonner, M. C., Yazdany, J., Trupin, L., Yelin, E., & Criswell, L. A. (2012). Physical activity, obesity, and cognitive impairment among women with systemic lupus erythematosus. *Arthritis Care & Research*, *64*(4), 502–510. doi: 10.1002/acr.21587

Keeling, D., Mackie, I., Moore, G. W., Greer, I. A., Greaves, M., & Haematology. (2012). Guidelines on the investigation and management of antiphospholipid syndrome. *British Journal of Haematology*, *157*(1), 47–58. doi: 10.1111/j.1365-2141.2012.09037

Kelly, M. C., & Denburg, J. A. (1987). Cerebrospinal fluid immunoglobulins and neuronal antibodies in neuropsychiatric systemic lupus erythematosus and related conditions. *The Journal of Rheumatology*, *14*(4), 740.

Kewman, D. G., Vaishampayan, N., Zald, D., & Han, B. (1991). Cognitive impairment in musculoskeletal pain patients. *International Journal of Psychiatry in Medicine*, *21*(3), 253–262. PMID: 1955277.

Kim, J. H., Choi, S.-J., Choi, C.-G., Lee, H. K., & Suh, D. C. (2000). Primary antiphospholipid antibody syndrome: Neuroradiologic findings in 11 patients. *Korean Journal of Radiology*, *1*(1), 5–10.

King, D., & Caine, E. D. (1996). Cognitive impairment and major depression: Beyond the pseudodementia syndrome. In I. Grant & K. M. Adams (Eds.), *Neuropsychological Assessment of Neuropsychiatric Disorders* (2nd ed., Vol. 14, pp. 200–217). New York: Oxford University Press.

Koffler, S. (1987). The role of neuropsychological testing in systemic lupus erythematosus. In R. G. Lahita (Ed.), *Systemic Lupus Erythematosus* (pp. 847–853). New York: John Wiley and Sons.

Komatsu, N., Kodama, K., Yamanouchi, N., Okada, S., Noda, S., Nawata, Y., . . . Sato, Y. (1999). Decreased regional cerebral metabolic rate for glucose in systemic lupuis erythematosus patients with psychiatric symptoms. *European Neurology*, *42*, 41–48.

Kowal, C., DeGiorgio, L. A., Nakaoka, T., Diamond, B., & Volpe, B. T. (2004, August). Cognition and immunity: Antibody inpairs memory. *Immunity*, *21*, 179–188. PMID: 15308099.

Kozora, E. (2008). Neuropsychological functioning in systemic lupus erythematosus. In J. E. Morgan & J. H. Ricker (Eds.), *Textbook of Clinical Neuropsychology* (pp. 636–649). New York: Taylor and Francis.

Kozora, E., Arciniegas, D. B., Duggan, E., West, S., Brown, M. S., & Filley, C. M. (2013). White matter abnormalities and working memory impairment in systemic lupus erythematosus. *Cognitvie and Behavioral Neurology*, *26*(2), 63–72.

Kozora, E., Arciniegas, D., et al. (2006). Brain abnormalities in SLE patients with cognitive impairment. *Arthritis & Rheumatism*, *54*(9S), S273.

Kozora, E., Arciniegas, D. B., Filley, C. M., Ellison, M. C., West, S. G., Brown, M. S., & Simon, J. H. (2005). Cognition, MRS neurometabolites, and MRI volumetrics in non-neuropsychiatric systemic lupus erythematosus: Preliminary data. *Cognitive and Behavioral Neurology: Official Journal of the Society for Behavioral and Cognitive Neurology*, *18*(3), 159–162. PMID: 16175019.

Kozora, E., Arciniegas, D. B., Filley, C. M., West, S. G., Brown, M., Miller, D., . . . Zhang, L. (2008). Cognitive and neurologic status in patients with systemic lupus erythematosus without major neuropsychiatric syndromes. *Arthritis and Rheumatism*, *59*(11), 1639–1646. PMID: 18975359. doi: 10.1002/art.24189

Kozora, E., Brown, M. S., Filley, C. M., Zhang, L., Miller, D. E., West, S. G., . . . Arciniegas, D. B. (2011). Memory impairment associated with neurometabolic abnormalities of the hippocampus in patients with non-neuropsychiatric systemic lupus erythematosus. *Lupus*, *20*(6), 598–606. doi: 10.1177/0961203310392425

Kozora, E., Ellison, M. C., & West, S. (2004). Reliability and validity of the proposed American College of Rheumatology neuropsychological battery for systemic lupus erythematosus. *Arthritis and Rheumatism*, *51*(5), 810–818. PMID: 15478145.

Kozora, E., Ellison, M. C., & West, S. (2006). Depression, fatigue, and pain in systemic lupus erythematosus (SLE): Relationship to the American College of Rheumatology SLE neuropsychological battery. *Arthritis and Rheumatism*, *55*(4), 628–635. PMID: 16874786.

Kozora, E., Erkan, D., West, S. G., Filley, S. M., Zhang, L., Ramon, G., . . . Lockshin, M. D. (2013). Site differences in mild cognitive dysfunction (MCD) among patients with systemic lupus erythematosus (SLE). *Lupus*, *22*(1), 73–80. doi: 10.1177/0961203312468963

Kozora, E., & Filley, C. M. (2011). Cognitive dysfunction and white matter abnormalities in systemic lupus erythematosus. *Journal of the International Neuropsychological Society: JINS*, 1–8. doi: 10.1017/S1355617711000191

Kozora, E., Filley, C. M., Zhang, L., Brown, M. S., Miller, D. E., Arciniegas, D. B., . . . West, S. G. (2012). Immune function and brain abnormalities in patients with systemic lupus erythematosus without overt neuropsychiatric manifestations. *Lupus*, *21*(4), 402–411. doi: 10.1177/0961203311429116

Kozora, E., Laudenslager, M., Lemieux, A., & West, S. G. (2001). Inflammatory and hormonal measures predict neuropsychological functioning in systemic lupus erythematosus and rheumatoid arthritis patients. *Journal of the International Neuropsychological Society: JINS*, *7*(6), 745–754.

Kozora, E., Swigris, J., Zell, J., Duggan, E. C., Strand, M., Burleson, A., & Make, B. (2013). Associations between exercise and cognitive impairment in patients with SLE and healthy controls. *Annual Meeting of American Psychosomatic Society Presentation*.

Kozora, E., Thompson, L. L., West, S. G., & Kotzin, B. L. (1996). Analysis of cognitive and psychological deficits in systemic lupus erythematosus patients without overt central nervous system disease. *Arthritis and Rheumatism*, *39*(12), 2035–2045. PMID: 8961909.

Kozora, E., West, S. G., Forrest, S., & Young, L. (2001, March 7–10). *Attention and depression in systemic lupus erythematosus*. Paper presented at the 59th Annual Meeting of American Psychosomatic Society, Monterey, CA.

Kozora, E., West, S. G., Kotzin, B. L., Julian, L., Porter, S., & Bigler, E. (1998). Magnetic resonance imaging abnormalities and cognitive deficits in systemic lupus erythematosus patients without overt central nervous system disease. *Arthritis and Rheumatism*, *41*(1), 41–47.

Kozora, E., West, S. G., Maier, S. F., Filley, C. M., Arciniegas, D. B., Brown, M., . . . Zhang, L. (2010). Antibodies against N-methyl-D-aspartate receptors in patients with systemic lupus erythematosus without major neuropsychiatric syndromes. *Journal of the Neurological Sciences*, *295*(1–2), 87–91. doi: S0022-510X(10)00197-8

Krupp, L. B., LaRocca, N. G., Muir, J., & Steinberg, A. D. (1990). A study of fatigue in systemic lupus erythematosus. *The Journal of Rheumatology*, *17*(11), 1450–1452. PMID: 2273484.

Krupp, L. B., LaRocca, N. G., Muir-Nash, J., & Steinberg, A. D. (1989). The fatigue severity scale: Application to patients with multiple sclerosis and systemic lupus erythematosus. *Archives of Neurology*, *46*(10), 1121–1123. PMID: 2803071.

Kutner, K. C., Busch, H. M., Mahmood, R., Racis, S. P., & Krey, P. R. (1988). Neuropsychological functioning in systemic lupus erythematosus. *Neuropsychology*, *2*, 119–126.

Laboni, A., Ibanez, D., Gladman, D. D., Urowitz, M. B., & Moldofsky, H. (2006). Fatigue in systemic lupus erythematosus: Contributions of disordered sleep, sleepiness, and depression. *The Journal of Rheumatology*, *33*(12), 2453–2457. PMID: 17143980. doi: 0315162X-33-2453

Lampropoulos, C. E., Koutroumanidis, M., Reynolds, P. P., Manidakis, I., Hughes, G. R., & D'Cruz, D. P. (2005). Electroencephalography in the assessment of neuropsychiatric manifestations in antiphospholipid syndrome and systemic lupus erythematosus. *Arthritis and Rheumatism*, *52*(3), 841–846.

Lapteva, L. (2004). *Cognitive Dysfunction (CDYSF) and Anti-N-Methyl-D-Asparate (NMDA) receptor antibodies in systemic lupus erythematosus SLE*. Paper presented at the The International Congress SLE and Related Conditions: Lupus, 2004, New York.

Lapteva, Nowak, M., Yarboro, C. H., Takada, K., Roebuck-Spencer, T., Weickert, T., . . . Illei, G. G. (2006). Anti-N-methyl-D-aspartate receptor antibodies, cognitive dysfunction, and depression in systemic lupus erythematosus. *Arthritis and Rheumatism*, *54*(8), 2505–2514.

Lapteva, L., Yarboro, C. H., & Roebuck-Spencer, T. (2006). Cognitive dysfunction and serum neuropeptides in systemic lupus erythematosus. *American College of Rheumatology Annual Scientific Meeting*, Abstract #631.

Lauvsnes, M. B., Maroni, S. S., Appenzeller, S., Beyer, M. K., Greve, O. J., Kvaløy, J. T., . . . Omdal, R. (2013). Memory dysfunction in primary Sjögren's syndrome is associated with anti-NR2 antibodies. *Arthritis and Rheumatism*, *65*(12), 3209–3217. doi: 10.1002/art.38127

Lawrence, R. C., Helmick, C. G., Arnett, F. C., Deyo, R. A., Felson, D. T., Giannini, E. H., . . . Wolfe, F. (1998). Estimates of the prevalence of arthritis and selected musculoskeletal disorders in the United States. *Arthritis and Rheumatism*, *41*(5), 778–799. PMID: 9588729. doi: 10.1002/1529-0131(199805)41:5<778::AID-ART4>3.0.CO;2-V

Leaven, S. R., & Welch, K. M. A. (1987). The spectrum of neurological disease associated with antiphospholipid antibodies. *Archives of Neurology*, *44*, 873–886.

Leblhuber, F., Neubauer, C., Peichl, M., Reisecker, F., Steinparz, F. X., Windhager, E., & Dienstl, E. (1993). Age and sex differences of dehydroepiandrosterone sulfate (DHEAS) and cortisol (CRT) plasma levels in normal controls and Alzheimer's disease (AD). *Psychopharmacology*, *111*(1), 23–26.

Leritz, E., Brandt, J., Minor, Reis-Jensen, F., & Petri, M. (2000). "Subcortical" cognitive impairment in patients with systemic lupus erythematosus. *Journal of the International Neuropsychological Society: JINS*, *6*(7), 821–825.

Leritz, E., Brandt, J., Minor, Reis-Jensen, F., & Petri, M. (2002). Neuropsychological functioning and its relationship to antiphospholipid antibodies in patients with systemic lupus erythematosus. *Journal of Clinical and Experimental Neuropsychology*, *24*(4), 527–533.

Levine, J. S., Branch, D. W., & Rauch, J. (2002). The antiphospholipid syndrome. *The New England Journal of Medicine*, *346*(10), 752–763.

Liang, M. H., Rogers, M., Larson, M., Eaton, H. M., Murawski, B. J., Taylor, J. E., . . . Schur, P. H. (1984). The psychosocial impact of systemic lupus erythematosus and rheumatoid arthritis. *Arthritis and Rheumatism*, *27*(1), 13–19. PMID: 6691857.

Liang, M. H., Socher, S. A., Larson, S. M. G., & Schur, P. H. (1989). Reliability and validity of six systems for the clinical assessment of disease activity in systemic lupus erythematosus. *Arthritis and Rheumatism*, *32*(9), 1107–1118.

Lijnen, H. R. (2001). Plasmin and matrix metalloproteinases in vascular remodeling. *Thrombosis and Haemostasis*, *86*(1), 324–333.

Lin, Y., Zou, Q. H., Wang, J., Wang, Y., Zhou, D. Q., Zhang, R. H., . . . Fang, Y. F. (2011). Localization of cerebral functional deficits in patients with non-neuropsychiatric systemic lupus erythematosus. *Human Brain Mapping*, *32*(11), 1847–1855. doi: 10.1002/hbm.21158

Linker-Israeli, M., Deans, R. J., Wallace, D. J., Prehn, J., Ozeri-Chen, T., & Klinenberg, J. R. (1991). Elevated levels of endogenous IL-6 in systemic lupus erythematosus: A putative role in pathogenesis. *Journal of Immunology*, *147*(1), 117–123.

Lipton, S. A., & Rosenberg, P. A. (1994). Excitatory amino acids as a final common pathway for neurologic disorders. *The New England Journal of Medicine*, *330*(9), 613–622. PMID: 7905600.

Long, A. A., Denburg, S. D., Carbotte, R. M., Singal, D. P., & Denburg, J. A. (1990). Serum lymphocytotoxic antibodies and neurocognitive function in systemic lupus erythematosus. *Annals of Rheumatic Diseases*, *49*(4), 249–253. PMID: 2339907.

Loukkola, J., Laine, M., Ainiala, H., Peltola, J., Metsanoja, R., Auvinen, A., & Hietaharju, A. (2003). Cognitive impairment in systemic lupus erythematosus and neuropsychiatric systemic lupus erythematosus: A population-based neuropsychological study. *Journal of Clinical and Experimental Neuropsychology*, *25*(1), 145–151.

Love, P. E., & Santoro, S. A. (1990a). Antiphospholipid antibodies: Anticardiolipin and the lupus anticoagulant in systemic lupus erythematosus (SLE) and in non-SLE disorders: Prevalence and clinical significance. *Annals of Internal Medicine*, *112*(9), 682–698.

Love, P. E., & Santoro, S. A. (1990b). Antiphospholipid antibodies: Anticardiolipin and the lupus anticoagulant in systemic lupus erythematosus (SLE) and in non-SLE disorders: Prevalence and clinical significance. *Annals of Internal Medicine*, *112*(9), 682–698.

Lu, X. Y., Zhu, C. Q., Qian, J., Chen, X. X., Ye, S., & Gu, Y. Y. (2010). Intrathecal cytokine and chemokine profiling in neuropsychiatric lupus or lupus complicated with central nervous system infection. *Lupus*, *19*(6), 689–695. doi: 0961203309357061

Mackay, M., Bussa, M. P., Aranow, C., Ulug, A. M., Volpe, B. T., Huerta, P. T., . . . Eidelberg, D. (2011). Differences in regional brain activation patterns assessed by functional magnetic resonance imaging in patients with systemic lupus erythematosus stratified by disease duration. *Molecular Medicine*, *17*, 11–12. doi: 10.2119/molmed.2011.00185

Maeshima, E., Yamada, Y., Yukawa, S., & Nomoto, H. (1992). Higher cortical dysfunction, antiphospholipid antibodies and neuroradiological examinations in systemic lupus erythematosis. *Internal Medicine*, *31*, 1169–1174.

Maier, S. F., & Watkins, L. R. (1998). Cytokines for psychologists: Implications of bidirectional immune-to-brain communication for understanding behavior, mood, and cognition. *Psychological Review*, *105*(1), 83–107.

Mak, A., Ren, T., Fu, E. H., Cheak, A. A., & Ho, R. C. (2012). A prospective functional MRI study for executive function in patients with systemic lupus erythematosus without neuropsychiatric symptoms. *Seminars in Arthritis and Rheumatism*, *41*(6), 849–858.

Malinow, K. L., Molina, R., Gordon, B., Selnes, O. A., Provost, I. T., & Alexander, E. L. (1985). Neuropsychiatric dysfunction in primary Sjogren's syndrome. *Annals of Internal Medicine*, *103*, 344–349.

Maneeton, B., Maneeton, N., & Louthrenoo, W. (2010). Cognitive deficit in patients with systemic lupus erythematosus. *Asian Pacific Journal of Allergy and Immunology*, *1*, 77–83.

McCune, W. J., MacGuire, A., Aisen, A., & Gebarski, S. (1988). Identification of brain lesions in neuropsychiatric systemic lupus erythematosus by magnetic resonance scanning. *Arthritis and Rheumatism*, *31*(2), 159–166.

McKinley, P. S., Ouellette, S. C., & Winkel, G. H. (1995). The contributions of disease activity, sleep patterns, and depression to fatigue in systemic lupus erythematosus: A proposed model. *Arthritis and Rheumatism*, *38*(6), 826–834. PMID: 777912.

McLaurin, E. Y., Holliday, S. L., Williams, P., & Brey, R. L. (2005). Predictors of cognitive dysfunction in patients with systemic lupus erythematosus. *Neurology*, *64*(2), 297–303.

Melchior, C. L., & Ritzmann, R. F. (1996). Neurosteroids block the memory-impairing effects of ethanol in mice. *Pharmacology, Biochemistry, and Behavior*, *53*(1), 51–56.

Melzak, R. (1975). The McGill pain questionnaire: Major properties and scoring methods. *Pain*, *1*(3), 277–299.

Menon, S., Jameson-Shortall, E., Newman, S. P., Hall-Craggs, M., Chinn, R., & Isenberg, D. A. (1999). A longitudinal study of anticardiolipin antibody levels and cognitive functioning in SLE. *Arthritis and Rheumatology*, *42*(4), 735–741. PMID: 10211888.

Middleton, G. D., McFarlin, J. E., & Lipsky, P. E. (1994). The prevalence and clinical impact of fibromyalgia in systemic lupus erythematosus. *Arthritis and Rheumatism*, *37*(8), 1181–1188. PMID: 8053957.

Mikdashi, J., & Handwerger, B. (2004). Predictors of neuropsychiatric damage in systemic lupus erythematosus: Data from the Maryland lupus cohort. *Rheumatology (Oxford)*, *12*, 1555–1560.

Miyakis, S., Lockshin, M. D., Atsumi, T., Branch, D. W., Brey, R. L., Cervera, R., . . . Krilis, S. A. (2006). International consensus statement on an update of the classification criteria for definite Antiphospholipid Syndrome (APS). *Journal of Thrombosis and Haemostasis*, *4*, 295–306.

Monastero, R., Bettini, P., Del Zotto, E., Cottini, E., Tincani, A., Balestrieri, B., . . . Padovani, A. (2001). Prevalence and pattern of cognitive impairment in systemic lupus erythematosus patients with and without overt neuropsychiatric manifestations. *Journal of the Neurological Sciences*, *184*(1), 33–39. PMID: 11231030.

Morgen, K., McFarland, H. F., & Pillemer, S. R. (2004). Central nervous sytem disease in primary sjogren' syndrome: The role of magnetic resonance imaging. *Seminars in Arthritis and Rheumatism*, *34*(3), 623–630.

Morreale, M., Marchione, P., Giacomini, P., Pontecorvo, S., Marianetti, M., Vento, C., . . . Francia, A. (2014). A: Neurological involvement in primary Sjogren's syndrome: A focus on central nervous system. *PloS One*. doi: 10.1371/journal.pone.0084605

Mortilla, M., Ermini, M., Nistri, M., Dal Pozzo, G., & Falcini, F. (2003). Brain study using magnetic resonance imaging and proton MR spectroscopy in pediatric onset systemic lupus erythematosus. *Clinical and Experimental Rheumatology*, *21*(1), 129–135.

Moutsopoulos, H. M., Sarmas, J. H., & Taland, N. (1993). Is central nervous system involvement a systemic manifestation of primary Sjorgrens syndrome. *Rheumatic Disease Clincs of America*, *19*, 909–912.

Naegele, B., Thouvard, V., Pepin, J. L., Levy, P., Bonnet, C., Perret, J. E., . . . Feuerstein, C. (1995). Deficits of cognitive executive functions in patients with sleep apnea syndrome. *Sleep*, *18*(1), 43–52. PMID: 7761742.

Naqibuddin, M., Wallace, D. J., Weisman, M. H., Brey, R. L., Sampedro, M., Carson, K. A., . . . Petri, M. (2005). Change in cognitive function in newly diagnosed systemic lupus erythematosus patients. *Arthritis and Rheumatism*, *52*(9), 975.

Nasman, B., Olsson, T., Backstrom, T., Eriksson, S., Grankvist, K., Viitanen, M., & Bucht, G. (1991). Serum dehydroepiandrosterone sulfate in Alzheimer's disease and in multi-infarct dementia. *Biological Psychiatry*, *30*(7), 684–690.

Nasreddine, Z. S., Phillipa, N. A., Bedirian, V., Charbonneau, S., Whitehead, V., Collin, I., . . . Chertkow, H. (2005). The Montreal Cognitive Assessment, MoCA: A brief screening tool for mild cognitive impairment. *Journal of the American Geriatrics Society*, *53*(4), 695–699.

Nelson, A., Fogel, B. S., & Faust, D. (1986). Bedside cognitive screening instruments: A critical assessment. *The Journal of Nervous and Mental Disease*, *174*(2), 73–83.

Nocturne, G., & Mariette, X. (2013). Advances in understanding the pathogenesis of primary Sjögren's syndrome. *Nature Reviews Rheumatology*, *9*(9), 544–556. doi: 10.1038/nrrheum.2013.110

Norwicka-Sauer, K., Czuszynska, Z., Smolenskda, Z., & Siebert, J. (2011). Neuropsychological assessment in systemic lupus erythematosus patients: Clinical usefulness of first-choice diagnostic tests in detecting cognitive impairment and preliminary diagnosis of neuropsychiatric lupus. *Clinical and Experimental Rheumatology*, *29*(2), 299–306.

Okamoto, H., Kobayashi, A., & Yamanaka, H. (2010). Cytokines and chemokines in neuropsychiatric syndromes of systemic lupus erythematosus. *Journal of Biomedicine and Biotechnology*, *2010*, 268436. doi: 10.1155/2010/268436

Omdal, R., Brokstad, K., Waterloo, K., Koldingsnes, W., Jonsson, R., & Mellgren, S. I. (2005). Neuropsychiatric disturbances in SLE are associated with antibodies against NMDA receptors. *European Journal of Neurology*, *12*(5), 392–398. PMID: 15804272.

Otte, A., Weiner, S. M., Peter, H. H., Mueller-Brand, J., Goetz, M., Moser, E., . . . Nitzsche, E. U. (1997). Brain glucose utilization in systemic lupus erythematosus with neuropsychiatric symptoms: A controlled positron emission tomography study. *European Journal of Nuclear Medicine*, *24*, 787–791.

Palagini, L., Tani, C., Gemignani, A., Mauri, M., Bombardieri, S., . . . Mosca, M. (2014). Sleep disorders and systemic lupus erythematosus. *Lupus*, *23*(2), 115–123. doi: 10.1177/0961203313518623

Papero, P. H., et al. (1990). Neuropsychologic deficits and antineuronal antibodies in pediatric sytemic lupus erythematosus. *Clinical and Experimental Rheumatology*, *8*(4), 417–424.

Paran, D., Litinsky, I., Shapira-Lichter, I., Navon, S., Hendler, T., Caspi, D., & Vakil, E. (2009). Impaired memory and learning abilities in patients with systemic lupus erythematosus as measured by the Rey Auditory Verbal Learning Test. *Annals of Rheumatic Diseases*, *68*(6), 812–816. doi: 10.1136/ard.2008.091538

Peretti, C. S., Peretti, C. R., Kozora, E., Papathanassiou, D., Chouinard, V. A., & Chouinard, G. (2012). Cognitive impairment in systemic lupus erythematosus women with elevated autoantibodies and normal single photon emission computerized tomography. *Psychotherapy and Pyshosomatics*, *81*(5), 276–285. doi: 10.1159/000336555

Perry, W., Hilsabeck, R. C., & Hassanein, T. I. (2008). Cognitive dysfunction in chronic hepatitis C: A review. *Digestive Diseases and Sciences*, *53*(2), 307–321. doi: 10.1007/s10620-007-9896-z

Petri, M. (2000). Epidemiology of the antiphospholipid antibody syndrome. *Journal of Autoimmunity*, *15*(2), 145–151.

Petri, M., Nagibuddin, M., Sampedro, M., Omdal, R., & Carson, K. A. (2011). Memantine in systemic lupus erythematosus: A randomized, double-blind placebo-controlled trial. *Seminars in Arthritis and Rheumatism*, *41*(2), 194–202. doi: 10.1016/j.semarthrit.2011.02.005

Petri, M., Naqibuddin, M., Carson, K. A., Sampedro, M., Wallace, D. J., Weisman, M. H., . . . Brey, R. L. (2008). Cognitive function in a systemic lupus erythematosus inception cohort. *The Journal of Rheumatology*, *35*(9), 1776–1781.

Petri, M., Naqibuddin, M., Carson, K. A., Wallace, D. J., Weisman, M. H., Holliday, S. L., . . . Brey, R. L. (2008). Brain magnetic resonance imaging in newly diagnosed systemic lupus erythematosus. *The Journal of Rheumatology*.

Pons-Estel, G. J., Alarcon, G. S., Scofield, L., Reinlib, L., & Cooper, G. S. (2010). Understanding the epidemiology and progression of systemic lupus erythematosus. *Seminars in Arthritis and Rheumatism*, *39*(4), 257–268. doi: S0049-0172(08)00197-2

Provenzale, J. M., Barboriak, D. P., Allen, N. B., & Ortel, T L. (1996). Patients with antiphospholipid antibodies: CT and MR findings of the brain. *AJR: American Journal of Roentgenology*, *167*(6), 1573–1578.

Reeves, D., Kane, R., & Winter, K. (1996). *Automated Neuropsychological Assessment Metrics (ANAM V3.11a/96) Users Manual: Clinical and Neurotoxicology Subset (Report No NCRF-SR-96–01)*. San Diego, CA: National Cognitive Foundation.

Rhiannon, J. J. (2008). Systemic lupus erythematosus involving the nervous system: Presentation, pathogenesis, and management. *Clinical Reviews in Allergy and Immunology*, *34*, 356–360. doi: 10.1007/s12016-007-8052-z

Ring, R. H. (2005). The central vasopressinergic system: Examining the opportunities for psychiatric drug development. *Current Pharmaceutical Design*, *11*(2), 205–225.

Robbins, M. L., Kornguth, S. E., Bell, C. L., Kalinke, T., England, D., Turski, P., & Graziano, F. M. (1988). Antineurofilament antibody evaluation in neuropsychiatric systemic lupus erythematosus: Combination with anticardiolipin antibody assay and magnetic resonance imaging. *Arthritis and Rheumatism*, *31*(5), 623–631.

Robb-Nicholson, L. C., Daltroy, L., Eaton, H., Gall, V., Wright, E., Hartley, L. H., . . . Liang, M. H. (1989). Effects of aerobic conditioning in lupus fatigue: A pilot study. *British Journal of Rheumatology*, *28*(6), 500–505. PMID: 2590802.

Rocca, M. A., Agosta, F., Mezzapesa, D. M., Ciboddo, G., Falini, A., Comi, G., & Filippi, M. (2006). An fMRI study of the motor system in patients with neuropsychiatric systemic lupus erythematosus. *NeuroImage*, *30*(2), 478–484.

Rodrigues, C. E., Carvalho, J. F., & Shoenfeld, Y. (2010). Neurological manifestations of antiphospholipid syndrome. *European Journal of Clinical Investigation*, *40*(4), 350–359. doi: 10.1111/j.1365-2362.2010.02263

Rodrigues, D. N., Hora, J. S. I., Sagado, M. C. F., Paes, R. A., Vasconcelos, C. C. F., Landeira-Fernandez, J., & Alvarenga, R. M. P. (2014). A short neuropsychological evaluation of patients with primary Sjogren's syndrome. *Arquivos De Neuro-Pisquiatr*, *72*(1), 38–43. doi: 10.1590/0004-282X20130195

Roebuck-Spencer, T. M., Yarboro, C., Nowak, M., Takada, K., Jacobs, G., Lapteva, L., . . . Bleiberg, J. (2006). Use of computerized assessment to predict neuropsychological functioning and emotional distress in patients with systemic lupus erythematosus. *Arthritis and Rheumatism*, *55*(3), 434–441. PMID: 16739211.

Roldan, J. F., & Brey, R. L. (2007). Neurologic manifestations of the antiphospholipid syndrome. *Current Rheumatology Reports*, *9*(2), 109–115.

Rozell, C. L., Sibbitt, W. L., Jr., & Brooks, W, M. (1998). Structural and neurochemical markers of brain injury in the migraine diathesis of systemic lupus erythematosus [see comments]. *Cephalalgia*, *18*(4), 209–215.

Rummelt, J. K., Sobota, W. L., Brickman, C. M., & Doyle, T. H. (1991). Memory and motor scores discriminate systemic lupus (SLE) patients from matched controls. *Journal of Clinical and Experimental Neuropsychology*, *13*(1).

Sabbadini, M. G., Manfredi, A. A., Bozzolo, E., Ferrario, L., Rugarli, C., Scorza, R., . . . Passaleva, A. (1999). Central nervous system involvement in systemic lupus erlythematosis patients without overt neuropsychiatric manifestations. *Lupus, Jan*, *8*(1), 11–19. PMID: 10025594.

Sabet, A., Sibbitt, W. L., Jr., Stidley, C. A., Danska, J., & Brooks, W. M. (1998). Neurometabolite markers of cerebral injury in the antiphospholipid antibody syndrome of systemic lupus erythematosus. *Stroke: A Journal of Cerebral Circulation*, *29*, 2254–2260. PMID: 9804631.

Sailer, M., Burchert, W., Ehrenheim, C., Smid, H. G., Haas, J., Wildhagen, K., . . . Deicher, H. (1997). Positron emission tomography and magnetic resonance imaging for cerebral involvement in patients with systemic lupus erythematosus. *Journal of Neurology*, *244*(3), 186–193. PMID: 9050960.

Sakic, B., Laflamme, N., Crnic, L. S., Szechtman, H., Denburg, J. A., & Rivest, S. (1999). Reduced corticotropin-releasing factor and enhanced vasopressin gene expression in brains of mice with autoimmunity-induced behavioral dysfunction. *Journal of Neuroimmunology*, *96*(1), 80–91.

Sakic, B., Szechtman, H., Denburg, J. A., Gorny, G., Kolb, B., & Whishaw, I. Q. (1998). Progressive atrophy of pyramidal neuron dendrites in autoimmune MRL-lpr mice. *Journal of Neuroimmunology*, *87*(1–2), 162–170.

Sanna, G., Bertolaccini, M. L., Cuadrado, M. J., Liang, H., Khamashta, M. A., Mathieu, A., & Hughes, G. R. (2003). Neuropsychiatric manifestations in systemic lupus erythematosus: Prevalence and association with antiphospholipid antibodies. *The Journal of Rheumatology*, *30*(5), 985–992. PMID: 12734893.

Santer, D. M., Yoshio, T., Minota, S., Moller, T., & Elkon, K. B. (2009). Potent induction of IFN-alpha and chemokines by autoantibodies in the cerebrospinal fluid of patients with neuropsychiatric lupus. *Journal of Immunology*, *182*(2), 1192–1201. doi: 182/2/1192 [pii]

Šarac, H., Markeljevič, J., Erdeljič, V., Josipovič-Jelič, Z., Hajnšek, S., Klapan, T., . . . Dobrila Dointinjana, R. (2013). Signal hyperintensities on brain magnetic resonance imaging in patients with primary Sjögren syndrome and frequent episodic tension-type headache: Relation to platelet serotonin level and disease activity. *The Journal of Rheumatology*, *40*(8), 1360–1366. doi: 10.3899/jrheum.121132

Schmidt, R., Auer-Grumbach, P., Fazekas, F., Offenbacher, H., & Kapeller, P. (1995). Anticardiolipin antibodies in normal subjects: Neuropsychological correlates and MRI findings. *Stroke: A Journal of Cerebral Circulation*, *26*(5), 749–754.

Schneebaum, A. B., Singleton, J. D., West, S. G., Blodgett, J. K., Allen, L. G., Cheronis, J. C., & Kotzin, B. L. (1991). Association of psychiatric manifestations with antibodies to ribosomal P proteins in systemic lupus erythematosus. *The American Journal of Medicine*, *90*(1), 54–62.

Schur, P. H. (1989). Clinical features of systemic lupus erythematosus. In W. N. Kelley, E. D. Harris, Jr., S. Ruddy, & R. B. Sledge (Eds.), *Textbook of Rheumatology* (pp. 1101–1129). Philadelphia, PA: WB Saunders.

Schwartz, D. P., Barth, J. T., & Done, J. R. (1987). Cognitive deficits in chronic pain patients with and without history of head/neck injury. *The Clnical Journal of Pain*, *3*, 94–101.

Scott, D. L., Wolfe, F., & Huizinga, T. W. (2010). Rheumatoid Arthritis. *Lancet*, *376*(9746), 1094–1108. doi: 10.1016/S0140-6736(10)60826-4

Segal, B. M., Pogatchnik, B., Holker, E., Liu, H., Sloan, J., Rhodus, N., & Moser, K. L. (2012). Primary Sjogren's syndrome: Cognitive symptoms, mood, and cognitive performance. *Acta Neurologica Scandinavica*, *125*(4), 272–278. doi: 10.1111/j.1600-0404.2011.01530.x

Selnes, O. A., Gordon, B., Malinow, K. L., & Alexander, E. L. (1985). Cognitive dysfunction in primary Sjogrens syndrome. *Neurology*, *35*(Suppl 1), 179.

Sewell, K. L., Livneh, A., Aranow, C. B., & Grayzel, A. I. (1989). Magnetic resonance imaging versus computed tomographic scanning in neuropsychiatric systemic lupus erythematosus. *The American Journal of Medicine*, *86*(5), 625–626.

Shapira-Lichter, I., Vakil, E., Litinsky, I., Oren, N., Glikmann-Johnston, Y., Caspi, D., . . . Paran, D. (2013). Learning and memory-related brain activity dynamics are altered in systemic lupus erythematosus: A functional magnetic resonance imaging study. *Lupus*, *22*(6), 562–573. doi: 10.1177/0961203313480399

Shin, S. Y., Katz, P., Wallhagen, M., & Julian, L. (2012). Cognitive impairment in persons with rheumatoid arthritis. *Arthritis Care and Research*, *64*(8), 1144–1150. doi: 10.1002/acr.21683

Shiozawa, S., Kuroki, Y., Kim, M., Hirohata, S., & Ogino, T. (1992). Interferon-alpha in lupus psychosis. *Arthritis and Rheumatism*, *35*(4), 417–422.

Shucard, J. L., Gaines, J. J., Ambrus, J., Jr., & Shucard, D. W. (2007). C-reactive protein and cognitive deficits in systemic lupus erythematosus. *Cognitive and Behavioral Neurology: Official Journal of the Society for Behavioral and Cognitive Neurology*, *20*(1), 31–37.

Shucard, J. L., Parrish, J., Shucard, D. W., McCabe, D. C., Benedict, R. H., & Ambrus, J., Jr. (2004). Working memory and processing speed deficits in systemic lupus erythematosus as measured by the paced auditory serial addition test. *Journal of the International Neuropsychological Society: JINS*, *10*(1), 35–45.

Sibbitt, W. L., Jr., Haseler, L. J., Griffey, R. R., Friedman, S. D., & Brooks, W. M. (1997). Neurometabolism of active neuropsychiatric lupus determined with proton MR spectroscopy. *AJNR: American Journal of Neuroradiology*, *18*(7), 1271–1277.

Sibbitt, W. L., Jr., Haseler, L. J., Griffey, R. H., Hart, B. L., Sibbitt, R. R., & Matwiyoff, N. A. (1994). Analysis of cerebral structural changes in systemic lupus erythematosus by proton MR spectroscopy. *AJNR: American Journal of Neuroradiology*, *15*(5), 923–928. PMID: 8059662.

Sibbitt, W. L., Jr., & Sibbitt, R. R. (1993). Magnetic resonance spectroscopy and positron emission tomography scanning in neuropsychiatric systemic lupus erythematosus. *Rheumatic Disease Clinics of North America*, *19*(4), 851–868. PMID: 8265826.

Sibbitt, W. L., Jr., Sibbitt, R. R., & Brooks, W. M. (1999). Neuroimaging in neuropsychiatric systemic lupus erythematosus. *Arthritis and Rheumatism*, *42*(10), 2026–2038.

Sibbitt, W. L., Jr., Sibbitt, R. R., Griffey, R. H., Eckel, C., & Bankhurst, A. D. (1989). Magnetic resonance and computed tomographic imaging in the evaluation of acute neuropsychiatric disease in systemic lupus erythematosus. *Annals of the Rheumatic Diseases*, *48*(12), 1014–1022.

Singh, A. K. (1992). Cytokines play a central role in the pathogenesis of systemic lupus erythematosus. *Medical Hypotheses*, *39*(4), 356–359.

Sonies, B., Klippel, J., Gerber, R., & Gerber, C. (1982). Cognitive performance in systemic lupus erythematosus, abstracted. *Arthritis and Rheumatism*, *25*(Suppl), S80.

Spezialetti, R., Bluestein, H. G., & Alexander, E. L. (1995). Neuropsychiatric disease in Sjogren's syndrome: Anti-ribosomal P and anti-neuronal antibodies. *The American Journal of Medicine*, *95*, 153–160.

Spreen, O., & Strauss, E. (1991). *A Compendium of Neuropsycholoigcal Tests*. New York: Oxford University Press.

Stanley, K., & Ghosh, R. (2013). Neuropsychiatric symptoms in a patient with primary antiphospholipid syndrome. *Progress in Neurology and Psychiatry*, *17*(2), 29–32. doi: 10.1002/pnp.277

Stein, H., Walters, K., Dillon, A., & Schulzer, M. (1986). Systemic lupus erythematosus--a medical and social profile. *The Journal of Rheumatology*, *13*(3), 570–576. PMID: 3735279.

Steup-Beekman, G., Steens, S., van Buchem, M., & Huizinga, T. (2007). Anti-NMDA receptor autoantibodies in patients with systemic lupus erythematosus and their first-degree relatives. *Lupus*, *16*(5), 329–334.

Stimmler, M. M., Coletti, P. M., & Quismorio, F. P., Jr. (1993). Magnetic resonance imaging of the brain in neuropsychiatric systemic lupus erythematosus. *Seminars in Arthritis and Rheumatism*, *22*(5), 335–349.

Stolt, P., Bengtsson, C., Nordmark, B., Lindblad, S., Lundberg, I., Klareskog, L., . . . Group. (2003). Quantification of the influence of cigarette smoking on rheumatoid arthritis: Results from a population based case-control study, using incident cases. *Annals of the Rheumatic Diseases*, *62*(9), 835–841.

Streifler, J. Y., & Molad, Y. (2014). Connective tissue disorders: Systemic lupus erythematosus, Sjögren's syndrome, and scleroderma. *Handbook of Clinical Neurology*, *119*, 463–473. doi: 10.1016/B978-0-7020-4086-3.00030-8

Sub-committee. (2007). Proposed response criteria for neurocognitive impairment in systemic lupus erythematosus trials. *Lupus*, *16*(6), 418–425.

Sundgren, P. C., Jennings, J., Attwood, J. T., Nan, B., Gebarski, S., McCune, W. J., . . . Maly, P. (2005). MRI and 2D-CSI MR spectroscopy of the brain in the evaluation of patients with acute onset of neuropsychiatric systemic lupus erythematosus. *Neuroradiology*, *47*(8), 576–585.

Suzuki, T., Suzuki, N., Engleman, Y., Mizushima, & Sakane, T. (1995). Low serum levels of dehydroepiandrosterone may cause deficient IL-2 production by lymphocytes in patients with systemic lupus erythematosus (SLE). *Clinical and Experimental Immunology*, *99*(2), 251–255.

Tajima, Y., Mito, Y., Owada, Y., Tsukishima, E., Moriwaka, F., & Tashiro, K. (1997). Neurologial manifestations of primary Sjogren's syndrome in Japanese patients. *Internal Medicine*, *36*, 690–693.

Taylor, J., Skan, J., Erb, N., Carruthers, D., Bowman, S., Gordon, C., & Isenberg, D. (2000). Lupus patients with fatigue-is there a link with fibromyalgia syndrome? *Rheumatology (Oxford)*, *39*(6), 620–623. PMID: 10888706.

Tektonidou, M. G., Varsou, N., Kotoulas, G., Antoniou, A., & Moutsopoulos, H. M. (2006). Cognitive deficits in patients with antiphospholipid syndrome: Association with clinical, laboratory, and brain magnetic resonance imaging findings. *Archives of Internal Medicine*, *166*(20), 2278–2284.

Temesvari, P., Denburg, J., Denburg, S., Carbotte, R., Bensen, W., & Singal, D. (1983). Serum lymphocytotoxic antibodies in neuropsychiatric lupus: A serial study. *Clinical Immunology and Immunopathology*, *28*(2), 243–251.

Tench, C., Bentley, D., Vleck, V., McCurdie, I., White, P., & D'Cruz, D. (2002). Aerobic fitness, fatigue, and physical disability in systemic lupus erythematosus. *The Journal of Rheumatology*, *29*(3), 474–481. PMID: 11908559.

Tench, C. M., McCurdie, I., White, P. D., & D'Cruz, D. P. (2000). The prevalence and associations of fatigue in systemic lupus erythematosus. *Rheumatology (Oxford)*, *39*(11), 1249–1254. PMID: 11085805.

Tobón, G. J., Pers, V., Devasuchelle-Pensec, V., & Youinou, P. (2012). Neurological disorders in primary Sjögren's syndrome: Autoimmune diseases. *Autoimmune Diseases*, *2012*.

Toledano, P., Sarbu, N., Espinosa, G., Bargallo, N., & Cervera, R. (2013). Neuropsychiatric systemic lupus erythematosus: Magnetic resonance imaging findings and correlation with clinical and immunological features. *Autoimmunity Reviews*, *12*(12), 1166–1170. doi: 10.1016/j.autrev.2013.07.004

Tomietto, P., Annese, V., D'Agostini, S., Venturini, P., La Torre, G., De Vita, S., & Ferraccioli, G. F. (2007). General and specific factors associated with severity of cognitive impairment in systemic lupus erythematosus. *Arthritis and Rheumatism*, *57*(8), 1461–1472. PMID: 18050188.

Tomita, M., Holman, B. J., & Santoro, T. J. (2001). Aberrant cytokine gene expression in the hippocampus in murine systemic lupus erythematosus. *Neuroscience Letters*, *302*(2–3), 129–132.

Trysberg, E., Blennow, K., Zachrisson, O., & Tarkowski, A. (2004). Intrathecal levels of matrix metalloproteinases in systemic lupus erythematosus with central nervous system engagement. *Arthritis Research and Therapy*, *6*(6), R551–R556.

Trysberg, E., Carlsten, H., & Tarkowski, A. (2000). Intrathecal cytokines in systemic lupus erythematosus with central nervous system involvement. *Lupus*, *9*, 498–503.

Tsai, C. Y., Wu, Tsai, S. T., Chen, K. H., Thajeb, P., Lin, W. M., . . . Yu, C. L. (1994). Cerebrospinal fluid interleukin-6, prostaglandin E2 and autoantibodies in patients with neuropsychiatric systemic lupus erythematosus and central nervous system infections. *Scandinavian Journal of Rheumatology*, *23*(2), 57–63.

Tzarouchi, L. C., Tsifetaki, N., Konitsiotis, S., Zikou, A., Astrakas, L., Drosos, A., & Argyropoulou, M. I. (2011). CNS involvement in primary Sjogren Syndrome: Assessment of gray and white matter changes with MRI and voxel-based morphometry. *AJR: American Journal of Roentgenology*, *197*(5), 1207–1212. doi: 10.2214/AJR.10.5984

Ulug, A. M., Vo, A., Kozora, E., Ramon, G., Vega, J., Zimmerman, R. D., . . . Lockshin, M. (2010). fMRI in systemic lupus erythematosus and antiphospholipid syndrome. *International Society for Magnetic Resonance in Medicine*, *18*, 4466A.

Unterman, A., Nolte, J. E., Boaz, M., Abady, M., Shoenfeld, Y., & Zandman-Goddard, G. (2011). Neuropsychiatric syndromes in systemic lupus erythematosus: A meta-analysis. *Seminars in Arthritis and Rheumatism*, *41*, 1–11.

Valencia-Flores, M., Resendiz, M., Castano, V. A., Santiago, V., Campos, R. M., Sandino, S., . . . Bliwise, D. L. (1999). Objective and subjective sleep disturbances in patients with systemic lupus erythematosus. *Arthritis and Rheumatism*, *42*(10), 2189–2193. PMID: 10524692. doi: 10.1002/1529-0131(199910)42:10<2189::AID-ANR21>3.0.CO;2-V

van der Woude, D., Houwing-Duistermaat, J. J., Toes, R. E., Huizinga, T. W., Thomson, W., Worthington, J., . . . de Vries, R. R. (2009). Quantitative heritability of anti-citrullinated protein antibody-positive and anti-citrullinated protein antibody-negative rheumatoid arthritis. *Arthritis and Rheumatism*, *60*(4), 916–923. doi: 10.1002/art.24385

Vitali, C., Bombardieri, S., Jonsson, R., Moutsopoulos, H. M., Alexander, E. L., Carsons, S. E., . . . Syndrome. (2002). Classification criteria for Sjogren's syndrome: A revised version of the European criteria proposed by the American-European consensus group. *Annals of Rheumatic Diseases*, *61*(6), 554–558.

Vogel, A., Bhattacharya, S., Larsen, J. L., & Jacobsen, S. (2011). Do subjective cognitive complaints correlate with cognitive impairment in systemic lupus erythematosus? A Danish outpatient study. *Lupus*, *20*(1), 35–43. doi: 10.1177/0961203310382430

Vogelweid, C. M., Wright, D. C., Johnson, J. C., Hewett, J. E., & Walker, S. E. (1994). Evaluation of memory, learning ability, and clinical neurologic function in pathogen-free mice with systemic lupus erythematosus. *Arthritis and Rheumatism*, *37*(6), 889–897.

Volk, C., Kratzsch, G., Krapf, H., Kornhuber, H. H., et al. (1994). Neurological and neuropsychiatric dysfunction in primary Sjogren's syndrome. *Acta Neurological Scandinavica*, *89*, 31–35.

Voss, E. V., & Stangel, M. (2012). Nervous system involvement of connective tissue disease: Mechanisms and diagnostic approach. *Current Opinion in Neurology*, *25*(3), 306–315. doi: 10.1097/WCO.0b013e328352ebfe

Voulgarelis, M., & Tzioufas, A. G. (2010). Pathogenetic mechanisms in the initiation and perpetuation of Sjögren's syndrome. *Nature Reviews Rheumatology*, *6*(9), 529–537. doi: 10.1038/nrrheum.2010.118

Walker, S. E., Wright, D. C., O'Sullivan, F. X., Johnson, G. C., Besch-Williford, C. L., & Vogelweid, C. M. (1997). Memory, learning ability, and neuropathologic status of mice with systemic lupus erythematosus. *Annals of the New York Academy of Sciences*, *823*, 107–115.

Waterloo, D., Omdal, R., Husby, G., & Mellgren, S. I. (2002). Neuropsychological function in systemic lupus erythematosus: A five-year longitudinal study. *Rheumatology (Oxford)*, *41*(4), 411–415. PMID: 11961171.

Waterloo, D., Omdal, R., Jacobsen, E. A., Klow, N. E., Husby, G., Torbergsen, G., & Mellgren, S. I. (1999). Cerebral computed tomography and electroencephalography compared with neuropsychological findings in systemic lupus erythematosus. *Journal of Neurology*, *246*(8), 706–711.

Waterloo, K., Omdal, R., Sjoholm, H., Koldingsnes, W., Jacobsen, E. A., Sundsfjord, J. A., . . . Mellgren, S. I. (2001). Neuropsychological dysfunction in systemic lupus erythematosus is not associated with changes in cerebral blood flow. *Journal of Neurology*, *248*(7), 595–602. PMID: 11518002.

Weiner, , S. I Otte, A., Schumacher, M., Klein, R., Gutfleisch, J., Brink, J., . . . Peter, H. (2000). Diagnosis and monitoring of central nervous system involvement in systemic lupus erythematosus: Value of F-18 fluorodeoxyglucose PET. *Annals of the Rheumatic Diseases*, *59*, 377–385.

Wekking, E. M. (1993). Psychiatric symptoms in systemic lupus erythematosus: An update. *Psychosomatic Medicine*, *55*(2), 219–228.

Wekking, E. M., Nossent, J. C., van Dam, A. P., & Swaak, A. J. (1991). Cognitive and emotional disturbances in systemic lupus erythematosus. *Psychotherapy and Psychosomatics*, *55*(2–4), 126–131. PMID: 1891558.

Wekking, E. M., Vingerhoets, A. J. J. M., van Dam, A. P., Nossent, J. C., & Swaak, A. J. J. G. (1991). Daily stressors and systemic lupus erythematosus: A longitudinal analysis--first findings. *Psychotherapy and Psychosomatics*, *55*(2–4), 108–113.

West, S. G. (1994). Neuropsychiatric lupus. *Rheumatic Disease Clinics of North America*, *20*(1), 129–158.

West, S. G. (2007). The nervous system. In D. J. Wallace & B. H. Hahn (Eds.), *Dubois' Lupus Erythematosus* (7th ed., pp. 707–746). Philadelphia, PA: Lippincott, Williams & Wilkins.

West, S. G., Emlen, W., Wener, M. H., & Kotzin, B. L. (1995). Neuropsychiatric lupus erythematosus: A 10-year prospective study on the value of diagnostic tests. *The American Journal of Medicine*, *99*(2), 153–163. PMID: 7625420.

Wolfe, F., & Michaud, K. (2004). Fatigue, rheumatoid arthritis, and anti-tumor necrosis factor therapy: An investigation in 24,831 patients. *The Journal of Rheumatology*, *31*(11), 2115–2120. doi: 0315162X-31-2115 [pii]

Wysenbeek, A. J., Leibovici, L., Weinberger, A., & Guedj, D. (1993). Fatigue in systemic lupus erythematosus: Prevalence and relation to disease expression. *British Journal of Rheumatology*, *32*(7), 633–635. PMID: 8339141.

Yazdany, J., Trupin, L., Gansky, S. A., Dall'Era, M., Yelin, E. H., Criswell, L. A., & Katz, P. P. (2011). Brief index of lupus damage: A patient-reported easure of damage in systemic lupus erythematosus. *Arthritis Care & Research*, *63*(8), 1170–1177. doi: 10.1002/acr.20503

Yeh, T. S., Wang, C. R., Jeng, G. W., Lee, G. L., Chen, M. Y., Wang, G. R., . . . Chen, C. Y. (1994). The study of anticardiolipin antibodies and interleukin-6 in cerebrospinal fluid and blood of Chinese patients with systemic lupus erythematosus and central nervous system involvement. *Autoimmunity*, *18*(3), 169–175.

Yoshio, T., Onda, K., Nara, H., & Minota, S. (2006). Association of IgG anti-NR2 glutamate receptor antibodies in cerebrospinal fluid with neuropsychiatric systemic lupus erythematosus. *Arthritis and Rheumatism*, *54*(2), 675–678.

Zhang, L., Harrison, M., Heier, L. A., Zimmerman, R. D., Ravdin, L., Lockshin, M., & Ulug, A. M. (2007). Diffusion changes in patients with systemic lupus erythematosus. *Magnetic Resonance Imaging*, *25*(3), 399–405.

Ziporen, L., Shoenfeld, Y., Levy, Y., & Korczyn, A. D. (1997). Neurological dysfunction and hyperactive behavior associated with antiphospholipid antibodies: A mouse model. *The Journal of Clinical Investigation*, *100*(3), 613–619.

Zivadinov, R., Shucard, J. L., Hussein, S., Durfee, J., Bergsland, N., Dwyer, M. G., . . . Shucard, D. W. (2013). Multimodal imaging in systemic lupus erythematosus patients with diffuse neuropsychiatric involvement. *Lupus*, *22*(7), 675–683. doi: 10.1177/0961203313486193

Zvaifler, N. J., & Bluestein, H. G. (1982). The pathogenesis of central nervous system manifestations of systemic lupus erythematosus. *Arthritis and Rheumatism*, *25*(7), 862–866.

27 Sports-Related Concussion

William B. Barr, Lindsay D. Nelson, and Michael A. McCrea

Introduction

Due to its extensive media coverage and public interest, sports-related concussion (SRC) continues as a major topic in the United States and worldwide (Pearce, Gallo, & McElvenny, 2015). The annual incidence of nonfatal traumatic brain injuries (TBIs) from sports and recreation activities in persons aged 19 years or younger is estimated to be more than 2.6 million per year in the United States and the numbers appear to be growing (Noble & Hesdorffer, 2013). A recent study indicated that from 1997 to 2007 emergency department visits for 8- to 13-year-old children affected by concussion in organized sports doubled and increased by more than 200% in the 14- to 19-year-old group (Bakhos, Lockhart, Myers, & Linakis, 2010). There are also indications that the reported incidence of SRC may even be higher than what was described in previous studies due to increased attention and awareness (LaBotz, Martin, Kimura, Hetzler, & Nichols, 2005; LaRoche, Nelson, Connelly, Walter, & McCrea, 2015; McCrea, Hammeke, Olsen, Leo, & Guskiewicz, 2004).

The increased incidence of SRC over the last several years may be driven, at least partially, by greater awareness and identification of SRC among current-era athletes relative to earlier generations (Hootman, Dick, & Agel, 2007). Because of the high incidence of concussion and concern for long-term neurologic consequences (DeKosky, Ikonomovic, & Gandy, 2010; Gilchrist, Thomas, Wald, & Langlois, 2007; Langlois, Rutland-Brown, & Wald, 2006), nearly all states have now enacted SRC management legislation. These laws require athletes, coaches, parents, and school organizations to be educated regarding the recognition, evaluation, and management of SRC and to have predefined return-to-play protocols.

In spite of a growing body of empirical research, sports medicine professionals continue to view the diagnosis of SRC and projection of postinjury recovery patterns among their most difficult clinical challenges. From the beginning, clinical neuropsychology, through its emphasis on standardized clinical testing, has made significant contributions to understanding the nature, severity, and recovery of symptoms observed in SRC (Belanger, Curtiss, Demery, Lebowitz, & Vanderploeg, 2005; Belanger & Vanderploeg, 2005; Echemendia et al., 2013; Erlanger, Kutner, Barth, & Barnes, 1999; Nelson, Janecek, & McCrea, 2013). Given their background in test construction and psychometrics, neuropsychologists have also been critically involved in developing new test methods for use exclusively in the sport setting. This chapter will provide a general review of the current status of SRC and provide an overview of the use of neuropsychological methods in sports, emphasizing an evidence-based approach to assessing and managing both acute and subacute symptoms.

Diagnosis Acute Recovery From SRC

Diagnostic Issues

The initial identification and management of the athlete with a suspected SRC begins on the field of play. This initial stage of evaluation is conducted most appropriately by individuals with specialized training in emergency medicine, such as licensed physicians and certified athletic trainers (ATCs). The primary aims of the initial assessment are to (a) recognize whether or not an injury to the brain or any other part of the body has occurred, and (b) determine whether transport to a medical facility is needed (Bailes & Hudson, 2001; Kelly & Rosenberg, 1997a, 1997b). It is extremely important to rule out whether there are any medical or neurological signs that would signal the presence of severe intracranial pathology or possibly serious injuries to the spinal cord or other parts of the body (Kelly & Rosenberg, 1997a). In spite of some initial controversy on same-day return to play, the emphatic approach used today is that any athlete with a suspected concussion should not return to play on the day of the injury and should not return to any form of practice or competition until he or she is evaluated and cleared by a qualified professional.

Controversies in concussion begin with definitions and diagnostic classifications. Most of the standard guidelines for defining and classifying levels of TBI have been of little use for diagnosing SRC. Systems commonly used by clinicians including the American Congress of Rehabilitation Medicine (ACRM) guidelines for mild TBI (MTBI; see Kay et al., 1993) place too much emphasis on duration of loss of consciousness (LOC) and posttraumatic amnesia (PTA) considering the fact that results from controlled investigations have now demonstrated that LOC occurs in less than 10% of the subjects with SRC, with no signs of either

LOC or PTA observed in more than 70% (Guskiewicz et al., 2003). For similar reasons, while scores on the Glasgow Coma Scale (GCS; see Teasdale & Jennett, 1974) may be useful for reconstructing injury severity from ambulance records following motor vehicle accidents, they are clearly less useful for making a diagnosis of SRC in an athletic setting.

For clinical purposes, many neuropsychologists in the athletic setting are now using the injury definitions provided in the sports medicine literature. While over the past 20 years there has been a plethora of definitions and grading scales developed for use in an athletic setting, there has been some movement towards use of the evolving set of definitions included consensus statements developed through a series of International Conferences on Concussion in Sport (Finch, Clapperton, & McCrory, 2013).

The definition developed in the most recent conference, held in Zurich in 2012, is provided in Table 27.1. In this definition, concussion is defined as "a complex pathophysiological process affecting the brain, induced by biomechanical forces" and extends to a brief description of possible causes and effects in addition to the expected course of recovery (McCrory, Meeuwisse, Aubry, Cantu, et al., 2013). In conjunction with a number of assessment tools outlined in the consensus statement, the criteria specified in this definition can be used in a model emphasizing a more empirical and multidimensional approach to documenting the signs and symptoms of injury.

Table 27.1 Definition of concussion: Consensus statement on concussion in sport from the the Third International Conference on Concussion in Sport held in Zurich, November 2012

Concussion is a brain injury and is defined as a complex pathophysiological process affecting the brain induced by traumatic biomechanical forces. Several common features that incorporate clinical pathologic and biomechanical injury constructs that may be utilized in defining the nature of a concussive head injury include:

1 Concussion may be caused either by a direct blow to the head face neck or elsewhere on the body with an "impulsive" force transmitted to the head.
2 Concussion typically results in the rapid onset of short-lived impairment of neurological function that resolves spontaneously. However in some cases symptoms and signs may evolve over a number of minutes to hours.
3 Concussion may result in neuropathological changes but the acute clinical symptoms largely reflect a functional disturbance rather than a structural injury and as such no abnormality is seen on standard structural neuroimaging studies.
4 Concussion results in a graded set of clinical symptoms that may or may not involve loss of consciousness. Resolution of the clinical and cognitive symptoms typically follows a sequential course. However it is important to note that in some cases symptoms may be prolonged.

(Used with permission from McCrory et al., 2013.)

Acute Clinical Effects and Recovery

The scientific literature supports a functional rather than a structural etiology for SRC (Signoretti, Lazzarino, Tavazzi, & Vagnozzi, 2011). The model commonly used to understand the neurophysiological basis of SRC and other forms of mild head injury, developed on the basis of animal models, is conceptualized as a multilayered neurometabolic cascade, involving a complex of interwoven cellular and vascular changes that occur following trauma to the brain (Giza & Hovda, 2001; Giza & Hovda, 2014). According to this model, the pathophysiology of SRC represents a temporary disruption of brain function secondary to ionic fluxes, abnormal energy transmission, diminished cerebral blood flow, and impaired neurotransmission rather than any readily identifiable form of structural brain damage.

Extensive research over the last 10–15 years has advanced our scientific understanding of the true natural history of SRC. The results show, in general, that the clinical recovery is favorable. A 2003 report was the first to plot the continuous time course of acute recovery immediately and within several days after SRC, indicating that more than 90% of athletes exhibited recovery within one week. Figure 27.1 displays the recovery curves for symptoms, cognitive performance, and postural stability from that study (McCrea et al., 2003). Since that time, several other prospective studies have confirmed the fact that most athletes achieve a complete recovery of symptoms, cognitive functioning, postural stability, and other functional impairments within a period of approximately one to two weeks following SRC (Belanger & Vanderploeg, 2005; Broglio & Puetz, 2008; Collins et al., 1999; Macciocchi, Barth, Alves, Rimel, & Jane, 1996).

Limited research findings haves suggested a lengthier recovery time in younger athletes (Field, Collins, Lovell, & Maroon, 2003), with some papers demonstrating that roughly half of all high school athletes require more than 14 days to recover (Henry, Elbin, Collins, Marchetti, & Kontos, 2015; Lau, Lovell, Collins, & Pardini, 2009; Lau, Collins, & Lovell, 2012). Unfortunately, these studies have not included control subjects and applied "recovery" criteria that may have resulted in high false-positive rates due to criterion contamination, complicating the interpretation of resulting data (Nelson et al., 2013). Other researchers have reported that female athletes experience more symptoms and greater cognitive impairment from SRC than male athletes, although findings from these studies are quite mixed (Covassin, Schatz, & Swanik, 2007; Dick, 2009; Zuckerman et al., 2012). Many of the studies reporting gender differences in recovery were hampered by small samples of female athletes, poorly matched groups, or lack of preinjury baseline data (Nelson et al., 2013).

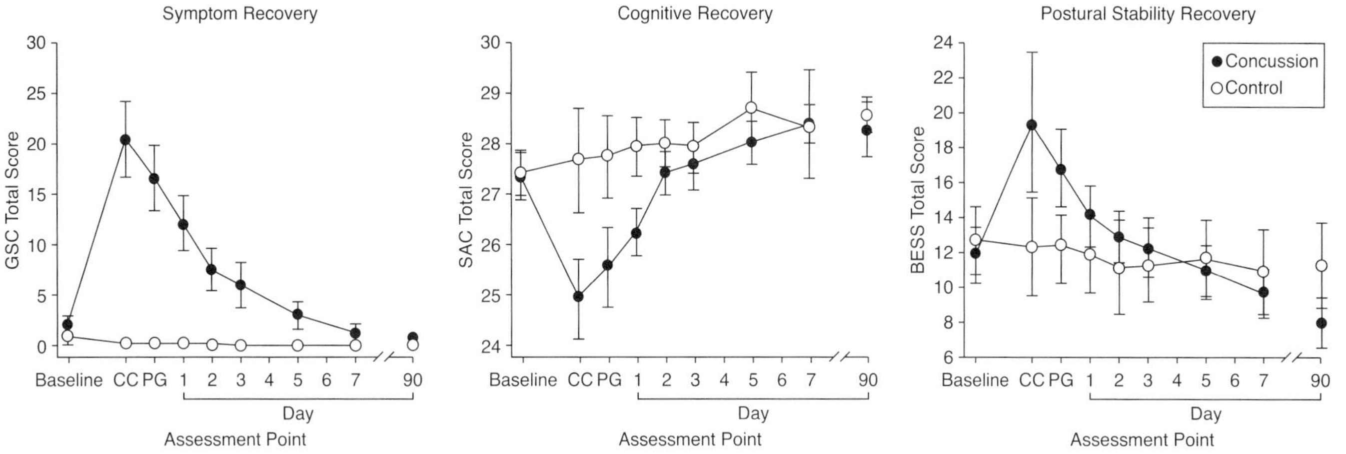

Figure 27.1 Recovery curves for clinical recovery from SRC in sample of 94 injured athletes and 56 controls (used with permission by McCrea et al., 2003.)

Assessment of Acute Injury Effects

Sideline Testing

The consensus opinion from a recent panel of experts in the field of sports injuries is that the sideline evaluation serves as an "essential component of the protocol" (Aubry et al., 2002). The timeline for formal assessment of an athlete using validated instruments begins right at the time of the injury. A comprehensive evaluation requires a multimodal approach, including information regarding subjective symptoms, examination of vestibular functions, and an assessment of neurocognitive status (McCrory, 1997). The immediate goal of the initial evaluation is to determine whether or not symptoms of SRC are present and to provide a means to track the course of recovery. For years, this critical evaluation was performed through informal examination methods, without any empirical evidence to support their validity (Maddocks, Dicker, & Saling, 1995; McCrea, Kelly, Kluge, Ackley, & Randolph, 1997; McCrory, 1997).

Over the years, a number of investigators have developed and validated a series of screening measures for use in evaluating athletes for SRC on the sideline (Collins & Hawn, 2002; Guskiewicz, Riemann, Perrin, & Nashner, 1997; McCrea et al., 1997). The requirements of these instruments are that they are portable, can be administered briefly, and can be used on multiple occasions. Since neuropsychologists are not typically present on the sideline for the initial assessment, it is important to utilize methods that can be administered and interpreted by team physicians and athletic trainers who have not received formal training in psychometric assessment. In the following, we present a multidimensional model of sideline assessment, comprised of measures that have been validated empirically for assessing symptoms, balance, and cognitive functioning.

Symptom Checklists

The subjective symptoms resulting from SRC are either reported spontaneously or are elicited through an examiner's questioning on the sidelines. Lovell and Collins (1998) introduced the Post-Concussion Scale–Revised (PCS-R) as a formal method of evaluating these symptoms in athletes, and this has gained rather wide acceptance for routine clinical use. The PCS-R consists of 21 symptoms commonly reported by individuals who have sustained a MTBI. The symptoms are rated individually on a 7-point Likert scale ranging from 0 (nonexistent) to 6 (severe). Ratings for each symptom are summed to obtain a total symptom score. Normative data on the original form of the instrument have been published (Lovell et al., 2006). Results from other investigations using modified versions of the instrument have demonstrated its utility in documenting symptoms of SRC (Guskiewicz & Broglio, 2011; McLeod & Leach, 2012).

The Concussion Symptom Inventory (CSI) is another brief 12-item instrument developed through psychometric methods that has proven to be sensitive to the effects of SRC (Randolph et al., 2009). This measure was developed from data obtained on more than 16,000 athletes receiving baseline testing and more than 600 athletes following SRC. A total of 12 of 27 symptoms were found to be most sensitive to detection of SRC in injured athletes. Each symptom is rated on a 7-point Likert scale ranging from 0 (nonexistent) to 6 (severe). Ratings for each symptom are summed to obtain a total symptom score. Studies on the validation sample indicated that this 12-item scale was as sensitive as prior measures composed of a larger number of items. At this point, this is the only empirically derived scale in existence for tracking SRC symptoms in injured athletes.

Neurocognitive Testing

The Standardized Assessment of Concussion (SAC) was developed by McCrea and colleagues as a brief and valid measure of neurocognitive functioning for use on the sideline for evaluating the immediate effects of SRC (McCrea, 2001; McCrea et al., 1997; McCrea et al., 1998). The instrument takes approximately five minutes to administer. It includes five orientation questions, a five-word list-learning test, digits backward, reversing the months of the year, and delayed recall of the word list. Summing scores from all of these tasks yields a 30-point composite score that can be used for aid in diagnosis and to guide immediate decision making. It also includes a standard neurologic screening, exertional maneuvers, and means for assessing LOC and posttraumatic amnesia. There are numerous studies demonstrating this measure's psychometric properties and its sensitivity to detecting symptoms of SRC in high school and college athletes (Barr & McCrea, 2001; M. McCrea et al., 2003; McCrea et al., 1998).

Balance Testing

Individuals sustaining a SRC are known to experience dizziness and resulting difficulties with balance. Positive Romberg signs can be elicited in up to two-thirds of athletes after the injury, making balance one of the most sensitive indices for assessing acute effects of SRC (Guskiewicz, Weaver, Padua, & Garrett, 2000). The Balance Error Score System (BESS) is a method developed by investigators at the University of North Carolina as a standardized measure of postural stability for assessment on the sideline (Guskiewicz, Ross, & Marshall, 2001; Riemann & Guskiewicz, 2000). The procedure requires the injured athlete to maintain three stances (double, single, and tandem) while resting on a firm surface or on a piece of 10-cm thick foam. Subjects are instructed to maintain their stance while keeping eyes closed and maintaining hands on their hips for 20 seconds. They are instructed to make any necessary adjustment to maintain their balance but to return to the original position as soon as possible. Examiners are trained to identify six types of errors. Scoring is based on the total number of errors observed over the six test trials. Psychometric properties and data demonstrating the reliability of this instrument have been reported in several research investigations (Guskiewicz & Broglio, 2011; Guskiewicz et al., 2001; Riemann, Guskiewicz, & Shields, 1999).

Other Sideline Instruments

The sports medicine literature includes descriptions of other standardized approaches to sideline testing of neurocognitive functioning (Collins & Hawn, 2002). In contrast to the SAC, many of these instruments provided structured guidelines for assessing mental status without computing a final test score. The subjective nature of these instruments limits their applicability in research settings and places restrictions on the ability to determine their validity and sensitivity to detecting the effects of SRC.

The Sports Concussion Assessment Tool, currently in its third revision (SCAT-3) is a measure that has been developed and modified over the years as part of the International Conference on Concussion in Sport (McCrory, Meeuwisse, Aubry, Cantu, et al., 2013). The intent has been to develop a standardized tool that could be used for patient education in addition to multidimensional clinical assessment of SRC. The original version included a combination of previously published tools, including lists of physical signs of concussion in combination with measures of clinical symptoms and cognitive functioning. More recent versions of this instrument (SCAT-2 and SCAT-3) incorporate a graded symptom checklist, SAC, modified (firm surface) BESS, and the Maddocks questions (Maddocks et al., 1995) in addition to providing a total score (Guskiewicz et al., 2013; Paul McCrory et al., 2009). While normative data on this instrument in its entirety were not available initially, a number of studies providing norms on subtests from various versions of the SCAT are appearing in the literature (Jinguji et al., 2012; Putukian et al., 2015), which should lead to more widespread adoption of this instrument in the sports medicine community.

Another measure used increasingly for assessment of acute concussion effects is the King-Devick test (KDT; see King, Clark, & Gissane, 2012). The KDT is a brief and portable test of visual functions that can be performed in less than one minute. The respondent reads a series of numbers whose placement on three cards requires saccadic (fast alternating) eye movements to fixed targets. Consistent with other standardized assessments that have been advocated recently for the assessment of SRC (e.g., the SCAT-2, SAC, BESS), there is evidence that the KDT is sensitive to the effects of SRC, although published samples have been small (Galetta et al., 2011; Galetta et al., 2013). However, at this point there is a relative lack of normative data on the KDT and limited information on its psychometric properties, such as test-retest reliability, when applied to athlete samples.

The Role of Neuropsychological Assessment

Neuropsychological assessment in the sports setting is utilized optimally for providing an objective basis for evaluating the effects of SRC, particularly at a point when athletes are no longer reporting subjective symptoms. The original intention was to use neuropsychological testing as the measure to officially mark when an otherwise "symptom free" individual is ready to return to play. Unfortunately, the data have not supported the use of neuropsychological testing for that purpose (Nelson et al., in press). While there is no doubt that neuropsychological testing has made a contribution to our ability to diagnose and manage SRC, valid questions regarding its usage for tracking acute injury effects have emerged over the past ten years (Broglio, Ferrara, Macciocchi,

Baumgartner, & Elliott, 2008; Guskiewicz et al., 2005; Guskiewicz et al., 2003; Randolph, McCrea, & Barr, 2005; Resch, McCrea, & Cullum, 2013). The aim of this section of the chapter is to critically evaluate the current use of neuropsychological assessment in a sports setting with the goal of moving towards an evidence-based model of practice.

Utility of Baseline Testing

At this point, many neuropsychologists have participated in baseline neuropsychological testing programs in the sports setting in a manner that is consistent with the model established by Barth, Alves, Ryan, Macciocchi, Rimel, and Jane (1989) with further refinement made by others for use with professional, collegiate, and high school athletes (Lovell & Collins, 1998). The overwhelming trend over the past several years has been to use computerized test batteries with team data obtained at preseason baseline, followed by testing performed on injured athletes within 48 hours of the injury. Additonal testing is performed subsequently until the athlete has demonstrated a "return" to his or her baseline level of performance. While this model holds much in terms of intuitive appeal, its success and wide acceptance appears to be based more on the effects of professional recommendations and opinion than the results of empirical research. Empirical findings supporting the utility of neuropsychological testing during the early stage of recovery from SRC are sorely lacking.

There are, indeed, a number of apparent advantages to the concept of performing neuropsychological testing on injured athletes when baseline test data are available for use as a comparison. The availability of this "within-subject" design enables the clinician to control for what might amount to confounding factors associated with premorbid intelligence, cultural factors, and the individual's neurodevelopmental background. However, what is tantamount to this model is an assumption that the clinician has a measure that is sensitive enough to detect a change in performance associated with the injury that can be detected over and above the noise associated with practice effects and the inherent reliability of the instrument. There are now a number of questions as to whether the neuropsychological tests currently used in the sport setting do indeed meet these criteria.

Over the past several years, a number of experts have begun to question whether the neuropsychological tests employed in most sports settings are actually sensitive enough to detect the effects of brain dysfunction underlying concussion. Randolph, McCrea, and Barr (2005) were the first to raise the issue of whether the neuropsychological tests used in both paper-and-pencil and computerized test batteries possessed the requisite reliability, validity, and sensitivity to the effects of SRC to warrant their use as part of a serial testing battery. Many of the arguments raised in this chapter have been supported by research findings published by other investigators demonstrating that tests contained in many of the commercially available computerized test batteries lacked the level of reliability needed to be sensitive to the effects of SRC (Broglio et al., 2008; Resch et al., 2013; Resch et al., 2013).

There is no doubt that obtaining baseline neuropsychological test data on a team of athletes requires large commitments of time, effort, and finances. The questions addressed regarding the reliability and sensitivity of the test instruments, raise further questions about whether baseline testing is actually necessary and essential to diagnosing the effects of SRC. At this point, there are no evidence-based research findings indicating that baseline neuropsychological testing provides a more sensitive means for detecting impairment associated with SRC in comparison to the "standard" clinical approach using a single cross-sectional assessment point combined with a psychometric definition of impairment based on a deviation from test norms (Echemendia et al., 2012; Schmidt, Register-Mihalik, Mihalik, Kerr, & Guskiewicz, 2012). Given the existing state of affairs, clinicians should consider revisiting the use of "standard" testing in conjunction with test norms in the sports setting.

Timing of Postinjury Testing

Another major question that arises with the use of neuropsychological testing is when to perform the postinjury assessment. Management models calling for routine assessment of the athlete within 24–48 hours of the injury run the risk of providing information that is redundant with data obtained through other sources such as the athlete's reporting of symptoms. There is also a potential for these results to introduce extra confounds in terms of practice effects.

Findings from a study performed on a large sample of collegiate athletes (see Figure 27.2) demonstrated that neuropsychological testing provides little unique information regarding abnormal test findings in relation to results obtained from sideline assessment methods used during the initial period of recovery (McCrea et al., 2005). Results from testing performed at seven days, in turn, provided some additional information regarding impairment relative to information from traditional sideline measures, although the overall contribution was rather small. These findings suggest that postinjury neuropsychological testing provide nothing unique in terms of information for tracking initial recovery from SRC, raising questions about whether this form of testing might be utilized most optimally when it is reserved for assessment of recovery in cases of a complicated pattern of recovery from SRC or a history of multiple previous concussions.

Computerized Versus Paper-and-Pencil Testing

The final question is whether computerized neuropsychological testing provides a more sensitive and efficient manner to assess cognitive functioning in injured athletes as compared to standard paper-and-pencil testing. Developers of

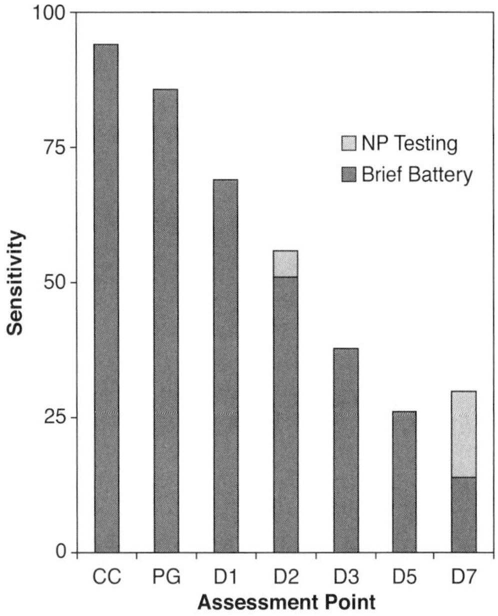

Figure 27.2 Percentage of concussion and control participants classified as "impaired" from time of injury through Day 7 on Brief Battery (GSC, BESS, and SAC) and NP Testing. GSC = Graded Symptom Checklist; BESS = Balance Error Scoring System; SAC = Standardized Assessment of Concussion; and NP Testing = Neuropsychological Test Battery. Assessment points: CC = time of concussion; PG = post-game/post-practice; D1 = postinjury Day 1, D2 = postinjury Day 2, etc. (adapted from by McCrea et al., 2005).

computerized test batteries have argued that the automated test platforms provide more efficient and accurate means for collecting data than standard paper-pencil batteries. The use of reaction time indices and randomized presentation of test items has been alleged to provide means for obtaining more reliable test data. However, those marketing claims have not been supported by results of empirical research.

At this point, the only study examining the sensitivity of computerized testing using prospective research designs has demonstrated no advantage to that form of testing relative to symptom checklists on injured athletes and matched controls compared with serial testing from baseline through the recovery of symptoms (Nelson et al., in press). There are no "head to head" studies demonstrating that any computerized test battery is more effective than standard paper-and-pencil testing for evaluating symptoms of SRC in this or any other population. The lack of empirical evidence supporting the use of neuropsychological tests of any kind in assessment of concussion symptoms raises questions about whether these measures should be used on a routine basis as part of a SRC management system.

Regarding other proposed advantages of computerized testing, there are no data supporting initial claims that these methods offer financial advantages to standard methods of testing. While the emphasis on reaction time as a dependent measure may be attractive from a theoretical standpoint, its proposed advantage over data obtained from traditional testing has not been demonstrated empirically. In fact, any claims of the precision added by the use of computers must be tempered by numerous technological questions that arise when using these test paradigms across different computer platforms and in varying conditions of traffic in local area networks and on the Internet (Rahman-Fillipiak & Woodard, 2013). There is a major disadvantage to testing memory on a computer, as the focus must be on recognition rather than recall, which research has been demonstrated to be among the most sensitive tasks for assessing the effects of concussion (Collins et al., 1999; Echemendia, Putukian, Mackin, Julian, & Shoss, 2001).

Finally, there are also concerns about the quality of data obtained when young athletes are tested on a computer in groups or under minimal supervision and when athletes are making an attempt to look bad on baseline testing (e.g., "sandbagging") in an attempt to mask detection of performance decline following injury (Erdal, 2012; Moser, Schatz, Neidzwski, & Ott, 2011). There is also an increasing sentiment that the growth of computer testing may lead to a decline in the role that neuropsychologists play in evaluating and tracking the effects of SRC (Echemendia, Herring, & Bailes, 2009).

Search for the Concussion "Biomarker"

Concussion causes temporary changes in brain function. The changes cannot be observed directly. They are typically inferred indirectly by scores from measures of behavior, symptoms, cognition, balance, and other functional abilities. Given the diagnostic difficulties associated with SRC, several lines of research are exploring the viability of using advanced imaging, electrophysiological techniques, and blood and cerebrospinal fluid (CSF) indices to arrive at a better understand of the physiologic effects of SRC. However, the clinical diagnosis of a SRC continue to be based on description of the acute injury characteristics, reported symptoms following the injury, and clinical measures of cognition or other functional activities. More recently, there is avid pursuit in the scientific community toward finding a definitive "biomarker" from a neurodiagnostic test or a blood sample that could enable a more objective diagnosis of SRC and indicate conclusively when an athlete has achieved a complete physiologic recovery and, therefore, is fit to safely return to play. To date, no such biomarker exists for clinical use, although some are considered viable candidates, as summarized below.

Structural Brain Imaging

The presence of structural brain pathology after concussion can have important diagnostic and prognostic implications.

To begin with, positive neuroimaging findings may signal the need for rapid intervention to avoid a catastrophic outcome. Additionally, when clinical neuroimaging reveals the presence of an observable abnormality, such as the presence of sudural or subarachnoid blood collection, the classification of the injury may change from a simple "concussion" to a more complicated form of MTBI. The expected course of recovery and return to play becomes very different when one experiences the effects of a complicated MTBI, as opposed to an uncomplicated form of concussion (Kashluba, Hanks, Casey, & Millis, 2008).

It is generally accepted that computed tomography (CT) scans have great value in detecting neurosurgical emergencies but also have the poorest sensitivity in detecting underlying abnormalities associated with milder forms of brain injury, including concussion (Yuh, Hawryluk, & Manley, 2014). The absence of focal findings on a CT scan is often equated incorrectly and inappropriately with a complete lack or nonexistence of brain injury, which then creates confusion amongst health care providers that often follows the patient throughout his or her clinical management after injury. There is a continual pursuit in the neurosciences to develop imaging techniques sensitive to detecting structural and functional abnormalities following milder forms of brain injury, even in the absence of traumatic abnormalities on head CT scan (Yuh et al., 2014).

When looking at all levels of TBI severity, magnetic resonance (MR) imaging provides a more sensitive means for detecting structural abnormalities associated with TBI than CT. MR methods has been found to be up to 25%–30% more sensitive than CT scanning in revealing diffuse axonal injury (Mittl et al., 1994) but both imaging modalities are found to be normal in most cases and have very weak correlation with clinical outcome after concussion (Hammoud & Wasserman, 2002). Cortical contusions, subdural hematomas, and hemorrhagic changes in the white matter are the most common findings on brain MRI after concussion, but as mentioned, are rarely seen as a result of SRC.

The potential utility of more sensitive imaging techniques is especially intriguing in cases where a patient remains symptomatic despite negative conventional imaging (e.g., CT, MR). Recent studies have investigated the utility of diffusion tensor MR imaging (DTI) in TBI, particularly in an attempt to detect and characterize underlying diffuse axonal injury (DAI) with more severe forms of injury. DTI is an application of MRI that capitalizes on the diffusion of water molecules for imaging the brain. While diffusion-weighted MR imaging measures the diffusion of water molecules in a particular direction, DTI extends this technology by imaging diffusion in several different directions (Belanger, Vanderploeg, Curtiss, & Warden, 2007). Many believe that DTI may be in a unique position to predict recovery in TBI patients, with particular relevance to concussion that results in axonal injury (not death) not identified on normal CT/MRI scans (Belanger et al., 2007). However, results from more recent reviews have demonstrated a range of disparate findings from DTI studies on concussion (Aoki, Inokuchi, Gunshin, Yahagi, & Suwa, 2012), indicating that its use for diagnosing brain effects of concussion on a clinical basis remain premature at this point.

Functional Brain Imaging

It has been suggested that functional MRI (fMRI) might be more sensitive to detecting brain changes in MTBI in symptomatic patients, in the absence of deficits on objective cognitive testing, as suggested by (McAllister et al., 1999). However, results from studies using fMRI in concussion subjects have varied widely, with findings across studies sometimes going in opposite directions. Some studies have reported decreased activation following the subacute phase of recovery in injured athletes (Gosselin et al., 2011) and still others have not shown any difference in brain activation patterns as measured by fMRI following the subacute recovery period (Elbin et al., 2012; Terry et al., 2012).

Hammeke and colleagues (2013) used an event-related fMRI design with a working memory task to investigate brain activation patterns in high school football players who had sustained two or three concussions. Injured athletes and control teammates (matched on a number of variables) were initially tested approximately 13 hours postinjury and then again during the subacute phase of the injury approximately seven weeks later. During the acute phase, the injured group showed the expected postconcussive symptoms and cognitive decline when compared to the healthy control subjects. Brain activation patterns showed decreases in the injured group compared to the control subjects in attention networks during this acute phase. During the subacute phase, the injured athletes showed the expected improvement in symptoms and cognitive performance. Brain activation patterns showed the reverse of the acute-phase activation patterns, in that the attention network of the concussed athletes was greater than the activation in the healthy control subjects. These results suggest that there is less activation during the acute symptomatic phase, which is indicative of underlying brain dysfunction. Conversely, after a period of recovery, the increase in brain activation is likely due to compensatory increases in brain activity to support normal behavioral performance.

The fMRI studies mentioned previously used a task-state fMRI design. The participant actively engages in a cognitive task, which is correlated with brain activity. Resting-state fMRI (R-fMRI) is another method to investigate brain function. R-fMRI involves data collection while the participant is at rest, rather than while the participant is performing a cognitive activation task. Work that began in the early 1990s showed that an individual's brain at rest demonstrates important information about functional organization (for a review, see Biswal, 2012). In that respect, there is a specific network of brain regions referred to as the *default network* that is consistently active during rest and has shown to be sensitive to a number of neurologic and psychiatric disorders (Buckner, 2012; Raichle et al., 2001). Further work is needed to determine whether a profile exists that can reliably distinguish R-fMRI abnormalities in concussion from those associated with a range of developmental neuropsychiatric conditions.

Electrophysiological Methods

While electrophysiological abnormalities can be demonstrated in a minority of concussed individuals through the use of routine EEG, the clinical significance of these findings have not been demonstrated in any reliable or scientifically rigorous manner (Nuwer, Hovda, Schrader, & Vespa, 2005).

A number of investigators have turned to the use of evoked related potentials (ERP) for the study of SRC. Some studies using small samples of athletes have demonstrated abnormalities of the P300 component with a suggestion that the abnormality corresponds in some way with symptom severity (Lavoie, Johnston, Leclerc, Lassonde, & Dupuis, 2004). Other findings have suggested abnormalities of certain ERP components extending beyond the athlete's reported recovery of symptoms (De Beaumont, Brisson, Lassonde, & Jolicoeur, 2007). Results from these studies indicate that electrophysiological indices hold promise as a means of identifying possible abnormalities in underlying brain function following concussion at a point when findings from other measures are negative.

Quantitative EEG (QEEG) investigations of concussion have reported abnormalities in many features reflecting changes in brain function, including reduced mean frequency of alpha, reduced power in the alpha and beta frequency bands, hypercoherence between frontal regions, and decreased gamma frequency (Tebano et al., 1988; Thatcher et al., 2001; Thatcher, Walker, Gerson, & Geisler, 1989; Thompson, Sebastianelli, & Slobounov, 2005; Watson et al., 1995) Using these features, normal controls have reportedly been discriminated from MTBI patients with high levels of sensitivity. The variables contributing to this discrimination include measures of coherence, phase and amplitude differences. It has been noted that frontal and fronto-temporal regions contributed more than other regions to such discrimination, suggesting increased vulnerability of these areas (Thompson et al., 2005). Much more work needs to be done in this area to demonstrate the specificity of the findings before these and other electrophysiological methods are ready for use in detecting abnormalities resulting from SRC.

The use of QEEG as a clinical tool to measure possible physiological vulnerability following concussion is of interest, but there are limited data on use of this methodology during the course of recovery following SRC. QEEG measures were recently used in a series of studies in conjunction with a number of clinical measures (Concussion Symptom Inventory, SAC, BESS, and Automated Neuropsychological Assessment Metrics) with athlete samples at the time of injury, at recovery Day 8 and recovery Day 45 (Barr, Prichep, Chabot, Powell, & McCrea, 2012; McCrea, Prichep, Powell, Chabot, & Barr, 2010; Prichep, McCrea, Barr, Powell, & Chabot, 2013). As expected, athletes with SRC demonstrated impairments on clinical measures at the time of injury, but these impairments resolved by Day 8 postinjury. The QEEG measure, however, showed abnormal findings in the concussed group when compared to control subjects on the day of injury that persisted through Day 8 (and resolved by Day 45). These data support the notion that a period of physiologic recovery persists beyond the point of full recovery on clinical measures.

Laboratory Biomarkers

Potential laboratory biomarkers include measures of a biological or pathological processes involving the brain that can be measured objectively in samples of blood or CSF. The theory behind the use of these measures in TBI research is based on a hypothesis that an injury to the brain causes a series of cellular processes affecting neurons and glia that result in a release of specific proteins and other biochemical products into the bloodstream, after crossing the blood-brain barrier (Mondello et al., 2014). The assumption is that these measures are associated with pathological processes induced by brain trauma and correlate in some manner with the magnitude of the underlying injury. Given the lack of any consistent imaging or electrophysiological findings associated with SRC, it is no surprise that there has been a surge of interest in finding a reliable biological index that can be used to determine the presence of SRC through a simple blood test.

The search for blood biomarkers has concentrated thus far on strategies for identifying disturbances of glial or neuronal processes. Most attention has focused on studies of S100B, a protein associated with neuronal and microglia processes that has been shown to be present in elevated levels in association with a number of neurological conditions (Zetterberg, Smith, & Blennow, 2013). While S100B has been demonstrated to be sensitive to the effects of TBI, its specificity has been questioned, as the protein is also present in a number of cell types independent of the central nervous system (CNS) (Schulte, Podlog, Hamson-Utley, Strathmann, & Struder, 2014). Its utility as a biomarker in athletic settings remains questionable, as elevations of S100B are commonly observed in athletes who have not sustained an SRC, indicating that its levels might be influenced by all types of bodily injuries, rather than injuries specific to the brain.

Other efforts to define a blood biomarker for SRC have examined the use of Neuron-Specific Enolase (NSE), a neuronally based enzyme that has been thought to provide a sensitive indicator of neuronal cell death. In contrast to the S100B protein, the issue with this enzyme has been its sensitivity, rather than specificity (Mondello et al., 2014). Studies on Glial Fibrillary Acidic Protein (GFAP) and Ubiquitin C-Terminal Hydrolase (UCH-L1) have generated some interest due to the fact that those compounds are found exclusively within the CNS and have been demonstrated to have associations with severity and outcome in more severe levels of TBI (Zetterberg et al., 2013). Substantial interest has also been placed on identification of the tau protein, a marker of axonal damage and degeneration (Gatson & Diaz-Arrastia, 2014). However, despite its purported association with neurodegenerative changes following SRC, there has been no consistent evidence that the tau protein has any diagnostic value in studies of MTBI or SRC or any sensitivity to detecting a risk for negative long-term outcome (Castellani, Perry, & Iverson, 2015; Mondello et al., 2014).

Many challenges thus remain to the identification of a blood biomarker that is sensitive and specific to the effects of SRC, and can be used effectively for diagnosis and prediction of outcome. Some argue that studies of CSF will provide measures of brain biochemistry that are less confounded than those obtained from blood samples (Neselius, Brisby, Granholm, Zetterberg, & Blennow, 2015). However, the more invasive methods of collecting such samples do not appear feasible in the athletic setting.

Other questions remain as to whether there will ever be any success in identifying a single biomarker that would be sufficient for diagnosis of SRC in addition to being useful for predicting clinical outcome and/or risk for subsequent injury. Due to variability in the biochemical processes underlying brain injury recovery, it appears very likely that a strategy based on use of a variety of different biomarkers will need to be developed, depending on whether one is attempting to study acute, subacute, or chronic stages of injury recovery (Mondello et al., 2014). In the meantime, there remain no empirical data to indicate that any identified blood or CSF biomarker is suitable for diagnosing or making predictions about long-term outcome of SRC.

Potential Complications in Recovery From SRC

Clinical strategies for management of SRC are based on an attempt to maintain the athlete's safety, by minimizing the possibility of sustaining a repeat injury, persistent symptoms, or more catastrophic or long-term effects. While it is known that the vast majority of athletes recover from concussion within a period of seven to ten days, there are beliefs that a window of cerebral vulnerability may extend beyond the point of clinical recovery after SRC, during which the brain remains physiologically compromised and athletes are at heightened risk of repetitive injury or complications (Nelson et al., 2013). The primary risk associated with repeat concussion is thought to be a slowed clinical recovery characterized by persistent symptoms or functional impairment. There are also significant concerns about prediction and prevention of more catastrophic effects of SRC, which appear to be exceedingly rare, and longer-term effects such as late-life dementia, which has been described in some individual athletes but has an incidence that remains unknown (Karantzoulis & Randolph, 2013).

Susceptibility to Repeat Injury and Catastrophic Outcome

There are indications that an athlete's risk of repeat concussion in the same sports season is essentially equivalent to the risk of a single concussion. In a large sample of collegiate football players investigated over three seasons (over 4,000 player seasons), it was found that 6.3% of players sustained a single concussion and 6.5% sustained a repeat concussion within the same season (Kevin M. Guskiewicz et al., 2003). Results from an expanded analysis of that sample demonstrated that 75%–90% of the same-season concussions occurred within seven to ten days of an initial concussion, during the period when there is a presumed increase in cerebral vulnerability (McCrea et al., 2009).

Prospective scientific studies on the effects of multiple concussions are difficult to perform, given the relatively low incidence of repeat injury. However, an emerging literature has begun to show that repeat concussions produce more severe symptoms, such as disorientation, LOC, and amnesia (Collins & Hawn, 2002; Guskiewicz, et al., 2003). Given the report of more severe symptoms, it is logical to expect longer periods of recovery postinjury following repeat concussions. Guskiewicz et al. (2003) showed that players with a self-reported history of multiple prior concussions take longer to recover, and there is also some evidence that athletes' performance on balance testing and some cognitive measures (e.g., verbal memory and reaction time) may recover more slowly after repeat concussions (Bruce & Echemendia, 2004; Covassin, Stearne, & Elbin, 2008). However, data capturing initial and repeated concussions prospectively have not revealed increased symptom duration between first and second concussions (McCrea et al., 2009).

There is also evidence to suggest that sustaining a concussion might increase an athlete's risk for subsequent injury. Studies have shown that individuals reporting a prior history of concussion are at three to six times the risk for sustaining subsequent concussions (Schulz, 2004; Zemper, 2003) in a given sports season and that there may be a dose-response type relationship, such that individuals reporting more concussions prior to study onset are at progressively increased risk for further injury (Guskiewicz, et al., 2003). There are also indications that a history of attention deficit/hyperactivity disorder (ADHD) or learning disability render one more susceptible to repeat concussion (Nelson et al., 2015).

Historically, the greatest concern linked to repetitive concussion centered on the risk of catastrophic outcomes (i.e., death or permanent disability) associated with diffuse cerebral swelling or second-impact syndrome (Cantu, 1998; Kelly, 1991; Saunders & Harbaugh, 1984). Occurrences of catastrophic outcome remain extremely rare and are presumed to be caused by a second injury event encountered while the brain is still in a state of vulnerability from an initial concussion days earlier. However, the pathophysiology of delayed cerebral swelling remains the subject of great debate and it remains unclear whether closely spaced injuries are the true underlying mechanism (Paul McCrory, 2001; McCrory & Berkovic, 1998; Randolph & Kirkwood, 2009).

Postconcussion Syndrome

There is little information regarding the rates of postconcussion syndrome (PCS) in athlete samples. Existing data indicate that concussed athletes, as a group, do not exhibit any significant differences from controls on neuropsychological testing performed at 90 days following the injury (McCrea et al., 2003). While injury factors such as LOC, posttraumatic amnesia, and more severe acute symptoms are found to predict prolonged recovery time (> seven days) in a minority of athletes (McCrea et al., 2013), there are no indications that any known injury factor, including LOC, renders an athlete at risk for development of more prolonged forms of PCS (Tator & Davis, 2014).

In spite of the relatively low number of complicated recoveries from SRC predicted by that study, persistent symptoms are believed to occur in 10%–15% of athletes (Makdissi, Cantu, Johnston, McCrory, & Meeuwisse, 2013; Morgan et al., 2015). Similar to what is estimated from studies of MTBI nonathlete samples, this prevalance estimate and factors responsible for the presence of PCS following SRC remains a topic of contention in head injury research. At this point, strategies for managing persistent PCS symptoms in athletes, as a group, are based primarily on anecdotal evidence or extrapolation of data from studies performed on more severe levels of TBI (Makdissi et al., 2013).

Based on reviews of the general literature, preinjury risk factors identified for development of PCS in adults include a number of personality variables and a prior history of psychiatric disturbance (Broshek, De Marco, & Freeman, 2015; Silverberg & Iverson, 2011). Predictive factors for PCS in children include learning difficulties, behavioral problems, and a previous history of head injury (Zemek, Farion, Sampson, & McGahern, 2013). Thus far, similar findings have been reported among the few studies examining PCS in athlete samples. One recent study found the risk of PCS to be increased in athletes with a personal and/or family history of mood disorder, other psychiatric illness, or migraine (Morgan et al., 2015). Interestingly, this study also found the rate of PCS to be increased in association with a postinjury risk factor, namely delayed symptom onset. Other researchers reported that more than 80% of their PCS cases in athletes had a history of at least one prior concussion (Tator & Davis, 2014). A high percentage of these cases reported a history of a premorbid psychiatric condition, ADHD, learning disability, and migraine.

There has been much interest over the past 20 years in identifying the psychological factors (e.g., misattribution, nocebo effect, "good-old-days" phenomena) underlying the tendency to report persisting symptoms following concussion in a range of settings, including sports (Gunstad & Suhr, 2001; Mittenberg, DiGiulio, Perrin, & Bass, 1992). As a group, athletes have been found to underestimate the level of baseline symptoms present before the injury and to overestimate changes in symptoms occurring after the injury, consistent with a model of expectation as etiology (Ferguson, Mittenberg, Barone, & Schneider, 1999; Mittenberg, DiGuilio, Perrin, & Bass, 1992). Another study found that athletes have a general expectation for a healthy recovery from concussion, which differs from the types of expectations observed in other groups (Gunstad & Suhr, 2001).

Chronic Traumatic Encephalopathy

Based on extensive media coverage, the public is now acutely aware of cases of former athletes who have died tragically and prematurely and have been reported to have exhibited features of a clinical syndrome labeled as Chronic Traumatic Encephalopathy (CTE; see McKee et al., 2009; Omalu, 2014). Features of this syndrome were initially described in retired boxers nearly a century ago, using the terms "punch drunk syndrome" or "*dementia pugilistica*" (Corsellis, Bruton, & Freeman-Browne, 1973; Critchley, 1957; Iverson, Gardner, McCrory, Zafonte, & Castellani, 2015; Jordan, 2000; Maroon et al., 2015; Martland, 1928; Millspaugh, 1937). The recent interest in this condition is based on results of autopsy reports on professional athletes following retirement from careers in American football, ice hockey, and other contact sports. The relationship between CTE and SRC remains unclear, leading to conclusions that the condition is the result of cumulative exposure to subconcussive blows to the brain over the course of one's career as an athlete, now referred to as repetitive brain injury (RBI) (Saigal & Berger, 2014; Stein, Alvarez, & McKee, 2015). The reported identification of CTE in a handful of younger athletes (< 25 years old) raises questions about the degree of exposure to RBI needed to produce CTE (McKee et al., 2009).

Proponents of CTE characterize it as a neurodegenerative disease distinguished from other forms of dementia by its widespread accumulation of hyperphosphorylated tau (p-tau; see McKee et al., 2009). Individuals with CTE have been described as exhibiting a number of characteristic behavioral features including mood changes, explosive behaviors, and cognitive disturbance (Stern et al., 2013). Based on results of autopsy studies, these individuals have been observed to exhibit extensive tau-immunoreactive neurofibrillary tangles throughout the brain, with a preferential involvement of superficial cortical layers and other characteristics that reportedly make it distinctive from all other known forms of dementia (McKee et al., 2009).

A number of reviews critical of the CTE literature have been published, with conclusions that there are no empirical data demonstrating a definitive association between concussion in sports and increased risk for late-life cognitive and neuropsychiatric impairment, including CTE (Castellani et al., 2015; Iverson et al., 2015; Karantzoulis & Randolph, 2013; Maroon et al., 2015; McCrory, Meeuwisse, Kutcher, Jordan, & Gardner, 2013; Wortzel, Brenner, & Arciniegas, 2013). The primary criticism is that the CTE studies are based on autopsy series of cases identified with a risk of ascertainment bias. Based on results from epidemiological studies, there are no indications of any conclusive link between concussion and any emerging late life conditions, including dementia, and no increased risk for dementia in retired athletes has been in studies examining larger numbers of retired athletes (Baron, Hein, Lehman, & Gersic, 2012; Savica, Parisi, Wold, Josephs, & Ahlskog, 2012).

In terms of clinical characteristics, it has been argued that many of the behavioral and cognitive features attributed to CTE can be seen in other forms of neurodegenerative and mood disorders common to individuals from similar age groups (Karantzoulis & Randolph, 2013). From a neuropathological standpoint, there has been a lack of consensus among CTE proponents regarding the observed pattern and location of histopathological abnormalities, raising questions on whether the existing data warrant identification of a new clinical disorder (Randolph, 2014). Studies examining neuropsychological performance and neuroimaging findings in retired football players have been unable to demonstrate any test findings that would distinguish that group from individuals exhibiting features of mild forms of neurocognitive or mood disorder (Hart et al., 2013; Randolph, Karantzoulis, & Guskiewicz, 2013; Strain et al., 2013; Strain et al., 2015).

There is no doubt that the identification of neurodegenerative conditions in association with long-term sports participation has raised legitimate concerns about long-term safety issues for professional athletes. However, based on the existing science, there are no indications that younger athletes playing contact sports in recreational leagues, high school, or at the collegiate level are at any increased risk for development of neurodegenerative changes in later life. In the meantime, the topic of CTE will remain one of most publicized and controversial topics in the neurosciences until definitive findings are obtained from more scientifically rigorous longitudinal and epidemiological studies.

Practice Recommendations for Neuropsychologists

Assessment and Management of Initial Recovery From SRC

As discussed in the initial sections of this chapter, the initial assessment and management of the athlete with a suspected SRC begins on the field of play and is conducted in most instances by ATCs or team physicians. While neuropsychologists are rarely called into action on the sideline, those who find themselves posted in those settings should nonetheless be equipped with methods for evaluating acute symptoms in addition to being aware of the team's protocol for dealing with emergency situations.

It is much more common for neuropsychologists consulting to sports teams to receive a call for evaluation of an athlete more than 48 hours after sustaining a SRC. For assessment of athletes during that time frame, we advocate a model using a multidimensional sideline battery consisting of a set of instruments discussed in this chapter, including a symptom checklist, testing of postural stability, and a screening of neurocognitive functions. All of those instruments can be found in the SCAT-3, the most recent revision of the sideline assessment tool (Guskiewicz et al., 2013). Over the course of the first week, symptoms should be evaluated on a daily basis by relevant staff members with the symptom checklist, until the athlete reports that he or she is symptom-free for a 24-hour period. Once the athlete is found to be symptom-free at rest, one can move on to a graduated return-to-play protocol.

As outlined in the most recent Zurich Consensus Statement on Concussion in Sport (McCrory, Meeuwisse, Aubry, Cantu, et al., 2013), a graduated return to play protocol is recommended, in which the athlete returns to full participation. According to the guidelines (listed in Table 27.3), athletes progress to subsequent stages of rehabilitation when they have been asymptomatic for at least 24 hours. There are a total of five stages, with the first stage being symptom-limited physical and cognitive rest. The second stage is

Table 27.2 Graduated return-to-play protocol from the consensus statement on concussion in sport: the Third International Conference on Concussion in Sport, held in Zurich, November 2012

Rehabilitation Stage	*Functional Exercise at Each Stage of Rehabilitation*	*Objective of Each Stage*
1 No activity	Symptom limited physical & cognitive	Recovery rest
2 Light aerobic exercise	Walking, swimming, or stationary cycling keeping intensity < 70% maximum permitted heart rate. No resistance training.	Increase heart rate
3 Sport-specific exercise	Skating drills in ice hockey, running drills in soccer. No head impact activities.	Add movement
4 Noncontact training drills	Progression to more complex training drills, e.g., passing drills in football and ice hockey. May start progressive resistance training.	Exercise, coordination, and cognitive load
5 Full-contact practice	Following medical clearance, participate in normal training activities.	Restore confidence and assess functional skills by coaching staff
6 Return to play	Normal game play.	

(Used with permission from McCrory et al., 2013.)

light aerobic activity, then sport-specific exercise (e.g., skating drills in hockey, running drills in soccer), noncontact training drills (e.g., passing drills in football), full contact practice, and then finally return to play. If at any time the athlete becomes symptomatic, he or she is to return to the previous stage until asymptomatic for a 24-hour period. As each step in this process should take approximately one day, the whole process is expected to take approximately one week (McCrory, Meeuwisse, Aubry, et al., 2013).

The issue of complete cognitive and physical rest has become a controversial topic in the clinical management of SRC (Craton & Leslie, 2014; Schneider et al., 2013). Recommendations for rest are based loosely on concepts obtained from animal studies where it is known that a premature activation of physiological activity during a period when the brain is undergoing a restorative process can have a negative effect on many of the neural factors important for recovery (Griesbach, 2011; Griesbach, Gomez-Pinilla, & Hovda, 2007). Based on this information, it makes sense to recommend a few days rest following an injury. However, the neuropsychologist must be careful not to overextend recommendations of rest, which could have the potential of placing the recovering athlete at risk for developing a maladaptive focus on their symptoms. In fact, the results of a recent randomized controlled trial on 88 athletes assigned to conditions of extreme rest (five days) or usual care (one to two days rest, followed by stepwise return to activity) found no difference in neurocognitve or balance outcome between the groups (Thomas, Apps, Hoffmann, McCrea, & Hammeke, 2015). However, the extreme rest group reported more symptoms and slower resolution times than the group receiving usual care, indicating that symptom reporting was somehow affected by the period of extreme rest.

A naturally occurring question is whether neuropsychological testing should be performed routinely with athletes during the initial stages of recovery from SRC. Whether testing is conducted with standard (paper-pencil) methods or through computers, there are an increasing number of questions about the validity of neuropsychological testing with athletes and whether the information provided by neuropsychological testing during the stage of initial recovery provides incremental value to what might otherwise be obtained through multidimensional evaluations using an instrument like the SCAT-3.

As stated earlier in this chapter, the routine use of neuropsychological testing during the first week of the injury runs the risk of providing redundant information and a potential for confounding the results of subsequent testing. For these reasons, we recommend against the routine use of neuropsychological testing during the initial stages of recovery from SRC, with the aim of reserving this form of testing for those cases exhibiting atypical patterns of recovery.

While the sports culture calls for athletes to remain "tough" in the face of injury, there is an increase in the appreciation of the level that psychological and motivational factors can influence prolonged symptom presentation in athletes as well as in other types of patients. With those factors in mind, neuropsychological consultation can add crucial information to developing plans for the athletes' return to play and to school. Psychoeducational sessions aimed at athletes and their families should focus significantly on a review of the evidence-based literature to help counteract much of the information they are likely to have received through the media and from clinicians who have apparently not kept up with the vast majority of findings indicating that recovery from SRC proceeds in a relatively uncomplicated manner in most athletes.

Assessment and Management of Longer-Term Effects of SRC

Clinicians involved in the diagnosis and treatment of sports concussion will undoubtedly encounter cases of complicated recovery, characterized by symptoms persisting beyond the period associated with a "normal" resolution of symptoms (Makdissi et al., 2013). In some cases, one might find that the prolonged recovery is attributed to underlying neurophysiological causes, including histories of recent or multiple concussions. In other cases, there will be no obvious physical causes, raising questions about the presence of a persistent PCS.

A focused approach to neuropsychological assessment can be very helpful to guide interventions aimed at athletes reporting symptoms for more than 14 days for SRC, which would take them beyond the window of vulnerability associated with physiological causes (Barr & McCrea, 2010; Nelson et al., 2013). Not faced with time constraints found in the setting of acute recovery, testing of cognitive functioning in patients with prolonged effects of SRC can be accomplished effectively with a medium-sized neuropsychological test battery focusing on assessment of a combination of cognitive and psychological symptoms. A test battery recommended for this purpose is listed in Table 27.3.

Table 27.3 Test battery for assessment of SRC symptoms

- Wechsler Abbreviated Scale of Intelligence (WASI-2)
- Test of Premorbid Functioning (TOPF)
- Digit Span (WAIS-IV)
- Symbol Digit Modalities Test (SDMT)
- Trail Making Test (TMT)
- Stroop Color Word Interference Test
- Controlled Oral Word Association Test (COWAT)
- Hopkins Verbal Learning Test (HVLT-R)
- Test of Memory Malingering
- Reliable Digit Span (RDS)
- Symptom Checklist (SCAT-3)
- Minnesota Multiphasic Personality Inventory (MMPI-2-RF)

While athletes might end up reporting a wide range of symptoms following SRC, findings from the evidence-based literature indicate that attention, processing speed, and memory are the functions most commonly affected and these are the functions that should receive the most attention through neuropsychological testing (Belanger et al., 2005). The tests recommended in Table 27.3 for assessment of these functions were chosen on the basis of their previous use in sports concussion assessment protocols and the availability of normative data for athletes across the age spectrum (Barr, 2003; McCrea et al., 2003; Oliaro, Guskiewicz, & Prentice, 1998; Solomon, Lovell, Casson, & Viano, 2015).

As mentioned throughout this chapter, the available evidence from controlled research studies does not support the existence of long-term effects on cognitive functioning directly resulting from the physiological effects of any lasting brain injury. In fact, given the effect sizes reported in meta-analyses, cognitive impairment attributable to the effects of SRC (Belanger & Vanderploeg, 2005), if present, would be undetectable using neuropsychological testing or any other known methodology.

Ironically, when assessing the chronic effects of SRC, the neuropsychologist should be more in a position of providing assurance and communication that the results of testing indicate no long-term cognitive consequences of brain injury, contrary to what might be reported by other health care professionals. The goal would be to provide the patient with evidence-based information on recovery that will help him or her return to school, sports, and other activities. The end result of the neuropsychological evaluation will be to provide the athlete, family, and others an explanation of factors other than the physiological effects of "brain damage" that are likely to be playing a role in the maintenance of persisting symptoms and how those factors can be addressed through appropriate psychological intervention or other forms of rehabilitation.

Symptom reporting is an important component of any evaluation of a patient following SRC, particularly since there are no independent means to confirm the presence of injury through other neurodiagnostic methods. A formal evaluation of symptoms through standardized and validated assessment methods is thus an essential component of the neuropsychological evaluation so that the clinician can determine whether symptom magnification might be playing a role or whether the reporting of postconcussion symptoms is affected by any comorbid conditions such as chronic pain, somatization, or mood disorder. A combination of brief illness focused measures of symptom reporting and larger scale psychological inventories, such as the Minnesota Multiphasic Personality Inventory (MMPI-2-RF) (Ben-Porath & Tellegen, 2008), are recommended for use in test batteries designed for assessment of athletes presenting with reported prolonged effects of SRC.

A formal evaluation of validity and response bias is critical in any test battery, particularly in one focusing on a condition such as SRC, where a combination of many physical, psychological, and motivational factors are likely to be in play. Evaluation of patients with prolonged effects of SRC requires tests of both performance and symptom validity (Larrabee, 2012). It is important to note that these measures are not only used for detection of malingering, which appears to be somewhat rare in athlete samples, but are also useful in helping to identify the influence that somatization, mood disorder, and other psychological disorders are having on the athlete's ability to maintain the level of effort that is necessary to obtain valid results on neuropsychological testing.

Researchers involved in studies of sports concussion are only beginning to address the problem of prolonged recovery and the issue of PCS (Morgan et al., 2015). One positive feature of making a diagnosis of PCS in athletes is that the clinician will have more information regarding the initial injury than what is typically available in nonathletes. The challenge is in how to evaluate and attribute the athlete's subjective symptoms, which are often nonspecific in nature and may represent the effects of other conditions, notably those involving disorders of mood and anxiety. This is the situation where neuropsychological testing can be most useful.

Research on effective intervention strategies for PCS in athletes is sorely lacking. While there is increasing evidence on the effectiveness of using cognitive behavioral therapy (CBT) for treatment of PCS (Al Sayegh, Sandford, & Carson, 2010), no controlled trials of this treatment modality have been attempted in a sports setting. Based on conclusions from a recent review, there is emerging evidence supporting the use of some forms of vestibular and oculomtor rehabilitation, although recommendations on these treatments remain at the consensus level (Broglio, Collins, Williams, Mucha, & Kontos, 2015). There is also some evidence that a graded approach to increasing exercise accompanied by close monitoring of physiological functions and symptoms can be useful in some athletes experiencing long-term effects of PCS (Leddy et al., 2013; Leddy, Sandhu, Sodhi, Baker, & Willer, 2012).

Conclusions

Major advances in the study of concussion have been made over the past 20 years and neuropsychologists, in particular, have made significant contributions to science and the practices established for assessment and management of SRC. The field's most valuable contributions have been in the development and validation of instruments for measuring symptoms and neurocognitive functions. Furthermore, based on the field's emphasis on science and methodology, neuropsychology has also played an essential role on establishing which methods and approaches are most effective for enabling an athlete to return to play and other activities in a safe and successful manner.

Over the past several years, protocols for assessment of early symptoms and return to play guidelines have become relatively well established, although these practices continue to be based on consensus recommendation rather than as a result of controlled clinical trials. While neuropsychologists play a critical consultative role to the management of SRC over the entire course of recovery, the issue of how and when to use neuropsychological testing in the sports setting remains somewhat controversial. Based on empirical findings, the current conclusion is that neuropsychological testing is used most effectively with those athletes who are reporting symptoms persisting for more than 14 days, at a point when the test findings can help identify whether prolonged symptom reporting is the result of previously unidentified psychological factors.

With continuing media coverage on the potential negative consequences of SRC and medical attempts to identify a biomarker for concussion effects, the view provided in this chapter is that neuropsychologists can play a major role in the sports setting by providing education to athletes, families, and other providers on the range of other "nonbiological" factors that can affect symptom reporting and recommendations for treatment. Keeping that role in mind, the goal in the coming years will be to further refine and develop methods for assessing the atypical long-term consequences of SRC and developing more effective methods for its treatment.

References

Al Sayegh, A., Sandford, D., & Carson, A. J. (2010). Psychological approaches to treatment of postconcussion syndrome: A systematic review. *Journal of Neurology, Neurosurgery & Psychiatry*, *81*(10), 1128–1134. doi: 10.1136/jnnp.2008.170092

Aoki, Y., Inokuchi, R., Gunshin, M., Yahagi, N., & Suwa, H. (2012). Diffusion tensor imaging studies of mild traumatic brain injury: A meta-analysis. *Journal of Neurology, Neurosurgery, and Psychiatry*, *83*(9), 870–876. doi: 10.1136/jnnp-2012-302742

Aubry, M., Cantu, R., Dvorak, J., Graf-Baumann, T., Johnston, K. M., Kelly, J., . . . Schamasch, P. (2002). Summary and agreement statement of the 1st International Symposium on Concussion in Sport, Vienna 2001. *Clinical Journal of Sport Medicine*, *12*(1), 6–11. Retrieved from www.ncbi.nlm.nih.gov/entrez/query.fcgi?cmd=Retrieve&db=PubMed&dopt=Citation&list_uids=11854582

Bailes, J. E., & Hudson, V. (2001). Classification of sport-related head trauma: A spectrum of mild to severe injury. *Journal of Athletic Training*, *36*(3), 236–243.

Bakhos, L. L., Lockhart, G. R., Myers, R., & Linakis, J. G. (2010). Emergency department visits for concussion in young child athletes. *Pediatrics*, *126*(3), e550–e556. doi: 10.1542/peds.2009-3101

Baron, S. L., Hein, M. J., Lehman, E., & Gersic, C. M. (2012). Body mass index, playing position, race, and the cardiovascular mortality of retired professional football players. *American Journal of Cardiology*, *109*(6), 889–896. doi: 10.1016/j.amjcard.2011.10.050

Barr, W. B. (2003). Neuropsychological testing of high school athletes: Preliminary norms and test-retest indices. *Archives of Clinical Neuropsychology*.

Barr, W. B., & McCrea, M. (2001). Sensitivity and specificity of standardized neurocognitive testing immediately following sports concussion. *Journal of the International Neuropsychological Society*.

Barr, W. B., & McCrea, M. (2010). Diagnosis and assessment of concussion. In F. M. Webbe (Ed.), *The Handbook of Sport Neuropsychology*. New York: Springer Publishing Corporation.

Barr, W. B., Prichep, L. S., Chabot, R., Powell, M. R., & McCrea, M. (2012). Measuring brain electrical activity to track recovery from sport-related concussion. *Brain Injury*, *26*(1), 58–66. doi: 10.3109/02699052.2011.608216

Barth, J. T., Alves, W., Ryan, T., Macciocchi, S., Rimel, R., & Jane, J. J. (1989). Mild head injury in sports: Neuropsychological sequelae and recovery of function. In H. Levin, J. Eisenberg, & A. Benton (Eds.), *Mild Head Injury* (pp. 257–275). New York: Oxford.

Belanger, H. G., Curtiss, G., Demery, J. A., Lebowitz, B. K., & Vanderploeg, R. D. (2005). Factors moderating neuropsychological outcomes following mild traumatic brain injury: A meta-analysis. *Journal of the International Neuropsychological Society*, *11*(3). doi: 10.1017/s1355617705050277

Belanger, H. G., & Vanderploeg, R. D. (2005). The neuropsychological impact of sports-related concussion: A meta-analysis. *Journal of the International Neuropsychological Society*, *11*(4), 345–357. doi: 10.1017/s1355617705050411. Retrieved from www.ncbi.nlm.nih.gov/entrez/query.fcgi?cmd=Retrieve&db=PubMed&dopt=Citation&list_uids=16209414

Belanger, H. G., Vanderploeg, R. D., Curtiss, G., & Warden, D. L. (2007). Recent neuroimaging techniques in mild traumatic brain injury. *Journal of Neuropsychiatry*, *19*(1), 5–20. doi: 10.1176/appi.neuropsych.19.1.5

Ben-Porath, Y. S., & Tellegen, A. M. (2008). *MMPI-2-RF: Manual for Administration, Scoring, and Interpretation*. Minneapolis, MN: University of Minnesota Press.

Biswal, B. B. (2012). Resting state fMRI: A personal history. *NeuroImage*, *62*(2), 938–944. doi: 10.1016/j.neuroimage.2012.01.090

Broglio, S. P., Collins, M. W., Williams, R. M., Mucha, A., & Kontos, A. P. (2015). Current and emerging rehabilitation for concussion: A review of the evidence. *Clinics in Sports Medicine*, *34*(2), 213–231. doi: 10.1016/j.csm.2014.12.005

Broglio, S. P., Ferrara, M. S., Macciocchi, S. N., Baumgartner, T., & Elliott, R. (2008). Stability of common computerized tests for concussion assessment. *Medicine & Science in Sports & Exercise*, *40*(Suppl), 33. doi: 10.1249/01.mss.0000320764.14496.bf

Broglio, S. P., & Puetz, T. W. (2008). The effect of sport concussion on neurocognitive function, self-report symptoms and postural control: A meta-analysis. *Sports Medicine*, *38*(1), 53–67.

Broshek, D. K., De Marco, A. P., & Freeman, J. R. (2015). A review of post-concussion syndrome and psychological factors associated with concussion. *Brain Injury*, *29*(2), 228–237. doi: 10.3109/02699052.2014.974674

Bruce, J. M., & Echemendia, R. J. (2004). Concussion history predicts self-reported symptoms before and following a concussive event. *Neurology*, *63*(8), 1516–1518. Retrieved from www.ncbi.nlm.nih.gov/entrez/query.fcgi?cmd=Retrieve&db=PubMed&dopt=Citation&list_uids=15505180

Buckner, R. L. (2012). The serendipitous discovery of the brain's default network. *NeuroImage*, *62*(2), 1137–1145. doi: 10.1016/j.neuroimage.2011.10.035

Cantu, R. C. (1998). Second-impact syndrome. [Review] [20 refs]. *Clinics in Sports Medicine*, *17*(1), 37–44.

Castellani, R. J., Perry, G., & Iverson, G. L. (2015). Chronic effects of mild neurotrauma: Putting the cart before the horse? *Journal of Neuropathology & Experimental Neurology*, *74*(6), 493–499. doi: 10.1097/nen.0000000000000193

Collins, M. W., Grindel, S. H., Lovell, M. R., Dede, D. E., Moser, D. J., Phalin, B. R., . . . McKeag, D. B. (1999). Relationship between concussion and neuropsychological performance in college football players. *Jama*, *282*(10), 964–970. Retrieved from www.ncbi.nlm.nih.gov/htbin-post/Entrez/query?db=m&form=6&dopt=r&uid=10485682

Collins, M. W., & Hawn, K. L. (2002). The clinical management of sports concussion. *Current Sports Medicine Reports*, *1*, 12–22.

Corsellis, J.A.N., Bruton, C. J., & Freeman-Browne, D. (1973). The aftermath of boxing. *Psychological Medicine*, *3*, 270–303.

Covassin, T., Schatz, P., & Swanik, C. B. (2007). Sex differences in neuropsychological function and post-concussion symptoms of concussed collegiate athletes. *Neurosurgery*, *61*(2), 345–350; discussion 350–341. doi: 10.1227/01.NEU.0000279972.95060.CB

Covassin, T., Stearne, D., & Elbin, R. (2008). Concussion history and postconcussion neurocognitive performance and symptoms in collegiate athletes. *Journal of Athletic Training*, *43*(2), 119–124. doi: 10.4085/1062-6050-43.2.119

Craton, N., & Leslie, O. (2014). Is rest the best intervention for concussion? Lessons learned from the whiplash model. *Current Sports Medicine Reports*, *13*(4), 201–204. doi: 10.1249/jsr.0000000000000072

Critchley, M. (1957). Medical aspects of boxing, particularly from neurological standpoint. *British Medical Journal*, *1*, 357–362.

De Beaumont, L., Brisson, B., Lassonde, M., & Jolicoeur, P. (2007). Long-term electrophysiological changes in athletes with a history of multiple concussions. *Brain Injury*, *21*(6), 631–644. doi: 10.1080/02699050701426931

DeKosky, S. T., Ikonomovic, M. D., & Gandy, S. (2010). Traumatic brain injury—football, warfare, and long-term effects. *New England Journal of Medicine*, *363*(14), 1293–1296. doi: 10.1056/nejmp1007051

Dick, R. W. (2009). Is there a gender difference in concussion incidence and outcomes? *British Journal of Sports Medicine*, *43*(Suppl 1), i46–i50. doi: 10.1136/bjsm.2009.058172

Echemendia, R. J., Bruce, J. M., Bailey, C. M., Sanders, J. F., Arnett, P., & Vargas, G. (2012). The utility of post-concussion neuropsychological data in identifying cognitive change following sports-related MTBI in the absence of baseline data. *Clinical Neuropsychologist*, *26*(7), 1077–1091. doi: 10.1080/13854046.2012.721006

Echemendia, R. J., Herring, S., & Bailes, J. (2009). Who should conduct and interpret the neuropsychological assessment in sports-related concussion? *British Journal of Sports Medicine*, *43*(Suppl 1), i32–i35. doi: 10.1136/bjsm.2009.058164

Echemendia, R. J., Iverson, G. L., McCrea, M., Macciocchi, S. N., Gioia, G. A., Putukian, M., & Comper, P. (2013). Advances in neuropsychological assessment of sport-related concussion. *British Journal of Sports Medicine*, *47*(5), 294–298. doi: 10.1136/bjsports-2013-092186

Echemendia, R. J., Putukian, M., Mackin, R. S., Julian, L., & Shoss, N. (2001). Neuropsychological test performance prior to and following sports-related mild traumatic brain injury. *Clinical Journal of Sport Medicine*, *11*(1), 23–31. Retrieved from www.ncbi.nlm.nih.gov/htbin-post/Entrez/query?db=m&form=6&dopt=r&uid=11176142

Elbin, R. J., Covassin, T., Hakun, J., Kontos, A. P., Berger, K., Pfeiffer, K., & Ravizza, S. (2012). Do brain activation changes persist in athletes with a history of multiple concussions who are asymptomatic? *Brain Injury*, *26*(10), 1217–1225. doi: 10.3109/02699052.2012.672788

Erdal, K. (2012). Neuropsychological testing for sports-related concussion: How athletes can sandbag their baseline testing without detection. *Archives of Clinical Neuropsychology*, *27*(5), 473–479. doi: 10.1093/arclin/acs050

Erlanger, D. M., Kutner, K. C., Barth, J. T., & Barnes, R. (1999). Neuropsychology of sports-related head injury: Dementia pugilistica to post concussion syndrome. *Clinical Neuropsychologist*, *13*(2), 193–209. Retrieved from www.ncbi.nlm.nih.gov/htbin-post/Entrez/query?db=m&form=6&dopt=r&uid=10949160

Ferguson, R. J., Mittenberg, W., Barone, D. F., & Schneider, B. (1999). Postconcussion syndrome following sports-related head injury: Expectation as etiology. *Neuropsychology*, *13*(4), 582–589.

Field, M., Collins, M. W., Lovell, M. R., & Maroon, J. (2003). Does age play a role in recovery from sports-related concussion? A comparison of high school and collegiate athletes. *Journal of Pediatrics*, *142*(5), 546–553. doi: 10.1067/mpd.2003.190

Finch, C. F., Clapperton, A. J., & McCrory, P. (2013). Increasing incidence of hospitalisation for sport-related concussion in Victoria, Australia. *Medical Journal of Australia*, *198*(8), 427–430. doi: 10.5694/mja12.11217

Galetta, K. M., Brandes, L. E., Maki, K., Dziemianowicz, M. S., Laudano, E., Allen, M., . . . Balcer, L. J. (2011). The King—Devick test and sports-related concussion: Study of a rapid visual screening tool in a collegiate cohort. *Journal of the Neurological Sciences*, *309*(1–2), 34–39. doi: 10.1016/j.jns.2011.07.039

Galetta, M. S., Galetta, K. M., McCrossin, J., Wilson, J. A., Moster, S., Galetta, S. L., . . . Master, C. L. (2013). Saccades and memory: Baseline associations of the King—Devick and SCAT2 SAC tests in professional ice hockey players. *Journal of the Neurological Sciences*, *328*(1–2), 28–31. doi: 10.1016/j.jns.2013.02.008

Gatson, J., & Diaz-Arrastia, R. (2014). Tau as a biomarker of concussion. *JAMA Neurology*, *71*(6), 677–678. doi: 10.1001/jamaneurol.2014.443

Gilchrist, J., Thomas, K. E., Wald, M., & Langlois, J. (2007). Nonfatal traumatic brain injuries from sports and recreation activities—United States, 2001–2005. Retrieved from http://dx.doi.org/10.1037/e660702007-001

Giza, C. C., & Hovda, D. A. (2001). The neurometabolic cascade of concussion. *Journal of Athletic Training*, *36*(3), 228–235. Retrieved from www.ncbi.nlm.nih.gov/entrez/query.fcgi?cmd=Retrieve&db=PubMed&dopt=Citation&list_uids=12937489

Giza, C. C., & Hovda, D. A. (2014). The new neurometabolic cascade of concussion. *Neurosurgery*, *75*, S24–S33. doi: 10.1227/neu.0000000000000505

Gosselin, N., Bottari, C., Chen, J.-K., Petrides, M., Tinawi, S., de Guise, É., & Ptito, A. (2011). Electrophysiology and functional MRI in post-acute mild traumatic brain injury. *Journal of Neurotrauma*, *28*(3), 329–341. doi: 10.1089/neu.2010.1493

Griesbach, G. S. (2011). Exercise after traumatic brain injury: Is it a double-edged sword? *PM R*, *3*(6 Suppl 1), S64–S72. doi: 10.1016/j.pmrj.2011.02.008

Griesbach, G. S., Gomez-Pinilla, F., & Hovda, D. A. (2007). Time window for voluntary exercise-induced increases in hippocampal neuroplasticity molecules after traumatic brain injury is severity dependent. *Journal of Neurotrauma*, *24*(7), 1161–1171. doi: 10.1089/neu.2006.0255

Gunstad, J., & Suhr, J. A. (2001). "Expectation as etiology" versus "the good old days": Postconcussion syndrome symptom reporting in athletes, headache sufferers, and depressed individuals. *Journal of the International Neuropsychological Society*, *7*, 323–333.

Guskiewicz, K. M., & Broglio, S. P. (2011). Sport-related concussion: On-field and sideline assessment. *Physical Medicine & Rehabilitation Clinics of North America*, *22*(4), 603–617, vii. doi: 10.1016/j.pmr.2011.08.003

Guskiewicz, K. M., Marshall, S. W., Bailes, J., McCrea, M., Cantu, R. C., Randolph, C., & Jordan, B. D. (2005). Association between recurrent concussion and late-life cognitive impairment in retired professional football players. *Neurosurgery*, *57*(4), 719–726; discussion 719–726. Retrieved from www.ncbi.nlm.nih.gov/entrez/query.fcgi?cmd=Rctricvc&db=PubMed&dopt=Citation&list_uids=16239884

Guskiewicz, K. M., McCrea, M., Marshall, S. W., Cantu, R. C., Randolph, C., Barr, W., . . . Kelly, J. P. (2003). Cumulative effects associated with recurrent concussion in collegiate football players: The NCAA concussion study. *Jama*, *290*(19), 2549–2555. doi: 10.1001/jama.290.19.2549. Retrieved from www.ncbi.nlm.nih.gov/entrez/query.fcgi?cmd=Retrieve&db=PubMed&dopt=Citation&list_uids=14625331

Guskiewicz, K. M., Register-Mihalik, J., McCrory, P., McCrea, M., Johnston, K., Makdissi, M., . . . Meeuwisse, W. (2013). Evidence-based approach to revising the SCAT2: Introducing the SCAT3. *British Journal of Sports Medicine*, *47*(5), 289–293. doi: 10.1136/bjsports-2013-092225

Guskiewicz, K. M., Riemann, B. L., Perrin, D. H., & Nashner, L. M. (1997). Alternative approaches to the assessment of mild head injury in athletes. *Medicine & Science in Sports & Exercise*, *29*(Suppl), S213–S221.

Guskiewicz, K. M., Ross, S. E., & Marshall, S. W. (2001). Postural stability and neuropsychological deficits after concussion in collegiate athletes. *Journal of Athletic Training*, *36*(3), 263–273.

Guskiewicz, K. M., Weaver, N. L., Padua, D. A., & Garrett, W. E., Jr. (2000). Epidemiology of concussion in collegiate and high school football players. *28*(5), 643–650.

Hammeke, T. A., McCrea, M., Coats, S. M., Verber, M. D., Durgerian, S., Flora, K., . . . Rao, S. M. (2013). Acute and subacute changes in neural activation during the recovery from sport-related concussion. *Journal of the International Neuropsychological Society*, *19*(8), 863–872. doi: 10.1017/s1355617713000702

Hammoud, D. A., & Wasserman, B. A. (2002). Diffuse axonal injuries: Pathophysiology and imaging. *Neuroimaging Clinics of North America*, *12*(2), 205–216. doi: 10.1016/s1052-5149(02)00011-4

Hart, J., Kraut, M. A., Womack, K. B., Strain, J., Didehbani, N., Bartz, E., . . . Cullum, C. M. (2013). Neuroimaging of cognitive dysfunction and depression in aging retired national football league players. *Jama Neurology*, *70*(3), 326. doi: 10.1001/2013.jamaneurol.340

Henry, L. C., Elbin, R. J., Collins, M. W., Marchetti, G., & Kontos, A. P. (2015). Examining recovery trajectories after sport-related concussion with a multimodal clinical assessment approach. *Neurosurgery*. doi: 10.1227/NEU.0000000000001041

Hootman, J. M., Dick, R., & Agel, J. (2007). Epidemiology of collegiate injuries for 15 sports: Summary and recommendations for injury prevention initiatives. *Journal of Athletic Training*, *42*(2), 311–319. Retrieved from www.ncbi.nlm.nih.gov/pmc/articles/PMC1941297/pdf/i1062-6050-42-2-311.pdf

Iverson, G. L., Gardner, A. J., McCrory, P., Zafonte, R., & Castellani, R. J. (2015). A critical review of chronic traumatic encephalopathy. *Neuroscience & Biobehavioral Reviews*, *56*, 276–293. doi: 10.1016/j.neubiorev.2015.05.008

Jinguji, T. M., Bompadre, V., Harmon, K. G., Satchell, E. K., Gilbert, K., Wild, J., & Eary, J. F. (2012). Sport concussion assessment tool-2: Baseline values for high school athletes. *British Journal of Sports Medicine*, *46*(5), 365–370. doi: 10.1136/bjsports-2011-090526

Jordan, B. D. (2000). Chronic traumatic brain injury associated with boxing. *Seminars in Neurology*, *20*, 179–185.

Karantzoulis, S., & Randolph, C. (2013). Modern chronic traumatic encephalopathy in retired athletes: What is the evidence? *Neuropsychology Review*, *23*(4), 350–360. doi: 10.1007/s11065-013-9243-4

Kashluba, S., Hanks, R. A., Casey, J. E., & Millis, S. R. (2008). Neuropsychologic and functional outcome after complicated mild traumatic brain injury. *Archives of Physical Medicine and Rehabilitation*, *89*(5), 904–911. doi: 10.1016/j.apmr.2007.12.029

Kay, T., Harrington, D. E., Adams, R. E., Anderson, T. W., Berrol, S., Cicerone, K., . . . Malec, J. (1993). Definition of mild traumatic brain injury: Report from the mild traumatic brain injury committee of the head injury interdisciplinary special interest group of the American congress of rehabilitation medicine. *Journal of Head Trauma Rehabilitation*, *8*(3), 86–87.

Kelly, J. P. (1991). Concussion in sports: Guidelines for the prevention of catastrophic outcome. *Jama: The Journal of the American Medical Association*, *266*(20), 2867–2869. doi: 10.1001/jama.266.20.2867

Kelly, J. P., & Rosenberg, J. H. (1997a). Diagnosis and management of concussion in sports. *Neurology*, *48*(3), 575–580. Retrieved from www.ncbi.nlm.nih.gov/htbin-post/Entrez/query?db=m&form=6&dopt=r&uid=9065529

Kelly, J. P., & Rosenberg, J. H. (1997b). Diagnosis and management of concussion in sports. *Neurology*, *48*(3), 575–580. doi: 10.1212/wnl.48.3.575

King, D., Clark, T., & Gissane, C. (2012). Use of a rapid visual screening tool for the assessment of concussion in amateur rugby league: A pilot study. *Journal of the Neurological Sciences*, *320*(1–2), 16–21. doi: 10.1016/j.jns.2012.05.049

LaBotz, M., Martin, M. R., Kimura, I. F., Hetzler, R. K., & Nichols, A. W. (2005). A comparison of a preparticipation evaluation history form and a symptom-based concussion survey in the identification of previous head injury in collegiate athletes. *Clinical Journal of Sport Medicine*, *15*(2), 73–78. Retrieved from www.ncbi.nlm.nih.gov/entrez/query.fcgi?cmd=Retrieve&db=PubMed&dopt=Citation&list_uids=15782050

Langlois, J. A., Rutland-Brown, W., & Wald, M. M. (2006). The epidemiology and impact of traumatic brain injury. *Journal of Head Trauma Rehabilitation*, *21*(5), 375–378. doi: 10.1097/00001199-200609000-00001

LaRoche, A. A., Nelson, L. D., Connelly, P. K., Walter, K. D., & McCrea, M. A. (2015). Sport-related concussion reporting and state legislative effects. *Clinical Journal of Sport Medicine*. doi: 10.1097/jsm.0000000000000192

Larrabee, G. J. (2012). Performance validity and symptom validity in neuropsychological assessment. *Journal of the International Neuropsychological Society*, *18*(4), 625–631. doi: 10.1017/s1355617712000240

Lau, B. C., Collins, M. W., & Lovell, M. R. (2012). Cutoff scores in neurocognitive testing and symptom clusters that predict protracted recovery from concussions in high school athletes. *Neurosurgery*, *70*(2), 371–379. doi: 10.1227/neu.0b013e31823150f0

Lau, B. C., Lovell, M. R., Collins, M. W., & Pardini, J. (2009). Neurocognitive and symptom predictors of recovery in high school athletes. *Clinical Journal of Sport Medicine*, *19*(3), 216–221. doi: 10.1097/jsm.0b013e31819d6edb

Lavoie, M. E., Johnston, K. M., Leclerc, S., Lassonde, M., & Dupuis, F. O. (2004). Visual P300 effects beyond symptoms in concussed college athletes. *Journal of Clinical and Experimental Neuropsychology (Neuropsychology, Development and Cognition: Section A)*, *26*(1), 55–73. doi: 10.1076/jcen.26.1.55.23936

Leddy, J. J., Cox, J. L., Baker, J. G., Wack, D. S., Pendergast, D. R., Zivadinov, R., & Willer, B. (2013). Exercise treatment for postconcussion syndrome: A pilot study of changes in functional magnetic resonance imaging activation, physiology, and symptoms. *Journal of Head Trauma Rehabilitation*, *28*(4), 241–249. doi: 10.1097/HTR.0b013e31826da964

Leddy, J. J., Sandhu, H., Sodhi, V., Baker, J. G., & Willer, B. (2012). Rehabilitation of concussion and post-concussion syndrome. *Sports Health*, *4*(2), 147–154. doi: 10.1177/1941738111433673

Lovell, M. R., & Collins, M. W. (1998). Neuropsychological assessment of the college football player. *Journal of Head Trauma Rehabilitation*, *13*(2), 9–26.

Lovell, M. R., Iverson, G. L., Collins, M. W., Podell, K., Johnston, K. M., Pardini, D., . . . Maroon, J. C. (2006). Measurement of symptoms following sports-related concussion: Reliability and normative data for the post-concussion scale. *Applied Neuropsychology*, *13*(3), 166–174. doi: 10.1207/s15324826an1303_4

Macciocchi, S. N., Barth, J. T., Alves, W., Rimel, R. W., & Jane, J. A. (1996). Neuropsychological functioning and recovery after mild head injury in collegiate athletes. *Neurosurgery*, *39*(3), 510–514. doi: 10.1097/00006123-199609000-00014

Maddocks, D. L., Dicker, G. D., & Saling, M. M. (1995). The assessment of orientation following concussion in athletes. *Clinical Journal of Sport Medicine*, *5*(1), 32–35.

Makdissi, M., Cantu, R. C., Johnston, K. M., McCrory, P., & Meeuwisse, W. H. (2013). The difficult concussion patient: What is the best approach to investigation and management of persistent (>10 days) postconcussive symptoms? *British Journal of Sports Medicine*, *47*(5), 308–313. doi: 10.1136/bjsports-2013-092255

Maroon, J. C., Winkelman, R., Bost, J., Amos, A., Mathyssek, C., & Miele, V. (2015). Chronic traumatic encephalopathy in contact sports: A systematic review of all reported pathological cases. *PLoS One*, *10*(2), e0117338. doi: 10.1371/journal.pone.0117338

Martland, H. S. (1928). Punch drunk. *Jama*, *91*, 1103–1107.

McAllister, T. W., Saykin, A. J., Flashman, L. A., Sparling, M. B., Johnson, S. C., Guerin, S. J., . . . Yanofsky, N. (1999). Brain activation during working memory 1 month after mild traumatic brain injury: A functional MRI study. *Neurology*, *53*(6), 1300–1300. doi: 10.1212/wnl.53.6.1300

McCrea, M. (2001). Standardized mental status testing on the sideline after sport-related concussion. *Journal of Athletic Training*, *36*(3), 274–279.

McCrea, M., Barr, W. B., Guskiewicz, K., Randolph, C., Marshall, S. W., Cantu, R., . . . Kelly, J. P. (2005). Standard regression-based methods for measuring recovery after sport-related concussion. *Journal of the International Neuropsychological Society*, *11*(1), 58–69. Retrieved from www.ncbi.nlm.nih.gov/entrez/query.fcgi?cmd=Retrieve&db=PubMed&dopt=Citation&list_uids=15686609

McCrea, M., Guskiewicz, K. M., Marshall, S. W., Barr, W., Randolph, C., Cantu, R. C., . . . Kelly, J. P. (2003). Acute effects and recovery time following concussion in collegiate football players. *Jama*, *290*(19), 2556–2563. doi: 10.1001/jama.290.19.2556

McCrea, M., Guskiewicz, K. M., Randolph, C., Barr, W. B., Hammeke, T. A., Marshall, S. W., & Kelly, J. P. (2009). Effects of a symptom-free waiting period on clinical outcome and risk of reinjury after sport-related concussion. *Neurosurgery*, *65*(5), 876–883. doi: 10.1227/01.neu.0000350155.89800.00

McCrea, M., Guskiewicz, K. M., Randolph, C., Barr, W. B., Hammeke, T. A., Marshall, S. W., . . . Kelly, J. P. (2013). Incidence, clinical course, and predictors of prolonged recovery time following sport-related concussion in high school and college athletes. *Journal of the International Neuropsychological Society*, *19*(1), 22–33. doi: 10.1017/s1355617712000872

McCrea, M., Hammeke, T., Olsen, G., Leo, P., & Guskiewicz, K. (2004). Unreported concussion in high school football players: Implications for prevention. *Clinical Journal of Sport Medicine*, *14*(1), 13–17. Retrieved from www.ncbi.nlm.nih.gov/entrez/query.fcgi?cmd=Retrieve&db=PubMed&dopt=Citation&list_uids=14712161

McCrea, M., Kelly, J. P., Kluge, J., Ackley, B., & Randolph, C. (1997). Standardized assessment of concussion in football players. *Neurology*, *48*(3), 586–588.

McCrea, M., Kelly, J. P., Randolph, C., Kluge, J., Bartolic, E., Finn, G., & Baxter, B. (1998). Standardized assessment of concussion (SAC): On-site mental status evaluation of the athlete. *Journal of Head Trauma Rehabilitation*, *13*(2), 27–35.

McCrea, M., Prichep, L., Powell, M. R., Chabot, R., & Barr, W. B. (2010). Acute effects and recovery after sport-related concussion: A neurocognitive and quantitative brain electrical activity study. *Journal of Head Trauma Rehabilitation*, *25*(4), 283–292. doi: 10.1097/HTR.0b013e3181e67923

McCrory, P. (2001). Does second impact syndrome exist? *Clinical Journal of Sport Medicine*, *11*(3), 144–149. doi: 10.1097/00042752-200107000-00004

McCrory, P., Meeuwisse, W. H., Aubry, M., Cantu, B., Dvorák, J. Í., Echemendia, R. J., . . . Turner, M. (2013a). Consensus statement on concussion in sport: The 4th international conference on concussion in sport held in Zurich, November 2012. *Journal of the American College of Surgeons*, *216*(5), e55–e71. doi: 10.1016/j.jamcollsurg.2013.02.020

McCrory, P., Meeuwisse, W. H., Aubry, M., Cantu, R. C., Dvorák, J. Í., Echemendia, R. J., . . . Turner, M. (2013b). Consensus statement on concussion in sport—the 4th international conference on concussion in sport held in Zurich, November 2012. *PM&R*, *5*(4), 255–279. doi: 10.1016/j.pmrj.2013.02.012

McCrory, P., Meeuwisse, W. H., Johnston, K., Dvorak, J., Aubry, M., Molloy, M., & Cantu, R. (2009). Consensus statement on concussion in sport 3rd international conference on concussion in sport held in Zurich, November 2008. *Clinical Journal of Sport Medicine*, *19*(3), 185–200. doi: 10.1097/jsm.0b013e3181a501db

McCrory, P., Meeuwisse, W. H., Kutcher, J. S., Jordan, B. D., & Gardner, A. (2013). What is the evidence for chronic concussion-related changes in retired athletes: Behavioural, pathological and clinical outcomes? *British Journal of Sports Medicine*, *47*(5), 327–330. doi: 10.1136/bjsports-2013-092248

McCrory, P. R. (1997). Were you knocked out? A team physician's approach to initial concussion management. *Medicine & Science in Sports & Exercise*, *29*(Suppl), S207–S212.

McCrory, P. R., & Berkovic, S. F. (1998). Second impact syndrome. *Neurology*, *50*(3), 677–683. Retrieved from www.ncbi.nlm.nih.gov/htbin-post/Entrez/query?db=m&form=6&dopt=r&uid=9521255

McKee, A. C., Cantu, R. C., Nowinski, C. J., Hedley-Whyte, E. T., Gavett, B. E., Budson, A. E., . . . Stern, R. A. (2009). Chronic traumatic encephalopathy in athletes. *Journal of Neuropathology and Experimental Neurology*, *68*(7), 709–735. doi: 10.1097/nen.0b013e3181a9d503

McLeod, T. C., & Leach, C. (2012). Psychometric properties of self-report concussion scales and checklists. *Journal of Athletic Training*, *47*(2), 221–223. Retrieved from www.ncbi.nlm.nih.gov/pmc/articles/PMC3418135/pdf/i1062-6050-47-2-221.pdf

Millspaugh, J. A. (1937). Dementia pugilistica. *U.S. Naval Medical Bulletin*, *35*, 297–303.

Mittenberg, W., DiGiulio, D. V., Perrin, S., & Bass, A. E. (1992). Symptoms following mild head injury: Expectation as aetiology. *Journal of Neurology, Neurosurgery & Psychiatry*, *55*(3), 200–204. doi: 10.1136/jnnp.55.3.200

Mittl, R. L., Grossman, R. I., Hiehle, J. F., Hurst, R. W., Kauder, D. R., Gennarelli, T. A., & Alburger, G. W. (1994). Prevalence of MR evidence of diffuse axonal injury in patients with mild head injury and normal head CT findings. *AJNR American Journal of Neuroradiology*, *15*(8), 1583–1589.

Mondello, S., Schmid, K., Berger, R. P., Kobeissy, F., Italiano, D., Jeromin, A., . . . Buki, A. (2014). The challenge of mild traumatic brain injury: Role of biochemical markers in diagnosis of brain damage. *Medicinal Research Reviews*, *34*(3), 503–531. doi: 10.1002/med.21295

Morgan, C. D., Zuckerman, S. L., Lee, Y. M., King, L., Beaird, S., Sills, A. K., & Solomon, G. S. (2015). Predictors of postconcussion syndrome after sports-related concussion in young athletes: A matched case-control study. *Journal of Neurosurgery: Pediatrics*, *15*(6), 589–598. doi: 10.3171/2014.10.PEDS14356

Moser, R. S., Schatz, P., Neidzwski, K., & Ott, S. D. (2011). Group versus individual administration affects baseline neurocognitive test performance. *American Journal of Sports Medicine*, *39*(11), 2325–2330. doi: 10.1177/0363546511417114

Nelson, L. D., Guskiewicz, K. M., Marshall, S. W., Hammeke, T., Barr, W., Randolph, C., & McCrea, M. A. (2015). Multiple self-reported concussions are more prevalent in athletes with ADHD and learning disability. *Clinical Journal of Sport Medicine*. doi: 10.1097/jsm.0000000000000207

Nelson, L. D., Janecek, J. K., & McCrea, M. A. (2013). Acute clinical recovery from sport-related concussion. *Neuropsychology Review*, *23*(4), 285–299. doi: 10.1007/s11065-013-9240-7

Nelson, L. D., LaRoche, A. A., Pfaller, A. Y., Lerner, E. Hammeke, T. A., Randolph, C., Barr, W.B., Guskiewicz, K., McCrea, M. A. (2016). Prospective, head-to-head study of three computerized neurocognitive assessment tools (CNTs): Reliability and validity for the assessment of sport-related concussion. *Journal of the International Neuropsychological Society*, *22*(1), 24–37.

Neselius, S., Brisby, H., Granholm, F., Zetterberg, H., & Blennow, K. (2015). Monitoring concussion in a knocked-out boxer by CSF biomarker analysis. *Knee Surgery, Sports Traumatology, Arthroscopy*, *23*(9), 2536–2539. doi: 10.1007/s00167-014-3066-6

Noble, J. M., & Hesdorffer, D. C. (2013). Sport-related concussions: A review of epidemiology, challenges in diagnosis, and potential risk factors. *Neuropsychology Review*, *23*(4), 273–284. doi: 10.1007/s11065-013-9239-0

Nuwer, M. R., Hovda, D. A., Schrader, L. M., & Vespa, P. M. (2005). Routine and quantitative EEG in mild traumatic brain injury. *Clinical Neurophysiology*, *116*(9), 2001–2025. doi: 10.1016/j.clinph.2005.05.008

Oliaro, S. M., Guskiewicz, K. M., & Prentice, W. E. (1998). Establishment of normative data on cognitive tests for comparison with athletes sustaining mild head injury. *Journal of Athletic Training*, *33*(1), 36–40. Retrieved from www.ncbi.nlm.nih.gov/pmc/articles/PMC1320373/pdf/jathtrain00009-0038.pdf

Omalu, B. (2014). Chronic traumatic encephalopathy. *Progress in Neurological Surgery*, *28*, 38–49. doi: 10.1159/000358761

Pearce, N., Gallo, V., & McElvenny, D. (2015). Head trauma in sport and neurodegenerative disease: An issue whose time has come? *Neurobiol Aging*, *36*(3), 1383–1389. doi: 10.1016/j.neurobiolaging.2014.12.024

Prichep, L. S., McCrea, M., Barr, W., Powell, M., & Chabot, R. J. (2013). Time course of clinical and electrophysiological recovery after sport-related concussion. *Journal of Head Trauma Rehabilitation*, *28*(4), 266–273. doi: 10.1097/HTR.0b013e318247b54e

Putukian, M., Echemendia, R., Dettwiler-Danspeckgruber, A., Duliba, T., Bruce, J., Furtado, J. L., & Murugavel, M. (2015). Prospective clinical assessment using sideline concussion assessment tool-2 testing in the evaluation of sport-related concussion in college athletes. *Clinical Journal of Sport Medicine*, *25*(1), 36–42. doi: 10.1097/jsm.0000000000000102

Raichle, M. E., MacLeod, A. M., Snyder, A. Z., Powers, W. J., Gusnard, D. A., & Shulman, G. L. (2001). A default mode of brain function. *Proceedings of the National Academy of Sciences*, *98*(2), 676–682. doi: 10.1073/pnas.98.2.676

Randolph, C. (2014). Is chronic traumatic encephalopathy a real disease? *Current Sports Medicine Reports*, *13*(1), 33–37. doi: 10.1097/opx.0000000000000170

Randolph, C., Karantzoulis, S., & Guskiewicz, K. (2013). Prevalence and characterization of mild cognitive impairment in retired National Football League players. *Journal of the International Neuropsychological Society*, *19*(8), 873–880. doi: 10.1017/S1355617713000805

Randolph, C., & Kirkwood, M. W. (2009). What are the real risks of sport-related concussion, and are they modifiable? *Journal of the International Neuropsychological Society*, *15*(4), 512. doi: 10.1017/s135561770909064x

Randolph, C., McCrea, M., & Barr, W. B. (2005). Is neuropsychological testing useful in the management of sport-related concussion? *Journal of Athletic Training*, *40*(3), 139–152. Retrieved from www.ncbi.nlm.nih.gov/pmc/articles/PMC1250250/pdf/i1062-6050-40-3-139.pdf

Randolph, C., Millis, S., Barr, W. B., McCrea, M., Guskiewicz, K. M., Hammeke, T. A., & Kelly, J. P. (2009). Concussion symptom inventory: An empirically derived scale for monitoring resolution of symptoms following sport-related concussion. *Archives of Clinical Neuropsychology*, *24*(3), 219–229. doi: 10.1093/arclin/acp025

Resch, J. E., Driscoll, A., McCaffrey, N., Brown, C., Ferrara, M. S., Macciocchi, S., . . . Walpert, K. (2013). ImPact test-retest reliability: Reliably unreliable? *Journal of Athletic Training*, *48*(4), 506–511. doi: 10.4085/1062-6050-48.3.09

Resch, J. E., McCrea, M. A., & Cullum, C. M. (2013). Computerized neurocognitive testing in the management of sport-related concussion: An update. *Neuropsychology Review*, *23*(4), 335–349. doi: 10.1007/s11065-013-9242-5

Riemann, B. L., & Guskiewicz, K. M. (2000). Effects of mild head injury on postural sway as measured through clinical balance test. *Journal of Athletic Training*, *35*, 19–25.

Riemann, B. L., Guskiewicz, K. M., & Shields, E. (1999). Relationship between clinical and forceplate measures of postural stability. *Journal of Sports Rehabilitation*, *8*, 71–82.

Saigal, R., & Berger, M. S. (2014). The long-term effects of repetitive mild head injuries in sports. *Neurosurgery*, *75*(Suppl 4), S149–S155. doi: 10.1227/NEU.0000000000000497

Saunders, R. L., & Harbaugh, R. E. (1984). The second impact in catastrophic contact-sports head trauma. *JAMA*, *252*(4), 538–539.

Savica, R., Parisi, J. E., Wold, L. E., Josephs, K. A., & Ahlskog, J. E. (2012). High school football and risk of neurodegeneration: A community-based study. *Mayo Clinic Proceedings*, *87*(4), 335–340. doi: 10.1016/j.mayocp.2011.12.016

Schmidt, J. D., Register-Mihalik, J. K., Mihalik, J. P., Kerr, Z. Y., & Guskiewicz, K. M. (2012). Identifying Impairments after concussion: Normative data versus individualized baselines. *Medicine and Science in Sports and Exercise*, *44*(9), 1621–1628. doi: 10.1249/MSS.0b013e318258a9fb

Schneider, K. J., Iverson, G. L., Emery, C. A., McCrory, P., Herring, S. A., & Meeuwisse, W. H. (2013). The effects of rest and treatment following sport-related concussion: A systematic review of the literature. *British Journal of Sports Medicine*, *47*(5), 304–307. doi: 10.1136/bjsports-2013-092190

Schulte, S., Podlog, L. W., Hamson-Utley, J. J., Strathmann, F. G., & Struder, H. K. (2014). A systematic review of the biomarker S100B: Implications for sport-related concussion management. *Journal of Athletic Training*, *49*(6), 830–850. doi: 10.4085/1062-6050-49.3.33

Schulz, M. R. (2004). Incidence and risk factors for concussion in high school athletes, North Carolina, 1996–1999. *American Journal of Epidemiology*, *160*(10), 937–944. doi: 10.1093/aje/kwh304

Signoretti, S., Lazzarino, G., Tavazzi, B., & Vagnozzi, R. (2011). The pathophysiology of concussion. *PM R*, *3*(10 Suppl 2), S359–S368. doi: 10.1016/j.pmrj.2011.07.018

Silverberg, N. D., & Iverson, G. L. (2011). Etiology of the post-concussion syndrome: Physiogenesis and Psychogenesis revisited. *NeuroRehabilitation*, *29*(4), 317–329. doi: 10.3233/NRE-2011-0708

Solomon, G. S., Lovell, M. R., Casson, I. R., & Viano, D. C. (2015). Normative neurocognitive data for National Football League players: An initial compendium. *Archives of Clinical Neuropsychology*, *30*(2), 161–173. doi: 10.1093/arclin/acv003

Stein, T. D., Alvarez, V. E., & McKee, A. C. (2015). Concussion in chronic traumatic encephalopathy. *Current Pain and Headache Reports*, *19*(10), 47. doi: 10.1007/s11916-015-0522-z

Stern, R. A., Daneshvar, D. H., Baugh, C. M., Seichepine, D. R., Montenigro, P. H., Riley, D. O., . . . McKee, A. C. (2013). Clinical presentation of chronic traumatic encephalopathy. *Neurology*, *81*(13), 1122–1129. doi: 10.1212/WNL.0b013e3182a55f7f

Strain, J. F., Didehbani, N., Cullum, C. M., Mansinghani, S., Conover, H., Kraut, M. A., . . . Womack, K. B. (2013). Depressive symptoms and white matter dysfunction in retired NFL players with concussion history. *Neurology*, *81*(1), 25–32. doi: 10.1212/WNL.0b013e318299ccf8

Strain, J. F., Womack, K. B., Didehbani, N., Spence, J. S., Conover, H., Hart, J., Jr., . . . Cullum, C. M. (2015). Imaging correlates of memory and concussion history in retired national football league athletes. *Jama Neurology*, *72*(7), 773–780. doi: 10.1001/jamaneurol.2015.0206

Tator, C. H., & Davis, H. (2014). The postconcussion syndrome in sports and recreation: Clinical features and demography in 138 athletes. *Neurosurgery*, *75*(Suppl 4), S106–S112. doi: 10.1227/NEU.0000000000000484

Teasdale, G., & Jennett, B. (1974). Assessment of coma and impaired consciousness: A practial scale. *Lancet*, *2*, 81–84.

Tebano, M. T., Cameroni, M., Gallozzi, G., Loizzo, A., Palazzino, G., Pezzini, G., & Ricci, G. F. (1988). EEG spectral analysis after minor head injury in man. *Electroencephalography and Clinical Neurophysiology*, *70*(2), 185–189. doi: 10.1016/0013-4694(88)90118-6

Terry, D. P., Faraco, C. C., Smith, D., Diddams, M. J., Puente, A. N., & Miller, L. S. (2012). Lack of long-term fMRI differences after multiple sports-related concussions. *Brain Injury*, *26*(13–14), 1684–1696. doi: 10.3109/02699052.2012.722259

Thatcher, R. W., North, D. M., Curtin, R. T., Walker, R. A., Biver, C. J., Gomez, J. F., & Salazar, A. M. (2001). An EEG severity index of traumatic brain injury. *JNP*, *13*(1), 77–87. doi: 10.1176/jnp.13.1.77

Thatcher, R. W., Walker, R. A., Gerson, I., & Geisler, F. H. (1989). EEG discriminant analyses of mild head trauma. *Electroencephalography and Clinical Neurophysiology*, *73*(2), 94–106. doi: 10.1016/0013-4694(89)90188-0

Thomas, D. G., Apps, J. N., Hoffmann, R. G., McCrea, M., & Hammeke, T. (2015). Benefits of strict rest after acute concussion: A randomized controlled trial. *Pediatrics*, *135*(2), 213–223. doi: 10.1542/peds.2014-0966

Thompson, J., Sebastianelli, W., & Slobounov, S. (2005). EEG and postural correlates of mild traumatic brain injury in athletes. *Neuroscience Letters*, *377*(3), 158–163. Retrieved from www.ncbi.nlm.nih.gov/entrez/query.fcgi?cmd=Retrieve&db=PubMed&dopt=Citation&list_uids=15755518

Watson, M. R., Fenton, G. W., McClelland, R. J., Lumsden, J., Headley, M., & Rutherford, W. H. (1995). The post-concussional state: Neurophysiological aspects. *The British Journal of Psychiatry*, *167*(4), 514–521. doi: 10.1192/bjp.167.4.514

Wortzel, H. S., Brenner, L. A., & Arciniegas, D. B. (2013). Traumatic brain injury and chronic traumatic encephalopathy: A forensic neuropsychiatric perspective. *Behavioral Sciences & the Law*, *31*(6), 721–738. doi: 10.1002/bsl.2079

Yuh, E. L., Hawryluk, G. W., & Manley, G. T. (2014). Imaging concussion: A review. *Neurosurgery*, *75*(Suppl 4), S50–S63. doi: 10.1227/NEU.0000000000000491

Zemek, R. L., Farion, K. J., Sampson, M., & McGahern, C. (2013). Prognosticators of persistent symptoms following pediatric concussion: A systematic review. *Jama Pediatrics*, *167*(3), 259–265. doi: 10.1001/2013.jamapediatrics.216

Zemper, E. D. (2003). Two-year prospective study of relative risk of a second cerebral concussion. *American Journal of Physical Medicine & Rehabilitation*, *82*(9), 653–659. doi: 10.1097/01.phm.0000083666.74494.ba

Zetterberg, H., Smith, D. H., & Blennow, K. (2013). Biomarkers of mild traumatic brain injury in cerebrospinal fluid and blood. *Nature Reviews Neurology*, *9*(4), 201–210. doi: 10.1038/nrneurol.2013.9

Zuckerman, S. L., Solomon, G. S., Forbes, J. A., Haase, R. F., Sills, A. K., & Lovell, M. R. (2012). Response to acute concussive injury in soccer players: Is gender a modifying factor? *Journal of Neurosurgery: Pediatrics*, *10*(6), 504–510. doi: 10.3171/2012.8.peds12139

28 The Three Amnesias

Russell M. Bauer and Breton Asken

During the past six decades, our understanding of memory and its disorders has increased dramatically. In 1950, very little was known about the localization of brain lesions causing amnesia. Despite a few clues in earlier literature, it came as a complete surprise in the early 1950s that bilateral medial temporal resection caused amnesia. The importance of the thalamus in memory was hardly suspected until the 1970s and the basal forebrain was an area virtually unknown to clinicians before the 1980s. An animal model of the amnesic syndrome was not developed until the 1970s. Thus, our understanding of amnesia is relatively recent, and is a remarkable testament to the power of translational research.

The famous case of Henry M. (H.M.), published by Scoville and Milner (1957), marked the beginning of what many have called the "Golden Age of Memory." Since that time, experimental analyses of amnesic patients, coupled with meticulous clinical description, pathological analysis, and, more recently, structural and functional imaging, has led to a better understanding of the nature and characteristics of the human amnesic syndrome. We now know that the amnesic syndrome does not affect all kinds of memory, and, conversely, that memory-disordered patients without full-blown amnesia (e.g., patients with frontal lesions) may have less severe impairment in critical cognitive processes that normally support remembering. It is now known that the amnesic syndrome can follow damage to three major functional systems of the brain: the medial temporal lobe/hippocampal memory system (Milner, 1972; Squire & Zola-Morgan, 1991), the diencephalon (Aggleton, 1986; Butters, 1981; Graff-Radford, Tranel, Van Hoesen, & Brandt, 1990), and the basal forebrain (Damasio, Graff-Radford, Eslinger, Damasio, & Kassell, 1985; DeLuca & Diamond, 1995; Hashimoto, Tanaka, & Nakano, 2000). In this chapter, we review the characteristics and anatomic bases for these "three amnesias." In a concluding section, we consider whether these three different disorders, or variations on a core amnesic syndrome.

Clinical Characteristics of the Amnesic Syndrome

The term *amnesic syndrome* describes patients with profound inability in day-to-day remembering and with varying degrees of remote or retrograde memory impairment whose memory-related disability exists in the context of comparatively spared cognitive and intellectual function. The disorder exists separately from generalized dementia, and from language or attentional disturbance, and has three distinct characteristics.

Anterograde Amnesia

The hallmark of the amnesic syndrome is a profound defect in new learning called *anterograde amnesia*. The deficit involves "recent" or "long-term" memory. The essential feature of the deficit is that that patient is impaired in the conscious, deliberate recall of information newly learned after illness onset. The defect primarily involves memory for events (episodic memory) and is apparent in practically any situation in which (a) the recall burden exceeds the immediate memory span, or (b) in which a substantial delay ensues between learning and retrieval. Amnesic patients are severely impaired in their daily functioning and their learning deficit is apparent on even casual observation. That is, the deficit is more than just a "memory problem." Such patients may fail to recognize or learn the names of newly encountered persons after even brief delays. They may appear disoriented in place or time because they have failed to update the details of their location or have lost the ability to monitor and keep track of ongoing events. Amnesic patients are frequently capable of engaging in routine conversation, but their deficit becomes obvious when they are asked to recall an event that occurred only hours or minutes before. Instructions to remember such events for later recall rarely result in measurable improvement. Formal neuropsychological assessment is usually not needed to reveal the deficit, but such assessment often helps in characterizing the deficit in quantitative and qualitative terms (Squire & Shimamura, 1986).

Retrograde Amnesia and Remote Memory Disturbance

The amnesic patient usually also has some difficulty in recalling information learned prior to illness onset, an impairment that is often worse for relatively recent events than for events that occurred in the very remote past. The deficit usually primarily involves "autobiographical" memories of the patient's specific past (e.g., the personally experienced circumstances surrounding an important relative's death), but also may involve memory for "public" information that has not been personally encountered (e.g., details about the most recent presidential election). Kapur (1999) suggests that autobiographical memory for past personal events is both anatomically and functionally distinct from remote semantic knowledge and fact memory, and some case studies, experimental data and recent functional neuroimaging studies (Cabeza & St Jaques, 2007; Soderlund, Moscovich, Kamar, Mandic, & Levine, 2012) support this distinction. Autobiographical defects are commonly seen after lesions to the medial temporal and diencephalic structures, while defects in remote semantic memory result more commonly from neocortical damage to the temporal lobe and other regions. Severity of retrograde and anterorgrade amnesia in the individual patient is typically correlated, and it has been argued that retrograde amnesia is often not measurable until anterograde amnesia reaches at least moderate severity (Smith, Frascino, Hopkins, & Squire, 2013).

Three patterns of remote memory impairment have been described in the literature (Albert, Butters, & Brandt, 1981). *Temporally limited remote memory disturbance is* an impairment that primarily involves the few years prior to the onset of amnesia with relative sparing of more remote time periods. This has been documented in the amnesic patient H.M. (Corkin, 1984; Marslen-Wilson and Teuber, 1974; Milner, Corkin, & Teuber, 1968), in patients receiving electroconvulsive therapy for depression (Squire, Slater, & Chace, 1975; Squire & Fox, 1980) and in recent cases of remote memory impairment after language-dominant temporal lobectomy (Barr, Goldberg, Wasserstein, & Novelly, 1990). This deficit pattern has been explained as a failure of consolidation. For example, H.M.'s remote memory defect is most severe for events taking place up to three years prior to his surgery in 1953. Consolidation accounts suggest that these more proximal remote memories are still in an unstable, not fully consolidated state, causing them to be more vulnerable to acquired brain injury than are more remote, firmly established memories. *Temporally graded remote memory disturbance* affects all time periods, with greater impairment of memories in the recent past. This pattern has been said to be typical of patients with alcoholic Korsakoff's (AK) syndrome (Albert, Butters, & Levin, 1979; Cohen & Squire, 1981; Meudell, Northern, Snowden, & Neary, 1980; Seltzer & Benson, 1974; Squire, Haist, and Shimamura, 1989), and has also been reported in patients with basal forebrain damage (Gade & Mortensen, 1990). At least in AK patients, an increasingly severe anterograde learning deficit associated with years of heavy drinking, coupled with an acute decade-nonspecific deficit coincident with the onset of Wernicke's encephalopathy, remain possible explanations of the temporally graded pattern. A recent study of remote episodic/autobiographical and semantic memory in AK and postencephalitic patients showed clear temporal gradients in episodic memory, but no evidence of a temporal gradient in semantic memory (Kopelman et al., 2009). A third pattern, a *decade-nonspecific, or pervasive remote memory disturbance* that affects all time periods equally, has been described in patients surviving herpes simplex encephalitis (Butters, Miliotis, Albert, & Sax, 1984; Cermak & O'Connor, 1983; Damasio et al., 1985; Kopelman, Stanhope, & Kingsley, 1999) and in certain other amnesic subjects (Sanders & Warrington, 1971) as well as in patients with Huntington's disease (Albert et al., 1981). This decade-nonspecific pattern has been primarily attributed to a retrieval deficit that impairs access to information from all time periods equally.

As suggested in the preceding section, recent studies have shown rather convincingly that retrieval of remote autobiographical information is distinct from retrieval of remote semantic material and facts, a finding that has led to the development of Multiple Trace Theory (MTT) as an alternative to standard consolidation theory (Moscovitch et al., 2005; Nadel, Samsonovich, Ryan, & Moscovitch, 2000). Standard consolidation theory would suggest that the hippocampus is involved in consolidation of new memories, but only for a relatively short period of time. In contrast, MTT suggests that, as time passes and memories are continually retrieved in different contexts, their episodic or autobiographical character can be blurred and, as a result, the corresponding trace can become more "semantic" (context-independent), and cortically based in nature. However, MTT states that, as long as a memory trace retains distinctive autobiographic qualities, the hippocampus remains strongly involved in its retrieval, regardless of its age. Recent data (Urbanowitsch, Gorenc, Herold, & Schröder, 2013) are clearly in favor of MTT, a major development in our theoretical understanding of the role played by the hippocampus and related structures in human memory performance.

Spared Abilities in Amnesic Patients

Despite significant impairments in new learning and remote memory, amnesics often perform normally or near-normally on psychometric tests of intelligence (e.g., Wechsler Scales) and on measures of immediate memory, provided that the amount of information is within their attention span (Drachman & Arbit, 1966) and that the recall test follows quickly after learning. Thus, amnesia cannot be explained on the basis of poor attention span or generalized intellectual loss. However, other cognitive deficits can be seen in some amnesic patients, and may contribute to their deficits in memory. Examples include visuoperceptual and executive skills deficits in AK syndrome (Kapur & Butters, 1977; Kopelman, 1995; Moscovitch, 1982; Squire, 1982b) and prominent frontal lobe-executive deficits in patients with basal forebrain amnesia (DeLuca & Diamond, 1995).

Remarkably, even densely amnesic patients show certain spared memory capacities. When memory is measured indirectly by evaluating changes in performance rather than by assessing conscious recollection ("what do you remember?"), amnesics often show normal or near-normal performance. These intact capabilities are reflected, for example, in (a) the acquisition of new motor, perceptual, and cognitive skills (Beaunieux et al., 1998; Cohen & Squire, 1980; Cohen, Poldrack, & Eichenbaum, 1997; Schmidtke, Handschu, & Vollmer, 1996); (b) the intact facilitation ("priming") of performance, as measured by increased accuracy or response speed when specific stimuli, or stimulus contexts, are repeated after initial presentation (e.g., Cermak, Talbot, Chandler, & Wolbarst, 1985; Gabrieli, Milberg, Keane, & Corkin, 1990; Hamann & Squire, 1997), and (c) intact "noncognitive" forms of learning such as classical conditioning in some amnesics but not others (Gabrieli, Fleischman, Keane, Reminger, & Morrell, 1995; Myers et al., 2001; Schugens & Daum, 1999; Woodruff Pak, 1993).

Anatomic Correlates of Amnesia

As indicated in the preceding section, amnesic syndrome can result from focal damage to the medial temporal lobes, the medial thalamus, or the basal forebrain. Anatomic, physiologic and behavioral studies in nonhuman primates have suggested why these regions may be important for memory. An understanding of the underlying circuitry provides a basis for understanding that these three regions are not discrete entities, but are parts of an integrated, distributed, memory system.

Temporal Lobe

The importance of the temporal lobes in memory was established in the 1950s by reports of severe and permanent amnesia after bilateral surgical resections of the medial aspects of the temporal lobes in humans (Scoville, 1954; Scoville & Milner, 1957). The aim of surgery was either to ameliorate psychotic behavior or to treat intractable epilepsy. H.M., who was treated for epilepsy, is the best studied of such patients, having been the subject of many reports and studies over nearly five decades.

H. M.'s intended lesions extended 8 to 9 CM back from the temporal poles, and included the amygdala, the hippocampus, and the parahippocampal cortex. An appreciation of the anatomic connections of these structures is key to understanding their role in memory function.

The Hippocampus and Parahippocampal Region

The hippocampus is a phylogenetically ancient cortical structure consisting of the dentate gyrus, the sectors of Ammon's horn (cornu Ammonis (CA) 1–4), and the subiculum. The internal connections of the hippocampus were identified by Ramón y Cajal and his student Lorrente de Nó, who first described the *trisynaptic circuit* (Van Hoesen, 1985). Neurons of the entorhinal cortex project via the *perforant pathway* to synapse on dendrites of granule cells in the dentate gyrus. Granule cell axons project to the dendrites of pyramidal cells in the CA3 region of Ammon's horn (*mossy fiber projection*). These pyramidal cells have axons that bifurcate, one branch projecting subcortically via the fimbria-fornix, and the other (*Shaffer collateral pathway*) to CA1. CA1 neurons project subcortically via the fimbria, but also to the subiculum, which is the major source of hippocampal efferent projections (Rosene & Van Hoesen, 1977). Efferent fibers from the subiculum project either to subcortical targets (via the fimbria and fornix) or to other cortical regions. The subiculum also projects back to the entorhinal cortex, completing a circuit. The connections described are unidirectional, suggesting an orderly progression of information through the hippocampus.

Although there are direct cortical connections to the hippocampus, the majority of hippocampal cortical inputs are from the adjacent parahippocampal region. The parahippocampal region consists of rhinal (entorhinal and perirhinal) cortex, pre- and parasubicular cortex, and parahippocampal cortex (Scharfman, Witter, & Schwarcz, 2000). The parahippocampal region is hierarchically organized, with the entorhinal cortex being the final common pathway to the hippocampus (Van Hoesen and Pandya, 1975). The entorhinal cortex receives afferents from perirhinal cortex and the parahippocampal gyrus (Insausti, Amaral, & Cowan, 1987a; Irle & Markowitsch, 1982; Rosene & Van Hoesen, 1977; Van Hoesen, Rosene, & Mesulam, 1979). These regions in turn receive projections from unimodal and polymodal association cortex, thus providing entorhinal cortex with indirect access to a variety of highly processed information (Amaral, Insausti, & Cowan, 1983; Insausti et al., 1987a; Van Hoesen, 1985; Van Hoesen, Pandya, & Butters, 1972). Unlike the intrinsic hippocampal connections, which are unidirectional, the connections of the parahippocampal region are reciprocal (Rosene & Van Hoesen, 1977). Both perirhinal and parahippocampal cortices are connected with visual and polymodal cortical regions, and, to a lesser extent, with somatosensory cortex; but only the parahippocampal cortex receives substantial input from parietal polysensory and auditory cortices (Suzuki & Eichenbaum, 2000).

Subcortical projections from the hippocampus travel in the fornix, a white matter structure that arches through the lateral ventricle and descends medial to the foramen of Munro into the lateral wall of the third ventricle, where it divides at the anterior commissure. Fibers from CA1, CA3 and the subiculum project in the precommissural fornix to the lateral septal nucleus (Swanson & Cowan, 1979). Other subicular projections travel in the postcommissural fornix and terminate in either the anterior nuclear complex of the thalamus or the mammillary bodies (Swanson & Cowan, 1979; Van Hoesen, 1985). There are also hippocampal projections to the amygdala, nucleus accumbens, and other regions in the basal forebrain, and to the ventromedial hypothalamus (Amaral & Insausti, 1990; Swanson & Cowan, 1979).

The hippocampal → post-commissural fornix → mammillary body projection was part of the "circuit" described by Papez in 1937 to explain how emotional expression and feeling, mediated by the hypothalamus, could be coordinated with cognition, mediated by the cortex. The hippocampus projects via the postcommissural fornix to the mammillary bodies, which, in turn, project via the mammillothalamic tract to the anterior nuclei of the thalamus. The circuit, which has since been referred to as the *medial limbic circuit,* is completed by thalamic projections to the cingulate gyrus and cingulate projections (via the cingulate bundle or cingulum) that extend back to the hippocampus.

The hippocampus also receives subcortical projections from the basal forebrain (medial septal nucleus and the nucleus of the diagonal band of Broca), from midline, anterior, and laterodorsal thalamic nuclei, and from the amygdala, hypothalamus, and brain stem, including the central gray, ventral tegmental area, raphé nuclei and locus coeruleus (Amaral & Cowan, 1980; Amaral & Insausti, 1990; Herkenham, 1978; Insausti, Amaral, & Cowan, 1987b; Van Hoesen, 1985).

The Amygdala

The amygdala is situated immediately anterior to the hippocampus and deep to the periamygdaloid and perirhinal cortices. It has two main parts: a large basolateral group of nuclei, with extensive connections to limbic and association cortex and to dorsomedial thalamus, and a smaller corticomedial segment, which extends into the basal forebrain and has extensive connections with basal forebrain, hypothalamus, and brain stem (DeOlmos, 1990; Heimer & Alheid, 1991; Scott, DeKosky, & Scheff, 1991). In a very general sense, the connections of amygdala and hippocampus are similar: both are strongly interconnected with frontal and temporal limbic cortex, and thus both have indirect access to polymodal and supramodal neocortical association areas (Herzog & Van Hoesen, 1976; Rosene & Van Hoesen, 1977). Both project to basal forebrain and hypothalamus. The amygdala and hippocampus also have direct connections with each other (Insausti et al., 1987b; Poletti, 1986; Saunders, Rosene, & Van Hoesen, 1988).

Although in the brains of higher mammals the amygdala is adjacent to the hippocampus, it differs radically from the hippocampus in structure and derivation. The amygdala is a subcortical structure, intimately related with the basal forebrain, and often classified as one of the basal ganglia. The amygdala is more closely related to limbic and neocortical regions that are of paleocortical derivation, whereas the hippocampus is archicortical, and is more closely related to cortex of archicortical derivation (Pandya & Yeterian, 1990). Thus, the amygdala is more closely related to orbitofrontal and anterior temporal cortex (Porrino, Crane, & Goldman-Rakic, 1981), and the hippocampus is more closely related to cingulate cortex. Abnormalities in emotional responsiveness and social interactions are associated with lesions in the amygdala and related anterior temporal and orbitofrontal cortex (Butter & Snyder, 1972).

The subcortical connections of the amygdala also differ from those of the hippocampus. Whereas the hippocampus is related through Papez's medial limbic circuit with the mammillary bodies and the anterior thalamic nuclei, the amygdala has projections (via the ventral amygdalofugal pathway) to the dorsomedial nucleus of the thalamus (Nauta, 1961). Basal forebrain connections also differ: The hippocampus is related to more ventral portions of the septal nuclei, and the amygdala has more extensive connections with the bed nucleus of the stria terminalis. Cholinergic projections to the amygdala are from the nucleus basalis of Meynert, whereas the hippocampus receives input from the septal region and diagonal band of Broca (Mesulam, Mufson, Levey, & Wainer, 1983). Finally, the amygdala has connections with brain stem autonomic centers (nucleus of the tractus solitarius), providing a direct pathway for limbic-autonomic interaction. In contrast to Papez's medial limbic circuit, the amygdala can be thought of as participating in a "lateral" limbic circuit: amygdala → dorsomedial nucleus of the thalamus → orbitofrontal cortex → uncus → amygdala.

The Anatomical Basis of Temporal Lobe Amnesia

Early studies of patients with bilateral temporal lobectomy supported the idea that damage to the hippocampus was necessary for medial temporal lesions to produce amnesia. Scoville and Milner (1957) reviewed ten patients with bilateral medial temporal resections. Removal of the uncus and amygdala (in one patient) caused no memory loss, but resections that extended posteriorly to involve the hippocampus and parahippocampal gyrus were associated with amnesia. Also, amnesia was more severe with more extensive resections. Scoville and Milner concluded that amnesia would not occur unless the surgery extended far enough back to involve the hippocampus.

The case for the importance of the hippocampus in memory was subsequently made even more convincingly by the study of patients who survived cardiopulmonary arrest with well-documented deficits in memory, and whose brains were examined after they died from other causes (Cummings, Tomiyasu, Read, & Benson, 1984; Victor & Agamanolis, 1990; Zola-Morgan, Squire & Amaral, 1986). In each case, damage was restricted almost entirely to the hippocampus, where the pyramidal neurons of CA1, exquisitely sensitive to hypoxia, were selectively destroyed. Global ischemia in monkeys causes similar lesions, with scores on memory tasks comparable to those of monkeys with surgical lesions restricted to the hippocampus (Squire & Zola-Morgan, 1991). It should be noted, however, that in these cases, memory loss was not as severe as that seen in H.M.

Our basic understanding of the anatomic substrate of temporal lobe amnesia was greatly enhanced in the 1970s by numerous investigations motivated by the original Scoville and Milner report on H.M., which eventually led to the development of animal models of amnesia. This advancement was facilitated by the development of tasks, including delayed matching-to-sample (DMS; Gaffan, 1974) and delayed nonmatching-to-sample (DNMS; Mishkin, 1978) that provided meaningful analogues to human memory paradigms. DNMS was learned more readily than DMS by normal monkeys, who presumably were drawn to novelty. Hundreds of different objects were used so that habits (or "familiarity") could not be used as a basis for recognition.

Monkeys with extensive medial temporal lesions, involving both amygdala and hippocampus, were more impaired on the DNMS task than were monkeys with damage to the hippocampus or amygdala alone. This critical observation led to the notion that *two parallel systems subserve memory, one involving the hippocampus and the other the amygdala* (Mishkin, 1978; Mishkin and Saunders, 1979; Mishkin, 1982; Mishkin, Spiegler, Saunders, & Malamut, 1982). Because either system can subserve memory in large part, lesions in both systems are required to produce severe amnesia. This has come to be known as the *dual system theory of amnesia*, and forms a core principle of understanding memory disorders regardless of lesion location. In a series of experiments, Mishkin and colleagues extended their observations to the subcortical projections of these two medial temporal structures, focusing on the circuits (medial and lateral limbic circuits) described in Figures 28.1 and 28.2.

The general principle that damage to both the medial and lateral limbic circuits is necessary for amnesia serves as a basis for understanding diencephalic and basal forebrain amnesias as well. Figure 28.2 depicts the basic anatomy of memory with a rudimentary representation of the basal forebrain contributions to the two limbic circuits added. Thus, for example, lesions that interrupt both the fornix (disrupting Papez's circuit) and the ventral amygdalofugal pathways (disrupting the lateral circuit) cause severe amnesia, whereas lesions restricted to either pathway alone cause

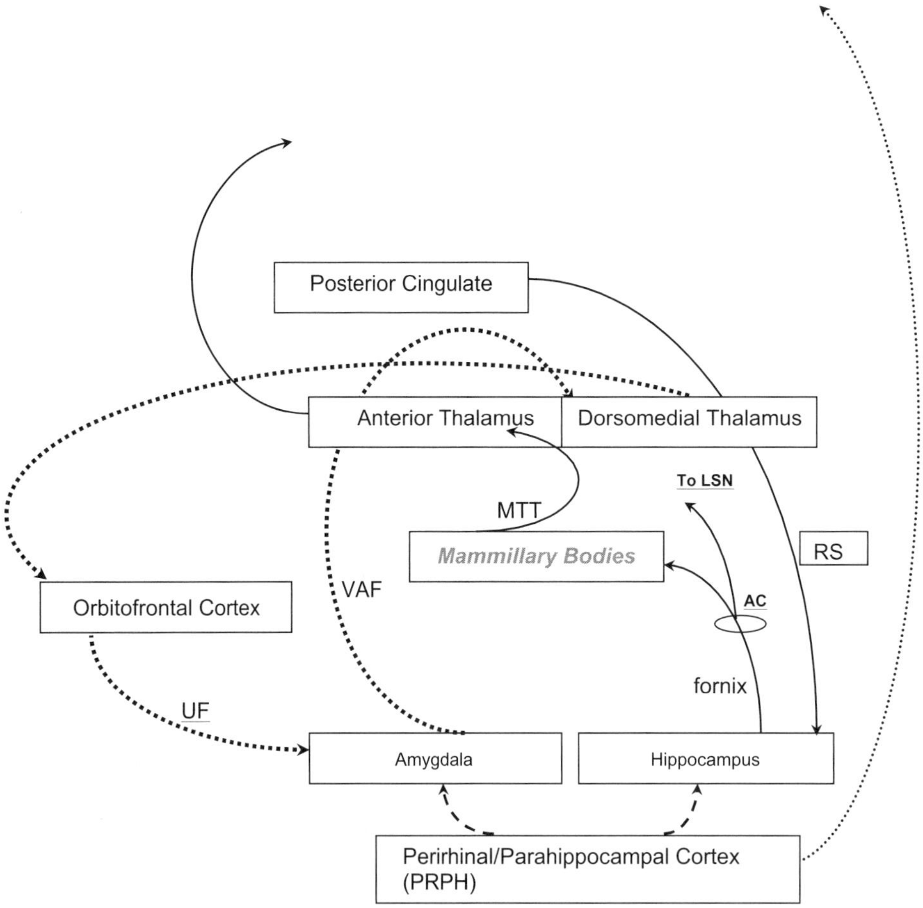

Figure 28.1 The dual-system theory of amnesia. The hippocampally based "medial" system is depicted by solid lines, while the amygdala-based "lateral" system is depicted by dotted lines. Perirhinal-parahippocampal cortex contributes to both systems by projecting to both amygdala and hippocampus, as well as to dorsomedial nucleus of the thalamus (right-most projection in the figure). AC, anterior commisure; LSN, lateral septal nucleus; MTT, mammillothalamic tract; VAF, ventral amygdalofugal pathway; RSA, retrosplenial area; UF, uncinate fasciculus.

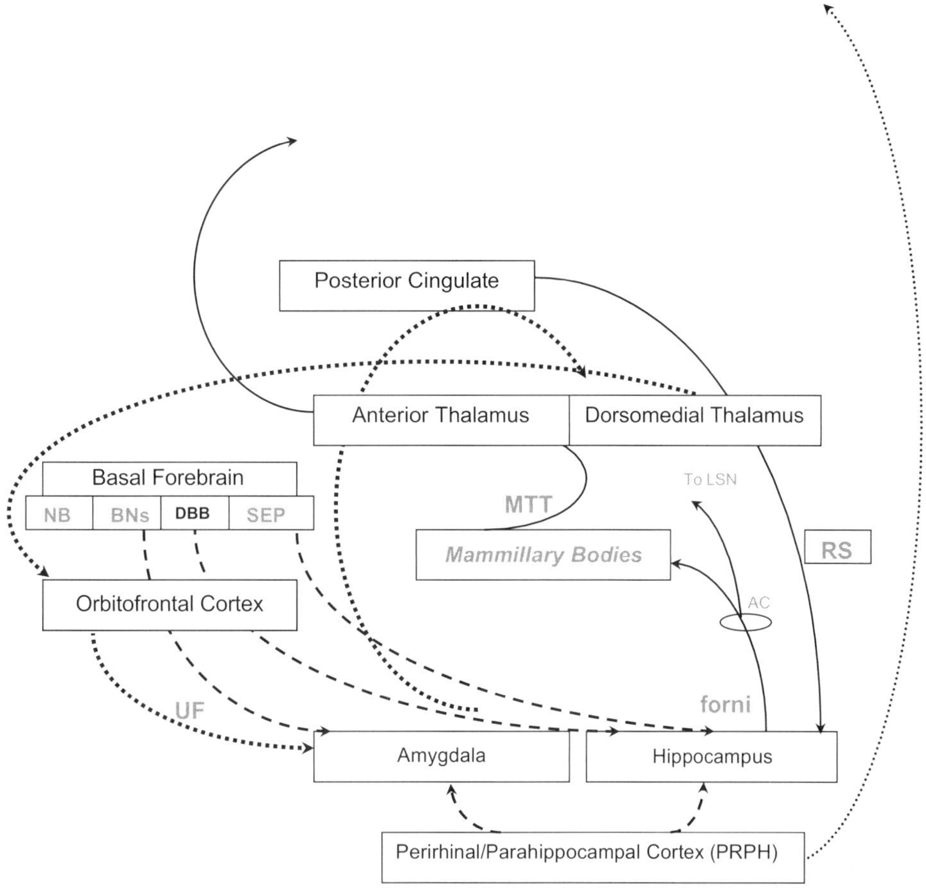

Figure 28.2 Dual system with basal forebrain inputs. Not all inputs from the basal forebrain are shown. Abbreviations within the two limbic circuits are as in Figure 28.1. NBM, nucleus basalis of Meynert; BNst, bed nucleus of the stria terminalis; DBB, diagonal band of Broca; SEP, septal nucleus.

less memory disturbance (Bachevalier, Saunders, & Mishkin, 1985; Bachevalier, Parkinson, & Mishkin, 1985). Many other combinations on this general theme are possible and have been documented in the literature.

Lesions that affect either the posteromedial or anteromedial aspect of the thalamus cause little memory disturbance; severe amnesia, comparable to that associated with medial temporal ablations, occurs only when *both* anterior and posterior medial thalamic regions are involved (Aggleton & Mishkin, 1983). Finally, lesions that affect the frontal projections of both Papez's circuit (anterior cingulate gyrus) and the lateral circuit (ventromedial frontal lobe) produce greater memory loss than lesions of either alone (Bachevalier & Mishkin, 1986). This series of studies on primates suggests (a) that structures within each memory system are highly interdependent, since damage to different parts of each system can cause apparently equivalent deficits; and (b) that each system can, to some extent, carry on the function of the other, since lesions affecting only one system result in memory loss that is far less severe than if both systems are damaged.

The dual-system theory, as first proposed, had to be modified when it was definitively shown that collateral damage to the perirhinal cortex was responsible for the memory deficits seen after amygdala lesions. In fact, stereotactic lesions of the amygdala sparing perirhinal cortex do not add to the memory deficit of animals with hippocampal and parahippocampal gyrus lesions (Zola-Morgan, Squire, & Amaral, 1989a). Zola-Morgan, Squire, Amaral, and Suzukiet al. (1989b) found that lesions involving both perirhinal and parahippocampal cortex *but not the hippocampus* cause severe memory impairment in the monkey. This is not explained entirely by interruption of cortical input to the hippocampus, because monkeys with this lesion had *more* severe memory deficits than monkeys with lesions that involved only the hippocampus and parahippocampal gyrus (Zola-Morgan & Squire, 1986; Squire & Zola-Morgan, 1991). This suggests that the perirhinal cortex not only conveys information to the hippocampus via entorhinal cortex, but that it also contributes to memory in its own right. Because both the amygdala and the perirhinal cortex project to dorsomedial thalamus, the dual-system theory could be easily modified by substituting perirhinal cortex for the amygdala (this connection is signified by the right-most line in Figure 28.1).

More recently the specific roles of these temporal lobe structures has been increasingly elucidated. The perirhinal cortex receives substantial cortical input from ventral temporal and occipital cortex concerned with the processing of objects. In contrast, the parahippocampal cortex receives widespread input from frontal and parietal association cortex that collectively code spatiotemporal context. It has been proposed that the perirhinal cortex codes item (object)–based memory, while the parahippocampal cortex codes contextual aspects of memory. By this view, both of these regions project to the hippocampus via separate pathways in the entorhinal cortex. The hippocampus then binds item and context through relational memory processing, producing an episodic memory trace.

In summary, the temporal lobes play a significant role in memory; however, the relative contribution of different temporal lobe structures remains to be worked out. At this point, one can argue on the basis of animal models that the hippocampus has a particular role in spatial memory, and that object memory may be more dependent upon perirhinal cortex. It is suggested that the hippocampus in humans may subserve episodic memory, and the perirhinal cortex may be necessary to establish semantic memories. The ability of children with hypoxic damage to the hippocampus to acquire semantic information (Vargha-Khadem et al., 1997) and of amnesic patients to acquire new vocabulary words (Verfaellie, Koseff, & Alexander, 2000) suggests some degree of independence between these kinds of memory; however, there is presently not enough evidence to support a neat anatomic parcellation of these functions. A related distinction between episodic recall and recognition memory is made by Aggleton and Brown (1999), who attribute the former to the hippocampal/diencephalic circuit of Papez, and the latter to the perirhinal cortex and dorsomedial thalamus. In humans, it has been proposed that the hippocampus mediates conscious, deliberate recall ("recollection"), while perirhinal cortex mediates "familiarity" based on item-based recognition (Diana, Yonelinas, & Ranganath, 2007; Eichenbaum, Yonelinas, & Ranganath, 2007). However, this viewpoint is controversial and considerable data from humans and animals suggest that the perirhinal-parahippocampal-entorhinal-hippocampal system is an integrated memory system that does not differentially represent these two subjective states of remembering (Squire & Wixted, 2011; Wixted & Squire, 2011).

Amnesia From Damage to Other Elements of the Medial Limbic Circuit

Having considered the importance of temporal lobe structures in amnesia, we now turn to consideration of whether amnesia can occur after damage to other components of the medial limbic circuit.

FORNIX

It was once widely held that surgical section of the columns of the fornix would not result in memory loss (Cairns & Mosberg, 1951; Dott, 1938; Garcia Bengochea, De La Torre, Esquivel, Vieta, & Fernandec, 1954; Woolsey & Nelson, 1975), although there was some early evidence to the contrary (Hassler & Riechert, 1957; Sweet, Talland, & Ervin, 1959). Heilman and Sypert (1977), reporting on a patient who had a tumor affecting fornix projections, argued that lesions of the fornix posterior to the anterior commissure affect not only fibers destined for the mammillary bodies, but also disrupt connections between the hippocampus and the basal forebrain and direct projections from the hippocampus to the anterior thalamic nuclei (Aggleton, Desimone, & Mishkin, 1986; Veazey, Amaral, & Cowan, 1982). They suggested that section of the columns of the fornix ventral to the anterior commissure might not cause amnesia, as it affects only projections to the mammillary bodies. Fornix damage usually results in some degree of amnesia both in animals (Bachevalier et al., 1985; Bachevalier et al., 1985; Carr, 1982; Gaffan, 1993, 1974; Moss, Mahut, & Zola-Morgan, 1981; Owen & Butler, 1981) and humans (Aggleton et al., 2000; Calabrese, Markowitsch, Harders, Scholz, & Gehlen, 1995; D'Esposito, Verfaellie, Alexander, & Katz, 1995; Gaffan, Gaffan, & Hodges, 1991; Gaffan & Gaffan, 1991; Grafman, Salazar, Weingartner, Vance, & Ludlow, 1985; McMackin, Cockburn, Anslow, & Gaffan, 1995; Moudgil, Azzouz, Al-Azzaz, Haut, & Guttmann, 2000; Park, Hahn, Kim, Na, & Huh, 2000). In primates, fornix damage, like hippocampal lesions, impairs spatial memory and memory for objects in a scene, a paradigm that Gaffan (Gaffan & Parker, 1996) suggests is related to episodic memory. In humans, fornix lesions have been found to affect recall more than recognition memory (Aggleton & Brown, 1999), and to cause anterograde but not retrograde amnesia (but see Yasuno et al., 1999).

MAMMILLARY BODIES

The anatomy of mammillary body connections is summarized by Aggleton and Sahgal (1993). This paired hypothalamic nucleus receives substantial input from the hippocampus. There are projections from the subicular complex of the hippocampus through the fornix to the medial mammillary nucleus, which is more affected than the lateral mammillary nucleus in Wernicke-Korsakoff disease. There are also hippocampal projections to the lateral mammillary nucleus and tuberomammillary nucleus. These hippocampal-mammillary body connections are not reciprocated. Mamillothalamic projections are also unidirectional. The mammillary bodies also project to the medial septum and midbrain.

The presence of prominent mammillary body damage in Wernicke-Korsakoff syndrome first suggested their importance in memory (Gamper, cited by Victor, Adams, & Collins, 1989). Victor et al. (1989) examined the mammillary bodies and the dorsomedial thalamic nucleus of 43 alcoholics. Five had suffered Wernicke's encephalopathy but had recovered without evidence of memory loss; 38 had Wernicke-Korsakoff disease, with persistent amnesia. At autopsy, all had lesions of the mammillary bodies; but only the 38 patients with persistent memory loss had concurrent lesions of the dorsomedial thalamic nucleus. Victor and colleagues concluded that memory loss could not be attributed solely to mammillary body damage, but was more likely to be associated with thalamic lesions. Mair, Warrington, and Weiskrantz (1979) and Mayes, Meudell, Mann, and Pickering (1988) each report two cases of Wernicke-Korsakoff syndrome with lesions in the thalamus restricted to a thin band of gliosis adjacent to the third ventricle affecting the midline nuclei but not the dorsomedial nucleus. Based on this, Mair et al. (1979) suggested that the mammillary body lesions (present in each of these patients) may account for the memory loss. Lesions restricted to the mammillary bodies have not been associated with deficits on DNMS tasks in monkeys (Aggleton & Mishkin, 1985). However, deficits on spatial memory tasks have been reported in monkeys (Parker & Gaffan, 1997) and in rats (Sziklas & Petrides, 1998). Human cases with selective mammillary body lesions are rare. Dusoir, Kapur, Byrnes, McKinstry, and Hoare et al. (1990) reported amnesia in a patient with MRI evidence of mammillary body lesions following a penetrating injury from a snooker cue. Loesch, Gilman, Del Dotto, and Rosenblum (1995) report memory deficits in a patient with a cavernous malformation of the mammillary bodies, and Tanaka, Miyazawa, Akaoka, and Yamada (1997) report memory loss with mammillary body damage following removal of a cystic craniopharyngioma. It is difficult to exclude extramammillary lesions in these cases, especially to adjacent portions of the hypothalamus or basal forebrain.

ANTERIOR THALAMIC NUCLEI

The anterior thalamic nuclei consist of anteromedial (am), anteroventral (av), anterodorsal (ad), and lateral dorsal (ld) nuclei. The medial mammillary nucleus projects ipsilaterally to am and av; whereas the lateral mammillary nucleus projects bilaterally to ad (see Aggleton & Sahgal, 1993). The anterior thalamic nuclei also receive a substantial direct projection from the hippocampus. Pre- and parasubiculum project to av, and subiculum to am, and the hippocampus also projects to ld. All of these hippocampal-thalamic projections are reciprocated.

The anterior thalamic nuclei project to the cingulate and retrosplenial cortices, among other locations. The lateral dorsal nucleus projects strongly to retrosplenial cortex, and shows specific degeneration in Alzheimer's disease (Xuereb et al., 1991).

Parker and Gaffan (1997) demonstrated deficits on a delayed-matching-to-place task in monkeys with anterior thalamic lesions. Ghika-Schmid and Bogousslavsky (2000) report a series of 12 patients with anterior thalamic infarcts, all of whom demonstrated anterograde amnesia (verbal with left and nonverbal with right hemisphere lesions) in combination with perseveration, transcortical motor aphasia, apathy, and executive dysfunction. The lesions involved the anterior thalamic nuclei and not the dorsomedial or ventrolateral nuclei. They also extended to involve the mammillothalamic tract and the internal medullary lamina. More often, thalamic lesions in humans associated with severe amnesia spare the anterior thalamic nuclei. DNMS deficits are reported only with more extensive thalamic involvement.

CINGULATE AND RETROSPLENIAL CORTEX

The major cortical connections of the anterior thalamic nuclei are with the cingulate gyrus. Bachevalier and Mishkin (1986) suggest that combined lesions of orbitofrontal and anterior cingulate cortex in monkeys damages both memory circuits, the orbitofrontal cortex being connected to the lateral limbic circuit, and the anterior cingulate to the medial circuit. But extensive frontal lesions in humans (Eslinger & Damasio, 1985) do not typically result in the classical amnesic syndrome. Meunier, Bachevalier, and Mishkin (1997) describe a spatial memory deficit in monkeys with anterior cingulate lesions; studies in rats (Aggleton, Neave, Nagle, & Sahgal, 1995) suggest that this may be due to damage to the underlying cingulate bundle. The anterior cingulate region appears to play a role in initiating movement, in motivation, and in goal-directed behaviors (Devinsky, Morrell, & Vogt, 1995), but anterior cingulate gyrus lesions have not been associated with amnesia in humans.

The principal projections of the anterior thalamic nuclei, however, are to posterior cingulate cortex, and especially retrosplenial cortex. These cortical regions are also interconnected with the hippocampus (Morris, Petrides, & Pandya, 1999). Lesions in humans that involve retrosplenial cortex can result in a classical amnesic syndrome (Valenstein et al., 1987) but there remains some debate whether the cause of the amnesia is interruption of cingulate/hippocampal connections via the cingulate bundle, damage to the retrosplenial cortex itself, or damage to hippocampal-thalamic, hippocampal-basal forebrain (septal nuclei) or frontal lobe connections traveling in the fornix (Rudge & Warrington, 1991; von Cramon & Schuri, 1992). Additional cases of amnesia with retrosplenial lesions have been reported in the Japanese literature by Arita et al., 1995; Iwasaki et al., 1993; Takayama, Kamo, Ohkawa, Akiguchi, & Kimura, 1991; Yasuda, Watanabe, & Ono, 1997). Takahashi et al. (1997) report pure topographic amnesia with a right retrosplenial lesion. Valenstein et al.'s case (1987) was left-sided, and the memory loss was predominately verbal.

Summary of Temporal Lobe Amnesia

The bulk of the evidence reviewed suggests that (a) damage to cortical and subcortical structures within the temporal lobe, whether focal or extensive, can result in amnesia; (b) amnesia most likely results from simultaneous damage to both the hippocampally based medial limbic circuit and the amygdala-based lateral limbic circuit; and (c) that damage to individual elements of these circuits can result in amnesia provided that it sufficiently impairs the functional integrity of this distributed memory system.

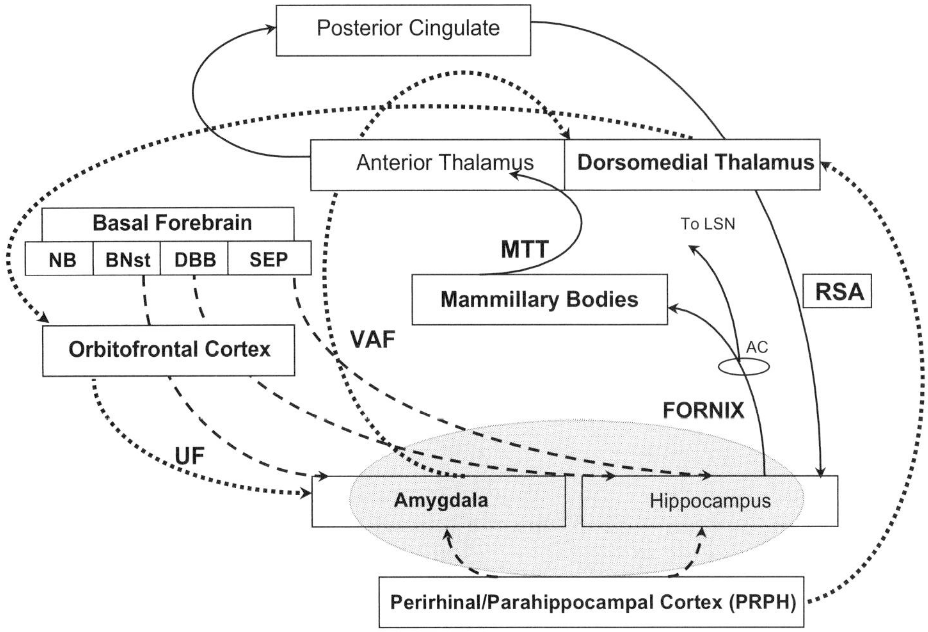

Figure 28.3 Two possible lesion Scenarios for bitemporal amnesia. In Panel A, a large lesion affects both amygdala and hippocampus and their connections with their respective circuits. In Panel B, a more restricted lesion affecting the PRPH affects inputs to both circuits including PRPH inputs to the dorsomedial thalamus.

Figure 28.3 depicts two possible lesion scenarios for bitemporal amnesia. In Panel A, an extensive lesion affects both hippocampus and amygdala, and their respective connections to the medial and lateral limbic circuits. In Panel B, a more restricted lesion of the perirhinal-parahippocampal (PRPH) region affects intrinsic functioning of this region and impairs its connectivity to amygdala, hippocampus, and dorsomedial thalamus. Both lesions would be expected to result in clinically significant amnesia.

Thalamic Amnesia

Amnesia associated with tumors in the walls of the third ventricle (Grünthal, 1939; Lhermitte, Doussinet, & Ajuriaguerra, 1937; Sprofkin & Sciarra, 1952; Williams & Pennybacker, 1954) provided early evidence that medial thalamic structures may be important in memory. The advent of neuroimaging made it possible to correlate memory deficits with restricted thalamic lesions in patients with thalamic strokes. Although initial reports appeared to confirm evidence from Wernicke-Korsakoff disease that dorsomedial thalamic lesions were associated with memory loss, subsequent studies cast doubt upon this. Early reports had suggested that N.A., a patient who became amnesic after a fencing foil passed through his nose into the brain (Teuber, Milner, & Vaughan, 1968), had a restricted lesion involving the left dorsomedial thalamic nucleus on CT scan (Squire & Moore, 1979), and that amnesic patients with thalamic strokes had CT evidence of restricted dorsomedial lesions (Bogousslavsky, Regli, & Assal, 1986; Choi, Sudarsky, Schachter, Biber, & Burke, 1983; Speedie & Heilman, 1983). High-resolution imaging in N.A., however, revealed that his lesion not only affected the ventral aspect of the dorsomedial nucleus, but also severely damaged the intralaminar nuclei, mammillothalamic tract, and internal medullary lamina (Squire et al., 1989). Such lesions impair connectivity between the mammillary bodies and the anterior nucleus, as well as between the amygdala and the dorsomedial nucleus. N.A. also had lesions affecting the postcommissural fornix, mammillary bodies, and the right temporal tip. More restricted lesions in patients with thalamic infarctions suggest that thalamic amnesia best correlates with anterior thalamic lesions affecting the internal medullary lamina and mammillothalamic tract (Gentilini, DeRenzi, & Crisi, 1987; Graff-Radford et al., 1990; Malamut, Graff-Radford, Chawluk, Grossman, & Gur, 1992, Winocur, Oxbury, Roberts, Agnetti, & Davis, 1984; von Cramon, Hebel & Schuri, 1985). More posterior lesions that involve portions of the dorsomedial nucleus but spare the internal medullary lamina and mammillothalamic tract do not produce amnesia (Graff-Radford et al., 1990; Kritchevsky, Graff-Radford, & Damasio, 1987; von Cramon et al., 1985). The association between anterior thalamic lesions and amnesia is entirely consistent with the dual-system theory. Graff-Radford et al. (1990) provided a clear anatomic demonstration in the monkey of the juxtaposition of components of both systems (the mammillothalamic tract and the ventral amygdalofugal pathway) in the internal medullary lamina.

Alternative explanations of thalamic amnesia suggest a role for the midline thalamic nuclei. These nuclei have connections with the hippocampus (Amaral & Cowan, 1980; Herkenham, 1978, Insausti et al., 1987b; Van Hoesen,

1985), and are quite consistently damaged in patients with Wernicke-Korsakoff disease (Mair et al., 1979; Mayes et al., 1988). Another proposal is that thalamic lesions may disconnect thalamic interactions with the frontal lobes. Warrington (Warrington and Weiskrantz, 1982; Warrington, 1985) proposed that restricted thalamic lesions found in their cases of Wernicke-Korsakoff disease (Mair et al., 1979) might disconnect mediodorsal-frontal connections important for coordinating posterior cortical regions subserving semantic memories with frontal structures that impose cognitive structure upon these memories.

Figure 28.4 depicts two possible lesion scenarios for diencephalic amnesia. In Panel A, an extensive lesion of the thalamus affecting both anterior and dorsomedial nuclei impairs both circuits. In Panel B, a more restricted lesion, meant to depict pathway disconnection in the internal medullary lamina, affects both the mammillothalamic tract (MTT), an intrinsic component of the medial circuit, and the ventral amygdalofugal (VAF) pathway, a component of the lateral circuit.

Basal Forebrain Amnesia

The basal forebrain is at the junction of the diencephalon and the cerebral hemispheres, and has, at minimum, the following components: the septal area, diagonal band of Broca, nucleus accumbens septi, olfactory tubercle, substantia

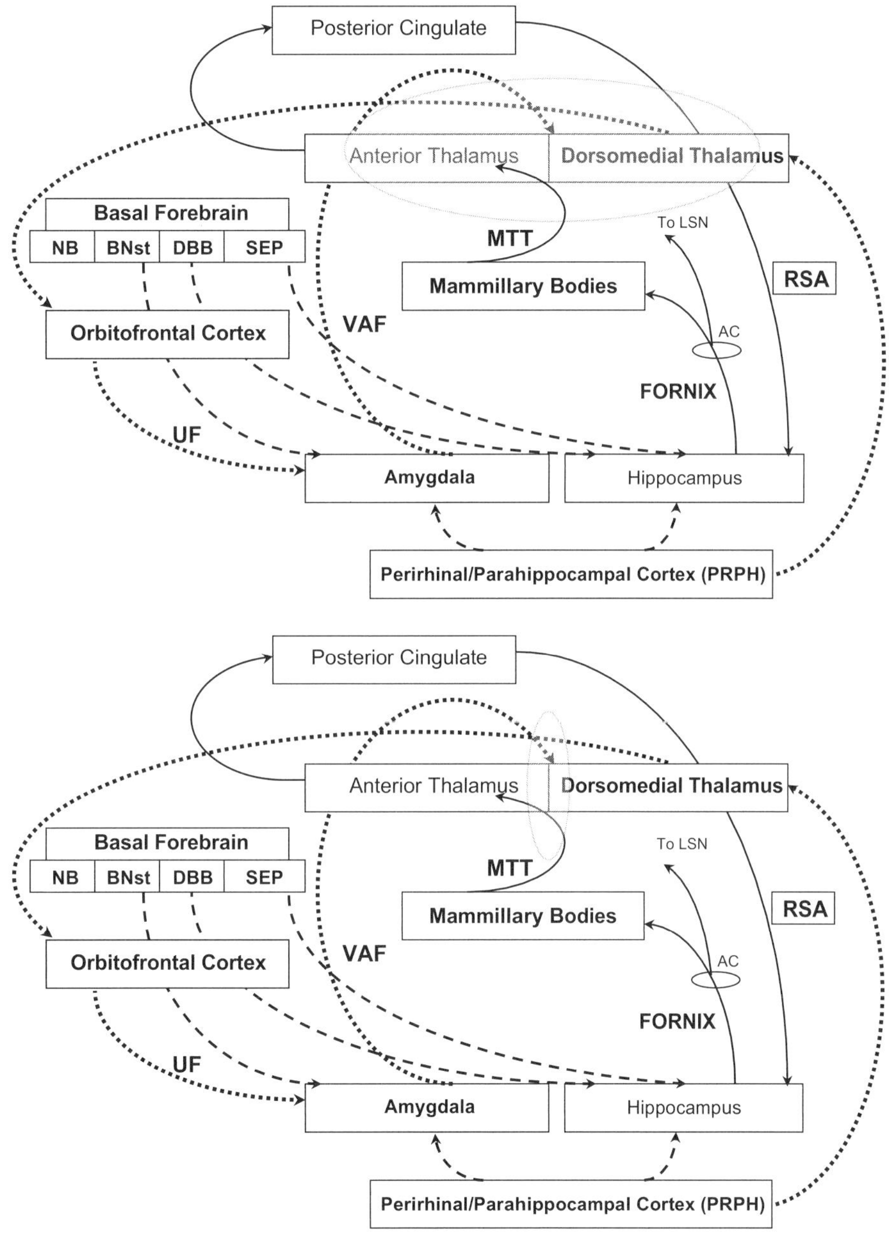

Figure 28.4 Two possible lesion scenarios for diencephalic amnesia. In Panel A, a large lesion affects both anterior and dorsomedial thalamic nuclei, thus impairing both circuits. In Panel B, a more restricted lesion affects the internal medullary lamina within the thalamus, impinging upon both the mammillothalamic tract and the ventral amygdalofugal pathway, thus impairing both circuits.

innominata (containing the nucleus basalis of Meynert), bed nucleus of the stria terminalis, and the preoptic area. It is the third major region, after the temporal lobes and diencephalon, to be considered essential for normal memory function in humans. It was known for many years that some patients developed memory loss after hemorrhage from rupture of anterior communicating artery aneurysms (Lindqvist & Norlen, 1966; Talland, Sweet, & Ballantine, 1967), but the pathogenesis of this amnesia was not understood.

One theory suggested that cholinergic neurons in the basal forebrain were involved in memory. Lewis and Shute (1967) documented a cholinergic projection from the medial septal region of the basal forebrain to the hippocampus. For many years, scopolamine, a centrally acting anticholinergic agent, had been used in obstetrics, in conjunction with analgesics, to induce a "twilight" state, after which women would have little recall of their deliveries. Drachman and Leavitt (1974) demonstrated that normal subjects had difficulty with free recall of words when given scopolamine, and that this effect was reversed by physostigmine, a centrally acting anticholinesterase agent that prevents inactivation of acetylcholine. Mesulam and Van Hoesen (1976) documented a cholinergic projection from the basal nucleus of Meynert, and in subsequent studies Mesulam and his colleagues (Mesulam et al., 1983; Mesulam & Mufson, 1984) defined the connections of basal forebrain cholinergic neurons. Neurons in the medial septal nucleus and diagonal band of Broca project strongly to the hippocampus, as had been documented by Lewis and Shute (1967). Cholinergic neurons in the substantia innominata (nucleus basalis of Meynert), however, project widely to limbic system and neocortex. In 1981, Whitehouse Price, Clark, Coyle, & DeLong documented selective loss of neurons in the nucleus basalis of Meynert in patients with Alzheimer's disease. Cell loss in cholinergic neurons of the basal forebrain (Arendt, Bigl, & Arendt, 1983) has also been found in Wernicke-Korsakoff syndrome (Butters, 1985; Butters & Cermak, 1980; Butters & Stuss, 1989). All of these lines of evidence suggested a role for the basal forebrain in memory, and more specifically, suggested that the cholinergic projections of the basal forebrain might be of particular importance. In this way, the structures of the basal forebrain can be thought of as key contributors to both the medial and lateral limbic circuits described earlier.

This "cholinergic hypothesis" (Bartus, Dean, Beer, Ponecorvo, & Flicker, 1985; Kopelman, 1986) has generated a large volume of research, but poses some continuing difficulty (Fibiger, 1991). Cholinergic medication provides only a very modest improvement in memory in patients with Alzheimer's disease (Johns, Greenwald, Mohs, & Davis, 1983; Peters & Levin, 1979, 1982; Thal, Fuld, Masure, & Sharpless, 1983). It may be the case, however, that acetylcholine replacement does not have the dramatic effect that dopamine treatment has in Parkinson's disease, since patients with Alzheimer's disease have degeneration in many other areas thought to be of importance in memory, including the target areas of basal forebrain cholinergic projections (the hippocampus, amygdala, and neocortex).

The complexity of basal forebrain anatomy makes it difficult to arrive at firm conclusions about the pathophysiology of amnesia associated with basal forebrain lesions. In addition to its role in cholinergic neurotransmission, the basal forebrain encompasses additional pathways and systems that could conceivably participate in memory. The anterior commissure crosses the midline just posterior to the septal nuclei. The columns of the fornix descend through the basal forebrain on their way to the hypothalamus. The ventral amygdalofugal pathway both projects to the basal forebrain and traverses it on its way to the thalamus. Thus structural lesions of the basal forebrain, if properly situated, may disrupt one or both of the pathways critical for memory. The medial forebrain bundle, which interconnects brain stem, hypothalamic and forebrain structures, travels through the lateral hypothalamus and the basal forebrain. Noradrenergic and dopaminergic pathways are represented in the median forebrain bundle. The *extended amygdala* refers to groups of neurons within the basal forebrain, including neurons in the bed nucleus of the stria terminalis and portions of the nucleus accumbens septi, that are anatomically considered to be related to the corticomedial amygdala, with which they are laterally confluent (Heimer & Alheid, 1991). The core of the nucleus accumbens and the olfactory tubercle closely resemble the caudate-putamen and form the *ventral striatum*, which, in turn, projects to the region of basal forebrain beneath the globus pallidus (the *ventral pallidum*). The *preoptic area* receives projections from amygdala, hippocampus, and other areas of the basal forebrain. It is involved in self-regulatory and species-specific behaviors (Swanson, 1987). It is not known if these areas contribute to memory function.

Most basal forebrain lesions reported in human cases of amnesia have been large, and probably affect all or many of the structures listed here. Often, they also affect areas outside the basal forebrain, such as the orbitofrontal and medial frontal cortices, and the caudate nucleus. Irle et al. (1992) studied 30 patients with brain lesions associated with anterior cerebral artery aneurysm rupture. Severe memory loss was associated with combined lesions in the striatum (caudate) and basal forebrain, whereas lesions restricted to basal forebrain were not associated with memory disturbance. Morris, Bowers, Chatterjee, and Heilman (1992), however, reported a patient with amnesia following removal of a very small glioma in the lamina terminalis, just posterior to the right gyrus rectus. Post-operative MRI scans demonstrated a lesion restricted to the diagonal band of Broca, anterior commissure, nucleus accumbens, and preoptic area. They postulated that destruction of the cholinergic projection to the hippocampus, most of which originates in the nucleus of the diagonal band of Broca, probably accounted for the amnesia, but they could not rule out contributions from other damaged areas. Although the cholinergic hypothesis has been popular, other neurotransmitter pathways (e.g., dopamine) may be of importance, and their contribution to memory remains to be elucidated.

Figure 28.5 depicts two possible lesion scenarios for basal forebrain amnesia. In Panel A, a large basal forebrain lesion affects both intrinsic information-processing within the basal forebrain as well as cholinergic input and fibers of passage that are components of both the medial and lateral limbic circuits. In Panel B, a more restricted lesion affects the cholinergic inputs to both circuits, thus impairing functional capacity of these two systems simultaneously.

Summary of the Anatomy of Memory

Earlier conceptions that memory was a localized function subserved by a specific structure such as the hippocampus or dorsomedial thalamus have given way to the view that memory is a distributed function of the human brain. The bulk of the evidence suggests that two functionally and anatomically integrated circuits, one involving the hippocampus and the other involving the amygdala form the basis of this distributed system. Amnesia is associated with medial temporal, thalamic, and basal forebrain damage to the extent that such

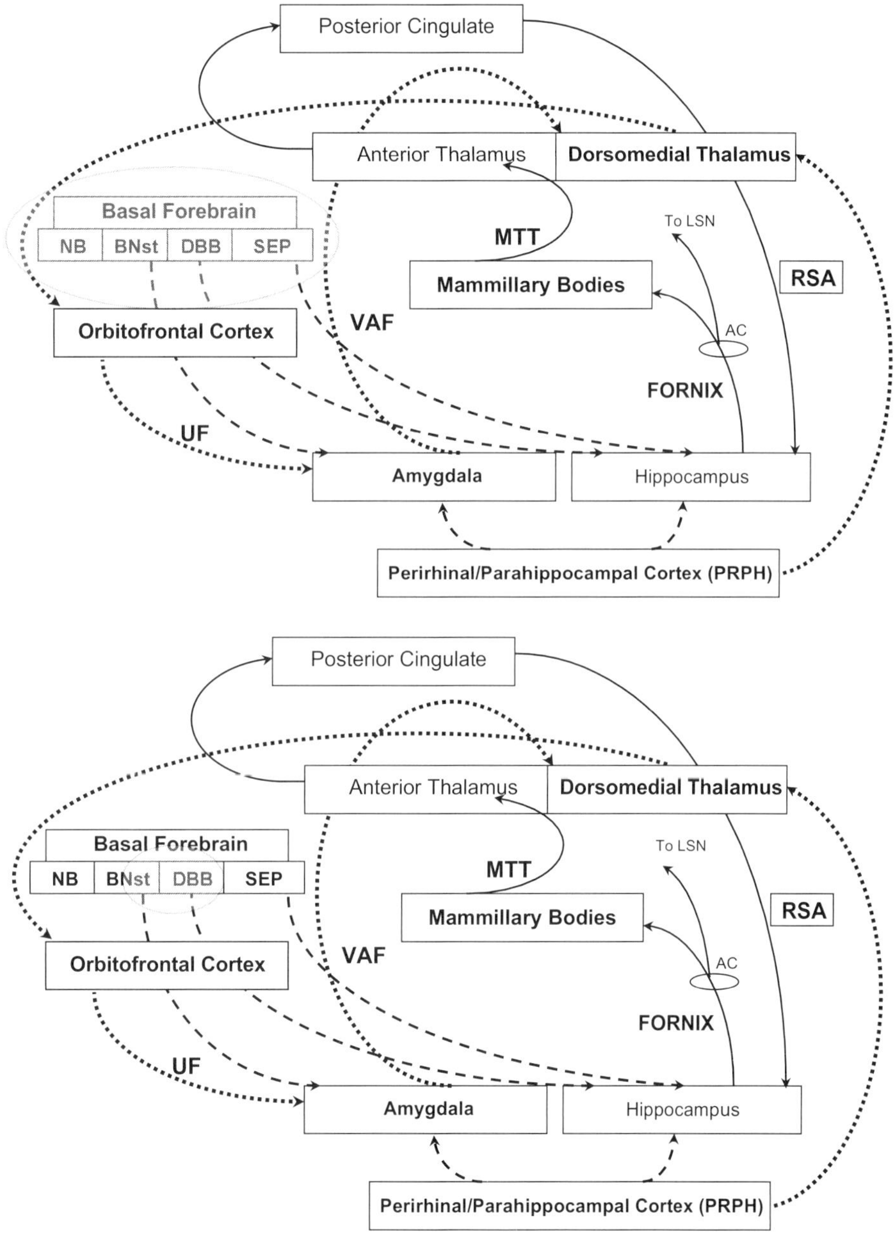

Figure 28.5 Two possible lesion scenarios for basal forebrain amnesia. In Panel A, a large lesion affects both structures within the basal forebrain (and their cholinergic projections to the two limbic circuits) as well as adjacent components of the limbic circuits themselves. In Panel B, a more restricted lesion affects cholinergic projections to both hippocampus and amygdala, thus functionally impairing both circuits.

damage either directly or indirectly impairs the functional integrity of these systems. Most existing evidence suggests that functional impairment of both circuits is necessary for full-blown amnesia to occur.

Amnesia Subtypes: Similarities and Differences Among Amnesics

The view that memory relies on a distributed system suggests the presence of a "core" amnesic syndrome that results when this system is damaged. Nonetheless, the clinical and neuropathologic heterogeneity in amnesics has suggested that profound memory loss following temporal, diencephalic, and basal forebrain damage may represent different *subtypes* of amnesia (Huppert & Piercy, 1979; Lhermitte & Signoret, 1972; Squire, 1981). Can these anatomic subtypes be distinguished on neuropsychological grounds? Data on this issue come from two main sources: studies evaluating rates of forgetting from long-term memory in diencephalic and bitemporal amnesics, and studies evaluating cognitive deficits specific to diencephalic amnesia, particularly AK syndrome.

Rate of Forgetting From Long-Term Memory

Rate of forgetting from long-term memory has been commonly assessed in experimental studies of amnesic patients. Using retention intervals from ten minutes to seven days, several authors have argued that bitemporal amnesics (e.g., H.M., herpes encephalitic, bilateral electroconvulsive therapy [ECT]) may show a more rapid rate of forgetting than diencephalic amnesics or controls (Huppert & Piercy, 1979; Martone, Butters, & Trauner, 1986; Squire, 1981). In most of these studies, diencephalic patients were given longer stimulus exposures than controls or bitemporals (to counteract an encoding deficit) in order to achieve comparable recognition performance at the shortest delays. This, coupled with faster forgetting for bitemporals, initially led to the conclusion that bitemporal amnesia involves a defect in "consolidation," while diencephalic amnesia involves an earlier defect in stimulus "registration" or encoding (Huppert & Piercy, 1979; Squire, 1982a; Winocur, 1984). By this reasoning, once the encoding deficit is circumvented by increased exposure to the stimuli, the normal forgetting in diencephalic amnesics has been taken to mean that their consolidation ability is intact, thus distinguishing them from bitemporals.

However, the view that bitemporal amnesia is distinctively characterized by abnormally rapid forgetting has been questioned by the results of more recent studies. One of the problems with the Huppert and Piercy study is that procedures for matching initial recognition levels (which required repeated exposures for the diencephalic group) resulted in longer study-test intervals in the bitemporal group than in the diencephalic group (Mayes, Downes, Symons, & Shoqeirat, 1994). Freed, Corkin, and Cohen (1987) retested H.M.'s recognition memory over intervals of 10 minutes, 24 hours, 72 hours and one week with two recognition paradigms, taking pains to precisely equate his 10-minute recall with that of normals. The first was a modified Huppert and Piercy (1979) rate-of-forgetting paradigm in which H.M. was given increased exposure to pictorial stimuli (10 sec. compared to one sec. for controls) and in which yes–no recognition was probed at the four retention intervals. H.M.'s performance was normal after 10 minutes, but dropped significantly below controls after 24 hours and remained at that level through the one-week recognition probe. The normal controls continued to forget over the entire week such that their recognition performance declined to H.M.'s level, and was not significantly better than his at 72 hours or one week. Freed et al. (1987: 467) suggested that their findings indicated a "normal rate of forgetting over a 1-week delay interval," though as Crosson (1992) has indicated, an alternative explanation of these results is that H.M.'s lowest level of performance for the one-week interval was raised above previous levels reported by Huppert and Piercy (1979) by virtue of additional stimulus exposure. That is, although Freed et al. focused on the equivalence between H.M. and normals at the 72-hour and one-week delays, the fact that H.M.'s performance leveled off more rapidly than controls may, in fact, be taken to support, rather than refute, the notion that bitemporal amnesics forget at an abnormally rapid rate (Crosson, 1992). In the second task reported by Freed et al., forgetting rate was assessed at the same intervals by a forced-choice recognition test rather than a yes–no recognition test. On this task, H.M.'s performance was not significantly different from controls at any interval, and in fact was slightly above that of the controls at 72 hours and one week. This is a more convincing demonstration that abnormally rapid forgetting caused by a consolidation defect does not necessarily characterize bitemporal amnesia.

McKee and Squire (1992) directly compared rate-of-forgetting from long-term memory in bitemporal and diencephalic amnesics equated for amnesia severity. Both groups of amnesics received eight seconds of exposure to each of 120 target pictures, while normal controls received one second of exposure. Ten minutes, two hours, and 30–32 hours after study, subjects were tested with four different recognition probes, including human analogues to paradigms (delayed nonmatching to sample, delayed matching to sample) used in the animal literature. There were no group differences for any of the recognition tests at any retention interval.

Thus, although initial studies differentiated bitemporal and diencephalic amnesia on the basis of long-term forgetting rate, recent studies have tended to emphasize the similarities, rather than the differences, in rate of forgetting in these two groups. Recent evidence suggests that rapid forgetting exists in many amnesics and may vary with the extent to which the memory test taps intentional ("recollection") versus automatic ("familiarity") aspects of memory (Green & Kopelman, 2002). Some recent studies suggest that there may be subtle differences in the shape of the forgetting curve when recognition probes are concentrated in the first 30 minutes, but there is little evidence of substantial differences thereafter (Downes, Holdstock, Symons, & Mayes, 1998; Mayes et al., 1994). McKee and Squire (1992: 3771) suggest that, although it is reasonable to suppose that the medial temporal lobe and diencephalic systems should have different contributions to normal memory, "each region might also be an essential component of a larger functional system such that a similar amnesia might result from damage to any portion of that system."

Patterns of Retrograde Amnesia

The three patterns of retrograde amnesia described in the "Retrograde Amnesia and Remote Memory Disturbance" section have been attributed at least in part to impairments in consolidation or retrieval that also produce anterograde learning deficits. Squire (1984) initially suggested that temporally limited retrograde amnesia was due to a defect in consolidation specifically related to dysfunction of the hippocampus (Zola-Morgan & Squire, 1990b), thus linking it specifically to bitemporal amnesia. However, Squire et al. (1989), using an updated version of Cohen and Squire's (1981) remote faces and events tests, found extensive, temporally limited retrograde amnesia in both AK patients (n = 7) and a group of patients with presumed medial temporal pathology secondary to anoxia or ischemia (n = 3). Although there were differences in the specific pattern exhibited by individual patients, their retrograde amnesia spanned a period of about 15 years and was not detectible in the more remote time periods. Gade and Mortensen (1990) found graded retrograde memory loss, supposedly typical of patients with bitemporal amnesia, in patients with basal forebrain and diencephalic amnesia (including five patients with AK syndrome). It is thus unlikely that differences in the degree or pattern of retrograde amnesia can reliably distinguish among basal forebrain, diencephalic, or medial temporal amnesics, though there may still be reason to distinguish between temporally graded, temporally limited, and decade-nonspecific patterns in the individual case. Some recent clinical and experimental evidence suggests that the degree and pattern of retrograde deficit may depend on concomitant involvement of temporal (Kapur & Brooks, 1999; Reed & Squire, 1998) or frontal (Kopelman, 1991; Kopelman et al., 1999; Winocur & Moscovitch, 1999) cortex that is regionally associated with temporal or diencephalic damage per se. (Kapur, 1999) suggests that, while lesions of the hippocampus and diencephalon can produce limited retrograde amnesia, more extensive episodic (autobiographical) or semantic (fact-based) retrograde amnesia generally requires neocortical damage. Kapur argues that those cases with extensive retrograde amnesia from ostensibly localized damage must be interpreted in light of the more widespread metabolic effects on brain function that result.

Deficits in the Spatiotemporal Context of Memory

Several studies have suggested that certain cognitive abilities might be disproportionately impaired in diencephalic amnesia, particularly in patients with AK syndrome. Early research on AK patients suggested that they may display disproportionate impairments in the spatiotemporal aspects of memory. A critical issue is whether such impairments are an obligatory part of the amnesia seen in these patients, or whether they result from concomitant frontal involvement.

Memory for Temporal Order

The ability to discriminate when a target item occurred in a study sequence is a critical memory function necessary to maintain order in the flow of events (Hirst & Volpe, 1982; Huppert & Piercy, 1976; McAndrews & Milner, 1991). In a typical temporal-order judgment paradigm, subjects are given a list discrimination task in which a target list is initially shown, followed after a brief delay by a second target list. During later testing, subjects are asked whether they had seen each stimulus before (recognition judgment) and, if so, whether it belonged to the first or second list (temporal order judgment). It is now clear that bitemporal and diencephalic amnesics can both show defects in temporal order judgments, but the issue of whether the underlying mechanisms are the same has not been fully resolved (Downes, Mayes, MacDonald, & Hunkin, 2002; Shimamura, Janowsky, & Squire, 1990). In an early study of this phenomenon, Squire, Nadel, and Slater (1981) examined temporal order judgments in bilateral ECT (bitemporal) patients, patient N.A. (diencephalic), and controls. They found that, though impairments in temporal order judgments were seen in both ECT patients and N.A., recognition judgments were also poor. When recognition performance was subsequently equated with normals, no temporal ordering deficit remained. Thus, in these patient groups, impaired temporal order judgments appeared to be similar and due to poor recognition memory. Hunkin, Awad, and Mayes (2015) compared temporal and diencephalic patients on within-list and between-list discrimination tests of temporal order memory and found that, while both groups performed poorly relative to controls, the diencephalic group was more impaired. Temporal order judgment correlated significantly with a composite measure of recognition memory.

However, the impairment in temporal order judgments exhibited by AK patients cannot, in most studies, be accounted for on the basis of their poor recognition performance (Bowers, Verfaellie, Valenstein, & Heilman, 1988; Meudell, Mayes, Ostergaard, & Pickering, 1985; Shuren, Jacobs, & Heilman, 1997; Squire, 1982b). Several authors (Moscovitch, 1982; Schacter, 1987b; Squire, 1982b) have attributed the temporal ordering impairment in these patients to concomitant frontal lobe pathology known to coexist with diencephalic damage (Jernigan et al., 1991a, 1991b;

Shimamura et al., 1990). By this view, impairments in judging temporal order is a "neighborhood sign" rather than a core symptom of amnesia. Indeed, *nonamnesic* patients with frontal lesions and basal ganglia disease show impairment in temporal order judgments (McAndrews & Milner, 1991; Milner, Petrides, & Smith, 1985; Sagar, Sullivan, Gabrieli, Corkin, & Growdon, 1988; Shimamura et al., 1990). Although the link to frontal lobe damage has been relatively consistent, there may be reasons to keep the book open on this issue. Results from a temporal-ordering study with a retrosplenial amnesic suggest that a defect in temporal ordering can exist independently of both recognition ability and frontal lobe dysfunction (Bowers et al., 1988, Parkin & Hunkin, 1993). Interestingly, this patient was dramatically impaired in temporal order judgments for newly acquired information, but had no difficulty judging the temporal order of remote events. He performed normally on tests of frontal lobe function, as did another patient with a hypothalamic glioma but no concomitant frontal damage (Parkin & Hunkin, 1993). These findings provide an initial clue that it may be important to distinguish between two kinds of temporal ordering deficits: (a) one which is a part of a more general, frontally mediated strategic deficit (as in AK syndrome; Shimamura et al., 1990; Squire, 1982b), and (b) another that reflects an anterograde impairment in "time tagging" new information that is independent of frontal pathology (Bowers et al., 1988; Parkin & Hunkin, 1993; Yasuno et al., 1999).

Source Monitoring and Source Amnesia

Successful retrieval from episodic memory has an autobiographical quality and is characterized by direct recollection of both the content and source of remembered information (Johnson, Hashtroudi, & Lindsay, 1993). The phenomenon of *source amnesia* illustrates that the content and source of recollected information are potentially dissociable (Shimamura & Squire, 1987). In source amnesia, recollection of the informational source of a memory item is lost despite intact memory for item content. For example, we might remember specific information about the *Hunger Games*, but be unable to recollect where that information was learned. Source attributions differentiate autobiographical event memories from more general factual knowledge.

Schacter, Harbluck, and McLachlan (1984) presented bogus facts (e.g., "Bob Hope's father was a fireman") to their patients and then gave a recall test. If a fact was recalled, patients were asked where they had learned it. Many patients demonstrated recall of at least some of the facts, but frequently asserted that they had learned them from a source other than the experimental session. This finding could not be explained by poor memory, since normal subjects whose recall was lowered by a one-week study-test interval did not commit source errors. Shimamura and Squire (1987) taught obscure (true) facts to a small group of AK patients and a smaller group of patients with amnesia secondary to anoxia. Severe source amnesia, in which recall was attributed to sources other than the experiment, was observed in three of the six AK patients and in one of the three anoxic patients. The level of fact memory performance did not predict the degree of source amnesia. Furthermore, patients with bitemporal amnesia (including H.M.) who display severe defects in fact memory often perform *better* at tests of recency and temporal order than do nonamnesic frontal patients (Milner, Corsi, & Leonard, 1991; Sagar, Gabrieli, Sullivan, & Corkin, 1990).

Some evidence suggests that, like temporal ordering, the severity of source amnesia varies as a function of frontal lobe impairment in both amnesic and nonamnesic subjects (Schacter et al., 1984; Janowsky, Shimamura, & Squire, 1989). Source monitoring tasks make variable demands on retrieval and cognitive estimation (Shallice & Evans, 1978), reality monitoring (Johnson, 1991), attribution (Jacoby, Kelly, & Dywan, 1989), and temporal order memory (Hirst & Volpe, 1982; Olton, 1989). Evidence suggests that distinctions between bitemporal and diencephalic amnesics that have emerged are due to the variable demands on such functions imposed by tests of source memory.

Deficits in Metamemory and "Feeling of Knowing"

Another cognitive domain that some have thought to be differentially impaired in AK syndrome has been referred to as *metamemory*. Metamemory involves knowledge about one's own memory capabilities, the memory demands of particular tasks or situations, and potentially useful strategies relevant to given tasks or situations (Flavell & Wellman, 1977; Gruneberg, 1983). It encompasses people's beliefs (e.g., "I will [or will not] be able to remember these words") as well as their knowledge about the memory system (e.g., rehearsal strategies that enhance recall). Hirst and Volpe (cited in Hirst, 1982) were among the first to report differentially impaired metamemory in AK patients when compared to other etiologies of amnesia. Based on interviews, they found that AK patients had less knowledge of mnemonic strategies than did patients with amnesia from other causes.

The most widely studied metamemorial capacity in amnesic patients is the feeling-of-knowing (FOK) phenomenon (cf. Gruneberg & Monks, 1974; Hart, 1965, 1967; Nelson, Leonesio, Shimamura, Landwehr, & Narens, 1982, Nelson, Gerler, & Narens, 1984). In a typical FOK experiment, subjects are asked to freely recall the answers to general information questions of varying difficulty (e.g., "What is the tallest mountain in South America?") until a certain number of failures occur. For these unrecalled items, subjects are then asked to judge the likelihood that they would be able to recognize the correct answer if it was presented along with other likely but incorrect choices. FOK predictions are then validated by a subsequent recognition test. In normal, recognition performance is better for questions eliciting strong FOK than for questions eliciting weak or no FOK.

Shimamura and Squire (1986) evaluated the ability of FOK judgments to predict subsequent recognition performance in patients with Korakoff's syndrome, psychiatric patients undergoing bilateral ECT, a mixed group of amnesics that included the diencephalic fencing victim N.A., and controls. Using general information questions (Study 1) and a sentence memory paradigm that assessed newly learned information (Study 2), they found that only the AK patients (and not the other diencephalic cases) displayed impairment in making FOK judgments. From these results, it appears that metamemory dysfunction is not an obligatory aspect of amnesia (or even diencephalic amnesia), since both can occur without any measurable impairment in FOK. The authors speculated that the disturbed FOK in AK patients might be a function of their frontal pathology, which would be expected to impair their ability on a variety of judgment and planning tasks.

Unique Characteristics of Basal Forebrain Amnesia

Amnesia due to basal forebrain lesions most commonly results from vascular lesion or aneurysm surgery in the region of the anterior communicating artery (Alexander & Freedman, 1983; Damasio et al., 1985; DeLuca & Cicerone, 1989; Gade, 1982; Okawa, Maeda, Nukui, & Kawafuchi, 1980; Volpe & Hirst, 1983; Vilkki, 1985; Phillips, Sangalang, & Sterns, 1987). After basal forebrain damage, the patient exhibits extensive anterograde but variable retrograde amnesia. Temporal gradients similar to that seen in AK syndrome have been described (Gade & Mortensen, 1990; Lindqvist & Norlen, 1966). Some authors have also described impairment in placing memories in proper chronological order (Damasio et al., 1985; Lindqvist & Norlen, 1966; Talland et al., 1967). Free, and sometimes wild, confabulation appears to be characteristic, particularly in the acute period (Alexander & Freedman, 1983; Damasio et al., 1985; Lindqvist & Norlen, 1966; Logue, Durward, Pratt, Piercy, & Nixon, 1968; Okawa et al., 1980; Talland et al., 1967) and probably relates to the extent of concomitant orbitofrontal involvement, particularly in those patients who show spontaneous or unprovoked confabulation (Damasio et al., 1985; DeLuca & Cicerone, 1989; Fischer, Alexander, D'Esposito, & Otto, 1995; Phillips et al., 1987; Turner, Cipolotti, Yousry, & Shallice, 2007; Turner, Cipolotti, Yousry, & Shallice, 2008); Vilkki, 1985). Some patients have difficulty distinguishing reality from dreaming. Although these behavioral abnormalities are distinctive, they may not be functionally related to the amnesia per se. Often, basal forebrain amnesia persists after dream–waking confusion and confabulation have subsided (Hashimoto et al., 2000; Morris et al., 1992).

Cueing seems to differentially improve memory performance in these patients, and anecdotal evidence suggests that many of these patients can recall specific information in one retrieval attempt, but not the next. These data have suggested that these patients have a problem in accessing information that does exist in long-term memory. However, further data is needed before accepting this proposition confidently. It has frequently been noted that these patients appear apathetic and unconcerned about their memory impairment (Alexander & Freedman, 1983; Phillips et al., 1987; Talland et al., 1967). Interestingly, Talland and colleagues regarded basal forebrain amnesics to show striking behavioral similarities to patients with AK syndrome, and Graff-Radford et al. (1990) saw similarities between these amnesics and those with memory loss secondary to paramedian thalamic infarctions. It may be that such similarities arise because the large, vascular lesions that characterize these cases also involve structures or pathways destined for components of the medial temporal or diencephalic memory systems (Gade, 1982; Crosson, 1992). Myers and colleagues (2001) have compared the performance of medial temporal and basal forebrain amnesics on delay eyeblink classical conditioning and found impairment in the basal forebrain (ACoA) patients but not the medial temporal (hypoxic) patients. In a subsequent study, these two groups were compared on performance in conditional discrimination and reversal tasks (Myers, DeLuca, Hopkins, & Gluck, 2006). The medial temporal patients showed spared acquisition but impaired reversal, while the ACoA patients showed the opposite pattern. Although quite suggestive, these studies did not rule out the possibility that such differences arose from differential involvement of neighborhood regions rather than damage to the memory system per se.

Conclusion

Four decades of research with amnesic subjects has led to an increased understanding of the role that specific brain regions and brain systems play in normal and disordered memory functions. It could be said that we now have a good understanding of the fundamental components of the brain's distributed memory system, and decades of experience with ammesic patients has led to an increased appreciation of the anatomic and symptomatic heterogeneity within the amnesic population. The focus of the next decade will likely be on building and testing more comprehensive models of memory function at the network level.

For now, we return to our original question: Are there really "three amnesias" or do the amnesias of medial temporal, diencephalic, or basal forebrain origin represent variations on a "core" amnesic syndrome? In our view, the weight of the current data favors the latter interpretation. To be sure, there are clinically significant differences between these three groups of amnesics, but many of these differences can be attributed to concomitant damage to cortical and subcortical structures adjacent to the integrated memory circuits. Distinctions among patients (and patient groups) on the basis of forgetting rates, encoding versus consolidation deficits, or on the basis of impairments in contextual or metamemorial aspects of memory are important on both clinical and experimental grounds, even though such distinctions do not thus far appear reliably reflective of lesion localization. Although the behavioral distinctions among amnesic subtypes are not that reliable or impressive, it still is reasonable to hypothesize that the different components of the distributed memory system have different functional contributions to memory performance and that such functions can be measured if sufficiently sensitive and specific behavioral probes are developed and implemented in clinical research.

The interprofessional neuroscientific study of memory and its disorders can be thought of as one of the most remarkable translational science love stories of our time. Surely our understanding of normal and impaired memory will continue to advance dramatically as increasingly sophisticated behavioral paradigms and neurodiagnostic technologies are brought to bear on this critically important area of brain function.

References

Aggleton, J. P. (1986). Memory impairments caused by experimental thalamic lesions in monkeys. *Revue Neurologique*, *142*(4), 418–424.

Aggleton, J. P., & Brown, M. W. (1999). Episodic memory, amnesia, and the hippocampal-anterior thalamic axis. *Behavioral and Brain Sciences*, *22*, 425–444.

Aggleton, J. P., Desimone, R., & Mishkin, M. (1986). The origin, course, and termination of the hippocampothalamic projections in the macaque. *Journal of Comparative Neurology*, *243*, 409–421.

Aggleton, J. P., McMackin, D., Carpenter, K., Hornak, J., Kapur, N., Halpin, S., . . . Gaffan, D. (2000). Differential cognitive effects of colloid cysts in the third ventricle that spare or compromise the fornix. *Brain*, *123*, 800–815.

Aggleton, J. P., & Mishkin, M. (1983). Memory impairments following restricted medial thalamic lesions in monkeys. *Experimental Brain Research*, *52*, 199–209.

Aggleton, J. P., & Mishkin, M. (1985). Mammillary-body lesions and visual recognition in monkeys. *Experimental Brain Research*, *58*, 190–197.

Aggleton, J. P., Neave, N., Nagle, S., & Sahgal, A. (1995). A comparison of the effects of medial prefrontal, cingulate cortex, and cingulum bundle lesions on tests of spatial memory: Evidence of a double dissociation between frontal and cingulum bundle contributions. *Journal of Neuroscience*, *15*, 7270–7281.

Aggleton, J. P., & Sahgal, A. (1993). The contribution of the anterior thalamic nuclei to anterograde amnesia. *Neuropsychologia*, *31*, 1001–1019.

Albert, M. S., Butters, N., & Brandt, J. (1981). Patterns of remote memory in amnesic and demented patients. *Archives of Neurology*, *38*, 495–500.

Albert, M. S., Butters, N., & Levin, J. (1979). Temporal gradients in the retrograde amnesia of patients with alcoholic Korsakoff's disease. *Archives of Neurology*, *36*, 211–216.

Alexander, M. P., & Freedman, M. (1983). Amnesia after anterior communicating artery rupture. *Neurology*, *33*(Suppl 2), 104.

Amaral, D. G., & Cowan, W. M. (1980). Subcortical afferents to the hippocampal formation in the monkey. *Journal of Comparative Neurology*, *189*, 573–591.

Amaral, D. G., & Insausti, R. (1990). Hippocampal formation. In G. Paxinos (Ed.), *The Human Nervous System* (pp. 711–755). San Diego: Academic Press.

Amaral, D. G., Insausti, R., & Cowan, W. M. (1983). Evidence for a direct projection from the superior temporal gyrus to the entorhinal cortex in the monkey. *Brain Research*, *275*, 263–277.

Arendt, T., Bigl., V., & Arendt, A. (1983). Loss of neurons in the nucleus basalis of Meynert in Alzheimer's disease, paralysis agitans and Korsakoff's disease. *Acta Neuropathologica*, *61*, 101–108.

Arita, K., Uozumi, T., Ogasawara, H., Sugiyama, K., Ohba, S., Pant, B., . . . Oshima, H. (1995). A case of pineal germinoma presenting with severe amnesia. *No Shinkei Geka*, *23*, 271–275.

Bachevalier, J., & Mishkin, M. (1986). Visual recognition impairment follows ventromedial but not dorsolateral prefrontal lesions in monkeys. *Behavioral Brain Research*, *20*, 249–261.

Bachevalier, J., Parkinson, J. K., & Mishkin, M. (1985). Visual recognition in monkeys: Effects of separate vs. combined transection of fornix and amygdalofugal pathways. *Experimental Brain Research*, *57*, 554–561.

Bachevalier, J., Saunders, R. C., & Mishkin, M. (1985). Visual recognition in monkeys: Effects of transection of the fornix. *Experimental Brain Research*, *57*, 547–553.

Barr, W. B., Goldberg, E., Wasserstein, J., & Novelly, R. A. (1990). Retrograde amnesia following unilateral temporal lobectomy. *Neuropsychologia*, *28*, 243–255.

Bartus, R. T., Dean, R. L., Beer, B., Ponecorvo, M. J., & Flicker, C. (1985). The cholinergic hypothesis: An historical overview, current perspective, and future directions. *Annals of the New York Academy of Sciences*, *444*, 332–358.

Beaunieux, H., Desgranges, B., Lalevee, C., de la Sayette, V., Lechevalier, B., & Eustache, F. (1998). Preservation of cognitive procedural memory in a case of Korsakoff's syndrome: Methodological and theoretical insights. *Perceptual and Motor Skills*, *86*, 1267–1287.

Bogousslavsky, J., Regli, F., & Assal, G. (1986). The syndrome of tuberothalamic artery territory infarction. *Stroke*, *17*, 434–441.

Bowers, D., Verfaellie, M., Valenstein, E., & Heilman, K. M. (1988). Impaired acquisition of temporal order information in amnesia. *Brain and Cognition*, *8*, 47–66.

Butter, C. M., & Snyder, D. R. (1972). Alterations in aversive and aggressive behaviors following orbital frontal lesions in rhesus monkeys. *Acta Neurobiologiae Experimentalis*, *32*, 525–565.

Butters, N. (1981). The Wernicke-Korsakoff syndrome: A review of psychological, neuropathological and etiological factors. *Currents in Alcohol*, *8*, 205–232.

Butters, N. (1985). Alcoholic Korsakoff syndrome: Some unresolved issues concerning etiology, neuropathology, and cognitive deficits. *Journal of Clinical and Experimental Neuropsychology*, *7*, 181–210.

Butters, N., & Cermak, L. S. (1980). *Alcoholic Korsakoff's Syndrome: An Information Processing Approach to Amnesia*. New York: Academic Press.

Butters, N., Miliotis, P., Albert, M. S., & Sax, D. S. (1984). Memory assessment: Evidence of the heterogeneity of amnesic symptoms. In G. Goldstein (Ed.), *Advances in Clinical Neuropsychology* (Vol. 1, pp. 127–159). New York: Plenum Press.

Butters, N., & Stuss, D. T. (1989). Diencephalic amnesia. In F. Boller & J. Grafman (Eds.), *Handbook of Neuropsychology* (Section Editor L. Squire) (Vol. 3, pp. 107–148). Amsterdam: Elsevier.

Cabeza, R., & St. Jaques, P. (2008). Functional neuroimaging of autobiographical memory. *Trends in Cognitive Science*, *11*, 219–227.

Cairns, H., & Mosberg, W. H. (1951). Colloid cyst of the third ventricle. *Surgery, Gynecology and Obstetrics*, *92*, 545–570.

Calabrese, P., Markowitsch, H. J., Harders, A. G., Scholz, M., & Gehlen, W. (1995). Fornix damage and memory: A case report. *Cortex*, *31*, 555–564.

Carr, A. C. (1982). Memory deficit after fornix section. *Neuropsychologia*, *20*, 95–98.

Cermak, L. S., & O'Connor, M. (1983). The anterograde and retrograde retrieval ability of a patient with amnesia due to encephalitis. *Neuropsychologia*, *21*, 213–234.

Cermak, L. S., Talbot, N., Chandler, K., & Wolbarst, L. R. (1985). The perceptual priming phenomenon in amnesia. *Neuropsychologia*, *23*, 615–622.

Choi, D., Sudarsky, L., Schachter, S., Biber, M., & Burke, P. (1983). Medial thalamic hemorrhage with amnesia. *Archives of Neurology*, *40*, 611–613.

Cohen, N. J., Poldrack, R. A., & Eichenbaum, H. (1997). Memory for items and memory for relations in the procedural/declarative memory framework. In A. R. Mayes & J. J. Downes (Eds.), *Theories of Organic Amnesia* (pp. 131–178). Hove, UK: Psychology Press/Erlbaum (UK) Taylor & Francis.

Cohen, N. J., & Squire, L. R. (1980). Preserved learning and retention of pattern analyzing skill in amnesia: Dissociation of knowing how and knowing that. *Science*, *210*, 207–209.

Cohen, N. J., & Squire, L. R. (1981). Retrograde amnesia and remote memory impairment. *Neuropsychologia*, *19*, 337–356.

Corkin, S. (1984). Lasting consequences of bilateral medial temporal lobectomy: Clinical course and experimental findings in H.M. *Seminars in Neurology*, *4*, 249–259.

Crosson, B. (1992). *Subcortical Functions in Language and Memory*. New York: Guilford Press.

Cummings, J. L., Tomiyasu, U., Read, S., & Benson, D. F. (1984). Amnesia with hippocampal lesions after cardiopulmonary arrest. *Neurology*, *42*, 263–271.

Damasio, A. R., Graff-Radford, N. R., Eslinger, P. J., Damasio, H., & Kassell, N. (1985). Amnesia following basal forebrain lesions. *Archives of Neurology*, *42*, 263–271.

DeLuca, J., & Cicerone, K. (1989). Cognitive impairments following anterior communicating artery aneurysm. *Journal of Clinical and Experimental Neuropsychology*, *11*, 47.

DeLuca, J., & Diamond, B. J. (1995). Aneurysm of the anterior communicating artery: A review of neuroanatomical and neuropsychological sequelae. *Journal of Clinical and Experimental Neuropsychology*, *17*, 100–121.

DeOlmos, J. S. (1990). Amygdala. In G. Paxinos (Ed.), *The Human Nervous System* (pp. 583–710). San Diego: Academic Press.

D'Esposito, M., Verfaellie, M., Alexander, M. P., & Katz, D. I. (1995). Amnesia following traumatic bilateral fornix transection. *Neurology*, *45*, 1546–1550.

Devinsky, O., Morrell, M. J., & Vogt, B. A. (1995). Contributions of anterior cingulate cortex to behaviour. *Brain*, *118*, 279–306.

Diana, R. A., Yonelinas, A. P., & Ranganath, C. (2007). Imaging recollection and familiarity in the medial temporal lobe: A three-component model. *Trends in Cognitive Science*, *11*, 379–386.

Dott, N. M. (1938). Surgical aspects of the hypothalamus. In W. E. Clark, G. Le, J. Beattie, G. Riddoch, & N. M. Dott (Eds.), *The Hypothalamus: Morphological, Functional, Clinical and Surgical Aspects* (pp. 131–185). Edinburgh: Oliver and Boyd.

Downes, J. J., Holdstock, J. S., Symons, V., & Mayes, A. R. (1998). Do amnesics forget colours pathologically fast? *Cortex*, *34*, 337–355.

Downes, J. J., Mayes, A. R., MacDonald, C., & Hunkin, N. M. (2002). Temporal order memory in patients with Korsakoff's syndrome and medial temporal amnesia. *Neuropsychologia*, *40*, 853–861.

Drachman, D. A., & Arbit, J. (1966). Memory and the hippocampal complex. *Archives of Neurology*, *15*, 52–61.

Drachman, D. A., & Leavitt, J. (1974). Human memory and the cholinergic system: A relationship to aging? *Archives of Neurology*, *30*, 113–121.

Dusoir, H., Kapur, N., Byrnes, D. P., McKinstry, S., & Hoare, R. D. (1990). The role of diencephalic pathology in human memory disorder: Evidence from a penetrating paranasal brain injury. *Brain*, *113*, 1695–1706.

Eichenbaum, H., Yonelinas, A. P., & Ranganath, C. (2007). The medial temporal lobe and recognition memory. *Annual Review of Neuroscience*, *30*, 123–152.

Eslinger, P. J., & Damasio, A. R. (1985). Severe disturbance of higher cognition after bilateral frontal lobe ablation: Patient EVR. *Neurology*, *35*, 1731–1741.

Fibiger, H. C. (1991). Cholinergic mechanisms in learning, memory and dementia: A review of recent evidence. *Trends in Neurosciences*, *14*, 220–223.

Fischer, R. S., Alexander, M. P., D'Esposito, M., & Otto, R. (1995). Neuropsychological and neuroanatomical correlates of confabulation. *Journal of Clinical and Experimental Neuropsychology*, *17*, 20–28.

Flavell, J. H., & Wellman, H. M. (1977). Metamemory. In R. V. Kail & J. W. Hagen (Eds.), *Perspectives on the Development of Memory and Cognition* (pp. 3–33). Hillsdale, NJ: Lawrence Erlbaum.

Freed, D. M., Corkin, S., & Cohen, N. J. (1987). Forgetting in H.M.: A second look. *Neuropsychologia*, *25*, 461–471.

Gabrieli, J.D.E., Fleischman, D. A., Keane, M. M., Reminger, S. L., & Morrell, F. (1995). Double dissociation between memory systems underlying explicit and implicit memory in the human brain. *Psychological Science*, *6*, 76–82.

Gabrieli, J.D.E., Milberg, W., Keane, M. M., & Corkin, S. (1990). Intact priming of patterns despite impaired memory. *Neuropsychologia*, *28*, 417–427.

Gade, A. (1982). Amnesia after operations on aneurysms of the anterior communicating artery. *Surgical Neurology*, *18*, 46–49.

Gade, A., & Mortensen, E. L. (1990). Temporal gradient in the remote memory impairment of amnesic patients with lesions in the basal forebrain. *Neuropsychologia*, *28*, 985–1001.

Gaffan, D. (1974). Recognition impaired and association intact in the memory of monkeys after transection of the fornix. *Journal of Comparative and Physiological Psychology*, *86*, 1100–1109.

Gaffan, D. (1993). Additive effects of forgetting and fornix transection in the temporal gradient of retrograde amnesia. *Neuropsychologia*, *31*, 1055–1066.

Gaffan, D., & Gaffan, E. A. (1991). Amnesia in man following transection of the fornix: A review. *Brain*, *114*, 2611–2618.

Gaffan, D., Parker, A. (1996). Interaction of perirhinal cortex with the fornix-fimbria: Memory for objects and "object-in-place" memory. *Journal of Neuroscience*, *16*, 5864–5869.

Gaffan, E. A., Gaffan, D., & Hodges, J. R. (1991). Amnesia following damage to the left fornix and to other sites: A comparative study. *Brain*, *114*, 1297–1313.

Garcia Bengochea, F., De La Torre, O., Esquivel, O., Vieta, R., & Fernandec, C. (1954). The section of the fornix in the surgical treatment of certain epilepsies: A preliminary report. *Transactions of the American Neurological Association*, *79*, 176–178.

Gentilini, M., DeRenzi, E., & Crisi, G. (1987). Bilateral paramedian thalamic artery infarcts: Report of eight cases. *Journal of Neurology, Neurosurgery, and Psychiatry*, *50*, 900–909.

Ghika-Schmid, F., & Bogousslavsky, J. (2000). The acute behavioral syndrome of anterior thalamic infarction: A prospective study of 12 cases. *Annals of Neurology*, *48*, 220–227.

Graff-Radford, N. R., Tranel, D., Van Hoesen, G. W., & Brandt, J. P. (1990). Diencephalic amnesia. *Brain*, *113*, 1–25.

Grafman, J., Salazar, A. M., Weingartner, J., Vance, S. C., & Ludlow, C. (1985). Isolated impairment of memory following a penetrating lesion of the fornix cerebri. *Archives of Neurology*, *42*, 1162–1168.

Green, R. E., & Kopelman, M. D. (2002). Contribution of recollection and familiarity judgements to rate of forgetting in organic amnesia. *Cortex*, *38*, 161–178.

Gruneberg, M. M. (1983). Memory processes unique to humans. In A. Mayes (Ed.), *Memory in Animals and Humans* (pp. 253–281). London: Van Nostrand Reinhold.

Gruneberg, M. M., & Monks, J. (1974). Feeling of knowing and cued recall. *Acta Psychologica*, *41*, 257–265.

Grünthal, E. (1939). Über das Corpus mamillare und den Korsakowshcen Symptomenkomplex. *Confinia Neurologica.*, *2*, 64–95.

Hamann, S. B., & Squire, L. R. (1997). Intact perceptual memory in the absence of conscious memory. *Behavioral Neuroscience*, *111*, 850–854.

Hart, J. T. (1965). Memory and the feeling-of-knowing experience. *Journal of Educational Psychology*, *56*, 208–216.

Hart, J. T. (1967). Memory and the memory-monitoring process. *Journal of Verbal Learning and Verbal Behavior*, *6*, 685–691.

Hashimoto, R., Tanaka, Y., & Nakano, I. (2000). Amnesic confabulatory syndrome after focal basal forebrain damage. *Neurology*, *54*, 978–980.

Hassler, R., & Riechert, T. (1957). Über einen Fall von doppelseitiger Fornicotomie bei sogenannter temporaler Epilepsie. *Acta Neurochirurgica*, *5*, 330–340.

Heilman, K. M., & Sypert, G. W. (1977). Korsakoff's syndrome resulting from bilateral fornix lesions. *Neurology*, *27*, 490–493.

Heimer, L., & Alheid, G. F. (1991). Piecing together the puzzle of basal forebrain anatomy. In T. C. Napier, P. W. Kalivas, & I. Hanin (Eds.), *The Basal Forebrain: Anatomy to Function* (pp. 1–42). New York: Plenum Press.

Herkenham, M. (1978). The connections of the nucleus reuniens thalami: Evidence for a direct thalamo-hippocampal pathway in the rat. *Journal of Comparative Neurology*, *177*, 589–610.

Herzog, A. G., & Van Hoesen, G. W. (1976). Temporal neocortical afferent connections to the amygdala in the rhesus monkey. *Brain Research*, *115*, 57–69.

Hirst, W. (1982). The amnesic syndrome: Descriptions of explanations. *Psychological Bulletin*, *91*, 435–462.

Hirst, W., & Volpe, B. T. (1982). Temporal order judgments with amnesia. *Brain and Cognition*, *1*, 294–306.

Hunkin, N. M., Awad, M., & Mayes, A. R. (2015). Memory for between-list and within-list information in amnesic patients with temporal lobe and diencephalic lesions. *Journal of Neuropsychology*, *9*, 137–156.

Huppert, F. A., & Piercy, M. (1976). Recognition memory in amnesic patients: Effect of temporal context and familiarity of material. *Cortex*, *12*, 3–20.

Huppert, F. A., & Piercy, M. (1979). Normal and abnormal forgetting in organic amnesia: Effect of locus of lesion. *Cortex*, *15*, 385–390.

Insausti, R., Amaral, D. G. and Cowan, W. M. (1987a). The entorhinal cortex of the monkey: II. Cortical afferents. *The Journal of Comparative Neurology*, *264*, 356–395.

Insausti, R., Amaral, D. G., & Cowan, W. M. (1987b). The entorhinal cortex of the monkey: III. Subcortical afferents. *The Journal of Comparative Neurology*, *264*, 396–408.

Irle, E., & Markowitsch, H. J. (1982). Widespread cortical projections of the hippocampal formation in the cat. *Neuroscience*, *7*, 2637–2647.

Irle, E., Wowra, B., Kunert, H. (1992). Memory disturbances following anterior communicating artery rupture. *Annals of Neurology*, *31*, 473–480.

Iwasaki, S., Arihara, T., Torii, H., Hiraguti, M., Kitamoto, F., Nakagawa, A., . . . Kurauchi, M. (1993). A case of splenial astrocytoma with various neuropsychological symptoms. *No To Shinkei*, *45*, 1067–1073.

Jacoby, L. L., Kelly, C. M., & Dywan, J. (1989). Memory attributions. In H. L. Roediger & F.I.M. Craik (Eds.), *Varieties of Memory and Consciousness: Essays in Honour of Endel Tulving* (pp. 391–422). Hillsdale, NJ: Lawrence Erlbaum Associates.

Janowsky, J. S., Shimamura, A. P., & Squire, L. R. (1989). Memory and metamemory: Comparisons between patients with frontal lobe lesions and amnesic patients. *Psychobiology*, *17*, 3–11.

Jernigan, T. L., Butters, N., DiTraglia, G., Schafer, K., Smith, T., Irwin, M., . . . Cermak, L. S. (1991b). Reduced cerebral grey matter observed in alcoholics using magnetic resonance imaging. *Alcoholism: Clinical and Experimental Research*, *15*, 418–427.

Jernigan, T. L., Schafer, K., Butters, N., & Cermak, L. S. (1991a). Magnetic-resonance-imaging of alcoholic korsakoff patients. *Neuropsychopharmacology*, *4*, 175–186.

Johns, C. A., Greenwald, B. S., Mohs, R. C., & Davis, K. L. (1983). The cholinergic treatment strategy in ageing and senile dementia. *Psychopharmacology. Bulletin*, *19*, 185–197.

Johnson, M. K. (1991). Reality monitoring: Evidence from confabulation in organic brain disease patients. In G. Prigatano & D. L. Schacter (Eds.), *Awareness of Deficit after Brain Injury* (pp. 176–197). New York: Oxford University Press.

Johnson, M. K., Hashtroudi, S., & Lindsay, D. S. (1993). Source monitoring. *Psychological Bulletin*, *114*, 3–28.

Kapur, N. (1999). Syndromes of retrograde amnesia: A conceptual and empirical synthesis. *Psychological Bulletin*, *125*, 800–825.

Kapur, N., & Brooks, D. J. (1999). Temporally specific retrograde amnesia in two cases of discrete bilateral hippocampal pathology. *Hippocampus*, *9*, 247–254.

Kapur, N., & Butters, N. (1977). Visuoperceptive deficits in long-term alcoholics with Korsakoff's psychosis. *Journal of Studies in Alcohol*, *38*, 2025–2035.

Kopelman, M. D. (1986). The cholinergic neurotransmitter system in human memory and dementia: A review. *Quarterly Journal of Experimental Psychology*, *38A*, 535–573.

Kopelman, M. D. (1991). Frontal dysfunction and memory deficits in the alcoholic Korsakoff syndrome and Alzheimer-type dementia. *Brain*, *114*, 117–137.

Kopelman, M. D. (1995). The Korsakoff syndrome. *British Journal of Psychiatry*, *166*, 154–173.

Kopelman, M. D., Bright, P., Fulker, H., Hinton, N., Morrison, A., & Verfaellie, M. (2009). Remote semantic memory in patients with Korsakoff's syndrome and herpes encephalitis. *Neuropsychology*, *23*, 144–157.

Kopelman, M. D., Stanhope, N., & Kingsley, D. (1999). Retrograde amnesia in patients with diencephalic, temporal lobe, or frontal lesions. *Neuropsychologia*, *37*, 939–958.

Kritchevsky, M., Graff-Radford, N. R., & Damasio, A. R. (1987). Normal memory after damage to medial thalamus. *Archives of Neurology*, *44*, 959–962.

Lewis, P. R., & Shute, C.C.D. (1967). The cholinergic limbic system: Projections of the hippocampal formation, medial cortex, nuclei of the ascending cholinergic reticular system, and the subfornical organ and supra-optic crest. *Brain*, *90*, 521–540.

Lhermitte, F., & Signoret, J.-L. (1972). Analyse neuropsychologique et differenciation des syndromes amnesiques. *Revue Neurologique*, *126*, 161–178.

Lhermitte, J., Doussinet, P., & Ajuriaguerra, J. (1937). Une observation de la forme Korsakowienne des tumeurs du 3d ventricule. *Revue Neurologique*, *68*, 709–711.

Lindqvist, G., & Norlen, G. (1966). Korsakoff's syndrome after operation on ruptured aneurysm of the anterior communicating artery. *Acta Psychiatrica Scandanavica*, *42*, 24–34.

Loesch, D. V., Gilman, S., Del Dotto, J., Rosenblum, M. L. (1995). Cavernous malformation of the mammillary bodies: Neuropsychological implications: Case report. *Journal of Neurosurgery*, *83*, 354–358.

Logue, V., Durward, M., Pratt, R.T.C., Piercy, M., & Nixon, W.L.B. (1968). The quality of survival after rupture of an anterior cerebral aneurysm. *British Journal of Psychiatry*, *114*, 137–160.

Mair, W.G.P., Warrington, E. K., & Weiskrantz, L. (1979). Memory disorder in Korsakoff's psychosis: A neuropathological and neuropsychological investigation of two cases. *Brain*, *102*, 749–783.

Malamut, B. L., Graff-Radford, N., Chawluk, J., Grossman, R. I., & Gur, R. C. (1992). Memory in a case of bilateral thalamic infarction. *Neurology*, *42*, 163–169.

Marslen-Wilson, W. D., & Teuber, H.-L. (1974). Memory for remote events in anterograde amnesia: Recognition of public figures from newsphotographs. *Neuropsychologia*, *13*, 353–364.

Martone, M., Butters, N., & Trauner, D. (1986). Some analyses of forgetting pictorial material in amnesic and demented patients. *Journal of Clinical and Experimental Neuropsychology*, *8*, 161–178.

Mayes, A. R., Downes, J. J., Symons, V., & Shoqeirat, M. (1994). Do amnesics forget faces pathologically fast? *Cortex*, *30*, 543–563.

Mayes, A. R., Meudell, P. R., Mann, D., & Pickering, A. (1988). Location of lesions in Korsakoff's syndrome: Neuropsychological and neuropathological data on two patients. *Cortex*, *24*, 367–388.

McAndrews, M. P., & Milner, B. (1991). The frontal cortex and memory for temporal order. *Neuropsychologia*, *29*, 849–859.

McKee, R. D., & Squire, L. R. (1992). Both hippocampal and diencephalic amnesia result in normal forgetting for complex visual material. *Journal of Clinical and Experimental Neuropsychology*, *14*, 103.

McMackin, D., Cockburn, J., Anslow, P., & Gaffan, D. (1995). Correlation of fornix damage with memory impairment in six cases of colloid cyst removal. *Acta Neurochir (Wien)*, *135*, 12–18.

Mesulam, M.-M., & Mufson, E. J. (1984). Neural inputs into the nucleus basalis of the substantia innominata (Ch4) in the rhesus monkey. *Brain*, *107*, 253–274.

Mesulam, M.-M., Mufson, E. J., Levey, E. J., Wainer, B. H. (1983). Cholinergic innervation of cortex by the basal forebrain: Cytochemistry and cortical connections of the septal area, diagonal band nuclei, nucleus basalis (substantia innominata) and hypothalamus in the rhesus monkey. *Journal of Comparative Neurology*, *214*, 170–197.

Mesulam, M.-M., & Van Hoesen, G. W. (1976). Acetylcholinesterase containing basal forebrain neurons in the rhesus monkey project to neocortex. *Brain Research*, *109*, 152–157.

Meudell, P. R., Mayes, A. R., Ostergaard, A., & Pickering, A. (1985). Recency and frequency judgments in alcoholic amnesics and normal people with poor memory. *Cortex*, *21*, 487–511.

Meudell, P. R., Northern, B., Snowden, J. S., & Neary, D. (1980). Long-term memory for famous voices in amnesic and normal subjects. *Neuropsychologia*, *18*, 133–139.

Meunier, M., Bachevalier, J., & Mishkin, M. (1997). Effects of orbitofrontal and anterior cingulate lesions on object and spatial memory in rhesus monkeys. *Neuropsychologia*, *35*, 999–1016.

Milner, B. (1972). Disorders of learning and memory after temporal lobe lesions in man. *Clinical Neurosurgery*, *19*, 421–446.

Milner, B., Corkin, S., & Teuber, H.-L. (1968). Further analysis of the hippocampal amnesic syndrome: 14-year follow-up study of H.M. *Neuropsychologia*, *6*, 215–234.

Milner, B., Corsi, P., & Leonard, G. (1991). Frontal lobe contribution to recency judgements. *Neuropsychologia*, *29*, 601–618.

Milner, B., Petrides, M., & Smith, M. L. (1985). Frontal lobes and the temporal organization of memory. *Human Neurobiology*, *4*, 137–142.

Mishkin, M. (1978). Memory in monkeys severely impaired by combined but not separate removal of the amygdala and hippocampus. *Nature*, *273*, 297–298.

Mishkin, M. (1982). A memory system in the monkey. *Philosophical Transactions of the Royal Society of London*, *298*, 85–95.

Mishkin, M., & Saunders, R. C. (1979). Degree of memory impairment in monkeys related to amount of conjoint damage to amygdaloid and hippocampal systems. *Society for Neuroscience Abstracts*, *5*, 320.

Mishkin, M., Spiegler, B. J., Saunders, R. C., & Malamut, B. L. (1982). An animal model of global amnesia. In S. Corkin, K. L. Davis, J. H. Growden, E. Usdin, & R. J. Wurtman (Eds.), *Alzheimer's Disease: A Report of Progress in Research Volume 19* (pp. 235–247). New York: Raven Press.

Morris, M. K., Bowers, D., Chatterjee, A., & Heilman, K. M. (1992). Amnesia following a discrete basal forebrain lesion. *Brain*, *115*, 1827–1847.

Morris, R., Petrides, M., & Pandya, D. N. (1999). Architecture and connections of retrosplenial area 30 in the rhesus monkey (Maccaca mulatta). *European Journal of Neuroscience*, *11*, 2506–2518.

Moscovitch, M. (1982). Multiple dissociations of function in amnesia. In L. S. Cermak (Ed.), *Human Memory and Amnesia* (pp. 337–370). Hillsdale, NJ: Lawrence Erlbaum.

Moscovitch, M., Rosenbaum, R. S., Gilboa, A., Addis, D. R., Westmacott, R., Grady, C., . . . Nadel, L. (2005). Functional neuroanatomy of remote episodic, semantic and spatial memory: A unified account based on multiple trace theory. *Journal of Anatomy*, *207*, 35–66.

Moss, M., Mahut, H., & Zola-Morgan, S. (1981). Concurrent discrimination learning of monkeys after hippocampal, entorhinal, or fornix lesions. *Journal of Neuroscience, 1*, 227–240.

Moudgil, S. S., Azzouz, M., Al-Azzaz, A., Haut, M., & Guttmann, L. (2000). Amnesia due to fornix infarction. *Stroke, 31*, 1418–1419.

Myers, C. E., DeLuca, J., Hopkins, R. O., & Gluck, M. S. (2006). Conditional discrimination and reversal in amnesia subsequent to hypoxic brain injury or anterior communicating artery aneurysm rupture. *Neuropsychologia, 44*, 130–139.

Myers, C. E., DeLuca, J., Schultheis, M. T., Schnirman, G. M., Ermita, B. R., Diamond, B., Warren, S. G., & Gluck, M. A. (2001). Impaired delay eyeblink classical conditioning in individuals with anterograde amnesia resulting from anterior communicating artery aneurysm rupture. *Behavioral Neuroscience, 115*, 560–570.

Nadel, L., Samsonovich, A., Ryan, L., & Moscovitch, M. (2000). Multiple trace theory of human memory: Computational, neuroimaging, and neuropsychological results. *Hippocampus, 10*, 352–368.

Nauta, W.J.H. (1961). Fibre degeneration following lesions of the amygdaloid complex in the monkey. *Journal of Anatomy, 95*, 515–531.

Nelson, T. O., Gerler, D., & Narens, L. (1984). Accuracy of feeling-of-knowing judgments for predicting perceptual identification and relearning. *Journal of Experimental Psychology: General, 113*, 282–300.

Nelson, T. O., Leonesio, R. J., Shimamura, A. P., Landwehr, R. F., & Narens, L. (1982). Overlearning and the feeling of knowing. *Journal of Experimental Psychology: Learning, Memory, and Cognition, 8*, 279–288.

Okawa, M., Maeda, S., Nukui, H., & Kawafuchi, J. (1980). Psychiatric symptoms in ruptured anterior communicating aneurysms: Social prognosis. *Acta Psychiatrica Scandinavica, 61*, 306–312.

Olton, D. S. (1989). Inferring psychological dissociations from experimental dissociations: The temporal context of episodic memory. In H. L. Roediger & F.I.M. Craik (Eds.), *Varieties of Memory and Consciousness: Essays in Honour of Endel Tulving* (pp. 161–177). Hillsdale, NJ: Lawrence Erlbaum.

Owen, M. J., & Butler, S. R. (1981). Amnesia after transection of the fornix in monkeys: Long-term memory impaired, short-term memory intact. *Behavioural Brain Research, 3*, 115–123.

Pandya, D. N., & Yeterian, E. H. (1990). Architecture and connections of cerebral cortex: Implications for brain evolution and function. In A. B. Schiebel & A. F. Wechsler (Eds.), *Neurobiology of Higher Cognitive Function* (pp. 53–84). New York: The Guilford Press.

Park, S. A., Hahn, J. H., Kim, J. I., Na, D. L., & Huh, K. (2000). Memory deficits after bilateral anterior fornix infarction. *Neurology, 54*, 1379–1382.

Parker, A., & Gaffan, D. (1997). Mammillary body lesions in monkeys impair object-in-place memory: Functional unity of the fornix-mammillary system. *Journal of Cognitive Neuroscience, 9*, 512–521.

Parkin, A. J., & Hunkin, N. M. (1993). Impaired temporal context memory on anterograde but not retrograde tests in the absence of frontal pathology. *Cortex, 29*, 267–280.

Peters, B. H., & Levin, H. S. (1979). Effects of physostigmine and lecithin on memory in Alzheimer disease. *Annals of Neurology, 6*, 219–221.

Peters, B. H., & Levin, H. S. (1982). Chronic oral physostigmine and lecithin administration in memory disorders of aging. In S. Corkin, J. H. Davis, E. Growdon, & R. J. Writman (Eds.), *Alzheimer's Disease: A Report of Progress in Research* (pp. 421–426). New York: Raven Press.

Phillips, S., Sangalang, V., & Sterns, G. (1987). Basal forebrain infarction: A clinicopathologic correlation. *Archives of Neurology, 44*, 1134–1138.

Poletti, C. E. (1986). Is the limbic system a limbic system? Studies of hippocampal efferents: Their functional and clinical implications. In B. K. Doane & K. E. Livingston (Eds.), *The Limbic System: Functional Organization and Clinical Disorders* (pp. 79–94). New York: Raven Press.

Porrino, L. J., Crane, A. M., & Goldman-Rakic, P. S. (1981). Direct and indirect pathways from the amygdala to the frontal lobe in rhesus monkeys. *Journal of Comparative Neurology, 198*, 121–136.

Reed, J. M., & Squire, L. R. (1998). Retrograde amnesia for facts and events: Findings from four new cases. *Journal of Neuroscience, 18*, 3943–3954.

Rosene, D. L., & Van Hoesen, G. W. (1977). Hippocampal efferents reach widespread areas of cerebral cortex and amygdala in the rhesus monkey. *Science, 198*, 315–317.

Rudge, P., & Warrington, E. K. (1991). Selective impairment of memory and visual perception in splenial tumours. *Brain, 114*, 349–360.

Sagar, H. J., Gabrieli, J. D., Sullivan, E. W., & Corkin, S. (1990). Recency and frequency discrimination in the amnesic patient H.M. *Brain, 113*, 581–602.

Sagar, H. J., Sullivan, E. V., Gabrieli, J. D., Corkin, S., & Growdon, J. H. (1988). Temporal ordering and short-term memory deficits in Parkinson's disease. *Brain, 111*, 525–539.

Sanders, H. I., & Warrington, E. K. (1971). Memory for remote events in amnesic patients. *Brain, 94*, 661–668.

Saunders, R. C., Rosene, D. L., & Van Hoesen, G. W. (1988). Comparison of the efferents of the amygdala and the hippocampal formation in the Rhesus monkey: II. Reciprocal and non-reciprocal connections. *The Journal of Comparative Neurology, 271*, 185–207.

Schacter, D. L. (1987b). Memory, amnesia, and frontal lobe dysfunction: A critique and interpretation. *Psychobiology, 15*, 21–36.

Schacter, D. L., Harbluck, J., & McLachlan, D. (1984). Retrieval without recollection: An experimental analysis of source amnesia. *Journal of Verbal Learning and Verbal Behavior, 23*, 593–611.

Scharfman, H. E., Witter, M. P., & Schwarcz, R. (2000). Preface to H. E. Scharfman, M. P. Witter, & R. Schwarcz (Eds.), *The Parahippocampal Region: Implications for Neurological and Psychiatric Diseases. Annals of the New York Academy of Sciences, 911*, ix–xii.

Schmidtke, K., Handschu, R., & Vollmer, H. (1996). Cognitive procedural learning in amnesia. *Brain and Cognition, 32*, 441–467.

Schugens, M. M., & Daum, I. (1999). Long-term retention of classical eyeblink conditioning in amnesia. *Neuroreport, 10*, 149–152.

Scott, S. A., DeKosky, S. T., & Scheff, S. W. (1991). Volumetric atrophy of the amygdala in Alzheimer's disease: Quantitative serial reconstruction. *Neurology, 41*, 351–356.

Scoville, W. B. (1954). The limbic lobe in man. *Journal of Neurosurgery, 11*, 64–66.

Scoville, W. B., & Milner, B. (1957). Loss of recent memory after bilateral hippocampal lesions. *Journal of Neurology, Neurosurgery, & Psychiatry*, *20*, 11–21.

Seltzer, B., & Benson, D. F. (1974). The temporal pattern of retrograde amnesia in Korsakoff's disease. *Neurology*, *24*, 527–530.

Shallice, T., & Evans, M. E. (1978). The involvement of the frontal lobes in cognitive estimation. *Cortex*, *14*, 294–303.

Shimamura, A. P., Janowsky, J. S., & Squire, L. R. (1990). Memory for the temporal order of events in patients with frontal lobe lesions and amnesic patients. *Neuropsychologia*, *28*, 803–813.

Shimamura, A. P., & Squire, L. R. (1986). Memory and metamemory: A study of the feeling-of-knowing phenomenon in amnesic patients. *Journal of Experimental Psychology: Learning, Memory, and Cognition*, *12*, 452–460.

Shimamura, A. P., & Squire, L. R. (1987). A neuropsychological study of fact memory and source amnesia. *Journal of Experimental Psychology: Learning, Memory, and Cognition*, *13*, 464–473.

Shuren, J. E., Jacobs, D. H., & Heilman, K. M. (1997). Diencephalic temporal order amnesia. *Journal of Neurology, Neurosurgery, and Psychiatry*, *62*, 163–168.

Smith, C. N., Frascino, J. C., Hopkins, R. O., & Squire, L. R. (2013). The nature of anterograde and retrograde memory impairment after damage to the medial temporal lobe. *Neuropsychologia*, *51*(13), 2709–2714.

Soderlund, H., Moscovich, M., Kamar, N., Mandic, M., & Levine, B. (2012). As time goes by: Hippocampal connectivity changes with remoteness of autobiographical memory retrieval. *Hippocampus*, *22*, 670–690.

Speedie, L., & Heilman, K. M. (1983). Anterograde memory deficits for visuospatial material after infarction of the right thalamus. *Archives of Neurology*, *40*, 183–186.

Sprofkin, B. E., & Sciarra, D. (1952). Korsakoff's psychosis associated with cerebral tumors. *Neurology*, *2*, 427–434.

Squire, L. R. (1981). Two forms of human amnesia: An analysis of forgetting. *Journal of Neuroscience*, *1*, 635–640.

Squire, L. R. (1982a). The neuropsychology of human memory. *Annual Review of Neuroscience*, *5*, 241–273.

Squire, L. R. (1982b). Comparison between forms of amnesia: Some deficits are unique to Korsakoff syndrome. *Journal of Experimental Psychology: Learning, Memory, and Cognition*, *8*, 560–571.

Squire, L. R. (1984). ECT and memory dysfunction. In B. Lerer, R. D. Weiner, & R. H. Belmaker (Eds.), *ECT: Basic Mechanisms* (pp. 156–163). Washington, DC: American Psychiatric Press.

Squire, L. R., Amaral, D. G., Zola-Morgan, S., Kritchevsky, M., & Press, G. (1989). Description of brain injury in the amnesic patient N.A. based on magnetic resonance imaging. *Experimental Neurology*, *105*, 23–35.

Squire, L. R., & Fox, M. M. (1980). Assessment of remote memory: Validation of the television test by repeated testing during a seven-day period. *Behavioral Research Methods and Instrumentation*, *12*, 583–586.

Squire, L. R., Haist, F., & Shimamura, A. P. (1989). The neurology of memory: Quantitative assessment of retrograde amnesia in two groups of amnesic patients. *Journal of Neuroscience*, *9*, 828–839.

Squire, L. R., & Moore, R. Y. (1979). Dorsal thalamic lesion in a noted case of chronic memory dysfunction. *Annals of Neurology*, *6*, 503–506.

Squire, L. R., Nadel, L., & Slater, P. C. (1981). Anterograde amnesia and memory for temporal order. *Neuropsychologia*, *19*, 141–145.

Squire, L. R., & Shimamura, A. P. (1986). Characterizing amnesic patients for neurobehavioral study. *Behavioral Neuroscience*, *100*, 866–877.

Squire, L. R., Slater, P., & Chace, P. M. (1975). Retrograde amnesia: Temporal gradient in very long-term memory following electroconvulsive therapy. *Science*, *187*, 77–79.

Squire, L. R., & Wixted, J. T. (2011). The cognitive neuroscience of human memory since H.M. *Annual Review of Neuroscience*, *34*, 259–288.

Squire, L. R., & Zola-Morgan, S. (1991). The medial temporal lobe memory system. *Science*, *253*, 1380–1386.

Suzuki, W. I., & Eichenbaum, H. (2000). The neurophysiology of memory. The neurophysiology of memory. *Annals of the New York Academy of Sciences*, *911*, 175–191.

Swanson, L. W. (1987). The hypothalamus. In A. Bjorklund, T. Hokfelt, & L. Swanson (Eds.), *Handbook of Chemical Neuroanatomy: Integrate Systems of the CNS: Part I—Hypothalamus, Hippocampus, Amygdala, Retina* (Vol. 5, pp. 1–124). Amsterdam: Elsevier.

Swanson, L. W., & Cowan, W. M. (1979). An autoradiographic study of the organization of the efferent connections of the hippocampal formation in the rat. *Journal of Comparative Neurology*, *172*, 49–84.

Sweet, W. H., Talland, G. A., & Ervin, F. R. (1959). Loss of recent memory following section of fornix. *Transactions of the American Neurological Association*, *84*, 76–82.

Sziklas, V., & Petrides, M. (1998). Memory and the region of the mammillary bodies. *Progress in Neurobiology*, *54*, 55–70.

Takahashi, N., Kawamura, M., Shiota, J., Kasahata, N., & Hirayama, K. (1997). Pure topographic disorientation due to right retrosplenial lesion. *Neurology*, *49*, 464–469.

Takayama, Y., Kamo, H., Ohkawa, Y., Akiguchi, I., & Kimura, J. (1991). A case of retrosplenial amnesia. *Rinsho Shinkeigaku*, *31*, 331–333.

Talland, G., Sweet, W. H., & Ballantine, H. T. (1967). Amnesic syndrome with anterior communicating artery aneurysm. *Journal of Nervous and Mental Disease*, *145*, 179–192.

Tanaka, Y., Miyazawa, Y., Akaoka, F., & Yamada, T. (1997). Amnesia following damage to the mammillary bodies. *Neurology*, *48*, 160–165.

Teuber, H.-L., Milner, B., & Vaughan, H. G. (1968). Persistent anterograde amnesia after stab wound to the basal brain. *Neuropsychologia*, *6*, 267–282.

Thal, L. J., Fuld, P. A., Masure, D. M., & Sharpless, N. S. (1983). Oral physostigmine and lecithin improves memory in Alzheimer's disease. *Annals of Neurology*, *113*, 491–496.

Turner, M. S., Cipolotti, L., Yousry, T., & Shallice, T. (2007). Qualitatively different memory impairments across frontal lobe subgroups. *Neuropsychologia*, *45*(7), 1540–1552.

Turner, M. S., Cipolotti, L., Yousry, T., & Shallice, T. (2008). Confabulation: Damage to a specific inferior medial prefrontal system. *Cortex*, *44*(6), 637–648.

Urbanowitsch, N., Gorenc, L., Herold, C.J., & Schröder, J. (2013). Autobiographical memory: A clinical perspective. *Frontiers in Behavioral Neuroscience*, *7*, 194.

Valenstein, E., Bowers, D., Verfaellie, M., Heilman, K. M., Day, A., & Watson, R. T. (1987). Retrosplenial amnesia. *Brain*, *110*, 1631–1646.

Van Hoesen, G. W. (1985). Neural systems of the non-human primate forebrain implicated in memory. *Annals of the New York Academy of Sciences*, *444*, 97–112.

Van Hoesen, G. W., & Pandya, D. N. (1975). Some connections of the entorhinal (area 28) and perirhinal (area 35) cortices of the rhesus monkey: I. Temporal lobe afferents. *Brain Research*, *95*, 25–38.

Van Hoesen, G. W., Pandya, D. N., & Butters, N. (1972). Cortical afferents to the entorhinal cortex of the rhesus monkey. *Science*, *175*, 1471–1473.

Van Hoesen, G. W., Rosene, D. L., & Mesulam, M.-M. (1979). Subicular input from temporal cortex in the rhesus monkey. *Science*, *205*, 608–610.

Vargha-Khadem, F., Gadian, D. G., Watkins, K. E., Connelly, A., Van Paesschen, W., & Mishkin, M. (1997). Differential effects of early hippocampal pathology on episodic and semantic memory. *Science*, *277*, 376–380.

Veazey, R. B., Amaral, D. G., & Cowan, W. M. (1982). The morphology and connections of the posterior hypothalamus in the cynomolgus monkey (Maccaca fascicularis): II. Efferent connections. *Journal of Comparative Neurology*, *207*, 135–156.

Verfaellie, M., Koseff, P., & Alexander, M. P. (2000). Acquisition of novel semantic information in amnesia: Effects of lesion location. *Neuropsychologia*, *38*, 484–492.

Victor, M., Adams, R. D., & Collins, G. H. (1989). *The Wernicke-Korsakoff syndrome and Related Neurologic Disorders Due to Alcoholism and Malnutrition* (2nd ed.). Philadelphia, PA: Davis.

Victor, M., & Agamanolis, D. (1990). Amnesia due to lesions confined to the hippocampus: A clinical-pathologic study. *Journal of Cognitive Neuroscience*, *2*, 246–257.

Vilkki, J. (1985). Amnesic syndromes after surgery of anterior communicating artery aneurysms. *Cortex*, *21*, 431–444.

Volpe, B. T., & Hirst, W. (1983). Amnesia following the rupture and repair of an anterior communicating artery aneurysm. *Journal of Neurology, Neurosurgery, and Psychiatry*, *46*, 704–709.

von Cramon, D. Y., Hebel, N., & Schuri, U. (1985). A contribution to the anatomical basis of thalamic amnesia. *Brain*, *108*, 993–1008.

von Cramon, D. Y., & Schuri, U. (1992). The septo-hippocampal pathways and their relevance to human memory: A case report. *Cortex*, *28*, 411–422.

Warrington, E. K. (1985). A disconnection analysis of amnesia. *Annals of the New York Academy of Sciences*, *444*, 72–77.

Warrington, E. K., & Weiskrantz, L. (1982). Amnesia: A disconnection syndrome? *Neuropsychologia*, *20*, 233–248.

Williams, M., & Pennybacker, J. (1954). Memory disturbances in third ventricle tumours. *Journal of Neurology, Neurosurgery and Psychiatry*, *17*, 115–123.

Whitehouse, P. J., Price, D. L., Clark, A. W., Coyle, J. T., & DeLong, M. R. (1981). Alzheimer disease: Evidence for selective loss of cholinergic neurons in the nucleus basalis. *Annals of Neurology*, *10*, 122–126.

Winocur, G. (1984). Memory localization in the brain. In L. R. Squire & N. Butters (Eds.), *Neuropsychology of Memory* (pp. 122–133). New York: Guilford Press.

Winocur, G., & Moscovitch, M. (1999). Anterograde and retrograde amnesia after lesions to frontal cortex in rats. *Journal of Neuroscience*, *19*, 9611–9617.

Winocur, G., Oxbury, S., Roberts, R., Agnetti, V., & Davis, C. (1984). Amnesia in a patient with bilateral lesions to the thalamus. *Neuropsychologia*, *22*, 123–143.

Wixted, J. T., & Squire, L. R. (2011). The medial temporal lobe and the attributes of memory. *Trends in Cognitive Science*, *15*, 210–217.

Woodruff Pak, D. S. (1993). Eyeblink classical conditioning in H.M.: Delay and trace paradigms. *Behavioral Neuroscience*, *107*, 911–925.

Woolsey, R. M., & Nelson, J. S. (1975). Asymptomatic destruction of the fornix in man. *Archives of Neurology*, *32*, 566–568.

Xuereb, J. H., Perry, R. H., Candy, J. M., Perry, E. K., Marshall, E., & Bonham, J. R. (1991). Nerve cell loss in the thalamus in Alzheimer's disease and Parkinson's disease. *Brain*, *114*, 1363–1379.

Yasuda, K., Watanabe, O., & Ono, Y. (1997). Dissociation between semantic and autobiographic memory: A case report. *Cortex*, *33*, 623–638.

Yasuno, F., Hirata, M., Takimoto, H., Taniguchi, M., Nakagawa, Y., Ikejiri, Y., . . . Takeda, M. (1999). Retrograde temporal order amnesia resulting from damage to the fornix. *Journal of Neurology, Neurosurgery, and Psychiatry*, *67*, 102–105.

Zola-Morgan, S., & Squire, L. R. (1986). Memory impairment in monkeys following lesions restricted to the hippocampus. *Behavioral Neuroscience*, *100*, 155–160.

Zola-Morgan, S., & Squire, L. R. (1990b). The primate hippocampal formation: Evidence for a time-limited role in memory storage. *Science*, *250*, 288–290.

Zola-Morgan, S., Squire, L. R., & Amaral, D. G. (1986). Human amnesia and the medial temporal region: Enduring memory impairment following a bilateral lesion limited to field CA1 of the hippocampus. *Journal of Neuroscience*, *6*, 2950–2967.

Zola-Morgan, S., Squire, L. R., & Amaral, D. G. (1989a). Lesions of the amygdala that spare adjacent cortical regions do not impair memory or exacerbate the impairment following lesions of the hippocampal formation. *The Journal of Neuroscience*, *9*, 1922–1936.

Zola-Morgan, S., Squire, L. R., Amaral, D. G., & Suzuki, W. A. (1989b). Lesions of perirhinal and parahippocampal cortex that spare the amygdala and hippocampal formation produce severe memory impairment. *The Journal of Neuroscience*, *9*, 4355–4370.

29 Neuropsychological Functioning in Affective and Anxiety-Spectrum Disorders in Adults and Children

Bernice A. Marcopulos

Neuropsychology in Psychiatry

Over the past 20 years, there has been a great expansion in the literature devoted to mental illness and neuropsychological functioning. A quick perusal of the major journals in psychiatry reveals a plethora of neuropsychology related articles, reflecting the intense interest in neurobiological mechanisms of mental illnesses. The National Institute of Mental Health (NIMH) has sponsored several initiatives, in collaboration with academic institutions and industry, to understand these neurocognitive mechanisms and more precisely devise new medications and behavioral treatments (Carter & Barch, 2007). Cognitive endophenotypes may advance our understanding of mental illness, placing neuropsychology in a prominent role in psychiatric research (Bilder et al., 2009; Bilder, Howe, & Sabb, 2013; also see Bilder, Chapter 8 in this volume). Grouping patients on the basis of core cognitive characteristics may be more productive than grouping by symptom characteristics which are based on subjective self-report. The World Health Organization (Mathers, Fat, & Boerma, 2008) lists mental disorders as a major source of disease burden. Cognitive impairment associated with these mental illnesses is believed to cause much of the burden (Whiteford et al., 2013). Neuropsychology is critical in evaluating the cognitive impairments that are present in nearly all the major mental illnesses because cognitive deficits are a strong predictor of functional outcome (Green, 1996; Keefe, 1995). Clinical neuropsychological interventions such as cognitive remediation have been specifically designed for psychiatric illness (see Medalia, Revheim, & Herlands, 2009) to address this burden.

Current training models in psychiatry emphasize neurobiology and neurochemistry and the logic of using medications to "correct" the underlying neurochemical defect. Perhaps as a result of their neurobiological focus, psychiatry has also recognized the importance of neurocognitive deficits in mental illness. Psychiatrists have devised their own screening methods to identify cognitive impairment (Gómez-Benito et al., 2013), but consult neuropsychologist colleagues for a more comprehensive evaluation. According to Sweet, Meyer, Nelson, and Moberget al. (2011) approximately 20% of neuropsychologists are employed in psychiatry departments, where they play an important role in the diagnosis, treatment, and clinical research of mental disorders.

Scope and Aim of This Chapter

There is a vast literature on mental illness and neurocognitive functioning, with several volumes dedicated to the neuropsychology of psychiatric disorders (e.g., Grant & Adams, 2009; Marcopulos & Kurtz, 2012; Wood, Allen & Pantelis, 2009). Since a chapter in the previous edition of this textbook covered schizophrenia in adults (Marcopulos et al., 2008), this chapter will focus on neuropsychological research on affective and anxiety disorders, which are more commonly encountered in any neuropsychologist's clinical practice. The goal of this chapter is to translate the research on bipolar, depressive, anxiety, and obsessive-compulsive disorders into a coherent summary that will be directly useful for the practicing clinician. The clinical presentation and epidemiology will be briefly described for each disorder, in addition to the nature of cognitive deficits and the mechanisms for impairment, if known. Since many, if not most, of the major psychiatric disorders have their origins in childhood and follow a developmental course, their neuropsychological manifestations will be considered across the life span. The incidence of psychiatric disorders peaks in late adolescence and young adulthood, with a significant number starting in childhood (Jones & Tarrant, 1999; Newman et al., 1996). There is some evidence that an early onset of a mental disorder may be associated with greater symptom morbidity and cognitive deficits that persist over the lifetime. Finally, and most importantly, the functional significance of cognitive deficits for daily functioning will be discussed.

An important question is whether the cognitive deficits associated with affective and anxiety disorders occur primarily during acute symptoms (state) or whether the cognitive deficits are evident even during stable phases (trait). In other words, are the cognitive deficits in a given mental disorder related to "state" or "trait"? These primary psychiatric disorders not only have their own neuropsychological manifestations, but also complicate neurological disorders such as stroke, dementia, or traumatic brain injury. Depression and anxiety, as a reaction to a brain injury, must be considered when interpreting neuropsychological test data. Understanding the unique impact of affective or anxiety disorders on neuropsychological functioning can help disentangle these psychiatric complications in primary neurological disorders.

Anxiety Disorders

Anxiety disorders are extremely commonplace, affecting approximately 11% of the U.S. population in any given year (12-month prevalence; Grant et al., 2004) and 28.8% experiencing an anxiety disorder over the lifetime (Kessler, Berglund et al., 2005). Anxiety disorders include a disparate array of clinical syndromes, including generalized anxiety disorder, obsessive-compulsive disorder (OCD), posttraumatic stress disorder, agoraphobia, and panic disorder. One of the primary symptoms of anxiety disorders is poor attention and concentration, which could negatively affect cognitive test performance. Some patients become extremely anxious during any medical procedures and in particular in response to cognitive testing. Acute situational anxiety can affect cognitive tests—even in patients without a diagnosis of anxiety—by impairing working memory (Darke, 1988). According to Attentional Control Theory (ACT; Eysenck, Derakshan, Santos, & Calvo, 2007), anxiety impacts working memory because of increased processing effort. Acute anxiety in healthy individuals impacts both verbal and visuospatial working memory by reducing executive resources needed to focus attention (Shackman et al., 2006). In patients with chronic anxiety, one might expect even more deficits, especially if they are taking medications to control their anxiety.

Airaksinen, Larsson, and Forsell (2005) examined the effects of anxiety disorders on neuropsychological functions. They tested a mixed clinical sample with panic disorder with and without agoraphobia, social phobia, generalized anxiety disorder, specific phobia, and OCD. The group as a whole exhibited deficits in executive and memory function. However, when the researchers examined the specific diagnoses, they found that individuals with generalized anxiety disorder and specific phobia did not show deficits, while individuals with panic disorder and OCD were impaired. Another study done in Finland (Castaneda et al., 2011) found that a history of anxiety disorder was not associated with neuropsychological impairment in a sample of young adults. However, the individuals in their sample with a current anxiety diagnosis, who were taking psychotropic medication, were impaired on tests measuring executive function (Trail Making Test A and B), psychomotor processing speed (Wechsler Adult Intelligence Scale–R [WAIS-R] Digit Symbol) and visual short-term memory (Visual Span Wechsler Memory Scale–R [WMS-R]). These patients also received lower ratings on a global rating of psychosocial functioning (Diagnostic and Statistical Manual Global Assessment of Functioning [DSM GAF] score). Acute administration of lorazepam has been found to negatively affect computerized cognitive test performance (CNS Vital Signs) in a small sample of 32 participants (Loring, Marino, Parfitt, Finney, & Meador, 2012). Older participants in the study were more affected than younger.

In summary, simple symptoms of anxiety do not seem to significantly affect neuropsychological function (O'Jile, Schrimsher & O'Bryant, 2005). However, there is some evidence that older patients might be more affected by anxiety and that medication to treat anxiety may impair functioning. More severe anxiety spectrum disorders such as OCD, panic disorder, and posttraumatic stress disorder are more likely to be associated with impairment than generalized anxiety or specific phobia.

Pediatric Considerations

Although anxiety disorders are quite common in children, far less clinical research has been conducted on the cognitive effects of anxiety on children suffering from the disorder. The cumulative prevalence of any anxiety disorder found in a longitudinal community study from age 9 through 16 years was 9.9% (Costello, Mustillo, Erkanli, Keeler, & Angold, 2003). In addition to primary anxiety disorders, children with brain injuries or disorders such as brain tumors are at risk of comorbid anxiety (Moitra & Armstrong, 2013). Approximately 25% of children diagnosed with attention deficit/hyperactivity disorder (ADHD) have a comorbid anxiety disorder (Jarrett & Ollendick, 2008).

Trait anxiety was found to impact working memory in preschoolers (Visu-Petra, Miclea, Cheie, & Benga, 2009; Visu-Petra, Cheie, Benga, & Packiam Alloway, 2011) affecting verbal more than visuospatial tasks. The results of these studies support the ACT model (Eysenck et al., 2007). Micco and colleagues (2009) found that children with current generalized anxiety showed poorer verbal memory and sustained attention, whereas children with social phobia had more omissions on a continuous performance task.

Toren and colleagues (2000) found that a small (N = 19) sample of drug-naive children and adolescents seeking treatment for anxiety disorders in a community outpatient clinic in Israel scored lower on the California Verbal Learning Test (CVLT) and made more errors on the Wisconsin Card Sorting Test (WCST) compared to healthy matched controls. They found no differences on the Rey Osterreith Complex Figure Test (ROCFT) or the Wechsler Intelligence Scale for Children–Revised (WISC-R). The authors concluded that anxiety inhibits encoding of linguistic information and tasks that require working memory.

The studies summarized so far did not specify how these cognitive findings impact children's functioning, particularly in academic settings. Since 25% of children with ADHD have a comorbid anxiety disorder, how do we account for the "extra" cognitive impairment due to anxiety?

Obsessive-Compulsive Disorder

Obsessive-compulsive and related disorders (OCRDs) comprise a varied constellation of disorders in the anxiety spectrum diagnoses. OCD consists of disturbing intrusive thoughts (obsessions) and repetitive thoughts or behaviors (compulsions) that a person feels compelled to perform (APA, 2013). Prevalence in the United States is estimated to be between 1.5% and 3% (American Epidemiologic Catchment Area [ECA] survey, Karno, Golding, Sorenson, & Burnam, 1988; National Co-morbidity Survey, Ruscio, Stein, Chiu, & Kessler, 2010) but varies across settings. For instance, a recent prevalence and incidence study done in Europe (Veldhuis et al., 2012) in a primary care setting found a one-year treatment-seeking incidence of 0.016% (95% CI: 0.014–0.018) and a treatment-seeking prevalence of 0.14% (95% CI: 0.126–0.145). The one-year prevalence of OCD was only 0.084% (95% CI 0.080–0.089) in primary care patients enrolled in a large U.S. health maintenance organization.

An extensive literature exists on the neuropsychology of OCD. The disorder sometimes emerges after damage to the basal ganglia and inferior frontal cortex. Psychosurgery to treat OCD involves severing fronto-subcortical connections. Structural and functional neuroimaging tends to find abnormalities in the orbitofrontal cortex, anterior cingulate cortex, and caudate nucleus (see review by Chamberlain, Blackwell, Fineberg, Robbins, & Sahakian, 2005). These studies implicate the cortico-striatal-thalamic-cortical (CSTC) loop in the etiology of OCD (Insel, 1992; Mataix-Cols & van den Heuvel, 2006; Milad & Rauch, 2012; Rauch & Baxter, 1998).

In individuals diagnosed with primary OCD, executive dysfunction tends to be the primary finding, with memory impairment surmised to be secondary to executive dysfunction (e.g., Harkin & Kessler, 2011). However, a recent meta-analysis found heterogeneity across neurocognitive domains and no specific OCD profile (Abramovitch, Abramowitz, & Mittelman, 2013). Many studies show impairment in executive functions and nonverbal memory (Fontenelle, Mendlowicz, & Versiani, 2004; Penades, Catalan, Andres, Salamero, & Gasto, 2005; Savage & Rauch, 2000; Savage et al., 2000). There has been controversy regarding the presence and source of working memory impairment in OCD in adults. Deficits in visuospatial memory may be attributed to difficulties in organizing material. Segalàs et al. (2008) found that patients with OCD differed from healthy controls on a Spanish verbal memory test similar to the CVLT, as well as the Rey Complex Figure Test (RCFT). Older onset of OCD, and severity of depressive and obsessive symptoms (as measured by the Yale-Brown Obsessive Compulsive Scale) were associated with more impairments. The authors hypothesized that differing neurocognitive profiles based on age of onset suggest different neurobiological substrates. Unlike other studies (e.g., Savage et al., 2000; Deckersbach, Otto, Savage, Baer, & Jenike, 2000) they did not find that organizational ability accounted for the poorer memory. There have been several ideas regarding the types of memory deficits in OCD: overall memory capacity impaired; modality specific, especially visuospatial, executive dysfunction, or metamemory. In addition, Simpson and colleagues (2006) did not find reliable neuropsychological deficits in OCD.

Researchers have found differences in cognitive functioning between OCD subtypes, with greater cognitive deficits for "checkers" (Nedelijkovic et al., 2009; Omori et al., 2007). Memory deficits might explain the compulsive checking behaviors (e.g., Woods, Vevea, Chambless, & Bayen, 2002). Grisham, Anderson, Poulton, Moffitt, and Andrews (2009) examined neuropsychological performance at age 13 and then followed individuals until age 32. The participants receiving a diagnosis of OCD at age 32 had shown impaired performance on visuospatial, visuoconstructive, and visuomotor skills, though findings regarding executive functioning were mixed, with deficits noted in planning and organization but not in other areas such as set shifting.

There is some disagreement in the literature as to whether the deficits seen in executive functioning represent a stable trait-like characteristic of the illness, an endophenotype, or to state variables such as severity of symptoms and effects of treatments. Moritiz et al. (2001) found that comorbid depression exacerbates executive deficits. Some studies have found persistent deficits even after pharmacological treatment (e.g., Kim, Park, Shin, & Kwon, 2002), while others have found improvement in cognition after a behavioral intervention (e.g., Mortiz, Kloss, Katenkamp, Birkner, & Hand, 1999; Kuelz et al., 2006).

Pediatric Considerations

Far less clinical research has been conducted on the cognitive effects of OCD on children suffering from the disorder. An earlier study did not see significant cognitive deficits in children newly diagnosed who were not on medications (Beers et al., 1999). But other studies find similar deficits in children as adults (Shin et al., 2008), such as executive function deficits and impairments in visual memory, visual organization, and processing speed (Andrés et al., 2007).

Brennan and Flessner (2015) conducted a comprehensive review of OCRD in adults and children. OCRDs include disorders like skin picking, hair pulling, hoarding, and body dysmorphic disorder. Brennan and Flessner (2015) summarized the cognitive risk factors across pediatric disorders marked by obsessive, compulsive, and repetitive or ritualistic behaviors. The difficulty with this literature, as well as much of the literature on cognitive effects of mental disorders, lies in studies with small sample sizes that are not replicated. Abramovitch et al. (2015) conducted a meta-analysis on 11 studies meeting their criteria, looking at attention, executive function, memory processing speed, visuospatial abilities, and working memory. They found small and insignificant effect sizes, concluding that there are no specific neuropsychological deficits in pediatric OCD.

Are the deficits seen in pediatric OCRD state or trait? A study by Andrés and colleagues (2008) contradicts the endophenotype (e.g., trait) hypothesis by showing that cognitive deficits resolve with treatment. They compared 29 children ages ranging from 7 to 18 years, with OCD and a score of at least 20 on the Children's Yale-Brown Obsessive-Compulsive Scale (CY-BOCS; Scahill et al., 1997) with healthy controls and found that the differences resolved after "naturalistic" treatment. The treatment consisted of either a Selective Serotonin Reuptake Inhibitor (SSRI) or clomipramine and individual and parental counseling. More than half the patients also received cognitive behavioral therapy in addition to medication. The children received neuropsychological testing before treatment and again after six months. At baseline, the OCD patients showed deficits relative to healthy controls on visual and verbal memory, speed of information processing, and executive functions. On follow-up, only deficits in verbal memory remained significant relative to controls. Practice effects and a between subjects rather than within subjects design limit the impact of these findings.

Affective Disorders

The 12-month prevalence of mood disorders in adults is approximately 9.21% (Grant et al., 2004). Lifetime prevalence is estimated at 20.8% (Kessler, Berglund et al., 2005). Neuropsychological deficits are very common in affective disorders and have functional significance. As in schizophrenia, neurocognitive deficits in affective disorders are not related to acute symptoms. The deficits persist even when symptoms have improved. This section will cover major depression and bipolar disorder in children and adults.

Major Depressive Disorder

The lifetime prevalence and 12-month prevalence for major depressive disorder are 16.5% and 6.7% respectively (Kessler, Chiu, Demler, & Walters, 2005). Women are much more likely to be diagnosed as depressed compared with men. The average age of onset is 32 years (Kessler et al., 2003) with younger adults having higher rates of depression than older adults (Husain et al., 2005). Depression frequently reoccurs in 50%–75% of diagnosed persons, and it is associated with more functional impairment (Kennedy & Paykel, 2004). Depression is an important cause of disease burden, and those individuals with a chronic disease and comorbid depression have the greatest health burden (Moussavi et al., 2007).

Since Kiloh's (1961) classic paper on "pseudo-dementia," clinicians have observed and remarked on the cognitive deficits related to depression. The relationship between depression and cognitive function is complex. Although psychotic depression has a more deleterious effect on cognition than nonpsychotic depression (Basso & Bornstein, 1999) and fits the pattern of neuropsychological deficits seen in schizophrenia (Hill, Keshavan, Thase, & Sweeney, 2004), the severity of a depressive episode is not necessarily correlated with cognitive dysfunction. Other aspects of depression such as number and duration of episodes, presence of psychotic features, age of onset, and treatment resistance, are more important to consider (McClintock, Husain, Greer, & Cullum, 2010).

Much of the research on cognitive impairment in depression has focused on older adult populations, but younger adults have also been found to have deficits on cognitive testing. In their review of the literature from 1990 through 2006, Castaneda, Tuulio-Henriksson, Marttunen, Suvisaari, and Lönnqvist (2008) found that executive function is most commonly affected in younger adults with depression. Problems in attention, working memory, and psychomotor impairments were also reported in some studies they reviewed. Other risk factors for greater cognitive impairment include having multiple episodes and a relative who has bipolar disorder (Smith, Muir, & Blackwood, 2006).

Beblo, Sinnamon, and Baune (2011) reviewed the literature on neurobiological, clinical, and demographic factors affecting cognitive functioning in depression. Mood disorders have been found to impact cognition in several ways. Decreased concentration and difficulty making decisions are part of the diagnostic criteria. There is the common finding of depressed persons negatively evaluating their cognition. The negative affective bias in depression has been well established in the literature (Clark, Chamberlain, & Sahakian, 2009). Antidepressants may act by ameliorating these negative biases directly (Roiser, Elliott, & Sahakian, 2012). The effects of depression vary, with most studies finding little effect on neuropsychological functioning.

Attention and memory appear to be most affected by major depressive disorder. Earlier studies suggested that speeded tasks and "effortful" tasks were most affected in depression (Christensen, Griffiths, MacKinnon, & Jacomb, 1997; Den Hartog, Derix, Van Bemmel, Kremer, & Jolles, 2003; Hasher & Zacks, 1979). Airaksinen, Larsson, Lundberg, and Forsell (2004) found that major depression and mixed anxiety and depression affected episodic memory and mental flexibility in a community sample of adults aged 10–64 in Sweden. Individuals in their sample had minor depression, dysthymia, and anxiety and depression. There were no effects of depression on verbal fluency (COWAT) or perceptual speed (Trail Making Test A). The depressed participants—particularly those with dysthymia—were slower, but not less accurate, on Trail Making B. Patients with minor depression did not differ from normal controls on any neuropsychological tests. They found that all groups benefitted from retrieval cues to the same degree to enhance episodic memory. Because the participants with major depression did not show more improvements with cues, they suggested that perhaps there are also encoding deficits. Airaksinen and colleagues (2004) found that psychotropic medications did not negatively impact episodic memory but had a negative effect on mental flexibility (Trail Making B). Depression severity, number of episodes, and symptom clusters have all been shown to be related to the cognitive deficits seen in depression. In general the cognitive deficits seen in depression have been characterized as fitting a subcortical profile with primary deficits in processing speed. Mesholam-Gately et al. (2012) found that a group of elders with mild depression were similar to normals on the CVLT, but those with major depressive disorder showed decrements like a subcortical profile.

State Versus Trait?

A number of studies have found residual cognitive deficits even when depression was in remission (Baune et al., 2010; Nagane et al., 2014), indicating that these deficits are not secondary to mood state. Gallasi, DiSarro, Morreale, and Amore (2006) concluded in their study of the effects of antidepressants on memory that the deficits in depression were both state and trait. They found anterograde deficits on the WMS Logical memory and Paired Associates. In younger patients, deficits in executive function, verbal learning, and memory can persist even in remission (Smith et al., 2006). This seems to depend upon depression severity as some studies of outpatients with mild depression show no residual deficits in remission (Wang et al., 2006). Lee, Hermens, Porter, and Redoblado-Hodge (2012), in their meta-analysis on first-episode depression in adults ages 16 and over, found small to medium effect sizes for cognitive deficits. Deficits in psychomotor speed and memory were related to clinical state, whereas attention and executive function were enduring trait markers. In those patients with continued dysfunction, neurocognitive deficits were more important predictors than depression symptoms (Jaeger, Berns, Uzelac, & Davis-Conway, 2006).

Pharmacological treatments for depression have been found to have negative effects on cognition. Tricyclic antidepressants (TCAs), which are much less often prescribed since the advent of SSRIs, have anticholinergic side effects that negatively impact memory (Nagane et al., 2014). Nagane and colleagues evaluated three groups of patients with major depressive disorder (medicated with TCA, SSRI or unmedicated) with a control group. All three groups were more impaired on the WMS Logical Memory and Verbal Paired Associates. On the Visual Reproduction subtest, the two medicated depressed groups were impaired relative to unmedicated and healthy controls. On the Stroop, the groups taking TCAs scored lower than controls and the other two depressed groups.

Electroconvulsive therapy (ECT) is highly effective for treating severe, treatment-resistant depression and it is relatively safe (Lisanby, 2007). However, it is controversial as patients report that it impairs memory, especially autobiographical memory. Patients typically experience temporary memory loss that recovers over time, although some patients have reported persistent impairment. McClintock and colleagues (2014) recently reviewed the literature on ECT and cognition. Unfortunately, since neuropsychological assessment is not a routine part of clinical ECT practice, data on cognitive outcome is sparse. Nevertheless, McClintock and colleagues were able to draw some conclusions and propose a model of the underlying factors mediating or moderating cognitive outcomes after ECT. The practice of ECT has changed over time in terms of type of treatment techniques and parameters for delivering the shock, such as electrode placement. McClintock and colleagues found that technique and electrode placement determines the extent of memory loss. Older methods for administering ECT, which used sine waves and bilateral electrode placement, have a much more persistent effect on cognition, particularly autobiographical memory, than more recent methods using ultra-brief pulse waveform and unilateral electrode placement. Age, education, premorbid intellectual ability, and cerebrovascular health are important moderator variables. In particular, patients with lower cognitive reserve and poor cognitive health are at higher risk for developing cognitive impairment post-ECT.

Pediatric Considerations

Children as young as 3 years have been diagnosed with depression (Luby, 2009). The cumulative prevalence of any depressive disorder in children ages 9–16 years in a longitudinal community study was 9.5% (Costello et al., 2003). The prevalence of depression in children younger than 13 has been reported as 2.8% but rises significantly during adolescence (Costello, Erkanli, & Angold, 2006). However, there is diagnostic uncertainly as some of these children presenting with unipolar depression will develop bipolar illness.

Livingston, Stark, Haak, and Jennings (1996) examined neuropsychological profiles in a small sample ($N = 56$) of children and young adolescents with diagnoses of unipolar depression, anxiety disorder, or comorbid anxiety/depressive disorder. All three groups displayed reduced attention abilities, but children with comorbid anxiety and depression generally performed worse than those with only anxiety or depression. Cataldo, Nobile, Lorusso, Battaglia, and Molteni (2005) found depressed children performed more poorly on a verbal fluency task, and on interference on the Stroop Color-Word Test compared to a healthy control group of children. They also had poorer sustained attention, slower reaction times, and greater omission errors on the Continuous Performance Test (CPT). The Stroop and CPT were significantly correlated with severity of current depressive symptoms. Micco and colleagues (2009) found that symptoms of major depression were associated with poorer performance on working memory and processing speed measures from the WISC III, and cognitive flexibility from the WCST.

Matthews, Coghill, and Rhodes (2008) studied neuropsychological functioning of a referred sample of medication-naive adolescent girls meeting criteria for a diagnosis of depressive episode. Depressed adolescent girls showed performance deficits on visual memory tasks (Pattern Recognition, Delayed Matching to Sample, and Paired Associates Learning), one measure of motor speed and on a test of Spatial Working Memory on the Cambridge Neuropsychological Test Automated Battery (CANTAB, a computerized assessment).

In summary, the few articles available on cognitive functioning in childhood depression suggest deficits similar to those found in adults. These studies must be viewed with caution as the sample sizes are small and they have not been replicated.

Bipolar Disorder

Bipolar I disorder, popularly referred to as "manic depression" is characterized by the cyclical pattern of manic and then depressive episodes. Some bipolar patients do not have mood swings but present with mixed features of depression and mania simultaneously, referred to as a *mixed episode* (Suppes et al., 2005). Bipolar II is characterized by major depression and at least one manic or hypomanic episode. Bipolar disorder can occur any time throughout an individual's lifetime but the mean age of onset is around age 18 (APA, 2013). The lifetime prevalence rate is 3.9% (Kessler & Wang, 2008). Using *Diagnostic and Statistical Manual of Mental Disorders,* fourth edition (DSM-IV criteria), the 12-month prevalence estimate in United States was 0.6% for Bipolar I with relatively equal prevalence for men and women (Merikangas et al., 2007). Bipolar disorder affects approximately 1% of the population (Birmaher, 2013). There is a very strong genetic component with a tenfold increase among close relatives (APA, 2013). Bipolar disorder and schizophrenia are thought to be genetically linked, as both serious mental disorders tend to run in families.

Bipolar disorder presents with extremes in mood that presumably could impact cognitive functioning directly. Bipolar illness has been associated with cognitive dysfunction, not only during the active phase of the illness (during a depressed or manic episode) but also when the patient is euthymic (e.g., Kurtz & Gerraty, 2009), consistent with trait abnormality. Thus, the neuropsychologist would be wise not to attribute an impaired profile to the current symptomatic affective state and expect that problems may resolve as the symptoms come under better control. More than half of individuals diagnosed with bipolar disorder have cognitive deficits. There is not a unique "bipolar profile" in terms of neurocognitive deficits, but commonly attention, working memory, verbal learning, and memory and executive functions are implicated (Torres, Boudreau, & Yatham, 2007).

Arts, Jabben, Krabbendam, and van Os (2011) followed a sample of bipolar patients over two years, testing them every two months. The patients performed more poorly than healthy controls, but effect sizes were small. Cognitive performance varied, but did not vary with mood. Sustained attention and motor speed did not vary across the study period. Second-generation antipsychotic medications were associated with cognitive decrement in motor speed and information processing. Bipolar patients typically score between patients with schizophrenia and healthy controls on neuropsychological tests. Although patients with bipolar illness are not as cognitively impaired as those with schizophrenia, the pattern is similar (Harvey, Wingo, Burdick, & Baldessarini, 2010; Krabbendam, Arts, van Os, & Aleman, 2005; Schretlen et al., 2007). The nature of cognitive impairment in bipolar disorder is similar to that seen in schizophrenia—with attention, memory, intelligence, and psychomotor function deficits—but differs in severity and course (Vöhringer et al., 2013). Vohringer and colleagues make the point in their review that negative symptoms are associated with poorer cognitive functioning in schizophrenia, but depression is not associated with poorer cognitive function in bipolar disorder. However, several studies have found just that. Cognitive difficulties in childhood are more common with schizophrenia than bipolar disorder. Cognitive difficulties in bipolar illness occur later in life after the onset of the illness and could exacerbate with each episode (Lewandowski, Cohen, & Öngur, 2011; Murray et al., 2004).

There have been several recent meta-analyses. Lee et al. (2014) reviewed 12 neuropsychological studies of patients with first onset bipolar disorder. They found medium to large effect sizes for psychomotor speed, attention, working memory, and cognitive flexibility. Small effect sizes were found in verbal learning and memory, attentional switching, and verbal fluency. Samamé, Martino, and Strejilevich (2014) performed a meta-analysis on longitudinal studies of cognition in bipolar illness. They found that cognitive functioning does not decline over time. The average retest interval for the 35 studies they included in the meta-analysis was 4.62 years. Robinson and Ferrier et al. (2006), Mann-Wrobel, Carreno, and Dickinson et al. (2011), and Torres et al. (2007) found cognitive impairment in euthymic bipolar patients, particularly in attention, processing speed, verbal memory, and executive functions. Mann-Wrobel and colleagues (2011) found that age and duration of illness were negatively correlated with deficits, and gender did not have an effect. More education was associated with fewer deficits. Vocabulary and word reading were preserved and did not differ from controls.

Like patients with schizophrenia, bipolar patients demonstrate deficits that impair social cognition. For instance, Van Rheenen and colleagues have found that persons with bipolar illness have difficulties processing facial affect. In a recent article Van Rheenen and Rossell (2014) found that bipolar patients were impaired in emotional processing and that this impairment was independent of mood state, again suggesting that neuropsychological deficits are "trait" rather than "state." The deficits tend to be subtle, however, with only modest effect sizes (Samamé, Martino, & Strejilevich, 2012; Samamé, 2013).

Older adults with euthymic bipolar disorder also show cognitive deficits, although not necessarily more than younger adults. Samamé, Martino and Strejilevich (2013) performed a meta-analysis looking at ten cognitive variables for euthymic older bipolar patients. There were no significant differences between older adults with or without bipolar disorder on global measures such as the Mini Mental State Examination (MMSE) or clock drawing, but bipolar patients showed moderate impairments (between 0.6 and 0.9 SDs) relative to controls in sustained attention tasks (i.e., Trail Making A, CPT), digit span (forwards and backwards), delayed recall (CVLT, CAMCOG, Signoret Memory Battery), serial learning (CVLT), cognitive flexibility (i.e., Trail Making B), and verbal fluency (category animal and letter). Bipolar disorder patients with later onset were more impaired relative to those with early onset. Compared to younger bipolar disorder patients, older euthymic patients did not show greater deficit, suggesting that there is no cognitive decline associated with the illness. Depp et al. (2008) found similar results, although they also found that the older bipolar patients showed more intraindividual variability.

Cognitive impairment contributes to disabilities in social and occupational functioning and ability to live independently (Depp, Mausbach, Bowie, 2012; Sanchez-Moreno et al., 2009; Torres et al., 2007). Depp and colleagues found that cognitive functioning was the strongest predictor variable for employment, followed by depressed mood. Similar to the research on schizophrenia, the functional outcome for bipolar illness is not well predicted on clinical variables such as number of manic episodes or severity of clinical symptoms. Rather, there is a closer association between neurocognitive variables and everyday functioning (e.g., (Depp, Mausbach, Harmell, 2012; Jaeger, Berns, Loftus, Gonzalez, & Czobor, 2007; Martínez-Arán et al., 2004; Torres et al., 2010; Wingo, Harvey, & Baldessarini, 2009).

Baseline cognitive functioning may predict later functioning, but the literature is not decisive on this point (Baune, Li, & Beblo, 2013). Baune et al. (2013) systematically reviewed the literature on neurocognitive impairment and general functioning in bipolar adults using PRISMA guidelines (Moher, Liberati, Tetzlaff, Altman, & Group, 2009). Baune and colleagues (2013) examined longitudinal and cross-sectional studies investigating a number of neurocognitive domains (attention, executive function, verbal learning and memory, verbal fluency, processing speed, working memory, visual learning and memory, psychomotor speed, and visuospatial ability) and activities of daily living, and social and occupational functioning. Depp, Mausbach, Harmell, (2012) also did a meta-analysis. They found that performance-based, real-world measures of functioning had higher correlation with neurocognitive variables than clinician or self-ratings. Gilbert and Marwaha (2013) utilized Meta-Analysis of Observations Studies in Epidemiology (MOOSE) guideline to do their systemic review of the predictors of employment for persons with bipolar illness. They found that depression and cognitive impairment were most associated with occupational outcome.

Langenecker, Saunders, Kade, Ransom, and McInnis (2010) found that illness severity as measured by number of hospitalizations and number of years of illness correlated with cognitive test scores. Euthymic bipolar patients performed more poorly than healthy controls on several cognitive factors including processing speed, fine motor dexterity, and speed and visual memory. Bipolar patients taking antipsychotic medication performed more poorly than those treated with Lithium and mood stabilizers. Patients on antipsychotic medication had more psychiatric hospitalizations and more severe illness. Langenecker and colleagues did not find that verbal learning and memory distinguished euthymic bipolar disorder from the healthy controls. Patients in the active phase of the illness performed more poorly on verbal memory. Langenecker and colleagues found more decrements in executive function in the manic state, which is consistent with clinical observations of more impulsivity. Executive factor scores included tests of verbal fluency, processing speed with interference resolution, conceptual reasoning, and set-shifting and inhibitory control. Langenecker and colleagues defined the deficits seen in executive dysfunction in bipolar disorder. In particular, they concluded that processing speed with interference resolution, as demonstrated on the Stroop color-word test, which is scored based on time, is impaired in all phases of the bipolar disorder, whereas inhibitory control is primarily affected during the hypomanic phase. During the depressed phase, Langenecker and colleagues found decreased verbal learning and memory, verbal fluency processing speed, and fine motor function. Interestingly, this profile has also been reported in major depressive disorder (Rogers et al., 2004). Langenecker and colleagues (2010) concluded that there were both trait and state cognitive features in bipolar disorder.

Other authors have suggested that executive dysfunction is more trait than state (Bora, Yucel, & Pantelis, 2009). According to Bora et al. (2011), persons with Bipolar I are more impaired on memory and semantic fluency than those with Bipolar II, but overall impairment is equivalent. Depp, Salva, Vergel de Dios, Mausbach, and Palmer (2012) followed 42 outpatients with bipolar disorder and tested them at 6, 12, and 26 weeks. Affective symptoms were measured along with cognitive function. They found that affective symptoms did not covary with cognitive changes, but patients with bipolar disorder showed more intra individuality than normal controls. Martínez-Arán and colleagues (2004) utilized a cross-sectional design, using three groups of bipolar patients: euthymic, depressed, and hypomanic. They tested the three groups with the WAIS Vocabulary test, WCST, Stroop Color Word, COWAT, Trail Making tests, CVLT, WMS-R Logical Memory, and Visual Reproduction. Compared to healthy controls, all three bipolar groups were impaired, especially on tests of verbal memory and executive functioning. Depressed patients had lower scores on verbal fluency, category fluency, and Trail Making A. Euthymic patients also scored lower on category fluency and Trail Making A. Psychosocial functioning correlated with neuropsychological variables but not clinical variables such as chronicity and number of hospitalizations. Social and occupational indicators were associated with cognitive variables, in particular the Stroop, WCST Digits Backwards, WMS-R, and CVLT.

Cognitive dysfunction has been studied as an intermediate endophenotype for mental illness. It is heritable, as first-degree relatives who do not have the diagnosis or clinical symptoms nevertheless show similar patterns on cognitive testing. For instance, verbal memory deficits are also present in relatives of bipolar patients (Quraishi et al., 2009). Memory, attention, executive functioning, and emotion processing tend to be most affected (Langenecker et al., 2010). Executive functioning, verbal learning, and memory have been proposed as viable endophenotypes (Glahn, Bearden, Niendam, & Escamilla, 2004). More recently, attention has been proposed as stable cognitive deficit in bipolar disorder (Burdick, Goldberg, Harrow, Faull, & Malhotra, 2006). Aminoff and colleagues (2013) described attempts to establish meaningful subtypes (endophenotypes) of bipolar disorder with characteristic cognitive features. For instance, they created subgroups based on presence of psychosis, and whether the primary feature is depression or mania, as well as age of onset. They found that the Bipolar I subgroup had lower scores on verbal learning and semantic fluency compared with Bipolar II. Bipolar I patients were more likely to take antipsychotic medications. Persons with bipolar disorder with psychosis performed more poorly on verbal memory and semantic fluency compared with patients without psychosis. Patients with depressive polarity performed better than elevated polarity on verbal learning and memory and had fewer intrusion errors on the CVLT. Age of onset had no bearing on cognitive test scores. They concluded that psychosis and mania had a more negative impact on cognitive than depression. Bipolar patients with psychotic features have more severe cognitive impairment, with executive processes being most affected (Allen et al., 2010). Solé et al. (2011) examined neuropsychological functioning in euthymic Bipolar II patients and found that attention, verbal memory, and executive functions were impaired.

Lithium, the oldest and most common medication used for bipolar disorder, has been found to affect cognition in some studies, but not others. Wingo, Wingo, Harvey, and Baldessarini (2009) performed a meta-analysis on studies done on lithium use between 1950 and 2008. They found small effect sizes (0.24) for immediate learning and memory. Attention, delayed verbal memory, visual memory, executive functions, psychomotor, and processing speed were relatively unaffected. More recently, López-Jaramillo and colleagues (2010) found that lithium had no effect on cognition. They found verbal and visual memory problems in bipolar patients compared with healthy controls independent of medication status. Findings for mood stabilizers have been mixed, with some finding cognitive effects, particularly with attention and concentration and psychomotor speed (e.g., Park & Kwon, 2008). Some authors have suggested that lithium may even have a protective effect on cognitive functions, while benzodiazepines and antipsychotics have deleterious effects (Torrent et al., 2011).

Cognitive remediation is a well-established and efficacious strategy for cognitive impairment in schizophrenia (e.g., Wykes, Huddy, Cellard, McGurk, & Czobor, 2011). Recently, there have been several trials of cognitive remediation for bipolar illness (Deckersbach et al., 2010; Torrent et al., 2013). Torrent, Martínez-Arán, and colleagues (Martínez-Arán et al., 2011; Torrent et al., 2013) developed a cognitive intervention for bipolar patients. This intervention focusses on improving the functional consequences of cognitive impairment. They utilized a number of paper-pencil and group exercises to address attention, executive functions, and verbal learning and memory. In their randomized control trial (Torrent et al., 2013), neuropsychological test scores did not improve, but functional outcome did improve after this intervention. Patients in the functional remediation intervention improved their psychosocial and occupational functioning compared to the treatment as usual group.

Pediatric Considerations

Pediatric bipolar disorder (PBD) is controversial, and diagnosis can be difficult. A full discussion of the diagnostic complexities of this disorder is beyond the scope of this chapter and the reader is directed to several recent comprehensive reviews (e.g., Birmaher, 2013). Briefly, however, young children often present in a rather undifferentiated way, typically exhibiting mood, behavioral, and cognitive symptoms. Psychotic symptoms may be present, as well as depression or elevated mood along with behavioral disturbance in the form of withdrawal and/or aggressive acting out. At a young age it is unclear whether such disturbances will evolve into a more differentiated bipolar disorder or schizophrenia.

There has been a dramatic increase in the diagnosis of bipolar disorder in children (Blader & Carlson, 2007; Moreno et al., 2007), with a concomitant increase in antipsychotic medication prescribed (Biederman, 2003; Biederman et al., 2003; Geller & Luby, 1997; Geller, Tillman, Craney, & Bolhofner, 2004). Bipolar illness in children is a heritable mental disorder characterized by extreme behavioral and affective dysregulation with aggression and severe irritability. A family history of bipolar disorder increases the risk 15-fold (Pavuluri, Henry et al., 2006). The risk of a child having bipolar disorder when one or both parents have the diagnosis ranges between 10% and 25% (Goldstein et al., 2010; Goodwin & Jamison, 2007). PBD has a chronic course and poor outcome, including higher rates of suicide and substance abuse (e.g., Geller et al., 2004). Neurocognitive deficits and poor school performance are common (Pavuluri et al., 2006). The earlier the onset, the greater the neurobehavioral and cognitive impairment and the more likely it will persist throughout adulthood (Lim et al., 2013; van Os, Jones, Lewis, Wadsworth, & Murray, 1997). Perinatal risk factors such as birth complications or exposure to maternal medication use further increase risk. More than half of adult patients with bipolar disorder worldwide report that their symptoms started before they were 21 years old (Baldessarini et al., 2010). Although the majority of children recover from manic and depressive episodes, most have recurrences of mood disorder, especially depression (Birmaher, 2007). Poor outcome is associated with risk factors such as earlier onset, longer duration of symptoms, low socioeconomic status, environmental stress, and family psychopathology. The risk of suicide is very high, with at least one-third attempting during their lifetime (Goldstein et al., 2010). Suicide attempt is another possible cause for cognitive impairment in these patients (drug overdose, asphyxiation, etc.).

There has been more research conducted on the cognitive effects of bipolar disorder in children than on other mental disorders such as anxiety and depression. Dickstein and colleagues (2004) used the CANTAB to examine cognitive functioning in 21 children and adolescents with bipolar disorder. They found deficits in attentional set-shifting and visuospatial memory. Pavuluri, Schenkel, and colleagues (2006) concluded that neurocognitive deficits in attention, executive functioning, working memory, and verbal memory were trait rather than state and were not due to medication effects. They compared three groups of 28 children (medicated, nonmedicated, healthy controls), matched on demographic variables, with an average age of 11.7 years. The medicated children were either on lithium plus risperidone or divalproex sodium plus risperidone. Tasks involving shifting attention, processing speed, and problem solving were most affected, implicating dorsolateral prefrontal cortex dysfunction, as shown in neuroimaging studies (e.g., Adleman et al., 2012). Unlike Dickstein et al., they did not find visuospatial deficits. Illness state as measured by the Young Mania Rating Scale, and medication use did not affect the results, but comorbid ADHD was associated with greater neurocognitive dysfunction.

Joseph, Frazier, Youngstrom, and Soares (2008) reviewed the literature on neurocognition in PBD. They performed a meta-analysis on ten studies examining cognitive deficits in PBD. Effect sizes for Full Scale Intelligence Quotient (FSIQ) were small to medium compared with healthy controls. No FSIQ differences were found compared to other psychiatric disorders. They surmised that comorbid ADHD and oppositional defiant disorder (ODD) most likely played a role in lower IQ. Reading achievement also fell in the small to medium range of effect sizes. Effect sizes for attention were in the medium range. Motor speed effect size was small. Executive functioning was moderate, corresponding with parent report of executive dysfunction in adolescents with bipolar disorder (Shear, DelBello, Rosenberg, & Strakowski, 2002). Working memory was in the medium to large range. Verbal fluency showed small to medium differences and visuoperceptual functions showed medium effect sizes, but they included only four studies. The effect size for visual memory was medium and verbal memory was large. Joseph et al. concluded that their meta-analysis was similar to those conducted with studies on adult bipolar disorder with verbal memory showing the largest effect. However, they cautioned that the presence of comorbid ADHD, which occurs in as much as 62% in pediatric bipolar disorder (Kowatch, Youngstrom, Danielyan, & Findling, 2005), may be a significant confound.

There is considerable comorbidity between ADHD and bipolar illness, which complicates the neurocognitive picture (e.g., West, McElroy, Strakowski, Keck, & McConville, 1995; Wozniak et al., 1995; also see the chapter by Wasserstein et al. in this volume). Co-morbid ADHD, ODD, and substance abuse makes it difficult to interpret manic and hypomanic symptoms (Birmaher, 2013; Klein, Pine, & Klein, 1998). Increased energy, distractibility, and pressured speech are the most common symptoms of bipolar disorder in children, but these symptoms are also common in ADHD (Kowatch et al., 2005). Like other mental disorders, the symptoms must exceed normal expectations for developmental stage, affect functioning across several settings (school, home, peers), and not be explained by cultural or environmental factors. Although bipolar disorder with ADHD might represent a distinct subgroup, Pavuluri, Henry, Nadimpalli, O'Connor, and Sweeney (2006), did not find differences in risk factors of neuropsychological functioning between bipolar disorder with or without ADHD. One study of stabilized adolescents with bipolar disorder found fewer attentional deficits than adults and no increased incidence of ADHD (Robertson, Kutcher, & Lagace, 2003). They examined the Freedom from Distractibility (FD) Composite Index of the WISC III, Conners Continuous Performance Test (CPT), WCST, and a subjective cognitive/attentional problems checklist. Doyle et al. (2005) examined neuropsychological functioning in a sample of 57 youth aged 10–18 years with bipolar disorder, while controlling for comorbid ADHD. They used a variety of neurocognitive measures of sustained attention, processing speed, working memory, interference control, abstract problem solving and set shifting, visuospatial organization, and verbal learning. After statistically controlling for ADHD, which was present in 74% of the sample, youth with bipolar disorder showed deficits in processing speed, sustained attention, and working memory and had lower academic achievement in arithmetic. Digit Symbol, and Stroop Color Word subtest showed the largest effect sizes.

In summary, children and adolescents with bipolar disorder are at risk for neurocognitive impairment that will impact academic and social functioning and have implications for future occupational achievement as well as independent living. Medications for bipolar disorder do not appear to either explain, or exacerbate these deficits. Early intervention is believed to mitigate some of these functional deficits and help these children and their families manage the disease and its implications over the long term. Educational interventions such as individual education plans (IEPs) or 504 plans that recognize and address the cognitive deficits in these children as well as their affective challenges will be most helpful in their academic success.

Conclusions

A neuropsychologist evaluating a patient with a psychiatric disorder or prominent psychiatric symptoms should be aware of associated cognitive deficits. As seen in this review, cognitive dysfunction is very common, but there are no unique cognitive profiles for specific affective and anxiety diagnoses. An important question is how acute symptoms impact test results. For example, depressed patients may be unwilling or unable to exert sufficient effort on tests, compromising validity. In most cases, it is advisable to wait until the patient is stable before starting a test battery. However, the research presented in this review shows that cognitive deficits are not merely epiphenomenon, but are enduring features of many psychiatric disorders. The cognitive effects are present even when the acute symptoms have abated. Not only do cognitive deficits persist, in some cases—especially in the more severe disorders like bipolar disorders—they impact daily functioning. In other cases, such as depression, cognitive issues might have minimal functional impact and primarily be subjectively experienced. Treatments for mental disorders can also negatively impact cognition although not as much as the illness itself. Except for ECT, which has been reported to impair memory, most medical treatments for mood disorders and anxiety disorders have only a modest effect and cannot entirely explain alterations on testing. An interesting question concerns how psychotherapy, behavioral therapy, or cognitive remediation may improve cognition in mental illness.

In many cases, symptoms of a serious mental disorder begin in childhood and persist into adulthood (Newman et al., 1996). Individuals whose mental illness starts in childhood are at greater risk for cognitive impairment. Disorders with a strong genetic component tend to start early in life, during predictable developmental epochs. These disorders tend to have more neurocognitive sequelae, particularly with executive functioning. The literature on children is sparse compared to the literature on adults, but suggests that there can be significant cognitive effects that impair learning. Also, childhood onset of major mental illness is also associated with poorer cognitive functioning and generally poorer prognosis.

Many primary psychiatric illnesses are associated with cognitive impairment that impacts social and occupational functioning. Given the functional impact of cognitive deficits, neuropsychological assessment should be an integral part of the management of psychiatric disorders. It is also important for neuropsychologists to appreciate how anxiety or mood symptoms can exacerbate cognitive test impairment in neurological disorders (e.g., Gillespie, 2015; Brown et al, 2014). Grosdemange et al. (2015) found that state anxiety was more deleterious to working memory for stroke patients compared with controls, although both groups were affected. Thus, state anxiety should be taken into account when evaluating patients with neurological disorders. It is critical that neuropsychologists have an appreciation of how psychiatric illness impacts cognition. Cognitive functioning impacts treatment adherence, community functioning, and employability.

References

Abramovitch, A., Abramowitz, J. S., & Mittelman, A. (2013). The neuropsychology of adult obsessive-compulsive disorder: A meta-analysis. *Clinical Psychology Review*, *33*(8), 1163–1171.

Abramovitch, A., Abramowitz, J. S., Mittelman, A., Stark, A., Ramsey, K., & Geller, D. A. (2015). Research review: Neuropsychological test performance in pediatric obsessive-compulsive disorder? A meta-analysis. *Journal of Child Psychology and Psychiatry*, *56*(8), 837–847. doi: 10.1111/jcpp.12414

Adleman, N. E., Fromm, S. J., Razdan, V., Kayser, R., Dickstein, D. P., Brotman, M. A., . . . Leibenluft, E. (2012). Cross-sectional and longitudinal abnormalities in brain structure in children with severe mood dysregulation or bipolar disorder. *Journal of Child Psychology and Psychiatry*, *53*(11), 1149–1156.

Airaksinen, E., Larsson, M., & Forsell, Y. (2005). Neuropsychological functions in anxiety disorders in population-based samples: Evidence of episodic memory dysfunction. *Journal of Psychiatric Research*, *39*(2), 207–214. doi: 10.1016/j.jpsychires.2004.06.001

Airaksinen, E., Larsson, M., Lundberg, I., & Forsell, Y. (2004). Cognitive functions in depressive disorders: Evidence from a population-based study. *Psychological Medicine*, *34*(1), 83–91.

Allen, D. N., Randall, C., Bello, D., Armstrong, C., Frantom, L., Cross, C., & Kinney, J. (2010). Are working memory deficits in bipolar disorder markers for psychosis? *Neuropsychology*, *24*(2), 244–254. doi: 10.1037/a0018159

American Psychiatric Association. (2013). *Diagnostic and Statistical Manual of Mental Disorders* (5th ed.). Arlington, VA, American Psychiatric Association. Retrieved June 1, 2013 from, dsm.psychiatryonline.org

Aminoff, S. R., Hellvin, T., Lagerberg, T. V., Berg, A. O., Andreassen, O. A., & Melle, I. (2013). Neurocognitive features in subgroups of bipolar disorder. *Bipolar Disorders*, *15*(3), 272–283. doi: 10.1111/bdi.12061

Andrés, S., Boget, T., Lázaro, L., Penadés, R., Morer, A., Salamero, M., & Castro-Fornieles, J. (2007). Neuropsychological performance in children and adolescents with obsessive-compulsive disorder and influence of clinical variables. *Biological Psychiatry*, *61*(8), 946–951. doi: 10.1016/j.biopsych.2006.07.027

Andrés, S., Lázaro, L., Salamero, M., Boget, T., Penadés, R., & Castro-Fornieles, J. (2008). Changes in cognitive dysfunction in children and adolescents with obsessive-compulsive disorder after treatment. *Journal of Psychiatric Research*, *42*(6), 507–514.

Arts, B., Jabben, N., Krabbendam, L., & van Os, J. (2011). A 2-year naturalistic study on cognitive functioning in bipolar disorder. *Acta Psychiatrica Scandinavica*, *123*(3), 190–205. doi: 10.1111/j.1600-0447.2010.01601.x

Atladottir, H. O., Gyllenberg, D., Langridge, A., Sandin, S., Hansen, S. N., Leonard, H., . . . Parner, E. T. (2015). The increasing prevalence of reported diagnoses of childhood psychiatric disorders: A descriptive multinational comparison. *European Child & Adolescent Psychiatry*, *24*(2), 173–183.

Baldessarini, R. J., Bolzani, L., Cruz, N., Jones, P. B., Lai, M., Lepri, B., . . . Vieta, E. (2010). Onset-age of bipolar disorders at six international sites. *Journal of Affective Disorders*, *121*(1), 143–146.

Basso, M. R., & Bornstein, R. A. (1999). Neuropsychological deficits in psychotic versus nonpsychotic unipolar depression. *Neuropsychology*, *13*(1), 69–75. doi: 10.1037/0894-4105.13.1.69

Baune, B. T., Li, X., & Beblo, T. (2013). Short- and long-term relationships between neurocognitive performance and general function in bipolar disorder. *Journal of Clinical and Experimental Neuropsychology*, *35*(7), 759–774. doi: 10.1080/13803395.2013.824071

Baune, B. T., Miller, R., McAfoose, J., Johnson, M., Quirk, F., & Mitchell, D. (2010). The role of cognitive impairment in general functioning in major depression. *Psychiatry Research*, *176*(2–3), 183–189. doi: http://dx.doi.org/10.1016/j.psychres.2008.12.001

Beblo, T., Sinnamon, G., & Baune, B. T. (2011). Specifying the neuropsychology of affective disorders: Clinical, demographic and neurobiological factors. *Neuropsychology Review*, *21*(4), 337–359. doi: 10.1007/s11065-011-9171-0

Beers, S. R., Rosenberg, D. R., Dick, E. L., Williams, T., O'Hearn, K. M., Birmaher, B., & Ryan, C. M. (1999). Neuropsychological study of frontal lobe function in psychotropic-naive children with obsessive-compulsive disorder. *American Journal of Psychiatry*, *157*, 1182–1183.

Biederman, J. (2003). Pediatric bipolar disorder coming of age. *Biological Psychiatry*, *53*, 931–934.

Biederman, J., Mick, E., Faraone, S. V., Spencer, T., Wilens, T., & Wozniak, J. (2003). Current concepts in validity, diagnosis and treatment of pediatric bipolar disorder. *International Journal of Neuropsychopharmacology*, *6*, 293–300.

Bilder, R. M., Howe, A. G., & Sabb, F. W. (2013). Multilevel models from biology to psychology: Mission impossible? *Journal of Abnormal Psychology*, *122*(3), 917–927. doi: 10.1037/a0032263

Bilder, R. M., Sabb, F. W., Parker, D. S., Kalar, D., Chu, W. W., Fox, J., . . . Poldrack, R. A. (2009). Cognitive ontologies for neuropsychiatric phenomics research. *Cognitive Neuropsychiatry*, *14*(4), 419–450. doi: http://doi.org/10.1080/13546800902787180

Birmaher, B. (2007). Longitudinal course of pediatric bipolar disorder. *American Journal of Psychiatry*, *164*, 537–539.

Birmaher, B. (2013). Bipolar disorder in children and adolescents. *Child and Adolescent Mental Health*, *18*(3), 140–148. doi: 10.1111/camh.12021

Blader, J. C., & Carlson, G. A. (2007). Increased rates of bipolar disorder diagnoses among U.S. child, adolescent, and adult inpatients, 1996–2004. *Biological Psychiatry*, *62*(2), 107–114. doi: http://dx.doi.org/10.1016/j.biopsych.2006.11.006

Bora, E., Yucel, M., & Pantelis, C. (2009). Cognitive endophenotypes of bipolar disorder: a meta-analysis of neuropsychological deficits in euthymic patients and their first-degree relatives. *Journal of Affective Disorders*, *113*(1), 1–20.

Bora, E., Yucel, M., Pantelis, C., & Berk, M. (2011). Meta-analytic review of neurocognition in bipolar II disorder. *Acta Psychiatrica Scandinavica*, *123*(3), 165–174.

Brennan, E., & Flessner, C. (2015). An interrogation of cognitive findings in pediatric obsessive-compulsive and related disorders. *Psychiatry Research*, *227*(2–3), 135–143. doi: 10.1016/j.psychres.2015.03.032

Brown, F. C., Westerveld, M., Langfitt, J. T., Hamberger, M., Hamid, H., Shinnar, S., . . . Spencer, S. S. (2014). Influence of anxiety on memory performance in temporal lobe epilepsy. *Epilepsy & Behavior*, *31*, 19–24. doi: 10.1016/j.yebeh.2013.10.009

Burdick, K. E., Goldberg, J. F., Harrow, M., Faull, R. N., & Malhotra, A. K. (2006). Neurocognition as a stable endophenotype in bipolar disorder and schizophrenia. *Journal of Nervous and Mental Disease*, *194*, 255–260. doi: 10.1097/01.nmd.0000207360.70337.7e

Carter, C. S., & Barch, D. M. (2007). Cognitive neuroscience-based approaches to measuring and improving treatment effects on cognition in schizophrenia: The CNTRICS initiative. *Schizophrenia Bulletin*, *33*(5), 1131–1137. doi: 10.1093/schbul/sbm081

Castaneda, A. E., Suvisaari, J., Marttunen, M., Perälä, J., Saarni, S. I., Aalto-Setälä, T., . . . Tuulio-Henriksson, A. (2011). Cognitive functioning in a population-based sample of young adults with anxiety disorders. *European Psychiatry*, *26*(6), 346–353. doi: http://dx.doi.org/10.1016/j.eurpsy.2009.11.006

Castaneda, A. E., Tuulio-Henriksson, A., Marttunen, M., Suvisaari, J., & Lönnqvist, J. (2008). A review on cognitive impairments in depressive and anxiety disorders with a focus on young adults. *Journal of Affective Disorders*, *106*(1–2), 1–27. doi: http://dx.doi.org/10.1016/j.jad.2007.06.006

Cataldo, M. G., Nobile, M., Lorusso, M. L., Battaglia, M., & Molteni, M. (2005). Impulsivity in depressed children and adolescents: A comparison between behavioral and neuropsychological data. *Psychiatry Research*, *136*, 123–133.

Chamberlain, S. R., Blackwell, A. D., Fineberg, N. A., Robbins, T. W., & Sahakian, B. J. (2005). The neuropsychology of obsessive-compulsive disorder: The importance of failures in cognitive and behavioural inhibition as candidate endophenotypic markers. *Neuroscience and Behavioural Reviews*, *29*, 399–419.

Christensen, H., Griffiths, K., Mackinnon, A., & Jacomb, P. (1997). A quantitative review of cognitive deficits in depression and alzheimer-type dementia. *Journal of the International Neuropsychological Society*, *3*(6), 631–651. doi: http://dx.doi.org/10.1017/S1355617797006310

Clark, L., Chamberlain, S. R., & Sahakian, B. J. (2009). Neurocognitive mechanisms in depression: Implications for treatment. *Annual Review of Neuroscience*, *32*, 57–74. doi: 10.1146/annurev.neuro.31.060407.125618

Costello, E. J., Erkanli, A., & Angold, A. (2006). Is there an epidemic of child or adolescent depression? *Journal of Child Psychology and Psychiatry*, *47*(12), 1263–1271.

Costello, E. J., Mustillo, S., Erkanli, A., Keeler, G., & Angold, A. (2003). Prevalence and development of psychiatric disorders in childhood and adolescence. *Archives of General Psychiatry*, *60*(8), 837–844. doi: 10.1001/archpsyc.60.8.837.

Darke, S. (1988). Anxiety and working memory capacity. *Cognition and Emotion*, *2*, 145–154.

Deckersbach, T., Nierenberg, A. A., Kessler, R., Lund, H. G., Ametrano, R. M., Sachs, G., . . . Dougherty, D. (2010). Cognitive rehabilitation for bipolar disorder: An open trial for employed patients with residual depressive symptoms. *CNS Neuroscience & Therapeutics*, *16*(5), 298–307. doi: 10.1111/j.1755-5949.2009.00110.x

Deckersbach, T., Otto, M. W., Savage, C. R., Baer, L., & Jenike, M. A. (2000). The relationship between semantic organization and memory in obsessive-compulsive disorder. *Psychotherapy and Psychosomatics*, *69*, 101–107.

Den Hartog, H., Derix, M., Van Bemmel, A., Kremer, B., & Jolles, J. (2003). Cognitive functioning in young and middle-aged unmedicated out-patients with major depression: Testing the effort and cognitive speed hypotheses. *Psychological Medicine*, *33*(8), 1443–1451.

Depp, C. A., Mausbach, B. T., Bowie, C., Wolyniec, P., Thornquist, M. H., Luke, J. R., . . . Patterson, T. L. (2012). Determinants of occupational and residential functioning in bipolar disorder. *Journal of Affective Disorders*, *136*(3), 812–818. doi: 10.1016/j.jad.2011.09.035

Depp, C. A., Mausbach, B. T., Harmell, A. L., Savla, G. N., Bowie, C. R., Harvey, P. D., & Patterson, T. L. (2012). Meta-analysis of the association between cognitive abilities and everyday functioning in bipolar disorder. *Bipolar Disorders*, *14*(3), 217–226. doi: 10.1111/j.1399-5618.2012.01011.x

Depp, C. A., Savla, G. N., de Dios, L.A.V., Mausbach, B. T., & Palmer, B. W. (2012). Affective symptoms and intra-individual variability in the short-term course of cognitive functioning in bipolar disorder. *Psychological Medicine*, *42*(7), 1409–1416. doi: 10.1017/S0033291711002662

Depp, C. A., Savla, G. N., Moore, D. J., Palmer, B. W., Stricker, J. L., Lebowitz, B. D., & Jeste, D. V. (2008). Short-term course of neuropsychological abilities in middle-aged and older adults with bipolar disorder. *Bipolar Disorders*, *10*(6), 684–690. doi: 10.1111/j.1399-5618.2008.00601.x

Dickstein, D. P., Treland, J. E., Snow, J., McClure, E. B., Mehta, M. S., Towbin, K. E., . . . Leibenluft, E. (2004). Neuropsychological performance in pediatric bipolar disorder. *Biological Psychiatry*, *55*(1), 32–39.

Doyle, A. E., Wilens, T. E., Kwon, A., Seidman, L. J., Faraone, S. V., Fried, R., . . . Biederman, J. (2005). Neuropsychological functioning in youth with bipolar disorder. *Biological Psychiatry*, *58*(7), 540–548. doi: 10.1016/j.biopsych.2005.07.019

Eysenck, M. W., Derakshan, N., Santos, R., & Calvo, M. G. (2007). Anxiety and cognitive performance: The attentional control theory. *Emotion*, *7*, 336–353.

Fontenelle, L. F., Mendlowicz, M. V., & Versiani, M. (2004). Patients with Obsessive Compulsive Disorder (OCD) displayed cognitive deficits consistent with a dorsolateral-striatal circuit. *Psychological Medicine*, *34*(1), 181–183.

Gallassi, R., Di Sarro, R., Morreale, A., & Amore, M. (2006). Memory impairment in patients with late-onset major depression: The effect of antidepressant therapy. *Journal of Affective Disorders*, *91*(2–3), 243–250. doi: http://dx.doi.org/10.1016/j.jad.2006.01.018

Geller, B., & Luby, J. (1997). Child and adolescent bipolar disorder: A review of the past 10 years. *Journal of the American Academy of Child and Adolescent Psychiatry*, *36*, 1168–1176.

Geller, B., Tillman, R., Craney, J. L., & Bolhofner, K. (2004). Four-year prospective outcome and natural history of mania in children with a prepubertal and early adolescent bipolar disorder phenotype. *Archives of General*, *61*, 459–467.

Gilbert, E., & Marwaha, S. (2013). Predictors of employment in bipolar disorder: A systematic review. *Journal of Affective Disorders*, *145*(2), 156–164. doi: 10.1016/j.jad.2012.07.009

Gillespie, D. C. (2015). Anxiety and working memory after stroke: Implications for norm-referenced methods of identifying cognitive deficits. *Journal of Neurology, Neurosurgery & Psychiatry*, *86*(5), 477–478. doi: 10.1136/jnnp-2014-309396

Glahn, D. C., Bearden, C. E., Niendam, T. A., & Escamilla, M. A. (2004). The feasibility of neuropsychological endophenotypes in the search for genes associated with bipolar affective disorder. *Bipolar Disorders*, *6*(3), 171–182. doi: 10.1111/j.1399-5618.2004.00113.x

Goldstein, B. I., Shamseddeen, W., Axelson, D. A., Kalas, C., Monk, K., Brent, D. A., . . . Birmaher, B. (2010). Clinical, Demographic, and Familial Correlates of Bipolar Spectrum Disorders among School-aged Offspring of Parents with Bipolar Disorder. *Journal of the American Academy of Child and Adolescent Psychiatry*, *49(4)*, 388–396.

Gómez-Benito, J., Guilera, G., Pino, Ó., Rojo, E., Tabarés-Seisdedos, R., Safont, G., . . . Rejas, J. (2013). The screen for cognitive impairment in psychiatry: Diagnostic-specific standardization in psychiatric ill patients. *BMC Psychiatry*, *13*, 137.

Goodwin, F. K., & Jamison, K. R. (2007). *Manic-Depressive Illness: Bipolar Disorders and Recurrent Depression*. Oxford: Oxford University Press.

Grant, B. F., Stinson, F. S., Dawson, D. A., Chou, S. P., Dufour, M. C., Compton, W., . . . Kaplan, K. (2004). Prevalence and co-occurrence of substance use disorders and independent mood and anxiety disorders: Results from the national epidemiologic survey on alcohol and related conditions. *Archives of General Psychiatry*, *61*(8), 807–816.

Grant, I., & Adams, K. M. (2009). *Neuropsychological Assessment of Neuropsychiatric and Neuromedical Disorders*. New York: Oxford University Press.

Green, M. F. (1996). What are the functional consequences of neurocognitive deficits in schizophrenia? *American Journal of Psychiatry*, *153*, 321–330.

Grisham, J. R., Anderson, T. M., Poulton, R., Moffitt, T. E., & Andrews, G. (2009). Childhood neuropsychological deficits associated with adult obsessive-compulsive disorder. *The British Journal of Psychiatry*, *195*(2), 138–141.

Grosdemange, A., Monfort, V., Richard, S., Toniolo, A., Ducrocq, X., & Bolmont, B. (2015). Impact of anxiety on verbal and visuospatial working memory in patients with acute stroke without severe cognitive impairment. *Journal of Neurology, Neurosurgery & Psychiatry*, *86*(5), 513–519. doi: 10.1136/jnnp-2014-308232

Harkin, B., & Kessler, K. (2011). The role of working memory in compulsive checking and OCD: A systematic classification of 58 experimental findings. *Clinical Psychology Review*, *31*, 1004–1021.

Harvey, P. D., Wingo, A. P., Burdick, K. E., & Baldessarini, R. J. (2010). Cognition and disability in bipolar disorder: Lessons from schizophrenia research. *Bipolar Disorders*, *12*(4), 364–375. doi: 10.1111/j.1399-5618.2010.00831.x

Hasher, L., & Zacks, R. T. (1979). Automatic and effortful processes in memory. *Journal of Experimental Psychology: General*, *108*(3), 356.

Hill, S. K., Keshavan, M. S., Thase, M. E., & Sweeney, J. A. (2004). Neuropsychological dysfunction in antipsychotic-naive first-episode unipolar psychotic depression. *The American Journal of Psychiatry*, *161*(6), 996–1003. doi: 10.1176/appi.ajp.161.6.996

Husain, M. M., Rush, A. J., Sackeim, H. A., Wisniewski, S. R., McClintock, S. M., Craven, N., . . . Hauger, R. (2005). Age-related characteristics of depression: A preliminary STAR*D report. *The American Journal of Geriatric Psychiatry*, *13*(10), 852–860. doi: 10.1176/appi.ajgp.13.10.852

Insel, T. R. (1992). Toward a neuroanatomy of obsessive—compulsive disorder. *Archives of General Psychiatry*, *49*, 739.

Jaeger, J., Berns, S., Loftus, S., Gonzalez, C., & Czobor, P. Á. (2007). Neurocognitive test performance predicts functional recovery from acute exacerbation leading to hospitalization in bipolar disorder. *Bipolar Disorders*, *9*(1), 93–102. doi: 10.1111/j.1399-5618.2007.00427.x

Jaeger, J., Berns, S., Uzelac, S., Davis-Conway, S., 2006. Neurocognitive deficits and disability in major depressive disorder. *Psychiatry Research*, *145*, 39–48.

Jarrett, M. A., & Ollendick, T. H. (2008). A conceptual review of the comorbidity of attention-deficit/hyperactivity disorder and anxiety: Implications for future research and practice. *Clinical Psychology Review*, *28*(7), 1266–1280. doi: http://dx.doi.org.proxy.its.virginia.edu/10.1016/j.cpr.2008.05.004

Jones, P. B., & Tarrant, C. J. (1999). Specificity of developmental precursors to schizophrenia and affective disorders. *Schizophrenia Research*, *39*, 121–125, discussion 161.

Joseph, M. F., Frazier, T. W., Youngstrom, E. A., & Soares, J. C. (2008). A quantitative and qualitative review of neurocognitive performance in pediatric bipolar disorder. *Journal of Child and Adolescent Psychopharmacology*, *18*(6), 595–605. doi: 10.1089/cap.2008.064

Karno, M., Golding, J. M., Sorenson, S. B., & Burnam, M. A. (1988). The epidemiology of obsessive-compulsive disorder in five US communities. *Archives of General Psychiatry*, *45*(12), 1094–1099.

Keefe, R.S.E. (1995). The contribution of neuropsychology to psychiatry. *The American Journal of Psychiatry*, *152*(1), 6–15.

Kennedy, N., & Paykel, E. S. (2004). Residual symptoms at remission from depression: Impact on long-term outcome. *Journal of Affective Disorders*, *80*(2–3), 135–144. doi: 10.1016/S0165-0327(03)00054-5

Kessler, R. C., Berglund, P. A., Demler, O., Jin, R., Koretz, D., Merikangas, K. R., . . . Wang, P. S. (2003). The epidemiology of major depressive disorder: Results from the National Comorbidity Survey Replication (NCS-R). *Journal of the American Medical Association*, *289*(23), 3095–3105.

Kessler, R. C., Berglund, P. A., Demler, O., Jin, R., & Walters, E. E. (2005). Lifetime prevalence and age-of-onset distributions of DSM-IV disorders in the National Comorbidity Survey Replication (NCS-R). *Archives of General Psychiatry*, *62*(6), 593–602.

Kessler, R. C., Chiu, W. T., Demler, O., & Walters, E. E. (2005). Prevalence, severity, and comorbidity of twelve-month DSM-IV disorders in the National Comorbidity Survey Replication (NCS-R). *Archives of General Psychiatry*, *62*(6), 617–627.

Kessler, R. C., & Wang, P. S. (2008). The descriptive epidemiology of commonly occurring mental disorders in the United States. *Annual Review of Public Health*, *29*, 115–129. doi: 10.1146/annurev.publhealth.29.020907.090847

Kiloh, L. G. (1961). Pseudo-dementia. *Acta Psychiatrica Scandinavica*, *37*(4), 336–351.

Kim, M. S., Park, S. J., Shin, M. S., & Kwon, J. S. (2002). Neuropsychological profile in patients with obsessive–compulsive disorder over a period of 4-month treatment. *Journal of Psychiatric Research*, *36*(4), 257–265.

Klein, R. G., Pine, D. S., & Klein, D. F. (1998). Resolved: Mania is mistaken for ADHD in prepubertal children. *Journal of the American Academy of Child and Adolescent Psychiatry*, *37*, 1093–1096.

Kowatch, R. A., Youngstrom, E. A., Danielyan, A., & Findling, R. L. (2005). Review and meta-analysis of the phenomenology and clinical characteristics of mania in children and adolescents. *Bipolar Disorders*, *7*(6), 483–496. doi: 10.1111/j.1399-5618.2005.00261.x

Krabbendam, L., Arts, B., van Os, J., & Aleman, A. (2005). Cognitive functioning in patients with schizophrenia and bipolar disorder: A quantitative review. *Schizophrenia Research*, *80*(2), 137–149.

Kuelz, A. K., Riemann, D., Halsband, U., Vielhaber, K., Unterrainer, J., Kordon, A., and Voderholzer, U. (2006). Neuropsychological impairment in obsessive-compulsive disorder—improvement over the course of cognitive behavioral treatment. *Journal of Clinical and Experimental Neuropsychology*, *28*, 1273–1287.

Kurtz, M. M., & Gerraty, R. T. (2009). A meta-analytic investigation of neurocognitive deficits in bipolar illness: Profile and effects of clinical state. *Neuropsychology*, *23*, 551–562.

Langenecker, S. A., Saunders, E.F.H., Kade, A. M., Ransom, M. T., & McInnis, M. G. (2010). Intermediate: Cognitive phenotypes in bipolar disorder. *Journal of Affective Disorders*, *122*(3), 285–293. doi: 10.1016/j.jad.2009.08.018

Lee, R.S.C., Hermens, D. F., Porter, M. A., & Redoblado-Hodge, M. A. (2012). A meta-analysis of cognitive deficits in first-episode major depressive disorder. *Journal of Affective Disorders*, *140*(2), 113–124.

Lee, R.S.C., Hermens, D. F., Scott, J., Redoblado-Hodge, M., Naismith, S. L., Lagopoulos, J., . . . Hickie, I. B. (2014). A meta-analysis of neuropsychological functioning in first-episode bipolar disorders. *Journal of Psychiatric Research*, *57*, 1–11. doi: 10.1016/j.jpsychires.2014.06.019

Lewandowski, K. E., Cohen, B. M., & Öngur, D. (2011). Evolution of neuropsychological dysfunction during the course of schizophrenia and bipolar disorder. *Psychological Medicine*, *41*(2), 225–241. doi: 10.1017/S0033291710001042

Lim, C. S., Baldessarini, R. J., Vieta, E., Yucel, M., Bora, E., & Sim, K. (2013). Longitudinal neuroimaging and neuropsychological changes in bipolar disorder patients: Review of the evidence. *Neuroscience & Biobehavioral Reviews*, *37*(3), 418–435.

Lisanby, S. H. (2007). Electroconvulsive therapy for depression. *New England Journal of Medicine*, *357*, 1939–1945.

Livingston, R. B., Stark, K. D., Haak, R. A., & Jennings, E. (1996). Neuropsychological profiles of children with depressive and anxiety disorders. *Child Neuropsychology*, *2*(1), 48–62. doi: 10.1080/09297049608401350

López-Jaramillo, C., Lopera-Vásquez, J., Ospina-Duque, J., García, J., Gallo, A., Cortez, V., . . . Vieta, E. (2010). Lithium treatment effects on the neuropsychological functioning of patients with bipolar I disorder. *Journal of Clinical Psychiatry*, *71*(8), 1055–1060. doi: 10.4088/JCP.08m04673yel

Loring, D. W., Marino, S. E., Parfitt, D., Finney, G. R., & Meador, K. J. (2012). Acute lorazepam effects on neurocognitive performance. *Epilepsy & Behavior*, *25*(3), 329–333. doi: http://dx.doi.org/10.1016/j.yebeh.2012.08.019

Luby, J. L. (2009). Early childhood depression. *The American Journal of Psychiatry*, *166*(9), 974–979. doi: 10.1176/appi.ajp.2009.08111709

Mann-Wrobel, M., Carreno, J. T., & Dickinson, D. (2011). Meta-analysis of neuropsychological functioning in euthymic bipolar disorder: An update and investigation of moderator variables. *Bipolar Disorders, 13*(4), 334–342. doi: 10.1111/j.1399-5618.2011.00935.x

Marcopulos, B. A., Fujii, D., O'Grady, J., Shaver, G., Manley, J., & Aucone, E. (2008). Providing neuropsychological services for persons with schizophrenia: A review of the literature and prescription for practice. In J. Morgan & J. Ricker (Eds.), *Textbook of Clinical Neuropsychology* (pp. 743–761). New York: Taylor & Francis.

Marcopulos, B. A., & Kurtz, M. (Eds.). (2012). *Clinical Neuropsychological Foundations of Schizophrenia*. New York: Psychology Press.

Martínez-Arán, A., Torrent, C., Solé, B., Bonnín, C. M., Rosa, A. R., Sánchez-Moreno, J., & Vieta, E. (2011). Functional remediation for bipolar disorder. *Clinical Practice and Epidemiology in Mental Health, 7*, 112–116. doi: 10.2174/1745017901107010112

Martínez-Arán, A., Vieta, E., Reinares, M., Colom, F., Torrent, C., Sánchez-Moreno, J., . . . Salamero, M. (2004). Cognitive function across manic or hypomanic, depressed, and euthymic states in bipolar disorder. *The American Journal of Psychiatry, 161*(2), 262–270. doi: 10.1176/appi.ajp.161.2.262

Mataix-Cols, D., & van den Heuvel, O. A. (2006). Common and distinct neural correlates of obsessive—compulsive and related disorders. *Psychiatric Clinics of North America, 29*, 391–410.

Mathers, C., Fat, D. M., & Boerma, J. T. (2008). *The Global Burden of Disease: 2004 Update*. Geneva, Switzerland: World Health Organization.

Matthews, K., Coghill, D., & Rhodes, S. (2008). Neuropsychological functioning in depressed adolescent girls. *Journal of Affective Disorders, 111*, 113–118.

McClintock, S. M., Choi, J., Deng, Z.-D., Appelbaum, L. G., Krystal, A. D., & Lisanby, S. H. (2014). Multifactorial determinants of the neurocognitive effects of electroconvulsive therapy. *Journal of ECT, 30*(2), 165–176.

McClintock, S. M., Husain, M. M., Greer, T. L., & Cullum, C. M. (2010). Association between depression severity and neurocognitive function in major depressive disorder: A review and synthesis. *Neuropsychology, 24*(1), 9–34. doi: 10.1037/a0017336

Medalia, A., Revheim, N., & Herlands, T. (2009). *Cognitive Remediation for Psychological Disorders: Therapist Guide*. Oxford: Oxford University Press.

Merikangas, K. R., Akiskal, H. S., Angst, J., Greenberg, P. E., Hirschfeld, R.M.A., Petukhova, M., & Kessler, R. C. (2007). Lifetime and 12-month prevalence of bipolar spectrum disorder in the national comorbidity survey replication. *Archives of General Psychiatry, 64*(5), 543–552. doi: 10.1001/archpsyc.64.5.543

Mesholam-Gately, R., Giuliano, A. J., Zillmer, E. A., Barakat, L. P., Kumar, A., Gur, R. C., . . . Moberg, P. J. (2012). Verbal learning and memory in older adults with minor and major depression. *Archives of Clinical Neuropsychology, 27*(2), 196–207. doi: 10.1093/arclin/acr106

Meyer-Baron, M., Blaszkewicz, M., Henke, H., Knapp, G., Muttray, A., Schaper, M., & van Thriel, C. (2008). The impact of solvent mixtures on neurobehavioral performance: conclusions from epidemiological data. *Neurotoxicology, 29*, 349–360.

Micco, J. A., Henin, A., Biederman, J., Rosenbaum, J. F., Petty, C., Rindlaub, L. A., . . . Hirshfeld-Becker, D. (2009). Executive functioning in offspring at risk for depression and anxiety. *Depression and Anxiety, 26*(9), 780–790. doi: 10.1002/da.20573

Milad, M. R., & Rauch, S. L. (2012). Obsessive-compulsive disorder: Beyond segregated cortico-striatal pathways. *Trends in Cognitive Sciences, 16*, 43–51.

Moher, D., Liberati, A., Tetzlaff, J., & Altman, D. G. (2009). Preferred reporting items for systematic reviews and meta-analyses: The PRISMA statement. *Annals of Internal Medicine, 151*(4), 264–269.

Moitra, E., & Armstrong, C. L. (2013). Neural substrates for heightened anxiety in children with brain tumors. *Developmental Neuropsychology, 38*(5), 337–351. doi: 10.1080/87565641.2013.799673

Moreno, C., Laje, G., Blanco, C., Jiang, H., Schmidt, A. B., & Olfson, M. (2007). National trends in the outpatient diagnosis and treatment of bipolar disorder in youth. *Archives of General Psychiatry, 64*(9), 1032–1039. doi: 10.1001/archpsyc.64.9.1032

Moritz, S., Birkner, C., Kloss, M., Jacobsen, D., Fricke, S., Böthern, A., & Hand, I. (2001). Impact of comorbid depressive symptoms on neuropsychological performance in obsessive-compulsive disorder. *Journal of Abnormal Psychology, 110*(4), 653–657. doi: 10.1037/0021-843X.110.4.653

Moritz, S., Kloss, M., Katenkamp, C., Birkner, C., & Hand, I. (1999). Neurocognitive functioning in OCD before and after treatment. *CNS Spectrums, 4*, 21–22.

Moussavi, S., Chatterji, S., Verdes, E., Tandon, A., Patel, V., & Ustun, B. (2007). Depression, chronic diseases, and decrements in health: Results from the world health surveys. *The Lancet, 370*(9590), 851–858. doi: http://dx.doi.org/10.1016/S0140-6736(07)61415-9

Murray, R. M., Sham, P., Van Os, J., Zanelli, J., Cannon, M., & McDonald, C. (2004). A developmental model for similarities and dissimilarities between schizophrenia and bipolar disorder. *Schizophrenia Research, 71*(2–3), 405–416. doi: 10.1016/j.schres.2004.03.002

Nagane, A., Baba, H., Nakano, Y., Maeshima, H., Hukatsu, M., Ozawa, K., . . . Arai, H. (2014). Comparative study of cognitive impairment between medicated and medication-free patients with remitted major depression: Class-specific influence by tricyclic antidepressants and newer antidepressants. *Psychiatry Research, 218*(1–2), 101–105. doi: http://dx.doi.org/10.1016/j.psychres.2014.04.013

Nedelijkovic, M., Kyrios, M., Moulding, R., Doron, G., Wainwright, K., Pantelis, C., . . . Maruff, P. (2009). Differences in neuropsychological performance between subtypes of obsessive—compulsive disorder. *Australian and New Zealand Journal of Psychiatry, 43*(3), 216–226.

Newman, D. L., Moffitt, T. E., Caspi, A., Magdol, L., Silva, P. A., & Stanton, W. R. (1996). Psychiatric disorder in a birth cohort of young adults: Prevalence, comorbidity, clinical significance, and new case incidence from ages 11–21. *Journal of Consulting and Clinical Psychology, 64*(3), 552–562. doi: 10.1037/0022-006X.64.3.552

O'Jile, J. R., Schrimsher, G. W., & O'Bryant, S. E. (2005). The relation of self-report of mood and anxiety to CVLT-C, CVLT, and CVLT-2 in a psychiatric sample. *Archives of Clinical Neuropsychology, 20*(4), 547–553. doi: 10.1016/j.acn.2004.12.001

Omori, I. M., Murata, Y., Yamanishi, T., Nakaaki, S., Akechi, T., Mikuni, M., Furukawa, T. A. (2007). The differential impact of executive function on episodic memory in obsessive—compulsive disorder patients with checking symptoms vs. those with washing symptoms. *Journal of Psychiatric Research*, *41*, 776–784.

Park, S., & Kwon, S. (2008). Cognitive effects of antiepileptic drugs. *Journal of Clinical Neurology*, *4*(3), 99–106. Retrieved from, http://synapse.koreamed.org/DOIx.php?id=10.3988%2Fjcn.2008.4.3.99

Pavuluri, M. N., Henry, D. B., Nadimpalli, S. S., O'Connor, M. M., & Sweeney, J. A. (2006). Biological risk factors in pediatric bipolar disorder. *Biological Psychiatry*, *60*(9), 936–941.

Pavuluri, M. N., Schenkel, L. S., Aryal, S., Harral, E. S., Hill, S. K., Herbener, E. S., & Sweeney, J. A. (2006). Neurocognitive function in unmedicated manic and medicated euthymic, pediatric bipolar patients. *American Journal of Psychiatry*, *163*, 286–293.

Penades, R., Catalan, R., Andres, S., Salamero, M., & Gasto, C. (2005). Executive function and nonverbal memory on obsessive-compulsive disorder. *Psychiatry Research*, *133*, 81–90.

Quraishi, S., Walshe, M., McDonald, C., Schulze, K., Kravariti, E., Bramon, E., . . . Toulopoulou, T. (2009). Memory functioning in familial bipolar I disorder patients and their relatives. *Bipolar Disorders*, *11*(2), 209–214. doi: 10.1111/j.1399-5618.2008.00661.x

Rauch, S., & Baxter, L. (1998). Neuroimaging in obsessive-compulsive disorder and related disorders. In M. A. Jenike, L. Baer, & W. E. Minichiello (Eds.), *Obsessive- Compulsive Disorders: Practical Management* (Vol. 289, pp. 289–317). Boston, MA: Mosby.

Robertson, H. A., Kutcher, S. P., & Lagace, D. C. (2003). No evidence of attentional deficits in stabilized bipolar youth relative to unipolar and control comparators. *Bipolar Disorders*, *5*, 330–339.

Robinson, L. J., & Ferrier, I. N. (2006). Evolution of cognitive impairment in bipolar disorder: A systematic review of cross-sectional evidence. *Bipolar Disorders*, *8*(2), 103–116. doi: 10.1111/j.1399-5618.2006.00277.x

Rogers, M. A., Kasai, K., Koji, M., Fukuda, R., Iwanami, A., Nakagome, K., . . . Kato, N. (2004). Executive and prefrontal dysfunction in unipolar depression: A review of neuropsychological and imaging evidence. *Neuroscience Research*, *50*, 1–11.

Roiser, J. P., Elliott, R., & Sahakian, B. J. (2012). Cognitive mechanisms of treatment in depression. *Neuropsychopharmacology*, *37*(1), 117–136.

Ruscio, A. M., Stein, D. J., Chiu, W. T., & Kessler, R. C. (2010). The epidemiology of obsessive-compulsive disorder in the National Comorbidity Survey Replication. *Molecular Psychiatry*, *15*, 53–63.

Samamé, C., Martino, D. J., & Strejilevich, S. A. (2012). Social cognition in euthymic bipolar disorder: Systematic review and meta-analytic approach. *Acta Psychiatrica Scandinavica*, *125*(4), 266–280. doi: 10.1111/j.1600-0447.2011.01808.x

Samamé, C., Martino, D. J., & Strejilevich, S. A. (2013). A quantitative review of neurocognition in euthymic late-life bipolar disorder. *Bipolar Disorders*, *15*(6), 633–644. doi: 10.1111/bdi.12077

Samamé, C., Martino, D. J., & Strejilevich, S. A. (2014). Longitudinal course of cognitive deficits in bipolar disorder: A meta-analytic study. *Journal of Affective Disorders*, *164*, 130–138. doi: 10.1016/j.jad.2014.04.028

Sanchez-Moreno, J., Martinez-Aran, A., Tabares-Seisdedos, R., Torrent, C., Vieta, E., & Ayuso-Mateos, J. L. (2009). Functioning and disability in bipolar disorder: An extensive review. *Psychotherapy and Psychosomatics*, *78*(5), 285–297. doi: 10.1159/000228249

Savage, C. R., Deckersbach, T., Wilhelm, S., Rauch, S. L., Baer, L., Reid, T., & Jenike, M. A. (2000). Strategic processing and episodic memory impairment in obsessive compulsive disorder. *Neuropsychology*, *14*(1), 141–151. doi: 10.1037/0894-4105.14.1.141

Savage, C. R., & Rauch, S. L. (2000). Cognitive deficits in obsessive-compulsive disorder. *American Journal of Psychiatry*, *157*, 7.

Scahill, L., Riddle, M. A., McSwiggin-Hardin, M., Ort, S. I., King, R. A., Goodman, W. K., . . . Leckman, J.F. (1997). Children's Yale-Brown Obsessive Compulsive Scale: Reliability and validity. *Journal of American Academy Children and Adolescents Psychiatry*, *36*(6), 844–852.

Schretlen, D. J., Cascella, N. G., Meyer, S. M., Kingery, L. R., Testa, S. M., Munro, C. A., . . . Pearlson, G. D. (2007). Neuropsychological functioning in bipolar disorder and schizophrenia. *Biological Psychiatry*, *62*(2), 179–186. doi: http://dx.doi.org/10.1016/j.biopsych.2006.09.025

Segalàs, C., Alonso, P., Labad, J., Jaurrieta, N., Real, E., Jiménez, S., . . . Vallejo, J. (2008). Verbal and nonverbal memory processing in patients with obsessive-compulsive disorder: Its relationship to clinical variables. *Neuropsychology*, *22*(2), 262–272. doi: 10.1037/0894-4105.22.2.262

Shackman, A. J., Sarinopoulos, I., Maxwell, J. S., Pizzagalli, D. A., Lavric, A., & Davidson, R. J. (2006). Anxiety selectively disrupts visuospatial working memory. *Emotion*, *6*, 40–61.

Shear, P. K., DelBello, M. P., Rosenberg, H. L., & Strakowski, S. M. (2002). Parental reports of executive dysfunction in adolescents with bipolar disorder. *Child Neuropsychology*, *8*(4), 285–295.

Shin, M.-S., Choi, H., Kim, H., Hwang, J.-W., Kim, B.-N., & Cho, S.-C. (2008). A study of neuropsychological deficit in children with obsessive-compulsive disorder. *European Psychiatry*, *23*, 512e520.

Simpson, H. B., Rosen, W., Huppert, J. D., Lin, S-H., Foa, E. B. & Liebowitz, M. R. (2006). Are there reliable neuropsychological deficits in obsessive-compulsive disorder? *Journal of Psychiatric Research*, *40*, 3, 247–257

Smith, D. J., Muir, W. J., & Blackwood, D.H.R. (2006). Neurocognitive impairment in euthymic young adults with bipolar spectrum disorder and recurrent major depressive disorder. *Bipolar Disorders*, *8*(1), 40–46. doi: 10.1111/j.1399-5618.2006.00275.x

Solé, B., Martínez-Arán, A., Torrent, C., Bonnin, C. M., Reinares, M., Popovic, D., . . . Vieta, E. (2011). Are bipolar II patients cognitively impaired? A systematic review. *Psychological Medicine*, *41*(9), 1791–1803. doi: 10.1017/S0033291711000018

Suppes, T., Mintz, J., McElroy, S. L., Altshuler, L. L., Kupka, R. W., Frye, M. A., . . . Post, R. M. (2005). Mixed hypomania in 908 patients with bipolar disorder evaluated prospectively in the stanley foundation bipolar treatment network: A sex-specific phenomenon. *Archives of General Psychiatry*, *62*(10), 1089–1096. doi: 10.1001/archpsyc.62.10.1089

Sweet, J. J., Meyer, D. G., Nelson, N. W., & Moberg, P. J. (2011). The TCN/AACN 2010 "salary survey": Professional practices, beliefs, and incomes of U.S. neuropsychologists. *The Clinical Neuropsychologist*, *25*(1), 12–61. doi: 10.1080/13854046.2010.544165

Toren, P., Sadeh, M., Wolmer, L., Eldar, S., Koren, S., Weizman, R., & Laor, N. (2000). Neurocognitive correlates of anxiety disorders in children: A preliminary report. *Journal of Anxiety Disorders*, *14*(3), 239–247. doi: 10.1016/S0887-6185(99)00036-5

Torrent, C., Bonnin, C.D.M., Martínez-Arán, A., Valle, J., Amann, B. L., González-Pinto, A., . . . Vieta, E. (2013). Efficacy of functional remediation in bipolar disorder: A multicenter randomized controlled study. *American Journal of Psychiatry*, *170*(8), 852–859. doi: 10.1176/appi.ajp.2012.12070971

Torrent, C., Martinez-Arán, A., Daban, C., Amann, B., Balanzá-Martínez, V., del Mar Bonnín, C., . . . Vieta, E. (2011). Effects of atypical antipsychotics on neurocognition in euthymic bipolar patients. *Comprehensive Psychiatry*, *52*(6), 613–622. doi: http://dx.doi.org/10.1016/j.comppsych.2010.12.009

Torres, I. J., Boudreau, V. G., & Yatham, L. N. (2007). Neuropsychological functioning in euthymic bipolar disorder: A meta-analysis. *Acta Psychiatrica Scandinavica*, *116*(Suppl), 17–26. doi: 10.1111/j.1600-0447.2007.01055.x

Torres, I. J., DeFreitas, V. G., DeFreitas, C. M., Kauer-Sant'Anna, M., Bond, D. J., Honer, W. G., . . . Yatham, L. N. (2010). Neurocognitive functioning in patients with bipolar I disorder recently recovered from a first manic episode. *Journal of Clinical Psychiatry*, *71*(9), 1234–1242. doi: 10.4088/JCP.08m04997yel

van Os, J., Jones, P., Lewis, G., Wadsworth, M., & Murray, R. (1997). Developmental precursors of affective illness in a general population birth cohort. *Archives of General Psychiatry*, *54*, 625–631.

Van Rheenen, T. E., & Rossell, S. L. (2014). Let's face it: Facial emotion processing is impaired in bipolar disorder. *Journal of the International Neuropsychological Society*, *20*(2), 200–208. doi: 10.1017/S1355617713001367

Veldhuis, J., Dieleman, J. P., Wohlfarth, T., Storosum, J. G., van Den Brink, W., Sturkenboom, M. C., & Denys, D. (2012). Incidence and prevalence of "diagnosed OCD" in a primary care, treatment seeking, population. *International Journal of Psychiatry in Clinical Practice*, *16*(2), 85–92.

Visu-Petra, L., Cheie, L., Benga, O., & Packiam Alloway, T. (2011). Effects of anxiety on memory storage and updating in young children. *International Journal of Behavioral Development*, *35*(1), 38–47. doi: 10.1177/0165025410368945

Visu-Petra, L., Miclea, M., Cheie, L., & Benga, O. (2009). Processing efficiency in preschoolers' memory span: Individual differences related to age and anxiety. *Journal of Experimental Child Psychology*, *103*(1), 30–48. doi: http://dx.doi.org.proxy.its.virginia.edu/10.1016/j.jecp.2008.09.002

Vöhringer, P. A., Barroilhet, S. A., Amerio, A., Reale, M. L., Alvear, K., Vergne, D., & Ghaemi, S. N. (2013). Cognitive impairment in bipolar disorder and schizophrenia: A systematic review. *Frontiers in Psychiatry*, *4*, 87–87. doi: 10.3389/fpsyt.2013.00087

Wang, C. E., Halvorsen, M., Sundet, K., Steffensen, A. L., Holte, A., & Waterloo, K. (2006). Verbal memory performance of mildly to moderately depressed outpatient younger adults. *Journal of Affective Disorders*, *92*(2–3), 283–286. doi: 10.1016/j.jad.2006.02.008

West, S. A., McElroy, S. L., Strakowski, S. M., Keck, P. E., & McConville, B. J. (1995). Attention deficit hyperactivity disorder in adolescent mania. *American Journal of Psychiatry*, *152*(2), 271–273.

Whiteford, H. A., Degenhardt, L., Rehm, J., Baxter, A. J., Ferrari, A. J., Erskine, H. E., . . . Vos, T. (2013). Global burden of disease attributable to mental and substance use disorders: Findings from the global burden of disease study 2010. *The Lancet*, *382*(9904), 1575–1586. doi: http://dx.doi.org/10.1016/S0140-6736(13)61611-6

Wingo, A. P., Wingo, T. S., Harvey, P. D., & Baldessarini, R. J. (2009). Effects of lithium on cognitive performance: A meta-analysis. *Journal of Clinical Psychiatry*, *70*(11), 1588–1597. doi: 10.4088/JCP.08r04972

Wood, S. J., Allen, N. B., & Pantelis, C. (2009). *The Neuropsychology of Mental Illness*. New York: Cambridge University Press.

Woods, C. M., Vevea, J. L., Chambless, D. L., & Bayen, U. J. (2002). Are compulsive checkers impaired in memory? A meta-analytic review. *Clinical Psychology: Science and Practice*, *9*(4), 353–366.

Wozniak, J., Biederman, J., Kiely, K., Ablon, J. S., Faraone, S. V., Mundy, E., & Mennin, D. (1995). Mania-like symptoms suggestive of childhood-onset bipolar disorder in clinically referred children. *Journal of the American Academy of Child & Adolescent Psychiatry*, *34*(7), 867–876. doi: 10.1097/00004583-199507000-00010

Wykes, T., Huddy, V., Cellard, C., McGurk, S. R., & Czobor, P. Á. (2011). A meta-analysis of cognitive remediation for schizophrenia: Methodology and effect sizes. *The American Journal of Psychiatry*, *168*(5), 472–485. doi: 10.1176/appi.ajp.2010.10060855

30 Dementia[1]

Glenn Smith and Alissa Butts

Overview

Recent scientific insights and technological advances in the field of dementia have provided compelling evidence that neurodegenerative diseases have a decades-long prodrome that includes reliably identifiable epochs preceding the manifestation of the full syndrome of dementia. These advances in science and technology have spurred demand for new consensus diagnoses. For example, Alzheimer's disease (AD) research criteria now recognize preclinical and prodromal periods in AD development. The syndromic phases of neurodegenerative dementing illnesses are not etiologically specific, thus most neurodegenerative dementias could be seen as having parallel syndromic stages. This chapter discusses these recent reformulations of clinical and research diagnostic criteria related to dementia generally and will use AD) in particular to demonstrate the trend of these reformulations. Newer clinical criteria for diagnosing dementia are presented in the *Diagnostic and Statistical Manual of Mental Disorders,* fifth edition (DSM-5) of the American Psychiatric Association. Updates to AD research criteria have been promulgated jointly by the National Institutes on Aging and the Alzheimer's Association. The criteria serve to more clearly delineate the distinction between syndromes (e.g., preclinical state, mild cognitive impairment and dementia) and etiologies (e.g., AD, vascular dementia, Lewy body disease frontotemporal dementia). After an overview of syndromes, we review etiology-specific criteria in separate sections that will also provide an overview of the neuropsychological phenotypes of each etiology. Last, we discuss behavioral interventions to improve outcomes in neurodegenerative disease. Note that these interventions align with the syndromes rather than the etiologies.

Syndromes

Clinical Criteria

The American Psychiatric Association panel on neurocognitive disorders decided to sunset the term *dementia* (Ganguli et al., 2011) and to elevate the concept of *mild cognitive impairment* (MCI) to more formal status in DSM-5. The respective terms *major neurocognitive disorder* (MND) was included in DSM-5 to replace the dementia and *mild neurocognitive disorder* (mND) and was elevated from use in research only to full clinical criteria. The DSM-5 criteria for major and mild neurocognitive disorder are as follows (American Psychiatric Association, 2010).

Major Neurocognitive Disorder

1. Evidence of significant cognitive *decline from a previous level of performance* in one or more cognitive domains (enumerated as complex attention, executive ability, learning and memory, language, visual constructional-perceptual ability, and social cognition) based on:
   - **a** reports by the patient or a knowledgeable informant, or observation by the clinician, of clear decline in specific cognitive abilities;
     AND
   - **b** clear deficits in objective assessment of the relevant domain, which is typically > 2.0 standard deviations below the mean (or below the 2.5th percentile) of an appropriate reference population (i.e., age, gender, education, premorbid intellect, and culturally adjusted).
2. The cognitive deficits are sufficient to interfere with independence; at a minimum requiring assistance with instrumental activities of daily living (ADLs; and i.e., more complex tasks such as finances or managing medications).
3. The cognitive deficits do not occur exclusively in the context of a delirium.
4. The cognitive deficits are not wholly or primarily attributable to another Axis I disorder (e.g., major depressive disorder, schizophrenia).

Mild Neurocognitive Disorder

1. Evidence of minor cognitive decline from a previous level of performance in one or more of the domains outlined above based on:
   - **a** reports by the patient or a knowledgeable informant, or observation by the clinician, of minor levels of decline in specific abilities as outlined for

the specific domains described in Item 1 in the Major Neurocognitive Disorder list;
AND

b mild deficits on objective cognitive assessment, typically 1.0 to 2.0 standard deviations below the mean (or in the 2.5th to 16th percentile) of an appropriate reference population (i.e., age, gender, education, premorbid intellect, and culturally adjusted). When serial measurements are available, a significant (e.g., 0.5 SD) decline from the patient's own baseline would serve as more definitive evidence of decline.

2 The cognitive deficits are not sufficient to interfere with independence (instrumental ADLs are preserved), but greater effort and compensatory strategies may be required to maintain independence.
3 The cognitive deficits do not occur exclusively in the context of a delirium.
4 The cognitive deficits are not wholly or primarily attributable to another Axis I disorder (e.g., major depressive disorder, schizophrenia).

These criteria underwent field testing to establish inter-rater and test-retest reliabilities at two primary sites: the University of California, Los Angeles, and Mayo Clinic in Minnesota (Regier et al., 2013). The primary author (GES) of this chapter led the field trial at Mayo. The inter-rater reliabilities obtained for these diagnoses are listed in Table 30.1.

Note that while both the UCLA and Mayo Clinic sites had acceptable and comparable inter-rater reliabilities for MND, kappa values were discrepant between the sites for mND. This may have resulted from several differences in the conduct of the field trial at each site, including the following:

- Mayo Clinic recruited predominantly from a neuropsychological assessment lab, whereas UCLA recruited from a geriatric psychiatry clinic.
- Therefore, Mayo Clinic had neuropsychological data in adjudication of a vast majority of its cases. UCLA used neuropsychological data to render diagnoses in far fewer cases.
- Two neuropsychologists were the clinicians independently applying the diagnostic criteria in the vast majority of cases at Mayo Clinic, whereas at UCLA a psychiatrist and a neuropsychologist generally were the independent raters.
- Because Mayo Clinic had two neuropsychologists as the independent clinicians, they could view the same neuropsychological data set, thus ensuring the kappa values were based on the reliability of the criteria rather than the reliability of neuropsychological measures. At UCLA even when neuropsychological data was available, the neuropsychologist was competent to view more and interpret this more extensive and sensitive data while the expertise of the psychiatrist limits the cognitive data set to only the mental status result.

Table 30.1 Field testing inter-rater reliability of DSM-5 neurocognitive disorder diagnoses (Regier et al., 2013)

	DX	*Kappa*	*CI*	*Interpretation*
Mayo Clinic	MND	.75	.59–.9	Very good
	mND	.76	.6–.88	Very good
UCLA	MND	.8	.65–.9	Very good
	mND	.18	.03–.32	Unacceptable
Dallas VA	mND	.43	.12–.66	Unsuccessful estimate

Ultimately, the differing kappa values between the two sites strongly suggests the importance of neuropsychological data in making a reliable DSM-5 diagnosis of mND. This is entirely expectable given that mND criterion 1b specifies a range of cognitive performance detectable on neuropsychological tests that is not likely to be discerned with simple mental status screening. Conversely, the kappa values suggest that extensive neuropsychological testing might not be required to make a reliable diagnosis of MND syndrome. Here, even though criterion 1b also specifies a range of cognitive performance, the degree of cognitive impairment is so substantial that simple mental status testing likely captures the impairments. In MND, neuropsychological data may have more value in determining etiology as opposed to the presence of the syndrome.

Research Criteria

A task force of experts from the United States and Europe empanelled by the National Institute on Aging (NIA) and the Alzheimer's Association convened to propose updated and revised guidelines for the evaluation of AD related diagnoses (Jack et al., 2011). Although the mission of these panels was to specifically advance research and clinical understanding of AD, the principles apply to other forms of dementia as well. By clearly specifying that the syndromic phases *may* be due to AD the criteria acknowledge that these same syndromes may not be due to AD but rather due to another etiology. The two most notable differences of the new criteria relative to the AD criteria published in 1984 (McKhann et al., 1984) are the incorporation of underlying disease biomarkers and the recognition of different syndromic phases of disease: preclinical AD, MCI, and dementia of the AD type.

Preclinical Stage

A variety of scientific advances are permitting the possibility of identifying biomarkers for neurodegenerative disease that can or might be detected years before symptoms arise. For several decades this has been true in Huntington's disease (HD) where detection of tri-nucleotide repeats predicted with accuracy who would eventually develop symptoms

(Snell et al., 1993). Causative genetic mutations have also been established for variants of fronto-temporal dementia (Baker et al., 2006), cerebral autosomal-dominant arteriopathy with subcortical infarcts and leukoencephalopathy (CADASIL) (Peters et al., 2005), as well as for AD (Hutton & Hardy, 1997). A variety of susceptibility genes for AD (Ertekin-Taner, 2007), particularly the apolipoprotein E (APOE) gene (Corder et al., 1993), and for Parkinson's disease (PD; see Lesage & Brice, 2009) have also been detected that appear to increase the risk of disease development.

In addition to genetic markers, neuroimaging technologies now permit identification of additional biomarkers, such as amyloid (Quigley, Colloby, & O'Brien, 2011) and phosphorylated tau accumulation (Zhang et al., 2012) in the brain, as well as cerebral hypometabolism (Mosconi et al., 2008) and disintegration of nodal network resting state function (Rombouts, Barkhof, Goekoop, Stam, & Scheltens, 2005) that have been shown to be associated with AD. These various technologies permit increasing accuracy at identifying people with a neurodegenerative process even if they are asymptomatic. An important analysis by Knopman suggests that more than 50% of a population-based sample of people over the age of 70 had indicators of neurodegeneration in spite of being found cognitively normal on full neurological and neuropsychological evaluation (Knopman et al., 2013).

Generic Mild Cognitive Impairment Criteria

The NIA Alzheimer's Association work group on MCI (Albert et al., 2011) proposed a two-step process as a clinical diagnosis of "generic" MCI, suggesting that MCI is identified first then biomarker information is used to consider the etiology (of AD) with increasing levels of confidence. The "generic" criteria for MCI are as follows.

1. Concern regarding a change in cognition: There should be evidence of concern about a change in cognition, in comparison to the person's prior level. This concern can be obtained from the patient, from an informant who knows the patient well, or from a skilled clinician observing the patient.
2. Impairment in one or more cognitive domains: There should be evidence of lower performance in one or more cognitive domains that is greater than would be expected for the patient's age and educational background. If repeated assessments are available, then a decline in performance should be evident over time. This change can occur in a variety of cognitive domains, including: memory, executive function, attention, language, and visuospatial skills.
3. Preservation of independence in functional abilities: Persons with MCI commonly have mild problems performing complex functional tasks they were once able to perform, such as paying bills, preparing a meal, or shopping at the store. An individual with MCI may take more time, be less efficient, and make more errors at performing such activities than in the past. Nevertheless, individuals with MCI generally maintain independence of function in daily life with minimal aids or assistance.
4. Not demented: These cognitive changes should be sufficiently mild that there is no evidence of a significant impairment in social or occupational functioning. It should be emphasized that the diagnosis of MCI requires evidence of intraindividual change. If an individual has only been evaluated once, change will need to be inferred from the history and/or evidence that cognitive performance is impaired beyond what would have been expected for that individual. Serial evaluations are optimal to document cognitive change over time, but may not be feasible in all circumstances.

Clinically, MCI has traditionally been further divided into four subtypes: amnestic MCI-single domain, amnestic MCI-multiple domains, nonamnestic MCI-single domain, and nonamnestic MCI-multiple domains based on the nature of the cognitive impairment (Petersen et al., 2004). While the amnestic and nonamnestic MCI types are roughly as prevalent, the MCI-single domain type is more prevalent than the MCI-multiple domains type (Busse, Hensel, Guhne, Angermeyer, & Riedel-Heller, 2006). Roughly 12% of patients diagnosed with MCI convert to dementia each year, whereas 1%–2% of the general population is thought to convert from cognitively intact to dementia in one year (Crutch et al., 2013). Many studies have examined the rate and patterns of conversion from the clinical syndrome of MCI to dementia. The exploration of models predicting conversion to dementia continues. It appears that the MCI subtype helps to inform the probability of converting to a certain dementia etiology (Busse et al., 2006; Ferman et al., 2013; Knopman, 2013; Petersen et al., 2001; Smith & Bondi, 2013). Because the different dementia etiologies are now thought to include prodromal stages of MCI, the nature of the mild cognitive impairments associated with the dementia syndromes will be discussed with the differing etiologies, respectively. Suffice it to say, if the generic criteria for MCI are met, the clinician then endeavors to determine the cause or etiology of the MCI.

Generic Dementia

The updated criteria for the syndrome of dementia (McKhann et al., 2011) remain much as they have since the McKhann criteria of 1984 (McKhann et al., 1984) and as generally stated in DSM-5 (American Psychological Association, 2011). Namely, dementia is diagnosed when there is evidence of the following.

- Impairment in two or more aspects of cognitive function that

- represent a decline from a previously higher level of cognitive functions and
- are sufficient to interfere with normal daily function and
- do not occur exclusively in the context of delirium.

Dementia syndromes broadly classified as "cortical" or "subcortical." This classification is a heuristic and it should be acknowledged that on autopsy "cortical" dementia will often include neuropathology in the subcortical regions and vice versa. The classification is largely based on the distribution and overall pattern of typical cognitive impairment (Crutch et al., 2012; Salmon & Filoteo, 2007). In general, "cortical" dementias tend to produce cognitive deficits affecting learning and memory, language, visuospatial skills, and executive functioning. "Subcortical" dementias, in addition to motor dysfunction, tend to produce slowness of thought, and also include early prominent deficits in executive function, and visuoperceptual and constructional abilities. Interestingly, the "subcortical" dementias tend to show only mild or moderate memory and language impairments that are both quantitatively and qualitatively different from those of cortical dementia patients. For example, compared to what can be seen in "cortical" dementias, such as AD, losses in semantic knowledge, or in its organization, do not occur in subcortical dementia syndromes, such as HD or PD. In addition, subcortical dementia patients appear to benefit more from phonemic cues because the cues help to obviate word retrieval difficulties whereas "cortical" dementias do not.

It is not uncommon for a patient to present with both "cortical" and "subcortical" features on neuropsychological testing, resulting in a mixed "cortical/subcortical" dementia picture. Typical AD is often considered a "cortical" dementia, whereas vascular dementia and PD are generally classified as "subcortical." Fronto-temporal dementia and dementia due to Lewy body disease commonly appear as with a mixed cortical/subcortical presentation. The specific neuropsychological profiles of these particular syndromes will be discussed later in this chapter, in the sections entitled the "Neuropsychological Profile of . . ." Subcortical dementias, such as PD dementia, in addition to the motor disorder, usually demonstrate slowness of thought and deficits in executive functions and visuoperceptual and constructional abilities.

Etiologies

Alzheimer's Disease

As discussed, updated guidelines now propose definitions for preclinical AD (Sperling et al., 2011). This asymptomatic stage is assumed to be present well before the development of dementia or even MCI. These operational research criteria for preclinical stages rely on different biomarkers, which are not yet validated for clinical use. These stages are described as follows:

1. Stage 1. Biomarker evidence of amyloid-β accumulation (asymptomatic cerebral amyloidosis), including
   - **a** elevated tracer retention on PET amyloid imaging, and/or
   - **b** low Aβ42 in cerebrospinal fluid (CSF) assay.
2. Stage 2. Additional biomarker evidence of synaptic dysfunction and/or early neurodegeneration (i.e., evidence of amyloid positivity + presence of one or more additional AD markers), including
   - **a** elevated CSF tau or phospho-tau,
   - **b** hypometabolism in an AD-like pattern (i.e., posterior cingulate, precuneus, and/or temporo-parietal cortices) on Fluorodeoxyglucose-Postitron Emission Tomography (FDG-PET), and
   - **c** cortical thinning/gray matter loss in AD-like anatomic distribution (i.e., lateral and medial parietal, posterior cingulate and lateral temporal cortices) and/or hippocampal atrophy on volumetric magnetic resonance imaging (MRI).
3. Stage 3. Evidence of subtle cognitive decline, but does not meet criteria for MCI or dementia (i.e., amyloid positivity + markers of neurodegeneration + very early cognitive symptoms), including
   - **a** demonstrated cognitive decline over time on standard cognitive tests, but not meeting criteria for MCI; and
   - **b** subtle impairment on challenging cognitive tests, particularly accounting for level of innate ability or cognitive reserve but not meeting criteria for MCI.

Criteria for the Diagnosis of MCI Due to AD

As discussed, directly preceding the dementia stage, the MCI stage is characterized by mild changes in cognition that are noticeable and measureable but do not disrupt day-to-day functioning. Biomarker ascertainment is used to establish level of confidence that the MCI is due to AD. Low confidence is reflected in the term *MCI with neurodegenerative etiology*. Intermediate confidence is described as MCI with presumed AD, and highest confidence is termed *prodromal AD* (Albert, et al., 2011).

MCI OF A NEURODEGENERATIVE ETIOLOGY

The criteria outlined on p. 717 for MCI with a presumed degenerative etiology represents the typical presentation of individuals who are at an increased risk of progressing to AD dementia (Petersen et al., 1999). These individuals typically have a prominent impairment in episodic memory (i.e., amnestic-MCI), but other patterns of cognitive impairment can also progress to AD dementia over time (e.g., executive dysfunction/nonamnestic MCI or multidomain MCI). Negative or ambiguous biomarker evidence (from either topographic or molecular biomarkers) is still consistent with the possibility that the patient with MCI has underlying AD pathology. However, if the biomarkers are negative for AD neuropathology, the likelihood that the diagnosis is due to AD, as opposed to an alternate cause, is low (Albert et al., 2011).

MCI OF THE ALZHEIMER TYPE

If the subject meets the MCI criteria on p. 717 but, in addition, has one or more topographic biomarkers associated with the "downstream" effects of AD pathology (e.g., MRI evidence of medial temporal atrophy, or FDG PET evidence of decreased temporoparietal metabolism, adjusting for age), then there is increased likelihood that the outcome will be AD dementia. In the absence of molecular biomarker information (or equivocal findings from molecular biomarkers) the presentation of cognitive impairment may still be consistent with an intermediate level of certainty that the individual will progress to AD dementia over time.

PRODROMAL ALZHEIMER'S DEMENTIA

If the subject meets the MCI criteria on p. 717, and in addition has a positive biomarker for the molecular neuropathology of AD (e.g., lower CSF Aß-42 and raised CSF tau measures), this provides the highest level of certainly that over time the individual will progress to AD dementia. This level of certainty would be increased even further if the individual has positive topographic biomarker evidence of AD. However, the absence of such topographic biomarker evidence (or equivocal or normal findings) is still consistent with the highest level of certainty that the individual will progress to AD dementia over time.

Dementia Due to Alzheimer's Disease

This stage is the most recognizable due to clear impairments in memory, cognition, and behavior that affect a person's ability to function independently in everyday life. The criteria for the diagnosis of AD dementia are based on the same criteria created almost three decades prior (McKhann et al., 1984) and attempt to update and clarify the diagnosis of dementia due to AD from other causes. These revised 2011 criteria (McKhann, 2011) include the following.

1 Insidious onset, in that symptoms have a gradual onset over months to years, and the onset was not sudden over hours or days; and,

2 clear-cut history of worsening cognition by report or observation; and

3 cognitive deficits are evident on history and examination in one of the two categories, including the following:
- **a** Amnestic presentation. The most common syndromic presentation of AD dementia. The deficits should include impairment in learning and recall of recently learned information. There should also be evidence of cognitive dysfunction in other cognitive domains.
- **b** Nonamnestic presentation:
  - **i** Language presentation: The most prominent deficits are in word-finding, but dysfunction in other cognitive domains should be present.
  - **ii** Visual presentation: The most prominent deficits are in spatial cognition, including object agnosia, impaired face recognition, simultanagnosia and alexia. Deficits in other cognitive domains should be present.
  - **iii** Executive presentation: The most prominent deficits are in impaired reasoning, judgment and problem solving. Deficits in other cognitive domains should be present.

In addition, characterization of AD dementia based on level of certainty was proposed with the introduction of a novel neuropathology qualifier (McKhann et al., 2011).

PATHOLOGICALLY PROVEN AD DEMENTIA

Meets clinical and cognitive criteria for probable AD dementia during life AND is proven AD by pathological examination.

CLINICAL AD DEMENTIA

The "Probable" and "Possible" qualifiers of the 1984 (McKhann et al., 1984) criteria were retained:

PROBABLE AD DEMENTIA

Meets clinical and cognitive criteria for AD dementia given on p. 719, AND without evidence of any alternative diagnoses, in particular, no significant cerebrovascular disease. In persons who meet the basic criteria for probable AD dementia, the diagnosis of probable AD dementia can be enhanced by one of these three features that increase certainty:

1 *Documented decline*: Has evidence of progressive cognitive decline on subsequent evaluations based on information from informants and cognitive testing in the context of either brief mental status examinations or formal neuropsychological evaluation;
OR

2 *Biomarker positive*: Has one or more of the following supporting biomarkers.
- **a** Low CSF Aβ42, elevated CSF tau or phospho tau

- **b** Positive amyloid PET imaging
- **c** Decreased FDG uptake on PET in temporoparietal cortex
- **d** Disproportionate atrophy on structural MRI in medial temporal lobe (especially hippocampus), basal and lateral temporal lobe, and medial parietal isocortex;

  OR

3 *Mutation carrier*: Meets clinical and cognitive criteria for AD dementia and has a proven AD autosomal dominant genetic mutation (PSEN1, PSEN2, APP).

POSSIBLE AD DEMENTIA

1 *Atypical Course*: Evidence for progressive decline is lacking or uncertain but meets other clinical and cognitive criteria for AD dementia;
OR
2 *Biomarkers Obtained and Negative*: Meets clinical and cognitive criteria for AD dementia but biomarkers (CSF, or structural or functional brain imaging) do not support the diagnosis;
OR
3 *Mixed Presentation*: Meets clinical and cognitive criteria for AD dementia but there is evidence of concomitant cerebrovascular disease; this would mean that there is more than one lacunar infarct; or a single large infarct; or extensive and severe white matter hyperintensity changes; or evidence for some features of dementia with Lewy bodies (DLB) that do not achieve a level of a diagnosis of probable DLB.

Not AD Dementia

1 Does not meet clinical criteria for AD dementia;
OR
2 Has sufficient evidence for an alternative diagnosis such as human immunodeficiency virus (HIV), HD, or others that rarely, if ever, overlap with AD.

A Note on Biomarkers

It has become increasingly clear that certain biomarkers, like those that associate with amyloid levels, are specific to etiology but do not associate well with disease burden (Knopman et al., 2013). Others, like levels of tau in CSF, are not etiologically specific but do associate with degree of brain involvement and therefore with cognitive, behavioral, and functional changes. Current etiological and disease burden biomarkers are listed in Table 30.2. Although used primarily to define syndrome phases, cognition itself can be thought of as a disease burden biomarker as neuropsychological measures meet the definition of a biomarker (Fields, Ferman, Boeve, & Smith, 2011).

Table 30.2 Etiological and disease burden biomarkers

Etiologic	*Burden of Disease*
Genes	Structural MRI
Amyloid Burden	Functional MRI
	CSF Tau
REM Sleep Behavior Disorder	Cognition

Neuropsychology of Alzheimer's Disease

Conventional wisdom holds that the pathophysiologic changes of AD begin years prior to the clinically evident manifestations of the disease (Crutch et al., 2013). As noted, more than 50% of older adults in a population-based sample with confirmed cognitive normality are positive for neurodegenerative biomarkers on neuroimaging (Knopman et al., 2013). The distribution of etiologic versus neurodegenerative biomarkers in this population-based sample is presented in Table 30.2. The significant number of older adults with positive biomarker findings but ostensibly normal cognition is used to suggest a late appearance of cognitive changes in AD (Jack et al., 2010). This proposed late staging of the cognitive decline in AD would appear to ignore the large body of literature on preclinical episodic memory changes and its predictive power for the development of AD some years later. In fact, data from the Alzheimer Disease Neuroimaging Initiative (ADNI) suggests that memory changes are the first measurable "biomarker" for AD (see Figure 30.1) (Jedynak et al., 2012).

Three other studies from ADNI compared the utility of genetic, CSF, neuroimaging biomarkers and neuropsychological measures, as well as their combinations, to predict progression from MCI to AD. Interestingly, these studies found cognitive, rather than the other biomarkers, had the strongest predictive power for progression to dementia (Gomar et al., 2011; Heister et al., 2011; Landau et al., 2010).

Earliest Neuropsychological Changes of Alzheimer's Disease

OVERVIEW

The pattern of performance on measures of episodic and semantic memory, visuospatial skills, and specific aspects of attention, working memory, and executive function, is important in the differential diagnosis of AD compared to other, predominantly subcortical, dementias. The general profile of impairment in the cortical dementia of typical AD is characterized by prominent deficits in new learning and delayed recall with additional challenges to language and semantic memory, abstract reasoning, executive functions, with possible later involvement of attention, constructional and visuospatial abilities (Salmon & Bondi, 2009; Salmon & Filoteo, 2007; Smith et al., 2007).

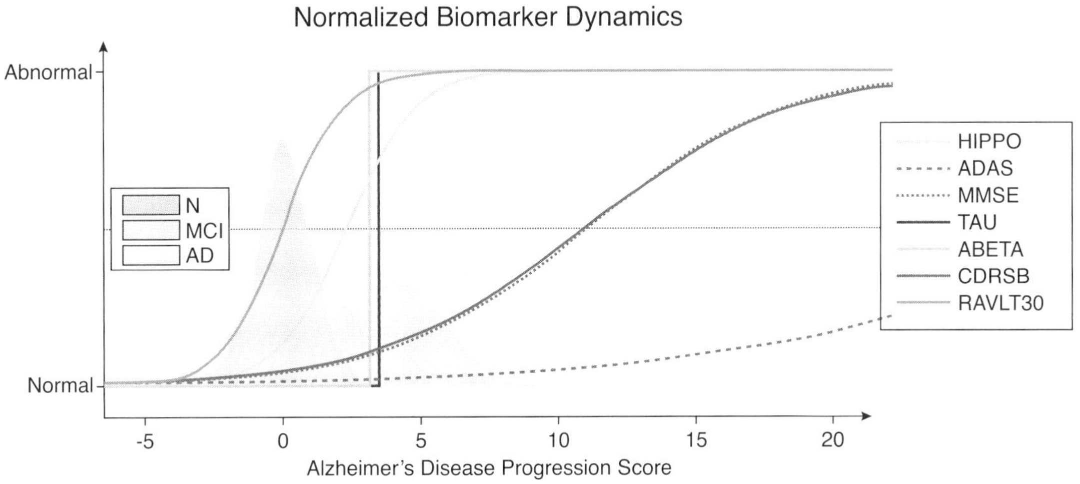

Figure 30.1 Estimated time course of disease progression. Hippo = MRI-measured hippocampal volume. ADAS = Alzheimer's Disease Assessment Score. MMSE = Mini-Mental State Exam. Tau and ABETA = Tau and Abeta42 levels in CSF. CDRSB = Clinical Dementia Rating Sum of Box scores. RAVLT30 = 30-minute delayed recall score for the Rey Auditory Verbal Learning Test. Reproduced from Jedynak et al. 2013 with permission.

MEMORY

Episodic memory changes have long been documented to appear in AD *prior* to the diagnosis of either dementia or MCI (Albert, Moss, Tanzi, & Jones, 2001; Bäckman, Small, & Fratiglioni, 2001; Chen et al., 2001; Fuld, Masur, Blau, Crystal, & Aronson, 1990; Grober & Kawas, 1997; Howieson et al., 1997; Jacobs et al., 1995; Lange et al., 2002). On average, individuals with preclinical AD show a significant decline in the retention aspects of episodic memory about four to five years prior to diagnosis (Chen et al., 2001; Lange et al., 2002). Following this decline in retention, retention stabilizes before it precipitously declines about one year prior to diagnosis of the dementia syndrome (Smith et al., 2007). In contrast to retention, encoding (or learning efficiency) appears to decline monotonically prior to diagnosis (Smith et al., 2007).

FLUENCY AND NAMING

AD patients exhibit a more pronounced impairment on category fluency than letter fluency, suggesting a breakdown in semantic knowledge access in AD (Henry, Crawford, & Phillips, 2004). AD patients also tend to make semantically based errors on confrontation naming (Salmon & Filoteo, 2007) though naming impairments are not consistently present in AD (Testa, Ivnik, & Smith, 2003).

EXECUTIVE FUNCTION

Early executive function impairments in AD occur in cognitive processes involved in divided attention, working memory, concept formation, and problem solving (Aretouli & Brandt, 2010; Salmon & Bondi, 2009).

VISUOSPATIAL SKILLS

Deficits in visuospatial skills and constructional praxis, though commonly observed in AD, tend to emerge later in the course of the disease (e.g., Mielke et al., 2007) except in the visual variant of AD, also known as posterior cortical atrophy (PCA) (Tang-Wai et al., 2004). That is, the PCA variant of AD differs from the typical AD neurocognitive profile in that the visuospatial deficits are most generally the presenting concern and most salient cognitive dysfunction causing disruption to ADLs, while memory and language skills are relatively preserved (Crutch et al., 2012; Crutch et al., 2013).

ASSOCIATED CLINICAL FEATURES

Behavioral disturbances are common in AD. Indeed, delusions of infidelity were the presenting complaint of Dr. Alzheimer's original AD patient, Auguste D (Alzheimer, 1906). Behavioral symptoms can contribute to differential diagnosis of dementia type, and it is often the absence or late onset of these symptoms that characterizes AD (McKeith et al., 2005). For example, disinhibition is often an early symptom of behavioral variant fronto-temporal dementia but a late symptom in AD. Moreover, late onset hallucinations is one feature distinguishing AD from Lewy body disease, in which hallucinations are an early phenomena (Ferman et al., 2003).

Rates (presumably point prevalence) of neuropsychiatric behavior in AD range from 57% for apathy, 28% for delusion, 13% for hallucination rates, and 5% for euphoria (Johnson, Watts, Chapin, Anderson, & Burns, 2011). Cumulative incidence of hallucinations and delusions is reported as 20% at one year, 36% at two, 50% at three, and 51% at four years post–baseline testing (Paulsen et al., 2000). However, the classification of neuropsychiatric symptoms using standard psychiatric nomenclature oversimplifies and often mislabels behavior. A person with dementia may forget storing valuables and deduce they have been stolen when he or she cannot find the items. Calling this paranoid or delusional ignores that the essence of this problem is memory and reasoning failure, not the persecutory bias or paranoia. Failure to identify the cognitive deficits of AD and/or apply psychiatric nomenclature that may ignore these deficits can lead family and health professionals to mislabel and mistreat behaviors. Furthermore, this misattribution of the cognitive deficits may lead to inflated prevalence estimates for psychosis in AD. Other behavioral disturbances that may occur throughout the different stages of AD are wandering, repetitive questioning, shadowing, aggressiveness, apathy, sleep disorder, hoarding, and resistance to help with daily activities (Johnson et al., 2011).

Behavioral and psychological disturbances in AD often also relate directly to the cognitive symptoms. Importantly, these noncognitive symptoms may be responsive to specific behavioral therapies and approaches (Rodda, Morgan, & Walker, 2009; Rovner, Steele, Shmuely, & Folstein, 1996; Schneider, Pollock, & Lyness, 1990; Small et al., 1997; Sultzer et al., 2008; Teri et al., 1992). Some specific examples and strategies are offered in the Intervention section.

Vascular Dementia

In 2011, a joint American Heart Association/American Stroke Association workgroup published consensus definitions and recommendations for the vascular contributions to cognitive impairment and dementia (Gorelick et al., 2011). This statement introduces vascular cognitive impairment (VCI) to include the range from MCI syndrome (denoted as VaMCI) to dementia (denoted as VaD). These criteria excluded persons with active drug or alcohol abuse/dependence in the last three months and those with delirium.

VaMCI

As discussed with the general criteria for MCI, the diagnosis of VaMCI may be further described as single domain amnestic, amnestic plus other domains, nonamnestic single domain, and nonamnestic multiple domains based on the cognitive domain(s) impaired by vasculopathy. These criteria require assessment of the same four domains listed earlier (executive/attention, memory, language, and visuospatial functions). Instrumental ADLs could be normal or mildly impaired, independent of the presence of motor/sensory symptoms.

PROBABLE VAMCI

1. There is cognitive impairment and imaging evidence of cerebrovascular disease, and
   - **a** There is a clear temporal relationship between a vascular event (e.g., clinical stroke) and onset of cognitive deficits; or,
   - **b** There is a clear relationship in the severity and pattern of cognitive impairment and the presence of diffuse, subcortical cerebrovascular disease pathology (e.g., as in CADASIL).
2. There is no history of gradually progressive cognitive deficits before or after the stroke that suggests the presence of a nonvascular neurodegenerative disorder.

POSSIBLE VAMCI

There is cognitive impairment and imaging evidence of cerebrovascular disease, but,

1. There is no clear relationship (temporal, severity, or cognitive pattern) between the vascular disease (e.g., silent infarcts, subcortical small-vessel disease) and onset of cognitive deficits.
2. There is insufficient information for the diagnosis of VaMCI (e.g., clinical symptoms suggest the presence of vascular disease, but no CT/MRI studies are available).
3. Severity of aphasia precludes proper cognitive assessment. However, patients with documented evidence of normal cognitive function (e.g., annual cognitive evaluations) before the clinical event that caused aphasia could be classified as having probable VaMCI.
4. There is evidence of other neurodegenerative diseases or conditions in addition to cerebrovascular disease that may affect cognition, such as the following.
   - **a** A history of other neurodegenerative disorders (e.g., Parkinson disease, progressive supranuclear palsy, dementia with Lewy bodies);
   - **b** The presence of AD pathology is confirmed by biomarkers (e.g., PET, CSF, amyloid ligands) or genetic studies (e.g., PS1 mutation); or,
   - **c** A history of active cancer or psychiatric or metabolic disorders that may affect cognitive function.

UNSTABLE VAMCI

Subjects with the diagnosis of probable or possible VaMCI whose symptoms revert to normal should be classified as having "unstable VaMCI."

Dementia

The 2011 criteria include the standard diagnosis of dementia, based on a decline in cognitive function from a prior baseline and a deficit in performance in two cognitive domains from among the set executive/attention, memory, language, and visuospatial function (Gorelick et al., 2011). The requirement that the deficits are of sufficient severity to affect a person's ADLs includes the caveat that the impairments in

ADLs are independent of the motor/sensory sequelae of a vascular event.

Criteria required to meet the respective stage and diagnostic confidence of VaD are:

PROBABLE VAD

1. There is cognitive impairment and imaging evidence of cerebrovascular disease.
2. There is a clear temporal relationship between a vascular event (e.g., clinical stroke) and onset of cognitive deficits, or there is a clear relationship in the severity and pattern of cognitive impairment and the presence of diffuse, subcortical cerebrovascular disease pathology (e.g., as in CADASIL).
3. There is no history of gradually progressive cognitive deficits before or after the stroke that suggests the presence of a nonvascular neurodegenerative disorder.

POSSIBLE VAD

There is cognitive impairment and imaging evidence of cerebrovascular disease, but:

1. There is no clear relationship (temporal, severity, or cognitive pattern) between the vascular disease (e.g., silent infarcts, subcortical small-vessel disease) and the cognitive impairment.
2. There is insufficient information for the diagnosis of VaD (e.g., clinical symptoms suggest the presence of vascular disease, but no CT/MRI studies are available).
3. Severity of aphasia precludes proper cognitive assessment. However, patients with documented evidence of normal cognitive function (e.g., annual cognitive evaluations) before the clinical event that caused aphasia could be classified as having probable VaD.
4. There is evidence of other neurodegenerative diseases or conditions in addition to cerebrovascular disease that may affect cognition, such as the following.
   a. A history of other neurodegenerative disorders (e.g., Parkinson disease, progressive supranuclear palsy, dementia with Lewy bodies);
   b. The presence of AD biology is confirmed by biomarkers (e.g., PET, CSF, amyloid ligands) or genetic studies (e.g., PS1 mutation); or
   c. A history of active cancer or psychiatric or metabolic disorders that may affect cognitive function.

Neuropsychology of Vascular Dementia

As noted in the AD section on p. 720, distinct patterns of performance on tests of episodic and semantic memory, visuospatial skills, and specific aspects of executive function, are important in the differential diagnosis of AD versus VaD. Some investigators express doubt that cognitive profiles are useful in separating AD from VaD (Schneider, Boyle, Arvanitakis, Bienias, & Bennett, 2007; Schneider, Wilson, Bienias, Evans, & Bennett, 2004; Wilson et al., 2011), not only because cerebrovascular disease contributes to some of the same domains of cognitive impairment as in AD (e.g., executive function), but also because of the common occurrence of mixed pathologic processes (Mielke et al., 2007) . Some authors suggest that many cases of dementia meeting the original criteria for the clinical diagnosis of probable AD (McKhann et al., 1984) have been shown to arise from mixed pathologies (Schneider, Arvanitakis, Leurgans, & Bennett, 2009; Sonnen et al., 2007).

The cortical versus subcortical neuropsychological patterns, as described on p. 718 (Salmon & Filoteo, 2007), are helpful in considering diagnoses of "pure" AD versus VCI versus "mixed" pathologies if there is sensitivity to the notion that cognitive domains may have subcomponents that are differentially impaired with the cortical/subcortical heuristic. For example, episodic memory includes learning efficiency and recall/retention. A simple difference drawn between impaired retention in the case of AD (i.e., rapid forgetting) versus impaired learning efficiency in the case of subcortical ischemic VaD (i.e., retrieval deficit) can help contribute to differential diagnosis.

EPISODIC MEMORY AND EXECUTIVE FUNCTIONS

Patients with subcortical VaD are generally more impaired than those with AD on tests of executive functions, whereas patients with AD are more impaired than those with subcortical VaD on tests of episodic memory (Desmond, 2004; Graham, Emery, & Hodges, 2004; Kertesz & Clydesdale, 1994; Lafosse et al., 1997; Lamar et al., 1997) but see Reed and colleagues (Reed et al., 2004; Reed et al., 2007) for a differing opinion. These studies also suggest that executive dysfunction is the most conspicuous deficit associated with subcortical VaD, perhaps because the subcortical pathology frequently interrupts fronto-subcortical circuits that mediate this aspect of cognition. VaD patients with significant white matter abnormalities on imaging demonstrate a profile of greater executive dysfunction and visuoconstructive impairments than impairment of memory and language abilities (Cosentino et al., 2004; Price, Jefferson, Merino, Heilman, & Libon, 2005; Reed et al., 2004; Reed et al., 2007). The executive dysfunction observed in small vessel ischemic VaD is also qualitatively distinct from that in AD (Seidel, Tiovannetti, & Libon, 2011). The executive control deficits seen in VaD tend to be ubiquitous not merely limited to the types of executive function problems noted in the AD section above.

VaD patients tend to demonstrate better episodic memory performance relative to patients with AD (Duke & Kaszniak, 2000) and the time course of the deficit profiles differ. That is, although executive function impairments are present in AD, they are less prominent than the episodic memory disorder during mild stages of AD and tend to become more pronounced later in the course of the illness. In contrast, patients with VaD may demonstrate executive dysfunction earlier in the disease progression and it tends to be greater than or at least equal to the degree of memory dysfunction (Reed et al., 2004; Reed et al., 2007).

FLUENCY AND NAMING

The output on tests of letter fluency produced by VaD patients is reduced relative to AD patients while the output on category (animal) fluency is similar to AD patients (Canning, Leach, Stuss, Ngo, & Black, 2004; Carew, Lamar, Cloud, Grossman, & Libon, 1997; Lafosse et al., 1997). The selective loss of semantic knowledge in AD impacts category fluency but mostly spares lexical fluency, whereas lexical fluency and other speed tests often are impaired in VaD due to "subcortical slowing" and not due to loss of semantic knowledge. Language disturbance is rarely specifically characterized in many studies of VaD, though one study failed to show group differences between AD and VaD on a confrontation-naming task (Laine, Vuorinen, & Rinne, 1997). Of course, in the absence of left middle cerebral artery infarction affecting language function, subcortical ischemic VaD would not be expected to impair object naming.

ATTENTION AND WORKING MEMORY

Patients with cerebral small vessel disease perform worse on processing speed measures (e.g., Digit Symbol) than patients with prodromal AD (Zhou & Jia, 2009). Those with cerebral small vessel disease also perform less accurately on tests designed to measure the capacity to establish and maintain a mental set through a series of tasks (Libon et al., 1997) and on measures of mental manipulation and temporal reordering (Lamar, Catani, Price, Heilman, & Libon, 2008; Lamar et al., 2007).

VISUOSPATIAL ABILITIES

Typical AD variant patients (i.e., not PCA) perform better than VaD patients on the Rey-Osterrieth Complex Figure Test (ROCF) copy portion, such that VaD patient drawings tend to be more fragmented and contain numerous perseverations and omissions (Freeman et al., 2000). VaD patients also make more clock drawing errors than AD patients (Cosentino, Jefferson, Chute, Kaplan, & Libon, 2004; Price et al., 2005).

Lewy Body Disease

Lewy body substrates are intraneuronal inclusions made of alpha-synuclein (McKeith et al., 2004). When seen in high enough concentration in the substantia nigra, these inclusions associate with parkinsonism (e.g., idiopathic PD). When also present in the cortex they can produce Lewy body disease. Often the acronyms LBD and DLB are used interchangeably. The subtle difference between these acronyms as used herein, is that LBD for Lewy body disease can be applied to any of the syndromes preclinical, MCI, or dementia, and while DLB applies only to the dementia syndrome due to Lewy body disease.

At the time of writing this chapter, the most recent consensus diagnostic criteria for Lewy body disease were updated in 2005 (McKeith et al., 2005), though revised criteria are anticipated in the near future. These 2005 criteria differed from the original with the inclusion of additional suggested features, most notably, REM sleep behavior disorder (RBD). Interestingly, in a more recent autopsy validation study, each of the three core features of LBD (parkinsonism, hallucinations, and fluctuations) increased the odds of autopsy-confirmed DLB up to twofold, while RBD increased the odds by sixfold (Ferman et al., 2011).

Preclinical Lewy Body Disease

In vivo imaging of the presence of alpha-synuclein in the brain is not yet available. There is emerging evidence that detection of abnormal dopamine transporter levels—currently via Iodine-123 fluoropropyl ([123I]FP-CIT) single photon emission computed tomography (SPECT)—scanning can identify people at risk to display cardinal features of LBD in the near future (Siepel et al., 2013). However, the most compelling "preclinical" marker for LBD is likely RBD (Ferman et al., 2011). Here, "preclinical" refers to the period preceding cognitive, behavioral, and functional change, but after the development of RBD.

As shown by case studies (Boeve et al., 2007; Turner, D'Amato, Chervin, & Blaivas, 2000), RBD may precede the onset of other symptoms of neurodegenerative diseases by years and even decades (Boeve et al., 1998; Plazzi et al., 1997; Schenck, Bundlie, & Mahowald, 1996; Turner, Chervin, Frey, Minoshima, & Kuhl, 1997). The estimated 5-year risk of developing PD or LBD in a cohort with idiopathic RBD is 17.7%, and the 12-year risk is 52.4% (Postuma et al., 2009). Twelve of 15 patients with a diagnosis of RBD and a neurodegenerative disorder that came to autopsy had Lewy body disease while the other three had multiple system atrophy (MSA), another known synucleinopathy. These findings provide compelling evidence that RBD reflects an underlying synucleinopathy (Boeve et al., 2003; Hulette et al., 1995). Therefore, RBD may serve as a valuable potential 'etiologic biomarker' identifying persons at high risk for MCI and ultimately dementia due to synucleinopathy.

MCI due to LBD

When people meet generic criteria for MCI, and RBD is present, no matter whether parkinsonism or visual hallucinations are present, the cognitive pattern is

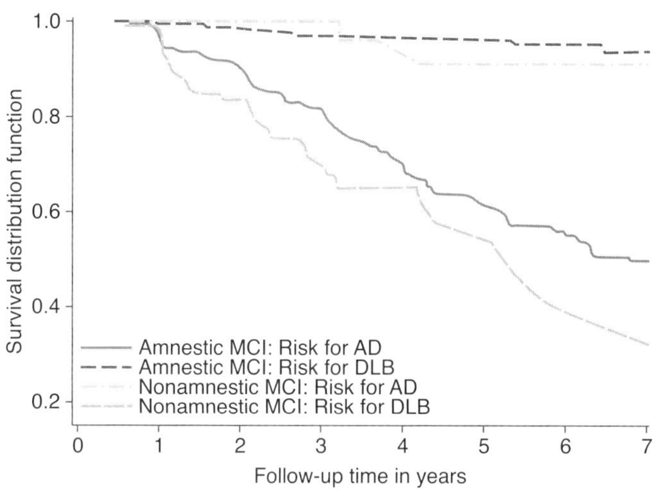

Figure 30.2 Progression of amnestic and nonamnestic MCI to dementia due to AD versus dementia due to Lewy body disease. Reproduced from (Ferman et al., 2013) with permission.

indistinguishable from LBD. Further, the cognitive profile of both those with MCI and RBD only and those with MCI plus the two or more cardinal symptoms of LBD significantly differs from AD (Ferman et al., 2002). In each case (RBD only or RBD plus cardinal features), Lewy bodies are present on autopsy (Molano et al., 2010). Thus RBD and cognitive change is one form of the MCI due to LBD.

The MCI phenotype for LBD tends to involve visuoperceptual and/or attention deficits (Ala, Hughes, Kyrouac, Ghobrial, & Elbie, 2001; Ballard et al., 1999; Calderon et al., 2001; Ferman et al., 1999) though memory impairments may also be present. This is understandable given that Lewy bodies and neuritic plaques and neurofibrillary tangles are all common in Lewy body dementia. Nevertheless relative to an amnestic MCI profile, a nonamnestic profile MCI is far more likely (Ferman et al., 2013). See Figure 30.2.

Criteria for Dementia Due to Lewy Body Disease (McKeith, et al., 2005)

1 Central feature (essential for a diagnosis of possible or probable DLB) is dementia defined as progressive cognitive decline of sufficient magnitude to interfere with normal social or occupational function.
   a Prominent or persistent memory impairment may not necessarily occur in the early stages but is usually evident with progression.
   b Deficits on tests of attention, executive function, and visuospatial ability may be especially prominent.

2 Core features (two core features are sufficient for a diagnosis of probable DLB, one for possible DLB):
   a Fluctuating cognition with pronounced variation in attention and alertness.
   b Recurrent visual hallucinations that are typically well formed and detailed.
   c Spontaneous features of parkinsonism.

3 Suggestive features (if one or more of these suggestive features is present in the presence of one or more core features, a diagnosis of probable DLB can be made. In the absence of any core features, one or more suggestive features is sufficient for possible DLB. Probable DLB should not be diagnosed on the basis of suggested features alone):
   a REM sleep behavior disorder.
   b Severe neuroleptic sensitivity.
   c Low dopamine transporter uptake in the basal ganglia demonstrated by SPECT or PET imaging.

4 Supportive features (commonly present but not proven to have diagnostic specificity):
   a Repeated falls and syncope.
   b Transient, unexplained loss of consciousness.
   c Severe autonomic dysfunction, e.g., orthostatic hypotension, urinary incontinence.
   d Hallucinations in other modalities.
   e Systematized delusions.
   f Depression.
   g Relative preservation of medial temporal lobe structures on CT/MRI scan.
   h Generalized low uptake on SPECT/PET perfusion scan with reduced occipital activity.
   i Abnormal (low uptake) metai-odobenzylguanidine (MIBG) myocardial scintigraphy.
   j Prominent slow wave activity on EEG with temporal lobe transient sharp waves.

5 A diagnosis of DLB is less likely in the following circumstances:
   a In the presence of cerebrovascular disease evident as focal neurologic signs or on brain imaging;
   b In the presence of any other physical illness or brain disorder sufficient to account in part, or in total for the clinical picture; or
   c If the parkinsonism only appears for the first time at a stage of severe dementia.

6 Temporal sequence of symptoms:
   a DLB should be diagnosed when dementia occurs before or concurrently with parkinsonism (if it is present). The term *Parkinson's disease dementia* (PDD) should be used to describe dementia that occurs in the context of well-established Parkinson's disease. In a clinical practice setting, the term that is most appropriate to the clinical situation should be used and generic terms such as *LB disease* are often helpful. In research studies in which distinction needs to be made between DLB

and PDD, the existing one-year rule between the onset of dementia and parkinsonism, DLB continues to be recommended. Adoption of other time periods will simply confound the data pooling or comparison between studies. In other research settings that may include clinicopathologic studies and clinical trials, both clinical phenotypes may be considered collectively under categories such as LB disease or alpha-synucleinopathy.

Neuropsychology of Lewy Body Disease

Impairment in basic attention, visual perception, visual construction and memory distinguish LBD from normal aging (sensitivity of 88.6%, specificity of 96.1%) (Ferman et al., 2006). However, impaired visual construction and attention plus relatively spared memory and naming skills can distinguish dementia due to DLB from AD (sensitivity of 83.3% and a specificity of 91.4% (Ferman et al., 1999; Ferman et al., 2002; Ferman et al., 2006). These findings highlight that the degree of visual perceptual and attentional impairment relative to memory impairment helps identify dementia due to LBD. In early typical AD, memory impairments are far more pronounced than attention or visual perception problems, but in LBD, attention and visual perception impairments are more salient.

Visuospatial Ability

LBD is associated with significant deficits in higher order visual processing, a finding that is not attributable to motor slowness associated with parkinsonism. Interestingly, people with LBD who experience visual hallucinations tend to do more poorly on visual tasks (Mosimann et al., 2004). Nonetheless, some studies have not found differences between AD and DLB on visual tasks (Forstl, Burns, Luthert, Ciarns, & Levy, 1993; Gnanalingham, Byrne, Thornton, Sambrook, & Bannister, 1997). One explanation is that the inclusion of patients in the advanced stages of dementia can obfuscate group differences due to generalized impairment.

Alternately, impaired performance on visual tasks may be the result of differential impairment of other task demands. For example, visual problem solving may be negatively affected by executive difficulties in AD, and by perceptual difficulties in DLB. Mori and colleagues examined this issue and revealed deficits in DLB but not AD on basic visual tasks that did not require executive function (Mori et al., 2000). Anatomical differences may also be contributing to poor performance on visual tasks. For example, reflexive saccadic eye movements responsible for shifting the fovea towards visual targets show greater impairment for the PD with dementia (PDD) and LBD groups compared to AD, PD without dementia groups, and normal controls (Mosimann et al., 2005). Also, flash electroretinography reveals abnormalities of the photoreceptors in the retina that may interfere with signal transmission to the bipolar cells (Devos et al., 2005). Regional blood flow has been shown to be lower in occipital regions in DLB but not AD (Imamura et al., 2001; Lobotesis et al., 2001). Overall, these findings suggest that the etiology of the visual impairment in DLB may not be entirely due to disruption of the cortical extra-striate association areas, but may also have an afferent or earlier neural contribution before reaching the cortex for further processing.

Episodic Memory

Memory difficulties, when present in early DLB, appear to be fairly mild and stand in direct contrast to the pronounced amnestic disturbance of AD. The memory problems are more likely to show a pattern of poor initial learning without the rapid forgetting that is typically observed in AD (Hamilton et al., 2004; Salmon, 2004). When people with pure AD (i.e., without concomitant Lewy bodies) were compared to those with pure LBD or mixed AD and LBD, they performed worse on tasks of verbal memory, while patients with pure LBD pathology performed worse on tasks of visual spatial skills. Those with combined pathology had poor visual spatial performance and nonverbal memory challenges but not verbal memory deficits (Johnson, Morris, & Galvin, 2005).

Fronto-temporal Lobar Degeneration

As is important for AD, vascular disease and LBD, there is need to distinguish the dementia syndromic phase of fronto-temporal lobar degeneration (FTLD) process. FTLD remains a heterogeneous collection of syndromes and associated neuropathologies, whereas the nomenclature *FTD* refers more specifically to the clinical aspects of the syndrome (Josephs, 2008). FTLD nosologies include different ranges of diagnoses (e.g., Pick's disease or primary progressive aphasia), syndromes (e.g., dementia with motor neuron disease), and etiologies (e.g., tauopathies vs. TDP-43 proteinopathies) (Josephs, 2008; Smith & Bondi, 2013). Currently, most nosologies include three main phenotypes: behavioral variant-FTD (bvFTD), semantic dementia, and primary progressive aphasia (PPA). PPA can be further subdivided into three variants, including logopenic (lvPPA), semantic (svPPA) and agrammatic (agPPA) (Gorno-Tempini et al., 2011), with the later sometimes referred to as *nonfluent progressive aphasia* (PNFA). The variant of PPA is classified based on clinical findings, with speech pathologists currently providing the most sensitive diagnostic differentiation. Recent pathology studies suggest that the svPPA and agPPA variants of PPA are more consistently predictive of FTLD spectrum disorders (i.e., tauopathies, TDP-43) while the lvPPA variant is strongly associated with AD pathology (Harris et al., 2013). Providing diagnostic criteria for all of these syndromes is beyond the scope of this chapter, in part because these criteria are dynamic and consensus remains a bit elusive. Indeed, with the rapidly progressive understanding of these clinical entities, there has been increasing incentive to update the diagnostic criteria of PPA (Mesulam & Weintraub, 2014; Wicklund et al., 2014). For a more extensive review of this topic, the reader is referred to other sources (see (Josephs, 2008; Miller, 2013).

Preclinical FTD

In the past five years several genetic mutations associated with FTD have been discovered. These include mutations in the MAPT, GRN, and C9ORF72 genes (Rohrer, Warren, Fox, & Rossor, 2013) . These genes provide etiological markers that can be identified in the presymptomatic state. In addition, PET imaging of tau is currently under study and *may* soon provide to be a biomarker of FTD-associated accumulation.

Mild Cognitive Impairment and FTLD

As the name, behavioral variant-FTD implies, the MCI phase of FTD often presents as impairments in "social cognition" with combinations of obsessions, disinhibition, apathy irritability, elation, lack of empathy or egocentrism, and aberrant motor behavior (de Mendonca, Ribeiro, Guerreiro, & Garcia, 2004; Miller et al., 2003). In contrast, the temporal variants of FTD, including the PPA variants, demonstrate early deficits in predominantly language, semantic knowledge or speech (Josephs, 2008; Machulda et al., 2013; Perry & Hodges, 2000; Wicklund, et al., 2014), though other neurocognitive deficits in the logopenic variant, in particular, may be affected though to a lesser degree than language (Rohrer et al., 2010, Butts et al., 2015). Yet most variants of FTLD show some similarities in behavioral disturbances, and significantly increased behavior disturbance when compared to AD patients matched on age and severity (Liu et al., 2004).

Neuropsychology of FTD

There are at least five challenges to describing "the" neuropsychology of FTD (Wittenberg et al., 2008). As previously described, (a) the diagnostic criteria for FTD have evolved and (b) remain confusing because (c) FTD is rare and sample sizes in descriptive studies are small, leading to variable findings, and (d) studies tend to lump bvFTD, semantic dementia, and PPA types to increase sample size, and finally, (e) to compare and contrast within FTLD syndromes and with other dementias, one must equate for severity. This is challenging since severity scales tend to be disease specific. Additionally, because many neuropsychological tests are mediated by language, assessing neurocognitive functioning beyond language in PPA patients can be particularly challenging. Thus, the known neuropsychological profiles associated with specific FTD syndromes are discussed in the rest of this section.

LEARNING AND MEMORY

FTD syndromes all contrast with AD in the relative preservation of memory early in the illness (Hutchinson & Mathias, 2007). In general, FTD patients have better free and cued recall, as well as better recognition memory than typical AD patients. A study examining learning and memory in PPA patients found evidence for impaired encoding and retrieval of verbal information in a pattern that differed from AD patients (Weintraub et al., 2013). Furthermore, we have also shown differing neuropsychological profiles among the three variants of PPA, including impaired learning and complex retention in lvPPA relative to svPPA and agPPA variants (Butts et al., 2015). Of course, as dementia worsens, all of the FTD variants show worsening memory performance, due not just to deterioration of attention and language skills, but due to eventual disease encroachment on mesial temporal structures. This highlights the notion that neuropsychological tests may have their greatest value in MCI and early dementia states and lose discriminative value as disease worsens.

FLUENCY AND LANGUAGE

There is, of course, variability in the regional atrophy of FTLD (Whitwell et al., 2009). As expected, this is associated with variable patterns of cognitive performance such that more frontal atrophy is associated with greater lexical fluency problems relative to more temporal patterns of atrophy that show greater challenges in naming. Overall, FTLD patients tend to display comparable deficits in semantic (category) and lexical (letter) fluencies (Rascovsky, Salmon, Hansen, Thal, & Galasko, 2007), whereas selective category fluency deficits commonly occur in AD (Monsch et al., 1992). While this impression may derive mostly from the inclusion of PNFA and semantic dementia patients in past FTLD studies, it also appears to hold for bvFTD cohorts (Rascovsky et al., 2007). While, the neurodegenerative syndrome of primary progressive apraxia of speech (PPAOS) is differentiated from primary progressive aphasia (Josephs et al., 2012), PPAOS is a known FTLD syndrome associated with tauopathy (Caso et al., 2014). This syndrome is characterized by impaired speech motor planning and/or organization resulting in dysfluent speech rather than a language deficit (Josephs et al., 2013; Josephs et al., 2012). Multiple neuroimaging modalities isolate PPAOS to the superior lateral premotor and supplementary motor area, which differentiates it from PPA that may affect additional frontal, temporal, parietal, and subcortical regions depending upon PPA variant (Josephs et al., 2013; Josephs et al., 2006; Whitwell et al., 2013).

LANGUAGE/SEMANTIC KNOWLEDGE

By definition (i.e., required for the diagnosis), the progressive aphasia variants of FTLD have deficits in aspects of language that cause disruption in daily function (Mesulam, 1982). In addition to fluency problems, lvPPA patients have problems with confrontation naming, repeating, and comprehending sentences, relatively preserved single word comprehension, with evidence of anomia, slowed rate of verbal expression due to pauses for word retrieval or verbal formulation, and possible phonemic paraphasias (Gorno-Tempini et al., 2011; Machulda et al., 2013). The aphasia in svPPA is dominated by anomia, poor word comprehension, and loss of single word and object meaning. Interestingly, the repetition and fluent speech is relatively preserved though the content may lack specificity (Gorno-Tempini et al., 2011).

EXECUTIVE FUNCTION

While FTLD patients have impairments on executive function tests, these tests have limited utility in differential diagnosis (Miller et al., 2003). FTLD and AD patients cannot be reliably distinguished by Trail Making Test Part B or the Stroop test (Hutchinson & Mathias, 2007). This may arise in part from the problem of mixing different FTLD syndromes, as described, but also may reflect that fairly early there is involvement of the frontal lobes in the typical AD process (Braak & Braak, 1997). However, studies also suggest that executive function tests may not be that good at distinguishing FTLD patients from normally aging samples. FTLD patients often score in the normal range on Wisconsin Card Sorting Test, Stroop, Digits Backwards from the Digit Span subtype, and on the Letter-Number Sequencing tasks (Wittenberg et al., 2008). Thus, traditional "frontal" measures have inconsistent sensitivity and poor differential specificity for the broad class of FTLD syndromes.

VISUOSPATIAL SKILLS

Tests of visuospatial skills tend to be preserved in FTLD syndromes, given the relative sparing of posterior cortices. For example, visuoconstructional deficits, but not memory deficits, have been shown to help distinguish AD from FTD (Razani, Boone, Miller, Lee, & Sherman, 2001). An earlier study from this group suggested AD and FTD groups differed on the discrepancy between nonverbal memory and letter fluency. Specifically, they found AD patients tended to have greater memory deficits relative to letter fluency problems, and FTD patients demonstrated the reverse pattern of greater fluency deficits relative to memory (Pachana, Boone, Miller, Cummings, & Berman, 1996).

Interventions

There are numerous strategies that can be deployed to try to prevent or delay progression from preclinical status to MCI to dementia. Table 30.3 provides a conceptual framework for these interventions.

Primary Prevention

The evidence supporting a role for primary prevention interventions in dementia is accumulating. Nearly all primary prevention models involve lifestyle modifications that improve overall health. A population-wide 25% reduction in midlife diabetes, obesity, hypertension, and physical and cognitive inactivity could potentially alleviate 500,000 cases of dementia (Barnes & Yaffe, 2011). The conceptual basis for these primary prevention strategies is likely the enhancement of cognitive reserve or resilience (Stern, 2006, 2009).

Two general approaches for maintaining or improving cognitive function in older adult have been studied. The first approach involves instruction in putatively useful strategies. This method yields improvement on cognitive test scores specific to the strategy instruction, but gains do not typically generalize to other tests or areas of function (Fillit et al., 2002). This ability to generalize a learned skill to other skills is a concept known as *transfer* (Rebok, Carlson, & Langbaum, 2007). Transferring from one skill to another may be "near" or "far" based on the relatedness of the tasks. Far transfer of putative techniques is poor (Zelinski et al., 2011), and older adults do not generally continue to use learned strategies over time (Rebok et al., 2007). Due to the relatively limited generalizability of "new" skills, strategy-training programs have not been widely adopted as a primary prevention approach. However, emerging literature suggests that information processing system improvement can occur via intensive learning and practice (Mahncke, Bronstone, & Merzenich, 2006). For example, computer training in information processing speed produces improvement in working memory related to neuropsychological tests (word list total score, digits backwards, letter-number sequencing) and in

Table 30.3 A conceptual framework for prevention and treatment interventions in AD

	Prevention		*Treatment*	
	Behavioralpsychological	*Pharmacological*	*Behavioralpsychological*	*Pharmacological*
Cognition	Brain fitness/physical fitness/ social engagement	–	–	Acetylcholinesterase Inhibitors ?
Daily Function		–	Compensation training	
Mood		–	Psychotherapy	SSRIs
Disruptive Behavior	Person centered, activity-based care	–	Person centered, activity-based care	Neuroleptics

participant-reported outcome measures (Smith et al., 2009; Zelinski et al., 2011). This improvement in working memory function may serve to enhance cognitive reserve.

The overall benefits of physical exercise are extensive, and there is growing evidence that physical exercise is an important factor in maintaining cognitive and cerebral health. For example, in healthy individuals, physical activity has been shown to help maintain healthy brain volume and provide protection against volume loss (Colcombe et al., 2003; Colcombe et al., 2006). Furthermore, higher levels of physical activity is correlated with larger volumes of the hippocampus, a region essential for memory (Erickson et al., 2009), and acts to increase hippocampal volume (Erickson et al., 2011). As assessed by a functional MRI (fMRI) paradigm examining patterns of activation during a semantic memory task, increased physical activity appears to be particularly beneficial for individuals who are at risk for AD (Smith et al., 2011).

Secondary Prevention

The focus on pre-clinical and MCI syndromes permits a concurrent focus on secondary prevention models aimed at delaying (or ideally preventing) progression to dementia. Interventions in the preclinical stage align with the primary prevention strategies noted in the previous section. The approaches that follow focus on different aspects of the MCI syndrome as described in Table 30.3.

BehavioralPsychological Interventions for MCI

COGNITIVE/FUNCTIONAL/MOOD SYMPTOMS

Memory rehabilitation can take two forms: (a) "memory building" or restorative techniques in which the goal is to regain memory function through repetitive training paradigms; or, (b) "memory compensation" or techniques focused on using external aids to help compensate for memory loss. Memory notebooks are a form of memory compensation with validated efficacy in TBI patients (Sohlberg & Mateer, 1989). There has been relatively little research regarding cognitive rehabilitation techniques in patients with MCI. Recent trials of a computer training program have suggested only modest benefit or no change in cognition and mood in patients with MCI (Barnes et al., 2009; Rozzini et al., 2007; Talassi et al., 2007; Unverzagt et al., 2007). However, in at least one study (Barnes et al., 2009), the observed effect size for those patients who completed a cognitive training intervention was nearly the same as the significant effect size reported for normal older adults (Smith et al., 2009). This suggests that some MCI studies may be underpowered to see the modest beneficial effect of computer training.

As noted, a second strategy involves using an external memory compensatory strategy for MCI patients comparable to that used in traumatic brain injury (Sohlberg & Mateer, 1989). There is emerging evidence that a memory compensatory strategy using external aides can benefit daily function and quality of life in persons with amnestic MCI (Greenaway, Duncan, & Smith, 2013; Greenaway, Hanna, Lepore, & Smith, 2008).

Physical activity interventions may also serve minimize cognitive decline in MCI (Ahlskog, Geda, Graff-Radford, & Petersen, 2011; Lautenschlager et al., 2008). Additionally, a brief 12-week exercise intervention for individuals with MCI showed normalization of brain activation during a semantic memory fMRI task, suggesting that exercise may help to improve neuronal efficiency in MCI (Smith et al., 2013). The emerging trend, however, is to provide multicomponent interventions for persons with MCI (Rapp, Brenes, & Marsh, 2002). Mayo Clinic investigators, including this chapter's lead author (GES), have created a program for MCI that includes five components: (a) memory compensation training with a calendar/journaling tool; (b) Brain Fitness with a well-studied computerized tool (Barnes et al., 2009; Smith et al., 2009); (c) physical fitness; (d) caregiver and patient support groups; and, (e) wellness education. This ten-day, 50-hour program is called Healthy Action to Benefit Independence and Thinking (HABIT). This intervention has had positive impact on self-efficacy and quality of life outcomes for patients and caregivers (Greenaway et al., 2013).

Tertiary Prevention: Nonpharmacological Interventions

Cognitive and Functional Symptoms

Memory rehabilitation in dementia has also focused on memory building techniques, with mixed results of effectiveness (Clare, Woods, Moniz Cook, Orrell, & Spector, 2003). Memory compensation in dementia using notebooks and calendars as a way of orienting significantly impaired individuals to date, basic schedules, and personal information has also showed mixed success (Loewenstein, Acevedo, Czaja, & Duara, 2004). A recent multicomponent rehabilitation approach demonstrated that individuals with MCI, but not early dementia, showed improvements in mood, memory, and functional abilities (Kurz, Pohl, Ramsenthaler, & Sorg, 2009). These data suggest primary and secondary prevention interventions may have more potential than tertiary interventions to impact cognition and function.

Mood

Diagnostic criteria for depression include dysphoria and vegetative changes in sleep, appetite, and activity level. There is a tendency to interpret the term *dysphoria* as "sad mood," but the term may also involve irritability. While DSM-5 (Association, 2013), specifically includes both sadness and irritability as components of depression in adolescents, this accommodation has not been applied to patients with cognitive impairment. A significant proportion of the cases of "agitation" in dementia are likely cases where the irritability of depression is present along with vegetative changes. Estimates suggest that 40% of AD patients may experience symptoms of depression at some point during the course of their illness (Burns, Jacoby, & Levy, 1990). Ascertaining depression can be difficult, even in MCI stages, because patients are challenged to reliably report mood over time. In dementia, the patient's ability to understand concepts like "feeling blue" or "having low self-esteem" also may deteriorate. Informant report, while typically reliable, may not be valid since the informant must infer the patient's subjective state. In dementia, the full range of evidence—including self- and informant-report and behavioral observations—needs to be considered when evaluating for mood disorder in dementia. Agitated patients often responded well to antidepressant medication in combination with behavioral activation.

Disruptive Behaviors

Behavioral disturbance is common in AD, and nonpharmacologic approaches to disruptive behaviors are the first-line treatment. These approaches can be effective in managing behavioral and psychological symptoms at home and in institutional settings. A recent meta-analysis of nonpharmacological interventions for neuropsychiatric symptoms of dementia revealed that studies generally used multiple types of interventions, including the following elements: (a) skills training for caregivers, (b) education for caregivers, (c) activity planning and environmental redesign, (d) enhancing support for caregivers, and (e) self-care techniques for caregivers, as well as (f) exercise for the patient and (g) collaborative care with a health professional (Brodaty & Arasaratnam, 2012). Given the range of interventions, it is clear why establishing efficacy on nonpharmacological interventions is difficult. Yet, it is evident from the list of available interventions that successful interventions are typically oriented towards the caregiver rather than the patient with dementia. Caregivers who learn what to expect as the disease progresses can anticipate cognitive and functional limitations and the expected behavioral effects as the dementia progresses.

One approach to conceptualizing management interventions for disruptive behaviors involves the following:

1. Understanding the etiology of the dementia syndrome
2. Assessing the severity of the illness
3. Recognizing that behavior is a form of communication and it is important to try to understand what is being communicated based by the behavior:
   - **a** Identifying environmental, physical, psychological, or social factors that may be the impetus for behavioral communication
4. Managing antecedents, not consequences
5. Using what the dementia "gives": taking advantage of the key features of the dementia syndrome to enhance contentment
6. Focusing on activity-based care
   - **a** Avoidance of efforts to create a behavioral vacuum

UNDERSTANDING THE ETIOLOGY OF THE DEMENTIA SYNDROME

Often, patients in care facilities have a generic dementia diagnosis without benefit of evaluation of the etiology of the dementia. Establishing etiology can avoid iatrogenic mistakes like oversedation from antipsychotic medications. Understanding that different behavioral profiles associate with dementia etiologies, (e.g., fully formed visual hallucinations are common early in LBD, but only later in AD) it is possible to more effectively consider whether comorbidities may be present. For example, observing visual hallucinations would raise concern about delirium early in AD, whereas these symptoms would be an expected part of the disorder in early DLB. Or, disrobing might be understood as simple disinhibition in an early FTD, versus communicating the need to use the bathroom in advanced AD. Understanding the nature and extent of the dementia can help provide the context for understanding what behavior may be communicating.

In dementia, understanding that new learning is often impossible helps caregivers understand why frequent reorientation is an exercise in futility and may well be agitating to the person with dementia (and her or his caregiver!). Understanding this cognitive deficit can also clarify behaviors that otherwise get mislabeled. The case of a person with AD forgetting where she placed valuables, like a purse, then assuming she is being robbed reframes "paranoia" to rather be poor memory and poor reasoning. Likely the most appropriate intervention here is to have caregivers unobtrusively search living quarters for the purse instead of giving psychotropic medication for psychosis. Understanding these patterns facilitates appropriate intervention plans. Helping caregivers understand these patterns aids their adherence to intervention plans.

ASSESSING THE SEVERITY OF THE ILLNESS

The severity of dementia may predispose people to different mediators of disruptive behavior. Persons with very mild dementia are often understimulated (i.e., bored) in typical long-term care settings where activities involved large groups and limited cognitive challenge. If bored, a patient may become restless and wander, attempt to escape, or become involved in self-stimulating behaviors, such as repeatedly calling out to caregivers (Hellen, 1992). Activities-based care may reduce understimulation. However, standard care center activities can also be overstimulating (i.e., agitating) to persons with severe dementia who can no longer understand verbal explanations, correctly interpret social interaction, or accommodate noise. Completing a simple but formal mental status evaluation can help to determine environmental mediators of disruptive behavior and assess for the appropriate level of activities-based care.

RECOGNIZING BEHAVIOR AS A KEY FORM OF COMMUNICATION

Communication is an adaptive means towards need fulfillment. In patients with dementia, as reasoning and language skills are lost, overt behavior will increasingly become a primary form of communication. Just as a preverbal child uses crying as a means of communicating hunger, pain, or fear, patients with dementia may use wandering, calling out, swearing, or other behaviors to communicate pain, anxiety, boredom, loneliness, etc. Even when speech is intact, verbal communication is often limited by difficulties in expressing desired thoughts correctly. The behavior of patients with advanced dementia often represents an attempt to express feelings and needs that cannot be verbalized adequately. These behaviors often represent an attempt to communicate regarding environmental, physical, psychological, or social factors that are distressing to the person with dementia. Calling such behaviors "inappropriate" or "disruptive" ignores the adaptation efforts reflected in that behavior.

IDENTIFYING ENVIRONMENTAL, PHYSICAL, PSYCHOLOGICAL, AND SOCIAL MEDIATORS

The same calling out, wandering, restlessness, aggression, and other difficult behaviors might be the expression of an inner emotional state in one patient, a long-standing behavioral pattern in another, an unrecognized physical need in a third patient, and a reaction to an external stimulus in a fourth. If clinicians observe only the behavior itself and ignore the complex mediators that may be at play, intervention is unlikely to be effective.

Environment

It is common for patients temporarily admitted from nursing homes to geriatric psychiatry units to have no problem behaviors while in the hospital but to have rapid re-emergence of the behaviors upon return to the nursing home. This A-B-A behavioral design routinely demonstrates that environmental factors are the primary mediators of that person's disruptive behavior. Often that admission could be avoided by considering environmental factors in the first place. This is more easily accomplished by evaluating the person in his or her typical living environment when possible. Multiple, simultaneous, or unnecessary stimuli may be difficult for the patient to interpret or may be overwhelming. For example, loud and repeated noise may lead to agitation (Robinson, Spencer, & White, 1988). Extraneous stimuli, such as television shows, may be misunderstood or mistaken for reality and cause patients with dementia to be frightened or angry. "Disembodied" voices from radios or overhead paging systems, or that result from whispering or laughing out of view, can similarly contribute to confusion, misperceptions, suspiciousness, and agitation. "Old-fashioned" music may be soothing to the patient, but modern music preferred by the young-adult care provider may be agitating. As a patient's language skills degenerate, he or she may become distressed in situations where there is high demand for language, such as congregate dining.

Familiar cues or personal belongings in the environment may reduce confusion, fear, and agitation. To compensate for sensory losses, environmental modifications such as reducing glare, increasing lighting, and using contrasting colors may enhance appropriate behavior (Whall et al., 1997). At latter stages, dementia patients may need to take meals and engage in activities in social settings with smaller groups and less talking. A simple, consistent, and predictable environment will provide familiarity and comfort for the patient. Conversely, an environment poorly adapted to cognitive losses may cause the patient to misinterpret surroundings and events and either behave in socially inappropriate ways or withdraw (Dawson, Kline, Wiancko, & Wells, 1986).

Physical Factors

Physical mediators of disruptive behavior can be iatrogenic and reflect a failure to consider palliative approaches in advanced dementia care. A patient with dementia place on salt restriction for blood pressure control may dislike the food in congregate dining and become agitated because he or she is left to sit in the dining hall though he or she has no interest in the food. The importance of tight blood pressure control in late-stage dementia may be dubious, and making more the food more palatable could reduce "agitation." It is worthwhile to analyze the benefits versus risks of tight hypertension control in people with advance dementia with the appropriate medical and family decision makers. One of the most helpful aspects of psychological consultation is simply to get all the care stakeholders together to facilitate such communications (Smith & Bondi, 2013).

Other physical factors include unrecognized infection (e.g., urinary tract infection) and pain. Dementia patients are often unable to describe the pain or physical symptoms that alert the care team to these factors. Although standard nursing home practices generally provide better support for assessing physical factors, compared to the environmental and social factors, it is still incumbent on the psychological consultant to consider physical factors during her or his assessment.

Social Factors

Social factors include the life experience of patients, their values, culture, family structure, history of preferences, etc. Despite progressive cognitive loss, older adults with dementia retain basic human needs, including the need to belong, to be loved, to be touched, to follow their values, and to feel useful. Unfortunately, meaningful relationships and appropriate social groups can be unavailable or insufficiently matched to the functional level of such patients. Psychologists can help family and facilities identify ways to help the person with dementia feel social connections.

MANAGING ANTECEDENTS, NOT CONSEQUENCES

Applied behavioral analysis reminds us that all behavior occurs in a context. This has been described as the ABCs of behavior management: antecedent, behavior, consequence. For each behavior, there are antecedent conditions that provide a setting for the behavior and, in many cases, may increase the probability of the behavior occurring. Then there is the behavior itself, followed by the consequences of behavior. Much of traditional behavior management has focused on controlling the consequences in order to shape behavior. However, the ability of an event happening after a behavior (consequence) to influence the future probability of that behavior requires the consequence to form a new association with the behavior. In other words, new learning must be possible. But in dementia, of course, the ability to form that association is increasingly impaired as the dementia progresses and the likelihood of behavioral disturbance increases. Thus, managing antecedents, as opposed to consequences, has the greater probability of success in dementia behavior management. Antecedent cues are an overlearned association between the cue and the behavior. For instance, the connection between silverware and eating does not dissipate until very late stage dementia. Managing antecedents requires being proactive, not reactive, and it requires an understanding of the intact abilities of the patient so that the cues result in behaviors within her or his capabilities.

USING WHAT THE DEMENTIA "GIVES"

Managing disruptive behavior in dementia is challenging. Successful intervention plans rarely eliminate disruptive behavior. Success involves reducing the frequency and/or intensity of the challenging behavior. Success is often predicated on putting the cognitive deficits of the dementia to use. For example, redirection is the most commonly used method of behavior management in most facilities. Redirection is often used when patients enter restricted areas, attempt to escape, or engage in problematic interpersonal exchanges. Bad redirection is often an antecedent to agitated or aggressive behavior, because bad redirection represents a thwarting of the goal-directed behavior. Good redirection will take advantage of the memory and attention impairments of the person with dementia and includes a three-step process. First, caregivers validate the apparent emotional state of the patient (e.g., "You look worried"); this involves assessing the feeling state the behavior is communicating (see "Recognizing Behavior as a Key Form of Communication"). It also helps to establish rapport. Next and critically, the caregiver joins in the patient's behavior. For example, "You want to go home? Well, I am ready to get out of here myself. Let's get our things together." Finally, once a common goal is established, distraction is easier (upon returning to the patient's room for his or her things the caregiver distracts, "Well, look at these pictures here, tell me about these people"). Distraction works best with patients who have substantial memory or attention problems. Most patients with dementia have such problems. This strategy may seem to require more time than simple redirection. However, facile caregivers can perform all steps quickly and ultimately save time because agitated behavior does not need to be managed.

FOCUSING ON ACTIVITY-BASED CARE

Adapting activities to the ability level of a person with dementia can address his or her desire to feel useful and serves to avoid unsuccessful attempts to create a behavioral vacuum (Hellen, 1992). Activities compete in real time to displace disruptive behavior and are thus a key part of a proactive approach. Planned activities should be "failure free," promoting a sense of success by accommodating the ability level of the patient. Meaningful activities should correspond to individual's life history, current abilities, and attention span when possible. Exercising existing abilities in a failure-free manner will provide reassurance and contribute to a sense of competence.

Conclusions and Future Directions

Modern nomenclature clearly recognizes different syndromes that occur across neurodegenerative diseases that lead to dementia. This includes new possibilities for identifying neurodegenerative diseases even when a person is asymptomatic (i.e., in the preclinical phase). There is now recognition of the MCI phase for all or nearly all neurodegenerative etiologies. The different etiologies produce different neuropsychological profiles in the MCI and early dementia stage. But late stages of dementia and cognitive, functional, and behavioral challenges converge and common strategies may aide in dementia management. The recognition of preclinical and MCI states are foundational to engaging prevention strategies in an effort to prevent or delay progression to dementia. Prevention strategies incorporating physical and cognitive exercise, social engagement and compensation strategies likely have greater near term potential than medication strategies for impacting the morbidity of neurodegenerative diseases.

Note

1 Parts of this work were supported by grants P50 AG16574, 1 R01NR12419, and CTSA Grant UL1 TR000135 from the National Center for Advancing Translational Science (NCATS). Its contents are solely the responsibility of the authors and do not necessarily represent the official views of the U.S. National Institutes of Health.

References

Ahlskog, J. E., Geda, Y. E., Graff-Radford, N. R., & Petersen, R. C. (2011). Physical exercise as a preventive or disease-modifying treatment of dementia and brain aging. *Mayo Clinic Proceedings*, *86*(9), 876–884. doi: 10.4065/mcp.2011.0252 S0025-6196(11)65219-1 [pii]

Albert, M., DeKosky, S., Dickson, D., Dubois, B., Feldman, H., Fox, N., . . . Phelps, C. (2011). The diagnosis of mild cognitive impairment due to Alzheimer's disease: Recommendations from the National Institute on Aging-Alzheimer's Association workgroups on diagnostic guidelines for Alzheimer's disease. *Alzheimer's & Dementia : The Journal of the Alzheimer's Association*, *7*(3), 270–279. doi: 10.1016/j.jalz.2011.03.008

Ala, T., Hughes, L., Kyrouac, G., Ghobrial, M., Elble, R. (2001). Pentagon copying is more impaired in dementia with Lewy bodies than in Alzheimer's disease. *Journal of Neurology, Neurosurgery & Psychiatry*, *70*(4), 483–488.

Albert, M., Moss, M., Tanzi, R., & Jones, K. (2001). Preclinical prediction of AD using neuropsychological tests. *Journal of the International Neuropsychological Society*, *7*, 631–639.

Alzheimer, A. (1906). Über einen eigenartigen schweren Erkrankungsprozeß der Hirnrinde. *Neurologisches Centralblatt*, *23*, 1129–1136.

American Psychiatric Association. (2010). S 24 Major Neurocognitive Disorder. Retrieved December 1, 2011, from www.dsm5.org/ProposedRevisions/Pages/proposedrevision.aspx?rid=419

American Psychological Association. (2011). Guidelines for the evaluation of dementia and age-related cognitive change. *The American Psychologist*, *67*, 1–9. doi: 10.1037/a0024643

Aretouli, E., & Brandt, J. (2010). Everyday functioning in mild cognitive impairment and its relationship with executive cognition. *International Journal of Geriatric Psychiatry*, *25*(3), 224–233.

American Psychiatric Association. (2013). *Diagnostic and Statistical Manual of Mental Disorders* (5th ed.). Arlington, VA: American Psychiatric Publishing.

Bäckman, L., Small, B., & Fratiglioni, L. (2001). Stability of the preclinical episodic memory deficit in Alzheimer's disease. *Brain*, *124*, 96–102.

Baker, M., Mackenzie, I. R., Pickering-Brown, S. M., Gass, J., Rademakers, R., Lindholm, C., . . . Hutton, M. (2006). Mutations in progranulin cause tau-negative frontotemporal dementia linked to chromosome 17. *Nature*, *442*(7105), 916–919. doi: 10.1038/nature05016

Ballard, C., Holmes, C., McKeith, I., Neill, D., O'Brien, J., Cairns, N., et al. (1999). Psychiatric morbidity in dementia with Lewy bodies: a prospective clinical and neuropathological comparative study with Alzheimer's disease. *American Journal of Psychiatry*, *156*,1039–1045.

Barnes, D. E., & Yaffe, K. (2011). The projected effect of risk factor reduction on Alzheimer's disease prevalence. *Lancet Neurolology*, *10*(9), 819–828. doi: 10.1016/S1474-4422(11)70072-2S1474-4422(11)70072-2 [pii]

Barnes, D. E., Yaffe, K., Belfor, N., Jagust, W., DeCarli, C., Reed, B., & Kramer, J. (2009). Computer-based cognitive training for mild cognitive impairment: Results from a pilot randomized, controlled trial. *Alzheimer Disease and Associated Disorders*, *23*(3), 205–210. doi: 10.1097/WAD.0b013e31819c6137

Boeve, B., Silber, M., Ferman, T., Kokmen, E., Smith, G., Ivnik, R., . . . Petersen, R. (1998). REM sleep behavior disorder and degenerative dementia: An association likely reflecting Lewy body disease. *Neurology*, *51*, 363–370.

Boeve, B., Silber, M., Parisi, J., Dickson, D., Ferman, T., Benarroch, E., . . . Mahowald, M. W. (2003). Synucleinopathy pathology and REM sleep behavior disorder plus dementia or parkinsonism. *Neurology*, *61*(1), 40–45.

Boeve, B., Silber, M., Saper, C., Ferman, T., Dickson, D., Parisi, J., . . . Braak, H. (2007). Pathophysiology of REM sleep behaviour disorder and relevance to neurodegenerative disease. *Brain: A Journal of Neurology*, *130*(Pt 11), 2770–2788. doi: 10.1093/brain/awm056

Braak, H., & Braak, E. (1997). Frequency of stages of Alzheimer-related lesions in different age categories. *Neurobiology of Aging*, *18*, 351–357.

Brodaty, H., & Arasaratnam, C. (2012). Meta-analysis of nonpharmacological interventions for neuropsychiatric symptoms of dementia. *American Journal of Psychiatry*, *169*(9), 946–953. doi: 10.1176/appi.ajp.2012.11101529 1356977 [pii]

Burns, A., Jacoby, R., & Levy, R. (1990). Psychiatric phenomena in Alzheimer's disease, III: Disorders of mood. *British Journal of Psychiatry*, *157*, 81–86, 92–84.

Busse, A., Hensel, A., Guhne, U., Angermeyer, M., & Riedel-Heller, S. (2006). Mild cognitive impairment: Long-term course of four clinical subtypes. *Neurology*, *67*, 2176–2185.

Butts, A. M., Machulda, M. M., Duffy, J. R., Strand, E. A., Whitwell, J. L. and Josephs, K. A. (2015). Neuropsychological profiles differ among the three variants of primary progressive aphasia. Doi:10.1017/S1355617715000399. *Journal of the International Neuropsychological Society*, *21*, 1–7

Calderon, J., Perry, R., Erzinclioglu, S., Berrios, G., Dening, T., Hodges, J. (2001). Perception, attention, and working memory are disproportionately impaired in dementia with Lewy bodies compared with Alzheimer's disease. *Journal of Neurology, Neurosurgery & Psychiatry*, *70*, 157–164.

Canning, S. J., Leach, L., Stuss, D., Ngo, L., & Black, S. E. (2004). Diagnostic utility of abbreviated fluency measures in Alzheimer disease and vascular dementia. *Neurology*, *62*(4), 556–562.

Carew, T. G., Lamar, M., Cloud, B. S., Grossman, M., & Libon, D. J. (1997). Impairment in category fluency in ischemic vascular dementia. *Neuropsychology*, *11*(3), 400–412.

Caso, F., Mandelli, M. L., Henry, M., Gesierich, B., Bettcher, B. M., Ogar, J., . . . Gorno-Tempini, M. L. (2014). In vivo signatures of nonfluent/agrammatic primary progressive aphasia caused by FTLD pathology. *Neurology*, *82*(3), 239–247. doi: 10.1212/wnl.0000000000000031

Chen, P., Ratcliff, G., Belle, S., Cauley, J., DeKosky, S., & Ganguli, M. (2001). Patterns of cognitive decline in presymptomatic Alzheimer disease: A prospective community study. *Archives of General Psychiatry*, *58*(9), 853–858.

Clare, L., Woods, R. T., Moniz Cook, E. D., Orrell, M., & Spector, A. (2003). Cognitive rehabilitation and cognitive training for early stage Alzheimer's disease and vascular dementia. *Cochrane Database of Systematic Reviews, 4*, CD003260. doi: 10.1002/14651858.CD003260

Colcombe, S. J., Erickson, K. I., Raz, N., Webb, A., Cohen, N., McAuely, E., & Kramer, A. (2003). Aerobic fitness reduces brain tissue loss in humans. *Journal of Gerontology Series A—Biological and Medical Sciences, 58*, 176–180.

Colcombe, S. J., Erickson, K. I., Scalf, P. E., Kim, J. S., Prakash, R., McAuley, E., . . . Kramer, A. F. (2006). Aerobic exercise training increases brain volume in aging humans. *Journal of Gerontology A: Biological Sciences and Medical Sciences, 61*(11), 1166–1170.

Corder, E., Saunders, A., Strittmatter, W., Schmechel, D., Gaskell, P., Small, W., . . . Pericak-Vance, M. (1993). Gene dose of apolipoprotein E type 4 allele and the risk of Alzheimer's disease in late onset families. *Science, 261*, 921–923.

Cosentino, S., Jefferson, A., Carey, M., Price, C., Davis-Garrett, K., Swenson, R., & Libon, D. (2004). The clinical diagnosis of vascular dementia: A comparison among four classification systems and a proposal for a new paradigm. *The Clinical Neuropsychologist, 18*(1), 6–21.

Cosentino, S., Jefferson, A., Chute, D., Kaplan, E., & Libon, D. (2004). Clock drawing errors in dementia: Neuropsychological and neuroanatomical considerations. *Cognitive and Behavioral Neurology, 17*(2), 74–84.

Crutch, S. J., Lehmann, M., Schott, J. M., Rabinovici, G. D., Rossor, M. N., & Fox, N. C. (2012). Posterior cortical atrophy. *Lancet Neurology, 11*(2), 170–178. doi: 10.1016/s1474-4422(11) 70289-7

Crutch, S. J., Schott, J. M., Rabinovici, G. D., Boeve, B. F., Cappa, S. F., Dickerson, B. C., . . . Fox, N. C. (2013). Shining a light on posterior cortical atrophy. *Alzheimer's & Dementia, 9*(4), 463–465. doi: http://dx.doi.org/10.1016/j.jalz.2012.11.004

Dawson, P., Kline, K., Wiancko, D., & Wells, D. (1986). Preventing excess disability in patients with Alzheimer's disease. *Geriatric Nursing, 7*, 298–301.

de Mendonca, A., Ribeiro, F., Guerreiro, M., & Garcia, C. (2004). Frontotemporal mild cognitive impairment. *Journal of Alzheimer's Disease, 6*(1), 1–9.

Desmond, D. (2004). The neuropsychology of vascular cognitive impairment: Is there a specific cognitive deficit? *Journal of Neurological Science, 226*(1–2), 3–7. doi: S0022-510X(04)00283-7 [pii] 10.1016/j.jns.2004.09.002

Devos, D., Tir, M., Maurage, C., Waucquier, N., Defebvre, L., Defoort-Dhellemmes, S., & Destee, A. (2005). ERG and anatomical abnormalities suggesting retinopathy in dementia with Lewy bodies. *Neurology, 65*, 1107–1110.

Duke, L., & Kaszniak, A. (2000). Executive control functions in degenerative dementias: A comparative review. *Neuropsychology Review, 10*(2), 75–99.

Erickson, K. I., Prakash, R. S., Voss, M. W., Chaddock, L., Hu, L., Morris, K. S., . . . Kramer, A. F. (2009). Aerobic fitness is associated with hippocampal volume in elderly humans. *Hippocampus, 19*(10), 1030–1039. doi: 10.1002/hipo.20547

Erickson, K. I., Voss, M. W., Prakash, R. S., Basak, C., Szabo, A., Chaddock, L., . . . Kramer, A. F. (2011). Exercise training increases size of hippocampus and improves memory. *Proceedings of the National Acadecmy of Sciences U S A, 108*(7), 3017–3022. doi: 10.1073/pnas.1015950108

Ertekin-Taner, N. (2007). Genetics of Alzheimer's disease: A centennial review. *Neurology Clinics, 25*(3), 611–667, v. doi: 10.1016/j.ncl.2007.03.009

Ferman, T., Boeve, B., Smith, G., Lin, S., Silber, M., Pedraza, O., . . . Dickson, D. (2011). Inclusion of RBD improves the diagnostic classification of dementia with Lewy bodies. *Neurology, 77*(9), 875–882. doi: 10.1212/WNL.0b013e31822c9148

Ferman, T., Boeve, B., Smith, G., Silber, M., Kokmen, E., Petersen, R., & Ivnik, R. (1999). REM sleep behavior disorder and dementia: Cognitive differences when compared with AD. *Neurology, 52*, 951–957.

Ferman, T., Boeve, B., Smith, G., Silber, M., Lucas, J., Graff-Radford, N., . . . Ivnik, R. (2002). Dementia with Lewy bodies may present as dementia and REM sleep behavior disorder without parkinsonism or hallucinations. *Journal of the International Neuropsychological Society, 8*, 907–914.

Ferman, T., Dickson, D., Graff-Radford, N., Arvanitakis, Z., DeLucia, M., Boeve, B., . . . Brassler, S. (2003). Early onset of visual hallucinations in dementia distinguishes pathologically confirmed Lewy body disease from AD. *Neurology, 60*(5), A264.

Ferman, T., Smith, G., Boeve, B., Graff-Radford, N., Lucas, J., Knopman, D., . . . Dickson, D. (2006). Neuropsychological differentiation of dementia with Lewy bodies from normal aging and Alzheimer's disease. *The Clinical Neuropsychologist, 20*(4), 623–636. doi: 10.1080/13854040500376831

Ferman, T. J., Smith, G. E., Kantarci, K., Boeve, B. F., Pankratz, V. S., Dickson, D. W., . . . Uitti, R. (2013). Nonamnestic mild cognitive impairment progresses to dementia with Lewy bodies. *Neurology, 81*(23), 2032–2038.

Fields, J., Ferman, T., Boeve, B., & Smith, G. (2011). Neuropsychological assessment of patients with dementing illness. *Nature Reviews Neurology, 7*, 677–687. doi: 10.1038/nrneurol.2011.173

Fillit, H., Butler, R., O'Connell, A., Albert, M., Birren, J., Cotman, C., . . . Tully, T. (2002). Achieving and maintaining cognitive vitality with aging. *Mayo Clinic Proceedings, 77*(7), 681–696.

Forstl, H., Burns, A., Luthert, P., Ciarns, N., & Levy, R. (1993). The Lewy-body variant of Alzheimer's disease: Clinical and pathological findings. *British Journal of Psychiatry, 162*, 385–392.

Freeman, R., Giovannetti, T., Lamar, M., Cloud, B., Stern, R., Kaplan, E., & Libon, D. (2000). Visuoconstructional problems in dementia: Contribution of executive systems functions. *Neuropsychology, 14*(3), 415–426.

Fuld, P., Masur, D., Blau, A., Crystal, H., & Aronson, M. (1990). Object-memory evaluation for prospective detection of dementia in normal functioning elderly: Predictive and normative data. *Journal of Clinical and Experimental Neuropsychology, 12*(4), 520–528.

Ganguli, M., Blacker, D., Blazer, D. G., Grant, I., Jeste, D. V., Paulsen, J. S., . . . Sachdev, P. S. (2011). Classification of neurocognitive disorders in DSM-5: A work in progress. *American Journal of Geriatric Psychiatry, 19*(3), 205–210.

Gnanalingham, K., Byrne, E., Thornton, A., Sambrook, M., & Bannister, P. (1997). Motor and cognitive function in Lewy body dementia: Comparison with Alzheimer's and Parkinson's diseases. *Journal of Neurology, Neurosurgery & Psychiatry, 62*(3), 243–252.

Gomar, J., Bobes-Bascaran, M., Conejero-Goldberg, C., Davies, P., Goldberg, T., & for the Alzheimer's Disease Neuroimaging Initiative. (2011). Utility of combinations of biomarkers, cognitive markers, and risk factors to predict conversion from mild cognitive impairment to Alzheimer disease in the Alzheimer's Disease Neuroimaging Initiative. *Archives of General Psychiatry*, *68*, 961–969.

Gorelick, P., Scuteri, A., Black, S., DeCarli, C., Greenberg, S., Iadecola, C., . . . Petersen, R. C. (2011). Vascular contributions to cognitive impairment and dementia: A statement for healtcare professionals from the American Heart Association/American Stroke Association. *Stroke*, *42*, 2672–2713.

Gorno-Tempini, M. L., Hillis, A. E., Weintraub, S., Kertesz, A., Mendez, M., Cappa, S. F., . . . Grossman, M. (2011). Classification of primary progressive aphasia and its variants. *Neurology*, *76*(11), 1006–1014. doi: WNL.0b013e31821103e6 [pii] 10.1212/WNL.0b013e31821103e6

Graham, N., Emery, T., & Hodges, J. (2004). Distinctive cognitive profiles in Alzheimer's disease and subcortical vascular dementia. *Journal of Neurology, Neurosurgery, and Psychiatry*, *75*(1), 61–71.

Greenaway, M. C., Duncan, N. L., & Smith, G. E. (2013). The memory support system for mild cognitive impairment: Randomized trial of a cognitive rehabilitation intervention. *International Journal of Geriatric Psychiatry*, *28*(4), 402–409. doi: 10.1002/gps.3838

Greenaway, M. C., Hanna, S. M., Lepore, S. W., & Smith, G. E. (2008). A behavioral rehabilitation intervention for amnestic mild cognitive impairment. *American Journal of Alzheimer's Disease and Other Dementias*, *23*(5), 451–461. doi: 10.1177/1533317508320352

Grober, E., & Kawas, C. (1997). Learning and retention in preclinical and early Alzheimer's disease. *Psychology & Aging*, *12*(1), 183–188.

Hamilton, J. M., Salmon, D. P., Galasko, D., Delis, D. C., Hansen, L. A., Masliah, E., . . . Thal, L. J. (2004). A comparison of episodic memory deficits in neuropathologically confirmed Dementia with Lewy bodies and Alzheimer's disease. *Journal of the International Neuropsychological Society*, *10*(5), 689–697. doi: 10.1017/s1355617704105043

Harris, J. M., Gall, C., Thompson, J. C., Richardson, A. M., Neary, D., du Plessis, D., . . . Jones, M. (2013). Classification and pathology of primary progressive aphasia. *Neurology*, *81*(21), 1832–1839. doi: 10.1212/01.wnl.0000436070.28137.7b

Heister, D., Brewer, J., Magda, S., Blennow, K., McEvoy, L., & for the Alzheimer's Disease Neuroimaging Initiative. (2011). Predicting MCI outcome with clinically available MRI and CSF biomarkers. *Neurology*, *77*, 1619–1628.

Hellen, C. (1992). *Alzheimer's Disease: Activity-Focused Care*. Boston, MA: Andover Medical Publishers.

Henry, J., Crawford, J., & Phillips, L. (2004). Verbal fluency performance in dementia of the Alzheimer's type: A meta-analysis. *Neuropsychologia*, *42*(9), 1212–1222. doi: 10.1016/j.neuropsychologia.2004.02.001

Howieson, D., Dame, A., Camicioli, R., Sexton, G., Payami, H., & Kaye, J. (1997). Cognitive markers preceding Alzheimer's dementia in the healthy oldest old. *Journal of the American Geriatrics Society*, *45*(5), 584–589.

Hulette, C., Mirra, S., Wilkinson, W., Heyman, A., Fillenbaum, G., & Clark, C. (1995). The Consortium to Establish a Registry for Alzheimer's Disease (CERAD), Part IX: A prospective clinico-neuropathologic study of Parkinson's features in Alzheimer's disease. *Neurology*, *45*(11), 1991–1995.

Hutchinson, A. D., & Mathias, J. L. (2007). Neuropsychological deficits in frontotemporal dementia and Alzheimer's disease: A meta-analytic review. *Journal of Neurology, Neurosurgery & Psychiatry*, *78*(9), 917–928. doi: 10.1136/jnnp.2006.100669

Hutton, M., & Hardy, J. (1997). The presenilins and Alzheimer's disease. *Human Molecular Genetics*, *6*(10), 1639–1646.

Imamura, T., Ishii, K., Hirono, N., Hashimoto, M., Tanimukai, S., Kazui, H., . . . Mori, E. (2001). Occipital glucose metabolism in dementia with lewy bodies with and without Parkinsonism: A study using positron emission tomography. *Dementia and Geriatric Cognitive Disorders*, *12*(3), 194–197.

Jack, C., Jr., Albert, M., Knopman, D., McKhann, G., Sperling, R., Carrillo, M., . . . Phelps, C. (2011). Introduction to the recommendations from the National Institute on Aging-Alzheimer's Association workgroups on diagnostic guidelines for Alzheimer's disease. *Alzheimer's & Dementia: The Journal of the Alzheimer's Association*, *7*(3), 257–262. doi: 10.1016/j.jalz.2011.03.004

Jack, C., Jr., Knopman, D., Jagust, W., Shaw, L., Aisen, P., Weiner, M., . . . Trojanowski, J. (2010). Hypothetical model of dynamic biomarkers of the Alzheimer's pathological cascade. *Lancet Neurology*, *9*(1), 119–128. doi: S1474-4422(09)70299-6 [pii] 10.1016/S1474-4422(09)70299-6

Jacobs, D., Sano, M., Dooneief, G., Marder, K., Bell, K., & Stern, Y. (1995). Neuropsychological detection and characterization of preclinical Alzheimer's disease. *Neurology*, *45*, 957–962.

Jedynak, B. M., Lang, A., Liu, B., Katz, E., Zhang, Y., Wyman, B. T., . . . Prince, J. L. (2012). A computational neurodegenerative disease progression score: Method and results with the Alzheimer's disease Neuroimaging Initiative cohort. *Neuroimage*, *63*(3), 1478–1486. doi: 10.1016/j.neuroimage.2012.07.059 S1053-8119(12)00789-6 [pii]

Johnson, D., Morris, J., & Galvin, J. (2005). Verbal and visuospatial deficits in dementia with Lewy bodies. *Neurology*, *65*, 1232–1238.

Johnson, D. K., Watts, A. S., Chapin, B. A., Anderson, R., & Burns, J. M. (2011). Neuropsychiatric profiles in dementia. *Alzheimer Disease and Associated Disorders*, *25*(4), 326–332. doi: 10.1097/WAD.0b013e31820d89b6 00002093-201110000-00006 [pii]

Josephs, K. (2008). Frontotemporal dementia and related disorders: Deciphering the enigma. *Annals of Neurology*, *64*(1), 4–14. doi: 10.1002/ana.21426

Josephs, K. A., Duffy, J. R., Strand, E. A., Machulda, M. M., Senjem, M. L., Lowe, V. J., . . . Whitwell, J. L. (2013). Syndromes dominated by apraxia of speech show distinct characteristics from agrammatic PPA. *Neurology*, *81*(4), 337–345. doi: 10.1212/WNL.0b013e31829c5ed5

Josephs, K. A., Duffy, J. R., Strand, E. A., Machulda, M. M., Senjem, M. L., Master, A. V., . . . Whitwell, J. L. (2012). Characterizing a neurodegenerative syndrome: Primary progressive apraxia of speech. *Brain*, *135*(Pt 5), 1522–1536. doi: 10.1093/brain/aws032

Josephs, K. A., Duffy, J. R., Strand, E. A., Whitwell, J. L., Layton, K. F., Parisi, J. E., . . . Petersen, R. C. (2006). Clinicopathological and imaging correlates of progressive aphasia and apraxia of speech. *Brain: A Journal of Neurology*, *129*(Pt 6), 1385–1398. doi: 10.1093/brain/awl078

Kertesz, A., & Clydesdale, S. (1994). Neuropsychological deficits in vascular dementia vs. Alzheimer's disease: Frontal lobe deficits prominent in vascular dementia. *Archives of Neurology*, *51*, 1226–1231.

Knopman, D. S. (2013). Alzheimer disease biomarkers and insights into mild cognitive impairment. *Neurology*, *80*(11), 978–980. doi: 10.1212/WNL.0b013e31828728ac

Knopman, D. S., Jack, C. R., Jr., Wiste, H. J., Weigand, S. D., Vemuri, P., Lowe, V. J., . . . Petersen, R. C. (2013). Brain injury biomarkers are not dependent on beta-amyloid in normal elderly. *Annals of Neurology*, *73*(4), 472–480. doi: 10.1002/ana.23816

Kurz, A., Pohl, C., Ramsenthaler, M., & Sorg, C. (2009). Cognitive rehabilitation in patients with mild cognitive impairment. *International Journal of Geriatric Psychiatry*, *24*(2), 163–168. doi: 10.1002/gps.2086

Lafosse, J., Reed, B., Mungas, D., Sterling, S., Wahbeh, H., & Jagust, W. (1997). Fluency and memory differences between ischemic vascular dementia and Alzheimer's disease. *Neuropsychology*, *11*, 514–522.

Laine, M., Vuorinen, E., & Rinne, J. (1997). Picture naming deficits in vascular dementia and Alzheimer's disease. *Journal of Clinical and Experimental Neuropsychology*, *19*(1), 126–140.

Lamar, M., Catani, M., Price, C., Heilman, K., & Libon, D. (2008). The impact of region-specific leukoaraiosis on working memory deficits in dementia. *Neuropsychologia*, *46*(10), 2597–2601. doi: S0028-3932(08)00125-5 [pii] 10.1016/j.neuropsychologia.2008.04.007

Lamar, M., Podell, K., Carew, T., Cloud, B., Resh, R., Kennedy, C., . . . Libon, D. (1997). Perseverative behavior in Alzheimer's disease and subcortical ischemic vascular dementia. *Neuropsychology*, *11*, 523–534.

Lamar, M., Price, C., Libon, D., Penney, D., Kaplan, E., Grossman, M., & Heilman, K. (2007). Alterations in working memory as a function of leukoaraiosis in dementia. *Neuropsychologia*, *45*, 245–254.

Landau, S., Harvey, D., Madison, C., Reiman, E., Foster, N., Aisen, P., . . . Jagust, W. (2010). Comparing predictors of conversion and decline in mild cognitive impairment. *Neurology*, *75*(3), 230–238. doi: WNL.0b013e3181e8e8b8 [pii] 10.1212/WNL.0b013e3181e8e8b8

Lange, K., Bondi, M., Salmon, D., Galasko, D., Delis, D., Thomas, R., & Thal, L. (2002). Decline in verbal memory during preclinical Alzheimer's disease: Examination of the effect of APOE genotype. *Journal of the International Neuropsychological Society: JINS*, *8*(7), 943–955.

Lautenschlager, N. T., Cox, K. L., Flicker, L., Foster, J. K., van Bockxmeer, F. M., Xiao, J., . . . Almeida, O. P. (2008). Effect of physical activity on cognitive function in older adults at risk for Alzheimer disease: A randomized trial. *JAMA: The Journal of the American Medical Association*, *300*(9), 1027–1037. doi: 10.1001/jama.300.9.1027

Lesage, S., & Brice, A. (2009). Parkinson's disease: From monogenic forms to genetic susceptibility factors. *Human Molecular Genetics*, *18*(R1), R48–59. doi: 10.1093/hmg/ddp012

Libon, D., Bogdanoff, B., Bonavita, J., Skalina, S., Cloud, B., Resh, R., . . . Ball, S. (1997). Dementia associated with periventricular and deep white matter alterations: A subtype of subcortical dementia. *Archives of Clinical Neuropsychology*, *12*(3), 239–250. doi: S0887-6177(96)00041-8 [pii]

Liu, W., Miller, B. L., Kramer, J. H., Rankin, K., Wyss-Coray, C., Gearhart, R., . . . Rosen, H. J. (2004). Behavioral disorders in the frontal and temporal variants of frontotemporal dementia. *Neurology*, *62*(5), 742–748.

Lobotesis, K., Fenwick, J., Phipps, A., Ryman, A., Swann, A., Ballard, C., . . . O'Brien, J. (2001). Occipital hypoperfusion on SPECT in dementia with Lewy bodies but not AD. *Neurology*, *56*, 643–649.

Loewenstein, D. A., Acevedo, A., Czaja, S. J., & Duara, R. (2004). Cognitive rehabilitation of mildly impaired Alzheimer disease patients on cholinesterase inhibitors. *The American Journal of Geriatric Psychiatry: Official Journal of the American Association for Geriatric Psychiatry*, *12*(4), 395–402. doi: 10.1176/appi.ajgp.12.4.395

Machulda, M. M., Whitwell, J. L., Duffy, J. R., Strand, E. A., Dean, P. M., Senjem, M. L., . . . Josephs, K. A. (2013). Identification of an atypical variant of logopenic progressive aphasia. *Brain and Language*, *127*(2), 139–144. doi: 10.1016/j.bandl.2013.02.007

Mahncke, H. W., Bronstone, A., & Merzenich, M. M. (2006). Brain plasticity and functional losses in the aged: Scientific bases for a novel intervention. *Progress in Brain Research*, *157*, 81–109. doi: 10.1016/S0079-6123(06)57006-2

McKeith, I., Dickson, D., Lowe, J., Emre, M., O'Brien, J., Feldman, H., . . . for the consortium on DLB. (2005). Diagnosis and management of dementia with Lewy bodies: Third report of the DLB consortium. [Review]. *Neurology*, *65*(12), 1863–1872.

McKeith, I., Mintzer, J., Aarsland, D., Burn, D., Chui, H., Cohen-Mansfield, J., . . . on behalf of the International Psychogeriatric Association Expert Meeting on DLB. (2004). Dementia with Lewy bodies. *Lancet Neurology*, *3*, 19–28.

McKhann, G. (2011). Changing concepts of Alzheimer disease. *Journal of the American Medical Association*, *305*, 2458–2459.

McKhann, G., Drachman, D., Folstein, M., Katzman, R., Price, D., & Stadlan, E. (1984). Clinical diagnosis of Alzheimer's disease: Report of the NINCDS-ADRDA work group under the auspices of department of health and human services task force on Alzheimer's disease. *Neurology*, *34*, 939–944.

McKhann, G., Knopman, D., Chertkow, H., Hyman, B., Jack, C., Jr., Kawas, C., . . . Phelps, C. (2011). The diagnosis of dementia due to Alzheimer's disease: Recommendations from the National Institute on Aging-Alzheimer's Association workgroups on diagnostic guidelines for Alzheimer's disease. *Alzheimer's & Dementia: The Journal of the Alzheimer's Association*, *7*(3), 263–269. doi: 10.1016/j.jalz.2011.03.005

Mesulam, M. M. (1982). Slowly progressive aphasia without generalized dementia. *Annals of Neurology*, *11*(6), 592–598. doi: 10.1002/ana.410110607

Mesulam, M. M., & Weintraub, S. (2014). Is it time to revisit the classification guidelines for primary progressive aphasia? *Neurology*, *82*(13), 1108–1109. doi: 10.1212/wnl.0000000000000272

Mielke, M. M., Rosenberg, P. B., Tschanz, J., Cook, L., Corcoran, C., Hayden, K. M., . . . Lyketsos, C. G. (2007). Vascular factors predict rate of progression in Alzheimer disease. *Neurology*, *69*(19), 1850–1858. doi: 10.1212/01.wnl.0000279520.59792.fe

Miller, B. (2013). *Frontotemporal Dementia* (Vol. 1). New York: Oxford University Press.

Miller, B. L., Diehl, J., Freedman, M., Kertesz, A., Mendez, M., & Rascovsky, K. (2003). International approaches to frontotemporal dementia diagnosis: From social cognition to neuropsychology. *Annals of Neurology*, *54*(Suppl 5), S7–S10. doi: 10.1002/ana.10568

Molano, J., Boeve, B., Ferman, T., Smith, G., Parisi, J., Dickson, D., . . . Petersen, R. (2010). Mild cognitive impairment associated with limbic and neocortical Lewy body disease: A clinicopathological study. *Brain: A Journal of Neurology*, *133*(Pt 2), 540–556. doi: 10.1093/brain/awp280

Monsch, A. U., Bondi, M. W., Butters, N., Salmon, D. P., Katzman, R., & Thal, L. J. (1992). Comparisons of verbal fluency tasks in the detection of dementia of the Alzheimer type. *Archives of Neurology*, *49*(12), 1253–1258.

Mori, E., Shimomura, T., Fujimori, M., Hirono, N., Imamura, T., Hashimoto, M., . . . Hanihara, T. (2000). Visuoperceptual impairment in dementia with Lewy bodies. *Archives of Neurology*, *57*(4), 489–493.

Mosconi, L., Tsui, W. H., Herholz, K., Pupi, A., Drzezga, A., Lucignani, G., . . . de Leon, M. J. (2008). Multicenter standardized 18F-FDG PET diagnosis of mild cognitive impairment, Alzheimer's disease, and other dementias. *Journal of Nuclear Medicine*, *49*(3), 390–398. doi: 10.2967/jnumed.107.045385

Mosimann, U., Mather, G., Wesnes, K., O'Brien, J., Burn, D., & McKeith, I. (2004). Visual perception in Parkinson disease dementia and dementia with Lewy bodies. *Neurology*, *63*(11), 2091–2096.

Mosimann, U., Muri, R., Burn, D., Felblinger, J., O'Brien, J., & McKeith, I. (2005). Saccadic eye movement changes in Parkinson's disease dementia and dementia with Lewy bodies. *Brain*, *128*, 1267–1276.

Pachana, N. A., Boone, K. B., Miller, B. L., Cummings, J. L., & Berman, N. (1996). Comparison of neuropsychological functioning in Alzheimer's disease and frontotemporal dementia. *Journal of the International Neuropsychological Society: JINS*, *2*(6), 505–510.

Paulsen, J., Salmon, D., Thal, L., Romero, R., Weisstein-Jenkins, C., Galasko, D., . . . Jeste, D. (2000). Incidence of and risk factors for hallucinations and delusions in patients with probable AD. *Neurology*, *54*(10), 1965–1971.

Perry, R., & Hodges, J. (2000). Differentiating frontal and temporal variant frontotemporal dementia from Alzheimer's disease. *Neurology*, *54*(12), 2277–2284.

Peters, N., Opherk, C., Bergmann, T., Castro, M., Herzog, J., & Dichgans, M. (2005). Spectrum of mutations in biopsy-proven CADASIL: Implications for diagnostic strategies. *Archives of Neurology*, *62*(7), 1091–1094. doi: 10.1001/archneur.62.7.1091

Petersen, R., Doody, R., Kurz, A., Mohs, R., Morris, J., Rabins, P., . . . Winblad, B. (2001). Current concepts in mild cognitive impairment. *Archives of Neurology*, *58*(12), 1985–1992.

Petersen, R., Ivnik, R., Boeve, B., Knopman, D., Smith, G., & Tangalos, E. (2004). Outcome of clinical substypes of MCI. *Neurology*, *62*, A29S.

Petersen, R. C., Smith, G. E., Waring, S. C., Ivnik, R. J., Tangalos, E. G., & Kokmen, E. (1999). Mild cognitive impairment: Clinical characterization and outcome. *Archives of Neurology*, *56*(3), 303–308.

Plazzi, G., Corsini, R., Provini, F., Pierangeli, G., Martinelli, P., Montagna, P., . . . Cortelli, P. (1997). REM sleep behavior disorders in multiple system atrophy. *Neurology*, *48*(4), 1094–1097.

Postuma, R., Gagnon, J., Vendette, M., Fantini, M., Massicotte-Marquez, J., & Montplaisir, J. (2009). Quantifying the risk of neurodegenerative disease in idiopathic REM sleep behavior disorder. *Neurology*, *72*, 1296–1300.

Price, C., Jefferson, A., Merino, J., Heilman, K., & Libon, D. (2005). Subcortical vascular dementia: Integrating neuropsychological and neuroradiologic data. *Neurology*, *65*(3), 376–382. doi: 65/3/376 [pii] 10.1212/01.wnl.0000168877.06011.15

Quigley, H., Colloby, S., & O'Brien, J. (2011). PET imaging of brain amyloid in dementia: A review. *International Journal of Geriatric Psychiatry*, *10*, 991–999.

Rapp, S., Brenes, G., & Marsh, A. (2002). Memory enhancement training for older adults with mild cognitive impairment: A preliminary study. *Aging Ment Health*, *6*(1), 5–11. doi: 10.1080/13607860120101077

Rascovsky, K., Salmon, D., Hansen, L., Thal, L., & Galasko, D. (2007). Disparate letter and semantic category fluency deficits in autopsy-confirmed frontotemporal dementia and Alzheimer's disease. *Neuropsychology*, *21*(1), 20–30. doi: 10.1037/0894-4105.21.1.20

Razani, J., Boone, K. B., Miller, B. L., Lee, A., & Sherman, D. (2001). Neuropsychological performance of right- and left-frontotemporal dementia compared to Alzheimer's disease. *Journal of the International Neuropsychological Society: JINS*, *7*(4), 468–480.

Rebok, G., Carlson, M., & Langbaum, J. (2007). Training and maintaining memory abilities in healthy older adults: Traditional and novel approaches. *The Journals of Gerontology. Series B, Psychological Sciences and Social Sciences*, *62*(Spec No 1), 53–61.

Reed, B., Mungas, D., Kramer, J., Betz, B., Ellis, W., Vinters, H., . . . Chui, H. (2004). Clinical and neuropsychological features in autopsy-defined vascular dementia. *The Clinical Neuropsychologist*, *18*(1), 63–74.

Reed, B., Mungas, D., Kramer, J., Ellis, W., Vinters, H., Zarow, C., . . . Chui, H. (2007). Profiles of neuropsychological impairment in autopsy-defined Alzheimer's disease and cerebrovascular disease. *Brain*, *130*(Pt 3), 731–739. doi: awl385 [pii] 10.1093/brain/awl385

Regier, D. A., Narrow, W. E., Clarke, D. E., Kraemer, H. C., Kuramoto, S. J., Kuhl, E. A., & Kupfer, D. J. (2013). DSM-5 field trials in the United States and Canada, Part II: Test-retest reliability of selected categorical diagnoses. *American Journal of Psychiatry*, *170*(1), 59–70. doi: 10.1176/appi.ajp.2012.12070999

Robinson, A., Spencer, B., & White, L. (1988). *Understanding Difficult Behaviors: Some Practical Suggestions for Coping With Alzheimer's Disease and Related Illnesses*. Ypsilanti: Geriatric Education Center of Michigan, Michigan State University.

Rodda, J., Morgan, S., & Walker, Z. (2009). Are cholinesterase inhibitors effective in the management of the behavioral and psychological symptoms of dementia in Alzheimer's disease? A systematic review of randomized, placebo-controlled trials of donepezil, rivastigmine and galantamine. *International Psychogeriatrics/IPA*, *21*(5), 813–824. doi: 10.1017/S1041610209990354

Rohrer, J. D., Ridgway, G. R., Crutch, S. J., Hailstone, J., Goll, J. C., Clarkson, M. J., . . . Warren, J. D. (2010). Progressive logopenic/phonological aphasia: Erosion of the language network. *Neuroimage*, *49*(1), 984–993. doi: 10.1016/j.neuroimage.2009.08.002

Rohrer, J. D., Warren, J. D., Fox, N. C., & Rossor, M. N. (2013). Presymptomatic studies in genetic frontotemporal dementia. *Revue Neurologique (Paris)*, *169*(10), 820–824. doi: 10.1016/j.neurol.2013.07.010

Rombouts, S., Barkhof, F., Goekoop, R., Stam, C., & Scheltens, P. (2005). Altered resting state networks in mild cognitive impairment and mild Alzheimer's disease: An FMRI study. *Human Brain Mapping*, *26*, 231–239.

Rovner, B., Steele, C., Shmuely, Y., & Folstein, M. (1996). A randomized trial of dementia care in nursing homes. *Journal of the American Geriatrics Society*, *44*(1), 7–13.

Rozzini, L., Costardi, D., Chilovi, B. V., Franzoni, S., Trabucchi, M., & Padovani, A. (2007). Efficacy of cognitive rehabilitation in patients with mild cognitive impairment treated with cholinesterase inhibitors. *International Journal of Geriatric Psychiatry*, *22*(4), 356–360.

Salmon, D. (2004, February 4, 2003). *Distinct patterns of cognitive deficits in neuropathologically confirmed dementia with Lewy bodies and pure Alzheimer's disease.* Paper presented at the 32nd Annual Meeting of the International Neuropsychological Society, Baltimore, MD.

Salmon, D., & Bondi, M. (2009). Neuropsychological assessment of dementia. *Annual Review of Psychology*, *60*, 257–282. doi: 10.1146/annurev.psych.57.102904.190024

Salmon, D., & Filoteo, J. (2007). Neuropsychology of cortical vs. subcortical dementia. *Seminars in Neurology*, *27*, 7–21.

Schenck, C., Bundlie, S., & Mahowald, M. (1996). Delayed emergence of a parkinsonian disorder in 38% of 29 older men initially diagnosed with idiopathic rapid eye movement sleep behaviour disorder. *Neurology*, *46*(2), 388–393.

Schneider, J., Arvanitakis, Z., Leurgans, S., & Bennett, D. (2009). The neuropathology of probable Alzheimer disease and mild cognitive impairment. *Annals of Neurology*, *66*, 200–208.

Schneider, J., Boyle, P., Arvanitakis, Z., Bienias, J., & Bennett, D. (2007). Subcortical cerebral infarcts, episodic memory, and AD pathology in older persons. *Annals of Neurology*, *62*, 59–66.

Schneider, J., Wilson, R., Bienias, J., Evans, D., & Bennett, D. (2004). Cerebral infarctions and the likelihood of dementia from Alzheimer disease pathology. *Neurology*, *62*, 1148–1155.

Schneider, L., Pollock, V., & Lyness, S. (1990). A meta-analysis of controlled trials of neuroleptic treatment in dementia. *Journal of the American Geriatrics Society*, *38*, 553–563.

Seidel, G., Tiovannetti, T., & Libon, D. (2011). Cerebrovascular disease and cognition in older adults. In M. Pardon & M. Bondi (Eds.), *Current Topics in Behavioral Neuroscience: Behavioral of Neurobiology of Aging* (pp. 213–231). New York: Springer-Verlag.

Siepel, F. J., Rongve, A., Buter, T. C., Beyer, M. K., Ballard, C. G., Booij, J., & Aarsland, D. (2013). (123I)FP-CIT SPECT in suspected dementia with Lewy bodies: A longitudinal case study. *Bmj Open*, *3*(4). doi: 10.1136/bmjopen-2013-002642

Small, G., Rabins, P., Barry, P., Buckholtz, N., DeKosky, S., Ferris, S., . . . Tune, L. (1997). Diagnosis and treatment of Alzheimer disease and related disorders: Consensus statement of the American Association for Geriatric Psychiatry, the Alzheimer's association, and the American Geriatrics Society. *JAMA*, *278*(16), 1363–1371.

Smith, G. E., & Bondi, M. W. (2013). *Mild Cognitive Impairment and Dementia: Definitions, Diagnosis, and Treatment*. Oxford, NY: Oxford University Press.

Smith, G. E., Housen, P., Yaffe, K., Ruff, R., Kennison, R. F., Mahncke, H. W., & Zelinski, E. M. (2009). A cognitive training program based on principles of brain plasticity: Results from the Improvement in Memory with Plasticity-based Adaptive Cognitive Training (IMPACT) study. *Journal of the American Geriatrics Society*, *57*(4), 594–603. doi: 10.1111/j.1532-5415.2008.02167.x

Smith, G. E., Pankratz, V. S., Negash, S., Machulda, M. M., Petersen, R. C., Boeve, B. F., . . . Ivnik, R. J. (2007). A plateau in pre-Alzheimer memory decline: Evidence for compensatory mechanisms? *Neurology*, *69*(2), 133–139. doi: 10.1212/01.wnl.0000265594.23511.16

Smith, J. C., Nielson, K. A., Antuono, P., Lyons, J. A., Hanson, R. J., Butts, A. M., . . . Verber, M. D. (2013). Semantic memory functional MRI and cognitive function after exercise intervention in mild cognitive impairment. *Journal of Alzheimer's Disease*, *37*(1), 197–215. doi: 10.3233/jad-130467

Smith, J. C., Nielson, K. A., Woodard, J. L., Seidenberg, M., Durgerian, S., Antuono, P., . . . Rao, S. M. (2011). Interactive effects of physical activity and APOE-epsilon4 on BOLD semantic memory activation in healthy elders. *Neuroimage*, *54*(1), 635–644. doi: 10.1016/j.neuroimage.2010.07.070

Snell, R. G., MacMillan, J. C., Cheadle, J. P., Fenton, I., Lazarou, L. P., Davies, P., . . . Shaw, D. J. (1993). Relationship between trinucleotide repeat expansion and phenotypic variation in Huntington's disease. *Nature Genetics*, *4*(4), 393–397. doi: 10.1038/ng0893-393

Sohlberg, M. M., & Mateer, C. A. (1989). Training use of compensatory memory books: A three stage behavioral approach. *Journal of Clinical and Experimental Neuropsychology*, *11*(6), 871–891. doi: 10.1080/01688638908400941

Sonnen, J., Larson, E., Crane, P., Haneuse, S., Li, G., Schellenberg, G., Craft, S., . . . Montine, T. J. (2007). Pathological correlates of dementia in a longitudinal, population-based sample of aging. *Annals of Neurology*, *62*, 406–413.

Sperling, R., Aisen, P., Beckett, L., Bennett, D., Craft, S., Fagan, A., . . . Phelps, C. (2011). Toward defining the preclinical stages of Alzheimer's disease: Recommendations from the National Institute on Aging-Alzheimer's Association workgroups on diagnostic guidelines for Alzheimer's disease. *Alzheimer's & Dementia: The Journal of the Alzheimer's Association*, *7*(3), 280–292. doi: 10.1016/j.jalz.2011.03.003

Stern, Y. (2006). Cognitive reserve and Alzheimer's disease. *Alzheimer Disease & Associated Disorders*, *20*(2), 112–117.

Stern, Y. (2009). Cognitive reserve. *Neuropsychologia*, *47*(10), 2015–2028. doi: S0028-3932(09)00123-7 [pii] 10.1016/j.neuropsychologia.2009.03.004

Sultzer, D. L., Davis, S. M., Tariot, P. N., Dagerman, K. S., Lebowitz, B. D., Lyketsos, C. G., . . . Schneider, L. S. (2008). Clinical symptom responses to atypical antipsychotic medications in Alzheimer's disease: Phase 1 outcomes from the CATIE-AD effectiveness trial. *The American Journal of Psychiatry*, *165*(7), 844–854. doi: 10.1176/appi.ajp.2008.07111779

Talassi, E., Guerreschi, M., Feriani, M., Fedi, V., Bianchetti, A., & Trabucchi, M. (2007). Effectiveness of a cognitive rehabilitation program in mild dementia (MD) and mild cognitive impairment (MCI): A case control study. *Archives of Gerontologic Geriatrics*, *44*(Suppl 1), 391–399.

Tang-Wai, D. F., Graff-Radford, N. R., Boeve, B. F., Dickson, D. W., Parisi, J. E., Crook, R., . . . Petersen, R. C. (2004). Clinical, genetic, and neuropathologic characteristics of posterior cortical atrophy. *Neurology*, *63*(7), 1168–1174.

Teri, L., Truax, P., Logsdon, R., Zarit, S., Uomoto, J., & Vitaliano, P. (1992). Assessment of behavioral problems in dementia: The revised memory and behavior problems checklist. *Psychology and Aging*, *7*, 622–631.

Testa, J., Ivnik, R., & Smith, G. (2003). Diagnostic utility of the Boston Naming Test in MCI and Alzheimer's disease. *Journal of the International Neuropsychological Society: JINS*, *9*, 306.

Turner, R., Chervin, R., Frey, K., Minoshima, S., & Kuhl, D. (1997). Probable diffuse Lewy body disease presenting as REM sleep behavior disorder. *Neurology*, *49*(2), 523–527.

Turner, R., D'Amato, C., Chervin, R., & Blaivas, M. (2000). The pathology of REM sleep behavior disorder with comorbid Lewy body dementia. *Neurology*, *55*(11), 1730–1732.

Unverzagt, F., Kasten, L., Johnson, K., Rebok, G., Marsiske, M., Koepke, K., . . . Tennstedt, S. (2007). Effect of memory impairment on training outcomes in ACTIVE. *Journal of the International Neuropsychological Society*, *13*, 953–960.

Weintraub, S., Rogalski, E., Shaw, E., Sawlani, S., Rademaker, A., Wieneke, C., & Mesulam, M. M. (2013). Verbal and nonverbal memory in primary progressive aphasia: The Three Words-Three Shapes Test. *Behavioural Neurology*, *26*(1–2), 67–76. doi: 10.3233/ben-2012-110239

Whall, A., Black, M., Groh, C., Yankou, D., Kupferschmid, B., & Foster, N. (1997). The effect of natural environments upon agitation and aggression in late stage dementia patients. *American Journal of Alzheimer's Disease and Other Dementias*, *12*, 216–220.

Whitwell, J. L., Duffy, J. R., Strand, E. A., Xia, R., Mandrekar, J., Machulda, M. M., . . . Josephs, K. A. (2013). Distinct regional anatomic and functional correlates of neurodegenerative apraxia of speech and aphasia: An MRI and FDG-PET study. *Brain and Language*, *125*(3), 245–252. doi: 10.1016/j.bandl.2013.02.005

Whitwell, J. L., Przybelski, S. A., Weigand, S. D., Ivnik, R. J., Vemuri, P., Gunter, J. L., . . . Josephs, K. A. (2009). Distinct anatomical subtypes of the behavioural variant of frontotemporal dementia: A cluster analysis study. *Brain*, *132*(11), 2932–2946. doi: awp232 [pii] 10.1093/brain/awp232

Wicklund, M. R., Duffy, J. R., Strand, E. A., Machulda, M. M., Whitwell, J. L., & Josephs, K. A. (2014). Quantitative application of the primary progressive aphasia consensus criteria. *Neurology*, *82*(13), 1119–1126. doi: 10.1212/wnl.0000000000000261

Wilson, R., Weir, D., Leurgans, S., Evans, D., Hebert, L., Langa, K., . . . Bennett, D. (2011). Sources of variability in estimates of the prevalence of Alzheimer's disease in the United States. *Alzheimer's & Dementia: The Journal of the Alzheimer's Association*, *7*(1), 74–79.

Wittenberg, D., Possin, K. L., Rascovsky, K., Rankin, K. P., Miller, B. L., & Kramer, J. H. (2008). The early neuropsychological and behavioral characteristics of frontotemporal dementia. *Neuropsychology Review*, *18*(1), 91–102. doi: 10.1007/s11065-008-9056-z

Zelinski, E. M., Dalton, S. E., & Smith, G. E. (2011). *Consumer Based Brain Fitness Programs*. New York: Springer.

Zelinski, E. M., Spina, L. M., Yaffe, K., Ruff, R., Kennison, R. F., Mahncke, H. W., & Smith, G. E. (2011). Improvement in memory with plasticity-based adaptive cognitive training: Results of the 3-month follow-up. *Journal of the American Geriatrics Society*, *59*(2), 258–265. doi: 10.1111/j.1532-5415.2010.03277.x

Zhang, W., Arteaga, J., Cashion, D. K., Chen, G., Gangadharmath, U., Gomez, L. F., . . . Kolb, H. C. (2012). A highly selective and specific PET tracer for imaging of tau pathologies. *Journal of Alzheimer's Disease*, *31*(3), 601–612. doi: 10.3233/JAD-2012-120712

Zhou, A., & Jia, J. (2009). Different cognitive profiles between mild cognitive impaire due to cerebral small vessel disease and mild cognitive impairment of Alzheimer's disease origin. *Journal of the International Neuropsychological Society: JINS*, *15*, 898–905.

31 Complexities of Metabolic Disorders

Marc A. Norman, Olivia Bjorkquist Harner, and S. Joshua Kenton

Metabolism is the breakdown of food into its more elementary components. These functions govern the transport, storage, and distribution of energy throughout the body, and abnormalities may not only create organ and tissue dysfunction, but also cognition may be altered. Complex chemical reactions create the processes that break down substances that the body no longer needs or make those it lacks. For this process to work efficiently, enzymes are needed to break down food into its constituent parts, so an enzyme deficiency can create metabolic abnormalities and dysfunction.

The majority of metabolic disorders are due to single genes that code for enzymes. While some metabolic dysfunction is relatively mild, other disorders can create severe changes. The course of the dysfunction can be acute or chronic, and the consequences can lead to the buildup of harmful substances if it is too low or if it is missing entirely. Disorders can occur in various ways, including inborn errors of metabolism, congenital metabolic disorders, and inherited metabolic disorders, although onset may occur in late life. In most disorders, problems arise due to the accumulation of substances that are toxic or interfere with normal function, or they may be due to the effects of reduced ability to synthesize essential compounds. One of the most common metabolic disorders in childhood is phenylketonuria (PKU) and in adulthood, diabetes.

With new and evolving technologies, tests, and science, the understanding and classification of metabolic disorders has changed. In the past, inherited metabolic diseases were categorized as disorders of carbohydrate metabolism, amino acid metabolism, organic acid metabolism, or lysosomal storage diseases; however, more recently hundreds of new inherited metabolic disorders have been discovered and the categories have expanded (see Table 31.1).

Inborn errors of metabolism affect about one in every 5,000 babies born, and some inborn errors of metabolism are more often found in certain racial and ethnic groups. Sickle cell anemia, for example, is found among those of African descent, and those of European heritage are more likely to pass on malfunctioning genes for cystic fibrosis. Children of women with inborn errors of metabolism are at risk because of exposure in the womb. Because of the wide range of metabolic disorders, there are myriad symptoms and syndromes that may be associated with specific conditions. These symptoms often present in childhood and almost any presenting complaint may have a congenital metabolic etiology (see Table 31.2).

Treatments for metabolic disorders vary by specific conditions and may include dietary restriction (i.e., phenylalanine), dietary supplementation or replacement (e.g., cornstarch for glycogen storage diseases), vitamins (e.g., for some disorders causing lactic acidosis), enzyme replacement, dialysis, medications, gene transfer, symptom treatment, or bone marrow or solid organ transplantation. Other treatments may focus on symptoms (i.e., antiepileptics, surgery, etc.).

While many etiologies are genetic, metabolic disorders can be secondary to other factors, such as a combination of inherited, environmental, or secondary medical factors. Examples of acute or chronic medical illnesses that may cause metabolic disorders include alcohol abuse, diabetes, diuretic abuse, gout, ingestion of poison or toxins—including excessive aspirin, bicarbonate, alkali, ethylene glycol, or methanol. Conversely, metabolic abnormalities may result from kidney failure, pneumonia, respiratory failure, collapsed lung, HIV/AIDS, or sepsis. This dynamic relationship between etiologies and symptoms may further result in complications including metabolic acidosis and kidney failure (with possible tertiary complications such as neuropathy, retinopathy, and nephropathy).

In addition to systemic dysfunction, metabolic abnormalities may cause changes in mental status and cause metabolic encephalopathies. These syndromes may vary along the continuum of acute versus chronic and reversible versus permanent. Examples of these metabolic encephalopathies include Wernicke's encephalopathy (deficiency of thiamine typically in setting of alcohol disorder), uremic encephalopathy (resulting from kidney toxins, but rare when dialysis is used), hepatic encephalopathy (resulting from liver dysfunction and possibly related to elevated ammonia), and mitochondrial encephalopathy (caused by mitochondrial DNA dysfunction).

Metabolic disorders constitute a large, heterogeneous group of medical conditions with high rates of comorbidities. In addition to physical effects on the body, many of these disorders impact cognition, behavior, and/or psychiatric

Table 31.1 Major classes of congenital metabolic diseases, with examples of each class

Disorders of carbohydrate metabolism
E.g., diabetes insipidus, hereditary fructose intolerance, galactosemia, pyruvate metabolism disorders, von Gierke's disease, McArdle disease, Pompe's disease, and Forbes' disease, glycogen storage disease
Disorders of amino acid metabolism
E.g., glutaric acidemia type 1, Tay-Sachs disease, PKU, tyrosinemia, maple syrup urine disease, and homocystinuria
Urea cycle defects/disorders
E.g., Carbamoyl phosphate synthetase I deficiency
Disorders of organic acid metabolism (organic acidurias)
E.g., alcaptonuria
Disorders of fatty acid oxidation and mitochondrial metabolism
E.g., Gaucher's disease, Niemann-Pick disease, Fabry's disease, and medium-chain acyl-coenzyme A dehydrogenase (MCAD) deficiency
Disorders of porphyrin metabolism
E.g., acute intermittent porphyria
Disorders of purine or pyrimidine metabolism
E.g., Lesch-Nyhan syndrome
Disorders of steroid metabolism
E.g., lipoid congenital adrenal hyperplasia, congenital adrenal hyperplasia
Disorders of mitochondrial function
E.g., Kearns-Sayre syndrome
Disorders of peroxisomal function
E.g., Zellweger syndrome
Lysosomal storage disorders
E.g., Gaucher's disease, Niemann Pick disease

status, and neuropsychological evaluation may be warranted. However, given etiological heterogeneity and comorbidity, elucidating the neuropsychological profiles of these disorders remains a challenge in the literature. The following describe neurocognition in select metabolic disorders that are more commonly seen in neuropsychology clinics, though this is not exhaustive.

Phenylketonuria

One of the most well-described metabolic disorders in children is PKU, a hereditary disorder characterized by inefficient metabolism of phenylalanine. It has multiple effects on the central nervous system, including dopamine deficiency and white matter abnormalities. Treatment of PKU involves early and continuous implementation of a low-phenylalanine diet. Left untreated, the disease causes structural brain damage with severe, irreversible cognitive decline. Even when treated early and continuously, children with PKU evidence generally average intelligence with subtle neuropsychological impairments, thought to reflect reduced dopamine and white matter abnormalities. The most prominent deficit reported in the literature is executive dysfunction (Janos, Grange, Steiner, & White, 2012; for review, see (Christ, Huijbregts, de Sonneville, & White, 2010; DeRoche & Welsh, 2008), but studies also report reduced processing speed, fine motor skills, and visuospatial abilities, with mixed results regarding language, learning, and memory in children with PKU (Albrecht, Garbade, & Burgard, 2009; Janzen & Nguyen, 2010). In adults with PKU, these deficits are more subtle, and reduced processing speed is thought to be the most prominent characteristic (Channon, Mockler, & Lee, 2005). The severity of neurocognitive impairment in PKU depends on a number of factors, including timing of initiation of treatment, duration of treatment, and blood phenylalanine levels.

Diabetes Mellitus

In adults, the most common disorder of metabolism is diabetes mellitus. This disease is characterized by elevated blood glucose levels related to insulin abnormality. Type 1 diabetes is an autoimmune disorder with destruction of pancreatic cells, leading to insulin deficiency, and treatment includes insulin, eating healthy foods, regular exercise, maintaining a healthy weight, blood sugar monitoring, and carbohydrate, fat, and protein counting. It typically presents in childhood

Table 31.2 Possible manifestations/presentations of metabolic disorders

Growth failure	Pain	Developmental delay	Deafness
Blindness	Stroke	Dementia	Failure to thrive
Delayed puberty	Agnosia	Encephalopathy	Lack of pigmentation
Precocious puberty	Hypothyroidism	Psychosis	Skin rash
Ambiguous Genitalia	Adrenal insufficiency	Immunodeficiency	Excessive hair growth
Congenital malformations	Diabetes mellitus	Seizures	Abnormal pigmentation
Dental abnormalities	Hypogonadism	Renal failure	Lumps and bumps
Unusual facial features	Weight loss	Enlarged spleen	Abnormal behavior
Dehydration	Hypotension	Enlarged lymph nodes	Enlarged heart
Edema	Thrombocytopenia	Many forms of cancer	Cardiac failure
Hypertension	Abdominal pain	Recurrent vomiting, diarrhea	Myocardial infarction
Hyperventilation	Anemia	Excessive urination	Hepatomegaly
Respiratory failure	Cramps	Depression	Liver failure
Joint pain	Muscle weakness		Jaundice

or early adulthood and accounts for approximately 5%–10% of diabetes cases. In contrast, Type 2 diabetes results from insensitivity to insulin with adult onset and increased prevalence with age, and treatment may include a healthy diet, regular exercise, blood sugar monitoring, and a diabetes medication or insulin. Diabetes mellitus may affect cognition via multiple pathways. First, insulin and insulin receptors are found throughout the brain, and insulin affects mechanisms related to neuronal activity and related cognitive functions. For example, insulin receptors are found in the hippocampus, and studies suggest insulin involvement in normal memory function (Craft & Watson, 2004). Second, disease characteristics such as chronic hyperglycemia and microvascular disease affect cognition in diabetes as well. Accordingly, neuropsychological impairment is reported in the diabetes literature.

In Type 1 diabetes, studies find subtle deficits in general intelligence, psychomotor efficiency, and mental flexibility, with smaller deficits in visual perception and sustained attention, and typically no impairment in learning and memory; cognitive dysfunction emerges early in the disease, effects are relatively consistent over time, and dementia risk is unclear (Brands, Biessels, de Haan, Kappelle, & Kessels, 2005; McCrimmon, Ryan, & Frier, 2012). In Type 2 diabetes, similar mild changes in attention, executive functions, and processing speed are reported, with one important difference: impaired learning and memory (e.g., McCrimmon et al., 2012; Palta, Schneider, Biessels, Touradji, & Hill-Briggs, 2014; Sadanand, Balachandar, & Bharath, 2015). Cognitive impairment may emerge in prediabetic stages and progresses over time (van den Berg et al., 2010), with some evidence of accelerated aging in those with more severe disease (Yaffe et al., 2012). Type 2 diabetes increases risk of dementia 1.5–2.5-fold (Strachan, Reynolds, Marioni, & Price, 2011), with increased rates of mild cognitive impairment, Alzheimer's disease, and vascular dementia (Cheng, Huang, Deng, & Wang, 2012).

Metabolic Syndrome

Metabolic syndrome is defined as co-occurrence of certain vascular risk factors, requiring three or more of the following: abdominal obesity, hypertriglyceridemia, low high-density lipoprotein level, hypertension, and hyperglycemia. Reduction of these risk factors may include maintaining a healthy weight and diet, smoking cessation, pharmacologic agents (e.g., statins, niacin, fibrates, etc.), anti-hypertensive agents, and diabetic medications. In addition to the previously described effects of diabetes on cognition, individual components of the syndrome have each been associated with impaired cognition, including hypertension (Novak & Hajjar, 2010; Peters & Beckett, 2009), obesity (Dahl et al., 2013), hypertriglyceridemia (Farr et al., 2008), and impaired glucose tolerance (Takahashi et al., 2011), with impairment ranging from subtle changes to dementia. Studies investigating metabolic syndrome as a whole have variable findings, including decreased intellectual functions, memory, executive functions, visuospatial abilities, and processing speed, although a few studies have reported no associations between metabolic syndrome and cognition (for review, see Yates, Sweat, Yau, Turchiano, & Convit, 2012). The heterogeneity of study results likely relates to differences in sample characteristics (e.g., comorbid medical conditions, demographics), sensitivity of test batteries, and differences in definition of metabolic syndrome. Metabolic syndrome poses an elevated risk for vascular dementia (Panza et al., 2010) and Alzheimer's disease (Kim & Feldman, 2015). The relative importance of each component varies across studies, though insulin resistance appears to play a central role in cognitive impairment and increased risk for dementia (Kim & Feldman, 2015). Additional proposed mechanisms include neuroinflammation, oxidative stress, abnormal brain lipid metabolism, and impaired vascular reactivity (Yates et al., 2012).

Thyroid Disease

The thyroid gland secretes hormones that act throughout the body and influence metabolism, amongst other functions. Thyroid hormone receptors are widely distributed throughout the brain, and proper function of this system is crucial for brain development. These hormones interact with multiple neurotransmitter systems throughout the life span, influencing cognition, mood, and behavior (Bauer, Goetz, Glenn, & Whybrow, 2008). Abnormal thyroid function has been shown to alter brain structure and function in rat models through a number of mechanisms, including reducing hippocampal granule cells and synaptic plasticity and altering neurotransmitter, neuromodulator, and growth factor systems (Samuels, 2014b). Dysfunction of the thyroid may arise from a number of etiologies, resulting in hypothyroid or hyperthyroid conditions. Hypothyroidism is characterized by low production of thyroid hormones, is most commonly caused by autoimmune-associated thyroid damage, and is treated with thyroid hormone medications. Hyperthyroidism involves excess thyroid hormones, is most commonly caused by Grave's disease, and is treated with antithyroid medications.

Without treatment, congenital hypothyroidism may be associated with profound mental retardation with severe cognitive impairment; although early identification and treatment improves cognitive outcome, studies report impaired attention, visuospatial abilities, motor dexterity, and comprehension that persist throughout childhood (Dugbartey, 1998). In adult-onset hypothyroidism, studies most consistently find impairment in verbal memory, in addition to deficits in general intelligence, psychomotor speed, and visuospatial abilities, with less impact on motor abilities, language, and sustained attention (Bauer et al., 2008; Dugbartey, 1998; Samuels, 2014a, 2014b). These deficits range from minimal to severe. Hypothyroidism is also commonly associated with depression and anxiety, although some studies fail to find this relationship (Samuels, 2014a). Generally, studies report reversal of cognitive and emotional symptoms with treatment, though subtle deficits may persist. In contrast, hyperthyroidism is not consistently associated with cognitive impairment, though some studies show subtle impairment in attention and executive functions, and patients often report cognitive problems (Bauer et al., 2008; Samuels, 2008). Increased rates of depression and anxiety are reported in hyperthyroidism as well. Controversy exists regarding subclinical hypo-and hyperthyroidism; patients often report cognitive and mood problems, but data are sparse and inconsistent, and it has been suggested that mood difficulties are likely unrelated to thyroid abnormality (Samuels, 2014a, 2014b).

Vitamin B12 Deficiency

Nutritional factors such as vitamin intake may affect neuropsychological functioning. Research suggests possible associations between cognition and levels of Vitamin D, folate, homocysteine, and B vitamins, for example (Etgen, Bickel, & Forstl, 2010). There is considerable overlap between vitamin deficiencies, as imbalance in one system may alter function in another. Vitamin B12, or cobalamin, is involved in a number of central nervous system functions, and its deficiency affects glial cells and myelin, and results in cytokine and growth factor imbalance (Scalabrino, 2009). B12 deficiency results from poor dietary intake (e.g., sometimes associated with vegetarianism), absorption or distribution (e.g., related to certain medical diseases such as Crohn's, or metformin use), and is more common in elderly patients.

Given its prevalence in the elderly, a majority of the literature on B12 focuses on older adults, though there is some evidence that early B12 deficiency may impair cognition in childhood and adolescence (Louwman et al., 2000). In healthy older adults, low B12 levels have been associated with impaired spatial copying (Riggs, Spiro, Tucker, & Rush, 1996) and information processing speed (Bohnen, Jolles, & Degenaar, 1992; Jelicic, Jonker, & Deeg, 2001); other studies showed no effect on memory (Goodwin, Goodwin, & Garry, 1983; Wahlin, Hill, Winblad, & Backman, 1996). Low levels of B12 are found in individuals with mild cognitive impairment, Alzheimer's disease, vascular dementia, and Parkinson's disease in cross-sectional studies (for review, see Moore et al., 2012), and one large longitudinal study found B12 deficiency preceded decline in MMSE score (Clarke et al., 2007).

While supplementation may normalize B12 levels, it is unclear whether or not it improves cognition. One literature review concluded that cognition may improve marginally in people with B12 deficiency who are cognitively impaired (Moore et al., 2012) while another concluded that B12 supplementation does not appreciably change cognitive function (Health Quality, 2013). Still, B12 deficiency is widely considered a reversible cause of dementia. One striking study found that, of 18 individuals with dementia and B12 deficiency who were treated with B12 supplements, 12 markedly improved and were cognitively equal to controls, while seven markedly declined after one year (Osimani, Berger, Friedman, Porat-Katz, & Abarbanel, 2005). In terms of psychiatric status, low B12 levels are associated with depression in the elderly (e.g., Hin et al., 2006), with no resolution of symptoms following B12 supplementation (Hin et al., 2006). Overall, the literature generally supports an association between B12 deficiency and neuropsychological impairment, though the exact nature of the relationship remains unclear.

As opposed to the direct affect of the aforementioned causes of metabolic dysfunction, the interrelationship between organ functioning and metabolic functioning is more complex. Metabolic disorder may result in organ failure (e.g., diabetic nephropathy), and organ failure may result in metabolic dysfunction (e.g., secondary hyperparathyroidism from renal disease). Additionally, there are many potential causes for organ failure, and these etiologies may exert different patterns of cognitive impairment.

Kidney Failure

The kidneys regulate the volume and composition of fluids. In addition to excreting metabolic waste, they have a pivotal role in regulating calcium, phosphorus, and parathyroid hormone levels, and they act as a stimulus for red blood cell production. Renal functioning is generally measured by creatinine (Cr), glomerular filtration rate (GFR), and creatinine clearance (CrCl). Creatinine is a breakdown product of creatinine phosphate, and it is a common indicator of kidney functioning. GFR measures kidney filtration and toxic substance clearance efficiency. The amount of creatinine excreted by the kidneys is measured by 24-hour creatinine clearance. Together, these markers in addition to others (e.g., serum urea nitrogen: BUN) estimate renal functioning. Individuals with compromised renal functioning may receive hemodialysis or peritoneal dialysis. Dialysis is a procedure to remove waste through either filtering blood through an external machine (hemodialysis) or filtering blood through the abdominal lining (peritoneal dialysis).

Most renal disease is secondary to other medical diseases and conditions (e.g., diabetes mellitus, hypertension, glomerulonephritis, polycystic kidney disease, etc.). The mechanisms of renal dysfunction on the brain vary as do the etiologies (Huber, 2008). Direct affects of toxin clearance or secondary complications and risk factors may affect cognition (i.e., vascular disease, anemia, hyperparathyroidism, sleep disturbance, dialysis hypotension etc.) (Madero, Gul, & Sarnak, 2008). For example, diabetes may affect vasculature resulting in microangiopathy or alterations in the blood-brain barrier, but lupus may result in cerebritis or vasculitis (Hailpern, Melamed, Cohen, & Hostetter, 2007; Kurella, Chertow, Luan, & Yaffe, 2004). Hypertension and diabetes mellitus are the leading causes of renal failure, and the onset of these disorders is typically later in life. Because of this, the affects of renal failure on cognition are interrelated to age. Research is further complicated by the lack of ethnicity studies. African Americans and Hispanics are at higher risk of developing diabetes, but they are generally underrepresented in research samples.

Several studies have found a relationship between chronic kidney disease and renal functioning, and it has been identified as an independent risk factor for cognitive impairment (Kurella et al., 2005; Kurella et al., 2004; Kurella, Yaffe, Shlipak, Wenger, & Chertow, 2005). Most studies use brief instruments that do not allow for detailed profile analysis (Kurella Tamura et al., 2011; Yaffe et al., 2010); however, more literature exists about some of the primary causes of renal failure. For example, diabetes is associated with microangiographic changes, which are related to deep white matter change (Huber, 2008). Overall, there are many cross-sectional and longitudinal studies, but they contain significant methodological limitations (i.e., limited screening, older adults, individuals with numerous coexisting illnesses, publication bias, poor demographic representation, etc.) (Madero et al., 2008).

Liver Failure

The liver is a life-sustaining organ that performs more than 500 functions, many of which are not fully understood. Metabolizing alcohol, toxins, medications, fats, and proteins as well as synthesizing clotting factors, bile production, and glycogen/glucose storage are among some its most important functions. Common causes of liver failure include viral infection (i.e., hepatitis B and hepatitis C), biliary dysfunction (primary biliary sclerosis, primary sclerosing cholangitis), autoimmune hepatitis, and nonalcoholic steatohepatitis (e.g., fatty liver).

Direct etiological factors on the liver and brain may cause cerebral compromise in addition to secondary hepatic failure on the brain. Direct causes such as viral infections (e.g., viral hepatitis) and alcohol may cause direct brain dysfunction, but they may also create liver compromise resulting in further cognitive impairment. Liver disease can cause systemic failure to clear toxins. In particular, the failure to clear ammonia, may cause acute cerebral dysfunction (i.e., hepatic encephalopathy) (Norman, 2011). Hepatic encephalopathy (HE) may occur as an acute, possibly reversible disorder or as a chronic disorder associated with chronic liver disease. Recent studies suggest that HE may be more persistent than once recognized, even after liver transplant (Campagna, Biancardi, Cillo, Gatta, & Amodio, 2010; Patel et al., 2015). Mild HE symptoms include irritability and sleep/wake difficulty, but this can progress to worsened mental status, confusion, coma, and death.

Because there are many causes of liver failure, no one pattern of neuropsychological function is specifically associated with liver-related cognitive dysfunction. It is difficult to measure the direct affects of liver failure on cognition because underlying etiologies may directly affect cognition (i.e., hepatitis C virus [HCV]). The most studied cognitively liver-related etiology is HCV. In a review, the most common areas of cognitive impairment were in attention and concentration, suggesting frontal-subcortical white matter involvement (Perry, Hilsabeck, & Hassanein, 2008).

The most common causes of acute liver failure in the United States are viruses and toxins. Possible viral causes include cytomegalovirus, Epstein-Barr, herpes simplex, human herpes virus 6, parvovirus B19, and varicella-zoster, viruses that cause hemorrhagic fever, and, rarely, aepatitis A or E. The most common toxin is acetaminophen/paracetamol toxicity, but other toxic causes include amoxicillin/clavulanate, halothane, iron compounds, isoniazid, nonsteroidal anti-inflammatory drugs, some ingredients in herbal drugs, and Amanita phalloides mushrooms. In contrast, alcohol, hepatitis B, hepatitis C, and nonalcoholic steatohepatitis are the most common chronic forms of failure and cirrhosis (Demir, Lang, & Steffen, 2015). The epidemiology is dramatically changing with an increase in nonalcoholic steatohepatitis (i.e., fatty liver disease) and better treatments to eradicate HCV viral load (Demir et al., 2015; Van Nuys et al., 2015).

Lung and Heart Failure

Similar to kidney and liver cognitive-related impairment, the interaction between lung and heart dysfunction and cognition is complex and not fully understood. Pulmonary and cardiac failure primarily compromise cerebral perfusion, although other conditions place individuals at higher risk for stroke (i.e., atrial fibrillation).

There are causes of pulmonary failure, but chronic obstructive pulmonary disease (COPD) is one of the leading causes of morbidity and mortality (Schou, Ostergaard, Rasmussen, Rydahl-Hansen, & Phanareth, 2012). Hypoxemia and hypercapnia have been associated with cognitive dysfunction in COPD (Antonelli-Incalzi et al., 2006). While low levels of oxygen in the blood and carbon dioxide retention are two possible causes of cognitive impairment, low blood flow (hypoperfusion) is another possible mechanism, and a direct effect of cognitive dysfunction has been described with hypoperfusion (Antonelli Incalzi et al., 2003; Hynninen, Breitve, Wiborg, Pallesen, & Nordhus, 2005). A significant complicating features of COPD is fatigue, and fatigue is known to have an relationship with cognitive impairment in COPD (Crews et al., 2001).

Cognitive impairment is estimated to occur in 30%–80% of persons with heart failure (Bennett & Sauve, 2003; Pressler, 2008). The pattern of cognitive impairment in heart failure is somewhat more clear than the kidneys and liver. The neuropsychological pattern appears to demonstrate subtle deficits in memory, attention, psychomotor speed, and executive functioning, and these are independent from age, sex, alcohol consumption, education and other comorbidities (Almeida & Tamai, 2001; Pressler et al., 2010; Vogels, Scheltens, Schroeder-Tanka, & Weinstein, 2007). This clearer pattern may be, in part, to there being less metabolic dysregulation attributed to cardiac functioning.

Case I.Z., later in this chapter, will highlight a relatively rare metabolic disorder, but in the larger picture, it will illustrate the medically complex interaction between metabolic functions and outcomes. Methylmalonic acidurias, also called *methylmalonic acidemias* (MMA), are a heterogeneous group of autosomal recessive inborn errors of organic acid metabolism. First described in 1967, MMA affects one in 50,000 to one in 8,000 births (Oberholzer, Levin, Burgess, & Young, 1967; Sniderman et al., 1999). MMA is characterized by deficient activity of methylmalonyl-CoA mutase, the B12-dependent enzyme responsible for converting methylmalonyl-CoA to succinyl-CoA (Fenton & Rosenberg, 2001). Seven distinct forms have been described on the basis of biochemical and somatic cell studies (Shevell, Matiaszuk, Ledley, & Rosenblatt, 1993). Dysfunction in this system causes the accumulation of MMA, which is most readily detected in urine, although elevated levels can be found in the blood and cerebrospinal fluid (Oberholzer et al., 1967; Stokke, Eldjarn, Norum, Steen-Johnsen, & Halvorsen, 1967). Children with MMA commonly present in the first year of life with recurrent episodes of vomiting, failure to thrive, muscular hypotonia, and encephalopathy (Nicolaides, Leonard, & Surtees, 1998). Other phenotypic expressions include ketoacidosis, developmental delay with mental retardation, and in severe cases, death (Fenton & Rosenberg, 2001; Matsui, Mahoney, & Rosenberg, 1983). Within this heterogeneous population, outcome is variable and plasma and urinary methylmalonate concentrations do not predict outcome well (Nicolaides et al., 1998).

MMA treatment may include vitamin B12 supplementation, but the majority of patients do not respond to this. Also, nutritional management includes high-energy diet with supplementary amino acids in some cases (Morioka et al., 2007). A less commonly used—and controversial—treatment has been liver transplant, because this offers only partial enzyme replacement and MMA fluid concentrations do not become normal, with no decrease in CSF MMA.

There is little literature on the cognitive affects of MMA, and most of this literature describes those in early life. Rarely, the less severe mut- form has been associated with normal neurodevelopment in asymptomatic cases or possibly mild to moderate cognitive deficits (Baumgarter & Viardot, 1995; Ledley, Levy, Shih, Benjamin, & Mahoney, 1984; O'Shea et al., 2012; Varvogli, Repetto, Waisbren, & Levy, 2000). In contrast, the mut0 form is seen neonatally and death occurs in early infancy, or children have very poor neurological outcomes (Matsui et al., 1983). O'Shea et al. (2012) found that early disease onset, presence of elevated ammonia, and history of seizures was associated with more greater impairment in aspects of processing speed (O'Shea et al., 2012). In a series of seven patients under age 8 (with one postoperative death), Morioka et al. (2007) described that all of the children undergoing living donor liver transplants had lethargy and cognitive deficits. These authors claim that cognitive deficits were "cured"; however, while the McCarthy General Cognitive Index significantly improved in their sample, the Denver Development Quotients improved slightly. All of these children were treated with pre- and postdietary restrictions and metabolism-correcting medications. Short of this study, there is little pre-/post-cognitive data in the literature, and none with adults who have undergone liver transplant.

The Case of I.Z.

The patient is a 30-year-old, right-handed bilingual Hispanic. His MMA resulted in a toxic buildup of amino acids that was thought to eventually lead to eventual coma and irreversible neurologic damage. He was referred by a liver transplant team as part of a liver transplant workup. This case will highlight the challenges of highly complex medical cases with primary and secondary metabolic issues.

Preoperative Evaluation

I.Z.'s preoperative liver transplant evaluation occurred when he was age 27, and his cognition waxed and waned frequently. It was unclear to what extent this was secondary to metabolic fluctuations, complications, or hepatic encephalopathy (Norman, 2011). According to his wife, he began to experience cognitive and functional decline within the preceding six months. The team questioned the potential efficacy of liver transplant, because there is limited outcome data in adults with MMA. The preponderance of data is in transplanting children to protect their neurologic status. In this case, this adult was already neurologically compromised, so the potential benefits of transplant were unknown.

Around the time of the work-up I.Z experienced increased episodes of acidosis and pancreatitis with numerous hospitalizations. Additionally, his functioning was variable. For instance, when he was doing well, he could shower, make his own food, and assist with other chores around his home. However, when not doing well, he reportedly was more withdrawn, aggravated and noncompliant. He expressed hesitation about following through with the liver transplant, because he questioned potential benefits of the procedure. At times he stated he did not want a transplant, so several evaluations for decision-making capacity were undertaken. I.Z. was able to explain basics about MMA, but did not appear to fully understand the transplant procedure and recovery process. In addition, he had limited insight into his cognitive dysfunction. Preoperatively, his medical history was significant for seizures of unclear etiology, gastritis, depression, hepatic encephalopathy, hypertension, ketoacidosis, pancreatitis, and bilateral ear surgery. His medications included megestrol, melatonin, allopurinol, amoxicillin/clavulanic acid, metoprolol, lisinopril, aspirin, lacosamide, levetiracetam, and albuterol. His MMA had been managed for many years with a low-protein diet with carnitine supplementation.

I.Z. reported a history of depression, but denied receiving mental health treatment. Following the neuropsychological evaluation, his depression improved with olanzapine 5mg. He reportedly smoked until age 20 and quite drinking alcohol at age 22. Also, he had a history of marijuana, methamphetamine, and cocaine use, with his last use of illicit drugs at the age of 23 or 24.

I.Z. graduated from high school and completed one year of college. He was two classes away from completing an Associate's Degree when he became ill and dropped out. He denied being diagnosed with a learning disorder, but acknowledged that he was a "slow learner." His education was interrupted by his frequent hospitalizations during his childhood and teen years. He worked for a brief time as an inventory clerk. He had not been employed since around age 25.

PREOPERATIVE TESTING RESULTS

During the first testing (following his noted cognitive decline), I.Z.'s affect was flat but became more irritable as testing progressed. He was a poor historian and had problems discussing complicated subjects such as his medical condition. His speech was hypophonic and slow in rate. He was noted to mumble to himself and displayed poor eye contact. His effort appeared to be good at the beginning of testing, but he displayed low frustration tolerance and wanted to quit.

I.Z. was administered a brief battery of neuropsychological tests and a clinical interview was conducted to assess compliance, social support, and mental health to determine his appropriateness for transplant. He was administered a brief cognitive screening, the Montreal Cognitive Assessment (MOCA), and his results were not scoreable secondary to comprehension problems and low frustration tolerance. On the Rey Osterrieth Complex Figure copy, he did not use a Gestalt approach or attend to details. He did not attempt to draw the figure following a 30-minute delay. On a test of fine motor dexterity, he refused to participate secondary to frustration during the test, and therefore the test was discontinued. Finally, his performance in semantic fluency was severely impaired. Computed tomography (CT) 18 months prior to the transplant demonstrated ventricular enlargement of uncertain significance, without increased intracerebral pressure (Figure 31.1—left image).

Even in the context of severely impaired cognition (with additional poor assessment effort), the patient was ultimately listed for liver transplant. It was believed that his liver was otherwise functioning normally (i.e., no cirrhosis), so the team elected to list I.Z. for a cadaveric transplant and implant his native liver into another individual needing a liver transplant. With more than 16,000 people waiting for liver transplants in the United States and 20% mortality while waiting, a "domino" liver transplant allowed two lives to be saved with one cadaveric organ. I.Z.'s liver had a genetic metabolic disorder, but a new recipient's body would be able to clear the amino acids and the person would be symptom free. A week prior to transplant I.Z. was admitted secondary to hypokalemia and dehydration.

Post-Operative

I.Z.'s posttransplantation course was complicated by multiple infections as well as vascular, renal, and metabolic abnormalities. Within a week following transplant he developed hypotension and low kidney output, and he was placed on

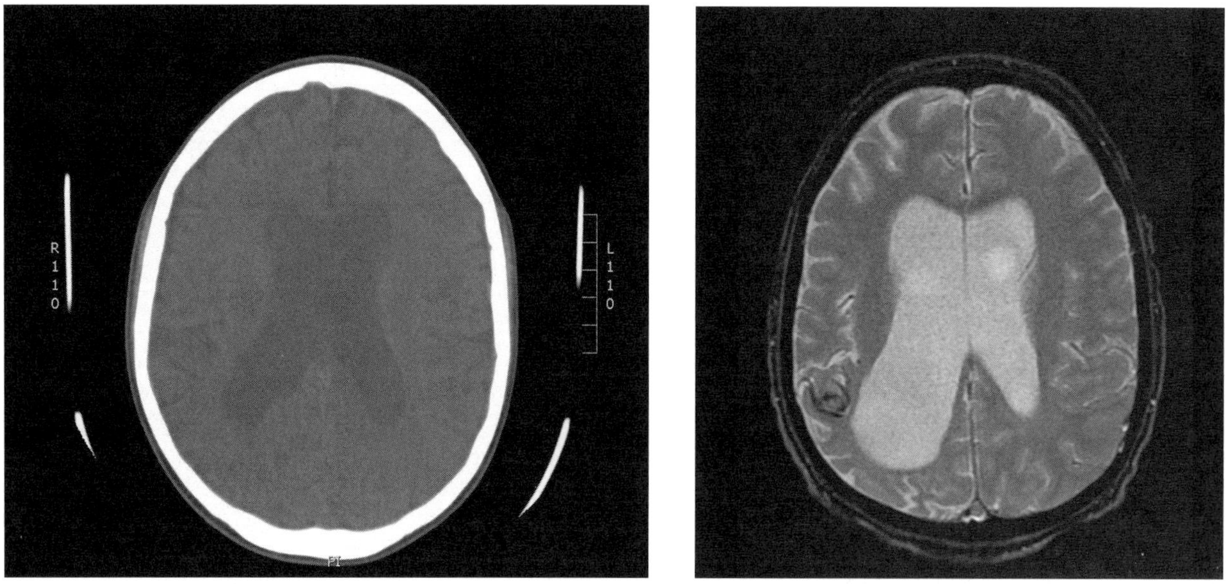

Figure 31.1 CT 18 months pretransplant (left), and T2 MRI 3 months posttransplant (right)

continuous veno-venous hemodialysis. He had (what ended up being recurrent) pseudomonas aeruginosa pneumonia and acute kidney injury secondary to dehydration and acute tubular necrosis. The following week he underwent a tracheostomy and was placed on a ventilator with a Glasgow Coma Scale (GCS) of 11T. His agitation was managed with benzodiazepines and aripiprazole, transitioning to olanzapine.

Two months posttransplant, while still hospitalized, he had a partial occlusion of the pulmonary artery and had large plural effusions and suspected chest abscesses. Two weeks later he underwent a balloon dilatation (and later angioplasty) to repair a stricture in the inferior vena cava and subsequently had further mental status deterioration. Over the following two months he was found to have multidrug resistant klebsiella, leukocytosis, and renal improvement.

Posttransplant month three, while still hospitalized, I.Z. experienced what was thought to be a partial seizure. While the etiology was unclear, two of his medications, tacrolimus and meropenem, were known to lower seizure threshold. He had bacteremia and hypercarbia. His GCS improved to 14, although his mental status continued to wax and wane. At 3.5 months following transplant, he was transferred to an acute rehabilitation unit. At that time he was off of dialysis but had continued hyperkalemia and ascites. His venricular dilation remained stable as demonsrated in the 3-month posttransplant MRI (Figure 31.1—right image).

About three weeks following admission to rehabilitation, I.Z. was again admitted with cardiomegaly, osteopenia, and persistent acidemia. The following month he was noted to have increased liver function tests and hypothyroidism, and a kidney transplant work-up was initiated. In the following months he had multiple readmissions with pneumonia.

Six months posttransplant, I.Z. experienced the next significant neurologic event. He was found to have cytomegalovirus (CMV) meningitis with intraparenchymal, subarachnoid, and intraventricular hemorrhages, and he had a cluster of seizures (Figure 31.2). The etiology of the meningitis was unclear; however, this is a known risk in immunosuppressed individuals. He continued to make slow improvement and was discharged about two weeks later. Over the following four months he had multiple admissions with leg pain, myalgias, weakness, shortness of breath, and hypoxia. Multiple episodes of respiratory failure led to brief periods of ventilator support.

I.Z. underwent postoperative evaluation approximately 20 months following his liver transplant. He was not confused and communicated appropriately. I.Z.'s primary complaint was worsening central vision, with relatively better peripheral vision. He was followed by a neuro-ophthalmologist for optical nerve damage and had been deemed legally blind one month prior to postoperative evaluation. He indicated that his mood had been affected by his visual problems, including episodes of feeling depressed, worthless, and inadequate because he was unable to do the things he previously enjoyed. He and his wife reported, however, that his mood had improved after he started to attend a vision rehabilitation

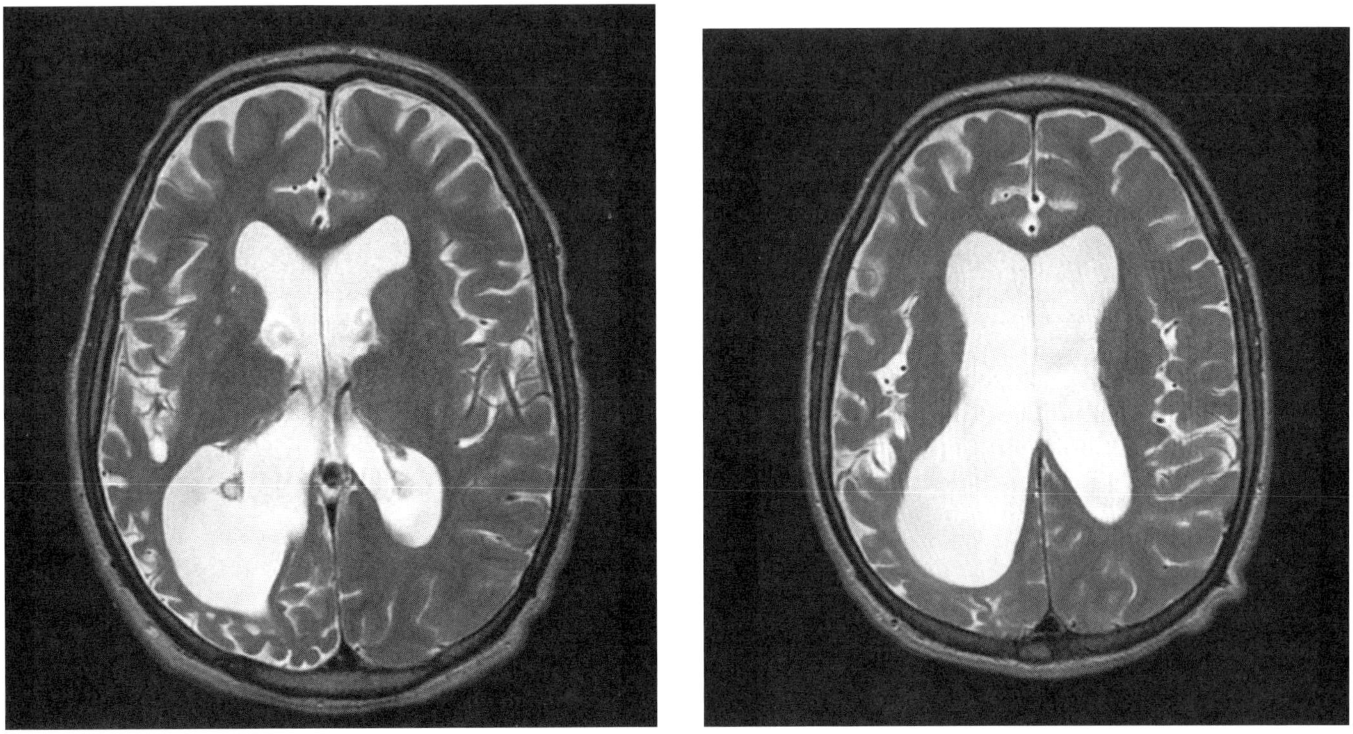

Figure 31.2 T2 (left) and gradient-echo (right) MRI demonstrating intraventricular and intraparenchymal hemorrhage six months posttransplant

service (two to three months prior). He indicated that the service was designed to improve independent living skills. He noted "I am really at a good point now" and that this has been the longest time span without a hospitalization.

The couple denied prominent changes in his cognition since the liver transplant. He had long-standing problems with speech (stutter) since age 6, but denied new problems with word finding or paraphasias. Functionally, he was assisted by his wife with household chores (e.g., laundry) and was responsible for his own hygiene. He required help from his wife to manage his medications, appointments, and finances. He did not drive. When he was not hospitalized or attending medical appointments, a typical day included taking walks, doing household chores, and listening to music.

I.Z. reported that he saw a psychiatrist between his preoperative testing and liver transplant. He was reportedly started on escitalopram and olanzapine. He was started on olanzapine based on episodes of altered mental status and "talking to himself." He denied frank psychotic symptoms. According to the couple, the escitalopram had been discontinued because his insurance did not cover it. I.Z. reported intermittent mild depressive symptoms (i.e., fatigue, frustration, feelings of worthlessness, sadness) and denied prominent emotional changes since liver transplant. He indicated that the mild depressive symptoms were exacerbated by his multiple medical conditions including his vision problems. He denied prominent symptoms of anxiety and indicated that his overall emotional condition had improved during the previous two to three months. He denied a history of suicidal or homicidal ideation, intent, or plans. He denied psychiatric hospitalizations.

I.Z. sometimes used a walker to ambulate, but at other times used a wheelchair to avoid episodes of shortness of breath associated with exertion. He complained of frequent fatigue, weakness in his legs/left hand, poor coordination, and problems with balance. He reported falls, but denied head injuries or loss of consciousness associated with the falls. He denied problems with numbness, dizziness, nausea, vomiting, or incontinence. He indicated that he had loss of hearing in his left ear, but it was unclear what percentage of hearing loss he sustained. He denied problems initiating sleep, but acknowledged that he slept more often, particularly if he had nothing scheduled for his day.

His posttransplant medications included sirolimus, cyclosporine, dapsone, nifedipine, metoprolol, lacosamide, levetiracetam, olanzapine, levothyroxine, levocarnitine, K-Phos Neutral, fludrocortisone, magnesium plus protein, sodium bicarbonate, ergocalciferol, Nephrocaps, omeprazole, albuterol, fluticasone, oxycodone hydrochloride, omega-3, and megestrol.

POST-OPERATIVE TESTING RESULTS

During the second testing he used a wheelchair. He was oriented to person, time, and situation, but not to place (an unfamiliar office). His recall was fair for recent events, but he requested that we ask his wife for specific details. Similar to the first testing, he appeared to become agitated as the tests progressed, but his frustration tolerance was better compared to his first testing session. He became somnolent at times. No psychotic symptoms or homicidal ideation was noted. His thought processes were logical, linear, and goal directed. His speech was characterized by slow rate with evidence of (pretransplant) stutter. He did not mumble or talk to himself. He displayed limited eye contact, and a vision pocket chart was used to estimate his vision. Based on his visual disturbance, some of the tests had to be administered in a nonstandardized manner for him to see the stimuli. His effort during testing was variable, though likely not intentional. His postoperative neuropsychological testing was more comprehensive than pre-transplant (Table 31.3).

Table 31.3 Summary of neuropsychological test scores

Wechsler Test of Adult Reading				
Full Scale IQ		78	T-score	35
Verbal IQ		78	T-score	35
Performance IQ		83	T-score	39
VISUOSPATIAL				
Rey-O Copy		9/36	T-score	19
LANGUAGE				
	Letter Fluency	29	T-score	42
	Category Fluency	14	T-score	37
	BNT Spont (1+3)	35/60	T-score	29
	W/Phonemic Cues	42		
WRAT-4		Std. Score		

Wechsler Test of Adult Reading				
Word Reading	66		T-score 27	
Spelling	83		T-score 39	
Math Comp	58		T-score 22	
TOMM				
Learning Trial 1		35/50		
Learning Trial 2		40/50		
Delayed Trial		44/50		
MEMORY				
CVLT-2		Raw	Z score	
List A 1–5 Total		35		36
List A Trial 1		5	−1.0	
List A Trial 2		6	−1.5	
List A Trial 3		7	−1.5	
List A Trial 4		9	−1.0	
List A Trial 5		8	−2.0	
List B		4	−1.0	
Short Delay Free		5	−2.0	
Short Delay Cued		6	−2.0	
Long Delay Free		7	−1.5	
Long Delay Cued		7	−1.5	
Semantic Cluster		0.6	0.0	
Serial Cluster (bi-direct)		0	-0.5	
% Primacy		40	2.0	
% Middle		34	−1.5	
% Recency		26	−0.5	
Slope (1–5)		0.9	−1.0	
Consistency		67%	−1.5	
Repetitions		6	0.5	
Total Free Recall Intrus.		0	−0.5	
Total Cued Recall Intrus.		9	3.0	
Recognition Hits		8	−5.0	
False Positive Errors		1	−0.5	
Total Recog Discrim		1.9	−1.5	
Source Recog Discrim		1.5	−1.5	
Total Response Bias **		0.9	2.5	
Forced Choice			16/16 100 cum%	
Rey-O Immed	9/36	T-score 19		
Rey-O Delay	6.5/36	T-score 19		
PSYCHOMOTOR				
Trails A	240.0	T-score 10	0.1%ile	
Trails B	Unable			
Beck Depression Inv. 2		15		

I.Z. did not perform above the established cutoffs on the TOMM (Trial 1 = 35/50, Trial 2 = 40/50; Retention Trial = 44/50). He did, however, score above the established cutoff on the CVLT-II Forced Choice (16/16). His performance on a premorbid intellectual estimate (Wechsler Test of Adult Reading; WTAR) predicted that his full scale IQ was in the mildly impaired range. His Montreal Cognitive Assessment (MOCA) total score was 11/30. On a task of psychomotor number sequencing (Trail Making Test Part A), I.Z. performed within the severely impaired range. On the Sensory Perceptual Exam, he did not demonstrate extinction from double simultaneous tactile, auditory, or visual stimulation,

Figure 31.3 Rey-Osterrieth complex figure copy

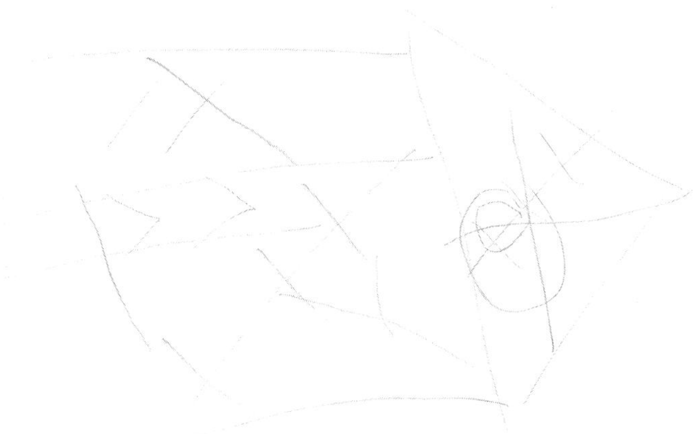

Figure 31.4 Rey-Osterrieth complex figure delay

but he did make multiple errors bilaterally on fingertip number writing and on tactile finger recognition. With regard to attention, he scored within the mildly to moderately impaired range on the Wechsler Adult Intelligence Scale–III (WAIS-III) Digit Span subtest. His complex figure drawing (Rey-O Copy; Figure 31.3) was within the severely impaired range (T < 20).

On a measure of confrontation naming, the Boston Naming Test, his performance was within the moderately impaired range. On a measure of lexical word generation, the Letter Fluency test, he performed within the low average range. His performance on the Category Fluency test was within the mildly impaired range. It should be noted that African American norms were used for fluency and Trail Making to take a conservative approach and because there were inadequate norms for a Hispanic individual. His academic skills, as measured by the Wide Range Achievement Test–fourth edition (WRAT-4), placed his word reading performance within the moderately impaired range and spelling within the mildly impaired range. His math computation subtest was discontinued after eight minutes after he indicated that he was having trouble seeing the items and that the items were becoming "too hard."

I.Z. completed the California Verbal Learning Test–II (CVLT-II), a measure of verbal list acquisition and memory. He recalled a total of 35 words from Trials 1–5, which was within the mildly impaired range. His Short Delayed Free Recall performance was within the mildly to moderately impaired range. His Long Delayed Free Recall performance was within the mildly impaired range (Figure 31.4). He committed no free recall intrusions and committed an average number of repetition errors. On recognition testing, he correctly identified eight out of 16 words, which was within the severely impaired range. He committed one false positive error. His overall recognition discriminability was within the mildly impaired range.

His immediate and delayed recall performances of a complex figure (Rey-O) were within the severely impaired range. On the Beck Depression Inventory-II, he scored a 15, which was within the mild range of depression.

Discussion

Because of the large number of metabolic disorders and even larger number of potential effects, this chapter provides an overview of the relationship between disorders of metabolism and cognition. The majority of metabolic disorders are due to single genes that code for enzyemes, but this seemingly simple fact belies the complexity and variability of metabolic disorders. A case example provided an illustration of these complexities.

The manifestations of metabolic disorders vary widely. Effects can be primary, secondary or tertiary, and a disturbance in one physiologic system may produce new metabolic or systemic dysfunction. The metabolic abnormalities may not exist in isolation, and multiple disorders can co-exist. Cognitive effects secondary to metabolic dysfunction may be insignificant to profound. For example, a short-term or mild blood sugar elevation may not affect cognition, but a metabolic abnormality leading to seizures with status epilepticus or repiratory failure with anoxia/hypoxia could produce severe cognitive impairment.

In addition to severity, a critical factor in how these disorders cognitively manifest is when the abnormality occurs. Inherited metabolic disorders may affect brain and cognitive development, so issues may be evident in early life. In other cases, brain development is normal, because the onset and effects of metabolic dysfunction is later in life. For example, PKU is associated with changes to the developing brain, while diabetes mellitus Type 2 is more likely to occur in later life. In the former example, effective treatment may still result in cognitive reduction, but in the the latter example

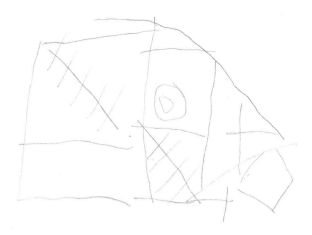

effective control of diabetes mellitus may not result in cognitive change.

Treatment of metabolic disorders vary by specific conditions. In the example of PKU, treatment involves a low-phenylalanine diet. In the case of diabetes mellitus, treatment involves dietary and medication management, in addition to maintaining a healthy weight. Even with adherent treatment, cognitive reduction may occur, but there is generally inadequate literature to describe a direct relationship between lab abnormalities or treatment with cognition. Even with this limitation, metabolic treatments often involve reducing secondary health risks. In the case of Metabolic Syndrome, the focus of treatment typically involves dietary, weight, medication, and lifestyle management. Managing obesity, triglicerides, lipoprotein, hypertensiona, and glycemia may reduce the risk of stroke and cardiovascular disease.

Another example of an inherited metabolic disorder that can lead to later life issues is Methylmalonic Aciduria.

The overall prognosis of MMA has improved over the last 30 years in part due to earlier diagnosis and better treatment options (Baumgarter & Viardot, 1995). Prognosis remains to be dependent on the mutant class and responsiveness to interventions. With this said, outcomes of children and adults with this specific disorder, and more generally, those with metabolic disorders, is complicated by complex metabolic interactions (i.e., body chemistry, neural chemistry, organ dysfunction with secondary features, etc. (Yohannes, Baldwin, & Connolly, 2006).

The chapter's case example highlights the complexity of metabolic disorders. This patient had cognitive impairment and psychiatric disturbance even prior to transplant, and he then had pulmonary, cerebrovascular, renal injury, additional metabolic changes, and infection complications. The interactions of these medical conditions render causal mechanisms difficult or impossible. Adding to this picture, there is existing, albeit limited, literature on the positive cognitive outcomes with liver transplantation in children, but not adults. It was hoped that liver transplantation would reverse the cognitive decline in I.Z, and it is unclear if it would have given his complicated posttransplant course.

The pretransplant work-up evaluated his medical and surgical risks, in addition to his social support, medication, and medical recommendation compliance. I.Z.'s substance use, depression, and anxiety were not considered to be contraindications to transplant. It was noted that his cognition was impaired prior to transplant, so concern was raised as to whether or not he would be able to manage his posttransplant medications. These medications, including immunosuppression, require complex scheduling (e.g., some medications on an empty stomach others with food, taken at specific times, refilling prescriptions etc.). Because his family and wife were considered to be well-informed, engaged, and supportive throughout his life-long illness, the team felt he would be able to appropriately take his medications. From a cognitive perspective, testing provided the transplant team with important information, but testing was limited because of the patient's significantly impaired mental status and effort.

The ultimate goal of transplant is to maximize successful outcomes. Had the patient not had strong family support, his impaired cognition would likely have been felt to be a contraindication to transplant. Generally, patients undergoing liver transplant do not have significant posttransplant cognitive improvement; however, pediatric literature with transplant in MMA suggests there might be cognitive benefit. This was unclear for an adult. Unfortunately, the current case does not shed definitive light into this question because of I.Z.'s complicated course (e.g., repeated hypoxia, intracerebral/intraventricular hemorrhage, etc.).

As in all transplant cases, the risks and benefits of transplant were weighed. Unlike most cases, the patient did not have end-stage liver disease, but the MMA was felt to contribute to significant problems (e.g., gastritis, vision, mental status, hearing) and worsening cognitive course. These risks were thoroughly discussed with the patient and his family. Because his mental status waxed and waned throughout his course, his decision-making capacity was evaluated multiple times to ensure his wishes were being met. There were times when the patient stated he did not want transplant, but these were at times of his greatest confusion. Ultimately, the patient and his family were agreeable to transplant and the domino procedure.

Another issue in this case, as with many metabolic presentations, is that I.Z.'s metabolic dysfunction is lifelong. There were likely unknown metabolic affects on cerebral development during critical neurodevelopmental periods. Although he had significant cognitive impairment when he was referred to the transplant team, this was not lifelong. I.Z. graduated from high school and attended some college, suggesting that his current status was a significant decline.

I. Z.'s testing results demonstrated global deficits across domains of language, attention, visuospatial skills, memory, and psychomotor functioning. From one perspective, he showed some signs of improvement when comparing his postoperative results to the brief initial testing session. For instance, his category fluency performance doubled in number of animals he named and his Rey-O copy was a more recognizable figure. Another significant factor to consider, as it relates to his overall profile, was I.Z's visual disturbance. During the postoperative testing some of the visual tests had to be administered in a nonstandardized way in order for him to see the stimuli. Despite these accommodations he still demonstrated impaired performances. One could argue that his overall performance may have been aided by use of measures that did not include a visual component, but his nonvisual test scores were also impaired. Also, he was more cooperative during the testing, showing better frustration tolerance. Overall, however, postoperative testing revealed persistent severe cognitive deficits, without appreciable improvement.

A striking issue with testing was I.Z.'s low scores on effort measures. The reasons for this were unclear and much debate revolves around this issue, especially in medically ill patients. During the postoperative testing his effort testing was not above the established cutoffs. It is unlikely that he was intentionally malingering or feigning impairment. Additionally, there was no identified secondary gain for I.Z. to perform poorly on the testing, and in fact, most transplant patients desire to be seen in the most positive light. A more plausible explanation is that his effort was affected by other cognitive and/or motivational factors (i.e., waxing and waning attention, fatigue etc.). Although he was on multiple mediations, including oxycodone, at the time of testing, his baseline cognitive status and months of cognitive decline did not suggest that these medications or intermittent depression significantly contributed to his cognitive profile. The role of metabolic syndromes and metabolic change is still poorly understood, and the timing (i.e., developmental vs. acquired), severity, and complicating factors make neuropsychological interpretations difficult, but important.

References

Albrecht, J., Garbade, S. F., & Burgard, P. (2009). Neuropsychological speed tests and blood phenylalanine levels in patients with phenylketonuria: A meta-analysis. *Neuroscience & Biobehavioral Reviews*, *33*(3), 414–421. doi: 10.1016/j.neubiorev.2008.11.001

Almeida, O. P., & Tamai, S. (2001). Congestive heart failure and cognitive functioning amongst older adults. *Arq Neuropsiquiatr*, *59*(2-B), 324–329. Retrieved from www.ncbi.nlm.nih.gov/pubmed/11460173

Antonelli-Incalzi, R., Corsonello, A., Pedone, C., Trojano, L., Acanfora, D., Spada, A., . . . Rengo, F. (2006). Drawing impairment predicts mortality in severe COPD. *Chest*, *130*(6), 1687–1694. doi: 10.1378/chest.130.6.1687

Antonelli Incalzi, R., Marra, C., Giordano, A., Calcagni, M. L., Cappa, A., Basso, S., . . . Fuso, L. (2003). Cognitive impairment in chronic obstructive pulmonary disease: A neuropsychological and spect study. *Journal of Neurology*, *250*(3), 325–332. doi: 10.1007/s00415-003-1005-4

Bauer, M., Goetz, T., Glenn, T., & Whybrow, P. C. (2008). The thyroid-brain interaction in thyroid disorders and mood disorders. *Journal of Neuroendocrinology*, *20*(10), 1101–1114. doi: 10.1111/j.1365–2826.2008.01774.x

Baumgarter, E. R., & Viardot, C. (1995). Long-term follow-up of 77 patients with isolated methylmalonic acidaemia. *Journal of Inherited Metabolic Disease*, *18*(2), 138–142. Retrieved from www.ncbi.nlm.nih.gov/pubmed/7564229

Bennett, S. J., & Sauve, M. J. (2003). Cognitive deficits in patients with heart failure: A review of the literature. *Journal of Cardiovascular Nursing*, *18*(3), 219–242. Retrieved from www.ncbi.nlm.nih.gov/pubmed/12837012

Bohnen, N., Jolles, J., & Degenaar, C. P. (1992). Lower blood levels of vitamin B12 are related to decreased performance of healthy subjects in the stroop color-word test. *Neuroscience Research Science*, *11*(1), 53–56.

Brands, A. M., Biessels, G. J., de Haan, E. H., Kappelle, L. J., & Kessels, R. P. (2005). The effects of type 1 diabetes on cognitive performance: A meta-analysis. *Diabetes Care*, *28*(3), 726–735. Retrieved from www.ncbi.nlm.nih.gov/pubmed/15735218

Campagna, F., Biancardi, A., Cillo, U., Gatta, A., & Amodio, P. (2010). Neurocognitive-neurological complications of liver transplantation: A review. *Metabolic Brain Disease*, *25*(1), 115–124. doi: 10.1007/s11011-010-9183-0

Channon, S., Mockler, C., & Lee, P. (2005). Executive functioning and speed of processing in phenylketonuria. *Neuropsychology*, *19*(5), 679–686. doi: 10.1037/0894-4105.19.5.679

Cheng, G., Huang, C., Deng, H., & Wang, H. (2012). Diabetes as a risk factor for dementia and mild cognitive impairment: A meta-analysis of longitudinal studies. *Internal Medicine Journal*, *42*(5), 484–491. doi: 10.1111/j.1445-5994.2012.02758.x

Christ, S. E., Huijbregts, S. C., de Sonneville, L. M., & White, D. A. (2010). Executive function in early treated phenylketonuria: Profile and underlying mechanisms. *Molecular Genetetics and Metabolism*, *99*(Suppl 1), S22–32. doi: 10.1016/j.ymgme.2009.10.007

Clarke, R., Birks, J., Nexo, E., Ueland, P. M., Schneede, J., Scott, J., . . . Evans, J. G. (2007). Low vitamin B-12 status and risk of cognitive decline in older adults. *The American Journal of Clinical Nutrition*, *86*(5), 1384–1391. Retrieved from www.ncbi.nlm.nih.gov/pubmed/17991650

Craft, S., & Watson, G. S. (2004). Insulin and neurodegenerative disease: Shared and specific mechanisms. *Lancet Neurology*, *3*(3), 169–178. doi: 10.1016/S1474-4422(04)00681-7

Crews, W. D., Jefferson, A. L., Bolduc, T., Elliott, J. B., Ferro, N. M., Broshek, D. K., . . . Robbins, M. K. (2001). Neuropsychological dysfunction in patients suffering from end-stage chronic obstructive pulmonary disease. *Archives of Clinical Neuropsychology*, *16*(7), 643–652. Retrieved from www.ncbi.nlm.nih.gov/pubmed/14589783

Dahl, A. K., Hassing, L. B., Fransson, E. I., Gatz, M., Reynolds, C. A., & Pedersen, N. L. (2013). Body mass index across midlife and cognitive change in late life. *International Journal of Obesity (Lond)*, *37*(2), 296–302. doi: 10.1038/ijo.2012.37

Demir, M., Lang, S., & Steffen, H. M. (2015). Nonalcoholic fatty liver disease: Current status and future directions. *Journal of Digestive Diseases*. doi: 10.1111/1751-2980.12291

DeRoche, K., & Welsh, M. (2008). Twenty-five years of research on neurocognitive outcomes in early treated phenylketonuria: Intelligence and executive function. *Developmental Neuropsycholology*, *33*(4), 474–504. doi: 10.1080/87565640802101482

Dugbartey, A. T. (1998). Neurocognitive aspects of hypothyroidism. *Archives of Internal Medicine*, *158*(13), 1413–1418. Retrieved from www.ncbi.nlm.nih.gov/pubmed/9665349

Etgen, T., Bickel, H., & Forstl, H. (2010). Metabolic and endocrine factors in mild cognitive impairment. *Ageing Research Reviews*, *9*(3), 280–288. doi: 10.1016/j.arr.2010.01.003

Farr, S. A., Yamada, K. A., Butterfield, D. A., Abdul, H. M., Xu, L., Miller, N. E., . . . Morley, J. E. (2008). Obesity and hypertriglyceridemia produce cognitive impairment. *Endocrinology*, *149*(5), 2628–2636. doi: 10.1210/en.2007-1722

Fenton, W., & Rosenberg, L. (2001). Disorders of propionate and methyl-malonate metabolism. In C. Scriver, A. Beaudet, W. Sly, D. Valle, B. Child, K. Zinzler, & B. Vogelstein (Eds.), *The Metabolic and Molecular Basics of Inherited Diseases* (8th ed., pp. 1423–1449). New York: McGraw Hill.

Goodwin, J. S., Goodwin, J. M., & Garry, P. J. (1983). Association between nutritional status and cognitive functioning in a healthy elderly population. *Journal of the American Medical Association*, *249*(21), 2917–2921. Retrieved from www.ncbi.nlm.nih.gov/pubmed/6842805

Hailpern, S. M., Melamed, M. L., Cohen, H. W., & Hostetter, T. H. (2007). Moderate chronic kidney disease and cognitive function in adults 20 to 59 years of age: Third National Health and Nutrition Examination Survey (NHANES III). *Journal of the American Society of Nephrology*, *18*(7), 2205–2213. doi: 10.1681/ASN.2006101165

Health Quality, O. (2013). Vitamin B12 and cognitive function: An evidence-based analysis. *Ontario Health Technology Assessment Series*, *13*(23), 1–45. Retrieved from www.ncbi.nlm.nih.gov/pubmed/24379897

Hin, H., Clarke, R., Sherliker, P., Atoyebi, W., Emmens, K., Birks, J., . . . Evans, J. G. (2006). Clinical relevance of low serum vitamin B12 concentrations in older people: The Banbury B12 study. *Age Ageing*, *35*(4), 416–422. doi: 10.1093/ageing/afl033

Huber, J. D. (2008). Diabetes, cognitive function, and the blood-brain barrier. *Current Pharmaceutical Design*, *14*(16), 1594–1600. Retrieved from www.ncbi.nlm.nih.gov/pubmed/18673200

Hynninen, K. M., Breitve, M. H., Wiborg, A. B., Pallesen, S., & Nordhus, I. H. (2005). Psychological characteristics of patients with chronic obstructive pulmonary disease: A review. *Journal of Psychosomatic Research*, *59*(6), 429–443. doi: 10.1016/j.jpsychores.2005.04.007

Janos, A. L., Grange, D. K., Steiner, R. D., & White, D. A. (2012). Processing speed and executive abilities in children with phenylketonuria. *Neuropsychology*, *26*(6), 735–743. doi: 10.1037/a0029419

Janzen, D., & Nguyen, M. (2010). Beyond executive function: Non-executive cognitive abilities in individuals with PKU. *Molecular Genetics and Metabolism*, *99*(Suppl 1), S47–51. doi: 10.1016/j.ymgme.2009.10.009

Jelicic, M., Jonker, C., & Deeg, D. J. (2001). Effect of low levels of serum vitamin B12 and folic acid on cognitive performance in old age: A population-based study. *Developmental Neuropsychology*, *20*(3), 565–571. doi: 10.1207/S15326942DN2003_1

Kim, B., & Feldman, E. L. (2015). Insulin resistance as a key link for the increased risk of cognitive impairment in the metabolic syndrome. *Experimental and Molecular Medicine*, *47*, e149. doi: 10.1038/emm.2015.3

Kurella, M., Chertow, G. M., Fried, L. F., Cummings, S. R., Harris, T., Simonsick, E., . . . Yaffe, K. (2005). Chronic kidney disease and cognitive impairment in the elderly: The health, aging, and body composition study. *Journal of the American Society of Nephrology*, *16*(7), 2127–2133. doi: 10.1681/ASN.2005010005

Kurella, M., Chertow, G. M., Luan, J., & Yaffe, K. (2004). Cognitive impairment in chronic kidney disease. *Journal of the American Geriatrics Society*, *52*(11), 1863–1869. doi: 10.1111/j.1532-5415.2004.52508.x

Kurella, M., Yaffe, K., Shlipak, M. G., Wenger, N. K., & Chertow, G. M. (2005). Chronic kidney disease and cognitive impairment in menopausal women. *Journal of the American Geriatrics Society*, *45*(1), 66–76. Retrieved from www.ncbi.nlm.nih.gov/pubmed/15696445

Kurella Tamura, M., Xie, D., Yaffe, K., Cohen, D. L., Teal, V., Kasner, S. E., . . . Go, A. S. (2011). Vascular risk factors and cognitive impairment in chronic kidney disease: The Chronic Renal Insufficiency Cohort (CRIC) study. *Clinical Journal of the American Society of Nephrology*, *6*(2), 248–256. doi: 10.2215/CJN.02660310

Ledley, F. D., Levy, H. L., Shih, V. E., Benjamin, R., & Mahoney, M. J. (1984). Benign methylmalonic aciduria. *The New England Journal of Medine,*, *311*(16), 1015–1018. doi: 10.1056/NEJM198410183111604

Louwman, M. W., van Dusseldorp, M., van de Vijver, F. J., Thomas, C. M., Schneede, J., Ueland, P. M., . . . van Staveren, W. A. (2000). Signs of impaired cognitive function in adolescents with marginal cobalamin status. *American Journal of Clinical Nutrition*, *72*(3), 762–769. Retrieved from www.ncbi.nlm.nih.gov/pubmed/10966896

Madero, M., Gul, A., & Sarnak, M. J. (2008). Cognitive function in chronic kidney disease. *Seminars in Dialysis*, *21*(1), 29–37. doi: 10.1111/j.1525-139X.2007.00384.x

Matsui, S. M., Mahoney, M. J., & Rosenberg, L. E. (1983). The natural history of the inherited methylmalonic acidemias. *The New England Journal of Medicine*, *308*(15), 857–861. doi: 10.1056/NEJM198304143081501

McCrimmon, R. J., Ryan, C. M., & Frier, B. M. (2012). Diabetes and cognitive dysfunction. *Lancet*, *379*(9833), 2291–2299. doi: 10.1016/S0140-6736(12)60360-2

Moore, E., Mander, A., Ames, D., Carne, R., Sanders, K., & Watters, D. (2012). Cognitive impairment and vitamin B12: A review. *International Psychogeriatriatrics*, *24*(4), 541–556. doi: 10.1017/S1041610211002511

Morioka, D., Kasahara, M., Horikawa, R., Yokoyama, S., Fukuda, A., & Nakagawa, A. (2007). Efficacy of living donor liver transplantation for patients with methylmalonic acidemia. *American Journal of Transplantation*, *7*(12), 2782–2787. doi: 10.1111/j.1600-6143.2007.01986.x

Nicolaides, P., Leonard, J., & Surtees, R. (1998). Neurological outcome of methylmalonic acidaemia. *Archives of Disease in Childhood*, *78*(6), 508–512. Retrieved from www.ncbi.nlm.nih.gov/pubmed/9713004

Norman, M. A. (2011). *A Case of Hepatic Encephalopathy in End-Stage Liver Disease Secondary to Alcoholic Cirrhosis* (J. E. Morgan, I. S. Baron, & J. H. Ricker Eds.). New York: Oxford Press.

Novak, V., & Hajjar, I. (2010). The relationship between blood pressure and cognitive function. *Nature Reviews Cardiology*, *7*(12), 686–698. doi: 10.1038/nrcardio.2010.161

Oberholzer, V. G., Levin, B., Burgess, E. A., & Young, W. F. (1967). Methylmalonic aciduria: An inborn error of metabolism leading to chronic metabolic acidosis. *Archives of Disease in Childhood*, *42*(225), 492–504. Retrieved from www.ncbi.nlm.nih.gov/pubmed/6061291

O'Shea, C. J., Sloan, J. L., Wiggs, E. A., Pao, M., Gropman, A., Baker, E. H., . . . Snow, J. (2012). Neurocognitive phenotype of isolated methylmalonic acidemia. *Pediatrics*, *129*(6), e1541–e1551. doi: 10.1542/peds.2011-1715

Osimani, A., Berger, A., Friedman, J., Porat-Katz, B. S., & Abarbanel, J. M. (2005). Neuropsychology of vitamin B12 deficiency in elderly dementia patients and control subjects. *Journal of Geriatric Psychiatry and Neurology*, *18*(1), 33–38. doi: 10.1177/0891988704272308

Palta, P., Schneider, A. L., Biessels, G. J., Touradji, P., & Hill-Briggs, F. (2014). Magnitude of cognitive dysfunction in adults with type 2 diabetes: A meta-analysis of six cognitive domains and the most frequently reported neuropsychological tests within domains. *Journal of the International Neuropsychological Society*, *20*(3), 278–291. doi: 10.1017/S1355617713001483

Panza, F., Frisardi, V., Capurso, C., Imbimbo, B. P., Vendemiale, G., Santamato, A., . . . Solfrizzi, V. (2010). Metabolic syndrome and cognitive impairment: Current epidemiology and possible underlying mechanisms. *Journal of Alzheimer's Disease*, *21*(3), 691–724. doi: 10.3233/JAD-2010-091669

Patel, A. V., Wade, J. B., Thacker, L. R., Sterling, R. K., Siddiqui, M. S., Stravitz, R. T., . . . Bajaj, J. S. (2015). Cognitive reserve is a determinant of health-related quality of life in patients with cirrhosis, independent of covert hepatic encephalopathy and model for end-stage liver disease score. *Clinical Gastroenterology and Hepatology*, *13*(5), 987–991. doi: 10.1016/j.cgh.2014.09.049

Perry, W., Hilsabeck, R. C., & Hassanein, T. I. (2008). Cognitive dysfunction in chronic hepatitis C: A review. *Digestive Diseases and Sciences*, *53*(2), 307–321. doi: 10.1007/s10620-007-9896-z

Peters, R., & Beckett, N. (2009). Hypertension, dementia, and antihypertensive treatment: Implications for the very elderly. *Current Hypertension Reports*, *11*(4), 277–282. Retrieved from www.ncbi.nlm.nih.gov/pubmed/19602329

Pressler, S. J. (2008). Cognitive functioning and chronic heart failure: A review of the literature (2002–July 2007). *Journal of Cardiovascular Nursing*, *23*(3), 239–249. doi: 10.1097/01.JCN.0000305096.09710.ec

Pressler, S. J., Subramanian, U., Kareken, D., Perkins, S. M., Gradus-Pizlo, I., Sauve, M. J., . . . Shaw, R. M. (2010). Cognitive deficits in chronic heart failure. *Nursing Research*, *59*(2), 127–139. doi: 10.1097/NNR.0b013e3181d1a747

Riggs, K. M., Spiro, A., 3rd, Tucker, K., & Rush, D. (1996). Relations of vitamin B-12, vitamin B-6, folate, and homocysteine to cognitive performance in the normative aging study. *American Journal of Clinical Nutrition*, *63*(3), 306–314. Retrieved from www.ncbi.nlm.nih.gov/pubmed/8602585

Sadanand, S., Balachandar, R., & Bharath, S. (2015). Memory and executive functions in persons with type 2 diabetes: A meta-analysis. *Diabetes/Metabolism Research and Reviews*. doi: 10.1002/dmrr.2664

Samuels, M. H. (2008). Cognitive function in untreated hypothyroidism and hyperthyroidism. *Current Opinions in Endocrinology Diabetes and Obesity*, *15*(5), 429–433. doi: 10.1097/MED.0b013e32830eb84c

Samuels, M. H. (2014a). Psychiatric and cognitive manifestations of hypothyroidism. *Current Opinions in Endocrinology Diabetes and Obesity*, *21*(5), 377–383. doi: 10.1097/MED.0000000000000089

Samuels, M. H. (2014b). Thyroid disease and cognition. *Endocrinology Metabolism Clinics of North America*, *43*(2), 529–543. doi: 10.1016/j.ecl.2014.02.006

Scalabrino, G. (2009). The multi-faceted basis of vitamin B12 (cobalamin) neurotrophism in adult central nervous system: Lessons learned from its deficiency. *Progress in Neurobiology*, *88*(3), 203–220. doi: 10.1016/j.pneurobio.2009.04.004

Schou, L., Ostergaard, B., Rasmussen, L. S., Rydahl-Hansen, S., & Phanareth, K. (2012). Cognitive dysfunction in patients with chronic obstructive pulmonary disease: A systematic review. *Respiratory Medicine*, *106*(8), 1071–1081. doi: 10.1016/j.rmed.2012.03.013

Shevell, M. I., Matiaszuk, N., Ledley, F. D., & Rosenblatt, D. S. (1993). Varying neurological phenotypes among muto and mut- patients with methylmalonylCoA mutase deficiency. *American Journal of Medical Genetetics*, *45*(5), 619–624. doi: 10.1002/ajmg.1320450521

Sniderman, L. C., Lambert, M., Giguere, R., Auray-Blais, C., Lemieux, B., Laframboise, R., . . . Treacy, E. P. (1999). Outcome of individuals with low-moderate methylmalonic aciduria detected through a neonatal screening program. *Journal of Pediatrics*, *134*(6), 675–680. Retrieved from www.ncbi.nlm.nih.gov/pubmed/10356133

Stokke, O., Eldjarn, L., Norum, K. R., Steen-Johnsen, J., & Halvorsen, S. (1967). Methylmalonic Acidemia a new inborn error of metabolism which may cause fatal acidosis in the neonatal period. *Scandinavian Journal of Clinical & Laboratory Investigation*, *20*(4), 313–328. doi: 10.3109/00365516709076961

Strachan, M. W., Reynolds, R. M., Marioni, R. E., & Price, J. F. (2011). Cognitive function, dementia and type 2 diabetes mellitus in the elderly. *Nature Reviews Endocrinology*, *7*(2), 108–114. doi: 10.1038/nrendo.2010.228

Takahashi, Y., Iseki, C., Wada, M., Momma, T., Ueki, M., Kawanami, T., . . . Kato, T. (2011). Impaired glucose metabolism slows executive function independent of cerebral ischemic lesions in Japanese elderly: The Takahata study. *Internal Medicine*, *50*(16), 1671–1678. Retrieved from www.ncbi.nlm.nih.gov/pubmed/21841324

van den Berg, E., Reijmer, Y. D., de Bresser, J., Kessels, R. P., Kappelle, L. J., Biessels, G. J., & Utrecht Diabetic Encephalopathy Study, G. (2010). A 4 year follow-up study of cognitive functioning in patients with type 2 diabetes mellitus. *Diabetologia*, *53*(1), 58–65. doi: 10.1007/s00125-009-1571-9

Van Nuys, K., Brookmeyer, R., Chou, J. W., Dreyfus, D., Dieterich, D., & Goldman, D. P. (2015). Broad hepatitis C treatment scenarios return substantial health gains, but capacity is a concern. *Health Affairs (Millwood)*, *34*(10), 1666–1674. doi: 10.1377/hlthaff.2014.1193

Varvogli, L., Repetto, G. M., Waisbren, S. E., & Levy, H. L. (2000). High cognitive outcome in an adolescent with mut- methylmalonic acidemia. *American Journal of Medical Genetics*, *96*(2), 192–195. Retrieved from www.ncbi.nlm.nih.gov/pubmed/10893496

Vogels, R. L., Scheltens, P., Schroeder-Tanka, J. M., & Weinstein, H. C. (2007). Cognitive impairment in heart failure: A systematic review of the literature. *European Journal of Heart Failure*, *9*(5), 440–449. doi: 10.1016/j.ejheart.2006.11.001

Wahlin, A., Hill, R. D., Winblad, B., & Backman, L. (1996). Effects of serum vitamin B12 and folate status on episodic memory performance in very old age: A population-based study. *Psychology and Aging*, *11*(3), 487–496. Retrieved from www.ncbi.nlm.nih.gov/pubmed/8893317

Yaffe, K., Ackerson, L., Kurella Tamura, M., Le Blanc, P., Kusek, J. W., Sehgal, A. R., . . . Chronic Renal Insufficiency Cohort, I. (2010). Chronic kidney disease and cognitive function in older adults: Findings from the chronic renal insufficiency cohort cognitive study. *Journal of the American Geriatrics Society*, *58*(2), 338–345. doi: 10.1111/j.1532-5415.2009.02670.x

Yaffe, K., Falvey, C., Hamilton, N., Schwartz, A. V., Simonsick, E. M., Satterfield, S., . . . Harris, T. B. (2012). Diabetes, glucose control, and 9-year cognitive decline among older adults without dementia. *Archives of Neurology*, *69*(9), 1170–1175. doi: 10.1001/archneurol.2012.1117

Yates, K. F., Sweat, V., Yau, P. L., Turchiano, M. M., & Convit, A. (2012). Impact of metabolic syndrome on cognition and brain: A selected review of the literature. *Arteriosclerosis Thrombosis and Vascular Biology*, *32*(9), 2060–2067. doi: 10.1161/ATVBAHA.112.252759

Yohannes, A. M., Baldwin, R. C., & Connolly, M. J. (2006). Depression and anxiety in elderly patients with chronic obstructive pulmonary disease. *Age Ageing*, *35*(5), 457–459. doi: 10.1093/ageing/afl011

32 Clinical Assessment of Posttraumatic Stress Disorder

Jim Andrikopoulos

Preface

> We conclude that the concept of PTSD has moved the mental health field away from, rather than towards a better understanding of the natural psychological responses to trauma. A return to prior standards of diagnostic practice and therapeutic planning would greatly benefit patient care.
>
> (McHugh & Treisman, 2007, p. 211)

Posttraumatic stress disorder (PTSD) has been plagued by more controversy than any other psychiatric disorder, at least in the United States. This comes as no surprise since it was coined in the aftermath of, and was a direct result of, an American event: the Vietnam War. While there is a pre-Vietnam historical precedent and clinical merit in having a disorder devoted to a stress syndrome, the profound social, legal, and political repercussions of the diagnosis have paradoxically had an iatrogenic consequence for the patient it was intended to benefit and for American society as a whole. The diagnosis has evolved in such a way that it now bears little resemblance to the definition first provided in the *Diagnostic and Statistical Manual,* third edition (DSM-III), of the American Psychiatric Association (APA, 1980). Because the diagnosis was originally an idiosyncratic by-product of an event in U.S. history, it is no surprise that our definition of PTSD might be dissimilar to that found in the *International Classification of Diseases* (ICD-10) as defined by the World Health Organization (WHO, 1992). If events that are generally "outside the range of usual human experience" (APA, 1980: 236) of non-Western cultures such as torture, terrorism, and war have a PTSD prevalence rate of 30% or less, why do some Western societies experience a comparable or higher PTSD prevalence rates from a motor vehicle accident? Is the disparity in prevalence from two very disparate human events a reflection of an ascertainment bias, assessment technique, cultural differences, or capricious views of what constitutes PTSD? It is the contention here that the last explanation is the most likely one.

Chapter Overview

> The ICD-10 proposals are thus a product of collaboration, in the true sense of the word, between very many individuals and agencies in numerous countries. They were produced in the hope that they will serve as a strong support to the work of the many who are concerned with caring for the mentally ill and their families.
>
> ICD-10 Classification of Mental and Behavioral Disorders (WHO, 1992, p. 6)

Let me outline the scope of the chapter. The assessment of PTSD will focus on the adult instead of the child. The discussion will be on the civilian literature and not PTSD arising out of military service. It is difficult to assess the nature, extent, and outcome of a condition when the possibility of compensation is omnipresent as is the case in the military. There is no requirement by the veteran to provide evidence of a stressor. The veteran's own testimony is sufficient evidence to make a claim of PTSD so long as a mental health care professional makes the diagnosis (Department of Veterans Affairs, 2008). Thus the burden of proof in the military is lower for the veteran than the civilian. In addition, there is a rather marked difference of opinion as to the prevalence of malingered PTSD in the military. The following is an illustration.

A study done at the National Center for PTSD at the Boston Veterans Administration (VA) using veterans to look at dissociation found 50% of the veterans currently had PTSD, but more surprising was that 20% of their spouses or intimate partners had current PTSD. The lifetime rates were 72% and 38%, respectively (Wolf et al., 2012). It is not clear how they were recruited or if they were treatment-seeking veterans. They were described as being "enrolled in recent studies." These rates equal or exceed the best of epidemiological studies done in other countries looking at events that are truly horrific (Bayer, Klasen, & Adam, 2007; North et al., 1999; Pham, Weinstein, & Longman, 2004; Verger et al., 2004). One has to question to what extent these incidence and prevalence rates are valid. Given the compensation context in which many of these veterans are seen there is no mention of this factor. The malingering prevalence rate falls closer to 40%, "plus or minus 10" (Larrabee, Millis, & Meyers, 2009; Mittenberg, Patton, Canyock, & Condit, 2002). In clinical neuropsychology there is an obligation outlined in practice guidelines to assess for malingering (Heilbronner et al., 2009).

With that said, no discussion of PTSD is complete without an understanding of the role the Vietnam War played in the introduction of the term into the psychiatric nomenclature. A historical discussion of PTSD in a military context is necessary. Without the Vietnam War, PTSD would not have found its way into DSM-III. This historical fact, however, does not diminish the clinical importance of the term.

The chapter will focus on the clinical assessment of PTSD with only a cursory overview of topics that deserve more attention than can be devoted to here. These topics are covered in more detail in our earlier chapter on PTSD (Andrikopoulos & Greiffenstein, 2012). In that chapter the task was to familiarize neuropsychologists with what they excel in, the clinical application of forensic principles, but to the context of a nonneuropsychological event, namely PTSD. Therefore, the medicolegal aspects of PTSD will not be covered here but instead commented on as needed. This chapter has the reverse goal in mind: to update the neuropsychologist on the important clinical issues surrounding PTSD outside a medicolegal context. At the risk of redundancy some population-based epidemiological studies will be repeated, while other sections that are more clinically relevant are new (i.e., cross-cultural issues). This leaves us with the two chief goals of this chapter.

The first is captured in the quote that leads off this section and is the heart of this chapter: to convince the reader that it is time to move from PTSD as defined by DSM-5 and transition to ICD. The evolution of the term *PTSD* as defined and shaped by U.S. psychiatry and psychology has radically changed from its initial inception 35 years ago. PTSD as currently defined by DSM-5 no longer captures the essence of the traumatic stress syndrome clinicians and researchers initially conceptualized as being a distinct psychiatric entity. The current ICD-10 definition of PTSD falls closer to what was envisioned when Gross Stress Reaction was introduced in DSM-I (APA, 1952) and PTSD in DSM-III. This chapter offers a modest proposal for assessing PTSD that conforms to the proposed ICD-11 definition. The proposal is "modest" to the extent that what is being proposed in regard to the assessment of PTSD is somewhat novel and not altogether empirically based. However, the same can be said regarding the updated assessment methods (i.e., the revised Clinical Administered PTSD Scale, or CAPS-5) of the new DSM-5 PTSD definition, which have been published but are in need of independent validation (Hoge, 2015). The proposed definition of PTSD in this chapter comes very close to what it will likely look like based on the current published ICD-11 literature. Additionally, practically speaking, if I were to focus on ICD-10 now, this chapter would be dated in 2018 when ICD-11 is scheduled to be released. The meaningful and important change to the definition of PTSD in ICD-11 deserves our attention now.

The second major goal is to propose a structured clinical interview that involves the application of the Clinical Administered PTSD Scale (CAPS), which is DSM-based, and how it might be applied to ICD-11. This is a chapter on clinical assessment. *The assessment of PTSD is the structured clinical interview.* Psychological testing is ancillary and cognitive testing is needed only in certain circumstances. Therefore, cognitive testing will be reviewed briefly. Formal testing in the case of PTSD is needed more in a medicolegal context. Finally, treatment should be something clinical neuropsychologists should know about, but it is not something they typically do. Nothing has changed in regard to the treatment of PTSD since the previous chapter was written. It will not be covered here. The treatment section is rather thorough, covering psychotherapy, psychopharmacology, and case consultation (Andrikopoulos & Greiffenstein, 2012).

The Harmony of Illusions: Inventing PTSD

> I will argue that this generally accepted picture of PTSD, and the traumatic memory that underlies it, is mistaken. The disorder is not timeless, nor does it possess an intrinsic unity. Rather it is glued together by the practices, technologies, and narratives with which it is diagnosed, studied, treated, and represented and by the various interests, institutions, and moral arguments that mobilized these efforts and resources.
>
> (Young, 1995, p. 5)

The book by Allan Young is one of a handful of books and multiple articles that tell the story of how PTSD came into existence. The title of this subsection and Young's quote are not meant to downplay the clinical significance the syndrome can have to an individual experiencing a genuinely traumatic event. Young states that his job as an ethnographer is not to deny the reality of PTSD but explain how it was made real. An accomplished PTSD researcher, Chris Brewin, phrased the history as a debate between the "Saviors" and the "Skeptics" (Brewin, 2003). In his book *Posttraumatic Stress Disorder: Malady or Myth*, Brewin states that the myth is not the unreality of the disorder but the argument of the Skeptics that already existing diagnoses capture the symptoms of PTSD, which are not unique to PTSD, with the possible exception of flashbacks. An anxiety or depressive disorder would suffice as a diagnosis without having to coin a new one. As a career-long student of neuroscience history, reading the history of PTSD, especially the history before the term was coined, has been the most enjoyable part of this project.

The criteria that eventually became part of DSM-III, more or less intact, were first published in the *New York Times* on May 6, 1972 in an article titled "The Post Vietnam Syndrome" (Shatan, 1972). The author, Chaim Shatan, was a New York University psychiatrist and codirector of its postdoctoral psychoanalytic training program. He outlined six basic themes he observed in the group psychotherapy sessions ("rap groups") he held with Vietnam veterans. Among those themes specifically mentioned were guilt, rage, numbing, and doubting their ability to love others (Nicosia, 2001). These were the symptoms that Dwight Johnson, a Medal of Honor winner, was said to be experiencing following his discharge from the service. He was shot in a robbery attempt and on

May 26, 1971 Johnson's story was told on the front page of the *New York Times* (Nordheimer, 1971): "From Dak to Detroit: The Life and Death of a Troubled Vietnam Hero." Shatan had been unsuccessful in getting his piece published earlier by the *New York Times*, but this event served as the impetus for its publication (Nicosia, 2001).

Shatan would eventually join forces with another psychiatrist, Robert Lifton. Lifton was an already accomplished Yale psychiatrist with a half-dozen books to his credit. He had as his mentor Erik Erickson, who was Anna Freud's student. Lifton, not unfamiliar with trauma, won the National Book Award for an earlier book, *Death in Life: Survivors of Hiroshima* (Lifton, 1968). In 1970 Lifton and Shatan started the first Vietnam rap-group session, unorthodox psychotherapy outside the confines of the VA system. The by-product of this work for Lifton was his book, *Home From the War* (Lifton, 1973). Lifton the theorist and Shatan the therapist were the nucleus of the movement to get PTSD in DSM-III.

In 1969 a Boston VA social worker named Sarah Haley reportedly met, in her first week on the job, a veteran who claimed to be at the March 1968 My Lai Massacre. She wrote in 1974 the most influential paper of the time in the *Archives of General Psychiatry*, "When the Patient Reports Atrocities: Specific Treatment Considerations of the Vietnam Veteran" (Haley, 1974). This caught the attention of many, but most importantly Shatan, who invited her in 1975 to be part of a symposium at the American Orthopsychiatry Association meeting. She was also invited that summer to be part of an American Psychiatric Association Vietnam veteran panel session. More importantly, at that latter meeting discussions were beginning regarding DSM-III. The chairperson for the DSM-III task force was Robert Spitzer. Shatan contacted Spitzer only to discover that Spitzer had no interest in including combat-related stress disorder in DSM-III (Nicosia, 2001). A confluence of events would change that.

There was a lawsuit following the Buffalo Creek dam break in West Virginia. A coal mining company built a dam that burst, killed 125 people, and injured over a thousand. The judge chastised the American Psychiatric Association for not having a more proper psychiatric diagnosis to assign to survivors that would be more fitting than anxiety or depressive reaction. At the same time Nazi concentration camp survivors were seeking war reparations for the trauma they endured. The American Psychiatric Association decided to hold a symposium at its1975 meeting. Researchers were invited to present their findings on the Buffalo Creek disaster. Shatan mobilized a team of 45 professionals from across the country to present data on Vietnam veterans. Jack Smith, a former Marine sergeant and Vietnam veteran, assisted Shatan (Nicosia, 2001). He was at the first rap session held by Shatan and Lipton and became the eventual president of the Vietnam Veterans Against the War (Scott, 1990). A Vietnam Veterans Working Group was formed (Nicosia, 2001). At that same meeting, opposite the "delayed-stress advocates," was the "St. Louis group" that included sociologist Lee Robins, a very influential epidemiology and clinical researcher from Washington University in St. Louis. She and her colleagues had already been publishing about Vietnam veterans. The alcohol and drug issues they were observing were for the most part minimal: While experimentation was common in the service, upon their return it was essentially at prewar levels (Robins, Helzer, & Davis, 1975). However, it was acknowledged that depression seemed a problem postdischarge (Helzer, Robins, & Davis, 1976). Spitzer invited some members of the Vietnam Veterans Working Group to join the Reactive Disorders Subcommittee of the DSM-III task force. University of Iowa psychiatrist Nancy Andreasen headed this latter committee. She was chosen partially because of her experience with burn victims. After a 1977 presentation by Shatan and his group at the American Psychiatric Association meeting, Spitzer agreed that a stress diagnosis should go into DSM-III (Nicosia, 2001).

The zealous advocacy and commitment more than anything else lead to the success of Shatan, Lifton, and Haley. Not only did they manage to get a stress disorder in DSM-III, but also—and more important—a delayed variant of the disorder. Shatan was tireless and an anti-Vietnam war campaigner. Shatan opened his most well-known Vietnam paper, "The Grief of Soldiers," with the following: "Atrocities perpetrated upon the Vietnamese while saving them from Communism are now almost as well known as those of Hitler's extermination camps" (Shatan, 1973, p. 640). Lifton's similar sentiments and academic credentials made him the perfect public relations representative for the group. He testified numerous times before Congress leading up to the publication of DSM-III. As for Haley, her professional experience up until DSM-III was devoted to the Vietnam veteran cause. The paper that lead to her national recognition as a PTSD clinician concluded in the second-to-last paragraph: "The only report that should not be accepted at face value, although one may choose not to challenge it initially, is the patient's report that combat in Vietnam had no effect on him" (Haley, 1974, p. 196). In the *Journal of Traumatic Stress Studies*, the official journal of the International Society for Traumatic Stress Studies, Shatan wrote her obituary, "A True Child of Trauma" (Shatan, 1990). The inclusion of Jack Smith, a non–health care professional, in the DSM-III deliberations was rather unprecedented. He eventually became a psychologist (Bloom, 2000). Two additional individuals merit special mention: Charles Figley and Mardi Horowitz.

Stress Disorder Among Vietnam Veterans represented the collective thoughts of the advocates at the time. Charles Figley edited this 1978 book and invited Shatan, Lifton, and Haley to contribute (Figley, 1978). Figley served in Vietnam in 1965 and later became a psychologist. He organized Vietnam symposia at the American Psychological Association and the American Sociological Association meetings (Bloom, 2000). He declined the offer to be the director of the newly formed national Vet Centers (Nicosia, 2001). In 1983, Figley sent out more than 60 letters to trauma researchers suggesting the formation of an organization devoted to assessment, treatment, and research in traumatic stress. This organization was formed in 1985 and eventually became the International Society for Traumatic Stress Studies, the principal organization devoted to stress disorders. Figley became the organization's first president (Bloom, 2000). While Figley, more so than the others, was a researcher, he was no less an advocate. When the controversial Report of Findings from the National Vietnam Veterans Readjustment Study was published suggesting that as many as 30% of Vietnam veterans had the full PTSD syndrome, Figley wrote the following editorial note as the editor of the book series that published the findings:

> Most important, perhaps when next confronted with the prospect of sending citizens to fight a war—the purpose of which is questionable—policymakers will consider these findings. Perhaps they will be moved to acknowledge the vast and enduring costs of such a war to an entire generation of this country's children. Perhaps.
>
> (Kulka et al., 1990, p. xxi)

Mardi Horowitz, another contributor to Figley's book, can reasonably be considered the father of modern stress studies. In 1976 he published *Stress Response Syndromes* (Horowitz, 1976). For the advocates, as crucial as getting any stress syndrome in DSM-III was including one that recognized that the symptoms could have a delayed onset of months to years. Shatan (1973) went so far as to say that it is "commonly not apparent until a considerable amount of time (nine to thirty months) after discharge" (p. 645). Part of the reason Shatan gave for forming the rap groups is that the veterans "had been told their disturbances manifested themselves too late to prove the 'service connection' required for VA treatment" (p. 641). Horowitz, like Lifton and Shatan, was heavily influenced by psychodynamic theory. Horowitz, in the first paper devoted to a delayed stress syndrome invoked a psychodynamic explanation, a "denial-numbing tendency" (Horowitz & Solomon, 1975: 68).

How much of an influence did the advocates have? If you believe the leading authority on the topic, Gerald Nicosia (2001), in his excellent book *Home From the War: A History of the Vietnam Veterans' Movement* (the title was given to him by Haley), he tells us the influence was immense:

> What occurred next was on the order of a major miracle. Andreasen, rather than writing the definition herself, invited Shatan, Smith, Haley and the other leading combat stress agitators to write whole sections for her, and agreed merely to "edit" their work. Shatan recalls that they were "practically dictating" the new definition of post-traumatic stress disorder into DSM-III.
>
> (p. 209)

From DSM-IV-TR to DSM-5

> In the first author's work on three DSMs over a period of 20 years, never once did he recall an expert make a suggestion that would reduce the boundary of his pet disorder. In contrast, they very often clamored for expansions.
>
> (Frances & Widiger, 2012, p. 118)

The harshest critic of DSM-5 is Duke University professor emeritus Allen Frances. Frances served as chairperson of the DSM-IV Task Force. In a series of commentaries posted to the *Psychology Today* website under the title series "DSM-5 in Distress," and in his book *Saving Normal* (Frances, 2013), Frances outlines the difficulties with DSM-5 in general; these go well beyond the problematic PTSD diagnosis. Frances maintains when he chaired the task force "the null position was always to keep things stable" via a three-stage process: a literature review, data reanalysis and field testing (Frances, 2009: 1). While beyond the scope of this review, his criticisms of DSM-5 can be summarized as follows: (a) the inclusion of new categories (i.e., major cognitive impairment when dementia would suffice) together with lowering of the threshold of existing disorders will result in higher rates of mental illness diagnoses; (b) there are significant forensic implications to the latter (Frances, 2010); (c) the DSM-5 process was not transparent (Frances, 2009); (d) field trials focused on reliability versus validity (Frances & Widiger, 2012); (e) and lowering the reliability standard—in the past, kappa values of 0.6 or above were "acceptable" whereas in DSM-5 kappa values at dramatically lower values of 0.2 to 0.4 were deemed acceptable (Frances, 2012a).

As DSM-5 was being developed, experts proposed changes in anticipation for what likely were to be more changes to the existing PTSD criteria. Before the reader is asked to adopt ICD-10 and the yet-unpublished ICD-11 PTSD definition in lieu of DSM-5, understanding the changes to DSM-5 will help to validate the need for the transition. Ironically, the best changes that were eventually proposed for DSM-5 but not adopted could be found in the already existing ICD-10 definition: namely, dropping symptoms that are not specific to PTSD. Table 32.1 lists the DSM-5 criteria in amended form. Let us begin by examining the changes that were recommended for PTSD in DSM-5, beginning with the suggestions of Robert Spitzer, the person who had been ultimately responsible for the introduction of the diagnosis. He has provided insightful and regular commentary on the DSM process over the years.

Proposed Changes to DSM-5

As with each release of the DSM, a spirited discussion preceded the release of DSM-5. What garnered the most attention, as has always been the case, were proposed changes to all aspects of Criterion A. Second, whether to exclude nonspecific PTSD symptoms (e.g., sleep problems, poor memory

Table 32.1 *DSM-5 criteria for posttraumatic stress disorder

A Exposure to actual or threatened death, serious injury, or sexual violence by:
- 1 Directly experiencing the traumatic event(s)
- 2 Witnessing, in person, the event(s) as it occurred to others
- 3 Learning a violent or accidental event(s) occurred to a close family member or close friend
- 4 Experiencing repeated or extreme exposure to aversive details of the event(s) but this does not apply to electronic media or TV unless work related

B Presence of one (or more) of the following intrusion symptoms associated with the event(s):
- 1 Recurrent, involuntary, and intrusive distressing memories of event(s)
- 2 Distressing trauma-related dreams
- 3 Dissociative reactions (e.g., flashbacks)
- 4 Distress at exposure to internal or external cues that symbolize or resemble the event(s)
- 5 Physiological reactions to internal or external cues that symbolize or resemble aspects of the event(s)

C Persistent avoidance of stimuli associated with the traumatic event(s), beginning after event(s) occurred, as evidenced by one or both of the following:
- 1 Avoidance or efforts to avoid distressing memories, thoughts, or feelings about or closely associated with the event(s)
- 2 Avoidance or efforts to avoid external reminders that arouse distressing memories, thoughts, or feelings associated with the event(s)

D Negative alterations in cognitions and mood associated with the event(s) as evidenced by two (or more) of the following:
- 1 Inability to remember an important aspect of the event(s)
- 2 Persistent and exaggerated negative beliefs or expectations about oneself, others, or the world
- 3 Persistent, distorted cognitions about the cause or consequences of the event(s) that lead the individual to blame self or others
- 4 Persistent negative emotional state (e.g., fear, horror, anger, guilt or shame)
- 5 Diminished interest or participation in significant activities
- 6 Feelings of detachment or estrangement from others
- 7 Persistent inability to experience positive emotions

E Marked alternations in arousal and reactivity associated with the event(s) as evidenced by two (or more) of the following:
- 1 Irritable behavior and angry outbursts (with little or no provocation) typically expressed as verbal or physical aggression toward people or objects
- 2 Reckless or self-destructive behavior
- 3 Hypervigilance
- 4 Exaggerated startle response
- 5 Problems with concentration
- 6 Sleep disturbance

F Duration of the disturbance (Criteria B, C, D, and E) is more than one month.

G Disturbance causes distress or impairment in social, occupational, or other important areas.

H Not attributable to the physiological effects of a substance or medical condition.

Specify whether:

With dissociative symptoms: Persistent or recurrent symptoms of either of the following:
- 1 *Depersonalization*: Persistent or recurrent experiences of feeling detached from, and as if one were an outside observer of, one's mental processes or body (e.g., feeling as if in a dream; feeling a sense of unreality of self or body or of time moving slowly).
- 2 *Derealization*: Persistent or recurrent experiences of unreality of surroundings (e.g., the world around the individual is experienced as unreal, dreamlike, distant, or distorted).

Specify if delayed expression: If the full diagnostic criteria are not met until at least six months after the event (although the onset and expression of some symptoms may be immediate).

* Modified from the DSM-5 (pp. 271–272).

for the event) in Criteria B, C, and D in DSM-IV-TR. This section summarizes these much-discussed pre-DSM-5 debate themes by reviewing some of the relevant literature. In doing so, the value of the PTSD literature cited to argue for or against these issues will be discussed by asking a rarely asked question in PTSD research: *Do PTSD studies, especially epidemiological research, help guide clinical practice?* It will be argued the generalizability and representativeness of some of this research has fallen short of the mark.

It is logical to assume that Spitzer would speak against the psychiatric nosological expansionism that Frances warned about, especially in reference to PTSD. The larger psychiatric community has come to accept PTSD—if not the term at least the concept—but has not universally embraced the manner in which it has evolved. Spitzer, in summarizing the proposed changes for DSM-5, understandably began with what to do with A1, the stressor criterion (Spitzer, First, & Wakefield, 2007). Adding the qualifier "directly experienced" in DSM-5 in reference to the event would strengthen Criterion A1. "The person experienced" terminology in DSM-IV-TR does not necessarily imply directly experiencing the event. Spitzer argued "being exposed" to an event might apply, for example, to witnessing 9/11 on television. Harvard psychologist Richard McNally (2009) suggested among a number of important recommended changes, requiring that the patient be present in the event. "Virtual trauma," he stated, does not cause PTSD (McNally & Breslau, 2008).

The historical precursor to PTSD, Gross Stress Reaction, was a disorder that was caused when the person was "under conditions of great or unusual stress" due to either combat or "civilian catastrophe" (APA, 1952: 40). DSM-III inherited that definition: "a psychologically traumatic event that is generally outside the range of usual human experience" (APA, 1980: 236). The "outside the range of usual human experience" terminology was omitted in DSM-IV (APA, 1994). The person needed only to be "exposed to a traumatic event," and not necessarily directly experience it. McNally called the evolution of the stressor criteria "conceptual bracket creep," the most often quoted phrase in the PTSD debate (McNally, 2003). Rosen (2004a) later modified the term to "criterion creep." It refers to the watering down of what constitutes a traumatic event from the initial "outside the realm of human experience" definition. The broadening of A1 diminishes the significance of the stressor by giving a concentration camp survivor and someone in a motor vehicle accident the same diagnosis (Andreasen, 2004). This is the core problem, whereas the other issues are of relatively less consequence.

Frances and Widiger (2012) make a related argument. The diagnostic system of psychiatry as defined by the organizers and developers of DSM is worried about false negatives. There is a preference for an inclusive diagnostic system, hence the broadening of A1. Weathers and Keane (2007) argued that A1 should be sensitive, casting a wide net to identify anyone who might have the diagnosis. It should minimize false negatives. This inclusivity is a synonym for criterion creep. McNally (2009), perhaps rhetorically, asks if we can "fix PTSD in DSM-V?" I believe we can if the A1 Criterion is fixed.

Brewin recommended a dramatic change: dropping A1 in toto. He suggested focusing instead on PTSD's central symptoms versus those that overlap with other disorders (Brewin, Lanius, Novac, Schnyder, & Galea, 2009). From the 17 core PTSD symptoms, Brewin proposed retaining only six. Reexperiencing would include recurrent nightmares and daytime images. Avoidance consists of avoiding internal (i.e., thoughts) and external (i.e., activities) reminders. Hyperarousal includes hypervigilance and the startle response. Brewin acknowledged that the two most valid reasons arguing against the elimination of Criterion A1 was that it would constitute a marked departure from the very spirit that defines PTSD (namely the stressor) and the absence of the gatekeeper criteria might trivialize the disorder. A fair but less compelling argument by Friedman (2013) was that removing the nonspecific symptoms (e.g., attention and sleep symptoms) would be analogous to removing pain and fever from a medical diagnosis because they are found in other diseases. The first study to test the Brewin criteria in an outpatient treatment-seeking sample found the overall PTSD prevalence rate did not change but an equal number of participants, 13%, had a change in diagnostic status, both losing and gaining the diagnosis (van Emmerik & Kamphuis, 2011).

While ridding A1 from PTSD practically eradicates the meaning of the disorder, the same cannot be said for dropping A2. Fear (to different degrees), helplessness, and horror have been part of the diagnosis from the start. In DSM-I, Gross Stress Reaction, "overwhelming fear" was a core feature of the condition (APA, 1952) and this has always been an important part of PTSD in every edition of DSM as a descriptor in the text. In DSM-IV fear, helplessness, and horror officially became Criterion A2 (APA, 1994). As will be discussed, while what defines the A1 Criterion is the core of the PTSD debate, there seems to be near universal agreement that it cannot be eliminated. As for A2, the definition is clear but there appears to be general agreement that it can be eliminated.

Studies employing both interview and self-report measures with various populations have concluded that A2 had very little effect on PTSD rates. This was found in a nonrandom community sample of non–treatment-seeking women using a structured interview (Anders, Frazier, & Frankfurt, 2011); a nonrandom community sample of non–treatment-seeking women responding to an advertisement reporting trauma histories using a PTSD checklist (Bedard-Gilligan & Zoellner, 2008); a randomly selected population based study using a structured interview (Breslau & Kessler, 2001); a random worldwide (21 countries) community sample of non–treatment-seeking subjects using a structured interview (Karam et al., 2010); consecutive hospital admissions following a traumatic injury using a structured interview (O'Donnell, Creamer, McFarlane, Silove, & Bryant, 2010); and a longitudinal cohort of nurses administered a PTSD checklist in the form of an interview (Roberts et al., 2012). This diverse literature would suggest removing the A2 Criterion would not impact PTSD rates.

There are two points to be made regarding the studies just listed. The first point requires a paradigm shift that asks the psychologist to query if certain kinds of research inform clinical practice. The second point involves A2 and the circumstances under which we can remove it.

This first point is captured by a title of a commentary piece by Williams (2005): "Does clinical epidemiology have a role in clinical practice?" Jelinek (2005) argues the term *clinical epidemiology* is an oxymoron. It is instead the study of a community in which average effects within that population are studied. Certain clinical questions can be answered only by studies that examine subjects that approximate the circumstances of an actual patient. The dual concerns regarding epidemiological research are representativeness and generalizability. Kukull and Ganguli (2012) discuss how these latter two principles may not apply to the epidemiological dementia literature. Having examined close to 1,000

Alzheimer patients, I believe the mild cognitive impairment literature and the registries throughout the world that track these patients will not inform me of what to do about a patient brought in by his or her daughter because of perceived cognitive symptoms. To illustrate, Hannaford and Owen-Smith (1998) sought to answer a commonly asked clinical question by reviewing the most sound methodological studies that might provide an answer to the following: "What is the risk of cardiovascular disease among users of currently available, low dose, combined oral contraceptives who are aged less than 35 years, do not smoke, and do not have a medical condition known to increase the risk of vascular disease?" They could not answer the question based on their review and suggested that this state of affairs is not likely unique to their clinical question. This is not to deny the importance of epidemiology research, as it is critical in informing us about the incidence and prevalence of a disease, possible causes, and risk factors.

The research-recruited subject who may in the remote past have had a questionable PTSD-causing event, whom the academician is now researching and writing about but never actually examined, is not the same patient arriving at the doctor's office seeking treatment for a psychological trauma. Who and what type of person might respond to a call for research subjects? To give an extraordinary example, in a very innovative PTSD study, McNally advertised for research subjects kidnapped by aliens so their physiological response, a biomarker of their PTSD, to the alien abduction could be measured. Results confirmed the hypothesis that alien abductees can generate emotional responses similar to that of combat veterans with PTSD (McNally, Lasko, Clancy, Macklin, Pitman, & Orr, 2004). Allen Frances, in his first commentary on the DSM-5 process, observed that those responsible for revising the DSM spent their careers in academic psychiatry. He maintained that a basic tenet of clinical epidemiology is that the research and clinical experience of tertiary-care centers may not generalize to the average clinic. "Experts are absolutely necessary to the development of a diagnostic system but are also a serious threat to its generalizability and safety" (Frances & Widiger, 2012, p. 118). This perception of disengagement of the PTSD academician from the clinical process was shared by enough clinician members of the International Society for Traumatic Stress Studies to cause a rift in the early 1990s resulting in some members resigning and forming their own organization, The Association for Traumatic Stress Specialists (Bloom, 2000). A large portion of PTSD research is conducted by recruiting subjects via advertisements or non–treatment-seeking subjects (e.g., undergraduate students reporting "traumas") and diagnosed with PTSD may not be generalizable. In one study (Pfaltz, Michael, Meyer, & Wilhelm, 2013), subjects recruited through newspaper advertisements reported an average of 17 traumatic memories. It is hard to imagine that there is any clinical generalizability in recruiting Alzheimer's disease patients from newspaper advertisements. This author cannot say if he has ever seen such a study in the neurology literature. In PTSD research this is common. Valid clinical research is examining a consecutive series of treatment-seeking patients.

The safety concerns Frances was referring to earlier are the iatrogenic consequences of an inclusive psychiatric diagnostic system that produce more patients than may actually exist (Frances, 2010). It has been argued, rather persuasively, that the sociology of psychiatric stigma is one in which psychiatry has not been an innocent bystander (Summerfield, 2001). Parenthetically, one also has to ask the question: Do researchers have an obligation to secure treatment for those patients diagnosed with PTSD in these epidemiological studies?

The studies previously reviewed that concluded A2 had very little effect on PTSD rates might look different in a patient sample. The first prospective longitudinal study to examine if A2 predicts PTSD was done by Brewin, Andrews, and Rose (2000). The patient sample was crime victims assaulted or threatened with assault by a nonhousehold member. They were recruited via police reports and hospitals. As predicted, all three emotions predicted the development of PTSD: fear, helplessness, or horror. The shortcoming of the study is that PTSD was diagnosed via a PTSD self-report measure versus an interview and that of the 2,161 eligible victims only 11% participated. One conclusion of the study is that it validated the new DSM-IV Criterion A2 (APA, 1994). In a population-based study, Creamer, McFarlane, and Burgess (2005) looked at the role of subjective experience via a structured interview in the development of various psychiatric disorders. Using DSM-IV, they identified ten A1 trauma categories. They concluded that meeting Criterion A2 varied with the type of trauma, with virtually anyone (97%) experiencing a rape meeting the A2 Criterion. Second, the prevalence rates of all psychiatric disorders are higher for those meeting both A1 and A2 versus just A1. A2 emotions at the time of the event not only predict PTSD, but psychiatric morbidity in general. In an aging study of well-adjusted (study entrance required good physical health and mental health at the time of admission) military veterans of World War II and the Korea War suggested that meeting A2 was a function of the nature of the A1 event. Sexual assault and war-zone exposure had the highest probability, between 75% and 80% meeting A2 criteria given A1 (Schnurr, Spiro, Vielhauer, Findler, & Hamblen, 2002). In summary, the first point addressed earlier concerned the epidemiological studies that are cited to support changes in DSM-5, especially in regard to Criterion A. These studies have to meet the litmus test of approximating the clinical situation. Second, in reference to Criterion A, the types of trauma should be identified since meeting A2 is a function of the type of A1 trauma.

The second point in regard to A2 comes from McNally (2009), who accurately phrased what should be the fate of A2: "In the language of behaviorism, it confounds the response with the stimulus. In the language of medicine, it confounds the host with the pathogen" (p. 598). On the surface it might ironically appear that the author of criterion creep might be advocating the further watering down of the stressor criteria by eliminating the fear, helplessness, and horror emotions that define trauma. However, McNally argues that the removing of A2 is contingent upon tightening up A1 by requiring that the person be physically present at the scene of the trauma. I would instead go further and argue that dropping A2 be contingent upon returning to the original definition of the type of event that constitutes trauma. If we stipulate that the A1 event must be beyond the realm of human experience as advocated by DSM-I and DSM-III, then the A2 criteria introduced in DSM-IV is indeed not necessary. A2 studies addressing the issue between A2 and the development of PTSD become obsolete. As the definition of the PTSD-producing events in A1 expands and the less representative the subjects are in terms of representing actual help-seeking patients, like university student volunteers responding to a PTSD checklist (Boals & Schuettler, 2009), the less likely the relevance of A2. The worse scenario is removing A2 and keeping A1 unaltered. That is what essentially happened in DSM-5. I say "essentially" because there has been at least some attempt to try and better operationally define the stressor in DSM-5. While applauded by some, it fails to resolve completely the Criterion A issue (Rosen, Lilienfeld, Frueh, McHugh & Spitzer, 2010).

Returning to the issue of the nonspecificity (i.e., irritability, anhedonia, attention problems, insomnia, and poor memory) of some PTSD criteria, one study with blinded raters found that 78.6% of patients enrolled in antidepressant clinical trials with an identified stressor met the B, C, and D DSM-IV PTSD criteria. However, an equal number, 80%, without trauma (or equivocal trauma), also met the criteria (Bodkin, Pope, Detke, & Hudson, 2007). This finding was repeated using a nationally stratified sample, the National Co-Morbidity Survey Replication and the DSM-IV definition (Elhai, Grubaugh, Kashdan, & Frueh, 2008). Following the deletion of nonspecific PTSD symptoms, they found the lifetime prevalence rate of PTSD changed very little (6.81% to 6.42%), but a sizable minority (13%) no longer met the DSM-IV criteria using the revised Spitzer criteria. One argument made by the authors for the lack of overall change in prevalence is that depression, a common comorbid condition, is part of PTSD, rather than a source of error in the diagnosis. Finally, a major problem in dropping Criterion A1 is its medicolegal implications. It does serve as a gatekeeper, albeit a weak one as currently defined.

PTSD Defined in DSM-5

The DSM-5 criteria are briefly summarized, and are listed in Table 32.1. Criterion A was maintained, requiring exposure to a trauma via four ways. As was expected, the A2 Criterion in DSM-IV-TR was dropped. Unlike the previous DSM, these four qualifiers are listed. The first would be exposure to an actual traumatic event (A1) or witnessing it in another person (A2). If the patient learned about the event it had to have happened to a close family member or friend and had to be of a violent or accidental nature (A3). Completely new is the addition of repeated exposure to traumatic events such as might be found in certain occupations, such as collecting human remains, or law enforcement personnel exposed repeatedly to traumatic events associated with their occupation (A4). This last criterion has potential medicolegal implications. This could assign a PTSD diagnosis to someone just by virtue of the everyday duties associated with his or her occupation.

A change welcomed by all was the splitting of the intrusion (Criterion B) and avoidance (Criterion C) symptoms. Only one symptom from each is needed to meet the criterion within each category. Criterion B requires the presence of recurrent, involuntary, and intrusive memories of the event (B1); recurrent dreams (B2); flashbacks (B3); distress to internal and external cues that symbolize the event (B4); and finally, a physiological reaction to those cues (B5). One or more of the criteria have to be met. Criterion C consists of avoiding internal and external reminders, respectively. Internal reminders are distressing memories, thoughts, and feelings about the event (C1) or the avoidance of external reminders (C2). At least one of the two criteria has to be met. Criterion D, negative alterations in cognitions and mood associated with the traumatic event, consists of organizing seven symptoms previously in DSM except for two that were added: exaggerated negative beliefs (D2) and distorted cognitions (D3). Two of the seven symptoms listed must be met. Two of six symptoms must be met in Criterion E. Unlike B and C, Criterion D and E symptoms are rather nonspecific in regard to PTSD with the exception of D1 (inability to recall important aspects of the event), E3 (hypervigilance), and exaggerated startle response (E4). Added to Criterion E (previously Criterion D) in the previous DSM was reckless or self-destructive behavior (E24, a symptom not in the previous DSM). Criterion F (duration of symptoms greater than one month), Criterion G (impairment in daily activities), and Criterion H (not due to another medical condition) remain relatively unaltered from the previous edition. The one change (Criterion F) is that there is no longer an acute (duration less than three months) versus chronic (longer than three months) subtype that needs to be specified. Instead of three clusters and 17 symptoms in the previous DSM, there are now four clusters and 20 symptoms.

Once the diagnosis is made the clinician would specify the dissociative subtype of PTSD: depersonalization or derealization is not included in the previous DSM. Finally, the clinician is asked to code if there is delayed onset PTSD present. Second only to the debate over what constitutes a trauma (Criterion A), delayed PTSD perhaps is the most problematic and remains problematic in DSM-5. The requirement to code a dissociative subtype now moves PTSD from the anxiety disorder camp, where some convincingly argue it should be, and makes it a dissociative disorder that is not in the Dissociative Disorders section but is instead in the new Trauma and Stressor-Related Disorders section. Despite arguable evidence that a dissociative subtype should be included, it is introduced and despite compelling evidence that delayed PTSD is rare it remains in DSM.

What to Do With Criterion A: The Stressor?

As has always been the case, the majority of the pre-DSM-5 debate centered on Criterion A: A1, the traumatic event and A2, fear, helplessness and horror. A review of the research that has been cited to justify revision of the criteria in DSM-5 is in order followed by an overview of the DSM-5 field trials that solidified these changes. As already noted, British psychologist Chris Brewin has commented extensively on what to do with the stressor criteria. His commentary has some empirical basis, but more importantly provides a perspective outside of North America, where the DSM has been viewed by some a chauvinistic, unpredictable, and proprietary enterprise.

What was novel about the new PTSD diagnosis in DSM-III was that a psychiatric syndrome was linked to a distinct class of stressors. The event more or less defined the syndrome. Furthermore an early critique of the DSM-III argued that there was no epidemiological evidence for linking a particular syndrome to extraordinary stressors versus ordinary stressors. It is the personal characteristics and social milieu of the individual that defines how a stressor will affect the individual (Breslau & Davis, 1987). Breslau and Davis argued that this notion in DSM-III had only face validity with no epidemiological studies to support the notion. I would argue that epidemiology is not a prerequisite for defining a syndrome. Alois Alzheimer was the first to link a neuropsychiatric syndrome to a neuropathology and he did this in one patient. While no seminal and or definitive epidemiological study was offered as evidence for the newly minted PTSD diagnosis, it is clear that exposure to extraordinary stressors can have a psychiatric consequence. What has been argued is if that psychiatric consequence needed a new label: PTSD. Some have suggested removing from the criteria the very definition of PTSD—the stressor criteria. Brewin and colleagues (2009) suggested that Criterion A be eliminated completely. An individual meeting a stringent DSM symptom cluster makes Criterion A unnecessary (Kraemer, Wittmann, Jenewein, Maier, & Schnyder, 2009; Maier, 2007). The counterargument is that this essentially eliminates the very essence of the diagnosis. PTSD does not occur spontaneously in nature. It must follow a stressor, and specifying the stressor informs us which stressors are likely to produce the diagnosis (Kilpatrick, Resnick, & Acierno, 2009). There is heuristic value in identifying stressors that produce symptoms independent of PTSD.

It is argued here that Criterion A needs to be maintained. First, the dropping of Criterion A is moot for clinicians in North America who have decided to continue using DSM-5. Second, the stressor criterion was present and preceded the debate that surrounded the new PTSD diagnosis. The stressor was the very definition of what Gross Stress Reaction was under DSM-II. Third, the ICD-10 PTSD criteria is consistent with the Gross Stress Reaction definition and what it means to have a stressor outside the realm of everyday experience as embodied in DSM-III. What is left to do is operationally define what those stressors might be.

The research regarding Criterion A2 (the fear, horror, and helplessness criteria) has been much more controversial. The biggest conceptual shift in the A1 and A2 criteria happened in DSM-IV. DSM III-R continued to define A1 as an extraordinary traumatic experience but the DSM-IV dropped the "outside the range of usual human experience" delineation. The DSM-IV field studies did not require the respondent to link symptoms to a traumatic event (Kilpatrick et al., 1998). To offset what would be perceived as a watering down of the stressor, A2 was added.

The standard was no longer an event that almost anyone would find traumatic, but the individual's subjective reaction to that event now became important. The field trials suggested this strongly correlated with PTSD (Kilpatrick et al., 1998). Since DSM-IV the tide has turned against the inclusion of A2 in DSM-5, so it was eliminated. Here I survey the evidence for its omission.

The Brewin study was the first longitudinal study to assess how the subjective reaction as to the intensity of the trauma predicted PTSD (Brewin et al. 2000). It largely supported the introduction of A2 in DSM-IV. Others have found a relationship as well. Creamer et al. (2005) persuasively argued that if we identify what constitutes a valid PTSD-producing A1 stressor the subjectivity of A2 is irrelevant. In this Australian population-based study virtually everyone experiencing rape as the A1 event also met criteria for A2 (97%). Next in line was sexual molestation and physical assault. This is in contrast to those who reported combat as the A1 event. Approximately 65% also met A2. While this may appear counterintuitive at first glance, this possibility was anticipated in DSM-III. The reason for including delayed PTSD was that in the course of combat, fear, helplessness, and horror are not very adaptive (Andreasen, 2004). It was only in the aftermath of battle that the emotional consequence would manifest itself. What delayed PTSD was not intended to do, and what makes little clinical sense, is for symptoms to be reported months or years after the precipitating event. Additionally, in the Creamer study, overall psychiatric morbidity (e.g., clinical depression) was higher for those that met both A1 and A2 criteria. The flipside to the A2 debate is that while A2 does not predict the presence of PTSD, the absence of it virtually rules out the presence of PTSD (Bedard-Gilligan & Zoellner, 2008; Breslau & Kessler, 2001). If it is not to be used as a core criterion, A2 is at least a risk factor (Karam et al., 2010). Since the absence of A2 strongly predicts the absence of PTSD, it should be retained in some form or another (Weathers &

Keane, 2007). A patient not volunteering horror, fear, and helplessness in response to an open-ended question means PTSD is unlikely.

The studies that argue against the utility of either A1 and A2, or both, in predicting PTSD are based on nongeneralizable samples of undergraduates and subjects responding to research advertisements reporting trauma histories (Bedard-Gilligan & Zoellner, 2008; Boals & Schuettler, 2009; Roemer, Orsillo, Borkovec, & Litz, 1998) or population or community-based studies in which subjects are asked to retrospectively recall potential trauma causing events from years ago (Anders et al., 2011; Breslau & Kessler, 2001; Karam et al., 2010). These studies are negligibly helpful in our clinical understanding of PTSD. Those that argue that the absence of fear, helplessness or horror do not predict PTSD use clinical samples that experience stressors that questionably meet the stressor criterion. A quarter of mild head injured patients who presumably have PTSD did not report A2 emotions (O'Donnell et ai., 2010).

One valid reason for removing both A1 and A2 is that the diagnosis would be based on the core symptoms without reference to an event—just like any other psychiatric disorder. Nielssen and Large (2011: e21) remind us doing this tends to ignore the fact "the diagnosis as it exists serves an important cultural purpose in acknowledging and compensating many forms of emotional distress."

The Dissociative Subtype

The Working Group Chair of ICD-11, Andreas Maercker, exclaimed in reference to DSM-5, "a new dissociative subtype with no research at all until last year has been included" in reference to the proposal to add this subtype (Maercker & Perkonigg, 2013: 561). Many of the major validity studies addressing Criterion A and dissociation appeared in close proximity to the release of the DSM-5 (Karam et al., 2010; O'Donnell et al., 2010; Stein et al., 2013, Steuwe, Lanius, & Frewen, 2012; Wolf et al., 2012) as did a number of review articles arguing for changes that eventually predicted most of the revisions that would occur (Carlson, Dalenberg, & McDade-Montez, 2012; Dalenberg & Carlson, 2012; Lanius, Brand, Vermetten, Frewen, & Spiegel, 2012). A review by Mathew Friedman, the then Executive Director for the National Center for PTSD, predicted some of these changes:

> A new set of diagnostic criteria is proposed for DSM-5 that: (a) attempts to sharpen the A1 criterion; (b) eliminates the A2 criterion; (c) proposes four rather than three symptom clusters; and (d) expands the scope of the B–E criteria beyond a fear-based context. The final sections of this review consider: (a) partial/subsyndromal PTSD; (b) disorders of extreme stress not otherwise specified (DESNOS)/complex PTSD; (c) cross-cultural factors; (d) developmental factors; and (e) subtypes of PTSD.
>
> (Friedman, Resick, Bryant, & Brewin, 2011 p. 750)

Dissociation is said to be a defense mechanism by which the dramatic experience is minimized by restricting the awareness of the experience. The most dramatic dissociative symptom to be introduced was when PTSD was introduced in DSM III: the flashback. DSM III-R introduced the second symptom: amnesia for the event. Peritraumatic dissociation may be important at the time of the trauma. It is said to be a risk factor for the development of PTSD (Ozer, Best, Lipsey, & Weiss, 2008). But Bryant (2007: 187) asks the provocative question, "Is dissociation necessarily bad?" He argued that it could be protective because it limits one's awareness of the experience.

Proponents have suggested that dissociation should be included as a subtype in DSM-5 (Dalenberg & Carlson, 2012). The same authors did a review of the literature and concluded there is a strong relationship between dissociation and trauma exposure, and the presence of dissociation is strongly related to the presence and severity of PTSD (Carlson et al., 2012). Despite this conclusion, the majority of the studies they cited were not PTSD samples per se but general psychiatric samples. A large sample of rape and sexual assault victims suggested that 13% evidenced a dissociative subtype of PTSD. This investigation was the first to be conducted in a European nonmilitary adult rape-victim sample (Armour, Elklit, Lauterbach, & Elhai, 2014). The largest study that involved a homogeneous clinical sample of rape victims found no association between dissociation and PTSD. This relationship is found instead in a comparison group of nonsexual assault victims (Dancu, Riggs, Hearst-Ikeda, Shoyer, & Foa, 1996). This would appear to be counterintuitive if it is true that dissociation is a PTSD risk factor and when considering that rape results in the highest rates of PTSD reported in the literature.

Since most studies on dissociation were done in Western countries, an international study was conducted, showing 14.4% of subjects have the dissociative subtype. This was the first large population-based study using layperson interviews (Stein et al., 2013). The authors acknowledge the use of layperson interviewers as a weakness given the very conceptual nature of dissociation. The presence of dissociation was based on answering two questions regarding depersonalization and one on derealization. Even before this most recent dissociation research, Bryant cautioned that these rates of dissociation are frequently obtained from questionnaires and checklists (Bryant, 2007). An additional problem with the later study is that the dissociation items were chosen post hoc versus for the purposes of operationalizing dissociation for DSM-5. Their finding that dissociation was more common in men contradicted previous studies that found it is higher in women or found no gender difference. In another study, a civilian sample was assessed for dissociative subtypes using the Dissociative Experiences Scale, the CAPS, and the Structured Clinical Interview for DSM Disorders. Depersonalization criteria were met by 25% of the sample and the same number met criteria for present derealization symptoms.

While the strength of the study was the use of structured interviews, the sample was recruited through advertisements posted in the community and in mental health centers (Steuwe et al., 2012). The DSM-5 field trials were equally controversial.

The DSM-5 Field Trials

Mathew Friedman was chairperson of the Trauma/Stress-Related and Dissociative Disorders Sub-Work Group for DSM-5. It consisted of five members and a subcommittee of 30 national experts in PTSD. The International Society for Traumatic Stress Studies was also well represented. The reason DSM "5" was chosen over DSM "V" is the expectation that over the next few years there may be updates (e.g., DSM-5.2; see Friedman, 2013). The DSM-5 field trials focused on test-retest reliability among clinicians, different than for the DSM-IV, which conducted field trials on the validity and reliability of the PTSD criteria. Two Internet surveys were designed to test the new criteria in order to compare with DSM-IV. The major findings were that prevalence was comparable to DSM-IV, the four-factor DSM-5 structure proved a better fit than the three-factor DSM-IV factor model, and symptoms within each diagnostic cluster loaded well together. Test-retest reliability for the PTSD criteria was examined at two VA sites in Dallas and Houston in veterans and not civilians. The kappa values at both sites were 0.63 and 0.69. These values were greater than for other DSM-5 conditions including major depression (Regier et al., 2013). The high kappa values for DSM-5 PTSD in the field trials were second only to major neurocognitive disorder. This was viewed as a "historic accomplishment" (Freedman et al., 2013).

Frances criticized these trials. His reasons include focusing on reliability versus how mental disorders will be diagnosed more often due to the lowering of diagnostic thresholds. Additionally, the kappa values for the present trials were different from past trials. Kappa values of 0.40 to 0.59 that would be considered poor in the past were now considered good (Frances, 2012b). These latter criticisms, in addition to others, were summarized by Jones (2012).

From DSM to ICD

"The American Psychiatric Association's classification is designed to meet the needs of one, or perhaps two, professions—psychiatrists and clinical psychologists—in a single country" (Kendell, 1991, p. 299). While it was always the intent that DSM and ICD would work toward a harmonized diagnostic system, the tension between the two was seen early. DSM-III, as innovative and as revolutionary as it was, broke ranks from the international community to put forth a system that was radically different from DSM-II. Regardless, the intent was for DSM-IV to be produced in conjunction with ICD-10. That did not occur as ICD-10 was practically completed before DSM-IV members met (Kendell, 1991). At present, the well-intended harmonization between the two diagnostic systems is no longer possible. PTSD as defined in ICD-10, and the further changes that will occur in ICD-11, will necessitate having to choose between the two (First & Pincus, 1999). The differences will be greater between DSM-5 and ICD-11 than they were between DSM-IV and ICD-10. In the United States many organizations are navigating away from DSM-5. The controversies that accompany each DSM, including DSM-III (Vaillant, 1984), have increased exponentially with each edition. DSM-5 is the crossroads. Legislation has provided much of the impetus for converting to ICD-11.

WHO member countries, including the United States, report health statistics to the WHO via the ICD classification system. Aside from impacting public health, two practical goals of the ICD have been to be a multilingual and multidisciplinary publication (Reed, 2010). The ICD should be multilingual because one of every five Americans over the age of 5 in the United States speaks another language other than English in the home (Camarota & Ziegler, 2015). As Zimmerman notes: "Ironically, a country as ethnically diverse as the United States is perhaps the most likely candidate for a system such as the ICD, which is designed for cross-cultural use" (Zimmerman, 1990: 975). The ICD should be multidisciplinary because, worldwide, less than 10% of patients will see a psychiatrist (Reed, 2010). Federal regulations in the United States (Medicare and the Health Insurance Portability and Accountability Act) require the use of ICD codes. By federal law, all entities and health care professionals are required to convert to ICD-10. Additional developments are precipitating the move away from DSM-5, but not necessarily toward ICD-10. The release of DSM-5 initiated at the National Institute of Mental Health (NIMH) a plan to introduce their own psychiatric classification (the Research Domain Criteria), adding that the project cannot succeed if DSM-5 criteria are used as the "gold standard" (Insel et al., 2010). The American Psychological Association is making the clinical transition to ICD (American Psychological Association, Practice Central, 2012). The National Alliance of Professional Psychology Providers, a professional practice organization that represents psychologists in the United States, has encouraged its members to adopt ICD-10, citing as one reason an effort to eliminate the political debates that adversely impact the frequent revision of DSM (Bradshaw, 2012). There are three versions to ICD-10: The ICD-10 *Clinical Descriptions and Diagnostic Guidelines* is the "conceptual core" that outlines the disorders (referred to as the *Blue Book*), the ICD-10 *Diagnostic Criteria for Research* operationally defines the disorders (the *Green Book*), and the WHO *Guide to Mental Health in Primary Care* is meant to be used in a primary care context to diagnose a handful of core disorders so the latter does not include PTSD (Jablensky, 2009). The clinical version of ICD-10 is difficult for researchers to use because the criteria are not operationally defined as they have been in the DSM since DSM-III.

Table 32.2 *F43.1 Posttraumatic stress disorder—research criteria

A	Exposure to a stressful event or situation of an exceptionally threatening or catastrophic nature, which is likely to cause pervasive distress in almost anyone
B	Persistent remembering or "reliving" the stressor by flashbacks, vivid memories, dreams, or by being exposed to circumstances resembling or associated with the stressor
C	Actual or preferred avoidance of circumstances resembling or associated with the stressor
D	Either (1) or (2):
	(1) Inability to recall, either partially or completely, some important aspects of the event
	(2) Symptoms of increased psychological sensitivity and arousal shown by two of the following:
	a difficulty in falling or staying asleep;
	b irritability or outbursts of anger;
	c difficulty in concentrating;
	d hyper-vigilance;
	e. exaggerated startle response.
E	Criteria B, C and D all occurred within six months of the stressful event (for some purposes delayed more than six months may be included but this should be clearly specified)

*Modified from ICD-10 (Green Book)

Table 32.3 Proposed diagnostic criteria for PTSD in ICD-11

Reexperiencing: either (i) or (ii)
(i) Recurrent distressing dreams related to an event now perceived as having severely threatened someone's physical or psychological well-being, from which the person wakes with marked fear or horror
(ii) Repeated daytime images related to an event now perceived as having severely threatened someone's physical or psychological well-being, experienced as recurring in the present and accompanied by marked fear or horror
Avoidance: either (i) or (ii)
(i) Efforts to avoid thoughts, feelings, conversations, or internal reminders associated with the reexperienced event(s)
(ii) Efforts to avoid activities, places, people, or external reminders associated with the reexperienced event(s)
Hyperarousal: either (i) or (ii)
(i) Hypervigilance
(ii) Exaggerated startle response
Impairment: The symptoms must last for at least several weeks and cause significant impairment in functioning

From Morina, van Emmerik, Andrews, and Brewin (2014)

Similar to DSM-I and DSM-II, the ICD-10 consists of clinical text descriptions that may be open to interpretation (Farmer & McGuffin, 1999). The PTSD ICD-10 research criteria operationally define PTSD (Table 32.2). Four things merit comment. First, the stressor should be "exceptionally threatening or catastrophic," similar to DSM-I and DSM-III. Second, the core features of the disorder of intrusive memories and avoidance of the event are prominent. Third, delayed PTSD is considered under special circumstances only. In ICD-10 delayed PTSD can be seen in a few weeks to months but "rarely exceeds six months." Finally, notable for its absence is the requirement that PTSD result in some functional impairment. On the one hand the requirement that the PTSD-causing event must be of an exceptional nature in some ways nullifies the need to include a functional impairment criterion. On the other hand, someone experiencing a catastrophic event may have had PTSD symptoms for some period of time, never felt the need for treatment, and had no appreciable functional consequence. Should such a person be included in a prevalence study? As with DSM-5, PTSD will be placed in a stress disorders section in ICD-11.

With each successive revision, the WHO is fine-tuning the PTSD definition to the approval of the majority of its users (Evans et al., 2013; Reed, Correia, Esparza, Saxena, & Maj, 2011). There have been considerable improvements when one considers that there was no PTSD diagnosis in ICD-9. ICD-9 was published in 1979, before PTSD was coined in 1980 for use in DSM-III. PTSD was introduced in ICD-10. The original release for ICD-11 that was meant for 2011/2012 (Frances, 2013) is now planned for release in 2018 (WHO, 2015a). Whereas there are now 20 core PTSD symptoms in DSM-5, ICD-11 is likely to have only six. Chris Brewin provided a convincing rationale for only six PTSD symptoms (Brewin et al. 2009). Table 32.3 outlines what at the time of this writing are the planned changes to the PTSD diagnosis in ICD-11. The essence of the change is removing the nonspecific PTSD symptoms as advocated by Brewin (Brewin et al., 2009). Spitzer et al. (2007) first directly advocated the removal of the nonspecific symptoms. Attention, sleep problems, irritability, and anhedonia should be eliminated as they overlap with mood and anxiety disorders. The fifth symptom (lack of or poor memory for the event) can occur for reasons other than repression or dissociation. While yet not finalized, it appears ICD-11 will have three core criteria: intrusions, avoidance, and hyperarousal. Intrusions will require the presence of one of two symptoms: nightmares and flashbacks. Avoidance will consist of avoiding either thoughts and/or feelings of the event or actual avoidance of people, places, or activities that remind the patient of the event. Finally, there will be two hyperarousal symptoms: startle response and hypervigilance. Meeting one of the two symptoms within each category will be required. It would appear that Criterion A will remain, while others have suggested that clinical judgment will play a role in defining the stressor more so than was the case in ICD-10 (Maercker et al., 2013; O'Donnell et al., 2014). At the time of this writing, the ICD-11 Beta Draft contains the language "extremely threatening or horrific event" (WHO, 2015b). Finally, functional impairment will be required in ICD-11 to differentiate it from normal reactions to extreme stress. The diagnosis should be made within a month. The focus will be on functional impairment rather than a specific class of stressors (Maercker et al., 2013). Like ICD-10, ICD-11 will have a section for specialty settings (Clinical Description and Diagnostic Guidelines) and a section for use in primary care, but it has not been decided if there will be a version for research purposes (Luciano, 2014).

ICD and DSM PTSD Studies

A logical place to start is the reliability of the PTSD diagnosis using the two diagnostic systems. The pivotal international ICD-10 field trial that included 568 clinicians and 2,460 patients from 39 countries yielded a modest kappa value for PTSD of 0.62. As a diagnostic group, the personality disorders yielded the lowest, a kappa value of 0.51 (Sartorius et al., 1993). When North American clinicians were compared to clinicians outside of Canada and the United States, the kappa value was 0.72 among North American clinicians versus 0.52 for the rest of the world. The Canadian and U.S. clinicians were more likely to assign more diagnoses (2.1 vs. 1.7). The caveat here is that the number of PTSD patients examined ($N = 19$) was far lower than other diagnostic categories, suggested that the kappa value might not be a reliable estimate of agreement (Regier, Kaelber, Roper, Rae, & Sartorius, 1994). The reliability of the PTSD diagnosis was not tested in the DSM-III field trials ($N = 400$), but in DSM-IV the kappa value was 0.71 (Kilpatrick et al., 1998). In the ICD-10 trials, the clinical and not research ICD-10 criteria were used. The ICD-10 field trial was repeated with an equally impressive sample using the ICD-10 research criteria for major disorders, but PTSD was not one of them. Kappa values in this study for major diagnostic categories were better for all major diagnostic categories (organic, schizophrenia, mood, dysthymia and anxiety disorders) when research criteria were used. Interestingly the largest difference was for the anxiety disorders: 0.74 when the research criteria were used versus 0.55 for the clinical criteria (Sartorius, Ustün, Korten, Cooper, & van Drimmelen, 1995). This suggests operationally defining the criteria increases reliability, especially for PTSD, and that this is most important for the anxiety disorders.

What are the prevalence rates of PTSD when comparing ICD-10 to DSM? Studies reporting prevalence within the last 12 months will be used. There are problems in making the comparison. Recalling traumatic events over a lifetime and what if any symptoms accompanied those events is subject to recall bias. A community based study ($N = 1,264$) used a structured interview, the Composite International Diagnostic Interview (CIDI), by comparing ICD-10 and DSM-IV (Peters, Slade, & Andrews, 1999). This resulted in a concordance rate of only 35%, with ICD-10 resulting in twice as many persons diagnosed with PTSD: 6.9% versus 3.0%. This was partially attributed to DSM-IV requiring functional impairment whereas ICD-10 did not. When the functional criteria were applied to ICD-10, the rate was 4%. Another problem is that numbing is a criterion of DSM-IV but not of ICD-10. The more criteria that are needed, the less likely the diagnosis is going to be made. This is further complicated by the fact that numbing is described in the ICD-10 clinical criteria, but it is not listed in the ICD-10 research criteria. It is not clear that the stressor criterion was adhered to in this study as applied to ICD-10. Per this study "exposure to a stressor" was required for both diagnostic criteria. Since DSM-IV requires an emotional response to the stressor (A2) and ICD-10 does not, this further accounts for the higher prevalence in ICD-10. In comparison the concurrence for major depression was 16.6% and 15.6% between ICD-10 and DSM-IV, respectively (Andrews, Slade, & Peters, 1999).

When we compare ICD-11 to DSM-5 we see the reverse pattern. O'Donnell and colleagues (2014) examined a clinical sample ($N = 510$) of trauma patients admitted to four hospitals following an accident or other injury. The CAPS was used to assess for the presence of PTSD. The PTSD definition followed by the prevalence of PTSD in parentheses was as follows: DSM-IV with A2 (5.9%), DSM-IV without A2 (8%), DSM-5 (6.7%), ICD-10 (9.0%) and ICD-11 (3.3%). The authors are operating under the assumption that the stressor as defined in ICD-11 would not be described as one that likely causes pervasive distress in almost anyone. The drop in prevalence from ICD-10 to ICD-11 was attributed to requiring that the patient meet one of the intrusion and hyperarousal symptoms. Again, requiring functional impairment also accounted for the decrease. More than 80% of the hospital admissions were following a motor vehicle accident or fall. Of these patients, 41% had a mild head injury. The ICD-10 stressor criteria would not appear to have been applied in this study. Were it applied, PTSD would be rare to nonexistent in this patient sample except for those with life-threatening injuries. This latter clinical study was the first comparing DSM-5 to ICD-11. The first large-scale international population-based study involving 13 countries employed the CIDI as administered by lay interviewers. It revealed the following prevalence rates: ICD-10 (4.4%), DSM-IV (3.3%), ICD-11 (3.2%), and DSM-5 (3.0%). Again, the reason given for the high ICD-10 prevalence rate is that it is the most narrowly defined criteria. The low prevalence in DSM-5 is likely a function of the opposite: a greater number of criteria that need to be met (four criteria and 20 symptoms) versus ICD-11 (three criteria and six symptoms). Again, what impact on how the stressor is defined in reference to the PTSD prevalence rates is not discussed.

Complex PTSD

The only major controversy surrounding ICD-11 is the introduction of complex PTSD (CPTSD). This was considered for inclusion in DSM-IV under Disorders of Extreme Stress Not Otherwise Specified (DESNOS) and more recently in DSM-5. It was not included in DSM-5. Whereas inside the United States there was enthusiasm for a dissociative subtype, internationally there was instead a keen interest in including CPTSD in ICD-11. CPTSD was in ICD-10 as "enduring personality change after catastrophic experiences"

(Maercker & Perkonigg, 2013: 199). It will be called CPTSD in ICD-11.

CPTSD was first clearly articulated by Herman (1992). Courtios (2004) summarized the work of Herman (1992) in reference to CTPD: The seven problem areas are poor regulation of affective impulses (e.g., anger); alterations in attention (e.g., dissociation); alterations in self-perception (e.g., guilt and shame); perception of the perpetrator (e.g., identification with their belief system); relationship with others (e.g., lack of trust and intimacy); somatization (e.g., can involve any body system); and alterations in a loss of meaning (e.g., feeling misunderstood). Unlike patients suffering from PTSD secondary to a discrete event such as rape, there are patients, Herman argues, who have a different clinical phenotype as a consequence of repeated and prolonged exposure to trauma. The most common and the one Herman focused on was repeated sexual and physical abuse. These are patients with persistent depression, suicidal thoughts, episodes of self-mutilation, substance abuse, and impulsivity. Somatization, dissociation, and the pathological relationship that they develop with their abuser alter their personality. The other class of traumas where CPTSD would be found includes refugees, victims of prolonged torture, or concentration- or labor-camp survivors. Herman notes Horowitz suggested a similar concept in the form of "post traumatic character disorder" (Horowitz, 1986, p. 49).

In order to appreciate the issues surrounding CPTSD, an overview of how the debate unfolded in the United States is in order. The June 2012 issue of the *Journal of Traumatic Stress Studies* was partially devoted to the topic. The lively and informative debate was around the merits of including CPTSD in DSM-5. The debate began with an invited article by Resick and colleagues (2012) that concluded that the weight of the evidence argues against inclusion in DSM-5. Resick provided a number of compelling arguments. The most salient is the most simple: First, there is no precedent in psychiatric diagnostic systems for splitting off a more severe form of the same disorder. Second, the DSM-IV field trials indicated that practically everyone (over 90%) who met criteria for complex PTSD also met criteria for PTSD (Roth, Newman, Pelcovitz, van der Kolk, & Mandel, 1997). Third, those meeting complex PTSD criteria overlap with borderline personality disorder (as well as major depression). The overlap with other disorders makes it less distinctive. Here one can just simply assign a comorbid diagnosis.

Some of the offered rebuttals raised issues that further confused the debate. CPTSD was originally conceptualized as being related to trauma that was prolonged and repeated versus an isolated traumatic event such as a rape event. Bryant (2012) argued that it is not necessary to focus on the nature of the event but instead on the symptoms. In response to Bryant, Resick argues that the nature of the stressor is the very basis for CPTSD. It is a different type of trauma than the one that typically produces PTSD. Finally, Resick takes issue with the arguments of Herman (2012) and Lindauer (2012) who make a plea for advocacy arguing that ."the scientific basis should be adequate but are we being a little too strict?" (Lindauer, 2012, p. 259). There has been an appeal to broad consensus opinion in support of the diagnosis. A small survey was undertaken of experts in CPTSD and PTSD regarding complex PTSD in which there was general agreement as to the symptoms and the type of treatment (Cloitre, 2011). Conspicuously absent in the discussion was the nature of the stressor needed to produce CPTSD. In ICD-10 the stressor for both PTSD and CPTSD is the foundation upon which the diagnosis rests.

CPTSD in ICD-10 (enduring personality change after catastrophic experiences) is very clear on the nature of the stressor: "The stress must be so extreme that it is unnecessary to consider personal vulnerability in order to explain its profound effect on the personality" (WHO, 1992, p. 163). The same descriptor of the stressor is provided in the ICD-10 research criteria. CPTSD as outlined in the research criteria is outlined in Table 32.4. Catastrophic events such as concentration camp exposure, torture, a refugee in a war zone,

Table 32.4 *F62.0 Enduring personality change after catastrophic experience

A A persistent change in perceiving, relating to, and thinking about the environment and oneself following catastrophic stress (i.e., concentration camp, torture, prolonged exposure to life-threatening situations).

B The personality change should be significant and represent inflexible and maladaptive features as indicated by the presence of at least two of the following:

1 Permanent hostile or distrustful attitude in a person without such traits premorbidly
2 Social withdrawal not due to another mental disorder
3 Constant feeling of emptiness and/or hopelessness, not limited to a discrete episode of mood disorder, and which was not present before the catastrophic stress experience
4 An enduring feeling threatened without cause as evidenced by an increased vigilance and irritability in a person who previously showed no such traits, which may be associated with substance abuse
5 Permanent feeling of being different from others (estrangement) and may be associated with emotional numbness

C The change should cause either significant interference with functioning.

D The personality develops after the catastrophic experience with no history of a preexisting personality disorder or trait accentuation that could explain the current personality traits.

E The personality change must have been present for at least three years and not related to other disorders.

F The personality change is often preceded by PTSD. The two conditions can overlap and the personality change may be a chronic outcome of PTSD. However, an enduring personality change should not be assumed in such cases unless, in addition to at least two years of PTSD there has been a further period of no less than two years during which the above criteria have been met.

*Modified from ICD-10 Research Criteria

and prolonged captivity are experiences outside the range of usual human experience in North America. This may be the reason CPTSD may not have been adopted in DSM-5. The very definition of CPTSD revisits an issue that has been officially settled in the opinion of some in the DSM, namely whether the stressor needs to be of a catastrophic nature. The ICD-10 definition of CPTSD considers "prolonged exposure to life-threatening circumstances" a catastrophic event. In North America that prolonged exposure leading to CPTSD, by default, is primarily repeated sexual and physical abuse of children. In the CPTSD survey study cited earlier eight treatment studies were identified, all of which involved childhood abuse (Cloitre, 2011). The other clinical scenario in which to diagnose CPTSD involves refugees and political prisoners with traumatic experiences who have relocated to North America. In the ICD-11 draft version "prolonged domestic violence and repeated childhood sexual or physical abuse" is specifically mentioned (WHO-ICD-11). In ICD-11 the name change will be official: from "enduring personality change after catastrophic experience" to CPTSD.

CPTSD was tested in the DSM-IV field trials (Roth et al., 1997) using criteria arising from the observations of Herman (1992). Kilpatrick et al. (1998) described the DSM-IV PTSD field trial. Most of the 400 treatment-seeking patients were being seen for exposure to a possible traumatic event. Of these patients, 234 reported physical and sexual abuse. Of these, 163 were diagnosed with PTSD (n = 45), PTSD or CPTSD (n = 113), or just CPTSD (n = 5). Given that the conditions are comorbid and it is rare to having just CTPSD without PTSD, the diagnosis was not included in DSM-IV. As to risk for CPTSD, women who suffered both sexual and physical abuse were 14.5 times more likely to be diagnosed with the disorder. Age of onset for both men and women did not predict CPTSD. A reanalysis of the DSM-IV field trial data yielded different results. The early onset abuse group was more likely to carry a dual diagnosis of PTSD and CPTSD versus PTSD alone. Surprisingly there was no attempt to reconcile these findings with the earlier findings of Roth et al. (1997)—this despite using the same patient sample and that Roth was one of the coauthors of the reanalysis (van der Kolk, Roth, Pelcovitz, Sunday, & Spinazzola, 2005). Elklit, Hyland, and Shelven (2014) carried out a larger and more representative study. The sample was composed of bereaved parents after the death of a child (n = 607), rape victims (n = 449), and victims of physical assault (n = 214). The major drawback was the diagnoses were made via self-report questionnaires: the Trauma Symptom Checklist and the Harvard Trauma Questionnaire Part IV. Sexual trauma victims, physical trauma victims, and bereaved parents had CPTSD rates of 20.7%, 13%, and 10.4%, respectively. Another study sought to provide support for the concept of CPTSD in ICD-11 by performing a latent class analysis on 280 females seeking treatment for childhood abuse to shore up support for including CPTSD in ICD-11. They identified four groups: a low-symptom group, a group high in PTSD symptoms but low in self-organization and borderline personality disorder symptoms, a CPTSD group with high PTSD symptoms and self-organization symptoms and low borderline personality symptoms, and a borderline personality group high on these symptoms in addition to PTSD and CPTSD. The discrimination among the groups was described as "acceptable." Of note is that these groups did not differ on any demographic variables, including age and employment status (Cloitre, Garvert, Brewin, Bryant, & Maercker, 2013). The major shortcoming was that CPTSD was measured by employing 21 questions across two structured interviews (CAPS and SCID-II) and a self-report instrument, the Brief Symptom Inventory. The proper method is to operationally define CPTSD using either the DSM-IV or ICD-10, which are very explicit, followed by a structured clinical interview to establish that these patients meet the clinical diagnosis of CPTSD before any statistical technique is applied to the sample. A similar approach was used by the same author in a sample of patients seeking treatment for interpersonal violence (Cloitre et al., 2013). A more extensive critique and possible solutions are suggested to the question of not only PTSD, but also CPTSD at a later point in this chapter ("PTSD Defined: A Hybrid Model").

The Epidemiology of PTSD

"Like mental retardation, posttraumatic stress disorder appears to be the extreme end of a normal distribution" (Robins, 1990: 1675).

In this section, the idea that the epidemiology of PTSD is problematical is elaborated upon. It is reasonable to ask if population-based epidemiological studies answer practical clinical questions. Among the many questions that can be asked, the most basic is that of the prevalence of PTSD. First, prevalence studies within the general population are discussed, followed by the prevalence in clinical samples. In the latter case, this will include treatment-seeking patients and cohorts of persons who have been exposed to an event truly outside the realm of every day experience (i.e., war, rape, torture, terrorism). Only when studying both types of populations can we answer the question of clinical relevancy. It will be argued that population-based studies magnify the prevalence of PTSD and ignore what is relevant to the clinician: the prevalence of disability and distress. With the transition to an international classification system and with the immigrant population of the United States increasing, we need to be more cross-culturally literate regarding PTSD in non–English speaking populations. Reviewing some of this literature is the second purpose of this section. The final purpose is to answer clinical questions that epidemiological studies are supposed to answer: risk factors, comorbid conditions and outcome. The outcome here is in reference to the chronicity of PTSD in these epidemiological studies as opposed to outcome following treatment.

Population Studies

With the support of the NIMH, a nationwide study was undertaken to look at the prevalence of psychiatric disorders in the United States: the National Comorbidity Survey (NCS). The results were published in 1994 (Kessler et al., 1994) with a ten-year follow-up (Kessler et al., 2005). The NCS was the first national population-based study, and it included 8,098 respondents (82.4% participation rate) from 48 states and 176 counties. The NCS included a separate publication on PTSD that used a subsample (n = 5,877) of participants (Kessler et al., 1995). Ronald Kessler, a sociologist by training, is the most often cited mental health researcher in the world (Horwitz & Gold, 2011).

To diagnose PTSD, a structured clinical interview was used that followed the DSM-III-R criteria (APA, 1987). The face-to-face interview was a modification of the Diagnostic Interview Schedule (DIS). Kessler et al. (1995) modified the DIS as follows. First, instead of asking a single question about a lifetime occurrence of a number of traumatic events to oneself (and others), they inquired about events with 12 different questions "in an effort to focus memory search" (Kessler et al., 1995: 1040). The 12th question asked about "any other terrible experience that most people never go through" (p. 1040). The answer was coded as meeting Criterion A or not. Second, because the participants might be embarrassed by the traumatizing events, the 12 events were presented in a checklist booklet format and the participant was asked about "event number 1" in the book, and so on. The third modification was that Criteria B through D were evaluated regardless whether Criterion A was met. This allowed researchers to assess if relaxing Criterion A affected prevalence. Finally, only one index event per respondent was assessed. If participants reported more than one trauma, they were asked to pick the most upsetting. The estimated lifetime prevalence of PTSD was 7.8% versus 8.4% if Criterion A was loosened. The most common traumas were witnessing someone being badly injured or killed; being involved in a fire, flood, or natural disaster; and experiencing a life-threatening accident. The study concluded that PTSD "is more prevalent than previously believed, and is often persistent" (p. 1048)—more than one third fail to recover after years of the disorder. This study had a profound influence not so much because of the scope of the survey, but because it contradicted earlier studies that found a significantly lower prevalence of PTSD.

The methodology of the NCS in reference to psychiatric disorders was actually first carried out by Lee Robins (coincidentally also a sociologist) and her colleagues from Washington University in St. Louis. In the Epidemiological Catchment Area (ECA) study they reported on the prevalence of 15 psychiatric disorders (Robins et al., 1984). Here we are going to take a brief detour to provide a brief historical synopsis of the research at Washington University that preceded the influential ECA study, which had a lasting influence on American psychiatry.

The psychiatric research done at Washington University group was influential for many reasons. First, as already reviewed, the Washington University group was engaged in the early controversy around the diagnosis of PTSD in DSM-III. In contrast to the PTSD advocates, they were actively researching the psychiatric adjustment of Vietnam veterans. I believe it is fair to say that the Washington University group ushered clinical psychiatry in the United States into the modern era. Their reputation in academic psychiatry was unmatched. First, in a seminal paper, Robins and Guze (1970) insisted we needed a rational and valid diagnostic classification system in psychiatry (I should note that the Robins in this study was Eli Robins, a psychiatrist at Washington University, and the spouse of Lee Robins). A second landmark paper operationally defined common psychiatric disorders with precise criteria. They provided criteria for 15 disorders (Feighner et al., 1972). Spitzer, inspired by what was popularly referred to as the "Feighner criteria," partnered with Eli Robins to develop the Research Diagnostic Criteria, which expanded the psychiatric disorders to 25 (Spitzer, Endicott, & Robins, 1978). In the midst of writing this paper, Spitzer was appointed DSM-III Task Force Chair. Spitzer would break fully from DSM-II by implementing the ideas of the Washington University group. The Research Diagnostic Criteria was the precursor to DSM-III (Decker, 2013). While on the one hand the Washington group conceded the inclusion of PTSD in DSM-III, on the other hand the field of psychiatry accepted their classification schema. A third paper by Lee Robins laid out the method by which not only the clinician, but also the lay interviewer, can collect clinical data and assign a diagnosis in a valid and reliable way: the structured clinical interview in the form of the DIS (Robins, Helzer, Croughan, & Ratcliff, 1981). Finally, they published, in *The New England Journal of Medicine*, a very influential PTSD study (Helzer, Robins, & McEvoy, 1987). In my opinion it remains the seminal epidemiological study.

This first population-based study, post DSM-III, looked at the prevalence of PTSD (Helzer et al., 1987). The researchers used their DIS to conduct three waves of interviews. The final wave consisted of 2,493 randomly selected St. Louis residents who were similar demographically to the rest of the nation based on the 1980 census. They were asked if they had experienced an event that had freighted them to the degree that they experienced one of the PTSD symptoms in DSM-III (APA, 1980). Consistent with the DSM-III definition, the event had to be outside the range of usual human experience. It had to fall into one of seven categories: combat, serious accident, physical attack (including rape), natural disaster, being threatened or almost seriously injured, witnessing someone being killed or injured, and "other." Onset, duration, and frequency of symptoms were ascertained. The lifetime prevalence was 1%. Chronic PTSD (greater than six months duration) was seen in half of that 1%, with one-third having symptoms more than three years. The researchers concluded: "This study of posttraumatic stress disorder in the general population has found that it exists but is uncommon except among wounded Vietnam veterans" (Helzer et al., 1987, p. 1633). It may not be a coincidence that Lee Robins chose mental retardation as the analogy for PTSD (Robins, 1990). The prevalence of mental retardation in the general population is said to be 1% per the DSM-5 (APA, 2013). To expand on the analogy, if we described PTSD to someone who has never heard of it, we would say it is an event that someone directly experienced or witnessed. That event was so traumatic that in the worse-case scenario, in the months and the years to come, a month does not go by (the CAPS requires the symptoms to be present over the last month) without it impacting his or her life in a clinically meaningful way. A description of the syndrome, without using the PTSD label per se, would suggest a truly catastrophic rare event (in DSM-II the examples were two: combat and "civilian catastrophe"). I suspect that the average person (including myself) is not likely to know personally more than one or two people out of 100 who are mentally retarded. Similarly, it is not likely that the average American would know one or two people who experienced such a life-altering stressor. The analogy between mental retardation and PTSD in regard to prevalence is apropos. PTSD should be a rare event, especially in civilians. Two additional early community studies, which also employed the DIS, yielded similar low prevalence rates.

The first study surveyed two rural northwest logging communities in the states of Washington and Oregon, one of which had been affected by the Mt. Saint Helens volcano eruption (Shore, Vollmer, & Tatum, 1989). The nonaffected community ($N = 477$) was compared with the affected community ($N = 548$). The latter group consisted of a high exposure group ($n = 138$). These were residents with $5,000 of property damage or those who experienced the death of a family member or close relative. The remainder ($n = 410$) was the low exposure group. They also required that at least one of the DSM-III symptoms interfere with the respondent's life or that they had told a doctor about the symptom. Using the DIS, lifetime prevalence was 3% and 2.5% if we exclude the Mt. Saint Helens residents with PTSD. The second early study surveyed 2,985 residents from five counties in North Carolina (Davidson, Hughes, Blazer, & George, 1991). Using the DIS, the lifetime prevalence was 1.3% and the six-month prevalence less than half a percent (0.44). In regard to outcome, for 46% of the sample, the symptoms were chronic (lasting greater than six months).

I now ask if population-based epidemiological studies answer practical clinical questions by using the Kessler study, the NCS, as an example. The most often quoted PTSD paper deserves a closer critical look. For the purposes of comparison I compare the Helzer ECA and Kessler NCS studies. What might explain the higher prevalence rate of PTSD in the NCS? The logical place to start is the interview instrument used and how the questions were phrased. In letters to the editor the ECA study was criticized primarily for its use of the DIS (Keane & Penk, 1988; Haber-Schaim, Solomon, Bleich, & Kottler, 1988). The validity of the instrument was questioned. All studies cited so far have used the DIS. In the ECA study the respondents were asked if they experienced an event that "frightened" them and was coded in one of nine categories that by definition are outside the realm of human experience. Not asking them directly about the nine categories may result in an underestimate of PTSD. Helzer and Robins (1988), in their response clarified that respondents were directly asked about each of the nine traumas. The NCS study asked about 12 types of traumas. DSM-III (used in the ECS study) and DSM-III-R (used in NCS) have similar definitions. How closely was Criterion A adhered to? This is the crux of the issue and the first major problem with epidemiological studies. In the NCS the most common causes of PTSD were the following: witnessing someone being badly injured or killed (25%), being involved in a life-threatening accident (19%), and being involved in a fire, flood, or natural disaster (17%). How "badly injured" must someone be to meet Criterion A? Can all car accidents that have rendered the vehicle inoperable be considered life threatening? If there was a fire in an empty house while someone was outside gardening, were they involved in a fire? Breslau and Kessler (2001) investigated the new two-part definition of PTSD introduced in DSM-IV. Criterion A2, the subjective component to PTSD, was now required. Nineteen events were used to operationalize Criterion A1. This resulted in a 59% increase in the number of events that can be used to diagnose PTSD leading them to conclude, "almost everyone has experienced a PTSD-level event" (Breslau & Kessler, 2001: 703). Even before Criterion A2 was added in DSM-IV, Breslau argued that within an urban setting (Detroit) PTSD-level events are common: 39% of young adults (21 to 30 years of age) are exposed to trauma. Of those 23.6% will develop PTSD, leading to a lifetime prevalence of 9.2%. Approximately 9.4% experienced at least three traumatic events.

Here is a possible worse-case scenario for a man raised in an urban setting. As early as grade school he witnessed violent fights among rival gangs after school let out. In high school he learned (but did not witness) that his brother was walking feet ahead of another student when that person was murdered in a drive-by shooting. In college he was held up at gunpoint while working at a sandwich shop. A few years later he was mugged walking home at night and his jewelry taken. At the age of 45 he was in a remote rural region in southern Europe that was ravaged by 3,000 fires that destroyed 1,000 square miles and killed approximately 80 people. The neighboring village five miles away was in danger but no fire could be seen due to poor visibility from the smoke. He put his mother in a cab with nothing else but his laptop so she could flee as he waited with his father for additional transportation to take them out of the village. These are my own experiences. Most would consider these traumas. If I were a subject in a research study, I would first have to recall what my reaction and symptoms were to events that happened years ago.

I experienced some fear. There was some avoidance of the neighborhood I was mugged in. I cannot recall any other symptoms. I could have been killed or badly injured but I was not. These traumas had no clinically meaningful adverse consequence.

Aside from the questionable adherence to Criterion A, the preceding clinical scenario suggests four problems with epidemiological research aside from what has already been mentioned. Using a rather loose definition of "trauma," we can say trauma is common and PTSD symptoms are common. In the ECA study, 15% of participants who had been exposed to trauma had some PTSD symptoms (Helzer et al., 1987). Traumatic events and PTSD symptoms are not synonymous with a PTSD diagnosis. So to solve the first problem, we should not equate the two. The second problem is deciding what constitutes a traumatic event. What is needed in epidemiological studies and in clinical practice is to explicitly say what traumatic events qualify for a PTSD diagnosis. Norris (1992: 409) provides a succinct answer (italics included): "Traumatic *events* are thus defined objectively leaving their consequences for subjective states of *stress* as an empirical question." The traumatic events need to be operationally defined, just like the criteria that define the disorder. Once the stressor-qualifying events are decided upon, the next step is determining their clinical impact on that patient's life, which leads us to what is probably the biggest shortcoming of in epidemiological research. The third problem is that the level of disability and distress must also be operationally defined. The Kessler NCS study does what few epidemiological studies do: It identifies what portion of patients actually sought treatment as a result of the PTSD. This indirectly tells us that the stressor was of sufficient severity to cause at the very least distress, if not disability. Of the 5,877 persons, 266 sought professional help. If help seeking is used as an indirect measure of significant distress and or impairment (Criterion F), the lifetime prevalence of PTSD is now cut by half (4.5%) in the NCS. Help seeking or reporting "a lot" of impairment cuts the PTSD prevalence by half (Beals et al., 2004). We could only assume that those studies finding a 1% prevalence rate, without any discussion of distress or disability, would likely lower the prevalence. The fourth problem of epidemiological studies is they do not provide the clinical context. Understanding the clinical context (in addition to fund of knowledge and clinical experience) is critical in making the correct clinical diagnosis (Bowen, 2006). The lay interviewer assisting in the study does not have the clinical acumen, or frankly the permission by virtue of the study design, to actually clinically diagnose PTSD in the study participant. The DIS follows a fixed algorithm specifically designed for epidemiological studies to be used by lay interviewers. This line of reasoning was offered by Robert Spitzer as the rationale for the development of the Structured Clinical Interview for DSM (Spitzer, Williams, Gibbon, & First, 1992). To address this fourth problem epidemiological studies must be complimented by prospective clinical studies.

Clinical Population and Cohort Studies

These first set of studies are not clinical per se because they do not originate in the clinic. They instead, as was originally intended per DSM-III, represent truly horrendous events that "would evoke significant symptoms of distress in most people." Unless otherwise mentioned, they employ structured clinical interviews to determine PTSD prevalence rates up to 12 months preceding the interview. This includes point prevalence rates (the presence of PTSD at the time of the interview). Five well-done large epidemiological studies employing a structured clinical interview indicate one-third of victims directly exposed to horrific, seldom-experienced events will develop PTSD: 34.9% of child soldiers (Bayer et al., 2007), 31% of terrorist bombing victims (Verger et al., 2004), 34.3% of those in the Oklahoma City bombing (North et al., 1999), 26.1% of those injured in September 11 (Bonanno, Galea, Bucciarelli, & Vlahov, 2006), and 24.8% of those surviving the Rwandan genocide (Pham et al., 2004).

Smaller studies employing interviews consisting of homogeneous clinical cohorts show similar prevalence rates: 31% of burn victims (Bryant, 1996) and 21% surviving the world's worse oil platform disaster (Hull, Alexander, & Klein, 2002). One month after a mass shooting in Killeen, Texas 136 survivors were interviewed (24 persons including the gunman were killed) and 28.8% were diagnosed with PTSD. A review of ten disasters compromising 712 survivors using similar methodology yielded a prevalence of 26% (North & Oliver, 2013). A meta-analytic review that surveyed refugees and conflict-affected populations yielded a PTSD prevalence rate of 24.9% (Steel, Chey, Silove, Maranen, Bryant, & Ommeren, 2009). This review was thorough to the extent that it looked at many data points. The most interesting include those that illustrate how methodology affects PTSD rates. The most important of these points is that PTSD prevalence was 10% higher when self-report instruments were used (34.6% vs. 24.9%). Additionally, studies with more than 1,000 respondents versus less than 100 produced prevalence rates of 15.7% and 39.4%, respectively. These were the two most important determinants of prevalence. Overall methodological characteristics between studies accounted for 13% of study variance. Less severe traumas yielded lower prevalence rates. A review of the literature in rescue workers was 9.30% (Berger et al., 2012). A literature review of refugees limited to those that have resettled in Western countries yielded a 9% prevalence rate (Fazel, Wheeler, & Danesh, 2005).

Population-based studies surveying all inhabitants that could have potentially, but not necessarily been exposed to trauma yield lesser numbers. A random survey of Manhattan residents living south of 110th Street suggested that 7.5% were suffering from PTSD one month post–September 11. Six months later it was 0.6% (Galea et al., 2003). Two locations in East Timor thought best to be representative of the country (no census data was available) found a point prevalence rate of PTSD of 1.47% (Silove et al., 2008). The lifetime prevalence of PTSD in a national sample of Iraqis carried out in 2006–2007 by lay interviewers using the CIDI was 2.5% (Alhasnawi et al., 2009). When considering that 1.5 million Iraqis were internally displaced within Iraq and 2.5 million were living in other countries, this number is quite small.

Cross-Cultural and Racial Issues

Here I begin with the population-based PTSD epidemiological studies from other countries and then differential provenance rates specific ethnic groups within the United States. Using a structured layperson or clinical interview of some type, the country followed by the current or 12-month estimated PTSD prevalence are listed: Australia, 1.3% (Creamer, Burgess, & McFarlane, 2001); Spain, 0.6% (Olaya, Alonso, Atwoli, Kessler, Vilagut, & Haro, 2015); and Canada, 2.4% (van Ameringen, Mancini, Patterson, & Boyle, 2008). The recent World Mental Health Survey assessed PTSD 12-month prevalence in 20 low, medium, and high-income countries (Karam et al., 2014). Twelve of these countries had a less than 1% prevalence rate. The highest, understandably so due to the civil strife, was Northern Ireland, with 3.8%. This was followed by the United States with 2.5%. High-income countries had twice the rate of PTSD: 1.5% versus 0.8 for low income and 0.7 for middle income. Looking at lifetime PTSD prevalence, developed countries have an almost three times higher prevalence rate than developing countries: 4.4% versus 1.6% (Kessler et al., 2011).

Population-based studies provide the best estimates for prevalence among different and racial and ethnic groups. In the National Comorbidity Survey, there was 11.4% African American and 9% Hispanic representation (Kessler et al., 1995). When controlling for age, gender, marital status, and the interaction among these potential predictions, no association was found between PTSD and racial group. This confirmed the findings of earlier population-based studies (Davidson et al., 1991; Helzer et al., 1987) and a subsequent study, the Detroit Area Survey of Trauma (Breslau, Kessler, Chilcoat, Schultz, Davis, & Andreski, 1998). Of note is that the Davidson et al. and Breslau et al. studies were regional, undertaken in the Piedmont region of North Carolina and in Detroit, Michigan, respectively, in which the samples included a high percentage of African Americans: 37.2% and 28.2%, respectively.

The National Survey on Alcohol and Related Conditions included a large national sample (N = 34,563) (Roberts, Gilman, Breslau, Breslau, & Koenen, 2011). The lifetime prevalence rates for PTSD are as follows: African Americans, 8.7%; Whites, 7.4%; Hispanics, 7%; and Asians, 0.7%. Whites had a lower prevalence than African Americans but a rate similar to Hispanics. It was noted however that while the conditional risk for developing PTSD once exposed to an event was statistically significant between African Americans and Whites, the difference was small (adjusted odds ratio =1.21 vs. 1) The higher socioeconomic status of Asian Americans is one explanation provided for the lower risk as is the possibility of underreporting stigmatizing events such as rape and sexual abuse (Roberts et al., 2011). What is of interest was the very low prevalence rate despite the facts that Asian Americans reported being more likely to be refugees and civilians in a war zone. Alcántara, Casement, and Lewis-Fernández (2013) found a higher risk for PTSD in Latinos versus non-Latinos in their review of 28 studies. The significance of using self-report instruments or layperson interviews versus clinician-administered interviews is illustrated best in their review. The three studies that used clinician-administered diagnostic interviews did not find an increased risk of PTSD in Latinos, consistent with Roberts et al. (2011). Of note, however, is that these later three were all in veteran samples. The remainder used layperson-administered structured diagnostic interviews or self-report instruments. Additionally, only a small percentage of the clinician and layperson interviews were done in Spanish (between 1% and 4%). Based on this review we can conclude very little about the risk of developing PTSD in Latinos versus non-Latinos in the United States other than they have higher rates of self-reported PTSD symptoms.

In another review American Indians and Alaskan Natives had a higher prevalence than Whites but whether this difference could be explained by the diagnostic method used (self-report versus structured interview) was not addressed. There were 16 comparison studies, but the diagnostic measure used in 11 was some version of the DSM without stating the specific diagnostic interview measure (Bassett, Buchwald, & Manson, 2014).

For a thorough assessment of cross-cultural issues, the reader is directed to an article by Hinton and Lewis-Fernández (2011) that was commissioned by one of the DSM-5 workgroups. They concluded what was suggested earlier: The results are mixed. Population-based studies are less likely to show differences (Breslau et al., 1998; Norris, 1992) while studies that compare groups experiencing the same trauma are more likely to find differences. Hispanics were more likely to be diagnosed with PTSD following September 11 than Whites, but there were no differences between African Americans, Whites, and Asians (Galea et al., 2002). Following Hurricane Andrew, Hispanics and African Americans had higher rates of PTSD. This was based on a self-report measure (Perilla, Norris, & Lavizzo, 2002). What was clear, however, from the Hinton and Lewis-Fernandez (2011) review is that there are clear differences in PTSD prevalence rates between countries, but they conclude by stating: "It is unclear why the U.S. prevalence is considerably higher" (p. 5). As noted in the Karam et al. (2014) multination study, the prevalence in the United States is 2.5%, exceeded only by Northern Ireland. Mexico and Colombia, which have a great deal of illicit drug and other civilian violence, have a rate of 0.3%. Lebanon, which has been in an almost constant state of war since the 1970s, has a rate of 1.6%. In Israel the rate is 0.4%.

A possible explanation is offered here for why the United States has such a high prevalence rate: "No diagnosis in the history of American psychiatry has had a more dramatic and pervasive impact on law and social justice than posttraumatic stress disorder" (Stone, 1993, p. 23). It has been argued herein that PTSD occupies a special place in the history of American psychiatry. It is as much a sociopolitical event as it is a psychiatric diagnosis. British psychiatrist Derek Summerfield, who has clinical experience with all forms of atrocity worldwide, has written scores of the most insightful commentary on this topic over the last two decades. His core argument: "Trauma is a growth industry in the West and thus fertile terrain for fashion." He wonders to what extent Western concepts of mental illness impute "inappropriate sick roles" to communities and cultures very different from our own (Summerfield, 1995: 509).

Risk Factors and Comorbid Conditions

To establish risk factors, I first begin with the epidemiological studies followed by two major reviews. The most consistent PTSD risk factor is female gender. In the NCS study, women were twice as likely to be diagnosed with lifetime PTSD: 10.5% versus 5% (Kessler et al., 1995). A doubling of PTSD (13% in women vs. 6.2% in men) was also found by Breslau et al. (1998). A literature review found this same doubling of PTSD rates in women regardless of type of study, population studies, or methodology that was employed (Tolin & Foa, 2006). This is contrary to other studies that may have found a higher rate in women but not at a level of statistical significance (Davidson et al., 1991; Helzer et al., 1987; Shore et al., 1989). The negative association in these latter studies is likely the result of the small number of cases that were actually diagnosed as PTSD, limiting the ability to detect a statistical difference. These gender differences were found in a consecutive series of patients (N = 1,132) seeking psychiatric treatment in an outpatient private practice within a hospital setting. A greater percentage of women (14.1%) were diagnosed with PTSD relative to men (9.1%; see Zlotnick, Zimmerman, Wolfsdorf, & Mattia, 2001).

Using the NCS sample, Bromet, Sonnega, and Kessler (1998) looked at nine risk factors. They found that there were many more risk factors in women than there were in men. In examining risk factors it is important to control for other variables that might affect PTSD prevalence. The first three factors were preexisting affective, anxiety and substance abuse disorders. This is followed by four indicators of childhood adversity which included parental aggression toward the patient, aggression between parents, lack of a confiding relationship with the mother and parental separation and/or divorce. The final two risk factors of PTSD were parental history of mental illness and substance abuse. Risk factors in both men and women included preexisting affective disorder and mental illness in the parents. A nonconfiding relationship with the mother was an additional risk factor in women. However, when trauma type was controlled, only a previous history of affective disorder remained significant in women and in men a previous history of anxiety disorder and mental illness in parents. For both men and women, the greater the number of risk factors, the greater the likelihood of PTSD. Taking sexual trauma as an example, in women PTSD was found in 11.7% in women and 5.1% in men who had no risk factors, but both genders had a similar risk of developing PTSD with one risk factor (approximately 30%), two risk factors (approximately 40%), and three or more risk factors (approximately 50%). In Davidson et al. (1991), those with PTSD were 2.7 to 3.3 times more likely to have experienced early childhood adversity characterized by parental poverty, mental illness in a family member, early parental separation, and child abuse.

Two meta-analytic studies have identified risk factors for the prediction of PTSD. Brewin, Andrews, and Valentine (2000) identified the following 14 risk factors followed by their respective effect size: gender (0.13), age at trauma (0.06), socioeconomic status (0.14), education (0.10), intelligence (0.18), race (.05), previous psychiatric history (0.11), childhood abuse (0.14), previous trauma (0.12), adverse childhood events (other than abuse) (0.12), family history of psychiatric illness (0.11), trauma severity (0.23), lack of social support (0.40), and life stress (0.32). While all were statistically significant, only the last three were associated with significant effect sizes. Brewin, Andrews, and Valentine (2000) then examined six sample and study characteristics (military versus civilian trauma, gender, retrospective or prospective study, PTSD diagnosis based on absence or presence of the disorder or continuous symptom scores, use of interview or questionnaire and if trauma occurred in childhood or adulthood) and how they might modify the 14 risk factors that were identified. Because of the many possible permutations (i.e., risk factor by study characteristic) the reader is directed to review the article for a detailed understanding of the results. With the Brewin, Andrews, and Rose (2000) review in mind, Ozer et al. (2008) decided to look at a separate set of variables with their own factor analysis. They found that peritraumatic dissociation, perceived support, peritraumatic emotions, and perceived life threat had the highest effect sizes (ranging from 0.35 to .026) while prior trauma, prior adjustment, and family psychiatric history were all equal predictors (0.17 effect size for all three).

It has been argued that, "There is perhaps no other Axis I disorder for which the issue of co-morbidity is more relevant than PTSD" (Spinazzola, Blaustein, & van der Kolk, 2005, p. 426). In the NCS study the comorbid psychiatric disorders included anxiety or depressive disorder, antisocial personality disorder, and alcohol and substance abuse and/or dependence.

Lifetime prevalence of at least one of these disorders was found in 88.3% of men and 79% of women (Kessler et al., 1995). Among those with PTSD, 14.9% carried one diagnosis; 14.4%, two diagnoses; and 59%, three diagnoses. Approximately 48% of men and women had a major depressive episode along with similar rates of dysthymia (21.4% of men and 23.3% of women).

The rate of substance-use disorders was higher in men—including both abuse and dependence—especially for alcohol (51.9% in men and 27.9% of women). For drug abuse and dependence, the rates were 34.5% in men and 26.9% in women. As might be expected, antisocial personality disorder was much more common in men than women (43.3% vs. 15.4%). In the ECS study, those with a PTSD diagnosis were twice as likely to have another disorder (Helzer et al., 1987). In Davidson et al. (1991), 62.3% of those with PTSD were likely to have another disorder. Anxiety disorders (social phobia, obsessive-compulsive disorder, and generalized anxiety disorder) and major depression were ten times more likely to occur in PTSD respondents. Panic disorder was 20 times more likely. Surprisingly, schizophrenia and schizophreniform were also found to co-occur with PTSD at this latter rate. Unlike in the NCS (Kessler et al., 1995), dysthymia, alcohol abuse/dependence, and mania were not found to be any more prevalent in Davidson et al. (1991). In a treatment-seeking sample, men diagnosed with PTSD are more likely to be diagnosed with a substance abuse or personality disorder (Zlotnick et al., 2001).

Of the comorbid disorders that might predict the development of PTSD, acute stress disorder (ASD) is of the most relevant. Australian psychologist and researcher Richard Bryant has been the most active in studying ASD. In a review in anticipation for DSM-5, Bryant (2011) reviewed all prospective ASD studies. He concluded that the ability of the ACS diagnosis to identify those who will eventually develop PTSD is poor. Of note, however, is that 13 of the 22 studies identified involved motor vehicle accidents, "brain injury," or injuries as measured by consecutive referral to a hospital, many of which were conducted by Bryant and his colleagues. These events would not be of sufficient severity to meet the stressor criteria under the definition of PTSD as proposed in this chapter. The only study that clearly met the stressor criteria assessed rape victims (Elklit & Christiansen, 2010). In this study, the sensitivity of the ASD diagnosis in predicting PTSD was 0.72.

I conclude by considering PTSD as a risk factor for the ultimate comorbid psychiatric condition, completed suicide. The first study to examine the association in a population-based sample was a nested case-control study of the whole population of Denmark (Gradus et al., 2010). Between 1994 and 2006, 9,612 cases of suicide were identified. Among suicide cases, 40% had been diagnosed with PTSD versus 5% of controls. As expected, the presence of depression modifies this risk by increasing suicide risk. As anticipated, suicide cases were primarily male (71%) and single (58%).

As for clinical outcome, two epidemiological studies suggested that PTSD could be chronic (Helzer et al., 1987; Kessler et al., 1995). The NCS study treated this subject more thoroughly, probably because of the significant higher prevalence rate that was found. Of note was a steep drop in PTSD prevalence in the first year in both those who did and those who did not seek treatment, but the median time to remission was 36 months in those who sought treatment and 64 months in those who did not. As already noted, about a third failed to remit after many years (Kessler et al., 1995). In the ECS study, about one-third of subjects had symptoms that lasted more than three years, particularly in combat veterans (Helzer et al., 1987).

The PTSD Interview

"If you have 30 minutes to see a patient, spend 29 on the history, one on the physical examination, and none on the x-rays": I first heard the advice above during neurology rounds from the director of the neurology clinic where I spent 15 years of my career. This simple axiom made an impression on me. It was taught to him during his neurology residency at the University of Iowa but he could not attribute it to any particular individual. I eventually tracked down the source: Adolph L. Sahs, the second chair of neurology at the University of Iowa from 1948 to 1974, and one of the four founders of the American Academy of Neurology (Joynt, 2001). It is of note that the diagnostic directive was made prior to the advent of computed tomography (CT). It continued to be followed long after the most sophisticated of neuroimaging techniques were introduced. The neuropsychology caveat relative to this quote is that we as neuropsychologists place disproportionate emphasis on tests, whereas in neurology, despite major advances in neurodiagnostic testing, it is implicit that the interview takes precedence. I regularly state in my medicolegal reports there are advantages of the interview over formal neuropsychological testing.

First, the interview narrative does not require any detailed explanation or prerequisite knowledge (e.g., testing procedures), only common sense. An interview is easier to explain and for a referral source, the reader, or for a jury to follow. The often technical and impenetrable narrative that characterizes most neuropsychological reports should be absent in an interview narrative. Second, while the cognitive impairment may have different etiologies that are beyond the control of the patient (e.g., medication effects, brain damage, pain, lack of motivation, etc.) the benefit of the interview is that the symptoms that the patient reports are under his or her control: They are volitional. While a borderline memory score may be due to pain symptoms beyond the patient's control, what the patient chooses to report in terms of symptoms is entirely under his or her control. That low verbal memory score may be due to many factors, yet there is only one explanation why a patient might report they now read at the fourth grade level as a result of their concussion: malingering. The patient just has to be provided the opportunity to report such improbable symptoms. Third, psychological and cognitive testing is often referred to as more "objective" than the clinical interview. What is objective is test administration and scoring. A score requires an interpretation that some might argue is subjective even though it should be based on the published literature. In the case of malingering, the test score is far from objective when the test is malingered.

This chapter can artificially be separated into two sections. This portion begins the second section: the PTSD evaluation, which is in essence the interview. As neuropsychology delves more into PTSD, what is needed is a clear conceptualization of the disorder. This was the chapter goal up to this point. The end goal, however, is to present how to conduct a competent PTSD evaluation.

DSM-III revolutionized clinical psychiatry by operationally defining syndromes. Among the "unintended consequences" was that it reduced the DSM to a symptom checklist (Andreasen, 2007). This accusation preceded DSM-III. The Feighner criteria and Research Diagnostic criteria were characterized as belonging to the "Chinese menu system of diagnosis" (Robins et al., 1981: 382). A neurologist would not simply record the absence or presence of a symptom without characterizing it. In clinical neuropsychology this has been referred to as the "bean counting" of symptoms (Bieliauskas, 1999). In my experience, it is rare in the evaluation of PTSD for the clinician to have at least inquired if each symptom is either present or absent, much less to conduct an exhaustive examination of each symptom similar to how a neurologist might examine the simplest of all movement disorders—tremor (i.e., onset, course, unilateral or bilateral, resting or intention, family history of tremor, any accompanying motor symptoms, etc.). The DSM criteria is no more than a grocery list that serves as a reminder to the examiner of what symptoms to inquire about, but to then do it in an exhaustive way, not in a binary fashion as might be found on a self-report depression screening. The goal of this section is to operationally define what is an exhaustive interview. The hallmark of any good clinical exam, psychiatric or otherwise, is a good interview. Before a new clinical interview for the diagnosis for PTSD is proposed, we need to define PTSD.

PTSD Defined: A Hybrid Model

One approach to harmonization of the ICD and DSM criteria suggested by First (2009) is to construct hybrid criteria that draw upon the best features of both. That is the approach being proposed here. First acknowledges that the drawback to this approach is that the new criteria are essentially untested. This can also be said for the CAPS-5 (Clinician-Administered PTSD Scale 5), which has been constructed to coincide with the new DSM-5 criteria, but studies have yet to be published.

The argument has been made to not adopt the DSM-5 PTSD definition but to instead move to ICD-10 and eventually, to the much-improved PTSD definition in ICD-11, which is due to be published in 2018. What the final product will look like is not precisely known. What follows is a very close approximation of the ICD-11 definition. First, the disorder must develop "following exposure to an extremely threatening or horrific event or series of events" (Maercker et al., 2013, p. 200). As Norris (1992) argues, "Traumatic events are thus defined objectively leaving their consequences for subjective states of stress as an empirical question. (p. 409)" The CIDI is a structured interview developed by the WHO that corresponds to both ICD-10 and DSM-IV. It assesses lifetime and 12-month prevalence and has been translated into other languages. It can be used by laypersons (Andrews & Peters, 1998). Since the current ICD-10 considers only events that are "exceptionally threatening or catastrophic in nature" the first step is to identify what those events should be for ICD-11.

There are 26 questions on the CIDI that correspond to traumatic events that could produce PTSD. Consistent with the international focus of the CIDI, some of these events are catastrophic experiences not seen in the United States (i.e., civilians in a war zone, being a refugee). These questions can be administered as a checklist. This is similar to the 17 questions that precede the administration of the CAPS: the Life Events Checklist. The neuropsychologist will know what the traumatic event is they are assessing. The purpose for the checklist is to see if there are any other traumas in addition to the one the patient is being examined for. In a medicolegal context this can be important. One referral seen by this writer had the patient claiming PTSD from a minor vehicle accident. On the CAPS checklist, however, he reported being a combat veteran yet never experiencing PTSD. In a clinical context, past trauma exposure is a risk factor for PTSD. We want the patient's complete trauma history.

As previously noted, the understanding is that ICD-11 will have six symptoms that belong to three clusters: reexperiencing, avoidance, and hyperarousal. Reexperiencing requires that the patient report either recurrent dreams or recurrent "daytime images." Of note is both of these symptoms are accompanied by both "fear and horror" (Morina, van Emmerik, Andrews & Brewin, 2014). Whether this wording will appear in ICD-11 is uncertain. Avoidance requires avoiding either thoughts about the events or activities or people that remind the patient of the event. Finally, hyperarousal requires either hypervigilance or an exaggerated startle response. One symptom in each category must be present to meet the diagnosis. The symptoms must last several weeks (here we are going to assume at least one month) and cause significant impairment in functioning (Maercker et al., 2013; Morina et al., 2014).

What about functional impairment or disability? If one were to meet all the criteria of a psychiatric diagnosis yet function without there being any impairment in social and occupational functioning one would be hard pressed to consider that to be a disorder. Functional impairment must also be included as this is a common question in a medicolegal context. DSM-5 requires that it be present, as will ICD-11.

In the past the most common method was found in DSM on Axis V, the Global Assessment of Functioning (GAF). For reasons that are arguably not convincing, both the Axis system and the GAF were dropped in DSM-5. Functional impairment needs to be operationally defined. The functional disability corollary to ICD is the WHODAS, the World Health Organization Disability Assessment Schedule 2.0. (WHOc, 2015a). Like ICD-11, DSM-5 supports the use of the WHODAS (APA, 2013, p. 16). Unfortunately, since the introduction in DSM-IV of Criterion F, the DSM does not necessarily require "impairment," "clinically significant distress" would also meet the criterion. The clinician should define *disability* or impairment while the patient can define *distress*, but the two should not be confused (Vázquez-Barquero, 2009; Ustün & Kennedy, 2009). The WHODAS has an interview version that takes five to ten minutes to complete, and also has a self-administered version. The time period to be evaluated is the past 30 days. The full version has 36 items. The 12-item short form is recommended as it explains 81% of the variance of the longer version. As for the choice of which structured PTSD interview to use, that decision is relatively straightforward: The CAPS is the most frequently used structured interview by both researchers and clinicians (Elhai, Gray, Kashdan, & Franklin, 2005).

The Clinical Interview

What DSM-III did was solve the problem of criterion variance, one major source of unreliability in psychiatric diagnosis. That is to say we need inclusion and exclusion criteria for a disorder. What the structured clinical interview does is to solve any problem, which is that of information variance. It gives clinicians the same amount and kind of information about the patient (Endicott & Spitzer, 1978). The DIS was the first instrument to make DSM-III diagnoses (Robins et al., 1981). Robins expanded on the latter interview by developing the CIDI for the WHO (Robins et al., 1988). One option is to simply adopt the questions from the CIDI that correspond to the six PTSD symptoms in the ICD-11 classification. In this proposed hybrid model we should instead incorporate a PTSD interview that has a long history and much research behind it: the CAPS (Weathers, Keane, & Davidson, 2001; Weathers et al., 2004). The CAPS has been updated (CAPS-5) to correspond to DSM-5 (Weathers et al., 2015). Since government employees created the CAPS-5, it is not copyrighted and can be obtained by writing to the National Center for PTSD. The CAPS has the advantage of assessing both frequency and severity of symptoms. The disadvantage is that it could take as long as an hour to give. With additional PTSD symptoms in DSM-5, the CAPS-5 could take longer. It is proposed here that a modified CAPS be used to assess ICD-11 PTSD criteria.

On the CAPS (not the CAPS-5) the six core criteria are already included. They are reexperiencing in the form of dreams (Item 2) and flashbacks (Item 3); avoidance in the form of thoughts (Item 6) and activities or places that are reminders of the event (Item 7); and hyperarousal in the form of hypervigilance (Item 16) and startle reaction (Item 17). The wording for each question would be the same as on the CAPS with additional modifications. A mock sample question accompanied by the frequency and intensity rating to be completed by the patient is shown in Table 32.5 and illustrates what an item might look like. The *first* modification is that for each symptom, the question of onset would be asked and if the symptom has gotten better, same or worse since it began. These two questions are rather basic with regard to any symptom inquiry. The *second* modification is adding questions to the six core symptoms. On the CAPS there is an Associated Features section that asks about additional PTSD symptoms (i.e., guilt) that can be features of PTSD but are not necessarily needed to make the diagnosis (Items 26–30). The following questions from the CAPS can be added in the following order: unwanted memories (Item 1), emotionally upset when reminded of the event (Item 4), and physical reactions (Item 5). At the time of this writing it is unclear how the "daytime images" will be defined in ICD-11. It will involve flashbacks but it is uncertain if simply reexperiencing memories, thoughts, and feelings about the event will qualify. A "flashback" is not the same as unwanted memories and reminders. Hence Items 1 and 4 from the CAPS can be retained. More important however is Item 5. In defining this hybrid model of PTSD, it is the contention here that PTSD is an anxiety disorder and should have remained in the anxiety disorders section of DSM. A trauma category of disorders was unnecessary. "Across the main theoretical models for understanding the development of PTSD is the centrality of classical conditioning of fear as a necessary, but not sufficient, mechanism for the development of PTSD" (Zoellner, Rothbaum, & Feeny, 2011, p. 853). In the family of anxiety disorders is panic disorder. Patients who report PTSD actually volunteer "panic attacks." The presence of the ten physical symptoms of panic needs to be assessed. The last three of the DSM panic symptoms (derealization, fear of losing control, or fear of dying) in my experience are rarely endorsed in a PTSD context. Items 26 and 27 of the CAPS are associated features and should be added when applicable to the individual case. They refer to guilt of what the patient did or did not do and survivor guilt, respectively. These two questions are very applicable as they are signature questions to be asked in rape victims and combat veterans (or any other trauma in which someone else was killed), respectively. There are then a total of 11 questions in the interview; six core questions needed for the diagnosis and five (Items 1, 4, 5, 26 and 27 of the CAPS) that I will term *ancillary questions*. The five ancillary questions are optional depending on the clinical circumstance. The *third* modification is adding additional follow-up questions beyond the core CAPS questions within each item to more thoroughly characterize the symptom. Nothing precludes a clinician from adding questions to clarify the symptom. This is not a research study or clinical trial but a clinical examination. The questions in italics are not CAPS questions but added to further clarify the symptom. The *fourth* modification is to record the emotional reaction that the patient volunteered at the time of the trauma. The presence of fear is a strong predictor of PTSD (Brewin et al., 2000). The *fifth* modification is to record if delayed onset is present, onset of PTSD six months after the incident event. Delayed onset has no practical clinical meaning (despite its continued use in DSM-5) but is practically pathognomonic for malingered PTSD. The *sixth* and final modification borrows the best feature of the CAPS and that is the assessment of the frequency and intensity of the symptom, which allows the examiner to then calculate a severity score. The major change here is allowing the patient to rate the severity and intensity of the six core PTSD symptom, instead of ratings by the examiner. After the full interview is complete the patient is asked to rate each symptom endorsed in the interview. As noted at the bottom of Table 32.5, the frequency question remains the same but intensity statements are reworded for this purpose and presented to the patient to complete. The item is scored in the standard way (Weathers et al., 2004). The frequency and intensity score are added to obtain a severity score. The frequency and intensity of the symptom conveys the patient's subjective distress similar to many of the PTSD checklists. This new six-item PTSD symptom checklist is directly tied to the CAPS questions. There is also nothing to preclude the examiner from doing the rating as per standard CAPS directions. However, both the examiner and patient rating may be affected by the additional questions that are asked in the interview. With the introduction of DSM-5, PTSD self-report instruments must be changed accordingly. Because the reliability and validity of the most common PTSD self-report instruments has yet to be established vis-à-vis the DSM-5, it is proposed to modify the CAPS interview to six questions accompanied by a six-item frequency and intensity rating, which will similarly need clinical validation.

Table 32.5 Mock CAPS interview question

Have you had hallucinations over the last month? Yes No
Onset:
Course: Better Same Worse
Do you hear or see things, or both?
Do you ever talk, yell or act out the hallucinations? Yes No
Describe your typical hallucination
Are the hallucinations exactly the same? Yes No
Frequency Rating
How often have you had hallucinations in the past month?
 0 None
 1 Once or twice a month
 2 Once or twice a week
 3 Several times a week
 4 Daily or almost every day
Intensity Rating by Examiner
How much did they interfere with your activities?
 0 None
 1 Mild, minimal distress or disruption of activities
 2 Moderate, distress present, some disruption of activities
 3 Severe, considerable distress, significant disruption of activities
 4 Extreme, incapacitating distress, unable to continue activities
Intensity Rating Reworded for Patient Rating
 1 These hallucinations cause minimal distress or disruption of my activities.
 2 These hallucinations are present but I can manage with some disruption of my activities.
 3 These hallucinations caused distress and significant disruption of my activities.
 4 These hallucinations caused distress making me unable to continue my activities.

Psychological Testing

A whole discipline within medicine, psychiatry, has essentially only the interview in its diagnostic armamentarium. While psychological testing is secondary, it provides supplementary information that can be important. The International Society for Traumatic Stress Studies has put out a practice guideline that emphasizes that multiple methods should be used to assess PTSD (Weathers, Keane, & Foa, 2008). There are essentially two additional methods: the self-report instrument and personality testing. The self-report instrument serves four purposes. First, while the clinician is formulating her or his diagnostic impressions of the patient, the patient is afforded an opportunity to do the same absent any input, bias, or preconceived notions of the examiner. We want the patient's diagnostic impression of himself or herself. Whether that impression does or does not coincide with the impression of the clinician is not relevant. Both convergence and divergence of opinion are sources of useful information. Second, self-report instruments help track treatment progress. Third, they help facilitate information across studies. Finally, the primary purpose for which they were designed was to serve as screening instruments. In regard to this last purpose, neuropsychologists—especially those who see forensic cases—are not unaware of the tendency to over-report on self-report instruments (Edens, Otto, & Dwyer, 1998). This inclination is also present in clinical cases (Mittenberg et al., 2002). In fact, as screening instruments, they fulfill the goal that they set out to meet: the minimization of false negatives. A negative screening negates the need for a clinical interview. The only instruction to giving any self-report instrument is when to give it relative to the interview. In a medicolegal context, all self-report instruments are given after the interview. The item content is obvious and there is the tendency to over-report. This is less of an issue with the clinical interview. In a clinical context, when used as a screening, it can be given first and shorten if not exclude the interview. Even in a clinical context, it is best to start with the interview. A checklist indirectly "coaches" the patient by providing them the test items in advance of the test (i.e., the interview).

In choosing a screening instrument we turn again to the practice survey of Elhai, Gray, Kashdan, and Franklin (2005). The most commonly preferred instruments among PTSD researchers are the PTSD Checklist, or PCL (Weathers, Litz, Herman, Huska, & Keane, 1993), and the Posttraumatic Stress Diagnostic Scale (PDS) by Foa (1995). The PCL has been updated by the National Center for PTSD, to the PCL-5, to mirror the DSM-5 criteria (Weathers, Marx, Friedman, & Schnurr, 2014). A critical review of the PCL provided generally favorable comments as a screening instrument (McDonald & Calhoun, 2010). Previously, Greiffenstein and I had recommended the PDS over the PCL (Andrikopoulos & Greiffenstein, 2012). The three advantages of the PDS are that the questions are tied directly to the 17 symptoms of DSM-IV-TR, and the instrument has quite a bit of research behind it, as does the PCL. But it measures functional impairment, making it preferable to the PCL. The PDS can be computer- or hand-scored. Unlike the PCL, which is free, the PDS is sold commercially (Foa, 1995). Foa has recently updated the PDS to coincide with DSM-5; the PDS-5 (Foa, 2013). This version has only 20 items that correspond directly to DSM-5, versus 49 items on the original version. The instrument will now be offered free of charge to qualified professionals by writing to Foa (Foa, 2013).

The PTSD instruments that are preferred here are those that have the most research. Referencing the research allows one to compare their patient's score to that of patients with similar traumas by comparing scores to assess severity and/or improvement. In a medicolegal context it allows for the assessment of a dose-response relationship (Bianchini, Curtis, & Greve, 2006). A head injury resulting in a Glasgow Coma Scale (GCS) 14 cannot result in a cognitive performance similar to a patient with an initial GCS of 6. Similarly, in a case that went to trial, the plaintiff that I evaluated was claiming PTSD from sexual harassment. Her somatic and cognitive complaints (as measured by the Somatic/Cognitive scales from the Minnesota Multiphasic Personality Inventory-2-Restructed Format [MMPI-2-RF]) exceeded that of a sample of multiple sclerosis patients with particularly bad disease who had not responded to the first-line multiple sclerosis drugs. The jury understood the point. This was much easier to explain than the Fake Bad Scale (Lees-Haley, English, & Glenn, 1991).

The most preferred instrument by clinicians (23%) was actually the Trauma Symptom Inventory (TSI; see Briere, 1995), followed by the PDS and PCL, both at 16%. However, for the reasons stated earlier, the instruments with the most research are preferred. Aside from the cost of purchasing the TSI there are other factors to consider. It is a 100-item questionnaire, with ten clinical scales and three validity scales. It can be computer scored. It takes longer to give. The TSI items are not directly tied to DSM-IV and functional impairment is not measured. It is considered more of a measure of traumatology versus a PTSD measure (Elhai et al., 2005). It covers a six-month time frame instead of the traditional one month of other scales. One perceived advantage is that the validity scales include a response bias scale. Per Elhai et al. (2005) the scale is a measure of general validity not specific for assessing malingered PTSD.

With the separation of PTSD in ICD-11 into three clusters, the preferred self-report instrument as part of any standard PTSD assessment should be the Impact of Events Scale (IES) (Horowitz, Wilner, & Alvarez, 1979). It is the perennial PTSD self-report instrument with over 35 years of research behind it tapping the core symptom cluster of PTSD. In the original version, avoidance and intrusion were the clusters measured. In the revised IES-R version, five hyperarousal symptoms were added (Weiss & Marmar, 1996) making this ideal for ICD-11. This is the second most commonly used instrument among researchers after the PCL (Elhai et al., 2005). It contains 22 items answered in a 5-point Likert format. It is freely available and has been translated into a number of languages. It does not, however, translate directly into a DSM diagnosis since at the time it was developed PTSD had not been coined.

Given the high prevalence of comorbid depression and anxiety disorders in PTSD, this should always be assessed with self-report measures. Spitzer and colleagues have developed the Patient Health Questionnaire–9 (Kroenke, Spitzer, & Williams, 2001) to screen for depression and the generalized anxiety disorder–7 (Spitzer, Kroenke, Williams, & Löwe, 2006). The advantages are threefold: they are publicly available, they are tied to the DSM-IV criteria, and they assess for the possibility that the DSM-IV criteria for depression and anxiety criteria may have been met. I give these two instruments to all patients, medicolegal or clinical, at the conclusion of the testing and interview.

The International Society for Traumatic Stress Studies mentioned the Minnesota Multiphasic Peronality Inventory-2 (MMPI-2) in the assessment guidelines when it recommends using multiple measures and when measuring response bias (Weathers et al., 2008). In the context of a PTSD forensic evaluation, the limitations of the MMPI-2 are as follows: there are few studies in PTSD civil litigants; many are simulation studies; most involve veterans; and the most robust litigant profile, that of somatic malingering (Larrabee, 1998), involves the assessment of exaggerated or malingered physical symptoms, not PTSD. In a previous chapter, Greiffenstein and I found no PTSD studies on the MMPI-2-RF (Andrikopoulos & Greiffenstein, 2012). For the present review, no studies could be located using a PTSD civilian sample in a nonlitigation context. We do not know what the MMPI-2-RF profile of a PTSD patient should look like. Ideally, the best place to start would be with the archetypal civilian PTSD patient, that of the rape victim. This state of affairs is not all that surprising since a traumatologist seeing a rape victim would have no useful reason to administer any personality testing if the goal is simply to diagnose and treat the PTSD. It might serve to identify some, as of yet unknown, personality profile or comorbid condition that might facilitate or hinder treatment. If there is a reluctance to administer personality testing when it is part of a guideline, there is little hope of administering cognitive testing if it is not recommended.

Cognitive Testing

The crux of the issue in regard to the administration of cognitive testing in the context of PTSD, (or any psychiatric disorder) was captured in the subheading of an editorial: "Case proven, but what is the significance?" (Hotopf & Wessely, 2006). U.S. soldiers returning from Iraq were found to have subtle neuropsychological impairment relative to nondeployed military personnel in sustained attention and visual and verbal memory. In fine motor speed, executive aspects of attention, and cognitive efficiency there were no differences (Vasterling, Proctor, Amoroso, Kane, Heeren, & White, 2006). No clear reason emerged that could explain these findings. Despite the absence of an explanation, the authors recommended that a post-deployment neuropsychological screening program be implemented, even in the absence of a negative medical workup. One might argue that this is an attempt to "neurologize" a psychiatric disorder (David, 1992).

There is no obvious reason to conduct neuropsychological testing on psychiatric patients as a matter of routine unless there is a compelling clinical and/or neurological reason. One legitimate reason might be to assess if a cognitive impairment might impact the psychiatric patient's academic or occupational functioning. In a medicolegal context, if cognitive impairment is what is forming the basis for the claimed disability, it needs to be assessed. The modal reason for cognitive testing in the context of a psychological or pain evaluation is that it affords the opportunity to administer malingering tests. An unequivocally failed malingering that takes five minutes to give might negate the need for an interview.

Because cognitive testing is more likely to be administered in a medicolegal context, this topic was addressed in my previous forensic chapter (Andrikopoulos & Greiffenstein, 2012) and will not be repeated here. The sparse literature in civilian nonlitigating PTSD patients was summarized there as follows: PTSD patients do cognitively worse than trauma patients without PTSD on most tests, trauma patients without PTSD do not differ from controls, PTSD patients do worse than normal controls, those with more PTSD symptoms do worse than those with fewer symptoms, and PTSD patients do not differ from non-PTSD psychiatric patients. The level of impairment is mild (i.e., low average scores). In reference to veterans that I examine in the context of a PTSD claim, I limit my cognitive evaluation to a screening (i.e., the Montreal Cognitive Assessment [MoCA], Nasreddine et al., 2005) and one malingering test. The remaining time, approximately two hours, is spent on a neuropsychological interview that covers a broad range of cognitive, motor, and sensory and psychiatric symptoms followed by a PTSD interview.

Concluding Commentary

> Our future success hinges upon acquiring a comparable clinical and research PTSD knowledge base on the accurate diagnosis of PTSD.
>
> (Andrikopoulos & Greiffenstein, 2012, p. 393)

To close this chapter there are five issues that deserve to be elaborated and commented upon: malingering, disparate cultural perspective of PTSD, "our clinical mind set," the neurobiology of PTSD, and a direction for neuropsychology in the study of PTSD.

The first issue is what Gerald Rosen has repeatedly voiced concern about—the "contaminated published rates of PTSD" (Rosen, 2004b, p. 1291). Epidemiology and clinical cohort studies are needed to understand any syndrome and disease process. Controlling for moderator variables that can affect prevalence rates is elemental research methodology. In 2008, the International Society for Traumatic Stress Studies published its second practice guideline (Weathers et al., 2008). Its ninth and final bullet point was that malingering "should be assessed routinely in *all* clinical and *research assessments* of PTSD" (p. 52, [emphasis added]), something not even mentioned in its first guideline (Foa, Keane, & Friedman, 2000). It has been my experience that the concept of malingering is foreign to our colleagues in medicine. It occupies no space in their journals. When unexplained symptoms are present, the response is to reflexively invoke the unconscious and diagnose conversion disorder. Only once have I seen the term *conversion* been critically questioned as a construct, and by none other than C. Miller Fisher, who until the time of his death in 2012, was arguably the most accomplished neurologist of our time (Fisher, 1995). In academic neurology, my unofficial survey of epileptologists (pseudoseizures) and movement disorder specialists (psychogenic movement disorders) at national meetings is that there is a consensus that malingering is rare (under 5%). The National Vietnam Veterans Readjustment Study has been revisited many times over the years, including a series of articles and editorials in *Science* (Dohrenwend et al., 2006; McNally, 2006). Recently a follow-up study was conducted wherein it was shown that 10.8% of male veterans still have PTSD (Marmar et al., 2015). After 40 years, most notable was that twice as many reported a worsening of symptoms rather than improvement (16% vs. 7.6%). Malingering or compensation status was not mentioned in a single instance in the article or in the accompanying editorial (Hoge, 2015). The National Center for PTSD is charged with addressing the clinical needs of veterans and conducting the research that provides for an evidence-based approach to meeting their needs. While Frueh, Grubaugh, Elhai, and Buckley (2007) suggest malingering is as high as 50% in veterans claiming PTSD, the contention of the Center is that malingering is practically nonexistent (0.6%) (Marx, Miller, Sloan, Litz, Kaloupek, & Keane, 2008). Clearly this contention is grossly inaccurate based on the literature within clinical neuropsychology, namely forensics, which occupies the largest space in our journals (Sweet, King, Malina, Bergman, & Simmons, 2002). Going forward, PTSD studies not assessing or addressing malingering in their methodology cannot be considered valid.

As has already been stated, the introduction of the term PTSD into the psychiatric nomenclature was a direct result of the Vietnam War. We must acknowledge this as a historical fact, then looking forward, be more cognizant of what forces unduly shape the science of PTSD. One such force is that of culture. The complete failure of the ICD/DSM harmonization process is culturally based (with some degree of politics to be sure). Trauma in the rest of the world may mean torture, civil war, genocide, and a regular flow of refugees fleeing from where the trauma happened. To fully capture the trauma associated with events that might be persistent, repeated, and outside everyday human experience, it is argued that something more than PTSD is needed. ICD-11 will be adopting CPTSD to serve this purpose because such events are not uncommon, while DSM will not be adopting the term, as such events are rare to nonexistent in the United States. The modal PTSD patient in the United States is the veteran; this is where resources and research are directed via the National Center for PTSD. The DSM-5 definition has arguably been altered so as to best accommodate this modal PTSD patient. Since blast injury is considered the "signature wound" of contemporary warfare, perhaps it should come as no surprise that traumatic brain injury is listed in the PTSD differential diagnosis, seemingly due to symptom overlap. It is hard to imagine that any neurologist could confuse the common cold with meningitis because fever can be present in both conditions. The literature in which mild head injury and PTSD coappear in the title has skyrocketed in the United Sates. The compensation implications of either disorder separately are known, much less the synergistic effect of combining both. It is hard to imagine in what possible clinical circumstance a clinician would consider head injury in the PTSD differential outside the idiosyncratic circumstance of serving in the U.S. military. More than 80% of mild head injuries in the military do not occur in the combat theatre (Tsao, Alphonso, Griffin, Yurkiewicz, & Ling, 2013). The arranged marriage between PTSD and mild head injury is unfortunate and iatrogenic. In the case of CPTSD and the mild head injury–PTSD amalgamation, culture shaped the science, more so in the latter case.

"Clinical Neuropsychology: It is not about the testing. The only prerequisite for conducting neuropsychological testing is literacy, while knowledge of the syndrome and disease requires an experienced and knowledgeable clinician." This adage, which I call *Reflection #3,* is part of a lecture I put together on the principles and myths in neuropsychology. I called it a reflection and not a principle, as there are probably very few things that a jury of neuropsychologists in a room can agree on when it comes to the brain. By the very nature of what we study, we are not as uniform in our clinical mindset as we should be as to how to assess the brain as are our neurology colleagues. Our focus is on the cognitive testing. To be sure, testing is of variable importance. The clearest dichotomy is between pediatric and adult neuropsychology. An accurate intelligence and achievement score in a child is more often necessary than it is in an adult. As an adult neuropsychologist, in an outpatient neurology setting where the goal is primarily diagnosis, the clinical approach is different. In the case of dementia, the majority of my clinic referrals, the testing can continue up until the point that you have answered the referral question. In the first minute of the exam, when the patient gives the wrong year, given the proper clinical context and reliable collateral history, a diagnosis is made and the remainder of the formal testing can be terminated. In behavioral neurology this occurs daily. Our testing mindset is best illustrated by how a neuropsychologist might present a case to colleagues versus a neurologist. We typically give a cryptic history that includes demographics and the listing of a handful of symptoms followed by a flurry of test scores (as is sometimes the case on our discussion list serves). A neurology resident in case conference asking or reporting the test results at the onset, absent the detailed history first, will not likely complete the residency successfully. The take-home message is we need to think more like clinicians and not terminally degreed psychometricians, even within the framework of traditional clinical neuropsychology. In the case of PTSD, we have no choice. There are no required tests.

A topic of interest is the neurobiology of PTSD. As a predoctoral intern in 1989, I recall a lecture in which I was shown a single positron emission computed tomography (SPECT) image of an Alzheimer's patient. I learned that hypoperfusion seen in the temporal and parietal areas is a biomarker of the disease. In 2004, a positron emission tomography (PET) imaging technique used a novel tracer that was able to image amyloid in the brain, one of the pathological hallmarks of Alzheimer's disease (Klunk et al., 2004). At the time of this writing, no advanced imaging technique is recommended as standard practice in the evaluation of dementia. The most elementary application of translational research is the biomarker. When used clinically, a biomarker is a laboratory finding that reflects disease activity (Katz, 2004). Let us take the example of magnetic resonance imaging (MRI), the most popular biomarker of multiple sclerosis activity. To the extent that the MRI is used in lieu of a clinically meaningful endpoint in multiple sclerosis, that biomarker becomes a validated biomarker (some call it a *validated surrogate marker*). The MRI should predict some clinically meaningful outcome, or in the case of a drug trial, predict the effect of therapy. So blood pressure is a validated biomarker of a disease process, namely hypertension. Antihypertension drugs have a direct effect on the validated biomarker, blood pressure, which if uncontrolled may lead to an adverse clinical outcome. We are not required to test that clinical outcome because the biomarker of high blood pressure does a good enough job. While some areas of medicine have validated biomarkers, the problem in neurology and psychiatry is there are no validated biomarkers that are used in lieu of a clinical outcome. The exception is in genetics when used to diagnose a disorder like Huntington's disease absent a clinical examination (MacDonald et al., 1993). No treatments for any neurological disorder have been approved based solely on the use of a biomarker. There are no valid biomarkers accurate enough to displace the clinical examination. The founder and first president of the International Society for Traumatic Stress Studies wrote in a book review on the neurobiology of PTSD that the topic may be more of interest to "neuroscientists and libraries" versus the clinician (Figley, 2010). There are nevertheless, some research findings (i.e., hippocampal volume, physiological reactivity, and cognitive function twin studies) that may be of interest to neuropsychologists (we previously covered these; see Andrikopoulos & Greiffenstein, 2012). The seminal studies in this area were recently reviewed and commented on by the National Center for PTSD (Rasmusson & Abdallah, 2015). The review of Roger Pitman, who has done a great deal of work in this area, is also recommended (Pitman et al., 2012). While there can be no advances in diagnosis and treatment without the prerequisite success in the basic sciences, Satel and Lilienfeld (2013) remind us in their appropriately subtitled book, "The Seductive Appeal of Mindless Neuroscience," to remain skeptical.

Where do we go from here? Armed with a little bit more conviction on the topic of PTSD than was the case a few years ago, I would like to offer a handful of remarks regarding the direction we might want to consider if we are going to enter the PTSD space. To be successful, we first need to acquire a comparable clinical and research PTSD knowledge base to that of our PTSD colleagues. Our medicolegal PTSD chapter (Andrikopoulos & Greiffenstein, 2012) had the title "Something to Talk About," perfectly chosen by Greiffenstein to reflect the trepidation we felt when asked to write on PTSD in a popular forensic neuropsychology text. After all, we are both neuropsychologists with a special interest in forensic neuropsychology, with some experience conducting PTSD medicolegal evaluations. Since that first writing project, I have become less timid. Neuropsychology should be doing more than just talking about PTSD. This perhaps false bravado is owing to a confluence of two factors: an understanding of the clinical context and acquiring a greater fund of knowledge (Bowen, 2006). As for context, the request for a PTSD evaluation nowadays is almost exclusively done within a medicolegal context, and nobody understands that context better than neuropsychologists. Unlike the history of clinical neuroscience (a personal avocation of mine), knowledge of the history of PTSD is a precondition for an informed clinical opinion. Knowing the history is just as important as knowing the PTSD literature. A neophyte clinical psychologist would have little reason to question the content of the DSM. Understanding that it was not entirely science that shaped the PTSD concept emboldens one to express opinions that otherwise might not be articulated. I think neuropsychologists are generally more skeptical of their science than the average clinical psychologist. When that skepticism involves a diagnosis that is almost exclusively forensic, our scientific contribution carries weight. Our opinions on this topic can be expressed more readily and with more conviction despite the fact that we are not traumatologists. Our advantage is that we bring to the table a critical mindset that puts us in a position to test some hypotheses about this very interesting and controversial topic.

Acknowledgment

The author wishes to thank Anthony Risser for his invaluable assistance with this chapter.

References

Alcántara, C., Casement, M. D., & Lewis-Fernández, R. (2013). Conditional risk for PTSD among Latinos: A systematic review of racial/ethnic differences and sociocultural explanations. *Clinical Psychology Review*, *33*, 107–119.

Alhasnawi, S., Sadik, S., Rasheed, M., Baban, A., Al-Alak, M. M., Othman, A. Y. . . . Kessler, R. C. (2009). Iraq mental health survey study group: The prevalence and correlates of DSM-IV disorders in the Iraq Mental Health Survey (IMHS). *World Psychiatry*, *8*, 97–109.

American Psychiatric Association. (1952). *Diagnostic and Statistical Manual of Mental Disorders*. Washington, DC: Author.

American Psychiatric Association. (1980). *Diagnostic and Statistical Manual of Mental Disorders* (3rd ed.). Washington, DC: Author.

American Psychiatric Association. (1987). *Diagnostic and Statistical Manual of Mental Disorders* (Rev. 3rd ed.). Washington, DC: Author.

American Psychiatric Association. (1994). *Diagnostic and Statistical Manual of Mental Disorders* (4th ed.). Washington, DC: Author.

American Psychiatric Association. (2013). *Diagnostic and Statistical Manual of Mental Disorders* (5th ed.). Washington, DC: Author.

American Psychological Association Practice Central. (2012). Transition to the ICD-10-CM: What does it mean for psychologists? Retrieved December 14, 2015 from www.apapracticecentral.org/update/2012/02-09/transition.aspx

Anders, S., Frazier, P., & Frankfurt, S. (2011). Variations in criterion A and PTSD rates in a community sample of women. *Journal of Anxiety Disorders*, *25*(1), 176–184.

Andreasen, N. C. (2004). Acute and delayed posttraumatic stress disorders: A history and some issues (editorial). *American Journal of Psychiatry*, *161*, 1321–1323.

Andreasen, N. C. (2007). DSM and the death of phenomenology in America: An example of unintended consequences. *Schizophrenia Bulletin*, *33*, 108–112.

Andrews, G., & Peters, L. (1998). The psychometric properties of the composite international diagnostic interview. *Social Psychiatry and Psychiatric Epidemiology*, *33*, 80–88.

Andrews, G., Slade, T., & Peters, L. (1999). Classification in psychiatry: ICD-10 versus DSM-IV. *British Journal of Psychiatry*, *174*, 3–5.

Andrikopoulos, J., & Greiffenstein, M. F. (2012). Something to talk about: The status of post-traumatic stress disorder in clinical neuropsychology. In G. J. Larrabee (Ed.), *Forensic Neuropsychology: A Scientific Approach* (2nd ed., pp. 365–400). New York: Oxford University Press.

Armour, C., Elklit, A., Lauterbach, D., & Elhai, J. D. (2014). The DSM-5 dissociative-PTSD subtype: Can levels of depression, anxiety, hostility, and sleeping difficulties differentiate between dissociative-PTSD and PTSD in rape and sexual assault victims? *Journal of Anxiety Disorders*, *28*, 418–426.

Bassett, D., Buchwald, D., & Manson, S. (2014). Posttraumatic stress disorder and symptoms among American Indians and Alaska Natives: A review of the literature. *Social Psychiatry and Psychiatric Epidemiology*, *49*, 417–433.

Bayer, C. P., Klasen, F., & Adam, H. (2007). Association of trauma and PTSD symptoms with openness to reconciliation and feelings of revenge among former Ugandan and Congolese child soldiers. *Journal of the American Medical Association*, *298*, 555–559.

Beals, J., Novins, D. K., Spicer, P., Orton, H. D., Mitchell, C. M., Barón, A. E., Manson, S. M., & the AI-SUPERPFP Team (2004). Challenges in operationalizing the DSM-IV clinical significance criterion. *Archives of General Psychiatry*, *61*, 1197–1207.

Bedard-Gilligan, M., & Zoellner, L. A. (2008). The utility of the A1 and A2 criteria in the diagnosis of PTSD. *Behaviour Research and Therapy*, *46*(9), 1062–1069.

Berger, W., Coutinho, E. S., Figueira, I., Marques-Portella, C., Luz, M. P., Neylan, T. C., . . . Mendlowicz, M. V. (2012). Rescuers at risk: A systematic review and meta-regression analysis of the worldwide current prevalence and correlates of PTSD in rescue workers. *Social Psychiatry and Psychiatric Epidemiology*, *47*, 1001–1011.

Bianchini, K. J., Curtis, K. L., & Greve, K. W. (2006). Compensation and malingering in traumatic brain injury: A dose-response relationship? *The Clinical Neuropsychologist*, *20*, 831–847.

Bieliauskas, L. A. (1999). Personality and emotional functioning. In J. Sweet (Ed.), *Forensic Neuropsychology: Fundamentals and Practice* (pp. 121–144). Amsterdam/Lisse: Swets & Zeitlinger.

Bloom, S. L. (2000). Our hearts and our hopes are turned to peace: Origins of the international society for traumatic stress studies. In A. Shalev, R. Yehuda, & S. McFarlene (Eds.), *International Handbook of Human Response to Trauma* (pp. 27–50). New York: Plenum.

Boals, A., & Schuettler, D. (2009). PTSD symptoms in response to traumatic and non-traumatic events: The role of respondent perception and A2 criterion. *Journal of Anxiety Disorders*, *23*, 458–462.

Bodkin, J. A., Pope, H. G., Detke, M. J., & Hudson, J. I. (2007). Is PTSD caused by traumatic stress? *Journal of Anxiety Disorders*, *21*, 176–182.

Bonanno, G. A., Galea, S., Bucciarelli, A., & Vlahov, D. (2006). Psychological resilience after disaster: New York City in the aftermath of the September 11th terrorist attack. *Psychological Science*, *17*, 181–186.

Bowen, J. L. (2006). Educational strategies to promote clinical diagnostic reasoning. *New England Journal of Medicine*, *355*, 2217–2225.

Bradshaw, J. (2012). Petition seeks to dump DSM and adopt ICD. *The National Psychologist*. Retrieved December 14, 2015 from http://nationalpsychologist.com/2012/09/petition-seeks-to-dump-dsm-and-adopt-icd/101764.html

Breslau, N., & Davis, G. C. (1987). Posttraumatic stress disorder: The etiologic specificity of wartime stressors. *American Journal of Psychiatry*, *144*, 578–583.

Breslau, N., & Kessler, R. C. (2001). The stressor criterion in DSM-IV posttraumatic stress disorder: An empirical investigation. *Biological Psychiatry*, *50*, 699–704.

Breslau, N., Kessler, R. C., Chilcoat, H. D., Schultz, L. R., Davis, G. C., & Andreski, P. (1998). Trauma and posttraumatic stress disorder in the community: The 1996 Detroit area survey of trauma. *Archives of General Psychiatry*, *55*, 626–632.

Brewin, C. R. (2003). *Post-Traumatic Stress Disorder: Malady or Myth?* New Haven, CT: Yale University Press.

Brewin, C. R., Andrews, B., & Rose, S. (2000). Fear, helplessness, and horror in posttraumatic stress disorder: Investigating *DSM-IV* criterion A2 in victims of violent crime. *Journal of Traumatic Stress*, *13*(3), 499–509.

Brewin, C. R., Andrews, B., & Valentine, J. D. (2000). Meta-analysis of risk factors for posttraumatic stress disorder in trauma-exposed adults. *Journal of Consulting and Clinical Psychology*, *68*, 748–766.

Brewin, C. R., Lanius, R. A., Novac, A., Schnyder, U., & Galea, S. (2009). Reformulating PTSD for DSM-V: Life after criterion A. *Journal of Traumatic Stress*, *22*(5), 366–373.

Briere, J. (1995). *Trauma Symptoms Inventory Professional Manual*. Odessa, FL: Psychological Assessment Resources.

Bromet, E., Sonnega, A., & Kessler, R. C. (1998). Risk factors for DSM-III-R posttraumatic stress disorder: Findings from the national comorbidity survey. *American Journal of Epidemiology*, *147*, 353–361.

Bryant, R. A. (1996). Predictors of post-traumatic stress disorder following burns injury. *Burns*, *22*, 89–92.

Bryant, R. A. (2007). Does dissociation further our understanding of PTSD? *Journal of Anxiety Disorders*, *21*(2), 183–191.

Bryant, R. A. (2011). Acute stress disorder as a predictor of posttraumatic stress disorder: A systematic review. *Journal of Clinical Psychiatry*, *72*, 233–239.

Bryant, R. A. (2012). Simplifying complex PTSD: Comment on Resick et al. (2012). *Journal of Traumatic Stress*, *25*, 252–253.

Camarota, S. A., & Zeigler, K. (2015). *One in Five US Residents Speaks Foreign Language at Home. Center for Immigration Studies.* Retrieved July 31, 2017 from http://cis. org/sites/cis. org/files/camarota-language-15.

Carlson, E. B., Dalenberg, C., & McDade-Montez, E. (2012). Dissociation in posttraumatic stress disorder part I: Definitions and review of research. *Psychological Trauma: Theory, Research, Practice, and Policy*, *4*, 479–489.

Cloitre, M. (2011). Treatment of complex PTSD: Results of the ISTSS expert clinician survey on best practices. *Journal of Traumatic Stress*, *24*, 615–627.

Cloitre, M., Garvert, D. W., Brewin, C. R., Bryant, R. A., & Maercker, A. (2013). Evidence for proposed ICD-11 PTSD and complex PTSD: A latent profile analysis. *European Journal of Psychotraumatology*, *4*(20706), 1–12.

Courtios, C. A. (2004). Complex trauma, complex reactions: Assessment and treatment. *Psychotherapy: Theory, Research, Practice, Training*, *41*, 412–425.

Creamer, M., Burgess, P., & McFarlane, A. C. (2001). Posttraumatic stress disorder: Findings from the Australian national survey of mental health and well-being. *Psychological Medicine*, *31*, 1237–1247.

Creamer, M., McFarlane, A. C., & Burgess, P. (2005). Psychopathology following trauma: The role of subjective experience. *Journal of Affective Disorders*, *86*, 175–182.

Dalenberg, C., & Carlson, E. B. (2012). Dissociation in posttraumatic stress disorder part II: How theoretical models fit the empirical evidence and recommendations for modifying the diagnostic criteria for PTSD. *Psychological Trauma: Theory, Research, Practice, and Policy*, *4*, 551–559.

Dancu, C. V., Riggs, D. S., Hearst-Ikeda, D., Shoyer, B. G., & Foa, E. B. (1996). Dissociative experiences and posttraumatic stress disorder among female victims of criminal assault and rape. *Journal of Traumatic Stress*, *9*(2), 253–267.

David, A. S. (1992). Frontal lobology: Psychiatry's new pseudoscience. *British Journal of Psychiatry*, *161*, 244–248.

Davidson, J.R.T., Hughes, D., Blazer, D. G., & George, L. K. (1991). Post-traumatic stress disorder in the community: An epidemiological study. *Psychological Medicine*, *21*, 713–721.

Decker, H. (2013). *The Making of DSM-III®: A Diagnostic Manual's Conquest of American Psychiatry*. New York: Oxford Press.

Department of Veterans Affairs. (2008). Posttraumatic stress disorder. *Federal Register*, *73*, 64208 (October 29, 2008, to be codified at 38 C.F.R., pt. 3).

Dohrenwend, B. P., Turner, J. B., Turse, N. A., Adams, B. G., Koenen, K. C., & Marshall, R. (2006). The psychological risks of Vietnam for U.S. veterans: A revisit with new data and methods. *Science*, *313*, 979–982.

Edens, J. F., Otto, R. K., & Dwyer, T. J. (1998). Susceptibility of the trauma symptom inventory to malingering. *Journal of Personality Assessment*, *71*, 379–392.

Elhai, J. D., Gray, M. J., Kashdan, T. B., & Franklin, C. L. (2005). Which instruments are most commonly used to assess traumatic event exposure and posttraumatic effects?: A survey of traumatic stress professionals. *Journal of Traumatic Stress*, *18*, 541–545.

Elhai, J. D., Gray, M. J., Naifeh, J. A., Butcher, J. J., Davis, J. L., Falsetti, S. A., & Best, C. L. (2005). Utility of the trauma symptom inventory's atypical response scale in detecting malingered post-traumatic stress disorder. *Assessment*, *12*, 210–219.

Elhai, J. D., Grubaugh, A. L., Kashdan, T. B., & Frueh, B. C. (2008). Empirical examination of a proposed refinement to DSM-IV posttraumatic stress disorder symptom criteria using the national comorbidity survey replication data. *Journal of Clinical Psychiatry*, *69*, 597–602.

Elklit, A., & Christiansen, D. M. (2010). ASD and PTSD in rape victims. *Journal of Interpersonal Violence*, *25*, 1470–1488.

Elklit, A., Hyland, P., & Shelven, M. (2014). Evidence of symptom profiles consistent with posttraumatic stress disorder and complex posttraumatic stress disorder in different trauma samples. *European Journal of Psychotraumatology*, *5*(24221), 1–10.

Endicott, J., & Spitzer, R. L. (1978). A diagnostic interview: The schedule for affective disorders and schizophrenia. *Archives of General Psychiatry*, *35*, 837–844.

Evans, S. C., Reed, G. M., Roberts, M. C., Esparza, P., Watts, A. D., Correia, J. M., . . . Saxena, S. (2013). Psychologists' perspectives on the diagnostic classification of mental disorders: Results from the WHO-IUPsyS global survey. *International Journal of Psychology*, *48*, 177–193.

Farmer, A., & McGuffin, A. (1999). Comparing ICD-10 and DSM-IV. *British Journal of Psychiatry*, *175*, 587–588.

Fazel, M., Wheeler, J., & Danesh, J. (2005). Prevalence of serious mental disorder in 7000 refugees resettled in Western countries: A systematic review. *Lancet*, *365*, 1309–1314.

Feighner, J. P., Robins, E., Guze, S. B., Woodruff, R. A, Jr., Winokur, G., & Munoz, R. (1972). Diagnostic criteria for use in psychiatric research. *Archives of General Psychiatry*, *26*, 57–63.

Figley, C. R. (1978). Psychosocial adjustment among Vietnam veterans: An overview of the research. In Figley, C. R. (Ed.), *Stress Disorders Among Vietnam Veterans* (pp. 57–70). New York: Brunner/Mazel.

Figley, C. R. (2010). Now we know much about the neurobiology of PTSD. So what? [Review of the book *stress disorder: Basic science and clinical practice*]. *PsycCRITQUES*, *55*.

First, M. B. (2009). Harmonisation of ICD-11 and DSM-V: Opportunities and challenges. *British Journal of Psychiatry*, *195*, 382–390.

First, M. B., & Pincus, H. A. (1999). "Classification in psychiatry: ICD-10 v. DSM-IV": A response [Peer commentary by M. B. First and H. A. Pincus]. *British Journal of Psychiatry*, *175*, 205–209.

Fisher, C. M. (1995). Similar disorders viewed with different perspectives (letter). *Archives of Neurology*, *52*, 743.

Foa, E. B. (1995). *Posttraumatic Diagnostic Scale Manual*. Minneapolis, MN: NCS Pearson.

Foa, E. B. (2013, unpublished). *Posttraumatic Diagnostic Scale-5 Manual*. Philadelphia, PA: Author.

Foa, E. B, Keane, T. M., & Friedman, M. J. (2000). *Effective Treatments for PTSD: Practice Guidelines from the International Society for Traumatic Stress Studies*. New York: Guilford Press.

Frances, A. (2009). A warning sign on the road to DSM-V: Beware of its unintended consequences. *Psychiatric Times*, *26*, 1–4.

Frances, A. (2010). The forensic risks of DSM-V and how to avoid them. *Journal of the American Academy of Psychiatry*, *38*, 11–14.

Frances, A. J. (2012a). DSM5: How reliable is reliable enough? *Psychology Today "DSM5 in Distress"* blog. Retrieved December 12, 2015 from www.psychologytoday.com/blog/dsm5-in-distress

Frances, A. J. (2012b). DSM 5 field trials discredit APA. *Psychology Today "DSM5 in Distress"* blog. Retrieved (Dec. 12, 2015) from www.psychologytoday.com/blog/dsm5-in-distress

Frances, A. (2013). *Saving Normal: An Insider's Revolt against Out-of-Control Psychiatric Diagnosis, DSM-5, Big Pharma, and the Medicalization of Ordinary Life*. New York: William Morrow.

Frances, A., & Widiger, T. (2012). Psychiatric diagnosis: Lessons from the DSM-IV past and cautions for the DSM-5 future. *Annual Review of Clinical Psychology*, *8*, 109–130.

Freedman, R., Lewis, D. A., Michels, R., Pine, D. S., Schultz, S. K., Tamminga, C. A., . . . Yager, J. (2013). The initial field trials of *DSM-5*: New blooms and old thorns. *American Journal of Psychiatry*, *170*, 1–5.

Friedman, M. J. (2013). Finalizing PTSD in DSM-5: Getting here from there and where to go next. *Journal of Traumatic Stress*, *26*, 548–556.

Friedman, M. J., Resick, P. A., Bryant, R. A., & Brewin, C. R. (2011). Considering PTSD for DSM-5. *Depression and Anxiety, 28*, 750–769.

Frueh, B. C., Grubaugh, A. L., Elhai, J. D., & Buckley, T. C. (2007). U.S. department of veterans affairs disability policies for posttraumatic stress disorder: Administrative trends and implications for treatment, rehabilitation, and research. *American Journal of Public Health, 97*, 2143–2145.

Galea, S., Ahern, J., Resnick, H., Kilpatrick, D., Bucuvalas, M., Gold, J., & Vlahov, D. (2002). Psychological sequelae of the September 11 terrorist attacks in New York City. *New England Journal of Medicine, 346*, 982–987.

Galea, S., Vlahov, D., Resnick, H., Ahern, J., Susser, E., Gold, J., . . . Kilpatrick, D. (2003). Trends of probable post-traumatic stress disorder in New York City after the September 11 terrorist attacks. *The American Journal of Epidemiology, 158*, 514–524.

Gradus, J. L., Qin, P., Lincoln, A. K., Miller, M., Lawler, E., Sorensen, H. T., & Lash, T. L. (2010). Posttraumatic stress disorder and completed suicide. *American Journal of Epidemiology, 171*, 721–727.

Haber-Schaim, N., Solomon, Z., Bleich, A., & Kottler, M. (1988). The prevalence of post-traumatic stress disorder (correspondence). *The New England Journal of Medicine, 318*, 1691.

Haley, S. A. (1974). When the patient reports atrocities: Specific treatment considerations of the Vietnam veteran. *Archives of General Psychiatry, 30*, 191–196.

Hannaford, P. C., & Owen-Smith, V. (1998). Using epidemiological data to guide clinical practice: Review of studies on cardiovascular disease and use of combined oral contraceptives. *British Medical Journal, 316*, 984–992.

Heilbronner, R. L., Sweet, J. J., Morgan, J. E., Larrabee, G. J., Millis, S. R., & Conference Participants. (2009). American academy of clinical neuropsychology consensus conference statement on the neuropsychological assessment of effort, response bias, and malingering. *The Clinical Neuropsychologist, 23*, 1–37.

Helzer, J. E., & Robins, L. N. (1988). The prevalence of post-traumatic stress disorder (correspondence). *The New England Journal of Medicine, 318*, 1692.

Helzer, J. E., Robins, L. N., & Davis, D. H. (1976). Depressive disorders in Vietnam returnees. *Journal of Nervous and Mental Disorders, 163*, 177–185.

Helzer, J. E., Robins, L. N., & McEvoy, L. (1987). Post-traumatic stress disorder in the general population: Findings of the epidemiologic catchment area survey. *New England Journal of Medicine, 317*, 1630–1634.

Herman, J. L. (1992). Complex PTSD: A syndrome in survivors of prolonged and repeated trauma. *Journal of Traumatic Stress, 5*, 377–391.

Herman, J. L. (2012). CPTSD is a distinct entity: Comment on Resick et al. (2012). *Journal of Traumatic Stress, 25*, 256–257.

Hinton, D. E., & Lewis-Fernández, R. (2011). The cross-cultural validity of posttraumatic stress disorder: Implications for DSM-5. *Depression and Anxiety, 28*, 783–801.

Hoge, C. W. (2015). Measuring the long-term impact of war-zone military service across generations and changing posttraumatic stress disorder definitions (editorial). *JAMA Psychiatry, 72*, 861–862.

Horwitz, A. V., & Gold, G. N. (2011). The checkered history of American psychiatric epidemiology. *The Milbank Quarterly, 89*, 628–657.

Horowitz, M. J. (1976). *Stress Response Syndromes (Classical Psychoanalysis and Its Applications)*. Lanham, MD: Jason Aronson Publishers.

Horowitz, M. J. (1986). *Stress Response Syndromes*. Lanham, MD: Jason Aronson Publishers.

Horowitz, M. J., & Solomon, G. F. (1975). A prediction of delayed stress response syndromes in Vietnam veterans. *Journal of Social Issues, 31*(4), 67–79.

Horowitz, M. J., Wilner, N., & Alvarez, W. (1979). Impact of event scale: A measure of subjective stress. *Psychosomatic Medicine, 41*, 209–218.

Hotopf, M., & Wessely, S. (2006). Neuropsychological changes following military service in Iraq: Case proven, but what is the significance? (editorial). *Journal of the American Medical Association, 296*, 574–575.

Hull, A. M., Alexander, D. A., & Klein, S. (2002). Survivors of the Piper Alpha oil platform disaster: Long-term follow-up study. *British Journal of Psychiatry, 181*, 433–438.

Insel, T., Cuthbert, B., Garvey, M., Heinssen, R., Pine, D. S., Quinn, K., . . . Wang, P. (2010). Research domain criteria (RdoC): Toward a new classification framework for research on mental disorders. *American Journal of Psychiatry, 167*, 748–751.

Jablensky, A. (2009). Towards ICD-11 and DSM-V: Issues beyond harmonisation. *British Journal of Psychiatry, 195*, 379–381.

Jelinek, M. (2005). Clinical epidemiology: A deconstruction. *Internal Medicine Journal, 35*, 104–105.

Jones, K. D. (2012). A critique of the DSM-5 field trials. *The Journal of Nervous and Mental Disease, 200*, 517–519.

Joynt, R. J. (2001) Changes · People · Comments. *Neurology, 77*(6) A31–A32.

Karam, E. G., Andrews, G., Bromet, E., Petukhova, M., Ruscio, A. M., Salamoun, M., . . . Kessler, R. C. (2010). The role of criterion A2 in the DSM-IV diagnosis of post-traumatic stress disorder. *Biological Psychiatry, 68*(5), 465–473.

Karam, E. G., Friedman, M. J., Hill, E. D., Kessler, R. C., McLaughlin, K. A., Petukhova, M., . . . Koenen, K. C. (2014). Cumulative traumas and risk thresholds: 12-month PTSD in the World Mental Health (WMH) surveys. *Depression and Anxiety, 31*(2), 130–142.

Katz, R. (2004). Biomarkers and surrogate markers: An FDA perspective. *NeuroRX, 1*, 189–195.

Keane, T. M., & Penk, W. E. (1988). The prevalence of post-traumatic stress disorder (correspondence). *The New England Journal of Medicine, 318*, 1690–1691.

Kendell, R. (1991). The relationship between DSM-IV and ICD-10. *Journal of Abnormal Psychology, 100*(3), 297–301.

Kessler, R. C., Berglund, P., Demler, O., Jin, R., Merikangas, K. R., & Walters, E. R. (2005). Lifetime prevalence and age-of-onset distributions of DSM-IV disorders in the national comorbidity survey replication. *Archives of General Psychiatry, 62*, 593–602.

Kessler, R. C., McGonagle, K. A., Zhao, S., Nelson, C. B., Hughes, M., Eshleman, S., . . . Kendler, K. S. (1994). Lifetime and 12-month prevalence of DSM-III-R psychiatric disorders in the United States: Results from the national comorbidity survey. *Archives of General Psychiatry, 51*, 8–19.

Kessler, R. C., Ormel, J., Petukhova, M., McLaughlin, K. A., Green, J. G., Russo, L. J., . . . Andrade, L. (2011). Development of lifetime comorbidity in the World Health Organization world mental health surveys. *Archives of General Psychiatry, 68*, 90–100.

Kessler, R. C., Sonnega, A., Bromet, E., Hughes, M., & Nelson, C. B. (1995). Posttraumatic stress disorder in the national comorbidity survey. *Archives of General Psychiatry*, *52*, 1048–1060.

Kilpatrick, D. G. (2013). The DSM-5 got PTSD right: Comment on Friedman (2013). *Journal of Traumatic Stress*, *26*(5), 563–566.

Kilpatrick, D. G., Resnick, H. S., & Acierno, R. E. (2009). Should PTSD criterion A be retained? *Journal of Traumatic Stress*, *22*, 374–383.

Kilpatrick, D. G., Resnick, H. S., Freedy, J. R., Pelcovitz, D., Resick, P., Roth, S., & van der Kolk, B. (1998). Posttraumatic stress disorder field trial: Evaluation of the PTSD construct- criteria A through E. In T. A. Widiger, A. J. Frances, H. A. Pincus, R. Ross, M. B. First, W. Davis, & Line, M. (Eds.), *DSM-IV Sourcebook* (Vol. 4, pp. 803–844). Washington, DC: American Psychiatric Association.

Klunk, W. E., Engler, H., Nordberg, A., Wang, Y., Blomqvist, G., Holt, D. P., . . . Långström, B. (2004). Imaging brain amyloid in Alzheimer's disease with Pittsburgh Compound-B. *Annals of Neurology*, *55*, 306–319.

Kraemer, B., Wittmann, L., Jenewein, J., Maier, T., & Schnyder, U. (2009). Is the stressor criterion dispensable? A contribution to the criterion A debate from a Swiss sample of survivors of the 2004 tsunami. *Psychopathology*, *42*, 333–336.

Kroenke, K., Spitzer, R. L., & Williams, J. B. (2001). The PHQ-9: Validity of a brief depression severity measure. *Journal of Internal Medicine*, *16*, 606–613.

Kukull, W. A., & Ganguli, M. (2012). Generalizability: The trees, the forest, and the low-hanging fruit. *Neurology*, *78*, 1886–1891.

Kulka, R. A., Schlenger, W. E., Fairbank, J. A., Hough, R. L., Jordan, B. K., Marmar, C. R., . . l. Weiss, D. L. (1990). *Trauma and the Vietnam War Generation*. New York: Brunner/Mazel Inc.

Lanius, R. A., Brand, B., Vermetten, E., Frewen, P. A., & Spiegel, D. (2012). The dissociative subtype of posttraumatic stress disorder: Rationale, clinical and neurobiological evidence, and implications. *Depression and Anxiety*, *29*, 701–708.

Larrabee, G. J. (1998). Somatic malingering on the MMPI and MMPI-2 in personal injury litigants. *The Clinical Neuropsychologist*, *12*, 179–188.

Larrabee, G. J., Millis, S. R., & Meyers, J. E. (2009). 40 plus or minus 10, a new magical number: Response to Russell. *The Clinical Neuropsychologist*, *23*, 841–849.

Lees-Haley, P. R., English, L. T., & Glenn, W. J. (1991). A fake bad scale on the MMPI-2 for personal injury claimants. *Psychological Reports*, *68*, 203–210.

Lifton, R. J. (1968). *Death in Life: Survivors of Hiroshima*. New York: Random House.

Lifton, R. J. (1973). *Home From the War: Vietnam Veterans: Neither Victims nor Executioners*. New York: Touchstone.

Lindauer, R.J.L. (2012). Child maltreatment—Clinical PTSD diagnosis not enough?!: Comment on Resick et al. 2012. *Journal of Traumatic Stress*, *25*, 258–259.

Luciano, M. (2014). Proposals for ICD-11: A report for WPA membership. *World Psychiatry*, *13*, 206–208.

MacDonald, M. E., Barnes, G., Srinidhi, J., Duyao, M. P., Ambrose, C. M., Myers, R. H., Gray, J., Conneally, P. M., Young, A., Penney, J., et al. (1993). Gametic but not somatic instability of CAG repeat length in Huntington's disease. *Journal of Medical Genetics*, *30*, 982–986.

Maercker, A., Brewin, C. R., Bryant, R. A., Cloitre, M., Reed, G. M., van Ommeren, M., . . . Saxena, S. (2013). Proposals for mental disorders specifically associated with stress in the international classification of diseases-11. *The Lancet*, *381*, 1683–1685.

Maercker, A., & Perkonigg, A. (2013). Applying an international perspective in defining PTSD and related disorders: Comment on Friedman (2013) [Peer commentary on "Finalizing PTSD in DSM-5: Getting here from there and where to go next" by A. Maercker and A. Perkonigg]. *Journal of Traumatic Stress*, *26*, 560–562.

Maier, T. (2007). Weathers' and Keane's, "The Criterion A problem revisited: Controversies and challenges in defining and measuring psychological trauma. *Journal of Traumatic Stress*, *20*(5), 915–916.

Marmar, C. R., Schlenger, W., Henn-Haase, C., Qian, M., Purchia, E., Li, M., . . . Kulka, R. A. (2015). Course of posttraumatic stress disorder 40 years after the Vietnam war: Findings from the national Vietnam veterans longitudinal study. *JAMA Psychiatry*, *72*, 875–881.

Marx, B. P., Miller, M. W., Sloan, D. M., Litz, B. T., Kaloupek, D. G., & Keane, T. M. (2008). Military-related PTSD, current disability policies, and malingering (letter). *American Journal of Public Health*, *98*(5), 773–774.

McDonald, S. D., & Calhoun, P. S. (2010). The diagnostic accuracy of the PTSD checklist: A critical review. *Clinical Psychology Review*, *30*, 976–987.

McHugh, P. R., & Treisman, G. (2007). PTSD: A problematic diagnostic category. *Journal of Anxiety Disorders*, *21*, 211–222.

McNally, R. J. (2003). Progress and controversy in the study of posttraumatic stress disorder. *Annual Review of Psychology*, *54*, 229–252.

McNally, R. J. (2006). Applying biological data in the forensic and policy areas. *Annals of New York Academy of Sciences*, *1071*, 267–276.

McNally, R. J. (2009). Can we fix PTSD in DSM-V? *Depression and Anxiety*, *26*, 597–600.

McNally, R. J., & Breslau, N. (2008). Does virtual trauma cause posttraumatic stress disorder? *American Psychologist*, *63*, 282–283.

McNally, R. J., Lasko, N. B., Clancy, S. A., Macklin, M. L., Pitman, R. K., & Orr, S. P. (2004). Psychophysiological responding during script-driven imagery in people reporting abduction by space aliens. *Psychological Science*, *15*, 493–497.

Mittenberg, W., Patton, C., Canyock, E. M., & Condit, D. C. (2002). Base rates of malingering and symptom exaggeration. *Journal of Clinical and Experimental Neuropsychology*, *24*, 1094–1102.

Morina, N., van Emmerik, A. A., Andrews, B., & Brewin, C. R. (2014). Comparison of DSM-IV and proposed ICD-11 formulations of PTSD among civilian survivors of war and war veterans. *Journal of Traumatic Stress*, *27*, 647–654.

Nasreddine, Z. S., Phillips, N. A., Bédirian, V., Charbonneau, S., Whitehead, V., Collin, I., . . . Chertkow, H. (2005). The montreal cognitive assessment, MoCA: A brief screening tool for mild cognitive impairment. *Journal of the American Geriatrics Society*, *53*, 695–699.

Nicosia, G. (2001). *Home to War: A History of the Vietnam Veterans' Movement*. New York: Crown Publishers.

Nielssen, O. B., & Large, M. M. (2011). Removing the A2 criteria will not rescue posttraumatic stress disorder (letter). *Biological Psychiatry*, *70*, e23.

Nordheimer, J. (1971, May 26). From Dak to Detroit. *New York Times*, p. A1.

Norris, F. H. (1992). Epidemiology of trauma: Frequency and impact of different potentially traumatic events on different demographic groups. *Journal of Consulting and Clinical Psychology*, *60*, 409–418.

North, C. S., Nixon, S. J., Shariat, S., Mallonee, S., McMillen, J. C., Spitznagel, E. L., & Smith, E. M. (1999). Psychiatric disorders among survivors of the Oklahoma City bombing. *Journal of the American Medical Association*, *282*, 755–762.

North, C. S., & Oliver, J. (2013). Analysis of the longitudinal course of PTSD in 716 survivors of 10 disasters. *Social Psychiatry and Psychiatric Epidemiology*, *48*(8), 1189–1197.

O'Donnell, M. L., Alkemade, N., Nickerson, A., Creamer, M., McFarlane, A. C., Silove, D., . . . Forbes, D. (2014). Impact of the diagnostic changes to post-traumatic stress disorder for DSM-5 and the proposed changes to ICD-11. *British Journal of Psychiatry*, *205*, 230–235.

O'Donnell, M. L., Creamer, M., McFarlane, A. C., Silove, D., & Bryant, R. A. (2010). Should A2 be a diagnostic requirement for posttraumatic stress disorder in DSM-V? *Psychiatry Research*, *176*, 257–260.

Olaya, B., Alonso, J., Atwoli, L., Kessler, R. C., Vilagut, G., & Haro, J. M. (2015). Association between traumatic events and post-traumatic stress disorder: Results from the ESEMeD-Spain study. *Epidemiology and Psychiatric Sciences*, *24*, 172–183.

Ozer, E. J., Best, S. R., Lipsey, T. L., & Weiss, D. S. (2008). Predictors of posttraumatic stress disorder and symptoms in adults: A meta-analysis. *Psychological Trauma: Theory, Research, Practice and Policy*, *1* (Suppl, S), 3–36.

Perilla, J. L., Norris, F. H., & Lavizzo, E. A. (2002). Ethnicity, culture, and disaster response: Identifying and explaining ethnic differences in PTSD six months after Hurricane Andrew. *Journal of Social and Clinical Psychology*, *21*, 20–45.

Peters, L., Slade, T., & Andrews, G. (1999). A comparison of ICD10 and DSM-IV criteria for posttraumatic stress disorder. *Journal of Traumatic Stress*, *12*, 335–343.

Pfaltz, M. C., Michael, T., Meyer, A. H., & Wilhelm, F. H. (2013). Reexperiencing symptoms, dissociation, and avoidance behaviors in daily life of patients with PTSD and patients with panic disorder with agoraphobia. *Journal of Traumatic Stress*, *26*, 443–450.

Pham, P. N., Weinstein, H. M., & Longman, T. (2004). Trauma and PTSD symptoms in Rwanda: Implications for attitudes toward justice and reconciliation. *Journal of the American Medical Association*, *292*, 602–612.

Pitman, R. K., Rasmusson, A. M., Koenen, K. C., Shin, L. M., Orr, S. P., Gilbertson, M. W., . . . Liberzon, I. (2012). Biological studies of post-traumatic stress disorder. *Nature Reviews Neuroscience*, *13*, 769–787.

Rasmusson, A. M., & Abdallah, C. G. (2015). Biomarkers for treatment and diagnosis. *PTSD Research Quarterly*, *26*(1), 1–4.

Reed, G. M. (2010). Toward ICD-11: Improving the clinical utility of WHO's international classification of mental disorders. *Professional Psychology: Research and Practice*, *41*, 457–464.

Reed, G. M., Correia, J. M., Esparza, P., Saxena, S., & Maj, M. (2011). The WPA-WHO global survey of psychiatrists' attitudes towards mental disorders classification. *World Psychiatry*, *10*, 118–131.

Regier, D. A., Kaelber, C. T., Roper, M. T., Rae, D. S., & Sartorius, N. (1994). The ICD-10 clinical field trial for mental and behavioral disorders: Results in Canada and the United States. *American Journal of Psychiatry*, *151*, 1340–1350.

Regier, D. A., Narrow, W. E., Clarke, D. E., Kraemer, H. C., Kuramoto, S. J., Kuhl, E. A., & Kupfer, D. J. (2013). DSM-5 field trials in the United Stated and Canada, Part II: Test-retest reliability of selected categorical diagnoses. *American Journal of Psychiatry*, *170*, 59–70.

Resick, P. A., Bovin, M. J., Calloway, A. L., Dick, A. M., King, M. W., Mitchell, K. S. . . . Wolfe, E. J. (2012). A critical evaluation of the complex PTSD literature: Implications for DSM-5. *Journal of Traumatic Stress*, *25*, 241–251.

Roberts, A. L., Dohrenwend, B. P., Aiello, A. E., Wright, R. J., Maercker, A., Galea, S., & Koenen, K. C. (2012). The stressor criterion for posttraumatic stress disorder: Does it matter? *Journal of Clinical Psychiatry*, *73*(2), e264–e270.

Roberts, A. L., Gilman, S. E., Breslau, J., Breslau, N., & Koenen, K. C. (2011). Race/ethnic differences in exposure to traumatic events, development of post-traumatic stress disorder, and treatment-seeking for post-traumatic stress disorder in the United States. *Psychological Medicine*, *41*, 71–83.

Robins, E., & Guze, S. B. (1970). Establishment of diagnostic validity in psychiatric illness: its application to schizophrenia. *American Journal of Psychiatry*, *126*, 983–987.

Robins, L. N. (1990). Steps toward evaluating post-traumatic stress reaction as a psychiatric disorder. *Journal of Applied Social Psychology*, *20*, 1674–1677.

Robins, L. N,. Helzer, J. E., Croughan, J., & Ratcliff, K. S. (1981). National institute of mental health diagnostic interview schedule: Its history, characteristics, and validity. *Archives of General Psychiatry*, *38*, 381–389.

Robins, L. N., Helzer, J. E., & Davis, D. H. (1975). Narcotic use in Southeast Asia and afterward: An interview study of 898 Vietnam returnees. *Archives of General Psychiatry*, *32*(8), 955–961.

Robins, L. N., Helzer, J. E., Weissman, M. M., Orvaschel, H., Gruenberg, E., Burke, J. D. Jr., & Regier, D. A. (1984). Lifetime prevalence of specific psychiatric disorders in three sites. *Archives of General Psychiatry*, *41*, 949–958.

Robins, L. N., Wing, J., Wittchen, H. U., Helzer, J. E., Babor, T. F., Burke, J., . . . Regier, D. A. (1988). The composite international diagnostic interview: An epidemiologic instrument suitable for use in conjunction with different diagnostic systems and in different cultures. *Archives of General Psychiatry*, *45*, 1069–1077.

Roemer, L., Orsillo, S. M., Borkovec, T. D., & Litz, B. T. (1998). Emotional response at the time of potentially traumatizing event and PTSD symptomatology: A preliminary retrospective analysis of the DSM-IV criterion A-2. *Journal of Behavior Therapy and Experimental Psychiatry*, *29*, 123–130.

Rosen, G. M. (2004a). Malingering and the PTSD database. In Gerald Rosen (Ed.), *Post-Traumatic Stress Disorder: Issues and Controversies* (pp. 85–99). New York: John Wiley and Sons.

Rosen, G. M. (2004b). Litigation and reported rates of posttraumatic stress disorder. *Personality and Individual Differences*, *36*, 1291–1294.

Rosen, G. M., Lilienfeld, S. O., Frueh, B. C., McHugh, P. R., & Spitzer, R. L. (2010). Reflections on PTSD's future in DSM-V. *British Journal of Psychiatry*, *197*, 343–344.

Roth, S., Newman, E., Pelcovitz, D., van der Kolk, B., & Mandel, F. S. (1997). Complex PTSD in victims exposed to sexual and physical abuse: Results from the DSM-IV field trial for posttraumatic stress disorder. *Journal of Traumatic Stress*, *10*, 539–555.

Sartorius, N., Kaelber, C. T., Cooper, J. E., Roper, M. T., Rae, D. S., Gulbinat, W., et al. (1993). Progress toward achieving a common language in psychiatry: Results from the field trial of the clinical guidelines accompanying the WHO classification of mental and behavioral disorders in ICD-10. *Archives of General Psychiatry*, *50*, 115–124.

Sartorius, N., Ustün, T. B., Korten, A., Cooper, J. E., & van Drimmelen, J. (1995). Progress toward achieving a common language in psychiatry, II: Results from the international field trials of the ICD-10 diagnostic criteria for research for mental and behavioral disorders. *American Journal of Psychiatry*, *152*, 1427–1437.

Satel, S., & Lilienfeld, S. (2013). *Brainwashed: The Seductive Appeal of Mindless Neuroscience*. New York: Basic Books.

Schnurr, P. P., Spiro III, A., Vielhauer, M. J., Findler, M. N., & Hamblen, J. L. (2002). Trauma in the lives of older men: Findings from the normative aging study. *Journal of Clinical Geropsychology*, *8*, 175–187.

Scott, W. J. (1990). PTSD in DSM-III: A case in the politics of diagnosis and disease. *Social Problems*, *37*(3), 294–310.

Shatan, C. F. (1972, May 6). Post-Vietnam syndrome. *The New York Times*, pp. 1971–1972.

Shatan, C. F. (1973). The grief of soldiers: Vietnam combat veterans' self-help movement. *American Journal of Orthopsychiatry*, *43*(4), 640–653.

Shatan, C. F. (1990). "A true child of trauma"—Sarah Haley: 1939–1989. *Journal of Traumatic Stress*, *3*(3), 477–481.

Shore, J. H., Vollmer, W. M., & Tatum, E. L. (1989). Community patterns of posttraumatic stress disorders. *Journal of Nervous and Mental Disorders*, *177*, 681–685.

Silove, D., Bateman, C. R., Brooks, R. T., Fonseca, C. A., Steel, Z., Rodger, J., . . . Bauman, A. (2008). Estimating clinically relevant mental disorders in a rural and an urban setting in postconflict Timor Leste. *Archives of General Psychiatry*, *65*, 1205–1212.

Spinazzola, J., Blaustein, M., & Van Der Kolk, B. A. (2005). Posttraumatic stress disorder treatment outcome research: The study of unrepresentative samples? *Journal of Traumatic Stress*, *18*, 425–436.

Spitzer, R. L., Endicott, J., & Robins, E. (1978). Research diagnostic criteria: Rationale and reliability. *Archives of General Psychiatry*, *35*, 773–782.

Spitzer, R. L., First, M. B., & Wakefield, J. C. (2007). Saving PTSD from itself in DSM-V. *Journal of Anxiety Disorders*, *21*, 233–241.

Spitzer, R. L., Kroenke, K., Williams, J. B., & Löwe, B. (2006). A brief measure for assessing generalized anxiety disorder: The GAD-7. *Archives of Internal Medicine*, *166*, 1092–1097.

Spitzer, R. L., Williams, J.B.W., Gibbon, M., & First, M. B. (1992). The structured clinical interview for DSM-III-R (SCID). I: History, rationale, and description. *Archives of General Psychiatry*, *49*, 624–629.

Steel, Z., Chey, T., Silove, D., Marnane, C., Bryant, R. A., & Van Ommeren, M. (2009). Association of torture and other potentially traumatic events with mental health outcomes among populations exposed to mass conflict and displacement: a systematic review and meta-analysis. *The Journal of the American Medical Association*, *302*, 537–549

Stein, D. J., Koenen, K. C., Friedman, M. J., Hill, E., McLaughlin, K. A., Petukhova, M., . . . Kessler, R. C. (2013). Dissociation in posttraumatic stress disorder: Evidence from the World Mental Health surveys. *Biological Psychiatry*, *73*, 302–312.

Steuwe, C., Lanius, R. A., & Frewen, P. A. (2012). Evidence for a dissociative subtype of PTSD by latent profile and confirmatory factor analyses in a civilian sample. *Depression and Anxiety*, *29*, 689–700.

Stone, A. A. (1993). Post-traumatic stress disorder and the law: Critical review of the new frontier. *The Bulletin of the American Academy of Psychiatry and the Law*, *21*, 23–36.

Summerfield, D. (1995). Debriefing after psychological trauma: Inappropriate exporting of Western culture may cause additional harm (letter to the editor). *British Medical Journal*, *311*, 509.

Summerfield, D. (2001). Does psychiatry stigmatize? *Journal of the Royal Society of Medicine*, *94*, 148–149.

Sweet, J. J., King, J. H., Malina, A. C., Bergman, M. A., & Simmons, A. (2002). Documenting the prominence of forensic neuropsychology at national meetings and in relevant professional journals from 1990 to 2000. *The Clinical Neuropsychologist*, *16*, 481–494.

Tolin, D. F., & Foa, E. B. (2006). Sex differences in trauma and posttraumatic stress disorder: A quantitative review of 25 years of research. *Psychological Bulletin*, *132*, 959–992.

Tsao, J. W., Alphonso, A. L., Griffin, S. C., Yurkiewicz, I. R., & Ling, G. S. (2013). Neurology and the military: Five new things. *Neurology: Clinical Practice*, *3*, 30–38.

Ustün, B., & Kennedy, C. (2009). What is "functional impairment"? Disentangling disability from clinical significance. *World Psychiatry*, *8*, 82–85.

van Ameringen, A., Mancini, C., Patterson, B., & Boyle, M. H. (2008). Post-traumatic stress disorder in Canada. *CNS Neuroscience & Therapeutics*, *14*, 171–181.

van der Kolk, B. A. (2013). Interview: What is PTSD really? Surprises, twists of history, and the politics of diagnosis and treatment [Interview by Lisa M Najavits]. *Journal of Clinical Psychology*, *69*(5), 516–522.

van der Kolk, B. A., Roth, S., Pelcovitz, D., Sunday, S., & Spinazzola, J. (2005). Disorders of extreme stress: The empirical foundation of a complex adaptation to trauma. *Journal of Traumatic Stress*, *18*, 389–399.

van Emmerik, A.A.P., & Kamphuis, J. H. (2011). Testing a DSM-5 reformulation of posttraumatic stress disorder: Impact on prevalence and comorbidity among treatment-seeking civilian trauma survivors. *Journal of Traumatic Stress*, *24*(2), 213–217.

Vasterling, J. J., Proctor, S. P., Amoroso, P., Kane, R., Heeren, T., & White, R. F. (2006). Neuropsychological outcomes of army personnel following deployment to the Iraq war. *Journal of the American Medical Association*, *296*, 519–529.

Vázquez-Barquero, L. J. (2009). The incorporation of the disability construct as an independent axis in the DSM-V and ICD-11 diagnostic systems. *World Psychiatry*, *8*, 92–94.

Verger, P., Dab, W., Lamping, D. L., Loze, J. Y., Deschaseaux-Voinet, C., Abenhaim, L., . . . Rouillion, F. (2004). The psychological impact of terrorism: An epidemiologic study of posttraumatic stress disorder and associated factors in victims of the 1995–1996 bombings in France. *The American Journal of Psychiatry*, *161*, 1384–1389.

Weathers, F. W., & Keane, T. M. (2007). The criterion A problem revisited: Controversies and challenges in defining and measuring psychological trauma. *Journal of Traumatic Stress*, *20*(2), 107–121.

Weathers, F. W., Keane, T. M., & Davidson, J. R. (2001). Clinician-administered PTSD scale: A review of the first ten years of research. *Depression and Anxiety*, *13*, 132–156.

Weathers, F. W., Keane, T. M., & Foa, E. B. (2008). Assessment of diagnosis of adults. In E. B. Foa, T. M. Keane, M. J. Friedman, & J. A. Cohen (Eds.), *Effective Treatments for PTSD: Practice Guidelines From the International Society for Traumatic Stress Studies* (2nd ed., pp. 23–61). New York: Guilford.

Weathers, F. W., Litz, B., Herman, D., Huska, J., & Keane, T. (1993). *The PTSD checklist (PCL): Reliability, validity, and diagnostic utility*. Paper presented at the annual meeting of the International Society for Traumatic Stress Studies, San Antonio, TX.

Weathers, F. W., Newman, E., Blake, D. D., Nagy, L. M., Schnurr, P. P., Kloupek, D. G., et al. (2004). *Clinician Administered PTSD Scale (CAPS)*. Los Angeles, CA: Western Psychological Services.

Weathers, F. W., Marx, B. P., Friedman, M. J., & Schnurr, P. P. (2014). Posttraumatic stress disorder in DSM-5: New criteria, new measures, and implications for assessment. *Psychological Injury and Law*, *7*, 93–107.

Weiss, D. S., & Marmar, C. R. (1996). The Impact of Event Scale - Revised. In J. Wilson & T. M. Keane (Eds.), *Assessing Psychological Trauma and PTSD* (pp. 399–411). New York: Guilford.

Williams, M. (2005). Does clinical epidemiology have a role in clinical practice? *Internal Medicine Journal*, *35*, 104.

Wolf, E. J., Miller, M. W., Reardon, A. F., Ryabchenko, K. A., Castillo, D., & Freund, R. (2012). A latent class analysis of dissociation and PTSD: Evidence for a dissociative subtype. *Archives of General Psychiatry*, *69*(7), 698–705.

World Health Organization. (1992). *International Classification of Mental Disorders and Related Health Problems (10th rev.)*. Geneva, Switzerland: Author.

World Health Organization. (2015a). The International Classification of Diseases 11th Revision is due by 2018. Retrieved (Dec. 14, 2015) from www.who.int/classifications/icd/revision/en/

World Health Organization. (2015b). ICD-11 beta draft: 7B20 Posttraumatic stress disorder. Retrieved (Dec. 14, 2015) from http://apps.who.int/classifications/icd11/browse/l-m/en#/http%3a%2f%2fid.who.int%2ficd%2fentity%2f2070699808

World Health Organization (2015c). WHO disability assessment schedule 2.0 (WHODAS 2.0). Retrieved (Dec. 14, 2015) from www.who.int/classifications/icf/whodasii/en/

Young, A. (1995). *The Harmony of Illusions: Inventing Post-Traumatic Stress Disorder*. Princeton, NJ: Princeton University Press.

Zimmerman, M. (1990). Is DSM-IV needed at all? (letter). *Archives of General Psychiatry*, *47*, 974–976.

Zlotnick, C., Zimmerman, M., Wolfsdorf, B. A., & Mattia, J. I. (2001). Gender differences in patients with posttraumatic stress disorder in a general psychiatric practice. *American Journal of Psychiatry*, *158*, 1923–1925.

Zoellner, L. A., Rothbaum, B. O., & Feeny, N. C. (2011). PTSD not an anxiety disorder? DSM committee proposal turns back the hands of time. *Depression and Anxiety*, *28*, 853–856.

33 Military Service–Related Traumatic Brain Injury

Louis M. French, Alison N. Cernich, and Laura L. Howe

Introduction

Traumatic brain injury (TBI) has been described as the "signature wound" of operations Enduring Freedom (OEF), Iraqi Freedom (OIF), and New Dawn (OND). The large number of military casualties in those conflicts coupled with the public's emerging interest in sports concussion, has fueled considerable interest in TBI and research related to its causes, treatment, and long-term effects. In the military, the most frequent cause of TBI in service members has been the explosive device. Explosive devices inflict injuries through a number of mechanisms, including dispersion of metallic fragments, the displacement of the individual through the air, the displacement of objects against the person, or the pressure and thermal blast wave itself. Other deployment-related health conditions such as stress or other emotional consequences, along with things like comorbid physical injuries, play a role in symptom expression and can complicate or mitigate the TBI recovery process.

TBI can be devastating for those affected and often places an enormous burden on their caregivers. TBI in civilians is considered a major public health concern. For example, the Centers for Disease Control and Prevention ("Surveillance for Traumatic Brain Injury-Related Deaths—United States, 1997–2007", 2011) estimates that about 1.1% of the U.S. civilian population, or roughly 3.2 million people, are living with long-term disability due to TBI. These estimates largely reflect those who have suffered more severe TBIs. However, much more common is mild TBI (mTBI; i.e., concussion), which is sometimes excluded from epidemiological studies concerning TBI. Although in the vast majority of cases, these mTBIs have no obvious enduring consequences, a minority of individuals will have persistent difficulties, which may relate to comorbid conditions.

TBI and its neuropsychological consequences are well described in Chapters 17 and 18 in this book. Our focus will be on TBI in a military population, including some typical injury mechanisms for this population, especially blast, comorbid conditions (including posttraumatic stress disorder) that are common, and long-term concerns in this group.

TBI Severity

TBI is typically defined as penetrating or closed. Penetrating TBI involves penetration of the dura by an object (e.g., bullet, metallic fragment, knife blade). These injuries, like more severe closed TBI, may require emergent neurosurgical intervention. The nature of these injuries is often very different from closed TBI (Carey, Sacco, & Merkler, 1982; Raymont et al., 2008), and have been the subject of extensive study in military settings (Grafman et al., 1996; Schwab, Grafman, Salazar, & Kraft, 1993; Sweeney & Smutok, 1983). Closed TBI can be differentiated as mild (also known as concussion), moderate, or severe, typically based upon acute injury characteristics that are used to determine the severity of the particular TBI. These injury characteristics include the duration of loss of consciousness (LOC), if any, Glasgow Coma Scale score (GCS; see Teasdale & Jennett, 1974), and the duration of posttraumatic amnesia (PTA), which is memory disruption following an injury that results in the inability to store or retrieve new information and ends when clear continuous memory encoding returns. There exists some slight variability in how practitioners differentiate the classifications (Ruff & Jurica, 1999). Very importantly, however, all the established severity level classification systems use characteristics determined at the time of injury and the postacute period. Characteristics or symptoms that emerge or endure weeks or years later are never utilized to determine the severity level classification. Additionally, the severity of symptoms manifested does not change the injury severity classification. While impairments years after an injury can characterize a person's current functioning, they cannot determine if an initial injury occurred or the severity of that injury, as many intervening personal or environmental factors contribute to a person's current level of functioning aside from the history remote TBI. In general, however, TBI severity correlates with recovery and long-term symptom expression, with those with more severe TBI having more long-term consequences of their injury. However, there are some individuals with catastrophic injuries who ultimately do quite well, while others with much more minor injuries report lasting consequences from the trauma.

There is generally good consensus on how practitioners define moderate and severe injuries. Acute injury

Table 33.1 TBI Severity Classification

Criteria	*Mild*	*Moderate*	*Severe*
Structural imaging	Normal	Normal or abnormal	Normal or abnormal
Loss of consciousness (LOC)	0–30 min	> 30 min and < 24 hrs	> 24 hrs
Alteration of consciousness/mental state (AOC) *	A moment up to 24 hrs	> 24 hours. Severity based on other criteria	
Posttraumatic amnesia (PTA)	0–1 day	> 1 and < 7 days	> 7 days
Glascow Coma Scale (best available score in first 24 hours)	13-15	9-12	< 9

characteristics such as prolonged coma make identification of the moderate to severe level injuries relatively apparent. Much less consensus exists on how mTBI is classified (McCrea, 2008). The mild classification severity level is more difficult to clearly and accurately identify because the boundary between hitting one's head and obtaining an actual mTBI is sometimes blurred. In addition, within the military milieu there exist many contextual variables (e.g., extreme stress or fatigue, adrenaline surge, physical injury) that can mimic some of the symptoms typically associated with mTBI (e.g., confusion). If one of the latter events occurs simultaneously while one is exposed to a blast or hits his or her head, there exists a risk that symptoms associated with the other event (e.g., dehydration, stress, fatigue, stress) may be attributed to the potential TBI when the symptoms are not actually caused by a brain-related event.

The American Congress of Rehabilitation Medicine defines mTBI as (a) associated diminished or altered state of, or loss of, consciousness for less than 30 minutes; (b) PTA for less than 24 hours, and (c) a GCS score of 13 or greater quantifying level of consciousness (Kay et al., 1993). How the U.S. Department of Defense (DoD) and Veterans Health Administration (VHA) categorize the three severity levels is presented in Table 33.1.

Brief History of Military TBI

TBI is as old as warfare. Its treatment has a remarkably long history too. The Egyptian Edwin Smith Papyrus from the 17th century B.C. describes the treatment of battlefield injuries, including a large number of TBI (Linley & Joseph, 2004). In modern military medicine much of the focus has been on the effects of bullets and metallic fragments upon the brain (French, 2010). In World War I, for example, the English neurologist Sir Gordon Holmes detailed his observations of more than 2,000 cases of head injury, including a detailed analysis of 23 cases involving penetrating injury to the visual cortex (McDonald, 2007). Teuber made significant contributions to our understanding of the effects of penetrating brain injury in warfare by studying those injured in World War II (Guy, Glover, & Cripps, 1998). Alexander Luria, whose work contributed much to the beginnings of what is now known as *neuropsychology*, also studied injured soldiers during World War II (Luria, 1976, 2004). His rehabilitation work centered on focal brain injury and how it affected cognition, language, and motor functioning. Later, the work of Grafman and colleagues through the groundbreaking Vietnam Head Injury study (Grafman et al., 1988; Raymont et al., 2008) and Carey (Carey et al., 1982) during the Vietnam era helped increase our understanding of both the acute effects and the late neurobehavioral changes of brain injuries. Partly because of the nature of current warfare and its weaponry (Owens et al., 2008) and partly because of increased awareness (and associated diagnosis) in the military, the health care community, and the public, much of the research and clinical focus has shifted to mTBI (concussion).

Epidemiology

With approximately 2.65 million deployments in support of OEF/OIF/OND through June of 2014 (OSD Press Office, 2014), there is a significant portion of the population that is placed at high risk for incurring a TBI (French, 2009). In addition, approximately 1.2 million individuals have had more than one deployment, increasing their risk for incurring a deployment related injury (OSD Press Office, 2014). Surveillance from the Defense and Veterans Brain Injury Center (DVBIC) reflects 313,816 incident TBIs coded in the military medical record from September of 2001 through the third quarter of 2014. The vast majority of those injuries have been mild (82.5%). Interestingly, the incident diagnosis of TBI is higher in nondeployed or noncombat settings (DVBIC, 2014).

Though larger numbers have been reported in the literature and in the media, these may be overestimates of the true incidence and prevalence of injury as they reflect screening data for TBI and likely include a number of false positives (Iverson, Langlois, McCrea, & Kelly, 2009a). Prevalence rates of TBI in service members are estimated to be between 10% and 20% of those who are currently serving in the military (Polusny et al., 2011a; Schneiderman, Braver, & Kang, 2008; Terrio et al., 2009) In many of these studies, there is some question as to whether the finding of continued symptoms associated with an injury event with either loss of, or alteration of, consciousness truly reflect mTBI and not another associated disorder (e.g., posttraumatic stress disorder, or

PTSD; pain related disorder; or depression) (Hoge et al., 2008b).

Returnees who report symptoms of mTBI through survey indicate being injured by a blast/explosion more so than any other mechanism (Hoge et al., 2008a; Owens et al., 2008). A blast TBI results from the service member being proximal to an explosive, such as an improvised explosive device (IED), rocket-propelled grenade, land mine, or other artillery or bombs (Okie, 2005a). Following blast-related TBI, the other major causes of deployment-related TBI are consistent with the major causes of TBI in the civilian population, with motor vehicle accidents or land transport accidents, falls, and sports and recreational injuries rounding out the major causes of TBI within the military population. In those with severe and penetrating TBI, the four most common etiologies are blast, motor vehicle accident, falls, and gunshots to the head or neck (Meyer, Helmick, Doncevic, & Park, 2008).

For those service members who were more severely injured, most injuries are related to combat activities (Galarneau, Woodruff, Dye, Mohrle, & Wade, 2008). A comprehensive review of records from OIF by the Naval Health Research Center for the period of March through September of 2004 noted ICD-9 codes consistent with TBI-related diagnoses in 115 personnel. Most of the injuries were due to combat activities (71%) with a smaller proportion related to nonbattle injuries (16%). Seven percent of the injuries were secondary to vehicle accidents. Thirteen percent of TBI patients were killed in action or died of their wounds. Concussion was the most common injury code, especially among the nonbattle injuries (94%). Skull fractures and other head wounds were prominently noted in those wounded in action or killed in action (26%–33%). The majority of injuries were caused by IED (52%); in those who died, gunshots and mortar rounds made up a larger proportion of this group (40%). The leading causes of noncombat injuries were blunt trauma and motor vehicle accidents. Most often those who were wounded in action had a higher percentage of other bodily injury, with face (50%) and extremity injuries (31%) representing the majority of other areas of injury. Return-to-duty rates were relatively high in the population, with 46% of those wounded in action returning to duty and 67% of those with nonbattle injuries returning to duty.

Though combat-related TBI is viewed as a common injury in the cohort of service members who have served in Iraq and Afghanistan, TBI has historically been a significant cause of hospitalization for service members prior to the current conflicts and remains a significant cause of hospitalization in the nondeployed population, with the rate exceeding that of combat-related TBI (74.6 vs. 50.3 per 100,000 service members; see Ivins, 2010a). In a ten-year study of TBI hospitalizations in the Continental United States (CONUS) or European MTF's conducted with records from 1997–2006, 110,392 service members had at least one medical encounter for TBI and there were 15,372 hospitalizations for TBI, with falls and land transport accidents representing the primary etiology for injury. Hospitalization rates have increased over the course of the conflict, vary by service branch and phase of the conflict, and reflect a higher rate of weapons related injuries. The service member hospitalized with TBI is generally a younger man, who is at the rank of junior enlisted or noncommissioned officer (E1–E5), and tends to serve in the Army or Marines. In examining the early stages of the conflict, Heltemes, Dougherty, MacGregor, and Galarneau (2011) determined an incident inpatient hospitalization rate for TBI of 10.4 service members per 10,000 troop strength (1,213 personnel in total) in either the Landstuhl Regional Medical Center (in Germany) or in the CONUS Regional Medical Center. This study found that of the sample, only 3% died of their injuries during hospitalization. The majority of the diagnoses were intracranial injury without skull fracture (59.7%), with 39.3% suffering a fracture of the skull. These data likely represent an underestimate of incident TBI hospitalizations as they did not account for in-theater deaths or hospitalization.

More recently, a study of all TBI hospitalizations in the U.S. Army for the period of September 2001 to September of 2007 documented that 46% of the hospitalizations were for severe TBI, 54% for moderate, and less than 1% were for mild (Wojcik, Stein, Bagg, Humphrey, & Orosco, 2010). Though 65% of the severe injuries were related to explosions, almost half of the injuries were related to noncombat causes. Overall, about 0.14% of service members in OEF and 0.31% of those serving in OIF had TBI-related hospitalizations. In a separate study of the Army hospitalization rates, Ivins and others (Ivins, 2010b) found a 105% increase in TBI hospitalizations in the Army from 2000 to 2006, with a 60-fold increase in those injuries attributed to weapons. Of the 2,959 cases that presented to an Army medical treatment facility, the majority of cases was mild in severity and was associated with extracranial injuries. Finally, studies that have assessed for TBI in those who were hospitalized for other conditions that warranted inpatient treatment noted about 20%–30% have TBI in addition to their other injuries (French, 2009; Gaylord et al., 2008). With reduced combat operations, there has been a related decrease in deployment related TBI, falling to a rate of 214 per month in 2013 to 92 per month in 2014. This is in contrast to a high of more than 564 per month in 2008 (Armed Forces Health Surveillance, 2014).

Data from the Department of Veterans Affairs (VA) reflect a high incidence of TBI in addition to other, significant bodily injury (Sayer et al., 2009) in its subacute rehabilitation facilities. Of 188 consecutive patients admitted to a VA Polytrauma Rehabilitation Center (PRC) between 2001 and 2006, 93% were diagnosed with a TBI in addition to their other injuries. In addition, pain disorders and mental health conditions were noted to have a high rate of co-occurrence (100% and 39%, respectively).

Both the Department of Defense (DoD) and the VA have active screening programs to detect potentially undiagnosed injury following deployment to enable treatment referral. In the DoD, screening data are usually obtained from the Post-Deployment Health Assessment/Post-Deployment Health Reassessment (PDHA/PDHRA). These measures are used to determine if the service member or veteran was involved in events that placed him or her at risk for TBI and if he or she continues to have symptoms at the time of screening; follow-up evaluations with a provider are used to determine presence of TBI and etiology of current symptoms. As the military continues to develop its care model in theater, there are now mandatory evaluations in place for those who are felt to be at risk for TBI with prescribed algorithms for follow-up care (Johnson, Hawley, & Theeler, 2014; Logan, Goldman, Zola, & Mackey, 2013). Screening data from the PDHA/PDHRA have not been published to date.

The Veterans Health Administration (VHA) TBI Screening Questionnaire (Brenner, Vanderploeg, & Terrio, 2009b) is utilized at the first visit for any individual who was in the military beginning September 11, 2001 and served in a combat environment. Approximately one out of five of the Iraq and Afghanistan war veterans who present to the VA screen positive for TBI. For the period from April of 2007 to March of 2011, the VA screened approximately 518,775 veterans of the current conflicts who have presented to VA medical facilities (DePalma, Cross, Beck, & Chandler, 2011). Of that number, 97,000 individuals have screened positive and were referred to secondary level evaluation. Of those, who screened positive, 72,623 individuals were referred for a secondary evaluation, during which their symptoms were examined in more detail and full clinical evaluation was performed. Following that secondary evaluation, 40,154, or 7% of the total of those screened, were found to have a symptom presentation and history consistent with mTBI.

Data from the VA's Polytrauma and Blast Related Injury Quality Enhance Research Program (PT/BRI QUERI) reflect that among 327,388 OEF/OIF veterans using VHA services in 2009, 6.7% were diagnosed with TBI. Among those with TBI diagnoses, 89% were diagnosed with a psychiatric diagnosis (the most frequent being PTSD at 73%), and 70% had a diagnosis of head, back, or neck pain. The rate of comorbid PTSD and pain among those with and without TBI was 54% and 11%, respectively. The median annual cost per patient was nearly four times higher for TBI-diagnosed veterans as compared with those without TBI ($5,831 vs. $1,547). Within the TBI group, cost increased as diagnostic complexity increased, such that those with TBI, pain, and PTSD demonstrated the highest median cost per patient ($7,974) (Taylor et al., 2012).

Blast Physics

Investigations have reported 78% to 88% of military injuries occurring in Afghanistan and Iraq result from explosive mechanisms such as IEDs and land mines (Hoge et al., 2008a; Murray et al., 2005; Owens et al., 2008). This injury mechanism has been the focus of significant speculation and scientific inquiry (Bhattacharjee, 2008; DePalma, Burris, Champion, & Hodgson, 2005). Given the importance of this issue, a review of basic blast physics is presented in this section.

Explosions are dynamic, with multiple events occurring both in succession and simultaneously. Initially, the blast wave created from an IED spreads from a point source and consists of a high-pressure shock wave (overpressurization) and a subsequent blast wind that closely follows the shock wave (DePalma et al., 2005). Then, as the outward spreading energy dissipates, there results a reversal wind back toward the point source, which ultimately causes underpressurization of the area (DePalma et al., 2005). Several factors including type of explosive, peak overpressure, duration of the overpressure, impulse (complex wave-forms), location of explosion, proximity of the person to the explosion, environmental hazards, body orientation to the blast, and barriers must be considered when evaluating what damage may have occurred due to a blast exposure (DePalma et al., 2005; Hirsch, 1968; Horrocks & Brett, 2000; Wightman & Gladish, 2001). Explosions result in four potential mechanisms of injury and are usually labeled as primary, secondary, tertiary, and quaternary effects. The primary effects include consequences directly attributable to the blast wave itself, which include the intense overpressurization and then underpressurization created by the blast waves. Primary blast injury can occur when direct or reflective waves impact body surfaces and potentially result in anatomical or physiological changes. Secondary effects include damage caused by projectiles such as flying debris and bomb fragments. IEDs used in the war in Iraq are often loaded with metallic objects to inflict penetrating injuries as well (DePalma et al., 2005). Body armor has been reported to be ineffective or even to potentially increase the severity of primary blast wave injuries because it provides a reflective surface even though it protects against secondary impacts of projectiles (Jensen & Bonding, 1993; Lipschutz, Pascuzzi, Bognanno, & Putty, 1991; Mayorga, 1997). Tertiary effects include effects due to structural collapse and effects directly attributable to the blast wind that follows closely behind the blast wave that may result in an individual being thrown resulting in a wide range of potential injuries such as fractures, traumatic amputations, crush injuries, or TBI (DePalma et al., 2005; Warden et al., 2006). Quaternary effects include all other explosion-related effects not accounted for within primary, secondary, and tertiary effects such as burns, asphyxia, and exposure to toxic inhalants as well as exacerbation of preexisting illnesses (DePalma et al., 2005; Taber, Warden, & Hurley, 2006).

In an outdoor setting, the intensity of the blast wave initially dissipates by a cubed root of the distance from the source (Cernak et al., 1996; Cernak et al., 1996). For example, a person who is 3 m from the point source experiences a ninefold increase in pressure compared to a person who is 6 m from the point source. At further distances, the dissipation transforms to a linear model of decay (Cernak et al., 1996). Solid surfaces reflect blast waves, which may result in someone being somewhat protected by a wall if he or she is on one side of it, and injuries may be compounded if he or she is on the other side because the wave would be reflected by the solid object and result in a more serious injury (Goh, 2009; Kaur et al., 1995). In enclosed spaces, the physics of blast waves are more complex (Cooper, Maynard, Cross, & Hill, 1983).

The secondary, tertiary, and quaternary mechanisms of blast injuries can be characterized as mechanical injuries, which would be expected to be similar to brain injuries sustained from falls or motor vehicle accidents (Belanger, Kretzmer, Yoash-Gantz, Pickett, & Tupler, 2009). The prognosis and recovery for moderate and severe TBIs sustained from secondary, tertiary, and quaternary impacts is similar to what the literature demonstrates for mechanical injuries such as motor vehicle accidents (Sayer, Chiros, et al., 2008). Controversy exists, however, surrounding the effects of the primary blast wave on the brain (Taber et al., 2006). Exposure to a blast wave is a unique aspect of explosion exposure. When considering the bulk of the scientific literature regarding the mechanism of injury of how TBIs occur (e.g., projectile missile, acceleration-deceleration forces, blunt force, something hitting the head), primary blast wave injury emerges as a different injury variable. It is important to note that blast exposure does not equate with blast-induced TBI. While researchers continue to examine the question of exposure, blast TBI is diagnosed only in the presence of traditional brain injury markers (i.e., alteration or LOC, etc.).

Physical Blast Effect and Barotrauma

Primary blast injuries are *barotraumas*. Barotraumas are injuries caused by pressure differences between the outer surface of the body and internal organs when the primary blast wave impacts the body (Bowen, Fletcher, Richmond, Hirsch, & White, 1968). Primary blast waves can cause injury by either overpressurization or underpressurization in relation to atmospheric pressure (DePalma et al., 2005).

When the blast wave reaches a living object three events occur at once: (a) part of the wave is reflected; (b) part of the wave is deflected; and (c) most of the wave is absorbed and propagated through the body as a stress wave, because the human body is a compliant surface (Cernak et al., 1996; Gruss, 2006). These dynamic pressure changes result in a high-frequency stress wave and a low-frequency shear wave at tissue-density interfaces (DePalma et al., 2005; Rahman, Timofeev, & Kleine, 2007). A shear wave results from compression of the body wall and structures underneath; this is hypothesized to be the main source of injury to solid abdominal viscera, mesenteries, and large bowel (Richmond, Yelverton, & Fletcher, 1981).

In contrast to shear waves, a stress wave has a high amplitude and travels at approximately the speed of sound. It can potentially injure tissue via spalling (i.e., cavitation created by reflections of a blast wave at the junction of media that consist of different densities or acoustic impedances), implosion (i.e., the process by which objects are destroyed by collapsing on themselves), and/or pressure differentials (Cernak et al., 1996). The pressure differential creates an external force that causes a sudden acceleration of a surface (e.g., tympanic membrane) (Cernak et al., 1996; Yang, Wang, Tang, & Ying, 1996). Air-filled organs and air-fluid interfaces within the body such as the middle ear, lungs, and gastrointestinal (GI) tract are the most susceptible to damage from high-force blast waves (DePalma et al., 2005; Glasser, 2007).

The body structure that is the most susceptible to injury due to minor increases in pressure, and therefore the most frequently injured structure in the human body via a primary blast wave mechanism, is the tympanic membrane (TM) (Bauman et al., 2009; DePalma et al., 2005). Because the eardrum is the most frequently impacted organ at the lowest pressure differential, it represents an ideal site for detecting minimum threshold effects from the primary blast wave alone. If the TM has not been ruptured, then the likelihood that the person experienced a significant blast is decreased (Argyros, 1997). Logically then, the likelihood that other air-filled organs have experienced any damage due to the primary effects of an explosion is also significantly decreased. For example, a study in 2000 investigated 647 bus explosion survivors and found that of the 193 with primary blast injuries, 142 (73.5%) experienced perforation of the eardrum only and 18 presented with isolated pulmonary injuries (9%). Likewise, when investigating injuries sustained during a train bombing, of 243 victims, Gutierrez de Ceballos, Turegano Fuentes, et al. (2005) found 99 (40.7%) who experienced TM ruptures and four who experienced pulmonary injuries without ruptured TMs (1.6%). Some interpret these data and similar studies to indicate that rupture of the TM is not a reliable marker as a threshold injury because studies have demonstrated other organ injuries in absence of TM rupture (Goh, 2009). Nevertheless, it appears that TM rupture may function as a guideline until a more robust and reliable marker is developed. Xydakis et al. (2007) found a significant association between TM perforation and LOC in the combat zone (relative risk, 2.76), although TBI occurred in some subjects in the absence of TM rupture and did not occur in some that did suffer TM rupture, limiting the predictive value of the measure. Because the TM is the most vulnerable structure and may be damaged even when other organs are not, sensory impairment may be an important part of the clinical picture in those injured (Lew et al., 2009).

The second body part most susceptible to primary explosion effects is the lungs, with pulmonary barotrauma being the most common critical injury of those close to the center point (DePalma et al., 2005). Primary blast injury to the brain has been hypothesized to include concussion and barotrauma from acute gas embolism (DePalma et al., 2005). With regards to the effects of the primary blast wave itself, it remains controversial whether brain injury occurs via the blast wave itself as it interacts with the brain or whether a brain injury occurs via a secondary process such as blast-induced dysfunction in the circulatory or pulmonary systems (Cernak et al., 1996). For example, it has been hypothesized that the primary blast effects (i.e., changes in pressure) can lead to cavitation in blood vessels, which can result in air or gas emboli causing a cerebral infarct (Kessler, Sonnega, Bromet, Hughes, & Nelson, 1995; Okie, 2005b). Air or gas emboli result when gas bubbles enter arteries, veins, and/or capillaries. An air or gas embolism results in reduced blood flow resulting in poor oxygen delivery to the areas supplied by the affected circulation. Potential symptoms can include weakness or paralysis of the limbs, impaired vision, and organ damage with the outcome ranging from death or severe, long-standing and irreversible physical and emotional disabilities at one end of the continuum to less severe symptoms at the other end of the continuum depending on what area is obstructed.

Animal Studies on Blast Injury

The majority of the research conducted regarding blast injury has been conducted on animals. Animal studies suggest primary blast waves by themselves without secondary, tertiary, and quaternary effects can cause damage to brain tissue and result in cognitive deficits (Breslau, Davis, Andreski, & Peterson, 1991). Contrary to the belief that the skull protects the brain from the primary blast wave impact, researchers have found that shock wave amplitude and waveform did not significantly decrease when passing through animal skulls (Chavko, Koller, Prusaczyk, & McCarron, 2007; Clemedson & Pettersson, 1956).

Enclosed spaces and reflective surfaces introduce numerous variables that can have an impact on the initial injury severity. The importance of the direction of impact was demonstrated in animal studies, which showed different blast energy dissipation mechanics depending on the orientation of the head to the blast (e.g., Chavko et al., 2007). Five repeated blast waves in succession have been shown in animal models using sheep and swine to reduce the injury threshold from peak overpressures as compared to one blast exposure (Cernak et al., 1996; Rosen et al., 2004).

Bauman and colleagues (Bauman et al., 2009; Macedonia, Zamisch, Judy, & Ling, 2012) developed a swine model of explosive blast injury to the brain during Phase I of the Defense Advanced Research Projects Agency (DARPA) Preventing Violent Explosive Neurotrauma (PREVENT) blast research program that could be used to "recreate the salient pathophysiological, neuropathological, neurological, and memory impairments of human TBI resulting from exposure to IED-explosions in simple and complex blast scenarios." Three situations were modeled: a blast tube that equated with a free-field blast situation, a humvee surrogate, and the four-sided building with an entrance and no roof. Each design took measures to minimize significant movement of the swine during blast exposure. They found that structure variables (e.g., size, percent enclosed) significantly impacted the amplitude, frequency, and time to decay of the blast waves and that the pressures were conducted into the brain as measured by fiber optic pressure transducers that were implanted within the brain and vasculature. Two weeks after blast exposure the swine demonstrated reduced coordination of the metacarpals of the forelimbs although it was not clear if the disruption in functioning was due to brain injury, peripheral neuromuscular injury, or a combination of both. Cernak, Wang, Jiang, Bian, and Savic, (2001) found the formation of cytoplasmic vacuoles and myelin alterations in the hippocampus of primary blast-exposed rodents, even when the blast was focused on the thorax and the head was protected. The extent of cognitive impairment and biochemical changes were correlated with blast injury severity.

Similarly, Bauman et al. (2009) found white matter fiber degeneration and astrocytosis in swine exposed to primary blast waves. Extrapolations from animal research to humans are limited by numerous factors including concerns regarding the blast wave generators themselves and anatomical differences such as skull size, shape, and geometry between animals and humans. Recent work (Marion & Regasa, 2014) suggests that human brain vulnerability to blast is actually higher than for any other mammalian species, which is in distinct contrast to previously proposed scaling laws based on body or brain mass. While animal models have distinct limitations (Panzer, Wood, & Bass, 2014) there is general consensus that many of the experimental TBI models demonstrate progressive changes in brain histopathology and behavior and contribute to our understanding of chronic TBI pathology in humans.

Differences in Blast Injury

Warden et al. (2009) report a case study of primary-blast-wave-associated TBI with no secondary and tertiary blast wave effects. The patient was exposed to multiple blast waves within a few hours. It is known that no secondary or tertiary blast effects co-occurred during her exposure to the primary blast waves because although she experienced altered awareness, she remained conscious throughout the event. She experienced concussive symptoms including headache, balance problems, dizziness, and vomiting. Magnetic resonance imaging (MRI) three months later was consistent with intracranial injury. In clinical practice, this is quite rare however, and most cases of blast injury involve blast with another mechanism.

It is unclear of the relative contribution of primary blast to symptom expression when it is coupled with mechanically induced brain injury. Taber and colleagues recently demonstrated brain changes in individuals exposed to blast even without associated TBI. In that study they conducted neuropsychological testing and MRI diffusion tensor imaging on 123 individuals who had been exposed to primary blast without TBI symptoms, six having primary blast with mTBI, and 16 unexposed blast. Those individuals exposed to primary blast both with and without mTBI it showed significantly lower functional anisotropy and higher radial diffusivity than those who experienced unexposed blast. More recently, one study examining functional connectivity to the posterior cingulate cortex in 134 military veterans demonstrated that exposure to a blast at close range (< 10 m) was associated with decreased connectivity of bilateral primary somatosensory and motor cortices, and these changes were not different from those seen in participants with blast-related mTBI. These results remained significant when clinical factors such as sleep quality, chronic pain, or PTSD were included in the statistical model. In contrast, differences in functional connectivity based on concussion history and blast exposures at greater distances were not seen (Robinson et al., 2014).

Relevant to this discussion is the examination of a unique group of military and law enforcement personnel called "breachers." Breachers are individuals who are routinely exposed to low-level blast during training and operations. As many of the blast events to which they are exposed are well quantified, they present a useful population for blast exposure studies. One recent study (Tate et al., 2013) of a group of breachers in the New Zealand Defense force selected those individuals who showed the greatest serum concentration of three biomarkers thought to be related to TBI. Those individuals showed poorer neurocognitive test performance and greater self-reported postconcussive symptoms than those with the lowest biomarker load following a two-week training course. The authors suggest that there is a measurable degree of brain dysfunction that can be linked to low-level blast exposure. Similar studies are ongoing in other breacher populations. In a study of Swedish military officers who were experimentally exposed to repeated detonating explosions or firing of heavy weapons (including repeated firing of a FH77B Howitzer or a bazooka or to 100 charges of detonating explosives of 180 dB) there was no neurochemical evidence of brain damage (Blennow et al., 2011) in the cerebrospinal fluid (CSF).

One difference in blast injuries is the high rate of comorbid physical injury. When comparing blast versus non-blast-induced injuries, Sayer, Chiros, et al. (2008) found that patients injured via a blast exposure had more soft tissue, eye, oral and maxillofacial, otologic, penetrating brain injuries, auditory impairments, and symptoms of PTSD than patients injured through another mechanism. However, mechanism of injury did not predict outcomes as measured by Functional Independence Measure (FIM) scores. Similarly, Warden (2006) found patients injured via blast were more likely to have acute stress disorder, lower limb amputations, seizures, and skull fracture.

In a review of military service members injured in 2001 through 2006 (87% of these by explosive device), 5.2% of all serious injuries and 7.4% of major limb injuries underwent amputation. This rate is similar to that of previous conflicts (e.g., 8.3% in Vietnam; see Stansbury, Lalliss, Branstetter, Bagg, & Holcomb, 2008). Individuals with traumatic limb amputations typically require extensive rehabilitation, and a variety of medical, emotional, and social issues can influence recovery (Messinger, 2009; Pasquina et al., 2008). Blast-induced limb loss with resulting loss of blood, as well as with high numbers of individuals who have sustained penetrating bodily injuries with at least some degree of hemorrhage, have raised concerns around some aspects of the trauma and its potential effects on outcome. More than 80% of the patients treated by one U.S. Marine forward resuscitation surgical unit were in hemorrhagic shock (Blanchard & Veazey, 2001). This raises the possibility of hemorrhagic or hypoxemic insults on the central nervous system. Inadequate cerebral blood flow can contribute to increased morbidity after TBI (DeWitt & Prough, 2009). Hypotension is a significant risk factor for death following trauma, even in the absence of a TBI (Shafi & Gentilello, 2005). Following TBI, the brain appears to be especially vulnerable to posttraumatic hypoxemia (DeWitt & Prough, 2009). Despite this, the long-term effects of severe hemorrhage (with or without co-occurring TBI) on cognition, emotion, or other neurobehavioral symptoms are largely unknown.

Modern body armor and advanced helmet design have dramatically reduced combat injuries. Casualties wearing a combat helmet are 2.7 times less likely to sustain a fragmentation wound to the head than those who were unprotected. Casualties wearing a body armor vest are 4.1 times less likely to sustain a fragmentation wound to the chest or abdomen than those who were unprotected, and casualties wearing pelvic protection are 10 times less likely to sustain a fragmentation wound to the pelvis (Blanchard et al., 2003). However, protection is not complete.

In a study of British service members, face and eye injuries were found in 33% and 10% of all battle-injured servicemen respectively, with 27% of eye wounds from explosions resulting in blindness and a further 17% in permanently reduced visual acuity. The lower third of the face was most commonly injured (60%), followed by the upper third (24%) (Blanchard et al., 2003). In a group of military polytrauma patients injured by blast (Goodrich, Kirby, Cockerham, Ingalla, & Lew, 2007) the rates of visual impairment were more than double compared to other causes of polytrauma. Overall, the rate of visual impairment in blast-related injury was 52% compared with 20% for all other sources of injury. Eye injuries are also connected to TBI. In a group of patients with TBI and comorbid combat ocular trauma at Walter Reed (Weichel, Colyer, Bautista, Bower, & French, 2009) (with blast accounting for 79% of the TBI-associated ocular

MACE

Military Acute Concussion Evaluation

DVBIC Defense and Veterans Brain Injury Center

Defense Centers of Excellence For Psychological Health & Traumatic Brain Injury

Patient Name: ______________________________

Service Member ID#: ________ Unit: ______________

Date of Injury: ______________ Time of Injury: __________

Examiner: ______________________________

Date of Evaluation: __________ Time of Evaluation: _______

CONCUSSION SCREENING

Complete this section to determine if there was both an injury event AND an alteration of consciousness.

1. Description of Incident

A. Record the event as described by the service member or witness.

Use open-ended questions to get as much detail as possible.

____

____

____

____

Key questions:

- Can you tell me what you remember?
- What happened?

B. Record the type of event.

Check all that apply:

☐ Explosion/Blast ☐ Fragment ☐ Motor Vehicle Crash

☐ Blunt Object ☐ Sports Injury ☐ Gunshot Wound

☐ Fall ☐ Other ______________________

C. Was there a head injury event?

☐ **YES** ☐ **NO**

Key questions:

- Did your head hit any objects?
- Did any objects strike your head?
- Did you feel a blast wave? (A blast wave that is felt striking the body/head is considered a blow to the head.)

Figure 33.1

Figure 33.2

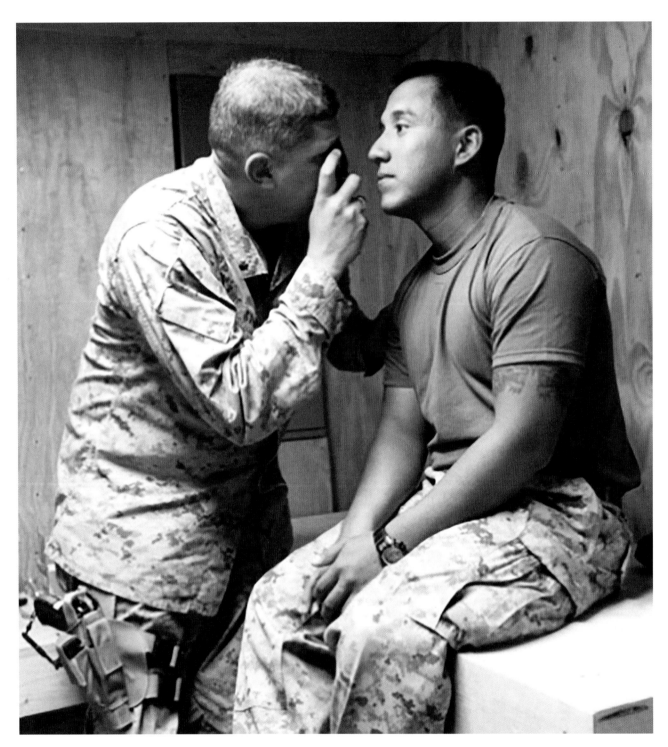

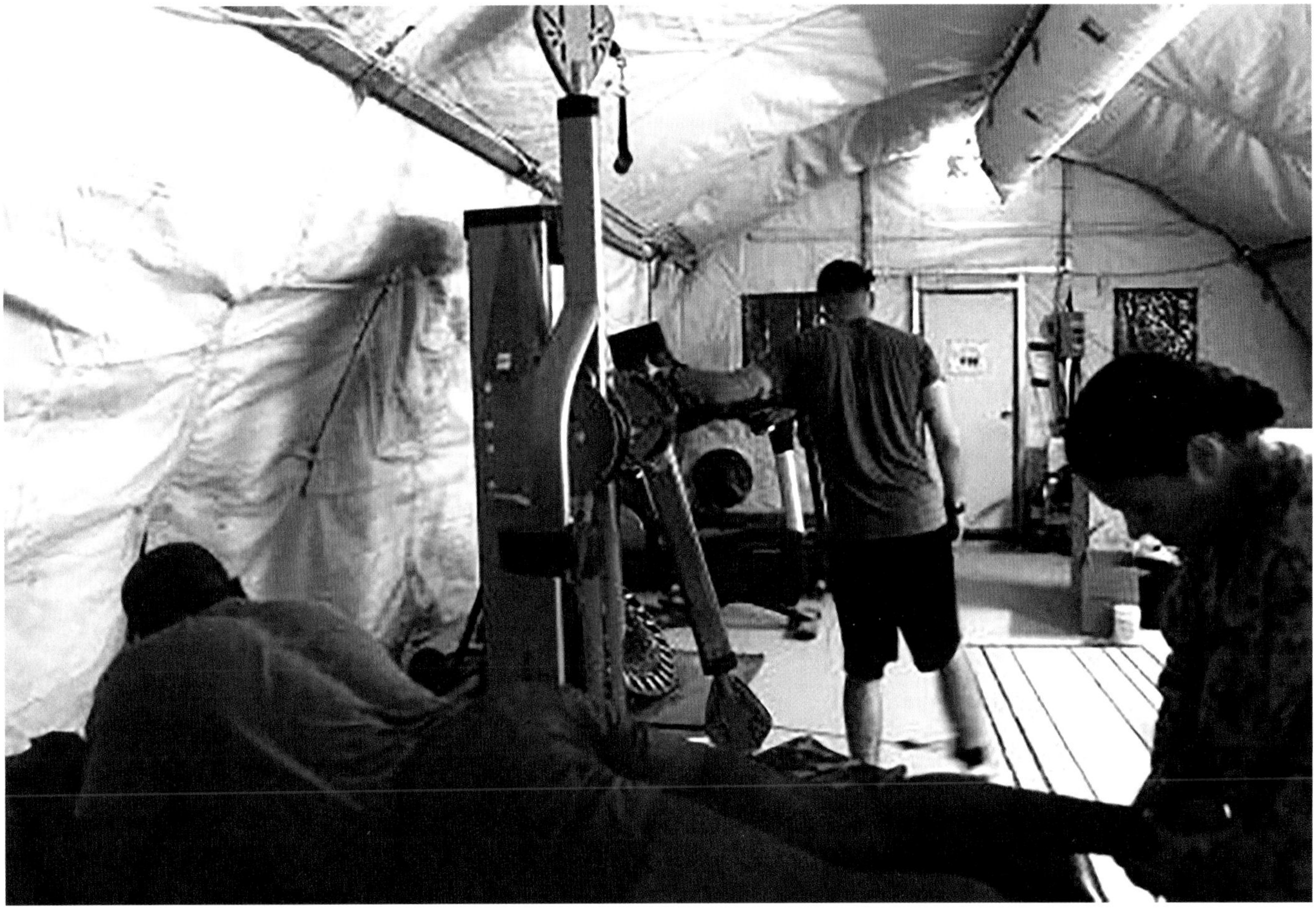

Figure 33.3

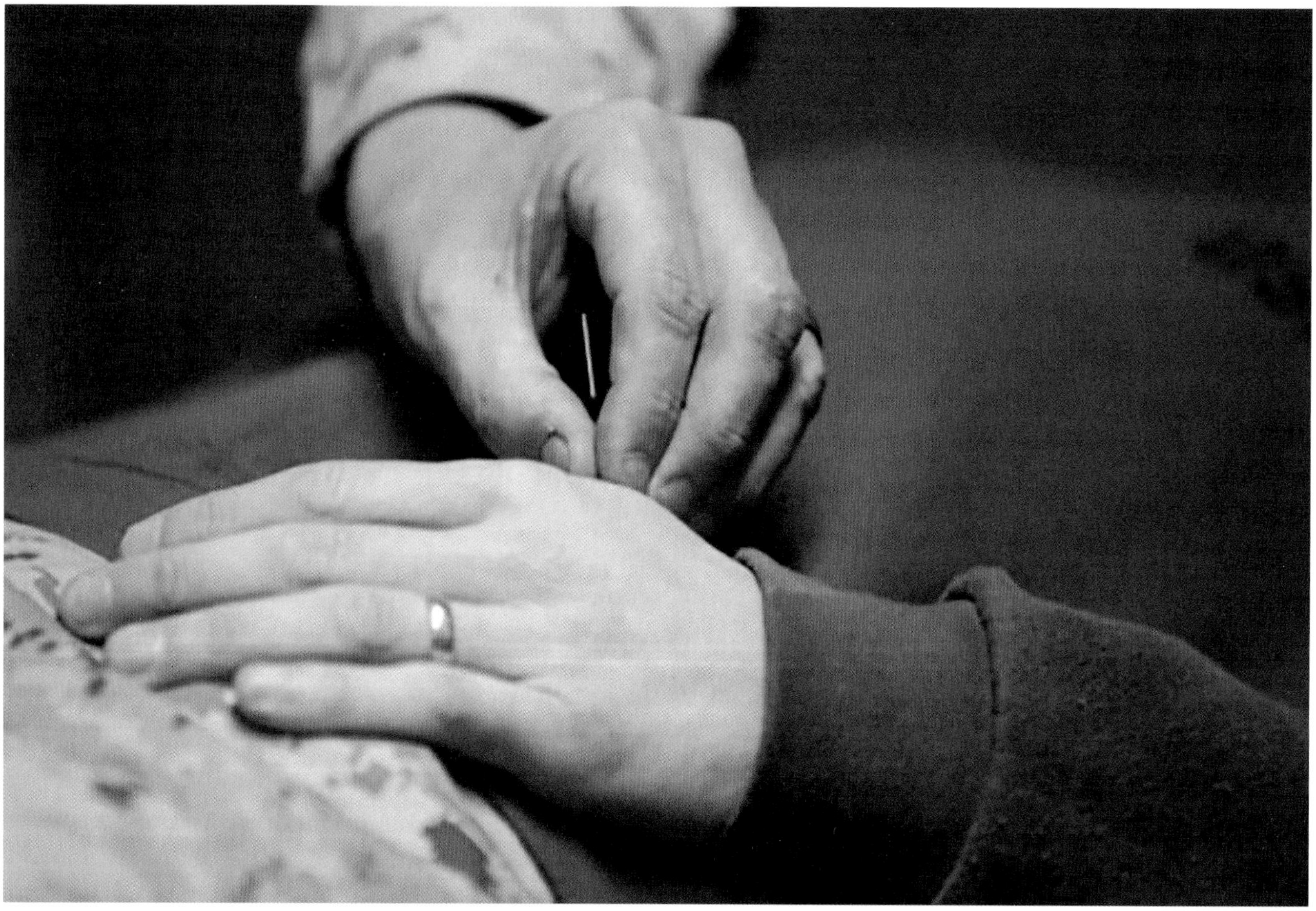

Figure 33.4

trauma), severe TBI was more frequently associated with combat ocular trauma than milder TBI. TBI occurred in two-thirds of all combat ocular trauma, and ocular trauma was a common finding in all TBI cases. In another sample of Iraq and Afghanistan veterans treated in a VA polytrauma center and injured by blast, 62% complained of hearing loss and 38% reported tinnitus. This compares to rates of 44% with hearing loss and 18% with tinnitus in those injured through some mechanism other than blast (Lew, Jerger, Guillory, & Henry, 2007).

For those with impairments in both hearing and vision, the difficulties may be even more significant. Dual sensory impairment has been associated with increased rates of depression (Bryant, Harvey, Dang, Sackville, & Basten, 1998) and lower overall health-related quality of life (Fecteau & Nicki, 1999). Lew (Lew et al., 2009) describes a VA sample in which hearing impairment was identified in 19% of the sample, visual impairment in 34% of the sample, and dual sensory impairment in 32% of the sample. Those with dual sensory impairment had difficulties participating in the rehabilitation process and showed an overall reduction in both FIM scores at discharge.

While it might be expected that greater comorbid physical injuries would be associated with greater symptom burden, two recent studies have shown that as the severity of bodily injuries increases, symptom burden decreases. In the first (French et al., 2012), 137 service members who had been evaluated and treated at Walter Reed Army Medical Center following medical evacuation from the combat theater of OEF and OIF were administered questionnaires measuring postconcussive symptoms and posttraumatic stress symptoms. All had sustained an uncomplicated mTBI and concurrent bodily injuries. The service members were divided into four groups based on severity of extracranial injury. The group with the most severe bodily injuries reported the fewest postconcussive and stress symptoms while the group with the bodily injuries of the least severity reported the greatest number of stress and postconcussive symptoms.

In an expansion of that study (Brickell, Lange, & French, 2014a), 579 individuals with uncomplicated mTBI and concurrent bodily injuries across two military medical centers were examined. Using linear regression to examine the relation between symptom reporting and injury severity across the six ISS body regions, three body regions were found to be significant predictors of the neurobehavioral symptom inventory total score (face, $p < 0.001$; abdomen, $p = 0.003$; extremities, $p < 0.001$). For the PTSD Checklist–Civilian, two body regions were significant predictors of the PCL-C total score (face, $p < 0.001$; extremities, $p < 0.001$). There was an inverse relation between bodily injury severity and symptom reporting in this sample. The reasons for this are unclear but may include underreporting of symptoms in those most severely injured, increased peer support for those with very visible wounds, disruption of fear conditioning because of acute morphine use in the acute injury period, or symptom expression may follow a different time course in those more severely injured.

Investigations of neuropsychological profiles after blast have failed to find differences for the most part. Belanger, Kretzmer, Yoash-Gantz, et al. (2009) compared individuals with TBI due to blast versus TBI due to nonblast-related mechanisms looking at select neuropsychological measures and found severity of injury and not mechanism of injury was predictive of performance on verbal learning and memory measures. This was replicated in a later study (Lange, Pancholi, Brickell, et al., 2012) in an active duty military population. In that study, subjects with "traditional" mTBI were compared to those who received an mTBI through a mechanism in which blast was a component on 14 clinical scales from the Personality Assessment Inventory (PAI) and 12 common neurocognitive measures. For the PAI, there were no significant differences between groups on all scales. However, medium effect sizes were found for the Depression ($d = .49$) and Stress ($d = .47$) scales (i.e., Blast Plus > Non-blast). On the neurocognitive measures, after controlling for the influence of depression and stress symptoms, there were no differences between the Non-blast and Blast Plus groups on all measures. This study suggested little evidence that blast exposure plus secondary blunt trauma results in worse cognitive or psychological recovery than blunt trauma alone.

Whether symptom profiles are different in those with a blast-related injury has also been investigated in a number of studies, both in acute and more chronic populations. One prospective cohort study (Macdonald et al., 2014) examined active duty U.S. military personnel evacuated from Iraq or Afghanistan to Landstuhl Regional Medical Center in Germany. Four groups of participants were enrolled from 2010 to 2013: (a) blast plus impact complex mTBI ($n = 53$), (b) non-blast-related mTBI with injury due to other mechanisms ($n = 29$), (c) blast-exposed controls evacuated for other medical reasons ($n = 27$), and (d) non-blast-exposed controls evacuated for other medical reasons ($n = 69$). Subjects were assessed 6–12 months following the injury with neurological exam, headache questionnaires, neuropsychological test battery, combat exposure and alcohol use surveys, and structured interview evaluations for PTSD and depression. Global outcomes, headache severity, cognitive performance, and PTSD severity and depression were indistinguishable between the two TBI groups. Both TBI groups had higher rates of overall disability than the control groups. Additionally, the blast-exposed controls had worse headaches and more severe PTSD than the non-blast-exposed controls. The authors concluded that overall outcomes were most strongly correlated with depression, headache severity, and number of abnormalities on neuropsychological testing. TBI itself, independent of injury mechanism and combat exposure intensity, was a primary cause of adverse outcomes. Overall disability was substantially greater than typically reported in civilian non-blast concussive patients with TBI, even with polytrauma.

Co-Occurring Disorders Including PTSD

PTSD and the anxiety spectrum disorders are another important high-base-rate differential in the combat-exposed population. It has been demonstrated that combat service may result in PTSD (Kang, Natelson, Mahan, Lee, & Murphy, 2003) and many studies have demonstrated the high prevalence of PTSD and other psychiatric illness resulting from OIF/OEF (Erbes, Westermeyer, Engdahl, & Johnsen, 2007; Grieger et al., 2006; Haagsma et al., 2012; Hoge, Auchterlonie, & Milliken, 2006; Hoge et al., 2004; McCarroll, Ursano, Fullerton, Liu, & Lundy, 2001; Milliken, Auchterlonie, & Hoge, 2007; Sundin, Forbes, Fear, Dandeker, & Wessely, 2011; Thomas et al., 2010; Verfaellie, Lafleche, Spiro, & Bousquet, 2013). PTSD symptoms in active duty military are around 5% prior to deployment (Hoge et al., 2004), however, estimates of PTSD after return from OIF are estimated to range from 13% to 17% (Hoge et al., 2004; Hoge, Terhakopian, Castro, Messer, & Engel, 2007). Physical injury while in combat is a risk factor for developing PTSD (Hoge et al., 2004; Hoge et al., 2007; Koren, Norman, Cohen, Berman, & Klein, 2005). Studies comparing injured versus noninjured soldiers from Vietnam found two to three times higher rates of PTSD in soldiers who were injured (Kulka et al., 1990; Pitman, Altman, & Macklin, 1989). Additionally, combat-related PTSD has been associated with more severe functional impairments in some studies (Prigerson, Maciejewski, & Rosenheck, 2001).

Similar to other studies, Schneiderman (Schneiderman et al., 2008) found reporting multiple injury mechanisms and combat mTBI were associated with PTSD. In fact, the strongest factor associated with postconcussional syndrome (PCS) was PTSD. Similarly, Hoge (Hoge et al., 2008a) found that 44% of soldiers with mTBI and associated LOC also met criteria for PTSD. After adjusting for PTSD and depression that mTBI was no longer significantly associated with PCS symptoms (except headache) or physical health outcomes. Patients with combat related PTSD often present with comorbidities (Brady, Killeen, Brewerton, & Lucerini, 2000; Hryvniak & Rosse, 1989) and PTSD, unlike mTBI, has been demonstrated to be associated with long-term negative health consequences such as cardiovascular disease and premature death (Ahmadi et al., 2011; Compare, Gondoni, & Molinari, 2006; Dirkzwager, van der Velden, Grievink, & Yzermans, 2007; Kang & Bullman, 1996). PTSD clearly needs to be considered in the differential diagnoses of soldiers returning from deployment.

Prevalence estimates of PTSD vary between studies. Based upon the DMS-III-R definition of PTSD, the National Comorbidity Survey (Turnbull, Campbell, & Swann, 2001) found that although the lifetime prevalence of exposure to traumatic events was 60.7% for men and 51.2% for women, the estimated lifetime prevalence of development of PTSD was overall only 7.8%. They found higher rates in women. The most common traumas associated with development of PTSD were combat exposure for men and rape and sexual molestation for women (Kessler et al., 1995). Likewise, Breslau et al. (1991) found the lifetime prevalence of exposure to traumatic events to be 39.1% but the lifetime prevalence of PTSD was only around 9%. This is consistent with the DSM-IV-TR, which reports the adult lifetime prevalence of PTSD to be around 8% in community-based studies (American Psychiatric Association, 2000).

It is important to note that PTSD develops in only a minority of individuals who are exposed to traumatic events (see e.g., Breslau et al., 1991). PTSD prevalence rates, however, have been shown to vary significantly according to the type of trauma experienced from as high as 80% in rape victims (Breslau et al., 1991) to 21%–24% for seeing someone killed or seriously hurt, news of sudden death or accident of a close relative or friend, experiencing a physical assault, or experiencing a threat to life (Breslau et al., 1991) to 15% in combat veterans (Kulka et al., 1990) to 9%–12% in motor vehicle accidents based upon epidemiological surveys (Breslau et al., 1991; Kessler et al., 1995). Epidemiological research has suggested MVAs are likely the leading cause of PTSD in the United States (Kessler et al., 1995; Norris, 1992) in part due to the high number of MVAs per year. Specific to MVAs, approximately 50% of the individuals who were injured and prospectively followed demonstrated a remission of symptoms within six months post-MVA (Blanchard & Hickling, 1997). Intervention consisting of cognitive behavioral techniques, and treatment or prolonged exposure has been shown to increase the rate of remittance of symptoms after an MVA even further (Bryant, Sackville, Dang, Moulds, & Guthrie, 1999; Price, Kearns, Houry, & Rothbaum, 2014).

There has been some debate in the literature regarding whether an individual can experience both PTSD and TBI with LOC from the same incident. Some have argued the presence of one precludes the development of the other; however, the majority of authors believe both diagnosis can develop from the same incident. For a review see (Hegde, Hegde, Parajuli, Kamath, & D, 2012; T, D, & V, 2012). On one side of the debate is the argument that individuals who cannot recall the traumatic event because of LOC or amnesia cannot "reexperience" the incident through flashbacks or intrusive memories. Therefore, individuals with significant amnesia around the time of the event are at low risk for developing PTSD (Bombardier et al., 2006; Levin et al., 2001; Sbordone & Liter, 1995).

Other researchers maintain that PTSD can occur despite memory impairment and can therefore exist as a comorbid condition with TBI (Harvey & Bryant, 2000; Mather, Tate, & Hannan, 2003; Mayou, Black, & Bryant, 2000). Several potential mechanisms have been postulated. Fear conditioning models of PTSD suggest that extreme fear at the time of trauma is conditioned with events and experiences occurring at the same time. These associations between the reminders of the emotional trauma and the anxiety responses cause subsequent PTSD (Balaji & D, 2011). It has been observed that people can reconstruct traumatic experiences in ways permitting them to compensate for impaired memory (Kress et al., 2010) (Singh, Srivastava, Kapoor, R, & R, 2009). Another possible mechanism is sustaining a TBI and later suffering traumatic experiences following the resolution of the PTA. A fourth possible mechanism involves dysfunctional neural functioning secondary to the TBI (Bryant, 2008). For example, damage to the medial prefrontal cortex may prevent inhibition of an exaggerated amygdala response (Balaji & D, 2011).

Turnbull et al. (2001) examined emergency department cases and demonstrated that having a memory of the trauma was not required for the development of symptoms associated with PTSD. In some studies, the level of PTSD-like symptoms that developed was associated with the length of PTA (less than one hour vs. greater than one hour) with a greater number of symptoms developing with a shorter PTA, but even extended periods of PTA of more than one week were associated with development of PTSD-like symptoms (Feinstein, Hershkop, Ouchterlony, Jardine, & McCullagh, 2002).

The continuing challenge for clinicians working with military service members with TBI is the high level of co-occurring disorders that are noted in the population, especially mental health difficulties, including PTSD and pain-related disorders. For example, in a sample of veterans who screened positive for TBI within the VA, those with clinically confirmed diagnosis of TBI were more likely than those without confirmed TBI to have clinical diagnoses of PTSD, other anxiety disorders, and adjustment disorders (Pizzo et al., 2008). Co-occurring mental health and TBI diagnoses in the VA setting varied by sex. Of those veterans with a confirmed TBI diagnosis, PTSD was the most common co-occurring psychiatric diagnosis, with men more likely to have a PTSD diagnosis than women (Neil, S, & Hanton, 2006). Women were two times more likely to have a depression diagnosis and 1.5 times more likely to have PTSD with co-occurring depression. In addition, women were noted to report more severe neurobehavioral symptoms than men. Screening-based survey data reflects a high overlap of TBI and mental health difficulties, especially PTSD, with overlap between the two estimated to be about 30% of all those who screen positive for TBI (Hoge et al., 2008b; Polusny et al., 2011b). The noted co-occurrence of PTSD tends to be associated with longer symptom duration following injury, especially in those with mTBI (Hoge et al., 2008b; Schneiderman et al., 2008).

With respect to other mental health diagnoses, there are fewer empirical studies. Veterans who have a history of clinically diagnosed TBI are 1.55 times more likely to die of suicide than those without TBI history and this rate was further increased in those with milder injuries (1.95) (Brenner et al., 2009b). Concurrent diagnosis of major depression was greater in those who died of suicide regardless of severity. Only one study specifically examined the rate of alcohol abuse following TBI in a military cohort: It found no relationship between alcohol abuse and TBI when other comorbid psychological health difficulties and demographics were controlled in a comparative model (Elsayed, Gorbunov, & Kagan, 1997). Finally, pain is a major complaint in this population, with a prevalence rate of pain disorders at 43.1% based on a meta-analysis of veterans. Though PTSD was thought to potentially mediate the relationship between TBI and pain, TBI continued to demonstrate an independent correlation with pain disorder diagnosis when mental health diagnoses were controlled for in the comparative model (Nampiaparampil, 2008).

Context of Injury

Additional factors that co-occur within the blast-exposure milieu within the military context at the time of potential injury and after need to be explored because the context in which any injury occurs may potentially impact symptom severity and course of recovery. The situational context in which blast exposures occur and the postdeployment environment are important in symptom creation, maintenance, and recovery. The contextual variables that add to the complexity of blast injuries and exposures will be reviewed. Some of these variables may account for why a percentage of individuals with blast related mTBI appear to be reporting symptoms in excess of what would be expected and for durations longer than would be expected.

One study has demonstrated a postdeployment effect on cognitive abilities within the first few months of return (Vasterling et al., 2006). The study administered select cognitive tests to 654 soldiers before and after deployment and compared them to a matched sample of 307 soldiers who were not deployed and found positive deployment status was associated with an increased negative affect state and decreased neuropsychological test scores on sustained attention, verbal learning, and visuospatial memory tasks with an increase in reaction time scores. Interestingly, experiencing a TBI between Time 1 and Time 2 testing and an increase in PTSD symptom levels *did not* have a significant impact on the neuropsychological findings. This study controlled for poor effort on testing; however, the mTBI were not differentiated based upon blast or other mechanism of injury, so conclusions cannot necessarily be extended to blast injuries.

A large web-based survey of Florida National Guard soldiers conducted an average of 31.8 months after deployment showed strong, statistically significant associations between self-reported military deployment-related factors and current adverse health status. Deployment-related mTBI was associated with depression, anxiety, PTSD, and postconcussive symptoms. Statistically significant increases in the frequency of depression, anxiety, PTSD, and a postconcussive symptom complex were seen comparing single to multiple TBIs. Associations between blast exposure and abdominal pain, pain on deep breathing, shortness of breath, hearing loss, and tinnitus suggested residual barotrauma. Combat exposures with and without physical injury were each associated with PTSD and numerous postconcussive and non-postconcussive symptoms. The experience of seeing others wounded or killed or experiencing the death of a comrade was associated with indigestion and headaches but not with depression, anxiety, or PTSD (Vanderploeg et al., 2012).

Postconcussional Syndrome

As described elsewhere in this volume, mTBI, even in the context of a combat environment, typically involves time-limited symptoms and complete recovery. Some individuals, for a variety of clinical reasons, show more persistent symptoms. The *Diagnostic and Statistical Manual of Mental Disorders,* fourth edition (DSM-IV), and *International Statistical Classification of Diseases and Related Health Problems,* 10th edition (WHO, 1992) clinical criteria for PCS are: a history of TBI with LOC and symptoms from three or more of the following categories developing within four weeks of the TBI: (a) headache, dizziness, malaise, fatigue, and noise intolerance; (b) irritability, depression, anxiety, and emotional lability; (c) subjective concentration and memory or intellectual difficulties without neuropsychological evidence of marked impairment; (d) insomnia; (e) reduced alcohol tolerance; and (f) preoccupation with the listed symptoms, and adoption of the sick role (WHO, 1992).

Studies have demonstrated that postconcussive symptoms are not specific and diagnostic of mTBI because patient groups without mTBI histories and the general population endorse PCS symptoms (e.g., Landre, Poppe, Davis, Schmaus, & Sobbs, 2006; Meares et al., 2006; Meares et al., 2008). For example, individuals in psychotherapy who do not have a history of head injury report elevated levels of PCS symptoms (Fox, Lees-Haley, Earnest, & Dolezal-Wood, 1995). Additionally, (Suhr & Gunstad, 2002) reported that a positive depression status accounted for elevated levels of PCS symptoms including cognitive symptoms more so than a history of head injury. Lees-Haley, Fox, and Courtney (2001) found symptoms associated with a mTBI diagnosis such as feeling dazed, confusion, and subjective memory complaints were endorsed in similar levels in patients exposed to traumatic events without TBI. Similarly, Iverson and McCracken (1997) found 39% of an outpatient pain sample met criteria for PCS even though none had a history of head injury.

Additionally, because cognitive complaints form part of the clinical picture, it is important to realize that subjective complaints of cognitive difficulties are often not related to actual performance on neuropsychological test measures (French, Lange, & Brickell, 2014; Schwartz, Kozora, & Zeng, 1996). Researchers have also reported a high correlation between self-reported cognitive symptoms and depression and anxiety in samples with (Maria, Pinkston, Miller, & Gouvier, 2001) and without history of head injury (Gfeller, Gripshover, & Chibnall, 1996; Tiersky, Johnson, Lange, Natelson, & Deluca, 1997). Frenisy (Frenisy et al., 2006) found that polytrauma patients who had not experienced a TBI endorsed high rates of neurobehavioral symptoms including attention and memory complaints, concept organization difficulties and mood symptoms such as irritability, mood swings, suspiciousness, decreased motivation, and guilt.

In a study of 1,600 U.S. service members who had sustained a mild-to-moderate TBI and who had been evaluated by the Defense and Veterans Brain Injury Center at one of six military medical centers, four of 22 factors were statistically and meaningfully associated with clinically elevated postconcussion symptoms: (a) low bodily injury severity, (b) posttraumatic stress, (c) depression, and (d) military operation where wounded. The combination of depression and posttraumatic stress symptoms accounted for the vast majority of unique variance and were strongly associated with, and predictive of, clinically elevated postconcussion symptoms. Five factors were statistically and meaningfully associated with clinically elevated posttraumatic stress symptoms: (a) low bodily injury severity, (b) depression, (c) a longer time from injury to evaluation, (d) military operation where wounded, and (e) current auditory deficits. Depression alone accounted for the vast majority of unique variance (60.0%) and was strongly associated with, and predictive of, clinically elevated posttraumatic stress symptoms (OR = 38.78; RR = 4.63). There was a very clear, strong, and clinically meaningful association between depression, posttraumatic stress, and postconcussion symptoms in this sample. Brain injury severity, however, was not associated with symptom reporting following TBI (Lange et al., 2014).

Sophisticated techniques of genetic analysis hold promise to increase our understanding of TBI and chronic postconcussive symptom reporting (Shen, Loo, Wanner, & Loo, 2014). Heinzelmann and colleagues (2014) examined expression profiles of transcripts across the genome to determine the role of gene activity in chronic symptoms following blast-TBI. There were 34 transcripts in 29 genes that were differentially regulated in blast-TBI participants compared to controls. Up-regulated genes included epithelial cell transforming sequence and zinc finger proteins, which are necessary for astrocyte differentiation following injury. Tensin-1, which has been implicated in neuronal recovery in preclinical TBI models, was down-regulated in blast-TBI participants. Protein ubiquitination genes, such as epidermal growth factor receptor, were also down-regulated.

Comorbid Deployment-Related Health Conditions and Concerns

Because many conditions and diagnoses can produce symptoms associated with PCS, it is important to know which conditions and situations occur within the postdeployment and blast-exposure milieu that may potentially account for the reported PCS symptoms that occur months to years postinjury. Differential diagnosis of persistent PCS symptoms in the blast exposure population includes (but is not limited to) brain injury; chronic pain secondary to physical injury (e.g., back pain, headaches); physical injury even without chronic pain (e.g., ear drum rupture, traumatic amputation); sleep disturbances; anxiety spectrum disorders, including but not limited to PTSD; depression; substance abuse disorders; somatoform disorders (e.g., conversion disorders, somatization disorders, hypochondriasis); factitious disorders; medication side effects; misattribution bias; diagnostic threat; symptom embellishment for secondary gain (i.e., malingering); and premorbid factors (e.g., learning disabilities). All these differentials may present with symptoms that overlap with PCS (Blennow et al., 2011; Gunstad & Suhr, 2004; Hoge et al., 2008a; Iverson & McCracken, 1997; McCauley, Boake, Levin, Contant, & Song, 2001; Melcer et al., 2014; Schneiderman et al., 2008; Smith-Seemiller, Fow, Kant, & Franzen, 2003; Vanderploeg et al., 2014).

For example, concussion, PTSD, and chronic pain share the same symptoms of fatigue, sleep disturbances, mood disturbances, psychosocial distress, and cognitive complaints (e.g., concentration and short-term memory), which can lead to role changes and impairments in everyday functioning. It is also important to realize the differential diagnoses are not all mutually exclusive. For example, a patient may have chronic pain due to physical injuries (e.g., knee pain or back injury), PTSD, a history of remote mTBI, and also embellish symptoms for secondary gain (e.g., to increase service connection).

Chronic pain is an important differential diagnosis when considering prolonged PCS symptom presentations. All of the mechanisms of blast exposure (e.g., primary, secondary, tertiary, and quaternary) can result in injuries that lead to transient or chronic pain (e.g., flying debris, falling, pressure changes). Significant transient pain can mimic symptoms associated with PCS and lead to a misdiagnosis of mTBI. Chronic pain can impact physical, social, cognitive, and emotional domains of functioning with resultant negative consequences for peer and family relationships. Chronic pain can disrupt sleep patterns and negatively impact sexual functioning. Patients with chronic pain may also potentially be taking medications that result in side effects, which could be incorrectly attributed to residual mTBI symptomology.

Substance abuse disorders, depressive disorders, conversion disorders, hypochondriasis, and factitious disorders can all produce symptoms associated with PCS. Sleep disturbances that co-occur or are caused by many of these diagnoses can produce PCS symptoms (e.g., irritability and fatigue) as well. Medication side effects can also produce symptoms associated with PCS. Even symptoms that some may believe are unique or indicative of mTBI—such as visual changes, vertigo or other balance problems, and auditory deficits and tinnitus—may actually be associated with some of the physical impacts of blasts and not even necessarily indicate a mTBI (e.g., tympanic membrane rupture). Iverson (2006) reported that substantial minorities of civilians with depression report "classic" postconcussion-like symptoms such as dizziness (31%), nausea (41%), and noise sensitivity (50%). As mentioned, symptoms of tympanic membrane rupture may mimic and be misidentified as symptoms related to an mTBI (e.g., dizziness, temporary hearing decrease).

It is important to realize that many of the diagnoses and symptoms are interrelated. For example, medication side effects may result in sleep disturbances, which negatively impact mood, which can intensify subjective distress related to chronic pain symptoms, which may result in increased doses of pain medication, which may further worsen sleep patterns. It is crucial to treat patients with a biopsychosocial or mechanism of injury approach (Scott, Belanger, Vanderploeg, Massengale, & Scholten, 2006) that does not solely treat the presenting symptoms but is mindful of the context and base rates of comorbidities, and views the patient holistically. When treating symptoms in isolation, there is a risk of decreasing one symptom (e.g., pain) while increasing others (e.g., sleep disturbances, mood disturbance, and cognitive complaints).

Due to the complexities of combat blast exposure, practitioners should be aware of the differential diagnoses, their associated symptoms, base rates, and the trajectory of recovery from each potential comorbid condition. This will aid the practitioner when diagnosing the patient and creating treatment plans.

External Incentives to Symptoms

External incentives are known to shape behavior. In legal and administrative situations where the possibility of external gain exists, fabrication and embellishment of symptoms and or situations have been widely reported. There are theoretically external incentives to claim an injury or embellish the severity of an injury while on active duty. In the combat environment an injury can excuse a service member from duty for a certain period of time or result in a change of duties. In extreme cases, an injury may result in the service member being medically boarded out of the service. Within the VHA and DoD, benefits vary depending on the nature and severity of the injuries sustained. Within the VHA system, recognition of an injury can result in a veteran obtaining a service-related disability rating ranging from 0% to 100%. The amount of disability awarded has an impact on disability payments, access to health care, copayments for services, and access to vocational training and educational expense reimbursement. New programs are developed to cater to the needs of the soldiers and veterans to make sure they are properly compensated for injuries obtained in the line of service. One example is the service members' Group Life Insurance Traumatic Injury Protection Program (TSGLI), which can result in a large one-time sum of money (up to $100,000) being dispersed to those who are injured.

Numerous researchers have reported that diagnoses that rely solely on self-report and subjective evidence can be feigned and misrepresented, and that symptom embellishment is a concern within a compensation context (Greiffenstein & Baker, 2008; Mittenberg, Canyock, Condit, & Patton, 2001). Some have argued the VHA disability program can have unintended consequences of promoting illness due to financial incentives and the structure of the system (Mossman, 1996). Veterans claiming disability status due to PTSD claims is one area that has raised concerns about secondary gain incentives in the VHA disability system (Sayer, Spoont, Nelson, Clothier, & Murdoch, 2008). Sayer et al. hypothesized this may have been due to the fact that a PTSD diagnosis depends heavily on self-report and there are no objective markers for PTSD. This is problematic even with honest reporting as individuals, including service members, have been shown to be poor judges of their objective deficits (Petit et al., 2014; Schiehser et al., 2011). Self-reported cognitive difficulties may be more related to mood or diminished insight than objective evidence would suggest. Based on review of military records, Burkett and Whitley (1998) estimated approximately 75% of Vietnam veterans who receive disability due to PTSD were never even exposed to combat. Symptoms associated with PTSD are widely known and readily accessible to the general public, and a diagnostic presentation of PTSD can be easily coached. Coaching is when an examinee is given information regarding a diagnosis that could result in his or her being able to alter his or her presentation to appear a certain way. Even if individuals are not coached, however, several investigators have demonstrated that individuals not familiar with the diagnostic criteria for PTSD can qualify for a diagnosis of PTSD 86%–94% of the time when instructed to do so on checklist questionnaires (Burges & McMillan, 2001; Lees-Haley & Dunn, 1994; Slovenko, 1994). PTSD can be completely fabricated and/or exaggerated due to the subjective nature of its diagnostic symptoms (Elhai & Frueh, 2001; Lees-Haley, 1986).

Burkett and Whitley (1998) suggested that some veterans use the VHA mental health system to establish a basis for their PTSD claims and then withdraw from services once their claim is finalized. Several studies have shown veterans who are seeking disability status for PTSD report more severe PTSD symptoms and show symptom exaggeration on MMPI-2 validity indices compared to veterans with PTSD who are not seeking disability status (Frueh, Gold, & de Arellano, 1997; Frueh, Hamner, Cahill, Gold, & Hamlin, 2000; Frueh, Smith, & Barker, 1996; Gold & Frueh, 1999). Studies investigating service utilization and disability-seeking status have shown mixed findings, with some studies finding a decrease in service use after an increase in PTSD service connection rating to 100% (Office of Inspector General, 2005), whereas another study found an increase in service usage after individuals became service connected for PTSD—but they did not control for continued compensation seeking (Sayer, Spoont, & Nelson, 2004). Sayer, Spoont, and colleagues (2008) investigated changes in reported symptoms, functioning, and service utilization as moderated by compensation-seeking status after their first PTSD claim was adjudicated in 101 participants. In their sample, reported symptom levels and mental health service utilization did not decrease when participants were no longer compensation seeking. In contrast, they found an increase in mental health service usage among participants who were no longer compensation seeking, which suggests services were not being used merely to justify a PTSD claim. In contrast, however, when administering symptom validity measures to Vietnam veterans with chronic combat-related PTSD diagnosis who presented for PTSD treatment in a VA residential setting, Freeman, Powell, and Kimbrell (2008) found a 53% clear symptom exaggeration rate on the SIRS, and the SIRS scores correlated significantly with self-reported PTSD symptom severity on the Clinician Administered PTSD scale (CAPS).

This is also a concern in mTBI diagnosis and compensation. As the diagnosis is often made based on self-report, it is important for clinicians and policy makers to be aware of the potential for symptom embellishment and malingering of mTBI. Researchers have reported that external incentives such as monetary gain from litigation correlate with persistent or worsening symptoms associated with PCS overtime (Belanger, Curtiss, Demery, Lebowitz, & Vanderploeg, 2005). In a meta-analysis, Binder and Rohling (1996) demonstrated that financial incentives had more of an impact on neuropsychological test performance than did mTBI. In a veteran population, one study showed that 17% (four of 23) of patients evaluated at a polytrauma network site performed below cutoffs on a symptom validity measure (Whitney, Shepard, Williams, Davis, & Adams, 2009). In another VA sample (Armistead-Jehle, 2010), 58% of 45 individuals assessed scored below the Medical Symptom Validity Test (MSVT) cut scores on subtests more sensitive to effort than to neurological insult. In that sample there were no differences among those who did and those who did not pass the MSVT as a function of gender, age, education, ethnicity, previous PTSD or substance use disorder diagnoses, or PAI validity scales designed to measure negative impression management. However, a higher number of those who were service connected and previously diagnosed with a depressive condition failed the measure at a higher rate than those who were not.

More recently, in Lange, Pancholi, Bhagwat, Anderson-Barnes, and French (2012) a sample of 143 U.S. service members who sustained a TBI were divided into three groups based on injury severity and performance on the Word Memory Test and four embedded markers of poor effort: mTBI-pass (n = 87), mTBI-fail (n = 21), and severe TBI-pass (n = 35). The patients in the mTBI-fail group performed worse on the majority of neurocognitive measures, followed by the severe TBI-pass group and then the mTBI-pass group. Likewise, on the PAI, the mTBI-fail group had higher scores on the majority of clinical scales ($p < .05$). The authors concluded that effort testing is an important component of postacute neuropsychological evaluations following combat-related mTBI, and those who fail effort testing are likely to be misdiagnosed as having severe cognitive impairment. Their symptom reporting is likely to be inaccurate if taken at face value (Lange et al., 2012). Studies have illustrated that when clinicians were made aware of potential threats to assessment validity this increased their detection of simulation (Hickling). It is important for clinicians to screen for poor effort and symptom validity and to be aware of the potential pull for symptom embellishment that is created by the system due to multiple external incentives when an injury can be established. Because knowledge of potential symptom embellishment can increase practitioners' ability to detect symptom embellishment (possible because they attend to the possibility) it stands to reason that education regarding this possibility should be provided to practitioners within the DoD and VHA system of care for all levels of practitioners, not just neuropsychologists and rehabilitation specialists. It is also important to clarify that stating clinicians should remain cognizant of potential symptom embellishment and malingering in no way infers individuals who sustained real injuries while on active duty should be denied benefits. It simply means individuals should be compensated at the level of injury they obtain and for what actually occurred to them.

Iatrogenic Illness, Diagnostic Threat, and Misattribution Bias

Several studies have found an increase in symptom endorsement over time (Belanger, Kretzmer, Vanderploeg, & French, 2009; Milliken et al., 2007). Various explanations have been advanced including (a) recovery from TBI may be associated with increased recovery of memories, (b) physiological changes that persist (e.g., vestibular changes, hearing loss, tinnitus) may result in increased anxiety responses overtime, and (c) awareness of symptoms may increase with time. While these are possibilities, it is also possible that the system and the public milieu may be functioning in a way to create, maintain, and/or accentuate the symptoms in some select cases.

As discussed, it is unlikely that persistent symptoms are related to a remote mTBI for the overwhelming majority of cases. Symptoms that are shared with other diagnoses such as substance abuse, sleep disorders, and mood disorders can persist, however, if not properly treated. Additionally, symptoms associated with mTBI can occur in normal healthy adults. These facts combined with the fact that misinformation about mTBI—including its base rate, recovery trajectory, and future implications—in the public domain creates a situation where expectations may result in individuals misattributing their symptoms to an improper source (e.g., remote mTBI) when they are actually caused by other comorbid conditions or everyday life fluctuates. Studies have investigated this phenomenon, which is called *misattribution bias* (Mittenberg, DiGiulio, Perrin, & Bass, 1992b).

Patients with a history of mTBI have been shown to under report preinjury levels of PCS symptoms (Mittenberg et al., 1992b). When study participants without a history of TBI were asked to imagine the symptoms of a mTBI, they reported symptoms typically endorsed by patients after a mTBI (Mittenberg et al., 1992b). With ambiguous stimuli such as internal states, individuals interpret the event based largely upon their expectation of that experience. Taken together, this suggests if there is an expectation of initial and continued symptoms that some individuals will in fact experience these symptoms (Mittenberg et al., 1992b). It has been suggested that Mittenberg's "expectation as etiology" hypothesis may be too specific and perhaps a "good old days" hypothesis would be more appropriate: After a negative event, people may attribute all symptoms to that negative event.

Misattributing symptoms to an incorrect etiology is problematic. Misdiagnosis can prevent the individual from obtaining the appropriate treatment. For example, if an individual's PCS symptoms are primarily due to an anxiety spectrum disorder, a sleep disorder, and narcotic use for chronic pain control, but the symptoms are misattributed completely to a remote mTBI, the individual may be misinformed the deficits are permanent and nothing can be done. In contrast, with proper differential diagnosis, evidence-based interventions such as cognitive behavioral therapy for anxiety symptoms, physical therapy for the pain disorder, alternatives to narcotic use for pain control, and sleep hygiene for the sleep disturbance can be attempted. A misdiagnosis could also potentially significantly reduce a person's quality of life and goal attainment. For instance, the belief that persistent symptoms are attributable to a remote mTBI that will not resolve may result in a person not attempting to get a job or obtain an advanced degree. This would limit the person's ability to engage in meaningful life activities that could be personally rewarding and self-fulfilling. This by itself could lead to isolation or depression.

Misinformation in the public domain that does not differentiate the severity levels of TBI and suggests mTBI has long-term deficits similar to a severe TBI is harmful to those who experience a blast exposure. Increased media attention has brought with it increased awareness around the occurrence of concussion and TBI, especially in the sports arena. There is also increased awareness around potential long-term effects. The DoD and VA have developed extensive screening and education programs around TBI for all service members, but not without a potential cost around stigma, misattribution, or other negative effects (Logan et al., 2013; Scholten, Cernich, Hurley, & Helmick, 2013).

Previous work (Mittenberg, DiGiulio, Perrin, & Bass, 1992a; Suhr & Gunstad, 2005) has shown that some individuals with mTBI may expect to have persistent problems even though they are showing a good recovery. While structured educational interventions have been shown to be effective in reducing postconcussive symptoms in both acute and more chronic TBI in active duty service members, veterans, and civilians (King et al., 2013), these interventions do not always reach the intended audience. In one study of veterans who screened positive for TBI (Spencer et al., 2013), "friends in the military" remained the most frequently source of information about TBI and its effects, with the second highest being the Internet. This heightens the possibility of misinformation about TBI and its possible consequences.

"Diagnostic threat" is similar but different than the "expectation as etiology" theory. Suhr and Gunstad (2002a, 2005) found when participants were randomly assigned to a group informed they were being assessed due to a history of mTBI, versus a group given neutral instructions that did not call attention to the remote mTBI, the group informed they were being assessed due to history of mTBI performed more poorly on neuropsychological test measures, which suggests a "diagnostic threat" when informing patients they are being evaluated for a particular reason. Expectations regarding a diagnosis can impact performance on some neuropsychological test measures (Suhr & Gunstad, 2005). This is especially problematic when the symptoms of the diagnosis are commonly occurring symptoms in the general public, because the experience of the symptoms—even though normal—can function to reinforce the thought the person is indeed "sick." As shown, PCS symptoms occur frequent in the healthy population (Mittenberg et al., 1992b). As stated in one study while overinclusive screenings assure individuals who need help are ascertained, overinclusive screenings also have several drawbacks such as dramatically increasing needed resources, potentially overinflating estimates of brain injury that might be based upon screening, and—as has been suggested previously—the screening itself may have adverse consequences for some false positives (e.g., iatrogenic illness).

TBI Programs Within the Departments of Defense and Veterans Affairs

In response to the number and types of injuries sustained during the conflicts, both the DoD and the Department of Veterans Affairs have established and expanded their systems of care to provide a network of services for individuals with brain injury. This includes protocols for care within the combat setting for those who do not require evacuation, and systematic stabilization and evacuation from theater for those who require more intensive surgical or medical services. Following the provision of acute care, each department provides acute and subacute rehabilitation, and in some cases, residential rehabilitation and community reintegration services.

An important part of these efforts has been the development of clinical practice guidelines, consensus papers, and literature reviews of important topics in military TBI care. Chief among these is the VA/DoD Clinical Practice Guideline for the treatment of mTBI (Group, 2009) which provides the foundation for clinical care of this population. Other guidelines, largely produced by the Defense and Veterans Brain Injury Program (DVBIC) have included "A Parent's Guide to Returning Your Child to School After a Concussion," "Assessment and Management of Dizziness Associated with mTBI Clinical Recommendation," "Assessment and Management of Visual Dysfunction Associated with mTBI," "Indications and Conditions for In-Theater Postinjury Neurocognitive Assessment Tool (NCAT)," "Testing Indications and Conditions for Neuroendocrine Dysfunction Screening Post mTBI," "Management of Sleep Disturbances Following Concussion/Mild Traumatic Brain Injury," "Neuroimaging following mTBI in the Non-Deployed Setting Clinical Recommendation," and "Progressive Return to Activity Following Acute Concussion/Mild Traumatic Brain Injury." Fact sheets and educational handouts for patients are also available in a large number of languages. As these are all government-funded projects, they are available free on the DVBIC website (DVBIC.DCOE.mil).

In-Theater Care

The DoD has rapidly evolved a system of trauma care services over the course of the current conflicts for those who received moderate, severe, and penetrating injuries as a result of combat engagement or accident. This includes a series of evidence-based trauma care guidelines to include stabilization of intracranial pressure, decompressive craniotomy, supportive use of whole blood and blood products, and protocols for stabilization of the patient prior to evacuation (www.usaisr.amedd.army.mil/clinical_practice_guidelines.html, 2014). Aeromedical evacuation procedures are tailored to flights of long duration at relatively high altitude with medical staff on hand for crisis management.

Many service members are wounded in theater and do not require evacuation to European or stateside hospitals, but instead receive triage and treatment services in the combat zone. A series of procedures have evolved to determine at what level an injury can be managed and by which types of providers. The immediate triage and treatment of a service member is often provided by a combat medic. The medic provides screening via the Military Acute Concussion Evaluation which consists of a brief neurological evaluation, documentation of the event and symptoms at the time of the event, and then, based on criteria related to those two evaluation portions, provides a brief mini-mental status examination and vestibular examination (balance evaluation and scoring system; see Guskiewicz, Ross, & Marshall, 2001) to assess other potential effects of the injury. If particular "red flags" are present during that evaluation (e.g., blown pupils) evacuation may be initiated. If no acute emergent needs are

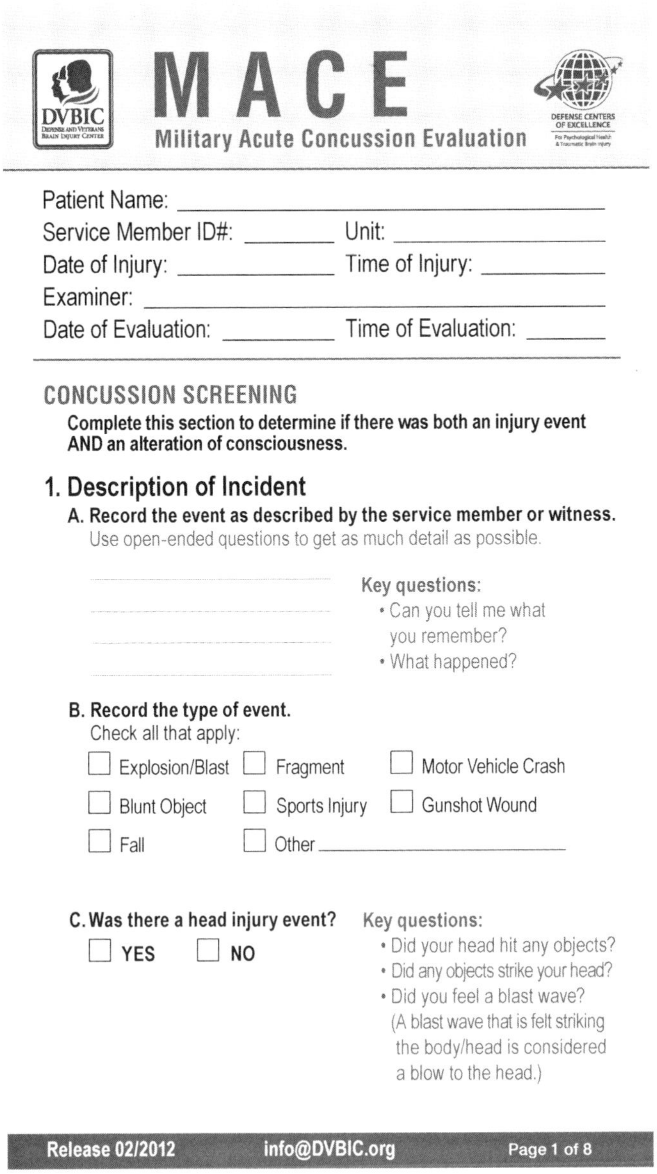

DVBIC Defense and Veterans Brain Injury Center

MACE

Military Acute Concussion Evaluation

Defense Centers of Excellence For Psychological Health & Traumatic Brain Injury

Patient Name: ______

Service Member ID#: ______ Unit: ______

Date of Injury: ______ Time of Injury: ______

Examiner: ______

Date of Evaluation: ______ Time of Evaluation: ______

CONCUSSION SCREENING

Complete this section to determine if there was both an injury event AND an alteration of consciousness.

1. Description of Incident

A. Record the event as described by the service member or witness.
Use open-ended questions to get as much detail as possible.

Key questions:
- Can you tell me what you remember?
- What happened?

B. Record the type of event.
Check all that apply:

☐ Explosion/Blast ☐ Fragment ☐ Motor Vehicle Crash

☐ Blunt Object ☐ Sports Injury ☐ Gunshot Wound

☐ Fall ☐ Other ______

C. Was there a head injury event?
☐ YES ☐ NO

Key questions:
- Did your head hit any objects?
- Did any objects strike your head?
- Did you feel a blast wave?
(A blast wave that is felt striking the body/head is considered a blow to the head.)

Release 02/2012 **info@DVBIC.org** **Page 1 of 8**

Figure 33.1 Military Acute Concussion Evaluation (MACE). *A color version of this figure can be found in Plate section 3*

Complete form can be downloaded at https://health.mil/Reference-Center/Forms/2015/04/30/MACE-2012

identified, an algorithm has been adopted to guide the treatment and referral process for a service member.

There are three levels of care in theater—referred to as Role 1, Role 2, and Role 3—which increase intensity of services systematically and require in theater transport to higher levels of medical services. Also included in the system of care are Concussion Recovery Centers (CRCs). At one time during the conflicts there were nine CRCs located in different areas of Afghanistan that provided systematic rest and rehabilitation protocols to allow for recovery and that allowed for the return of approximately 97% of service members to full duty status (Logan et al., 2013).

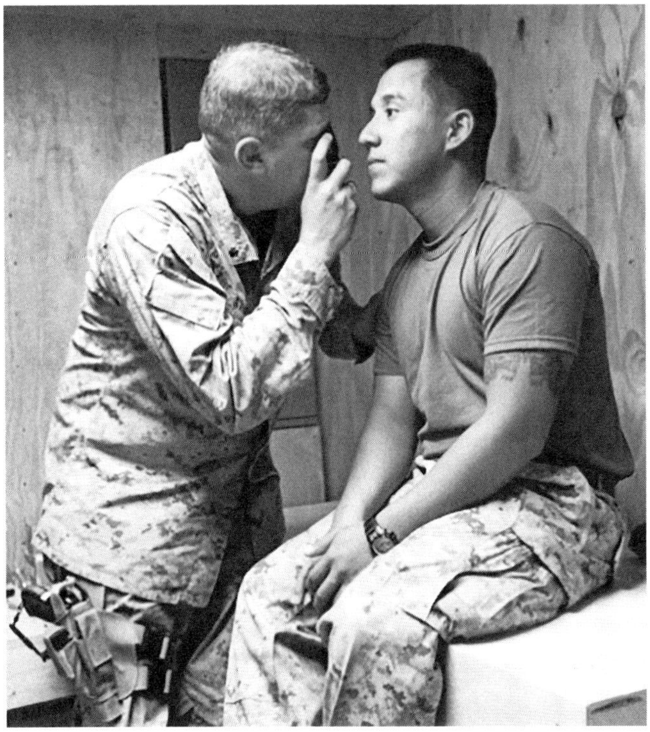

Figure 33.2 Combat medic administers MACE to a Service Member in theater. *A color version of this figure can be found in Plate section 3*

Acute and Subacute Rehabilitation

Acute medical stabilization and surgical interventions continue upon arrival to medical centers that are based primarily in Germany (Jaffee & Meyer, 2009). At this point, the service member receives additional surgical services, may require addition stabilization of intracranial pressure to enable transport stateside, or may initiate rehabilitation care. Though some service members return to duty from the European medical support hospitals, most are transferred to hospitals in the CONUS.

The primary sites of care for service members who have moderate to severe brain injuries when they arrive stateside are Walter Reed National Military Medical Center in Bethesda, Maryland; Brooke Army Medical Center in San Antonio, Texas; and Balboa Naval Hospital in San Diego, California. The site of care is based on a number of factors, including the type and severity of associated injuries co-occurring with the brain injury (e.g., injury to the extremity/amputation, burn, severe eye/visual injury, or genitourinary injury), proximity to post or home, and bed availability. Following acute stabilization and initiation of rehabilitation in the acute-care setting, a plan of care is established for each individual that includes disposition and potential referral within the military health system to a medical setting nearer the patient's military assignment or home, a private care setting that would be funded through a purchased care arrangement, or to the Department of Veterans Affairs Polytrauma System of Care.

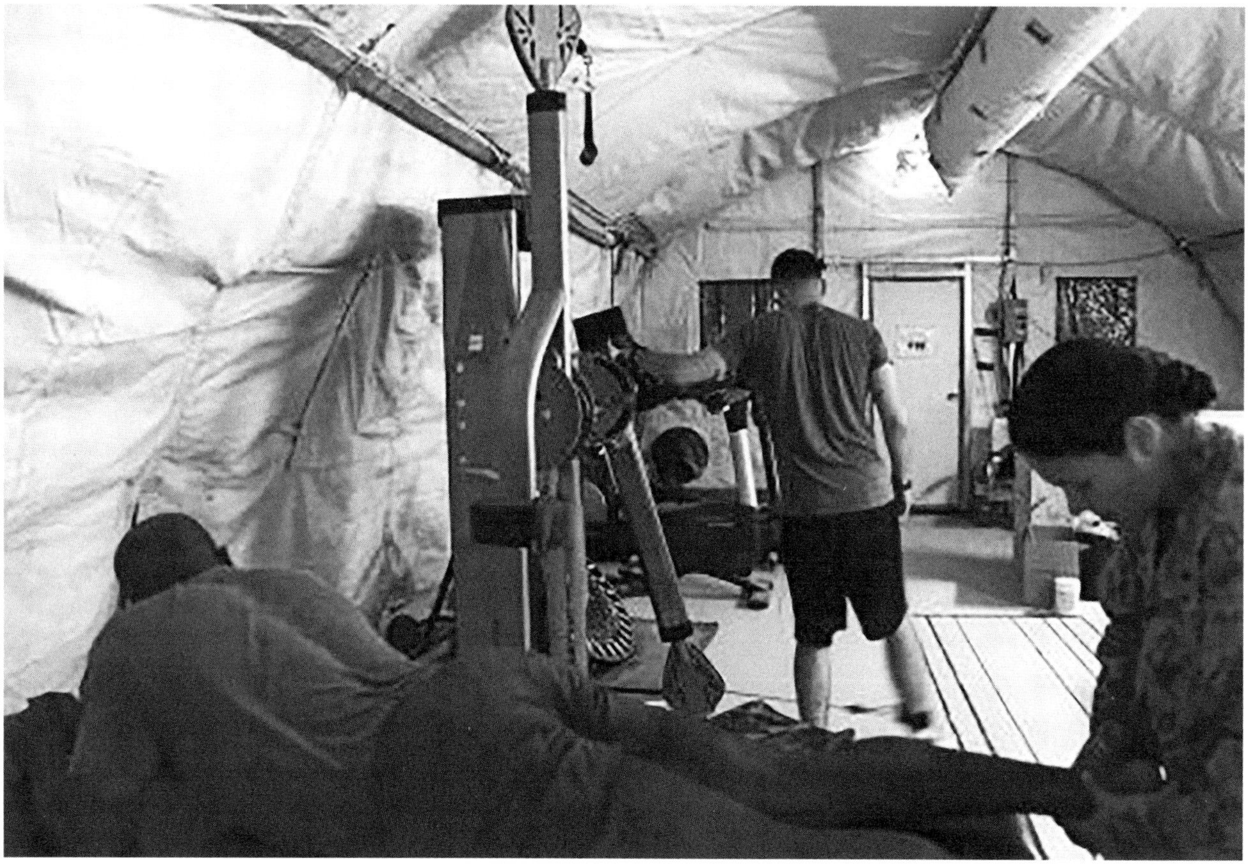

Figure 33.3 Service Member receives rehabilitation treatment in theater. *A color version of this figure can be found in Plate section 3*

The VA Polytrauma System of Care consists of four levels of care that are dispersed throughout the nation (Sigford, 2008). The most intensive care is provided at Level I facilities, which provide acute and subacute management of brain and other major bodily injuries and serve as the hubs for the Polytrauma System of Care in their regions. The five Level I facilities are located in Richmond, Virginia; Tampa, Florida; San Antonio, Texas; Minneapolis, Minnesota; and Palo Alto, California. Each program provides 10–15 inpatient beds and has step-down programs that provide for outpatient day programs and residential rehabilitation programs.

The Polytrauma Network Sites, or Level II facilities, offer structured outpatient day programs and comprehensive outpatient services, as well as a limited number of inpatient beds for continuation of care within each of the VA's 21 Integrated Service Networks (VISNs). There is a full complement of rehabilitation staff, care management services, and augmented rehabilitation services to enable community reintegration and continuation of rehabilitation support.

At the Polytrauma Support Clinics, or Level III facilities, comprehensive rehabilitation services are offered on an outpatient basis. These services are tailored to patient needs and potential consultation or referral to Level II facilities is considered where needed. The Polytrauma Points of Contact are primarily care managers who can facilitate care in the area in which the Veteran resides or coordinate care with higher levels of treatment located in the region.

Emerging Consciousness

All Level I facilities provide services for those individuals who remain in coma, a persistent vegetative state, or a minimally conscious state (McNamee. Howe, Nakase-Richardson, & Peterson, 2012). Known as the Emerging Consciousness Program, these services are geared toward promoting optimal stimulation and rehabilitation aimed at returning the individual to the highest possible level of function. They include: skilled nursing and rehabilitation medical services; individualized multimodal stimulation program; active therapy involvement; weekly monitoring of objective functional status; intensive social work and case management; and psychological support services, training and education to support families and caregivers (McNamee et al., 2012; Nakase-Richardson et al., 2013). There have been a relatively small number (fewer than 200) of individuals admitted to the Polytrauma Rehabilitation

System of Care with disorders of consciousness who have been enrolled in this program (Nakase-Richardson et al., 2013). Individuals admitted are primarily active duty men who entered the program with a median GCS of 3 on acute admission; 91% were on a ventilator during acute stay. Individuals in the program had a median acute length of stay of 51 days and a median rehabilitation stay of 132 days, with longer lengths of stay noted in individuals with blast injury. Many of the individuals had a high level of medical comorbidities including spasticity, autonomic nervous system dysregulation, and seizure. Of those enrolled, 64% have emerged to regain consciousness at the minimally conscious state as defined by coma recovery scale—revised or evidence of interaction communication, functional object use, or Rancho LCFS greater than or equal to 4. Thirty-eight percent of the sample regained full orientation. Functional improvement was noted in the sample in cognitive and motor domains of the FIM, though these were improvements above the rating scale floor in the other trauma group (non-blast or combat-related trauma). Those with neurotrauma secondary to blast were less likely to recover to full orientation, had higher levels of medical comorbidity, and had fewer functional gains.

Residential Programs

The VA offers residential rehabilitation programming at its Polytrauma Transitional Rehabilitation Programs. Located at each of the Level I facilities, they offer 15–20 residential beds in tiered levels of medical supervision to promote community reintegration and independent living skills through an intensive program. This includes vocational rehabilitation, driving rehabilitation, recreational therapy, compensated work therapy programs, and comprehensive rehabilitation services.

The National Intrepid Center of Excellence

The National Intrepid Center of Excellence (NICoE) for Psychological Health and Traumatic Brain Injury at Walter Reed National Military Medical Center specializes in treating service members with mTBI and co-occurring psychological health issues that have failed in more traditional treatment settings (Miller, 2011; Wesolowski, 2010). This four-week program relies heavily on an intensive, comprehensive assessment in a healing environment with a heavy emphasis on complementary and alternative medicine interventions to include acupuncture, art therapy, service dog programs, and other techniques (Foote & Schwartz, 2012; Garrison & Stewart, 2014; Yount, Olmert, & Lee, 2012). These techniques are not intended to supplant traditional interventions but to provide an alternative that may be useful for some who have failed other treatments, or need to pursue medication alternatives because of existing polypharmacy (Koffman & Helms, 2013).

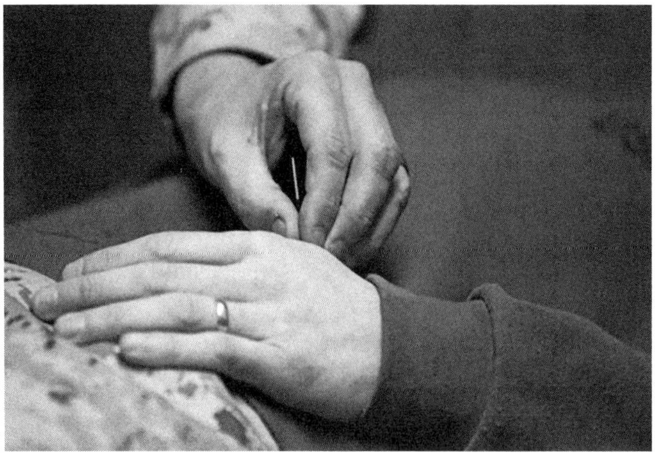

Figure 33.4 Service Member receives acupuncture at the National Intrepid Center of Excellence (NICoE). *A color version of this figure can be found in Plate section 3*

Screening and Evaluation

In contrast to moderate to severe TBI, the immediate symptoms of mTBI can be subtle and difficult to detect. This is particularly true within a combat situation when symptoms of mTBI may be mistaken for the stresses of deployment or other psychological trauma/shock. In the deployed environment, the DoD enacted a policy to require screening following potentially concussive events, standardized evaluation of symptoms, and documentation of the event, symptoms, and resultant diagnosis (Helmick, Baugh, Lattimore, & Goldman, 2012). Following the enactment of this policy, the DoD increased training of medics in appropriate screening for concussion and modified its clinical care algorithms to reflect recent evidence from theater-based research. The DoD continues to emphasize detection of mTBI by requiring screening at multiple time points (e.g., point of injury, prior to medical evacuation to the United States, and before redeployment). Survey questions targeting TBI detection at postdeployment and at postdeployment reassessment were recently refined to encourage symptom reporting in order to connect service members to care (Helmick et al., 2012). Looking forward, research efforts are under way to evaluate the efficacy of biomarkers, neuroimaging, and other novel approaches for unequivocal diagnosis of TBI (Maruta, Lee, Jacobs, & Ghajar, 2010; Mondello et al., 2011; Svetlov et al., 2009).

Due to the growing concern over the health consequences of TBI, all service members returning from combat are screened for TBI using the PDHA/PDHRA from the DoD or the VHA's TBI Screening Questionnaire (Brenner, Vanderploeg, & Terrio, 2009a). These measures screen for potential exposure to risk events and ongoing symptomology. However, the timing of administration of these measures can play an important role in what the service member is willing to report. Some service members may minimize symptoms so as not to delay their return home with lengthy follow-up evaluations (Brenner et al., 2009a; Schneiderman et al., 2008). Others may not recognize the extent of their symptoms or may minimize the impact of their symptoms until they return home to their regular activities. Any delays in the initiation of treatment can negatively affect the path of symptom resolution and recovery; therefore, continued efforts to better identify injuries as close to the time of injury as possible are critical.

As the DoD continues to develop its care model in theater, there are now mandatory evaluations in place for those who are felt to be at risk for TBI (Ling & Ecklund, 2011), with prescribed algorithms for follow-up care. Refinements of the questions asked during the PDHA/PDHRA are also focused to address underreporting and to encourage acknowledgment of symptoms to connect service members to care (Helmick et al., 2012). The attention to screening and follow-up evaluation provides documentation of diagnosis of TBI, records multiple exposures and/or injuries in the population, and provides a better basis from which one can evaluate long-term outcomes and dementia risk.

Since 2007, VA provides screening and evaluation for all veterans accessing care who served in the Global War on Terror and separated from active duty service after September 11, 2001(Scholten et al., 2013). This four-question screen is similar to the one used during the PDHA/PDHRA process and identifies events that place the individual at risk for TBI, a history of symptoms following injury if identified, and the presence of current symptoms. Following a positive screen the individual is referred to the Polytrauma System of Care and receives a comprehensive TBI evaluation that includes a history of the injury event, a physical evaluation, and a 22-item symptom questionnaire (the Neurobehavioral Symptom Inventory; see Cicerone & Kalmar, 1995) to determine current symptoms that are impacting functional ability. Diagnosis is provided at that time (if it is not specified in available records) and if concordant with history of injury and presence of symptoms at time of injury. In a recent analysis, of those 49,962 veterans with completed TBI evaluations, 59% (29,534) received a clinician-confirmed TBI diagnosis (Carlson et al., 2013). Among those diagnosed, 81% met criteria for mTBI, and clinicians' diagnoses reflected a high rate of comorbidity of behavioral health symptoms with current symptoms of mTBI (58%).

In the VA an integrated individual care plan is required for all patients and is entered into the medical record in a standardized format to allow for retrieval and analysis. In a recent evaluation of the presenting symptoms indicated on the initial evaluation and care plan, more than three-quarters of veterans reported moderate to very severe difficulty with irritability, sleep disturbance, forgetfulness, and anxiety (Scholten et al., 2013). The types of injury noted were blast exposure (36%), other trauma (19%) and both blast and non-blast for those remaining (44%). Thirty-eight percent of this sample did sustain their injury during deployment. Of note, about 23% of the population that had symptoms and also were assigned a TBI diagnosis were felt to have symptoms more attributable to behavioral health conditions than to TBI.

Screening in the VA has not been universally accepted as beneficial. One recent paper concluded that the core conditions essential for beneficial medical screening-progressive disease, symptoms related to the identified disease, suitable tests or examinations for accurate diagnosis, and accepted and effective treatment were not present within the context of TBI screening, and that the potential harms/costs outweigh any potential benefits of population-based screening for TBI. As postconcussion-like symptoms can be effectively treated in a symptom-specific manner, tying them to concussion through a screening and evaluation process is wasteful and potentially harmful (Vanderploeg & Belanger, 2013). This view has been countered by other clinicians in the VA system, saying that such screening identifies those who would have otherwise been missed and allows for individualized care (Scholten et al., 2013).

There has been some research indicating that informational techniques providing psychoeducation regarding the expected symptoms and trajectory of recovery from mTBI may minimize potential iatrogenic impacts from postdeployment screening for mTBI. Mittenberg, Tremont, Zielinski, Fichera, and Rayls (1996) investigated outcomes between two conditions and found that an intervention of extensive written instructions and a meeting with a therapist for information and to advise to gradually return to premorbid activities before discharge ($n = 29$) versus routine discharge information with advice to rest ($n = 29$) resulted in reduced symptoms and disability at six months postinjury via interview. Other studies have found that providing patients with information regarding the normal course and recovery trajectory expected for mTBI can decrease symptom prevalence in children (Ponsford et al., 2001) and adults (Ponsford et al., 2002).

Ponsford et al. (2002) compared the standard emergency department treatment, which did not include an informational booklet regarding the symptoms and expected recovery trajectory from mTBI ($n = 123$), to a group who obtained an assessment and an information booklet outlining common symptoms associated with mild head injury, their likely time course, and suggested coping strategies, within one week after mTBI ($n = 79$). They found that at a three-month follow-up looking at symptoms, psychological adjustment, and concurrent life stresses that the provision of an information booklet reduced anxiety and decreased reported level of ongoing problems. These and similar studies suggest that interventions that inform individuals of the expected symptoms, the trajectory of recovery along with suggested coping strategies within one week of sustaining a concussion will at later follow-ups result in patients reporting fewer symptoms and reduced anxiety (Mittenberg et al., 1996; Paniak, Toller-Lobe, Reynolds, Melnyk, & Nagy, 2000; Wade, Crawford, Wenden, King, & Moss, 1997).

These studies investigated informational interventions close in time to the actual injury. Few studies have investigated informational interventions with patients who have persistent symptoms several years post mTBI. It is not known if these approaches would work as well at a later time point (Belanger, Uomoto, & Vanderploeg, 2009). There are several reasons simple informational interventions may not be as helpful with persistent PCS symptoms in the blast exposure population as they have been in acute mTBI situations.

First, it is possible that misattribution over an extended period of time may lead to a psychological investment in the symptoms on multiple levels. Social roles, financial compensation, perceived self-efficacy, and personal life expectations may all be altered by prolonged periods of misattributed persistent PCS symptoms.

Second, in many cases, the persistent PCS symptoms may be due to comorbid condition(s) and simply informing the patients that they should not have symptoms due to a remote mTBI will not alleviate symptoms stemming from a different source. This underscores the importance of appropriate differential assessment and diagnosis based upon a mechanism of injury approach (Scott, Belanger, Vanderploeg, Massengale, & Scholten, 2006). In either situation, if symptoms stem from a different etiology or iatrogenic symptoms were created, symptom resolution will require a mental paradigm shift in the individual. It is important for clinicians treating these patients to get them "treatment ready," which means aiding them with the mental paradigm shift and helping them to be willing to consider that persistent symptoms may be related to psychological or physical factors and not organically based. This process will likely take more than one discussion and individuals and their families may go through a range of emotions during and after these discussions. Expecting a solider to easily transition the mindset would be naive on the part of the treatment provider. The reallocation of the long-standing misattribution of symptoms to a different cause requires some recreation of personal identity.

Tiersky et al. (2005) compared wait-listed controls (n = 9) with patients enrolled in an 11-week program consisting of 33 sessions of individualized cognitive remediation and cognitive behavioral psychotherapy and found the intervention resulted in lowered levels of depression and anxiety, and improved performance on a measure of divided auditory attention, suggesting interventional techniques with more long-standing misattribution of symptoms is possible as well.

The Role of Neurocognitive Testing

To aid in the detection of mTBI and its sequelae in the deployed environment, multiple policies and programs were initiated by the DoD, including the implementation of a neurocognitive baseline assessment program at predeployment that allows for postinjury comparison (USD P&R DoD 6490.13; U.S. House of Representatives H.R. 4986, NDAA 2008, Sec 1618). In 2008 Congress mandated a baseline predeployment neurocognitive assessment for all U.S. service members to address increasing concern surrounding the risk of cognitive insult during military deployment (Cole et al., 2013; Ivins, Kane, & Schwab, 2009; Seegmiller & Kane, 2010). However, the empirical validity of baseline cognitive testing within concussion monitoring and management programs for preventing or mitigating concussion risk has been questioned (Kirkwood, Randolph, & Yeates, 2009).

Although some studies (Echemendia et al., 2012; Schmidt, Register-Mihalik, Mihalik, Kerr, & Guskiewicz, 2012) have suggested no added value of baseline testing in civilian concussion monitoring programs, there is evidence that baseline testing reduces the possibility of false positive detection of concussion in healthy service members. A large study of military service members (N = 8,002) found that when norm-referenced postdeployment scores were considered in isolation, 66% of individuals classified as "atypical" actually showed no change from baseline. Baseline testing, especially testing that can be repeated over the life span, allows for longitudinal tracking of an individual's cognitive trajectory and detection of factors that cause a change from baseline. Monitoring of these results over time, controlling for effects of aging, or other normative causes of cognitive change, could improve the sensitivity of dementia monitoring protocols (Roebuck-Spencer, Vincent, Schlegel, & Gilliland, 2013).

The Intersection of Service Members and the Criminal Justice System

In the years following the war in Vietnam, popular perception linked military combat, PTSD, and criminal behavior. The veteran was perceived as more likely to commit crime because of high rates of unemployment, mental health issues, substance abuse, thrill-seeking behaviors, or other reasons (Sparr, Reaves, & Atkinson, 1987). In 1951 Lunden wrote:

> In the aftermath of every major war certain people and some organizations give considerable credence to the idea that military service tends to create criminality in the men who have served in the armed forces of the nation after they return to civilian life. In some instances novels and movies popularize the notion that military duty fosters crime and disorder among men in arms after a war. After World War I such novels and plays as "What Price Glory?," "They Put a Gun in My Hand," "All Quiet on the Western Front" and "The Road Back" more than suggested that soldiering resulted in crime. Since World War II there has been less evidence of this idea, but when newspapers report a crime committed by some ex-G.I. his war record often appears in the account in such a manner as to intimate that military duty had something to do with the violation.
>
> (Lunden, 1951, p. 766)

In reality, identifying whether there is a relationship between combat exposure or injuries and civilian violence on return from deployment is complicated by differences in reactions of individuals to combat exposure, the overlapping effects of TBI and PTSD, and the low base rate of civilian violence after combat exposure (Sreenivasan et al., 2013). In a large cohort study of UK military personnel, 17.0% of 12,359 male UK military personnel had a criminal record for any offense during their lifetime. The prevalence was highest in men under 30 years old. Deployment was not independently associated with increased risk of violent offending, but serving in a combat role conferred an additional risk. Increased exposure to traumatic events during deployment also increased risk of violent offending. Violent offending was strongly associated with postdeployment alcohol misuse, PTSD (especially hyperarousal symptoms), and high levels of self-reported aggressive behavior (Macmanus et al., 2013). In a national survey of 1,388 Iraq and Afghanistan war era veterans, 9% of respondents reported arrests after returning home from deployment. Most arrests were associated with nonviolent criminal behavior resulting in incarceration for less than two weeks. Those who reported anger/irritability were more likely to be arrested than were other veterans. Arrests were found to be significantly related to younger age, male gender, having witnessed family violence, prior history of arrest, alcohol/drug misuse, and PTSD with high anger/irritability but were not significantly related to combat exposure or TBI (Elbogen et al., 2012).

A few high-profile cases, including that of SSG Robert Bales, have increased public perception that there is a link between PTSD and war atrocities. Bales is a former U.S. Army soldier who murdered 16 Afghan civilians in Kandahar, Afghanistan, in March, 2012. He later pleaded guilty to 16 counts of murder and six counts of assault and attempted murder, and was sentenced to life in prison without parole. His lawyer claimed that he suffered from PTSD symptoms (Leonnig, 2012). One recent study (Wilk et al., 2013) examined whether unethical battlefield conduct is a proxy for aggression and whether specific combat experiences and PTSD are independently associated with unethical behavior. The results of this study showed that aggression and specific combat experiences (particularly, witnessing war atrocities and fighting) were much more strongly associated with unethical conduct than was PTSD.

In response to concerns about military veterans entering the criminal justice because of actions related to deployment related health conditions (especially PTSD and TBI) many jurisdictions established Veterans Courts, intended to funnel those committed nonviolent offenses to treatment programs rather than punishment if appropriate (Hawkins, 2010; Holbrook, 2010; Pratt, 2010). This has not been without controversy, however. In some cases, there is concern over whether veterans courts unfairly shift the focus of justice away from the interests of victims to the rehabilitative interests of perpetrators (Holbrook, 2010).

Research and Longitudinal Follow-Up

In 2013 the White House announced that the University of Texas Health Science Center–San Antonio and Virginia Commonwealth University would each lead new research consortia with more than $100 million of support from DoD and VA to help better recognize and treat PTSD and the links between TBI and other mental health issues. More broadly, however, both the DoD and the VA are actively following service members with TBI longitudinally, in empirical studies to include the 15 Year Study by the Defense and Veterans Brain Injury Center (U.S. House of Representatives NDAA 2007, Sec 721) and the TBI Model Systems effort within VA (Brickell et al., 2014a; Brickell, Lange, & French, 2014b; Lamberty et al., 2014; Lange, Brickell, French, et al., 2012; Lange, Brickell, Ivins, Vanderploeg, & French, 2012; McGarity et al., 2013). Longitudinal follow-up and data monitoring is intended to help to clarify initial care that helped to improve outcome and the natural course of brain injury and polytrauma over the life span. This systematic monitoring of service members and veterans over their life span will lay the groundwork for tracking of cost of care and health care utilization for those individuals with premorbid brain injury, track the development of dementia and CNS illnesses, and monitor the efficacy of treatment programs among other things.

Primary to any major longitudinal monitoring effort is definition of key data elements that allow for integration of data from multiple studies and shared ontologies associated with that data to allow for reliable analysis and interpretation. DoD, VA, the National Institute on Disability and Rehabilitation Research (NIDRR), and the National Institutes of Health (NIH) have contributed to the development of common data elements for use in research related to TBI (Thurmond et al., 2010; Whyte, Vasterling, & Manley, 2010; Wilde et al., 2010). Many of these agencies now require the use of those data elements for their funded research. In addition, the NIH and DoD have sponsored a collaborative database aimed to integrate findings from funded research, especially clinical trials, which are available upon request for aggregated analysis and publication (https://fitbir.nih.gov). Similar to efforts in aging and autism, this increases available data to examine effective treatments, novel contributors to positive outcome, or evaluation of devices or methods for diagnosis and detection.

Other efforts under way include the Defense and Veterans Brain Injury Center's evaluation of the computerized cognitive tests available for postinjury assessment (Cole et al., 2013), a randomized controlled trial of cognitive rehabilitation in the military population, and an evaluation of the incidence and prevalence of multiple concussions in the military. In the VA, the Quality Enhancement Research Initiative in Polytrauma and Blast Related Injury (PT/BRI QUERI); Cifu, Cohen, Lew, Jaffee, & Sigford, 2010) is in the process of evaluating its screening and evaluation procedures, the effect of comorbidities on the utilization of care for mTBI patients, and the impact of these injuries on the caregiver and family. In addition, the VA has funded VA Epilepsy Centers of Excellence to study and provide services for those individuals with epilepsy, including those who have posttraumatic seizures following mild to severe TBI.

Chronic Traumatic Encephalopathy

One recently recognized long-term effect of repeated TBI is chronic traumatic encephalopathy (CTE). CTE is a progressive neurodegenerative disorder characterized by accumulation of hyper-phosphorylated tau deposits in neurons along with atrophy of brain tissue. CTE has been described primarily in professional athletes, although recently Goldstein and colleagues (2012) found CTE-like neuropathologic characteristics in the postmortem examination of brains from three military personnel who had been exposed to blast. Another study identified CTE in 21 military veterans (McKee et al., 2012). These studies have led some to suggest that there is a large emerging public health threat (Stern et al., 2011) for those in the military. However, a recent conclusion by the Institute of Medicine was that there is limited evidence of an association between recurrent blast TBI and chronic traumatic encephalopathy with progressive cognitive and behavioral decline (Medicine, 2014). While there are an increasing number of journal articles discussing the potential threat for service members, the studies of pathological changes in military service members are scant. Newly developed PET ligands (Gandy et al., 2014) that bind to tau will soon increase the number of potential subjects that can be examined for CTE-like brain changes after military service.

PTSD and Aging

The Department of Veterans Affairs conducted a large, retrospective cohort study of over 181,000 veterans 55 years or older without dementia from fiscal years 1997 through 2000. In the follow-up period from 2000 to 2007, 17.2% veterans had diagnosed dementia. Patients with PTSD were more than twice as likely to develop dementia compared with those without PTSD. After multivariable adjustment, patients with PTSD were still more likely to develop dementia (hazard ratio, 1.77; 95% confidence interval, 1.70–1.85), even when those with a history of head injury, substance abuse, or clinical depression were excluded (Yaffe et al., 2010).

In a study of 637 veterans without known coronary artery disease (CAD), screening showed that in subjects with PTSD, coronary artery calcium (CAC) was more prevalent than in the non-PTSD cohort (76.1% vs. 59%, $p = 0.001$) and their CAC scores were significantly higher in each Framingham risk score category compared to the non-PTSD group. PTSD was an independent predictor of the presence and extent of atherosclerotic CAD. During a mean follow-up of 42 months, the death rate was higher in the PTSD compared to the non-PTSD group. The authors concluded that PTSD is associated with the presence and severity of coronary atherosclerosis and predicts mortality independent of age, gender, and other conventional risk factors (Ahmadi et al., 2011).

Conclusion

TBI is an important concern in the military, both in peace and wartime. Because of the demographics of the military, mostly young men, there is an inherent risk for TBI. This risk is increased by combat operations and training. In both military conflicts and terrorism, the explosive device has emerged as a major cause of injury, including TBI.

In assessing or treating an individual injured in a military context, especially through blast, it is important to think in a comprehensive fashion taking into account the full range of possible consequences of that injury to include TBI, sensory impairment, pain issues, effort and motivation, and the emotional context in which the injury occurred. PTSD, mood changes, substance abuse, family dynamics, the disability process, and individual personality characteristics of the injured individual all have an impact on symptom presentation, rehabilitation, and recovery.

References

Ahmadi, N., Hajsadeghi, F., Mirshkarlo, H. B., Budoff, M., Yehuda, R., & Ebrahimi, R. (2011). Posttraumatic stress disorder, coronary atherosclerosis, and mortality. *The American Journal of Cardiology*, *108*(1), 29–33. doi: 10.1016/j.amjcard.2011.02.340

American Psychiatric Association. (2000). *Diagnostic and Statistical Manual of Mental Disorders* (4th ed.—Text Revision ed.).

Argyros, G. J. (1997). Management of primary blast injury. *Toxicology*, *121*(1), 105–115.

Armed Forces Health Surveillance, C. (2014). Deployment-related conditions of special surveillance interest, U.S. armed forces, by month and service, January 2003–October 2014. *Medical Surveillance Monthly Report*, *21*(11), 17.

Armistead-Jehle, P. (2010). Symptom validity test performance in U.S. veterans referred for evaluation of mild TBI. *Applied Neuropsychology*, *17*, 52–59.

Balaji, J., & D, M. (2011). Clinical and radiological profile of neurocysticercosis in South Indian children. *Indian Journal of Pediatrics*, *78*(8), 1019–1020. doi: 10.1007/s12098-011-0406-0

Bauman, R. A., Ling, G., Tong, L., Januszkiewicz, A., Agoston, D., Delanerolle, N., . . . Ecklund, J. (2009). An introductory characterization of a combat-casualty-care relevant swine model of closed head injury resulting from exposure to explosive blast. *Journal of Neurotrauma*, *26*(6), 841–860.

Bauman, R. A., Ling, G., Tong, L., Januszkiewicz, A., Agoston, D., Delanerolle, N., . . . Parks, S. (2009). An introductory characterization of a combat-casualty-care relevant swine model of closed head injury resulting from exposure to explosive blast. *Journal of Neurotrauma*, *26*(6), 841–860. doi: 10.1089/neu.2009-0898

Belanger, H. G., Curtiss, G., Demery, J. A., Lebowitz, B. K., & Vanderploeg, R. D. (2005). Factors moderating neuropsychological outcomes following mild traumatic brain injury: A meta-analysis. *Journal of the International Neuropsychological Society*, *11*(3), 215–227.

Belanger, H. G., Kretzmer, T., Vanderploeg, R. D., & French, L. M. (2009). Symptom complaints following combat-related traumatic brain injury: Relationship to traumatic brain injury severity and posttraumatic stress disorder. *Journal of the International Neuropsychological Society*, 1–6.

Belanger, H. G., Kretzmer, T., Yoash-Gantz, R., Pickett, T., & Tupler, L. A. (2009). Cognitive sequelae of blast-related versus other mechanisms of brain trauma. *Journal of the International Neuropsychological Society*, *15*(1), 1–8. doi: S1355617708090036 [pii] 10.1017/S1355617708090036

Belanger, H. G., Uomoto, J. M., & Vanderploeg, R. D. (2009). The veterans health administration system of care for mild traumatic brain injury: Costs, benefits, and controversies. *Journal of Head Trauma and Rehabiliation*, *24*(1), 4–13.

Bhattacharjee, Y. (2008). Neuroscience: Shell shock revisited: Solving the puzzle of blast trauma. *Science*, *319*(5862), 406–408. doi: 10.1126/science.319.5862.406

Binder, L. M., & Rohling, M. L. (1996). Money matters: A meta-analytic review of the effects of financial incentives on recovery after closed-head injury. *American Journal of Psychiatry*, *153*(1), 7–10.

Blanchard, E. B., & Hickling, E. J. (1997). *After the Crash: Assessment and Treatment of Motor Vehicle Accident Survivors*. Washington, DC: American Psychological Association.

Blanchard, E. B., Hickling, E. J., Devineni, T., Veazey, C. H., Galovski, T. E., Mundy, E., . . . Buckley, T. C. (2003). A controlled evaluation of cognitive behavioural therapy for posttraumatic stress in motor vehicle accident survivors. *Behaviour Research and Therapy*, *41*(1), 79–96.

Blanchard, E. B., Hickling, E. J., Forneris, C. A., Taylor, A. E., Buckley, T. C., Loos, W. R., & Jaccard, J. (1997). Prediction of remission of acute posttraumatic stress disorder in motor vehicle accident victims. *Journal of Traumatic Stress*, *10*(2), 215–234.

Blanchard, E. B., & Veazey, C. H. (2001). Mental disorders resulting from road traffic accidents. *Current Opinion in Psychiatry*, *14*(2), 143–147.

Blennow, K., Jonsson, M., Andreasen, N., Rosengren, L., Wallin, A., Hellstrom, P. A., & Zetterberg, H. (2011). No neurochemical evidence of brain injury after blast overpressure by repeated explosions or firing heavy weapons. *Acta Neurologica Scandinavica*, *123*(4), 245–251. doi: 10.1111/j.1600-0404.2010.01408.x

Bombardier, C. H., Fann, J. R., Temkin, N., Esselman, P. C., Pelzer, E., Keough, M., & Dikmen, S. (2006). Posttraumatic stress disorder symptoms during the first six months after traumatic brain injury. *Journal of Neuropsychiatry and Clinical Neurosciences*, *18*(4), 501–508. doi: 18/4/501 [pii] 10.1176/appi.neuropsych.18.4.501

Bowen, I. G., Fletcher, E. R., Richmond, D. R., Hirsch, F. G., & White, C. S. (1968). Biophysical mechanisms and scaling procedures applicable in assessing responses of the thorax energized by air-blast overpressures or by nonpenetrating missiles. *Annals of the New York Academy of Sciences*, *152*(1), 122–146.

Brady, K. T., Killeen, T. K., Brewerton, T., & Lucerini, S. (2000). Comorbidity of psychiatric disorders and posttraumatic stress disorder. *Journal of Clinical Psychiatry*.

Brenner, L. A., Vanderploeg, R. D., & Terrio, H. (2009a). Assessment and diagnosis of mild traumatic brain injury, posttraumatic stress disorder, and other polytrauma conditions: Burden of adversity hypothesis. *Rehabilitation Psychology*, *54*(3), 239–246. doi: 2009-12547-001 [pii] 10.1037/a0016908

Brenner, L. A., Vanderploeg, R. D., & Terrio, H. (2009b). Assessment and diagnosis of mild traumatic brain injury, posttraumatic stress disorder, and other polytrauma conditions: Burden of adversity hypothesis. *Rehabilitation Psychology*, *54*(3), 239–246. doi: 10.1037/a0016908 [doi]

Breslau, N., Davis, G. C., Andreski, P., & Peterson, E. (1991). Traumatic events and posttraumatic stress disorder in an urban population of young adults. *Archives of General Psychiatry*, *48*(3), 216–222.

Brickell, T. A., Lange, R. T., & French, L. M. (2014a). Health-related quality of life within the first 5 years following military-related concurrent mild traumatic brain injury and polytrauma. *Military Medicine*, *179*(8), 827–838. doi: 10.7205/milmed-d-13-00506

Brickell, T. A., Lange, R. T., & French, L. M. (2014b). Three-year outcome following moderate-to-severe TBI in U.S. military service members: A descriptive cross-sectional study. *Military Medicine*, *179*(8), 839–848. doi: 10.7205/milmed-d-14-00016

Bryant, R. A. (2008). Disentangling mild traumatic brain injury and stress reactions. *The New England Journal of Medicine*, *358*(5), 525–527.

Bryant, R. A., Harvey, A. G., Dang, S. T., Sackville, T., & Basten, C. (1998). Treatment of acute stress disorder: A comparison of cognitive-behavioral therapy and supportive counseling. *Journal of Consulting and Clinical Psychology*, *66*(5), 862–866.

Bryant, R. A., Sackville, T., Dang, S. T., Moulds, M., & Guthrie, R. (1999). Treating acute stress disorder: An evaluation of cognitive behavior therapy and supportive counseling techniques. *American Journal of Psychiatry*, *156*(11), 1780–1786.

Burges, C., & McMillan, T. (2001). The ability of naive participants to report symptoms of post-traumatic stress disorder. *British Journal of Clinical Psychology*, *40*(2), 209–214.

Burkett, B. G., & Whitley, G. (1998). *Stolen Valor: How the Vietnam Generation Was Robbed of Its Heroes and Its History*. Dallas, TX: Verity Press.

Carey, M. E., Sacco, W., & Merkler, J. (1982). An analysis of fatal and non-fatal head wounds incurred during combat in Vietnam by U.S. forces. *Acta Chirugica Scandinavica Supplementum*, *508*, 351–356.

Carlson, K. F., Barnes, J. E., Hagel, E. M., Taylor, B. C., Cifu, D. X., & Sayer, N. A. (2013). Sensitivity and specificity of traumatic brain injury diagnosis codes in United States Department of veterans affairs administrative data. *Brain Injury*, *27*(6), 640–650. doi: 10.3109/02699052.2013.771795

Cernak, I., Savic, J., Malicevic, Z., Zunic, G., Radosevic, P., & Ivanovic, I. (1996). Leukotrienes in the pathogenesis of pulmonary blast injury. *Journal of Trauma-Injury Infection and Critical Care*, *40*(3 Suppl), S148–S151.

Cernak, I., Savic, J., Malicevic, Z., Zunic, G., Radosevic, P., Ivanovic, I., & Davidovic, L. (1996). Involvement of the central nervous system in the general response to pulmonary blast injury. *Journal of Trauma-Injury Infection and Critical Care*, *40*(3 Suppl), S100–S104.

Cernak, I., Wang, Z., Jiang, J., Bian, X., & Savic, J. (2001). Ultrastructural and functional characteristics of blast injury-induced neurotrauma. *Journal of Trauma-Injury Infection and Critical Care*, *50*(4), 695–706.

Chavko, M., Koller, W. A., Prusaczyk, W. K., & McCarron, R. M. (2007). Measurement of blast wave by a miniature fiber optic pressure transducer in the rat brain. *Journal of Neuroscience Methods*, *159*(2), 277–281. doi: 10.1016/j.jneumeth.2006.07.018

Cicerone, K., & Kalmar, K. (1995). Persistent postconcussion syndrome: The structure of subjective complaints after mild traumatic brain injury. *Journal of Head Trauma and Rehabiliation*, *10*, 1–7.

Cifu, D. X., Cohen, S. I., Lew, H. L., Jaffee, M., & Sigford, B. (2010). The history and evolution of traumatic brain injury rehabilitation in military service members and veterans. *American Journal of Physical Medicine & Rehabilitation*, *89*(8), 688–694. doi: 10.1097/PHM.0b013e3181e722ad

Clemedson, C. J., & Pettersson, H. (1956). Propagation of a high explosive air shock wave through different parts of an animal body. *American Journal of Physiology*, *184*(1), 119–126.

Cole, W. R., Arrieux, J. P., Schwab, K., Ivins, B. J., Qashu, F. M., & Lewis, S. C. (2013). Test—retest reliability of four computerized neurocognitive assessment tools in an active duty military population. *Archives of Clinical Neuropsychology*, *28*(7), 732–742.

Compare, A., Gondoni, L., & Molinari, E. (2006). Psychological risk factors for cardiac disease and pathophysiological mechanisms: An overview. In *Clinical Psychology and Heart Disease* (pp. 21–32). New York: Springer.

Cooper, G. J., Maynard, R. L., Cross, N. L., & Hill, J. F. (1983). Casualties from terrorist bombings. *Journal of Trauma-Injury Infection and Critical Care*, *23*(11), 955–967.

DePalma, R. G., Burris, D. G., Champion, H. R., & Hodgson, M. J. (2005). Blast injuries. *The New England Journal of Medicine*, *352*(13), 1335–1342.

DePalma, R. G., Cross, G. M., Beck, L., & Chandler, D. (2011). *Epidemiology of mTBI (mild traumatic brain injury) due to blast: History, DOD/VA databases: Challenges and opportunities*. Paper presented at the Proc NATO RTO-MP-HFM-207 Symposium on A Survey of Blast Injury across the Full Landscape of Military Science.

DeWitt, D. S., & Prough, D. S. (2009). Blast-induced brain injury and posttraumatic hypotension and hypoxemia. *Journal of Neurotrauma*, *26*(6), 877–887. doi: 10.1089/neu.2007.0439

Dirkzwager, A. J., van der Velden, P. G., Grievink, L., & Yzermans, C. J. (2007). Disaster-related posttraumatic stress disorder and physical health. *Psychosomatic Medicine*, *69*(5), 435–440.

DVBIC. (2014). DoD worldwide numbers for TBI. Retrieved December 21, 2014, from http://dvbic.dcoe.mil/dod-worldwide-numbers-tbi

Echemendia, R. J., Bruce, J. M., Bailey, C. M., Sanders, J. F., Arnett, P., & Vargas, G. (2012). The utility of post-concussion neuropsychological data in identifying cognitive change following sports-related MTBI in the absence of baseline data. *Clinical Neuropsychologist*, *26*(7), 1077–1091. doi: 10.1080/13854046.2012.721006

Elbogen, E. B., Johnson, S. C., Newton, V. M., Straits-Troster, K., Vasterling, J. J., Wagner, H. R., & Beckham, J. C. (2012). Criminal justice involvement, trauma, and negative affect in Iraq and Afghanistan war era veterans. *Journal of Consulting and Clinical Psychology*, *80*(6), 1097–1102. doi: 10.1037/a0029967

Elhai, J. D., & Frueh, B. C. (2001). Subtypes of clinical presentations in malingerers of posttraumatic stress disorder: An MMPI-2 cluster analysis. *Assessment*, *8*(1), 75–84.

Elsayed, N. M., Gorbunov, N. V., & Kagan, V. E. (1997). A proposed biochemical mechanism involving hemoglobin for blast overpressure-induced injury. *Toxicology*, *121*(1), 81–90.

Erbes, C., Westermeyer, J., Engdahl, B., & Johnsen, E. (2007). Posttraumatic stress disorder and service utilization in a sample of service members from Iraq and Afghanistan. *Military Medicine*.

Fecteau, G., & Nicki, R. (1999). Cognitive behavioural treatment of post traumatic stress disorder after motor vehicle accident. *Behavioural and Cognitive Psychotherapy*, *27*(3), 201–214.

Feinstein, A., Hershkop, S., Ouchterlony, D., Jardine, A., & McCullagh, S. (2002). Posttraumatic amnesia and recall of a traumatic event following traumatic brain injury. *Journal of Neuropsychiatry and Clinical Neurosciences*, *14*(1), 25–30.

Foote, F. O., & Schwartz, L. (2012). Holism at the National Intrepid Center of Excellence (NICoE). *Explore: The Journal of Science and Healing*, *8*(5), 282–290.

Fox, D. D., Lees-Haley, P. R., Earnest, K., & Dolezal-Wood, S. (1995). Base rates of postconcussive symptoms in health maintenance organization patients and controls. *Neuropsychology*, *9*(4), 606.

Freeman, T., Powell, M., & Kimbrell, T. (2008). Measuring symptom exaggeration in veterans with chronic posttraumatic stress disorder. *Psychiatry Research*, *158*(3), 374–380.

French, L. M. (2009). TBI in the military: Preface. *Journal of Head Trauma Rehabilitation*, *24*(1), 1–3. doi: 10.1097/HTR.0b013e318197a14c00001199-200901000-00001 [pii]

French, L. M. (2010). Military traumatic brain injury: An examination of important differences. *Annals of the New York Academy of Sciences*, *1208*, 38–45. doi: 10.1111/j.1749-6632.2010.05696.x

French, L. M., Lange, R. T., & Brickell, T. (2014). Subjective cognitive complaints and neuropsychological test performance following military-related traumatic brain injury. *Journal of Rehabilitation Research & Development*, *51*(6), 933–950. doi: 10.1682/JRRD.2013.10.0226

French, L. M., Lange, R. T., Iverson, G. L., Ivins, B., Marshall, K., & Schwab, K. (2012). Influence of bodily injuries on symptom reporting following uncomplicated mild traumatic brain injury in U.S. military service members. *Journal of Head Trauma Rehabilitation*, *27*(1), 63–74. doi: 10.1097/HTR.0b013e3182248344

Frenisy, M.-C., Benony, H., Chahraoui, K., Minot, D., d'Arthis, P., Pinoit, J.-M., & Freysz, M. (2006). Brain injured patients versus multiple trauma patients: Some neurobehavioral and psychopathological aspects. *The Journal of Trauma Injury, Infection, and Critical Care*, *60*, 1018–1026.

Frueh, B. C., Gold, P. B., & de Arellano, M. A. (1997). Symptom overreporting in combat veterans evaluated for PTSD: Differentiation on the basis of compensation seeking status. *Journal of Personality Assessment*, *68*(2), 369–384. doi: 10.1207/s15327752jpa6802_8

Frueh, B. C., Hamner, M. B., Cahill, S. P., Gold, P. B., & Hamlin, K. L. (2000). Apparent symptom overreporting in combat veterans evaluated for PTSD. *Clinical Psychology Review*, *20*(7), 853–885.

Frueh, B. C., Smith, D. W., & Barker, S. E. (1996). Compensation seeking status and psychometric assessment of combat veterans seeking treatment for PTSD. *Journal of Traumatic Stress*, *9*(3), 427–439.

Galarneau, M. R., Woodruff, S. I., Dye, J. L., Mohrle, C. R., & Wade, A. L. (2008). Traumatic brain injury during operation Iraqi freedom: Findings from the United States navy-marine corps combat trauma registry. *Journal of Neurosurgery*, *108*(5), 950–957. doi: 10.3171/JNS/2008/108/5/0950

Gandy, S., Ikonomovic, M. D., Mitsis, E., Elder, G., Ahlers, S. T., Barth, J., . . . DeKosky, S. T. (2014). Chronic traumatic encephalopathy: Clinical-biomarker correlations and current concepts in pathogenesis. *Molecular Neurodegeneration*, *9*, 37.

Garrison, J., & Stewart, F. (2014). *The influence of music therapy on heart rate variability at the national intrepid center of excellence*. Paper presented at the Applied Psychophysiology and Biofeedback.

Gaylord, K. M., Cooper, D. B., Mercado, J. M., Kennedy, J. E., Yoder, L. H., & Holcomb, J. B. (2008). Incidence of posttraumatic stress disorder and mild traumatic brain injury in burned service members: Preliminary report. *Journal of Trauma-Injury Infection and Critical Care*, *64*(2 Suppl), S200–S205; discussion S205–206. doi: 10.1097/TA.0b013e318160ba42 00005373-200802001-00030 [pii]

Gfeller, J. D., Gripshover, D. L., & Chibnall, J. T. (1996). Assessing self-rated memory impairment in persons with posttraumatic headache. *Assessment*, *3*(4), 393–402.

Glasser, R. (2007). A shock wave of brain injuries. *Washington Post*, B01.

Goh, S. H. (2009). Bomb blast mass casualty incidents: Initial triage and management of injuries. *Singapore Medical Journal*, *50*(1), 101–106.

Gold, P. B., & Frueh, B. C. (1999). Compensation-seeking and extreme exaggeration of psychopathology among combat veterans evaluated for posttraumatic stress disorder. *Journal of Nervous and Mental Disease*, *187*(11), 680–684.

Goldstein, L. E., Fisher, A. M., Tagge, C. A., Zhang, X.-L., Velisek, L., Sullivan, J. A., . . . Wojnarowicz, M. W. (2012). Chronic traumatic encephalopathy in blast-exposed military veterans and a blast neurotrauma mouse model. *Science Translational Medicine*, *4*(134), 134ra160–134ra160.

Goodrich, G. L., Kirby, J., Cockerham, G., Ingalla, S. P., & Lew, H. L. (2007). Visual function in patients of a polytrauma rehabilitation center: A descriptive study. *Journal of Rehabilitation Research & Development*, *44*(7), 929–936.

Grafman, J., Jonas, B. S., Martin, A., Salazar, A. M., Weingartner, H., Ludlow, C., . . . Vance, S. C. (1988). Intellectual function following penetrating head injury in Vietnam veterans. *Brain*, *111*(Pt 1), 169–184.

Grafman, J., Schwab, K., Warden, D. L., Pridgen, A., Brown, H. R., & Salazar, A. M. (1996). Frontal lobe injuries, violence, and agression: A report of the Vietnam head injury study. *Neurology*, *46*(5), 1231–1238.

Greiffenstein, M. F., & Baker, W. J. (2008). Validity testing in dually diagnosed posttraumatic stress disorder and mild closed head injury. *The Clinical Neuropsychologist*, *22*(3), 565–582.

Grieger, T. A., Cozza, S. J., Ursano, R. J., Hoge, C., Martinez, P. E., Engel, C. C., & Wain, H. J. (2006). Posttraumatic stress disorder and depression in battle-injured soldiers. *American Journal of Psychiatry*, *163*(10), 1777–1783; quiz 1860.

Group, T. M. o. C. m. W. (2009). *VA/DoD Clinical Practice Guideline for Management of Concussion/Mild Traumatic Brain Injury*. Washington, DC.

Gruss, E. (2006). A correction for primary blast injury criteria. *Journal of Trauma-Injury Infection and Critical Care*, *60*(6), 1284–1289. doi: 10.1097/01.ta.0000220015.21948.ec

Gunstad, J., & Suhr, J. A. (2004). Cognitive factors in postconcussion syndrome symptom report. *Archives of Clinical Neuropsychology*, *19*(3), 391–405.

Guskiewicz, K. M., Ross, S. E., & Marshall, S. W. (2001). Postural stability and neuropsychological deficits after concussion in collegiate athletes. *Journal of Athletic Training*, *36*(3), 263.

Gutierrez de Ceballos, J. P., Turegano Fuentes, F., Perez Diaz, D., Sanz Sanchez, M., Martin Llorente, C., & Guerrero Sanz, J. E. (2005). Casualties treated at the closest hospital in the Madrid, March 11, terrorist bombings. *Critical Care Medicine*, *33*(1 Suppl), S107–S112.

Guy, R. J., Glover, M. A., & Cripps, N. P. (1998). The pathophysiology of primary blast injury and its implications for treatment. Part I: The thorax. *Journal of the Royal Naval Medical Service*, *84*(2), 79–86.

Haagsma, J. A., Polinder, S., Olff, M., Toet, H., Bonsel, G. J., & van Beeck, E. F. (2012). Posttraumatic stress symptoms and health-related quality of life: A two year follow up study of injury treated at the emergency department. *BMC Psychiatry*, *12*, 1. doi: 10.1186/1471-244X-12-1

Harvey, A. G., & Bryant, R. A. (2000). Two-year prospective evaluation of the relationship between acute stress disorder and posttraumatic stress disorder following mild traumatic brain injury. *American Journal of Psychiatry*, *157*(4), 626–628.

Hawkins, M. D. (2010). Coming home: Accomodating the special needs of military veterans to the criminal justice system. *Ohio State Journal of Criminal Law*, *7*, 563–573.

Hegde, M., Hegde, C., Parajuli, U., Kamath, P., & D, M. R. (2012). Combined orthodontic and surgical correction of an adolescent patient with thin palatal cortex and vertical maxillary excess. *Kathmandu University Medical Journal (KUMJ)*, *10*(39), 88–92.

Heinzelmann, M., Reddy, S. Y., French, L. M., Wang, D., Lee, H., Barr, T., . . . Gill, J. (2014). Military personnel with chronic symptoms following blast traumatic brain injury have differential expression of neuronal recovery and epidermal growth factor receptor genes. *Frontiers in Neurology*, *5*, 198.

Helmick, K., Baugh, L., Lattimore, T., & Goldman, S. (2012). Traumatic brain injury: Next steps, research needed, and priority focus areas. *Military Medicine*, *177*(8S), 86–92.

Heltemes, K. J., Dougherty, A. L., MacGregor, A. J., & Galarneau, M. R. (2011). Inpatient hospitalizations of U.S. military personnel medically evacuated from Iraq and Afghanistan with combat-related traumatic brain injury. *Military Medicine*, *176*(2), 132–135.

Hickling, E. J., Blanchard, E. B., Mundy, E., & Galovski, T. E. (2002). Detection of malingered MVA related posttraumatic stress disorder: An investigation of the ability to detect professional actors by experienced clinicians, psychological tests and psychophysiological assessment. *Journal of Forensic Psychology Practice*, *2*(1), 33–53.

Hirsch, F. G. (1968). Effects of overpressure on the ear: A review. *Annals of the New York Academy of Sciences*, *152*(1), 147–162.

Hoge, C. W., Auchterlonie, J. L., & Milliken, C. S. (2006). Mental health problems, use of mental health services, and attrition from military service after returning from deployment to Iraq or Afghanistan. *Jama*, *295*(9), 1023–1032.

Hoge, C. W., Castro, C. A., Messer, S. C., McGurk, D., Cotting, D. I., & Koffman, R. L. (2004). Combat duty in Iraq and Afghanistan, mental health problems, and barriers to care. *The New England Journal of Medicine*, *351*(1), 13–22.

Hoge, C. W., McGurk, D., Thomas, J. L., Cox, A. L., Engel, C. C., & Castro, C. A. (2008a). Mild traumatic brain injury in U.S. soldiers returning from Iraq. *The New England Journal of Medicine*, *358*(5), 453–463.

Hoge, C. W., McGurk, D., Thomas, J. L., Cox, A. L., Engel, C. C., & Castro, C. A. (2008b). Mild traumatic brain injury in U.S. soldiers returning from Iraq. *New England Journal of Medicine, 358*(5), 453–463. doi: 10.1056/NEJMoa072972

Hoge, C. W., Terhakopian, A., Castro, C. A., Messer, S. C., & Engel, C. C. (2007). Association of posttraumatic stress disorder with somatic symptoms, health care visits, and absenteeism among Iraq war veterans. *American Journal of Psychiatry, 164*(1), 150–153. doi: 164/1/150 [pii] 10.1176/appi.ajp.164.1.150

Holbrook, J. G. (2010). Veterans court and criminal responsibility: A problem solving history & approach to the liminality of combat trauma. In D. C. Kelly, D. Gitelson & S. H. Barksdale (Eds.), *Young Veterans: A Resilient Community of Honor, Duty and Need* (Vol. Widender Law School Legal Studies Research Paper, pp. 1–52). Wilmington, DE: Widener University School of Law.

Horrocks, C., & Brett, S. (2000). Blast injury. *Current Anaesthesia & Critical Care, 11*(2), 113–119. doi: http://dx.doi.org/10.1054/cacc.2000.0260

Hryvniak, M., & Rosse, R. (1989). Concurrent psychiatric illness in inpatients with posttraumatic stress disorder. *Military Medicine, 154*(8), 399–401.

Iverson, G. L. (2006). Misdiagnosis of the persistent postconcussion syndrome in patients with depression. *Archives of Clinical Neuropsychology, 21*(4), 303–310.

Iverson, G. L., Langlois, J. A., McCrea, M. A., & Kelly, J. P. (2009a). Challenges associated with post-deployment screening for mild traumatic brain injury in military personnel. *Clinical Neuropsychologist, 23*(8), 1299–1314. doi: 916359595 [pii] 10.1080/13854040903153902

Iverson, G. L., Langlois, J. A., McCrea, M. A., & Kelly, J. P. (2009b). Challenges associated with post-deployment screening for mild traumatic brain injury in military personnel. *The Clinical Neuropsychologist, 23*(8), 1299–1314.

Iverson, G. L., & McCracken, L. M. (1997). "Postconcussive" symptoms in persons with chronic pain. *Brain Injury, 11*(11), 783–790.

Ivins, B. J. (2010a). Hospitalization associated with traumatic brain injury in the active duty U.S. Army: 2000–2006. *NeuroRehabilitation, 26*, 199–212.

Ivins, B. J. (2010b). Hospitalization associated with traumatic brain injury in the active duty U.S. Army: 2000–2006. *NeuroRehabilitation, 26*(3), 199–212. doi: 10.3233/nre-2010-0556

Ivins, B. J., Kane, R., & Schwab, K. A. (2009). Performance on the automated neuropsychological assessment metrics in a nonclinical sample of soldiers screened for mild TBI after returning from Iraq and Afghanistan: A descriptive analysis. *The Journal of Head Trauma Rehabilitation, 24*(1), 24–31.

J, D. M. (2011). Exploring personality—personality disorder relations and their implications for DSM-5. *World Psychiatry, 10*(2), 110–111.

Jaffee, C.M.S., & Meyer, K. S. (2009). A brief overview of traumatic brain injury (TBI) and posttraumatic stress disorder (PTSD) within the department of defense. *The Clinical Neuropsychologist, 23*(8), 1291–1298. doi: 10.1080/13854040903307250

Jensen, J. H., & Bonding, P. (1993). Experimental pressure induced rupture of the tympanic membrane in man. *Acta Otolaryngolica, 113*(1), 62–67.

Johnson, M. A., Hawley, J. S., & Theeler, B. J. (2014). Management of acute concussion in a deployed military setting. *Current Treatment Options in Neurology, 16*(9), 1–16.

Kang, H. K., & Bullman, T. A. (1996). Mortality among U.S. veterans of the Persian Gulf War. *New England Journal of Medicine, 335*(20), 1498–1504.

Kang, H. K., Natelson, B. H., Mahan, C. M., Lee, K. Y., & Murphy, F. M. (2003). Posttraumatic stress disorder and chronic fatigue syndrome-like illness among Gulf War veterans: A population-based survey of 30,000 veterans. *American Journal of Epidemiology, 157*(2), 141–148.

Kaur, C., Singh, J., Lim, M. K., Ng, B. L., Yap, E. P., & Ling, E. A. (1995). The response of neurons and microglia to blast injury in the rat brain. *Neuropathology and Applied Neurobiology, 21*(5), 369–377.

Kay, T., Harrington, D. E., Adams, R., Anderson, T., Berrol, S., Cicerone, K., . . . Malec, J. (1993). Definition of mild traumatic brain injury. *Journal of Head Trauma Rehabilitation, 8*(3), 86–87.

Kessler, R. C., Sonnega, A., Bromet, E., Hughes, M., & Nelson, C. B. (1995). Posttraumatic stress disorder in the national comorbidity survey. *Archives of General Psychiatry, 52*(12), 1048–1060.

King, E. G., Kretzmer, T. S., Vanderploeg, R. D., Asmussen, S. B., Clement, V. L., & Belanger, H. G. (2013). Pilot of a novel intervention for postconcussive symptoms in active duty, veterans, and civilians. *Rehabilitation Psychology, 58*(3), 272–279. doi: 10.1037/a0033116

Kirkwood, M., Randolph, C., & Yeates, K. (2009). Returning pediatric athletes to play after concussion: The evidence (or lack thereof) behind baseline neuropsychological testing. *Acta Paediatrica, 98*(9), 1409.

Koffman, R. L., & Helms, J. M. (2013). Acupuncture and PTSD: "Come for the needles, stay for the therapy". *Psychiatric Annals, 43*(5), 236–239.

Koren, D., Norman, D., Cohen, A., Berman, J., & Klein, E. M. (2005). Increased PTSD risk with combat-related injury: A matched comparison study of injured and uninjured soldiers experiencing the same combat events. *American Journal of Psychiatry, 162*(2), 276–282. doi: 162/2/276[pii] 10.1176/appi.ajp.162.2.276

Kress, W. J., J, D. M., Sabu, M., Prince, L. M., Dey, S., & Sanoj, E. (2010). Larsenianthus: A new Asian genus of Gingers (Zingiberaceae) with four species. *PhytoKeys*, (1), 15–32. doi: 10.3897/phytokeys.1.658

Kulka, R., Schlenger, W., Fairbank, J., Hough, R., Jordan, K., & Marmar, C. (1990). PTSD among Vietnam veterans: A family perspective. *Trauma and the Vietnam War Generation; Report of Findings from the National Vietnam Veterans Readjustment Study*, 236–257.

Lamberty, G. J., Nakase-Richardson, R., Farrell-Carnahan, L., McGarity, S., Bidelspach, D., Harrison-Felix, C., & Cifu, D. X. (2014). Development of a traumatic brain injury model system within the department of veterans affairs polytrauma system of care. *The Journal of Head Trauma Rehabilitation, 29*(3), E1–E7.

Landre, N., Poppe, C. J., Davis, N., Schmaus, B., & Sobbs, S. E. (2006). Cognitive functioning and postconcussive symptoms in trauma patients with and without mild TBI. *Archives of Clinical Neuropsychology, 21*(4), 255–273.

Lange, R. T., Brickell, T. A., French, L. M., Merritt, V. C., Bhagwat, A., Pancholi, S., & Iverson, G. L. (2012). Neuropsychological outcome from uncomplicated mild, complicated mild, and moderate traumatic brain injury in U.S. military personnel.

Archives of Clinical Neuropsychology, *27*(5), 480–494. doi: acs059 [pii] 10.1093/arclin/acs059

Lange, R. T., Brickell, T. A., Ivins, B., Vanderploeg, R., & French, L. M. (2012). Variable, not always persistent, postconcussion symptoms following mild TBI in U.S. military service members: A 5-year cross-sectional outcome study. *Journal of Neurotrauma*. doi: 10.1089/neu.2012.2743

Lange, R. T., Brickell, T. A., Kennedy, J. E., Bailie, J. M., Sills, C., Asmussen, S., . . . French, L. M. (2014). Factors influencing postconcussion and posttraumatic stress symptom reporting following military-related concurrent polytrauma and traumatic brain injury. *Archives of Clinical Neuropsychology*, *29*(4), 329–347. doi: 10.1093/arclin/acu013

Lange, R. T., Pancholi, S., Bhagwat, A., Anderson-Barnes, V., & French, L. M. (2012). Influence of poor effort on neuropsychological test performance in U.S. military personnel following mild traumatic brain injury. *Journal of Clinical and Experimental Neuropsychology*, *34*(5), 453–466. doi: 10.1080/13803395.2011.648175

Lange, R. T., Pancholi, S., Brickell, T. A., Sakura, S., Bhagwat, A., Merritt, V., & French, L. M. (2012). Neuropsychological outcome from blast versus non-blast: Mild traumatic brain injury in U.S. military service members. *Journal of the International Neuropsychological Society*, *18*(3), 595–605. doi: 10.1017/S1355617712000239

Lees-Haley, P. R. (1986). Pseudo-posttraumatic stress disorder. *Trial Diplomacy Journal*.

Lees-Haley, P. R., & Dunn, J. T. (1994). The ability of naive subjects to report symptoms of mild brain injury, posttraumatic stress disorder, major depression, and generalized anxiety disorder. *Journal of Clinical Psychology*, *50*(2), 252–256.

Lees-Haley, P. R., Fox, D. D., & Courtney, J. C. (2001). A comparison of complaints by mild brain injury claimants and other claimants describing subjective experiences immediately following their injury. *Archives of Clinical Neuropsychology*, *16*(7), 689–695.

Leonnig, C. D. (2012). Staff Sgt. Robert Bales describes PTSD-like symptoms, lawyer says. *The Washington Post*, *28*.

Levin, H. S., Brown, S. A., Song, J. X., McCauley, S. R., Boake, C., Contant, C. F., . . . Kotrla, K. J. (2001). Depression and posttraumatic stress disorder at three months after mild to moderate traumatic brain injury. *Journal of Clinical and Experimental Neuropsychology*, *23*(6), 754–769.

Lew, H. L., Garvert, D. W., Pogoda, T. K., Hsu, P. T., Devine, J. M., White, D. K., . . . Goodrich, G. L. (2009). Auditory and visual impairments in patients with blast-related traumatic brain injury: Effect of dual sensory impairment on Functional Independence Measure. *Journal of Rehabilitation Research and Development*, *46*(6), 819–826. doi: 10.1682/JRRD.2008.09.0129

Lew, H. L., Jerger, J. F., Guillory, S. B., & Henry, J. A. (2007). Auditory dysfunction in traumatic brain injury. *Journal of Rehabilitation Research & Development*, *44*(7), 921–928.

Ling, G. S., & Ecklund, J. M. (2011). Traumatic brain injury in modern war. *Current Opinion in Anesthesiology*, *24*(2), 124–130. doi: 10.1097/ACO.0b013e32834458da

Linley, P. A., & Joseph, S. (2004). Positive change following trauma and adversity: A review. *Journal of Traumatic Stress*, *17*(1), 11–21. doi: 10.1023/B:JOTS.0000014671.27856.7e

Lipschutz, J. H., Pascuzzi, R. M., Bognanno, J., & Putty, T. (1991). Bilateral anterior cerebral artery infarction resulting from explosion-type injury to the head and neck. *Stroke*, *22*(6), 813–815.

Logan, B. W., Goldman, S., Zola, M., & Mackey, A. (2013). Concussive brain injury in the military: September 2001 to the present. *Behavioral Sciences & the Law*, *31*(6), 803–813. doi: 10.1002/bsl.2092

Lunden, W. A. (1951). Military service and criminality. *Journal of Criminal Law, Criminology and Police Science*, *42*, 766.

Luria, A. R. (1976). *The Working Brain: An Introduction to Neuropsychology*. New York: Basic Books.

Luria, A. R. (2004). *The Man With a Shattered World: The History of a Brain Wound*. Boston: Harvard Press.

Macdonald, C. L., Johnson, A. M., Nelson, E. C., Werner, N. J., Fang, R., Flaherty, S. F., & Brody, D. L. (2014). Functional status after blast-plus-impact complex concussive traumatic brain injury in evacuated United States military Personnel. *Journal of Neurotrauma*. doi: 10.1089/neu.2013.3173

Macedonia, C., Zamisch, M., Judy, J., & Ling, G. (2012). *DARPA challenge: Developing new technologies for brain and spinal injuries*. Paper presented at the SPIE Defense, Security, and Sensing.

Macmanus, D., Dean, K., Jones, M., Rona, R. J., Greenberg, N., Hull, L., . . . Fear, N. T. (2013). Violent offending by UK military personnel deployed to Iraq and Afghanistan: A data linkage cohort study. *Lancet*, *381*(9870), 907–917. doi: 10.1016/s0140-6736(13)60354-2

Maria, M.P.S., Pinkston, J. B., Miller, S. R., & Gouvier, W. D. (2001). Stability of postconcussion symptomatology differs between high and low responders and by gender but not by mild head injury status. *Archives of Clinical Neuropsychology*, *16*(2), 133–140.

Marion, D. W., & Regasa, L. E. (2014). Revisiting therapeutic hypothermia for severe traumatic brain injury. . . again. *Critical Care*, *18*(3), 160. doi: 10.1186/cc13955

Maruta, J., Lee, S. W., Jacobs, E. F., & Ghajar, J. (2010). A unified science of concussion. *Annals of the New York Academy of Sciences*, *1208*, 58–66. doi: 10.1111/j.1749-6632.2010.05695.x

Mather, F. J., Tate, R. L., & Hannan, T. J. (2003). Posttraumatic stress disorder in children following road traffic accidents: A comparison of those with and without mild traumatic brain injury. *Brain Injury*, *17*(12), 1077–1087.

Mayorga, M. A. (1997). The pathology of primary blast overpressure injury. *Toxicology*, *121*(1), 17–28.

Mayou, R. A., Black, J., & Bryant, B. (2000). Unconsciousness, amnesia and psychiatric symptoms following road traffic accident injury. *British Journal of Psychiatry*, *177*, 540–545.

McCarroll, J. E., Ursano, R. J., Fullerton, C. S., Liu, X., & Lundy, A. (2001). Effects of exposure to death in a war mortuary on posttraumatic stress disorder symptoms of intrusion and avoidance. *Journal of Nervous and Mental Disease*, *189*(1), 44–48.

McCauley, S. R., Boake, C., Levin, H. S., Contant, C. F., & Song, J. X. (2001). Postconcussional disorder following mild to moderate traumatic brain injury: Anxiety, depression, and social support as risk factors and comorbidities. *Journal of Clinical and Experimental Neuropsychology*, *23*(6), 792–808.

McCrea, M. (2008). *Mild Traumatic Brain Injury and Postconcussion Syndrome: The New Evidence Base for Diagnosis and Treatment*. New York: Oxford University Press.

McDonald, I. (2007). Gordon Holmes lecture: Gordon Holmes and the neurological heritage. *Brain*, *130*(Pt 1), 288–298. doi: 130/1/288 [pii] 10.1093/brain/awl335

McGarity, S., Nakase-Richardson, R., Lamberty, G. J., Farrell-Carnahan, L., Howe, L. L., Chung, J., . . . Kretzmer, T. (2013). Poster

100 the VA PRC traumatic brain injury model system program. *Archives of Physical Medicine and Rehabilitation*, *94*(10), e45.

McKee, A. C., Stein, T. D., Nowinski, C. J., Stern, R. A., Daneshvar, D. H., Alvarez, V. E., . . . Baugh, C. M. (2012). The spectrum of disease in chronic traumatic encephalopathy. *Brain*, aws307.

McNamee, S., Howe, L., Nakase-Richardson, R., & Peterson, M. (2012). Treatment of disorders of consciousness in the veterans health administration polytrauma centers. *The Journal of Head Trauma Rehabilitation*, *27*(4), 244–252.

Meares, S., Shores, E. A., Batchelor, J., Baguley, I. J., Chapman, J., Gurka, J., & Marosszeky, J. E. (2006). The relationship of psychological and cognitive factors and opioids in the development of the postconcussion syndrome in general trauma patients with mild traumatic brain injury. *Journal of the International Neuropsychological Society*, *12*(6), 792–801.

Meares, S., Shores, E. A., Taylor, A. J., Batchelor, J., Bryant, R. A., Baguley, I. J., . . . Marosszeky, J. E. (2008). Mild traumatic brain injury does not predict acute postconcussion syndrome. *Journal of Neurology, Neurosurgery, and Psychiatry*, *79*(3), 300–306.

Medicine, I. o. (2014). *Gulf War and Health, Volume 9: Long-Term Effects of Blast Exposures*. Washington, DC: The National Academies Press.

Melcer, T., Walker, J., Sechriest, V. F., Lebedda, M., Quinn, K., & Galarneau, M. (2014). Glasgow coma scores, early opioids, and posttraumatic stress disorder among combat amputees. *Journal of Traumatic Stress*, *27*, 1–8.

Messinger, S. D. (2009). Incorporating the prosthetic: Traumatic, limb-loss, rehabilitation and refigured military bodies. *Disability and Rehabilitation*, 1–5. doi: 911800061 [pii] 10.1080/09638280902943223

Meyer, K., Helmick, K., Doncevic, S., & Park, R. (2008). Severe and penetrating traumatic brain injury in the context of war. *Journal of Trauma Nursing*, *15*(4), 185–189; quiz 190–181. doi: 10.1097/01.JTN.0000343324.55087.de

Miller, G. (2011). Healing the brain, healing the mind. *Science*, *333*(6042), 514–517.

Milliken, C. S., Auchterlonie, J. L., & Hoge, C. W. (2007). Longitudinal assessment of mental health problems among active and reserve component soldiers returning from the Iraq war. *Jama*, *298*(18), 2141–2148. doi: 298/18/2141 [pii] 10.1001/jama.298.18.2141

Mittenberg, W., Canyock, E. M., Condit, D., & Patton, C. (2001). Treatment of post-concussion syndrome following mild head injury. *Journal of Clinical and Experimental Neuropsychology*, *23*(6), 829–836.

Mittenberg, W., DiGiulio, D. V., Perrin, S., & Bass, A. E. (1992a). Symptoms following mild head injury: Expectation as aetiology. *Journal of Neurology, Neurosurgery, and Psychiatry*, *55*(3), 200–204.

Mittenberg, W., DiGiulio, D. V., Perrin, S., & Bass, A. E. (1992b). Symptoms following mild head injury: Expectation as aetiology. *Journal of Neurology, Neurosurgery and Psychiatry*, *55*, 200–204.

Mittenberg, W., Tremont, G., Zielinski, R. E., Fichera, S., & Rayls, K. R. (1996). Cognitive-behavioral prevention of postconcussion syndrome. *Archives of Clinical Neuropsychology*, *11*(2), 139–145.

Mondello, S., Muller, U., Jeromin, A., Streeter, J., Hayes, R. L., & Wang, K. K. (2011). Blood-based diagnostics of traumatic brain injuries. *Expert Review of Molecular Diagnostics*, *11*(1), 65–78.

Mossman, D. (1996). Veterans affairs disability compensation: A case study in countertherapeutic jurisprudence. *Journal of the American Academy of Psychiatry and the Law Online*, *24*(1), 27–44.

Murray, C. K., Reynolds, J. C., Schroeder, J. M., Harrison, M. B., Evans, O. M., & Hospenthal, D. R. (2005). Spectrum of care provided at an echelon II medical unit during operation Iraqi freedom. *Military Medicine*, *170*(6), 516–520.

Nakase-Richardson, R., McNamee, S., Howe, L. L., Massengale, J., Peterson, M., Barnett, S. D., . . . Scott, S. (2013). Descriptive characteristics and rehabilitation outcomes in active duty military personnel and veterans with disorders of consciousness with combat-and noncombat-related brain injury. *Archives of Physical Medicine and Rehabilitation*, *94*(10), 1861–1869.

Nampiaparampil, D. E. (2008). Prevalence of chronic pain after traumatic brain injury: A systematic review. *Jama*, *300*(6), 711–719.

Neil, R., S, D. M., & Hanton, S. (2006). Psychological skills usage and the competitive anxiety response as a function of skill level in rugby union. *Journal of Sports Science and Medicine*, *5*(3), 415–423.

Norris, F. H. (1992). Epidemiology of trauma: Frequency and impact of different potentially traumatic events on different demographic groups. *Journal of Consulting and Clinical Psychology*, *60*(3), 409–418.

Okie, S. (2005a). Traumatic brain injury in the war zone. *New England Journal of Medicine*, *352*(20), 2043–2047. doi: 352/20/2043 [pii] 10.1056/NEJMp058102

Okie, S. (2005b). Traumatic brain injury in the war zone. *The New England Journal of Medicine*, *352*(20), 2043–2047.

Owens, B. D., Kragh, J. F., Jr., Wenke, J. C., Macaitis, J., Wade, C. E., & Holcomb, J. B. (2008). Combat wounds in operation Iraqi freedom and operation enduring freedom. *The Journal of Trauma Injury, Infection, and Critical Care*, *64*(2), 295–299.

Paniak, C., Toller-Lobe, G., Reynolds, S., Melnyk, A., & Nagy, J. (2000). A randomized trial of two treatments for mild traumatic brain injury: 1 year follow-up. *Brain Injury*, *14*(3), 219–226.

Panzer, M. B., Wood, G. W., & Bass, C. R. (2014). Scaling in neurotrauma: How do we apply animal experiments to people? *Experimental Neurology*, *261*, 120–126. doi: 10.1016/j.expneurol.2014.07.002

Pasquina, P. F., Tsao, J. W., Collins, D. M., Chan, B. L., Charrow, A., Karmarkar, A. M., & Cooper, R. A. (2008). Quality of medical care provided to service members with combat-related limb amputations: Report of patient satisfaction. *Journal of Rehabilitation Research & Development*, *45*(7), 953–960.

Petit, J., Bres, C., Just, D., Garcia, V., Mauxion, J. P., Marion, D., . . . Rothan, C. (2014). Analyses of tomato fruit brightness mutants uncover both cutin-deficient and cutin-abundant mutants and a new hypomorphic allele of GDSL lipase. *Plant Physiology*, *164*(2), 888–906. doi: 10.1104/pp.113.232645

Pitman, R. K., Altman, B., & Macklin, M. L. (1989). Prevalence of posttraumatic stress disorder in wounded Vietnam veterans. *The American Journal of Psychiatry*.

Pizzo, E., Varcamonti, M., Di Maro, A., Zanfardino, A., Giancola, C., & D'Alessio, G. (2008). Ribonucleases with angiogenic and bactericidal activities from the Atlantic salmon. *FEBS J*, *275*(6), 1283–1295. doi: 10.1111/j.1742-4658.2008.06289.x

Polusny, M. A., Kehle, S. M., Nelson, N. W., Erbes, C. R., Arbisi, P. A., & Thuras, P. (2011a). Longitudinal effects of mild traumatic brain injury and posttraumatic stress disorder comorbidity on postdeployment outcomes in national guard soldiers deployed to Iraq. *Archives of General Psychiatry*, *68*(1), 79–89. doi: 10.1001/archgenpsychiatry.2010.172

Polusny, M. A., Kehle, S. M., Nelson, N. W., Erbes, C. R., Arbisi, P. A., & Thuras, P. (2011b). Longitudinal effects of mild traumatic brain injury and posttraumatic stress disorder comorbidity on postdeployment outcomes in national guard soldiers deployed to Iraq. *Archives of General Psychiatry*, *68*(1), 79–89. doi: 10.1001/archgenpsychiatry.2010.172

Ponsford, J., Willmott, C., Rothwell, A., Cameron, P., Ayton, G., Nelms, R., . . . Ng, K. (2001). Impact of early intervention on outcome after mild traumatic brain injury in children. *Pediatrics*, *108*(6), 1297–1303.

Ponsford, J., Willmott, C., Rothwell, A., Cameron, P., Kelly, A. M., Nelms, R., & Curran, C. (2002). Impact of early intervention on outcome following mild head injury in adults. *Journal of Neurology, Neurosurgery, and Psychiatry*, *73*(3), 330–332.

Pratt, M. (2010). New courts on the block: Specialized criminal courts for veterans in the United States. *Appeal*, *39*, 1–19.

Price, M., Kearns, M., Houry, D., & Rothbaum, B. O. (2014). Emergency department predictors of posttraumatic stress reduction for trauma-exposed individuals with and without an early intervention. *Journal of Consulting and Clinical Psychology*, *82*(2), 336–341. doi: 10.1037/a0035537

Prigerson, H. G., Maciejewski, P. K., & Rosenheck, R. A. (2001). Combat trauma: Trauma with highest risk of delayed onset and unresolved posttraumatic stress disorder symptoms, unemployment, and abuse among men. *The Journal of Nervous and Mental Disease*, *189*(2), 99–108.

Rahman, S., Timofeev, E., & Kleine, H. (2007). Pressure measurements in laboratory-scale blast wave flow fields. *Review of Scientific Instruments* , *78*(12), 125106. doi: 10.1063/1.2818807

Raymont, V., Greathouse, A., Reding, K., Lipsky, R., Salazar, A., & Grafman, J. (2008). Demographic, structural and genetic predictors of late cognitive decline after penetrating head injury. *Brain*, *131*(Pt 2), 543–558. doi: awm300 [pii] 10.1093/brain/awm300

Richmond, D. R., Yelverton, J. T., & Fletcher, E. R. (1981). The biological effects of repeated blasts: DTIC Document.

Robinson, M. E., Lindemer, E. R., Fonda, J. R., Milberg, W. P., McGlinchey, R. E., & Salat, D. H. (2014). Close-range blast exposure is associated with altered functional connectivity in Veterans independent of concussion symptoms at time of exposure. *Human Brain Mapping*. doi: 10.1002/hbm.22675

Roebuck-Spencer, T. M., Vincent, A. S., Schlegel, R. E., & Gilliland, K. (2013). Evidence for added value of baseline testing in computer-based cognitive assessment. *Journal of Athletic Training*, *48*(4), 499–505.

Rosen, C. S., Chow, H. C., Finney, J. F., Greenbaum, M. A., Moos, R. H., Sheikh, J. I., & Yesavage, J. A. (2004). VA practice patterns and practice guidelines for treating posttraumatic stress disorder. *Journal of Traumatic Stress*, *17*(3), 213–222. doi: 10.1023/b:jots.0000029264.23878.53

Ruff, R. M., & Jurica, P. (1999). In search of a unified definition for mild traumatic brain injury. *Brain Injury*, *13*(12), 943–952.

Sayer, N. A., Chiros, C. E., Sigford, B., Scott, S., Clothier, B., Pickett, T., & Lew, H. L. (2008). Characteristics and rehabilitation outcomes among patients with blast and other injuries sustained during the global war on terror. *Archives of Physical Medicine and Rehabilitation*, *89*(1), 163–170.

Sayer, N. A., Cifu, D. X., McNamee, S., Chiros, C. E., Sigford, B. J., Scott, S., & Lew, H. L. (2009). Rehabilitation needs of combat-injured service members admitted to the VA polytrauma rehabilitation centers: The role of PM&R in the care of wounded warriors. *PM R*, *1*(1), 23–28. doi: 10.1016/j.pmrj.2008.10.003

Sayer, N. A., Spoont, M., & Nelson, D. (2004). Veterans seeking disability benefits for posttraumatic stress disorder: Who applies and the self-reported meaning of disability compensation. *Social Science & Medicine*, *58*(11), 2133–2143. doi: 10.1016/j.socscimed.2003.08.009

Sayer, N. A., Spoont, M., Nelson, D. B., Clothier, B., & Murdoch, M. (2008). Changes in psychiatric status and service use associated with continued compensation seeking after claim determinations for posttraumatic stress disorder. *Journal of Traumatic Stress*, *21*(1), 40–48. doi: 10.1002/jts.20309

Sbordone, R. J., & Liter, J. C. (1995). Mild traumatic brain injury does not produce posttraumatic stress disorder. *Brain Injury*, *9*, 405–412.

Schiehser, D. M., Delis, D. C., Filoteo, J. V., Delano-Wood, L., Han, S. D., Jak, A. J., . . . Bondi, M. W. (2011). Are self-reported symptoms of executive dysfunction associated with objective executive function performance following mild to moderate traumatic brain injury? *Journal of Clinical and Experimental Neuropsychology*, *33*(6), 704–714. doi: 10.1080/13803395.2011.553587

Schmidt, J. D., Register-Mihalik, J. K., Mihalik, J. P., Kerr, Z. Y., & Guskiewicz, K. M. (2012). Identifying impairments after concussion: Normative data versus individualized baselines. *Medicine and Science in Sports and Exercise*, *44*(9), 1621–1628. doi: 10.1249/MSS.0b013e318258a9fb

Schneiderman, A. I., Braver, E. R., & Kang, H. K. (2008). Understanding sequelae of injury mechanisms and mild traumatic brain injury incurred during the conflicts in Iraq and Afghanistan: Persistent postconcussive symptoms and posttraumatic stress disorder. *American Journal of Epidemiology*, *167*(12), 1446–1452.

Scholten, J., Cernich, A., Hurley, R. A., & Helmick, K. (2013). Department of veterans affairs's traumatic brain injury screening and evaluation program: Promoting individualized interdisciplinary care for symptomatic veterans. *Journal of Head Trauma Rehabilitation*, *28*(3), 219–222. doi: 10.1097/HTR.0b013e318291daca

Schwab, K., Grafman, J., Salazar, A. M., & Kraft, J. (1993). Residual impairments and work status 15 years after penetrating head injury: Report from the Vietnam head injury study. *Neurology*, *43*(1), 95–103.

Schwartz, C. E., Kozora, E., & Zeng, Q. (1996). Towards patient collaboration in cognitive assessment: Specificity, sensitivity, and incremental validity of self-report. *Annals of Behavioral Medicine*, *18*(3), 177–184.

Scott, S. G., Belanger, H. G., Vanderploeg, R. D., Massengale, J., & Scholten, J. (2006). Mechanism-of-injury approach to evaluating patients with blast-related polytrauma. *Journal of the American Osteopathic Association*, *106*(5), 265–270. doi: 106/5/265 [pii]

Seegmiller, A., & Kane, R. L. (2010). The future of military neuropsychology. *Military Neuropsychology*, 383.

Shafi, S., & Gentilello, L. (2005). Hypotension does not increase mortality in brain-injured patients more than it does in non-brain-injured Patients. *Journal of Trauma-Injury Infection and Critical Care*, *59*(4), 830–834; discussion 834–835. doi: 00005373-200510000-00004 [pii]

Shen, S., Loo, R. R., Wanner, I. B., & Loo, J. A. (2014). Addressing the needs of traumatic brain injury with clinical proteomics. *Clinical Proteomics*, *11*(1), 11.

Sigford, B. J. (2008). "To care for him who shall have borne the battle and for his widow and his orphan"(Abraham Lincoln): The department of veterans affairs polytrauma system of care. *Archives of Physical Medicine and Rehabilitation*, *89*(1), 160–162.

Singh, R., Srivastava, A., Kapoor, R., R, K. S., & R, D. M. (2009). Impact of CYP3A5 and CYP3A4 gene polymorphisms on dose requirement of calcineurin inhibitors, cyclosporine and tacrolimus, in renal allograft recipients of North India. *Naunyn-Schmiedeberg's Archives of Pharmacology*, *380*(2), 169–177. doi: 10.1007/s00210-009-0415-y

Slovenko, R. (1994). Legal aspects of posttraumatic stress disorder. *Psychiatric Clinics of North America*.

Smith-Seemiller, L., Fow, N. R., Kant, R., & Franzen, M. D. (2003). Presence of post-concussion syndrome symptoms in patients with chronic pain vs. mild traumatic brain injury. *Brain Injury*, *17*(3), 199–206.

Sparr, L. F., Reaves, M. E., & Atkinson, R. M. (1987). Military combat, posttraumatic stress disorder, and criminal behavior in Vietnam veterans. *Journal of the American Academy of Psychiatry and the Law Online*, *15*(2), 141–162.

Spencer, R. J., McGuire, A. P., Tree, H. A., Waldron-Perrine, B., Pangilinan, P. H., & Bieliauskas, L. A. (2013). Report of traumatic brain injury information sources among OIF/OEF Veterans undergoing polytrauma evaluations. *Journal of Rehabilitation Research & Development*, *50*(1), 1–6.

Sreenivasan, S., Garrick, T., McGuire, J., Smee, D. E., Dow, D., & Woehl, D. (2013). Critical concerns in Iraq/Afghanistan war veteran-forensic interface: Combat-related postdeployment criminal violence. *Journal of the American Academy of Psychiatry and the Law*, *41*(2), 263–273.

Stansbury, L. G., Lalliss, S. J., Branstetter, J. G., Bagg, M. R., & Holcomb, J. B. (2008). Amputations in U.S. military personnel in the current conflicts in Afghanistan and Iraq. *Journal of Orthopaedic Trauma*, *22*(1), 43–46. doi: 10.1097/BOT.0b013e31815b35aa00005131-200801000-00009 [pii]

Stern, R. A., Riley, D. O., Daneshvar, D. H., Nowinski, C. J., Cantu, R. C., & McKee, A. C. (2011). Long-term consequences of repetitive brain trauma: Chronic traumatic encephalopathy. *PM&R*, *3*(10), S460–S467.

Suhr, J. A., & Gunstad, J. (2002a). "Diagnosis threat": The effect of negative expectations on cognitive performance in head injury. *Journal of Clinical and Experimental Neuropsychology*, *24*(4), 448–457.

Suhr, J. A., & Gunstad, J. (2002b). Postconcussive symptom report: The relative influence of head injury and depression. *Journal of Clinical and Experimental Neuropsychology*, *24*(8), 981–993.

Suhr, J. A., & Gunstad, J. (2005). Further exploration of the effect of "diagnosis threat" on cognitive performance in individuals with mild head injury. *Journal of the International Neuropsychological Society*, *11*(1), 23–29. doi: 10.1017/S1355617705050010

Sundin, J., Forbes, H., Fear, N. T., Dandeker, C., & Wessely, S. (2011). The impact of the conflicts of Iraq and Afghanistan: A UK perspective. *International Review of Psychiatry*, *23*(2), 153–159. doi: 10.3109/09540261.2011.561303

Surveillance for traumatic brain injury-related deaths—United States,1997–2007 (2011). In M. E. a. P. Staff (Ed.), *Morbidity and Morality Weekly Report* (Vol. 60, pp. 1–33). Atlanta, GA: Centers for Disease Control and Prevention.

Svetlov, S. I., Larner, S. F., Kirk, D. R., Atkinson, J., Hayes, R. L., & Wang, K. K. (2009). Biomarkers of blast-induced neurotrauma: Profiling molecular and cellular mechanisms of blast brain injury. *Journal of Neurotrauma*, *26*(6), 913–921. doi: 10.1089/neu.2008.0609

Sweeney, J. K., & Smutok, M. A. (1983). Vietnam head injury study: Preliminary analysis of the functional and anatomical sequelae of penetrating head trauma. *Physical Therapy*, *63*(12), 2018–2025.

T, M. K., D, M., & V, R. M. (2012). Cysticercus of the breast which mimicked a fibroadenoma: A rare presentation. *Journal of Clinical and Diagnostic Research*, *6*(9), 1555–1556. doi: 10.7860/JCDR/2012/4184.2559

Taber, K. H., Warden, D. L., & Hurley, R. A. (2006). Blast-related traumatic brain injury: What is known? *Journal of Neuropsychiatry and Clinical Neurosciences*, *18*(2), 141–145.

Tate, C. M., Wang, K. K., Eonta, S., Zhang, Y., Carr, W., Tortella, F. C., . . . Kamimori, G. H. (2013). Serum brain biomarker level, neurocognitive performance, and self-reported symptom changes in soldiers repeatedly exposed to low-level blast: A breacher pilot study. *Journal of Neurotrauma*. doi: 10.1089/neu.2012.2683

Taylor, B. C., Hagel, E. M., Carlson, K. F., Cifu, D. X., Cutting, A., Bidelspach, D. E., & Sayer, N. A. (2012). Prevalence and costs of co-occurring traumatic brain injury with and without psychiatric disturbance and pain among Afghanistan and Iraq War veteran VA users. *Medical Care*, *50*(4), 342–346.

Teasdale, G., & Jennett, B. (1974). Assessment of coma and impaired consciousness: A practical scale. *Lancet*, *2*(81–84).

Terrio, H., Brenner, L. A., Ivins, B. J., Cho, J. M., Helmick, K., Schwab, K., . . . Warden, D. (2009). Traumatic brain injury screening: Preliminary findings in a U.S. army brigade combat team. *Journal of Head Trauma Rehabilitation*, *24*(1), 14–23.

Thomas, J. L., Wilk, J. E., Riviere, L. A., McGurk, D., Castro, C. A., & Hoge, C. W. (2010). Prevalence of mental health problems and functional impairment among active component and national guard soldiers 3 and 12 months following combat in Iraq. *Archives of General Psychiatry*, *67*(6), 614–623. doi: 67/6/614 [pii] 10.1001/archgenpsychiatry.2010.54

Thurmond, V. A., Hicks, R., Gleason, T., Miller, A. C., Szuflita, N., Orman, J., & Schwab, K. (2010). Advancing integrated research in psychological health and traumatic brain injury: Common data elements. *Archives of Physical Medicine and Rehabilitation*, *91*(11), 1633–1636. doi: S0003-9993(10)00672-6 [pii] 10.1016/j.apmr.2010.06.034

Tiersky, L. A., Anselmi, V., Johnston, M. V., Kurtyka, J., Roosen, E., Schwartz, T., & Deluca, J. (2005). A trial of neuropsychologic rehabilitation in mild-spectrum traumatic brain injury. *Archives of Physical Medicine and Rehabilitation*, *86*(8), 1565–1574.

Tiersky, L. A., Johnson, S. K., Lange, G., Natelson, B. H., & Deluca, J. (1997). Neuropsychology of chronic fatigue syndrome: A critical review. *Journal of Clinical and Experimental Neuropsychology*, *19*(4), 560–586.

Turnbull, S. J., Campbell, E. A., & Swann, I. J. (2001). Posttraumatic stress disorder symptoms following a head injury: Does amnesia for the event influence the development of symptoms? *Brain Injury*, *15*(9), 775–785. doi: 10.1080/02699050110034334

Vanderploeg, R. D., & Belanger, H. G. (2013). Screening for a remote history of mild traumatic brain injury: When a good idea is bad. *Journal of Head Trauma Rehabilitation*, *28*(3), 211–218. doi: 10.1097/HTR.0b013e31828b50db

Vanderploeg, R. D., Belanger, H. G., Horner, R. D., Spehar, A. M., Powell-Cope, G., Luther, S. L., & Scott, S. G. (2012). Health outcomes associated with military deployment: Mild traumatic brain injury, blast, trauma, and combat associations in the Florida National Guard. *Archives of Physical Medicine and Rehabilitation, 93*(11), 1887–1895. doi: 10.1016/j.apmr.2012.05.024

Vanderploeg, R. D., Cooper, D. B., Belanger, H. G., Donnell, A. J., Kennedy, J. E., Hopewell, C. A., & Scott, S. G. (2014). Screening for postdeployment conditions: Development and cross-validation of an embedded validity scale in the neurobehavioral symptom inventory. *Journal of Head Trauma Rehabilitation, 29*(1), 1–10. doi: 10.1097/HTR.0b013e318281966e

Vasterling, J. J., Proctor, S. P., Amoroso, P., Kane, R., Heeren, T., & White, R. F. (2006). Neuropsychological outcomes of army personnel following deployment to the Iraq War. *Jama, 296*(5), 519–529.

Verfaellie, M., Lafleche, G., Spiro, A., & Bousquet, K. (2013). Neuropsychological outcomes in OEF/OIF veterans with self-report of blast exposure: Associations with mental health, but not mTBI. *Neuropsychology*. doi: 10.1037/neu0000027

Wade, D., Crawford, S., Wenden, F., King, N., & Moss, N. (1997). Does routine follow up after head injury help? A randomised controlled trial. *Journal of Neurology, Neurosurgery & Psychiatry, 62*(5), 478–484.

Warden, D. L. (2006). Military TBI during the Iraq and Afghanistan wars. *Journal of Head Trauma Rehabilitation, 21*(5), 398–402. doi: 00001199-200609000-00004 [pii]

Warden, D. L., French, L. M., Shupenko, L., Fargus, J., Riedy, G., Erickson, M. E., . . . Moore, D. F. (2009). Case report of a soldier with primary blast brain injury. *Neuroimage, 47*(Suppl 2), T152–T153.

Warden, D. L., Gordon, B., McAllister, T. W., Silver, J. M., Barth, J. T., Bruns, J., . . . Zitnay, G. (2006). Guidelines for the pharmacologic treatment of neurobehavioral sequelae of traumatic brain injury. *Journal of Neurotrauma, 23*(10), 1468–1501.

Weichel, E. D., Colyer, M. H., Bautista, C., Bower, K. S., & French, L. M. (2009). Traumatic brain injury associated with combat ocular trauma. *Journal of Head Trauma Rehabilitation, 24*(1), 41–50.

Wesolowski, K. (2010). New national treatment center for soldiers with TBI and PTSD opens. *Neurology Today*.

Whitney, K. A., Shepard, P. H., Williams, A. L., Davis, J. J., & Adams, K. M. (2009). The Medical symptom validity test in the evaluation of operation Iraqi freedom/operation enduring freedom soldiers: A preliminary study. *Archives of Clinical Neuropsychology, 24*(2), 145–152. doi: acp020 [pii] 10.1093/arclin/acp020

WHO. (1992). The ICD-10 classification of mental and behavioural disorders: Clinical descriptions and diagnostic guidelines.

Whyte, J., Vasterling, J., & Manley, G. T. (2010). Common data elements for research on traumatic brain injury and psychological health: Current status and future development. *Archives of Physical Medicine and Rehabilitation, 91*(11), 1692–1696. doi: S0003-9993(10)00651-9 [pii] 10.1016/j.apmr.2010.06.031

Wightman, J. M., & Gladish, S. L. (2001). Explosions and blast injuries. *Annals of Emergency Medicine, 37*(6), 664–678. doi: 10.1067/mem.2001.114906

Wilde, E. A., Whiteneck, G. G., Bogner, J., Bushnik, T., Cifu, D. X., Dikmen, S., . . . Steinbuechel, N. v. (2010). Recommendations for the use of common outcome measures in traumatic brain injury research. *Archives of Physical Medicine and Rehabilitation, 91*(11), 1650–1660.

Wilk, J. E., Bliese, P. D., Thomas, J. L., Wood, M. D., McGurk, D., Castro, C. A., & Hoge, C. W. (2013). Unethical battlefield conduct reported by soldiers serving in the Iraq war. *Journal of Nervous and Mental Disease, 201*(4), 259–265.

Wojcik, B. E., Stein, C. R., Bagg, K., Humphrey, R. J., & Orosco, J. (2010). Traumatic brain injury hospitalizations of U.S. army soldiers deployed to Afghanistan and Iraq. *American Journal of Preventive Medicine, 38*(1 Suppl), S108–S116. doi: 10.1016/j.amepre.2009.10.006

Xydakis, M. S., Bebarta, V. S., Harrison, C. D., Conner, J. C., Grant, G. A., & Robbins, A. S. (2007). Tympanic-membrane perforation as a marker of concussive brain injury in Iraq. *The New England Journal of Medicine, 357*(8), 830–831. doi: 357/8/830 [pii] 10.1056/NEJMc076071

Yaffe, K., Vittinghoff, E., Lindquist, K., Barnes, D., Covinsky, K. E., Neylan, T., . . . Marmar, C. (2010). Posttraumatic stress disorder and risk of dementia among U.S. veterans. *Archives of General Psychiatry, 67*(6), 608–613. doi: 10.1001/archgenpsychiatry.2010.61

Yang, Z., Wang, Z., Tang, C., & Ying, Y. (1996). Biological effects of weak blast waves and safety limits for internal organ injury in the human body. *Journal of Trauma-Injury Infection and Critical Care, 40*(3 Suppl), S81–S84.

Yount, R. A., Olmert, M. D., & Lee, M. R. (2012). Service dog training program for treatment of posttraumatic stress in service members. *U.S. Army Medical Department Journal*, 63–69.

34 Pain and Pain-Related Disability

Kevin W. Greve, Kevin J. Bianchini, and Steven T. Brewer

Introduction

Neuropsychologists will almost inevitably be confronted with issues of pain and pain-related disability in their practice. Pain is a feature of a variety of conditions commonly encountered by neuropsychologists such as multiple sclerosis, Parkinson's disease, and traumatic brain injury (TBI). Chronic pain after TBI, for example, occurs in 75% of mild TBI patients and 32% of moderate–severe TBI patients (Nampiaparampil, 2008). Pain is an important prognostic indicator for TBI recovery (Alexander, 1995; Mooney, Speed, & Sheppard, 2005) and should be addressed in order to reduce residual disability and maximize functional outcomes. Moreover, the same psychosocial factors that influence disability and recovery from pain likely complicate the management of neuropsychological conditions. Therefore, it is essential for the neuropsychologist to have an understanding of pain and the factors that influence pain-related disability.

Pain affects more than 50 million Americans, incurring a cost of over $70 billion annually in health care and lost productivity, and accounts for more than 80% of all clinical visits (Gatchel, 2004). Approximately 57% of adult Americans report experiencing recurring or chronic pain, 62% of whom were in pain for more than one year with 40% reporting constant pain (American Academy of Pain Management, 2003). Pain has a large impact on health-related quality of life (Morken et al., 2002) and back pain alone is thought to contribute to more than 100 million lost workdays yearly (Guo, Tanaka, Halperin, & Cameron, 1999). The total economic burden of pain-related health care and disability has been estimated to exceed $150 billion a year (Gatchel & Okifuji, 2006; Mayer, Gatchel, & Polatin, 2000).

Pain is defined as "an unpleasant sensory and emotional experience associated with actual or potential tissue damage, or described in terms of such damage" (International Association for the Study of Pain, 1994: 209-214). The experience of pain is influenced by both psychological and contextual factors that are not necessarily dependent on tissue damage or specific nociceptive activation (Merskey & Bogduk, 1994). Loeser and Melzack (1999) describe three broad categories of pain: (a) transient, (b) acute, and (c) chronic. "Acute pain ordinarily has a useful purpose, such as signaling damage or that something is wrong. By contrast, chronic pain has no such value, but is a disease in its own right, causing widespread suffering, distress, and disability" (Pappagallo & Werner, 2008, p. 17). Pain is termed *chronic* when symptoms do not follow the natural course of healing after injury or persist for longer than three months without biological value (Merskey & Bogduk, 1994). Psychological factors are important in the transition from acute to chronic pain Linton (2000). Chronic pain is due to stress as well as environmental and affective factors that may be superimposed on the original damaged tissue (Gatchel, Peng, Fuchs, Peters, & Turk, 2007; Loeser & Melzack, 1999).

Pathological findings from commonly used medical diagnostic techniques—e.g., magnetic resonance imaging (MRI) of the spine—are not sufficient to explain current or future pain-related symptoms or disability. For example, objective evidence of physical pathology does not always correlate with pain symptoms or disability, nor does it reliably predict who will become symptomatic in the future. Cervical and lumbar disc abnormalities, including some that would be considered surgical lesions, have been found in the cervical and lumbar spines of asymptomatic patients (Boden, Davis, Dina, Patronas, & Wiesel, 1990; Boden et al., 1990; Jarvik, Hollingworth, Heagerty, Haynor, & Deyo, 2001). Additionally, the presence of an identifiable abnormality of the disc or spinal canal in the lumbar spine of asymptomatic patients does not predict subsequent low back pain seven years later (Borenstein et al., 2001). What does predict the development of low back pain after three years in cases asymptomatic at baseline is self-reported depression at baseline (Jarvik et al., 2005). This applies not just to spinal pain. Incidental meniscal findings on MRI of the knee are common in the general population (Englund et al., 2008) and more than 60% of persons with one or more meniscal tears are asymptomatic. Further, a finding of meniscal pathology without frequent symptoms at baseline did not have a significant relationship with the development of knee symptomology 15 months later (Englund et al., 2007). Similarly, among persons with carpal tunnel syndrome there was no association between electrodiagnostic findings and symptoms/disability (Chan et al., 2007). In short, objective physical findings do not fully explain the symptom presentation of a large proportion of patients seen by physicians for complaints of pain. In fact, psychosocial factors may predict important outcomes (e.g., return to work) better than physical variables such as MRI-identified morphologic abnormalities (Schade, Semmer, Main, Hora, & Boos, 1999).

Conversely, many people present to physicians with a variety of physical symptoms for which no medical explanation can be found. For example, 75% of the Englund et al. (2008) sample without meniscal pathology or radiographic evidence of osteoarthritis were symptomatic. Nearly 20% of patients seen in primary care clinics present with medically unexplained symptoms, a finding not explained by comorbid depression or anxiety (Barsky, Orav, & Bates, 2005). Among first-time referrals to a neurology service, 61% (59% of females, 63% of males) had at least one medically unexplained symptom (Fink, Steen Hansen, & Sondergaard, 2005). Thirty-four percent (41.3% of females, 27.7% of males; 20.5% of inpatients, 43.2% of outpatients) of the Fink et al. (2005) cases met the diagnostic ICD-10 criteria for a somatoform disorder. Neuropsychologists are familiar with psychogenic nonepileptic seizures, which are diagnosed in approximately 30% of patients evaluated using video-EEG monitoring (Benbadis, O'Neill, Tatum, & Heriaud, 2004; Gates, Ramani, Whalen, & Loewenson, 1985; Martin, Burneo, Prasad, et al., 2003).

In short, pain and pain-related disability are complex biopsychosocial phenomena, and consideration of psychosocial factors is essential for a comprehensive understanding and appropriate treatment of pain and patients with pain (Gatchel & Okifuji, 2006). This chapter will review the science of pain and pain-related disability including the neuroanatomy/neurophysiology of pain as well as the psychosocial/person factors and context/system factors that influence pain-related disability. Assessment of the patient with chronic pain will then be reviewed followed by a discussion of behavioral approaches to the management of pain-related disability.

Neuroanatomy and Physiology

Pain is the unpleasant experience associated with tissue damage or potential tissue damage. As such, it is a neurobiological phenomenon. However, by its very nature, pain is a cognitive and emotional phenomenon as well. This section is intended to provide the neuropsychologist with some understanding of the neurobiology of pain and the neural mechanisms linking pain to important psychological factors such as anxiety and depression. A full discussion of the neurobiology of pain is beyond the scope of this chapter. The interested reader is referred to Deer et al. (2013), McMahon, Koltzenburg, Tracey, and Turk (2013) and Millan (1999), for a more in-depth review of this topic.

Neural Systems of Pain

Nociception is the neural mechanism that allows the organism to detect possible tissue damage (Jaggar, 2005). Once a nociceptive event is detected, the neural signal is transmitted primarily by two types of neuronal fibers, Aδ and C fibers. Aδ fibers are larger and more myelinated than C-fibers, which are generally unmyelinated but make up the majority of afferent nociceptive input (Cafferty, 2005; Millan, 1999). These two fiber systems transmit information of different types at different speeds. Aδ signals are received as a first wave of pain and perceived as sharp in nature, while the unmyelinated C-fibers conduct a slower second wave of pain signals that are perceived as dull in nature (Cafferty, 2005; Millan, 1999).

This information is transmitted to the dorsal horn of the spinal cord and from there it is transmitted from the spinal cord to the thalamus primarily along a spinothalamic pathway (Hoffman, Harrington, & Fields, 2005). The thalamus projects to sensory areas (S1 and S2) of the cortex (Wager, 2005; Hoffman et al., 2005). Spinal cord and sensory area neurons also project to the anterior insula (AINS), and the anterior cingulate cortex (ACC), which are believed to be involved in the affective qualities of pain (Craig, Chen, Bandy, & Reiman, 2000; Wager, 2005). These pain signals are believed to be further processed and evaluated through complex interconnections within the orbitofrontal cortex (OFC), AINS, and ACC. These signals may be maintained and elaborated upon through cognitive processes (e.g., attention) in the dorsolateral prefrontal cortex (DLPFC) and ventrolateral prefrontal cortex (VLPFC) (Wager, 2005).

This emotional/affective information and attention-enhanced information is then transmitted back to the periaqueductal gray (PAG) and then to rostral ventromedial medulla (RVM), particularly the RVM's nucleus raphe magnus (NRM). The NRM, which is rich in serotonergic neurons, connects to interneurons in the dorsal horn of the spinal cord, forming a descending pain control pathway that can influence ascending pain signals (Hoffman et al., 2005). This has been referred to as the *Gate Control Theory of Pain* (Melzack & Wall, 1965). Thus, these higher level cortical/neurocognitive processes can inhibit or enhance ascending pain signals and thus influence the experience of pain.

In addition to providing a mechanism for pain relief, it also appears that aspects of this system can influence descending input that can increase pain sensitivity through mechanisms like anxiety and depression. Anxiety specifically is known to activate the hypothalamic-pituitary-adrenal (HPA) axis. The anticipation of pain is known to activate a pro-nociceptive neuropeptide known as cholecystokinin (CCK) and to be associated with a reduction in dopamine levels (Benedetti, 2009). These neurotransmitters will be briefly discussed in the next section; for a more in-depth discussion of dopamine, CCK, and anxiety the reader is referred to Benedetti (2009).

Pain-related Neurotransmitters

Opioids

Opioids are powerful analgesics that can be classified generally into two categories, weak (e.g., codeine) and strong (e.g., morphine), which describe their relative efficacy and receptor site affinity (Twycross, 1994). Opiates (derivatives of the poppy plant) and opioids (synthetic molecules) bind to opioid receptors producing an analgesic response relative to the category in which they belong. Opioid receptors are found throughout the brain, brain stem, and the spinal cord (Benedetti, 2009). Receptors are found to be particularly dense in the cingulate cortex, prefrontal cortex (Pfeiffer, Pasi, Mehraein, & Herz, 1982), PAG, and RVM (Fields, 2004). The latter two areas, as mentioned earlier, are particularly important for the blockade of ascending pain signals. The neurotransmitters described in the following subsections work through the opioid system by inhibiting or facilitating the release of endorphins and enkephalins, the brain's endogenous opioids.

Cholecystokinin (CCK)

Cholecystokinin (CCK) is an endogenous peptide. Its receptors are found in the same structures as opioid receptors and in approximately the same density. In the central nervous system, CCK is considered to be a pro-nociceptive neurotransmitter, increasing pain perception and exacerbating symptoms (Enck, Benedetti, & Schedlowski, 2008). CCK, for example, has been experimentally shown to reverse opioid analgesia (Mitchell, Lowe, & Fields, 1998; Heinricher, McGaraughty, & Tortorici, 2001) by acting on the pain-facilitating neurons within RVM (Heinricher & Neubert, 2004). CCK is also involved with the anticipatory anxiety specifically associated with impending pain rather than a global anxiogenic event (Benedetti et al., 2006; Koyama, Tanaka, & Mikami, 1998; Sawamoto et al., 2000).

Dopamine

There are two primary dopamine (DA) cell groups—the substantia nigra pars compacta and the ventral tegmental area—and each has disparate neuronal projections (Alexander, Delong, & Strick, 1986; de la Fuente-Fernandez & Stoessl, 2002). The substantia nigra, which projects primarily to the dorsal striatum, is primarily involved in motor function (de la Fuente-Fernandez & Stoessl, 2002) and is not relevant for pain. The second major group of DA neurons originates in the ventral tegmental area (VTA) and projects to other brains structures via two pathways. The first projects via the mesolimbic pathway to subcortical limbic structures (ventral striatum, amygdala, hippocampus, olfactory tubercle, and septal region). The second projects via the mesocortical pathway from lateral regions of the VTA to frontal cortical regions (de la Fuente-Fernandez & Stoessl, 2002). Both the pathways are associated with pain sensitivity and inhibition. The limbic and prefrontal cortex can influence opioid release via DA input directly into the PAG (Christie, James, & Beart, 1986). The VTA also has direct projections to the PAG (Beitz, 1982). The nucleus accumbens (NA), which is involved in pain-related placebo responses (de la Fuente-Fernandez & Stoessl, 2002; Scott et al., 2008), influences PAG via the hypothalamus (Yu & Han, 1989). In addition, the PAG has projections back to limbic structures including the VTA, NA, amygdala and limbic frontal areas (Cameron, Khan, Westlund, Cliffer, & Willis, 1995). These reciprocal connections indicate a relationship between dopamine release and the *perception* of pain (de la Fuente-Fernandez & Stoessl, 2002). There are DA-related pain systems separate from these cortical-subcortical pathways. The dorsal horn of the spinal cord is the site at which ascending sensory information, including pain signals, enters the spinal cord. Dopaminergic networks there have the capacity to inhibit or facilitate pain signaling in complex ways depending on the amount of DA released (Millan, 1999).

Serotonin/Norepinephrine

Serotonin (5-hydroxtryptamine, 5-HT) and norepinephrine (NE) are monoamine neurotransmitters whose association with depression is well known. In addition to the role 5-HT plays in depression, its role in the inhibition and promotion of pain is also well known, if less well understood. Moreover, depression and pain appear to be closely linked. There is a growing body of literature regarding what some have referred to as the "depression-pain syndrome" (Bair, Robinson, Katon, & Kroenke, 2003). Serotonin-containing neurons are found in the RVM (in particular, the NRM). These neurons project to dorsal horn interneurons and are involved in the inhibition of ascending pain signals (Sommer, 2004). Like 5-HT, NE is involved in the suppression of ascending pain signals from the dorsal horn of the spinal cord. The NE neurons that influence ascending pain signals originate in the dorsolateral pontine tegmentum (DLPT) and project to the RVM as well as directly to the dorsal horn (Bair et al., 2003). It appears that NE and 5-HT have a complex relationship in the inhibition of ascending nociceptive information. In this context, it is necessary to discuss two types of RVM interneuron: on-cells and off-cells. On-cells facilitate pain transmission from the periphery to the spinal cord; off-cells inhibit pain signals that are ascending from the spinal cord to higher levels of the nervous system. Both are activated by stimulation of PAG (Bair et al., 2003; Benarroch, 2008). It is thought that the role of this system is to prioritize attentional resources to external painful events and minimize attention to internal pain signals (Bair et al., 2003; Okada, Murase, & Kawakita, 1999). However, disrupting serotonergic and noradrenergic activity as occurs during depression may result in the amplification of internal pain states and increased perception of normally suppressed pain signals (Bair et al., 2003). This research offers a potential biological mechanism underlying the well-documented link between depression and pain. Therapeutically, selective serotonin reuptake inhibitor (SSRI) and serotonin-norepinephrine reuptake inhibitor (SNRI) drugs have differential effects on pain (Zhao et al.,

2007) with SNRIs being more effective than SSRIs (Benarroch, 2008).

Summary

One of the take-home messages from this section is that complex ascending and descending neural systems can modulate nociceptive signals associated with specific injury so that the pain experienced is greater than that produced by the pathophysiology of the actual injury itself. Research using a placebo/nocebo methodology has contributed to the elucidation of the complex neurobiological systems that underpin pain experience. Moreover, this methodology has demonstrated how nonbiological factors can exert a powerful influence on these neurobiological systems. While there is debate over precise definitions (see for example, Stewart-Williams & Podd, 2004), for purposes of the following discussion, a placebo or nocebo, generally, is a substance or procedure that has no inherent power to produce the effect that is sought or expected. A placebo effect is a genuine *positive*/beneficial psychological or physiological response that is attributable to receiving a substance or undergoing a procedure, but is not due to the inherent powers of that substance or procedure. A nocebo effect is a genuine *negative*/adverse psychological or physiological response that is attributable to receiving a substance or undergoing a procedure, but is not due to the inherent powers of that substance or procedure.

Expectancy and classical conditioning are believed to the principal processes responsible for the placebo/nocebo effect (Benedetti, 2008, 2009; Evans, 2004; Finniss, Kaptchuk, Miller, & Benedetti, 2010; Hoffman et al., 2005; Kirsch, 1999; Moerman, 2002; Montgomery & Kirsch, 1996, 1997; Price et al. 1999; Price, Finiss, & Benedetti, 2008; Stewart-Williams, 2004; Stewart-Williams & Podd, 2004; Voudouris, Peck, & Coleman, 1989, 1990). Expectancy is thought to be acquired in a number of ways including direct personal experience, verbal instructions (suggestion), observational learning, and contextual factors (Stewart-Williams, 2004). The use of the term *expectancy* does not imply a cognitive process of which the individual is aware; "expectancy" effects are also observed in animals. How do expectancies manifest? There can be a dose response in which two placebo pills are better than one and in which the color and a suggested meaning of the color (sedative vs. stimulant) of the pills influence perceived effects (Blackwell, Bloomfield, & Buncher, 1972). Placebo injections may be perceived as more powerful than oral placebos (de Craen, Tijssen, de Gans, & Kleijnen, 2000). Surgical intervention can have the most profound effect of all.

A surgical procedure of ligating internal mammary arteries to relieve angina pectoris in the 1950s was a common practice. This practice was called into question, and two independent teams of surgeons and cardiologists explored the practice by conducting double-blind trials (Cobb, Thomas, Dillard, & Marendino, & Bruce, 1959; Dimond, Kittle, & Crockett, 1960). The surgeons performing the procedure were not informed until the moment of surgery whether the patient would receive the real or sham procedure, which involved everything except ligating the internal mammary arteries. A six-month follow-up by blinded cardiologists indicated 67% of patients receiving the full surgery reported substantial improvement while 82% of patients receiving the sham surgery reported substantial improvement. Improvement was measured as longer exercise times, fewer nitroglycerine tablets, reduction in pain, and in some cases improved ECG readings (Wall, 1996). In another surgical example, Moseley, Wray, and Kuykendall (1996) and Moseley et al. (2002) conducted two randomized controlled placebo trials using patients with osteoarthritis of the knee. Placebo patients were put to sleep, draped, injected with a local anesthetic and given three stab wounds to the skin, as would have been done in an arthroscopic debridement. The arthroscopic instruments were inserted and a debridement was simulated in case the patient was aware during the surgical procedure. Results measured at several time points for two years indicated placebo treatment was significantly better then debridement for up to a year and at two years there was no significant difference, although placebo still outperformed debridement. In addition the 2002 study included psychological measures evaluating anxiety, depression, optimism, health satisfaction, somatization, stress, and vitality. There were no differences between groups on any of these measures. It is worth highlighting the duration of perceived benefit here as placebos are often considered to be transient occurrences.

Can expectancy enhance effective therapy? Analysis of five widely administered postoperative analgesics (morphine, buprenorphine, tramadol, ketorolac, metamizole) using an open versus hidden paradigm have been conducted (Amanzio, Pollo, Maggi, & Benedetti, 2001; Colloca, Lopiano, Lanotte, & Benedetti, 2004). In these evaluations doctors would carry out an open administration (bedside) for each of these drugs, telling patients the injection was a powerful analgesic and the pain would subside after a few minutes. This was compared to an automatic infusion pump administering the same dose of each of the medications without patient awareness. The analyses found the dose required to achieve 50% pain reduction (ED50) was significantly increased when the administration was hidden for each of the five drugs. The only difference between groups was the presence of medical practitioners and verbal assurance.

Expectancy not only lends itself to symptom improvement but importantly to symptom worsening as well. Verbal suggestion alone can influence the perception of analgesia from nitrous oxide to that of hyperalgesia (Dworkin, Chen, LeResche, & Clark, 1983). Nocebo designed open/hidden paradigms have been explored as well. In a study of post-operative patients receiving morphine for 48 hours, some patients were told that their morphine had been stopped (open condition) and some patients were told nothing about their morphine being discontinued (hidden condition). At 10 hours after morphine interruption, a significantly larger number of patients in the open condition requested more morphine than the hidden condition (Benedetti et al. 2003; Colloca et al. 2004).

Voudouris, Peck and Coleman (1989, 1990) conditioned subjects to painful electronic stimulation over a period of three days. On Day 1 a tolerance level was established. On Day 2, participants received a placebo cream and were told that it was an analgesic. In addition, they were told that the electrical stimulation intensity was the same as the day before; when in reality the voltage had been turned down or turned up. On Day 3, voltage was returned to Day 1 levels. Subjects who had experienced a lessened voltage on Day 2 reported much less pain, while subjects exposed to more voltage experienced heightened pain. In another study, Benedetti et al. (2003) conditioned two groups of subjects pharmacologically with ketorolac (a nonopioid analgesic) for two days while two other groups received no conditioning and a natural history group was included for comparative purposes. On Day 3 the conditioned groups were given a saline injection and were told it was a powerful analgesic or were told it was hyperalgesic. The unconditioned groups were simply given a saline injection and told that it was a powerful analgesic or hyperalgesic. Results indicated that for the conditioned analgesia group, they experienced a dramatic reduction in pain. The unconditioned analgesia group experienced a reduction in pain compared to the natural history group, but was nowhere near the magnitude of the conditioned group. The second conditioned group when administered saline and the suggestion of pain worsening experienced a complete reversal of all conditioned analgesia. A number of other studies have observed similar conditioning/abolishment results (Kirsch, 1999; Montgomery & Kirsch, 1996; Price, Milling, Kirsch, Duff, Montgomery et al., 1999).

Analgesia and hyperalgesia can be conditioned, and if verbal expectancy is combined with the conditioning process, analgesia can be greatly increased or conditioning can be completely abolished. In short, placebo/nocebo effects demonstrate how external factors can influence the activity of the neurobiological pain system such that experienced pain can be magnified or suppressed. This research offers a physiological mechanism by which nonbiological factors including personality style, psychological distress, psychosocial stress, and sociodemographic variables can influence the experience of pain and the degree of pain-related disability. The following sections review the research on the role of person-centered variables and system-centered variables in the clinical management of pain.

Psychosocial/Person Factors

Consideration of person-centered psychosocial factors is essential for a comprehensive understanding and appropriate treatment of patients with pain (see the following for detailed reviews: Gatchel, 2004; Keefe, Rumble, Scipio, Giordano, & Perri, 2004; Linton, 2000). Injury recovery is affected by person-centered physical characteristics such as age and weight as well as demographic factors such as education and income (Crook & Moldofsky, 1994; Rubin, 2007; Stover, Wickizer, Zimmerman, Fulton-Kehoe, & Franklin, 2007). Psychosocial factors serve as important prognostic indicators of cases that transition from acute to chronic pain (Carragee, Alamin, Miller, & Carragee, 2005; Dersh, Gatchel, & Polatin, 2001; Keefe et al., 2004; Linton, 2000; Pincus, Burton, Vogel, & Field, 2002). Psychopathology can increase perceived pain intensity, hamper rehabilitation efforts, and magnify perceived disabilities—all of which serve to reinforce and perpetuate pain-related dysfunction (Gatchel & Dersh, 2002; Holzberg, Robinson, Geisser, & Gremillion, 1996; Leeuw et al., 2007).

The relationship between psychosocial factors and pain-related disability is not simple cause-and-effect but is instead reciprocal and complex. Linton (2000) concluded that these factors are related to every aspect and phase of neck and back pain, and are particularly important in the transition between acute and chronic pain. The following subsection will review several of these factors and their relationship to outcome in pain-related conditions. The subsequent subsection will review the influence of socioeconomic factors in pain. While this chapter presents these factors in discrete sections, this should not imply independence. Many of the factors are closely linked conceptually and functionally, and recognition of their interrelatedness is important.

Childhood Adversity

Childhood adversity in the form of abuse, neglect, and abandonment has proven an important predictor of current and future mental health (Arnow, 2004; Taylor & Jason, 2002; Widom, DuMont, & Czaja, 2007). Childhood sexual abuse in particular is associated with the presence of medically unexplained symptoms such as irritable bowel syndrome and chronic pain, and with high health care use (Nelson, Baldwin, & Taylor, 2012). Brown, Schrag, and Trimble (2005) found that physical/emotional abuse was more common and more extreme in patients with unexplained neurological symptoms who met *Diagnostic and Statistical Manual of Mental Disorders* (DSM) criteria for somatization disorder than in those with a neurologically based dystonia. A higher degree of family conflict was present in the somatization group; however, there were no group differences for neglect, sexual abuse, or witnessing violence. Exposure to emotional abuse accounted for 50% of the variance in unexplained symptoms. These effects are not simply explained by psychiatric comorbidity. Spitzer, Barnow, Gau, Freyberger, and Grabe (2008) found that the odds of having been sexually abused in childhood were nine times higher in persons who met DSM criteria for somatization disorder than in those meeting criteria for major depressive disorder.

Childhood adversity is also an important predictor of pain symptoms (Davis, Luecken, & Zautra, 2005). For example, Walker, Gelfand, Gelfand, Green, and Katon (1996) found that women with both irritable bowel syndrome and chronic pelvic pain were significantly more likely to have a history of childhood sexual abuse as well as a variety of mood and anxiety disorders, somatization disorder, and hysterectomy. Childhood adversities are more common in somatoform pain disorder, and fibromyalgia is particularly associated with severe maltreatment in childhood (Imbierowicz & Egle, 2003; Walker et al., 1997; Wolfe & Hawley, 1998). Brown, Berenson, and Cohen (2005) surveyed a community sample and found that adult chronic pain was associated with a history of sexual abuse, and that this effect was not attributable to the presence of depression at the time the survey was completed. Walsh, Jamieson, Macmillan, and Boyle (2007) found that a history of physical and sexual abuse differentiated adult chronic pain patients with disability in some aspect of their life from those with pain but without disability.

A history of childhood adversity is also associated with outcomes in the treatment of pain (Linton, 2000). Two studies are particularly revealing. In the first study, Schofferman, Anderson, Hines, Smith, and White (1992) retrospectively examined 86 patients who underwent lumbar spine surgery. Five types of childhood trauma were considered: (a) physical abuse, (b) sexual abuse, (c) emotional neglect or abuse, (d) abandonment, and (d) a chemically dependent caregiver. Of patients who had experienced three or more of these types of trauma, 85% had unsuccessful surgical outcomes. In contrast, only 5% of the patients who had experienced none of these traumas had unsuccessful surgery. A similar study of patients who had undergone multidisciplinary evaluation for refractory back pain also found a high incidence of childhood traumas, especially in patients with minimal signs of pathology (Schofferman, Anderson, Hines, Smith, & Keane, 1993). Not surprisingly, health care utilization is greater in persons with a history of abuse, neglect, or serious family dysfunction in childhood (Arnow, 2004; Arnow, Hart, Hayward, Dea, & Barr-Taylor, 2000). Even disability retirement is associated with childhood adversity. Of nearly 9,000 community survey respondents ranging in age from 40 to 54, those with multiple childhood adversities were more than three times as likely to take disability retirement compared to those with no history of such adversity (Harkonmaki et al., 2007). Spitzer et al. (2008) concluded "childhood sexual abuse is an important factor in the multifactorial aetiopathogenesis of somatization disorder" (p. 335) and Arnow (2004) stated that "the more severe the abuse, the stronger the association with poor outcomes in adulthood" (p. 10).

The mechanisms underlying the translation of adverse childhood experiences into health-related phenomena are complex and multifactorial (Spitzer et al., 2008). Physiologically, childhood adversity is known to cause acute and chronic disruption of the HPA axis (Bremner & Vermetten, 2001; Tarullo & Gunnar, 2006; Teicher et al., 2003). It is also associated with the development of psychopathology and certain pain syndromes (i.e., chronic pelvic pain; see Heim, Ehlert, Hanker, & Hellhammer, 1998). Behaviorally, Waldinger, Schulz, Barsky, and Ahernet al. (2006) found that in women, fearful attachment mediated the link between childhood trauma and somatization. In men, attachment style and trauma each contributed independently to the development of somatization. The authors concluded that "childhood trauma shapes patients' styles of relating to others in times of need, and these styles, in turn, influence the somatization process" (Waldinger et al., 2006, p. 129). The process of somatization may be one link between childhood psychological trauma and problematic pain outcomes (Roelofs & Spinhoven, 2007).

Somatization

Somatization and related terms (e.g., somatoform disorder) have a complex and sometimes controversial history (Lamberty, 2008). Nonetheless, as a narrow concept, somatization is a central factor in understanding disability attributed to chronic pain. Somatization refers to the way

> certain patients use their physical symptoms as a way of dealing with, and communicating about, their emotional lives . . . in this type of symptom magnification, physical symptoms may be easier to accept as causing current unhappiness and discontent than admitting that some psychological reason is contributing to it.
>
> (Gatchel, 2004, p. 204)

In short, somatization reflects the expression of psychological problems through physical symptoms and complaints, a tendency to complain of or develop physical symptoms and illness when under emotional stress, and be excessively focused on one's physical functioning. Somatization may be best viewed as a potentially maladaptive personality and/or coping style. As used here, *somatization* refers not to a diagnostic entity but to a mode of thinking about one's self and world that contributes to medically unexplained illness and excess disability. Somatoform tendencies include cognitive, perceptual, and behavioral features. Elements include excessive worry about serious illness (i.e., hypochondriasis), hypervigilence towards bodily sensations, negative interpretations or disease attributions for benign sensations, sensitivity to unpleasant somatic sensations, and excessive care seeking or need for illness validation. These factors are often viewed as a cycle in which cognitions, perceptions, and behaviors mutually reinforce and strengthen each other (Barsky & Borus, 1999). It is important to recognize that patients with somatoform tendencies and/or disorders are not necessarily consciously magnifying their symptoms, as is seen with factitious disorders and malingering, but instead hold a conviction that they are physically ill.

Among patients with chronic pain, somatization is associated with more medically unexplained symptoms, poorer response to treatment, and future development of disability. Elevations on scales 1 (Hypochondriasis) and 3 (Hysteria) of the Minnesota Multiphasic Personality Inventory (MMPI; Butcher, Dahlstrom, Graham, Tellegen, & Kaemmer, 1989; Hathaway & McKinley, 1943) are considered indicators of somatization (Block, Gatchel, Deardorff, & Guyer, 2003; Blumetti & Modesti, 1976; Friedman, Gleser, Smeltzer, Wakefield, & Schwartz, 1983; Marks & Seeman, 1963). Block, Vanharanta, Ohnmeiss, and Guyer (1996) found a higher incidence of nonorganic symptom responses on discograms in patients with elevation on MMPI Scales 1 and 3. also found that these MMPI elevations were associated with poorer response to both surgery and conservative care (e.g., Block et al., 1996). Gatchel, Polatin, Mayer, and Garcy (1994) found that among acute back pain patients, elevations on MMPI Scale 3 predicted higher levels of disability one year later. Bigos et al. (1991) and Applegate et al. (2005) showed that early (preinjury) tendencies or predispositions for somatization, as measured by the MMPI, are linked to subsequent development of physical symptoms including back pain. Bigos et al. (1991) conducted a longitudinal study of 3,020 aircraft employees to identify risk factors for reporting acute back pain at work. About 16% of these workers developed back problems over the four-year follow-up period. The 20% of participants with the highest Scale 3 scores were twice as likely to report back problems as those with lower scores. Applegate et al. (2005) found that the MMPI at college admission ($N = 2{,}332$) predicted pain-related conditions at 30-year follow up. Among men, MMPI Scales 1, 3, and 5 were most predictive of the number of chronic pain conditions. Among women, Scales 1, 3, and 6 were most predictive. For both men and women, Scales 1 and 3 predict chronic pain 30 years later.

Catastrophizing

Over the past 25 years "pain catastrophizing" has emerged as an important predictor of pain experience and pain-related disability (Sullivan et al., 2001). Pain catastrophizing has been defined as a tendency to fear pain, have a fear-inducing understanding of the meaning of pain (e.g., the presence of pain is an indication of harm), and/or a tendency to allow pain to be a dominant focus of one's life (Proctor, Gatchel, & Robinson, 2000). More simply, it is the interpretation of pain as being extremely threatening (Crombez, Eccleston, Baeyens, & Eelen, 1998). Psychometrically, pain catastrophizing has proven to be a stable construct that is related to but not redundant with depression and other forms of psychological distress (Sullivan et al., 2001).

Turner and Aaron (2001) suggest that catastrophizing reflects a relatively stable personality disposition whose manifestation may be influenced by situational variables such as changes in physical condition or implementation of specific cognitive interventions. Theoretical formulations to explain pain catastrophizing and hypotheses regarding the mechanisms by which pain catastrophizing influence reports of pain and pain-related disability have only begun to emerge (Sullivan et al., 2001; Turner & Aaron, 2001). Edwards, Bingham, Bathon, and Haythornthwaite (2006) reviewed four mechanisms by which pain catastrophizing may act: (a) interfering with pain coping and beneficial health behaviors, (b) increasing attention to pain, (c) amplifying pain processing in the central nervous system, and (d) maladaptive impacts on the social environment.

Pain catastrophizing predicts the development of chronic pain complaints in the general population. Pain catastrophizing is associated with greater pain vigilance and preoccupation with pain and physical problems (Goubert, Crombez, & Van Damme, 2004), and it may mediate the reduced activity level seen in some clinical patients (Sullivan, Stanish, Sullivan, & Tripp, 2002). Pain catastrophizing is also related to a variety of important functional and outcome variables, pain intensity, psychological distress, and level of disability (Severeijns, Vlaeyen, van den Hout, & Weber, 2001; Turner, Jensen, Warms, & Cardenas, 2002; Woby, Watson, Roach, and Urmston (2004). This relationship is independent of the level of physical injury or impairment (Severeijns et al., 2001). For reviews of pain catastrophizing, see Sullivan et al. (2001) and Edwards et al. (2006). There is evidence that pain catastrophizing is a precursor to the development of pain-related fear (Leeuw et al., 2007).

Depression and Anxiety

Depression and anxiety disorders are common in patients with chronic pain. In a large survey of the general population, approximately 18% of persons reporting chronic spinal pain were diagnosed with a comorbid mood disorder, while approximately 27% were diagnosed with some form of anxiety disorder (Von Korff et al., 2005). Patients seeking treatment for pain-related conditions are particularly likely to report symptoms of depression, as the prevalence of major depression in this population has been reported to be more than 50% (Dersh, Gatchel, Mayer, Polatin, & Temple, 2006; Mayer, Towns, Neblett, Theodore, & Gatchel, 2008).

Depression is a particularly important consideration in patients with chronic pain as studies have shown a near linear association between self-reported pain intensity and depressive symptoms (Carroll, Cassidy, & Côté, 2000; Currie & Wang, 2004). However, depression and chronic pain have a complex, reciprocal, relationship: (a) there is some overlap between symptoms (e.g., sleep disturbances or reduced activity levels); (b) they may share physiological mechanisms, specifically NE and 5-HT dysregulation (Bair et al., 2003); (c) the presence of either predicts future development of the other (Gureje, Simon, & Von Korff, 2001); and (d) comorbidity complicates treatment for both conditions (Moultry & Poon,

2009). Depression may be a particularly important predictor of pain-related disability (Alshuler, Theisen-Goodvich, Haig, & Geisser, 2008), with studies suggesting that it may serve as a moderator for the relationships between other psychological vulnerabilities discussed in this section and self-perceived disability (Boersma & Linton, 2005, 2006).

Anxiety can also influence perceptions of pain and response to treatment. Anxious expectations have been found to significantly increase the perceived intensity of painful stimuli by directly facilitating nociceptive transmission (Colloca & Benedetti, 2007). Anxiety also impacts outcome following surgery, as higher presurgical anxiety is associated with slower recovery and more complications postsurgery (Kiecolt-Glaser, Page, Marucha, MacCallum, & Glaser, 1998). Similarly, Trief, Grant, and Fredrickson (2000) found that higher levels of presurgical anxiety significantly predicted poorer functional outcome one year after receiving lumbar spine surgery to relieve pain. The negative effects of anxiety on patient outcome may be explained in part by the relationship between anxiety sensitivity and fear of pain (Martin, McGrath, Brown, & Katz, 2007).

Education

Lower education is associated with the presence of chronic pain (Rashiq & Dick, 2009) and has been identified as a prognostic indicator of work-related disability (Abásolo et al., 2012; Breslin et al., 2008; Hagen, Holte, Tambs, & Bjerkedal, 2000). Lower education is associated with longer pain duration following back injury and a higher rate of pain recurrence (Dionne et al., 2001). Even after controlling for age, pain duration, sex, and incentive status, lower education is significant associated with higher self-perceived disability (Janowski, Steuden, & Kuryłowicz, 2010; Moffett, Underwood, & Gardiner, 2009; Roth & Geisser, 2002). Lower education is also associated with more misconceptions about back pain (Goubert, Crombez, & De Bourdeaudhuij, 2004). Roth and Geisser (2002) concluded that the relationship between education and disability was mediated by maladaptive pain beliefs and coping strategies. Arts, Kols, Onderwater, and Peul (2012) found that education was the only baseline characteristic associated (negative correlation) with outcome from spine surgery. To the extent that educational achievement and measured intelligence are correlated, measured intelligence would also likely be an important variable to consider.

Fear Avoidance

Fear is a reaction that occurs in the presence of a specific, identifiable, immediate threat and often leads to escape or avoidance behaviors (Rachman, 1998). Fear-avoidance models of chronic pain-related disability hypothesize that the emotional, cognitive, and behavioral factors discussed earlier interact with the pain experience to contribute to a reinforcing cycle of fear and anxiety towards pain-related stimuli (see Asmundson, Vlaeyen, & Crombez, 2004; Vlaeyen, Kole-Snijders, Boeren, & van Eek, 1995; Vlaeyen & Linton, 2000). Fears can be directed towards pain itself, reinjury, or specific activities such as movement (i.e., kinesiophobia). Avoidance of activities, in turn, contributes to the development and maintenance of functional disability (Leeuw et al., 2007; Woby et al., 2004). Fear-avoidance models of pain-related disability are similar to models of the development and maintenance of panic disorder and agoraphobia (Klein & Gorman, 1987). The maladaptive element of the Fear-Avoidance Model is reciprocal, which allows for increasing disability and the development of comorbid depression. Pain catastrophizing appears to be a critical element, or trigger, in the development of pain-related fear and anxiety (Vlaeyen et al., 1995). It is the emotional and coping response to the injury which determines whether recovery will be complicated. Coping strategies account for adjustment to chronic pain above and beyond what is predicted by pain-related history and tendency to somaticize (Rosenstiel & Keefe, 1983). Regardless of the specific trigger, fear avoidance is an obstacle to functional improvement in chronic pain patients (Smeets, van Geel, & Verbunt, 2009; Turner et al., 2006; Vlaeyen et al., 1995; Vlaeyen & Linton, 2000). The presence of the various factors of the Fear-Avoidance Model are associated with poor outcome following spine surgery (Alodaibi, Minick, & Fritz, 2013) and with increased disability in patients with chronic pain (Zale, Lange, Fields, & Ditre, 2013).

Context/System Factors

The focus of the previous section was on the role of person-centered psychosocial factors associated with a complicated clinical pain presentation. However, when injuries are sustained on the job, treatment and recovery from injury occur within a complex social network (e.g., employers, insurance adjusters, and attorneys). In this context, complications can arise from a number of sources, including the injured worker's attitudes about his or her work or company, the relationship with the insurance company and claims adjusters, treatment delays, attorney involvement, and litigation. These contextual effects are not limited to persons whose presentation is complicated by the person-centered psychosocial factors already described. Rather, contextual factors are known to impact injury recovery even in patients with well-described and documented physical injuries who might otherwise lack psychological complication. These context effects have been shown in patients with significant and objectively documented physical injuries and in patients whose injuries are more ambiguous (Atlas et al., 2006; Carroll et al., 2008; Cassidy, Carroll, Cote, Berglund, & Nygren, 2003; Cassidy et al., 2000). In the past 20 years a sizeable literature has developed examining noninjury characteristics/risk factors associated with the injury context and how these factors affect symptomatic and functional outcomes.

Occupation and Work-Related Factors

Physical work load and job satisfaction both are prognostic indicators of back pain-related work absences and disability (Bigos et al., 1991; Hagen et al., 2002; Hoogendoorn et al., 2002; Shaw et al., 2005). Hagen et al. (2000) found that unskilled workers are two to three times more likely to retire due to disability than professionals. McIntosh, Frank, Hogg-Johnson, Bombardier, and Hall (2000) and Stover, Wickizer, Zimmerman, Fulton-Kehoe, and Franklin (2007) found that working in the construction industry to be among several factors that predicted work disability. Volinn, Van Koevering, and Loeser (1991) found that lower pay is associated with longer back pain chronicity. Similarly, Tate (1992) found that younger workers with higher preinjury wages, greater seniority, and less severe injuries were more likely to return to work postinjury.

Elements of the relationship between the worker and the company, including job satisfaction and availability of accommodations can also impact outcome and even the initiation of symptom reports. For example, in a study of 3,020 aircraft industry employees, those who reported that they "hardly ever" enjoyed their work were 2.5 times more likely to report a back injury than those who reported more positive feelings about their job/work (Bigos et al., 1991). Shaw, Pransky, Patterson, & Winters (2005) examined psychosocial factors in patients referred to an occupational medicine clinic for back pain and found that job characteristics including job tenure, physical work demands, availability of modified duty, and earlier reporting to employer, were more predictive of outcome than physical examination. Similarly, Turner et al. (2007) found that baseline demographic variables, symptom severity, functional limitations, lack of job accommodation, job physical demands, job psychosocial conditions, and psychosocial characteristics predicted chronic disability following a claim for carpal tunnel syndrome. Each domain of variables (sociodemographic, clinical, psychosocial, work related) added significantly to the prediction of chronic disability.

Aside from the complexities of these interactions, the injured worker who is attempting to return to work may encounter obstacles. For the subset of patients who have performed heavy physical labor, returning to their previous level of work may no longer be possible and a return to even modified work can pose considerable challenges. The sometimes daunting obstacles for a worker to return to work include insufficient training or education to do work other than heavy work, advanced age, a feeling of uncertainty about other job tasks, poor information or misinformation about what would be required for a work return, unavailability of vocational rehabilitation, and financial disincentives for returning to work.

Delays in Treatment

When a work injury occurs there are a number of different sources of delay in the ultimate rehabilitation of the patient. For example, in many state worker's compensation systems second opinions can be required before surgeries or rehabilitation can be funded. Conversely, when the worker has attorney representation the duration claim is longer, suggesting some mechanism of delay (Bernanki & Tao, 2008; Olney, Quenzer, & Makowsky, 1999). Olney, Quenzer, and Makowsky (1999) found that among patients undergoing carpal tunnel release, contested worker's compensation claims (those requiring the intervention of an attorney) were associated with a higher risk of poor outcome while patients with uncontested worker's compensation claims had outcomes nearly as good as noncompensation patients. Following the switch from a tort-compensation system to a no-fault system in Canada, the average time between injury and claim resolution for whiplash was more than halved (Cassidy et al., 2000). This finding implies that delayed recovery, to the extent that it is reflected in time to claim resolution, is often a function of the compensation system.

The effects of these delays are not minor or inconsequential: The longer the delay between injury and treatment, the greater the probability of disability. Crook and Moldofsky (1994) conducted a prospective, longitudinal, cohort study of patients with musculoskeletal soft tissue impairment following a work-related injury. Among their findings was a strong relationship between the passage of time and persistent disability. Moreover, early attempts at work return contributed to a decrease in overall work disability. McIntosh, Frank, Hogg-Johnson, Bombardier, and Hall (2000) also found that the lag time from injury to treatment was a strong predictor of chronicity. Interestingly, they also found that workers with a previous history of back problems who had returned to work were more likely to return to work than first-time injured workers. In a population-based retrospective inception cohort study of 81,077 workers who had four or more days of work disability resulting from workplace injuries over six years (Stover, Wickizer, Zimmerman, Fulton-Kehoe, & Franklin, 2007), the length of time from claim filing to medical treatment was among several factors predicting long-term disability.

Satisfaction With Care

The satisfaction of injured workers with their medical care has important implications for recovery and return to work. Wickizer, Franklin, Fulton-Kehoe, et al. (2004) studied 681 workers who had ongoing follow-up care after initial treatment and examined their satisfaction with interpersonal and technical aspects of care. They found that satisfaction was strongly and positively associated with their ratings of their overall treatment experience, explaining 38% of the observed variance. Injured workers who were less satisfied with their treatment experiences were 3.5 times more likely to still be out of work six or 12 months after filing the claim compared to patients whose treatment experience was more positive. The authors observed that it was not clear whether "dissatisfaction leads to poorer outcomes, or whether the types of people most likely to have poor outcomes are most likely to be dissatisfied with care" (Wickizer, Franklin, Fulton-Kehoe, et al., 2004: 743). The same group (Wickizer, Franklin, Turner, et al., 2004) found that satisfaction with claims administration procedures was a significant predictor of attorney retention or appeal filing by an injured worker. However, Wickizer, Franklin, Turner, et al. (2004b) found that attorney retention occurred about one year on average after the initiation of the claim. This lead them to conclude that attorney retention was a correlate rather than a predictor of disability. This is important because it shows not only the relationship with the company but also that the relationship with treatment providers can be important for understanding and predicting outcome in injured workers.

Financial Incentive Effects

It is not uncommon for chronic pain cases to be seen in a context involving financial compensation such as personal injury litigation, workers' compensation, or disability determinations. The presence of financial incentive is a robust predictor of outcome in patients with pain. Patients seen in a compensated context report significantly more pain, depression, and disability than patients not involved in compensation (Chibnall & Tait, 1994; Rainville, Sobel, Hartigan, & Wright, 1997; Rohling, Binder, & Langhinrichsen-Rohling, 1995). Further, compensation status is associated with overall decreased treatment efficacy (Gatchel, Polatin, & Mayer, 1995; Rainville et al., 1997; Rohling et al., 1995), including worse surgical outcomes (Harris, Mulford, Solomon, van Gelder, & Young, 2005) even for clearly defined spinal pathology (Atlas et al., 2006; Atlas et al., 2006; Voorhies, Jiang, & Thomas, 2007). As an example of the systemic effects of compensated context, recent changes to a "no fault" compensation system in Canada were found to result in a lower incidence of lower-back pain and whiplash injuries following accidents and better prognosis for recovery (Cameron et al., 2008; Cassidy et al., 2003). Overland et al. (2008) found that reports of pain, anxiety, depression, sleep disturbances, and somatic symptoms steadily increased as a financial disability determination neared and then steadily decreased after the determination was made.

Pain often occurs in the context of a legally compensable event such as a work-related injury or incident in which some other party is potentially liable and there are financial incentives to appear disabled. Therefore, malingering is a potential issue. The prevalence of malingering in patients with pain who are referred for psychological evaluation is between 20% and 50% (Mittenberg, Patton, Canyock, & Condit, 2002; Greve, Ord, Bianchini, & Curtis, 2009; Kay & Morris-Jones, 1998) depending on the method of assessment and case-specific factors. These rates are consistent with those reported in other compensable conditions and contexts such as criminal forensic settings (Ardolf, Denney, & Houston, 2007), Social Security disability evaluations (Chafetz, 2008), toxic exposure (Greve, Bianchini, Black, et al., 2006), TBI (Larrabee, 2003), and among Vietnam-era veterans receiving services within the Veterans Administration system (Larrabee, Millis, & Meyers, 2008). These studies demonstrate that overall malingering, including in patients with pain, is not a rare event or trivial phenomenon despite earlier claims to the contrary (e.g., Fishbain, Cutler, Rosomoff, & Rosomoff, 1999; Sears, Wickizer, & Franklin, 2008). Using published base rates of malingering, Chafetz and Underhill (2013) estimated the cost of malingering on Social Security disability examinations to be about $20 billion in 2011. Given the prevalence of pain-related complaints in the general population, malingering in patients with pain potentially has a very significant economic impact.

Many indicators of malingered cognitive, emotional, and physical disability have now been validated in patients with chronic pain (for reviews, see Greve, Bianchini, & Brewer, 2013; Greve, Curtis, & Bianchini, 2013). A striking feature of some of these data is that the rate of positive findings (i.e., test failure) is associated in a dose-response fashion with increasing objective evidence of malingering but not with injury characteristics (Ben-Porath, Greve, Bianchini, & Kaufmann, 2009; Greve et al., 2010; Greve, Bianchini, Etherton, Ord, & Curtis, 2009; Greve, Etherton, Ord, Bianchini, & Curtis, 2009). This finding in pain patients is complemented by the finding in TBI patients that the magnitude of potential compensation is associated with malingering test failures (Bianchini, Curtis, & Greve, 2006). Interestingly, in Canada, a change in personal injury liability law was followed by a nearly 50% decline in disability claims related to back pain (Cassidy et al., 2003). Taken together, these findings support the conclusion that empirically defined "improbable" test performance is motivated by financial incentive and reinforce the need to consider the potential role of malingering in patients whose persisting disability is poorly explained by objective medical factors.

Clinical Applications

The influence of these psychosocial and system factors on pain-related disability has implications for psychological assessment and treatment of the patient with pain, and for behavioral approaches to treatment. The psychological pain evaluation has the potential to illuminate the clinical circumstances of a given patient in a way and to a degree that is not possible in the evaluations of other clinicians. In fact, it is not uncommon for a patient with pain to be referred for a psychological evaluation after years of failed medical treatment efforts that have often frustrated multiple treaters. Other times the evaluation is initiated because of concerns about depression, though this is still usually in the context of slow or atypical recovery. Sometimes a case is referred specifically because the treater has suspicions of malingering. Regardless of the specific referral question, the psychological evaluation can clarify the case and lead to treatment recommendations that can improve overall treatment efficacy, functional capacity, and quality of life.

Psychological Pain Evaluation

The psychological pain evaluation requires a comprehensive approach, one that actively considers all of the factors that can complicate the management of pain. The assessment approach recommended in this chapter is one that most neuropsychologists will find familiar. It is flexible in scope and test battery composition while still assessing the multiple behavioral domains relevant to the referral question. This multidimensional approach allows a comprehensive assessment of an individual's functional status that can lead to detailed recommendations regarding the management of his or her pain and pain-related disability and supply valuable information to vocational experts and life-care planners. The specific procedures selected (especially the inclusion of cognitive measures) will depend on the context of the evaluation and likely future uses of the data (e.g., ability testing data has significant value for vocational rehabilitation). This section is intended to provide an overview of the conceptual approach to the assessment of the chronic pain patient and not to review comprehensively or in detail the many psychological tests that might be included in such an evaluation. Examples will be provided and a table of some of available questionnaires is included (see Appendix on p. 845).

A careful review of all available medical records and, when possible, any other records that may have bearing on subsequent conclusions (e.g., accident reports, personnel records, depositions) is a central part of the psychological pain evaluation. It is recognized that some records may not be available or be incomplete, in other cases the records may be voluminous, and in still others there may be no or limited reimbursement for record review. Nonetheless, these records provide important context including the nature of the injury, treatment efforts and complications (e.g., infection at a surgical site, overuse of pain medications), indications of complicating behavioral factors (e.g., symptom magnification, nonphysiological responses to diagnostic testing), and evidence of the influence of extrainjury stressors that can have an adverse effect on the clinical presentation (e.g., death of a loved one, legal problems). The records can also reveal inconsistencies in symptom report between different doctors (e.g., reporting a decrease in pain to the spine surgeon while reporting the same or worsening pain to the pain management doctor who is writing the narcotic prescriptions) and changes in the description of the accident over time.

Like any psychological evaluation, the pain psychological evaluation will typically begin with a clinical interview. This will generally address the nature of the accident, efforts at treatment, and current status including symptoms and complaints. However, the interview should also assess the variety of complicating factors such as recent and ongoing psychosocial stressors, past psychiatric history, childhood psychological trauma, and job factors that might predict poor outcome from treatments. Ideally, patients should not be given information regarding pain-related symptoms, including symptom checklists and direct questioning about symptoms, until after they have been asked to spontaneously report all of their symptoms in all domains so as to reduce the risk of suggesting symptoms that may bias subjective report.

After the clinical interview the patient is administered standardized psychological and neuropsychological tests and procedures. The composition of the test battery will depend on the referral question and context of the evaluation. Typically, patients referred in a clinical (noncompensate) context for psychological screening prior to some form of invasive surgical procedure (e.g., spinal fusion, implantation of a dorsal column stimulator or intrathecal morphine pump) will be the most streamlined and may include only questionnaires. In contrast, patients seen as part of their workers' compensation or personality injury litigation claims may require more comprehensive batteries. Pain patients may report disabling problems in multiple functional domains (e.g., physical, emotional, and cognitive; see Schnurr & MacDonald, 1995; Meyers & Diep, 2000; Ericsson et al., 2002; Wilson, Eriksson, D'Eon, Mikail, & Emery, 2002), all of which may have important implications for the decision making of various clinicians (Gatchel, 2004).

Therefore, the psychological pain evaluation should be designed to objectively assess the common cognitive, psychological, emotional, and physical complaints of patients with pain and pain-related disability. Among cognitive domains that are functionally important are attention and concentration, processing speed, learning and memory, general knowledge, intelligence, and problem solving skills. These cognitive domains have implications for return to work (e.g., poor attention would potentially limit the ability of a person to return to work in a safety-sensitive position such as a crane operator) and alternative work placement/retraining (e.g., a laborer with average intelligence who is limited to light duty by his or her injury will have more retraining options that if he or she had low average/borderline intelligence). Moreover, lower educational achievement/measured intelligence is a risk factor for increased disability. Thus, it is helpful to use broad measures of intelligence such as the Wechsler Adult Intelligence Scale–IV or Wechsler Abbreviated Scale of Intelligence as well as well-validated neuropsychological tests of memory (e.g., California Verbal Learning Test or subtests from the Wechsler Memory Scale or Neuropsychological Assessment Battery).

Typically, current emotional state and personality style as well as physical complaints and perceived pain-related disability are evaluated in the clinical interview as well as with questionnaires. The Minnesota Multiphasic Personality Inventory (MMPI; see Hathaway & McKinley, 1943) in its modern forms (MMPI-2, Butcher et al., 1989; MMPI-2-RF,

Ben-Porath & Tellegen, 2008), are the most widely used psychological assessment instruments (Lubin, Larsen, & Matarazzo, 1984; Rabin, Barr, & Burton, 2005; Sharland & Gfeller, 2007). They are among also the most commonly used in evaluating chronic pain patients in general (e.g., Robinson, Swimmer, & Rallof, 1989; Keller & Butcher, 1991; Deardorff, Chino, & Scott, 1993; Slesinger, Archer, & Duane, 2002) and to predict response to pain management interventions (Love & Peck, 1987), the likelihood of return to work (e. g., Bigos et al., 1991; Vendrig, Derksen, & de Mey, 1999), and outcome from spinal surgery (Block et al., 2003). It is also helpful to include specific behavioral health measures such as the Battery for Health Improvement–2 (BHI-2; see Bruns & Disorbio, 2003), the Millon Behavioral Health Inventory (MBHI; see Millon, Green, & Meagher, 1982). The BHI-2 (a 217-item multiple choice test normed on physical rehabilitation patients) is particularly useful because it was developed specifically to assess many of the psychosocial and contextual factors already discussed as relevant for pain management and functional outcome. This part of the evaluation is often supplemented by specific measures of pain and pain-related disability.

Finally, there must also be a comprehensive assessment of response and performance validity because the results of psychological tests can be invalidated by biased responding and/or poor effort. Malingering is an obvious risk when a patient is seen in a compensated context. However, even in cases not seen in a compensation-seeking context magnification of pain-related disability may also be motivated by the desire to obtain pain medication. The MMPI-2 has scales whose accuracy in detecting symptom magnification and malingering has been documented (Greve et al., 2013). The accuracy of validity scales of the BHI-2 has been examined in rehabilitation patients responding honestly and in patients asked to exaggerate their problems. Among specialty pain questionnaires, lack of validity scales tends to be the rule. If cognitive tests are included then it will be necessary to include performance validity measures as well. We have recently outlined our approach to the assessment of validity in the psychological pain evaluation (Greve et al., 2013).

The Preprocedure Psychological Screen

The preprocedure psychological screen is a special case of the psychological pain evaluation, but one that contains the critical elements of any psychological pain evaluation. This chapter has already summarized the literature showing that psychosocial factors influence pain complaints and pain-related disability. The importance of considering such factors in the context of invasive medical efforts to relieve pain, which involve damaging tissue and thus have the potential to do harm, is essential.

> Spine surgery's ultimate effectiveness . . . depends on much more than the surgeons' diagnostic acumen and technological skill. Psychological factors exert very strong influences—ones that can improve, or inhibit, the patient's ultimate recovery . . . surgical results can be greatly augmented by the inclusion of psychological components in the assessment and preparation of patients for spine surgery, as well as in post-operative rehabilitation.
>
> (Block et al., 2003, p. 4)

Block et al. (2003) have argued that preprocedure psychological screening is an essential component in the medical diagnostic process of spine surgery candidates, especially when the major goal is symptomatic pain reduction. Further emphasizing this point, Lebovits (2000) has stated that

> although the treatment of a patient with chronic pain mandates a comprehensive evaluation of the medical as well as psychological contributions to the etiology, maintenance, and exacerbation of pain, evaluating and treating patients with chronic pain with a unimodal, strictly medical approach still occurs. This, unfortunately, often leads to iatrogenic effects, such as failed surgical interventions and activity restriction.
>
> (Lebovits, 2000, p. 126)

The psychological assessment of surgical risk is not simply a matter of determining if a patient is psychotic, has a pathological body image, has somatic delusions, or is depressed. While the presence of significant psychopathology that might lead to postsurgical psychological instability or problems with medical compliance is an issue of importance, this type of problem may be a minority in presurgical pain cases, particularly those seen in a medicolegal context. Nelson, Novy, Averill, and Berry (1996) have argued that in addition to active psychosis, suicidality, untreated major depression, and substance dependence, factors such as somatization, lack of social support, and cognitive deficits should exclude patients from receiving a spinal cord stimulator. They also noted that disincentive to recover related to compensation or litigation issues was a factor that would require exclusion.

There is now strong empirical research regarding what psychological factors predict outcome from surgery (e.g., Block, 1996; Block et al., 2003; Bruns & Disorbio, 2009; Voorhies, Jiang, & Thomas, 2007). See Bruns and Disorbio (2009) for a review of a number of preprocedure psychological screening methods. Block and colleagues (Block et al., 2001; Epker & Block, 2001) have demonstrated that the presence of certain psychosocial factors predicts poor outcome from lumbar disc surgery. Among these factors are financial incentive, history of abuse or abandonment, job dissatisfaction, problems with social support, substance abuse, preexisting psychopathology, depression/anxiety, and pain catastrophizing as well as compliance problems and deception. These psychosocial risk factors have been summarized and integrated into a presurgical screen risk factor checklist by Block et al. (2001). A similar medical risk factor checklist is part of their comprehensive presurgical screen.

The presurgical screening approach developed by Block et al. (2001) has been thoroughly explicated (Block et al., 2003; Block, 2013; Block, Ben-Porath, & Marek, 2013) and the ultimate process is laid out in the form of an easy-to-use flowchart. The Block algorithm has recently been revised for use with the MMPI-2-RF (Block et al., 2013) and expanded to include spinal cord stimulator implantation. This latest screening model is particularly helpful because it provides specific cut scores for all the psychometric variables. While the original risk factor checklist allowed for a determination of high risk of poor surgical outcome due to psychosocial and medical risk factors, it did not offer other guidance. In contrast, the more recent methods offer treatment guidance ranging from "good prognosis, no psychological treatment needed" to "poor prognosis, discharge recommended," with specific forms of intervention recommended for intermediate levels of risk.

Similar approaches have been reported for screening of patients being considered for intrathecal morphine pump and dorsal column stimulator implantation (Bruns & Disorbio, 2009; Jamison & Edwards, 2013). The model outlined by Bruns and Disorbio (2009) is based on data derived from the BHI-2 (Bruns & Disorbio, 2003). "Exclusionary" and "Cautionary" risk scores based on BHI-2 responses have been identified. The "exclusionary" criteria include such things as active suicidal or homicidal ideation, active delusional thinking, active substance abuse, and litigation. The "cautionary" scores include depression, cognitive disorder or low education, diffuse somatic complaints, job or doctor dissatisfaction, and history of abuse. Higher scores were required for an "exclusionary" factor to be positive (i.e., score level observed in about 1% of patients) than for a "cautionary" factor to be positive (i.e., score level observed in about 16% of patients). However, the method also includes information derived from medical examination (e.g., medically impossible symptoms, major inconsistencies, noncompliance), history (e.g., multiple failures of the same treatment, violation of opioid contract), and science (i.e., evidence that the proposed medical treatment would be injurious or ineffective given the circumstances). The numbers of positive "exclusionary" and "cautionary" can be compared to those of patients and healthy community members. However, specific guidance regarding surgical risk and advisability of other forms of intervention like that found in the Block algorithms has not been provided for the Bruns and Disorbio model.

At a conceptual level, Bruns and Disorbio (2009: 143) have emphasized that the preprocedure screen is a "collaborative biopsychosocial decision-making process" involving both the psychologist and physician. They caution against setting up an adversarial process in which the surgeon sees the psychological screen as an obstacle imposed from the outside (e.g., insurance company). At the same time, the psychologist needs to recognize that certain factors related to medical necessity may trump the psychosocial risk factors (e.g., when there is imminent risk to life or function). For example, while depression is a negative predictor of surgical outcome, a successful spinal cord stimulator implantation (defined as a 50% reduction in pain) can lead to improvement in depressive symptoms (Jamison, 2008). At this point, the research literature on predicting outcome in individual patients undergoing treatment with pumps or stimulators remains relatively small (Jamison & Edwards, 2013). Nonetheless, outcome related to pumps and stimulators is related to the same factors as outcome from spine surgery. In general, preprocedure psychological screening like that proposed by Block should identify those patients who would be expected to have a complicated course and delayed outcomes regardless of the specific intervention procedure being proposed. At the same time, it is also important to recognize that the medical risks of major spine surgery (e.g., spinal fusion) are different from those associated with a pump or stimulator, so the psychosocial risk may need to be weighed differently. The same may be true for the minimally invasive discectomy-fusion procedures that are becoming more common.

Even when specific surgical procedures are not being proposed, the psychological pain evaluations and preprocedure psychological screening have broad clinical utility and may provide significant benefits for those managing a pain case. Psychosocial factors are important to surgery outcome even in the context of clear and objective indications for surgery (Voorhies et al., 2007). In cases where there is disagreement or ambiguity related to the physical indications for surgery, the results of a preprocedure psychological screen may provide even more valuable guidance. Specifically, a psychological evaluation that identifies factors in a patient that would predict higher risk of poor outcome from surgical intervention may encourage continued conservative interventions and even a shift to functional restoration that incorporates active management of psychological risk factors and comorbidities. Finally, the variables assessed by these methods are relevant beyond preprocedure screening and even in patient groups whose primary complaint is not pain (e.g., concussion patients). In short, the preprocedure psychological screen model provides information about the complex psychosocial factors that can adversely affect treatment and recovery, and thus have value even when no specific "procedure" is being contemplated.

Biopsychosocial Intervention Models

As has been demonstrated, chronic pain is a complex biopsychosocial phenomenon. Biomedical interventions that focus solely on nociceptive mechanisms and pain symptoms are incomplete and unlikely to provide lasting benefit to persons with delayed recovery or chronic pain (Feinberg, Gatchel, Stanos, Feinberg, & Johnson-Montieth, 2013; Waddell, 2006). Currently, the most therapeutically and cost-effective method for treating chronic pain is functional restoration (Feinberg et al., 2013; Gatchel & Okifuji, 2006; Guzman et al., 2002). The features of functional restoration include multidisciplinary treatment including physical therapy and psychological assessment/treatment for psychological comorbidities, an assessment of psychological and other risk factors for poor outcome, the systematic management of the risk factors, and an organized and systematic approach to work return (Westman et al., 2006). Excellent resources include *Clinical Essentials of Pain Management* (Gatchel, 2005), *Interdisciplinary Functional Restoration and Pain Programs* (Feinberg et al., 2013), and *Evidence-based Scientific Data Documenting the Treatment and Cost-effectiveness of Comprehensive Pain Programs for Chronic Non-malignant Pain* (Gatchel & Okifuji, 2006).

The critical feature of the functional restoration approach is a focus on whole-person rehabilitation and restoration of function, not necessarily symptom amelioration. In fact, the functional restoration approach is rehabilitative. This key feature is philosophical and practical. Ideally, functional restoration would be provided in an interdisciplinary setting housed under one roof, much like rehabilitation programs with which neuropsychologists are familiar. The absence of an integrated pain rehabilitation program does not mean that functional restoration is not possible as long as the necessary treating disciplines (e.g., physical medicine, psychology, physical therapy, occupational therapy) are involved. This multidisciplinary approach is, by nature, not as collaborative as an interdisciplinary program, and is thus likely to be less effective. Feinberg et al. (2013) and Gatchel and Okifuji (2006) present the outcome data on functional restoration. Overall, when dealing with motivated patients, the functional restoration approach is superior to symptom-focused treatment alone in reducing pain, increasing functional status including return to work, and decreasing lifetime medical costs. Moreover, interdisciplinary pain rehabilitation may obviate the need for surgical treatment of pain symptoms.

The ultimate goal of functional restoration is maximizing functional independence to the extent possible given the individual's objective physical impairments. As part of the comprehensive biopsychosocial assessment required to develop an appropriate functional restoration plan, determination of the individual's understanding of his or her condition is essential and misunderstandings should be corrected. Proper information and expectations should be developed. Often misinformation and misunderstanding can lead to unnecessary fear of reinjury, pain fear, and pain catastrophizing. This fear may be more disabling than the biomedical aspects of the injury itself. Learning to pace activities so as to not overdo, or reinjure, or to otherwise punish oneself for increasing activity is important. Patients commonly report trying to be "normal" when they are feeling good and then being laid up with increased symptoms for days after. Moreover, flare-ups of intense pain often occur and guidance in the management of these flare-ups is important. All treating disciplines can contribute to this educational process. The need for the treating disciplines to be on the same page regarding the status and needs of the patient and the necessity to share information about progress and obstacles emphasizes the value of the single setting interdisciplinary program. This type of routine communication is possible, but it is more difficult when the treatment providers are in separate physical locations. The psychologist will be involved in these various functions and will also have the responsibility for direct treatment of affective and other comorbid psychological disorders and in providing stress management/coping skills training.

Functional restoration emphasizes improving functional capacity and encourages, to the extent possible, early work return. Early work return may be a particularly critical factor in the rehabilitation of patients with pain. Injured workers who stayed at work ("presentees") after their injuries were more likely than "absentees" (those who remained off work) to complete a functional restoration treatment program, to return to work, to retain work one-year posttreatment, and to not have a decreasing job demand from preinjury to posttreatment time periods (Howard, Mayer, & Gatchel, 2009). Among persons who failed to complete functional restoration, opioid dependence and personality disorder were the most important risk factors (Howard, Mayer, Theodore, & Gatchel, 2009). Ultimately, consideration of psychosocial and socioeconomic complexities of patients with pain in a comprehensive pain management program with a functional restoration focus can lead to a reduction in the need for invasive treatment procedures and overall improved outcomes (Gatchel & Okifuji, 2006).

Psychological Pain Management

Psychological treatments, including cognitive behavioral therapy (CBT) and behavior therapy (BT), have been studied for their efficacy in dealing with pain, pain disability, and affective comorbidities, including depression. In early studies (e.g., Block et al., 2003; Gatchel et al., 2006), CBT has been demonstrated to be effective in improving clinical outcomes in clinical pain cases. Applied in isolation, these treatments have a weak effect on pain and disability, although they may be some help in altering mood outcomes (Eccleston, Williams, & Morley, 2009). However, recent reviews on the efficacy of psychological treatments is more promising.

Eccleston, Morley, and Williams (2009) conducted a systematic review of psychological interventions for pain, finding a benefit of CBT in comparison to other therapies (e.g., behavior therapy). Effect sizes of 0.48 were found for musculoskeletal pain and 0.34 for cancer pain, thus demonstrating an effective therapeutic benefit in adults. The most marked improvements were in quality of life issues (disability, psychological distress, depression) and to some extent the pain itself. In children and adolescents, psychological treatments for pain secondary to a variety of medical conditions (i.e., headache, abdominal pain, mixed pain, fibromyalgia, sickle cell disease, and juvenile idiopathic arthritis) have also proven effective. All treatment types (relaxation, hypnosis, coping-skills training, biofeedback, CBT) were consolidated into one general class of "psychological therapies." Overall, 49% of children receiving treatment experienced improvement contrasted to 17% improvement in children who did not receive therapy. Significant improvement in mood of the headache group was seen at follow-up and posttreatment disability significantly improved in nonheadache groups.

Eccleston et al. (2009) concluded that there is sufficient evidence showing that CBT does work in patients with pain and that research focus should shift to identifying those for whom it works most effectively and under what circumstances. Combining therapies in a multidisciplinary rehabilitation format has shown promise, particularly for treating patients at higher risk for poor outcome (Westman et al., 2006). The studies show that CBT contributes to lower levels of pain symptoms and higher levels of adaptive functioning, particularly when employed along with rehabilitation medicine and physical therapy as part of a functional restoration treatment model.

The presence of psychosocial risk factors argues for incorporating CBT into the treatment plan of patients whose chronic pain has failed to respond to medical/surgical interventions. CBT would reduce depression, increase self-efficacy, foster accurate and realistic beliefs regarding surgery and/or other medical pain management approaches and their possible outcomes, and develop and practice effective pain-coping strategies. Typically, the CBT component could be completed within 10–12 weekly appointments. It would emphasize observable, quantifiable behavior change, and be guided by the establishment and tracking of specific goals to be achieved on a week-to-week basis and over the course of the entire treatment program (including a plan for returning to work). With appropriate treatment compliance, the patient would be expected to gain an increased understanding of the psychological facets of chronic pain, master relaxation techniques, learn to identify and modify pain-magnifying thoughts, reduce depression, learn to better pace his or her behavior to avoid a cycle of overexertion and deactivation, manage stress and anger more effectively, improve sleep, and plan for and cope more effectively with intermittent flare-ups in pain.

The patient's motivation and suitability for CBT treatment should be assessed over the course of a three-session trial focusing on goal setting, education, practice of basic relaxation techniques, and record keeping. If significant compliance problems are observed during the trial, no additional sessions would be recommended. If he or she demonstrated good compliance and was benefitting from treatment, an additional eight to nine sessions could be conducted to complete the entire treatment protocol. Regardless of the outcome, there is no indication for open-ended, supportive counseling secondary to the index injury. In a work-related context, if, at the conclusion of the CBT program for chronic pain, residual symptoms unrelated to the work injury remain, treatment should be arranged outside the worker's compensation system if the patient is interested in addressing those other issues.

Psychiatric Management

Patients with pain conditions, particularly chronic conditions, have a higher incidence of affective disorders than the general public (Dersh, Gatchel, Mayer, Polatin, & Temple, 2006; Mayer, Towns, Neblett, Theodore, & Gatchel, 2008), and pain increases pain sensitivity and perception of disability. This recognition has led to the utilization of a variety of psychiatric and psychological therapies for the treatment of pain, pain related disability, and psychiatric comorbidities to pain conditions. Selective serotonin reuptake inhibitor (SSRI) and serotonin-norepinephrine reuptake inhibitor (SNRI) drugs, both antidepressants, have differential effects on pain (Zhao et al., 2007) with SNRIs being more effective than SSRIs (Benarroch, 2008). A full review of the role of psychopharmacology management strategies for pain and pain-related affective disorders is beyond the scope of this chapter. The reader is referred to Polatin and Dersh (2004) for a review of relevant issues and applications of these interventions. It is important to recognize that while treatment with psychiatric medications may be helpful for the management of psychiatric symptoms (especially affective symptoms) and even pain, traditional psychiatric care alone is insufficient to address the psychosocial issues that often complicate chronic pain cases.

Conclusion

Pain is a complex biopsychosocial phenomenon that, for many persons, cannot be effectively and efficiently addressed by medical/surgical interventions alone. Failure of patients to progress is often confounding to clinicians, but psychological methods exist to identify persons at risk for chronic pain and to characterize the specific factors that are contributing to a specific individual's slow or absent recovery. Psychosocial interventions can facilitate recovery and improved function, and reduce the risk of unnecessary physical and psychological morbidity secondary to difficulty recovering. It is essential that all clinicians involved in the treatment of persons with pain recognize the significant impact psychosocial factors can have on treatment outcome and quality of life.

References

Abásolo, L., Lajas, C., León, L., Carmona, L., Macarrón, P., Candelas, G., . . . Jover, J. (2012). Prognostic factors for long-term work disability due to musculoskeletal disorders. *Rheumatology International*, *32*(12), 3831–3839.

Alexander, G. E., DeLong, M. R., & Strick, P. L. (1986). Parallel organization of functionally segregated circuits linking basal ganglia and cortex. *Annual Review of Neuroscience*, *9*, 357–381.

Alexander, M. P. (1995). Mild traumatic brain injury: Pathophysiology, natural history, and clinical management. *Neurology*, *45*(7), 1253–1260.

Alodaibi, F. A., Minick, K. I., & Fritz, J. M. (2013). Do preoperative fear avoidance model factors predict outcomes after lumbar disc herniation surgery? A systematic review. *Chiropractic & Manual Therapies*, *21*(1), 40.

Alschuler, K. N., Theisen-Goodvich, M. E., Haig, A. J., & Geisser, M. E. (2008). A comparison of the relationship between depression, perceived disability, and physical performance in persons with chronic pain. *European Journal of Pain*, *12*(6), 757–764.

Amanzio, M., Pollo, A., Maggi, G., & Benedetti, F. (2001). Response variability to analgesics: A role for non-specific activation of endogenous opioids. *Pain*, *90*, 205–215.

American Academy of Pain Management. (2003). *Proceedings of the 2003 annual meeting of the American Chronic Pain Association*. Denver, CO.

Applegate, K. L., Keefe, F. J., Siegler, I. C., Bradley, L. A., McKee, D. C., Cooper, K. S., et al. (2005). Does personality at college entry predict number of reported pain conditions at mid-life? A longitudinal study. *Journal of Pain*, *6*(2), 92–97.

Ardolf, B. R., Denney, R. L., & Houston, C. M. (2007). Base rates of negative response bias and malingered neurocognitive dysfunction among criminal defendants referred for neuropsychological evaluation. *The Clinical Neuropsychologist*, *21*(6), 899–916.

Arnow, B. A. (2004). Relationships between childhood maltreatment, adult health and psychiatric outcomes, and medical utilization. *Journal of Clinical Psychiatry*, *65*(Suppl 12), 10–15.

Arnow, B. A., Hart, S., Hayward, C., Dea, R., & Barr Taylor, C. (2000). Severity of child maltreatment, pain complaints and medical utilization among women. *Journal of Psychiatric Research*, *34*(6), 413–421.

Arts, M. P., Kols, N. I., Onderwater, S. M., & Peul, W. C. (2012). Clinical outcome of instrumented fusion for the treatment of failed back surgery syndrome: A case series of 100 patients. *Acta Neurochirurgica*, *154*(7), 1213–1217.

Asmundson, G. J., Vlaeyen, J. W., & Crombez, G. (Eds.). (2004). *Understanding and Treating Fear of Pain*. Oxford: Oxford Press.

Atlas, S. J., Chang, Y., Keller, R. B., Singer, D. E., Wu, Y. A., & Deyo, R. A. (2006). The impact of disability compensation on long-term treatment outcomes of patients with sciatica due to a lumbar disc herniation. *Spine*, *31*(26), 3061–3069.

Bair, M. J., Robinson, R. L., Katon, W., & Kroenke, K. (2003). Depression and pain comorbidity: A literature review. *Archives of Internal Medicine*, *163*(20), 2433–2445.

Barsky, A. J., & Borus, J. F. (1999). Functional somatic syndromes. *Annals of Internal Medicine*, *130*(11), 910–921.

Barsky, A. J., Orav, E. J., & Bates, D. W. (2005). Somatization increases medical utilization and costs independent of psychiatric and medical comorbidity. *Archives of General Psychiatry*, *62*(8), 903–910.

Beitz, A. J. (1982). The organization of afferent projections to the midbrain periaqueductal gray of the rat. *Neuroscience*, *7*, 133–159.

Benarroch, E. E. (2008). Descending monoaminergic pain modulation: Bidirectional control and clinical relevance. *Neurology*, *71*(3), 217–221.

Benbadis, S. R., O'Neill, E., Tatum, W. O., & Heriaud, L. (2004). Outcome of prolonged video-EEG monitoring at a typical referral epilepsy center. *Epilepsia*, *45*(9), 1150–1153.

Benedetti, F. (2008). Mechanisms of placebo-related effects across diseases and treatments. *Annual Review of Pharmacology Toxicology*, *48*, 33–60.

Benedetti, F. (2009). *Placebo Effects: Understanding the Mechanisms in Health and Disease*. Oxford: Oxford University Press.

Benedetti, F., Manzio, M., Vighetti, S., & Asteggiano, G. (2006). The biochemical and neuroendocrine bases of the hyperalgesic nocebo effect. *Journal of Neuroscience*, *26*(46), 12014–12022.

Benedetti, F., Pollo, A., Lopiano, L., Lanotte, M., Vighetti, S., & Rainero, I. (2003). Conscious expectations and unconscious conditioning in analgesic, motor and hormonal placebo/nocebo responses. *Journal of Neuroscience*, *23*(10), ef4315–ef4323.

Ben-Porath, Y. S., Greve, K. W., Bianchini, K. J., & Kaufmann, P. M. (2009). The MMPI-2 symptom validity scale (FBS) is an empirically validated measure of over-reporting in personal injury litigants and claimants: Reply to Butcher et al. (2008). *Psychological Injury and the Law*, *1*, 62–85.

Ben-Porath, Y. S., & Tellegen, A. (2008). *MMPI-2-RF: Manual for Administration, Scoring and Interpretation*. Minneapolis, MN: University of Minnesota Press.

Bernacki, E. J., & Tao, X. G. (2008). The relationship between attorney involvement, claim duration, and workers' compensation costs. *Journal of Occupational and Environmental Medicine*, *50*(9), 1013–1018.

Bianchini, K. J., Curtis, K. L., & Greve, K. W. (2006). Compensation and malingering in traumatic brain injury: A dose-response relationship? *The Clinical Neuropsychologist*, *20*(4), 831–847.

Bigos, S. J., Battie, M. C., Spengler, D. M., Fisher, L. D., Fordyce, W. E., Hansson, T. H., . . . Wortley, M. D. (1991). A prospective study of work perceptions and psychosocial factors affecting the report of back injury. *Spine*, *16*(1), 1–6.

Blackwell, B., Bloomfield, S. S., & Buncher, C. R. (1972). Demonstration to medical students of placebo responses and non-drug factors. *Lancet*, *763*, 1279–1282.

Block, A. R., Ben-Porath, Y. S., & Marek, R. J. (2013). Psychological risk factors for poor outcome of spine surgery and spinal cord stimulator implant: A review of the literature and their assessment with the MMPI-2-RF. *The Clinical Neuropsychologist*, *27*(1), 81–107.

Block, A. R., Gatchel, R. J., Deardorff, W. W., & Guyer, R. D. (2003). *The Psychology of Spine Surgery*. Washington, DC: American Psychological Association.

Block, A. R., Ohnmeiss, D. D., Guyer, R. D., Rashbaum, R. F., & Hochschuler, S. H. (2001). The use of presurgical psychological screening to predict the outcome of spine surgery. *Spine Journal*, *1*(4), 274–282.

Block, A. R., Vanharanta, H., Ohnmeiss, D. D., & Guyer, R. D. (1996). Discographic pain report: Influence of psychological factors. *Spine*, *21*(3), 334–338.

Blumetti, A., & Modesti, L. (1976). Psychological predictors of success or failure of surgical intervention for intractable back pain. In J. J. Bonica & D. Albe-Fessard (Eds.), *Advances in Pain Research and Therapy* (pp. 323–325). New York: Raven Press.

Boden, S. D., Davis, D. O., Dina, T. S., Patronas, N. J., & Wiesel, S. W. (1990). Abnormal magnetic-resonance scans of the lumbar spine in asymptomatic subjects: A prospective investigation. *Journal of Bone and Joint Surgery: American Volume*, *72*(3), 403–408.

Boden, S. D., McCowin, P. R., Davis, D. O., Dina, T. S., Mark, A. S., & Wiesel, S. (1990). Abnormal magnetic-resonance scans of the cervical spine in asymptomatic subjects: A prospective investigation. *Journal of Bone and Joint Surgery1: American Volume*, *72*(8), 1178–1184.

Boersma, K., & Linton, S. J. (2005). Screening to identify patients at risk: Profiles of psychological risk factors for early intervention. *The Clinical Journal of Pain*, *21*(1), 38–43.

Boersma, K., & Linton, S. J. (2006). Expectancy, fear and pain in the prediction of chronic pain and disability: A prospective analysis. *European Journal of Pain*, *10*(6), 551–551.

Borenstein, D. G., O'Mara, J. W., Jr., Boden, S. D., Lauerman, W. C., Jacobson, A., Platenberg, C., . . . Wiesel, S. W. (2001). The value of magnetic resonance imaging of the lumbar spine to predict low-back pain in asymptomatic subjects: A seven-year follow-up study. *Journal of Bone and Joint Surgery: American Volume*, *83-A*(9), 1306–1311.

Bremner, J. D., & Vermetten, E. (2001). Stress and development: Behavioral and biological consequences. *Development and Psychopathology*, *13*, 473–489.

Breslin, F. C., Tompa, E., Zhao, R., Pole, J. D., Amick Iii, B. C., Smith, P. M., & Hogg-Johnson, S. (2008). The relationship between job tenure and work disability absence among adults: A prospective study. *Accident Analysis & Prevention*, *40*(1), 368–375.

Brown, J., Berenson, K., & Cohen, P. (2005). Documented and self-reported child abuse and adult pain in a community sample. *Clinical Journal of Pain*, *21*(5), 374–377.

Brown, R. J., Schrag, A., & Trimble, M. R. (2005). Dissociation, childhood interpersonal trauma, and family functioning in patients with somatization disorder. *American Journal of Psychiatry*, *162*(5), 899–905.

Bruns, D., & Disorbio, J. M. (2003). *Battery for Health Improvement 2 Manual.* Minneapolis, MN: Pearson.

Bruns, D., & Disorbio, J. M. (2009). Assessment of biopsychosocial risk factors for medical treatment: A collaborative approach. *Journal of Clinical Psychology in Medical Settings*, *16*(2), 127–147.

Butcher, J. N., Dahlstrom, W. G., Graham, J. R., Tellegen, A., & Kaemmer, B. (1989). *MMPI-2: Manual for Administration and Scoring*. Minneapolis, MN: University of Minnesota Press.

Cafferty, W. (2005). Peripheral mechanisms. In A. Holdcroft & S. Jaggar (Eds.), *Core Topics in Pain* (pp. 7–16). New York: Cambridge University Press.

Cameron, A. A., Khan, I. A., Westlund, K. N., Cliffer, K. D., & Willis, W. D. (1995). The efferent projections of the periaqueductal gray in the rat: Aphaseolus vulgaris-leucoagglutinin study: I. Ascending projections. *Journal of Comparative Neurology*, *351*, 568–584.

Cameron, I. D., Rebbeck, T., Sindhusake, D., Rubin, G., Feyer, A. M., Walsh, J., . . . Schofield, W. N. (2008). Legislative change is associated with improved health status in people with whiplash. *Spine*.

Carragee, E. J., Alamin, T. F., Miller, J. L., & Carragee, J. M. (2005). Discographic, MRI and psychosocial determinants of low back pain disability and remission: A prospective study in subjects with benign persistent back pain. *Spine Journal*, *5*(1), 24–35.

Carroll, L. J., Cassidy, J. D., & Côté, P. (2004). Depression as a risk factor for onset of an episode of troublesome neck and low back pain. *Pain*, *107*(1), 134–139.

Carroll, L. J., Holm, L. W., Hogg-Johnson, S., Cote, P., Cassidy, J. D., Haldeman, S., . . . Bone and Joint Decade 2000-2010 Task Force on Neck Pain and Its Associated Disorders (2008). Course and prognostic factors for neck pain in whiplash-associated disorders (WAD): Results of the bone and joint decade 2000–2010 task force on neck pain and its associated disorders. *Spine*, *33*(4 Suppl), S83–S92.

Cassidy, J. D., Carroll, L. J., Cote, P., Berglund, A., & Nygren, A. (2003). Low back pain after traffic collisions: A population-based cohort study. *Spine (Phila Pa 1976)*, *28*(10), 1002–1009.

Cassidy, J. D., Carroll, L. J., Cote, P., Lemstra, M., Berglund, A., & Nygren, A. (2000). Effect of eliminating compensation for pain and suffering on the outcome of insurance claims for whiplash injury. *New England Journal of Medicine*, *342*(16), 1179–1186.

Chafetz, M. D. (2008). Malingering on the social security disability consultative exam: Predictors and base rates. *The Clinical Neuropsychologist*, *22*(3), 529–546.

Chafetz, M., & Underhill, J. (2013). Estimated costs of malingered disability. *Archives of Clinical Neuropsychology*, *28*(7), 633–639.

Chan, L., Turner, J. A., Comstock, B. A., Levenson, L. M., Hollingworth, W., Heagerty, P. J., . . . Jarvik, J. G. (2007). The relationship between electrodiagnostic findings and patient symptoms and function in carpal tunnel syndrome. *Archives of Physical Medicine and Rehabilitation*, *88*(1), 19–24.

Chibnall, J. T., & Tait, R. C. (1994). The pain disability index: Factor structure and normative data. *Archives of Physical Medicine and Rehabilitation*, *75*(10), 1082–1086.

Christie, M. J., James, L. B., & Beart, P. M. (1986). An excitatory amino acid projection from rat prefrontal cortex to periaqueductal gray. *Brain Research Bulletin*, *16*, 127–129.

Cobb, L., Thomas, G. I., Dillard, D. H., Merendino, K. A., & Bruce, R. A. (1959). An evaluation of internal-mammary artery ligation by a double blind technique. *New England Journal of Medicine*, *260*(22), 1115–1118.

Colloca, L., & Benedetti, F. (2007). Nocebo hyperalgesia: How anxiety is turned into pain. *Current Opinion in Anaesthesionlogy*, *20*(5), 435–439.

Colloca, L., Lopiano, L., Lanotte, M., & Benedetti, F. (2004). Overt versus covert treatment for pain, anxiety and parkinson's disease. *Lancet Neurology*, *3*(11), 679–684

Craig, A. D., Chen, K., Bandy, D., & Reiman, E. M. (2000). Thermosensory activation of insular cortex. *Nature Neuroscience*, *3*, 184–190.

Crombez, G., Eccleston, C., Baeyens, F., & Eelen, P. (1998). When somatic information threatens, catastrophic thinking enhances attentional interference. *Pain*, *75*(2–3), 187–198.

Crook, J., & Moldofsky, H. (1994). The probability of recovery and return to work from work disability as a function of time. *Quality of Life Research*, *3*(Suppl 1), S97–S109.

Currie, S. R., & Wang, J. (2004). Chronic back pain and major depression in the general Canadian population. *Pain*, *107*(1), 54–60.

Davis, D. A., Luecken, L. J., & Zautra, A. J. (2005). Are reports of childhood abuse related to the experience of chronic pain in adulthood? A meta-analytic review of the literature. *Clinical Journal of Pain*, *21*(5), 398–405.

Deardorff, W. W., Chino, A. F., & Scott, D. W. (1993). Characteristics of chronic pain patients: Factor analysis of the MMPI-2. *Pain*, *54*(2), 153–158.

De Craen, A. J., Tijssen, J. G., de Gans, J., & Kleijnen, J. (2000). Placebo effect in the acute treatment of migraine: Subcutaneous placebos are better than oral placebos. *Journal of Neurology*, *247*(3), 183–188.

Deer, T. R., Grigsby, E., Weiner, R. L., Wilcosky, B., & Kramer, J. M. (2013). A prospective study of dorsal root ganglion stimulation for the relief of chronic pain. *Neuromodulation: Technology at the Neural Interface*, *16*(1), 67–72.

de la Fuente-Fernandez, R., & Stoessl, A. J. (2002). The biochemical bases for reward: Implications for the placebo effect. *Evaluation & the Health Professions*, *25*, 387–398.

Dersh, J., Gatchel, R. J., Mayer, T., Polatin, P., & Temple, O. R. (2006). Prevalence of psychiatric disorders in patients with chronic disabling occupational spinal disorders. *Spine*, *31*(10), 1156–1162.

Dersh, J., Gatchel, R. J., & Polatin, P. (2001). Chronic spinal disorders and psychopathology: Research findings and theoretical considerations. *Spine Journal*, *1*(2), 88–94.

Dimond, E. G., Kittle, C. F., & Crockett, J. E. (1960). Comparison of internal mammary ligation and sham operation for angina pectoris. *American Journal of Cardiology*, *5*, 483–486.

Dionne, C. E., Von Korff, M., Koepsell, T. D., Deyo, R. A., Barlow, W. E., & Checkoway, H. (2001). Formal education and back pain: A review. *Journal of Epidemiology and Community Health*, *55*(7), 455–468.

Dworkin, S. F., Chen, A. C., LeResche, L., & Clark, D. W. (1983). Cognitive reversal of expected nitrous oxide analgesia for acute pain. *Anesthesia and Analgesia*, *62*, 1079–1077.

Eccleston, C., Williams, A. C., & Morley, S. (2009). Psychological therapies for the management of chronic pain (excluding headache) in adults. *Cochrane Database of Systematic Reviews*, (2), CD007407.

Edwards, R. R., Smith, M. T., Stonerock, G., & Haythornthwaite, J. A. (2006). Pain-related catastrophizing in healthy women is associated with greater temporal summation of and reduced habituation to thermal pain. *Clinical Journal of Pain*, *22*(8), 730–737.

Enck, P., Benedetti, F., & Schedlowski, M. (2008). New insights into the placebo and nocebo responses. *Neuron Review*, *59*, 195–206.

Englund, M., Guermazi, A., Gale, D., Hunter, D. J., Aliabadi, P., Clancy, M., . . . Felson, D. T. (2008). Incidental meniscal findings on knee MRI in middle-aged and elderly persons. *New England Journal of Medicine*, *359*(11), 1108–1115.

Englund, M., Niu, J., Guermazi, A., Roemer, F. W., Hunter, D. J., Lynch, J. A., . . . Felson, D. T. (2007). Effect of meniscal damage on the development of frequent knee pain, aching, or stiffness. *Arthritis and Rheumatism*, *56*(12), 4048–4054.

Epker, J., & Block, A. R. (2001). Presurgical psychological screening in back pain patients: A review. *Clinical Journal of Pain*, *17*(3), 200–205.

Ericsson, M., Poston, W. S., Linder, J., Taylor, J. E., Haddock, C. K., & Foreyt, J. P. (2002). Depression predicts disability in long-term chronic pain patients. *Disability and Rehabilitation*, *24*(6), 334–340.

Evans, D. (2004). *Placebo: Mind Over Matter in Modern Medicine*. Oxford: Oxford University Press.

Fields, H. (2004). State-dependent opioid control of pain. *Nature Reviews Neuroscience*, *5*, 565–575.

Fink, P., Steen Hansen, M., & Sondergaard, L. (2005). Somatoform disorders among first-time referrals to a neurology service. *Psychosomatics*, *46*(6), 540–548.

Finniss, D. G., Kaptchuk, T. J., Miller, F., & Benedetti, F. (2010). Biological, clinical, and ethical advances of placebo effects. *The Lancet*, *375*(9715), 686–695.

Fishbain, D. A., Cutler, R., Rosomoff, H. L., & Rosomoff, R. S. (1999). Chronic pain disability exaggeration/malingering and submaximal effort research. *Clinical Journal of Pain*, *15*(4), 244–274.

Friedman, A. F., Gleser, G. C., Smeltzer, D. J., Wakefield, J. A., Jr., & Schwartz, M. S. (1983). MMPI overlap item scales for differentiating psychotics, neurotics, and nonpsychiatric groups. *Journal of Consulting and Clinical Psychology*, *51*(4), 629–631.

Gatchel, R. J. (2004). Psychosocial factors that can influence the self-assessment of function. *Journal of Occupational Rehabilitation*, *14*(3), 197–206.

Gatchel, R. J., & Dersh, J. (2002). Psychological disorders and chronic pain: Are there cause and effect relationships? In D. C. Turk & R. J. Gatchel (Eds.), *Psychological Approaches to Pain Management: A Practitioners Handbook* (2nd ed., pp. 30–51). New York: Guilford Press.

Gatchel, R. J., & Okifuji, A. (2006). Evidence-based scientific data documenting the treatment and cost-effectiveness of comprehensive pain programs for chronic nonmalignant pain. *Journal of Pain*, *7*(11), 779–793.

Gatchel, R. J., Peng, Y. B., Fuchs, P. N., Peters, M. L., & Turk, D. C. (2007). The biopsychosocial approach to chronic pain: Scientific advances and future directions. *Psychological Bulletin*, *133*(4), 581–624.

Gatchel, R. J., Polatin, P. B., & Mayer, T. G. (1995). The dominant role of psychosocial risk factors in the development of chronic low back pain disability. *Spine*, *20*(24), 2702–2709.

Gatchel, R. J., Polatin, P. B., Mayer, T. G., & Garcy, P. D. (1994). Psychopathology and the rehabilitation of patients with chronic low back pain disability. *Archives of Physical Medicine and Rehabilitation*, *75*(6), 666–670.

Gates, J. R., Ramani, V., Whalen, S., & Loewenson, R. (1985). Ictal characteristics of pseudoseizures. *Archives of Neurology*, *42*(12), 1183–1187.

Goubert, L., Crombez, G., & De Bourdeaudhuij, I. (2004). Low back pain, disability and back pain myths in a community sample: Prevalence and interrelationships. *European Journal of Pain*, *8*(4), 385–394.

Greve, K. W., Bianchini, K. J., Black, F. W., Heinly, M. T., Love, J. M., Swift, D. A., . . . Ciota, M. A. (2006). The prevalence of cognitive malingering in persons reporting exposure to occupational and environmental substances. *Neurotoxicology*, *27*(6), 940–950.

Greve, K. W., Bianchini, K. J., & Brewer, S. T. (2013). The assessment of performance and self-report validity in persons claiming pain-related disability. *The Clinical Neuropsychologist*, *27*(1), 108–137.

Greve, K. W., Bianchini, K. J., Etherton, J. L., Meyers, J. E., Curtis, K. L., & Ord, J. S. (2010). The reliable digit span test in chronic pain: Classification accuracy in detecting malingered pain-related disability. *The Clinical Neuropsychologist*, *24*(1), 137–152.

Greve, K. W., Curtis, K. L., & Bianchini, K. J. (2013). Symptom validity testing: A summary of recent research. *Neuropsychology Science and Practice*, *1*, 61–94.

Greve, K. W., Etherton, J. L., Ord, J., Bianchini, K. J., & Curtis, K. L. (2009). Detecting malingered pain-related disability: Classification accuracy of the test of memory malingering. *The Clinical Neuropsychologist*, *23*(7), 1250–1271.

Greve, K. W., Ord, J. S., Bianchini, K. J., & Curtis, K. L. (2009). Prevalence of malingering in patients with chronic pain referred for psychologic evaluation in a medico-legal context. *Archives of Physical Medicine and Rehabilitation*, *90*(7), 1117–1126.

Gureje, O., Simon, G. E., & Von Korff, M. (2001). A cross-national study of the course of persistent pain in primary care. *Pain*, *92*(1), 195–200.

Guo, H. R., Tanaka, S., Halperin, W. E., & Cameron, L. L. (1999). Back pain prevalence in U.S. industry and estimates of lost workdays. *American Journal of Public Health*, *89*(7), 1029–1035.

Guzman, J., Esmail, R., Karjalainen, K., Malmivaara, A., Irvin, E., & Bombardier, C. (2002). Multidisciplinary bio-psycho-social rehabilitation for chronic low back pain. *Cochrane Database of Systematic Reviews*, 1, CD000963.

Hagen, K. B., Holte, H. H., Tambs, K., & Bjerkedal, T. (2000). Socioeconomic factors and disability retirement from back pain: A 1983–1993 population-based prospective study in Norway. *Spine*, *25*(19), 2480–2487.

Hagen, K. B., Tambs, K., & Bjerkedal, T. (2002). A prospective cohort study of risk factors for disability retirement because of back pain in the general working population. *Spine (Phila Pa 1976)*, *27*(16), 1790–1796.

Harkonmaki, K., Korkeila, K., Vahtera, J., Kivimaki, M., Suominen, S., Sillanmaki, L., . . . Koskenvuo M. (2007). Childhood adversities as a predictor of disability retirement. *Journal of Epidemiology and Community Health*, *61*(6), 479–484.

Harris, I., Mulford, J., Solomon, M., van Gelder, J. M., & Young, J. (2005). Association between compensation status and outcome after surgery: A meta-analysis. *JAMA*, *293*(13), 1644–1652.

Hathaway, S. R., & McKinley, J. C. (1943). *MMPI Manual*. New York: Psychological Corporation.

Heim, C., Ehlert, U., Hanker, J. P., & Hellhammer, D. H. (1998). Abuse-related posttraumatic stress disorder and alterations of the hypothalamic-pituitary-adrenal axis in women with chronic pelvic pain. *Psychosomatic Medicine*, *60*(3), 309–318.

Heinricher, M. M., McGaraughty, S., & Tortorici, V. (2001). Circuitry underlying antiopioid actions of cholecystokinin within the rostral ventromedial medulla. *Journal of Neurophysiology*, *85*, 280–286.

Heinricher, M. M., & Neurbert, M. J. (2004). Neural basis for the hyperalgesic of cholecystokinin in the rostral ventromedial medulla. *Journal of Neurophysiology*, *92*, 1982–1989.

Hoffman, G. A., Harrington, A., & Fields, H. L. (2005). Pain and the placebo: What we have learned. *Perspectives in Biology and Medicine*, *48*(2), 248–265.

Holzberg, A. D., Robinson, M. E., Geisser, M. E., & Gremillion, H. A. (1996). The effects of depression and chronic pain on psychosocial and physical functioning. *Clinical Journal of Pain*, *12*(2), 118–125.

Hoogendoorn, W. E., Bongers, P. M., de Vet, H. C., Ariens, G. A., van Mechelen, W., & Bouter, L. M. (2002). High physical work load and low job satisfaction increase the risk of sickness absence due to low back pain: Results of a prospective cohort study. *Occupational and Environmental Medicine*, *59*(5), 323–328.

Howard, K. J., Mayer, T. G., & Gatchel, R. J. (2009). Effects of presenteeism in chronic occupational musculoskeletal disorders: Stay at work is validated. *Journal of Occupational and Environmental Medicine*, *51*(6), 724–731.

Imbierowicz, K., & Egle, U. T. (2003). Childhood adversities in patients with fibromyalgia and somatoform pain disorder. *European Journal of Pain*, *7*(2), 113–119.

International Association for the Study of Pain. Pain, IASP Pain Terminology. 1994. Retrieved from www.iasp-pain.org/AM/Template.cfm?Section=Pain_Definitions&Template=/CM/HTMLDisplay. cfm&ContentID=1728#Pain

Jaggar, S. I. (2005). Overview of pain pathways. In A. Holdcroft & S. Jaggar (Eds.), *Core Topics in Pain* (pp. 3–6). New York: Cambridge University Press.

Jamison, R. N., & Edwards, R. R. (2013). Risk factor assessment for problematic use of opioids for chronic pain. *The Clinical Neuropsychologist*, *27*(1), 60–80.

Janowski, K., Steuden, S., & Kuryłowicz, J. (2010). Factors accounting for psychosocial functioning in patients with low back pain. *European Spine Journal*, *19*(4), 613–623.

Jarvik, J. G., Hollingworth, W., Heagerty, P. J., Haynor, D. R., Boyko, E. J., & Deyo, R. A. (2005). Three-year incidence of low back pain in an initially asymptomatic cohort: Clinical and imaging risk factors. *Spine*, *30*(13), 1541–1548; discussion 1549.

Jarvik, J. J., Hollingworth, W., Heagerty, P., Haynor, D. R., & Deyo, R. A. (2001). The Longitudinal Assessment of Imaging and Disability of the Back (LAIDBack) study: Baseline data. *Spine (Phila Pa 1976)*, *26*(10), 1158–1166.

Kay, N. R., & Morris-Jones, H. (1998). Pain clinic management of medico-legal litigants. *Injury*, *29*(4), 305–308.

Keefe, F. J., Rumble, M. E., Scipio, C. D., Giordano, L. A., & Perri, L. M. (2004). Psychological aspects of persistent pain: Current state of the science. *Journal of Pain*, *5*(4), 195–211.

Keller, L. S., & Butcher, J. N. (1991). *Assessment of Chronic Pain Patients With the MMPI-2*. Minneapolis, MN: University of Minnesota Press.

Kiecolt-Glaser, J. K., Page, G. G., Marucha, P. T., MacCallum, R. C., & Glaser, R. (1998). Psychological influences on surgical recovery: Perspectives from psychoneuroimmunology. *American Psychologist*, *53*(11), 1209–1218.

Kirsch, I. E. (1999). *How Expectancies Shape Experience*. Washington, DC: American Psychological Association.

Klein, D. F., & Gorman, J. M. (1987). A model of panic and agoraphobic development. *Acta Psychiatrica Scandinavica. Supplementum*, *335*, 87–95.

Koyama, T., Tanaka, Y. Z., & Mikami, A. (1998). Nociceptive neurons in the macaque anterior cingulated activate during anticipation of pain. *Neuroreport*, *9*, 2663–2667.

Lamberty, G. J. (2008). *Understanding Somatization in the Practice of Clinical Neuropsychology*. New York: Oxford University Press.

Larrabee, G. J. (2003). Detection of malingering using atypical performance patterns on standard neuropsychological tests. *The Clinical Neuropsychologist*, *17*(3), 410–425.

Larrabee, G. J., Millis, S. R., & Meyers, J. E. (2008). Sensitivity to brain dysfunction of the Halstead-Reitan vs. an ability-focused neuropsychological battery. *The Clinical Neuropsychologist*, *22*(5), 813–825.

Lebovits, A. H. (2000). The psychological assessment of patients with chronic pain. *Current Review of Pain*, *4*(2), 122–126.

Leeuw, M., Goossens, M. E., Linton, S. J., Crombez, G., Boersma, K., & Vlaeyen, J. W. (2007). The fear-avoidance model of musculoskeletal pain: Current state of scientific evidence. *Journal of Behavioral Medicine*, *30*(1), 77–94.

Linton, S. J. (2000). A review of psychological risk factors in back and neck pain. *Spine*, *25*(9), 1148–1156.

Loeser, J. D., & Melzack, R. (1999). Pain: An overview. *The Lancet*, *353*, 1607–1609.

Love, A. W., & Peck, C. L. (1987). The MMPI and psychological factors in chronic low back pain: A review. *Pain, 28*(1), 1–12.

Lubin, B., Larsen, R. M., & Matarazzo, J. D. (1984). Patterns of psychological test usage in the United States: 1935–1982. *American Psychologist, 39*, 451–455.

Marks, P. A., & Seeman, W. (1963). *The Actuarial Description of Abnormal Personality*. Baltimore: Williams & Wilkins.

Martin, A. L., McGrath, P. A., Brown, S. C., & Katz, J. (2007). Anxiety sensitivity, fear of pain and pain-related disability in children and adolescents with chronic pain. *Pain Research & Management: The Journal of the Canadian Pain Society, 12*(4), 267.

Martin, R., Burneo, J. G., Prasad, A., Powell, T., Faught, E., Knowlton, R., . . . Kuzniecky, R. (2003). Frequency of epilepsy in patients with psychogenic seizures monitored by video-EEG. *Neurology, 61*(12), 1791–1792.

Mayer, T. G., Gatchel, R. J., & Polatin, P. B. (Eds.). (2000). *Occupational Musculoskeletal Disorders: Function, Outcomes and Evidence*. Philadelphia, PA: Lippincott Williams & Wilkins.

Mayer, T. G., Towns, B. L., Neblett, R., Theodore, B. R., & Gatchel, R. J. (2008). Chronic widespread pain in patients with occupational spinal disorders: Prevalence, psychiatric comorbidity, and association with outcomes. *Spine (Phila Pa 1976), 33*(17), 1889–1897.

McIntosh, G., Frank, J., Hogg-Johnson, S., Bombardier, C., & Hall, H. (2000). Prognostic factors for time receiving workers' compensation benefits in a cohort of patients with low back pain. *Spine, 25*(2), 147–157.

McMahon, S., Koltzenburg, M., Tracey, I., & Turk, D. C. (2013). *Wall & Melzack's Textbook of Pain: Expert Consult-Online*. Milton, Ontario: Elsevier Health Sciences.

Melzack, R., & Wall, P. D. (1965). Pain mechanisms: A new theory. *Science, 150*, 971–979.

Merskey, H. M., & Bogduk, N. (1994). *Classification of Chronic Pain* (2nd ed.). Seattle: IASP Press.

Meyers, J. E., & Diep, A. (2000). Assessment of malingering in chronic pain patients using neuropsychological tests. *Applied Neuropsychology, 7*(3), 133–139.

Millan, M. J. (1999). The induction of pain: An integrative review. *Progress in Neurobiology, 57*, 1–164.

Millon, T., Green, C. J., & Meagher, R. B. (1982). *Millon Behavioral Health Inventory Manual*. Minneapolis, MN: Interpretive Scoring Systems.

Mitchell, J. M., Lowe, D., & Fields, H. L. (1998). The contribution of the rostral ventromedial medulla to the antinociceptive effects of systemic morphine in restrained and unrestrained rats. *Neuroscience, 87*, 123–133.

Mittenberg, W., Patton, C., Canyock, E. M., & Condit, D. C. (2002). Base rates of malingering and symptom exaggeration. *Journal of Clinical and Experimental Neuropsychology, 24*(8), 1094–1102.

Moerman, D. (2002). *Meaning, Medicine and the 'Placebo Effect'*. Cambridge: Cambridge University Press.

Moffett, J. A., Underwood, M. R., & Gardiner, E. D. (2009). Socioeconomic status predicts functional disability in patients participating in a back pain trial. *Disability & Rehabilitation, 31*(10), 783–790.

Montgomery, G. H., & Kirsch, I. (1996). Mechanisms of placebo pain reduction: An empirical investigation. *Psychological Science, 7*, 174–176.

Montgomery, G. H., & Kirsch, I. (1997). Classical conditioning and the placebo effect. *Pain, 72*, 107–113.

Mooney, G., Speed, J., & Sheppard, S. (2005). Factors related to recovery after mild traumatic brain injury. *Brain Injury, 19*(12), 975–987.

Morken, T., Riise, T., Moen, B., Bergum, O., Hauge, S. H., Holien, S., . . . Thoppil, V. (2002). Frequent musculoskeletal symptoms and reduced health-related quality of life among industrial workers. *Occupational Medicine, 52*(2), 91–98.

Moseley, J. B., O'Malley, K., Peterson, N. J., Menke, T. J., Brody, B. A. . . . Wray, N. P. (2002). A controlled trail of arthroscopic surgery for osteoarthritis of the knee. *New England Journal of Medicine, 347*(2), 81–88.

Moseley, J. B., Wray, J., & Kuykendall, D. (1996). Arthroscopic treatment of osteoarthritis of the knee: A prospective randomized, placebo-controlled trial: Results of a pilot study. *American Journal of Sports Medicine, 24*, 28–34.

Moultry, M. A., & Poon, I. O. (2009). The use of antidepressants for chronic pain. *U.S. Pharmacist, 34*(5), 26–34.

Nampiaparampil, D. E. (2008). Prevalence of chronic pain after traumatic brain injury: A systematic review. *Jama, 300*(6), 711–719.

Nelson, D. V., Novy, D. M., Averill, P. M., & Berry, L. A. (1996). Ethnic comparability of the MMPI in pain patients. *Journal of Clinical Psychology, 52*(5), 485–497.

Nelson, S., Baldwin, N., & Taylor, J. (2012). Mental health problems and medically unexplained physical symptoms in adult survivors of childhood sexual abuse: An integrative literature review. *Journal of Psychiatric and Mental Health Nursing, 19*(3), 211–220.

Okada, K., Murase, K., & Kawakita, K. (1999). Effects of electrical stimulation of thalamic nucleus submedius and periaqueductal gray on the visceral nociceptive responses of spinal dorsal horn neurons in the rat. *Brain research, 834*(1), 112–121.

Olney, J. R., Quenzer, D. E., & Makowsky, M. (1999). Contested claims in carpal tunnel surgery: Outcome study of worker's compensation factors. *Iowa Orthopaedic Journal, 19*, 111–121.

Overland, S., Glozier, N., Henderson, M., Maeland, J. G., Hotopf, M., & Mykletun, A. (2008). Health status before, during and after disability pension award: The Hordaland Health Study (HUSK). *Occupational and Environmental Medicine, 65*(11), 769–773.

Pappagallo, M., & Werner, M. (2008). *Chronic Pain: A Primer for Physicians*. London: Remedica.

Pfeiffer, A., Pasi, A., Mehraein, P., & Herz, Q. (1982). Opiate receptor binding sites in human brain. *Brain Research, 248*, 87–96.

Pincus, T., Burton, A. K., Vogel, S., & Field, A. P. (2002). A systematic review of psychological factors as predictors of chronicity/disability in prospective cohorts of low back pain. *Spine, 27*(5), E109–E120.

Polatin, P. B., & Dersh, J. (2004). Psychotropic medication in chronic spinal disorders. *The Spine Journal, 4*(4), 436–450.

Price, D. D., Finiss, D. G., & Benedetti, F. (2008). A comprehensive Review of the placebo effect: Recent advances and current thought. *Annual Review of Psychology, 59*, 565–590.

Price, D. D., Milling, L. S., Kirsch, I., Duff, A., Montgomery, G. H., & Nicholls, S. S. (1999). An analysis of factors that contribute to the magnitude of placebo analgesia in an experimental paradigm. *Pain*, *83*(2), 147–156.

Proctor, T., Gatchel, R. J., & Robinson, R. C. (2000). Psychosocial factors and risk of pain and disability. *Occupational Medicine*, *15*(4), 803–812.

Rabin, L. A., Barr, W. B., & Burton, L. A. (2005). Assessment practices of clinical neuropsychologists in the United States and Canada: A survey of INS, NAN, and APA division 40 members. *Archives of Clinical Neuropsychology*, *20*(1), 33–65.

Rachman, S. (1998). *Anxiety*. Hove, UK: Psychological Press.

Rainville, J., Sobel, J. B., Hartigan, C., & Wright, A. (1997). The effect of compensation involvement on the reporting of pain and disability by patients referred for rehabilitation of chronic low back pain. *Spine*, *22*(17), 2016–2024.

Rashiq, S., & Dick, B. D. (2009). Factors associated with chronic noncancer pain in the Canadian population. *Pain Research & Management: The Journal of the Canadian Pain Society*, *14*(6), 454.

Robinson, M. E., Swimmer, G. I., & Rallof, D. (1989). The P-A-I-N MMPI classification system: A critical review. *Pain*, *37*(2), 211–214.

Roelofs, K., & Spinhoven, P. (2007). Trauma and medically unexplained symptoms towards an integration of cognitive and neuro-biological accounts. *Clinical Psychology Review*, *27*(7), 798–820.

Rohling, M. L., Binder, L. M., & Langhinrichsen-Rohling, J. (1995). Money matters: A meta-analytic review of the association between financial compensation and the experience and treatment of chronic pain. *Health Psychology*, *14*(6), 537–547.

Rosenstiel, A. K., & Keefe, F. J. (1983). The use of coping strategies in chronic low back pain patients: Relationship to patient characteristics and current adjustment. *Pain*, *17*(1), 33–44.

Roth, R. S., & Geisser, M. E. (2002). Educational achievement and chronic pain disability: Mediating role of pain-related cognitions. *Clinical Journal of Pain*, *18*(5), 286–296.

Rubin, D. I. (2007). Epidemiology and risk factors for spine pain. *Neurologic Clinics*, *25*(2), 353–371.

Sawamoto, N., Honda, M., Okada, T., Hanakawa, T., Kanda, M., Fukuyama, H., . . . Shibasaki, H. (2000). Expectation of pain enhances responses to nonpainful somatosensory stimulation in the anterior cingulated cortex and parietal operculum/posterior insula: An event-related functional magnetic resonance imaging study. *Journal of Neuroscience*, *20*, 7438–7445.

Schade, V., Semmer, N., Main, C. J., Hora, J., & Boos, N. (1999). The impact of clinical, morphological, psychosocial and work-related factors on the outcome of lumbar discectomy. *Pain*, *80*(1–2), 239–249.

Schnurr, R. F., & MacDonald, M. R. (1995). Memory complaints in chronic pain. *Clinical Journal of Pain*, *11*(2), 103–111.

Schofferman, J., Anderson, D., Hines, R., Smith, G., & White, A. (1992). Childhood psychological trauma correlates with unsuccessful lumbar spine surgery. *Spine*, *17*(6 Suppl), S138–S144.

Schofferman, J., Anderson, D., Hines, R., Smith, G., & Keane, G. (1993). Childhood psychological trauma and chronic refractory low-back pain. *Clinical Journal of Pain*, *9*(4), 260–265.

Scott, D. J., Stohler, C. S., Egnatuk, C. M., Wang, H., Koeppe, R. A., & Zubieta, J. K. (2008). Placebo and nocebo effects are defined by opposite opioid and dopaminergic responses. *Archives of General Psychiatry*, *65*, 220–231.

Sears, J. M., Wickizer, T. M., & Franklin, G. M. (2008). Overstating the prevalence of symptom exaggeration in workers' compensation cases. *Journal of Hand Surgery: American Volume*, *33*(6), 1014–1015; author reply 1015–1017.

Severeijns, R., Vlaeyen, J. W., van den Hout, M. A., & Weber, W. E. (2001). Pain catastrophizing predicts pain intensity, disability, and psychological distress independent of the level of physical impairment. *Clinical Journal of Pain*, *17*(2), 165–172.

Sharland, M. J., & Gfeller, J. D. (2007). A survey of neuropsychologists' beliefs and practices with respect to the assessment of effort. *Archives of Clinical Neuropsychology*, *22*(2), 213–223.

Shaw, W. S., Pransky, G., Patterson, W., & Winters, T. (2005). Early disability risk factors for low back pain assessed at outpatient occupational health clinics. *Spine*, *30*(5), 572–580.

Slesinger, D., Archer, R. P., & Duane, W. (2002). MMPI-2 characteristics in a chronic pain population. *Assessment*, *9*(4), 406–414.

Smeets, R. J., van Geel, K. D., & Verbunt, J. A. (2009). Is the fear avoidance model associated with the reduced level of aerobic fitness in patients with chronic low back pain? *Archives of Physical Medicine and Rehabilitation*, *90*(1), 109–117.

Sommer, C. (2004). Serotonin in pain and analgesia. *Molecular Neurobiology*, *30*(2), 117–125.

Spitzer, C., Barnow, S., Gau, K., Freyberger, H. J., & Grabe, H. J. (2008). Childhood maltreatment in patients with somatization disorder. *Australian and New Zealand Journal of Psychiatry*, *42*(4), 335–341.

Stewart-Williams, S. (2004). The placebo puzzle: Putting together the pieces. *Health Psychology*, *23*(2), 198–206.

Stewart-Williams, S., & Podd, J. (2004). The placebo effect: Dissolving the expectancy versus conditioning debate. *Psychological Bulletin*, *130*(2), 324–340.

Stover, B., Wickizer, T. M., Zimmerman, F., Fulton-Kehoe, D., & Franklin, G. (2007). Prognostic factors of long-term disability in a workers' compensation system. *Journal of Occupational and Environmental Medicine*, *49*(1), 31–40.

Sullivan, M. J., Stanish, W., Sullivan, M. E., & Tripp, D. (2002). Differential predictors of pain and disability in patients with whiplash injuries. *Pain Research and Management*, *7*(2), 68–74.

Sullivan, M. J., Thorn, B., Haythornthwaite, J. A., Keefe, F., Martin, M., Bradley, L. A., & Lefebvre, J. C. (2001). Theoretical perspectives on the relation between catastrophizing and pain. *Clinical Journal of Pain*, *17*(1), 52–64.

Tarullo, A. R., & Gunnar, M. R. (2006). Child maltreatment and the developing HPA axis. *Hormones and Behavior*, *50*(4), 632–639.

Tate, D. G. (1992). Workers' disability and return to work. *American Journal of Physical Medicine and Rehabilitation*, *71*(2), 92–96.

Taylor, R. R., & Jason, L. A. (2002). Chronic fatigue, abuse-related traumatization, and psychiatric disorders in a community-based sample. *Social Science and Medicine*, *55*(2), 247–256.

Teicher, M. H., Andersen, S. L., Polcari, A., Anderson, C. M., Navalta, C. P., & Kim, D. M. (2003). The neurobiological consequences of early stress and childhood maltreatment. *Neuroscience and Biobehavioral Reviews*, *27*(1–2), 33–44.

Trief, P. M., Grant, W., & Fredrickson, B. (2000). A prospective study of psychological predictors of lumbar surgery outcome. *Spine*, *25*(20), 2616–2621.

Turner, J. A., & Aaron, L. A. (2001). Pain-related catastrophizing: What is it? *Clinical Journal of Pain*, *17*(1), 65–71.

Turner, J. A., Franklin, G., Fulton-Kehoe, D., Sheppard, L., Wickizer, T. M., Wu, R., et al. (2006). Worker recovery expectations and fear-avoidance predict work disability in a population-based workers' compensation back pain sample. *Spine*, *31*(6), 682–689.

Turner, J. A., Franklin, G., Fulton-Kehoe, D., Sheppard, L., Wickizer, T. M., Wu, R., . . . Egan, K. (2007). Early predictors of chronic work disability associated with carpal tunnel syndrome: A longitudinal workers' compensation cohort study. *American Journal of Industrial Medicine*, *50*(7), 489–500.

Turner, J. A., Jensen, M. P., Warms, C. A., & Cardenas, D. D. (2002). Catastrophizing is associated with pain intensity, psychological distress, and pain-related disability among individuals with chronic pain after spinal cord injury. *Pain*, *98*(1–2), 127–134.

Twycross, R. G. (1994). Opiods. In P. D. Wall & R. Melzack (Eds.), *Textbook of Pain* (3rd ed., pp. 943–962). New York: Chuchhill Livingstone.

Vendrig, A. A., Derksen, J. L., & de Mey, H. R. (1999). Utility of selected MMPI-2 scales in the outcome prediction for patients with chronic back pain. *Psychological Assessment*, *11*, 381–385.

Vlaeyen, J. W., Kole-Snijders, A. M., Boeren, R. G., & van Eek, H. (1995). Fear of movement/(re)injury in chronic low back pain and its relation to behavioral performance. *Pain*, *62*(3), 363–372.

Vlaeyen, J. W., & Linton, S. J. (2000). Fear-avoidance and its consequences in chronic musculoskeletal pain: A state of the art. *Pain*, *85*(3), 317–332.

Volinn, E., Van Koevering, D., & Loeser, J. D. (1991). Back sprain in industry: The role of socioeconomic factors in chronicity. *Spine*, *16*(5), 542–548.

Von Korff, M., Crane, P., Lane, M., Miglioretti, D. L., Simon, G., Saunders, K., . . . Kessler, R. (2005). Chronic spinal pain and physical-mental comorbidity in the United States: Results from the national comorbidity survey replication. *Pain*, *113*(3), 331–339.

Voorhies, R. M., Jiang, X., & Thomas, N. (2007). Predicting outcome in the surgical treatment of lumbar radiculopathy using the pain drawing score, McGill short form pain questionnaire, and risk factors including psychosocial issues and axial joint pain. *Spine Journal*, *7*(5), 516–524.

Voudouris, N. J., Peck, C. L., & Coleman, G. (1989). Conditioned response models of placebo phenomena: Further support. *Pain*, *38*, 109–116.

Voudouris, N. J., Peck, C. L., & Coleman, G. (1990). The role of conditioning and verbal expectancy in the placebo response. *Pain*, *43*, 121–128.

Wager, T. D. (2005). The neural bases of placebo effects in pain. *Current Directions in Psychological Science*, *14*(4), 176–179.

Waldinger, R. J., Schulz, M. S., Barsky, A. J., & Ahern, D. K. (2006). Mapping the road from childhood trauma to adult somatization: The role of attachment. *Psychosomatic Medicine*, *68*(1), 129–135.

Walker, E. A., Gelfand, A. N., Gelfand, M. D., Green, C., & Katon, W. J. (1996). Chronic pelvic pain and gynecological symptoms in women with irritable bowel syndrome. *Journal of Psychosomatic Obstetrics and Gynaecology*, *17*(1), 39–46.

Walker, E. A., Keegan, D., Gardner, G., Sullivan, M., Bernstein, D., & Katon, W. J. (1997). Psychosocial factors in fibromyalgia compared with rheumatoid arthritis: II. Sexual, physical, and emotional abuse and neglect. *Psychosomatic Medicine*, *59*(6), 572–577.

Wall, P. D. (1994). The placebo and the placebo response. In P. D. Wall & R. Melzack (Eds.), *Textbook of Pain* (3rd ed., pp. 1297–1308). New York: Churchhill Livingstone.

Walsh, C. A., Jamieson, E., Macmillan, H., & Boyle, M. (2007). Child abuse and chronic pain in a community survey of women. *Journal of Interpersonal Violence*, *22*(12), 1536–1554.

Westman, A., Linton, S. J., Theorell, T., Ohrvik, J., Wahlen, P., & Leppert, J. (2006). Quality of life and maintenance of improvements after early multimodal rehabilitation: A 5-year follow-up. *Disability and Rehabilitation*, *28*(7), 437–446.

Wickizer, T. M., Franklin, G., Fulton-Kehoe, D., Turner, J. A., Mootz, R., & Smith-Weller, T. (2004). Patient satisfaction, treatment experience, and disability outcomes in a population-based cohort of injured workers in Washington State: Implications for quality improvement. *Health Services Research*, *39*(4 Pt 1), 727–748.

Wickizer, T. M., Franklin, G., Turner, J., Fulton-Kehoe, D., Mootz, R., & Smith-Weller, T. (2004). Use of attorneys and appeal filing in the Washington State workers' compensation program: Does patient satisfaction matter? *Journal of Occupational and Environmental Medicine*, *46*(4), 331–339.

Widom, C. S., DuMont, K., & Czaja, S. J. (2007). A prospective investigation of major depressive disorder and comorbidity in abused and neglected children grown up. *Archives of General Psychiatry*, *64*(1), 49–56.

Wilson, K. G., Eriksson, M. Y., D'Eon, J. L., Mikail, S. F., & Emery, P. C. (2002). Major depression and insomnia in chronic pain. *Clinical Journal of Pain*, *18*(2), 77–83.

Woby, S. R., Watson, P. J., Roach, N. K., & Urmston, M. (2004). Adjustment to chronic low back pain: The relative influence of fear-avoidance beliefs, catastrophizing, and appraisals of control. *Behaviour Research and Therapy*, *42*(7), 761–774.

Wolfe, F., & Hawley, D. J. (1998). Psychosocial factors and the fibromyalgia syndrome. *Zeitschrift fur Rheumatologie*, *57*(Suppl 2), 88–91.

Yu, L. C., & Han, J. S. (1989). Involvement of arcuate nucleus of hypothalamus in the descending pathway from nucleus accumbens to periaqueductal grey subserving an antinociceptive effect. *International Journal of Neuroscience*, *48*, 71–78.

Zale, E. L., Lange, K. L., Fields, S. A., & Ditre, J. W. (2013). The relation between pain-related fear and disability: A meta-analysis. *The Journal of Pain*, *14*(10), 1019–1030.

Zhao, Z. Q., Chiechio, S., Sun, Y. G., Zhang, K. H., Zhao, C. S., Scott, M., . . . Chen, Z. F. (2007). Mice lacking central serotonergic neurons show enhanced inflammatory pain and an impaired analgesic response to antidepressant drugs. *The Journal of Neuroscience*, *27*(22), 6045–6053.

Appendix: Table of common tests and measures

Test	*Purpose*
Ominibus Measures	
Millon Clinical Multiaxial Inventory-III (MCMI-III)	175 item measure. Assesses personality disorders and clinical syndromes.
Minnesota Multiphasic Inventory-2 (MMPI-2)	567 item personality inventory, symptom validity.
Minnesota Multiphasic Inventory-2-RF (MMPI-2-RF)	338 item personality inventory, revised form.
Personality Assessment Inventory (PAI)	344 Item measure. Assesses personality disorders and psychopathological syndromes.
Specific Pain Measures	
Brief Pain Inventory (BPI)	32 item measure. Assesses pain severity, location and global functioning.
Chronic Pain Coping Inventory (CPCI)	65 item measure. Assesses coping strategies.
Coping Strategies Questionnaire (CSQ)	50 item measure. Assesses behavior and cognitive pain coping strategies.
Dallas Pain Questionnaire (DPQ)	16 item measure. Assesses functional and emotional aspect of chronic low back pain.
McGill Pain Questionnaire(MPQ)	Scale of sensory, affective and evaluative pain dimensions
SF-McGill Pain Questionnaire (SF-MPQ)	15 item short form version
Modified Somatic Perception Questionnaire (MSPQ)	13 item scale of somatic and autonomic perception/coping style
Multidimensional Pain Inventory (MPI)	60 item measure. Assesses psychosocial functioning.
Neck Pain And Disability Scale (NPAD)	20 item measure. Assesses neck pain and associated disability.
Oswestry Pain Disability (OPD)	60 item measure. Assesses daily global functioning.
Pain Anxiety Sensitivity Scale-20 (PASS-20)	20 item measure. Assesses pain specific anxiety
Pain Catastrophizing Scale (PCS)	13 item scale of catastrophic thinking/coping style
Pain Coping Inventory (PCI)	92 Item measure. Assesses behavioral, cognitive and psychological dimensions of chronic pan.
Pain Disability Index (PDI)	7 item self-report that measures 7 areas of functioning.
Pain patient profile (P-3)	132 item measure. Assesses the depression, anxiety, somatization and validity index of pain patients.
Survey of Pain Attitudes (SOPA)	57 item measure. Assesses belief sets about pain.
Tampa Scale for Kenisiophobia (TSK)	17 item measure. Fear of movement scale.
Vanderbilt Pain Management Inventory (VPMI)	18 item measure. Assesses coping strategies of chronic pain patients.
West Haven-Yale Multidimensional Pain Inventory (WHYMPI)	52 item measure. Assesses pain perception and functioning among 12 scales.
Other pain related measures	
Battery for Health Improvement-2 (BHI-2)	31 item measure. Assesses biopsychosocial factors.
Millon Behavioral Health Inventory	150 items. provide information regarding a patient's likely style of relating to health-care personnel, problematic psychosocial attitudes and stressors, as well as an individual's similarity to patients with psychosomatic complications or poor responses to either illness or treatment interventions.
Beck Anxiety Inventory (BAI)	21 item measure. Assesses anxiety symptomology.
Beck Depression Inventory (BDI)	21 item measure. Assesses depression symptomology.
Short Form-36 Health Survey (SF-36)	36 item measure. Assesses general health perceptions.

35 Neuropsychological and Psychological Assessment of Somatic Symptom Disorders

Greg J. Lamberty and Ivy N. Miller

Introduction

The neuropsychological tradition of characterizing disorders by describing patterns of deficit or impairment has not been edifying in the case of somatic symptom disorders. There is often a surfeit of self-reported cognitive dysfunction in individuals with such diagnoses, but quality studies identifying specific neurocognitive difficulties are rare. Attention has been paid to putative underlying mechanisms in disorders that have, at turns, been called *somatoform disorders, functional somatic syndromes,* and now *somatic symptom disorders.* What has *not* emerged is a clear pattern of neurocognitive dysfunction associated with any such syndrome (Suhr & Spickard, 2007). As the goals of the neuropsychological evaluation have evolved, localizing dysfunction has become less relevant, while determinations about the nature and extent of demonstrated difficulties has taken precedence. In particular, symptom and performance validity measures have assisted clinicians and researchers in identifying plausible and implausible performances. Thus, in the case of individuals with somatic symptom disorders, the neuropsychological evaluation is most often concerned with identifying a lack of cognitive dysfunction and describing the nature of the individual's numerous other symptoms, particularly those of a psychological or emotional nature.

Somatic Symptom and Related Disorders in the *Diagnostic and Statistical Manual of Mental Disorders*, fifth edition (DSM-5; American Psychiatric Association, 2013) represents a substantial revision of the Somatoform Disorders category that was initially introduced in the DSM-III (1980) and modified slightly in subsequent versions of the DSM-IV (1994, 2000). In practice environs and the clinical literature, references to somatization, conversion, and hysteria have abounded, but the accuracy and utility of such diagnoses has been vigorously debated (Engel, 2006; Mayou, Kirmayer, Simon, Kroenke, & Sharpe, 2005; Noyes, Stuart, & Watson, 2008; Voigt et al., 2010). Pre–DSM-5 deliberations resulted in clinical diagnostic criteria that are substantially more inclusive than their predecessors. Given that the Somatoform Disorders were never highly regarded as a diagnostic category (Lamberty, 2008), research efforts focused on more specific characterization of various debated clinical diagnoses such as chronic fatigue syndrome (CFS, see Deluca, Johnson, & Natelson, 1993) and psychogenic nonepileptic seizures (Driver-Dunckley, Stonnington, Locke, & Noe, 2011), while others have discussed the impact of "medically unexplained symptoms" on neuropsychological assessment measures more broadly (Binder, 2005; Binder & Campbell, 2004).

Neuropsychologists are not typically asked to conduct neuropsychological assessments to characterize individuals identified as having a somatoform disorder. However, the presence of medically unexplained symptoms is increasingly recognized as common (Lamberty, 2008) and can often end up being a primary diagnosis. Thus, while the main purpose of an assessment may not involve the identification and delineation of a somatic symptom disorder, attention to a variety of unexplained symptoms is a very important element of the neuropsychological assessment. This is particularly true when individuals present with myriad concerns that have not been adequately ruled in or out by primary care providers or other specialists. Therefore, in clinical practice, knowledge of somatic symptom disorders and how they impact the gathering of assessment data is essential for all practitioners.

Pathology and Clinical Presentations

In the time that elapsed between the publication of Briquet's (1859) monograph on hysteria and the inclusion of somatization disorder in the DSM-III, a significant shift in the understanding about what underlies the presentation occurred. Briquet and Charcot were of the opinion that the there was a primary neurologic cause for hysteria, while the DSM-III was clear in indicating that somatization was characterized by *a lack of* underlying biological etiology. Absolute either/or distinctions are rare in clinical settings, but it is generally understood that patients with a primary diagnosis of somatoform or somatic symptom disorders do not have a characteristic underlying neuropathology (APA, 2013; Lamberty, 2008). Complicating things further is the occasional finding that patients with clear central nervous system disorders can also present with prominent unexplained somatic symptoms. Therefore, it important to assess a wide range of cognitive and emotional/psychological symptoms in all assessments, irrespective of the presumed etiology of a patient's primary diagnosis.

Over the past 30 to 40 years the approach to studying somatoform disorders has varied and evolved. After DSM-III, investigators sought to validate the new construct of somatization. When it became clear that there was not a unitary etiology or presentation, attention shifted to different disorders that basically had medically unexplained symptoms as their hallmark (e.g., Binder, 2005). While we will not provide an extensive review of these conditions, it is important for the practicing clinician to be aware of such disorders. Individuals who present with these diagnoses often have strong biases and an expectation that their doctors will be similarly informed and oriented. An awareness of these dynamics can better prepare the neuropsychologist for a productive interview and assessment experience.

Medically Unexplained Symptoms and Associated Disorders

Among the more commonly diagnosed and long-standing disorders associated with medically unexplained symptoms are fibromyalgia, CFS (aka myalgic encephalomyelitis, post-viral fatigue syndrome, chronic fatigue immune dysfunction syndrome), idiopathic environmental intolerances (IEI; aka multiple chemical sensitivities), postconcussive syndrome (PCS), psychogenic movement disorders (PMD), and psychogenic nonepileptic seizures (PNES). Fatigue and chronic pain disorders in particular are more common in women (Jason et al., 1999) and are associated with a history of trauma/abuse (Walker et al., 1997). Mood and anxiety disorders are commonly comorbid with these diagnoses (Bagayogo, Interian, & Escobar, 2013; Mariman et al., 2013; Walker et al., 1997; Yalcin & Barrot, 2014). Neuropsychological studies of fibromyalgia, CFS, and IEI have failed to find consistent deficits that cannot be accounted for by psychological/emotional distress (Suhr, 2003). Methodological issues such as lack of symptom validity test (SVT) inclusion in test batteries have been highlighted across studies (Lamberty, 2008; Lamberty & Sim, 2014). As suggested by the cognitive symptom validity literature for all somatoform disorders, subjective cognitive complaints of fatigue and chronic pain disorders significantly outweigh documented impairments on neuropsychological measures (Binder & Campbell, 2004; Suhr, 2003). Brooks, Johnson-Greene, Lattie, and Ference (2012) found that SVT performance was significantly correlated with scores on the somatoform, depression, and anxiety subscales of the Millon Clinical Multiaxial Inventory (MCMI-III) in individuals with a fibromyalgia diagnosis. Cognitive and psychological symptom validity scores were significantly related, and authors suggested that neuropsychological evaluation of both cognitive and psychological symptom validity should be a part of a comprehensive diagnostic assessment for fibromyalgia (Brooks et al., 2012). Johnson-Greene, Brooks, and Ference (2013) found that 37% of fibromyalgia patients failed one or both of two performance validity tests (PVTs; Green's Word Memory Test/Test of Memory Malingering and Reliable Digit Span) in a standard neuropsychological assessment. When analyses were conducted comparing individuals who exhibited two versus one, versus no failures, results were significant for daily and weekly pain, and sleep but not fatigue. Analysis of disability status (on disability, applying for disability, and not on disability) was significant for daily and weekly pain and fatigue but not sleep. The authors suggested that PVT performance and disability status was associated with exaggeration of noncognitive symptoms (Johnson-Greene et al., 2013).

Attention has been paid to pseudoneurological disorders such as PNES and PMD, with a goal of understanding possible relationships between PNES and PMD populations and in attempting to differentiate PNES from electric seizures (ES). In a retrospective study, Driver-Dunckley et al. (2011) found that there are more similarities than differences among PNES and PMD patients, suggesting that they are manifestations of the same psychopathology. For example, they had similar family histories (psychiatric disorders, drug and alcohol abuse), similar rates of unemployment/disability status, and prolonged time to diagnosis including multiple evaluations and unnecessary interventions. PNES patients were younger, more likely to have intermittent symptoms associated with altered consciousness, and had lower levels of education. Neuropsychological testing was part of the medical evaluation process for 82% of PNES but only 9% of PMD. Neuropsychological and personality assessment results were suggested in this study to be helpful in determining accurate diagnosis and in helping patients accept the somatoform diagnosis (Driver-Dunckley et al., 2011). Across studies, inclusion of PVTs, SVTs and personality inventories have been shown to help differentiate PNES and ES (Binder, Kindermann, Heaton, & Salinsky, 1998; Binder, Storzbach, & Salinsky, 2006; Drane et al., 2006). With regard to neuropsychological deficits, multiple studies have found that PNES patients may appear similarly impaired to ES patients (Lamberty, 2008), though one study found that PNES patients who passed Green's Word Memory Test exhibited less impairment on neuropsychological tests, imaging, and video-EEG monitoring (Drane et al., 2006). Similarly, in a PMD sample, individuals did not show worse performance on most neuropsychological tests from healthy control participants and patients with Gilles de la Tourette syndrome, but did report more cognitive complaints in daily life and performed worse on SVTs than the other two groups (Heintz et al., 2013).

Assessment

Cognitive Symptom and Performance Validity Tests

Indistinct cognitive complaints are common among individuals with somatoform and other psychological and medical disorders, but they have been conceived of as a proxy for distress rather than objective cognitive difficulties (Binder, 2005; Heintz et al., 2013; Lamberty, 2008; Lamberty & Sim, 2014;

Wilson, Arnold, Schneider, Li, & Bennett, 2007). While various studies have reported cognitive deficits in attention/concentration, information processing speed, working memory, motor speed, and agility (Ambrose, Gracely, & Glass, 2012; Libon et al., 2010; Sjøgren, Christrup, Petersen, & Højsted, 2005), underlying mechanisms are not understood and there is little indication of neuropsychological deficits that are directly linked to central nervous system dysfunction in individuals with somatoform disorders (Heintz et al., 2013; Inamura et al., 2014; Lamberty, 2008; Lamberty & Sim, 2014). Previous reviews have highlighted the importance of inclusion of symptom and performance validity tests (SVTs, PVTs) and consideration of motivational factors (e.g., disability status) in neuropsychological assessment with patients with somatoform symptoms (Iverson & McCracken, 1997; Lamberty, 2008; Landrø, Stiles, & Sletvold, 1997; Suhr, 2003; Suhr & Spickard, 2007). Studies using the Minnesota Multiphasic Personality Inventory, second edition (MMPI-2) have described a relationship between cognitive effort measures and somatic personality configurations (Brauer Boone & Lu, 1999; Jones, Ingram, & Ben-Porath, 2012; Larrabee, 1998; Sellbom, Wygant, & Bagby, 2012).

Previous estimates of SVT failure in individuals with somatoform disorders vary based on disability and litigation status, with individuals with secondary gain likely to produce SVT failures (Gervais, Rohling, Green, & Ford, 2004). For example, a minority of nonlitigant patients with medically unexplained symptoms (11%) presenting to a neurology clinic fail effort tests (Kemp et al., 2008). It is possible that there are conscious and nonconscious reasons for failures in such patients. Other studies of patients and disability litigants have estimated SVT failure rates of 31%–35% (Gervais et al., 2004; Mittenberg, Patton, Canyock, & Condit, 2002). Roberson and colleagues (2013) found that b Test failures in credible patients with somatoform disorders (defined as nonlitigant, nondisability claimants who failed less than two PVTs) were common and attributable to slow processing and commission errors, indicating that this test may be valuable in detecting nonconsciously created cognitive dysfunction (Roberson et al., 2013). The mechanism behind nonconscious symptom reporting was recently explored in a series of experiments based on the residual effects of feigning (Merckelbach, Jelicic, & Pieters, 2011). Undergraduate students who had previously been asked to exaggerate symptoms continued to exaggerate even when later asked to respond honestly. Students then completed a symptom list of psychiatric complaints and were asked to explain why they had endorsed two target symptoms that they did not actually endorse. Fifty-seven percent of participants in this study did not detect the discrepancy between actual and manipulated symptom endorsement and tended to agree with the manipulated symptoms. The authors suggested that these studies might help to explain the susceptibility of individuals to suggestion and overreporting of somatic symptoms.

Despite significant evidence supporting inclusion of SVTs/PVTs in neuropsychological evaluations, particularly in assessing patients with medically unexplained symptoms, a recent survey of neuropsychologists in six European countries found that while most individuals had technical knowledge about symptom validity, there was little consensus about how to handle test failure (Dandachi-FitzGerald, Ponds, & Merten, 2013). There continues to be variability in the inclusion of SVTs in the research literature as well. Studies that do not include SVTs/PVTs when exploring neuropsychological impairments in somatoform disorders (e.g., Al-Adawi, Al-Zakwani, Obeid, & Zaidan, 2010; Onofrj, Bonanni, Manzoli, & Thomas, 2010) are limited in their ability to draw conclusions about reasons for cognitive differences and changes in somatoform populations.

Psychological/Personality Tests

The relationship between psychological disturbance and somatoform disorders is well supported in the literature (Grover et al., 2015; Lahmann et al., 2015; Röhricht & Elanjithara, 2014). Diagnostically, the most basic feature of somatoform disorders is the acknowledgement of numerous physical symptoms, along with a high level of distress related to these symptoms. While a basic clinical interview will usually uncover this, psychological assessment measures are useful for a more nuanced understanding of psychopathology. Further, in addition to the performance validity measures previously noted, it is also important to assess the validity of symptom reporting. Finally, tracking outcomes can be useful in the clinical intervention context, though this may not require a thorough personality assessment measure.

The Patient Health Questionnaire–15 (PHQ-15; Kroenke, Spitzer, & Williams, 2002) is used frequently as an index of the severity of somatoform symptoms in treatment outcome and epidemiological studies. It samples from a number of different somatic complaints including pain, dizziness, fatigue, and gastrointestinal complaints. In the clinical environment, the PHQ-15 can also serve as a screening measure for patients with multiple and difficult to characterize somatic concerns. While there is not an extensive literature on the PHQ-15 in the context of neuropsychological assessment, it is a freely available measure that is easy to administer and score. Such measures are useful adjuncts that can assist in decisions about referrals and more extensive personality assessment, especially in environments where time and resources are limited.

The MMPI-2 (Butcher, Dahlstrom, Graham, Tellegen, & Kaemmer, 1989) has been used widely in the identification of somatoform disorders. Elevations on Clinical Scales 1 (Hypochondriasis) and 3 (Hysteria) from the MMPI-2 are associated with somatoform disorders, and with conversion disorder when Scale 2 (Depression) is considerably lower ("Conversion V"; Graham, 2012). A study describing prototypical somatoform validity score patterns on the MMPI-2 in a sample of litigants with idiopathic environmental intolerance (aka multiple chemical sensitivities) found that most validity scales, with the exception of L (the deliberate attempt to portray oneself in an unrealistically favorable way) and K (more subtle defensiveness/presentation of oneself in a favorable light), were not elevated, while one-fourth to one-half of participants exhibited elevations on the FBS (referred to as the Symptom Validity scale; Staudenmayer & Philips, 2008).

The utility of the MMPI-2 and MMPI-2-RF is well recognized in a number of assessment contexts and this is particularly true for somatoform disorders (Lamberty, 2008). The use of validity scales was an important advance in personality assessment and this tradition has been exemplified in the development and refinement of the MMPI over the years. The three original validity scales—Lie (L), Infrequency (F), and Defensiveness (K)—allowed insights into response bias that were unique in personality assessment, but were limited in scope. With successive revisions of the MMPI, additional scales were added to provide more specific and accurate information about response bias and its effects on profile validity and interpretation.

When the Restructured Clinical (RC) scales were introduced in 2003, Somatic Complaints (RC1) was the index that indicated overall level of physical symptom reporting. Elevations on RC1 are associated with preoccupation with physical symptoms, the development of symptoms in response to stressors and fatigue (Ben-Porath, 2012), and a diagnosis of somatoform disorders (Simms, Casillas, Clark, Watson, & Doebbeling, 2005), but not to any one specific somatoform diagnosis (Ben-Porath, 2012). Thomas and Locke (2010) found that RC1 scale is most precise for T score estimates between 55 and 90, and that the scale is well suited for the assessment of somatization (Thomas & Locke, 2010). Studies examining different samples have validated the utility of RC1 in distinguishing between samples (epilepsy and PNES) as well as characterizing what elevations mean in different samples (e.g., Arbisi, Sellbom, & Ben-Porath, 2008). The RC scales limited the need for and utility of codetype interpretation that became popular with the MMPI and MMPI-2. Improved psychometrics and a general lessening of the impact of distress or demoralization on the main clinical scales has reduced the need to combine scale elevations as a means of making important interpretations with the MMPI-2-RF.

The MMPI-2-Restructured Form (MMPI-2-RF; Ben Porath & Tellegen, 2011) is now in wide use and includes additional validity scales with direct relevance to individuals reporting high levels of somatic and cognitive symptoms (Ben-Porath, 2012; Ben-Porath & Tellegen, 2011). Of particular interest is the Infrequent Somatic Responses (Fs) scale, which is recommended as a general index of the credibility of somatic symptom reporting (Ben-Porath, 2012). Elevations of $T \geq 100$ on Fs suggest exaggeration of symptoms at a level that is unrealistic under most circumstances and thus not likely valid. As a result, scores on the other somatically oriented indices should not be included in the interpretive profile. Whether or not such elevations are associated with malingering is not yet clear, though certainly the validity of assessments with these kinds of elevations would seem questionable. A recent study attempted to use the MMPI-2-RF to differentiate between individuals with somatoform disorders and other individuals endorsing somatic complaints, a difficult task. For example, Sellbom et al. (2012) found that Fs and Fp-r were best at differentiating between individuals feigning physical health problems, patients with somatoform disorders, and medical patients without mental health disorders. The clearest distinctions were made by these scales in differentiating somatic malingering from somatoform and medical illness groups. MMPI-2-RF scales of interest could not distinguish between somatic malingering and somatoform patients (Sellbom et al., 2012), highlighting the need for evaluation of motivational/secondary gain factors during the clinical interview portion of a psychological assessment.

Two additional scales that emanated largely from the clinical neuropsychology literature: the Symptom Validity Scale (FBS, or FBS-r in the MMPI-2-RF) and the Response Bias Scale (RBS; Gervais, Ben-Porath, Wygant, & Sellbom, 2010), which are both sensitive to symptom overreporting (Ben-Porath, 2012). FBS-r is sensitive to general elevations in somatic symptoms, while RBS is elevated primarily by acknowledgement of memory and cognitive difficulties. All such symptom reporting is important in the context of neuropsychological exams. In his interpretive book on the MMPI-RF, Ben-Porath noted that overreporting on these validity scales does not necessarily mean the test taker is intentionally overreporting and may represent a somatoform disorder (Ben-Porath, 2012). A few papers have examined the extent to which these indices impact profile validity and cognitive test performances, though a more general understanding of such patterns remains to be elucidated. For example, in an investigation of the stability of FBS-r in a nonforensic Veterans Administration sample of neuropsychological referrals, Gass and Odland (2012) found two latent constructs within FBS-r—Somatic Complaints and Optimism/Virtue—that together accounted for 95% of the variance in FBS-r scores. They noted that FBS-r contains 15 items that were empirically keyed with conversion disorder and 13 items with hypochondriasis, and that scores are influenced by a denial of socially undesirable behavior and a rejection of cynical interpretations of people's motivations. Authors suggested that FBS-r is potentially unstable because it lacks a statistically coherent factor structure, though it does provide a rough estimate of anxiety severity and opinions about one's personal values and human nature (Gass & Odland, 2012). Jones and Ingram (2011) found that in a sample of military members the Henry-Heilbronner Index (HHI), RBS, FBS and FBS-r outperformed the F-family scales in classification accuracy analyses in predicting effort status on cognitive tests, with moderate effect sizes. Fs performed at the same level as F, the best performing F-family scale (Jones &

Ingram, 2011). RBS showed the strongest relationship with memory complaints in a sample of non-head-injury disability related referrals, and provided incremental contribution above and beyond the F-r, Fp-r, Fs, and FBS-r in predicting memory complaints (Gervais et al., 2010). Authors suggested that subjective memory complaints in the context of elevated RBS scores are unlikely to indicate objective memory deficits (Gervais et al., 2010). RBS also showed the largest effect size of all overreporting scales in a military sample completing neuropsychological evaluations for mild TBI, in which SVT failure was associated with linear increases in MMPI-2-RF overreporting scales and most substantive scales (Jones et al., 2012). With regard to the substantive scale analyses in this study, Cognitive Complaints (COG) had the largest effect size, followed by Somatic Complaints (RC1), Head Pain Complaints (HPC), Malaise (MLS), and Neurological Complaints (NUC). Participants who passed SVTs had clinically significant elevations only on COG and NUC. In another sample of TBI litigants, elevations on the Somatic/Cognitive scales profile were significant predictors of effort test failure, and were better predictors of effort test failure than the MMPI-2-RF validity scales. MLS arose as the single best predictor of effort test failure. Authors noted that all items on MLS were part of the MMPI-2 Hy scale. FBS-r was also significantly related to passing or failing effort tests, and there was only a modest, nonsignificant association with poor effort for Fs (Youngjohn, Wershba, Stevenson, Sturgeon, & Thomas, 2011). In a study using the Forensic Disability Claimant Sample from the MMPI-2-RF Technical Manual, SVT failure was associated with significant elevations throughout the MMPI-2-RF overreporting and substantive scales, including COG. Authors concluded that claimants appear to use both personality and SVT tests to communicate their claimed neurocognitive impairment, physical complaints, and emotional dysfunction (Gervais, Wygant, Sellbom, & Ben-Porath, 2011).

Among the newly developed Specific Problems Scales are the Somatic/Cognitive Scales, which are brief and focused indices of physical complaints including MLS, HPC, Gastrointestinal Complaints (GIC), NUC, and COG. In contrast to the overreporting validity scales and RC1, the Somatic/Cognitive scales assess more specific symptoms that might reasonably be associated with different kinds of clinical or medical problems. These scales should be interpreted in light of Fs, the validity score noting overreporting of somatic symptoms, as well as FBS and RBS, which note overreporting of cognitive symptoms. Literature on these scales is limited, though in the clinical context valuable descriptive information can be obtained through a careful review of the indices. Overall, studies utilizing the MMPI-2-RF to assess for somatic symptoms provide more detailed information than was previously available through earlier editions of the MMPI.

Outside of the MMPI literature, several other psychological studies have attempted to better characterize individuals with somatic symptoms. For example, in comparing patients with somatization to control patients in an outpatient setting, Stonnington, Locke, Hsu, Ritenbaugh, and Lane (2013) found that somatizing patients exhibited a deficit in the experience of positive emotions and a tendency to not immediately make emotional attributions to their physical symptoms, which may explain the tendency to reject psychological explanations for symptoms (Stonnington et al., 2013). In another study, depression, anxiety, and somatization patients showed deficits in the ability to forget illness-related stimuli relative to neutral material (Wingenfeld, Terfehr, Meyer, Löwe, & Spitzer, 2013), suggesting a cognitive bias in these individuals. Other studies have related depressive symptoms to somatic presentations as well. In a sample of mild to moderate TBI patients, somatic symptoms and chronic stress explained variation in depressive symptoms (Bay & Covassin, 2012). Compared with nondepressed patients with medically unexplained symptoms, depressed patients had more severe somatic symptoms, more psychological symptoms, and more functional impairment (Hilderink et al., 2009). Alexithymia was strongly associated with the number of somatic symptoms and negative affect in patients with somatoform disorder (Tominaga, Choi, Nagoshi, Wada, & Fukui, 2014). Compared with patients with nonsomatoform mental disorders as well as patients with "organic" illness, somatoform patients reported greater frustration with ill health and higher utilization of care (Schmid et al., 2014). Less attention has been paid to the prevalence and characterization of somatoform disorders and medically unexplained symptoms in older adults (Lamberty & Bares, 2013). A recent review on this topic found that these symptoms are common in elderly individuals, but prevalence rates of somatoform disorders appear lower than in younger populations. Authors suggested that like depression in the elderly, it may be that subsyndromal somatoform disorders are more common than disorders that meet the full criteria (Hilderink, Collard, Rosmalen, & Oude Voshaar, 2013). These studies highlight potentially important characteristics of individuals with somatoform disorders and may provide insight into treatment potential for these complex patients.

Intervention

Treating patients with somatic symptom disorders can be a challenge for even skilled therapists, though the nihilism associated with treating such patients appears to have lessened considerably in recent times (Lamberty, 2008). This is likely due to the emergence of empirically supported treatments that involve cognitive behavioral therapy (CBT), mindfulness-based approaches, complementary and alternative interventions, and physically oriented interventions like physical therapy and yoga (Lamberty & Sim, 2014; Lamberty, 2014; Lamberty & Bares, 2013). A recent Cochrane review examining the effectiveness of pharmacological treatments for somatoform disorders indicated that the quality of evidence for new-generation antidepressants was very low, while evidence for natural products was low (Kleinstäuber et al., 2014). Further, to the extent that there were significant effects for antidepressants, these needed to be balanced against the high rates of adverse effects with those drugs (Kleinstäuber et al., 2014). In slight contrast, a Cochrane review of nonpharmacological interventions for somatoform disorders and medically unexplained physical symptoms (MUPS) indicated that psychological therapies were superior to usual care in terms of reduction of symptoms (van Dessel et al., 2014). Effect sizes were small and the highest quality studies were conducted with CBT (van Dessel et al., 2014). Showing strong evidence via comparative effectiveness reviews is a gold standard that is difficult for many interventions to achieve. The fact that "work needs to be done" should not be discouraging and it is impressive that there are studies of adequate quality to be reviewed in this often murky area.

Most neuropsychologists do not identify themselves as participating regularly in the provision of psychotherapy or intervention services (Sweet, Giuffre Meyer, Nelson, & Moberg, 2011). The ascendance of empirically supported treatment makes some forms of intervention seemingly more straightforward and applicable for neuropsychologists that might be reluctant to engage in intervention services. This may be particularly true for groups that have traditionally been perceived as clinically challenging and not likely to benefit from psychotherapy. Lamberty and Nelson (2012) note that empirically supported treatments such as motivational interviewing (MI; Rollnick, Miller, & Butler, 2008) and other approaches like *therapeutic assessment* (Finn & Kamphuis, 2006) or *collaborative therapeutic neuropsychological assessment* (Gorske & Smith, 2009) might realistically fit into the practice models of some neuropsychologists. In the absence of taking on intervention cases, there is clear value in improving one's awareness of efficacious treatments for challenging patients. At the very least, a strong knowledge base of appropriate and empirically supported interventions will bolster the neuropsychologist's ability to remain responsive to his or her patients and referral sources and assure his or her practice viability into the future.

Summary

Neuropsychologists frequently encounter individuals who meet criteria for a somatic symptom disorder, particularly since DSM criteria have changed substantially and are more inclusive. Traditional neuropsychological assessment does not reveal a characteristic pattern of cognitive difficulties in patients with somatoform concerns. Despite frequently expressed concerns about cognitive functioning in such patients, neuropsychological evaluations are most useful in identifying patterns of variable or suspect effort and symptom reporting that are associated with somatoform presentations. Elucidation of psychological and personality features is an especially important element of the neuropsychological evaluation as this information can be used to guide patients and referral sources to more productive courses of treatment. The challenging qualities of such patients can lead to quick and dismissive encounters with providers, resulting in the common attribution that their doctors think their problems are "all in their head." A thorough neuropsychological evaluation can serve as a useful intervention that assures a patient that his or her concerns have been extensively assessed and considered. The delineation of what are often multiple comorbid issues is an important part of a process that can lead to an integrated and interdisciplinary approach that is emerging as an evidence-based standard for managing complex patients.

References

Al-Adawi, S., Al-Zakwani, I., Obeid, Y. A., & Zaidan, Z. (2010). Neurocognitive functioning in women presenting with undifferentiated somatoform disorders in Oman. *Psychiatry and Clinical Neurosciences*, *64*(5), 555–564. doi: 10.1111/j.1440-1819.2010.02117.x

Ambrose, K. R., Gracely, R. H., Glass, J. M. (2012). Fibromyalgia dyscognition: Concepts and issues. *Reumatismo*, *64*(4), 206–215. doi: 10.4081/reumatismo.2012.206

American Psychiatric Association. (2013). *Diagnostic and Statistical Manual of Mental Disorders* (5th ed., pp. 5–25). Arlington, VA: American Psychiatric Publishing. ISBN 978-0-89042-555-8.

Arbisi, P. A., Sellbom, M., & Ben-Porath, Y. S. (2008). Empirical correlates of the MMPI-2 restructured clinical scales in psychiatric inpatients. *Journal of Personality Assessment*, *90*, 122–128.

Bagayogo, I. P., Interian, A., & Escobar, J. I. (2013). Transcultural aspects of somatic symptoms in the context of depressive disorders. *Advances in Psychosomatic Medicine*, *33*, 64–74. doi: 10.1159/000350057. Epub 2013 Jun 25.

Bay, E., & Covassin, T. (2012). Chronic stress, somatic and depressive symptoms following mild to moderate traumatic brain injury. *Archives of Psychiatric Nursing*, *26*(6), 477–486. doi: 10.1016/j.apnu.2012.06.002

Ben-Porath, Y. S. (2012). *Interpreting the MMPI-2-RF*. Minneapolis, MN: University of Minnesota Press.

Ben-Porath, Y. S., & Tellegen, A. (2011). *MMPI-2-RF (Minnesota Multiphasic Personality Inventory—2 Restructured Form): Manual for Administration, Scoring, and Interpretation*. Minneapolis, MN: University of Minnesota Press. (Original work published 2008).

Binder, L. M. (2005). Forensic assessment of medically unexplained symptoms. In G. J. Larrabee (Ed.), *Forensic Neuropsychology: A Scientific Approach* (pp. 298–333). New York: Oxford University Press.

Binder, L. M., & Campbell, K. A. (2004). Medically unexplained symptoms and neuropsychological assessment. *Journal of Clinical and Experimental Neuropsychology*, *26*(3), 369–392. doi: 10.1080/13803390490510095

Binder, L. M., Kindermann, S. S., Heaton, R. K., & Salinsky, M. C. (1998). Neuropsychologic impairment in patients with nonepileptic seizures. *Archives of Clinical Neuropsychology*, *13*(6), 513–522. doi: 10.1093/arclin/13.6.513

Binder, L. M., Storzbach, D., & Salinsky, M. C. (2006). MMPI-2 profiles of persons with multiple chemical sensitivity. *The Clinical Neuropsychologist*, *20*(4), 848–857. doi: 10.1080/13854040500246927

Brauer Boone, K., & Lu, P. H. (1999). Impact of somatoform symptomatology on credibility of cognitive performance. *The Clinical Neuropsychologist*, *13*(4), 414–419. doi: 10.1076/1385-4046(199911)13:04;1-Y;FT414

Briquet, P. (1859). *Traité de l'Hystérie*. Paris: JB Baillière et Fils.

Brooks, L., Johnson-Greene, D., Lattie, E., & Ference, T. (2012). The relationship between performances on neuropsychological symptom validity testing and the MCMI-III in patients with fibromyalgia. *The Clinical Neuropsychologist*, *26*(5), 816–831. doi: 10.1080/13854046.2012.662999

Butcher, J. N., Dahlstrom, W. G., Graham, J. R., Tellegen, A., & Kaemmer, B. (1989). *The Minnesota Multiphasic Personality Inventory-2 (MMPI-2): Manual for Administration and Scoring*. Minneapolis, MN: University of Minnesota Press.

Dandachi-FitzGerald, B., Ponds, R. W., & Merten, T. (2013). Symptom validity and neuropsychological assessment: A survey of practices and beliefs of neuropsychologists in six European countries. *Archives of Clinical Neuropsychology*, *28*(8), 771–783. doi: 10.1093/arclin/act073

DeLuca, J., Johnson, S. K., & Natelson, B. H. (1993). Information processing efficiency in chronic fatigue syndrome and multiple sclerosis. *Archives of Neurology*, *50*, 301–304.

Drane, D. L., Williamson, D. J., Stroup, E. S., Holmes, M. D., Jung, M., Koerner, E., . . . Miller, J. W. (2006). Cognitive impairment is not equal in patients with epileptic and psychogenic nonepileptic seizures. *Epilepsia*, *47*(11), 1879–1886. doi: 10.1111/j.1528-1167.2006.00611.x

Driver-Dunckley, E., Stonnington, C. M., Locke, D. E., & Noe, K. (2011). Comparison of psychogenic movement disorders and psychogenic nonepileptic seizures: Is phenotype clinically important? *Psychosomatics*, *52*(4), 337–345. doi: 10.1016/j.psym.2011.01.008

Engel, C. C. (2006). Explanatory and pragmatic perspectives regarding idiopathic physical symptoms and related syndromes. *CNS Spectrums*, *11*(3), 225–232.

Finn, S. E., & Kamphuis, J. H. (2006). Therapeutic assessment with the MMPI-2. In J. N. Butcher (Ed.), *MMPI-2: A Practitioner's Guide* (pp. 165–191). Washington, DC: American Psychological Association.

Gass, C. S., & Odland, A. P. (2012). Minnesota multiphasic personality inventory-2 revised form symptom validity scale-revised (MMPI-2-RF FBS-r; also known as fake bad scale): Psychometric characteristics in a nonlitigation neuropsychological setting. *Journal of Clinical and Experimental Neuropsychology*, *34*(6), 561–570. doi: 10.1080/13803395.2012.666228

Gervais, R. O., Ben-Porath, Y. S., Wygant, D. B., & Sellbom, M. (2010). Incremental validity of the MMPI-2-RF over-reporting scales and RBS in assessing the veracity of memory complaints. *Archives of Clinical Neuropsychology*, *25*(4), 274–284. doi: 10.1093/arclin/acq018

Gervais, R. O., Rohling, M. L., Green, P., & Ford, W. (2004). A comparison of WMT, CARB and TOMM failure rates in non-head injury disability claimants. *Archives of Clinical Neuropsychology*, *19*, 475–487. doi: 10.1016/j.acn.2003.05.001

Gervais, R. O., Wygant, D. B., Sellbom, M., & Ben-Porath, Y. S. (2011). Associations between symptom validity test failure and scores on the MMPI-2-RF validity and substantive scales. *Journal of Personality Assessment*, *93*(5), 508–517. doi: 10.1080/00223891.2011.594132

Gorske, T. T., & Smith, S. R. (2009). *Collaborative Therapeutic Neuropsychological Assessment*. New York: Springer.

Graham, J. R. (2012). *MMPI-2: Assessing Personality and Psychopathology* (5th ed.). New York: Oxford University Press.

Grover, S., Aneja, J., Sharma, A., Malhotra, R., Varma, S., Basu, D., & Avasthi, A. (2015). Do the various categories of somatoform disorders differ from each other in symptom profile and psychological correlates? *International Journal of Social Psychiatry*, *61*(2), 148–156.

Heintz, C. E., van Tricht, M. J., van der Salm, S. M., van Rootselaar, A. F., Cath, D., Schmand, B., & Tijssen, M. A. (2013). Neuropsychological profile of psychogenic jerky movement disorders: Importance of evaluating non-credible cognitive performance and psychopathology. *Journal of Neurology, Neurosurgery, and Psychiatry*, *84*(8), 862–867. doi: 10.1136/jnnp-2012-304397

Hilderink, P. H., Benraad, C. E., van Driel, D., Buitelaar, J. K., Speckens, A. E., Olde, Rikkert, M. G., & Voshaar, R. C. (2009). Medically unexplained physical symptoms in elderly people: A pilot study of psychiatric geriatric characteristics. *American Journal of Geriatric Psychiatry*, *17*(12), 1085–1088. doi: 10.1097/JGP.0b013e3181b975a1

Hilderink, P. H., Collard, R., Rosmalen, J. G., & Oude Voshaar, R. C. (2013). Prevalence of somatoform disorders and medically unexplained symptoms in old age populations in comparison with younger age groups: A systematic review. *Ageing Research Reviews*, *12*(1), 151–156. doi: 10.1016/j.arr.2012.04.004

Inamura, K., Tsuno, N., Shinagawa, S., Nagata, T., Tagai, K., & Nakayama, K. (2014). Correlation between cognition and symptomatic severity in patients with late-life somatoform disorders. *Aging & Mental Health*, *29*, 1–6.

Iverson, G. L., & McCracken, L. M. (1997). "Postconcussive" symptoms in persons with chronic pain. *Brain Injury*, *11*(11), 783–790.

Jason, L. A., Richman, J. A., Rademaker, A. W., Jordan, K. M., Plioplys, A. V., Taylor, R. R., . . . Plioplys, S. (1999). A community-based study of chronic fatigue syndrome. *Archives of Internal Medicine*, *159*(18), 2129–2137. doi: 10.1001/archinte.159.18.2129

Johnson-Greene, D., Brooks, L., & Ference, T. (2013). Relationship between performance validity testing, disability status, and somatic complaints in patients with fibromyalgia. *The Clinical Neuropsychologist*, *27*(1), 148–158. doi: 10.1080/13854046.2012.733732

Jones, A., & Ingram, M. V. (2011). A comparison of selected MMPI-2 and MMPI-2-RF validity scales in assessing effort on cognitive tests in a military sample. *The Clinical Neuropsychologist*, *25*(7), 1207–1227. doi: 10.1080/13854046.2011.600726

Jones, A., Ingram, M. V., & Ben-Porath, Y. S. (2012). Scores on the MMPI-2-RF scales as a function of increasing levels of failure on cognitive symptom validity tests in a military sample. *The Clinical Neuropsychologist*, *26*(5), 790–815. doi: 10.1080/13854046.2012.693202

Kemp, S., Coughlan, A. K., Rowbottom, C., Wilkinson, K., Teggart, V., & Baker, G. (2008). The base rate of effort test failure in patients with medically unexplained symptoms. *Journal of Psychosomatic Research*, *65*(4), 319–325. doi: 10.1016/j.jpsychores.2008.02.010

Kleinstäuber, M., Witthöft, M., Steffanowski, A., van Marwijk, H., Hiller, W., & Lambert, M. J. (2014). Pharmacological interventions for somatoform disorders in adults. *Cochrane Database of Systematic Reviews, 11*. Art. No.: CD010628. doi: 10.1002/14651858.CD010628.pub2

Kroenke, K., Spitzer, R. L., & Williams, J. B. (2002). The PHQ-15: Validity of a new measure for evaluating the severity of somatic symptoms. *Psychosomatic Medicine*, *64*(2), 258–266.

Lahmann, C., Henningsen, P., Brandt, T., Strupp, M., Jahn, K., Dieterich, M., . . . Schmid, G. (2015). Psychiatric comorbidity and psychosocial impairment among patients with vertigo and dizziness. *Journal of Neurology, Neurosurgery, & Psychiatry*, *86*(3), 302–308. pii: jnnp-2014-307601. doi: 10.1136/jnnp-2014307601

Lamberty, G. J. (2008). *Understanding Somatization in the Practice of Clinical Neuropsychology*. New York: Oxford University Press.

Lamberty, G. J. (2014). Biopsychosocial approaches to chronic health conditions. In K. Stucky, M. Kirkwood, & J. Donders (Eds.), *Clinical Neuropsychology Study Guide and Board Review* (pp. 576–588). New York: Oxford University Press.

Lamberty, G. J., & Bares, K. (2013). Neuropsychological assessment and management of older adults with multiple somatic symptoms. In L. D. Ravdin & H. L. Katzen (Eds.), *Clinical Handbook on the Neuropsychology of Aging and Dementia* (Vol. 2, pp. 121–134). New York: Springer.

Lamberty, G. J., & Nelson, N. W. (2012). *Specialty Competencies in Clinical Neuropsychology*. New York: Oxford University Press.

Lamberty, G. J., & Sim, A. H. (2014). Somatic symptom disorders. In M. W. Parsons & T. A. Hammeke (Eds.), *Clinical Neuropsychology: A Pocket Handbook for Assessment* (pp. 659–676). Washington, DC: American Psychological Association.

Landrø, N. I., Stiles, T. C., & Sletvold, H. (1997). Memory functioning in patients with primary fibromyalgia and major depression and healthy controls. *Journal of Psychosomatic Research*, *42*(3), 297–306.

Larrabee, G. J. (1998). Somatic malingering on the MMPI and MMPI-2 in personal injury litigants. *The Clinical Neuropsychologist*, *12*, 179–188. doi: 10.1076/clin.12.2.179.2008

Libon, D. J., Schwartzman, R. J., Eppig, J., Wambach, D., Brahin, E., Peterlin, B. L., . . . Kalanuria, A. (2010). Neuropsychological deficits associated with complex regional pain syndrome. *Journal of the International Neuropsychological Society*, *16*(3), 566–573. doi: 10.1017/S1355617710000214. Epub 2010 Mar 19.

Mariman, A., Delesie, L., Tobback, E., Hanoulle, I., Sermijn, E., Vermeir, P., . . . Vogelaers, D. (2013). Undiagnosed and comorbid disorders in patients with presumed chronic fatigue syndrome. *Journal of Psychosomatic Research*, *75*(5), 491–496. doi: 10.1016/j.jpsychores.2013.07.010. Epub 2013 Aug 20.

Mayou, R., Kirmayer, L. J., Simon, G., Kroenke, K., Sharpe, M. (2005). Somatoform disorders: Time for a new approach in DSM-V. *American Journal of Psychiatry*, *162*(5), 847–855.

Merckelbach, H., Jelicic, M., & Pieters, M. (2011). The residual effect of feigning: How intentional faking may evolve into a less conscious form of symptom reporting. *Journal of Clinical and Experimental Neuropsychology*, *33*(1), 131–139. doi: 10.1080/13803395.2010.495055

Mittenberg, W., Patton, C., Canyock, E. M., & Condit, D. C. (2002). Base rates of malingering and symptom exaggeration. *Journal of Clinical and Experimental Neuropsychology*, *24*, 1092–1102. doi: 10.1076/jcen.24.8.1094.8379

Noyes, R. R., Stuart, S., & Watson, D. (2008). A reconceptualization of the somatoform disorders. *Psychosomatics*, *49*, 14–22.

Onofrj, M., Bonanni, L., Manzoli, L., & Thomas, A. (2010). Cohort study on somatoform disorders in Parkinson disease and dementia with Lewy bodies. *Neurology*, *74*(20), 1598–1606. doi: 10.1212/WNL.0b013e3181df09dd

Roberson, C. J., Boone, K. B., Goldberg, H., Miora, D., Cottingham, M., Victor, T., . . . Wright, M. (2013). Cross validation of the b test in a large known groups sample. *The Clinical Neuropsychologist*, *27*(3), 495–508. doi: 10.1080/13854046.2012.737027

Röhricht, F., & Elanjithara, T. (2014). Management of medically unexplained symptoms: Outcomes of a specialty liason clinic. *Psychiatric Bulletin*, *38*(3), 102–107.

Rollnick, S., Miller, W. R., & Butler, C. C. (2008). *Motivational Interviewing in Health Care: Helping Patients Change Behavior*. New York: Guilford.

Schmid, G., Dinkel, A., Henningsen, P., Dieterich, M., Hopfner, A., Pieh, C., & Lahmann, C. (2014). Assessment of psychological aspects of somatoform disorders: A study on the German version of the Health Attitude Survey (HAS). *Comprehensive Psychiatry*, *55*(1), 155–164. doi: 10.1016/j.comppsych.2013.08.013

Sellbom, M., Wygant, D., & Bagby, M. (2012). Utility of the MMPI-2-RF in detecting non-credible somatic complaints. *Psychiatry Research*, *197*(3), 295–301. doi: 10.1016/j.psychres.2011.12.043

Simms, L. J., Casillas, A., Clark, L. A., Watson, D., & Doebbeling, B. N. (2005). Psychometric evaluation of the restructured clinical scales of the MMPI-2. *Psychological Assessment*, *17*(3), 345–358.

Sjøgren, P., Christrup, L. L., Petersen, M. A., & Højsted, J. (2005). Neuropsychological assessment of chronic non-malignant pain patients treated in a multidisciplinary pain centre. *European Journal of Pain*, *9*(4), 453–462. Epub 2004 Nov 5.

Staudenmayer, H., & Phillips, S. (2008). MMPI-2 validity, clinical and content scales, and the fake bad scale for personal injury litigants claiming idiopathic environmental intolerance. *Journal of Psychosomatic Research*, *62*, 61–72. doi: 10.1016/j.jpsychores.2006.01.013

Stonnington, C. M., Locke, D. E., Hsu, C. H., Ritenbaugh, C., & Lane, R. D. (2013). Somatization is associated with deficits in affective theory of mind. *Journal of Psychosomatic Research*, *74*(6), 479–485. doi: 10.1016/j.jpsychores.2013.04.004

Suhr, J. A. (2003). Neuropsychological impairment in fibromyalgia: Relation to depression, fatigue, and pain. *Journal of Psychosomatic Research*, *55*(4), 321–329. doi: 10.1016/S0022-3999(02)00628-1

Suhr, J. A., & Spickard, B. (2007). Including measures of effort in neuropsychological assessment of pain-and fatigue-related medical disorders. In K. B. Boone (Ed.), *Assessment of Feigned Cognitive Impairment: A Neuropsychological Perspective* (pp. 259–280). New York: Guilford Press.

Sweet, J., Giuffre Meyer, D., Nelson, N., & Moberg, P. (2011). The TCN/AACN "salary survey": Professional practices, beliefs, and incomes of U.S. neuropsychologists. *The Clinical Neuropsychologist*, *25*, 12–61.

Thomas, M. L., & Locke, D. E. (2010). Psychometric properties of the MMPI-2-RF somatic complaints (RC1) scale. *Psychological Assessment*, *22*(3), 492–503. doi: 10.1037/a0019229

Tominaga, T., Choi, H., Nagoshi, Y., Wada, Y., & Fukui, K. (2014). Relationship between alexithymia and coping strategies in patients with somatoform disorder. *Neuropsychiatric Disease and Treatment*, *10*, 55–62. doi: 10.2147/NDT.S55956

van Dessel, N., den Boeft, M., van der Wouden, J. C., Kleinstäuber, M., Leone, S. S., Terluin, B., Numans, M. E., van der Horst, H. E., vanMarwijk, H. (2014). Non-pharmacological interventions for somatoform disorders and medically unexplained physical symptoms (MUPS) in adults. *Cochrane Database of Systematic Reviews*, *11*. Art. No.: CD011142. doi: 10.1002/14651858.CD011142.pub2

Voigt, K., Nagel, A., Meyer, B., Langs, G., Braukhaus, C., & Löwe, B. J. (2010). Towards positive diagnostic criteria: A systematic review of somatoform disorder diagnoses and suggestions for future classification. *Journal of Psychosomatic Research*, *68*(5), 403–414. doi: 10.1016/j.jpsychores.2010.01.015. Epub 2010 Mar 12

Walker, E. A., Keegan, D., Gardner, G., Sullivan, M., Katon, W. J., & Bernstein, D. (1997). Psychosocial factors in fibromyalgia compared with rheumatoid arthritis: I. Psychiatric diagnoses and functional disability. *Psychosomatic Medicine*, *59*(6), 565–571. doi: 10.1097/00006842-199711000-00002

Wilson, R. S., Arnold, S. E., Schneider, J. A., Li, Y., & Bennett, D. A. (2007). Chronic distress, age-related neuropathology, and late-life dementia. *Psychosomatic Medicine*, *69*(1), 47–53. doi: 10.1097/01.psy.0000250264.25017.21

Wingenfeld, K., Terfehr, K., Meyer, B., Löwe, B., & Spitzer, C. (2013). Memory bias for emotional and illness-related words in patients with depression, anxiety and somatization disorders: An investigation with the directed forgetting task. *Psychopathology*, *46*(1), 22–27. doi: 10.1159/000338609

Yalcin, I., & Barrot, M. (2014). The anxiodepressive comorbidity in chronic pain. *Current Opinion in Anaesthesiology*, *27*(5), 520–527. doi: 10.1097/ACO.0000000000000116. PubMed PMID: 25188218.

Youngjohn, J. R., Wershba, R., Stevenson, M., Sturgeon, J., & Thomas, M. L. (2011). Independent validation of the MMPI-2-RF somatic/cognitive and validity scales in TBI litigants tested for effort. *The Clinical Neuropsychologist*, *25*(3), 463–476. doi: 10.1080/13854046.2010.550635

Part III

Forensic, Ethical, and Practice Issues

36 Forensic Neuropsychology

An Overview of Issues, Admissibility, and Directions

Jerry J. Sweet, Paul M. Kaufmann, Eric Ecklund-Johnson, and Aaron C. Malina

Introduction

Professional surveys show that involvement in forensic activities has become a common part of professional practice for clinical neuropsychologists (e.g., Sweet, Peck, Abramowitz, & Etzweiler, 2003). For example, a survey by Sweet, Moberg, and Suchy (2000) found that attorneys are the number one referral source for private practice neuropsychologists, who now represent the majority of the field. As a specialty practice of psychology, clinical neuropsychology applies unique methods and legally protected test materials (Kaufmann, 2009) in conjunction with the brain-behavior knowledge base to evaluate, diagnose, and treat individuals with known or suspected neurological disease and/or injury (Kaufmann, 2012). Lawyers increasingly seek consultation with neuropsychologist experts on an expanding set of legal issues, in part, because neuropsychologists apply scientific approaches that meet judicial standards for expert testimony (Larrabee, 2012).

Forensic neuropsychology has also become prominent within the neuropsychological literature and at relevant professional meetings. More specifically, examination of publication content within the most important clinical neuropsychology journals from 1990 through 2000 has demonstrated that forensic neuropsychology is a common topic within journal articles and at professional meetings (Sweet, King, Malina, Bergman, & Simmons, 2002), accounting for up to 16% of journal content and 11% of conference presentations. Thus, because of its increasing prominence, presumably associated with increasing influence, it is appropriate within this comprehensive handbook on the practice of clinical neuropsychology to consider important issues and directions of forensic neuropsychology. The present chapter will describe the historical background, major activities, key issues, admissibility challenges, and future directions of forensic neuropsychology.

For the purposes of the present chapter, we will consider *forensic neuropsychology* to include all neuropsychological practice in which a clinician provides evaluation or consultative services to an individual involved in a proceeding that is potentially *adversarial* in nature. Adversarial proceedings are those that involve two or more interested parties who must reach a resolution of a common concern or disagreement from potentially antagonistic positions. Adversarial proceedings may be either *formal*, often taking place in a courtroom and involving criminal, civil (including personal injury and medical malpractice), or family (including divorce and child custody) law, or *informal*, often involving administrative matters, such as disability determination, fitness for duty, and due process educational hearings. Greiffenstein and Kaufmann (2012) note the criminal, civil, administrative, probate, and alternative dispute resolution settings in which neuropsychologists are commonly asked to consult. In all these proceedings, the offering of specialty knowledge by the clinical neuropsychologist is to inform a "trier of fact" or a less-formal process regarding an individual who is designated a *litigant*, if involved in formal court proceedings, or as a *claimant*, if involved in less formal proceedings (e.g., seeking disability status or seeking special considerations in an educational system). As such, a forensic opinion occurs within a context that can be distinguished from the normal clinical routine in which a health care service is provided to a "patient" who is seeking treatment for a malady. Stated differently, forensic services are viewed as outside routine health care, which explains why these services are not reimbursed under health insurance benefits.

Historical Background

As noted earlier, there is strong evidence from professional surveys that involvement in forensic neuropsychology has increased substantially over time, such that it is a common part of practice for most clinical neuropsychologists and a major portion of practice for some. The growth of forensic consulting in neuropsychology is well documented (Sweet et. al., 2002; Heilbronner, 2004; Kaufmann, 2009), including pediatric populations (Sherman & Brooks, 2012). Braun et al. (2011) noted a 6% average rate of annual growth in Lexis cases referencing neuropsychology from 2005 to 2009, and an unprecedented 20% increase in 2010. Kaufmann has closely tracked these trends for the past decade, most recently showing how neuropsychology is outpacing every related area of brain-behavior expertise (Kaufmann & Greiffenstein, 2013). Recently, Kaufmann (2016) noted a 97% increase in time devoted to forensic consulting over the past decade when comparing professional practice survey data

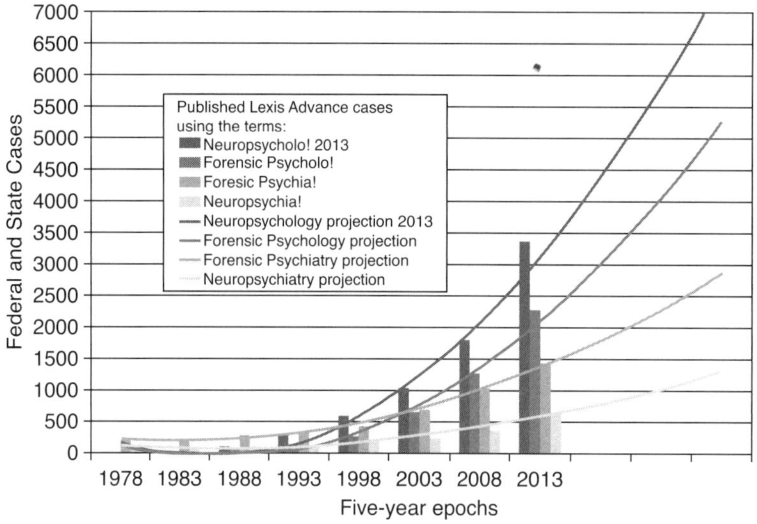

Figure 36.1 Number of U.S. federal and state cases using the root terms *Neuropsycholo!*, *Forensic Psycholo!*, *Forensic Psychia!*, and *Neuropsychia!* in five-year epochs for the past 35 years, used as a basis for polynomial regression projections for the next 15 years. These frequency counts represent the "tip of the iceberg" because the Lexis Advance database includes only appellate cases and narrowly selected trials introducing novel legal concepts. The interested reader may review the first references to these disciplines in published legal cases. See *Smith v. Metropolitan Life Ins., Co.* (1943) for neuropsychology, *Hovey v. Hobson* (1867) for forensic psychology, *State v. Knight* (1901) for forensic psychiatry, and *Hines v. Welch* (1928) for neuropsychiatry.

from Sweet and his colleagues (2006, 2011, and 2015). Figure 36.1 shows a steady upward trend in forensic consulting for neuropsychologists.

It is likely that these historical data pertaining to formal litigation proceedings are paralleled by equally impressive growth in separate informal adversarial proceedings, such as disability determination and due process educational hearings.

An interesting question is, what caused this impressive practice growth? In the sections immediately following, we explore possible causative factors.

Health Care Advances and Resulting Societal Change

In discussing reasons for the growth of forensic neuropsychology, Taylor (1999) offered five factors that were deemed significant in explaining the emergence of neuropsychologists as litigation experts. These factors were (a) an increasing traumatic brain injury (TBI) population, (b) development of advocacy organizations, (c) advent of *neurolaw* (Taylor's approach to proceedings involving neurological injury), (d) increasing supply of neuropsychologists, and (e) response of the legal system. In Taylor's view, increased TBI survival rates stem directly from medical advances, which in turn impact society and result in items (a) through (c). Common causes of TBI include vehicular accidents and accidents in the workplace, which are often associated with subsequent litigation. Whereas if TBI results in death, neuropsychologists are an unlikely expert witness, TBI survivors can have cognitive, emotional, and behavioral changes that are best assessed by neuropsychologists, who therefore become key witnesses in resulting litigation. Thus, a sizeable TBI survivor cohort leads to development of advocacy groups, such as the Brain Injury Association of America, which in turn leads to greater consciousness raising among the general public and politicians, and greater allocation of societal resources, such as resources for rehabilitation and residential living. Lawyers develop greater interest in the unique aspects of brain injury as pertains to litigation and increasingly need relevant expert witnesses. Demand for clinical neuropsychologists arises then out of both the clinical need and the litigation need to deal expertly with TBI survivors. These factors influence one another in a positive and synergistic fashion. As clinical neuropsychologists played a greater clinical role in dealing with TBI survivors, such that physicians and other health care providers relied upon them to assist in evaluating and treating TBI patients, ultimately, the court system acknowledged their role in the courtroom by promulgating common law (i.e., the rulings of judges) and statutory law that facilitate their involvement. As Taylor (1999) notes, "the law encourages that which it permits" (p. 424).

Health Care Market Forces

In the same interval of time in which forensic neuropsychology has grown substantially, health care reimbursement models changed meaningfully. The era of *managed care* in U.S. health care greatly changed the means and amounts of reimbursements for routine clinical services, including those of clinical neuropsychologists. Instead of indemnity insurance, managed care became a dominant force in U.S. health care. In a 2000 national survey of clinical neuropsychologists, managed care was identified as the number one reimbursement source for clinical services (Sweet et al., 2003). In response to the increased paperwork and reduced reimbursement associated with managed care, many U.S. clinicians, including neuropsychologists, pursued *self-pay* opportunities. Self-pay refers to non-insurance-based reimbursement, which of course includes forensic activities, which, as unrelated to health services, do not rely upon insurance. At this point, although varying greatly from one individual to another, forensic activities constitute a sizeable source of income to the field in general (cf. Sweet et al., 2000, 2003), to the point that some private practices are entirely based on forensic consultations.

Scientist-Practitioner Model

Based on the previous discussion of factors that may explain the growth of forensic neuropsychology, it already seems likely that multiple factors are involved. Sweet (1999a) has argued that a predominant factor in this growth is the scientist-practitioner conceptual foundation of the field. This viewpoint suggests that the well-recognized scientist-practitioner model (cf. Barlow, Hayes, & Nelson, 1984), which was originally developed to conceptualize the training of clinical psychologists and their subsequent idealized clinical practice methods, has resulted in neuropsychologist subspecialists being attractive and valuable experts for adversarial proceedings. Specifically, Sweet opines that among the "relevant by-products of a scientist-practitioner approach are: familiarity with disciplined scrutiny (i.e., peer review), clinical procedures emphasizing data-based decision-making (i.e., accountability), and comfort with hypothesis-testing (i.e., objective differential diagnosis)" (Sweet, 1999a, p. xviii).

As Lees-Haley and Cohen (1999) have noted, the fundamental contributions of experts, including neuropsychologists, to forensic adversarial proceedings are embodied in being a *scientific expert*. The empirical foundation, ability to entertain reasonable alternative hypotheses, ability to acknowledge limitations of method and research literature, and also to be open to reasoned criticism, among other characteristics, are the hallmarks of both a good scientist and a good expert witness. That clinical neuropsychology is rooted in science appears salient in making practitioners in the field attractive to triers-of-fact. It may well be that this scientific foundation in describing cognition, behavior, and emotion provides the essential attractive feature to attorneys, which when coupled with societal and health care changes that provided motivation for individual practitioners, explain the growth of forensic neuropsychology in the last two decades.

Judicial Standards for Admissibility

Although forensic consulting in neuropsychology began in the 1970s, Figure 36.1 shows that the rapid growth in preference for neuropsychologist experts did not appear in published legal cases until the early 1990s. Coincidentally, the U.S. Supreme Court handed down its landmark ruling in *Daubert v. Merrell Dow Pharm., Inc.* (1993) that changed the admissibility standards for expert witnesses. Even as some feared that *Daubert* might be used to exclude psychologist experts, the nonexclusive factors suggested by the Court have been favorable for neuropsychologist experts and likely contributed to increased utilization. Psychologists evaluate clinical impressions from an interview, behavioral observations, and informal assessment, with the added benefit of comparing the individual's test performance to norms. Indeed, it is the integration of divergent sources of information with test findings that draws upon the unique skills of professional psychologists. The competent practice of modern neuropsychology requires current understanding and reasonable fluency in the behavioral and cognitive neurosciences. This brain-behavior knowledge base from the neurosciences, used in conjunction with standardized psychometric tests, neuroimaging results, neurodiagnostic findings, neurologic history, interviewing, behavioral observations, and informal assessment means that neuropsychological formulations and expert opinions are scientifically informed and refined by objective test results. These techniques easily fulfill state and federal legal standards for scientific methodology because psychological tests and neurodiagnostic techniques are widely accepted and, more importantly, experimentally verified. Kaufmann (2005) argued this practice distinguishes clinical neuropsychology in forensic settings, such that it has little or no redundancy with other health care disciplines or mental health expertise. Neuropsychologist experts who conduct evaluations using standardized, reliable, valid, and norm-referenced psychological tests with technical manuals easily fulfill *Daubert's* nonexclusive evidentiary standards.

Assessment of Response Bias, Effort, and Malingering

The publication of Faust and Ziskin's (1988: 33) blistering critique that experts in psychology and psychiatry "will most likely move the jury further from the truth, not closer to it," highlighted the questionable methods used by mental health experts and set off alarm bells among consulting neuropsychologists. There were predictable rebuttals offered to the methods skeptics (Matarazzo, 1990; Barth, Ryan, & Hawk, 1991) and obligatory surrebuttals (Faust, 1991; Faust, Ziskin, & Hiers, 1991; Matarazzo, 1991). However, when methods skeptics suggested that "MMPI indices for malingering may sometimes aid the court" (Faust & Ziskin, 1988: 34) neuropsychologists took the criticisms seriously and began devising new methods to improve the relevance and reliability of expert options. Shortly thereafter, the Minnesota Multiphasic Personality Inventory (MMPI) "fake bad" scale was introduced (Lees-Haley, English, & Glenn, 1991). The last two decades have witnessed an unprecedented effort by the neuropsychology community to develop and implement symptom validity and performance validity techniques to detect response bias, suboptimal effort, and malingering (Slick, Sherman, & Iverson, 1999; Bianchini, Greve, & Glynn, 2005), culminating in the American Academy of Clinical Neuropsychology (AACN) Consensus Conference statement (Heilbronner et al., 2009). In the 1980s, neuropsychologists were trained to give mild TBI patients the benefit of the doubt; but now they apply symptom and performance validity techniques, and work to reduce doubt. The increasingly successful neuropsychological methods for detecting malingering have captured the attention of the judiciary and contributed substantially to the preference for forensic neuropsychologist consultants in court.

Key Issues in Forensic Neuropsychology

There are a number of important issues that relate to the practice of clinical neuropsychology within a forensic context. Many of these issues relate to the interface between the field of neuropsychology and the legal profession. Differences exist between the two disciplines in their underlying philosophies and expectations, and it is important that neuropsychologists understand how these differences are likely to affect their interactions with the legal system.

Empirical Bases for Conclusions Based on Neuropsychological Tests

Although empirically grounded practice is important for all neuropsychological activities, issues regarding the scientific bases for conclusions take on particular importance within the forensic context. This is largely because of standards for admissibility of evidence that have been developed to protect the legal system from the influence of "junk science" (i.e., pseudoscientific theories derived from unreliable methods; see Huber, 1991). While clinical neuropsychology enjoys a firm grounding in empirical research, issues remain with respect to the validity of our methods for forensic purposes.

Evidentiary Standards

For many years, the Frye standard (*Frye v. United States*, 1923), which stated that evidence provided by experts must be "generally accepted" within the particular field from which it was derived, was the prevailing standard governing the admissibility of expert testimony (Laing & Fisher, 1997). More recently, several U.S. Supreme Court rulings have addressed the issue of admissibility of expert evidence, beginning with *Daubert v. Merrell Dow Pharm., Inc.* (1993).

Under federal rules, courts must examine expert qualifications to determine the relevance of the expert opinions to the issue in dispute and the reliability of the bases for those opinions, before those opinions are admitted into evidence and heard by a jury. Judges must decide whether special experience is required to develop expert opinions that will assist the jury in resolving an issue in the case at bar.[1] Therefore, consulting neuropsychologists should understand the court standards for evaluating expert qualifications and the admissibility of testimony as addressed in FED. R. EVID. 104 Preliminary Questions and FED. R. EVID. 403 Relevance. Then, experts should understand how jurisdictions use *Frye*, *Daubert* and its progeny, and FED. R. EVID. 702 Testimony of Experts to make final determinations.

Although state Rules of Evidence vary somewhat, the legal basis for judicial review of expert methodology and testimony begins with FED. R. EVID. 104 (a) Preliminary Questions of Admissibility, and (b) Relevancy Conditioned on Fact, as follows:

- **a** The court must decide any preliminary question about whether a witness is qualified, a privilege exists, or evidence is admissible. In so deciding, the court is not bound by evidence rules, except those on privilege.
- **b** "When the relevance of evidence depends on whether a fact exists, proof must be introduced sufficient to support a finding that the fact does exist. The court may admit the proposed evidence on the condition that the proof be introduced later."

Some courts refer generically to Rule 104 hearings when hearing *Daubert* or *Frye* challenges to expert testimony. Rule 104(b) refers to FED. R. EVID. 403, as follows:

> Although relevant, evidence may be excluded if its probative value is substantially outweighed by the danger of unfair prejudice, confusion of the issues, or misleading the jury, or by considerations of undue delay, waste of time, or needless presentation of cumulative evidence.
>
> (Fed. R. Evid. 403)

These federal rules (and state equivalents) set the stage for challenging expert testimony. However, not all state courts have adopted the *Daubert* framework, and a few still rely on *Frye*.[2]

The second-degree murder conviction in *Frye* was appealed, claiming the trial court erred when it excluded expert testimony on a "systolic blood pressure deception test" (*Frye v. United States,* 1923: 1013). Defense efforts to conduct the test in the court and admit expert opinions were denied. The *Frye* court affirmed the trial judge and created the following rule by quoting from the government's brief:

> when the question involved does not lie within the range of common experience or common knowledge, but requires

> special experience or special knowledge, then the opinions of witnesses skilled in that particular science, art, or trade to which the question relates are admissible in evidence.
>
> (*Frye v. United States,* 1923: 1014)

In a two-page unanimous opinion, the appellate court found that the deception test did not have "standing and scientific recognition among physiological and psychological authorities as would justify the courts in admitting expert testimony" (*Frye v. United States,* 1923: 1014). Essentially, the test was not admitted because it was not *generally accepted* in the relevant scientific community. *Frye* was the law governing experts for the next 70 years, and it is still used today to exclude evidence that is not generally accepted in the scientific community (e.g., restricting behavioral genetics evidence in federal and *habeas corpus* review; *Cullen v. Pinholster*, 2011).

In *Daubert v. Merrell Dow Pharm., Inc.* (1989), infants and guardians sued to recover for limb reduction birth defects caused by ingestion of the anti-nausea "morning sickness" drug Bendectin during pregnancy. Merrell Dow won on summary judgment[3] under *Frye* with the trial judge noting the "prevailing school of thought" (*Daubert v. Merrell Dow Pharm., Inc.,* 1989: 572) about Bendectin and legal authority that epidemiological studies are the most reliable causation evidence in this field of study. The plaintiffs failed to present "statistically significant epidemiological proof that Bendectin causes limb reduction defects" because their expert relied, in part, on in vitro animal and chemical studies (*Daubert v. Merrell Dow Pharm., Inc.,* 1989: 575). The plaintiffs appealed, arguing the trial court erred when excluding the scientific studies and reanalysis of the epidemiological data by their experts. The three-judge Ninth Circuit Appellate Court unanimously affirmed the trial court, *Daubert v. Merrell Dow Pharm., Inc.* (1992), citing *Frye* and following the precedent, referencing

> a well-founded skepticism of the scientific value of the reanalysis methodology employed by plaintiffs' experts; they recognize that "[t]he best test of certainty we have is good science—the science of publication, replication, and verification, the science of consensus and peer review." P. Huber, Galileo's Revenge: Junk Science in the Courtroom 228 (1991).
>
> (*Daubert v. Merrell Dow Pharm., Inc.,* 1989: 1131)

The Ninth Circuit suggested in vitro studies were junk science, affirming the trial court decision to ignore this new scientific evidence because it failed *Frye's* general acceptance test. The plaintiffs appealed and the U.S. Supreme Court granted *Certiorari*.[4]

In a landmark decision regarding expert testimony, the U.S. Supreme Court held that Fed. R. Evid. 702 superseded *Frye's* general acceptance test, thereby requiring all federal courts to admit any "scientific, technical, or other specialized knowledge" that assists the trier of fact to understand the evidence (*Daubert v. Merrell Dow Pharm., Inc.,* 1989: 580). "General acceptance" was no longer required to admit scientific evidence in federal court. A 7–2 majority also found that District Court judges (gatekeepers) must evaluate the admissibility of expert testimony, although Honorable Chief Justice William Rehnquist disagreed on the trial judge's role, writing

> I do not doubt that Rule 702 confides to the judge some gatekeeping responsibility in deciding questions of the admissibility of proffered expert testimony. But I do not think it imposes on them either the obligation or the authority to become amateur scientists in order to perform that role.
>
> (*Daubert v. Merrell Dow Pharm., Inc.,* 1989: 600–601)

Chief Justice Rehnquist was "at a loss" in understanding what "falsifiability" meant when applied to a scientific theory and he predicted other federal judges would too. Nevertheless, the Ninth Circuit decision was reversed and remanded for further proceedings.

For efficient justice, the Ninth Circuit conducted the "brave new world" of *Daubert* analysis of Fed. R. Evid. 702, framing the question as follows: "How do we figure out whether scientists have derived their findings through the scientific method or whether their testimony is based on scientifically valid principles?" (*Daubert v. Merrell Dow Pharm., Inc.,* 1989: 1316). A unanimous Ninth Circuit affirmed the original summary judgment under Rule 702 and *Daubert* because the plaintiff presented only experts' qualifications, their conclusions, and their assurances of reliability. *Daubert* plaintiffs received due process, equal protection, and justice, but no compensation, because the expert scientific evidence failed to show, with a preponderance of the evidence, that Bendectin caused the birth defects.

Two subsequent U.S. Supreme Court cases, *General Electric Co. v. Joiner* (1997) and *Kumho Tire Co. v. Carmichael* (1999), refined *Daubert* and extended its holding. In *Joiner*, a city electrician with lung cancer brought suit against the manufacturer of polychlorinated biphenyls (PCBs) and the manufacturers of electrical transformers and dielectric fluid, alleging his exposure to these materials caused his cancer. Joiner relied on an expert to prove his case. The District Court judge excluded the expert testimony, finding it "subjective belief or unsupported speculation" (*General Electric Co. v. Joiner*,1997: 140) and Joiner appealed. Under a stringent standard of review, the 11th Circuit Appellate Court reversed the trial court, finding the judge erred in excluding the expert testimony. The U.S. Supreme Court reversed the 11th Circuit, thereby affirming and strengthening the gatekeeping function of the trial court, and directing appellate courts not to review admissibility of expert opinions unless the trial judge committed a clear abuse of discretion. Basically, appellate courts were ordered to show great deference to the gatekeeping judges in District Courts and to not disturb the decisions of the trial judge regarding the admissibility of expert testimony absent gross error.

In *Kumho Tire*, a vehicle overturned when a right rear tire blew out, killing one passenger and injuring others. The plaintiffs sought to admit a tire analyst's visual and tactile tire inspection testimony, under the theory that the absence of at least two of four specific physical indicators meant a tire defect caused failure. The defendant moved to exclude the tire analyst testimony, claiming the methodology failed Fed. R. Evid. 702 requirements. The trial court applied *Daubert* and the judge excluded the tire analyst after finding the methodology employed was insufficiently reliable. Carmichael appealed. The 11th Circuit held that the trial court erred in applying *Daubert*, believing that it only applied to scientific testimony. The U.S. Supreme Court reversed the 11th Circuit and clarified that *Daubert* factors apply to the testimony of engineers and other experts who are not scientists. Experts may also be evaluated and admitted to testify based on skill, experience, and other specialized knowledge, not only scientific knowledge. Even after broadening the criteria, the tire expert opinion was excluded.

In 2002, the U.S. Supreme Court holdings from the *Daubert* "trilogy" were codified into an amendment to Rule 702 governing expert testimony. Rule 702 reads as follows:

> If scientific, technical, or other specialized knowledge will assist the trier of fact to understand the evidence or to determine a fact in issue, a witness qualified as an expert by knowledge, skill, experience, training, or education, may testify thereto in the form of an opinion or otherwise, if (1) the testimony is based upon sufficient facts or data, (2) the testimony is the product of reliable principles and methods, and (3) the witness has applied the principles and methods reliably to the facts of the case.
>
> (Fed. R. Evid. 702)

In summary, *Daubert* incorporated the *Frye* "general acceptance" test and added other factors that federal court gatekeepers may consider when evaluating expert testimony. After general acceptance within the relevant scientific community, *Daubert* also encouraged judges to consider whether the methodology employed by the expert was subject to peer review, testable (falsifiable), and had a known error rate. Generally, psychologist experts have fared well under *Daubert* because standardized methods supported by data in a technical manual are favored. However, these factors are neither exhaustive nor exclusive, and subsequent federal courts have departed from the original *Daubert* list to consider more factors, such as

- Whether experts are proposing to testify about matters growing naturally and directly out of research they have conducted independent of the litigation, or whether they have developed their opinions expressly for purposes of testifying. *Daubert v. Merrell Dow Pharm., Inc.* (1995).
- Whether the expert has unjustifiably extrapolated from an accepted premise to an unfounded conclusion. *General Elec. Co. v. Joiner* (1997).
- Whether the expert has adequately accounted for obvious alternative explanations. *Claar v. Burlington N.R.R.* (1994).
- Whether the expert "is being as careful as he would be in his regular professional work outside his paid litigation consulting." *Sheehan v. Daily Racing Form, Inc.* (1997).
- Whether the field of expertise claimed by the expert is known to reach reliable results for the type of opinion the expert would give. *Kumho Tire Co. v. Carmichael* (1999).

Daubert clearly provides the court greater flexibility in its analysis of new science and although it offers courts greater protection against junk science, it also places a greater burden on trial court judges. Chief Justice Rehnquist described that burden when noting the "amateur scientist" role implicit in the gatekeeping function. Nevertheless, *Daubert* flexibility is considered to have liberated courts to seek relevant and reliable expert opinions to assist the trier of fact. With each passing year, more jurisdictions adopt its basic framework, while restricting or completely abandoning *Frye*.

Early legal experts believed that *Daubert* would tighten the evidentiary standards for admissibility (Dixon & Gill, 2002; Grove & Barden, 1999), and there has been some empirical evidence to suggest that it has had or is beginning to have the desired effect (Dixon & Gill, 2002; Johnson, Krafka, & Cecil, 2000; Krafka, Dunn, Treadway Johnson, Cecil, & Miletich, 2002). For instance, Dixon and Gill (2002) found that the proportion of cases in which the reliability of expert evidence from various types of experts was challenged, including health care/medicine and social/behavioral science, appears to have increased significantly since the *Daubert* ruling to 62% and 84%, respectively during the most recent period examined, which was July 1997 to June 1999, as compared to 23% and 56% during the period immediately prior to *Daubert*, which was July 1989 to June 1993. Furthermore, Dixon and Gill (2002) found that the proportion of *successful* challenges to social and behavioral science evidence also increased significantly during the same time period, from 8% of cases challenged between July 1989 and June 1993 to 47% between July 1997 and June 1999 (although the period of July 1989 to June 1993 appears to be somewhat of a statistical outlier, as 43% of challenges were successful during the decade of the 1980s). Interestingly, the proportion and success rate of challenges to physical science evidence were highest relative to all other types of evidence (health care/medicine, engineering/technology, social/behavioral science, and business/law/public administration) during most of the time periods examined by Dixon and Gill (2002). In spite of these apparent changes, it appears that the *Daubert* standard may not be applied consistently to behavioral science evidence (Shuman & Sales, 1999; Tenopyr, 1999), and that judges in many jurisdictions may continue to rely primarily on the *Frye* standard (Krafka et al., 2002). Furthermore, individual judges and attorneys vary considerably in their level of sophistication in dealing with issues of admissibility and their knowledge of scientific methods. These issues highlight what might appear to be a confusing state of affairs confronting the neuropsychological expert witness. A table of admissibility decisions that pertain to *Daubert* and related federal and state standards involving neuropsychological testimony, taken from the Daubert Tracker online database (MDEX Online, 2017), have been included, and provide some idea of the challenges facing neuropsychologists who serve as expert witnesses (see Table 36.1).

Table 36.1 Results of Daubert and other related evidentiary challenges to testimony of neuropsychologists

Case	*Year*	*Court*	*Plaintiff/ Defense*	*Outcome*	*Reason for Challenge*	*Other expert testimony admitted/denied*
Hutchison v. American Family Mutual Insurance Co.	1994	Iowa, Supreme Court	Defense	Testimony admitted	Neuropsychologist not qualified to testify regarding causation	Neuropsychologist was only expert challenged
Maritime Overseas Corp. v. Ellis	1994[a]	Texas, Court of Appeals	Defense	Testimony admitted in two separate hearings	Admissibility not an issue, but Daubert cited in dissenting opinion	Medical and other psychological testimony also admitted
Goewey v. United States	1995/ 1997[a]	South Carolina/ 4th Circuit	Plaintiff	Testimony denied	Neuropsychologist unable to make clear causal link	Medical and scientific testimony also denied
Hose v. Chicago Northwestern Transport Co.	1995	8th Circuit	Plaintiff	Testimony admitted	Neuropsychologist not qualified to determine medical causation	Medical testimony also admitted
Summers v. Missouri Pacific Railroad System	1995/ 1997[a]	Oklahoma Eastern District/ 10th Circuit	Plaintiff	Testimony denied	Neuropsychologist not expert in medicine or toxicology	Medical testimony also denied
Sanderson v. International Flavors & Fragrances	1996	California, Central District	Plaintiff	Testimony denied	Neuropsychologist unable to make clear causal link	Medical and scientific testimony also denied
Valentine v. Pioneer Chlor Alkali Co.	1996	Nevada	Plaintiff	Testimony denied	Neuropsychologist unable to make clear causal link	Medical testimony also denied
Brafford v. Brafford's Construction Co.	1997	North Carolina, Court of Appeals	Plaintiff	Affirmed lower court ruling to admit testimony	Neuropsychologist inappropriately based opinion on plaintiff's self-report of premorbid function	Neuropsychologist was only expert challenged
Doe v. Provident Life and Accident Insurance Co.	1997	Pennsylvania, Eastern District	Defense	Testimony Admitted	Neuropsychologist not qualified to comment on appropriateness of medical treatment	Neuropsychologist was only expert challenged
Huntoon v. Cablevision	1997	Colorado, Court of Appeals	Plaintiff	Lower court should have excluded testimony	Neuropsychologist not qualified to determine cause of physical injury	Neuropsychologist was only expert challenged
Nations v. State of Texas	1997	Texas, Court of Appeals	Defense	Testimony admitted	Neuropsychologist's testimony based on unreliable methods	Neuropsychologist was only expert challenged
United States v. Gigante	1997[a]	New York, Eastern District	Both	Testimony denied/ later Admitted	Neuropsychologist's testimony speculative	Medical and other psychological testimony initially denied/ admitted in later hearings
Chrissafis v. Continental Airlines	1998	Illinois, Northern District	Defense	Testimony admitted in part	Daubert cited by defense in response to plaintiff attempt to exclude testimony as not relevant	Neuropsychologist was only expert challenged
Louderback v. Orkin Exterminating Co.	1998	Kansas	Plaintiff	Testimony admitted in part	Neuropsychologist not qualified to testify about cause	Scientific testimony also admitted
Johnson Electric Co. v. Wiley	1999	Texas, Court of Appeals	Plaintiff	Testimony admitted	Testimony based on unreliable methods and insufficient to show causation	Neuropsychologist was only expert challenged

(*Continued*)

Table 36.1—Continued

Case	*Year*	*Court*	*Plaintiff/ Defense*	*Outcome*	*Reason for Challenge*	*Other expert testimony admitted/denied*
Miller v. Conrail	1999	Pennsylvania, Eastern District	Defense	Set up a pre-trial voir dire	Neuropsychologist not an expert on Lyme disease	Medical and scientific testimony also subjected to voir dire
United States v. Willis	1999	6th Circuit	Defense	Testimony denied	Testimony not relevant	Neuropsychologist was only expert challenged
Young v. American Reliable Insurance Co.	1999	Louisiana, Eastern District	Defense	Pre-trial hearing to determine whether admissible	Opinion based on unreliable methods	Other professional testimony admitted or admitted in part
Anello v. Shaw Industries	2000	Massachusetts	Plaintiff	Testimony admitted	Opinion based on unreliable methods	Medical and scientific testimony admitted, admitted in part, or denied
Coe v. State of Tennessee	2000	Tennessee, Supreme Court	Court appointed	Testimony admitted	Opinion based on unreliable methods—tests not normed for death row inmates	Neuropsychologist was only expert challenged
Minner v. American Mortgage & Guaranty Co.	2000	Delaware, Superior Court	Both	Testimony admitted in part	Flexible battery approach challenged; neuropsychologist not qualified to testify regarding causation	Medical testimony admitted or admitted in part
In Re: New Orleans train car leakage fire litigation	2000	Louisiana, Court of Appeal	Plaintiff	Testimony admitted	Study of psychological effects of event conducted by expert not submitted to peer review	Medical testimony also admitted
Ruckman v. State of Texas	2000	Texas, Court of Appeals	Plaintiff	Upheld lower court exclusion	Opinion based on unreliable methods	Neuropsychologist was only expert challenged
United States v. Bridges	2000	4th Circuit	Defense	Testimony denied	Testimony not relevant	Neuropsychologist was only expert challenged
Villalba v. Consolidated Freightways Corp.	2000	Illinois, Northern District	Defense	Testimony admitted	Neuropsychologist did not disclose norms on which decisions were based	Neuropsychologist was only expert challenged
Walker v. Conrail	2000	Indiana, Northern District	Plaintiff	Testimony admitted	Neuropsychological test results not sufficient to determine that TBI was sustained	Medical testimony also admitted
Walker v. Soo Line Railroad	2000	7th Circuit	Plaintiff	Testimony Admitted	Opinion based on unreliable methods—relied partially on inaccurate educational history	Medical and scientific testimony also admitted
Bonner v. ISP Techs., Inc.	2001	8th Circuit	Plaintiff	Testimony Admitted	Scientific basis for neuropsychologist's testimony challenged	Scientific testimony also admitted
New Haverford Partnership v. Stroot	2001	Delaware, Supreme Court	Plaintiff	Testimony admitted	Neuropsychologist did not "scientifically eliminate" other possible causes of injury	Medical and scientific testimony also admitted
Sea Robin Pipeline Co. v. Mew Medico Head Clinic Facility	2001	Louisiana, Court of Appeal	Plaintiff	Reversed lower court exclusion	Dissenting opinion suggested expert opinions were speculative and not based on reliable evidence	Medical and other psychological testimony also should not have been excluded
Abron v. Dean Lumber Co.	2002	Texas, Eastern District	Plaintiff	Motion to exclude testimony denied	Neuropsychologist's opinion did not meet Daubert standard	Motion to exclude medical and other expert testimony also denied
Alder v. Bayer Corp.	2002	Utah, Supreme Court	Plaintiff	Reversed lower court exclusion	Opinion regarding cause of injury based on unreliable methods	Medical and scientific testimony also admitted
Allison v. Fire Insurance Exchange	2002	Texas, Court of Appeals	Plaintiff	Upheld lower court exclusion	Neuropsychologist's opinion based on unreliable methods	Medical testimony also denied
Blansett v. BP Exploration & Oil, Inc.	2002	Ohio, Court of Appeals	Both	Testimony admitted	Some of the tests used in forming opinion regarding malingering have been "scientifically discredited"	Medical, other psychological, and scientific testimony also admitted

Case	*Year*	*Court*	*Plaintiff/ Defense*	*Outcome*	*Reason for Challenge*	*Other expert testimony admitted/denied*
Chu v. American Airlines	2002[a]	8th Circuit	Plaintiff	Case settled without ruling on admission	Defendant appealed failure of lower court to submit expert testimony to test of evidentiary standards	Medical, scientific, and other testimony also challenged in prior case, which was dismissed prior to ruling on admissibility
Commonwealth of Massachusetts v. Montanez	2002	Massachusetts, Appeals Court	Defense	Testimony should not have been excluded at original trial	Diagnostic category (dissociative trance disorder) not scientifically reliable	Neuropsychologist was only expert challenged
Floyd v. McGill	2002	North Carolina, Court of Appeals	Plaintiff	Affirmed lower court ruling to admit testimony	Neuropsychologist lacked expertise on biomechanics of closed head injury to determine cause	Medical and other experts also ruled appropriately admitted by lower court
Akers v. United States	2003	Oregon	Plaintiff	Testimony admitted—methods not challenged	Defendant raised question of admissibility, but did not specifically challenge underlying methods	Medical and other experts also admitted
Fini v. General Motors Corp.	2003	Michigan, Court of Appeals	Plaintiff	Testimony admitted	Functional neuroimaging on which expert relied not a reliable means of diagnosing injury	Neuropsychologist was only expert challenged
Grenitz v. Tomlian	2003	Florida, Supreme Court	Plaintiff	Upheld lower court's exclusion	Neuropsychologist not qualified to determine cause of birth defect	Neuropsychologist was only expert challenged
Martinez v. Dretke	2003	Texas, Southern District	Defense	Testimony admitted	Neuropsychologist did not have scientific basis for conclusions and was not qualified at time of initial examination of defendant	Psychological and other experts also admitted
Roberti v. Andy's Termite and Pest Control, Inc.	2003	California, Court of appeals	Plaintiff	Testimony should not have been excluded at original trial—Daubert not applicable under CA law	Methods used in forming opinion not supported by peer-reviewed research	Medical and other experts were also improperly excluded in lower court trial
Taylor v. American Fabritech, Inc.	2004	Texas, Court of Appeals	Plaintiff	Affirmed lower court ruling to admit testimony	Defendant challenged scientific basis for neuropsychologist's conclusions admitted in lower court	Medical and other experts also admitted
Amos v. Keller Transfer Line, Inc.	2005	Michigan, Court of Appeals	Plaintiff	Affirmed lower court ruling to admit testimony	Neuropsychologist formed opinion without obtaining records to establish premorbid function	Neuropsychologist was only expert challenged
Bado-Santana v. Ford Motor Co.	2005	Puerto Rico	Plaintiff	Testimony excluded pending Daubert hearing	Neuropsychologist not qualified to determine causation	Medical experts excluded or partially excluded; scientific and other experts admitted
Hufford v. Harris Corp.	2005	Florida, Middle District	Defense	Testimony admitted	Neuropsychologist who performed an IME did not base opinion on scientific evidence and was biased by virtue of being paid by defendant	Medical and other experts also admitted
Marmo vs. IBP, Inc.	2005	Nebraska	Defense	Testimony moot in part, admitted for certain issues	Neuropsychologist failed to consider possible alternative explanations in reaching opinion	Medical, scientific, and other experts' testimony either admitted or considered moot

(*Continued*)

Table 36.1—Continued

Case	*Year*	*Court*	*Plaintiff/ Defense*	*Outcome*	*Reason for Challenge*	*Other expert testimony admitted/denied*
McCarthy v. Atwood	2005	Virginia, Circuit Court	Defense	Testimony admitted in part (not allowed to comment on cause)	Neuropsychologist not qualified to determine causation	Neuropsychologist was only expert challenged
Blair et al. v. U.S. Steel Corp.	2005	Indiana, Superior Court of Lake County	Plaintiff	Testimony denied	Neuropsychologist's opinion not sufficiently based on reliable factual/scientific principles	Neuropsychologist was only expert challenged
Baxter v. Temple	2005[b]	New Hampshire, Merrimack County Superior Court	Plaintiff	Testimony denied	Boston Process Approach as employed by neuropsychologist deemed unreliable for forensic purposes	Neuropsychologist was only expert challenged

[a] Denotes a case in which multiple evidentiary decisions were rendered (e.g., initial rulings appealed to higher courts).

[b] This case was not yet listed in the *Daubert* Tracker database at the time the other cases were reviewed, but came to the attention of the authors and was included because of its obvious relevance.

Note: Information within this table was used with permission and derived from a proprietary legal database called MDEX Online Daubert Tracker© at www.dauberttracker.com. IME = Independent Medical Examination.

The *Daubert* decision and other similar rulings have caused some concern among neuropsychologists that such standards might lead to the exclusion of neuropsychological tests and expert witnesses. However, Table 36.1 shows that this is not the case, as neuropsychologists do not appear to have fared worse than other experts. It is important to recognize that decisions involving evidentiary standards are case-specific and are influenced by the individual expert, the procedures he or she uses, and the underlying scientific evidence in a particular case. Thus, it is quite possible that a particular expert's testimony might be accepted in one instance and denied in another, depending on whether his or her assertions in each specific case are judged to have a valid scientific basis. Mainstream scientist-practitioner neuropsychologists have never been threatened by the need to provide empirical justification for their work, and should applaud such standards, as they target witnesses from fields without a firm grounding in science.

Since publication of the first edition, two civil cases heard by state supreme courts illustrate the nature of admissibility challenges confronting expert neuropsychologists under *Daubert*. The first case showed how neuropsychologist opinions may be wrongfully excluded (*Baxter v. Temple*, 2008); the second suggested that expert opinions about brain-behavior relations may be wrongfully admitted (*Bennett v. Richmond*, 2012).

In *Baxter v. Temple* (2005), the defense filed a motion *in limine*[5] to exclude the testimony of Barbara Bruno-Golden, Ed.D. as insufficiently reliable under *Daubert*. During the evidentiary hearing Bruno-Golden described the Boston Process Approach (BPA) she employed in the neuropsychological evaluation of a child exposed allegedly to lead poisoning. The defendants argued successfully that her testimony should be excluded because her BPA methodology is not generally accepted in the appropriate scientific literature, has not been subject to peer review and publication, and has no known or potential error rate. Hearing testimony reveals how a trial judge used *Daubert* factors to exclude expert neuropsychological evidence and how such outcomes may be avoided (Desmond, 2007).

All three neuropsychologists, Bruno-Golden, Sandra Shaheen, and David Faust, testified that the BPA methodology employed was untested (*Baxter v. Temple*, 2005, p. 8). Bruno-Golden added that the BPA she used in this evaluation, "has never been . . . and *cannot be* tested, because it varies from practitioner to practitioner" (p. 9) [*emphasis added*]. In fact, Bruno-Golden testified that she "could not recall if she had ever administered the same test battery" (p. 9) on the thousands of other patients she evaluated during her career. The trial judge ruled that Bruno-Golden's BPA cannot be and was not tested in this case.

The neuropsychologist experts also agreed that the BPA methodology employed was not subjected to peer review, nor described in published articles. Although Bruno-Golden offered a professional position paper supporting the BPA, Faust noted it was not in a peer-reviewed publication. Shaheen noted learned treatises on BPA general acceptance in clinical neuropsychology practice, yet admitted that Bruno-Golden's specific methodology had not been subject to peer review or described in published articles. Finally, Bruno-Golden admitted she had not previously used the methodology employed and it was likely that no other clinician had either. Therefore, the trial judge found the BPA as employed in this case had not been subject to peer review and publication.

The BPA error rate was essentially unknowable and no evidence was offered. Bruno-Golden testified that she disregarded standardized time constraints in order to "test the limits" of the child's performance on selected tests. No experts offered any evidence on the reliability of testing the limits. Faust noted that variations in the standardized instructions interfere with test interpretation and destroy the normative comparisons of the child's performance to like-aged peers, making it impossible to determine an error rate. Faust testified that when Bruno-Golden modified the BPA she created an "idiosyncratic combination, if not hodgepodge of multiple influences" (p. 11). The court detailed some departures from standardized techniques. Faust concluded, the methodology employed was "not scientifically validated . . . founded on guesswork, speculation, and conjecture, which sometimes flies directly in the face of scientific literature" (p. 11). Hence, the judge ruled the methodology employed by Bruno-Golden did not have a known or potential error rate.

The *Baxter* trial court concluded its analysis by distinguishing between appropriate scientific literature for clinical assessment and "a 'forensic' approach to assessing children with lead poisoning" (p. 13). Faust explained how a clinical or forensic referral changes the expert neuropsychologist role. This important distinction between the clinical provider and forensic examiner has been described often (Greenberg & Shuman, 1997; Heilbrun, 2001). Although most authorities agree that clinical and forensic roles are irreconcilable and every effort should be made to avoid conflicts of interest (Greenberg & Shuman, 2007), others' approaches are more situational (Woody, 2009), and a minority even suggest that the roles are potentially compatible (Heltzel, 2007). In the end, neuropsychologists in forensic practice must employ objective methods that allow them to be unbiased truth seekers.

Upon reviewing the *Daubert* hearing testimony, the *Baxter* trial court seemingly had overwhelming undisputed evidence that Bruno-Golden's methodology was not sufficiently reliable for forensic analysis (Desmond, 2007). The trial court judge found her methodology failed to meet any *Daubert* factors. Therefore, the motion *in limine* was granted, Bruno-Golden's testimony was excluded, and the jury never heard her opinions in the case. The plaintiff appealed and the New Hampshire Supreme Court certified three questions for judicial review, asking whether the trial court erred when excluding: (a) the neuropsychologist's testimony based on the BPA, (b) the IQ test testimony, and (c) the pediatrician's testimony that reasonably relied upon the neuropsychologist's report.

In a unanimous decision that includes a thorough analysis of neuropsychological test administration errors, the New Hampshire Supreme Court reversed the trial court on the first question and vacated the subsequent questions as moot. The *Baxter* court reasoned, "the *Daubert* test does not stand for the proposition that scientific knowledge must be absolute or irrefutable" (citing *State v. Dahood*, 2002). Referring to the trial court's conclusion, it

> focused upon the plaintiff's failure to demonstrate that the specific battery—the entire series of tests viewed as a whole—employed by Dr. Bruno-Golden in this case was, or could not be, tested, was subject to peer review and publication, or has a known or potential error rate.
>
> (*Baxter*, p. 174)

The high court cited *Kumho Tire* language that *Daubert* factors "do not constitute a definitive checklist or test," but even if they did, "the BPA meets three of four *Daubert* factors." (p. 184). The *Baxter* court expressly rejected the battery as a whole argument, finding "that the individual tests he or she administered as part of the battery, not the battery as a whole, have been tested, have been subject to peer review and publication, and have a known or potential error rate" (p. 184). The *Baxter* court wrote, "we reject the defendant's assertion that Dr. Bruno-Golden's methodology, the BPA as a flexible battery approach, is not a sufficiently reliable methodology to assist the fact finder in understanding the plaintiff's neuropsychological status" (p. 187). The case was remanded back to the trial court with the instruction to admit Dr. Bruno-Golden's opinions based on the BPA.

The *Baxter* court relied, in part, on an Amicus Brief from the AACN. Justices referred to the AACN brief during oral arguments, raising questions about the standard of care for clinical neuropsychology. AACN drew an analogy between the specialty practices of clinical neuropsychology and neurology, arguing that neurologists do not "conduct either an invariant exam procedure or order an invariant set of diagnostic tests for each and every patient" (p. 9). AACN asserted "that administering the same set of tests to all patients and litigants, regardless of the known or suspected condition is uninformed and inappropriate practice" (p. 9). Further, AACN noted "a standardized battery runs counter to an acceptable standard of care in neurology" and "we know of no area of specialty or subspecialty in clinical medicine in which a routine, invariant battery of tests across all medical conditions being evaluated would be acceptable practice" (p. 9). Although not explicitly written, AACN was seemingly advocating for a flexible battery standard of care for clinical neuropsychology. For most referral questions, a flexible battery approach is the predominant form of practice, even as the fixed battery method remains a respectable minority practice in clinical neuropsychology. In what is probably the best example of the application of *Daubert* factors to neuropsychological methodology, *Baxter* illustrates how federal courts and most state courts would address admissibility based on battery selection. *Baxter* also illustrates how neuropsychology is approaching early questions about standards of care for the profession.

Although *Baxter* resolved admissibility questions of flexible batteries in forensic practice for New Hampshire, Dr. Bruno-Golden withdrew and her testimony was never heard, in what was the oldest pending case in New Hampshire (McCrystal, September 23, 2012). Indeed, *Baxter* was a plaintiff in a second lawsuit alleging that state budget cuts resulted in an unconstitutional delay of justice (*Baxter et al. v. State*, 2010). The second lawsuit was promptly dismissed and a retrial took place in September 2012. In the end, the Temples were negligent landlords in not providing notice of lead paint to the Baxters, but no money damages were awarded to Shelby Baxter or her parents. Despite elevated lead levels as an infant, the jury found that the negligence identified did not cause any damages. This case was the first lead case in New Hampshire that went to trial.

On May 24, 2004, John Richmond was sitting in his van, stopped for a school bus, when it was rear-ended by Henry Bennett, who was driving a 42,000-pound roll-off container truck for his employer. Upon collision, Richmond's one-ton van was propelled 300 feet from a stopped position. Richmond sustained head and neck injuries. In December 2004, Richmond sustained a back injury in the course of employment that exacerbated injuries incurred during the May 2004 accident. Apparently, he was a self-employed builder-contractor. In December 2005, Richmond and his wife sued Bennett and his employer for injuries Richmond sustained to his neck and back in the collision. Upon referral by his attorney, Richmond underwent a neuropsychological evaluation with Dr. Sheridan McCabe in October, 2006.

McCabe obtained a M.A. degree in General Psychology in 1956 and a PhD in Counseling Psychology in 1958. McCabe testified that Counseling Psychology was an applied field "working with people who were not psychiatric patients, but rather kind of regular people who had some sort of problem and counseling dealt with that," and that it involved "the assessment of a patient's psychological well-being." (Appellant's App., p. 235). He attended continuing education workshops specializing in forensic applications of psychology that "touched on subjects that relate to evaluation of traumatic brain injuries" (p. 69). McCabe reported that two neurologists referred cases to him for "specific aspects of brain behavior relationship questions" (p. 70), and other general practitioners referred cases to him for insight into the "relationship between the presenting psychological problems and . . . underlying medical issues" (p. 70). McCabe's route to clinical neuropsychology practice reflects a bygone era of exclusive reliance upon workshop training that does not meet modern standards for neuropsychology training (Hannay et al., 1998).

The defense hired a board-certified clinical neuropsychologist, David Kareken, PhD, ABPP, to conduct an independent neuropsychological evaluation of Richmond. Kareken's evaluation used modern approaches to forensic neuropsychology (e.g., using symptom validity techniques), which disputed McCabe's findings. Both parties filed motions to exclude the opposing experts. The trial court denied both motions. However, Kareken did not testify as an expert witness, presumably because the defense decided to challenge whether a psychologist could render an opinion about the cause of brain damage. If the defense strategy was to argue that psychologists cannot render causation opinions, then it would not make sense to call a psychologist expert to rebut such opinions.

The court denied defense motions to exclude McCabe's opinion before and during the trial. McCabe testified that Richmond suffered a TBI in the accident and the jury returned a $200,000 judgment in his favor. Bennett appealed the judgment, claiming the trial court abused its discretion by permitting a psychologist to testify as to the cause of a brain injury. In a unanimous opinion, the appellate court agreed with Bennett, and reversed and remanded for a new trial (*Bennett v. Richmond*, 2010). The court added,

> no medical doctor or other qualified practitioner diagnosed Richmond with a brain injury. Rather, based upon neuropsychological testing given more than two years after the accident, Dr. McCabe opined that Richmond had sustained a brain injury as a result of the accident. The trial court should have exercised its discretion as gatekeeper prior to trial to exclude Dr. McCabe's proffered causation testimony based upon his lack of qualifications to give such testimony.
>
> And the evidence regarding Richmond's damages other than the alleged brain injury is not sufficient to support the $ 200,000 jury verdict.
>
> (*Bennet v. Richmond*, 2010: 712)

The defense strategy worked, then Richmond appealed.

In a stunning reversal, a unanimous Indiana Supreme Court vacated the appellate court opinion and affirmed the trial court's determination that McCabe's opinion testimony was admissible. That is, it was not an abuse of discretion for the trial court to admit, as sufficiently reliable, a psychologist's opinion that the rear-end collision caused the motorist to suffer TBI. (*Bennett v. Richmond*, 2012). Such dramatic swings in judicial opinion warrant further consideration of McCabe's credentials, methodology, and bases for his expert opinions.

Dr. McCabe denied being a neuropsychologist, yet clearly asserted his expertise regarding TBI. He reviewed medical records before and after the accident, including a radiologist's impressions of a December 13, 2007 brain magnetic resonance imaging (MRI) report, as follows:

> The MRI report indicates small chronic lacunar infarction in the head of the left caudate nucleus. While this type of finding is more indicative of ischemic episodes, it does not rule out the possibility of other causes such as the closed head injury that I suggested in my report . . . [T]his MRI finding is consistent with the sort of brain damage that could produce memory problems.
>
> (Appellant's App., p. 255)

Despite these equivocal impressions, McCabe concluded that the MRI results "were consistent with *his* findings of brain injury." [emphasis added] (Appellant's App., p. 252.). However, other brain structures, such as the frontal/temporal poles or the corpus callosum, are more commonly vulnerable to damage following closed head injury than the head of one caudate nucleus. McCabe selectively misconstrued the radiologist's opinion.

What was the basis for McCabe's findings of brain injury? McCabe administered, scored, and interpreted a battery of neuropsychological tests. However, his opinion also relied upon clinical and collateral interviews, that is, the self-report of interested parties. Specifically, the trial court heard McCabe's impressions based on clinical interviews, but also testimony provided by Richmond's wife, Jennifer, and Richmond's brother, Andrew. Richmond also relied on the testimony of a treating chiropractor, Gary McLeod. All of these witnesses testified about injuries sustained in the accident and problems that evolved after the accident. For example, Richmond called his wife Jennifer from the accident scene and she reported he "sounded shaken-up and was slurring at the time and sounded like he was hesitating on what he was trying to say" (Appellee's App., p. 120; Tr. 447). After the accident, Jennifer also noticed that her husband "was always forgetting things and leaving sticky notes all over the place to remind him of things" (Appellee's App., p. 122; Tr. 449). Richmond also complained of persistent headache.

McCabe administered the Wechsler Adult Intelligence Scale, Third Edition (WAIS-III), the Wechsler Memory Scale, Third Edition (WMS-III), and the Halstead-Reitan Neuropsychological Test Battery (HRB). His brain injury findings were inferred from discrepancies noted among subtest scores on the WAIS-III and the WMS-III that he characterized as "cognitive inefficiency" and "some sort of interference with [Richmond's] cognitive process" (Appellant's App., pp. 89–90; Tr. 331/24–25; 332/1 5). Dr. McCabe also found a mild to moderate impairment on the HRB with special emphasis on category test performance, noting "the first test . . . is a test of problem-solving thinking ability, very sensitive to brain damage" (Appellant's Appendix, p. 91; Tr. 333/1–10). From these findings, McCabe inferred that Richmond

> sustained a diffuse axonal injury [in the course of the rear-end accident in which he was involved]: that is to say, that kind of motion to the head caused damage to the connections between the cells of the brain through the axons. They were sufficiently messed up to provide him with these processing problems that he has manifested—by the time I saw him two years later.
>
> (Appellant's App., p. 92; Tr. 334/6–13)

However, McCabe also agreed that depression and/or anxiety could have caused the cognitive inefficiency noted in his evaluation (Appellant's App., p. 154; Tr. 396).

McCabe testified that Richmond sustained a diffuse axonal injury, which he offered, "as a kind of explanation of the damage [Richmond] sustained" (Appellant's App., p. 145; Tr. 387). However, when asked what he meant by diffuse brain damage, McCabe responded, in part, that

> the pattern of functioning revealed by the tests is that the damage that underlies it is of a diffuse character. That is, its across various areas of the brain . . . I would infer, not assert, but suggest that the damage is in the axonal connections in the frontal lobe between the cortex and the lower brain centers, providing this kind of inefficiency: not localized to the visual cortex or the auditory cortex or so on.
>
> (Appellant's App., p. 145; Tr. 387)

McCabe expressly refused to testify to a reasonable degree of medical certainty. Similarly, when asked whether he could testify to a reasonable degree of psychological certainty, McCabe responded, "No. I am asserting it upon the pattern of functioning." (Appellant's App., pp. 146–147; Tr. 388–389).

When asked to further explain his opinion that Richmond sustained a diffuse axonal injury, McCabe said that it was an inference he drew from "the pattern of what I call 'cognitive inefficiency' that I saw in the test results" (Appellants App., p. 172; Tr. 414). In commenting on the physician's impression about a "small chronic lacunar infarction in the head of the left caudate nucleus" on the MRI, McCabe agreed that such a finding was more often indicative of ischemic episodes and not a closed head injury. However, McCabe maintained that the MRI results did not rule out the possibility of other causes, such as the closed head injury he suggested (Appellant's App., pp. 254–255).

McCabe did not testify about symptom or performance validity. There was no reference to EMT records from the accident scene and there was no description of Richmond's acute neurologic status following the collision. Again, as a counseling psychologist, McCabe's evaluation and inferences about brain damage causation reflected a bygone era of neuropsychological test interpretation. His conclusions were not consistent with those of a board certified clinical neuropsychologist who had conducted an evaluation that defense counsel elected not to file. Ultimately, defense counsel made two strategic errors. First, the defense failed to call for a *Daubert* hearing to challenge the reliability and relevance of McCabe's credentials, methodology, and basis for his expert opinions. Second, the defense should have called a board certified neuropsychologist to dispute McCabe's testimony at trial.

Baxter and *Richmond* are not easily harmonized, in part, because the defense strategies were so different. In *Baxter*, the defense aggressively attacked the plaintiff expert by retaining an opposing expert to testify at a pretrial *Daubert* hearing about the inadequacies of her methodology. This strategy was initially successful in excluding the plaintiff expert. Even though the trial court erred in excluding Bruno-Golden, in the final analysis, she withdrew and never testified. Even though the defendant landlord was found negligent, this was a defense verdict because the insurance company was not required to pay any damages.

Defense counsel in *Richmond* took a very different approach. Rather than attack the specific methodology of the plaintiff expert in a *Daubert* hearing, the defense elected to pursue a failed attack on the profession of psychology as a whole on appeal. Initially, that strategy was successful and the defense may have felt they simply needed to shore up a win. Basically, the defense argued that psychologists and neuropsychologists are not qualified to render expert opinions about the causes of brain damage. No *Daubert* hearing was conducted and no opposing neuropsychologist testified, even though a defense neuropsychological evaluation consistent with modern practice was performed and readily available. By failing to call an opposing board certified neuropsychologist at trial to detail the inadequacies in McCabe's methods, the *Richmond* defense missed an opportunity to distinguish the outdated methods of a counseling psychologist using a fixed battery from the modern methods of a board-certified neuropsychologist using a flexible battery with symptom validity techniques. Moreover, there was no record developed by the defense to show the plaintiff's acute neurologic status immediately after the collision. Appeals can only review facts presented at trial.

The heterogeneity that exists in the application of evidentiary standards makes it difficult to draw general conclusions about admissibility of neuropsychological evidence. However, it is clearly in the best interest of neuropsychologists who engage in forensic activities to have solid empirical support for their opinions and to resist the temptation to speculate beyond what is apparent and can reasonably be inferred from the data. As clinical neuropsychologists, we often take great pride in the scientist-practitioner tradition embodied in our field, but there are a number of challenges related to the validity of our methodology that must continue to be addressed through research and continued refinement of methods, including the quality and applicability of available norms for many neuropsychological instruments, inferences about changes in cognitive functioning, and current limitations of neuropsychological tests in predicting functional outcome.

Quality and Applicability of Norms

Normative studies provide empirical reference points for comparisons of patient performances, and are thus crucial to our ability to understand the meaning of test scores. Given the important role of norms for clinical (and forensic) decision making, it is perhaps surprising that relatively few neuropsychological tests have had large-scale normative studies performed on them (Mitrushina, Boone, & D'Elia, 1999). With the exception of a few very-well-researched measures, neuropsychologists are often forced to rely on converging evidence from multiple less well-normed instruments, as well as patient history and behavioral observations. Even when relatively large normative studies are available, the validity of conclusions based on test performance may be attenuated if individuals tested are dissimilar to the normative sample in some way (e.g., in terms of age, education, racial/ethnic background), which can limit the conclusions that can be made based on test scores (Joint Committee on Standards for Educational and Psychological Testing, 1999). Furthermore, it is important to remember that no test is a pure measure of a particular neuropsychological function or neurological disorder, and most tests encompass a number of different functions (Rankin & Adams, 1999). For example, a low score on the learning trials of a verbal list-learning task could reflect poor encoding of information, poor attention span, language disturbance, or poor effort, among other possibilities. Thus, it is incumbent upon the forensic neuropsychologist to demonstrate that his or her conclusions fit the data better than plausible alternative explanations (Kay, 1999). This is best achieved through rational interpretation based on careful integration of various test results and other available data (e.g., behavioral, historical, collateral).

Inferences About Premorbid Functioning

In addition to comparing individuals' test performances to appropriate norms, conclusions about the impact of injuries on an individual's cognitive functioning also require comparison of current performance to inferred premorbid levels of performance. For example, simply relying on patient self-report of academic achievement is likely to be problematic and can lead to erroneous conclusions about the impact of injuries suffered (Greiffenstein, Baker, & Johnson-Greene, 2002). Several objective methods have been derived that can assist the clinician in estimating premorbid functioning, including regression equations based on demographic and/or test performance variables, and tests that are known to be relatively insensitive to brain injury (Franzen, Burgess, & Smith-Seemiller, 1997; Kareken, 1997). However, these methods give an estimate of the general level of intellectual functioning, and care must be taken in making inferences about premorbid abilities within more specific domains of cognitive functioning (Franzen et al., 1997). Furthermore, they fail to account for premorbid personality characteristics that might impact performance (Putnam, Ricker, Ross, & Kurtz, 1999).

Limitations of Tests in Predicting Functional Outcome

Neuropsychological test results, when interpreted by an adequately trained clinician, clearly improve the prediction and understanding of real world deficits relative to the level of prediction and understanding that would be possible without objective data (Bieliauskas, Fasteneau, Lacy, & Roper, 1997; Bowman, 1997). However, neuropsychological performances often fall short of achieving fully accurate prediction of everyday functioning within the complexity of the real world environment outside of the testing context (LeBlanc, Hayden, & Paulman, 2000; Long & Collins, 1997; Sbordone, 2001; Sbordone & Long, 1996).

One particularly illustrative example of the difficulty in predicting functional outcome from neuropsychological test performance comes from the domain of executive functioning. Existing tests of executive functions often fail to provide an adequate representation of the novelty and complexity of the real world (Burgess, Alderman, Evans, Emslie, & Wilson, 1998; Goldberg & Podell, 2000). According to Goldberg and Podell (2000), the shortcomings are due in large part to the fact that objective tests are scored according to correctness/incorrectness of responses in an absolute sense, while decision making in a real-world context involves an ordering of possible choices according to priorities intrinsic to the individual. Another source of difficulty relates to the still incompletely understood and multifaceted nature of the domain of executive functioning itself. Within the domain of executive functioning, a given test may be sensitive to deficits within a particular subdomain only (e.g., shifting of attention or abstract reasoning) and may be insensitive to deficits in other subdomains (Burgess et al., 1998; Osmon, 1999). The imperfect relationship between test performance and real-world functioning underscores the need for caution in interpretation when performing forensic evaluations, as well as a need for further research on ecological validity within the field.

Detection of Insufficient Effort and Malingering

A major challenge to the forensic neuropsychologist's ability to draw conclusions based on test performance is the potential influence of insufficient effort or deliberate feigning, which in compensation-seeking populations is characterized as malingering. In fact, recent research suggests that insufficient effort can account for more variance in neuropsychological test performance among compensation-seeking individuals than objectively confirmed neurological injury (Green, Rohling, Lees-Haley, & Allen, 2001). Clinical observation, even by an experienced professional, has proven to be an inadequate method of detecting invalid test performance, necessitating the prospective assessment of the validity of test performance in all adversarial cases in which external motivating factors are present (Sweet, 1999b). Kaufmann (2012) summarized cases challenging the admissibility of some symptom validity techniques commonly used by neuropsychologists. Because the issue of malingering is discussed in detail in Millis and Kaufmann (Chapter 38 in this volume), only a brief overview is provided here.

Slick and colleagues (1999) have provided criteria to facilitate the clinical detection and empirical study of malingering. They suggest categorizing suspected malingering into *definite, probable,* and *possible* malingering based on various types of evidence, including the existence of extrinsic motivating factors and demonstration of insufficient effort during testing. While it is often (although certainly not always) apparent when external motivating factors are present, neuropsychologists have only recently begun to develop sophisticated techniques for the objective assessment of effort during a neuropsychological evaluation. These techniques include a number of tests designed for the specific purpose of detecting insufficient effort (e.g., Green, Iverson, & Allen, 1999; Slick, Hopp, Strauss, & Spellacy, 1996) and examination of indicators derived from neurocognitive test performance (e.g., Demakis et al., 2001; Sweet & King, 2002). Indices have also been derived to detect overreporting of symptomatology by litigating populations on psychological inventories (e.g., Lees-Haley, English, & Glenn, 1991). In addition to Chapter 38 in this volume, numerous reviews have documented developments in the assessment of poor effort/malingering (Bordini, Chaknis, Ekman-Turner, & Perna, 2002; Franzen, Iverson, & McCracken, 1990; Haines & Norris, 1995; Hayes, Hilsabeck, & Gouvier, 1999; Iverson & Binder, 2000; Miller & Miller, 1992; Millis & Putnam, 1996; Nies & Sweet, 1994; Rogers, Harrell, & Liff, 1993; Sweet, 1999b; Vanderploeg & Curtiss, 2001).

Expert Witness Role

A major role that is played by neuropsychologists within the forensic setting is that of expert witness or expert independent examiner. Neuropsychologists are often asked to perform evaluations and render opinions about the existence and probable cause of cognitive impairments in litigants or claimants. This may require the neuropsychologist to provide testimony regarding his or her opinion, sometimes subjecting him or her to intense cross-examination from opposing attorneys (Bick, 1999). Another aspect of forensic neuropsychological practice that may be unfamiliar to many is the absence of a typical psychologist-patient relationship (Sweet, Grote, & van Gorp, 2002). The neuropsychologist who performs a forensic evaluation and/or provides expert testimony serves in a consultant role, rather than an assessing/treating clinician role, and it is important that this be made clear from the outset to all parties involved, particularly the litigant or claimant. A list of items that address the nonclinical aspect of the neuropsychologist's role can be found in Table 36.2. The individual should be informed that the usual expectation of confidentiality does not apply in this situation, and that he or she should not provide any information to the neuropsychologist that he or she does not want revealed to all parties involved. This role is very dissimilar to traditional clinical roles played by neuropsychologists, and may become uncomfortable if approached without careful thought. Because neuropsychologists have special expertise that can allow them to assist triers-of-fact in understanding complex issues related to cognitive dysfunction, and therefore can be of help to the

Table 36.2 Points that can be discussed at the outset of a forensic examination to ensure that the claimant or litigant is fully informed about the nature of the examination about to be undertaken

1	Clarification of the reasons for the evaluation
2	Identification of the referral source and any relationship, or lack thereof, with the examiner
3	A general description of the types of information that will be gathered during the evaluation
4	A description of the lack of confidentiality within the examination, making it different from the normal "doctor-patient" relationship
5	Clarification that no treatment will be offered to the examinee
6	The intent of maintaining objectivity on the part of the examiner and clarification that the examiner is not acting as an interested party regarding the outcome of the claim or litigation
7	The importance of the examinee being honest in providing information and also putting forth full effort on the formal testing

decision-making process in such cases, their forensic activities make an important contribution. Neuropsychologists may also be retained as consultants to review the work of colleagues in cases where they do not evaluate the litigating patient directly, an area of practice that has received relatively little consideration from a perspective of ethical standards (Guilmette & Hagan, 1997; Johnson-Greene & Bechtold, 2002; McSweeny, 1997). Whether retained as an expert witness or to provide consultation to attorneys, the best way to accomplish the goal of assisting the courts is through maintaining objectivity and relying on the empirical foundations of the field (Guilmette & Hagan, 1997; Martelli, Zasler, & Grayson, 1999b; McSweeny, 1997). Issues involved in working within the legal system are covered in greater depth in Greiffenstein and Kaufmann (Chapter 37 in this volume), but an overview of major issues related to the expert witness role will be provided here.

Covert and Overt Pressures and Deceptive Attorney Behaviors

In contrast to the more familiar clinical setting, forensic work often introduces pressures on the neuropsychologist to arrive at an opinion that is favorable to one side or another. In fact, some of the values and ethics of attorneys and psychologists are fundamentally in conflict with one another (Gutheil & Simon, 1999; Martelli, Bush, & Zasler, 2003; Melton, Petrila, Poythress, & Slobogin, 1997). Psychologists tend to value detached objectivity in their assessments of patients, believing that this is the best method of arriving at an accurate understanding of an individual's functioning (i.e., detached objectivity is the best method for discovering the truth). In contrast, attorneys have an obligation to advocate vigorously for their clients, with the underlying assumption that the truth is best sought through adversarial proceedings.

In spite of the pressures placed on attorneys by this adversarial system, most treat expert witnesses in an ethical manner. Nonetheless, a minority of attorneys use unscrupulous methods to exert pressure on expert witnesses. These methods can range from subtle (e.g., profuse praise of the expert's work) to more overt means (e.g., bribery, threats) to influence experts to produce opinions favorable to the attorney's side (Gutheil & Simon, 1999; Gutheil, Commons, & Miller, 2001; Hess, 1998). Although most attorneys do not engage in such practices, it is apparently not unusual for experts who practice frequently in the forensic arena to experience them from time to time. In a pilot study of expert witnesses' experiences with such pressures, Gutheil and colleagues (2001) found that more than one-third of their sample said they had had an attorney attempt to influence them to provide a favorable opinion and almost one-fifth said they had been threatened (e.g., with a complaint about the expert to a state licensing board).

Some attorneys may attempt to influence the results of evaluations not through pressuring the evaluating expert, but by coaching patients to report selected information during the clinical interview or to perform on cognitive tests in a manner consistent with injury (Lees-Haley, 1997a; Wetter & Corrigan, 1995). Coached deficits may allow more sophisticated faking of deficits than would be possible without attorney input and can affect the ability to reach valid conclusions based on testing (Coleman et al., 1998; Youngjohn, Lees-Haley, & Binder, 1999). Information about neuropsychological methods is widely available through various textbooks and the Internet, and it is naive to think that this information will not be exploited by some individuals given the incentives and pressures associated with proving that an injury has occurred. In fact, some attorneys believe such preparations are consistent with their role as zealous advocates under ABA Model Rules of Professional Conduct 1.3 Diligence (American Bar Asoociation, 2002). However, the requirement for diligent representation of clients must be reasonably balanced with Rule 3.3 Candor Toward the Tribunal (Ben-Porath, Greve, Bianchini, & Kaufmann, 2009).

Importance of Maintaining Objectivity to the Individual and Field

As unpleasant as it may be to confront perceived attempts at influencing the expert, and as difficult as it may be to maintain objectivity steadfastly in the presence of numerous pressures to the contrary, doing so is extremely important to the long-term viability of the expert's career, as well as to the broader field. Just as a minority of attorneys may compromise their ethics in the face of various pressures and incentives, it is generally recognized that some experts act as "hired guns," offering to advocate the desired opinion for the right price (Fisher, 1997; Gutheil & Simon, 1999). While it is clear that such behavior impacts the perception of the individual by his or her peers, it is also likely to be detrimental to the view of neuropsychologists and the field of psychology in general if we are perceived by those in the legal profession as experts for hire (Boccaccini & Brodsky, 2002; Fisher, 1997). While it is relatively easy to detect and criticize obvious abuses, such as opinions for hire, the influence of the various pressures and incentives involved in the expert witness role are often much more subtle, and therefore more difficult to defend against. A number of strategies for debiasing, including self-examination regarding objectivity, have been proposed that can be helpful in ensuring the maintenance of a high level of objectivity for neuropsychologists involved in adversarial proceedings (Sweet & Moulthrop, 1999).

Forensic Neuropsychology and Ethics

In addition to the ethical principles and standards that apply to all activities of psychologists, there are a number of issues that arise frequently in the forensic neuropsychological context that merit discussion. As mentioned in the previous section, because of the interactions with individuals from other professions that occur in the forensic arena, maintaining high ethical standards is important not only to the individual, but to the reputation of the field as a whole.

Relevant Standards

The American Psychological Association's code of ethics (APA, 2017) includes a number of ethical standards that are of particular relevance to the practice of forensic neuropsychology (for a more extensive review of standards relevant to forensic neuropsychological practice, see Martelli et al., 2003; Sweet et al., 2002; Grote et al., 2005). One of these is Standard 2.01 (Boundaries of Competence). Psychologists are admonished to practice only within those areas for which they are appropriately trained. Clearly, this standard speaks to the importance of obtaining appropriate training in clinical neuropsychology. However, the standard goes on to specify "when assuming forensic roles, psychologists are or become reasonably familiar with the judicial or administrative rules governing their roles" (APA, 2017: 5). The APA has also published *Specialty Guidelines for Forensic Psychology*, which was most recently updated in 2013.

There is continued debate about the appropriate definition of a neuropsychologist and the accompanying training trajectory, but there is currently general agreement that training in clinical neuropsychology should include (a) a doctoral degree in psychology from an accredited program, (b) a clinically relevant internship, (c) two years (at least one being postdoctoral) of supervised experience in neuropsychology, and (d) psychology and/or neuropsychology licensure in the state in which one practices. Furthermore, although it is not required to meet the definition of a neuropsychologist, board certification is recognized as the best method of establishing competence to practice clinical neuropsychology (NAN Policy and Planning Committee, 2003). It is also important to recognize one's areas of competence within the broader field (e.g., areas in which the clinician has received supervised training and/or published original research). Attempts by neuropsychologists to extend these boundaries to include areas in which the neuropsychologist is not experienced are not only ethically dangerous, but also may open the clinician to unwelcome scrutiny in the courtroom. It should be noted that there are currently very few, if any, graduate programs that provide extensive formal training in the practice of forensic neuropsychology, forcing those wishing to acquire competence in the area to seek out less-formal training experiences and making it somewhat difficult to assess the competence of neuropsychologists to practice in the forensic context.

Also particularly relevant to forensic neuropsychology is Standard 2.04 (Bases for Scientific and Professional Judgments). As mentioned previously, while it is always important to have a solid empirical foundation, it is especially important to avoid speculating beyond the data within the forensic arena. Another important standard is Standard 4.02 (Discussing the Limits of Confidentiality), particularly as it applies to the lack of a typical doctor-patient relationship in forensic evaluations. Other important standards include 9.01 (Bases for Assessments), 9.02 (Use of Assessments), and 9.06 (Interpreting Assessment Results), which again underscore the importance of competence and the need for empirically sound bases for interpretations based on assessment instruments.

Two other standards, 9.04 (Release of Test Data) and 9.11 (Maintaining Test Security), merit discussion. The former is intended to allow appropriate access by patients to results of psychological tests that they have undergone, while the latter is intended to protect the integrity of test stimuli. Many psychologists agree that releasing raw test data that include test stimuli to nonpsychologists is inappropriate and breaches the security of these tests (Knapp & VandeCreek, 2001; Sweet et al., 2002; Kaufmann, 2005). Since the first edition of this book, Attix et al. (2007) provided an Official Position on Disclosure of Test Data from APA Division 40, AACN, and APPCN. Kaufmann (2009) framed the public policy debate and detailed legal and other persuasive strategies to protect test security and prevent wrongful release of psychological test materials to nonpsychologists. Possible negative outcomes of breaching test security include infringement on the rights of companies that develop and sell the tests and facilitation of future coaching by attorneys. Forensic neuropsychologists receive frequent requests for the release of raw data, sometimes in the form of a subpoena or even a court order. The National Academy of Neuropsychology (NAN) has provided a decision tree to aid in dealing with such requests in a manner that strives to maintain test security and prevent the misuse of raw test data (NAN Policy and Planning Committee, 2000). In brief, requests should be written, include a signed release from the patient, and include assurances that test security will be protected. If a request is made in the form of a court order, neuropsychologists must respond in a timely manner, although strategies to preserve test security even in this instance are included in the decision tree. Importantly, both sides of an adversarial proceeding must and can have access and still maintain test security, and neuropsychologists should strive to balance this concern with the interests of test developers and users in preventing invalidation of tests.

Responding to Ethical Dilemmas and Perceived Unethical Practices

Despite the best efforts to develop broad and well-articulated ethical standards, situations arise in the course of day-to-day practice for which ethical standards do not provide a clear answer. This can be especially true when one is involved in forensic activities. One issue that forensic neuropsychologists may face is the confrontation of perceived unethical practices by colleagues. While general guidelines provided by the APA ethics code for responding to perceived ethical violations (Standards 1.04, Informal Resolution of Ethical Violations, and 1.05, Reporting Ethical Violations) are helpful, responding to perceived unethical practices of colleagues can be particularly delicate within a forensic context, given its adversarial and emotionally charged nature (Brodsky & McKinzey, 2002; Johnson-Greene & Bechtold, 2002; Sweet, 2003). In fact, the American Academy of Clinical Neuropsychology (AACN; the membership organization of neuropsychologists who are board-certified by the American Board of Professional Psychology) has published an official position paper regarding an unfortunate outcome related to involvement in adversarial proceedings as an expert witness, namely, having specious ethics complaints filed against the expert witness (AACN, 2003). It is important that forensic neuropsychologists consider these issues. In instances in which they believe an ethical violation has occurred, it is wise to consider waiting to pursue a decision regarding action until the conclusion of the litigation that brought the possible ethical violation to light. At such a time, when it is determined that an ethical violation has occurred (i.e., ethical principles/standards have been violated and harm has been done as a result), and it is clear that the confidentiality of individuals involved will not be compromised by addressing the perceived violation, it is incumbent upon the neuropsychologist to address it (Grote, Lewin, Sweet, & van Gorp, 2000). As suggested by the APA ethics code, an attempt should first be made to resolve the issue informally before registering a formal complaint.

Examples of Major Forensic Activities and Roles

This section will cover some of the major roles for neuropsychologists within the forensic arena. We will begin by discussing two common areas of acquired brain injury civil litigation (e.g., TBI and toxic exposure). We will then discuss two common settings within which neuropsychologists frequently play a role (i.e., disability examinations and school consultations). Finally, this section considers the possible involvement of neuropsychologists in evaluation of competence and determinations specific to criminal litigation.

Traumatic Brain Injury and Neurotoxin Litigation

In the role of forensic evaluator/expert witness in the context of civil litigation, TBI and neurotoxin related injury are generally the most common referrals. Issues related to evaluation of these two types of referrals are discussed in this section.

Traumatic Brain Injury

Since the early 1990s, TBI civil litigation has increased dramatically with a related increase in referrals to neuropsychologists (Ruff & Richardson, 1999; Stern, 1997).

In cases of moderate to severe brain trauma with prolonged loss of consciousness, medical records documenting the extent of injury, and evidence of specific cerebral insult on neuroimaging, there is often no question whether a brain injury occurred. For these cases, the forensic issue is not the presence of injury, as it is clearly documented prior to the neuropsychologist becoming involved with the case, but rather the presence and severity of cognitive impairment, the functional implications, and ramifications for the person's quality of life.

With milder trauma, in which there is possible brief or transient alteration in consciousness with no clear signs of injury on imaging, the existence of brain damage is less clear (American Congress of Rehabilitation Medicine, 1993). The role of the neuropsychologist in litigation of milder brain injury is not just to clarify the effects of the injury, but additionally—and often more importantly—to clarify the existence of a brain injury. The determination of an initial injury is separate from the determination of persistent problems. Attorneys sometimes lose sight of this (Hartlage, 1997; Silver & McAllister, 1997).

Neurotoxin Litigation

Neuropsychological toxicology is the study of "human neurological, behavioral, cognitive and emotional concomitants of toxic and neurotoxic exposures" (Hartman, 1999, p. 339). Individuals who sustain toxin related neuropsychological injuries are often referred for an evaluation in the context of a toxic tort, "a legal cause of action after a plaintiff develops an injury or illness in response to a chemical, industrial product, metal, drug or other exogenous agent" (Hartman, 1999, p. 340).

For the neuropsychologist working within the arena of toxic torts, a thorough understanding of some of the more common toxicants (e.g., metals, lead, mercury, carbon monoxide, organic solvents, pesticides, prescription drugs, etc.), their effect on the central nervous system, and cognition specifically, are essential. The reader is referred to other excellent sources for relevant description of such agents (Hartman, 1999; Miller, 1993).

Unlike brain injury, in which at least the more severe injuries and related deficits can be relatively focal and often are associated with well-documented acute effects in medical records and possibly even neuroimaging findings, the neuropsychological effects of toxicants are often more subtle and generalized, with the litigant/claimant frequently presenting with diffuse neurological and cognitive complaints. Neurotoxic exposure can impact the central nervous system on a neurochemical or cellular level that is less evident on broad examination. The role of the neuropsychologist in a toxic tort case is to clarify if there has been a neurotoxic injury and to quantify the effects of the injury, as well as emotional factors, directly due to the effects of the agents (Hartman, 1999; Lees-Haley, 1997b).

After exposure is confirmed, the expert seeks to determine whether the level and type of neuropsychological symptoms reported are consistent with the level of exposure. That is, are the claims credible or sensible from a toxicologic and neuropsychological perspective? Based on findings, common conclusions can include that symptoms are consistent/inconsistent with the type of exposure, symptoms are an emotional reaction to central nervous system changes, or symptoms are a reaction to the stress of being exposed even without central nervous system injury. As with TBI, other factors such as emotional functioning at the time of the evaluation, effects of pain and pain medications, fatigue, and external factors such as secondary gain and effort must be considered. (Hartman, 1995; Lees-Haley, 1997b).

Commonalities in the Expert Role in TBI and Neurotoxin Litigation

Prior to seeing the litigant, it is important to obtain records. When the neuropsychologist is working with an experienced attorney familiar with forensic neuropsychological evaluations, relevant records are often prepared and sent to the neuropsychologist as soon as he or she is retained. However, many attorneys are newer to the areas of TBI and neurotoxin litigation and less aware of what a neuropsychologist may need. Part of the neuropsychologist's role is to educate the attorney about relevant information and the types of records needed for the neuropsychologist to proceed effectively.

The overriding question presented to the neuropsychologist is whether there has been a decline in functioning related to the alleged injury and/or exposure. Understanding premorbid (e.g., preinjury/accident) factors is crucial in understanding the client's current presentation. Are reported deficits due to the injury or better explained by preexisting factors? Important information to obtain includes:

1. Records related to the injury including how the purported injury or exposure was sustained (motor vehicle accident, assault, work related, etc.). Was a loss of consciousness noted? What evaluations/tests were conducted and treatments/surgeries performed? The emergency room records are especially important. In reviewing records, those closest to the time of injury/exposure tend to be most valid with fewer effects of bias and rehearsal. Over time, incorrect information can be introduced into the chart.
2. Preinjury school and occupational history to establish gross baseline functioning (e.g., grade school, secondary and post secondary education, work history).
3. Premorbid medical history, including any previous brain injury or neurological illness.
4. Premorbid psychiatric history including that related to other traumas. Previous psychological/neuropsychological evaluations.
5. Premorbid alcohol and substance use history, including history of any chemical dependency treatments.

In conducting the clinical interview, the expert can assess the patient's account of the incident that caused the reported injury or exposure (being aware of any inconsistencies with the available records), as well as level of functioning, perceived cognitive strengths and weaknesses, emotional reactions to the incident, and pre- and postinjury stressors. It is important to be aware of secondary gain issues and, whenever possible, attempt to verify the validity of the interview information through collateral sources.

In conducting testing, one should consider the impact of noncerebral injury variables such as peripheral injury, pain, headache, and behavioral evidence of current emotional difficulties, fatigue, and the effects of medications. It is important to use well-accepted, standardized, and valid measures and use the most appropriate and accepted norms (Klonoff & Lamb, 1998; Murrey, 2000; Silver & McAllister, 1997; Williams, 1997; Zasler & Martelli, 2003).

A forensic evaluation should be a broad-based assessment of a range of cognitive and emotional functions in order to allow for a thorough differential diagnosis. That is, it is not only the deficits and intact abilities that are expected, but those that are not expected to be deficient or intact that must be considered, if one is to be able to "prove" cause and effect with regard to the forensic matter at issue. In litigation and other adversarial proceedings, large sums of money or other external incentives are often at stake. Inclusion of measures of effort is essential to clarify the client's level of engagement in the evaluation. In fact, the omission of effort testing when evaluating a possible neuropsychological injury with ability tests is no longer acceptable; such an omission is clearly not in keeping with current practice expectations expressed in the extensive literature on forensic neuropsychology (cf. Sweet et al., 2002). Similarly, forensic psychologists evaluating emotional injury cases have been found to prefer instruments that contain validity scales (Boccaccini & Brodsky, 1999), which also has relevance to forensic neuropsychological evaluations.

In addition to the primary role of conducting an evaluation, the role of the neuropsychologist in a forensic brain injury case can include assisting the retaining attorney in evaluating the strengths and weaknesses of a case by reviewing records, advising on the expertise of other experts, quality of reports, and basis for findings. The neuropsychologist can perform these roles on behalf of either the plaintiff or defense; the goals are the same irrespective of which side retains the neuropsychologist. Examples of questions often asked of the neuropsychologist who conducts a forensic evaluation include: (a) Does the event at issue in the proceeding appear to be a credible cause of claimed problems? (b) Does the plaintiff present with relevant neuropsychological deficits on testing? (c) If deficits exist, are they proportional (i.e., reasonably expected) relative to the specific event at issue? (d) What is the functional impact of the injury and related deficits on the individual? (e) Are the identified deficits neurogenic, psychogenic, or due to other factors such as secondary gain? (f) What is the role of premorbid and comorbid factors?

These are complicated questions, but they are also very familiar as the common questions that can occur in routine clinical evaluations, in which the referral source, or consumer of the evaluation results, is typically a physician. As is the case with such clinical work, the neuropsychologist who participates as an expert in TBI or neurotoxic litigation needs to have knowledge of the relevant literature and practices within the field (Hartlage, 1997; Ruff & Richardson, 1999).

Retained Expert for Independent Medical Evaluations

Neuropsychologists are often asked to render an objective opinion on the diagnosis, status and/or prognosis of a patient by a third party, such as an insurance company or disability carrier, in an independent medical evaluation (IME). Although sometimes referred to as independent psychological evaluations (IPE), they are often referred to as IMEs regardless of the clinician's discipline.

There appear to be some differential applications of the term *IME* that also might prove confusing to the reader. Whereas all disability evaluations for a third party can be called IMEs, in some areas of the country, litigation-related evaluations, even though unrelated to determination of disability benefits, may also be referred to as IMEs. For the purpose of the present chapter, IME is used to refer more narrowly to evaluations for the purpose of determination of disability benefits.

The goal of an IME is to provide an objective assessment of the patient for some purpose, usually clarification of a diagnosis, need for additional testing or evaluation, need for additional treatment, determination of functional limitations, likely impact of cognitive impairment on job performance, assessment of the severity of impairment, need for (continuation of) disability compensation, or to determine if maximal medical improvement (MMI; the person having received optimal treatment without expectation of further recovery through additional conventional treatment) has occurred. An IME must be objective, which therefore excludes a claimant's treating doctor from carrying out such an evaluation (Kraus, 1997). Although the content of the evaluation is often comparable to that of an extensive clinical evaluation, there are a number of unique issues involved in performing IMEs, and in this respect the earlier information pertaining to informed consent of litigants applies.

Within clinical settings, the clinician develops a relationship with the patient for the purpose of assessment and treatment. However, in an IME, the primary relationship is between the neuropsychologist and referring third party (e.g., insurance company, state agency etc.), who requested and is paying for the evaluation. The goal is *not* to provide treatment or treatment-oriented assessment for a patient, but instead to provide an objective evaluation of the factors underlying the claimant's functioning to the third party. Related to this goal, confidentiality is between the third-party referent and examiner. All information obtained during the record review, clinical interview, and testing will be communicated in the report to the third party. In most cases, the claimant will not be granted direct access to the report, and instead will receive this information from either the third party or his or her own lawyer, if the matter is being formally disputed. Additionally, no treatment will be offered to the patient—and even if treatment recommendations are part of the report, the examinee will not be made aware of these recommendations by the examiner directly (Grant, 1997; Martelli, Zasler, & Grayson, 1999a, 1999b; Perlo, 1996; Silver & McAllister, 1997).

The APA has no specific guidelines for psychologists/neuropsychologists involved in doing IMEs, but other organizations have developed guidelines and standards. An association of psychologists involved in IMEs and disability assessments in Canada, the Canadian Academy of Psychologists in Disability Assessment (CAPDA), has developed a set of standards entitled *Practice Standards for the Psychological Assessment of Disability and Impairment* (CAPDA, 2000). The reader is encouraged to review these standards, as they provide sound guidance. Similar to some of the matters described earlier, the standards deal with issues including the relationship with third-party referents and the role of the compensation process, need for objectivity, unique nature of confidentiality, competency of providers, importance of considering all relevant factors, components of an appropriate evaluation, and how findings are communicated.

Although not specifically applicable to neuropsychologists, the American Medical Association (AMA) also has IME-specific guidelines, such as those related to the patient-physician relationship (i.e., Code 1.2.6: Work-Related and Independent Medical Examinations) and confidentiality (i.e., Code 3.2.3: Industry-Employed Physicians and Independent Medical Examiners) within IME contexts (American Medical Association, 2016a, 2016b). The AMA criteria are similar in many ways to common psychological practice, but differ in the nature of the clinical relationship viewing it as a limited doctor-patient relationship with release of confidential information still requiring patient consent, even in the context of a third-party payor.

Readers are encouraged to familiarize themselves with these guidelines and ways in which they differ from general neuropsychological practice. Attorneys may not be aware of differences between medical and neuropsychological practice, and it may be incumbent upon the neuropsychologist to clarify these differences.

Many aspects of conducting IMEs are still areas of discussion and controversy within the field. Although common practices do exist, the need for a well-defined set of standards and guidelines, such as those offered by the CAPDA, is clearly indicated. Although not as formal as standards and guidelines, both AACN and NAN have recently published position papers on issues related to IMEs (AACN, 2003; Bush et al., 2005).

Retained Expert for Independent School Evaluations

It may seem strange to include a section on the role of neuropsychologists in schools in a chapter on forensics. However, much of the activity of a neuropsychologist within the school system is directly related to federal legislation and court decisions. This section will briefly discuss the most pertinent legislation, specifically the Individuals with Disabilities Education Act (IDEA) and Section 504 of the Rehabilitation Act, as well as the some of the roles of neuropsychologists within the schools.

IDEA (originally the Education Act of All Handicapped Children) was initially passed in 1975, and modifications were made over time. The reader is encouraged to review the most current version of IDEA, amended in 1997 (20 U.S.C. Sec 1401). The purpose of IDEA is to provide children with disabilities, from age 3 to 21, with the same education as nondisabled students, providing a "free appropriate public education" in the "least restrictive environment" (Braden, 2003; Melton, Petrila, Poythress, & Slobogin, 1997). According to IDEA, children with the following 13 disabilities are covered: Autism; Deaf-Blindness; Deafness; Emotional Disturbance; Hearing Impairment; Mental Retardation; Multiple Disabilities; Orthopedic Impairment; Other Health Impairment; Specific Learning Disability; Speech and Language Impairment; Traumatic Brain Injury; and Visual Impairment.

Children who are eligible to receive services under IDEA are also eligible for "related services," which are intended to assist a disabled child to benefit from special education and can include developmental services, psychological services, social work, counseling, therapeutic recreation, rehabilitation counseling, and some limited medical services. The student is eligible for related services only as they aid him or her in benefiting from special education. The act also requires that the student be educated in the least restrictive environment possible, emphasizing mainstreaming. Under the act, specific procedures are elucidated, including: (a) identification of the disabled child, the burden of which falls upon the school system or local educational agency (LEA); (b) evaluation of the child by a multidisciplinary team and development of the individual education plan (IEP), which includes a description of current levels, annual goals, educational services to be provided, the expected date when services will be started and expected duration, and criteria for evaluation on at least an annual basis; and (c) review. If parents are dissatisfied with the findings of the evaluation process, they can seek an independent evaluation, often with a neuropsychologist, for which (depending on circumstances) the school may be required to pay.

The questions to be answered by the evaluation include whether the child has one of the IDEA-listed disabilities that requires special education, what would constitute an appropriate education, what related services are necessary, and whether services can be provided within a regular classroom setting. The child's placement must be determined annually, based on his or her IEP, and should be located as close to the child's home as possible (Lorber & Yurk, 1999; Melton et al., 1997).

Section 504 of the Rehabilitation Act, a predecessor of the IDEA, enacted almost 25 years ago, is another major piece of school-related legislation. Section 504 is an antidiscrimination statute. Unlike IDEA, it is not a grant statute and does not have mandates for federal funding (U.S. Department of Education, 2003). Section 504 was designed to eliminate impediments or barriers to students with disabilities in the classroom, and requires that schools not discriminate against students with disabilities. Section 504 has a much broader definition of disability than the IDEA (Rosenfeld, 2003). It protects all individuals with a disability who have a physical or mental impairment that substantially limits one or more major life activities, a record of such impairment, and are regarded as having such an impairment.

The primary question under Section 504 is whether the student has an impairment that is limiting his or her ability to learn. Schools are required to provide a free appropriate public education to qualified students with determined disabilities (U.S. Department of Education, 2003).

Within both IDEA and Section 504, schools are responsible for identifying students who have disabilities and are in need of services. The initial screening evaluations are often accomplished by a multidisciplinary team at the school (Braden, 2003).

Neuropsychologists can play a significant role in the evaluation of and advocacy for students with disabilities under both acts. Neuropsychologists can become involved in the process through referral from the school or child's parents. Through evaluations, neuropsychologists can help to clarify a student's cognitive achievement and emotional functioning, identifying learning strengths and weaknesses, and needs for remediation. The neuropsychologist, often in working with a multidisciplinary team, can help to diagnose and/or clarify if the student is in one of the protected categories and if so, in need of special education and related services. If the school and family are unable to agree on the need for services, a Due Process hearing, considered a federal hearing and adjudicated by an appointed and trained hearing officer, can be requested by either party. In these hearings, the neuropsychologist can advocate for the appropriate services dependent on evaluation results and also act as a consultant to either the family or school.

Another area under these acts in which the neuropsychologist can play a role is school disciplinary codes. All schools maintain disciplinary codes, often with predetermined consequences. Although these rules are appropriate for the general student body, they may not be appropriate for a child with a disability. When a child with a disability who is receiving special services breaks a school rule that requires disciplinary action, a multidisciplinary team must first meet to determine if the violation was related to the disability and if the student can understand the rule and consequences of the violation. In their role as experts in the assessment of cognition and behavior, neuropsychologists are uniquely suited to assist the team in determining if the rule violation was related to the disability (Lorber & Yurk, 1999).

IDEA and Section 504 of the Rehabilitation Act have significantly changed educational opportunities for students with disabilities. Under both acts, there are varied roles for neuropsychologists. Pediatric practice, especially within the school system, requires a broad understanding of the relevant legislation and related court decisions.

Referrals for Evaluations of Civil Competence

The notion of competency is grounded in the societal ideals of autonomy versus beneficence, in which the independence of the individual is countered by the greater society's role of caring for those in need. Doctors have historically worked with patients from a *parens patriae* viewpoint, as if a parent and child. However, over time the relationship and decision-making process have become more collaborative (Melton et al., 1997), and in general there has been a societal trend toward maintaining the autonomy of the individual. In this context, neuropsychologists are often consulted to assess a patient's capacity to help medical staff, and at times, the courts, in clarifying his or her level of competence.

The terms *competency* and *capacity* are often used interchangeably, but in reality they differ significantly. *Capacity* is a nonlegal, clinical determination assessed by a health professional, such as a neuropsychologist or psychiatrist, and is concerned with functional abilities. *Competency* is determined by a judge or other legal body, with capacity being only part of the consideration. A person is assumed competent unless proven otherwise. Although competency is ultimately a legal decision that varies under state law, in common practice, clinicians are regularly called upon to make decisions regarding patient capacity without a formal legal determination of competency ever occurring (Fellows, 1998; Kim, Karlawish, & Caine, 2002). Recently, Demakis (2016) edited a special section on civil capacities, including representative cases (Kaufmann, 2016). There are numerous capacities that have been differentiated (see Table 36.3).

For a finding of incompetence, there must be evidence of a clinical condition that is causative. At one time, psychiatric illness or significant cognitive impairment equaled incompetence, but this is no longer the case. The mere presence of a psychiatric illness or a neurological illness such as Alzheimer's disease or Parkinson's disease does not warrant a determination of incompetence (Department of Veterans Affairs, 1997; Haffey, 1989). If a disorder has been established, the question for the clinician is whether the person is sufficiently impaired as a result of it to be considered incompetent.

Capacity is not a static concept. Although some disorders, such as dementias, are progressive, in other conditions (e.g., delirium, acute brain injury, psychosis), the person may lack capacity at one point, but not at another (Hart & Nagele, 1996). With such conditions, serial assessments are often necessary.

Capacity can be brought into question in an individual of any age or diagnostic group (e.g., mental retardation, psychiatric illness, brain injury, etc.), but the group most commonly associated with the assessment of capacity is older adults. Older adults have a higher incidence of medical illnesses and therefore need to make more medically relevant decisions, and are most vulnerable to disorders impacting cognition (Marson & Harrell, 1999).

At this time, physician judgment is still the most common means of determining competence. However, physicians

Table 36.3 Types of capacities (i.e., nonlegal, functional ability areas, the status of which is determined by clinical means)

1	Medical decision making
2	Consent to treatment (informed consent)
3	Refusal of medications
4	Driving
5	Financial (capacity to manage own monetary funds)
6	Activities of daily living and instrumental activities of daily living
7	Manage medications
8	Testamentary (i.e., wills)
9	Contracts
10	Parenting
11	Return to work
12	Live independently
13	Consent to be a research subject

generally receive little training in this area and most judgments are impressionistic or based on brief assessment such as the Mini Mental Status Examination (MMSE; Folstein, Folstein, & McHugh, 1975). However, there has been greater appreciation over time for the need to develop more specific, valid, and reliable means for assessing competence (Department of Veterans Affairs, 1997).

The assessment of capacity and competency is an increasing area of involvement for neuropsychologists. As defined by Baker, Lichtenberg, and Moye (1998: 151), competency assessment is the "clinical assessment process to supply a cognitive, mental health, and functional evaluation when questions of legal competencies or capacities are raised." There is a lack of consensus for neuropsychologists involved in these endeavors. As a result, clinicians often need to rely on clinical experience and varied research findings.

However, at least in the assessment of the older adult, guidelines have been developed that can generalize to other populations. *Assessment of Competency and Capacity of the Older Adult: A Practice Guideline for Psychologists* was developed by the Department of Veterans Affairs to assist clinicians with these evaluations (Department of Veterans Affairs, 1997). These guidelines, as well as other sources, recommend a multistep process in capacity assessment (Baker et al. 1998; Department of Veterans Affairs, 1997; Haffey, 1989; Hart & Nagele, 1996; Melton et al., 1997).

Referral questions are often vague, so first it is important to clarify the specific issue(s) to be addressed. The clinician must ask—competency or capacity for what? Second, informed consent and confidentiality need to be discussed. Patients have to be aware of the purpose of the evaluation. A thorough review of case history, not only including normal medical, psychiatric and social information, but also history specific to the question at hand should be completed.

The assessment should then include a clinical interview and evaluations of cognitive skills, mental health, and functional abilities. The mental health assessment should cover a broad range of psychological conditions with the understanding that limitations due to some conditions may be temporary. The cognitive and functional evaluations should focus on abilities/tasks specific to the capacity being questioned. Commonly relevant areas include perception and ability to understand relevant information without distortion, ability to retain and recall relevant information, ability to identify options and to logically reason and problem solve among them, and ability to make a decision based on deliberation regarding options.

In selecting measures for competency evaluations, clinicians should choose measures that tap the underlying skills that are relevant for the question being asked and also appropriate to assess the condition that may be compromising the patient's capacity (Department of Veterans Affairs, 1997). Relevant areas may include any cognitive domain but especially language (receptive and expressive), new learning and memory, and executive functioning. An evaluation should be broad-based to understand the person's ability level specific to the question at hand.

The report should clearly delineate the referral for a capacity evaluation, relevant history, test results, and a rationale as to how the results support a finding of full or diminished capacity. Often, especially with conditions that can change or vary over time, follow-up is necessary to monitor the person's capacity.

Retained Expert Witness for Criminal Proceedings

Within the forensic arena, neuropsychologists play a prominent role in civil and educational proceedings, as previously described. Within the criminal arena, although a less common area of practice for neuropsychologists, there are a number of areas in which clinicians regularly contribute. This section will review some relevant areas of law related to criminal proceedings and the role of neuropsychologists within the criminal justice system.

In clinical practice, neuropsychologists objectively assess and describe the cognitive, behavioral, and functional aspects of brain injury and brain disease. In some criminal proceedings, attorneys need an objective means of explaining to a trier of fact that their client's thinking or behavior has been or is currently being impacted by brain dysfunction. If during a criminal proceeding, there is suspicion by either the prosecution or defense that brain dysfunction had an adverse impact on the defendant's behavior, a neuropsychologist may be called in as a consultant to provide quantifiable objective information about the defendant. In general, when a neuropsychologist is retained by an attorney who handles criminal cases, three main areas need to be addressed (Kirkish & Sreenivasan, 1999; Martell, 1992):

1. What are the appropriate diagnoses?
2. If present, what effects have the brain damage or disease had on the defendant either at the time of the alleged incident or within the court proceeding?
3. Is the defendant malingering?

There are nine primary areas in which the mental health or competence of a defendant can be of issue, and which therefore may merit a neuropsychological evaluation, including: (a) competence to waive Miranda, (b) competence to waive right to counsel, (c) competence to stand trial, (d) advisement of rights and validity of confessions, (e) entry of a plea, (f) determination of criminal responsibility, (g) advisability of defendant testifying, (h) sentencing, and (i) competence for execution.

Competence to Stand Trial

Assessments related to competency to stand trial are one of the most common reasons for mental health evaluations within the criminal justice system. The courts recognize that a defendant's cognitive, mental, or emotional difficulties might interfere with the defendant's right to a fair trial. A U.S. Supreme Court decision, *Dusky v. United States* (1960) laid out the parameters to assess whether a defendant is competent to proceed to trial. There is a two-pronged test, consisting of a cognitive prong and an interpersonal/communication prong. Under the cognitive prong the question is: Does the defendant, as a result of mental disease or defect, lack the capacity to understand the proceedings against him or her? This can involve an assessment of cognitive functions, including orientation, attention, comprehension, and memory. The question under the interpersonal/behavioral cooperation prong is: Does the defendant lack the capacity to meaningfully assist in his or her own defense? The issue here is to determine if the defendant maintains adequate communication and reasoning skills to communicate with his or her attorney to participate in the proceeding: Can the defendant participate in his or her defense? Are the requisite receptive and expressive language skills, memory, and executive functioning (including reasoning) skills present for the defendant to work with his or her counsel? (Grisso, 2003; Kirkish & Sreenivasan, 1999; Martell, 1992; Nestor, Daggett, Haycock, & Price, 1999).

Entry of a Plea/Not Guilty by Reason of Insanity

To be tried for a crime, the law requires that an individual engaged in an unlawful act and did so with unlawful intent. The law assumes free will, but also recognizes that there are individuals who have impaired cognitive or volitional abilities. If this is so, then their culpability may be diminished (Grisso, 2003). The purpose of the "not guilty by reason of insanity" defense is to prevent imposition of criminal sanctions on an individual who may not be fully responsible for his or her actions (Diaz, 1995).

"Insanity" is not a psychiatric term, but is instead defined by the legal system. Depending on the jurisdiction, there are different "tests" that are applied to determine if a person is legally insane, but the primary question involves determining if the person has a mental illness that resulted in decreased capacity to appreciate the wrongfulness of his or her action. Depending on the test, issues around impaired cognition and/or impulse control come into play. The neuropsychologist's role in these proceedings is to quantify the degree of impairment and assist the trier of fact in determining whether the deficits constitute a lack of capacity. It is not the role of the neuropsychologist to determine if the defendant is insane.

A related area is diminished capacity. Different from not guilty by reason of insanity, the defense tries to argue that the defendant lacked capacity to form the criminal intent for the crime for which he is being charged, but instead should be convicted of a lesser charge (e.g., manslaughter vs. murder). In this case, neuropsychological evaluation results could help the trier of fact to understand the cognitive limitations of the defendant with regard to the cognitive skills needed to commit the relevant crime (Martell, 1992; Rehkopf & Fisher, 1997).

Other Areas

Advisement and waiver of rights and validity of confessions relates to the defendant's ability to understand his or her Miranda rights and knowingly consent, without coercion, to a police search. If the defendant's attorney questions whether his or her client lacked adequate mental skills at the time rights were waived or a search was done, a neuropsychologist may be asked to provide data to support this supposition. A neuropsychologist may be called in to determine if a defendant's cognitive or behavioral impairment limits his or her ability to testify. If the defense wants the defendant to testify, information about impairments (e.g., limited vocabulary, expressive speech impairments etc.) may help the trier of fact better understand the behaviors they are seeing on the stand. This information can also help the defense lawyer in preparing to examine his or her client on the stand.

Once a defendant is found guilty or not guilty by reason of insanity, the results of the neuropsychological evaluation can assist the trier of fact in determining the appropriate sentence by providing information on how the person may react in certain settings based on brain disease and, at times, assist with appropriate placement.

In *Ford v. Wainwright* (1986), the U.S. Supreme Court determined that the condemned, in order to be executed, must first understand that he has been sentenced to death and why. The neuropsychologist can again play a role in assessing the defendant's cognitive abilities to assist the trier of fact with answering the question of competency to be executed (Grisso, 2003; Rehkopf & Fisher, 1997).

In all proceedings related to the criminal system, it is essential for the neuropsychologist to remember that issues of insanity or incompetence are for the courts to decide. The neuropsychologist's role is to provide objective, quantifiable information to assist the trier of fact with this decision.

Future Directions

There is no reason to believe that interest in retaining clinical neuropsychologists to render expert opinions in adversarial proceedings will wane. In fact, because neuropsychologists offer unique information that is scientifically grounded, the trend is more likely to continue in the direction of increased interest. This may be especially true in the area of pediatric neuropsychology, which is beginning to receive the degree of attention shown in the area of adult neuropsychology (Wills & Sweet, 2006).

Key Areas of Forensic Research

Within pediatric and adult neuropsychology there are specific areas of knowledge that bear directly on issues commonly addressed. Most, but not all, are areas within which clinical neuropsychologists have inherent, substantial interests. Areas in which continued research investigations are needed and likely to continue are: (a) continued development of techniques for evaluating effort, especially for use with children and adolescents, (b) improved normative studies that elucidate important variables such as minority status, influence of culture, and educational deprivation, (c) more specific research related to ecological validity that might enable more precise correlations between test findings and expectations of daily functioning, and (d) greater specificity in ruling in or ruling out the etiology of patterns of strengths and weaknesses found on formal ability and emotional testing. To be sure, there will never be a point at which further research will not be helpful in almost any health care or forensic endeavor. However, there are some areas, such as those listed here, in which the forensic questions neuropsychologists are often asked, and assuredly will continue to be asked, frequently seem to outdistance our ability to respond with empirically based answers.

Need for Formal Training of Future Neuropsychologists

The academic preparation of clinical neuropsychologists for participation in forensic activities remains generally absent. Almost all clinical psychology doctoral programs offer one or more courses pertaining to clinical neuropsychology, which has been true for many years (Wedding & Williams, 1983). However, at present, very few programs have substantive coursework preparing clinical neuropsychology practitioners for their inevitable involvement in forensic work. Because neuropsychologists have clinical interactions with individuals whose disorders stem from situations (e.g., accidents, assaults, environmental exposure, or medical errors) in which someone can be accused of being at fault, plus numerous individuals who because of possible disability are applying for some type of benefit, there is almost no way that a practitioner can avoid requests to provide relevant information to triers-of-fact. Academic preparation is necessary for the nearly unavoidable involvement in forensic activities. Kaufmann and Greiffenstein (2013) recently called upon neuropsychology to revisit and revise training requirements to respond to the growing demand for forensic consultation. It seems quite likely that clinical psychology training programs at the graduate school and internship levels with a strong commitment to training clinical psychologists will begin to develop curricula to facilitate knowledge and skill acquisition in this important practice area. Minimally, a graduate school curriculum for all doctoral students intending to enter clinical neuropsychology could include a required course in the fundamentals of forensic neuropsychology followed by an advanced seminar of special topics and controversial issues. Practicum experiences may be difficult to find at the graduate student level, both because of scarcity in practicum sites and also because involving students in such evaluations is almost always contraindicated as mistakes by beginners should not be entered into such evaluations. Those practicum sites at which forensic cases are seen by staff can provide didactic exposure to students in case conference and group supervision formats. Actual practical experience in forensic neuropsychology can be included within clinical internships and residencies, many of which are housed in medical settings at which practitioners become involved in conducting IMEs or as retained experts in litigation cases.

Notes

1 Meaning the current case being heard by the court.
2 Jurisdictions relying on a *Frye* standard include California, the District of Columbia, Florida, Illinois, Kansas, Maryland, Minnesota, New Jersey, New York, Pennsylvania, and Washington. Most recently, Arizona, Alabama, and Wisconsin abandoned *Frye*. California is likely next; see *Sargon Enters., Inc. v. Univ. of S. Cal.* (2012).
3 There is no genuine issue of material fact upon which the plaintiff could prevail as a matter of law. The trial judge rendered a verdict for Merrell Dow based on briefs without a trial.
4 The most common mechanism used by the U.S. Supreme Court chooses to hear a case by order directing a lower court to deliver the case record.
5 A motion to limit or exclude allegedly prejudicial evidence presented to the judge or during a trial.

References

American Academy of Clinical Neuropsychology. (2003). Official position of the American academy of clinical neuropsychology on ethical complaints made against clinical neuropsychologists during adversarial proceedings. *The Clinical Neuropsychologist, 17*, 443–445. [Online]. Retrieved from www.tandfonline.com/doi/pdf/10.1076/clin.17.4.443.27943. (last visited November 30, 2013).

American Bar Association. (2002). Model rules of professional conduct, [Online]. Retrieved from www.Americanbar.org/groups/professional_responsibility/publications/model_rules_of_professional_conduct.html (last visited November 30, 2013).

American Congress of Rehabilitation Medicine (ACRM). (1993). Definition of mild traumatic brain injury. *Journal of Head Trauma and Rehabilitation, 8*(3), 86–87.

American Medical Association. (2016a). *Chapter 1: Opinions on patient-physician relationships,* [Online]. Retrieved from https://www.ama-assn.org/delivering-care/ama-code-medical-ethics

American Medical Association. (2016b). *Chapter 3: Opinions on privacy, confidentiality & medical records,* [Online]. Retrieved from https://www.ama-assn.org/delivering-care/ama-code-medical-ethics

American Psychological Association. (2017). *Ethical principles of psychologists and code of conduct.* [Online]. Retrieved from www.apa.org/ethics/code/principles.pdf

American Psychological Association. (2013). Specialty guidelines for forensic psychology. *American Psychologist, 68*(1), 7–19. [Online]. Retrieved from www.apa.org/pubs/journals/features/forensic-psychology.pdf

Attix, D. K., Donders, J., Johnson-Greene, D., Grote, C. L., Harris, J. G., & Bauer, R. (2007). Disclosure of neuropsychological test data: Official position of division 40 (Clinical Neuropsychology) of the American Psychological Association, Association of Postdoctoral Programs in Clinical Neuropsychology, and the American Academy of Clinical Neuropsychology. *The Clinical Neuropsychologist*, *21*, 232–238, [Online]. Retrieved from www.tandfonline.com/doi/pdf/10.1080/13854040601042928 (last visited November 30, 2013).

Baker, R. R., Lichtenberg, P. A., & Moye, J. (1998). A practice guideline for assessment of competency and capacity of the older adult. *Professional Psychology: Research and Practice*, *29*(2), 149–154.

Barlow, D. H., Hayes, S. C., & Nelson, R. O. (1984). *The Scientist Practitioner: Research and Accountability in Clinical and Educational Settings*. New York: Pergamon.

Barth, J. T., Ryan, T. V., & Hawk, G. L. (1991). Forensic neuropsychology: A reply to the method skeptics. *Neuropsychology Review*, *2*(3), 251–266.

Baxter et al. v. State, No. 217–2010—CV—00683 (N.H. Sup. Ct., October 29, 2010) (order dismissing claim alleging unconstitutional delay of justice).

Baxter v. Temple, No.01—C—0567 (N.H. Sup. Ct. Aug. 8, 2005) (order granting motion *in limine*).

Baxter v. Temple, 949 A.2d 167 (N.H., 2008).

Baxter v. Temple, unpublished second trial (2012).

Bennett v. Richmond, 932 N.E.2nd 704 (Ind. Ct. Ap., 2010).

Bennett v. Richmond, 960 N.E.2nd 782 (Ind., 2012).

Ben-Porath, Y. S., Greve, K. W., Bianchini, K. J., & Kaufmann, P. M. (2009). The MMPI symptom validity scale (FBS) is an empirically validated measure of over-reporting in personal injury litigants and claimants: Reply to Butcher, et al. (2008). *Psychological Injury and the Law*, *2*(1), 62–85.

Bianchini, K. J., Greve, K. W., & Glynn, G. (2005). On the diagnosis of malingered pain-related disability: Lessons from cognitive malingering research. *The Spine Journal*, *5*(4), 404–417.

Bick, R. L. (1999). The expert witness in litigation and legal matters. In M. A. Shiffman (Ed.), *Ethics in Forensic Science and Medicine: Guidelines for the Forensic Expert and the Attorney* (pp. 19–28). Springfield, IL: Charles C. Thomas.

Bieliauskas, L. A., Fasteneau, P. S., Lacy, M. A., & Roper, B. L. (1997). Use of the odds ratio to translate neuropsychological test scores into real-world outcomes: From statistical significance to clinical significance. *Journal of Clinical & Experimental Neuropsychology*, *19*(6), 889–896.

Boccaccini, M. T., & Brodsky, S. L. (1999). Diagnostic test usage by forensic psychologists in emotional injury cases. *Professional Psychology: Research and Practice*, *30*, 253–259.

Boccaccini, M. T., & Brodsky, S. L. (2002). Believability of expert and lay witnesses: Implications for trial consultation. *Professional Psychology: Research and Practice*, *33*(4), 384–388.

Bordini, E. J., Chaknis, M. M., Ekman-Turner, R. M., & Perna, R. B. (2002). Advances and issues in the diagnostic differential of malingering versus brain injury. *Neurorehabilitation*, *17*, 93–104.

Bowman, M. L. (1997). Ecological validity of neuropsychological and other predictors following head injury. *The Clinical Neuropsychologist*, *10*(4), 382–396.

Braden, J. P. (2003). Psychological assessment in school settings. In J. R. Graham & J. A. Naglieri (Vol. Eds.), *Handbook of Psychology* (pp. 261–290). New York: Wiley.

Braun, M., Tupper, D., Kaufmann, P., McCrea, M., Postal, K., Westerveld, M., . . . Deer, T. (2011). Neuropsychological assessment: A valuable tool in the diagnosis and management of neurological, neurodevelopmental, medical, and psychiatric disorders. *Cognitive and Behavioral Neurology*, *24*(3), 107–114.

Brief for Amicus Curiae American Academy of Clinical Neuropsychology. *Baxter v. Temple* (N.H., 2008).

Brodsky, S. L., & McKinzey, R. K. (2002). The ethical confrontation of the unethical forensic colleague. *Professional Psychology: Research and Practice*, *33*(3), 307–309.

Burgess, P. W., Alderman, N., Evans, J., Emslie, H., & Wilson, B. A. (1998). The ecological validity of tests of executive function. *Journal of the International Neuropsychological Society*, *4*(6), 547–558.

Bush, S. S., Barth, J. T., Pliskin, N. H., Arffa, S., Axelrod, B. N., Blackburn, L. A., . . . Silver, C. H. (2005). Independent and court-ordered forensic neuropsychological examinations: Official NAN position. *Archives of Clinical Neuropsychology*, *20*, 997–1007. [Online]. Retrieved from www.nanonline.org/docs/PAIC/PDFs/NANIMEpaper.pdf (last visited November 30, 2013).

Canadian Academy of Psychologists in Disability Assessment. (2000). Practice standards for the psychological assessment of disability and impairment. [Online]. Retrieved from www.capda.ca/docs/resources/practice-standards-for-the-psychological-assessment-of-disability-and-impairment.pdf?sfvrsn=2 (last visited November 30, 2013).

Claar v. Burlington N.R.R., 29 F.3d 499 (9th Cir. 1994).

Coleman, R. D., Rapport, L. J., Millis, S. R., Ricker, J. H., & Farchione, T. J. (1998). Effects of coaching on detection of malingering on the California Verbal Learning Test. *Journal of Clinical and Experimental Neuropsychology*, *20*(2), 201–210.

Cullen v. Pinholster, 131 S. Ct. 1388 (U.S. 2011).

Daubert v. Merrell Dow Pharm., Inc., 43 F.3d 1311 (9th Cir., 1995).

Daubert v. Merrell Dow Pharm., Inc., 509 U.S. 579 (U.S. 1993).

Daubert v. Merrell Dow Pharm., Inc., 727 F. Supp. 570, 575 (S.D. Cal. 1989).

Daubert v. Merrell Dow Pharm., Inc., 951 F.2d 1128 (9th Cir. 1992).

Demakis, G. J. (2016). Special issue on civil capacity assessment in clinical neuropsychology. *Archives of Clinical Neuropsychology*, *31*(6), 485–569.

Demakis, G. J., Sweet, J. J., Sawyer, T. P., Moulthrop, M., Nies, K., & Clingerman, S. (2001). Discrepancy between predicted and obtained WAIS-R IQ scores discriminates between traumatic brain injury and insufficient effort. *Psychological Assessment*, *13*(2), 240–248.

Department of Veterans Affairs. (1997). *Assessment of Competency and Capacity of the Older Adult: A Practice Guideline for Psychologists*. Milwaukee, WI: National Center for Cost Containment. (NTIS No. PB970147904).

Desmond, J. M. (Winter, 2007). Admissibility of neuropsychological evidence in New Hampshire. *New Hampshire Bar Journal*, *47*(4), 12–17, [Online]. Retrieved from www.nhbar.org/publications/display-journal-issue.asp?id=347 (last visited November 30, 2013).

Diaz, F. G. (1995). Traumatic injury and criminal behaviour. *Medicine and the Law*, *14*, 131–140.

Dixon, L., & Gill, B. (2002). Changes in the standards for admitting expert evidence in federal civil cases since the *Daubert* decision. *Psychology, Public Policy, and Law*, *8*(3), 251–308.

Dusky v. United States, 362 U.S. 402 (1960).

Faust, D. (1991). Forensic neuropsychology: The art of practicing a science that does not yet exist. *Neuropsychology Review*, *2*(3), 205–231.

Faust, D., & Ziskin, J. (1988). The expert witness in psychology and psychiatry. *Science*, *241*, 31–35.

Faust, D., Ziskin, J., & Hiers, J. (1991). *Brain Damage Claims: Coping With Neuropsychological Evidence*. Los Angeles: Law and Psychology Press.

Fellows, L. K. (1998). Competency and consent in dementia. *Journal of the American Geriatrics Society*, *46*, 922–926.

Fisher, M. (1997). The psychologist as "hired gun." *The American Journal of Forensic Psychology*, *15*(2), 25–30.

Folstein, M. F., Folstein, S. E., & McHugh, P. R. (1975). "Mini-mental state": A practical method for grading the cognitive state of patients for the clinician. *Journal of Psychiatric Research*, *12*, 189–198.

Ford v. Wainwright, 477 U.S. 399 (1986).

Franzen, M. D., Burgess, E. J., & Smith-Seemiller, L. (1997). Methods of estimating premorbid functioning. *Archives of Clinical Neuropsychology*, *12*(8), 711–738.

Franzen, M. D., Iverson, G., & McCracken, L. (1990). The detection of malingering in neuropsychological assessment. *Neuropsychology Review*, *1*, 247–279.

Frye v. United States, 293 F. 1013 (D.C. Cir. 1923).

General Electric Co. v. Joiner, 522 U.S. 136 (1997).

Goldberg, E., & Podell, K. (2000). Adaptive decision making, ecological validity, and the frontal lobes. *Journal of Clinical and Experimental Neuropsychology*, *22*(1), 56–68.

Grant, D. (1997). Independent medical examinations and the fuzzy politics of disclosure. *Canadian Medical Association Journal*, *156*(1), 73–75.

Green, P., Iverson, G. L., & Allen, L. (1999). Detecting malingering in head injury litigation with the word memory test. *Brain Injury*, *13*(10), 813–819.

Green, P., Rohling, M. L., Lees-Haley, P. R., & Allen, L. M. (2001). Effort has a greater effect on test scores than severe brain injury in compensation claimants. *Brain Injury*, *15*(12), 1045–1060.

Greiffenstein, M. F., Baker, W. J., & Johnson-Greene, D. (2002). Actual versus self-reported scholastic achievement of litigating postconcussion and severe closed injury claimants. *Psychological Assessment*, *14*(2), 202–208.

Greiffenstein, M. F., & Kaufmann, P. M. (2012). Neuropsychology and the law: Principles of productive attorney-neuropsychologist relations. In G. Larrabee (Ed.), *Forensic Neuropsychology: A Scientific Approach* (2nd ed., pp. 23–69). New York: Oxford University Press.

Greenberg, S. A., & Shuman, D. W. (1997). Irreconcilable conflict between therapeutic and forensic roles. *Professional Psychology: Research and Practice*, *28*, 50–57.

Greenberg, S. A., & Shuman, D. W. (2007). When worlds collide: Therapeutic and forensic roles. *Professional Psychology: Research and Practice*, *38*(2), 129–132.

Grisso, T. (2003). *Evaluating Competencies: Forensic Assessments and Instruments* (2nd ed.). New York: Kluwer Academic/Plenum Publishers.

Grote, C. (2005). Ethical practice of forensic neuropsychology. In G. Larrabee (Ed.), *Forensic Neuropsychology: A Scientific Approach* (pp. 92–114). New York: Oxford University Press.

Grote, C. L., Lewin, J. L., Sweet, J. J., & van Gorp, W. G. (2000). Responses to perceived unethical practices in clinical neuropsychology: Ethical and legal considerations. *The Clinical Neuropsychologist*, *14*(1), 119–134.

Grove, W. M., & Barden, R. C. (1999). Protecting the integrity of the legal system: The admissibility of testimony from mental health experts under *Daubert/Kumho* analyses. *Psychology, Public Policy, and Law*, *5*(1), 224–242.

Guilmet-De Simone, H., & Greenspan, L. (1997). Disclosure and independent medical examinations. *Canadian Medical Association Journal*, *157*(7), 977.

Guilmette, T. J., & Hagan, L. D. (1997). Ethical considerations in forensic neuropsychological consultation. *The Clinical Neuropsychologist*, *11*(3), 287–290.

Gutheil, T. G., Commons, M. L., & Miller, P. M. (2001). Withholding, seducing, and threatening: A pilot study of further attorney pressures on expert witnesses. *Journal of the American Academy of Psychiatry and Law*, *29*, 336–339.

Gutheil, T. G., & Simon, R. I. (1999). Attorneys' pressures on the expert witness: Early warning signs of endangered honesty, objectivity, and fair compensation. *Journal of the American Academy of Psychiatry and Law*, *27*, 546–553.

Haffey, W. J. (1989). The assessment of clinical competency to consent to medical rehabilitative interventions. *Journal of Head Trauma and Rehabilitation*, *4*(1), 43–56.

Haines, M., & Norris, M. (1995). Detecting the malingering of cognitive deficits: An update. *Neuropsychology Review*, *5*, 125–148.

Hannay, H. J., Bieliauskas, L. A., Crosson, B. A., Hammeke, T. A., Hamsher, K. deS., & Koffler, S. P. (1998). Proceedings of the Houston conference on specialty education and training in clinical neuropsychology. *Archives of Clinical Neuropsychology, Special Issue*, *13*(2), 157–250.

Hart, T., & Nagele, D. (1996). The assessment of competency in traumatic brain injury. *Neurorehabilitation*, *7*, 27–38.

Hartlage, L. C. (1997). Forensic aspects of mild brain injury. *Applied Neuropsychology*, *4*(1), 69–74.

Hartman, D. E. (1995). *Neuropsychological Toxicology: Identification and Assessment of Neurotoxic Syndromes*. New York: Plenum.

Hartman, D. E. (1999). Neuropsychology and the (neuro)toxic tort. In J. Sweet (Ed.), *Forensic Neuropsychology: Fundamentals and Practice* (pp. 339–367). Lisse, Netherlands: Swets & Zeitlinger.

Hayes, J. S., Hilsabeck, R. C., & Gouvier, W. D. (1999). Malingering traumatic brain injury: Current issues and caveats in assessment and classification. In N. R. Varney & R. J. Roberts (Eds.), *The Evaluation and Treatment of Mild Traumatic Brain Injury* (pp. 249–290). Mahwah, NJ: Lawrence Erlbaum Associates.

Heilbronner, R. L. (2004). A status report on the practice of forensic neuropsychology. *The Clinical Neuropsychologist*, *18*, 312–326.

Heilbronner, R. L., Sweet, J. J., Morgan, J. E., Larrabee, G. J., Millis, S. R., & Conference Participants. (2009). American academy of clinical neuropsychology consensus conference statement on the neuropsychological assessment of effort, response bias, and malingering. *The Clinical Neuropsychologist*, *23*(7), 1093–1129.

Heilbrun, K. (2001). *Principles of Forensic Mental Health Assessment*. New York: Kluwer Academic/Plenum.

Heltzel, T. (2007). Compatibility of therapeutic and forensic roles. *Professional Psychology: Research and Practice*, *38*(2), 122–128.

Hess, A. K. (1998). Accepting forensic case referrals: Ethical and professional considerations. *Professional Psychology: Research and Practice*, *29*(2), 109–114.

Hines v. Welch, 23 F.2d 979 (D.C. Cir. 1928).
Hovey v. Hobson, 55 Me. 256 (Me. 1867).
Huber, P. W. (1991). *Galileo's Revenge: Junk Science in the Courtroom*. New York: Basic Books.
Iverson, G., & Binder, L. (2000). Detecting exaggeration and malingering in neuropsychological assessment. *Journal of Head Trauma Rehabilitation*, *15*, 829–858.
Johnson, M. T., Krafka, C., & Cecil, J. S. (2000). *Expert Testimony in Federal Civil Trials: A Preliminary Analysis.* Washington, DC: Federal Judicial Center.
Johnson-Greene, D., & Bechtold, K. T. (2002). Ethical considerations for peer review in forensic neuropsychology. *The Clinical Neuropsychologist*, *16*(1), 97–104.
Joint Committee on Standards for Educational and Psychological Testing. (1999). *Standards for Educational and Psychological Testing*. Washington DC: American Educational Resource Association.
Kareken, D. A. (1997). Judgment pitfalls in estimating premorbid intellectual function. *Archives of Clinical Neuropsychology*, *12*(8), 701–709.
Kaufmann, P. M. (2005). Protecting the objectivity, fairness, and integrity of neuropsychological evaluations in litigation: A privilege second to none? *Journal of Legal Medicine*, *26*, 95–131.
Kaufmann, P. M. (2009). Protecting raw data and psychological tests from wrongful disclosure: A primer on the law and other persuasive strategies. *The Clinical Neuropsychologist*, *23*(7), 1130–1159.
Kaufmann, P. M. (2012). Admissibility of expert opinions based on neuropsychological evidence. In G. Larrabee (Ed.), *Forensic Neuropsychology: A Scientific Approach* (2nd ed., pp. 70–100). New York: Oxford University Press.
Kaufmann, P. M., & Greiffenstein, M. F. (2013). Forensic neuropsychology: Training, scope of practice, and quality control. *NAN Bulletin*, *27*(1), 11–15.
Kaufmann, P. M. (2016). Neuropsychologist experts and civil capacity evaluations: Representative cases. *Archives of Clinical Neuropsychology*, *31*(6), 487–494.
Kay, T. (1999). Interpreting apparent neuropsychological deficits: What is really wrong? In J. J. Sweet (Ed.), *Forensic Neuropsychology: Fundamentals and Practice* (pp. 145–183). Lisse, Netherlands: Swets & Zeitlinger.
Kim, S.Y.H., Karlawish, J.H.T., & Caine, E. D. (2002). Current state of research on decision-making competence of cognitively impaired elderly persons. *American Journal of Geriatric Psychiatry*, *10*(2), 151–165.
Kirkish, P., & Sreenivasan, S. (1999). Neuropsychological assessment of competency to stand trial evaluations: A practical conceptual model. *Journal of the American Academy of Psychiatry and the Law*, *27*(1), 101–113.
Klonoff, P. S., & Lamb, D. G. (1998). Mild head injury, significant impairment on neuropsychological test scores, and psychiatric disability. *The Clinical Neuropsychologist*, *12*(1), 31–42.
Knapp, S., & VandeCreek, L. (2001). Ethical issues in personality assessment in forensic psychology. *Journal of Personality Assessment*, *77*(2), 242–254.
Krafka, C., Dunn, M. A., Treadway Johnson, M., Cecil, J. S., & Miletich, D. (2002). Judge and attorney experiences, practices, and concerns regarding expert testimony in federal civil trials. *Psychology, Public Policy, and Law*, *8*(3), 309–332.
Kraus, J. (1997). The independent medical examination and the functional capacity evaluation. *Occupational Medicine*, *12*, 525–556.
Kumho Tire Co. v. Carmichael, 526 U.S. 137 (1999).
Laing, L. C., & Fisher, J. M. (1997). Neuropsychology in civil proceedings. In R. J. McCaffrey, A. D. Williams, J. M. Fisher, & L. C. Laing (Eds.), *The Practice of Forensic Neuropsychology: Meeting Challenges in the Courtroom* (pp. 117–133). New York: Plenum Press.
Larrabee, G. J. (2012). *Forensic Neuropsychology: A Scientific Approach* (2nd ed.). New York: Oxford University Press.
LeBlanc, J. M., Hayden, M. E., & Paulman, R. G. (2000). A comparison of neuropsychological and situational assessment for predicting employability after closed head injury. *Journal of Head Trauma Rehabilitation*, *15*, 1022–1040.
Lees-Haley, P. R. (1997a). Attorneys influence expert evidence in forensic psychological and neuropsychological cases. *Assessment*, *4*(4), 321–324.
Lees-Haley, P. R. (1997b). Neurobehavioral assessment in toxic injury evaluations. *Applied Neuropsychology*, *4*(3), 180–190.
Lees-Haley, P. R., & Cohen, L. (1999). The neuropsychologist as expert witness: Toward credible science in the courtroom. In J. Sweet (Ed.), *Forensic Neuropsychology: Fundamentals and Practice* (pp. 443–468). Lisse, Netherlands: Swets & Zeitlinger.
Lees-Haley, P. R., English, L. T., & Glenn, W. J. (1991). A fake bad scale on the MMPI-2 for personal injury claimants. *Psychological Reports*, *68*(1), 203–210.
Long, C. J., & Collins, L. F. (1997). Ecological validity and forensic neuropsychological assessment. In R. McCaffrey, A. Williams, J. Fisher, & L. Laing (Eds.), *The Practice of Forensic Neuropsychology: Meeting Challenges in the Courtroom* (pp. 153–164). New York: Plenum Press.
Lorber, R., & Yurk, H. (1999). Special pediatric issues: Neuropsychological applications and consultations in schools. In J. Sweet (Ed.), *Forensic Neuropsychology: Fundamentals and Practice* (pp. 369–418). Lisse, Netherlands: Swets & Zeitlinger.
Marson, D. C. (2001). Loss of financial competency in dementia: Conceptual and empirical approaches. *Aging, Neuropsychology and Cognition*, *8*(3), 164–181.
Marson, D. C., & Harrell, L. (1999). Neurocognitive changes associated with loss of capacity to consent to medical treatment in patients with Alzheimer's Disease. In D. C. Park, R. W. Morrell, & K. Shifren (Eds.), *Processing of Medical Information in Aging Patients* (pp. 117–136). Mahwah, NJ: Lawrence Erlbaum Associates.
Martell, D. A. (1992). Forensic neuropsychology and the criminal law. *Law and Human Behavior*, *16*(3), 313–336.
Martelli, M. M., Bush, S. S., & Zasler, N. D. (2003). Identifying, avoiding, and addressing ethical misconduct in neuropsychological medicolegal practice. *International Journal of Forensic Psychology*, *1*(1), 26–44.
Martelli, M. F., Zasler, N. D., & Grayson, R. (1999a). Ethical considerations in medicolegal evaluation of neurologic injury and impairment following acquired brain injury. *Neurorehabilitation*, *13*, 45–66.
Martelli, M. M., Zasler, N. D., & Grayson, R. L. (1999b). Medicolegal evaluation of impairment after brain injury. In M. Shiffman (Ed.), *Ethics in Forensic Science and Medicine* (pp. 194–235). Springfield, IL: Charles C. Thomas.

Matarazzo, J. D. (1990). Psychological assessment versus psychological testing: Validation from Binet to the school, clinic, and courtroom. *American Psychologist*, *45*(9), 999–1017.

Matarazzo, J. D. (1991). Psychological assessment is reliable and valid: Reply to Ziskin and Faust. *American Psychologist*, *46*(8), 882–884.

McCrystal, L. (2012, September 23). Concord/Wakefield 11 years on, verdict in lead case. *Concord Monitor*. Retrieved November 30, 2013 from www.concordmonitor.com/news/

MDEX Online. (2017). *Daubert Tracker* [website]. Retrieved from www.dauberttracker.com.

Melton, G. B., Petrila, J., Poythress, N. G., & Slobogin, C. (1997). *Psychological Evaluations for the Courts: A Handbook for Mental Health Professionals and Lawyers* (2nd ed.). New York: Guilford Press.

Miller, L. (1993). Toxic torts: Clinical, neuropsychological and forensic aspects of chemical and electrical injuries. *The Journal of Cognitive Rehabilitation*, *11*(1), 6–18.

Miller, W., & Miller, E. (1992). Malingering and neuropsychological assessment. *Physical Medicine and Rehabilitation: State of the Art Reviews*, *6*, 547–563.

Millis, S., & Putnam, S. (1996). Detection of malingering in postconcussive syndrome. In M. Rizzo & D. Tranel (Eds.), *Head Injury and Postconcussive Disorder* (pp. 481–498). New York: Churchill Livingston.

Mitrushina, M. N., Boone, K. B., & D'Elia, L. F. (1999). *Handbook of Normative Data for Neuropsychological Assessment*. New York: Oxford University Press.

Murrey, G. J. (2000). Overview of traumatic brain injury: Issues in the forensic assessment. In G. J. Murrey (Ed.), *The Forensic Evaluation of Traumatic Brain Injury* (pp. 1–22). Boca Raton, FL: CRC Press LLC.

NAN Policy and Planning Committee. (2000). Test security: Official position statement of the National Academy of Neuropsychology. *Archives of Clinical Neuropsychology*, *15*(5), 383–386.

NAN Policy and Planning Committee (Barth, J. T., Pliskin, N., Axelrod, B., Faust, D., Fisher, J., Harley, H. J., . . . Silver, C.). (2003). Introduction to the NAN 2001 definition of a clinical neuropsychologist: NAN policy and planning committee. *Archives of Clinical Neuropsychology*, *18*(5), 551–555.

Nestor, P. G., Daggett, D., Haycock, J., & Price, M. (1999). Competence to stand trial: A neuropsychological inquiry. *Law and Human Behavior*, *23*(4), 397–412.

Nies, K., & Sweet, J. (1994). Neuropsychological assessment and malingering: A critical review of past and present strategies. *Archives of Clinical Neuropsychology*, *9*, 501–552.

Osmon, D. C. (1999). Complexities in the evaluation of executive functions. In J. J. Sweet (Ed.), *Forensic Neuropsychology: Fundamentals and Practice* (pp. 185–226). Lisse, Netherlands: Swets & Zeitlinger.

Perlo, S. (1996). The ABCs of psychiatric disability evaluations. *Occupational Medicine*, *11*(4), 747–765.

Putnam, S. H., Ricker, J. H., Ross, S. R., & Kurtz, J. E. (1999). Considering premorbid functioning: Beyond cognition to a conceptualization of personality in postinjury functioning. In J. J. Sweet (Ed.), *Forensic Neuropsychology: Fundamentals and Practice* (pp. 39–81). Lisse, Netherlands: Swets & Zeitlinger.

Rankin, E. J., & Adams, R. L. (1999). The neuropsychological evaluation: Clinical and scientific foundations. In J. J. Sweet (Ed.), *Forensic Neuropsychology: Fundamentals and Practice* (pp. 83–119). Lisse, Netherlands: Swets & Zeitlinger.

Rehkopf, D. G., & Fisher, J. M. (1997). Neuropsychology in criminal proceedings. In R. J. McCaffrey, A. D. Williams, J. M. Fisher, & L. C. Laing (Eds.), *The Practice of Forensic Neuropsychology: Meetings Challenges in the Courtroom* (pp. 135–151). New York: Plenum Press.

Rogers, R., Harrell, E., & Liff, C. (1993). Feigning neuropsychological impairment: A critical review of methodological and clinical considerations. *Clinical Psychology Review*, *13*, 255–275.

Rosenfeld, S. J. (2003). Section 504 and IDEA: Basic similarities and differences. [Online]. Retrieved from www.ldonline.org/ld_indepth/legal_legislative/edlaw504.html

Ruff, R. M., & Richardson, A. M. (1999). Mild traumatic brain injury. In J. Sweet (Ed.), *Forensic Neuropsychology: Fundamentals and Practice* (pp. 315–338). Lisse, Netherlands: Swets & Zeitlinger.

Sargon Enters., Inc. v. Univ. of S. Cal., 288 P. 3d 1237 (Cal. 2012).

Sbordone, R. J. (2001). Limitations of neuropsychological testing to predict the cognitive and behavioral functioning of persons with brain injury in real-word settings. *Neurorehabilitation*, *16*(4), 199–201.

Sbordone, R. J., & Long, C. J. (1996). *Ecological Validity of Neuropsychological Testing*. Delray Beach, FL: GR Press/St. Lucie Press.

Sheehan v. Daily Racing Form, Inc., 104 F.3d 940, 942 (7th Cir. 1997).

Sherman, E. S., & Brooks, B. L. (2012). *Pediatric Forensic Neuropsychology*. New York: Oxford University Press.

Shuman, D. W., & Sales, B. D. (1999). The impact of *Daubert* and its progeny on the admissibility of behavioral and social science evidence. *Psychology, Public Policy, and Law*, *5*(1), 3–15.

Silver, J. M., & McAllister, T. W. (1997). Forensic issues in the neuropsychiatric evaluation of the patient with mild traumatic brain injury. *Journal of Neuropsychiatry*, *9*(1), 102–113.

Slick, D. J., Hopp, G., Strauss, E., & Spellacy, F. J. (1996). Victoria symptom validity test: Efficiency for detecting feigned memory impairment and relationship to neuropsychological tests and MMPI-2 validity scales. *Journal of Clinical and Experimental Neuropsychology*, *18*(6), 911–922.

Slick, D. J., Sherman, E.M.S., & Iverson, G. L. (1999). Diagnostic criteria for malingered neurocognitive dysfunction: Proposed standards for clinical practice and research. *The Clinical Neuropsychologist*, *13*(4), 545–561.

Smith v. Metropolitan Life Insurance Company, 317 Ill. App. 624 (Ill. App. Ct. 1943).

State v. Dahood, 814 A.2d 159 (N.H., 2002).

State v. Knight, 95 Me. 467, (Me. 1901).

Stern, B. H. (1997). Approach to handling brain injury cases. *Trial Diplomacy Journal*, *20*, 201–205.

Sweet, J. J. (Ed.). (1999a). *Forensic Neuropsychology: Fundamentals and Practice*. Lisse, Netherlands: Swets & Zeitlinger.

Sweet, J. J. (1999b). Malingering: Differential diagnosis. In J. Sweet (Ed.), *Forensic Neuropsychology: Fundamentals and Practice* (pp. 255–285). Lisse, Netherlands: Swets & Zeitlinger.

Sweet, J. J. (2003). Ethics cases: Forensic neuropsychology. In S. Bush (Ed.), *Ethics Casebook for Neuropsychologists* (pp. 51–61). Lisse, Netherlands: Swets & Zeitlinger.

Sweet, J. J., Benson, L. M., Nelson, N. W., & Moberg, P. J. (2015). The American Academy of Clinical Neuropsychology, National Academy of Neuropsychology, and Society for Neuropsychology (APA Division 40) 2015 TCN Professional Practice and "Salary Survey": Professional Practices, Beliefs, and Incomes of U.S. Neuropsychologists. *The Clinical Neuropsychologist*, *29*(8), 1069–1162.

Sweet, J. J., Grote, C., & van Gorp, W. (2002). Ethical issues in forensic neuropsychology. In S. Bush & M. Drexler (Eds.), *Ethical Issues in Clinical Neuropsychology* (pp. 103–133). Lisse, Netherlands: Swets & Zeitlinger.

Sweet, J. J., & King, J. H. (2002). Category test validity indicators: Overview and practice recommendations. *Journal of Forensic Neuropsychology*, *3*, 241–274.

Sweet, J. J., King, J. H., Malina, A., Bergman, M., & Simmons, A. (2002). Documenting the prominence of forensic neuropsychology at national meetings and in relevant professional journals from 1990–2000. *The Clinical Neuropsychologist*, *16*, 481–494.

Sweet, J. J., Meyer, D. G., Nelson, N. W., & Moberg, P. J. (2011). The TCN/AACN 2010 "Salary Survey": Professional Practices, Beliefs, and Incomes of U.S. Neuropsychologists. *The Clinical Neuropsychologist*, *25*(1), 12–61.

Sweet, J. J., Moberg, P., & Suchy, Y. (2000). Ten-year follow-up survey of clinical neuropsychologists: Part II: Private practice and economics. *The Clinical Neuropsychologist*, *14*, 479–495.

Sweet, J. J., & Moulthrop, M. (1999). Self-examination questions as a means of identifying bias in adversarial assessments. *Journal of Forensic Neuropsychology*, *1*, 73–88.

Sweet, J. J., Nelson, N. W., & Moberg, P. J. (2006). The TCN/AACN "Salary Survey": Professional Practices, Beliefs, and Incomes of U.S. Neuropsychologists. *The Clinical Neuropsychologist*, *20*(3), 325–364.

Sweet, J. J., Peck, E., Abramowitz, C., & Etzweiler, S. (2003). National Academy of Neuropsychology/Division 40 (American Psychological Association) Practice Survey of Clinical Neuropsychology in the United States, Part II: Reimbursement experiences, practice economics, billing practices, and incomes. *Archives of Clinical Neuropsychology*, *18*(6), 557–582.

Taylor, J. S. (1999). The legal environment pertaining to clinical neuropsychology. In J. Sweet (Ed.), *Forensic Neuropsychology: Fundamentals and Practice* (pp. 419–442). Lisse, Netherlands: Swets & Zeitlinger.

Tenopyr, M. L. (1999). A scientist-practitioner's viewpoint on the admissibility of behavioral and social scientific information. *Psychology, Public Policy, and Law*, *5*(1), 194–202.

Vanderploeg, R. D., & Curtiss, G. (2001). Malingering assessment: Evaluation of validity of performance. *Neurorehabilitation*, *16*, 245–251.

Wedding, D., & Williams, J. (1983). Training options in behavioral medicine and clinical neuropsychology. *Clinical Neuropsychology*, *5*, 100–102.

Wetter, M. W., & Corrigan, S. K. (1995). Providing information to clients about psychological tests: A survey of attorneys' and law students' attitudes. *Professional Psychology: Research and Practice*, *26*(5), 474–477.

Williams, A. D. (1997). The forensic evaluation of adult traumatic brain injury. In R. J. McCaffrey, A. D. Williams, J. M. Fisher, & L. C. Laing (Eds.), *The Practice of Forensic Neuropsychology: Meeting Challenges in the Courtroom* (pp. 37–56). New York: Plenum Press.

Wills, K., & Sweet, J. (2006). Neuropsychological considerations in forensic child assessment. In J. Sparta & G. Koocher (Eds.), *Forensic Mental Health Assessment of Children and Adolescents* (pp. 260–284). New York: Guilford.

Woody, R. H. (2009). Ethical considerations of multiple roles in Forensic Services. *Ethics and Behavior*, *19*(1), 79–87.

Youngjohn, J. R., Less-Haley, P. R., & Binder, L. M. (1999). Comment: Warning malingerers produces more sophisticated malingering. *Archives of Clinical Neuropsychology*, *14*(6), 511–515.

Zasler, N. D., & Martelli, M. F. (2003). Mild traumatic brain injury: Impairment and disability assessment caveats. *Neuropsychological Rehabilitation*, *13*(1/2), 31–41.

37 Basics of Forensic Neuropsychology

Manfred F. Greiffenstein and Paul M. Kaufmann

Forensic neuropsychology is the practice of providing neuropsychological evidence and opinions for court systems on issues involving cognitive status. In almost all jurisdictions, neuropsychological assessment is recognized as assisting the trier of fact in resolving legal issues such as criminal culpability, mental injury, and competence to conduct affairs independently (Slobogin, 2003). In Shapiro's (1991) view, legal applications of neuropsychology have arrived and are here to stay.

Most neuropsychologists should agree with Sweet's (1999) observation that neuropsychologists neither anticipated nor prepared for courtroom involvement during their training. Bush (2003) argues neuropsychologists are naturally suited for legal activity. Perceived strengths of clinical neuropsychologists include multifaceted analytic abilities (nomothetic, quantitative, idiographic), a nonadversarial and objective ethos, and a multidisciplinary knowledge base (e.g., neuroanatomy, clinical neurology, medical terminology, psychometric methods). The neuroscience knowledge base, used in conjunction with standardized psychometric tests, neuroimaging results, neurodiagnostic findings, neurologic history, interviewing, behavioral observations, and informal assessment means that neuropsychological formulations and expert opinions are scientifically informed and refined by objective test results. As detailed in Sweet, Kaufmann, Ecklund-Johnson, and Malina (Chapter 36 in this volume), neuropsychological techniques easily fulfill state and federal legal standards for scientific methodology because psychological tests and neurodiagnostic techniques are widely accepted and, more importantly, experimentally verified. Kaufmann (2005) argued this practice distinguishes clinical neuropsychology in forensic settings, such that it has little or no redundancy with other health care disciplines or mental health expertise. The cognitive activity of the neuropsychologist underlying differential diagnosis may even be a microcosm of the jury process of sifting through competing hypotheses.

Forensic activities represent a growing percent of neuropsychology private practice (Sweet, Guiffre Meyer, Nelson, & Moberg, 2010). Kaufmann (2016) reported a 97% increase in time devoted to forensic consulting based on his analysis of sequential surveys. Many factors drive interest in forensic neuropsychology, including more income in a managed care era, intellectual curiosity, revenue diversification, and ego gratification. However, there are also perceived impediments that inhibit involvement in forensic activity. These factors include perceptions that the adversarial system is too complex, ignorance of the law and courtroom practices, reluctance to criticize others, and fears of intense public scrutiny. After all, the term *forensic* derives from the Greek word *forensis*, meaning public debate.

The main goal of this chapter is to reduce the perceived complexity of the adversarial system into terms understandable to most neuropsychologists. Involvement in the legal system does not require encyclopedic knowledge of the law and court rulings. Goals of this chapter include describing differences between pure clinical and forensic neuropsychological evaluations, summarizing the empirical foundations of forensic neuropsychology and psychology, briefly describing the history of psychological evidence in the courts, and reviewing landmark rulings as they relate to neuropsychological practice. Other goals include discussion of ethical considerations unique to forensic practice, enumeration of the general and case-specific challenges of forensic work, and to provide practical guidelines for offering testimony. An earlier chapter (Greiffenstein & Kaufmann, 2012) emphasized purely practical aspects of forensic neuropsychology; this chapter better emphasizes the scientific and knowledge bases of the forensic neuropsychology endeavor.

Basic Legal Terminology

Adjustment to any new intellectual endeavor requires a working vocabulary shared by persons engaging in that effort. Whole dictionaries are devoted to legal terminology, but the neuropsychologist should familiarize himself with a small set of terms. The following nomenclature is often encountered in legal filings, depositions, and case law.

Admissibility and *weight* are concepts referring to the legal treatment of evidence. Admissibility rules dictate what evidence is allowed before a jury and is strictly a matter of law decided by the judge. Weight is a jury issue and refers to the relative value assigned to a piece of evidence. Two different neuropsychological approaches may be legally admissible but viewed quite differently by the jury. Confusions between weight and admissibility are common, even among experienced attorneys.

Prejudicial and *probative* are related concepts referring to the relevance of evidence. Prejudicial evidence refers to facts potentially causing strong emotional reactions and is not admissible because of a negative halo effect coloring perception of all the evidence. Probative means the evidence is relevant because it has greater probability to affect a juror's ultimate decision than its presence. Probative evidence is always admissible. At times a piece of evidence may have both qualities, requiring a judge to weigh the probative versus prejudicial value. For example, the information that a plaintiff was imprisoned for a violent crime prior to a compensable head injury may be probative if he claims "dysexecutive and emotional dyscontrol syndrome due to frontal lobe damage" but could be more prejudicial if the damages claim was only headaches. Criminal history may be probative to the claim, but is highly prejudicial to most juries.

Tort and *administrative actions* describe the nature of the legal action. A tort is a civil wrong that justifies initiation of a lawsuit. The elements of a tort are duty, foreseeability, negligence, causation, and damages. A car accident is a tort. Administrative actions refer to legal compensation seeking where tort rights are suspended because fault is not an issue. The plaintiff makes an application for benefits to a government agency rather than civil court (e.g., workers' compensation). *Published* and *unpublished* court opinions denote the scope of a court's decision. Published opinions mean a broad scope of application that is binding on trial judges in future. An unpublished opinion typically means a ruling that is limited to a particular case. The case of *Daubert v. Merrell Dow Pharm, Inc.* (1993) is a U.S. Supreme Court published opinion, meaning it is the law of the land. The case of *Chapelle v. Ganger* (1998; discussed in depth in a later section) is an unpublished opinion about a trial judge's finding of fact applied to a single case. There is no generalizable law derived from an unpublished case.

Most legal research is a search for authority, law that prompts in a more favorable outcome for one party or the other in a dispute. The inherent structure of the law—hierarchy of legal authority—is not readily apparent, even to first-year law students. Legal authority takes several forms: primary and secondary, controlling (binding), and persuasive. *Primary* legal authority (case law, statutes, regulations, administrative agency decisions, executive orders, and treaties) comes directly from a governmental entity in the discharge of its official duties. Courts are constitutionally required to interpret law; for example, case law often requires statutory and regulatory interpretation as applied to specific facts. *Secondary* authority includes other legal research found in attorney general opinions, agency interpretations, law review articles, restatements, treatises, or other commentary. Although courts may accept guidance from a wide range of sources, only primary authority is *controlling* in its application. Whether primary authority is, or is not, controlling, depends on case-specific facts and the jurisdiction in which the case is being heard. That is, courts are bound only by legal authority from the same jurisdiction (federal, state, county, or municipality) that is controlling for that particular type of case. Finally, the decisions of a particular court are controlling for any court lower in the same jurisdictional hierarchy. However, common errors in legal analysis include the mistaken notions that federal cases control state courts, or that federal law always preempts state law. Some federal law does not apply in state courts and is, therefore, not controlling. However, federal law may be *persuasive* in state courts. Case law from other states may be highly persuasive. There are numerous factors that make court decisions persuasive beyond its controlling jurisdiction: factual similarity, sound reasoning, judicial reputation, and level of the court.

Ultimate legal questions refer to those that can be answered by the trier of fact only ("This car accident caused this plaintiff's brain damage"), while *penultimate* testimony refers to opinions just short of the ultimate questions ("The plaintiff's scores are consistent with closed head injury"). There is considerable controversy in the forensic psychology literature as to whether psychologists allow themselves ultimate or penultimate testimony (Melton, Petrila, Poythress, & Slobogin, 1997). Ogloff (1990) discussed methods for testifying on malingering issues in a light of a penultimate-only requirement.

Burdens of proof vary in civil and criminal proceedings. Most civil proceedings use the preponderance of evidence (lowest) standard of proof. However, some probate proceedings require clear and convincing evidence. Criminal cases require proof beyond a reasonable doubt. Kagehiro (1990) estimated confidence levels for each standard as follows: preponderance (> 50%), clear and convincing (~ 75%), and beyond reasonable doubt (~ 90%). However, judges, jurors, and laypersons do not systematically apply such probabilities when rendering judgments (Wright, 2008) and most trial consultants advise that jurors will never decide cases on the basis of probabilities (Ball, 2008). It is also important to recognize which party carries the *burden of persuasion* to meet the burden of proof. In criminal proceedings, the defendant enters court with the presumption of innocence and the state has the burden of persuading the trier of fact that the defendant committed the crime beyond a reasonable doubt. However, when claiming insanity, the defendant must persuade the trier of fact that he or she was insane at the time of the crime. In many jurisdictions, insanity need only meet a clear and convincing standard of proof.

Latin terms are commonly used because much of the adversarial system stems from medieval law. *Stare decisis* is a legal principle dating from the Renaissance and means courts must apply past decisions (precedent) to current cases. *Certiorari* is an order issued by a superior court to a lower court, asking for a certified record of a case the superior court wishes to review. This is the method used by the U.S. Supreme Court to review cases. *In camera* and *in limine* refer to evidentiary hearings without the jury present. They are literally held in the judge's chambers and usually involve admissibility issues. The concurrence of *mens rea* and *actus reus* refer to elements necessary to prove a serious crime: *Mens rea* refers to the mental state preceding a crime and *actus reus* refers to the physical act of the crime. *Mens rea* evidence is challenged in legal insanity defenses. *Amicus curiae* literally means "friend of the court," a person or organization not party to an issue who provides information relevant to the case before bar. The American Psychological Association (APA) may file *amicus briefs* if organized psychology's interests are at stake.

Differences Between Clinical and Forensic Assessments

There is much overlap between forensic and clinical neuropsychology insofar as both rely on the same measurement and scientific bases, neurocognitive constructs, differential diagnosis of generally accepted disorders (Rankin & Adams, 1999), and balanced integration of actuarial (base rate) versus idiographic (clinical) considerations (Berent & Swartz, 1999; Rankin & Adams, 1999; Slobogin, 2003). However, the forensic examination is not just a clinical exam in a legal setting. Instead, there are differences that shape the data collection process, reporting style, interpretation, and dispositional options. An understanding of differences between neuropsychology in clinical and forensic settings is necessary for an effective courtroom role.

Social Context of Evaluation: Expectancies

Symptom expectancies affect self-report and are associated with legal culture. Good arguments can be made that some disorders typically encountered in forensic neuropsychology settings are socially constructed, not disorders of the natural kind. Symptom report differs in societies offering few prospects for compensation or civil litigation. Mickeviciene, Schrader, Nestvold, Surkiene, Kunickas, et al. (2002) found little difference in symptom base rates between concussed and nonconcussed Lithuanian injury victims. Canadians, residing in an adversarial legal culture, reported expectations of more chronic symptoms following concussion than Greek (Ferrari, Constantoyannis, & Papadakis, 2001) and Lithuanian cohorts (Ferrari et al., 2001).

Symptom expectancies may have quantifiable impact on psychometric measures. The stereotype threat is that literature suggests negative expectations can lower test scores compared to groups given neutral invitations for examinations (Brown & Pinel, 2003; Steele, 1997). Suhr and Gunstad (2002) applied this methodology to undergraduates selected for histories of remote concussion. Undergraduates offered pretest neurocognitive expectancies for head injury performed worse on intelligence and memory measures than injured undergraduates given customary instructions. Terming this phenomenon "diagnosis threat," Suhr and Gunstad (2005) later reported brain damage expectancies also negatively influenced attention, psychomotor speed, and working memory tasks. Effort and self-report mood measures did not correlate with group differences. Although only speculative, one theory is that diagnostic threats activate behavioral and/or cognitive schema for acting out "brain damaged" behavior (Wheeler & Petty, 2001). More research is necessary to determine whether compensability augments diagnosis threat.

Social Context: Postincident Exposures

A major contextual difference in forensic matters is postincident influences that are less frequent or prominent than in clinical situations (Greiffenstein & Kaufmann, 2012). There is good empirical evidence for Lees-Haley's (2003) assertion that persons pursuing litigation act differently than nonlitigating patients undergoing evaluations for the same underlying disease. Postincident influences can create genuine-appearing syndromes at the level of clinical history in persons without residual injury, or postincident influences can distort the clinical picture in persons with genuine residual brain damage (Boone & Lu, 2003). Specific postincident influences include compensation, symptom education, forewarning, and coaching.

Compensation is an especially powerful reinforcer of postincident adaptive and illness behavior (Rogers, 1990). Inception cohort studies of patients matched in mild traumatic brain injury (mTBI) severity show those patients pursuing compensation take longer to return to work (Carroll et al., 2004); they also get more medications. However, they continue reporting nearly twice the symptoms of nonlitigating cohorts (Reynolds, Paniak, Toller-Lobe, & Nagy, 2003). The effect size relationship between subjective postincident pain and compensation ranged from 0.48 to 0.60 in a sample of 3,000 inpatients (Binder & Rohling, 1996). In a later meta-analysis of 211 surgery outcome studies, Harris, Mulford, Solomon, van Gelder, and Young (2005) reported poor outcome associated with compensation in a nearly 4:1 ratio relative to noncompensable causation. Pobereskin (2005) followed more than 1,000 whiplash patients and found that preaccident pain and compensation pursuit were the best predictors of one-year symptom status but initial injury severity the weakest.

Another potential influence is symptom education. Volunteer simulators given minimal information about concussion cannot be distinguished from genuinely injured patients on symptom self-report (Martin, Hayes, & Gouvier, 1996). One form of symptom education includes diagnosis-specific attorney coaching (Rosen, 1995; Youngjohn, 1995). The Internet provides another means of symptom information (Risser, 2003). Some attorneys pay fees to Internet companies so public searches of the term <traumatic brain injury> prioritize links to law firm websites. A search on the exact phrase <closed head injury> at Dell Computer's My Way search engine conducted November 2, 2005, produced ten law firm websites at the top of the results screen (e.g., www.

BrainDamageAttorneys.com). All ten offered aggressive pursuit of brain injury claims irrespective of accident severity. A more direct Internet-facilitated threat compromising neuropsychological validity is test-specific information offering forewarning. Ruiz, Drake, Glass, Marcotte, & van Gorp (2002) demonstrated the ease with which focused Internet searches allow nonpsychologists to educate themselves on specific psychological tests such as the Minnesota Multiphasic Personality Inventory–2 (MMPI-2). Empirically, asking volunteers to simulate psychopathology after receiving sensitive task information lowers the diagnostic efficiency of the MMPI-2 validity scales (Lamb, Berry, Wetter, & Baer, 1994; Martin et al., 1996; Storm & Graham, 2000).

These postincident conditions can also make the plaintiff hypervigilant for minor cognitive errors and lead him or her to misattribute these errors to brain dysfunction. Yartz, Zvolensky, Gregor, Feldner, & Leen-Feldner (2005) showed that persons with poor health perception were more likely to engage in bodily oriented catastrophic thinking and symptom vigilance. That is not to say that symptom education is a blanketly negative influence. Indeed, such a psychoeducational approach can truly be helpful to legitimately injured persons (Miller & Mittenberg, 1998).

Status of Self-Report

The self-reported history provides a wealth of information regarding causation and injury impact (Spreen & Strauss, 1998), drives the assessment process, and contributes to diagnosis (Othmer & Othmer, 1989). In clinical settings, there is an assumption of veridicality: The patient is assumed to accurately report his or her inner state. In administrative or forensic settings however, there are stronger incentives to misrepresent one's psychological state, and much depends on the accuracy, honesty, and insight of the claimant (or criminal defendant). A bestselling book, *Stolen Valor*, documented frequent and gross misrepresentation of combat experience in pursuit of veteran's benefits (Burkett & Whitley, 1998). Self-report in litigation should be taken seriously but cannot be relied upon in the same uncritical way as in a pure clinical setting.

Retrospective or present self-report in compensable contexts may show strong perceptual bias. One form of biased reporting is mischaracterization of injury and health history. Schrag, Brown, and Trimble (2004) compared retrospective histories supplied by disability seekers with actual medical records and found so many inaccuracies, they warned, "reported previous diagnoses should not be taken at face value" (p. 608). As an illustration from the neurotoxicology literature, Korgeski and Leon (1983) showed an Agent Orange exposure effect on the MMPI (i.e., more elevated MMPI profiles) when based on veteran-reported estimates of exposure times. This effect disappeared when subjects were regrouped based on records showing actual deployment in areas where Agent Orange exposure was highest.

Other forms of skewed reporting include positive and negative bias. Positive bias refers to exaggeration of preincident attributes and virtues. The claimant may exaggerate his or her educational achievements (Greiffenstein, Baker, & Johnson-Greene, 2002) or report fewer premorbid forgetting episodes than uninjured controls (Mittenberg, Diguilio, Perrin, & Bass, 1992). In contrast, most clinical patients demonstrate conformity between self-report and school records, with the exception of substance abusers (Johnson-Greene et. al., 1997). Negative bias refers to exaggeration of postincident symptoms relative to patients with the same claimed etiology. By way of illustration, the Fake Bad Scale (FBS) is an MMPI-based measure of symptom magnification designed for personal injury contexts to overcome drawbacks of traditional MMPI validity indicators (Lees-Haley, English, & Glenn, 1991). Persons with severe brain injuries seen clinically score very low on the FBS (Miller & Donders, 2001; Woltersdorf, 2005), but mildly injured groups pursuing financial benefits score very high (Greiffenstein, Baker, Donders, & Miller, 2002). Ross, Millis, Krukowski, Putnam, and Adams (2004) reported strong associations between the FBS and objective measures of incomplete effort on memory tests but found weaker association with MMPI-2 infrequency indicators.

Threats to Validity

Neuropsychologists in both clinical and forensic settings are trained to be cognizant of threats to validity. A threat to validity is defined as any nonneurological factor that affects performance on a neuropsychological measure and gives a misleading picture of brain-behavior relationships (Suhr & Gunstad, 2002). The major threat to validity in both settings is physical problems peripheral to the central nervous system that affect input (sensory) or output (motor) modalities (Reitan, 2001). Examples of peripheral problems include carpal tunnel syndrome or arthritis affecting upper extremity motor skills tests and hearing loss affecting auditory processing tasks.

The main validity threat in the forensic setting is test-taking motivation (Heaton, Smith, Lehman, & Vogt, 1978). The forensic setting provides stronger incentives to underperform or distort responses (Rogers, 1997). Motivational distortions take the form of either insufficient effort or motivated distortion (malingering). Estimates vary as to the exact base rate of poor effort and/or malingering, but the weight of peer-reviewed studies indicate prevalence is high in persons persistently pursuing monetary and social benefits. Mittenberg, Patton, Canyock, and Condit (2002) surveyed board-certified neuropsychologists with a combined experience of more than 33,000 legal cases and reported a 40% base rate of suspiciously poor performance. Greiffenstein, Baker and Gola (1994) estimated prevalence ranging from 33% to 66% depending on definitional stringency. Writing in a neurotoxic compensability context, van Hout, Schmand,

Wekking, Hageman, and Deelman (2003) reported 46% of 145 litigants failed either the Amsterdam Short-Term Memory Test or the Test of Memory Malingering. Greiffenstein and Baker (2006) conducted a prevalence study considering both malingering type (memory, motor, and psychiatric) and criterion stringency (possible, probable noncredibility) in two large cohorts of persons claiming permanent disability following minor neck/head trauma. They found 80% prevalence of at least *one* atypical psychometric sign under a liberal "possible" rule and 60% prevalence under a stringent "probable" rule.

These threats to validity can only be addressed by reliance on (a) extra-test medical data and (b) symptom validity tests (SVTs). The use of SVTs should be standard in every forensic examination or in any clinical evaluation with a high risk of forensic involvement (Hartman, 2002; Greiffenstein & Kaufmann, 2012; Sweet, 1999b).

Conflicting Paradigms

The law involves an epistemology differing markedly from the neuropsychology scientist-practitioner's outlook (Greiffenstein & Kaufmann, 2012). Productive attorney-neuropsychologist relations and useful testimony require the forensic specialist to adjust to the inevitable conflicts between these professions (Blau, 1998). Table 37.1 summarizes the best-known structural conflicts, termed *structural* because they are endemic to every legal case and not subject to alteration.

The main conflict endemic to the forensic context is partisanship versus objectivity. Attorneys play an adversarial role, have no affirmative obligation to the complete truth, and strive to ignore or minimize evidence inconvenient to their medical-legal theories. In contrast, neuropsychologists operate under the ethos of objectivity, choosing clinical theories that best fit the facts irrespective of the social or financial implications of their conclusions.

The legal principle most antithetical to scientific psychology is *stare decisis*: Attorneys and courts consider past legal decisions fundamentally determinative of current issues. It took a half-century to overturn the legal precedent of separate-but-equal schools for minorities. But under the canons of modern science, the goal is attempted falsification of scientific precedent (Larrabee, 2012a). Evidentiary thresholds and standards of proof differ under the law depending on case gravity. In civil cases, a preponderance of the evidence model is applied; meaning the prevailing party's version of facts having at more than 50% of the evidence in its favor, while in criminal cases, the evidentiary threshold is "beyond a reasonable doubt," which has been interpreted as a 90% confidence level (Kagehiro, 1990). In contrast, neuropsychologists use instruments derived from quasi-experimental research showing findings associated with 95%–99% confidence group differences are not due to chance. The courtroom also relies on anecdotal, single-case methodology, in which each side offers specific hypotheses to be tested, although the critical p value threshold is $p > 0.50$.

Causation Analysis

Forensic neuropsychologists concern themselves with issues of causation to a degree not present clinically. Mental illness is multifactorial in nature, and clinicians rarely concern themselves with ultimate causation. With the exception of a few organic brain syndromes, the causes of mental illness in general and most cognitive disorders in particular are unknown. The forensic neuropsychologist, however, is required to state whether the legal cause of action (work or car accident, toxic exposure) is a factor in explaining abnormalities in test scores or subjective complaints. The law requires only that psychologists be reasonably confident in their conclusions.

Admissibility of Neuropsychological Testimony

Neuropsychologists anticipating involvement in adjudicated cases need to have a core forensic knowledge database. This supports both understanding the legal process and

Table 37.1 Structural conflicts between the law and neuropsychology

Issue	*Courtroom Practice*	*Neuropsychology Practice*
Historical Approach	*Stare decisis*: Legal precedent is either dispositive or given dominant consideration	Prior studies provide pretext for research only; science advances by trying to falsify precedent
Role Orientation	Partisanship, zealous advocacy	Objectivity, unconcern over legal outcome
Goal Orientation	Winning a case; justice over truth	Truth over justice: Finding best fitting neuropsychological theory
Evidentiary Model	Variable evidentiary thresholds differing across legal setting	Conservative evidentiary thresholds constant across settings
Methodology model	Anecdotal, single case methodology	Experimental or quasi-experimental group studies, replicated over long time periods
Rhetorical approach	Persuasion through emotional impact	Persuasion by means of logic, facts, and supportable theory
Typical Audience	Judge and jury	Physicians and other professionally educated medical professionals

productively interacting with the retaining attorney (Greiffenstein & Kaufmann, 2012). Kaufmann (2012) describes and explains admissibility standards and a careful understanding of how these standards operate is important. Admissibility refers to the rules that govern admission and disqualification of evidence. The admissibility guidelines applicable to neuropsychologists cover three broad issues: (a) competence to testify, (b) scope of neuropsychological testimony, and (c) specific methodologies relied upon by neuropsychologists.

General Competence to Testify

For most of the 20th century, courts took a dim view of psychological evidence (Blau, 1998). *Jenkins v. U.S.* (1962) was a watershed case for qualifying psychologists to testify. Vincent E. Jenkins mounted an insanity defense, introducing the testimony of psychiatrists and psychologists that he was suffering mental disease (schizophrenia) at the time of a sexual assault. The trial court instructed the jury to disregard psychometric evidence on the grounds that psychologists were disqualified from testifying about mental disease for lack of medical training. The appeals court for the Second District (Washington, DC) reversed the trial judge, ordering the new trial to include psychological testimony and psychometric findings. The appeals court noted a diverse array of nonphysicians regularly offered opinions, such as electricians and doctoral-level toxicologists. Judge Bazelon wrote the majority opinion, offering a two-pronged test of admissibility for psychologists' testimony: "The critical factors in respect to admissibility is the actual experience of the witness and the probative value of his opinion" (*Jenkins,* p. 646). This opinion implies a medical degree is neither sufficient nor necessary to testify as to mental state. The trial judge must determine a particular psychologist's qualifications through a context-specific, fact-intensive exploration of background, training, education, and knowledge.

Subsequent legal cases dealt specifically with the competence of neuropsychologists to testify on issues before a court. An early case involving testimonial competence is *Simmons v. Mullins* (1975). The minor plaintiff proffered neuropsychological evidence in support of a brain injury claim arising out of a car accident. The defendant objected to admission of this testimony, but both trial and appellate courts disagreed, ruling that neuropsychologists are competent to testify on cognitive damages associated with organic brain syndrome. As in *Jenkins* (1962), the courts noted that nonmedical persons have always been allowed to testify within their special knowledge, additionally pointing out the necessity of consultation with neuropsychologists in brain damage cases. Overall, the weight of legal authority strongly recognizes neuropsychologists as generally competent to testify, contingent on adequate demonstration of academic coursework, peer reviewed research, and supervised training experiences (Greiffenstein & Kaufmann, 2012; Shapiro, 1991).

Neuropsychologists' Scope of Testimony

The scope of testimony refers to the range of subject matter that neuropsychologists may address in front of a jury (e.g., causation of deficits). Neuropsychologists offer testimony whether the cause of action is a contributing factor to weak test scores. In general, both trial and appellate court rulings appear to be divided on the issue of whether neuropsychologists can comment on general causation (the physical state of the brain) or specific causation (e.g., car accident).

A number of causation testimony cases challenged by civil defendants drew amicus briefs from the APA. In *Horne v. Goodson Logging* (1986), a neuropsychologist offered psychometric evidence of a logger's disabling brain injury. On appeal, both Workers' Compensation (WC) commission and appellate boards ruled that neuropsychologists are not competent to render opinions about physical bases. On higher appeal, the APA successfully petitioned a North Carolina appeals court to reverse the WC commission and rule neuropsychologists competent to render judgments about disability. *Landers v. Chrysler Corp.* (1997) and *Huntoon v. TCI Cablevision* (1998) had similar facts and allowed psychologist expert testimony on organic causation. In a role reversal, plaintiffs in *Martin v. Benson* (1998) argued neuropsychologists are categorically unqualified to render causation testimony regarding brain dysfunction, because a defendant's neuropsychologist convinced a jury that mood and medication effects better explained the plaintiff's presentation. The divided state appeals court overrode its own decision in *Horne v. Goodson Logging* and ruled neuropsychological testimony inadmissible. Defendants prevailed at the North Carolina Supreme Court only on narrow procedural grounds of the plaintiff failing to preserve his objection at trial.

Other jurisdictions provided stronger grounds supporting testimony about physical brain state. In the case of *Valiulis v. Scheffeos* (1989), an Illinois appeals court strengthened the logical basis for allowing neuropsychological testimony by noting:

> It would be somewhat anomalous to conclude that [the neuropsychologist] would not be qualified to testify as to cause of plaintiffs injury when the neurologist and psychologist who sought out his expertise and assistance in diagnosing the disease would likely be qualified to do so.
>
> (pp. 1267–1297)

The Iowa Supreme Court directly dealt with neuropsychologists' causation testimony in *Hutchison v. Am. Family Mut. Ins.* (1994). This court conducted a wide-ranging survey of practices in many jurisdictions and determined "there seems little dispute that a psychologist may testify as to the existence of a brain injury or at least the condition of the brain in general" (p. 886). However, this court fractionated the causation testimony issue into two parts: neuropsychologists' ability to testify on physical state of the brain versus causation of altered brain state. The *Hutchison* court acknowledged that the causation issue divided most courts, but in general, such causation testimony was allowed.

Some courts drew different conclusions in contexts not involving closed head injury. The Ninth Circuit appeals court took up the issue of toxic causation in *Schudel v. General Elec.* (1995), a case involving the alleged poisoning of workers by organic solvents, detergents, and polychlorinated biphenyls (PCBs). The trial court ruled neuropsychologists could testify as to test scores and cognitive levels but could not infer physical causation. On appeal, the APA again filed an amicus brief arguing that Federal Rules of Evidence (FRE) 702 established relaxed standards biased towards admission of scientific evidence. Nevertheless, the Ninth Circuit affirmed the trial judge's ruling, limiting neuropsychology testimony to issues of (cognitive) damages but not causation. Neuropsychologists have also been barred from inferring neurophysiological causation of EEG patterns (*John v. Im*, 2002) and cerebral palsy (*Grenitz v. Tomlian*, 2003). Courts have properly limited neuropsychologist causation testimony in cases involving head trauma inflicted in distinctly separated incidents in the medical history (*Guzman v. 4030 Bronx Blvd. Assoc., L.L.C.*, 2008).

Enter *Daubert*: Admissibility of Neuropsychological Methodology

The well-qualified neuropsychologist allowed broad scope of testimony might nonetheless be required to defend his or her particular selection of test instruments. Although neuropsychologists have no greater obligation to validate an entire assessment process than a physician, there is important admissibility law that addresses the methodologies neuropsychologists rely upon in drawing conclusions. This is perhaps the most critical component of the forensic knowledge base with which neuropsychologists should be familiar. These important bases include the Federal Rules of Evidence and a trilogy of U.S. Supreme Court decisions.

Frye (1923) Dominates

For 70 years, a federal appellate court's *Frye* decision (1923) provided judges a simple analytic tool for guiding admission of scientific testimony. James Frye was convicted of murder and appealed a court's refusal to admit scientifically based exculpatory evidence. This evidence was an early polygraph that relied on blood pressure changes to detect the sympathetic arousal theoretically associated with lying. The *Frye* court affirmed the trial judges *in limine* ruling, reasoning that the psychophysiological principle underlying the technique had not yet gained "evidential force" in the transition from "the experimental" towards the "demonstrable" stages. Although recognizing the ambiguity in determining the evolutionary stage of a principle or technique ("twilight zone" in this court's words), the court issued what is now known as the *Frye* rule to help resolve the ambiguity: Only scientific principles or techniques achieving general acceptance within a specific scientific community developing the technique are admissible (see Table 37.2 for full language of decision). The *Frye* rule is commonly named the "general acceptance" standard.

Table 37.2 Summaries of the Frye and Daubert trilogy decisions controlling admission of neuropsychological evidence

Frye Test (1923)

"While the courts will go a long way in admitting expert testimony, deduced from a well-recognized scientific principle or discovery, the thing from which the deduction is made must be sufficiently established to have gained *general acceptance* in the particular field in which it belongs." (Emphasis added)

Daubert (1993)

The admissibility of scientific principles or assessment methods is based on the following criteria.

General criteria: Whether the reasoning or methodology underlying the testimony is scientifically *valid* and whether that reasoning or methodology is *relevant* to the facts at issue.

Suggested logical characteristics:

- Falsifiability: In practice, the test or method can be disproved
- The principle or technique has been subjected to peer review and publication
- Known or potential error rate in classification
- Technique or principle generally accepted in the relevant field

Joiner (1997)

- Reiteration of Daubert's relevance requirement: Whether scientific evidence (theory and method) fits the legal question presented
- Reinforces the role of trial judge as gatekeeper of scientific evidence
- Extrapolation from existing data to particular case requires a link more lucid than an *ipse dixit* (subjective speculation) argument

Kumho (1999)

- Extends Daubert to areas of technical and specialized knowledge
- Includes behavioral science
- The four main *Daubert* factors are not exhaustive; they are polythetic: one or more are sufficient grounds for admitting/rejecting scientific evidence

Frye is widely (but not universally) considered a conservative rule that bars "junk science" in that it rejects speculative approaches. But the general acceptance rule also bars recent or novel advances that are undeniably valid but not yet general knowledge (Melton et al., 1997). Other criticisms of the *Frye* rule include admission of invalid techniques just because a majority of scientists believes in them (see section on Myths of Forensic Neuropsychology that begins on p. 914), plus difficulties in determining which scientific community applies or degree of scientific consensus based on a small sample of expert witnesses in a particular case.

Increasingly few states still rely on *Frye* and its hybrids to regulate scientific admission. There is little published case law involving *Frye* challenges to neuropsychologist testimony. Anecdotal evidence suggests that attempts to find certain neuropsychological measures inadmissible have failed. McKinzey and Ziegler (1999) drafted a *Frye* challenge to a "flexible test battery" but the trial judge still allowed such a battery into evidence. It is reasonable to argue that most neuropsychological procedures easily pass the *Frye* rule of general acceptance. General acceptance is easily shown by peer-reviewed reports. The American Academy of Neurology (AAN) Therapeutics and Technology Subcommittee Report (1996b) amply demonstrates the acceptance of neuropsychological measurement by a respected scientific body independent of self-interested neuropsychologists. The AAN (1996b) report is especially powerful evidence when one considers the same committee rejected use of some medical procedures in detection of remote mild brain injury and advised against use in the courts (AAN, 1996a). Thus, it is likely that neuropsychological test procedures pass *Frye* because neurologists as well as neuropsychologists generally accept them. Other methods for supporting neuropsychological instrumentation under *Frye* include reliance on surveys of test usage patterns (Boccaccini & Brodsky, 1999; Lees-Haley, Smith, Williams, & Dunn, 1996), test encyclopedias summarizing multiple validation studies of commonly used instruments (Spreen and Strauss, 1998), or the validation studies cited in standardized test manuals.

But certain neuro-medical procedures have a history of inadmissibility under *Frye*, such as quantitative EEG (QEEG; Nuwer, 1997) and brain single photon emission computed tomography (SPECT; AAN, 1996a). QEEG evidence has consistently been ruled inadmissible in many jurisdictions. Good examples include *John v. Im* (2002) and *Nadel v. Las Vegas Metro* (2001). Generally, courts have refused to admit QEEG results as proof of any diagnosis, physical or psychological. This outcome is noted early in civil (*Head v. Lithonia Corp.*, 1989) and criminal (*State v. Zimmerman*, 1990) cases and continues throughout the past two decades (*Ross v. Schrantz*, 1995; *Tran v. Hilburn*, 1997; *In re: Breast Implant Litigation*, 1998; *Craig v. Orkin Exterminating Co.*, 2000; *Feria v. Dynagraphics Co.*, 2004; *LaMasa v. Bachman*, 2005), despite claims of improved QEEG technology, data processing, and reliability. Additionally, *Craig* notes a similar result for brain electrical activity mapping (BEAM) technology and *LaMasa* also reports on the exclusion of positron emission tomography (PET). Brain SPECT has also been ruled inadmissible insofar as diagnosis of multiple chemical sensitivities is concerned (*Summers v. Missouri Pac R.R.*, 1997). Although SPECT cannot be used for causation opinions and is routinely excluded for diagnostic purposes, some courts have admitted opinions, under *Frye*, based on SPECT used for more narrow purposes. For example, these *Frye* jurisdiction courts allowed experts to use SPECT to supplement opinions with findings "consistent with" diagnoses made using other tests. (*Fini v. General Motors Corp.*, 2003; *People v. Urdiales*, 2007; *Matuszak v. Cerniak*, 2004; *Donnellan v. First Student, Inc.*, 2008).

Federal Rules of Evidence

Starting in the late 1960s, Congress rewrote evidence law for use in federal courts and in 1975 codified the new FRE and the Federal Rules of Civil Procedure (FRCP, 1975). The states slowly adopted FRE into their own evidentiary statutes and are now substantially in force in the court systems of 35 states. FRE articles 401, 402, and 702–705 (see Table 37.3) describe the rules permitting expert testimony. One caveat about the FRE is important to consider. The rules have a generally liberal thrust, designed to admit a broad range of evidence to ensure fairness and to avoid orthodoxy.

The federal rules in the 400 series define the relationship between proffered evidence and the legal issues involved in litigation. Rule 401 defines "relevant" evidence as any item introducing a fact having potential impact on legal decisions raised by a trial. In scientific terminology, FRE 401 is a Bayesian statement that a given piece of evidence has a nonzero probability of affecting a trial's outcome (Mossman, 2000). It is Bayesian in the sense that the trial judge makes a determination based on what is already known about the case ("prior probability") to assign a zero (irrelevant) or nonzero (probative) weight to proffered evidence ("posterior probability"). This means that any two neuropsychological methodologies of significant but different validities for a given diagnosis are given equal footing in an admissibility determination, as long as validities are not zero (see the Myths of Forensic Neuropsychology section in this chapter). Rule 402 qualifies that 401 requires probative evidence not be overly prejudicial. In criminal contexts, self-incriminating material inappropriately elicited by a neuropsychologist would be barred irrespective of whether this fact is relevant to brain-behavior relationships.

The rules in the 700 series define the vehicle (witnesses) for proffering evidence at trial. There are two types of witnesses: fact ("lay") and expert witnesses. Rule 701 defines a lay witness as someone who conveys information gleaned through the senses only, also known as a fact witness. For example, "I saw Jones shoot Smith in the head." Some limited inferences by lay witnesses are allowed, e.g., "Smith looked really

Table 37.3 Federal rules of evidence relevant to neuropsychological testimony

Rule 401

Definition of "Relevant Evidence"

"'Relevant evidence' means evidence having any tendency to make the existence of any fact that is of consequence to the determination of the action more probable or less probable than it would be without the evidence."

Rule 402

Relevant Evidence Generally Admissible; Irrelevant Evidence Inadmissible

"All relevant evidence is admissible, except as otherwise provided by the Constitution of the United States, by Act of Congress, by these rules, or by other rules prescribed by the Supreme Court pursuant to statutory authority. Evidence which is not relevant is not admissible."

Rule 701

Opinion Testimony by Lay Witnesses

"If the witness is not testifying as an expert, the witness' testimony in the form of opinions or inferences is limited to those opinions or inferences which are (a) rationally based on the perception of the witness and (b) helpful to a clear understanding of the witness' testimony or the determination of a fact in issue. "

Rule 702

Testimony by Experts

"If scientific, technical, or other specialized knowledge will assist the trier of fact to understand the evidence or to determine a fact in issue, a witness qualified as an expert by knowledge, skill, experience, training, or education, may testify thereto in the form of an opinion or otherwise."

Rule 703

Bases of Opinion Testimony by Experts

"The facts or data in the particular case upon which an expert bases an opinion or inference may be those perceived by or made known to the expert at or before the hearing. If of a type reasonably relied upon by experts in the particular field in forming opinions or inferences upon the subject, the facts or data need not be admissible in evidence."

Rule 704

Opinion on Ultimate Issue

"(A) Except as provided in subdivision (b), testimony in the form of an opinion or inference otherwise admissible is not objectionable because it embraces an ultimate issue to be decided by the trier of fact. (B) No expert witness testifying with respect to the mental state or condition of a defendant in a criminal case may state an opinion or inference as to whether the defendant did or did not have the mental state or condition constituting an element of the crime charged or of a defense thereto. Such ultimate issues are matters for the trier of fact alone."

Rule 705

Disclosure of Facts or Data Underlying Expert Opinion

"The expert may testify in terms of opinion or inference and give reasons therefore without first testifying to the underlying facts or data, unless the court requires otherwise. The expert may in any event be required to disclose the underlying facts or data on cross-examination."

scared." A treating psychologist is technically considered a fact witness.

An expert witness is one who offers an opinion about what the evidence means. Rule 702 defines an expert witness as someone with "specialized knowledge" who helps the trier of fact in either one of two basic ways: (a) to understand the evidence, or (b) determine a fact at issue. In regards to (a), the forensic neuropsychologist could provide definitions of neuropsychological testing, discuss cognitive test development, or summarize functional organization of the brain. In regards to element (b), a fact at issue could be the permanency of cognitive deficits in the hypothetical victim Smith. The neuropsychologist could opine, "The gunshot wound to Smith's brain damaged his ventro-medial frontal lobes and took away his ability to judge risk or make appropriate decisions." Rule 702 also addresses the issue of bases for judging expertise: not only scientific training or a higher degree but also experience and technical knowledge. Note the liberal thrust of the definition, especially by the term *experience*. Interestingly, the legislative reporter's notes to this rule do not even mention *Frye* (Sanders, Diamond, & Vidmar, 2002), while making reference to the *Daubert* factor of general acceptance.

Rule 703 provides a liberal definition of the bases on which experts can base their opinions. Some legal scholars term 703 the *hearsay* rule. Essentially, the neuropsychology expert is not limited to basing opinions of neuropsychological measures or procedures, but may also opine on other data as long as such data is "reasonably relied upon" by experts in a particular field. Essentially, Rule 703 permits opinions based on hearsay ("The plaintiff told me his memory is only bad for what his wife tells him") or evidence not gleaned from direct observation (e.g., outside records). Rule 703 is especially important for mental health professionals, as their work depends on hearsay (what the examinee said during a diagnostic interview). Neuropsychologists also rely on medical records or medical opinions they themselves did not produce (e.g., EEG and computed tomography, or CT, scan reports). According to Rule 703, the neuropsychologist may integrate such outside neurological studies, as well as verbal behavior of the plaintiff, into an opinion.

Rule 704 dictates the boundaries of expert opinion and addresses the issue of penultimate versus ultimate opinions. Part A (see Table 37.3) allows the expert to give opinions similar to legal decisions made by the trier of fact. Part B offers the exception that experts may not offer ultimate opinions on a criminal defendant's state of mind. Under this rubric, a neuropsychologist can testify that an accident caused (or did not cause) permanent cognitive deficits but may not opine regarding the impact of neuropsychological deficits on criminal culpability. A neuropsychologist could answer a penultimate question, such as "He was suffering severe cognitive deficits around the time of the crime." Part B was added by Congress in the early 1980s and is known as the "Hinckley" exception.

Landmark Ruling: Daubert

Much of modern scientific admissibility law stems from a trilogy of cases, beginning with *Daubert*. The landmark U.S. Supreme Court case of *Daubert v. Merrell Dow Pharm., Inc.* (1993) and its two follow-on rulings are summarized in Table 37.2. *Dauber*t has been adopted by the majority of states.

In *Daubert*, plaintiff alleged that the antiemesis drug Benedectin induced birth defects. Using a relatively new quantitative method known as *meta-analysis,* plaintiff's experts reanalyzed previously published data and offered a countervailing conclusion that the drug caused mutagenesis. The trial court granted the defense motion for summary disposition, ruling plaintiff's reanalysis of earlier data was novel and unpublished, therefore violating the "general acceptance" provision of *Frye*. The plaintiff appealed, arguing the FRE were designed to supplant *Frye*, were the law of the land, and offered more relaxed admissibility standards. The U.S. Supreme Court agreed with the plaintiff: The *Daubert* Court ruled that expert evidence must meet only two general prongs: *reliability*[1] and *relevance*. The court went on to provide trial judges with suggested, nonbinding indicia for reliability and relevance by further elaborating on FRE 702.

The *Daubert* factors, described more fully in Table 37.2, contain four basic elements: (a) falsifiability, (b) peer review, (c) known or potential error rate, and (d) general acceptance. Parsing of the principles suggest the *Daubert* court was guided by many different logical, practical, and philosophical sources. The "falsifiability" element obviously stems from Karl Popper's reasoning that no theory can ever be proven, one can only "fail to disprove." Thus, "falsifiability" means an admissible scientific principle must be expressed in terms of the conditions under which it can be disproved. An explanation that cannot be disproved is a pseudotheory and not admissible—a sufficiently obtuse factor that the Honorable Chief Justice Rehnquist was "at a loss" to understand. The peer review element means that a neuropsychological technique or principle was published in a print journal with a peer review process. Either the "error rate" can refer to a zero-order validity study or it can refer to errors in diagnostic classification. The final element is the *Frye* general acceptance rule. Beliefs to the contrary, *Daubert* did not invalidate the general acceptance standard. Instead, the *Daubert* court incorporated "general acceptance" as one element to consider among many.

The *Daubert* court provided some general contours of admissibility analysis. The court stressed that science admissibility should be based on the *existence* of studies, manuals, and desirable logical characteristics; admissibility should be not guided by the conclusions of any study. In other words, the mere existence of a validation study may be sufficient to gain admission into evidence of a neuropsychological measure, but the conclusions of the published study are not to be considered until trial, as they go to the weight of the evidence (see the Myths of Forensic Neuropsychology section on confusion between admissibility and weight). Chief Justice Rehnquist concurred in the outcome but issued a partial dissent warning the *Daubert* ruling restricted itself to the term *scientific* from FRE 702, ignoring the other key language of "experience" and "technical knowledge." This dissent was prescient.

Kumho Decision

The *Daubert* decision contained some ambiguities begging for clarification. One issue was the necessary and sufficient features of the guidelines. Were they polythetic criteria requiring flexible combination of a minimal number of elements, or were the *Daubert* guidelines a checklist of exhaustive criteria, meaning every element had to be present?

The issue in *Kumho* (*Kumho Tire v. Carmichael*, 1999) was whether *Daubert* applies to scientific ideas only. Carmichael, the survivor of a deadly car crash, sued a tire manufacturer. The plaintiff's main witness was a self-described tire expert who asserted the defendant's tire was defective based on simple palpation ("tactile and visual exploration") of the blown tire, hence representing a combination of experiential and technological testimony. Using the *Daubert* analysis, the trial court excluded this form of engineering testimony as unreliable. The appeals court reversed, holding that a *Daubert* analysis was restricted to purely scientific testimony mentioned in FRE 702. The U.S. Supreme Court granted *certiorari*, ultimately reinstating the trial court's determination. The *Kumho* court reasoned that the trial judge's gatekeeper function extended to experiential and technical evidence, and that the same analytic tools used to determine scientific reliability should be used to determine reliability of other methods. The Supreme Court also reaffirmed the flexibility of the *Daubert* criteria and ruled the trial judge appropriately rejected the expert even after a very liberal application of *Daubert*.

Joiner Decision

While the *Daubert* and *Kumho* decisions dealt exclusively with methodological bases underlying an opinion, the U.S. Supreme Court used the *Joiner* matter (*General Elec. v. Joiner*, 1997) to further expand the gatekeeper role to include admissibility of expert's *conclusions*. Electrician Robert Joiner developed lung cancer and sued the manufacturer of PCBs on the theory that exposure to mineral spirits caused his condition. The plaintiff's experts offered epidemiological and animals studies in support of their causation and damages theories. The trial judge ruled this testimony irrelevant because the conditions of the animal studies could not be generalized to humans, and the epidemiologic studies involved multiple chemical exposures in addition to PCB. The judge ruled that generalization from epidemiological studies to the plaintiff's condition was too large an analytical gap that was "bridged only by subjective belief or unsupported speculation." The plaintiff appealed, arguing *Daubert* required focus only on the scientific and logical characteristics of research (falsifiability, peer review, etc.) but explicitly barred admissibility judgments based on any study's conclusions (cf. *Daubert*, 1993, p. 595). The *Joiner* court disagreed, ruling it was within a trial court's discretion to disqualify *opinion evidence* based on no more than the fact the expert said it *(ipse dixit)*, irrespective if the extrapolated-from studies were themselves scientifically sound and reliable. Any extrapolation from literature to individual legal cases has to be bridged by lucid links other than the expert's belief there is a link. This is simply a restatement of the *Daubert* court's requirement that the basis for expert testimony had to be relevant in addition to being reliable (valid). In neuropsychology terms, this could mean that introduction of valid and replicated neuropsychological principles could still be barred if not generalizable. For example, the finding that the General Neuropsychological Deficit Scale is sensitive to metastasized brain cancer (Wolfson & Reitan, 1995) is not automatically generalizable to remote mTBI cases.

Empirical Impact of Daubert

The impact of *Daubert* on trial court and appellate behavior has undergone quantified scrutiny. Groscup, Penrod, Studebaker, Huss, & O'Neil (2002) examined expert admission rates documented in published opinions before and after *Daubert*. They found little overall change in admission of expert evidence at either the trial or appellate levels. Even *Joiner,* with its emphasis on the relevance of an expert's conclusions, did not lower admission rates. Interestingly, trial and appellate changes devoted the least number of words to four *Daubert* elements, but devoted more discussion to the FRE. Groscup, Penrod, Studebaker, Huss, & O'Neil (2002) concluded judges gave little more than passing attention to *Daubert*'s analytic tools. Dahir et al. (2005) directly surveyed judge's treatment of mental health evidence following *Daubert*. They came to similar conclusions as Groscup et al.: Judges rarely made decisions based on falsifiability or error rate, expressing greater comfort with pre-Daubert guidelines, namely *Frye* and general acceptance.

There is case law bearing on *Daubert* challenges to neuropsychological measures. In *Villalba v. Consol. Freightways* (2000), the plaintiff lost a brain injury tort in part due to failing neurocognitive validity tests such as the Computerized Assessment of Response Bias (CARB) and Tests of Memory Malingering (TOMM). Plaintiff appealed, arguing this SVT evidence should have been excluded because of the witness's refusal to photocopy and disclose TOMM items or normative data. The appeals court found no factual basis for the appeal (the neuropsychologist presented bar charts at trial) and further noted that the plaintiff had not proven the unscientific basis for SVTs through application of the *Daubert* factors. In *Coe v. Tennessee* (2000), a death row inmate appealed the admission of malingering measures for lack of peer-reviewed studies demonstrating sensitivity to malingering among death row inmates specifically. The Tennessee Supreme Court affirmed the trial court, ruling that malingering measures are generally accepted and reasonably generalizable to a criminal context. Ironically, this court also noted the defense's own neuropsychologist used SVTs, rendering the appeal internally inconsistent.

Third-Party Observers

No issue highlights science–law conflicts in neuropsychology like third-party observation (TPO). Most jurisdictions allow observers to be present during independent medical examinations (IMEs). Statutory language refers to having the plaintiff's "physician" or an attorney present during a "medical examination." For example, the Michigan Compiled Laws Annotated 600.1445(1) reads:

> Whenever in any proceeding before any court, board or commission, or other public body or officer, requiring and commanding that a person shall submit to a physical examination, the order shall also provide that the attorney for such person may be present at such physical examination of the party to such examination desires than an attorney representing him be present.

Trial judges have considerable latitude in determining whether this language applies narrowly to physical examinations or broadly to any type of examination, including neuropsychological. Under Rule 36 of the Federal Rule of Civil Procedure (FRCP, 1975), an attorney can ask the court to place restrictions on an examination, including the time, place, manner, conditions, and scope of the assessment; most states adopted this language. In some cases, the trial judge may even agree and allow for videotaping or TPO of the neuropsychological testing.

The neuropsychology community typically resists such requests on multiple scientific and practical grounds. Two major neuropsychology organizations have published official positions on TPO (Axelrod et al., 2000; American Academy of Clinical Neuropsychology, 2001). Empirically, the scientific evidence generated by social psychologists overwhelming shows TPO negatively affects performance (see McCaffrey, Fisher, Gold, and Lynch (1996) for review of social facilitation literature). Kehrer, Sanchez, Habif, Rosenbaum, and Townes (2000) and Constantinou, Ashendorf, and McCaffrey (2002) both showed negative impact on attention and speed measures. Butler and Baumeister (1998) reported that even warm, *supportive* third-party observers caused decrements on skilled tasks relative to unmonitored performance, disproving the common legal position that plaintiff-friendly observers are necessary. An entire issue of *Journal of Forensic Neuropsychology* was devoted to scientific studies of TPO (McCaffrey, 2005): All studies showed experimental evidence for significant, in some cases robust, effects for observers on neuropsychological domains.

There is considerable case law on this issue, although most decisions are unpublished, having little far-ranging application. The weight of authority of these cases recognizes the validity of psychological test responses are more affected by TPO than physical responses are in medical examinations. A number of appellate rulings barring plaintiff's intrusion into neuropsychological testing include *Cline v. Firestone Tire* (1988) and *Tomlin v. Holecek* (1993). In *Troiano v. John Hancock* (2003), the court ruled that the plaintiff did not show good cause why an observer should be present for neuropsychological testing. In *Ragge v. MCA/Universal Studios*, (1995), a California Federal District Court denied the plaintiff's request for both TPO and advance notification of which tests would be given. However, TPO is allowed in California state court by statute ("The examiner and examinee shall have the right to record a mental examination by audio technology" (C.C.C.P. § 2032.530(a), as directly applied to neuropsychological evaluations; see *Golfland Entm't Ctrs. v. Sup. Ct.*, 2003). Although this is not a comprehensive list, New York, Florida, Oregon, Washington, Kentucky, Alabama, and Alaska allow TPO for mental examinations under specified circumstances. States vary considerably on tolerance for third-party observers and practitioners are encouraged to understand appropriate jurisdictional rules.

Common Settings for Forensic Neuropsychologists

There are four basic legal forums in which neuropsychologists can be asked to offer opinions: administrative, civil, probate, and criminal.

Administrative Law

Administrative law courts represent a hybrid between a civil court and a governmental agency. Typically, a governmental agency is empowered to hold hearings in which magistrates or hearing officers determine findings of fact and law. The setting is more informal, and evidentiary rules are commonly relaxed. The government may be a party to this dispute, such as in license revocation and restoration.

WC disputes fall into this category and are a frequent source of neuropsychological damage claims in industrialized areas. WC cases involve two private parties, but are distinguished from civil actions by the absence of tort law: Both parties give up tort rights, so negligence and liability are not issues of fact to dissect. WC was historically adjudicated in civil court until the World War I era, but employers' strong liability defenses left severely injured workers and their families destitute, resulting in sweeping legal reform (Melton et al., 1997). Another distinguishing characteristic is the burden of proof: Although mostly equivalent to "preponderance of the evidence" model, the standard is even lower in some states. In Michigan, for example, the workplace incident must form a "vital component" of the claimant's present problems, meaning it can be a contributing factor, even if the workplace injury does not contribute more than 50% to symptoms.

Civil Court

Civil courts involve disputes between two private parties where both liability and damages are the key issues. The government merely provides the forum for resolving the disputes. Typical civil suits encountered by neuropsychologists involve claims of psychological and cognitive damages stemming from motor vehicle accidents, toxic exposure, or medical malpractice. The issues of fact determined by the jury are (a) whether there was a neurological injury to begin with and (b) whether it resulted in cognitive or emotional deficits. The evidentiary threshold is the lower "preponderance of the evidence" model, because there are no liberty interests at stake as in probate or criminal matters (Melton et al., 1997). That is, the prevailing party is the one whose version of events is perceived at least 51% correct. Over the years, discovery rules have been broadened to avoid "surprise" at trial and to ensure verdicts are more strongly linked to objective evidence than to differences in lawyerly skill or resources (Lees-Haley & Cohen, 1999).

Probate Proceedings

Probate proceedings originally evolved to certify wills and manage postmortem disposition of estates. *Probate* is derived from "probe," meaning to examine or test a will. Private parties may dispute the disposition of a decedent's property, and the dispute is adjudicated in a probate court much like a civil trial. Probate courts evolved to serve a second function, namely assignment of guardians and conservators to physically or mentally incompetent persons. Competency is defined as an individual's legal capacity to make certain decisions and to perform certain acts (Marson & Hebert, 2005). Liberty interests are at stake here, as probate proceedings deal with the "taking" of property against the earlier wishes of a decedent, or the removal of a living person's rights as in a guardianship proceeding. Marson and Hebert (2005) identified three civil competency issues in which neuropsychologists can play roles: Capacity for medical consent, mental state of a will's creator, and capacity to manage financial affairs.

Testamentary competence (TC) is the legal term for the validity of a will as it relates to minimum cognitive capacity for wills creation. Most definitions of TC make some reference to mental ability, implying an ideal area for neuropsychologists' involvement. Opinions about TC may be requested antemortem, but more often questions about competence arise postmortem (Spar & Garb, 1992). Because liberty interests are at stake, the threshold for testamentary competence is set low, or put differently, the burden of proving lack of capacity is high (Greiffenstein, 2003a). Exclusive of some variants, the concept of testamentary competence is generally uniform across jurisdictions and consists of these four elements: (a) knowledge of the will's existence, (b) memory and comprehension of personal assets, (c) knowledge of potential heirs, and (d) anticipation of the will's effects on the heirs. Mapping these terms into neuropsychological terms suggest the following scheme: (a) recent and long-term memory, (b) object recognition and long-term memory, (c) facial recognition and long-term memory, and (d) executive-cognitive capacity. From a neuropsychological standpoint, some state variants are interesting. Minnesota law seems to require direct evidence of intact working and recent memory: The testator "must be able to hold [nature and extent of property] in his mind long enough to form a rational judgment concerning them" (*Estate of Congdon*, 1981). Kaufmann (2016) recently provided some representative cases illustrating the impact of neuropsychologist experts in probate cases.

A valid will also requires absence both "insane delusions" and "undue influence" (UI). UI means the testator's volition was undermined by an individual exercising inappropriate control. A neuropsychologist may for example provide evidence that the testator's neuropsychological deficits rendered him or her suggestible or controllable by adverse parties. There are many indicia for UI, which are discussed elsewhere in detail (Greiffenstein, 2003a). Antemortem assessment and postmortem inferential methods are offered by Heinik, Werner, and Lin (1999); Marson (2001); Marson, Annis, McInturff, Bartolucci, and Harrell (1999); Spar and Garb (1992); and Greiffenstein (1996, 2003a).

Criminal

The government initiates a criminal proceeding when it charges a person with crime punishable by imprisonment and/or fine (Denney, 2003). Because of strong liberty interests at stake (loss of life, freedom, or property), the evidentiary model for determining outcome is set high and the stages highly formalized. The burden of proof lies with the government prosecution, and the government must meet the familiar standard of "beyond a reasonable doubt," which to some is interpreted as 90% confidence that evidence shows guilt (Kagehiro, 1990).

Many legal decisions in criminal cases revolve around the cognitive, social, and behavioral capacities of the defendants. Competencies specific to criminal proceedings include competency to stand trial, confess, plead guilty, waive Miranda rights, waive right to counsel, receive a sentence, understand execution, and appreciate criminal responsibility (Grisso, 1986, 1988; Marson & Hebert, 2005). Neuropsychological testing can fulfill the law's needs by offering objective and quantified assessments that measure cognitive, social, and affective constructs linked to legal concepts of competence.

The most common criminal application for neuropsychologists addresses criminal responsibility. The most serious crimes require proof of concurrence between the mental element and the physical act of the crime. *Mens rea* is the mental capacity to plan a crime and foresee its consequences, and *actus reus*, is the physical criminal act itself. Concurrence requires that *actus reus* and *mens rea* occur at the same time. Persons pleading not guilty by reason of insanity (NGRI) seek acquittal, arguing they did not have the mental capacity to form intent. Neuropsychologists may determine that defendants' cognitive weaknesses do or don't relate to mental state at the time of the crime. Many courts may allow neuropsychologists to testify about criminal capacity, but a common complaint about forensic psychologists is that they do not understand the difference between legal insanity and clinical psychopathology. Not all states share the same legal definitions.

The earliest legal insanity test and one still used in nearly half the states is the *M'Naghten* (1843: 720) insanity test:

> At the time of the act, the party accused was laboring under such a defect of reason from disease of the mind, as not to know the nature and quality of the act he was doing; or, if he did know it, that he did not know he was doing what was wrong.

Often termed a "knowing right from wrong test" (Sullivan & Denney, 2003: 210), *M'Naghten* is a simple polythetic (either–or) definition that focuses strictly on general cognitive ability isolated from other elements of cognitive and psychological-emotional functioning. Some have argued the rule's general contour demands a *profound* general cognitive defect ("from *such* a defect"), implying only mental retardation fits the definition. Mapping this insanity test's terms onto neuropsychological concepts suggests the following. *Disease of the mind* refers to a recognized form of mental illness or organic brain disease. Not *knowing* the "quality or nature of the act" and the word *wrong* appear to emphasize profound deficit in semantic memory and fund of general knowledge to the point the person did not know the behavior was unlawful even if they could appreciate the lethality of their actions. A more liberal interpretation of *M'Naghten* is the terms could also refer to a serious defect in any one of other cognitive systems, including poor executive-cognitive skills (unable to foresee the immediate outcome) and visual perception (did not know he or she had a weapon).

The *M'Naghten* test came under criticism from some legal scholars and psychiatrists in the late 1800s because the test appeared limited to profound cognitive defects, while ignoring less severe cognitive deficits and completely ignoring behavioral and affective/emotional problems. The "irresistible impulse" and *Durham* (1954) tests were a response to the perceived inadequacies of *M'Naghten's* "knowing" test. The *Durham* (1954) test, authored by Judge Bazelon, states "An accused is not criminally responsible if his unlawful act was the product of mental disease or defect" (pp. 874–875).

Legal scholars refer to *Durham* (1954) as a "products test," meaning the criminal act was a product of mental illness. This vague rule created many problems with unwelcome social outcomes. Unlike earlier or later insanity tests, the *Durham* test did not suggest a threshold for the magnitude of mental illness necessary for application. Hence, many health professionals assumed the mere existence of a diagnosable disorder was sufficient to support legal insanity. It was also easy to show that any criminal act would have some connection to mental illness (Shapiro, 1991). Worst of all, psychopathy had recently been recognized as a mental illness, making antisocial behavior easily excusable. In neuropsychological terms, even a mild impairment could support a NGRI defense under *Durham*.

The American Law Institute (ALI, 1962: 4) tried to resolve these problems by formulating a model insanity test that is now in use in most states.

> A person is not responsible for criminal conduct if at the time of such conduct as a result of mental disease or defect he lacks substantial capacity either to appreciate the criminality [wrongfulness] of his conduct or to conform his conduct to the requirements of the law. The term mental disease or defect does not include an abnormality manifested only by repeated criminal or otherwise antisocial conduct.

The ALI insanity test indicates the presence of a proven brain disorder or recognizable neurocognitive deficit as necessary but not sufficient to meet the test. This overcomes the wideness of the *Durham* test, which implied any mental disorder was sufficient. The exclusion of antisocial personality also defeated the efforts of psychopathic offenders to win NGRI cases. The ALI test replaces the *M'Naghten* rule's "such a defect" language with *substantial incapacity* as the criterion.[2] The ALI definition does however move beyond *M'Naghten's* purely cognitive insanity test and adds a volitional prong by stressing inability to conform behavior to the law. This addition may be critical for neuropsychologists.

Neuropsychologists continue to make contributions to criminal courts, both as researchers and testifying experts (Denney & Wynkoop, 2000), and legal decisions stimulate their work. The volitional prong of the ALI definition implies executive-cognitive dysfunction. Persons with abnormal frontal lobe physiology, theoretically, could commit crimes because of inability to inhibit behavior (Damasio, Tranel, & Damasio, 1990). Neuropsychologists involvement in criminal matters also include classification of aggressive behavior into primary and secondary types (Houston, Stanford, Villemarette-Pittman, Conklin, & Helfritz, 2003), juvenile adjudicative competence (Wynkoop, 2003), malingering to evade criminal culpability (Wynkoop & Denney, 1999), and restoration to competence through use of medication (Stanford et al., 2005).

In 1984, Congress passed the Insanity Defense Reform Act (IDRA) after John Hinckley was found to be NGRI in his attempt to assassinate President Ronald Reagan (*United States v. Hinckley*, 1981). *Hinckley* was the first case to introduce neuroimages (computerized axial tomography [CAT] scans) as evidence of a psychiatric condition. Reaction to the verdict fueled the IDRA effort to narrow the circumstances when an "otherwise culpable defendant is excused for his conduct because of mental disease or defect" (18 U.S.C. § 17). Subsequent case law attempted to delineate the proper use of mental health evidence related to legal excuse and criminal culpability (*United States v. Cameron*, 1990).

Cameron explained how IDRA narrowed the use of mental health evidence in federal criminal trials:

1. Removing the volitional "diminished capacity" element of the insanity defense (§ 17(a)),
2. Ending all other affirmative defenses or excuses based on mental disease or defect (§ 17(a)),
3. Requiring defendants to show clear and convincing evidence of insanity (§ 17(b)),
4. Limiting expert psychological testimony regarding ultimate issues (FED. R. EVID. 704(b)), and
5. Linking a NGRI verdict directly to federal civil commitment proceedings (§ 4242(b)).

Notwithstanding the statutory language or congressional intent behind IDRA, federal courts have struggled with statutory interpretation and its application to criminal cases (*Cameron*, 1990, p. 1062).

When a defendant who is found competent to stand trial fails to show clear and convincing evidence of insanity, or cannot prove that diminished capacity negated the *mens rea* component of a crime, his or her mental condition may still be relevant in mitigating punishment. Consequently, when the battle of neuropsychologists experts does not yield a favorable verdict for the defendant, testimony used by the defense to argue incompetence, insanity, or diminished capacity may be resurrected to reduce a sentence or avoid the death penalty. Testimony about brain damage may be an important factor mitigating against the death penalty for competent defendants found guilty of capital murder. Failure to call a neuropsychologist expert to present evidence of brain damage at trial has been the basis for ineffective assistance of counsel claims.

Common Issues for Neuropsychological Analysis of Damage Claims

There is no known limit to the number of neurologic and pseudoneurologic conditions that neuropsychologists could address in forensic examinations, but there are a narrower set of damage and causation claims that neuropsychologists routinely encounter. Certain generalizations apply to all neurologic damages claims, but each claim has its own unique set of challenges, issues, and empirical bases.

Head Injury and Postconcussion Syndrome

A key element of a tort is proving the existence of damages. The most common damages issue encountered by neuropsychologists is the effects of remote head–neck injury (Ruff & Richardson, 1999). The specific issues are whether remote mTBI, adult common whiplash, or uncomplicated concussion can explain multiyear subjective disability or present cognitive profile (Alexander, 1998, 2003). Do late postconcussion syndrome (LPCS) claims represent a disorder of the "natural kind" (neurobiologically real, independent of culture; see McNally, 2005). mTBI is an objective, self-limiting, acute neurologic disease that resolves rapidly (Alexander, 1995; McCrea et al., 2003), hence a disorder of the natural kind. LPCS appears in part to be a social construction because of its historical association with compensability legislation and social upheavals (Erichsen, 1866). Boake et al. (2004) showed limited agreement on postconcussion incidence between the *Diagnostic and Statistical Manual of Mental Disorder*, fourth edition (DSM-IV) and *International Classification of Diseases* (ICD) definitions in persons with mTBI, although there was *no difference in neurocognitive or health outcome under either definition*. Failure of a subjective syndromal definition to predict some clinical endpoint means that definition is invalid as a disease concept.

In LPCS cases, the forensic neuropsychologist assists the trier of fact by (a) staging of initial injury severity based on objective indices, (b) background review of LPCS literature, and (c) assessment of the factors contributing to the plaintiff's current neuropsychological presentation (Greiffenstein, 2000). The necessary first step is to stage initial head-neck injury severity with generally accepted criteria for objective injury, based on emergency room or paramedic records. Although published criteria for mTBI vary (Paniak, MacDonald, Toller-Lobe, Durand, & Nagy, 1998; Ruff & Richardson, 1999), the overlap of definitions allows a distillation into a uniform set of core characteristics: mTBI is diagnosed when there is (a) *brief* loss of consciousness (LOC) or *brief* posttraumatic amnesia (PTA) (b) induced by rapid acceleration/deceleration of the head (c) after blunt force trauma (Shaw, 2002). Neurophysiologically, mTBI represents a transient disruption of intracellular and intercellular communication, not a structural lesion. There is no scientific dispute that these are sufficient conditions representing a fundamental definition of mTBI.

A good quantitative method that puts the testifying expert on solid scientific grounds is the core mTBI definition offered by the American Academy of Neurology (AAN) (1997). These graded criteria for sports concussion are both time and symptom weighted: Grade I concussion (no LOC with < 15 minutes PTA), Grade II (no LOC with one hour PTA), and Grade III (+LOC "seconds to minutes"). The AAN (1997) criteria deemphasize reliance on subjective mental changes although there is no way to eliminate all self-reports. The AAN criteria are also supported by the classical mTBI literature, which rely on participants with LOC duration of less than 30 minutes and PTA durations in the one-hour range (Gronwall & Wrightson, 1974; Gronwall, 1977; Newcombe, Rabbitt, & Briggs, 1994). The cognitive effects of mTBI are short-lasting, on the order of days to weeks (Dikmen, McLean, Temkin, & Wyler, 1986; McCrea et al., 2003; McCrea, Kelly, Randolph, Cisler, & Berger, 2002).

The second step is providing conceptual background for juries to understand the facts of a case should include well-established facts. One critical point is that LPCS symptoms are nonspecific. A reasonable distillation comprises nine proposed symptoms: headaches, dizziness, somatic preoccupation, memory loss, concentration lapses, irritability, mood disturbance, pain (excluding headaches), and sensory hyperacuity (Brown, Fann, & Grant, 1994). These symptoms' nonspecificity is proven by their high frequency in personal injury litigants not claiming brain injury or in medical outpatients (Fox, Lees-Haley, Earnest, & Dolezal-Wood, 1995). LPCS does not demonstrate any objective neurologic findings (Alexander, 1995). It is associated with extremely elevated MMPI-2 profiles disproportionate to injury characteristics (Youngjohn, Davis, & Wolf, 1997), atypical motor findings on standardized neurocognitive measures (Greiffenstein, Baker & Gola, 1996a), higher symptom report than acute brain injury (Miller & Donders, 2001), and positive findings on symptom validity tests (Greiffenstein et al. 1994; Greiffenstein, Baker, & Gola, 1996b; Greiffenstein & Baker, 2006). LPCS patients are very similar to other persons with poorly defined, chronic complaints (viz., chronic fatigue syndrome, chronic insomnia) whose interpersonal style draws attention to their disability (Greiffenstein, 2000). Differences of opinion among some neuropsychologists yield different scholarly approaches regarding the scope (width) of the mTBI criteria. The scope of any definition is critical because it determines the mTBI prevalence rates (McCauley et al., 2005) and further unlocks access to financial benefits, treatment, and social validation of disability. The well-grounded forensic neuropsychologist should emphasize mTBI and its variants *should not be diagnosed at random postinjury intervals on the basis of subjective symptom severity*. The American Congress of Rehabilitation (1993) criteria are problematic because of their overly broad scope: One criterion of this definition allows *any* "altered mental state" in the absence of blunt head trauma to qualify as brain injury, implying that any car accident involving a subjective state of being caught off-guard justifies diagnosing mTBI. Kibby and Long (1996) and Paniak et al. (1998) commented on the vagueness of the "altered mental status" feature and the false positive diagnoses it creates. When testifying in court on such matters, the forensic neuropsychologists may succinctly explain to the jury what false positive and negative errors are.

The third step, determination of causative factors, requires reasonable certainty of neurological, social, intellectual, and temperamental correlates of LPCS. There is no reasonable debate that initial head injury severity is the chief determinant of neurologic and neuropsychological outcome (Dikmen, Machamer, Winn, & Temkin, 1995; Rohling, Meyers, & Millis, 2003; Volbrecht, Meyers, & Kaster-Bundgaard, 2000), so persons with no emergency room evidence for amnesia, delirium, unresponsivity, or blunt head trauma are not likely to have acutely injured brains. The neuropsychologist may conclude by acknowledging there is no generally accepted single explanation for LPCS, but *it is generally accepted that LPCS is multifactorial and cannot be explained by a single discrete or systemic neurological problem* (Greiffenstein, 2000; Lishman, 1988; Luis, Vanderploeg, & Curtiss, 2003). LPCS likely represents the final common pathway of many preinjury and postinjury environmental, neurological, academic, social class, medical, and personality risk factors unrelated to traumatic brain (TBI) changes (Greiffenstein, 2000; Greiffenstein & Baker, 2003; Lishman, 1988; Ruff & Richardson, 1999). McCauley, Boake, Levin, Contant, & Song, (2001) showed LPCS correlates with gender, ethnicity, and social support networks. Clearly, social factors contribute heavily to the phenomenology of LPCS. Hence, the scientific literature justifies a greater focus on studying preinjury and postinjury social and situational factors in understanding current LPCS presentations. But one should always be open to new and objective case-specific information that may "trump" base rates and provide compelling contrary evidence for residual posttraumatic brain damage.

Neurotoxic Torts

A steadily growing area of legal contention is the purported role of environmental toxins in central nervous dysfunction (Bolla, 2005). The issue of fact is whether plaintiffs' brains were permanently damaged following exposure to various neurotoxins. The list includes organic solvents (e.g., Toluene, halides), organometals (e.g., lead, manganese), microorganisms ("black mold"; Lees-Haley, 2003), and even common chemicals ("multiple chemical sensitivity"). Research into neuropsychological correlates of claimed and proven toxic exposure is growing. There have been investigations of neuropsychological correlates of exposure to neurotoxicants such as manganese (Bowler, Mergler, Sassine, Larribe, & Hudnell, 1999; Deschamps, Guillaumot, & Raux, 2001), mercury (Meyer-Baron, Schaeper, Van Thriel, & Seeber, 2003), organic solvents (Albers & Berent, 2000; Colvin, Myers, Nell, Rees, & Cronje, 1993), and PCB (Jacobson & Jacobson, 2002, 2003; Schantz et al., 1996).

A special case of neurotoxic torts is lead poisoning in children and adolescents. Unlike toxic claims for which there is no reliable somatic marker, there are objective measures of body lead levels. Lead is easily absorbed by the body and is measured in micrograms per deciliter (mcg/dl). Per suggested guidelines by the Centers for Disease Control (CDC, 1991), < 10 mcg/dl is inconsequential, 10–19 mcg/del is of indeterminate medical meaning, > 20 requires a medical evaluation, and > 70 mcg/dl is a medical emergency. Empirically, Goldstein's (1984) review of empirical literature suggested > 80 mcg/dl is associated with proven brain tissue damage. The forensic controversy centers on whether *low blood lead levels*, defined by the CDC (1991) as 10–20 mcg/dl, has any impact on general neuropsychological functioning. For example, the 14-month-old plaintiff in *Baxter v. Temple* (2008) had a lead level of 36 mcg/del, although the jury eventually found no evidence of damage caused by lead (*Baxter v. Temple*, 2012; see Chapter 36 in this volume for extended discussion). Proponents of a lead–cognition link argue that even low blood levels in the 10–20 mcg range have severe consequences for intellectual functioning (Needleman, 1979; Needleman & Leviton, 1979). More refined dose-response investigations showed lead–IQ effect sizes were small, with the best-designed studies showing group differences of three IQ points (Pocock, Smith, & Baghurst, 1994; Tong, Baghurst, McMichael, Sawyer, & Mudge, 1996), equivalent to a small effect size around 0.20.

Typically, these claims have a similar logical structure to LCPS, asserting that (a) exposure (trauma) levels below recognized disease-inducing thresholds causes occult brain damage not detectable through standard medical testing, (b) subjective disability and cognitive weakness are evidence for such brain damage, and (c) "syndromes" are defined by many nonspecific complaints. Circular reasoning problems endemic to many chronic low-dose claims remain a major methodological issue: "The exposure to solvents prove the plaintiff's memory complaints are organic, but the memory complaints prove he or she must have had damaging solvent exposure." Some neuropsychologists rely on this reasoning to support their arguments. For example, Bowler et al. (2003) judged manganese neurotoxicity to be present based on the plaintiff's (a welder) 25-year retrospective recall of how often windows were open in the identified plants. Questionable reliance on post hoc evidence or the strongly held personal beliefs of litigants does not disprove manganese-cognition claims; it only means such evidence is insufficient and potentially misleading.

The issue of fact that neuropsychologists cope with is which of multiple competing explanations best fits the facts of the individual case. Taking lead as an example, the modest associations between lead and cognition do not yet meet accepted standards of causality (Hill, 1965). Like other neurotoxic claims and LPCS, lead poisoning cases are confounded by powerful social comorbidities: Lead research studies and claims are strongly associated with covariate imbalances in socioeconomic status, parental cognitive aptitudes, and ethnic status. Hebben (2001) cited literature showing lead accounts for less intellectual variance than sociodemographic and other factors. In Kaufman's (2001) view, 26 of the best-designed lead-cognition studies still displayed marked shortcomings, including: uncontrolled variables clouding conclusion, insufficient assessment of parental IQ, failure to control for multiple comparisons, inappropriate comparison of extreme groups, and variable examiner characteristics. Most important, Kaufman's (2001) review failed to show any linear relationships between lead levels and IQ in the low range. Needleman and Bellinger's (2001) response to Kaufman (2001) offers a good example of unscholarly responses that testifying neuropsychologists should avoid: dismissal of any possible criticism, accusing critics of offering "weary" arguments, and joining "spokespersons for (fill in the blank) industry." Needleman went on to argue that even tiny effects could still have practical actuarial impact on intelligence levels depending on the population scale. But Needleman et al. (2002) later reported low lead levels caused executive-cognitive dysfunction in adjudicated delinquents, but no intellectual effects.

Needleman and Bellinger's (2001) visceral investment in lead-cognition effects aside, the challenge for the serious neuropsychologist in neurotoxic cases remains one of disentangling the brain effects of neurotoxins from the nonproximate, enduring, and situational characteristics of the person bringing a lead-cognition claim. This may be impossible in some cases and is certainly a difficulty in most. One should always recognize that lead can have a deleterious effect on brain tissue but the focus in the individual litigant should be on the reasonable impact of subclinical doses of lead.

Suboptimal Effort and Malingering

An important difference between clinical and forensic settings is the element of secondary gain. Secondary gain is defined as any external incentive for sustaining subjective disability inconsistent with the natural history of the claimed disorder. Secondary gain can take the form of positive reinforcements (compensation, attention, access to narcotics) or negative reinforcement (release from work obligations, inhibition of an abusive spouse). The mere existence of a lawsuit or compensable injury is insufficient to diagnose malingering, but it is sufficient grounds for justifying effort testing. Rogers (1997) systematized forms of noncredible presentations. Invalidity may take the form of suboptimal effort (not trying hard enough), exaggeration of minor complaints (embellishment), dissimulation (exaggerating virtue and pre-accident adjustment), and effortful distortion of responses (malingering). As discussed earlier, diagnoses of malingering may not be allowed in some jurisdictions or by some judges, but acceptable alternate language is available, e.g., effort testing indicates scores not consistent with genuine brain injury (Ogloff, 1990; Tombaugh, 1995).

Traditional SVTs embedded in personality scales are insufficient for detecting malingered neurocognitive deficits. The Infrequency (F) scale of the MMPI-2 may capture simulation of psychotic syndromes, but it is insensitive to implausible pseudoneurologic histories (Greiffenstein et al., 2002), exaggerated cognitive deficit (Greiffenstein, Baker, & Gola, 1995; Larrabee, 2003c; Ross et al., 2004), exaggerated trauma syndromes (Greiffenstein, Baker, Axelrod, Peck, & Gervais, 2004) or exaggerated posttraumatic pain (Larrabee, 2003a, 2003b).

There are many methods for detecting response distortion, some grounded in logic and others in empirical findings. Sweet (1999b) classifies invalid neuropsychological performances into three basic types: (a) poor performance on specific validity tests; (b) atypical score patterns on genuine neuropsychological measures; and (c) poor ecological validity, which is defined as marked incongruence between scores and observed behavior. Use of specific validity tests is a purely objective approach and the other two a mixture of objective findings and clinical judgment.

Specific Validity Tests

Specific tests designed for detection of response bias were termed SVTs. More recently, Larrabee (2012c) distinguished performance validity tests (PVTs) as the validity of test performance from symptom validity as the validity of symptom report. PVTs typically target implausible memory and attention deficits, although any implausible performance from any neurobehavioral domain can be measured. The most effective PVTs are simple verbal or visual two-alternative recognition memory tests passed with ease by all but the most profoundly impaired neurological patients. Examples of two-choice verbal PVTs include the CARB (Allen, Iversen, & Green, 2002), the Word Memory Test (Green, Iverson, & Allen, 1999; Green, Lees-Haley, & Allen, 2002; Green, 2003), the Medical Symptom Validity Test (Green, 2004); the Non-Verbal Medical Symptom Validity Test (Green, 2008), and the Warrington Recognition Memory Test verbal condition (Millis, 2002). Examples of two-choice visual memory tests include the TOMM (Rees, Tombaugh, Gansler, & Moczynski, 1998; Tombaugh, 1995; Tombaugh, 2002) and the Warrington faces condition (Millis, 2002). Another validity determination method is a floor effects strategy, where the cutting score is based on a lower performance limit of clinical groups with known brain disease (Frederick, 2003; Taylor, Kreutzer, & West, 2003; van Gorp et. al., 1999). Minor injury litigants scoring "below" the floor of persons with substantial brain damage are probably putting forth insufficient effort. A good example of this is the Rey 15-Item Memory Test, a visual immediate recall task (Rey, cited in Lezak, 1995). Persons with moderate to severe closed head injury obtain a group mean of 12 items (four rows) with a lower limit of ten items; they rarely produce intrusion errors. Persons seeking compensation with a mean of 2.2 years postinjury often score < 10 (Greiffenstein et al., 1994; Greiffenstein et al., 1996b).

Atypical Patterns

Pairs or groups of test scores inconsistent with neuropsychological or neuroanatomical first principles should be viewed with suspicion. Atypical patterns include (a) violations of test difficulty hierarchy, (b) extreme variability on tests measuring the same underlying cognitive processes, (c) incompatibility of test pairs, or (d) disease-deficit incompatibility (Larrabee, 2012b). A violation of the difficulty hierarchy means the claimant fails easy items but passes more difficult items in the same conceptual domain. Extreme variability refers to large discrepancies between test scores measuring the same underlying construct. Incompatibility of test pairs refers to tests with unidirectional relationship where the direction of dependence is violated. For example, recent memory depends on adequate attention, but attention does not depend on memory. Mittenberg, Azrin, Millsaps, and Heilbronner (1993) showed student simulators performed more poorly on the Attention/Concentration Index than the General Memory Index of the Wechsler Memory Scale–Revised, the opposite of genuine brain injury. Disease-deficit incompatibility means an abnormal score is not consistent with the claimed disease. For example, brief working memory tasks are not affected by nondementing brain disorders with the exception of conduction aphasia. Persons feigning brain injury are not aware of this and perform poorly on digit span tasks (Mittenberg et al., 2001; Greiffenstein et al., 1994; Greve, Bianchini, Mathias, Houston, & Crouch, 2003). Another example is implausible motor dysfunction: Damage to motor control centers of the brain results in a gradient of increasing impairment as a function of task complexity (Haaland, Harrington, & Yeo, 1987; Haaland, Temkin, Randahl, & Dikmen, 1994), but Greiffenstein, Baker, and Gola (1996a) showed compensation seekers with minor traumas show the inverse pattern, with grip strength performance worst, finger tapping intermediate, and small parts dexterity best.

Lack of ecological validity is the neuropsychologist's judgment that a respondent's scores or history are not consistent with observable behavior (Larrabee, 1990; Sweet, 1999b). This is a subjective judgment that requires a comparison of the informal mental status evaluation (MSE) to the deficits implied by neurocognitive test scores. Persons with extremely low cognitive scores should display obvious problems during an interview. For example, a person with genuine organic amnesia will exhibit considerable difficulty recalling postaccident information and a true aphasic will have great difficulty communicating thoughts. But persons feigning brain damage have to prove their claims through two clashing paradigms: (a) relying on intact cognitive processes to communicate disability beliefs during the interview but (b) proving cognitive defects by underperforming on neurocognitive measures. A good example of poor ecological validity is the person who performs < three standard deviations below expectations on memory and language tests, but who spontaneously and fluently verbalizes many symptoms during face-to-face interview. Greiffenstein et al. (1994) and Slick, Sherman, and Iverson (1999) offer behavioral criteria for judging unusual symptom reports. It has been empirically demonstrated that persons with genuine memory disorders report fewer complaints than normal controls (Feher, Larrabee, Sudilovsky, & Crook, 1994; Prigatano, Altman, & O'Brien, 1990). But neurologically normal persons with LPCS voice many complaints, and those who feign disability may offer dozens of symptoms. Such overreporting behavior is the opposite that expected in persons with genuine brain disease. Greiffenstein and Baker (2006) showed that malingering was more frequent in persons voicing the most LPCS complaints and nonexistent in those voicing the fewest.

The Process of Forensic Neuropsychological Assessment

There are many phases to the neuropsychologist-attorney and neuropsychologist-court interaction. The assessment phase is the most crucial, because it is here that the bases for creating opinion are developed. Opinions and testimony develop easily if one has performed an adequate assessment.

General Contours of Assessment

The neuropsychologist answers legal questions, not clinical ones. The assessment phase starts when the neuropsychologist begins collecting the data upon which answers to hypothetical questions (opinions) will be based. The evaluation of the neuropsychological injury claim requires selection of neurocognitive measures shaped by the legal context. The following principles constitute the structure of the forensic neuropsychological assessment. These principles are not independent, overlapping to some extent.

First, it is critical to recognize at the outset that *forensic neuropsychological assessment is a process*, of which formal test instruments are only one component. The entire process requires a multimethod, convergent evidence model. Neuropsychologists have no greater requirement to validate the entire process than physicians do to combining physical findings with "records and history." Neuropsychology, like medicine, is an inexact science that combines subjective art with objective measures.

Second, extratest data provide the enriched context for disentangling the many confounds present in individual brain damage claim cases, improving interpretation of nonspecific findings (Bolla, 2005; Guirguis, 1997; Matarazzo & Herman, 1985). In addition to neuropsychological test data, the three additional forms of extratest data constituting the entire assessment process are:

- Interview data (history, current self-reported symptoms, etc.)
- The MSE (Speech, affect, etc.)
- Collateral sources (medical records, neuroimaging studies, etc.)

Third, blind interpretation of isolated test scores is not a viable practice in neuropsychology. There is no such thing as a neuropsychological test with universal sensitivity and specificity across all possible pairings of target and control groups; reliability and validity of tests are *always contingent* and need to incorporate data on gender, ethnicity, demographics, and cultural factors (Hunsley & Mash, 2005). A convergent evidentiary model further recognizes there is no single, foolproof method or battery for differentiating organic posttraumatic changes forms nonneurological factors (Pope, Butcher, & Seelen, 1993). A good example is the ubiquitous Performance IQ < Verbal IQ difference scores on Wechsler intelligence tests (Matarazzo & Herman, 1985). This pattern can be associated with acute right brain injury, but is also seen in persons with visual problems, motor deficits, low motivation, and preinjury developmental learning disabilities (Greiffenstein & Baker, 2002). There is always some potential nonneurological condition associated with low scores on a given measure.

Fourth, test selection for the assessment *relies on multiple standardized measures of effort and function that have (a) sound scientific and normative bases and (b) are relevant to the legal context.* Because the legal issues are broader than clinical ones, the legal contexts so variable, and the environment after various neurologic insults so much different, there is no legal (or scientific) requirement for a "fixed" or universal test battery.

Extratest Elements of the Assessment Process

Interview

The clinical interview and accompanying behavior observations usually take place before the administration of tests. Clinical history and MSE observations help provide a context that may substantially affect the interpretation of scores (Lezak, 1995; Vanderploeg, 1994). The history is divided into two groupings: presenting complaints and past personal histories. The history of presenting complaints pursues key case information regarding the date(s) of the incident, initial injury severity; symptom mode of evolution (clinical course), present symptoms, claimant's attribution of complaints, subjective functional status, and treatment related to the current problems. The past personal history gathers information extending into the past as far as necessary to consider *reasonable* nonincident-related explanations of a claimant's current presentation (Melton et al., 1997). An intense analysis of dynamics in the family of origin is usually unnecessary in a neuropsychological context. This initial phase is critical in collecting demographic information that shapes performance expectations of the claimant. This is often termed the *estimation of premorbid cognitive levels* (Greiffenstein & Baker, 2003). Variables that help estimate premorbid functioning include years of education (Heaton, Grant, & Matthews, 1991), quality of educational attainment (Greiffenstein & Baker, 2003; Manly, Jacobs, Touradji, Small, & Stern, 2002), special education, age (Heaton, Ryan, Grant, & Matthews, 1996), gender (Dodrill, 1979), employment history (Heaton, Chelune, & Lehman, 1978), and intellectual level (Tremont, Hoffman, Scott, & Adams, 1998).

A symptom timeline documenting the appearance and disappearance of symptoms can be indispensable. Civil War neurologist Weir Mitchell noted, "Time is the great diagnostician!"[3] The symptom mode of evolution should follow a pattern generally consistent with the natural history of the claimed disease. mTBI typically resolves on the order of days to one week, reflecting restabilization of neuronal chemical processes (Guskiewicz et al., 2003; McCrea et al., 2003; McCrea et al., 2002). Factors that influence symptom evolution may also include symptom suggestion through Internet research, symptom suggestion by financially interested family members, changed socioeconomic circumstances, reinforcement of the illness role, and implantation of diagnoses by aggressive treaters. The neuropsychologist weighs what combination of psychogenic, reinforcement, and/or neurogenic factors best explains the symptom evolution.

There is no generally accepted history form, although forensic specialists should develop a standardized form to promote comparison across individuals within a specific legal context. The interview should balance open-ended and close-ended questions (Othmer & Othmer, 1989). The open-ended questions allow the claimant to prioritize their complaints and provide an injury narrative. Open-ended inquiry allows the neuropsychologist to make initial observations of the claimant's memory function and discourse organization at a conversational level. The close-ended questions ("systems review") provide opportunity to voice additional complaints. In this phase, the neuropsychologist may evaluate symptom suggestibility (false positive symptoms), assist patients who have genuine memory problems, or encourage productivity in minimally responsive persons. The neuropsychologist must ask follow-up questions about each complaint and never passively accept the claimant's self-diagnoses. Lees-Haley (1995) noted there is a widespread tendency for clinicians to presume etiology or diagnosis based on lay patient's conclusions about these issues. For example, the complaint of "confusion" should not be interpreted as evidence for organic delirium. This complaint should be followed by questions. Good memory for one's own confusion is likely nonorganic.

Mental Status Evaluation

The MSE includes categorization of the claimant's speech and language, affect, reported mood, motor behavior, cognitive organization, and speech content. Behavior observation provides another source of confirmatory (or refuting) evidence to correlate with test scores. The good historian who produces poor memory scores and the talkative patient who reports severe depression while smiling tentatively raises incongruence issues. However, some incongruities can be clinically meaningful: Schizophrenics may show incongruity between affect (laughing) and speech content (discussing a recent funeral), those with orbital-medial frontal damage appear unconcerned, and those with conversion features may appear bland while discussing their pseudoparesis. Again, such incongruities must never be viewed in isolation from other data.

Review of Records

Medical records are critical in forming the extratest context that shapes neuropsychological test interpretations. For example, field, ambulance, and emergency department records allow reasonable estimates of initial severity. They may also provide the only objective evidence that a physical injury to the brain injury occurred, e.g., neuroimaging studies, observations of an exposed brain made by a neurosurgeon, coma status. A single negative neuroimaging study cannot rule out a closed head injury, but serial negative neurodiagnostic evaluations make brain injury less likely. Of the three methods, records are probably the most fallible because records are created by somebody else, and hence represent the perceptions, judgments, and interpretations of somebody who is not available for questioning. Cripe's (2002) excellent critical review points out the limitations of analyzing records, which include unverifiable assumption of diagnostic accuracy. A preexisting diagnosis of anxiety disorder by a general practitioner may be insufficiently documented to support the conclusion. Conversely, the absence of medical records is not evidence for absence of mental illness. Persons with personality disorders are especially vulnerable to poor postaccident coping, but are also prone to misattribute long-standing coping difficulties to a single pivotal accident (Greiffenstein, 2002). One of the defining characteristics of persons with disordered personalities is poor insight and refusal to seek treatment.

Neuropsychological Test Selection

The battery should contain core tests of functions and modalities in sensory, motor, and cognitive domains, with additional tests showing clear relevance to the legal issues at hand. A neuropsychological battery that is reliable, valid, standardized, and well normed is not necessarily a logical choice in a given legal issue. The error of giving a fixed battery to all legal situations is easily evident: There would be no reason to give the Mattis Dementia Rating Scale (MDRS) in an mTBI tort, although the MDRS might be acceptable in a civil competence matter. The *Joiner* (1997) legal decision allows a trial judge to disqualify even sound methods if they have no lucid link to the case at hand. In general, a flexible test battery routinely administered to persons with the same claimed etiology or the same legal context is sufficient to draw defensible conclusions and gain admission to court. Single tests of "organicity," although they may show modest sensitivity to some forms of cerebral dysfunction (Frankle, 1995; Lacks, 1982), are not likely to answer all questions before the court or may even miss severe neuropathology (Bigler & Ehrfurth, 1980).

The forensic neuropsychologist should always give symptom validity tests. Forensic settings contain strong incentives for distorting test scores or interview data. There is no legitimate reason for avoiding these measures in a forensic context. The base rate for invalid response styles in litigated brain damage claims is high, even when stringent criteria for malingering are applied.

The *Daubert* factors may be used as an aspirational guideline to assist in test selection. It is important to again emphasize that *Daubert* has a generally liberal thrust, and requires the existence of certain salutary scientific or logical characteristics. Again, *Daubert* addresses probative value for admissibility decisions. Hence, two measures with nonzero but different validities are both admissible. The *Daubert* criteria are assessed against individual tests, not batteries or groupings (see section of forensic neuropsychology myths, this chapter). The Halstead-Reitan Battery (HRB) and Luria-Nebraska Neuropsychological Battery (LNNB) are undoubtedly acceptable in court. They meet all criteria except for general acceptance, when this is defined in terms of community use. Per Sweet, Meyer, Nelson, and Moberg (2010), HRB and LNNB adherents are a shrinking minority (5%) of neuropsychology practitioners. Use by a minority does not make them poor measures; it only makes general acceptance difficult to prove.

Interpretation and Report Writing

Virtually all cases referred by legal sources require a written report (Melton, Petrilla, Poythress, & Slobogin, 1997). Forensic neuropsychological reporting overlaps with written communication in clinical settings but distinguishes itself in a number of ways.

General Contours of the Interpretive Process

First, the hypothetical legal question must be combined with what Larrabee (2012a) termed a *four-component consistency analysis*:

1. Are the data consistent within and between neuropsychological domains?

2 Is the score profile consistent with the claimed etiology?
3 Are the cognitive scores consistent with the documented injury severity?
4 Are the data consistent with behavioral presentation?

Scores are only initial data that need to be interpreted in light of other extratest data (Matarazzo & Hermann, 1985; Matarazzo, Bornstein, McDermott, & Noon, 1986). At best, neurocognitive measures give only an indirect picture of brain functioning.

Second, consider both nomothetic (general scientific laws) and idiographic (personal and context specific) factors. Much of the perceived conflict between academic and clinical neuropsychologists boils down to the tension between the nomothetic and idiographic approaches, also known as the *clinical versus actuarial controversy* (Meehl, 1954). The place of psychology in a nomothetic-idiographic dimension has been the cause of much controversy (Holt, 1998). However, these two methods have mistakenly been treated as irreconcilable and antithetical, when the fact is they are customarily integrated in everyday clinical sciences, such as forensic psychology (Slobogin, 2003). A good example of nomothetic considerations in neuropsychology is the *dose-response relationship* in head injury, the generalization that brain injury severity is the chief determinant of outcome in adults (Dikmen et al., 1995; Volbrecht et al., 2000) and children (Schwartz et al., 2003; Yeates et al., 2002). Another example of a nomothetic principle is the *inverse dose-response* relationship in litigated neurological damage claims: The more minor the remote injury in litigated cases, the greater the symptom production (Miller & Cartlidge, 1972). Inverse slopes were shown in protracted head injury litigation (Greiffenstein & Baker, 2006; Youngjohn et al., 1997), minor electrical injury (Pliskin et al., 1998), and organic solvent exposure (Albers & Berent, 2000). The dose-response generalization provides the crucial nexus when neuropsychologists correlate neuropsychological test scores, interval since injury, and present complaints. Idiographic considerations come into play when extratest data could substantially modify the interpretation. For example, in a two-year-old case of moderate-severe closed head injury, one would not expect poor Wisconsin Card Sorting Test (WCST) scores, but if one claimant shows encephalomalacia in the frontal lobes, this would be compelling evidence to ignore the outcome base rates and link poor WCST scores deficits to the accident. The maxim to be drawn is this: (a) Always consider base rates in forensic cases but do not let them rule you and (b) it takes powerful case-specific facts to ignore the base rates (Gouvier, 1998).

Crucial Elements of Forensic Neuropsychology Report

The remainder of this section describes the crucial elements of the forensic neuropsychology report that differentiate it from the common clinical report.

The crucial elements are:

- Causation analysis through sound reasoning
- Functional analysis
- Accurate attribution of facts

Causal Reasoning

The law is very concerned with antecedent causal connections that weigh which of several earlier conditions best account for the current state of affairs. The law recognizes two forms of causation: general causation (e.g., Could the accident cause cognitive problems?) and specific causation (e.g., Did this toxic exposure cause cognitive deficits?) (Sanders et al., 2002). The forensic specialist assesses the likelihood of neuropsychological damages acquired as a result of the legal cause of action. The law requires only reasonable likelihood, not experimental certainty of $p < .05$ for every conclusion (Greiffenstein & Kaufmann, 2012). There is no formula or mathematical algorithm for drawing cause-effect conclusions; again, forensic neuropsychological analysis is an *entire assessment process* whose totality does not require sensitivity and specificity values. This reasoning process combines generally accepted principles and instruments (nomothetic, scientific knowledge) with idiographic data (case-specific facts). Hartman (1999) provides the most concise snapshot: The forensic reasoning process is *developing a chain of logical causation that considers the influence of a traumatic event or exposure in the context of a broad life history*.

There are three classes of variables that form this life history context: predisposing (risk), precipitating, and perpetuating variables (Greiffenstein, 2000). Put simply, the injury characteristics are weighed against nonproximate preinjury and postinjury variables as reasonable explanation for findings. Table 37.4 summarizes variables to consider within each of these three categories. Preinjury (risk) variables are nonneurological, sociodemographic, or other features of the individual that have proven association with cognition (Rankin & Adams, 1999). Large portions of neurocognitive score variance, sometimes up to 40%, can be explained by factors such as intelligence, education, grade point average, culture, age, and gender (Anger et al., 1997; Greiffenstein & Baker, 2003). In mTBI there is greater strength of association of scores with education than initial injury severity (Dikmen, Machamer, & Tempkin, 2001). Other preinjury variables that affect symptom reporting include premorbid personality style (Luis, Vanderploeg, & Curtiss, 2003; Ruff & Richardson, 1999), and premorbid body-oriented catastrophic thinking (Greiffenstein & Baker, 2001). Precipitating (periaccidental) factors include the severity of the brain trauma and any consequent medical complications influencing integrity of the central nervous system. Common symptom postaccident perpetuating factors suggestion, reinforcement of illness behaviors, and litigation.

Table 37.4 Tripartite list of moderator variables to consider in causation analysis of neuropsychological scores

Preaccident (Predisposing)
Congenital and/or experiential aptitude (IQ, academic achievement)
Demographics associated with neurocognitive patterns (e.g., age, gender, handedness)
Low education and poor academic achievement
Learning disability (dyslexia, nonverbal learning problems, perceptual-motor incoordination)
Nonneurological medical disorders with systemic effects (e.g., liver dysfunction)
Peripheral nervous system dysfunction (e.g., carpal tunnel syndrome)
Personality organization (e.g., dependent, histrionic, borderline, antisocial, narcissistic)
Vocational history (type of occupation, complexity, stability, downward drift)
Periaccidental (Precipitating)
Acute effects of medication (e.g., narcotics, mood stabilizers such as Depakote)
Neurological trauma severity (e.g., Glasgow Coma Scale (GCS); Grade I–III concussion, days to follow commands)
Electrodiagnostic findings (e.g., evoked potentials, EEG)
Internal distraction by pain (e.g., neuropathic pain, radiculopathy)
Posttraumatic psychiatric disorder (e.g., posttraumatic stress disorder, sleep adjustment disorder, acute stress)
Radiographic findings (e.g., CT/MRI, PET/SPECT imaging)
Topographic features of lesion (e.g., laterality, caudality, focal vs. diffuse)
Traumatic peripheral nervous system injury (e.g., neuropathic pain)
Postaccident (Perpetuating)
Acute + chronic effects of strong psychotropic and narcotic medication
Chronicity of brain lesion and complications (e.g., seizures, encephalomalacia)
Compensation and litigation
Negative reinforcement of illness behaviors (e.g., avoidance of unrewarding preinjury job)
Poor physical stamina (e.g., deconditioning, inactivity due to low postaccident expectations)
Positive reinforcement of illness behaviors (e.g., narcotic medications for pain, compensation)
Suboptimal motivation and deliberate feigning of deficits
Symptom suggestion (e.g., Internet, attorney, aggressive treater implanting diagnoses)

The process of weighing preaccident, periaccidental, and postaccident factors must be grounded in sound judgment. Hill (1965), writing in the context of epidemiological research, offered multifaceted causation analysis guidelines easily generalizable to the forensic setting. Table 37.5 summarizes Hill's (1965) factors used in support of causation judgments. "Plausibility" and "biological gradient" are the most pertinent factors for neuropsychologists to consider in judging the impact of periaccidental variables (e.g., brain injury severity). A documented history of mTBI with brief amnesia is not a plausible explanation for uniformly poor test scores one year later. The role of intervention (named "experimental evidence" by Hill, 1965) is useful in weighing causation factors: Posttreatment score improvements in severe brain injury adds weight to a neurogenic causation theory, but such causation is less likely in a person whose posttreatment scores show declines absent intervening neurological insult. The "coherence" factor refers to the consistency between a person's clinical course and the natural history of the claimed etiology (see also Larrabee, 1990).

Important caveats include never relying on post hoc symptoms alone to draw inferences about brain injury. One does not diagnose TBI on the basis of symptom severity at random intervals after accidents; it is determined by quantifiable variables closest to the injury date. Claims that individuals can recall alterations in conscious more clearly after longer delay, assumes that retrospective recall is more accurate than in situ recall. This belief is unsupported nonsense best described as "junk science" (Worthington, Stallard, Price, & Goss, 2002). The dangers of post hoc reliance are shown by Varney, Kubu, and Morrow (1998), who used self-report alone to diagnose "intermediate" central nervous system damage after alleged organic solvent exposure. One needs a quantifiable somatic marker independent of self-report. In toxic cases where such markers are not readily apparent, Hartman (1999) recommends a minimum requirement of objective evidence for excessive toxins in a defined geographic area in the absence of evidence for somatic markers in a particular individual. Such conditions would fit a general causation model, but more is needed for a specific causation argument. In view of the *Joiner* (1997) decision, it is unclear whether Hartman's (1999) method is admissible.

Functional Analysis

The law concerns itself greatly with the functional capacities of individuals. Functional capacity refers to what activities a person can carry out in everyday life and what knowledge is necessary to accomplish such activities (Grisso, 1986). Legal decisions are based on the mental and social capacities of

Table 37.5 Sir Bradford Hill's (1965) nine factors for analyzing causal statements

Hill's Factors	*Description in neuropsychological context*
Specificity	Exposure associated with specific set of deficits not seen with other diseases or different chemical exposures. Is plaintiff's cognitive profile similar to profiles reported in good research papers?
Strength	Association so strong that competing factors are easily ruled out. Effect size calculations and correlation coefficients large. Example: Age and education no longer moderators in dementia patients (Tombaugh et al., 1996)
Consistency	Replication. Other researchers demonstrate same pattern of scores in similar disease group or similar litigating group. Example: Reliable Digit Span repeatedly shown sensitive and specific to feigned cognitive disorder
Temporality	A strong temporal link. Merely showing "B followed A" at a random time interval does not meet this criterion. Example: Plaintiff's memory complaints starting day after head injury versus six months later.
Biological gradient	Increased exposure correlates with deficit; identical to dose-response law. Example: Bullet wound to frontal lobe correlates with poor WCST score.
Plausibility	Is there a credible neurologic mechanism that explains associated deficit pattern? Example: A pattern of diffusely poor test scores is implausible in mTBI but more plausible in a dementia claim.
Coherence	Is deficit pattern consistent with natural history of disease? A major deviation from the expected course is evidence against coherence. Example: Worsening cognitive complaints not consistent with mTBI.
Experimental evidence	Does known intervention remediate deficits? Example: Neurocognitive scores worsening after "cognitive rehabilitation" is evidence against neurogenic causes in nondementing cases.
Analogy	Is there a similar exposure we can compare we can draw a relationship with? Example: Workers with organic solvent exposure in one industry (railroad) should look the same as similar exposure in a different industry (munitions).

individuals, and it is here that forensic neuropsychology can make its greatest contribution. A probate court may be interested whether an aged person can make a will, a civil court whether a plaintiff can work, and a criminal court whether a defendant could plan a crime.

A common mistake of psychologists in general is to equate neuropsychological diagnosis with functional disability. A remote diagnosis of mTBI does not automatically mean the person is not able to function, nor does a learning disability equate to legal insanity. The DSM-V (American Psychiatric Association, 2013) criteria require some evidence for functional problems in order to warrant a mental illness diagnosis, but some psychologists stop the inferential process after a patient fulfills symptom criteria. Similarly, neuropsychologists may find weakness, abnormalities, deficits, etc., on their tests then go on to conclude these findings imply inability to work, socially interact, or function around the house. The maxim should be *an abnormal test score is not the end of the diagnostic process but the beginning*. How exactly can "subtle" neurocognitive deficits (assuming they exist) impact driving or work? One must be careful to differentiate self-imposed disability from objectively manifested disability.

Empirically, the research suggests that pervasive cognitive impairments in combination with motor deficits are the only supportable grounds for finding functional disability. Dikmen, Temkin, Machamer, Holubkov, et al. (1994) attempted point predictions by calculating work return rates in a large sample of brain-injured persons. Relative to a preinjury employment base rate of 80%, the poorest return rates (46%) were only associated with Halstead Impairment Index scores of 0.80–1.0, meaning impairment on nearly all tests of the HRB. The only single measure best associated with lower rates was dominant name-writing speed of > one minute. Searight et al. (1989) reported significant association between HRB scores and general competence in a geriatric sample, but poor prediction of individual living tasks as rated by caregivers of early dementia patients. LeBlanc, Hayden, and Paulman (2000) and Sbordone (2001) did not identify any single useful test in predicting in vivo situational behaviors, although general level of performance is useful.

Attribution of Facts

Clinical report writing is designed to achieve economy of expression. To achieve this, there is an assumption of veridical reporting by the patient. A patient states "I am supposed to get neuropsychological testing for my closed head injury" and the clinician writes, "Patient is 35 year old female currently 5 months status-post closed head injury." However, in forensic writing, source attribution is critical in separating fact from allegation. The forensic neuropsychologist should write "The claimant is a 35 year old female who (believes/states/represents) she sustained a closed head injury five months ago." In this manner, the neuropsychologist avoids basing test interpretations on a scaffold of uncritically accepted and possibly false allegations.

Neuropsychological Testimony

The neuropsychologist enters the testimony phase when he or she is asked to give opinions under oath in a number of response formats. These response formats include interrogatories (written answers to questions), affidavits (sworn and signed declarations of opinions), discovery depositions (*duces tecum*), trial depositions (*bene esse*), or live testimony in front of the trier of fact.

Trial depositions and live testimony are the main vehicles for proffering neuropsychologist's opinions in court. A deposition is a pretrial procedure given under oath and used to (a) narrow legal disputes down to core ideas, (b) cement expert opinions, and (c) to discover whether the opposing expert is helpful to one's own client (Pope et al., 1993). Depositions are broken into two phases: direct examination by the retaining attorney and cross-examination by the opposing attorney. Both phases are different in character and purpose. The direct examination is conducted by the retaining attorney and consists of open-ended questions designed to establish the neuropsychologist's (a) credentials, (b) data collection methods, (c) case-specific findings, and (b) final opinion. Cross-examination is the questioning by opposing counsel about matters brought up during direct examination. The object of cross-examination is challenging the neuropsychologist's credibility, competency, and logical basis for opinions. There are a number of general principles for effective neuropsychological testimony and coping with cross-examination. The first, and overriding, principle is preparation: A good neuropsychological examination interpreted in the context of extratest information (demographics, medical records) and behavior observations helps adjustment to the most aggressive cross-examination. "Blind interpretation" of fixed batteries or brain damage diagnoses based on history alone are easily exploited and usually fatal. A second principle is acknowledging weaknesses in one's approach or conclusions when confronted with questions raising genuine issues. "Courtroom unfamiliar" (Brodsky, 1991) neuropsychologists view every question as a trap or contrivance; they strive to defend every statement in their report against every question, thereby eroding expert credibility. The third important principle is to always maintain the mental set that the neuropsychologist is there *to educate the jury* in general in principles of neuropsychology and the basis for one's opinion. This mental set fits the two prongs of FRE 702: providing background knowledge so the jury can understand evidence or providing a case-specific cognitive interpretation of evidence.

Not all cross-examination questions are genuine efforts to understand the neuropsychologist's position. Some questions are designed to undermine the neuropsychologist's credibility, others to manufacture pseudo-issues, blur important distinctions, or to create misimpressions. A general feature of cross-examinations is the use of ambiguity and imprecision present in all human discourse to parse opinions and impeach testimony. In depositions, most attorneys are interested in observing the expert's professional demeanor and poise when confronting subtle changes in wording of questions. One's prior testimony may be slightly paraphrased in such a way to convey meaning different than was originally intended. Coping with cross-examination requires (a) attentive listening for imprecision/ambiguity, (b) calm professionalism, and (c) preparation for the most common approaches, termed *gambits.*

The most common gambit is the "learned treatise" (LT) approach; an effort to undermine the neuropsychologist's credibility by showing inconsistencies between the neuropsychologist's opinions from that held by the (purportedly) unimpeachable authority (Babitsky & Mangraviti, 1997). The LT is a completely legal construction that has no true parallel in science. It stems from the religious origins of the adversarial system: Religious canon was the foundation of all opinion and could not be questioned. Scientist-practitioners eschew attribution of perfection to any source. The gambit always begins by getting the witness to agree a certain person, text, excerpt, or pamphlet is a "reliable authority." The response is to deny any text the voice of *complete* authority (Brodsky, 1991). Instead, answers should qualify the limits of authority. For example, witness this interchange with a series of proposed answers:

Q: Isn't Muriel Lezak's book *Neuropsychological Assessment* a standard authority in your field?"

A(1): If you are asking if I agree with everything Dr. Lezak wrote in her book, no, but it is a useful resource.

A(2): Dr. Lezak's book is an excellent resource providing brief summaries of almost all neuropsychological tests, but I don't consider it the final word.

A(3): Some chapters and insights from the book are very reliable statements, but other chapters or insights are weaker. Which section did you have in mind?

A list of common cross-examination gambits is summarized in Table 37.6. A common gambit with many variants is "lumping." The questioner uses imprecise language to blur graded phenomena into a single category, implying the magnitude of a neurological condition is irrelevant. This method is often combined with the "yes-no" pigeonhole. A typical question may be, "Isn't head injury commonly associated with symptoms like (personality change/memory loss/attention deficits/headaches)?" The careful listener immediately notes imprecision as to (a) severity of the initial injury and (b) the postinjury interval at which the symptom is reported. The answer is quite different if you see an mTBI versus severe TBI patient within days postinjury versus years. When dealing with imprecise questions, the best strategy is *active answering*. This means you address both the surface and latent (unspoken) content. There is no statutory requirement or rule of court procedure that requires experts to limit answers to yes and no. The following interchange is an example of active answering:

Q: My client said she has terrible short-term memory. Isn't that complaint consistent with a head injury, yes or no, doctor?

Table 37.6 Common cross-examination gambits

Gambit	*Description*	*Typical Question*
Learned Treatise	Try to show neuropsychologist's conclusions differ from that of a famous neuropsychologist or key textbook.	"Would it change your opinion if Dr. Ima Legend published a position against the test you used?"
Isolate and Trap (The Hypothetical)	Takes one fact or finding out of context and asks the neuropsychologist to reformat his or her opinion. Tries to highlight isolated fact for jury as if critical/dispositive.	"Would it change your opinion if . . .?" or "Did you know . . .?"
Hired Gun	Proving the expert's opinion is offered on basis of money rather than objectivity.	"How much are you being paid for your testimony"?
General Pigeonhole	Witness is asked to place answers in overly simplified scheme. Witness forced into self-imposed halo effect when minor mistakes pointed out.	"Would you say you were X% accurate in your opinions offered today?" or "What letter grade would you assigned your practices, A? B? C?"
Yes-No Pigeonhole	Demands that answers be limited to Yes–No–I Don't Know; questioner implies this answer format is statutory.	"Head injury will cause headaches, yes or no, doctor?"
False Alternative Pigeonhole	A pigeonhole technique where neuropsychologist is asked to choose between two polar options.	"So if my client isn't faking, that leaves only brain damage?"
Subtle Restatement	Questioner paraphrases witness's earlier testimony in a subtle way. This is used to manufacture inconsistencies in testimony.	"Earlier you said that nearly all litigants are (malingerers/brain damaged)?"
Unreliable Examination	The attorney asks questions about the uncertainty of findings and opinions, often by exaggerating the virtues of any test *not* given by the witness.	"Doctor, isn't it true that only the complete Halstead-Reitan Battery shows excellent sensitivity and specificity?"
False Conceit Gambit	Attorney (typically for the plaintiff) portrays client as special/unique and hence not subject to general expectations of most persons with claimed etiology; this is often combined with the Unreliable Examination gambit to exaggerate virtues of opposing expert.	"My expert spent 25 hours testing my client, but you spent only five hours. Doesn't that make my expert's diagnosis of permanent brain damage more accurate?" (Context = three-year-old whiplash case)
Blurring	Questions blur important distinctions among graded phenomenon, leaving impression that "all injuries are the same."	"Head injuries can cause permanent memory problems?"

A: Memory deficits depend on the severity and the length of time since injury. In your client's case, a two-year-old head trauma without any immediate memory loss cannot explain her current belief in a memory disorder.

This answer addresses the imprecision of the question, educates the jury in dose-response thinking, stresses the subjectivity of memory complaints, and links a general principle (dose-response relations) to the instant case.

Brodsky (1991, 1999) provides generally useful techniques for resisting problematic gambits designed only to leave misimpressions. Two useful techniques include the Admit-Deny and Push-Pull tactics. With Admit-Deny, the neuropsychologist provides a two-clause answer; the first (dependent) clause acknowledges a kernel of truth to the question. The second clause, the "deny" step, strongly refutes the fact implied by the question. Note the following interchange between a plaintiff attorney and a neuropsychologist:

Q: Isn't it true that malingering measures are very controversial and not generally accepted?

A: Although there are some neuropsychologists who believe people never fake, considerable research has shown certain tests are very good at detecting persons not behaving like truly brain injured patients.

The dependent structure requires the questioner to wait for the full sentence. In this example, the dependent clause starts with "although," holding the listener in abeyance, making it difficult to interrupt.

Another form of cross-examination includes questions designed to put neuropsychologists on the defensive by inquiring into known weaknesses of the field. The "unreliable examination" gambit highlighted in Table 37.6 is very common and manifests in two variants: (a) questioning the status of the tests given by the witness, or (b) touting the superiority of tests not given. The latter variant is commonly seen when the cross-examiner retains a neuropsychologist using different tests. The witness should readily concede weaknesses and limitations without appearing defensive. The Push-Pull tactic helps the neuropsychologist take control of the issue that is raised. The technique works by not only conceding the point made, but also amplifying the allegation as if the witness owned the point. Witness the following exchanges:

Q: Isn't it true, Dr. Greiffenstein, that you did not give all the tests given by my expert?

A: You have no idea how many tests I could have given but did not. Judging the appropriateness of any test battery is always an issue neuropsychologists wrestle with.

Q: Wouldn't you agree the (clinical neuropsychological interview/records review) is subjective and may vary from examiner to examiner? (Asked by both plaintiff and defense attorneys.)

A: The (interview/records review) is *very* subjective and the weakest part of the examination. That's why we give tests to correlate with the more subjective data to see if they match.

Q: Isn't it true that weak neuropsychological test scores can be due to things other than brain damage?

A: The list of explanations for abnormal test scores may be *very* long. No test score can tell you its own cause. I always aim to consider reasonable explanations.

Ethical Issues in Forensic Practice

The courtroom setting brings an intense focus on ethical issues, as ethics and the law are tightly intertwined concepts that evolved together. Fair or unfair, it is inevitable that the testifying neuropsychologist will be confronted with the ethical ramifications of his or her practices. It is important to keep key ethical standards in mind, and know the ethical principles embedded in each phase of the forensic assessment. There are two main authorities for ethical conduct: the code of conduct for psychologists published in 1992 (American Psychological Association, 1992; hereinafter the 1992 Code) and the new conduct code (American Psychological Association, 2002; hereinafter the 2002 Code) as amended in 2010 and applicable to current practice. The 1992 Code is still of historical interest, and may continue to influence the thinking of some neuropsychologists. The 2002 Code includes modifications important for forensic neuropsychologists that reflect the evolving relations between psychology and the law (Fisher, 2003). The main change between 1992 and 2002 was the elimination of "specialty" language such as a separate section on forensic practices. The 2002 Code subsumes forensic considerations into more general standards. All subsequent discussion of ethical principles in this chapter will rely primarily on the 2002 Code.

Under Standard 2.01 (Boundaries of Competence), the 2002 Code requires that psychologists practice within areas in which they have appropriate experience and training. Most relevant: "when assuming forensic roles, psychologists are or become reasonably familiar with the judicial or administrative rules governing their roles" (Standard 2.01(f)). The reader may also appreciate the history of "aspirational" Specialty Guidelines for Forensic Psychologists (Committee on Ethical Guidelines for Forensic Psychologists, 1991). These are nonbinding on most neuropsychologists except those who are members of the American Board of Forensic Psychology, an ABPP specialty. Binder and Thompson (1995) proposed similar nonbinding guidelines specific to forensic neuropsychology. APA published updated Specialty Guidelines for Forensic Psychology (2013). These guidelines are good sources for ideas in areas where the 2002 Code may be silent. For example, the 2002 APA Code is silent on the issue of liens and contingency fees for doing plaintiff's work, but the Specialty Guidelines strictly prohibit taking any financial interest in the outcome of a trial. The next section provides a partial listing of ethical guidelines associated with steps in the assessment process. The reader is referred to Grote and Pyykkonen (2012) for a comprehensive treatment of ethical issues in the forensic neuropsychology setting.

Ethics of the Assessment Phase

Test selection is guided by a number of standards, foremost of which are 9.08 (Obsolete Tests and Outdated Test Results). *Obsolete* does not mean "old" tests; it means tests that are outdated for the current purpose. Older tests relying on very old normative tables should not be used. For example, some fixed battery proponents recommend using the old Wechsler-Bellevue and Wechsler Adult Intelligence Scale (WAIS) tests, but these tests rely on standardization samples that are more than 60 years old. Cohort effects can be important in neuropsychology, and a 48-year-old plaintiff should be compared to only persons who are currently 48, not those who were 48 years old in 1950.

There are legal circumstances when neuropsychologists may be asked to offer opinions based on records review only. For example, repeat neuropsychological testing may not be warranted because the claimant underwent numerous prior examinations. In other cases, an attorney may successfully block an examination or the discovery period may lapse. Basing one's opinions on records only is ethically allowable as indicated by 9.01 (Bases for Assessments). Subsections 9.01(b) and (c) require the testifying neuropsychologist to state the impact of limited information on the reliability and validity of his or her opinions and acknowledge records were the only basis for opinions. Further suggestions are provided in Specialty Guideline 9.03 (Opinions Regarding Persons Not Examined).

Litigation Consultation

The trial consulting role poses special ethical risks. Typically, the consultant is anonymous. Anonymity may disinhibit aggressive behavior by removing typical consequences for inappropriate behavior. The absence of "moral hazard" can be an invitation to mischief. The 1992 Code did warn about situations where no "corrective mechanism" was in place (McSweeny, 1997). There are no specific guidelines addressing litigation consultation in the 2002 Code, but some ethical standards provide self-direction for anonymous experts. Standard 1.01 (Misuse of Psychologist's Work) recommends "correcting or minimizing misuse or misrepresentation" of psychologist's work. Further, Specialty Guideline 4.01 urges psychologists serving as litigation consultants to clarify role expectations and "any limitations to privacy, confidentiality, or privilege" that may apply. Here, it may be important for the consultant to understand attorney work product rules in the jurisdiction in which the case is filed.

A good approach to behaving ethically in a background consultant role is to *raise only genuinely debatable issues*; see Specialty Guidelines 10.01 (Focus on Legally Relevant Factors). There are core positions within neuropsychology over which there is no reasonable debate. For example, it is undebatable that factors such as age, education, gender, social class, culture, and aptitude contribute to individual differences on neuropsychological measures (Greiffenstein & Baker, 2003; Heaton et al., 1991). Hence, telling the retaining attorney that age and education are inconsequential is unprofessional behavior. In contrast, a genuinely debatable issue in this situation might be the particular choice of normative table in the case of measures with multiple normative studies: for example, the choice of IQ-based normative table (Tremont et al., 1998) versus a strictly age-based table (Mitrushina, Boone, & D'Elia, 1999). Challenging these core positions is nothing more than nihilistic method skepticism. Similarly, the need for SVTs and PVTs in litigated contexts is beyond dispute. A genuinely debatable issue is the interpretation of SVTs and PVTs in a given case, or the strengths and weaknesses of a particular SVT or PVT.

Discovery: Raw Data Disclosure

A chronically contentious issue is the extent to which neuropsychological evidence is discoverable by opposing counsel. The 1992 Code (APA, 1992) contained conflicting imperatives. Neuropsychologists were required to provide documentation of their work for "reasonable scrutiny in an adjudicative forum" (per Standard 1.23 (b)), but also required avoidance of disseminating test data to "persons unqualified" (Standard 2.02 (b)). Historically, some neuropsychologists took an "exceptionalist" posture, emphasizing the public policy of test security and asserting that neuropsychological data were so unique they were not subject to the same scrutiny as any other legal evidence (Tranel, 1994). Others took what may be termed a "legal primacy" posture based on discovery rules, arguing that withholding raw test data violates due process rights, creates a special class of experts, protects psychologists from normal courtroom stresses, and allows neuropsychologists the de facto right to dictate cross-examination procedures (Lees-Haley & Courtney, 2000).

The 2002 Code (APA, 2002), however, eliminates forensic specialty guidelines and tries to resolve the 2002 Code's ambiguities by dividing test material into two categories: (a) an individual respondent's scored test protocols, commonly referred to as "raw data" (described in Standard 9.04); and (2) test instrumentation such as manuals and stimuli (described in 9.11, Maintaining Test Security). Test data can be disseminated to nonpsychologists under two clear conditions: a signed release from the patient (Standard 9.04(a)) or requirements dictated *by local law* (Standard 9.04 (b)). To the extent that placing one's neurocognitive status into legal contention via lawsuit voids the doctor–patient privilege, an implicit patient waiver is present in most lawsuits. Hence, one reasonable interpretation is that a valid subpoena is sufficient grounds for releasing raw data to an attorney.

Kaufmann (2009) outlined the public policy debate and detailed legal and other persuasive strategies to protect test security and prevent wrongful release of psychological test materials to nonpsychologists. Possible negative outcomes of breaching test security include infringement on the rights of companies that develop and sell the tests and facilitation of future coaching by attorneys. Standard 9.11 offers the exception for test instrumentation and stimuli. In this case, proliferation of test manuals are a realistic public threat and the neuropsychologist is required to take "reasonable steps" to protect these materials. Although no concrete examples are offered, a protective order limiting scrutiny of the test instrumentation is a reasonable interpretation of this standard. Professional psychology has not set forth a workable standard to resolve the raw data problem arising in forensic consultation. Both sides of an adversarial proceeding must and can have access while maintaining test security, and neuropsychologists should strive to balance this concern with the interests of test developers and users in preventing invalidation of tests. Greiffenstein and Kaufmann (2012) favor security of test manuals, stimuli, and items because it is consistent with law and best record-release in psychology practice. Some attorneys get court orders allowing videotaping of a neuropsychological evaluation. Depending upon jurisdictional law, the neuropsychologist should either refuse participation or petition the court to destroy or return all videotapes at the conclusion of litigation.

Testimony Phase

The testimony phase begins when the neuropsychologist is asked to offer opinions under oath. Opinions can be offered through discovery depositions, affidavits, interrogatories, *de bene esse* (trial) depositions, and live courtroom testimony. Testifying provides the only public face of forensic neuropsychology and is regulated by Standard 5.0 (Advertising and Other Public Statements), and Specialty Guidelines 2.05 (Knowledge of the Scientific Foundation for Opinions and Testimony) and 11.04 (Comprehensive and Accurate Presentation of Opinions in Reports and Testimony). Testimony usually begins with the neuropsychologist presenting her or his credentials qualifying her or him to testify as an expert. Accurate summaries of training, background, and research are required in legal proceedings and are required by Standard 5.01 (a) (Avoidance of False and Deceptive Statements) and Specialty Guideline 11.01 (Accuracy, Fairness, and Avoidance of Deception). Omission of crucial details gives a misleading picture of competence and training. Drawing on case files, a testifying neuropsychologist limited his description of postdoctoral experience to include "University of Michigan 1980–1982." But cross-examination uncovered mere attendance at irregular group supervision meetings with a retired professor in the Ann Arbor area. This willful omission on his *vitae* left the impression of two years of postdoctoral training in an organized health care setting.

After the credentials phase of testimony, neuropsychologists offer opinions on the meaning of their test results as they relate to the case. The ethical treatment of presentation and basis for opinions is described in Standard 9.10 (Explaining Assessment Results). Standard 2.04 (Bases for Scientific and Professional Judgments) further requires opinions to be grounded in both nomothetic psychological knowledge and customary practices (termed "professional knowledge").

Responses to Ethical Issues

Psychologists typically operate under an ethos of collegiality, conferring with each other to reach points of agreement. Nevertheless, colleagues may be asked to critique each other's work in the forensic arena. This scrutiny of others' work and professional behavior may uncover ethical lapses from time to time. Suggested responses to perceived ethical lapses by other psychologists are grouped under Ethical Standard 1.0 (Resolving Ethical Issues) and Specialty Guideline 7.03 (Resolving Ethical Issues with Fellow Professionals). Standard 1.05 (Reporting Ethical Violations) suggests a threshold for deciding whether to report behavior to an ethics board: evidence for past public harms or clear future prospects for such harm. Disagreements over ultimate opinions or test selection are common and do not constitute public harm. If there is a perceived lapse that does not rise to the level of harm, an informal resolution between neuropsychologists is recommended by Standard 1.04 (Informal Resolution). Brodsky and McKinzey (2002) provide guidance on raising and responding to ethical issues arising in the course of litigation consultation. They offer the following formula: (a) polite introductory language, (b) the specifics of the concern, and (c) polite concluding comments requesting some action. Nonetheless, some neuropsychologists take great offense to any criticism or disagreement. Plaintiff advocates may become enraged if the defense expert does not find the "catastrophic brain damage" they diagnosed, and some defense experts charge incompetence when another expert misdiagnoses somebody with TBI. Threatening to bring ethical charges against a disagreeing neuropsychologist is unethical behavior if the complainant makes allegations "with reckless disregard for or willful ignorance of facts that would disprove the allegation "(Standard 1.07, Improper Complaints). Some neuropsychologists acting as dual treater-experts may passive-aggressively vent their hostility by proxy, subtly manipulating their "patients" to file the ethics charge, but Standard 1.07 also bars "encouraging others" to file a complaint.

Myths of Forensic Neuropsychology

Gaps between science and everyday practice are often filled by clinical myths (McNally, 2005). Myth-driven practices are defined as psychological or medical concepts that influence clinical decision making but for which there is little to no empirical support. Myths originate in face valid reasoning ("A memory complaint must mean there is brain damage"); overgeneralizations from a single anecdotal report (Paauw, 1999); unfalsifiable psychodynamic theories ("His malingering can only be unconscious"); uncritically accepted insights passed down from instructors to students; or illusory correlation based on cultural associations (Chapman and Chapman, 1969). Although forensic neuropsychology is relatively new, a set of myths is already emerging.

Myth: "Only Fixed Battery Is Admissible Under **Daubert"**

Some advocates for narrower sets of neurocognitive procedures interpret the *Daubert* ruling to support reliance on commercially available "fixed" test batteries such as the HRB (version unknown) or LNNB in courtroom settings. In this scheme, "flexible test batteries" are not or should not be admissible. A number of commentators expressed doubt that test groupings other than fixed batteries would be admissible under *Daubert* (Posthuma, Podrouzek, & Crisp, 2002; Reitan & Wolfson, 2002). The common source for this myth is a commentary article by Reed (1996), who cited the TBI case of *Chapple v. Ganger* (1998) to draw the following conclusion: "The *Daubert* standard was applied for the very first time to the use of fixed (standardized) versus flexible neuropsychological test batteries in the federal court" (p. 315). Reed understood the trial judge to bar admission of flexible test battery evidence because of "lack of medical and scientific evidence to support the conclusions" (p. 315) made from the flexible batteries.

Contrary to Reed's (1996) characterization, even a cursory reading of the *Chapple* opinion reveals the following facts: There was *no* Daubert challenge to a "flexible" test battery; both the flexible test battery (plaintiff expert) and fixed battery data (defense expert) were admitted into evidence; and even testimony based on *partial* HRBs were admitted. Instead, the judge's verdict was based on the *weight* of neuropsychological testimony: The court merely preferred the testimony of one "fixed battery" specialist because that expert integrated outside records into his opinion. Hence, it was the thoroughness of the reasoning process, not the type of test battery, that swayed the judge. Reed (1996) likely confused the different issues of *admissibility* versus the *weight* of evidence, not recognizing that *Daubert* goes only to admissibility.[4] In summary, the "*Daubert* requires fixed battery only" recommendation is a myth based on overgeneralization from a mischaracterized and unpublished (nonbinding) single case ruling.

As noted in the lengthy discussion of *Baxter v. Temple* (2008) in Sweet et al. (Chapter 36 in this volume), fixed battery superiority in forensic consulting is a myth that lives on in the minds of a few practitioners (Russell, 2012) as critiqued by Greiffenstein (2013).

Myth: "Practice Effects Must Always Be Avoided"

A recurring forensic issue is the impact of "practice effects" on cognitive scores. Practice effects (PEs) refer to gains in neurocognitive scores when a person is retested on the same instrument (Kaufman, 1994). PE issues are often raised in forensic cases, because parties undergo examination by two or more neuropsychologists retained by opposing sides. Some neuropsychologists assert a *blanket* prohibition against any repeat testing for a "protected" period after their own testing. Proponents for minimum test-retest intervals justify the prohibition by arguing that PEs may "mask" or "hide" underlying neurocognitive deficits they believe are present. It is difficult to identify any influential research citation for this belief, suggesting it rose *de novo* on a face valid basis. One psychologist's website (United Psychological Services, www.brainevaluation.com, accessed on August 4, 2017) makes the assertion that the APA advises against retesting within a six-month interval. However, there is no such position statement during a restricted field search of the term <practice effects> at the APA website.

The "PE avoidance" belief can be labeled a myth for many reasons. First, and contrary to this belief, PEs provide much useful information to clinicians (Lezak, 1995; McCaffrey & Westervelt, 1995). PE is not methodological artifact from which no conclusions can be drawn. PEs are reliably *unidirectional* (better scores) in motivated subjects, meaning they cannot be error or random occurrence (Theisen, Rapport, Axelrod, & Brines, 1998), so they must represent the operation of memory retrieval.

The second objection is logical: The myth places its advocate in the contradictory position of claiming organic memory loss but refusing to consider score improvement as evidence for functional or improving memory systems. Third, stable and severe organic deficits do not improve with retesting (Shatz, 1981). Fourth, an examination of the review literature indicates no empirically mandated length of test-retest interval. Putnam, Adams, and Schneider (1992) found equivalent results with a one-day retest interval in an injured scuba diver, based on application of the standard error of measurement (SEM; standard deviation divided by the square root of *N*). Finally, a rich empirical literature on repeat testing strongly contradicts the blanket prohibition notion (Lezak, 1995). PEs depend on many factors, including demographics, the length of interval, baseline performance level, the severity of the brain disease in question, and the cognitive domain tested (McCaffrey & Westervelt, 1995). PEs are greater in younger participants than older ones (Horton, 1992), smaller in persons with severe baseline deficits (Shatz, 1981), and depend on the cognitive domain being tested (Mitrushina & Satz, 1991) and brain lesion severity (Shatz, 1981). For example, Dodrill and Troupin (1975) showed negligible PEs for most tests in the HRB except for the Category Test. Further, the absence of PEs where they are expected can sometimes be crucial evidence favoring a plaintiff's position. Chelune et al. (1993) found small decrements in post-lobectomy memory scores compared to presurgical baseline; decrements on tasks with known high PE must represent substantial learning loss.

In conclusion, there is no authority for the view that retesting is harmful or artifactual (McCaffrey & Westervelt, 1995). The "meaning of PE depends solely on the generalization sought or needed" (Kaufman, 1994, p. 828). Neuropsychologists can offer opinions on any psychological phenomenon relevant to understanding an individual's capacity for memory and new learning. Hence, the presence (or even absence) of PEs is just another important psychological datum that needs to be explained in the context of other case-specific knowledge. Lezak (1995) sagely advises a careful analytical approach to interpreting change (or its absence). Whether a robust PE represents intact memory or whether it represents recovery from a brain injury cannot be answered in isolation from extratest data (e.g., initial injury severity) and statistical considerations (SEM). More recently, the AACN (2010) provided guidance on repeat test administrations in clinical and forensic settings.

Myth: Forewarning Improves Motivation and Validity of Deficits

A universal procedural concern is obtaining maximal performance. Many manuals and texts offer general guidelines for encouraging best performances (Lezak, 1995), suggestions tempered by standardized administration rules. Most neuropsychologists try to find the balance between obtaining optimal performance and allowing deficits to emerge (Vanderploeg, 1994). Nevertheless, some neuropsychologists have drawn unsupportable conclusions from these guides, creating the following myth: Forewarning the respondent about specific effort tests safeguards the examination from insufficient effort or malingering. Put differently, warning otherwise deceptive persons guarantees effortful responding.

This belief achieves mythical status because there is no logical or empirical evidence that explicit forewarnings suppress response bias in persons otherwise intending to feign deficits. The "forewarning" myth is linked to a role-play simulation study by Johnson and Lesniak-Karpiak (1997), who compared undergraduate controls to student simulators asked to feign deficits for hypothetical compensation. Two groups of simulators were either forewarned about effort tests or not forewarned. Johnson and Lesniak-Karpiak reported an effect for warning: The warned group showed higher motor and memory scores than the naive simulation group on memory and motor tests, with 45% of the warned group achieving classification as normal controls. Despite reporting that 55% of warned simulators still produced implausible scores, Johnson and Lesniak-Karpiak (1997: 321) made the blanket conclusion that "(the) results provide support for effectiveness of warning in reducing malingering behavior on selected measures." Further, "use of a warning in cases of personal injury litigation will likely provide a more accurate cognitive profile" (p. 236). Youngjohn, Lees-Haley, and Binder (1999) criticized Johnson and Lesniak-Karpiak's conclusions as unsupported by the data. Their reanalysis showed the coached group's general level of performance was still well below that of a good effort control.

There is no empirical support for the forewarning myth: No study of coaching has *ever* demonstrated normalization of scores in all simulators with forewarning. Johnson was unable to replicate her initial findings in a study of feigned intellectual and memory deficits (Johnson, Bellah, Dodge, Kelley, & Livingston, 1998). Wong, Lerner-Poppen, and Durham (1998) were also unable to diminish exaggerated motor deficit with forewarnings. The work of Julie Suhr and her colleagues suggests forewarning changes only the style of malingering memory deficits (Suhr & Gunstad, 2000). Suhr (2002) further showed that naive and warned simulator groups still showed suspiciously low primacy scores on Rey's Auditory Verbal Learning Test (RAVLT; Lezak, 1995), suggesting forewarning, fortunately, does not correct fakers' erroneous internal stereotypes of brain-injured performance.

In conclusion, warning litigants about upcoming "specific malingering measures" is not an effective way of improving motivation in persons intending to feign deficits. Instead, the relevant body of research indicates "tipping off" changes only the preferred malingering style, making it less extreme (Storm & Graham, 2000).

Summary Conclusions

Kaufmann and Greffenstein (2013) note that neuropsychologists are becoming the preferred brain–mental state behavior experts in our courts, not just our medical clinics; the LEXIS database cases noted by Sweet et.al (Chapter 36 in this volume) clearly show that trend. Expert neuropsychologists who understand the principles and spirit of communicating in a legal setting are now positioned to make valuable contributions to our clients, our society, and the judicial system. Neuropsychology–law interactions are bidirectional. Our opinions can influence legal decisions and even public policy. Alternatively, legal considerations can stimulate neuropsychological research or improve ways to think about what we are doing. The evidentiary demands of the legal system can be similar to the rigors of science: Both are crucibles that separate workable from unworkable, bad from good ideas.

A distillation of this chapter's main ideas is presented in Table 37.7. This table of "Rules of the Road" is presented in the style of the late Ted Blau (1998). A number of general themes are interwoven throughout this list. First, these proposed rules treat the *Daubert* guidelines as an aspirational template, not a threat. The *Daubert* decision should be viewed as an ideal in conducting research and improving objective decision aids. All courts recognize that clinical inference (subjectivity) in the absence of an on-point study will always be part of every opinion. The threatened demise of psychology and neuropsychology after *Daubert* has yet to materialize. If anything, *Daubert* has strengthened the hand of scientist-practitioners: Neuropsychologists can more easily differentiate themselves from psychiatrists, counselors, and social workers who diagnose on the basis of history and intuitive impression (Lally, 2003). Unlike other mental health professionals, psychologists use objective psychological tests to refine clinical impressions when formulating working diagnoses, initial treatment plans, and expert opinions. Neuropsychology adds the brain–behavior knowledge base and incorporates neuroimaging, neurodiagnostic, and other neurologic findings to the history and clinical interview, thereby creating the unique practice of forensic neuropsychology consulting (Kaufmann, 2009). Kaufmann (2013) recently reviewed admissibility challenges to neuropsychologist testimony and called for greater interdisciplinary dialog among law, medicine, and psychology about neuropsychological evidence.

Another interwoven theme is principled forensic neuropsychology. This requires the integration of two attitudes: the ethical and the aspirational. Both are necessary conditions for the image of the profession and for personal development. The ethical attitude demands that forensic neuropsychologists always be aware of the multiple ethical issues embedded in every phase of neuropsychology-law interactions. The legal environment contains many pressures to deviate from both professional and societal codes of conduct. Being retained by one side rather than being hired by the court by itself creates a pull to affiliate with the retaining advocate. Seeing one's courtroom role as the educator of the jury helps resist the pull of affiliation. It should be clear that morality, righteousness, and justness do not reside in a particular retaining side, be it plaintiff, defense, or prosecution. These characteristics reside in individuals, not situations. The posttrial phase of every examination requires some self-scrutiny. This process is similar to reviewing manuscripts submitted for publication: Questions such as "Have I (Has the author) considered statements (literature) at odds with my opinion (the mainstream literature) on this subject?" Sweet and Moulthrop (1999) provide a comprehensive program for self-scrutiny.

The aspirational arm of principled behavior means holding ideals that go beyond the individual legal case. One ideal is inductive: generalizing societal consequences from the individual case. Hess (1999) advises considering the wider ramifications in every single case one encounters. Opinions can have major consequences with effects that can persist after the jury verdict. This attitude is especially critical in legal cases where liberty interests are at stake, such as death

Table 37.7 Some rules of the road for forensic neuropsychologists

Admissibility Issues

- Keep up on admissibility developments in state and federal law.
- Use a flexible test battery organized around a core battery that is specific to legal issue.
- Select tests and procedures that meet general acceptance (*Frye*) rule + one other *Daubert* factor.
- Maintain a minimum document set to oppose the rare *Frye* or *Daubert* challenge.
- Be prepared for challenges to symptom and performance validity measures.

Assessment/Data Collection

- Remember that *Daubert* factors may be used as aspirational framework for choosing tests.
- Recognize and accept the nonspecificity problem for neuropsychological tests.
- Use converging evidence model based on three prongs: interview and mental status observations, neuropsychology test scores, key outside records.
- Use a multistrategy, multidomain approach to assess for validity of memory, somatic-motor and psychiatric malingering, consistent with the AACN Consensus Conference Statement.

Interpretation Phase

- An abnormal test score is the beginning, not the end of the inferential process. Respect that ecological validity and nonspecificity of neurocognitive measures is resolvable only with extratext data.
- Consider the influence of a traumatic event or exposure in the context of a broad life history.
- Be aware that neuropsychological interpretation works best on a nomothetic (lawful) foundation modified by idiographic (case-specific) data depending on the legal question. Nomothetic considerations include useful generalizations such as dose-response effects in brain injury; idiographic considerations may include an abnormal CT scan.
- Create a causal model that is plausible, coherent, fitted to a biological gradient, and consistent with postinjury interventions.

Report Writing

- Separate inferences and opinions from fact.
- Minimize clinical jargon and use plain language when offering testimony.
- Provide a logical link (nexus) between findings and opinions.
- Provide a functional analysis: Neuro- or psychodiagnosis does not automatically entail disability.

Testimony Phase

- Educate the jury on general background and the neuropsychologist's opinion.
- Refrain from giving opinions as to ultimate legal issues unless otherwise allowed by the court or statute.
- Apply a standard of reasonable probability to offered opinions.
- Use Push-Pull and Admit-Deny tactics selectively but do not overuse. It is more important to be genuine than clever.

Post-Trial Phase

- Conduct self-analysis of objectivity and ethics.
- Consider implications of individual opinions for profession, individuals, and society.
- Consider heuristic value of cases for generating research ideas.
- Actively combat "junk science" and misrepresentation of credentials.

penalty mitigation, legal insanity, and civil competence. If a neuropsychologist opines that "subtle" cognitive deficits either justify legal guardianship or support legal insanity, other individuals are made less safe from the government in the former and from amoral predators in the latter. Another facet of aspirational behavior is to combat "junk science." Junk science occurs when expert witnesses either employ questionable methodology to reach unsupported conclusions or present grossly fallacious interpretations of published data. Fox, Greiffenstein, and Lees-Haley (2005) showed how design and reasoning absurdities produce unsupportable conclusions about household mold and cognition. Finally, consider how a case may contain at least one heuristic issue stimulating future research (Greiffenstein, 2003b).

Notes

1 The use of the term *reliability* may be confusing to psychologists because they define it narrowly as referring to the consistency and stability of observation. The *Daubert* Court's uses of the term *reliability* is synonymous with the scientific term *reliability.*

2 This does not seem like much of an improvement, as both the ALI and *M'Naghten* rules imply a threshold set at severe defects.

3 Weir Mitchell was writing in the context of pseudocyesis (false pregnancies). He meant that women might initially convince earnest physicians they are truly pregnant. The progressive accumulation of irregularities eventually prompts skepticism, and the absence of a baby in the delivery room seals the diagnosis.

4 There was a *Daubert* challenge in this case, but it involved testimony from a vocational specialist who merely speculated about the future job prospects of the minor plaintiff. The judge excluded that intuitive testimony prior to trial.

References

Albers, J. W., & Berent, S. (2000). Controversies in neurotoxicology: Current status. *Neurology Clinics, 18*, 741–764.

Alexander, M. P. (1995). Mild traumatic brain injury: Pathophysiology, natural history and clinical management. *Neurology, 45*, 1253–1260.

Alexander, M. P. (1998). In the pursuit of proof of brain damage after whiplash injury. *Neurology, 51*, 336–340.

Alexander, M. P. (2003). The evidence for brain injury in whiplash injuries. *Pain Research & Management, 8*, 19–23.

Allen, L. M., III, Iversen, G. L., & Green, P. (2002). Computerized Assessment of Response bias in forensic neuropsychology. *Journal of Forensic Neuropsychology, 3*, 205–225.

American Academy of Clinical Neuropsychology. (2001). Policy statement on the presence of third party observers in neuropsychological assessments. *The Clinical Neuropsychologist, 15*, 433–439. [Online]. Retrieved from www.tandfonline.com/doi/pdf/10.1076/clin.15.4.433.1888 (last visited November 30, 2013).

American Academy of Clinical Neuropsychology. (2003). Official position of the American Academy of Clinical Neuropsychology on ethical complaints made against clinical neuropsychologists during adversarial proceedings. *The Clinical Neuropsychologist, 17*, 443–445. [Online]. Retrieved from www.tandfonline.com/doi/pdf/10.1076/clin.17.4.443.27943 (last visited November 30, 2013).

American Academy of Neurology. (1997). Practice parameter: The management of concussion in sports (summary statement from the Quality Standards Subcommittee). *Neurology, 48*, 581–585.

American Academy of Neurology, Therapeutics and Technology Assessment Subcommittee. (1996a). Assessment of brain SPECT: Report of the Therapeutics and Technology Assessment Subcommittee of the American Academy of Neurology. *Neurology, 46*, 278–85.

American Academy of Neurology, Therapeutics and Technology Assessment Subcommittee. (1996b). Assessment: Neuropsychological testing of adults: Considerations for neurologists. *Neurology, 47*, 592–599.

American Law Institute. (1962). *Model Penal Code* (Section 4.01). Philadelphia, PA: Author.

American Psychiatric Association. (1994). *Diagnostic and Statistical Manual of Mental Disorders* (4th ed.). Washington, DC: Author.

American Psychological Association. (1992). Ethical principles of psychologists and code of conduct. *American Psychologist, 47*, 1597–1611.

American Psychological Association. (2002). Ethical principles of psychologists and code of conduct. *American Psychologist, 57*, 1060–1073.

American Psychological Association. (2013). Specialty guidelines for forensic psychology. *American Psychologist, 68*(1), 7–19. Preliminary and final APA authorized drafts, [Online]. Retrieved from www.ap-ls.org/aboutpsychlaw/SpecialtyGuidelines.php (last visited November 30, 2013).

American Psychological Association. (2017). *Ethical principles and code of conduct* (2002, Amended June 1, 2010 and January 1, 2017).

Anger, W. K., Sizemore, O. J., Grossmann, S. J., Glasser, J. A., Letz, R., & Bowler, R. (1997). Human neurobehavioral research methods: Impact of subject variables. *Environmental Research, 73*(1–2), 18–41.

Axelrod, B., Barth, J., Faust, D., Fisher, J., Heilbronner, R., Larrabee, G., et al. (2000). Presence of third party observers during neuropsychological testing: Official statement of the National Academy of Neuropsychology. *Archives of Clinical Neuropsychology, 15*, 379–380.

Babitsky, S., & Mangraviti, J. J. (1997). *How to Excel During Cross-Examination: Techniques for Experts That Work*. Falmouth, MA: S.E.A.K, Inc. Press.

Ball, D. (2008). Making preponderance work. *Trial, 44*, 35–44.

Baxter v. Temple, 949 A.2d 167 (N.H., 2008).

Baxter v. Temple, unpublished second trial (2012).

Berent, S., & Swartz, C. L. (1999). Essential psychometrics. In J. J. Sweet (Ed.), *Forensic Neuropsychology: Foundations and Practice* (pp. 1–26). Lisse, the Netherlands: Swets and Zeitlinger.

Bigler, E. D., & Ehrfurth, J. W. (1980). Critical limitations of the Bender Gestalt Test in clinical neuropsychology: Response to Lacks. *International Journal of Clinical Neuropsychology, 2*, 88–90.

Binder, L. M., & Rohling, M. L. (1996). Money matters: A meta-analytic review of the effects of financial incentives on recovery after closed-head injury. *American Journal of Psychiatry, 153*(1), 7–10.

Binder, L. M., & Thompson, L. L. (1995). Ethics code and neuropsychological assessment practices. *Archives of Clinical Neuropsychology, 10*, 27–46.

Blau, T. H. (1998). *The Psychologist as Expert Witness* (2nd ed.). New York: Wiley.

Boake, C., McCauley, S. R., Levin, H. S., Contant, C. F., Song, J. X., Brown, S. A., et al. (2004). Limited agreement between criteria-based diagnoses of postconcussional syndrome. *Journal of Neuropsychiatry Clinical Neurosciences, 16*(4), 493–499.

Boccaccini, M. T., & Brodsky, S. L. (1999). Diagnostic test usage by forensic psychologists in emotional injury cases. *Professional Psychology: Research & Practice, 30*, 253–259.

Bolla, K. (2005). Neurotoxic injury. In G. J. Larrabee (Ed.), *Forensic Neuropsychology: A Scientific Approach* (pp. 271–297). New York: Oxford University Press.

Boone, K. B., & Lu, P. (2003). Noncredible cognitive performance in the context of severe brain injury. *Clinical Neuropsychologist, 17*(2), 244.

Bowler, R. M., Gysens, S., Diamond, E., Booty, A., Hartney, C., & Roels, H. A. (2003). Neuropsychological sequelae of exposure to welding fumes in a group of occupationally exposed men. *International Journal of Hygiene and Environment Health, 206*, 517–529.

Bowler, R. M., Mergler, D., Sassine, M. P., Larribe, F., & Hudnell, K. (1999). Neuropsychiatric effects of manganese on mood. *Neurotoxicology, 20*, 367–378.

Brodsky, S. L. (1991). *Testifying in Court: Guidelines and Maxims for the Expert Witness*. Washington, DC: American Psychological Association Press.

Brodsky, S. L. (1999). *The Expert Expert Witness: More Maxims and Guidelines for Testifying in Court*. Washington, DC: American Psychological Association.

Brodsky, S. L., & McKinzey, R. K. (2002). The ethical confrontation of the unethical forensic colleague. *Professional Psychology: Research & Practice, 33*, 307–309.

Brown, R. P., & Pinel, E. C. (2003). Stigma on my mind: Individual differences in the experience of stereotype threat. *Journal of Experimental Social Psychology, 39*(6), 626.

Brown, S. J., Fann, J. R., & Grant, I. (1994). Postconcussional disorder: Time to acknowledge a common source of neurobehavioral morbidity. *Journal of Neuropsychiatry & Clinical Neuroscience, 6*, 15–22.

Burkett, B. G., & Whitley, G. (1998). *Stolen Valor*. Dallas: Verity Press.
Butler, J. L., & Baumeister, R. F. (1998). The trouble with friendly faces: Skilled performance with a supportive audience. *Journal of Personality and Social Psychology*, *75*(5), 1213–1230.
Bush, D. S. (2003). On the practice of forensic neuropsychology. In G. L. Lamberty, R. L. Heilbronner, & J. C. Courtney (Eds.), *The Practice of Clinical Neuropsychology* (pp. 197–211). Lisse, The Netherlands: Swets & Zeitlinger.
Cal. Civ. Proc. Code § 2032.530 (2013).
Carroll, L. J., Cassidy, J. D., Peloso, P. M., Borg, J., von Holst, H., Holm, L., et al. (2004). Prognosis for mild traumatic brain injury: Results of the WHO collaborating centre task force on mild traumatic brain injury. *Journal of Rehabilitation Medicine*, (43 Suppl), 84–105.
Centers for Disease Control. (1991). Preventing lead poisoning in young children. In *Statement of the Centers for Disease Control* (p. 3). Atlanta, GA: Author.
Chapman, L. J., & Chapman, J. P. (1969). Illusory correlation as an obstacle to the use of valid psychodiagnostic signs. *Journal of Abnormal Psychology*, *74*, 271–280.
Chapple v. Ganger, 851 F. Supp. 1481 (E.D. Wash., 1998).
Chelune, G. J., Naugle, R. I., Lueders, H., Sedlak, J., et al. (1993). Individual change after epilepsy surgery: Practice effects and base-rate information. *Neuropsychology*, *7*, 41–52.
Cline v. Firestone Tire and Rubber Co., 118 F.R.D. 588 (S.D. W. Va. 1988).
Coe v. State, 17 S.W.3d 193 (Tenn. 2000).
Colvin, M., Myers, J., Nell, V., Rees, D., & Cronje, R. (1993). A cross-sectional survey of neurobehavioral effects of chronic solvent exposure on workers in a paint manufacturing plant. *Environmental Research*, *63*, 122–132.
Committee on Ethical Guidelines for Forensic Psychologists. (1991). Specialty guidelines for forensic psychologists. *Law and Human Behavior*, *15*, 655–665.
Constantinou, M., Ashendorf, L., & McCaffrey, R. J. (2002). When the third party observer of a neuropsychological evaluation is an audio-recorder. *Clinical Neuropsychologist*, *16*, 407–412.
Craig v. Orkin Exterminating Co., Inc., 2000 U.S. LEXIS 19240 (S.D. Fl., 2000).
Cripe, L. I. (2002). Limitations of records reviews. *Division of Clinical Neuropsychology Newsletter*, *40*(20), 7–8.
Dahir, V. B., Richardson, J. T., Ginsburg, G. P., Gatowski, S. I., Dobbin, S. A., & Merlino, M. L. (2005). Judicial application of Daubert to psychological syndrome and profile evidence: A research note. *Psychology, Public Policy, & Law*, *11*(1), 62.
Damasio, A. R., Tranel, D., & Damasio, H. (1990). Individuals with sociopathic behavior caused by frontal damage fail to respond autonomically to social stimuli. *Behavior & Brain Research*, *41*, 81–94.
Daubert v. Merrell Dow Pharm., Inc., 509 U.S. 579 (1993).
Denney, R. L. (2003). Introduction: Criminal forensic neuropsychology. *Journal of Forensic Neuropsychology*, *3*, 1.
Denney, R. L., & Wynkoop, T. F. (2000). Clinical neuropsychology in the criminal forensic setting. *Journal of Head Trauma Rehabilitation*, *15*(2), 804.
Deschamps, F. J., Guillaumot, M., & Raux, S. (2001). Neurological effects in workers exposed to manganese. *Journal of Occupational & Environmental Medicine*, *43*, 127–132.
Dikmen, S. S., Machamer, J. E., & Temkin, N. (2001). Mild head injury: Facts and artifacts. *Journal of Clinical and Experimental Neuropsychology*, *23*, 729–738.
Dikmen, S. S., Machamer, J. E., Winn, H. R., & Temkin, N. R. (1995). Neuropsychological outcome at 1-year post head injury. *Neuropsychology*, *8*(1), 80–90.
Dikmen, S. S, McLean, A., Jr., Temkin, N. R., & Wyler, A. R. (1986). Neuropsychologic outcome at one-month postinjury. *Archives of Physical Medicine & Rehabilitation*, *67*, 507–513.
Dikmen, S. S., Temkin, N. R., Machamer, J. E., Holubkov, A. L., et al. (1994). Employment following traumatic head injuries. *Archives of Neurology*, *51*, 177–186.
Dodrill, C. B. (1979). Sex differences on the Halstead-Reitan Neuropsychological Battery and on other neuropsychological measures. *Journal of Clinical Psychology*, *35*, 236–241.
Dodrill, C. B., & Troupin, A. S. (1975). Effects of repeated administrations of a comprehensive neuropsychological battery among chronic epileptics. *Journal of Nervous & Mental Disease*, *161*, 185–190.
Donnellan v. First Student, Inc., 891 N.E.2d 463 (Ill Ap. Ct. 2000).
Durham v. United States, 214 F.2d 862 (D.C. Cir, 1954).
Erichsen, J. E. (1866). *On Railway and Other Injuries of the Nervous System*. London: Walton & Maberly.
Estate of Congdon, 309 NW.2d 261, 265 (Minn. 1981).
Federal Rule of Civil Procedure (1975). St. Paul, MN: West Publishing.
Federal Rules of Evidence for United States Courts and Magistrates (1975). St. Paul, MN: West Publishing.
Feher, E. P., Larrabee, G. J., Sudilovsky, A., & Crook, T. H. (1994). Memory self-report in Alzheimer's disease and in age-associated memory impairment. *Journal of Geriatric Psychiatry & Neurology*, *7*, 58–65.
Feria v. Dynagraphics Co., 2004 Tex. App. LEXIS 2366 (Tx. App. Ct. 2004).
Ferrari, R., Constantoyannis, C., & Papadakis, N. (2001). Cross-sectional study of symptom expectation following minor head injury in Canada and Greece. *Clinical Neurology & Neurosurgery*, *103*, 254–259.
Ferrari, R., Obelieniene, D., Russell, A. S., Darlington, P., Gervais, R., & Green, P. (2001). Symptom expectation after minor head injury: A comparative study between Canada and Lithuania. *Clinical Neurology & Neurosurgery*, *103*, 184–190.
Fini v. General Mot. Corp., 3002 Mich. App. LEXIS 884 (Mich App. Ct. 2003).
Fisher, C. B. (2003). Release of test data and the new APA ethics code. *American Psychology Law Society News*, *23*, 1–6.
Fox, D. D., Greiffenstein, M. F., & Lees-Haley, P. R. (2005). Commentary on cognitive impairment with toxigenic fungal exposure. *Applied Neuropsychology*, *12*, 129–133.
Fox, D. D., Lees-Haley, P. R., Earnest, K., & Dolezal-Wood, S. (1995). Base rates of postconcussive symptoms in health maintenance organization patients and controls. *Neuropsychology*, *9*, 606–611.
Frankle, A. H. (1995). A new method for detecting brain disorder by measuring perseveration in personality responses. *Journal of Personality Assessment*, *64*, 63–85.
Frederick, R. I. (2003). A review of Rey's strategies for detecting malingered neuropsychological impairment. *Journal of Forensic Neuropsychology*, *2*, 1–25.
Frye v. U.S., (D.C. Cir. 1923) 293 F. 1013.
General Elec. v. Joiner, 522 U.S. 136 (1997).
Goldstein, G. W. (1984). Brain capillaries: A target for inorganic lead poisoning. *Neurotoxicology*, *5*, 167–175.
Golfland Entm't Ctrs, Inc. v. Sup. Ct., 108 Cal.4th. 739 (Cal. App. 4th 2003).

Gouvier, W. D. (1998). Base rates and clinical decision making. In J. J. Sweet (Ed.), *Forensic Neuropsychology: Fundamentals and Practice* (pp. 27–38). Lisse, the Netherlands: Swets & Zeitlinger.

Green, P. (2003). *Word Memory Test for Windows: User's Manual and Program*. Edmonton, Alberta, Canada: Green Publishing.

Green, P. (2004). *Medical Symptom Validity Test for Windows: User's Manual and Program*. Edmonton, Alberta, Canada: Green Publishing.

Green, P. (2008). *Non-Verbal Medical Symptom Validity Test for Windows: User's Manual and Program*. Edmonton, Alberta, Canada: Green Publishing.

Green, P., Iverson, G. L., & Allen, L. (1999). Detecting malingering in head injury litigation with the Word Memory Test. *Brain Injury*, *13*, 813–819.

Green, P., Lees-Haley, P. R., & Allen, L. M., III. (2002). The Word Memory Test and the validity of neuropsychological test scores. *Journal of Forensic Neuropsychology*, *2*, 97–124.

Greiffenstein, M. F. (1996). The neuropsychological autopsy. *Michigan Bar Journal*.

Greiffenstein, M. F. (2000). Late Post-concussion syndrome as learned illness behavior: Proposal for a multifactorial model. *Brain Injury Source*, *4*(Fall issue), 26–27.

Greiffenstein, M. F. (2002). An analysis of premorbid MMPI profiles in 28 late postconcussion claimants. *Division 40 (Clinical Neuropsychology) Newsletter*, *20*, 9–14.

Greiffenstein, M. F. (2003a). Testamentary competence: Antemortem and postmortem neuropsychological analysis. *Division 40 (Clinical Neuropsychology) Newsletter*, *21*, 7–9, 33–36.

Greiffenstein, M. F. (2003b). Research out of a private practice setting. In G. L. Lamberty, R. Heilbronner, & J. Courtney (Eds.), *The Practice of Neuropsychology* (pp. 125–142). Lisse, the Netherlands: Swets & Zeitlinger.

Greiffenstein, M. F. (2013). Hagiography masquerading as scientific neuropsychology. *Psyccritiques*, *58*(3), 1–4.

Greiffenstein, M. F., & Baker, W. J. (2001). Comparison of premorbid and postinjury MMPI-2 profiles in late postconcussion claimants. *Clinical Neuropsychologist*, *15*, 162–170.

Greiffenstein, M. F., & Baker, W. J. (2002). Neuropsychological and psychosocial correlates of adult arithmetic deficiency. *Neuropsychology*, *16*, 451–458.

Greiffenstein, M. F., & Baker, W. J. (2003). Premorbid clues? Preinjury scholastic performance and present neuropsychological functioning in late postconcussion syndrome. *Clinical Neuropsychologist*, *17*, 561–573.

Greiffenstein, M. F., & Baker, W. J. (2006). Miller was (mostly) right: Simulation inversely related to injury severity. *British Journal of Legal and Criminological Psychology*, *20*, xx–xx.

Greiffenstein, M. F., Baker, W. J., Axelrod, B. A., Peck, T. E., & Gervais, R. (2004). The Fake Bad Scale and MMPI-2 F-Family in the detection of implausible psychological trauma Claims. *The Clinical Neuropsychologist*, in press.

Greiffenstein, M. F., Baker, W. J., Donders, J., & Miller, L. (2002). The Fake Bad Scale in atypical and severe closed head injury litigants. *Journal of Clinical Psychology*, *58*, 1591–1600.

Greiffenstein, M. F., Baker, W. J., & Gola, T. (1994). Validation of measures of malingered amnesia with a large clinical sample. *Psychological Assessment*, *6*, 218–224.

Greiffenstein, M. F., Baker, W. J., & Gola, T. (1995). MMPI-2 vs. domain specific measures in the detection of factitious traumatic brain injury. *The Clinical Neuropsychologist*, *9*, 230–240.

Greiffenstein, M. F., Baker, W. J., & Gola, T. (1996a). Motor dysfunction profiles in documented TBI and postconcussion syndrome. *Neuropsychology*, *2*, 477–485.

Greiffenstein, M. F., Baker, W. J., & Gola, T. (1996b). Comparison of multiple scoring methods for Rey's malingered amnesia measures. *Archives of Clinical Neuropsychology*, *11*, 283–293.

Greiffenstein, M. F., Baker, W. J., & Gola, T. (2001). Epidemiology of invalid performances in a large postconcussion sample. *Journal of the International Neuropsychology Society*, *7*, 148.

Greiffenstein, M. F., Baker, W. J., & Johnson-Greene, D. (2002). Actual versus self-reported scholastic achievement of litigating postconcussion and severe closed head injury claimants. *Psychological Assessment*, *14*, 202–208.

Greiffenstein, M. F., & Kaufmann, P. M. (2012). Neuropsychology and the law: Principles of productive neuropsychologist-attorney interactions. In G. L. Larrabee (Ed.), *Forensic Neuropsychology: Scientific Foundations* (2nd ed., pp. 23–69). New York: Oxford University Press.

Grenitz v. Tomlian, 858 So. 2d 999 (2003 Fla).

Greve, K. W., Bianchini, K. J., Mathias, C. W., Houston, R. J., & Crouch, J. A. (2003). Detecting malingered performance on the Wechsler Adult Intelligence Scale: Validation of Mittenberg's approach in traumatic brain injury. *Archives of Clinical Neuropsychology*, *18*, 245–260.

Grisso, T. (1986). *Evaluating Competencies: Forensic Assessments and Instruments*. New York: Plenum.

Grisso, T. (1988). *Competency to Stand trial: A Manual for Practice*. Sarasota, FL: Professional Resources Exchange, Inc.

Gronwall, D., & Wrightson, P. (1974). Delayed recovery of intellectual function after minor head injury. *Lancet*, *2*(7881), 605–609.

Gronwall, D. M. (1977). Paced auditory serial-addition task: A measure of recovery from concussion. *Perceptual & Motor Skills*, *44*, 367–373.

Groscup, J. L., Penrod, S. D., Studebaker, C. A., Huss, M. T., & O'Neil, K. M. (2002). The effects of Daubert on the admissibility of expert testimony in state and federal criminal cases. *Psychology, Public Policy, & Law*, *8*(4), 339.

Grote, C. L., & Pyykkonen, B. A. (2012). Ethical practice of forensic neuropsychology. In G. Larrabee (Ed.), *Forensic Neuropsychology: Scientific Foundations* (2nd ed., pp. 101–115). New York: Oxford University Press.

Guirguis, S. (1997). Neurobehavioral tests as a medical surveillance procedure: Applying evaluative criteria. *Environmental Research*, *73*, 63–69.

Guskiewicz, K. M., McCrea, M., Marshall, S. W., Cantu, R. C., Randolph, C., Barr, W., et al. (2003). Cumulative effects associated with recurrent concussion in collegiate football players: The NCAA concussion study. *Journal of the American Medical Association*, *290*, 2549–2555.

Guzman `v. 4030 Bronx Blvd. Assoc. L.L.C., 54 A.D.3d 42 (N.Y. App. Div. 2008).

Haaland, K. Y., Harrington, D. L., & Yeo, R. (1987). The effects of task complexity on motor performance in left and right CVA patients. *Neuropsychologia*, *25*, 783–794.

Haaland, K. Y., Temkin, N., Randahl, G., & Dikmen, S. (1994). Recovery of simple motor skills after head injury. *Journal of Clinical & Experimental Neuropsychology*, *16*, 448–456.

Harris, I., Mulford, J., Solomon, M., van Gelder, J. M., & Young, J. (2005). Association between compensation status and outcome after surgery: A meta-analysis. *JAMA*, *293*(13), 1644–1652.

Hartman, D. E. (1999). Neuropsychology and the (neuro)-toxic tort. In J. J. Sweet (Ed.), *Forensic Neuropsychology: Fundamentals and Practice* (pp. 339–367). Lisse, Netherlands: Swets and Zeitlinger.

Hartman, D. E. (2002). The unexamined lie is a lie worth fibbing: Neuropsychological malingering and the Word Memory Test. *Archives of Clinical Neuropsychology*, *17*, 709–714.

Head v. Lithonia Corp., 881 F.2d 941 (10th Cir. 1989).

Heaton, R. K., Chelune, G. J., & Lehman, R. A. (1978). Using neuropsychological and personality tests to assess the likelihood of patient employment. *Journal of Nervous and Mental Disease*, *166*, 408–416.

Heaton, R. K., Chelune, G. J., Talley, J. L., Kay, G. G., & Curtis, G. (1993). *Wisconsin Card Sorting Test (WCST) Manual Revised and Expanded*. Odessa, FL: Psychological Assessment Resources.

Heaton, R. K., Grant, I., & Matthews, C. G. (1991). *Comprehensive Norms for an Extended Halsted-Reitan Neuropsychological Test Battery*. Odessa, FL: Psychological Assessment Resources, Inc.

Heaton, R. K., Ryan, L., Grant, I., & Matthews, C. G. (1996). Demographic influences on neuropsychological test performance. In I. Grant & K. M. Adams (Eds.), *Neuropsychological Assessment of Neuropsychiatric Disorders*. New York: Oxford University Press.

Heaton, R. K., Smith, H. H., Lehman, R. A., & Vogt, A. T. (1978). Prospects for faking believable deficits on neuropsychological testing. *Journal of Consulting & Clinical Psychology*, *46*(5), 892–900.

Hebben, N. (2001). Low lead levels and neuropsychological assessment: Let us not be mislead. *Archives of Clinical Neuropsychology*, *16*, 353–357.

Heilbronner, R. L., Sweet, J. J., Attix, D. K., Kroll, K. R., Henry, G. K., & Hart, R. P. (2003). Official position of the American Academy of Clinical Neuropsychology on serial neuropsychological assessments: The utility and challenges of repeat test administrations in clinical and forensic contexts. *The Clinical Neuropsychologist*, *24*, 1267–1278. [Online]. Retrieved from www.tandfonline.com/doi/pdf/10.1080/13854046.2010.526785 (last visited November 30, 2013).

Heinik, J., Werner, P., & Lin, R. (1999). How do cognitively impaired elderly patients define "testament": Reliability and validity of the testament definition scale. *Israeli Journal of Psychiatry & Related Sciences*, *36*, 23 28.

Hess, A. K. (1999). Practicing principled forensic psychology: Legal, ethical and moral considerations. In A. K. Hess & I. B. Weiner (Eds.), *The Handbook of Forensic Psychology* (2nd ed., pp. 673–699). New York: John Wiley & Sons.

Hill, A. B. (1965). The environment and disease: Association or causation? *Proceedings of the Royal Society of Medicine*, *58*, 295–300.

Holt, R. R. (1998). Individuality and generalization in the Psychology of Personality: A theoretical rationale for personality assessment and research. Retrieved April 5, 2004, from www.priory.com/ital/docum6-i.htm.

Horne v. Goodson Logging Co., 349 S.E.2d 293 (N.C. Ct. App. 1986).

Horton, A. M. (1992). Neuropsychological practice effects and age: A brief note. *Perceptual & Motor Skills*, *75*, 257–258.

Houston, R. J., Stanford, M. S., Villemarette-Pittman, N. R., Conklin, S. M., & Helfritz, L. E. (2003). Neurobiological correlates and clinical implications of aggressive subtypes. *Journal of Forensic Neuropsychology*, *3*(4), 67.

Hunsley, J., & Mash, E. J. (2005). Introduction to the special section on developing guidelines for the evidence-based assessment (EBA) of adult disorders. *Psychological Assessment*, *17*, 251–255.

Huntoon v. TCI Cablevision of Colorado, 969 P. 2d 681 (1998).

Hutchison v. Am. Family Mut. Ins., 514 N.W., 2d 882 (Iowa 1994).

In re: Breast Implant Litigation, 11 F. Supp. 2d 1217, (D. Colo. 1998).

Insanity Defense Reform Act of 1984. ("IDRA") 18 U.S.C. §§ 17, 4244, 4245 (2013).

Jacobson, J. L., & Jacobson, S. W. (2002). Association of prenatal exposure to an environmental contaminant with intellectual function in childhood. *Journal of Toxicology & Clinical Toxicology*, *40*, 467–475.

Jacobson, J. L., & Jacobson, S. W. (2003). Prenatal exposure to polychlorinated biphenyls and attention at school age. *Journal of Pediatrics*, *143*, 780–788.

Jenkins v. U.S., 307 F.2d 637 (1962).

John v. Im (2002). 263 Va. 315; 559 S.E.2d 694 (Virginia Supreme Court, 2002).

Johnson, J. L., Bellah, C. G., Dodge, T., Kelley, W., & Livingston, M. M. (1998). Effect of warning on feigned malingering on the WAIS-R in college samples. *Perceptual & Motor Skills*, *87*, 152–154.

Johnson, J. L., & Lesniak-Karpiak, K. (1997). The effect of warning on malingering on memory and motor tasks in college samples. *Archives of Clinical Neuropsychology*, *12*, 231–238.

Johnson-Greene, D., Dehring, M., Adams, K. M., Miller, T., Arora, S., Beylin, A., & Brandon, R. (1997). Accuracy of self-reported educational attainment among diverse patient populations: A preliminary investigation. *Archives of Clinical Neuropsychology*, *12*, 635–643.

Kagehiro, D. (1990). Defining the standard of proof in jury instructions. *Psychological Science*, *1*, 194–200.

Kalechstein, A. D., Newton, T. F., & van Gorp, W. G. (2003). Neurocognitive functioning is associated with employment status: A quantitative review. *Journal of Clinical & Experimental Neuropsychology*, *25*, 1186–1191.

Kaufman, A. S. (1994). Practice effects. In R. J. Sternberg (Ed.), *Encyclopedia of Human Intelligence* (Vol. 2, pp. 828–833). New York: Macmillan Publishing Company.

Kaufman, A. S. (2001). How dangerous are low (not moderate or high) doses of lead for children's intellectual development? *Archives of Clinical Neuropsychology*, *16*, 403–431.

Kaufmann, P. M. (2005). Protecting the objectivity, fairness, and integrity of neuropsychological evaluations in litigation: A privilege second to none? *The Journal of Legal Medicine*, *26*, 95–131.

Kaufmann, P. M. (2009). Protecting raw data and psychological tests from wrongful disclosure: A primer on the law and other persuasive strategies. *The Clinical Neuropsychologist*, *23*(7), 1130–1159.

Kaufmann, P. M. (2012). Admissibility of expert opinions based on neuropsychological evidence. In G. Larrabee (Ed.), *Forensic Neuropsychology: A Scientific Approach*. (2nd ed., pp. 70–100). New York: Oxford University Press.

Kaufmann, P. M. (2013). Neuropsychologist experts and neurolaw: Cases, controversies, and admissibility challenges. *Behavioral Sciences and the Law*, *31*(6), 739–755.

Kaufmann, P.M. (2016). Neuropsychologist experts and civil capacity evaluations: Representative cases. *Archives of Clinical Neuropsychology*, 31(6), 487–494.

Kaufmann, P. M., & Greffenstein, M. F. (2013). Forensic neuropsychology: Training, scope of practice, and quality control. *National Academy of Neuropsychology Bulletin*, *27*, 11–14.

Kehrer, C. A., Sanchez, P. N., Habif, U., Rosenbaum, J. G., & Townes, B. D. (2000). Effects of a significant-other observer on neuropsychological test performance. *Clinical Neuropsychologist*, *14*, 67–71.

Kibby, M. Y., & Long, C. J. (1996). Minor head injury: Attempts at clarifying the confusion. *Brain Injury*, *10*, 159–186.

Korgeski, G. P., & Leon, G. R. (1983). Correlates of self-reported and objectively determined exposure to Agent Orange. *American Journal of Psychiatry*, *140*, 1443–1449.

Kumho Tire v. Carmichael, 526 U.S. 137 (1999).

Lacks, P. (1982). Continued clinical popularity of the Bender-Gestalt Test: Response to Bigler and Ehrfurth. *Professional Psychology: Research & Practice*, *13*, 677–680.

Lally, S. J. (2003). What tests are acceptable for use in forensic evaluations? A survey of experts. *Professional Psychology: Research and Practice*, *34*, 491–498.

Lamasa v. Bachman, N.Y. Misc. LEXIS 1164 (N.Y Sup. Ct. 2005).

Lamb, D. G., Berry, D.T.R., Wetter, M. W., & Baer, R. A. (1994). Effects of two types of information on malingering of closed head injury on the MMPI-2: An analog investigation. *Psychological Assessment*, *6*(1), 8.

Landers v. Chrysler Corp., 963 S.W.2d 275 (1997).

Larrabee, G. J. (1990). Cautions in the use of neuropsychological evaluation in legal settings. *Neuropsychology*, *4*, 239–247.

Larrabee, G. J. (2003a). Exaggerated pain report in litigants with malingered neurocognitive dysfunction. *Clinical Neuropsychologist*, *17*, 395–401.

Larrabee, G. J. (2003b). Exaggerated MMPI-2 symptom report in personal injury litigants with malingered neurocognitive deficit. *Archives of Clinical Neuropsychology*, *18*, 673–686.

Larrabee, G. J. (2003c). Detection of malingering using atypical performance patterns on standard neuropsychological tests. *Clinical Neuropsychologist*, *17*, 410–425.

Larrabee, G. J. (2012a). A scientific approach to forensic psychology. In G. Larrabee (Ed.), *Forensic Neuropsychology: A Scientific Approach* (2nd ed., pp. 3–22). New York: Oxford University Press.

Larrabee, G. J. (2012b). Assessment of malingering. In G. Larrabee (Ed.), *Forensic Neuropsychology: A Scientific Approach* (2nd ed., pp. 116–159). New York: Oxford University Press.

Larrabee, G. J. (2012c). Performance validity and symptom validity in neuropsychological assessment. *Journal of the International Neuropsychological Society*, *18*, 625–630.

LeBlanc, J. M., Hayden, M. E., & Paulman, R. G. (2000). A comparison of neuropsychological and situational assessment for predicting employability after closed head injury. *Journal of Head Trauma Rehabilitation*, *15*, 1022–1040.

Lees-Haley, P. R. (2003). Toxic mold and mycotoxins in neurotoxicity cases: Stachybotrys, fusarium, trichoderma, aspergillus, penicillin, cladosporium, alternaria, trichothecenes. *Psychological Reports*, *93*, 561–584.

Lees-Haley, P. R., & Cohen, L. J. (1999). The neuropsychologist as expert witness: Towards credible science in the courtroom. In J. J. Sweet (Ed.), *Forensic Neuropsychology: Fundamentals and Practice* (pp. 443–468). Lisse, the Netherlands: Swets & Zeitlinger.

Lees-Haley, P. R., & Courtney, J. C. (2000). Reply to the commentary on "Disclosure of tests and raw test data to the courts." *Neuropsychology Review*, *10*, 181–182.

Lees-Haley, P. R., English, L. T., & Glenn, W. J. (1991). A Fake Bad Scale on the MMPI-2 for personal injury claimants. *Psychological Reports*, *68*, 203–210.

Lees-Haley, P. R., Smith, H. H., Williams, C. W., & Dunn, J. T. (1996). Forensic neuropsychological test usage: An empirical survey. *Archives of Clinical Neuropsychology*, *11*, 45–51.

Lezak, M. (1995). *Neuropsychological Assessment* (3rd ed.). New York: Oxford University Press.

Lishman, W. A. (1988). Physiogenesis and psychogenesis in the 'Post-Concussional Syndrome'. *British Journal of Psychiatry*, *153*, 460–469.

Luis, C. A., Vanderploeg, R. D., & Curtiss, G. (2003). Predictors of postconcussion symptom complex in community dwelling male veterans. *Journal of the International Neuropsychology Society*, *9*(7), 1001–1015.

Manly, J. J., Jacobs, D. M., Touradji, P., Small, S. A., & Stern, Y. (2002). Reading level attenuates differences in neuropsychological test performance between African American and White elders. *Journal of the International Neuropsychological Society*, *8*, 341–348.

Marson, D. C. (2001). Loss of financial competency in dementia: Conceptual and empirical approaches. *Aging, Neuropsychology, & Cognition*, *8*, 164–181.

Marson, D. C., Annis, S. M., McInturff, B., Bartolucci, A., & Harrell, L. E. (1999). Error behaviors associated with loss of competency in Alzheimer's disease. *Neurology*, *53*, 1983–1992.

Marson, D. C., & Hebert, K. (2005). Assessing civil competencies in older adults with dementia. In G. J. Larrabee (Ed.), *Forensic Neuropsychology: A Scientific Approach* (pp. 334–377). New York: Oxford University Press.

Martin, R. C., Hayes, J. S., & Gouvier, W. D. (1996). Differential vulnerability between postconcussion self-report and objective malingering tests in identifying simulated mild head injury. *Journal of Clinical Neuropsychology*, *18*(2), 265.

Martin v. Benson. 348 NC 684 (North Carolina Supreme Court, 1988).

Matarazzo, J. D., Bornstein, R. A., McDermott, P. A., & Noonan, J. V. (1986). Verbal IQ versus Performance IQ difference scores in males and females from the WAIS-R standardization sample. *Journal of Clinical Psychology*, *42*, 965–974.

Matarazzo, J. D., & Herman, D. O. (1985). Clinical uses of the WAIS-R: Base rates of differences between VIQ and PIQ in the WAIS-R standardization sample. In B. B. Wolfman (Ed.), *Handbook of Intelligence* (pp. 899–932). New York: Wiley.

Matuszak v. Cerniak, 805 N.E.2d 681 (Ill. Ap. Ct. 2004).

M'Naghten's Case, 10 Cl. F. 200, 8 Eng Rep. 718 (H.L. 1843).

McCaffrey, R. J. (2005). Third party observers. *Journal of Forensic Neuropsychology*, *4*, 1–91.

McCaffrey, R. J., Fisher, J. M., Gold, B. A., & Lynch, J. K. (1996). Presence of third parties during neuropsychological evaluations: Who is evaluating whom? *The Clinical Neuropsychologist*, *10*, 435–449.

McCaffrey, R. J., & Westervelt, H. J. (1995). Issues associated with repeated neuropsychological assessments. *Neuropsychology Review*, *5*, 203–221.

McCauley, S. R., Boake, C., Levin, H. S., Contant, C. F., & Song, J. X. (2001). Postconcussional disorder following mild to moderate traumatic brain injury: Anxiety, depression, and social support as risk factors and comorbidities. *Journal of Clinical and Experimental Neuropsychology*, *23*(6), 792–808.

McCauley, S. R., Boake, C., Pedroza, C., Brown, S. A., Levin, H. S., Goodman, H. S., et al. (2005). Postconcussional disorder: Are the DSM-IV criteria an improvement over the icd-10? *Journal of Nervous & Mental Disorders*, *193*(8), 540–550.

McCrea, M., Guskiewicz, K. M., Marshall, S. W., Barr, W., Randolph, C., Cantu, R. C., et al. (2003). Acute effects and recovery time following concussion in collegiate football players: The NCAA Concussion Study. *Journal of the American Medical Association*, *290*, 2556–2563.

McCrea, M., Kelly, J. P., Randolph, C., Cisler, R., & Berger, L. (2002). Immediate neurocognitive effects of concussion. *Neurosurgery*, *50*, 1032–1040.

McKinzey, R. K., & Ziegler, T. (1999). Challenging a flexible neuropsychological battery under Kelly/Frye: A case study. *Behavioral Sciences & the Law*, *17*, 543–551.

McNally, R. J. (2005). The science and controversy of traumatic memory. *American Journal of Psychology*, *118*(1), 152.

McSweeny, A. J. (1997). Regarding ethics in forensic neuropsychological consultation: A comment on Guilmette and Hagan. *Clinical Neuropsychologist*, *11*, 291–293.

Meehl, P. (1954). *Clinical and Actuarial Prediction*. Minneapolis, MN: University of Minnesota Press.

Melton, G. B., Petrila, J., Poythress, N. G., & Slobogin, C. (1997). *Psychological Evaluations for the Courts. A Handbook for Mental Health Professionals and Lawyers* (2nd ed., p. 794). New York: Guilford Press.

Meyer-Baron, M., Schaeper, M., Van Thriel, C., & Seeber, A. (2003). Neurobehavioral test results and exposure to inorganic mercury: In search of dose-response relations. *Archives of Toxicology*.

Mickeviciene, D., Schrader, H., Nestvold, K., Surkiene, D., Kunickas, R., Stovner, L. J., & Sand, T. (2002). A controlled historical cohort study on the post-concussion syndrome. *European Journal of Neurology*, *9*, 581–587.

Miller, H., & Cartlidge, N. (1972). Simulation and malingering after injuries to the brain and spinal cord. *Lancet*, *1*(7750), 580–585.

Miller, L. J., & Donders, J. (2001). Subjective symptomatology after traumatic head injury. *Brain Injury*, *15*, 297–304.

Miller, L. J., & Mittenberg, W. (1998). Brief cognitive behavioral interventions in mild traumatic brain injury. *Applied Neuropsychology*, *5*, 172–183.

Millis, S. R. (2002). Warrington's Recognition Memory Test in the detection of response bias. *Journal of Forensic Neuropsychology*, *2*(3–4), 147–166.

Mitrushina, M. N., Boone, K. B., & D'Elia, L. F. (1999). *Handbook of Normative Data for Neuropsychological Assessment*. London: Oxford University Press.

Mitrushina, M. N., & Satz, P. (1991). Effect of repeated administration of a neuropsychological battery in the elderly. *Journal of Clinical Psychology*, *47*, 790–801.

Mittenberg, W., Azrin, R., Millsaps, C., & Heilbronner, R. (1993). Identification of malingered head injury on the Wechsler Memory Scale—Revised. *Psychological Assessment*, *5*, 34–40.

Mittenberg, W., Diguilio, D., Perrin, S., & Bass, A. (1992). Symptoms following mild head injury: Expectation as aetiology. *Journal of Neurology, Neurosurgery and Psychiatry*, *55*, 200–214.

Mittenberg, W., Patton, C., Canyock, E. M., & Condit, D. C. (2002). Base rates of malingering and symptom exaggeration. *Journal of Clinical & Experimental Neuropsychology*, *24*, 1094–1102.

Mittenberg, W., Theroux, S., Aguila-Puentes, G., Bianchini, K., Greve, K., & Rayls, K. (2001). Identification of malingered head injury on the wechsler adult intelligence scale—3rd edition. *The Clinical Neuropsychologist*, *15*, 440–445.

Mossman, D. (2000). The meaning of malingering data: Further applications of Bayes' theorem. *Behavioral Sciences & Law*, *18*, 761–779.

Nadell v. Las Vegas Metro. Police Dep't, 268 F.3d 924 (9th Cir. 2001), *cert. denied*, 535 U.S. 1057 (2002).

Needleman, H. L. (1979). Lead levels and children's psychologic performance. *New England Journal of Medicine*, *301*, 163.

Needleman, H. L., & Bellinger, D. (2001). Studies of lead exposure and the developing central nervous system: A reply to Kaufman. *Archives of Clinical Neuropsychology*, *16*, 359–374.

Needleman, H. L., & Leviton, A. (1979). Lead and neurobehavioral deficit in children. *Lancet*, *14*, 8133.

Needleman, H. L., McFarland, C., Ness, R. B., Fienberg, S. E., & Tobin, M. J. (2002). Bone lead levels in adjudicated delinquents: A case control study. *Neurotoxicology and Teratology*, *24*, 711–717.

Newcombe, F., Rabbitt, P., & Briggs, M. (1994). Minor head injury: Pathophysiological or iatrogenic sequelae? *Journal of Neurology, Neurosurgery, & Psychiatry*, *57*, 709–716.

Nuwer, M. (1997). Assessment of digital EEG, quantitative EEG, and EEG brain mapping: Report of the American Academy of Neurology and the American Clinical Neurophysiology Society. *Neurology*, *49*, 277–292.

Ogloff, J. R. (1990). The admissibility of expert testimony regarding malingering and deception. *Behavioral Sciences & the Law*, *8*, 27–43.

Othmer, E., & Othmer, S. C. (1989). *The Clinical Interview Using the DSM-III-R*. Washington, DC: American Psychiatric Press.

Paauw, D. S. (1999). Did we learn evidence-based medicine in medical school? Some common medical mythology. *Journal of the American Board of Family Practice*, *12*, 143–149.

Paniak, C., MacDonald, J., Toller-Lobe, G., Durand, A., & Nagy, J. (1998). A preliminary normative profile of mild traumatic brain injury diagnostic criteria. *Journal of Clinical & Experimental Neuropsychology*, *20*, 852–855.

People v. Urdiales, 871 N.E.2d, 669 (Ill. 2007).

Pliskin, N. H., Capelli-Schellpfeffer, M., Law, R. T., Malina, A. C., Kelley, K. M., & Lee, R. C. (1998). Neuropsychological symptom presentation after electrical injury. *Journal of Trauma*, *44*, 709–715.

Pobereskin, L. H. (2005). Whiplash following rear end collisions: A prospective cohort study. *Journal of Neurology Neurosurgery & Psychiatry*, *76*(8), 1146–1151.

Pocock, S. J., Smith, M., & Baghurst, P. (1994). Environmental lead and children's intelligence: A systematic review of the epidemiological evidence. *British Medical Journal*, *309*, 1189–1197.

Pope, K. S., Butcher, J. N., & Seelen, J. (1993). *MMPI, MMPI-2, & MMPI-A in court*. Washington: American Psychological Association.

Posthuma, A., Podrouzek, W., & Crisp, D. (2002). The implications of Daubert on neuropsychological evidence in the assessment of remote mild traumatic brain injury. *American Journal of Forensic Psychology*, *20*, 21–38.

Prigatano, G. P., Altman, I. M., & O'Brien, K. P. (1990). Behavioral limitations that traumatic-brain-injured patients tend to underestimate. *Clinical Neuropsychologist*, *4*, 163–176.

Putnam, S. H., Adams, K. M., & Schneider, A. M. (1992). One-day test-retest reliability of neuropsychological tests in a personal injury case. *Psychological Assessment*, *4*, 312–316.

Ragge v. MCA/Universal Studios, 165 FRD 605 (1995).

Rankin, E. J., & Adams, R. L. (1999). The neuropsychological evaluation: Clinical and scientific foundations. In J. J. Sweet (Ed.), *Forensic Neuropsychology: Foundations and Practice* (pp. 83–120). Lisse, the Netherlands: Swets and Zeitlinger.

Rapport, L. J., Farchione, T. J., Coleman, R. D., & Axelrod, B. N. (1998). Effects of coaching on malingered motor function profiles. *Journal of Clinical & Experimental Neuropsychology*, *20*, 89–97.

Reed, J. E. (1996). Fixed vs. flexible neuropsychological test batteries under the Daubert standard for the admissibility of scientific evidence. *Behavioral Sciences & the Law*, *14*, 315–322.

Rees, L. M., Tombaugh, T. N., Gansler, D. A., & Moczynski, N. P. (1998). Five validation experiments of the Test of Memory Malingering (TOMM). *Psychological Assessment*, *10*, 10–20.

Reitan, R. M. (2001). Differentiating between peripheral and central lateralized neuropsychological deficits. *Journal of Forensic Neuropsychology*, *2*, 21–27.

Reitan, R. M., & Wolfson, D. (2002). Detection of malingering and invalid test results using the Halstead-Reitan Battery. *Journal of Forensic Neuropsychology*, *3*, 275–314.

Reynolds, S., Paniak, C., Toller-Lobe, G., & Nagy, J. (2003). A longitudinal study of compensation-seeking and return to work in a treated mild traumatic brain injury sample. *Journal of Head Trauma & Rehabilitation*, *18*(2), 139–147.

Risser, A. (2003). The <E-practice>. Internet resources for the practicing neuropsychologist. In G. Lamberty, R. L. Heilbronner, & J. C. Courtney (Eds.), *The Practice of Clinical Neuropsychology* (pp. 143–172). Lisse, Netherlands: Swets-Zeitlinger.

Rogers, R. (1990). Models of feigned mental illness. *Professional Psychology: Research & Practice*, *21*, 182–188.

Rogers, R. (1997). Introduction. In R. Rogers (Ed.), *Clinical Assessment of Malingering and Deception* (pp. 1–19). New York: Guilford.

Rohling, M. L., Meyers, J. E., & Millis, S. R. (2003). Neuropsychological impairment following traumatic brain injury: A dose-response analysis. *The Clinical Neuropsychologist*, *17*, 289–302.

Rosen, G. M. (1995). The Aleutian Enterprise sinking and posttraumatic stress disorder: Misdiagnosis in clinical and forensic settings. *Professional Psychology: Research & Practice*, *26*, 82–87.

Ross, S. R., Millis, S. R., Krukowski, R. A., Putnam, S. H., & Adams, K. M. (2004). Detecting incomplete effort on the MMPI-2: An examination of the Fake-Bad Scale in mild head injury. *Journal of Clinical & Experimental Neuropsychology*, *26*, 115–124.

Ross v. Schrantz, 1995 Minn. App. LEXIS 586 (Minn, App. Ct. 1995).

Ruff, R., & Richardson, A. M. (1999). Mild traumatic brain injury. In J. J. Sweet (Ed.), *Forensic Neuropsychology* (pp. 313–338). Lisse, Netherlands: Swets & Zeitlinger.

Ruiz, M. A., Drake, E. B., Glass, A., Marcotte, D., & van Gorp, W. G. (2002). Trying to beat the system: Misuse of the Internet to assist in avoiding the detection of psychological symptom dissimulation. *Professional Psychology: Research & Practice*, *33*(3), 294.

Russell, E. W. (2012). *The Scientific Foundation of Neuropsychological Assessment*. Amsterdam, Netherlands: Elsevier.

Sanders, J., Diamond, S. S., & Vidmar, N. (2002). Legal perceptions of science and expert knowledge. *Psychology, Public Policy, and Law*, *8*, 139–153.

Sbordone, R. J. (2001). Limitations of neuropsychological testing to predict the cognitive and behavioral functioning of persons with brain injury in real-world settings. *Neuro Rehabilitation*, *16*, 199–201.

Schantz, S. L., Sweeney, A. M., Gardiner, J. C., Humphrey, H. E., McCaffrey, R. J., Gasior, D. M., Srikanth K. R., & Budd M. L. (1996). Neuropsychological assessment of an aging population of Great Lakes fisheaters. *Toxicology & Industrial Health*, *12*(3–4), 403–417.

Schrag, A., Brown, R. J., & Trimble, M. R. (2004). Reliability of self-reported diagnoses in patients with neurologically unexplained symptoms. *Journal of Neurology, Neurosurgery & Psychiatry*, *75*, 608–611.

Schudel v. General Elec., 120 F.3d 991 (1995).

Schwartz, L., Taylor, H. G., Drotar, D., Yeates, K. O., Wade, S. L., & Stancin, T. (2003). Long-term behavior problems following pediatric traumatic brain injury: Prevalence, predictors, and correlates. *Journal of Pediatric Psychology*, *28*, 251–263.

Searight, H. R., Dunn, E. J., Grisso, T., Margolis, R. B., & Gibbons, J. L. (1989). The relation of the Halstead-Reitan Neuropsychological Battery to ratings of everyday functioning in a geriatric sample. *Neuropsychology*, *3*, 135–145.

Shapiro, D. L. (1991). *Forensic Psychological Assessment: An Integrative Approach*. Boston: Allyn & Bacon.

Shatz, M. W. (1981). WAIS practice effects in clinical neuropsychology. *Journal of Clinical Neuropsychology*, *3*, 171–179.

Shaw, N. A. (2002). The neurophysiology of concussion. *Progress in Neurobiology*, *67*, 281–344.

Simmons v. Mullins, 231 Pa. Super. 199, 331 A.2d 892 (Pa. Super. 1975).

Slick, D. J., Sherman, E.M.S., & Iverson, G. L. (1999). Diagnostic criteria for malingered neurocognitive dysfunction: Proposed standards for clinical practice and research. *Clinical Neuropsychologist*, *13*, 545–561.

Slobogin, C. (2003). Pragmatic forensic psychology: A means of "scientizing" expert testimony from mental health professionals? *Psychology, Public Policy, & Law*, *9*(3–4), 275.

Spar, J. E., & Garb, A. S. (1992). Assessing competency to make a will. *American Journal of Psychiatry*, *149*, 169–174.

Spreen, O., & Strauss, E. (1998). *A Compendium of Neuropsychological Tests: Administration, Norms, and Commentary* (2nd ed.). New York: Oxford University Press.

Stanford, M. S., Helfritz, L. E., Conklin, S. M., Villemarette-Pittman, N. R., Greve, K. W., Adams, D., & Houston, R. J. (2005). A comparison of anticonvulsants in the treatment of impulsive aggression. *Experimental & Clinical Psychopharmacology*, *13*(1), 72.

State v. Zimmerman, 802 P. 2d 1024 (Az. App. Ct., 1990).

Steele, C. M. (1997). A threat in the air: How stereotypes shape intellectual identity and performance. *American Psychologist*, *52*(6), 613.

Stokes v. State (1989), 548 So. 2d (Fla.) 188, 193.

Storm, J., & Graham, J. R. (2000). Detection of coached general malingering on the mmpi—2. *Psychological Assessment*, *12*(2), 158.

Suhr, J. A. (2002). Malingering, coaching, and the serial position effect. *Archives of Clinical Neuropsychology*, *17*, 69–77.

Suhr, J. A., & Gunstad, J. (2000). The effects of coaching on the sensitivity and specificity of malingering measures. *Archives of Clinical Neuropsychology*, *15*, 415–424.

Suhr, J. A., & Gunstad, J. (2002). "Diagnosis threat": The effect of negative expectations on cognitive performance in head injury. *Journal of Clinical & Experimental Neuropsychology*, *24*(4), 448.

Suhr, J. A., & Gunstad, J. (2005). Further exploration of the effect of "diagnosis threat" on cognitive performance in individuals with mild head injury. *Journal of the International Neuropsychological Society*, *11*(1), 23.

Sullivan, J. P., & Denney, R. L. (2003). Constitutional and judicial foundations in criminal forensic neuropsychology. *Journal of Forensic Neuropsychology*, *3*(4), 13.

Summers v. Missouri Pac. R.R., No. 94–468-P, United States District Court for the Eastern District of Oklahoma, 897 F. Supp. 533; 1997.

Sweet, J. J. (1999a). Introduction. In J. J. Sweet (Ed.), *Forensic Neuropsychology: Fundamentals and Practice* (pp. xvii–xix). Lisse, the Netherlands: Swets and Zeitlinger.

Sweet, J. J. (1999b). Malingering: Differential diagnosis. In J. J. Sweet (Ed.), *Forensic Neuropsychology: Fundamentals and Practice* (pp. 255–285). Lisse, Netherlands: Swets and Zeitlinger.

Sweet, J. J., Guiffre Meyer, D., Nelson, N. W., & Moberg, P. J. (2010). The TCN/AACN 2010 "salary survey": Professional practices, beliefs, and incomes of U.S. neuropsychologists. *The Clinical Neuropsychologist*, *25*, 12–61.

Sweet, J. J., & Moulthrop, M. A. (1999). Self-examination questions as a means of identifying bias in adversarial assessments. *Journal of Forensic Neuropsychology*, *1*, 73–88.

Taylor, L. A., Kreutzer, J. S., & West, D. D. (2003). Evaluation of malingering cut-off scores for the Rey 15-Item Test: A brain injury case study series. *Brain Injury*, *17*, 295–308.

Theisen, M. E., Rapport, L. J., Axelrod, B. N., & Brines, D. B. (1998). Effects of practice in repeated administrations of the Wechsler Memory Scale—Revised in normal adults. *Assessment*, *5*, 85–92.

Tombaugh, T. N. (1995). *The Test of Memory Malingering*. Toronto, Canada: Multi-Health Systems.

Tombaugh, T. N. (2002). The Test of Memory Malingering (TOMM) in forensic psychology. *Journal of Forensic Neuropsychology*, *2*(3–4), 69–96.

Tomlin v. Holecek, 150 FRD 628 (1993).

Tong, S., Baghurst, P., McMichael, A., Sawyer, M., & Mudge, J. (1996). Lifetime exposure to environmental lead and children's intelligence at 11–13 years: The Port Pirie cohort study. *British Medical Journal*, *312*, 1569–1575.

Tran v. Hilburn, 948 P. 2d (Colo. App., 1997).

Tranel, D. (1994). The release of psychological data to nonexperts: Ethical and legal considerations. *Professional Psychology: Research & Practice*, *25*, 33–38.

Tremont, G., Hoffman, R. G., Scott, J. G., & Adams, R. L. (1998). Effect of intellectual level on neuropsychological test performance: A response to Dodrill (1997). *The Clinical Neuropsychologist*, *12*, 560–567.

Troiano v. John Hancock Mutual, Life Ins. Co., 02 Civ. 2921 (2003).

United States v. Cameron, 907 F.2d 1051 (11th Cir. 1990).

United States v. Hinckley, 525 F. Supp. 1342 (D.D.C. 1981), *clarified* 529 F. Supp. 520 (D.D.C. 1981), *aff'd* 672 F.2d 115 (D.C. Cir. 1982).

Valiulis v. Scheffeos, 191 Ill. App. 3d 775, 547 N.E. 2d 1290 (Ill. App. 2 Dist. 1989).

Vanderploeg, R. D. (1994). Interview and testing: The data collection phase of neuropsychological evaluations. In R. D. Vanderploeg (Ed.), *Clinician's Guide to Neuropsychological Assessment* (pp. 1–42). New York: Lawrence Erlbaum & Associates.

Van Gorp, W. G., Humphrey, L. A., Kalechstein, A., Brumm, V. L., McMullen, W. J., Stoddard, M., & Pachana, N. A. (1999). How well do standard clinical neuropsychological tests identify malingering? A preliminary analysis. *Journal of Clinical & Experimental Neuropsychology*, *21*, 245–250.

Van Hout, M. S., Schmand, B., Wekking, E. M., Hageman, G., & Deelman, B. G. (2003). Suboptimal performance on neuropsychological tests in patients with suspected chronic toxic encephalopathy. *Neurotoxicology*, *24*, 547–551.

Varney, N. R., Kubu, C. S., & Morrow, L. A. (1998). Dichotic listening performances of patients with chronic exposure to organic solvents. *Clinical Neuropsychologist*, *12*, 107–112.

Villalba v. Consolidated Freightways Corp., Case No. 98 C 5347, USDC for the Northern District of Illinois, Eastern Division.

Volbrecht, M. E., Meyers, J. E., & Kaster-Bundgaard, J. (2000). Neuropsychological outcome of head injury using a short battery. *Archives of Clinical Neuropsychology*, *15*, 251–265.

Wheeler, S. C., & Petty, R. E. (2001). The effects of stereotype activation on behavior: A review of possible mechanisms. *Psychological Bulletin*, *127*(6), 797.

Wolfson, D., & Reitan, R. M. (1995). Cross-validation of the general neuropsychological deficit scale (GNDS). *Archives Clinical Neuropsychology*, *10*(2), 125–131.

Woltersdorf, M. A. (2005, October). *FBS in clinical and forensic practice sample in Midwest*. Poster session presented at annual meeting of the National Academy of Neuropsychology, Tampa, FL.

Wong, J. L., Lerner-Poppen, L., & Durham, J. (1998). Does warning reduce obvious malingering on memory and motor tasks in college samples? *International Journal of Rehabilitation & Health*, *4*, 153–165.

Worthington, D. L., Stallard, M. J., Price, J. M., & Goss, P. J. (2002, June). Hindsight bias, Daubert, and the silicone breast implant litigation: Making the case for court-appointed experts in complex medical and scientific litigation. *Psychology, Public Policy, and Law*, *8*(2), 154–179.

Wright, R. W. (2008). Symposium: Liability for possible wrongs: Causation, probability, and the burden of proof. *Loyola of Los Angeles Law Review*, *41*, 1295–1343.

Wynkoop, T. F. (2003). Neuropsychology of juvenile adjudicative competence. *Journal of Forensic Neuropsychology*, *3*(4), 45.

Wynkoop, T. F., & Denney, R. L. (1999). Exaggeration of neuropsychological deficit in competency to stand trial. *Journal of Forensic Neuropsychology*, *1*(2), 29.

Yartz, A. R., Zvolensky, M. J., Gregor, K., Feldner, M. T., & Leen-Feldner, E. W. (2005). Health perception is a unique predictor of anxiety symptoms in non-clinical participants. *Cognitive Behaviour Therapy*, *34*(2), 65.

Yeates, K. O., Taylor, H. G., Wade, S. L., Drotar, D., Stancin, T., & Minich, N. (2002). A prospective study of short- and long-term neuropsychological outcomes after traumatic brain injury in children. *Neuropsychology*, *16*, 514–523.

Youngjohn, J. R. (1995). Confirmed attorney coaching prior to neuropsychological evaluation. *Assessment*, *2*, 279–283.

Youngjohn, J. R., Davis, D., & Wolf, I. (1997). Head injury and the MMPI-2: Paradoxical severity effects and the influence of litigation. *Psychological Assessment*, *9*, 177–184.

Youngjohn, J. R., Lees-Haley, P. R., & Binder, L. M. (1999). Comment: Warning malingerers produces more sophisticated malingering. *Archives of Clinical Neuropsychology*, *14*, 511–515.

38 Assessment of Incomplete Effort and Malingering in the Neuropsychological Examination

Scott R. Millis and Paul M. Kaufmann

If it can't be expressed in figures, it is not science; it is opinion.
—*Robert A. Heinlein (1907–1988)*

Neuropsychological tests require the cooperation and effort of examinees to complete the tests to the best of their abilities. As Demakis, Sweet, Sawyer, Moulthrop, Nies, and Clingerman (2001) have observed, "If effort is fully applied throughout testing, the resulting test data can be considered valid, but if incompletely or insufficiently applied (whether because of psychopathology, malingering, or some other cause), test data may be invalid" (p. 240). One type of incomplete effort is malingering. Malingering has been defined as "the volitional exaggeration or fabrication of cognitive dysfunction for the purpose of obtaining substantial material gain, or avoiding for escaping formal duty or responsibility" (Slick, Sherman, & Iverson, 1999, p. 552). However, incomplete effort can occur in the absence of external incentives. Hence, the assessment of incomplete effort needs to be conducted within in the larger context of the differential diagnosis in which several diagnoses need to be considered. Therein lays the challenge. Malingering has no virus or bacteria associated with it. Its neuroimaging correlates are unknown. The behavior of malingering may be observed in other disorders as well. Although a veritable cottage industry has sprung up over the past decade offering a plethora of malingering tests, interest is this topic is quite old.

Historical Context

In 1788, Samuel Farr's *Elements of Medical Jurisprudence* was published in Great Britain, which dealt with the clinical detection of malingering (Geller, Erlen, Kaye, & Fisher, 1990). The 18th- and 19th-century papers that followed focused primarily on malingering of psychiatric disorders. A wide variety of methods were used to detect malingering such as flagellation, emetics, beef tea enemas, the "whirling chair," and electrical shocks to the tongue from galvanic batteries (Geller et al., 1990). Although these methods have largely been abandoned, behavioral observation, clinical interview, and patient history are still central elements in assessing for malingering. Ray's observation in 1838 remains relevant today, "In simulated madness, the common error is to imagine that nothing must be remembered correctly, and that the more inconsistent and absurd the discourse, the better is the attempt at deception sustained" (Geller et al., 1990, p. 12).

Neuropsychology's chief contribution in the assessment of malingering arguably has been the application of the psychometric and actuarial approach to diagnosis. This is not to imply that a single test in isolation should be used to diagnose a disorder. The perspective of this chapter is that the evaluation of malingering and incomplete effort will, by necessity, require the collection and integration of several types of information in addition to any test data obtained from the latest malingering test du jour. In addition, a bias of this chapter is that this diagnostic process should use quantitative actuarial formulas when available. Data can be systematically collected and integrated in a logically coherent and transparent fashion such that an external observer would be able to repeat the steps of the process. The external observer may disagree with the specific decision rules but will be in the position to empirically test any of the decision rules. This diagnostic process can be divided into several steps:

1. Assessing the role of external incentives;
2. Determining injury severity;
3. Evaluating the impact of psychosocial factors on patient behavior;
4. Using tests to refine diagnostic hypotheses;
5. Applying specialized tests;
6. Analyzing test performance patterns;
7. Integrating all sources of information; and
8. Applying new statistical methods to assist in decision making.

This chapter will consider the assessment of incomplete effort in the context of mild head injury (MHI). It is difficult to separate a discussion of malingering assessment from MHI. First, most effort tests and indices were developed from samples of persons with different severities of traumatic brain injury (TBI). Second, the incidence of mild and moderate brain injury is relatively high in the United States and most neuropsychologists will encounter head injury cases in the course of their practice. In an analysis of the National Health Interview Survey, Sosin, Sniezek, and Thurman (1996) estimated that

1.5 million U.S. civilians each year sustain a nonfatal brain injury that does not result in institutionalization. Third, litigation involving head injury claims is common, e.g., brain injury claims accounted for 7% of total plaintiff verdicts in vehicular accidents for the period between 1992 and 1998 (Jury Verdict Research, 2000). Fourth, neuropsychological data often play a central role in the litigated MHI case.

Taking these factors into consideration, it likely that most neuropsychologists will confront the assessment of malingering and incomplete effort in context of the MHI case. However, the general guidelines and procedures presented in this chapter may be applicable in other diagnostic settings where malingering and cognitive impairment are at issue, e.g., toxic exposure, multiple chemical sensitivity, or electrical injuries. However, the generalizability of specific cutoff scores from effort measures to disorders other than those conditions from which they were derived remains an empirical question.

The Role of External Incentives

By virtue of their training, neuropsychologists may tend to focus primarily on individual factors that influence behavior while ignoring environmental and situational factors. Yet, environmental contingencies have considerable impact on neuropsychological test performance. In a meta-analysis of 17 studies involving 2,353 participants, Binder and Rohling (1996) found a significant effect of financial incentives on disability and symptoms after head injury. A moderate overall effect size of 0.47 was reported. Persons with financial incentives showed greater *apparent* disability despite less severe injuries. Paniak, Reynolds, Toller-Lobe, Melnyk, Nagy, and Schmidt (2002) compared 50 persons with mild TBI without financial incentives with 18 who were seeking or receiving financial compensation at treatment intake, three months postinjury, and 12 months postinjury. The study participants volunteered to participate in a treatment study. The financial incentive group consistently reported a significantly higher number of symptoms (about one standard) and greater symptom severity at all intervals. There were no injury-related or demographic differences between the groups. Paniak et al. (2002) concluded that,

> The correspondence between compensation status and symptoms level is suggestive of negative effects on functioning related to (though not necessarily caused by) aspects of the compensation process. This is the first time that this finding has been demonstrated in a 'treated' MTBI sample. It illustrates that even treatment that is highly rated by patients (Paniak, Toller-Lobe, et al., 1998) cannot overcome the strong relationship between compensation status and symptom report that has been previously reported in primarily 'untreated' MTBI samples (Binder & Rohling, 1996). (p. 192)

This is not to imply that all patients who are involved in litigation, receiving compensation, on disability, or seeking compensation are malingering. However, the compensation process may be associated with an increased prevalence of malingering or symptoms endorsement. First, the litigation and disability proceedings can be protracted. In 1999, the median number of months from accident date to trial in vehicular liability cases in the United State was 37 months (Jury Verdict Research, 2000). During this period, plaintiffs will have undergone multiple medical examinations, recalled their accident and symptoms dozens of times, and undergone extensive treatment. This process may selectively reinforce attitudes and behaviors associated with a disability lifestyle. Second, the jury awards in brain injury litigation can be substantial. The median awards for mild TBI and moderate TBI were $271,350 and $1,375,000, respectively for the period of 1993–2001 (Kaiman, 2003). Third, state auto insurance systems offer different incentives for nonexistent or exaggerated claims. A study by the Rand Corporation (Abrahamse & Carroll, 1999) found that tort and dollar-threshold states have a higher frequency of excess soft-tissue injury claims than no-fault states. The study concluded that 42% of reported soft-injury claims in the tort and dollar-threshold states were for nonexistent or preexisting injuries.

These factors may differentially elicit and maintain illness behavior or malingering. As a starting point in the neuropsychological examination, it is essential for the neuropsychologist to determine whether external incentives for illness behavior exist for the persons they are evaluating. In addition, familiarity with one's state's automobile insurance and workers' compensation systems may help in assessing environmental contingencies that reinforce or discourage excess claims.

Injury Severity in the Assessment of Effort

Having determined whether external incentives exist for illness behavior, knowledge of a patient's initial injury is the next essential step in the diagnostic process. Injury or illness severity can help in determining whether neuropsychological test scores "make sense." For example, there is a dose-response relationship between initial TBI injury severity and the degree of associated cognitive impairment (Dikmen, Machamer, Winn, & Temkin, 1995) that tends to be linear (Rohling, 2000). As severity of head injury increases, so do the extent and severity of neuropsychological impairment. Dikmen et al. (1995) found that "significant neuropsychological impairment due to a mild head injury is as unlikely as is escaping an impairment in the case of a very severe head injury" (p. 87).

Evidence from well-designed studies is quite compelling that the neuropsychological deficits from a single uncomplicated MHI are relatively subtle. Dikmen, Machamer, and Temkin (2001) examined a subgroup of persons with MHI from two earlier longitudinal studies of TBI. This subgroup met stringent criteria for MHI: posttraumatic amnesia of 24 hours or less, time to follow commands of less than one hour, and no computed tomography (CT) abnormalities. This group was compared to a matched group of participants with injuries to other parts of the body (trauma control group) on the Selective Reminding Test, Seashore Rhythm Test, Trail Making Test B, and Wechsler Adult Intelligence Scale (WAIS) Performance IQ (PIQ). At one-month postinjury, there were no statistically significant differences between the MHI and trauma control (TC) groups on these measures. In fact, the MHI performed slightly better on three of the measures. On the Selective Reminding Test, the MHI group recalled about two fewer words on the sum of recall index, a difference that is associated with a small effect size (Hedges' $g = 0.17$).

In an Australian study, Ponsford et al. (2000) also employed a trauma control group in comparison with consecutively enrolled patients with head injury. At one week postinjury, the mild TBI participants performed worse on complex attention tasks compared to trauma controls. At three months, there were no statistically significant differences between the groups on neuropsychological measures. Viewed from a broader perspective, Binder, Rohling, and Larrabee (1997) found a small effect size of mild TBI on cognitive functioning (Hedges's $g = 0.07$) in a meta-analysis of 11 studies involving 622 subjects.

Neuropsychologists can establish initial brain injury severity with measures that assess alteration in consciousness, e.g., the Glasgow Coma Scale (GCS), Revised Trauma Score, time to follow commands (derived from the motor score on the GCS), or length of posttraumatic amnesia as determined by the Galveston Orientation and Amnesia Scale. These measures are commonly available from emergency department, acute hospitalization, or inpatient rehabilitation medical records. Estimates of initial injury severity can be compared with a given patient's neuropsychological test results to determine if the panel of results deviates significantly from expected patterns of neuropsychological test performance. Numerous studies are available that provide data on typical neuropsychological test performances of persons from different backgrounds with varying levels of TBI severity; see Dikmen et al. (1995); Kreutzer, Gordon, Rosenthal, and Marwitz (1993); Levin et al. (1987); Millis (2002); Millis et al. (2001) and Ponsford et al. (2000).

Excessively impaired neuropsychological test scores in MHI cases alone do not necessarily indicate malingering or incomplete effort. Conversely, reflexively attributing poor test scores to a MHI is also unwarranted. The diagnostic challenge is to detect the small neuropsychological effect of MHI in a sea of substantial variability in cognitive performance in the general population without acquired brain injury. In an analysis of their data, Dikmen et al. (2001) noted, "With this much variability, one would expect that 35% of those without brain injury would score at least as badly as the average person with stringently defined mild TBI 1 month after injury" (p. 736). Hence, the issue is much broader than malingering versus brain dysfunction cause by MHI. In order to clarify the diagnosis, it is necessary to consider the individual differences that might account for the cognitive variability among examinees. In addition to external incentives, and initial injury severity characteristics, psychosocial factors provide important data regarding individual differences.

Psychosocial Influences

Anxiety, dizziness, headache, memory and concentration problems, fatigue, irritability, depression, and noise sensitivity may occur following MHI (Alexander, 1995). Yet, these symptoms are not diagnostically specific for MHI. They are common in the general population and are also associated with other medical and psychological disorders (Fox, Lees-Haley, Earnest, & Dolezal-Wood, 1995; Gouvier, Uddo-Crane, & Brown, 1988; Lees-Haley & Brown, 1993; Lees-Haley, Fox, & Courtney, 2001; Sawchyn, Brulot, & Strauss, 1999; Suhr & Gunstad, 2002; Trahan, Ross, & Trahan, 2001). In one sample of healthy individuals, 90% reported various somatic symptoms during a one-week period (Kellner & Sheffield, 1973), such as headache, fatigue, muscle pain, and irritability. Fox et al. (1995) found the following rates of symptom endorsement in a sample of persons seeking outpatient psychotherapy: headache (52%), memory problems (31%), dizziness (30%), concentration problems (45%), fatigue (55%), and irritability (55%). Paniak, Reynolds, Phillips, Toller-Lobe, Melnyk, and Nagy (2002) compared symptom complaints of a patient with MHI within one month of injury with a matched control group of healthy participants. Interestingly, they found that subjective complaints did not adequately differentiate persons with MHI from the normal controls even soon after injury. Clearly, subjective complaints should not be used to diagnose head injury in the absence of other evidence.

In addition to the high prevalence of somatic and cognitive symptoms in normal and clinical groups, there appears to be an association between persisting symptoms following MHI and preexisting emotional distress and mental disorders, concurrent distress, and chronic social difficulties (Fenton, McClelland, Montgomery, MacFlynn & Rutherford, 1993; Klonoff & Lamb, 1998; Ponsford et al., 2000). Stogner (1999) administered a battery of personality tests to consecutively admitted patients with MHI at two hospital emergency departments within ten days of injury. Patients high on neuroticism at baseline were more likely to develop symptoms of postconcussive syndrome at three months postinjury. Greiffenstein and Baker (2001) examined premorbid and postinjury Minnesota Multiphasic Personality Inventory–2 (MMPI-2) profiles in a sample of compensation-seeking individuals with persistent concussion symptoms following MHI. The premorbid MMPI-2 modal profile indicated somatoform psychopathology. The postinjury MMPI-2 profiles also showed continued somatization but with a decrease in global psychopathology.

These findings suggest that the assessment of malingering should also involve determining whether psychopathology or situational stressors are present. The MHI cases that come to litigation are invariably persons with persistent symptoms. It is possible that an individual can have both a mental disorder and be malingering, a mental disorder alone, or be malingering. The prevalence of mental disorders in this country is high. The Epidemiologic Catchment Survey (ECA; Robins & Regier, 1991) and the National Comorbidity Survey (Kessler, 1994) estimated that about 20% of the people in the United States are affected by mental disorders during a given year, including anxiety, mood, somatoform, and schizophrenic disorders. It has also been estimated that up to three of every 50 patients seen by primary care providers may have somatoform disorder or a subsyndromal form of somatization (NIMH, 1990).

Screening for mental disorders is inadequate (Butler, Jenkins, & Braff, 1993). Taking a comprehensive history and using standardized personality assessment instruments like the MMPI-2 (Butcher, Dahlstrom, Graham, Tellegen, & Kaemmer, 1989) or the Personality Assessment Inventory (Morey, 1991) can be recommended.

Using Tests to Refine Diagnostic Hypotheses

Up to this point, the discussion has focused on obtaining a good history from the patient: i.e., presenting complaints, past medical and psychological history, and environmental factors. Consideration of malingering or incomplete effort occurs in this broader diagnostic process. The neuropsychologist develops diagnostic hypotheses based on this information, but substantial uncertainty may still exist without the use of tests.

> Testing is used in the process of hypothesis refinement to help formulate a working diagnostic hypothesis, defined previously as one that is sufficiently unambiguous to set the stage for making decisions about further invasive testing, treatment, or judgments about prognosis.
>
> (Kassirer & Kopelman, 1991, p. 17)

The fundamental diagnostic question is, "Given a positive test score, what is the probability that the patient has the disorder or condition?" This question is answered by combining test results with the information obtained in the history and related materials. Formally, this can be done by using the information from the patient's history to estimate the prior probability of the disorder. Prior probability is also known as *prevalence* or *base rate*. It can also be expressed as the pretest odds. A diagnostic test result can be summarized as a single number, the likelihood ratio (LR) (Sackett, Straus, Richardson, Rosenberg, & Haynes, 2000).

$$LR = \frac{sensitivity}{(1 - specificity)}$$

The LR is the likelihood that a given test result would be expected in a person with the disorder compared to the likelihood that the same result would be expected in a person without the disorder (Greenhalgh, 1997). The LR is then multiplied by the pretest odds to obtain the posttest odds, i.e., the probability that the person has the disorder given a positive test result. The larger the LR, the greater the diagnostic power of the test.

To use an obvious case for an example, let's suppose that a 30-year-old man presents six months status-post-TBI with an initial GCS score of 5, 15 days to follow commands, and cranial CT within 48 hours of injury showing midline shift of 5.5 mm. When examined, the patient was not litigating. Given this presentation, most neuropsychologists would estimate the prior probability that this man's performance on cognitive testing would be consistent with a diagnosis of TBI would be high, say 0.75. This is equal to a pretest odds of 0.75 / (1–0.75) or 3.0. To convert a probability to odds, we use the following formula:

$$odds = \frac{probability}{(1 - probability)}$$

The patient was given the Halstead-Reitan Battery (HRB) and obtained an Average Impairment Rating (AIR) T score of 30, based on the Heaton, Grant, and Adams (1991) norms. The AIR has a sensitivity of 0.80 and a specificity of 0.88, when using a T-score cutoff of less than 40 to define impairment, which yields a LR of 6.7. Combing the pretest odds with the LR from the AIR, the posttest odds would be (3.0) * (6.7) = 20.1 in favor of the diagnosis of brain injury. Converting odds to a posttest probability, we obtain a probability of 0.95 of a diagnosis of brain injury through the use of the following formula:

$$probability = \frac{odds}{(1 + odds)}$$

This approach can also be applied in the assessment of malingering. Estimates of LRs for several response bias measures can be calculated from studies in the literature. Table 38.1 contains estimated LRs for several measures.

Table 38.1 Likelihood ratios for selected measures

Test or Index	*Likelihood Ratio*
Symptom Validity Tests (Portland Digit Recognition Test and Hiscock Forced-Choice Procedure	15
Word Memory Test	4.6
Reliable Digit Span	19.5
Mittenberg WAIS-R Discriminant Function	5.8
California Verbal Learning Test (CVLT) Discriminate Function	6.9
CVLT Recognition Hits	8.6
Victoria Symptom Validity Test	7.4
Warrington Recognition Memory Test–Words	16.5

Several stipulations are in order: This is neither an exhaustive review of available response bias measures nor a meta-analysis of diagnostic efficiency statistics for selected measures. In addition, the measures were based on different samples and there is the possibility of spectrum bias. That is, a test will have a larger LR when extreme groups are studied (e.g., very ill vs. healthy controls). Hence, the LRs presented in this table cannot be used to determine which is the "best" effort test.

In a second example, let's say that a 35-year-old woman is being evaluated who reported having sustained a MHI two years earlier. She reported no loss of consciousness and did not seek medical care following the motor vehicle accident. She saw her family physician a month later with complaints of headache, memory problems, language disturbance, and the inability to return to work as a cashier. She is receiving chiropractic care three days a week and is in civil litigation. Binder and Rohling (1996) estimated the prevalence of biased responding following mild TBI to be 0.26, based on a weighted mean effect size from a meta-analysis. This estimate yields a pretest odds of 0.35. Let's suppose that this patient was given the WAIS-R. Mittenberg, Theroux-Fichera, Zielinski, and Heilbronner (1995) developed a seven-subtest WAIS-R discriminant function that was designed to detect incomplete effort. Based on several studies, the LR is estimated to be 5.76. Thus, if our hypothetical litigant's score on the WAIS-R discriminant function was in the response bias range, the posttest odds would be 2.02 or 67% in favor of the diagnosis of biased responding.

Several issues arise when using this approach to weigh diagnostic evidence. First, it is based on the assumption that reasonably accurate estimates of prior probabilities of the target disorder are available. We would argue that any system of diagnosis, whether explicitly quantitative or not, depends on prevalence rates. It is inescapable. The accuracy of all diagnostic decisions depends on the estimates or assumptions that one makes about prevalence rates. When clinicians do not explicitly consider a disorder's prior probability, they implicitly assume that the prevalence is 50%. This is often not the case. Consequently, the diagnostic value of the test result is overstated. This quantitative system simply forces the diagnostician to be explicit about the assumptions underlying the decision making process.

A second issue is the used of single cutoff scores for diagnosis and the derivation of LRs. Neuropsychologists are urged to abandon rigid diagnostic cutoff scores for any test. Diagnosis occurs in different contexts such that the relative costs of false positive and false negative errors will not be constant across situations. Raising or lowering a test's cutoff score will increase or decrease the test's sensitivity and specificity in an inverse fashion. In other words, when sensitivity is increased, specificity decreases. Hence, when a cutoff score yields high *sensitivity* and the test result is a *negative*, the disorder is more easily *ruled out*. Conversely, when a cutoff score yield high *specificity* and the test result is *positive*, the disorder is more easily *ruled in*. Sackett et al. (2000) developed the mnemonics, SnOut (when a test has high **Sensi**tivity, a **N**egative result rules **OUT** the disorder) and SpPin (when a test has high **Sp**ecificity, a **P**ositive result rule **IN** the disorder).

A third issue that is less easily resolved is the multiplicity problem. That is, we rarely use a single test to make a diagnosis. Moreover, there is no "gold standard" test for either brain dysfunction or response bias. If the tests were statistically independent, one could simply multiply the running product by the LR generated by each subsequent test. However, it is likely that there is some degree of collinearity among tests that preclude us from doing this. In later sections of this chapter, approaches to the multiplicity problem will be discussed. In the next section, the application of specialized tests to assess effort will be considered.

Applying Specialized Tests

Forced-choice tests (FCTs), also known as *symptom validity tests,* are, by far, the most extensively studied and validated single measures designed to detect malingering or incomplete effort (Slick et al., 1999). In FCTs, target stimuli are presented, followed by a two-choice recognition task in which the target item is paired with a foil. Some FCTs present the recognition task immediately following each target item while other FCTs present an entire set of target items (e.g., 50 items) before the recognition trial. The examinee's task is to identify the target item. Stimuli have included words, digits, photographs, and line drawings. The premise of FCTs is that examinees would score at chance level even if the test items were never seen. A performance that departs significantly below chance (e.g., $p < .05$) is considered to be a rare event that would be unlikely to have occurred by chance. It is inferred that the examinee was purposely choosing incorrect items, i.e., is malingering. The probability of obtaining a particular score can be calculated with the normal approximation to the binomial distribution (Altman, 1999), where x is the observed score and n is the total number of test items:

$$z = \frac{|x - (0.5 \times n)| - 0.5}{\sqrt{0.25 \times n}}$$

For example, the probability of obtaining score of less than 19 on a 50-item test is 0.03. In addition to determining the probability of chance level performance, most FCTs are extremely easy tasks. Even persons with significant cognitive impairment tend to score well above chance on FCTs.

Of the digit recognition FCTs, the 72-item Portland Digit Recognition Test (PDRT; Binder & Willis, 1991) is one of the best validated FCTs (Efcoff & Kampfer, 1996). Binder (2002) presents a current review of the PDRT. Depending on the cutoff score, sensitivity to incomplete effort can range from 39% to 77%. Using a cutoff of 39 for the total score, no patient with brain dysfunction was misclassified, i.e., 100%

specificity (Binder, 2002). In a sample of 120 persons with brain dysfunction, total scores below 46 occurred in 4% of the sample (Binder, 2002).

Other FCTs having empirical support include the Computerized Assessment of Response Bias (CARB; Conder, Allen, & Cox, 1992), the Test of Memory Malingering (TOMM; Tombaugh, 2002), the Victoria Symptom Validity Test (VSVT; Slick, Hopp, Strauss, & Thompson, 1997), and the Word Memory Test (WMT; see Green, Allen, & Astner, 1996). The CARB is a computerized version of the forced-choice digit recognition paradigm. A recent review of the CARB's psychometric and diagnostic properties was conducted by Allen, Iverson, and Green (2002). Various patient groups have been given the CARB and Allen et al. (2002) reported a combined total CARB score of 97.8% correct. Hence, it is an extremely easy test to perform. Although the probability of below chance performance can be calculated for performance scores on the CARB, cutoff scores above chance can be used to detect incomplete effort. The VSVT is also a computer-administered and scored, dichotomous, forced-choice digit recognition task. It has 48 items and response latency is considered along with the total number correct. Thompson (2002) provided a review of recent studies of the VSVT.

The TOMM is a FCT that uses 50 line-drawn pictures as stimuli (Tombaugh, 2002). Similar to the CARB and VSVT, the TOMM is an easy test and a criterion score above chance can be used to classify examinees with regard to effort. Very low failure rates have been observed for persons with TBI, dementia, aphasia, and depression (Tombaugh, 2002). The WMT employs a slightly different format in which the examinee is first presented with 20 pairs of words auditorily or on a computer screen. The examinee is asked to choose the correct words from target-foil pairs in both immediate and delayed recognition conditions. Again, the WMT is an easy task even for patients with pronounced cognitive dysfunction. Green, Lees-Haley, and Allen (2002) provided a comprehensive review of the WMT's psychometric and diagnostic properties.

Standard neuropsychological tests with a forced-choice recognition format have also been used to assess effort and motivation. The Recognition Memory Test's (RMT; Warrington, 1984) sensitivity to incomplete effort has been reported to range from 70% to 95% and specificity to TBI, 90% to 100%, for its Words subtest (Iverson & Franzen, 1994; Iverson & Franzen, 1998; Millis, 1992; Millis, 1994; Millis, 2002; Millis & Putnam, 1994). Similarly, the Seashore Rhythm Test, Speech-sounds Perception Test (SSPT) (Gfeller & Cradock, 1998; Goebel, 1983; Heaton, Smith, Lehman, & Vogt, 1978; Mittenberg, Rotholc, Russell, & Heilbronner, 1996; Millis, Putnam, & Adams, 1996; Trueblood & Schmidt, 1993), and Category Test (Sweet & King, 2002) can be used to assess effort.

It should be stressed, however, that these standard neuropsychological measures do differ from the CARB, PDRT, TOMM, VSVT, and WMT in the sense that they are sensitive in varying degrees to cognitive impairment, i.e., persons with genuine impairment may, of course, perform poorly on the Category Test, RMT, Seashore Rhythm Test, or SSPT. Tests like the CARB are more resistant to the effects of brain dysfunction. Nonetheless, it is instructive to note that the mean performance on the RMT Words subtest was 40.8 out of 50 in a sample of *acute* rehabilitation inpatients with *severe* traumatic brain injuries (GCS 3 to 8) (Millis, 2002).

Although the MMPI-2 requires examinees to answer "true" or "false" to items, it is, of course, not a symptom validity test like the PDRT or TOMM. However, a rationally derived scale composed of 43 MMPI-2 items, the Fake Bad Scale (Lees-Haley, English, & Glenn, 1991), has been found to be superior to the standard MMPI-2 validity scales in characterizing symptom endorsement patterns associated with incomplete effort (Greiffenstein, Baker, Gola, Donders, & Miller, 2002; Larrabee, 1998; Martens, Donders, & Millis, 2001; Slick, Hopp, Strauss, & Spellacy, 1996). Scores in excess of 22 on the FBS may suggest response bias in litigated mild TBI cases.

FCTs represent a major advancement in the assessment of malingering and incomplete effort. Nonetheless, the majority of malingerers will not perform below chance. In a survey of studies, Hiscock, Branham, and Hiscock (1994) found that no greater than 34% of the cases performed below chance. As noted earlier, investigators using the CARB, PDRT, TOMM, VSVT, and WMT have derived cutoff scores that are above chance but still have acceptable diagnostic efficiency. In addition, there is the question whether FCTs they will "lose" their capacity over time to detect response bias as laypersons become more familiar with them. Some FCTs may be easily recognizable such that examinees can be warned to perform them to the best of their ability while performing other tests suboptimally.

A third issue is test redundancy. With the proliferation of effort measures and indices, how should the results be combined? Should some tests be given more weight? For example, Finger Tapping Test (FTT) has been found to be useful in detecting incomplete effort (e.g., Binder, 1990; Binder & Willis, 1991; Larrabee, 2002). A logistic regression model was fitted using the data set from Millis and Volinsky (2001) for participants having data for the FTT. Indeed, the FTT was a significant predictor of incomplete effort ($p = 0.002$). It had high specificity (96% of the 93 persons with TBI were correctly classified) but low sensitivity (15% of the 44 litigants with MHI were correctly classified). Previous investigations have also identified Recognition Hits from the CLVT and digit span as sensitive to incomplete effort (e.g., Meyers & Volbrecht, 1998; Millis, Putnam, Adams, and Ricker, 1995). A second logistic regression model was fitted that included FTT, Recognition Hits, and forward digit span from the WAIS-R. Parameter estimates appear in Table 38.2. Now, FTT is no longer a significant predictor of incomplete effort in the presence of Hits and digits forward. Sensitivity to

Table 38.2 Logistic regression model parameter estimates

	B	*S.E.*	*Wald*	*df*	*Sig.*	*Odds Ratio*
FTT	−0.021	0.027	0.559	1	.455	.980
Digits Forward	−0.485	0.189	6.612	1	.010	.616
CVLT Hits	−0.803	0.219	13.498	1	.000	.448

incomplete effort increased to 75% and specificity to TBI was 95%. Although the development of better tests should not cease, there is a pressing need to determine how effort tests relate to each other and to standard cognitive measures in order to derive efficient diagnostic algorithms. The examination of performance patterns among several tests is one approach to this challenge.

Analysis of Test Performance Patterns

Pattern analysis to detect incomplete effort is not new. In the late 1970s, Heaton et al. (1978) used discriminant function analysis with the HRB to differentiate persons with head injuries from people instructed to feign neuropsychological impairment. The study's findings were limited by a model that had too few subjects for the number of predictor variables. Nonetheless, the methodology inspired dozens of studies that followed.

Discriminant function analysis (DFA) and logistic regression have been the most commonly used statistical techniques for pattern analysis and group classification. For reasons unknown to us, DFA has been used more frequently in psychological research, yet logistic regression has clear advantages over DFA. Logistic regression has fewer restrictive assumptions, e.g., it does not require multivariate normality and homogeneous covariance matrices as does DFA (Long, 1997). In addition, interpretation of the relative importance of individual predictor variables is more straightforward. The logistic regression function can also be used to calculate the probability that an individual belong to one of the groups in the following manner. A linear composite known as the *logit* (also known as the *logged odds* or *linear predictor*) is calculated by multiplying each predictor variable's raw score by its respective coefficient (e.g., $\beta_1 x_1 + \beta_2 x_1$) and then a constant is added. The logit is exponentiated in the following manner to yield the probability of an individual belonging to one of two groups, based on the raw scores entered into this formula:

$$p = \frac{e^{\alpha + \beta 1x1 + \beta 2x2}}{1 + e^{\alpha + \beta 1x1 + \beta 2x2}}$$

Generally, the cutoff for p is 0.50, i.e., greater than 50% probability of membership in one of the two groups. However, the cutoff score can be adjusted in light of the relative costs of making either a false positive or false negative error.

Tests that have been used in subsequent pattern analysis of incomplete effort include the HRB, WAIS, and CVLT. Extending the original work of Heaton et al. (1978), Mittenberg et al. (1996) used stepwise discriminant function analysis to differentiate persons with TBI from normal volunteers instructed to simulate cognitive impairment. The ten-variable HRB function correctly classified 89% of the cases. When applied to a sample of Veterans Administration patients with TBI, the discriminant function correctly classified 78% of the sample (McKinzey & Russell, 1997).

Mittenberg et al. (1995) also derived a seven-subtest WAIS-R discriminant function that accurately classified 79% persons with TBI and uninjured persons instructed to malinger. Millis, Ross and Ricker (1998) cross-validated the function: 92% of persons with moderate to severe TBI were correctly classified as were 88% of mild TBI litigants who had performed within chance on the RMT. Axelrod and Rawlings (1999) also applied this WAIS-R to a sample of persons with TBI who had received the WAIS-R two to four times over the course of one year postinjury. Rates of correct classification ranged from 76% to 93%. Mittenberg, Theroux, Aguila-Puentes, Bianchini, Greve, and Rayls (2001) applied the WAIS-R function on a new sample of persons given the WAIS-III. That is, a new function based on the WAIS-III was not derived. Rather, the original discriminant function derived from the WAIS-R was applied to WAIS-III data. This function and cutoff score accurately classified 83% of persons with TBI and 72% of persons simulating head injury. Mittenberg et al. (2001) provide alternative cutoff scores for the discriminant function that may improve diagnostic accuracy.

Several studies have used the CVLT (Delis, Kramer, Kaplan, & Ober, 1987) to examine incomplete effort. Millis et al. (1995) found that a three-variable CVLT discriminant function correctly classified 91% of persons with moderate to severe brain injuries and a groups of litigants with MHI who scored below chance on Warrington's RMT. Millis et al. (1995) also examined CVLT Recognition Hits as a single variable. Sensitivity to incomplete effort was 83% and specificity to TBI was 96%. Subsequent studies by Baker, Donders, and Thompson (2000), Coleman, Rapport, Millis, Ricker, and Farchione (1998), and Sweet et al. (2000) applied the original cutoff scores derived by Millis et al. (1995) to other groups of persons with TBI and to groups of analog and probable clinical malingerers. Sensitivity to response bias has been lower than the findings reported by Millis et al. (1995), e.g., 63% to 80% for Hits and 74% for the discriminant function, but specificity for TBI has remained high, e.g., 87% to 94% for Hits and 83% to 93% for the discriminant function. More broadly, biased responding appears to be associated with disproportionate impairment on recognition tasks in an absolute sense and in relationship to free recall performance on list learning tasks.

Although pattern analysis has made important contributions in the assessment of malingering, it is not without its limitations. It suffers from the same multiplicity problem as the single test approach. That is, how are tests selected for inclusion in the logistic regression function? There are potentially dozens of effort tests and indices from which to choose. Yet, it is often not reasonable to include all potential measures because sample sizes may not be sufficiently large to avoid overfitting the model. Even when a moderate number of tests are chosen, the number of potential models is huge. For example, if one considers 15 different tests, there are 32,768 potential subsets of tests to evaluate (i.e., 2^{15})! Moreover, theory and past research findings may not provide enough guidance for variable selection. We return to this issue with a discussion of approaches to this problem in "Challenge of Test Selection: New Statistical Methods." In the next section, a strategy for combining data is covered.

Integration of Information

Having completed the examination, the neuropsychologist will have information from the history and related sources along with test data. Slick et al. (1999) have developed a strategy for combining and interpreting these data. Acknowledging that there are various degrees of diagnostic certainty, the guidelines proposed by Slick et al. have specific criteria for *definite*, *probable*, and *possible* malingered neurocognitive disorder (MND). For example, if there are external incentives in a given case and the examinee performs below chance on an FCT, and there are no psychiatric or neurologic disorders to account for this performance, there is sufficient evidence for *definite* MND. As noted earlier, the majority of litigants will not score below chance on FCTs. Accordingly, these criteria do allow the use of other validated effort tests or indices along with an analysis of discrepancies between test results and patient behavior:

- "*Discrepancy between test data and known patterns of brain functioning*" (e.g., patient performs in the profoundly impaired range on measures of attention but within normal limits on memory measures).
- "*Discrepancy between test data and observed behavior*" (e.g., patient is unable to perform confrontation naming test but has no visuoperceptual deficits and spontaneous speech is fluent and without paraphasic errors).
- "*Discrepancy between test data and reliable collateral reports*" (e.g., patient handles financial affairs like balancing check book but is unable to perform simple arithmetic problems in the clinical examination).
- "*Discrepancy between test data and documented background history*" (e.g., patient with history of mild TBI who obtains memory test scores in the profoundly impaired range).

(Slick et al. 1999, pp. 553–554)

Two or more types of evidence from effort indices or test-behavior discrepancies would warrant a diagnosis of *probable* MNC, given the presence of external incentives and the absence of psychiatric or neurologic disorders to account for this behavior.

The criteria also allow the use of patient self-report data in examining for discrepancies:

- "*Self-reported history is discrepant with documented history*" (e.g., patient reports an exaggerated length of loss of consciousness).
- "*Self-reported symptoms are discrepant with known patterns of brain functioning*" (e.g., patient claims inability to recall own birthdate and address following mild TBI).
- "*Self-reported symptoms are discrepant with behavioral observations*" (e.g., patient reports severe cognitive impairment yet lives independently, manages own financial affairs, and drove self to office).
- "*Self-reported symptoms are discrepant with information obtained from collateral informants*" (e.g., patient acts cognitively impaired but spouse or job supervisor report that patient experiences no functional difficulties).
- "*Evidence of exaggerated or fabricated psychological dysfunction*" (e.g., validity scales from the MMPI-2 or Personality Assessment Inventory indicate "fake bad" profile).

(Slick et al., 1999, p. 554)

A diagnosis of *probable* MND can also be made on the basis of one type of psychometric evidence and one type of self-report discrepancy. In the absence of psychometric evidence, one or more self-report discrepancies is sufficient for a diagnosis of *possible* MND.

The Challenge of Test Selection: New Statistical Methods in Assist in Decision Making

It could be argued that there are now enough effort tests and indices to assess for malingering and incomplete effort. At this point, the next step in the evolution of malingering assessment is to determine which effort tests and indices should be combined and weighted to yield optimal diagnostic accuracy. Moreover, the task is broader in terms of possibly combining effort tests with standard neuropsychological measures to derive the actuarial diagnostic algorithms. In the past, stepwise regression methods have been used for selecting sets of tests for use in prediction. However, there are many problems with the stepwise method. Harrell (2001) has summarized the flaws: It yields inflated R-squared values; the F and chi-squared tests do not have the claimed distribution; it produces confidence intervals that are falsely narrow; it produces biased regression coefficients that need shrinkage; and it has severe problems in the presence of collinearity. Increasing the sample size does not overcome these problems. Fortunately, several new statistical methods are now available to assist in selecting sets of predictor variables.

Bayesian Modeling Averaging

Bayesian model averaging (BMA; Hoeting, Madigan, Raftery, & Volinsky, 1999) approaches the problem of variable and model selection by averaging over the best models according to posterior probabilities. Unlike stepwise methods, BMA searches the entire model space and evaluates every possible model. Averaging over many models in this manner has been found to provide superior out-of-sample predictive performance compared to the typical approach of evaluating a single model (Madigan & Raftery, 1994). More detailed discussions of applied statistical and mathematical aspects of BMA can be found in Hoeting et al. (1999) and Millis and Volinsky (2001).

Millis and Volinsky (2001) used BMA to select and evaluate models composed of variables from the CVLT for the detection of incomplete effort. The BMA attempts to differentiate persons with documented moderate to severe TBIs from persons with mild injuries in litigation who show evidence of incomplete effort. The CVLT has over a dozen variables and, although previous studies identified CVLT variables that are sensitive to incomplete effort, an unresolved question was whether there are optimal sets of CVLT variables to predict incomplete effort. Millis and Volinsky's BMA identified four models with different combinations of CVLT variables that appeared optimal (Table 38.3). Bayesian modeling requires the specification of a reference set of prior probabilities, which are indexed by the ϕ parameter. Different prior probabilities were selected to perform a sensitivity analysis. All models performed in a similar fashion under different prior probabilities. As can be observed in Table 38.3, Model 1 (SDFR, LDFR, Hits, and Bias) had the greatest support but there remained some degree of statistical uncertainty so that additional models were included. In terms of decision making, each model is used in a logistic regression model and its contribution is weighted according to its posterior probability. A spreadsheet that performs the mathematical calculations is available from the first author. If an examinee produced the following panel of results (Short Delay Free Recall, or SDFR = 3; Short Delay Cued Recall, or SDCR = 4; Long Delay Free Recall, or LDFR = 4; Primacy = 32; Hits = 5, False Positives = 1; and Bias = −.83), the probability is incomplete effort is 99%, based on averaging over the four best models appearing in Table 38.3.

The computational and conceptual complexities of Bayesian modeling may dissuade some investigators from using it. There are additional approaches that can be used to select and simplify models.

Stepdown Analysis

In stepdown analysis, a prognostic index is constructed, which is a linear combination of the variables in the model. It is used to determine what variables may be dropped from a model. The mathematical details can be found in Ambler, Brady, and Royston (2002). The same data used in the BMA study (Millis & Volinsky, 2001) were used in this stepdown analysis. Interestingly, the variables identified as important predictors of incomplete effort by the stepdown analysis were the same ones found to be important in the BMA except for False Positive errors (Table 38.4). This logistic regression prediction formula would need to be validated on independent samples before it should be used clinically. For each case, the CVLT raw scores for the respective variables would be multiplied by their respective coefficients to obtain the probability of incomplete effort, e.g., SDFR * 0.404, etc. To illustrate with an example, let's say an examinee obtains the following scores on these CVLT variables: SDFR = 3; SDCR = 4; LDFR = 4; Primacy = 32; Hits = 5; and Bias = −.83). The following linear composite (i.e., logit) is obtained:

$$(3) * (0.404) + (4) * (0.287) + (4) * (-0.502) + (32) * (-0.061) + (5) * (-1.05) + (-0.83) * (2.281) + 13.232 = 4.489$$

Hence, the probability of incomplete effort is $[e^{4.489} / (1 + e^{4.489})] = 0.99$. For greater ease of application of a logistic regression function, a nomogram (Figure 38.1) can be drawn that converts each CVLT variable in the model to a 0–100 scale that is proportional to the log odds (i.e., logit). One goes vertically from the variable to the top to the "Points" line. These points are added across the CVLT variables to calculate the Total Points. Going vertically from the "Total Points" line down to the "Linear Predictor," the total points are converted to the logit and then to the predicted probability. For example, an examinee gets about 7 points for recalling three words on SDFR, 7 points for recalling four words on SDCR, 35 point for recalling four words on LDFR, 14 points for a Primacy

Table 38.3 Logistic regression models and model posterior probabilities following BMA—CLVT *

Model	*Variables*	*Posterior Probabilities (%)* $f = 1.00$	$f = 1.65$	$f = 5.00$
1	SDFR, LDFR, Hits, Bias	42	43	44
2	SDFR, LDFR, Primacy, Hits	25	24	24
3	SDCR, LDFR, Hits, Bias	25	26	26
4	SDCR, LDFR, Hits, False Positives	7	7	6

* SDFR = Short Delay Free Recall. SDCR = Short Delay Cued Recall. LDFR = Long Delay Free Recall. Hits = Recognition Hits. Bias = Response Bias.

Table 38.4 Stepdown analysis model—CLVT*

Variables	*Coef.*	*SE*	*Z*	*P*
SDFR	0.404	0.187	2.17	.030
SDCR	0.287	0.848	1.55	.121
LDFR	−0.502	0.172	−2.92	.004
Primacy	−0.061	0.0318	−1.92	.055
Hits	−1.05	0.220	−4.77	.000
Bias	2.281	0.926	2.46	.014
Constant	13.232	2.647		

* SDFR = Short Delay Free Recall. SDCR = Short Delay Cued Recall. LDFR = Long Delay Free Recall. Hits = Recognition Hits. Bias = Response Bias.

score of 32, 70 points for five Recognition Hits, and 1 point for a Response Bias score of −0.83. This total score of 134 points corresponds to a linear predictor score (i.e., logit) of approximately 4.8 and a probability of 0.99. These estimates are quite close to the formal calculation with the formula, which yielded a logit of 4.489 and a probability of 0.99. Once a model has been validated, nomograms provide a convenient tool for clinicians to apply complex algorithms in day-to-day practice. This nomogram was produced using a function in Harrell's (2001) *Design* library that is available in S-Plus 6.1 (Insightful Corporation, 2002). Stepdown analysis can be performed with Stata Version 8.0 (Stata Corporation, 2003) and S-Plus Version 6.1 (Insightful Corporation, 2002) statistical software.

Recursive Partitioning

The methods described thus far are parametric methods. A nonparametric alternative is recursive partitioning (RP). RP can be particularly useful for examining relationships among variables in the absence of a well-developed model. In this approach, a "tree structure" is created by dividing the sample recursively into a number of subgroups. The divisions are selected so as to maximize the difference in the response variable in the resulting two groups. RP has additional advantages over parametric methods. Parametric methods are based on specific statistical assumptions. When they are violated, the parameter estimates may be inefficient or biased. Recursive partitioning has some advantages over parametric methods: (a) they may be easier to interpret when there is a mix of categorical and continuous predictors; (b) they are invariant to monotone re-expressions of predictor variables; and (c) they can handle missing values and nonadditive behavior (Chambers & Hastie, 1992).

RP was applied to the sample data from Millis and Volinsky (2001). For simplicity, three CVLT variables were selected: Recognition Hits, Long Delay Free Recall, and Short Delay Free Recall. A decision tree was derived (Figure 38.2). At the top of the tree, all 160 participants begin in one group. The statistic G^2 refers to the LR chi-square, which is the criterion used to select variables. The "Level" column refers to the groups (0 = persons with TBI, 1 = persons showing

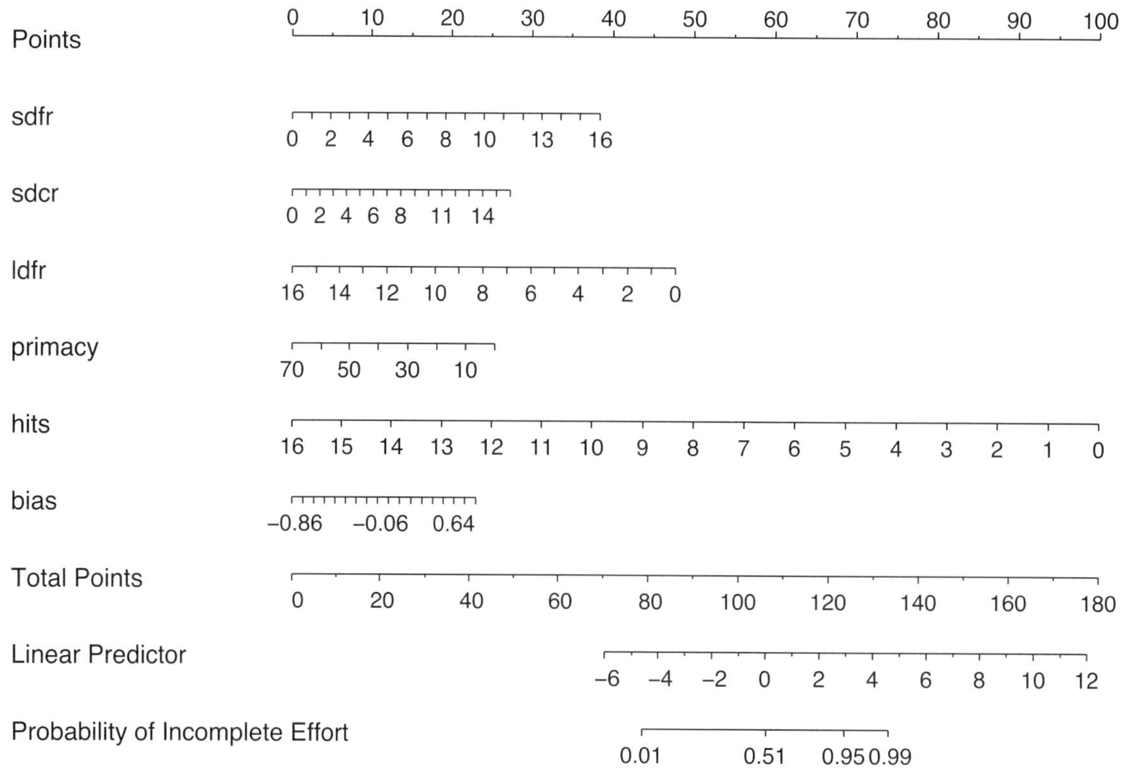

Figure 38.1 Nomogram to calculate probability of incomplete effort

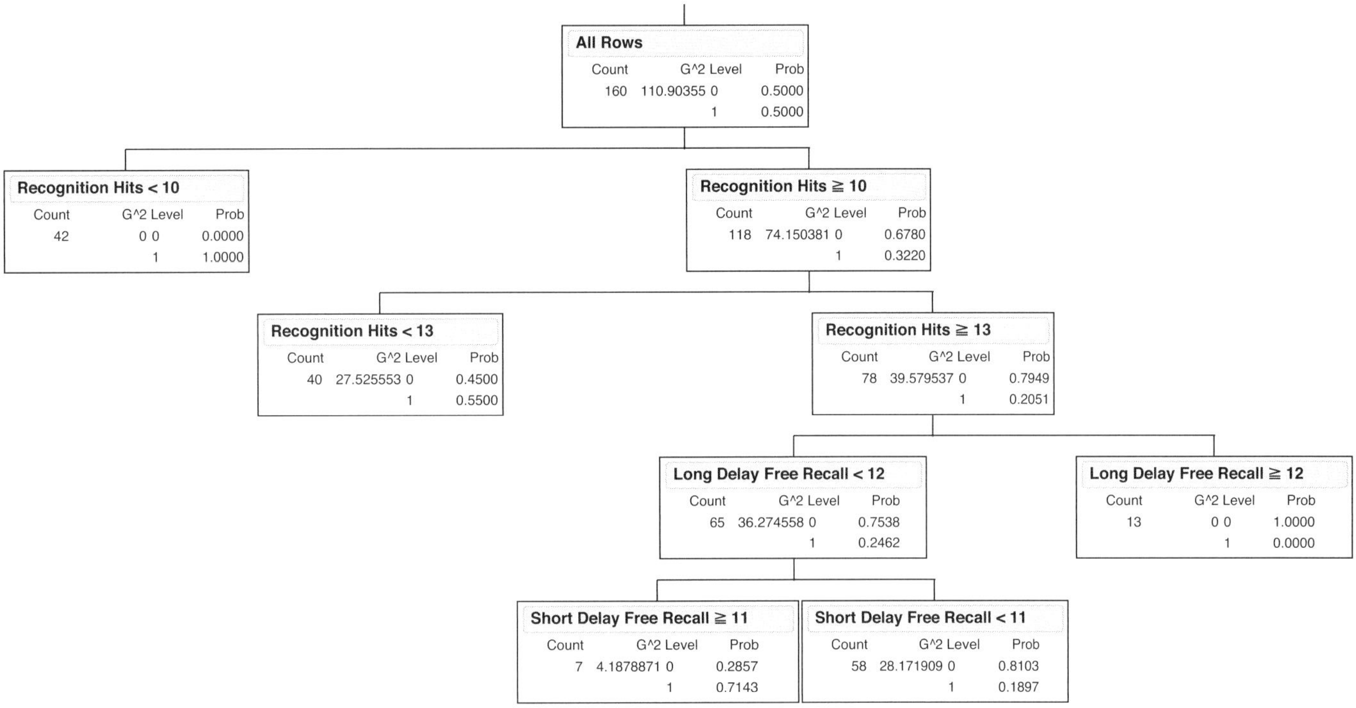

Figure 38.2 Recursive partitioning tree diagram—CLVT

incomplete effort). At the first split, Hits less than ten results in a subgroup of 42 persons showing incomplete effort (Effort). No persons with TBI are in that subgroup. All of the TBI participants and the remaining 38 from the Effort group are in the subgroup with Hits greater than or equal to 10. From this point, another advantage of RP becomes apparent (i.e., subtypes may be able to be identified). It appears that one type of incomplete effort is characterized primarily by atypically low recognition scores. Another possible subtype might be marked by mildly impaired or normal recognition in combination with SDFR performance being relatively better than LDFR. As with the stepdown derived-model, this RP model needs to be validated on independent samples before being used clinically. RP can be done with a number of statistical packages. JMP Version 5 (SAS Institute, 2002) was used for this example.

A variable can be useful for prediction in different ways. For example, further analysis of SDFR suggested that it may be a suppressor variable in that it suppresses variance that is actually irrelevant in the prediction of incomplete effort. In this case, it may be enhancing the effect of LDFR. Evidence pointing to SDFR being a suppressor variable is that its point biserial correlation with the grouping variable (−0.34) and beta weight (0.46) have opposite signs (Tabachnick & Fidell, 2001). In contrast, the correlations of Hits and LDFR with the grouping variable and regression coefficients are consistent in size and direction. When LDFR is dropped from the equation, SDFR is no longer a significant predictor of incomplete effort. This is not to imply SDFR is unimportant but rather that its usefulness in predicting incomplete effort is indirect and emerges is in combination with of LDFR.

Legal Implications

Scientific innovation always precedes the law. No published legal cases have considered these statistical methods, nor base rates, nor LRs, as applied to malingering in forensic neuropsychological evaluations. Many judges would not recognize the relevance of these topics and would likely exclude such evidence out of fear that it would "confuse of the issues, or misleading the jury" (Fed. R. of Evid. 403). When there are no cases on point, legal scholars attempt to generalize by analogy to consider how courts may rule when an appropriate case or controversy is heard. Here, courts have considerable experience with the application of population frequency statistics to DNA evidence as first introduced in the 1987 rape convictions of Robert Melias (England) and Tommy Lee Andrews (Alabama) (Connors, Lundregan, Miller, & McEwen, 1996). Population frequency statistics used for DNA evidence are generally admissible and analogous to the base rate and LRs—the point of departure for the statistical methods described in this chapter.

This chapter sets forth, with mathematical precision, the scientific principles of assessment of incomplete effort and malingering in neuropsychological examination. It is only a matter of time until a defendant or plaintiff challenges the admissibility of the actuarial methods used, in part, to render a malingering diagnosis. Although no neuropsychological evaluation was performed, *Berry v. CSX Transp., Inc.* (1998) addresses population frequency statistics and neuropsychological methods when rendering expert testimony about causation in a toxic tort case. No psychologist testified, even though a neuropsychiatrist found severe cognitive deficits that other physician experts attempted to link to the exposure to organic solvents trichloroethane (TCA), trichloroethylene (TCE), perchloroethylene (PCE), and mineral spirits. The *Berry* appellate panel found that the trial court erred when excluding population frequency statistics proposed to bolster epidemiological studies in support of the plaintiff's claim. Essentially, if an expert's opinion is well-founded and based upon generally accepted scientific principles and methodology, it will be admitted and weighed by a trier of fact, whether or not the expert's opinion is generally accepted. By analogy, this legal principle applies to neuropsychologists rendering expert opinions about response bias, suboptimal effort, or malingering.

This chapter considered such expert testimony in the context of MHI and highlighted the frequency of brain injury claims in civil litigation. Courts hear and consider expert opinions about malingering without necessarily appreciating the underlying probabilistic framework upon which such opinions are based. In *Reiner v. Warren Resort Hotels, Inc.* (2008), the plaintiff alleged a brain injury over two years after she slipped, fell, and struck her head while exiting the hotel hot tub. Preinjury medical and psychological history were complicated by preexisting conditions. Of particular interest was a preinjury neuropsychological evaluation in 1985 for complaints about memory and concentration. Reiner's injury occurred on May 1, 2005 and her occipital and basilar skull fractures were never in dispute. Moreover, there was no loss of consciousness, no amnesia, and no confusion. A CT scan was negative and magnetic resonance imaging (MRI) identified a preexisting 12 mm anomaly consistent with left posterior frontal meningioma. Neuropsychologists identified suboptimal effort on three measures—TOMM, CARB, and the MMPI-2 FBS—but expert opinions about effort diverged significantly. Among various motions *in limine*, the plaintiff moved to exclude FBS and a *Daubert* hearing ensued.

The plaintiff argued that FBS assigns malingering points to honest answers a subject provides, and this is especially true when the subject is a woman. Further, the defense neuropsychologist opined, "there is a lot of controversy surrounding the test." The plaintiff entered two articles highlighting the controversy over this method of testing for malingering. Defense countered that the plaintiff opened the door to this evidence by relying on a neuropsychologist who administered two tests for malingering and planned to use the test results to bolster the plaintiff's credibility with respect to her brain-injury claim. Moreover, the defense noted 11 articles recognizing FBS and several state and federal cases in which FBS results were admitted in evidence.

The defense in *Reiner* argued that the FBS is reliable enough, when considered together with other factors. This practice is consistent with the AACN Consensus Conference Statement (2009) encouraging practitioners to not rely on a single symptom validity test, but multiple measures administered throughout the assessment day(s). Further, neuropsychologists must be mindful of the important difference between scientifically based clinical decisions and legal adjudication, while showing respect to the laws and customs of the jurisdiction in which they practice when describing the behavioral presentation at issue. In the end, the *Reiner* judge admitted FBS and all other symptom and performance validity measures. Readers are directed to Kaufmann (2012, 2013) for more lengthy discussion of admissibility challenges to neuropsychological evidence of suboptimal effort. Most recently, challenges to symptom and performance validity measures are taking place in consultative examinations of Social Security litigation (*Bradley v. Astrue*, 2012; *Taylor v. Astrue*, 2012; *Pratt v. Astrue*, 2009).

Closing Remarks

We rely on our clinical judgment to generate hypotheses. However, in an earlier discussion, Millis and Volinsky (2001) reflected on the limitations of clinical judgment in making accurate diagnoses:

> As humans, we often have a low tolerance for ambiguity, which impels us to impose meaning on experience. This tendency carries over into the diagnostic realm. If we rely on our clinical judgment alone, our diagnostic accuracy can be abysmal. Humans tend to ignore prevalence rates, assign non-optimal weights to predictor variables, disregard regression toward the mean, improperly assess covariation, and over-weigh vivid data (Grove, Zald, Lebow, Snitz, & Nelson, 2000). Meehl (1954) was among the first to alert psychologists to the superiority of statistical prediction compared to clinical judgment. Little has changed in this regard over the last 46 years.
>
> (p. 823)

Further advances in the assessment of malingering and incomplete effort will likely be fueled by human intuition and creativity and tempered by quantitative rigor.

References

Abrahamse, A. F., & Carroll, S. J. (1999). *The Frequency of Excess Claims for Automobile Personal Injuries*. Santa Monica, CA: Rand.

Alexander, M. P. (1995). Mild traumatic brain injury: Pathophysiology, natural history, and clinical management. *Neurology*, *45*, 1253–1260.

Allen, L. M., III, Iverson, G. L., & Green, P. (2002). Computerized Assessment of Response Bias in forensic neuropsychology. *Journal of Forensic Neuropsychology*, *3*, 205–225.

Altman, D. G. (1999). *Practical Statistics for Medical Research*. Boca Raton, FL: Chapman and Hall/CRC.

Ambler, G., Brady, A. R., & Royston, P. (2002). Simplifying a prognostic model: A simulation study based on clinical data. *Statistics in Medicine*, *21*, 3803–3822.

Axelrod, B. N., & Rawlings, D. B. (1999). Clinical utility of incomplete effort WAIS-R Formulas: A longitudinal examination of individuals with traumatic brain injuries. *Journal of Forensic Neuropsychology*, *1*, 15–27.

Baker, R., Donders, J., & Thompson, E. (2000). Assessment of incomplete effort with the California Verbal Learning Test. *Applied Neuropsychology*, *7*, 111–114.

Berry v. CSX Transp., Inc., 709 So.2d 552 (Fla. Dist. Ct. Ap. 1998).

Binder, L. M. (1990). Malingering following minor head trauma. *The Clinical Neuropsychologist*, *4*, 25–36.

Binder, L. M. (2002). The Portland Digit Recognition Test: A review of validation data and clinical use. *Journal of Forensic Neuropsychology*, *2*, 27–41.

Binder, L. M, & Rohling, M. L. (1996). Money matters: A meta-analytic review of the effect of financial incentives on recovery after closed head injury. *American Journal of Psychiatry*, *153*, 7–10.

Binder, L. M., Rohling, M. L., & Larrabee, G. J. (1997). A review of mild head trauma. Part I: Meta-analysis review of neuropsychological studies. *Journal of Clinical and Experimental Neuropsychology*, *19*, 421–431.

Binder, L. M., & Willis, S. C. (1991). Assessment of motivation after financially compensable minor head injury. *Psychological Assessment*, *3*, 175–181.

Bradley v. Astrue, 2012 U.S. Dist. LEXIS 166084 (D. Kan. 2012).

Butcher, J. N., Dahlstrom, W. G., Graham, J. R., Tellegen, A., & Kaemmer, B. (1989). *Minnesota Multiphasic Personality Inventory (MMPI-2): Manual for Administration and Scoring*. Minneapolis, MN: University of Minnesota Press.

Butler, R. W., Jenkins, M. A., & Braff, D. L. (1993). The abnormality of normal comparison groups: The identification of psychosis proneness and substance abuse in putatively normal research subjects. *American Journal of Psychiatry*, *150*, 1386–1391.

Chambers, J. M., & Hastie, T. J. (Eds.). (1992). *Statistical Models in S*. London: Chapman and Hall.

Coleman, R., Rapport, L., Millis, S., Ricker, J., & Farchione, T. (1998). Effects of coaching on the detection of malingering on the California Verbal Learning Test: An analog study of malingered head injury. *The Clinical Neuropsychologist*, *20*, 201–210.

Conder, R., Allen, L., & Cox, D. (1992). *Computerized Assessment of Response Bias Test Manual*. Durham, NC: Cognisyst.

Connors, E., Lundregan, T., Miller, N., & McEwen, T. (1996). *Convicted by Juries, Exonerated by Science: Case Studies in the Use of DNA Evidence to Establish Innocence After Trial*. U.S. Department of Justice Research Report.

Delis, D. C., Kramer, J. H., Kaplan, E., & Ober, B. A. (1987). *California Verbal Learning Test: Adult Version*. San Antonio, TX: The Psychological Corporation.

Demakis, G. J., Sweet, J. J., Sawyer, T. P., Moulthrop, M., Nies, K., & Clingerman, S. (2001). Discrepancy between predicted and obtained WAIS-R IQ scores discriminates between traumatic brain injury and insufficient effort. *Psychological Assessment*, *13*, 240–248.

Dikmen, S. S., Machamer, J. E., & Temkin, N. (2001). Mild head injury: Facts and artifacts. *Journal of Clinical and Experimental Neuropsychology*, *23*, 729–738.

Dikmen, S. S., Machamer, J. E., Winn, H. R., & Temkin, N. R. (1995). Neuropsychological outcome at one-year post head injury. *Neuropsychology*, *9*, 80–90.

Efcoff, L. M., & Kampfer, K. M. (1996). Practical guidelines in the use of symptom validity and other psychological tests to measure malingering and symptom exaggeration in traumatic brain injury cases. *Neuropsychology Review*, *6*, 171–201.

Federal Rule of Evidence 403 (2014).

Fenton, G., McClelland, R., Montgomery, A., MacFlynn, G., & Rutherford, W. (1993). The postconcussional syndrome: Social antecedents and psychological sequelae. *British Journal of Psychiatry*, *162*, 493–497.

Fox, D. D., Lees-Haley, P. R., Earnest, K., Dolezal-Wood, S. (1995). Base rates of postconcussive symptoms in health maintenance organization patients and controls. *Neuropsychology*, *9*, 606–611.

Geller, J. L., Erlen, J., Kaye, N. S., & Fisher, W. H. (1990). Feigned insanity in nineteenth-century America: Tactics, trials, and truth. *Behavioral Sciences and the Law*, *8*, 3–26.

Gfeller, J. D., & Cradock, M. M. (1998). Detecting feigned neuropsychological impairment with the Seashore Rhythm Test. *Journal of Clinical Psychology*, *54*, 431–438.

Goebel, R. A. (1983). Detection of faking on the Halstead-Reitan Neuropsychological Test Battery. *Journal of Clinical Psychology*, *39*, 731–742.

Gouvier, W. D., Uddo-Crane, M., & Brown, L. M. (1988). Base rates of post-concussional symptoms. *Archives of Clinical Neuropsychology*, *3*, 273–278.

Green, P., Allen, L. M., & Astner, K. (1996). *The Word Memory Test: A User's Guide to the Oral and Computer Administered Forms, U.S. Version 1.1*. Durham, NC: CogniSyst.

Green, P., Lees-Haley, P. R., & Allen, L. M., III. (2002). The Word Memory Test and the validity of neuropsychological test scores. *Journal of Forensic Neuropsychology*, *2*, 97–124.

Greenhalgh, T. (1997). How to read a paper: Papers that report diagnostic or screening tests. *British Medical Journal*, *315*, 540–543.

Greiffenstein, M. F., & Baker, W. J. (2001). Comparison of premorbid and post injury MMPI-2 profiles in late postconcussion claimants. *The Clinical Neuropsychologist*, *15*, 162–170.

Greiffenstein, M. F., Baker, W. J., Gola, T., Donders, J., & Miller, L. (2002). The Fake Bad Scale in atypical and severe closed head injury litigants. *Journal of Clinical Psychology*, *58*, 1591–1600.

Harrell, F. E., Jr. (2001). *Regression Modeling Strategies*. New York: Springer.

Heaton, R. K., Grant, I., & Matthews, C. G. (1991). *Comprehensive Norms for an Expanded Halstead-Reitan Battery*. Odessa, FL: Psychological Assessment Resources.

Heaton, R. K., Smith, H. H., Lehman, R.A.W., & Vogt, A. T. (1978). Prospects for faking believable deficits on neuropsychological testing. *Journal of Consulting and Clinical Psychology*, *46*, 892–900.

Heilbronner, R. L., Sweet, J. J., Attix, D. K., Kroll, K. R., Henry, G. K., & Hart, R. P. (2003). Official position of the American Academy of Clinical Neuropsychology on serial neuropsychological assessments: The utility and challenges of repeat test administrations in clinical and forensic contexts. *The Clinical Neuropsychologist*, *24*, 1267–1278. [Online]. Retrieved from www.tandfonline.com/doi/pdf/10.1080/13854046.2010.526785 (last visited November 30, 2013).

Hiscock, C. K., Branham, J. D., & Hiscock, M. (1994). Detection of feigned cognitive impairment: The two-alternative forced-choice method compared with selected conventional tests. *Journal of Psychopathologic Behavior*, *16*, 95–110.

Hoeting, J. A., Madigan, D., Raftery, A. E., & Volinsky, C. T. (1999). Bayesian model averaging: A tutorial (with discussion). *Statistical Science*, *14*, 382–417. (a corrected version of the paper is retrieved from www.stat.colostate.edu/~jah/documents/bma2.ps).

Insightful Corporation. (2002). *S-Plus 6.1*. Seattle: Insightful Corporation.

Iverson, G. L., & Franzen, M. D. (1994). The Recognition Memory Test, Digit Span, and Knox Cube Test as markers of malingered memory impairment. *Assessment*, *1*, 323–334.

Iverson, G. L., & Franzen, M. D. (1998). Detecting malingered memory deficits with the Recognition Memory Test. *Brain Injury*, *12*, 275–282.

Jury Verdict Research. (2000). *2000 Current Award Trends in Personal Injury*. Horsham, PA: LRP Publications.

Kaiman, R. (2003). Median award for mild brain injuries is $271,350. *Personal Injury Verdict Reviews*, *11*, 3.

Kassirer, J. P., & Kopelman, R. I. (1991). *Learning Clinical Reasoning*. Philadelphia, PA: Lippincott, Williams & Wilkins.

Kaufmann, P. M. (2012). Admissibility of expert opinions based on neuropsychological evidence. In G. Larrabee (Ed.), *Forensic Neuropsychology: A Scientific Approach*. (2nd ed., pp. 70–100). New York: Oxford University Press.

Kaufmann, P. M. (2013). Neuropsychologist experts and neurolaw: Cases, controversies, and admissibility challenges. *Behavioral Sciences and the Law*, *31*(6), 739–755.

Kellner, R., & Sheffield, B. F. (1973). The one-week prevalence of symptoms in neurotic patients and normals. *American Journal of Psychiatry*, *130*, 102–105.

Kessler, R. C., McGonagle, K. A., Zhao, S., Nelson, C. B., Hughes, M., Eshleman, S., Wittchen, H. U., & Kendler, K. S. (1994). Lifetime and 12-month prevalence of DSM-III-R psychiatric disorders in the United States: Results from the National Comorbidity Survey. *Archives of General Psychiatry*, *51*, 8–19.

Klonoff, P. S., & Lamb, D. G. (1998). Mild head injury, significant impairment on neuropsychological test scores, and psychiatric disability. *The Clinical Neuropsychologist*, *12*, 31–42.

Kreutzer, J. S., Gordon, W. A., Rosenthal, M., & Marwitz, J. (1993). Neuropsychological characteristics of patients with brain injury: Preliminary findings from a multicenter investigation. *Journal of Head Trauma Rehabilitation*, *8*(2), 47–59.

Larrabee, G. J. (1998). Somatic malingering on the MMPI and MMPI-2 in personal injury litigants. *The Clinical Neuropsychologist*, *12*, 179–188.

Larrabee, G. J. (2002, April). *Identification of personal injury malingerers using the MMPI-2 and patterns of atypical neuropsychological test performance*. Paper presented at the 12th Annual Nelson Butter' West Coast Neuropsychology Conference, San Diego, CA.

Lees-Haley, P. R., & Brown, R. S. (1993). Neuropsychological complaint base rates of 170 personal injury claimants. *Archives of Clinical Neuropsychology*, *8*, 203–209.

Lees-Haley, P. R., English, L. T., & Glenn, W. J. (1991). A fake bade scale on the MMPI-2 for personal injury claimants. *Psychological Reports*, *68*, 208–210.

Lees-Haley, P. R., Fox, D. D., & Courtney, J. C. (2001). A comparison of complaints by mild injury claimants and other claimants describing subjective experiences immediately following their injury. *Archives of Clinical Neuropsychology*, *16*, 689–695.

Levin, H. S., Mattis, S., Ruff, R. M., Eisenberg, H. M., Marshall, L. F., & Tabaddor, K. (1987). Neurobehavioral outcome following minor head injury: A 3-center study. *Journal of Neurosurgery*, *66*, 234–243.

Long, J. S. (1997). *Regression Models for Categorical and Limited Dependent Variables*. Thousand Oaks, CA: Sage.

Madigan, D., & Raftery, A. E. (1994). Model selection and accounting for model uncertainty in graphical models using Occam's window. *Journal of the American Statistical Association*, *89*, 1535–1546.

Martens, M., Donders, J., & Millis, S. R. (2001). Evaluation of invalid response set after traumatic brain injury. *Journal of Forensic Neuropsychology*, *2*, 1–18.

McKinzey, R. K., & Russell, E. W. (1997). Detection of malingering on the Halstead-Reitan Battery: A cross-validation. *Archives of Clinical Neuropsychology*, *12*, 585–589.

Meyers, J. E., & Volbrecht, M. (1998). Validation of reliable digits for detection of malingering. *Assessment*, *5*, 303–307.

Millis, S. R. (1992). The Recognition Memory Test in the detection of malingered and exaggerated memory deficits. *The Clinical Neuropsychologist*, *6*, 406–414.

Millis, S. R. (1994). Assessment of motivation and memory with the Recognition Memory Test after financially compensable mild head injury. *Journal of Clinical Psychology*, *50*, 601–605.

Millis, S. R. (2002). Warrington's Recognition Memory Test in the detection of response bias. *Journal of Forensic Neuropsychology*, *2*, 147–166.

Millis, S. R., & Putnam, S. H. (1994). The Recognition Memory Test in the assessment of memory impairment after financially compensable mild head injury: A replication. *Perceptual and Motor Skills*, *79*, 384–386.

Millis, S. R., Putnam, S. H., & Adams, K. M. (1996). Speech-sounds Perception Test and Seashore Rhythm Test as validity indicators in the neuropsychological evaluation of mild head injury [abstract]. *Archives of Clinical Neuropsychology*, *11*, 425.

Millis, S. R., Putnam, S. H., Adams, K. M., & Ricker, J. H. (1995). The California Verbal Learning Test in the detection of incomplete effort in neuropsychological evaluation. *Psychological Assessment*, *7*, 463–471.

Millis, S. R., Rosenthal, M., Novack, T. A., Sherer, M., Nick, T. G., Kreutzer, J. S., . . . Ricker, J. H. (2001). Long-term neuropsychological outcome following traumatic brain injury. *Journal of Head Trauma Rehabilitation*, *16*(4), 343–355.

Millis, S. R., Ross, S. R., & Ricker, J. H. (1998). Detection of incomplete effort on the Wechsler Adult Intelligence Scale-Revised: A cross-validation. *Journal of Clinical and Experimental Neuropsychology*, *20*, 167–173.

Millis, S. R., & Volinsky, C. T. (2001). Assessment of response bias in mild head injury: Beyond malingering test. *Journal of Clinical and Experimental Neuropsychology*, *23*, 809–828.

Mittenberg, W., Rotholc, A., Russell, E., & Heilbronner, R. (1996). Identification of malingered head injury on the Halstead-Reitan Battery. *Archives of Clinical Neuropsychology*, *11*, 271–281.

Mittenberg, W., Theroux, S., Aguila-Puentes, G., Bianchini, K., Greve, K., & Rayls, K. (2001). Identification of malingered head injury on the Wechsler Adult Intelligence Scale—3rd Edition. *The Clinical Neuropsychologist*, *15*, 440–445.

Mittenberg, W., Theroux-Fichera, S., Zielinski, R. E., & Heilbronner, R. (1995). Identification of malingered head injury on the Wechsler Adult Intelligence Scale-Revised. *Professional Psychology: Research and Practice*, *26*, 491–498.

Morey, L. C. (1991). *Personality Assessment Inventory*. Odessa, FL: Personality Assessment Resources.

Paniak, C., Reynolds, S., Phillips, K., Toller-Lobe, G., Melnyk, A., & Nagy, J. (2002). Patient complaints within 1 month of mild traumatic brain injury: A controlled study. *Archives of Clinical Neuropsychology*, *17*, 319–334.

Paniak, C., Reynolds, S., Toller-Lobe, G., Melnyk, A., Nagy, J., & Schmidt, D. (2002). A longitudinal study of the relationship between financial compensation and symptoms after treated mild traumatic brain injury. *Journal of Clinical and Experimental Neuropsychology*, *24*, 187–194.

Ponsford, J., Willmot, C., Rothwell, A., Cameron, P., Kelly, A., Nelms, R., . . . Ng, K. (2000). Factors influencing outcome following mild traumatic brain injury in adults. *Journal of the International Neuropsychological Society*, *6*, 568–570.

Pratt v. Astrue, 2009 U.S. Dist. LEXIS 72090 (E.D. Tenn. 2009).

Reiner v. Warren Resort Hotels, Inc., 2008 WL 5120682 (D. Mont. 2008).

Robins, L. N., & Regier, D. A. (1991). *Psychiatric Disorders in America: The Epidemiologic Catchment Area Study*. New York: Free Press.

Rohling, M. L. (2000). Generating a linear function for residual impairment for TBI: A comparison of the HRB and a flexible battery approach. *Archives of Clinical Neuropsychology*, *15*, 821–822.

Sackett, D. L., Straus, S. E., Richardson, W. S., Rosenberg, W., & Haynes, R. B. (2000). *Evidence-Based Medicine*. New York: Churchill Livingstone.

SAS Institute. (2002). *JMP 5*. Cary, NC: SAS Institute, Inc.

Sawchyn, J. M., Brulot, M. M., & Strauss, E. (1999). Note on use of the Postconcussion Syndrome Checklist. *Archives of Clinical Neuropsychology*, *15*, 1–8.

Slick, D. J., Hopp, G., Strauss, E., & Spellacy, F. J. (1996). Victoria Symptom Validity Test: Efficiency for detecting feigned memory impairment and relationship to neuropsychological tests and MMPI-2 validity scales. *Journal of Clinical and Experimental Neuropsychology*, *18*, 911–922.

Slick, D. J., Hopp, G., Strauss, E., & Thompson, G. B. (1997). *Victoria Symptom Validity Test: Professional Manual*. Odessa, FL: Psychological Assessment Resources, Inc.

Slick, D. J., Sherman, E.M.S., & Iverson, G. L. (1999). Diagnostic criteria for malingered neurocognitive dysfunction: Proposed standards for clinical practice and research. *The Clinical Neuropsychologist*, *13*, 545–561.

Sosin, D. M., Sniezek, J. E., & Thurman, D. J. (1996). Incident of mild and moderate brain injury in the United States, 1991. *Brain Injury*, *10*, 47–54.

Stata Corporation. (2003). *Stata 8.0*. College Station, TX: Stata Corporation.

Stogner, B. L. (1999). Prediction of postconcussional syndrome from personality and health psychology variables. *Dissertation Abstracts International*, *60*. (UMI No. 9954220).

Suhr, J. A., & Gunstad, J. (2002). Postconcussive symptom report: The relative influence of head injury and depression. *Journal of Clinical and Experimental Neuropsychology*, *24*, 981–993.

Sweet, J. J., & King, J. H. (2002). Category Test validity indicators: Overview and practice recommendation. *Journal of Forensic Neuropsychology*, *3*, 241–274.

Sweet, J. J., Wolf, P., Sattlberger, E., Numan, B., Rosenfeld, J. P., Clingerman, S., & Nies, K. J. (2000). Further investigation of traumatic brain injury versus insufficient effort with the California Verbal Learning Test. *Archives of Clinical Neuropsychology*, *15*, 105–113.

Tabachnick, B. G., & Fidell, L. S. (2001). *Using Multivariate Statistics* (4th ed.). Boston: Allyn & Bacon.

Taylor v. Astrue, U.S. Dist. LEXIS 113220 (N.D. Okla. 2012).

Thompson, G. B., III. (2002). The Victoria Symptoms Validity Test: An enhanced test of symptom validity. *Journal of Forensic Neuropsychology*, *2*, 43–67.

Tombaugh, T. N. (2002). The Test of Memory Malingering (TOMM) in forensic psychology. *Journal of Forensic Neuropsychology*, *2*, 69–96.

Trahan, D. E., Ross, C. E., & Trahan, S. L. (2001). Relationships among postconcussional-type symptoms, depression, and anxiety in neurologically normal young adults and victims of mild brain injury. *Archives of Clinical Neuropsychology*, *16*, 435–445.

Trueblood, W., & Schmidt, M. (1993). Malingering and other validity considerations in the neuropsychological evaluation of mild head injury. *Journal of Clinical and Experimental Neuropsychology*, *15*, 578–590.

Warrington, E. K. (1984). *Recognition Memory Test*. Windsor: NFER-Nelson.

39 Pediatric Forensic Neuropsychology

Jacobus Donders, Brian L. Brooks, Elisabeth M. S. Sherman, and Michael W. Kirkwood

The mainstay of the practice of most pediatric neuropsychologists (PNs) involves clinical evaluations of children who are referred by a physician, parent, or teacher, and with whom an advocating and/or treating clinician-patient relationship is established. This chapter, however, will deal with forensic contexts, where the client is an attorney representing a child, and which can range from personal injury litigation to disputes about eligibility for special education services to allegations about medical malpractice. We will review some of the variables that need to be considered routinely in the context of forensic neuropsychological evaluations of children. The term *forensic* is used here specifically as pertaining to a civic medicolegal or educational context and is not intended to apply to cases involving child custody or criminal responsibility. In addition, the term *child(ren)* is used with the understanding that this covers any person under the age of 18, unless the individual has become an emancipated minor. Throughout the chapter, the role of the PN will be assumed to be that of an independent expert, as opposed to some other potential role (e.g., litigation consultant to an attorney).

In this chapter, we will first review some basic aspects of legal procedures and contingencies that the PN needs to be familiar with before considering or performing a forensic evaluation. Next, we discuss several issues that are pertinent to the interpretation of assessment results, including definition of impairment and base rates of low scores. Specific attention will be paid to the evaluation of validity, as well as to malingered neuropsychological deficits and other conditions associated with under-performance or over-reporting of symptoms. Finally, some illustrative case examples will be provided with regard to options for documentation and sworn testimony.

Forensic Context

Doing a forensic neuropsychological evaluation of a child is quite different from regular clinical practice, in a number of ways. Some of these differences are summarized in Table 39.1. It is important to have unequivocal common ground with the retaining attorney about these differences *before* agreeing to do the evaluation. At the time of the initial contact with the attorney, the PN also needs to have a good understanding of the purpose of the evaluation. When considering a forensic referral, the PN must (a) only accept cases that are actually within his or her boundaries of professional competence (as is true with any referral), and (b) be reasonably familiar with judicial and administrative rules affecting local forensic work, as documented in standards 2.01(a) and 2.01(f) of the American Psychological Association (APA) Ethics code (2002). Therefore, a person with little or no continuing education in, or experience with, lead poisoning should most likely decline a request for an independent medicolegal evaluation of a child with such an alleged history. At the same time, a PN with considerable experience with the condition or area of interest should still make sure that he or she understands how the local legal system works.

Once the nature of the case has been established and it has been determined that it is within the boundaries of expertise of the PN, it needs to be ascertained that he or she can conduct an unbiased and objective examination, with access to relevant documents (including medical and school records) as well as the child. If the child has already undergone a prior neuropsychological or educational evaluation with a different provider, it is standard of care to request the associated report as well as the raw data. Fees and/or retainers for services should also be made explicit at the time of the initial contact with the attorney.

Any potential conflicts of interest dual-role situations should be ruled out prior to accepting a forensic case, as stated in Standard 3.05(a) of the APA ethics code (2002). For example, a PN who had at one time completed a clinical evaluation at the request of the child's pediatrician should definitely not later accept a referral from the attorney who represents the parents of the child in a personal injury lawsuit for another "expert" evaluation. As yet another example, if that same child had been clinically evaluated by PN A in the same department of which PN B was the director, it would most likely behoove PN B to decline doing an "independent" evaluation of that child.

Prior to the evaluation, it is advisable to obtain a specific set of questions from the retaining attorney to identify the main issues relevant to the case that need to be addressed. Sometimes, the PN will be asked to do a records review only. This is permissible as long as the limits this places on the ability to make specific diagnostic impressions are documented,

Table 39.1 Differences between clinical and forensic pediatric neuropsychology

Neuropsychologist Variable	*Clinical Evaluation*	*Forensic Evaluation*
Typical referral agent	Physician, parent, or teacher	Attorney
The client	Patient and parents/legal representative	Referring agent
Professional role with child	Treating clinician, patient advocate	Objective/independent expert
Relationship with other professionals	Collegial	Adversarial
Confidentiality	Maintained unless under extreme conditions (e.g., suspicion of child abuse)	Privilege has been waived; "private" information becomes a matter of public record
HIPAA/FERPA rules	Applicable	Superseded by discovery rules
Obtaining details about family medical and psychosocial history	Standard of care	Highly desirable but may be subject to legal/privacy objections
Necessity of performance/symptom validity testing	Recommended	Indispensable
Level of certainty required in interpretation of the data	Based on definition of impairment, base rates, and confidence intervals	More likely than not *or* with a reasonable degree of scientific certainty
Audience for the report	Treating professionals, school teachers	Attorneys, judges, and juries
Handling of raw data	Must attempt to maintain test security	Must often be made available in most states
Feedback to or follow-up with patient	Routine	Typically not allowed if retained by opposing counsel
Witness during deposition or trial	Fact witness	Expert witness

Note: Adapted (with permission) from Donders, J. (2012).
HIPAA = Health Insurance Portability and Accountability Act. FERPA = Family Educational Rights and Privacy Act.

consistent with standards 9.01(b) and 9.01(c) of the APA ethics code (2002). More commonly, the attorney will ask for an actual neuropsychological evaluation. Details of that process, including consideration of general psychometric issues and specific performance validity as well as symptom validity, will be discussed later, in the section on Identifying Cognitive Impairment. In general, though, it is important that the PN uses procedures that are ethical, widely accepted in the professional community, and grounded in psychometric and neurobehavioral science. This would also be an important proactive defense against any potential later challenges to the admissibility of the PN's report or sworn testimony.

When the parents or guardians bring a child in for a forensic evaluation, it is of utmost importance that the PN explains to them at the very beginning what the contingencies are and how these differ from a traditional clinical context. This starts with disclosing who retained the PN and what the nature and purpose of the evaluation are. Informed consent from the parent or guardian, as well as assent from the child, must be obtained in a language that they can understand, consistent with Standard 3.10(a–d) of the APA ethics code (2002). Sample consent forms are available from the website of the National Academy of Neuropsychology (www.nanonline.org). Normally, the Health Insurance Portability and Accountability Act (HIPAA) would apply to a traditional health care environment, and the less-restrictive Family Educational Rights and Privacy Act (FERPA) to educational evaluations; in both cases, the child and parent are the client. Although the PN does not need to go into details about those laws, it needs to be made explicit to the parents that the rights that these laws offer are not in effect during independent forensic evaluations. For example, they need to understand that the usual rules of confidentiality do not apply, that they may not have direct access to the report, and that follow-up is not routinely available. Nevertheless, the PN should conduct the evaluation in a respectful and evidence-based manner, with the goal of discerning information that will ultimately help the trier of fact (i.e., a judge or a jury).

It is distinctly not the role of the PN to try to "win the case" for either side in a pending legal dispute. During the entire forensic evaluation process, the PN should make every attempt at maintaining personal neutrality and scientific objectivity. Several authors have provided practical suggestions for self-screening by neuropsychologists for potential bias during the forensic evaluation process (Sweet & Moulthrop, 1999; Van Gorp & McMullen, 1997).

The reader is referred to Chapters 36 and 37 of this volume for a thorough review of all the legal terms, rules of evidence, and procedural issues that may arise in the context of a forensic neuropsychological evaluation. However, a few issues that arise commonly merit some further discussion. The first of these is that, at all times, the PN should aspire to the highest ethical, professional, and scientific standards, consistent with the ethics code of the APA (2002). At the same time, it needs to be realized that state or federal law may have different standards that will typically trump those of APA in case of conflict between them. For example, when faced with a subpoena for the raw data to be sent to the opposing attorney, the PN may and should express a preference to send those data directly to another PN, citing issues of test security and the like; consistent with the standards of practice in the field. However, except in cases where state law prohibits such direct disclosure or when the PN can clearly demonstrate the likelihood of substantial harm to the child, a judge may ultimately order release of the raw data to the opposing attorney, anyway. In that case, the PN will most likely need to comply, or risk being held in contempt of court and face the legal consequences. The official joint position of various professional neuropsychological organizations with regard to test data disclosure has been described by Attix and colleagues (2007).

Another notable difference in standards between the traditional clinical environment and the forensic context pertains to the degree of certainty that is required for an opinion. The traditional $p < 0.05$ criterion from the null hypothesis test context that is familiar to most PNs is typically not the evidentiary standard in a legal arena. In forensic cases, the PN may be asked whether something is "more likely than not," which essentially means anything that is > 51% likely. A more stringent standard is applied if the PN is asked to offer an opinion with a "reasonable degree of scientific/neuropsychological certainty," in which case a 90% likelihood level may be assumed.

Regardless of the type of certainty that is asked for, it is typically a good idea for PNs to qualify their professional opinions with reference to a level of probability, or a degree to which the phenomenon deviates from expected patterns. For example, if it is known from independent empirical studies that test A has a specificity of 88% and test B a specificity of 86%, then "positive" findings on both tests in the same child would typically be expected less than 2% of the time ($[1 - 0.88] \times [1 - 0.86] = 0.0168$) if the tests were largely uncorrelated. Phrasing this in the report or during testimony as something that would most likely occur in fewer than two out of every 100 patients would place the information in a context that is intelligible to those who are typically not experts in psychometrics, such as judges and juries.

It is also possible that PNs find themselves in a deposition or courtroom as a treating doctor who had originally seen the child for standard clinical reasons at the request of a physician, but is now asked to testify as part of legal procedures involving the same child. In such cases he or she will most likely be called as a fact witness, who can technically speak directly to the actual assessment findings only, whereas an independent expert witness has more leeway to offer professional opinions that include attribution of causality and discussion of the consensus in the literature. In reality, though, these lines are often blurred, and treating neuropsychologists are typically viewed as experts by most attorneys and judges. Requests from the opposing attorney for presence of a third-party observer during the evaluation present a unique challenge. Judges have leeway in the degree to which they may allow such presence but this varies considerably from state to state, which highlights the importance of familiarity with local jurisdictions. With that reservation in mind, the PN should object to the presence of third-party observers during the actual psychometric assessment process, because of the deviation from standardized procedures and the likely confounding impact on the behavior of the examinee. Several professional organizations, including the National Academy of Clinical Neuropsychology (2000) and the American Academy of Clinical Neuropsychology (2001), have issued position papers on this matter, and there are also empirical studies that have documented the invalidating influences associated with third-party observers, even when the "observer" is a recording device (e.g., Constantinou, Ashendorf, & McCaffrey, 2005; Lynch, 2005). It is advisable to submit these references as part of a notarized affidavit. Most often, attorneys are agreeable to limiting the presence of a third person to the interview, but this is not universal. Howe and McCaffrey (2010) provide further suggestions about how to deal with third-party observer requests.

Some opposing attorneys may request, prior to the evaluation, a list of all the tests that the PN plans to administer. It is advisable to decline such a request on the grounds that (a) the choice of specific tests may not be made until after the completion of the interview and history, and (b) potentially providing the opportunity to review specific tests or items in advance would likely jeopardize the validity of the evaluation. Often, a reasonable compromise is that specific cognitive domains of assessment can be provided (i.e., memory, attention, etc.). Alternatively, a complete list of every possible test that is available in the PN's arsenal and that could reasonably be considered for a child of this specific age and background can be offered, with the understanding that not all those tests will be given but that selections will be made from them.

Another barrier that PNs may face when preparing for a forensic evaluation is that the opposing attorney may object to the inquiry about any kind of family medical history, even though this would be the standard of care in clinical practice. Families may consequently decline to answer such questions, or a judge may even prohibit such inquiry. Under such circumstances, the PN must (a) respect any boundaries imposed by a judge, (b) decide if he or she still wants to proceed or withdraw from the case, (c) if the choice is made to proceed, then clearly note the nature and extent of the imposed restrictions in the report, and (d) explain in the same report how those restrictions limit the scope of the conclusions that can be made.

After completion of the records review, interview, and testing, the PN will typically be expected to prepare a report. In some cases, the retaining attorney may request that this be deferred until he or she and the PN have verbally discussed the findings. This should be determined before commencing the actual evaluation. When a written report is desired, the PN usually sends this to the retaining attorney only, but it still needs to be understood that any written documentation of this kind is "discoverable" in a forensic context. In fact, the

PN's entire file may need to be made available for inspection by opposing counsel as part of a later deposition or trial process. This highlights the importance of making sure that the file is complete and that the report is evidence-based, and addresses in professional yet intelligible language if the child has any current neuropsychological deficits and to what degree those are related to a neurological condition of interest (e.g., traumatic brain injury; or TBI) or other factors. It is very important in this context that the PN offers only professional opinions that are based on his or her expertise and not engage in speculation. For example, in the case of an allegation of malpractice by an obstetrician during a pregnancy and/or delivery, the PN can most likely comment on the degree to which the child's current neurobehavioral functioning at the age of 4 years deviates from normal, and potentially even relate it causally to known brain damage that was visualized on neuroimaging, but comments about whether or not the obstetrician acted negligently during the perinatal process should be avoided.

At some point—which can occur weeks to months after the evaluation—the PN may be asked to provide some kind of sworn testimony about the case. This can be in the form of a deposition, where only attorneys from both sides of the case plus a court recorder are present, or an actual courtroom appearance during trial in front of a judge and/or jury. Some depositions are videotaped for later presentation at trial in lieu of live testimony. It is far more common for PNs to participate in depositions than testifying in court because many cases get settled out of court.

Prior to a deposition or trial testimony, the PN should confer with the retaining attorney about the procedures and the specific issues that may come up. New information that was not available previously (e.g., what another expert had testified to or new records that became available) may be provided. If this alters the PN's opinions or conclusions about the case in any way, this should be made explicit at that time. Subsequently, during the actual deposition or trial, it is important to understand that the PN is primarily there to assist the jury or judge, during both direct and cross examination. Attorneys are supposed to argue a case for their client in a vigorous manner. Therefore, tough or challenging questions are to be expected and should most often not to be taken personally. The most effective report or testimony comes from PNs who are (a) thoroughly prepared, with recent review of their own case file as well as awareness of the current state of the scientific literature on the condition of interest, (b) capable of prompt and active answering in a way that is responsive to the question while also addressing ambiguities or possible misperceptions, (c) calm and professional without being completely devoid of emotion, and (d) familiar with common courtroom strategies or gambits (see the "Documentation and Testimony" section). Part of being thoroughly prepared includes a good understanding of psychometric issues when considering a group of neuropsychological test results. One common mistake is to overinterpret isolated "abnormal" findings that would be commonly found in the general population. The next section will address these issues and related pitfalls.

Identifying Cognitive Impairment Using (Multiple) Neuropsychological Tests

Neuropsychological assessment most often entails the administration of multiple tests, which shifts the interpretation of test scores from a Gaussian or univariate distribution (used for considering performance on a single test score in isolation) to a multivariate one (used for simultaneously considering performance on multiple test scores). The need for a multivariate interpretation of test scores has risen from the knowledge that obtaining some low scores on a neuropsychological assessment is common and expected in a substantial minority of healthy people (Binder, Iverson, & Brooks, 2009), which has been repeatedly demonstrated using neuropsychological measures with children (Brooks, 2010; Brooks et al., 2013b; Brooks, Iverson, Sherman, & Roberge, 2010a; Brooks, Iverson, Sherman, & Holdnack, 2009; Brooks & Sherman, 2012; Brooks, Sherman, & Iverson, 2010b; Crawford, Garthwaite, & Gault, 2007; Hurks, Hendriksen, Dek, & Kooij, 2013).

When interpreting multiple test scores, the PN needs to understand several key concepts that differ from interpreting a single score in isolation. Five key concepts of multivariate test interpretation are presented in the following sections (see also Brooks & Iverson, 2012 for a thorough review). Understanding and incorporating these concepts is beneficial for diagnostic judgment. Failing to appreciate or consider these five multivariate concepts may lead to increased chances of misdiagnosis of cognitive impairment.

Test-Score Variability (Scatter) Is Common

There is classic thinking in the field of neuropsychology that a healthy brain has consistency across all cognitive domains, whereas an injured brain has variability. In contrast, existing research indicates that healthy children and adolescents commonly display variability (or "scatter") across their test scores and considerable differences between their highest and lowest scores. Indeed, it is actually uncommon to *not* have scatter among test scores. For example, having all ten primary subtests from the Wechsler Intelligence Scale for Children–IV (WISC-IV; see Wechsler, 2003) fall within one standard deviation (SD) is found in only 0.4% of healthy children from the standardization sample. Having at least a six-scaled-score spread (i.e., ≥ two SDs) is found in as much as 73.4% of healthy children from the WISC–IV standardization sample. Even a nine-scaled-score spread (i.e., ≥ three SDs) is found in 22.5% of this sample. Interestingly, the amount of scatter may increase with more tests being administered (see Figure 2 in Brooks & Iverson, 2012) and may differ based on demographic characteristics, with boys and those with higher full-scale IQs having more intersubtest scatter than girls and those with lower full-scale IQs (Hurks et al., 2013).

The Number of Low Scores Depends on Where a PN Sets the Cutoff

There is no single universally accepted definition of what constitutes cognitive impairment on objective neuropsychological tests. Without clear direction on what is cognitive impairment or how to quantify it, PNs are left to arbitrarily determine and use various cutoff scores as interpretive guidelines for identifying a score that is in the "impaired" range. As might be expected, the more stringent a cutoff score (i.e., further from the mean in a negative direction), the less likely it is for an obtained score to be considered in the range of impairment. The same principle holds true for interpretation of multiple test scores: The prevalence of low scores on a battery of tests will depend on where the cutoff for "impairment" is set, with more stringent cutoffs resulting in fewer scores in the "impaired" range.

Figure 39.1 presents a simple example of the inverse relation between cutoff score and prevalence of healthy youth with low scores. When considering the ten primary subtests from the WISC–IV, 61% of children have two or more subtest scores ≤ 25th percentile. The prevalence rate drops as the cutoff is set further from the mean, with only about 8% having two or more scores ≤ 2nd percentile.

The Number of Low Scores Depends on the Number of Tests Administered

A simple principle exists for neuropsychologists in any setting: The more tests administered, the more likely one will obtain low scores. This does not argue against a thorough and lengthy assessment when warranted, but it does argue for the inclusion of multivariate base rates (whenever available) as part of the interpretation of the battery of tests.

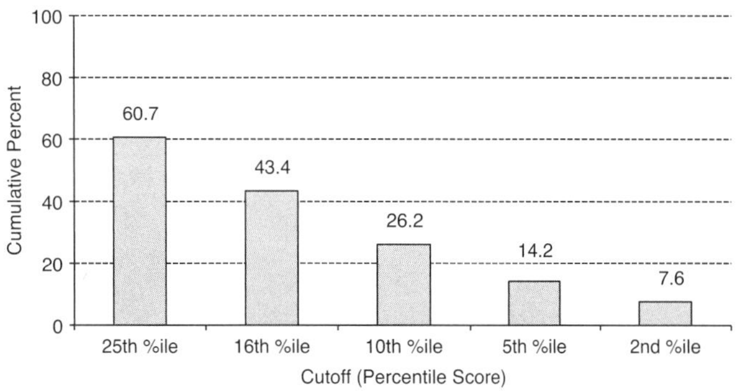

Figure 39.1 Percentage of healthy youth with two or more low WISC-IV subtest scores across various cutoffs

Note: Values were calculated from data provided in Table 1 in Brooks (2010)

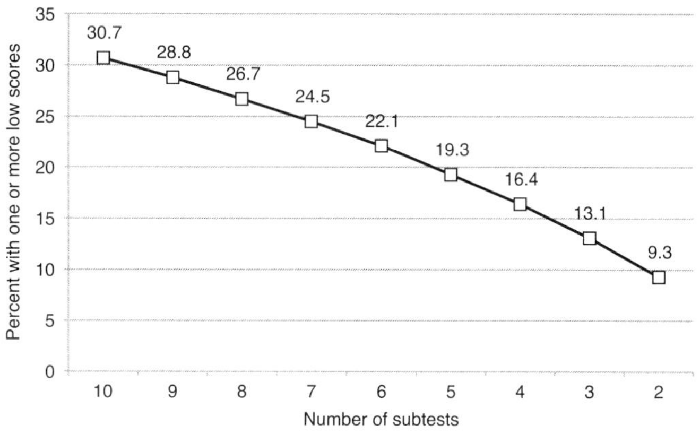

Figure 39.2 Estimated percent of people with at least one low subtest score (< fifth percentile) when varying the length of a battery

Note: Percent of people with low scores was estimated using the Crawford et al. (2007) Monte Carlo program and an average intersubtest correlation of 0.3.

Figure 39.2 illustrates the prevalence of low scores across a battery with varying numbers of subtests, when considering all scores simultaneously. In this example, which was derived using a Monte Carlo estimation (Crawford et al., 2007) and an average intersubtest correlation of 0.3, having one or more scores below the fifth percentile is found in nearly 31% when considering ten subtests but only 9% when considering two subtests.

The Number of Low Scores Varies by Examinee Characteristics

Neuropsychological test performance relates to multiple examinee characteristics including age, gender, culture, language, and socioeconomic status. These relations partially form the basis for census-matched normative samples and demographic adjustments to standard scores. There are some factors, however, that are not accounted for in standard scores but can have an impact on the prevalence of low scores. For example, a child's level of intellectual functioning and a parent's level of education (which is related to a child's intelligence and socioeconomic status) can impact multivariate base rates.

As noted previously, a study by Hurks and colleagues (Hurks et al., 2013) revealed that children with higher intelligence had more subtest variability or scatter on the Dutch Wechsler Preschool and Primary Scale of Intelligence–third edition (Wechsler, 2010) than children with lesser intelligence. However, children with lesser intelligence are expected to get more low scores than children with higher intelligence. For example, Brooks et al. (2009) showed that the prevalence of low memory scores increases as intellectual levels decrease. In those with below average intellectual scores, having one or more Children's Memory Scale (CMS; Cohen, 1997) index score fall ≤ fifth percentile is found in 33% of healthy youth. This is contrasted with only 3.5% of healthy youth with above average intellectual abilities having one or more CMS index scores ≤ fifth percentile.

Parental education also has a relation with child neurocognitive functioning (e.g., Devlin, Daniels, & Roeder, 1997; Schoenberg, Lange, Brickell, & Saklofske, 2007; Schoenberg, Lange, & Saklofske, 2007; Thomas, Sukumaran, Lukose, George, & Sarma, 2007), which in turn has an impact on the prevalence of low scores found in youth. Brooks et al. (2010b) illustrated that 67.2% of 7–16-year-olds with parents having less than high school education had one or more low NEPSY-II scores (≤ fifth percentile) compared to 33.9% of those children with average parental education of at least an undergraduate degree. Similar findings with more low scores in those with lesser intellectual abilities were also reported for the WISC-IV (Brooks, 2010).

Low Scores Are Common Across All Neuropsychological Tests

No neuropsychological test is immune to the presence of some low scores, even when administered to healthy children and adolescents. Several examples of multivariate base rates in pediatric neuropsychological batteries have been published (Brooks, 2010; Brooks et al., 2013b; Brooks et al., 2009; Brooks et al., 2010b; Crawford et al., 2007). Having some low scores is not an artifact of a specific standardization sample or a specific type of neurocognitive test. There are, however, differences in the prevalence rates of low scores depending on how strong the subtests are correlated. Figure 39.3 demonstrates an example of the percent of healthy people who would obtain one or more scores ≤ fifth percentile if the mean intercorrelation (r) was set at 0.1, = 0.5, or 0.9. When considering the multivariate base rates for 20 subtests, having one or more low scores is found in 57% when

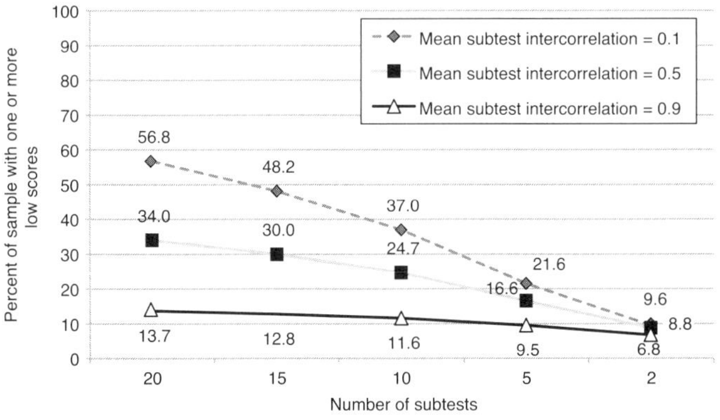

Figure 39.3 Estimated percent of healthy people who would obtain at least one low subtest score (<5th percentile) across different subtest intercorrelations

Note: Percent of people with low scores was estimated using the Crawford et al. (2007) Monte Carlo program

the mean r = 0.1, in 34% when the mean r = 0.5, and in 14% when the mean r = 0.9. Overall, the prevalence of low scores is higher when subtests have weaker intercorrelations, particularly when more tests are administered and interpreted (e.g., the prevalence rates start to converge with fewer subtests).

Currently, only a limited number of publications exist that can help the PN determine the multivariate base rates in a pediatric forensic assessment (Brooks, 2010; Brooks, Holdnack, & Iverson, 2011; Brooks, Iverson, & Holdnack, 2013a; Brooks et al., 2013b; Brooks et al., 2009; Brooks et al., 2010b). As such, the onus should be placed on test publishers to start producing this information as part of technical manuals and/or scoring programs. Some guidelines for the PN follow (Brooks & Iverson, 2012).

- The information on the prevalence of low scores is specific to the tests included in the analyses (i.e., one cannot substitute tests or index scores or apply a table to a different battery of tests) and to the number of tests included in the analyses (i.e., one cannot use the tables for more or fewer scores).
- When stratification by level of intelligence, parental education, or other demographic variable is not available, the PN may consider the prevalence of low scores in the entire sample. However, the PN needs to be aware that the prevalence rates are likely higher for lower functioning children and lower for higher functioning children.
- Some caution is warranted when interpreting the prevalence of low scores for a single battery or a single domain in isolation from the rest of the measures in a lengthy neuropsychological assessment (i.e., the base rates increase with more tests administered).
- Knowing the prevalence of low scores is designed to supplement, *not replace*, clinical judgment. Like any other psychometric information that is provided for test-score interpretation, the PN needs to make a determination based on all pieces of information and in the context of the specific details of the case.
- Having a common number of low scores does not mean that a low score cannot represent a relative weakness for a patient.

Consideration of these fundamental psychometric issues is not the only thing that is important in the interpretation of test results during a pediatric forensic neuropsychological evaluation. Consideration of validity issues is another crucial step.

Validity Testing

Neuropsychological test interpretation rests upon the assumption that the examinee responded in an unbiased fashion during the exam. If a child provides noncredible effort during testing or overreports symptoms, the resulting data will represent an inaccurate representation of the child's true abilities and/or difficulties. Reliance on such data can lead to a host of problems for the PN, including interpretive errors, inaccurate diagnostic and etiologic conclusions, mischaracterization of brain-behavior relationships, and possibly inappropriate recommendations. Thus, the incorporation of objective validity tests to detect invalid responding is crucial during all forensic evaluations. PNs should keep in mind, however, that the motivation to feign or exaggerate is typically complex in children, and failure on a validity test cannot be equated simplistically with "malingering." Motivations for invalid responding can be driven by both conscious and unconscious processes and include attempts to obtain external incentives and/or to fulfill internal psychological needs (Boone, 2007). In children, the motivations underlying noncredible performance are quite diverse, even in clinical populations (Kirkwood, Kirk, Blaha, & Wilson, 2010). In forensic settings, motivations are likely to be even more challenging to discern, with some children likely feigning in an attempt to seek indirect approval or attention from family members and others acting more directly to achieve an external incentive, either on their own accord or after explicit caregiver coaching or coercion (see section on Malingering, later in this chapter).

The frequency with which adults provide invalid test results during forensic evaluations is well studied, with rates as high as 40% across a variety of compensation-seeking contexts (Mittenberg, Patton, Canyock, & Condit, 2002). Relatively little attention was paid historically to how often noncredible presentations occurred during pediatric neuropsychological evaluations. However, over the last ten years, individual case reports and larger case series have documented clearly that children can, and do, underperform or even feign and/or exaggerate problems during both clinical and forensic neuropsychological evaluations.

In clinical settings, multiple case series across a host of populations have consistently found that a small percentage (~5%) of general pediatric outpatients perform suboptimally because of effort-related problems (Brooks, 2012; Carone, 2008; Donders, 2005; Kirk et al., 2011; MacAllister, Nakhutina, Bender, Karantzoulis, & Carlson, 2009). Certain pediatric clinical populations are apt to present in a noncredible fashion more frequently. For example, in a mild TBI case series consisting of children and adolescents referred exclusively for clinical evaluation, 17% of the sample failed an objective validity test, which was the same percentage estimated to have put forth noncredible effort more broadly across the exam once possible false positives and false negatives were taken into account (Kirkwood & Kirk, 2010).

In forensic settings, multiple authors have also presented individual cases of children providing noncredible effort, both when the child was likely acting independently and at the behest of a caregiver (Chafetz & Prentkowski, 2011; Flaro & Boone, 2009; Henry, 2005; Lu & Boone, 2002; McCaffrey & Lynch, 2009). No identified case series have reported how often biased responding occurs in pediatric civil litigation contexts but a surprisingly high rate of validity test failure has been found in the only compensation seeking context that has been studied. During determination evaluations for U.S. Social Security Disability benefits, Chafetz and colleagues found that 28% to 37% of children failed objective validity tests (Chafetz, 2008; Chafetz, Abrahams, & Kohlmaier, 2007). Similarly, no identified studies have examined the base rate of response bias during pediatric independent educational evaluations. However, studies with university students seeking accommodations for learning disabilities or attention deficit/hyperactivity disorder (ADHD) raise serious questions for PNs conducting such evaluations, as the rate of invalid responding in these young adults has been found to be between 15% and 30% (Harrison, Rosenblum, & Currie, 2010; Suhr, Hammers, Dobbins-Buckland, Zimak, & Hughes, 2008; Suhr, Sullivan, & Rodriguez, 2011; Sullivan, May, & Galbally, 2007).

The incorporation of validity tests into neuropsychological evaluations has been endorsed strongly by various professional neuropsychological organizations (Bush et al., 2005; Heilbronner, Sweet, Morgan, Larrabee, & Millis, 2009), although an endorsement specifically for PNs has yet to be provided. Variance in pediatric neuropsychological ability-based test performance is also known to be accounted for to a considerable degree by validity test results. For example, in a pediatric mild TBI sample, validity test performance was correlated significantly with performance on all ability-based tests and explained more than a third (38%) of the variance on an ability-based test summary index (Kirkwood, Yeates, Randolph, & Kirk, 2012).

The two primary objective methods to evaluate the validity of an individual's neuropsychological data are (a) stand-alone or embedded performance validity tests (PVTs) that measure response validity using performance-based tests and (b) symptom validity tests (SVTs) that measure response validity during self-report instruments (Larrabee, 2012). Of course, responses from any validity test depend in part on the particular demands of the task and can vary for a multitude of reasons, including true cognitive impairment and temporary fluctuations in arousal, attention, emotional state, and effort. Determining whether a child is responding more broadly in an invalid fashion not only requires careful examination of validity test performance but also a solid understanding of the natural history of the presenting condition; scrutiny of the child's developmental, medical, educational, and environmental background; and thorough consideration of the consistency and neuropsychological plausibility of the behavioral, self-report, and test data.

Performance Validity Tests

A review of all PVTs that have been studied with children is beyond the scope of this chapter. However, as highlighted in Table 39.2, and discussed in more detail in Kirkwood (2012),

Table 39.2 Empirical evidence estimates for performance validity tests in pediatric populations

Test	*Strength of Empirical Evidence in Various Pediatric Samples*			
	Community samples	*Clinical samples*	*Secondary gain samples*	*Simulation samples*
Amsterdam Short-Term Memory Test (ASTM)	+	–	–	–
Automatized Sequencing Task	–	+	–	–
California Verbal Learning Test–Children's Version	–	+	–	–
Computerized Assessment of Response Bias (CARB)		+	–	–
Fifteen Item Test (FIT)	+	+	–	–
Medical Symptom Validity Test (MSVT)	+	++	+	++
Nonverbal Medical Symptom Validity Test (NV-MSVT)	–	+	–	–
Test of Memory Malingering (TOMM)	++	++	+	+
Symptom Validity Scale for Low Functioning Individuals	–	–	+	–
Victoria Symptom Validity Test (VSVT)	–	+	–	–
Word Memory Test (WMT)	+	++	–	+

Note: ++ adequate evidence base;
+ modest evidence base;
– no or conflicting evidence
Adapted (with permission) from Kirkwood (2012).

at least two of them have received enough empirical attention in children that they could be justified for use by the PN during a forensic evaluation, at least with certain populations. Specifically, the Test of Memory Malingering (TOMM; Tombaugh, 1996) and the Medical Symptom Validity Test (MSVT; Green, 2004) have the most validation evidence for this specific purpose, at this time.

The TOMM has been investigated in child samples more than any other PVT including with community-based populations (Constantinou & McCaffrey, 2003; Rienstra, Spaan, & Schmand, 2010), a wide variety of clinical samples (Brooks, Sherman, & Krol, 2012; Donders, 2005; Gast & Hart, 2010; Kirk et al., 2011; MacAllister et al., 2009; Perna & Loughan, 2013), a secondary gain sample (Chafetz et al., 2007), and children asked to simulate impairment (Blaskewitz, Merten, & Kathmann, 2008; Gunn, Batchelor, & Jones, 2010; Nagle, Everhart, Durham, McCammon, & Walker, 2006). Collectively, these studies indicate that TOMM performance may be very modestly affected by age or IQ but that the vast majority of school-aged children can score above "adult" pass/fail cutoffs when providing adequate effort. Recent work indicates that administering only Trial 1 of the TOMM may be sufficient in certain clinical situations (Brooks et al., 2012; Perna & Loughan, 2013), although more work is probably needed in this regard before Trial 2 can be comfortably disregarded during forensic evaluations.

Several independent studies have also included the MSVT in pediatric samples. One focused on a clinical population of children with significant neurologic or developmental problems (Carone, 2008), several have been from an overlapping case series of patients with mild TBI (Kirkwood & Kirk, 2010; Kirkwood, Connery, Kirk, & Baker, 2014; Kirkwood, Yeates, Randolph, & Kirk, 2012), one has included a secondary gain context (Chafetz et al., 2007), and one used a simulation design (Blaskewitz et al., 2008). One of the MSVT's clear strengths is its brief administration time, which makes it a good candidate for a screening validity test. Normative data and a growing body of independent work suggest that the vast majority of children who can read at a third-grade level or higher can pass using adult cutoffs. Some pediatric data (Blaskewitz et al., 2008; Nagle et al., 2006) indicate that it may be more sensitive than the TOMM. Further independent research will be necessary to examine specificity in pediatric patients with significant deficits and to establish the classification utility of profile analysis in child samples.

Self-Report Validity Tests

Numerous pediatric self-report instruments include validity scales designed to detect symptom exaggeration. Commonly used measures in pediatric neuropsychological evaluations that contain a "fake bad" scale include general personality instruments such as the Minnesota Multiphasic Personality Inventory–Adolescent (MMPI-A, Infrequency scale), Personality Inventory for Youth (PIY; Dissimulation Scale), and Behavior Assessment System for Children–second edition (BASC-2, F Index), as well as domain- and disorder-specific scales such as the Behavior Rating Inventory of Executive Function–Self-Report (Negativity scale) and Trauma Symptom Checklist for Children (Hyperresponse scale). Each of these scales has solid normative data and at least adequate psychometric properties. Nevertheless, to date, very little to no independent research has focused on the utility of the validity indices in particular.

A few studies have provided initial support for the MMPI-A in identifying feigned psychopathology (Baer, Kroll, Rinaldo, & Ballenger, 1999; Lucio, Duran, Graham, & Ben-Porath, 2002; Rogers, Hinds, Sewell, 1996; Stein, Graham, & Williams, 1995). One study also provided support for the PIY Dissimulation Scale in identifying feigned emotional distress and psychosis (Wrobel, Lachar, Wrobel, Morgan, & Gruber, 1999). However, these studies have focused on simulators, so the value of the scales to detect exaggerated or feigned complaints in real-world examinees remains largely unknown. Moreover, none of the studies were conducted with individuals presenting for neuropsychological evaluation, so their applicability to children who may be more likely to present with physical or cognitive complaints, rather than psychiatric problems, is uncertain.

The only identified study that has focused on the value of an SVT in a neuropsychological setting examined the relationship between the BASC-2 Self-Report of Personality validity scales and the MSVT in a pediatric mild TBI sample (Kirk, Hutaff-Lee, Connery, Baker, & Kirkwood, 2014). Somewhat unexpectedly, no relationship was found between those children identified as responding invalidly via the BASC-2 and those failing the MSVT. The results of this pediatric study indicate that relying exclusively on the BASC-2 validity scales as an indication of the validity of the overall neuropsychological data will almost certainly significantly underestimate the percentage of patients providing invalid data during evaluation. Thus, the study reinforces the value of adding objective PVTs to the neuropsychological evaluation of school-age patients and also highlights the importance of future research into SVTs for nonpsychiatric pediatric populations. Unfortunately, at this point, PNs simply do not have any empirically backed SVTs to choose from when they want to detect the overreporting of health-related problems rather than psychiatric concerns.

In general, it is advisable to include both PVTs and SVTs during pediatric forensic neuropsychological evaluations. However, one of the most significant challenges that the PN may face pertains to the identification and reporting of deliberate poor performance, and the possibility of malingering.

Malingering

Malingering is a behavior, not a clinical disorder. In *the Diagnostic and Statistical Manual of Mental Disorders*, fifth edition (DSM-5; American Psychiatric Association, 2013), it can be found with other behaviors classified under "Nonadherence to Medical Treatment." Conceptualizing malingering as a form of nonadherence to neuropsychological assessment is also a useful way of helping clinicians maintain a behavioral, nonjudgmental approach to detection and interpretation. DSM-5 notes that malingering can at times be an adaptive behavior; the reality is that examinees may malinger for a variety of reasons that may or may not be available to the PN, whose job is to maintain professionalism and objectivity at all times.

Over the last two decades, various definitions and criteria for malingering of cognitive problems have been proposed for application in neuropsychology. However, the Slick, Sherman, and Iverson (1999) criteria continue to stand the test of time as the most commonly used definition, and the definition with the most empirical basis (e.g., Larrabee, 2012). In the Slick et al. framework, the term *malingered neuropsychological dysfunction* (MND) was defined as "the volitional exaggeration or fabrication of cognitive dysfunction for the purpose of obtaining substantial material gain, or avoiding or escaping formal duty or responsibility" (Slick et al., 1999, p. 552).

From a pediatric perspective, the Slick et al. (1999) criteria posed some problems. First, the criteria made only a cursory reference to situations involving malingering behavior in vulnerable examinees. Children or adolescents may exaggerate symptoms for material gain, but they do not necessarily have the ability to appreciate the consequences of their actions, whether a coercing adult is involved or not. On a more general level, the criteria were unclear regarding situations where malingering and bona fide impairment coexisted and whether the presence of another disorder would invalidate the presence of malingering. Finally, there was a need for more coverage regarding the diagnostic utility of self-reported symptoms and more explicit inclusion of compelling inconsistencies (Bianchini, Greve, & Glynn, 2005).

Slick and Sherman (2012) therefore proposed an update of these criteria (Table 39.3). The main changes were to divide malingering into three subcategories, namely, (a) *primary MND*, which essentially reflects the 1999 definition of MND; (b) *secondary MND*, for situations where MND is attributable to immaturity or developmental, neurological or psychiatric disorder; and (c) *MND by proxy*, where MND is attributable to the influence of another person on a vulnerable examinee, typically a child.

MND by proxy is poorly understood. To date, three cases of malingering of cognitive problems by proxy have been reported in the literature, two litigating and one seen as part of a Social Security Disability evaluation (Chafetz & Prentkowski, 2011; Lu & Boone, 2002; McCaffrey & Lynch, 2009). However, some settings may be associated with high rates. Chafetz and Prentkowski (2011) stressed that it is parents who arrange and carry out the plan to deceive in order to gain monetary awards on their children's behalf, presumably by coaching children.

As in the earlier 1999 criteria, MND, secondary MND, and MND by proxy can be coded in terms of certainty, namely *definite*, *probable*, and *possible* MND. Definite MND is defined by the presence of either (a) below-chance performance on forced-choice measures, (b) high posterior probability (≥ 0.95 that performance is substantially below actual ability level) on one or more well-validated psychometric indices, and (c) self-reported symptoms that are

Table 39.3 Proposed diagnostic criteria for malingered neuropsychological dysfunction, a revision and extension of the Slick et al. (1999) criteria for Malingered Neuropsychological Dysfunction

Primary MND

Definite

1 Presence of a substantial external incentive for exaggeration/fabrication of symptoms (Criterion 1)

2 One or more very strong indicators of exaggeration/fabrication of neuropsychological problems or deficits (one or more of Criteria 2.1–2.3)

3 Behaviors meeting necessary criteria are not substantially accounted for by psychiatric, neurological, or developmental factors

Probable

1 Presence of a substantial external incentive for exaggeration/fabrication of symptoms (medical-legal secondary gain)

2 Three or more indicators of possible exaggeration/fabrication of neuropsychological problems or deficits (three or more of Criteria 3.1–3.7)

Secondary MND (Definite and Probable)

Criteria for definite or probable malingered neuropsychological dysfunction (MND) are otherwise met, but there are compelling grounds to believe that at the time of assessment the examinee did not have the cognitive capacity to understand the moral/ethical/legal implications of his or her behavior, and/or was unable to control his or her behavior, secondary to immaturity (i.e., in childhood) or bona fide developmental, psychiatric, or neurological disorders or injuries of *at least* moderate severity. Secondary malingering cannot be diagnosed in persons with mild conditions such as mild TBI.

MND by Proxy (Definite and Probable)

Criteria for definite or probable MND are otherwise met, but there are compelling grounds to believe that a vulnerable examinee acted primarily under the guidance, direction, influence, or control of another individual. Examinees may be vulnerable to the influence of others by virtue of immaturity, neurodevelopmental and cognitive disabilities, and psychiatric illness, or by perceived inability to escape or avoid substantial coercion such as threats of physical harm for failure to behave as directed.

Specific Criteria

1 Presence of a substantial external incentive for exaggeration/fabrication of symptoms (medical-legal secondary gain)

2 Very strong indicators of exaggeration/fabrication of neuropsychological problems or deficits

2.1 Below chance performance (≤ 0.05) on one or more forced choice measures

2.2 High posterior probability (≥ 0.95 that performance is substantially below actual ability level) on one or more well-validated psychometric indices

2.3 Self-reported symptoms are unambiguously incompatible with or directly contradicted by directly observed behavior and/or test performance

3 Possible indicators of exaggeration/fabrication of neuropsychological problems or deficits

3.1 Data from one or more well-validated psychometric measures, while not sufficient to meet Criteria 2a or 2b, are on balance more consistent with non-compliance than compliance

3.2 Marked and implausible discrepancy between test performance and level of function expected based on developmental and medical history

3.3 Marked and implausible discrepancy between test performance and directly observed behavior and capabilities

3.4 Marked and implausible discrepancy between test performance and reliable collateral reports concerning behavior and capabilities

3.5 Marked and implausible discrepancy between self-reported and documented history, consistent with exaggeration of preinjury level of function and capabilities, minimization or preexisting injuries or neuropsychological problems, and/or exaggeration of the severity of new injuries

3.6 Marked and implausible discrepancy between self-reported symptoms and level of function expected based on developmental and medical history

3.7 Marked and implausible discrepancy between self-reported symptoms and information obtained from reliable collateral informants

unambiguously incompatible or directly contradicted by directly observed behavior and/or test performance. In practical terms, this means that *definite malingering* can be defined only by below-chance performance on a PVT or observation of behaviors incompatible with reported symptoms (e.g., surveillance video of a child walking despite complaints of complete paralysis). Presumably an actual confession by the child would also be sufficient. The term can also be applied when a well-validated Bayesian model that uses multivariable input, such as scores from one or more tests that provide positive predictive values of malingering, indicates that the positive predictive power for a given examinee is equal to or greater than 0.95. Any compelling evidence for malingering that falls short of these possibilities must therefore be termed *possible malingering*.

Importantly, avoiding false positives should be the goal in identifying cases of MND, as it should be when using PVTs and SVTs. In adults, failure on two PVTs is associated with exceedingly low rates of false positive errors, with failure on three PVTs associated with essentially nil chance of a false positive identification of MND (Larrabee, 2012). In children, this has yet to be empirically determined. However, a good rule of thumb would be to identify MND only when at least two PVTs are failed, at minimum. Ideally, PNs would use measures with embedded validity indicators, in addition to stand-alone validity tests. In the end, the PN must identify a *reason* for the questionable or invalid test results. This is where the differentiation of MND from other conditions occurs. A number of different conditions should be considered before attributing underperformance to malingering.

Conversion Disorder or Functional Neurological Symptom Disorder

Conversion disorder, also known in DSM-5 as "Functional Neurological Symptom Disorder" and included under the broad category of "Somatic Symptom and Related Disorders," involves voluntary motor or sensory symptoms that are incompatible with recognized neurological or medical conditions, are not better explained by another condition, and cause impairment and distress. The earlier criterion from DSM-IV that symptoms not be feigned, or not intentionally produced, is no longer needed in DSM-5—likely because establishing causality and veracity was too fraught with difficulty. Children with conversion disorder will rarely be encountered in clinical practice by most PNs most of the time, unless they work in settings where unexplained medical symptoms are more common, such as movement disorder clinics or epilepsy-monitoring units, where a subgroup of children may present with unexplained paralysis or nonepileptic seizures. Most importantly, cognitive symptoms are *not* included under the diagnosis of conversion disorder, although some experts believe they should have been (Stone et al., 2011). Because of this, conversion disorder is no longer a condition that needs to be frequently considered in the differential diagnosis of feigned/implausible cognitive deficits or self-reported cognitive symptoms, although it can certainly co-occur with feigned or intentionally produced symptoms, according to the DSM-5 reformulation.

Factitious Disorder Imposed on Self, and Factitious Disorder Imposed on Another

Factitious disorder is the fabrication of physical or psychological symptoms, in order to deceive, without the necessary presence of external rewards. The DSM-5 formulation divides factitious disorder into two separate subcategories: *factitious disorder imposed on self*, and *factitious disorder imposed on another*. The latter replaces "factitious disorder by proxy." Of note, the presence of material gain or external incentives does not rule out factitious disorder, and so this may be a diagnosis to consider in cases where internal as well as external incentives are involved. Factitious disorder should not be diagnosed in the presence of another mental disorder that better accounts for symptoms (e.g., delusional or psychotic disorders).

Illness Anxiety Disorder

Illness anxiety disorder bears considering here as well, even though it does not technically involve exaggerated or feigned cognitive problems. Instead, persons presenting with illness anxiety disorder have an intense fear about having a disorder. DSM-5 defines illness anxiety disorder as a preoccupation with having or acquiring a serious illness, without any physical symptoms, or else preoccupation in excess to symptoms. The main symptom is excessive preoccupation with health, not accounted for by other disorders such as generalized anxiety disorder or obsessive-compulsive disorder. For example, illness anxiety disorder may involve overreporting of cognitive symptoms due to overvigilance and anxiety, rather than deception or feigning, and therefore children with this condition may produce invalid or questionable results on SVTs due to excessive symptom reporting. Other reasons for overreporting of symptoms may involve attention seeking, hypervigilance, or catastrophizing of symptoms. The prevalence of illness anxiety disorder in children and adolescents is unknown.

Determination of whether or not the test data are valid, and whether or not the criteria are met for either malingered neuropsychological deficit or another condition associated with underperformance or overreporting of symptoms, is a key responsibility of the PN. The next step is to develop the ability to convey information about the validity and implications of the assessment findings in a report and during deposition or trial testimony.

Documentation and Testimony

No deposition or trial is the same. However, we want to illustrate some common questions, tasks and scenarios that the PN often has to deal with when doing forensic work. As neuropsychologists, we do not presume to offer formal legal advice. In addition, our intent is not to provide tips for how to "win." Instead, we simply offer options for various strategies that respect the integrity of the legal process while also assuring that the judge or jury is presented with the most accurate and complete information. The following is not an exhaustive list of suggestions for dealing with every possible forensic deposition or courtroom strategy or dilemma that a PN may encounter. Only some of the most common ones that often arise in the context of civil litigation regarding personal injury, special education eligibility, and/or medical malpractice involving children are reviewed. For more specific suggestions about testifying during depositions or trials, the reader is referred to Greiffenstein and Kaufmann (2012), Tsushima and Anderson (1996) and the series of books by Brodsky (1991, 1999, 2004).

1 *Be clear about who, what, and when.*
A report should state who retained the PN and which side of the legal dispute this attorney represented. Sometimes listing all the records that were made available can be helpful, but at a minimum, specific records should be identified when information is included in the report (e.g., that the Glasgow Coma Scale score was mentioned in the emergency room report of a certain date). If potentially important information is not available (e.g., school records from before alleged mold exposure), it should be explained how this limits the ability to draw firm conclusions about the available data. If information becomes available at some later point and if that alters the PN's opinions (e.g., a novel record pertaining to a history of bacterial meningitis, well before any lead was detected in the blood of the child), this should be documented in an addendum to the report. Documentation of informed consent/assent should also be included at the beginning of the report.

2 *Keep written documentation objective.*
The PN should maintain a neutral tone in the report, avoiding "crusader" comments to bolster one side of the case, and also avoiding emotional overtones, particularly when expressing disagreement with the opinions of another expert, or when pointing out discrepancies between objective documents and observed examinee behaviors. For example, instead of saying:

> "The mother denied any history of premorbid adjustment problems, which is a lie."

The PN would likely be better off stating that:

> "John's mother reported no premorbid problems with John. However, this was inconsistent with the available school records, which documented a long history of detentions, preceding the motor vehicle accident in question by more than a year."

Similarly, instead of attacking another provider with pejorative remarks about his or her level of training, board certification status, or experience, the PN should, both in documentation and during sworn testimony, maintain the high road. For example, instead of saying:

> "Dr. Jones was certified by a vanity board, plus I have ten more publications than he does about lead poisoning, so my opinion should weigh more."

a preferred approach might be:

> "I will leave it up to the jury to decide about Dr. Jones' credentials, but I feel very confident about mine, as I do about my conclusions, which are simply based on the objective facts of the case."

3 *Keep the written documentation intelligible.*
A report should offer scientifically sound interpretations and conclusions, not speculation to favor one side of the case. In addition, it should be phrased in a manner that is empirically accurate but clear to the judge or jury, who most likely do not have a background in clinical neuropsychology. For example, about an examinee who failed the MSVT, a PN who is used to communicating with other psychologists could write:

> "The examinee's performance on a standardized forced-choice performance validity measure was not consistent with veracious effort because of the violation of empirical criteria and therefore indicative of a high probability of deliberate symptom magnification for secondary gain."

However, a more effective way of documenting this for a judge or jury might be:

> "On a task where the chance of getting the right answer was equal to the flip of a coin, Jane answered correctly only 25% of the time. A person who had never seen the words on the computer screen, and just guessed, would most likely have done better than that. Therefore, I must conclude that Jane's test results do not show her true mental ability."

4 *Be well-prepared.*
One of the worst mistakes a PN can make with regard to sworn testimony is to not be intimately familiar with the facts of the case, the contents of his or her file, and the standard of care and consensus literature regarding the condition of interest. Particularly if the examination was done a considerable time in the past, the PN should again review relevant case information. Meeting with the retaining attorney prior to the deposition or trial is highly advisable. The PN should always make available a copy of his or her current CV. Particularly in federal cases, it is also advisable to have access to a list of all the depositions/trial testimonies that the PN has given over the past several years, along with a breakdown of plaintiff *v.* defense, when possible.

5 *Set limits.*
The time required for a deposition should be made clear in advance, in order not to jeopardize other professional activities that the PN has that day. It is perfectly reasonable for the PN to limit this to anywhere from 2 to 4 hours. When called to testify in court, it is the responsibility of the retaining attorney to make the time schedule as convenient as possible. It is also advisable to request a nonrefundable retainer fee before depositions, because sometimes these get cancelled on very short notice. During sworn testimony, the PN will be expected to answer any reasonable questions about the case at hand. However, in the rare event that questions are viewed as entirely irrelevant or objectionable (e.g., about the PN's private life), then the PN can ask for a decision

from the judge before answering. In court, this can be done by turning directly to the judge. During a deposition, the PN may decline to answer any further questions on the topic at hand until a ruling from the judge on the need to answer has been issued.

6 *Understand that it is not about you.*

Although there is no universal agreement on courtroom dress code, standard business or business casual is typically advisable. The PN should realize that typically, he or she is only one of a number of experts to be called and that the deposition or trial is not for purposes of bringing attention to his or her appearance or for puffing up one's own ego but about helping the trier of fact. This may be particularly important when, at the beginning of the testimony, a review of the PN's credentials is sought. Although the entire 20+ page resume may be very interesting to the PN, the jury will likely only need to hear something like:

> "I obtained my PhD from the University of X, did my internship at Y hospital, and my residency at Z medical center. I am licensed as a psychologist, and am board-certified in the specialty of clinical neuropsychology, which deals with brain-behavior relationships. TBI is an area of subspecialty for me because it is the condition I see relatively most often."

7 *Don't come across as defensive.*

It is common to be asked in what percentage of cases the PN testifies for the defense or plaintiff. It is best to simply provide that breakdown, and not to elaborate too much about it. However, if forensic work is only a relatively small proportion of the PN's activity, this can be explained as well. It is a myth that only those who have a 50/50 balance in plaintiff *v.* defense work will be seen as believable. However, it may help to put the information in context. For example:

> "More than 85% of all the clinical work that I do is based on referrals by doctors. Of the 15% of medicolegal work that I do, I am retained by the defense in the majority of cases."

Or:

> "In all the depositions over the last three years, I testified as a treating doctor by plaintiff request ten times, and as an expert witness upon request by the defense 20 times. Keep in mind that when, as an expert witness, I arrive at an opinion that does not support their side, they often settle the case instead of having me testify."

When the PN does not know the answer to a question, it is best to simply acknowledge this. Long-winded, extemporaneous answers should be avoided. The PN may also be asked about fees. Again, it is simply best to provide those. However, if insinuations are made about objectivity, the PN should deal with those while answering in a matter-of-fact manner. For example, assume a treating clinician/fact witness was asked: "You would say anything here to help your patient, right?" An unfortunate answer would be something like:

> "I am her doctor and I have been taking care of her for years, so of course I want what's best for her!"

Instead, a more effective answer would be:

> "I have sworn to tell the truth, and I take that oath seriously. I will answer any reasonable questions to the best of my ability. What specific question do you have for me about Jane?"

Similarly, assume an independent examiner/expert witness was asked: "You are being paid for your opinion here, today, right?" An unsatisfactory answer would be:

> "Well, yeah, I guess—I mean, I hope so. And there's nothing wrong with charging more for depositions because everybody does that!"

In contrast, a more convincing answer would be:

> "I expect to get paid today for my time. I have been hired for my expertise, not for a specific opinion."

8 *Listen and answer actively.*

When attorneys pose questions or rephrase previous statements made, the PN should start by listening very carefully. If the question is not clear or too convoluted, ask that it be clarified. Any inaccuracies or mischaracterizations of previous testimony or about the consensus in the field should be immediately corrected, in a neutral voice. The PN should look at the attorney during the question but at the camera or jury when answering. The answer should be given with confidence, avoiding terms like "I believe" or "I suppose." Instead, calmly state one's objective, professional opinion. The latter should also be done succinctly. A common mistake for those PNs who are new to the process is that they talk too much, and lose the interest of the jury. Instead, they should just answer the question, elaborating only to make a crucial point of clarification. Referencing scientific literature can be helpful, as long as it is done objectively and not too broadly. For example, rather than stating that:

> "The literature suggests that there are no long-term sequelae whatsoever of mild TBI."

It may be better to be more specific by saying:

> "The most comprehensive, recent reviews in the literature, such as done by Babikian and colleagues out of UCLA, suggest that the vast majority of children with uncomplicated mild TBI do not have any long-term deficits, and that in those who do, there are almost always preexisting or other factors that are unrelated to the brain and that influenced recovery."

Humor can be used occasionally during answering questions but only very sparingly, and preferably not at the expense of the opposing attorney (i.e., no lawyer jokes) or anything that might be construed as derogative with regard to the child or parents. It is acceptable to repeat something to make a specific point, but again this should be done sparingly, in order to avoid coming across as argumentative or closed-minded. If opposing counsels argue amongst themselves about particular objections or other legal procedures, the PN should stay out of it and let them come to an agreement. In a courtroom, it is perfectly permissible to turn to the judge for guidance before answering a question.

9 *Stay within your areas of expertise.*

If the PN is asked about data or records that are not within his or her area of expertise, this should be simply stated and further comment should be refused. For example, it is permissible to acknowledge that the child broke multiple bones in the accident but the PN should not offer expert opinions about measures of bone density or the surgical technique used to repair the fractures. Sometimes, peripherally related information may be introduced that has the potential to confuse or mislead the judge or jury. In that case, the PN should address this by bringing the focus back on topics related to neuropsychology. For example, pictures of the car may be shown in which the child sustained an uncomplicated TBI, along with close-ups of specific damage to the car, in an apparent attempt to suggest the presence of a more significant neurological injury. One proper way to address this would be:

> "These pictures tell me a lot about that car; it looks pretty banged up and I doubt that it is still drivable. But then again, I am not an expert on cars. More importantly, these pictures tell me nothing about the child or how serious the injuries were that he sustained. For that, I have to rely on the emergency room records."

10 *Be aware of binary questions.*

It is not uncommon for a PN to be asked to answer a question with "yes" or "no." If this can be done easily and unequivocally, then the requested type of answer should be provided. If not, then the PN should say so and express a need to elaborate briefly. In addition, a specific way of answering such questions in an active manner would be to use dependent clauses at the beginning of the answer, such as "although" or "whereas." For example, let's assume the question is phrased as: "Are there a lot of children who were never exposed to lead who have learning disabilities—yes or no?" A passive answer would be:

> "Yes."

Instead, an active answer would be:

> "Although it is indeed possible for children to have a learning disability in the absence of any lead poisoning, my review of John's school records—both before and after the lead exposure—clearly suggests a significant drop in standardized test scores. Given the fact that there were no other complicating factors, I consider it most likely that the lead poisoning was responsible for that decline."

This is what Brodsky (1991) calls the admit/deny technique. The first part of the answer specifically admits the true component of the question but the second part confidently denies any untrue implications that might result from a passive or binary answer. A related way of answering is what Brodsky calls the push/pull technique, which means that when the attorney pushes, the PN answers by pulling in the same direction while immediately providing important additional information. For example, the PN may be asked: "Did you even bother to talk to this child's teacher, or to her coach, who will both be called to testify in this case? Did you?" A defensive and likely ineffective reaction would be:

> "Well no, there really was not any time for that. I had a lot of tests to do."

Instead, a more effective way of answering would be to "pull" the example in a more extreme direction and then to "push" back by qualifying the statement. Something like:

> "Not only did I not talk to her teacher or her coach, I also did not call her grandmother or her parish priest. I talked to her, and to her parents, and I read her school and medical records, just like I would with any other child I saw in my office."

11 *Address successive yes/no questions.*

Sometimes, the PN may be asked a series of questions that may seem innocent and then get into a pattern of responding "yes" or "no" to each one. It remains important to listen carefully to each new alternative because it would not be unusual for one term or possibility to be thrown in that the PN would otherwise not agree with. In addition, it may be prudent to preface one's answer by putting it in context. For example, if a PN were asked: "Can children with TBI have problems with amnesia? With intense headaches? With gross irritability? With . . . ?" it would be inadvisable to simply answer "Yes" to each item. Instead, a more active and effective way of answering might be:

> "Let's first be clear about what we're talking about—severe TBI or mild TBI, which is what Jane had? And are we talking about right after injury or more than a year later, like we are now? I ask, because my answers would be different."

12 *Deal with the alleged superiority of the treating doctor.*
Sometimes, an independent expert PN for the defense may be challenged by plaintiff's counsel that "their" doctor has been seeing the child for medical care or psychotherapy on multiple occasions, instead of only a one-time evaluation by the PN. Again, the PN should not get defensive about this but simply restate the basis for his or her professional opinion. For example:

> "I respectfully disagree that just because Dr. Jones has seen John more than once makes him a better judge of his current status. Two different radiologists have read John's CT and MRI scans as entirely unremarkable. That makes no difference, regardless of whether or not they knew John from before the accident. Furthermore, Dr. Jones did not perform the comprehensive assessment of John's mental abilities that I did. Those data were objectively compared to John's peers and they pretty much speak for themselves: They are all within normal limits."

13 *Answer the question: "Is it authoritative?"*
A PN may be asked during cross-examination whether the work of a particular author is familiar and whether it would be considered "authoritative." Simply saying "yes" to that question can be misconstrued as deferring to any opinions that are stated in that particularly referenced work, with excerpts sometimes presented out of context. Instead, the author or the work can be acknowledged, while still making it clear that this does not mean that the PN simply defers to it. An effective answer might be:

> "I have Dr. Jones' book in my office. I have even found it occasionally helpful, just like I rely on many other books and articles to stay informed about the field of lead poisoning, but that does not mean that I necessarily agree with everything Dr. Jones has written. Which particular part of her book do you want me to comment on? I would just need a minute to read that part again."

14 *Answer the question: "Is it possible?"*
Another common scenario is that the PN is asked if it is "possible" that this particular child might have a certain symptom or condition. Simply acknowledging that something is "possible," without further qualification, may be perceived or misconstrued as supporting a position that may not actually be the PN's opinion. For example, in response to the question: "Isn't it possible, doctor, to have neuropsychological problems for several years after TBI?" the PN might answer:

> "This would be common with severe TBI but not with uncomplicated mild TBI, which is what we are dealing with here. I cannot rule it out with 100% certainty but I would consider it extremely unlikely unless there were other factors, like prior behavioral problems or family stress, that could have hindered recovery."

15 *Leave in a dignified manner.*
After conclusion of any deposition or trial testimony, the PN should leave the proceedings in a professional manner. Shaking hands, not only with the retaining attorney but also with the opposing attorney, would show courtesy at the end of a deposition. In a courtroom, the PN should wait until after having been excused by the judge, after which he or she may simply say "Thank you, Your Honor," briefly nod to the jury, and then walk out. The PN should not try to find out later who received a favorable verdict or how much money was awarded. That would have nothing to do with the business of evidence-based forensic work, and might cloud the PN's level of professional and scientific objectivity in future cases. If the retaining attorney is pleased with the PN's work, increased future referrals will likely result, anyway. For the novice PN who is deposed or appearing in court for the first time, however, it may be helpful to have the testimony observed by a senior colleague, to receive constructive performance feedback at some later point.

Conclusion

PNs can make important contributions to the accurate evaluation of children in a forensic context, as long as they adhere to an ethical and scientifically defensible approach, without personalized investment in the outcome of the legal proceedings. It is important to be aware of not only the current state of the literature on the condition of interest but also of basic legal contingencies and proceedings as well as of general psychometric and specific performance/symptom validity issues. The PN who offers clear, intelligible, and evidence-based written and oral reports to the legal system serves not only the neuropsychological profession but also the public.

References

American Academy of Clinical Neuropsychology. (2001). Policy statement on the presence of third party observers in neuropsychological assessment. *The Clinical Neuropsychologist*, *15*, 433–439.

American Psychiatric Association. (2013). *Diagnostic and Statistical Manual of Mental Disorders* (5th ed.). Arlington, VA: American Psychiatric Association.

American Psychological Association. (2002). Ethical principles of psychologists and code of conduct. *American Psychologist*, *57*, 1060–1073.

Attix, D. K., Donders, J., Johnson-Greene, D., Grote, C. L., Harris, J. G., & Bauer, R. M. (2007). Disclosure of neuropsychological test data: Official position of division 40 (Clinical

Neuropsychology) of the American Psychological Association, Association of Postdoctoral Programs in Clinical Neuropsychology, and American Academy of Clinical Neuropsychology. *The Clinical Neuropsychologist*, *21*, 232–238.

Baer, R. A., Kroll, L. S., Rinaldo, J., & Ballenger, J. (1999). Detecting and discriminating between random responding and overreporting on the MMPI—A. *Journal of Personality Assessment*, *72*, 308–320.

Bianchini, K. J., Greve, K. W., & Glynn, G. (2005). On the diagnosis of malingered pain-related disability: Lessons from cognitive malingering research. *The Spine Journal*, *5*, 404–417.

Binder, L. M., Iverson, G. L., & Brooks, B. L. (2009). To err is human: "abnormal" neuropsychological scores and variability are common in healthy adults. *Archives of Clinical Neuropsychology*, *24*, 31–46.

Blaskewitz, N., Merten, T., & Kathmann, N. (2008). Performance of children on symptom validity tests: TOMM, MSVT, and FIT. *Archives of Clinical Neuropsychology*, *23*, 379–391.

Boone, K. B. (2007). *Assessment of Feigned Cognitive Impairment: A Neuropsychological Perspective*. New York: Guilford.

Brodsky, S. L. (1991). *Testifying in Court: Guidelines and Maxims for the Expert Witness*. Washington, DC: American Psychological Association.

Brodsky, S. L. (1999). *The Expert Witness: More Maxims and Guidelines for Testifying in Court*. Washington, DC: American Psychological Association.

Brodsky, S. L. (2004). *Coping With Cross-Examination and Other Pathways to Effective Testimony*. Washington, DC: American Psychological Association.

Brooks, B. L. (2010). Seeing the forest for the trees: Prevalence of low scores on the Wechsler Intelligence Scale for Children, Fourth Edition (WISC-IV). *Psychological Assessment*, *22*, 650–656.

Brooks, B. L. (2012). Victoria symptom validity test performance in children and adolescents with neurological disorders. *Archives of Clinical Neuropsychology*, *27*(8), 858–868.

Brooks, B. L., Holdnack, J. A., & Iverson, G. L. (2011). Advanced clinical interpretation of the WAIS-IV and WMS-IV: Prevalence of low scores varies by level of intelligence and years of education. *Assessment*, *18*, 156–167.

Brooks, B. L., & Iverson, G. L. (2012). Improving accuracy when identifying cognitive impairment in pediatric neuropsychological assessments. In E.M.S. Sherman & B. L. Brooks (Eds.), *Pediatric Forensic Neuropsychology* (pp. 66–88). New York: Oxford.

Brooks, B. L., Iverson, G. L., & Holdnack, J. A. (2013a). Understanding multivariate base rates. In J. A. Holdnack, L. Drozdick, L. G. Weiss, & G. L. Iverson (Eds.), *WAIS-IV, WMS-IV, & ACS: Clinical Use and Interpretation* (pp. 75–102). New York: Elsevier.

Brooks, B. L., Iverson, G. L., Koushik, N. S., Mazur-Mosiewicz, A., Horton, A. M., Jr., & Reynolds, C. R. (2013b). Prevalence of low scores in children and adolescents on the test of verbal conceptualization and fluency. *Applied Neuropsychology: Child*, *2*, 70–77.

Brooks, B. L., Iverson, G. L., Sherman, E. M., & Holdnack, J. A. (2009). Healthy children and adolescents obtain some low scores across a battery of memory tests. *Journal of the International Neuropsychological Society*, *15*, 613–617.

Brooks, B. L., Iverson, G. L., Sherman, E. M., & Roberge, M. C. (2010a). Identifying cognitive problems in children and adolescents with depression using computerized neuropsychological testing. *Applied Neuropsychology*, *17*, 37–43.

Brooks, B. L., & Sherman, E. M. (2012). Computerized neuropsychological testing to rapidly evaluate cognition in pediatric patients with neurologic disorders. *Journal of Child Neurology*, *27*, 982–991.

Brooks, B. L., Sherman, E.M.S., & Iverson, G. L. (2010b). Healthy children get some low scores too: Prevalence of low scores on the NEPSY-II in preschoolers, children, and adolescents. *Archives of Clinical Neuropsychology*, *25*, 182–190.

Brooks, B. L., Sherman, E.M.S., & Krol, A. L. (2012). Utility of TOMM Trial 1 as an indicator of effort in children and adolescents. *Archives of Clinical Neuropsychology*, *27*, 23–29.

Bush, S. S., Ruff, R. M., Troster, A. I., Barth, J. T., Koffler, S. P., Pliskin, N. H., . . . Silver, C. H. (2005). Symptom validity assessment: Practice issues and medical necessity NAN policy & planning committee. *Archives of Clinical Neuropsychology*, *20*, 419–426.

Carone, D. A. (2008). Children with moderate/severe brain damage/dysfunction outperform adults with mild-to-no brain damage on the Medical Symptom Validity Test. *Brain Injury*, *22*, 960–971.

Chafetz, M. D. (2008). Malingering on the Social Security disability consultative exam: Predictors and base rates. *The Clinical Neuropsychologist*, *22*, 529–546.

Chafetz, M. D., Abrahams, J. P., & Kohlmaier, J. (2007). Malingering on the Social Security disability consultative exam: A new rating scale. *Archives of Clinical Neuropsychology*, *22*, 1–14.

Chafetz, M. D., & Prentkowski, E. (2011). A case of malingering by proxy in a Social Security disability psychological consultative examination. *Applied Neuropsychology*, *18*, 143–149.

Cohen, M. J. (1997). *Children's Memory Scale*. San Antonio, TX: Psychological Corporation.

Constantinou, M., Ashendorf, L., & McCaffrey, R. J. (2005). Effects of a third party observer during neuropsychological assessment: When the observer is a video camera. *Journal of Forensic Neuropsychology*, *4*, 39–48.

Constantinou, M., & McCaffrey, R. J. (2003). Using the TOMM for evaluating children's effort to perform optimally on neuropsychological measures. *Child Neuropsychology*, *9*, 81–90.

Crawford, J. R., Garthwaite, P. H., & Gault, C. B. (2007). Estimating the percentage of the population with abnormally low scores (or abnormally large score differences) on standardized neuropsychological test batteries: A generic method with applications. *Neuropsychology*, *21*, 419–430.

Devlin, B., Daniels, M., & Roeder, K. (1997). The heritability of IQ. *Nature*, *388*, 468–471.

Donders, J. (2005). Performance on the Test of Memory Malingering in a mixed pediatric sample. *Child Neuropsychology*, *11*, 221–227.

Donders, J. (2012). Forensic considerations. In M. W. Kirkwood & K. O. Yeates (Eds.), *Mild Traumatic Brain Injury in Children and Adolescents* (pp. 374–390). New York: Guilford.

Flaro, L., & Boone, K. (2009). Using objective effort measures to detect noncredible cognitive test performance in children and adolescents. In J. Morgan & J. Sweet (Eds.), *Neuropsychology of Malingering Casebook* (pp. 369–376). New York: Psychology Press.

Gast, J., & Hart, K. J. (2010). The performance of juvenile offenders on the Test of Memory Malingering. *Journal of Forensic Psychology Practice*, *10*, 53–68.

Green, P. (2004). *Manual for the Medical Symptom Validity Test*. Edmonton: Green's Publishing.

Greiffenstein, M. F., & Kaufmann, P. M. (2012). Neuropsychology and the law: Principles of productive attorney-neuropsychologist relations. In G. L. Larrabee (Ed.), *Forensic Neuropsychology: A Scientific Approach* (2nd ed., pp. 23–69). New York: Oxford.

Gunn, D., Batchelor, J., & Jones, M. (2010). Detection of simulated memory impairment in 6- to 11-year-old children. *Child Neuropsychology*, *16*, 105–118.

Harrison, A. G., Rosenblum, Y., & Currie, S. (2010). Examining unusual digit span performance in a population of postsecondary students assessed for academic difficulties. *Assessment*, *17*, 283–293.

Heilbronner, R. L., Sweet, J. J., Morgan, J. E., Larrabee, G. J., & Millis, S. R. (2009). American Academy of Clinical Neuropsychology consensus conference statement on the neuropsychological assessment of effort, response bias, and malingering. *The Clinical Neuropsychologist*, *23*, 1093–1129.

Henry, G. K. (2005). Childhood malingering: Faking neuropsychological impairment in an 8-year-old. In J. Morgan & J. Sweet (Eds.), *Neuropsychology of Malingering Casebook* (pp. 205–217). New York: Guilford.

Howe, L. L. S., & McCaffrey, R. J. (2010). Third party observation during neuropsychological evaluation: An update on the literature, practical advice for practitioners, and future directions. *The Clinical Neuropsychologist*, *24*, 518–537.

Hurks, P. P., Hendriksen, J. G., Dek, J. E., & Kooij, A. P. (2013). Normal variability of children's scaled scores on subtests of the Dutch Wechsler Preschool and Primary scale of Intelligence—third edition. *The Clinical Neuropsychologist*, *27*, 988–1003.

Kirk, J. W., Harris, B., Hutaff-Lee, C. F., Koelemay, S. W., Dinkins, J. P., & Kirkwood, M. W. (2011). Performance on the Test Of Memory Malingering (TOMM) among a large clinic-referred pediatric sample. *Child Neuropsychology*, *17*, 242–254.

Kirk, J. W., Hutaff-Lee, C., Connery, A. K., Baker, D. A., & Kirkwood, M. W. (2014). The relationship between the self-report BASC-2 validity indicators and performance validity test failure after pediatric mild traumatic brain injury. *Assessment*, *21*, 562–569.

Kirkwood, M. W. (2012). Overview of tests and techniques to detect negative response bias in children. In E. Sherman & B. Brooks (Eds.), *Pediatric Forensic Neuropsychology* (pp. 136–161). New York: Oxford.

Kirkwood, M. W., Connery, A. K., Kirk, J. W., & Baker, D. A. (2014). Detecting performance invalidity in children: Not quite as easy as A, B, C, 1, 2, 3 but automatized sequences appears promising. *Child Neuropsychology*, *20*, 245–252. doi: 10.1080/09297049.2012.759553

Kirkwood, M. W., & Kirk, J. W. (2010). The base rate of suboptimal effort in a pediatric mild TBI sample: Performance on the Medical Symptom Validity Test. *The Clinical Neuropsychologist*, *24*, 860–872.

Kirkwood, M. W., Kirk, J. W., Blaha, R. Z., & Wilson, P. E. (2010). Noncredible effort during pediatric neuropsychological exam: A case series and literature review. *Child Neuropsychology*, *16*, 604–618.

Kirkwood, M. W., Yeates, K. O., Randolph, C., & Kirk, J. W. (2012). The implications of symptom validity test failure for ability-based test performance in a pediatric sample. *Psychological Assessment*, *24*, 36–45.

Larrabee, G. J. (2012). Performance validity and symptom validity in neuropsychological assessment. *Journal of the International Neuropsychological Society*, *18*, 625–630.

Lu, P. H., & Boone, K. B. (2002). Suspect cognitive symptoms in a 9-year-old child: Malingering by proxy? *The Clinical Neuropsychologist*, *16*, 90–96.

Lucio, E., Duran, C., Graham, J. R., & Ben-Porath, Y. S. (2002). Identifying faking bad on the Minnesota Multiphasic Personality Inventory—Adolescent with Mexican adolescents. *Assessment*, *9*, 62–69.

Lynch, J. K. (2005). Effects of a third party observer on neuropsychological test performance following closed head injury. *Journal of Forensic Neuropsychology*, *4*, 17–25.

MacAllister, W. S., Nakhutina, L., Bender, H. A., Karantzoulis, S., & Carlson, C. (2009). Assessing effort during neuropsychological evaluation with the TOMM in children and adolescents with epilepsy. *Child Neuropsychology*, *15*, 521–531.

McCaffrey, R. J., & Lynch, J. K. (2009). Malingering following documented brain injury: Neuropsychological evaluation of children in a forensic setting. In J. Morgan & J. Sweet (Eds.), *Neuropsychology of Malingering Casebook* (pp. 377–385). New York: Psychology Press.

Mittenberg, W., Patton, C., Canyock, E. M., & Condit, D. C. (2002). Base rates of malingering and symptom exaggeration. *Journal of Clinical and Experimental Neuropsychology*, *24*, 1094–1102.

Nagle, A. M., Everhart, D. E., Durham, T. W., McCammon, S. L., & Walker, M. (2006). Deception strategies in children: Examination of forced choice recognition and verbal learning and memory techniques. *Archives of Clinical Neuropsychology*, *21*, 777–785.

National Academy of Clinical Neuropsychology. (2000). Presence of third party observers during neuropsychological testing: Official statement of the National Academy of Neuropsychology. *Archives of Clinical Neuropsychology*, *15*, 379–380.

Perna, R. B., & Loughan, A. R. (2013). Children and the Test of Memory Malingering: Is one trial enough? *Child Neuropsychology*, *19*, 438–447.

Rienstra, A., Spaan, P. E., & Schmand, B. (2010). Validation of symptom validity tests using a "child-model" of adult cognitive impairments. *Archives of Clinical Neuropsychology*, *25*, 371–382.

Rogers, R., Hinds, J. D., & Sewell, K. W. (1996, October). Feigning psychopathology among adolescent offenders: Validation of the SIRS, MMPI-A, and SIMS. *Journal of Personality Assessment*, *67*, 244–257.

Schoenberg, M. R., Lange, R. T., Brickell, T. A., & Saklofske, D. H. (2007). Estimating premorbid general cognitive functioning for children and adolescents using the American Wechsler Intelligence Scale for Children-Fourth Edition: Demographic and current performance approaches. *Journal of Child Neurology*, *22*, 379–388.

Schoenberg, M. R., Lange, R. T., & Saklofske, D. H. (2007). A proposed method to estimate premorbid Full Scale Intelligence Quotient (FSIQ) for the Canadian Wechsler Intelligence Scale for Children-Fourth Edition (WISC-IV) using demographic and combined estimation procedures. *Journal of Clinical and Experimental Neuropsychology*, *29*, 867–878.

Slick, D. J., Sherman, E., & Iverson, G. (1999). Diagnostic criteria for malingered neurocognitive dysfunction: Proposed standards for clinical practice and research. *The Clinical Neuropsychologist*, *13*, 545–561.

Slick, D. J., & Sherman, E.M.S. (2012). Differential diagnosis of malingering and related clinical presentations. In E.M.S. Sherman & B. L. Brooks (Eds.), *Pediatric Forensic Neuropsychology* (pp. 113–135). New York: Oxford.

Stein, L. A., Graham, J. R., & Williams, C. L. (1995). Detecting fake-bad MMPI-A profiles. *Journal of Personality Assessment*, *65*, 415–427.

Stone, J., LaFrance, W. C., Brown, R., Spiegel, D., Levenson, J. L., & Sharpe, M. (2011). Conversion disorder: Current problems and potential solutions for DSM—5. *Journal of Psychosomatic Research*, *71*, 369–376.

Suhr, J., Hammers, D., Dobbins-Buckland, K., Zimak, E., & Hughes, C. (2008). The relationship of malingering test failure to self-reported symptoms and neuropsychological findings in adults referred for ADHD evaluation. *Archives of Clinical Neuropsychology*, *23*, 521–530.

Suhr, J. A., Sullivan, B. K., & Rodriguez, J. L. (2011). The relationship of noncredible performance to continuous performance test scores in adults referred for attention-deficit/hyperactivity disorder evaluation. *Archives of Clinical Neuropsychology*, *26*, 1–7.

Sullivan, B. K., May, K., & Galbally, L. (2007). Symptom exaggeration by college adults in attention-deficit hyperactivity disorder and learning disorder assessments. *Applied Neuropsychology*, *14*, 189–207.

Sweet, J. J., & Moulthrop, M. A. (1999). Self-examination questions as a means of identifying bias in adversarial assessments. *Journal of Forensic Neuropsychology*, *1*, 73–88.

Thomas, S. V., Sukumaran, S., Lukose, N., George, A., & Sarma, P. S. (2007). Intellectual and language functions in children of mothers with epilepsy. *Epilepsia*, *48*, 2234–2240.

Tombaugh, T. N. (1996). *Test of Memory Malingering*. North Tonawanda, NY: Multi-Health Systems.

Tsushima, W. T., & Anderson, R. M. (1996). *Mastering Expert Testimony: A Courtroom Handbook for Mental Health Professionals*. Mahwah, NJ: Lawrence Erlbaum.

Van Gorp, W. G., & McMullen, W. J. (1997). Potential sources of bias in forensic neuropsychological evaluations. *The Clinical Neuropsychologist*, *11*, 180–187.

Wechsler, D. (2003). *Wechsler Intelligence Scale for Children, Fourth Edition: Technical and Interpretive Manual*. San Antonio, TX: Psychological Corporation.

Wechsler, D. (2010). *WPPSI-III-NL Nederlandstalige Bewerking: Technische Handleiding [Dutch Version of the WPPSI-III-NL: Technical and Interpretive Manual] (Dutch Adaptation by: Hendriksen, J., & Hurks, P., 2010)* (2nd ed.). Amsterdam, Netherlands: Pearson.

Wrobel, T. A., Lachar, D., Wrobel, N. H., Morgan, S. T., & Gruber, C. P. (1999). Performance of the Personality Inventory for Youth validity scales. *Assessment*, *6*, 367–380.

40 Clinical Neuropsychology in Criminal Forensics

Robert L. Denney, Rachel L. Fazio, and Manfred F. Greiffenstein

The inclusion of this chapter within the second edition of the *Textbook of Clinical Neuropsychology* reflects the increased awareness of neuropsychology's role and increasing presence within the criminal forensic setting. In the first book devoted solely to this subject, Kaufmann (2008) noted the 54% of published legal cases citing expert testimony from neuropsychologists over the preceding decade were criminal cases. This finding suggests neuropsychologists are, indeed, commonly involved in criminal matters. It should create no surprise then that neuropsychologists are involved in the assessment of criminal forensic issues as the demands placed on criminal defendants are largely cognitive. When liberty and due process interests are at stake, as is the case in criminal proceedings, the law demands a specific level of functional ability of defendants. They need to be able to understand their situation, their rights, and make knowing decisions for themselves. Neuropsychologists are positioned quite well to address these issues for the trier of fact, that is, either a judge or jury. Neuropsychologists are only helpful, however, when they understand the nature of the presented questions, which are rather unique in the criminal forensic setting.

The application of neuropsychological principles to criminal forensic issues requires knowledge outside the standard venue of clinical practice because issues before the trier of fact in the criminal setting generally have specific standards in law (Melton et al., 2007). Consequently, it is incumbent for neuropsychologists who choose to practice in this area to gain additional familiarity of the legal issues involved in order to practice competently (Sullivan & Denney, 2008). With that caveat in mind, this chapter will highlight the most common aspects of criminal forensics in which neuropsychologists become involved.

We will initially present the important theoretical and methodological differences between forensic neuropsychology compared to clinical neuropsychology, particularly as it relates to criminal matters, and touch on the assessment process. We will then review specific content areas and criminal legal standards. These topics include criminal competencies, criminal responsibility, diminished capacity and responsibility, dangerousness, and death penalty issues. We will then close by addressing common ethical concerns.

Theoretically Driven Practice of Criminal Forensic Neuropsychology

There are striking differences inherent within the context of forensic psychology compared to clinical psychology. These differences are equally present when considering clinical neuropsychology and forensic neuropsychology. The goal in good clinical evaluation is most commonly the alleviation of human suffering through proper diagnosis and establishment of intervention plans. The goal in forensic assessment is most commonly whether or not an examinee's mental status meets a particular legal standard. It is not unusual for experts to provide information that may assist the court in obtaining proper treatment for the examinee; however, the end goal even in this situation is the improvement of the examinee's mental status in order for the defendant to complete a specific legal process or answer a legal question—*nothing more*. The issue is almost always about answering a specific question for the trier of fact. Forensic examinations are not primarily about helping the examinee, but rather, answering the question posed by the referral source. This different goal creates a different set of assumptions, roles, alliances, and methods.

Assumptions

The assumption in clinical practice is that patients want to get better. They seek services from psychologists because they are having emotional hurt (symptoms) or functional impairment and want help in either dealing with them or making them go away. It is often presumed that they have a diagnosable condition because they would not have made the effort to seek help if the difficulty was not clinically significant. However, in criminal forensics, the defendants are not self-referred, or even voluntary in many instances. Additionally, the possibility of harsh criminal punishment creates a significant incentive for criminal defendants to manipulate the evaluator in order to alter the course of the adjudicative process. It is counterproductive to assume criminal defendants want to be freed from difficult symptoms or neurocognitive impairments; research suggests that many manipulate in order to improve their life situations (Ardolf, Denney, & Houston, 2007). The difference in assumptions between clinical and forensic assessment directly relates to different roles for neuropsychologists.

Roles

The clinical evaluator seeks to maintain a helper role based on the assumption the patient is in distress and is seeking help. If fact, this is oftentimes the reason psychologists entered the mental health field in the first place, to serve in the role of patient-helper. In contrast, the forensic evaluator attempts to maintain a role consistent with a "seeker of truth" and educator to the trier of fact. As a seeker of truth, the evaluator cannot be biased by the desire to help the criminal defendant, but as a goal must maintain objectivity in seeking the truth in the situation (Saks, 1990). In many instances the findings of the neuropsychologist may not help the criminal defendant and indeed, the findings may actually do more "harm" to the defendant than good. In many instances the consequences are great as is demonstrated in the situation of evaluating a defendant facing a life sentence or even a potential death penalty. The roles can too easily become blurred when clinicians who are used to performing in the clinical setting enter the forensic setting; forensic evaluators must understand and remain true to the role for which they have been called (Bush, Connell, & Denney, 2006). The unique role of the forensic evaluator requires maintaining the proper alliance.

Alliance

Although a therapeutic alliance is at the core of providing excellent clinical services, forensic neuropsychological examinations are not therapeutic endeavors. Hence, developing a therapeutic alliance is not appropriate during forensic examinations. The forensic examiner's allegiance should remain with seeking the truth, not creating a therapeutic alliance with the defendant. On more than one occasion we have seen well-intended psychologists abandon the role of objective evaluator and act like the primary emotional support for the defendant—even having an arm around the defendant in an emotionally supportive manner during courtroom proceedings! Dispensing with the therapeutic alliance does not obviate the need to develop a working rapport with the defendant. Forensic examiners must develop and maintain a professional relationship with the defendant based upon dignity and respect. Rapport is needed in order to foster disclosure and help motivate the criminal defendant to perform his or her best during cognitive testing. It is possible to maintain the strict boundaries inherent in a forensic examination while at the same time maintaining a professional and ethical relationship with the criminal defendant.

Methodology

The proper assumptions lead the way for a proper role and alliance, which set the stage for proper methodology. The common and acceptable practice in the clinical setting is rarely appropriate methodology within the criminal forensic setting. A clinical interview and testing is sufficient in many clinical settings, but such simple methods are ineffectual in a setting where one cannot place the same weight of credibility on self-report. Those methods may be adequate to assist the patient, his or her caregivers, medical managers, and family in a timely fashion, but they do not correspond with the assumptions, roles, and goals inherent with forensic examinations. Clinical neuropsychologists who start to practice in the forensic setting must understand the differences between clinical practice and criminal forensic practice.

Similarities and Differences Between Clinical and Criminal Forensic Practice

Some of the issues mentioned so far are likely not entirely novel to the clinical neuropsychologist; for example, variable effort or malingering is also present in other contexts. While clinical and criminal forensic practices have substantial overlap, there are also substantial differences. As illustrated in Table 40.1, the differences may be quite striking to those unfamiliar with criminal forensic work.

Table 40.1 Similarities and differences between clinical and criminal forensic practice

Similarities	*Differences*
Avoid conflicts of interest and dual relationships	• The individual being evaluated is typically not the client; there is no "feedback session." • Typically all communication is through the court or lawyers rather than with the individual being assessed. • One should take care to avoid fee arrangements which could create bias towards one party.
Appreciate individual and group differences	• A higher standard exists for test selection and administration in light of cultural issues given the weight of the matters involved.
Evaluees must be notified of the nature and purpose of the evaluation, including limits to confidentiality	• Many evaluees are not voluntary, and they may not have to participate for the evaluation to proceed. • There is limited confidentiality.
The referral question should be answered	• *Only* the referral question should be addressed—to open other issues would be problematic both ethically and for the court. • In clinical evaluations, there is a focus on diagnosis—in forensic evaluations, it may not be necessary to include a diagnosis in the report. • The evaluator may or may not be allowed to answer the "ultimate issue" depending on what the issue is and the jurisdiction.
Appropriate records should be maintained and only disclosed to appropriate parties	• It may be necessary to retain records for a much longer period of time for criminal forensic cases, as appeals can take decades. • One must typically comply with subpoenas and other requests for information while ensuring it is used in the appropriate manner.

Forensic Evaluation Process

The practice of criminal forensic neuropsychology is particularly unique because it is not uncommon for experts to be asked to formulate an opinion that deals with a criminal defendant's past behavior. The most common of such instances is criminal responsibility (also known as an evaluation of sanity). Evaluations of past events can also include the ability to form prerequisite intent to perform the alleged criminal behavior and retrospective competencies, such as understanding *Miranda* warning, waiving the right to remain silent and confessing to a crime, and competency to stand trial, enter a guilty plea, or be sentenced. All of these particular evaluations require the examiner to understand a past mental state of the defendant.

Although we will discuss each of the specific legal criteria related to the evaluations described in the upcoming sections, each of them require the same methodological process to ensure a thorough examination and proper outcome. Figure 40.1 provides a graphic display of sources of information commonly needed to provide retrospective forensic formulations. The model highlights the key issue that information should come from self-report and corroborative information specific to each period of time: present, historical, and at the time in question. The first two columns represent necessary information from both the defendant and corroborative sources. Each row represents a different period in time. Information from each box in a particular column should make some logical sense as far as consistency with information from other sources in other boxes within that column, just as each row should have some logical consistency from left to right. Self-report and corroborative information for the present should be reasonably consistent. Self-report and corroborative information for the defendant's past should be reasonably consistent. Self-report and corroborative information for the specific time in question should be reasonably consistent as well. The examiner can have significantly more confidence regarding the clinical opinion when both self-report and corroborative information coincides. For example when a defendant is behaving in a manner presently that suggests a severe mental illness such as

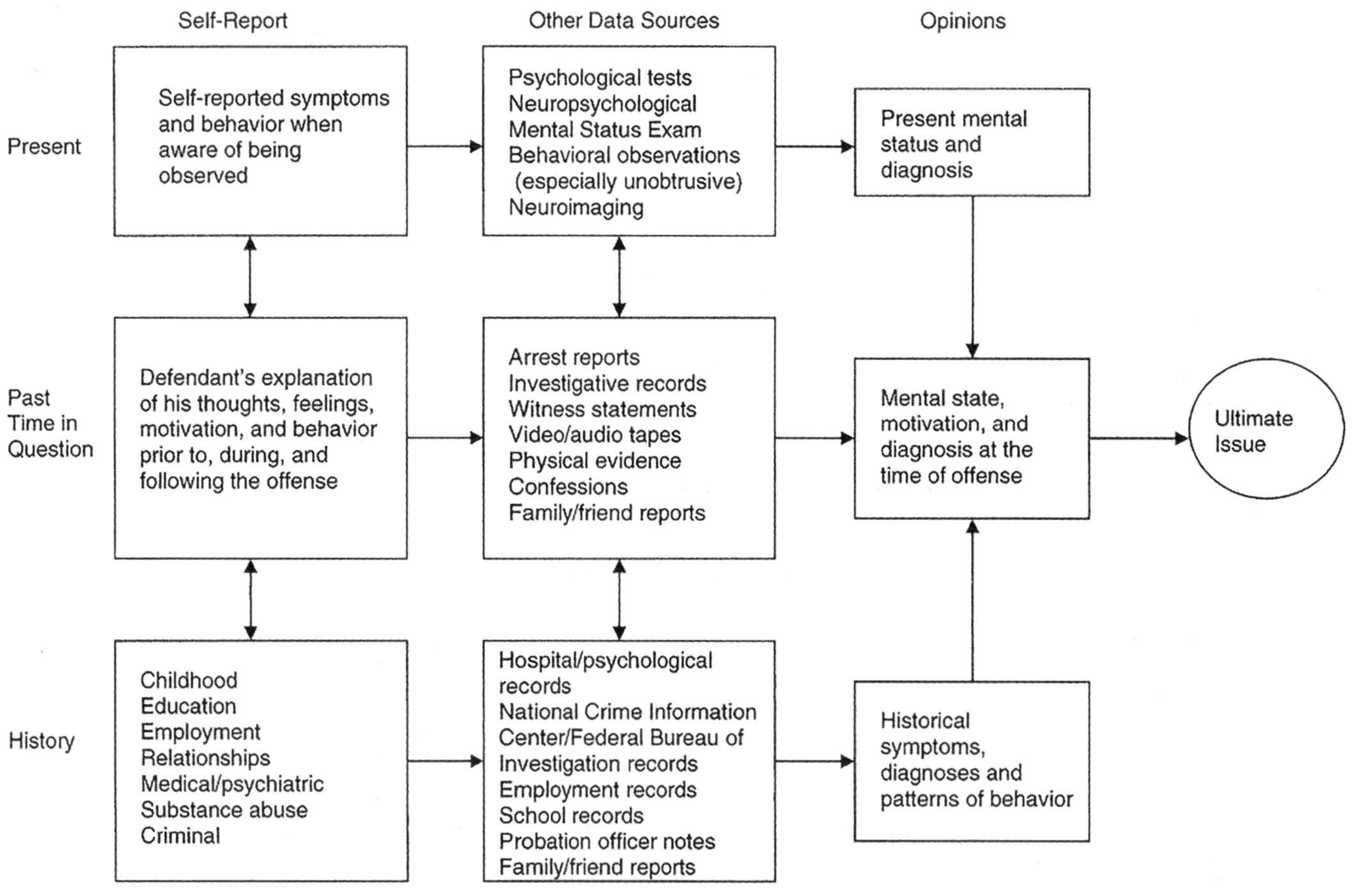

Figure 40.1 Multiple data source model for the assessment of past mental states. The left-hand column indicates period of time in question. Connecting lines represent avenues of expected consistency, with arrows leading toward opinions. The ultimate issue signifies the expert's opinion on the sanity (it could also represent an opinion on other *mens rea* defenses or retrospective competencies such as the *Miranda* waiver, competency to confess or stand trial). Reproduced with permission of David Mrad, PhD.

schizophrenia, the self-report and corroborative information regarding the defendant's history should be consistent with the proper age of onset for that condition. Those two specific rows then also support what the defendant's mental state was like at the time in question, such as during an alleged offense, but corroborative information regarding his or her behavior at that time in question must also be consistent with that clinical picture. The examiner can only provide a competent opinion regarding the ultimate issue after arriving at a clinical opinion pertaining to each of these three periods in time. This multiple data source model was originally conceptualized by Mrad (1996) then adapted to neuropsychology (Denney & Wynkoop, 2000) and personal injury assessment (McLearen, Pietz, & Denney, 2004). One of us (RLD) has also presented this model in the criminal arena elsewhere (Denney, 2005, 2012b; Yates & Denney, 2008).

Criminal Competencies

Competency is the ability to understand and make reasonably knowledgeable decisions, and it is the question forensic neuropsychologists (FNs) will be asked to answer most often in the criminal setting. While those decisions do not necessarily need to reflect what one might consider the best judgment, they must reflect a knowing and intelligent choice among alternatives. The minimal level of understanding includes some sense of appreciation for the nature of the procedure, risks, a sense of likelihood of success, available alternatives, and the relative advantages and disadvantages of any available course of action (Denney, 2012a). It has been a long held requirement within the United States that criminal defendants must be competent to face criminal prosecution (Youtsey, 1899). In other words, defendants cannot progress through the criminal adjudication process unless they understand the nature of the proceedings and can assist in their own defense. The only exception to this rule is when the Court must stop the proceedings to determine competency and facilitate appropriate treatment to restore competency in the event the defendant is determined not competent to proceed.

The question of a defendant's competency to proceed can arise at any point in the adjudicative process from hearing a *Miranda* warning from a police officer, standing trial, waiving the appeals process, to even facing a lethal injection. Table 40.2 highlights common points when competency to proceed is often questioned as well as the general competency related principle in question for that period of time.

The reader may notice that "understand and appreciate" are the prevailing concepts pertaining to competency to proceed regardless of the specifics in question. These concepts derive, in large part, from the primary source of competency determination, *Dusky v. United States* (1960).

Table 40.2 Specific competencies in criminal adjudication

Competency To:	*General Concept at Issue*
Confess (or to Waive Rights at Pretrial Investigations)	Understanding and appreciation of rights to silence and legal counsel when the rights may be waived at the request of law enforcement investigators seeking a self-incriminating statement
Plead Guilty	Understanding and appreciating of above, and of the right to a jury trial, the right to confront one's accusers, and the consequences of a conviction
Waive Right to Counsel	Understanding and appreciation of the dangers of self-representation at trial
Stand Trial	Ability to assist an attorney in developing and presenting a defense, and to understand the nature of the trial and its potential consequences
Acting as One's Own Counsel During Trial	Understanding and appreciating of above, and ability to interact properly with courtroom participants, generally act with proper decorum in the courtroom while in front of a jury, and present a defense without assistance of counsel
Be Sentenced	Understanding and appreciation of nature of the sentence to be imposed (after trial has resulted in conviction or the entering of a guilty plea)
Waive Further Appeal (when Facing Execution)	Understanding and appreciation of right for additional appeal and potential consequences of waiving it
Be Executed	Understanding and appreciation of nature and purpose of the punishment, and ability to assist counsel in any available appeal

Note: The wording of these definitions does not conform to prevailing legal terminology. They are intended only to convey the general issues raised in each specific situation. Updated and adapted from *Competency to Stand Trial Evaluations, by* Grisso, 1988, p. 3. With permission of Professional Resource Press.

DUSKY V. UNITED STATES

Youtsey (1899) established that defendant competence was a U.S. Constitutional requirement in order for the government to prosecute someone; however, it did not spell out the difference between competence and incompetence. The Supreme Court of the United States established that standard in the 1960 ruling of *Dusky v. United States*.

Milton Dusky was arrested in 1958 for kidnapping a 15-year old girl, transporting her from Kansas to Missouri, and raping her. He received a mental health evaluation, and the psychiatrist testified before the presiding U.S. District Court judge that, as a result of severe mental illness, he was "unable to properly understand the proceedings against him and unable to adequately assist counsel in his defense" (Dusky, 1960: 402). The judge determined that he was competent to proceed, nonetheless, because he was oriented and had some recollection of the events in question. He was convicted of kidnapping. The defense appealed to the U.S.

Court of Appeals for the Eighth Circuit, but the conviction was upheld.

The U.S. Supreme Court reviewed the case and overturned the conviction, sending the case back to the trial judge for a new competency assessment, and making the point that the trial court's standard of competency was not adequate. The high court opinion indicated: "It is not enough for the district judge to find that the defendant is oriented to time and place and has some recollection of events" (p. 402). The trial court held a new hearing and found him competent under the new standard. The U.S. Supreme Court's decision has become known as the *Dusky standard* and is the primary rule of law for competency to proceed in all U.S. jurisdictions ever since. Although courts in the United States can provide additional safe guard pertaining to a defendant's competency to proceed, they cannot provide less than the *Dusky* standard: "[The] test must be whether he has sufficient present ability to consult with his lawyer with a reasonable degree of rational understanding—and whether he has a rational as well as factual understanding of the proceedings against him" (p. 402).

Several key points regarding this standard need highlighting. The decision makes it clear that competency is an issue of *current* ability, which is contrasted with formulations pertaining to mental state at the time of the crime. Occasionally, courts need to determine competency pertaining to a time in the past, such as during a past confession, trial, or guilty plea, but typically competency pertains to current mental state, and to some degree mental state in the foreseeable future (i.e., upcoming legal proceedings). The phrase "*ability* to consult with his lawyer" in the standard indicates *capacity* to cooperate rather than *desire* to cooperate. It is not uncommon for criminal defendants to choose to not cooperate with the proceedings, but improper motivation does not meet the standard unless it is considered caused by a severe mental illness (e.g., psychosis, as opposed to maladaptive personality disorder). Evaluators must also keep in mind that *ability to consult with* in no way means a "meaningful attorney-client relationship" (*Morris v. Slappy*, 1983). Additionally, the standard also includes the phrase "*reasonable* level of understanding"—that is, not necessarily a complete understanding. Criminal defendants are not expected to have a perfect understanding.

The core aspect of the *Dusky* standard can be reduced to "rational as well as factual understanding." *Factual* understanding is viewed as strict understanding, such as the ability to repeat information provided, paraphrasing it in the defendant's own words, and demonstrating the ability to put the understanding to use by making a decision. *Rational* understanding pertains to understanding that can be compromised by severe mental illness or defect. Although a person could understand the underlying facts of the case, such as expected roles of courtroom participants, the basic adjudication process, and the fact that he or she is a criminal defendant facing specific charges related to his or her alleged behavior, it is possible that the person's rational understanding is compromised by psychotic mentation. The following case, evaluated by one of us (RLD) demonstrates this very issue.

> Mr. Defendant was found standing next to FBI agents, dressed in a dark suit, when the FBI were acting security for Governor William Clinton, when he was in Little Rock, Arkansas. Governor Clinton was under federal protection because he had formally entered his run for U.S. president. When the FBI noticed one among them who did not belong, they began questioning him and searched his vehicle. They found a high powered rifle with a telescope sight attached resting in the trunk.
>
> Mr. Defendant was referred for a competency to proceed mental health evaluation because of unusual ideas he voiced to his lawyer. During the evaluation, he voiced his belief that Governor Clinton ran a clandestine sex trade network focused on minors. He believed the only reason he was charged with his current offense was because he had special knowledge regarding Governor Clinton and was arrested and sent to a forensic hospital to keep him quiet and keep him from derailing the governor's bid for president.
>
> The details of his beliefs and presentation indicated he held grandiose and paranoid delusional beliefs. He was diagnosed with Delusional Disorder. The evaluator considered him not competent to proceed not because of impaired factual understanding, but because of impaired rational understanding due to genuine psychotic delusional beliefs. He was able to describe adequately the roles of courtroom participants, the nature of his charges and their potential outcomes, and plea options available to him. Although he acknowledged those facts were supposed to be true for him, he believed that no matter what he did or said, he would be held in order to keep him quiet and away from the media because of his special knowledge. In essence, he did not believe he would get a fair and impartial trial, and that belief was due to a severe mental illness.

The case highlights the difference between a factual understanding and a rational understanding. I (RLD) have evaluated other cases where defendants believed the presiding judge on the case was not actually human but Satan in human form, a belief stemming from schizophrenia. Although individuals who have lost their rational ability to consider facts can sometimes still acknowledge those facts, it does not necessarily make them competent to the point that they have a rational as well as a factual understanding and can assist properly in their defense. Oftentimes, they are so focused on explaining their psychotic beliefs to the judge, jury, or media that they are not able to assist properly in their defense, even with a skilled lawyer. This case also demonstrates that the abnormal ideation or understanding must stem from severe mental illness. The *Dusky v. United States* case document does not make it clear that Milton Dusky's problem was due to psychosis, but he was in fact diagnosed with schizophrenia (Frederick, DeMier, & Towers, 2004). There can be cases where defendants are so incapacitated by physical disease that they become incompetent, but under most circumstances the question of incompetency deals with mental illness. As is also true in most jurisdictions, the federal statute (Title 18, U.S.C., Section 4241a) makes this clear: "The defendant, as a result of mental disease or defect, is unable to understand the nature and consequences of the proceedings against him or assist properly in his defense." The federal statute also highlights an issue by substituting the word *consult* with the phrase *assist properly* in regarding working with a defense lawyer. There is no case law of which we are aware that spells out the exact meaning of "assisting properly." The level of assistance needed for a particular case depends on the specific situation. In this regard, there is a sense that competence is, to some degree, context based.

Competency in Context

Grisso (1988) presented a theoretical structure for how we can consider criminal competence within a context. By this perspective the level of competence needed varies based on the demands required. There is clear U.S. Supreme Court guidance that the standard of competence does not vary between waiving one's right to a trial or to an attorney, as all competencies are benchmarked by *Dusky v. United States* (1960; see *Godinez v. Moran, 1993*); however, there is common sense and a practical aspect to how a judge determines competence to proceed as well. We will address this issue when we touch on the complicated matter of letting a criminal defendant act as his or her own lawyer during a trial before a jury shortly.

Grisso presented five areas of analysis that are helpful for the forensic evaluator: (a) functional description of specific abilities, (b) causal explanations for deficits in competency abilities, (c) interactive significance of deficits in competency ability, (d) conclusory opinions about legal competency, and (e) prescriptive remediation for deficits in competency abilities. Functional description of specific abilities in competency is the act of presenting defendant strengths and weaknesses as they relate to competency requirements. The causal explanation is the direct linking of those competency deficits to mental illness or defect. The facts of the case described earlier could be changed some to demonstrate this point. Rather than a psychotic-illness-based delusion, the defendant could have believed he would not be treated fairly because his past experience with the government had never turned out well for him, and he simply expected the same outcome. Such beliefs are common among repeat offenders, particularly if they have significant antisocial personality characteristics. The point of the causal link is for the evaluator to specifically address whether or not the presumed deficits in competency are directly related to a mental illness (which most jurisdictions require to be severe) rather than ignorance, culturally based beliefs that are not considered an indication of mental illness, or volitional behaviors from the defendant.

The interactive significance of the deficits forces the evaluator to make a judgment of the demands required of the defendant by his or her specific situation. This focus of analysis is difficult for the clinician to fulfill because it takes competent understanding of the legal demands placed on a defendant, and the demands placed on the defendant could change depending on future decisions the defendant makes through the process. The best judge of the demands placed on a defendant at any specific time in the adjudicative process is the judge. Nonetheless, some jurisdictions (e.g., federal) require evaluators to provide an answer to the referral questions. In those instances, it is best for the evaluator to describe his or her reasoning related to perceived demands based on the nature of the criminal case (e.g., simple bank robbery or a multibank, multiaccount embezzlement scheme), what the defendant plans to do for a defense, and whether or not the defendant plans on utilizing the assistance of a lawyer.

The conclusory opinion about competency and prescriptive remediation often go hand in hand. The conclusory opinion is simply answering the ultimate issue question, in this case, competency to proceed. Some authors (Grisso, 1986, 1988; Grisso, Borum, Edens, Moye, & Otto, 2003) suggest it is more proper for the evaluator to not provide the answer to the ultimate issue. This view implies that a judge may be overly influenced by the testimony or report of an expert, a view that we have found unrealistic as related to competency. Typically, judges seek opinions when they want opinions and recognize them as opinions only. Evaluators are best served, however, to remember they are not generally experts in the law; they are simply consultants to the legal system, and the judge is in the best situation to take all facts into account when rendering a ruling on competency.

Prescriptive remediation for deficits in competency refers to providing education and guidance on the nature of the pathology involved and what it will specifically take from a treatment perspective to restore competency to proceed. Judges require this information to provide disposition for the defendant that will best serve the goal of the state as well as the defendant's U.S. Constitutional rights. If the condition is treatable, prescriptive recommendations can include such information as what treatment is needed, the likely duration of treatment, and local facilities that might be available to provide the treatment (Grisso, 1988).

As mentioned, different competency questions such as competency to stand trial, waive right to trial and plead guilty, waive rights to have assistance of counsel, and other nexus points in the process as listed in Table 40.2 are based on the same *Dusky v. United States* (1960) standard (*Godinez v. Moran*, 1993). Those issues are the most common types of questions asked regarding competency to proceed and generally have straightforward analyses as part of the conceptual formulation. For more detail regarding competency at those specific points in time, we recommend Grisso and colleagues (2003), Denney (2012a, 2012b), and of course, Melton and colleagues (2007). For now, we will turn briefly to two unique issues within the subject of competency to proceed and then address death penalty related competency under the death penalty section.

Miranda Warning and Competency to Confess

The requirement for criminal defendants to be competent to proceed begins before they are actually criminal defendants. It certainly begins by the time law enforcement personnel provide a suspect with his or her *Miranda* warning (*Miranda v. Arizona*, 1966), a point where the suspect should be competent such that he or she can knowingly, intelligently, and voluntarily make the decision to remain silent or confess. FNs can become involved in evaluations related to past competence to waive the right to remain silent as well as whether or not a mental aberration existed at the time the suspect was questioned that might make plausible the possibility he or she provided a false or "involuntary" confession. Some mental abnormalities make it possible that a suspect might have been unduly influenced to confess, not because of overreaching police behavior during interrogation, but because of characteristics inherent within the suspect. Covering the nuances of these concerns from a practice standpoint is beyond the scope of this chapter. The area is relatively complicated, and there are specialized assessment tools clinicians can use to assess both *Miranda* comprehension as well as suspect susceptibility to influence and suggestion. We recommend Frumkin (2008) for a good primer to the area.

A Unique Trial Competency

We need to add an additional word regarding the contextual demands placed on a defendant as a result of an interesting U.S. Supreme Court decision. In *Indiana v. Edwards* (2008), the High Court chose to not maintain a single rule when comparing a defendant who is competent to proceed to trial with aid of counsel to a defendant proceeding to trial without the aid of counsel. Thus, the court has split the issue such that a criminal defendant could be found competent to proceed to trial with aid of counsel, but not competent to represent him- or herself without the aid of counsel. Consequently, FNs may find themselves in a situation where they are asked to opine on the issue of whether or not an otherwise competent defendant is also able to represent him- or herself during a trial without the assistance of counsel. For a more detailed discussion of this interesting case and the conceptual background for the U.S. Supreme Court's conclusion, see Denney (2012a).

Competency-Related Measures

Many competency questions can be assessed without any formal, structured instrument, and frequently are by seasoned evaluators. The competency-related measures discussed in this section are primarily structured interviews designed to help evaluators ensure they have covered the essential features of competency rather than to produce a score that determines whether the defendant is competent. It should be noted that there are also instruments dedicated to assessing competency related to *Miranda* (Standardized Assessment of Miranda Abilities; Rogers, Sewell, Drogin, & Fiduccia, 2012), those with low intelligence and intellectual disability (Competency Assessment for Standing Trial for Defendants with Mental Retardation; Everington & Luckasson, 1992), and an instrument designed specifically to assess malingering of competency-related deficits (Inventory of Legal Knowledge; Otto, Musick, & Sherrod, 2010).

Revised Competency Assessment Instrument

The Competency Assessment Instrument (CAI) was originally developed by the Laboratory of Community Psychiatry in 1973 (McGarry, Lelos, & Lipsitt, 1973), and later revised (Riley, 1998). The Revised CAI (R-CAI) is an approximately 45-minute semistructured interview that should be administered in a flexible fashion, emphasizing questions that are relevant to the particular defendant.

Georgia Court Competency Test–Mississippi State Hospital Revision

Originally developed by Wildman et al. (1978) and consisting of 17 items, the most recent edition of the Georgia Court Competency Test (GCCT), the GCCT–Mississippi State Hospital Revision (GCCT-MSH) has 21 items. The test includes items asking the defendant to identify various figures in the courtroom using a line drawing of a courtroom, questions regarding the function of the various individuals in a courtroom, what charges the defendant is facing, and questions regarding the defendant's relationship with his attorney. The GCCT-MSH's strength is its use of a visual aide in the assessment of competency; its primary weakness is that it essentially assesses foundational competency only with little information gleaned about decisional competencies (Zapf, Roesch, & Pirelli, 2013).

MacArthur Competency Assessment Tool–Criminal Adjudication

The MacArthur Competency Assessment Tool–Criminal Adjudication (MacCAT-CA; Poythress et al., 1999) is the only instrument discussed here to use a hypothetical vignette in order to evaluate a defendant's competency. This has the benefit of perhaps better being able to assess the competency of a cautious defendant who does not want to discuss his or her own case; alternately, this instrument requires a higher level of cognitive capacity for the defendant to be able to comprehend the story, remember the details, and then be able to apply legal knowledge to a case that is not his or her own.

The MacCAT-CA uses the vignette and the first eight items to assess the defendant's understanding of the legal system and process, and the vignette and an additional eight questions to assess his or her ability to reason. The final questions assess the defendant's knowledge of his or her own case and beliefs about how things will go as opposed to his or her more generalized knowledge and beliefs, hopefully allowing for any assessment of delusional belief systems.

Evaluation of Competency to Stand Trial–Revised

The Evaluation of Competency to Stand Trial—Revised (ECST-R; see Rogers, Tillbrook, & Sewell, 2004) was designed to assess domains of knowledge consistent with the *Dusky* standard. Specifically, its subscales consist of Consult with Counsel, Factual Understanding of the Courtroom Proceedings, and Rational Understanding of the Courtroom Proceedings. It is unique, however, in that it includes a scale (Atypical Presentation) that assesses response style; evaluators who have not administered this instrument before may want to practice reading these questions in a serious fashion prior to actual test administration as they are quite unusual. Items on the ECST-R are scored on a Likert scale and normative data is provided both in terms of T-scores as well as level of certainty (i.e., preponderance, probable, etc.).

Readers may wish to refer to Denney (2012a) as these competency related measures are reviewed in more detail and with a focus on their application to neurocognitive disorders. We will now turn to the unique situation where criminal defendants have self-reported amnesia for the alleged crime.

Competency and Amnesia

The *Dusky* standard makes no reference to a defendant's memory capabilities directly. While anterograde amnesia would likely impair a defendant's current abilities to consult with counsel and understand the proceedings against him or her, retrograde amnesia for the time of the offense has *not* been considered a sufficient basis for a finding of incompetency in an otherwise competent defendant. Indeed, no court to date has found amnesia for the crime alone as a barrier to competency (Tysse, 2005). While a number of courts have stated, hypothetically, that amnesia alone could preclude competency in certain circumstances, no court has come upon such a set of hypothetical circumstances (*U.S. v. Andrews*, 2006).

History of Competency and Amnesia

This issue was examined by the DC Circuit Court in 1968, in *Wilson v. United States*. In this case, Robert Wilson was involved in a high speed chase in a stolen yellow Mustang that subsequently crashed into a tree, leading Mr. Wilson to incur a severe traumatic brain injury (TBI). This case was unique in that there was no argument to the fact that Mr. Wilson indeed had permanent retrograde amnesia for the events of that day due to his verified brain injury. While initially found incompetent due to his amnesia impacting his ability to consult with counsel, this finding was eventually reversed. The reasoning was that, in this case, Mr. Wilson had sufficient *present* abilities to consult with counsel, as well as the

> ability to construct a knowledge of what happened from other sources . . . a loss of memory should bar prosecution only when its presence would in fact be crucial to the construction and presentation of a defense and hence essential to the fairness and accuracy of proceedings.
>
> (*Wilson v United States*, 1968: 463)

On Mr. Wilson's later appeal, the appellate court essentially agreed, but also indicated that a posttrial review was necessary in order to determine if the defendant's amnesia did impact his competency as evidenced during the proceedings. In this review, it was stated that the court should consider how the defendant's amnesia affected his ability to assist his lawyer and testify on his own behalf, how well the evidence could be extrinsically reconstructed, how much the government assisted with that reconstruction, the strength of the prosecution's case, and any other circumstances which would indicate whether the defendant had a fair trial. If the trial was deemed to be unfair due to the defendant's amnesia, the court should vacate the conviction and a retrial may occur; after such retrial, if the trial remained unfair, the indictment should be dismissed.

Other Findings Regarding Amnesia

A more recent discussion of how retrograde amnesia may impact competency can be found in *U.S. v. Andrews* (2006). In this case, the court points out that only the DC Circuit Court has held that a posttrial review of competency is necessary when amnesia is an issue. In *Andrews*, the court instead indicated that, as in any case, the issue of competency can be raised *sua sponte* (at the judge's own accord) at any point throughout the proceedings; if this issue is not raised in the normal course of the trial by a concerned party, it is apparently not of sufficient concern to warrant a posttrial review specifically due to the issue of amnesia.

Practical Considerations Regarding Competency and Amnesia

As stated in *U.S. v. Swanson* (1978), the trier of fact "is in the best position to make a determination between allowing amnesia to become an unjustified safe haven for a defendant and, on the other hand, requiring an incompetent person to stand trial." Several of the issues outlined in *Wilson* (1968) and reaffirmed in *U.S. v. Rinchack* (1987) pertain to issues outside the expertise of mental health professionals, such as the extent the evidence can be extrinsically constructed including evidence of the crime itself and any potential alibi as well as the overall strength of the prosecution's case against the defendant and "any other facts and circumstances" (p. 464) pertaining to the defendant getting a fair trial. See Denney (2012b) or more detail regarding this issue and also for methods to potentially determine when the claimed amnesia is feigned. Although amnesia for the crime can affect a defendant's competency to proceed, it has nothing to do with whether or not he or she is criminally responsible.

Criminal Responsibility

Criminal responsibility has to do with one's mental state at the time of the offense, and is commonly known as "the insanity defense." The criminal court system has long recognized that individuals are not necessarily responsible for, and therefore should not be punished for, things done while they are not truly cognizant of what they are doing, and would not have done except for their mental state at the time of the offense. Given that two of the primary purposes of the criminal justice system are deterrence and retribution, what purpose would be served by punishing someone who was insane at the time of the offense? That is the key point—insanity has only to do with *mental state at the time of the offense.* This stands in contrast to issues of competency, which have nothing to do with mental state at the time of the offense, but pertain only to the defendant's current cognitive abilities and mental state.

A defendant can be sane at the time of the offense but yet not competent to stand trial. For example, if a man with a delusional belief system pertaining to the government happens to seriously injure another man in a bar fight over something said about his girlfriend, there is no evidence to believe he was not sane at the time of the offense. If, however, his delusional belief system regarding the government then hindered his ability to work with his court-appointed public defender, he may very well not be competent to stand trial. Alternately, many individuals who were psychotic at the time of the offense subsequently receive treatment with antipsychotic medication once they are arrested and otherwise involved with the legal system; while they may meet legal criteria for insanity at the time of the offense, once treated with antipsychotic medication, they will hopefully be restored to competency to stand trial. The ability to view these as two separate, often entirely unrelated issues is typically one of the most difficult concepts to grasp for those just entering the criminal forensic area.

Brief History of the Insanity Defense

The criteria for the insanity defense have varied substantially over the years and continue to vary widely between jurisdictions. Historically, evidence of some form of an insanity defense can be found even in ancient Egyptian and Hebrew civilizations, although most U.S. law has its roots in English case law (Melton et al., 2007). In the 1700s various definitions of insanity were used; perhaps the best known of these was put forth by Justice Tracy, who stated that to be insane, "a man must be totally deprived of his understanding and memory so as not to know what he is doing, no more than an infant, brute or a wild beast" (*Arnold's Case*, 1723). The definition then shifted, however, from an emphasis on lack of awareness to a more nuanced test, involving whether the defendant was able to distinguish right from wrong. This became known as the *M'Naghten test.* The ruling in this case (*Rex v. M'Naghten*, 1843) defined insanity as that, at the time of the offense, "the party accused was laboring under such a defect of reason . . . as not to know the nature and quality of the act he was doing; or, if he did know it, that he did not know he was doing what was wrong."

The *M'Naghten* test held in the United States until 1887, at which point an additional facet was added—that of one's ability to control one's impulses (Melton et al., 2007). In *Parsons v. State,* the court concluded that a person was insane at the time of the offense if, due to mental disease, the defendant "had so far lost the power to choose between the right and wrong, and to avoid doing the act in question, as that his free agency was at the time destroyed" (*Parsons v. State*, 1887). The definition of insanity continued to evolve, later leading to various iterations such as the "product test" and a number of cases further defining those criteria (Melton et al., 2007).

The next major shift in the definition of insanity came when the American Law Institute (ALI) proposed a new rule. It read:

> A person is not responsible for criminal conduct if at the time of such conduct as a result of mental disease or defect he lacks substantial capacity either to appreciate the criminality [wrongfulness] of his conduct or to conform his conduct to the requirements of the law.
>
> (ALI, 1955)

This definition also included a statement specifically prohibiting the inclusion of antisocial personality or psychopathy. The ALI rule was adopted by many jurisdictions from its proposal in 1955 (Melton et al., 2007) until the Insanity Defense Reform Act (IDRA) of 1984.

In 1984, John Hinckley, Jr., was found to be not guilty by reason of insanity (NGRI) in his assassination attempt of President Ronald Regan. This verdict was not well received by the public, causing the IDRA to be enacted, substantially narrowing the legal definition of insanity. The current federal definition of insanity reads: "at the time of the commission of the acts constituting the offense, the defendant, as a result of a severe mental disease or defect, was unable to appreciate the nature and quality or the wrongfulness of his acts" (United States Code, Title 18, Section 17). The following case vignette highlights how a criminal defendant's beliefs can meet the sanity standard for some aspects of a crime, but not necessarily all aspects of the crime:

> A 53-year old man was pulled over at night by state police because his van tail light had burned out. The man acted oddly in the van, and the police called for backup. The man was asked to exit his van and speak with the police. After he exited the van he attempted to injure the police officer with his bare hands when the officer asked him for his identification. He was taken into custody. Found in the van were numerous wired contraptions that appeared to be booby traps for the van, and it was apparent he had been living in the van. Also found was a homemade white gas device that was classified as a bomb by the Bureau of Alcohol, Tobacco, Firearms, and Explosives, but which he later said was simply a homemade heater for his van. He was charged with possession of explosives and for assaulting an officer.
>
> During his mental health evaluation, he disclosed his beliefs that the government could track people through their identification cards and that they were systematically collecting people's identification cards in order to control and kill them. His ideas became increasingly paranoid and psychotic. Information from his daughter verified that he had long held quite psychotic beliefs, lived in his van, and traveled the country, but had never been known to harm anyone.
>
> One of us (RLD) evaluated this man and diagnosed him with schizophrenia. The report provided the opinion that the man's psychotic beliefs caused him to act in immediate self-defense when the officer asked him to hand over his identification card because he believed he was going to be killed. For this charge, he was considered insane because he did not appreciate the nature, quality, or wrongfulness of his act. Because the gas heater/bomb was not included in any psychotic thinking, he was not considered insane regarding possession of the device. He simply denied that it was a bomb, in what amounted to an "I did not do it" assertion.

Current State of the Defense

As the U.S. Supreme Court presented in *Clark v. Arizona* (2006), states are not required under the U.S. constitution to offer an insanity defense in any form; despite this, most do. At that time, the federal government and 17 states defined insanity as some form of the *M'Naghten* test (both prongs), one only *M'Naghten's* cognitive test, and for ten, the moral test alone. Fourteen states were using the ALI rule or a variation thereof, and three a combination of *M'Naghten* plus volitional capacity. One state continued to use the "product test." Three states had no insanity defense, and one offered no insanity defense but the option of a "guilty but mentally ill" plea. A very nice table of the relevant statutes and information about the "variations" they contain is presented in Packer (2009).

Other Points Regarding Insanity

The insanity defense is rarely used and even less often successful. When it is successful, however, acquittees are typically remanded for evaluation of dangerousness, and if found dangerous, can be committed indefinitely for purposes of treatment. A number of defendants, if made aware of the ramifications of pleading NGRI, may opt not to use the defense, as they would rather have a defined sentence and release date, particularly if the sentence would not be overly lengthy. It should also be noted that a defendant is not eligible for the insanity defense (or at least would likely not be found NGRI) if his or her "insanity" at the time of the offense was due to substance abuse, as this is also specifically excluded in most definitions.

Diminished Capacity and Responsibility

The issue of diminished capacity may arise when a defendant does not meet the jurisdiction's standards for a finding of NGRI, or when a jurisdiction lacks an insanity defense altogether. One scenario in which "diminished capacity" may occur is when the defendant committed a crime while under the substantial influence of drugs or alcohol. In this scenario, the issue is not the defendant's ultimate guilt, but rather that of which crime they are guilty. Put simply, due to their altered mental status, they may not have had the mental abilities to act with *malice aforethought*, which is a necessary precondition to be convicted of what are typically classified as first degree offenses, that is, those which are both deliberate and premeditated.

Alternately, diminished responsibility implies that the defendant is less culpable for a crime committed due to a mental abnormality, but does not imply that the defendant did not have the capacity to form the requisite intent (Clark, 2013). An example of a circumstance where the concept of diminished responsibility may be important is in a jurisdiction where there is no volitional prong to the insanity defense, and a deficit in cognitive, emotional, or behavioral control secondary to a neurological condition may be relevant, whether during trial or sentencing (Denney, 2012b). It should be noted, however, that while diminished responsibility is a formal legal concept in several European countries, there is currently no formally defined U.S. equivalent; in the United States, the concepts of diminished capacity and NGRI have frequently metamorphosed to include more or less of the concept of diminished responsibility over the past few decades (Clark, 2013). The IDRA essentially ended the concept of diminished responsibility in the United States with its statement that there shall be no affirmative defense other than insanity that relates to a mental disease or defect.

Mens Rea

Mens rea is essentially the intent to commit a criminal act. Whereas a finding of NGRI absolves the defendant of responsibility entirely, diminished capacity does not negate all criminal responsibility, but is only a finding that the defendant was not capable of forming the *mens rea* for a specific criminal charge (Clark, 2013). Therefore, the defendant may be convicted of a lesser offense amongst the original charges. As an example, say that a mother, while in a drunken stupor, beat her child to death. She may be charged with crimes such as first degree murder, second degree murder, and manslaughter. In this case, her capacity to form the intent and plan to murder her child was likely compromised due to her severe intoxication, making a conviction for first degree murder less likely should the defense present evidence relating to diminished capacity.

It should be noted that a string of cases in various jurisdictions have clarified the statement in the IDRA that short of insanity, "mental disease or defect does not otherwise constitute a defense." While at first, this seems to eliminate the ability of a trier of fact to consider diminished capacity, all subsequent district and appellate cases have agreed that the purpose of the IDRA was not to prohibit the appropriate consideration of *mens rea* (Clark, 2013). As best summarized in *U.S. v. Pohlot* (1987), the phrasing of the IDRA was interpreted as leaving "no doubt that Congress intended . . . to bar only 'affirmative defenses' that 'excuse' misconduct but not evidence that disproves an element of the crime itself" (p. 897). Simply stated, demonstrating *mens rea* is essential for the prosecution to meet its burden of proof for all necessary elements of a crime (Clark, 2013), making diminished capacity a valid issue open for expert testimony.

Assessment of Dangerousness

Neuropsychologists can be called upon to provide an assessment of the dangerousness of a defendant or inmate in a number of scenarios. For example, if a defendant is found noncompetent and nonrestorable, his or her dangerousness must be assessed; if he or she does not pose a serious risk of violence towards persons or property, the charges may be dropped. Alternately, if the defendant is dangerous due to mental disease or defect, he or she can be civilly committed, potentially indefinitely. This issue of dangerousness due to mental disease or defect is also relevant for those found NGRI and inmates at the end of their sentences if they are mentally ill or meet certain criteria regarding sexual offenses. While neuropsychologists may be able to provide special expertise in cases where dangerousness is an issue due to a neuropathological condition, they must also be familiar with the general principles of risk assessment as well as the broader static and dynamic risk factors.

Methods of Risk Assessment

Just as in neuropsychology some clinicians prefer fixed batteries and some flexible, those performing risk assessments have a number of approaches from which to choose. The four most common are clinical judgment, structured professional judgment, actuarial, and adjusted actuarial. Clinical judgment is just that—based entirely on the clinician's own judgment and experience, which may or may not have any empirical underpinnings. Clinical judgment was essentially the only method of assessment until more scientific studies of risk assessment were performed and actuarial methods began to be produced. One early seminal study in risk assessment that used clinical judgment (Kozol, Boucher, & Garofalo, 1972) has been—somewhat erroneously—interpreted as resulting in the clinicians' predictions being wrong two-thirds of the time, in other words, worse than chance (Douglas, Hart, Groscup, & Litwack, 2013). This method is not recommended as it is unlikely to meet legal standards regarding the scientific basis of expert testimony.

At the far end of the spectrum from clinical judgment would be actuarial assessment, which involves deriving a formula for considering and weighting risk factors from a known-groups population; this formula then allows the clinician to make a probabilistic prediction of the examinee's future dangerousness. While the highly scientific appearance of actuarial instruments is attractive, they do have some weaknesses. Many actuarial instruments are not well cross-validated: Clinicians must keep in mind there may be "shrinkage" of classification accuracies when the instruments are used in different populations. For example, many of the popular actuarial instruments were designed in an incarcerated Canadian population, which may have very different sociodemographic characteristics than that of an urban metropolitan detention center or state prison.

Another critique of the actuarial risk assessment method is that it entirely disallows for clinical judgment, even in exceptional cases. So, for example, an inmate produces the highest score possible on an actuarial risk assessment method—but was seriously assaulted by another inmate while in prison and is now a quadriplegic. Regardless, this individual would be high risk using a strictly actuarial method. This is why some clinicians prefer an adjusted actuarial method, where they essentially administer and consider actuarial methods, but also use their own common sense and empirical knowledge of violence risk factors to sometimes modify the level of risk predicted by the actuarial instrument.

The previous example also illustrates a further limitation of the actuarial method; that is, actuarial methods rely largely on static as opposed to dynamic risk factors. Static risk factors are risk factors that are unmodifiable, such as the number of past victims and the examinee's age. Alternately, dynamic risk factors are more fluid risk factors, which can also be targets for intervention to prevent future violence. These can include factors such as substance use, coping skills, education, employment, and a stable living situation. Clinicians' desire to be able to account for both static and dynamic risk factors has led to increasing use of a *structured professional judgment* (SPJ) approach. This method is where clinicians base their assessment of an examinee's dangerousness based upon the current empirical research and make their own judgment regarding overall level of risk. There are instruments that can guide the clinician's SPJ as well,

Table 40.3 Common risk assessment tools

Instrument	*Type*	*Citation*
Classification of Violence Risk (COVR)	Violence–Actuarial	Monahan et al. (2005)
Violence Risk Appraisal Guide (VRAG)	Violence–Actuarial	Harris, Rice, and Quinsey (1993)
Violence Risk Scale (VRS)	Violence–Actuarial	Wong and Gordon (1999)
Sex Offender Risk Appraisal Guide (SORAG)	Sexual–Actuarial	Quinsey, Harris, Rice, and Cormier (2006)
Static-99	Sexual–Actuarial	Hanson and Thronton (1999)
Historical-Clinical-Risk Management (HCR-20; version 3)	Violence–SPJ	Douglas, Hart, Webster, and Belfrage (2013)
Risk for Sexual Violence Protocol (RSVP)	Sexual–SPJ	Hart et al. (2003)

although the final determination is still the clinician's own. See Table 40.3 for a list of some common risk assessment tools.

Dangerousness and Neuropathology

While the risk assessment tools in Table 40.3 will provide an adequate guide for those assessing dangerousness in a general sense, neuropsychologists may be called in when the standard methodology would not be entirely accurate due to issues involving neuropathology. For example, a convicted offender with known frontal lobe pathology may be at higher risk for affective or impulsive violence than one without. It is important to keep in mind that in this context civil commitment for dangerousness hinges upon dangerousness *due to a mental disease or defect.* What happens, for example, when an offender who was clearly already dangerous due to his past criminal history acquires neuropathology during the course of his detainment or incarceration? If a detainee is pending trial for a first degree murder charge, has a history of gang membership and similar charges, and then incurs a severe case of herpes simplex virus encephalitis during his detainment, does this now make him dangerous due to a mental disease or defect? How might his relatively dense amnesia increase or decrease his propensity for future acts of violence? These are cases that must be assessed cautiously when using standardized actuarial risk assessment instruments and empirically based SPJ measures, as neurocognitive and neuropathological features are simply not included in the extant instruments. For a detailed discussion of affective and predatory violence and the neurobiological underpinnings of such, which may be of relevance to neuropsychologists performing these assessments of dangerousness, see Fazio and Denney (2015).

Death-Penalty-Related Matters

FNs are commonly utilized as experts in death penalty litigation. Because a human life is at stake in death penalty litigation, the process undergoes a higher level of scrutiny at every level than other more routine criminal adjudication. FNs participate in the same issues such as *Miranda* competency, competency to stand trial or enter a guilty plea, and be sentenced; however, there are unique points of entry for FNs as well, such as the issue of potential intellectual disability at the early stage, mitigation at the sentencing phase, and competency to be executed at the late stage.

Atkins v. Virginia *(2002)*

The U.S. Supreme Court decision in *Atkins v. Virginia* (2002) is particularly significant for FNs involved in death penalty proceedings. Daryl Atkins and an accomplice abducted a man, robbed him, forced him to withdraw cash from an ATM, drove him to an isolated location, and then shot and killed him. Atkins was convicted of abduction, armed robbery, and capital murder. During the penalty phase, the defense-selected psychologist testified that Atkins achieved an IQ of 59, and concluded the defendant was mentally retarded. Rebuttal testimony by the government's psychiatrist painted a picture of psychopathic personality. The jury sentenced Atkins to death, the state supreme court affirmed the judgment, and the case was appealed to the U.S. Supreme Court.

The U.S. Supreme Court reviewed the various state standards across the union and determined that the number of states banning execution had increased substantially since the issue of executing the mentally retarded was last raised (*Penry v. Lynaugh*, 1989). This observed trend was a significant factor in the legal analysis. However, more significant for forensic neuropsychological analysis was the High Court's conclusion that developmental intellectual disability was associated with several cognitive limitations. They are detailed in Table 40.4.

Table 40.4 Cognitive domains relevant to mental retardation determination, per *Atkins v. Virginia* (2002)

- Comprehend information
- Process information
- Communicate
- Learn and remember
- Profit from mistakes and experience
- Engage in logical reasoning
- Control impulses
- Understand the reaction of others

The High Court also addressed the historical justification for the death penalty: retribution and deterrence of future capital crimes. It reached two conclusions: the diagnosis of retardation (now termed *intellectual disability,* or ID) implied both reduced culpability and lowered prospects for deterrence. In other words, persons with ID are less likely to understand and profit from an understanding of the deterrence value of the death penalty, and hence cannot control their conduct through the verbal mediation of a deterrence concept. Finally, the court expressed concern that offenders with ID may face an increased risk for wrongful execution because they may unwittingly provide false confessions. The idea is that those with ID are less able to resist persuasion and deceptive police tactics.

The *Atkins* decision had many ramifications, both positive and negative, for forensic examiners. The decision showed positive awareness of the unspoken criminal responsibility issue, as the court concluded that mental retardation did not necessarily eliminate a person's ability to appreciate right from wrong. Presciently, and of importance to FNs who also evaluate for feigned deficits, Justice Scalia writing the dissenting opinion in the Atkins case expressed concern that manipulative defendants would eagerly seek a mental retardation label long before a trial's penalty phase, to enhance chances of not only avoiding the ultimate penalty, but winning a legal insanity defense during the guilt phase.

More problematic for future examiners was poor guidance on defining retardation. The High Court neither dictated the exact manner in which ID was defined (thus leaving it up to the states), nor did it offer guidance on the severity of ID necessary to remove execution risk. All subsequent case law of which we are aware has settled on the conclusion that any level of ID will meet the Atkins standard.

We offer the following best practice. A reasonable interpretation of *Atkins* is that in order to be proven intellectually disabled, the FN should rely on the most contemporary *Diagnostic and Statistical Manual* (DSM). DSM-IV (American Psychiatric Association, 1994) was current at the time of Atkins, but was replaced by *DSM-5* in 2013 (American Psychiatric Association, 2013).

The defendant must show (a) subaverage intelligence during an individualized assessment, (b) impairment in daily adaptive functioning, and (c) evidence that the condition existed prior to the age of 18 years. Although some erroneously believe DSM-5 criteria no longer concerns itself with an IQ score (*Hall v. Florida*, 2014, Alito Dissenting), the preeminent criterion soundly remains in place. The authors simply removed the reference to an IQ score of 70 in Criterion A page, but retained it in the text:

> Individuals with intellectual disability have scores of approximately two standard deviations or more below the population mean, including a margin for measurement error . . . On tests with a standard deviation of 15 and a mean of 100, this involves a score of 65–75 (70 ± 5).
>
> (p. 37)

It must be noted, however, that this five-point confidence interval varies depending on the test, the IQ score, and the age of the individual. Adaptive functioning (solving everyday problems) was divided into 11 categories in DSM-IV, but reduced to three general categories in DSM-5, because of the clear influence from the American Association on Mental Retardation (AAMR), now called the American Association on Intellectual and Developmental Disabilities (AAIDD). Although not relevant to *Atkins* decisions because the litigation focuses on whether or not a defendant has ID, DSM-5 raised the significance of adaptive functioning within the diagnosis by using it to determine the difference between mild, moderate, severe, and profound ID, rather than the IQ score.

Since *Atkins*, courts and psychologist experts retained in the litigation continually struggle with four issues: the standard error of measurement (SEM), test-retest effects, whether IQ scores should be corrected for the so-called Flynn effect, and measurement of adaptive functioning.

Standard Error of Measurement

Although the mental health field has long understood that IQ scores are estimates of intellectual ability in which inherent error is contained, the legal system has not always appreciated this reality. Recently, the U.S. Supreme Court overturned a Florida court's decision to limit intellectual disability for purposes of death penalty litigation to those individuals who score 70 or below on IQ testing irrespective of the test's SEM (*Hall v. Florida*, 2014). The High Court concluded that it was a violation of the Eighth Amendment against cruel and unusual punishment for trial courts to limit the consideration for intellectual disability to a strict 70 cutoff without considering the SEM.

When testifying about the confidence interval derived from the SEM, FNs need to remember that the confidence interval developed from the SEM does not remain a bell-shaped (Gaussian) curve once the score deviates significantly from the mean (Nunnally & Bernstein, 1994). In other words, the distribution becomes increasingly positively skewed as the score falls closer to 70 and below as a result of regression toward the mean. The practical ramification of this fact is that courts can have increased confidence that the true score is more likely to fall at the obtained score or higher in the confidence interval rather than the lower end of the interval. It is exceedingly unlikely that the true score would fall at the lowest point of the confidence interval.

Test-Retest Effects

Criminal defendants progressing through death penalty litigation are likely to undergo multiple examinations regarding their intelligence. Additionally, they will likely have a history of previous intellectual assessment. When comparing results of multiple IQ tests, not only differences between tests need consideration, but it is proper to consider potential test-retest effects as well. This issue almost always arises during an *Atkins* hearing. FNs need to be aware of how different versions of intelligence tests compare (if research of that comparison exists) and also how scores change with retesting using the same test. For the Wechsler Adult Intelligence Test, fourth edition (WAIS-IV), the technical manual (Wechsler, 2008) indicates the test was administered twice to the same healthy people, with retest intervals ranging from 8 to 82 days (mean = 22). Results indicated the Full Scale IQ increased by an average of 4.3 points over the entirety of the four age bands (ages 16–90 years). This sample was stratified by race/ethnicity, region of the country, and education (< 9 years to > 17 years). The greatest Index increase was 4.4 for Processing Speed, while Perceptual Reasoning was 3.9, Working Memory was 3.1, and Verbal Comprehension was 2.5. Overall, one should expect about a four-point increase in IQ with retesting if it was done within about three months of the initial testing. It is illogical to expect much greater differences as the delay interval increases beyond three months. Catron and Thompson (1979) administered the WAIS to college students on two occasions with intervals of one week, one month, two months, or four months. They found the average increase in FSIQ was 8.0, 5.7, 5.4, and 4.2 points for each interval, respectively. These findings support the belief that retest gains lessen as the interval increases, at least with college students.

Estevis, Basso, and Combs (2012), in contrast to the WAIS-IV validation study, highlighted the effects of IQ and education. They found an average increase in FSIQ on the WAIS-IV of seven points with healthy, educated (M = 14.9, SD = 0.9), young adults (M = 20.9, SD = 2.5) who were intellectually high average (FSIQ M = 111.6, SD = 12.1). There was no statistically significant difference between three-month and six-month intervals. Such a large increase was likely due to uniformly higher education and intellectual levels as well as smaller percentage of racial/ethnic minorities than that present in the WAIS-IV validation studies. Less extreme increases would be expected with individuals having lower IQs, particularly those falling in the range of intellectual disability. Rapport, Brines, Axelrod, and Theisen (1997) revealed this very finding that practice effects were smaller for those with IQs falling in the low-average range (80–90) than for those in the average (95–105) and high average (110–120) ranges when tested repeatedly with the WAIS-R (Wechsler, 1981) at two-week intervals. Results for the low-average IQ group more closely approximated findings from the WAIS-IV validation studies (i.e., FSIQ average increase of 5.6 points). We are not aware of any practice effect studies with individuals having intellectual disability.

One of us (RLD) has repeatedly faced cross-examination where the defense attorney presents a copied section out of Kaufman and Lichtenberger (2006) dealing with "progressive error" (p. 163). Progressive error refers to the compounding effect of test-retest error over the course of more than two IQ test administrations. Kaufman and Lichtenberger cite Kausler's (1982, 1991) work as the originator of the concept. They then highlight two longitudinal studies dealing with IQ testing among the elderly as examples of how this effect is revealed (Schmitz-Scherzer & Thomae, 1983; Siegler, 1983). The fact that performances did not decrease as expected during the studies was interpreted to indicate the age effects were being countered by the effect of progressive error. The answer to this interesting finding is presented by Kaufman and Lichtenberger on the pages following shortly thereafter. The section is called "Selective Attrition" and refers to the interesting finding that participants do not uniformly return for follow-up assessments during longitudinal studies. However, this attrition is not uniform across the IQ distribution. Interestingly, those who do return for follow-up assessments have, on average, higher IQs than those who do not return. The sum effect of this selective attrition is to increase the mean IQ scores during subsequent test administrations. In effect the follow-up groups are not the same as the initial group. Kaufman and Lichtenberger (2006) conclude, "Hence, generalizations from longitudinal studies must be made quite cautiously because of the considerable selective attrition factor" (p. 167).

Empirical data pertaining to multiple IQ administrations among those with very low IQs is lacking. Rawlings and Crewe (1992), in a retrospective study, compared repeated IQ test administrations among TBI survivors who were matched on variables thought to have "confounding influences" (p. 418). The "experimental" group of patients was tested at two-month, four-month, eight-month, and 12-month intervals. The other group of patients was tested at two and 12 months. Both groups were compared at 12 months to determine the effect of four multiple assessments over two assessments. The group that was administered four assessments increased the FSIQs an average of 2.97 points over and above the two assessment group at 12 months. Although the experimental group had a greater change effect size than the control group, these findings suggested the effect of an increased number of assessments over just two assessments was clinically negligible as scores fell well within the confidence interval. While progressive error is raised as a concern, empirical data to support the concept appears lacking. At this point, we consider selective attrition to be the more parsimonious explanation for so-called progressive error.

Flynn Effect: The Phenomenon

The Flynn Effect (FE) refers to a large secular increase in aggregate intelligence scores since the 1930s, and it is a generally accepted phenomena (Neisser, 1998). The eponymic label became widespread because of political scientist James Flynn's prolific writing on the topic (Flynn, 1984), although he was not the first to observe and theorize about the rise. Greiffenstein (2011) reviewed earlier literature that showed rising IQ scores since World War I.

The trend line across many studies suggests a rate of 0.3 IQ points per year (three per decade), if the baseline is set in the 1930s. The parameters of the rise include increases in many different industrialized countries and a greater rise in measures of "fluid intelligence" versus "crystallized," with a more recent leveling off (possibly pausing) in IQ gains (Sundet, Barlaug, & Torjussen, 2004). The best evidence comes from national military records. Such samples are massive, and especially representative of the population in countries with conscription (Flynn, 1987a, 1987b).

Flynn Effect: Theory

There is no widely accepted explanation of the intergenerational IQ trends. There are disagreements whether the increase represents actual changes in underlying *g* or ordinary facultative changes (learning and rote memorization); or whether methodological artifact (e.g., differences in recruitment bias between standardization cohorts), changes in subtest instructions and constructs (Kaufman, 2010), and/or if epigenetics (factors turning genes off/on) play roles (Greiffenstein, 2011). In 1998, the American Psychological Association published a monograph on the topic, with several authorities on intelligence weighing on with theories (Neisser, 1998).

There are single-process explanations of rising IQ. They include improved nutrition, learning to solve abstract problems without increased *g*, compulsory education since 1900, and increasing cultural complexity. However, the intermediate steps between the proposed single causes and rising IQs have not been specified in any concrete way. The short timescale of the massive secular IQ gains is inconsistent with positive selection of a recent gene mutation, but other genetic mechanisms are possible.

Greiffenstein (2011) theorized an epigenetic mechanism. He applied life-history theory as a conceptual tool, and argued that secular trends (primarily improved nutrition) changed the phenotypic expression of the genotype that controls the neurophysiology of problem solving. More resources ("energetics") were committed to reasoning than other bodily functions, because the environment was more resource-rich and dependable. Essentially, Greiffenstein (2011) argued for earlier cognitive maturation than in prior generations, and mandatory education had a multiplier effect, increasing IQ scores.

Flynn Effect: Practical Considerations

Moving from group to individual data, the FE is evident in everyday practice. Persons who take old IQ tests today score much higher than persons of the same age when that IQ test was first published, a fact reflected in data tables in some test manuals. The standardization group for the WAIS-R (Wechsler, 1981) also took the 1950 WAIS, and scored 11 points higher on average. Hence, the WAIS-R had to be recalibrated to a mean of 100. In death penalty venues, however, standardized intelligence test administration, as memorialized in the test manuals, is considered inadequate by some forensic psychologists. These psychologists are proponents of making downward adjustments to current IQ scores, to "correct" for the age of the test norms, in criminal cases (Fletcher, Stuebing, & Hughes, 2010; Reynolds, Niland, Wright, & Rosenn, 2010). They typically subtract a fractional IQ unit from the current score to elucidate the "true" IQ score, arguing that this practice removes the test-age bias that is presumed to be systematic. As stated earlier, the rise has been a remarkably consistent 0.3/year when one smooths aggregated testing data bases that in some cases are separated by decades. This simple formula has been proposed:

$$\text{Adjusted IQ} = \text{Observed IQ} - [0.3 \times \text{years since test norming}]$$

Take, for example, a criminal defendant who is tested with the WAIS-R in 2000 and earns a Full Scale IQ of 75. Taking measurement error into account, the score is in a range consistent with V62.89, Borderline Intellectual Functioning per the DSM-IV-TR (APA, 2013). The WAIS-R was normed in 1980 (Wechsler, 1981). The forensic psychologist reports a "Flynn adjusted" score of 69, by subtracting 6 (0.3×20) from 75, and concludes that the defendant exhibits mild intellectual disability, rendering him ineligible for the death penalty.[1]

Proponents of "Flynn corrections" support their position with some reasonable arguments. The most compelling one is that the FE stands for increasing inaccuracy of Full Scale IQs as a function of test age. The older an IQ test is, the greater the upward bias in scoring error (i.e., IQ inflation). A psychologist needs to consider the alleged bias of an aging IQ test, because overestimating IQ has profound consequences. The death penalty is one of them, but outside of criminal law, special education services may be denied because "the IQ is too high." Kanaya (2004) conducted a longitudinal test-retest study of children in special education and found large decreases in IQ when retested on new norms, when compared to old norms. Hence, children who may have qualified for special education services earlier may have been denied them because scores were inflated by the older first test.

Fletcher and colleagues (2010), proponents of applying FE, add that "correcting an IQ score is not a violation of test administration, rather it is selecting an appropriate normative comparison" (p. 4570). They give the example of a pediatrician relying on current national height/weight norms rather than old or foreign ones. Additionally, Fletcher et al. counter critics by making the aggressive argument that all practice standards should be ignored except for one: the manual published by the American Association of Intellectual and Developmental Disabilities, which advises correcting IQ scores in death penalty cases. Unfortunately, Fletcher et al. do not offer any norms for Flynn-corrected scores, or any data on the reliability and validity of adjusted scores.

Not all proponents are reasonable. The justification for making corrections is hotly debated, and sometimes rancorously. For example, Reynolds and colleagues (2010) acknowledged that adherence to the test manual is "standard practice," but threatened future charges of "malpractice" against those who do not make score adjustments that those authors demand.

Critics of making adjustments reasonably point out several problems with "Flynn" corrections. One problem is lack of general acceptance. The practice of adjustments is so far limited to a small cadre of psychologists who are usually hired by defense attorneys and specialize in pretrial evaluations in capital cases. Hagan, Drogin, and Guilmette (2008) used two methods to evaluate general acceptance: (a) a survey of doctoral training program directors and (b) a systematic review of relevant source material (test manuals, textbooks on IQ testing, and sources of legal/ethical guidance). Both survey and textual evidence demonstrated that IQ adjustments deviated markedly from the prevailing standards of psychological practice. Of further consequence to admissibility and ethics is the fact that downward corrections are never used in other contexts where IQ is critical, such as Social Security Disability evaluations.

The concern that aggregated cohort differences in IQ standardization causes inflated scores is valid. Nonetheless, there are serious logical problems with making adjustments in the *individual case*. It is unknown, for example, whether the 0.3/year increase applies universally to all examinees (Sternberg, 2010). More serious is the unproven assumption that increases are uniform across time and individuals. The annual 0.3 rate is just a convenient extrapolation from aggregated data separated by many years. In other words, it remains unknown whether the leap in IQ scores was densely clustered in a past generation followed by periods of dormancy ("lumpiness"), or if the trend was perfectly linear as implied by the FE correction formula. This question is not trivial, because if the IQ increase was both "lumpy" and remote in time (e.g., the 1930s to 1970s), then correcting more modern tests could distort scoring. There is, in fact, good evidence that the FE ended by the mid-1990s—interestingly, at the same time that height gains stopped (Sundet et al., 2004; also see Greiffenstein, 2011, regarding nutrition as a "prime mover" for FE). Equally unknown is the reliability and validity of Flynn-corrected scores, an issue ignored by corrections proponents. A Flynn correction is technically a change score, and change scores have more error than individual scores (Nunnally & Bernstein, 1994).

The hazards of applying corrections to the individual case are demonstrated in a critical study by Zhou, Zhu, and Weiss (2010). They administered pairs of old-new tests to large samples of children and adults. Their aggregate data showed the classic FE of 0.3/year, but the magnitude of the difference was not evenly distributed across ability level. Those with subaverage IQs (< 89) showed the largest mean inflation on the older test, but 40% still showed either a *decrease* (newer IQ score below older one) or little to no change. Applying a downward correction to a person's subaverage IQ score would be wrong at least 40% of the time, and of unknown exactitude in the other 60% percent. This adds even more error, beyond the SEM.

Flynn Effect: Best Forensic Neuropsychology Practice

We strongly recommend against making FE corrections. There are several reasons to avoid the practice. The reliability and validity of corrected scores is unknown and likely to contain more error; the contemporary (ongoing) existence of secular increases in IQ is scientifically disputable, because the trend may have ended decades ago; and it is unknown whether the corrections can universally be applied or whether further adjustments have to be made to the adjustment, based on the characteristics of examines (race, age, gender); and Zhou et al. (2010) proved that the FE magnitude varies widely across and within ability levels. Finally, assigning a number in this fashion is pseudoscientific, because it gives the misleading impression of mathematical accuracy, when the assumption of underlying linearity is just speculative.

We recommend, however, including some consideration of the FE in the interpretive section of FN reports as mandatory practice. The FE is a real phenomenon, and the historical need to recalibrate IQ to center on 100 is all the proof needed to reflect that the "true" score could potentially deviate from an observed score with an aging test. We agree with Hagan et al. (2010) that, when there is legitimate concern about a difference in "true" versus observed scores on an intelligence test, psychologists are "justified in sharing this perspective in *narrative* form" (p. 475, emphasis added), not in pseudoscientific numerical form. Consider this excerpt from a FN report from one of us (MFG):

> Defendant's expert opined that the defendant should be viewed as mentally retarded, after 'Flynn-effect correcting' the 1980 WAIS and later 2010 WAIS-III scores, with a static formula. In my professional opinion, it is possible that the defendant's true IQ is below the scores calculated according to older test manuals. Nonetheless, the size of the score inflation is unknown, even assuming that the FE ever touched this individual. For example, the Verbal IQ of 80 obtained with the Wechsler Adult Intelligence Scale in 1980, was based on persons who were defendant's age in 1950. His old verbal IQ can reasonably be viewed as an over-estimate. However, no number reflective of his "true" verbal IQ can be calculated. The calculation formula is unreliable because it is based on unsupported premises, one falsifiable premise being that the Flynn Effect has been linear and uniform for everybody.
>
> In summary of my professional opinion, defendant's past IQ scores reasonably reflect *some* degree of overestimation. But IQ is not the sole basis for evaluating MR, and the totality of the evidence shows ordinary levels of adaptive function in several domains. His adaptive functioning skills appear more in line with the observed IQ scores, and not in line with the much lower "Flynn corrected IQ scores." His

> leadership qualities in running gangs inside and outside of prison are impressive, he taught himself to read, and there is no evidence that he was mentally retarded before age 18, except for his mother's belated insight that he was "retarded as a child" after the defendant was charged with a capital crime.

Measurement of Adaptive Function

It is well understood that the assessment of adaptive function must be multidimensional. Olley and Cox (2008) provided this conclusion:

> By using multiple sources of information and thoroughly understanding the nature of mental retardation, the expert can reach a conclusion that has consensual validity. Ideally, many sources of information are congruent and lead to a single conclusion . . . the expert who relies on multiple sources is better equipped to use his or her judgment to draw a valid conclusion.
>
> (p. 387)

Use of a multidimensional model of adaptive functioning that incorporates multiple interviews as well as standardized scales is consistent with the Multi-Data Source Model (Denney, 2005, 2012b). The model is particularly relevant in *Atkins* litigation because the assessment of adaptive function should take into consideration adaptive function currently (or at the time of the crime) as well as retrospectively, to when the defendant was in the developmental period (defined as prior to 18 years of age). Added to the complexity is the need to consider atypical motivations not only for the defendant, but also for family members and spouses because of the forensic context. Examiners who use standardized scales such as the Vineland Adaptive Behavior Scales, third edition (Sparrow, Cicchetti, & Saulnier, 2016), and Adaptive Behavior Assessment System, third edition (Harrison & Oakland, 2015) to obtain information need to be aware that such scales have no validity scales within them and are relatively easy for examinees to manipulate (Doane & Salekin, 2009). An important issue to keep in mind in this regard is consistency across domains. It is clear that individuals with ID can have strengths and weakness, but adaptive function deficits that are significant will cut across multiple functional domains. The overall clinical picture must make sense with the facts of the person's life.

Mitigation Expertise at Sentencing

Any and all mental-health-related issues can be presented to the jury at the sentencing phase providing they are considered relevant by the trial judge. FNs are often called upon to examine the defendant and testify to developmental issues, learning issues, current emotional and cognitive issues, and basically any relevant issue within the scope of practice for a neuropsychologist that might help a jury consider the uniqueness of this particular defendant before determining whether or not to impose a death sentence. The U.S. Supreme Court has made it rather plainly clear that virtually any relevant individualized mitigating information pertaining to the convicted individual should be allowed (*Eddings v. Oklahoma*, 1982; *Lockett v. Ohio*, 1978; *Rompilla v. Beard*, 2005; *Skipper v. South Carolina*, 1986; *Wiggins v. Smith*, 2003). For a more detailed review of issues relevant for the FN and the evaluation process, see Heilbronner and Waller (2008) and Cunningham and Goldstein (2012).

Ethical Considerations

When one enters the forensic arena, particularly the criminal forensic arena, where questions of loss of liberty or even life or death are at issue, one must be certain to practice with high ethical standards. Above all, psychologists will be held to the American Psychological Association's Ethical Code of Conduct for Psychologists (American Psychological Association, 2002), with which most clinical neuropsychologists should already be familiar. The code no longer includes a special section of forensics, but many standards continue to apply. For example, this ethics code mandates that one should not practice outside of their realm of competency. Entering the criminal forensic arena raises a number of clinical and ethical considerations with which most clinical neuropsychologists are *not* familiar, and can easily thrust them outside the realm in which they are competent and into the area of malpractice. As such, this decision should not be made lightly, and extensive training and supervision should be pursued. For example, when neuropsychologists enter this area of practice, they must always be aware of issues such as in which jurisdiction they are practicing, who is their client, and what is the actual legal standard or question that they are assessing. For many clinical neuropsychologists, this raises the unfortunate scenario of *professional anosognosia*—they are not even aware of what they do not know. To paraphrase a former defense secretary, novices can be hampered with too many "unknown unknowns."

Another important consideration is to determine one's temperament and adjustment capacity, when exposed to criminal forensic scenarios. Clinical neuropsychologists must ask themselves if they can cope with the emotional costs of giving important testimony in a death penalty case (e.g., insomnia), if they can remain an impartial evaluator after exposure to documented details of heinous crimes, and if they can maintain their composure when dealing with quite aggressive cross-examination. The next section offers aspirational guidelines for ideal professional behavior in the forensic arena.

Specialty Guidelines for Forensic Psychology

Perhaps more so than in the civil area, the criminal forensic neuropsychologist should be familiar with the *Specialty*

Guidelines for Forensic Psychology (American Psychological Association, 2013). In addition to the aforementioned issues of competency and impartiality, these guidelines also emphasize issues such as having an adequate understanding of the scientific foundation of one's opinions and testimony, cultural sensitivity, and avoiding conflicts of interest and multiple relationships. For example, one should not perform a clinical evaluation for therapeutic purposes and then also serve as an expert witness in a criminal matter; one should only serve as a fact witness in this scenario.

Conclusions Regarding Ethical Issues

It is appropriate that we conclude this chapter on the subject of ethics; it is undoubtedly one of the most important subjects for clinical neuropsychologists practicing in criminal forensics (Sullivan & Denney, 2008). One cannot obtain a level of advance professional competency in this arena without a willingness to maintain the highest level of integrity and remain fixed to the genuine conclusions raised by the facts of the case, regardless of whether or not those conclusions favor the neuropsychologist's referral source. Maintaining a higher standard for one's level of expertise regarding the tests and procedures used helps ensure the most accurate testimony possible for the trier of fact and readies the neuropsychologist to face the corresponding level of scrutiny seen in the courtroom.

Note

1 Some argue that the calculation should not be based on the publication year of the manual, but should instead reflect the actual year of norming, which takes place in 1-2 years prior to official test publication and marketing.

References

American Law Institute. (1955). *Model Penal Code*, Section 4.01(1)(2), (Tent. Draft No. 4). Philadelphia, PA: Author.

American Psychiatric Association. (1994). *Diagnostic and Statistical Manual* (4th ed). Washington, DC: Author.

American Psychiatric Association. (2013). *Diagnostic and Statistical Manual* (5th ed). Washington, DC: Author.

American Psychological Association. (2002). American Psychological Association ethical principles of psychologists and code of conduct. *American Psychologist*, *57*, 1060–1073.

American Psychological Association. (2013). Specialty guidelines for forensic psychology. *American Psychologist*, *68*(1), 7.

Ardolf, B. R., Denney, R. L., & Houston, C. M. (2007). Base rates of negative response bias and malingered neurocognitive dysfunction among criminal defendants referred for neuropsychological evaluation. *The Clinical Neuropsychologist*, *21*(6), 899–916. doi: 10.1080/13825580600966391

Rex v. Arnold, 16 St. Tr. 695, 765 (1724).

Atkins v. Virginia, 536 U.S 304 (2002).

Bush, S. S., Connell, M. A., & Denney, R. L. (2006). *Ethical Practice in Forensic Psychology: A Systematic Model for Decision Making*. Washington, DC: American Psychological Association.

Catron, D. W., & Thompson, C. C. (1979). Test-retest gains in WAIS scores after four retest intervals. *Journal of Clinical Psychology*, *35*, 352–357.

Clark, C. R. (2013). Specific intent and diminished capacity. In I. B. Weiner & R. K. Otto (Eds.), *Handbook of Forensic Psychology* (4th ed., pp. 353–381). Hoboken, NJ: Wiley.

Clark v. Arizona, 548 U.S. 735 (2006).

Cunningham, M. D., & Goldstein, A. M. (2012). Sentencing determinations in death penalty cases. In R. K. Otto (Vol. Ed.) & I. B. Weiner (Series Ed.), *Handbook of Psychology: Vol. 11. Forensic Psychology* (2nd ed., pp. 473–514). Hoboken, NJ: Wiley.

Denney, R. L. (2005). Criminal responsibility and other criminal forensic issues. In G. J. Larrabee (Ed.), *Forensic Neuropsychology: A Scientific Approach*. (pp. 425–465). New York: Oxford University Press.

Denney, R. L. (2012a). Criminal forensic neuropsychology and assessment of competency. In G. J. Larrabee (Ed.), *Forensic Neuropsychology: A Scientific Approach* (2nd ed., pp. 438–472). New York: Oxford University Press.

Denney, R. L. (2012b). Criminal responsibility and other criminal forensic issues. In G. J. Larrabee (Ed.), *Forensic Neuropsychology: A Scientific Approach* (pp. 473–500). New York: Oxford University Press.

Denney, R. L., & Wynkoop, T. F. (2000). Clinical neuropsychology in the criminal forensic setting. *Journal of Head Trauma Rehabilitation*, *15*(2), 804–828.

Doane, B. M., & Salekin, K. L. (2009). Susceptibility of current adaptive behavior measures to feigned deficits. *Law & Human Behavior*, *33*, 329–343. doi: 10.1007/s10979-008-9157-5

Douglas, K. S., Hart, S. D., Groscup, J. L., & Litwack, T. R. (2013). Assessing violence Risk. In I. B. Weiner & R. K. Otto (Eds.), *Handbook of Forensic Psychology* (4th ed., pp. 385–441). Hoboken, NJ: Wiley.

Douglas, K. S., Hart, S. D., Webster, C. D., & Belfrage, H. (2013). *Historical-Clinical-Risk Management-20 (Version 3): Violence Risk Assessment Guidelines (HCR-20 V3)*. Burnaby, Canada: Mental Health, Law, and Policy Institute, Simon Fraser University.

Dusky v. United States, 362 U.S. 402 (1960).

Eddings v. Oklahoma, 455 U.S. 104 (1982).

Everington, C. T., & Luckasson, R. (1992). *Competence Assessment for Standing Trial for Defendants With Mental Retardation (CAST*MR): Test Manual*. Worthington, OH: IDS.

Estevis, E., Basso, M. R., & Combs, D. (2012). Effects of practice on the Wechsler Adult Intelligence Scale-IV across 3- and 6-month intervals. *The Clinical Neuropsychologist*, *26*, 239–254. doi: 10.1080/13854046.2012.659219

Fazio, R. L., & Denney, R. L. (2015). Assessment of neurophysiological and neuropsychological bases for violence. In C. A. Pietz & C. A. Mattson (Eds.) *Violent Offenders: Understanding and Assessment* (pp. 425-451). New York: Oxford University Press.

Fletcher, J. M., Stuebing, K. K., & Hughes, L. C. (2010). IQ scores should be corrected for the Flynn effect in high-stakes decisions. *Journal of Psychoeducational Assessment*, *28*(5), 469–473. doi: 10.1177/0734282910373341

Flynn, J. R. (1984). The mean IQ of Americans: Massive gains 1932 to 1978. *Psychological Bulletin*, *95*(1), 29.

Flynn, J. R. (1987a). Massive IQ gains in 14 nations: What IQ tests really measure. *Psychological Bulletin*, *101*(2), 171.

Flynn, J. R. (1987b). "Massive IQ gains in 14 nations: What IQ tests really measure": Correction to Flynn. *Psychological Bulletin, 101*(3), 427.

Frederick, R. I., DeMier, R. L., & Towers, K. (2004). *Assessing Competency to Stand Trial: Foundations in Case Law*. Sarasota, FL: Professional Resource Press.

Frumkin, I. B. (2008). Psychological evaluation in *Miranda* waiver and confession cases. In R. L. Denney & J. P. Sullivan (Eds.). *Clinical Neuropsychology in the Criminal Forensic Setting* (pp. 135–175). New York: Guilford Press.

Godinez v. Moran, 125 L. Ed. 2d, 509 U.S. 389 (1993).

Gresham, F. M. (2009). Interpretation of intelligence test scores in *Atkins* cases: Conceptual and psychometric issues. *Applied Neuropsychology, 16*, 91–97.

Greiffenstein, M. (2011). Secular IQ increases by Epigenesis? The hypothesis of cognitive genotype optimization. *Psychological Reports, 109*(2), 353–366.

Grisso, T. (1986). *Evaluating Competencies: Forensic Assessments and Instruments*. New York: Plenum Press.

Grisso, T. (1988). *Competency to Stand Trial Evaluations: A Manual for Practice*. Sarasota, FL: Professional Resource Exchange.

Grisso, T., Borum, R., Edens, J. F., Moye, J., & Otto, R. K. (2003). *Evaluating Competencies: Forensic Assessments and Instruments* (2nd ed.). New York: Kluwer Academic/Plenum.

Hagan, L. D., Drogin, E. Y., & Guilmette, T. J. (2008). Adjusting IQ scores for the Flynn effect: Consistent with the standard of practice? *Professional Psychology: Research and Practice, 39*(6), 619.

Hagan, L. D., Drogin, E. Y., & Guilmette, T. J. (2010). IQ scores should not be adjusted for the Flynn effect in capital punishment cases. *Journal of Psychoeducational Assessment, 28*(5), 474–476.

Hall v. Florida, 572 U.S., 134 S. Ct. 1986 (2014).

Hanson, R. K., & Thronton, D. (1999). *Static-99: Improving Actuarial Risk Assessments for Sex Offenders*. User Report 99–02. Ottawa, Canada: Department of the Solicitor General.

Harris, G. T., Rice, M. E., & Quinsey, V. (1993). Violent recidivism of mentally disordered offenders: The development of a statistical prediction instrument. *Criminal Justice and Behavior, 20*, 315–335.

Harrison, P. L., & Oakland, T. (2015). *Adaptive Behavior Assessment System* (3rd ed.). Los Angeles, CA: Western Psychological Services.

Hart, S. D., Kropp, P. R., Laws, D. R., Klaver, J., Logan, C., & Watt, K. A. (2003). *The Risk for Sexual Violence Protocol (RSVP): Structured Professional Guidelines for Assessing Risk of Sexual Violence*. Burnaby, Canada: Mental Health, Law, and Policy Institute, Simon Fraser University.

Heilbronner, R. L., & Waller, D. (2008). Neuropsychological consultation in the sentencing phase of capital cases. In R. L. Denney & J. P. Sullivan (Eds.), *Clinical Neuropsychology in the Criminal Forensic Setting* (pp. 273–294). New York: Guilford.

Indiana v. Edwards, 544 U.S. 164 (2008).

Kanaya, T. (2004). *Age Differences in IQ Trends: Unpacking the Flynn Effect*. Doctoral Dissertation. Cornell University, Ithaca, NY.

Kanaya, T., Ceci, S. J., & Scullin, M. H. (2005). Age differences within secular IQ trends An individual growth modeling approach. *Intelligence, 33*(6), 613–621.

Kaufman, A. S. (2010). "In what way are apples and oranges alike?" A critique of Flynn's interpretation of the Flynn Effect. *Journal of Psychoeducational Research, 28*, 382–398.

Kaufman, A. S., & Lichtenberger, E. O. (2006). *Assessing Adolescent and Adult Intelligence* (3rd ed.). Hoboken, NJ: Wiley & Sons.

Kaufmann, P. M. (2008). Admissibility of neuropsychological evidence in criminal cases. In R. L. Denney & J. P. Sullivan (Eds.), *Clinical Neuropsychology in the Criminal Forensic Setting* (pp. 55–90). New York: Guilford Press.

Kausler, D. H. (1991). *Experimental Psychology, Cognition, and Human Aging*. New York: Springer-Verlag.

Kausler, D. H. (1982). *Experimental Psychology and Human Aging*. New York: Wiley.

Kozol, H. L., Boucher, R. J., & Garofalo, R. F. (1972). The diagnosis and treatment of dangerousness. *Crime and Delinquency, 18*, 371–392.

Lockett v. Ohio, 438 U.S. 586 (1978).

McGarry, A. L., Lelos, D., & Lipsitt, P. D. (1973). *Competency to Stand Trial and Mental Illness*. Washington, DC: U.S. Government Printing Office.

McLearen, A. M., Pietz, C. A., & Denney, R. L. (2004). Evaluation of psychological damages. In W. O'Donohue & E. Levensky (Eds.), *Forensic Psychology* (pp. 267–299). New York: Academic.

Melton, G. B., Petrila, J., Poythress, N. G., Slobogin, C., Lyons, P. M., & Otto, R. K. (2007). *Psychological Evaluations for the Courts: A Handbook for Mental Health Professional and Lawyers* (3rd ed.). New York: Guilford Press.

Miranda v. Arizona, 384 U.S. 436 (1966).

Monahan, J., Steadman, H., Appelbaum, P., Grisso, T., Mulvey, E., Roth, L., . . . Silver, E. (2005). *The Classification of Violence Risk*. Lutz, FL: Psychological Assessment Resources.

Morris v. Slappy, 461 U.S. 1 (1983).

Mrad, D. (1996, September). *Criminal responsibility evaluations*. Paper presented at Issues in Forensic Assessment Symposium, Federal Bureau of Prisons, Atlanta, GA.

Neisser, U. (1998). Introduction: Rising test scores and what they mean. In U. Neisser (Ed.), *The Rising Curve: Long-Term Gains in IQ and Related Measures* (pp. 3–22). Washington, DC: American Psychological Association.

Nunnally, J. C., & Bernstein, I. H. (1994). *Psychometric Theory* (3rd ed.). New York: McGraw Hill.

Olley, J. G., & Cox, A. W. (2008). Assessment of adaptive behavior in adult forensic cases: The use of the Adaptive Behavior Assessment System-II. In T. Oakland & P. L. Harrison (Eds.), *ABAS-II: Clinical Use and Interpretation* (pp. 381–398). New York: Academic.

Otto, R. K., Musick, J. E., & Sherrod, C. B. (2010). *Inventory of Legal Knowledge: Professional Manual.* Lutz, FL: Psychologial Assessment Resources.

Packer, I. K. (2009). *Best Practices in Forensic Mental Health Assessment: Evaluation of Criminal Responsibility*. New York: Oxford University Press.

Parsons v. State, 81 Ala. 577, 2 So. 854, 2 So. 2d 854 (1887).

Penry v. Lynaugh, 492 U.S. 1 (1989).

Poythress, N. G., Nicholson, R., Otto, R. K., Edens, J. F., Bonnie, R. J., Monahan, J., & Hoge, S. K. (1999). *The MacArthur Competence Assessment Tool—Criminal Adjudication: Professional manual*. Lutz, FL: Psychological Assessment Resources.

Quinsey, V. L., Harris, G. T., Rice, M. E., & Cormier, C. (2006). *Violent Offenders: Appraising and Managing Risk* (2nd ed.). Washington, DC: American Psychological Association.

Rapport, L. J., Brines, D. B., Axelrod, B. N., & Theisen, M. E. (1997). Full scale IQ as mediator of practice effects: The rich get richer. *The Clinical Neuropsychologist, 11*, 375–380. doi: 10.1080/13854049708400455

Rawlings, D. B., & Crewe, N. M. (1992). Test-retest practice effects and the test score changes of the WAIS-R in recovering traumatically brain-injured survivors. *The Clinical Neuropsychologist, 6*, 415–430. doi: 10.1080/13854049208401868

Rex v. M'Naghten, 8 Eng. Rep. 718 (H.L. 1843).

Reynolds, C. R., Niland, J., Wright, J. E., & Rosenn, M. (2010). Failure to apply the Flynn Correction in death penalty litigation: Standard practice of today maybe, but certainly malpractice of tomorrow. *Journal of Psychoeducational Assessment, 28*(1), 477–481.

Riley, J. A. (1998, March) Introducing the Revised-CAI and assessment of trial competency—Use of the *Revised-Competency Assessment Instrument Handbook*. Presentation at American Psychology–Law Society Biennial Conference, Redondo Beach, CA.

Rogers, R., Sewell, K. W., Drogin, E. Y., & Fidduccia, C. E. (2012). *Standardized Assessment of Miranda Abilities: Professional Manual*. Lutz, FL: Psychological Assessment Resources.

Rogers, R., Tillbrook, C. E., & Sewell, K. W. (2004). *Evaluation of Competency to Stand Trial–Revised*. Lutz, FL: Psychological Assessment Resources.

Rompilla v. Beard, 545 U.S. 374 (2005).

Saks, M. J. (1990). Exert witnesses, nonexpert witnesses, and nonwitness experts. *Law and Human Behavior, 14*, 291–313.

Schmitz-Scherzer, R., & Thomae, H. (1983). Constancy and change of behavior in old age: Findings from the Bonn longitudinal study on aging. In K. W. Schaie (Ed.), *Longitudinal Studies of Adult Psychological Development* (pp. 191–221). New York: Guilford.

Siegler, I. (1983). Psychological aspects of the Duke longitudinal studies. In K. W. Schaie (Ed.), *Longitudinal Studies of Adult Psychological Development* (pp. 136–190). New York: Guilford.

Skipper v. South Carolina, 476 U.S. 1 (1986).

Sparrow, S. S., Cicchetti, D. V., & Saulnier, C. A. (2016). *Vineland Adaptive Behavior Scales* (3rd ed.). Bloomington, MN: Pearson.

Sternberg, R. J. (2010). The Flynn effect: So what? *Journal of Psychoeducational Assessment, 28*, 434–440. doi: 10.1177/0734282910373349

Sullivan, J. P., & Denney, R. L. (2008). A final word on authentic professional competence in criminal forensic neuropsychology. In R. L. Denney & J. P. Sullivan (Eds.), *Clinical Neuropsychology in the Criminal Forensic Setting* (pp. 391–400). New York: Guilford Press.

Sundet, J. M., Barlaug, D. G., & Torjussen, T. M. (2004). The end of the Flynn effect? A study of secular trends in mean intelligence test scores of Norwegian conscripts during half a century. *Intelligence, 32*(4), 349.

Tysse, J. E. (2005). Note: The right to an "imperfect" trial—Amnesia, malingering, and competency to stand trial. *William Mitchell Law Review, 32*, 353–387.

United States Code (2011). Title 18, Section 17, Insanity Defense.

United States v. Andrews, 469 F.3d 1113 (7th Cir. 2006).

United States v. Pohlot, 827 F. 2d 889 (3rd Cir. 1987).

United States v. Rinchack, 820 F.2d 1557 (11th Cir., 1987).

United States v. Swanson, 572 F.2d 523 (5th Cir. 1978).

Wechsler, D. (1981). *Wechsler Adult Intelligence Scale* (Revised). New York: Psychological Corporation.

Wechsler, D. (2008). *Wechsler Adult Intelligence Scale* (4th ed.). San Antonio, TX: NCS Pearson.

Wildman, R. W., Batchelor, E. S., Thompson, L., Nelson, R. R., Moore, J. T., Patterson, M. E., & de Laosa, M. (1978). *The Georgia Court Competency Test: An Attempt to Develop a Rapid, Quantitative Measure of Fitness for Trial*. (Unpublished manuscript). Forensic Services Division, Central State Hospital, Midgeville, GA.

Wiggins v. Smith, 539 U.S. 510 (2003).

Wildman, R. W., Batchelor, E. S., Thompson, L., Nelson, R. R., Moore, J. T., Patterson, M. E., & deLaosa, M. (1978). *The Georgia Court Competency Test: An Attempt to Develop a Rapid, Quantitative Measure of Fitness for Trial*. (Unpublished manuscript). Forensic Services Division, Central State Hospital, Midgeville, GA.

Wilson v. United States, 391 F.2d 460 (D.C. Cir. 1968).

Wong, S., & Gordon, A. E. (1999–2003). *The Violence Risk Scale*. Saskatoon, Canada: University of Saskatchewan, Department of Psychology.

Yates, K. F., & Denney, R. L. (2008). Neuropsychology in the assessment of mental state at the time of the offense. In R. L. Denney & J. P. Sullivan (Eds.). *Clinical Neuropsychology in the Criminal Forensic Setting* (pp. 204–237). New York: Guilford Press.

Youtsey v. United States, 97 F. 937, 940 (6th Circ.1899).

Zapf, P. A., Roesch, R., & Pirelli, G. (2013). Assessing competency to stand trial. In I. B. Weiner & R. K. Otto (Eds.), *Handbook of Forensic Psychology* (4th ed., pp. 281–314). Hoboken, NJ: Wiley.

Zhou, X., Zhu, J., & Weiss, L. G. (2010). Peeking inside the "black box" of the Flynn effect: Evidence from three Wechsler instruments. *Journal of Psychoeducational Assessment, 28*(5), 399–411.

41 Disability

Michael Chafetz

Disability Terminology and Constructs

The term *disability* is defined in a broad way by advocacy and professional groups and typically has a distinct meaning from legal terminology one sees in public (Social Security) and private (insurance) disability evaluation settings. For example, the World Health Organization (WHO) World Health Report (2001) invokes *disability* to describe limitations from many different sources of impairment. WHO (2001) used a Global Burden of Disease (GBD) metric called the *disability-adjusted life year* (DALY). One DALY unit can be thought of as one lost year of healthy life due to premature death or disability. WHO (2001) reported that mental and neurological disorders accounted for 10.5% of the total DALYs lost due to all diseases and injuries. According to WHO (2001), the GBD 2000 estimates indicated that mental and neurological conditions account for 30.8% of all years lived with disability.

The American Psychological Association in its *Guidelines for Assessment of and Interventions With Persons With Disabilities* (2012) cited the U.S. Department of Health and Human Services (2005) construct that *disabilities* are physical, mental, and/or sensory characteristics that affect a person's ability to engage in activities of daily life. Similarly, in the Americans With Disabilities Act (ADA) Amendments Act of 2008, *disability* is defined as a physical or mental impairment that substantially limits a person's ability to engage in a life activity. These definitions are of great importance in both public and private evaluations for disability in which assessment of daily living activities takes on significance in the understanding of limitations caused by the impairments. WHO (2001) calls for a public health approach linking biological, psychological, and social factors to reduce the overall burden of mental disorders.

Rosa's Law (2010) amended all federal public laws that use *mental retardation* terminology, replacing the older term with *intellectual disability* (ID). The American Association on Intellectual and Developmental Disabilities (AAIDD), formerly the American Association on Mental Retardation (AAMR) has taken a disability-based environmental perspective in redefining *mental retardation.* AAIDD now states that the basis for helping and defining the levels of persons with ID is by the supports necessary to achieve optimal functioning (Schalock, Borthwick-Duffy, Bradley, Buntinx, Coulter, et al., 2010). AAIDD promoted the adoption of Rosa's Law. According to AAIDD, the construct of *disability* has evolved from a *deficit*, which is person-centered, into a *human phenomenon* with origins that lie in organic and social factors. It is no longer an absolute and unvarying trait of a person, but now an interaction of a person and the environment. With appropriate personalized supports over a continuous and sustained period, the functioning of a person with ID will improve.

Under the Social Security definition of disability, the claimant must be unable to engage in any substantial gainful activity (SGA) because of a medically determinable physical or mental impairment. This impairment must last (or be expected to last) 12 months continuously or be expected to result in death (Social Security Administration [SSA], 2013a). Under this definition, the claimant must prove inability to work in any job for money; under the Supplemental Security Income (SSI) program, a means-tested program, the claimant must not be able to earn more than a legal limit (about $1,000/month), which is the SGA amount (unless the claimant is blind). This is a strict legal definition of disability under which SSA determines whether an applicant is eligible for benefits. A claimant must meet the particular listing requirements from the Blue Book (SSA, 2013b) for benefits for any particular disability (e.g., mental disorders). For children, *disability* means that the child has a medically determinable physical or mental impairment that causes marked or severe functional limitations (Morton, 2010).

Under private disability contracts with a disability insurance carrier (e.g., Unum, Northwestern Mutual, Liberty Mutual), an individual may obtain disability benefits for partial or total disability, whereas Social Security has benefits for total disability only. Private disability carriers may also define contracts for short-term or long-term disability benefits. Some contracts may provide benefits if the individual is unable to work in his own occupation, while others are for any occupation for which the individual has training or skills (as with Social Security). As with Social Security, private disability carriers define the particular disabilities in specific terms, and are interested in how the impairments limit the person's activities, particularly work activities. Social Security benefits are funded by general tax revenues (SSI) or the

Federal Insurance Contributions Act (FICA) tax withdrawals from paychecks of workers for Social Security Disability Insurance (SSDI). Private disability premiums are paid for by the individual, the employer, or both.

The SSA has two basic disability programs: SSDI for workers and their dependents who have paid into the Social Security Trust Fund through the FICA tax; and SSI for disabled individuals and dependents with limited income and assets.

The Disability Determinations Services (DDSs) are state agencies funded by SSA that administer these disability programs. Through a professional liaison, the DDSs find and credential qualified psychologists. The schedulers arrange consultative examinations (CEs) with psychologists who have already been qualified, and the psychologists will then perform psychological consultative examinations (PCEs) for the referred cases. The DDSs will also obtain medical evidence about the claimant, attempting to catalogue impairments from claimed symptoms and the obtained evidence. As part of making a disability determination, the DDS personnel will have to look at all the evidence and determine whether the claim meets the legal definition of Disability according to the Blue Book listings for each mental impairment (SSA, 2008).

Legislative History

On August 14, 1935, President Franklin Delano Roosevelt signed the Social Security Act into law, providing an old-age retirement pension (Old Age and Survivors Program) as income for those who were no longer working. This law saved millions from becoming impoverished when they were no longer able to work, thus setting the stage for the disability compensation laws in the 1950s. In 1954, amendments to the Social Security Act led to the Disability Insurance program, and in 1955 a "freeze" was placed on records during the periods a person was unable to work, which prevented the disability from reducing or eliminating retirement benefits (SSA, 2012). On August 1, 1956, President Dwight Eisenhower signed the new disability legislation, which delivered cash benefits to disabled workers aged 50–64 after a six-month waiting period.

Over the next four years, Congress broadened the scope of this new disability program, allowing benefits for dependents and for workers under the age of 50 who became disabled. The Civil Rights Act of 1964 protected women and minorities from discrimination in employment, and in the same period Congress passed legislation benefitting people with disabilities, including Medicare, the Elementary and Secondary Education Act, and the expansion of the Vocational Rehabilitation Act (Winegar, 2006). However, it was not until 1972 that President Richard Nixon signed into law the needs-based SSI program established to provide a true social safety net for disabled individuals who were never able to work, and for children with disabilities.

The next stage for disability legislation occurred with the ADA in 1990. The ADA was based on the Education for the Handicapped Act of 1975 (Colker, 2005; Chafetz, 2015), which in a newer version in 1997 was called the Individuals With Disabilities Education Act (IDEA, 1997). This law specified that in order to receive federal funds, states must develop and implement policies that ensure that all children with disabilities receive a free appropriate public education. The original act is known as Public Law 94–142. The Individuals With Disabilities Education Improvement Act (IDEIA) of 2004 provided additional procedural safeguards for students with disabilities.

The ADA (Title I) prohibited discrimination against a qualified individual with a disability concerning any aspect of the employment. Employers cannot discriminate against disabled individuals who, with appropriate accommodations, could perform the essential functions of their positions (Colker, 2001, 2005).

The ADA was heralded as becoming potentially one of the great civil rights laws for disabled individuals, but the next 15 years were seen as a time during which disabled plaintiffs frequently lost cases in favor of employer-defendants (Colker, 2001, 2005; Winegar, 2006). The ADA did not provide the intended relief during this period, and Colker (2001) has indicated that appellate litigation has not been an effective vehicle for ADA enforcement. Colker (2001) chided Shalit's (1997) characterization ("buffet of perks") as being inaccurate and misleading.

For a summary of various disability statutes and laws, including the Telecommunications Act, Fair Housing Act, Voting Accessibility for the Elderly and Handicapped Act, etc., see the U.S. Department of Justice Guide to Disability Rights (www.ada.gov/cguide.htm#anchor64984).

Social-Political Climate

It is interesting to note the political climate of the times. In 1972, the Democrat nominee for president, Senator George McGovern, had to replace Senator Thomas Eagleton (D-Mo) in the vice presidential slot on the ticket when it was disclosed that Senator Eagleton had been treated for depression, and there was a negative public reaction (Colker, 2005). In the 1988 presidential race between Michael Dukakis and the senior George Bush, there were rumors about mental illness flying when Governor Dukakis refused to disclose his medical records. When President Reagan, who was finishing his term and not running further for office, was asked about these rumors, he replied: "Look, I'm not going to pick on an invalid."

However, at about the same time, in August 1988, Vice President Bush was urging Congress to enact the ADA, and bills were introduced in the Senate and House of Representatives. The Senate bill passed 76:8 in September 1989, and the House bill passed 403:20 in May 1990. George Bush's son Neil had struggled with dyslexia. As president, George Bush commanded Attorney General Dick Thornburgh, whose own son had experienced a traumatic brain injury (TBI) in a 1960 motor vehicle accident, to work with Congress on the legislation (Colker, 2005). As so often happens, the legislation was pushed by those who had directly experienced struggles with disabling conditions.

A Medicolegal Arena: Ethics and Boundaries

Whether performing public or private disability evaluations, military compensation and pension, fitness-for-duty assessments, or for workers' compensation (WC), evaluators must understand that they are working in a medicolegal arena. Evaluations for accommodations for testing or for the schools fall under the same rubric, as the goal of the client is not necessarily to be helped clinically but to obtain a compensation or benefit under the law.

The typical training for a clinician involves developing knowledge of the consultation in which a patient comes to the clinician seeking help for a mental or cognitive condition. The psychologist's role in a clinical consultation is to offer assessment, diagnosis, recommendations, or forms of intervention and treatment. The client in this scenario is the patient, whether self-referred or referred by another provider. Payment in some form is usually expected, by the patient or from a third party (e.g., insurance company or parents), except when the psychologist accepts the case pro bono (work undertaken for the public good without charge). No matter what form or source of payment, however, the psychologist is expected to attempt to help the patient-client concerning the presenting condition. The psychologist has a fiduciary duty to this person (and/or parents or guardians). Privacy rights extend to this person under the relevant Health Insurance Portability and Accountability Act (HIPAA) of 1996 provisions. A treatment alliance is expected, and there exists a typical doctor–patient relationship, with appropriate clinical boundaries to avoid harm and exploitation of this relationship (American Psychological Association, 2002).

Concerning a medicolegal evaluation, the evaluator should fully understand that the motivations of claimants and patients are different (Greenberg & Shuman, 1997, 2007; Strasburger, Gutheil, & Brodsky, 1997). While the patient is seeking understanding and help regarding an uncomfortable condition, the claimant is seeking to have the disability or worker's compensation claim approved. These motivations are widely disparate, and frequently lead to different presentations. Claimants are often uncomfortable about doing anything that might lead to a denial of the claim. There may be an active attempt by the claimant to mislead the evaluator about the condition being claimed. The evaluator should not treat this behavior as a personal affront. It is always wise for the evaluator to be respectful toward the claimant, which may alleviate discomfort, but the evaluator is not expected to provide treatment or any intervention.

In a medicolegal workup for public disability (Social Security Disability), the client may be the local DDS, one of the state agencies funded by SSA to apply the rules and listings of disabilities to the determination of each claim. A Social Security private attorney may contract with the evaluator for a psychiatric, psychological, or neuropsychological examination. In this case, the claimant (through his or her attorney) is indeed the client. The motivation, however, is the same: That is, to prove to the DDS that the claimant has met the listing requirements to be awarded disability benefits. The evaluation is not about diagnosis or impairment per se, but about the claim for an inability to work (Puente, 1987).

These boundary conditions will also be seen in a WC setting. The evaluator may be seen at the request of the claimant (often through his or her attorney), or can be retained directly by the WC carrier. Again, the motivation by the claimant, no matter which "side" retaining the evaluator, is to obtain the legally appropriate benefits or compensation under the law. In WC cases, it is interesting that the payment to the evaluator usually comes from the WC carrier, no matter which "side" is consulting with the evaluator.

In both public and private disability cases, the evaluator is frequently asked to perform an IME, which can take the form of an independent psychological or neuropsychological evaluation. The term *independent* in these cases is taken to mean that the evaluator has not formed the doctor–patient relationship with the claimant, and is indeed *independent* of that relationship. As a practical matter, the evaluator who performs all, or predominantly, IMEs may be challenged as to "sidedness," with the criticism that the evaluator's opinions are shaped by the income coming largely from one "side."

This form of criticism, coming usually from lawyers, rests on the assumption that a 50–50 split of consultation from the plaintiff and defense (IME) sides would preclude bias, but this reasoning is faulty. For example, if the 50–50 evaluator always decides for the defense when the defense is paying, and always for the plaintiff when the plaintiff is paying, then the evaluator is perfectly biased toward where the money is coming from. This scenario presents the ultimate condition of bias.

The truly unbiased examiner should understand that integrity comes from the willingness (and actual behavior) to call the case exactly as the data findings show. When performing a disability IME, if the claimant is impaired and the scores are valid, then the conclusions and questions answered should accurately reflect the findings. If, in a plaintiff's case, the individual is found to be malingering, the examiner should inform the lawyer about the facts. While the retaining party may not be pleased, it is the duty of the examiner to follow the findings of the examination. Moreover, it is considered a myth that performing a defense-retained IME causes poor effort by the claimant (Greiffenstein, 2009). Indeed, the source of forensic referral (plaintiff vs. defense) does not affect any domain of neuropsychological test performance in those who pass validity tests or those who fail validity tests (Meyers, Reinsch-Boothby, Miller, Rohling, & Axelrod, 2011).

In a PCE for the DDS, the DDS is the client of the psychologist/neuropsychologist. Indeed, the PCE can be considered as a psychological IME in which SSA is sending the claimant for an independent examination as part of the evidence gathering for a disability determination. The psychologist conducting the PCE neither works for the DDS nor for the claimant, and should fully embrace the independence. The job is to be objective and accurate, and to avoid bias in favor of the DDS or the claimant.

Concerning private disability evaluations, there is now a cottage industry of IME companies positioned between the disability insurance carrier and the evaluators. Typically, the IME companies have a number of examiners nationwide who have been vetted carefully and whose reports can be trusted to provide an accurate accounting of the findings and to answer the referral questions. Concerning the issue of bias, these IME companies provide a buffer between the disability carrier, who is paying the fee, and the examiner providing the IME service. In this way, the IME companies help ensure that the focus of the evaluation is on the accurate answering of the referral questions.

Informed Consent

Under the American Psychological Association ethics code (3.10, 9.03), it is necessary for the psychologist to obtain informed consent for assessments except where testing is mandated by law. In criminal law (e.g., *Atkins* defense), when a defendant raises the defense of ID (formerly, *mental retardation*), the state has a right to its own examination of the individual. In litigation generally, as a practical matter, the lawyers (on both sides) will agree to the evaluation, and thus the plaintiff's attorney has already provided consent for the individual. When a claimant applies for Social Security Disability (SSD)[1], the claimant agrees to be evaluated at the request of the DDS officials. Private disability contracts usually have a provision for evaluation at the request of the disability carrier. Nevertheless, under the American Psychological Association ethics code (3.10), at the time of assessment the evaluator should convey to the claimant in language that is reasonably understandable to that person the nature and boundaries of the evaluation.

The informed consent should contain information on the additional limits on confidentiality inherent in an IME, and may even restate the traditional limits on confidentiality under applicable state law (e.g., abuse of vulnerable persons). A statement that there is no doctor–patient relationship is important, and it is helpful to include that this examination does not replace psychiatric, psychological, or neuropsychological examination or treatment. A listing of points to include in a disability IME is shown on pp. 981 and 982.

A question often arises whether or what kind of warning about malingering should be provided in the informed consent. When this writer was performing psychological CEs, the local DDS required the following warning: "Failure to do your best on these tests may result in an unfavorable decision on your claim." This warning is reportedly still being given. The debate about warnings concerns whether malingerers may attempt to cover their tracks when warned (Schenk & Sullivan, 2010; Boone, 2013).

As Boone (2013) has reviewed, there are studies showing reduced sensitivity of validity tests when a warning is given. Boone (2013) further argues that no warning is necessary when embedded validity indicators are administered, as these are an integral part of tests normally given in a neuropsychological evaluation. For example, the Minnesota Multiphasic Personality Inventory–2 (MMPI-2 or MMPI-RF) has validity scales by which one can determine the validity of the examination, but there is no tradition of warning about specific scales on the MMPI.

Points to Include in Disability IME Informed Consent

- An insurance company is requesting an examination of you and will pay the fee.
- This insurance company is regarded as the client of the examiner.
- The examiner will prepare a written report that details the findings, and answers the questions asked by the insurance company.
- If you decide to withhold the report, you must send a request in writing to the examiner. This request will be effective only insofar the examiner has not already relied upon this release of the report.
- The examiner cannot foresee the consequences of any decision not to participate in the examination or to withhold the report.
- Because of your relationship with the insurance company, any findings that you are entitled to [note: be sure to check your state's applicable law] should be obtained directly from the insurance company.
- The examiner is an independent practitioner who does not work for this insurance company and is not employed by them.
- The examiner does not participate in any decision concerning your claim.
- To maintain the integrity of the evaluation, the examiner does not permit any recording of the evaluation, either secretly or openly. By your signature, you agree not to record this evaluation yourself or permit this evaluation to be recorded by others.
- The examiner has [check applicable state law] a duty to warn anyone to whom you express a violent threat, which duty is discharged by calling the police. The examiner is also required by law to report abuse of vulnerable persons.
- This is an objective evaluation. You are warned to do your best on everything, and to provide accurate responding, as the examiner cannot foresee the consequences if there is any finding to the contrary.

- Please understand that you are not the examiner's patient, and the examiner cannot offer you treatment or advice. The examiner will certainly offer you respect for your dignity and person, but if you need treatment or advice you must obtain this from your own doctor(s).
- This examination does not replace regular psychological or neuropsychological examination or treatment.

Bush (2013), in discussing ethics in validity assessment, argued that justification for examiner deception in validity assessment can be found in the American Psychological Association ethics code (8.07) on "Deception in Research" in which deception is prohibited unless the techniques have a significant scientific, educational, or applied value and that effective nondeceptive procedures are not feasible. Indeed, providing claimants with accurate information that a particular test is not a real neuropsychological test but in fact measures their quality of effort would defeat the purpose of the test. Bush (2013) also argues that the other point that permits ethical use of deception is the informed consent process in which the examinees are told before the examination that measures to determine the validity of the examination (i.e., effort and accuracy of reporting) will be administered. Thus, warnings are ethically appropriate and even necessary in a general way at the outset of the examination.

Concerns About Cheating

Stevens (1986) cited Rabbi Jerome Folkman's observation that in Judea in the middle of the second century B.C. rabbis discovered people taking advantage of relief programs of the era. According to Pratico (2001: 78), as the SSDI program was being debated in 1954, Elmer Hess, president of the American Medical Association (AMA) warned that "being on the federal dole would be crippling to the psyche of workers," that it was "tantamount to the government bribing them to stay out of the workforce," and that the program provided "an institutionalized reason to avoid vocational rehabilitation." Cyrus Anderson also warned that there would be doctors who would not be above certifying a dubious disability, and that there would be other doctors who lose patients because they refuse to cooperate with malingerers.

To be sure, the Office of the Inspector General (OIG) Fraud Unit for the SSA has traditionally been concerned with individuals who "purposely withhold, exaggerate, or fabricate work or medical information" (OIG, 2013) to collect disability benefits for which they are not eligible. The OIG's Cooperative Disability Investigations program and SSA's continuing disability reviews are noted to be highly effective in guarding against disability overpayments. However, in Congressional testimony dated March 20, 2013, OIG noted that increasing numbers of disability claims and beneficiaries have strained resources (OIG, 2013). In his own investigation, Senator Tom Coburn (Social Security Benefits, 2013) uncovered numerous abuses in the system.

The Issue of Malingering

The form of cheating to which disability evaluators will be most exposed is *malingering*, defined as the intentional production or exaggeration of false or misleading symptoms for compensation or the avoidance of punishment or duty (American Psychiatric Association; 2000; 2013). Malingering is also defined behaviorally as performance invalidity (Larrabee, 2012) in which an examinee intentionally underperforms on a cognitive test to demonstrate impaired memory processes, mental slowing, perceptual distortion, etc., for compensation or avoidance of punishment.

Malingering is widespread in medicolegal examinations. Summing more than 11 studies of base-rates of malingering, Larrabee (2003) showed an overall frequency of 548/1,363 subjects (40.2%), most claiming mild TBI, who were identified with performance deficits consistent with malingering. Appreciating the consistency in base-rate estimates of malingering in numerous studies over a wide review, Larrabee, Millis, and Meyers (2009) proposed a "new magic number" of 40% ± 10% to indicate the average base rate (prevalence) of malingering being about 30%–50% in individuals who have an external incentive.

Whether a claimant is malingering is an inference by the examiner based upon a probability analysis with strict knowledge of guidelines in the field. Generally accepted guidelines for malingered neurocognitive dysfunction were developed by Slick, Sherman, and Iverson (1999), and updated by Slick and Sherman (2013). The guidelines for probable malingered cognitive dysfunction require an external incentive (A), with two or more types of evidence from neuropsychological testing (B). The latter could include two failures on established validity tests (Larrabee, Greiffenstein, Greve, & Bianchini, 2007), or be a matter of atypical performance patterns on cognitive testing (Larrabee, 2003). The Slick et al. (1999) guidelines also include evidence from inconsistencies in self-report (C); probable malingering can also be defined with one inconsistency from testing (B) and one from self-report (C). In these guidelines, definite malingering is defined as involving clear and compelling evidence of volitional exaggeration or fabrication of cognitive dysfunction absent plausible alternative explanations, as when someone performs significantly below chance ($p < 0.05$) on a test of validity. Significantly below chance performance on forced-choice validity testing has also been termed "the smoking gun of intent" (Pankratz & Erickson, 1990: 385). If the individual had been blindfolded, and thus unable to see the test stimuli, the performance would have been at chance levels, and therefore higher. In these guidelines, alternative explanations of test performance must be ruled out (D-criterion), as when developmental or neurological conditions would also cause the poor validity test performance. In these cases, the conclusion of *probable* malingering would be mitigated to *possible* malingering.

Another area in which helpful guidelines have been proposed is malingered pain-related disability (MPRD; see Bianchini, Greve, & Glynn, 2005; Greve, Bianchini, & Brewer, 2013). In disability evaluations that involve pain conditions, malingering has been difficult to assess, largely because pain is multifaceted and appreciated mostly by self-report. Moreover, in disability evaluations, the pain is not the target of the assessment; it is about whether the pain is disabling, preventing the individual from working (Greve et al., 2013). While there are sometimes compelling inconsistencies that provide for straightforward assessment of malingering (e.g., as when someone with "debilitating lower back pain" is caught on surveillance performing a brake job for a neighbor), it has been difficult without guidelines to assess MPRD. Therefore, Bianchini et al. (2005), citing evidence from symptom and performance validity assessments of pain claimants, showed that in pain cases with significant external incentive (Criterion A), evidence from inconsistencies in the physical evaluation (B), and inconsistencies in cognitive-perceptual neuropsychological testing (C), along with evidence from inconsistencies in self-report (D) can be used to adduce the inference of malingering. Similar exclusion criteria (E) are used so that the inference points toward volitional evidence.

One readily sees the probabilities involved when multiple failure of validity tests is considered. The error term of special interest is the false-positive (FP) error rate (1-Specificity). If the appropriate classification accuracy study is performed, one can identify the specificity of any test, which is the probability of correct rejection of an individual who does not have the diagnosis of interest. For validity tests when malingering is the construct of interest, specificity is the probability of correctly identifying an honest claimant—one who is not malingering. For this particular test, the FP rate is the chance of misidentifying this individual as a malingerer (and the true positive [TP] rate is the chance of correctly identifying this person as a malingerer). As an examiner wishes not to harm the claimant by misidentifying the validity status, the examiner desires to have as low a FP rate as possible.

If multiple validity test failures are considered, one can show considerable diminishing of the FP rate. The pretest probability of malingering is the base rate (BR; Larrabee, 2008). The posttest, or posterior, probability when the validity test is positive depends upon the classification accuracy characteristics of the test. A likelihood ratio, dividing sensitivity by the FP rate, is multiplied by the pretest odds (formed from the pretest probability by dividing the BR by 1 − BR) to give the posttest odds, from which the posterior probability is calculated by Odds / Odds + 1. When a test is positive, the examiner can be more positive about the finding, as the probability (of malingering) rises from the base-rate level to a new higher level based upon the characteristics of the test.

Larrabee (2008) demonstrated that if two or more results from nonsignificantly correlated validity tests are chained by taking the posterior odds from the first as the pretest odds for the second, the posterior probability for the second positive validity test then rises substantially. The posterior probabilities for three or more positive validity tests approach 1.0. This joint posterior probability is identical to the joint positive predictive value (PPV). Given that PPV = TP / (TP + FP), one can easily see that as the joint posterior probability is approaching 1.00 with multiple validity test failure, the FP rate is approaching 0.0, leaving PPV = TP / (TP + ~0.0). Thus, with two or more positive results on validity tests, the examiner can be more certain that there is no mislabeling of the claimant.

The same findings of joint high posterior probabilities of malingering can be shown whether one uses the calculated method (Larrabee, 2008), or by strictly empirical methods (Victor, Boone, Serpa, Buehler, & Ziegler, 2009) in which the joint classification accuracy statistics are simply derived from the data set. In a combined SSD data set, Chafetz (2011a) showed high and almost identical posterior probabilities for two or more embedded validity indicators, with occasional small differences. The posterior probabilities depend largely on the specificities of the individual test or embedded indicator, but rise to 0.99+ with three positive embedded indicators in this SSD data set (Chafetz, 2011a). Thus, with multiple validity test or embedded indicator failure, the evaluator can be more confident in the determination of malingering.

Expert Consensus on Malingering

As expressed in the American Academy of Clinical Neuropsychology (AACN) Consensus Conference statement (Heilbronner et al., 2009), neuropsychologists are concerned with cognitive and emotional symptoms, and physical capacities. Examinees who are seeking compensation or avoiding punishment employ strategies that involve attempts to intentionally create the appearance of disability or dysfunction. They do so by exaggerating symptoms or intentionally reducing their abilities. This behavior is not simply a matter of poor effort. When an evaluator considers the diagnosis of malingering, there is an explicit determination of intent, and evaluators can use the current body of knowledge on validity testing to differentiate intentionally produced noncredible presentations (e.g., malingering and factitious disorder) from unintentional noncredible presentations (e.g., somatoform pain disorders or cogniform disorders). The AACN Conference statement recognized that malingering can be adaptive, and that the best way to assess intent was to rule out other conditions (e.g., psychological, neurological, developmental) that might better explain the noncredible presentation.

Before this consensus statement, the National Academy of Neuropsychology (NAN) Policy and Planning Committee had produced a position paper on symptom validity assessment (Bush et al., 2005). This policy paper noted that noncredible symptom exaggeration or production occurs in a large minority of neuropsychological examinees, with a higher base rate in medicolegal or forensic contexts. They noted a number of terms in current use, including *symptom validity*, the accuracy or truthfulness of the symptom presentation; *response bias*, an attempt to mislead the examiner through the use of incomplete responses; *effort*, the investment in performing at capacity; *malingering*, the intentional production of false or exaggerated symptoms, motivated by external incentives; and *dissimulation*, the intentional misrepresentation or falsification of symptoms to appear dissimilar from one's true state. In this context, Larrabee (2012) has more recently distinguished between symptom validity tests (SVTs), which examine the validity of the claimant's symptom presentation, and performance validity tests (PVTs), which determine the validity of the claimant's behavioral performance on cognitive testing. The NAN policy paper asserts that validity testing is an essential part of a neuropsychological examination, and that the evaluator should be prepared to justify any decision *not* to use these tests.

Base Rates of Malingering in Disability Examinations

More than 25 years ago, Puente (1987) considered the issue of malingering in the PCE for SSD, but the tools back then were limited mostly to an analysis of inconsistencies in the presentation and history. More recently, Chafetz (2008) showed widespread validity failure by adults and child claimants. In this study, the archived records of claimants were apportioned into separate graded effort groups. The Definite group was defined by most egregious validity test failure—significantly below chance performance (Slick et al., 1999). The next level was defined as Chance performance, which could as easily be obtained if the claimant had simply closed his or her eyes, not able to see any of the stimuli. This level of performance is obtained only by the most impaired of individuals—who cannot possibly track a conversation well enough to provide a history, or even make it to the evaluation without much help. As Chafetz (2008) discussed, Chance failure was the more egregious level of validity test failure, though not as bad as Below-Chance failure. The next level was Fail Two validity tests, which also satisfies the Slick et al. (1999) criteria for Probable malingering. The next graded level of effort was Fail One validity test; then there was Fail Indicators (embedded) without failing any one validity test; and then there were those who did Not Fail any test or embedded indicator.

Because of the absence of records and the overall unreliable nature of self-report in these examinations, Chafetz (2008) did not use the C criteria (self-report) from Slick et al. (1999). Moreover, because most of the Full Scale IQ scores were in the ID range, the question naturally arose whether these "developmental disabilities" mitigated Probable malingering to Possible malingering per Slick et al. (1999) guidelines. However, it was considered that if indeed these individuals were malingering, then the obtained IQ scores would not be valid indicators of their true abilities. Thus, the D criteria were left as an open question, and indeed it was later discovered that low IQ itself was not a likely cause of validity failure in these examinations (Chafetz & Biondolillo, 2012; Chafetz, Prentkowski, & Rao, 2011).

Table 41.1 Rates of SSD validity failure and IQ levels from Chafetz (2008)

	TOMM		*MSVT*	
	n (% of N)	*FSIQ M(SD)*	*n (% of N)*	*FSIQ M(SD)*
Definite	16 (13.6%)	52.4 (4.4)	7 (12.3%)	50.7 (4.1)
Chance	27 (22.9%)	57.2 (8.0)	20 (35.1%)	59.9 (8.1)
Fail 2	11 (9.3%)	60.0 (3.8)	7 (12.3%)	62.1 (5.7)
Fail 1	26 (22%)	63.9 (6.1)	5 (8.8%)	64.6 (4.0)

Note: MSVT = Medical Symptom Validity Test; TOMM = Test of Memory Malingering.

Table 41.1 shows the rates of validity failure in a SSD claimant sample using the Test of Memory Malingering (TOMM; Tombaugh, 1996) and a sample using Green's Medical Symptom Validity Test (MSVT; Green, 2004). In the archives for all SSD claimants, the total score from the Symptom Validity Scale (SVS) for low-functioning individuals (renamed from Chafetz, Abrahams, & Kohlmaier, 2007) was calculated.

We keep in mind that each graded level of validity failure is independent of the other. These rates of validity failure show that 45.8% of SSD claimants in the TOMM study fail two validity tests (TOMM and SVS) or worse, failing the TOMM at chance levels, or significantly below chance levels. In the MSVT study, 59.7% at least fail two validity tests (MSVT and SVS) or worse (chance or below chance). The difference lies largely in how many fail at chance levels of performance, as the rates of Definite (below-chance) failure (13.6% TOMM; and 12.3% MSVT) are about the same, and the rates of Fail Two tests (9.3% TOMM; 12.3% MSVT) are similar.

In both Adult samples (TOMM and MSVT samples), the correlation between the SVS total score (validity scale) and Full Scale IQ was $r = -0.83$, accounting for about 69% of the shared variance between invalidity and IQ. In both Child samples (TOMM and MSVT), the correlation between the SVS total score and Full Scale IQ was $r = -0.75$, accounting for about 56% of the shared variance between invalidity and IQ.

As can be seen in Table 41.1, mean IQ scores progress linearly from very low levels in the Definite group, to levels on the transition between Extremely Low and Borderline ranges in the Not Fail group. The interpretation of these groups is straightforward, graded from those who clearly have intent to fail testing up to those who do not fail validity testing. Thus, the interpretation of the corresponding IQ scores is that they are dependent on the validity levels, and not the other way around. In a later section on low IQ individuals, more data will be shown illustrating that the failure of validity testing, particularly on the SVS, is not due to low IQ levels.

Data from other researchers show similar rates of validity failure in SSD samples. For example, Miller, Boyd, Cohn, Wilson, and McFarland (2006) showed 50+% validity test failure in an SSD sample in Georgia. Jason King also showed 50+% validity test failure in his sample (personal communication). Research presented at the 2012 NAN convention scientific session by Buddin, Schroeder, Teichner, and Waid (2012) showed that 35% of those applying for disability in South Carolina and 50% of those receiving disability failed the MSVT. Many consider that the turning point for the modern guidelines for the diagnosis of malingering occurred with the Slick et al. (1999) publication. Before these guidelines, Griffin, Normington, May, and Glassmire (1996) showed that 19% of DDS claimants had evidence of malingering when a Composite Disability Malingering Index was used. In this writer's invited address at the local state DDS (April 28, 2003), data were presented showing that before this writer used validity testing in DDS claimants, only 5% of DDS claimants were determined as having clear evidence of malingering, while 20% had some evidence. Clearly, without the use of validity testing, the DDSs have many false positives for disability benefits.

Costs of Malingered Disability

Chafetz and Underhill (2013) have calculated the potentially staggering costs of SSA's failing to detect malingering. Considering the most widely accepted base rate of malingering in medicolegal cases of 40% ± 10% (Larrabee et al., 2009), the costs range from \$20 billion in one year considering mental disabilities alone up to \$180 billion in one year considering everything, including secondary costs (e.g., Medicare and Medicaid benefits) and all possible claim categories (Chafetz, 2011b).

Other Claimant-Centered Challenges to Validity

When people have considerable internal distress or conflict, somatoform symptoms may be produced (American Psychiatric Association, 2000, 2013). Somatization disorder typically starts before age 30, has multiple symptoms, and involves a combination of pain, gastrointestinal, sexual, and pseudoneurological symptoms that are not fully explained by a general medical condition, effects of a substance, or by another mental disorder (American Psychiatric Association, 2000). Somatization disorder, which is more broadly called *Somatic Symptom Disorder* in DSM-5 (American Psychiatric Association, 2013), and requires only one or more somatic symptoms, is not typically considered volitional. It occurs when the person, not realizing the distress or admitting to the conflict, starts having stomachaches and headaches, and becomes "sick." The reader will recognize this presentation in a child who knows he must take the math test but does not feel he has mastered the material and does not wish to let his parents down or invite their censure. Being "sick" is okay, and "resolves" the conflict. Conversion disorder describes the production of medically unexplained neurological (motor or sensory) symptoms such as numbness or paralysis, often out of guilt or conflict.

Delis and Wetter (2007) proposed a "cogniform disorder," which is the mental-cognitive equivalent. In a cogniform disorder, there is a production of medically unexplained cognitive problems (e.g., memory loss) when the person has unrealized internal distress or conflict. This writer once had a 74-year-old patient who was convinced she had Alzheimer's disease. When the examination revealed no neuropsychological problems, and feedback led to psychological therapy, it was discovered that she had boyfriend problems with a traveling salesman. Her "memory problems" arose from his unexpected arrivals or nonarrivals, prompting her to turn the anger on herself and complain of a memory disorder.

Boone (2009) analyzed the Delis and Wetter (2007) algorithm, suggesting that while it was a substantial advance in identifying individuals with noncredible cognitive symptoms and/or implausibly low cognitive scores, it did not distinguish between implausible cognitive complaints and implausibly low test scores. Boone (2009) presented the construct of neurocognitive hypochondriasis, which is a fixed belief in cognitive dysfunction despite normal cognitive test scores. It is likely that the example of the 74-year-old patient given earlier would fit neatly into this paradigm.

Factitious disorder is a volitional form of noncredible presentation in which the person plays a sick role, seeking treatment for medically unexplained symptoms to gain attention by doctors (American Psychiatric Association, 2000, 2013; Delis & Wetter, 2007). Factitious disorder has been called *Munchausen Syndrome* in the extreme case in which the individual begins introducing more harmful and invasive medical problems (American Psychiatric Association, 2000; but not 2013).

In this context of symptoms without a physical basis, one must consider "diagnosis threat" (Suhr & Gunstad, 2002), a form of self-fulfilling prophecy in which the individual "learns" that there is a disorder consistent with a diagnosis that has just been received. Consider, for example, the patient who comes to the emergency department of a major hospital with a "concussion." Despite that the head injury may not have been severe enough to cause damage, and there is no evidence of brain damage upon examination, hospital personnel will likely act in a conservative say, providing a warning sheet to be helpful to the patient. The warning sheet will discuss "management of your TBI," and may discuss legitimate signs of a TBI, including memory and concentration problems. A fixed belief may then develop concerning the effects of the TBI, and this belief may persist for long periods.

Chafetz (2011b) has discussed these problems in the context of a claimant who is seeking disability. Considering the motivational differences in the Chafetz et al. (2011) study, in which disability claimants, compared to state rehabilitation or child protection claimants, were the only ones to show high rates of validity test failure, we have to view the possibility of other noncredible presentations in this context. In disability claims, these other nonvolitional forms of noncredible symptom presentation are not likely to be good explanations of the noncredible findings. Indeed, SSD claimants are aware of the burden of proving disability under the strict Social Security definition of disability. Having the burden of proving one's disability requires considerable deliberation and undergoing many hurdles, and indeed it is not unusual in a private disability examination to see letters from claimants to their doctors (while attempting to get SSD) asking for a doctor's note with specific disability language (e.g., "severe limitations" or "marked impairment"). This deliberation is clearly volitional. Moreover, the claim by Dan Allsup, communications director of Allsup, Inc., a company that helps disability applicants, that these hurdles help weed out malingerers (Ohlemacher, 2010) cannot possibly be true, as it is likely that these hurdles only increase the incentives to feign more believable symptomology.

The Use of Validity Testing in Low-IQ Individuals

Validity testing in low IQ individuals has been criticized largely because of lower specificity, but also because validity tests had not traditionally been developed in low IQ samples (Salekin & Doane, 2009; Shandera, Berry, Clark, Schipper, Grau, & Harp, 2010; Smith et al., 2014; Victor & Boone, 2007).

Chafetz et al. (2011) conducted a study comparing individuals with low IQ in three groups with differing motivations for assessment. The SSD group were composed of individuals seeking monetary benefits for an inability to work; the state rehabilitation service (SRS) group were composed of individuals seeking to make money by going to work; and the child protection (CP) group were individuals seeking to have their children returned from state custody. In the CP group, these individuals were motivated to look good on testing, wanting to do everything in their power to have their children returned. IQ and validity test scores were obtained on all claimants. Individuals were defined as malingering if they failed the MSVT at significantly below chance levels, or if they failed the MSVT and the A-Test (Chafetz, 2012), which was developed on SSD claimants as a test of feigned auditory inattention. Profile analysis was used on the MSVT to remove individuals who were truly impaired (Howe & Loring, 2009).

Considering only the claimants who passed validity testing, the mean IQ scores of the SSD (67.5 ± 6.0), SRS (69.2 ± 8.3), and CP (71.7 ± 7.7) groups were not significantly different. However, 45.5% of the SSD group, 6.7% of the SRS group, and 0.0% of the CP group met criteria for malingering. Thus, validity test failure in low-IQ individuals depended only upon the identified motivation of the group: Those seeking benefits for an inability to work showed a high rate of malingering (45.5%); those seeking to work for compensation showed a low rate (6.7%); and those seeking the return of their children from state custody showed no validity failure (0.0%). Moreover, concerning those few who failed validity testing in the SRS group, further investigation revealed that due to agency cooperation the local DDS office for Social Security had sent these claimants to the local state rehabilitation office to determine work status. It was therefore possible that these few individuals who failed validity testing when ostensibly seeking to work were indeed protecting disability status. After all, similarly low-IQ individuals motivated to look good to have their children returned showed no validity test failure.

In an extension of this study for other purposes, Chafetz and Biondolillo (2012) obtained a larger sample of CP claimants, all with IQ < 76. In all of these individuals, 35 of 37 (95%) passed Immediate Recognition (IR) of the MSVT, 34 of 37 (92%) passed Delayed Recognition (DR), and 35 of 37 (95%) passed Consistency (Cn). On the SVS, 94% passed at a more stringent cutoff (> 7). On the A-Test (cutoff > 2), 100% passed, and on Reliable Digit Span (RDS; Greiffenstein, Baker, & Gola, 1994), 32 of 35 (91%) passed a more stringent cutoff (< 6). When considering only those CP claimants with IQ = 60–75, 100% passed all the MSVT effort variables, 100% passed the more stringent SVS cutoff (> 7), 100% passed the A-Test, and 30 of 32 (94%) passed the more stringent RDS cutoff (< 6). Thus, IQ < 60 appears to be the tipping point for more validity failure, though in this well-motivated group there was no validity test failure above 10% (pass rates 90%+).

Considering the issue of validity tests designed for low-IQ functioning individuals, Shandera et al. (2010) and Musso, Barker, Jones, Roid, and Gouvier (2011) acknowledged the Symptom Validity Scale (SVS) for Low Functioning Individuals (renamed from Chafetz et al., 2007) as the first validity scale specifically designed for working with low-IQ individuals. The SVS was analyzed for use in disability examinees for Social Security. Most of these cases were from SSI referrals, mostly with low intellectual functioning. One of the advantages of using the SVS is that the examination can be done as it is usually done, and then the evidence from the examination can be entered into the scale afterwards; no additional testing is necessary. Embedded indicators such as coding errors or Ganser-like answers (where the numerical answer provided is immediately adjacent to the correct answer: 2 + 3 = *6*; 3 + 4 = *8*) are given score weights depending upon their value. As indicated in the Chafetz and Biondolillo (2012) study, a cutoff of > 7 on the SVS has no false positives in well-motivated individuals with IQ between 60 and 75.

The A-Test (Chafetz, 2012) has been redesigned as a test of feigned auditory vigilance embedded within the mental-cognitive status examination (Strub & Black, 1993). It was also developed in the SSD sample. As shown in Chafetz and Biondolillo (2012), it has a 100% pass rate (0% false positives) in a well-motivated sample of low-IQ individuals, even when IQ dips below 60. Chafetz (2008) showed that the mean scores follow the graded effort groups with good precision, accounting for 35% of the differences (eta^2) between the separate effort groups.

The Musso et al. (2011) work developed a Rarely Missed Index on the Stanford-Binet-5 with a high pass rate in the ID group of the standardization sample. They developed a "floor" of nonverbal items that are infrequently missed by identified ID subjects plus additional standardization sample subjects with IQ < 71. The sensitivity of this index was determined by using college students as simulators, which does not present an adequate real-life comparison. Thus, this index awaits validation in a criterion group of identified malingerers, preferably with low IQ. Also, no one in the standardization sample completed validity testing during the standardization process, and so it is unknown whether the "floor" might be lower than necessary and therefore less sensitive. Nevertheless, overall classification was 77.6% accurate, with 74.1% of analog malingerers and 83.9% of low-IQ individuals correctly identified with a logistics regression equation.

Principles for Validity Testing in Low-Functioning Individuals

- Below-chance performance is still definite malingering: Approximately 10%–13% of low-IQ individuals obtain significantly below-chance performance on validity testing (Chafetz, 2008), termed "the smoking gun of intent" (Pankratz & Erickson, 1990).
- Understand the difference between lower and higher IQ levels in ID: In well-motivated low-IQ individuals (IQ between 60 and 75), there is little failure on validity tests (Chafetz & Biondolillo, 2012).
- Account for motivation: Well-motivated low-IQ individuals (IQ 60–75) do not fail certain validity tests. There may be hidden secondary-gain issues in individuals who are apparently motivated to do well, including protection of disability benefits.
- Accommodate for executive dysfunction or reading difficulties: A combined computer–oral administration, with the examiner operating the mouse (or keys) removes errors due to executive dysfunction, leaving only the choices to be made.
- Use appropriate cutoff scores for validity tests that have an ability component: More stringent cutoffs are needed for low-ability individuals.
- Use appropriate test selection: People with particular impairments should not be tested on validity measures whose task demands require those abilities (e.g., a person with acalculia should not be tested on the Dot Counting Test, which requires multiplication).
- Where possible, use validity tests designed for low-IQ individuals: A few have been developed.

Chafetz and Biondolillo (2012) and Chafetz (2015) have proposed principles for dealing with validity issues in low-functioning individuals, including the necessity for understanding the level of impairment, the choice of tests, and the knowledge of studies showing pass rates in low-functioning individuals. It is also important to understand that the aggregation of three or more positive results can show high posterior probabilities for malingering in low-IQ individuals (Chafetz, 2011a).

Other Reasons for Poor Performance on Validity Tests?

It is natural to question whether other syndromes can cause validity test failure on their own. One might question, for example, whether people who are affected by pain might fail validity testing due to the distracting nature of pain. However, cold-pressor pain that produces considerable discomfort does not by itself reduce scores below cutoffs on validity tests (Etherton, Bianchini, Greve, & Ciota, 2005). Yanez, Fremouw, Tennant, Strunk, and Coker (2006) showed that severely depressed individuals did not significantly differ from controls on TOMM performance. Only one of 20 of these severely depressed individuals failed Trial 2 of the TOMM and only one failed the retention trial. Indeed, Rohling, Green, Allen, and Iverson (2002) showed that when highly depressed individuals pass validity testing, they do not score below controls on neurocognitive testing, indicating that the only reason for depressed individuals to have reduced scores on neurocognitive testing is because of poor quality of effort.

Performance validity accounts for the largest proportion of variance in a neurocognitive examination, even more than moderate to severe TBI (Green, Rohling, Lees-Haley, & Allen, 2001). Ord, Greve, Bianchini, and Aguerrevere (2010) also found that performance validity had a larger effect on neurocognitive measures than TBI severity.

Meeting the Requirements for Disability

In the box, the reader will see an example of the Social Security listing requirements for disability from a depressive disorder. For disability benefits from depression, a claimant must have five of the typical symptoms of depression (e.g., depressed mood, appetite disturbance, sleep disturbance, decreased energy, suicidal thoughts), resulting in extreme limitation of one or marked limitation of two of the following: (a) understanding, remembering, or applying information, (b) interacting with others, (c) concentrating, persisting, or maintaining pace, or (d) adapting or managing oneself; or the depressive disorder is serious and persistent (that is, the claimant has a medically documented history of the existence of the disorder over a period of at least two years, and there is evidence of both treatment, intervention, or supports that are ongoing and that diminish the signs and symptoms of the disorder; and marginal adjustment, with minimal capacity to adapt to changes in the environment or to demands that are not already a part of daily life).

Blue Book Listing 12.04 Depressive, Bipolar, and Related disorders

- Meets listing with documented depression symptoms (at least five); AND extreme limitation in one or marked limitation in two of the following:
  - Understand, remember, or apply information;
  - Interact with others;
  - Concentrate, persist, or maintain pace;
  - Adapt or manage oneself.
- Or the depressive disorder is serious and persistent; that is, the claimant has a medically documented history of the existence of the disorder over a period of at least two years, and there is evidence of both:
  - Treatment, intervention, or supports that are ongoing and that diminish the signs and symptoms of the disorder; and
  - Marginal adjustment, with minimal capacity to adapt to changes in the environment or to demands that are not already a part of daily life.

Applicants for SSD may be turned down at any stage of the application process. They might have demonstrated SGA, making more money than allowed for SSI under the law. They might have gone through a consultative examination, and have not demonstrated sufficiently disabling problems to meet one of the listing requirements. Applicants who are denied may appeal by taking their own case further down the process, by hiring a disability attorney, or by seeking services through a disability company such as Allsup, Inc. Allsup Inc. boasts a 97% award rate compared to a 33% national average for those who apply without assistance (How It Works At Allsup, n.d.).

Appeals are handled through the Office of Disability Adjudication Review (ODAR) in hearings before an Administrative Law Judge (ALJ). The federal ALJs involved in these hearings are paid by the SSA. They must follow administrative law, which is public law that deals with the rules set forth by the administrative agency, in this case the SSA. The appeals hearing involves an ALJ and a court reporter. The ALJ is the fact-finder and decider. The claimant appears either alone or with representation (e.g., a disability attorney). There is no counsel to represent the people (government). ALJ decisions are public, and disability attorneys often display their decision records on the attorney website, thus telling the public to watch out about "certain judges."

The ALJ obtains consultation by having medical experts present and sworn in. The expert can be present by phone. The medical expert is called according to the professional field involved in the claimed disability. For example, a psychologist might be called if the claim is for ID (listing 12.05). The ALJ typically asks the expert questions about whether the evidence meets the listing requirements. It is incumbent upon the expert to have read the records and history supplied by the ODAR office. The expert may be cross-examined by the disability attorney, but there is no "direct" examination, as there is no government lawyer. Typically, what stands for the "direct" examination are the questions put forth by the ALJ.

Military Disability Examinations

The Veterans Administration is composed of three organizations: (a) the Veterans Health Administration (VHA), which is one of the largest health care systems in the world; (b) the Veterans Benefits Administration (VBA), which manages compensation and vocational assistance to disabled veterans; and (c) the National Cemetery Administration (NCA), which honors veterans with a final resting place and memorials to commemorate their service. This chapter is especially concerned with the disability activities of the VBA, which also provides home loan guaranty, education, and insurance programs (for more information, visit the VBA website, www.benefits.va.gov/BENEFITS/). The VBA has 57 regional offices in 50 states, Puerto Rico, and the Philippines.

According to the VBA, disability compensation is a tax-free monetary benefit paid to veterans with documented disabilities resulting from disease or injury while in active military service. The injury or illness may also have been aggravated during active military service. Even after discharge, compensation may be paid for disabilities considered related or secondary to those that occurred while in service. There is also payment for dependents of service members who die while on active duty. For specific disabilities (e.g., loss of use of a limb), there is special monthly compensation, including an additional higher rate for aid and attendance by another person. The VA also provides housing and insurance benefits to veterans with disabilities. Once a disability has been determined to be service connected, the veteran may also get access to programs for an automobile and clothing allowance, hospitalization, and convalescence.

The rating of the degree of disability is designed to compensate for the loss of working time from the disabling problem. Thus, as with any other disability program, the compensation is provided for an inability to work. The benefit amount is scaled in 10% increments from 10% to 100% according to the degree of the veteran's disability. The VA will attempt to determine a service connection for all the claimed disabilities, and it is not uncommon to see a VA determination of service connection (or not) for posttraumatic stress disorder (PTSD), hypertension, sleep apnea, knee injury, liver disease, and TBI all in the same veteran. Service connection is granted for a disease or injury incurred during active military service or active duty for training. Service connection by law is also granted for conditions that existed before the veteran entered the service if the condition is shown to be aggravated by the service.

It is instructive to compare military compensation to SSD compensation. As Buddin and Kapur (2005) have indicated, the Code of Federal Regulations focuses the percentage rankings of VA disability compensation on the earnings loss of veterans who are disabled. These rankings are based on the average impairment in earning capacity. The analysis involves comparing what the veteran could have earned without the disability to the (reduced) earnings with the disability. Chafetz (2013) compared these rules to those in SSD, where disability is conditioned on the total inability to work. This is an extreme definition of disability that has been viewed as contrary to work motivation, as it disincentivizes those who might otherwise work part-time (see Chafetz, 2010). Indeed, this writer has been asked many times by claimants for other agencies (e.g., child protection, state vocational rehabilitation) not to mention to Social Security side income from hidden jobs. One claimant for state vocational rehabilitation mentioned that he worked at his uncle's business without pay to avoid interfering with his SSI, which of course belied his claim to Social Security that he could not work. Veterans do not have to claim "total disability." While this disincentive might not carry forward into the VA claim (Chafetz, 2013), veterans might see fabrication or exaggeration of symptoms as a pathway to a higher percentage rating. Thus, there is still an issue of the validity of the claim.

While private disability compensation (and to some extent SSDI) is tied to an individual's earnings, the rating in VBA compensation is based upon the disability. In Buddin and Kapur's (2005) example, a private and a major who both lose a foot are entitled to the same benefit, regardless of experience and earning potential. Moreover, earnings in civilian life do not affect disability compensation from the VA.

Psychologists who become involved with providing disability examinations for veterans frequently do so through IME companies (e.g., QTC or VES) who have contracts with the VA. The psychologist is instructed to fill out a Disability Benefits Questionnaire (DBQ) on (proprietary) software provided by the IME company. With experience, many examinations take approximately one hour, though some programs require more extensive detail and additional assessment, requiring at least two hours. With veterans who have combat experience, or who otherwise were stationed in a war zone, the consultation is frequently about PTSD or about TBI. However, any mental or cognitive problem may be the target of examination, or may be uncovered by the examination. The contract may be for examinations of veterans awaiting discharge, or for veterans who have already been discharged. Essentially, the VA wants to leave no veteran behind, and it is recognized that many older veterans (e.g., Vietnam era) had problems that went unrecognized during their service. This writer once evaluated a 92-year-old veteran of World War II whose job it was to retrieve the remains of the dead. Although he had a long and fruitful life, he still could not get the odor of decay and death out of his system. The odor was with him everywhere. He was making a disability claim to be able to leave benefits for his family.

This method of using proprietary software does not permit thorough assessment of cognitive problems or of validity. For additional cognitive assessment, the psychologist may be asked to administer the Mini-Mental State Examination (MMSE; Folstein, Folstein, & McHugh, 1975), the Montreal Cognitive Assessment (MoCA; Nasreddine et al., 2005), or the St. Louis University Mental Status (SLUMS) examination (Tariq, Tumosa, Chibnall, Perry, & Morley, 2006). None of these instruments is ideal for assessing the cognitive problems of veterans who have had a brain injury. For one, the MoCA, SLUMS, and the MMSE were developed in older individuals suspected of mild neurocognitive impairment or dementia; indeed, these are screening instruments for dementia. Thus, older veterans (who were involved in Vietnam or Korea) may score lower than expected, but the older veterans may also have complicating problems due to brain disease, poor health, or dementing illness that have nothing to do with a mild TBI suspected 45 years earlier. Ultimately, the evaluator may have to rely on an evaluation of the claimant's history as compared with the medical records provided, plus knowledge of the neuropsychological record on TBI (Iverson & Lange, 2011).

Moreover, the proprietary software is limited in guidance, frequently not distinguishing between problems associated with mild TBI versus moderate to severe TBI. The VA likely did not provide neuropsychological guidance to these IME companies. As Iverson, Langlois, McCrea, and Kelly (2009) have indicated, the VA has been deliberately overinclusive about TBI in postdeployment screenings, not wanting to miss any deserving case. Thus, the evaluator may see a case of TBI in the records, and the proprietary software will ask the evaluator to determine (many years after the event) if cognitive problems from this TBI have interfered with the veteran's social and occupational functioning. It is up to the evaluator to know the literature on TBI (Iverson & Lange, 2011; McCrea, 2008), be able to discriminate mild from moderate to severe TBI, and to determine whether it is possible that this particular injury left the residue of cognitive problems that are being claimed several years later.

The proprietary software does not ask the psychologist to determine the validity of these symptom reports. The style is medical: Self-reported symptoms are supposed to indicate to the clinician the nature and extent of the problems. In disability examinations, however, self-report is fraught with difficulty when it comes to determining the validity of the claims (Chafetz, 2010, 2011; Guilmette, 2013). With claims of psychiatric problems such as PTSD, it is up to the psychologist to carefully sort out the claim from the history. It is helpful to ask about the content of nightmares, comparing that with the history of involvement in combat-related activities. There is more veracity to the claim when the nightmares are about convoy explosions and the veteran was involved as a driver in convoys in Afghanistan or Iraq. If the veteran was a driver, he or she may report being hypervigilant about objects in the road when he or she is driving at home. If the veteran was in the back of the truck, there may be no such avoidance. Alternatively, if the veteran did not experience combat first-hand, but only heard about others being killed, and dreams about problems at home that are unrelated to combat, the veracity of the PTSD claim is less likely.

To determine the validity of cognitive complaints, a similar analysis of potential inconsistencies in the history may be used. For example, recovery of function from an injury is the norm, and mild TBI without complication is known to show little or no significant clinical effect beyond three months after the injury (Iverson & Lange, 2011; McCrea, 2008). The claim that memory problems from an established mild TBI have been worsening yearly for the past five years to the point where the claimant can remember almost nothing lacks credibility. It is helpful for the examiner, at another point in the examination in which memory is not being discussed, to ask the veteran what he or she had for breakfast, for dinner the night before, and to tell the examiner what he or she has been most interested recently in the news. This information can be enlightening. The veteran who goes on at length concerning a recent news story about military policy is exhibiting intact recent memory, not worsening memory.

Concerning performance validity on the MoCA, the enterprising examiner will realize there are several opportunities for validity assessment. For one, there is a somewhat reduced A-Random Letter Test of Auditory Vigilance (Strub & Black, 1993), which has been shown to be an adequate measure of performance validity on SSD examinations (Chafetz, 2012). Given that veterans are typically higher functioning than Social Security claimants (Chafetz et al., 2007), and that the test on the MoCA has fewer items, it is likely that a cutoff of two or more errors on this reduced-item test would suffice to indicate validity problems. Moreover, the examiner could extend the testing of digit span to achieve a Reliable Digit Span (Greiffenstein et al., 1994), another well-known indicator of validity. The MoCA also has a multiple forced choice recognition trial as part of the delayed recall of five words, which may offer other clues as to the validity of the veteran's performance.

An excellent review of the compensation and pension (C&P) examinations for the VA and practical guide for psychologists can be found in Worthen and Moering (2011). These authors help psychologists understand the legal framework and roles involved in C&P examinations, detailing the specific language of the opinion. For example, if the examiner finds that the veteran is probably suffering from PTSD as a result of his traumatic experiences, the language of the opinion must include: "It is more likely than not that the veteran's PTSD was caused by the specific traumatic stressor." This language tells the VA that there is more than a 50% probability that the veteran has PTSD from the stated trauma. Worthen and Moering (2011) discuss the difficulties involved in arriving at that opinion from using the DBQ, as outlined above. They also discuss the general rating formula for mental disorders, the way VA records are used, how the veterans statements are taken into account, and the difficulties involved with noncredible findings.

As with SSD (Chafetz & Underhill, 2013), it is instructive to calculate the costs of malingered disability in the VA system. According to Buddin and Kapur (2005), the total amount spent on all veterans receiving disability compensation in 2003 was $19.536 billion. Using the same assumptions as in Chafetz and Underhill (2013), this would mean that $7.81 billion was spent on malingered disability in the VA system in 2003.

If the psychologist can tolerate some uncertainty about the claim, and is content to work with proprietary software rather than using typical psychological or neuropsychological assessment tools, these examinations can provide considerable satisfaction. Veterans who have experienced combat have undergone extreme human conditions unlike that of most others psychologists will have the chance to work with. The contrast between the clarity of mission and purpose and the "tedium" of home life is something that is difficult for combat veterans to convey. This is a chance for the astute psychologist to provide insightful assessment and recommendations that can ultimately have an impact on the veteran's life and recovery. It is also a chance for the psychologist to learn about military technology, policy, and the human condition under extreme circumstances.

Private Disability Examinations

Private disability carriers may offer disability policies tailored to the claimant's own work, or for any work for which the claimant is qualified by training or experience. There may be short-term or long-term policies. As with SSA, private disability carriers are interested in the claimant's residual strengths, as well as limitations in the abilities to perform tasks. Typically, the examiner is not being asked whether the claimant can perform a job, but whether there are limitations in job-related tasks: mental focus, understanding instructions, explaining things from different points of view, multitasking, influencing others, working alone, working with others, and remembering instructions or customer information. If the policy is specific for the claimant's line of work, there may be questions about limitations related to that line of work. For example, the examiner for a claimant who is a lawyer may be asked whether there are limitations on conceptualizing and writing. A thorough review of the examiner's role in handling a disability independent examination can be found in Oakes, Lovejoy, and Bush (2017).

Some disability carriers may ask about maximum medical improvement (MMI), inquiring whether the claimant's psychological or neuropsychological condition has become stable such that further treatment will not improve the condition, or result in significant changes to the claimant's abilities for occupational functioning. There may be a question whether the condition permanently prevents the claimant from working.

The carrier is usually interested in different analyses of limitations, comparing self-reported limitations with those observed during the examination, indicated by cognitive testing, and documented by collateral interviews or in the medical record. Note that these limitations are not the same thing as psychological symptoms and problems, although knowledge and findings about these symptoms and problems can inform the analysis of limitations. For example, emotional lability and frequent crying may suggest social and emotional limitations that might carry over into the workplace. Moreover, limitations may indicate workplace restrictions; for example, fatigue that indicates limitations in the workplace may also indicate a restriction for not working more than four hours in a workday.

A thorough analysis of activities of daily living, both before and after the claimant stopped work, can be especially enlightening, as the examiner is frequently able to get information about social interactions and other abilities and limitations. For example, the parent who is not working but is very active in a child's schooling may demonstrate abilities to interact and influence others (e.g., teachers, child), handle phone calls, drive, remember and coordinate information, and understand spoken and written language. Alternatively, if there are documented memory problems (valid on neuropsychological testing), and the claimant requires others to handle these chores, the examiner may adduce evidence for limitations in remembering spoken instructions, and this finding may help elucidate the claim. The examiner might be directly asked whether there is psychologically or neuropsychologically based impairment in the claimant's abilities to carry out tasks.

Typically, the disability carrier is clear that these are independent examinations (independent of the claimant's own doctors). Whether the carrier uses an IME company or consults with the neuropsychologist (or psychologist) directly, there is an expressed need to assess the validity of the claims, and the consistency of the claimant's self-report. In this, the private disability claim evaluation stands apart from the public (SSD or VBA) disability. Indeed, the examiner will frequently get a written request to examine for "motivation," "secondary gain" issues, "insufficient effort," "symptom exaggeration," or to frankly determine whether there is malingering. The examiner might be asked whether the sources of information obtained are consistent or inconsistent with each other, recognizing that one of the time-honored methods of determining validity is an analysis of inconsistencies (Slick et al., 1999).

While there is a high base rate of malingering in medicolegal examinations (Larrabee et al., 2009), the examiner should be alert to other sources of noncredible complaints and behavior. Diagnosis threat (Suhr & Gunstad, 2002) occurs when a claimant has been diagnosed with an impairing condition and begins acting consistently with the predicted outcomes of that condition. For example, the individual who is unwittingly (and inaccurately) told that she has a dementing condition, and then who looks up that condition on the Internet,[2] may be extremely scared to find that in a few short years she might need full supervised care. Her spouse will be appropriately concerned and engaged when they come in for the disability examination. If you, the examiner, find that no such condition exists, the claimant is then confronted with the potential denial of disability benefits and the uncomfortable feeling of having been misdiagnosed. Good reviews of other noncredible behaviors and problems can be found in Boone (2007, 2009, 2013).

Use of the MMPI-2 (Butcher, Dahlstrom, Graham, Tellegen, & Kaemmer, 1989), or MMPI-2-RF (Ben-Porath & Tellegen, 2008/2011), or the Personality Assessment Inventory (PAI; Morey, 1991), will frequently be required in these examinations, whether neuropsychological or purely psychological. The validity scales on the MMPI-2 (or RF) have been well established. The Variable Response Inconsistency (VRIN) scale evaluates the consistency of responding. Random or otherwise inconsistent responding will produce an elevation on this scale, which will invalidate the other validity scales, as well as all the clinical scales. The True Response Inconsistency (TRIN) scale shows content-irrelevant true or false responding. TRIN thus evaluates whether the claimant tended to mostly respond true or most respond false regardless of what the items said. If TRIN is elevated in either direction (true or false), it also invalidates the validity scales and the clinical scales.

The F-Family scales (F, Fb, and Fp on the MMPI-2; F, Fp, and Fs on the RF) measure whether the claimant endorses items that people infrequently endorse. These scales provide an index of overreporting of psychopathology and of somatic symptoms (Fs). A symptom validity scale (the Fake Bad Scale [FBS]) was developed by Lees-Haley, English, and Glenn (1991) to assess noncredible neurocognitive and somatic complaints. The Response Bias Scale (RBS), developed by Gervais, Ben-Porath, Wygant, and Green (2007), utilized a series of multiple regression analyses to identify items that discriminate individuals passing and failing well-established freestanding validity tests. Both RBS and FBS discriminate well those who pass and those who fail validity tests (Gervais, Wygant, Sellbom, & Ben-Porath, 2011; Wygant et al., 2009).

In a study of non-head-injury disability claimants (Tarescavage, Wygant, Gervais, & Ben-Porath, 2013), higher scores on the MMPI-2-RF validity scales, especially the RBS, were associated with probable and definite malingered neurocognitive dysfunction (Slick et al., 1999). RBS was likely the best discriminator in this study, as it was originally defined by being able to discriminate those who passed and failed performance validity tests. In the Tarescavage et al. (2013)

study of disability claimants, the effect sizes for discriminating incentive only, suspect malingering, and probable malingering groups were greatest on clinical and content measures of reporting of cognitive complaints ($d = 1.10$), low positive emotions ($d = 0.86$), neurological complaints ($d = 0.79$), and malaise ($d = 0.78$).

In this writer's experience, the request by disability carriers for the use of the PAI has been diminishing, but it is still occasionally an option. The validity scales on the PAI include inconsistency (ICN), infrequency (INF), negative impression management (NIM), and positive impression management (PIM). The NIM scale was designed to indicate the probability that the test taker was portraying a more negative impression than was otherwise warranted. NIM items have low frequencies of endorsement in normal and clinical populations. Significant elevations on NIM are associated with higher reporting of pathology. Individuals with severe emotional problems will also get high NIM scores, as individuals with mental disorders frequently self-report more negative items. For example, a depressed person might report herself as worthless and incompetent, where others might see her as worthwhile and competent (Morey, 1991). While NIM is not to be interpreted in a straightforward manner as an indicator of malingering, Hopwood, Morey, Rogers, and Sewell (2007) provided evidence that the differences between actual and NIM-predicted clinical scales provides information about the type of symptoms being feigned (e.g., anxiety, depression, psychosis). Hammond (2006) showed that in SSD claimants, there was a 50% rate of claimants exceeding the cutoff on NIM. However, Sellbom and Bagby (2008) showed that NIM, the malingering index (MAL; Morey, 1991), and the Rogers Discriminant Function (RDF; Rogers, Sewell, Morey, & Ustad, 1996) had unacceptably high false-positive rates for the classification of malingering.

Workers' Compensation

WC laws generally protect people who are injured on the job. Federal WC law (visit the Cornel Law School's Legal Information Institute website, www.law.cornell.edu/uscode/text/5/8102) specifies compensation for disability or death of an employee resulting from a personal injury while on duty. The U.S. Department of Labor, Office of Workers' Compensation lists four major disability compensation programs: (a) wage replacement benefits, (b) medical treatment, (c) vocational rehabilitation, and (d) other benefits (visit the U.S. Department of Labor Workers' Compensation website for more information: www.dol.gov/dol/topic/workcomp/). There are also other specific groups that provide compensation, including Energy Employees Occupational Illness Compensation, the Federal Employees Compensation program, the Longshore and Harbor Workers Compensation program, and the Black Lung Benefits Program.

The states have their own departments or commissions devoted to labor issues. For example, the North Carolina Industrial Commission (www.ic.nc.gov) provides steps for injured workers:

1. Report the injury to the employer and seek medical treatment.
2. Tell the medical provider that the injury is related to work, and have them bill WC for the service.
3. Tell the manager that you have initiated a work-related claim.
4. Provide written notice about the claim and describe the accident.
5. Follow the physician's instructions for medical treatment.

The state commission also provides advice to attorneys concerning a compromise settlement agreement. There is also advice to medical providers, and providers can also see a fee schedule.

As a practical matter, WC evaluations involve providing details about symptoms and problems that require appropriate treatment. There may be a determination of skills and capacities that underlie the ability to perform a job. There may also be a determination of whether the employee has reached MMI. This means that further treatment would not be expected to provide any further improvement in the employee's condition concerning his or her occupational abilities.

Thus, boundaries may be blurred. On one hand, this is inherently medicolegal work in which a hurt individual is seeking diagnosis and treatment for a disabling problem. On the other hand, the psychologist may be providing information about MMI and about the person's psychological abilities to perform their work.

However, psychologists may be retained directly by the WC carrier in which a typical IME is performed. Sometimes the Department of Labor may retain the psychologist for a second-opinion IME to decide on the differences found in the original WC evaluation versus the IME sought by the carrier.

Frequently, especially in industrial areas, the issues involve pain-related disability (Greve et al., 2013). As Greve et al. (2013) indicate, about one-third of all people will experience spinal pain in their lifetimes; half of these individuals will have chronic pain. In these cases, knowledge about how to evaluate pain looms large.

The Battery for Health Improvement–2 (Bruns & Disorbio, 2003) is a multiscale inventory that provides a validity assessment of whether the claimant is overdisclosing, and therefore inflating the self-report, or whether the claimant is responding defensively, and underdisclosing his or her conditions. Four scales are related to pain: Somatic Complaints, Pain Complaints, Functional Complaints, and Muscular Bracing. The Muscular Bracing scale indicates whether there is a high level of muscle tension in reaction to pain, which serves to increase the level of perceived pain. There are also scales of Depression, Anxiety, and Hostility. These, together with the

Table 41.2 Hypothetical example of CPCI findings

Scale	*T-Score*
Illness Focused	
Guarding	**70**
Resting	50
Asking for Assistance	*37*
Wellness-Focused	
Exercise/stretch	58
Relaxation	49
Task persistence	41
Coping self-statements	*38*
Pacing	49
Seeking social support	*39*

MMPI-2 (RF) and/or the PAI can be used to evaluate Axis I conditions that may be interfering with work. There are also scales of long-existing chronic maladjustment, and a Borderline scale that indicates personality characteristics showing emotionality that would interfere with work. There are also helpful practical scales of family dysfunction, survivor of violence, doctor dissatisfaction, and job dissatisfaction, all of which provide predictors about a claimant's interest in and problems in the workplace.

The Chronic Pain Coping Inventory (CPCI; Jensen, Turner, Romano, & Strom, 1995) is a 64-item questionnaire with nine scales divided into categories of Illness-Focused Coping (Guarding, Resting, and Asking for Assistance) and Wellness-Focused Coping (Exercise/Stretch, Relaxation, Task Persistence, Coping Self-Statements, Pacing, and Seeking Social Support). The CPCI emphasizes the importance of reducing maladaptive behaviors and increasing adaptive coping behaviors, and is therefore useful in a direct and practical way for treatment. An example of a CPCI result is given in Table 41.2, and an interpretation follows.

In this example, there is a significant level of guarding behavior, which is illness focused. The individual has fear that movement will lead to pain and further injury, and thus restricts or limits his or her movements. This can lead to deconditioning and further impairment. There is also a low level of coping self-statements. With improvement in these thoughts about pain and injury, the person can develop a more positive outlook. This individual is also rather isolated and is not seeking much social support. In this case, asking for assistance is also low. While the person is not facilitating disability by getting others to wait on him or her, this person is rather isolated and generally without much support.

It's Also About Work

Fitness For Duty

While this chapter is focused on disability, which involves the inability to work, it is important to contrast a disability examination with other types of assessment that are focused on work. For example, a Fitness-For-Duty (FFD) examination involves an individual whose employer is concerned whether he or she can work. In these cases, the individual typically wants to be back at work, but there has been a problem: a threat, an altercation, an angry and inappropriate outburst, or an emotional setback. Sometimes there are cognitive problems. Frequently, management wants to know whether the person is a risk to him- or herself or others. While the concerns about a postal employee "going postal" have become a cliché, indeed the U.S. Postal Service is one of those employers who will want a FFD examination when a worker is displaying unstable or inappropriate behaviors. This writer was involved in a FFD evaluation in which a postal employee bought an AR-15 when many gun lovers were buying them right before the legislation banning assault rifles was voted on. The employee had bragged about his new purchase in the workplace, prompting a FFD evaluation.

In FFD examinations, it is frequently helpful for an IME company to arrange the evaluation, which facilitates a well-controlled environment. While a full interview will be conducted, and appropriate psychological testing will be administered, the employer should not see this information, as it could be prejudicial. Indeed, the employer should see only the answers to the referral questions, which involve whether there is any increased health or safety risk in the workplace, there is any potential risk, there are psychological problems that need treatment, the workplace environment needs to be changed to decrease any potential problems, accommodations are needed, the employee needs time off from work, and whether there are any suggestions for management. There are many cautions, as it is usually difficult to predict dangerousness or violence with any certainty. The reporting is typically short, as the employer should see only the assurances that the psychological or neuropsychological work was done, and then the answers to the questions (leaving out prejudicial background information and findings). For these examinations, collateral interviews with supervisors and managers are most helpful.

Examples of FFD evaluations include (in addition to the postal worker example) an individual with paranoid personality disorder who was blaming everyone in the workplace for his problems, a hospital concerned about an elderly surgeon blowing up at his nurse, management being concerned about an elderly financial manager's skills, a university concerned with an elderly professor who was noncompliant with his medications for bipolar disorder, a case in which suicidal ideation was expressed in the workplace, and the deterioration of an employee's safety-sensitive work in a high-stress job.

Regulatory Evaluations

Regulatory agencies such as the Federal Aviation Administration (FAA) will have specific fitness for duty requirements when a pilot or prospective pilot has used psychostimulants for attention deficit/hyperactivity disorder (ADHD), is using an antidepressant, has substance abuse problems, or has any form of cognitive problem needing assessment. The FAA will issue specification sheets for each of these types of evaluation. Frequently, there is a need for the use of Cogscreen Aeromedical Edition (Kay, 1995), a computer-based touch-screen evaluation of attention, problem solving, and processing speed that has been validated specifically for pilots. See Kay (2013) for a review of psychological and neuropsychological issues involved in aeromedical evaluations.

Licensing Board Evaluations

Each licensing board has a mission of public trust to protect the public from licensees who may be doing a disservice from unscrupulous, ill-advised, illegal, or impaired practice. Psychologists and neuropsychologists may be asked to evaluate possibly impaired practitioners to help the board determine whether they are safe to practice in their specialties. For example, a neuropsychologist may be asked to evaluate an elderly physician to determine whether there is a dementing illness that is causing problems with practice of the specialty. Frequently, substance abuse is an issue in licensing board evaluations.

State Vocational Rehabilitation

These are state agencies (e.g., Louisiana Rehabilitation services, www.laworks.net/WorkforceDev/LRS/LRS_Main.asp) to assist those with disabilities in their desire to obtain or maintain employment. Frequently, there is a goal for independence in the community, and the agency will help with independent living. Agencies will work cooperatively with businesses and other community resources to help an individual with employment. Psychologists and neuropsychologists may be asked to provide an evaluation focused on helping the individual with work in spite of a disability. Thus, as with disability evaluations, an analysis of strengths and limitations is useful. Compared with disability evaluations, however, the motivation of these claimants is to find or maintain work (Chafetz et al., 2011).

Acknowledgments

The author would like to thank Paige Haley for her due diligence in helping with references, formatting, and APA style.

Notes

1 In this chapter, SSD will be used to refer to both of the disability programs under Social Security: SSDI or SSI.

2 Alternatively, the examiner should be aware that it is easy to look up symptoms to provide an authentic-sounding case during the interview. For example, see the Centers for Disease Control's Traumatic Brain Injury Signs & Symptoms page (https://www.cdc.gov/traumaticbraininjury/symptoms.html).

References

American Academy of Clinical Neuropsychology (AACN). (2007). American Academy of Clinical Neuropsychology (AACN) practice guidelines for neuropsychological assessment and consultation. *The Clinical Neuropsychologist*, *21*, 209–231.

American Psychiatric Association. (2000). *Diagnostic and Statistical Manual of Mental Disorders—Text Revision* (4th ed.). Washington, DC: Author.

American Psychiatric Association. (2013). *Diagnostic and Statistical Manual of Mental Disorders-5* (5th ed.). Arlington, VA: Author.

American Psychological Association. (2002). Ethical principles of psychologists and code of conduct. *American Psychologist*, *57*, 1060–1073.

American Psychological Association. (2012). Guidelines for assessment of and interventions with persons with disabilities. *American Psychologist*, *67*, 43–62.

Americans with Disabilities Act (ADA) Amendments Act of 2008. 42 U.S.C. § 12101 (2008).

Americans with Disabilities Act (ADA) of 1990. Pub. L. No. 101–336, § 2, 104 Stat 328 (1991).

Ben-Porath, Y. S., & Tellegen, A. (2008/2011). *The Minnesota Multiphasic Personality Inventory-2 Restructured Form: Manual for Administration, Scoring, and Interpretation*. Minneapolis, MN: University of Minnesota Press.

Bianchini, K. J., Greve, K. W., & Glynn, G. (2005). On the diagnosis of malingered pain-related disability: Lessons from cognitive malingering research. *The Spine Journal*, *5*, 404–417.

Boone, K. B. (2007). *Assessment of Feigned Cognitive Impairment*. New York: The Guilford Press.

Boone, K. B. (2009). Fixed belief in cognitive dysfunction despite normal neuropsychological scores: Neurocognitive hypochondriasis? *The Clinical Neuropsychologist*, *23*, 1016–1036.

Boone, K. B. (2013). *Clinical Practice of Forensic Neuropsychology: An Evidence Based Approach*. New York: Guilford Press.

Bruns, D., & Disorbio, J. M. (2003). *Battery for Health Improvement-2: Manual*. Minneapolis, MN: Pearson.

Buddin, R., & Kapur, K. (2005). *An Analysis of Military Disability Compensation*. Santa Monica, CA: Research and Development Corporation.

Buddin, W., Schroeder, R., Teichner, G., & Waid, R. (2012). Patients applying for disability versus patients already receiving disability: Is there a difference in medical symptom validity test failure rates? National Academy of Neuropsychology scientific session, B-55. *Archives of Clinical Neuropsychology*, *27*, 636.

Bush, S. S. (2013). Ethical considerations in mild traumatic brain injury cases and symptom validity assessment. In D. A. Carone & S. S. Bush (Eds.), *Mild Traumatic Brain Injury: Symptom Validity Assessment and Malingering* (pp. 45–56). New York: Springer Publishing Company.

Bush, S. S., Ruff, R. M., Troster, A. I., Barth, J. T., Koffler, S. P., Pliskin, N. H., Reynolds, C. R., & Silver, C. H. (2005). Symptom validity assessment: Practice issues and medical necessity. *Archives of Clinical Neuropsychology*, *20*, 419–426.

Butcher, J. N., Dahlstrom, W. G., Graham, J. R., Tellegen, A., & Kaemmer, B. (1989). *Minnesota Multiphasic Personality Inventory-2 Manual for Administration and Scoring*. Minneapolis, MN: University of Minnesota Press.

Chafetz, M. D. (2008). Malingering on the Social Security disability consultative examination: Predictors and base rates. *The Clinical Neuropsychologist*, *22*, 529–546.
Chafetz, M. D. (2010). Symptom validity issues in the psychological consultative examination for Social Security disability. *The Clinical Neuropsychologist*, *24*, 1045–1063.
Chafetz, M. D. (2011a). Reducing the probability of false positives in malingering detection of Social Security disability claimants. *The Clinical Neuropsychologist*, *25*, 1239–1252.
Chafetz, M. D. (2011b). The psychological consultative examination for social security disability. *Psychological Injury & Law*, *4*, 235–244.
Chafetz, M. D. (2012). The A-test: A symptom validity indicator embedded within a mental status examination for Social Security disability. *Applied Neuropsychology*, *19*, 121–126.
Chafetz, M. D. (2013). Symptom validity assessment of mild traumatic brain injury cases in disability and civil litigation contexts. In D. Carone & S. Bush (Eds.), *Mild Traumatic Brain Injury: Symptom Validity Assessment and Malingering*, (pp. 347–356). New York: Springer Publishing.
Chafetz, M. D. (2015). *Intellectual Disability: Criminal and Civil Forensic Issues (AACN Workshop Series)*. New York: Oxford University Press.
Chafetz, M. D., Abrahams, J. P., & Kohlmaier, J. (2007). Malingering on the Social Security disability consultative examination: A new rating scale. *Archives of Clinical Neuropsychology*, *22*, 1–14.
Chafetz, M. D., & Biondolillo, A. M. (2012). Validity issues in Atkins death cases. *The Clinical Neuropsychologist*, *26*, 1358–1376.
Chafetz, M. D., Prentkowski, E., & Rao, A. (2011). To work or not to work: Motivation (not low IQ) determines SVT findings. *Archives of Clinical Neuropsychology*, *26*, 306–313.
Chafetz, M. D., & Underhill, J. (2013). Estimated costs of malingered disability. *Archives of Clinical Neuropsychology*, *28*(7), 633–639. doi: 10.1093/arclin/act038
Colker, R. (2001, October 17). *The Americans with disabilities act: The first decade of enforcement*. Columbus: The Ohio State University Distinguished Lecture.
Colker, R. (2005). *The Disability Pendulum: The First Decade of the Americans with Disabilities Act*. New York: New York University Press.
Delis, D. C., & Wetter, S. R. (2007). Cogniform disorder and cogniform condition: Proposed diagnoses for excessive cognitive symptoms. *Archives of Clinical Neuropsychology*, *22*, 589–604.
Etherton, J., Bianchini, K., Greve, K., & Ciota, M. (2005). Test of memory malingering is unaffected by laboratory induced pain: Implications for clinical use. *Archives of Clinical Neuropsychology*, *20*, 375–384.
Folstein, M., Folstein, S., & McHugh, P. (1975). Mini-mental state. A practical method for grading the cognitive state of patients for the clinician. *Journal of Psychiatric Research*, *12*, 189–198.
Gervais, R. O., Ben-Porath, Y. S., Wygant, D. B., & Green, P. (2007). Development and validation of a Response Bias Scale (RBS) for the MMPI-2. *Assessment*, *14*, 196–208.
Gervais, R. O., Wygant, D. B., Sellbom, M., & Ben-Porath, Y. S. (2011). Associations between SVT failure and scores on the MMPI-2-RF validity and substantive scales. *Journal of Personality Assessment*, *93*, 508–517.
Green, P. (2004). *Manual for the Medical Symptom Validity Test*. Edmonton: Green's Publishing, Inc.
Green, P., Rohling, M. L., Lees-Haley, P. R., & Allen, L. A. (2001). Effort has a greater effect on test scores than severe brain injury in compensation claimants. *Brain Injury*, *15*, 1045–1060.
Greenberg, S. A., & Shuman, D. W. (1997). Irreconcilable conflict between therapeutic and forensic roles. *Professional Psychology: Research and Practice*, *28*, 50–57.
Greenberg, S. A., & Shuman, D. W. (2007). When worlds collide: Therapeutic and forensic roles. *Professional Psychology: Research and Practice*, *38*, 129–132.
Greiffenstein, M. F. (2009). Clinical myths of forensic neuropsychology. *The Clinical Neuropsychologist*, *23*(2), 286–296.
Greiffenstein, M. F., Baker, W. J., & Gola, T. (1994). Validation of malingered amnesia measures with a large clinical sample. *Psychological Assessment*, *6*, 218–224.
Greve, K. W., Bianchini, K. J., & Brewer, S. T. (2013). The assessment of performance and self-report validity in persons claiming pain-related disability. *The Clinical Neuropsychologist*, *27*, 108–137.
Griffin, G.A.E., Normington, J., May, R., & Glassmire, D. (1996). Assessing dissimulation among Social Security disability income claimants. *Journal of Consulting and Clinical Psychology*, *64*, 1425–1430.
Guilmette, T. (2013). The role of clinical judgment in symptom validity assessment. In D. Carone, & S. Bush (Eds.), *Mild Traumatic Brain Injury: Symptom Validity Assessment and Malingering* (pp. 31–44). New York: Springer Publishing.
Hammond, J. (2006, October 15). *Symptom validity and cognition among claimants for social security disability benefits: Utility of the Structured Inventory of Malingered Symptoms (SIMS) and effect of warning*. Poster presented at the Annual Meeting of the National Academy of Neuropsychology, San Antonio, TX, USA.
Health Insurance Portability and Accountability Act (HIPAA) of 1996, 42 U.S.C. ∮ 201 (1996).
Heilbronner, R. L., Sweet, J. J., Morgan, J. E., Larrabee, G. J., Millis, S. R., & Conference Participants. (2009). American academy of clinical neuropsychology consensus conference statement on the neuropsychological assessment of effort, response bias, and malingering. *The Clinical Neuropsychologist*, *23*, 1093–1129.
Hopwood, C. J., Morey, L. C., Rogers, R., & Sewell, K. (2007). Malingering on the personality assessment inventory: Identification of specific feigned disorders. *Journal of Personality Assessment*, *88*, 43–48.
How it works at Allsup-The Allsup SSDI application process. (n.d.). Retrieved from https://www.allsup.com/allsup-representation/how-it-works-at-allsup
Howe, L.L.S., & Loring, D. W. (2009). Classification accuracy and predictive ability of the medical symptom validity test's dementia profile and general memory impairment profile. *The Clinical Neuropsychologist*, *23*, 329–342.
Individuals with Disabilities Education Act of 1997, Pub. L. No. 105-17, ∮ 111 Stat. 107 (1997).
Individuals with Disabilities Education Improvement Act of 2004, 20 U.S.C. ∮ 1400 (2004)
Iverson, G. L., & Lange, R. T. (2011). Mild traumatic brain injury. In M. R. Schoenberg & J. G. Scott (Eds.), *The Little Black Book of Neuropsychology: A Syndrome-Based Approach* (pp. 697–720). New York: Springer Publishing.
Iverson, G. L., Langlois, J .A., McCrea, M. A., & Kelly, J. P. (2009). Challenges associated with postdeployment screening for mild traumatic brain injury in military personnel. *The Clinical Neuropsychologist*, *23*(8), 1299–1314.

Jensen, M. P., Turner, J. A., Romano, J. M., and Strom, S. E. (1995). The chronic pain coping inventory: Development and preliminary validation. *Pain, 60*, 203–216.

Kay, G. G. (1995). *Cog Screen: Professional Manual.* Odessa, FL: Psychological Assessment Resources, Inc.

Kay, G. G. (2013). Aviation neuropsychology. In C. H. Kennedy & G. G. Kay (Eds.), *Aeromedical Psychology* (pp. 239–268). Burlington, VT: Ashgate Publishing Company.

Larrabee, G. J. (2003). Detection of malingering using atypical performance patterns on standard neuropsychological tests. *The Clinical Neuropsychologist, 17*, 410–425.

Larrabee, G. J. (2008). Aggregation across multiple indicators improves the detection of malingering: Relationship to likelihood ratios. *The Clinical Neuropsychologist, 22*, 666–679.

Larrabee, G. J. (2012). Performance validity and symptom validity in neuropsychological assessment. *Journal of the International Neuropsychological Society, 18*, 1–7.

Larrabee, G. J., Greiffenstein, M. F., Greve, K. W., & Bianchini, K. J. (2007). Redefining diagnostic criteria for malingering. In G. J. Larrabee (Ed.), *Assessment of Malingered Neuropsychological Deficits* (pp. 334–371). New York: Oxford University Press.

Larrabee, G. J., Millis, S. R., & Meyers, J. E. (2009). 40 Plus or Minus 10, a new magical number: Reply to Russell. *The Clinical Neuropsychologist, 23*, 841–849.

Lees-Haley, P. R., English, L. T., & Glenn, W. J. (1991). A fake bad scale on the MMPI-2 for personal injury claimants. *Psychological Reports, 68*, 203–210.

McCrea, M. (2008). *Mild Traumatic Brain Injury and Post-concussion Syndrome: The New Evidence Base for Diagnosis and Treatment.* New York: Oxford University Press.

Meyers, J., Reinsch-Boothby, L., Miller, R., Rohling, M., & Axelrod, B. (2011). Does the source of forensic referral affect neuropsychological test performance on a standardized battery of tests? *The Clinical Neuropsychologist, 25*, 477–487.

Miller, L. S., Boyd, M. C., Cohn, A., Wilson, J. S., & McFarland, M. (2006, February). *Prevalence of sub-optimal effort in disability applicants.* Poster session presented at the Annual Meeting of the International Neuropsychological Society, Boston, MA.

Morey, L. (1991). *The Personality Assessment Inventory Professional Manual.* Odessa, FL: Psychological Assessment Resources.

Morton III, D. A. (2010). *Nolo's Guide to Social Security Disability* (5th ed.). Berkeley, CA: Nolo.

Musso, M. W., Barker, A. A., Jones, G. N., Roid, G. H., & Gouvier, W. D. (2011). Development and validation of the tanford binet-5 rarely missed items-nonverbal index for the detection of malingered mental retardation. *Archives of Clinical Neuropsychology, 26*, 756–767.

Nasreddine, Z., Phillips, N., Bedirian, V., Charbonneau, S., Whitehead, V., Collin, I., . . . Chertkow, H. (2005). The Montreal cognitive assessment, MoCA: A brief screening tool for mild cognitive impairment. *Journal of the American Geriatric Society, 53*, 695–699.

Oakes, H. J., Lovejoy, D. W., & Bush, S. S. (2017). *The Independent Neuropsychological Evaluation (AACN Workshop Series).* New York: Oxford University Press.

Office of the Inspector General. (2013). *Challenges of achieving fair and consistent disability decisions.* Retrieved from: http://oig.ssa.gov/sites/default/files/ testimony/March%2020%20Written%20 Statement%20Final.pdf

Ohlemacher, S. (2010, May 9). Social Security disability system bogged down with requests. *Oneida Dispatch.* Retrieved from http://www.oneidadispatch.com/general-news/20100509/social-security-disability-system-bogged-down-with-requests?viewmode=fullstory

Ord, J. S., Greve, K. W., Bianchini, K. J., & Aguerrevere, L. E. (2010). Executive dysfunction in traumatic brain injury: The effects of injury severity and effort on the Wisconsin Card Sorting Test. *Journal of Clinical and Experimental Neuropsychology, 32*(2), 132–140.

Pankratz, L., & Erickson, R. D. (1990). Two views of malingering. *The Clinical Neuropsychologist, 4*, 379–389.

Pratico, D. (2001). *Eisenhower and Social Security: The Origins of the Disability Program.* New York: Writers Club Press.

Puente, A. (1987). Social Security disability and clinical neuropsychological assessment. *The Clinical Neuropsychologist, 4*, 353–363.

Rogers, R., Sewell, K. W., Morey, L. C., & Ustad, K. W. (1996). Detection of feigned mental disorders on the personality assessment inventory: A discriminant analysis. *Journal of Personality Assessment, 67*, 629–640.

Rohling, M. L., Green, P., Allen, L. M., & Iverson, G. L. (2002). Depressive symptoms and neurocognitive test scores in patients passing symptom validity tests. *Archives of Clinical Neuropsychology, 17*, 205–222.

Rosa's Law, Pub. L. No. 111–256, 124 Stat. 2643–2645 (2010).

Salekin, K. L., & Doane, B. M. (2009). Malingered intellectual disability: The value of available measures and methods. *Applied Neuropsychology, 16*, 105–113.

Schalock, R. L., Borthwick-Duffy, S. A/, Bradley, V. J., Buntinx, W.H.E., Coulter, D. L., Craig, E. M., . . . Yeager, M. H. (2010). *Intellectual Disability: Definition, Classification, and Systems of Supports* (11th ed.). Washington, DC: American Association on Intellectual and Developmental Disabilities.

Schenk, K., & Sullivan, K. A. (2010). Do warnings deter rather than produce more sophisticated malingering? *Journal of Clinical and Experimental Neuropsychology, 32*, 752–762.

Sellbom, M., & Bagby, R. M. (2008). Response styles on multiscale inventories. In R. Rogers (Ed.), *Clinical Assessment of Malingering and Deception* (3rd ed., pp. 182–206). New York: Guilford Press.

Shalit, R. (1997, August 25). Defining disability down: Why Johnny can't read, write, or sit still. *The New Republic, 16*, 22.

Shandera, A. L., Berry, D.T.R., Clark, J. A., Schipper, L. J., Grau, L. O., & Harp, J. P. (2010). Detection of malingered mental retardation. *Psychological Assessment, 22*, 50–56.

Slick, D. J., & Sherman, E.M.S. (2013). Differential diagnosis of malingering. In D. Carone & S. Bush (Eds.), *Mild Traumatic Brain Injury: Symptom Validity Assessment and Malingering* (pp. 57–72). New York: Springer Publishing.

Slick, D. J., Sherman, E.M.S., & Iverson, G. L. (1999). Diagnostic criteria for malingered neurocognitive dysfunction: Proposed standards for clinical practice and research. *The Clinical Neuropsychologist, 13*, 545–561.

Smith, K., Boone, K., Victor, T., Miora, D., Cottingham, M., Ziegler, E., . . . Wright, M. (2014). Comparison of credible patients of very low intelligence and non-credible patients on neurocognitive performance validity indicators. *The Clinical Neuropsychologist, 28*(6), 1048–1070.

Social Security Administration. (2008). Disability evaluation under Social Security (Blue Book). (SSA Publication No. 64–039). Retrieved from www.ssa.gov/disability/professionals/bluebook/.

Social Security Administration. (2012). *Annual Statistical Report on the Social Security Disability Insurance Program, 2011*. Washington, DC: SSA Publication No. 13–11827.

Social Security Administration. (2013a). Red book: How do we define disability? Retrieved from http://1.usa.gov/15Gkwtj.

Social Security Administration. (2013b). Disability evaluation under Social Security: 12.00 mental disorders—Adult. Retrieved from http://1.usa.gov/bl3ewE.

Social security disability benefits: Did a group of judges, doctors, and lawyers abuse programs for the country's most vulnerable: Hearings before the Committee on Homeland Security and Governmental Affairs, 113th Cong. 2 (2013) (testimony of Tom Coburn).

Stevens, J. (1986). Is it organic or is it functional: Is it hysterical or is it malingering? *Psychiatric Clinics of North America*, *9*, 241–254.

Strasburger, L. H., Gutheil, T. G., & Brodsky, A. (1997). On wearing two hats: Role conflict in serving as both psychotherapist and expert witness. *American Journal of Psychiatry*, *154*, 448–456.

Strub, R. L., & Black, F. W. (1993). *The Mental Status Examination in Neurology* (3rd ed.). Philadelphia, PA: F. A. Davis Co.

Suhr, J. A., & Gunstad, J. (2002). "Diagnosis threat": The effect of negative expectations on cognitive performance in head injury. *Journal of Clinical and Experimental Neuropsychology*, *24*, 448–457.

Tarescavage, A. M., Wygant, D. B., Gervais, R. O., & Ben-Porath, Y. S. (2013). Association between the MMPI-2 restructured form (MMPI-2-RF) and malingered neurocognitive dysfunction among non-head injury disability claimants. *The Clinical Neuropsychologist*, *27*, 313–335.

Tariq, S. H., Tumosa, N., Chibnall, J. T., Perry III, H. M., & Morley, J. E. (2006). The Saint Louis University Mental Status (SLUMS) examination for detecting mild cognitive impairment and dementia is more sensitive than the Mini-Mental Status Examination (MMSE)—A pilot study. *American Journal of Geriatric Psychiatry*, *14*, 900–910.

Tombaugh, T. N. (1996). *TOMM. Test of Memory Malingering*. North Tonawanda, NY: Multi-Health Systems.

United States. (1975). Public Law 94–142 - Education of All Handicapped Children Act. Title 20, Section 1400. Retrieved from www.scn.org/~bk269/94-142.html.

U.S. Department of Health and Human Services. (2005). *The surgeon general's call to action to improve the health and wellness of persons with disabilities.* Retrieved from https://www.ncbi.nlm.nih.gov/books/NBK44667/pdf/Bookshelf_NBK44667.pdf.

Victor, T. L., & Boone, K. B. (2007). Identification of feigned mental retardation. In K. B. Boone (Ed.), *Assessment of Feigned Cognitive Impairment* (pp. 310–345). New York: The Guilford Press.

Victor, T. L., Boone, K. B., Serpa, J. G., Buehler, J., & Ziegler, E. A. (2009). Interpreting the meaning of multiple symptom validity test failure. *The Clinical Neuropsychologist*, *23*(2), 297–313.

Winegar, M. D. (2006). Big talk, broken promises: How title I of the Americans with disabilities act failed disabled workers. *Hofstra Law Review*, *34*, 1267–1317.

World Health Organization. (2001). *The World Health Report 2001: Mental Health: New Understanding, New Hope*. Geneva, Switzerland: World Health Organization.

Worthen, M. D., & Moering, R. G. (2011). A practical guide to conducting VA compensation and pension exams for PTSD and other mental disorders. *Psychological Injury and Law*, *4*, 187–216.

Wygant, D. B., Ben-Porath, Y. S., Arbisi, P. A., Berry, D.T.R., Freeman, D. B., & Heilbronner, R. L. (2009). Examination of the MMPI-2 restructured form (MMPI-2-RF) validity scales in civil forensic settings: Findings from simulation and known group samples. *Archives of Clinical Neuropsychology*, *24*, 671–680.

Yanez, Y. T., Fremouw, W., Tennant, J., Strunk, J., & Coker, K. (2006). Effects of severe depression on TOMM performance among disability-seeking outpatients. *Archives of Clinical Neuropsychology*, *21*, 161–165.

42 Ethical Practice of Clinical Neuropsychology

Shane S. Bush

Do I need to use the most recent version of a test as soon as it is published? Do I allow family members to serve as interpreters for neuropsychological evaluations of patients who cannot speak English? Do I have to use performance validity measures in routine clinical evaluations? Is it best to use the normative data that comes with the test when it is published? Do I release raw test data to attorneys? Do I need to be board certified in neuropsychology? This brief series of questions reflects a sample of issues that lie at the intersection of ethics, laws, and clinical practice. Although these specific issues have been addressed in the neuropsychology literature, they nevertheless pose challenges for many practitioners. Even more complex issues with unique elements and no clear solution are routinely encountered in neuropsychological practice, requiring practitioners to be or become familiar with a variety of resources and a structured approach to ethical decision making.

It has been more than 20 years since the discussion of ethical issues in clinical neuropsychology began expanding from the classroom and clinic into the published literature (Binder & Thompson, 1995; Brittain, Francis, & Barth, 1995; Fowles & Fox, 1995). The initial articles specific to ethical issues in neuropsychology were published on the heels of early publications on policy and legal issues (Woody, 1989) and ethics in closely related specialties such as rehabilitation medicine (Ackerman & Banks, 1990; Banja, 1989; Banja & Johnston, 1994; Malec, 1993). These early neuropsychology ethics articles were immediately followed in the literature by additional application of professional ethics to various aspects of neuropsychological and neurorehabilitation research and practice (Anderson & Shields, 1998; Argarwal, Ferran, Ost, & Wilson, 1996; Artiola i Fortuny & Mullaney, 1998; Banja, 1996; Banja & Rosenthal, 1996; Banja, Adler, & Stringer, 1996; Guilmette & Hagan, 1997; Johnson-Greene, Hardy-Morais, Adams, Hardy, & Bergloff, 1997; Malec, 1996; Rosenthal, 1996; Rosenthal & Lourie, 1996; Sim, 1998; van Gorp & McMullen, 1997; Wong, 1998; Woody, 1997).

The period from the late 1980s to the turn of the century also brought publications on professional practice issues that have direct ethical implications involving professional competence; selection, use, and interpretation of tests; test security; and preservation of the examiner–examinee diad (Binder & Johnson-Greene, 1995; Bornstein, 1991; DeLuca, 1989; Donders, 1999; Freides, 1993; Grote, Lewin, Sweet, & van Gorp, 2000; Macartney-Filgate & Snow, 2000; Martelli, Zasler, & Grayon, 1999; Matthews, Harley, & Malec, 1991; McCaffrey, Fisher, Gold, & Lynch, 1996; McSweeny, Becker, Naugle, Snow, Binder, & Thompson, 1998; van Gorp & McMullen, 1997; Youngjohn, Spector, & Mapou, 1998). Some publications during this time resulted in engaging commentary and discussion, which helped to refine the ethical and professional aspects of common practice issues (e.g., Barth, 2000; Freides, 1993, 1995; Lees-Haley, 1999; Lees-Haley & Courtney, 2000a, 2000b; Matarazzo, 1995; Naugle & McSweeny, 1995; Naugle & McSweeny, 1996; Sweet & Moulthrop, 1999a, 1999b; Tranel, 2000). These publications provided the foundation for the position papers from professional organizations such as the American Academy of Clinical Neuropsychology and the National Academy of Neuropsychology that began emerging in the late 1990s and early 21st century and help define standards of practice in clinical neuropsychology.

With these early articles, chapters, and position papers as the foundation, neuropsychology has seen steady growth in publications on ethical, legal, and professional aspects of practice. Edited books on ethical practice in neuropsychology provided coverage of ethical issues with various patient populations across multiple clinical settings (Bush, 2005a; Bush & Drexler, 2002). Subsequent publications have emphasized the importance of addressing ethical challenges with a structured decision-making model, pursuing high standards of ethical conduct beyond risk management, and striving to anticipate and avoid ethical challenges before they become dilemmas (e.g., Bush, 2007, 2009). Johnson-Greene and Nissley (2008) noted that knowledge of ethical standards and doctrine is not synonymous with sound ethical decision making; rather, knowledge of both ethical content and the decision-making process are essential for making good decisions in ethical matters.

The primary purpose of the present chapter is to provide an updated overview of ethical issues and decision making in clinical neuropsychology. Recently published ethical, legal, and professional resources are reviewed, an ethical decision-making model is presented, and the importance of a personal commitment to ethical practice is emphasized.

Ethical Challenges and Ideals

If one were to consider complaints and notices filed with the American Psychological Association (APA) Ethics Committee when determining which ethical issues are most important for neuropsychologists and how seriously ethical issues should be taken, it would be easy to conclude that there is little to worry about as long as harmful dual relationships, particularly those of a sexual nature, are avoided. In 2011, complaints were filed with the APA Ethics Committee against 0.07% of the membership, and the Ethics Committee received notices of inappropriate behavior from licensing boards and other entities for 0.09% of the APA membership (APA Ethics Committee, 2012). Of the nine ethics cases that were opened in 2011, none came from complaints filed with the committee. The categories of ethics cases opened by the APA Ethics Committee in 2011 were as follows: Dual Relationship (Sexual Misconduct–Adult), $N = 5$ (55.6% of cases); Dual Relationship (nonsexual), $N = 2$ (22.2% of cases); Inappropriate Professional Practice (Insurance/Fee Problems), $N = 1$ (11.1% of cases); and Inappropriate Research, Teaching, or Administrative Practice (Other), $N = 1$ (11.1% of cases) (APA Ethics Committee, 2012).

Similar figures were reported for 2012 (APA Ethics Committee, 2013). That year, complaints were filed with the APA Ethics Committee against 0.08% of the membership, and the Ethics Committee received notices of inappropriate behavior from licensing boards and other entities for 0.05% of the APA membership. Just two (15.4%) of the 13 ethics cases that were opened in 2012 came from complaints filed with the committee. The categories of ethics cases opened by the APA Ethics Committee in 2012 were as follows: Dual Relationship (Sexual Misconduct–Adult), $N = 5$ (38.5% of cases); Dual Relationship (Nonsexual), $N = 2$ (15.4% of cases); Inappropriate Professional Practice (Child Custody), $N = 3$ (23.1% of cases); and Inappropriate Professional Practice (Insurance/Fee Problems), $N = 2$ (15.4% of cases) (APA Ethics Committee, 2013).

However, ethical practice in clinical neuropsychology extends well beyond the avoidance of complaints filed with the APA Ethics Committee. Psychological ethics, designed to prevent harm and to promote the well-being of consumers of psychological services, require practitioners to be aware of each aspect of their professional behavior and how those behaviors impact others, leading to choices that are consistent with the goals of professional ethics. While all ethical standards and principles are applicable to various neuropsychological activities, certain standards are more relevant than others for common neuropsychological practices (Brittain, Frances, & Barth, 1995; Bush, 2007; Bush, Grote, Johnson-Greene, & Macartney-Filgate, 2008). Based on a review of the literature and personal experience, 12 common sources of ethical conflict were identified, in the following order of importance: professional competence, roles and relationships (dual/multiple), test security and release of raw test data, third-party observers, confidentiality, assessment, conflicts between ethics and laws, false or deceptive statements, objectivity, cooperation with other professionals, informed consent and third-party requests for services, and record keeping and fees (Bush, 2007). Practitioners working in various subspecialties within neuropsychology will place different degrees of emphasis on the various ethical standards depending on the needs of the patients or practice setting.

For each of these ethical standards, there are actions that can be taken to minimally satisfy the ethical requirement, and there are actions that can be taken that reflect the pursuit of higher standards of ethical practice. Aspiring to high ethical standards of professional behavior or ethical ideals, referred to as *positive ethics* (Knapp & VandeCreek, 2006), often requires more time and effort than is required to satisfy minimum requirements. Nevertheless, patients, other consumers of neuropsychological services, and the profession are typically better served by the practitioner's extra investment.

For example, regarding the first area of ethical importance (professional competence), obtaining board certification readily identifies a neuropsychologist to patients, the public, and others as meeting a certain level of professional competence. However, the board certification process can be time- and labor-intensive, as well as an added expense and source of stress in one's professional life. Some qualified clinicians choose not to undergo the examination process because of its challenges, time requirements, and expense, particularly given that it is not required for practice in most contexts; yet it can be difficult to distinguish those qualified clinicians from those not providing competent services.

To address the question "Do I need to be board certified in neuropsychology," the short answer, consistent with minimal ethical standards and legal requirements, is "no." However, at this point in the evolution of the profession, clinicians who perform neuropsychological services but have not obtained, or are not pursuing, board certification would be hard pressed to defend the decision to not demonstrate their knowledge and skills through formal peer review. Knapp, Younggren, VandeCreek, Harris, and Martin (2013) noted:

> A continual danger is that psychologists' perceived personal skill inventory almost always will be greater than their actual skill inventory. Psychologists can reduce the gap between their perceived and actual skill inventories by ongoing contact and feedback with other mental health professionals.
>
> (p. 13)

Board certification is ideal for determining whether one's actual skill inventory corresponds with one's perceived skill inventory and whether the actual skill inventory reflects competence in neuropsychology.

The value of board certification to the public, the profession, and practitioners has long been acknowledged and repeatedly emphasized (e.g., Cox, 2010). Evidence indicates that board certification in neuropsychology is increasing (e.g., McCrea, 2011) and is achieving higher numbers than other specialties within psychology (Cox, 2010). Obtaining the highest credential offered in the specialty is consistent with the pursuit of the highest standards of ethical practice in the area of professional competence.

Similar examples can be provided for each of the 12 common sources of ethical conflict that were previously described. The important point is that there typically exists a range of ethically appropriate actions that practitioners can take when confronted with ethical issues and dilemmas, and the easiest option may not be the best option. A personal commitment to the pursuit of ethical ideals benefits patients and the profession.

Ethics Resources and Preparation

Neuropsychologists practicing in the United States are aware of the APA ethics code (APA, 2010) and likely turn to the code first when confronting ethical questions or conflicts. In some circumstances, the code may not fully address the issue being confronted by the clinician. In other circumstances, the issue being addressed may be more of a legal, clinical, or risk management issue than an ethical issue per se (Behnke, 2014). Determining whether the issue of concern is an ethical, legal, professional, or risk management issue or some combination of these issues will dictate which resources will be useful for addressing the issue. Thus, familiarity with multiple resources can facilitate decision making when faced with challenging situations.

The following list provides some of the primary resources that can help neuropsychologists with ethical and legal decision making: (a) general bioethical principles; (b) ethics codes of organizations other than APA; (c) Code of Conduct of the Association of State and Provincial Psychology Boards; (d) jurisdictional laws; (e) position papers and practice guidelines from professional organizations; (f) scholarly publications such as books, articles, and chapters; (g) ethics committees; (h) professional liability insurance carriers; (i) institutional guidelines and resources; and (j) experienced and knowledgeable colleagues. These types of resources tend to provide more specific guidance than can typically be offered by a general ethics code.

Savvy practitioners do not wait until confronted with a challenging ethical matter before obtaining and familiarizing themselves with ethical and legal resources. They *anticipate* the types of issues and challenges that are most likely to be encountered in their practice and strive to *avoid* ethical dilemmas by reviewing relevant resources and establishing appropriate practices and routines. Although not all ethical challenges can be avoided, such practitioners are typically well prepared to *address* ethical challenges when they arise, taking the steps necessary as they *aspire* to the highest standards of ethical practice. These four words (anticipate, avoid, address, and aspire), known as the *Four A's of ethical practice* (Bush, 2009), can cue practitioners to be mindful of the importance of regularly attending to ethical issues across the span of professional activities. Holding ethics rounds or seminars, or making a commitment to become familiar with one ethics resource per month, promotes the type of focus on professional behavior that is consistent with high standards of ethical practice.

Practitioners are also well served by understanding factors that tend to predispose them to, and protect them from, ethical misconduct (Johnson-Greene & Nissley, 2008; Knapp et al., 2013). Predisposing risk factors include (a) practicing in isolation where there tends to be little direct oversight of one's work and more limited availability of peer consultation; (b) practicing outside of one's boundaries of competence; (c) being an impaired provider, due to psychological, cognitive, or social problems; (d) working with certain patient populations (e.g., serious personality disorders, complex posttraumatic stress disorder) or in certain practice contexts (e.g., forensics); and (e) having limited awareness of, or corrective response to, personal and professional biases. Factors that help protect practitioners from ethical misconduct are essentially the opposite of predisposing factors and include (a) maintaining a system of protection, including membership in professional organizations and a network of colleagues for consultation when needed; (b) appreciating the limits of one's skill inventory and practicing within one's boundaries of competency; (c) establishing and maintaining familiarity with ethical issues, resources, and decision making; (d) engaging in self-examination so that maladaptive actions can be changed. Periodically reviewing these precipitating and protective factors with the goal of improving one's professional services reflects the pursuit of high standards of ethical practice.

Application of Resources to Ethical Challenges

Familiarity with ethical and legal resources is usually necessary but not sufficient for addressing complex ethics questions. The information must be organized and applied in a manner that promotes sound decision making, with consideration of personal and situational factors and the dynamic nature of any complex decision making process. A structured ethical decision-making model can help in that regard. Such models help clarify the nature of the problem, identify requirements and guidelines from relevant resources, and generate possible solutions. Detailed models (e.g., Bush, 2007) break the process down into multiple steps, each of which can influence the decision making process and choices made.

Johnson-Greene and Nissley (2008) emphasized the importance of a process-oriented model in which

> there is an appreciation for the dynamic nature of the model, acknowledgement of the multitude of predisposing

> and protective factors, sources of ethical standards and variation in experiences and skills, and an understanding that all ethical issues start and end within the patient—provider relationship and the provider's emphasis on the three ethical foundations of patient autonomy, beneficence, and nonmalfeasance.
>
> (p. 955)

Use of ethical decision-making models reduces the likelihood that complex ethical decisions are made on the basis of personal judgment alone.

To address the questions posed at the beginning of this chapter, neuropsychologists have considered the various possible solutions, often applying the decision-making model with a variety of resources, and arrived at the following conclusions.

1 Do I need to use the most recent version of a test as soon as it is published? No.

> Determining whether or when to transition to a new version of a test can be particularly difficult for clinicians in psychological specialties because it can take years after publication of a revised test for research with special patient populations to be performed and published. As a result, different clinicians may adopt newer versions of tests at different times or elect not to use the newest version, depending on the specific patient population and referral questions. Decisions regarding transitioning to new test revisions should be based on the scientific merits of the tests, not on an arbitrarily defined time frame. Clinicians ultimately must use their judgment regarding which test version is best for a given patient at a given point in time.
>
> (Bush, 2010, p. 7)

2 Do I allow family members to serve as interpreters for neuropsychological evaluations of patients who cannot speak English? Typically, no.

> When providing service directly in the examinee's preferred language is not feasible, neuropsychologists should make efforts to use professional interpreters and translators. . . . Whenever possible, neuropsychologists should avoid using family members, attorneys, and other persons known to the client as interpreters, unless circumstances dictate and permit such use.
>
> (Judd et al., 2009, p. 131)

3 Do I need to use performance validity measures in routine clinical evaluations? Yes.

> Adequate assessment of response validity is essential in order to maximize confidence in the results of neurocognitive and personality measures and in the diagnoses and recommendations that are based on the results. Symptom validity assessment may include specific tests, indices, and observations. The manner in which symptom validity is assessed may vary depending on context but must include a thorough examination of cultural factors. Assessment of response validity, as a component of a medically necessary evaluation, is medically necessary.
>
> (Bush et al., 2005, p. 419)

Additionally, a consensus conference on the neuropsychological assessment of effort, response bias, and malingering (Heilbronner et al., 2009) concluded, "Even in a routine clinical context the presence of problematic effort and response bias can potentially invalidate results. The assessment of effort and genuine reporting of symptoms is important in all evaluations" (p. 1121).

4 Is it best to use the normative data that comes with the test when it is published? The answer to this question depends entirely on the specific test and the patient being evaluated. For some new tests or new versions of older tests, the accompanying normative data is an improvement over that of preexisting tests for certain patient populations; however, the same data set may not be the most appropriate option for patients with certain disorders for whom a large body of published data exists for a prior test. Similarly, for older tests, research and normative data published subsequent to the publication of the tests are often preferred over the original normative data.

5 Do I release raw test data to attorneys? Typically this is not done as a first option and not without requesting safeguards. This question has been covered extensively in the neuropsychology literature (e.g., Bush & Martin, 2006; Bush, Rapp, & Ferber, 2010; Kaufmann, 2009) and by professional organizations (e.g., American Psychological Association & Committee on Legal Issues, 2006; Attix et al., 2007; National Academy of Neuropsychology, 2000, National Academy of Neuropsychology Policy and Planning Committee, 2003). Despite a lack of clear or rational guidance from the APA ethics code, multiple ethical and legal resources describe the potential problems associated with reproducing and releasing raw test data to nonpsychologists who do not have the education or training to understand and appropriately use and protect the materials. For example:

> Threats to test security by release of test data to nonpsychologists are significant. . . . the National Academy of Neuropsychology fully endorses the need to maintain test security, views the duty to do so as a basic professional and ethical obligation, strongly discourages the release of materials when requests do not contain appropriate safeguards, and, when indicated, urges the neuropsychologist to take appropriate and reasonable steps to arrange conditions for release that ensure adequate safeguards.
>
> (National Academy of Neuropsychology, 2000, pp. 383–384).

These questions reflect a very small sample of the types of questions that neuropsychologists have commonly found challenging over the years. More challenging for practitioners at this time are those that involve unique situations that have not yet received extensive attention by professional organizations or extensive coverage in the literature. It is in such situations that familiarity with a variety of resources, awareness of a decision-making model, and access to knowledgeable and experienced colleagues can be of greatest value.

Changes Over Time and Future Directions

Since articles on ethical issues in neuropsychology began appearing the literature about 20 years ago, nearly every aspect of clinical practice and professional behavior has been dissected from the perspective of professional ethics and laws. Articles and book chapters on ethics pertaining to various subspecialties, patient populations, practice contexts, and emerging issues have been published, including, but not limited to, pediatrics, geriatrics, sport, forensics, military and veterans, and technology. Numerous resources that extend beyond the APA ethics code have been identified, decision-making models have been proposed, and professional organizations have taken positions on issues.

Despite these advances, unique situations continue to arise that challenge practitioners to make sound ethical decisions despite the absence of a clearly preferred course of action. It is in such situations that reliance on the core bioethical principles that have always been the foundation of good clinical practice can be of most value. A commitment to promoting understanding and welfare of patients, avoiding actions that are likely to be harmful to patients, respecting patient autonomy, and practicing in a manner that promotes fairness and justice can help practitioners maintain high standards of ethical practice, avoid ethical misconduct, and address dilemmas when they arise.

There seems to be little doubt that technology will continue to play an increasing role in neuropsychological practice, from electronic medical records to more extensive computer administration, scoring, and interpretation, to imaging, to telemedicine, and to options that practitioners have not yet considered. While some of these practices are already under way in some contexts, they are likely to be adopted more widely, and the range of activities will expand. In the rush to adopt new technologies and to apply technology to neuropsychology in new ways that can better serve patients and the profession, care must be taken to determine that quality is not lost and that patient care and the profession do not suffer. The following conclusion, drawn more than ten years ago, seems even more relevant today: "Neuropsychologists will minimize chances for ethical misconduct by increasing their sensitivity to the relevant ethical issues associated with ITT as well as by ensuring competence in those technologies used in clinical practice and/or research" (Bush, Naugle, & Johnson-Greene, 2002, p. 543; note: "ITT" is "information technology and telecommunications"). When both technology-based and traditional options are available, informing patients and allowing them to choose reflects respect for patient autonomy.

A trend toward greater involvement in forensic cases has also been observed in recent years and is likely to continue (Kaufmann, 2009). With passage and recent implementation of the Patient Care and Affordable Care Act [P.L. 111–148] (ACA), some neuropsychologists are already experiencing an adverse impact on their hospital-based practices. Although the broader and longer-term impact of the ACA on neuropsychological practice remains unknown, and new opportunities are certain to arise for some clinicians, other clinicians may use this time of transition and uncertainty to begin or increase forensic work. Thus, the trend toward increased forensic work for neuropsychologists that was observed prior to implementation of the ACA may be further accelerated in the coming years, bringing to more practitioners the ethical issues and challenges encountered more commonly in forensic practice (e.g., Bush, 2005b).

As the practice of clinical neuropsychology continues to evolve, the application of professional ethics to clinical practice will need to keep pace. Maintaining open discussion of ethical questions, challenges, and solutions, and sharing experiences with colleagues, will promote ethical practice and be particularly valuable during times of transition. A personal commitment to the shared values of the profession, reflected in general bioethical principles and a variety of published resources, helps position neuropsychologists to understand ethical issues, anticipate and avoid ethical challenges, and successfully resolve ethical dilemmas when they arise. And, most importantly, those served by neuropsychologists benefit.

References

Ackerman, R. J., & Banks, M. E. (1990). Computers and ethical treatment for brain-injured patients. *Social Science Computer Review*, *8*, 83–95.

American Psychological Association. (2010). Ethical principles of psychologists and code of conduct. Retrieved November 7, 2012 from www.apa.org/ethics/code/index.aspx

American Psychological Association, Committee on Legal Issues. (2006). Strategies for private practitioners coping with subpoenas or compelled testimony for client records or test data. *Professional Psychology: Research and Practice*, *37*, 215–222.

American Psychological Association Ethics Committee. (2012). Report of the Ethics Committee, 2011. *American Psychologist*, *67*, 398–408.

American Psychological Association Ethics Committee. (2013). Report of the Ethics Committee, 2012. *American Psychologist*, *68*, 370–379.

Anderson, R. M. Jr., & Shields, H. (1998). Ethical issues in neuropsychological assessment. In R. M. Anderson, Jr., T. L. Needels, & H. V. Hall (Eds.), *Avoiding Ethical Misconduct in Psychology Specialty Areas* (pp. 131–141). Springfield, IL: Charles C. Thomas Publisher.

Argarwal, M. R., Ferran, J., Ost, K., & Wilson, K. (1996). Ethics of informed consent in dementia research-the debate continues. *International Journal of Geriatric Psychiatry*, *11*, 801–806.

Artiola i Fortuny, L., & Mullaney, H. A. (1998). Assessing patients whose language you do not know: Can the absurd be ethical? *The Clinical Neuropsychologist*, *12*, 113–126.

Attix, D. K., Donders, J., Johnson-Greene, D., Grote, C. L., Harris, J. G., & Bauer, R. M. (2007). Disclosure of neuropsychological test data: Official position of Division 40 (Clinical Neuropsychology) of the American Psychological Association, Association of Postdoctoral Programs in Clinical Neuropsychology, and American Academy of Clinical Neuropsychology. *The Clinical Neuropsychologist*, *21*, 232–238.

Banja, J. D. (Ed.). (1989). Ethical and legal issues (Special issue). *Journal of Head Trauma Rehabilitation*, *4*(1).

Banja, J. D. (1996). Ethics, values, and world culture: The impact on rehabilitation. *Disability Rehabilitation*, *18*, 279–284.

Banja, J. D., Adler, R. K., & Stringer, A. Y. (1996). Ethical dimensions of caring for defiant patients: A case study. *Journal of Head Trauma Rehabilitation*, *11*, 93–97.

Banja, J. D., & Johnston, M. V. (1994). Outcomes evaluation in TBI rehabilitation. Part III: Ethical perspectives and social policy. *Archives of Physical Medicine and Rehabilitation*, *75*(12 Spec No), SC 19–26; discussion SC 27–28.

Banja, J. D., & Rosenthal, M. (guest editors). (1996). Ethics. *NeuroRehabilitation*, *6*(2), special issue.

Barth, J. T. (2000). Commentary on "Disclosure of tests and raw test data to the courts" by Paul Lees-Haley and John Courtney. *Neuropsychology Review*, *10*, 179–180.

Behnke, S. (2014). What kind of issue is it? A "four-bin" approach to ethics consultation is helpful in practice settings. *Monitor on Psychology*, *45*, 62–63.

Binder, L. M., & Johnson-Greene, D. (1995). Observer effects on neuropsychological performance: A case report. *The Clinical Neuropsychologist*, *9*, 74–78.

Binder, L. M., & Thompson, L. L. (1995). The ethics code and neuropsychological assessment practices. *Archives of Clinical Neuropsychology*, *10*, 27–46.

Bornstein, R. A. (1991). Report of the division 40 task force on education, accreditation and credentialing: Recommendations for education and training of nondoctoral personnel in clinical neuropsychology. *The Clinical Neuropsychologist*, *5*, 20–23.

Brittain, J. L., Frances, J. P., & Barth, J. T. (1995). Ethical issues and dilemmas in neuropsychological practice reported by ABCN diplomates. *Advances in Medical Psychotherapy*, *8*, 1–22.

Bush, S. S. (Ed.). (2005a). *A Casebook of Ethical Challenges in Neuropsychology*. New York: Psychology Press.

Bush, S. S. (guest editor). (2005b). Ethical issues in forensic neuropsychology. *Journal of Forensic Neuropsychology*, *4*(3), special issue.

Bush, S. S. (2007). *Ethical Decision Making in Clinical Neuropsychology*. New York: Oxford University Press.

Bush, S. S. (2009). *Geriatric Mental Health Ethics: A Casebook*. New York: Springer Publishing Company.

Bush, S. S. (2010). Determining whether or when to adopt new versions of psychological and neuropsychological tests. *The Clinical Neuropsychologist*, *24*, 7–16.

Bush, S. S., & Drexler, M. L. (Eds.). (2002). *Ethical Issues in Clinical Neuropsychology*. Lisse, NL: Swets & Zeitlinger Publishers.

Bush, S. S., Grote, C., Johnson-Greene, D., & Macartney-Filgate, M. (2008). A panel interview on the ethical practice of neuropsychology. *The Clinical Neuropsychologist*, *22*, 321–344.

Bush, S. S., & Martin, T. A. (2006). The ethical and clinical practice of disclosing raw test data: Addressing the ongoing debate. *Applied Neuropsychology*, *13*(2), 115–124.

Bush, S., Naugle, R., & Johnson-Greene, D. (2002). The interface of information technology and neuropsychology: Ethical issues and recommendations. *The Clinical Neuropsychologist*, *16*, 536–547.

Bush, S. S., Rapp, D. L., & Ferber, P. S. (2010). Maximizing test security in forensic neuropsychology. In A. M. Horton, Jr. & L. C. Hartlage (Eds.), *Handbook of Forensic Neuropsychology* (2nd ed., pp. 177–195). New York: Springer Publishing Co.

Bush, S. S., Ruff, R. M., Tröster, A. I., Barth, J. T., Koffler, S. P., Pliskin, N. H., . . . Silver, C. H. (2005). Symptom validity assessment: Practice issues and medical necessity: Official position of the National Academy of Neuropsychology. *Archives of Clinical Neuropsychology*, *20*(4), 419–426.

Cox, D. (2010). Board certification in professional psychology: Promoting competency and consumer protection. *The Clinical Neuropsychologist*, *24*, 493–505.

DeLuca, J. W. (1989). Neuropsychology technicians in clinical practice: Precedents, rationale and current deployment. *The Clinical Neuropsychologist*, *3*, 3–21.

Donders, J. (1999). Pediatric neuropsychological reports: Do they really have to be so long? *Child Neuropsychology*, *5*, 70–78.

Fowles, G. P., & Fox, B. A. (1995). Competency to consent to treatment and informed consent in neurobehavioral rehabilitation. *The Clinical Neuropsychologist*, *9*, 251–257.

Freides, D. (1993). Proposed standard of professional practice: Neuropsychological reports display all quantitative data. *The Clinical Neuropsychologist*, *7*, 234–235.

Freides, D. (1995). Interpretations are more benign than data. *The Clinical Neuropsychologist*, *9*, 248.

Grote, C. L., Lewin, J. L., Sweet, J. J., & van Gorp, W. G. (2000). Responses to perceived unethical practices in clinical neuropsychology: Ethical and legal considerations. *The Clinical Neuropsychologist*, *14*, 119–134.

Guilmette, T. J., & Hagan, L. D. (1997). Ethical considerations in forensic neuro-psychological consultation. *The Clinical Neuropsychologist*, *11*, 287–290.

Heilbronner, R. L., Sweet, J. J., Morgan, J. E., Larrabee, G. J., Millis, S., & Conference Participants. (2009). American Academy of Clinical Neuropsychology consensus conference statement on the neuropsychological assessment of effort, response bias, and malingering. *The Clinical Neuropsychologist*, *23*, 1093–1129.

Johnson-Greene, D., Hardy-Morais, C., Adams, K. M., Hardy, C., & Bergloff, P. (1997). Informed consent and neuropsychological assessment: Ethical considerations and proposed guidelines. *The Clinical Psychologist*, *11*, 454–460.

Johnson-Greene, D., & Nissley, H. (2008). Ethical challenges in neuropsychology. In J. E. Morgan & J. H. Ricker (Eds.), *Textbook of Clinical Neuropsychology* (pp. 945–959). New York: Psychology Press.

Judd, T., Capetillo, D., Carrion-Baralt, J., Marmol, L. M., San Miguel-Montes, L., Navarrete, M. G., . . . Silver, C. H. (2009). Professional considerations for improving the neuropsychological evaluation of Hispanics: A National Academy of Neuropsychology Education Paper. *Archives of Clinical Neuropsychology*, *24*, 127–135.

Kaufmann, P. M. (2009). Protecting raw data and psychological tests from wrongful disclosure: A primer on the law and other persuasive strategies. *The Clinical Neuropsychologist, 23*, 1130–1159.

Knapp, S., & VandeCreek, L. (2006). *Practical Ethics for Psychologists: A Positive Approach*. Washington, DC: American Psychological Association.

Knapp, S., Younggren, J. N., VandeCreek, L., Harris, E., & Martin, J. N. (2013). *Assessing and Managing Risk in Psychological Practice: An Individualized Approach* (2nd ed.). Rockville, MD: The Trust.

Lees-Haley, P. (1999). Commentary on Sweet and Moulthrop's debiasing procedures. *Journal of Forensic Neuropsychology, 1*, 43–57.

Lees-Haley, P. R., & Courtney, J. C. (2000a). Disclosure of tests and raw test data to the courts: A need for reform. *Neuropsychology Review, 10*, 169–175.

Lees-Haley, P. R., & Courtney, J. C. (2000b). Reply to the commentary on "Disclosure of tests and raw test data to the courts." *Neuropsychology Review, 10*, 181–182.

Macartney-Filgate, M., & Snow, W. (2000). Forensic assessments and professional relations. *Division 40 Newsletter, 18*, 28–31.

Malec, J. F. (1993). Ethics in brain injury rehabilitation: Existential choices among western cultural beliefs. *Brain Injury, 7*, 383–400.

Malec, J. F. (1996). Ethical conflict resolution based on an ethics of relationships for brain injury rehabilitation. *Brain Injury, 10*, 781–795.

Martelli, M., Zasler, N., & Grayon, R. (1999). Ethical considerations in medicolegal evaluations of neurologic injury and impairment following acquired brain injury. *NeuroRehabilitation: An Interdisciplinary Journal, 13*, 45–66.

Matarazzo, R. G. (1995). Psychological report standards in neuropsychology. *The Clinical Neuropsychologist, 9*, 249–250.

Matthews, C. G., Harley, J. P., & Malec, J. F. (1991). Guidelines for computer-assisted neuropsychological rehabilitation and cognitive remediation. *The Clinical Neuropsychologist, 5*, 3–19.

McCaffrey, R. J., Fisher, J. M., Gold, B. A., & Lynch, J. K. (1996). Presence of third parties during neuropsychological evaluation: Who is evaluating whom? *The Clinical Neuropsychologist, 10*, 435–449.

McCrea, M. (2011). President's annual state of the Academy report. *The Clinical Neuropsychologist, 25*, 3–11.

McSweeny, A. J., Becker, B. C., Naugle, R. I., Snow, W. G., Binder, L. M., & Thompson, L. L. (1998). Ethical issues related to presence of third party observers in clinical neuropsychological evaluations. *The Clinical Neuropsychologist, 12*, 552–560.

National Academy of Neuropsychology. (2000). Test security: Official position statement of the National Academy of Neuropsychology. *Archives of Clinical Neuropsychology, 15*, 383–386.

National Academy of Neuropsychology Policy and Planning Committee. (2003). Test security: An update. *Official Statement of the National Academy of Neuropsychology*. Retrieved February 17, 2004 from http://nanonline.org/paio/security_update.shtm.

Naugle, R. I., & McSweeny, A. J. (1995). On the practice of routinely appending neuropsychological data to reports. *The Clinical Neuropsychologist, 9*, 245–247.

Naugle, R. I., & McSweeny, A. J. (1996). More thoughts on the practice of routinely appending raw data to reports: Response to Freides and Matarazzo. *The Clinical Neuropsychologist, 10*, 313–314.

Rosenthal, M. (1996). 1995 Sheldon Berrol, MD senior lectureship: The ethics and efficacy of traumatic brain injury rehabilitation-myths, measurements, and meaning. *Journal of Head Trauma Rehabilitation, 11*, 88–95.

Rosenthal, M., & Lourie, I. (1996). Ethical issues in the evaluation of competence in persons with acquired brain injuries. *NeuroRehabilitation, 6*, 113–121.

Sim, J. (1998). Respect for autonomy: Issues in neurological rehabilitation. *Clinical Rehabilitation, 12*, 3–10.

Sweet, J. J., & Moulthrop, M. A. (1999a). Self-examination questions as a means of identifying bias in adversarial assessments. *Journal of Forensic Neuropsychology, 1*, 73–88.

Sweet, J. J., & Moulthrop, M. A. (1999b). Response to Lees-Haley's commentary: Debiasing techniques cannot be completely curative. *Journal of Forensic Neuropsychology, 1*, 49–57.

Tranel, D. (2000). Commentary on Lees-Haley and Courtney: There is a need for reform. *Neuropsychology Review, 10*, 177–178.

van Gorp, W., & McMullen, W. (1997). Potential sources of bias in forensic neuropsychological evaluations. *The Clinical Neuropsychologist, 11*, 180–187.

Wong, T. M. (1998). Ethical issues in the evaluation and treatment of brain injury. In R. M. Anderson, Jr., T. L. Needles, & H. V. Hall (Eds.), *Avoiding Ethical Misconduct in Psychology Specialty Areas* (pp. 187–200). Springfield, IL: Charles C. Thomas Publisher.

Woody, R. H. (1989). Public policy and legal issues for clinical child neuropsychology. In C. R. Reynolds & E. Fletcher-Janzen (Eds.), *Handbook of Clinical Child Neuropsychology* (pp. 573–583). New York: Plenum Press.

Woody, R. H. (1997). Psycholegal issues for clinical child neuropsychology. In C. R. Reynolds & E. Fletcher-Janzen (Eds.), *Handbook of Clinical Child Neuropsychology* (2nd ed., pp. 712–725). New York: Plenum Press.

Youngjohn, J., Spector, J., & Mapou, R. (1998). Failure to assess motivation, need to consider psychiatric disturbance, and absence of objectively verified physical pathology: Some common pitfalls in the practice of forensic neuropsychology. *The Clinical Neuropsychologist, 12*, 233–236.

43 Evidence-Based Practice in Clinical Neuropsychology

Jerry J. Sweet, Daniel J. Goldman, and Leslie M. Guidotti Breting

Introduction

Health care practice is constantly evolving. Although health care in the United States has a very long history of aspiring to have clinical science as its seminal basis, there have been numerous critics who have claimed that medical practice is not scientific enough (cf. Institute of Medicine, 2001). In fact, critics of nonscientific medical practice within organized medicine at an international level reacted by initiating a high level, explicit process of supporting assessment and treatment procedures that are *evidence-based* nearly 20 years ago. At the outset of this era, Sackett, Rosenberg, Gray, Haynes, and Richardson (1996) published a frequently cited article that described some essential features of evidence-based medicine (EBM). These authors noted that in fact EBM had been a "hot topic" for years, attributing the foundation to "ancient origins," while also suggesting that the approach had been misunderstood and in their view had not reached the practice mainstream. A brief quote from Sackett et al. (1996) captures their view on the central thrust of EBM:

> Evidence based medicine is the conscientious, explicit, and judicious use of current best evidence in making decisions about the care of individual patients. The practice of evidence based medicine means integrating individual clinical expertise with the best available external clinical evidence from systematic research.
>
> (p. 71)

More recently, the Agency for Healthcare Research and Quality (AHRQ), which sponsors Evidence-Based Practice Centers (EPCs), has opined that a "quality gap" remains (i.e., a gap between best available clinical research evidence and practice; see Shojania, McDonald, Wachter, & Owens, 2004). In the words of Shojania et al. (2004), "Substantial evidence suggests that there is a wide gap between evidence-based best practices and those treatment practices actually used in day-to-day clinical medicine" (p. v).

In recent years, the visibility of EBM initiatives has been impressive. As of 2014, the *Journal of Evidence-Based Medicine* is in its seventh year of publication, the journal of *Evidence-Based Dental Practice* is in its 14th year of publication, and the journal of *Evidence-Based Mental Health* is in its 17th year of publication. The term itself, *evidence-based,* has been applied to numerous specialties within medicine, as well as separate practice disciplines, such as social work, nursing, physical therapy, and psychology, to name but a few. Indeed, a search of documents within the website of the U.S. Department of Health and Human Services that houses AHRQ's National Guidelines Clearinghouse returns approximately 1,700 documents that use the term *evidence-based.* Similarly, a search of the inventory of books listed on the Academic section of the Oxford University Press website (http://global.oup.com/academic) using the term *evidence-based* results in identification of dozens of books across multiple disciplines with the term in the title and a total of 11,720 books that apparently contain the term. Of this larger sum, surely some have mentioned the term only in passing, but the point is made that the term is now widely known and broadly applied across specialties and disciplines.

Over time, with such widespread application beyond the discipline of medicine, the more general term that has been applied across health care specialties and disciplines has been *evidence-based practice* (EBP), which will be used throughout the remainder of this chapter.

Similar to medicine, the history of aspiring to base practice on research evidence is not new to psychology. In fact, nearly 70 years ago the American Psychological Association (APA) recommended training guidelines specifying that the desired model for doctoral-level graduate training is the "scientist-practitioner" model (Shakow et al., 1947). Even with such a long history of emphasizing and promoting science as the basis for practice, it was not until 2006 that the APA published an official policy statement as an appendix to its 2005 Presidential Task Force on Evidence-Based Practice (American Psychological Association Presidential Task Force on Evidence-Based Practice, 2006). This evolution to more explicit commitment to practice based on best available research by organized psychology mirrors the evolution in the discipline of medicine; in fact, the official positions of these disciplines (n.b., medicine's position has often been attributed to the 2001 Institute of Medicine report) are noted in APA's document as quite similar. Relevant to promoting and disseminating relevant psychological research, billions of dollars have been made available for EBP psychological research funding, which will strongly promote a more complete shift to EBP in psychology (McHugh & Barlow, 2010).

Perhaps more so than any other psychology practice specialty, scientific research and empiricism have been the bedrock foundation of clinical neuropsychology. For many decades, clinical neuropsychologists have produced practice-specific assessment research demonstrating scientifically the clinical merit of its procedures. For the last three decades, such research has been published in journals devoted entirely to neuropsychological practice research (e.g., *Archives of Clinical Neuropsychology*, *The Clinical Neuropsychologist*). Authors have credited the subspecialty growth of forensic neuropsychology practice to the very fact that neuropsychological practice was scientifically based, and thus able to offer evidence for consideration in legal proceedings that is objective, rather than impressionistic or based solely on clinician opinion (Larrabee, 2012; Sweet, 1999; Sweet, Ecklund-Johnson, & Malina, 2008). In this sense, EBP is not a new concept for clinical neuropsychologists, but rather a movement well fitted to a preexisting philosophy and easily endorsed. However, as Chelune (2010) has pointed out, true outcomes-based research that demonstrates the economic value and value to society of neuropsychological consultation is only now emerging, with related advocacy regarding the import of decades of clinical research and service also in its infancy.

National policy has explicitly promoted EBP within the Patient Protection and Affordable Care Act (Public Law No: 111–148, Mar 23, 2010), which is known simply as the Affordable Care Act (ACA) and more colloquially as "Obamacare." In a detailed discussion for psychology, Rozensky (2014) has noted the intent of the ACA to disseminate evidence-based health care research to practitioners and within the government's own services to rely only on such information when determining payment coverage for health care services. Having become literally required by law, it seems clear that the EBP movement will continue. In sections that follow, more specific information will be provided and the "goodness of fit" with regard to neuropsychology practice will be explored.

Overview of Evidence-Based Practice

In an influential 2001 report, the Institute of Medicine (IOM) identified six dimensions of ideal health care in the 21st century: safe, effective, patient-centered, timely, efficient, and equitable (IOM, 2001). In the subsequent recommendations regarding how present-day health care could be redesigned to fulfill this description, a central recommendation was the following: "*Evidence-based decision making*. Patients should receive care based on the best available scientific knowledge. Care should not vary illogically from clinician to clinician or from place to place" (IOM, 2001: 8).

In searching for information pertaining to EBP, one can quickly develop the impression that the term *evidence-based* is overused and may have lost some meaning. Among the numerous authors who have provided guidance, Sackett et al. (1996) plainly describe what it is and what it is *not*. The EBP approach takes into account that at times the best available evidence is not the result of quintessential research methods, such as randomized clinical trials, when either none exist or the clinical problem at hand does not lend itself to such a research design. However, when high-quality clinical research evidence is available, clinicians are to rely on this information in applying related assessment and treatment procedures to individual patients. The EBP approach is not meant to represent a purely sterile, scientific approach; explicit consideration of the application of best available evidence involves consideration and respect of patient-specific values.

What then defines "best available scientific knowledge?" Research methodologists have described in detail the research methods and specific criteria for research publishing that can produce greater generalizability, replication studies, and clinical applications of research findings. The *APA Presidential Task Force on Evidence-Based Practice* report (2006) identified multiple types of research evidence that can be considered in determining EBP:

> *Clinical observation* **(including individual case studies) and basic psychological science are valuable sources of innovations and hypotheses (the context of scientific discovery).**
>
> *Qualitative research* **can be used to describe the subjective, lived experiences of people, including participants in psychotherapy.**
>
> *Systematic case studies* **are particularly useful when aggregated—as in the form of practice research networks—for comparing individual patients with others with similar characteristics.**
>
> *Single-case experimental designs* **are particularly useful for establishing causal relationships in the context of an individual.**
>
> *Public health and ethnographic research* **are especially useful for tracking the availability, utilization, and acceptance of mental health treatments as well as suggesting ways of altering these treatments to maximize their utility in a given social context.**
>
> *Process–outcome studies* **are especially valuable for identifying mechanisms of change.**
>
> *Studies of interventions* **as these are delivered in naturalistic settings (effectiveness research) are well suited for assessing the ecological validity of treatments.**
>
> *Randomized clinical trials and their logical equivalents* **(efficacy research) are the standard for drawing causal inferences about the effects of interventions (context of scientific verification).**
>
> *Meta-analysis* **is a systematic means to synthesize results from multiple studies, test hypotheses, and quantitatively estimate the size of effects.**
>
> (p. 274)

Efforts to improve the quality of published clinical research studies are ongoing. Various professional organizations, some of which are multidisciplinary and international, have promulgated recommendations and guidelines that foster promotion and dissemination of high quality health care research. Generally referred to as journal *reporting guidelines*, a listing and brief description of current key guidelines are shown in Table 43.1. These efforts have become so prominent in academic health care that guidance on the development of guidelines has also been offered (Moher, Schulz, Simera, & Altman, 2010). Minimally, guidelines such as these are intended to facilitate critical analysis of the results during the prepublication peer-review process, and, in some instances, replication and extension (perhaps to different types of patients) after studies are published. Additionally, inclusion of key research methodology information and clinical sample characteristics allows practitioners, as consumers of the research studies, to determine with whom and under what conditions the study results may apply to their own patients.

Of the currently available reporting guidelines, one of the first was the Consolidated Standards of Reporting Trials (CONSORT), which first appeared in 1996 (Begg et al.) and is now in its third iteration (Schulz, Altman, Moher, & for the CONSORT Group, 2010). For a discussion of CONSORT as it pertains to neuropsychological research, see Miller, Schoenberg, and Bilder (2014). The acceptance and influence of such reporting guidelines is evident in the fact that with CONSORT alone there have been, to date, nine specialized versions of CONSORT for such specific clinical research applications as how to conduct clinical trials related to acupuncture, herbal treatments, and nonpharmacological interventions. Moreover, as of the writing of this manuscript, the EQUATOR (Enhancing the Quality and Transparency Of health Research)-network website indicates that there are presently CONSORT extensions underway for social and psychological interventions, as well as for N-of-1 trials. In total, the EQUATOR-network website lists 21 new reporting guidelines currently in development. The net intended effect of the resources listed in Tables 43.2 and 43.3 is to improve the quality and specificity of clinical research, which is a key component of EBP.

To facilitate understanding and use of reporting guidelines by clinical researchers, a group of researchers founded the EQUATOR Network in 2006, which is self-described as "an international initiative that seeks to improve the reliability and value of published health research literature by promoting transparent and accurate reporting and wider use of robust reporting guidelines" (EQUATOR Network, 2006). This organization provides downloadable checklists that clinical researchers can use as a means of self-monitoring regarding study execution and manuscript preparation prior to submission to a peer-reviewed journal. In turn, peer-reviewed health care journals have gradually adopted one or more specific reporting guidelines. An international subset of journal editors themselves have organized to form the International Committee of Medical Journal Editors (ICMJE), which has created and, at intervals, updates recommendations regarding the means of conducting, reviewing, and publishing biomedical research that are viewed as increasing the likelihood of "accurate, clear, and unbiased" journal articles (www.icmje.org). More than 500 journals have endorsed and attested to following the ICMJE recommendations. In keeping with the EBP movement, these recommendations include

Table 43.1 Select research reporting guidelines and resources

Guideline or Resource	*Description*	*Website*
STROBE Statement (Strengthening the Reporting of Observational Studies in Epidemiology)	• International research reporting guidelines for the conduct and dissemination of observational studies	www.strobe-statement.org
STARD Statement (Standards For The Reporting Of Diagnostic Accuracy Studies)	• Guidelines for improving the accuracy and completeness of the reporting of studies of diagnostic accuracy	www.stard-statement.org
CONSORT Statement (Consolidated Standards of Reporting Trials)	• Guidelines and recommendations for reporting the results of randomized controlled trials (RCTs)	www.consort-statement.org
PRISMA Statement (Preferred Reporting Items for Systematic Reviews and Meta-Analyses)	• Guidelines and recommendations for reporting in systematic reviews and meta-analyses	http://www.prisma-statement.org
EQUATOR Network	• An international initiative that promotes the broader use of research reporting guidelines and, more generally, transparent and accurate reporting • Contains links to and information about each of the major reporting guidelines	http://equator-network.org
International Committee of Medical Journal Editors	• Provides recommendations and guidelines related to conducting, reviewing, editing, and publishing research in medical journals	www.icmje.org
World Association of Medical Editors	• Provides broad and detailed guidelines and recommendations to promote honesty, transparency, and accuracy in biomedical publishing	www.wame.org

Table 43.2 General evidence-based practice resources

Resource	*Description*	*Website*
Centre for Evidence-Based Medicine	• Develops, teaches, and promotes evidence-based health care. • Holds conferences and workshops, and provides tools for all healthcare fields.	www.cebm.net
Centre for Evidence-Based Mental Health (CEBMH)	• Promotes the teaching and practice of evidence-based care within the mental health field • Develops, evaluates, and disseminates methods for using research in practice	http://www.cebmh.net
American Psychological Association (APA) Evidence-Based Practice in Psychology Resource Web Site	• Provides access to the APA's report and policy statement on evidence-based practice in psychology	http://www.apa.org/practice/resources/evidence/index.aspx
Institute of Medicine's (2001) report regarding evidence-based Medicine, titled "Crossing the Quality Chasm: A New Health System for the 21st Century"	• Free public access to the full report and report brief in PDF format	http://www.nationalacademies.org/hmd/~/media/Files/Report%20Files/2001/Crossing-the-Quality-Chasm/Quality%20Chasm%202001%20%20report%20brief.pdf
Substance Abuse and Mental Health Services Administration (SAMHSA) Guide to Evidence-Based Practices on the Web	• Provides, among other resources, a list of web sites with information regarding specific EBPs or comprehensive reviews of research findings	http://www.samhsa.gov/ebp-web-guide/index.asp
KT Clearinghouse Centre for Evidence-Based Medicine Toronto	• Develops, disseminates, and evaluates resources for the practice and teaching of evidence-based health care in a many disciplines • Resources and tools for undergraduate, graduate, and continuing education for professionals	http://ktclearinghouse.ca/cebm
Duke University Evidence-Based Medicine Tutorial	• Offers a basic introduction to the principles of EBP • Appropriate for students and professionals	http://guides.mclibrary.duke.edu/ebmtutorial
University of Illinois at Chicago (UIC) Evidence-Based Medicine Guide	• Facilitates effective and efficient use of the medical literature by students and healthcare professionals	http://researchguides.uic.edu/ebm
Dartmouth College's Evidence-Based Medicine: Teaching Materials	• Provides a variety of resources for learning about and teaching EBP	http://www.dartmouth.edu/~library/biomed/guides/research/ebm-teach.html

Table 43.3 Additional evidence-based practice resources and tools

Resource or Tool	*Description*	*Website*
Critically-Appraised Topics Worksheets	• Complements major research reporting guidelines by helping clinicians routinely apply criteria for evaluating research evidence and utilize such evidence to answer patient-specific questions	www.cebmh.com
QUADAS-2 (Quality Assessment of Diagnostic Accuracy Studies)	• Quality assessment tool for diagnostic accuracy studies	http://www.bris.ac.uk/quadas
AGREE II (Appraisal of Guidelines Research & Evaluation II)	• Assesses the quality and reporting of practice guidelines • Provides relevant publications, training tools, and practice guidelines	http://www.agreetrust.org/resource-centre/agree-ii
Cochrane Collaboration	• International network that organizes and synthesizes published evidence to make it useful for healthcare decision making	www.cochrane.org
Evidence-Based Mental Health	• Journal that surveys international medical journals and evaluates the quality and validity of research findings • Provides summaries and commentaries on the best studies	http://ebmh.bmj.com
Psychological Database for Brain Impairment Treatment Efficacy (PsycBITE)	• Database of studies, rated for methodological quality, related to cognitive, behavioral, and other treatments for the psychological and other sequelae of acquired brain injuries	http://www.psycbite.com

Resource or Tool	*Description*	*Website*
Psychdisclosure.org	• Platform for authors of recently published articles to publicly disclose methodological details in four categories that are not disclosed under current reporting standards	http://psychdisclosure.org
Agency for Healthcare Research and Quality (AHRQ)	• U.S. government agency that produces evidence to improve the safety, quality, accessibility, equity, and affordability of healthcare • Sponsors a number of initiatives, centers, grants, and tools to achieve this mission	www.ahrq.gov
National Guideline Clearinghouse	• Searchable public resource for evidence-based clinical practice guidelines • One of the many projects of the AHRQ	http://www.guideline.gov/index.aspx

endorsement of reporting guidelines by journals, as well as transparency of author, peer review, and journal procedures and responsibility for the publication outcome, as well as sponsor involvement and inclusion of sufficient methods and sample information to allow replication and clear application of results in clinical settings. In similar fashion, the World Association of Medical Editors (WAME) has provided broad and detailed guidance for researchers and editors regarding honesty, transparency, and accuracy at all levels of the biomedical publishing enterprise (WAME, 2017).

Evidence-Based Practice in Mental Health

As described earlier, EBP has a relatively long history in the field of medicine. Many of the principles described have been modified to apply specifically to the field of mental health. In 1998, one of the first major steps supportive of EBP within mental health was the establishment of the journal *Evidence-Based Mental Health*, which informs clinicians regarding important advances in treatment, diagnosis, etiology, prognosis, continuing education, economic evaluation, and qualitative research in mental health by selecting and summarizing high quality original and review articles from other peer-reviewed journals.

Importantly, the 1999 U.S. Department of Health and Human Services Surgeon General Report on mental health marks a turning point related to EBP in mental health. This report noted that "a variety of treatments of well-documented efficacy exist for the array of clearly defined mental and behavioral disorders that occur across the life span" and that the mental health field should make these EBPs available to all who seek treatment (U.S. Department of Health and Human Services, 1999: 3). A few years later, in 2003, President George W. Bush's New Freedom Commission on Mental Health reported on the need to develop, implement, and expand EBPs; and it even formed a subcommittee to examine and offer policy recommendations on EBPs. Despite these efforts dating back to 1999 a gap continues to exist between the EBP research and clinical applications currently.

Oddly, despite clinical psychologists' history of strong training in research and statistical methods, psychology was one of the last health care disciplines to formally adopt and support EBP. Due to the need to shift toward EBP, in 2005 the APA organized a Presidential Task Force on EBP and in 2006 released a statement on EBP in Psychology. The 2006 report from this task force agreed upon a definition: "Evidence-based practice in psychology (EBPP) is the integration of the best available research with clinical expertise in the context of patient characteristics, culture, and preferences" (APA Presidential Task Force on EBP, 2006: 273). The Task Force also designated that: "The purpose of EBPP is to promote effective psychological practice and enhance public health by applying empirically supported principles of psychological assessment, case formulation, therapeutic relationship, and intervention." (p. 273)

To continue these efforts, the APA later established a task force specifically related to EBP within the child and adolescent population (APA Task Force on EBP for Children and Adolescents, 2008). Even prior to the formation of this task force, psychologists had been examining EBP within children and adolescents to illustrate the challenges of implementation within this population (Kazdin, 2004; Kratochwill & Hoagwood, 2006).

Spring (2007) proposed a three-legged stool model for EBPs within the practice of psychology. This article is one of many cited within the present chapter that was a part of a special issue on Evidence-Based Practice in Clinical Psychology: Education and Training Issues within the *Journal of Clinical Psychology* in 2007. Spring's model of EBP emphasizes:

> (a) the best available research evidence; (b) clinical expertise; and (c) patient values, preferences, characteristics, and circumstances. Evidence-based practice is the process of integrating the circles or tying together the three legs via a process of clinical decision-making.
>
> (Spring, 2007, p. 613)

Rapp and Goscha (2005) describe six basic features that are common to EBP within psychology regardless of diagnosis, setting, or other factors. These six features include: (a) primary focus on recovery, (b) facilitating empowerment and choice, (c) recognizing the role of relationship, (d) importance of in-vivo service delivery, (e) utilization of the environment as a resource, and (f) primary focus on teamwork and integration of helping.

In a 2005 textbook, Azrin and Goldman stated that "evidence-based practice has emerged as the dominant practice model for mental health care" (p. 67). The 21st century has seen a clear shift from systems and practices having been based on theory and clinical opinions to guidance from research on EBPs.

Challenges to Implementing Evidence-Based Practices in Psychology

Many challenges currently exist when attempting to implement EBPs within the practice of psychology. There are too many challenges to list all of them in this chapter, but a few include resistance at the level of the psychologist or client; inconsistent construct definitions within the research; insufficient training; lack of infrastructure to support EBPs; complex presentations with comorbidities and social or family confounds; and even the complexities of designing, implementing, and testing EBPs. The majority of the evidence-based treatment models have been designed and researched for only a single diagnosis or similar symptom manifestations. As EBPs continue to be studied and implemented these challenges should continue to dissipate. Additionally, within a busy clinical practice it is difficult to find the time to keep up with the most recent EBPs, which is one of the reasons why continuing education for psychologists is required, and lifelong learning is so important.

Lilienfeld, Ritschel, Lynn, Cautin, and Latzman (2013) discussed survey data on psychologists' attitudes toward EBP, finding six sources underpinning the misunderstandings of those psychologists who are resistant:

> (a) naïve realism, which can lead clinicians to conclude erroneously that client change is due to an intervention itself rather than to a host of competing explanations; (b) deep-seated misconceptions regarding human nature (e.g., mistaken beliefs regarding the causal primacy of early experiences) that can hinder the adoption of evidence-based treatments; (c) statistical misunderstandings regarding the application of group probabilities to individuals; (d) erroneous apportioning of the burden of proof on skeptics rather than proponents of untested therapies; (e) widespread mischaracterizations of what EBP entails; and (f) pragmatic, educational, and attitudinal obstacles, such as the discomfort of many practitioners with evaluating the increasingly technical psychotherapy outcome literature.
>
> (p. 883)

As mentioned earlier, some psychologists continue to be resistant to the idea of EBP. However, many studies have demonstrated that most mental health professionals hold reasonably positive views of EBP (Borntrager, Chorpita, Higa-McMillan, & Weisz, 2009; Sheldon & Chilvers, 2002). The varying levels of support and implementation of EBP in clinical practice have been discussed (Pagoto et al., 2007) and even those who support EBP may have hesitations or negative attitudes toward fully utilizing EBP. Lilienfeld and colleagues (2013) conclude that it is important for the field to advance educational proposals for articulating the importance of EBP to future clinical practitioners and researchers to assist with changing the current psychologists' objections to EBP. The importance of utilizing education to advance EBP within psychology has been described and this education should specifically recommended that educators "inject significant new content into research, design, and methodology courses and to further integrate research and practicum training" (Bauer, 2007: 685). Toward this effort by psychologists to better educate about EBP at the graduate level, several EBP textbooks were published between 2005 and 2008 (Drake, Lynde, & Merrens, 2005; Norcross, Hogan, & Koocher, 2008; Sturmey & Hersen, 2012).

Kazdin (2008) discussed some of the issues related to the gap between science and clinical practice within the field of mental health related to EBPs and made specific recommendations related to research and practice. Related to research, Kazdin proposed that

> more work is needed on the mechanisms of change—not correlates of change alone but explanations of precisely how therapy works. . . . This is different from disseminating treatment manuals and prescribing specific interventions as our primary focus.
>
> (p. 157)

Kazdin also recommended refocusing the emphases in clinical practice, which included monitoring treatment with systematic assessment and the important of integrating research and practice for clinical care, which would include assessment in the context of clinical care.

Despite the work toward using EBPs within the mental health field, research continues to demonstrate low rates of dissemination of these interventions within clinical practice (Stewart & Chambless, 2007) and at the training level within graduate and internship programs (Weissman et al., 2006). Responding to the similar status of a number of disciplines, the government has continued to allot funds toward better dissemination of EBPs within the mental health field. McHugh and Barlow (2010) have discussed the leading efforts at the national, state, and individual treatment developer levels to integrate psychology's EBP into service delivery settings, as well as offer recommendations for future implementation strategies.

Evidence-Based Practice in Clinical Neuropsychology

As described earlier, the field of clinical neuropsychology has been a relative latecomer to EBPs in the formal sense described previously in this chapter (i.e., Sackett et al., 1996). However, clinical neuropsychologists have always emphasized evidence-based approaches to clinical practice and research in less explicit ways, including through the use of empirically validated and standardized testing procedures, knowledge and application of psychometrics to test selection and interpretation, utilization of the best available normative data for each patient, and reporting of statistics such as sensitivity, specificity, positive predictive power, and negative predictive power in research findings. In an effort to guide the continuation of such EBPs, the American Academy of Clinical Neuropsychology (AACN) has published a number of relevant position papers that are based on the most rigorous available research data, including on topics such as serial neuropsychological assessment (Heilbronner et al., 2010) and the assessment of effort, response bias, and malingering (Heilbronner et al., 2009). Related, clinical neuropsychology's evidence-based roots and high-quality research data clearly played crucial roles in the American Academy of Neurology's (AAN) practice guideline recommending the utilization of neuropsychological assessment for identifying patients with dementia (Peterson et al., 2001). This history, combined with training in the scientist-practitioner model, has positioned the specialty of clinical neuropsychology to effectively adopt the principles of EBP more formally in training, research, and clinical practice.

In keeping with the movement toward EBP in other health-related fields, there has been a recent push within clinical neuropsychology to adopt the principles of EBP (e.g., Bilder, 2011; Bowden, Harrison, & Loring, 2013; Chelune, 2010; Loring & Bowden, 2013). In fact, in 2014, a special issue entitled "Improving Neuropsychological Research Through Use of Reporting Guidelines" was published in *The Clinical Neuropsychologist*, the official journal of the American Academy of Clinical Neuropsychology (Schoenberg, 2014). Although there is no consensus definition for EBP of clinical neuropsychology (EBP-CN), Chelune (2010) proposed that the definition should include the integration of clinical expertise, best outcomes research, and the unique characteristics of the patient. Inclusion of these principles would keep the definition of EBP-CN consistent with the definition of EBM put forth by Sackett et al. (1996) and with the definition of EBP in psychology (EBPP) put forth by APA Presidential Task Force on EBP (2006). Additionally, given the consultative nature of clinical neuropsychology practice, the definition of EBP-CN must include consideration of the concerns and needs of the referral source. That is, determining the meaning of best practices with regard to each patient must involve being responsive to the specific referral question. In doing so, as Chelune (2010) has noted, the clinical neuropsychologist is required

> to do only what is necessary to answer the specific questions asked while continuing to use their clinical judgment and expertise to know when to clarify or expand the referral question to explore alternative hypotheses and to meet the needs of the patient.
>
> (p. 455)

Adopting a definition of EBP-CN that incorporates the principles addressed earlier will lead clinical neuropsychologists through essentially the same steps as those involved in evidence practice in other areas of health care. Adapting from Chelune (2010), the steps are as follows:

1. Generate answerable questions based on a careful evaluation of the presenting problems and complaints.
2. Gather relevant psychosocial and medical background information in order to integrate it with the best available outcomes research specific to the questions just formulated.
3. Obtain relevant data for the patient and specific questions by selecting germane test protocols.
4. Analyze the data with respect to the unique characteristics of the given patient.
5. Apply the results of this analysis to the patient in question, for example in making a diagnostic decision and formulating specific recommendations.
6. Objectively monitor the outcomes of the evaluation. It is important to note that in this context, outcomes refer to discrete, measurable events that impact a patient's condition, can be tracked at the individual and aggregate level, and are publicly verifiable (i.e., they are explicit in our reports).

Chelune (2010) further argues that the advancement of EBP-CN in both the clinical and research domains requires neuropsychologists to adopt two broad tenets. The first tenet is that "clinical outcomes are individual events characterized by a change in status, performance, or other objectively defined endpoint" (p. 456). The second tenet is that "to be useful in the care of patients, data from outcomes research must be analyzed and packaged in such a way that they can be directly evaluated and 'used' by the end-user, namely the clinician" (p. 456). Although the remainder of this chapter separates how EBP-CN can be achieved in the clinical and research domains, it is clear that the two are inseparably intertwined. In the tradition of the scientist-practitioner, clinical questions should inform outcomes research and outcomes research should guide best clinical practices.

Research Applications of Evidence-Based Practice of Clinical Neuropsychology

A key component of advancing outcomes research for EBP-CN is moving away from simple null-hypothesis significance testing of mean differences (e.g., Chelune, 2010; Bowden et al., 2013). These authors and many others have made the compelling case (which will not be detailed here) for adoption of more clinically applicable statistics, including effect sizes, positive/negative predictive power, base rates, and odds ratios. Briefly, such statistics allow for clinicians and other researchers to critically evaluate the *clinical* significance of findings beyond the fact that statistical significance has been observed with respect to the null hypothesis (for more regarding the difference between statistical and clinical significance, see Meehl, 1973).

Chelune (2010) outlines three specific steps for researchers that may increase the potential that their outcomes data will be more useful to clinical practice. First, neuropsychological outcomes should be defined in a manner that can be applied clinically. For example, by determining and reporting the magnitude of a difference on some measure(s) between individuals with and without a condition of interest. Reporting data in this way can also facilitate reporting of base rate information with regard to such outcomes. Second, researchers should report base rate information whenever possible in order to calculate relevant statistics that will increase the accuracy of clinicians' inferences in a given case. Third, researchers should provide contingency table analyses that are supplemented with base rates. This will allow end-users (i.e., clinicians) to calculate and/or access sensitivity, specificity, positive and negative predictive power, optimal cutoff scores, odds ratios, likelihood ratios, and pre- and posttest odds, all of which are critical to making optimal inferences regarding test results and are consistent with the superior methods of reporting results described above.

These goals can be more broadly achieved by adopting the appropriate research reporting guidelines (e.g., STROBE, CONSORT, and STARD) that have been established for EBP in neuropsychology's peer-reviewed literature. STROBE, for example, is particularly relevant for neuropsychology. Much of our literature is inherently biased because it consists of unfunded studies that rely on convenient patient populations and use quasi-experimental or observational study designs, and the STROBE reporting criteria explicitly improve transparency, which reduces the impact of such bias (Loring & Bowden, 2013). In addition, STROBE emphasizes reporting of effect sizes and practical implications (such as diagnostic accuracy classification statistics), rather than just statistical significance. For a detailed explanation of how each of the STROBE criteria apply to research in neuropsychology, which is beyond the scope of this chapter, see Loring and Bowden (2013).

In a related, but separate, endeavor, it has been proposed that researchers and/or clinicians create collaborative neuropsychological databases (e.g., Bilder, 2011). Given the relatively standardized data types and homogeneity of collected variables, neuropsychologists should be able to efficiently create such centralized resources using both individual case data and published group-level data. With shared access to data from a multitude of populations located across the country (or even the world), neuropsychologist researchers could generate substantially larger groups of participants in order to generate high-quality research related to a wider range of disorders, tests, and patient populations than is currently feasible. Additionally, normative data for commonly used tests could be dynamically updated for specific populations beyond the timetables of test updates provided by publishers, possibly even in real time. In turn, such collaborative databases could facilitate the formulation of new research questions, data analyses, and, ultimately, clinical decision making to advance EBP-CN.

Consistent with such ideas, the National Academy of Neuropsychology (NAN) is developing the HONE-In (Health Outcomes and Neuropsychology Efficacy Initiative) project, with the goal of creating a centralized source of information regarding the utility and cost effectiveness of clinical neuropsychological services. The project was started in response to the ongoing need of clinical neuropsychologists to justify the effectiveness of neuropsychological services, often related to reimbursement challenges. The HONE-In team is compiling a listing of citations, including summaries of the articles and comments regarding outcome utilities of neuropsychological services. These will address general utility, as well as specific patient populations, including brain injury, concussion, and rehabilitation; employment; multiple sclerosis; Parkinson's disease; pediatrics; primary care; and seizure disorders.

Clinical Applications of Evidence-Based Practice in Clinical Neuropsychology

Chelune (2010) offers three broad clinical practice guidelines that are incorporated into all EBP. First, referral questions must be converted into answerable questions, such as, Does this patient have attention and memory deficits after sustaining a moderate traumatic brain injury three months ago? To answer such a question, the neuropsychologist must know the specific characteristics of the patient as well as the relevant outcomes literature, including the best assessment tools for answering the question, and the test findings needed to make a positive versus negative determination. Second, clinicians should use base-rate information when describing test results in their reports. This includes describing base rates appropriately depending on whether the data from which they are derived are normally distributed and may include describing a patient's performances in terms of how far they deviate from expectations. And third, clinicians should incorporate and use the best available information, in the form of outcomes research, to guide assessments. This may be difficult, at times, given that there is no single repository for neuropsychological outcomes data and that it is rare to find relevant studies that sufficiently meet criteria of good quality research for EBP purposes (such as those defined by STROBE, CONSORT, or STARD). At present, the most useful data often comes from meta-analyses and review articles. In addition, clinicians can become outcomes researchers by monitoring and tracking outcomes within their own practices in order to improve the accuracy of test interpretation and diagnostic decision making.

To aid in the implementation of EBP, clinical neuropsychologists reading research articles and evaluating outcomes data can utilize Critically Appraised Topics (CAT) toolkits, which are available online through the Centre for Evidence Based Medicine (www.cebm.net/critical-appraisal/). CATs have been developed as compliments to the major research reporting guidelines to assist in evaluating the quality of systematic review/meta-analytic, treatment, diagnostic, and prognostic studies. Bowden et al. (2013) argue that routine practice of critical appraisal gives clinicians the skills needed to "(1) evaluate the clinical relevance of new or unfamiliar research findings with a focus on patient benefit, (2) help focus on research quality, and (3) incorporate evaluation of clinical impact into educational and professional development activities" (p. 1). That is, employing the CAT method helps clinicians learn to routinely apply criteria for evaluating research evidence and to utilize such evidence in answering patient-specific questions, the latter of which is absent from the research guidelines. The techniques contained in the CAT process capitalize on the clinician's knowledge and expertise by guiding him or her to a focused answer to a particular clinical question. While not necessarily needed for all cases, the approach can be particularly useful for unfamiliar areas and topics.

Given the nature of clinical neuropsychology practice, clinicians are likely to find the diagnostic CAT worksheet to be the most useful. Bowden et al. (2013) provide a detailed walkthrough of the use of the diagnostic CAT within clinical neuropsychology through a hypothetical example involving the use of a dementia-screening tool in making a diagnostic decision. With its emphasis on study design and accounting for base rates, the diagnostic CAT worksheet can be used as a framework for evaluating test utility and criterion-related validity, thereby making diagnostic decision processes more explicit. The worksheet is broken down into three parts, two of which contain subquestions to help focus critical appraisal of the research in question. Part 1 guides the clinician in determining whether the results of a diagnostic study are valid. Part 2 asks the clinician to then evaluate whether the results of the study are important (i.e., not just statistically significant). If the overall answers to Parts 1 and 2 are yes, Part 3 consists of a series of questions to help the clinician assess whether the evidence about the test in question can be directly applied to the patient the clinician is evaluating.

Of course, many specific clinical questions remain that cannot be clearly answered by applying EBP-CN principles, due to limited evidence or, at times, a lack of directly applicable evidence of sufficient quality. Such situations may be related to given neuropsychiatric conditions, patient characteristics, evaluation contexts, or other factors specific to individual patients. In such situations, APA Presidential Task Force on EBP (2006) broadly suggests that clinicians rely on clinical expertise in interpreting and applying the best available evidence, continually monitor patient progress, and adapt the assessment or intervention as appropriate. For EBP-CN, this requires (at a minimum) including appropriate caveats in the report about difficulties with test interpretation and, perhaps, uncertainty regarding diagnostic conclusions in certain cases in which the empirical support is sparse for the use and interpretation of our tests or normative data.

Select Examples of Neuropsychology Research That Can Directly Influence EBP-CN

The ability to engage in the EBP-CN continues to grow rapidly, as high-quality data that are readily applicable to specific clinical questions are more available than ever before. For example, evidence regarding the value of clinical neuropsychological test data as they relate to the diagnosis and treatment of mild cognitive impairment (MCI) and Alzheimer's dementia (AD) is increasingly strong. Bondi and Smith (2014) review the neuropsychological literature as it relates to the diagnosis of MCI and conclude that careful neuropsychological assessment improves the reliability of MCI diagnoses over and above commonly used screening measures, rating scales, and limited test batteries. When comprehensive neuropsychological assessments are utilized, test results turn out to be strongly related to relevant biomarkers and can at times be shown to represent pathologies other than, or in addition to, AD. Additionally, neuropsychological research data demonstrate that mild, but identifiable, functional difficulties are present in individuals with MCI. Bondi and Smith (2014) conclude that neuropsychological tests should play a key diagnostic role in studies of MCI and clinical practice.

Related, Schmand et al. (2014) compared the effectiveness of various MRI measures and neuropsychological tests as outcome measures for intervention studies of AD and MCI at baseline and after two years. Results demonstrated that the sample sizes needed to detect a 50% reduction in the rate of change in the respective outcome measures were substantially larger using hippocampal atrophy ($n = 131$) or cortical thickness ($n = 488$) versus change scores on neuropsychological tests ($n = 62$). The authors concluded that in memory clinic patients, neuropsychological assessment is more sensitive than MRI measures of brain atrophy for measuring disease progression. In a similar vein, Gomar, Bobes-Bascaran, Conejero-Goldberg, Davies, and Goldberg (2011) examined the effectiveness of various biomarkers and neuropsychological tests as predictors of conversion from MCI to AD over a two-year period. Effect size analyses demonstrated that neuropsychological tests and a rating scale assessing daily functioning were more robust predictors of conversion from MCI to AD than most biomarkers. In addition, declines in executive functioning and daily functioning appeared to drive conversion more than neurobiological changes, indicating that neuropsychological testing is best positioned to provide data that can predict conversion of MCI to AD. Studies such as these continue to support clinical neuropsychology's key role in the assessment and management of dementing conditions.

Similar evidence regarding the utility of neuropsychological assessment for other conditions is also increasingly available. For example, Williams, Rapport, Hanks, Millis, and Greene (2013) demonstrated that clinical neuropsychological assessment following mild complicated, moderate, and severe traumatic brain injury was uniquely predictive of functional disability two years postinjury, even after accounting for injury severity and demographic characteristics, including computed tomography (CT) scan data. As another example, neuropsychological assessment has also been shown to add uniquely to the treatment and behavioral management of attention deficit/hyperactivity disorder following diagnosis. Specifically, Pritchard, Koriakin, Jacobson, and Mahone (2014) found that in families whose children received neuropsychological assessment services, there was more behavior management training, special education services, and medication management of symptoms over the follow-up period. While unrelated, studies of these types continue to demonstrate the evidence-based added value of neuropsychological assessment for a variety of relevant conditions.

Beyond clinical practice, it is important to also acknowledge the rapidly growing, robust, high-quality evidence regarding the practice of clinical neuropsychology in forensic, or medical-legal, settings. This is an area of research and practice that continues to grow rapidly, with neuropsychological evidence and neuropsychologist experts being widely accepted in legal proceedings (e.g., Sweet & Goldman, 2015). The concrete data neuropsychologists can provide regarding cognitive functioning has repeatedly proven to be valuable to the courts. For more information, also see Sweet, Kaufman, Ecklund-Johnson, and Malina (Chapter 36 in this volume).

Future Directions

Kaufman, Boxer, and Bilder (2013) persuasively argued that clinical neuropsychology needs to continue to produce quality evidence to demonstrate the field's value in making differential diagnoses, predicting functional treatment outcomes, and measuring the effectiveness of various treatments. In order to do so, clinical neuropsychology must adopt higher standards for reporting research results in our journals, consistent with the various resources described earlier in this book, including STROBE, EQUATOR, and STARD.

Bilder (2011) and Kaufman, Boxer, & Bilder (2013) further argue that EBP-CN would be well served if researchers and clinicians shared group level and individual case data, respectively, in central databases, such as the one described above that is being considered by NAN or the one being proposed to Division 40 of the APA (Pliskin, personal communication). EBP is the other primary area for future growth within clinical neuropsychology. As the field pushes forward in adopting the principles of EBP, the teaching of EBP-CN must be incorporated into doctoral programs, internships, and postdoctoral training programs. Such training should encompass how to report research results consistent with the relevant guidelines, how to search out and critically appraise published evidence, and how to apply the principles of EBP as a graduate-level practicum student, intern, and postdoctoral resident. Of course, education in EBP should not end during formal training. Continuing education for licensed neuropsychologists should include refreshers in the basics and updates in EBP advances.

References

American Psychological Association Presidential Task Force on Evidence-Based Practice. (2006). Evidence-based practice in psychology. *American Psychological Association*, *61*, 271–285.

American Psychological Association Task Force on Evidence-Based Practice for Children and Adolescents. (2008). *Disseminating Evidence-Based Practice for Children and Adolescents: A Systems Approach to Enhancing Care*. Washington, DC: American Psychological Association.

Azrin, S. T., & Goldman, H. H. (2005). Evidence-based practice emerges. In R. E. Drake, D. W. Lynde, & M. R. Merrens (Eds.), *Evidence-Based Mental Health Practice: A Textbook* (pp. 67–93). New York: W.W. Norton & Company.

Bauer, R. M. (2007). Evidence-based practice in psychology: Implications for research and research training. *Journal of Clinical Psychology*, *63*(7), 685–694.

Begg, C., Cho, M., Eastwood, S., Horton, R., Moher, D., Olkin, I., . . . Stroup, D.F. (1996). Improving the quality of reporting of randomized controlled trials: The CONSORT statement. *Journal of the American Medical Association*, *276*, 637–639.

Bilder, R. M. (2011). Neuropsychology 3.0: Evidence-based science and practice. *Journal of the International Neuropsychological Society*, *17*, 7–13.

Bondi, M. W., & Smith, G. E. (2014). Mild cognitive impairment: A concept and diagnostic entity in need of input from neuropsychology. *Journal of the International Neuropsychological Society*, *20*, 129–134.

Borntrager, C., Chorpita, B., Higa-McMillan, C., & Weisz, J. (2009). Provider attitudes toward evidence-based practices: Are the concerns with the evidence or with the manuals? *Psychiatric Services*, *60*, 677–681.

Bowden, S. C., Harrison, E. J., & Loring, D. W. (2013). Evaluating research for clinical significance: Using critically appraised topics to enhance evidence-based neuropsychology. *The Clinical Neuropsychologist*, *28*, 653–668. doi: 10.1080/13854046.2013.776636

Chelune, G. J. (2010). Evidence-based research and practice in clinical neuropsychology. *The Clinical Neuropsychologist*, *24*, 454–467.

Drake, R. E., Lynde, D. W., & Merrens, M. R. (Eds.). (2005). *Evidence-Based Mental Health Practice: A Textbook*. New York: W.W. Norton & Company.

EQUATOR network. (2006). *Enhancing the QUAlity and Transparency Of health Research*. Centre for Statistics in Medicine, NDORMS, University of Oxford. Information retrieved from www.equator-network.org.

Gomar, J. J., Bobes-Bascaran, M. T., Conejero-Goldberg, C., Davies, P., & Goldberg, T. E. (2011). Utility of combinations of biomarkers, cognitive markers, and risk factors to predict conversion from mild cognitive impairment to Alzheimer disease in patients in the Alzheimer's disease neuroimaging initiative. *Archives of General Psychiatry*, *68*, 961–969.

Heilbronner, R. L., Sweet, J. J., Attix, D. K., Krull, K. R., Henry, G. K., & Hart, R. P. (2010). Official position of the American Academy of Clinical Neuropsychology on serial neuropsychological assessments: The utility and challenges of repeat test administrations in clinical and forensic contexts. *The Clinical Neuropsychologist*, *24*, 1267–1278.

Heilbronner, R. L., Sweet, J. J., Morgan, J. E., Larrabee, G. J., Millis, S. R., & Conference Participants. (2009). American Academy of Clinical Neuropsychology consensus conference statement on the neuropsychological assessment of effort, response bias, and malingering. *The Clinical Neuropsychologist*, *23*, 1093–1129.

Institute of Medicine. (2001). *Crossing the Quality Chasm: A New Health System for the 21st Century*. Washington, DC: National Academy of Sciences Press.

Kaufman, D.A.S., Boxer, O., & Bilder, R. M. (2013). Evidence-based science and practice in neuropsychology: A review. In S. Koffler, J. Morgan, I. S. Baron, & M. F. Greiffenstein (Eds.), *Neuropsychology: Science and Practice*, *I* (pp. 1–38). New York: Oxford University Press.

Kazdin, A. E. (2004). Evidence-based treatments: Challenges and priorities for practice and research. *Child and Adolescent Psychiatric Clinics of North America*, *13*(4), 923–940.

Kazdin, A. E. (2008). Evidence-based treatment and practice: New opportunities to bridge clinical research and practice, enhance the knowledge base, and improve patient care. *American Psychologist*, *63*(3), 146–159.

Kratochwill, T. R., & Hoagwood, K. E. (2006). Evidence-based interventions and system change: Concepts, methods and challenges in implementing evidence-based practices in children's mental health. *Child and Family Policy and Practice Review*, *2*, 12–17.

Larrabee, G. J. (Ed.). (2012). *Forensic Neuropsychology: A Scientific Approach* (2nd ed.). New York: Oxford University Press.

Lilienfeld, S. O., Ritschel, L. A., Lynn, S. J., Cautin, R. L., & Latzman, R. D. (2013). Why many clinical psychologists are resistant to evidence-based practice: Root causes and constructive remedies. *Clinical Psychology Review*, *33*(7), 883–900.

Loring, D. W., & Bowden, S. C. (2013). The STROBE statement and neuropsychology: Lighting the way toward evidence-based practice. *The Clinical Neuropsychologist*, *28*, 556–574. doi: 10.1080/13854046.2012.762552

McHugh, R. K., & Barlow, D. H. (2010). The dissemination and implementation of evidence based psychological treatments: A review of current efforts. *American Psychologist*, *65*(2), 73–84.

Meehl, P. E. (1973). *Psychodiagnosis: Selected Papers*. Minneapolis, MN: University of Minnesota Press.

Miller, J. B., Schoenberg, M. R., & Bilder, R. M. (2014). Consolidated Standards of Reporting Trials (CONSORT): Considerations for neuropsychological research. *The Clinical Neuropsychologist*, *28*, 575–599.

Moher, D., Schulz, K. F., Simera, I., & Altman, D. G. (2010). Guidance for developers of health research reporting guidelines. *PLoS Medicine*, *7*(2), e1000217. doi: 10.1371/journal.pmed.1000217

National Academy of Neuropsychology Legislative Action & Advocacy Committee. (n.d.). *HONE-In*. Retrieved from http://nanonline.org/nan/Professional_Resources/LAAC/HONE-In/NAN/_ProfessionalResources/_LAAC/HONE_IN.aspx

Norcross, J. C., Hogan, T. P., & Koocher, G. P. (2008). *Clinician's Guide to Evidence Based Practices: Mental Health and the Addictions*. Oxford University Press: New York.

Pagoto, S. L., Spring, B., Coups, E. J., Mulvaney, S., Coutu, M., & Ozakinci, G. (2007). Barriers and facilitators of evidence-based practice perceived by behavioral science health professionals. *Journal of Clinical Psychology*, *63*, 695–705.

Peterson, R. P., Stevens, J. C., Ganguli, M., Tangalos, E. G., Cummings, J. L., & DeKosky, S. T. (2001). Practice parameter: Early detection of dementia: Mild cognitive impairment (an evidence-based review): Report of the quality standards subcommittee of the American Academy of Neurology. *Neurology*, *56*, 1133 1142.

President's New Freedom Commission on Mental Health. (2003). *Achieving the Promise: Transforming Mental Health Care in America: Final Report*. Rockville, MD: U.S. Government Printing Office.

Pritchard, A. E., Koriakin, T., Jacobson, L. A., & Mahone, E. M. (2014). Incremental validity of neuropsychological assessment in the identification and treatment of youth with ADHD. *The Clinical Neuropsychologist*, *28*, 26–48.

Rapp, C. A., & Goscha, R. J. (2005). *What are the Common Features of Evidence-Based Practices?* In R. E. Drake, D. W. Lynde, & M. R. Merrens (Eds.), *Evidence-Based Mental Health Practice: A Textbook* (pp. 189–215). New York: W.W. Norton & Company.

Rozensky, R. H. (2014). Implications of the *Affordable Care Act* for education and training in professional psychology. *Training and Education in Professional Psychology*, *8*, 1–12. doi: 10.1037/tep0000021

Sackett, D. L., Rosenberg, W.M.C., Gray, J. M., Haynes, R. B., & Richardson, W. S. (1996). Evidence based medicine: What it is and what it isn't. *British Medical Journal*, *312*, 71–72.

Shakow, D., Hilgard, E. R., Kelly, E. L., Luckey, B., Sanford, R. N., & Shaffer, L. F. (1947). Recommended graduate training program in clinical psychology. *American Psychologist*, *2*, 539–558.

Schmand, B., Rienstra, A., Tamminga, H., Richard, E., van Gool, W. A., Caan, M.W.A., & Majoie, C. B. (2014). Responsiveness of magnetic resonance imaging and neuropsychological assessment in memory clinic patients. *Journal of Alzheimer's Disease*, *40*(2), 409–418. doi: 10.3233/JAD-131484

Schoenberg, M. R. (2014). Introduction to the special issue on Improving neuropsychological research through use of reporting guidelines. *The Clinical Neuropsychologist*, *28*, 549–555.

Schulz, K. F., Altman, D. G., Moher, D., & the CONSORT Group. (2010). CONSORT 2010 statement: Updated guidelines for reporting parallel group randomized trials. *Annals of Internal Medicine*, *152*, 1–7.

Sheldon, B., & Chilvers, R. (2002). An empirical study of the obstacles to evidence-based practice. *Social Work and Social Sciences Review*, *10*, 6–26.

Shojania, K. G., McDonald, K. M., Wachter, R. M., & Owens, D. K. (2004). *Closing the Quality Gap: A Critical Analysis of Quality Improvement Strategies, Volume 1—Series Overview and Methodology*. Agency for Healthcare Research and Quality Publication No. 04–0051–1. Rockville, MD.

Spring, B. (2007). Evidence-based practice in clinical psychology: What it is; why it matters; what you need to know. *Journal of Clinical Psychology*, *63*, 611–631.

Stewart, R. E., & Chambless, D. L. (2007). Does psychotherapy research inform treatment decision in private practice? *Journal of Clinical Psychology*, *63*, 267–281.

Sturmey, P., & Hersen, M. (2012). *Handbook of Evidence-Based Practice in Clinical Psychology*. Hoboken, NJ: John Wiley and Sons.

Sweet, J. J. (Ed.). (1999). *Forensic Neuropsychology: Fundamentals and Practice*. Lisse, Netherlands: Swets & Zeitlinger (Reprinted and currently distributed by Taylor & Francis).

Sweet, J. J., Ecklund-Johnson, E., & Malina, A. (2008). Overview of forensic neuropsychology. In J. Morgan & J. Ricker (Eds.), *Textbook of Clinical Neuropsychology* (pp. 869–890). New York: Taylor & Francis.

Sweet, J. J., & Goldman, D. J. (2015). Forensic neuropsychology: Annual review. In S. Kofler, J. Morgan, M. Greiffenstein, & B. Marcopolous (Eds.), *Neuropsychology: A Review of Science and Practice* (2nd ed.). New York: Oxford University Press.

Sweet, J. J, Kaufman, P. M., Ecklund-Johnson, E., & Malina, A. (2017). Forensic neuropsychology: An overview of issues, admissibility and directions. In J. E. Morgan & J. H. Ricker (Eds.), *Textbook of Clinical Neuropsychology*. New York: Taylor & Francis.

U.S. Department of Health and Human Services (DHHS). (1999). *Mental Health: A Report of the Surgeon General*. Rockville, MD: U.S. Department of Health and Human Services.

Weissman, M. M., Verdeli, H., Gameroff, M. J., Beldsoe, S. E., Betts, K., Mufson, L., & Wickramaratne, P. (2006). National survey of psychotherapy training in psychiatry, psychology, and social work. *Archives of General Psychiatry*, *63*, 925–934.

Williams, M. W., Rapport, L. J., Hanks, R. A., Millis, S. R., & Greene, H. A. (2013). Incremental validity of neuropsychological evaluations to computed tomography in predicting long-term outcomes after traumatic brain injury. *The Clinical Neuropsychologist*, *27*, 356–375.

The World Association of Medical Editors. (2017). Information retrieved from www.wame.org

44 Medical and Psychological Iatrogenesis in Neuropsychological Assessment

Dominic A. Carone

Today, we are frequently required to relieve our patients of their diagnoses so that the path is clear for them to understand and address their problems.

—Martyn Patfield (2011)

Health care providers have long been familiar with the basic tenet of the Hippocratic Oath, which is to do no harm to patients. This tenet is expressed in the original language of the oath, which states: "And I will use regimens for the benefit of the ill in accordance with my ability and judgment, but from [what is] to their harm or injustice I will keep [them]" (Miles, 2005, p. xiii). A later section of the oath makes mention of not causing *intentional* harm and that is generally how the oath is conceptualized. However, despite the best of intentions, treatment and information provided to patients by their health care providers can sometimes prolong or worsen existing physical and/or mental health problems or cause new ones. When this happens it is known as *iatrogenesis*. The term has its roots in the Greek word *iatros* meaning "physician/healer" and the Greek word *genesis* meaning "origin," meaning that the health care provider is the source of the creation of additional problems. The problem is so rampant in some medical settings (e.g., intensive care units, nursing homes) that it is referred to as "The I word" (Dunn & Murphy, 2010; Mitty, 2010).

In the most literal sense, *iatrogenesis* can be used to refer to any outcome (positive or negative) brought on by the health care provider although the term is mostly used to refer to negative outcomes, which has been criticized by some (Jacobs, Benavidez, Bacha, Walters, & Jacobs, 2008). For the purposes of this chapter, the term *iatrogenesis* is used to describe negative health outcomes caused by the health care provider.

There are two broad categories of iatrogenesis based on the underlying mechanism: medical and psychological. In psychological iatrogenesis, the patient develops new and/or worsening health problems due to negative expectations and beliefs that are either introduced or reinforced by the health care provider during the diagnostic and/or treatment process. In some cases, the information provided (e.g., prognosis, treatment needs) about the diagnosis may be incorrect and/or the actual diagnosis (or lack thereof) may be wrong. There are three main types of iatrogenic diagnostic errors: (a) diagnosing the wrong condition when an actual condition exists, (b) diagnosing a condition when none actually exists, and (c) not providing a diagnosis when an actual condition exists. Each diagnostic error introduces the risk of adverse psychological and medical outcomes.

With the increasing availability of medical information to the layperson (e.g., Internet searches, TV shows, radio, print media), patients are increasingly comfortable with applying definitive diagnoses to themselves or family members that may or may not be accurate (Patfield, 2011), and pressuring their health care provider to agree. There can be various reasons such pressure is exerted, including the following: the patient or family is a known advocate for people with the condition; the diagnostic term is comforting for the patient in some way (e.g., providing an external locus of control and a feeling of validation); or the person needs the diagnosis for secondary gain purposes (e.g., disability application, litigation, obtaining prescription drugs for abusive purposes). In some cases, a provider may feel pressured *not* to provide the actual diagnosis because the patient or family member voices opposition to it—e.g., a parent stating that he or she does not believe attention deficit/hyperactivity disorder exists (ADHD). Sometimes, the pressure is self-exerted due to the provider's belief systems (e.g., not wanting to provide a mental health diagnosis due to fearing that the patient may feel he or she is being blamed for his or her problems) as opposed to being based on anything the patient explicitly stated. These types of false positive and false negative diagnostic errors are likely to occur in situations in which diagnoses are based solely on subjective symptom reporting rather than objective data (e.g., biomarkers, test scores). This is particularly the case when the patient is evaluated by health care providers who see their role as a patient advocate first and as an objective scientist practitioner second.

In medical iatrogenesis, the patient develops new and/or worsening health problems due to the physical effects of treatment. Examples include medication side effects, medication overdose, prescription errors, and adverse outcomes from surgical procedures. In many conditions, psychological and medical iatrogenesis co-occur. This chapter will focus on psychological and medical aspects of iatrogenesis, particularly as they relate to conditions that neuropsychologists frequently encounter or need to rule out (although covering all such conditions is beyond the scope of this chapter). This is followed by a discussion on how to reduce iatrogenesis and address it once it is suspected or identified.

Mild Traumatic Brain Injury and "Post Concussion Syndrome"

There is perhaps no condition where the risks of iatrogenesis are greater than during the assessment and management of patients with known or suspected mild traumatic brain injury (mTBI; also known as concussion). In a now-classic study, Mittenberg, DiGiulio, Perrin, and Bass (1992) showed how expectations about the effects of brain injury led a healthy control group to endorse virtually identical symptom rates compared to an mTBI group reporting persisting symptoms after being provided an imaginary vignette about suffering an mTBI. This led to the "expectations as etiology" hypothesis for chronic symptom reporting (e.g., three months or longer) after mTBI. Another interesting finding from the aforementioned study was that the mTBI group significantly underestimated the base rate of premorbid symptoms when compared to the control group. This is partly because people begin to focus more on symptoms once a salient negative event has occurred.

In mTBI and other medical conditions, psychological iatrogenesis can begin before the patient is evaluated by a health care provider, based on beliefs the patient has developed through sociocultural influences (e.g., movies, television shows, the media). A common example derived from the movies is the unrealistic portrayal of profound retrograde amnesia after head injury (Baxendale, 2004). Another example is the patient who suffered one concussion who then misapplies information (e.g., risk of prolonged symptoms) to him or herself from popular news stories about professional athletes suffering a career worth of multiple concussions. For a detailed review of the media's influence on the course and prognosis of recovery after sports concussion, see Carone (2014).

With these beliefs established, mTBI patients experiencing either (a) normal symptoms during the acute phase of recovery and/or (b) normal everyday cognitive lapses and physical symptoms can begin to misinterpret normal everyday symptoms (e.g., forgetting keys in the car) as reflective of concussion or misinterpret genuine concussion symptoms as reflective of a more severe neurological condition. It is at this point where it is most helpful for health care providers to intervene by normalizing symptoms and providing patients with *proper* (e.g., nonalarmist) education about treatment, expected prognosis, and instructions on resuming premorbid activities. For example, Mittenberg et al. (1996) found that by doing the latter in an emergency room setting with mTBI patients as opposed to providing routine hospital discharge and treatment instructions (mTBI control group) that the experimental group experienced significantly shorter symptom duration, fewer symptoms, and fewer symptomatic days. The results indicated that a brief, psychoeducational intervention could reduce the incidence of those reporting persisting symptoms after mTBI. These general findings have been extended and replicated by others (Miller & Mittenberg, 1998; Mittenberg, Canyock, Condit, & Patton, 2001; Ponsford et al., 2001; Ponsford et al., 2002).

Providing an early positive and normalizing message after mTBI helps to counter incorrect beliefs that a patient may have developed before interacting with a health care provider. However, logic dictates that a well-meaning but incorrect opposite message could increase the incidence of symptom persistence or worsen the presentations of those who are already reporting symptom persistence. A common example would be telling a patient with a single mTBI on the initial visit that he or she is expected to have a long and unpredictable recovery, that some symptoms may never improve, and/or that extensive rehabilitative efforts and medication treatment is needed. There are no evidence-based data to support such statements. In this sort of scenario, a patient's incorrect beliefs may be unintentionally reinforced or created by the health care provider, sometimes causing significant distress in the process. While the health care provider may be attempting to be helpful by "validating" the patient's subjective experiences, this validation can ultimately be counterproductive if not accompanied by accurate information.

Another commonly encountered iatrogenic cause of persisting problems in mTBI is the advice for excessive bed rest and withdrawal from all stimulating activities including school and work. While rest may be indicated for a very brief period (e.g., a few days) there is no evidence to support that chronic bed rest and excessive withdrawal from school and work is a helpful intervention. In fact, it is much more likely to be harmful due to facilitating the disability role, increasing feelings of depression, anxiety, frustration, and isolation (Allen, Glasziou, & Del Mar, 1999; Asher, 1947; de Kruijk, Leffers, Meerhoff, Rutten, & Twijnstra, 2002; Kouyanou, Pither, & Wessely, 1997a). Newer research has shown that making patients more physically active with controlled aerobic exercise soon after mTBI can be helpful in the recovery process (Leddy et al., 2012; Schneider et al., 2013), although the evidence base is sparse at this point. A similar iatrogenic problem emerges for mTBI patients advised to wear sunglass chronically and most of the day due to reported photophobia. Wearing such glasses excessively has two main iatrogenic effects: it serves as a visual prop to reinforce disability beliefs, and it causes the eyes to be more sensitive to any incoming light (falsely reinforcing the concept that the glasses are still needed due to brain injury).

Neuropsychologists particularly need to be mindful of the effects that communications from themselves or others about a neuropsychological assessment can have on the evaluation results. For example, Suhr and Gunstad (Suhr & Gunstad, 2002, 2005) have documented the effects of "diagnosis threat" when neuropsychologically evaluating patients with mTBI.

Specifically, when mTBI patients were randomly assigned to the diagnosis threat group, attention was called to their head injury and they were informed that many patients with mTBI show evidence of cognitive deficits on neuropsychological testing. Those assigned to the neutral group did not have any attention brought to their head injury and no mention was made of cognitive deficits. They were essentially told that they would take cognitive tests of varying difficulty and to do their best. Both studies showed that the diagnosis threat group performed worse than the neutral group in various cognitive domains, and the 2005 study showed that these effects were not caused by differing levels of depression, anxiety, or effort between the two groups. The results served as an important reminder of the powerful effects that communications by health care providers have on the behaviors of their patients.

Whiplash Injuries

Whiplash injuries are injuries to the neck caused by sudden acceleration of the trunk with abnormal extension and/or flexion of the neck, and are most often caused by motor vehicle accidents (Storaci et al., 2006). Because whiplash injuries often occur after such accidents and involve acceleration/deceleration forces, they often co-occur with mTBI. Much like research has shown with patients complaining of chronic postconcussive symptoms, subjective complaints in whiplash patients are associated with somatization and poor coping, especially in chronic cases (Guez, Brannstrom, Nyberg, Toolanen, & Hildingsson, 2005). Whiplash and mTBI also share many symptoms, making it possible that symptoms related to neck injury may be falsely attributed to brain injury by patients and their providers. No patho-anatomical foundation has been found for whiplash injury (Cote & Soklaridis, 2011) similar to many known or suspected mTBI patients who present with negative objective biomarkers.

Cote and Soklaridis (2011) found that overtreating patients during the early stages of recovery after whiplash can lead to iatrogenesis by promoting the development of chronic illness behaviors through emphasizing the use of passive coping behaviors. These authors also criticized whiplash becoming a medicalized concept, in which nonmedical problems or ordinary ailments are defined and treated as medical problems (e.g., diseases, disorders, illness), often resulting in mild symptoms being viewed as serious. Identical problems are known to occur in mTBI management.

Multiple Chemical Sensitivities

Multiple chemical sensitivities (MCS), which is also known as *idiopathic environmental intolerance* is a set of nonspecific symptoms affecting many possible organ systems after low-level exposures to chemicals commonly found in the environment. The similarities between MCS and "postconcussion syndrome" are striking. First, both involve claims of persisting nonspecific symptoms after exposure to a mild event that does not cause chronic problems in the vast majority of people. Second, many people claiming to be affected by these conditions report being chronically disabled. Third, many are pursuing some type of compensation such as medical disability and/or personal injury litigation (Binder, Storzbach, & Salinsky, 2006; Mittenberg, Patton, Canyock, & Condit, 2002; Staudenmayer & Phillips, 2007). Fourth, there are no proven reliable and valid objective biomarkers to confirm that the etiology of persisting symptoms is due to a prior concussion or mild chemical exposure (Baines, McKeown-Eyssen, Riley, Marshall, & Jazmaji, 2007). Fifth, both conditions are associated with a high degree of psychiatric comorbidity, neuroticism, and premorbid psychiatric problems (Black et al., 2000; Carone, 2008; Osterberg, Persson, Karlson, Carlsson Eek, & Orbaek, 2007; Reid et al., 2001) although patients may be more defensive about acknowledging this (Staudenmayer & Phillips, 2007). Sixth, both are typically reported in high levels in Western countries but are virtually unknown or rarely reported in other countries (e.g., Lithuania, Eastern Europe) (Bornschein, Forstl, & Zilker, 2001; Bornschein, Hausteiner, Zilker, & Forstl, 2002; Mickeviciene et al., 2002; Mickeviciene et al., 2004; Stovner, Schrader, Mickeviciene, Surkiene, & Sand, 2009), particularly if there are minimal opportunities for monetary compensation in the country. Seventh, both involve patients who are typically convinced that there is no other possible explanation for their symptoms besides the alleged triggering event (Staudenmayer, 2000). Eighth, both are associated with high levels of exaggerated responsiveness that can sometimes be caused by psychiatric factors (Leznoff, 1997) but sometimes can be caused by malingering (Mittenberg et al., 2002). Ninth, both conditions typically involve the use of lengthy and/or expensive treatments with a limited-to-nonexistent evidence base that rarely demonstrate effectiveness (Das-Munshi, Rubin, & Wessely, 2007), particularly in terms of meaningful outcome data (e.g., return to work, symptom reduction). Tenth, a cottage industry of self-proclaimed specialists have emerged to treat these conditions, claiming unique expertise outside of the scientific mainstream, which many patients tend to gravitate towards as they feel misunderstood by the mainstream medical community (Dumit, 2006; Lipson & Doiron, 2006). Eleventh, symptoms can be reduced in both conditions with psychoeducational approaches designed to minimize attributions to organic causes and by providing simple psychoeducational approaches designed to reassure patients (Herr et al., 2004; Miller & Mittenberg, 1998; Mittenberg et al., 2001; Mittenberg et al., 1996; Ponsford et al., 2001; Ponsford et al., 2002).

Given these common features, the risk of iatrogenesis in patients reporting MCS is particularly high, and health care providers need to be mindful of how the type of information they provide to their patients can affect them in undesirable ways. For example, Dalton (1999) found that telling patients that an odor to be presented is going to be harmful resulted in them reporting significantly more symptoms and more intense irritation upon odor exposure compared to when patients were told that the identical odor will be neutral or healthful. The authors concluded that the actual odor exposure was not responsible for the reported health-related effects but was rather caused by the person's beliefs about the relationship between the environment and their health. Similarly, Leznoff (1997) showed dramatic and severe responses to nonchemicals when patients were led to believe they were real chemicals (cf., "expectations as etiology" in concussion described earlier). Another study found that painters reporting MCS actually reported more sensitivity to nonchemicals (i.e., coffee fumes) than chemicals (i.e., acetone), which the authors stated may be due to less familiarity with the former than the latter (Georgellis, Lindelof, Lundin, Arnetz, & Hillert, 2003). In these studies, patient beliefs—sometimes influenced by the examiner—caused more symptom reporting. However, negative belief systems can also be created and fostered by the media and lead to higher symptom reporting compared to patients who are not exposed to negative media reports (Winters et al., 2003). Thus, health care providers must be careful when discussing media stories (particularly those designed to raise awareness or to grab sensationalistic headlines) with patients because the message they send has the potential to contribute to iatrogenesis, negatively affecting patient outcomes (Carone, 2014).

Health care providers must also be aware that using unproven explanations for symptoms can sometimes lead to treatments with iatrogenic effects, some of which can be severe and can affect neuropsychological functioning. A good example is the case of a 39-year-old woman with multiple environmental sensitivities reported by Brusko and Marten (1991) who developed hepatic encephalopathy after being prescribed ketoconazole (an antifungal medication) by a "clinical ecologist" for systemic candidiasis (a type of fungal infection) despite no actual documentation of a fungal infection. Rather, it appears that the diagnosis (and subsequent treatment suggestions) was based purely on subjective reporting of symptom persistence for ten years. Liver function test results progressively worsened after treatment was initiated. She became extremely jaundiced, lethargic, slow to answer questions, developed worsening asterixis (hand tremor), and was transferred to a hospital for possible liver transplant. Although her reaction to the medication was rare and idiosyncratic, the case presentation suggests that it could have been avoided because she may not have had the treated condition to begin with. Making this case directly relevant to neuropsychology is the fact that hepatic encephalopathy is a well-known cause of cognitive impairment (Munoz, 2008).

As some have noted, patients with environmental sensitivities who feel abandoned and isolated by conventional medicine will likely turn to alternative/nonconventional treatments in a search for answers (Taylor, Krondl, Spidel, & Csima, 2002). However, it is important to note that many of these patients have not truly been abandoned by conventional scientific approaches. Rather, some may be resisting what are indeed accurate findings and explanations (e.g., negative test findings, psychological etiology, medical comorbidities other than the one the patient is focused on). Anger and resistance towards conventional medicine can lead to further psychological distress and symptom exacerbation that perpetuates itself in a reciprocal feedback cycle along with exaggeration, assumption of a chronic disability role, and adherence to scientifically unproven nonconventional treatments. As Das-Munshi et al. (2007) noted, "Eventually, a protracted course of avoidance may lead to chronic disability, in part perpetuated by the iatrogenesis of unproven therapies which the sufferer may have sought from numerous 'experts'" (p. 277).

Although it is beyond the scope of this chapter to review all such conditions that can be caused by iatrogenesis, it should be noted that similar iatrogenic concerns are present for other conditions (e.g., fibromyalgia, chronic fatigue syndrome, sick building syndrome, Gulf war syndrome, electrical sensitivity) that are also poorly defined, controversial, and/or characterized by chronic nonspecific symptom reporting with few to no associated objective biomarkers. Other have found that patients with medically unexplained symptoms were more likely to experience higher frequencies of psychiatric morbidity and iatrogenesis than patients with medically explained symptoms (Kouyanou, Pither, Rabe-Hesketh, & Wessely, 1998).

Dissociative Identity Disorder

Another area in neuropsychology where the role of iatrogenesis is highly debated is dissociative identity disorder (DID; formerly known as *multiple personality disorder*). This is of interest to neuropsychologists who often work in forensic settings but also due to the differential diagnosis in clinical settings that sometimes needs to be made between DID, schizophrenia, epilepsy, and psychogenic nonepileptic seizures (Bowman & Coons, 2000; Foote & Park, 2008). DID is a highly controversial diagnosis, which some conceptualize as a psychological defense mechanism to avoid conscious processing of significantly traumatic memories (e.g., severe childhood physical, sexual, and/or emotional abuse) while others conceptualize it as a culture-bound phenomenon caused by treatment providers eliciting the personalities through suggestion, leading questions, and techniques (e.g., hypnosis, memory retrieval) geared towards suggestible individuals (Boysen, 2011; Piper & Merskey, 2004). These two etiologies are known as the *posttraumatic model* (PTM) and *sociocognitive model* (SCM), respectively.

There is no greater example to highlight the contrast between these two explanations of DID than *Sybil*, which was published in 1973 (selling more than 6 million copies) and made into a television movie in 1976. The public was fascinated by what was presented as a true story (PTM model), but recent documents have shown that Sybil's case was worsened significantly through iatrogenesis (SCM model). Since

Sybil is now the most well-known case of doctor-induced iatrogenesis, and it is described in more detail here, based on a summary of events detailed in Nathan (2012).

Sybil (real name = Shirley Mason) began treatment with a psychiatrist (Cornelia Wilbur) in 1954 for a multitude of problems that included "blackouts," anorexia, anxiety, and depression. The treatment initially consisted of psychotherapy, but over time, personal and professional boundaries were crossed, which increased the risk of iatrogenesis. Examples include: (a) Sybil falling in love with Wilbur due to feeling that she understood her like no one else; (b) Wilbur over-indulging details about her own personal life to Sybil; (c) Wilbur offering to get Sybil a job as an art therapist, get her into classes at a college she taught in, get her into medical school, and to sell her paintings for her, later paying for her apartment and giving her numerous gifts; and (d) telling her that further therapy was needed so she (Sybil) could become a psychoanalyst.

Despite this "treatment," Sybil reported worsening symptoms. Wilbur responded by prescribing medications in higher doses than were necessary. Sybil began reporting fugue states and multiple personalities (four). Wilbur diagnosed her with multiple personality disorder, which was met with relief by Sybil. Further treatments continued, which included electrical shocks and injections with "truth serums" such as sodium pentothal, which she became addicted to. Attempts to wean her from the drug resulted in aggressive and regressive behaviors.

After four years of "treatment," Sybil had become much worse, developing new problems, worsening problems, and (reportedly) ten personalities. In 1958, Sybil wrote a letter to Wilbur stating that she had problems but that she did not actually have multiple personalities or fugue states, and that she had been lying for attention and excitement (i.e., factitious disorder). Sybil admitted that Wilbur's unwavering devotion and belief in her stories led her to continue them and exaggerate them via sodium pentothal. Wilbur, who believed she had an important patient who could advance her career, refused to accept the recantation, labeling it a defense mechanism to avoid therapy. This created a nonscientific scenario, as there was no evidence that Wilbur would accept that would scientifically falsify the original claims. Sybil then wrote a new letter claiming that Wilbur knew better and that the person who confessed to lying was actually a new personality. Five new therapy sessions a week followed with additional sodium pentothal, fostering apparently false memories of abuse. Despite the additional treatment, she added six more personalities. Wilbur eventually proclaimed her as cured in 1965 and the two eventually moved in with one another.

Since the popularization of the Sybil story in the late 1970s, there was a significant rise in the number of people claiming to have this condition, including criminal defendants claiming that the condition rendered them not criminally responsible for their actions. Specifically, by 1980, 200 cases of DID were reported worldwide (Bliss, 1980), whereas only 14 cases were reported worldwide between 1944 and 1969 (Greaves, 1980). The cultural popularization of DID thus makes it ripe for malingering attempts as a way to avoid criminal responsibility or as a form of factitious disorder to gain attention (Coons, 1991).

For the purposes of this chapter, the more salient issue is whether the Sybil case not only reflected the effects of iatrogenesis upon Shirley Mason, but also whether popularization of the case in society, related media coverage, administration of self-report scales with dissociative content, and suggestions of dissociative symptoms by therapists and influential others have led vulnerable (e.g., suggestible, attention seeking, traumatized) individuals to present with multiple distinct fully elaborated personalities when they otherwise would not have (Merskey, 1992; Scroppo, Drob, Weinberger, & Eagle, 1998; Weissberg, 1993). Of course, an iatrogenic explanation of some DID cases does not mean that the condition does not legitimately exist in some people, but only that some presentations may be caused or exacerbated by improper treatment. There has been long-standing continued controversy in the trauma literature as to the role (or extent of the role) that iatrogenesis has in DID, with some strongly making the case for the iatrogenic role (Lilienfeld et al., 1999; Merskey, 1992; Spanos, 1994) and others strongly refuting it (Gleaves, 1996; Reinders, Willemsen, Vos, den Boer, & Nijenhuis, 2012; Scroppo et al., 1998). More recently, a scientific review of the childhood DID literature supported the iatrogenic model more than the posttraumatic model because DID was found to be extremely rare outside of therapy, unevenly distributed across clinicians (with 65% of cases coming from four research groups), and mostly a Western phenomenon (Boysen, 2011).

Iatrogenesis From Medications and Medical Procedures

Iatrogenesis resulting from inpatient hospital stays is a common problem, affecting between 3% and 20% of patients across the world (Baker et al., 2004; Brennan et al., 1991; Davis et al., 2002, 2003; Schimmel, 2003; Thomas et al., 2000; Wilson et al., 1995). In one study, up to half of the adverse events leading to hospital admissions were preventable and 7%–19% resulted in death. The problems in these studies were deemed to result from the health care management itself as opposed to the underlying disease process. Some problems in these studies are caused by medication iatrogenesis and/or iatrogenesis from medical procedures, some of which is classified as negligent.

In medication iatrogenesis, medications unintentionally exacerbate existing signs and symptoms, create new signs and symptoms (e.g., memory and concentration problems, weight changes), and/or can cause death (Dunn & Murphy, 2010; Ksouri et al., 2010; McAllister et al., 2009). Some refer to this as an adverse drug reaction (ADE) and it is the most common form of medical iatrogenesis (Mitty, 2010). ADEs can be reactions to a normal medication dose but can also be the result of medical errors such as an incorrectly written prescription or a filling error at the pharmacy (e.g., wrong medications or higher-dose pills filled). Topiramate is an example of a medication neuropsychologists encounter frequently that is well-known to have particularly negative effects on cognition in its use in treating migraines, headaches, and seizures, particularly as the dose increases (Fritz et al., 2005; Loring, Williamson, Meador, Wiegand, & Hulihan, 2011). Psychiatric effects can occur as well such as psychosis (e.g., visual hallucinations) caused by medications to treat movement disorders such as Parkinson's disease (Friedman, 2002).

Medication iatrogenesis is particularly relevant for neuropsychologists to consider when assessing (a) the cause of chronic nonspecific symptoms such as headache (e.g., rebound headaches caused by excessive use of ibuprofen in a patient reporting chronic worsening headaches after concussion) (b) the cause of a new health conditions (e.g., neuroleptic malignant syndrome; delirium caused by excessive sedation on an inpatient unit, cancer treatment, immobilization, sleep deprivation, dehydration, and complications from indwelling catheters; see Inouye, Schlesinger, & Lydon, 1999; Jeste & Krull, 1990; van Steijn, Nieboer, Hospers, de Vries, & Mulder, 2001; Vasilevskis et al., 2010), and (c) the cause of poor neuropsychological test performance (e.g., cognitive impairment due to excessive chronic opioid use for low back pain; Pransky, Borkan, Young, & Cherkin, 2011; or from an incorrectly written prescription/pharmacy filling error resulting in an accidental overdose). Iatrogenesis is known to play a significant role in maintenance of chronic pain in subsets of patients through misdiagnosis, overinvestigation, overtreatment, inappropriate medication prescriptions, and conveying inappropriate information and advice to patients that legitimizes incorrect beliefs about the medical basis of symptoms (Kouyanou et al., 1998; Kouyanou et al., 1997a; Kouyanou, Pither, & Wessely, 1997b).

Lack of knowledge about iatrogenic treatment effects can lead to circular reasoning and persistent harmful treatment. An example would be a patient with chronic headaches 18 months postconcussion who is treated with high-dose topiramate. At the next visit, the patient reports continued headaches, "confusion," and other cognitive changes (e.g., attention and memory problems). Rather than recognizing this as a potential iatrogenic treatment effect, the provider attributes this change to concussion as well, increases the topiramate dose, and adds a neurostimulant, which then triggers significant weight loss and irritability. Thus, rather than tapering the patient off of the medication, the treatment is increased further. Despite the provider's good intentions, the patient worsens from the intervention.

Neuropsychologists also need to be mindful of iatrogenesis that can result from medical procedures that can impact neuropsychological functioning as they will sometimes be asked to evaluate patients after this has occurred. One example is blood pressure changes leading to hypoxia/stroke during a surgical or diagnostic procedure either due to the effects of the surgery itself on the cardiovascular system and/or an adverse reaction to medications used at the time of surgery (including anesthesia). Other examples include delirium caused by hospital-acquired infection as well as severe impairments in speech and/or memory after an anterior lobectomy to treat intractable seizures. Another example is prion disease (e.g., Creutzfeld-Jakob disease), which has been transmitted to more than 400 patients through the use of neurosurgical instruments, intracerebral EEG electrodes, human pituitary hormone, dura mater grafts, corneal transplants, and blood transfusions (Hamaguchi et al., 2009). Many patients who neurologists evaluate are being treated by chiropractors, and cervical manipulation can result in increased pain and headache in 30% of cases (Hurwitz, Morgenstern, Vassilaki, & Chiang, 2004). There is also controversy as to whether cervical chiropractic manipulation can lead to a vertebro-basilar stroke (Cassidy et al., 2008; Ernst, 2002).

Elderly patients (≥ age 65) are at high risk of iatrogenesis because they often require multiple treatments and have a higher incidence of cognitive difficulties (Fantino et al., 2006). In working with elderly patients, neuropsychologists and other health care providers must be aware of the potential for *cascade iatrogenesis*. Cascade iatrogenesis is the serial development of multiple medical complications triggered by an initial medical intervention and is associated with reduced mechanisms for coping with external stresses (Potts et al., 1993; Rothschild, Bates, & Leape, 2000). An example would be an elderly patient who is oversedated with analgesics for arthritis, falls due to imbalance, breaks a hip, becomes immobile, develops pneumonia, and experiences adverse medication reactions and side effects, followed by delirium. In cascade iatrogenesis, one adverse medical problem follows (cascades) from the other and is associated with decreased cognitive and/or physical reserve (e.g., less-effective kidney and liver functioning) (Rothschild et al., 2000). The elderly have a tenfold increase in falls (Rothschild et al., 2000) which increases their risk for traumatic brain injury (TBI). In fact, TBI hospital discharge rates for falls are highest for patients aged 65 and above (Langlois et al., 2003).

On the other end of the spectrum, medical iatrogenesis is common in neonatal intensive care units (NICUs). For example, Kugelman et al. (2008) found a 19% prevalence rate of iatrogenic events in NICUs, with 83% as preventable, 7.9% as life threatening, and 45.1% as harmful. They also found that the prevalence rate was much higher in younger infants (e.g., 57% for those at 24–27-week gestations compared to 3% born at term) and that the effects were more severe and harmful. Some of the iatrogenic effects have the potential to impact neuropsychological functioning such as hypoxia/anoxia from tracheal tube malpositioning, perforation of the inferior vena cava due to umbilical venous catheter use, and late-onset sepsis.

Finally, in some instances, it should be noted that determining whether certain medications patients are using have iatrogenic effects is controversial. Perhaps the best example is the controversy surrounding an alleged increased risk of suicidality when patients are treated with antidepressant medication. These concerns surfaced in 2004 when the U.S. Food and Drug Administration mandated strong "black box" suicide warnings on all antidepressant medications based on the antidepressant arm of randomized controlled studies with a placebo (Check, 2004). However, a subsequent comprehensive review showed that antidepressant medication actually serves to effectively treat and protect patients from suicide, especially if they follow up regularly with their providers (Rihmer & Akiskal, 2006).

E-Iatrogenesis (Technological Iatrogenesis)

As technology has progressed and health care reform is implemented, more health care providers are being required to use electronic medical record (EMR) systems. Such programs are often integrated with computerized clinical decision support systems (CDSS) to improve compliance with best-practice guidelines (Seroussi, Falcoff, Sauquet, Julien, & Bouaud, 2010). While this technology certainly has benefits, it also creates the risk of what has been termed *e-iatrogenesis* (or *technological iatrogenesis*), which is when patient harm is caused at least in part by the use (or misuse) of health care information technology (Palmieri, Peterson, & Ford, 2007; Weiner, Kfuri, Chan, & Fowles, 2007). Such risk can be broadly divided into commission errors (e.g., false positive diagnosis; prescribing the wrong treatment; death) or omission errors (false negative diagnosis; not prescribing a needed treatment).

Health care providers should be aware that in some health care systems, EMR systems includes non-evidence-based clinical protocols and provider order sets in order to get as many clinicians to "buy in" to the system as possible (i.e., keep them happy) (Simpson, 2010). This is important to know because the use of non-evidence-based protocols and treatments increase the risk of iatrogenesis. In addition, EMR systems have been shown to decrease the efficiency of health care providers (Furukawa, Raghu, & Shao, 2010). This can lead to efforts to bypass time-consuming safety features and has even resulted in patient fatality (Smetzer, Baker, Byrne, & Cohen, 2010).

Computerized CDSS technology is also used in clinical neuropsychology in which automated interpretations are provided for some symptom validity, personality, and cognitive tests. This often results in diagnostic *possibilities* and treatment *considerations*. As with physicians, such technology has the capacity to both decrease and increase iatrogenesis in neuropsychological practice, depending on how the technology is used. Specifically, the risk of iatrogenesis will be increased with such technology when the data gathered is used in a rigid cookbook-like fashion without taking other factors into consideration such as data from clinical interview/medical records review (e.g., history of treatment responses), medical comorbidities, behavioral observations, and convergence with published diagnostic criteria. Neuropsychologists should pay attention to disclaimer statements published in automated reports. For example, in the diagnostic possibilities section of the Personality Assessment Inventory–Adolescent (Morey, 2007) interpretive printout it states that "A diagnosis should be made only after careful examination of the specific DSM-IV diagnostic criteria and should be informed by clinical judgment."

Preventing/Reducing and Addressing Iatrogenesis

Some suggestions for preventing/reducing iatrogenesis were discussed in the preceding sections and are discussed more fully in this section.

Objective Corroboration of Subjective Reporting and Resisting Patient Pressure

Health care providers must be especially cautious about the role and effects of iatrogenesis when assessing patients whose presentation is solely based on subjective symptom reporting. In such cases, the health care provider should seek objective information to corroborate the patient complaints (e.g., neuropsychological testing, objective biomarkers, physical exam findings that cannot be influenced by the patient) and should become increasingly concerned about the reliability and validity of these complaints (or at least their potential neurological basis) the more results come back as negative. Careful review of patient medical records should be used to verify patient reports (Doty & Crastnopol, 2010). The more discrepancy there is between self-report and statements in the medical record (pre- and postsymptom onset) the more that similar concerns should emerge (Slick et al., 1999). Health care providers should be especially cautious in such cases when diagnosing a neurological condition without converging objective evidence that the condition is actually present.

A significant cause of unnecessary medical procedures and inaccurate explanations that can cause patient harm is a response to significant pressure placed on treating providers by patients to agree with their conceptualization of the problem; to order requested procedures, therapies, and medications; and to write disability or out of school notes *ad infinitum*. In a desire to please the patient in a helping profession, along with a desire not to engender complaints, treating providers may sometimes go against their better judgment and write disability notes or order tests and treatments that are of no genuine benefit to the patient and may actually cause harm. Indeed, Little et al. (2004) found that doctors' perception of patient pressure was a strong predictor of prescribing, examinations, referrals, and examination, even in cases where there was slight to no actual medical need.

In order to prevent unnecessary utilization of health care resources and reduce iatrogenesis, the authors encouraged doctors to have a direct conversation with their patient about their expectations. As Kouyanou et al. (1997a) describe, the pressure that the doctor feels to help the desperate-appearing patient and search excessively for an organic cause when none likely exists can add to patient anxiety and impede the development of coping skills that could have helped resolve the problem.

Undiagnosis

As discussed earlier, misdiagnosis is a common theme in many forms of iatrogenesis because it leads to incorrect treatment and can cause patients to develop a false belief system regarding their symptoms, each of which can lead to adverse outcomes. It has been argued recently that misdiagnosis has increased (Patfield, 2011), and this increase will likely continue as policy changes in the health care system (e.g., insurance companies, hospitals) and will lead to pressures to evaluate more patients in less time and with fewer resources. Since neuropsychologists have more time to interview patients/collaterals and review medical records to gather a proper history and integrate this information with objective test data, they are in a unique position to review the evidence in a comprehensive manner that should increase diagnostic accuracy. It is not uncommon for a neuropsychologist to conclude that the sum of the evidence indicates that the presumptive diagnosis is incorrect (referred to as "undiagnosis"; see Patfield, 2011). In some cases, the patient may be informed that a different diagnosis appears to be more appropriate or that no diagnosis is appropriate.

A common example of undiagnosis in neuropsychology would be informing a patient that the cause of his or her problems 18 months postinjury is not "postconcussion syndrome" as he or she has been told by numerous health care providers. In fact, the patient may also be told that he or she does not even meet liberal criteria (Mild Traumatic Brain Injury Committee of the Head Injury Interdisciplinary Special Interest Group of the American Congress of Rehabilitation Medicine, 1993) for a diagnosis of a concussion because review of medical records and interview data does not indicate the presence of altered mental status or a focal neurological deficit. The patient may be informed that an undifferentiated somatoform disorder is a far more appropriate diagnosis and that treatment with cognitive behavioral therapy is indicated rather than chronic treatment with medications (some of which can cause cognitive dysfunction), physical therapy, occupational therapy, vision therapy, and/or chiropractic services.

While undiagnosis is a role that neuropsychologists are highly qualified to address, clinicians must be aware that it comes at the risk of upsetting a referral source (who may have made an incorrect diagnosis) or patient/family members (who may be psychologically invested in the diagnosis). To mitigate this, it is important to use an informed consent form with patients before the evaluation informing them that a second opinion may result and by being careful in the report not to specifically attack other health care providers. Rather, it is best to simply provide a clearly stated independent opinion that is based on data, national practice standards, high-quality published research, and published diagnostic criteria. It is important to emphasize to patients how undiagnosis and a possible replacement diagnosis can lead to new and better treatment approaches (e.g., cognitive behavioral therapy) and a higher likelihood of functional improvement (e.g., return to work). In other cases it is helpful to explain to patients that there is "good news" that no underlying illness appears to be present and that the problems present are modifiable and not beyond their control to fix. Clinicians are urged not to provide a diagnosis merely because it provides patients relief that they have an answer for their problems, because that relief is often short-lived and can lead to adverse treatment effects if the diagnosis is incorrect (Patfield, 2011). However, clinicians must also be empathic and convey that they are trying to help people. Thus, it is best to avoid using terms that will alienate the patient such as that their symptoms are "imaginary" or "in your head" so that the patient does not attempt to prove the doctor wrong by producing more illness-behavior (Kouyanou et al., 1998). For more information on feedback approaches in such circumstances, see Carone, Bush, and Iverson (2013) and Carone, Iverson, and Bush (2010).

Use of Evidence-Based Treatments

The use of evidence-based treatments needs to become more commonplace in health care. If health care providers do not voluntary treat patients with such approaches, there will be increasing pressure (if not mandates) for them to do so based on modern-day health care reform. As a panel of international health care experts recently concluded, many countries (particularly the United States) have more of a medical industrial complex that is focused more on economics (e.g., billing for services) rather than actually improving health care (Pransky et al., 2011). Such approaches are ultimately more harmful to the patient, scientifically unjustifiable, and economically unsustainable. By using evidence-based treatment approaches, patients and providers can embark from the outset on clearly specified expectations, a clear understanding of risks and benefits, and a plan of action to change the treatment plan if it is not working by a certain time. Related to the latter, health care reimbursement will increasingly be tied to evidence that the patient is making improvements.

Measuring treatment effectiveness will require the use of outcome assessment measures during the course of treatment or before and after treatment. If a patient is not showing improvement in functioning (e.g., symptoms are the same or worsening, remains out of work) then the treatment is not working and should not be maintained indefinitely. It is important to note that some health care providers may justify excessive treatments by pointing to times when the patient subjectively reported an improvement in symptoms across a few sessions. However, without objectively measuring such improvements, determining if the improvements are sustained, and simultaneously examining improvement in functional abilities (e.g., return to work, school, and/or driving), indefinite treatments are not well justified. Finally, as per Simpson's (2010) recommendation, EMR systems should not include protocols and order sets that are not evidence-based merely to please the health care provider.

Reducing Medical Iatrogenesis

Scott, Gray, Martin, and Mitchell (2012) proposed a ten-step model to minimize iatrogenesis related to inappropriate medication use. Of these, the step where neuropsychologists can have the greatest input is defining and confirming current indications for ongoing treatment. For example, if a patient had been using donepezil or memantine for presumed Alzheimer's disease but evaluation results revealed that the patient was actually cognitively normal (e.g., "worried well") or had mild cognitive declines related to poor effort in the context of major depressive disorder, these medications would no longer be indicated. Sometimes, these medications are also inappropriately used to treat persisting self-reported memory deficits after mild head injury/concussion even though no good scientific evidence exists to support this practice.

Another step where neuropsychologists can have partial input is estimating the magnitude of benefit versus harm in relation to each medication. Of course, neuropsychologists vary with regards to their expertise on certain medications and should modify their input accordingly, particularly focusing on medications that have known deleterious cognitive side effects. Thus, neuropsychologists may not be able to provide input on each medication depending on the number and type. In some cases, neuropsychologists may comment broadly on the cognitive effects of certain classes of medications (e.g., opioid analgesics) but in other cases may comment on the cognitive side effects of a particular medication (e.g., topiramate). See Stein and Strickland (1998) for a review of the cognitive effect of numerous prescription medications.

Neuropsychologists can provide input on another step, which is to review the relative utility of different medications. Again, input here will be limited to the neuropsychologist's experience, the type of medication(s) used, and the condition being treated. However, for many medications, neuropsychologists can usually provide some input. The last step of relevance to neuropsychologists is to implement and monitor a drug minimization plan (e.g., reducing polypharmacy when possible) with ongoing reappraisal of drug utility and patient adherence by a single nominated clinician. While neuropsychologists cannot implement and monitor such a plan or serve as the single nominated clinician, they are often in a position to strongly advocate that such a plan be put in place, particularly in cases where it is evident that numerous health care providers are prescribing various medications without communicating with one another. This is most common in cases of polypharmacy in the elderly.

In inpatient settings, neuropsychologists may be able to provide input or advocate for fall prevention strategies that can cause or exacerbate a brain injury. An example would be recommending a sitter for an impulsive patient with a severe traumatic brain injury or an elderly patient with unstable gait. In such settings, neuropsychologists can also play a useful role in helping medical staff identify the early signs of hypoactive delirium so that it can be treated properly and not worsened by iatrogenic treatments. Neuropsychologists working in integrated care settings can also help facilitate communication among a patient's health care providers to reduce iatrogenic errors. They can also assist in routine cognitive screenings of elderly patients to detect acute changes suggestive of delirium.

While neuropsychologists can be helpful in reducing medical iatrogenesis, physicians and other health care providers will ultimately take the lead role in addressing factors contributing to it. Examples include utilizing evidence-based interventions to reduce the risk of preventable delirium (Bell, 2009; Inouye et al., 1999), improving the attitudes of health care staff towards the elderly to prevent delirium (Inouye et al., 1999), implementing fall prevention strategies (Reading, 2009), reducing delayed hospital discharges in the elderly after acute illness (Haeck, 2009), adequate follow-up of abnormal physical findings and test results (Nemergut, 2009), more patient education on the effective and safe use of medication (Kouyanou et al., 1997b), implementing methods to reduce unnecessary transfer of patients from a nursing home to the hospital (Brooks, Warshaw, Hasse, & Kues, 1994), and reducing the risk of prion disease by using disposable instruments (Hamaguchi et al., 2009). In addition, the use of electronic prescribing can decrease some types of prescribing errors, and being familiar with drug formularies can decrease the chance of dosing errors when a provider must prescribe an alternative medication because the first choice is not covered by the insurance company (Olson-Garewal, 2001). Robinson and Weitzel (2009) discussed numerous ways to reduce cascade iatrogenesis in the elderly such as reviewing and minimizing the use of high-risk drugs, starting at the lowest reasonable medication dose and increasing the dose slowly as needed ("start low and go slow"), making sure they are wearing properly functioning sensory assistance devices (e.g., hearing aids), closely monitoring for pressure sores (which can lead to infection and altered cognitive functioning), and openly communicating with caregivers.

After finding far from optimal prescribing patterns towards the elderly among physicians, Fantino et al. (2006) also urged more cautious prescribing practices in the elderly to reduce iatrogenesis, which can further be accomplished by full access to the patient's medical history, obtaining therapeutic data and setting treatment goals, utilizing good communication skills to decrease improper medication use, encouraging communication by the patient to the provider, and understanding the social and psychological status of their patients. The latter was noted by these authors to be an area that physicians appeared to have a general lack of interest in obtaining themselves, which makes it all the more important for neuropsychologists to bring significant psychosocial factors to their attention. An example would be depression or cognitive impairment interfering with the ability to understand medication directions.

In a study by Kugelman et al. (2008), NICU staff hired an iatrogenesis advocate who monitored and recorded iatrogenic events, and made the staff aware of them through open discussions but in an anonymous fashion to avoid individual blame. This intervention reduced the iatrogenic incidence rate slightly but not the prevalence rate. Government-sponsored initiatives (e.g., public ads, mandated continuing education on the topic) are another way to increase awareness on iatrogenesis among the public and health care providers. Also, as Johnson (2010) noted, devoting more time to quality assurance programs in hospitals is another way to try to reduce iatrogenesis. With regards to alternative and complementary therapies, Biley (2002) suggested developing an adverse events register to monitor for iatrogenic treatment effects.

Summary and Conclusions

In summary, iatrogenesis is a serious problem that neuropsychologists will frequently encounter when working with patients. Iatrogenic effects are more likely to occur in cases where there is a lack of objective biomarkers and when patients are being treated by health care providers who view themselves and/or practice more as patient advocates than as scientific practitioners. However, psychological and medical iatrogenesis can theoretically present in any condition where a neuropsychologist evaluates and no health care provider is immune from causing iatrogenic effects. Although not all iatrogenic complications are avoidable and some are expected from standard therapies (e.g., neurological and neuropsychological impairments from cancer treatments such as radiation, chemotherapy, and other medication) many can be avoided by implementing some of the suggestions discussed in this chapter.

References

Allen, C., Glasziou, P., & Del Mar, C. (1999). Bed rest: A potentially harmful treatment needing more careful evaluation. *Lancet*, *354*(9186), 1229–1233.

Asher, R. A. (1947). The dangers of going to bed. *British Medical Journal*, *2*(4536), 967.

Baines, C. J., McKeown-Eyssen, G. E., Riley, N., Marshall, L., & Jazmaji, V. (2007). University of Toronto case-control study of multiple chemical sensitivity-3: Intra-erythrocytic mineral levels. *Occupational Medicine(London)*, *57*(2), 137–140. doi: 10.1093/occmed/kql104

Baker, G. R., Norton, P. G., Flintoft, V., Blais, R., Brown, A., Cox, J., . . . Tamblyn, R. (2004). The Canadian adverse events study: The incidence of adverse events among hospital patients in Canada. *CMAJ*, *170*(11), 1678–1686.

Baxendale, S. (2004). Memories aren't made of this: Amnesia at the movies. *BMJ (Clinical Research Ed.)*, *329*(7480), 1480–1483. doi: 10.1136/bmj.329.7480.1480

Bell, G. (2009). State adopts nation's toughest sports concussion law. Retrieved August 6, 2009, from www.komonews.com/news/local/45059357.html.

Biley, F. C. (2002). Primum non nocere: Thoughts on the need to develop an 'adverse events' register for complementary and alternative therapies. *Complementary Therapies in Nursing and Midwifery*, *8*(2), 57–61. doi: 10.1054/ctnm.2002.0612

Binder, L. M., Storzbach, D., & Salinsky, M. C. (2006). MMPI-2 profiles of persons with multiple chemical sensitivity. *Clinical Neuropsychology*, *20*(4), 848–857. doi: 10.1080/13854040500246927

Black, D. W., Doebbeling, B. N., Voelker, M. D., Clarke, W. R., Woolson, R. F., Barrett, D. H., & Schwartz, D. A. (2000). Multiple chemical sensitivity syndrome: Symptom prevalence and risk factors in a military population. *Archives of Internal Medicine*, *160*(8), 1169–1176.

Bliss, E. L. (1980). Multiple personalities: A report of 14 cases with implications for Schizophrenia and hysteria. *Archives of General Psychiatry*, *37*(12), 1388–1397.

Bornschein, S., Forstl, H., & Zilker, T. (2001). Idiopathic environmental intolerances (formerly multiple chemical sensitivity) psychiatric perspectives. *Journal of Internal Medicine*, *250*(4), 309–321.

Bornschein, S., Hausteiner, C., Zilker, T., & Forstl, H. (2002). Psychiatric and somatic disorders and multiple chemical sensitivity (MCS) in 264 'environmental patients'. *Psychological Medicine*, *32*(8), 1387–1394.

Bowman, E. S., & Coons, P. M. (2000). The differential diagnosis of epilepsy, pseudoseizures, dissociative identity disorder, and dissociative disorder not otherwise specified. *Bulletin of the Menninger Clinic*, *64*(2), 164–180.

Boysen, G. A. (2011). The scientific status of childhood dissociative identity disorder: A review of published research. *Psychotherapy and Psychosomatics*, *80*(6), 329–334. doi: 10.1159/000323403

Brennan, T. A., Leape, L. L., Laird, N. M., Hebert, L., Localio, A. R., Lawthers, A. G., . . . Hiatt, H. H. (1991). Incidence of adverse events and negligence in hospitalized patients: Results of the Harvard Medical Practice Study I. *New England Journal of Medicine*, *324*(6), 370–376. doi: 10.1056/nejm199102073240604

Brooks, S., Warshaw, G., Hasse, L., & Kues, J. R. (1994). The physician decision-making process in transferring nursing home patients to the hospital. *Archives of Internal Medicine*, *154*(8), 902–908.

Brusko, C. S., & Marten, J. T. (1991). Ketoconazole hepatotoxicity in a patient treated for environmental illness and systemic candidiasis. *DICP*, *25*(12), 1321–1325.

Carone, D. A. (2014). The role and ramifications of the media's reporting on concussions. In R. J. Echemendia & G. L. Iverson (Eds.), *Oxford Handbook of Sport-Related Concussion* (pp. 1–15). New York: Oxford University Press.

Carone, D. A., Bush, S. S., & Iverson, G. L. (2013). Providing feedback on symptom validity, mental health, and treatment in mild traumatic brain injury. In D. A. Carone & S. S. Bush (Eds.), *Mild traumatic Brain Injury: Symptom Validity Assessment and Malingering* (pp. 101–118). New York: Springer Publishing, Company Inc.

Carone, D. A., Iverson, G. L., & Bush, S. S. (2010). A model to approaching and providing feedback to patients regarding invalid test performance in clinical neuropsychological evaluations. *Clinical Neuropsychology*, *24*(5), 759–778. doi: 922328119 [pii] 10.1080/13854041003712951 [doi]

Carone, D. A., & Shah, A. (2008). *A five factor personality profile analysis of patients with persisting symptoms after mild traumatic brain/head injury*. Paper presented at the National Academy of Neuropsychology, New York City, New York.

Cassidy, J. D., Boyle, E., Cote, P., He, Y., Hogg-Johnson, S., Silver, F. L., & Bondy, S. J. (2008). Risk of vertebrobasilar stroke and chiropractic care: Results of a population-based case-control and case-crossover study. *Spine (Phila Pa 1976)*, *33*(Suppl 4), S176–S183. doi: 10.1097/BRS.0b013e3181644600

Check, E. (2004). U.S. antidepressants to carry suicide warnings. *Nature*. Retrieved from www.nature.com/news/2004/041018/full/news041018-2.html

Coons, P. M. (1991). Iatrogenesis and malingering of multiple personality disorder in the forensic evaluation of homicide defendants. *Psychiatric Clinics of North America*, *14*(3), 757–768.

Cote, P., & Soklaridis, S. (2011). Does early management of whiplash-associated disorders assist or impede recovery? *Spine (Phila Pa 1976)*, *36*(Suppl 25), S275–S279. doi: 10.1097/BRS.0b013e3182388d32

Dalton, P. (1999). Cognitive influences on health symptoms from acute chemical exposure. *Health Psychology*, *18*(6), 579–590.

Das-Munshi, J., Rubin, G. J., & Wessely, S. (2007). Multiple chemical sensitivities: Review. *Current Opinion in Otolaryngology & Head and Neck Surgery*, *15*(4), 274–280. doi: 10.1097/MOO.0b013e328259c360

Davis, P., Lay-Yee, R., Briant, R., Ali, W., Scott, A., & Schug, S. (2002). Adverse events in New Zealand public hospitals I: Occurrence and impact. *New Zealand Medical Journal*, *115*(1167), U271.

Davis, P., Lay-Yee, R., Briant, R., Ali, W., Scott, A., & Schug, S. (2003). Adverse events in New Zealand public hospitals II: Preventability and clinical context. *New Zealand Medical Journal*, *116*(1183), U624.

de Kruijk, J. R., Leffers, P., Meerhoff, S., Rutten, J., & Twijnstra, A. (2002). Effectiveness of bed rest after mild traumatic brain injury: A randomised trial of no versus six days of bed rest. *Journal of Neurology, Neurosurgery and Psychiatry*, *73*(2), 167–172.

Doty, R. L., & Crastnopol, B. (2010). Correlates of chemosensory malingering. *Laryngoscope*, *120*(4), 707–711. doi: 10.1002/lary.20827

Dumit, J. (2006). Illnesses you have to fight to get: Facts as forces in uncertain, emergent illnesses. *Social Science and Medicine*, *62*(3), 577–590. doi: 10.1016/j.socscimed.2005.06.018

Dunn, W. F., & Murphy, J. (2010). Death by compassion—dilemmas and opportunities in sedation delivery: Iatrogenesis within a profession in denial. *Chest*, *138*(5), 1034–1035. doi: 10.1378/chest.10-1731

Ernst, E. (2002). Manipulation of the cervical spine: A systematic review of case reports of serious adverse events, 1995–2001. *Medical Journal of Australia*, *176*(8), 376–380.

Fantino, B., Voirin, N., Laforest, L., Fantino, F., Chretin, S., & Van Ganse, E. (2006). Primary care physicians' behaviors towards risk of iatrogenesis in elderly patients. *European Journal of Clinical Pharmacology*, *62*(7), 563–570. doi: 10.1007/s00228-006-0125-z

Foote, B., & Park, J. (2008). Dissociative identity disorder and schizophrenia: Differential diagnosis and theoretical issues. *Current Psychiatry Reports*, *10*(3), 217–222.

Friedman, J. H. (2002). Iatrogenesis imperfecta. *Medicine and Health, Rhode Island*, *85*(7), 198.

Fritz, N., Glogau, S., Hoffmann, J., Rademacher, M., Elger, C. E., & Helmstaedter, C. (2005). Efficacy and cognitive side effects of tiagabine and topiramate in patients with epilepsy. *Epilepsy and Behavior*, *6*(3), 373–381. doi: 10.1016/j.yebeh.2005.01.002

Furukawa, M. F., Raghu, T. S., & Shao, B. B. (2010). Electronic medical records, nurse staffing, and nurse-sensitive patient outcomes: Evidence from California hospitals, 1998–2007. *Health Services Research*, *45*(4), 941–962. doi: 10.1111/j.1475-6773.2010.01110.x

Georgellis, A., Lindelof, B., Lundin, A., Arnetz, B., & Hillert, L. (2003). Multiple chemical sensitivity in male painters; a controlled provocation study. *International Journal of Hygiene and Environmental Health*, *206*(6), 531–538. doi: 10.1078/1438-4639-00253

Gleaves, D. H. (1996). The sociocognitive model of dissociative identity disorder: A reexamination of the evidence. *Psychological Bulletin*, *120*(1), 42–59.

Greaves, G. B. (1980). Multiple personality: 165 years after Mary Reynolds. *Journal of Nervous and Mental Disease*, *168*(10), 577–596.

Guez, M., Brannstrom, R., Nyberg, L., Toolanen, G., & Hildingsson, C. (2005). Neuropsychological functioning and MMPI-2 profiles in chronic neck pain: A comparison of whiplash and non-traumatic groups. *Journal of Clinical and Experimental Neuropsychology*, *27*(2), 151–163. doi: 10.1080/13803390490515487

Haeck, T. (2009). Maple Valley parents settle with school district after son's injury. Retrieved August 5, 2009, from www.mynorthwest.com/?nid=11&sid=213328.

Hamaguchi, T., Noguchi-Shinohara, M., Nozaki, I., Nakamura, Y., Sato, T., Kitamoto, T., . . . Yamada, M. (2009). The risk of iatrogenic Creutzfeldt-Jakob disease through medical and surgical procedures. *Neuropathology*, *29*(5), 625–631. doi: 10.1111/j.1440-1789.2009.01023.x

Herr, C. E., Kopka, I., Mach, J., Runkel, B., Schill, W. B., Gieler, U., & Eikmann, T. F. (2004). Interdisciplinary diagnostics in environmental medicine—findings and follow-up in patients with chronic medically unexplained health complaints. *International Journal of Hygiene and Environmental Health*, *207*(1), 31–44. doi: 10.1078/1438-4639-00263

Hurwitz, E. L., Morgenstern, H., Vassilaki, M., & Chiang, L. M. (2004). Adverse reactions to chiropractic treatment and their effects on satisfaction and clinical outcomes among patients enrolled in the UCLA Neck Pain Study. *Journal of Manipulative and Physiological Therapeutics*, *27*(1), 16–25. doi: 10.1016/j.jmpt.2003.11.002

Inouye, S. K., Schlesinger, M. J., & Lydon, T. J. (1999). Delirium: A symptom of how hospital care is failing older persons and a window to improve quality of hospital care. *American Journal of Medicine*, *106*(5), 565–573.

Jacobs, J. P., Benavidez, O. J., Bacha, E. A., Walters, H. L., & Jacobs, M. L. (2008). The nomenclature of safety and quality of care for patients with congenital cardiac disease: A report of the Society of Thoracic Surgeons Congenital Database Taskforce Subcommittee on Patient Safety. *Cardiology in the Young*, *18*(Suppl 2), 81–91. doi: 10.1017/s1047951108003041

Jeste, D. V., & Krull, A. J. (1990). Neuroleptics and tardive dyskinesia—a case of iatrogenesis. *Western Journal of Medicine*, *153*(5), 560–561.

Johnson, G. (2010). Second impact syndrome—from CDC. Retrieved August 9, 2010, from http://waiting.com/blog/2010/06/second-impact-syndrome-from-cdc.html

Kouyanou, K., Pither, C. E., Rabe-Hesketh, S., & Wessely, S. (1998). A comparative study of iatrogenesis, medication abuse, and psychiatric morbidity in chronic pain patients with and without medically explained symptoms. *Pain*, *76*(3), 417–426.

Kouyanou, K., Pither, C. E., & Wessely, S. (1997a). Iatrogenic factors and chronic pain. *Psychosomatic Medicine*, *59*(6), 597–604.

Kouyanou, K., Pither, C. E., & Wessely, S. (1997b). Medication misuse, abuse and dependence in chronic pain patients. *Journal of Psychosomatic Research*, *43*(5), 497–504.

Ksouri, H., Balanant, P. Y., Tadie, J. M., Heraud, G., Abboud, I., Lerolle, N., . . . Faisy, C. (2010). Impact of morbidity and mortality conferences on analysis of mortality and critical events in intensive care practice. *American Journal of Critical Care*, *19*(2), 135–145; quiz 146. doi: 10.4037/ajcc2010590

Kugelman, A., Inbar-Sanado, E., Shinwell, E. S., Makhoul, I. R., Leshem, M., Zangen, S., . . . Bader, D. (2008). Iatrogenesis in neonatal intensive care units: Observational and interventional, prospective, multicenter study. *Pediatrics*, *122*(3), 550–555. doi: 10.1542/peds.2007-2729

Langlois, J. A., Kegler, S. R., Butler, J. A., Gotsch, K. E., Johnson, R. L., Reichard, A. A., . . . Thurman, D. J. (2003). Traumatic brain injury-related hospital discharges: Results from a 14-state surveillance system, 1997. *MMWR Surveillance Summaries: Morbidity and Mortality Weekly Report*, *52*(4), 1–20.

Leddy, J. J., Cox, J. L., Baker, J. G., Wack, D. S., Pendergast, D. R., Zivadinov, R., & Willer, B. (2012). Exercise treatment for postconcussion syndrome: A pilot study of changes in functional magnetic resonance imaging activation, physiology, and symptoms. *Journal of Head Trauma Rehabilitation*. doi: 10.1097/HTR.0b013e31826da964

Leznoff, A. (1997). Provocative challenges in patients with multiple chemical sensitivity. *Journal of Allergy and Clinical Immunology*, *99*(4), 438–442.

Lilienfeld, S. O., Lynn, S. J., Kirsch, I., Chaves, J. F., Sarbin, T. R., Ganaway, G. K., & Powell, R. A. (1999). Dissociative identity disorder and the sociocognitive model: Recalling the lessons of the past. *Psychological Bulletin*, *125*(5), 507–523.

Lipson, J. G., & Doiron, N. (2006). Environmental issues and work: Women with multiple chemical sensitivities. *Health Care for Women International*, *27*(7), 571–584. doi: 10.1080/07399330600803709

Little, P., Dorward, M., Warner, G., Stephens, K., Senior, J., & Moore, M. (2004). Importance of patient pressure and perceived pressure and perceived medical need for investigations, referral, and prescribing in primary care: Nested observational study. *BMJ (Clinical Research Ed.)*, *328*(7437), 444. doi: 10.1136/bmj.38013.644086.7C

Loring, D. W., Williamson, D. J., Meador, K. J., Wiegand, F., & Hulihan, J. (2011). Topiramate dose effects on cognition: A randomized double-blind study. *Neurology*, *76*(2), 131–137. doi: WNL.0b013e318206ca02 [pii] 10.1212/WNL.0b013e318206ca02 [doi]

McAllister, E. J., Dhurandhar, N. V., Keith, S. W., Aronne, L. J., Barger, J., Baskin, M., . . . Allison, D. B. (2009). Ten putative contributors to the obesity epidemic. *Critical Reviews in Food Science and Nutrition*, *49*(10), 868–913. doi: 10.1080/10408390903372599

Merskey, H. (1992). The manufacture of personalities: The production of multiple personality disorder. *British Journal of Psychiatry*, *160*, 327–340.

Mickeviciene, D., Schrader, H., Nestvold, K., Surkiene, D., Kunickas, R., Stovner, L. J., & Sand, T. (2002). A controlled historical cohort study on the post-concussion syndrome. *European Journal of Neurology*, *9*(6), 581–587. doi: 497 [pii]

Mickeviciene, D., Schrader, H., Obelieniene, D., Surkiene, D., Kunickas, R., Stovner, L. J., & Sand, T. (2004). A controlled prospective inception cohort study on the post-concussion syndrome outside the medicolegal context. *European Journal of Neurology*, *11*(6), 411–419. doi: 10.1111/j.1468-1331.2004.00816.x [doi] ENE816 [pii]

Mild Traumatic Brain Injury Committee of the Head Injury Interdisciplinary Special Interest Group of the American Congress of Rehabilitation Medicine. (1993). Definition of mild traumatic brain injury. *Journal of Head Trauma Rehabilitation*, *8*(3), 86–87.

Miles, S. H. (2005). *The Hippocratic Oath and the Ethics of Medicine*. New York: Oxford University Press.

Miller, L. J., & Mittenberg, W. (1998). Brief cognitive behavioral interventions in mild traumatic brain injury. *Applied Neuropsychology*, *5*(4), 172–183. doi: 10.1207/s15324826an0504_2 [doi]

Mittenberg, W., Canyock, E. M., Condit, D., & Patton, C. (2001). Treatment of post-concussion syndrome following mild head injury. *Journal of Clinical and Experimental Neuropsychology*, *23*(6), 829–836.

Mittenberg, W., DiGiulio, D. V., Perrin, S., & Bass, A. E. (1992). Symptoms following mild head injury: Expectation as aetiology. *Journal of Neurology, Neurosurgery and Psychiatry*, *55*(3), 200–204.

Mittenberg, W., Patton, C., Canyock, E. M., & Condit, D. C. (2002). Base rates of malingering and symptom exaggeration. *Journal of Clinical and Experimental Neuropsychology*, *24*(8), 1094–1102.

Mittenberg, W., Tremont, G., Zielinski, R. E., Fichera, S., & Rayls, K. R. (1996). Cognitive-behavioral prevention of postconcussion syndrome. *Archives of Clinical Neuropsychology*, *11*(2), 139–145. doi: 0887-6177(95)00006-2 [pii]

Mitty, E. (2010). Iatrogenesis, frailty, and geriatric syndromes. *Geriatric Nursing*, *31*(5), 368–374. doi: 10.1016/j.gerinurse.2010.08.004

Morey, L. C. (2007). *Personality Assessment Inventory-Adolsecent: Professional Manual*. Lutz, FL: Psychological Assessment Resources.

Munoz, S. J. (2008). Hepatic encephalopathy. *Medical Clinics of North America*, *92*(4), 795–812, viii. doi: 10.1016/j.mcna.2008.03.009

Nathan, D. M. (2012). *Sybil Exposed: The Extraordinary Story Behind the Famous Multiple Personality Case*. New York: Free Press.

Nemergut, L. (2009). Concussions and the new impact test. Retrieved August 5, 2010, from www.argorps.com/?p=487

Olson-Garewal, J. K. (2001). Making sense of outpatient pharmacy management: How to control pharmacy costs while delivering quality care. *Postgraduate Medicine*, *110*(1), 7–10.

Osterberg, K., Persson, R., Karlson, B., Carlsson Eek, F., & Orbaek, P. (2007). Personality, mental distress, and subjective health complaints among persons with environmental annoyance. *Human and Experimental Toxicology*, *26*(3), 231–241. doi: 10.1177/0960327107070575

Palmieri, P. A., Peterson, L. T., & Ford, E. W. (2007). Technological iatrogenesis: New risks force heightened management awareness. *Journal of Healthcare Risk Management*, *27*(4), 19–24. doi: 10.1002/jhrm.5600270405

Patfield, M. (2011). Undiagnosis: An important new role for psychiatry. *Australasian Psychiatry*, *19*(2), 107–109. doi: 10.3109/10398562.2010.539226

Piper, A., & Merskey, H. (2004). The persistence of folly: A critical examination of dissociative identity disorder. Part I: The excesses of an improbable concept. *Canadian Journal of Psychiatry*, *49*(9), 592–600.

Ponsford, J., Willmott, C., Rothwell, A., Cameron, P., Ayton, G., Nelms, R., . . . Ng, K. (2001). Impact of early intervention on outcome after mild traumatic brain injury in children. *Pediatrics*, *108*(6), 1297–1303.

Ponsford, J., Willmott, C., Rothwell, A., Cameron, P., Kelly, A. M., Nelms, R., & Curran, C. (2002). Impact of early intervention on outcome following mild head injury in adults. *Journal of Neurology, Neurosurgery, and Psychiatry*, *73*(3), 330–332.

Potts, S., Feinglass, J., Lefevere, F., Kadah, H., Branson, C., & Webster, J. (1993). A quality-of-care analysis of cascade iatrogenesis in frail elderly hospital patients. *QRB: Quality Review Bulletin*, *19*(6), 199–205.

Pransky, G., Borkan, J. M., Young, A. E., & Cherkin, D. C. (2011). Are we making progress?: The tenth international forum for primary care research on low back pain. *Spine (Phila Pa 1976)*, *36*(19), 1608–1614. doi: 10.1097/BRS.0b013e3181f6114e

Reading, N. (2009). House passes bill to prevent youth concussions. Retrieved August 5, 2010, from www.tvw.org/capitolrecord/index.php/2009/03/house-passes-bill-to-prevent-youth-concussions/

Reid, S., Hotopf, M., Hull, L., Ismail, K., Unwin, C., & Wessely, S. (2001). Multiple chemical sensitivity and chronic fatigue syndrome in British Gulf War veterans. *American Journal of Epidemiology*, *153*(6), 604–609.

Reinders, A. A., Willemsen, A. T., Vos, H. P., den Boer, J. A., & Nijenhuis, E. R. (2012). Fact or factitious? A psychobiological study of authentic and simulated dissociative identity states. *PLoS One*, *7*(6), e39279. doi: 10.1371/journal.pone.0039279

Rihmer, Z., & Akiskal, H. (2006). Do antidepressants t(h)reat(en) depressives? Toward a clinically judicious formulation of the antidepressant-suicidality FDA advisory in light of declining national suicide statistics from many countries. *Journal of Affective Disorders*, *94*(1–3), 3–13. doi: 10.1016/j.jad.2006.04.003

Rothschild, J. M., Bates, D. W., & Leape, L. L. (2000). Preventable medical injuries in older patients. *Archives of Internal Medicine*, *160*(18), 2717–2728.

Schimmel, E. M. (2003). The hazards of hospitalization, 1964. *Quality and Safety in Health Care*, *12*(1), 58–63; discussion 63–54.

Schneider, K. J., Iverson, G. L., Emery, C. A., McCrory, P., Herring, S. A., & Meeuwisse, W. H. (2013). The effects of rest and treatment following sport-related concussion: A systematic review of the literature. *British Journal of Sports Medicine*, *47*(5), 304–307. doi: 10.1136/bjsports-2013-092190

Scott, I. A., Gray, L. C., Martin, J. H., & Mitchell, C. A. (2012). Minimizing inappropriate medications in older populations: A 10-step conceptual framework. *American Journal of Medicine*, *125*(6), 529–537, e524. doi: 10.1016/j.amjmed.2011.09.021

Scroppo, J. C., Drob, S. L., Weinberger, J. L., & Eagle, P. (1998). Identifying dissociative identity disorder: A self-report and projective study. *Journal of Abnormal Psychology*, *107*(2), 272–284.

Seroussi, B., Falcoff, H., Sauquet, D., Julien, J., & Bouaud, J. (2010). Role of physicians' reactance in e-iatrogenesis: A case study with ASTI guiding mode on the management of hypertension. *AMIA Annual Symposium Proceedings*, *2010*, 737–741.

Simpson, K. R. (2010). e-Iatrogenesis. *MCN: American Journal of Maternal Child Nursing*, *35*(5), 308. doi: 10.1097/NMC.0b013e3181e6f0e8

Slick, D. J., Sherman, E. M., & Iverson, G. L. (1999). Diagnostic criteria for malingered neurocognitive dysfunction: Proposed standards for clinical practice and research. *Clinical Neuropsychology*, *13*(4), 545–561.

Smetzer, J., Baker, C., Byrne, F. D., & Cohen, M. R. (2010). Shaping systems for better behavioral choices: Lessons learned from a fatal medication error. *Joint Commission Journal on Quality and Patient Safety*, *36*(4), 152–163.

Spanos, N. P. (1994). Multiple identity enactments and multiple personality disorder: A sociocognitive perspective. *Psychological Bulletin*, *116*(1), 143–165.

Staudenmayer, H. (2000). Psychological treatment of psychogenic idiopathic environmental intolerance. *Occupational Medicine*, *15*(3), 627–646.

Staudenmayer, H., & Phillips, S. (2007). MMPI-2 validity, clinical and content scales, and the Fake Bad Scale for personal injury litigants claiming idiopathic environmental intolerance. *Journal of Psychosomatic Research*, *62*(1), 61–72. doi: 10.1016/j.jpsychores.2006.01.013

Stein, R. A., & Strickland, T. L. (1998). A review of the neuropsychological effects of commonly used prescription medications. *Archives of Clinical Neuropsychology*, *13*(3), 259–284.

Storaci, R., Manelli, A., Schiavone, N., Mangia, L., Prigione, G., & Sangiorgi, S. (2006). Whiplash injury and oculomotor dysfunctions: Clinical-posturographic correlations. *European Spine Journal*, *15*(12), 1811–1816. doi: 10.1007/s00586-006-0085-0

Stovner, L. J., Schrader, H., Mickeviciene, D., Surkiene, D., & Sand, T. (2009). Headache after concussion. *European Journal of Neurology*, *16*(1), 112–120. doi: 10.1111/j.1468-1331.2008.02363.x

Suhr, J. A., & Gunstad, J. (2002). "Diagnosis Threat": The effect of negative expectations on cognitive performance in head injury. *Journal of Clinical and Experimental Neuropsychology*, *24*(4), 448–457. doi: 10.1076/jcen.24.4.448.1039

Suhr, J. A., & Gunstad, J. (2005). Further exploration of the effect of "diagnosis threat" on cognitive performance in individuals with mild head injury. *Journal of the International Neuropsychological Society*, *11*(1), 23–29. doi: 10.1017/s1355617705050010

Taylor, J. P., Krondl, M. M., Spidel, M., & Csima, A. C. (2002). Dietary adequacy of the rotary diversified diet as a treatment for "Environmental Illness." *Canadian Journal of Dietetic Practice and Research*, *63*(4), 198–201.

Thomas, E. J., Studdert, D. M., Burstin, H. R., Orav, E. J., Zeena, T., Williams, E. J., . . . Brennan, T. A. (2000). Incidence and types of adverse events and negligent care in Utah and Colorado. *Medical Care*, *38*(3), 261–271.

van Steijn, J. H., Nieboer, P., Hospers, G. A., de Vries, E. G., & Mulder, N. H. (2001). Delirium after interleukin-2 and alpha-interferon therapy for renal cell carcinoma. *Anticancer Research*, *21*(5), 3699–3700.

Vasilevskis, E. E., Ely, E. W., Speroff, T., Pun, B. T., Boehm, L., & Dittus, R. S. (2010). Reducing iatrogenic risks: ICU-acquired delirium and weakness—crossing the quality chasm. *Chest*, *138*(5), 1224–1233. doi: 10.1378/chest.10-0466

Weiner, J. P., Kfuri, T., Chan, K., & Fowles, J. B. (2007). "e-Iatrogenesis": The most critical unintended consequence of CPOE and other HIT. *Journal of the American Medical Informatics Association*, *14*(3), 387–388; discussion 389. doi: 10.1197/jamia.M2338

Weissberg, M. (1993). Multiple personality disorder and iatrogenesis: The cautionary tale of Anna O. *International Journal of Clinical and Experimental Hypnosis*, *41*(1), 15–34. doi: 10.1080/00207149308414535

Wilson, R. M., Runciman, W. B., Gibberd, R. W., Harrison, B. T., Newby, L., & Hamilton, J. D. (1995). The quality in Australian Health Care Study. *Medical Journal of Australia*, *163*(9), 458–471.

Winters, W., Devriese, S., Van Diest, I., Nemery, B., Veulemans, H., Eelen, P., . . . Van den Bergh, O. (2003). Media warnings about environmental pollution facilitate the acquisition of symptoms in response to chemical substances. *Psychosomatic Medicine*, *65*(3), 332–338.

45 Complementary and Alternative Medicine for Children With Developmental Disabilities

Karen E. Wills

Adequate evidence is lacking for the efficacy of complementary and alternative medicine treatments (CAM) over placebo in children with developmental disabilities, for symptoms other than pain or insomnia (Golnik & Ireland, 2009; Harrington & Allen, 2014; Perrin et al., 2012). This has been the case for a century or more, during which the popularity of CAM has steadily grown, particularly for children with autism and attention deficit/hyperactivity disorder (ADHD), and increasingly for children with Down syndrome and other developmental disabilities (Kemper, Vohra, & Walls, 2008). Rather than redo existing comprehensive scientific reviews of CAM techniques and efficacy—an approach that clearly would conclude with the summary statement that this chapter begins with, as every other neutral review has done—the present chapter will address practical questions for pediatric neuropsychologists, specifically:

- What types of treatment are considered CAM?
- What problems does CAM offer to treat?
- Which patients and families are most likely to engage with CAM practitioners?
- Does any type of CAM work?
- What harm can scientifically unsupported CAM do? Can it do any good?
- Why are so many types of CAM popular if they don't work?
- What should neuropsychologists consider when discussing CAM?

What Types of Treatment Are Considered CAM?

As shown in Table 45.1, allopathic (mainstream) medicine encompasses procedures of a nature similar to CAM procedures—the difference being an assumption that procedures should be subject to scientific validation of efficacy. That is not to say that in fact all of the procedures used in mainstream medicine have been validated, merely that it is assumed they ought to be, and that if scientifically unsupported, they should be discontinued.

Thus, CAM refers to a wide array of procedures usually defined by exclusion as being not subjected to scientific inquiry, "not scientifically proven," or "not mainstream" medicine or surgery. The most commonly used procedures including massage, breathing, relaxation exercises, yoga, and guided meditation. The more intrusive or elaborate CAM treatments are much less commonly used, although they get more press. Sometimes a treatment that starts out as CAM becomes validated and then may no longer be considered CAM—for example, the use of melatonin to enhance sleep onset has been excluded from CAM in some recent studies (Perrin et al., 2012).

What is considered CAM varies across studies and over time, which makes it hard to compare studies that reference CAM as an "umbrella" term for a range of procedures. For instance, massage therapy may be included as one type of CAM by one investigator, but as a mainstream palliative treatment by others. Whether or not an approach is CAM may depend, in part, on whether there is scientific support for its efficacy as a treatment for the particular symptom or outcome to which it is being applied—for example, massage as a treatment for pain or spasticity may be considered mainstream, whereas massage to enhance sustained attention among children with ADHD may be considered CAM. The list of CAM procedures changes over time, as well, because adverse events, changing fads, updated technology, or popularized research results may make particular techniques obsolete as new ones emerge.

CAM in some sense has existed for centuries but by definition could not exist without a formally established medical mainstream that endorses treatments based on scientific research with clinical trials. Since the 1930s, organized medicine dominated the available interventions, which were focused mostly on relief of life-threatening illnesses. Beginning in the 1970s, as many infectious diseases were nearly eradicated, there was increasing emphasis within the medical community on health and wellness, rather than illness. Benson (1975) in "The Relaxation Response" emphasized the use of breathing, meditation, and relaxation strategies to relieve pain, anxiety, insomnia, and hypertension. David Eisenberg (1993) learned Chinese medicine and helped popularize it within the United States. Subsequently, these strategies have been used to deal with anxiety, nausea, medical anorexia, pain, and insomnia, in adults and children with serious chronic illnesses such as cancer, heart disease, and arthritis. The idea that such treatments augmented

Table 45.1 Treatments for childhood behavioral or developmental problems

Dietary manipulations and supplements (efforts to eliminate perceived toxins, supplement perceived missing substances, or add perceived beneficial nutrients)
Elimination (e.g., sugar-free, gluten-free, casein-free, preservative-free, food "allergies")
Supplements (e.g., herbs, vitamins, oils, minerals, enzymes, probiotics, antifungals)
Special food preparation (e.g., raw foods, green smoothies)
Homeopathic treatments, naturopathic treatments (Atwood, 2003)
Melatonin (for sleep onset; see Bendz & Scates, 2010)
Psychopharmacology (allopathic)
Biomechanical (passive movement) therapies (touching, moving, piercing or adjusting the child's body as an effort to improve motor function and response to physical sensation, or to ameliorate pain or physical discomfort)
Massage therapies (Khilnani et al., 2003)
Sensory integration therapy: compression, brushing
Chiropractic (Synovitz & Larson, 2013)
Acupuncture/acupressure
Orthopedics (surgery, bracing, casting; allopathic)
Mind/body, expressive, and active movement therapies (to improve mood, behavior, and well-being or ameliorate a broad spectrum of symptoms)
Art, music, dance, movement therapies (e.g., Interactive Metronome)
Sensory integration: gross motor/vestibular stimulation (swinging, spinning)
Yoga, therapeutic horseback riding, martial arts, swimming, other exercise/sports
Play therapy, sand play, other interpretive play techniques
Psychotherapy (allopathic)
Mind/body, relaxation and spiritual energy therapies (to improve mood, behavior, and well-being or ameliorate a broad spectrum of symptoms)
Relaxation, eye muscle Desensitization with relaxation
Hypnosis
Meditation
Biofeedback (muscle relaxation, galvanic skin response)
EEG biofeedback (for concentration and/or memory and learning; Steiner et al.)
Cranio-sacral healing (Gray et al., 2011), Qi Gong, therapeutic touch
Prayer healing/faith healing/shaman ritual
Listening/fostering the doctor–patient relationship (Allopathic)
Physical/respiratory environment
Hyperbaric oxygen chamber
Salt caves
Erlen lenses; colored overlays (effort to improve reading)
Eliminate florescent lights; use broad-spectrum "natural" light
Control acoustics (echo reduction) and light touch (soft clothing)
Filter air and water (effort to remove perceived irritants or toxins)
Aromatherapy (effort to combat nausea and pain of chemotherapy and other procedures)
Chelation (allopathic to treat lead poisoning; otherwise, risky: Brown et al., 2006)
Exposure to "green space" (spending time in nature; Kuo & Taylor,)
Exposure to magnets or magnetic fields
Sensory-motor training therapies
Behavioral optometry (vision therapy; effort to improve functional vision for reading)
Auditory Integration Therapy, Fast Forward, other "listening" therapies (effort to improve functional listening and communication skills, for speech and reading)
Speech/language therapies (allopathic)
Occupational therapies (allopathic when used to train specific skills)

conventional medicine, rather than substituted for it, took hold as mainstream hospitals hired practitioners of "complementary" or "integrative" medicine. In 1992, an Office of Alternative Medicine was established at the National Institutes of Health. In 1999, the name was officially changed to The National Consortium on Complementary and Alternative Medicine. A major conference on use of CAM with children took place in 2000. Going forward, the U.S. federal government may play an increasing role in regulating CAM, although the involvement of CAM practitioners in directing the NCCAM has been critically challenged (Atwood, 2003).

What Problems Does CAM Offer to Treat?

Rather than objectively measureable signs of illness (such as fever), most symptoms and conditions addressed by CAM for adults and adolescents involve subjective distress, such as pain, malaise, nausea, fatigue, dizziness, anxiety, and depression. For children, including those with developmental disabilities, CAM is most commonly used to try to alleviate the following symptoms:

- Externalizing behavior problems such as irritability, aggression, impulsivity, and hyperactivity;
- Repetitive autistic-like behaviors such as self-injurious behavior, tics, stereotyped movements ("self-stimming"), and inflexible or perseverative behaviors;
- Anxious/agitated behavior such as agitation, anxiety, fearfulness, and "meltdowns";
- Inattention, distractibility, and learning and memory problems;
- Insomnia, including settling to sleep and staying asleep through the night;
- GI symptoms such as cramps, gas, encopresis, diarrhea, and constipation;
- Pain such as headache, stomachache, cramps, and other aches and pains; and
- Seizures and staring spells.

Children with motor dyspraxias or cerebral palsy are subject to a range of interventions in an effort to improve their posture, gait, hand control, and speech that tend to be far more physically intrusive but no more effective than most of the common CAM treatments for autism and ADHD—for example, hyperbaric oxygen and stem cell injection—though the most common therapies are massage and hydrotherapy (Wray REF).

Which Patients and Families Are Most Likely to Engage With CAM Practitioners?

CAM may be marketed or perceived as an alternative to mainstream treatments. It is viewed by some as avoiding adverse effects of medications or surgeries; offering a cure or symptom alleviation for problems when traditional medicine has proven insufficient or offers no recourse; sometimes providing less-expensive, more-comprehensive, or more-lasting treatment; emphasizing wellness and holistic health rather than mere symptom relief; providing more "natural" forms of intervention rather than synthetic chemical solutions; or as a more respectful "person-centered" approach rather than one that coerces or subjugates patients to a doctor's authority.

While this "medicine avoidant" use of CAM might be more common among adults treating themselves, surveys consistently find that most parents who use CAM are not abjuring standard medical treatments for their children. For children, CAM seems to be more often "complementary" than "alternative." While for most studies this finding could result from an ascertainment bias (because parents often are interviewed in the waiting room of a clinic or hospital), the same pattern was found in a very large sample drawn from a national autism advocacy group (Perrin et al., 2012) and in a population-based Canadian survey (Adams et al., 2013). Most families who use CAM for children also are using traditional mainstream pediatric care, as well as educational interventions. It is less clear how often CAM is utilized in conjunction with scientifically tested psychological therapies for autism, ADHD, anxiety, and other behavior problems in children, although these are not intrinsically incompatible. CAM is seen by some medical providers as truly "complementary"—a useful adjunct to medication or standard physical or mental health care (Golnik & Ireland, 2009). In this context, it is used primarily for relaxation, distraction, desensitization, mindfulness, managing disruptive or risky behaviors, and lifestyle changes such as ceasing harmful habits or establishing health-promoting habits. CAM of this sort has been incorporated as a service or freestanding program into many major medical centers and is very popular with patients. It may be prescribed for children with cancer, diabetes, asthma, and other chronic illnesses. Hospital- and clinic-based CAM or Integrative Medicine services, and pediatric psychology services, may overlap, coexist, or sometimes conflict. Some hospital ethicists have cautioned that standards of informed consent, evidence-based treatment, and outcome evaluation of CAM do not equal those to which traditional medicine and psychological interventions are held (Ernst, 2009; Nissen, Weidenhammer, Schunder-Tatzber, & Johannessen, 2013).

Pediatricians at the Boston Children's Hospital (Perrin et al., 2012) analyzed use of CAM by children with autism who were included in the Autism Speaks treatment network registry as of April 2011. The participants self-reported their choices of treatment in an organizational survey. This is one of few studies to date that avoided the problem of recruiting bias; that is, most studies estimate CAM use based on a sample of families who expressed interest in participating in a study about CAM and/or who were being treated already in a mainstream pediatric clinic—which may increase estimated prevalence of CAM use, and particularly increase the estimation of CAM use as a supplement rather than as an alternative to "standard" treatment. The psychometric properties of most surveys of CAM use, which are designed informally and unvalidated for the most part, also have been criticized (Toupin et al., 2012). Despite these problems and differences in study design, surveys of patterns of CAM utilization for children have yielded some remarkably consistent findings across countries (Adams et al., 2013; Akins et al., 2006; Akins, Krakowiak, Angkustsiri, Hertz-Picciotto, & Hansen, n.d.; Chugh, Erickson, & Fermin, 2006; Italia, Wolfenstetter, &

Teuner, 2014; Treat et al., 2014; Wray et al., 2014). CAM is used much more often for children with developmental disabilities (autism, ADHD, ID) than for other children. Parents who use CAM for children with developmental-behavioral disorders such as autism or ADHD tend to be more affluent, with higher educational attainment, than those who do not. Parents who use CAM themselves also are more likely to use it for their children. White families generally are more likely to use CAM than Latino or African American families (Akins, Krakowiak, Angkustsiri, Hertz-Picciotto, & Hansen, 2014; Perrin et al., 2012), although a Philadelphia survey of parents using CAM with newly diagnosed autistic children found an increased prevalence among Latino parents (Levy, Mandell, Merhar, Ittenbach, & Pinto-Martin, 2003). There may be some differences across ethnic or cultural groups in what kinds of CAM are most popular; for example, prayer was uncommon among Anglo American parents but a preferred approach for Latina mothers in New York (Chugh et al., 2006; Fortier et al., 2014) and Muslim mothers in Jordan (Aburahma, Khader, Alzoubi, & Sawalha, 2010).

The prevalence of CAM use and preferred types of CAM vary widely across regions of Canada or the United States, as well as across countries. Several large surveys have found more prevalent use of CAM for children with autism than for children with intellectual disabilities, attention deficit disorder, cerebral palsy, or behavioral disorders. More severe and persistent symptoms are associated with greater likelihood of CAM use. In Perrin's U.S. national sample of children with autism (N = 3,413), 17% of the families reported use of special diets and 20% reported use of other CAM approaches (Perrin et al., 2012). That study did *not* include sensory integration therapy, massage, or melatonin in its definition of CAM treatments. Studies that do include those treatments in the definition of CAM yield much higher estimates of use, ranging to 90% of families affected by autism (Kemper et al., 2008). Use of CAM was associated with the presence of gastrointestinal symptoms, seizures, and clinically significant parent-rated behavior problems. Children who were using medications, and those with milder forms of autism (Asperger's disorder or pervasive developmental disorder), were less likely to be using CAM. Perrin and associates also reviewed previous work on CAM in children with autism, indicating that families report having tried an average of seven different types of CAM therapies, either sequentially or simultaneously. Dietary interventions were the most commonly tried. Valicenti-McDermott and colleagues (2014) also reported an association between use of CAM gastrointestinal, behavior, and sleep problems, as well as higher self-reported parental stress, among children with autism whose families were using CAM.

CAM treatments for ADHD are similar, and often the same, as for autism. Just as for children with autism, for the 50% or more of children with ADHD whose families use CAM, the most common treatments are dietary changes or oral supplements (Chan, Rapoport, & Kemper, 2003. For example, the Feingold diet restricts synthetic coloring, flavoring, preservatives, and artificial sweeteners, as well as certain salicylate-containing fruits (apples, grapes). It does not involve restricting sugar. Repeated double-blind studies have shown no effect of sugar on children's behavior. Kemper (2015) cites some studies suggesting decreased hyperactivity or impulsivity among some children with ADHD treated by the Feingold diet, though changes tend to be minimal and impermanent. The Australian Guidelines report no benefit of the Feingold diet based on several well-controlled studies.

The findings that vitamin and mineral deficiencies were more common among children with ADHD than in the general population, and also that children with nutritional deficiencies are more restless and distractible than others, contributed to the idea that adding vitamin and mineral supplements might normalize behavior in children with nutritional deficiencies and ADHD. Megavitamin treatments have been shown to have significant negative side effects, as acknowledged in popular press and websites, and their use has diminished (Christison & Ivany, 2006). This shows that some scientific evidence does get shared in the popular press—particularly when children are made ill by a treatment. Several reviews have concluded that adding standard daily vitamin supplements to a standard balanced diet provides sufficient nutrients, vitamins and minerals, without need for additional supplementation. The strongest clinical evidence of benefit for any nutritional supplement is for zinc supplementation, which may potentiate the effect of methylphenidate treatment for ADHD (Rucklidge, Johnstone, Gorman, Boggis, & Frampton, 2014; Sarris, Kean, Schweitzer, & Lake, 2011; Searight, Robertson, Smith, Perkins, & Searight, 2012). Zinc deficiency contributes to problems of growth and development among malnourished children, although in infants with adequate general nutrition, zinc supplementation does not enhance their development (Gogia & Sachdev, 2012).

There are a few studies about the use of CAM within particular ethnic, cultural, or demographic groups, showing differences in the prevalence and preferences for children, as has been shown for adults (Hsiao et al., 2006). Chugh, Erickson, & Fermin (2005) reported an interview study of 101 low-income Hispanic mothers of general pediatric clinic patients in New York City. Those with higher education, and those who used CAM themselves, reported using CAM to treat their children. Childhood asthma was common, but not associated with any increased use of CAM treatments. Home remedies (30%), herbs (18%), and prayer (12%) were most commonly used. Other strategies were rare (including chiropractic, massage, acupuncture, naturopathy and spiritual healing). Immigration status and acculturation were not found to have an effect on CAM use in this sample.

Why Are So Many Types of CAM Popular If They Don't Work?

CAM Is Big Business With Successful Marketing

There has been significant increase in patient interest in CAM as the cost of traditional medical care has skyrocketed, so some have suggested that CAM is a less costly alternative to allopathic medicine. That might be true for strategies such as prayer or home remedies, but CAM for children doesn't typically save any expense for families of children with neurodevelopmental disorders such as autism or ADHD. Supplements and treatment procedures can be expensive. In 2009, $34 billion was spent on CAM in the United States, including two-thirds for adult self-care and about one third for care of children (Briggs & Killen, 2013). With the exception of acupuncture, chiropractic, and massage therapy, CAM approaches rarely are covered by medical insurance. Moreover, as mentioned earlier, most parents use CAM to complement mainstream medical treatments for their children, not as an alternative.

In some communities, CAM providers advertise and market their services far more heavily and effectively than providers of scientifically supported treatments. Free-market traditions and concerns about restraint of trade make it difficult to inhibit any practice that stays outside of mainstream medicine and does not result in direct physical harm to the patient, even when substantial evidence shows the practice is ineffective. Miller, Shreck, Mulick, and Butter (2012) found that parents' choice of initial treatment for children with autism was heavily influenced by popular media, anecdotal stories of other parents, and nonmedical professionals (most often educators). Educators were somewhat more likely to recommend popular but unsupported treatments for autism (such as sensory integration therapy) than scientifically supported treatments (such as behavioral therapies). Stephenson, Carter, and Kemp (2012) reported that the major national autism websites—a major source of information for parents of newly diagnosed autism—listed 33 treatments, of which only three were scientifically supported. Descriptions of all treatments generally were positive and uncritical. Paradoxically, even negative information about a particular treatment may increase exposure, familiarity, and public awareness of that treatment, and thereby may increase parents' interest in trying it (Skurnik, Yoon, Park, & Schwarz, 2005).

CAM Often Is Marketed and Perceived as "The Natural Choice"

CAM typically is perceived as more "natural," less physically invasive, and less likely to cause unwanted adverse effects, in contrast to allopathic medicine's use of synthetic chemicals or surgical procedures. Concern about adverse effects of environmental toxins and chemicals has extended to worries about vaccines and prescribed medications such as Ritalin, and to the notion that childhood conditions may be cured by removing "bad" chemicals from the body, via dietary restriction, environmental accommodations (such as air filters or avoiding florescent lights), or chelation. Preference for a "natural therapy" differentiated CAM users from nonusers in a large sample of Boston parents of children with ADHD (Chan et al., 2003). Interest in CAM also has been fueled by public awareness that traditional medicine has flaws and limitations, may offer unnecessary invasive treatments or medications with adverse effects, and may sometimes be regulated for profit rather than for quality outcomes.

CAM Often Addresses Symptoms That Bother Parents

The most popular CAM treatments for children address problems such as diarrhea, biting, and sleeplessness, which create tremendous stress for families but generally are not addressed by mainstream pediatric or psychological treatments. Pediatricians may class these as behavior problems rather than "health problems," and may not be aware of resources or strategies to address such issues. The promise of a cure or significant symptomatic improvement is bound to be highly attractive, particularly if it entails no direct adverse consequences.

CAM Often Offers a "Homey" Care Environment

CAM practitioners may emphasize listening and establishing a personal relationship with patients who experience mainstream practitioners as too busy or indifferent to their specific concerns. Meeting in a more "homelike" setting, rather than having to deal with a large clinic or hospital staff, may appeal to some families. The social and physical context of a typical medical center visit—driving into a city, parking, taking elevators, sitting in a waiting room crowded with other children who have medical conditions, talking with a receptionist and nurse before visiting with a uniformed doctor for a strictly limited time period—often is stressful for parents and aversive to children with disabilities, no matter how good the quality of care provided. CAM may be perceived as more compatible with personal, cultural, religious, or spiritual values and beliefs, particularly when parents can select culturally congruent CAM providers.

Providers' Familiarity With Effective Treatment May Be Limited

The popularity of scientifically unsupported CAM is partly due to parents and treating professionals (physicians and educators, in particular) having inadequate information about scientifically supported, effective treatment of autism and other developmental disabilities. Golnik and Ireland (2009) surveyed primary care physicians (each of whom treats, on average, ten children with autism; Dosreis et al., 2006). They found much uncertainty and willingness to endorse whatever the parents already had initiated, as long as it was not directly harmful. Some physicians, educators, and parents may be unaware that there is good-quality evidence for improved function and reduced symptoms associated with mainstream medical and psychological treatment (e.g., Fein, 2011; Floet, Scheiner, & Grossman, 2010).

Parents Face Systemic Obstacles to Choosing Optimal Treatment

Even when providers are well informed, the structure of a typical pediatric practice may not allow adequate time or resources for parent guidance and care coordination. Children with autism are somewhat more likely to find a "medical home" than those with other conditions, and those who do find care coordination tend to do better, but such wrap-around care is not routine (Golnik, Scal, Wey, & Gaillard, 2012; Kogan et al., 2009). Parents are largely on their own to identify, evaluate, access, and coordinate providers and care options for children with developmental disabilities and special health care needs. "Gabe's Care Map" (Figure 45.1) illustrates the caregivers coordinated by one mother of a child with autism (Antonelli & Lind, 2012; this figure is available online at www.childrenshospital.org/care-coordination-curriculum/care-mapping).

Finally, for many children, availability of effective treatment may be limited by financial costs, lack of transportation, and poor interface among the administrative systems of medical care, social services, and special education. For example, early intensive behavioral intervention has been shown to benefit children with autism (Peters-Scheffer, Didden, Korzilius, & Sturmey, 2011) but access to such services varies greatly with income, place of residence, and type of health insurance (Liptak et al., 2008).

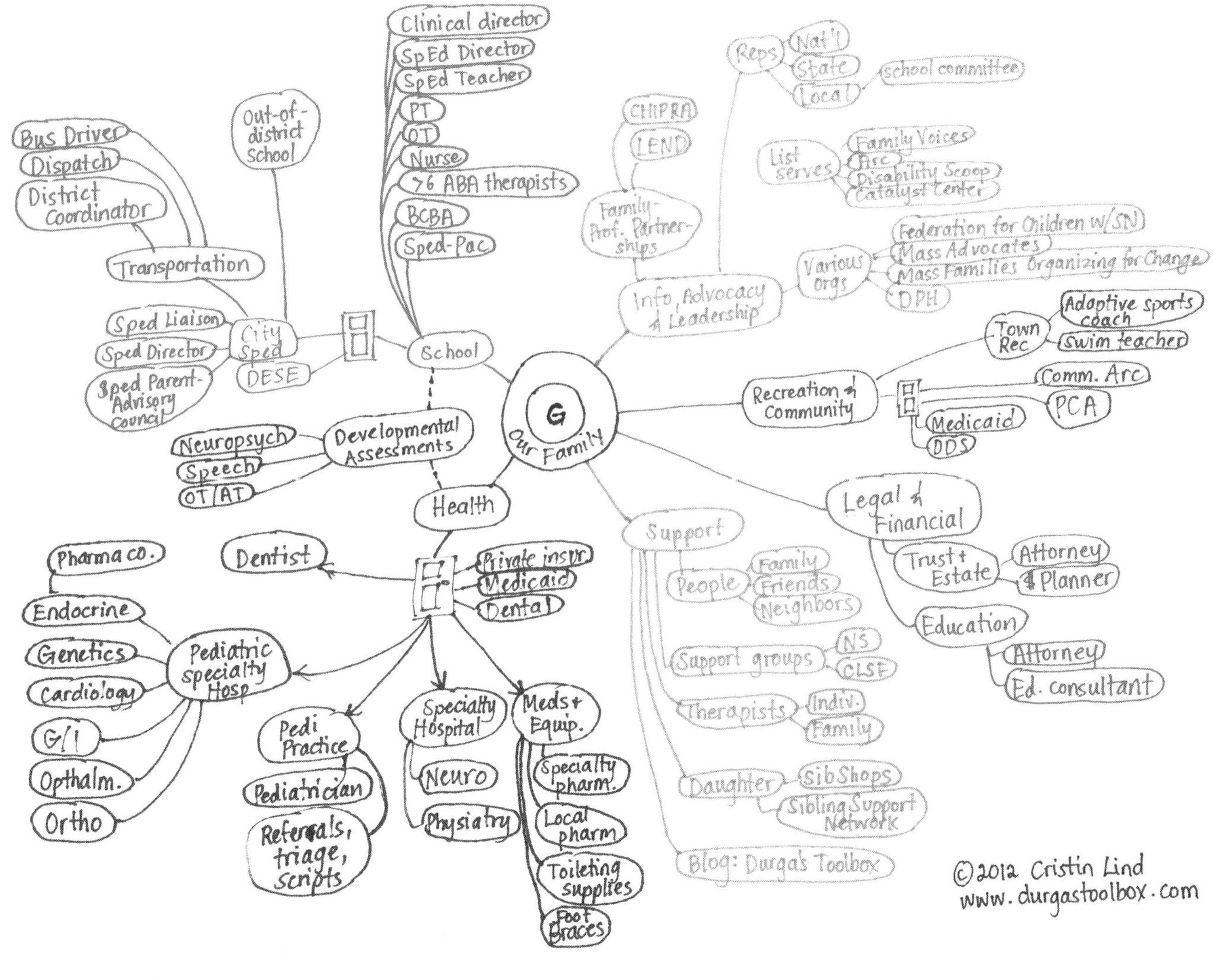

Figure 45.1 Care mapping for a child with autism

Does CAM Work?

As with any heterogeneous group of treatments, a better question is: which, if any, type of CAM works for which problems in which children? Unfortunately, with the exceptions of treating pain and insomnia, there is no consistent evidence of a lasting, substantial, positive effect of any sort of CAM for behavioral or developmental problems in children of any age with any diagnosis. Several studies report a positive effect of melatonin to help regulate sleep onset (Bendz & Scates, 2010; Levy & Hyman, 2002). Relaxation, hypnosis, and massage are effective in managing pain, at least in the short term (see, for example, Rutten, Korterink, Venmans, Benninga, & Tabbers, 2015), but have not been shown to reduce hyperactivity or autistic symptoms in controlled trials. Zinc supplementation, which is better researched than most other oral supplements, may augment the effects of methylphenidate and help sustain concentration, particularly if children are zinc-deficient (Arnold et al., 2011).

The majority of studies of CAM are so poorly designed as to be uninterpretable. A Cochrane review of effects of acupuncture for children with ADHD concludes the following:

> Further well-designed trials are required to confirm or refute its efficacy. Future trials should avoid methodological limitations. In particular, they should include enough participants to detect at least a modest effect; they should ensure adequate concealment of allocation and blinding of participants and outcome assessors; objective and quantifiable tools should be used to assess the short-term outcomes; and participants should be followed up for at least six months to assess the clinically important outcomes.

These conclusions apply to the majority of studies of CAM approaches.

In addition, studies of CAM should specify and measure behavioral targets of intervention more precisely. Recent studies of ADHD treatment outcomes in response to medication and behavioral therapy concluded that changes in symptoms were related to functional, adaptive improvements, but some children showed improved function despite little or no change in clinical symptoms (Karpenko, Owens, Evangelista, & Dodds, 2009).

One of the most interesting things about CAM is that despite widespread negative results and generally discouraging advice from professionals, many parents who use CAM tend to express satisfaction, believe it is helpful, and tell other parents to try it. Perhaps CAM does not actually change the child, but does change the parent, in some meaningful way. Professionals tend to assume that parents simply see what they hope to see, rating improvement unrealistically in its absence. Alternatively, perhaps the perception of "being in treatment" changes parents' levels of intrusiveness or disengagement, frustration versus patience, anxiety versus acceptance, such that the child does respond positively to momentary changes in parental behavior, but doesn't show measureable changes in symptoms or function when observed alone or in school settings, or rated on global measures. If that were true, then there should be observable changes in parent and/or child dyadic interactions when the parent thinks that an effective CAM (or other) treatment has been given, versus when the parent believes the child has had only placebo. This type of study was done using methylphenidate, showing that changes in the child's impulsivity decreased command/control utterances by the mother, but this sort of approach has not yet been used to study how CAM treatments affect parent-child behavioral interactions.

What Harm Does CAM Do?

The financial cost of CAM, which can be high, generally is out-of-pocket because few procedures are covered by medical insurance. Therefore, CAM treatments most commonly are accessed by higher income, higher educated families whose children have conditions that are chronic but not life-threatening. Though many people are very credulous about CAM, many also are skeptical about its efficacy, and well aware there is limited evidence of positive outcomes. Some procedures clearly entailed significant risk of harm, which has been publicized in public media. For example, chelation therapy, wrapping or extreme compression of children with autism, "regression therapy," and use of high-dose megavitamins, have caused serious illness or even death in children and therefore are widely discredited. Some herbal products may be teratogens; may affect breastfeeding infants; or may potentiate, diminish, or conflict with effects of prescribed medications (Buehler, 2007). The consistency, purity, potency, and safety of nutritional supplements, vitamins, and minerals vary and are not regulated (Chan, 2002).

Harm has gradations, however, including costs of time, money, and energy invested in therapies of questionable value, and lost in pursuit of treatments that have a greater likelihood of success. Some treatments (e.g., ABA therapy for autism) may be maximally effective within a particular time window and less effective once that "sensitive period" has passed. Spending hours on scientifically unsupported treatment, such as Sensory Integration Therapy's "sensory diet" (e.g., joint compression, brushing, swinging, and spinning) may block or restrict the onset, duration, frequency, or intensity of more effective treatments (American Academy of Pediatrics, 2012; Hoehn & Baumeister, 1994; Stephenson & Carter, 2009).

From a public health perspective, an ethical response to the proliferation of CAM providers would include building parents' health literacy, skills for critical thinking about treatment options, and support for choosing and coordinating care, as well as regulating the quality and safety of CAM options in the same way that mainstream medical options are regulated (Kennedy, Mercer, Mohr, & Huffine, 2002; Nissen et al., 2013).

What Should Neuropsychologists Consider When Discussing CAM?

Gupta (2010) advises that physicians' communication styles affect parents' trust and willingness to be guided by medical advice about autism treatment:

> The American Academy on Physician and Patient suggests a pneumonic, PEARLS, for this relationship building: partnership, empathy, apology, respect, legitimization, and support. Acknowledging that you will ride with the family in their predicament, supporting and respecting their views and decisions even if they are at variance with your opinions and suggestions as long they do not harm the child; acknowledging the scientific uncertainty about the cause, management, and outcome of autism; asking parents about their view of their child's condition and their expectations; respecting the parents' view of their child's symptoms and causation, acknowledging their suffering, anger, and frustration and assuring them that you will not abandon them even as they seek solutions that you do not agree with, as long as they do not harm the child. Words should be matched by appropriate nonverbal behavior.
>
> (p. 344)

Pappas and Perlman (2002) suggested those exploring parents' reasons for seeking CAM treatments might help to identify concerns about standard treatments that, once aired, could be addressed and resolved. Continuing to monitor the child's response to treatment may provide later opportunities to revisit the decision to pursue an unsupported therapy (Bell, Wallace, Chouinard, Shevel, & Racine, 2011).

Advising families about treatment options for behavioral and developmental problems may involve a pediatric psychologist or neuropsychologist in consultation with the child's primary care provider, other specialists, and educators. How can we help parents make an informed choice? Researchers in education and library science have tested different strategies for teaching people how to critically evaluate what they glean from the Internet or television. One approach involves providing a "checklist" of attributes, typically referencing authoritative sources. To review current knowledge about particular CAM approaches, some resources include: The Physician's Desk Reference for Herbal Medications, the National Center for Complementary and Integrative Health (https://nccam.nih.gov), Quackwatch (www.quackwatch.org), and ConsumerLab.com (www.consumerlab.com) (Buehler, 2007). However, "checking the data" may be insufficient to help with health care decision making, since approximately two-thirds of patients find the scientific data irrelevant, as stated in the May issue of *Mayo Clinic Proceedings* (Bardia, 2007). Another approach to assessing media claims is "contextual" (Meola, 2004)—weighing one source of information against others to seek corroboration or disconfirmation. Figure 45.2 outlines an approach that

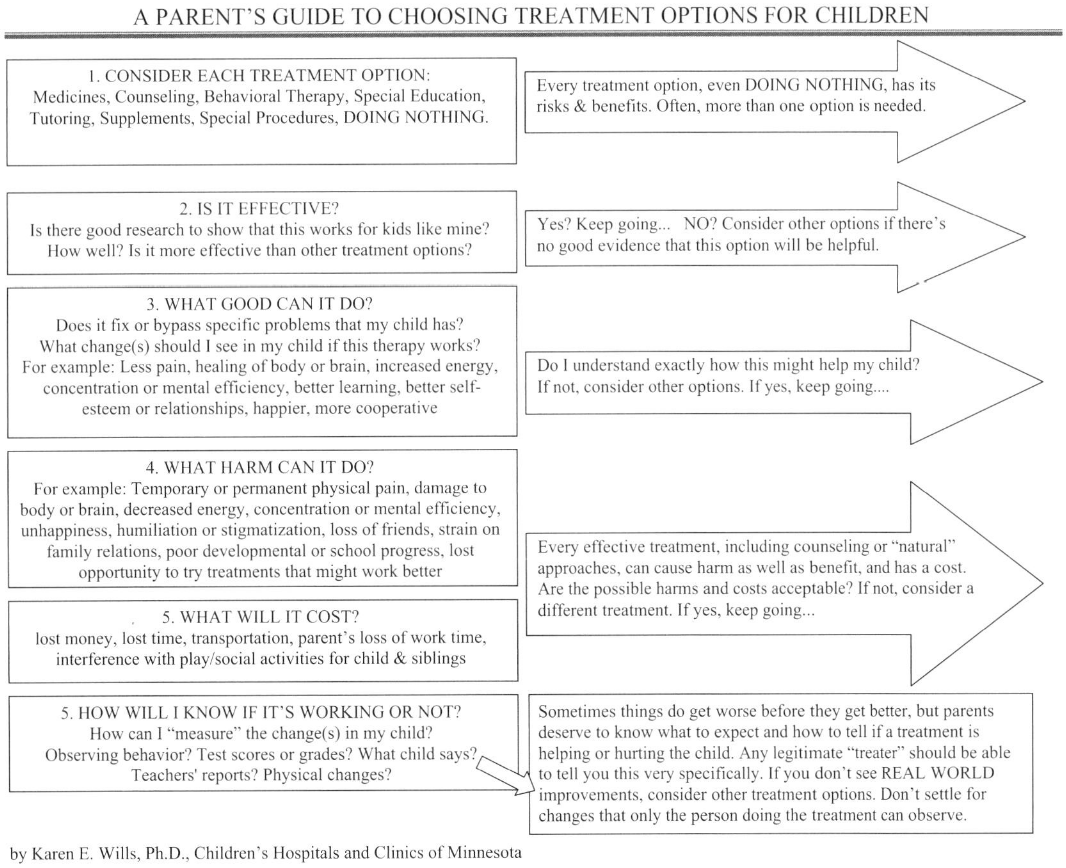

A PARENT'S GUIDE TO CHOOSING TREATMENT OPTIONS FOR CHILDREN
1. CONSIDER EACH TREATMENT OPTION: Medicines, Counseling, Behavioral Therapy, Special Education, Tutoring, Supplements, Special Procedures, DOING NOTHING.
Every treatment option, even DOING NOTHING, has its risks & benefits. Often, more than one option is needed.
2. IS IT EFFECTIVE? Is there good research to show that this works for kids like mine? How well? Is it more effective than other treatment options?
Yes? Keep going... NO? Consider other options if there's no good evidence that this option will be helpful.
3. WHAT GOOD CAN IT DO? Does it fix or bypass specific problems that my child has? What change(s) should I see in my child if this therapy works? For example: Less pain, healing of body or brain, increased energy, concentration or mental efficiency, better learning, better self-esteem or relationships, happier, more cooperative
Do I understand exactly how this might help my child? If not, consider other options. If yes, keep going....
4. WHAT HARM CAN IT DO? For example: Temporary or permanent physical pain, damage to body or brain, decreased energy, concentration or mental efficiency, unhappiness, humiliation or stigmatization, loss of friends, strain on family relations, poor developmental or school progress, lost opportunity to try treatments that might work better
5. WHAT WILL IT COST? lost money, lost time, transportation, parent's loss of work time, interference with play/social activities for child & siblings
Every effective treatment, including counseling or "natural" approaches, can cause harm as well as benefit, and has a cost. Are the possible harms and costs acceptable? If not, consider a different treatment. If yes, keep going...
5. HOW WILL I KNOW IF IT'S WORKING OR NOT? How can I "measure" the change(s) in my child? Observing behavior? Test scores or grades? What child says? Teachers' reports? Physical changes?
Sometimes things do get worse before they get better, but parents deserve to know what to expect and how to tell if a treatment is helping or hurting the child. Any legitimate "treater" should be able to tell you this very specifically. If you don't see REAL WORLD improvements, consider other treatment options. Don't settle for changes that only the person doing the treatment can observe.
by Karen E. Wills, Ph.D., Children's Hospitals and Clinics of Minnesota

Figure 45.2 A parents' guide to choosing treatments

may be useful in assisting parents to critically evaluate CAM treatments, by providing them with a set of questions that can be used to evaluate any treatment—including those of mainstream medicine. This approach honors the autonomy of parents to select their own strategies, while responsibly offering information about the risks and benefits of different treatment options.

Rather than evaluating one particular treatment, parents are encouraged to "chuck the checklist" (Meola, 2004) and consider their various options—conventional and CAM treatments—with regard to relative efficacy, benefit, harm, costs (in money, time, effort, and lost opportunities), desired effects, and measured outcomes. Processing this information with a parent may fulfill some functions that may make CAM attractive, namely, listening to and identifying what is bothering the parent, defining specific targets of intervention according to the family's needs as well as the child's condition, and considering emotional well-being and functional capabilities as well as clinical symptoms and disabilities (Karpenko et al., 2009; Pappas & Perlman, 2002).

References

Aburahma, S. K., Khader, Y. S., Alzoubi, K., & Sawalha, N. (2010). Complementary and alternative medicine use in a pediatric neurology clinic. *Complementary Therapies in Clinical Practice*, *16*(3), 117–120.

Adams, D., Dagenais, S., Clifford, T., Baydala, L., King, W. J., Hervas-Malo, M., . . . Vohra, S. (2013). Complementary and alternative medicine use by pediatric specialty outpatients. *Pediatrics*, *131*(2), 225–232.

Akins, R. S., Krakowiak, P., Angkustsiri, K., Hertz-Picciotto, I., & Hansen, R. L. (2014). Utilization patterns of conventional and complementary/alternative treatments in children with autism spectrum disorders and developmental disabilities in a population-based study. *Journal of Developmental and Behavioral Pediatrics: JDBP*, *35*(1), 1–10.

American Academy of Pediatrics. (2012). Sensory integration therapies for children with developmental and behavioral disorders. *Pediatrics*, *129*(6), 1186–1189.

Antonelli, R., & Lind, C. (2012, October). Care Mapping: An Innovative Tool and Process to Support Family-Centered, Comprehensive Care Coordination. In Poster session presented at the annual Primary Care Innovation Conference of the Harvard Medical School Primary Care Center, Boston, MA.

Arnold, L. E., Disilvestro, R. A., Bozzolo, D., Bozzolo, H., Crowl, L., Fernandez, S., . . . Joseph, E. (2011). Zinc for attention-deficit/hyperactivity disorder: Placebo-controlled double-blind pilot trial alone and combined with amphetamine. *Journal of Child and Adolescent Psychopharmacology*, *21*(1), 1–19.

Atwood, K. (2003). Homeopathy and naturopathy. *Medscape General Medicine*, *5*.

Bardia, A., Nisly, N.L., Zimmerman, M.B., Gryzlak, B.M., & Wallace, R.B. (2007). *Mayo Clinic Proceedings*, 82, 561–566.

Bell, E., Wallace, T., Chouinard, I., Shevel, M., & Racine, E. (2011). Responding to requests of families for unproven interventions in neurodevelopmental disorders: Hyperbaric oxygen "treatment" and stem cell "therapy" in cerebral palsy. *Developmental Disabilities Research Reviews*, *17*(1), 19–26.

Bendz, L. M., & Scates, A. C. (2010). Melatonin treatment for insomnia in pediatric patients with attention-deficit/hyperactivity disorder. *The Annals of Pharmacotherapy*, *44*(1), 185–191.

Benson, H., Greenwood, M., & Klemchuk, H. (1975). The relaxation response: psychophysiologic aspects and clinical applications. *International Journal of Psychiatry and Medicine*, 6, 87–98.

Briggs, J. P. & Killen, J. (2013). Perspectives on complementary and alternative medicine research. *Journal of the American Medical Association*, 310, 691–692.

Buehler, B. A. (2007). Complementary and alternative medicine (CAM) in genetics. *American Journal of Medical Genetics*, 143A, 2889–2892.

Chan, E., Rappaport, L., & Kemper, K.(2003). Complementary and alternative therapies in childhood attention and hyperactivity problems. *Journal of Developmental and Behavioral Pediatrics*, 24, 4–8.

Christison, G. W., & Ivany, K. (2006). Elimination diets in autism spectrum disorders: Any wheat amidst the chaff? *Journal of Developmental and Behavioral Pediatrics: JDBP*, *27*(2 Suppl), S162–S171.

Chugh, R., Erickson, C., & Fermin, M. (2006). Use of complementary and alternative therapies in an Hispanic immigrant inner city population. *Developmental and Behavioral Pediatrics*, *27*(5)444.

DosReis, S., Weiner, C. L., Johnson, L., & Newschaffer, C.J. (2006). Autism spectrum disorder screening and management practices among general pediatric providers. *Journal of Developmental and Behavioral Pediatrics*, *27*:S88–S94.

Eisenberg, D. M., Kessler, R. C., Foster, C., Norlock, F. E., Calkins, D. R., & Delbanco, T. L. (1993). Unconventional medicine in the United States: Prevalence, costs, and patterns of use. *New England Journal of Medicine*, *328*, 246–252.

Ernst, E. (2009). Ethics of complementary medicine: practical issues. *British Journal of General Practice*, 59, 517–519.

Fein, D. (2011). *The Neuropsychology of Autism*. New York: Oxford University Press.

Fortier, M. A., Gillis, S., Gomez, S. H., Wang, S.-M., Tan, E. T., & Kain, Z. N. (2014). Attitudes toward and use of complementary and alternative medicine among Hispanic and white mothers. *Alternative Therapies in Health and Medicine*, *20*(1), 13–19.

Gogia, S., & Sachdev, H. (2012). Zinc supplementation for mental and motor development in children. *Cochrane Database of Systematic Reviews (Online)*, *12*, 1–52.

Golnik, A.E. & Ireland, M. (2009). Complementary alternative medicine for children with autism: a physician survey. *Journal of Autism and Developmental Disorders*, *39*, 996–1005.

Golnik, A., Scal, P., Wey, A., & Gaillard, P. (2012). Autism-specific primary care medical home intervention. *Journal of Autism and Developmental Disorders*, *42*, 1087–1093.

Gupta, V. B. (2010). Communicating with parents of children with autism about vaccines and complementary and alternative approaches. *Journal of Developmental and Behavioral Pediatrics*, *31*, 343–345.

Harrington, J. W., & Allen, K. (2014). The clinician's guide to autism. *Pediatrics in Review/American Academy of Pediatrics*, *35*(2), 62–78.

Hoehn, T.P. & Baumeister, A.A. (1994). A critique of the application of sensory integration therapy to children with learning disabilities. *Journal of Learning Disabilities*, *27*, 338–350.

Hsiao, A.-F., Wong, M. D., Goldstein, M. S., Yu, H.-J., Andersen, R. M., Brown, E. R., . . . Wenger, N. S. (2006). Variation in complementary and alternative medicine (CAM) use across racial/ethnic groups and the development of ethnic-specific measures of CAM use. *Journal of Alternative and Complementary Medicine (New York, N.Y.)*, *12*(3), 281–290.

Kogan M.D., Blumberg S. J., Schieve L. A., Boyle C. A., Perrin JM, Ghandour R. M., Singh G. K., Strickland B. B., Trevathan E, & van Dyck P. C. (2009). Prevalence of parent-reported diagnosis of autism spectrum disorder among children in the US 2007. *Pediatrics*, *124*, 1395–1403.

Italia, S., Wolfenstetter, S. B., & Teuner, C. M. (2014). Patterns of Complementary and Alternative Medicine (CAM) use in children: A systematic review. *European Journal of Pediatrics*.

Karpenko, V., Owens, J. S., Evangelista, N. M., & Dodds, C. (2009). Clinically significant symptom change in children with attention-deficit/hyperactivity disorder: Does it correspond with reliable improvement in functioning? *Journal of Clinical Psychology*, *65*(1), 76–93.

Kemper, K. J., Vohra, S., & Walls, R. (2008). American Academy of Pediatrics: The use of complementary and alternative medicine in pediatrics. *Pediatrics*, *122*(6), 1374–1386.

Kennedy, S. S., Mercer, J., Mohr, W., & Huffine, C. W. (2002). Snake oil, ethics, and the first amendment: What's a profession to do? *The American Journal of Orthopsychiatry*, *72*(1), 5–15.

Levy, S. E., & Hyman, S. L. (2002). Alternative/complementary approaches to treatment of children with autistic spectrum disorders. *Infants & Young Children: An Interdisciplinary Journal of Special Care Practices*, *14*(3), 33–43.

Levy, S. E., Mandell, D. S., Merhar, S., Ittenbach, R. F., & Pinto-Martin, J. A. (2003). Use of complementary and alternative medicine among children recently diagnosed with autistic spectrum disorder. *Journal of Developmental and Behavioral Pediatrics: JDBP*, *24*(6), 418–423.

Liptak, G. S., Benzoni, L. B., Mruzek, D. W., Nolan, K. W., Thingvoll, M. A., Wade, C. M., & Fryer, G. E. (2008). Disparities in diagnosis and access to health services for children with autism: Data from the National Survey of Children's Health. *Journal of Developmental and Behavioral Pediatrics: JDBP*, *29*(3), 152–160.

Meola, M. (2004). Chucking the checklist: A contextual approach to teaching undergraduates web-site evaluation. *Portal: Libraries and the Academy*.

Miller, V. A., Schreck, K. A., Mulick, J. A., & Butter, E. (2012). Factors related to parents' choice of treatments for their children with autism spectrum disorders. *Research in Autism Spectrum Disorders*, *6*, 87–95.

Nissen, N., Weidenhammer, W., Schunder-Tatzber, S., & Johannessen, H. (2013). Public health ethics for complementary and alternative medicine. *European Journal of Integrative Medicine*, *5*(1), 62–67.

Pappas, S. & Perman, A. (2002). Complementary and alternative medicine: the importance of doctor-patient communication. *Medical Clinics of North America*, *86*, 1–10.

Perrin, J. M., Coury, D. L., Hyman, S. L., Cole, L., Reynolds, A. M., & Clemons, T. (2012). Complementary and alternative medicine use in a large pediatric autism sample. *Pediatrics*, *130* (Suppl 2), S77–S82.

Peters-Scheffer, N., Didden, R., Korzilius, H., & Sturmey, P. (2011). A meta-analytic study on the effectiveness of comprehensive ABA-based early intervention programs for children with autism spectrum disorders. *Research in Autism Spectrum Disorders*.

Rucklidge, J. J., Johnstone, J., Gorman, B., Boggis, A., & Frampton, C. M. (2014). Moderators of treatment response in adults with ADHD treated with a vitamin-mineral supplement. *Progress in Neuro-Psychopharmacology and Biological Psychiatry*, *50*, 163–171.

Rutten, J.M.T.M., Korterink, J. J., Venmans, L.M.A. J., Benninga, M. A., & Tabbers, M. M. (2015). Nonpharmacologic treatment of functional abdominal pain disorders: A systematic review. *Pediatrics*, *135*(3), 522–535.

Sarris, J., Kean, J., Schweitzer, I., & Lake, J. (2011). Complementary medicines (herbal and nutritional products) in the treatment of Attention Deficit Hyperactivity Disorder (ADHD): A systematic review of the evidence. *Complementary Therapies in Medicine*.

Searight, H. R., Robertson, K., Smith, T., Perkins, S., & Searight, B. K. (2012). Complementary and alternative therapies for pediatric attention deficit hyperactivity disorder: A descriptive review. *ISRN Psychiatry*, *2012*, 804127.

Skurnik, I., Yoon, C., Park, D. C., & Schwarz, N. (2005). How warnings about false claims become recommendations. *Journal of Consumer Research*, *31*, 713–724.

Stephenson, J. & Carter, M. (2009). The use of weighted vests with children with autism spectrum disorders and other disabilities. *Journal of Autism and Developmental Disorders, 39*, 105–114.

Stephenson, J., Carter, M., & Kemp, C. (2012). Quality of the information on educational and therapy interventions provided on the web sites of national autism associations. *Research in Autism Spectrum Disorders*, *6*, 11–18.

Synovitz, L., & Larson, K. (2013). *Complementary and Alternative Medicine for Health Professionals*. Burlington, MA: Jones & Bartlett.

Toupin, A. K., Rader T, Hawker G. A., Stacey D, O'Connor A. M., Welch V, Lyddiatt A, McGowan J, Thorne J. C., Bennett C, Pardo Pardo J, Wells G. A., Tugwell P. (2012). Development and alpha-testing of a stepped decision aid for patients considering nonsurgical options for knee and hip osteoarthritis management. *Journal of Rheumatology, 43*, 1891–1896.

Treat, L., Liesinger, J., Ziegenfuss, J. Y., Humeniuk, K., Prasad, K., & Tilburt, J. C. (2014). Patterns of complementary and alternative medicine use in children with common neurological conditions. *Global Advances In Health and Medicine*, *3*(1), 18–24.

Valicenti-McDermott, M., Burrows, B., Bernstein, L., Hottinger, K., Lawson, K., Seijo, R., . . . Shinnar, S. (2014). Use of complementary and alternative medicine in children with autism and other developmental disabilities: Associations with ethnicity, child comorbid symptoms, and parental stress. *Journal of Child Neurology*, *29*(3), 360–367.

Wray, J., Edwards, V., Wyatt, K., Maddick, A., Logan, S., & Franck, L. (2014). Parents' attitudes toward the use of complementary therapy by their children with moderate or severe cerebral palsy. *Journal of Alternative and Complementary Medicine (New York, N.Y.)*, *20*(2), 130–135.

Part IV

Interventions

46 Psychotherapy and the Practice of Clinical Neuropsychology

George P. Prigatano

Introduction

In the first edition of this book, this chapter focused on neuropsychological rehabilitation and the role psychodynamic psychotherapy can play in facilitating a positive rehabilitation outcome (Prigatano, 2008). Since that time, several other clinical neuropsychologists have discussed the role of psychotherapy in the care of brain-dysfunctional patients (e.g., Klonoff, 2010; Laaksonen & Ranta, 2013; Ruff & Chester, 2014). Providing effective psychotherapeutic interventions for patients is an important clinical skill that will help maintain the viability of our profession in the present health care marketplace (Prigatano & Morrone-Strupinsky, 2010). Approximately three-fours of practicing clinical neuropsychologists have their doctorate degree in clinical psychology (Sweet, Meyer, Nelson, & Moberg, 2011) and therefore are indeed in a unique position to provide such services. This chapter attempts to broaden the discussion of the role that psychotherapy may play in the general practice of clinical neuropsychology, where the emphasis is primarily on neuropsychological assessment and secondarily on providing individual psychotherapy for patients who might benefit from such services. It reviews empirical findings and presents case vignettes that illustrate the potential value of psychotherapy (in its different formats) to help reduce depression after stroke as well as to lessen anxiety and depression in patients with multiple sclerosis (MS). It also discusses common issues encountered when attempting to provide psychotherapy for patients who have a reduced awareness of their neuropsychological disturbances following severe traumatic brain injury (TBI). This chapter does not provide an extensive review of the literature on psychotherapy with brain dysfunctional patients or their family members.

A Definition of Psychotherapy

Psychotherapy is an intensely personal dialogue between two individuals that results in a working (or therapeutic) relationship in which one person (the therapist) attempts to help another (the patient or client) cope with a personal problem or problems the latter individual seems to have difficulty managing on his or her own. The personal problem(s) may clearly vary, but often centers on some type of emotional disturbance or severe dissatisfaction with life. Coetzer (2007) has emphasized that many patients with a brain disorder struggle with feelings of loss and grief. Klonoff (2010) has emphasized the need of patients to be realistic about their neuropsychological disturbance and acceptant of those changes. Salas, Vaughan, Shanker, and Turnbull (2013) point out there is a complicated interaction between the cognitive and emotional deficits/changes that a patient experiences. This issue has to be addressed when working with brain dysfunctional patients from a psychotherapeutic perspective. Judd and Wilson (2005) have made a similar point when using the term *neuropsychotherapy* for brain dysfunctional patients (also see the work of Laaksonen & Ranta, 2013). Whatever the personal struggles are for a given patient, ultimately his or her emotional/motivational disturbance frequently interfere with establishing and maintaining mutually satisfying interpersonal relationships. They also can affect multiple domains of functioning include sleep, appetite, automatic control of bodily functions (such as the ability to maintain consciousness in patients with psychogenic seizures or involuntary movements in patients with psychogenic motor disorders), sexual activity, socially appropriate management of angry or aggressive feelings, and the capacity to remain productive (e.g., work) at a level appropriate to the person's abilities throughout the life cycle. They disrupt the person's sense of meaning to his or her life and deprive the person of an inner peace and sense of joy from living (Prigatano, 1991).

For psychotherapeutic dialogue to be successful, the therapist needs professional training in understanding the nature of the patient's personal struggles as well as his or her neuropsychological strengths and limitations. The therapist must have the capacity to form a therapeutic relationship and skill at guiding this learning process. Finally, the therapist must have the time and willingness to help the patient. The patient (or client) needs the financial resources to pay for this service, adequate cognitive and emotional/motivational skills to learn from the dialogue, and the willingness to "face the truths" in his or her life.

This learning process can be approached in different ways. Helping patients understand how certain thoughts and feelings aid or hinder their adjustment to their personal problems is crucial. Thus, different forms or approaches to psychotherapy have appeared over the years.

Data on the Efficacy of Psychotherapy for Persons Without Brain Disorders

Before attempting a discussion of whether or not psychotherapy can help brain dysfunctional patients, the broader question of whether psychotherapy can help non-brain-dysfunctional individuals' needs to be considered. Several review papers have documented the potential value of cognitive behavioral therapy (CBT) for treatment of a depression and anxiety in non-brain-dysfunctional patients (Beltman, Oude Voshaar, & Speckens, 2010; Covin, Ouimet, Seeds, & Dozois, 2008; Gould, Coulson, & Howard, 2012; Hofmann & Smits, 2008; Jakobsen, Hansen, Storebo, Simonsen, & Gluud, 2011; Mitte, 2005; Spek et al., 2007; Stewart & Chambless, 2009). This form of psychotherapy is presently quite popular and has been applied to various patient groups. Psychodynamic psychotherapy is often seen as less effective and clearly not cost-effective. There is a common misconception that there is a lack of empirical support for this form of psychotherapy.

In an extremely useful and frequently cited review paper, Shedler (2010) presents convincing evidence for the efficacy of psychodynamic psychotherapy. He notes that many of the features of CBT are actually based on psychodynamic approaches to psychotherapy. This may contribute to both forms of psychological treatment being useful in reducing anxiety and depression in non-brain-dysfunctional individuals. They include the establishment of a good working or therapeutic alliance and having the patient experience how emotions can influence the thinking process and vice versa. Both forms of therapy note that the patient's enhanced awareness of how implicit feelings and beliefs (i.e., meanings) greatly influence behavior and mood can contribute to a good treatment outcome.

An important observation of Shedler (2010) that is relevant to the psychological care of brain-dysfunctional individuals is that: "The goals of psychodynamic therapy include, but extend beyond, symptom remission. Successful treatment should not only relieve symptoms (i.e., get rid of something), but also foster the positive presence of psychological capacities and resources" (p.100). This is often the goal when helping individuals adjust to the permanent effects of brain disorder.

Shedler's (2010) meta-analytic review notes a consistent trend in which psychodynamic therapy with non-brain-dysfunctional patients leads to continue improved psychological adjustment after therapy has ended. Under what conditions this may be accomplished when working with patients with brain disorders is an important question that clinical neuropsychologists, who are trained in psychodynamic psychotherapy, may well help to answer in the future.

Finally, Shedler (2010) notes that various meta-analyses reveal that the overall effect sizes of psychotherapy for treating depression can be substantial. It is not uncommon to demonstrate a size effect of 0.73 (see Robinson, Berman, & Neimeyer, 1990). In contrast, "the overall mean effect size for antidepressant medications approved by the FDA between 1987 and 2004 was 0.31" (Turner, Matthews, Linardatos, Tell, and Rosenthal, 2008, p. 100). These observations should help clinical neuropsychologists who want evidence-based treatments to serious consider the potential role of psychodynamic psychotherapy, as well as CBTs when helping their patients with symptom relief and improving their long-term adjustment to neuropsychological consequences of their brain disorder.

Neuropsychological Assessment and the Beginnings of a Psychotherapeutic Dialogue

In the course of interviewing patients and conducting clinical neuropsychological examinations, patients often reveal their personal concerns and emotional reactions to their neuropsychological disturbances. If the examining clinical neuropsychologist shows an interest in them and not just the patient's test scores, the professional relationship is enhanced (Prigatano, 1999a). Within the confines of that relationship, the patient and/or family may directly or indirectly express a need for psychotherapeutic consultation to help them deal with the neuropsychological disturbances in everyday life.

Repeatedly, patients report increased irritability, anxiety, and depression as they attempt to cope with their cognitive limitations (e.g., Sherer & Sander, 2014). After the neuropsychological examination is completed, it is not uncommon for patients (or family members) to ask what can be done to improve their cognitive status and reduce emotional distress. Depending on the extent of their cognitive impairments and degree of impaired "executive functions or ego functions," different forms of psychological interventions may be attempted (Prigatano, 2016). If a patient has adequate impulsive control and a basic capacity and willingness to observe and understand his or her own cognitions, feelings, and behavior, then psychotherapy should be attempted by the clinical neuropsychologist, who understands the patient's brain-behavior difficulties and has a willingness and professional training to help the patient improve his or her psychological adjustment to the effects of the brain disorder. This requires time, patience, and clinical skill on the part of the clinical neuropsychologist.

Depression and Psychotherapy After Cerebral Vascular Accident (or Stroke)

Clinically defined depression is common after stroke (Robinson, 2003). Prevalence rates vary depending on the measurement techniques and the time of assessment following stroke.

Estimates of major depressive disorder are in the range of 20%, while estimates of minor depression range from 9% to 18%. During the acute phases following stroke (i.e., one to two months), left frontal and left basal ganglia lesions are frequently observed in severely depressed individuals (Starkstein & Robinson, 1993) Prolonged depression, several months or years poststroke, is associated with multiple factors. They include a history of previous psychiatric disorder as well as dependence in activities of daily living (Robertson, 1997).

Literature reviews (e.g., Eldred & Sykes, 2008) frequently report that various forms of psychosocial support for the patient with a stroke and family caregivers helps improve psychological health, which includes reducing depression. The nature of "effective interventions," however, is often not clearly specified, which is understandable giving this diverse patient population.

The most recent Cochrane review on "Interventions for treating depression after stroke" (Hackett, Anderson, House, & Xia, 2008) concluded:

> There was some evidence of benefit of pharmacotherapy in terms of complete remission of depression and a reduction (improvement) in scores on depression rating scales, but there was also evidence of an associated increase in adverse events. There was no evidence of benefit of psychotherapy.
>
> (p.1)

The last conclusion was rather surprising in light of the clinical experience of psychotherapists that depression can be reduced via psychotherapy (e.g., Robinson et al., 1990). A close reading of this Cochrane review highlights some important methodological limitations that can be easily glossed over if one is not an experienced psychotherapist.

Hackett et al. (2008) limited their review to randomized controlled trials only (RCTs) and had rather strict exclusion criteria. Consequently, only three clinical trials were evaluated regarding the impact of psychotherapy on depression. Four studies, however, were reviewed. While the sample size of 445 patients was relatively impressive, the studies that Hackett and colleagues cite were not. One study was described as offering a counseling approach to problem solving conducted by social workers. A second study was described as a structured CBT program offered by nurses. A third study was on motivational interviewing that was "delivered by nurses and non-clinical psychologists" (p. 8).The fourth study was described as "a supportive psychological intervention including education delivery by special personnel" (p. 8).

Most experienced psychotherapists would hardly consider this a test of the efficacy of psychotherapy for depression after stroke. Too often such reviews (which can be quite influential from an academic and insurance coverage point of view) focus on strict methodology, without fully understanding the phenomena that is being studied or reported to being studied (see Prigatano, 1999b). Consequently, erroneous conclusions can be put forward which are damaging to patient care.

What is actually involved in the psychotherapy of patients who suffer some form of intracranial hemorrhage? First, a careful assessment of lesion type, location, and resultant neurocognitive and neuroaffective disorders is necessary. Second, the acuteness of the patient's clinical condition is considered before deciding on whether some form of psychotherapy is warrant. Acute and severely aphasic patients following left hemisphere stroke or acute confusional patients with hemineglect or anosognosia following right hemisphere (AHP) stroke should be made comfortable, but attempts at psychotherapeutic interventions would seem premature. As patients recover and start to communicate about their clinical condition, depression can then be assessed. This can be done through an interview or having the patient complete various brief questionnaires concerning behavior, mood, and thought patterns.

Dialogue with the patient and the family is aimed at providing supportive diagnostic and at times prognostic information in the hopes of developing a therapeutic or working alliance. Once a trusting relationship is established, then gentle probes regarding how one might best help the person (and family members) fully engage rehabilitation activities and reduce the potential adverse effects of severe depression on recovery and social interactions are considered. This is a highly individual process that keeps in mind the patient's age, educational level, occupational history, psychiatric history, gender, cultural and religious values, aspirations in life, and traditional methods of coping with loss or tragedy in life. While these are variables that any experienced psychotherapist would consider, other important variables need to be assessed and worked into a treatment plan.

An understanding of the direct and indirect effects of a brain disorder for a given patient is crucial (Goldstein, 1952; Prigatano, 1999a). Helping the patient make adaptive choices in face of permanent neuropsychological deficits is perhaps one of the most useful services that a clinical neuropsychologist can provide, especially during the postacute and chronic phases following a brain disorder (as Goldstein, 1952 noted several years ago). Educating the patient regarding the effects of a stroke on certain higher integrative brain functions is crucial in this regard. If the patient does not know "what is wrong," he or she cannot take steps to cope with impairments. Likewise, the clinical neuropsychologist, if properly trained in psychotherapy, can help patients made adaptive choices that restore, in part, their sense of dignity as they relate to key family members (see Prigatano, 2011a). Finally, the treating psychotherapist needs to be clinically sensible, as well as clinically sensitive (see Prigatano, 1999a). Considerations as to where in life a patient is, what his or her psychosocial situation consists of, what his or her premorbid psychological adjustment history was like, and the extent of present neuropsychological strengths and limitations, must guide any attempt at psychotherapeutic interventions. There is no easy formula for guiding the psychotherapy process with different patients. The first goal, of course, is to do no harm to patients, followed by the goal of helping them cope with the effects of a brain injury in light of the variables noted above. The clinical neuropsychologist must be able to draw on large bodies of knowledge found in clinical psychology and psychiatry when attempting this work (Prigatano, 2011b).

Research on psychotherapy for depression after right and left hemisphere stroke should continue to clarify how to best describe the specific and general effects of such lesions on the patient's mood, behavior and cognitive capacities. Such studies are needed before global studies on its effectiveness of psychotherapy can be meaningfully assessed. Specific case examples provide clues on how to best treat these patients from a psychotherapeutic perspective.

Pinhasi-Vittorio (2007) eloquently describes work with an aphasic patient that reflects the confusion and frustration of many aphasic individuals. When the patient came to the point of wanting to give up on a therapeutic exercise because he felt so incompetent, the therapist recalled Luria's (1972) book, *Man with a Shattered World.* She asked the patient to write ten to 20 minutes each day because writing consisted of "kinetic melodies" that may facilitate the recovery of certain aspects of language. The patient did this and it was a "turning point" in helping him. He now wrote poetry that conveyed his authentic experiences (not just a boring speech and language exercise). As a result, he became more "proactive in his healing process" (Pinhasi-Vittorio, 2007, p. 118). This is a realistic description of how a psychotherapeutic experience (provided by linguist/therapist) with an aphasic patient makes a real difference in that patient's life.

Patients with right hemisphere lesions often have adequate language function, but can suffer with ill-defined visual spatial deficits that impact their lives in unpredictable fashions and can lead to significant depression. Several years ago, a 33-year-old woman was referred to me for treatment of depression. She was approximately three years post a ruptured arteriouvenous malformation (AVM) involving the right parietal lobe. To my surprise, she was a physician, but she did not refer to herself as a doctor. She stopped using the MD initials after her name and now worked as a statistician in a hospital.

She never received a neuropsychological examination after surgical resection of her AVM. She attempted to return to her residency program in radiology after she made an apparently good neurological recovery. She was not knowledgeable about why she had difficulty perceiving different "shadows" on the imaging films and consequently left her residency program because she could not meet academic requirements. She was understandably very depressed because her one aspiration in life was to be a doctor.

Her psychotherapy brought to light the importance of Freudian and Jungian ideas when helping brain dysfunctional patients cope with their personal losses (e.g., the phenomena of transference, the relationship between anger and depression, and the underlying and at times unconscious motivations to pursue certain careers). Moreover, her dreams and poetry revealed all of the frustrations and psychodynamics of not living up to one's personal aspirations in life. In the context of dealing with her anger toward life and resultant depression, a therapeutic "turning point" also occurred for her. I want to emphasize this turning point occurred only after a strong therapeutic alliance was established as a result of intensive discussions regarding multiple feelings she had toward me, her husband, and her parents. The patient struggled about whether she should return to some practice of medicine or not, given that she could not be a radiologist.

In the course of psychotherapeutic dialogue, it came up that the patient loved golf. I asked the patient the following question: Suppose you were playing professional golf and found that after attempting to hit the ball, you miss it after several swings. This occurred daily after your intracranial hemorrhage and your doctor's release to go back to playing. Angered and embarrassed you are faced with an existential question: Should you leave the game (i.e., the aspiration to be a radiologist) or play miniature golf on the weekends with friends (be a doctor in a substantially reduced capacity) since you love the "game" so much.

She chose to work for an insurance company conducting histories and physicals. She enjoyed patient care (it gave her a sense of meaning in life) and as a consequence her depression slowly resolved into predictable human sadness over a major loss in life. Her neuropsychological rehabilitation was successful in large part due to the impact of psychotherapy.

These two case vignettes highlight the notion that understanding the patients' cognitive deficits (the direct effect of a brain injury) and their personality prior to their brain disorder can substantially help reduce their reactionary depression (an indirect effect of a brain lesion). Note these patients had posterior brain lesions not directly affecting frontal mediated cognitive processes.

Multiple Sclerosis, Anxiety, and Depression

MS is a common neurological disorder that results in demyelination of axons and the formulation of sclerotic plagues. The neurocognitive impairments include deceased speed of information processing and problem solving, impaired verbal and visuospatial learning, and a reduction in working memory (Thornton & DeFreitas, 2009). Emotional disturbances are also common, especially depression. Feinstein (2011) suggests that significant depression can affect up to 50% of patients with MS. Anxiety is also very common in depressed MS patients (Burns, Siddique, Fokuo, & Mohr, 2010).

A Cochrane review (Thomas, Thomas, Hillier, Galvin, & Baker, 2006) cautiously recommended that various sources of psychological interventions potentially could help MS patients with their anxiety and depression. They specially noted that the variable and unpredictable nature of symptoms could certainly increase the psychological distress level of patients.

Brief relaxation training has been showed to reduce anxiety in MS patients (Artemiadis et al., 2012). Small group exercises to help MS patients maintain an active life style also appear to be of help (Nordin & Rorsman, 2012). Grossman et al. (2010), in a randomized trial, demonstrated that mindfulness-based intervention improved not only the quality of life of MS patients, but resulted in substantial declines in depression, anxiety, and fatigue.

In a recent randomized trial, MS patients were taught behavioral stress management therapies to improve their coping skills (Mohr et al., 2012). Participants who received such training not only reported a reduction in their stress levels, but also their magnetic resonance imaging (MRI) scans of the brain revealed fewer new gadolinium-enhancing lesions. The effect was present only when actually receiving the therapies. While the effect did not sustain itself after the therapies were concluded, the findings suggest a very interesting possibility. Not only do the patients feel better during their time of their psychological treatment, but fewer lesions develop during this time. Sustained efforts at treatment may prove clinically helpful for some individuals.

While sustained efforts at cognitive behavioral strategies may be very helpful, also helping the individuals understand how their approach to life (i.e., their basic psychodynamics) may aid or hinder their adjustment to MS should be seriously considered. For example, a 32-year-old professional man who was diagnosed as having MS was constantly fatigued. His wife had very unrealistic expectations of what she considered he should do at home despite his MS and associated fatigue. Given his dependence on maternal approval (which was only partly recognized by him), it was very difficult for him to set appropriate boundaries with his wife. His fatigue worsened as did his depression. These realities are seldom discussed when evaluating the effectiveness of psychotherapy in helping MS patients. Individual psychodynamic insights do not lend themselves to randomized control studies. Yet, they may be crucial ingredients to the effectiveness of psychotherapeutic interventions.

In the early 1970s, I was asked to examine a 50-year-old male who had been diagnosed as having MS for at least ten years. He was now complaining of memory difficulties. At that time, many neurologists did not believe that MS patients should have memory difficulties. Using the old Wechsler Memory Scale, I demonstrated to the patient and his neurologist that he indeed had memory difficulties relative to his intelligence. Also, during that time in my career, I administered the Rorschach. When I got to Card VIII, he refused to offer any response to this card. He turned it over and asked to see the next card.

After the neurologist got my neuropsychological report, he acknowledged to the patient that indeed the patient did have memory difficulties. The patient felt vindicated in his complaints and asked to see me again. He wanted to know if I could help him with his depression and anger over having MS. We begin talking in weekly psychotherapy sessions about his life. He told me some general facts about his childhood and why he choose to be an engineer. With time he also spoke about how he often was uncomfortable with women, but eventually married his wife of some 30 years.

In conjoint sessions with his wife, she talked about her husband getting very angry, very quickly over what appeared to be slight frustrations in life. After several other individual sessions with this patient, he asked me to pull out the Rorschach cards and specially show him Card VIII. He then gave me his perceptions of what the card looked like to him and stated that when he looked at this card he was reminded of his mother. As an adolescent boy his mother would approach him in a negligee and ask him to rub her back. He was both sexually excited and scared by these repeated experiences. This always occurred when his father was not home. He did not want to be alone with his mother (and now knew why he probably was uncomfortable as a man when being alone with women). This is a prime example frequently observed in psychodynamic psychotherapy. The goal is not to simply focus on the past, but to understand how the past sheds light on current psychological difficulties (see Shedler, 2010).

With the help of psychotherapy, he began to be less angry and less frightened about his disease. He accepted his wife's help with his physical limitations and could also accept he could no longer function as an engineer in light of his memory difficulties. He experienced a certain internal peace of mind and his anger was substantially reduced.

While both of these MS patients had diffuse white matter lesions, their "executive" or "ego" functions remained intact. Clinically, this seemed to help them reflect on the psychotherapeutic dialogue and benefit from discussions about how previous relationships, recurring themes in their life, and how powerful emotions that they did not seem to fully understand influenced their behavior in a maladaptive fashion. These are key topics frequently discussed in psychodynamic psychotherapy (Shedler, 2010).

Denial/Unawareness of Impaired Neuropsychological Functioning after Severe Traumatic Brain Injury

Early efforts at neuropsychological rehabilitation of patients with moderate to severe TBI noted the importance of impaired self-awareness (ISA) as a deterrent to successful outcomes, particularly the ability to maintain gainful employment (Prigatano et al., 1984). Subsequent and recent reviews have also identified ISA in TBI patients as an important predictor of rehabilitation outcome (see Sherer & Sander, 2014). Sherer and Fleming (2014) provide a comprehensive review of various treatment approaches to improve self-awareness after TBI. Psychotherapy is considered as one possible alternative, and they provide a case example of how it might be approached.

A key issue when providing psychotherapy for patients with moderate or severe TBI who show poor self-awareness of their residual neuropsychological disturbances, is obtaining a realistic understanding of what is causing their apparent lack of awareness. In some instances, significant frontal contusions in the presence of diffuse axonal injury seem to underlie the disturbances. These patients often show many neuropsychological signs of severe executive dysfunction. In other instances, the picture is more complex. The patient may show not only signs of "organically" based ISA, but behave in a manner suggestive of denial of disability (see Prigatano & Klonoff, 1997; Prigatano, 2014). The psychotherapeutic approach to patients with these two conditions can be different.

In the former case in which significant executive dysfunction is present, traditional forms of psychodynamic therapy may not be especially helpful, as noted in our early work (Prigatano, Fordyce, Roueche, Pepping, & Wood, 1986) and as recently emphasized by Ben-Yishay and Diller (2016). These patients present with significant disturbances in what psychodynamic therapists refer to as "ego-functions" and what Goldstein (1952) referred to as disturbance in the "abstract attitude." These patients may have a difficult time introspecting and understanding how past relationships with significant others may influence their behavior in the present. More importantly, their behavioral and associated emotional and motivation reactions may be a direct effect of severe bilaterial frontal-temporal lobe damage (not psychodynamic conflicts). Thus, their behavioral and personal adjustment issues may be best treated by providing them carefully constructed feedback concerning their behaviors (particularly within the context of a milieu rehabilitation program) in a manner they can "concretely" understand (see Ben-Yishay & Diller, 2016). Within the context of a therapeutic environment, they can be taught specific methods of copy that result in improved social integration and adjustment. They do require, however, a therapist who can deal with the broader issues of establishing meaning in life despite their severe cognitive impairments (see Prigatano, 1999a). Table 46.1 summarizes key components when attempting psychotherapy with this group of patients.

Patients with less severe brain injuries and more intact ego-functions, however, potentially may benefit from traditional forms of psychotherapy, including psychodynamic-oriented psychotherapy. This appears to be especially true when the problem is mediated more by psychological denial than severe ISA. One example is that of a young man who had a moderate TBI and who refused to admit to any substantial cognitive difficulties. He was frequently belligerent and argued that whatever difficulties he had performing neuropsychological tests were irrelevant or existed prior to his injury. He showed many of the behaviors that Klonoff and Lage (1991) described as "narcissistic injuries." Helping him face his tendency for risk taking and propensity to engage in addictive behaviors slowly resulted in his acknowledging that his memory was indeed compromised. After several years of psychotherapy, he began to make more adaptive choices regarding work and interpersonal relationships. These types of patients are perhaps the most difficult to treat, but helping them understand the psychological basis of their denial is crucial for a successful outcome. Working closely with a psychiatrist who can provide psychotropic mediations as needed is also very important when working with these individuals.

Table 46.2 provides some guidelines when attempting psychodynamic psychotherapy with brain-dysfunctional patients who have relatively intact ego or executive functions.

Table 46.1 Suggestions for conducting psychotherapy after brain injury when there has been significant disruption of higher integrative brain functions and patient requires a holistic, milieu-oriented neuropsychological rehabilitation program (adapted from Prigatano et al., 1986)

1	Provide a model or models that help the patient understand what has happened to him or her.
2	Help the patient deal with the meaning of the brain injury in his or her life.
3	Help the patient achieve a sense of self-acceptance and forgiveness for himself or herself and others who may have caused the accident.
4	Help the patient make realistic commitments to work and interpersonal relations.
5	Teach the patient how to behave in different social situations (to improve competence).
6	Provide specific behavioral strategies for compensating for neuropsychological deficits.
7	Foster a sense of realistic hope.

Table 46.2 General considerations relevant to successful psychotherapy with persons who have a brain injury, but relatively preserved executive or ego functions

1	The psychotherapist should help the patient understand "basic facts" about all human beings and how they apply their particular background and psychodynamics (Prigatano, 2011b) (e.g., the role of sex and aggression in animal and human behavior; the struggle to find meaning in life; parental influences in forming social attitudes and choices of a partner and work preferences, etc.)
2	The psychotherapist must understand the nature of the patient's neuropsychological strengths and limitations and focus the psychotherapeutic dialogue in a manner that is understandable to him or her (Prigatano, 2012).
3	The patient's life history should be explored and the psychotherapist should encourage introspection on the patient's part as to what has most influenced his or her behavior, thought processes, decisions in life, and methods of copying with adversity.
4	The psychotherapist should gently point out or make explicit how recurring themes/perceptions in the patient's life have helped him or her to adapt to certain situations or conversely resulted in repeated poor adaptations with increased anxiety, depression, and/or anger. This should be done in an empathetic, nonjudgmental fashion.
5	The psychotherapist should listen carefully to what the patient says about him- or herself and restate it back in a manner that allows them "to hear" what exactly he or she is saying (i.e., experiencing) (Rogers, 1961; Prigatano, 2011b). This often helps the patient consciously experience ambivalent or even contradictory subjective feeling states.
6	The psychotherapist must understand the important symbols that guide a given patient's life before and after brain injury and use those symbols (including metaphors) to help the patient cope with his or her daily problems and adjust to the long-term effects of the brain injuries (Prigatano, 1999a, 2012).
7	The psychotherapist should encourage the patient to discuss dreams that come up at certain points in the psychotherapy and what they may mean as he or she faces different issues/problems in the "here and now."
8	The psychotherapist should encourage the patient to use various art forms (writing poetry, storytelling, painting, drawings, etc.) to help clarify his or her subjective experience. The patient's favorite songs and fairy tales provide rich insights into core features of the patient's personality that the patient may not be able to verbally identify.
9	The psychotherapist should encourage the patient to view anxiety and depression as behavioral reactions to life's problems. Since life always presents problems, anxiety and depression will never go away, but they can be reduced as the patient better understands themselves and what is the best plan of action for them when dealing with their struggles in life.
10	The psychotherapist should help the patient remain as productive as possible and work at establishing and maintaining love relationships. This has to be done with a full recognition of the individuality of the patient and his or her long-term struggle to deal with their sense of "lost normality" (Prigatano, 1991, 1999a).

The Strength and Limitation of the Therapeutic Alliance in Psychotherapy

While the therapeutic alliance is clearly an important component to various forms of psychotherapy, it is crucial to recognize it is often not a sufficient condition to produce meaningful change in the patient's life. This error is frequently made and is reflected in the title of Schofield's (1964) book: *Psychotherapy: The Purchase of Friendship.* For example, a strong therapeutic alliance does relate to work productivity after neuropsychological rehabilitation (Prigatano et al., 1994; Klonoff, Lamb, & Henderson, 2001), but not necessarily to job satisfaction (Lustig, Strauser, Weems, Donnell, & Smith, 2003). Job and interpersonal satisfaction often requires the patient to have greater insight into his or her motivations, past and present.

Martin, Garske, and Davis (2000) define the therapeutic alliance "as the collaborative and affective bond between therapist and patient" (p. 438). Their meta-analytic review on the role of the therapeutic alliance on treatment outcome is informative. First, there are many scales for measuring the therapeutic alliance, and the reliability of these scales is good (average reliability was 0.79 based on 93 reliability indices). It is a "real" phenomenon that can be consistently measured. Second, and most importantly, Martin et al. (2000) reports a conservative estimate of the effect size on psychotherapeutic outcome to be 0.22 when reviewing 79 studies. They emphasize that this is a conservative estimate because of the heterogeneity of the study samples. They conclude that the therapeutic alliance has moderate—not mild or minor—effect on treatment outcome. This has been my clinical experience as well. The therapeutic alliance is a necessary, but not sufficient condition for successful psychotherapy outcomes in many patient groups, including those with brain disorders. Successful psychotherapy with brain-dysfunctional patients requires a broad knowledge of learning theory and practices, the biological basis of behavior (and cognition), psychodynamic theory in its psychoanalytic and analytic forms (Prigatano, 2012), and an appreciation of how a particular patient's developmental and cultural history influences his or her view of life and what makes it meaningful or meaningless (Prigatano, 2011a). Insight—yoked with practical suggestions for behavioral changes—is often necessary for meaningful emotional/motivational change. In this latter regard, patients must have the desire, and the cognitive and behavioral skills, to implement change given the support and the relationship they experience with their psychotherapist.

Summary Observations and Conclusions

Clinical neuropsychologists, who have expert knowledge regarding brain-behavior relationships, are in a unique position to provide psychotherapy services for some of their assessment patients. The neuropsychological examination provides a unique opportunity to provide feedback to patients (and their family members) that helps clarify the cognitive, behavioral, and affective disturbances that are directly or indirectly related to a known or suspected underlying brain disorder. This process fosters an initial sense of trust and understanding that is crucial to begin psychotherapeutic dialogue. This chapter attempts to highlight how this may proceed when working with the problems of depression after stroke; the depression and anxiety associated with MS; and the complex disturbances of ISA and denial of disability often encountered in persons who have a history of severe TBI. There are also many other brain-dysfunctional patient groups that could also benefit from psychotherapy that are not considered in this chapter. The major point of this chapter, however, is that if the clinical neuropsychologist has training in various forms of psychotherapy, and the time and patience to work with these patients, the process of providing psychotherapy for brain-dysfunctional patients can be an extremely important and rewarding professional activity (Klonoff, 2010; Laaksonen & Ranta, 2013; Ruff & Chester, 2014). It requires, however, that the clinical neuropsychologist has adequate skill and knowledge to understand the patient's subjective experiences that fuel anxiety and depression. It also requires the clinical neuropsychologist to understand how patients' psychological development and present neuropsychological status must be considered when talking to them and guiding them when dealing with their life's problems and decisions.

References

Artemiadis, A. K., Vervainioti, A. A., Alexopoulos, E. C., Rombos, A., Anagnostouli, M. C., & Darviri, C. (2012). Stress management and multiple sclerosis: A randomized controlled trial. *Archives of Clinical Neuropsychology*, *27*(4), 406–416.

Beltman, M. W., Oude Voshaar, R. C., & Speckens, A. E. (2010). Cognitive-behavioral therapy for depression in people with a somatic disease: Meta-analysis of randomized controlled trials. *The British Journal of Psychiatry*, *197*, 11–19.

Ben-Yishay, Y., & Diller, L. (2016). *Turning Points*. Youngsville, NC: Lash & Associates Publishing/Training Inc.

Burns, M. N., Siddique, J., Fokuo, J. K., & Mohr, D. C. (2010). Comorbid anxiety disorders and treatment of depression in people with multiple sclerosis. *Rehabilitation Psychology*, *55*(3), 255–262.

Coetzer, R. (2007). Psychotherapy following traumatic brain injury: Integrating theory and practice. *Journal of Head Trauma Rehabilitation*, *22*(1), 39–47.

Covin, R., Ouimet, A. J., Seeds, P. M., & Dozois, D. J. (2008). A meta-analysis of CBT for pathological worry among clients with GAD. *Journal of Anxiety Disorders*, *22*, 108–116.

Eldred, C., & Sykes, C. (2008). Psychosocial interventions for carers of survivors of stroke: A systematic review of interventions based on psychological principles and theoretical frameworks. *British Journal of Health Psychology*, *13*, 563–581.

Feinstein, A. (2011). Multiple sclerosis and depression. *Multiple Sclerosis Journal*, *17*(11), 1276–1281.

Goldstein, K. (1952). The effect of brain damage on the personality. *Psychiatry*, *15*, 245–260.

Gould, R. L., Coulson, M. C., & Howard, R. J. (2012). Efficacy of cognitive behavioral therapy for anxiety disorders in older people: A meta-analysis and meta-regression of randomized controlled trials. *Journal of the American Geriatrics Society*, *60*, 218–229.

Grossman, P., Kappos, L., Gensicke, H., D'Souza, M., Penner, I. K., & Steiner, C. (2010). MS quality of life, depression, and fatigue improve after mindfulness training: A randomized trial. *Neurology*, *75*, 1141–1149.

Hackett, M. L., Anderson, C. S., House, A., & Xia, J. (2008). Interventions for treating depression after stroke (review). *Cochrane Database of Systematic Reviews*, *1*, 1–21. doi: 10.1002/14651858.CD003437.pub3/full

Hofmann, S. G., & Smits, J. A. (2008). Cognitive-behavioral therapy for adult anxiety disorders: A meta-analysis of randomized placebo-controlled trials. *Journal of Clinical Psychiatry*, *69*(4), 621–632.

Jakobsen, J. C., Hansen, J. L., Storebo, O. J., Simonsen, E., & Gluud, C. (2011). The effects of cognitive therapy versus "treatment as usual" in patients with major depressive disorder. *PLoS One*, *6*, 1–11.

Judd, D., & Wilson, S. L. (2005). Psychotherapy with brain injury survivors: An investigation of the challenges encountered by clinicians and their modifications to therapeutic practice. *Brain Injury*, *19*(6), 437–449.

Klonoff, P. S. (2010). *Psychotherapy After Brain Injury: Principles and Techniques*. New York: The Guilford Press.

Klonoff, P. S., & Lage, G. A. (1991). Narcissistic injury in patients with traumatic brain injury. *Journal of Head Trauma Rehabilitation*, *6*(4), 11–21.

Klonoff, P. S., Lamb, D. G., & Henderson, S. W. (2001). Outcomes from milieu-based neurorehabilitation at up to 11 year post-discharge. *Brain Injury*, *15*, 413–428.

Laaksonen, R., & Ranta, M. (2013). *Introduction to Neuropsychotherapy*. New York: Psychology Press.

Luria, A. R. (1972). *The Man With a Shattered World*. New York: Basic Books.

Lustig, D. C., Strauser, D. R., Weems, G. H., Donnell, C. M., & Smith, L. D. (2003). Traumatic brain injury and rehabilitation outcomes: Does the working alliance making a difference? *Journal of Applied Rehabilitation Counseling*, *34*(4), 30–37.

Martin, D. J., Garske, J. P., & Davis, M. K. (2000). Relation of the therapeutic alliance with outcome and other variables: A meta-analytic review. *Journal of Consulting and Clinical Psychology*, *68*(3), 438–450.

Mitte, K. (2005). Meta-analysis of cognitive-behavioral treatments for generalized anxiety disorder: A comparison with pharmacotherapy. *Psychological Bulletin*, *131*(5), 785–795.

Mohr, D. C., Lovera, J., Brown, T., Cohen, B., Neylan, T., & Henry, R. (2012). A randomized trial of stress management of the prevention of new brain lesions in MS. *Neurology*, *79*, 412–419.

Nordin, L., & Rorsman, I. (2012). Cognitive behavioural therapy in multiple sclerosis: A randomized controlled pilot study of acceptance and commitmennt therapy. *Journal of Rehabilitative Medicine*, *44*, 87–90.

Pinhasi-Vittorio, L. (2007). The role of written language in the rehabilitation process of brain injury and aphasia: The memory of the movement in the reacquisition of language. *Topics in Stroke Rehabilitation*, *14*(1), 115–122.

Prigatano, G. P. (1991). Disordered mind, wounded soul: The emerging role of psychotherapy in rehabilitation after brain injury. *Journal of Head Trauma Rehabilitation*, *6*(4), 1–10.

Prigatano, G. P. (1999a). *Principles of Neuropsychological Rehabilitation*. New York: Oxford University Press.

Prigatano, G. P. (1999b). Commentary: Beyond statistics and research: A critique of the Carney et al. review paper. *Journal of Head Trauma Rehabilitation*, *14*(3), 308–311.

Prigatano, G. P. (2008). Neuropsychological rehabilitation and psychodynamic psychotherapy. In *Handbook of Clinical Neuropsychology* (pp. 985–995). New York: Taylor & Francis Group.

Prigatano, G. P. (2011a). The importance of the patient's subjective experience in stroke rehabilitation. *Topics in Stroke Rehabilitation*, *18*(1), 30–34.

Prigatano, G. P. (2011b). Psychotherapy. In J. M. Silver, T. W. McAllister, & S. C. Yudofsky (Eds.), *Textbook of Traumatic Brain Injury* (2nd ed., pp. 571–577). Washington, DC: American Psychiatric Association Press.

Prigatano, G. P. (2012). Jungian contributions to successful neuropsychological rehabilitation. *Psychoanalysis*, *14*(2), 175–185.

Prigatano, G. P. (2014). Anosognosia and patterns of impaired self-awareness observed in clinical practice. *Cortex*, *61*, 81–92.

Prigatano, G. (2016). Positive and negative turning points after neuropsychological rehabilitation ended. In Y. Ben-Yishay & L. Diller (Eds.), *Turning Points* (pp. 56–63). Youngsville, NC: Lash & Associates Publishing/Training Inc.

Prigatano, G. P., Fordyce, D. J., Roueche, J. R., Pepping, M., & Wood, B. C. (1986). *Neuropsychological Rehabilitation After Brain Injury*. Baltimore, MD: The Johns Hopkins University Press.

Prigatano, G. P., Fordyce, D. J., Zeiner, H. K., Roueche, J. R., Pepping, M., & Wood, B. (1984). Neuropsychological rehabilitation after closed head injury in young adults. *Journal of Neurology, Neurosurgery, and Psychiatry*, *47*, 505–513.

Prigatano, G. P., & Klonoff, P. S. (1997). A clinician's rating scale for evaluating impaired self-awareness and denial of disability following brain injury. *The Clinical Neuropsychologist*, *11*(1), 1–12.

Prigatano, G. P., Klonoff, P. S., O'Brien, K. P., Altman, I., Amin, K., Chiapello, D. A., . . . Mora, M. (1994). Productivity after neuropsychologically oriented, milieu rehabilitation. *Journal of Head Trauma Rehabilitation*, *9*(1), 91–102.

Prigatano, G. P., & Morrone-Strupinsky, J. (2010). Advancing the profession of clinical neuropsychology with appropriate outcome studies and demonstrated clinical skills. *The Clinical Neuropsychologist*, *24*(3), 468–480.

Robertson, M. M. (1997). Depression in neurological disorders. In M. M. Robertson & C.L.E. Katona (Eds.), *Depression and Physical Illness* (Vol. 6, pp. 305–340). West Sussex, UK: John Wiley & Sons, Ltd.

Robinson, L. A., Berman, J. S., & Neimeyer, R. A. (1990). Psychotherapy for the treatment of depression: A comprehensive review of controlled outcome research. *Psychological Bulletin*, *108*(1), 30–49.

Robinson, R. G. (2003). Poststroke depression: Prevalence, diagnosis, treatment, and disease progression. *Biological Psychiatry*, *54*(3), 376–387.

Rogers, C. R. (1961). *On Becoming a Person*. Boston: Houghton Mifflin Company.

Ruff, R. M., & Chester, S. K. (2014). *Effective Psychotherapy for Individuals With Brain Injury*. New York: The Guilford Press.

Salas, C. E., Vaughan, F. L., Shanker, S., & Turnbull, O. H. (2013). Stuck in a moment: Concreteness and psychotherapy after acquired brain injury. *Neuro-Disability and Psychotherapy*, *1*(1), 1–38.

Schofield, W. (1964). *Psychotherapy: The Purchase of Friendship*. Englewood Cliffs, NJ: Prentice-Hall Inc.

Shedler, J. (2010). The efficacy of psychodynamic psychotherapy. *American Psychologist*, *65*(2), 98–109.

Sherer, M., & Fleming, J. (2014). Impaired self-awareness. In M. Sherer & A. M. Sander (Eds.), *Handbook on the Neuropsychology of Traumatic Brain Injury*. New York: Springer.

Sherer, M., & Sander, A. M. (Eds.). (2014). *Handbook on the Neuropsychology of Traumatic Brain Injury* (pp. 233–255). New York: Springer.

Spek, V., Cuijpers, P., Nyklicek, I., Riper, H., Keyzer, J., & Pop, V. (2007). Internet-based cognitive behavior therapy for symptoms of depression and anxiety: A meta-analysis. *Psychological Medicine*, *37*, 319–328.

Starkstein, S. E., & Robinson, R. G. (1993). *Depression in Neurologic Disease*. Baltimore, MD: The Johns Hopkins University Press.

Stewart, R. E., & Chambless, D. L. (2009). Cognitive-behavioral therapy for adult anxiety disorders in clinical practice: A meta-analysis of effectiveness studies. *Journal of Consulting and Clinical Psychology*, *77*(4), 595–606.

Sweet, J. J., Meyer, D. G., Nelson, N. W., & Moberg, P. J. (2011). The TCN/AACN 2010 "Salary Survey": Professional practices, beliefs, and incomes of U.S. neuropsychologists. *The Clinical Neuropsychologist*, *25*(1), 12–61.

Thomas, P. W., Thomas, S., Hillier, C., Galvin, K., & Baker, R. (2006). Psychological interventions for multiple sclerosis. *Cochrane Database of Systematic Reviews*, *1*, 1–55.

Thornton, A. E., & DeFreitas, V. G. (2009). The neuropsychology of multiple sclerosis. In I. Grant & K. M. Adams (Eds.), *Neuropsychological Assessment of Neuropsychiatric Disorders* (3rd ed., pp. 280–305). New York: Oxford University Press.

Turner, E. H., Matthews, A. M., Linardatos, E., Tell, R. A., & Rosenthal, R. (2008). Selective publication of antidepressant trials and its influence on apparent efficacy. *New England Journal of Medicine*, *358*, 252–260.

47 Mindfulness-Based Interventions in Neuropsychology

Patricia M. Arenth

Introduction

The aim of this chapter is to discuss the developing literature regarding mindfulness meditation as it relates to the field of neuropsychology. The research literature in the field of mindfulness study has grown exponentially in the past 20 years. In fact, based on citations in a recently formed database of the published literature (Black, 2010; American Mindfulness Research Association, https://goamra.org/), after the first listed publication of mindfulness meditation in 1966, 17 additional publications are recorded during the 1970s, with increased rates of publications beginning in the 1980s and continued acceleration to the present. Currently, updates to the database are occurring monthly at a rate of approximately 50 new studies per month. As a result of the breadth and high volume, a full review of the mindfulness literature is beyond the scope of this chapter. It should be noted, however, that in comparison to other fields of study, the scientific study of mindfulness is still relatively young. That stated, the emerging findings suggest that mindfulness-based interventions (MBIs) have the potential to positively impact multiple aspects of emotional, behavioral, biological, and neuropsychological functioning in ways that may be of benefit to individuals with many of the diagnoses discussed in the other chapters of this book. As a result, the review and discussion in this chapter will focus on the potential utility of these types of practices for the rehabilitation and training of individuals with neurologically based injuries and illnesses. While globally, the literature in this area should be considered preliminary, with more rigorous study needed, the employment of mindfulness training with clinical groups may prove to offer neuropsychologists tools with which to train patients and clients in methods with broad, as well as targeted benefits, which are nonpharmaceutical, and which can be taught at relatively low cost in a group setting. Most importantly, these skills, once learned, can potentially be used by patients and clients for positive self-care in the long-term.

Defining Meditation

In the broad sense, meditation has been present, in many forms and across world cultures and religions, for thousands of years. While meditation is most commonly associated with Eastern cultures, it could be asserted that even some denominations of Western Christianity include meditation practices in certain forms of contemplative prayer. As a result of this broad use of the term *meditation,* there have been challenges in attaining a consensus definition for the purposes of scientific study. In an effort to do so, the Agency for Healthcare Research and Quality (www.ahrq.gov) proposed a definition that includes three essential principles (Ospina et al., 2008): (a) a defined technique allowing for a describable set of instructions for practice; (b) an element described as "logic relaxation," meaning that there is a lack of intent to make judgments, create expectations, or analyze the practice itself; and (c) a self-induced state or mode, indicating that a person is not under the direct instruction of another person (i.e., as in hypnosis). This definition was later modified further (Goyal et al., 2014) to differentiate forms of meditation during which one remains stationary (i.e., transcendental meditation or other sitting practices) from forms of meditation that involve awareness during meditative movement (i.e., yoga, Tai Chi).

Mindfulness Meditation

Mindfulness is a specific form of meditation with basic philosophical foundations in Asian Buddhist practices, although ascribing to a specific cultural or religious belief system is not required. In fact, it has been argued that the basic tenets of mindfulness are anchored in universal principles rather than specific religious or cultural ideas (Kabat-Zinn, 2003). Many traditions and practices are often included under the umbrella of mindfulness meditation; some familiar traditions may include Zen, Hatha yoga, and Insight meditation. Clinical training and treatments using mindfulness approaches or mixing various practices are often included in a general category of MBIs in the literature. The differences in specific training and traditions pose some challenges in the study of mindfulness, and it has been suggested that different approaches may impact various psychological, cognitive, and brain changes in different manners, as will be discussed later in the chapter (i.e., Fox et. al., 2014). All forms of mindfulness meditation do share some basic tenets, as suggested by this straight-forward definition of mindfulness offered by Jon Kabat-Zinn (1994), the founder of the Mindfulness-Based

Stress Reduction (MBSR) program: "Mindfulness means paying attention in a particular way: on purpose, in the present moment, and non-judgmentally." This simple definition meets the formal criteria set forth by the Agency for Healthcare Research and Quality, and can be engaged in during both sitting and active movement practices. At the most basic levels of training, mindfulness involves focus on the breath and other bodily sensations, as well as any thoughts and emotions that may arise during a practice session. The aim is to attend without judgment, but with simple awareness. Through practicing this form of meditation, and observing thoughts, feelings, and emotions as they occur in the moment, practitioners may gain greater awareness of how they are interacting, and may choose to mentally position themselves differently in relation or response. In addition, as will be described later in this chapter, positive changes in emotional, cognitive and physiological health appear to be by-products of even relatively brief periods of practice.

To some degree, mindfulness practice is deceptively easy. In its basic form, it is concrete, simple, and focused on the present moment. The initial attention to the physical awareness of the breath and bodily sensations allows for disengagement from the higher level processing of emotions and thoughts, with a focus only on experiencing, rather than judging, analyzing, or responding. There is scientific evidence that this initial focus on the body may neurologically precede changes in emotion and cognition (i.e., Kerr et al., 2013). This simplicity and "unplugging" from all but the basic sensations may at least partially account for the increased interest and popularity of mindfulness in Western cultures, where stress related to the intensity of fast-paced jobs, activities, and lifestyles, as well as "information overload" from electronic media and devices is becoming a common complaint (i.e., Ludwig & Kabat-Zinn, 2008). In fact, the term *mindfulness* has become much more a part of the popular literature in recent years. Just as yoga has become more widely accepted, so the ideas of meditation, and in particular, mindful forms of practice, have become much more widely available and accepted. In fact, mindfulness has graced the cover of major magazines (for examples, see www.scientificAmerican.com/article/neuroscience-reveals-the-secrets-of-meditation-s-benefits/ and http://time.com/1556/the-mindful-revolution/), has been a topic on popular talk shows such as Oprah Winfrey's *SuperSoul Sunday* (watch "The Difference Between Mindfulness and Meditation?" at www.youtube.com/watch?v=Nigoy8rIuT4) and trainings have been offered to executives and employees of major U.S. corporations (see the Visionary Insights website at https://visionaryinsights.wordpress.com/category/popular-culture/ and www.huffingtonpost.com/2014/01/02/will-2014-be-the-year-of-_0_n_4523975.html) .

Just as yoga that has become "Westernized" as a form of exercise, some would argue that the philosophical underpinnings of mindfulness are in danger of being diluted or lost completely (for example, see Rapgay & Bystrisky, 2009), as mindfulness training has been touted as a potential method for gaining an "edge" or improving productivity in our competitive American culture, or as a "quick fix" for the stress of our hectic lifestyles (i.e., www.theatlantic.com/business/archive/2015/03/corporations-newest-productivity-hack-meditation/387286/). Indeed, although it is sometimes misunderstood, the goal of mindfulness meditation is not to shut the world out, or to gain a competitive edge, but rather, through slowing down to focus on the moment, the aim is to experience the moment clearly, with the opportunity to respond deliberately, rather than reactively via the increased awareness gained over slow and deliberate daily practice.

One significant positive impact of the increased interest and acceptance of mindfulness in the United States and other Western countries is that this has produced a surge in science and research in this area. In addition, clinical adaptations and protocol programs have created unique opportunities in psychology, medicine, and education. There has been a growing acceptance of the teaching of mindfulness to many groups, and it has been employed with reportedly positive results in the treatment of a wide range of problems and diverse treatment groups—from incarcerated individuals (i.e., Leonard et al., 2013; Barnert et al., 2014; Samuelson et al., 2007), to schoolchildren (i.e., Napoli, Krech, & Holley, 2005; Wisner, Jones, & Gwin, 2010), soldiers and veterans (i.e., Trousselard et al., 2012; Serpa, Taylor, & Tillisch, 2014; Serpa, 2014), professionals (i.e., Galantino et al., 2005; Kelley & Lambert, 2012), and to individuals with chronic health conditions and diseases (i.e., Baer, Carmondy, & Hunsinger, 2012). While the current "hype" around mindfulness in the popular media will certainly wane with time, in the area of neuropsychology, the ideas of mindfulness practice, in both theory and philosophy, fit well with the focus of rehabilitation and provide skills training that research suggests may positively impact cognition and emotion. In addition to behavioral studies, more recent neuroimaging research has suggested that brief periods of mindfulness training have the potential to physically alter brain function and structure in ways which positively impact attention, memory, and frontal lobe functioning, as well as improve emotional regulation (i.e., Tang et al., 2015).

The remainder of this chapter will be focused on elucidating the current state of the literature related to mindfulness and MBIs, with particular attention paid to the multifaceted ways in which this form of practice has the potential to benefit individuals who have sustained neurological injuries and diseases. Given the preliminary nature of the overall literature in this area, an exhaustive review of the literature will not be undertaken; however key exemplars and reviews will be utilized in order to elucidate, along with discussion of our aims in the field of rehabilitation with the goal of highlighting the potential opportunities for additional study and clinical exploration within our field.

Mindfulness-Based Stress Reduction

Although there are many forms of mindfulness meditation, MBSR is a program that is particularly notable in the sense that, from the time of its founding, the primary focus has been on providing mindfulness training and interventions to individuals with health issues in a medical setting. For example, the first studies or MBSR indicated positive results for use with individuals diagnosed with chronic pain (Kabat-Zinn et al., 1985, 1987), increased response to light therapy for patients with psoriasis (Kabat-Zinn et al., 1998), and improvements for individuals with anxiety (Kabat-Zinn, 1992). In addition to the focus on medically related issues, over time the program has been protocolized in a manner that has made it useful for study via research paradigms.

MBSR was formulated by Jon Kabat-Zinn in 1979 as a program for a newly formed outpatient stress reduction clinic at the University of Massachusetts Medical Center (Kabat-Zinn, 1982). The program began as a consult service to assist patients in managing symptoms associated with chronic pain and various medical diagnoses, as well as other life stressors. The intention of the program from the onset was to compliment medical care, not to replace it. Over time, MBSR has evolved into the current design, in which the intervention is administered as an eight-week group program (for a full description of the program, refer to the book entitled *Full Catastrophe Living: Using the Wisdom of Your Body and Mind to Face Stress, Pain, and Illness,* by Jon Kabat-Zinn, 1991). Individuals in the program are required to participate in group education and practice for two-hour sessions weekly, and are asked to engage in individual practice at home on a daily basis.

The initial components of this program are focused on body awareness, which is practiced through sitting and supine mindfulness meditation practices involving focusing on the breath, and engaging in the "Body Scan," which entails bringing awareness to successive body areas in a sequential manner with the aim of focused attention and awareness of sensations occurring with each body area. As the eight-week course progresses, sessions include didactic presentations, movement (mindful Hatha yoga and mindful walking), as well as specific exercises in mindful eating and observation of positive and negative thoughts. An all-day silent retreat is part of the program as well. It should be noted that, from its inception, while MBSR practices are derived from Eastern traditions of meditation and yoga, Kabat-Zinn intentionally removed specific cultural or philosophical language from the program in a concerted effort to make it universally accessible to clinical patients of all backgrounds (i.e., Kabat-Zinn, 2003). This program has grown exponentially in recent years and is now known as the Center for Mindfulness in Medicine, Healthcare, and Society. Kabat-Zinn and colleagues have now trained practitioners worldwide to teach the eight-week course, with more than 20,000 individuals participating up to this point (for information about the program and training, visit the Center for Mindfulness website at: www.umassmed.edu/cfm/).

Over the course of the MBSR course, weekly themes are introduced that are incorporated into didactic presentations and group discussions. Although meditation practices are conducted with a focus on attentional awareness without judgment or response, the weekly themes provide a context with which to consider the information gained through observation during practice. Weekly themes build over the course of the program and are designed to provide information about how stress impacts health and the body, as well as to assist participants in gaining insight and perspective regarding choices available to them in responding to pain, illness, and chronic life stressors.

It is worth noting that, with the increasing popularity of mindfulness research, there are efforts to differentiate and identify types of practices studied in an effort to clarify how the use of different practices or methods may lead to distinct findings in the literature. For example, there has become a growing interest in adapting the eight-week MBSR protocol to meet the needs of various groups and programs. In an effort to preserve the authenticity of the program and clarity in research literature, an effort has been made in the literature to designate that only programs and studies implementing the full eight-week course with trained instructors and the protocolized format should be described as MBSR. Any changes in characteristics, such as variations in the number of weeks, length of sessions, themes, or practices, are designated as various MBIs in order to differentiate and evaluate emerging studies. It should be noted that MBIs are not considered to be inferior to MBSR, but are valid and important tools that can be quite useful and studied in their own right. The differentiation is made merely for clarity in the literature. An example of a specific MBI, which will be discussed at a later point in this chapter, is Mindfulness-Based Cognitive Therapy (MBCT; see Teasdale, Segal, & Williams, 1995). Other examples include the alteration of the MBSR program in the length of sessions for number of sessions to accommodate individuals with chronic illness who may fatigue easily or require additional time and repetition due to cognitive limitations. As the scientific study of mindfulness has continued to grow, additional efforts in the larger literature have also been made to more clearly define which types of meditation practices are being used across various studies, due to increased awareness that different types of meditation may produce distinct findings due to variations in active processes across types. Higher-level studies of individual practices and traditions may allow for increased clarity regarding the key components of activation. For example, as we explore MBSR in the next section, efforts to evaluate the active components involve study of the order in which changes occur through practice, behavioral considerations, as well as various brain structures and functions may be altered via participation in MBSR. It should be noted that there some (i.e., Rapgay & Bystrisky, 2009) who argue that, despite its higher level of protocolization as compared to some paradigms, there still may be too many "moving parts" in MBSR due to the mixed forms of practice (i.e., sitting, yoga, breath awareness, body scan). These authors assert that research may be better served by studying more classic mindfulness paradigms.

Following are some examples of studies evaluating outcomes from MBSR programs on physical and mental health in individuals with stress and chronic medical issues.

Early in the development of MBSR, Kabat-Zinn and colleagues (1985) used a ten-week course of mindfulness meditation to train 90 individuals with chronic pain, compared to a group of pain patients receiving traditional treatment protocols. Measures evaluating self-report of present-moment pain, negative body image, inhibition of activity due to pain, symptoms, mood disturbance and psychological symptoms, including those related to anxiety and depression symptoms were measured. The utilization of pain medications, activity levels and self-esteem reports were also monitored over the course of treatment. Results indicated statistically significant positive changes in all measures, including physical and emotional symptoms and pain-related behaviors when pre- and posttreatment assessments were compared. In addition, utilization of pain-related medications was significantly decreased. Results indicated that findings of improvement appeared to be independent of gender, referral source, and type of pain. In comparison, participants in the traditional treatment protocols did not show significant improvement on the same measures. Follow-up indicated that improvements for those receiving mindfulness training persisted up to 15 months after participation in the program for all measures, except present-moment pain. In addition, the majority of participants in mindfulness training reported continued to use mindfulness practice in daily life.

From the behavioral perspective, a study by Baer, Carmody, and Hunsinger (2012) evaluated the weekly changes in self-reported mindfulness and perceived stress in a group of 87 adults with chronic illness, pain, and life stressors who were engaged in an MBSR program. The aims of the study were not only to evaluate changes occurring overall between pre- and post-MBSR participation, but also to look at patterns for the development of change. Via evaluation of weekly questionnaires, significant increases in the acquisition of mindfulness skills, as well as significantly decreased reports of perceived stress were reported from pretreatment to posttreatment overall. Regarding timing and patterns of change, however, subjects reported significant changes in mindfulness occurring by the second week of the program, where significant decreases in perceived stress were not noted until the fourth week. Additional evaluation of these differences indicated that the extent of change in mindfulness skills during the first three weeks of the program was predictive of the extent of perceived stress reduction over the course of the intervention. Conclusions of this study were that the improvement of mindfulness skills may predict and mediate the effects of mindfulness training on positive outcomes reported as stress reduction.

In 2010, Merkes conducted a review article of 15 studies reporting outcomes of MBSR programs for adults with chronic diseases. Outcomes reported in these studies were regarding physical and mental health, well-being, and quality of life. The articles evaluated used both self-report and physiological outcome measures. Clinical diagnoses included chronic pain, rheumatoid arthritis, Type 2 Diabetes, chronic fatigue syndrome, multiple chemical sensitivity, cardiovascular diagnoses and fibromyalgia. Due to the inclusion of multiple and variable measures, specific outcomes of studies were difficult to compare, however, improvements were reported in all 15 studies, with no negative changes reported in any study between baseline and follow-up.

In additional study of individuals with chronic pain and a diagnosis of "Failed Back Surgery Syndrome," Esmer and colleagues (2010) completed a randomized, single-blind, parallel-group clinical trial in which 25 participants were randomly assigned to MBSR therapy plus traditional therapy or traditional therapy alone. Final analysis was completed at the time of a 12-week follow up. Results indicated that the addition of MBSR to traditional treatment produced statistically and clinically significant increases in measures of pain acceptance and quality of life, decreases in functional limitations, decreased visual analog pain scale reports, and reduced frequency of use and potency of pain medications, as well as resulting in improvements on a self-reported measure of sleep quality.

Taken together, these studies suggest that participation in MBSR is unlikely to be associated with negative outcomes, and that positive outcomes such as improved coping, well-being, and quality of life are likely to be reported by individuals with chronic health issues who participate in MBSR groups. As we consider the populations who are followed in our inpatient and outpatient rehabilitation settings, many individuals are working to manage with chronic disability, health issues, and often pain. At this very basic level, as we work to provide treatments that are cost-effective and efficacious in training patients and clients to engage in self-care for the purposes of managing current health issues and perhaps reducing exacerbation or future issues, MBSR or related mindfulness practices—which can be presented relatively inexpensively as a nonpharmacological group treatment—may be worth consideration.

Frequency and Length of Practice: Impact on Brain and Behavior

Neuroimaging studies of Buddhist monks and other master practitioners of meditation have shown significantly altered brain structure and function. For example, in a structural neuroimaging study of 22 long-term meditators as compared to 22 nonexperienced control participants using voxel-based morphometry, Luders and colleagues (2009) found gray matter volumes to be significantly larger in the right orbitofrontal cortex and the right hippocampus for meditators as compared to controls. The authors stated that both areas were associated with response control and emotional regulation. Of note is that this was a study of practitioners of various forms of meditation, as compared to other studies focusing on one method of practice. The authors assert that these findings may be representative of overall changes related to meditation in general, while variations in practice types may have additional specific regional findings not supported by this less specific, yet broader study.

Clearly, in studies of long-term practitioners, the question arises about what other sorts of personality and lifestyle factors may play a role in these alterations as compared to nonpractitioners. In addition, the question of how long one has to practice in order to achieve noticeable changes is a consideration for training individuals who are patients and clients. Of interest is the fact that several studies have now been conducted with results suggesting that novice practitioners of mindful practice may show positive functional and structural changes in the brain after just eight weeks of mindfulness training. For example, Hölzel and colleagues (2011) completed a study in which changes in gray matter concentrations were investigated using voxel-based morphometry and compared with a wait list control group. Sixteen healthy participants who were naive to meditation and 17 wait list controls completed neuroimaging before and after the eight-week period during which the treatment group participated in MBSR. Findings indicated increases in gray matter concentration within the left hippocampus (the a priori region of interest). Whole-brain analysis identified increases in the posterior cingulate cortex, the temporo-parietal junction, and the cerebellum. The authors note that these findings represent gray matter regions involved in learning and memory processing, emotional regulation, self-referential processing and perspective taking.

Hölzel and colleagues (2010) also completed an additional longitudinal evaluation of the relationship between changes in amygdala gray matter density following an eight-week MBSR intervention. The aim of this study was to evaluate if a psychological variable (perceived stress) may be associated with changes in the brain following mindfulness practice. The amygdala was chosen as the brain structure of interest, as it is known to be involved in the response to stress, and previous studies had reported increases in activity during functional studies of stress conditions. Following the intervention, participants in this study reported significant reductions in perceived stress and these reductions correlated positively with decreases in the right basolateral amygdala gray matter density.

Kilpatrick et al. (2011) applied functional magnetic resonance imaging (fMRI) to evaluate whether participation in MBSR was associated with alternations in intrinsic connectivity networks. Healthy female subjects were randomly assigned to participation in either MBSR or a wait-list control group. After eight weeks, fMRI data were acquired while subjects rested with eyes closed and were instructed to attend to the sounds of the scanner environment. Results indicated that, as compared to controls, individuals participating in MBSR showed increased functional connectivity within auditory and visual networks, and increased functional connectivity between the auditory cortex and areas associated with attentional and self-referential processes. Stronger anticorrelations between auditory and visual cortex, and between visual cortex and areas associated with attentional and self-referential processes were also noted. The conclusion of this study was that eight weeks of participation in mindful meditation training alters intrinsic functional connectivity in ways that may reflect a more consistent attentional focus, enhanced sensory processing, and reflective awareness of sensory experience.

In all, at least 21 studies have been conducted to examine structural changes related to mindfulness meditation. It should be noted, however, that various traditions of mindfulness meditation were included, and designs and measures differ across studies, precluding the full comparison across all studies. In addition, the majority of these studies have had small sample sizes and many have employed post-hoc explorations of changes, which reflects the "young" nature of this literature. As a result, many studies in these areas should be considered preliminary, although these early findings have implications that are potentially quite interesting for clinical practice. For example, such studies have indicated changes in cortical thickness (i.e., Lazar et al., 2005; Grant et al., 2010), gray matter volume and density (i.e., Vestergaard-Poulsen et. al., 2009; Hozel et al., 2011), and white matter changes (Tang et al., 2010; Tang et al., 2012). In at least some of these studies, structural changes in the brain have been associated with psychological variables, such as self-reports of stress reduction (Hölzel et al., 2011), emotional regulation (i.e., Tang et al., 2012), or an increased sense of well-being (Singleton et al., 2014). In a recent review of the neuroscience findings associated with mindfulness, Tang, Hölzel, and Posner (2015) conclude that there is "emerging evidence" of neuroplasticity in brain structure and functional regions associated with emotion, self-awareness, and attention regulation; however, they indicate the need for additional rigorous research with larger sample sizes for further scientific study. In an addition, Fox and colleagues (2014) concluded conservatively that the results most concurrent across studies of morphological differences associated with meditation indicated positive changes in the left rostrolateral prefrontal cortex, the anterior/mid-cingulate cortex, the anterior insula, primary/secondary somatomotor cortices, left inferior temporal gyrus, and the hippocampus.

Given these findings, further studies and consideration of correlations between structural and functional brain changes associated with mindful practices, along with evaluations of how these alterations may impact areas such as memory, attention, executive functioning, as well as emotional response will be of interest, as these areas have the potential to significantly impact outcomes for individuals in our clinical rehabilitation populations with neurologically based illnesses or injuries.

Biophysiological Functioning

In addition to brain-based alterations, significant changes in immune function, inflammatory markers and physical health have been reported with MBSR and other mindfulness training. For example, Davidson and colleagues (2003) conducted a randomized controlled trial of MBSR to evaluate how reported changes in mental and physical health reported with mindfulness training may be associated with biological changes. This group measured electrical activity in the brain prior to participation in an eight-week MBSR course, immediately following completion of the course, and at a follow up session four months after completion of the program. Twenty-five subjects completed the MBSR arm of the study, while 16 subjects in a wait-list control group were assessed at the same time points as the MBSR group. At the end of the eight-week MBSR versus wait-list control period, individuals in both groups were given an influenza vaccine. Results of the study indicated that individuals participating in the MBSR arm, as compared to controls, displayed an increase in electrical activation of the left-sided anterior areas of the brain, a pattern previously shown to be associated with positive affect. Subjects in the MBSR group also were found to have significant increases in antibody titers to the influenza vaccine as compared to nonmeditators. In addition, the magnitude of increases in brain activation associated with positive affect predicted the magnitude of antibody titer rise in response to the vaccine.

Studies have also been conducted to look at how participation in mindfulness practice might modulate neurogenic inflammation. In one study (Rosenkranz et al., 2013), evaluated MBSR compared to the Health Enhancement Program (HEP), a recently validated active control intervention (MacCoon et al., 2012). Stress response was measured using a paradigm in which participants engaged in a standardized socially stressful situation (a five-minute speech and mental arithmetic—a modified version of the Trier Social Stress Test, or TSST; see Kirschbaum et al., 1993) and a local neurogenic inflammatory response (capsaicin cream topically applied to the forearm), after which baseline self-report, saliva cortisol, and molecular (blister fluid cytokines—TNF-α), and skin inflammatory (flare) measures collected. Subjects then participated in one of the two groups for eight weeks, after which the experimental stress paradigm was repeated. Findings indicated that both groups had equivalently reduced reports of psychological distress and physical symptoms and comparable stress-evoked cortisol levels. Despite similar levels of stress hormones (cortisol), however, individuals in the MBSR group did have significantly smaller inflammatory response at postintervention testing as compared to HEP. The main difference between MBSR and HEP is that MBSR focuses on reducing emotional reactivity as compared to HEP, which has a focus on well-being-promoting activities. The authors suggest that reduced emotional reactivity may be the active ingredient of MBSR associated with reduced inflammatory response to stress. In an additional study of elderly individuals, Creswell and colleagues (2012) noted that older adults who are lonely have been shown to have an increase in expression of proinflammatory genes, as well as an increased risk for morbidity and mortality. They assessed whether participation in an MBSR program might impact these factors. They compared 40 older adults (aged 55–85) who were randomly assigned to MBSR or a wait-list control group. Participants were asked to complete measures including a loneliness scale and also provided a blood sample at baseline and after the end of the eight-week period. Findings indicated significantly decreased reports of loneliness in the MBSR group as compared to the control group, as well as a down-regulation of the specific proinflammatory gene expression profile.

In an additional study of psychological and physiological outcomes with a clinical group, breast and prostate cancer patients, Carlson and colleagues (2007) completed baseline and follow-up measures immediately postparticipation, and again at six and 12 months after completion. Measures of quality of life, mood, stress symptoms, salivary cortisol levels, immune cell counts, intracellular cytokine production, blood pressure, and heart rate were included. Results indicated that improvements in stress maintained over the follow-up period. In addition, decreased cortisol levels, continued reduction of proinflammatory cytokines, and systolic blood pressure decreased from baseline to post-group. Heart rate was also positively associated with self-reported symptoms of stress.

Mindfulness and Cognition

In the American Mindfulness Research Association database, there are listed 177 citations for publications related to attention and meditation. This level of scientific inquiry in the literature is not surprising as the focus of attention is one of the hallmark components of definitions of various forms of meditation practice. Although the literature in this area is fairly sizable, it should be noted that findings related to attention remain somewhat mixed. While the general consensus is that mindfulness practice does seem to have a positive impact on performance on some attentional tasks, and brain areas associated with regulation of attention do seem to be impacted by participation in mindfulness-based practice, there is not yet scientific evidence to definitively conclude that alterations in attention are responsible for the changes observed (i.e., for a review, see Tang Hölzel & Posner, 2015). In part, this is due to the fact that there are multiple types of attention, and multiple types of training that may impact attention differently, as well as other confounding factors making it difficult to tease out causation and effect. Further studies are needed in this area to more fully elucidate the relationship between mindfulness and attentional functioning. Of potential significant interest to rehabilitation practitioners, a study by Kerr and colleagues (2013) provides a theoretical framework suggesting that the initial weeks of standardized practices of focusing on the sensory experiences of the breath and learning to control the focus of attention on various parts of the body in a systematic way through the body scan provide training in sensory attention that leads to later positive changes in seemingly unrelated cognitive and affective measures (i.e., mood, rumination, working memory, and pain-related distress). This framework lays out a predictable sensory-cognitive sequence of practice-related gains whereby localized attention to body sensations enables subsequent gains in emotional and cognitive regulation by enhancing sensory information processing in the brain.

As with attention, the literature related to the associations memory functioning and mindfulness training are not entirely clear. This is also in part due to the fact that there are multiple types of memory and multiple ways in which memory may be targeted. Available studies do suggest positive associations between mindfulness training and working memory capacity (Mrazek et al., 2015; Jha et al., 2010). Of particular interest for the current discussion is a systematic review of meditation associations with age-related decline (Gard, Hölzel, & Lazar, 2014) that indicated preliminary findings of positive effects of mindfulness on general cognition, including attention, memory, executive functioning, and processing speed in relation to aging and cognitive decline. An additional study (Marciniak et al., 2014) evaluated mindfulness in the context of neurogenerative disease and aging. Seven studies were analyzed and also suggested positive effects of mindfulness on cognition, in particular in the areas of attention, memory, verbal fluency, and cognitive flexibility. Of note, however, is that both studies included in the analysis utilized various forms of meditation, and the authors concluded that further longitudinal and stringent designs were needed for results to be declared more than preliminary.

A thorough review of 23 studies of mindfulness-based practices and cognitive functioning (Chiesa, Calati, & Serretti, 2011)—including attention, memory, executive functioning, and other cognitive measures—suggested that practices of mindfulness training (often early in training) in which the aim is to build focused attention may have a positive impact on selective and executive attention, where open monitoring practices focusing on internal and external stimuli may be positively associated with unfocused sustained attention. Participation in mindfulness-based practices was also associated with improvements in working memory and some executive functions such as improved verbal fluency and reduced cognitive proponent responses on set tasks. As with other reviews of the literature, this group cautioned that further higher quality studies were needed for scientific validation of these preliminary findings.

Mindfulness and Affective Disorders

In a recent review article evaluating the potential effects of meditation for the treatment of affective dysregulation, Leung, Lo, and Lee (2014) asserted that affective dysregulation is the root cause of emotional illness, including poor response to stress, as well as anxiety and depression. The authors reviewed the empirical evidence for the neural impact of mindfulness meditation and compassion meditation. These two forms of meditation were chosen as the authors assert that each form of meditation engages different cognitive processes, and are therefore interesting to compare from a neuroscience standpoint. Mindfulness meditation focuses on engaging and practicing attention for the purpose of nonjudgmental monitoring of present-moment thoughts and sensations. In comparison, compassion meditation engages the emotional regulation and response system in the brain. The authors of this review conclude that both mindfulness meditation and compassion meditation have a positive impact on attention and emotional regulation, and that practice in these forms of meditation can produce lasting morphological changes in the corresponding neural regions—specifically the prefrontal regions and amygdala. They assert that healthy regulation of affect requires top-down cognitive control in which the prefrontal regions modulate the bottom-up processing of the subcortical regions, and that mood disorders result from the weakening of cognitive control due to activation of the limbic system over the prefrontal control system, thus allowing for heightened response to emotional stimuli and creating vulnerability to mood disorder. They suggest that mindfulness meditation can be considered as an exercise that may have potential for both prevention of and intervention in mood and affective disorders. They state that further study is needed to evaluate the use of meditation in general as a clinical treatment.

Jain, Walsh, Eisendrath, Christensen, and Cahn (2015) conducted a clinical review of 18 studies of meditation trials for depression. The studies reviewed included a mix of meditation modalities. The authors' overall conclusion was that the use of meditation interventions in the clinical setting as a primary or adjunct treatment for depression appears to be promising, especially as there is little risk of negative side effects and potential benefits that far outweigh any risks. While pointing out significant limitations in the literature, the authors indicated that data from randomized controlled trials suggest that meditation-based meditative interventions may have substantial effects on depressive symptoms in patients with clinically diagnosed depressive disorders, including both patients with major depressive disorder as well as those in partial remission. Variations among subcomponents of different types of meditation therapies did not allow for derivation of a common effect size—although, overall, data from the reviewed studies suggest that meditative interventions may have substantial effects on depressive symptoms in patients with clinically diagnosed depressive disorders, including those having diagnoses of acute major depressive disorder, as well as those in partial remission. Variations among subcomponents of different types of meditation therapies did not allow for derivation of a common effect size. The authors made specific recommendations for further carefully designed studies, including differentiating groups with various distinct levels of affective disorders. Additionally they recommended the inclusion of individuals with significant medical comorbidities, as the benefits of efficacious, yet nonpharmacological interventions for depression may be of even greater benefit to individuals at higher risk for negative side effects or polypharmacy interactions.

Mindfulness-Based Cognitive Therapy

One MBI of particular interest in the treatment of affective disorders is MBCT (Teasdale, Segal, & Williams, 1995). This intervention was specifically designed as a clinical treatment for depression and anxiety. Both MBCT and MBSR employ a standardized protocol for practice, including an almost identical eight-week instructional format that involves three somatically focused meditative techniques (body scan, sitting meditation, mindful yoga), however MBCT modifies traditional MBSR to incorporate components of cognitive behavioral therapy (CBT), which is widely accepted as an efficacious treatment for anxiety and mood disorders.

Maj van der Velden and colleagues (2015) reviewed 23 studies evaluating the mechanisms of change in MBCT in the treatment of major depressive disorder. Of the studies included in their analysis, the authors report that 12 studies found alterations in mindfulness, rumination, worry, compassion or meta-awareness that were associated with, predicted, or mediated MBCT's effect on treatment outcome. In addition, preliminary studies indicated that alterations in attention, memory specificity, self-discrepancy, emotional reactivity, and momentary positive and negative affect might play a role in how MBCT exerts its clinical effects. The authors called for more rigorous designs to assess greater levels of causal specificity.

Neuropsychology and Rehabilitation

Chapters in this book provide examples of the many sorts of diagnoses for which clinical neuropsychologists are often asked to provide evaluations. Neuropsychological deficits may be the result of newly acquired injuries or medical events, gradual declines in function associated with chronic conditions or aging, or other disease processes that impact neurological functioning. The ultimate aim of neuropsychological assessment in rehabilitation is to evaluate which areas of limitation may be amenable to therapeutic interactions for improvement, to identify the types of cues and methods that might be most helpful in providing treatments, and to determine how the areas of remaining strength may be used to assist in restoration of function or accommodation. The overarching aim of the rehabilitation process is to ultimately allow each individual to attain and maintain the highest degree of function and independence possible. In addition to evaluating and treating physical, cognitive, and sensory processes, neuropsychologists also often evaluate and treat emotional and behavioral issues, some of which may be the direct result of neurological injury or disease process, and some of which may be due to challenges with adjustment to disability, and, including significant anxiety and depression.

Where Neuropsychology, Rehabilitation and Mindfulness Meet

Following acute injury or a sudden decline in neurological status, simple movements that were once conducted with little thought, such as standing, walking, and grooming, may require conscious effort. In rehabilitation, we are often helping patients to "relearn" these previously automatic tasks. Many patients in the early stages of recovery report that significant cognitive, emotional energy, and physical energy is expended to produce even small coordinated movements, or to sequence or place limbs properly for activity. In order to work most effectively within therapy sessions, patients are truly asked to ascribe to the basic definition of mindfulness put forward by Jon Kabat-Zinn: "Paying attention in a particular way: on purpose, in the present moment, and non-judgmentally" (Kabat-Zinn, 1994). In working with our patients on these therapeutic tasks, we are asking them to bring new awareness to their bodies in ways that are consistent with the focus on body sensation, movement, balance, and proprioception practiced in mindful meditation practices. Working with them to engage in these therapeutic tasks mindfully and assisting them with suspending judgment fits naturally with our daily work in rehabilitation.

In addition, neuropsychologists are often working with individuals with neurological illnesses or injuries impacting brain functioning and causing significant deficits in attention, memory, and executive functioning. Our role as neuropsychologists is often to work to find methods of remediation or compensation for cognitive disability. As we have discussed in this chapter, it appears that engaging in MBIs may be associated with structural and functional changes in the brain and with positive general changes in attention, memory, and executive functioning. As practitioners, it seems possible that any small positive changes in brain structure associated with some of the very cognitive components most often impacted by neurological issues has the potential for real functional changes in cognition. As a clinical example, it is well known that after traumatic brain injury (TBI) attentional, memory, and executive functioning are commonly impaired. Based on this, as well as the literature previously discussed, it is likely that an individual with TBI may require some alterations in a traditional MBSR program (for example extra repetition, shorter sessions to manage attention and fatigue, extra practice, and additional cues). As will be elucidated in the following section, the literature suggests that, with some small changes, individuals with TBI are able to learn and benefit from MBIs. If, for example, key components of attention are shown to improve with mindfulness training, it is possible that increased attention could significantly impact encoding and memory, leading to significant improvements in cognitive functioning and, ultimately, to improved outcomes for individuals with cognitive issues associated with TBI.

From an emotional standpoint, in rehabilitation, we are often asking patients to simultaneously participate fully in therapies designed to optimize their recovery during relatively brief inpatient rehabilitation stays or a set number of outpatient therapy sessions, while also asking them to adjust to significant changes in health and function. Patients and families are often dealing with stress related to multiple—potentially overwhelming—factors, including acute and chronic disability, acute and chronic pain, cognitive limitations associated with injury, illness, emotional adjustment, anxiety, depression, potential changes in roles at work and home, financial security, and often likely permanent changes in independence, mobility and lifestyle. Ultimately, we work with individuals to assist them in positively adjusting to new changes in function and ability. As part of this process, mindfulness-based practices are based in themes that resonate with positive emotional adjustment. For example, for positive adjustment to occur, it is necessary for individuals with newly acquired disability to overcome the tendency to focus on the way things were before injury, and to move towards living and finding meaning in the present life as it is. The mindful approach of focusing on and accepting the present moment, as well as the didactic themes that are part of MBSR programs, including discussion about accepting ourselves as "whole" as we are in the present moment, may be very powerful and meaningful to individuals working to adapt to new life circumstances. In addition, the aim of experiencing and examining the present moment, and making choices about relating to the present in order to move towards future choices, also fits well with the immediate needs of individuals after injury or illness, as life plans and goals must often be altered based on the new circumstances presented to the patient in the form of new disability.

From a long-term perspective, it is also worth noting that individuals with significant neurological illnesses or injuries often follow up with their rehabilitation physicians and team for many years after injury. Given the chronic health and disability issues of many of our rehabilitation populations, therapeutic interventions that can be employed efficiently and have lasting effects are of significant interest. In addition, our goal is for individuals to attain the highest level of recovery and independence as possible. Based on these factors, there are a number of potential advantages of teaching mindfulness to patients and clients: We are empowering patients to participate in the management of their own physical, emotional, and cognitive symptoms. Skills can be taught efficiently in a group program. Once learned, skills can be practiced anywhere and employed over a lifetime, making the teaching of these skills both efficient and cost effective. In addition, due to the increased awareness of bodily sensations and functioning that may be associated with mindfulness practice, patients may have an improved ability to recognize and report new symptoms and changes to their medical team. Ultimately, this may enhance self-management and increase appropriate use of medical services, potentially reducing complications or other additional medical problems. It a sense, mindfulness practice has the potential to empower patients and clients to more fully engage in a partnership with health care providers as they participate in their own care.

Finally, for consideration, following TBI—as well as other diseases impacting frontal lobe functioning in particular—impulsive behaviors and difficulty with controlling emotional responses such as anger are sometimes concerns and can have a significant impact on outcome, as "frontal lobe symptoms" may cause significant difficulties in interpersonal relationships and in work and community re-entry. Training individuals with frontal behaviors to focus on triggers and to learn to recognize increases in anxiety or irritation prior to explosive behaviors occurring is part of the efforts that are often employed in treatment. Based on the available literature as presented in this chapter, it is possible that mindfulness-based interactions may assist individuals with frontal lobe symptoms to more readily engage in "top-down" management of emotions as suggested by Leung et al. (2014).

As an example of a mindfulness-based approach, let's consider the management of chronic pain related to illness or injury: Mindfulness practice can be used to assist with pain management by teaching patients to pay attention to the present moment in order to manage or work through pain. For example, patients may learn to experience the thoughts that accompany pain, so that they can later determine the veracity of those thoughts or make conscious efforts to evaluate and change them. Patients can be taught to breathe through painful moments, and to learn more about their pain through observation (i.e., attention to the sensations of pain in detail may allow an individual to notice that the pain is not actually constant, but may come in waves or wax and wane with various circumstances or timing). This observation of and facing of the pain directly rather than avoidance can assist patients in changing their relationship with the pain and ultimately in managing pain more effectively while regaining an increased sense of control and self-efficacy. Breathing techniques, use of the body scan, and evaluation of the thoughts and emotions associated with the pain can be associated with significant gains in pain management.

Traumatic Brain Injury

Efforts have been made to create programs tailored to individuals with specific limitations. For example, an earlier randomized controlled trial of the use of a brief mindfulness training paradigm with individuals with TBI (McMillan et al., 2002) did not result in positive findings. The authors indicated that the brevity of training may have been a factor. In contrast, a later pilot of an MBI for individuals with mild TBI was conducted by Azulay and colleagues (2012) in which a traditional MBSR course was modified with recognition that individuals with brain injury may require additional considerations for training due to limitations in attention and memory, mental fatigue, and other cognitive issues. Modifications included a ten-week rather than eight-week course with weekly two-hour sessions. Main outcome measures included the Perceived Quality of Life Scale, the Perceived Self-Efficacy Scale, and the Neurobehavioral Symptom Inventory. Secondary measures included neuropsychological testing results and self-report measures of mindfulness and problem solving. Although this was a pilot study, the results indicated that it is possible to adapt the MBSR program for the inclusion of individuals with mild TBI. Clinically relevant improvements in measures of quality of life and perceived self-efficacy were reported, with smaller (but still significant) effects on measures of the central executive aspects of working memory and the regulation of attention. The authors concluded that additional comparative effectiveness research is warranted regarding the use of MBIs with this population.

In another pilot study with individuals with TBI, Bédard and colleagues (2003) 12 weekly sessions, which included a form of mindfulness-based meditation called Insight Meditation, breathing exercises, guided visualization, and group discussion focusing on altering perceptions of disability, increasing acceptance, and moving beyond limiting beliefs. Subjects were ten individuals with mild to moderate TBI who were at least one year postinjury. Findings of this pilot indicated improvements in self-reports of quality of life and on the cognitive-affective domain of the Beck Depression Inventory II (BDI II). Changes in the overall BDI II and positive symptom distress inventory of the SCL-90R approached significance. The authors concluded that the intervention was simple and had improved quality of life after other treatment options were exhausted.

Bédard and colleagues (2012) evaluated the use of MBCT in a group of 20 individuals with diagnosed clinical depression after TBI. Subjects participated in an eight-week course of 90-minute weekly MBCT sessions using materials that combined MBCT and MBSR manualized programs. Measures of depression, pain frequency and intensity, energy levels, health status, and function were collected pre- and postparticipation. Findings indicated that participation in the intervention significantly reduced depressive symptoms on all scales. Medium to large effect sizes for each depression measure were indicated. Significant reductions in pain intensity and significant increases in energy levels were also reported. No significant changes were reported in anxiety symptoms, pain frequency, or level of functioning. The authors concluded that MBCT was efficacious in decreasing depression symptomology after TBI, and that further studies with more robust designs were warranted.

Individuals with a history of TBI often report ongoing issues with focused and/or sustained attention. McHugh and Wood (2013) reported positive findings in a study in which they completed in which 24 individuals with ongoing issues with focused or sustained attention were divided between a mindfulness intervention and control (no treatment) group. Individuals in both groups were asked to participate in a task designed to measure stimulus overselectivity (i.e., paying attention to one environmental stimulus disproportionally to other salient stimuli, suggesting difficulties with attentional control). Per the results of this study, stimulus overselectivity was indicated in individuals with TBI participating in the study at baseline, however, this was significantly reduced after mindfulness training as compared to those who participated in the no-intervention control group.

One group has produced multiple studies of the utilization of mindfulness-based practices with individuals with a history of TBI, with results indicating significant benefits for reducing self-reported symptoms of depression (Bédard et al., 2003) and depression and anxiety (Bédard et al., 2014) after TBI via treatment with MBCT. An additional study by the same group indicated reductions in self-reported symptoms of depression, with maintenance of improvement at the time of a three-month follow-up (Bédard et al., 2014).

Stroke

Lawrence and colleagues (2013) conducted a review of four studies of the use of MBIs with individuals with a history of stroke. In total, 160 participants were involved across the four studies. Three interventions were delivered via a group format and one was delivered one-to-one. The authors report a positive trend in findings, suggesting benefits ranging across multiple psychological and physiological outcomes, including depression, fatigue, blood pressure, perceived health, anxiety, and quality of life. They concluded, however, that further study is needed with enhanced scientific methodology in order to validate results. An additional review article (Lazaridou, Philbrook, & Tzika, 2013) evaluated the use of yoga and mindfulness in stroke rehabilitation. The review evaluated five clinical trials, four case studies, and one qualitative design. Again citing the need for additional research, the authors indicated preliminary findings suggesting improvements in cognition, mood stress reduction, and balance associated with the therapeutic use of MBIs after stroke.

Johansson, Bjuhr, and Rönnbäck, conducted a series of studies regarding mental fatigue following acquired brain injury. In the first study, (2012), 18 individuals with stroke and 11 with TBI, who had no residual significant physical or cognitive impairments aside from mental fatigue, were randomized to a MBSR course or a wait-list control group. Results indicated that statistically significant positive changes in self-assessments of mental fatigue were reported by individuals engaged in MBSR. Secondarily, improvements were noted on neuropsychological tests (digit symbol-coding, and the Trail Making Test). Conclusions of the study were that MBSR may be a promising nonpharmacological treatment for mental fatigue after stroke or TBI. Johansson and colleagues were also able to obtain positive outcomes in an additional advanced mindfulness program with the same population (2015) and in delivering an online MBSR program to individuals with ongoing issues of fatigue after stroke or TBI in a live and interactive format to enhance care and participation (2015).

These findings showcase just a few of the studies suggesting benefits of MBIs for populations with diagnoses that are commonly followed by neuropsychologists engaged in the rehabilitative evaluation and treatment of individuals with neurologically based injuries or illnesses. It is worth noting that, in addition to stroke and TBI, studies have indicated benefits associated with the use of mindfulness for emotional adjustment and coping associated with diagnostic groups including of Parkinson's disease (i.e., Advocat et al., 2013; Pickuta et al., 2013), multiple sclerosis (Agha-Bagheri et al., 2013; Pakenham et al., 2013; Simpson et al., 2014; Senders et al., 2014), and other chronic and disabling diagnoses, including a fairly large literature on fibromyalgia (see, for example: Henke & Chur-Hansen (2014) and cancer (see, for example: Zainal, Booth, & Huppert, 2013).

Methodological Considerations: Summary and Recommendations for Future Study

In most available reviews of the mindfulness literature, authors have continually asserted that additional scientific study of mindfulness is warranted and necessary. Most recently, Tang, Hözel, and Posner (2015), in a review of the neuroscience literature, summed up nicely what has been repeatedly stated. In discussing the current challenges, the authors caution readers to be vigilant of the fact that research in this field, although promising, is relatively preliminary. They note that further replication and validation are needed via studies that are larger and more stringent in methodology. We are reminded that mindfulness research, in general, is a relatively young field. While findings in the past 20 years have been supportive of the beneficial effects of mindfulness on physical and emotional health, as well as on improved cognition, the neuroscience findings are more recent. In general, neuroimaging studies and neurobiological studies have had relatively small sample sizes, with few longitudinal studies. The authors point out the limitations of cross-sectional designs comparing individuals or groups with various experience in meditation to control groups with no exposure or practice. In some cases, long-term meditators have been compared to individuals with no experience (i.e., Luders et al., 2011), while other studies have compared novices who undergo training for variable periods of time to wait-list control groups (i.e., Hölzel et al., 2011; Kilpatrick et al., 2011). Although behavioral as well as structural and functional changes in the brain have been reported in many of the early studies reviewed, Tang and colleagues (2015) point out that it is possible that there are other factors outside of the meditation experience that may play a role in the findings observed. For example, it is possible that other personality or lifestyle characteristics may make it more likely for an individual to practice or persist in meditation. In addition, the authors point out that it may be necessary to control for other factors that may be active ingredients in the changes noted, such as dietary changes made during the practice period due to greater awareness of or desire to make healthy lifestyle changes, or other factors associated with social participation in a group. Tang and colleagues (2015) also assert that control conditions within neuroimaging sessions may be difficult to control for, as it may not always be possible to monitor true resting-state periods in individuals who may be practiced meditators and may naturally fall into a meditative state during rest periods. Active distraction, however, may be hard to differentiate from brain activity due to target tasks. Overall, the authors conclude that evidence from these early studies suggests that mindfulness meditation may cause structural and functional changes in the brain. The current evidence indicates changes in specific areas associated with regulation of attention, self-awareness, and emotion. The authors assert that further, more rigorously controlled, studies with larger sample sizes are necessary for further validation of the current findings.

A Few Final Considerations

Modern medicine and modern society often focus on "cures" and "quick fixes" that are often desired to alleviate pain and medical issues. As the landscape of medicine and health care continue to shift towards increased focus on patient satisfaction and outcomes after injury or illness, it becomes even more important for professionals working with individuals with chronic health conditions to seek interventions with the potential for significant potency and long-term impact. Individuals who are often seen in rehabilitation settings due to neurological injuries, illnesses, or diseases often present with a complex constellation of challenges and needs. In our work with them, it is likely that physical, cognitive, and emotional aspects of care will be important to consider. The research reviewed in this chapter suggests that the literature regarding MBSR and other MBIs requires additional scientific validation. That said, the interventions available via mindfulness-based programs have the potential to address patient and client concerns in a multifaceted fashion, and to have a positive impact on areas of significant concern for our clinical populations. As a result, mindfulness appears to be a field worth following, with an awareness that as neuropsychologists we may be in a unique position to further study and apply mindfulness techniques and practices in our work in the rehabilitation of individuals with neurologically based injuries or illnesses.

References

Advocat, J., Russell, G., Enticott, J., Hassed, C., Hester, J., & Vandenberg, B. (2013). The effects of a mindfulness-based lifestyle programme for adults with Parkinsons disease: protocol for a mixed methods, randomised two-group control study. *BMJ Open*, *3*(10), e003326.

Agha-Bagheri, H., Mohammad-Khani, P., Emrani, S., & Farahmand, V. (2012). The Efficacy of Mindfulness-Based Cognitive Therapy Group on the Increase of Subjective Well-Being and Hope in Patients with Multiple Sclerosis. *Journal of Clinical Psychology*, *4*(1), 23–31.

Azulay, J., Smart, C. M., Mott, T., & Cicerone, K. D. (2013). A Pilot Study Examining the Effect of Mindfulness-Based Stress Reduction on Symptoms of Chronic Mild Traumatic Brain Injury/Postconcussive Syndrome. *Journal of Head Trauma Rehabilitation*, *28*(4), 323-331. doi: Doi 10.1097/Htr.0b013e318250ebda

Baer, R. A., Carmody, J., & Hunsinger, M. (2012). Weekly change in mindfulness and perceived stress in a mindfulness-based stress reduction program. *Journal of Clinical Psychology*, *68*(7), 755–765. doi: 10.1002/jclp.21865

Barnert, E. S., Himelstein, S., Herbert, S., Garcia-Romeu, A., & Chamberlain, L. J. (2014). Innovations in Practice: Exploring an intensive meditation intervention for incarcerated youth. *Child and Adolescent Mental Health*, *19*(1), 69–73. doi: Doi 10.1111/Camh.12019

Bédard, M., Felteau, M., Mazmanian, D., Fedyk, K., Klein, R., Richardson, J., Parkinson, W., & Minthorn-Biggs, M. B. (2003). Pilot evaluation of a mindfulness-based intervention to improve quality of life among individuals who sustained traumatic brain injuries. *Disability & Rehabilitation*, *25*(13), 722–731.

Bédard, M., Felteau, M., Marshall, S., Cullen, N., Gibbons, C., Dubois, S., Maxwell, H., Mazmanian, D., Weaver, B., Rees, L., Gainer, R., Klein, R., & Moustgaard, A. (2014). Mindfulness-based cognitive therapy reduces symptoms of depression in people with a traumatic brain injury: results from a randomized controlled trial. *The Journal of Head Trauma Rehabilitation*, *29*(4), E13–E22.

Black, S. (2010). Mindfulness research guide: A new paradigm for managing empirical health information. *Mindfulness, 1*(3), 174–176. doi:10.1007/s12671 010 0019 0.

Carlson, L. E., Speca, M., Faris, P., & Patel, K. D. (2007). One year pre–post intervention follow-up of psychological, immune, endocrine and blood pressure outcomes of mindfulness-based stress reduction (MBSR) in breast and prostate cancer outpatients. *Brain, Behavior and Immunity*, *21*(8), 1038–1049.

Chiesa, A., Calati, R., & Serretti, A. (2011). Does mindfulness training improve cognitive abilities? A systematic review of neuropsychological findings. *Clinical Psychology Review*, *31*(3), 449–464.

Creswell, J. D., Irwin, M. R., Burklund, L. J., Lieberman, M. D., Arevalo, J. M., Ma, J., Crabb Breen, E., Cole, S. W. (2012). Mindfulness-Based Stress Reduction training reduces loneliness and pro-inflammatory gene expression in older adults: a small randomized controlled trial. *Brain Behavior and Immunity*, *26*(7), 1095–1101. doi: 10.1016/j.bbi.2012.07.006

Davidson, R. J., Kabat-Zinn, J., Schumacher, J., Rosenkranz, M., Muller, D., Santorelli, S. F., Urbanowski, F., Harrington, A., Bonus, K., Sheridan, J. F. (2003). Alterations in brain and immune function produced by mindfulness meditation. *Psychosomatic Medicine*, *65* (4) , 564–570. doi: 10.1097/01.PSY.0000077505.67574.E3

Esmer, G., Blum, J., Rulf, J., & Pier, J. (2010). Mindfulness-based stress reduction for failed back surgery syndrome: a randomized controlled trial. *Journal of the American Osteopathy Association*, *110*(11), 646–652.

Fox, K. C., Nijeboer, S., Dixon, M. L., Floman, J. L., Ellamil, M., Rumak, S. P., Christoff, K. (2014). Is meditation associated with altered brain structure? A systematic review and meta-analysis of morphometric neuroimaging in meditation practitioners. *Neuroscience Biobehavior Review*, *43*, 48–73. doi: 10.1016/j.neubiorev.2014.03.016

Galantino, M. L., Baime, M., Maguire, M., Szapary, P. O., & Farrar, J. T. (2005). Association of psychological and physiological measures of stress in health-care professionals during an 8-week mindfulness meditation program: Mindfulness in practice. *Stress and Health*, *21*(4), 255–261.

Gard, T., Hölzel, B. K., & Lazar, S. W. (2014). The potential effects of meditation on age-related cognitive decline: a systematic review. *Annals of the New York Academy of Sciences*, *1307*(1), 89–103.

Garland, E. L., & Howard, M. O. (2013). Mindfulness-oriented recovery enhancement reduces pain attentional bias in chronic pain patients. *Psychotherapy Psychosom*, *82*(5), 311–318. doi: 10.1159/000348868

Goyal M, Singh S., Sibinga, E., Gould, N., Rowland-Seymour, A., Sharma, R., Berger, Z., Sleicher, D., Maron, D., Shihab, H., Ranasinghe, P, Linn, S., Saha, S., Bass, E., Haythornthwaite, J., (2014) Meditation Programs for Psychological Stress and Well-being: A Systematic Review and Meta-analysis. *JAMA Internal Medicine*, *174*(3):357–368. doi:10.1001/jamainternmed.2013.13018.

Grant, J. A., Courtemanche, J., Duerden, E. G.,Duncan, G. H. & Rainville, P. (2010) Cortical thickness and pain sensitivity in zen meditators. *Emotion 10*, 43–53.

Henke, M., & Chur-Hansen, A. (2014). The effectiveness of mindfulness-based programs on physical symptoms and psychological distress in patients with fibromyalgia: A systematic review. *International Journal of Wellbeing*, *4*(1).

Hölzel , B. K., Carmody, J., Evans, K. C., Hoge, E. A., Dusek, J. A., Morgan, L., Pitman, R., Lazar, S. W. (2010). Stress reduction correlates with structural changes in the amygdala. *Social Cognitive and Affective Neuroscience*, *5*(1), 11–17. doi: 10.1093/scan/nsp034

Hölzel, B. K., Carmody, J., Vangel, M., Congleton, C., Yerramsetti, S. M., Gard, T., & Lazar, S. W. (2011). Mindfulness practice leads to increases in regional brain gray matter density. *Psychiatry Research*, *191*(1), 36-43. doi: 10.1016/j.pscychresns.2010.08.006

Jain, F. A., Walsh, R. N., Eisendrath, S. J., Christensen, S., & Cahn, B. R. (2014). Critical analysis of the efficacy of meditation therapies for acute and subacute phase treatment of depressive disorders: A systematic review. *Psychosomatics*, *56*(2).

Jha, A. P., Stanley, E. A., Kiyonaga, A., Wong, L., & Gelfand, L. (2010). Examining the protective effects of mindfulness training on working memory capacity and affective experience. *Emotion*, *10*(1), 54.

Johansson, B., Bjuhr H. & Rönnbäck. (2012). Mindfulness-based stress reduction (MBSR) improves long-term mental fatigue after stroke or traumatic brain injury. *Brain Injury, 26* , Issue 13–14.

Johansson, B., Bjuhr, H., Karlsson, M., Karlsson, J-O., Rönnbäck, L., (2015). Mindfulness-Based Stress Reduction (MBSR) delivered live on the internet to individuals suffering from mental fatigue after an acquired brain Injury. *Mindfulness, 6*, 1356. https://doi.org/10.1007/s12671-015-0406-

Johansson, B., Bjuhr, H. & Rönnbäck, L. (2015). Evaluation of an Advanced Mindfulness Program Following a Mindfulness-Based Stress Reduction Program for Participants Suffering from Mental Fatigue After Acquired Brain Injury. *Mindfulness, 6*, 227. https://doi.org/10.1007/s12671-013-0249-z

Kabat-Zinn, J. (1982). An outpatient program in behavioral medicine for chronic pain patients based on the practice of mindfulness meditation: theoretical considerations and preliminary results. *General Hospital Psychiatry*, *4*(1), 33–47.

Kabat-Zinn, J., Lipworth, L., & Burney, R. (1985). The clinical use of mindfulness meditation for the self-regulation of chronic pain. *Journal of Behavioral Medicine*, *8*(2), 163–190.

Kabat-Zinn, J., Lipworth, L., Burncy, R., & Sellers, W. (1987). Four-Year Follow-Up of a Meditation-based program for the self-regulation of chronic pain: treatment outcomes and compliance. *Clinical Journal of Pain*, *2*(3), 159–173.

Kabat-Zinn, J., & University of Massachusetts Medical Center/Worcester. (1991). *Full Catastrophe Living: Using the Wisdom of your Body and Mind to Face Stress, Pain, and Illness*. New York, N.Y: Dell Pub.

Kabat-Zinn, J., Massion, A. O., Kristeller, J., Peterson, L. G., Fletcher, K. E., Pbert, L., Lenderking, W., Santorelli, S. F. (1992). Effectiveness of a meditation-based stress reduction program in the treatment of anxiety disorders. *American Journal of Psychiatry*, *149*(7), 936–943.

Kabat-Zinn, J. (1994). Wherever you go, there you are: Mindfulness meditation in everyday life.

Kabat-Zinn, J., Wheeler, E., Light, T., Skillings, A., Scharf, M. J., Cropley, T. G., Hosmer, D., Bernhard, J. D. (1998). Influence of a mindfulness meditation-based stress reduction intervention on rates of skin clearing in patients with moderate to severe psoriasis undergoing phototherapy (UVB) and photochemotherapy (PUVA). *Psychosomatic Medicine*, *60*(5), 625–632.

Kabat-Zinn, J. (2003). Mindfulness-based interventions in context: Past, present, and future. *Clinical Psychology: Science and Practice, 10* (2): DOI: 10.1093/clipsy/bpg016

Kelley, T. M., & Lambert, E. G. (2012). Mindfulness as a Potential Means of Attenuating Anger and Aggression for Prospective Criminal Justice Professionals. *Mindfulness*, *3*(4), 261–274. doi: Doi 10.1007/S12671-012-0090-9

Kerr, C. E., Sacchet, M. D., Lazar, S. W., Moore, C. I., & Jones, S. R. (2013). Mindfulness starts with the body: somatosensory attention and top-down modulation of cortical alpha rhythms in mindfulness meditation. *Frontiers in Human Neuroscience*, *7*, doi:10.3389/fnhum.2013.00012

Kilpatrick, L. A., Suyenobu, B. Y., Smith, S. R., Bueller, J. A., Goodman, T., Creswell, J. D., Tillish, K., Mayer E. A., & Naliboff, B. D. (2011). Impact of mindfulness-based stress reduction training on intrinsic brain connectivity. *NeuroImage*, *56*(1), 290–298. doi: 10.1016/j.neuroimage.2011.02.034

Kirschbaum, C., Pirke, K., & Hellhammer, D.H. (1993). The 'Trier Social Stress Test' – a tool for investigating psychobiological stress responses in a laboratory setting. *Neuropsychobiology*, *28*:76–81

Lawrence, M., Booth, J., Mercer, S., & Crawford, E. (2013). A systematic review of the benefits of mindfulness-based interventions following transient ischemic attack and stroke. *International Journal of Stroke*, *8*(6), 465–474. doi: 10.1111/ijs.12135

Lazar, S. W. et al. (2005) Meditation experience is associated with increased cortical thickness. *Neuroreport* 16,1893–1897.

Lazarindou, A., Philbrook, P., Tzika, A. A. (2013). Yoga and mindfulness as therapeutic interventions for stroke rehabilitation: A systematic review. *Evidence-Based Complementary and Alternative Medicine*, 1–7.

Leonard, N. R., Jha, A. P., Casarjian, B., Goolsarran, M., Garcia, C., Cleland, C. M., Gwadz. M., Massey, Z. (2013). Mindfulness training improves attentional task performance in incarcerated youth: a group randomized controlled intervention trial. *Frontiers in Psychology*, *4*, 792. doi: 10.3389/fpsyg.2013.00792

Leung, N. T. Y., Lo, M. M., & Lee, T. M. C. (2014). Potential therapeutic effects of meditation for treating affective dysregulation. *Evidence Based Complementary Alternative Medicine*.

Luders, E., Clark, K., Narr, K. L., & Toga, A. W. (2011). Enhanced brain connectivity in long-term meditation practitioners. *NeuroImage*, *57*(4), 1308-1316. doi: 10.1016/j.neuroimage.2011.05.075

Ludwig, D. S., & Kabat-Zinn, J. (2008). Mindfulness in medicine. *The Journal of the American Medical Association*, *300*(11), 1350–1352. doi: 10.1001/jama.300.11.1350

MacCoon, D. G., Imel, Z. E., Rosenkranz, M. A., Sheften, J. G., Weng, H. Y., Sullivan, J. C., Bonus, K. A., Stoney, C. M., Salomons, J. C., Davidson, R. J., Lutz, A. L. (2012). The validation of an active control intervention for mindfulness based stress reduction (MBSR). *Behaviour Research and Therapy*, *50* (1), 3–12.

Maj van der Velden, A. M., Kuyken, W., Wattar, U., Crane, C., Pallesen, K. J., Dahlgaard, J., Fjorbac, L. O. & Piet, J. (2015). A systematic review of mechanisms of change in mindfulness-based cognitive therapy in the treatment of recurrent major depressive disorder. *Clinical Psychology Review*, *37*, 26–39.

Marciniak, R., Sheardova, K., Čermáková, P., Hudeček, D., Šumec, R., & Hort, J. (2014). Effect of meditation on cognitive functions in context of aging and neurodegenerative diseases. *Frontiers in Behavioral Neuroscience*, *8*:17.

McHugh, L., & Wood, R. (2013). Stimulus over-selectivity in temporal brain injury: Mindfulness as a potential intervention. *Brain Injury*, *27*(13-14), 1595–1599.

McMillan, T., Robertson, I. H., Brock, D., & Chorlton, L. (2002). Brief mindfulness training for attentional problems after traumatic brain injury: A randomised control treatment trial. *Neuropsychological Rehabilitation*, *12*(2), 117–125. doi: 10.1080/09602010143000202

Merkes, M. (2010). Mindfulness-based stress reduction for people with chronic diseases. *Australian Journal of Primary Health*, *16*(3), 200–210. doi: 10.1071/PY09063

Mrazek, M. D., Franklin, M. S., Phillips, D. T., Baird, B., & Schooler, J. W. (2013). Mindfulness training improves working memory capacity and GRE performance while reducing mind wandering. *Psychological Science*, 0956797612459659.

Napoli, M., Krech, P. R., & Holley, L. C. (2005). Mindfulness Training for Elementary School Students: The Attention Academy. *Journal of Applied School Psychology*, *21*(1), 99–123. New York: Hyperion.

Ospina, M. B., Bond, K, Karkhaneh, M., Buscemi, N., Dryden, D. M., Barnes, V., Carlson, L.E., Dusek, J.A., and David

Shannahoff-Khalsa, D. (2008). Clinical trials of meditation practices in health care: Characteristics and quality. *The Journal of Alternative and Complementary Medicine*, *14*(10): 1199–1213. doi:10.1089/acm.2008.0307.

Pakenham, K. I., & Samios, C. (2013). Couples coping with multiple sclerosis: a dyadic perspective on the roles of mindfulness and acceptance. *Journal of Behavorial Medicine*, *36*(4), 389–400. doi: 10.1007/s10865-012-9434-0

Pickuta, B.A.,Van Heckea, W., Kerckhofsd E., Mariëne, P., Vannestea, S., Crasa, P., Parizela, P. M., (2013). Mindfulness based intervention in Parkinson's disease leads to structural brain changes on MRI: A randomized controlled longitudinal trial. *Clinical Neurology and Neurosurgery*, *115* (12) 2419–2425.

Rapgay and Bystrisky (2009). Classical Mindfulness: An Introduction to its theory and practice for clinical application, Longevity, Regeneration, and Optimal Health: *Annals of the New York Academy of Sciences*, *1172*, 148–162

Rosenkranz, M. A., Davidson, R. J., Maccoon, D. G., Sheridan, J. F., Kalin, N. H., & Lutz, A. (2013). A comparison of mindfulness-based stress reduction and an active control in modulation of neurogenic inflammation. *Brain, Behavior, and Immunity*, *27*(1), 174–184. doi: 10.1016/j.bbi.2012.10.013

Samuelson, M., Carmody, J., Kabat-Zinn, J., & Bratt, M. A. (2007). Mindfulness-based stress reduction in Massachusetts correctional facilities. *Prison Journal*, *87*(2), 254–268. doi: Doi 10.1177/0032885507303753

Senders, A., Bourdette, D., Hanes, D., Yadav, V., & Shinto, L. (2014). Perceived stress in multiple sclerosis: the potential role of mindfulness in health and well-being. *Journal of Evidence Based Complementary Alternative Medicine*, *19*(2), 104–111. doi: 10.1177/2156587214523291

Serpa, J. G., Taylor, S. L., & Tillisch, K. (2014). Mindfulness-based Stress Reduction (MBSR) reduces anxiety, depression, and suicidal ideation in veterans. *Medical Care*, *52*, S19–S24.

Simpson, R., Booth, J., Lawrence, M., Byrne, S., Mair, F., & Mercer, S. (2014). Mindfulness based interventions in multiple sclerosis--a systematic review. *BMC Neurology*, *14*, 15. doi: 10.1186/1471-2377-14-15

Singleton, O. et al. (2014). Change in brainstem grey matter concentration following a mindfulness-based intervention is correlated with improvement in psychological well-being. *Frontiers in Human Neuroscience*, *8*, 33

Tang, Y. Y., Hölzel, B. K., & Posner, M. I. (2015). The neuroscience of mindfulness meditation. *Nature Reviews Neuroscience*, *16*(4), 213–225.

Tang, Y. Y. et al. (2010). Short-term meditation induces white matter changes in the anterior cingulate. *Proc. Natl Acad. Sci. USA*, *107*, 15649–15652 (2010).

Tang, Y. Y., Lu, Q., Fan, M., Yang, Y. & Posner, M. I. (2012). Mechanisms of white matter changes induced by meditation. *Proceedings of the National Academy of Sciences of the USA*, *109*, 10570–10574.

Teasdale, J. D., Segal, Z. V., & Williams, J. M. G. (1995). How does cognitive therapy prevent depressive relapse and why should attentional control (mindfulness) training help? *Behaviour Research and Therapy*, *33*, 25–39.

Trousselard, M., Steiler, D., Claverie, D., & Canini, F. (2012). Relationship between mindfulness and psychological adjustment in soldiers according to their confrontation with repeated deployments and stressors. *Psychology*, *3*(1), 100–115.

Vestergaard-Poulsen, P. et al. (2009). Long-term meditation is associated with increased grey matter density in the brain stem. *Neuroreport 20*, 170–174, 115, 12, 2419–2425.

Wisner, B. L., Jones, B., & Gwin, D. (2010). School-based meditation practices for adolescents: A resource for strengthening self-regulation, emotional coping, and self-esteem. *Children and Schools*, *32*(3), 150–159.

Zainal, N. Z., Booth, S., & Huppert, F. A. (2013). The efficacy of mindfulness-based stress reduction on mental health of breast cancer patients: a meta-analysis. *Psychooncology*, *22*(7), 1457–1465. doi: 10.1002/pon.3171

48 Collaborative Therapeutic Neuropsychological Assessment

Tad T. Gorske

Collaborative Therapeutic Neuropsychological Assessment (CTNA) is a method for giving feedback from neuropsychological test results that is based on client-centered principles (Gorske & Smith, 2009). This chapter will provide an overview of CTNA principles and methods as well as developments in collaborative neuropsychology, and will describe two cases where CTNA feedback methods were used.

Roots of Collaborative Therapeutic Neuropsychological Assessment

CTNA's roots are most directly tied to Finn's Therapeutic Assessment (TA) and Fischer's Collaborative Individualized Assessment (Gorske & Smith, 2009). However, the history of psychological testing as a therapeutic intervention can be traced to the late 1940s and 1950s, when practitioners used performance-based tests as precursors to psychotherapy and, in some cases, as part of the therapy encounter (Aronow & Reznikoff, 1971; Bellack, Pasquarelli, & Braverman, 1949; Berg, 1985; Harrower, 1956; Luborsky, 1953: Mosak & Gushurst, 1972). Fischer developed these approaches further into Collaborative Individualized Assessment (CIA). CIA reflected a "human-science" assessment process that emphasized humanistic and existential principles of psychological assessment into a collaborative "man-as-co-constitutor" experience (Fischer, 1970, 1994). Beginning in the 1990s, Finn used the Minnesota Multiphasic Personality Inventory–2 (MMPI-2) and other performance-based tests as therapeutic interventions and developed guidelines for conducting a TA (Finn, 1996a, 1996b, Finn, 2007). Over time TA and CIA mutually influenced each other. Since the initial publications, TA has developed increasing empirical support (Finn, Fischer, & Handler, 2012). TA and CIA methods traditionally employ personality-assessment measures and occasionally intelligence and cognitive tests; however, there has been little application of TA and CIA in neuropsychology (Finn, 1996a, 2003).

Feedback in Neuropsychology

There is limited empirical literature about neuropsychological assessment feedback methods. Gass and Brown (1992) were the first authors to emphasize the importance of feedback in neuropsychological assessment and to provide a framework for conducting a feedback session. Prior to their 1992 article there was almost no information on a neuropsychological feedback process or its value in patient care. Luria's Neuropsychological Investigation (LNI) emphasized a phenomenological analysis of the patients' cognitive life and a qualitative analysis of patient functioning (Christensen & Caetano, 1996). The preliminary conversation in Luria's method emphasized a positive therapeutic atmosphere with a flexible and interactive examination that included a feedback process (Christensen & Caetano, 1999; Christensen, Goldberg, & Bougakov, 2009). However, LNI in and of itself was not a formal feedback method.

Following Gass and Brown's article, authors wrote about the utility of neuropsychological test feedback and emphasized its importance, but no formal studies or methods were offered (Armengol, Kaplan, & Moes, 2001; Bennett-Levy, Klein-Boonschate, Batchelor, McCarter, & Walton, 1994; Malla et al., 1997). In 2005 Pegg and colleagues published what could arguably be the first article looking at the utility of providing medical and neuropsychological information to traumatic brain injury (TBI) patients (Pegg, Auerback, Seel, Buenaver, Kiesler, and Plybon, 2005). The results indicate that patients who received feedback about their medical and neuropsychological information in a person-centered style of interaction were more empowered and informed consumers of a TBI rehabilitation program (Pegg et al., 2005). Pegg noted that patients who received this information tended to be more assertive and inquisitive about their condition and treatments (Pegg, P., personal communication, 2004).

Development of Collaborative Therapeutic Neuropsychological Assessment

CTNA developed from the work of the present author and Steven Smith from the University of California, Santa Barbara, along with guidance and mentoring from Finn, Fischer, and Diane Engelmann. The present author had been working in an extended joint postdoctoral placement in addiction medicine and clinical neuropsychology, under the mentorship of Christopher Ryan, at Western Psychiatric Institute and Clinic in Pittsburgh, Pennsylvania. At the time, this author was working with patients diagnosed with substance abuse and psychiatric disorders (dual disorders) in a specialized Dual Diagnosis Clinic. This author and Ryan developed a method for giving patients feedback from neuropsychological test results. Initially the feedback method was based on the Motivational Interviewing Personal Feedback Report and adapted to include neuropsychological assessment results only (Gorske & Smith, 2009; Miller, Zweben, DiClemente, & Rychtarik, 1999). Positive feedback was received from patients about the neuropsychological feedback sessions and the utility of the method was explored more formally. Following collection of pilot data, a Career Development Award Grant through the National Institute on Drug Abuse was awarded in 2004 (NIDA–DA017273–01). It was during that time that the author had formal contact with Finn, Fischer, Smith, and Engelman during the Spring 2006 annual convention at the Society for Personality Assessment, where methods were presented. Smith had been developing Collaborative Neuropsychological Assessment (CNA) with adolescents and their families at UC Santa Barbara. Eventually methods were combined into a CTNA model that was presented at the National Academy of Neuropsychology in 2006. The model was continually developed and refined and led to the Gorske and Smith publication in 2009.

Collaborative Therapeutic Neuropsychological Assessment Model

CTNA begins with seven basic assumptions, which will be summarized here (Gorske & Smith, 2009). These assumptions guide the CTNA process and provide a conceptual framework for which a clinician approaches the feedback process.

1. The patient/caregiver/referral source has noticed a change in the patient's cognitive and/or behavioral functioning and would like a professional to determine if there is a true change.
2. The patient/family members are distressed because of a change in the patient's cognitive/behavioral functioning.
3. Patients would like to learn potential ameliorative strategies so that they are able to perform better in school, work, and social spheres.
4. Patients want to be respected and empowered as active and autonomous participants in treatment and decision making.
5. Neuropsychological tests provide objective, concrete information about patients' cognitive and behavioral functioning as it applies to their daily life and problems they may be experiencing.
6. Feedback from neuropsychological tests can help answer questions regarding changes in cognitive and behavioral functioning, provide hypotheses as to causes of change, and give direction for treatment.
7. Feedback presented in a patient-centered manner can enlist the patient as an active collaborator, empower the individual in the treatment and decision making process, and lower resistance to hearing difficult or discrepant information. This will motivate the patient to work more closely with professionals to alleviate his or her problems and distress.

The Initial Interview: Collaborative Information Gathering

Collaborative information gathering is an interviewing style that emphasizes listening to the patient's story in addition to collecting important clinical information necessary for understanding what will later be called the patient's *Central Cognitive-Emotional Complaint* (Gorske & Smith, 2009). Collaborative information gathering emphasizes a directive–nondirective approach similar to that found in Motivational Interviewing methods (Miller & Rollnick, 1991/2002). The clinician uses person-centered skills such as empathy, summarization, open-ended questions, and skilled reflections to elicit and elaborate upon the patient's story. Throughout this process the clinician is also guiding the interview in a direction that helps clarify the nature of the patient's cognitive and functional difficulties. This style is especially helpful when the patient is scared, confused, or unclear as to the nature of the problem. Skilled empathic direction and elaboration can help to crystallize the problem more succinctly. This is a skill I emphasize when working with neuropsychology students. I encourage students to learn a person centered-directive style of interviewing versus following a checklist approach. By modeling this in actual patient interviews, one hopes to show how this style can elicit more information about a patient's clinical history and cognitive difficulties that will ultimately help with the neuropsychological interpretation after testing.

In conducting a collaborative interview, there are five phases (Gorske & Smith, 2009). The first, Understanding the Problem, is a gathering of background information while seeking to understand symptoms and problem in context of day-to-day life. Second, Understanding the Emotional Experience of the Problem is when the clinician seeks to understand his or her patients' emotional experience of the problem and its effect on their experience of themselves, their life, relationships, and future. Third is the identification of the Central Cognitive-Emotional Complaint (CCEC). Based on Lester Luborsky's (1984) model, this is a conceptual framework in which the clinician seeks to understand (a) the patients' wish or desire for themselves and their lives, (b) a behavioral or cognitive reaction, (c) an emotional response to that difficulty. Fourth is an understanding of the patient's wishes for the assessment, results, and outcomes. This helps to guide the testing and subsequent feedback process. Finally, the fifth phase is a summarization of topics discussed in order to set the stage for the upcoming tasks of assessment and consequent feedback. The neuropsychological testing session then proceeds in the standard manner based on whatever procedure(s) and battery the clinician chooses. The hope is that by fully elucidating the concerns of patients (and family members), CCEC, wishes and hopes for the future through an open ended/directive collaborative style, the clinician feels he or she has a roadmap for the best way to proceed with testing in order to answer the questions as fully as possible.

Collaborative Therapeutic Neuropsychological Assessment Feedback Session

CTNA is based on three primary approaches: therapeutic/individualized models of psychological assessment; recommendations from previous authors on the provision of neuropsychological test feedback; and Motivational Interviewing principles as reflected in the format for providing information and advice, which is termed "elicit-provide-elicit" (Miller & Rollnick, 1991/2002).

The first step of the CTNA feedback session is Setting the Agenda and Introducing the Feedback Report. This is where the clinician sets the agenda with the patient/family members by outlining the goals and structure of the feedback session. This is followed by a "check in" where the clinician assesses how the patient's life has been since the initial assessment and testing. Part of the check in is to remind the patient of the CCEC as in order to establish a focus for the feedback. The second step is to develop Life Implication Questions, which is where the clinician guides the patient in developing well-formed and specific questions that guide the CTNA feedback session. The third step is the determination of a Personal Skill Profile. This is where the clinician describes to the patient how different cognitive skills are rated and determined to be normal, above normal, or below normal. Essentially, the clinician is describing in lay terms how norm-based scores are obtained. The fourth step is the provision of individual test results. At this stage the clinician revisits the tests given and the skills assessed, and then provides information and feedback in the "elicit-provide-elicit" format. The clinician summarizes a patient's strengths and weaknesses, all the while eliciting patient thoughts, reactions, and understanding of the information provided. Throughout this process the clinician is continually interacting with the patient in a person-centered manner using skills reflected in the acronym "OARS," which stands for "open-ended questions, affirmation, reflections, and summaries." The clinician is always aware of times when resistance may occur in response to the information given. Consistent with Motivational Interviewing principles, the clinician deals with resistance with understanding, empathy, and inviting the patient to consider alternative viewpoints (Miller & Rollnick, 1991/2002). The fifth step is the summarization of the information provided and the relationship between the results and the patient's questions and life goals. Essentially, this step is the bridge between the assessment and the patient's concerns for the future. During this stage the clinician provides a general summary of information provided, gives information and advice, and elicits the patient's thoughts on how he or she would like to use the information for his or her benefit. This stage leads to the final phase of the CTNA session, which is the development of recommendations and a change plan. Here the clinician and patient further develop their partnership in the CTNA process by negotiating and developing concrete change plans. Part of this process is assessing the patient's level of readiness to follow through with change plan recommendations.

At this point the CTNA session focuses on change planning and the implementation of goals and recommendations. Clinical experience suggests that patients who undergo a neuropsychological test feedback session have greater levels of satisfaction with the services provided and are more likely to follow through with goals and recommendations. From a research perspective there is limited information on the effectiveness of feedback on outcomes and goal attainment. The pilot study conducted with dual diagnosis clients at the University of Pittsburgh, Western Psychiatric Institute and Clinic, demonstrated the effectiveness of the Neuropsychological Assessment Feedback Intervention (NAFI) in increasing patients' compliance with a partial hospital group program (Gorske & Smith, 2009). Other research has examined both clinician and patient perceptions of a neuropsychological feedback process with generally positive results (Bennett-Levy et al., 1994; Donofrio, Piatt, Whelihan, & DiCarlo, 1999; Smith, Wiggins, & Gorske, 2007). To date, no formal study has utilized the CTNA approach to assess clinical outcomes. However, there have been further developments in collaborative neuropsychology feedback methods.

Contemporary Developments and Adaptations

Since CTNA was published in 2009, other authors have developed guidelines about the neuropsychological feedback process in clinical situations. However, this line is increasingly blurred when patients referred by a physician for a clinical evaluation often have current or pending litigation, disability, or workman's compensation claims. Carone, Iverson, and Bush (2010) provide guidelines on the provision of feedback to patients in clinical settings when there is evidence of suboptimal effort and response bias. This issue is important given the increased use of symptom validity testing in clinical settings. Carone and colleagues reiterate the widely held belief that it is not advisable, and in fact discouraged, to give patients feedback in forensic settings because the typical doctor–patient relationship does not exist in these circumstances. While a clinical question may be at the forefront of the referral, there will likely be an underlying forensic matter that will surface immediately or in the near future. Carone and colleagues provide sound suggestions on ways to address evidence of suboptimal effort and response bias with patients in a way that maintains a positive therapeutic relationship.

They propose a three-phase model. The first phase involves building rapport and obtaining informed consent. Here the clinician sets the tone and ground rules for the clinical interaction by laying expectations on the table and making sure a client is fully informed, and all the while establishing and maintaining an effective working relationship. The second phase involves completing the evaluation and laying the groundwork for an open discussion of results. If there is sufficient evidence of invalid performance, the authors suggest exploring the patients' willingness to acknowledge poor or variable effort. The authors appropriately caution on the language used to describe suboptimal effort in patients (i.e., framing poor effort as "not fully invested" vs. "lying"). The third and final phase is the feedback session. Carone and colleagues emphasize many sound clinical skills such as maintaining objectivity and professionalism while framing results in terms of strengths and weaknesses. The authors recommend comparing the performance of "poor effort" patients to known clinical groups for comparison. This avoids judgment and labeling and simply points out a discrepancy for patients to consider. The article goes on to address other clinical issues that may be present with patients who give suboptimal effort such as identification of specific effort tests, caution on using terms such as exaggeration and malingering, managing resistance, whether or not to provide a report copy, and handling complaints by patients (Carone et al., 2010; Carone & Bush, 2013). The authors' model contains methods and principles highly consistent with the CTNA approach and is an excellent guideline for providing difficult feedback to patients about effort and motivation in the neuropsychological testing process.

More recently, Postal and Armstrong published *Feedback that Sticks: The Art of Effectively Communicating Neuropsychological Assessment Results* (Postal & Armstrong, 2013). They interviewed 85 neuropsychologists to learn ways these clinicians communicate results from neuropsychological tests in ways that "stick" with patients. The authors identified "pearls" of communicative wisdom from each clinician. The pearls were "ways of explaining clinical phenomenon and findings that engage patients in ways that can alter their lives" (c.f. Postal & Armstrong, 2013: xxxi). The first part of the book discusses what feedback is and what makes it effective and memorable. They also discuss feedback protocols and theoretical issues, concluding with specifics about how feedback is presented. The second part reviews the way feedback is utilized in various clinical populations. Each chapter reviews issues that may arise during a feedback session with different clinical groups. The authors then illustrate examples of feedback that clinicians have given patients in ways that help them understand and learn complex neuropsychological phenomenon. For example, in explaining mild cognitive impairment (MCI; see Postal & Armstrong, 2013, p. 92), Postal and Armstrong provide examples of how clinicians have used down-to-earth and simple language and metaphors to describe the concept of MCI and its relationship to dementia (pp. 92–94). The goal of the book is to provide readers examples of how to give feedback to patients in ways that facilitates learning and understanding. The third and final section of the book is about communicating information beyond the feedback session to other professionals and in report writing (Postal & Armstrong, 2013). The book is an excellent contribution in the effort to help make neuropsychological test feedback meaningful and applicable to the daily lives of patients.

Since the publication of CTNA in 2009, its methods have been recommended by authors for different clinical situations and populations. Pachana, Squelch, and Paton (2010) described the application of CTNA, more specifically Therapeutic Neuropsychological Assessment (TNA) and CNA, which are precursors to CTNA, in giving feedback to older adults in a collaborative and therapeutic manner. In Schoenberg and Scott (2011), *The Little Black Book of Neuropsychology: A Syndrome Based Approach*, Suarez discusses the application of Motivational Interviewing in neuropsychology in the rehabilitation process (Suarez, 2011). An interesting article by Lucas in the *African Journal of Psychiatry* discusses the possible role of CTNA approaches in situations where intervention is required for patients with deteriorating decision-making processes (Lucas, 2010).

Since 2009, very few studies have examined the effects of neuropsychological test feedback on clinical outcomes. Tharinger and Pilgrim (2012) investigated the effects of receiving neuropsychological assessment findings in the form of therapeutic "fables" on clinical outcomes with children and their families. A "fable" is an individualized story developed for a child based on guidelines from Tharinger et al. (2008). The results were that children who received the experimental neuropsychological feedback intervention reported a greater sense of having learned new things about themselves and perceived their parents as understanding their problems better. Both children and parents in the experimental group reported a significantly more positive relationship with the assessor, a greater sense of collaboration with the assessment process, and greater overall satisfaction with the clinical service.

Longley, Tate, and Brown (2012) investigated the psychological benefit of neuropsychological test feedback to patients with multiple sclerosis while looking at the type of patients who benefitted most from feedback. The intervention was described as a semistructured, collaborative, and interactive feedback session based on Gorske (2008); Gass and Brown (1992); and Pachana et al. (2010). They measured treatment fidelity with audio recordings and a feedback checklist reviewed by a blind observer. They examined a number of outcomes, including improvements in client knowledge and use of adaptive strategies, improved caregiver knowledge and decreased burden, improvement in various *patient* psycho-emotional factors and relationship quality, and improvement in *caregiver* psycho-emotional status and relationship quality. The paper concluded that the study design was realistic and feasible, with results pending at the time of its publication (Longley et al., 2012). Since this initial paper, the authors have conducted a randomized controlled trial of neuropsychological assessment with feedback as a therapeutic intervention to improve psychological well-being in patients with multiple sclerosis. Preliminary results showed that patients who received the intervention had reduced levels of distress, increased social confidence, and a high level of satisfaction with the neuropsychological assessment process. Caregiver satisfaction with the assessment process was also high. Caregivers also reported a reduced need to provide psychological support to patients (implying the issue of caregiver burnout) (Longley, Tate, Brown, & Contini, 2013).

In reviewing the developments discussed in this section, there appears to be a burgeoning interest in a collaborative neuropsychology approach among clinicians who wish to blend the scientific discipline of neuropsychology with patient-centered and collaborative methods designed to enhance the working alliance with patients seeking guidance and answers about various neuropsychological conditions. The challenge will be to find the best practice model for the CTNA approach. Neuropsychological practitioners will need to ask the same questions that psychotherapists have asked in regard to the efficacy and effectiveness of psychotherapy interventions: "What treatment, by whom, is most effective for this individual with that specific problem, and under which set of circumstances?" (Paul, 1967: 111). The outcome studies mentioned in this chapter may provide some preliminary information as to how CTNA approaches are best utilized from a research perspective. The case studies presented in the next section will provide examples of how CTNA may be used clinically.

Case Examples

The two cases presented in this section provide contrasting examples of how CTNA may be used. The first is a deidentified TBI case where CTNA was used with a gentleman who suffered a TBI, and had made a reasonably good recovery by the time he was seen for neuropsychological assessment, but continued to experience various deficits including anosognosia and a need to get back to his former life as quickly as possible. However, his intense desire to "be cured" was actually moving his TBI recovery backward. The CTNA session was able to disrupt his regression and help him get his recovery back on track. The second is a continuation of a case presented in Gorske (2008) on "Amy," a young woman diagnosed with a grade IV glioblastoma in the right temporal lobe and her struggle to retain her sense of identity in the face of brain cancer and physically taxing treatments. The case not only shows the importance of goal development in the CTNA approach, but also the ways in which highly motivated patients can use the assessment and feedback process for their benefit. In these situations it is important for the clinician to listen to patients and follow their lead as they struggle on a journey of healing and wholeness in the face of fear and uncertainty.

Case 1: Traumatic Brain Injury Recovery

The first case is a Caucasian gentleman in his late 40s who was an avid bicyclist and was struck by an automobile while riding in the streets. He had no memory for the events and local bystanders contacted Emergency Medical Services (EMS) who took him to the emergency room. He had a Glasgow Coma Score of 8, and exams revealed right frontal, subdural, subarachnoid, and intraparenchymal hemorrhaging. He required a posterior craniectomy due to developing hydrocephalus and a compressive cerebellar hematoma. His course was also complicated by seizure activity. He was eventually stabilized and transferred to inpatient brain injury rehabilitation. When inpatient neuropsychology saw him, he was determined to be just emerging from the posttraumatic amnesia phase (the period of confusion and inability to form new memories after sustaining a brain injury) of recovery about 20 days post injury. Due to ongoing symptoms and recurring hydrocephalus he required a ventriculoperitoneal shunt, which allowed symptoms to resolve. He was eventually discharged about 50 days postinjury. He had to go back to the emergency room within a month after hospital discharge due to a reoccurrence of symptoms, also suffering a seizure and shunt malfunction. This was successfully treated and he was discharged home. He was followed up by outpatient brain injury psychiatrists, neurosurgery, and rehabilitation specialists with reported good progress.

I saw the patient for an outpatient neuropsychological assessment about seven months postinjury. By all accounts he was doing reasonably well and had "graduated" from outpatient physical, occupational, and speech therapies. He was continuing to struggle with nausea and occasional dizziness that seemed to improve with rest. Cognitively the most notable differences were difficulty sustaining attention without becoming distracted and becoming overwhelmed with large amounts of stimulation, such as a busy shopping area, driving in traffic, or being around people where there are multiple simultaneous conversations. Another issue was that the patient was very anxious to get back to his normal activities, particularly exercising. He was an avid bicyclist and loved to exercise. Both the patient and his spouse admitted a tendency toward impatience, particularly when doctors set limits on his activities. He stated that he was trying to take walks and use a stationary bike but found these to be unfulfilling compared to his previous level of activity.

From a neuropsychological perspective, the patient demonstrated average intellectual functioning and was performing normally on tests of attention, working memory, visuomotor tracking, verbal learning and immediate recall, retention, and recognition. He also performed normally on tests of visual recognition, expressive language, and response inhibition. Thus, he had likely made a reasonably good cognitive recovery at the time. He was demonstrating moderate deficits in psychomotor speed, mild deficits in verbal encoding and delayed verbal memory, significant visuoconstructional deficits with low average visual free recall, moderately impaired cognitive flexibility, mildly impaired higher level executive functions, and mildly impaired processing speed.

I met with the patient and his wife about a month later to review the neuropsychological test results and discuss recommendations. Following the introduction and overview of the feedback process, the patient's individual test results were discussed. Although the patient had made a reasonably good cognitive recovery at the time of the assessment, he continued to have deficits and became easily overwhelmed with large amounts of stimulation, a common impairment seen in TBI patients. Therefore, it was important to present the information in small chunks and use strategies to ensure understanding. Fortunately, his wife was present for the feedback—which would help should they decide to review information from our session at a later time. An example of the dialogue is as follows:

GORSKE: "Do you remember the test that required you to draw a line connecting numbers and letters? Like 1-A, 2-B, etc.?"

PATIENT: "Oh yes, I remember that. I think I started off OK but then I got lost?"

GORSKE: "That's right, you started off pretty well but then lost track about half way through. Do you remember what it was like to do that test?"

PATIENT: "I'm not entirely sure. I think I remember just saying it in my head (1-A, 2-B, 3-C) but then at some point I kind of blanked and forgot what I was doing. I'm not sure I can explain it any better." (The patient's wife is sitting behind him and nodding vigorously).

GORSKE: "So it seems like when it comes to activities where you have to move your attention from one thing to another as quick as you can, you might do OK for a while but then find yourself lost. It looks like you wife has something to add to this."

PATIENT'S WIFE: "Yes, this is what happens throughout the day. He tries very hard to help out around the house, which is fine if I give him one thing to do and he sticks with it, but then he tries to do more than one thing at a time; he starts out OK but then there are times I'll see him just standing there looking lost."

GORSKE: (To patient) "Did what she said make sense and have you noticed this yourself?"

PATIENT: "I don't really notice when I *blank* out until someone sort of *wakes me up*. Then I realize that I haven't done what I set out to do. It's frustrating because I'm really trying to get better. It's been what, eight months now? I feel like I should be back to normal now and that's what gets me more depressed than anything. I'm not depressed like sleeping all day or want to kill myself, I just get impatient and down."

PATIENT'S WIFE: "Honestly, you're trying too hard I think."

This interaction brought up some important issues for the patient's recovery. One of the issues he struggled with was multitasking, which was reflected in his reduced executive functioning scores in addition to lower processing speed. This is a common cognitive deficit following a TBI, and ways were discussed to help the patient identify situations he is most likely to try and multitask, learn to slow down and break tasks into smaller and more manageable "chunks," and ways his wife could remind him to follow this plan so he doesn't try to manage too much at one time. However the larger issue was the patient's frustration and impatience with his perceived lack of progress and intense desire to "get better" and get back to normal activities. This tendency was consistent with his personality. Prior to the TBI he was very active—almost obsessive—about exercising and working, and easily managed multiple tasks at one time. The patient tended to minimize the intensity with which he approached activities, but his wife stated that he would often work himself to exhaustion in an effort to convince himself and others that he was back to normal. As a result he would be exhausted and nonfunctional the next day. In fact, through further exploration it was discovered that the day before he suffered the seizure he had been extremely active on a stationary bike, and doing activities in and outside the house, and likely did not drink enough fluids. From this conversation a plan was developed that included (a) frequent planned rest breaks throughout the day, (b) counseling with a rehabilitation psychologist on learning the physiological and mental signs that he may be pushing himself too hard and needs to stop and rest, (c) general brain injury recovery education about timelines and reasonable expectations for progress. The patient's psychiatrist and neurosurgeon reinforced these suggestions, and over time plans were developed for gradual supervised re-entry into activities such as bill paying and other household activities. Counseling helped him cope with his frustrations and impatience.

This case illustrates some of the ways CTNA can be used in neurological disorder cases.

1 Awareness and insight: In this patient's case, there was evidence of anosognosia that was keeping him from being fully aware of his cognitive and functional deficits. However, there was also an element of emotional denial given his premorbid personality was one of very high activity that was almost obsessive in nature yet functional. Now that same premorbid tendency was a detriment to recovery because the patient became overwhelmed easily and his insistence on pushing through actually caused him to regress. The objective data, combined with an empathic and inquisitive approach presented in small and understandable points, allowed the patient to gradually integrate the information and, with the help of his spouse, use the information to enhance his recovery.

2 Providing information about cognition that is applicable and relevant: In order to make the cognitive information understandable and relevant, a continual give and take occurred between the neuropsychologist, patient, and family member about what skills the tests are assessing and how those skills apply to the patients' daily life. One method for this is using plain and simple language. A second method is finding an example in the patient's daily life that he or she can relate to and use that situation to illustrate a cognitive skill. Another method is the use of story or metaphor, as illustrated in Postal and Armstrong (2013). For this patient, biking was used to explain the concept of cognitive set shifting:

"Do you remember a time when you would be riding on a road behind a car and the car would come to a sudden stop? What kind of things did you have to do to avoid hitting the car? First, you had to sense that the car had abruptly stopped and judge your distance from the car; second, you had to apply the brakes; third, you had to shift your body weight back so you wouldn't fly over the handlebars; fourth, you had to unclip your feet so you could put them on the ground so you wouldn't fall. Those four basic things used to be automatic and your brain easily shifted from one task to another rapidly and almost effortlessly. However, now the brain becomes confused and it doesn't send messages as quickly. It's as if your brain needs to relearn how to do this."

3 Developing recovery plans: From one test (Trail Making B) two important recovery issues were identified, including (a) the need to break up multitasking activities into smaller parts, and (b) the need to increase rest breaks and learn to listen to his mind and body to avoid exhausting himself and compromising his health and recovery.

This case illustrates ways to develop goals and objectives that can guide TBI rehabilitation and assess progress at a later date. The next case shows how a young woman used the neuropsychological assessment experience to help her cope with an existential crisis in her fight with brain cancer. This case shows how the CTNA approach can go beyond educating patients about cognitive functioning for goal development and delve more deeply into their daily struggles and life stories (Finn, 2003).

Case 2: The Case of Amy, Continued

In 2008, I wrote an article that was published in the *Journal of Humanistic Psychology,* "Therapeutic Neuropsychological Assessment: A Humanistic Model and Case Example" (Gorske, 2008). This article introduced "The Case of Amy" (p. 327). Amy was a young woman diagnosed with brain cancer who underwent neuropsychological testing and feedback in July 2006. Meetings together illustrated the spirit of CTNA, which is the use of neuropsychological test results as a tool to understand and form a patient's "life story" to promote healing and growth. Amy's real name, published here with permission from her estate, was Marisa Muscarella, and sadly she died on April 2, 2012 after becoming sick and suffering a seizure presumptively related to her brain cancer. This case study conveys more of Marisa's life story following the initial meeting in 2006.[1]

Marisa was born in 1976 to a Sicilian father and a mother from the island of Malta. Marisa was described as a very intelligent, passionate, and strong-willed young woman who had an intense zest for life and was not afraid to express her opinions to others. She described herself as someone who "loved to wake up in the morning" (Gorske, 2008, p. 329) and her family described her as the "go-to" person when it came to knowing the latest activities and events around the city. She was especially passionate about good food and restaurants in Pittsburgh, Pennsylvania, and had high standards as to how food should be cooked, served, and savored. She earned a Master's Degree in Social Work in 2001 and was working with children in the Pittsburgh public schools. She brought the same passion and zest for life to her work and it was said that she treated the children she worked with as if they were her own.

Marisa was diagnosed with brain cancer in April 2006. The details of her diagnosis and treatment are in Gorske (2008) but will be briefly summarized. She experienced her first symptoms around April 26, 2006 when she became ill and suffered a grand mal seizure. Following treatments and evaluations she was initially diagnosed with a grade I pilocytic astrocytoma in the right temporal lobe and underwent surgery on May 23, 2006, which was by all accounts successful at the time. However, later testing revealed that she actually had a grade IV glioblastoma and she began radiation and chemotherapy. I first met Marisa on July 15, 2006 for neuropsychological testing, which was broken up over two days with a feedback session a few weeks after. The details of the testing and feedback session can be found in Gorske (2008). The predominant theme that arose from the meetings and feedback session was Marisa's strong and intense desire to hold onto her sense of self, which she felt was being robbed of by the tumor and consequent treatments. Her neuropsychological test results revealed some expected, mostly mild, deficits consistent with the location of the tumor in her brain and compounded by the effects from chemotherapy and radiation treatments. What was most impressive was how the neuropsychological tests became a "battleground" for Marisa where she was going to prove to herself and others that she would reclaim the life that the cancer was trying to take from her. This was most evident on the Digit Span Subtest of the Wechsler Adult Intelligence Scale, third edition (WAIS-III) where despite her obvious exhaustion she managed to perform in the 96th percentile for Digits Forward and the 92nd percentile for Digits Backward (Gorske, 2008). Another theme that emerged was the need for Marisa to create balance in her life. Although her desire to "beat" the cancer energized her and pushed her to heal herself, this also took an immense toll on her in that she was frequently exhausted and could not be at her best. This was illustrated by her performance on the Rey Complex Figure Test. On this test she was so intent on performing "perfectly" that she was tense, anxious, and not processing the information efficiently. The fact that she experienced peripheral vision loss made it even more difficult. Her experience of that subtest became a teaching moment when I encouraged her to relax, breathe, and just try to "soak in" the whole picture without trying to be perfect. This "perfectionistic tendency" became a second theme wherein Marisa needed to find a balance between fighting and giving herself permission to rest and heal (Gorske, 2008). The recommendations generated from the CTNA feedback session reflected these two themes: (a) Marisa was going to continually search for ways to battle the cancer and reclaim her sense of herself; and (b) that she would learn to listen to her mind and body, and give herself permission to rest and to heal so she can re-energize and be at her best to continue the battle.

Once the diagnosis of brain cancer became a reality, Marisa experienced sadness, depression, and grief, but in the same turn her family described her as being happier with the simple things in life. Her basic personality remained the same. She was still passionate, strong willed, and had an intense zest for life—but her focus changed. Her family described it as changing from focusing on worldly things to simpler things. She became stronger in her faith and found comfort in Bible passages such as Philippians 4:11–13: "I am not saying this because I am in need, for I have learned to be content whatever the circumstances. I know what it is to be in need, and I know what it is to have plenty. I have learned the secret of being content in any and every situation, whether w*ell fed or hungry, whether living in plenty or in want. I can do all this through him who gives me strength."* She joined a brain cancer survivors group and support group, which would go on trips—including a rock climbing excursion (being a brain injury specialist, I was a bit concerned about this, but she was adamant). She became involved with Gilda's Club in Pittsburgh; she took college classes and was working on a Master's Degree in Food Studies; she took both Salsa and Belly Dancing lessons; and she learned Italian at The Chautauqua Institute in addition to many other new endeavors. She was "in her glory" when she visited Sicily with her father, Giovanni Muscarella, because she was very proud of her heritage. Sadly, her father died in November 2009. Most of all, her family described Marisa as someone who wanted to be around others. She would confide in and talk with someone whenever she could and was always ready to express her thoughts, her fears, and her hopes.

I met with Marisa two other times, in May 2007 and September 2010. She shared many of the things described earlier. She talked about all the activities she was involved in, how her treatments were progressing, and how she felt on a day-to-day basis. She shared all the positive things that were happening, but also the painful things such as the physical toll, relationship challenges, and fears about the future. After testing, there were feedback sessions that always revisited the themes developed in the first meeting. Marisa admitted that she often struggled with the "resting" part, but was getting better at listening to her body and knowing when it was time to stop, regroup, rest, and heal. She also had a black Labrador Retriever mix who was a source of love and comfort for her and was described as a dog who would "take Marisa for a walk."

Marisa was stable and doing well even up through January 2012. She was among the few people who had survived more than five years having been diagnosed with a grade IV glioblastoma. She continued to follow up with neurology and Duke University Medical Center in addition to all her other activities. In March 2012 she had been experiencing migraine headaches and nausea. On April 1, 2012 she experienced severe bouts of headache, nausea, and vomiting and was taken to the emergency room in Pittsburgh. Her computed tomography (CT) scans were essentially unchanged at the time. She was admitted to the hospital and during the night was found on the floor of her room unresponsive. Attempts to revive her were unsuccessful and her time of death was recorded 5:15 am on April 2, 2012, at age 36. A later autopsy would reveal the cause to be a seizure leading to unexpected death.

During the time before her death her family described her as suffering but compassionate. She was described as kind and sweet to everyone, and appreciative of all they had done and continued to do for her. In the last few weeks and months before her death she was also described as frequently disoriented, fatigued, and nauseous. Despite these symptoms she continued to try to do things for her family in an effort to feel normal, such as help with the laundry and drive her mother places, even though they would plead for her to rest. The day before she became very sick and had to go to the emergency room, her mother was sitting on a chair, exhausted from caregiving. Her mother thought to herself out loud, "I wish someone would make me a cup of tea." Marisa did just that. This reminded her mother of when Marisa was a little girl, she would do things like put a blanket on her mother when she was lying or sitting on the couch. Even up to the very end, Marisa was doing things that were true to her sense of self.

After Marisa's death and funeral there were many changes in her family. Her mother moved from Jamestown, New York to live closer to her family in Pittsburgh. Her mother, sister, and other family members became more involved in the church Marisa had been attending. Marisa's mother became involved in a church ministry to women in prison. In doing so she reached out to a particularly troubled woman by giving her a bible that had belonged to Marisa. It was somewhat worn with writing and highlights throughout the book. This gesture was a transformational experience in her mother's relationship with this woman, and her mother stated that she felt Marisa's presence during the encounter. Marisa's sister made some bold changes of her own. One in particular involved a plot of land that Marisa had wanted her sister to have for a garden. Sometime after her death, Marisa's brother-in-law created "Marisa's Garden" where they grow herbs and vegetables that they use to feed and share with others. Marisa's family says that people come up to them almost every day and tell stories of how Marisa touched their lives. One time Marisa's mother recalled the movie *The Blue Butterfly,* which was the story of a terminally ill boy who travels with an entomologist to South America to find and catch an elusive and mythic blue butterfly. During a time when Marisa's mother was grieving and holding a picture of Marisa, she saw a butterfly near the house and felt Marisa's presence—Marisa also loved butterflies. Even after her death, Marisa's sense of self was inspiring, moving her family to take risks, make changes, and connect with something larger than themselves.

My last meeting with Marisa was September 27, 2010. Her family stated that Marisa spoke of the neuropsychological testing and feedback sessions, saying that they were very positive points in her life, and that she used them to prove that she would not be affected by the tumor, chemo, and radiation treatments. Of course, I have no misconceptions that the testing and feedback sessions were *pivotal points* for Marisa that were dramatically life altering. What I would like to believe is that these meetings were brief *pit stops* where Marisa could see how she was doing from a cognitive and emotional perspective in terms of the goals and themes developed from the initial meeting in July 2006. Marisa had always feared losing her sense of herself as a person and that the tumor and treatments had somehow changed who she was. One would like to think that the neuropsychological assessments and feedback sessions were small microcosms of her greater struggle that allowed her to gauge where she stood in her fight against cancer to reclaim her sense of self and make any needed changes from discussing the results and the implications for her life. Based on everything observed and heard from her family, Marisa's personality and sense of self were never lost, but instead redirected and refocused to where she touched people's lives in a deeper and more meaningful way than even she may have imagined. Not only was her sense of self retained, but it actually grew and flourished to where Marisa became even more like the person she wanted to be. She always remained energetic, a "type A go-getter," passionate, and strong willed. This was who she was before the cancer, during her fight against the cancer, and even beyond death when she continued to touch the lives of others and most importantly her family. Given that Marisa's goal was to claim her sense of self in her fight with cancer, one thing is clear: She won.

Note

1 The author would like to thank Michelle Ulrich, the executor of Marisa Muscarella's estate, for giving express written permission to use Marisa's name and other identifying medical information in the writing of this chapter.

References

Armengol, C. G., Kaplan, E., & Moes, E. (Eds.). (2001). *The Consumer Oriented Neuropsychological Report*. Lutz, FL: Psychological Assessment Resources, Inc.

Aronow, E., & Reznikoff, M. (1971). Application of projective tests to psychotherapy: A case study. *Journal of Personality Assessment, 35*, 379–393.

Bellack, L., Pasquarelli, B. A., & Braverman, S. (1949). The use of the thematic apperception test in psychotherapy. *Journal of Nervous & Mental Disease, 110*, 51–65.

Bennett-Levy, J., Klein-Boonschate, M. A., Batchelor, J., McCarter, R., & Walton, N. (1994). Encounters with Anna Thompson: The consumer's experience of neuropsychological assessment. *The Clinical Neuropsychologist, 8*(2), 219–238.

Berg, M. (1985). The feedback process in diagnostic psychological testing. *Bulletin of the Menninger Clinic, 49*(1), 52–69.

Carone, D. A., & Bush, S. S. (Eds.). (2013). *Mild Traumatic Brain Injury: Symptom Validity Assessment and Malingering*. New York: Springer Publishing Company, LLC.

Carone, D. A., Iverson, G. L., & Bush, S. S. (2010). A model to approaching and providing feedback to patients regarding invalid test performance in clinical neuropsychological evaluations. *The Clinical Neuropsychologist, 24*(5), 759–778.

Christensen, A. L., & Caetano, C. (1996). Alexandr Romanovich Luria (1902–1977): Contributions to neuropsychological rehabilitation. *Neuropsychological Rehabilitation, 6*(4), 279–303.

Christensen, A. L., & Caetano, C. (1999). Luria's neuropsychological investigation in the Nordic countries. *Neuropsychology Review, 9*(2), 71–78.

Christensen, A. L., Goldberg, E., & Bougakov, D. (2009). *Luria's Legacy in the 21st Century*. New York: Oxford University Press, Inc.

Donofrio, N., Piatt, A., Whelihan, W., & DiCarlo, M. (1999). Neuropsychological test feedback: Consumer evaluation and perceptions. *Archives of Clinical Neuropsychology, 14*(8), 721.

Finn, S. E. (1996a). Assessment and feedback integrating MMPI-2 and Rorschach findings. *Journal of Personality Assessment, 67*(3), 543–557.

Finn, S. E. (1996b). *Using the MMPI-2 as a Therapeutic Intervention*. Minneapolis, MN: University of Minnesota Press.

Finn, S. E. (2003). Therapeutic assessment of a Man with "ADD." *Journal of Personality Assessment, 80*(2), 115–129.

Finn, S. E. (2007). *In Our Clients' Shoes: Theory and Techniques of Therapeutic Assessment*. Mahwah, NJ: Lawrence Erlbaum Associates.

Finn, S. E., Fischer, C. T., & Handler, L. (Eds.). (2012). *Collaborative/Therapeutic Assessment: A Casebook and Guide*. Hoboken, NJ: John Wiley and Sons, Inc.

Fischer, C. T. (1970). The testee as co-evaluator. *Journal of Counseling Psychology, 17*(1), 70–76.

Fischer, C. T. (1994). *Individualizing Psychological Assessment* (2nd ed.). Hillsdale, NJ: Lawrence Erlbaum Associates.

Gass, C. S., & Brown, M. C. (1992). Neuropsychological test feedback to patients with brain dysfunction. *Psychological Assessment, 4*(3), 272–277.

Gorske, T. (2008). Therapeutic neuropsychological assessment: A humanistic model and case example. *Journal of Humanistic Psychology, 48*(3), 320–339.

Gorske, T. T., & Smith, S. R. (2009). *Collaborative Therapeutic Neuropsychological Assessment*. New York: Springer Science + Business Media, LLC.

Harrower, M. (1956). Projective counseling: A psychotherapeutic technique. *American Journal of Psychotherapy*, *10*, 74–86.

Longley, W. A., Tate, R., & Brown, R. (2012). A protocol for measuring the direct psychological benefit of neuropsychological assessment with feedback in multiple sclerosis. *Brain Impairment*, *13*(2), 238–255.

Longley, W. A., Tate, R., Brown, R., & Contini, E. (2013, November 14–15). *Neuropsychological assessment with feedback tends to reduce distress and improve social confidence in patients with multiple sclerosis: Preliminary results from a randomised controlled trial*. Abstract submitted to Progress in MS Research Conference, Sydney Australia.

Luborsky, L. (1953). Self-interpretation of the TAT as a clinical technique. *Journal of Projective Techniques*, *17*, 217–223.

Luborsky, L. (1984). *Principles of Psychoanalytic Psychotherapy: A Manual for Supportive-Expressive (SE) Treatment*. New York: Basic Books.

Lucas, M. (2010). The role of the neuropsychological assessment in relinquishing decision making rights. *African Journal of Psychiatry*, *13*, 245–247.

Malla, A. K., Lazosky, A., McLean, T., Rickwood, A., Cheng, S., & Norman, R.M.G. (1997). Neuropsychological assessment as an aid to psychosocial rehabilitation in severe mental disorders. *Psychiatric Rehabilitation Journal*, *21*(2), 169–173.

Miller, W. R., & Rollnick, S. (1991/2002). *Motivational Interviewing: Preparing People to Change*. New York: Guilford Press.

Miller, W. R., Zweben, A., DiClemente, C. C., & Rychtarik, R. G. (1999). *Motivational Enhancement Therapy Manual: A Clinical Research Guide for Therapists Treating Individuals With Alcohol Abuse and Dependence*. Rockville, MD: National Institute on Alcohol Abuse and Alcoholism.

Mosak, H. H., & Gushurst, R. S. (1972). Some therapeutic uses of psychological testing. *American Journal of Psychotherapy*, *26*, 539–546.

Pachana, N. A., Squelch, N. S., & Paton, H. (2010). The importance of feedback and communication strategies with older adults: Therapeutic and ethical considerations. In N. Pachana, K. Laidlaw, & B. Knight (Eds.), *Casebook of Clinical Geropsychology: International Perspective on Practice* (pp. 155–176). New York: Oxford University Press, Inc.

Paul, G. L. (1967). Strategy of outcome research in psychotherapy. *Journal of Consulting Psychology*, *31*, 109–118.

Pegg, P., Auerbach, S., Seel, R., Buenaver, L., Kiesler, D., & Plybon, L. (2005). The impact of patient-centered information on patients' treatment satisfaction and outcomes in traumatic brain injury rehabilitation. *Rehabilitation Psychology*, *50*(4), 366–374.

Postal, K., & Armstrong, K. (2013). *Feedback That Sticks: The Art of Effectively Communicating Neuropsychological Assessment Results*. New York: Oxford University Press.

Schoenberg, M.R. & Scott, J.G. (2011). *The Little Black Book of Neuropsychology: A Syndrome-Based Approach*. New York: Springer Science & Business Media.

Smith, S., Wiggins, C., & Gorske, T. (2007). A survey of psychological assessment feedback practices. *Assessment*, *14*(3), 310–319.

Suarez, M. (2011). Application of motivational interviewing to neuropsychology practice: A new frontier for evaluation and rehabilitation. In M. R. Schoenberg & J. G. Scot (Eds.), *The Little Black Book of Neuropsychology* (pp. 863–871). New York: Springer Science + Business Media, LLC.

Tharinger, D. J., Finn, S. E., Wilkinson, A. D., DeHay, T., Parton, V., Bailey, K., & Tran, A. (2008). Providing psychological assessment feedback to children through individualized fables. *Professional Psychology: Research and Practice*, *39*, 610–618.

Tharinger, D. J., & Pilgrim, S. (2012). Parent and child experiences of neuropsychological assessment as a function of child feedback by individualized fable. *Child Neuropsychology*, *18*(3), 228–241.

49 Empirically Based Rehabilitation of Neurocognitive Disorder

Anthony Y. Stringer

I am convinced that considerable results can be obtained with restoring to aphémiques the part of their intellect that perished with a part of their brain.

—Paul Broca

A Short History of Cognitive Rehabilitation

In his seminal 1865 paper, Paul Broca (transl. Berker, Berker, & Smith, 1986) not only solidified a new era in our understanding of aphasia, but he also introduced the idea that, with training, aphasic patients could regain aspects of their compromised oral and written language ability. Arguably, cognitive rehabilitation therapy (CRT) has been practiced since at least this early observation. The large number of World War I and II soldiers who, thanks to medical and surgical advances, survived what formerly were fatal penetrating missile wounds to the brain, gave further impetus to this burgeoning field and expanded its reach beyond language disorder (Prigatano, 2009). In the 1940s, Aleksandr Luria, then a member of the Russian National Volunteer Corps, organized a hospital in the Southern Urals dedicated to the rehabilitation of recovering soldiers (Homskaya, 2001). Luria's wide-ranging clinical investigations encompassed pharmacological and rehabilitative interventions for both motor and cognitive disorders. Always an integrative thinker, Luria postulated that these interventions worked by: (a) releasing a temporarily inhibited function, (b) recruiting the participation of the spared hemisphere in task performance, and (c) reorganizing functional systems in the brain. Not surprisingly, given the scope of Luria's insights, this early rubric encapsulates most contemporary CRT approaches.

More recent growth in CRT practice is due more to carnage on the roadway than the battlefield. The postwar era brought vehicle ownership, longer driving distances from home to work, and more opportunities for vehicular injury. The 1970s and 1980s saw an expansion of CRT for traumatic brain injury (TBI), often with little demonstrated empirical support. CRT became standard care in rehabilitation hospitals throughout the United States and Europe, before outcome studies were performed. With clinical need driving this expansion, clinical science did its best to catch up. Several hundred CRT outcome studies have been completed since the 1980s. While methodological rigor has varied across these studies, sufficient data have been collected, analyzed, and meta-analyzed to permit the establishment of practice standards and guidelines (see Cicerone et al., 2000, 2005, 2011; Rohling, Faust, Beverly, & Demakis, 2008).

The field of cognitive rehabilitation is no longer in its infancy. Since Broca's early musings about aphasia rehabilitation, CRT has matured into a multidisciplinary field grounded in the science of neuroplasticity and the art of clinical rehabilitation. This chapter provides a short overview of the practice of CRT, characterizes the various approaches utilized to rehabilitate patients with neurocognitive impairment, and summarizes the evidence on CRT outcome. The chapter closes with some projections on what this now mature field will accomplish in the decades ahead.

Definition and Overview of Cognitive Rehabilitation Therapy Practice

The American Congress of Rehabilitation Medicine Brain Injury Special Interest Group (Harley et al., 1992) broadly defines CRT as "systematic, functionally oriented . . . therapeutic cognitive activities, based on an assessment and understanding of the person's brain-behavior deficits" (p. 62). This definition encompasses *remediation techniques* intended to restore a damaged cognitive ability, as well as *compensatory techniques* that aim to maximize functioning irrespective of whether a cognitive deficit remains. Remediation techniques generally employ a rehearsal or "mental exercise" approach to rehabilitation. They treat the brain as if it were a muscle that can be strengthened through the exercise of weakened cognitive abilities. Compensatory approaches are largely agnostic with regards to what happens to underlying cognitive abilities. Their goal is to improve functioning using any technique that allows a patient to circumvent cognitive limitations. Such techniques may be internal, as when patients are taught a mnemonic strategy to aid recall of information, or external as when patients use a notebook or calendar to store information they would otherwise forget. Rehearsal and practice remain an important aspect of compensatory CRT, but the goal of rehearsal is to make patients proficient in the use of a strategy rather than to restore a cognitive ability.

Surveys of cognitive rehabilitation practice patterns are few and far between. Unfortunately the most recent surveys are more than a decade old. Blundon and Smits (2000) surveyed Canadian occupational therapists at 27 nonrandomly selected sites to identify therapeutic modalities used to treat brain injury survivors. With a 74% response rate, these investigators reported memory impairment was the most common cognitive domain treated. Interventions included both compensatory and remediation approaches.

Stringer (2003) sent surveys to 270 randomly selected rehabilitation hospitals and programs within all nine American Hospital Association regions (covering the United States, Puerto Rico, and Canada), yielding a 45% response rate. Cognitive compensation approaches were being utilized only slightly more often than rehearsal approaches. The most common areas of cognition addressed (in order of highest to lowest frequency) were attention, memory, reasoning/executive function, and visual perception. Rehearsal techniques utilized (again in order of frequency) included practice of activities of daily living, paper-and-pencil exercises, practice of vocational tasks, board games that involved cognitive skill, computerized cognitive exercises, and computer games. The most common compensatory strategies in rank order were written aids, problem-solving strategies, mnemonics, and electronic aids.

Patients with strokes or traumatic brain injuries were the most common patients being treated in the Stringer survey, but CRT was also attempted with patients diagnosed with brain tumors, dementia, anoxic brain damage, demyelinating diseases, and cerebral infection. The CRT field was truly interdisciplinary, with (in order of frequency of involvement) speech therapists, occupational therapists, neuropsychologists, recreation therapists, physical therapists, and nurses all delivering care. The overwhelming majority of patients in the programs responding to this survey were in individual CRT, with group sessions rarely utilized. Most patients were in therapy from one to six months, with relatively few programs reporting patients finishing therapy in less or more than this period of time.

Much has doubtlessly changed in the years since these surveys were collected. Lumosity, the leader in Internet-based computer games intended to improve cognitive function, reports on its website (www.lumosity.com/) having 50 million users from 182 countries. While the vast majority of these are healthy individuals with no discernable cognitive impairment, the 50 million users doubtlessly include people with neurocognitive impairment who are attempting to improve their abilities independently or with the guidance of a therapist. Even more striking, since smartphones were first marketed in 1996, users have grown to 1 billion worldwide (Business Wire, 2012). With their ease of use and countless applications that store information, remind users of appointments and tasks, and provide organizational tools, these almost ubiquitous devices cannot help but find use as compensatory aids for cognitively impaired patients. A contemporary survey would likely find a very different profile of remediation and compensatory-based rehabilitation strategies in use in North America.

Cognitive Rehabilitation Therapy Approaches

Both remedial and compensatory CRT approaches are available for the three most commonly treated cognitive domains of attention, memory, and executive function/problem solving. Before turning to the outcome research, I'll briefly illustrate each approach with respect to these three cognitive domains.

Attention

Attention Process Training (APT) (Sohlberg & Mateer, 1989) attempts to remediate deficits in sustained attention, working memory, selective attention, suppression of response to competing inputs, and alternating attention through the use of progressively more difficult cognitive exercises. The earliest version of APT utilized paper-and-pencil exercises; however, the latest version uses computer administration with the assistance of a therapist. The patient moves from relatively easy exercises to more complex tasks as performance improves. Both visual and auditory stimuli are incorporated, although most of the activities are fairly artificial and would not be encountered in everyday life. The therapist plays a vital role in treatment, and the program is not intended for unaided patient use.

Lumosity and PositScience Brain HQ are more recent Internet-based examples of the remedial approach to attention; however, these programs also target the much larger healthy population by promulgating the idea that neurologically healthy people need to exercise their brains. PositScience (www.positscience.com/why-brainhq), for example, draws a direct analogy to the "revolution" in physical fitness that took place in the 1980s and 1990s when more people began going to the gym. "Brain fitness" is supposedly the "next step in that revolution." Physical fitness, however, became a contemporary priority in the United States as a consequence of increasingly sedentary work, high-calorie fast-food diets, and a growing rate of obesity. In contrast to this physically sedentary lifestyle, contemporary life does provide ample cognitive exercise for neurological healthy people, leaving little need for a "brain workout."

While not well-researched in adults, excessive time spent playing computer games is associated with eye strain (Gillespie, 2002) and obesity (Carvalhal, Padez, Moreira, & Rosado, 2006) in nonclinical pediatric samples, and may provoke seizures in pediatric epilepsy patients (Shoja et al., 2007). Hence, it is a bit ironic to posit that computerized games can lead to fitness of any kind in presumably healthy individuals.

These Internet-based approaches to attention make little use of a therapist. This may arise from the fact that their primary market is comprised of healthy individuals. Active involvement of an actual therapist may be critical to the success of cognitive rehabilitation. This may give APT an advantage over most of the Internet programs. However, it should be noted that one such program—Scientific Brain Training Pro (SBTP; at www.scientificbraintrainingpro.com)—does incorporate a therapist and allows the therapist to select exercises, monitor performance, and guide participation even when the patient is playing the games on a home computer.

Compensatory approaches to attention are largely absent from the clinical and research literature, however, in our clinic (Stringer, Denham, & White, in press) we utilize a technique called DIRECT. This approach teaches a patient to "direct" attention by manipulating the environment. DIRECT is an acronym that cues the patient to manipulate six factors in the environment in order to compensate for attention impairment. These six factors are (a) *D*istractions and (b) *I*nterruptions (both of which the patient should eliminate), (c) *R*ate of performance (which the patient increases or decreases to maximize attention), (d) *E*arnings (which the patient tries to increase, as we tend to pay more attention when there is a tangible and immediate payoff, (e) *C*omplexity (which the patient tries to decrease as attention wanes when tasks are too complex), and (f) *T*iredness (which the patient uses as a cue to take a break as attention tends to wane with fatigue). The intent of therapy is to give the patient tools that can be used in everyday home and work settings to maximize attention. The techniques are intended to improve performance in attentionally demanding situations, without necessarily improving actual attention abilities. What hopefully does improve is the patient's ability to recognize what in the environment can be changed to facilitate attentiveness.

Memory

Lumosity, PositScience, and SBTP also include Internet-based games to improve memory. Lumosity, for example, includes games that require the recall of spatial positions, associations between stimuli, and associations between names and faces. In contrast, the BrainTrain program (www.braintrain.com/), provides cognitive remediation software that runs on a desktop computer or network, with optional cloud data storage for remote access. BrainTrain, one of the earliest exemplars of the mental exercise remedial approach, has been continuously updated since 1989 to now include hundreds of exercises in its "Memory Gym." The program also incorporates EEG monitoring and brainwave feedback to develop what the program refers to as "CHARM"—a calm, happy, alert, and relaxed mental state. Regardless of whether the approach is Internet or desktop-based, the basic premise continues to be that an impaired mental ability can be repaired through exercise and practice. BrainTrain and SBTP incorporate a therapist, while as already noted, Lumosity and PositScience do not. All programs target both the cognitively impaired and the cognitively healthy who want to improve functioning from a current baseline.

Compensatory approaches to memory provide internal mnemonic aids or external means of storing and retrieving information with the intent of improving memory performance, if not actual memory ability. Mnemonic strategies are as old as ancient Greece. Cicero (Sutton & Rackham, 1942) relates the legend of Simonides (circa 556–468 B.C.), a Greek poet who narrowly escaped the collapse of a banquet hall roof and subsequently discovered he could identify the physically unrecognizable corpses of the diners by recalling where they were positioned around the banquet table. From this experience came the "method of loci," a strategy for mentally associating an image of something to be recalled with a location along an already known path. Once the association is learned, the information is recalled by taking a mental "walk" along the path to see what image has been placed in each location.

These and other mnemonic techniques were originally intended to enhance the performance of healthy individuals whose work demanded a prodigious memory. Clinicians have adapted them for use by patients with memory impairment. The "peg system," another imagery mnemonic, makes use of high-imagery words that rhyme with numbers 1–12 (systems developed for healthy individuals expand the number of peg words well into the hundreds, but clinicians typically make use of only 10–12 peg words). The rhyme makes it easy for even people with memory impairment to learn the number-word association (e.g., "one-bun," "two-shoe," "three-tree"). Once the association is learned, an image of the peg word can serve as a substitute for the associated number. Chains of such images provide a means of learning a series of digits such as a phone number or address. These imagery chains are often humorous or bizarre, which enhances their memorability. A patient who recalls the image chain can back-translate it to retrieve the desired number.

While many mnemonics are imagery based, verbal strategies are also common. In an acronym, each letter of a word represents a piece of information to be remembered. Similarly, in an acrostic, the first letter of each word of a sentence represents the target information. Such techniques rely on the memorability of the word or sentence, which then cues recall of the embedded information. Beginning piano students, for example, learn to associate notes with the lines and spaces of a musical stave using such acrostics as "Every good band draws fans," with the first letter of each word ("E," "G," "B," etc.) representing a musical note.

Some verbal mnemonics enhance depth of information processing, rather than providing a means of storing and retrieving information. "PQRST," a strategy for learning narrative information, guides the reader to first *p*review text, develop *q*uestions about the content, *r*ead the text to answer the questions, *s*tudy the questions and answers to memorize the content, and *t*est memory by attempting to recall the answers to the questions. PQRST fosters a deeper engagement and depth of processing of the narrative in order to facilitate retention of content. While not providing a specific mnemonic strategy, it uses an acronym to help the reader remember the steps in the process.

External memory aids attempt to put information at a patient's fingertips in an easy to retrieve format. Low-technology examples include memory notebooks and appointment calendars. The advent of personal digital assistants and wearable technology has made available many new ways of storing and retrieving information. A smartphone can provide a calendar of appointments and scheduled activities, an alarm to cue a patient to keep the appointment or perform the activity, multiple applications for storing information that might be needed at home or in the community, a global positioning system application and maps to assist with navigation to a destination, applications for storing information (including a photograph) about people, and a means of summoning help via text or voice when all else fails. Smartphones and portable tablet computers are, in essence, all-purpose external memory aids for both the cognitively well and the cognitively impaired.

Even people with intact memories struggle to retain all the information that comes at them in the course of a day and utilize a combination of internal and external memory aids. Consequently, it makes sense to incorporate both types of aids in working with memory-impaired patients. One difficulty, however, is that patients often mix up which aids to use with which type of information. The Ecologically Oriented Neurorehabilitation of Memory (EON-Mem) program (Stringer, 2007) makes use of both internal and external memory aids, and attempts to reduce patient confusion by using the same four-step method (Write-Organize-Picture-Rehearse) for all types of memory content.

A final compensatory approach to memory should be included here, known as "domain-specific learning" (DSL; see Schacter & Glisky, 1986). This approach, developed for severely amnestic patients, utilizes memory strategies without *explicitly* teaching them to the patients. Instead, often severely amnestic patients, are taught specific content utilizing *implicit* memory strategies. For example, the DSL approach may use "errorless learning," in which maximum cues are provided on every trial so that the patient never makes a mistake during the acquisition of a skill or information. Cues are gradually faded, but never so rapidly as to produce a performance error, until the patient has mastered the skill or acquired the information. Incorrect responses are thought to compete in one's memory with correct responses, hence by avoiding errors, learning is enhanced even in an amnestic patient. Another common strategy utilizes "spaced retrieval," in which the time between study and recall is systematically increased, but again at a rate at which recall accuracy is maintained. Using these and other implicit strategies, even amnestic patients can learn complex skills, despite having no recollection of ever undergoing training (Glisky & Schacter, 1987; Glisky, Schacter, & Tulving, 1986a, 1986b; Schacter, Rich, & Stampp, 1985).

DSL is compensatory in the sense that it attempts to enhance performance through a learning strategy, but it does not attempt to improve memory ability. It has some unique limitations. Human beings seem to naturally learn through trial and error, and it can be a challenge to design a rehabilitation intervention in which errors are eliminated. As patients are taught specific content, rather than a strategy they can independently use across content, the technique may not generalize to new content and the patient may never be independent in use of the technique. In addition, learning can be hyperspecific. In amnestic patients, even a minor change (e.g., switching keyboards when patients were being taught to operate a computer) is sufficient to eliminate the benefits of training (Glisky et al., 1986a). Despite these limitations, DSL can improve performance in amnestic patients who do not respond to any other remedial or compensatory approach.

Problem Solving

To varying degrees, the Internet and desktop computer remediation programs already discussed include exercises that target problem solving, reasoning, and related abilities. PositScience has fewer exercises in this area. It includes what it refers to as "Intelligence Exercises," but these consist primarily of variations on the "n-back" task in which a player tries to determine whether a current stimulus matches a previous stimulus presented a specified number of trials back. Lumosity, in contrast, makes use of a number of arithmetic games to provide practice in problem solving. SBTP uses "Tower of Hanoi" games in which patients must follow preset rules for moving stimuli from one location to another, word puzzles (e.g., cracking a code in order to decipher a famous quotation in which letters have been replaced by coded symbols), and sequencing exercises. These are all computerized versions of an earlier generation of paper-and-pencil "brain teaser" games in which people attempt to solve riddles. Often the solution involves paying attention to the wording of the riddle in order to discover a clever resolution.

The compensatory approach typically utilizes a problem-solving algorithm that can be applied across different problems. These algorithms variously emphasize slowing down decision making, thinking flexibly, brainstorming, and being systematic. Goal Management Training™ (GMT) teaches five problem-solving steps: Stop (become aware of the problem situation), Define (set a goal), List (divide the problem solving task into substeps), Learn (remember the steps for completing the task), and Check (compare the result to the goal). In our clinic, we employ the Ecologically Oriented Neurorehabilitation Executive (EON-Exec; see Stringer et al., in press) program, which makes use of the acronym "GO-AS" to teach four problem solving steps: setting a *G*oal, developing *O*ptions for achieving the goal, *A*nticipating and rating the outcomes associated with each of these options, and *S*electing the option that leads to the best anticipated outcomes. We have also adapted GO-AS for modern times by developing a "smart form" version that runs on tablet computers. In contrast, GMT is designed to run on a desktop computer system only. Both programs utilize a variety of problem scenarios to train patients in use of the respective algorithms.

Cognitive Rehabilitation Therapy Outcome Studies

Having characterized remedial and compensatory approaches to attention, memory, and problem solving impairment, in this section I will review evidence on the outcome of cognitive rehabilitation. Specifically, the following three questions will be addressed: (a) For what neurological conditions is CRT effective? (b) For which cognitive domains is it effective? (c) Is there an outcome difference for remediation versus compensatory CRT approaches? In answering these three questions, we will consider the results of available evidence-based reviews and meta-analytic studies, updated with more recently published studies not included in these reviews.

For What Neurological Conditions Is Cognitive Rehabilitation Therapy Effective?

The overwhelming majority of research on CRT outcome has been in patients with stroke or TBI. For these two patient populations, the evidence for CRT effectiveness is quite strong. Cicerone and colleagues (Cicerone et al., 2000, 2005, 2011) on the Brain Injury Interdisciplinary Special Interest Group of the American Congress of Rehabilitation Medicine have reviewed a combined 60 prospective, randomized controlled trials (RCT) and an additional five quasi-randomized studies of cognitive rehabilitation in stroke or TBI. Across these studies, CRT was found to improve cognitive performance in stroke and TBI. The European Federation of Neurological Societies Task Force on Cognitive Rehabilitation came to a similar conclusion (Cappa et al., 2005) as the Cicerone group with regards to the benefits of CRT in stroke and TBI.

Rohling et al. (2008), however, came to more tempered conclusions about CRT outcome in TBI and stroke after conducting a meta-analysis of the RCTs, nonrandomized control group studies, and single group pre- and posttreatment comparisons included in the first two of the Cicerone et al. (2000, 2005) reviews. Many of the studies included in the Rohling et al. meta-analysis were also included in the Cappa et al. (2005) paper, so their less sanguine conclusions apply to the European review as well. Rohling and his colleagues found that effect sizes tended to be small in true RCTs. Effect sizes were larger in single group, pretreatment, and posttreatment comparison studies. These larger effect sizes in single-group designs were thought to be due to practice effects from repeated test administration.

Stringer (2011) directly compared CRT outcome across stroke, TBI, and a mixed neurological group in a nonrandomized clinical trial and found all three groups showed comparable improvements in memory performance with a strategy training program. Effect sizes were 0.65, 0.73, and 0.89 respectively for stroke, TBI, and the mixed neurological groups. Importantly, this study controlled for practice effects in many of the pre- and posttreatment comparisons by utilizing alternate test forms when available. Effect sizes remained high even when practice effects were controlled in this manner, and the average effect size across patient groups did not differ significantly when the same (effect size of 0.75) or an alternate (effect size of 0.72) form was used.

Stringer's (2011) mixed neurological group was too small for findings to be considered robust, but it included patients diagnosed with epilepsy, brain neoplasm, or cerebral infection. The fact that the effect size was highest in this group suggests that CRT may be effective in patients with neurological diagnoses beyond stroke and TBI. Though fewer studies have been conducted in patient populations other than TBI and stroke, results have generally supported CRT effectiveness.

Given their often prominent anterograde memory impairment, temporal lobe epilepsy (TLE) surgery patients have been the target of several CRT studies. In one of the earliest studies of CRT in this population, Jones (1974) reported improved verbal memory performance when left temporal lobectomy patients used an imagery mnemonic. Engelberts et al. (2002) contrasted patients randomly assigned to compensatory training, remediation, and a wait-list control group. Both CRT groups showed improved performance on neuropsychological tests, decreased cognitive complaints, and higher quality of life scores after treatment and at a six-month follow-up. However, the patients undergoing compensatory training improved more in word memory, while patients undergoing the remediation approach showed increased response rates.

Helmstaedter et al. (2008) compared treatment and no treatment control patients (matched on demographic and seizure-related variables), in a nonrandomized clinical trial. Postsurgical CRT was multifactorial and included computer exercises, group interventions, and occupational therapy. CRT resulted in better verbal learning (with less impact on retention). Visuospatial memory did not show improvement and attention improved in all patients regardless of whether they received CRT.

A weakness of both wait-list and no-treatment control studies is that the control group gets less attention and has fewer opportunities to interact with a therapist, so that treatment effects could result simply from greater contact. It is reasonable to expect these nonspecific factors to impact all cognitive functions equally. The differential effect of CRT on verbal versus visuospatial memory in the Helmstaedter et al.

(2008) study and the different effects of remediation versus compensatory training in the Engelberts et al. (2002) study support, but do not prove, the hypothesis that the effects were due to the interventions rather than the greater attention that treated patients receive.

Taking a somewhat different approach, Koorenhof, Baxendale, Smith, and Thompson (2011) compared pre and postsurgical CRT in TLE patients. Presurgical CRT did not lead to a better outcome than did postsurgical CRT and improvements on outcome measures were associated with improved mood. While not providing strong support for CRT in TLE, the study highlights the importance of considering the impact of affective status in CRT outcome research.

Butler and Copeland (2002) combined elements of the APT remediation program for attention (described on p. 1074), strategy training, and cognitive behavior therapy and found better attention performance in a group of treated brain tumor patients (n = 21) compared to wait-list controls (n = 10). In a larger, multicenter study, Butler et al. (2008) randomly assigned brain tumor patients to the treatment combination described earlier (n = 108) or to a wait-list condition (n = 53). Outcomes were evaluated by examiners blind to treatment condition at multiple time points from six weeks to six months after study enrollment. This study found significantly better performance on academic measures and better observer ratings of attention in the treated patients. Despite Butler's inclusion of a number of methodological controls in the second study (i.e., random assignment, multicenter recruitment, blind evaluation, and outcome assessment at multiple time points), the combination treatment used in both studies does not allow us to determine what led to improved cognitive performance. This problem is again compounded by the use of a wait-list control.

Poppelreuter, Weis, Mumm, Orth, and Bartsch, (2008) randomly assigned cancer patients (= 157) undergoing stem cell transplant to two groups receiving compensatory attention and memory training, or computerized attention and memory remediation. A third, nonrandomized no-treatment control group was subsequently recruited for comparison. All three groups improved significantly in outcome performance, but did not differ from one another. While studying a different cancer population than Butler and colleagues (2008) and utilizing less rigorous methodological control, these findings raise further questions about the efficacy of CRT in cancer patients with cognitive dysfunction.

A small number of studies have explored CRT in various other medical populations, also with mixed results. Hypoxemic patients did not improve significantly when given CRT compared to a control group (Incalzi et al., 2008). Similarly, toxic encephalopathy patients showed no statistically significant improvement in memory performance in a study that compared training in compensatory memory strategies and psychosocial treatment (control condition) in a study using a counterbalanced crossover design (van Hout, Wekking, Berg, & Deelman, 2008). In contrast, Parkinson's disease patients receiving practice-based remediation showed better executive functioning compared to controls receiving standard medical care only (Sammer, Reuter, Hullman, Kaps, & Vaitl, 2006); however, both groups included only 13 subjects.

As is the case with CRT research in other patient populations, attempts to demonstrate an impact in patients with early dementia or mild cognitive impairment (MCI) have struggled to show improvement in treated patients beyond what occurs in active control interventions (Martin, Clare, Altgassen, Cameron, & Zehnder, 2011). Recently, I have collaborated on a series of studies exploring CRT in patients diagnosed with amnestic MCI (aMCI). While sample sizes have been small, these studies have incorporated randomization to treatment versus active control conditions, posttreatment follow-up assessment, cognitive outcome measures, and both structural and functional magnetic resonance imaging (fMRI).

The first in this series of studies (Hampstead, Sathian, Moore, Nalisnick, & Stringer, 2008) was a pilot investigation that attempted to see whether memory strategy training was even feasible with an aMCI sample (N = 8) given the expectation that many would progress towards dementia. Patients attempted to learn 90 face-name pairs, during three 1-hour long training sessions. Gender-appropriate names were randomly paired with the faces. The 90 training stimuli were divided into two sets of 45 face-name pairs, with each set of faces matched for gender, race, and age, and each set of names matched for length and popularity of the name. For half the pairs we trained patients to associate the sound of the name with a distinctive facial feature (i.e., the memory strategy condition). Patients rehearsed the other 45 face–name pairs without benefit of a strategy (the control condition). No differences in recognition accuracy for the two sets of face–name pairs was present before training. At the end of training and at one-month follow-up, recognition accuracy was significantly higher and response latencies were shorter for face–name pairs in the strategy training condition compared to the control condition. Patients also showed greater left temporal, parietal, anterior cingulate, insular and frontal opercular cortex activation to strategy trained stimuli, with the differences in activation magnitude for trained and untrained stimuli significantly correlated with recognition accuracy (Hampstead et al., 2011).

The second of these studies (Hampstead, Sathian, et al., 2012) randomly assigned healthy controls (n = 21) and aMCI patients (n = 28) to mnemonic strategy training to learn object locations within a pictured room or a control condition involving matched exposure to the object location training stimuli. While controls were always superior to aMCI patients, for both groups, strategy training led to better retention of object locations than matched exposure, a difference that persisted at one month follow-up. The ability to benefit from strategy training was positively correlated with baseline memory and executive function test performance, suggesting that the patients who benefitted the most had less initial impairment. Structural imaging results also supported this conclusion as greater inferior lateral ventricular volume (an index of hippocampal atrophy) was negatively correlated with improvement after strategy training.

We also obtained fMRI in healthy elderly and aMCI patients undergoing strategy training or matched exposure to learn object locations (Hampstead, Stringer, Stilla, Giddens, & Sathian, 2012). Prior to training, aMCI patients showed reduced hippocampal activity during both encoding and retrieval of object locations relative to healthy controls. After strategy training, hippocampal activation increased in the aMCI strategy training group during encoding and retrieval of object locations, partially reversing the initial hypoactivation. Statistically greater activation was seen in the aMCI patients who received strategy training compared to those given matched exposure to object locations. This difference was especially evident in the right hippocampus during retrieval of object locations from memory.

Consistent with these investigations, there is an emerging consensus that CRT can improve functioning in MCI in the short term (Belleville, 2008; Cotelli, Menenti, Zanetti, & Miniussi, 2012; Jean, Bergeron, Thivierge, & Simard, 2010; Li et al., 2011; Rejinders, van Heugten, & van Boxtel, 2013; Simon, Yokomizo, & Bottino, 2012). To date, there is no evidence that CRT significantly impacts the progression of MCI patients towards dementia, although it may be neuroprotective in the healthy elderly.

A longitudinal study of cognitive training in a cohort of 2,832 older, independent, community-dwelling adults showed that groups who received training functioned better at ten-year follow-up compared to no-contact controls in the areas of reasoning and processing speed, but not memory (Rebok et al., 2014). While this project has the weakness of using a no-contact control, it remains impressive that ten initial and four booster sessions of cognitive training yields benefits evident a decade later. It is hard to attribute such a difference to treatment group contact with the experimenters in this community dwelling cohort. This project suggests there may be value in studying further the long-term effects of CRT in MCI.

Broadly speaking, the strongest evidence is for the efficacy of CRT following TBI and stroke, and indeed it is now standard of care in these patients, particularly when they have vocational and community reentry goals that require a level of independent functioning. Evidence for CRT efficacy in other diagnostic conditions is emerging, though further research is required. For example, there is beginning support for CRT in epilepsy surgery, brain tumor, Parkinson's disease, and MCI patients. While perhaps not at the point where CRT is standard care in conditions beyond TBI and stroke, the accumulating evidence makes it a reasonable intervention to attempt with any patient whose cognitive impairment is stable over at least the short term and whose quality of life may be enhanced through cognitive intervention. The decision to initiate CRT, therefore, should be focused less on etiological diagnosis, and more on other factors that may determine treatment outcome. Such factors will be highlighted in the remainder of this chapter.

For Which Cognitive Domains Is Cognitive Rehabilitation Therapy Effective and Is There a Difference Between Remediation and Compensation Approaches?

Cognitive domain is an obvious factor that could influence CRT outcome. Is CRT effective for all or only some cognitive domains? Similarly, it is obvious to ask whether both remedial and compensatory approaches are equally effective across cognitive domains. To avoid confounding the effects of etiology and cognitive domain, in answering these questions about factors moderating outcome, it is necessary to hold etiology constant. As CRT outcome has been most thoroughly researched in TBI and stroke, we will look to research in these populations to address these questions about what moderates outcome.

RCTs and other (including nonrandomized) control group investigations in TBI and stroke have demonstrated improved memory following CRT using compensatory training (Kaschel et al., 2002; Ownsworth & McFarland, 1999; Schmitter-Edgecombe, Fahy, Whelan, & Long, 1995). Studies incorporating a direct comparison have shown compensatory training to be more effective than remedial approaches to memory (Berg, Konning-Haanstra, & Deelman, 1991; Doornhein & de Haan, 1998; Fish, Manly, Emslie, Evans, & Wilson, 2008; Kalla, Downes, & van den Broek, 2001; Wilson, Emslie, Quirk, & Evans, 2001; Wilson, Emslie, Quirk, Evans, & Watson, 2005), with the exception of one early study that failed to find a difference in the two approaches (Ryan & Ruff, 1988). Similarly, various domain-specific learning strategies appear to improve performance more than trial-and-error learning/rote rehearsal or no treatment control conditions (Baddeley & Wilson, 1994; Dou, Man, Ou, Zheng, & Tam, 2006; Hunkin, Squires, Parkin, & Tidy, 1998; Squires, Hunkin, & Parkin, 1997).

CRT therefore has yielded positive results for TBI and stroke patients with memory impairment. Memory compensation and domain-specific learning appear to be the better approaches to memory rehabilitation following TBI or stroke, a conclusion also supported by evidence-based reviews that included studies lacking adequate control groups in addition to the RCTs reviewed here (Cicerone et al., 2000, 2005, 2011). The Rohling et al. (2008) meta-analysis, however, found only a moderate (though statistically significant) effect size for memory rehabilitation in TBI, and the effect size became even weaker, and statistically nonsignificant, when the meta-analysis included only studies employing independent group pre- and posttest designs.

Rohling et al. (2008) found more support in their meta-analysis for an impact of CRT on attention. Attention training produced medium range, statistically significant effect sizes across RCTs and single group research designs. Specifically, computer-aided compensatory strategy training has produced greater and more stable improvements in TBI and stroke patients compared to control interventions (Gray, Robertson, Pentland, & Anderson, 1992; Niemann, Ruff, & Baser, 1990). As expected with a computerized program, the interventions also incorporated considerable practice of attention skills. Hence, while they involved compensatory training, they may also have had a remedial effect on attention. Accordingly, automated computerized attention remediation programs requiring little therapist contact, and therapist-intensive programs like the APT remedial program, both improve attention performance compared to control conditions (Sohlberg, McLaughlin, Pavese, Heidrich, & Posner, 2000; Westerberg et al., 2007). Some studies, however, combine these remedial approaches with strategy training (Tiersky et al., 2005), again obscuring the active therapeutic ingredient. Direct comparison of compensatory and remedial approaches to attention, however, do appear to favor compensatory CRT (Fasotti, Kovacs, Eling, & Brouwer, 2000).

In summary, there is evidence for positive effects of both compensatory and remedial approaches to CRT for attention. Direct comparisons of the two approaches are limited, but appear to favor compensation. Typically the two approaches are combined when treating attention, so that it remains unclear whether one is truly more effective than the other. The effectiveness of attention training survives even the Rohling et al. (2008) meta-analysis, with the one notable study that failed to show a difference between attention training and a control intervention confounded by spontaneous recovery in an acute TBI sample (Novak, Caldwell, Duke, & Berquist, 1996).

Strategy training, including the GMT program described on p. 1076, improved problem-solving performance compared to control conditions in two TBI and stroke clinical trials (Levine et al., 2000; von Cramen, Mathes-von Cramen, & Mai, 1991). Hewitt, Evans, and Dritschel (2006) used an interesting combination of memory and problem solving training in an additional clinical trial. Patients were taught to use autobiographical memory (i.e., examples from their past experience) to guide them in a new planning task. This approach improved planning performance compared to a group that did not receive training in the autobiographical memory strategy.

A final study combined training in problem solving and emotional self-regulation strategies and found that, compared to "standard" neuropsychological rehabilitation, this experimental group intervention improved performance more on executive function tests, problem-solving self-ratings, and observer ratings of problem solving during role-play situations (Rath, Simon, Langenbahn, Sherr, & Diller, 2003). Interestingly, patients who processed information the slowest at baseline showed the most benefit from the experimental treatment. They did not improve on timed attention tests, despite showing improved performance after treatment and at follow-up. The authors interpreted this as reflecting the patients' successful use of compensatory strategies despite having ongoing executive dysfunction.

As reviewed in this section, research on problem-solving CRT is quite limited. Strategy training has been tested alone, or in combination with other strategies, and has consistently resulted in improved problem solving. Despite the number of available computerized remedial approaches that provide practice of executive functions, there is little well-designed research on the effectiveness of this approach.

The Future of a Now-Mature Field

Given the amount of research conducted across multiple cognitive domains and diagnostic etiologies, CRT is arguably now a mature field of practice and research. Compensatory approaches to CRT have been shown to be effective in addressing attention, memory, and problem solving though the size and robustness of the effect varies by cognitive domain. Practice-based remedial approaches also are of benefit in treating attention and memory deficits, but have not been well-studied in the problem solving domain. In most direct comparisons, the compensatory approach appears to have an edge over the remedial approach, but in reality strategy training never occurs in isolation. Compensatory treatments always involve rehearsal of cognitive skills, and part of their effectiveness may derive from this remedial aspect of the intervention.

Given the state of the research, questions about CRT effectiveness seem less urgent than they were even a decade ago. While the most solid data on efficacy and effectiveness comes from studies of TBI and stroke patients, CRT is being used and is producing positive outcomes with a widening spectrum of medical conditions (Langenbahn, Ashman, Cantor, & Trott, 2013). CRT is standard care in the treatment of TBI and stroke, and when cognition is a factor in the patient's quality of life, CRT is becoming standard care regardless of etiology.

Some questions, however, remain perpetual in the field of CRT. Since its inception, CRT has fallen short in proving the generalization of its benefits beyond the clinic and laboratory. This is less the fault of CRT itself, than a limitation of assessment methodologies. With neuropsychological testing itself not always able to demonstrate its ecological validity (Spooner & Pachana, 2006), it is not surprising that CRT would have a similar weakness. Given the limited ability of neuropsychological tests to predict everyday functioning, they are not the best outcome measures for a treatment study. Alternative measures include self and observer rating scales, but these are heavily influenced by rater biases. One promising approach is to use simulations of everyday cognitive activities or role-play scenarios that can be administered in the clinic (Rath et al., 2003; Stringer, 2007), but such procedures are few and far between. The best approach may be to use a combination of neuropsychological tests, rating scales, and simulated everyday activities to evaluate CRT effectiveness, both in the clinic and the research laboratory. Without such a combined assessment strategy, generalization of training will remain an uncertain proposition.

Technology has played and will continue to play an important role in CRT. The cost of technology decreases as it pervades the societal landscape. The cognitive rehabilitation field can be expected to make increasing use of smartphones, tablet computers, and all manner of wearable technologies (Gillespie, Best, & O'Neill, 2012). The risk will be that the hype of technological innovation will exceed the substance. Commercialization of cognitive games via the Internet is a good example of this problem of exaggerated results (Owen et al., 2010), and the best antidote is the insistence on randomized control group investigations to support all claims of effectiveness. While one cannot prevent a commercial entity from making claims that outstrip the science, clinicians should insist upon a higher standard of evidence before they prescribe and use such interventions.

None of this is intended to stifle innovation and creativity. While there is little evidence supporting entire suites of cognitive exercises, there is support for the potential of specific computerized exercises to improve selected aspects of cognition (Glass, Maddox, & Love, 2013). While innovation is important, new CRT programs should minimally be based upon the science of CRT and should limit their claims to what the science actually supports. Available therapies should follow the evidence, rather than the evidence perpetually having to catch up with the available therapies.

Finally, almost no work has been done combining CRT with interventions that more directly impact brain physiology and function. Psychiatric disorders such as depression and anxiety often respond best to the combination of pharmacologic and psychotherapeutic interventions. The synergistic effect of CRT and pharmacotherapy remains unexplored, even in populations such as Alzheimer's disease where a number of drugs are available, but with only limited, short-duration benefit. It should be a priority to change this state of affairs, particularly within the drug companies that fund the majority of research in this area. Likewise, Transcranial Direct Current Stimulation, a recent innovation that alters cortical excitability by passing a current between electrodes placed on the scalp, may have a future role in rehabilitation by inducing neuroplasticity (Halko et al., 2011). Unknown is whether such techniques might also work synergistically with CRT in improving cognitive function.

Mature fields of research can stagnate if new directions of research and practice do not continuously evolve from existing protocols. While arguably mature, the field of CRT is far from stagnant. There is far more work to be done in the future than has been done up to the present. One could not ask for better future prospects for cognitive rehabilitation.

References

Baddeley, A., & Wilson, B. A. (1994). When implicit learning fails: Amnesia and the problem of error elimination. *Neuropsychologia, 42*, 1223–1234.

Belleville, S. (2008). Cognitive training for persons with mild cognitive impairment. *International Psychogeriatric, 20*, 57–66.

Berg, I., Konning-Haanstra, M., & Deelman, B. (1991). Long term effects of memory rehabilitation: A controlled study. *Neuropsychological Rehabilitation, 1*, 97–111.

Berker, E. A., Berker, A. H., & Smith, A. (1986). Translation of Broca's 1865 report: Localization of speech in the third frontal convolution. *Archives of Neurology, 43*, 1065–1072. doi: 10.1001/archneur.1986.00520100069017

Blundon, G., & Smits, E. (2000). Cognitive rehabilitation: A pilot survey of therapeutic modalities used by Canadian occupational therapists with survivors of traumatic brain injury. *Canadian Jouranl of Occupational Therapy, 67*(3), 184–196.

Business Wire. (2012, October 17). Strategy analytics: Worldwide smartphone population tops 1 billion in Q3 2012. Retrieved from www.businesswire.com/news/home/20121017005479/en/Strategy-Analytics-Worldwide-Smartphone-Population-Tops-1#.UsrrafRDt8G

Butler, R. W., & Copeland, D. R. (2002). Attentional processes and their remediation in children treated for cancer: A literature review and the development of a therapeutic approach. *Journal of the International Neuropsychological Society, 8*, 115–124.

Butler, R. W., Copeland, D. R., Fairclough, D. L., Mulhern, R. K., Katz, E. R., Kazak, A. E, . . . Sahler, O. J. (2008). A multicenter, randomized clinical trial of a cognitive remediation program for childhood survivors of a pediatric malignancy. *Journal of Consulting and Clinical Psychology, 76*, 367–378. doi: 10.1037/0022-006X.76.3.367

Cappa, S. F., Benke, T., Clarke, S., Rossi, B., Stemmer, B., & van Heugten, C. M. (2005). EFNS guidelines on cognitive rehabilitation: Report of the EFNS task force. *European Journal of Neurology, 12*, 665–680.

Carvalhal, M. M., Padez, M. C., Moreira, P. A., & Rosado, V. M. (2006). Overweight and obesity related to activities in Portuguese children, 7–9 year. *European Journal of Public Health, 17*(1), 42–46.

Cicerone, K. D., Dahlberg, C., Kalmar, K., Langenbahn, D. M., Malec, J. F., Bergquist, T. F, . . . Kneipp, S. (2000). Evidence-based cognitive rehabilitation: Recommendations for clinical practice. *Archives of Physical Medicine and Rehabilitation, 81*, 1596–1615.

Cicerone, K. D., Dahlberg, C., Malec, J. F., Langenbahn, D. M., Felicetti, T., Kneipp, S, . . . Laatsch, L. (2005). Evidence-based cognitive rehabilitation: Updated review of the literature from 1998 through 2002. *Archives of Physical Medicine and Rehabilitation, 86*, 1681–1692.

Cicerone, K. D., Langenbahn, D. M., Braden, C., Malec, J. F., Kalmar, K., Fraas, M, . . . Cantor, J. (2011). Evidence-based cognitive rehabilitation: Udated review of the literature from 2003 through 2008. *Archives of Physical Medicine and Rehabilitation, 92*, 519–530.

Cotelli, M., Menenti, R., Zanetti, O., & Miniussi, C. (2012). Non-pharmacological intervention for memory decline. *Frontiers in Human Neuroscience, 6*(article 46), 1–17.

Doornhein, K., & de Haan, E.H.F. (1998). Cognitive training for memory deficits in stroke patients. *Neuropsychological Rehabilitation, 8*, 393–400.

Dou, Z. L., Man, D. W., Ou, H. N., Zheng, J. L., & Tam, S. F. (2006). Computerized errorless learning-based memory rehabilitation for Chinese patients with brain injury: A preliminary quasi-experimental clinical design study. *Brain Injury*, *20*, 219–225.

Engelberts, N. H., Klein, M., Ader, H. J., Heimans, J. J., Trenite, D. G., & van der Ploeg, H. M. (2002). The effectiveness of cognitive rehabilitation for attention deficits in focal seizures: A randomized controlled study. *Epilepsia*, *43*, 587–595.

Fasotti, L., Kovacs, F., Eling, P. A., & Brouwer, W. H. (2000). Time pressure management as a compensatory strategy training after closed head injury. *Neuropsychological Rehabilitation*, *10*, 47–65.

Fish, J., Manly, T., Emslie, H., Evans, J. J., & Wilson, B. A., (2008). Compensatory strategies for acquired disorders of memory and planning: Differential effects of a paging system for patients with brain injury of traumatic versus cerebrovascular aetiology. *Journal of Neurology, Neurosurgery, and Psychiatry*, *79*, 930–935.

Gillespie, A., Best, C., & O'Neill, B. (2012). Cognitive function and assistive technology for cognition: A systematic review. *Journal of the International Neuropsychological Society*, *18*, 1–19. doi: 10.1017/S1355617711001548

Gillespie, R. M. (2002). The physical impact of computers and electronic game use on children and adolescents, a review of current literature. *Work*, *18*, 249–259.

Glass, B. D., Maddox, W. T., & Love, B. C. (2013). Real-time strategy game training: Emergence of a cognitive flexibility trait. *PLOS One*, *8*(8), 1–7.

Glisky, E. L., & Schacter, D. L. (1987). Acquisition of domain-specific knowledge in organic amnesia: Training for computer-related work. *Neuropsychologia*, *25*, 893–906.

Glisky, E. L., Schacter, D. L., & Tulving, E. (1986a). Computer learning by memory-impaired patients: Acquisition and retention of complex knowledge. *Neuropsychologia*, *24*, 313–328.

Glisky, E. L., Schacter, D. L., & Tulving, E. (1986b). Learning and retention of computer related vocabulary in memory-impaired patients: Method of vanishing cues. *Journal of Clinical and Experimental Neuropsychology*, *8*, 292–312.

Gray, J. M., Robertson, I., Pentland, B., & Anderson, S. (1992). Microcomputer-based attentional retraining after brain damage: A randomized group controlled trial. *Neuropsychological Rehabilitation*, *2*, 97 115.

Halko, M. A., Datta, A., Plow, E. B., Scaturro, J., Bikson, M., & Merabet, L. B. (2011). Neuroplastic changes following rehabilitation training correlate with regional electrical field induced with tDCS. *NeuroImage*, *57*, 885–891.

Hampstead, B. M., Sathian, K., Moore, A. B., Nalisnick, C., & Stringer, A. Y. (2008). Explicit memory training leads to improved memory for face-name pairs in patients with mild cognitive impairment: Results of a pilot investigation. *Journal of the International Neuropsychological Society*, *14*, 883–889. doi: 10.1017/S1355617708081009

Hampstead, B. M., Sathian, K., Phillips, P. A., Amaraneni, A., Dalaune, W. R., & Stringer, A. Y. (2012). Mnemonic strategy training improves memory for object location associations in both healthy elderly and patients with amnestic mild cognitive impairment: A randomized, single-blind study. *Neuropsychology*, *26*, 385–399. doi: 10.1037a0027545

Hampstead, B. M., Stringer, A. Y., Stilla, R. F., Deshpande, G., Hu, X., Moore, A. B., & Sathian, K. (2011). Activation and effective connectivity changes following explicit-memory training for face-name pairs in patients with mild cognitive impairment: A pilot study. *Neurorehabilitation and Neural Repair*, *25*, 210–222.

Hampstead, B. M., Stringer, A. Y., Stilla, R. F., Giddens, M., & Sathian, K. (2012). Mnemonic strategy training partially restores hippocampal activity in patients with mild cognitive impairment. *Hippocampus*, *22*, 1652–1658.

Harley, J. P., Allen, C. Braciszewski, T. L., Cicerone, K. D., Dahlberg, C., Evans, S, . . . Smigelski, J. S. (1992). Guidelines for cognitive rehabilitation. *NeuroRehabilitation*, *2*, 62–67.

Helmstaedter, C., Loer, B., Wohlfahrt, R., Hammen, A., Saar, J., Steinhoff, B. J, . . . Schulze-Bonhage, A. (2008). The effect of cognitive rehabilitation on memory outcome after temporal lobe epilepsy surgery. *Epilepsy and Behavior*, *12*, 402–409.

Hewitt, J., Evans, J. J., & Dritschel, B. (2006). Theory driven rehabilitation of executive functioning: Improving planning skills in people with traumatic brain injury through the ue of an autobiographical memory cueing procedure. *Neuropsychologia*, *44*, 1468–1474.

Homskaya, E. D. (2001). *Alexander Romanovich Luria: A Scientific Biography*. New York: Plenum Publishers.

Hunkin, N. M., Squires, E. J., Parkin, A. J., & Tidy, J. A. (1998). Are the benefits of errorless learning dependent on implicit memory? *Neuropsychologia*, *36*, 25–36.

Incalzi, R. A., Corsonello, A., Trojano, L., Pedone, C., Acanfora, D., Spada, A, . . . Rengo, F. (2008). Cognitive training is ineffective in hypoxemic COPD: A six-month randomized controlled trial. *Rejuvenation Research*, *111*, 239–250. doi: 10.1089/rej.2007.0607

Jean, L., Bergeron, M.-E., Thivierge, S., & Simard, M. (2010). Cognitive intervention programs for individuals with mild cognitive impairment: Systematic review of the literature. *The American Journal of Geriatric Psychiatry*, *18*(4), 281–296.

Jones, M. K. (1974). Imagery as a mnemonic aid after left temporal lobectomy: Contrast between material specific and generalized memory disorders. *Neuropsychologia*, *12*, 21–24.

Kalla, T., Downes, J. J., & van den Broek, M. (2001). The pre-exposure technique: Enhancing the effects of errorless learning in the acquisition of face-name associations. *Neuropsychological Rehabilitation*, *11*, 1–16.

Kaschel, R., Della Sala, S., Cantagallo, A., Fahlbock, A., Laaksonen, R., & Kazen, M. (2002). Imagery mnemonics for the rehabilitation of memory: A randomized group controlled trial. *Neuropsychological Rehabilitation*, *12*, 127–153.

Koorenhof, L., Baxendale, S., Smith, N., & Thompson, P. (2011). Memory rehabilitation and brain training for surgical temporal lobe epilepsy patients: A preliminary report. *Seizure*, *21*, 178–182. doi: 10.1016/j.seizure.2011.12.001

Langenbahn, D. M., Ashman, T., Cantor, J., & Trott, C. (2013). An evidence-based review of cognitive rehabilitation in medical conditions affecting cognitive function. *Archives of Physical Medicine and Rehabilitation*, *94*, 271–286.

Levine, B., Robertson, I. H., Clare, L., Carter, G., Hong, J., Wilson, B. A, . . . Stuss, D. T. (2000). Rehabilitation of executive functioning: An experimental-clinical validation of goal management training. *Journal of the International Neuropsychological Society*, *6*, 296–312.

Li, H., Li, J., Li, N., Li, B., Wang, P., & Zhou, T. (2011). Cognitive intervention for persons with mild cognitive impairment: A meta-analysis. *Ageing Research Reviews*, *10*, 285–296.

Martin, M., Clare, L., Altgassen, A. M., Cameron, M. H., & Zehnder, F. (2011). Cognition-based interventions for healthy older people and people with mild cognitive impairment. *Cochrane Database of Systematic Reviews, 19*(1), 1–51.

Niemann, H. Ruff, R. M., & Baser, C. A. (1990). Computer assisted attention retraining in head injured individuals: A controlled efficacy study of an out-patient program. *Journal of Consulting and Clinical Psychology, 58*, 811–817.

Novak, T. A., Caldwell, S. G., Duke, L. W., & Berquist, T. (1996). Focused versus unstructured intervention for attention deficits after traumatic brain injury. *Journal of Head Trauma Rehabilitation, 11*, 52–60.

Owen, A. M., Hampshire, A., Grahn, J. A., Stenton, R., Dajani, S., Burns, A. S, . . . Ballard, C. G. (2010). Putting brain training to the test. *Nature, 465*, 775–779. doi: 10.1038/nature09042

Ownsworth, T. L., & McFarland, K. (1999). Memory remediation in long-term acquired brain injury: Two approaches in diary training. *Brain Injury, 13*, 605–626.

Poppelreuter, M., Weis, J., Mumm, A., Orth, H. B., & Bartsch, H. H. (2008). Rehabilitation of therapy-related cognitive deficits in patients after hematopoietic stem cell transplantation. *Bone Marrow Transplant, 41*, 79–90.

Prigatano, G. P. (2009). A history of cognitive rehabilitation. In P. W. Halligan & D. T. Wade (Eds.), *The Effectiveness of Rehabilitation for Cognitive Deficits* (pp. 3–10). New York: Oxford University Press.

Rath, J. F., Simon, D., Langenbahn, D. M., Sherr, R. L., & Diller, L. (2003). Group treatment of problems-solving deficits in outpatients with traumatic brain injury: A randomized outcome study. *Neuropsychological Rehabilitation, 13*, 341–488.

Rebok, G. W., Ball, K., Guey, L. T., Jones, R. N., Kim, H.-Y., King, J. W., . . . Willis, S. L. for the ACTIVE Study Group. (2014). Ten-year effects of the advanced cognitive training for independent and vital elderly cognitive training trial on cognition and everyday functioning in older adults. *Journal of the American Geriatrics Society, 62*, 16–24. doi: 10.1111/jgs.12607

Reijnders, J., van Heugten, C., & van Boxtel, M. (2013). Cognitive interventions in healthy older adults and people with mild cognitive impairment: A systematic review. *Ageing Research Reviews, 12*, 263–275.

Rohling, M. L., Faust, M. E., Beverly, B., & Demakis, G. (2008). Effectiveness of cognitive rehabilitation following acquired brain injury: A meta-analytic re-examination of Cicerone et al.'s (2002, 2005) systematic reviews. *Neuropsychology, 23*, 20–39. doi: 10.1037/a0013659

Ryan, T. V., & Ruff, R. M. (1988). The efficacy of structured memory retraining in a group comparision of head trauma patients. *Archives of Clinical Neuropsychology, 3*, 165–179.

Sammer, G., Reuter, J., Hullmann, K., Kaps, M., & Vaitl, D. (2006). Training of executive function in Parkinson's disease. *Journal of Neurological Science, 248*, 115–119.

Schacter, D. L., & Glisky, E. L. (1986). Memory remediation: Restoration, alleviation, and the acquisition of domain-specific knowledge. In B. Uzzell & Y. Gross (Eds.), *Clinical Neuropsychology of Intervention* (pp. 257–282). Boston: Martinus Nijhoff.

Schacter, D. L., Rich, S. A., & Stampp, M. S. (1985). Remediation of memory disorders: Experimental evaluation of the spaced retrieval technique. *Journal of Clinical and Experimental Neuropsychology, 7*, 79–96.

Schmitter-Edgecombe, M., Fahy, J., Whelan, J., & Long, C. (1995). Memory remediation after severe closed head injury: Notebook training versus supportive therapy. *Journal of Consulting and Clinical Psychology, 63*, 484–489.

Shoja, M. M., Tubbs, R. S., Malekian, A., Jafari Rouhi, A. H., Barzgar, M., & Oakes, W. J. (2007). Video game epilepsy in the twentieth century: A review. *Child's Nervous System, 23*(3), 265–267.

Simon, S. S., Yokomizo, J. E., & Bottino, C.M.C. (2012). Cognitive intervention in amnestic mild cognitive impairment: A sustematic review. *Neuroscience and Biobehavioral Reviews, 36*, 1163–1178.

Sohlberg, M. M., & Mateer, C. A. (1989). *Introduction to Cognitive Rehabilitation: Theory and Practice*. New York: Guilford Press.

Sohlberg, M. M., McLauglin, K. A., Pavese, A., Heidrich, A., & Posner, M. I. (2000). Evaluation of attention process training and brain injury education in persons with acquired brain injury. *Journal of Clinical and Experimental Neuropsychology, 22*, 656–676.

Spooner, D. M., & Pachana, N. A. (2006). Ecological validity in neuropsychological assessment: A case for greater consideration in research with neurologically intact populations. *Archives of Clinical Neuropsychology, 21*, 327–337.

Squires, E. J., Hunkin, N. M., & Parkin, A. J. (1997). Errorless learning of novel associations in amnesia. *Neuropsychologia, 35*, 1103–1111.

Stringer, A. Y. (2003). Cognitive rehabilitation practice patterns: A survey of American Hospital Association Rehabilitation Programs. *The Clinical Neuropsychologist, 17*, 34–44.

Stringer, A. Y. (2007). *Ecologically Oriented Neurorehabilitation of Memory Therapist Guide*. Los Angeles, CA: Western Psychological Services.

Stringer, A. Y. (2011). Ecologically oriented neurorehabilitation of memory: Robustness of outcome across diagnosis and severity. *Brain Injury, 25*, 169–178.

Stringer, A. Y., Denham, M., & White, A. K. (in press). *Ecologically Oriented Neurorehabilitation of Executive Function Therapist Guide*. Los Angeles, CA: Western Psychological Services.

Sutton, E. W., & Rackham, H. (Trans.). (1942). *Cicero: On the Orator, Books I-II (Loeb Classical Library No. 348)* (English and Latin ed.). London: William Heinemann.

Tiersky, L. A., Anselmi, V., Johnston, M. V., Kurtyka, J., Roosen, E., Schwartz, T., & Deluca, J. (2005). A trial of neuropsychologic rehabilitation in mild-spectrum traumatic brain injury. *Archives of Physical Medicine and Rehabilitation, 86*, 1565–1574.

van Hout, M.S.E., Wekking, E. M., Berg, U., & Deelman, B. G. (2008). Psychosocial and cognitive rehabilitation of patients with solvent-induced chronic toxic encephalopathy: A randomized controlled study. *Psychotherapy and Psychosomatics, 77*, 289–297. doi: 10.1159/000140088

von Cramen, D. Y., Mathes-von Cramen, G., & Mai, N. (1991). Problem solving deficits in brain injured patients: A therapeutic approach. *Neuropsychological Rehabilitation, 1*, 45–64.

Westerberg, H., Jacobaeus, H., Hirvikoski, T., Clevberger, P., Ostensson, M. L., Bartfai, A., & Klingberg, T. (2007). Computerized working memory training after stroke-a pilot study. *Brain Injury, 21*, 21–29.

Wilson, B. A., Emslie, H. C., Quirk, K., & Evans, J. J. (2001). Reducing everyday memory and planning problems by means of a paging system: A randomized control crossover study. *Journal of Neurology, Neurosurgery, and Psychiatry, 70*, 477–482.

Wilson, B. A., Emslie, H., Quirk, K., Evans, J., & Watson, P. (2005). A randomized control trial to evaluate a paging system for people with traumatic brain injury. *Brain Injury, 19*, 891–894.

50 Clinical Psychopharmacology

Samuel Alperin and Lenard A. Adler

This chapter will provide an overview of major psychiatric disorders, including presenting symptoms, pathophysiology, and treatment options. Given space limitations, the discussion is not meant to be exhaustive or complete, but rather to provide a background for the reader that may be helpful in understanding other chapters. The treatment recommendations are not meant to be specific to any patient and treatment decisions must be tailored for each individual patient by the providers.

Schizophrenia

Schizophrenia spectrum disorders are defined by abnormalities in at least one of the five domains: delusions, hallucinations, disorganized thinking (speech), grossly disorganized or abnormal motor behavior (including catatonia), and negative symptoms (American Psychiatric Association, 2013). Negative symptoms include the absence of normal behavior as seen with flattened affect, alogia, apathy, avolition and social withdrawal (American Psychiatric Association, 2013). According to DSM-5, schizophrenia is diagnosed by the presence of the following (American Psychiatric Association, 2013).:

- Criterion A: At least two of the previous five domains (one of which must be either delusions, hallucinations, or disorganized speech)
- Criterion B: Impairment for a significant portion of time in a major area of functioning
- Criterion C: Signs of the disturbance continuously for at least six months
- Criterion D: Schizoaffective, depressive, or bipolar disorder with psychotic features have been ruled out
- Criterion E: The symptoms are not attributed to the effects of some substance (medications) or medical condition
- Criterion F: There is no history of autism spectrum disorder or a communication disorder during childhood

There are five types of schizophrenia: paranoid, disorganized, catatonic, undifferentiated, and residual. The majority of individuals manifest with symptoms in their 20s (American Psychiatric Association, 2013; Davis, Charney, Coyle, & Nemeroff, 2002; Schultz, North, & Shields, 2007). Risk factors include family history of psychoses, older age of father, autoimmune disorders, and viral infections during the first or second trimester (Schultz et al., 2007). The worldwide prevalence of schizophrenia is about 1%, and is equally prevalent amongst men and women, although men usually present slightly earlier than women (American Psychiatric Association, 2013; Schultz et al., 2007). Furthermore, most patients go through a prodromal phase, where there is a slow onset of developing symptoms, including social withdrawal, worsening of hygiene and grooming, unusual behaviors like outburst of anger, and deterioration and loss of interest in school or work (American Psychiatric Association, 2013; Davis et al., 2002).

Cognitive impairments in schizophrenic patients include deficits in memory, abstraction, and attention. With impaired activation of the prefrontal cortex (PFC), they generally have reduced intelligence measures along with delays in early developmental milestones. Unlike many of the other major psychiatric disorders, schizophrenia generally presents with "global" cognitive impairments that include difficulty with everything from attention, to memory, to fluency, executive function, and verbal ability (Lepage, Bodnar, & Bowie, 2014; Millan et al., 2012; Schaefer, Giangrande, Weinberger, & Dickinson, 2013). Nonetheless, schizophrenia commonly leads to an especially significant decline in processing speed and episodic memory. Furthermore, the impairment in verbal memory has been posited as a strong marker of outcome of schizophrenic symptoms (Lepage et al., 2014).

Although the pathophysiology of the disorder is not fully established, it is believed that symptoms of schizophrenia are attributable to dysregulation within the dopaminergic tracts of the brain. There are four main tracts, namely the mesolimbic, mesocortical, nigrostriatal, and tuberoinfundibular (Purves et al., 2007). It is hypothesized that there is excess dopaminergic activity within the mesolimbic pathway leading to the positive symptoms, with a simultaneous reduced dopaminergic activity in the mesocortical pathway, resulting in the negative symptoms (Davis et al., 2002; Miyamoto, Miyake, Jarskog, Fleischhacker, & Lieberman, 2012). The mesolimbic dopaminergic pathway includes the connections between the ventral tegmental area (VTA) and the nucleus accumbens and mostly the D1 and D2 receptors. The mesocortical pathway includes connections from the VTA to the temporal cortex, frontal cortex, and PFC, and mostly D1 receptors with some presence of D2 and D5 receptors (Purves et al., 2007). The last two dopaminergic pathways consist of connections from the substantia nigra to the corpus striatum (the nigrostriatal) and from the hypothalamus to the anterior pituitary (the tuberoinfundibular) (Purves et al., 2007).

There are two main categories of antipsychotics: first generation (FGA, also known as the *typical*) and second generation (SGA, also known as the *atypical*) (Davis et al., 2002; Ellenbroek, 2012; Golan, Tashjian, Armstrong, & Armstrong, 2011). It is believed that FGAs, like chlorpromazine and haloperidol, have high affinity for dopamine receptors, specifically the D2, especially within the mesolimbic pathway, thereby decreasing the presence of positive symptoms (Ellenbroek, 2012; Golan et al., 2011; Miyamoto et al., 2012). Conversely, SGAs (like clozapine, risperidone, olanzapine, quetiapine, and aripiprazole) have slightly decreased affinity for the D2 receptors, but are believed to have some serotonin antagonism (Ellenbroek, 2012; Golan et al., 2011; Miyamoto et al., 2012). Furthermore, SGAs have an increased disassociation constant than dopamine (Golan et al., 2011).

The main side effects from FGAs include extrapyramidal side effects (EPS) from acute use and tardive dyskinesia (TD) from more chronic use (Davis et al., 2002; Ellenbroek, 2012; Schultz et al., 2007). EPS is defined as parkinsonism (rigidity, bradykinesia, shuffling gait, tremor), dystonia (fixed upper gaze, neck twisting, facial muscle spasms), and akathisia (inability to sit still, restlessness, tapping of feet). Studies have shown that while about 65%–70% receptor occupancy of D2 allow for the antipsychotic effects of the FGAs, above 80% occupancy leads to the increased risk of EPS (Davis et al., 2002; Golan et al., 2011; Miyamoto et al., 2012). It is believed that it is D2 inhibition within the basal ganglia that leads to EPS, as is similar to Parkinson's disease (Golan et al., 2011). EPS is mostly treated with anticholinergic drugs, although some studies have shown that these may lead to further cognitive impairment (e.g., verbal memory or confusion; see Golan et al., 2011). Akathisia has been shown to be responsive to low doses of beta blockers (Adler, Angrist, Reiter, & Rotrosen, 1989). Furthermore, it is important to keep in mind that while decreasing the dose of FGAs helps to decrease EPS, lower doses have increased probability of relapse (Golan et al., 2011). TD is defined as involuntary movements, especially of the lower face. One proposed etiology of TD is an adaptive hypersensitivity of D2 receptors in the striatum.

The main benefit of SGAs over the FGAs is their decreased risk of EPS and TD (Davis et al., 2002; Golan et al., 2011). Decreased presence of these side effects is believed to be a result of the increased serotonergic inhibition (Miyamoto et al., 2012) of a relatively lower level of dopaminergic blockade. Nonetheless, SGAs come along with their own set of side effects, including sedation, weight gain, and diabetes mellitus type II (DMII; this risk is separate from the weight gain) (Davis et al., 2002; Schultz et al., 2007).

Depression

Depression, as defined in the DSM-5 (American Psychiatric Association, 2013), consists of a pervasive feeling of sadness or irritability that results in significant disturbances in energy, sleep, appetite, sexual drive, weight, or the ability to express or seek pleasure. Major depressive disorder (MDD) is defined as depression that lasts for at least a two-week period, with symptoms that cause clinically significant impairment at work, with the family, or in other important areas. There are three types of MDD: typical (melancholic), atypical, and psychotic (American Psychiatric Association, 2013). MDD can present at any age, but has an increased likelihood during puberty (Kessler et al., 2003). Furthermore, the 12-month prevalence of MDD in the United States is about 7% (about 4.7% worldwide; see Ferrari, 2013), with a prevalence of twice as much in women than in men (Kupfer, Frank, & Phillips, 2012). MDD is also highly associated with many other health issues, including coronary artery disease, metabolic syndrome, diabetes, and other chronic illness (American Psychiatric Association, 2013; Kupfer et al., 2012). MDD also shows some heritability, of about 40% (American Psychiatric Association, 2013; Belmaker & Agam, 2008).

While depression usually leads to overall poor performance on cognitive tests (Millan et al., 2012), studies have found specific deficits in some areas. In one meta-analysis of those presenting with their first episode of MDD, significant impairment was found in psychomotor speed, attention, and visual learning and memory (Lee, Hermens, Porter, & Redoblado-Hodge, 2012). Furthermore, executive dysfunction was specific to attentional switching, verbal fluency performance, and cognitive flexibility (Lee et al., 2012). When considering lifetime impairment from MDD, significant impairment was found in executive function, processing speed, and episodic memory (Trivedi & Greer, 2014). Furthermore, these impairments have been found to persist even after symptoms have remitted (McIntyre, Cha, Soczynska, et al., 2013).

The main theory of depression is known as the "monoamine" theory, which postulates that depression is due to decreased serotonergic and/or noradrenergic neurotransmission within the brain (Belmaker & Agam, 2008; Golan et al., 2011; Krishnan & Nestler, 2008). Norepinephrine, on the one hand, is a molecule mostly produced in the locus ceruleus (LC) and is involved in vigilance, stress response, neuroendocrine function, pain control, and the sympathetic nervous system (Golan et al., 2011). Serotonin, on the other hand, is produced within the raphe nucleus, and is involved in modulation of mood, the sleep–wake cycle, motivation and reward, cognition function, and pain perception, as well as neuroendocrine function (Golan et al., 2011). After being released into the synaptic cleft, these molecules are then transported back through a nonspecific transporter, vesicular monoamine transporter (VMAT), or through specific serotonin transporter (SERT) and norepinephrine transporters (NET). Both of these molecules then get degraded intracellulary by an enzyme called *monoamine oxidase* (MAO), of which there are two types: MAO-A degrades serotonin, norepinephrine, and dopamine, while MAO-B degrades dopamine only. Another enzyme, catechol-O-methyltransferase (COMT), is involved in monoamine degradation extracellularly, but is only found more peripherally outside the brain (Purves et al., 2007).

The norepinephrine from the LC innervates a wide variety of structures throughout the brain, including the amygdala, the hippocampus, prefrontal and frontal cortices, and the raphe nuclei and VTA (thereby, controlling the release of 5-HT and DA, respectively). The dopamine release from the VTA helps to modulate the reward network of the ventral striatum, orbitofrontal cortex, and the medial PFC, while the serotonin helps to modulate the limbic or emotional system of the amygdala, medial PFC, and anterior cingulate cortex (Krishnan & Nestler, 2008; Davis et al., 2002). Some studies have shown that those with depression have increased activity in the amygdala, ventral striatum, and medial PFC in reaction to negative emotion, while decreased activity in the ventral striatum in response to positive emotions and reward (Kupfer et al., 2012). The theory is, therefore, that those who are depressed have an increased emotional reaction (as seen with increased activity in the amygdala and medial PFC), with decreased voluntary control over the emotion (as seen with activity in the dorsolateral PFC; see Kupfer et al., 2012). Studies have shown that there is decreased gray matter volume and glial density in the PFC and hippocampus in those with diagnosed MDD, while imaging studies have shown increased activity on fMRI and PET in the amygdala and subgenual cingulate cortex (a small portion of the PFC) (Krishnan & Nestler, 2008).

There are three main types of medications that treat depression: the classical MAO inhibitors, reuptake inhibitors, and the atypicals (Golan et al., 2011). Reuptake inhibitors fall into four categories: tricyclic antagonists (TCAs), selective serotonin reuptake inhibitors (SSRIs), serotonin-norepinephrine reuptake inhibitors (SNRIs), and heterocyclics.

MAO inhibitors (MAO-Is) inhibit the breakdown of the monoamines once they have been taken back up by the presynaptic cell, thereby increasing their availability for release back into the synapse. The irreversible MAO-Is include iproniazid, phenylzine, and isocarboxazid (Davis et al., 2002; Golan et al., 2011). The newer MAO-Is are reversible and also selective for MAO-A (which degrades all three, 5-HT, NE, and DA), and includes moclebemide, befloxatone, and brofaromine (Davis et al., 2002; Golan et al., 2011). The older, irreversible MAO-Is have a higher risk of tyramine toxicity (tyramine comes from products like wine and cheese and is also metabolized by the liver version of MAO), leading to sympathomimetic side effects like hypertension, headache, tachycardia, nausea, cardiac arrhythmias, and stroke (Golan et al., 2011). The newer MAO-Is are easily replaced by tyramine, and therefore have a decreased risk of this toxicity; however, nonetheless the risk of this toxicity has limited the clinical utility of all MAO-Is.

TCAs are broken up into secondary amines and tertiary amines. The former is more selective for NE and the latter for 5-HT (Davis et al., 2002; Golan et al., 2011). Nonetheless, TCAs block SERT, NET, and dopamine active transporter (DAT), resulting in increased levels of 5-HT, NE and DA in the synaptic cleft, respectively. The list of TCAs includes imipramine, desipramine, clomipramine, amitriptyline, and nortriptyline, among others (Davis et al., 2002; Golan et al., 2011). Common side effects of TCAs include their anticholinergic effects of nausea, vomiting, orthostatic hypotension, anorexia, dry mouth, blurred vision, confusion, constipation, tachycardia, and urinary retention (Golan et al., 2011). The potential for orthostatic hypotension is important to consider when using TCAs in the elderly as it may increase the risk for serious falls (Glassman, 1984). Furthermore, TCAs also have some antihistaminergic effects of sedation, weight gain, and confusion in the elderly (Golan et al., 2011). Finally, TCAs have some antiadrenergic effects such as reflex tachycardia, drowsiness, and dizziness (Golan et al., 2011). The pharmacologic class has also shown to have some Type I antiarrythmic effects that can predispose to cardiac conduction problems, especially in patients with underlying cardiovascular disease (Glassman & Bigger, 1981). SSRIs have more selectivity for the SERT receptors and therefore are associated with less adverse events (compared to TCAs), and are therefore generally considered the first-line medications for MDD (with specifically increased effectiveness for typical, melancholic-type depression) (Golan et al., 2011; Timonen & Liukkonen, 2008). In addition to treatment of MDD, SSRIs are also used to treat panic syndrome, obsessive-compulsive disorder (OCD), premature ejaculation, and PTSD (Golan et al., 2011). Their major limiting factor is dosage: while increased dose shows increased effect, it also shows increased binding to NET receptors. Major side effects of SSRIs include sexual dysfunction and gastrointestinal (GI) problems. The list of SSRIs includes fluoxetine, citalopram, fluvoxamine, paroxetine, sertraline, and escitalopram. Although the evidence has been debated, there is some that shows there is an increased risk of suicide with SSRI treatment, warranting clinicians to be watchful (Golan et al., 2011; Kupfer et al., 2012). There are specific warnings regarding the risk of new onset suicidal ideation in children, adolescents, and young adults (Hetrick, McKenzie, Cox, Simmons, & Merry, 2012).

Unlike TCAs, SNRIs inhibit only SERT and NET, thereby decreasing the reuptake of serotonin and norepinephrine (Davis et al., 2002; Golan et al., 2011). SNRIs are generally considered second-line after SSRIs, due to their more limited receptor selectivity than TCAs (Golan et al., 2011). The list of SNRIs includes venlafaxine, desvenlafaxine (a metabolite of venlafaxine), and duloxetine. Side effects of SNRIs include hypertension, sweating, weight loss, GI distress, blurred vision, nervousness, and sexual dysfunction (Golan et al., 2011).

The last class of antidepressants is the atypicals, which includes bupropion, mirtazapine, and trazodone (Davis et al., 2002; Golan et al., 2011; _Kupfer et al., 2012). Bupropion increases the levels of serotonin and dopamine in the synaptic cleft (in a similar manner to the amphetamines; see Golan et al., 2011) and is a modest dopamine and norepinephrine reuptake inhibitor (Carroll et al., 2014). Side effects include seizures (generally thought to occur in doses > 450 mg/day), insomnia, and electrolyte abnormalities (and there is a noted contraindication in patients with eating disorders). Bupropion has also been shown to be helpful in smoking cessation (Cahill, Stevens, Perera, & Lancaster, 2013). Mirtazapine blocks the postsynaptic serotonin receptors, as well as the α_2-adrenergic autoreceptors, thereby decreasing serotonin neurotransmission (Golan et al., 2011). Due to its appetite-stimulating effects (possibly from its antihistaminic properties), mirtazapine is particularly effective for elderly patients suffering from weight loss and eating problems. Trazodone is thought to exert its mechanism of action through effects on serotonin; the most common adverse events noted are sedation, headache, and dizziness (Fagiolini, Comandini, Catena Dell'Osso, & Kasper, 2012). The sedative properties of trazodone have led to its off-label use as a hypnotic in a variety of conditions, including antidepressant-associated insomnia (Nierenberg, Adler, Peselow, Zornberg, & Rosenthal, 1994).

Drugs within the SSRI category usually do not show any effect for about two to three weeks. These effects take a while to take hold due to the fact that they are due to more chronic changes at the synaptic level, which are secondary to the increase in monoamines in the cleft (Davis et al., 2002; Golan et al., 2011; Krishnan & Nestler, 2008). Finally, it is important that a misdiagnosis of MDD, with an underlying bipolar disorder (BPD), and treatment with MAO-Is, SSRIs, and TCAs (and some heterocyclics) can precipitate manic and hypomanic symptoms (Golan et al., 2011).

Bipolar Disorder

BPD is characterized by three stages: periods of mania that percolate periods of depression, surrounded by periods of euthymia (mood defined as neither depressed nor excessively elevated). Mania is defined in the *Diagnostic and Statistical Manual of Mental Disorders,* fifth edition (DSM-5) by elevated levels of euphoria or mood and energy that last at least one week (American Psychiatric Association, 2013). These periods of mania are characterized with an inflated self-esteem, little need for sleep, inability to stop talking, racing thoughts, distractibility, involvement in dangerous or negative activities, and an increase in goal-directed activity. BPD requires that these manic periods cause impairment in social and occupational realms. BPD is most frequently diagnosed prior to the age of 30, usually around 18 years old, and most patients present during periods of depression, and so it is important to probe for previous manic or hypomanic episodes (American Psychiatric Association, 2013; Connolly & Thase, 2011). This disorder has a lifetime prevalence of about 1%–2% worldwide (American Psychiatric Association, 2013; Geddes & Miklowitz, 2013). Those with BPD have some residual depressive symptoms that present for about one-third of their life (Geddes & Miklowitz, 2013).

Cognitive impairments of BPD depend on the specific stage. The manic and depressed stages are associated with moderate deficits in executive function, memory, and attention (Malhi et al., 2007; Miklowitz, 2011). The depressive stage is further associated with impairment in fine motor skills. Some studies have also found deficits in verbal learning and processing speed (Miklowitz, 2011). As has been seen with MDD, absence of symptoms does not lead to improvement in impairment. Memory deficits, especially those with verbal recall, have been observed in euthymic bipolar subjects (Malhi et al., 2007).

The neurobiology of BPD centers around the limbic system and especially the amygdala. A model recently put forth by a consensus group shows that it is most likely a dysregulation of two networks that results in the symptoms seen with BPD (Strakowski et al., 2012). The first network, the so-called *external emotional control* network arises from the ventrolateral PFC. This external control includes functions such as understanding facial emotion. The second network originates in the orbitofrontal cortex and is called the *internal emotional control* network, as it is more involved in the emotional response to certain cues. Both of these networks are connected with the limbic system, which involves the hippocampus, thalamus, cingulate gyrus, limbic cortex, and hypothalamus. It is believed, therefore, that there is impaired regulation of the amygdala from both networks, allowing overactivation of the amygdala and its control over the limbic system (Blond, Fredericks, & Blumberg, 2012; Strakowski et al., 2012). This increased amygdala activity is usually only seen during manic episodes, and disappears when anticonvulsants are used (Blond et al., 2012).

Historically, the most common medication used for treatment of mania associated with BPD has been lithium carbonate. Lithium is believed to block regeneration of PIP2, a second messenger that is involved in the intracellular signaling initiated by neurotransmitters within the adrenergic, muscarinic and serotonergic systems (Davis et al., 2002; Golan et al., 2011; Oruch, Elderbi, Khattab, Pryme, & Lund, 2014). Other mechanisms thought to be involved in lithium's actions include affecting the synthesis and degradation of dopamine and norepinephrine, affecting glutamate neurotransmission, and increasing serotonin release from the raphe nucleus (Oruch et al, 2014). The dosing of lithium is titrating according to blood levels, which should be maintained within a therapeutic range. While lithium has been shown to be effective for acute mania, psychotic symptoms associated with BPD, and even perhaps maintenance therapy (it helps to decrease manic and depressive relapse between 28% and 38%, (Geddes & Miklowitz, 2013), it has been shown to have less of an effect with bipolar depressive symptoms (Davis et al., 2002). Lithium is associated with adverse events, including dangerous effects on the thyroid, cardiac abnormalities, and GI dysfunction, along with many others (Golan et al., 2011; Oruch et al, 2014). Furthermore, hyponatremia and concomitant treatment with NSAIDs can lead to acute lithium toxicity, which includes symptoms of tremor, ataxia, dysarthria, renal insufficiency, confusion, delirium, neuromuscular dysfunction, and seizures (Golan et al., 2011; Oruch et al, 2014).

Another effective treatment has been valproate or divalproex, which was initially marketed as an antiepileptic. Divalproex acts to slow down sodium channel recovery from an inactivated state after an action potential as well as to limit activity of T-type calcium channels. Finally, divalproex has been shown to increase availability of GABA within neurons, both through decreased degradation and increased synthesis (Golan et al., 2011). Divalproex has been shown to be effective for acute manic and psychotic symptoms of bipolar and may be more effective for depressive symptoms than lithium (Davis et al., 2002).

The third major drug used in treatment of bipolar is carbamazepine, another antiepileptic that also slows sodium channel recovery from an inactive state. Carbamazepine has been shown to be more effective than placebo and about as effective as lithium. Lamotrigine is another antiepileptic that has similar mechanism of action as carbamazepine, but there is little evidence of its efficacy in acute mania (Geddes & Miklowitz, 2013); lamotrigine is more commonly used in maintenance therapy of BPD with prominent depressive symptoms (Reid, Gitlin, & Altshuler, 2013). It is believed that antiepileptics (divalproex, carbamazepine and lamotrigine) may help restore the balance between glutamate and GABA inputs, thereby decreasing the postulated overactivity in the amygdala (Blond et al., 2012).

Recently, there has been evidence that antipsychotics, both FGAs and SGAs, have also been effective in treatment of acute mania (Geddes & Miklowitz, 2013; Golan et al., 2011; Oruch et al, 2014). Specifically, the FGAs most frequently used have been chlorpromazine and haloperidol, and olanzapine, risperidone, and quetiapine have been the effective SGAs used. Antipsychotics have been shown to have more frequent and more severe side effects in the long run, but have a faster onset of action, and therefore may have greater efficacy in acute mania, while lithium and other mainstay treatments take time to take effect (Geddes & Miklowitz, 2013; Golan et al., 2011).

In bipolar depression, the symptoms have been shown to be different from those seen in unipolar depression (like in MDD). This conclusion comes from the fact that antidepressants used to treat MDD have not been as effective, although there is definite heterogeneity (Geddes & Miklowitz, 2013). Combination treatments of antidepressant and antipsychotic (e.g., fluoxetine and olanzapine) have shown some positive effects (Geddes & Miklowitz, 2013). Recently, SGAs like quetiapine and lurasidone have been used with some positive benefits for bipolar depression (McIntyre, Cha, Kim, & Mansur, 2013). Lurasidone can be used in addition to the treatment of the manic symptoms (i.e., lithium or divalproex). Some of the drawbacks of these medications are the potential for weight gain and metabolic disruption (McIntyre, Cha, Kim, et al., 2013). Lamotrigine is also FDA approved for the treatment of bipolar depression (Vasquez, Holtzman, Tondo, & Baldessarini, 2015).

Anxiety Disorders

Anxiety disorders are mental disorders that are characterized by anxiety and fear. Anxiety is defined as the fearful behavioral response to a potential future threat and the uncertainty of the effects of the threat, whereas fear is related to the emotional response to current events. Anxiety disorders can be broken up into about six different major sub-categories; namely, panic disorders (PD), generalized anxiety disorders (GAD), social anxiety disorder (SAD), PTSD, OCD, and specific phobias. The 12-month prevalence of anxiety disorders in the United States is around 18%, with 12-month prevalence of each of the anxiety disorders as follows: PD (2.4%), GAD (2.0%), SAD (7.4%), PTSD (3.7%), OCD (1.2%), and specific phobias (12.1%) (Kessler, Chiu, Demler, Merikangas, & Walters, 2005; Kessler, Petukhova, Sampson, Zaslavsky, & Wittchen, 2012). Most of the anxiety disorders can present at childhood and continue to present into adulthood (American Psychiatric Association, 2013). Females are twice as likely to have anxiety disorders than males (American Psychiatric Association, 2013).

Each anxiety disorder presents with its own unique list of cognitive impairments, but overall, the anxiety disorders present with impairments in executive function and verbal episodic memory (although GAD usually presents with very little overall impairment; see Millan et al., 2012). OCD mostly presents with executive dysfunction but also impairments in long- and short-term visual memory, and processing speed (Castaneda, Tuulio-Henriksson, Marttunen, Suvisaari, & Lonnqvist; Millan et al., 2012). Similarly, PTSD presents with short- and long-term verbal and visual memory impairment and executive dysfunction. However, PD, while presenting with processing speed impairment, executive dysfunction, and issues with divided attention (but not selective attention), only presents with short-term verbal memory impairment, and without any visual memory impairment (Castaneda et al., 2008). It is interesting to note that most of the anxiety disorders (i.e., PTSD, OCD, and PD) actually have improvement in attention, mostly due to their increased vigilance (Millan et al., 2012).

While each of the individual anxiety disorders have their own unique neural correlates, most of them center around the amygdala–PFC circuitry (Martin, Ressler, Binder, & Nemeroff, 2009; Mohler, 2012). While the amygdala is associated with detection of threat and gives rise to the emotion of fear, the PFC controls the amygdala in top-down manner. Most studies of anxiety have shown that there is hyperreactivity in the amygdala to stimuli and hypoactivity in the PFC. Specifically within the PFC, the orbitofrontal cortex and the medial PFC have been associated with the assessment and integration of stimuli (Mohler, 2012). Unlike MDD, where there is also hyperactivity of the amygdala, this increased activity results only when provoked by environmental stimuli that are considered neutral by those not suffering from the anxiety disorders (Martin et al., 2009).

The hyperactivity in the amygdala and hypoactivity in the PFC are most likely due to decreased inhibition of the fear circuitry due to dysfunction of the GABAergic system. GABA (γ-aminobutyric acid) is the main inhibitory neurotransmitter in the central nervous system (CNS). There are two types of GABA receptors: Type A and Type C, both of which are ligand-gated ion channel (although $GABA_A$ is the main one found in the CNS), and Type B, a metabotropic G-protein coupled receptor. Deficits in the number of $GABA_A$ receptors have been found in various anxiety disorders such as PTSD, and have been correlated with anxiety symptoms (Mohler, 2012).

One main class of medications used to treat this impaired inhibition of the fear circuitry has been the benzodiazepines, which act to enhance the GABA transmission in the CNS (Davis et al., 2002; Golan et al., 2011; Griebel & Holmes, 2013; Mohler, 2012). Benzodiazepines—such as diazapem, alprazolam, lorazepam, and clorazepate—have mainly anxiolytic, sedative, hypnotic, amnestic, and muscle-relaxant effects. Their main mechanism of action is to bind to $GABA_A$ receptors and to increase the chance of the channel being open at low GABA concentrations as well as slowing down the receptor deactivation (Golan et al., 2011). There is also evidence that benzodiazepines increase the affinity of GABA to the receptor. Benzodiazepines range in their duration of action from short-acting (e.g., three to eight hours for clorazepate) to long-acting (e.g., one to three days for diazepam). Nonetheless, while benzodiazepines are effective in the treatment of anxiety, they are limited by their potential for tolerance, dependence, and addiction, and are therefore best used intermittently (Golan et al., 2011; Griebel & Holmes, 2013; Mohler, 2012). The tolerance is believed to be either due to decreased expression of the $GABA_A$ receptor at the synapse or due to the uncoupling of the binding site of the benzodiazepines from the GABA site (Golan et al., 2011). Furthermore, they should not be used concomitantly with other sedatives like alcohol, CNS depressants, opioid analgesics, and TCAs, due to the possible synergistic effect on the $GABA_A$ receptor (Golan et al., 2011). Benzodiazepines should be tapered slowly due to potential for a withdrawal syndrome that includes symptoms of confusion, seizures, anxiety, agitation, and insomnia (Davis et al., 2002; Golan et al., 2011).

SSRIs like sertraline, paroxetine, and fluvoxamine have also been shown to be efficacious in treating anxiety disorders. See the "Depression" section for a description of SSRIs. SSRIs have been prescribed more for long-term treatment as their initial anxiogenic effects can be somewhat problematic, while their long-term adverse effects are more tolerable than other classes (although they include sexual dysfunction and weight gain; see Davis et al., 2002). Serotonergic fibers from the raphe nucleus are believed to modulate both the GABA interneurons that modulate the fear circuitry and the neurons within the lateral amygdala.

Tricyclic antidepressants like imipramine and clomipramine have also been shown to be effective, most likely due to their serotoninergic effects, although they have the same list of adverse events as discussed with MDD. Similarly, MAO inhibitors like moclobemide have similar effects but are only used after other classes are found to be ineffective due to MAO-I's poor drug–drug and food interactions.

Buspirone is a nonbenzodiazepine anxiolytic that is an agonist at the $5\text{-}HT_{1A}$ receptor and has nonaddictive and nonsedative properties that make it more attractive than benzodiazepines (Golan et al., 2011). Buspirone, however, has been found to be most useful for GAD and not as helpful for other anxiety disorders like PD and OCD (Griebel & Holmes, 2013).

Glutamatergic signaling has also been implicated in various anxiety disorders. Glutamate, another amino acid neurotransmitter (like GABA), is critical in associative learning as seen with the hippocampus and amygdala association during fear learning (Griebel & Holmes, 2013; Martin et al., 2009; Mathew, Price, & Charney, 2008). As with GABA, there are ionotropic and metabotropic glutamate receptors. Ionotropic receptors include AMPA, NMDA, and kainate, the first two of which are implicated in associative learning during long-term potentiation and long-term depression (Davis et al., 2002; Purves et al., 2007). It has been hypothesized that there is elevated glutamatergic signaling, allowing for easier association of anxious and fearful response to neutral stimuli (Davis et al., 2002; Martin et al., 2009; Mathew et al., 2008).

Finally, other drugs used to treat disorders like bipolar and depression, including pregabablin and gabapentin, have found some off-label use in treatment of some of the anxiety disorders (see previous sections on BPD and MDD for descriptions) (Frampton, 2014).

Attention Deficit/Hyperactivity Disorder

Attention deficit/hyperactivity disorder (ADHD) is characterized by symptoms of poor impulse control, impaired attention regulation, excessive motor activity, and restlessness. The DSM-5 lists nine symptoms of inattention and nine symptoms of hyperactivity/impulsivity. It divides ADHD into three Presentations: Predominantly Inattentive (those with at least six of the former group of symptoms), Predominantly Hyperactive/Impulsive (those with at least six of the latter group of symptoms), and Combined (with at least six in both groups of symptoms for patients under the age of 17 years; the required symptom threshold is five and not six symptoms for patients 17 and older; see the American Psychiatric Association, 2013). ADHD is considered a childhood and adult disorder, though at least some of the symptoms must present by the age of 12. Significant impairment must be noted in two out of three domains (work/school, home, and/or social). Additionally, the childhood symptoms must be multidimensional and the symptoms and impairments must be from ADHD and not another mental health disorder (Adler & Alperin, 2014). Studies have shown that as many as 60% of adolescents continue to have symptoms of ADHD into their adulthood (Floet, Scheiner, & Grossman, 2010). Prevalence of the disorder range from about 6%–9% in childhood to about 4.4% in adults (Faraone, Sergeant, Billberg, & Biederman, 2003; Kessler et al., 2003). While boys are much more likely to have the disorder during childhood, the ratios even out within the adult population (Floet, Scheiner, & Grossman 2010; Kessler et al., 2003). ADHD commonly presents comorbidly with other disorders including conduct disorder, BPD, anxiety disorders, and depression.

Cognitive impairments in ADHD are not limited to issues with attention. ADHD also leads to impairment in working memory and processing speed (Millan et al., 2012). ADHD commonly cotravels with deficits in executive function and with difficulties in organization, planning, initiating, and completing tasks, shifting tasks, self-monitoring and self-inhibition (Barkley & Murphy, 2010; Brown, 2013).

The PFC is involved in regulation of attention and thought, and is therefore implicated in ADHD. Specifically, the dorsal and lateral PFC help to monitor attention and activity; while the ventral (orbital) and medial structures monitor emotion (Arnsten & Berridge, 2014). Furthermore, the PFC has many connections with the temporal and parietal cortices and therefore is involved in behaviors initiated in those loci (Arnsten & Berridge, 2014). The PFC has also been implicated in inhibition of inappropriate behaviors, and especially in the right hemisphere (Arnsten & Berridge, 2014). There are two neurotransmitters that play an important role in the PFC: the adrenergic and the dopaminergic system (Arnsten & Berridge, 2014; Golan et al., 2011). Of note, all marketed medications for ADHD have been shown to mediate their effects through these two neurotransmitters. Within the PFC, norepinephrine has a high affinity for the α_2 receptors, and dopamine binds to the two main receptors found in the PFC, D1, and D5 (Arnsten & Berridge, 2014). The dopaminergic system is believed to be involved in weakening and suppressing irrelevant signals, while the adrenergic system may help enhance and strengthen behaviorally appropriate systems. Not only have studies shown that the PFC in ADHD subjects is reduced, but also that is has reduced functional activity, most likely due to decreased signaling from these two systems (Arnsten & Berridge, 2014; Davis et al., 2002).

Therefore, pharmacological treatment of ADHD generally aims to enhance or mimic catecholaminergic signaling, specifically within the PFC. The medications fall into three categories: stimulants, nonstimulants, and atypical. The stimulants can be further broken into two main groups: methylphenidate and amphetamine. Stimulants block dopamine and norepinephrine reuptake into presynaptic neurons (Arnsten & Berridge, 2014; Davis et al., 2002; Golan et al., 2011). Unlike amphetamine, methylphenidate increases the release of dopamine (and norepinephrine at higher doses) from the presynaptic neuron (Arnsten & Berridge, 2014; Davis et al., 2002; Prince, Morrison, & Wilens, 2014). Although some stimulants also have an inhibitory effect on serotonin reuptake, this is not thought to play a major role mediating their therapeutic effect (Arnsten & Berridge, 2014; Prince et al., 2014). Furthermore, the effect on symptoms is generally thought to be a result of stimulant effect on catecholamines, specifically within the PFC and not outside the PFC (Arnsten & Berridge, 2014; Prince et al., 2014). Stimulants come in a variety of different formulations, from immediate-release to sustained and extended-release. There are four extended release stimulants that are FDA approved for adults with ADHD: two methylphenidate (dexmethylphenidate XR, OROS methylphenidate) and two amphetamine (mixed amphetamine salts XR and lisdexamfetamine) preparations. Potential side effects include nausea, difficulty falling asleep, anorexia, obsessiveness, headaches, dry mouth, rebound phenomena, anxiety, nightmares, dizziness, irritability, dysphoria, and weight loss (Prince et al., 2014). There is also misuse and diversion of stimulants, which appears to be greater with the immediate-release preparations (Prince et al., 2014), further highlighting the preference for treatment with extended-release preparations.

The main nonstimulant medication is atomoxetine, which acts as a selective norepinephrine reuptake inhibitor. Although it has no direct effect on dopamine transporters, it is believed that there is some effect on dopamine concentration within the synapse, since NET channels have increased affinity or dopamine, especially in the PFC, which has limited density of DAT channels (Arnsten & Berridge, 2014; Swanson et al., 2006). Atomoxetine may be particularly useful with adults with substance abuse issues (a common comorbid disorder) due to its lack of abuse liability (Prince et al., 2014). The overall magnitude of effect of atomoxetine is less than seen with stimulants (Prince et al., 2014). Both stimulants and atomoxetine can have cardiovascular effects, with modest elevations of blood pressure and pulse, suggesting the need to monitor these measures during treatment.

Other categories of effective medications that have been shown to be effective in off-label studies in adults with ADHD (and generally have not been extensively studied, as stimulants or atomoxetine) include antidepressants (specifically TCAs and bupropion) and the adrenergic agonists (specifically α_2) (Davis et al., 2002).

References

Adler, L. A., & Alperin, S. (2014). Diagnosing ADHD in adults in the primary care setting. In R. A. Barkley (Ed.), *Attention-Deficit Hyperactivity Disorder: A Handbook for Diagnosis and Treatment* (pp. 501—511). New York: Guilford Press.

Adler, L. A., Angrist, B., Reiter, S., & Rotrosen, J. (1989). Neuroleptic-induced akathisia: A review. *Psychopharmacology*, *97*(1), 1–11.

American Psychiatric Association. (2013). *Diagnostic and Statistical Manual of Mental Disorders* (5th ed.). Arlington, VA: American Psychiatric Publishing.

Arnsten, A. F., & Berridge, C. W. (2014). Catecholamine influences on the PFC. In L. A. Adler, T. J. Spencer, & T. E. Wilens (Eds.), *Attention-Deficit Hyperactivity Disorder in Adults and Children* (pp. 161–173). Cambridge: Cambridge University Press.

Barkley, R. A., & Murphy, K. R. (2010). Impairment in occupational functioning and adult ADHD: The predictive utility of executive function (EF) ratings versus EF tests. *Archives of Clinical Neuropsychology*, *25*(3), 157–173.

Belmaker, R. H., & Agam, G. (2008). Major depressive disorder. *New England Journal of Medicine*, *358*(1), 55–68. doi: 10.1056/NEJMra073096

Blond, B. N., Fredericks, C. A., & Blumberg, H. P. (2012). Functional neuroanatomy of bipolar disorder: Structure, function, and connectivity in an amygdala-anterior paralimbic neural system. *Bipolar Disorders*, *14*(4), 340–355. doi: 10.1111/j.1399-5618.2012.01015.x

Brown, T. E. (2013). *A New Understanding of ADHD in Children and Adults: Executive Function Impairments*. New York: Routledge.

Cahill, K., Stevens, S., Perera, R., & Lancaster, T. (2013). Pharmacological interventions for smoking cessation: An overview and network meta-analysis. *Cochrane Database of Systematic Reviews*, *5*, Cd009329. doi: 10.1002/14651858.CD009329.pub2

Carroll, F. I., Blough, B. E., Mascarella, S. W., Navarro, H. A., Lukas, R. J., & Damaj, M. I. (2014). Bupropion and bupropion analogs as treatments for CNS disorders. *Advances in Pharmacology*, *69*, 177–216. doi: 10.1016/b978-0-12-420118-7.00005-6

Castaneda, A. E., Tuulio-Henriksson, A., Marttunen, M., Suvisaari, J., & Lonnqvist, J. (2008). A review on cognitive impairments in depressive and anxiety disorders with a focus on young adults. *Journal of Affective Disorders*, *106*(1–2), 1–27. doi: 10.1016/j.jad.2007.06.006

Connolly, K. R., & Thase, M. E. (2011). The clinical management of bipolar disorder: A review of evidence-based guidelines. *Primary Care Companion CNS Disorders*, *13*(4). doi: 10.4088/PCC.10r01097

Davis, K. L., Charney, D., Coyle, J. T., & Nemeroff, C. (Eds.). (2002). *Neuropsychopharmacology: The Fifth Generation of Progress*. Philadelphia, PA: Lippincott Williams & Wilkins.

Ellenbroek, B. A. (2012). Psychopharmacological treatment of schizophrenia: What do we have, and what could we get? *Neuropharmacology*, *62*(3), 1371–1380. doi: 10.1016/j.neuropharm.2011.03.013

Fagiolini, A., Comandini, A., Catena Dell'Osso, M., & Kasper, S. (2012). Rediscovering trazodone for the treatment of major depressive disorder. *CNS Drugs*, *26*(12), 1033–1049. doi: 10.1007/s40263-012-0010-5

Faraone, S. V., Sergeant, J., Billberg, C., & Biederman, J. (2003). The worldwide prevalence of ADHD: Is it an American condition? *World Psychiatry*, *2*(2), 104–113.

Ferrari, A. J., Somerville, A. J., Baxter, A. J., Norman, R., Patten, S. B., Vos, T., & Whiteford, H. A. (2013). Global variation in the prevalence and incidence of major depressive disorder: a systematic review of the epidemiological literature. *Psychological Medicine*, *43*(3), 471–481. doi: 10.1017/S0033291712001511.

Floet, A. M., Scheiner, C., & Grossman, L. (2010). Attention-deficit/hyperactivity disorder. *Pediatrics in Review*, *31*(2), 56–69. doi: 10.1542/pir.31-2-56

Frampton, J. E. (2014). Pregabalin: A review of its use in adults with generalized anxiety disorder. *CNS Drugs*, *28*(9), 835–854. doi: 10.1007/s40263-014-0192-0

Geddes, J. R., & Miklowitz, D. J. (2013). Treatment of bipolar disorder. *Lancet*, *381*(9878), 1672–1682. doi: 10.1016/s0140-6736(13)60857-0

Glassman, A. H. (1984). Cardiovascular effects of tricyclic antidepressants. *Annual Review of Medicine*, *35*, 503–511. doi: 10.1146/annurev.me.35.020184.002443

Glassman, A. H., & Bigger, J. T., Jr. (1981). Cardiovascular effects of therapeutic doses of tricyclic antidepressants: A review. *Archives of General Psychiatry*, *38*(7), 815–820.

Golan, D. E., Tashjian, A. H., Armstrong, E. J., & Armstrong, A. W. (Eds.). (2011). *Principles of Pharmacology: The Pathophysiologic Basis of Drug Therapy* (3rd ed.). Philadelphia, PA: Lippincott Williams & Wilkins.

Griebel, G., & Holmes, A. (2013). 50 years of hurdles and hope in anxiolytic drug discovery. *Nature Reviews: Drug Discovery*, *12*(9), 667–687. doi: 10.1038/nrd4075

Hetrick, S. E., McKenzie, J. E., Cox, G. R., Simmons, M. B., & Merry, S. N. (2012). Newer generation antidepressants for depressive disorders in children and adolescents. *Cochrane Database of Systematic Reviews*, *11*, Cd004851. doi: 10.1002/14651858.CD004851.pub3

Kessler, R. C., Adler, L., Barkley, R., Biederman, J., Conners, C. K., Demler, O., . . . Howes, M. J. (2006). The prevalence and correlates of adult ADHD in the United States: Results from the National Comorbidity Survey Replication. *American Journal of Psychiatry*, *163*(4), 716–723.

Kessler, R. C., Berglund, P., Demler, O., Jin, R., Koretz, D., Merikangas, K. R., . . . Wang, P. S. (2003). The epidemiology of major depressive disorder: Results from the National Comorbidity Survey Replication (NCS-R). *JAMA*, *289*(23), 3095–3105. doi: 10.1001/jama.289.23.3095

Kessler, R. C., Chiu, W. T., Demler, O., Merikangas, K. R., & Walters, E. E. (2005). Prevalence, severity, and comorbidity of 12-month DSM-IV disorders in the National Comorbidity Survey Replication. *Archives of General Psychiatry*, *62*(6), 617–627. doi: 10.1001/archpsyc.62.6.617

Kessler, R. C., Petukhova, M., Sampson, N. A., Zaslavsky, A. M., & Wittchen, H. U. (2012). Twelve-month and lifetime prevalence and lifetime morbid risk of anxiety and mood disorders in the United States. *International Journal of Methods in Psychiatric Research*, *21*(3), 169–184. doi: 10.1002/mpr.1359

Krishnan, V., & Nestler, E. J. (2008). The molecular neurobiology of depression. *Nature*, *455*(7215), 894–902. doi: 10.1038/nature07455

Kupfer, D. J., Frank, E., & Phillips, M. L. (2012). Major depressive disorder: New clinical, neurobiological, and treatment perspectives. *Lancet*, *379*(9820), 1045–1055. doi: 10.1016/s0140-6736(11)60602-8

Lee, R. S., Hermens, D. F., Porter, M. A., & Redoblado-Hodge, M. A. (2012). A meta-analysis of cognitive deficits in first-episode major depressive disorder. *Journal of Affective Disorders*, *140*(2), 113–124. doi: 10.1016/j.jad.2011.10.023

Lepage, M., Bodnar, M., & Bowie, C. R. (2014). Neurocognition: Clinical and functional outcomes in schizophrenia. *Canadian Journal of Psychiatry/Revue Canadienne de Psychiatrie*, *59*(1), 5–12.

Malhi, G. S., Ivanovski, B., Hadzi-Pavlovic, D., Mitchell, P. B., Vieta, E., & Sachdev, P. (2007). Neuropsychological deficits and functional impairment in bipolar depression, hypomania and euthymia. *Bipolar Disorders*, *9*(1–2), 114–125. doi: 10.1111/j.1399-5618.2007.00324.x

Martin, E. I., Ressler, K. J., Binder, E., & Nemeroff, C. B. (2009). The neurobiology of anxiety disorders: Brain imaging, genetics, and psychoneuroendocrinology. *Psychiatric Clinics of North America*, *32*(3), 549–575. doi: 10.1016/j.psc.2009.05.004

Mathew, S. J., Price, R. B., & Charney, D. S. (2008). Recent advances in the neurobiology of anxiety disorders: Implications for novel therapeutics. *American Journal of Medical Genetics: Part C, Seminars in Medical Genetics*, *148c*(2), 89–98. doi: 10.1002/ajmg.c.30172

McIntyre, R. S., Cha, D. S., Kim, R. D., & Mansur, R. B. (2013). A review of FDA-approved treatment options in bipolar depression. *CNS Spectrums*, *18*(Suppl 1), 4–20; quiz 21. doi: 10.1017/s1092852913000746

McIntyre, R. S., Cha, D. S., Soczynska, J. K., Woldeyohannes, H. O., Gallaugher, L. A., Kudlow, P., . . . Baskaran, A. (2013). Cognitive deficits and functional outcomes in major depressive disorder: Determinants, substrates, and treatment interventions. *Depression and Anxiety*, *30*(6), 515–527. doi: 10.1002/da.22063

Miklowitz, D. J. (2011). Functional impairment, stress, and psychosocial intervention in bipolar disorder. *Current Psychiatry Reports*, *13*(6), 504–512. doi: 10.1007/s11920-011-0227-x

Millan, M. J., Agid, Y., Brune, M., Bullmore, E. T., Carter, C. S., Clayton, N. S., . . . Young, L. J. (2012). Cognitive dysfunction in psychiatric disorders: Characteristics, causes and the quest for improved therapy. *Nature Reviews: Drug Discovery*, *11*(2), 141–168. doi: 10.1038/nrd3628

Miyamoto, S., Miyake, N., Jarskog, L. F., Fleischhacker, W. W., & Lieberman, J. A. (2012). Pharmacological treatment of schizophrenia: A critical review of the pharmacology and clinical effects of current and future therapeutic agents. *Molecular Psychiatry*, *17*(12), 1206–1227. doi: 10.1038/mp.2012.47

Mohler, H. (2012). The GABA system in anxiety and depression and its therapeutic potential. *Neuropharmacology*, *62*(1), 42–53. doi: 10.1016/j.neuropharm.2011.08.040

Nierenberg, A. A., Adler, L. A., Peselow, E., Zornberg, G., & Rosenthal, M. (1994). Trazodone for antidepressant-associated insomnia. *American Journal of Psychiatry*, *151*(7), 1069–1072.

Oruch, R., Elderbi, M. A., Khattab, H. A., Pryme, I. F., & Lund, A. (2014). Lithium: A review of pharmacology, clinical uses, and toxicity. *European Journal of Pharmacology*, *740*, 464–473. doi: 10.1016/j.ejphar.2014.06.042

Prince, J. B., Morrison, N. R., & Wilens, T. E. (2014). Pharmacotherapy of ADHD in adults. In L. A. Adler, T. J. Spencer, & T. E. Wilens (Eds.), *Attention-Deficit Hyperactivity Disorder in Adults and Children* (pp. 276–297). Cambridge: Cambridge University Press.

Purves, D., Augustine, G. J., Fitzpatrick, D., Hall, W. C., LaMantia, A., McNamara, J. O., & White, L. E. (Eds.). (2007). *Neuroscience* (4th ed.). Sunderland, MA: Sinauer Associates, Inc.

Reid, J. G., Gitlin, M. J., & Altshuler, L. L. (2013). Lamotrigine in psychiatric disorders. *Journal of Clinical Psychiatry*, *74*(7), 675–684. doi: 10.4088/JCP.12r08046

Schaefer, J., Giangrande, E., Weinberger, D. R., & Dickinson, D. (2013). The global cognitive impairment in schizophrenia: Consistent over decades and around the world. *Schizophrenia Research*, *150*(1), 42–50. doi: 10.1016/j.schres.2013.07.009

Schultz, S. H., North, S. W., & Shields, C. G. (2007). Schizophrenia: A review. *American Family Physician*, *75*(12), 1821–1829.

Strakowski, S. M., Adler, C. M., Almeida, J., Altshuler, L. L., Blumberg, H. P., Chang, K. D., . . . Townsend, J. D. (2012). The functional neuroanatomy of bipolar disorder: A consensus model. *Bipolar Disorders*, *14*(4), 313–325. doi: 10.1111/j.1399-5618.2012.01022.x

Swanson, C. J., Perry, K. W., Koch-Krueger, S., Katner, J., Svensson, K. A., & Bymaster, F. P. (2006). Effect of the attention deficit/hyperactivity disorder drug atomoxetine on extracellular concentrations of norepinephrine and dopamine in several brain regions of the rat. *Neuropharmacology*, *50*(6), 755–760. doi: 10.1016/j.neuropharm.2005.11.022

Timonen, M., & Liukkonen, T. (2008). Management of depression in adults. *BMJ*, *336*(7641), 435–439. doi: 10.1136/bmj.39478.609097.BE

Trivedi, M. H., & Greer, T. L. (2014). Cognitive dysfunction in unipolar depression: Implications for treatment. *Journal of Affective Disorders*, *152–154*, 19–27. doi: 10.1016/j.jad.2013.09.012

Vázquez, G. H., Holtzman, J. N., Tondo, L., & Baldessarini, R. J. (2015). Efficacy and tolerability of treatments for bipolar depression. *Journal of Affective Disorders*, *183*, 258–262. doi: 10.1016/j.jad.2015.05.016

Author Index

Aaron, L. A. 829
Abbott, R. D. 296
Abrahams, B. S. 196
Abramovitch, A. 703–704
Abramowitz, J. S. 794
Adamo, M. 227
Adams, K. M. 890, 915
Adamson, G. J. 435
Adamson, L. B. 233
Adler, R. K. 794
Aggleton, J. P. 684
Aguerrevere, L. E. 989
Aguila-Puentes, G. 933
Ahern, D. K. 828
Ahles, T. A. 570–572
Airaksinen, E. 702, 704–705
Akaoka, F. 685
Akinwuntan, A. E. 608
Albert, M. L. 530
Albertsson, M. 571
Alcántara, C. 773
Aldridge, F. 189
Alegret, M. 516
Alessio, A. 452
Alexander, D. A. 643
Alexopoulos, A. V. 457
Alinaghizadeh, H. 571
Allen, L. 638
Allsup, D. 988
Alper, K. 508
Alpherts, W. C. 465
Alves, W. 663
Aman, C. J. 301
Amaral, D. G. 185, 208, 683
Amato, M. P. 607
Ambler, G. 935
Aminoff, S. R. 708
Amore, M. 705
Anastasi, A. 23–25
Anderson-Barnes, V. 804
Anderson, D. 828
Anderson-Roswall, L. 465
Anderson, R. M. 701
Anderson, C. 984
Anderson, S. 434
Andrés, S. 704
Andrews, K. 701
Andrews, B. 776
Andrews, T. L. 937
Anney, R. 197
Annis, S. M. 899
Antoniou, A. 637
Appenzeller, S. 633–634, 640–641
Applegate, K. L. 829
Arango-Lasprilla, J. 609
Arbisi, P. A. 24
Arciniegas, D. B. 434
Armengol, C. G. 502
Armstrong, C. L. 566
Armstrong, K. 19, 1071, 1074
Arnett, P. A. 611–612
Arnold, S. 456
Arts, B. 706
Ashendorf, L. 898
Ashkenazi, S. 295
Ashlton, V. L. 426
Ashwin, C. 234
Ashwin, E. 234
Asperger, H., 185
Atladottir, H. O. 202
Atlis, M. M. 24
Attix, D. K. 873, 944
Attwood, J. T. 633
Averill, P. M. 834
Awad, I. A. 25
Awad, M. 691
Axelrod, B. N. 933, 973
Azrin, R. 904
Azrin, S. T. 1011–1012

Baade, L. E. 47
Bachevalier, J. 685
Bachman, D. L. 46
Baciu, M. 451
Bacon, A. M. 293
Baer, L. 1055
Bagby, R. M. 994
Bailey, A. 205
Baird, G. 222
Bak, T. H. 535
Bakeman, R. 233
Baker, R. 933
Baker, R. R. 879
Baker, W. J. 890–891, 904, 929
Baldessarini, R. J. 708
Bales, R. 812
Ballard, C. G. 525
Bandini, L. G. 235
Banich, M. T., 301
Bansal, R. 304
Baranek, G. T. 233, 243
Barboriak, B. P. 638
Barghout, N. K. 47
Barker, A. A. 988
Barker, M. D. 389
Barkley, R. A. 287, 289
Barlow, D. H. 1012
Barnes, J. 296
Barnes, M. A. 296
Barnow, S. 827
Baron-Cohen, S. 191, 222, 230, 234, 236
Baron, I. S. 15
Barr, W. B. 663
Barsky, A. J. 828
Barth, J. T. 663
Bartolini, M. 640
Bartolucci, A. 899
Barton, M. L. 189, 232
Bartsch, H. H. 576, 1083
Barwick, F. H. 426
Bass, A. E. 1019
Basso, M. R. 973
Battaglia, M. 705
Bauman, M. L. 208
Bauman, R. A. 797
Baumeister, R. F. 896
Baune, B. T. 704, 707
Baxendale, S. 1083
Baxter, S. 868
Bazarian, J. J. 425
Beblo, T. 704
Bédard, M. 1061
Beebe, D. 19
Belanger, H. G. 426–428, 799
Belger, A. 243
Bellinger, D. 903
Bell, M. A. 98
Belmonte, M. K. 227
Bender, M. 7–8
Benedetti, F. 824, 827
Benedict, H. 623
Benedict, R.H.B. 604–606, 611
Bengner, T. 47
Bennett, H. 868
Bennetto, L. 230–231, 236–237
Ben-Porath, Y. S. 993
Benson, D. F. 1030
Benton, A. L. 30–31
Benton, A. 7, 14
Ben-Yishay, Y. 1050
Berch, D. B. 295
Berenson, K. 828
Berger, H. 294

Berkson, G. 233
Berlin, R. 282
Bernardin, L. 604
Berninger, V. W. 293, 296
Bernstein, I. H. 22
Berry, L. A. 834
Berthelson, L. 41
Bertone, A. 234–235
Bhagwat, A. 804
Bhan, V. 611
Bianchini, K. 933
Bianchini, K. J. 28, 985, 989
Bian, X. 797
Bidwell, L. C., 301
Bieliauskas, L. A. 14–15
Bigham, S. 229
Bigler, E. D. 498
Biglia, N. 571
Bigos, S. J. 829
Bilder, R. M. 1016
Biley, F. C. 1027
Bilo, L. 457
Binder, D. K. 465
Binder, L. M. 34, 428, 916, 928–929, 931
Biondolillo, A. M. 46, 988–989
Birch, S. 292
Bisarya, D. 191
Bjuhr, H. 1061
Black, L. 225
Blake, R. 234
Blatter, D. D. 498
Blau, T. 916
Block, A. R. 829, 834–835
Bloomfield, D. 571
Blumenfeld, H. 456
Blumstein, S. 9
Boake, C. 420, 902
Bobes-Bascaran, M. T. 1015
Bogousslavsky, J. 685
Bolte, S. 234–235
Bombardier, C. 831
Bonelli, S. B. 461
Boone, K. B. 32, 40, 983, 987
Bora, E. 707
Borg, J. 411
Boringa, J. B. 607
Bortnik, K. E. 46
Bosma, I. 564
Boucher, J. 229, 235
Bouix, S. 418
Bowden, S. C. 1013–1015
Bower, J. H. 534
Bowers, D. 688
Bowler, D. M. 230–231
Bowler, R. M. 902
Boxer, O. 1016
Boyd, M. C. 987
Boyle, M. 828
Braak, H. 510
Braakman, H. M. 457
Brady, A. R. 935
Brandeis, D. 303
Branham, J. D. 932
Braun, M. 857
Brennan, A. 28
Brennan, E. 703
Brenner, L. A. 434
Breslau, N. 773, 776
Brewin, C. 758, 762, 765, 776
Brines, D. B. 973
Briquet, P. 846
Broca, P. 281, 1078
Brock, J. 235
Brodmann, K. 81
Brodsky, S. L. 911, 914, 955
Bromet, E. 776
Brooks, B. L. 426, 946–947
Brooks, L. 34, 847
Brooks, N. 399
Brothers, L. 244
Brown, C. C. 235
Brown, J. 828
Brown, M. C. 1068, 1071
Brown, M. W. 684
Brown, P. D. 561, 564
Brown, R. 1071
Brown, R. G. 514
Brown, R. J. 827, 890
Bruno-Golden, B. 866–868
Bruns, D. 835
Brusko, C. S. 1021
Bryant, R. A. 432, 766, 770, 777
Buckley, T. C. 783
Bucy, P. 4, 479
Buddin, R. 986, 991
Buddin, W. H. 47
Buelow, M. T. 295
Buitelaar, J. K. 204, 302
Burgess, D. C., 301
Burgess, P. 763
Burkett, B. G., 804
Burton, R. L. 46
Bush, B. A., 401
Bush, D. S. 887
Bush, G. W. 981–982, 1011
Bush, N. 981
Bush, S. S. 984, 1025, 1070
Busl, K. M. 495
Butcher, J. N. 24
Butler, R. W. 172–173, 1083
Butters, N. 1034
Butters, N. 9–10
Butterworth, B. 295
Buxbaum, J. D. 185
Byrnes, D. P. 685

Cahn, D. A. 1058
Caine, D. 496
Calamia, M. 23
Calhoun, S. L. 225
Calloway, J. 46
Caltagirone, C. 344
Campbell, D. T. 26
Campbell, R. 305
Campbell, S. 296
Canitano, R. 221
Canyock, E. M. 890
Cappa, S. F. 1082
Carbotte, R. M. 621, 626–628, 635
Cardoner, N. 210
Carey, M. E. 793
Carlomagno, S. 625
Carlson, G. A. 1057
Carlsten, H. 630
Carmody, J. 1055
Carone, D. 1025
Carone, D. A. 1019, 1070
Carpenter, P. A. 229
Carper, R. A. 211
Carroll, J. B. 27
Carson, K. A. 624
Carter, S. 1034
Carvell, S. 515
Casanova, M. F. 209
Casement, M. D. 773
Casey, B. J., 300
Casey, P. H. 207
Cassell, K. 625
Cassidy, J. D. 428
Castaneda, A. E. 704
Cataldo, M. G. 705
Catani, M. 211
Cattell, J. M. 4
Cauda, F. 211
Cautin, R. L. 1012
Centeno, M. 457
Cermak, L. 9–10
Cermak, L. S. 478
Cermak, S. A. 235
Cernak, I. 797
Chabris, C. F. 105
Chafetz, M. 46, 832
Chafetz, M. D. 985–990, 992
Chaix, Y. 306
Chalela, J. A. 498
Chambers, C. A. 591
Chamelian, L. 433
Chandler, F. 189
Chan, F. 455
Chapman, J. 639
Chapman, C. H. 562
Charcot, J.-M. 6
Charcot, J. M. 508
Chase, C. 292
Chatterjee, A. 688
Chee, M.W.L. 58
Chelune, G. 464–465
Chelune, G. J. 25, 915, 1008, 1013–1014
Chen, N. C. 591
Cherrier, M. M. 576
Cheung, Y. T. 160
Chiaravalloti, N. 609
Choi, H. 639
Christakou, A. 228
Christensen, S. 1058
Cicero 1080
Cicerone, K. D. 1082
Cirino, P. T. 294
Clark, A. W. 688
Clingerman, S. 927
Cody, H. A. 31
Coghill, D. 706
Cohen, J. 28
Cohen, L. 308, 859
Cohen, M. 305
Cohen, N. J. 690–691
Cohen, P. 828
Cohn, A. 987

Cole, J. 451
Coleman, G. 827
Coleman, K. 637
Coleman, R. 933
Colker, R. 981
Collins, B. 571–572
Collins, M. W. 661
Combs, D. 973
Comi, A. M. 203
Condes, F. 640–641
Condit, D. C. 890
Conejero-Goldberg, C. 1015
Conklin, H. M. 172
Connelly, V. 296
Connolly, D. A. 47
Constantinou, M. 898
Contant, C. F. 902
Cooper, B. A. 571
Copeland, D. R. 1083
Corkin, S. 690
Corn, B. W. 564
Correa, D. D. 565
Costallat, L. T. 640–641
Cotard, J. 281
Cote, P. 1020
Courchesne, E. 206, 208–209, 211, 227–228
Cousin, E. 451
Cousins, R. 515
Covey, T. J. 623
Cox, A. 222
Cox, A. W. 976
Coyle, J. T. 688
Crawford, J. R. 34
Creamer, M. 763
Crewe, N. M. 973
Cripe, L. I. 906
Cronbach, L. J. 22, 25
Crook, J. 831
Crosson, B. 690
Crowley, D. J. 204
Cuddy, L. L. 47
Cullum, C. M. 376
Cummings, J. L. 287
Curtin, C. 235
Curtis, K. L. 28
Cuthbert, B. N. 108
Czernecki, V. 514

Dallison, A. 458
Dalton, P. 1020
Damasio, A. R. 238
Das-Munshi, J. 1021
Davidson, R. J. 1057
Davidson, J.R.T. 777
Davies, A. D. 515
Davies, P. 1015
Davis, J. J. 41
Davis, M. K. 1051
Dawson, G. 185, 225, 235, 237
Dean, A. C. 42, 46–47
Debess, J. 572
de Dios, L.A.V. 707
Deelman, B. G. 890–891
Deer, T. R. 824
Dehaene, S. 308
Del Dotto, J. 685
Delis, D. C. 987
DeLong, M. R. 688
DeLuca, J. 609
Demakis, G. J. 878, 927
Demonet, J. F. 306
Denburg, N. L. 622, 626–628, 631, 635
Denckla, M. B. 292–293
Denney, R. L. 46, 965–968, 971
Dennis, M. 167
Deona, T. 219
Depp, C. A. 707
Depue, B. E. 301, 304
Descartes, R. 62, 76, 332–333, 336
Desoete, A. 295
Deutsch, G. 571
De Win, M.M.L. 593
Diamond, A. 95
Dichter, G. S. 243
Dickstein, D. P. 709
Dicks, W. 24
Diehl, J. J. 236–237
DiGiulio, D. V. 1019
Dikmen, S. S. 35, 394, 399, 909, 928–929
DiLalla, D. L. 219
Diller, L. 1050
Di Sarro, R. 705
Disorbio, J. M. 835
Dixon, L. 862
Doctor, J. N. 399
Dodd, M. J. 571
Dodrill, C. B. 915
Doehnert, M. 303
Dolan, R. J. 452
Donders, J. 933
Donders, J. 19
Dougherty, A. L. 794
Downes, J. J. 525
Drachman, D. A. 688
Drag, L. L. 423
Drake, E. B. 890
Drechsler, R. 303
Drislane, F. W. 308
Dritschel, B. 1085
Driver-Dunckley, E. 847
Drogin, E. Y. 975
Duffin, J. 47
Duff, K. 25, 46
Duffy, F. H. 204
Dukakis, M. 981
Dulay, M. F. 464
Duncan, J. S. 452
Dunham, K. J. 46
Durham, J. 916
Durston, S. 311
Dusky, M. 963
Dusoir, H. 685

Earnst, K. S. 32
Eccleston, C. 836–837
Ecklund-Johnson, E. 887, 1016
Eden, G. F. 307
Edge-Booth, H. 498
Edmed, S. L. 426
Edwards, R. R. 829
Eickhoff, S. B. 302
Eigsti, I. M. 235, 237
Eisenberg, D. 1032
Eisendrath, S. J. 1058
Elger, C. E. 461
Elhai, J. D. 781, 783
Elia, J. 299
Elklit, A. 771
Emmer, B. J. 642
Engeland, H. 234
Engelberts, N. H. 1082
English, L. T. 993
Engman, E. 465
Enright, J. 46
Ent, D. V. 311
Epstein, L. C. 643
Erickson, Erik 759
Erlanger, D. 423
Esmer, G. 1055
Estes, A. 225
Estevis, E. 973
Evans, J. J. 1085
Ewertz, M. 572

Fama, R. 516
Farchione, T. 933
Farewell, V. 624
Farmer, J. E. 225
Farr, S. 927
Fatemi, S. H. 202–203
Faubert, J. 234
Faust, D. 859, 866–867
Fazio, R. L. 971
Feinberg, T. E. 834
Fein, D. 185, 233, 235, 237–238
Fein, D. A. 235
Feinstein, A. 433, 612
Feldman, R. G. 530
Feldner, M. T. 890
Ference, T. 847
Ferrier, I. N. 706
Ferstl, R. 626–627
Fichera, S. 810
Fichtenberg, N. L. 30, 46, 424
Figley, C. 759–760
Figueiredo, P. 452
Filliter, J. H. 230
Fine, J. G. 232
Finn, S. E. 1068
Finton, M. J. 516
First, M. B. 778
Fischer, C. T. 1068
Fisher, C. M. 782
Fisher, S. E. 289
Fiske, D. W. 26
Fisk, J. D. 611
Fleissbach, K. 567
Fletcher, C. 703
Fletcher, H. M. 204
Fletcher, J. M. 296, 974
Foa, E. B. 781
Folkman, J. 984
Fombonne, E. 190, 205
Forsell, Y. 702
Foster, L. G. 233
Fox, D. D. 929
Fox, N. A. 98
Frakey, L. L. 295

Frances, A. 760–763, 767
Frank, J. 831–832
Franklin, C. L. 781
Franklin, G. 831
Franz, S. I. 4
Frazier, T. W. 709
Fredrickson, B. 830
Freed, D. M. 690
Freeman, R. Q. 516
Freeman, T. 804
Freimer, N. 107
Freitag, C. M. 234
French, L. M. 804
Freud, S. 62
Freyberger, H. J. 827
Friedman, M. 767
Friedman, M. J. 762
Froklage, F. E. 564
Frueh, B. C. 783
Frumkin, I. B. 966
Frye, V. H. 203
Fuchs, L. S. 296
Fulton-Kehoe, D. 831

Gabig, C. S. 238
Gade, A. 691
Gaffan, D. 684–685
Gaigg, S. B. 230–231
Galaburda, A. M. 305, 308
Galarneau, M. R. 794
Galen 62
Gale, S. D. 500
Gallasi, R. 705
Gall, F. J. 84
Ganguli, M. 762
Garb, A. S. 899
Garcy, P. D. 829
Gardiner, J. M. 230
Garnett, E. S. 635
Garretson, H. B. 228
Garske, J. P. 1051
Garthwaite, P. H. 34
Gary, H. E., Jr. 393
Gass, C. S. 849, 1068, 1071
Gatchel, R. J. 829, 835
Gatlin, R. 434
Gau, K. 827
Gault, C. B. 34
Gazzaniga, M. S. 336
Gehring, K. 569
Geisser, M. E. 830
Gelb, A. 6
Gelfand, A. N. 828
Gelfand, M. D. 828
Geller, E. 204
Gerber, E. 204
Gerstmann, J. 294
Gervais, R. O. 993
Geschwind, D. 185
Geschwind, D. H. 196
Geschwind, N. 9, 86, 305
Ghia, A. 568
Ghika-Schmid, F. 685
Gibbon, F. 237
Gibbs, V. 189
Gilbert, E. 707
Gill, B. 862
Gilman, S. 685
Ginsberg, M. D. 628
Gladman, D. D. 627, 632
Glass, A. 890
Glassmire, D. 987
Glenn, W. J. 993
Gnanalingham, K. K. 525
Goethe, K. E. 31
Goh, J.O.S. 58
Gola, T. 890
Goldberg, E. 871
Goldberg, M. C. 228
Goldberg, T. E., 1015
Goldman, H. H. 1011–1012
Goldstein, G. 225, 229, 231
Goldstein, G. W. 902
Goldstein, J. 230–231
Goldstein, K. 6–7, 10, 14, 1050
Gollomp, S. 515
Gomar, J. J. 1015
Gomez-Puerta, J. A. 639
Goodglass, H. 9–10
Goodlin-Jones, B. L. 225
Gordon, B. 643
Gordon, W. A. 929
Gorrindo, P. 234
Gorske, T. 1071–1073
Goscha, R. J. 1011
Gottlieb, M. C. 376
Gouider-Khouja, N. 534
Gould, J. 185, 232
Gouvier, W. D. 988
Grabe, H. J. 827
Graff-Radford, N. R. 516, 686, 693
Grafman, J. 47, 793
Graham, N. L. 535
Grant, W. 830
Gray, J. M. 1007
Gray, L. C. 1026
Gray, M. J. 781
Greenberg, D. A. 192
Green, C. 828
Greene, H. A. 31, 1015
Green, P. 993
Greer, D. M. 495
Gregoire, J. 295
Gregor, K. 890
Greiffenstein, M. 973–974
Greiffenstein, M. F. 857, 872, 881, 890–891, 899, 904, 915–917, 929
Greve, K. 933
Greve, K. W. 28, 989, 994
Grice, S. J. 230
Griffin, G.A.E. 987
Griffith, H. R. 31–32
Grigorenko, E. L. 304
Grisham, J. R. 701
Grisso, T. 965
Grosch, M. C. 376
Groscup, J. L. 897
Grosdemange, A. 710
Gross, D. 487
Grossman, M. 515
Gross, R. 201
Groswasser, Z. 502
Grote, C. L. 912
Grover, W. 204
Grubaugh, A. L. 783
Guiffre Meyer, D. 906
Guilmette, T. J. 975
Gunlogson, C. 236–237
Gunstad, J. 429, 805–806, 889, 1019
Guo, M. F. 495
Guo, S. S. 207
Gupta, V. B. 1037
Gurunathan, N. 191
Guskiewicz, K. M. 427, 667
Gutheil, T. G. 872
Guthrie, R. 432
Gutierrez des Ceballos, J. P. 796
Guyer, R. D. 829
Guze, S. B. 772
Gwin, J. T. 434
Gysland, S. M. 435

Haak, R. A. 705
Habif, U. 898
Hachulla, E. 639
Hackett, M. L. 1047
Hagan, L. D. 975
Hagen, K. B. 831
Hagerman, G. 890–891
Haggerty, N. 24
Haist, F. 227
Hala, S. 230
Haley, S. 759
Hall, H. 831
Halperin, J. M. 287
Halstead, W. 4–6
Hamberger, M. J. 451
Hamed, S. A. 641
Hameroff, S. 332
Hammeke, T. A. 665
Hammond, J. 994
Handley, S. J. 293
Hanks, R. A. 31, 1015
Hanley, J. R. 515
Hanlon, R. E. 423
Hanly, J. G. 624–629
Hannaford, P. C. 763
Hanna-Pladdy, B. 432
Hao, X. 304
Happé, F. 210, 244
Harbluck, J. 692
Harder, H. 566
Hardy, K. K. 173
Harmell, A. L. 707
Harrell, F. E., Jr. 934, 936
Harrell, L. E. 31, 899
Harris, E. 1001
Harris, I. 889
Harrower, M. 7–8
Hart, H. 304
Hart, T. 400
Hartman, D. E. 907–908
Harvey, P. D. 708
Hashimoto, T. 517
Haskins, E. C. 343
Hay, E. M. 625, 631
Hayden, M. E. 909
Haynes, R. B. 1007

Hay-smith, E. J. 426
Hazlett, H. C. 212
Hazrati, L. N. 433–434
Head, H. 6
Heaton, R. K. 32, 34–35, 933
Hebb, D. O. 4, 8
Hebben, N. 903
Hedayati, E. 571
Heilbronner, R. 904, 931
Heilbronner, R. L. 976
Heilman, K. M. 684, 688
Heinik, J. 899
Heinlein, R. A. 927
Heinzelmann, M. 802
Heirichs, R. J. 47
Hellweg, R. 47
Helmstaedter, C. 461, 1082–1083
Heltemes, K. J. 794
Helzer, J. E. 773
Henderson, A. M. 230
Henik, A. 295
Henriksen, T. B. 202
Henry, D. B. 709
Henschen, S. E. 294
Hepburn, S. 233
Herman, J. L. 770
Hermann, B. P. 455
Hermelink, K. 572
Hermens, D. F. 705
Heslenfeld, D. J. 302
Hess, A. K. 916
Hess, E. 984
Hessen, E. 416
Hetherington, R. 167
Hewitt, J. 1085
High, W. M., Jr. 393
Hill, A. B. 908
Hilsabeck, R. C. 47
Hilsabeck, R. 19
Hilverda, K. 564
Himanen, L. 416
Hinckley, J., Jr. 900, 968
Hines, R. 828
Hinkle, J. L. 430
Hinton, D. E. 775
Hippocrates 51, 62
Hirst, W. 692
Hiscock, C. K. 932
Hiscock, M. 235, 932
Hoare, R. D. 685
Hodge, S. E. 192
Hodges, J. R. 535
Hoeting, J. A. 935
Hoffman, H. 282
Hof, P. R. 185
Hoge, C. W. 423
Hogg-Johnson, S. 831
Holdnack, J. A. 33
Holland, S. K. 452
Holliday, S. 625
Holmes, G. 793
Holubkov, A. L. 909
Hölzel, B. K. 1056
Honarmand, K. 608–609, 612
Hopkins, R. O. 498–500
Hopwood, C. J. 994
Horner, M. D. 46
Horowitz, M. 759–760
Horton, K. D. 47
Hou, R. 426
Howe, L.L.S. 944
Howells, J. 234
Hsu, C. H. 850
Huang, C. W. 591
Huang, E. 204
Huber, B. T. 487
Huettel, S. A. 115
Hughes, C. P. 637
Huizinga, M. 628
Hulme, C. 292
Hulst, H. E. 610
Hultman, C. M. 191
Hunkin, N. M. 691
Hunsinger, M. 1055
Huppert, F. A. 690
Hurks, P. P. 946
Hurtig, H. I. 515
Huss, M. T. 897
Hutt, C. 231
Hyland, P. 771
Hynd, G. W. 305

Iao, L. S. 239
Ibanez, D. 632
Ikeda, S. 517
Imhof, K. 303
Ingram, K. K. 31
Ingram, M. V. 849
Innocenti, G. 219
Insel, T. R. 108
Ioannidis, J. P. 104
Ireland, M. 1034–1035
Irle, E. 688
Ivanov, I. 304
Ivers, H. 571
Iverson, G. 950
Iverson, G. L. 34, 424, 426, 802, 803, 904, 984, 986, 991, 1025, 1070

Jabben, N. 706
Jacobson, L. A. 1015
Jacobson, M. 637–638
Jacobson, N. S. 25
Jacot-Descombes, S. 208
Jahansham, M. 514
Jain, N. 1058
Jamieson, E. 828
Jane, J. J. 663
Jansen, C. E. 571
Jelenic, P. 234
Jelinek, M. 762
Jenkins, V. 571
Jenkins, V. E. 892
Jennings, D. 633
Jennings, E. 705
Jensen, A. B. 572
Jiang, J. 797
Johansson, M. 1061–1062
Johnson, D. J. 296
Johnson, D. 758–759
Johnson, G. 1027
Johnson-Greene, D. 847, 1002–1003
Johnson, J. L. 915–916
Johnson, S. A. 230
Joiner, R. 897
Jones, A. 849
Jones, A. M. 233
Jones, E.J.H. 765
Jones, G. N. 988
Jones, M. K. 1082
Jones, W. 217, 234
Joseph, M. F. 709
Judd, D. 1045

Kabat-Zinn, J. 1052, 1054–1057
Kadan-Lottick, N. S. 162
Kade, A. M. 707
Kagehiro, D. 888
Kahane, P. 451
Kakela, M. 291
Kamio, Y. 230–231, 237
Kanaya, T. 974
Kane, R. L. 29
Kanner, L. 184, 191, 204–205, 216–218, 226, 231
Kanne, S. M. 225
Kaplan, E. 9–10
Kaplan, E. E. 28–29
Kapur, K. 991
Kapur, N. 479, 679, 685, 691
Karam, E. G. 775
Karantzoulis, S. 46, 427
Kareken, D. 868
Kashdan, T. B. 781
Kasner, S. E. 498
Katai, S. 517
Katon, W. J. 828
Katz, I. R. 794
Kaufman, A. S. 973
Kaufmann, P. M. 857, 859, 871–873, 881, 887, 892, 903, 913, 916, 938, 960, 1016
Kausler, D. H. 973
Kay, G. G. 996
Kay, T. 421
Kazdin, A. E. 1012
Keane, T. M. 762
Keddache, M. 220
Keenan, K. 637
Kehrer, C. A. 898
Keita, L. 235
Kelley, E. 237–238
Kellison, I. L. 35
Kelly, J. P. 804, 991
Kelser, S. R. 173
Kemner, C. 234
Kemp, J. 1034
Kemper, K. J. 1035
Kemper, T. L. 208
Kenet, T. 234–235
Kennedy, D. P. 228
Kern, J. K. 233
Kerr, L. 1058
Kesler, S. R. 167, 498, 576
Kessler, R. C. 772–773, 776
Kibby, M. Y. 902
Kiloh, L. G. 704
Kilpatrick, D. 1056
Kilpatrick, D. G. 771

Kim, D. M. 639
Kimbrell, T. 804
Kinney, D. K. 204
Kinsbourne, M. 233, 235, 294
Kip, D. E. 426
Kirk, S. A. 283
Kirkwood, M. 19
Kissler, J. 47
Kjelgaard, M. M. 237
Klein, M. 564
Klein, P. 293
Klin, A. 217, 234
Klinger, L. G. 229, 237
Klinger, M. R. 229
Klonoff, P. S. 1045, 1050
Kluver, H. 4, 479
Knapp, S. 1001
Knopman, A. A. 457
Koenig, K. A. 610
Koffka, K. 7
Köhler, W. 8
Kolb, B. 458
Kolevzon, A. 201
Koltzenburg, M. 824
Komatsu, N. 635–636
Konrad, K. 302
Koontz, K. L. 295
Koorenhof, L. 1083
Korgeski, G. P. 890
Koriakin, T. 1015
Kosc, L. 294
Koshino, H. 231
Kotoulas, G. 637
Kouyanou, K. 1025
Koylu, B. 452
Krabbendam, L. 706
Kraepelin, E. 4
Kramer, F. 282
Kratz, A. L. 613
Kraus, J. 794
Kretzmer, T. 426, 799
Kreutzer, J. S. 929
Krishnan, C. 203
Kroger, A. 234
Krukowski, R. A. 890
Krull, K. R. 160
Krupp, L. B. 486
Kubu, C. S. 908
Kuder, G. F. 23
Kugelman, A. 1023, 1027
Kuhl, K.-P. 47
Kukull, W. A. 762
Kulisevksy, J. 527
Kunickas, R. 889
Kurita, H. 219
Kussmaul, A. 282
Kutner, K. C. 621–622, 640
Kuykendall, D. 826

Laasonen, M. 293
Laboni, A. 632
Lage, G. A. 1050
Lainhart, J. E. 220
Lamberty, G. J. 851
Lamme, V. A. 234
Lampropoulos, C. E. 639
Lane, R. D. 850
Lange, K. W. 534
Langenecker, S. A. 707
Langen, M. 243
Lange, R. T. 426, 804
Langlois, J. A. 804, 991
Lanting, S. 46
Lapteva, L. 628, 630
Large, M. M. 766
Larrabee, G. J. 30–32, 41, 428, 906–907, 929, 984–986
Larson, E. B. 426
Larsson, M. 702
Lashley, K. 4, 6, 84
Lattie, E. 847
Latzman, R. D. 1012
Laurence, J. A. 203
Law, P. A. 203
Lawrence, R. C. 1061
Leach, L. 28–29
Leader, G. 201
Leavitt, J. 688
Le Bas, J. F. 451
LeBlanc, J. M. 909
Lebovits, A. H. 834
LeCompte, D. C. 47
Lee, E. J. 455
Lee, H. K. 638, 1058
Leekam, S. R. 232, 239
Leen-Feldner, E. W. 890
Lee, R.S.C. 705–706
Lees-Haley, P. R. 24, 859, 889, 916–917, 993
Lehtinen, L. E. 282
Lencz, T. 105–106
Lengenfelder, J. 609
Leo, G. J. 604
Leon, G. R. 890
Lepisto, T. 235
Lerner-Poppen, L. 916
Lesniak-Karpiak, K. 915–916
Leung, N.T.Y. 1058
Levin, D. 499
Levine, S. Z. 191
Levin, H. S. 393, 902, 929
Levitsky, W. 305
Lewis-Fernández, R. 775
Lewis, P. R. 688
Lewy, A. 235
Lewy, F. 508
Lezak, M. 910, 915
Lezak, M. D. 390
Leznoff, A. 1021
Libby, S. J. 232
Lichtenberg, P. A. 879
Lichtenberger, E. O. 973
Lichtenstein, P. 191
Lifton, R. 759
Lilenfeld, S. O. 1012
Lilienfeld, S. 784
Lindauer, R.J.L. 770
Lindenberger, U. 96
Lin, D. J. 234
Lind, S. E. 230
Lin, R. 899
Linton, S. J. 827
Liss, M. 233
Little, P. 1024
Litvan, I. 535
Livingstone, M. S. 308
Livingston, R. B. 705
Llufriu, S. 610
Locke, D. E. 569, 850
Locke, J. 333–334
Lockyer, L. 219
Loesch, D. V. 685
Loeser, J. D. 823, 831
Lombardo, M. V. 230
Long, C. J. 902
Longley, W. A. 1071
Lönnqvist, J. 704
López-Jaramillo, C. 708
Loring, D. W. 28, 1013
Lorusso, M. L. 705
Lotter, V. 219
Lovell, M. R. 423, 661
Luborsky, L. 1069
Lucas, J. A. 15, 516
Lucas, M. 1071
Luchetti, A. 221
Luders, E. 1055–1056
Luders, H. 25
Luis, C. A. 425
Lunden, W. A. 811
Luria, A. R. 9, 294, 793, 1048
Lynn, S. J. 1012
Lyon, G. R. 296

Ma, C. G. 495
Mabbott, D. J. 172
McAllister, L. D. 567
McAllister, T. W. 435
McCabe, S. 868–869
McCaffrey, R. J. 898, 944
McCann, J. 237
MacCarthy, B. 514
McCauley, S. R. 420, 902
Macciocchi, S. 663
McClintock, S. M. 705
McCracken, L. M. 802
McCrea, M. 663
McCrea, M. A. 804, 991
McCune, W. J. 633
McDonald, B. C. 573
McDonald, W. I. 604
McDonough, J. 236–237
McFarland, M. 987
McFarlane, A. C. 763
McGovern, G. 981
McGrath, W. M. 204
MacGregor, A. J. 794
Machamer, J. E. 909, 928
McHugh, N. J. 1061
McHugh, R. K. 1012
McInnis, M. G. 707
McIntosh, G. 831
McInturff, B. 899
McKee, A. C. 433–434
McKee, R. D. 690
MacKenzie, J. 571

McKhann, G. 719
McKinsey, R. K. 894
McKinstry, S. 685
McKinzey, R. K. 914
McLachlan, D. 692
McLaurin, E. Y. 629
MacLean, M. 296
MacLean, P. D. 83
McLeod, G. 869
McMahon, S. 824
Macmillan, H. 828
McNally, R. 762–764
McNulty, J. L. 24
McSweeney, A. J. 25
Mahone, E. M. 135, 301, 1015
Mahone, M. 15
Mair, W.G.P. 685
Makowsky, M. 831
Maldjian, J. A. 498
Malina, A. C. 887, 1016
Malinow, K. L. 643
Malmgren, K. 465
Maly, P. 633
Manjaly, Z. M. 227
Mann, D. 685
Mannon, A. 201
Mann-Wrobel, M. 706
Marcotte, D. 890
Mar Fan, H. G. 572
Markon, K. 23
Marks, A. R. 47
Marsden, C. D. 514
Marshall, P. S. 41
Marson, D. C. 31, 899
Marten, J. T. 1021
Martin, C. R. 185
Martin, D. J. 1051
Martinez-Arán, A. 707–708
Martin, J. H. 1026
Martin, J. N. 1001
Martin, L. J. 220
Martino, D. J. 706–707
Marttunen, M. 704
Maruyama, T. 517
Marwaha, S. 707
Marwitz, J. 929
Mason-Brothers, A. 205
Mason, S. 1021–1022
Mataix-Cols, D. 210–211
Matthews, C. 706
Maurer, R. G. 238
Mausbach, B. T. 707
Mayer, T. G. 829
Mayes, A. 229
Mayes, A. R. 685, 691
Mayes, S. D. 225
May, R. 987
Mazerolle, E. L. 611
Meares, S. 424
Meehl, P. E. 25
Mehlsen, M. 572
Meier, M. J. 14
Meissner, C. 495
Melias, R. 937
Melnyk, A. 928–929
Melton, G. B. 965
Melzack, R. 823
Menci, E. 237
Mendel, G. 103
Merkes, M. 1055
Mesulam, M.-M. 688
Meudell, P. R. 685
Meunier, M. 685
Meyer, A. L. 487
Meyer, D. G. 701
Meyers, C. A. 561, 568
Miaskowski, C. A. 571
Micco, J. A. 705
Mickeviciene, D. 889
Milis, S. R. 1015
Miller, A. M. 204
Miller, J. B. 30
Miller, J. N. 185
Miller, J. R. 435
Miller, L. J. 41
Miller, L. S. 987
Millis, S. 871, 933
Millis, S. R. 30–31, 35, 41, 890, 929, 932–933, 935–936, 938
Millspas, C. 904
Milner, B. 8–9, 678, 681–682
Minshew, N. J. 225, 227, 229–231
Mishkin, M. 685
Mitchell, C. A. 1026
Mitchell, W. 905
Mittenberg, W. 41, 806, 890, 904, 931, 933, 1019
Miyazawqa, Y. 685
Moberg, P. J. 701, 857, 906
Modahl, C. 235
Moffitt, T. E. 701
Moldofsky, H. 831
Molloy, C. A. 220–222
Molteni, M. 705
Molyneux, W. 333–334
Monza, D. 534
Mooney, G. 428
Moore, I. M. 173
Morey, L. C. 993
Morgan, D. 46
Morgan, J. T. 203
Morgan, V. L. 458
Morgan, W. P. 281–282
Morioka, D. 747
Moritz, S. 703
Morley, S. 836
Morreale, A. 705
Morris, E. B. 161
Morris, M. K. 294, 688
Morris, R. 571
Morris, R. D. 294
Morrow, L. A. 908
Mortensen, E. L. 691
Moseley, J. B. 826
Mostow, A. J. 228
Mottron, L. 234–235
Moulds, M. 432
Moulthrop, M. 927
Moulthrop, M. A. 59, 916
Moura-Serra, J. 219
Moutsopoulos, H. M. 637
Moye, J. 879
Mrad, D. 963
Mulchan, S. S. 41
Mulford, J. 889
Mulick, J. A. 1034
Mumm, A. 1083
Muratori, F. 207
Murphy, K. R. 287, 289
Murrough, J. W. 304
Musielak, K. A. 232
Musso, M. W. 988–989
Myers, C. E. 693
Myklebust, H. R. 296

Nadel, L. 691
Nadimpalli, S. S. 709
Nagy, J. 928–929
Nahmias, C. 635
Najm, I. M. 457
Nakase-Richardson, R. 341, 390, 393
Nakase-Thompson, R. 390, 393
Naqibuddin, M. 624–626
Nascimbene, C. 203
Naugle, R. I. 25
Naville, F. 508
Needleman, H. L. 903
Nellaus, G. 207
Nelson, D. V. 834
Nelson, N. W. 701, 851, 906
Nestvold, K. 889
Nick, T. G. 393
Nicoll, D. 192
Nicosia, G. 760
Nielsen, K. H. 296
Nielssen, O. B. 766
Nies, K. 927
Nieto, C. 232
Nighingale, N., 222
Nissley, H. 1002–1003
Nixon, R. 981
Nixon, R. D. 432
Nobilex, M. 705
Noe, E. 525
Nordahl, C. W. 208
Normington, J. 987
Norris, F. H. 778
Nossent, J. C. 622, 640
Novack, T. 396, 401
Novitski, J. 46
Novy, D. M. 834
Nowak, M. 628
Nunnally, J. C. 22
Nyman, H. 571

O'Brien, A. 609
O'Connell, M. E. 46
O'Connor, M. M. 709
Odland, A. P. 41, 849
O'Donnell, M. L. 769
Oechmichen, M. 495
Ogloff, J. R. 888
O'Hare, A. 237
Ohnmeiss, D. D. 829
Okifuji, A. 836

Olley, J. G. 976
Olney, J. R. 831
Omalu, B. 433
Omisade, A. 624
O'Neil, K. M. 897
Oosterlaan, J. 302
Ord, J. 28
Ord, J. S. 989
Ore, G. D. 479
Orfei, M. D. 344
Ornitz, E. M. 231
Ortel, T. L. 638
Orth, H. B. 1083
O'Shea, A. G. 230
Overland, S. 832
Owen, A. M. 527
Owen-Smith, V. 763
Oyegbile, T. 455
Ozonoff, S. 185, 225, 229, 231–233, 235, 239

Pachana, N. A. 1071
Padilla-Medina, J. A. 234
Palmer, B. W. 707
Pancholi, S. 804
Paniak, C. 432, 902, 928–929
Papero, P. H. 626
Papez, J. 78
Pappas, S. 1037
Pardo, C. A. 203
Parisi, L. 610
Park, D. 58
Parker, A. 685
Parkinson, J. 508
Parner, E. T. 202
Parr, L. A. 220
Pascualvaca, D. M. 229
Passamonti, L. 614
Patel, V. B. 185
Patfield, M. 1018–1019
Patterson, W. 831
Patton, C. 890
Paulman, R. G. 909
Paul, R. 237
Paus, T. 96
Pavuluri, M. N. 709
Peck, C. L. 827
Peck, C. P. 47
Pedersen, A. D. 572
Peeden, J. N. 203
Pels, H. 567
Penfield, W. 7–8
Pennington, B. F. 230, 239, 301
Penrod, S. D. 897
Penrose, R. 332
Peppe, S. 237
Perlman, T. 1037
Perrin, J. M. 1035
Perrin, S. 1019
Peterson, B. S. 304
Petri, J. 624
Phelan, H. L. 230
Philips, L. 291
Phillips, K. 929
Pichat, C. 451
Pickering, A. 685
Piercy, M. 690
Pilgrim, S. 1071
Pillon, B. 534
Pinhasi-Vittorio, L. 1048
Pink, M. M. 435
Playfer, J. R. 515
Podell, K. 871
Polatin, P. B. 829
Pollnow, H. 282
Ponsford, J. 423, 425, 810, 929
Ponziani, G. 607
Poppelreuter, M. 576, 1083
Porter, M. A. 705
Posner, M. I. 1056, 1062
Postal, K. 1071, 1074
Poulton, R. 701
Pound, C. M. 162
Powell, M. 804
Pozdol, S. L. 234
Pransky, G. 831
Pratico, D. 984
Preedy, V. R. 185
Pribram, K. H. 332
Price, D. L. 688
Prigatano, G. P. 499
Pritchard, A. E. 1015
Privitera, M. D. 452
Proctor, B. 294
Provenzale, J. M. 638
Puente, A. 986
Putnam, S. H. 890, 915
Pyykkonen, B. A. 912

Quadfasel, F. 9
Quenzer, D. E. 831
Quesnel, C. 571
Quintana, J. W. 31

Radua, J. 210–211
Ramsay, G. 234
Randolph, C. 46, 427, 663
Randolph, J. K. 225
Ransom, M. T. 707
Rao, S. M. 604–607
Rapin, I. 219
Rapp, C. A. 1011
Rapport, L. J. 31, 973, 1015
Raskind, W. 296
Rasmussen, C. 230
Rawlings, D. B. 933, 973
Rayls, K. 933
Rayls, K. R. 810
Raznahan, A. 207
Reagan, R. 968, 981
Reber, M. 185
Redoblado-Hodge, M. A. 705
Reed, J. E. 914
Rehnquist, W. 861–862, 896
Reichenberg, A. 191, 201
Reis, M. 433
Reitan, R. 5–6, 14, 28
Relander, M. 431
Rendell, P. G. 609
Renner, P. 229
Resick, P. A. 770
Reynolds, S. 928–929
Rhodes, S. 706
Rhydderch, D. 234
Richardson, M. P. 452
Richardson, M. W. 23
Richardson, W. S. 1007
Richler, J. 191
Richmond, A. 869
Richmond, J. 869
Richmond, J. 868–870
Ricker, J. 933
Ricker, J. H. 933
Riis, J. O. 572
Rimel, R. 663
Rimland, B. 227–228, 231
Rippon, G. 235
Ristic, A. J. 457
Ritenbaugh, C. 850
Ritschel, L. A. 1012
Riva, D. 216
Rizzo, M. 38
Roberson, C. J. 848
Roberts, A. L. 775
Roberts, R. J. 301
Robins, D. L. 233
Robins, L. 759, 772
Robinson, L. J. 706
Robinson, R. G. 1024
Roche, A. F. 207
Rodrigues, C. E. 643
Roebuck-Spencer, T. M. 624
Rogers, R. 903, 994
Rogers, S. J. 219, 230–233, 235
Rohling, M. L. 428, 928–929, 931, 1082, 1084–1085
Roid, G. H. 988
Ronald, A. 244
Rosenbaum, J. G. 898
Rosenberger, L. R. 451
Rosenberg, W.M.C. 1007
Rosenblum, M. L. 685
Rosen, G. 782
Rosen, G. D. 308
Rosen, G. M. 762
Rosenhan, D. 52
Rosenthal, M. 929
Rose, S. 776
Rossell, S. L. 706
Ross, S. R. 890, 933
Rothbart, M. K. 93–94
Roth, R. S. 830
Roth, S. 771
Rourke, B. P. 294, 296
Rovee-Collier, C. 94, 98
Royston, P. 935
Rozensky, R. H. 1008
Rubin, G. J. 429
Rudel, R. G. 292
Rudman, N. 46–47
Rudnick, E. 170
Ruff, H. A. 93–94
Ruff, R. M. 423
Ruiz, M. A. 890
Russell, W. R. 390

Rutecki, P. 455
Rutherford, M. 237
Rutter, M. 185, 219
Ryan, C. 1068
Ryan, T. 663
Rzezak, P. 456

Sabatti, C. 107
Sabb, F. W. 105
Sackett, D. L. 931, 1007–1008
Sahgal, A. 684
Sahs, A. L. 777
Sailer, M. 635
Salas, C. E. 1045
Salva, G. N. 707
Samamé, C. 706–707
Samuelsson, H. 465
Sanchez-Marin, F. J. 234
Sanchez, P. N. 898
Sanders, J. F. 46
Sandin, S. 191
Sand, T. 889
Sanna, G. 628
Satel, S. 784
Saulnier, C. 233
Saunders, E.F.H. 707
Savard, J. 571
Savic, J. 797
Sawyer, T. P. 927
Sbordone, R. J. 909
Schacter, D. L. 692
Schagen, S. B. 571
Schain, R. J. 207–208
Schedin, A. 571
Scheerer, M. 6–7, 9–10
Schefft, B. K. 452
Schendel, D. E. 202
Schenkel, L. S. 709
Scherling, C. 571
Schieve, L. A. 201
Schindler, S. 47
Schmand, B. 890–891, 1015
Schmidt, D. 928
Schnebel, B. 434
Schneider, A. M. 915
Schneiderman, A. I. 800
Schoenberg, M. R. 1066
Schofferman, J. 828
Schofield, W. 1051
Scholte, H. S. 234
Schrader, H. 889
Schrag, A. 827, 890
Schreiber, S. 425
Schroeder, R. 987
Schroeder, R. W. 41, 47
Schuh, J. 237
Schulte, F. 174
Schultheis, M. T. 608
Schultz, R. T. 237
Schulz, K. P. 287
Schulz, M. S. 828
Schumann, C. M. 208, 212
Scott, I. A. 1026
Scott-Van Zeeland, A. A. 215
Scoville, W. B. 678, 681–682
Searle, J. R. 335–336
Sedlak, J. 25
Seel, R. T. 339
Segalàsk, C. 703
Seidenberg, M. 455
Sellbom, M. 849, 994
Selnes, O. A. 643
Semrud-Clikeman, M. 232
Sewell, K. 994
Shadi, S. 46
Shafritz, K. M. 243
Shaheen, S. 866
Shalev, R. S. 308
Shalit, R. 981
Shalom, D. B. 229
Shandera, A. L. 988
Shanker, S. 1045
Shapiro, D. L. 887
Shaskin, D. 508
Shatan, C. 758–760
Shaw, P. 304
Shaw, W. S. 831
Shaywitz, S. E. 307
Shedler, J. 1046
Shelven, M. 771
Sherer, M. 29, 341, 390, 393, 396, 401
Sherman, E. 950
Sherman, E.M.S. 33, 904, 950, 984, 986
Shilling, V. 571
Shimamura, A. P. 692–693
Shing, Y. L. 96
Shojania, K. G. 1007
Shucard, J. L. 623
Shute, C.C.D. 688
Siegert, R. G. 426
Sigurdardottir, S. 422, 425
Silverberg, N. D. 35, 46
Silver, J. M. 421
Siman, R. 432
Simpson, K. R. 1026
Singal, D. 627
Sinnamon, G. 704
Siracusa, G. 507
Sivan, A. B. 31
Skefos, J. 242
Slater, P. C. 691
Slick, D. J. 871, 904, 934, 950, 984, 986–987
Smith, A. 390, 571
Smith, A. M. 610–611
Smith, G. 828
Smith, K. 47, 189
Smith, N. 1083
Smith, S. 1068
Smith, S. A. 47
Smoski, M. J. 234
Snell, D. L. 426
Sniezek, J. E. 927–928
Snowling, M. J. 292
Soares, J. C. 709
Sofko, C. A. 46
Soklaridis, S. 1020
Solé, B. 708
Soliveri, P. 534
Solomon, M. 225, 889
So, N. 457
Song, J. X. 902
Sonnega, A. 776
Sorbi, S. 607
Sosin, D. M. 927–928
Sowinski, J. 192
Spalletta, G. 344
Spar, J. E. 899
Sperry, R. W. 336
Spiegler, B. J. 167
Spitzer, C. 827–828
Spitzer, R. 759, 761, 764, 768, 772
Spreen, O. 33, 296–297
Spring, B. 1011
Squire, L. R. 683, 690–693
Stanfield, A. C. 210
Stark, K. D. 705
Staunton, R. 236
Steele, C. M. 530
Steele, S. 46
Steens, S. C. 628
Steere, A. C. 487
Stefanatos, G. A. 204, 219, 221, 225, 287
Stegen, S. 623
Steinberg, B. A. 14
Steinhausen, H. 303
Stein, R. A. 1026
Stephenson, J. 1034
Stern, M. B. 515
Stern, R. A. 434
Stern, W. 9
Steup-Beekman, G. M. 628
Stevens, J. 984
Stevens, S. S. 22
Still, G. 282
Stogner, B. L. 929
Stoltenberg, C. 206
Stone, W. L. 234
Stonnington, C. M. 850
Stothers, M. 293
Stover, B. 831
Stovner, L. J. 889
Strange, B. A. 452
Strauss, A. A. 282
Strauss, E. 33
Strejilevich, S. A. 706–707
Strickland, T. L. 1026
Stringer, A. Y. 1079, 1082
Strober, L. B. 611–612
Stroup, E. 465
Struchen, M. A. 390
Stucky, Kirk 19
Studebaker, C. A. 897
Stuss, D. T. 341, 344, 393
Suchy, Y. 857
Suh, J. 238, 639
Suhr, J. A. 429, 806, 889, 916, 1019
Sullivan, K. A. 426
Summerfield, D. 776
Sumowski, J. F. 609
Sundgren, P. C. 633
Sundstrom, A. 433
Suren, P. 206
Surgenor, L. J. 426
Surkiene, D. 889

Surma-aho, O. 565
Sutton, B. P. 58
Suvisaari, J. 704
Suzuki, W. A. 683
Swanson, H. L. 293
Sweeney, J. A. 709
Sweetet, J. C. 435
Sweettenham, J. 222
Sweet, J. J. 59, 701, 857–859, 887, 903, 906, 915–916, 927, 1016
Sypert, G. W. 684
Szaflarski, J. P. 452

Taber, K. H. 797–798
Tager, F. A. 572
Tager-Flusberg, H. 237
Talland, G. 693
Tanaka, Y. 685
Tang, C. 1056, 1062
Tanner, J. M. 207
Tarazi, R. 135
Tarescavage, A. M. 993
Tarkowski, A. 630
Tasca, G. A. 571
Tate, D. G. 831
Tate, R. 1071
Tate, R. L. 394
Taylor, J. S. 858
Taylor, M. J. 306
Teichner, G. 987
Tektonidou, M. G. 637–639
Temkin, N. 928
Temkin, N. R. 909
Terrell, T. R. 433
Terzian, H. 479
Teuber, H. L. 7–8
Thakkar, K. N. 243
Tharinger, D. J. 1071
Theisen, M. E. 973
Theroux Fichera, S. 931
Theroux, S. 933
Thompson, E. 933
Thompson, P. 1083
Thornburgh, D. 982
Thurman, D. J. 927–928
Thurstone, L. L. 5
Tiersky, L. A. 811
Tietjen, G. E. 637
Toichi, M. 230–231
Toller-Lobe, G. 928–929
Tomietto, P. 626, 629
Toren, P. 702
Torrent, C. 708
Townes, B. D. 898
Townsend, J. 227
Tracey, I. 824
Trahan, D. E. 31
Tranel, D. 23
Tremont, G. 810
Trief, P. M. 830
Tremblay, S. 427
Trimble, M. R. 827, 890
Tröster, A. I. 540
Troupin, A. S. 915
Truax, P. 25
Trysberg, E. 630
Turegano Fuentes, F. 796
Turk, D. C. 824
Turnbull, C. J. 515
Turnbull, O. H. 1045
Turnbull, S. J. 801
Turner, C. A. 225
Turner, J. 832
Turner, J. A. 829, 831
Turner, L. M. 234
Tuulio-Henriksson, A. 704
Tyson, K. 238

Uitti, R. J. 516
Underhill, J. 832, 987, 992
Universagt, F. 604
Unterman, A. 619
Urbina, S. 23–25
Urowitz, M. B. 632

Vaessen, M J. 457
Valencia-Flores, M. 632
Valentine, J. D. 776
van Buchem, M. A. 628
VandeCreek, L. 1001
Vandenbroucke, M. W. 234
Vanderploeg, R. D. 426–427
van Ewijk, H. 302
van Gelder, J. M. 889
van Gorp, W. G. 890
Vanharanta, H. 829
Van Hoesen, G. W. 688
van Hout, M. S. 890–891
Van Koevering, D. 831
Vannest, J. 452
van Os, J. 706
Van Rheenen, T. E. 706
Vargas, D. L. 203
Varney, N. R. 908
Varsou, N. 637
Vasterling, J. J. 424
Vaughan, F. L. 1045
Vearncombe, K. J. 571
Vesalius 62
Via, E. 210–211
Victor, M. 684
Victor, T. L. 40–41
Vohringer, P. A. 706
Volinn, E. 831
Volinsky, C. T. 932, 935–936, 938
Volk, C. 643
Volkmar, F. R. 185, 220
Volpe, B. T. 692
Von Ah, D. 576
Voudouris, N. J. 827
Vulpian, A. 508
Vygotsky, L. 9

Wagner, K. 454
Waid, R. 987
Waldinger, R. I. 828
Walker, E. A. 828
Wallace, D. J. 624
Waller, D. 976
Walsh, C. A. 828
Wang, Z. 458, 797
Ward, A. J. 204
Warden, D. L. 797–798
Warrington, E. K. 294, 685
Wasserstein, J. 287, 293
Waterhouse, L. 232, 235, 635–636
Waterloo, D. 625, 627
Watson, D. 236–237
Watson, J. D. 496
Weathers, F. W. 762
Weaver, L. K. 500
Wefel, J. S. 570–572
Wegiel, J. 208
Wehner, E. 233
Weis, J. 576, 1083
Weiskrantz, L. 685
Weiss, G. L. 287
Weiss, L. G. 33, 975
Wekking, E. M. 890–891
Welzel, G. 568
Werner, P. 899
Wernicke, K. 6
Wertheimer, J. C. 46
Westerfield, M. 227
Westerveld, M. 15
Wetter, S. R. 987
Wheelwright, S. 191
White, A. 828
Whitehouse, P. J. 688
Whitely, G. 804
Whittaker, R. 426
Wholihan, K. 207
Wickizer, T. M. 831–832
Widiger, T. 762
Wiggins, L. D. 233
Wijsman, E. M. 296
Wilke, M. 451
Willcut, E. G. 301
Williams, A. C. 836
Williams, D. L. 229, 231
Williams, M. 762
Williams, M. W. 31, 1015
Willingham, A. C. 31
Willis, A. L. 530
Wilson, J. S. 987
Wilson, K. 204
Wilson, R. 967
Wilson, S. L. 1045
Wing, L. 185, 232
Wingo, A. P. 708
Wingo, T. S. 708
Winston, G. P. 466
Winters, T. 831
Witte, R. H. 291
Witthoft, M. 429
Witzlsperger, E. 189
Wojtowicz, M. 611
Wolf, R. L. 498
Wolff, J. J. 212
Wong, C. 457
Wong, J. L. 916
Woods, S. P. 540
Wortzel, H. S. 434
Wray, J. 826
Wright, E. C. 499

Wundt, W. 3–4
Wygant, D. B. 993
Wygant, D. P. 993

Xydakis, M. S. 796

Yablon, S. 390, 393
Yablon, S. A. 341
Yaghmai, F. 305
Yamada, T. 685
Yarboro, C. H. 630
Yannet, H. 207–208
Yarnell, H. 508
Yartz, A. R. 890
Yeates, K. O. 15
Yoash-Gantz, R. 799
Young, A. 758
Young, J. 889
Younggren, J. N. 1001
Youngjohn, J. R. 916
Youngstrom, E. A. 709
Yu, J. Z. 495
Yurgelun-Todd, D. A. 227

Zabel, T. A. 135
Zachariae, R. 572
Zakzanis, K. K. 28–29
Zangwill, Ol 8
Zappella, M. 221
Zheng, H. 58
Zhou, X. 975
Zhu, J. 975
Ziegler, A. L. 219
Ziegler, T. 894
Zielinski, R. E. 810, 931
Zimmerman, A. W. 203
Zimmerman, F. 831
Ziskin, J. 859
Zola-Morgan, S. 683
Zurif, E. 9
Zvolensky, M. J. 890
Zwiers, M. P. 302

Subject Index

Boldface page references indicate tables and boxed text. Italic references indicate figures and photographs.

ABA Model Rules of Professional Conduct 872
ABCDE of differential diagnosis 59–60
abdominal obesity 372
ablative surgery 463–465, 528, **528**
accredited programs 17–19
acquired immunodeficiency syndrome (AIDS): clinical considerations 480–482; neuropathology 482–483; neuropsychological implications 483–484; presentation 479–480
activated studies paradigm 111
activator 102
active answering 910–911
actus reus principle 889, 899
acute liver failure 746
acute lymphoblastic leukemia (ALL): chemotherapy 159–160, *161*; cranial radiation therapy 159–160; incidence 159, *159*; in infants 170–171; methotrexate-related neurotoxicity and 160–162; neuroimaging *161*; risk factors in neuropsychological outcomes 160; steroid treatment 162; survival rate 158–159, *158*, 169, *169*; treatment 159–160, 162
acute respiratory distress syndrome (ARDS) 499
acute stress disorder (ASD) 777
adaptive function measurement 976
additive processes 92
adenine 102, 195
adenosine triphosphate (ATP) 494
Ad Hoc Cognition Sub-committee for the Committee on Lupus Response Criteria 620
administrative actions 888
administrative law and forensic neuropsychology 898
Administrative Law Judge (ALJ) 990
admissibility in forensic neuropsychology 859–860, 891–897, 914–915
Admit-Deny tactic 911
adult-onset hypothyroidism 744
adversarial proceedings 857; *see also* forensic neuropsychology
adverse events, pre- and perinatal 201–202
adversity in childhood 827–828
affective disorders: bipolar disorder 706–710; cognitive impairment and 701–702; major depressive disorder 704–706; mindfulness-based interventions and 1060–1061; overview 701, 710; prevalence 704; *see also specific type*
Afghanistan war veterans 812, 991–992
Agency for Healthcare Research and Quality (AHRQ) 1007, 1054
Agent Orange exposure 890
AIDS *see* acquired immunodeficiency syndrome
alcohol 593
alexithymia 850
alleles 103, 290, 510
allocortex 80
ALS and NFL football players 427
altered mental status 902
alternate form reliability 23
Alzheimer Disease Neuroimaging Initiative (ADNI) 722
Alzheimer's disease (AD): associated clinical features 723–724; behavioral disturbance in 732; delayed recall effect and 29; dementia due to 721–724; diagnostic terminology, evolution of **718**; episodic memory and 723; etiology 720–724; executive function and 723; fluency and naming and 723; framework for preventing and treating **730**; genetics and 105; mild cognitive impairment due to 720–721; neuropsychological testing 26, 30–32; neuropsychology of 722–724, *723*; periods in development of 717; prodromal 720–721; traumatic brain injury and 421, 427; visuospatial skills and 723
American Academy of Clinical Neuropsychology (AACN) 15–16, 867, 874, 944, 985, 1012
American Academy of Neurology (AAN) 19, 337, 354, 894, 901, 1013
American Academy of Pediatrics 222
American Association on Intellectual and Developmental Disabilities (AAIDD) (formerly American Association of Mental Retardation) 972, 980
American Association on Mental Retardation (AAMR) (now American Association on Intellectual and Developmental Disabilities) 972, 980
American Board of Clinical Neuropsychology (ABCN) 3, 14, 16–17, 19
American Board of Professional Psychology (ABPP) 3, 15–17, 19
American College of Emergency Physicians 432
American College of Obstetricians and Gynecologists 132
American Congress of Rehabilitation Medicine 347, 412, **412**, 659, 793, 1078, 1082
American Heart Association 354, 375, 724
American Law Institute (ALI) 900, 968
American Medical Association (AMA) 876–877, 984
American Mindfulness Research Association 1059
American Psychiatric Association 759
American Psychological Association (APA): accredited programs in neuropsychology 17–19; *amicus briefs* and 889; dementia term and 717; disability and 980; Division 40 and 3, 14–16, **16**; *Ethical Principles of Psychologists and Code of Conduct* 58; ethics code 58, 873, 912–913, 942–943, 976, 983–984; Ethics Committee 1001; evidence-based practice in clinical neuropsychology and 1007–1009; Flynn effect and 974; independent medical evaluation and 876; Presidential Task Force on Evidenced-Based Practice 1008–1009, 1015
Americans with Disabilities Act (ADA) (1990) 980–981
American Stroke Association 375, 724
amicus curiae principle 889
amnesia: anatomic correlates of 680–690; anterograde 678; anterior temporal nuclei and 685; autism spectrum disorder and 229; basal forebrain 687–690, *689*, 693–694; bitemporal 686, *686*; case studies, famous 678; cingulate gyrus and 685; clinical characteristics of 678–680; competency and 967–968; diencephalic 687, *687*, 691, 693–694; dual system theory of 682, *682–683*; fornix and 684; infantile 93; mammillary bodies and 684–685; memory anatomy and 689–690; overview 693–694; posttraumatic 340–341, 389–390, 392–393, 396; remote memory disturbance and 678–679; retrograde 678–679, 691;

retrosplenial cortex and 685; similarities and differences among subtypes 690–693; source 692; spared abilities in 679–680; temporal lobe and 680–686, *682–683*, *686*, 693–694; thalamic 686–687, *687*
amnesic syndrome 678
amphetamines 592–593, 1095
Amsterdam Short-Term Memory Test 891
amygdala 78, 681, 688
Anaplasma phagocytophilum 487
aneurysm 361–364, *361*, **361**, *362*, 376
angiography 373–374
angular gyrus 309, 311
anisotropy 634
anosognosia 344–346, 976
anoxia 494
anterior cerebral arteries (ACAs) 351–352, *352*
anterior cingulate cortex (ACC) 824
anterior insula (AINS) 824
anterior temporal lobectomy (ATL) 454, 463
anterior thalamic nuclei 685
anterograde amnesia 678
anticholinergic medications 527, **527**
anticipatory awareness 345, **346**
anticoagulants 363, 375
antidepressants 1090–1092, 1094
antiepileptic drugs (AEDs) 376, 459–460, **460**, 561
antiepileptic polytherapy 565–566
antihypertension drugs 784
antineuronal antibodies 628
antiphospholipid antibodies (APL) 629
antiphospholipid syndrome: biobehavioral mechanisms of cognitive impairment and 638–639; cognitive impairment and 638–639; defining 637; epidemiology 637; neuroimaging 639–640; neuropsychiatric 637–638; overview 640; treatment studies 639
antiplatelet agents 363, 375
antipsychotic drugs 1090, 1093
anti-ribosomal P antibodies 629
antisocial behavior 287, 289
anxiety 824
anxiety disorders: attention deficit/hyperactivity disorder and 289; cerebrovascular disease and 372; cognitive impairment and 701–702; epilepsy and 461, *462*; illness anxiety disorder 952; incidence 702; multiple sclerosis and 614; neuropsychological function and 702; obsessive-compulsive disorder 703–704; overview 701, 710; Parkinson's disease and 520; pediatric considerations 702; pharmacological interventions 1093–1094; subcategories of 1093; trait anxiety 702; *see also specific type*
apathy and Parkinson's disease 520
aphasia 354, **355**
apolipoprotein (APOE) gene 147, 371
apolipoprotein 4 (APOE4) gene 105–106, 160, 369, 371, 433, 563, 719
apolipoprotein E (APOE) gene 371, 719
apoptosis 495
arachnoid 64
arachnoid villi 70
archicortex 80
arcuate fasciculus 80
arcutate fibers 80
area under curve (AUC) 28, 30
arousal 333
arousal disorders 337–340, **337**
arterial spin labeling (ASL) 115
arteries 65
arteriovenous malformations (AVM) 356–360, *357–358*, 359–360, *359–360*
ascending reticular activating system (ARAS) 72, 75
Aspen Neurobehavioral Conference 337
Asperger's disorder (AspD) 185
assessment: baseline 134; multiple 136–137; neuropsychological screening 135; planned follow-up 134–135; problem-focused 135; *see also* diagnosis; historical trends in assessment; *specific disorder and test*
Assessment of Competency and Capacity of the Older Adult 879
Association for Doctoral Education in Clinical Neuropsychology (ADECN) 15–16
Association of Internship Training in Clinical Neuropsychology (AITCN) 15–16
Association of Neuropsychology Students in Training (ANST) 16
Association of Postdoctoral Programs in Clinical Neuropsychology (APPCN) 15, 18–19
Association of Psychology Postdoctoral and Internship Centers (APPIC) 18
astrocytes 66
astroglia 203
ataxia 73
atherosclerosis 371
athletic trainers, certified (ATCs) 659
Atkins v. Virginia (2002) 971–972, **971**, 976
atomoxetine 1095
atrial fibrillation (AF) 371
atrophy measures 610
attention: autism spectrum disorder and 227–228; at 2 to 3 months 94; at 8 to 12 months 95; at 16 to 24 months 95; at birth 93–94; cognitive rehabilitation therapy and 1079–1080; consciousness and 336; focus of 227–228; at 4 years through adolescence 96–97; major depressive disorder and 704; moderate and severe traumatic brain injury and disorder of 395; multiple sclerosis and 605; Parkinson's disease and 513; sustained 228; systemic lupus erythematosus and 624; tests, listing of 27, 32–33; vascular memory and 726
attention deficit disorder 283
attention deficit/hyperactivity disorder (ADHD): antisocial behavior and 287, 289; anxiety disorders and 289; autism spectrum disorder and 289–290; candidate gene studies and 298; clinical profiles 285–297; cognitive impairment and 1095; comorbidity in 287–289; complementary and alternative medicine for 1035; deficits, underlying 285–287; diagnosis 134, 283, 286; in DMS-5 130; epigenetics 299–300; epilepsy and 291; etiological models 287, **288**; functional implications of 302–304; functional neuroimaging and 303; gender and 286; genetic disorders and 290; genetics and 297–298; genome-wide association studies and 298–299; heritability studies and 297–298; historical perspective 281–283; language disorders and 289–290; lead exposure and 588; learning disability and 281, 286; learning problems and 286; mood disorders and 289; motor disorders and 290–291; neural correlates of 300–302; neurodevelopment disorders and 289–291; neuroimaging *130*, 303; neuroscience of 297–311; overview 310–311; personality disorders and 289; pharmacological intervention 1094–1095; presentations 285–287; psychiatric disorders and 287; repeat concussions and 667; seizure disorders and 291; structural variants in 298–299; substance abuse and 287, 289; subtyping 108; symptoms 129–130; validity testing and 948
attention impairment disorders and conscious access 340–341
Attention Process Training (APT) 1079
atypical antidepressants 1091–1092
atypical antipsychotics 1090
atypical drugs 1090–1092, 1095
audition (hearing) 71–72
Auditory Memory Index (AMI) 24–25
autism spectrum disorder (ASD): adverse events and, pre- and perinatal 201–202; amnesia and 229; assessment 222–240; attention and 289–290; broader autism phenotype and 192–193; central coherence and 227–228; classification of 186, **187**; clinical features of 216–222; complementary and alternative medicine and 1039; complementary and alternative medicine for 1034–1035, *1037*; criteria for diagnosis, current 186, **187**, 188–189; defining 184; developmental course 216–222; diagnosis 184–186, **187**, 222, **223–225**; in DSM-5 184, 189; dysmorphogenesis in 191–192; early infant autism and 184; endophenotypes 200–201; environmental influences on 203–204; epidemiology 189–190; epigenetics and *194*, 200; episodic memory and 230; etiology 191–201, *194*; executive function and 238–240; focus of attention and 227–228; functional connectivity and 213–216; functional neuroimaging and 213–216; gender and 190–191, 203–204; genetic/environmental interactions and 203–204; genetic influences and 191–201, *194*, ***198***, 203–204, 222; genetic influences on neurodevelopment in 197–200; genomic perspectives on 130, 194–197; head circumference and 204–207; heritability and 192; hypersensitivities and 188–189, 232; immunological factors and 202–203; implications, broader 201; inhibition and 228; intellectual functioning and 225; language disorders and 236–238, 289–290; memory and 229–231; metabolic neuroimaging and 213; motor disorders and 226–227; neuroimaging 213–216;

neuropathological studies on 207–210; neuroscience of 204–216; orienting and, exogenous and endogenous 227; overview 184, 201, 204, 243–244; parental age and 191; patterns of onset and 218–222; perceptual abilities and 231–236; race and 191; regressive 204, 219–222; restricted and repetitive patterns of behavior and 185–186, 188–189, 217–218, 242–243; risk for **198**, 222; screening 222–225, **223–224**; set-shifting and 228–229; social class and 191; social communication and 185–186, 188, 217–218, 240–242; stress and 204; structural neuroimaging and 210–213; sustained attention and 228; symptoms 130, 184; syndrome forms of 193–194; tactile defensiveness and 188; vision and 189; Von Economo neurons and 336
autoantibodies 628
autobiographical memory 230
autoimmune disorders: antiphospholipid syndrome 637–640; cognitive impairment and 618; overview 618, 645; primary Sjögrens syndrome 643–645; rheumatoid arthritis 640–643; symptoms 618; systemic lupus erythematosus 618–637; *see also specific type*
Automated Neuropsychological Assessment Metrics (ANAM) 625
automaticity of numerical processing 295
autonoetic consciousness 336
autonomic nervous system 63, **63**
"autopilot" 343
autoregulation 353
Average Impairment Rating (AIR) 34, 930
awareness impairments 344–346, **345–346**
awareness interventions 345–346, **346**
axons 66, 603

Babesia microti 487
Balance Error Score System (BESS) 662
balance system 71
balance testing 662
barotraumas 796–797
basal forebrain amnesia 687–690, *689*, 693–694
basal ganglia 76–77
baseline assessment 134
baseline testing in sports-related concussion 663–664
base rate, defining 930
Battery for Health Improvement-2 994
Baxter v. State (2010) 868–869
Baxter v. Temple (2005) 866–867, 902
Bayesian model averaging (BMA) 935, **935**
Beck Anxiety Inventory (BAI) 520
behavioral intervention for pediatric cancer 172
behaviorally defined neurodevelopment disorders: attention deficit/hyperactivity disorder 129–130, *130*; autism spectrum disorder 130; in DSM-5 129; intellectual disability 129; learning disorders 129; *see also specific type*
behavior and brain 81–86, 127–128
behavior therapy (BT) 836
Bell curve 58
benign epilepsy with centrotemporal spikes (BECTS) 458
Bennett v. Richmond (2010) 868–870
Benton's neuropsychological tests **7**
benzodiazepines 1094
berry aneurysm 361
Berry v. CSX Transp. (1998) 938
bevacizumba 568
bias in genotyping 104
biochemical changes and hypoxia of the central nervous system 495
biological gradient and forensic neuropsychology 908
biology, central dogma of 102–104
biomarkers: concussion 664–667; disease burden 722, **722**; etiologic 722, **722**; Huntington's disease 718–719; inflammatory 371; laboratory 666–667; magnetic resonance spectroscopy and 116; mild traumatic brain injury 432; posttraumatic stress disorder 783–784; traumatic brain injury 798
biophysiological functioning and mindfulness 1059
biopsychosocial intervention models 835–837
biopsychosocial questions and differential diagnosis **59**
bipolar disorder: bipolar I 706; bipolar II 706; cognitive impairment and 706–708, 1092; cognitive remediation and 708; depression and 1092; in DSM-5706, 1092; euthymia and 707, 1092; executive function and 707–708; mania and 1092; meta-analyses of 706; mixed episode and 706; neurobiology of 1092; neuropsychological function and 57; pediatric considerations 708–710; pharmacological intervention 707–708, 1092–1093; severity of illness 707; stages of 1092; symptoms 1092–1093; terms for 706
bitemporal amnesia 686, *686*
blast injury 783, 794, 797–799; *see also* military service-related traumatic brain injury
blast physics 795
Blast Related Injury Quality Enhance Research Program 795
blood-brain barrier (BBB) permeability/disruption 561–563, 567, 628
blood oxygen level dependent (BOLD) effect 114–115, 213, 235, 458, 466
blood supply to brain 66, *67*, 68, *68*
blood tests 374
Borrelia burgdorferi 484, 486–487
Boston Children's Hospital 1034
Boston Diagnostic Aphasia Examination (BDAE) 10
Boston Process Approach (BPA) 9–10, 866
Boston VA test battery 10, **10**
brain: amygdala 78; basal ganglia 76–77; behavior and 81–86, 127–128; bilateral activation 97; blood supply to 66, *67*, 68, *68*; Broca's area 83; cerebellum 72–74, *74–75*; cerebral cortex 80–81, *82*; cerebrospinal fluid 65, 68, 70; cerebrum 64, **64**, 84, **85**; changes in 91, 97; competition among structures of 127; corpus callosum 80; cranial nerves 70–71, *71*; "crowding" in 127; diencephalon 74–76; epilepsy and 449–450; formation of basic structures of 91; gross anatomy 64–65; hippocampus 78; horizontal organization of 83–84; left hemisphere 84; limbic system 76–78, *77*, *79–81*; longitudinal organization of 83; microscopic anatomy 65–66, *65*; mindfulness-based intervention and 1057–1059; neomammalian 83; neural networks 84; occipital lobe 85; paleomammalian 83; parietal lobe 85; philosophy of 62; plasticity of 92–93; reptilian 83; right hemisphere 83–84; stem 72; stimulation 340; temporal lobe 85; "triune" 83; ventricles 68, *69*, 70; vertical organization of 83; white matter 65, 73, 78, 80
brain attack/stroke 350
brain-computer interfaces (BCI) 378
"brain damage" 28; *see also* traumatic brain injury (TBI)
brain-derived neurotrophic factor (BDNF) 510
Brain electrical Activity Mapping (BEAM) 307
BRAIN group 19
Brain Injury Association of America 858
brain-machine interfaces (BMI) 378
brain stem 72, 498–499
brain tumors: adult versus children 162; chemotherapy for 162–163, 563, 567; classification of 560; cognitive impairment and 569; cognitive rehabilitation therapy and 569; high-grade 563–656; incidence 162; in infants 170–171; low-grade 164–165, *164*, 565–566; metastatic 567–569; neuroimaging *164–166*, *560*, *562*; neuropsychological studies 563–569; pharmacological interventions 568–569; radiation therapy for 162, 561–563, 566–568; risk factors 162–164; surgery for 162; symptoms 561; treatment 162–163, 561–563, 566–691; treatment effects 561–563; types of 164–165, *164–166*
brainwave technology 378
Brief International Cognitive Assessment for MS (BICAMS) 608
Brief Repeatable Battery (BRB) 604, 607
Broca's area 83
Brodmann Area 85, 209
bundles 78
burden of persuasion 888
burdens of proof 888
buspirone 1094

C20 antigen 639
California Verbal Learning Test (CVLT) 10, 935, **935**
calpain-cleaved all-spectrin N-terminal fragment (SNTF) 432
Cameron case (1990) 900
Canadian Academy of Psychologists in Disability Assessment (CAPDA) 876
cancer and polychlorinated biphenyls 861, 893; *see also* central nervous system cancers; non-central nervous system cancers; pediatric cancer
candidate gene/SNPs 103, 196

candidate studies 298
cannabis 592
capacity 878, 969–970
capillaries 66
CAPS checklist 778, 779–780, **780**
carbamazepine 376, 1093
carbon monoxide (CO) exposure 590–592
care mapping 1037, *1037*
cascade iatrogenesis 1023
case-control research design 103
catastrophic experience 770–771; *see also* posttraumatic stress disorder (PTSD)
catastrophizing 829
catechol-O-methyl-transferase (COMT) inhibitors 510, 527, 1091
causal reasoning 907–908, **908–909**
cavernous malformation 356–357, 360–361
CD4 cells 480–481
cell damage 495
cell death 495
Centers for Disease Control and Prevention (CDC) 130, 142, 190, 285, 792, 902
central auditory processing disorder (CAPD) 290
central coherence 227–228
central executive network (CEN) 215
central nervous system (CNS): 2 to 3 months 94; 8 to 12 months 94–95; 16 to 24 months 95–96; adulthood 97–98, 451; aging 97–98; birth 93–94; brain changes and 91; cerebrospinal fluid and 68, 70; challenges in development and 97–98; four years through adolescence 96–97; injury, mechanism of 561–562; neuroanatomy 63, **63**; neurodevelopmental disorders and alterations to 127; overview 91, 98; plaques and 603; prenatal 91–93; principles, basic 91–93; reorganization of 127; timing of disruption to 127; tumors 158; *see also* central nervous system cancers; hypoxia of the central nervous system; non-central nervous system cancers; toxins in the central nervous system
central nervous system cancers: brain tumors 560–569, *560*, *562*; cognitive impairment and 560, 569; non-central nervous system cancers and 569–573, **574–575**, 576; overview 560, 576–577; primary lymphoma 560, 566–567; research 560; *see also specific type*
cerebella mutism 163
cerebellar abnormalities in dyslexia 305, 311
cerebellar atrophy 498
cerebellum 72–74, *74–75*, 208, 302, 498
cerebral amyloid angiopathy (CAA) 364–365
cerebral angiography 373
cerebral aqueduct 70
cerebral autosomal dominant arteriopathy with subcortical infarcts and leukoencephalopathy (CADASIL) 365–366, *365*
cerebral cortex 80–81, *82*
cerebral dominance 459
cerebral hyperperfusion syndrome 376
cerebral lateralization 83
cerebral palsy 131–132
cerebral vasculature 351–352, *352*
cerebrospinal fluid (CSF) 65, 68, 70, 478, 511, 630
cerebrovascular accident (CVA) 350, 1045–1048
cerebrovascular disease 350, 353, 371, 376–379; aneurysm 361–364, *361*, **361**, *362*, 376; anxiety and 372; APOE4 gene and 371; arteriovenous malformation 356–357, *357–358*, 359–360, *359–360*; atherosclerosis and 371; cavernous malformation 356–357, 360–361; cerebral amyloid angiopathy 364–365; cerebral autosomal dominant arteriopathy with subcortical infarcts and leukoencephalopathy 365–366, *365*; cerebral hyperperfusion syndrome and 376; cognitive impairment and 377; complications 376–377; depression and 343, 372, 1045–1048; diabetes and 370; dyslipidemia and 371; edema and 376; epidemiology 350–353; hallucinations and 372–373; heart disease and 371; hemorrhagic conversion and 376; hemorrhagic stroke 356–357, **356–357**; homocysteine and 371; hydrocephalus and 376; hypertension and 370–371; inflammatory biomarkers and 371; intracranial pressure and 376; ischemic stroke 353–354; management, acute 374–376, **375**; metabolic syndrome and 370–371; mixed dementia 369–370; mortality 350, *351*; moyamoya disease 366–367, *366*; neuroimaging 373–374, 377; obesity and 372; obstructive sleep apnea and 372; overview 350, 379; pathology 353–367; pharmacological intervention 375; prevention 377–378; psychiatric considerations 372–373; rehabilitation 377–378, *378*; risk factors 370–372; seizure and 376; smoking and 371–372; telestroke 375–376; terminology, general 350; transient ischemic attack 354–356; treatment 374–376; vascular cognitive impairment 367–369, **368**; vascular dementia 367–369; vasospasm and 376; web resources **351**, **370**, **374**, **379**; *see also specific type*
cerebrum 64, *64*, 83, **85**
certiorari principle 888
change scores, reliable 25
Chapelle v. Ganger (1998) 888, 914
Checklist for Autism and Toddlers (CHAT) 222
chelating therapies 589–590
chemo-brain 569, 594–595
chemo-fog 569, 594
chemotherapy: acute lymphoblastic leukemia 159–160, *161*; brain tumor risk factor and 164; for brain tumors 162–163, 563, 567; cognitive impairment and 569, 594–595; mood disorders and 594; neuroimaging effects of 594; non-central nervous system cancers 569, 587; pediatric cancer 159–160; toxins in the central nervous system and 587, 593–595
Chicago Multiscale Depression Inventory (CMDI) 611
Childhood Cancer Survivor Study (CCSS) 166–167
childhood disintegrative disorder (CDD) 185
Children's Memory Scale (CMS) 946–947
Children's Oncology Group clinical trial 172
Children's Orientation and Amnesia Test (COAT) 146
Children's Yale-Brown Obsessive-Compulsive Scale (CY-BOCS) 704
cholecystokinin (CCK) 824–825
cholesterol levels 370
choline (Ch) 634
cholinergic hypothesis 688
cholinergic neurons 688
cholinesterase inhibitors 527
chorda tympani 71
choroid plexus 66
chromosomes 195, 290, 304
chronic cluster headaches 54
chronic Lyme disease 486
chronic obstructive pulmonary disease (COPD) 494, 499–500, 746
Chronic Pain Coping Inventory (CPCI) 995, **995**
chronic traumatic encephalopathy (CTE) 52, 429, 433–434, 668–669, 813
cigarette smoking 371–372
cingulate gyrus 685
cingulum 80
circle of Willis 65–66, 68
cisterna magna 70
civil competence, referrals for evaluating 878–879, **878**
civil court and forensic neuropsychology 898
Civil Rights Act (1964) 981
claimant 857
Clark v. Arizona (2006) 969
Cline v. Firestone Tire (1988) 898
clinical approaches 3
clinical judgments 938
clinically definite diagnosis 539
clinically established diagnosis 539
Clinical Neuropsychology Synarchy (CNS) 15–16
clinical psychopharmacology *see* pharmacological intervention
clinical significance 1013
clinical versus actuarial controversy 907
Clinician Global Impression of Change ratings 528
clomipramime 704
cochlear division 71
Cochrane review 528, 1038, 1047, 1049
Coe v. Tennessee (2000) 897
Cogmed Working Memory Training 173
cogniform disorder 987
cognitive behavioral therapy (CBT) 595, 671, 836, 850, 1046, 1061; *see also* psychotherapy
cognitive changes 91, 97
cognitive development: 2 to 3 months 94; 4 years through adolescence 96–97; 8 to 12 months 94–95; 16 to 24 months 95–96; adulthood 97–98; aging 97–98; birth 93–94; brain changes and 91; challenges to 97–98; gains in 98; overview 91, 98; principles, basic 91–93; sensitive periods in 127; traumatic brain injury and 145–146

cognitive functioning: defining 63; genetics and 104–106; mindfulness-based interventions and 1059–1060; multiple sclerosis and 604–608; obsessive-compulsive disorder and 703; systemic lupus erythematosus and 625; visuospatial functioning and 606; *see also* cognitive development; cognitive impairment
Cognitive Genomics consorTium (COGENTI) 105–106
cognitive impairment: affect disorders and 701–702; antiphospholipid syndrome and 637–638; anxiety disorders and 701–702; attention deficit/hyperactivity disorder and 1095; bipolar disorder and 706–708, 1092; brain tumors 569; central nervous system cancers and 560, 569; cerebrovascular disease and 377; chemotherapy and 569, 594–595; depression and 705; epilepsy and 449–450, 460–461; genetics and 104–106; heart failure and 746–747; mild traumatic brain injury and 416, **416–417**; moderate and severe traumatic brain injury and 394–396; multiple sclerosis and 606–607, 609–610; non-central nervous system cancers and 569–570; Parkinson's disease and 513–518; pediatric forensic neuropsychology and identifying 945–947, *946–947*; primary Sjögren's syndrome and 643; rheumatoid arthritis and 641–642; surgical resection and 561; systemic lupus erythematosus and 619–622, *621*, **622**; toxins in the central nervous system and 595; vascular 367–369, **368**, 724; *see also* cognitive functioning; mild cognitive impairment (MCI)
cognitive phenotypes 107
Cognitive Rehabilitation Manual 343
cognitive rehabilitation therapy (CRT): approaches 1079–1082; attention 1079–1080; brain tumors and 569; defining 1078–1079; efficacy of 1082–1085; future directions 1085–1086; historical perspective 1078; memory 1080–1081; mild cognitive impairment and 1083; multiple sclerosis and 610; outcome studies 1082–1085; overview 1078–1079; Parkinson's disease and 529, 1083; problem solving 1081–1082; stroke and 1084–1085; systemic lupus erythematosus and 633; traumatic brain injury and 1084–1085; *see also* rehabilitation
cognitive reserve 167
cognitive testing 782
cognitive training for pediatric cancer 172–173
coherence factor 908
Collaborative Individualized Assessment (CIA) 1068
Collaborative Therapeutic Neuropsychological Assessment (CTNA): assumptions of 1069; case examples 1072–1076; contemporary developments and adaptations in 1070–1072; defining 1068; development of 1068–1069; feedback in neuropsychology and 1068; feedback session 1070; information gathering and 1069–1070; interview, initial 1069–1070; knowledge of, acquiring 851; model 1069; roots of 1068; traumatic brain injury recovery example 1072–1076
Colorado Family Reading study 304
coma 338–340, 392
Coma Recovery Scale—Revised (CRS-R) 338, 396
combined antiretroviral therapy (CART) 480, 483
communication and traumatic brain injury 395; *see also* language disorders
Community Integration Questionnaire (CIQ) 397
comorbid deployment-related health conditions 802–803
comparative judgment 295
compensatory techniques 1078
competence to stand trial 879–880, 892, 967
competency: ability to consult and 964; amnesia and 967–968; capacity versus 878; to confess 966; in context 965–966; criminal 963–966, **963**; factual understanding and 964; forensic neuropsychology and 878–879; measures of 966–967; rational understanding and 964; standing trial and 879–880, 892, 967; unique trial 966
Competency Assessment Instrument (CAI) 966
complementary and alternative medicine (CAM) for children with developmental disabilities: attention deficit/hyperactivity disorder 1035; autism spectrum disorder 1034–1035, *1037*, 1039; business of 1036; care mapping and 1037, *1037*; considerations in 1039–1040, **1039**; efficacy of 1038; evidence of efficacy 1032; families likely to engage in 1034–1035; harm caused by 1038; "homey" care environment promoted by 1036; marketing of 1036; as "natural choice"1036; parents' decisions and 1037; popularity of 1036–1037; prevalence of 1035; problems treated by 1034; providers' knowledge of effect treatment and 1036–1037; symptoms addressed by 1036; treatment 1032–1033, **1033**; types of 1032–1033, **1033**
complex posttraumatic stress disorder (CPTSD) 769–771
computed tomography (CT) 63, 373
Computerized Assessment of Response Bias (CARB) 897, 932
computerized clinical decision support systems (CDSS) 1024
Computerized Test of Information Processing 610–611
concussion: biomarker 664–667; defining 411, 413, 415, 660, **660**; in sports literature 415; *see also* mild traumatic brain injury; sports-related concussion (SRC)
Concussion Recovery Centers (CRCs) 807, **807**
Concussion Symptom Inventory (CSI) 661
cones 70
Conference on Internship Training (1989) 16
Conference on Postdoctoral Training (1993) 16
Conference on Postdoctoral Training in Professional Psychology (1992) 20
confirmatory bias 52
confirmatory factor analysis 27
conformal radiotherapy 561–563
confusional states **337**, 340–341, **342**
Confusion Assessment Metrics (CAM) 341
Confusion Assessment Protocol (CAP) 342, 396
co-normed batteries 34–35
conscious access 336, **337**, 340–341
consciousness: access and 334, **337**, 340–341; arousal disorders and 337–340, **337**; arousal/vigilance and 333; attention and 336; attention impairment disorders 340–341; autonoetic 336; awareness impairments 344–346, **345–346**; complexity of 332; conscious access and 336, **337**, 340–341; defining 333; Descartes and 332–333; disorders of 336–346; elements of 333–335, *333*; episodic memory and 336–337, 342–343; historical perspective 332–333, *332*; inner speech and 335; intransitive 333; level of 72; loss of 411, 423, 659–660, 792, 901; memory and 342–343; neuroimaging 339; neuropsychology's role in understanding 346; neuroscience of 335–336; overview 346; self-awareness and 335; self-monitoring and 335; self-monitoring impairments and 343–344; semantic memory and 336; sensory perception and 333–334
Consolidated Standards of Reporting Trials (CONSORT) 1009
construct validity 25–26
consultative examinations (CEs) 981
continuous performance test (CPT) 39
contusions 391
conversion 782
conversion disorder 952
co-occurring disorders 800–801
copy number variants/variation (CNV) 195–196
core amnesic syndrome 690, 693
core zone 353
corpus callosum 64–65, 80, 211
cortex 208–209
cortical dementia 720
cortical dysplasia-focal epilepsy syndrome (CDFE) 199
corticobasal degeneration (CBD) 534
corticobasalganglionic degeneration (CBGD) 534–535
corticobasal syndrome (CBS) 534
corticobulbar fibers 80
corticobulbar tract 72, 83
corticospinal fibers 78
corticospinal tract 72
corticosteroids 561
Craig v. Orkin Exterminating Co., Inc. (2000) 894
cranial nerves (CNs) 70–72, *71*
cranial radiation therapy (CRT) 158–160
craniopharyngioma 165, *165*
C-reactive protein (CRP) 371, 630
creatine (CR) 634
criminal competencies 963–966, **966**
criminal forensics: ability to consult and 964; amnesia and competency and 967–968;

clinical practice versus 960–961, **961**; competency to confess and 966; criminal competencies and 963–966, **963**; criminal responsibility and 968–969; dangerousness assessment and 970–971, **971**; death-penalty-related issues and 971–976; diminished capacity and responsibility and 969–970; *Dusky v. United States* and 963–965; ethics and 976–977; evaluation process 962–963, *962*; factual understanding and 964; insanity defense and 968–969; malice of aforethought and 969; measures of competency and 966–967; *Miranda* warning and 962–963, 966; neuropsychological principles applied to 960; overview 960; rational understanding and 964; unique trial competency and 966
criminal justice system and military service-related traumatic brain injury 811–812
criminal proceedings and forensic neuropsychology 879–880, 899–901
criminal responsibility 968–969
criterion validity 25, 28–32
Cronbach's α 24
"crowding" effects 127, 458
cueing 693
cultural differences and differential diagnosis 58–59
cytoarchitectural abnormalities in dyslexia 305
cytokines 202, 630
cytomegalovirus (CMV) 749
cytosine 102, 195, 299

damage claims, neuropsychological analysis of: generalizations about 901; head injury and postconcussion syndrome 901–902; neurotoxic torts 902–903; suboptimal effort and malingering 903–904
dangerousness, assessing criminal 970–971, **971**
Daubert v. Merrell Dow Pharm., Inc. (1993) 10, 859–862, 866–867, 870, 888, 893–897, **893**, 906, 914, 916, 938
DBS 528–529, **528**
death-penalty-related issues: adaptive function measurement 976; *Atkins v. Virginia* 971–972, **971**; Flynn effect 973–976; forensic neuropsychologists and 971; mitigation expertise at sentencing 976; standard error of measurement 972; test-retest effects 972–973
decade-nonspecific remote memory disturbance 679
declarative memory 78
deep brain stimulation (DBS) 340, 508
default mode network (DMN) 116, 214, 452, 665–666
Defense Advanced Research Projects Agency (DARPA) 797
Defense and Veterans Brain Injury Center (DVBIC) 793, 802, 806, 812
deficit, defining 136
delay, defining 136
delayed recall effect 29
deletion syndrome 133–134, 290
delirium 340
Delis-Kaplan Executive Function System (DKEFS) 10
dementia: activity-based care and 734; Alzheimer's disease as cause of 720–724; APA and term of 717; behavioral disturbances in 732–734; clinical criteria 717; cortical 720; in DSM-5717; environment and 733; etiologies 720–730, 732; fronto-temporal 336; fronto-temporal lobar degeneration 728–730; future directions 734; generic 719–720; interventions 730–734; with Lewy bodies 507, 525; Lewy body disease 726–728; major neurocognitive disorder 717; mild neurocognitive disorder 717–718; mild traumatic brain injury and 421; mixed 369–370; moderate and severe traumatic brain injury and 394; overview 717, 734; paralysis agitans and 508; Parkinson's disease with 507, 509, 525; physical factors and 733; primary prevention 730–731; redirection and 734; research criteria 718–720; secondary prevention 731; severity of, assessing 732–733; social factors and 734; subcortical 530, 720; syndromes 717–720; tertiary prevention 731–734; traumatic brain injury and 29, 394; vascular 367–369, 724–726; *see also* Alzheimer's disease (AD); mild cognitive impairment (MCI)
dementia with Lewy bodies (DLB) 507, 525
dementia pugilistica 668; *see also* chronic traumatic encephalopathy (CTE)
Dementia Rating Scale (DRS) 510
demyelinating conditions 603; *see also* multiple sclerosis (MS)
demyelination 562
dendrites 65
denial 344–346
denial/unawareness of impaired neuropsychological functioning 1045, 1050, **1050–1051**
de novo mutations 197
dentate gyrus 78
dentate nuclei 73
Department of Defense (DoD) 793–795, 806–809, 812
Department of Health and Human Services 980, 1011
Department of Labor 994
dephasing 90
depression: bipolar disorder and 1092; after cerebrovascular accident 1045–1048; cerebrovascular disease and 372, 1046–1048; cognitive impairment and 705; electroconvulsive therapy for 705; epilepsy and 461; long-term 450; major depressive disorder 704–706; monoamine theory and 1090; multiple sclerosis and 611–614, *612*; neuropathology 614; pain and pain-related disability and 829–830; Parkinson's disease and 518–520, **519**; pharmacological intervention 705, 1090–1092; after stroke 372; trunk and branch model of, in multiple sclerosis 611, *612*
descriptive diagnosis 51–52
desychronization 90
developmental delay, defining 136
developmental dyscalculia (DD) 294–295
diabetes/diabetes mellitus 370, 743–744
diagnosis: clinically definite 539; clinically established 539; descriptive 51–52; documented 539; laboratory-supported definite 539; medical 56; neuropsychological, meaning of 51; presumptive 52; *see also* differential diagnosis; *specific disorder*
diagnostic delay 170
Diagnostic and Statistical Manual for Mental Disorders, fifth edition (DSM-5): attention deficit/hyperactivity disorder in 130; autism spectrum disorder in 130, 184, 189; bipolar disorder in 706, 1092; dementia in 717; depressive disorders in 518; educational disability definitions and 136; evidence for mental illness diagnosis and 909; learning disability in 285; learning disorders in 129; malingering in 950; mild cognitive impairment in 717; neurodevelopmental disorders in 129; postconcussion syndrome in 420, 802, 901; posttraumatic stress disorder in 757, 760–771, **761**; schizophrenia in 1090; somatic symptom disorders in 846; somatization in 827; vascular dementia in 367
diagnostic threat 426, 429, 805–806, 987, 993
diaschisis 353
diencephalic amnesia 687, *687*, 691, 693–694
diencephalon 65, 74–76
differential diagnosis: ABCDE of 59–60; biopsychosocial questions and **59**; confirmatory bias and 52; cultural differences and 58–59; with dementia and dementia with Lewy bodies 525; descriptive 51–52; domain-specific differential 53; effort and 57; etymology of 51; factitious disorder and 58; justifying 59; medical history and 54, **54–56**; motivation and 57–58, *58*; multidomain neuropsychological 53; practice of 51; psychiatric disorders and 56–57; recommendations for 59–60; syndrome analysis and *51*, 53, *53*
diffuse axonal injury (DAI) 391–392, 411
diffusion tensor imaging (DTI) 70, 80, 212, 302, 356, 373, 391–392, 457, 466, 562, 634–635
diffusion-weighted imaging (DWI) 354, 373
DiGeorge syndrome 290
diminished capacity 969–970
DIRECT technique 1079
disability: APA and 980; cheating concerns and 984–987; for children 980; cogniform disorder 987; constructs 980–981; consultative examinations and 981; deficit and, evolution from 980; defining 129; disability-adjusted life year and 980; factitious disorder and 987; Federal Insurance Contributions Act and 981; Global Burden of Disease metric and 980; informed consent and 983–984, **983–984**; intellectual 105, 129, 972; legislative history and 981; malingering and 984–987, *986*, **987**; medicolegal area and 982–983;

military examinations 990–992; other challenges to validity and 987–988; other work-related assessments versus 995–996; in posttraumatic stress disorder, defining 779; private examinations 992–994; private insurance contracts 980; requirements for 989–990, **990**; socio-political climate and 981–982; somatic symptom disorders 987; Supplemental Security Income and 980–981; terminology 980–981; validity testing and 988–989, **989**; workers' compensation and 982, 994–995
disability-adjusted life year (DALY) 980
Disability Benefits Questionnaire (DBQ) 991
Disability Determinations Services (DSSs) 981
Disability Rating Scale (DRS) 397
discrepancy between test data 934
discriminant function analysis (DFA) 933
dishabituation 93
disorders of consciousness (DOC) 399; *see also* consciousness
dissociative identity disorder (formerly multiple personality disorder) 1021–1022
distress 779
divalproex 1093
Division 40 3, 14–16, **16**
DNA 102–103, 195–196, 562; *see also* genetics
domain-specific differential diagnosis 53
domain-specific hypothesis 106
DOMINION study 521
Donezepil 172
dopamine (DA) 298, 510, 525, 527, 825, 1091, 1095
dopaminergic dysregulation syndrome 521
dorsolateral prefrontal cortex (DLPFC) 92, 824
dose-response relationship 907
double association 8
Down syndrome 131, 195
drugs *see* pharmacological intervention; *specific type*
DSM-IV-TR 760–771
dualism 62
dual system theory of amnesia 682, *682–683*
Due Process hearing 878
Dunedin Multidisciplinary Health and Development Study 592
Dunn's Sensory Profile 233
dura mater 64
Durham tests 900
Dusky standard 964
Dusky v. United States (1960) 880, 963–965
dysarthria 73
dyscalculia 294–295, 308–310
dysgraphia 295–296
dyslexia: cerebellar abnormalities in 305, 311; cytoarchitectural abnormalities in 305; electroencephalography and 307–308; event-related potentials and 307–308; functional neuroimaging and 306–307; genetics of 304–305; magnetoencephalography and 307–308; neural correlates of 305–308; neurobiology of 304–308; neuroimaging 306–307; overview 311; as reading disorder 292–294; structural findings and 305; structural neuroimaging and 306; symptoms 292–294; "triangular" model of 292; types of 292; visual evoked potentials and 308; word blindness and 282
dyslipidemia 370
dysmorphogenesis in autism spectrum disorder 191–192
dysphoria 731
dystonia 539

early infant autism 184
echocardiography 354
Ecologically Oriented Neurorehabilitation Executive (EON-Exec) 1081–1082
Ecologically Oriented Neurorehabilitation of Memory (EON-Mem) program 1081
ecologic validity 31
edema 376
educational intervention 173
Education for All Handicapped Children Act 283
educational testing 136
effective connectivity 213
effort: defining 986; differential diagnosis and 57; forensic neuropsychology and assessment of 859–860, 871, 903–904; suboptimal 871, 903–904; tests of 428
ehrlichiosis 487
e-iatrogenesis 1024
electric seizure (ES) 847
electroconvulsive therapy (ECT) 705
electrocortical stimulation (ECS)/ electrocorticography 465, 467
electro-cortical stimulation mapping (ESM) 467
electroencephalography (EEG) 116–117, 307–308, 339
electronic medical record (EMR) 1024
electrophysiological abnormalities and sports-related concussion 666
electrophysiological brain mapping 116–117, *117*
embolic shower 354
emboliform nuclei 73
embolism 354
embolization 359
emergent awareness 345, **346**
Emerging Consciousness Program 808–809
emotional valence 609
endocrine function 76
endophenotypes 200–201
endovascular treatment 359, 363
enhancers 102
environmental influences on autism spectrum disorder 203–204
enzyme-linked immunosorbent assay (ELISA) 480
ependymal cells 66
Epidemiologic/Epidemiological Catchment Area (ECA) survey 772, 930
epigenetics *194*, 200, 299–300
epilepsy: age of onset and 457–458, *459*; anterior temporal lobectomy and 454, 463; anxiety and 461, *462*; attention deficit/ hyperactivity disorder and 291; benign 458; brain and 449–450; cerebral dominance and 459; chronicity and 458–459; chronological age and 457–458; cognitive impairment and 449–450, 460–461; depression and 461; factors mediating cognitive network reorganization in 457–459, *459*; frontal-lobe 456–457; interaction between cognitive and emotional/behavioral disruptions in 461, *462*, 463; medications, cognitive and behavioral impact of 459–460; mesial temporal lobe 450, 461, 463; multifocal deficits in focal 455–457, *455*; neuroimaging 465–467; neuropathology of seizure and 449, *451*; occipital lobe 457; overview 449; parietal lobe 457; pharmacological intervention 459–460, **460**; plasticity and 449–450; progression of cognitive deficits and 460–461; research insights 449; seizure-induced reorganization of cognitive networks and 451–455, *453–454*; surgery for, predicting neuropsychological status after 463–465, *463*; symptoms 449; temporal lobe 451–452, *453*, 454, 456, 459, 463, *463*, 1082; *see also* seizure
epileptic encephalopathies 221
episodic memory: Alzheimer's disease and 723; autism spectrum disorder and 230; consciousness and 336–337, 342–343; Lewy body disease and 728; vascular dementia and 725–726
EQUATOR Network website 1009
equipotential theory 84
erethism 589
error rate, known or potential 896
essential tumor 539
estimation of premorbid cognitive levels 905
ethical practice of clinical neuropsychology: application of resources to challenges 1002–1004; board certification and 1001–1002; challenges 1001–1002; discussions about, increasing 1000; evolution of 1004; Four As of 1002; future directions 1004; ideals 1001–1002; overview 1000; resources 1002
Ethical Principles of Psychologists and Code of Conduct (APA) 58
ethics: APA's code of 58, 873, 912–913, 942–943, 976, 983–984; criminal forensics and 976–977; expert witness and 873–874; forensic neuropsychology and 873–874, 912–914; pediatric forensic neuropsychology and 942–943; positive 1001; *see also* ethical practice of clinical neuropsychology
Ethyl Cysteinate Dimer (ECD) 112
euthymia 707, 1092
Evaluation of Competency to Stand Trial-Revised (ECST-R) 967
event-free survival (EFS) 170
event-related potentials (ERPs) 94–95, 303–304, 307–308, 339
evidence-based decision making 1008
evidence-based medicine 1007
evidence-based practice (EBP) in clinical neuropsychology: APA and 1007–1009; APA Presidential Task Force on 1008–1009, 1015; clinical applications of 1014–1015; dimensions of ideal health care and 1008; evidence-based medicine and 1007; examples of neuropsychology

research influencing 1015–1016; future directions 1016; health care practice and, evolving 1007–1008; historical perspective of 1007; implementation 1012–1013; in mental health 1011–1012; overview 1007–1016; in psychology 1011; research applications of 1013–1014; resources 1009, **1009**; scientific research and 1008
Evidence-Based Practice Centers (EPCs) 1007
evidence-based treatments 1025–1026
evidentiary standards 860–863, **863–866**, 866–870
evoked related potentials (ERPs) 666
excitation 114
excitatory amino acids (EEA) neurotransmitters 495
exclusionary criteria 835
executive function: Alzheimer's disease and 723; at 2 to 3 months 94; at 4 years through adolescence 96–97; at 8 to 12 months 95; at 16 to 24 months 95; autism spectrum disorder and 238–240; bipolar disorder and 707–708; at birth 93–94; fronto-temporal lobar degeneration and 730; moderate and severe traumatic brain injury and 395–396; multiple sclerosis and 606; Parkinson's disease and 513–514; systemic lupus erythematosus and 624; tests, listing of 27; vascular dementia and 725–726
exercise endurance 633
exons 102
Expanded Paired Associate Test (EPAT) 31
expectancy 826, 889
experimental evidence 908
expert witness: in criminal proceedings 879–880; deceptive attorney behaviors and 872; ethical dilemmas and, responding to 874; ethics and 873–874; for independent medical evaluations 876–877; for independent school evaluations 877–878; in neurotoxin litigation 875–876; objectivity of, importance of maintaining 872–873; other areas of 880; referrals for evaluations of civil competence and 878–879, **879**; role of 871–873, **872**; sentencing mitigation and 976
explicit memory 230
extended amygdala 688
external capsules 76
external incentives and neuropsychological examination 928
extrapyramidal side effects (EPS) 1090

facial nerves 70–71
Facial Recognition Test 30–31
factitious disorder 58, 952, 987
factor analyses 26–28
Factor C 5
factual understanding 964
failure to keep pace, defining 136
Fake Bad Scale (FBS) 57, 781, 860, 890
false discovery rate (FDR) 104
falsibility 896
familial intracranial aneurysm 362–363
Family Educational Rights and Privacy Act (FERPA) 943
family practice model 134
fasciculi 78
fashionable illnesses 52
fastigial nuclei 73
fasting glucose levels 370–371
fatigue 632
Fatigue Severity Scale 632
fear avoidance 830
Federal Insurance Contributions Act (FICA) 981
Federal Rules of Civil Procedure (FRCP) 894
Federal Rules of Evidence (FRE) 893–896, **895**
Feighner criteria 772
fetal alcohol spectrum disorder 133
fetal alcohol syndrome (FAS) 133
fetal mesencephalic cell transplantation **528**, 529
F-Family scales 993
first generation antipsychotics (FGA) 1090
fissures 64
Fitness-For-Duty (FDD) examination 995
flight or fight response 76, 78
flocculonodular lobe 73
Florida National Guard survey 801
fluency and naming 723, 726, 729
fluid attenuated inversion recovery (FLAIR) 90, 478, 480, 639
Flynn effect (FE) 137, 973–976
focal anoxic brain injury **500**
focal brain ischemia 350
folate deficiency 132
Food and Drug Administration 132, 589, 1024
foramen of Magendie 70
foramen magnum 64
foramen of Monro 70
foramina of Luschka 70
forced-choice tests (FCTs) 931–932; *see also* symptom validity tests (SVTs)
Ford v. Wainwright (1986) 880
forensic neuropsychologist (FN) 971; *see also* criminal forensics; forensic neuropsychology
forensic neuropsychology: active answering and 910–911; administrative law and 898; admissibility 859–860, 891–897, 914–915; Admit-Deny tactic 911; adversarial aspect of 857; applicability of norms 870; areas of, key 880–881; assessment process 859–860, 904–906; attribution of facts and 909; biological gradient and 908; capacity and 878; causation analysis and 891; civil court and 898; claimant and 857; clinical versus forensic assessments 889–891; coherence factor and 908; competence to stand trial and 879–880, 892; competency and 878–879; criminal proceedings and 879–880, 899–901; cross-examination 910–911, **911**; damage claims and, common issues of 901–904; *Daubert* case and 893–897; deceptive attorney behaviors and 872; defining 887; discovery and 913; effort assessment and 859–860, 871, 903–904; elements of assessment process 905–906; empirical bases for conclusions based on 860–871; ethics and 873–874, 912–914; evidentiary standards and 860–863, **863–866**, 866–870; examples of major activities and roles 874–880; expectancy and 889; experimental evidence and 908; expert witness role in 871–873, **872**; factors influencing emergence of 858; Flynn effect and 975–976; forewarning respondents and 915–916; functional analysis and 908–909; future directions 880–881; health care advances and resulting societal change 858; health care market forces 858–859; hearsay rule and 895; historical perspective 857–860; independent medical evaluations, retained expert for 876–877, 897; independent school evaluations, retained expert for 877–878; insanity plea 880; interpretive process 906–907; interview and 905–906; issues in, key 860–874; law and conflicts with 891, **891**; learned treatise and 910, **911**; limitations of tests predicting functional outcome 870–871; litigant and 857; litigation consultation and 912–913; malingering assessment and 859–860, 871, 903–904; mental state evaluation and 906; myths of 914–916; normative studies and 870; objectivity and, importance of maintaining 872–873; overview 857, 887, 916–917; performance validity tests and 903; plausibility and 908; plea entry 880; posterior probability and 894; postincident exposures and 889–890; practice effects and 915; premorbid functioning, inferences about 870; prior probability and 894; probate proceedings and 898–989; prominence of, increasing 857, *858*, 887; Push-Pull tactic 911; quality of norms 870; raw data disclosure and 913; referrals for evaluations of civil competence 878–879, **878**; report writing 907–909; research areas, key 880–881; response bias assessment and 859–860; Rules of the Road for 916, **917**; scientist-practitioner model 859; self-report and 890; settings for neuropsychologists, common 898–901; social context of evaluation 889–890; Specialty Guidelines for 976–977; suboptimal effort and 871, 903–904; terminology, basic 887–889; testamentary competence and 899; testimony 892, 909–914, **911**; test selection and 906; third-party observers and 897–898; training, need for formal 881; traumatic brain injury and neurotoxin litigation 874–876; traumatic brain injury and rise of 858; validity and, threats to 890–891; weight of evidence and 887, 896; *see also* pediatric forensic neuropsychology; *specific case*
forensic, term of 887, 942; *see also* criminal forensics; forensic neuropsychology; pediatric forensic neuropsychology
forewarning respondents and forensic neuropsychology 915–916
forgetting, rate of 690–691; *see also* amnesia
fornix 78, 80, 680, 684
Four As of ethical practice 1002
fractional anisotropy (FA) 302, 454, 593
Fragile X mental retardation 1 (FMR 1) gene 131, 193
Fragile X spectrum disorder 131

Fragile X syndrome 105, 131, 233
Franz test battery 4, **4**
free recall 230
free will 335
frontal lobe epilepsy (FLE) 456–457
fronto-striatal system 300–301
fronto-temporal dementia(FTD) 336
fronto-temporal lobar degeneration (FTLD) 728–730
Frye v. United States (1923) 860–863, 893–896, **893**
functional adaptation 377
functional analysis 908–909
functional connectivity 213–216
functional connectivity magnetic resonance imaging 115–116, 466–467
functional magnetic resonance imaging (fMRI) 114–115, 466
functional and molecular neuroimaging: attention deficit/hyperactivity and 303; autism spectrum disorder and 213–216; caution about 111; dyslexia and 306–307; electrophysiological brain mapping techniques 116–117, *117*; functional transcranial Doppler ultrasonography 118; future directions 119; illness characteristics and 118–119; injury characteristics and 118–119; interpreting, methodological considerations in 118–119; magnetic resonance-based 114–116; multiple sclerosis and 610–611; optical (near-infrared) imaging 118; other technologies 118; overview 111, 119; radioisotope-based 111–114; resting versus activated studies and 111; sports-related concussion and 665–666; *see also specific test*
functional neurological symptom disorder 952
functional neuronal changes and hypoxia of the central nervous system 495
functional reorganization 377
functional somatic syndromes *see* somatic symptom disorders
functional transcranial Doppler ultrasonography 118
funiculi 78

GABA receptors 449–450
Galveston Orientation and Amnesia Scale (GOAT) 390, 396
Gate Control Theory of Pain 824
gender: attention deficit/hyperactivity and 286; autism spectrum disorder and 190–191, 203–204; mild traumatic brain injury and 425; traumatic brain injury and 141
gene networks 106
General Ability Index (GAI) 24–25
general acceptance 896
General Electric Co. v. Joiner (1997) 861–862, 897, 906, 908
Generalist Gene hypothesis 106
generalized anxiety disorder (GAD) 1093–1094
generalized tonic-clonic seizure (GTCS) 458
genes 103, 195, 298; *see also* genetics; genomics and phenomics
genetic correlations 106
genetic disorders: attention deficit/hyperactivity disorder and 290; cerebral palsy 131–132; deletion syndrome 133–134; Down syndrome 131; fetal alcohol syndrome 133; Fragile X syndrome 131; prematurity 132, *132*; spina bifida 132–133; *see also specific type*
genetics: Alzheimer's disease and 105; attention deficit/hyperactivity and 297–298; autism spectrum disorder and 192–201, *194*, ***198***, 203–204, 222; classical research 103; cognitive functioning and 104–106; cognitive impairment and 104–106; corticobasalganglionic degeneration and 534–535; dyslexia and 304–305; Huntington's disease and 536; mild traumatic brain injury and 432–433; Parkinson's disease and 509–510
genome-wide association studies (GWAS) 103–104, 107, 196–197, 298–299
genomics and phenomics: Alzheimer's disease and 105; cognitive function/dysfunction and 104–106; domain-specific hypothesis and 106; gene networks and 106; Generalist Gene hypothesis and 106; genetic correlations and 106; Human Connectome Project and 107; overview 102; precision medicine and 108; principles, basic 102–104
Geographic and Racial Differences in Stroke (REGARDS) Study 356
Georgia Court Competency Test (GCCT) 966
Georgia Court Competency Test-Mississippi State Hospital Revision (GCCT-MSH) 966
Geriatric Depression Scale (GDS) 519–520
Gerstmann syndrome 294
giant aneurysms 361–362
Glasgow Coma Scale (GCS) 35, 144–146, 338, 388–389, 411–412, 660, 749, 781
Glasgow Outcome Scale (GOS) 147, 397, **397–398**, 433
glia cells 65–66
Glial Fibrillary Acidic Protein (GFAP) 666–667
gliomas 164–165, *164*, 560, 563–566; *see also* brain tumors
Global Burden of Disease (GBD) metric 980
Global War on Terror 810
globose nuclei 73
glutamatergic signaling 1094
Goal Management Training (GMT) 1081
Goldstein-Scheerer test battery 6–7, **6**
gradient echo (GRE) 90
grammar 237; *see also* language disorders
gray matter (GM) 65, 210–211, 633
great vessels to the neck 66
Gross Stress Reaction 762; *see also* posttraumatic stress disorder (PTSD)
Group Life Insurance Traumatic Injury Protection Program (TSGLI) 803
guanine 102, 195
gyri 64, 80, 85, 91, 309, 685

hallucinations 372–373
Halstead Impairment Index 28
Halstead-Reitan battery (HRB) 4–6, **5**, 906, 909, 914, 930
Harvard Trauma Questionnaire 771
headaches 54
head circumference 204–207
health care advances and resulting societal changes 858
health care market forces 858–859
Health Environment Program (HEP) 1059
Health Insurance Portability and Accountability Act (HIPAA) 943, 982
health-related quality of life (HRQOL) 463–464
hearing 71–72
hearsay rule 895
heart disease 371
heart failure 746–747
heavy metals: defining 587; impact of, general 587; lead 587–588, 902; mercury 588–590
hedonistic homeostatic dysregulation syndrome 521, 525
hematomas 376, 391
hemispatial neglect 31
hemodynamics 352–353
hemorrhage 356
hemorrhagic conversion/transformation 376
hemorrhagic stroke 356–357, **356–357**
Henry-Heilbronner Index (HHI) 849
Henry M. (H. M.) case study 678, 680, 682
hepatic encephalopathy (HE) 746
hepatitis C virus (HCV) 482
heritability studies 297–298
herpes simplex encephalitis (HSE): clinical considerations 478; neuropathology 478; neuropsychological implications 478–479; presentation 477–478, *477*
heterocyclics 1091
Hexamethyl-propylene Amine Oxime (HMPAO) 112
high blood pressure 53–54, 356, 370–371
high density lipoprotein (HDL) 370
high-grade glioma 563–565
hippocampal sclerosis (HS) 452, 464, *464*
hippocampus 78, 680–681
hippocampus proper 78
historical trends in assessment: background information 3; Benton's tests 6, **7**; Boston Process Approach and 9–10; Boston VA test battery and 10, **10**; development of methods 3; Franz test battery and 4, **4**; Goldstein-Scheerer battery 6–7, **6**; Halstead-Reitan battery and 4–6, *5*; Montreal Neurological Institute test battery and 9, **9**; qualitative approaches 6–10, **7–10**; quantitative approaches 3–6, **4–6**; Teuber's battery **9**; update on current trends and 10–11
HIV infection *see* acquired immunodeficiency syndrome
H. M. case study 678, 680, 682
holonomic brain theory 332
homocysteine 371
HONE-In (Health Outcomes and Neuropsychology Efficacy Initiatives) 1014
Hopkins Verbal Learning Test (HVLT) 30
horizontal organization of brain 83–84
hormonal factors and systemic lupus erythematosus 631

hormonal therapies 569–570
Horne v. Goodson Logging (1986) 892
Houston Conference 16–18
HRB Impairment Index 29, 34
Human Connectome Project 107
human genome 195, 299
human granulocytic anaplasmosis (HGA) 487
Huntington's disease (HD): biomarkers 718–719; case example of 537–538, **538**; cause of 536; epidemiology 536; genetics and 536; neurobehavioral features of 537; neuropathology 537
Huntoon v. TCI Cablevision (1998) 892
Hurricane Andrew and posttraumatic stress disorder 775
Hutchison v. Am. Family Mut Ins. (1994) 892–893
hydrocephalus 163, 376
hyperactivity 282; *see also* attention deficit/hyperactivity disorder
hyperacusis 188
hypercapnia 746
hyperkinesis 282
hyperkinetic disease 282
hypersensitivities 188–189, 232
hypertension 53–54, 356, 370–371
hyperthyroidism 744
hypothalamic dysfunction 165
hypothalamic-pituitary-adrenal (HPA) axis and anxiety 824
hypothalamus 65, 75–76
hypothesis 52
hypothetical ability-focused neuropsychological battery 32
hypothyroidism 744
hypoxemia 494
hypoxia 494, 746
hypoxia of the central nervous system: affective changes and 500; apoptosis and 495; biochemical changes and 495; causes of 494; cognitive impairment and, characterization and treatment of 501–502; focal anoxic brain injury and **500**; functional neuronal changes and 495; hypoxic brain injury and 494–495; incidence 494; mechanisms of brain injury and 495, **496**; necrosis and 495; neuroimaging 496–499, *497–498*; neuropsychological implications 499–500, **501**; overview 502; psychiatric changes and 500; reoxygenation injury and 495; reperfusion injury and 495
hypoxic brain injury 494–495

iatrogenesis in neuropsychological assessment: cascade 1023; categories of 1018–1019; defining 1018; dissociative identity disorder and 1021–1022; evidence-based treatments and 1025–1026; medical, reducing 1026–1027; from medications and medical procedures 1022–1024; mild traumatic brain injury and 1019–1020; multiple chemical sensitivities and 1020–1021; objective corroboration of subjective reporting and 1024–1025; overview 1018, 1027; patient pressure and, resisting 1024–1025; postconcussion syndrome and 1019–1020; preventing 1024–1027; technological 1024; undiagnosis and 1025; whiplash injuries and 1020
iatrogenic illness 805–806
idiopathic environmental intolerance 1020–1021
illness anxiety disorder 952
immunoglobulins 202–203
immunological factors and autism spectrum disorder 202–203
Impact of Events Scale (IES) 781
impaired self-awareness (ISA) 1045, 1050, **1050–1051**
improvised explosive device (IED) 794–795, 797; *see also* blast injury
impulse control disorders (ICDs) 521
impulsive and related behaviors 521
inattentional blindness 336
in camera evidentiary hearings 888–889
independent medical evaluation (IME) 876–877, 897
independent psychological evaluation (IPE) 876
independent school evaluations 877–878
Index of the Conners Teacher Rating Scale 172
Indiana v. Edwards (2008) 966
individual education plan (IEP) 136, 283, 710, 877
individualized quantitative behavioral assessment (IQBA) 338
Individuals with Disabilities Education Act (IDEA) (formerly Education Act of All Handicapped Children) 877–878, 981
Individuals with Disability Act (1990) 189
infantile amnesia 93
inferior occipitofrontal fasciculus 80
inferior prefrontal cortex 309
inflammation 630–631
inflammatory biomarkers 371
informed consent 983–984, **983–984**
inhibition and autism spectrum disorder 228
in limine evidentiary hearings 888–889, 893
inner speech 335
in-phase precession 90
Insanity Defense Reform Act (IDRA) (1984) 900, 968–969
insanity plea/defense 880, 909, 968–969
INS/APA Guidelines Report (1987) 14
in silica modeling 107
Institute of Medicine (IOM) 1008
instrumental activities of daily living (IADLs) 514
insula 81
intellectual awareness 345, **346**
intellectual development disorder 105, 129
intellectual disability 105, 129, 972
intellectual functioning 137, 225, 513, 606, 973–976; *see also* IQ scores
interdisciplinary model 134–135
interitem consistency 23
interleukin-18 (IL-18) 371
internal capsules 76
internal consistency reliability 23
International Classification of Diseases (tenth edition) (ICD-10) 367, 757, 767–769, 778, 802, 901
International Committee of Medical Journal Editors (ICMJE) 1009
International Conference on Concussion in Sports 662
International Neuropsychological Society (INS) 14
International Primary CNS Lymphoma Collaborative Group (IPCG) 566
International Society for Traumatic Stress Studies 760, 767, 781–782
International Working Party 337
interneurons 65
Interorganizational Council (IOC) for Accreditation of Postdoctoral Programs in Psychology 16
interpretive process in forensic neuropsychology 906–907
interview, clinical 905–906
intracerebral hemorrhage (ICH) 356
intraclass correlation 24
intracranial hematomas 391
intracranial pressure (ICP) 356, 376
intransitive consciousness 333
intraparietal sulcus (IPS) 308–310
introns 102
inverse dose-response relationship 907
"invisible gorilla" experiment 334
Iowa Gambling Task (IGT) 514
IQ scores 34, 58, 129, 143; *see also* intellectual functioning
Iraq war(s) veterans 428–429, 792, 812, 991–992, 1021
irresistible impulse test 900
ischemia 350, 494, 499
ischemic stroke 353–354
island of Reil 81

Jenkins v. U.S. (1962) 892
John v. Im (2002) 894
"junk" DNA 102
"junk science" 860

Kappa values 767
kidney failure 745–746
Killeen (Texas) shooting 774
King-Devick test (KDT) 662
KLOTHO gene 105
Kluver-Bucy syndrome 479
"knock out" test paradigm 465
knowing *see* semantic memory
knowing right from wrong test 899–900
knowledge base thought of training 17
Kuder-Richardson Formula 20 and 21 23–24
Kumho Tire Co. v. Carmichael (1999) 861–862, 867, 896–897

laboratory-supported definite diagnosis 539
lacunar infarct 350
lacune 350
Lamasa v. Bachman (2005) 894
Landau-Kleffner syndrome (LKS) 221
Landers v. Chrysler Corporation (1997) 892
Landstuhl Regional Medical Center 799
language development: at 2 to 3 months 94; at 4 years through adolescence 97; at 8 to

12 months 95; at 16 to 24 months 95–96; at birth 94
language disorders: attention deficit/hyperactivity disorder and 289–290; autism spectrum disorder and 236–238, 289–290; fronto-temporal lobar degeneration and 729–730; grammar 237; moderate and severe traumatic brain injury and 395; multiple sclerosis and 606; orthography 292; Parkinson's disease and 514–515; phonology 236, 292; pragmatics 238; prosody 236–237; semantics 237–238, 292; source 230; systemic lupus erythematosus and 625
late postconcussion syndrome (LPCS) 901–903
lead exposure 587–588, 902
learned treatise (LT) 910
learning: Parkinson's disease and 516–517; self-generated 609; systemic lupus erythematosus and 623–624; tests, listing of 27, 32–33
learning difference 282
learning disability (LD): attention deficit/hyperactivity disorder and 281, 286; clinical profile 285–297; deficits, underlying 291–297; diagnosis 283–285; in DSM-5 285; dyscalculia and 294–295, 308–310; dysgraphia and 295–296; historical perspective 281–283; math disorders and 294–295; neurobiology of 304–310; neuroscience of 297–311; nonverbal 296–297; overview 310–311; presentations 291–297; reading disorders and 292–294; repeat concussions and 667; *see also* dyslexia
learning disorders 129, 282
left hemisphere of brain 83
left-hemisphere damage (LHD) 30–31
lemnisci 78
lenticular nucleus 76
lesions 391, 497–498, *497*, 498, *498*, 603, 682–683
levodopa 525
Lewy body disease (LBD) 726–728
licensing board evaluations 996
likelihood ratio (LR) 930, **930**
Likert scale 661
limbic system 76–78, *78–81*, 208, 498
linear predictor 933, 935
Line Orientation Test 31
lithium 707–708, 1092–1093
litigant 857
litigation consultation 912–913
liver failure 746
liver transplant case study 747–754, *748–749*, **750–751**, *752*
local education agency (LEA) 877
localizationist theory 84
locatable region 102
logged odds 933
logic relaxation 1054
logistic regression analysis 196
logit 933
longitudinal organization of brain 83
long-term depression (LTD) 450
long-term potentiation (LTP) 450
loss of consciousness (LOC) 411, 423, 659–660, 792, 901
low density lipoprotein (LDL) 370
low-grade glioma 164–165, *164*, 565–566
Luminosity 1079–1080
lung failure 746–747
lupus anticoagulant (LAC) 628
Luria-Nebraska Neuropsychological Battery (LNNB) 906, 914
Lyme arthritis 487
Lyme disease and related disorders: clinical considerations 484, *485*; neuropsychological implications 484, 486–487; presentation 484

MacArthur Competency Assessment Tool-Criminal Adjudication (MacCAT-CA) 966–967
M'Naghten's Case (1843) 899–900, 968–969
macroencephaly 191–192, 204–207
Mad Hatter's disease 589
magnetic resonance angiography (MRA) 373–374, 633–634
magnetic resonance-based imaging: biophysics and 114; functional connectivity magnetic resonance imaging 115–116; functional magnetic resonance imaging 114–115; molecular imaging with MRI 116; overview 114
magnetic resonance imaging (MRI) 63, 373, 465
magnetic resonance spectroscopy (MRS) 116, 374, 634
magnetoencephalography (MEG) 117, *117*, 307–308, 310
major depressive disorder (MDD) 704–706, 1090
major neurocognitive disorder (MND) 717, 934
malice of aforethought 969
malingering: definite 950–951; disability and 984–987, *986*, **987**; in DSM-5950; forensic neuropsychology and assessment of 859–860, 871, 903–904; pain and 834; pediatric forensic neuropsychology assessment of 950–952, **951**; possible 950–951; probable 950–951; testing memory 39, 891, 897, 932, 949, 989
malingering neuropsychological dysfunction (MND) 950–952, **951**
mammillary bodies 684–685
mammillothalamic tract (MMT) 687, *687*
managed health care 858–859
mania 1092
marijuana 592
material-specific deficits 230–231
math disorders 294–295
matrix metalloproteinases (MMPs) 630
Mattis Dementia Rating Scale (MDRS) 906
maximal medical improvement (MMI) 876, 992
MDMA 592–593
measurement 51–52
measurement error 24–25
medial forebrain bundle 80
medial lemniscus 72
medial limbic circuit 681
medical diagnosis 56
medical history 54, **54–56**
medical iatrogenesis 1018, 1026–1027; *see also* iatrogenesis in neuropsychological assessment
medically unexplained symptoms (MUPS) 847, 851
Medical Symptom Validity Test (MSVT) 804, 949
meditation 1054–1055, 1057–1058
medulla 65
medulloblastoma 165–166, *166*
megalencephaly 204–207
megencephaly 192
melancholia 508
melatonin 76, 1038
Memantine 633
memory: 2 to 3 months 94; at 4 years through adolescence 96; at 8 to 12 months 94–95; at 16 to 24 months 95; anatomy of 689–690; autism spectrum disorder and 229–231; autobiographical 230; awareness of impairment 344–346; at birth 93; cognitive rehabilitation therapy and 1080–1081; consciousness and 342–343; cueing and 693; declarative 78; denial of impairment 344–346; explicit 230; free recall 230; major depressive disorder and 704; metamemory and 692–693; moderate and severe traumatic brain injury and disorders of 395; multiple sclerosis and 605; Parkinson's disease and 516–517; processes 229–230; prospective 517, 609; rehabilitation 731; seizure and 452; self-monitoring and 343–344; semantic 336, 342–343; short-term 97; spatiotemporal context deficits of 691–693; systemic lupus erythematosus and 623–624; temporal lobe and 680–686; for temporal order 691–692; tests, listing of 27, 32–33; *see also* episodic memory; working memory
Memory and Attention Adaptation Training (MAAT) 576
meningitis 477
mens rea principle 889, 899, 969–970
mental health and evidence-based practice 1011–1012
mental retardation (now intellectual disabilities) 105, 129, 980
mental state evaluation (MSE) 904, 906
mental tests, first use of term 4
mercury exposure 588–590
mesial temporal lobe epilepsy(MTL) 450, 461, 463
messenger RNA (mRNA) 102, 195; *see also* genetics
Meta-Analysis Of Observations Studies in Epidemiology (MOOSE) guidelines 707
metabolic autoregulation 353
metabolic disorders: causes of 742; classes of 742, **743**; diabetes mellitus 743–744; heart failure 746–747; kidney failure 745–746; liver failure 746; liver transplant case study 747–754, *748–749*, **750–751**, *752*; lung failure 746–747; manifestations of, possible 742, **743**; metabolic syndrome 744; phenylketonuria 742–743; prognosis

753; symptoms 742–743; thyroid disease 744–745; vitamin B12 deficiency 745
metabolic neuroimaging 213
metabolic syndrome 370–371, 744
metabolism 742
metamemory 692–693
metastatic brain tumors 567–569
methamphetamine 592
methotrexate (MTX) 160
methotrexate-related neurotoxicity 160–162
methylation 299
methylmalonic acidemias (MMA) 747
methylphenidate (MPH) 171–172, 1095
Meyers loop damage 466
Meyers Neuropsychological Battery (MNB) 32
Michigan Compiled Laws Annotated 897
microcephaly 205
microglia 66, 203
micro RNAs (miRNAs) 300
microtubule-associated protein tau (MAPT) 510
midbrain 65
middle cerebral arteries (MCAs) 68, 351–352, *352*
Midwest Consortium of Postdoctoral Programs in Clinical Neuropsychology 15
migraine headaches 54
mild cognitive impairment (MCI): Alzheimer's disease causing 720–721; behavioral disturbance in 732–734; behavioral interventions for 731; cognitive and functional symptoms of 731; cognitive rehabilitation therapy and 1083; in DSM-5717; fronto-temporal lobar degeneration and 729; Lewy body disease and 726–727, *727*; mood and 731–732; in Parkinson's disease 507, 517–518, *518*; psychological interventions for 731; systemic lupus erythematosus and 618, 620–622
mild head injury (MHI) neuropsychological examination 927–938; external incentives 928; incidence 927–928; integrating information 934; legal implications 937–938; psychosocial influences 929–930; refining diagnostic hypothesis and 930–931; severity of injury 928–929; specialized tests, applying 931–933; test performance patterns, analyzing 933–934; test selection challenges 934–937
mild neurocognitive disorder (mND) 717–718
mild traumatic brain injury: beliefs/expectations and 425–427; biomarkers 432; chronic traumatic encephalopathy and 433–434; cognitive impairment outcomes 416, **416–417**; comorbidities 424–425; complicated 413; context of 427–429; controversies 432–436; dementia and 421; demographics 425; diagnosis 412–415, **412**, 901; epidemiology of 412; factors affecting outcomes 421–429, *422*; functional outcomes 416–419; future directions 432–436; gender and 425; genetics and 432–433; hospitalization and 794; iatrogenesis in neuropsychological assessment and 1019–1020; litigation and 428; media and 429; medical history and 425; military and 428–429; mood disorders and 419, 424; neuroimaging and 411–412, 417–419; number of injuries and 426–427; overview 436; overview of outcomes 415–416; pathophysiology of 411–412; politics and 429; posttraumatic stress disorder and 415; psychological outcomes 419; severity of 421–423; sleep and 424; sports and 427–428; structural outcomes 416–419; studies on outcomes 413, **413–415**; subconcussions 434–436; symptom-related outcomes 419–421, *420*; terminology 411; testing and 39; treatment 429–432, **430–431**
Military Acute Concussion Evaluation *807*
military disability examination 990–992
military service-related traumatic brain injury: aging and 813; animal studies on blast injury and 797; barotraumas and 796–797; blast injury 783, 794, 797–799; blast physics and 795–796; chronic traumatic encephalopathy and 813; context of injury 801–802; co-occurring disorders and 800–801; criminal justice system and 811–812; diagnostic threat and 805–806; differences in blast injury 797–799; Emerging Consciousness Program and 808–809; epidemiology 793–795; evaluation 809–811; external incentives to symptoms and 803–805; follow-up, longitudinal 812–813; historical perspective 793; iatrogenic illness and 805–806; impact of 792; in-theater care 806–807; misattribution bias and 805–806; National Intrepid Center of Excellence and 809; neurocognitive testing and 811; overview 813; physical blast effect and 796–797; postconcussion syndrome and 802–803; programs for 806–809; rehabilitation, acute and subacute 807–809; research 812–813; residential programs and 809; screening 809–811; severity of injury 792–793, **793**; symptoms 792
Millon Clinical Multiaxial Inventory (MCMI-III) 847
Minamata disease 589
mindfulness 335, 343–344, 1055
Mindfulness-Based Cognitive Therapy (MBCT) 1056, 1062
mindfulness-based interventions (MBIs): in affective disorders 1060–1061; behavior and 1057–1059; biophysiological functioning and 1059; brain and 1057–1059; cognitive functioning and 1059–1060; cognitive therapy based on 1056, 1062; future research 1064; impact of 1054; meditation 1054–1055, 1057–1058; methodological considerations 1064; neuropsychology and 1062–1064; overview 1054, 1064; rehabilitation and 1062–1064; in stress reduction 1054–1059; stroke and 1062–1063; traumatic brain injury and 1061–1063
Mindfulness-Based Stress Reduction (MBSR) 1054–1059
mind reading 239
minicolumns 206
Minimal Assessment of Cognitive Function in MS (MACFIMS) 607–608
minimally conscious state (MCS) 338–340
Mini-mental State Exam (MMSE) 356, 377, 510, 528, 564, 625, 707, 991
Minnesota Multiphasic Personality Inventory (MMPI) 671, 781, 833–834, 848, 860, 983
Minnesota Multiphasic Personality Inventory-2-Restructured Form (MMPI-2-RF) 848–849, 1068
Miranda warning 962–963, 966, 971
misattribution bias 805–806
mismatch negativity (MMN) 307
mitigation expertise at sentencing 976
mixed dementia 369–370
mixed episode 706
moderate and severe traumatic brain injury: attention disorders and 395; classification of severity 388–390, **389**; cognitive impairment and 394–396; communication and 395; defining 387; dementia and 394; employment after 399; executive function and 395–396; incidence 387–388; independent living outcomes and 400; language disorders and 395; link between 393; memory disorders and 395; motor disorders and 393; neuroanatomical findings following 390–392; neurobehavioral functioning after 394–396; neuropsychological assessment of moderate and severe 396–397; neuropsychological functioning after 394–396; new-onset disability incidence and 141, 387–388; overview 387, 401; posttraumatic amnesia and 389–390, 392–393, 396, 901; predictors of death after 398; predictors of functions after 400, **400**; prevalence 387–388; recovery from 392–394, *392*; risk factors 387–388
molecular biology/genetics 108, 195–196
molecular imaging with MRI 116
molecular imaging with SPECT and PET 113–114
molecular neuroimaging *see* functional and molecular neuroimaging
Molyneux's problem 333–334, **333**
monoamine (MAO) inhibitors 1091
monoamine oxidase (MAO) enzyme 1091
monoamine theory 1090
Monte Carlo estimation 946
Montreal Cognitive Assessment (MoCA) 356, 377, 625, 748, 751
Montreal Neurological Institute test battery 9, **9**
mood disorders: attention deficit/hyperactivity disorder and 289; chemotherapy and 594; mild traumatic brain injury and 419, 424; Parkinson's disease and 518–525
mood disorders; *see also specific type*
morphometry 310, 456
mossy fiber protection 680
motivation and differential diagnosis 57–58, *58*
motor disorders: attention deficit/hyperactivity disorder and 290–291; autism spectrum disorder and 226–227; moderate and severe traumatic brain injury and 393; *see also specific type*
movement disorders: clinical considerations 540–541, **541**; dystonia 539; essential

tremor 539; psychogenic 539–540; *see also* Huntington's disease (HD); Parkinson's disease (PD)
Movement Disorder Society (MDS) **521**
moyamoya disease 366–367, *366*
Multi-Data Source Model 976
multidomain neuropsychological diagnosis 53
multifocal axonal injury 411
multiple chemical injuries (MCS) 1020–1021
multiple personality disorder (now dissociative identity disorder) 1021–1022
multiple sclerosis (MS): anxiety disorders and 614; attention and 605; Brief International Cognitive Assessment for MS and 608; Brief Repeatable Battery and 604, 607; Chronic Progressive 604, 607; clinically isolated syndrome and 606; cognitive functioning and 604–608; cognitive impairment and 606–607, 609–610; cognitive rehabilitation therapy and 610; depression and 611–614, *612*; diagnosis 603–604; driving and 608; emotional valence and 609; employment and 608–609; epidemiology 603; executive functioning and 606; functional neuroimaging and 610–611; incidence 603; intellectual functioning and 606; language disorders and 606; measurement 607–608; Minimal Assessment of Cognitive Function in MS and 607–608; neuroimaging and 610–611; neuropathology 603; neuropsychological tests in 608–609; overview 614; patterns 604–606; prevalence 604–606; prospective memory and 609; psychiatric issues and 611–614; psychotherapy for 1045, 1048–1049; Relapsing-Remitting 604, 607–608, 610; self-generated learning and 609; symptom onset 603–604; testing effect and 609–610; types of 604; visuospatial functioning and 606
multiple system atrophy: epidemiology 533; genetics and 533; neurobehavioral features of 534; neuropathology 533, *533*; parkinsonian form of (MSA-P) 531; preclinical Lewy body disease and 726; symptoms 532; terminology 532
Multiple Trace Theory (MTT) 679
multitasking 343
Munchausen Syndrome 987
myelination 94–95

N-acetyle aspartate (NAA) 634
Nadel v. Las Vegas Metro (2001) 894
nadir CD4 cell 480
National Academy of Clinical Neuropsychology 944
National Academy of Neuropsychology (NAN) 16, 57–58, 873, 985–986, 1014
National Alliance of Professional Psychology Providers 767
National Cancer Institute (NCI) 561
National Consortium on Complementary and Alternative Medicine 1033
National Comorbidity Survey (NCS) 772
National Football League (NFL) players study 427
National Health and Nutrition Examination Survey (NHANES) 53
National Institute on Aging (NIA) 718–719
National Institute of Mental Health (NIMH) 107–108, 701, 767
National Institute of Neurological Disorders and Stroke—Association International pour la Recherche et l'Enseignement en Neurosciences (NINDS-AIREN) 367, **368**
National Institute of Neurological Disorders and Stroke—Canadian Stroke Network Vascular Cognitive Impairment Harmonization Standards 368
National Intrepid Center for Excellence (NCoE) 809
National Joint Committee on Learning Disabilities 284
National Survey on Alcohol and Related Conditions 775
National Vietnam Veterans Readjustment Study 760, 782
necrosis 495
neglect 31
neocortex 80
neomammalian brain 83
nerve cells 65
neural correlates 305–310
neural networks 84
neuroanatomy: central nervous system 63, **63**; cognitive functions and 63; divisions, major 63, **63**; of higher function 63, **63**, 84; historical perspective 62; neuroimaging and 63–64, *63*, 87–90, *87–90*; overview 62; peripheral nervous system 63, **63**; *see also* brain
neurobiology of learning disability: dyscalculia 308–310; dyslexia 304–308
neurodegenerative etiology 720
neurodevelopmental disorders: assessment of 134–135; attention deficit/hyperactivity disorder 289–291; behaviorally defined 129–130; brain-behavior relationships and 127–128; central nervous system alterations and 127; challenges to conceptualization and service provision and 135–137; classification of 128–129, **128**; defining 127; developmental neuropsychological formulation for 135; educational testing and, high-stakes 136; Flynn effect and 137; framework for conceptualization of 134; multiple assessments and 136–137; with neurological conditions 130–137; overview 137; practice effects and 137; terminology 136; time-referenced symptom and 127; transition into adulthood and 128; *see also specific type*
neurofibromatosis 105
neuroimaging: acute lymphoblastic leukemia *161*; alcohol use 593; antiphospholipid syndrome 639–640; attention deficit/hyperactivity disorder *130*, 303; autism spectrum disorder 213–216; blast injury 797–798; brain tumors *164–166*, *560*, *562*; carbon monoxide exposure 591; cerebrovascular disease 373–374, 377; chemotherapy effects 594; consciousness 339; dyslexia 306–307; epilepsy 465–467; functional 213–216, 306–307, 610–611, 665–666; hypoxia of the central nervous system 496–499, *497–498*; meditation 1057–1058; mercury intoxication 589; metabolic 213; mild traumatic brain injury 411–412, 417–419; multiple sclerosis 610–611; neuroanatomy 63–64, *63*, 87–90, *87–89*; non-central nervous system cancers 573, **574–575**, 576; opiate use 593; optic nerves 70, *71*; organic solvents exposure 590; posttraumatic stress disorder 783–784; prematurity *132*; primary Sjögren's syndrome 644–645; rheumatoid arthritis 642; sports-related concussion 664–666; structural 210–213, 306, 610, 664–665; systemic lupus erythematosus 633–637; traumatic brain injury 145; white matter 80; *see also* functional and molecular neuroimaging; *specific test*
neurolaw 858
neurological conditions with neurodevelopment disorders: background information 130; cerebral palsy syndrome 131–132; deletion syndrome 133–134; Down syndrome 131; fetal alcohol syndrome 133; Fragile X syndrome 131; prematurity 132, *132*; spina bifida 132–133
neurons 65, 70, 208
Neuron-Specific Enolase (NSE) 666
neuropeptide factors and systemic lupus erythematosus 631
neuroplasticity 449–450
Neuropsychiatric Inventory (NPI) 535
neuropsychiatric manifestations: of antiphospholipid syndrome 637–638; of rheumatoid arthritis 643; of systemic lupus erythematosus 618–619, **620–622**
Neuropsychological Assessment Battery (NAB) 32, 397
Neuropsychological Assessment Feedback Intervention (NAFI) 1070
neuropsychological diagnosis, meaning of 51
neuropsychological examination: clinical judgments and 938; diagnostic hypothesis and, refining 930–931; discrepancy between data and 934; external incentives and 928; historical perspective 927–928; injury severity in assessment of effort 928–929; integrating information and 934; legal implications of 937–938; malingering and 927; mild head injury 927–938; overview 927–928; parameter estimates 932–933, **933**; performance patterns and, analyzing 933–934; psychosocial influences on 929–930; selecting test, challenge of 934–937; specialized, applying 931–933
neuropsychological implications: of acquired immunodeficiency syndrome 483–484; of aneurysm 363–364; of arteriovenous malformation 359–360; of cavernous malformation 361; of cerebral amyloid angiopathy 364–365; of cerebral autosomal dominant arteriopathy with subcortical infarcts and leukoencephalopathy 365–366; of herpes simplex encephalitis 478–479;

of hypoxia of the central nervous system 499–500, **501**; of lead exposure 588; of Lyme disease and related disorders 484, 486–487; of mercury exposure 589; of moyamoya disease 367; of transient ischemic attack 356; of vascular cognitive impairment 369; of vascular dementia 369
neuropsychological screening 135
Neuropsychological Working Group 368
Neuropsychology Task Force of MDS Multiple System Atrophy (MODIMSA) Study 534
neuropsychotherapy 1045
neuroscience: of attention deficit/hyperactivity disorder 297–311; of autism spectrum disorder 204–216; of learning disability 297–311
neurotoxicity 563
neurotoxin litigation 874–876, 902–903
neurotransmitters 66, 450, 495, 824–827
neurotropic infections: acquired immunodeficiency syndrome 479–484; background information 477; herpes simplex encephalitis *473*, 477–479; Lyme disease and related disorders 484, *485*, 486–487; meningitis 477; overview 477, 487; viral infections and 477
New Freedom Commission 1011
NIH Toolbox 397
nitric oxide synthase (NOS) 495
N-Methyl-D-Aspartate (NMDA) receptor 450, 478, 628–629
nociception 824
non-central nervous system cancers: chemotherapy for 569, 587; cognitive impairment and 569–570; cross-sectional neuropsychological studies posttreatment 570; findings overview 573–574; longitudinal neuropsychological studies pre- and posttreatment 570–573; neuroimaging 573, **574–575**, 576; overview 577; treatment 569–570, 576, 587
nonfluent progressive aphasia (PNFA) 728
noninvasive vascular imaging 354
nonstimulants 1095
nonverbal learning disability 296–297
norepinephrine (NE) 825–826, 1090–1091
normative studies 870
nucleotides 102, 195
numerical cognition 294

OARS (open-ended questions, affirmations, reflections, and summaries) 1070
obesity 372, 627, 632–633
obsessive-compulsive disorder (OCD) 703–704, 1093
obstructive hydrocephalus 133
obstructive sleep apnea (OSA) 372, 494, 499–500
occipital-frontal head circumference (OFHC) 205
occipital lobe of brain 85
occipital lobe epilepsy(OLE) 457
occluded carotid artery 353
Office of Disability Adjudication Review (ODAR) 990
Office of the Inspector General (OIG) Fraud Unit 984
Oklahoma City bombings 774
Oklahoma Pre-morbid Intelligence Estimate (OPIE) 33
olfaction 70
olfactory epithelium 70
oligodendrocytes 66
Online Mendelian Inheritance in Man (OMIM) 105
opiates 593
opioids 824 825
oppositional defiant disorder (ODD) 144
opsoclonus myoclonus ataxia (OMA) syndrome 169–170
optical (near-infrared) imaging 118
optic images of letters 282
optic nerves 70, *71*
optic radiations 78
orbitofrontal cortex (OFC) 824
Orch-OR theory 332
organic solvents, exposure to 590
orienting, exogenous and endogenous 227
orthnography 292; *see also* language disorders
Overall Test Battery Mean 34
oxygen deprivation, effects of 494; *see also* hypoxia of the central nervous system
oxygen extraction fraction (OEF) 353, *353*

pain and pain-related disability: anxiety disorders and 829–830; autoimmune disorders and 632; biopsychosocial intervention models 835–837; catastrophizing and 829; childhood adversity and 827–828; chronic 823; clinical applications 832–837; context factors 830–832; defining pain and 823; depression and 829–830; education 830; fear avoidance and 830; financial incentive effects and 832; Gate Control Theory of Pain and 824; iatrogensis in managing 1023; incidence 823; malingering and 834; neural systems of pain and 824; neuroanatomy 824–827; neurotransmitters and 824–827; occupation and work-related factors 831; overview 823–824, 837; perception of pain and 825; person factors 827–830; physiology 824–827; preprocedure psychological screen and 834–835; psychological management of 836–837; psychological pain evaluations 833–834; psychosocial factors 827–830; satisfaction with care and 831–832; somatization and 827–829; system factors 830–832; treatment delays and 831
paleocortex 80
paleomammalian brain 83
panic disorder (PD) 1093–1094
Papez circuit 78, *78*, 80, 684
paraenchymal hematomas 376
parahippocampal region 680–681
paralimbic system 208
parallel form of reliability 23
paralysis agitans 508
parens patriae viewpoint of doctors 878
parental age and autism spectrum disorder 191
parietal lobe 85, 301–302
parietal lobe epilepsy 457
Parkinsonian disorders, atypical: corticobasalganglionic degeneration 534–535; multiple system atrophy 532–534, *533*; neuropsychological tests in differentiating among 535–536, **536**; progressive supranuclear palsy 529–532, *530–531*; *see also specific type*
parkinsonism 507–509
Parkinson's disease (PD): anxiety disorders and 520; apathy and 520; attention and 513; case example 522–525, *523*, **523**, *524*; cerebrospinal fluid and 511; cognitive impairment and 513–518; cognitive rehabilitation therapy and 529, 1083; with dementia 507, 509, 525; with dementia with Lewy bodies 507, 525; depression and 518–520, **519**; diagnosis 507, **507**; differential diagnosis with dementia and dementia with Lewy bodies 507, 525; epidemiology 508–509; executive function and 513–514; genetics and 509–510; historical perspective 508; impulsive and related behaviors and 521; intellectual functioning and 513; language disorders and 514–515; learning and 516–517; measuring severity of 51; memory and 516–517; mild cognitive impairment in 507, 517–518, **518**; mood disorders and 518–522, **519**; multiple system atrophy and 531; neurobehavioral features of 511–517; neuropathology 510–512, **510**; NFL football players and 427; overview 507; parkinsonism versus 507–509; pathophysiology 510–512, *512–513*; pharmacological intervention 525, **526**, 527–528; psychiatric disturbances and 518–522, **521–522**; psychosis and 522; spatial functions and 515–516; surgery for 528–529, **528**; Sydney Multicenter Study of 511; visuoperceptual functions and 515–516; working memory and 513; *see also* Parkinsonian disorders, atypical
Parkinson's disease with dementia (PDD) 507, 509, 525
Parsons v. State (2007) 968
Participation Assessment with Recombined Tools—Objective (PART-O) 397
parvocellular system 308
Patient Health Questionnaire (PHQ) 781, 848
patterns in test performance 933–934
pediatric bipolar disorder (PBD) 708–710
pediatric cancer: acute lymphoblastic leukemia 157–162, *159*, *161*; adolescence and 168–169; adult outcomes 166–168; aging and, early 167–168; behavioral intervention 172; brain tumors 162–166, *164–166*; chemotherapy 159–160; cognitive reserve and 167; cognitive training for 172–173; educational intervention 173; field of 158; future directions 171; infant ALL and brain tumors 170–171; methotrexate for 160; opsoclonus myoclonus ataxia syndrome 169–170; overview 158; pharmacological intervention 171–172; social intervention 174; survival rates 158, *158*, 169, *169*; treatment 171–174

pediatric forensic neuropsychology: cognitive impairment and, identifying 945–947, *946–947*; documentation 952–956; ethics and 942–943; forensic context of 942–945, **943**; as mainstay of discipline 942; malingering and 950–952, **951**; overview 942, 956; performance validity tests and 948–949; self-report validity tests and 949–950; testimony 952–956; validity testing 947–950, **949**
pediatric neuropsychologist (PN) 942; *see also* pediatric forensic neuropsychology
peduncles 78
peer review 896
penultimate testimony 888
penumbra zone 353
perceptual abilities and autism spectrum disorder 231–236
perforant pathway 680
performance validity tests (PVTs): background information 39; case studies 39–40; defining 39; differential diagnosis of actual versus feigned dementia and 42, **43–44**, 45–48, **45**; evidence from 42; forensic neuropsychology and 903; inconsistency in test scores across cognitive exams **44**, 45–48, **45**; interpretation of data from multiple 40–42; mismatch between test scores and demonstrated functionality and 45; pediatric forensic neuropsychology and 948; somatic symptom disorders and 847–848; symptom validity tests versus 32; *see also specific test*
perikaryon 65
peripheral nervous system (PNS) 63, **63**, 66
Personality Assessment Inventory (PAI) 799, 993
personality disorders 289
personality tests 848–850; *see also specific name*
pervasive development disorder (PDD) 185
pervasive development disorder—not otherwise specified (PDD-NOS) 185
pervasive remote memory disturbance 679
pharmacological intervention: aneurysms 363; anxiety disorders 1093–1094; attention deficit/hyperactivity disorder 1094–1095; bipolar disorder 707–708, 1092–1093; brain tumors 568–569; cerebrovascular disease 375; delirium 341; depression 705, 1090–1092; epilepsy 459–460, **460**; extrapyramidal side effects and 1090; iatrogenesis and 1022–1024; Parkinson's disease 525, **526**, 527–528; pediatric cancer 171–172; schizophrenia 1089–1090; seizures 376; systemic lupus erythematosus 633; *see also specific drug*
phenomics 107; *see also* genomics and phenomics
phenylketonuria (PKU) 742–743
phenytoin 376
phonology 236, 292; *see also* language disorders
photons 113
Physical Activity Recall Interview 613–614
pia mater 64
"pick and choose" tests 39
placebo effect 826
planned follow-up assessment 134–135
planum temporale 84
plaques 371, 603
plasticity 92–93, 449–450
plausibility and forensic neuropsychology 908
pleas, entering in criminal proceedings 880
polychlorinated biphenyls (PCBs) 861, 893
polygraph 893
polymerase chain reaction (PCR) 477
polymorphisms 103
Polytrauma Network Sites 808
Polytrauma Rehabilitation Center (PRC) 794
Polytrauma Support Clinics 808
Polytrauma System of Care 808–809
Polytrauma Transitional Rehabilitation Programs 809
pons 65
population stratification 104
positive ethics 1001
positive predictive value (PPV) 985
Positive Romberg signs 662
positron emission tomography (PET) 93, 113, 213, 374, 465, 635
PositScience 1079–1080
postconcussion disorder (PCD) 419
postconcussion/postconcussional/postconcussive syndrome (PCS) 52, 419–420, 422–423, 425–427, 436, 668, 671, 802–803, 901
Post-Concussion Scale-Revised (PCS-R) 661
Post-Deployment Health Assessment/Post-Deployment Health Reassessment (PDH/PDHRA) 795
postdoctoral residency 17–19
posterior cerebral arteries (PCAs) 351–352, *352*
posterior communicating arteries (PCoAs) 67
posterior fossa syndrome (PFS) 163
posterior probability 894
posterior reversible encephalopathy syndrome(PRES) 161–162, *161*
postincident exposures 889–890
postinjury testing in sports-related concussion 663, *664*
post-Lyme disease syndrome 486
poststroke depression 372
posttraumatic amnesia (PTA): external symptoms 803–805; moderate and severe traumatic brain injury and 389–390, 392–393, 396, 901; symptoms 340–341, 803–805
posttraumatic confusional state (PTCS) 340–342, 390, 393
posttraumatic model (PTM) 1021
posttraumatic stress disorder (PTSD): biomarkers 783–784; blast injury and 783; clinical interview 779–780; clinical population studies 774–775; cognitive testing 782; cohort studies 774–775; comorbid conditions 776–777; complex 769–771; controversy 757; cross-cultural issues 775–776; defining 764–767, 778–779; diagnostic criteria **768**; disability in defining 779; dissociative subtype 766–767; in DSM-5757, 760–771, **761**; from DSM-IV-TR to DSM-5760–771; epidemiology 771–775; establishing 758–760; evaluation 809–811; field trials 767; Hurricane Andrew and 775; hybrid model 778–779; in *International Classification of Diseases* 757, 767–769, 778; interview 758, 777–782; mild traumatic brain injury and 415; National Center for PTSD study and 757; neurobiology of 783; neuroimaging 783–784; overview 757–760, 782–784; personality changes and 770–771, **770**; population studies 772–775; precursor to 762; prevalence 769, 800; psychological testing 780–782; racial issues 775–776; research criteria **768**; risk factors 776–777; screening 809–811; stressor and 765–766; as subcategory of anxiety disorders 1093
practice effects (PEs) 137, 915
Prader-Willi syndrome 165
pragmatics 238
precentral gyrus 83, 85
precision medicine 108
prefrontal cortex (PFC) 91, 309
prejudicial relevance of evidence 888
prematurity 132, *132*
premorbid functioning, inferences about 870
pre-optic area 688
pre- and perinatal adverse events 201–202
preprocedure psychological screen 834–835
prespecified genes 298
presumptive diagnosis 52
prevalence, defining 930
Preventing Violent Explosive Neurotrauma (PREVENT) 797
primary central nervous system lymphoma (PCNSL) 560, 566–567
primary dyscalculia 294
primary injuries 142
primary legal authority 888
primary progressive aphasia (PPA) 728
primary Sjögren's syndrome (PSS): biobehavioral correlates of cognitive impairment and 644; cognitive impairment and 643–644; defining 643; epidemiology 643; neuroimaging 644–645; neuropsychiatric 643
prior probability 894
private disability examination 992–994
probate proceedings and forensic neuropsychology 898–899
probative relevance of evidence 888
problem-focused assessment 135
problem solving 1081–1082
process approach 10
processing speed tests 27, 32–33
prodromal Alzheimer's disease 720–721
professional anosognosia 976
Profile of Mood States (POMS) 520
progressive apraxia of speech (PPAOS) 729
progressive supranuclear palsy (PSP): case study 531–532; epidemiology 529–530; genetics and 529–530; neurobehavioral features 530–531; neuropathology 530, *530–531*; neuropsychological testing 532, **532**
proliferative zones 92
prosody 236–237; *see also* language disorders
prospective memory (PM) 517, 609
proton density sequences 90
pseudo-dementia 704

psychiatric disorders: attention deficit/hyperactivity disorder and 287; differential diagnosis and 56–57; neuropsychology and 701–702; *see also specific type*
psychiatric disturbances and Parkinson's disease: anxiety 520; apathy 520; depression 518–520, **519**; impulsive and related behaviors 521
psychogenic movement disorder (PMD) 539–540, 847
psychogenic nonepileptic seizures (PNES) 847
psychological iatrogenesis 1018; *see also* iatrogenesis in neuropsychological assessment
psychological pain management 836–837; *see also* pain and pain-related disability
psychological tests and somatic symptom disorders 848–850; *see also specific test name*
psychometric testing: change scores and, reliable 25; defining 22–23; factor analyses of 26–28; interpretation of scores and 32–35; measurement error and 24–25; overview 22, 35; reliability and 23–24; traumatic brain injury and 147; validity and 25–32
psychosis 372–373, 522
psychotherapy: defining 1045–1046; for denial/unawareness of impaired neuropsychological functioning 1045, 1050, **1050–1051**; for depression after cerebral vascular accident 1045–1048; dialogue 1045–1046; efficacy of, with patients without brain disorders 1046; importance of 1045; limitations of alliance in 1051; for multiple sclerosis 1045, 1048–1049; overview 1045, 1051–1052; strength of alliance in 1051; *see also* cognitive behavioral therapy (CBT)
published court opinions 888
punch drunk syndrome 433, 668; *see also* chronic traumatic encephalopathy (CTE)
Push-Pull tactic 911

qualitative approaches 6–10, **7–10**
Quality Enhancement Research Initiative in Polytrauma and Blast-Related Injury 812–813
quality of life (QoL) evaluations 561
quantitative approaches 3–6, **4–6**
quantitative EEG (QEEG) 117–118, 307, 666, 894
quantitative electroencephalography 116–117
quantitative trait loci (QTL) 311
quantity, understanding 308–309
Questionnaire for Impulsive-Compulsive Disorders in Parkinson's disease (QUIP) 521

race and autism spectrum disorder 191
radial diffusion (RD) 212
radiation encephalopathy 562
radiation therapy: brain tumor risk and 163; for brain tumors 162, 561–563, 566–568; for craniopharyngioma 165
Radiation Therapy Oncology Group (RTOG) 561
radioisotope-based imaging 111–114
Ragge v. MCA/Universal Studios (1995) 898
Rand Corporation study of tort and dollar-threshold states 928
rapid automatic naming (RAN) 292
raw data disclosure 913
Raynaud's phenomenon 627
RBANS Effort Scale (ES) 46
reactive oxygen species (ROS) 562
reading disorders 292–294
reasonable understanding 964
receiver operating characteristic (ROC) 28, 30
Recognition Memory Test (RMT) 932
records, review of 906
recursive partitioning (RP) 936–937, *937*
regions of interest (ROI) 300
regression 136
regressive autism spectrum disorder (RASD) 204, 219–222
regulatory agency evaluations 995–996
rehabilitation: cerebrovascular disease 377–378, *378*; memory 731; mindfulness-based interventions and 1062–1064; neuropsychology and 1062–1064; state vocational 996; stroke 376–377; *see also* cognitive rehabilitation therapy (CRT)
Rehabilitation Act 877–878
Rehabilitation Services Administration (RSA) 284
Reiner v. Warren Resort Hotels, Inc. (2008) 938
relative standing, defining 136
reliability 23–24
remediation techniques 1078
remembering *see* episodic memory; memory
remote memory disturbance 678–679
REM sleep behavior disorder (RBD) 726
renal disease 745–746
reoxygenation injury 495
reperfusion injury 495
repetitive transcranial magnetic stimulation (rTMS) 340
reporting guidelines 1009
report writing 907–909
repressors 102
reptilian brain 83
Research Diagnostic Criteria 772
Research Domains Criteria (RDoC) (NIMH) 107–108
resective surgery 463–465
residential programs for military service-related traumatic brain injury 809
Response Assessment in Neuro-Oncology (RANO) group 565, 568
response bias 428, 859–860, 986
Response Bias Scale (RBS) 849–850, 993
resting-state networks (RSNs) 452
resting studies paradigm 111
restricted and repetitive patterns of behavior (RRBIAs) 185–186, 188–189, 242–243
Restructured Clinical (RC) scales 849
reticular formation 72
retinal ischemia 350
retrograde amnesia 678–679, 691
retrosplenial cortex 685
Rett's disorder (RD) 185
reuptake inhibitors 1091
reversible ischemic neurologic deficit (RIND) 354
Revised Competency Assessment Instrument (R-CAI) 966
Rey-Osterrieth Complex Figure and Clock Drawing Test 10
rheumatoid arthritis (RA): biobehavioral mechanisms of cognitive dysfunction and 642; cognitive impairment and 641–642; defining 640; epidemiology 640; flares 640; neuroimaging 642; neurologic 640–641; overview 642–643
right hemisphere of brain 84
risk assessment methods of dangerousness 970–971, **971**
RNA 102
rods 70
Rohling Interpretive Method (RIM) 34–35
Rolandic fissure 81
Romberg sign 498
Rosa's Law 980
Rules of Evidence 860, 862, 893–896, **895**

St. Jude Children's Research Hospital studies 165
salience network (SN) 215
SBTP 1080
scanning speech 73
scatter 945–946
schizophrenia 57, 708, 906, 1089–1090
Schudel v. General Electric (1995) 893
Schwann cells 66
Scientific Brain Training Pro (SBTP) program 1080
scientific expert 859; *see also* expert witness
scientist-practitioner model 859
Scoville and Milner case study 678
secondary injuries 142
secondary legal authority 888
secondary Sjögren's syndrome 643
second generation of antipsychotics (SGA) 1090
seizure: chronic 458–459; disorders 291; electric 847; generalized tonic-clonic 458; hemorrhagic stroke and 376; memory and 452; neuropathology 449, *451*; neurotransmitters associated with 450; pathophysiology of 449; prophylaxis 376; psychogenic nonepileptic 847; *see also* epilepsy
selective reporting bias 104
selective serotonin reuptake inhibitor (SSRI) 704–705, 825, 837, 1091, 1094
self-awareness 335–336
self-generated learning 609
self-monitoring 335
self-monitoring impairments 343–344
self-pay health care 859
self-report 890
self-report validity tests 949–950
self, sense of 334–335
semantic memory 336, 342–343
semantics 237–238, 292; *see also* language disorders
sensorimotor function tests 26–27
sensorimotor regulation 339–340
sensory function 71

Sensory Integration Therapy 1038
sensory perception 333–334
sentencing, mitigation expertise at 976
serotonin 72, 825, 1090–1091
serotonin-norepinephrine reuptake inhibitor (SNRI) 825, 837, 1091
serum IgG 202
serum versus CSF studies 630–631
set-shifting and autism spectrum disorder 228–229
severe traumatic brain injury *see* moderate and severe traumatic brain injury
Shaffer collateral pathways 680
Sheehan v. Daily Racing Form, Inc. (1997) 862
Sheperd Center rehabilitation program for arousal disorders 339
short association fibers 80
short-term memory 97
sideline testing in sports-related concussion 661–662
significance, statistical 103–104
silencers 102
silent stroke 350
Simmons v. Mullins (1975) 892
single nucleotide polymorphism (SNP) 103–104, 195–196
single photon emission computed emission tomography (SPECT) 111–113, 374, 465, 635
sinks 117
Sjögren's Syndrome Foundation 643
skill base thought of training 17
sleep 424, 632, 1038
smoking cigarettes 371–372
social abilities 94
social anxiety disorder (SAD) 1093–1094
social class and autism spectrum disorder 191
social communication and autism spectrum disorder 185–186, 188, 217–218, 240–242
social intervention 174
Social Security Act (1935) 981
Social Security Disability (SSD) 983
Society of Clinical Neuropsychology (formerly Division 40) 14
Society of Neuropsychology (Division 40) 3, 14–16, **16**
Society for Traumatic Stress Studies 780
sociocognitive model (SCM) 1021
sodium MR imaging 116
soma 65
somatic symptom disorders: assessment 846–850; associated disorders with 847; cognitive symptoms 847–848; disability and 987; in DSM-5846; intervention 850–851; medically unexplained symptoms and 847, 851; overview 846, 851; pathology 846–847; performance validity tests and 847–848; presentations 846–847; psychological/personality tests and 848–850; terms for 846
somatization 828–829
somatoform disorders *see* somatic symptom disorders
somatoform tendencies 828
source amnesia 692
source memory 230
sources 117
space, understanding 308–309
spatial functions and Parkinson's disease 515–516
specialized knowledge 895; *see also* expert witness
Specialty Guidelines for Forensic Psychology 873, 912–914
Specific Problems Scales 850
specific validity tests 903–904
spina bifida 97–98, 132–133
spinothalamic tract 72
split-half reliability 23
Sports Concussion Assessment Tool (SCAT-3) 662, 670
sports-related concussion (SRC): assessment of acute injury effects 661–662; balance testing 662; baseline testing 663–664; biomarker for concussion and, search for 664–667; chronic traumatic encephalopathy and 668–669; clinical effects, acute 660; complications in recovery from 667–669; computerized versus paper-and-pencil testing 663–664; diagnostic challenges and issues 659–660; electrophysiological abnormalities and 666; functional neuroimaging 665–666; incidence 659; initial recovery from 669–670; King-Devick test and 662; laboratory biomarkers 666–667; longer-term effects of 670–671, **670**; media and 659; neuroimaging 664–666; neuropsychological assessment 662–664; overview 659, 671–672; postconcussion syndrome 668; postinjury testing, timing of 663, *664*; practice recommendations 669–671, **669**; recovery from 659–660, 669–670; repeat injury and 667–668; sideline testing 661–662; Sports Concussion Assessment Tool and 662; symptom checklists 661–662
standard error of measurement (SEM) 24, 972
Standardized Assessment of Concussion (SAC) 662
standardized mean effect size 28
stare decisis principle 888, 891
State of California Alzheimer Disease Diagnostic and Treatment Centers (ADDTC) 367
state vocational rehabilitation 996
statistical approaches 3
Steele-Richardson-Olszewski syndrome *see* progressive supranuclear palsy (PSP)
stepdown analysis 935, *935*, **936**
sterioids 561
steroid treatment 162
stimulants 1095
STrengthening the REporting of Genetic Association (STREGA) studies 103
Strengthening the Reporting of Observational Studies in Epidemiology (STROBE) 103
stress and autism spectrum disorder 204
stressor 765–766, 774
striatonigral degeneration (SND) 531
striatum 76
stroke: brain dysfunction analysis and 29; cognitive rehabilitation therapy 1084–1085; complications 376–377; defining 350; depression after 372; hemorrhagic 356–357, **356–357**; ischemic 353–354; mindfulness-based intervention and 1062–1161; prevention 377–378; rehabilitation 376–377; risk factors 370–372; telestroke 375–376; *see also* cerebrovascular disease
structural neuroimaging 210–213, 306, 610, 664–665
structural variations 298–299
structured professional judgment (SPJ) 970–971
subarachnoid hemorrhage (SAH) 361–362, 376
subconcussions 434–436
subcortical dementia 530, 720
subdural hematoma (SDH) 391
subiculum 78
substances of abuse: alcohol 593; amphetamines 592–593; cannabis 592; MDMA 592–593; opiates 593
substance use 287, 289
substantial gainful activity (SGA) 980
subthalamus 76
subtractive processes 92
sulci 64, 91, 308–310
superconducting quantum-interference devices (SQUIDs) 117
superior occipitofrontal fasciculus 80
Supervision Rating Scale (SRS) 397
Supplemental Security Income (SSI) 980–981
supplementary motor cortex (SMC) 301
surgery: ablative 463–465, 528, **528**; aneurysms 363; arteriovenous malformation 359; cavernous malformation 360–361; epilepsy 463–465; Parkinson's disease 528–529; for Parkinson's disease 528–529, **528**; resective 463–465
surgical hematoma evacuation 364
susceptibility-weighted sequence (SWI) 90
Sybil's case 1021–1022
Sydney Multicenter Study of Parkinson's disease 511
Sylvian fissure 81
symptom checklists 661–662
symptom validity 986
Symptom Validity Scale (FBS) 849
symptom validity tests (SVTs) 32, 848, 891, 931, 948, 986
synapses 65
synaptogenesis 92
synarchy 16
syndrome analysis *51*, 53, *53*
systemic lupus erythematosus (SLE): activity of disease and 627; antineuronal antibodies and 628; antiphospholipid antibodies and 629; anti-ribosomal P and 629; attention and 624; autoantibodies and 628; behavioral mechanisms of cognitive impairment 626–633; behavioral mechanisms of 631–633; biobehavioral mechanisms of cognitive impairment and 620, **622**; characteristics of disease and 626–629; cognitive functioning and 625; cognitive impairment and 619–625, *621*, **622**; cognitive rehabilitation therapy and 633; cytokines and 630; defining 618; duration of disease and 626; epidemiology 618; executive function and 624; exercise

endurance and 632–633; fatigue and 632; hormonal factors and 631; inflammation mediators and 630–631; information processing and 624; language disorders and 625; learning and 623–624; matrix metalloproteinases and 630; medications and 627; memory and 623–624; mild cognitive dysfunction and 618, 620–622; neuroimaging 633–637; neuropeptide factors and 631; neuropsychological screening and 625–626; NMDA receptor antibodies and 628–629; neuropsychiatric 618–619, **620**, **622**; obesity and 632–633; overview 637; pain and 632; problem solving and 624; psychological factors and 631–632; serum versus CSF studies and 630–631; sleep and 632; treatment 633; visuoconstruction and 624; visuospatial functioning and 624

tactile defensiveness 188, 212
tactile hypersensitivities 188–189
TBI Model Systems 388
T cells 487
technological iatrogenesis 1024
telestroke 375–376
temporal lobe 85, 680–686
temporal lobe amnesia 681–684, *682–683*, *686*, 693–694
temporal lobe epilepsy (TLE) 451–452, *453*, 454, 456, 459, 463, *463*, 1082
temporal lobe-limbic system 78
temporally graded remote memory disturbance 679
temporally limited remote memory disturbance 679
temporolimbic system 78
testamentary competence (TC) 899
testing effect 609–610
testing the limits 9
Test of Memory Malingering (TOMM) 39, 891, 897, 932, 949, 989
test performance patterns 933–934
test retest reliability 23, 767, 972–973
test scores, interpreting 32–35; *see also specific test*
thalamic amnesia 686–687, *687*
thalamic radiations 78
thalamus 65, 75, *76*, 824
theory of mind (ToM) 239
Therapeutic Assessment (TA) 851, 1068; *see also* Collaborative Therapeutic Neuropsychological Assessment (CTNA)
third-party observers (TPO) 897–898
threshold effect 426, 434–435
threshold of viability 132
thrombolytic therapy 374
thrombosis 354
thrombotic infarcts 354
thymine 102, 195
thyroid disease 744–745
thyroid hormones 744
tick-borne infections 484, 486–487
time-referenced symptoms 127
tissue plasminogen activator (tPA) 375
Tomlin v. Holecek (1993) 898
Toronto Test of Acute Recovery After TBI 396
tort 888, 902–903
toxins in the central nervous system: alcohol 593; amphetamines 592–593; cannabis 592; carbon monoxide 590–592; chemotherapy 587, 593–595; cognitive impairment and 595; heavy metals 587–589; lead 587–588; MDMA 592–593; mercury 588–590; opiates 593; organic solvents 590; overview 587, 595; substances of abuse 592–593
tracts 78, 80
training in clinical neuropsychology: APA accreditation and 17–19; APA Division 40 and 14, 16, **16**; controversies in 19–20; current developments 19–20; Houston Conference and 16–18; knowledge base thought of 17; in 1980s 14–15; in 1990s 15–16; organizations involved in 14–16, 20; overview 20; postdoctoral residency 17–19; skill base thought of 17
trait anxiety 702
Transcranial Direct Current Stimulation 1086
transcranial Doppler (TCD) sonography 118, 374
transcranial magnetic stimulation (TMS) 377
transcription 102
transcription factors 300, 450
transfer 730
transient ischemic attack (TIA) 350, 354–356
transplantation **528**, 529
Trauma Symptom Checklist 771
Trauma Symptom Inventory (TSI) 781
traumatic axonal injury (TAI) 411
traumatic brain injury (TBI): advocacy groups 858; Alzheimer's disease and 421, 427; assessment 149–150, **149**; biomarkers 798; case illustration 148–150, *148*, **149**; causes of 141, 388; closed 792; cognitive abilities and 143; cognitive development and 145–146; cognitive rehabilitation therapy and 1084–1085; Collaborative Therapeutic Neuropsychological Assessment and recovery from 1072–1076; communication and 395; dementia and 29, 394; demographics and 141; epidemiology 141–143; forensic neuropsychology and rise of 858; functional outcomes 143–144; future directions 150; gender and 141; general outcomes 143–144; incidence 659; injury characteristics and 144; Iraq war veterans and 792; late effects of 142–143; methodological critique 146–148; mild 792; mindfulness-based interventions and 1061–1063; mortality 141–142; neurochemical mechanisms and 142; neuroimaging 145; neurometabolic mechanisms and 142; neuropathology 142–143, **142**; neuropsychological testing and 25–26, 29–30; neurotoxin litigation and 874–876; non-injury-related influences 145; pathophysiology 142–143; penetrating 792; predictors of outcomes 144–146, 148; prevalence 141; primary injuries and 142; programs 806–809; psychometric testing 147; recovery from 147; Screening Questionnaire 795; secondary injuries 142; severity of 792–793; *see also* mild traumatic brain injury; military service-related traumatic brain injury; moderate and severe brain injury
traumatic events 774
treatment *see specific type*
tricyclic antagonists/antidepressants (TCAs) 705, 1091, 1094
trisomy 21 131
trisynaptic circuit 680
"triune" brain 83
Trolano v. John Hancock (2003) 898
True Response Inconsistency (TRIN) scale 993
truncal ataxia 73
trunk and branch model of depression in multiple sclerosis 611, *612*
Twins Early Development Study (UK) 298
Type I diabetes 370, 744
Type I error 104
Type II diabetes 370, 744
typical antipsychotics 1090

Ubiquitin C-Terminal Hydrolase (UCH-L1) 666–667
U fibers 80
ultimate legal questions 888
ultrasonography 118
uncinate fasciculus 80
unconsciousness 333
undiagnosis 1025
United States v. Cameron (1990) 900
unpublished court opinions 888
unresponsive wakefulness syndrome 338
Updated Sapporo Classification Criteria 637
U.S. v. Andrews (2006) 967
U.S. v. Pohlot (1987) 970
U.S. v. Rinchack (1987) 967
U.S. v. Swanson (1978) 967

validated surrogate marker 783
validity: construct 25–26; criterion 25, 28–32; ecologic 31; psychometric testing and 25–32; testing 947–950, 988–989, **989**; *see also* performance validity tests (PVTs)
Valiulis v. Scheffeos (1989) 892
valproate 1093
variability of test scores 945–946
Variable Response Inconsistency (VRIN) scale 993
vascular cognitive impairment (VCI) 367–369, **368**, 724
vascular dementia (VaD) 367–369, 724–726
vasospasm 376
vegetative state (VS) 338–340, 392, 398
velocardiofacial syndrome 290
ventral anterior (VA) nuclei 73, 75
ventral lateral (VL) nuclei 73, 75
ventral pallidum 688
ventral posterior medial (VPM) 71
ventral striatum 688
ventrical amygdalaofugal (VAF) pathway 687, *687*

ventricles 65, 68, *69*, 70
Ventricle-to-Brain Ratio 499
ventrolateral prefrontal cortex (VLPFC) 824
verbal symbolic abilities tests 26, 32–33
vermis 73
vertical organization of brain 83
very low density lipoprotein (VLDL) 370
vestibular division 71
vestibulocochlear nerve 71
Veterans Affairs 794–795, 806–809, 812–813
Veterans Benefits Administration (VBA) 990
Veterans Health Administration (VHA) 795
Vietnam Veterans Against the War 759
Vietnam Veterans Working Group 759
Vietnam war veterans 429, 758–760
vigilance 333
Villalba v. Consol. Freightways (2000) 897
Vineland Adaptive Behavior Scales 233, 976
viral infections 477
vision 70, 189
visual evoked potentials (VEPs) 308, 311
visual field deficit (VFD) 466
Visual Form Discrimination Test 31
visualization of the analysis of variance (VISOVA) 107
visualization of variance (ViVA) 107
visual learning tests 27
visuoperceptual functions and Parkinson's disease 515–516
visuoperceptual judgment tests 26–27, 32–33
visuospatial functioning: Alzheimer's disease and 723; fronto-temporal lobar degeneration and 730; Lewy body disease and 728; multiple sclerosis and 606; systemic lupus erythematosus and 624; vascular memory and 726
visuospatial judgment tests 26–27, 32–33
vitamin B12 deficiency 745
Von Economo neurons (VENs) 336
voxel-based morphometry (VBM) 300, 456

Walter Reed Army Medical Center 798–799, 809
Washington University group 772
watershed zone 356
Wechsleer Memory Scale (WMS) 10
Wechsler Adult Intelligence Scale (WAIS) 10; WAIS-IV index 33; WAIS Verbal and Performance IQ 30–31
weight of evidence 887, 896
Wernicke-Korsakoff syndrome 684–685, 687
Weschsler Test of Premorbid Function (TOPF) 33
Western Blot Test 484
whiplash injuries 1020
white matter (WM) 65, 73, 78, 80, 210–212, 302, 369, 392, 454, 457, 633
white matter hyperintensities (WMH) 480, 562, 633, 642
WHOADAS (World Health Organization Disability Assessment) 779
whole-brain radiotherapy 561–563
Wilson v. United States (1968) 967
Winnie Dunn's Sensory Profile 233
WMS-IV Indexes 24–25
Woodcock-Johnson tests 294
word blindness 282
workers' compensation (WC) 982, 994–995
working memory: at 8 to 12 months 95; autism spectrum disorder and 229; cognitive construct of, hypotheses for 107; Parkinson's disease and 513; tests, listing of 27, 32–33; trait anxiety and 702; vascular memory and 726
World Association of Medical Editors (WAME) 1011
World Health Organization (WHO) 52, 370, 412, 701, 767, 779, 980

yoga 1054

zinc supplementation 1038
zone of proximal development 9
Zurich Consensus Statement on Concussion in Sport 669, **669**